D1311472

5 Griffith's -MINUTE CLINICAL CONSULT 2005

Contributing Authors

David J. Framm, MD
Directory of Echocardiography
Mecklenburg Medical Group
Charlotte, NC

Anatoli Freiman, MD
Resident, Division of Dermatology
McGill University Health Center
Montreal, Quebec CANADA

Gregory G. Gaar, MD
Senior Vice-President, Senior Medical Director
Florida Poison Information and Toxicology Resource Center
Tampa General Hospital
Tampa, FL

Eric P. Gall, MD
Professor and Chairman
Department of Medicine
Rosalind Franklin University of Medicine & Science
Chicago Medical School
North Chicago, IL

Leonard Ganz, MD
Director of Cardiac Electrophysiology
Cardiovascular Institute
University of Pittsburgh Medical Center
Pittsburgh, PA

Gale Gardner, MD
Clinical Professor
Department of Otolaryngology
University of Tennessee, Memphis
Memphis, TN

William G. Gardner, MD
Chairman, Department of Medicine
Northeastern Ohio Universities College of Medicine
Akron, OH

Mark Gerstberger, DO
Private Practice
Ulysses, KS

Jeff Ray Gibson, Jr., MD
Department of Anesthesiology
Scott and White Clinic
Temple, TX

Bruce C. Gilliland, MD
Professor of Medicine and Laboratory Medicine
School of Medicine
University of Washington
Seattle, WA

Gary A. Goforth, MD
Professor of Family Medicine
Medical University of South Carolina
Program Director, Self Regional Healthcare
Family Practice Residency Program
Greenwood, SC

Neal S. Gold, MD
Great Northwest Medical Group
Buffalo Grove, IL

Leonard G. Gomella, MD
Chairman, Department of Urology
Professor
Thomas Jefferson University
Philadelphia, PA

Paul R. Gordon, MD
Department of Family & Community Medicine
University of Arizona College of Medicine
Tucson, AZ

R. Scott Gorman, MD
Community Internal Medicine
Mayo Clinic
Scottsdale, AZ

Oren N. Gottfried, MD
Department of Neurosurgery
University of Utah Health Sciences Center
Salt Lake City, UT

Steven Eisenstein, MD
Private Practice
The Family Doctors of Northbrook
Northbrook, IL

Nancy C. Elder, MD, MSPH
Associate Professor, Family Medicine
University of Cincinnati
Cincinnati, OH

J. Gregory Elders, MD
Family Practice
Baxter Regional Medical Center
Mountain Home, AR

Pamela I. Ellsworth, MD
Chief, Division of Urology
U Mass Memorial Medical Center
Worcester, MA

Kurt Elward, MD, MPH
Family Medicine of Albemarle
Research Assistant Professor, Department of Family Medicine
University of Virginia
Charlottesville, VA

Joseph G. Ewing, MD
Assistant Professor of Family Practice
Family Practice Residency Program at Conroe
University of Texas Medical Branch, Galveston
Conroe, TX

Fady Faddoul, DDS, MSD
Director, Advanced Education in General Dentistry
Case Western Reserve University
School of Dentistry
Mayfield Village, OH

Robert G. Fante, MD
Clinical Assistant Professor
University of Colorado
Denver, CO

Andrew H. Fenton, MD
Associate Professor of Surgery
Northeastern Ohio Universities College of Medicine
Akron General Medical Center
Akron, OH

Scott A. Fields, MD
Professor and Vice Chair
Family Medicine
Oregon Health and Science University
Portland, OR

Stanley Fineman, MD
Clinical Associate Professor
Department of Pediatrics
Emory University School of Medicine
Marietta, GA

Gene S. Fisch, PhD
Senior Research Statistician and Investigator
North Shore/LIJ Research Institute
New York, NY

Daniel B. Fishbein, MD
Medical Epidemiologist, Adult Section
National Immunization Program
Centers for Disease Control
Atlanta, GA

Jonathan M. Flacker, MD
Director, Emma I Darnell Geriatrics Center
Emory University School of Medicine
Atlanta, GA

Joseph A. Florence, MD
Director, Division of Rural Programs
Department of Family Medicine
East Tennessee State University
Johnson City, TN

Grant C. Fowler, MD
Professor and Vice Chair
Family Practice and Community Medicine
The University of Texas-Houston Medical School
Houston, TX

Contributing Authors

Marc Darr, MD
Clinical Associate Professor
University of Arizona College of Medicine
Prescott, AZ

Mark D. Darrow, MD
Associate Professor
Medical Director ECU Physicians
Department of Family Medicine
Brody School of Medicine
East Carolina University
Greenville, NC

Janice E. Daugherty, MD
Associate Professor of Family Medicine
Director of Predoctoral Education
Brody School of Medicine, East Carolina University
Greenville, NC

Tim DeBlieck, MD
Faculty
Family Practice Residency of Idaho
Boise, ID

Bart Demaerschalk, MD
Assistant Professor of Neurology,
Cerebrovascular Divison
Department of Neurology
Mayo Clinic, Scottsdale
Scottsdale, AZ

Robert DeMarco, MD
Professor of Internal Medicine
Northeastern Ohio Universities College of Medicine
Youngstown, OH

Milind Deogaonkar, MD
Post-Doctoral Research Fellow
Neural Transplantation and Gene Therapy Program
Department of Neuroscience
Cleveland Clinic Foundation
Cleveland, OH

David deVlaming, DDS
Private Practice
Fort Worth, TX

Emil S. Dickstein, MD
Associate Professor of Medicine
Northeastern Ohio Universities College of Medicine
Youngstown, OH

Nuhad D. Dinno, MD
Emeritus Clinical Professor
Center on Human Development and Disability
Department of Pediatrics
University of Washington School of Medicine
Seattle, WA

William Dobak, DO
Fellow
Emory University
Atlanta, GA

Michel J. Dodard, MD
Associate Professor
Family Medicine and Community Health
University of Miami School of Medicine
Miami, FL

David Donahue, MD
Private Practice
Neurosurgery
Cook Children's Medical Center
Fort Worth, TX

Michael Donahue, MD
Resurrection Family Practice Residency
Chicago, IL

Dan Doss, DDS
Private Practice
Fort Worth, TX

S. Shevaun Duiker, MD
Private Practice
Indian Peaks Family Medicine
Lafayette, CO

Terence S. Edgar, MD
Department of Pediatric Neurology
Prevea Pediatric Neurology
Green Bay, WI

J. C. Chava-Zimmerman, MD
Medical Director
St. Francis Family Practice Residency
Lincolnwood, IL

Robert A. Cheney, MD
Associate Clinical Instructor
Orthopaedic Surgery
Albany Medical College
Albany, NY

Anthony W. Chow, MD
Professor of Medicine
Division of Infectious Diseases
Vancouver Hospital
Vancouver, British Columbia CANADA

S. Lindsey Clarke, MD
Assistant Professor of Family Medicine
Medical University of South Carolina
Self Regional Healthcare
Family Practice Residency Program
Ware Shoals, SC

Kathi Clement, MD
St. John's - St. James Clinic
St. James, MO

William W. Cleveland, MD
Professor and Chairman Emeritus
Department of Pediatrics
University of Miami
Miami, FL

Richard D. Clover, MD
School of Public Health and Information Sciences
University of Louisville
Louisville, KY

Dana Collaguazo, MD
Department of Emergency Medicine
The University of Iowa
Iowa City, IA

Douglas Collins, MD
Private Practice
Bonifay, FL

Michael A. Cooper, MD
Greater Cincinnati Associated Physicians
Cincinnati, OH

Carol Cordy, MD
Family Physician
Clinical Associate Professor, UW S.O.M.
Residency Site Director
45th St. Clinic
Seattle, WA

Alan J. Cropp, MD
Professor of Internal Medicine
Northeastern Ohio Universities College of Medicine
Youngstown, OH

Paul T. Cullen, MD
Director, Family Practice Residency Program
The Washington Hospital
Washington, PA

M. Beatriz Currier, MD
Department of Psychiatry
University of Miami School of Medicine
Miami, FL

James E. Dalen, MD, MPH
Professor Emeritus of Medicine and Public Health
University of Arizona
Tucson, AZ

Mark R. Dambro, MD
Family Medicine
Fort Worth, TX

Nancy N. Dambro, MD
Pediatric Pulmonology
Cook Children's Medical Center
Fort Worth, TX

Contributing Authors

Stoney A. Abercrombie, MD
Professor, Family Medicine
Anderson Family Practice Residency Program
Anderson, SC

Abdulrazak Abyad, MD, MPH
Director, Abyad Medical Center & Middle-East Longevity Institute
Editor, Middle-East Journal of Family Medicine
Editor, Middle-East Journal of Age & Aging
Abyad Medical Center
Middle-East Longevity Institute
Tripoli, Lebanon

Rodney D. Adam, MD
Professor of Medicine & Microbiology/Immunology
University of Arizona College of Medicine
Tucson, AZ

Stephen M. Adams, MD
Assistant Professor
Department of Family Medicine
University of Tennessee College of Medicine
Chattanooga Unit
Chattanooga, TN

Alan Adelman, MD, MS
Department of Family and Community Medicine
Milton S. Hershey Medical Center
Hershey, PA

Augusto Aguirre, MD
Medical Director, Microbiology Department
Grant-Riverside Hospitals
Columbus, OH

Richard W. Allinson, MD
Senior Staff Physician
Scott & White Clinic, Waco
Associate Professor
The Texas A & M University System Health Science Center
Waco, TX

Aarthi Anand, MD
Resident
Resurrection Family Practice Residency
Chicago, IL

Watson C. Arnold, MD
Director, Pediatric Nephrology
Cook Children's Medical Center
Fort Worth, TX

Vernan Atienza, MD
Private Practice
Des Plaines, IL

Robert L. Atmar, MD
Department of Medicine
Baylor College of Medicine
Houston, TX

Colin R. Bamford, MD
Department of Neurology
University of Arizona College of Medicine
Tucson, AZ

Benjamin Barankin, MD
Dept. of Medicine, Division of Dermatology
University of Alberta
Edmonton, Alberta CANADA

Chandramohan Batra, MD
Director, Women & Children's Services
East Kentucky Family Practice Residency Program
University of Kentucky
Hazard, KY

Robert P. Baughman, MD
Professor of Medicine, Internal Medicine
University of Cincinnati Medical Center
Cincinnati, OH

K. J. Oommen, MD

Associate Professor
Department of Neurology
University of Oklahoma College of Medicine
Oklahoma City, OK

Steven M. Shaw, MD

Private Practice
Tucson, AZ

Robert W. Snyder, MD, PhD

Department of Ophthalmology
University of Arizona College of Medicine
Tucson, AZ

Daniel K. Winstead, MD

Department of Psychiatry & Neurology
Tulane University School of Medicine
New Orleans, LA

Ralph M. Wynn, MD

Former Professor of Obstetrics & Gynecology & Pathology
State University of New York Health Science Center at Brooklyn
New York, NY

Contributing Authors

Caroline K. Buckway, MD
Private practice
Providence Alaska Medical Center
Pediatric Subspecialty Clinic
Anchorage, AK

Robert Burgos, MD
Private Practice
Gastroenterology
Huguley Memorial Medical Center
Fort Worth, TX

John R. Burk, MD
Private Practice
Pulmonology
Fort Worth, TX

David E. Burtner, MD
Vice Chairman and Professor
Department of Family & Community Medicine
Mercer University School of Medicine
Macon, GA

Roger Cady, MD
Medical Director
Headache Care Center
Springfield, MO

Cynthia Gail Carmichael, MD
Staff Physician
North Richmond Center for Health
Contra Costa Health Services
Richmond, CA

Kevin Carmichael, MD
Unit Chief
El Rio Special Immunology Associates
Tucson, AZ

Todd S. Carran, MD
Adjunct Assistant Professor of Clinical Family Medicine
University of Cincinnati
Cincinnati, OH

John Z. Carter, MD
Private Practice
Family Practice/Geriatrics
Tucson, AZ

L. Philip Carter, MD
Western Neurological, Ltd.
Tucson, AZ

Roy R. Casiano, MD
Professor and Vice-Chair, Dept of Otolaryngology
Director, Division of General Otolaryngology
University of Miami School of Medicine
Miami, FL

Mary Cataletto, MD
Associate Director, Pediatric Pulmonary Medicine
Associate Professor of Clinical Pediatrics
SUNY Stonybrook
Winthrop University Hospital, Mineola NY
Mineola, NY

A. Peter Catinella, MD
Associate Professor and Vice Chairman
Department of Family & Preventive Medicine
University of Utah
Salt Lake City, UT

Frank 'Chip' Celestino, MD
Associate Professor
Department of Family & Community Medicine
Wake Forest University School of Medicine
Winston-Salem, NC

Jasmine Chao, DO
Clinical Instructor
McGaw Medical Center of Northwestern Family Practice Residency
Northwestern University Medical School
Skokie, IL

Jason Chao, MD, MS
Professor, Dept. of Family Medicine
Case Western Reserve Univ and Univ Hospitals of Cleveland
Cleveland, OH

Kay A. Bauman, MD, MPH
Medical Director, Department of Public Safety
Professor, Department of Psychiatry
University of Hawaii
John A. Burns School of Medicine
Department of Public Safety, State of Hawaii
Honolulu, HI

Bruce G. Bellamy, MD
Saint Luke's Medical
Clinton, MO

Paul J. Benke, MD, PhD
University of Miami School of Medicine
Miami, FL

George R. Bergus, MD
Associate Professor, Dept of Family Medicine
University of Iowa
Iowa City, IA

Alexander Berry, MD
Division of Urology
University of Mass Memorial Medical Center
Worcester, MA

Frances Biagioli, MD
Assistant Professor Family Health Center
Oregon Health Sciences University
Portland, OR

Linda Bigi, DO
Clinical Instructor, Department of Family Practice
Northwestern University Medical School
Glenview, IL

William H. Billica, MD
Assistant Director
Family Practice Residency Program
Good Samaritan Medical Center
Phoenix, AZ

Timothy L. Black, MD
Pediatric Surgery
Cook Children's Medical Center
Fort Worth, TX

Shawn H. Blanchard, MD
Assistant Professor
Department of Family Medicine
Oregon Health & Science University
Portland, OR

Bruce Block, MD
Director, Primary Care Institute
UPMC - Shadyside Hospital
Pittsburgh, PA

Jess G. Bond, MD, MPH
Assistant Professor of Internal Medicine
Northeastern Ohio Universities College of Medicine
Akron, OH

Patricia Borman, MD
Director Advanced Training in Geriatrics
Swedish Family Medicine
Clinical Assistant Professor
University of Washington
Seattle, WA

Marjorie A. Bowman, MD, MPA
Department of Family Practice & Community Medicine
University of Pennsylvania Health System
Philadelphia, PA

Jack Bradford, DO
Department of Emergency Medicine
Akron General Medical Center
Akron, OH

Steven M. Bromley, MD
Research Affiliate
Smell and Taste Center
University of Pennsylvania
Philadelphia, PA

James F. Broomfield, MD
Assistant Professor of Family Practice
University of Wyoming Family Practice Residency Program at Cheyenne
Cheyenne, WY

Consultant Board

the reference citations for every topic will be available on the web site. And citations for a few lengthy topics that benefit from extra space will be available only on the web site. The web site has provided helpful information to many and it is my hope that as it matures it will continue as a reliable source of reviewed, dependable clinical information. Renovations to the web site are underway to include more information, more links, and additional formats. Keep checking back for the latest.

The web site also delivers up-to-date information on the hand-held versions of the 5-Minute. This year, The 5-Minute has been made available in several handheld formats — review them all to find the one best for your needs.

A Developer's Page helps bring the database to those who create the truly remarkable software and hardware devices that bring The 5-Minute to the clinician. Included are general comments regarding the database structure and a subset sample suitable for downloading and initial prototype work.

The book, handhelds, and web site are a compilation of many people's efforts, including the contributing authors and the consultants who review the topics — each deserves a special thanks for their time. I'd especially like to also thank Mrs. Danette Somers, for her support; the staff at Lippincott Williams & Wilkins who have done so much to keep the book and the concept of "The 5-Minute Consult" alive; my family for their patience and support; Mrs. Rose W. Cummings for her diligence in coordinating the many aspects of the project; and finally, Mrs. Jo Griffith, whose late husband is recognized in the book's title. Her hard work and persistent search for that elusive goal, perfection, has greatly improved the book.

I wish to make this work continuously responsive to the needs of its readers, and I thank those who have taken their time to write reviews and suggestions. I take your comments seriously and hope you will find many of them in this year's edition. As always, I invite you to express your wishes regarding chapters or changes you would like to appear in future editions. Send your comments and suggestions to:

Mark R. Dambro, MD
email: editor@5mcc.com

Griffith's: 5-Minute Clinical Consult aims to bring current and relevant clinical data to:

- Busy practitioners who need to quickly refresh their memory of diagnostic or treatment alternatives
- Students who need a quick update on the basics (description, genetics, prevalence, signs and symptoms, etc.)
- Patients who want to review their particular disease

To all these, and others, I hope this 5-Minute brings the kind of data they find useful. It has been, and continues to be, my desire that the database of information, collected and updated by so many clinicians, be easily accessible to its readers. Toward this end I strive to help all who share this goal to obtain and use the database for helping clinicians help their patients.

Last year, in response to several requests and in an effort to reflect changing terminology, the possessive eponym forms were changed to their singular forms. Some of these seem very straightforward: Legionnaires' disease to Legionnaires disease is hardly a cause for pause, and Kartagener's syndrome to Kartagener syndrome may even be easier to speak. On the other hand, Crohn's disease to Crohn disease is downright awkward! For consistency, however, all eponyms have been changed — such is the price of change.

This year, new material has been added.

- **Algorithms**. Dr. Douglas Collins (author of many titles dealing with the interpretation of signs and symptoms) has created over 100 new flowcharts or algorithms to help the reader in the diagnostic process. The flowcharts are primarily organized by a symptom or sign — the way patients tend to present themselves. The algorithms lead the reader through a series of questions helping to resolve the presenting complaint or finding into a diagnostic entity. The algorithms are not meant to be complete nor exhaustive lists of diseases. In fact, the physician, in even a brief review, will easily find diseases not represented. However, the clinician will find that following an algorithm will jog the memory, uncovering important questions or bringing back a forgotten case which is relevant today.

- **Medications**. Another new section, Medications, has been added to help the 5-Minute become a more complete all-in-one reference. Most of the medications noted in the text will be found in this section. The following information headings are presented: Therapeutic class, Warnings, Indications, Interactions and Formulations/Trade names.

- **U.S. Preventive Services Task Force Recommendations**. This third new section brings together the most current recommendations for Screening, Counseling, Chemophylaxis, and Immunizations. The recommendations include the rating (A for highly recommended to D, not recommended). I've added a Clinical Guide (R for relevant in many practice settings; NR for not as relevant in most settings) allowing the reader to quickly find those measures of high relevance and with good evidence for implementation in most practices.

A companion work, *The 5-Minute Patient Advisor*, links patient education topics, to the topics in this book. Look for the "link" symbol ▯ indicating a matching topic for your patient.

To bring the data to even more people, the book's web site (http://www.5mcc.com), which initially contained the table of contents and summaries of each topic, continues to evolve. This year,

Griffith's: 5-Minute Clincial Consult — 2005 represents the 13th annual edition of a quick medical reference for current diagnosis and treatment. The key features are:

- **Scope**

  Over 1000 topics arranged alphabetically and cross-indexed to synonyms: 610 expanded topics in a format that contains enough detail to confirm the diagnosis and treat the problem; 433 short topics in a brief format. ICD-9-CM entries for every topic make coding easier.

  Additional sections help make the 5-Minute a complete clinical guide: Medications, U.S. Preventive Services Task Force Recommendations, Signs & Symptoms Algorithms, and ICD-9-CM index.

- **Contributing Authors**

  Over 300 experienced clinicians writing on medical and surgical problems within their areas of interest and expertise. Authors make a final review of their topics just a few months before the book is published — insuring timeliness.

- **Consultants**

  Nearly 40 authorities in general and specialty practice. Consultants review the topics for accuracy, currency, appropriateness, completeness, and safety. Medication entries and dosages were reviewed by a Doctor of Pharmacy and contributing authors just prior to publication.

- **Updates**

  Annual updates assure inclusion of the most recent norms of practice and consensus of the majority of experts.

- **Format**

  For the expanded topics, a consistent, two-page, graphic, chart-like format, similar to the skeleton format presented below. The 6 major divisions and 38 information blocks cover the major aspects of each disorder. The remaining topics are presented in an abbreviated format reserved for those needing a shorter discussion.

  If you find the symbol, , in the PATIENT EDUCATION section of a topic, check for related patient education material in *The 5-Minute Patient Advisor*.

Basics	Diagnosis	Treatment	Medication	Followup	Miscellaneous
Description	Differential	Appropriate healthcare	Drug(s) of choice	Monitoring	Associated conditions
System(s) affected	Laboratory	General measures	Contra-indications	Prevention	Age-related factors
Genetics	Pathological findings	Surgical measures	Precautions	Complications	Pregnancy
Incidence/Prevalence	Special tests	Activity	Interactions	Prognosis	Synonyms
Age/Gender	Imaging	Diet	Alternative drugs		ICD-9-CM
Signs and symptoms	Diagnostic procedures	Patient education			See also
Causes					Other notes
Risk factors					Abbreviations
					References

Acquisitions Editor: Danette Somers
Senior Managing Editor: Stacey Sebring
Production Editor: Bridgett Dougherty, David Murphy
Manufacturing Manager: Benjamin Rivera
Marketing Manager: Kathleen Neely
Printer: Quebecor World - Taunton

530 Walnut Street
Philadelphia, PA 19106 USA
LWW.com

Printed in the United States of America

0-7817-5182-9

10 9 8 7 6 5 4 3 2 1

Griffith's 5-MINUTE CLINICAL CONSULT 2005

Mark R. Dambro, MD

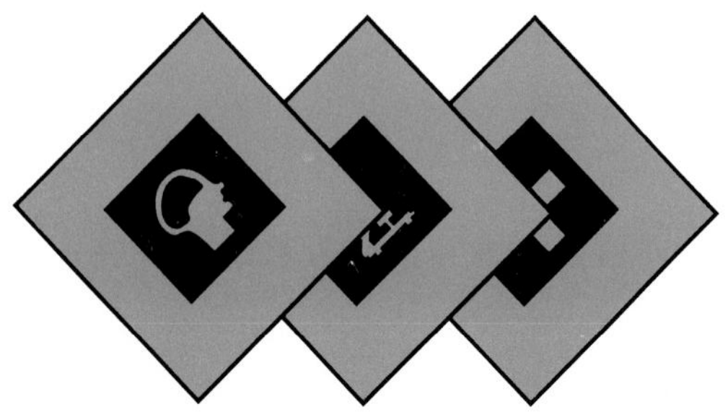

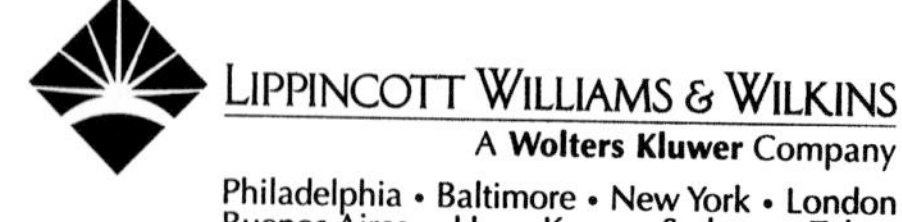

LIPPINCOTT WILLIAMS & WILKINS
A Wolters Kluwer Company
Philadelphia • Baltimore • New York • London
Buenos Aires • Hong Kong • Sydney • Tokyo

J. Christopher Graves, MD
Associate Professor
Department of Family Medicine
University of Tennessee
Chattanooga Unit of the College of Medicine
Chattanooga, TN

David S. Gray, MD
Sonoma Developmental Center
Eldridge, CA

J. Thomas Grayston, MD
Professor Emeritus of Epidemiology
Dept of Epidemiology
University of Washington
School of Public Health and Community Medicine
Seattle, WA

Ronald A. Greenfield, MD
Professor of Medicine & Chief, Infectious Diseases Section
University of Oklahoma Health Sciences Center
Oklahoma City, OK

David A. Griesemer, MD
Chairman, Department of Neurology
Medical University of South Carolina
Charleston, SC

John Guisto, MD
Associate Professor of Clinical Emergency Medicine,
Department of Emergency Medicine
University of Arizona College of Medicine
Tucson, AZ

Vladimir Hachinski, MD, DSc
Professor and Chair
Department of Clinical Neurological Sciences
The University of Western Ontario
London, Ontario CANADA

David E. Hall, MD
Clinical Associate Professor of Pediatrics
Emory University School of Medicine
Children's Healthcare of Atlanta at Scottish Rite
Atlanta, GA

R. Bruce Hall, MD
Private Practice, Orthopedics
Southern Bone & Joint Specialists
Dothan, AL

Larry W. Halverson, MD
Director, Cox Family Practice Residency Program
Cox Health
Springfield, MO

Clyde L. Harris, MD
Private Practice
Hospitalist
New Hanover Regional Medical Center
Wilmington, NC

Kristyna Hartse, PhD
Clinical Director
Baylor University Medical Center
Dallas, TX

Fern R. Hauck, MD, MS
Associate Professor and Director of Research
Department of Family Medicine
University of Virginia Health System
Charlottesville, VA

Cathryn Heath, MD
Professor of Family Medicine
UMDNJ Robert Wood Johnson Medical School
New Brunswick, NJ

Darell E. Heiselman, DO
Chief, Critical Care Medicine, Akron General Medical Center
Professor, Northeastern Ohio Universities College of Medicine
Clinical Professor, Ohio University, Athens, Ohio
Clinical Adjunct Professor, Lake Erie College of Osteopathic Medicine
Akron, OH

Thomas W. Hejkal, MD, PhD
Associate Professor
Department of Ophthalmology
University of Nebraska Medical Center
Omaha, NE

Patrick C. Henderson, MD
Department of Orthopedic Surgery
University of Arizona
Tucson, AZ

Scott T. Henderson, MD
Program Director
Mercy Family Medicine Residency
Mason City, IA

Eric Henley, MD, MPH
Associate Professor and Chair
Department of Family & Community Medicine
University of Illinois College of Medicine at Rockford
Rockford, IL

Sean Herrington, MD
Private Practice
Salina Clinic, LLC
Salina, KS

Mark Hickman, MD
Private Practice
Delaware, OH

Matthew Hintz, MD
Department of Family Practice
Grant Medical Center
Columbus, OH

Doreen L. Hock, MD
Reproductive Endocrinology & Infertility
Reproductive Medicine Associates of New Jersey
Somerset, NJ

Ira N. Hollander, MD
Private Practice
Urology Clinics of North Texas
Fort Worth, TX

Michael P. Hopkins, MD, MEd
Director, Department of Obstetrics & Gynecology
Aultman Health Foundation
Professor, Northeastern Ohio Universities College of Medicine
Canton, OH

Mark Horattas, MD
Professor of Surgery
Department of Surgery
Northeastern Ohio Universities College of Medicine
Akron, OH

Hans House, MD
Assistant Professor
Department of Emergency Medicine
University of Iowa
Iowa City, IA

Douglas M. Hoy, MD
Associate Clinical Professor
Department of Family Medicine
Medical College of Ohio
Bellevue, OH

Dennis E. Hughes, DO
Medical Director
Cox-Monett Emergency Department
Cox Health Systems
Springfield , MO

Wendy Humphrey, MD
Clinical Professor of Obstetrics and Gynecology
Northeastern Ohio Universities College of Medicine
Naples, FL

John J. Hutter, Jr., MD
Professor of Pediatrics
Chief, Pediatric Hematology/Oncology
University of Arizona College of Medicine
Tucson, AZ

Frank L. Iber, MD
Emeritus Professor of Medicine
Loyola University
Department of Gastroenterology
Department of Veterans Affairs
Riverside, IL

Mark C. Iber, PA
Physician's Assistant
Department of Medicine
New Hampshire Hospital
Concord, NH

Charles N. Jacobs, MD
Nephrologist
Waterville, ME

Philip E. Jaffe, MD
Associate Professor of Medicine
University of Connecticut Health Center
GI Division
Farmington, CT

Vivek Jain, MD
The University of Western Ontario
London, Ontario CANADA

Carrie A. Jaworski, MD
Associate Director
Resurrection Family Practice Residency
Resurrection Medical Center
Chicago, IL

Eric L. Jenison, MD
Professor of Obstetrics & Gynecology
Northeastern Ohio Universities College of Medicine
Chairman and Program Director OB-GYN Residency
Akron General Medical Center
Akron, OH

Smith L. Johnston, III, MD, MS
NASA Medical Officer/Flight Surgeon
Flight Medicine Clinic/CD26
NASA Johnson Space Center
Houston, TX

Morton S. Kahlenberg, MD
Chief, Division of Surgical Oncology
Department of Surgery
Univ. of Texas Health Science Center San Antonio
San Antonio, TX

Marc Jeffrey Kahn, MD
Associate Dean of Student Affairs
Professor of Medicine
Section of Hematology and Medical Oncology
Tulane University Health Sciences Center
School of Medicine
New Orleans, LA

Paul E. Kaplan, MD
Medical Director
Rehabilitation Management Systems
Citrus Heights, CA

Wayne J. Katon, MD
Professor of Psychiatry, Vice Chair
Department of Psychiatry, School of Medicine
University of Washington Medical School
Seattle, WA

Rick Kellerman, MD
Professor and Chair
Department of Family and Community Medicine
University of Kansas School of Medicine-Wichita
Wichita, KS

Robert M. Kershner, MD
Clinical Professor, University of Utah Medical Center
Visiting Professor of Ophthalmology
Chinese University of Hong Kong
Tucson, AZ

Ejaz Khan, MD
Resurrection Family Practice Residency
Chicago, IL

George E. Kikano, MD
Chairman & Professor
Dept of Family Medicine
Case Western Reserve University
University Hospitals of Cleveland
Cleveland, OH

Contributing Authors

Jane S. Kim, MD
Geriatrician
Total Longterm Care
Lone Tree, CO

Scott A. Kincaid, MD
Assistant Clinical Professor of Family Medicine
University of Virginia, Charlottesville, VA
Radford, VA

Mitchell S. King, MD
Associate Professor, Dept. of Family Medicine
Northwestern University Medical School
Northbrook, IL

Jeffery T. Kirchner, DO
Associate Director
Family Practice Residency Program
Lancaster General Hospital
Temple University School of Medicine
Lancaster, PA

Julienne K. Kirk, PharmD
Associate Professor
Department of Family & Community Medicine
Wake Forest University Baptist Medical Center
School of Medicine
Winston-Salem, NC

Evan W. Kligman, MD
Professor
Public Health, Medicine, Family and Community Medicine
Co-Director, Center on Aging
University of Arizona
Tucson, AZ

Mary E. Klink, MD
University of Wisconsin Medical Foundation
Medical Director, Sleep Disorders Center
Meriter Hospital
Madison, WI

Sandra Knaur, MSN
Private Practice
Sleep Consultants, Inc.
Fort Worth, TX

Aubrey L. Knight, MD
Director of Geriatric Education
Carilion Health Systems
Roanoke, VA

Peter Kozisek, MD
Family Practice Residency of Idaho
Boise, ID

Michael Krew, MD
Co-Director MFM
Aultman Hospital
Associate Professor Clinical OB/Gyn
Northeastern Ohio Universities College of Medicine
Canton, OH

Pushpa Krishnasami, MD
Resident
St. Francis Family Practice Residency
Lincolnwood, IL

Lars C. Larsen, MD
Professor
Department of Family Medicine
The Brody School of Medicine
at East Carolina University
Greenville, NC

Richard A. Larson, MD
Professor of Medicine
Director, Hematologic Malignancies
The University of Chicago
Chicago, IL

Mark C. Leeson, MD
Professor of Orthopedic Surgery
Northeastern Ohio Universities College of Medicine
Akron, OH

Matthew R Leibowitz, MD
Assistant Clinical Professor
Division of Infectious Diseases
David Geffen School of Medicine at UCLA
Los Angles, CA

Gary Levine, MD
Associate Professor, Dept. of Family Medicine
In-Patient Service Coordinator
Brody School of Medicine at East Carolina University
Greenville, NC

Richard P. Levy, MD
Adjunct Professor of Medicine
Dartmouth Medical School
Quechee, VT

James H. Lewis, MD
Professor of Medicine
Division of Gastroenterology
Georgetown University Medical Center
Washington, DC

Mian Li, MD, PhD
Clinical Co-Director
War-Related illness and Injury Center
Department of Veterans Affairs
National Institutes of Health
Potomac, MD

Leonard S. Lilly, MD
Associate Professor of Medicine
Harvard Medical School
Brigham and Women's Hospital
Boston, MA

Carol B. Lindsley, MD
Professor of Pediatrics and Chair
Director, Pediatric Rheumatology
University of Kansas School of Medicine
Kansas City, KS

Phil Lobstein, MD
Private Practice
Cardiology
Fort Worth, TX

Rich Londo, MD
Assistant Professor of Clinical Family Medicine
Department of Family and Community Medicine
University of Illinois College of Medicine-Rockford
Rockford, IL

Edgar A. Lucas, PhD
Private Practice
Sleep Consultants, Inc.
Fort Worth, TX

Brock D. Lutz, MD
East Texas Infectious Disease Consultants
Tyler, TX

Linda J. Machado, MD
Assistant Professor, Infectious Diseases
University of Oklahoma Health Sciences Center
Oklahoma City, OK

D. W. MacPherson, MD
McMaster University
Hamilton, Canada
Gatineau, Quebec CANADA

Barbara A. Majeroni, MD
Associate Clinical Professor
Department of Family Medicine
State University of New York at Buffalo
Buffalo, NY

Ronald L. Malm, DO
Assistant Professor
University of Wyoming Family Practice Residency Program at Cheyenne
Cheyenne, WY

Dannen D. Mannschreck, MD
Regional Chairman
Department of Family & Community Medicine
Texas Tech University
Health Sciences Center, Odessa
Odessa, TX

Robert A. Marlow, MD, MA
Associate Director/Director of Research
Family Practice Residency Program
Scottsdale Healthcare
Scottsdale, AZ

Anna N. Maxey, MD
Assistant Director
Family Practice Residency Program
Saint Elizabeth Medical Center
Edgewood, KY

Susana May, MD, MPH
Private Practice
University of Miami
Department of Family Medicine
Tavernier, FL

Sumner T. McAllister, MD
Family Practice
Salt Lake City, UT

Mark McConnell, MD
Medical Director, PICU
San Jose Medical Center and Good Samaritan Hospital
San Jose, CA

Timothy McCurry, MD
Program Director
Resurrection Family Practice Residency
Chicago, IL

K. Patricia McGann, MD, MSPH
Palo Alto Medical Foundation
and Associate Professor of Clinical Medicine
Stanford University School of Medicine
Los Altos, CA

Don McHard, MD
Retired
Phoenix, AZ

William Merriam, MD
Division of Urology
U Mass Memorial Medical Center
Worcester, MA

Eric S. Miller, MD
Clinical Assistant Professor
Director, Family Practice Residency OB/GYN
Program at Shadyside Hospital
University of Pittsburgh Medical Center
Shadyside Hospital
Pittsburgh, PA

Gary M. Miller, MD
Pediatric Neurology of Georgia
Woodstock, GA

James P. Miller, MD
Pediatric Surgery
Pediatric Surgical Associates of Fort Worth
Fort Worth, TX

Karl E. Miller, MD
Professor
Department of Family Medicine
University of Tennessee College of Medicine
Chattanooga Unit
Chattanooga, TN

Sandra Miller, MD
Assistant Director, Residency
Family Practice Center
Good Samaritan Regional Medical Center
Phoenix, AZ

Larry Millikan, MD
Chairman, Department of Dermatology
Tulane University School of Medicine
New Orleans, LA

Jeffrey F. Minteer, MD
Associate Director
Family Practice Residency Program
The Washington Hospital
Washington, PA

Charles D. Mitchell, MD
Division of Immunology & Infectious Diseases
Department of Pediatrics
University of Miami School of Medicine
Miami, FL

Reza Moattari, MD
Professor of Medicine and Head,
Endocrinology Division
Northeastern Ohio Universities College of Medicine
Chief, Endocrinology Section, Akron General Hospital
Akron, OH

Susan Louisa Montauk, MD
Professor of Clinical Family Medicine
Department of Family Medicine
University of Cincinnati College of Medicine
Cincinnati, OH

Phyllis Montellese, MD
Associate Director
Sports Medicine Fellowship
University of Pittsburg Medical Center Shadyside
Pittsburgh, PA

T. Glendon Moody, MD
Clinical Lecturer
Department of Ophthalmology
University of Arizona College of Medicine-Tucson
Tempe, AZ

William J. Moran, DO
Affiliate Clinical Instructor
Department of Family Medicine
Chicago College of Osteopathic Medicine
Elmhurst, IL

Samuel L. Moschella, MD
Clinical Professor Dermatology (Emeritus)
Harvard Medical School
Senior Consultant, Lahey Clinic
Burlington, MA

Brian J. Murray, MD
Director, Student Health & Wellness Center
University of California at San Diego
La Jolla, CA

Eleftherios Mylonakis, MD
Infectious Disease Division
Massachusetts General Hospital
Boston, MA

Gabriel Neal, MD
Resident, Family Practice
Grant Family Practice Residency
Grant Medical Center
Columbus, OH

Donald A. F. Nelson, MD
Director of Medical Informatics
Cedar Rapids Medical Education Foundation
Family Practice Center
Cedar Rapids, IA

Peter T. Nieh, MD
Associate Professor, Department of Urology
Emory University
The Emory Clinic
Atlanta, GA

Laura L. Novak, MD
Barberton Citizens Hospital
Barberton, OH

Olatoyosi Odenike, MD
University of Chicago
Chicago, IL

Tadao Okada, MD, MPH
Director & Interim Chief
Family Medicine Residency
Department of Family Medicine
Kameda Medical Center
Kamogawa, Chiba Japan

Edwin J. Olsen, MD, MBA
Department of Psychiatry
University of Miami School of Medicine
Miami, FL

Brenda Oshea-Robinson, RPAC
Bayside, NY

Tejal Parikh, MD
Clinical Assistant Professor
Department of Family & Community Medicine
University of Arizona
Campus Health
Tucson, AZ

Douglas S. Parks, MD
Associate Professor
Family Practice Residency Program at Cheyenne
University of Wyoming
Cheyenne, WY

Deogracias R. Peña, MD
Pediatric Nephrology
Cook Children's Medical Center
Fort Worth, TX

John R. Person, MD
Fallon Clinic
Auburn, MA

Bobby Peters, MD
Assistant Clinical Professor
Program in Emergency Medicine
University of Iowa Hospitals & Clinics
Iowa City, IA

Claudia A. Peters, MD
Queen's Student Health Service
Queen's University
Kingston, Ontario CANADA

Nicole Pilevsky, MD
Private Practice
Columbia, MD

David G. Pocock, MBBS
Shappert Primary Care Clinic at Belvidere
Belvidere, IL

Gregory A. Poland, MD
Professor
Department of Internal Medicine
Mayo Vaccine Research Group
The Mayo Clinic and Foundation
Rochester, MN

David A. Pope, MD
Private Practice
Mayo Health System
Janesville, MN

Laurel Powers, MD
Associate Director for Women's Health and Pre-Doctoral Education
St Francis Family Practice Residency Program
Lincolnwood, IL

William A. Primack, MD
Professor of Clinical Pediatrics
University of North Carolina
Chapel Hill, NC

Ronald E. Pust, MD
Professor and Director, Predoctoral Program
Department of Family and Community Medicine
University of Arizona College of Medicine
Tucson, AZ

James K. Radike, MD
Infectious Disease Consultant/ ID Section
Naval Medical Center Portsmouth
Portsmouth, VA

Kathryn Reilly, MD, MPH
Director, Graduate Medical Education
Family Practice Residency Programs
University of Oklahoma Health Sciences Center
Oklahoma City, OK

Rick Ricer, MD
Department of Family Medicine
University of Cincinnati College of Medicine
Cincinnati, OH

J. Randall Richard, MD
Professor of Clinical Family Medicine
Northeastern Ohio Universities College of Medicine
Director, Family Practice Residency
Barberton Citizens Hospital
Barberton, OH

Michel E. Rivlin, MD
Department of Obstetrics & Gynecology
University of Mississippi Medical Center
Jackson, MS

Milisa Rizer, MD
Vice Chair for Clinical Affairs
Associate Professor of Clinical Family Medicine
Ohio State University Dept. of Family Medicine
Rardin Family Practice Center
Columbus, OH

Timothy Robinson, DO
Bayside, NY

Duane C. Roe, MD
Professor of Clinical Internal Medicine
Northeastern Ohio Universities College of Medicine
Akron, OH

Lewis C. Rose, MD
Coordinator of Procedural Training
Department of Family and Community Medicine
University of Texas Health Sciences Center at San Antonio
San Antonio, TX

Bruce M. Rothschild, MD
Professor, Northeastern Ohio Universities College of Medicine
Director, Arthritis Center of Northeast Ohio
Youngstown, OH

Marc Rucquoi, MD
Family Medicine
The Family Healthcare Center
Clinton, SC

James H. Rudick, MD
Assistant Professor of Internal Medicine
Northeastern Ohio Universities College of Medicine
Canton, OH

Glenn Russo, MD
Professor, Department of Dermatology
Tulane University Medical Center
New Orleans, LA

Kia Saeian, MD
Assistant Professor
Division of Gastroenterology and Hepatology
Medical College of Wisconsin
Froedtert Hospital
Milwaukee, WI

Shagun Saggar, MD
Resident
Resurrection Family Practice Residency
Chicago, IL

Richard F. Salmon, DO
Scottish Rite Pediatric and Adolescent Consultants
Children's Healthcare of Atlanta at Scottish Rite
Atlanta, GA

Ricardo Samson, MD
Associate Professor, Cardiology Section
Department of Pediatrics
University of Arizona
Health Sciences Center
Tucson, AZ

Arthur Sanders, MD
Professor, Department of Emergency Medicine
University of Arizona College of Medicine
Tucson, AZ

Daniel T. Schelble, MD
Chairman, Department of Emergency Medicine
Akron General Medical Center
Professor of Clinical Emergency Mecicine
Northeastern Ohio Universities College of Medicine
Akron, OH

Karl M. Schmitt, MD
Assistant Director
Family Practice Residency Program
Saint Elizabeth Medical Center
Edgewood, KY

F. David Schneider, MD, MSPH
Associate Professor
Department of Family and Community Medicine
University of Texas Health Science Center at San Antonio
San Antonio, TX

Lisa M. Schroeder, MD
Assistant Director
Barberton Family Practice Residency Program
Barberton, OH

Robert M. Schultz, MD
Pediatric Endocrine Associates, PC
Director, Pediatric Endocrinology
Children's Hospital of Atlanta at Scottish Rite
Atlanta, GA

Wayne H. Schwesinger, MD
Head, Section of General Surgery
Department of Surgery
The University of Texas Health Science Center at San Antonio
San Antonio, TX

Jon C. Seager, MD
Hartville Family Physicians
Hartville, OH

David P. Sealy, MD
Director, Sports Medicine
Clinical Professor & Director, Resident Education
Self Memorial Hospital Family Medicine Residency
Greenwood, SC

W. Franklin Sease, Jr, MD
Assistant Director, UPMC-St. Margaret
Primary Care Sports Medicine Fellowship
Department of Family Medicine
University of Pittsburgh Medical Center
Pittsburgh, PA

Shefali K. Shah, MD
Resident
Resurrection Family Practice Residency
Resurrection Medical Center
Chicago, IL

Mark M. Shelton, MD
Director, Infectious Diseases
Cook Children's Medical Center
Fort Worth, TX

Albert T. Shiu, MD
Professor of Clinical Obstetrics and Gynecology
Director of Obstetrics and Gynecology Residency Program
Northeastern Ohio Universities College of Medicine
St. Elizabeth Health Center
Canfield, OH

Joseph Shrum, MD
Professor of Dermatology
Department of Dermatology
Tulane University Medical Center
New Orleans, LA

Aamir Siddiqi, MD
Associate Director, St Lukes's Family Practice Residency Program
Assistant Professor, Department of Family Medicine
University of Wisconsin Medical School
Milwaukee, WI

Gary J. Silko, MD, MS
Director, Family Practice Residency Program
Saint Vincent Health Center
Erie, PA

Richard J. Simensen, PhD
Neuropsychologist
Greenwood Genetic Center
Columbia, SC

Janelle D. Simpson, MD
Instructor, Department of Family Medicine
University of Tennessee College of Medicine
Chattanooga Unit
Chattanooga, TN

Violet Siwik, MD
Assistant Medical Director
Department of Family and Community Medicine
University of Arizona
Tucson, AZ

Leonard N. Slater, MD
Professor of Medicine, Infectious Diseases Section
University of Oklahoma Health Sciences Center
& Veterans Affairs Medical Center
Oklahoma City, OK

Arthur R. Slaughter, MD
Associate Director, Family Practice Education
Carilion Family Practice Residency Program
Roanoke, VA

W. Paul Slomiany, MD
Assistant Director
Family Practice Residency Program
Washington Hospital
Washington, PA

H. Gratin Smith, MD
Director of Pediatric Education
Family Practice Residency Program
Self Regional Healthcare
Greenwood, SC

Hugh S. Smith, MD
Department of Family Practice
Cheyenne, WY

Michael J. Smith, MD
Assistant Professor of Orthopedic Surgery
Northeastern Ohio Universities College of Medicine
Akron, OH

Stanley G. Smith, MA, MB
Professor Emeritus
University of Western Ontario
Southwest Middlesex Health Centre
Mt. Brydges, Ontario CANADA

John C. Smulian, MD, MPH
Associate Professor of Obstetrics, Gynecology, &
Reproductive Sciences
Acting Director, Maternal & Fetal Medicine
UMDNJ-Robert Wood Johnson Medical School
Robert Wood Johnson University Hospital
New Brunswick, NJ

Nancy Snapp, MD, MPH
International Community Health Services
Assistant Clinical Professor
Department of Family Medicine
University of Washington School of Medicine
Seattle, WA

Gregory Snyder, MD
Department of Family Medicine
State University of New York at Buffalo
Buffalo, NY

Beck Soderberg, MD
Staff Physician
Pinnacle Health Care
San Jose, CA

Vera Y. Soong, MD
Baptist Princeton Medical Center
Birmingham, AL

John Spangler, MD, MPH
Associate Professor
Department of Family and Community Medicine
Wake Forest University School of Medicine
Winston-Salem, NC

Kevin Spear, MD
Assistant Professor, Urology
Northeastern Ohio Universities College of Medicine
Akron, OH

Nicholas J. Spirtos, DO
Associate Professor, NEOUCOM
Director, Northeastern Ohio Fertility Center
Northeastern Ohio Universities College of Medicine
& Summa Health System
Akron, OH

Sukanya Srinivasan, MD, MPH
Associate Professor
Department of Family Medicine
University of Pittsburgh, School of Medicine
Pittsburgh, PA

Thomas R. Strigle, MD
Private Practice
Findlay Surgical Associates
Findlay, OH

David H. Stubbs, MD
The Iowa Clinic
Heart & Vascular Care
Iowa Methodist Medical Center
Des Moines, IA

Gregg W. Suits, MD
Private Practice
Hillsboro, OR

Sandra M. Sulik, MD
Associate Professor of Family Medicine
St. Joseph's Family Practice Residency
Upstate Medical Center
Fayetteville, NY

Geoffrey R. Swain, MD, MPH
Visiting Associate Professor
Department of Family Medicine
University of Wisconsin Medical School
Center Scientist, Center for Urban Population Health
Associate Medical Director
City of Milwaukee Health Department
Milwaukee, WI

Vassiliki Syriopoulou, MD
Associate Professor of Pediatrics, Athens University
Aghia Sophia Children's Hospital
Chief, Division of Pediatrics, First Department of Pediatrics
Athens, GREECE

David H. Thom, MD, PhD
Associate Professor, Dept of Family and Community Medicine
University of California at San Francisco School of Medicine
San Francisco, CA

Rob Tiller, MD
Family Medicine Faculty Physician
Rural Medicine Director
Self Regional Healthcare
Montgomery Center for Family Medicine
Greenwood, SC

William L. Toffler, MD
Professor
Department of Family Medicine
Oregon Health & Science University
Portland, OR

Moshe S. Torem, MD
Professor, Department of Psychiatry
Northeastern Ohio Universities College of Medicine
Medical Director
The Center for Mind-Body Medicine
Akron, OH

Peter P. Toth, MD, PhD
Director of Preventive Cardiology
Sterling Rock Falls Clinic, Ltd.
Visiting Clinical Associate Professor
University of Illinois School of Medicine, Peoria
Sterling, IL

Michael Tutt, MD
Internal Medicine
Fort Defiance Hospital
Fort Defiance, AZ

Rohit Uppal, MD
Department of Family Practice
Grant Medical Center
Columbus, OH

Francisco G. Valencia, MD
University Orthopedic Specialists
Tucson, AZ

Michael M. Van Ness, MD
Gastroenterology Specialists, Inc.
Aultman Hospital
Canton, OH

Bruce T. Vanderhoff, MD
Co-Chair, Department of Family Medicine &
Residency Director
Clinical Assistant Professor
Grant Medical Center
Ohio State Univ. College of Medicine & Public Health
Columbus, OH

Lisa Vantrease, MD
Beavercreek Family Physicians
Beavercreek, OH

Jacob Varghese, MD
Resident, Family Practice
Grant Family Practice Residency
Clinical Instructor, Family Medicine
Ohio State University School of Medicine
Columbus, OH

Rajiv R. Varma, MD
Associate Professor
Division of Gastroenterology and Hepatology
Medical College of Wisconsin
Froedtert Hospital
Milwaukee, WI

V. Vasudeviah, BSc, MBBS
Consultant
Villivakam, Chennai INDIA

Richard Viken, MD
Chairman, Department of Family Practice
The University of Texas Health Center at Tyler
Tyler, TX

Chris Vincent, MD
Faculty, Family Practice Residency
Swedish Family Medicine
Seattle, WA

Jonathan Vinson, MD
Captain, USAF
1st Medical Group
United States Air Force
Langley AFB, VA

Kenton Voorhees, MD
Assistant Prof., Department of Family Medicine
Residency Program Director
Swedish Family Medicine Residency
Littleton, CO

Kimberle Vore, MD
Clinical Instructor
Washington Hospital
Washington, PA

Gene W. Voskuhl, MD
Infectious Disease Section
University of Oklahoma Health Sciences Center
Oklahoma City, OK

Amy Y. Wang, MD
Family Practice
Chicago, IL

John R Waterson, MD, PhD
Medical Geneticist
Director, Medical Genetics Division
Children's Hospital & Research Center at Oakland
Oakland, CA

Kurt J. Wegner, MD
Professor of Pediatrics
Neonatologist, Geneticist and Pediatric Consultant
Northeastern Ohio Universities College of Medicine
Tod Children's Hospital
Youngstown, OH

Martin E. Weinand, MD
Professor of Surgery
Division of Neurosurgery
University of Arizona College of Medicine
Tucson, AZ

Barry D. Weiss, MD
Professor, Department of Family and Community Medicine
University of Arizona College of Medicine
Tucson, AZ

Gary B. Williams, MD
Associate Professor of Surgery
Northeastern Ohio Universities College of Medicine
Akron, OH

Fremont P. Wirth, MD
Neurological Institute of Savannah
Savannah, GA

Christopher M. Wise, MD
W. Robert Irby Professor Medicine
Division of Rheumatology, Allergy & Immunology
Medical College of Virginia/Virginia Commonwealth University
Richmond, VA

Jeffrey D. Wolfrey, MD
Program Director, Family Practice Residency Program
Banner Good Samaritan Medical Center
Phoenix, AZ

Douglas C. Woolley, MD
Associate Professor
Family and Community Medicine
Kansas University School of Medicine - Wichita
Wichita, KS

Frances Y. Wu, MD
Assistant Director
Somerset Family Practice Residency Program
Somerville, NJ

Alayne Yates, MD
Department of Psychiatry
John A. Burns School of Medicine
University of Hawaii
Honolulu, HI

Solomon Yigazu, MD
Resident
St Francis Family Practice Residency Program
Lincolnwood, IL

William F. Young, Jr, MD
Professor of Medicine, Division of Endocrinology & Metabolism
Mayo Clinic and Foundation
Rochester, MN

Aaron T Yu, MD
Puyallup, WA

Richard Kent Zimmerman, MD, MPH
Associate Professor, Departments of Family Medicine & Clinical Epidemiology & Behavioral and Community Health Sciences
University of Pittsburgh
Pittsburgh, PA

TABLE OF CONTENTS

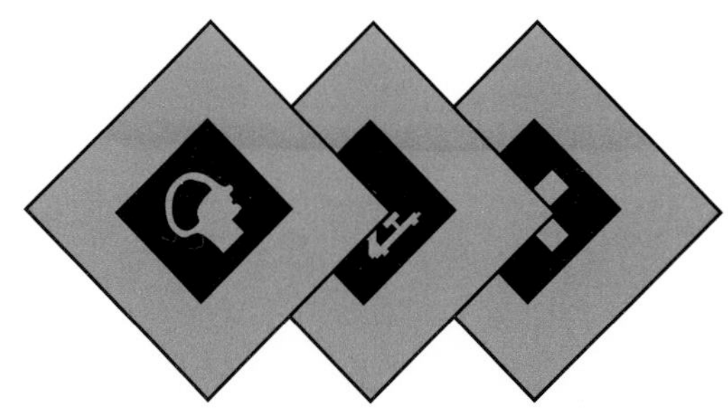

Expanded Topics

Expanded Topics

Expanded Topics

Short Topics

Signs & Symptoms: An Algorithmic Approach

Section 1

Expanded Topics

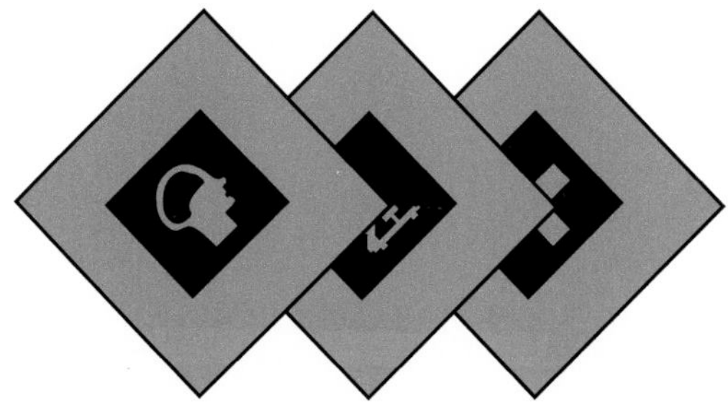

BASICS

DESCRIPTION The Papanicolaou (Pap) smear is a screening test for cervical cellular pathology. The abnormal Pap smear can range from benign cellular changes to suggestion of invasive cancer.
System(s) affected: Reproductive
Genetics: N/A
Incidence/Prevalence in USA: SIL (squamous intraepithelial lesion) low grade ranges from 10-50% of all Pap smears. SIL High grade and invasive cancer is present on 4% of all Pap smears. Other reactive, reparative and ASC-US (atypical squamous cells of undetermined significance) results are difficult to assess because of the lack of reporting mechanisms.
Predominant age: Can range from when a female becomes sexually active into the geriatric age group
Predominant sex: Female only

SIGNS & SYMPTOMS
- Frequently there are no symptoms
- Occasionally will have external genital HPV lesions
- Occasionally will have vaginal discharge related to STDs
- Rarely can have vaginal bleeding related to a malignant lesion

CAUSES Strong link to HPV infections. HPV viral types 16, 18, 31, 35, 45, 51, 52, 56, 58 are common high-risk or oncogenic virus types for cervical cancer. HPV viral types 6, 11, 42, 43, and 44 are considered low-risk.

RISK FACTORS
- Multiple sexual partners
- Cigarette smoking
- Early age of intercourse
- Intercourse with a high risk male partner
- HPV infection
- Human immunodeficiency virus infection
- Immunosuppression

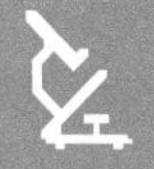

DIAGNOSIS

DIFFERENTIAL DIAGNOSIS
- Cervical SIL
- Acute or chronic cervicitis
- Vaginitis
- HPV infection
- Invasive cervical malignancy

LABORATORY
Bethesda System for Reporting Pap Smear Results
- Specimen adequacy
- Negative for Intraepithelial Lesion or Malignancy
- Epithelial cell abnormalities:
  - ◊ Atypical squamous cells (ASC)
  - ◊ Atypical squamous cells of undetermined significance (ASC-US)
  - ◊ Atypical cells cannot exclude high grade SIL (ASC-H)
  - ◊ Low-grade squamous intraepithelial lesion (LSIL)
  - ◊ High-grade squamous intraepithelial lesion (HSIL)
  - ◊ Squamous cell carcinoma
- Glandular cells:
  - ◊ Atypical glandular cells (AGS)
  - ◊ Atypical glandular cells, favor neoplasia
  - ◊ Endocervical adenocarcinoma in situ
  - ◊ Adenocarcinoma
- Thin-Preparation is a sampling technique that uses a liquid collection device and preparation. The advantage to this technique is that it improves the sensitivity of Pap smears. The disadvantage is that this technique is more expensive.

Drugs that may alter lab results: N/A

Disorders that may alter lab results: N/A

PATHOLOGICAL FINDINGS
- Atypical squamous or columnar cells
- Coarse nuclear material
- Increases nuclear diameter
- Koilocytosis

SPECIAL TESTS
- Colposcopy - generally recommended when any of these are present:
  - ◊ Initial Pap smear with HSIL or worse
  - ◊ ASC or ASC-US present on two Pap smears 4-6 months apart
  - ◊ ASC-H needs colposcopic evaluation
  - ◊ Any abnormal or suspicious lesion of the cervix or vagina that can be visualized by the naked eye
  - ◊ Atypical endocervical cells
- HPV viral typing: Hybrid capture 2 test has two viral type probes, a low-risk and high-risk probe. This high-risk probe can be used to identify patients with ASC-US or low-grade SIL that need colposcopy follow-up.

IMAGING N/A

DIAGNOSTIC PROCEDURES
- Colposcopy with visually directed biopsy
- Loop electrosurgical excision procedure (LEEP)
- Cone biopsy
- Cervicography

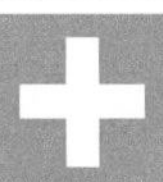

TREATMENT

APPROPRIATE HEALTH CARE Outpatient

GENERAL MEASURES Office evaluation and observation

SURGICAL MEASURES
- SIL Low, High grade, and CIS can be treated with outpatient surgery - cryotherapy, laser ablation, LEEP/LLETZ, or conization
- If cervical malignancy, see separate topic

ACTIVITY N/A

DIET No restrictions

PATIENT EDUCATION N/A

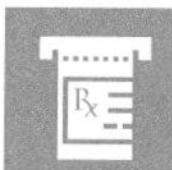

MEDICATIONS

DRUG(S) OF CHOICE
- Infective/reactive Pap smear
  - ◊ Metronidazole 250 mg tid x 7 days
- Condyloma acuminatum
  - ◊ Cryotherapy
  - ◊ Podophyllin
  - ◊ Trichloroacetic acid (TCA)

Contraindications: N/A
Precautions: N/A
Significant possible interactions: N/A

ALTERNATIVE DRUGS N/A

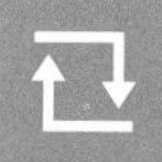

FOLLOWUP

PATIENT MONITORING
- ASC-US can be followed with HPV hybrid capture 2 test. If positive for high risk viral type - colposcopy. If negative for high risk viral type - repeat pap smear in one year.
- SIL low or high grade, ASC-H, invasive squamous or adenocarcinoma - colposcopy

PREVENTION/AVOIDANCE
- Delay first intercourse to age 20
- Monogamous relationship for both partners
- Smoking cessation
- Routine Pap smears
- Use barrier methods of birth control if nonmonogamous relationship

POSSIBLE COMPLICATIONS
- Minor abnormalities on Pap smears can mask more advanced lesions
- High grade SIL can progress to invasive cancer

EXPECTED COURSE/PROGNOSIS
- Generally excellent
- Less than half of the persistent infective, reactive, reparative or ASC-US Pap smears will have more advanced lesions
- Only a small percentage of SIL low grade will progress to more advanced lesion
- Lesions discovered early are very amenable to treatment with excellent results and few recurrences

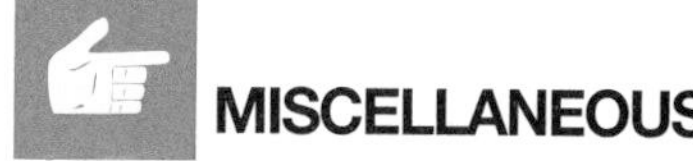

MISCELLANEOUS

ASSOCIATED CONDITIONS N/A

AGE-RELATED FACTORS
Pediatric: Very rare
Geriatric: Less frequent except in the unscreened population
Others: Abnormal Pap smears can occur at any age. The more advanced the abnormality, the more likely the patient is 25-45 years of age.

PREGNANCY
SIL lesions can progress during pregnancy

SYNONYMS N/A

ICD-9-CM
622.1 Dysplasia of cervix (uteri)

SEE ALSO
Cervical malignancy
Condyloma acuminata
Failure to thrive (FTT)
Trichomoniasis
Vulvovaginitis, bacterial

OTHER NOTES N/A

ABBREVIATIONS
HPV = human papilloma virus
ASC-US = atypical squamous cells of undetermined significance
SIL = squamous intraepithelial lesion
LEEP = loop electrosurgical excision procedure
CIS = carcinoma in situ
LLETZ = large loop excision of transition zone

REFERENCES

- Wright TC Jr, Cox JT, Massad LS, et al. ASCCP-Sponsored Consensus Conference. 2001 Consensus Guidelines for the management of women with cervical cytological abnormalities. JAMA 2002;287(16):2120-9
- Melnikow J, Kuppermann M, Birch S, Chan BK, Nuovo J. Management of the low-grade abnormal Pap smear: What are women's preferences? J Fam Pract 2002;51(10):849-55
- Canavan TP, Doshi NR. Cervical cancer. Am Fam Phys 2000;61(5):1369-76
- Guide to Clinical Preventive Services: Report of the US Preventive Services Task Force, 2nd ed. Baltimore: Williams and Wilkins, 1996:105-17
- Apgar BS, Brotzman G. HPV testing in the evaluation of the minimally abnormal Papanicolaou smear. Am Fam Physician 1999;59(10):2794-801
- Bishop JW, Marshall CJ, Bentz JS. New technologies in gynecologic cytology. J Reprod Med 2000;45(9):701-19
- Solomon S, Davey D, Kurman R, et al. The 2001 Bethesda System: terminology for reporting results of cervical cytology. JAMA 2002;287:2114-19

Web references: 2 available at www.5mcc.com
Illustrations N/A

Author(s):
Karl E. Miller, MD
Janelle D. Simpson, MD

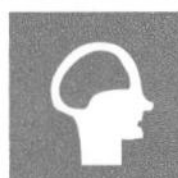

BASICS

DESCRIPTION Abortion is the separation of products of conception from the uterus prior to the potential for fetal survival outside the uterus. Gestationally, the point at which potential fetal viability exists has been the subject of much legal and scientific debate, and definitions vary from state to state; however, a "potentially viable" fetus generally weighs at least 500 grams and/or has a gestational age over 20 weeks.

- Spontaneous abortion: refers to expulsion of all (complete abortion) or part (incomplete abortion) of the products of conception from the uterus prior to the 20th completed week of gestation. The placenta, either in whole or in part, can be retained and leads to continuing vaginal bleeding (sometimes profuse). Abortion is "threatened" when vaginal bleeding occurs early in pregnancy, with or without uterine contractions, but without dilatation of the cervix, rupture of the membranes, or expulsion of products of conception. Cervical dilation, rupture of membranes or expulsion of products in the presence of vaginal bleeding portends "inevitable abortion." Differentiation between threatened and inevitable abortion is desirable since management differs.
- Missed abortion: Failed first trimester pregnancy but without the usual signs and symptoms such as bleeding or cramping. Term blighted ovum replaced with anembryonic gestation. Ultrasound findings of "empty sac."
- Induced abortion: refers to the evacuation of uterine contents/products of conception by either medical or surgical methodology
- Infected abortion: infection involving the products of conception and the maternal reproductive organs
- Septic abortion: dissemination of bacteria (and/or their toxins) into the maternal circulatory and organ system
- Habitual spontaneous abortion: three or more consecutive spontaneous abortions. Risk of another spontaneous abortion is approximately 25-30% with 70% rate of successful pregnancy in subsequent pregnancy.

System(s) affected: Endocrine/Metabolic, Reproductive

Genetics: Approximately 2/3 of first trimester spontaneous abortions have significant chromosomal anomalies with 1/2 of these being autosomal trisomies and the remainder being triploidy, tetraploidy, or 45X monosomies

Incidence/Prevalence in USA:

- Approximately 10-15% of all clinically recognized pregnancies end in spontaneous abortion
- Biochemical pregnancy manifests itself by the presence of ß-HCG in the blood 7-10 days after conception. When both clinical and biochemical pregnancies are considered, more than 50% of conceptions are spontaneous aborted.

Predominant age: Increases with advancing age, especially after 35 years of age. At age 40, the loss rate is 2 times that of age 20.

Predominant sex: Female only

SIGNS & SYMPTOMS

- In a previously diagnosed intrauterine pregnancy
  - ◊ Vaginal bleeding
  - ◊ Uterine cramping
  - ◊ Cervical dilation
  - ◊ Ruptured membranes
  - ◊ Passage of non-viable products of conception

CAUSES See Risk Factors

RISK FACTORS

- Chromosomal abnormalities
- Luteal phase defect
- Leiomyomas
- Incompetent cervix
- Infections
- Antifetal antibodies
- Autoimmune disease - phospholipid syndrome
- Alloimmune disease (shared paternal antigens)
- Drugs, chemicals, noxious agents (alcohol, smoking, caffeine)
- X-irradiation
- Contraceptive IUD

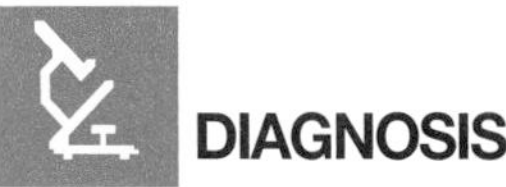

DIAGNOSIS

DIFFERENTIAL DIAGNOSIS

- Ectopic pregnancy: a potentially life-threatening complication, difficult to distinguish from threatened abortion. Transvaginal ultrasonography can identify intrauterine gestational sacs at 32 days of gestation (at serum HCG levels of 1500-2000 IU). The absence of transvaginal ultrasound evidence of an intrauterine gestation with serum HCG over 2000 IU/L should be considered an ectopic pregnancy until proven otherwise.
- Cervical polyps, neoplasias, and/or inflammatory conditions can cause vaginal bleeding. This bleeding is not usually associated with pain/cramping and is apparent on speculum exam.
- Hydatidiform mole pregnancy usually ends in abortion prior to the 20th week of pregnancy. Bloody discharge prior to abortion is common. An intrauterine grape-like appearing mass on the ultrasound is diagnostic (a "snow storm" appearance). Human chorionic gonadotropin (HCG) is often high.
- Membranous dysmenorrhea: characterized by bleeding, cramps and passage of endometrial casts can mimic spontaneous abortion. HCG is negative.
- HCG secreting ovarian tumor

LABORATORY

- Cultures - gonorrhea and chlamydia
- CBC
- Rh type
- Human chorionic gonadotropin (HCG)
- Serial ß-HCG measurements can assess viability of the pregnancy. Normal gestations have an approximate 67% increase over 2-day interval. Abnormal gestations do not rise appropriately, plateau, or decrease in level before the eighth week of gestation.

Drugs that may alter lab results: N/A

Disorders that may alter lab results: N/A

PATHOLOGICAL FINDINGS Products of conception, placental villi

SPECIAL TESTS Progesterone levels > 25 ng/mL are consistent with normal intrauterine pregnancy and are rarely seen in ectopic and/or non-viable pregnancy. A progesterone of < 5 ng/mL is an indicator of a nonviable intrauterine gestation or an ectopic pregnancy.

IMAGING

- Ultrasound examination for fetal viability and to rule out ectopic pregnancy
- Ultrasound imaging can be sensitive enough to confirm an intrauterine pregnancy in the fourth or fifth gestational week from last menstrual period

DIAGNOSTIC PROCEDURES

- Viable intrauterine pregnancy with fetal cardiac activity detected between 5-8 weeks from last menstrual period on transvaginal ultrasound
- Transvaginal ultrasound criteria for nonviable intrauterine gestation include:
  - ◊ 5 mm fetal pole without cardiac activity, or
  - ◊ 16 mm gestational sac without a fetal pole
- Fetal heart tones can be auscultated with doppler starting between 10-12 weeks gestation from last menstrual period for a viable pregnancy
- Consider a diagnosis of spontaneous abortion in a woman, of childbearing age, presenting with abnormal vaginal bleeding

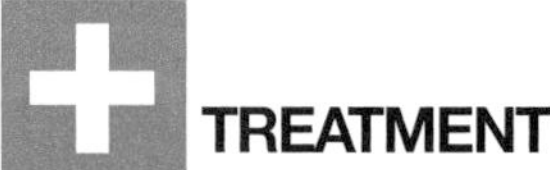

TREATMENT

APPROPRIATE HEALTH CARE Outpatient or inpatient, depending on severity of symptoms (bleeding or pain)

GENERAL MEASURES

- Explore any first trimester vaginal bleeding
- Serial quantitative ß-HCG determination and progesterone assay
- Transvaginal ultrasonography

SURGICAL MEASURES

- Inevitable or incomplete abortion: Dilatation and curettage (D&C) (usually suction)
- When completeness of an abortion is uncertain, a D&C for retained products should be performed

ACTIVITY If appropriate, bed rest; probably no effect on eventual outcome

DIET No special diet

PATIENT EDUCATION American College of Obstetricians & Gynecologists, 409 12th St., SW, Washington, DC 20090-6290 (800)762-2264, pamphlet #AP090

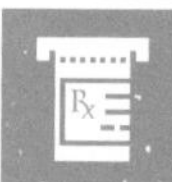

MEDICATIONS

DRUG(S) OF CHOICE

- Bleeding following uncomplicated D&C or spontaneous abortion usually controlled by:
  - ◊ Carboprost (Hemabate) 250 mcg IM
  - ◊ Oxytocin (Pitocin) 10 units IM, or IV
  - ◊ Methylergonovine (Methergine) 0.2 mg IM
- Analgesics if needed
- Rho(D) immune globulin if mother is Rh negative
- Progesterone, if deficiency confirmed prior to pregnancy

Contraindications: None

Precautions: Do not give methylergonovine IV. Refer to manufacturer's literature.

Significant possible interactions: Refer to manufacturer's literature

ALTERNATIVE DRUGS N/A

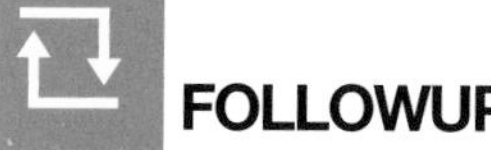

FOLLOWUP

PATIENT MONITORING

- Identification of products of conception within material expelled from the uterus or D&C specimen
- If abortion is complete, observe the patient for further bleeding
- Complete abortion usually indicated by decreased bleeding, closed cervix, intact or complete products of conception passed, and ultrasound findings of empty uterus and endometrial stripe. Follow HCG's weekly to zero to confirm complete evacuation of products of conception. Can take 2 weeks. If levels plateau, suspect retained products of conception or ectopic pregnancy.

PREVENTION/AVOIDANCE

- Any vaginal bleeding in intrauterine pregnancy is abnormal and should be considered a "threatened" abortion. In reality, vaginal bleeding in early pregnancy is common (occurring in up to 1/3 of pregnancies) and often the bleeding source eludes diagnosis.
- In habitual abortion, the abortus should be sent for karyotyping. Explore other causes of habitual abortion with the couple to determine the best therapy.
- Special care and attention for the patient who has a subsequent pregnancy

POSSIBLE COMPLICATIONS

- Complications of D&C include uterine perforation, infection and bleeding
- Possibly retained products of conception
- Depression and feelings of guilt (patient may need education and reassurance that she did not cause the miscarriage)

EXPECTED COURSE/PROGNOSIS

- If bleeding ceases, prognosis is excellent.
- Habitual abortion: prognosis is dependent on etiology. After a 2 consecutive abortions, most couples want some investigation of the problem. After 3 spontaneous abortions, evaluation is usually indicated. Prognosis is still excellent with up to 70% rate of success with subsequent pregnancy.

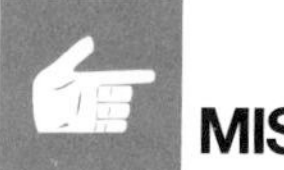

MISCELLANEOUS

ASSOCIATED CONDITIONS N/A

AGE-RELATED FACTORS

Pediatric: N/A
Geriatric: N/A
Others: N/A

PREGNANCY Confined to pregnancy

SYNONYMS

- Miscarriage
- Habitual abortion
- Recurrent abortion

ICD-9-CM

632 Missed abortion
629.9 Unspecified disorder of female genital organs
634.92 Spontaneous abortion without mention of complication, complete
634.91 Spontaneous abortion without mention of complication, incomplete
640.03 Threatened abortion, antepartum condition or complication

SEE ALSO

Ectopic pregnancy

OTHER NOTES N/A

ABBREVIATIONS N/A

REFERENCES

- Rempen A. Diagnosis and viability of early pregnancy with vaginal sonography. J Ultrasound Med 1990; 9:711-716
- Daily CA, et al. The prognostic value of serum progesterone and quantitative ß-Human Chorionic Gonadotropin in early human pregnancy. Am J Obstet Gynecol 1994;171:380-384
- Ohno M, et al. A Cytogenic study of spontaneous abortion with direct analysis of chorionic villi. Obstet Gynecol 1991;77(3):394-398
- Benne H, Michael J. Abortion. In: Hacker & Moore, eds. Essentials of Obstetrics and Gynecology. 3rd ed. Philadelphia, WB Saunders Co., 1998
- Palmieri A, Moore G, et al. Ectopic pregnancy. In: Hacker & Moore, eds. Essentials of Obstetrics and Gynecology. 3rd ed. Philadelphia, WB Saunders Co., 1998
- Simpson JL. Fetal wastage. In: Gabbe S, Niebyl J, et al, eds. Obstetrics: Normal and Problem Pregnancies. 3rd ed. New York, Churchill Livingstone, 1996
- Genovese S. Antepartal hemorrhagic disorders. In: Lowdermilk D, Perry S, eds. Maternity and Women's Health. 8th ed. St Louis: Mosby; 2004
- Garmel S. Early pregnancy risks. In: DeCherney A, Pernall M, eds. Current Obstetric and Gynecologic Diagnosis and Treatment. 9th ed. New York: McGraw-Hill; 2003

Web references: 1 available at www.5mcc.com
Illustrations N/A

Author(s):

Wendy Humphrey, MD

BASICS

DESCRIPTION Premature separation of otherwise normally implanted placenta. Sher's grades:
1: Minimal or no bleeding; detected as retroplacental clot after delivery of viable fetus
2: Viable fetus with bleeding and tender irritable uterus
3: Type A with dead fetus and no coagulopathy; type B with dead fetus and coagulopathy (about 30% of grade 3's)

System(s) affected: Cardiovascular, Reproductive

Genetics: N/A

Incidence/Prevalence in USA:
- 1% of all deliveries
- 15% if one prior episode
- 25% if ≥ 2 prior episodes

Predominant age: All childbearing ages

Predominant sex: Female only

SIGNS & SYMPTOMS
- Second or third trimester vaginal bleeding greater than one pad or tampon per hour
- Back pain, abdominal pain
- Uterine tenderness, hypertonia, or high frequency contractions
- Blood loss may be concealed; clinical signs of shock may occur with little vaginal bleeding
- Since blood volumes increase in pregnancy, volume lost may exceed 30% before signs of shock or hypovolemia. Vital signs may be preserved even with significant loss.
- Fetal distress or demise
- Idiopathic preterm labor with or without fetal distress

CAUSES
- Cocaine use and abuse
- Trauma of variable amounts; especially blunt abdominal trauma in which external signs of trauma may be incongruent with fetal injury (motor vehicle accidents or domestic violence)
- Sudden decompression of over-distended uterus as in hydramnios or twin gestation

RISK FACTORS
- Prior abruption (increases risk 10-fold)
- Maternal smoking
- Severe small for gestational age birth
- Alcohol abuse
- Hypertension: pregnancy-induced and chronic
- Uterine anomalies
- Advanced maternal age
- Increased risk if hypertensive and parity > 3
- Preterm rupture of membranes, especially if bleeding occurs during observation interval
- Vaginal bleeding before spontaneous rupture of membranes

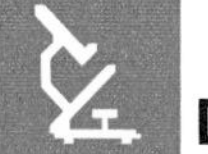

DIAGNOSIS

DIFFERENTIAL DIAGNOSIS Uterine rupture, placenta previa, vasa previa, marked bloody show, cervical and vaginal causes (e.g., chlamydia or gonorrhea with bloody, friable cervix), masses, other painful conditions (e.g., appendicitis, pyelonephritis), and labor.

LABORATORY
- Blood type, Rh, Coombs
- CBC with platelet count
- Prothrombin time (PT) , partial thromboplastin time (PTT), fibrinogen levels
- Cross match at least three units

Drugs that may alter lab results:
- Those affecting clotting parameters
- RHoD immune globulin less than 12 weeks prior may affect antibody test

Disorders that may alter lab results:
- Fibrinogen levels climb to 350-550 mg/dl (3.5-5.5 g/L) in third trimester and must fall to 100-150 mg/dl (1.0-1.5 g/L) before PTT will rise
- Fibrin split or degradation products are elevated in pregnancy and are not very helpful in assessing disseminated intravascular coagulation (DIC)

PATHOLOGICAL FINDINGS
- Normocytic normochromic anemia with acute bleeding
- Elevated PT, PTT, fibrinogen levels below 100-150 mg/dl (1.0-1.5 g/L), platelets 20,000-50,000 if DIC active
- Positive Kleihauer-Betke reaction if fetal-maternal transfusion has occurred
- Positive antibody if RhoD isosensitization has occurred

SPECIAL TESTS
- Kleihauer-Betke for fetal-maternal transfusion
- Bedside clot test with red top tube of maternal blood with poor or non-clotting blood after 7-10 minutes indicating coagulopathy
- Apt test for fetal blood origin: mix vaginal blood with small amount tap water to cause hemolysis, centrifuge several minutes, mix pink hemoglobin containing supernatant with 1 cc 1% sodium hydroxide (NaOH) for each 5 cc supernatant, reading color in two minutes with fetal Hgb staying pink and adult turning yellow-brown
- Wright stain vaginal blood, observe for nucleated RBC's - usually of fetal origin
- Lecithin/sphingomyelin (L/S) ratio if delay of delivery is an option and length of pregnancy is preterm

IMAGING
- Although ultrasound may show sonolucent retroplacental clot, rounded placenta margin or thickened placenta, it is often not definitive - especially with posterior placement or mild abruption

DIAGNOSTIC PROCEDURES
- External uterine monitoring often shows elevated baseline pressure and frequent low amplitude contractions

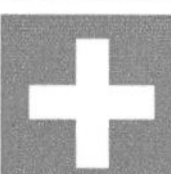

TREATMENT

APPROPRIATE HEALTH CARE Hospitalize until stable

GENERAL MEASURES
- History and physical exam with past medical history, allergies, prior ultrasounds this gestation, and time of last meal
- In general, severe abruption best managed by delivery of fetus
- Sher's grade 1 - usual labor protocol
- Sher's grade 2 - rapid delivery most often by cesarean section
- Sher's grade 3 - vaginal delivery preferable if mother stable
- In trauma monitor inpatient at least 4 hours for evidence of fetal insult, abruption, fetal-maternal transfusion
- Early aggressive restoration of maternal physiology to protect fetus and maternal organs from hypoperfusion/DIC
- Stabilize vitals, keep Hct >30, urine output >30 cc/hr
- Bedrest with external fetal and labor monitoring, if fetus is viable
- Large bore 16-18 gauge IV crystalloid infusion, central line placement only after coagulation status has been assessed
- Transfusions of whole blood may be necessary
- Follow hemoglobin/hematocrit (H/H) and coagulation status every 1-2 hours
- Place intrauterine pressure catheter (IUPC) since fetal risk climbs with elevated pressure
- Role of amniotomy to prevent amniotic fluid embolism is debatable but will speed delivery
- Positioning on left side may enhance venous return and cardiac output
- Oxygen for all patients
- If trauma without compromise after observation or small abruption and preterm may observe outpatient encouraging reduction of risk factors

SURGICAL MEASURES May need cesarean section after maternal stabilization if fetus viable and situation urgent

ACTIVITY Bedrest until status defined

DIET NPO until status defined and cesarean section possibility ruled out

PATIENT EDUCATION Call physician or proceed to hospital whenever bleeding more than one pad occurs, or if severe uterine or back pain occurs
- Mayo Health; http://mayohealth.org/mayo/baby/htm/bab_3_6.htm#Placenta

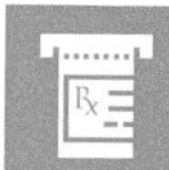

MEDICATIONS

DRUG(S) OF CHOICE
- Oxygen
- Saline or Ringer's lactate
- Whole blood and packed RBC's to keep hematocrit > 30
- May use oxytocin (Pitocin) augmentation to speed delivery
- Tocolytics like terbutaline may be used in mild non-compromising preterm abruption
- Rho(D) immune globulin for RhoD negative mother if undelivered or indicated after delivery
- 300 mcg RhoD immune globulin/15 cc fetal blood transfused, if Kleihauer-Betke test returns positive
- Fresh frozen plasma and platelet transfusions for coagulopathy with cryoprecipitate and fibrinogen given if indicated

Contraindications: Tocolytics should be withheld in preterm labor until abruption ruled out and fetal status defined

Precautions:
- Suffusion of blood into myometrium with weakening may increase risk of uterine rupture with oxytocin (Pitocin) augmentation
- Cryoprecipitate and fibrinogen may represent greater transfusion infection transmission risk

Significant possible interactions: Refer to manufacturer's profile of each drug

ALTERNATIVE DRUGS N/A

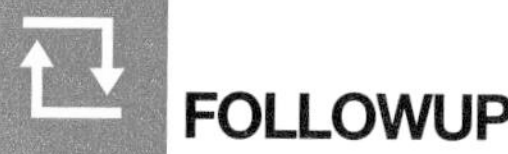

FOLLOWUP

PATIENT MONITORING
- If not delivered, monitor for intrauterine growth retardation (IUGR)
- See regularly and assess for preterm labor

PREVENTION/AVOIDANCE
Eliminate risk factors when possible

POSSIBLE COMPLICATIONS
- Infection transfusion risks: Hepatitis, cytomegalovirus infection, HIV and others
- Sensitization from blood product transfusion

EXPECTED COURSE/PROGNOSIS
- 0.5% to 1% fetal mortality and 30-50% perinatal mortality
- With trauma and abruption 1% maternal and 30-70% fetal mortality
- Labor typically more rapid but hypotonus from blood suffusion may occur

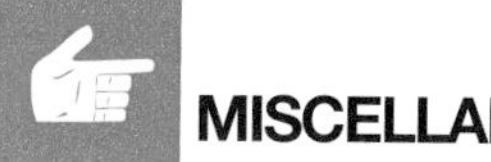

MISCELLANEOUS

ASSOCIATED CONDITIONS
- Preeclampsia and other forms of hypertension in pregnancy
- Hypertension
- Postpartum hemorrhage
- Maternal and fetal organ damage from hypoperfusion

AGE-RELATED FACTORS
Pediatric: N/A
Geriatric: N/A
Others: Multiparity, advanced maternal age - more at risk

PREGNANCY
This problem limited to pregnancy

SYNONYMS
- Placental abruption
- Premature separation of the placenta
- Couvelaire placenta

ICD-9-CM
641.20 Premature separation of placenta, unspecified

SEE ALSO
Placenta previa

OTHER NOTES
- Increased pelvic blood flow of pregnancy may enhance blood loss
- Amniotic fluid embolism is rare but may present with DIC and severe respiratory distress
- Increased risk of fetal-maternal transfusion with trauma of anterior placenta location

ABBREVIATIONS N/A

REFERENCES

- Scott JR. Placenta previa and abruption. In: Danforth DN, editor. Danforth's Obstetrics and Gynecology. 8th ed. Baltimore: Lippincott Williams & Wilkins; 1999
- Toivonen S, Heinonen S, Anttila M, Kosma VM, Saarikoski S. Reproductive risk factors, Doppler findings, and outcome of affected births in placental abruption: a population-based analysis. Am J Perinatol 2002;19(8):451-60

Web references: 0 available at www.5mcc.com
Illustrations N/A

Author(s):
Cathryn Heath, MD

Acetaminophen poisoning

BASICS

DESCRIPTION
- A disorder characterized by hepatic necrosis following large ingestions of acetaminophen. Symptoms may vary from initial nausea, vomiting, diaphoresis, and malaise to jaundice, confusion, somnolence, coma, and death. The clinical hallmark is the onset of symptoms within 24 hours of ingestion of acetaminophen-only or combination products.
- Acetaminophen poisoning is most often encountered following large single ingestions of acetaminophen-containing medications. Usual toxic doses are > 7.5 g in adults and 150 mg/kg in children. However, poisoning also occurs following acute and chronic ingestions of lesser amounts in susceptible individuals including those who regularly abuse alcohol, are chronically malnourished, or take medications which affect hepatic metabolism of acetaminophen.
- Therapeutic adult doses are 0.5-1.0 g every 4-6 hours, up to a maximum of 4 g/day. Therapeutic pediatric doses are 10-15 mg/kg every 4-6 hours, not to exceed 5 doses in 24 hours.

System(s) affected: Cardiovascular, Gastrointestinal, Renal/Urologic

Genetics: N/A

Incidence/Prevalence in USA:
- Over 118,900 ingestions of acetaminophen-containing medications reported by poison control centers in 2002
- 285 deaths in 2002, none in children < 6

Predominant age:
- Occurs in children and adults at any age
- Approximately 30% of exposures are in children under 6 years

Predominant sex: No reported association

SIGNS & SYMPTOMS
- Develop over the first 24 hours following large ingestions and may last as long as 8 days
- Severe symptoms indicate large ingestions or co-ingestants
- Fulminant hepatic failure occurs in less than 1% of adults and is very rare in children under 6 years
- Stage 1, first 24 hours
  - ◊ Nausea
  - ◊ Vomiting
  - ◊ Diaphoresis
- Stage 2, 24-48 hours
  - ◊ Right upper quadrant pain
  - ◊ Typically less nausea, vomiting, diaphoresis, and malaise than in stage 1
- Stage 3, 72-96 hours
  - ◊ Nausea, vomiting, malaise reappear
  - ◊ Severe poisonings may result in jaundice, confusion, somnolence, and coma
- Stage 4, 7-8 days
  - ◊ Resolution of clinical signs in survivors
- May develop gradually following long-term ingestion of near-therapeutic amounts of acetaminophen. Such patients may present in any stage 1-3 without a history of ingestion of the usual toxic doses.

CAUSES Accidental or intentional ingestion of acetaminophen or combination medications containing acetaminophen

RISK FACTORS
- Age less than 6 years
- Concurrent oral poisoning with other substances
- Psychiatric illness
- History of previous toxic ingestions or suicide attempts
- Regular ingestion of large amounts of alcohol

DIAGNOSIS

DIFFERENTIAL DIAGNOSIS
- Consider presence of co-ingestants, especially alcohol
- Other ingested toxins which produce severe acute hepatic injury, including the mushroom Amanita phalloides and products containing yellow phosphorus or carbon tetrachloride

LABORATORY
- Plasma acetaminophen levels should be drawn on all patients 4 or more hours after ingestion (levels prior to 4 hours not helpful)
- At least one additional acetaminophen level drawn 4-6 hours after the first level is recommended if the ingested acetaminophen is an extended release product (e.g., Tylenol Extended Relief) or is not known to be an immediate release product
  - ◊ If the second level is higher than the first level or is close to the "possible risk" level on the Rumack-Matthew nomogram, it may be prudent to obtain additional acetaminophen levels every 2 hours until the levels stabilize or decline
  - ◊ If co-ingestants include drugs that slow gastrointestinal motility, an acetaminophen level drawn 4-6 hours after the second level may detect a late increase in serum acetaminophen concentration
- Screens for suspected co-ingestants (aspirin, iron, others) may be positive (especially when suicide is a possibility)
- With toxic ingestions, aspartate transaminase (AST; SGOT), alanine transaminase (ALT; SGPT), and bilirubin levels begin to rise in Stage 2 and peak in Stage 3. In severe poisonings, the PT will parallel these changes.
- AST levels over 1000 IU/L are consistent with the diagnosis and levels of 20,000 IU/L are not uncommon
- Laboratory abnormalities usually resolve by stage 4
- Renal function abnormalities are common in patients with hepatotoxicity
- Evidence of damage to the pancreas and heart may present following severe poisonings

Drugs that may alter lab results: None with clinically significant cross-reactivity with plasma acetaminophen assay

Disorders that may alter lab results: Diseases or toxic substances which damage the liver, particularly alcohol

PATHOLOGICAL FINDINGS Centrilobular hepatic necrosis

SPECIAL TESTS N/A

IMAGING N/A

DIAGNOSTIC PROCEDURES None other than correlating plasma acetaminophen levels with the clinical presentation

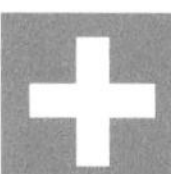

TREATMENT

APPROPRIATE HEALTH CARE
- Contact a regional poison control center for management recommendations. In the United States, a local poison control center can be reached by calling (800)222-1222.
- All patients should be evaluated at a health care facility
- Outpatient for non-toxic accidental ingestions
- Inpatient for toxic and intentional ingestions

GENERAL MEASURES
- Activated charcoal should be used, but preferably not within 1 hour of administration of the antidote N-acetylcysteine (NAC)
- The stomach of untreated patients may be emptied by gastric lavage if within 1 hour of ingestion
- Ipecac is no longer recommended for routine use at home or in health care facilities
- NAC should be given when plasma acetaminophen concentrations measured 4 or more hours after ingestion are in the "possible risk" or higher levels on the Rumack-Matthew nomogram. This corresponds to acetaminophen levels greater than 150 μg/mL (993 μmol/L), 75 μg/mL (497 μmol/L), and 40 μg/mL (265 μmol/L) at 4 hours, 8 hours, and 12 hours after ingestion, respectively.
- NAC therapy may be effective up to 36 hours or more after ingestion

SURGICAL MEASURES N/A

ACTIVITY Restricted if significant hepatic damage has occurred

DIET No special diet except with severe hepatic damage

PATIENT EDUCATION
- Education of parents/caregivers during well child visits
- Anticipatory guidance for caregivers, family, and cohabitants of potentially suicidal patients
- Patient brochure (item 1515): Child Safety: Keeping your home safe for your baby. American Academy of Family Physicians, 11400 Tomahawk Creek Parkway, Leawood, KS 66211-2672
- Education of patients taking long-term acetaminophen therapy

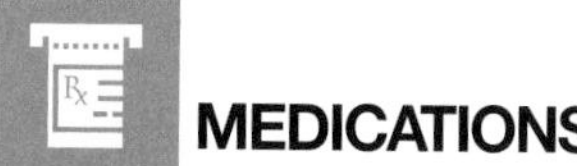

MEDICATIONS

DRUG(S) OF CHOICE

- Two classes of medicine:
  - ◊ Activated charcoal
  - ◊ Acetylcysteine (N-acetylcysteine, NAC, Mucomyst)
- Emergency facility/hospital:
  - ◊ Patients evaluated within 1 hour of ingestion may have their stomachs evacuated by gastric lavage
  - ◊ Activated charcoal: 1 g/kg for initial dose; preferably not within 1 hour of NAC administration. Additional concurrent use during NAC therapy is controversial.
  - ◊ Acetylcysteine: oral loading dose of 140 mg/kg, followed by 70 mg/kg every 4 hours for 17 additional doses. Whenever possible, NAC therapy should be initiated within 8 hours following the toxic ingestion.

Contraindications: Medication allergies

Precautions: NAC may cause significant nausea and vomiting due to its sulfur content; consider administration by nasogastric tube. Nausea can be treated with metoclopramide (Reglan) 0.5-1 mg/kg IV or ondansetron (Zofran) 0.15 mg/kg IV, for age > 4 years; usually 4 mg/dose.

Significant possible interactions: Activated charcoal given within 1 hour of NAC may adsorb the NAC, thereby limiting its effectiveness

ALTERNATIVE DRUGS

- IV NAC outside US; in approved trials within US
- Oral racemethionine (methionine)

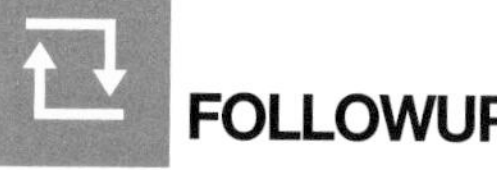

FOLLOWUP

PATIENT MONITORING Psychiatric follow-up after intentional ingestions

PREVENTION/AVOIDANCE

- Parent/caregiver education essential
  - ◊ Education during well child exams regarding poisoning prevention
  - ◊ Emergency telephone numbers

POSSIBLE COMPLICATIONS Rare following recovery from acute poisoning

EXPECTED COURSE/PROGNOSIS

- Complete recovery with early therapy
- Fewer than 1% of adult patients develop hepatic failure
- Hepatic failure is very rare in children under 6 years

MISCELLANEOUS

ASSOCIATED CONDITIONS N/A

AGE-RELATED FACTORS

Pediatric: Hepatic damage at toxic acetaminophen levels is decreased in children less than 6 years

Geriatric: Hepatic damage may be increased if taking hepatotoxic medications chronically

Others: N/A

PREGNANCY

- Increased incidence of spontaneous abortion, especially with overdose at early gestational age
- Incidence of spontaneous abortion or fetal death appears increased when NAC treatment is delayed

SYNONYMS

- Paracetamol poisoning

ICD-9-CM

965.4 Poisoning by aromatic analgesics, NEC

SEE ALSO

OTHER NOTES N/A

ABBREVIATIONS

NAC = N-acetylcysteine

REFERENCES

- Shannon M. Ingestion of toxic substances by children. N Engl J Med 2000;342(3):186-91
- American Academy of Pediatrics Committee on Injury, Violence, and Poison Prevention. Poison treatment in the home. American Academy of Pediatrics Committee on Injury, Violence, and Poison Prevention. Pediatrics 2003;112(5):1182-5
- Zed PJ, Krenzelok EP. Treatment of acetaminophen overdose. Am J Health-Syst Pharm 1999;56:1081-91
- Watson WA, Litovitz TL, Rodgers GC Jr, et al. 2002 annual report of the American Association of Poison Control Centers Toxic Exposure Surveillance System. Am J Emerg Med 2003;21(5):353-421

Web references: 0 available at www.5mcc.com

Illustrations N/A

Author(s):

Lars C. Larsen, MD

BASICS

DESCRIPTION Chronic skin eruption with flushing and dilation of small blood vessels in the face, especially nose and cheeks. Sometimes associated with ocular symptoms (ocular rosacea).
System(s) affected: Skin/Exocrine
Genetics: People of Northern European and Celtic background commonly afflicted
Incidence/Prevalence in USA: Common
Predominant age: 30-50
Predominant sex: Female > Male

SIGNS & SYMPTOMS
- Skin flush - prominent at onset
- Redness - lower half of nose, sometimes whole nose, forehead, cheeks, chin
- Conjunctivae red - (sometimes)
- Erythema, dusky - (in advanced cases)
- Blood vessels in involved area collapse under pressure
- Acne lesions form papules, pustules, and nodules; comedones are rare
- Telangiectasia
- Rhinophyma (sometimes) more common in males

CAUSES
- No proven cause. Possibilities include:
  - ◊ Thyroid and gonadal disturbance
  - ◊ Alcohol, coffee, tea, spiced food overindulgence (unproven)
  - ◊ Demodex follicular parasite (suspected)
  - ◊ Exposure to cold, heat, hot drinks
  - ◊ Emotional stress
  - ◊ Dysfunction of the gastrointestinal tract
  - ◊ Environmental trigger factors - sun, wind, cold

RISK FACTORS N/A

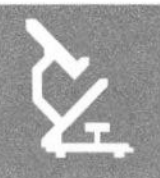

DIAGNOSIS

DIFFERENTIAL DIAGNOSIS
- Drug eruptions (iodides and bromides)
- Granulomas of the skin
- Cutaneous lupus erythematosus
- Carcinoid syndrome
- Deep fungal infection
- Acne vulgaris
- Seborrheic dermatitis
- Steroid rosacea (abuse)

LABORATORY N/A

Drugs that may alter lab results: N/A

Disorders that may alter lab results: N/A

PATHOLOGICAL FINDINGS
- Inflammation around hypertrophied sebaceous glands, producing papules, pustules and cysts
- Absence of comedones and blocked ducts
- Vascular dilatation and dermal lymphocytic infiltrate

SPECIAL TESTS N/A

IMAGING N/A

DIAGNOSTIC PROCEDURES N/A

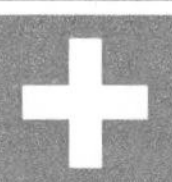

TREATMENT

APPROPRIATE HEALTH CARE Outpatient

GENERAL MEASURES
- Reassurance
- Treat psychological stress if present
- Avoid oil based cosmetics. Others are acceptable and may help women tolerate the symptoms.
- Electrodesiccation or chemical sclerosis of permanently dilated blood vessels
- Possible evolving laser therapy

SURGICAL MEASURES Surgical treatment of rhinophyma

ACTIVITY No restrictions. Support physical fitness.

DIET Avoid any food or drink that causes facial flushing, e.g., hot drinks, spiced food, alcohol

PATIENT EDUCATION
- American Academy of Dermatology (708)330-0230

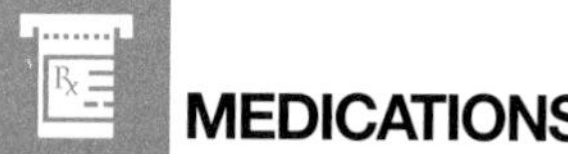

MEDICATIONS

DRUG(S) OF CHOICE
- Low dose oral tetracycline 500-1000 mg/day or doxycycline 20 mg bid (persistant), 50-150 mg/day or minocycline 75-200 mg/day
- Sulfur-containing local applications
  - ◊ Alcohol-sulfur (Liquimat)
  - ◊ Sulfur (Fostril)
  - ◊ Resorcinol-sulfur (Rezamid)
  - ◊ Sulfacetamide-sulfur (Sulfacet-R, Nicosyn, Avar Gel Avar Cleanser, Avar Green, Rosanil Cleanser, Plexion Cleanser, Ovace Wash, Clenia Emollient Cream, Clenia Foam Wash)
  - ◊ Urea-sulfacetamide-sulfur (Rosula)
- Azelaic acid (Finacea)
- Topical metronidazole (MetroGel) 0.75% gel - apply each morning and at bedtime after cleansing skin; also available as a cream and lotion which may be better tolerated by some patients; or 1% cream formulation of metronidazole (Noritate) used in a once daily manner
- Topical erythromycin
- Topical clindamycin lotion preferred
- Possible utility of calcineurin inhibitors (tacrolimus - 0.1%, pimecrolimus 0.1%
- Topical steroids should not be used as they may aggravate rosacea

Contraindications:
- Tetracycline: not for use in pregnancy or children < 8 years
- Isotretinoin: teratogenic; not for use in pregnancy or in women or reproductive age who are not using a reliable birth control method

Precautions:
- Tetracycline: may cause photosensitivity; sunscreen recommended

Significant possible interactions:
- Tetracycline: avoid concurrent administration with antacids, dairy products, or iron
- Broad-spectrum antibiotics: may reduce the effectiveness of oral contraceptives; barrier method recommended

ALTERNATIVE DRUGS
- For severe cases, isotretinoin orally for 4 months.

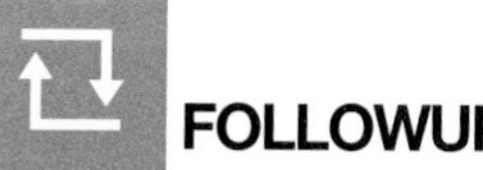

FOLLOWUP

PATIENT MONITORING Occasional and as needed. Close follow-up for women using isotretinoin.

PREVENTION/AVOIDANCE No preventive measure known

POSSIBLE COMPLICATIONS
- Rhinophyma (dilated follicles and thickened bulbous skin on nose), especially in men
- Conjunctivitis
- Blepharitis
- Keratitis

EXPECTED COURSE/PROGNOSIS
- Slowly progressive
- Subsides spontaneously (sometimes)

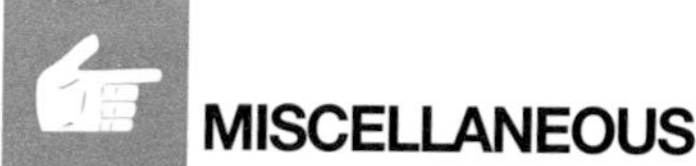

MISCELLANEOUS

ASSOCIATED CONDITIONS
- Seborrheic dermatitis of scalp and eyelids
- Keratitis with photophobia, lacrimation, visual disturbance
- Corneal lesions
- Blepharitis
- Uveitis

AGE-RELATED FACTORS
Pediatric: Unlikely in this age group
Geriatric: Uncommon after age 60
Others: N/A

PREGNANCY Use of oral isotretinoin contraindicated

SYNONYMS Rosacea

ICD-9-CM
695.3 Rosacea

SEE ALSO
Acne vulgaris
Blepharitis
Dermatitis, seborrheic
Lupus erythematosus, discoid
Uveitis

OTHER NOTES N/A

ABBREVIATIONS N/A

REFERENCES

- Fitzpatrick TB, et al, eds. Dermatology in General Medicine. 5th Ed. New York, McGraw-Hill, 1999
- Habif T. Clinical Dermatology. 4th Ed. St. Louis, CV Mosby, 2004

Web references: 1 available at www.5mcc.com
Illustrations 8 available

Author(s):
Larry Millikan, MD

BASICS

DESCRIPTION Acne is an androgenically stimulated, inflammatory disorder of the sebaceous glands, resulting in comedones, papules, inflammatory pustules and, occasionally, scarring.
System(s) affected: Skin/Exocrine
Genetics: Approximately 50% of affected individuals have a family history of acne; higher prevalence in Caucasians
Incidence/Prevalence in USA: 50 million; virtually 100% of adolescents are affected to some degree. 15% will seek medical advice.
Predominant age: Early-late puberty, may persist into 3rd-4th decade. Affected ages: 16, 100%; 25-34, 8% ; 35-44, 3%
Predominant sex: Male > Female (adolescence), Female > Male (adult)

SIGNS & SYMPTOMS
- Closed comedones (whiteheads)
- Open comedones (blackheads)
- Nodules or papules
- Pustules, with or without redness and edema ("cysts")
- Scars - ice pick, rolling, boxcar, atrophic macules, hypertrophic, depressed, sinus tracts
- Lesions occur on forehead, cheeks and nose, may extend over central chest and back (greatest concentration of sebaceous glands)
- Factors influencing symptomatology
  - ◊ Sex: males: later onset, greater severity; females: earlier onset, lesser severity
  - ◊ Seasonal: less severe in summer
  - ◊ May worsen immediately prior to menses
- Grading system (numerical)
  - ◊ 1: Comedonal - closed/open
  - ◊ 2: Papular >25 lesions on face & trunk
  - ◊ 3: Pustular >25 lesions, mild scarring
  - ◊ 4: Nodulocystic - inflammatory nodules and cysts, extensive scarring
- Grading system (presence of inflammatory lesions); severity:
  - ◊ Mild: papules/pustules = few; nodules = none
  - ◊ Moderate: papules/pustules = several/many; nodules = few
  - ◊ Severe: papules/pustules = numerous; nodules = many

CAUSES
- Overproduction of androgens
- Hyperresponsiveness of follicle/sebaceous gland (concentrated in face, upper neck, chest) to androgens (most affected individuals have normal androgen levels)
- Hypersensitivity to P. acnes & its metabolic products
- Pathogenesis
  - ◊ Androgens - dihydroxytestosterone DHT), dehydroepiandrosterone (DHEA) stimulate sebum production & proliferation of keratinocytes in hair follicles
  - ◊ Keratin plug obstructs follicle opening; causes sebum accumulation and follicular distention
  - ◊ Propionibacterium acnes, an anaerobe, colonizes & proliferates in the plugged follicle
  - ◊ P. acnes hydrolyzes sebum triglycerides into free fatty acids, produces chemotactic factors and pro-inflammatory mediators, and activates complement; causes follicle and surrounding dermis inflammation

RISK FACTORS
- Adolescence; male sex
- Androgenic steroids, e.g., steroid abuse, some birth control pills
- Oily cosmetics, including cleansing creams, moisturizers, oil-based foundations
- Rubbing or occluding skin surface (eg, sports equipment - helmets and shoulder pads), holding the telephone or hands against the skin
- Drugs - iodides or bromides, lithium, phenytoin, isoniazid, methotrexate, vitamin B-12, long acting progestins, phenobarbital, ethionamide, azathioprine, disulfiram, cyclosporine
- Systemic corticosteroids
- Virilization disorders (POS)
- Hot, humid climate

DIAGNOSIS

DIFFERENTIAL DIAGNOSIS
- Occupational exposure to tars, oils, grease
- Folliculitis
- Acne (rosacea, cosmetica, steroid induced)
- Perioral dermatitis
- Chloracne
- Pseudo-folliculitis barbae
- Drug eruption
- Sarcoidosis
- Verruca vulgaris and plana
- Trichoepithelioma
- Angiofibroma
- Keratosis pilaris

LABORATORY N/A

Drugs that may alter lab results: N/A

Disorders that may alter lab results: N/A

PATHOLOGICAL FINDINGS
- Oiliness, thickening of the skin
- Hypertrophy of the sebaceous glands
- Perifolliculitis
- Scarring

SPECIAL TESTS Testosterone, DHEA-S, LH, & FSH can be measured in those rare cases when acne arises de novo in previously unaffected adult. FSH/LH > 2-3 - polycystic ovary syndrome, testosterone > 150-200 ng/mL- polycystic ovary syndrome, testosterone > 200 ng/ml - ovarian tumor, DHEA-S > 800 microg/dL - adrenal tumor.

IMAGING N/A

DIAGNOSTIC PROCEDURES History and physical exam

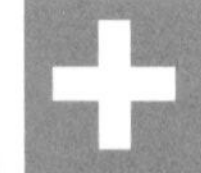

TREATMENT

APPROPRIATE HEALTH CARE Outpatient

GENERAL MEASURES
- Therapy goals - lessen physical discomfort, minimize scarring, improve appearance, avoid adverse psychological impact
- Cleansing: mild soap twice a day will control surface oiliness
- Avoid drying agents in combination with keratinolytics
- Skin type/recommended vehicle type: dry/sensitive - cream; oily - gel/solution; hairy - lotion
- Apply topicals to lesions and surrounding area
- Topical retinoid + antibiotic better than antibiotic alone
- Stop antibiotic therapy when lesions resolve
- Oil-free sun screens
- Stress management helpful if acne flares with stress

SURGICAL MEASURES
- Comedo extraction
- Injection of large cystic lesions with 0.05-0.3 mL of triamcinolone (Kenalog 2-5 mg/mL), use 30-gauge needle, slightly distend cyst
- Acne scar treatment

ACTIVITY Full activity. Physical conditioning important.

DIET Good nutrition. Special diets do not diminish acne. Chocolate/fatty foods do not aggravate acne.

PATIENT EDUCATION
- No cure for acne
- Treatment takes a minimum of 4 weeks to show results
- Topical agents can cause redness and drying
- Do not pick at or pop lesions

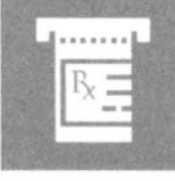

MEDICATIONS

DRUG(S) OF CHOICE
- Comedonal acne (grade 1) - keratinolytic agent
  - ◊ Tretinoin (Retin-A, Avita): 0.025%, 0.05%, and 0.1% cream, 0.01% and 0.025% gel, 0.1% microemulsion, 0.05% solution, Retin-A Micro (0.1% gel microsphere), Avita (0.025% cream/gel with PP-2); apply hs; wash skin & let skin dry 30 min before application
    - Cream - better in cold/dry weather; gel - more drying, better in hot/humid weather, better for chest/back
    - Inactivated by UV light and oxidized by benzoyl peroxide
    - Retin-A Micro and Avita less irritating, less phototoxic
    - May cause an initial pustular flare, indicating a good response;preventby 14 day course of oral antibiotics
    - Start with lowest strength cream and increase as tolerated to effective dose
    - Thins stratum corneum layer- avoid excessive sun exposure/use sunscreens; pregnancy class C
  - ◊ Adapalene (Differin): 0.1% gel & hydroalcoholic solution, cream, pledgets, apply hs. As effective and better tolerated than tretinoin; side effects - erythema, dryness, scaling, pruritus; pregnancy class C.
  - ◊ Azelaic acid (Azelex): 20% cream bid
    - Keratinolytic, antibacterial, and anti-inflammatory; side effects - erythema, dryness, scaling, hypopigmentation; pregnancy class B
    - Reduces post-inflammatory hyperpigmentation in dark-skinned individuals
  - ◊ Salicylic acid 0.5-5.0% hydroalcoholic, apply daily or bid; less effective than tretinoin

◊ Tazarotene (Tazorac): 0.05-0.1% gel, 0.05% and 0.10% cream, pregnancy class X, apply hs; can use on alternate days, can use short contact method (apply for 2-5 min bid x 12 weeks); highly effective
◊ Alpha-hydroxy acids, 5-10% glycolic acid available OTC
- Mild Inflammatory acne (grade 2) - keratinolytic agent plus (benzoyl peroxide or topical antibiotic)
◊ Topical benzoyl peroxide 2.5-5% and 10% gel; 2.5%, 5% and 10% wash; apply hs
  - Bactericidal through direct toxic effect; no *P. acnes* resistance
  - 2.5% as effective as stronger preparations
  - With tretinoin, apply BP in AM & tretinoin hs; when used simultaneously, degrades tretinoin by 50% in 2 hrs and 80-90% in 24 hrs; sde effects - skin irritation, may bleach clothes
◊ Topical antibiotic
  - Erythromycin (A/T/S, Emgel, Erycette, EryDerm): 2% gel or solution, bid
  - Clindamycin (Cleocin-T, Clindaderm, Dalacin T, Clindets): 1% gel, solution, lotion, pledgets bid
  - Metronidazole gel, once daily
  - Azelaic acid (Azelex): 20% cream, bid; enhanced bactericidal effect and decreased risk of resistant *P. acnes* when used with zinc and benzoyl peroxide
  - Benzoyl peroxide-erythromycin (Benzamycin): 5%/3% gel bid; very effective topical antibiotic; especially in combination with azelaic acid
  - Benzoyl peroxide-clindamycin (BenzaClin, DUAC, Clindoxyl) 5%/1% gel bid
  - Sodium sulfacetamide (Sulfacet-R, Novacet, Klaron): 5-10% lotion, qd or bid, may contain sulfur, useful in acne with seborrheic dermatitis or rosacea
◊ Zinc 200 mg daily, somewhat effective vs. inflammatory lesions
- Moderate inflammatory acne (grade 3) - keratinolytic agent plus ([benzoyl peroxide or topical antibiotic] and/or systemic antibiotic). Maintain keratinolytic agent after completion of antibiotic.
◊ Topical tretinoin, and topical antibiotic/benzoyl peroxide, or systemic (oral) antibiotic
  - Tetracycline: 500-2,000 mg daily; begin at high dose, then taper in 4-6 months if good response; avoid in children < 8 & pregnancy; side effects - photosensitivity, esophagitis
  - Minocycline 50-200 mg daily; side effects - photosensitivity, urticaria, gray-blue skin color, vertigo, autoimmune hepatitis, pseudotumor cerebri, lupus-like syndrome
  - Doxycycline 50-200 mg daily; side effects - photosensitivity
  - Erythromycin: 500-1000 mg daily; decreasing effectiveness as a result of increasing *P. acnes* resistance
  - Trimethoprim-sulfamethoxazole (Bactrim-DS, Septra-DS) 160/800 mg, qday or bid
  - Trimethoprim 300 mg bid
- Severe Inflammatory acne (grade 4)
◊ Isotretinoin (Accutane): 0.5-1.0 mg/kg day bid; 60-90% cure rate; 20% of patients relapse and require retreatment - given after 8 week drug free interval. Usually given for 12-20 weeks, total dose 120-150 mg/kg.
  - Consider polycystic ovary syndrome in women who fail to respond to isotretinoin
  - Indications- severe nodular (cystic) acne with scarring, improves < 50% after 6 months of topical + systemic antibiotics, moderate acne persisting with significant atrophic scarring or significant psychological distress
  - Side effects: cheilitis, arthralgias, tendinitis, hyperlipidemia, pseudotumor cerebri, depression/suicide, poor wound healing, highly teratogenic
  - Monitor lipids, LFTs at baseline, 4 and 8 weeks
- Other medications:
◊ Oral contraceptives (females): most effective when estrogen = 50 mg; progestin = norgestimate or desogestrel (Ortho Tri-Cyclen, Ortho-Cyclen, Desogen) or ethynodiol diacetate-ethinyl estradiol (Zovia)
◊ Spironolactone (Aldactone) women only; 25-200 mg/day; anti-androgen that reduces sebum production
◊ Corticosteroids: low dose, give hs, suppresses adrenal androgens
  - Prednisone 2.5 - 7.5 mg/day
  - Dexamethasone 0.25 - 0.75 mg/day

Contraindications:
- Allergy
- Severe hepatic dysfunction - all oral agents
- Tetracyclines: not for use in pregnancy or children < 8 years
- Isotretinoin: teratogenic; not for use in pregnancy or in women of reproductive age who are not using a reliable birth control

Precautions: Tetracycline(s) photosensitivity

Significant possible interactions:
- Tetracycline(s): antacids, iron.
- Broad-spectrum antibiotics: may reduce the effectiveness of oral contraceptives; barrier method recommended
- Avoid tetracyclines or vitamin A preparations during isotretinoin therapy

ALTERNATIVE DRUGS N/A

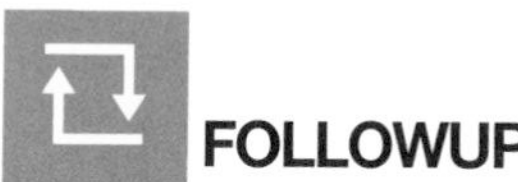

FOLLOWUP

PATIENT MONITORING
- Monthly visits until adequate response
- Pre-treatment and monthly serum lipids, liver function tests, and pregnancy tests for patients on isotretinoin
- Consider antibiotic resistance (60% overall) or gram-negative folliculitis if treatment fails despite patient compliance
- Dermatology consultation recommended - refractory lesions despite appropriate therapy, consideration of isotretinoin therapy, management of acne scars

PREVENTION/AVOIDANCE N/A

POSSIBLE COMPLICATIONS
- Acne conglobata - a severe confluent inflammatory acne with systemic symptoms
- Facial- and psychological scarring
- Gram-negative folliculitis - superinfection due to long term oral antibiotic use, treatment with ampicillin, trimethoprim-sulfa, isotretinoin

EXPECTED COURSE/PROGNOSIS
Gradual improvement over 4-8 weeks

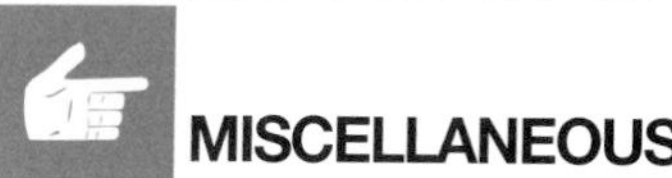

MISCELLANEOUS

ASSOCIATED CONDITIONS
- Acne fulminans, acne conglobata
- Pyoderma faciale
- Hidradenitis suppurativa
- Acne excoriee des jeunes filles
- Acne mechanica; acne aestivalis
- Pomade acne
- SAPHO syndrome - synovitis, acne, pustulosis, hyperostosis, osteitis
- PAPA syndrome - pyogenic sterile arthritis, pyoderma gangrenosum, cystic acne

AGE-RELATED FACTORS
Pediatric:
- Neonatal acne: mostly closed comedones
- Infantile acne: inflammatory papules, beginning at 3-6 months of age, may be due to excessive androgens, increased risk for severe teenage acne vulgaris, treat with topical agents
- Rare in age 1-7; check for hyperandrogenemia

Geriatric: Favre-Racouchot syndrome - comedones on face and head, due to sun exposure

Others: N/A

PREGNANCY
- May result in a flare, or remission, of acne
- Isotretinoin: causes severe fetal malformations; ensure effective contraception
- Erythromycin can be used in pregnancy; use topical agents when possible
- Avoid topical tretinoin; although there is no good evidence that its use is teratogenic
- Contraindicated - isotretinoin, tazarotene, tetracycline, doxycycline, minocycline

SYNONYMS N/A

ICD-9-CM
706.1 Other acne

SEE ALSO
Acne rosacea

OTHER NOTES
- Acne often more significant to adolescent than to doctor; often "entry ticket;" for other advice
- High intensity (blue and red) light is effective
- Dark skinned individuals (SPT IV - VI): keloidal scarring seen in 50% of individuals; pomade use highly associated with forehead lesions; acne hyperpigmented macules (AHM) in > 50% of individuals; hydroquinones (1.5-10%), azelaic acid, and topical retinoids effective treatment of AHM

ABBREVIATIONS N/A

REFERENCES

- Oberemok SS, Shalita AR. Acne vulgaris I - pathogenesis and diagnosis. Cutis 2002;70:101-105
- Oberemok SS, Shalita AR. Acne vulgaris II - treatment. Cutis 2002;70:111-114

Web references: 2 available at www.5mcc.com
Illustrations 12 available

Author(s):
Gary Levine, MD

BASICS

DESCRIPTION Adrenal hypofunction from primary disease (partial or complete destruction) of the adrenal gland with inadequate secretion of glucocorticoids and mineralocorticoids. An autoimmune process is the most common cause (80% of the cases) followed by tuberculosis. AIDS is becoming a more frequent cause.

- Addison disease (primary adrenocortical insufficiency) is differentiated from secondary (pituitary failure) and tertiary (hypothalamic failure) causes of adrenocortical insufficiency (see Differential Diagnosis). Mineral corticoid function usually remains intact in secondary and tertiary adrenocorticoid insufficiency.
- Addisonian (adrenal) crisis - acute complication of adrenal insufficiency (circulatory collapse, dehydration, hypotension, nausea, vomiting, hypoglycemia); usually precipitated by acute physiologic stressor such as surgery, illness, exacerbation of co-morbid process, acute withdrawal of long term corticosteroid therapy

System(s) affected: Endocrine/Metabolic

Genetics: Autoimmune adrenal insufficiency shows some hereditary disposition. Familial glucocorticoid insufficiency may have recessive pattern; adrenomyeloneuropathy is X-linked. Frequent association with other autoimmune disorders.

Incidence/Prevalence in USA: Prevalence 4:100,000; incidence 0.6:100,000

Predominant age: All ages; usually 3rd to 5th decade

Predominant sex: Females > Males (slight)

SIGNS & SYMPTOMS

- Weakness, fatigue, tiredness
- Weight loss
- Dizziness; low blood pressure, orthostatic hypotension
- Increased pigmentation (extensor surfaces, hand creases, dental-gingival margins, buccal and vaginal mucosa, lips, areola, pressure points, scars; "tanning"; freckles; vitiligo)
- Anorexia; nausea; vomiting
- Chronic diarrhea
- Abdominal pain
- Decreased cold tolerance
- Salt craving
- Hair loss in females
- Depression (60-80% of patients)
- Vitiligo

CAUSES

- Autoimmune adrenal insufficiency (≈80% of cases in USA)
- Tuberculosis (most common infectious cause worldwide)
- HIV (most common infectious cause in USA)
- Waterhouse-Friderichsen syndrome (disseminated adrenal infection and subsequent infarction; meningococcemia most common; Pseudomonas aeruginosa common in children; atypical pathogens, CMV, Cryptococcus, MAC in immunosuppressed and AIDS)
- Fungal disease (histoplasmosis, blastomycosis, coccidioidomycosis)
- Bilateral adrenal hemorrhage and infarction (anticoagulants; 50% are in therapeutic range at time of hemorrhage)
- Antiphospholipid syndrome
- Metastatic (lung, breast, kidney, colon, melanoma), lymphoma, Kaposi sarcoma (tumor must destroy 90% of gland to produce hypofunction)
- Drugs (ketoconazole, etomidate)
- Shock
- Surgical adrenalectomy
- Radiation therapy
- Sarcoidosis
- Hemochromatosis
- Amyloidosis
- Adrenoleukodystrophy
- Adrenomyelodystrophy
- Polyglandular autoimmune endocrine syndromes
  - ◊ APS I (autoimmune polyglandular syndrome 1)
    - Childhood onset
    - HLA-DR not associated
    - Single gene mutation in APECED gene (APECED = autoimmune polyendocrinopathy-candidiasis-ectodermal dystrophy)
  - ◊ APS II (autoimmune polyglandular syndrome II)
    - Schmidt syndrome (50% of patients with Addison disease have Schmidt syndrome)
    - Adult onset
    - HLA-DR associated
    - Adrenal failure with type I diabetes mellitus and/or autoimmune thyroid disease (Hashimoto's or Graves')
- Congenital (enzyme defects; hypoplasia; familial glucocorticoid insufficiency)
- Idiopathic

RISK FACTORS

- Family history of autoimmune adrenal insufficiency. About 40% of patients have a first- or second-degree relative with one of the associated disorders.
- Taking steroids for prolonged periods, then experiencing severe infection, trauma or surgical procedures

DIAGNOSIS

DIFFERENTIAL DIAGNOSIS

- Secondary adrenocortical insufficiency (pituitary failure)
  - ◊ Withdrawal of long-term corticosteroid use. Adrenal insufficiency from hypothalamic-pituitary axis depression from long-term corticosteroid use is much more common than Addison disease.
  - ◊ Sheehan syndrome (postpartum necrosis of pituitary)
  - ◊ Empty sella syndrome
  - ◊ Surgical excision of pituitary
  - ◊ Radiation to pituitary
  - ◊ Pituitary adenomas, carcinomas (rare), craniopharyngiomas
  - ◊ Infiltrative disorders of pituitary (sarcoidosis, hemochromatosis, amyloidosis, histiocytosis X)
  - ◊ Megestrol
- Tertiary adrenocortical insufficiency (hypothalamic failure)
  - ◊ Pituitary stalk transection
  - ◊ Trauma
  - ◊ Disruption of production of corticotropic releasing factor (CRF)
  - ◊ Hypothalamic tumors
- Myopathies
- Syndrome of inappropriate antidiuretic hormone (SIADH)
- Heavy metal ingestion
- Severe nutritional deficiencies
- Sprue syndrome
- Hyperparathyroidism
- Neurofibromatosis
- Peutz-Jeghers syndrome
- Porphyria cutanea tarda
- Salt-losing nephritis
- Bronchogenic carcinoma
- Anorexia nervosa
- Other causes of hypoglycemia
- Depression

LABORATORY

- Low serum sodium
- Elevated serum potassium
- Elevated BUN, creatinine
- Elevated serum calcium
- Hypoglycemia when fasted
- Metabolic acidosis
- Low cortisol level (between 8 and 9 a.m.)
- Elevated ACTH level
- Moderate neutropenia
- Eosinophilia
- Relative lymphocytosis
- Anemia, normochromic, normocytic
- Adrenal-cortex autoantibody (ACA/21-hydroxylase)
- Low aldosterone levels
- TSH - repeat when condition has stabilized. Thyroid hormone levels may normalize with treatment of Addison disease.

Drugs that may alter lab results: Digitalis

Disorders that may alter lab results: Diabetes mellitus

PATHOLOGICAL FINDINGS Atrophic adrenals in autoimmune adrenalitis. Infiltrative and hemorrhagic disorders produce enlargement with destruction of entire gland.

SPECIAL TESTS

- Rapid ACTH stimulation test: Cosyntropin 0.25 mg IV, measure pre-injection and 60 minute post-injection cortisol levels. Patients with Addison disease have low to normal values that do not rise
- Metapyrone test
- Insulin-induced hypoglycemia test
- CRH may help distinguish secondary from tertiary adrenal insufficiency
- Autoantibody tests
  - ◊ 21-Hydroxylase (most common and specific)
  - ◊ 17-Hydroxylase
  - ◊ 17-alfa-Hydroxylase (may not be associated)
  - ◊ Adrenomedullin

IMAGING

- Abdominal CT scan
  - ◊ Small adrenal glands in autoimmune adrenalitis
  - ◊ Enlarged adrenal glands in infiltrative and hemorrhagic disorders
- Abdominal x-ray: may show adrenal calcifications
- CXR: may show adrenal calcifications, small heart size, calcification of cartilage

DIAGNOSTIC PROCEDURES A work-up to determine the cause of Addison disease. CT guided fine-needle biopsy of adrenal masses may be helpful.

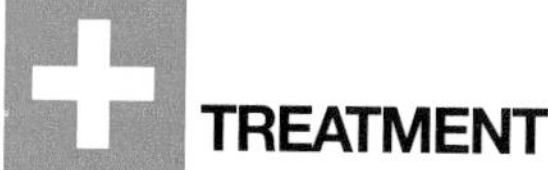

TREATMENT

APPROPRIATE HEALTH CARE
- Outpatient
- Inpatient during adrenal crisis

GENERAL MEASURES
- Treatment for adrenal insufficiency is with glucocorticoid and mineralocorticoid replacement
  - ◊ 5 S's of management of adrenal crisis: salt, sugar, steroids, support, search for precipitating illness
- Appropriate treatment for underlying cause (e.g., tuberculosis)

SURGICAL MEASURES N/A

ACTIVITY As tolerated

DIET Arrange for a diet that maintains water, sodium and potassium balances

PATIENT EDUCATION
- For patient education materials, contact: National Addison Disease Foundation, 505 Northern Blvd., Suite 200, Great Neck, NY 11021, (516)487-4992
- Patient should wear or carry medical identification with information about the disease and the need for hydrocortisone or other replacement therapy
- Instruct patient in self-administering of parenteral hydrocortisone for emergency situations (e.g., traveling in remote areas away from medical help)

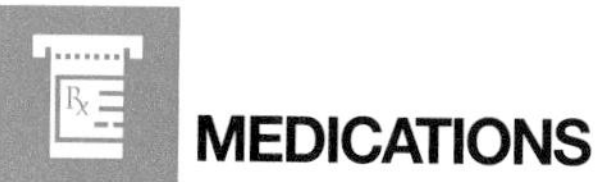

MEDICATIONS

DRUG(S) OF CHOICE
- For chronic adrenal insufficiency:
  - ◊ Hydrocortisone 15-20 mg orally each morning upon arising and 10 mg at 4-5 each afternoon is usual dosage (dosage may vary and is usually less in children's) PLUS
  - ◊ Fludrocortisone 0.05-0.2 mg orally once/day plus
  - ◊ Dehydroepiandrosterone 25-50 mg orally once a day (monitor lipid profile, breast or prostate cancer)
  - ◊ May require salt supplementation
- Acute adrenal insufficiency
  - ◊ Hydrocortisone 100 mg IV followed by 10 mg/hr infusion
  - ◊ IV glucose, saline, plasma expanders
  - ◊ Fludrocortisone 0.05 mg qd
- For acute illnesses (fever, stress, minor trauma)
  - ◊ Double the patient's usual steroid dose. Taper gradually over a week or more, monitor VS and serum sodium.
- Supplement for surgical procedures: 25-150 mg hydrocortisone or 5-30 mg methylprednisolone IV on day of procedure in addition to maintenance therapy. Taper gradually to usual dose over 1-2 days.

Contraindications: Refer to manufacturer's literature

Precautions:
- Patients with hepatic disease may need a reduced dose
- Elderly should have a slightly reduced dose
- Excessive corticosteroid doses or excessive duration of supplemental treatment of those who are acutely ill or undergoing surgery may increase the mortality rate
- Refer to manufacturer's literature for other precautions

Significant possible interactions: Refer to manufacturer's literature. Rifampin, phenytoin, and barbiturates may precipitate adrenal insufficiency in addisonian patients by inducing steroid-metabolizing liver enzymes. Patients on these drugs may require higher doses of corticosteroid due to increased steroid metabolism.

ALTERNATIVE DRUGS Prednisone 5 mg in AM and 2.5 mg at hs plus fludrocortisone, and DHEA; dexamethasone 0.5 mg in AM plus fludrocortisone plus DHEA

FOLLOWUP

PATIENT MONITORING
- Verify adequacy of therapy - normal blood pressure, serum electrolytes normal, normal plasma renin, improvement of appetite and strength, increase in heart size to normal, normal fasting blood glucose level
- Lifelong medical supervision for signs of continued adequate therapy and avoidance of overdose

PREVENTION/AVOIDANCE
- No preventive measures known for Addison disease
- Prevention of complications
  - ◊ Anticipate adrenal crisis and treat before symptoms begin
  - ◊ If nausea and vomiting preclude oral therapy, patient should seek medical help to start parenteral therapy
  - ◊ Elective surgical procedures require upward adjustment in steroid dose
  - ◊ Prevent exposure to infections

POSSIBLE COMPLICATIONS
- Hyperpyrexia
- Psychotic reactions
- Complications from underlying disease
- Over- or under-steroid treatment
- Hyperkalemic paralysis (rare)
- Addisonian crisis

EXPECTED COURSE/PROGNOSIS
- Requires lifetime treatment
- Good outlook with appropriate treatment. With adequate replacement therapy, life expectancy approximates normal.
- 100% lethal without treatment

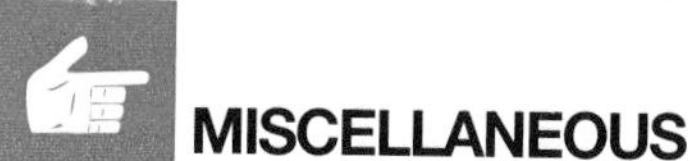

MISCELLANEOUS

ASSOCIATED CONDITIONS
- Diabetes mellitus
- Grave disease
- Hashimoto thyroiditis
- Hypoparathyroidism
- Hypercalcemia
- Ovarian failure
- Pernicious anemia
- Myasthenia gravis
- Vitiligo
- Chronic moniliasis
- Sarcoidosis
- Sjögren syndrome
- Chronic active hepatitis
- Schmidt syndrome (multiple endocrine deficiency syndrome)
- Adrenoleukodystrophy

AGE-RELATED FACTORS
Pediatric:
- Hydrocortisone and fludrocortisone doses are lower than adults
- More difficult to diagnose
- Occurs in siblings

Geriatric: Acute adrenal crisis more likely

Others: N/A

PREGNANCY N/A

SYNONYMS
- Adrenocortical insufficiency
- Waterhouse-Friderichsen syndrome (adrenal crisis)
- Corticoadrenal insufficiency
- Primary adrenocortical insufficiency

ICD-9-CM
255.4 Corticoadrenal insufficiency

SEE ALSO
Sjögren syndrome

OTHER NOTES N/A

ABBREVIATIONS N/A

REFERENCES

- Coursin DB, Wood KE. Corticosteroid supplementation for adrenal insufficiency. JAMA 2002;287(2):236-40
- Dale DC, Federman DD, eds. Scientific American Medicine. New York, Scientific American, Inc., 1997
- Oelkers W. Adrenal insufficiency. NEJM 1996;335(16):1206-12
- Oelkers W. Dehydroepiandrosterone for adrenal insufficiency. NEJM 1999;341(14):1073-4
- King MS. Adrenal insufficiency: an uncommon cause of fatigue. J Am Board Fam Pract 1999;12(5):386-90

Web references: 6 available at www.5mcc.com

Illustrations N/A

Author(s):
Rick Kellerman, MD
Mark Gerstberger, DO

BASICS

DESCRIPTION Usually self-limited febrile illnesses characterized by inflammation of conjunctivae and the respiratory tract. Adenovirus infections occur in epidemic and endemic situations.

- Common types
  - ◊ Acute febrile respiratory illness (AFRI) affecting primarily children
  - ◊ Acute respiratory disease (ARD) affecting adults
  - ◊ Viral pneumonia affecting children and adults
  - ◊ Acute pharyngoconjunctival fever (APC) affecting children, particularly after summer swimming
  - ◊ Acute follicular conjunctivitis affecting all ages
  - ◊ Epidemic keratoconjunctivitis (EKC) affecting adults
  - ◊ Intestinal infections leading to enteritis, mesenteric adenitis and intussusception

System(s) affected: Cardiovascular, Gastrointestinal, Hemic/Lymphatic/Immunologic, Musculoskeletal, Nervous, Pulmonary, Renal/Urologic
Genetics: N/A
Incidence/Prevalence in USA: Very common infection, estimated at 2-5% of all respiratory infections. More common in infants and children.
Predominant age: All ages
Predominant sex: Male = Female

SIGNS & SYMPTOMS

- Depends on type (see "Differential diagnosis")

In common with most respiratory forms:

- Headache
- Malaise
- Sore throat
- Cough
- Fever (moderate to high)
- Vomiting
- Diarrhea
- Mucosa exhibits patches of white exudate

CAUSES

- Adenovirus (DNA viruses 60-90 nm in size with 47 known serotypes; 3 types cause gastroenteritis); difficult to eliminate from skin and environmental surfaces
- Different serotypes have different epidemiologies
- Most common known pathogens are:
  - ◊ Types 1, 2, 3, 5, 7 cause respiratory illness
  - ◊ Type 3 causes pharyngoconjunctival fever
  - ◊ Types 4, 7, 21 cause acute respiratory disease
  - ◊ Several other types may cause epidemic keratoconjunctivitis

RISK FACTORS

- Large number of people gathered in a small area (military recruits, college students at the beginning of the school year, daycare centers, community swimming pools, etc.)
- Immunocompromised at risk for severe disease

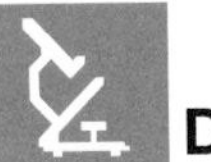

DIAGNOSIS

DIFFERENTIAL DIAGNOSIS

Early diagnosis depends on clinical evaluation. The following are the primary characteristics of the major adenovirus infections:

- Acute febrile respiratory illness:
  - ◊ Nonspecific cold-like symptoms, similar to other viral respiratory illnesses (fever, pharyngitis, tracheitis, bronchitis, pneumonitis)
  - ◊ Mostly in children
  - ◊ Incubation period 2 to 5 days
  - ◊ May be pertussis-like syndrome rarely
- Acute respiratory disease:
  - ◊ Malaise, fever, chills, headache, pharyngitis, hoarseness and dry cough
  - ◊ Fever lasts 2 to 4 days
  - ◊ Illness subsides in 10 to 14 days
- Viral pneumonia
  - ◊ Sudden onset of high fever, rapid infection of upper and lower respiratory tracts, skin rash, diarrhea
  - ◊ Occurs in children aged a few days up to 3 years
  - ◊ Common; severe illness occurs in subset
- Acute pharyngoconjunctival fever
  - ◊ Spiking fever lasting several days, headache, pharyngitis, conjunctivitis, rhinitis, cervical adenitis
  - ◊ Conjunctivitis is usually unilateral
  - ◊ Subsides in about 1 week
- Epidemic keratoconjunctivitis
  - ◊ Usually unilateral onset of ocular redness and edema, periorbital edema, periorbital swelling, local discomfort suggestive of foreign body
  - ◊ Lasts 3 or 4 weeks

LABORATORY

- Viral cultures from respiratory, ocular or fecal sources can establish diagnosis. Pharyngeal isolate suggests recent infection.
- Antigen detection in stool for enteric serotypes is available
- Serologic procedures such as complement fixation with a four fold rise in serum antibody titer identifies recent adenoviral infection

Drugs that may alter lab results: N/A

Disorders that may alter lab results: N/A

PATHOLOGICAL FINDINGS

- Varies with each virus, severe pneumonia may be reflected by extensive intranuclear inclusions
- Bronchiolitis obliterans may occur

SPECIAL TESTS Cultures and serologic studies if appropriate

IMAGING X-ray: bronchopneumonia in severe respiratory infections

DIAGNOSTIC PROCEDURES

- Biopsy (lung or other) may be needed in severe or unusual cases

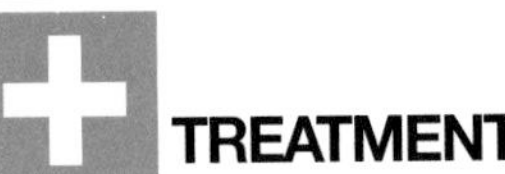

TREATMENT

APPROPRIATE HEALTH CARE Ambulatory except for severely ill infants or those with epidemic keratoconjunctivitis or infants with severe pneumonia. Contact and droplet precautions during a hospitalization are indicated.

GENERAL MEASURES Treatment is supportive and symptomatic. Infections are usually benign and of short duration.

SURGICAL MEASURES N/A

ACTIVITY Rest during febrile phases

DIET No special diet

PATIENT EDUCATION Avoid aspirin in children. Give instructions for nasal spray, cough preparations, frequent hand washing.

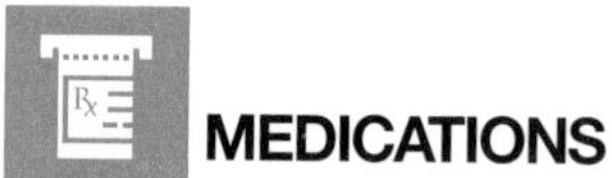

MEDICATIONS

DRUG(S) OF CHOICE
- Acetaminophen, 10-15 mg/kg/dose, for analgesia (avoid aspirin)
- Topical corticosteroids for conjunctivitis (after consulting an ophthalmologist)
- Cough suppressants and/or expectorants

Contraindications: Refer to manufacturer's literature
Precautions: Refer to manufacturer's literature
Significant possible interactions: Refer to manufacturer's literature

ALTERNATIVE DRUGS N/A

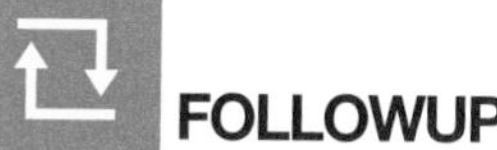

FOLLOWUP

PATIENT MONITORING
For severe infantile pneumonia and conjunctivitis: daily physical exam until well

PREVENTION/AVOIDANCE
- Live types 4 and 7 adenovirus vaccine orally in enteric coated capsule reduces incidence of acute respiratory disease
- Frequent hand washing among office personnel and family members

POSSIBLE COMPLICATIONS
- Few if any recognizable long-term problems

EXPECTED COURSE/PROGNOSIS
- Self-limited, usually without sequelae
- Severe illness and death in very young and in immunocompromised hosts

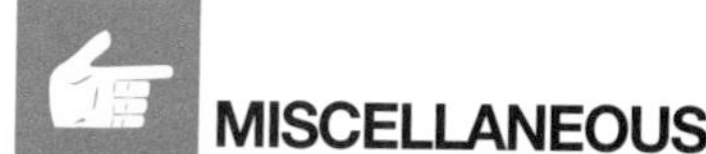

MISCELLANEOUS

ASSOCIATED CONDITIONS
- Hemorrhagic cystitis (can be caused by adenovirus)
- Viral enteritis
- Intussusception and mesenteric adenitis

AGE-RELATED FACTORS
Pediatric: Viral pneumonia in infants may be fatal
Geriatric: Complications more likely
Others: N/A

PREGNANCY
No special precautions

SYNONYMS N/A

ICD-9-CM
079.0 Adenovirus
462 Acute pharyngitis
480.0 Pneumonia due to adenovirus

SEE ALSO
Conjunctivitis, acute
Intussusception
Pneumonia, viral

OTHER NOTES
Conjunctivitis sometimes called "pink eye"

ABBREVIATIONS N/A

REFERENCES

- Mandell GL, et al, eds: Principles and Practice of Infectious Diseases. 5th Ed. New York, Churchill Livingstone, 2000
- Fields BN, Knipe DM, eds: Fundamental Virology. 3rd Ed. New York, Raven Press, 1995

Web references: 0 available at www.5mcc.com
Illustrations N/A

Author(s):
Ronald L. Malm, DO

BASICS

DESCRIPTION Any pattern of alcohol use causing significant physical, mental, or social dysfunction; key features are tolerance, withdrawal, and persistent use despite problems; for DSM-IV criteria see chapter on Substance use disorders.

System(s) affected: Gastrointestinal, Nervous

Genetics: 50-60% of risk is genetic, based on twin and adoption studies

Incidence/Prevalence in USA:
- Lifetime prevalence 13.6%
- 20% in primary care setting

Predominant age:
- 18-25, but all ages affected

Predominant sex: Male > Female (3:1)

SIGNS & SYMPTOMS
- Behavioral
  - ◊ Psychological and social dysfunction
  - ◊ Marital problems (divorce or separation)
  - ◊ Anxiety, depression, insomnia
  - ◊ Social isolation or withdrawal
  - ◊ Child or spouse abuse
  - ◊ Alcohol-related arrests or legal problems
  - ◊ Preoccupation with recreational drinking
  - ◊ Repeated attempts to stop or reduce drinking
  - ◊ Loss of interest in non-drinking activities
  - ◊ Employment problems (tardiness, absenteeism, decreased productivity, interpersonal problems at work, frequent job changes)
  - ◊ Blackouts (not remembering what happened during drinking spells)
  - ◊ Complaints by family members or friends about alcohol-related behavior
- Physical
  - ◊ Gastrointestinal: anorexia, nausea, vomiting, abdominal pain, stigmata of chronic liver disease, peptic ulcer disease, pancreatitis, esophageal malignancies, varices
  - ◊ Cardiovascular: hypertension, dilated cardiomyopathy, palpitations
  - ◊ Respiratory: aspiration pneumonia
  - ◊ Genitourinary: impotence, menstrual irregularities, testicular atrophy, infertility
  - ◊ Endocrine/metabolic: hyperlipidemias, cushingoid appearance, gynecomastia
  - ◊ Dermatologic: burns (e.g., cigarettes), bruises in various stages of healing, poor hygiene, palmar erythema, spider telangiectasias, caput medusa, jaundice, hyperpigmentation
  - ◊ Musculoskeletal: old fractures and fractures in various stages of healing, myopathy, osteopenia, bone marrow suppression
  - ◊ Neurologic: cognitive deficits (e.g., memory impairment), peripheral neuropathy, Wernicke-Korsakoff syndrome, grand-mal seizures, delirium tremors
  - ◊ HEENT: plethoric facies, parotid hypertrophy, poor oral hygiene, oropharyngeal malignancies

CAUSES Multifactorial including genetic, environmental

RISK FACTORS
- Family history
- Depression, anxiety
- Other substance use disorders
- Male gender
- Low socioeconomic status
- Unemployment
- Peer, social approval
- Accessibility of alcohol
- Family dysfunction or trauma
- Antisocial personality disorder
- Academic problems, school dropout
- Criminal involvement

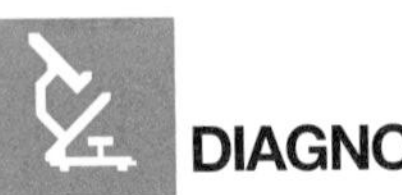

DIAGNOSIS

DIFFERENTIAL DIAGNOSIS
- Other substance use disorders
- Depression
- Dementia
- Cerebellar ataxia
- Benign essential tremor
- Seizure disorder
- Hypoglycemia, diabetic ketoacidosis
- Viral hepatitis

LABORATORY
- Blood alcohol concentration:
  - ◊ >100 mg/dL (22 mmol/L) as outpatient
  - ◊ >150 mg/dL (33 mmol/L) without obvious signs of intoxication
  - ◊ >300 mg/dL (65 mmol/L) at any time
- Suggestive - if increased:
  - ◊ Gamma-glutamyl transferase (GGT)
  - ◊ Aspartate aminotransferase (AST)
  - ◊ Alanine aminotransferase (ALT)
  - ◊ Alkaline phosphatase
  - ◊ Bilirubin (total)
  - ◊ AST/ALT > 2.0
  - ◊ Uric acid
  - ◊ Triglycerides
  - ◊ Cholesterol (total, HDL)
  - ◊ Mean corpuscular volume (MCV)
  - ◊ Prothrombin time (PT)
- Suggestive - if decreased:
  - ◊ Calcium, magnesium, phosphorus
  - ◊ Blood urea nitrogen
  - ◊ White blood cell count
  - ◊ Platelet count
  - ◊ Hematocrit, hemoglobin
  - ◊ Serum protein, albumin

Drugs that may alter lab results: See manufacturer's profile for each drug patient takes

Disorders that may alter lab results: Liver, heart, and kidney diseases

PATHOLOGICAL FINDINGS
- Liver: inflammation or fatty infiltration (alcoholic hepatitis), periportal fibrosis (alcoholic cirrhosis - occurs in only 10-20% of alcoholics)
- Gastric mucosa: inflammation, ulceration
- Pancreas: inflammation, liquefaction necrosis
- Intestine: flattening of villi, loss of enzymes
- Heart: interstitial fibrosis and myofibril atrophy (dilated cardiomyopathy)
- Immune system: decreased granulocyte production
- Endocrine organs: elevated plasma cortisol levels, testicular atrophy, suppression of reproductive hormones in women
- Brain: cortical atrophy, enlarged ventricles

SPECIAL TESTS
- CAGE questionnaire:
  - ◊ Have you ever felt you should cut down on your drinking?
  - ◊ Have people annoyed you by criticizing your drinking?
  - ◊ Have you ever felt bad or guilty about your drinking?
  - ◊ Have you ever had a drink first thing in the morning to steady your nerves or to get rid of a hangover (eye-opener)?

More than 2 "yes" answers is 74-89% sensitive, 79-95% specific for alcohol use disorder; less sensitive for early problem drinking or heavy drinking
- AUDIT (Alcohol Use Disorders Identification Test): 10 items, score > 4 is 70-92% sensitive, 73-94% specific
- 1 and 2 - item screening tests also effective for identifying problem drinking

IMAGING
- X-ray: multiple old rib fractures
- CT scan, MRI of brain: cortical atrophy, structural lesions in the thalamic nucleus and basal forebrain

DIAGNOSTIC PROCEDURES Liver biopsy: alcoholic hepatitis, cirrhosis

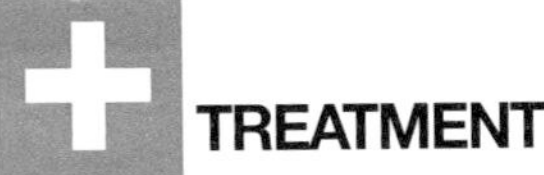

TREATMENT

APPROPRIATE HEALTH CARE
- Indications for inpatient detoxification:
  - ◊ Severe withdrawal symptoms
  - ◊ Prior delirium tremens, withdrawal seizures
  - ◊ Coexisting acute or chronic illness
  - ◊ Strong craving for alcohol or lack of commitment to abstinence
  - ◊ Suicidal ideation or significant psychiatric symptoms
  - ◊ Obstacles to close monitoring (follow-up not feasible)
  - ◊ Pregnancy

GENERAL MEASURES
- Supportive, non-judgmental attitude helpful
- Brief interventions by primary care physicians are highly effective for problem drinking
- Consider addiction specialist consult

SURGICAL MEASURES N/A

ACTIVITY Fall preventions or restrictions if delirious

DIET Alcoholics tend to have adequate caloric intake but deficiencies in folate; vitamins B1, B6, B12; magnesium, phosphate and zinc

PATIENT EDUCATION
- National Clearinghouse for Alcohol and Drug Information: (800) 729-6686
- Alcoholics Anonymous: literature, crisis hot line through a local chapter

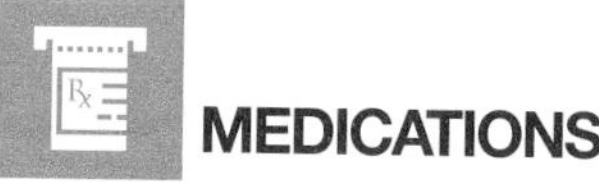

MEDICATIONS

DRUG(S) OF CHOICE

- For detoxification and management of alcohol withdrawal syndrome: (multiple regimens)
  - ◊ For treatment of acute withdrawal, first dose of benzodiazepine should achieve sedation without respiratory compromise; drugs then are tapered daily as long as withdrawal symptoms are stable
  - ◊ Chlordiazepoxide 25-100 mg PO/IM qd-tid
  - ◊ Diazepam 5-20 mg PO/IM/IV tid
  - ◊ Lorazepam 1-4 mg PO/IM/IV q 2-6 hrs; lorazepam preferred in elderly, severe liver disease, or for IV drip
  - ◊ Phenobarbital 60-120 mg PO/IM/IV tid-qid may be safer in pregnancy
  - ◊ Carbamazepine 200 mg bid-qid
- Adjuncts to detoxification:
  - ◊ Beta blockers for tachycardia
  - ◊ Clonidine 0.1-0.2 mg PO tid for autonomic hyperactivity
  - ◊ Haloperidol for psychosis, agitation
- Adjuncts to rehabilitation:
  - ◊ Naltrexone 50 mg PO qd, opiate antagonist shown to reduce craving and chance of heavy drinking with relapse; may improve abstinence rate
  - ◊ Disulfiram 250-500 mg PO qd, lack of proven efficacy, may provide psychologic deterrent to drinking
- Supplements to all:
  - ◊ Thiamine 100 mg PO/IV qd (first dose IV)
  - ◊ Folic acid 1 mg PO/IV qd
  - ◊ Multivitamin PO qd
  - ◊ Magnesium sulfate 1 gm IM/IV q4-6hr (especially if history of delirium tremens or withdrawal seizure)

Contraindications:
- All: persistent alcohol use
- Naltrexone: pregnancy, acute hepatitis, hepatic failure
- Disulfiram: pregnancy, ischemic heart disease

Precautions:
- Severe liver disease, organic pain, organic brain syndromes
- Monitor for nystagmus, ataxia, excessive somnolence, slurred speech, other signs of intoxication

Significant possible interactions:
- Alcohol and benzodiazepines, sedatives, hypnotics
- Naltrexone and narcotics
- Disulfiram and metronidazole, phenytoin, isoniazid, anticoagulants

ALTERNATIVE DRUGS

- Anticonvulsants gabapentin (Neurontin) and vigabatrin (Sabril) are being studied for use in detoxification
- Acamprosate, a glutamate antagonist used in Europe and currently being tested in U.S.. appears to reduce craving and improve abstinence rate

FOLLOWUP

PATIENT MONITORING

- Inpatient detoxification: monitor withdrawal symptoms, vital signs at least every 4 hours
  - ◊ Clinical Institute Withdrawal Assessment Scale for Alcohol (CIWA-Ar) very helpful
- Outpatient detoxification: daily visits
- Early outpatient rehabilitation: weekly visits
- First 3 months critical to long term sobriety

PREVENTION/AVOIDANCE

- Preventive counseling of patients with a family history of alcoholism
- Public health and education measures

POSSIBLE COMPLICATIONS

- Cirrhosis (women sooner than men)
- Gastrointestinal malignancies
- Neuropathy, dementia
- Wernicke-Korsakoff syndrome
- Cerebrovascular accident
- Increased susceptibility to infection
- Aseptic necrosis of the hip
- Relapse of drinking
- Depression, suicide
- Trauma
- Death

EXPECTED COURSE/PROGNOSIS

- Chronic relapsing disease
- Alcoholics have mortality rate more than twice that of general population and die an average of 10-15 years earlier
- Alcohol causes 100,000 excess deaths per year
- Abstinence has documented benefits for survival, mental health, marriage, parenting, and employment

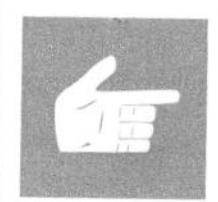

MISCELLANEOUS

ASSOCIATED CONDITIONS

- Tobacco, substance use disorders
- Depression, affective disorders
- Anxiety disorders
- Antisocial personality disorder
- Dilated cardiomyopathy
- Hypertension
- Peptic ulcer disease
- Gastritis
- Hepatic cirrhosis
- Fatty liver infiltration
- Cholelithiasis
- Viral hepatitis
- Diabetes
- Pancreatitis
- Hyperlipidemia
- Malnutrition
- Upper gastrointestinal malignancies
- Peripheral neuropathy
- Primary seizure disorder
- Sexual abuse
- Domestic violence
- Trauma (falls, motor vehicle accidents)

AGE-RELATED FACTORS

Pediatric:
- Children of alcoholics at high risk
- In 2000, 27.5% persons age 12-20 reported use in past month, and 1 in 5 was a binge drinker; bingers 7 times more likely to report illicit drug use
- Negative impact on normal maturation and development and on attainment of social, educational and occupational skills
- Watch for depression, suicidal behavior, family disruption, disorderly behavior, violence or destruction of property, poor school or work performance, sexual promiscuity, social immaturity, lack of hobbies or interests, isolation, moodiness

Geriatric:
- Drug interactions
- Alcoholism often missed; signs and symptoms may be different or attributed to chronic medical problem or dementia
- Assessment tools standardized on younger populations often inappropriate

Others: Women experience harmful effects at lower levels of alcohol consumption than men

PREGNANCY

- Alcohol is highly teratogenic, especially during early weeks of fetal development.
- Women should abstain when planning conception and throughout pregnancy

SYNONYMS

- Alcoholism
- Alcohol abuse
- Alcohol dependence

ICD-9-CM

303.90 Other and unspecified alcohol dependence, unspecified
305.00 Alcohol abuse, unspecified
303.00 Acute alcoholic intoxication, unspecified
291.81 Alcohol Withdrawal

SEE ALSO

Substance use disorders

OTHER NOTES N/A

ABBREVIATIONS

DSM-IV = Diagnostic and Statistical Manual of Mental Disorders, 4th edition

REFERENCES

- National Institute on Alcohol Abuse and Alcoholism: Tenth Special Report to the US Congress on Alcohol and Health. DHHS, 2000
- Mersy DJ. Recognition of alcohol and substance abuse. Am Fam Physician 2003;67(7):1529-32
- Enoch MA, Goldman D. Problem drinking and alcoholism: diagnosis and treatment. Am Fam Physician 2002;65(3):441-8
- Kosten TR, O'Connor PG. Management of drug and alcohol withdrawal. N Engl J Med 2003;348(18):1786-95
- Center for Substance Abuse Treatment. Treatment Improvement Protocol Series 24: A Guide to Substance Abuse Services for Primary Care Clinicians. Substance Abuse and Mental Health Services, DHHS, 1997
- Saitz R, O'Malley SS. Pharmacotherapies for alcohol abuse. Med Clin of North Am 1997;81(4):881-907
- Franklin JE, Frances RJ. Alcohol and other psychoactive substance use disorders. In: Hales RE, Yudofsky SC, Talbott JA, editors. Textbook of Psychiatry. 3rd Ed. Washington, DC: American Psychiatric Press; 1999
- The National Household Survey on Drug Abuse. Substance Abuse and Mental Health Services Administration, DHHS, 2000

Web references: 6 available at www.5mcc.com
Illustrations 4 available

Author(s):
S. Lindsey Clarke, MD

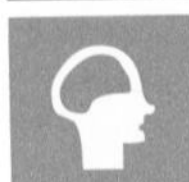

BASICS

DESCRIPTION The clinical syndrome of hypertension, hypokalemia, low plasma renin activity, and increased aldosterone secretion.
- Unilateral aldosterone-producing adenoma (APA) - cured with unilateral adrenalectomy
- Idiopathic hyperaldosteronism (IHA) due to bilateral zona glomerulosa hyperplasia - not cured with surgery. Chronic medical therapy is treatment of choice.

System(s) affected: Endocrine/Metabolic
Genetics: Unknown
Incidence/Prevalence in USA:
- 5-10% of the hypertensive population

Predominant age: Usually diagnosed third to sixth decades
Predominant sex: APA more common in women

SIGNS & SYMPTOMS
- Usually asymptomatic
- Most patients are normokalemic
- Marked hypokalemia may be associated with muscle weakness and cramping, headaches, palpitations, polydipsia, polyuria, or nocturia
- Mild to severe hypertension
- Funduscopy - benign or grade 1-2
- Edema (rare)
- Hypokalemia (not required)
- Metabolic alkalosis
- Relative "hypernatremia"
- Impaired glucose tolerance
- Increased incidence of renal cysts

CAUSES
- Unilateral aldosterone-producing adrenal adenoma (APA)
- Idiopathic hyperaldosteronism (IHA)
- Aldosterone-producing adrenocortical carcinoma
- Other rare subtypes

RISK FACTORS N/A

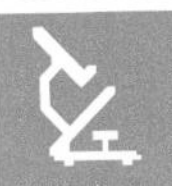

DIAGNOSIS

DIFFERENTIAL DIAGNOSIS
- Diuretic use
- Renovascular hypertension
- Pheochromocytoma
- Renin-secreting tumor
- Malignant hypertension
- Congenital adrenal hyperplasia
- Deoxycorticosterone-producing tumor
- Exogenous mineralocorticoid
- High dose glucocorticoid therapy
- Apparent mineralocorticoid excess syndrome (congenital or acquired due to licorice ingestion)
- Liddle syndrome

LABORATORY
- Hypokalemia with inappropriate kaliuresis
- Unsuppressible urine or plasma aldosterone levels
- Low ambulatory plasma renin activity
- High plasma aldosterone to renin ratio (> 20 in ng/dL [> 55 nmol/L] and ng/mL/h, respectively)
- Normal glucocorticoid excretion

Drugs that may alter lab results: Spironolactone

Disorders that may alter lab results: Malignant hypertension

PATHOLOGICAL FINDINGS Unilateral aldosterone-producing adrenal adenoma (APA), bilateral idiopathic adrenal hyperplasia (IHA), aldosterone-producing adrenocortical carcinoma

SPECIAL TESTS
- Aldosterone suppression test with either a high salt diet or saline infusion
- Spironolactone treatment trial
- Adrenal venous sampling (for aldosterone and cortisol)

IMAGING Adrenal computerized tomography (CT preferred over MRI). Use 3 mm cuts.

DIAGNOSTIC PROCEDURES Adrenal venous sampling

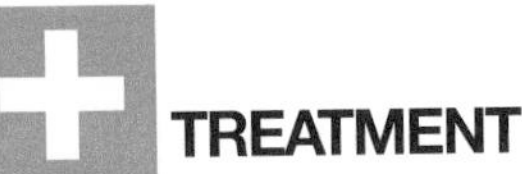

TREATMENT

APPROPRIATE HEALTH CARE
- Unilateral APA - unilateral adrenalectomy
- Bilateral IHA - chronic medical therapy

GENERAL MEASURES
- Unilateral APA - correct hypokalemia preoperatively with spironolactone
- Bilateral IHA - low sodium diet, regular isotonic exercise, maintenance of ideal body weight, tobacco avoidance, mineralocorticoid receptor antagonist, antihypertensive agent (e.g., calcium channel antagonist, ACE-inhibitor, low-dose thiazide diuretic)

SURGICAL MEASURES The treatment of choice for patients with an unilateral APA is adrenalectomy. Patients with bilateral IHA are treated medically.

ACTIVITY No limitations

DIET Low sodium

PATIENT EDUCATION N/A

MEDICATIONS

DRUG(S) OF CHOICE

- Potassium-sparing agent - spironolactone (Aldactone)or amiloride (Midamor)
- Antihypertensive agent - calcium channel antagonist, ACE-inhibitor, angiotensin-II receptor antagonist or low-dose thiazide diuretic

Contraindications: Potassium-sparing agent and ACE-inhibitors in renal failure, hyperkalemia, and pregnancy

Precautions: Monitor serum potassium closely after any adjustment in potassium replacement or potassium-sparing agent

Significant possible interactions: Lithium and diuretics, non-steroidal anti-inflammatory agents with diuretics and ACE-inhibitors

ALTERNATIVE DRUGS N/A

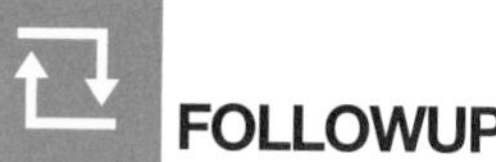

FOLLOWUP

PATIENT MONITORING

- Blood pressure checks
- Serum potassium check
- 24-hour urine aldosterone following surgery

PREVENTION/AVOIDANCE N/A

POSSIBLE COMPLICATIONS Cardiac arrhythmia associated with severe hypokalemia

EXPECTED COURSE/PROGNOSIS

Surgical removal of an APA results in cure of hypertension in approximately 30-60% of cases. Hypertension does not resolve immediately post operatively, but rather over 1 to 4 months.

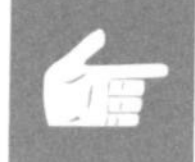

MISCELLANEOUS

ASSOCIATED CONDITIONS Cystic renal disease

AGE-RELATED FACTORS

Pediatric: Bilateral adrenal idiopathic hyperplasia is the most common form in children

Geriatric: N/A

Others: N/A

PREGNANCY Treat hypertension with agents proven to be safe during pregnancy; avoid spironolactone and ACE-inhibitors

SYNONYMS

- Conn syndrome
- Hyperaldosteronism

ICD-9-CM

255.10 Primary aldosteronism

SEE ALSO

Hypertension, essential
Hypokalemia
Liddle syndrome

OTHER NOTES

- Who should be screened for primary aldosteronism?

1) All patients with hypertension and spontaneous hypokalemia
2) All patients with treatment-resistant hypertension

ABBREVIATIONS

APA = aldosterone-producing adenoma
IHA = idiopathic hyperaldosteronism

REFERENCES

- Young WF Jr, Stanson AW, Grant CS, et al: Primary aldosteronism: adrenal venous sampling. Surgery 1996;120:913-920
- Young WF Jr, Hogan MJ: Renin-independent hypermineralocorticoidism. Trends Endocrinol Metab 1994;5:97
- Weinberger MH, Fineberg NS: The diagnosis of primary aldosteronism and separation of the two major subtypes. Arch Int Med 1993;153:2125-2129

Web references: 0 available at www.5mcc.com

Illustrations N/A

Author(s):

William F. Young, Jr, MD

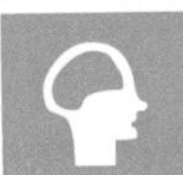

BASICS

DESCRIPTION Absence of the hair from skin areas where it normally is present
- Telogen effluvium - diffuse hair loss that results in decreased hair density but does not progress to complete baldness
- Anagen effluvium - diffuse shedding of hairs, including growing hairs, that may progress to complete baldness
- Cicatricial alopecia - also known as scarring alopecia and characterized by slick, smooth scalp without any evidence of follicular openings of hair
- Androgenic alopecia - hair loss occurring in either sex, caused by stimulation of the hair roots by male hormones
- Alopecia areata - patchy, non-scarring hair loss
- Traction alopecia - patchy, initially non-scarring hair loss
- Tinea capitis - patches of hair broken off close to the scalp, with or without associated inflammation, caused by fungus infection

System(s) affected: Skin/Exocrine
Genetics: In Caucasians, androgenic alopecia follows a dominant trait with incomplete penetrance. The hereditary incidence is notable not only in men but also in women with a strong family history of baldness.
Incidence/Prevalence in USA: 50% of Caucasian males by 50 years of age have noticeable male-pattern baldness. 37% of postmenopausal females show some evidence of hair loss.
Predominant age: The incidence of androgenic alopecia increases with increasing age. Tinea capitis and traction alopecia are more common in children.
Predominant sex: Male > Female

SIGNS & SYMPTOMS
- Hair loss
- Pruritus (in tinea capitis)
- Scaling of the scalp (in tinea capitis)
- Broken hairs (in tinea capitis and traction alopecia)
- Tapered hair at the borders of the patch of alopecia (in alopecia areata)
- Easily removable hairs at the periphery of the patch of alopecia (in alopecia areata)
- Inflammation (in tinea capitis)

CAUSES
- Telogen effluvium
  - ◊ Postpartum
  - ◊ Drugs (oral contraceptives, anticoagulants, retinoids, beta blockers, chemotherapeutic agents, interferon)
  - ◊ Stress (physical or psychological)
  - ◊ Hormonal (hypo- or hyperthyroidism, hypopituitarism)
  - ◊ Nutritional (malnutrition, iron deficiency, zinc deficiency)
  - ◊ Diffuse alopecia areata
- Anagen effluvium
  - ◊ Mycosis fungoides
  - ◊ X-ray treatment
  - ◊ Drugs (chemotherapeutic agents, allopurinol, levodopa, bromocriptine)
  - ◊ Poisoning (bismuth, arsenic, gold, boric acid, thallium)
- Cicatricial alopecia
  - ◊ Congenital and developmental defects
  - ◊ Infection (leprosy, syphilis, varicella-zoster, cutaneous leishmaniasis)
  - ◊ Basal cell carcinoma
  - ◊ Epidermal nevi
  - ◊ Physical agents (acids and alkali, burns, freezing, radiodermatitis)
  - ◊ Cicatricial pemphigoid
  - ◊ Lichen planus
  - ◊ Discoid lupus erythematosus
  - ◊ Sarcoidosis
- Androgenic alopecia
  - ◊ Adrenal hyperplasia
  - ◊ Polycystic ovaries
  - ◊ Ovarian hyperplasia
  - ◊ Carcinoid
  - ◊ Pituitary hyperplasia
  - ◊ Drugs (testosterone, danazol, ACTH, anabolic steroids, progesterones)
- Alopecia areata
  - ◊ Unknown, but possibly autoimmune
- Traction alopecia
  - ◊ Trichotillomania (direct self-pulling of the hair)
  - ◊ Tight rollers or braids
- Tinea capitis
  - ◊ Microsporum species
  - ◊ Trichophyton species

RISK FACTORS
- Positive family history of baldness
- Physical or psychological stress
- Pregnancy
- Poor nutrition

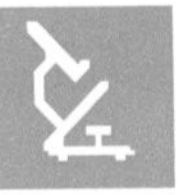

DIAGNOSIS

DIFFERENTIAL DIAGNOSIS Search for type of alopecia and then for possible reversible causes

LABORATORY
- Thyroid function tests
- Complete blood count (may reflect an underlying immunologic disorder)
- Free testosterone and dehydroepiandrosterone sulfate (DHEA-S) in women with androgenic alopecia
- Serum ferritin
- VDRL or RPR for syphilis
- Lymphocyte T and B cell number (sometimes low in patients with alopecia areata)

Drugs that may alter lab results:
- Antifungal drugs may make KOH examination falsely negative
- Thyroid drugs and iodine preparations (including topicals) will alter thyroid function tests

Disorders that may alter lab results: N/A

PATHOLOGICAL FINDINGS Scalp biopsy with routine microscopy and direct immunofluorescence will aid in the diagnosis of tinea capitis, diffuse alopecia areata, and the scarring alopecias due to lupus erythematosus, lichen planus, and sarcoidosis

SPECIAL TESTS
- Light hair-pull test (positive in alopecia areata)
- Direct microscopic examination of the hair shaft
- Potassium hydroxide (KOH) examination of the scale, if present (positive in tinea capitis)
- Fungal culture of the scale, if present

IMAGING N/A

DIAGNOSTIC PROCEDURES Scalp biopsy (sometimes)

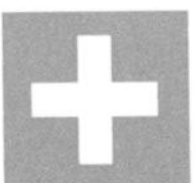

TREATMENT

APPROPRIATE HEALTH CARE Outpatient

GENERAL MEASURES
- Telogen effluvium - maximum shedding 3 months after the inciting event (medication, stress, nutritional deficiency) and recovery following correction of the cause. Rarely permanent baldness.
- Anagen effluvium - shedding begins days to a few weeks after the inciting event with recovery following correction of the cause. Rarely permanent baldness.
- Cicatricial alopecia - hair follicles are permanently damaged. Only effective treatment is surgical (graft transplantation, flap transplantation, or excision of the scarred area).
- Androgenic alopecia - by 12 months of using topical minoxidil, 39% of subjects reported moderate to marked hair growth. Other treatments for androgenic alopecia are surgical (hair transplantation, scalp reduction, transposition flap, and soft tissue expansion).
- Alopecia areata - usually the disease resolves within three years without treatment. Recurrences are, however, common.
- Traction alopecia - only with discontinuation of the hair pulling will the disorder resolve. Psychologic or psychiatric intervention may be necessary. Successful therapeutic approaches have included medications, behavior modification, and hypnosis.
- Tinea capitis - six to eight weeks of therapy are often necessary. Careful handwashing and laundering of head wear and towels.

SURGICAL MEASURES N/A

ACTIVITY Fully active

DIET No special diet

PATIENT EDUCATION National Alopecia Areata Foundation, 714 C Street, San Rafael, CA 94901

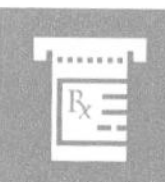

MEDICATIONS

DRUG(S) OF CHOICE

- Androgenic alopecia - topical minoxidil (Rogaine) 2%; finasteride (Propecia), 1 mg once daily
- Alopecia areata - high potency topical steroids, topical anthralin, intralesional steroids, PUVA, cyclosporine
- Tinea capitis - griseofulvin [ultramicrosize] 250-375 mg/day in adults, 5.5-7.3 mg/kg/day in children. Alternatively, ketoconazole 200 mg once daily. Treatment for 6-8 weeks.

Contraindications:

- Griseofulvin - pregnancy, porphyria, hepatocellular failure
- Ketoconazole and cisapride (Propulsid) should not be used together
- Itraconazole and cisapride should not be used together

Precautions:

- Topical minoxidil
  - ◊ Burning and irritation of the eyes
  - ◊ Salt and water retention
  - ◊ Tachycardia
  - ◊ Angina (rare)
- Topical steroids
  - ◊ Local burning and stinging
  - ◊ Pruritus
  - ◊ Skin atrophy
  - ◊ Telangiectasias
  - ◊ Hypothalamic-pituitary-adrenal (HPA) suppression if high-potency steroids used for prolonged duration
- Griseofulvin
  - ◊ Photosensitivity reaction
  - ◊ Lupus-like syndrome
  - ◊ Oral thrush
  - ◊ Granulocytopenia
- Ketoconazole
  - ◊ Anaphylaxis
  - ◊ Hepatotoxicity
  - ◊ Oligospermia
  - ◊ Neuropsychiatric disturbances
  - ◊ Gynecomastia
- Itraconazole
  - ◊ Hepatotoxicity
  - ◊ Nausea, vomiting
- Finasteride
  - ◊ Not indicated for use in women
  - ◊ Caution when there is liver disease

Significant possible interactions:

- Topical minoxidil-guanethidine: may potentiate orthostatic hypotension (rare)
- Griseofulvin and warfarin: decreased activity of warfarin
- Griseofulvin and barbiturates: depressed activity of griseofulvin
- Ketoconazole and warfarin: may enhance the activity of warfarin
- Ketoconazole and isoniazid, rifampin: decreased activity of ketoconazole
- Ketoconazole and phenytoin: may alter the metabolism of either drug
- Itraconazole and terfenadine: prolonged QT and ventricular arrhythmias
- Itraconazole and astemizole: prolonged QT and ventricular arrhythmias
- Itraconazole and cisapride: contraindicated
- Itraconazole and digoxin: may result in elevated levels of digoxin
- H2 blockers or antacids and ketoconazole: decreased absorption of ketoconazole. If concomitant therapy needed, give H2 blocker or antacids at least 2 hours after ketoconazole dose. Avoid using the proton pump inhibitor omeprazole for the same reason.

ALTERNATIVE DRUGS N/A

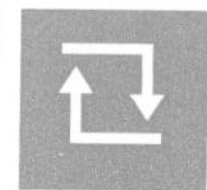

FOLLOWUP

PATIENT MONITORING With ketoconazole, monitor liver enzymes

PREVENTION/AVOIDANCE N/A

POSSIBLE COMPLICATIONS N/A

EXPECTED COURSE/PROGNOSIS

- Telogen effluvium - rarely permanent baldness
- Anagen effluvium - rarely permanent baldness
- Cicatricial alopecia - the hair follicles are permanently damaged
- Androgenic alopecia - depends on treatment
- Alopecia areata - recurrences are common
- Traction alopecia - depends on behavior modification
- Tinea capitis - usually complete recovery

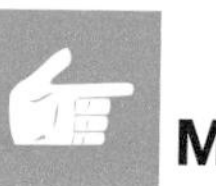

MISCELLANEOUS

ASSOCIATED CONDITIONS Alopecia areata - Down syndrome, vitiligo, diabetes

AGE-RELATED FACTORS

Pediatric: Tinea capitis only common form of alopecia

Geriatric: Androgenic alopecia more common after 50

Others: N/A

PREGNANCY Post partum hair loss is due to altered physiology during pregnancy

SYNONYMS

- Androgenic alopecia

ICD-9-CM

704.00 Alopecia, unspecified
704.01 Alopecia areata
704.09 Diseases of hair and hair follicles, other
110.0 Dermatophytosis of scalp and beard

SEE ALSO

Acrodermatitis enteropathica
Cutaneous T cell lymphoma
Lichen planus
Syphilis
Tinea capitis
Werner syndrome

OTHER NOTES N/A

ABBREVIATIONS

RPR = rapid plasma reagin
HPA = hypothalamic-pituitary axis

REFERENCES

- Rietschel RL. A simplified approach to the diagnosis of alopecia. Dermatol Clin 1996;14:691-5
- Whiting DA. Chronic telogen effluvium. Dermatol Clin 1996;14:723-31
- Fiedler VC, Alaiti S. Treatment of alopecia areata. Dermatol Clin 1996;14:733-8
- Habif TP: Hair diseases. Clinical Dermatology. 4th edition; 2004
- Sperling LC. Hair and systemic disease. Dermatol Clin 2001;19(4):711-26
- Jackson EA. Hair disorders. Prim Care 2000;27(2):319-32

Web references: 4 available at www.5mcc.com
Illustrations 14 available

Author(s):

Aubrey L. Knight, MD

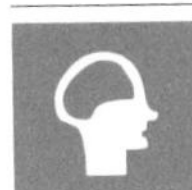

BASICS

DESCRIPTION Altitude illness is a spectrum of medical problems ranging from mild discomfort to fatal illness that may occur on ascent to higher altitude. It can affect anyone, including the most experienced and fit individual, who ascends to more than about 8,000 feet (2438 m). Several factors appear to be important in adaptation to altitude: How long the ascent takes, how high, and length of stay. There is a great deal of variation between people and an individual's response may vary from ascent to ascent.

- Acute mountain sickness (AMS): Begins within 4 to 6 hours after arrival at altitude, rare below 8,000 feet (2438 m), and affects most above 10,000 (3048 m)
- High altitude pulmonary edema (HAPE): Abnormal accumulation of fluid in the lungs. Begins 24 to 96 hours after arrival at altitude. Rare below 8,000 (2438 m) feet but affects more than 10% of individuals above 14,500 feet (4420 m).
- High altitude cerebral edema (HACE): Indicates swelling of the brain. It is the least common but most severe of the high altitude illnesses since it can result in permanent injury or death. Occurs 48 to 72 hours after arrival at altitude. Rare below 12,000 feet (3656 m).

System(s) affected: Cardiovascular, Nervous, Pulmonary
Genetics: N/A
Incidence/Prevalence in USA: Unknown
Predominant age: Any age (young, well-conditioned climbers have a higher incidence of altitude illness, probably because they push themselves more)
Predominant sex: Male = Female

SIGNS & SYMPTOMS

- AMS mild to moderately severe symptoms:
  - ◊ Headache, plus at least one of the following:
  - ◊ Lack of energy and appetite
  - ◊ Mild nausea, vomiting or anorexia
  - ◊ Dizziness
  - ◊ Weakness
  - ◊ Insomnia
- AMS severe symptoms:
  - ◊ Increased headache
  - ◊ Irritability
  - ◊ Marked fatigue
  - ◊ Shortness of breath with exercise
  - ◊ Nausea and vomiting
  - ◊ Irregular or periodic breathing at night (Cheyne-Stokes)
  - ◊ Breathing apnea
- HAPE symptoms:
  - ◊ Excessive shortness of breath on exertion
  - ◊ Severe respiratory distress
  - ◊ Shortness of breath at rest
  - ◊ Dry cough and/or wheezing
  - ◊ Heart rate and respiratory rate increased
  - ◊ Marked periodic breathing present at night
  - ◊ Gurgling breathing
  - ◊ Frothy cough
  - ◊ Wet crackling sounds in the lungs
  - ◊ Confusion
  - ◊ Coma
- HACE symptoms:
  - ◊ Progressive headache that is unrelieved by mild pain relievers
  - ◊ Lack of coordination (e.g., unable to perform a heel-to-toe walk)
  - ◊ Confusion and bizarre behavior followed by unconsciousness
  - ◊ Other symptoms of moderate AMS, such as dizziness, vomiting, and irritability, are usually present

CAUSES The physiology of altitude illness is still not completely understood. The fundamental problem results from the fact that with increasing altitude there is a progressive decrease in barometric pressure and a corresponding lower partial pressure of oxygen in inspired air, resulting in less oxygen delivery to the body.

RISK FACTORS

- In general, the faster the ascent and the higher, the more likely a person will experience symptoms of altitude illness
- Chronic illness
- Lack of conditioning

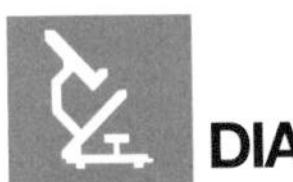

DIAGNOSIS

DIFFERENTIAL DIAGNOSIS

- Viral upper respiratory infection
- Gastroenteritis
- Pneumonia
- Other infections
- Cerebral vascular accident
- Ketoacidosis
- Pulmonary emboli
- Congestive heart failure

LABORATORY

- AMS: Laboratory studies are nonspecific and rarely required for diagnosis
- HAPE: WBC - often slightly elevated, erythrocyte sedimentation rate normal
- Arterial blood gas - may show hypoxia, hypocapnia, alkalosis

Drugs that may alter lab results: N/A

Disorders that may alter lab results: N/A

PATHOLOGICAL FINDINGS N/A

SPECIAL TESTS ECG may show only sinus tachycardia, possibly right heart strain

IMAGING CXR (in HAPE) shows Kerley's lines and a patchy distribution of edema

DIAGNOSTIC PROCEDURES N/A

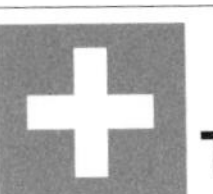

TREATMENT

APPROPRIATE HEALTH CARE Outpatient for mild cases, inpatient for severe cases

GENERAL MEASURES

- Therapy must be tailored to fit severity of disease and may be constrained by the environment
- Definitive treatment is to descend to a lower altitude. Dramatic improvement accompanies even modest reductions in altitude (as little as 1,000 feet [305 m]).
- Oxygen, given continuously at 1-2 liters per minute helps relieve symptoms. For severe symptoms, continuous oxygen should be administered and descent to a lower altitude is mandatory.
- AMS
  - ◊ Stop ascent. Acclimatize at the same altitude; give acetazolamide 125 -250 mg orally two times a day, or descend 460 m (1500 ft) or more until symptoms resolved
- HAPE and HACE
  - ◊ Patient must be treated by immediate evacuation to a lower altitude. Occasionally, however, foul weather, lack of transportation or long distances prevent immediate evacuation. In these cases, supportive measures, such as bedrest and oxygen, will help.
  - ◊ Hyperbaric therapy is another effective and practical alternative when descent is not possible. A portable hyperbaric chamber, the "Gamow bag," made of fabric and weighing only 8 pounds (3.6 kg) can be inflated to 2 pounds per square inch (13.8 kPa) using a foot pump. This is equivalent to a drop in altitude of about 5,000 feet (1524 m). Improvement is usually immediate after being placed in the hyperbaric chamber.
  - ◊ If patient is hospitalized, rule out any other pulmonary disease first, provide adequate oxygen (possibly by intubation or positive end-expiratory pressure [PEEP]), bed rest, diuresis if needed and postural drainage

SURGICAL MEASURES N/A

ACTIVITY Rest until symptoms clear

DIET Increased intake of fluids, a light diet, and avoidance of alcohol

PATIENT EDUCATION See guidelines in Prevention/Avoidance

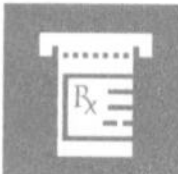

MEDICATIONS

DRUG(S) OF CHOICE

- Aspirin or codeine can be used to relieve the headache. Antibiotics, if infection is present.
- Both dexamethasone and acetazolamide have been used to treat patients with severe symptoms of AMS. Dosage of dexamethasone is 8 mg initially, followed by 4 mg every six hours by mouth. Doses of acetazolamide of up to 1.0 g/day may be required for effective treatment.
- Dexamethasone may be effective in mild cases of HAPE, but this has not been proven
- Diuretics have not been useful
- Corticosteroids should be given even though their effectiveness is questionable

Contraindications: Refer to manufacturer's profile of each drug

Precautions: Refer to manufacturer's profile of each drug

Significant possible interactions: Refer to manufacturer's profile of each drug

ALTERNATIVE DRUGS N/A

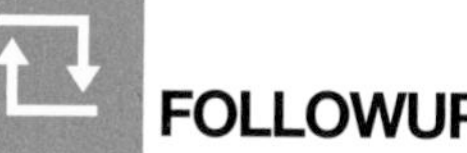

FOLLOWUP

PATIENT MONITORING

- For mild cases, no follow-up needed
- For more severe cases, follow until symptoms subside
- If underlying cardiopulmonary or cardiovascular disease, follow as needed

PREVENTION/AVOIDANCE

- General guidelines
  - ◊ Staged ascent: "Staging" is the process of remaining at an intermediate altitude (6600 to 9800 feet [2012 to 2988 m]) for a few days before attempting the ultimate altitude
  - ◊ Conventional prescription for avoiding altitude illness is to allow one day to ascend and acclimatize each 1,000 feet (305 m) from elevations of 10,000 to 14,000 feet (3,048 to 4,267 m). Two days per 1,000 feet (305 m) at elevations above 14,000 feet (4267 m.
  - ◊ Sleeping elevation - climber's maximum "climb high and sleep low" is a prudent practice for anyone going above 12,000 feet (3656 m)
  - ◊ Adequate hydration - dehydration increases the likelihood of and worsens the symptoms of AMS
  - ◊ Good physical conditioning
  - ◊ Consider carrying a supply of oxygen
- Drug prophylaxis
  - ◊ Acetazolamide (if patient has a history of problems at altitude and/or plans a rapid ascent to above 8,000 feet [2438 m] in a car or airplane). Dosage is usually 250 mg orally twice daily, starting 24 hours before ascent and continuing for two to three days while at altitude. Anyone with a known drug allergy to sulfa should avoid acetazolamide.
  - ◊ Dexamethasone may significantly reduce the incidence and severity of acute mountain sickness. The dosage is 2 to 4 mg every six hours, begun the day of the ascent, continued for three days at the higher altitude, then tapered over five days. Adverse side effects are uncommon.

POSSIBLE COMPLICATIONS

- Without treatment, HACE can cause motor and sensory deficits, seizures and coma
- HAPE may progress to cyanosis and respiratory distress syndrome
- Patient may experience high altitude retinal hemorrhage (HARH) - can cause visual changes, but is usually asymptomatic

EXPECTED COURSE/PROGNOSIS

- Mild to moderate AMS resolves over 1-3 days. Patients may resume ascent once symptoms subside.
- HAPE and HACE patients can expect complete recovery, if there is no underlying disease. Should not resume ascent.
- Problems are more likely to recur in people who have had one or more attacks

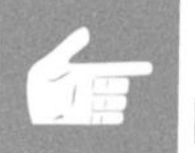

MISCELLANEOUS

ASSOCIATED CONDITIONS N/A

AGE-RELATED FACTORS

Pediatric: Children under 6 are more susceptible than adults

Geriatric: Elderly more likely to have chronic conditions (coronary artery disease, congestive heart failure, chronic obstructive pulmonary disease) that may be exacerbated at altitudes of 6000-8000 feet (1829-2438 m)

Others: Women in premenstrual phase are more vulnerable

PREGNANCY N/A

SYNONYMS Mountain sickness

ICD-9-CM

993.2 Other and unspecified effects of high altitude

SEE ALSO

OTHER NOTES N/A

ABBREVIATIONS

- AMS = acute mountain sickness
- HACE = high altitude cerebral edema
- HAPE = high altitude pulmonary edema

REFERENCES

- Zell SC, Goodman PH: Acetazolamide and dexamethasone in the prevention of acute mountain sickness. West J Med 1988;148:541
- Johnson TS, Rock PB: Current concepts, acute mountain sickness. New Engl J Med 1988;319:841

Web references: 0 available at www.5mcc.com

Illustrations N/A

Author(s):

Tejal Parikh, MD

Kevin Carmichael, MD

BASICS

DESCRIPTION A degenerative organic mental disease characterized by progressive intellectual deterioration and dementia; usually occurring after age 65. The diagnosis is made on clinical grounds after ruling out treatable disorders with similar characteristics. Long-term care cost to the nation is approximately $100 billion/year.
Usual course - progressive; chronic.
System(s) affected: Nervous
Genetics: Positive family history in 50% of cases. Markers on chromosomes: 1 and 14 (early onset disease); 12,19 (late onset); 21 (onset age 50-65).
Incidence/Prevalence in USA: 1100/100,000 people. 40% of those over age 85 are affected.
Predominant age: > 60
Predominant sex: Female > Male (slightly)

SIGNS & SYMPTOMS
- Acalculia
- Agnosia
- Anhedonia
- Anxiety
- Apathy
- Aphasia
- Apraxia
- Confabulation
- Delusions
- Dementia
- Depression
- Impaired abstraction
- Intellectual decline
- Loss of interest
- Occupational dysfunction
- Personality change
- Progressive cognitive impairment
- Recent memory loss (key finding)
- Restlessness
- Sleep disturbances
- Social withdrawal
- Visuospatial distortion
- Weight loss
- Late signs - seizures, myoclonus, extrapyramidal dysfunction, incontinence

CAUSES
- Unknown, but toxic beta-amyloid deposits in neuritic plaques and arteriolar walls appear critical to pathogenesis. Beta-amyloid precursor gene localized to chromosome 21.
- Unsubstantiated possibilities - slow virus, bacterial infection (*Chlamydia pneumoniae*), metals (aluminum), accelerated aging, autoimmune attack

RISK FACTORS
- Aging
- Head trauma
- Low education level
- Down syndrome
- Positive family history
- Inheritance of the E4 allele of apolipoprotein E gene on chromosome 19 (E4 is much less of a risk factor for African Americans and Hispanics)
- Smoking (2-4fold increases)

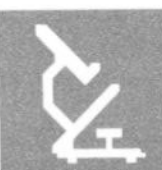

DIAGNOSIS

DIFFERENTIAL DIAGNOSIS
- Vascular dementia
- Multi-infarct dementia
- Dementia associated with Parkinson
- Normal pressure hydrocephalus
- Creutzfeldt-Jakob disease
- End-stage multiple sclerosis
- Brain tumor - primary or metastatic
- Subdural hematoma
- Progressive multifocal leukoencephalopathy
- Metabolic dementia (hypothyroidism)
- Drug reactions
- Alcoholism and other addictions
- Dementia pugilistica
- Subcortical dementias
- Depression (persistent diminished interest and pleasure, insomnia or hyposomnia, psychomotor retardation, feelings of hopelessness and helplessness, thoughts of death, decreased ability to concentrate)
- Toxicity from liver or kidney failure
- Vitamin and other nutritional deficiencies
- Vasculitis
- Lewy body disease
- Neurosyphilis

LABORATORY
- To help rule out other causes of dementia:
  - ◊ CBC
  - ◊ Chemistry panel
  - ◊ Thyroid function studies
  - ◊ Folate and B-12 levels
  - ◊ VDRL
  - ◊ Sedimentation rate
  - ◊ HIV antibody (selected cases)

Drugs that may alter lab results: N/A

Disorders that may alter lab results: N/A

PATHOLOGICAL FINDINGS
- Gross - diffuse cerebral atrophy in association areas, hippocampus, amygdala and some subcortical nuclei
- Micro - pyramidal cell loss
- Micro - decreased cholinergic innervation (other neurotransmitters variably decreased)
- Micro - neuritic senile plaques
- Micro - degeneration of locus ceruleus and basal forebrain nuclei of Meynert
- Neurofibrillary tangles
- Amyloid angiopathy common
- Inflammatory cells present

SPECIAL TESTS
- Lumbar puncture (depending on circumstances and clinical information)
- Extensive neuropsychological battery - only needed if clinical picture is confusing
- Controversy exists about need for routine cerebral imaging. MRI or CT clearly needed if cognitive decline is recent, there is history of stroke, or focal neurologic signs are present.

IMAGING
- Head CT/MRI - moderate cortical atrophy, ventricular enlargement - to rule out infarcts, subdural hematomas, normal pressure hydrocephalus, neoplasm
- MRI-based hippocampal volumetry, positron emission tomography (PET) and single photon emission computed tomography (SPECT) have not yet reached clinical reality as tools to distinguish early Alzheimer disease from other dementias but show promise

DIAGNOSTIC PROCEDURES
- This is a clinical diagnosis - history, physical examination, tests (neurological and memory)
- More specific tests (CSF beta-amyloid, tau, AD7C levels; urinary AD7C; serum beta-amyloid precursor protein; excessive pupillary dilatation to mydriatics; 3-item smell test) still investigational
- Testing for E4 allele of apolipoprotein E gene is available (but is not officially recommended) for assessing prognosis of early memory loss or predicting risk of dementia in at-risk individuals or patient's relatives

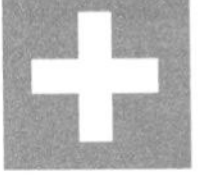

TREATMENT

APPROPRIATE HEALTH CARE Outpatient, day care, assisted living center, nursing home (when necessary)

GENERAL MEASURES
- Supportive
- Optimize treatment of associated co-morbidities
- Exercises to reduce restlessness
- Occupational therapy
- Music therapy
- Continued cognitive challenge - shown to slow deterioration rate
- Analyze environment for safety and security
- Consider day care centers
- Assess needs of spouse/care giver
- Consider nursing home
- Referrals to:
  - ◊ Visiting nurse
  - ◊ Social worker
  - ◊ Physical therapist
  - ◊ Occupational therapist
  - ◊ Lawyer
  - ◊ Support groups for patient and family
  - ◊ Assess driving safety

SURGICAL MEASURES N/A

ACTIVITY To whatever extent possible

DIET No special diet

PATIENT EDUCATION
- Printed patient and family information available from: Alzheimer Association, 919 N. Michigan Ave., Suite 1000, Chicago, IL, (312)335-8700, (800)272-3900
- Help family understand the progressive nature of the disease
- Arrange durable power of attorney
- Advance directives planning as early as possible

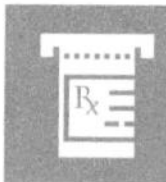

MEDICATIONS

DRUG(S) OF CHOICE

- No specific drug therapy available for halting disease. Clinical studies are ongoing.
- Use as few drugs as possible
- No drugs are helpful for - wandering, restlessness, fidgeting, uncooperativeness, hoarding, irritability. Use behavioral techniques, environmental modification.
- For depression (which occurs in 1/3 of patients), use selective serotonin reuptake inhibitors. Start with half the usual adult dose.
- For insomnia - can try trazodone 25-100 mg qhs, zolpidem (Ambien) 5 mg qhs, zaleplon (Sonata) 5-10 mg qhs, or temazepam (Restoril) 7.5-15 mg qhs
- For moderate anxiety/restlessness - can try low dose, short-acting benzodiazepines or buspirone, but efficacy unproven
- For severe aggressive agitation, especially if psychotic features present (delusions, hallucinations) - risperidone (Risperdal) 0.25 -1.0 mg bid, olanzapine 2.5 mg q day bid, and other newer atypical antipsychotic agents now preferred in this setting due to better side effect profile. Anticholinesterase inhibitors also help behavioral symptoms. Remember to attempt periodic dose reductions or discontinuation, especially in nursing home patient (see OBRA [Omnibus Reconciliation Act] 1987).
- Carbamazepine (Tegretol) 100 mg bid-tid, propranolol (Inderal) 10-40 mg bid-tid, trazodone 200 mg/day and valproic acid 250-1,500 mg/day also may help to reduce severe aggressive agitation. SSRIs also being tried.
- For memory enhancement - donepezil (Aricept) 5-10 mg qd, rivastigmine (Exelon) 3-6 mg bid or galantamine (Reminyl) 8-12 mg bid. Best in mild to moderate disease (Folstein's MMSE scores 10-24), but may also show modest benefit in more severe disease. Rivastigmine found effective in more severe cases and in Lewy body dementia. Only 30-40% of patients will respond - either by modest improvement or minimal decline over 1-2 years. Unlike tacrine, no liver toxicity seen. Most common side effects are gastrointestinal.
- Memantine (Namenda), first of new class of NMDA receptor antagonists, can be used as monotherapy or in combination with acetylcholinesterase inhibitors to enhance or preserve memory. Start 5 mg qd titrating to target dose of 10 mg bid after 4 weeks. Shows efficacy in severe disease (MMSE 5-14).
- A recent study supported modest efficacy of selegiline 5 mg bid and/or vitamin E, 1000 IU bid in slowing progression of disease (vitamin E is cheaper and preferred)

Contraindications:
- Avoid anticholinergic drugs, such as tricyclic antidepressants (TCA) and antihistamines
- Ginkgo biloba - avoid anticoagulants and aspirin

Precautions:
- Benzodiazepines may produce paradoxical excitation or daytime drowsiness
- Triazolam (Halcion) can produce confusion, memory loss and psychotic reactions in the elderly
- Risperidone may be associated with hyperglycemia and ketoacidosis

Significant possible interactions:
- Antipsychotics: lithium may induce extrapyramidal symptoms and disorientation
- Benzodiazepines: increased serum phenytoin concentration. Cimetidine may increase the benzodiazepine concentration.
- Donepezil (Aricept): use with caution with anticholinergic medication or in patients with sick sinus syndrome or a history of peptic ulcers. Avoid paroxetine (Paxil) - causes increased donepezil levels.

ALTERNATIVE DRUGS Randomized trials of ginkgo biloba, 40 mg tid have produced conflicting results. This drug may have modest benefit, but can be associated with prolonged bleeding time.

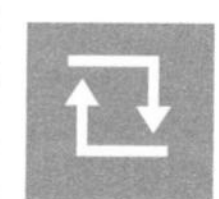

FOLLOWUP

PATIENT MONITORING

- As often as necessary to treat poor nutrition, medical complications, monitor drug use, provide support for family, assess need for placement
- Serial mental status testing potentially helpful, but bedside tests (MMSE) offer wide variability and lack sensitivity.
- Monitor caregiver burnout

Manifesitation of Alzheimer's disease by year:

Problem with:	Onset (yrs)
Cognition	0 - 5
Financial management	1 - 5
Behavior	2 - 12
Self-bathing	4 - 7
Urinary continence	5 - 8
Death†	3 - 8

†6-8 years if diagnosed before age 65

PREVENTION/AVOIDANCE

- NSAIDs and vitamin E show promise in early studies of delaying onset of AD in high risk patients
- Family members may seek genetic screening for presence of E4 allele of apolipoprotein E gene (kits already marketed), but such screening is not recommended

POSSIBLE COMPLICATIONS

- Behavioral - hostility, agitation, wandering, uncooperativeness
- Metabolic - infection, dehydration, drug toxicity, malnutrition
- Others - falls, "sundowning"
- Family or caregiver burnout
- Depression occurs in third of patients
- Suicide - in early stages, especially if depression present

EXPECTED COURSE/PROGNOSIS

Poor; 4-6 year average survival

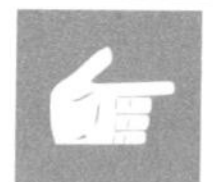

MISCELLANEOUS

ASSOCIATED CONDITIONS

- Down syndrome
- Depression
- Insomnia

AGE-RELATED FACTORS

Pediatric: N/A
Geriatric: A frequent and serious problem
Others: N/A

PREGNANCY N/A

SYNONYMS

- Presenile dementia
- Senile dementia of the Alzheimer type (SDAT)
- Primary degenerative dementia

ICD-9-CM

290.0 Senile dementia, uncomplicated
290.10 Presenile dementia, uncomplicated
331.0 Alzheimer disease

SEE ALSO

Alcohol use disorders
Anemia, pernicious
Creutzfeldt-Jakob disease
Dementia
Depression
Hypothyroidism, adult

OTHER NOTES N/A

ABBREVIATIONS

DAT = dementia of Alzheimer type

REFERENCES

- Tariot PN, Farlow MR, Grossberg GT, et al. Memantine treatment in patients with moderate to severe Alzheimer disease already receiving donepezil: a randomized controlled trial. JAMA 2004;291(3):317-24
- Trinh NH, Hoblyn J, Mohanty S, Yaffe K. Efficacy of cholinesterase inhibitors in the treatment of neuropsychiatric symptoms and functional impairment in Alzheimer disease: a meta-analysis. JAMA 2003;289(2):210-6
- Tariot PN. Medical management of advanced dementia. J Am Geriatr Soc 2003;51(5 Suppl Dementia):S305-13
- Kawas CH. Clinical practice. Early Alzheimer's disease. N Engl J Med 2003;349(11):1056-63
- Alva G, Potkin SG. Alzheimer disease and other dementias. Clin Geriatr Med 2003;19(4):763-76
- Grossberg GT, Desai AK. Management of Alzheimer's disease. J Gerontol A Biol Sci Med Sci 2003;58(4):331-53
- Clark CM, Karlawish JH. Alzheimer disease: current concepts and emerging diagnostic and therapeutic strategies. Ann Intern Med 2003;138(5):400-10
- Cummings JL, Frank JC, Cherry D, et al. Guidelines for managing Alzheimer's disease: Alzheimer's disease: part I. Assessment. Am Fam Physician 2002;65(11):2263-72; Part II. Treatment. Am Fam Physician 2002;65(12):2525-34
- Galasko D, editor. Alzheimer's disease/dementia. Geriatr Clin 2001;May:entire volume
- AMA. Diagnosis, management and treatment of dementia - a practical guide for primary care physicians. Guttman R, Seleski M (eds.), AMA, Chicago, 1999

Web references: 6 available at www.5mcc.com
Illustrations N/A

Author(s):
Frank 'Chip' Celestino, MD

BASICS

DESCRIPTION Amblyopia describes a reduction in visual acuity that cannot be corrected by eyeglasses or contact lenses in the absence of a structural or pathological abnormality of the eye.
System(s) affected: Nervous
Genetics: There is an increased incidence in children where one parent has a history of amblyopia
Incidence/Prevalence in USA: Approximately 2-2.5% in the general population
Predominant age: May be present from birth or may be detected at any age
Predominant sex: Male = Female

SIGNS & SYMPTOMS
- Rubbing the eyes
- Sitting close to TV or computer screen
- Problems in sports
- Preference for front row seating
- Covering or closing an eye
- Squinting eye in bright light
- Eye turns "in" or "out"; wandering eye
- Poor vision in one eye without apparent explanation
- Poor vision that does not correct with glasses

CAUSES
- Strabismic amblyopia is a loss of visual acuity in an individual due to suppression of the images in eye which turns out or in
- Anisometropic amblyopia is present when one eye has a significantly different refractive error than the fellow eye and leads to visual blurring
- Refractive amblyopia is due to uncorrected high refractive error resulting in visual blurring in either or both eyes
- Deprivation amblyopia (amblyopia ex anopsia) is due to relative complete visual deprivation in one eye that can be caused by a congenital abnormality such as a corneal scar or cataract

RISK FACTORS None identified

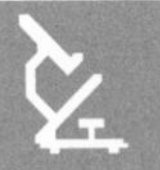

DIAGNOSIS

DIFFERENTIAL DIAGNOSIS The diagnosis of amblyopia can be confused with an organic lesion causing decreased visual acuity and this must always be excluded before the diagnosis of amblyopia is considered

LABORATORY N/A

Drugs that may alter lab results: N/A

Disorders that may alter lab results: N/A

PATHOLOGICAL FINDINGS N/A

SPECIAL TESTS Examination by an ophthalmologist to screen for unequal refractive error, outward turning, or inward turning of the eye (strabismic amblyopia) and proper vision testing of the eye under monocular conditions. A complete slit lamp and dilated funduscopic examination is necessary to exclude an organic cause for the decreased visual acuity.

IMAGING N/A

DIAGNOSTIC PROCEDURES N/A

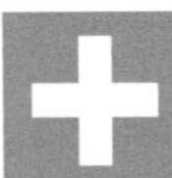

TREATMENT

APPROPRIATE HEALTH CARE All children should have complete visual examinations prior to starting school with each eye tested individually. Those children from families with a known history of amblyopia or strabismus should have special exams by an ophthalmologist.

GENERAL MEASURES
- Correction of the underlying disorder should be instituted at the earliest opportunity
- Full refractive correction and/or patching of the stronger eye to encourage visual development of the amblyopic eye is warranted
- Amblyopia never corrects itself spontaneously and will always require treatment. Children do not outgrow amblyopia.
- Surgical correction of an abnormal eye position may also be required

SURGICAL MEASURES N/A

ACTIVITY No restrictions

DIET No special diet

PATIENT EDUCATION All parents should be made aware of the need to have their children's eyes examined prior to starting school

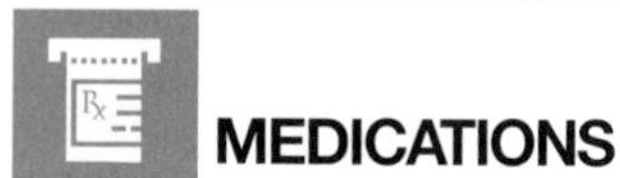

MEDICATIONS

DRUG(S) OF CHOICE N/A
Contraindications: N/A
Precautions: N/A
Significant possible interactions: N/A

ALTERNATIVE DRUGS N/A

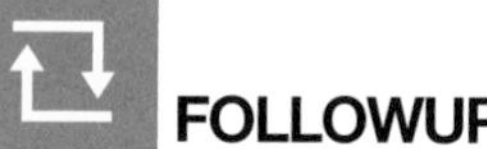

FOLLOWUP

PATIENT MONITORING Once the diagnosis of amblyopia is made, the patient needs to be seen frequently at the discretion of the ophthalmologist until complete resolution of the problem occurs

PREVENTION/AVOIDANCE None

POSSIBLE COMPLICATIONS If there is failure to institute proper therapy early, permanent and profound visual loss can be expected

EXPECTED COURSE/PROGNOSIS
Amblyopia is a treatable condition in most cases if the diagnosis is made early. Patching therapy, eyeglasses, and surgical correction of abnormal eye positions can result in near normalcy of vision when instituted early. Visual development occurs during the first several years of life and amblyopia therapy can be effective until approximately age 12.

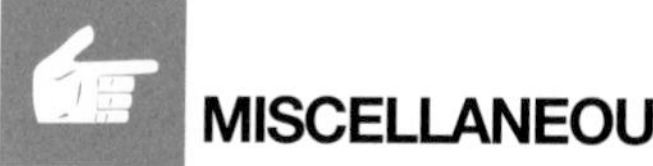

MISCELLANEOUS

ASSOCIATED CONDITIONS Amblyopia is more common in families with a history of unequal refractive errors, high uncorrected refractive errors, and strabismus

AGE-RELATED FACTORS
Pediatric: More commonly seen in the pediatric age group early in life
Geriatric: When seen in the geriatric population, the diagnosis has usually been made early in childhood
Others: N/A

PREGNANCY N/A

SYNONYMS Lazy eye

ICD-9-CM
368.00 Amblyopia, unspecified

SEE ALSO
Refractive errors
Strabismus

OTHER NOTES
- Deficiency amblyopia: Also known as nutritional optic neuropathy or tobacco-alcohol amblyopia. Deficiencies of B1, B12, or riboflavin may be responsible. Treatment consists of balanced diet, vitamins, and avoidance of alcohol and tobacco.

ABBREVIATIONS N/A

REFERENCES

- Binocular Vision And Ocular Motility. In Ophthalmology Basic and Clinical Science Course. (American Academy of Ophthalmology)
- Harley RD: Pediatric Ophthalmology. Philadelphia, W.B. Saunders Co., 1983

Web references: 0 available at www.5mcc.com
Illustrations N/A

Author(s):
Robert M. Kershner, MD

BASICS

DESCRIPTION Amebiasis is caused by the intestinal protozoan, *Entamoeba histolytica*. Infection results from ingestion of fecally contaminated food, such as garden vegetables or by direct fecal-oral transmission. Most persons are asymptomatic or have minimal diarrheal symptoms. In a few patients, invasive intestinal or extraintestinal (e.g., liver, and less commonly kidney, bladder, male or female genitalia, skin, lung, brain) infection results. Amebic abscess of the liver may develop during the acute attack or 1-3 months later; symptoms may be abrupt or insidious. Entamoeba histolytica has been divided into "pathogenic" and "nonpathogenic" strains. The pathogenic strains commonly cause invasive infection while the noninvasive strains cause only asymptomatic intestinal infection. More recently, the nonpathogenic strains have been assigned to a separate species, E. dispar. Unfortunately, the species cannot be distinguished in a routine clinical laboratory.
System(s) affected: Gastrointestinal, Nervous, Renal/Urologic, Reproductive, Skin/Exocrine
Genetics: N/A
Incidence/Prevalence in USA: Probably <1% overall, but much higher in some risk groups, such as areas with large immigrant populations
Predominant age: All
Predominant sex: Male > Female; probably because of greater occupational exposure

SIGNS & SYMPTOMS
- Noninvasive infection (up to 99%)
  - ◊ Asymptomatic (90%)
  - ◊ Mild diarrhea
  - ◊ Abdominal discomfort
- Invasive intestinal infection
  - ◊ Abdominal pain and tenderness
  - ◊ Rectal pain
  - ◊ Diarrhea
  - ◊ Bloody stools
  - ◊ Fever (30%)
  - ◊ Systemic toxicity
- Extraintestinal infection
  - ◊ Fever
  - ◊ Systemic toxicity
  - ◊ RUQ abdominal pain and tenderness
  - ◊ Nausea and vomiting
  - ◊ Diarrhea (50%)
  - ◊ Hematuria, dysuria, urinary frequency and urgency

CAUSES Infection with *Entamoeba histolytica* is transmitted through contaminated food or water, or through person-to-person contact

RISK FACTORS
- Low socioeconomic status
- Institutional living
- Male homosexuality
- Invasive disease is more common in certain geographic locations, including some parts of Mexico, South Africa, and India

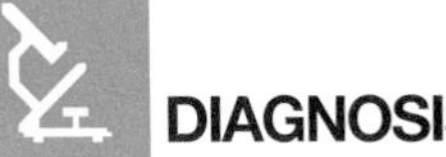

DIAGNOSIS

DIFFERENTIAL DIAGNOSIS
- Other infectious causes of colitis, including shigellosis, Campylobacter infection, pseudomembranous colitis, and occasionally salmonellosis or Yersinia infection
- Noninfectious causes of colitis include ulcerative colitis, Crohn colitis and ischemic colitis
- Hepatic amebiasis must be distinguished from pyogenic liver abscess or superinfection of amebic abscess

LABORATORY
- Stool for ova and parasites (unfortunately, the sensitivity of this exam is poor). Diarrheal stool should be examined immediately for trophozoites in addition to fixed stool specimens (repeated as necessary). In invasive intestinal infection, stools are bloody, but fecal leukocytes are usually absent.
- Serologic tests (especially indirect hemagglutination (IHA), positive in 85% of colitis patients and most patients with extraintestinal disease. Serologic tests should be done in patients with idiopathic inflammatory bowel disease to rule out amebiasis.
- In bladder infections - amoebae and/or cysts in urine
- Liver enzymes and alkaline phosphatase may be elevated in hepatic disease

Drugs that may alter lab results: Many drugs interfere with stool exams

Disorders that may alter lab results: N/A

PATHOLOGICAL FINDINGS
- Colon biopsy
  - ◊ Lysis of mucosal cells (flask ulcers)
  - ◊ PAS-stained trophozoites
  - ◊ Neutrophils at the periphery
- Liver biopsy
  - ◊ Necrosis surrounded by a rim of trophozoites
- Liver aspirate - red-brown material (anchovy paste)

SPECIAL TESTS N/A

IMAGING CT scan or ultrasound for hepatic infection

DIAGNOSTIC PROCEDURES
- Rectosigmoidoscopy with biopsy
- Needle aspirate of hepatic lesions may be needed to rule out pyogenic infection or superinfection

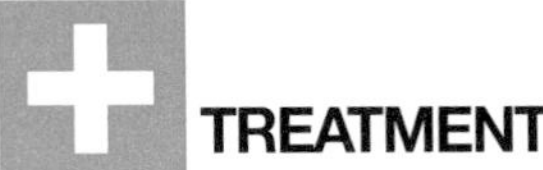

TREATMENT

APPROPRIATE HEALTH CARE Outpatient

GENERAL MEASURES
- Fluids and nutrition
- Electrolyte management

SURGICAL MEASURES With severe amebic colitis, surgery may be necessary

ACTIVITY In accordance with illness of patient

DIET As tolerated

PATIENT EDUCATION Avoid conditions of re-exposure

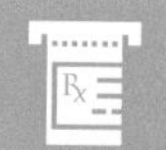

MEDICATIONS

DRUG(S) OF CHOICE
- Noninvasive infection
  - ◊ Diiodohydroxyquin [also called iodoquinol] 650 mg tid for 20 days
- Invasive infection
  - ◊ Metronidazole (Flagyl) 750 mg tid for 5-10 days, followed by a 20 day course of diiodohydroxyquin to eliminate intestinal carriage

Contraindications:
- Diiodohydroxyquin - use cautiously in patients with thyroid diseases. Contraindicated in hepatic or renal dysfunction. May cause optic neuritis or peripheral neuropathy.
- Known allergy to given medication

Precautions: None of the agents are proven safe in pregnancy, but pregnant women with invasive disease should still be treated

Significant possible interactions:
- Metronidazole-ethanol: disulfiram reaction

ALTERNATIVE DRUGS
- Noninvasive infection
  - ◊ Diloxanide 500 mg tid for 10 days
  - ◊ Paromomycin 500 mg tid for 10 days
- Invasive infection
  - ◊ Dehydroemetine (as effective as metronidazole, but cardiotoxic) 1-1.5 mg/kg/day IM for 5 days
  - ◊ Chloroquine (less effective) 600 mg base/day for 2 days, then 200 mg/day for 2-3 weeks. Children 10 mg/kg/day up to maximum of 300 mg/day.
  - ◊ Tinidazole 600-800 mg tid for 5 days (not available in US)

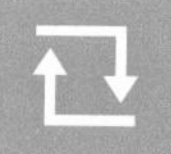

FOLLOWUP

PATIENT MONITORING Patient signs and symptoms, stool for ova and parasite

PREVENTION/AVOIDANCE Avoid risk factors when possible

POSSIBLE COMPLICATIONS
- Toxic megacolon with rupture
- Rupture of hepatic abscess which may perforate into subphrenic space, right pleural cavity or other nearby organs
- Bladder perforation, urethral strictures, vesicointestinal fistula

EXPECTED COURSE/PROGNOSIS
Untreated invasive amebiasis is frequently fatal. With treatment, improvement usually occurs within a few days. Some patients with amebic colitis have irritable bowel symptoms for weeks after successful treatment. Relapses possible.

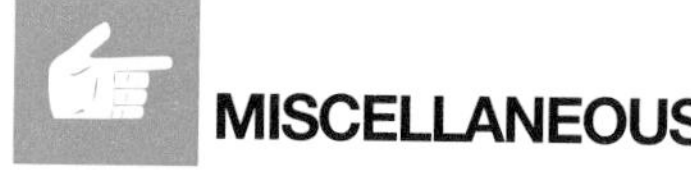

MISCELLANEOUS

ASSOCIATED CONDITIONS N/A

AGE-RELATED FACTORS
Pediatric: More severe in neonates
Geriatric: More severe in elderly
Others: More severe in patients on corticosteroids and other immunocompromised patients

PREGNANCY More severe in pregnancy. Most agents are avoided in pregnancy (especially first trimester) because of concerns of teratogenicity, but invasive disease must still be treated. Paromomycin is sometimes recommended for noninvasive disease because it is not absorbed. Infectious disease consultation should be obtained.

SYNONYMS
- Amebic colitis
- Amebic dysentery

ICD-9-CM
006.0 Acute amebic dysentery without mention of abscess
006.3 Amebic liver abscess
006.4 Amebic lung abscess
006.5 Amebic brain abscess
006.6 Amebic skin ulceration
006.8 Amebic infection of other sites
006.9 Amebiasis, unspecified

SEE ALSO
Diarrhea, acute
Diarrhea, chronic

OTHER NOTES N/A

ABBREVIATIONS N/A

REFERENCES

- Petri WA Jr, Singh U. Diagnosis and management of amebiasis. Clinical Infect Dis 1999;29:1117-25
- Bruckner DA. Amebiasis. Clin Microbiol Rev 1992;5:356-369
- Ravdin JI. <I>Entamoeba histolytica</I> (amebiasis). In: Mandell GL, Bennett JE, Dolin R, eds. Principles and Practice of Infectious Diseases. 5th Ed. New York, Churchill Livingstone, 2000

Web references: 0 available at www.5mcc.com
Illustrations N/A

Author(s):
Rodney D. Adam, MD

BASICS

DESCRIPTION The absence of menses.

- Primary amenorrhea - no menses by age 14 with absence of secondary sexual characteristics, or no menses by age 16 with normal secondary characteristics
- Secondary amenorrhea - the cessation of menses for three cycles or 6 months of amenorrhea

System(s) affected: Endocrine/Metabolic, Reproductive

Genetics: No known genetic pattern

Incidence/Prevalence in USA:

- Incidence of primary amenorrhea 0.3%
- Incidence of secondary amenorrhea 3.3%

Predominant age: Menarche to menopause

Predominant sex: Female only

SIGNS & SYMPTOMS

- The absence of periods
- Galactorrhea
- Symptoms of hypothyroidism
- Symptoms of early pregnancy
- Signs of androgen excess
- Signs of estrogen deficiency

CAUSES

- Primary amenorrhea
  - ◊ Imperforate hymen
  - ◊ Agenesis of the uterus and upper 2/3 of the vagina (Müllerian agenesis)
  - ◊ Turner syndrome
  - ◊ Constitutional delay
- Secondary amenorrhea
  - ◊ Physiological - pregnancy, corpus luteal cyst, breast-feeding, menopause
  - ◊ Suppression of the hypothalamic-pituitary axis - post pill amenorrhea, stress, intercurrent illness, weight loss, low body mass index
  - ◊ Pituitary disease - ablation of the pituitary gland, Sheehan syndrome, prolactinoma
  - ◊ Uncontrolled endocrinopathies - diabetes, hypo- or hyperthyroidism
  - ◊ Polycystic ovarian disease (PCOD), (Stein-Leventhal syndrome)
  - ◊ Chemotherapy
  - ◊ Pelvic irradiation
  - ◊ Endometrial ablation (inducing Asherman syndrome)
  - ◊ Drug therapy - systemic steroids, danazol, GRH-RH analogs, antipsychotics, OCP's
  - ◊ Premature ovarian failure

RISK FACTORS

- Over-training (e.g., long-distance runner, ballet dancer)
- Eating disorders
- Psycho-social crisis

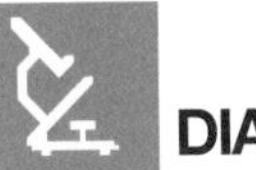

DIAGNOSIS

DIFFERENTIAL DIAGNOSIS Includes all of the causes listed above. The most common cause of secondary amenorrhea is early pregnancy.

LABORATORY

- Pregnancy test if negative, obtain:
  - ◊ Serum prolactin
  - ◊ FSH
  - ◊ TSH
  - ◊ Blood sugar

Drugs that may alter lab results: N/A

Disorders that may alter lab results: Pregnancy, menopause, hyperprolactinemia, ovarian suppression, endocrinopathy

PATHOLOGICAL FINDINGS Due to underlying disease

SPECIAL TESTS

- Progesterone challenge test - 10 mg of medroxyprogesterone acetate orally for 5 days
  - ◊ If withdrawal bleeding occurs, amenorrhea most likely due to chronic anovulation with estrogen (PCOD)
  - ◊ If no bleeding, evaluate estrogen status with FSH
    - FSH high: ovarian failure
    - FSH low or normal: give cyclic estrogen and progesterone and if menses start diagnose chronic anovulation, estrogen absent (functional hypothalamic amenorrhea) or if menses don't start diagnose Mullerian agenesis
- Prolactin elevated
  - ◊ Suspect prolactinoma, proceed with imaging the sella turcica

IMAGING

- Ultrasound may show cysts undetectable on pelvic examination
- Radiologic evaluation of the sella turcica if
  - ◊ prolactinoma suspected (elevated serum prolactin) OR
  - ◊ functional hypothalamic amenorrhea suspected since adenomas can occur even with normal prolactin levels

DIAGNOSTIC PROCEDURES

- Laparoscopy - diagnosis of the streak ovaries of Turner syndrome, or polycystic ovarian disease (not often done)
- Hysterosalpingogram - to rule out Asherman syndrome if appropriate clinical situation

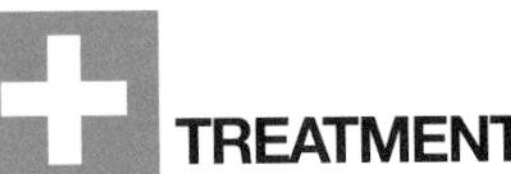

TREATMENT

APPROPRIATE HEALTH CARE Outpatient

GENERAL MEASURES Definitive treatment depends on determining the cause of the amenorrhea. May not be necessary to treat all cases especially if just temporary amenorrhea.

SURGICAL MEASURES

- Hymenectomy, done as a day surgery, will be required for those whose primary amenorrhea is due to imperforate hymen
- Lysis adhesions in Asherman syndrome

ACTIVITY No restrictions

DIET Correct overweight or underweight by dietary management

PATIENT EDUCATION

- Consists of fully informing the patient of your findings, including the presence or absence of pregnancy, and of the underlying cause
- Specific educational resources can be utilized as necessary, e.g., prenatal classes, menopause support groups
- Specific information should be given about the expected duration of amenorrhea (temporary or permanent), effect on fertility, and the long-term sequelae of untreated amenorrhea (e.g., osteoporosis, vaginal dryness)
- Appropriate contraceptive advice should be given, as fertility returns before menses
- Additional support may be needed if the amenorrhea is associated with a reduction in, or loss of, fertility
- Society for Menstrual Cycle Research, 10559 N. 104th Place, Scottsdale, AZ 85258, (602)451-9731

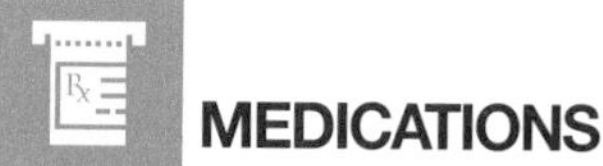

MEDICATIONS

DRUG(S) OF CHOICE

- Progesterone replacement - medroxyprogesterone (Provera) 5 mg bid for 5 days, will result in a withdrawal bleed if the hypothalamopituitary-ovarian axis is intact and there is some endogenous estrogen production
- Estrogen replacement - conjugated estrogen, conjugated (Premarin) 0.625 mg for 25 days with progesterone added as above for the last 10 days will result in a withdrawal bleed if the uterus and lower genital tract are normal
- Use of hormonal therapies will not correct underlying problem. Other drugs might be required to treat specific conditions, e.g., bromocriptine for hyperprolactinemia.
- Use of hormonal replacement therapy is recommended after 6 months of amenorrhea (regardless of the primary cause) in order to reduce the risks of osteoporosis and hypercholesterolemia secondary to hypoestrogenism
- Calcium supplementation 1500 mg/day if cause is hypoestrogenism
- Oral contraceptive pills or patches replace estrogen and prevent pregnancy and are probably first line drugs unless contraindicated

Contraindications:

- Pregnancy
- Thromboembolic disease
- Previous myocardial infarct, cerebrovascular accident
- Estrogen-dependent malignancy
- Severe hepatic impairment or disease

Precautions:

- Diabetes
- Seizure disorder
- Migraine headache
- Smoker over 35

Significant possible interactions: Barbiturates, phenytoin, rifampin, corticosteroids, theophyllines, tricyclics, oral anticoagulants (anticoagulant effect may be decreased)

ALTERNATIVE DRUGS Use of oral contraceptives for hormonal replacement if patient has difficulty following above regimen

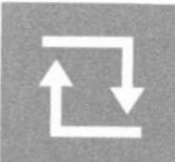

FOLLOWUP

PATIENT MONITORING Depends on the cause, and the treatment chosen. If hormonal replacement is used, discontinuation after six months is advised, to assess spontaneous resumption of menses.

PREVENTION/AVOIDANCE Maintenance of proper body mass index (BMI)

POSSIBLE COMPLICATIONS

- Estrogen deficiency symptoms, e.g., hot flushes, vaginal dryness
- Osteoporosis, in prolonged hypoestrogenic amenorrhea
- Increased risk of endometrial cancer in hyperestrogenism without progestin

EXPECTED COURSE/PROGNOSIS Reflects the underlying cause. In secondary amenorrhea from hypothalamopituitary suppression, spontaneous resumption of menses with time (99% within 6 months) and correction of body mass index.

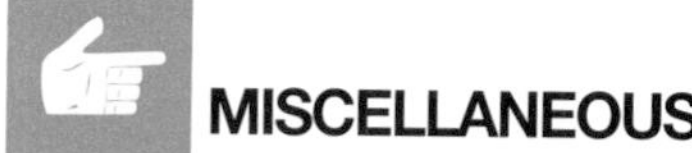

MISCELLANEOUS

ASSOCIATED CONDITIONS N/A

AGE-RELATED FACTORS

Pediatric: Primary amenorrhea commonly diagnosed in this group
Geriatric: N/A
Others: N/A

PREGNANCY One of the primary causes

SYNONYMS N/A

ICD-9-CM

626.0 Absence of menstruation

SEE ALSO

Diabetes mellitus, Type 1
Diabetes mellitus, Type 2
Hyperthyroidism
Hypothyroidism, adult
Osteoporosis
Polycystic ovarian disease

OTHER NOTES

- Use of hormonal replacement therapy is symptomatic and is discretionary if amenorrhea is temporary (e.g., hypothalamopituitary suppression)
- Patients who are amenorrheic and wish to become pregnant should not be given hormone replacement therapy, but should receive treatment for infertility based on specific cause
- Women less than age 30 with ovarian failure should have karyotype analysis

ABBREVIATIONS

PCOD = polycystic ovarian disease

REFERENCES

- Yen SSC, Jaffe RB, eds. Reproductive Endocrinology. 4th ed. Philadelphia: W.B. Saunders Co; 1999
- Speroff L, Glass R, Kase N, eds. Clinical Gynecology, Endocrinology and Infertility. 6th Ed. Baltimore: Williams & Wilkins; 1999
- Kiningham R, Apgar B, Schwenk T. Evaluation of amenorrhea. Am Fam Physician 1996;53:1185-94

Web references: 0 available at www.5mcc.com
Illustrations N/A

Author(s):

Kathryn Reilly, MD, MPH

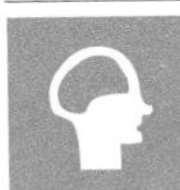

BASICS

DESCRIPTION A group of diseases characterized by increased deposition of amyloid fibrils in the tissues. Several different proteins may give rise to amyloid. These proteins are present due to their overproduction or decreased clearance. Their deposition may lead to compromise of vital organ function. Specific amyloid proteins aggregate mostly in specific organs. The most common types of amyloidosis are:
- Primary amyloidosis: usually associated with the plasma cell disorders multiple myeloma and MGUS (monoclonal gammopathy of undetermined significance)
- Secondary amyloidosis: associated with several chronic inflammatory diseases such as rheumatoid arthritis, osteomyelitis, malaria, tuberculosis, leprosy and familial Mediterranean fever
- Familial (hereditary) amyloidosis: may occur in almost every ethnic group
- Hemodialysis amyloidosis: associated with renal hemodialysis
- Localized amyloidosis: associated with Alzheimer disease

System(s) affected: Cardiovascular, Endocrine/Metabolic, Gastrointestinal, Musculoskeletal, Nervous, Pulmonary, Renal/Urologic, Skin/Exocrine

Genetics: Only hereditary amyloidosis can be inherited. The genetics are variable but usually autosomal dominant.

Incidence/Prevalence in USA:
- Primary amyloidosis: 1 per 100,000 person years
- Secondary amyloidosis: very rare
- Familial amyloidosis: 1 per million person years

Predominant age: 60-70

Predominant sex: Male > Female (2:1)

SIGNS & SYMPTOMS

May be highly variable depending upon which organ system is affected and to what degree:
- Fatigue, weight loss, gastroparesis, pseudo-obstruction, malabsorption, diarrhea, macroglossia
- Peripheral neuropathy, carpal tunnel syndrome
- Ascites, hepatomegaly
- Dyspnea, interstitial lung disease, congestive heart failure, arrhythmia, angina pectoris, sudden death
- Hilar adenopathy, mediastinal adenopathy
- Symmetrical polyarthritis, rubbery periarticular soft tissue swelling
- Translucent/waxy skin papules, purpura (especially periorbital purpura), edema
- Renal failure, nephrotic syndrome
- Dementia (may play a role in development of Alzheimer disease)

CAUSES

- Substitution of a single amino acid transforms proteins to become amyloidogenic
- Primary amyloidosis: The amyloid consists of immunoglobulin light chains (AL) which are overproduced in plasma cell disorders
- Secondary amyloidosis: The amyloid consists of amyloid fibrillary protein (AA) formed from serum amyloid protein (SAA), which is overproduced in chronic inflammatory conditions
- Familial (hereditary) amyloidosis: The amyloid consists of abnormal transthyretin protein (ATTR) or lysozyme protein (ALys) produced in the liver
- Hemodialysis amyloidosis: The amyloid consists of beta-2-microglobulin which is normally cleared by the kidney, but cannot be cleared by hemodialysis
- Localized amyloidosis: associated with hormonal proteins or aging such as beta amyloid proteins in Alzheimer disease and other neurodegenerative diseases

RISK FACTORS

- Underlying plasma cell dyscrasia
- Underlying chronic inflammatory disease
- Familial Mediterranean fever
- Hemodialysis

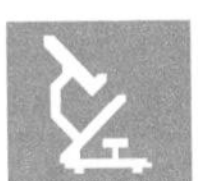

DIAGNOSIS

DIFFERENTIAL DIAGNOSIS

- Peripheral neuropathy - diabetes mellitus, alcoholism, vitamin deficiencies
- Carpal tunnel syndrome - hypothyroidism, trauma, rheumatoid arthritis, etc.
- Restrictive cardiomyopathy: acute viral myocarditis, endomyocardial fibrosis, sarcoidosis, hemochromatosis
- Nephrotic syndrome - glomerulonephritis, renal vein thrombosis
- Renal failure - glomerulonephritis, obstructive uropathy, toxin or drug-induced, acute tubular necrosis
- Symmetric polyarthritis - rheumatoid arthritis, psoriatic arthritis, SLE
- Interstitial lung disease - connective tissue diseases, infectious, sarcoidosis, drug-induced, pneumoconiosis
- Demential - Alzheimer disease and multi-infarct dementia

LABORATORY

- Anemia may be present
- Hypothyroidism may be present due to amyloidosis of the thyroid
- Renal insufficiency present in ≈50%
- Proteinuria present in almost 80%
- In primary amyloidosis, an elevated monoclonal protein level will be found in the serum and/or urine
- In secondary amyloidosis, tests to assess the underlying inflammatory disease will be useful. In familial amyloidosis, an abnormal transthyretin protein may be isolated.

Drugs that may alter lab results: N/A

Disorders that may alter lab results: N/A

PATHOLOGICAL FINDINGS

- Demonstration of amyloid deposits in tissues
- With Congo red staining, amyloid produces a green birefringence under polarized light
- Electron microscopy is the definitive diagnostic tool

SPECIAL TESTS Specialized screening for mutant transthyretin

IMAGING Echocardiography (if cardiac involvement is suspected)

DIAGNOSTIC PROCEDURES

- Rectal biopsy (70% positive)
- Bone marrow biopsy (20% positive)
- Abdominal fat pad biopsy (up to 85% positive)
- Endomyocardial biopsy
- Renal biopsy

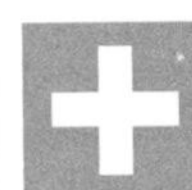

TREATMENT

APPROPRIATE HEALTH CARE Outpatient except for serious complications (congestive heart failure, renal failure)

GENERAL MEASURES Change from hemodialysis to peritoneal dialysis, which clears beta-2-microglobulin, in those with hemodialysis amyloidosis

SURGICAL MEASURES

- Splenectomy may ameliorate this condition by decreasing the amount of amyloid produced
- Renal transplantation may improve the status of renal amyloidosis
- Liver transplantation or partial liver transplantation may cure familial (hereditary) amyloidosis
- Other measures: Treatment of multiple myeloma with bone marrow transplantation is an option for some patients
- Pacemaker may be indicated in those with amyloid-induced conduction defects

ACTIVITY

- Fully active as tolerated
- Fatigue and shortness of breath may limit activity

DIET

- Low protein, low salt for renal failure patients
- Low salt for congestive heart failure patients

PATIENT EDUCATION

- For more information:
  - ◊ National Organization for Rare Disorders (NORD), Box 8923, New Fairfield, CT 06812
  - ◊ National Institute of Diabetes, Digestive and Kidney Disorders Information Clearinghouse, Bldg 31, Rm 9A04, Bethesda, MD 20892
  - ◊ Amyloid Treatment and Research Program, Boston University School of Medicine. 715 Albany St., EB33, Boston, MA 02118
- For genetic information and counseling referrals:
  - ◊ March of Dimes Birth Defects Foundation, 1275 Mamaroneck Ave., White Plains, NY 10605
  - ◊ National Center for Education in Maternal and Child Health

MEDICATIONS

DRUG(S) OF CHOICE
- Primary amyloidosis
  - ◊ Treatment of the underlying plasma cell disorder may or may not affect the outcome
  - ◊ Melphalan and prednisone are among the drugs of choice for plasma cell disorders. Thalidomide is also effective. The role of Colchicine is now considered less important; although it may slow amyloid deposition.
- Secondary amyloidosis
  - ◊ Treatment of the underlying inflammatory process with disease-specific medications usually improves the outcome (i.e., isoniazid and rifampin for M. Tuberculosis, methotrexate for rheumatoid arthritis)
  - ◊ Donepezil, galantamine and memantine have been approved for mild to moderate dementia caused by Alzheimer disease
  - ◊ Colchicine, 0.6 mg two or three times a day may improve familial Mediterranean fever
- Familial amyloidosis
  - ◊ None
- Hemodialysis amyloidosis
  - ◊ None

Contraindications: Refer to manufacturer's literature

Precautions:
- Melphalan - bone marrow depression, including agranulocytosis, pancytopenia, thrombocytopenia, or aplastic anemia, may occur with prolonged administration. Monitor CBC periodically. Counsel patient to report symptoms/signs of infection promptly (headache, sore throat, fever).
- Thalidomide - severe birth defects
- Colchicine - nausea and diarrhea

Significant possible interactions: Refer to manufacturer's literature

ALTERNATIVE DRUGS N/A

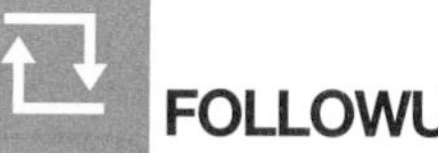

FOLLOWUP

PATIENT MONITORING
- Primary amyloidosis
  - ◊ Regular testing of monoclonal protein levels to assess response to therapy
  - ◊ Regular testing of renal function to assess response to therapy
- Secondary and hemodialysis amyloidosis
  - ◊ Follow-up to assess control of the underlying disease process
  - ◊ Regular testing of renal function to assess degree of impairment

PREVENTION/AVOIDANCE Unknown

POSSIBLE COMPLICATIONS Despite intervention, worsening renal failure, heart failure, arthropathy, interstitial lung disease, and neuropathy are common

EXPECTED COURSE/PROGNOSIS
- Primary amyloidosis
  - ◊ The prognosis is dependent upon the underlying disease
  - ◊ Once renal failure has developed, the prognosis is usually less than one year
  - ◊ Congestive heart failure has a four month prognosis
  - ◊ Overall prognosis is poor; reported survival rates are 51% at 1 year and 16% at 5 years
- Secondary amyloidosis
  - ◊ The prognosis is much better, depending upon the ability to control the underlying inflammatory process
- Familial and hemodialysis amyloidosis
  - ◊ Highly variable
  - ◊ Liver transplant may be curative, but is linked to duration and severity of pre-transplant illness
  - ◊ Deposition of amyloid in the heart may continue even after successful transplantation

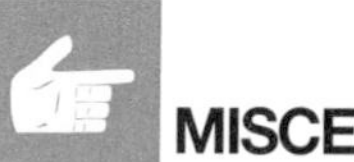

MISCELLANEOUS

ASSOCIATED CONDITIONS
- Amyloid may bind Factor X leading to bleeding problems

AGE-RELATED FACTORS
Pediatric: Not reported
Geriatric: In general, older individuals do less well. Age may precipitate familial amyloidosis suggesting an age-related trigger.
Others: N/A

PREGNANCY No information available

SYNONYMS N/A

ICD-9-CM
277.3 Amyloidosis

SEE ALSO
Multiple myeloma

OTHER NOTES N/A

ABBREVIATIONS N/A

REFERENCES

- Dember L, et al. Effect of dose-intensive melphalan and autologous blood stem-cell transplantation on AL amyloidosis-associated renal disease. Ann Int Med 2001;134(9):746-53
- Kyle RA, et al. Primary Systemic Amyloidosis: multivariate analysis for prognostic factors in 168 cases. Blood 1986;68(1):220-4
- Cohen AS, et al. Survival of patients with primary (AL) amyloidosis. Colchicine-treated cases from 1976-1983 compared with cases seen in previous years (1961-1973). Am J Med 1987;82(6):1182-90
- Fiter J, et al. Methotrexate treatment of amyloidosis secondary to rheumatoid arthritis. Clin Rev of Spain 1995;195(6):390-392
- Falk RH, et al. The systemic amyloidosis. NEJM 1997;337(13):898-909
- Skinner M. Amyloidosis. In: Kelley WN, Harris ED, et al, editors. The Textbook of Rheumatology. Philadelphia, WB Saunders, 1996. p.1409-17
- Kyle RA, Gertz MA, Greipp PR, et al. Long-term survival (10 years or more) in 30 patients with primary amyloidosis. Blood 1999;93(3):1062-6
- Merlini G, Bellotti V. Molecular mechanisms of amyloidosis. NEJM 2003;349(6):583-596

Web references: 2 available at www.5mcc.com
Illustrations 1 available

Author(s):
R. Scott Gorman, MD

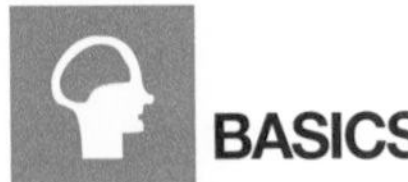

BASICS

DESCRIPTION A degenerative disease (or group of diseases) which affects the upper and lower motor neurons.

- Amyotrophic lateral sclerosis: the term applied to the sporadic and most common form of the disease. Includes a number of overlapping syndromes such as pseudobulbar palsy, progressive bulbar palsy, progressive muscular atrophy and primary lateral sclerosis.
- Familial ALS: an autosomal dominant or recessive disease which is clinically similar to sporadic ALS but probably represents a distinct entity pathologically and biochemically.
- ALS-Parkinson-dementia complex of Guam: an ALS like syndrome, often, but not always, associated with Parkinson syndrome and dementia, which is prevalent amongst the Chamorro Indians of Guam (very rare in the USA).

System(s) affected: Nervous
Genetics: Familial ALS
Incidence/Prevalence in USA: 0.4-2.0/100,000 incidence; 5.0-8.0/100,000 prevalence
Predominant age: Uncommon before age 40
Predominant sex: Male > Female

SIGNS & SYMPTOMS

- Variable combinations of:
  - ◊ Unexplained weight loss
  - ◊ Focal wasting of muscle groups
  - ◊ Limb weakness with variable symmetry and distribution
  - ◊ Difficulty walking
  - ◊ Difficulty swallowing
  - ◊ Slurring of speech
  - ◊ Inability to control affect
  - ◊ Atrophy of muscle groups, initially in a myotomal distribution
  - ◊ Fasciculations (other than calves)
  - ◊ Hyperactive deep tendon reflexes (including jaw jerk)
  - ◊ Spares cognitive, oculomotor, sensory and autonomic functions

CAUSES

- Sporadic ALS - degeneration of the upper and lower motor neurons with their respective axons. Cause is unknown, but elevated levels of glutamate have been found in serum and CSF. High levels of glutamate are toxic. 90-95% of cases of ALS are sporadic.
- Familial ALS - a genetically transmitted degenerative disease. Gene locus has been localized to the long arm of chromosome 21 and encodes the enzyme superoxide dismutase (SOD1) in 20% of familial ALS cases. 5-10% of cases of ALS are familial.
- ALS-Parkinson-dementia complex of Guam - possible relationship to ingestion of the cycad nut or to some other environmental toxin

RISK FACTORS

- Age over 40
- Family history of ALS

DIAGNOSIS

DIFFERENTIAL DIAGNOSIS

- Focal motor neuropathy
- Cervical spondylosis
- Lead intoxication
- Spinal muscular atrophy (adult form)
- Primary lateral sclerosis
- Familial spastic paraparesis
- Spinal multiple sclerosis
- Tropical spastic paraparesis

LABORATORY

- Elevated levels of glutamate in CSF and serum
- Anti-GM1 autoantibodies in low titer commonly found (of unclear significance)
- Possibly reduced levels of nerve growth factor
- There is no simple reliable laboratory test available that confirms the diagnosis of ALS

Drugs that may alter lab results: N/A

Disorders that may alter lab results: N/A

PATHOLOGICAL FINDINGS

- Loss of Betz's cells in the motor cortex
- Atrophic or absent anterior horn cells of spinal cord
- Atrophic or absent neurons within the motor nuclei of the medulla and pons
- Degeneration of the lateral columns of the spinal cord
- Atrophy of the ventral roots
- Grouped atrophy of muscle (motor units)

SPECIAL TESTS N/A

IMAGING N/A

DIAGNOSTIC PROCEDURES

- Electromyography: denervation potentials (fibrillations, positive sharp waves) and often doublets are associated with prominent fasciculations (which suggest anterior horn cell dysfunction). Voluntary motor unit potentials have increased amplitude, long duration and/or polyphasic pattern. The recruitment pattern is reduced for the force generated and individual motor units have a high rate of discharge.
- Muscle biopsy - will show groups of shrunken angulated muscle fibers (grouped atrophy) amid other groups of fibers with a uniform fiber type (fiber type grouping).

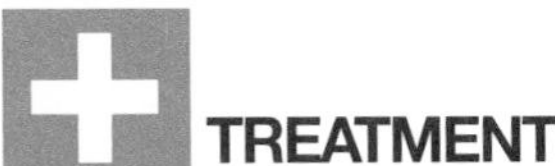

TREATMENT

APPROPRIATE HEALTH CARE

- Outpatient initially, may ultimately need nursing home placement and/or hospice
- Supportive care for complicating emergencies (aspiration, respiratory failure). Use of a respirator is a major ethical dilemma. Consideration should be given to those with selective respiratory dysfunction.

GENERAL MEASURES Prosthetic devices, e.g., wheelchair, etc.

SURGICAL MEASURES N/A

ACTIVITY As tolerated

DIET Modify as tolerated. May need tube feedings.

PATIENT EDUCATION

- Printed material for patients (and reference lists for physicians) available from the Muscular Dystrophy Association, (520)529-2000, (800)572-1717; www.mdausa.org
- The ALS Association - (800)782-4747; www.alsa.org
- Families of spinal muscular atrophy - www.fsma.org

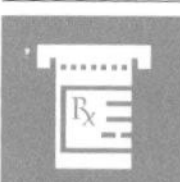

MEDICATIONS

DRUG(S) OF CHOICE Riluzole produces a slight prolongation in life expectancy by decreasing the release of glutamate
Contraindications: N/A
Precautions: N/A
Significant possible interactions: N/A

ALTERNATIVE DRUGS Therapeutic trials of the efficacy of antioxidants (vitamins E, C, and beta-carotene), nerve growth factor, gabapentin, myotrophin and thyrotropin releasing hormone have been undertaken. Reports are not encouraging.

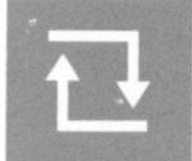

FOLLOWUP

PATIENT MONITORING
- Initially every three months, frequency to be increased as need for symptomatic therapy develops
- Patients with a presumed diagnosis of ALS should have imaging of the cervical spine and electrodiagnostic studies

PREVENTION/AVOIDANCE N/A

POSSIBLE COMPLICATIONS
- Aspiration pneumonia
- Decubitus ulcers
- Pulmonary embolism
- Nutritional deficiency

EXPECTED COURSE/PROGNOSIS
- ALS usually terminates in death within five years
- Patients predominantly manifesting progressive muscular atrophy have a better prognosis
- There have been reports of spontaneous arrest of the disease

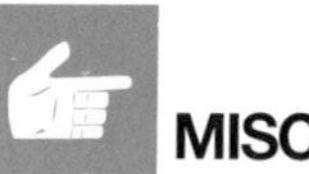

MISCELLANEOUS

ASSOCIATED CONDITIONS None

AGE-RELATED FACTORS
Pediatric: Infantile and juvenile spinal muscular atrophies are conditions which are distinct from amyotrophic lateral sclerosis clinically and pathologically
Geriatric: Symptoms of ALS may inappropriately be attributed to age
Others: N/A

PREGNANCY Pregnancy is uncommon among affected individuals. Pregnancy would be unwise in any individual suffering from a disease with so poor a prognosis. If pregnancy did occur, the only foreseeable difficulties would be related to weakness.

SYNONYMS
- Motor neuron disease
- Lou Gehrig disease
- ALS

ICD-9-CM
335.29 Motor neuron disease, other
335.20 Amyotrophic lateral sclerosis

SEE ALSO

OTHER NOTES Also referred to as Mill's variant (unilateral involvement)

ABBREVIATIONS N/A

REFERENCES

- Rowland LD, ed. Merritt's Textbook of Neurology. 9th ed. Philadelphia: Williams & Wilkins; 1995
- Brown WF, Botton CF. Clinical Electromyography. 2nd ed. Boston, Butterworth-Heinemann; 1993

Web references: 2 available at www.5mcc.com
Illustrations N/A

Author(s):
Colin R. Bamford, MD

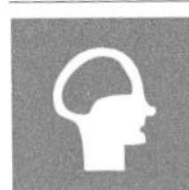

BASICS

DESCRIPTION Gangrene is local death of soft tissues due to disease or injury and is associated with loss of blood supply. Anaerobic and necrotizing infections may be associated with gas.
System(s) affected: Cardiovascular, Skin/Exocrine
Genetics: N/A
Incidence/Prevalence in USA: Rare
Predominant age: Any
Predominant sex: Male = Female

SIGNS & SYMPTOMS
- Local pain
- Foul odor
- Abnormally dark skin and tissues under skin (dark green to black)
- Crepitation (gas)
- Fever
- Rapid pulse
- Fulminant course leading to death without treatment

CAUSES
- Local injury
- Superimposed infection (surface or deep; local or distant)
- Carcinoma of large intestine
- Hematologic malignancies
- Severe neutropenia, related or not related to chemotherapy
- Burns
- Liposuction

RISK FACTORS
- Poor blood supply (arteriosclerosis)
- Old age
- Trauma
- Diabetes mellitus
- Malnutrition
- Immune suppression
- Chickenpox

DIAGNOSIS

DIFFERENTIAL DIAGNOSIS
- Deep infections with muscle involvement
  - ◊ Gas gangrene
    - Gas gangrene resulting from soft tissue trauma with multiple aerobic and anaerobic organisms; synergistic necrotizing sepsis, synergistic necrotizing cellulitis; clostridial myositis; clostridial myonecrosis
    - Abdominal wall gas gangrene; postoperative clostridial sepsis of the abdominal wall; clostridial myonecrosis of the abdominal wall
    - Nontraumatic, metastatic, clostridial myonecrosis; metastatic clostridial myositis; metastatic gas gangrene; gas gangrene without a visible wound; spontaneous gas gangrene
    - Uterine clostridial infections
    - Gas gangrene of the heart
    - Gas gangrene of the brain
  - ◊ Streptococcal myositis: anaerobic streptococcal myonecrosis; anaerobic streptococcal myositis
  - ◊ Infected vascular gas gangrene; non-clostridial gas gangrene; non-clostridial myositis
- Superficial infections - with or without abscess
  - ◊ Hemolytic streptococcal gangrene
  - ◊ Acute, infectious staphylococcal gangrene
  - ◊ Anaerobic cellulitis; crepitant phlegmon; clostridial cellulitis
  - ◊ Necrotizing fasciitis due to multiple aerobic and anaerobic organisms; synergistic gangrene; non-clostridial anaerobic cellulitis; anaerobic cutaneous gangrene; perineal phlegmon; Fournier gangrene. (Note: If there is extension to the tissues of the abdominal wall below the deep fascia, such as the anterior sheath of the rectus muscle, perineal phlegmon or Fournier gangrene is a synergistic necrotizing sepsis rather than just a necrotizing fasciitis. These are similar infections but are in different locations.)
  - ◊ Necrotizing fasciitis due to group A streptococcus (there may be very rapid extension to structures deep to the deep fascia)
  - ◊ Panophthalmitis
- Simple clostridial contamination of wounds
- Infiltration or injection or aspiration of gas into wounds
  - ◊ Wounds with gas not produced by bacteria
  - ◊ Injection of gas into wounds
    - Therapy (e.g., hydrogen peroxide)
    - Pranksters' jokes
    - Malingerers
    - Psychiatric problems
  - ◊ Aspiration and dissemination of air into wounds by muscular activity
  - ◊ Subcutaneous emphysema related to air leak syndrome or trauma
- Gas in tissues after industrial accidents
  - ◊ *Magnesiogenous pneumogranuloma*
- Gas in tissues after injections of chemicals
  - ◊ Injection of drugs
  - ◊ Accidental injection of a foreign agent, such as benzene
- Gas in tissues after laparoscopic examination and treatment

LABORATORY
- With severe gangrene, studies will reveal anemia and leukocytosis
- Gram smears for many possible organisms
- Daily serum creatine kinase determinations

Drugs that may alter lab results: Antibiotics prior to culture

Disorders that may alter lab results: N/A

PATHOLOGICAL FINDINGS
- Necrosis of tissues with foul odor
- Sometimes, gas in tissues
- Microorganisms

SPECIAL TESTS
- Cultures and sensitivity tests for microorganisms reported to produce gas in human tissues:
  - ◊ Gram-positive anaerobes: Cocci - Peptostreptococcus (anaerobic Streptococcus) (usually with group A Streptococcus [Streptococcus pyogenes, beta-hemolytic Streptococcus] or Staphylococcus aureus)
  - ◊ Gram-positive anaerobes: Bacilli - Clostridium perfringens and other clostridia
  - ◊ Gram-negative aerobes: Bacilli - Escherichia coli, Klebsiella pneumoniae, Enterobacter species, Proteus species (all usually in mixed infections)
  - ◊ Gram-negative anaerobes: Bacilli - Bacteroides fragilis (usually with other gram-negative bacilli)

IMAGING Plain radiographs, gas in tissues; with MRI, edema

DIAGNOSTIC PROCEDURES
IMMEDIATE SURGICAL INTERVENTION with longitudinal incisions of skin, superficial fascia, deep fascia, and muscles to look for necrotic tissue and/or foreign bodies and with removal of necrotic tissue or foreign bodies. Daily repetition if indicated. Repeated physical examinations for another, similar, focal infection.

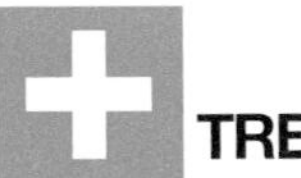

TREATMENT

APPROPRIATE HEALTH CARE
Hospital inpatient

GENERAL MEASURES
- Infectious disease consultation if available
- Intravenous fluids with glucose, electrolytes, blood, vitamins
- Daily CBC and electrolytes in acute phase
- Prophylaxis for tetanus
- Hyperbaric oxygen: unclear therapeutic value; no delay of surgical intervention for hyperbaric oxygen therapy

SURGICAL MEASURES
- Surgical intervention for diagnosis and débridement of necrotic tissues; possibly daily
- Re-operation if possibility of spreading or unrecognized necrosis and/or foreign bodies (with abnormal daily CPK determination)
- Surgical repair for loss of skin and subcutaneous tissues

ACTIVITY Bedrest

DIET By mouth, as tolerated

PATIENT EDUCATION N/A

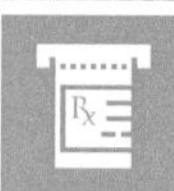

MEDICATIONS

DRUG(S) OF CHOICE

- Initially broad spectrum, antibiotic regimen; then specific antibiotic regime as determined by stained smears, cultures, and sensitivity tests with particular reference to the sensitivities of the hospital where the patient is being treated (although anaerobic organisms are difficult to culture and identify). Dosage will vary according to clinical circumstances; refer to manufacturer's literature and suggestions of infectious disease consultant. Important: don't delay treatment if smear, cultures and tests negative.

Gram stain and prsumptive organism:

Gram stain	Presumed organism
+ cocci	Streptococcus
+ cocci	Staph. aureus
+ bacilli	Clostridium spp
- bacilli	Bacteroides spp
- bacilli	Coliforms

- ◊ Gram-positive cocci: penicillin G, nafcillin (Unipen), clindamycin (Cleocin), metronidazole (Flagyl), or cephalosporins
- ◊ Gram-positive bacilli: penicillin G, clindamycin, metronidazole or cephalosporins
- ◊ Gram-negative bacilli (Bacteroides): clindamycin, metronidazole, cefoxitin (Mefoxin) [many B. fragilis are resistant], ticarcillin (Ticar) or mezlocillin (Mezlin)
- ◊ Gram-negative bacilli (Coliforms): gentamicin (Garamycin), tobramycin (Nebcin), amikacin (Amikin), cephalosporins, ampicillin, mezlocillin, or ticarcillin
- Intravenous calcium gluconate if extensive fat necrosis

Contraindications: Sensitivity to drugs

Precautions:

- Sedatives and analgesics (both before and after exploratory and therapeutic operations) may make recognition of spreading gangrene more difficult
- Repeated gram smears, culture and sensitivity tests for the best antibiotic(s)

Significant possible interactions: See manufacturer's profile of each drug.

ALTERNATIVE DRUGS

As above

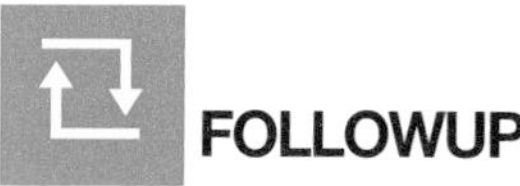

FOLLOWUP

PATIENT MONITORING

- Diligence required to recognize spreading gangrene
- Monitor effective blood levels of prescribed antibiotics
- Electrolytes
- Nutrition
- CPK determinations daily for myonecrosis
- Progress notes in charts daily or as often as every 4 hours

PREVENTION/AVOIDANCE

- Avoidance of trauma
- Good care of skin
- Avoidance of tight orthopedic casts

POSSIBLE COMPLICATIONS

- Tissue and functional losses
- Amputation
- Death

EXPECTED COURSE/PROGNOSIS

- Fair if early diagnosis and treatment, and if gangrene arrested at an early stage
- Fatal without treatment and possibly with treatment
- Fair if large intestine disease is recognized and removed immediately or if hematologic malignancy is recognized and treated immediately

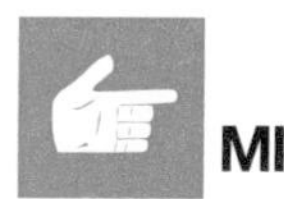

MISCELLANEOUS

ASSOCIATED CONDITIONS

- Diabetes mellitus with impaired blood flow
- Altered immunocompetence: Depressed immunocompetence may require an alteration of treatment, especially with tumor treatments

AGE-RELATED FACTORS

Pediatric: N/A

Geriatric: Diseases of the aged with debility and poor blood supply

Others: N/A

PREGNANCY

Treatment as for nonpregnant, but consider the pregnancy

SYNONYMS

N/A

ICD-9-CM

785.4 Gangrene
040.0 Gas gangrene
136.9 Unspecified infectious and parasitic diseases
682.9 Cellulitis and abscess at unspecified site

SEE ALSO

Tetanus

OTHER NOTES

- Group A Streptococcus: "flesh eating bacterium"

ABBREVIATIONS

CBC = complete blood count
MRI = magnetic resonance imaging
CPK = serum creatinine phosphokinase

REFERENCES

- van der Horst CM. Complications following liposuction. Ned Tijdschr Geneeskd 2002;146(50):2405-6
- Nagelvoort RW, Hulstaert PF, Kon M, Schuurman AH. Necrotising fasciitis and myositis as serious complications after liposuction. Ned Tijdschr Geneeskd 2002;146(50):2430-5
- Sharma M, Khatib R, Fakih M. Clinical characteristics of necrotizing fasciitis caused by group G Streptococcus: case report and review of the literature. Scand J Infect Dis 2002;34(6):468-71
- Bryant P, Carapetis J, Matussek J, Curtis N. Recurrent crepitant cellulitis caused by Clostridium perfringens. Pediatr Infect Dis J 2002;21(12):1173-4
- Clark P, Davidson D, Letts M, Lawton L, Jawadi A. Necrotizing fasciitis secondary to chickenpox infection in children. Can J Surg. 2003;46(1):9-14
- Furste W, Lobe TE, Botros NM: Gangrenous soft tissue infections. Inf in Surgery 1985;4:837-878
- Furste W, Dolor MC, Rothstein LB, Vest CR: Carcinoma of the large intestine and nontraumatic metastatic clostridial myonecrosis. Diseases of Colon & Rectum 1986;29:899-904
- Furste W, Wheeler WL: Tetanus: a team disease. Curr Prob in Surg 1972;9:1-72
- Rice B: $15 million deep. Med Econ 1995;14:47-50
- Golshani S, Simons AJ, Der R, et al: Necrotizing fasciitis following laparoscopic surgery. Surg Endosc 1996;10:751-754
- Tibbles PM, Edelsberg JS: Hyperbaric-oxygen therapy. New Engl J Med 1996;334:1642-1648
- Bury TF: Clostridial gas gangrene of the spleen presenting as pneumoperitoneum. Contemp Surg 1997;51:312-316
- Furste W: A golden opportunity, review of tetanus prophylaxis (1890-1998). J Trauma 1998;44:1110-1112
- Sobolewski AP, Welling RE: Management of Fournier's gangrene. Surg Rounds 1997;20:285-287
- Rai RK, Londhe S, Sinha S, et al. Spontaneous bifocal Clostridium septicum gas gangrene. J Bone Joint Surg Br 2001;83(1):115-6
- Faucher LD, Morris SE, Edelman, LS et al. Burn center management of necrotizing soft-tissue in unburned patients. Amer J Surg 2001;182:563-9
- Furste W. Tetanus: a new threat. J Trauma 2001;51(2):416-7
- Halpin TF, Molinari JA. Diagnosis and management of Clostridium perfringens sepsis and uterine gas. Obstet Surv 2002;57(l):53-57
- Bhatti MA, Seville MTA. Hematogenous anaerobic osteomyelitis. New Eng J Med 2002;346:1060
- Moses AE, Goldberg S, Konenman Z et al. Invasive group A streptococcal infections, Israel. Emerg Inf Dis 2002;88(4):421-4
- Garcia-Suarez J, de Miguel D, Krsnik I, et al. Spontaneous gas gangrene in malignant lymphoma: an under-reported complication? Am J Hematol 2002;70(2):145-8

Web references: 0 available at www.5mcc.com

Illustrations N/A

Author(s):

Augusto Aguirre, MD

BASICS

DESCRIPTION
- An IgE mediated acute, systemic reaction following antigen exposure in a sensitized person.
- A non-IgE mediated idiopathic anaphylactoid reaction also may occur. Anaphylactoid reactions are clinically indistinguishable from anaphylaxis and are treated in the same manner.

System(s) affected: Cardiovascular, Endocrine/Metabolic, Gastrointestinal, Hemic/Lymphatic/Immunologic, Pulmonary, Skin/Exocrine
Genetics: Genetic predisposition for sensitization to certain antigens
Incidence/Prevalence in USA:
- Between 20,592 and 47,024 cases of idiopathic anaphylaxis occur per year (no identifiable cause)
- Drug-induced anaphylaxis in 1/2,700 hospitalized patients
- 0.3-0.7/100,000/yr anaphylaxis deaths

Predominant age: All ages
Predominant sex: Male = Female

SIGNS & SYMPTOMS
- Pruritus, flushing, urticaria, angioedema
- Dyspnea, cough, rhonchi
- Rhinorrhea, bronchorrhea, wheezing
- Difficulty swallowing
- Nausea, vomiting, diarrhea, cramps, bloating
- Tachycardia, hypotension, shock, syncope
- Malaise, shivering
- Mydriasis

CAUSES
- IgE mediated mast cell degranulation
- Complement activation (C3a, C4a, C5a) by antigen-antibody complexes that contain complement fixing antibodies
- Other non-IgE dependent anaphylaxis-like syndromes may be caused by modulators of arachidonic acid metabolism, sulfiting agents, exercise induced anaphylaxis, and idiopathic recurrent anaphylaxis
- Some important causes of anaphylaxis are:
  - ◊ Antimicrobials (e.g., penicillin)
  - ◊ Blood products (especially in IgA deficient patients)
  - ◊ Diagnostic chemicals (iodinated contrast media)
  - ◊ Ethylene oxide gas (dialysis tubing, other sterilized products)
  - ◊ Exercise
  - ◊ Foods (e.g., peanuts, nuts, fish, crustaceans, mollusks, cow milk, eggs, soybean most common)
  - ◊ Immunotherapy
  - ◊ Insect stings (e.g., honeybees, wasps, kissing bugs, deer flies)
  - ◊ Latex rubber (gloves, catheters)
  - ◊ Macromolecules (e.g., chymopapain, insulin, dextran, glucocorticoid, protamine)
  - ◊ Vaccines

RISK FACTORS Previous anaphylaxis; history of atopy or asthma

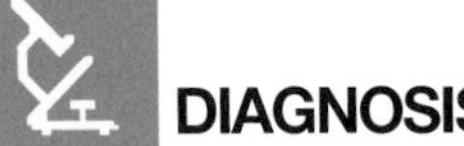

DIAGNOSIS

DIFFERENTIAL DIAGNOSIS
- Anaphylactoid reactions: May occur after the first contact with substance, such as polymyxin, pentamidine, radiographic contrast media, aspirin
- Carcinoid syndrome
- Globus hystericus: may mimic pharyngeal edema.
- Hereditary angioedema: C1q esterase deficiency with painless, pruritus-free angioedema without urticaria, flushing or wheezing.
- Pheochromocytoma: Paradoxically, because of beta-2 stimulation, some patients have hypotensive attacks accompanied by tachycardia. Urticaria, angioedema, and wheezing absent.
- Pseudoanaphylactic reaction: After injection of procaine penicillin. Is a drug effect of procaine and not a penicillin allergy.
- Scombroid poisoning: From ingestion of dark meat fish (e.g., tuna, mackerel, mahi-mahi). Histamine-like mediator - symptoms include flushing, sweating, nausea, vomiting, diarrhea, headache, palpitations, dizziness, rash, swelling of face and tongue, respiratory distress, vasodilatory shock.
- Serum sickness: Occurs several days after exposure to inciting agent
- Systemic mastocytosis: Benign or malignant overgrowth of mast cells. Urticaria pigmentosa seen in benign form and the presence of reddish brown macular-papular cutaneous lesions which urticate after trauma - Darier's sign.
- Vasovagal reactions: Bradycardia and hypotension without tachycardia, flushing, urticaria, angioedema, pruritus, and wheezing
- Pulmonary embolism, foreign body aspiration, arrhythmia

LABORATORY
- Hypoxemia, hypercarbia, acidosis. Acidosis may cause apparent hyperkalemia by moving potassium extracellularly.
- Elevated serum and urine histamine (short-lived in circulation)
- Elevated serum tryptase, a mast cell enzyme marker for allergic and anaphylactic reactions. Peak level: 30-90 minutes after reaction onset.

Drugs that may alter lab results: Epinephrine and albuterol may cause apparent hypokalemia by shifting K+ intracellularly

Disorders that may alter lab results: N/A

PATHOLOGICAL FINDINGS N/A

SPECIAL TESTS N/A

IMAGING N/A

DIAGNOSTIC PROCEDURES N/A

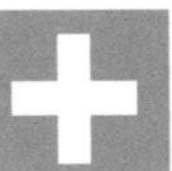

TREATMENT

APPROPRIATE HEALTH CARE
- Outpatient: Patients with cutaneous angioedema, urticaria, and minimal bronchospasm may be released when symptoms and signs have cleared. Continue antihistamines (diphenhydramine/cimetidine) and oral steroids for 72 hours.
- Moderate-severe anaphylaxis, admit observation; may need ventilatory support.
- Allergist referral, if anaphylaxis cause unclear
- Patients with anaphylaxis from insect stings benefit from desensitization immunotherapy

GENERAL MEASURES
- Treatment depends on severity
- Maintain a patent airway - endotracheal intubation and assisted ventilation may be necessary; possibly tracheostomy, or needle cricothyrotomy in kids under age 12
- Oxygen
- Tourniquet placed proximal to injected or stung site if possible, to occlude lymphatic and venous drainage (but not arterial flow)
- IV fluids (normal saline/lactated ringers) restores intravascular volume; avoid precipitating CHF
- Monitor vital signs

SURGICAL MEASURES N/A

ACTIVITY Bedrest until anaphylaxis clears and patient hemodynamically stable

DIET Nothing until acute symptoms are controlled

PATIENT EDUCATION
- Printed patient information available from: Asthma & Allergy Foundation of America, 1717 Massachusetts Avenue, Suite 305, Washington, DC 20036,(800)7-Asthma or American Allergy Association, P.O. Box 7273, Menlo Park, CA 94026, (415)322-1663
- Medic-Alert type tags (Medic-Alert Foundation, Turlock, CA 95381-1009
- Avoid beta-blockers if possible
- Instruct patient in use of bee sting kit

MEDICATIONS

DRUG(S) OF CHOICE

- Epinephrine
  - ◊ Less severe reaction: 0.3-0.5 mg (0.01 mg/kg in children)= (0.3-0.5 mL of a 1:1000 solution, 0.01 mL/kg in children), SQ q 20-30 minutes as needed up to 3 doses
  - ◊ Life-threatening reactions: 0.5 mg (5 mL of a 1:10,000 solution)(for children: 0.05-0.1 mL/kg/dose) given IV slowly q 5-10 minutes as needed. If IV access not possible, endotracheal or intraosseous may be effective.
- Diphenhydramine, an H1 blocker 25-50 mg IV (IM or PO) immediately and then, q6h for 72 hours (children 1.25 mg/kg to 25 mg)
- Cimetidine, an H2 blocker, 300 mg IV over 3-5 minutes (children 5-10 mg/kg/dose) and then 400 mg PO bid is helpful and may be more effective than diphenhydramine.
- Corticosteroids: No immediate effect and no good evidence that they prevent recurrence - can be administered if desired.
  - ◊ Hydrocortisone sodium succinate 250-500 mg IV q 4-6 h (4-8 mg/kg for children), or
  - ◊ Prednisone, 1 mg/kg in children, up to 60 mg, or
  - ◊ Methylprednisolone 60-125 mg IV in adults. 1-2 mg/kg in children.
- Bronchodilator, if persistent bronchospasm
  - ◊ Inhaled beta-2 agonists. Continuous nebulized albuterol of 10 mg/hr or 2.5 mg q 15-20 minutes is safe, effective and preferable to aminophylline as first line therapy.
- Laryngeal edema:
  - ◊ Epinephrine 5 mL 1:1000 by nebulizer. More effective than racemic epinephrine and usually available.
- Persistent hypotension
  - ◊ Dopamine 200 mg in 500 mL of dextrose in water given by infusion pump. Titrate to blood pressure (3-20 mcg/kg/min)
  - ◊ Glucagon: May be beneficial for resistant hypotension caused by concurrent beta-blockade therapy 50 mcg/kg IV bolus over 1 minute, or alternatively, because of short half-life, can give as continuous infusion at 5-15 mcg/min
- Normal saline or Ringer's lactate: As necessary to maintain tissue perfusion
- Oral antihistamines and steroids for 72 hours

Contraindications:
Refer to manufacturer's literature

Precautions:
Refer to manufacturer's literature

Significant possible interactions: None

ALTERNATIVE DRUGS

- Several reports of tranexamic acid-1000 mg IV or sigma-aminocaproic acid for refractory anaphylaxis. Reserve for last resort in patient not responding to other therapy; these drugs not considered standard of care! Not to be used in pregnant women, or known vascular thrombosis.
- Aminophylline 5-6 mg/kg IV in 100 cc D5W over 20 minutes, then maintenance at 1 mg/kg/hr drip

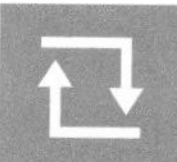

FOLLOWUP

PATIENT MONITORING Follow vital signs closely during treatment and for several hours after anaphylaxis has resolved. Symptoms can recur for up to 72 hours.

PREVENTION/AVOIDANCE

- Avoid drugs, foods that cause the reaction
- Carry a pre-filled epinephrine syringe; avoid areas where insect exposure likely. Avoid wearing things that attract insects (e.g., perfumes, bright-colored clothing); avoid bare feet outdoors.
- Carry/wear medical alert ID about anaphylaxis-causing substance or event
- When radiologic contrast is unavoidable, use of low osmolar contrast agents (e.g., iothalamate) reduces risk of contrast reactions in those with previous contrast reaction to 3.1%; only 0.22% were considered severe. Stop beta-blockers before administering contrast materials; pre-treat with diphenhydramine (50 mg IV) and steroid (e.g., methylprednisolone 60 mg IV). If possible, start methylprednisolone the day before the procedure is scheduled and administer every 6 hours until the procedure.
- Those with frequent (>6/year) episodes of idiopathic anaphylaxis should be treated prophylactically with prednisone 40-60 mg/day in a single a.m. dose, hydroxyzine-25 mg tid, and albuterol 2 mg po tid. The prednisone should be rapidly tapered to a qod regimen.
- Have latex-free kit (gloves, IVs, etc) available for treatment of latex allergic patients; some latex allergic patients will react to tropical fruits (e.g., kiwi, bananas) also avocados, chestnuts
- Avoid beta blockers

POSSIBLE COMPLICATIONS Hypoxemia; cardiac arrest; death

EXPECTED COURSE/PROGNOSIS

- Good prognosis if treated immediately; worse outcome with a delay of >30 minutes in administration of epinephrine
- Of those with idiopathic anaphylaxis - 60% are free of anaphylactic episodes at 2.5 years; most others were steroid free with a decrease in the number of episodes

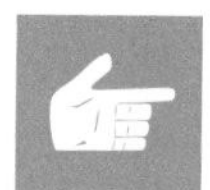

MISCELLANEOUS

ASSOCIATED CONDITIONS Asthma; atopy

AGE-RELATED FACTORS

Pediatric: N/A

Geriatric: Epinephrine may induce ischemia and myocardial infarction in those with cardiac disease; still the drug of choice. Be alert for anti-cholinergic and CNS side effects after giving diphenhydramine or cimetidine.

Others: N/A

PREGNANCY Epinephrine, other pressors may reduce placental blood flow; but may save life of mother and fetus. It also increases incidence of congenital malformation.

SYNONYMS

- Anaphylactoid reactions

ICD-9-CM

995.0 Other anaphylactic shock
E947.8 Adverse effects in therapeutic use of other drugs and medicinal substances
E947.9 Adverse effects in therapeutic use of unspecified drug or medicinal substance

SEE ALSO

Food allergy
Insect bites & stings

OTHER NOTES

- Allergy to one species of legume (e.g., peanuts) or one type of seafood (e.g., shrimp) doesn't mean allergy to all products in that category. Skin testing is prudent.
- MMR vaccine can be safely administered to those with a history of egg allergy since most egg allergies are related to the albumin.
- Penicillin allergic patients can generally tolerate second and third generation cephalosporins as well as monobactams (e.g., aztreonam); generally will be allergic to carbapenems (e.g., imipenem) and first generation cephalosporins
- IgA deficient patients should have washed RBCs for transfusion
- Those allergic to seafood are not allergic to iodine-based radiocontrast. Shellfish allergy is protein related.

ABBREVIATIONS N/A

REFERENCES

- Tintinalli JE, et al. Emergency Medicine, A Comprehensive Study Guide. 4th ed. New York: McGraw-Hill; 1995
- Patterson R, Hogan MB, Yarnold PR, Harris KE. Idiopathic anaphylaxis: An attempt to estimate the incidence in the United States. Archives of Internal Medicine 1995;155(8):869-71
- Freeman TM. Allergy and Immunology. Anaphylaxis: Diagnosis and treatment. Primary Care; Clinics in Office Practice, 1998;25:809
- The Diagnosis and Management of Anaphylaxis. Joint Task Force on Practice Parameters, American Academy of Allergy, Asthma and Immunology, American College of Allergy, Asthma and Immunology, and the Joint Council of Allergy. Asthma and Immunology. Journal of Allergy and Clinical Immunology 1998;6(101)
- Sloop GD, Friedberg RC. Complications of blood transfusion: How to recognize and respond to noninfectious reactions. Postgrad Med 1995;98(1):159-62,166,169-72
- Tanus T, Mines D, Atkins PC, Levinson AL. Serum tryptase in idiopathic anaphylaxis: A case report and review of the literature. Annals Of Emergency Medicine 1994;24(1):104-7
- Wittbrodt ET, Spinler SA. Prevention of anaphylactoid reactions in high-risk patients receiving radiographic contrast media. Annals Of Pharmacotherapy 1994;28(2):236-41
- Anne S, et al. Risk of administering cephalosporin antibiotics to patients with histories of penicillin allergy. Ann Allergy Asthma Immun 1995;74:167
- Hoste S, Van Aken H, Stevens E. Tranexamic acid in the treatment of anaphylactic shock. Acta Anaesthesiologica Belgica 1991;42(2):113-16
- Sandler SG, Mallory D, Malamut D, Eckrich R. IgA anaphylactic transfusion reactions. Transfusion Medicine Reviews 1995;9(1):1-8

Web references: 2 available at www.5mcc.com
Illustrations N/A

Author(s):

Bobby Peters, MD

BASICS

DESCRIPTION An anemia in which the bone marrow fails to produce adequate numbers of peripheral blood elements. Usual course - insidious. Pure red cell aplasia is a related syndrome that is caused by a selective failure of the production of erythroid elements. It can be associated with thymomas. Constitutional (Fanconi) anemia is associated with congenital anomalies.

System(s) affected: Hemic/Lymphatic/Immunologic

Genetics:
- Genetic pattern undetermined in acquired
- Autosomal recessive in constitutional

Incidence/Prevalence in USA: Not very common

Predominant age:
- Constitutional - children and young adults
- Acquired - all ages

Predominant sex: Male = Female

SIGNS & SYMPTOMS
- Dyspnea
- Ecchymoses, petechiae
- Fatigue, fever
- Hemorrhage, menorrhagia, occult stool blood, melena, epistaxis
- Pallor
- Palpitations
- Progressive weakness
- Retinal flame hemorrhages
- Systolic ejection murmur
- Weight loss
- Constitutional:
  - ◊ Short stature
  - ◊ Microcephaly
  - ◊ Radius and thumb anomalies
  - ◊ Renal anomalies
  - ◊ Hypospadias
  - ◊ Hyperpigmentation

CAUSES
- Idiopathic (about 50% of the cases)
- Injury to pluripotential stem cells
- Destruction of pluripotential stem cells
- Immunologic injury
- Toxic exposure, e.g., benzene, inorganic arsenic
- Infectious hepatitis
- Radiation exposure
- Drugs - especially antibiotics, anticonvulsants, gold
- Pregnancy (rare)
- Inherited (constitutional anemia)

RISK FACTORS
- Viral illness
- Toxin exposure
- Tumors of thymus (red cell aplasia)

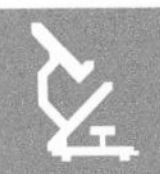

DIAGNOSIS

DIFFERENTIAL DIAGNOSIS
- Other causes of pancytopenia
- Myelodysplastic disorders
- Paroxysmal nocturnal hemoglobinuria
- Acute leukemia
- Hairy cell leukemia
- Systemic lupus erythematosus
- Disseminated infection
- Hypersplenism
- Transient erythroblastopenia of childhood

LABORATORY
- Pancytopenia
- Anemia
- Leukopenia
- Neutropenia
- Thrombocytopenia
- Decreased reticulocytes
- Increased serum iron secondary to transfusion
- Normal total iron binding capacity (TIBC)
- Borderline high mean corpuscular volume (MCV) > 104
- Hematuria
- Abnormal liver function tests (hepatitis)
- Increased fetal hemoglobin (Fanconi)
- Increased chromosomal breaks under specialized conditions (Fanconi)
- Molecular determination of abnormal gene (Fanconi)

Drugs that may alter lab results: N/A

Disorders that may alter lab results: N/A

PATHOLOGICAL FINDINGS
- Normochromic RBC
- Bone marrow:
  - ◊ Decreased cellularity (< 10%)
  - ◊ Decreased megakaryocytes
  - ◊ Decreased myelocytes
  - ◊ Decreased erythroid precursors

SPECIAL TESTS Chromosome breakage (Fanconi); fetal hemoglobin; red cell adenosine deaminase (pure red cell aplasia); molecular determination of abnormal genes

IMAGING
- CT of thymus region if thymoma-associated RBC aplasia suspected
- Radiographs of radius and thumbs (constitutional anemia)
- Renal ultrasound (constitutional anemia)

DIAGNOSTIC PROCEDURES Bone marrow biopsy

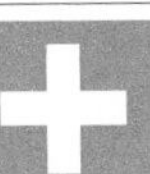

TREATMENT

APPROPRIATE HEALTH CARE Inpatient. Referral to an institution that has experience in treating these patients is recommended.

GENERAL MEASURES
- Vigorous supportive measures
- Oxygen therapy for severe anemia
- Good oral hygiene
- Avoid causative agents
- Human leukocyte antigen (HLA) testing on all patients and their immediate families
- Transfusion support (judiciously prescribed RBCs for severe anemia, consider leukocyte depleted units; platelets for severe thrombocytopenia; WBCs)
- Immunosuppressive therapy (cyclosporine, corticosteroids, antithymocyte globulin [ATG]) if no suitable donor
- Androgen therapy if less severe

SURGICAL MEASURES
- Bone marrow transplantation for patients with severe aplastic anemia and an HLA-identical donor. Upper age restrictions on transplantations varies among institutions that perform them.
- Unrelated donor transplants, if other therapy fails
- Thymectomy for thymoma

ACTIVITY Isolation procedures if neutropenic

DIET No special diet, but nutritious diet important to improve resistance to infection

PATIENT EDUCATION Printed patient information available from: Aplastic Anemia Foundation of America, P.O. Box 22689, Baltimore, MD 21203, (410)955-2803

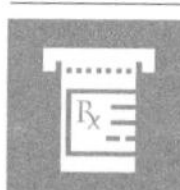

MEDICATIONS

DRUG(S) OF CHOICE
- Antithymocyte globulin (ATG)
  - ◊ It is a horse serum containing polyclonal antibodies against human T cells. Skin test patients to determine any hypersensitivity.
  - ◊ Treatment for older patients and patients without a compatible donor
  - ◊ May be used as a single agent or in combination with corticosteroids
- Cyclosporine
  - ◊ Monitor trough blood levels. Normal values for assays vary.
  - ◊ 3-6 months trial may be necessary
- Androgens
  - ◊ Clinical trials inconclusive
  - ◊ Useful for some patients lacking other options and less severe patients
  - ◊ Oxymetholone - 1-2 mg/kg/day orally
  - ◊ 2-3 month trial usually necessary to assess response
- Prednisone for pure red cell anemia

Note: Relapses may occur after initial response to immunosuppressive therapy

Contraindications: Refer to manufacturer's literature

Precautions: Refer to manufacturer's literature

Significant possible interactions: Refer to manufacturer's literature

ALTERNATIVE DRUGS Granulocyte colony stimulating factor (G-CSF)

FOLLOWUP

PATIENT MONITORING Close monitoring for all treatments. Drugs and other forms of treatment have numerous and severe side effects.

PREVENTION/AVOIDANCE
- Avoid possible toxic agents
- Use safety measures when working with radiation

POSSIBLE COMPLICATIONS
- Hemorrhage
- Infection
- Transfusion hemosiderosis
- Transfusion hepatitis
- Heart failure
- Complications of therapy
- Development of acute leukemia
- Neoplasm may complicate constitutional anemia

EXPECTED COURSE/PROGNOSIS
Depending on age and treatment available - guardedly favorable

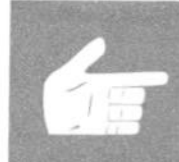

MISCELLANEOUS

ASSOCIATED CONDITIONS N/A

AGE-RELATED FACTORS
Pediatric:
- Pure red cell anemia (Diamond-Blackfan) and constitutional anemia are seen more often in children
- Idiopathic aplastic anemia is more common in adolescents
- Secondary aplastic anemia seen in children exposed to ionizing radiation or treated with cytotoxic chemotherapeutic agents

Geriatric: The elderly are more exposed to large numbers of drugs and therefore more susceptible to secondary aplastic anemia

Others: N/A

PREGNANCY Pregnancy may, rarely, be associated with aplastic anemia

SYNONYMS
- Hypoplastic anemia
- Panmyelophthisis
- Refractory anemia
- Aleukia hemorrhagica
- Toxic paralytic anemia

ICD-9-CM
284.9 Aplastic anemia, unspecified

SEE ALSO
Leukemia, hairy cell
Myelodysplastic syndromes (MDS)
Paroxysmal nocturnal hemoglobinuria
Systemic lupus erythematosus (SLE)

OTHER NOTES N/A

ABBREVIATIONS N/A

REFERENCES

- Williams WJ, et al. Hematology. 4th Ed. New York, McGraw-Hill, 1990
- Lee GR, et al. Wintrobe's Clinical Hematology. 9th Ed. Philadelphia, Lea & Febiger, 1993

Web references: 0 available at www.5mcc.com

Illustrations N/A

Author(s):
John J. Hutter, Jr., MD

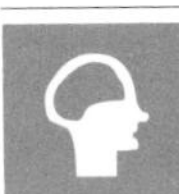

BASICS

DESCRIPTION Acquired anemia induced by binding of autoantibodies and/or complement to the red cells
- Three main types
  - ◊ Warm (37°C) antibody (80-90%)
  - ◊ Cold reacting antibody (10%)
  - ◊ Drug-induced

System(s) affected: Hemic/Lymphatic/Immunologic
Genetics: Unknown
Incidence/Prevalence in USA:
- Incidence: 4/100,000 per year
- Prevalence: N/A

Predominant age: < 50 years
Predominant sex: Female > Male

SIGNS & SYMPTOMS
- Weakness
- Fatigue
- Exertional dyspnea
- Dizziness
- Palpitations
- Malaise
- Dyspnea
- Pallor
- Jaundice
- Splenomegaly
- Hepatomegaly
- Tachycardia
- Anemia (may be sudden and life threatening)

CAUSES
- Warm antibody
  - ◊ Idiopathic (50%)
  - ◊ Neoplasia (Leukemia, myeloma, lymphoma, thymoma)
  - ◊ Collagen vascular disease
  - ◊ Viral infection: e.g., hepatitis
- Cold antibody
  - ◊ Idiopathic (50%)
  - ◊ Infection (Mycoplasma, mononucleosis, viral)
  - ◊ Neoplasia (lymphoma)
  - ◊ Cold agglutinin disease
- Drug induced
  - ◊ Methyldopa, quinidine, penicillin

RISK FACTORS Listed with Causes

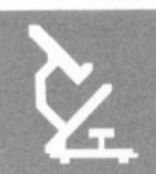

DIAGNOSIS

DIFFERENTIAL DIAGNOSIS Other hemolytic anemias

LABORATORY
- Direct Coombs' (antiglobulin test) - positive
- CBC
  - ◊ Anemia (normocytic, normochromic)
  - ◊ Mild to moderate increase in mean corpuscular volume (MCV) depending on level of reticulocystosis
  - ◊ Increased mean cell hemoglobin concentration (MCHC)
  - ◊ Spherocytosis
  - ◊ Poikilocytosis
  - ◊ Anisocytosis
  - ◊ Rouleaux
  - ◊ Reticulocytosis
  - ◊ Nucleated RBC
  - ◊ Large polychromatophilic reticulocytes
- Hyperbilirubinemia
- Decreased haptoglobin
- Hemoglobinemia

Drugs that may alter lab results: N/A

Disorders that may alter lab results: N/A

PATHOLOGICAL FINDINGS
- Bone marrow hyperplasia
- Increased marrow hemosiderin

SPECIAL TESTS
- IgG antibody (warm)
- IgM antibody (cold)

IMAGING N/A

DIAGNOSTIC PROCEDURES N/A

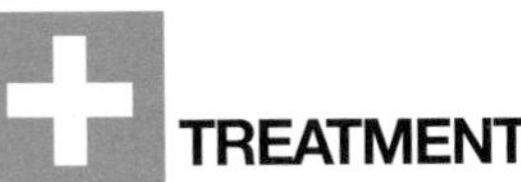

TREATMENT

APPROPRIATE HEALTH CARE Inpatient

GENERAL MEASURES
- Warm antibody
  - ◊ Mild - conservative therapy
  - ◊ Moderate - prednisone
  - ◊ Severe - high dose prednisone, danazol (Danocrine), immunosuppressant, packed red cell transfusion (which is difficult to crossmatch - need special blood bank techniques; in emergency, use most compatible crossmatch), splenectomy
- Cold antibody
  - ◊ Supportive
  - ◊ Avoid cold
  - ◊ Red cell transfusion (which is difficult to crossmatch - need special blood bank techniques; in emergency, use most compatible crossmatch)
  - ◊ Consider high dose prednisone
- Drug induced
  - ◊ Stop the offending drug
- Plasmapheresis/exchange transfusion for severe life-threatening cases

SURGICAL MEASURES In severe warm antibody splenectomy may be needed

ACTIVITY Rest until asymptomatic

DIET No special diet

PATIENT EDUCATION Griffith, H.W.: Instructions for Patients; Philadelphia, 1998 W.B. Saunders Co

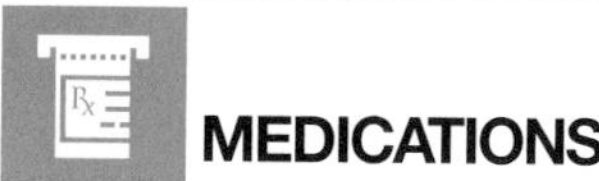

MEDICATIONS

DRUG(S) OF CHOICE

- Glucocorticoids - prednisone 1 mg/kg each day in divided doses. Adjust downward for longer term treatment.

Contraindications: Refer to manufacturer's literature
Precautions: Refer to manufacturer's literature
Significant possible interactions: Refer to manufacturer's literature

ALTERNATIVE DRUGS

- Immunosuppressive drugs (if prednisone and splenectomy do not cure)
  - ◊ Azathioprine (Imuran) up to 125 mg/day for up to 6 months
- Danazol 400-600 mg/day
- Immune globulin IV

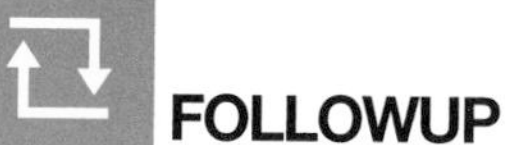

FOLLOWUP

PATIENT MONITORING Monitor carefully if transfusion essential

PREVENTION/AVOIDANCE No preventive measures known

POSSIBLE COMPLICATIONS

- Shock (severe anemia)
- Thromboembolism
- Thrombocytopenic purpura (Evans's syndrome)

EXPECTED COURSE/PROGNOSIS

- Good with appropriate treatment
- If secondary to an underlying disorder, the prognosis is determined by the course of the primary disease

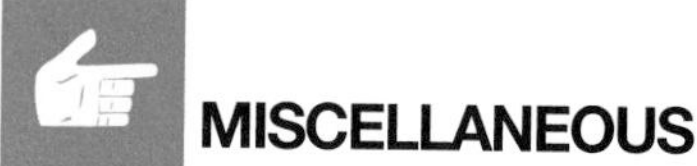

MISCELLANEOUS

ASSOCIATED CONDITIONS

- Systemic lupus erythematosus
- Chronic lymphocytic anemia
- Diffuse lymphomas

AGE-RELATED FACTORS

Pediatric: May occur in pediatric age group
Geriatric: Unusual in this age group; rule out neoplasia
Others: N/A

PREGNANCY N/A

SYNONYMS N/A

ICD-9-CM

283.0 Autoimmune hemolytic anemias

SEE ALSO

Leukemia
Lymphoma, non-Hodgkin
Systemic lupus erythematosus (SLE)

OTHER NOTES N/A

ABBREVIATIONS N/A

REFERENCES

- Hashimoto C. Autoimmune hemolytic anemia. Clinical reviews. Allergy Immunology 1998;16(3):285-295
- Rosenwasser LJ, Joseph BZ. Immunohematologic Disorders. JAMA 1992;268:2940-5
- Gehrs BC, Friedberg RC. Autoimmune hemolytic anemia. Am J. Hematol 2002;69:258-71
- Dhaliwal G, et al. Hemolytic anemia. Am F Phys 2004;69:2599-606

Web references: 0 available at www.5mcc.com
Illustrations N/A

Author(s):
Brian J. Murray, MD

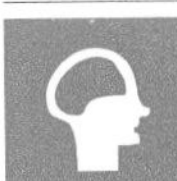

BASICS

DESCRIPTION A disorder due to vitamin B12 deficiency. Pernicious anemia is invariably associated with atrophic gastritis and histamine-fast achlorhydria. Vitamin B12 cannot be absorbed in the terminal ileum without intrinsic factor (a secretion of the parietal cells of the gastric mucosa). Usual course - slowly progressive.
System(s) affected: Gastrointestinal, Hemic/Lymphatic/Immunologic, Nervous
Genetics: HLA-DR2; HLA-DR4. Present in the rare form of pernicious anemia that is hereditary. Endemic areas - northern Europe, including Scandinavia.
Incidence/Prevalence in USA: Unknown
Predominant age: Older adults (> 60 years)
Predominant sex: Male = Female

SIGNS & SYMPTOMS
- Abnormal reflexes
- Anorexia; weight loss
- Ataxia
- Atrophic glossitis
- Babinski's sign - positive
- Confusion
- Congestive heart failure
- Dementia
- Depression
- Exertional dyspnea
- Extremity numbness
- Extremity paresthesias
- Hepatomegaly
- Pallor
- Palpitations
- Poor finger coordination
- Position sense - decreased
- Prematurely gray-haired
- Purpura
- Romberg's sign, positive
- Skin pigmentation increased
- Sore tongue
- Splenomegaly
- Tachycardia
- Tinnitus
- Vertigo
- Vibration sense - decreased
- Vitiligo
- Weakness

CAUSES
- Atrophic gastric mucosa
- Intrinsic factor deficiency
- Probable autoimmunity against gastric parietal cells
- Autoimmunity against intrinsic factor

RISK FACTORS
- Vegetarian diet, without B12 supplementation
- Gastrectomy
- Blind loop syndrome
- Fish-tapeworm infestation
- Malabsorption syndromes
- Drugs: oral calcium-chelating drugs, aminosalicylic acid, biguanides
- Chronic pancreatitis
- Alcoholism

DIAGNOSIS

DIFFERENTIAL DIAGNOSIS
- Folic acid deficiency
- Myelodysplasia
- Neurological disorders without B12 deficiency
- Liver dysfunction
- Hypothyroidism
- Hemolysis or bleeding
- Drug effects
- Alcoholism

LABORATORY
- Achlorhydria
- Anisocytosis
- Anti-intrinsic poikilocytosis factor antibody
- Anti-parietal cell antibody
- Direct hyperbilirubinemia
- Haptoglobin decreased
- Howell-Jolly bodies
- Hypergastrinemia
- Hypersegmented neutrophils
- LDH increased
- Leukopenia
- Macrocytic anemia
- Mean corpuscular volume - 110-140
- Pentagastrin stimulation - stomach pH > 6
- Peripheral blood smear - macro-ovalocytes
- Poikilocytes
- Serum ferritin increased
- Serum vitamin B12 level < 100 pg/mL (< 74 pmol/L)
- Thrombocytopenia

Drugs that may alter lab results: N/A

Disorders that may alter lab results:
- Falsely elevated MCV
  - ◊ Cold agglutinins
  - ◊ Hyperglycemia
  - ◊ Marked hyperleukocytosis
- Falsely normal serum vitamin B12 level
  - ◊ Myeloproliferative disorders
  - ◊ Liver disease
- Falsely low serum B12 level
  - ◊ Multiple myeloma
  - ◊ Oral contraceptive intake
  - ◊ Pregnancy
  - ◊ Folate deficiency
  - ◊ Transcobalamin I deficiency
  - ◊ Recent isotope administration

PATHOLOGICAL FINDINGS
- Bone marrow - hypercellular, macrocytes, iron stores increased
- Nests of megaloblasts
- Giant metamyelocytes
- Macro-polymorpho-leukocytes
- Hypersegmented neutrophils
- Stomach - atrophic gastritis, goblet cells increased
- Parietal cell atrophy
- Chief cell atrophy
- Gastric cytology - cellular atypia
- Spinal cord - myelin degeneration of the dorsal and lateral tracts
- Peripheral nerve degeneration
- Degenerative changes of the posterior root ganglia

SPECIAL TESTS
- Schilling test plus intrinsic factor - normal vitamin B12 absorption
- Schilling test - decreased vitamin B12 absorption
- Gastric analysis - achlorhydria

IMAGING N/A:

DIAGNOSTIC PROCEDURES
- Bone marrow aspiration
- Detailed history and physical exam

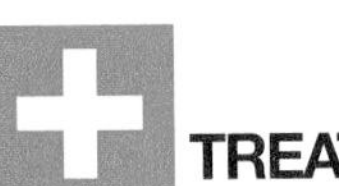

TREATMENT

APPROPRIATE HEALTH CARE Outpatient

GENERAL MEASURES
- Treatment must be continued for life
- Identification and treatment of the underlying disorder

SURGICAL MEASURES N/A

ACTIVITY Unlimited

DIET Emphasize meat, animal protein foods, legumes unless contraindicated

PATIENT EDUCATION Griffith, H.W.: Instructions for Patients, W.B. Saunders Co, Philadelphia (instructions to photocopy for patient)

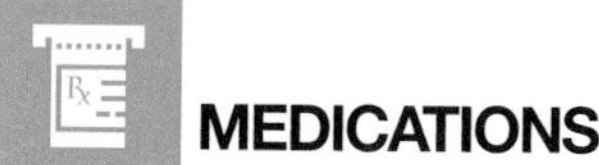

MEDICATIONS

DRUG(S) OF CHOICE
- Parenteral Vitamin B12 (cyanocobalamin)
  - ◊ 100 mcg subcutaneously for each dose
  - ◊ Administer daily for the first week
  - ◊ Administer weekly for one month
  - ◊ Monthly injections for remainder of life (patients may be taught to give self-injection)

Contraindications: None
Precautions: Do not give folic acid supplements without vitamin B12 - may cause fulminant neurological deficit
Significant possible interactions: N/A

ALTERNATIVE DRUGS
None

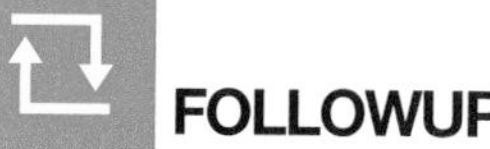

FOLLOWUP

PATIENT MONITORING
- Monthly injections of vitamin B12
- Endoscopy every 5 years to rule out gastric carcinoma

PREVENTION/AVOIDANCE
Early detection of anemia; workup of anemia

POSSIBLE COMPLICATIONS
- Hypokalemia may complicate first week of treatment
- Central nervous system symptoms may be permanent if patient is not treated in less than six months after symptoms begin
- Gastric polyps
- Stomach cancer

EXPECTED COURSE/PROGNOSIS
Anemia reversible with parenteral vitamin B12; neurologic effects not reversible with parenteral vitamin B12

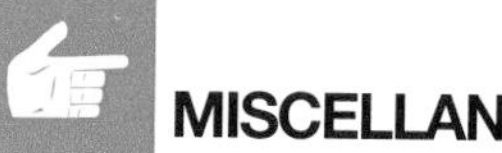

MISCELLANEOUS

ASSOCIATED CONDITIONS
- Autoimmune diseases including rheumatoid arthritis, IgA deficiency
- Graves' disease
- Myxedema
- Iron deficiency
- Thyroiditis
- Vitiligo
- Idiopathic adrenocortical insufficiency
- Hypoparathyroidism
- Agammaglobulinemia
- Tropical sprue
- Celiac disease
- Crohn disease
- Infiltrate disorders of the ileum and small intestine

AGE-RELATED FACTORS
Pediatric:
- Juvenile pernicious anemia occurs in older children and is the same in most respects as in adults
- Congenital pernicious anemia - usually evident before 3 years of age

Geriatric: More common in this age group and often in association with other autoimmune disorders, depression, and dementia
Others: N/A

PREGNANCY
N/A

SYNONYMS
- Addison anemia
- Megaloblastic anemia due to B12 deficiency

ICD-9-CM
281.0 Pernicious anemia
281.1 Other vitamin B12 deficiency anemia

SEE ALSO
Tropical sprue

OTHER NOTES
- There is a 3-fold likelihood of developing gastric carcinoma. Suggest endoscopy approximately every 5 years even if asymptomatic.
- Folic acid treatment in patients with pernicious anemia is contraindicated

ABBREVIATIONS
N/A

REFERENCES

- Bennett JC, Plum F, eds. Cecil Textbook of Medicine. 20th Ed. Philadelphia, W.B. Saunders Co., 1996
- Williams WJ, Beutler E, Erslev AJ, et al, eds. Hematology. 4th Ed. New York, McGraw-Hill, 1990
- Munseys W, ed. The Medical Clinic of North America 1992;76(3)
- Chui CH, Lau FY, Wong R, et al. Vitamin B12 deficiency--need for a new guideline. Nutrition 2001;17(11-12):917-20

Web references: 0 available at www.5mcc.com
Illustrations 1 available

Author(s):
Abdulrazak Abyad, MD, MPH

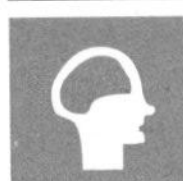

BASICS

DESCRIPTION A chronic hemoglobinopathy transmitted genetically, marked by moderately severe chronic hemolytic anemia, periodic acute episodes of painful "crises," and increased susceptibility to intercurrent infections, especially S. pneumoniae. The heterozygous condition (Hb A/S) is called sickle cell trait and is usually asymptomatic, with no anemia.
System(s) affected: Hemic/Lymphatic/Immunologic, Musculoskeletal
Genetics: Autosomal recessive, mostly in blacks. Homozygous presence of a variant hemoglobin, HbS or sickle hemoglobin. Heterozygous condition Hb A/S.
Incidence/Prevalence in USA: Approximately 1/500 black Americans and 1/1000 Hispanics have sickle cell anemia; 10% black Americans have sickle trait
Predominant age: All ages
Predominant sex: Male = Female

SIGNS & SYMPTOMS
- Often asymptomatic in early months of life
- After 6 months of age, earliest symptoms are pallor and symmetric, painful swelling of the hands and feet (hand-foot syndrome)
- Chronic hemolytic anemia
- Painful "crises" in bones, joints, abdomen, back, and viscera (account for 90% of all hospital admissions)
- Mild scleral icterus
- Increased susceptibility to infections, especially pneumococcal sepsis and Salmonella osteomyelitis
- Functional asplenia by age 5-6
- Delayed physical/sexual maturation, especially boys
- Many multi-system complications, especially in later childhood and adolescence
- Acute chest syndrome (clinical picture consistent with pneumonia and/or infection)

CAUSES
- At molecular level: Hb S is produced by substitution of valine for glutamic acid in the sixth amino acid position of the beta chains of the hemoglobin molecule. When deoxygenated, Hb S polymerizes and forms long rods that change RBC from biconcave to sickle shape.
- At cellular level: Sickle RBCs are inflexible; odd shape and cell rigidity cause increased blood viscosity, stasis, and mechanical obstruction of small arterioles and capillaries, leading to distal ischemia. Sickle RBCs are also more fragile than normal, leading to hemolytic destruction in blood and reticuloendothelial system.
- At clinical level: Chronic anemia; a variety of "crises"; infections
  - ◊ Vaso-occlusive crisis ("painful crisis"): Most common; pain results from tissue necrosis secondary to vascular occlusion and tissue hypoxia. Progressive organ failure and acute tissue damage results from repeated vaso-occlusive episodes.
  - ◊ Aplastic crisis: Temporary suppression of RBC production in bone marrow by severe infection
  - ◊ Hyperhemolytic crisis: Accelerated hemolysis; increased RBC fragility/shortened life span
  - ◊ Sequestration crisis: Splenic sequestration of blood (only in infants/young children)
  - ◊ Susceptibility to infection: Impaired/absent splenic function; defect in the alternate pathway of complement activation

RISK FACTORS
- Vaso-occlusive crisis
  - ◊ Hypoxia
  - ◊ Dehydration
  - ◊ Infection
  - ◊ Fever
  - ◊ Acidosis
  - ◊ Cold
  - ◊ Anesthesia
  - ◊ Strenuous physical exercise
  - ◊ Smoking
- Aplastic crisis
  - ◊ Severe infections
  - ◊ Human parvovirus B19 infection
  - ◊ Folic acid deficiency
- Hyperhemolytic crisis
  - ◊ Acute bacterial infections
  - ◊ Exposure to oxidant drugs

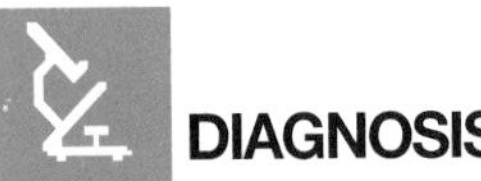

DIAGNOSIS

DIFFERENTIAL DIAGNOSIS
- Anemia: Other hemoglobinopathies, e.g., Hb SC disease, Hb C disease, Sickle cell-beta thalassemia
- Painful crisis: Other causes of acute pain in bones, joints, and abdomen. Seek infection and other precipitating causes.

LABORATORY
- Hb electrophoresis: Hb S predominates, variable amount Hb F, no Hb A. (In sickle cell trait, both Hb S and A are present).
- Screening tests: Sodium metabisulfite reduction-test; "Sickledex" test
- Anemia; hemoglobin approximately 8 g/dL (1.24 mmol/L); RBC indices usually normal but mean corpuscular volume (MCV) > 75 μm3 (> 75 fL)
- Reticulocytosis of 10-20%
- Leukocytosis; bands normal in absence of infection
- Thrombocytosis
- Peripheral smear: few sickled RBC's, polychromasia, nucleated RBC's, Howell-Jolly bodies
- Serum bilirubin mildly elevated (2-4 mg/dL [34-68 μmol/L]); fecal/urinary urobilinogen high
- ESR low
- Serum LDH elevated
- Haptoglobin absent or very low

Drugs that may alter lab results: N/A

Disorders that may alter lab results:
- Infection
- Other anemias (e.g., iron deficiency)

PATHOLOGICAL FINDINGS
- In moderate to severe cases, hyposplenism due to autosplenectomy is common
- Hypoxia/infarction in multiple organs

SPECIAL TESTS N/A

IMAGING
- Bone scan (to rule out osteomyelitis)
- CT/MRI (to rule out CVA)
- CXR: may show enlarged heart; diffuse alveolar infiltrates in acute chest syndrome

DIAGNOSTIC PROCEDURES N/A

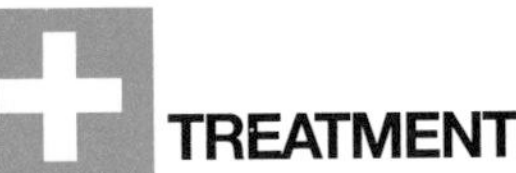

TREATMENT

APPROPRIATE HEALTH CARE
- General health maintenance: Assessment of growth/development, regular immunizations, vision/hearing screening, and regular dental care
- Hospitalization for many crises and complications

GENERAL MEASURES
- Infections/fever - prompt treatment with antibiotics
- Minimize factors that enhance sickling
- Painful crises - hydration (2 X maintenance fluids); analgesics (narcotic and nonnarcotic); oxygen if hypoxic
- Transfusion needed with aplastic crises, severe complications (i.e., CVA), before surgery, and with recurrent debilitating painful crises
- Retinal evaluation starting at school age to detect proliferative sickle retinopathy
- Special immunizations:
  - ◊ Influenza vaccine yearly starting at age 2
  - ◊ Heptavalent conjugated pneumococcal vaccine at 2, 4, 6 months; booster at 15 months
  - ◊ 23-valent pneumococcal vaccine at 2 years; booster at age 5
  - ◊ Meningococcal vaccine after age 2; need for booster unknown

SURGICAL MEASURES Bone marrow transplantation is curative but availability is limited

ACTIVITY
- Bedrest with crises
- Activity as tolerated; often limited due to chronic anemia and poor muscular development

DIET Balanced diet; folic acid supplementation; avoid alcohol (leads to dehydration)

PATIENT EDUCATION
- Guidelines for prompt management of fever, infections, pain, and specific complications should be reviewed at each visit
- Stress importance of keeping well-hydrated
- Teach early recognition of possible complications, especially priapism
- Genetic counseling
- Avoidance of alcohol and smoking

MEDICATIONS

DRUG(S) OF CHOICE

- Painful crises (mild, outpatient): nonnarcotic analgesics (ibuprofen, acetaminophen or tramadol)
- Painful crises (severe, hospitalized): parenteral narcotics, e.g., morphine, meperidine (Demerol) on fixed schedule; (PCA pump may be useful way of delivering narcotics); gradually lower dose and replace with oral medication as soon as possible (acetaminophen-codeine, ibuprofen). Correct dehydration and acidosis.
- Ketorolac and tramadol have shown excellent efficacy (in recent trials) of painful crisis. Ketorolac proved superior to meperidine.
- Corticosteroids (dexamethasone 0.3 mg/kg q 12 hours for 4 doses in children) have shown promise in reducing need for analgesia, oxygen, transfusions, and hospitalization in setting of painful crisis or chest syndrome
- Poloxamer 188, an artificial nonionic surfactant, appears promising in early studies for speeding resolution of painful crisis
- Prevention of painful crisis:
  - ◊ Hydroxyurea (Droxia) in adult patients with ≥ 3 crisis/year. Start with 15 mg/kg day single daily dose; titrate upward every 12 weeks if blood counts satisfactory. Increase in 5 mg/kg increments to maximum of 35 mg/kg/day. Reduces crisis and chest syndrome 50%; long term safety unknown. Contraindicated in pregnancy.
  - ◊ Nitric oxide, arginine butyrate, pentoxifylline, clotrimazole, and combination of erythropoietin with hydroxyurea show promise
  - ◊ Oral magnesium, 0.6 meq/kg/day has been shown to decrease frequency of painful crisis in one study
- Priapism prevention - stilbestrol possibly helpful
- Infections: prior to culture results, give antibiotic that covers S. pneumoniae, H. influenzae, mycoplasma pneumoniae and Chlamydia pneumoniae. If bone infection suspected, cover for staphylococcus aureus and salmonella.
- Prophylactic penicillin is indicated in all infants and children starting at 2 mos
  - ◊ 2-6 mos 62.5 mg bid; 6 mos-3 yrs 125 mg bid; 3-5 yrs 250 mg bid
  - ◊ If no pneumococcal infections and no splenectomy, stop prophylaxis at 5-6 years. If high risk remains, continue until puberty
  - ◊ Alternative penicillin, benzathine IM 300,000 units a month ages 4 mos-3 yrs and 600,000 units monthly ages 3-5 yrs
  - ◊ Rising pneumococcal resistance to penicillin may change future recommendations

Contraindications: None

Precautions: Avoid high-dose estrogen oral contraceptives; consider Depo-Provera as alternate contraceptive

Significant possible interactions: None

ALTERNATIVE DRUGS

- Other NSAIDs
- Folic acid supplements (recommended by most authorities) 0.1 mg/day from 0-6 mos; 0.25 mg/day from 6-12 mos; 0.5 mg/day from 1-2 yrs; 1 mg/day beyond age 2

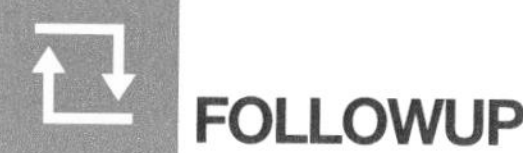

FOLLOWUP

PATIENT MONITORING

- Frequency determined by number/severity of crises and complications
- Early recognition/early treatment of infections. Parents/patient should be instructed that temperature of 101° F (38.3°C) or above requires immediate medical attention.
- All febrile patients require cultures (blood/urine), CXR, CBC/reticulocytes
- For patients who receive chronic transfusions - monitor for hepatitis and hemosiderosis
- Begin periodic evaluations at age 5 to detect early proliferative sickle retinopathy

PREVENTION/AVOIDANCE

- Avoid conditions that precipitate sickling (hypoxia, dehydration, cold, infection, fever, acidosis, anesthesia)
- Use of granulocyte colony-stimulating factor is absolutely contraindicated because it may cause crisis and acute chest syndrome
- Based on STOP trial, many authorities recommend periodically screening all children age 2-16 with transcranial Doppler ultrasound prior to any CVA. If blood velocity elevated, begin monthly transfusions which reduce CVA incidence 90%.

POSSIBLE COMPLICATIONS

- Alloimmunization
- Bone infarct
- Aseptic necrosis of femoral head
- Cerebrovascular accidents with neurologic sequelae (peak age 3-10). In the 10% of patients who suffer these, transfusions q 3-4 weeks will reduce risk by 90%. With this therapy, most patients require iron chelation therapy.
- Cardiac enlargement
- Cholelithiasis/abnormal liver function
- Chronic leg ulcers
- Priapism
- Hematuria/hyposthenuria
- Renal concentrating and acidifying defects
- Retinopathy
- Acute chest syndrome (infection/infarction), leading to chronic pulmonary disease
- Infections (pneumonia, osteomyelitis, meningitis, pyelonephritis). Increased risk of sepsis with each.
- Hemosiderosis (2° to multiple transfusions)
- Decreased intellectual function - even without clinical stroke

EXPECTED COURSE/PROGNOSIS

Anemia is lifelong. In second decade, number of crises diminish but complications more frequent. Some patients die in childhood, of CVA or sepsis. Most patients live to early-mid adulthood; median age of death is 42 for men and 48 for women. Common causes of death are infections, thrombosis, pulmonary emboli, or renal failure. Prognosis may be modified in future when gene therapy and/or messenger RNA repair become a reality

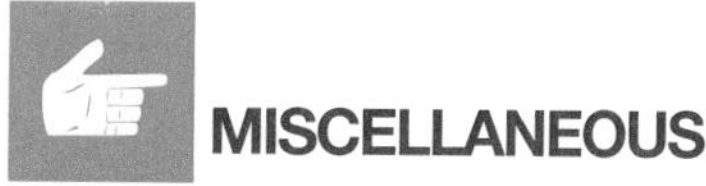

MISCELLANEOUS

ASSOCIATED CONDITIONS

Psychosocial effects of chronic illness, especially low self-esteem, depression, and dependency. May need counseling, tutoring, antidepressants and/or vocational training.

AGE-RELATED FACTORS

Pediatric:

- Sequestration crises and hand-foot syndrome seen only in infants/young children
- Functional asplenia in later childhood
- Adolescence/young adulthood:
  - ◊ Frequency of complications and secondary organ/tissue damage increase with age; except for strokes which occur mostly in childhood
  - ◊ Psychological complications, including body-image and sexual identity problems, interrupted schooling/career training, restriction of activities, stigma of chronic disease, low self-esteem, fear of future

Geriatric: N/A

Others: N/A

PREGNANCY

- Usually complicated and hazardous, especially 3rd trimester and delivery
- Complications include increased number/severity of crises, toxemia, infection, pulmonary infarction, phlebitis
- Fetal mortality 35-40%; abortions/stillbirths, prematurity
- Prophylactic partial exchange transfusion in 3rd trimester reduces maternal morbidity and fetal mortality

SYNONYMS

- Sickle cell disease
- Hb S disease

ICD-9-CM

282.60 Sickle cell disease, unspecified

SEE ALSO

OTHER NOTES N/A

ABBREVIATIONS N/A

REFERENCES

- Steinberg MH, Barton F, Castro O, et al. Effect of hydroxyurea on mortality and morbidity in adult sickle cell anemia: risks and benefits up to 9 years of treatment. JAMA 2003;289(13):1645-51
- Halsey C, Roberts IA. The role of hydroxyurea in sickle cell disease. Br J Haematol 2003;120(2):177-86
- Wilson RE, Krishnamurti L, Kamat D. Management of sickle cell disease in primary care. Clin Pediatr (Phila) 2003;42(9):753-61
- Claster S, Vichinsky EP. Managing sickle cell disease. BMJ 2003;327(7424):1151-5
- Ballas SK. Sickle cell anaemia: progress in pathogenesis and treatment. Drugs 2002;62(8):1143-72
- Fixler J, Styles L. Sickle cell disease. Pediatr Clin North Am 2002;49(6):1193-210
- Adams RJ. Lessons from the Stroke Prevention Trial in Sickle Cell Anemia (STOP) study. J Child Neurol 2000;15(5):344-9
- Wethers DL. Sickle cell disease in childhood: Part I. Laboratory diagnosis, pathophysiology and health maintenance. Am Fam Physician 2000;62(5):1013-20, 1027-8

Web references: 4 available at www.5mcc.com

Illustrations 1 available

Author(s):
Frank 'Chip' Celestino, MD

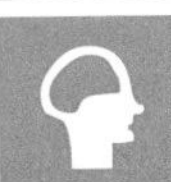

BASICS

DESCRIPTION A permanent localized (i.e., focal) dilatation of the abdominal aorta having at least a 50% increase in diameter compared to the expected diameter of the artery. The clinical presentation of aneurysms relates to location, size, type, and comorbid factors affecting the patient. The majority of aneurysms are asymptomatic. Some present with rupture, others with embolism or thrombosis. The management and indications for surgical repair is dictated by the natural history of the aneurysm, the type, the consequences of repair, and the general status of the patient. Types: infrarenal (90%) and thoracoabdominal.

System(s) affected: Cardiovascular, Hemic/Lymphatic/Immunologic

Genetics: Familial aggregations exist, but pathogenesis relates to interaction of genetics, environmental, and biochemical factors.

- Marfan syndrome
- Ehlers-Danlos syndrome

Incidence/Prevalence in USA:

- >15,000 deaths per year
- 10th leading cause of death in males over 55
- 2 to 5% of men > 60 years; 6% of men > 65; 11% of men > 75
- 4% of women > 65

Predominant age: Elderly

Predominant sex: Male > Female (4:1)

SIGNS & SYMPTOMS Majority of patients with abdominal aortic aneurysm (AAA) are asymptomatic. Many are discovered during radiologic procedures performed for other reasons.

- Pulsatile epigastric mass
- Vague abdominal pain
  - ◊ May radiate to the back of flank
- Encroachment by aneurysm
  - ◊ Vertebral body erosion
  - ◊ Gastric outlet obstruction
  - ◊ Ureteral obstruction
- Lower extremity ischemia secondary to micro or macro embolization of mural thrombus
- The triad of shock, pulsatile mass, and abdominal pain should always suggest rupture of AAA:
  - ◊ Shock may be absent if the rupture is contained
  - ◊ Palpable pulsatile mass may be absent in up to 50% with rupture
  - ◊ Pain may radiate to back or into groin
- Unusual presentations
  - ◊ Primary aortoenteric fistula--erosion/rupture of AAA into duodenum
  - ◊ Aortocaval fistula-- erosion/rupture of AAA into vena cava or left renal vein
  - ◊ Inflammatory aneurysm--encasement of aneurysm by thick inflammatory rind associated with chronic abdominal pain, weight loss, and elevated ESR. Surrounding viscera are densely adherent.

CAUSES

- Atherosclerosis
- Inflammatory (5-10%)
- Traumatic
- Genetic predisposition (Marfan, Ehlers-Danlos)

RISK FACTORS

- Hypertension
- Nicotine
- COPD
- Familial: siblings of patients with AAA
  - ◊ Males = 40% risk
  - ◊ Females = 15% risk

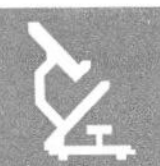

DIAGNOSIS

DIFFERENTIAL DIAGNOSIS

- Abdominal masses transmitting aortic pulse
- Other causes of abdominal pain (e.g., peptic ulcer disease)
- Other causes of back pain (e.g., arthritis, metastatic disease)

LABORATORY N/A

Drugs that may alter lab results: N/A

Disorders that may alter lab results: N/A

PATHOLOGICAL FINDINGS N/A

SPECIAL TESTS

- Evaluation for concomitant CAD
  - ◊ Selective evaluation for CAD is appropriate prior to elective AAA repair:
  - ◊ Mild, stable cardiac symptoms should have non invasive cardiac stress study
  - ◊ Coronary revascularization should be performed when the CAD would merit intervention on its own

IMAGING N/A

DIAGNOSTIC PROCEDURES

- Clinical examination
- Ultrasonography. Preferred initial diagnostic tool in suspected AAA, but is not reliable for diagnosis of rupture.
- CT scans. Preferred preoperative study. Avoid contrast if patient has significant renal insufficiency. Diagnostic for inflammatory aneurysm.
- MRI. Similar to CT and avoids contrast. MR angiography may replace arteriograms.
- Aortography. Does not define outside dimensions of aneurysms. Indications for aortography:
  - ◊ Associated renovascular hypertension
  - ◊ Symptoms of visceral angina
  - ◊ Significant iliofemoral occlusive disease
  - ◊ Peripheral aneurysms
  - ◊ Horseshoe or pelvic kidney
  - ◊ Prior colectomy

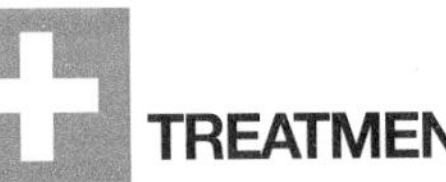

TREATMENT

APPROPRIATE HEALTH CARE

- The treatment of AAA is elective repair
- The prevention of RAAA is elective repair

GENERAL MEASURES

- Control hypertension
- Treat atherosclerotic risk factors

SURGICAL MEASURES

- Repair when:
  - ◊ Rupture occurs
  - ◊ Size > 5.5 cm (or > 6 cm in poor surgical risk patients)
  - ◊ Expansion > 0.5 cm/6 months
  - ◊ Symptoms occur
- Poor surgical risk patients:
  - ◊ Class III - IV angina; LVEF < 30%; recent CHF or MI; severe valve disease
  - ◊ Serum creatinine > 3 mg/dL
  - ◊ PaO2 < 50 mmHg; FEV1< IL
  - ◊ Cirrhosis with ascites
  - ◊ Diffuse retroperitoneal fibrosis; hostile abdomen
  - ◊ Physiologic age > chronological age
- Endovascular aneurysm repair
  - ◊ There are currently 3 devices approved by the FDA for marketing. Late complications of these devices continues to occur.
  - ◊ Long term CT surveillance is required
    - Adequate iliac/femoral access
    - Infrarenal non-aneurysmal neck length of at least 1 cm at the proximal and distal ends of the aneurysm
    - Morphology suitable for endovascular repair
    - One of the following: a diameter > 5 cm; a diameter of 4-5 cm and an increase in size by 0.5 cm in the past 6 months
    - Health status adequate to undergo the 2 hour plus implementation procedure

ACTIVITY Ad lib

DIET Low fat

PATIENT EDUCATION N/A

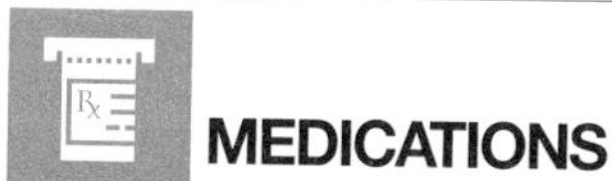

MEDICATIONS

DRUG(S) OF CHOICE N/A
Contraindications: N/A
Precautions: N/A
Significant possible interactions: N/A

ALTERNATIVE DRUGS N/A

FOLLOWUP

PATIENT MONITORING
- Hypertension control
- Lipid control
- Perioperative complications
  - ◊ MI = 5%
  - ◊ Renal failure =6%, chronic dialysis = 1%
  - ◊ Pulmonary failure = 5-8%
  - ◊ Microembolism (trash foot) = 1-4%
  - ◊ Ischemic colitis = 0.5-1%
  - ◊ Wound infection = 2%
  - ◊ Graft infection = < 0.5%
  - ◊ Stroke = 0.5-1%
  - ◊ Paraplegia = 0.2%
- Post-surgical monitoring
  - ◊ Anastomotic aneurysm
  - ◊ Graft infections
  - ◊ Aortoenteric fistula
  - ◊ Graft limb occlusion
  - ◊ Additional aneurysms - thoracic, thoracoabdominal, femoral

PREVENTION/AVOIDANCE
- Screening not cost effective
- High risk groups and incidence
  - ◊ Coronary disease: 5-9%
  - ◊ Peripheral vascular disease: 10-15%
  - ◊ First degree relative with AAA: 25%
  - ◊ Obese patients > 65 yrs
  - ◊ Presence of peripheral aneurysms

POSSIBLE COMPLICATIONS
- Rupture
- Associated dissection
- Thrombosis
- Embolization distally

EXPECTED COURSE/PROGNOSIS
- Usually expand over time (Laplace's Law: T=pr. Wall tension is directly related to blood pressure and the radius of the artery.) When wall tension exceeds wall tensile strength rupture occurs.
- Mean expansion is 0.4 cm/year
- Rupture risk is increased by
  - ◊ Diastolic hypertension
  - ◊ Tobacco use
  - ◊ Diameter > 6 cm
  - ◊ COPD
  - ◊ Familial history
- Ruptured aneurysms
  - ◊ 80% die before receiving definitive care and 50% of the remaining die during their treatment or hospitalization

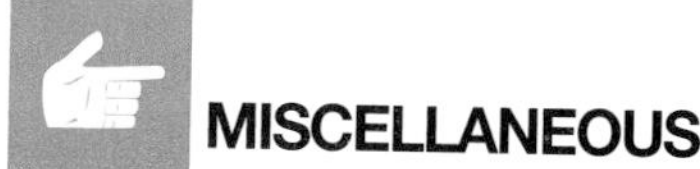

MISCELLANEOUS

ASSOCIATED CONDITIONS
- Marfan syndrome
- Ehlers-Danlos syndrome

AGE-RELATED FACTORS
Pediatric: Etiology more likely infectious or collagen disorders
Geriatric: More common in this age group and may present atypically
Others: N/A

PREGNANCY N/A

SYNONYMS
- Aortic aneurysms

ICD-9-CM
441.00 Dissection of aorta, unspecified site
441.4 Abdominal aneurysm without mention of rupture

SEE ALSO
Aortic dissection
Ehlers-Danlos syndrome
Giant cell arteritis
Marfan syndrome
Polyarteritis nodosa
Takayasu syndrome
Turner syndrome

OTHER NOTES N/A

ABBREVIATIONS
CAD = coronary artery disease
CHF = congestive heart failure
COPD = chronic obstructive pulmonary disease
LVEF = left ventricular ejection fraction
MI = myocardial infarction

REFERENCES

- Irvin TT, Abdominal pain: A surgical audit of 1190 emergency admissions. Brit J Surg 1989;76:1121
- Johnston W, et al, Suggested standards for reporting on arterial aneurysms. J Vasc Surg 1991;13:452
- Mason JJ, et al, The role of coronary angiography and coronary revascularization before non cardiac vascular surgery. JAMA 1995;273:1919
- Porter JM, ed, The Year Book of Vascular Surgery. New York, Mosby - Year Book, Inc. 1997
- Rutherford B, ed, Vascular Surgery. 14th Ed. Philadelphia, WB Saunders Co., 1995
- Szilagyi DE, et al, Contribution of abdominal aortic aneurysmectomy to prolongation of life. Ann Surg 1966;164:678
- Lederle FA, Wilson SE, Johnson GR, et al. Aneurysm Detection and Management Veterans Affairs Cooperative Study Group. Immediate repair compared with surveillance of small abdominal aortic aneurysms.
- N Engl J Med 2002;346(19):1437-44

Web references: 0 available at www.5mcc.com
Illustrations N/A

Author(s):
David H. Stubbs, MD

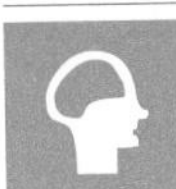

BASICS

DESCRIPTION Symptom complex resulting from mismatch of myocardial oxygen demand and supply

- Classic angina - a sense of choking or of pressure or heaviness deep to the precordium, usually brought on by exertion or anxiety and relieved by rest.
- Anginal equivalent - exertional dyspnea or exertional fatigue which results from myocardial ischemia and is relieved by rest or nitroglycerin
- Variant angina - also referred to as Prinzmetal angina describes angina occurring at rest of in atypical patterns such as after exercise or nocturnally. Prinzmetal angina is caused by coronary artery spasm and is associated with ECG changes (usually ST elevation) during symptoms
- Unstable angina - pain which is new or which is changed in character to become more frequent, more severe or both. Unstable angina portends myocardial infarction in a certain percentage of patients.

System(s) affected: Cardiovascular
Genetics: Coronary artery disease has genetic implications.
Incidence/Prevalence in USA: The presenting symptom of coronary artery disease in 38% of men and 61% of women.
Predominant age: Most common in middle age and older men; postmenopausal women
Predominant sex: Male > Female

SIGNS & SYMPTOMS

- Precordial pressure or heaviness, radiating to the back, neck or arms, brought on by exercise, emotional stress, meals, cold air or smoking, and relieved by rest or nitrates
- Discomfort may radiate to neck, lower jaw, teeth, shoulders, inner aspects of the arms or back
- Discomfort may be described with a clinched fist over the sternum (Levine's sign)
- Dyspnea on exertion may present as the only symptom
- A choking sensation on exertion is a classic symptom

CAUSES

- Atherosclerosis of the coronary arteries
- Coronary artery spasm
- Aortic stenosis
- Hypertrophic cardiomyopathy
- Severe hypertension
- Aortic insufficiency
- Primary pulmonary hypertension

RISK FACTORS

- Family history of premature coronary artery disease (CAD)
- Hypercholesterolemia
- Hypertension
- Tobacco abuse
- Diabetes mellitus
- Male gender
- Advanced age
- Morbid obesity

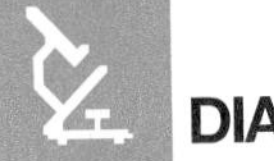

DIAGNOSIS

DIFFERENTIAL DIAGNOSIS

- Esophagitis (GERD)
- Esophageal spasm
- Peptic ulcer disease
- Gastritis
- Cholecystitis
- Costochondritis
- Pericarditis
- Aortic dissection
- Pleurisy
- Pulmonary embolus
- Pulmonary hypertension
- Pneumothorax
- Radiculopathy
- Shoulder arthropathy
- Psychological - anxiety and panic disorders

LABORATORY

- Total cholesterol - frequently elevated
- HDL cholesterol - frequently reduced
- LDL cholesterol - frequently elevated

Drugs that may alter lab results: N/A

Disorders that may alter lab results: N/A

PATHOLOGICAL FINDINGS Atherosclerosis of the coronary arteries

SPECIAL TESTS

- ECG - may show evidence of ischemia or prior myocardial infarction. Other findings are nonspecific and tracings are frequently normal. Bundle branch block, Wolff-Parkinson-White syndrome or intraventricular conduction delay may make the ECG unreliable.
- Exercise stress testing

IMAGING

- Radionuclide scintigraphy
- Stress echocardiography
- Stress scintigraphy
- Coronary angiography

DIAGNOSTIC PROCEDURES

- Rapid sequence MRI may show coronary artery calcification and thereby identify coronary artery disease. It does not identify obstructive coronary lesions however.
- Definitive evaluation and therapy involves coronary arteriography, necessary for confirmation and delineation of coronary disease, and direction of interventional therapy or surgery. Coronary artery stenting has proven very effective, with restenosis rates (in skilled hands) often below 10%, eliminating need for surgery in many cases. Surgery in CAD not amenable to intervention has proven long term benefit.

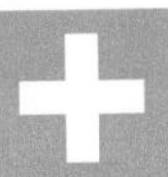

TREATMENT

APPROPRIATE HEALTH CARE The patient's symptoms should be brought under control medically. If symptoms are unstable, hospitalization is warranted.

GENERAL MEASURES

- Treatment goal - involves reducing myocardial oxygen demand or to increase oxygen supply
- Noninvasive testing is often indicated as a means of stratifying the patient's risk for an event that might seriously compromise myocardial function
- Quit smoking
- Minimize emotional stress

SURGICAL MEASURES Coronary artery bypass graft surgery, angioplasty, stent placement, atherectomy in selected cases

ACTIVITY

- As tolerated after consulting physician
- Exercise program after physician's approval; very effective if consistent

DIET Low fat, low cholesterol diet

PATIENT EDUCATION American Heart Association, 7320 Greenville Avenue, Dallas, TX 75231, (214)373-6300

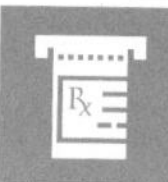

MEDICATIONS

DRUG(S) OF CHOICE
- Aspirin, 81-325 mg qd
- Beta-blockers: atenolol 25-100 mg qd, metoprolol 25-100 mg bid or bisoprolol 2.5-10 mg day. Beta-blockers are effective in reducing heart rate and thereby decreasing oxygen consumption and reducing angina. Adjust doses according to the clinical response. Aim to maintain resting heart rate of 50-60 beats per minute. Side effects are infrequent but include fatigue, erectile dysfunction, exacerbation of peripheral vascular and obstructive pulmonary disease, depression.
- Nitroglycerin 0.4 mg SL is the most effective therapy for acute anginal episodes. Repeat 2-3 times over a 10-15 minute time period; if no relief patient should seek immediate medical attention.
- Long acting nitrates (mononitrates or transdermal nitrates): should be used with a drug free interval of 10-14 hours to prevent tolerance. Tachyphylaxis occurs rapidly. Act through preload reduction and coronary vasodilatation. Side effects which include headaches and hypotension, tend to clear with continued usage. A beta-blocker or calcium channel blocker should be used in conjunction with the nitrates during the drug free interval.
- Long acting calcium channel blockers: verapamil 160-480 mg qd or diltiazem 90-360 mg qd or nifedipine 30-120 mg qd or amlodipine 5-20 mg qd. The various agents have their own individual side effects (i.e., verapamil - constipation; nifedipine - peripheral edema).
- HMC CoA reductase inhibitors (e.g., atorvastatin, pravastatin, lovastatin) for hypercholesterolemia. These drugs decrease incidence of symptomatic CAD, and reduce both myocardial infarction and death from MI.
- Heparin: low molecular weight heparin should be initiated in patients hospitalized with unstable angina
- Combination therapy: especially nitrates plus calcium antagonists with or without beta-blockers may be used.

Contraindications:
- Sildenafil (Viagra) with nitrates should be avoided due to hypotension and possible death

Precautions:
- Avoid verapamil and diltiazem with compromised ventricular function (left ventricular ejection fraction < 40%) especially in conjunction with beta-blockers.

Significant possible interactions:
- Combination therapies may impair LV function and precipitate heart failure
- Beta-blockers and calcium channel blockers
  - ◊ May combine to produce symptomatic heart block although either class of drug may act alone in producing this side effect
- Niacin may worsen glucose intolerance

ALTERNATIVE DRUGS
- Lipid lowering drugs are often initiated in patients with unfavorable lipid profiles, whether symptomatic from CAD or not
- Consider adding clopidogrel (Plavix) to ASA for severe diffuse CAD

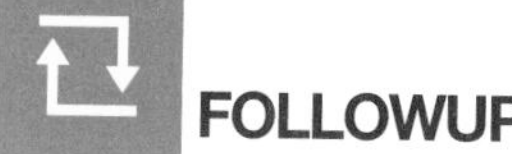

FOLLOWUP

PATIENT MONITORING
- Depends on the frequency and severity of the complaints
- Hospitalization is indicated in patients diagnosed with unstable angina

PREVENTION/AVOIDANCE
- Discontinue tobacco, adherence to low fat/low cholesterol diet, regular aerobic exercise program
- Anti-lipidemics

POSSIBLE COMPLICATIONS
- Related to myocardial damage occurring during infarction
- Arrhythmia
- Cardiac arrest
- Congestive heart failure

EXPECTED COURSE/PROGNOSIS
- Variable and depending on the extent of coronary artery disease as well as left ventricular function
- Annual mortality is 3-4% overall

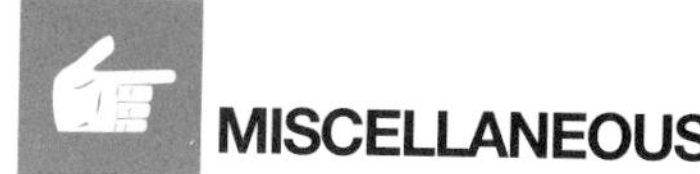

MISCELLANEOUS

ASSOCIATED CONDITIONS
- Hypercholesterolemia
- Claudication
- Peripheral vascular occlusion disease
- Arterial aneurysms
- Mitral regurgitation
- Papillary muscle dysfunction
- Ventricular aneurysm
- Abdominal aortic aneurysm
- Hypertrophic subaortic stenosis
- Primary hyperthyroidism
- Pernicious anemia and other high output states

AGE-RELATED FACTORS
Pediatric: Suspect familial dyslipidemias in children presenting with manifestations of coronary artery disease

Geriatric: Patients may be very sensitive to the side effects of medications (i.e., beta-blockers - depression)

Others: N/A

PREGNANCY
Other diagnosis should be excluded and the patient managed closely by an obstetrician and cardiologist as the metabolic demands of pregnancy will exacerbate symptoms and directly interfere with treatment

SYNONYMS
- Heberden syndrome

ICD-9-CM
411.1 Intermediate coronary syndrome
413 Angina pectoris
413.1 Prinzmetal angina
413.9 Other and unspecified angina pectoris

SEE ALSO

OTHER NOTES
N/A

ABBREVIATIONS
N/A

REFERENCES

- Topol E, editor. Textbook of Cardiovascular Medicine. Philadelphia: Lippincott-Raven; 1997
- Gibbons RJ, et al. ACC/AHA/ACP-ASIM guidelines for the management of patients with chronic stable angina: executive summary and recommendations. Circ 1999;99:2829-48
- Mehta SR, Yusuf S. Clopidogrel in Unstable angina to prevent Recurrent Events (CURE) Study Investigators. The Clopidogrel in Unstable angina to prevent Recurrent Events (CURE) trial programme; rationale, design and baseline characteristics including a meta-analysis of the effects of thienopyridines in vascular disease. Eur Heart J 2000;21(24):2033-41

Web references: 0 available at www.5mcc.com

Illustrations N/A

Author(s):
Phil Lobstein, MD

BASICS

DESCRIPTION

- Dermal (subcutaneous or submucosal) extravasation of fluid, leading to localized edema. Release of inflammatory vasoactive mediators increases vascular permeability.
- Skin, gastrointestinal tract and respiratory tract most commonly involved. Life threatening if upper airway is affected. Resolves in hours to days.
- Can be idiopathic or induced by medications, allergens (e.g., food) or physical agents (e.g., vibration, cold).
- Two rare but well described categories result from deficiency of C1 esterase inhibitor (C1 INH) of the compliment and kallikrein-kinin systems: hereditary angioedema (HAE) and acquired angioedema (AAE).
  - ◊ HAE type I (80-85%): Due to hereditary deficiency of C1-INH. Recurrent episodes of angioedema, involving both skin and mucous membranes or intestinal mucosa. 25% mortality.
  - ◊ HAE type II (15-20%): Normal or elevated quantities of functionally impaired C1-INH.
  - ◊ HAE type III: Rare, recently described form, observed in women.
  - ◊ AAE type I: Increased destruction of C1-INH. Occurs in patients with rheumatologic disorders and B-cell lymphoproliferative malignancies, such as leukemia, T-cell lymphoma, multiple myeloma, and essential cryoglobulinemia. Also reported with carcinomas, infections and vasculitides. Immune complexes continuously activate C1, leading to consumption of C1-INH and precipitating angioedema.
  - ◊ AAE type II: B cells secrete autoantibodies against C1-INH, leading to its inactivation.
- Medication-induced angioedema:
  - ◊ Immunologic hypersensitivity, as in penicillin reaction
  - ◊ Non-immunologic, as in reactions to NSAIDs (e.g., aspirin)
  - ◊ Angiotensin converting enzyme (ACE) inhibitors decrease levels of angiotensin II and stimulate production of bradykinin, a potent vasodilator, thus leading to angioedema. May occur immediately, or months after starting the drug.

System(s) affected: Skin/Exocrine
Genetics: HAE types I and II are inherited in autosomal dominant mode, while type III is X-linked. 25% of HAE occur as a result of spontaneous mutations.
Incidence/Prevalence in USA: 1 in 5,000. Accompanies urticaria 40-50% of time.
Predominant age: HAE - infancy to second decade of life. AAE - typically patients over 40yrs old.
Predominant sex: Male = Female (idiopathic)

SIGNS & SYMPTOMS

- Occurs alone or is associated with urticaria in 50% of cases
- Angioedema usually does not cause itching in comparison to urticaria, but can cause burning
- Relatively rapid onset of presentation; usually resolves spontaneously in < 72 hours
- Skin: may occur anywhere on body; usually face, extremities, genitalia; often asymmetric. Frequently disfiguring and frightening to the patient.
- Gastrointestinal: may present with intermittent unexplained abdominal pain
- Respiratory: may be associated with generalized anaphylactic reaction, potentially fatal if upper airway is compromised

CAUSES

- Idiopathic
- Medication-induced: ACE inhibitors, NSAIDs, antibiotics
  - ◊ ACE inhibitors (ACEI) are ascribed to 10-25% of angioedema cases mostly occurring within the first 3-4 weeks of use. However, first onset may be delayed years. Failure to react to re-challenge with drug does not rule out a cause-effect relation between the ACEI and angioedema.
  - ◊ Losartan (Cozaar) and valsartan (Diovan), both angiotensin II receptor blockers, can also cause angioedema. It can occur within 24 hours to 16 months after initiating losartan therapy.
- Allergen-induced: food allergens, such as fish, nuts and preservatives
- Physically-induced: cold, pressure, vibration
- Hereditary or acquired C1-INH deficiency
- Thyroid autoimmunity has been reported to be associated with angioedema

RISK FACTORS

- Medications and foods that can cause allergic reactions
- ACE inhibitors are contraindicated in patients with C1-INH deficiency

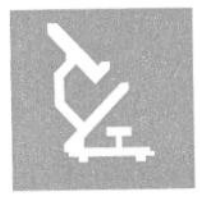

DIAGNOSIS

DIFFERENTIAL DIAGNOSIS

- Urticaria
- Allergic contact dermatitis
- Connective tissue disease: lupus, dermatomyositis
- Anaphylaxis
- Cellulitis, erysipelas
- Lymphedema
- Diffuse subcutaneous infiltrative process
- Localized edema

LABORATORY

- Testing for low serum C4 is a very sensitive but non-specific screening test for hereditary and acquired C1-INH deficiency. If C4 is normal, urticaria work-up is recommended.
- If C4 is low, C1-INH assay (immunoreactive) is performed for HAE type I, and C1-INH assay (functional) for HAE type II
- C1q is decreased in acquired C1-INH deficiency
- If C4 and C1q are low (as in AAE), neoplastic and autoimmune work-up are warranted. Routine blood tests, a smear, protein electrophoresis, immunophenotyping of lymphocytes and imaging studies are often undertaken to rule out hematological malignancies or cancer.

Drugs that may alter lab results: Antihistamines, H2-blockers, tricyclic antidepressants

Disorders that may alter lab results: N/A

PATHOLOGICAL FINDINGS Edema, vasculitis and/or perivasculitis involving subcutaneous tissues or dermis

SPECIAL TESTS N/A

IMAGING As part of neoplastic work-up if relevant

DIAGNOSTIC PROCEDURES Skin biopsy (poor correlation with clinical picture)

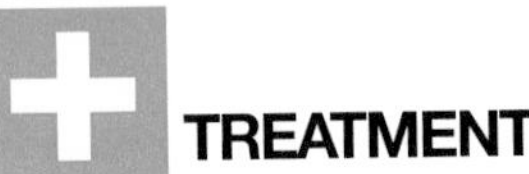

TREATMENT

APPROPRIATE HEALTH CARE

- Symptomatic, supportive management
- Ensure airway patency first! Protect airway if mouth, tongue, throat are involved
- CPR and transport to emergency facility, if necessary

GENERAL MEASURES

- Avoid known triggers
- Cool, moist compresses to control itching or burning

SURGICAL MEASURES N/A

ACTIVITY As desired. HAE patients should avoid violent exercise and trauma.

DIET Avoidance of known trigger foods

PATIENT EDUCATION Educate HAE and AAE patients to inform health care providers of their disease

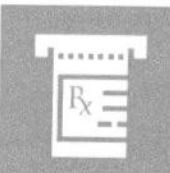

MEDICATIONS

DRUG(S) OF CHOICE
- First generation antihistamines for acute angioedema
  - ◊ Older children and adults: hydroxyzine (Vistaril) 10-25mg TID or diphenhydramine (Benadryl) 25-50mg q6h
  - ◊ Children under six: diphenhydramine 12.5mg (elixir) q6-8h (5mg/kg/day)
- Second generation H1 blockers are more expensive, about as effective as older antihistamines, but are less sedating (14% of patients, still less than 1st generation drugs), because they do not cross the blood-brain barrier
  - ◊ Fexofenadine (Allegra) 60mg bid
  - ◊ Loratadine (Claritin) 10mg daily
  - ◊ Acrivastine (Semprex) 8mg tid
  - ◊ Cetirizine (Zyrtec)10mg daily. More sedating than others in this class
- Anaphylaxis: Intubation if airway is threatened. Epinephrine 1:1000, 0.2-0.3mL IV or SC.
- Specific HAE and AAE therapy:
  - ◊ C1-INH concentrate
  - ◊ Attenuated androgens - danazol or stanozolol particularly effective for prevention of HAE. They increase amount of active C1-INH. Give 200-600mg daily for 1 month, then 5 days on, 5 days off. Side effects: headaches, weight gain, hematuria.
  - ◊ Antifibrinolytic agents (plasmin inhibitors), such as tranexamic acid and aminocaproic acid may also be used, but are not as effective as attenuated androgens in the management of HAE. Rarely can cause thrombophlebitis, embolism, myositis.

Contraindications: Danazol not to be used in childhood, pregnancy, lactation and prostate cancer

Precautions:
- Drowsiness with first generation drugs
- Second generation H1 blockers should be used with caution in pregnancy and the elderly

Significant possible interactions: Refer to manufacturer's profile of each drug

ALTERNATIVE DRUGS
Doxepin (Sinequan) may be effective for angioedema (10-25mg at bedtime)

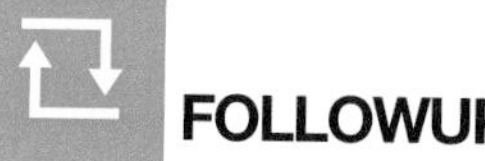

FOLLOWUP

PATIENT MONITORING
- Diagnostic work-up if symptoms severe, persistent or recurrent
- Protect airway if mouth, tongue, throat involved

PREVENTION/AVOIDANCE
- If etiology known, avoidance
- Avoid ACE inhibitors in patients with history of angioedema

POSSIBLE COMPLICATIONS
Anaphylaxis, respiratory compromise

EXPECTED COURSE/PROGNOSIS
Most patients with idiopathic angioedema do well. Chronic forms dependent on nature of pathology.

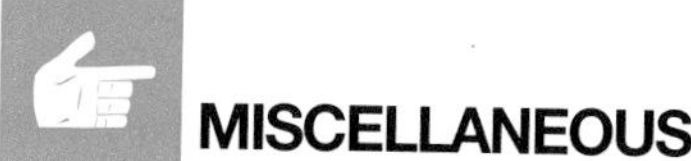

MISCELLANEOUS

ASSOCIATED CONDITIONS
- Urticaria
- Anaphylaxis

AGE-RELATED FACTORS
Pediatric: N/A
Geriatric: N/A
Others: N/A

PREGNANCY

SYNONYMS
- Angioneurotic edema
- Quincke's edema

ICD-9-CM
995.1 Angioneurotic edema
277.6 Other deficiencies of circulating enzymes

SEE ALSO

OTHER NOTES
Similar pathophysiology for urticaria and angioedema - localized anaphylaxis causes vasodilatation and vascular permeability of superficial (urticaria) or subcutaneous/deeper dermal tissue (angioedema)

ABBREVIATIONS
HAE = hereditary angioedema
AAE = acquired angioedema
C1-INH = C1-esterase inhibitor

REFERENCES

- Nzeako UC et al. Hereditary Angioedema. Arch Intern Med 2001;161:2417-29
- Heymann WR. Acquired angioedema. J Am Acad Dermatol 1997;26(4):611-5
- Frigas E, Nzeako UC. Angioedema. Clin Rev All Immunol 2002;23:217-31
- Charlesworth EN. Differential diagnosis of angioedema. Allergy and Asthma Proc 2002;23: 337-9
- Cooper KD: Urticaria and angioedema: Diagnosis and evaluation. J Am Acad Dermatol 1991;25:166
- Greaves M, Lawlor F: Angioedema: Manifestations and management. J Am Acad Dermatol 1991;25:155

Web references: 1 available at www.5mcc.com
Illustrations 1 available

Author(s):
Anatoli Freiman, MD

BASICS

DESCRIPTION Bite wounds to humans from dogs, cats, other animals including humans
System(s) affected: Endocrine/Metabolic, Hemic/Lymphatic/Immunologic, Nervous, Skin/Exocrine
Genetics: N/A
Incidence/Prevalence in USA:
- Dog bites: 1200/100,000
- Cat bites: 160/100,000
- Snake bites: 15/100,000 non-venomous bites and 3/100,000 venomous bites per year. Lifetime prevalence for animal bite 50,000/100,000.
- Dog bites are responsible for 1/3 million ER visits per year

Predominant age: All ages, but children more likely to be affected
Predominant sex: Male > Female

SIGNS & SYMPTOMS
- Bite wounds can be tears, punctures, scratches, avulsions or crush injuries
- Dog bites (80-90% of bites)
  - ◊ Hands are most commonly affected for adults
  - ◊ The face is the most common site of injury for children, and involvement of the trunk is uncommon
- Cat bites (10% of bites)
  - ◊ Predominantly involve the hands, followed by lower extremities, face and trunk
  - ◊ Are more likely to become infected because of puncture type of wounds

CAUSES
- Most bite wounds are from a domestic pet known to the victim. Large dogs are the most common source.
- Human bites are often the result of one person striking another in the mouth with a clenched fist

RISK FACTORS
- Dog bites are more common during warm weather. Male dogs more likely to bite.
- Clenched fist injuries are frequently associated with the use of alcohol

DIAGNOSIS

DIFFERENTIAL DIAGNOSIS The diagnosis is straight forward. What is of concern is judging the risk to the patient from the injury and resulting infection.

LABORATORY
- 85% of bite wounds will yield a positive culture, but culturing at time of injury is of little benefit
- Wound culture is essential in directing therapy of infected wounds. Some pathogens are slow growing so cultures should be kept for 7-10 days. Gram stain is sensitive but not specific for infecting organism.
- Dog bites - *Pasteurella multocida* is present in 25% of bites. *Streptococcus viridans*, *Staphylococcus aureus*, coagulase-negative Staphylococcus, *Bacteroides*, *C. canimorsus*, and *Fusobacterium* can also be found.
- Cat bites - *Pasteurella multocida* is present in 50% of bites. The wound is often contaminated by other mixed bacteria, including several species of both aerobic and anaerobic organisms.
- Human bites - Streptococcus species, *Staphylococcus aureus*, *Eikenella corrodens* and various anaerobic bacteria are common
- Other animal bites - scant information on the pathogens of these

Drugs that may alter lab results: Previous antibiotic therapy

Disorders that may alter lab results: N/A

PATHOLOGICAL FINDINGS N/A

SPECIAL TESTS N/A

IMAGING
- If bite wound is near a bone or joint, a plain radiograph is needed to check for bone injury and to use for comparison later if osteomyelitis is suspected
- In human bite wounds from clenched fist injuries, order plain film radiographs to check for metacarpal or phalanx fracture

DIAGNOSTIC PROCEDURES Surgical exploration might be needed to ascertain extent of injuries. Exploration should be performed on all serious hand wounds, especially clenched-fist injuries involving a joint.

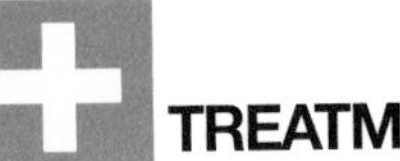

TREATMENT

APPROPRIATE HEALTH CARE Outpatient setting unless patient has fulminant infection requiring systemic antibiotics, close observation, or surgery

GENERAL MEASURES Elevation of the injured extremity to prevent swelling. Contact the local health department and consult about the prevalence of rabies in the species of animal involved.

SURGICAL MEASURES
- Copious irrigation of the wound with normal saline via a catheter tip is needed to reduce risk of infection
- Devitalized tissue needs débridement
- Débridement of puncture wounds not advised
- Consider surgical closure if the wound is clean after irrigation and bite is less than 12 hours old. Puncture wounds should be left open.
- Delayed primary closure in 3-5 days is an option for infected wounds
- Splint hand if it is injured
- Human bite wounds on the hands should not be primarily closed due to the high risk of infection. Large, gaping wounds should be reapproximated with widely space sutures or Steri-Strips.

ACTIVITY No restriction

DIET No special diet

PATIENT EDUCATION
- Discussion with parents at "well child checks" should include education on how to avoid animal bites
- KidsHealth at the AMA - www.ama-assn.org/insight/h_focus/nemours/emer/whattodo/bites.htm
- AAFP - www.aafp.org/patientinfo/dogbite.html

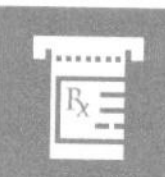

MEDICATIONS

DRUG(S) OF CHOICE

- Consider antirabies therapy
- Use tetanus toxoid in those previously immunized, but more than 5 years since their last dose
- Consider tetanus immune globulin (TIG) in patients without a full primary series of immunizations
- Prophylactic therapy if wound seen in first 12 hours:
  - ◊ Dog, cat, human - amoxicillin-clavulanate 250-500 mg tid po; child 20-40 mg/kg/day po given tid
  - ◊ Snake bite - if venomous, the patient needs rapid transport to facility capable of definitive evaluation. If an envenomation has occurred, the patient will need to receive antivenin unless envenomation was only minimal. Be sure patient is stable for transport; consider measuring and or treating coagulation and renal status along with any anaphylactic reactions before transport.
  - ◊ Other bites - amoxicillin-clavulanate (Augmentin) potassium - dosage - adult 250-500 mg po tid; child 20-40 mg/kg/day given tid
- Established infection
  - ◊ Once patient has developed a clinical infection, amoxicillin-clavulanate potassium (Augmentin) can be used pending culture reports

Contraindications: Do not use penicillin-derived antibiotics in those with penicillin allergy

Precautions: Prescribe dosage of antibiotics by body weight and renal function

Significant possible interactions: Antibiotics may decrease efficacy of oral contraceptives

ALTERNATIVE DRUGS

- Alternative therapy for penicillin allergic patients: (for prophylaxis or empiric treatment):
  - ◊ Approximately 10% cross reactivity with cephalosporins in penicillin allergic patients
  - ◊ Dog bite - Moxifloxacin 400 mg qd x 7 days in adults. In children trimethoprim-sulfamethoxazole along with clindamycin. Avoid cephalexin due to resistant strains of *P. Multocida*.
  - ◊ Cat bite - as for dog bite
  - ◊ Human bite - cefuroxime 500 mg bid
- If hospitalized with established infection, ampicillin-sulbactam (Unasyn) 1-2 gm IV q 6 hours or ticarcillin-clavulanate (Timentin) 3.1gm IV q 4-6 hours

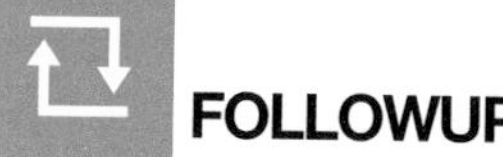

FOLLOWUP

PATIENT MONITORING

- Patient should be rechecked in 24-48 hours if not infected at time of first encounter
- Daily followup is warranted with active infections
- If antibiotics are used for an active infection, the duration of therapy should be 7-14 days depending on the severity of the infection and the clinical response

PREVENTION/AVOIDANCE

Instruct children and adults about animal hazards. Education of dog owners about responsible dog ownership. Stronger enforcement of animal control laws.

POSSIBLE COMPLICATIONS

Complications from bites can include septic arthritis, osteomyelitis, extensive soft tissue injuries with scarring, sepsis, hemorrhage, death. Gas gangrene can take an exceedingly rapid course and should be treated very aggressively.

EXPECTED COURSE/PROGNOSIS

Wounds should steadily improve and close over by 7-10 days

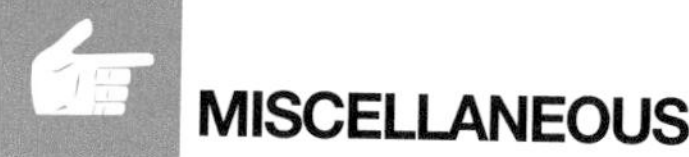

MISCELLANEOUS

ASSOCIATED CONDITIONS

N/A

AGE-RELATED FACTORS

Pediatric: Young children are more likely to have severe bites

Geriatric:

- Serious injury from any bite wound is more common in persons greater than 50 years old, those with wounds in the upper extremities or those with puncture wounds
- Increased risk of infection in those greater than 50 years old

Others: N/A

PREGNANCY

No special precautions

SYNONYMS

N/A

ICD-9-CM

879.8 Open wound(s) of unspecified site(s) without mention of complications

882.0 Open wound of hand except finger(s) alone without mention of complication

873.40 Open wound of face without mention of complications, unspecified site

SEE ALSO

Bartonella infections

Cellulitis

Rabies

Snake envenomations: Crotalidae

Snake envenomations: Elapidae

OTHER NOTES

Rabies: Contact your local health department for information about the risk of rabies

ABBREVIATIONS

N/A

REFERENCES

- Griego RD, et al. Dog, cat and human bites: A review. J AM Acad Dermatol 1995;33:1019-1029
- Cummings P. Antibiotics to prevent infection in patients with dog bite wounds: A meta-analysis. Ann Emerg Med 1994;23:535-540
- Presutti RJ. Prevention and treatment of dog bites. Am Fam Physician 2001;63(8):1567-72, 1573-74
- Sacks JJ, et al. Fatal dog attacks 1989-1994. Pediatrics 1996;97:891-895
- Fleisher GR. The management of bite wounds. NEJM 1999:340;138-140

Web references: 0 available at www.5mcc.com

Illustrations N/A

Author(s):

George R. Bergus, MD

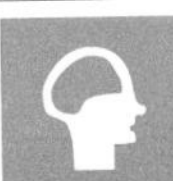

BASICS

DESCRIPTION A chronic, usually progressive, condition in which inflammatory changes and new bone formation occurs at the attachment of tendons and ligaments to bone (enthesopathy)
- Sacroiliac joint involvement is the hallmark of ankylosing spondylitis (AS) with variable degrees of spinal involvement. However, 20-30% of patients also have larger peripheral joint involvement

System(s) affected: Musculoskeletal
Genetics: Familial clustering and higher than expected frequency of HLA-B27 tissue antigen. Frequency of HLA-B27 in North American Caucasians = 7%. Frequency of HLA-B27 in African Americans = 1-2%.
Incidence/Prevalence in USA:
- 0.5-5 per 1000 in white males
- Less common in women and Blacks

Predominant age:
- Usually symptoms begin in early twenties
- Onset of symptoms - rarely occurs after age 40

Predominant sex: Male > Female (2-5:1)

SIGNS & SYMPTOMS
- Subgluteal or low back pain and/or stiffness
- Insidious onset
- Duration greater than 3 months
- Morning stiffness
- Frequently awaken at night to "walk off" stiffness
- Improvement in stiffness with activity
- Increased symptoms with rest
- Pleuritic chest pain is often an early feature
- Hip, shoulder, or knee complaints
- Diminished range of motion in the lumbar spine in all three planes of motion
- Loss of lumbar lordosis
- Thoracocervical kyphosis (rarely occurs before ten years of symptoms)
- Aortic root dilatation (1%)
- Aortic regurgitation murmur (1%)
- Acute anterior uveitis (25-30%)
- Osteoporosis
- Constitutional symptoms (fatigue, weight loss, low-grade fever)
- Plantar fasciitis

CAUSES Unknown

RISK FACTORS
- HLA-B27 (1-7% of HLA-B27 positive adults likely to have AS)
- Positive family history
- 10% risk of developing AS for HLA-B27 positive child of spondylitic parent

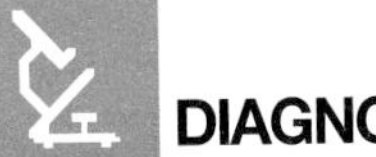

DIAGNOSIS

DIFFERENTIAL DIAGNOSIS
- Reactive arthritis
- Psoriatic arthritis
- Diffuse idiopathic skeletal hypertrophy (DISH)
- Spondylitis associated with inflammatory bowel disease
- Rheumatoid arthritis

LABORATORY
- HLA-B27 tissue antigen is present in 90% of white AS patients compared to 5-8% incidence in general population
- Erythrocyte sedimentation rate (ESR) is elevated in 80% of cases, but correlates poorly with disease activity and prognosis
- Absent rheumatoid factor
- Mild normochromic anemia (15%)

Drugs that may alter lab results: N/A

Disorders that may alter lab results: N/A

PATHOLOGICAL FINDINGS
- Erosive changes coupled with new bone formation at attachment of tendons and ligaments to bone resulting in ossification of periarticular soft-tissues
- Synovial changes are indistinguishable from rheumatoid arthritis. Erosion of articular cartilage is less severe than in rheumatoid arthritis.

SPECIAL TESTS
- Synovial fluid - mild leukocytosis, decreased viscosity
- EKG - conduction defects
- Measurement of respiratory excursion of chest wall - less than 5 cm maximal respiratory excursion of chest wall measured at fourth intercostal space. Less than 2.5 cm is virtually diagnostic of ankylosing spondylitis.
- Wright-Schober test for lumbar spine flexion is abnormal

IMAGING
- Sacroiliac joint early - sclerosis on both sides of joint not extending more than 1 cm from articular surface
- Sacroiliac joint late - ankylosis of sacroiliac joint; osteopenia
- Spine - "squaring" of vertebral bodies and ossification of annulus fibrosis giving appearance of "bamboo spine". Ankylosis of facet joints.
- Peripheral joint - symmetric erosive changes in larger joints. Pericapsular ossification, sclerosis, loss of joint space.

DIAGNOSTIC PROCEDURES
- Physical examination
- Radiographs - sacroiliac joint films, lumbar spine series

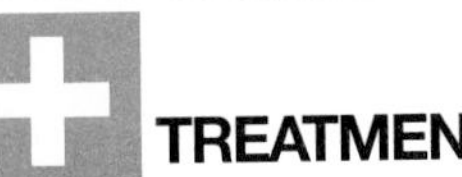

TREATMENT

APPROPRIATE HEALTH CARE Outpatient

GENERAL MEASURES
- Posture training and range of motion exercises for spine are essential
- Firm bed
- Sleep in prone position or supine without a pillow
- Breathing exercises 2-3 times/day
- Swimming
- Physical therapy
- Stop smoking, if a smoker
- Avoidance of trauma/contact sports
- Avoidance of prolonged standing

SURGICAL MEASURES Total hip replacement should be considered to restore upright posture and to control pain

ACTIVITY Encourage active lifestyle

DIET No special diet

PATIENT EDUCATION
- For a listing of sources for patient education materials favorably reviewed on this topic, physicians may contact: American Academy of Family Physicians Foundation, P.O. Box 8418, Kansas City, MO 64114, (800)274-2237, ext. 4400

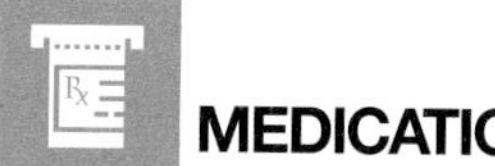

MEDICATIONS

DRUG(S) OF CHOICE
- Nonsteroidal anti-inflammatory drugs provide symptomatic relief
- Selection is empiric, but traditionally indomethacin 50 mg tid or qid has been used
- Osteoporosis prophylaxis and treatment

Contraindications: See Precautions

Precautions:
- All patients on long term NSAIDs should have renal function monitored
- NSAIDs may aggravate peptic ulcer disease or cause gastritis
- Don't use NSAIDs for patients with a bleeding diathesis or patients requiring anticoagulants

Significant possible interactions: Refer to manufacturer's profile of each drug

ALTERNATIVE DRUGS
- Etanercept (anti-tumor necrosis factor alpha agent) showed rapid, significant and sustained improvement
- Thalidomide shows promise
- Infliximab may be efficacious

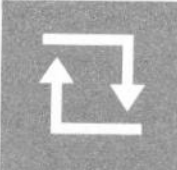

FOLLOWUP

PATIENT MONITORING Visits every six to twelve months to monitor posture and range of motion

PREVENTION/AVOIDANCE N/A

POSSIBLE COMPLICATIONS
- Spine: Pseudarthrosis, cervical spine fracture (high mortality rate), C1-C2 subluxation, spondylodiscitis, cauda equina syndrome (rare)
- Peripheral joint ankylosis
- Pulmonary: Restrictive lung disease, diaphragmatic breathing, upper lobe fibrosis (rare)
- Cardiac: Conduction defects, aortic insufficiency (2%), aortitis, pericarditis
- Uveitis
- Renal: IgA nephropathy, amyloidosis (rare)
- Cutaneous LCV (rare)

EXPECTED COURSE/PROGNOSIS
- Unpredictable course
- Prognosis good if mobility and upright posture maintained. Usually progressive disability.

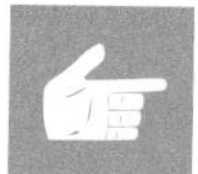

MISCELLANEOUS

ASSOCIATED CONDITIONS
- Inflammatory bowel disease
- Uveitis
- Iritis
- Psoriasis

AGE-RELATED FACTORS
Pediatric: N/A

Geriatric: N/A

Others: N/A

PREGNANCY N/A

SYNONYMS
- Rheumatoid spondylitis
- Marie-Strumpell disease

ICD-9-CM
720.0 Ankylosing spondylitis

SEE ALSO
Arthritis, psoriatic
Arthritis, rheumatoid (RA)
Crohn disease
Reiter syndrome
Ulcerative colitis

OTHER NOTES N/A

ABBREVIATIONS N/A

REFERENCES

- van der Linden S, van der Heijde D. Ankylosing spondylitis. Clinical features. Rheum Dis Clin North Am 1998;24(4):663-76, vii
- Klippel J, ed. Primer on the Rheumatic Diseases. 12th Ed. Atlanta, Arthritis Foundation, 2001
- Ruddy S, Kelley S. Textbook of Rheumatology. 6th ed. Philadelphia: WB Saunders Co; 2001
- Gorman JD, Sack KE, Davis JC Jr. Treatment of ankylosing spondylitis by inhibition of tumor necrosis factor alpha. N Engl J Med 2002;346(18):1349-56
- Davis JC Jr, Huang F, Maksymowych W. New therapies for ankylosing spondylitis: etanercept, thalidomide, and pamidronate. Rheum Dis Clin North Am 2003;29(3):481-94

Web references: 2 available at www.5mcc.com

Illustrations N/A

Author(s):
Jane S. Kim, MD

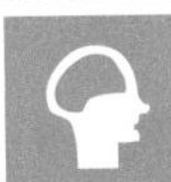

BASICS

DESCRIPTION Localized induration and fluctuance due to inflammation of the soft tissue near the rectum or anus. 80% are perianal, the remainder are intrasphincteric or supra-levator.
System(s) affected: Gastrointestinal, Skin/Exocrine
Genetics: No known genetic pattern
Incidence/Prevalence in USA: Common
Predominant age: All ages (most common in infants)
Predominant sex: Male > Female (4:1)

SIGNS & SYMPTOMS
- Perirectal swelling for superficial abscesses
- Perirectal redness
- Perirectal tenderness
- Perirectal throbbing pain
- Fever and other toxic symptoms with deep abscesses
- If abscess is not accompanied by external swelling, digital exam will reveal a swollen tender mass
- Pain on defecation

CAUSES
- Bacterial invasion of the anal glands found in the intersphincteric space which may begin with an abrasion or tear in lining of anal canal, rectum or perianal skin
- Organisms: usually mixed, E. coli, Proteus vulgaris, streptococci, staphylococci, bacteroides, pseudomonas aeruginosa

RISK FACTORS
- Inciting trauma
  - ◊ Injections for internal hemorrhoids
  - ◊ Enema tip abrasions
  - ◊ Puncture wounds from eggshells or fish bones
  - ◊ Foreign objects
  - ◊ Prolapsed hemorrhoid
- Inflammatory bowel disease
- Chronic granulomatous disease
- Immunodeficiency disorders
- Hematologic malignancies (5-8% of these patients will have abscess at some time)

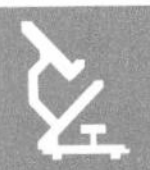

DIAGNOSIS

DIFFERENTIAL DIAGNOSIS
- Carcinoma
- Retrorectal tumors
- Crohn disease
- Primary lesions of syphilis
- Tuberculous ulceration

LABORATORY CBC - leukocytosis

Drugs that may alter lab results: N/A

Disorders that may alter lab results: N/A

PATHOLOGICAL FINDINGS
- Inflammation of anal mucosa
- Pus
- Inflammatory tissue

SPECIAL TESTS N/A

IMAGING Barium enema (rarely needed)

DIAGNOSTIC PROCEDURES
Only indicated if diagnosis in doubt:
- Sigmoidoscopy - rule out unusual causes
- Proctoscopy - redness, induration of anus; tender mass

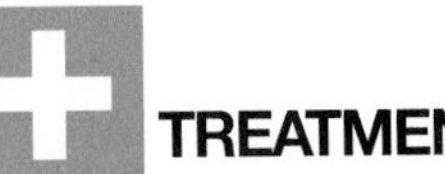

TREATMENT

APPROPRIATE HEALTH CARE
- Outpatient surgery
- Inpatient surgery with IV antibiotics for supra-levator abscess or toxicity

GENERAL MEASURES N/A

SURGICAL MEASURES
- Perianal abscess
  - ◊ Incise and drain abscess
  - ◊ Local anesthetic frequently appropriate
  - ◊ Pack wound with lodoform gauze (24-48 hours)
- Ischiorectal abscess
  - ◊ Incise and drain abscess
  - ◊ General anesthetic usually required
  - ◊ Pack wound with lodoform gauze (removed gradually over several days)
  - ◊ Fistulectomy may be done at same time in selected cases
- After surgery:
  - ◊ Sitz baths q 2-4 hours
  - ◊ Heating pad, heat lamp or warm compress as needed for pain
  - ◊ Encourage moving legs as soon as possible
  - ◊ Prevent constipation

ACTIVITY Resume work and normal activity as soon as possible

DIET Increase fiber and fluid intake

PATIENT EDUCATION
- Sitz bath instruction
- Diet instructions
- Dressing change instructions
- Stress length of time to heal
- Stress physical cleanliness
- Possible development of fistula-in-ano
- Stress stool regularity

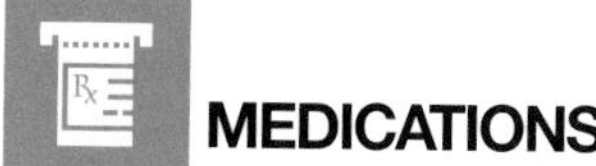

MEDICATIONS

DRUG(S) OF CHOICE
- Antibiotics
- Stool softening laxatives

Contraindications: Refer to manufacturer's literature
Precautions: Refer to manufacturer's literature
Significant possible interactions: Refer to manufacturer's literature

ALTERNATIVE DRUGS N/A

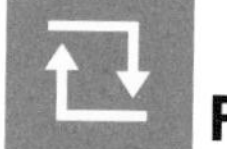

FOLLOWUP

PATIENT MONITORING Routine postoperative care with attention to wound healing which should progress from the inside out

PREVENTION/AVOIDANCE
- Avoid constipation
- Don't use enemas
- Avoid rectal temperatures or medicines in immunocompromised patients

POSSIBLE COMPLICATIONS
- Possible anorectal fistula (in 25% of patients)
- Possible rectovaginal fistula
- Fecal incontinence due to rupture through sphincter muscle
- Recurrence of abscess if underlying cause not corrected
- Necrotizing and infection with rapid progression and sepsis

EXPECTED COURSE/PROGNOSIS
- Slow healing depending on extent of disease and concurrent illnesses, complete healing by 6 months if no complications
- Healing in infants may be complete in 1-3 weeks
- Drainage alone results in cure of 50% or more

MISCELLANEOUS

ASSOCIATED CONDITIONS
- Crohn disease
- Other inflammatory disease such as appendicitis, salpingitis, diverticulitis
- Possibly perianal hidradenitis suppurativa, or HIV infection in patients with recurring perianal or ischiorectal abscesses

AGE-RELATED FACTORS
Pediatric: Common in first year of life
Geriatric: In elderly patients, a high pelvirectal abscess may cause no symptoms except lower abdominal pain and fever
Others: N/A

PREGNANCY N/A

SYNONYMS N/A

ICD-9-CM
566 Abscess of anal and rectal regions

SEE ALSO
Anorectal fistula

OTHER NOTES N/A

ABBREVIATIONS N/A

REFERENCES

- Schwartz SI, Shires GT, Spencer FC, et al, editors. Principles of Surgery. 7th ed. New York: McGraw-Hill Book Co; 1999
- Ashcraft KW, Murphy JP, Sharp RJ, editors. Pediatric Surgery. 3rd ed. Philadelphia: WB Saunders Co; 2000
- Fazio VW. Anorectal Disorders. In: Gastroenterology Clinics of North America. Philadelphia: WB Saunders Co; 1987
- Ziegler M, Azizkhan R, Weber T, et al, editors. Operative Pediatric Surgery. New York: McGraw-Hill Companies; 2003

Web references: 1 available at www.5mcc.com
Illustrations N/A

Author(s):
Timothy L. Black, MD

BASICS

DESCRIPTION Inflammatory track with one opening in the anal canal and another in perianal skin. Fistulas occur spontaneously or secondary to perirectal abscess. Most fistulas originate in the anal crypts at the anorectal juncture.

- Goodsall's rule
  - ◊ If external opening is anterior to an imaginary line drawn horizontally through anal canal, fistula usually runs directly into anal canal
  - ◊ If external opening is posterior to line, the fistula usually curves to posterior midline of anal canal
  - ◊ In children, track is usually straight
- Classification
  - ◊ Intersphincteric
  - ◊ Transsphincteric
  - ◊ Suprasphincteric
  - ◊ Extrasphincteric

System(s) affected: Gastrointestinal, Skin/Exocrine
Genetics: No known genetic pattern
Incidence/Prevalence in USA: Common
Predominant age: All ages
Predominant sex: Male = Female

SIGNS & SYMPTOMS

- Constant or intermittent drainage or discharge
- Firm tender perianal lump
- External anal sphincter pain during and after defecation
- Spasm of external anal sphincter during and after defecation
- Anal bleeding
- Discoloration of skin surrounding the fistula
- Fistulous opening frequently granulose or scarred
- Possible fever

CAUSES

- Erosion of anal canal
- Extension from infection from a tear in lining in anal canal
- Infecting organism is commonly Escherichia coli

RISK FACTORS

- Injection of internal hemorrhoids, puncture wound from eggshells or fish bones, foreign objects, enema tip injuries
- Ruptured anal hematoma
- Prolapsed internal hemorrhoid
- Acute appendicitis, salpingitis, diverticulitis
- Inflammatory bowel disease (chronic ulcerative colitis, Crohn disease)
- Previous perirectal abscess
- Radiation treatment to perineum/pelvis

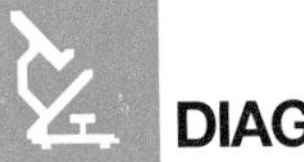

DIAGNOSIS

DIFFERENTIAL DIAGNOSIS

- Pilonidal sinus
- Perianal abscess
- Urethroperineal fistulas
- Ischiorectal abscess
- Submucous or high muscular abscess
- Pelvirectal abscess (rare)
- Rule out: Crohn disease; carcinoma; retrorectal tumors

LABORATORY

- CBC (usually not indicated)
- Prometheus IBD First Step serology (if Crohn disease suspected)

Drugs that may alter lab results: N/A

Disorders that may alter lab results: N/A

PATHOLOGICAL FINDINGS

- Fistulous tract may be simple or multiple
- Fistulous tract has primary opening in anal crypt; secondary opening in anal skin, para-anal skin, perineal skin, or in rectal mucus membrane
- Anal sinus - opens in anal crypt
- Termination of sinus is blind and located in para-anal or pararectal tissue

SPECIAL TESTS N/A

IMAGING Lower GI series if inflammatory bowel disease suspected

DIAGNOSTIC PROCEDURES

- Proctoscopy
- Sigmoidoscopy
- Probe inserted into tract to determine its course (be careful not to create an artificial opening)
- Injection of dilute methylene blue into abscess cavity may be helpful in demonstrating fistula

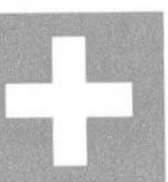

TREATMENT

APPROPRIATE HEALTH CARE Outpatient surgery

GENERAL MEASURES Sitz baths 3-4 times per day until definitive surgery

SURGICAL MEASURES

- Fistulotomy - surgical incision of entire length of fistula (unroofing). Mucosal tract may be cauterized or curetted. Sphincterotomy.
- Fistulectomy - complete excision of tract (rarely indicated due to extensive tissue loss). Sphincterotomy.
- General anesthesia or regional anesthesia usually required
- Postoperative - hot sitz baths
- Avoid constipation

ACTIVITY Resume work and normal activity as soon as possible

DIET Clear liquid diet until gastrointestinal function returns

PATIENT EDUCATION

- Stress perianal cleanliness
- Sitz baths

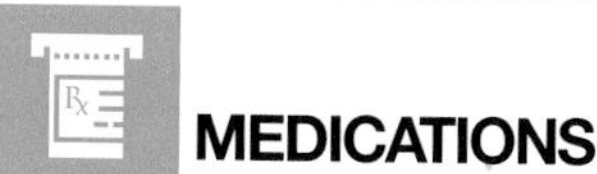

MEDICATIONS

DRUG(S) OF CHOICE
- Broad spectrum antibiotic if active infection
  - ◊ Cephalexin (Keflex)
  - ◊ Cefadroxil (Duricef)
  - ◊ Ampicillin-sulbactam (Unasyn)
  - ◊ Amoxicillin-clavulanate (Augmentin)
- Stool-softening laxative

Contraindications: Refer to manufacturer's literature
Precautions: Refer to manufacturer's literature
Significant possible interactions: Refer to manufacturer's literature

ALTERNATIVE DRUGS N/A

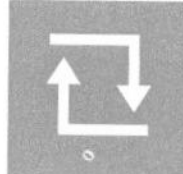

FOLLOWUP

PATIENT MONITORING Frequent follow-up examinations following surgery to ensure complete healing and assess continence

PREVENTION/AVOIDANCE N/A

POSSIBLE COMPLICATIONS
- Constipation (urge to defecate may be suppressed due to pain)
- Rectovaginal fistula
- Partial incontinence of fecal material if sphincter is divided
- Delayed wound healing
- Low grade carcinoma may develop in long-standing fistulas
- Recurrent anorectal fistula if fistula is incompletely opened or excised
- Chronic intermittent infections
- Sepsis (rarely)

EXPECTED COURSE/PROGNOSIS
- Surgical results usually excellent
- Postoperative healing requires 4-5 weeks for perianal fistulas; 12-16 weeks for deeper fistulas
- Postoperative healing may occur within 2-3 weeks in children

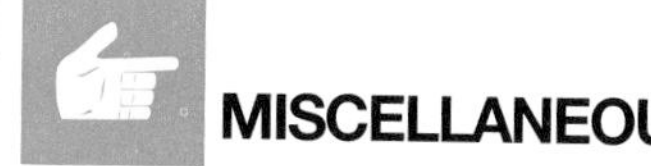

MISCELLANEOUS

ASSOCIATED CONDITIONS
- Possibly associated with penetrating injury, intestinal tuberculosis, ulcerative colitis
- Hidradenitis suppurativa
- Crohn disease

AGE-RELATED FACTORS
Pediatric: Most common in infants. More frequent in males.
Geriatric: Constipation is a common complication
Others: N/A

PREGNANCY N/A

SYNONYMS
- Fistula-in-ano
- Anal fistula

ICD-9-CM
565.1 Anal fistula

SEE ALSO
Anorectal abscess
Crohn disease

OTHER NOTES N/A

ABBREVIATIONS N/A

REFERENCES

- Kirsner JB, Shorter G, editors. Diseases of the Colon, Rectum and Anal Canal. Baltimore: Williams & Wilkins; 1989
- Sleisenger MH, Fordtran JS, editors. Gastrointestinal Disease: Pathophysiology, Diagnosis, Management. 5th ed. Philadelphia: WB Saunders Co; 1994
- Schwartz SI, Shires GT, Spencer FC, et al, editors. Principles of Surgery. 7th ed. New York: McGraw-Hill Book Co; 1999
- O'Neill JA, Rowe MI, Grosfeld JL, et al. Pediatric Surgery. 5th ed. St Louis: Mosby; 1998

Web references: 1 available at www.5mcc.com
Illustrations N/A

Author(s):
Timothy L. Black, MD

BASICS

DESCRIPTION Anorexia (AN) always involves refusal to maintain a reasonable body weight. AN is divided into restricting and binge-eating/purging subtypes.
System(s) affected: Cardiovascular, Endocrine/Metabolic, Gastrointestinal, Nervous, Reproductive
Genetics: First degree female relatives contribute; perfectionism
Incidence/Prevalence in USA: Approximately 1% of females; males comprise 10-50% of cases
Predominant age: Usually adolescents or young adults, but can occur at any age
Predominant sex: Female > Male

SIGNS & SYMPTOMS
- Usually insidious in onset
- Amenorrhea
- Onset may be stress related
- Deny seriousness of problem
- Claim to feel fat even when emaciated
- Preoccupation with body size, weight control
- Elaborate food preparation and eating rituals
- Extensive exercise, especially running or use of stair stepper
- Stress fractures
- Sexual disinterest; social isolation
- Cracked, dry skin, sparse scalp hair
- Fine, downy lanugo hair on extremities, face, and trunk
- Growth arrest
- Decreased pain sensitivity
- Hypotension and bradycardia
- Hypothermia, cold intolerance
- Peripheral edema
- Cognitive impairment
- Constipation

CAUSES Serotoninergic dysregulation commonly implicated. Thought to be genetic and emotional. Comorbid major depression and/or dysthymia in 50-75% of patients. Obsessive-compulsive disorder in 10-13% of patients.

RISK FACTORS
- Perfectionistic personality, compulsivity
- Low self-esteem, body dissatisfaction
- Achievement pressure; high self-expectations
- Acceptance of the culturally condoned ideal of slimness
- Ambivalence about dependence/independence
- Stress due to multiple responsibilities, tight schedules
- Early puberty
- Diabetes
- History of sexual abuse is equivalent to other psychiatric patient populations

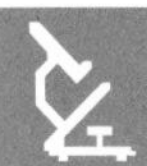

DIAGNOSIS

DIFFERENTIAL DIAGNOSIS Kluver-Bucy, Kleine-Levin, Crohn disease, Addison disease; brain tumor; bulimia; depressive disorders with loss of appetite; food phobia; conversion disorder; schizophrenic disorder; body dysmorphic disorder; hyperthyroidism

LABORATORY
- Most findings are directly related to starvation, dehydration: no biological test is specific for anorexia. All findings may be within normal limits.
- Diminished plasma LH, FSH, T3, leptin
- Elevated growth hormone, cortisol, cholesterol, vasopressin
- Abnormal liver enzymes
- Diminished BUN, creatinine clearance
- Flat glucose tolerance curve, depressed fasting blood sugar
- Anemia, low B-12 level
- Low resting metabolic rate
- Low CD4/CD8 ratio
- Electrolyte disturbance; prolonged QT interval
- Neutropenia with relative lymphocytosis
- Hypercarotenemia
- Low serum zinc
- Abnormal CT, MRI (ventricular enlargement)
- Osteoporosis
- Blunted prolactin response to serotonin agonists
- Decreased binding of serotonin uptake inhibitors

Drugs that may alter lab results: N/A

Disorders that may alter lab results: N/A

PATHOLOGICAL FINDINGS All are directly related to starvation
- Arrested maturation
- Pathological fractures
- Cognitive deficits

SPECIAL TESTS Measure percent body fat and bone density (DEXA)

IMAGING
- Not indicated in most cases
- CT shows ventricular enlargement during starvation
- MRI shows decrease in grey and white matter; grey matter deficit may persist

DIAGNOSTIC PROCEDURES
- Psychological screening
- Symptom assessment scale (EAT, EDI, SCANS)

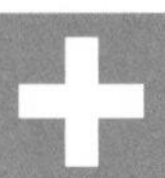

TREATMENT

APPROPRIATE HEALTH CARE
- Hospitalize if weight less than 75% of normal for height and age; if marked orthostatic hypotension, bradycardia less than 40, tachycardia more than 100 or inability to sustain core body temperature of 98.6°, if patient is suicidal; or if there has been no response to outpatient therapy.
- Initial goal geared to weight restoration
- Partial hospitalization if patient more than 70% of ideal body weight, motivated and capable of interpersonal; relatedness

GENERAL MEASURES
- Inpatient:
  - ◊ If possible admit to specialized eating disorders unit
  - ◊ Monitor vital signs, cardiac function, watch for edema, rapid weight gain (fluid overload)
  - ◊ Initial bedrest with supervised meals may be necessary
  - ◊ Stepwise gradual increase in calories consumed
  - ◊ Stepwise increase in activity
  - ◊ Involve patient in establishing target weight
  - ◊ Weigh daily at first, then 3 x per week
  - ◊ Achieve 1-2 pound (0.45-0.91 kg) per week weight gain
  - ◊ Supportive therapy
  - ◊ Behavioral approach to provide positive and negative reinforcement, plus feedback about progress and problems encountered
  - ◊ Tube feeding only as last resort
- Outpatient:
  - ◊ Build trust, treatment alliance
  - ◊ Involve patient in establishing target weight
  - ◊ Achieve gradual weight gain
  - ◊ Weigh weekly at first, monthly when progress is evident
  - ◊ Focus on overall indices of health, rather than weight gain alone
  - ◊ Challenge fear of uncontrolled weight gain
  - ◊ When initial weight gain achieved, consider cognitive-behavioral, educational-behavioral, individual
  - ◊ Family therapy for adolescents; couples therapy for older patients
  - ◊ Medicate for symptom relief
  - ◊ When condition is chronic, goal may be to achieve a safe weight rather than a healthy weight

SURGICAL MEASURES N/A

ACTIVITY
- Monitor activity
- Stepwise increase as patient gains weight
- Focus on playful rather than goal oriented activities

DIET
- Goal is stabilization at a healthy weight on a balanced diet with normal eating pattern
- Diminished ruminations about calories, weight; increased enjoyment

PATIENT EDUCATION
- Provide information on nutrition, metabolic balance, natural history of the disorder
- Ask patient to keep a "food diary" listing feelings and foods eaten
- For patient education materials see Internet References

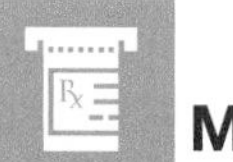

MEDICATIONS

DRUG(S) OF CHOICE
- Medications should not be used as sole or primary treatment of this disorder
- Fluoxetine (Prozac) 10-60 mg relieves symptoms and helps prevent relapse after weight gain
- Olanzapine - 2.5-5 mg daily. May diminish anxiety and core symptoms.
- Ondansetron, a SHT-3 antagonist, 4 mg tid has been used in case reports; insufficient data available

Contraindications: Refer to manufacturer's literature

Precautions: Starved patients are more sensitive to medication, likely to suffer dangerous or lethal side effects due to compromised cardiac, liver and kidney function; caution is indicated

Significant possible interactions: Refer to manufacturer's literature

ALTERNATIVE DRUGS
- Estrogen - estradiol 0.5-1 mg - does not enhance bone density in underweight patients
- Alendronate 35-70 mg weekly, has been used to treat osteoporosis, but no research on use in anorexia
- Psyllium (Metamucil) preparations (1 tbsp hs) to prevent constipation
- Therapeutic vitamin-mineral supplement

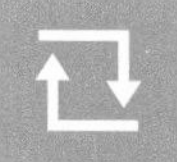

FOLLOWUP

PATIENT MONITORING
- Level of activity. Is the activity driven?
- Weigh weekly until stable, then monthly
- Depression, self-esteem, suicidal ideation
- Ruminations and rituals
- Repeat any abnormal lab values weekly or monthly
- Hypophosphatemia common during refeeding

PREVENTION/AVOIDANCE
- Efficacy not demonstrated
- Encourage rational attitude about weight
- Moderate overly high self-expectations
- Enhance self-esteem
- Diminish stress

POSSIBLE COMPLICATIONS
- Hypophosphatemia can generate short runs of ventricular tachycardia
- Potassium depletion; cardiac arrhythmia; cardiac arrest in purging patients
- Nitrogen depletion, exhaustion, collapse
- Cardiomyopathy, congestive heart failure
- Delayed gastric emptying
- Necrotizing colitis
- Convulsions, peripheral neuropathy
- Osteoporosis, bone loss
- Too rapid initial weight gain can cause fluid retention and congestive heart failure
- Infertility, perinatal complications

EXPECTED COURSE/PROGNOSIS
- Prognosis: less than 50% recover; 1/3 improved; 20% chronically ill
- Overall treatment efficacy not convincingly demonstrated
- Mortality - 5%
- Better outcome if patient hospitalized until weight in normal range
- Speed of weight gain does not predict treatment success
- Greater weight gain in trunk initially
- Poor prognosis indicated by repeated hospitalization, failed treatment, initial low weight, vomiting, being married, poor maturation, disordered relationships
- Substance abuse may need to be treated first
- Early adolescent onset short duration indicates more favorable prognosis
- Many symptoms resolve spontaneously with weight gain
- Ruminations, rituals, social isolation, and abnormal attitudes toward food and the body often persist after weight gain
- Patients often become depressed after they recover
- May need 200-400 more calories per day than anticipated in order to maintain weight

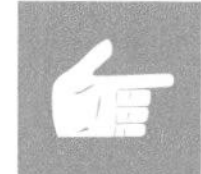

MISCELLANEOUS

ASSOCIATED CONDITIONS
- Major depression or dysthymia
- Social phobia
- Obsessive-compulsive disorder
- Other anxiety disorders
- Substance abuse disorder
- Borderline or avoidant personality disorder

AGE-RELATED FACTORS
Pediatric: Growth can be compromised in preadolescence and early adolescence

Geriatric: Difficult to diagnose in elderly

Others:
- High risk
  - ◊ Ballet dancers, models, cheerleaders
  - ◊ Athletes, especially runners, gymnasts, weight lifters, body builders, jockeys, divers, wrestlers, figure skaters, field hockey players
  - ◊ Japanese, Caucasian

PREGNANCY
Unlikely due to amenorrhea

SYNONYMS
N/A

ICD-9-CM
307.1 Anorexia nervosa

SEE ALSO
Amenorrhea
Idiopathic edema
Osteoporosis

OTHER NOTES
N/A

ABBREVIATIONS
N/A

REFERENCES

- Striegel-Moore R, Smolak L. Eating Disorders: Innovative Directions in Research and Practice. Washington DC: Am Psychiatry Assn: 2001
- Fairburn CG, Harrison PJ. Eating disorders. Lancet 2003;361(9355):407-16
- Casper RC. How useful are pharmacological treatments in eating disorders? Psychopharmacol Bull 2002;36(2):88-104
- Ben-Tovin. Eating disorders: outcome, prevention and treatment. Curr Opin Psychiatry 2003;16:65-9
- Lewinsohn PM, Striegel-Moore RH, Seeley JR. Epidemiology and natural course of eating disorders in young women from adolescence to young adulthood. J Am Acad Child Adolesc Psychiatry 2000;39(10):1284-92

Web references: 4 available at www.5mcc.com

Illustrations N/A

Author(s):
Alayne Yates, MD

BASICS

DESCRIPTION A common acute or chronic, fearful emotion with associated physical symptoms. DSM-IV-R recognizes the following sub types:
- Acute situational anxiety: Response to recent stressful event, usually transient symptoms
- Adjustment disorder with anxious mood: Persistent, maladaptive reaction following psychosocial stress and lasting up to six months
- Generalized anxiety disorder: Persistent underlying anxiety or adjustment disorder with anxious mood and significant symptoms of motor tension, autonomic hyperactivity and hypervigilance, lasting more than six months
- Panic disorder: Recurrent unexpected attacks with at least one attack (or more) associated with persistent concern about additional attacks, worries about implications of the attack (losing control, having a heart attack) or a significant change in behavior related to the attack; often leads to agoraphobia
- Post-traumatic stress disorder: Recurrent flashbacks or nightmares of catastrophic event by survivors, often associated with panic attacks and major depression
- Specific phobias: Intense recurrent fear of, and avoidance of, an object or situation
- Social phobia: Marked and persistent fear and avoidance of performance or social situations in which the person is exposed to unfamiliar people or scrutiny
- Obsessive-compulsive disorder: Persistent unwanted and disturbing thoughts and recurrent behavioral patterns (i.e., hand washing) which interfere with daily life

System(s) affected: Nervous
Genetics: Panic disorder - increased concordance in monozygotic versus dizygotic twins
Incidence/Prevalence in USA: 40 million (the most common psychiatric disorder in US)
- 12 month prevalence rate
  - ◊ Panic disorder - female 3.2%, male 1.3%
  - ◊ Obsessive compulsive disorder - female 2.6-3.1%, male 1.1-2.6%
  - ◊ Agoraphobia - female 3.8%, male 1.7%
  - ◊ Generalized anxiety disorder - female 4.3%, male 2.0%
  - ◊ Social phobia - female 5.2%, male 3.8%
- Lifetime prevalence PTSD - female 10.4%, male 5.0%

Predominant age: Mainly adults, highest prevalence in 20 to 45 year age group
Predominant sex: Female > Male (social phobia female 5.27:male 3.87)

SIGNS & SYMPTOMS Patterns vary with subtype of anxiety; not all present in each case
- Unrealistic or excessive anxiety or worry
- Sense of impending doom
- Nervousness
- Instability
- Tachycardia; palpitations
- Systolic click murmur
- Hyperventilation, choking sensation
- Labile hypertension
- Sighing respiration
- Nausea or abdominal distress
- Paresthesias
- Diaphoresis
- Dizziness or syncope
- Flushing
- Muscle tension
- Tremulousness
- Restlessness
- Chest tightness, pressure (pseudoangina)
- Headache, backaches, muscle spasm

CAUSES
- Panic disorder, social phobia and obsessive compulsive disorder are associated with genetic factors
- Psychosocial stressors commonly trigger anxiety disorders and may provoke a genetic diathesis
- Trauma such as physical assault, rape, conflict experience provoke PTSD symptoms
- Mediated by abnormalities of neurotransmitter systems (serotonin, norepinephrine and gamma-aminobutyric acid [GABA])

RISK FACTORS
- Social and financial problems
- Medical illness
- Family history
- Lack of social support

DIAGNOSIS

DIFFERENTIAL DIAGNOSIS
- Cardiovascular:
  - ◊ Ischemic heart disease
  - ◊ Valvular heart disease
  - ◊ Cardiomyopathies
  - ◊ Myocarditis
  - ◊ Arrhythmias
  - ◊ Mitral valve prolapse (most symptomatic cases are associated with panic disorder)
- Respiratory:
  - ◊ Asthma
  - ◊ Emphysema
  - ◊ Pulmonary embolism
  - ◊ Hamman-Rich syndrome
  - ◊ Scleroderma
- CNS:
  - ◊ Transient cerebral insufficiency
  - ◊ Psychomotor epilepsy
  - ◊ Essential tremor
- Metabolic and Hormonal:
  - ◊ Hyperthyroidism
  - ◊ Pheochromocytoma
  - ◊ Adrenal insufficiency
  - ◊ Cushing syndrome
  - ◊ Hypokalemia, hypoglycemia
  - ◊ Hyperparathyroidism
  - ◊ Myasthenia gravis
- Nutritional:
  - ◊ Thiamine, pyridoxine, or folate deficiency
  - ◊ Iron deficiency anemia
- Intoxication:
  - ◊ Caffeine
  - ◊ Alcohol
  - ◊ Cocaine
  - ◊ Sympathomimetics
  - ◊ Amphetamines
- Withdrawal:
  - ◊ Alcohol
  - ◊ Sedative-hypnotics
- Other:
  - ◊ Depression
  - ◊ Panic disorder is associated with several physical disorders including:
    - Mitral valve prolapse (systolic click-murmur)
    - Labile hypertension
    - Migraine headaches
    - Irritable bowel syndrome
    - Asthma (COPD)
    - Interstitial cystitis

LABORATORY
- Selective use of laboratory tests, (with minimal to more extensive workup depending on clinical picture). Laboratory tests often normal in anxiety disorders.
- CBC and urinalysis
- Sequential serial multiple analysis (SMA-12 panel)
- Thyroid function studies

Drugs that may alter lab results: SSRIs may raise serum levels of other medications such as warfarin (Coumadin) and tricyclic antidepressants

Disorders that may alter lab results: N/A

PATHOLOGICAL FINDINGS N/A

SPECIAL TESTS EEG, ECG, etc.

IMAGING Usually none; chest x-ray possibly

DIAGNOSTIC PROCEDURES
- Psychologic testing (e.g., Spitzer's Patient Health Questionnaire, Hamilton's anxiety scale)
- DSM-IV based interview

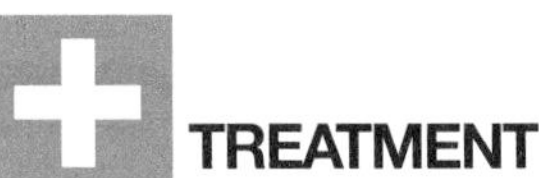

TREATMENT

APPROPRIATE HEALTH CARE Outpatient

GENERAL MEASURES
- Should be based on careful workup and identification of etiology and subtype of anxiety disorders
- Adequate workup
- Identify co-existent substance abuse
- Counseling or psychotherapy along with medications
- Regular exercise program
- Biofeedback in selected cases
- Serial office visits
- Judicious reassurance after other medical disorders ruled out

SURGICAL MEASURES N/A

ACTIVITY Fully active

DIET No special diet

PATIENT EDUCATION
- AAFP - 800-274-2237, ext 4400
- National Institute of Mental Health (NIMH) - National Anxiety Awareness Program, 9000 Rockville Pike, Bethesda, MD 20892
- Anxiety Disorders Association of America - www.adaa.org

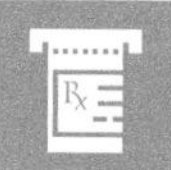

MEDICATIONS

DRUG(S) OF CHOICE

- Conditions
  - ◊ Acute situational anxiety:
    - Short-term (up to 1 month) treatment with benzodiazepines
  - ◊ Adjustment disorder with anxiety mood:
    - Benzodiazepines
  - ◊ Generalized anxiety disorder:
    - Azapirones - e.g., buspirone
    - SSRIs
    - Venlafaxine (Effexor)
  - ◊ Panic disorder and social phobia:
    - SSRIs
    - TCAs - e.g., imipramine
  - ◊ Obsessive-compulsive disorder:
    - TCAs - e.g., clomipramine
    - SSRIs also effective
- Drug doses
  - ◊ SSRIs:
    - Citalopram (Celexa) 10 mg q/day; increase by 10 mg q 7 days to maximum of 20-40 mg q/day
    - Fluoxetine (Prozac) 10 mg; increase by 10 mg q 7 days to maximum daily dosage of 20-40 mg
    - Paroxetine (Paxil) 10 mg; increase by 10 mg q 5 days
    - Sertraline (Zoloft) 25 mg; increase by 25 mg q 5 days
    - Venlafaxine (Effexor) SR 37.5 mg; increase by 37.5 mg q 5-7 days
  - ◊ Benzodiazepines
    - Alprazolam (Xanax) 0.25 mg bid-tid; increase by 0.25 mg if needed
    - Clonazepam (Klonopin) 0.5 mg po tid, to maximum of 1.5-4.5 mg/day
    - Diazepam (Valium) 2-5 mg bid; increase by 2 mg if needed
    - Lorazepam (Ativan) 0.5 mg bid-tid; increase by 0.5 mg if needed (response, if any is slow, often 4-6 weeks)
  - ◊ Azapirones
    - Buspirone (BuSpar) 5 mg bid-tid; increase 5 mg q 2-3 days to maximum of 60 mg/day in divided doses
  - ◊ Tricyclics
    - Clomipramine (Anafranil) 25 mg bid; increase gradually to maximum of 250 mg/day
    - Imipramine (Tofranil) 10-25 mg qhs; increase by 10-25

Contraindications:

- Benzodiazepines - 1st-trimester pregnancy, acute alcohol intoxication with depressed vital signs, acute angle-closure glaucoma, sleep apnea, history of personality disorder or substance abuse. Avoid long-term/prn use.
- Buspirone - concurrent MAO inhibitor use
- TCAs - acute myocardial infarction, bundle branch block

Precautions:

- Benzodiazepines - advanced age, renal insufficiency, suicidal tendency, open-angle glaucoma. Sudden discontinuation increases risk of seizures, especially with alprazolam
- Benzodiazepines with short half-lives (e.g., alprazolam) increase potential for dependency and protracted withdrawal symptoms; extreme caution with severe panic disorder who are taking other CNS sedatives or who have a history of substance abuse/dependence
- Buspirone - hepatic and/or renal dysfunction. Buspirone will not protect against benzodiazepine withdrawal seizures; taper benzodiazepines.
- TCAs - advanced age, glaucoma, benign prostate hypertrophy, hyperthyroidism, cardiovascular disease, liver disease, urinary retention, MAO inhibitor treatment

Significant possible interactions:

- Benzodiazepines - cimetidine, ethanol, oral contraceptives, disulfiram, levodopa, rifampin
- Buspirone - MAO inhibitors
- TCAs - amphetamines, barbiturates, guanethidine, clonidine, epinephrine, ethanol, norepinephrine, MAO inhibitors, propoxyphene
- SSRIs - MAO inhibitors (may cause fatal serotonin syndrome [confusion, hyperthermia, etc.]), may raise serum levels of other medications

ALTERNATIVE DRUGS

- Generalized anxiety disorder: Short-term use of benzodiazepine or TCAs
- Panic disorder: Although TCAs or SSRIs are the drugs of choice for panic disorder, they are slow in onset of action (2-3 weeks). Benzodiazepines may be helpful for initial control of symptoms until the SSRIs or TCAs are effective. Also, 10-20% of patients with panic do not tolerate side effects of SSRIs or TCAs. High potency benzodiazepines (alprazolam, clonazepam, lorazepam) or MAO inhibitors are effective alternatives.
- Social phobia: phenelzine - initial dose 15 mg bid, increase by 15 mg every week to a total dose of 45-90 mg. Need to be on MAOI diet and avoid stimulant medications (pseudoephedrine, SSRIs). Benzodiazepines: clonazepam.

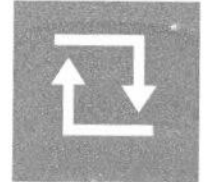

FOLLOWUP

PATIENT MONITORING

- Follow-up by regular office visits
- Watch for and treat associated depression
- Monitor mental status on benzodiazepines and avoid drug dependence
- Monitor blood pressure, heart rate, anticholinergic side effects on TCAs
- Periodic serum levels, if indicated, for TCAs

PREVENTION/AVOIDANCE

Management of stress, to extent possible, relaxation techniques, meditation

POSSIBLE COMPLICATIONS

- Impaired social/occupational functioning
- Drug dependence (benzodiazepines)
- Cardiac arrhythmias (TCAs)
- Alcohol dependence

EXPECTED COURSE/PROGNOSIS

- With active treatment, excellent results can often be obtained, especially with short-term anxiety disorders, including panic disorder
- Obsessive-compulsive disorder, and post-traumatic stress disorder are more difficult to treat, often requiring long-term psychotherapy and medication (combination treatment)

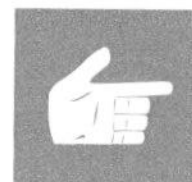

MISCELLANEOUS

ASSOCIATED CONDITIONS

- Depression (commonly)
- Agoraphobia
- Alcohol or substance abuse
- Somatoform disorders

AGE-RELATED FACTORS

Pediatric: Reduced dosage of medications in adolescent

Geriatric: Reduced dosage of medications

Others: N/A

PREGNANCY

- Benzodiazepines - contraindicated in first-trimester of pregnancy, and with caution later in pregnancy and during lactation. May cause lethargy and weight loss in nursing infants; avoid breast feeding if mother taking benzodiazepines chronically or in high doses.
- TCAs - some evidence of fetal risk, especially in first trimester
- SSRIs - taper and discontinue, if possible, in first trimester; may be used later in pregnancy

SYNONYMS

- Hyperventilation syndrome
- Panic disorder

ICD-9-CM

300.00 Anxiety state, unspecified

SEE ALSO

OTHER NOTES N/A

ABBREVIATIONS

DSM-IV-R = Diagnostic and Statistical Manual of Mental Disorders, 4th edition

TCA = tricyclic antidepressant

SSRI = selective serotonin reuptake inhibitor

REFERENCES

- Ciechanowski P, Katon W. Overview of Anxiety. In: Rose BD, editor. UpToDate. Wellesley, M: UpToDate; 2003
- Katon W. Panic Disorder in the Medical Setting. Washington, D.C., American Psychiatric Press, 1991
- Stein M, Liebowitz M, Lydiard R, et al. Paroxetine treatment of generalized social phobia (social anxiety disorder): a randomized controlled trial. JAMA 1998;280:708-13
- Brady K, Pearlstein T, Asnis G, et al. Efficacy and safety of sertraline treatment of post-traumatic stress disorder: a randomized controlled trial. JAMA 2000;283:1837-44
- Lydiard RB, Brawman-Mintzor O, et al. Recent developments in the psychopharmacology of anxiety disorders. J Consult Clin Psychol 1996;64:660-668
- Roy-Byrne P, Stein M, Bystrisky A, Katon W. Pharmacotherapy of panic disorder. J Am Board Fam Pract 1998;11:282-90
- Katon W, Geyman JP: Anxiety. In: Rakel RE, ed. Textbook of Family Practice. 6th Ed. Philadelphia: W.B. Saunders Co., 2002:1438-1454
- Johnson GE: Essentials of Drug Therapy. Philadelphia: W.B. Saunders Co., 1991

Web references: 1 available at www.5mcc.com

Illustrations N/A

Author(s):

Wayne J. Katon, MD

BASICS

DESCRIPTION Intimal tear in the aorta propagated via hematoma formation causing further dissection and separation producing a false lumen in the arterial wall.

- The Debakey classification:
  - ◊ Type I: Involves the aortic root, aortic arch, and the descending aorta
  - ◊ Type II: Involves only the ascending aorta
  - ◊ Type III: Involves only the distal aorta beyond the origin of the left subclavian artery
- Stanford classification:
  - ◊ Type A: ascending and aortic arch
  - ◊ Type B: descending aorta

System(s) affected: Cardiovascular
Genetics: Increased incidence among family members
Incidence/Prevalence in USA:
- 1 in 10,000 patients admitted to hospital; found 1 in 350 patients at autopsy
- 2000 new cases diagnosed annually

Predominant age: Dependent on etiology; Marfan commonly present in the third and fourth decade; most common between the 6th and 8th decades
Predominant sex: Male > Female (3:1)

SIGNS & SYMPTOMS
- Abrupt onset of tearing pain
- Shearing anterior chest pain which radiates to the interscapular region
- Back pain
- Syncope
- Symptoms of congestive heart failure
- Stroke
- Limb ischemia
- Abdominal pain
- Acute myocardial infarction/angina
- Spinal cord syndromes/deficits
- Hypotension or hypertension
- Wide pulse pressure
- Murmur of aortic insufficiency
- Features of tamponade
- Dullness in left lung base (effusion)
- Pulse deficits or asymmetry
- Fever

CAUSES
- Cystic medionecrosis
- Iatrogenic during arterial catheterization

RISK FACTORS
- Hypertension
- Pregnancy
- Chest trauma
- Cocaine use
- Cardiovascular surgery
- Age
- Marfan syndrome
- Ehlers-Danlos syndrome
- MDMA (ecstasy use)
- Alpha1 antitrypsin deficiency

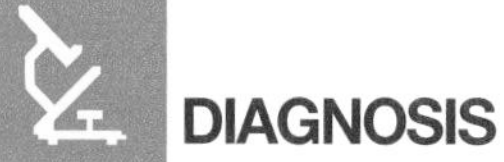

DIAGNOSIS

DIFFERENTIAL DIAGNOSIS
- Myocardial infarction
- Pulmonary embolism
- Pneumonia
- Pleurisy
- Pericarditis
- Pneumothorax
- Angina
- Acute pancreatitis
- Penetrating duodenal ulcer

LABORATORY No special studies required

Drugs that may alter lab results: N/A

Disorders that may alter lab results: N/A

PATHOLOGICAL FINDINGS Approximately 60% of intimal tears occur in the proximal ascending aorta. The remainder are found between the origin of the left subclavian artery and ligamentum arteriosum, descending aorta (20%), aortic arch (10%), and the abdominal aorta. Although medionecrosis is found in normal aging aortas, it appears to be more extensive in patients who develop aortic dissection. Cystic medionecrosis is seen in patients with defects in elastin and connective tissue organization i.e., Marfan, Ehlers-Danlos, etc. Death usually due to rupture and tamponade.

SPECIAL TESTS
- Electrocardiogram: LVH, nonspecific ST-T changes, electrical alternans with associated tamponade
- Echocardiogram: dilated aortic root, increased aortic posterior or anterior wall thickness, pericardial effusion, oscillating intimal flap

IMAGING Chest x-ray: widening of the superior mediastinum, left pleural effusion, haziness or enlargement of the aortic knob, double density of the descending aorta, irregular aortic contour, > 5 mm separation of intimal calcification from outer aortic contour, rightward displacement of the trachea, cardiomegaly.

DIAGNOSTIC PROCEDURES
[Sensitivity/Specificity indicated for each]
- CT chest - demonstration of two lumens with hematoma formation, detection of intimal flap, differential flow between two lumens, compression of true lumen by false lumen [88/100%]
- Spiral CT aortography may be more sensitive and specific (99/99)
- Aortogram - demonstration of two lumens, detection of intimal flap, compression of true lumen, ulcer-like projections of contrast, arterial compromise, altered flow patterns, aortic insufficiency (not as sensitive as previous thought) [88/94%]
- Transesophageal echocardiography (TEE) - test of choice for hemodynamically unstable patients [99/98%]
- MRI - if available and patient hemodynamically stable, test of choice for delineation of vascular anatomy
- Intravascular ultrasonography - may detect dissections even with negative TEE

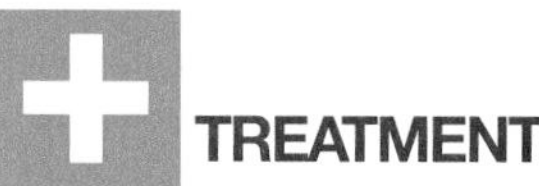

TREATMENT

APPROPRIATE HEALTH CARE Admission to intensive care unit or transfer to operative suite

GENERAL MEASURES
- Treatment of choice - surgical for all ascending aortic dissections and medical for descending dissections without complications (Type III)
- Medical therapy is based on decreasing blood pressure and the "shearing" forces of myocardial contractility (dp/dt) to attempt to decrease intimal tear and hematoma propagation
- Arterial blood pressure monitoring is critical
- Careful observation for changes in mentation, neurological signs, or evidence of organ dysfunction
- A Foley catheter should be used to follow urine output
- Swan-Ganz catheterization may be very helpful to monitor cardiac performance and filling pressures during the use of vasoactive and cardio-depressive drugs
- Pain control may be difficult despite use of narcotics

SURGICAL MEASURES
- Surgical indications for Type III
  - ◊ Increasing size of hematoma
  - ◊ Impending rupture
  - ◊ Inability to control pain
  - ◊ Bleeding into pleural space
- Endovascular stents, fenestration, and stent-grafting

ACTIVITY Bedrest

DIET NPO until surgical evaluation is complete and patient classified as medical therapy only

PATIENT EDUCATION Depending on etiology, emphasis must be placed on risk factors and recurrence of symptoms

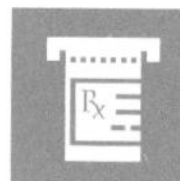

MEDICATIONS

DRUG(S) OF CHOICE Propranolol in 0.5-1 mg IV doses every 5 minutes until the heart rate is 60-70 beats per minute plus nitroprusside titrated to reduce systolic blood pressure to 100-110 mm Hg (13.3-14.6 kPa)

Contraindications:
- Propranolol - in bronchial asthma, diabetes mellitus, Raynaud disease, sinus bradycardia, A-V heart block greater than first degree, in presence of monoamine oxidase inhibitors, cardiogenic shock, congestive heart failure or right ventricular failure from pulmonary hypertension
- Nitroprusside - in treatment of compensatory hypertension, i.e., arteriovenous shunt, in patients with inadequate cerebral circulation, and for use during emergency surgery in moribund patients

Precautions:
- Use propranolol cautiously in patients with angina pectoris, cardiac failure, impaired renal or hepatic function, thyrotoxicosis, pre-excitation syndromes, diabetes, hypoglycemia or nonallergic bronchospasm. Propranolol may produce significant bradycardia, heart block or hypotension. Patients should not be suddenly withdrawn from beta blockers.
- Nitroprusside:
  - ◊ May not lower blood pressure adequately, another agent may be required
  - ◊ In patients with renal or hepatic insufficiency, may cause cyanide toxicity, through excessive production of serum thiocyanate. Confusion and hyperreflexia are the early signs of thiocyanate toxicity. Thiocyanate inhibits the uptake and binding of iodine, use caution in the presence of hypothyroidism. Check thiocyanate levels after 48 hours of nitroprusside use.
  - ◊ Because of the rapid onset and potency, administration should be with the use of an infusion pump
  - ◊ Methemoglobinemia may be seen rarely

Significant possible interactions:
- Propranolol with adenosine, albuterol, alfentanil, amiodarone, barbiturates, bromazepam, chlorothiazide, chlorpromazine, chlorpropamide, chlorprothixene, cimetidine, clonidine, dextroamphetamine, diazoxide, dihydroergotamine, diltiazem, disopyramide, tricyclic antidepressants, encainide, epinephrine, flecainide, fluvoxamine, furosemide, glipizide, halofenate, haloperidol, heparin, ibuprofen, indomethacin, insulin, isoniazid, isoproterenol, lidocaine, lidoflazine, methacholine, methyldopa, metoclopramide, naproxen, nifedipine, phenylpropanolamine, procainamide, quinidine, reserpine, rifampin, ritodrine, sulfonylureas, theophylline, thioridazine, tocainide, tubocurarine, verapamil, warfarin.
- Nitroprusside with clonidine and other antihypertensives to make their hypotensive effects cumulative

ALTERNATIVE DRUGS
- Labetalol, 10-20 mg IV bolus to a maximum of 300 mg total, then titrated to response with an infusion
- Trimethaphan, at an infusion rate of 1-2 mg/min
- Reserpine 0.5-2 mg intramuscularly every 4-8 hours. Onset of action is 1-3 hours.
- Methyldopa 250-500 mg every 6 hours. Unfortunately, it has a delayed onset of action of 4 to 6 hours and prolonged duration of 10 to 12 hours.

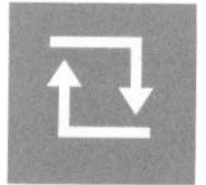

FOLLOWUP

PATIENT MONITORING
- Systolic blood pressure should be maintained at 120 mm Hg (16 kPa) or below as tolerated
- Routine chest x-rays and/or chest CT may be helpful in following the progress of any long-term medically treated patient
- Patients should have a one month follow-up visit, and then at three month intervals. During the follow-up, careful attention should be placed on signs and symptoms of aortic insufficiency, chest or back pain, and development of saccular aneurysms as displayed on CXR.

PREVENTION/AVOIDANCE Long-term control of hypertension

POSSIBLE COMPLICATIONS Redissection, localized saccular aneurysm, cardiac tamponade, aortic valvular insufficiency and progressive aortic enlargement

EXPECTED COURSE/PROGNOSIS
- Mortality of patients left untreated is: 33% in 24 hours, 60% in 2 weeks, approximately 90% in three months
- Hospital survival is estimated at approximately 70% in patients treated both medically and surgically
- Patients with ascending dissection treated early with surgery still have a mortality of 29-38%
- 10 year survival of all operated patients is 40%
- Redissection risk is 13% at 5 years; 23% at 10 years

MISCELLANEOUS

ASSOCIATED CONDITIONS
- Ehlers-Danlos syndrome
- Marfan syndrome
- Aortic stenosis
- Coarctation of aorta
- Bicuspid valve
- Turner syndrome
- Osteogenesis imperfecta
- Syphilis
- Relapsing polychondritis

AGE-RELATED FACTORS N/A

Pediatric: N/A

Geriatric: N/A

Others: N/A

PREGNANCY Aortic dissection may be associated with cystic medionecrosis of pregnancy and appears to have an increased associated risk with pregnancy. It is still unclear whether pregnancy itself is the originating factor or that it simply contributes to the worsening of an already pre-existing condition.

SYNONYMS
- Dissecting aneurysm

ICD-9-CM

441.00 Dissection of aorta, unspecified site

SEE ALSO

Ehlers-Danlos syndrome

Marfan syndrome

OTHER NOTES N/A

ABBREVIATIONS N/A

REFERENCES

- Rogers FB, et al. Aortic dissection after trauma: Case report and review of literature. J Trauma 1996;41:906-908
- Pretre R, et al. Aortic dissection. Lancet 1997;May17;349:1461-64
- Lindsay JJ. Diagnosis and treatment of diseases of the aorta. Curr Probl Cardiol 1997;Oct 22(70) 485-542
- Summer T, Fehska W, et al. Aortic dissection: a comparative study of diagnosis with spiral CT, multiplanar transesophageal echocardiography, and MR imaging. Radiology 1996;199(2):347-52
- Manninen HI, Rasanen H. Intravascular ultrasound in interventional radiology Eur Radiol 2000;10(11):1754-62
- Penco M, Paparoni S, Dagianti A, et al. Usefulness of transesophageal echocardiography in the assessment of aortic dissection. Amer J of Cardiology 2000;86(4A):53G-56G
- Hartnell GG. Imaging of aortic aneurysms and dissection: CT and MRI. J of Thoracic Imaging 2001;16(1):35-46
- Umana JP, Mitchell RS. Endovascular treatment of aortic dissections and thoracic aortic aneurysms. Sem in Vascular Surg 2000;13(4):290-8
- Beckman JA, O'Gara PT. Diseases of the aorta. Advances. Inter Med 1999;44:267-91

Web references: 2 available at www.5mcc.com

Illustrations N/A

Author(s):

Darell E. Heiselman, DO

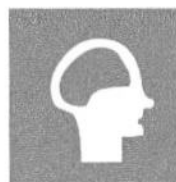

BASICS

DESCRIPTION An acquired or congenital obstruction to systolic left ventricular outflow across the aortic valve

System(s) affected: Cardiovascular

Genetics: N/A

Incidence/Prevalence in USA:
- Except for mitral regurgitation due to myocardial disease, valvular aortic stenosis is the most common fatal cardiac valve lesion
- Bicuspid aortic valve has a frequency of 400 per 100,000 live births

Predominant age:
- Age < 30 years - predominantly congenital
- Age 30 to 70 years - most commonly congenital or rheumatic
- Age > 70 years - most commonly degenerative calcification of the aortic valve

Predominant sex:
- Congenital bicuspid valves: Male > Female (4:1)
- Congenital unicuspid valves: Male > Female (3:1)

SIGNS & SYMPTOMS
- Angina pectoris (most frequent symptom, occurring in 50-70% of patients with severe aortic stenosis)
- Near syncope
- Syncope (often exertional, occurs in 15-30% of patients with severe aortic stenosis)
- Exertional dyspnea
- Orthopnea
- Paroxysmal nocturnal dyspnea
- Palpitations
- Fatigue
- Neurologic events (transient ischemic attack or cerebrovascular accident) due to embolization
- Systolic crescendo-decrescendo murmur, usually best heard at the second right sternal border (may have associated thrill) and may radiate into the carotid arteries
- Ejection (early systolic) click
- Prolonged ejection time
- Delayed, small carotid upstroke
- Delayed/decreased intensity of A2
- Paradoxical splitting of S2
- Left ventricular heave
- A high pitched diastolic blow may be present at the left sternal border (associated aortic regurgitation)

CAUSES
- Congenital etiologies
  - ◊ Unicuspid valve
  - ◊ Bicuspid valve (not inherently stenotic, but becomes so as a result of 'wear and tear' thickening and calcification; a calcified bicuspid valve is the most common cause of isolated aortic stenosis in adults)
  - ◊ 3 cusped valve with fusion of commissures
  - ◊ Hypoplastic annulus
- Acquired etiologies
  - ◊ Rheumatic (or, rarely, other inflammatory disease)
  - ◊ Degenerative calcific aortic stenosis in the elderly

RISK FACTORS Prior rheumatic fever

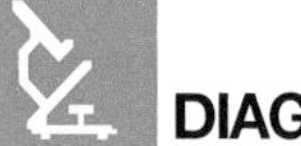

DIAGNOSIS

DIFFERENTIAL DIAGNOSIS
- Mitral regurgitation, either primary or secondary to underlying coronary artery disease or dilated cardiomyopathy. Mitral regurgitation, however, is usually an apical, high frequency, pansystolic murmur, often radiating to the axilla.
- Hypertrophic obstructive cardiomyopathy. This murmur is also a systolic crescendo-decrescendo murmur, but is best heard at the left sternal border and may radiate into the axilla. However, this murmur characteristically is intensified by moving from squatting to standing position and/or Valsalva maneuver, and lessened by changing from standing to squatting.
- Aortic supravalvular stenosis
- Discrete subaortic stenosis

LABORATORY N/A

Drugs that may alter lab results: N/A

Disorders that may alter lab results: N/A

PATHOLOGICAL FINDINGS
- Left ventricular hypertrophy
- Myocardial interstitial fibrosis
- Aortic valvular calcification in older patients
- 50% incidence of concomitant coronary artery disease

SPECIAL TESTS ECG: Left ventricular hypertrophy, often with associated ST segment depression, conduction defects, left atrial enlargement, ventricular arrhythmias

IMAGING
- Chest x-ray
  - ◊ May be normal in compensated, isolated valvular aortic stenosis
  - ◊ Cardiac hypertrophy early, later cardiomegaly
  - ◊ Post stenotic dilatation of the ascending aorta
  - ◊ Calcification of aortic valve cusps (may require fluoroscopy to visualize)

DIAGNOSTIC PROCEDURES
- Echocardiography:
  - ◊ Aortic valve morphology, thickening, calcifications
  - ◊ Decreased aortic valve excursion
  - ◊ Planimetry of aortic valve area
  - ◊ Left ventricular hypertrophy
  - ◊ Left ventricular ejection fraction
  - ◊ Chamber dimensions
  - ◊ Presence or absence of wall motion abnormalities suggestive of coronary artery disease
- With Doppler echocardiography:
  - ◊ Transvalvular gradient
  - ◊ Valve area
  - ◊ Diastolic function
  - ◊ Associated aortic regurgitation
- Cardiac catheterization:
  - ◊ Transvalvular gradient
  - ◊ Valve area
  - ◊ Left ventricle ejection fraction
  - ◊ Concomitant coronary artery disease

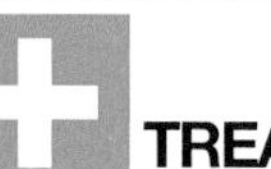

TREATMENT

APPROPRIATE HEALTH CARE Outpatient except for surgical intervention

GENERAL MEASURES
- Aortic stenosis is a progressive disease. The asymptomatic patient with non-critical aortic stenosis can be closely followed with appropriate evaluation.
- All patients with valvular aortic stenosis should receive endocarditis prophylaxis, prior to dental work or invasive procedures regardless of age, etiology or severity of the stenosis (as recommended by the American Heart Association in Circulation, 1997; 96: 358-366)
- Patients with a rheumatic etiology should receive (in addition to endocarditis prophylaxis prior to dental work or invasive procedures) rheumatic fever prophylaxis, especially if less than 35 years of age, or continue to be in close contact with young children

SURGICAL MEASURES
- Prompt aortic valve replacement is clearly indicated in patients with symptomatic severe aortic stenosis
- Consider aortic valve replacement in asymptomatic patients with critical aortic stenosis (aortic valve area < 1.0 cm2 or gradient > 50 mm Hg [> 6.6 kPa]) particularly if there is left ventricular dysfunction, increasing cardiomegaly, and clinical symptoms
- Surgical valve replacement consists of the removal of the stenotic, native valve and placement of a prosthetic mechanical or tissue valve
- Balloon angioplasty of stenotic aortic valves may be of benefit in the pediatric patient with congenital disease. Also feasible (although one must expect suboptimal results) in the elderly, debilitated patient who may not tolerate valve replacement.

ACTIVITY In known or suspected severe aortic stenosis, vigorous physical activity is contraindicated

DIET No restrictions except sodium restriction in presence of congestive heart failure

PATIENT EDUCATION
- Educate the patient about the symptoms of symptomatic aortic stenosis and to report these promptly should they occur
- If moderate or severe aortic stenosis is known or suspected, instruct the patient to avoid vigorous physical activity
- Instruct the patient when prophylactic antibiotics are needed for medical or dental procedures

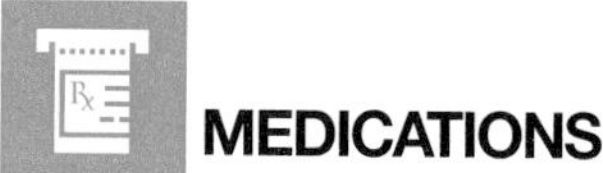

MEDICATIONS

DRUG(S) OF CHOICE

- None for treatment. Prophylactic antibiotics when needed.
- The use of vasodilators, nitrates, calcium channel blockers, beta blockers as well as diuretics are potentially hazardous in aortic stenosis and should be used cautiously, if at all

Contraindications: N/A
Precautions: N/A
Significant possible interactions: N/A

ALTERNATIVE DRUGS N/A

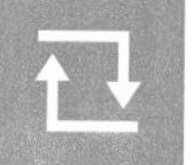

FOLLOWUP

PATIENT MONITORING

- Asymptomatic patients without critical aortic stenosis should be followed with a history and physical examination every 3-6 months
- An echocardiogram should be performed every 6-12 months to assess progression
- Advise the patient to immediately report any symptoms referable to the aortic stenosis

PREVENTION/AVOIDANCE

- Bacterial endocarditis prophylaxis
- Rheumatic fever prophylaxis, where indicated
- Avoidance of vigorous physical activity

POSSIBLE COMPLICATIONS

- Progressive stenosis
- Sudden death
- Congestive heart failure
- Angina
- Syncope
- Hemolytic anemia
- Infective endocarditis

EXPECTED COURSE/PROGNOSIS

- Mean life expectancy without intervention in patients with aortic stenosis is 5 years after the onset of exertional chest discomfort, 3 years after the onset of syncope, 2 years after the development of heart failure
- Sudden death occurs in 15 to 20% of patients with symptomatic aortic stenosis

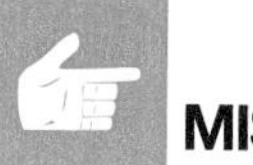

MISCELLANEOUS

ASSOCIATED CONDITIONS

- Coronary artery disease is present in 50% of patients with aortic stenosis
- Aortic regurgitation (particularly seen in calcified bicuspid valves and rheumatic disease)
- Mitral valve disease (primarily in rheumatic heart disease)

AGE-RELATED FACTORS

Pediatric: N/A
Geriatric: Increased incidence of degenerative calcific aortic stenosis
Others: N/A

PREGNANCY Severe critical aortic stenosis tolerates poorly the hemodynamic changes in pregnancy, labor and delivery. Pregnancy should be avoided with critical aortic stenosis.

SYNONYMS N/A

ICD-9-CM

424.90 Endocarditis, valve unspecified, unspecified cause

SEE ALSO

OTHER NOTES As the left ventricle is relatively noncompliant in aortic stenosis, atrial contraction is an important component of diastolic filling. The loss of this component with the onset of atrial fibrillation can cause acute clinical and hemodynamic deterioration.

ABBREVIATIONS N/A

REFERENCES

- Brandenburg RO, et al: Cardiology: Fundamentals and Practice. New York, Year Book Publishers, 1987
- Dalen JE, Alpert JS: Valvular Heart Disease. 2nd Ed. New York, Little Brown & Co, 1987
- Hurst JW, et al: The Heart. 8th Ed. New York, McGraw-Hill, 1994
- Isselbacher KJ, et al, eds: Harrison's Principles of Internal Medicine. 13th Ed. New York, McGraw-Hill, 1994

Web references: 1 available at www.5mcc.com
Illustrations N/A

Author(s):
Mark R. Dambro, MD

BASICS

DESCRIPTION Acute inflammation of the vermiform appendix
- First described by Fitz in 1886
- McBurney described the point of maximal tenderness

System(s) affected: Gastrointestinal
Genetics: Unknown.
Incidence/Prevalence in USA:
- 10/100,000
- Most common acute surgical condition of abdomen
- 1 in every 15 persons (7%) at some time in their life

Predominant age:
- Ages 10-30 - Male > Female (3:2)
- Over age 30 - Male = Female

Predominant sex: Slight male predominance

SIGNS & SYMPTOMS
- Abdominal pain (100%) - periumbilical then right-lower-quadrant (RLQ). Pain lessened with flexion of thigh.
- Muscle guarding
- Anorexia (almost 100%)
- Nausea (90%)
- Vomiting (75%)-mild
- Obstipation
- Diarrhea-mild
- Sequence of symptom appearance (95%) - anorexia, then abdominal pain, then vomiting
- Slight temperature (one degree centigrade) elevation
- Slight tachycardia
- Patient frequently lies motionless with right thigh drawn up
- Maximal tenderness at "McBurney's point"
- Direct and referred RLQ tenderness
- Voluntary and involuntary guarding
- Cutaneous hyperesthesia at T10-12
- Rovsing's sign - RLQ pain with palpatory pressure in LLQ
- Psoas sign-pain with right thigh extension
- Obturator sign-pain with internal rotation of flexed right thigh
- Retrocecal appendix-flank tenderness in RLQ
- Pelvic appendix-local and suprapubic pain on rectal exam

CAUSES
- Obstruction of appendiceal lumen
  - ◊ Fecaliths (most common)
  - ◊ Lymphoid tissue hypertrophy
  - ◊ Inspissated barium
  - ◊ Vegetable, fruit seeds and other foreign bodies
  - ◊ Intestinal worms (ascarids)
  - ◊ Strictures

RISK FACTORS
- Adolescent males
- Familial tendency
- Intra-abdominal tumors

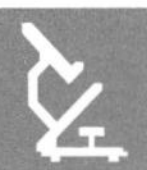

DIAGNOSIS

DIFFERENTIAL DIAGNOSIS
- Any cause of the "acute abdomen"
- 75% of erroneous diagnoses accounted for by acute mesenteric lymphadenitis, no organic pathologic condition, acute PID, twisted ovarian cyst, ruptured graafian follicle, acute gastroenteritis
- Also consider urologic causes, inflammatory bowel disease, colonic disorders, and other gynecologic diseases

LABORATORY
- Moderate leukocytosis - 10,000 to 18,000/mm3 in 75%
- Moderate polymorphonuclear predominance
- Urinalysis-elevated specific gravity, hematuria (sometimes), pyuria (sometimes), albuminuria (sometimes)

Drugs that may alter lab results:
- Antibiotics
- Steroids

Disorders that may alter lab results: N/A

PATHOLOGICAL FINDINGS
- Acute inflammation of the appendix
- Local vascular congestion
- Obstruction
- Gangrene
- Perforation with abscess (15-30%)

SPECIAL TESTS N/A

IMAGING (Used in differential diagnosis and to detect complications)
- KUB: gas-filled appendix; radiopaque fecalith; deformed cecum; fluid level; ileus; free air
- Barium enema-non-filling appendix; RLQ mass effect
- Ultrasound-appendiceal inflammation; other pelvic pathology, such as inflammatory mass
- CT scan - diagnostic test of choice; also for abscess

DIAGNOSTIC PROCEDURES
- Cornerstone of diagnosis is history and clinical findings
- Diagnostic laparoscopy - consider in young adult females
- Rectal and pelvic examinations
- Intensive in-hospital observation

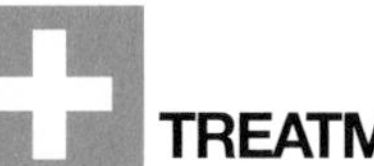

TREATMENT

APPROPRIATE HEALTH CARE
- Inpatient surgery

GENERAL MEASURES
- Preoperative preparation
  - ◊ Correction of fluid and electrolyte deficits
  - ◊ Consider broad-spectrum antibiotic coverage
- For non-surgical patients, antibiotic coverage (e.g. quinolone + metronidazole)

SURGICAL MEASURES
- Immediate appendectomy; open or laparoscopic
- Drainage of abscess, if present

ACTIVITY
- Early postoperative ambulation
- Return to full activity by 4 to 6 weeks postop

DIET Regular diet with return of bowel function, usually within 24 to 48 hours postop

PATIENT EDUCATION
- Restricted activity for 4 to 6 weeks postop
- Contact physician for development of postop anorexia, nausea, vomiting, abdominal pain, fever, or chills

MEDICATIONS

DRUG(S) OF CHOICE
- Uncomplicated acute appendicitis - one preoperative dose of broad spectrum antibiotic; cefoxitin (Mefoxin), cefotetan (Cefotan)
- Gangrenous or perforating appendicitis - broadened antibiotic coverage for aerobic and anaerobic enteric pathogens, dosage and choice of antibiotic should be adjusted based on intraoperative cultures. Continue antibiotics for 7 days postop or until patient becomes afebrile with normal white count. Pathogens usually sensitive to ampicillin, gentamicin, and clindamycin.

Contraindications: Documented allergy to specific antibiotic

Precautions: Adjust antibiotic dosages for elderly and renal failure patients

Significant possible interactions: Refer to manufacturer's literature for each drug

ALTERNATIVE DRUGS
- Metronidazole (Flagyl) - anaerobic coverage only
- Ampicillin-sulbactam (Unasyn)
- Ticarcillin-clavulanate (Timentin)
- Piperacillin-tazobactam (Zosyn)

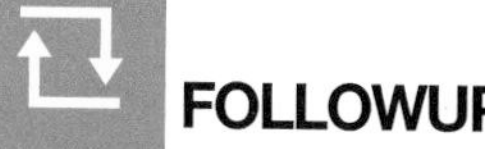

FOLLOWUP

PATIENT MONITORING Routine visits at 2 and 6 weeks postoperatively

PREVENTION/AVOIDANCE N/A

POSSIBLE COMPLICATIONS
- Wound infection
- Intra-abdominal abscess, sometimes diaphragmatic
- Fecal fistula
- Intestinal obstruction
- Incisional hernia
- Liver abscess (rare)
- Peritonitis with paralytic ileus

EXPECTED COURSE/PROGNOSIS
- Generally uncomplicated course in young adults with non-ruptured appendicitis.
- Factors increasing morbidity and mortality are extremes of age and appendiceal rupture.
- Morbidity rates:
  - ◊ 3% with non-perforated appendicitis
  - ◊ 47% with perforated appendicitis
- Mortality rates:
  - ◊ 0.1% unruptured acute appendicitis
  - ◊ 3% ruptured acute appendicitis
  - ◊ 15% elderly patient with ruptured appendix

MISCELLANEOUS

ASSOCIATED CONDITIONS N/A

AGE-RELATED FACTORS
Pediatric:
- Rare in infancy
- Decreased diagnostic accuracy
- Higher fever, more vomiting
- Rupture earlier
- Rupture rate: 15 to 50%
- May return to full activities earlier

Geriatric:
- Decreased diagnostic accuracy
- Rupture rate: 67 to 90%
- Patients over 60 years of age account for 50% of deaths from acute appendicitis

Others: N/A

PREGNANCY
- Most common extra-uterine surgical emergency
- 1 in 2000 pregnancies
- Difficult diagnosis
- Appendix displaced superolaterally by gravid uterus
- Fetal mortality rate: 2 to 8.5%

SYNONYMS N/A

ICD-9-CM
540.0 Acute appendicitis with generalized peritonitis
540.9 Acute appendicitis without mention of peritonitis

SEE ALSO

OTHER NOTES
- In a non-surgical candidate, antibiotic therapy can be used - recurrence rate is too high to recommend as a primary therapy in other patients.

ABBREVIATIONS
KUB = kidney, ureter, bladder

REFERENCES
- Schwartz SI, ed. Principles of Surgery. 5th Ed. New York, McGraw-Hill, 1989
- Moody FG, ed. Surgical Treatment of Digestive Disease. 2nd Ed. Chicago, Year Book Medical Publishers, 1990
- Horattas MC, Guyton DP, Wu DA. Reappraisal of appendicitis in the elderly. Amer J of Surg 1990;160:291-293

Web references: 1 available at www.5mcc.com
Illustrations N/A

Author(s):
Andrew H. Fenton, MD

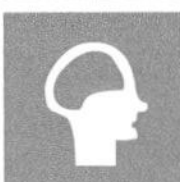

BASICS

DESCRIPTION The acute loss of perfusion distal to an occlusion of a major artery due to an embolus which migrates to the point of occlusion or a clot intrinsic to the point of occlusion (thrombosis). Both are true emergencies. Following obstruction of an artery, a soft coagulum forms both proximally and distally in the areas of stagnant flow. As the clot extends, collateral pathways are involved and the process becomes self-propagating. Ultimately, the venous circulation can be involved. The extent of vascular compromise is critical and determines the "golden" period of four to six hours. After this time, the profound ischemia leads to cellular death and is irreversible.

System(s) affected: Cardiovascular, Hemic/Lymphatic/Immunologic

Genetics: Can be associated with inheritable hypercoagulable and premature atherosclerotic syndromes

Incidence/Prevalence in USA: 50-100/100,000 hospital admissions. A leading cause of death and limb loss in the elderly.

Predominant age: Elderly

Predominant sex: Male > Female

SIGNS & SYMPTOMS

- To estimate occlusion location
  - ◊ Symptoms typically start one joint below occlusion
  - ◊ Palpable pulses are absent below an occlusion and are accentuated above
- The five "P's": Pain, Pulselessness, Pallor, Paresthesias, and Paralysis. If any one is present, frequent re-evaluations indicated. Proximal occlusions lead to a more rapid progression of findings. Occlusion at the aortic bifurcation can produce bilateral findings.
  - ◊ Pain: Diffuse in distal area. If persists, crescendo in nature. Predominates as first symptom in embolism. Not alleviated by change of position.
  - ◊ Pulselessness: Mandatory for the diagnosis of embolism or thrombosis. Pedal pulses subject to observer error. Always compare to the opposite limb.
  - ◊ Pallor: Skin color pale early, cyanotic later. Check extremity temperature left to right and top to bottom. Look for signs of chronic ischemia - skin atrophy, loss of hair, thick nails.
  - ◊ Paresthesia: Numbness early with thrombosis. Light touch first to be lost. Not reliable in diabetics. Loss of pain and pressure indicate advanced ischemia.
  - ◊ Paralysis: Motor defect occurs after sensory and indicates profound ischemia
- Distribution of emboli
  - ◊ Femoral artery 30%
  - ◊ Iliac artery 15%
  - ◊ Aortic bifurcation 10%
  - ◊ Popliteal artery 10%
  - ◊ Brachial 10%
  - ◊ Mesenteric arteries 5%
  - ◊ Renal 5%
  - ◊ Cerebral - estimated 15-20%

CAUSES

- Emboli
  - ◊ Cardiac
    - Atrial flutter/fibrillation
    - Valve disease
    - Myocardial infarction
    - Cardiomyopathy
    - Cardiac tumors
    - Endocarditis
  - ◊ Aneurysms - cardiac, aortic, peripheral
  - ◊ Paradoxical
- Thrombosis:
  - ◊ Atherosclerotic occlusive disease
  - ◊ Aortic and peripheral aneurysms - especially popliteal
  - ◊ Hypercoagulable states
  - ◊ Venous gangrene
  - ◊ Drug abuse
  - ◊ Heparin allergy
  - ◊ Vascular bypass
- Trauma:
  - ◊ Blunt
  - ◊ Penetrating
  - ◊ Vascular and cardiac interventional procedures

RISK FACTORS

- Drug abuse

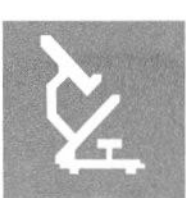

DIAGNOSIS

DIFFERENTIAL DIAGNOSIS

Emboli vs thrombosis

- Emboli
  - ◊ Myocardial diseases - myocardial infarction, arrhythmias - atrial fibrillation
  - ◊ Aneurysms
  - ◊ Pain as first symptom
- Thrombosis
  - ◊ Absence of heart disease - arrhythmias/infarction
  - ◊ Chronic vascular history
  - ◊ Bilateral changes of chronic ischemia
  - ◊ Numbness rather than pain as first symptom
  - ◊ Vascular procedures - bypass/interventional
- Acute aortic dissection; chest or back pain
- Acute deep vein thrombosis; massive swelling and warm skin
- Low flow states

LABORATORY

- Acute diagnosis is by history and exam: Laboratory data is for preoperative evaluation, elucidation of etiology, or documentation of severity of ischemia.
  - ◊ EKG
  - ◊ Myocardial/muscle isoenzymes
  - ◊ Coagulation parameters
  - ◊ Blood pH/bicarbonate
  - ◊ Urine myoglobin
  - ◊ Electrolytes

Drugs that may alter lab results: N/A

Disorders that may alter lab results: N/A

PATHOLOGICAL FINDINGS N/A

SPECIAL TESTS

- Noninvasive - indirect:
  - ◊ Doppler: presence or absence of flow
  - ◊ A/ai (ankle/arm index): dorsal pedal/posterior tibial pressure divided by brachial pressure; a/ai > 0.30 favorable
- Noninvasive - direct
  - ◊ Duplex imaging if time permits

IMAGING N/A

DIAGNOSTIC PROCEDURES

- Arteriography
  - ◊ Rarely indicated preoperatively in threatened limb
  - ◊ May help differentiate thrombosis from embolus in non-threatened limb
  - ◊ Useful with occluded grafts

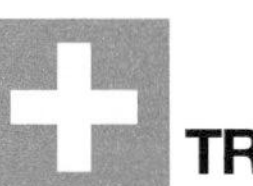

TREATMENT

APPROPRIATE HEALTH CARE Based on detailed exam, history, and Doppler exam. Triage determines appropriate therapy.

- Viable
  - ◊ Mild ischemic pain
  - ◊ Normal neurologic exam
  - ◊ Capillary refill present
  - ◊ Arterial signals present by Doppler in distal extremity
  - ◊ A/ai > 0.30
- Threatened
  - ◊ Ischemic pain
  - ◊ Mild neurologic deficit
    - Weakness of dorsiflexion
    - Minimal sensory loss - light touch and/or vibratory
  - ◊ No pulsatile flow by Doppler
  - ◊ Venous flow present
- Major ischemic changes - irreversible
  - ◊ Profound sensory loss
  - ◊ Muscle paralysis
  - ◊ Absent capillary refill
  - ◊ Skin marbling
  - ◊ Muscle rigor
  - ◊ No arterial or venous signals by Doppler

GENERAL MEASURES

- Time is of the essence
- In the threatened category nothing should delay appropriate therapy
- Unless contraindicated, systemic heparinization to decrease clot propagation and prophylaxis against further emboli
- Resuscitation and stabilization of patient to extent permitted by time
- Viable - symptomatic
  - Heparin (see Medications)
  - Arteriography
  - Embolism
  - Surgical removal if acceptable operative risk, e.g., balloon embolectomy
  - Anticoagulation vs intraarterial thrombolytics if prohibitive risk
  - ◊ Thrombosis
    - Trial of thrombolytics and correction of arterial defect if good risk
    - Anticoagulation if poor risk or thrombolytics contraindicated
- Threatened - salvageable
  - ◊ Heparin (see Medications)
  - ◊ Minimal delay to definitive therapy
  - ◊ Arteriography
  - ◊ Individualized thrombolysis and/or operative procedure (depending on extent of thrombosis and amenability for surgical removal)
  - ◊ Thrombolysis to optimize alternatives
  - ◊ Adjunctive operative therapy
    - Intraoperative lytic therapy
    - Bypass
    - Patch angioplasty
- Major ischemia - irreversible
  - ◊ Arteriography usually not warranted
  - ◊ Attempts at reperfusion contraindicated
  - ◊ Anticoagulation
  - ◊ Definitive amputation if possible

SURGICAL MEASURES See General Measures

ACTIVITY N/A

DIET N/A

PATIENT EDUCATION N/A

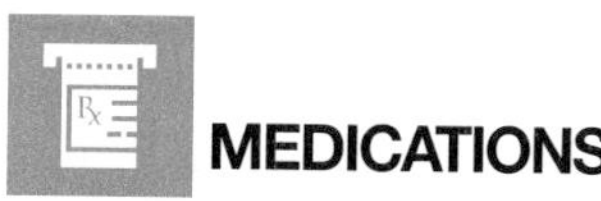

MEDICATIONS

DRUG(S) OF CHOICE

- Heparin
  - ◊ 100 units/kg IV loading dose (approximately 5,000-10,000 units)
  - ◊ Continuous heparin infusion sufficient to double the PTT, generally 1000 to 1500 units/hour
- TPA/Urokinase
  - ◊ Refer to manufacturer's literature

Contraindications:

- Heparin:
  - ◊ Allergy
  - ◊ Bleeding diathesis
  - ◊ Trauma (e.g., head injury)
  - ◊ Hematuria/hemoptysis
  - ◊ Acute aortic dissection
- Tissue plasminogen activator (TPA/Urokinase)
  - ◊ Non-salvageable ischemia
  - ◊ Recent MI
  - ◊ Aneurysm
  - ◊ Aortic dissection
  - ◊ Trauma
  - ◊ Uncontrolled hypertension
  - ◊ Recent operative procedure

Precautions: N/A

Significant possible interactions: N/A

ALTERNATIVE DRUGS

- Multiple thrombolytics in development

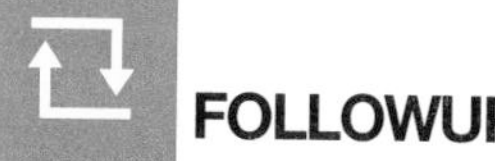

FOLLOWUP

PATIENT MONITORING

- Post operative monitoring:
  - ◊ Anticoagulation
  - ◊ Establish brisk diuresis
  - ◊ Continued resuscitation and diagnosis including echocardiography and other studies (see Causes and Risk Factors)
  - ◊ Monitor perfusion stability
  - ◊ Treat/eliminate causative factors

PREVENTION/AVOIDANCE

- Chronic anticoagulation in atrial arrhythmia
- Reduction of risk factors for atherosclerosis

POSSIBLE COMPLICATIONS

- Acidosis
- Myoglobinuria
- Hyperkalemia
- Recurrent occlusion
- Failure to remove clot/obstruction
- Compartment syndromes/reperfusion syndrome; delayed or instant
  - ◊ Predisposing factors include: combined arterial injury, profound and prolonged ischemia, hypotension
  - ◊ Occurs both in upper and lower extremities
  - ◊ Clinical findings
    - Severe pain
    - Pain with passive muscle movement
    - Hypesthesias of nerves in compartment
    - Paralysis of nerves especially peroneal - foot drop
    - Tender, tense edema
    - Compartment pressure > 30-45 mm Hg
  - ◊ Consequences of unrecognized compartment syndrome - acute
    - Amputation
    - Sepsis
    - Myoglobin renal failure
    - Shock
    - Multiple organ failure
  - ◊ Delayed
    - Ischemic contracture
    - Infection
    - Causalgia
    - Gangrene
  - ◊ Treatment
    - Fasciotomy

EXPECTED COURSE/PROGNOSIS

- 90% good outcome with prompt treatment
- Delayed/untreated associated with high mortality and limb loss
- 20-30% hospital mortality associated with causative factors

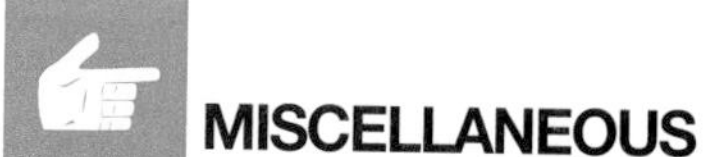

MISCELLANEOUS

ASSOCIATED CONDITIONS

- Acute mesenteric ischemia
- Renal infarction
- Carotid/CVA
- Multiple emboli
- Digital microembolization

AGE-RELATED FACTORS

Pediatric: Rare in children
Geriatric: Most common age affected
Others: N/A

PREGNANCY Rare

SYNONYMS N/A

ICD-9-CM

444.0 Arterial embolism and thrombosis of abdominal aorta
444.21 Arterial embolism and thrombosis of arteries of upper extremity
444.22 Arterial embolism and thrombosis of arteries of lower extremity
444.81 Arterial embolism and thrombosis of iliac artery
444.9 Arterial embolism and thrombosis of unspecified artery

SEE ALSO

OTHER NOTES N/A

ABBREVIATIONS

A/ai = Ankle/arm index

REFERENCES

- Rutherford RB, Flannigan DP, Gupta SK, et al: Suggested standards of reports dealing with lower extremity ischemia. J Vasc Surg 1986;64:80-94
- Brewster DC, Chin AK, Fogarty TJ: Arterial Thrombosis. In: Rutherford RB, ed. Vascular Surgery. 3rd Ed. Philadelphia, W.B. Saunders Co., 1989
- Miller DC., Roon AJ, eds: Diagnosis and Management of Peripheral Vascular Diseases. Menlo Park, CA., Addison-Wesley Co., 1982

Web references: 0 available at www.5mcc.com
Illustrations N/A

Author(s):
David H. Stubbs, MD

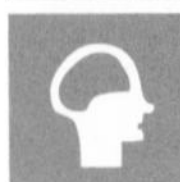

BASICS

DESCRIPTION Air released from an over-pressurized alveolus enters the pulmonary capillaries then travels through the arterial circulation causing occlusion of the cerebral and/or coronary circulation.

- Arterial gas embolism is the most serious and rapidly fatal of all SCUBA diving injuries and is second only to drowning as the leading cause of death associated with sport diving.
- Arterial gas embolism occurs on ascent and the time from alveolar rupture to the manifestation of symptoms is nearly always less than ten minutes.

System(s) affected: Cardiovascular, Musculoskeletal, Nervous
Genetics: N/A
Incidence/Prevalence in USA: It is estimated (based on injury/mortality reports collected by Divers Alert Network) to occur in approximately 4 per 100,000 sport divers per year.
Predominant age: Young adult
Predominant sex: Male > Female

SIGNS & SYMPTOMS

- Group 1: Neurologic symptoms only. Divers presenting with neurologic symptoms but without impairment of spontaneous respirations and cardiac function. May be impossible to clinically distinguish from severe decompression sickness.
  - ◊ Asymmetrical multiplegia or paralysis
  - ◊ Tingling or numbness
  - ◊ Blindness or other visual disturbances
  - ◊ Deafness
  - ◊ Vertigo
  - ◊ Dizziness
  - ◊ Headache
  - ◊ Confusion
  - ◊ Convulsions
  - ◊ Aphasia
  - ◊ Personality change; from subtle changes to unconsciousness
- Group 2: Loss of consciousness, apnea, and cardiac arrest or dysrhythmia. Divers presenting with both neurologic and cardiac impairments. All of the above signs and symptoms plus those below are possible.
  - ◊ Dysrhythmias
  - ◊ Cardiac arrest

CAUSES

- Group 1: Localized obstruction of cerebral blood flow by an embolus of air. Local capillary endothelial damage with vasogenic edema leading to a rise in intracranial pressure and ischemia.
- Group 2: This is thought to be due to localized obstruction of both cerebral and coronary blood flow by an embolus of air

RISK FACTORS

- History of a rapid ascent
- History of panic during dive
- History of holding breath while diving
- History of loss of consciousness (or with other noted symptoms) within seconds to minutes after or during a dive
- History of patent foramen ovale has been associated with a 4.5-fold increase in decompression illness events and 2 times more ischemic brain lesions than divers without this condition

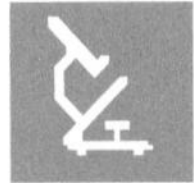

DIAGNOSIS

DIFFERENTIAL DIAGNOSIS Decompression sickness

LABORATORY

- Hematocrit - increased indicating volume depletion
- Serum creatine kinase - the correlation between serum kinase activity and outcome suggest that elevated serum level of this enzyme may be a marker for size and severity of arterial gas embolism
- Urinalysis - increased specific gravity indicating volume depletion

Drugs that may alter lab results: N/A

Disorders that may alter lab results: N/A

PATHOLOGICAL FINDINGS N/A

SPECIAL TESTS

- ECG

IMAGING

- Chest x-ray to rule out pneumothorax

DIAGNOSTIC PROCEDURES N/A

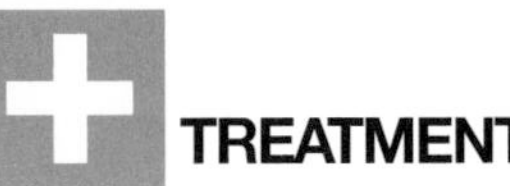

TREATMENT

APPROPRIATE HEALTH CARE

- Hospital based hyperbaric chamber capable of performing a U.S. Navy Table 6A recompression (165 feet of seawater [FSW]).

GENERAL MEASURES

- Immediate transport to a suitable hyperbaric chamber for recompression as soon as possible; do not delay with nonessential procedures.
- Transport by aircraft is justifiable if it will save a significant amount of time (aircraft must fly at low altitudes or be capable of maintaining cabin pressure at about one atmosphere)
- Life-saving measures (CPR) must take precedence to sustain life
- Administration of high flow maximum concentration oxygen therapy by a tight fitting mask or by intubation and mechanical ventilation during transport
- Keep patient in recumbent position while maintaining airway
- Maintain hydration with IV fluids
- For assistance and advice in locating the nearest treatment chamber in your area (world-wide) call DIVERS ALERT NETWORK (DAN) at any hour (919) 684-8111

SURGICAL MEASURES N/A

ACTIVITY None until after treatment

DIET None until after treatment

PATIENT EDUCATION

- Divers Alert Network (DAN)
  - ◊ Diving emergency hotline for medical emergencies only - 919-684-8111 or 919-684-4DAN (collect); 24 hours, 365 days a year
  - ◊ Medical information line for nonemergency questions - 919-684-2948 M-F (9-5 EST)
  - ◊ DAN America information line - 800-446-2671 or 919-684-2948 M-F (9-5 EST); website www.diversalert-network.org
  - ◊ On-Site neurological exam by Ed Thalmann, MD; website www.diversalertnetwork.org/medical/neuro-exam.asp

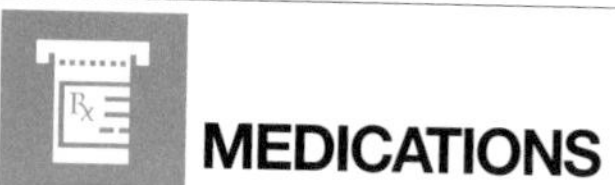

MEDICATIONS

DRUG(S) OF CHOICE
- Oxygen

Contraindications: N/A
Precautions: N/A
Significant possible interactions: N/A

ALTERNATIVE DRUGS
None

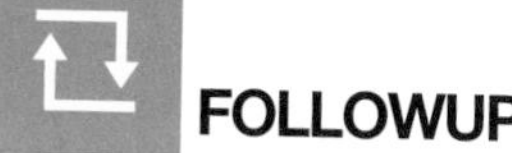

FOLLOWUP

PATIENT MONITORING
- Frequent neurological checks in the acute pre-treatment and treatment phase
- Complete neurological assessment at one, three, six and twelve at months

PREVENTION/AVOIDANCE
- Strict adherence to diver safety protocols, especially including the buddy system
- No diving after any dive injury or with any medical condition until evaluated and approved by a physician knowledgeable in diving medicine

POSSIBLE COMPLICATIONS
- Long term serious neurologic impairments
- Death

EXPECTED COURSE/PROGNOSIS
- Complete to partial resolution with adequate treatment

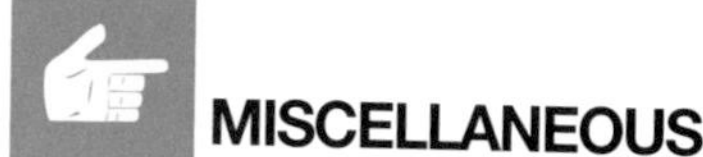

MISCELLANEOUS

ASSOCIATED CONDITIONS
- Pulmonary barotrauma leading to arterial gas embolism, can also cause pneumomediastinum, subcutaneous emphysema, pneumopericardium, pneumothorax, and pneumoperitoneum
- Always consider the possibility of decompression sickness in addition to arterial gas embolism in any SCUBA diver who has recently completed a dive
- Patent foramen ovale and diving has been associated with ischemic brain lesions

AGE-RELATED FACTORS
Pediatric: N/A
Geriatric: N/A
Others: N/A

PREGNANCY
N/A

SYNONYMS
- Gas embolism
- Air embolism

ICD-9-CM
958.0 Air embolism

SEE ALSO

OTHER NOTES
- Any diver who has an onset of new symptom(s) or sign(s) after recently completing a SCUBA dive of any type, to any depth, for any period of time - serious consideration must be given as having sustained a dive related injury

ABBREVIATIONS
DAN = Divers Alert Network
AGE = arterial gas embolism
FSW = feet of seawater

REFERENCES

- Schwerzmann M, Seller C, Lipp E. Relation between directly detected patent foramen ovale and ischemic brain lesions in sport divers. Ann InternMed 2001;134(1):21-4
- van Hulst RA, Klein J, Lachmann B. Gas embolism: pathophysiology and treatment. Clin Physiol Funct Imaging 2003 Sep;23(5):237-46
- Davis J. Medical Examination of Sport Scuba Divers. 2nd ed. Medical Seminars, Inc; 1986
- Bove A, Davis J. Bove and Davis Diving Medicine. 4th ed. Philadelphia: WB Saunders Co; 2003
- Edmonds C, Lowry C, Pennefather J. Diving and Subaquatic Medicine 3rd ed. Boston: Butterworth-Heinemann Medical; 1994

Web references: 2 available at www.5mcc.com
Illustrations N/A

Author(s):
Jess G. Bond, MD, MPH

BASICS

DESCRIPTION Arteriosclerosis is a group of diseases characterized by thickening and loss of elasticity of the arterial walls which progressively blocks the coronary arteries and their branches. Arteriosclerosis is the most common form of coronary arteriosclerosis. The process is chronic, occurring over many years, and is the most common cause of cardiovascular disability and death. Other forms of arteriosclerosis include arteriolosclerosis and medial calcific stenosis, both of which are uncommon in the coronary vasculature.
System(s) affected: Cardiovascular
Genetics: Tendency is inheritable
Incidence/Prevalence in USA: Common. Causes 35% of deaths in men age 35-50. Death rate age 55-64 - 1:100.
Predominant age: Men 50-60, women 60-70, for peak clinical manifestations
Predominant sex: Male > Female

SIGNS & SYMPTOMS
- Variable. May remain clinically asymptomatic even in advanced disease states, eg, silent ischemia.
- Clinical manifestations
  - ◊ Substernal chest pain
  - ◊ Exertional dyspnea
  - ◊ Orthopnea
  - ◊ Paroxysmal nocturnal dyspnea
  - ◊ Cardiac arrhythmias
  - ◊ Systolic murmur
  - ◊ Cardiomegaly
  - ◊ Pedal edema

CAUSES
- Atherosclerosis
- Narrowing of coronary arteries
- Embolism compromising coronary arteries at orifices
- Subintimal atheromas in large and medium vessels

RISK FACTORS
- Elevated low density lipoprotein (LDL)
- Decreased high density lipoprotein (HDL)
- Elevated triglycerides
- Smoking
- Family history of premature arteriosclerosis
- Obesity
- Hypertension
- Stress
- Sedentary life style
- Increasing age
- Male sex
- Diabetes mellitus

DIAGNOSIS

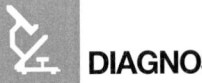

DIFFERENTIAL DIAGNOSIS N/A

LABORATORY
- Elevated triglycerides
- Elevated total cholesterol
- Elevated low density lipoproteins
- Decreased high density lipoproteins
- Elevated cholesterol/HDL ratio

Drugs that may alter lab results: N/A

Disorders that may alter lab results: N/A

PATHOLOGICAL FINDINGS
- Gross - narrowed coronary arteries
- Micro - cholesterol plaques on intima of coronary vessels
- Fibrotic subendothelial connective tissue of intima with plaque

SPECIAL TESTS
- ECG - variable. May be normal or may see ST segment elevation/depression and/or T wave inversion.
- Exercise stress test - positive

IMAGING
- Angiography - narrowed coronary arteries
- Echocardiography - wall motion abnormalities
- Pharmacologic stress tests (dobutamine, dipyridamole, adenosine) - positive
- Stress thallium test - positive

DIAGNOSTIC PROCEDURES N/A

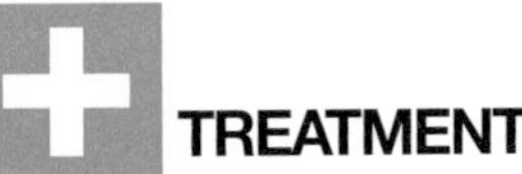

TREATMENT

APPROPRIATE HEALTH CARE
- Outpatient for management of risk factors
- Inpatient for acute ischemic syndromes

GENERAL MEASURES
- Prevention of further progression of the disease
  - ◊ Smoking cessation
  - ◊ Treatment of hypercholesterolemia (diet, drugs)
  - ◊ Increase high density lipoprotein (diet, exercise)
  - ◊ Control of blood pressure
  - ◊ Diabetes mellitus treated early and adequately
  - ◊ Exercise
  - ◊ Prophylactic aspirin
  - ◊ Stress reduction
  - ◊ Diet changes
  - ◊ Weight loss
  - ◊ Estrogen replacement therapy in postmenopausal women is currently controversial
- Treatment of complications
  - ◊ Covered elsewhere under the individual topics (e.g., angina pectoris, myocardial infarction, heart failure, stroke, peripheral arterial occlusion, etc.)

SURGICAL MEASURES N/A

ACTIVITY Exercise may be helpful in preventing clinical coronary disease and useful for therapeutic measures

DIET
- Low-fat (20-30 grams of fat/day total intake)
- Weight-loss diet, if obesity a problem
- Increase soluble fiber

PATIENT EDUCATION For patient education materials favorably reviewed on this topic, contact: American Heart Association, 7320 Greenville Avenue, Dallas, TX 75231, (214)373-6300

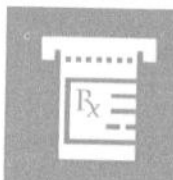

MEDICATIONS

DRUG(S) OF CHOICE
- Aspirin, 160-325 mg/day, unless contraindicated
- Cholesterol-lowering agents
  - ◊ Cholestyramine or colestipol, (bile acid sequestrants) 12-32 gm orally BID-QID
  - ◊ Niacin 2-6 gm daily in divided doses (highly efficacious, but side effects restrict use)
  - ◊ Gemfibrozil 600 mg bid
  - ◊ Fenofibrate 67-200 mg/day
  - ◊ Probucol 500 mg bid
  - ◊ Colesevelam 3.75-4.375 g/day
  - ◊ Ezetimibe 10 mg/day
  - ◊ HMG-CoA reductase inhibitors (dose varies with product): atorvastatin (Lipitor), fluvastatin (Lescol), lovastatin (Mevacor), pravastatin (Pravachol), simvastatin (Zocor), rosuvastatin (Crestor)

Contraindications: Refer to manufacturer's literature

Precautions: SR form of niacin may be linked to hepatotoxicity. Refer to manufacturer's literature.

Significant possible interactions: Refer to manufacturer's literature

ALTERNATIVE DRUGS Ticlopidine - antiplatelet activity

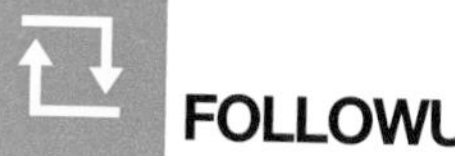

FOLLOWUP

PATIENT MONITORING Monitor cholesterol, triglyceride levels, other preventive programs (weight loss, smoking cessation)

PREVENTION/AVOIDANCE See General measures

POSSIBLE COMPLICATIONS
- Myocardial infarction
- Ventricular fibrillation
- Congestive heart failure
- Angina pectoris
- Sudden cardiac death

EXPECTED COURSE/PROGNOSIS
Guardedly favorable. Many risk factors can be modified.

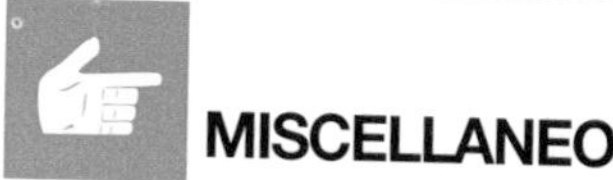

MISCELLANEOUS

ASSOCIATED CONDITIONS
- Obesity
- Hypertension
- Diabetes
- Hypercholesterolemia

AGE-RELATED FACTORS
Pediatric: Preventive measures can begin early (proper nutrition, exercise, weight control, smoking deterrent programs, etc.)

Geriatric: Greatest incidence in this age group

Others: N/A

PREGNANCY Rare in pregnant women

SYNONYMS
- Coronary artery disease (CAD)
- Coronary heart disease
- Coronary arteriosclerosis

ICD-9-CM
414.00 Coronary atherosclerosis of unspecified type of vessel, native or graft

SEE ALSO
Angina
Atherosclerosis
Myocardial infarction

OTHER NOTES N/A

ABBREVIATIONS N/A

REFERENCES

- Hurst JW, et al. The Heart. 10th ed. New York: McGraw-Hill; 2001
- Braunwald E, editor. Heart Disease: A Textbook of Cardiovascular Medicine. 6th ed. Philadelphia: WB Saunders Co; 2001
- Goldman L, Braunwald E. Primary Cardiology. 2nd ed. Philadelphia: WB Saunders Co; 2003

Web references: 0 available at www.5mcc.com

Illustrations N/A

Author(s):
Peter Kozisek, MD

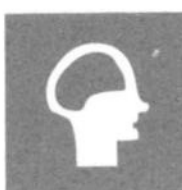

BASICS

DESCRIPTION Invasion of joints by live micro-organisms or their fragments. One of the few curable causes of arthritis. May allow early recognition of systemic infection/disease.

System(s) affected: Musculoskeletal

Genetics: N/A

Incidence/Prevalence in USA:
- Neisserial:
  - ◊ Responsible for 50% of infectious arthritis
  - ◊ Arthritis occurs in 0.6% of the 3% of women with gonorrhea
  - ◊ Arthritis occurs in 0.1% of the 0.7% of men with gonorrhea
  - ◊ Arthritis occurs in 7% of individuals with N. meningitidis
- Non-Neisserial:
  - ◊ Half as frequent as Neisserial

Predominant age:
- Neisserial:
  - ◊ Especially 15-40, can occur at any age
- Non-Neisserial:
  - ◊ Prior to age 2: 27% Staphylococcus, 20% Streptococcus, 33% Haemophilus, and 13% other gram negative rods, 7% miscellaneous
  - ◊ Age 2-14: 34% Staphylococcus, 29% Streptococcus, 13% Haemophilus, and 13 % other gram negative rods, 11% miscellaneous
  - ◊ Adult: 34% Staphylococcus, 38% Streptococcus, 2% Haemophilus, and 26% other gram negative rods

Predominant sex:
- Neisserial: Female > Male (4:1)
- Non-Neisserial: Male > Female (2:1)
- Subacute bacterial endocarditis-related: Male = Female

SIGNS & SYMPTOMS
- Predominantly monoarticular (90%). (Haemophilus may be pauciarticular and Mycoplasma often presents as a migratory polyarthritis).
- Limited joint use/motion (especially in children)
- Joint effusion, tenderness
- Joint warmth - present in less than 50%
- Joint redness- present in less than 50%
- Loss of joint motion
- Tenosynovitis
- Sudden flare of one or two joints in a patient with underlying joint disease
- Fever - in 90% at some time during the course of the infection
- Chills, malaise
- Cutaneous lesions
- Peripheral neuropathy
- Back pain - especially in subacute bacterial endocarditis (SBE)
- Hypertrophic osteoarthropathy - rare, secondary to endocarditis
- Fretfulness - especially in children
- Dermato-arthritis - usually pustular skin lesions in gonorrhea - usually petechial rash in meningococcemia
- Bacteremic phase - migratory polyarthritis, tenosynovitis, high fever, chills, pustules
- Localized phase - usually monoarticular, low grade fever (80%)

CAUSES
- Hematogenous invasion by microorganisms (80-90%)
- Contiguous spread (10-15%) from adjacent osteomyelitis in children
- Direct penetration of micro-organisms secondary to trauma or joint injection

RISK FACTORS
- Young patient with venereal exposure
- Concurrent extra-articular infection
- Prior arthritis in infected joint
- Trauma
- Joint puncture or surgery
- Prosthetic joint
- Prior antibiotic, corticosteroid, or immunosuppressive therapy
- Serious chronic illness (e.g., diabetes, liver disease, malignancy, primary immunodeficiency)
- Defective phagocytic mechanisms (e.g., chronic granulomatous disease)
- Intravenous drug abuse
- Travel/habitat history
- Sickle cell anemia
- C8 deficiency

DIAGNOSIS

DIFFERENTIAL DIAGNOSIS
- Gout
- Pseudogout (calcium pyrophosphate deposition disease)
- Spondyloarthropathy (Reiter syndrome, psoriatic arthritis, ankylosing spondylitis, the arthritis of inflammatory bowel disease)
- Juvenile rheumatoid arthritis
- Type IIa hyperlipoproteinemia
- Foreign body synovitis
- Rheumatoid arthritis
- Rheumatic fever
- AIDS
- Cellulitis
- Palindromic rheumatism
- Neuropathic arthropathy
- Lyme arthritis
- Sarcoidosis
- Granulomatous arthritis

LABORATORY
- Synovial fluid usually cloudy with > 50,000 WBC/HPF (high power field), but may have fewer white blood cells present or over 100,000. (Caveat - cell count must be performed within 1 hour of obtaining specimen to be valid).
- Synovial fluid white count can be recognized as elevated (in presence of trauma) if RBC:WBC ratio significantly less than 700
- Polymorphonuclear leukocytes usually predominate in synovial fluid
- Synovial fluid glucose often more than 40 mg/dL (2.22 mmol/L) less than in a simultaneously obtained serum glucose value (in fasting patient). However, arthrocentesis should not be delayed simply to obtain fasting synovial fluid glucose level.
- Westergren erythrocyte sedimentation rate - often elevated, but normal in 20%
- Rheumatoid factor positive in 50% - if endocarditis present and in viral arthritis
- Anti-teichoic acid antibodies - with Staphylococcus infection
- Elevated peripheral white blood cell count (in 50-90%)
- Cryoglobulins
- Immune complexes
- Febrile agglutinins (to include Brucella and rickettsial-related titers)
- Antistreptolysin O (ASO) titer is usually normal, exclusive of streptococcal infections
- Depressed synovial fluid and occasionally depressed serum levels of complement
- Microscopic hematuria in subacute bacterial endocarditis (SBE)
- Presence of crystals (e.g., urate or calcium pyrophosphate) does not exclude infectious arthritis

Drugs that may alter lab results: Antibiotics

Disorders that may alter lab results: N/A

PATHOLOGICAL FINDINGS Synovial biopsy will reveal polymorphonuclear leukocytes and possibly the causative organism - if cultures are negative of fluid

SPECIAL TESTS
- Joint fluid - for gram stain (positive in 50%); culture (positive in 50-70%)
- Serum cidal level assessment of antibiotic adequacy is suggested with virulent organisms or therapeutic unresponsiveness (tenfold margin suggested)
- Blood, orifice, urine cultures. "Bedside culture" is recommended to enhance isolation of fastidious organisms.
- All cultures should be preserved and observed for at least 3 days and preferably 2 weeks. Observing synovial fluid cultures for at least 3 days allows isolation of fastidious organisms such as those of rat bite fever (Streptobacillus moniliformis and Spirillum minus).
- Neisserial infection generally requires use of special agars (e.g., chocolate or Thayer Martin) and relative anaerobic culturing conditions
- Countercurrent immunoelectrophoresis or complement fixation for specific bacterial antigens
- Polymerase chain reaction for specific bacterial DNA

IMAGING
- X-ray
  - ◊ Soft tissue swelling
  - ◊ Juxta-articular osteoporosis
  - ◊ Radiolucent area (gas) in a joint space from gas forming organisms. (Caveat - may also occur normally as a "vacuum phenomenon").
  - ◊ Effacement of the obturator fat pad (with hip involvement)
  - ◊ X-ray changes are usually a late phenomenon
  - ◊ Rarefaction of subchondral bone may occur as early as 2-7 days
  - ◊ Joint space loss (secondary to cartilage destruction) may be seen as early as 4-10 days
  - ◊ Erosions
  - ◊ Joint destruction with ankylosis may occur as early as 2 weeks

- Other imaging techniques
  - ◊ Technetium joint scans - reveal distribution of inflammation - sensitive, not specific
  - ◊ Gallium or Ceretec WBC scan-Indium scans - reveal inflammation as well as infection
  - ◊ CT - to identify sequestration
  - ◊ MRI - effusion, perhaps early cartilage damage, osteomyelitis

DIAGNOSTIC PROCEDURES
- Arthrocentesis with gram stain and culture - only positive in 50-70% dependent on organism. Must be done in all patients when possibility of infectious arthritis is considered. Arthrocentesis should probably be performed within 12 hours of suspicion.
- Arthrocentesis approach must avoid contaminated tissue (e.g., overlying cellulitis)

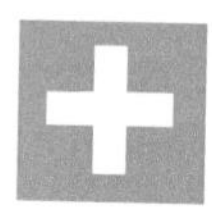

TREATMENT

APPROPRIATE HEALTH CARE
- Hospitalization for parenteral therapy
- Rarely an extremely compliant patient with a very sensitive organism might be treated as an outpatient

GENERAL MEASURES
- Repeat arthrocentesis to drain the joint, as fluid re-accumulates
- Avoid adding anti-inflammatory therapy so as not to compromise assessment of therapeutic response to antibiotic
- If a joint prosthesis is present in an infection, the infection is very difficult to eradicate, without removal of the prosthesis
- Treatment is continued for 1-2 weeks after total resolution of all signs of inflammation, 3-4 weeks for gram negative organisms, and 6-8 weeks if the joint was previously diseased (e.g., involved by arthritis)
- Intra-articular antibiotics are not required and may actually aggravate the arthritis

SURGICAL MEASURES Arthrotomy indicated only if fluid accumulated is loculated and/or not amenable to needle drainage, or if antibiotics fail

ACTIVITY Limit activity or splint the joint initially. Continuous passive motion may be used as an alternative approach.

DIET No special diet

PATIENT EDUCATION
- Rothschild, B.: Diagnosing and treating infectious arthritis. Geriatric Consultant. 5:14-15, 1986
- Arthritis Foundation pamphlet

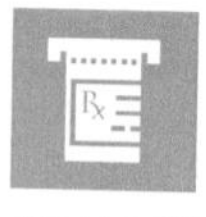

MEDICATIONS

DRUG(S) OF CHOICE
- Neisserial
  - ◊ Ceftriaxone 1 gm IM or IV every day for 14 days (but at least 7 days after symptoms resolve)
  - ◊ Spectinomycin 2 gm IM every 12 hours for 10 days
- Non-Neisserial:
  - ◊ Gram positive cocci in chains or clumps - nafcillin 150 mg/kg/day q 4-6 h IV/IM
  - ◊ Gram positive diplococci - penicillin G 1.4 million units q6h
  - ◊ Gram negative bacilli: In neonates - penicillin and gentamicin; in children age 6 months to 4 years - cefuroxime; in adult - penicillin or cephalosporin plus gentamicin, all at full dose. Add clindamycin, at full dose, in the presence of retroperitoneal or pelvic abscess.
  - ◊ Gram negative pleomorphic organisms - clindamycin at full dose (clindamycin has gram negative activity only against anaerobes)
  - ◊ No bacteria seen on smear - penicillin or cephalosporin plus gentamicin, all at full dose

Contraindications:
- Tetracycline: not for use in pregnancy or children < 8 years.

Precautions:
- Observe for allergic reactions/serum sickness
- Tetracycline: may cause photosensitivity; sunscreen recommended.

Significant possible interactions:
- Tetracycline: avoid concurrent administration with antacids, dairy products, or iron.
- Broad-spectrum antibiotics: may reduce the effectiveness of oral contraceptives; barrier method recommended.

ALTERNATIVE DRUGS
- Non-Neisserial
  - ◊ In children age 6 months to 4 years - ampicillin; chloramphenicol may be required to cover resistant Haemophilus
  - ◊ Infectious disease consult strongly advised to supplement rheumatologist input for Haemophilus infections
- Quinolones (e.g., ciprofloxacin)

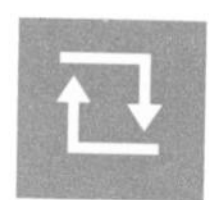

FOLLOWUP

PATIENT MONITORING
- Recurrent arthrocentesis, as fluid re-accumulates - to verify sterilization of the joint and to verify reversion of inflammatory signs to normal
- If no definitive improvement within 48 hours, re-evaluate completely
- Complete blood count, liver and kidney function and urinalysis twice a week, while on antibiotics (perhaps with creatinine every other day when gentamicin used)
- Gentamicin levels
- It is essential to followup one week and a month after stopping antibiotics to detect any relapse

PREVENTION/AVOIDANCE
- Prophylaxis in presence of predisposing joint condition
- Condoms and discretion for STD protection for Neisseria

POSSIBLE COMPLICATIONS
- Death (9-33% in elderly)
- Limited joint range of motion
- Flail or fused or dislocated joint
- Carpal tunnel syndrome
- Septic necrosis
- Sinus formation
- Ankylosis
- Osteomyelitis
- Postinfectious synovitis
- Shortening of the limb (in children)

EXPECTED COURSE/PROGNOSIS
- Early treatment should allow cure
- Delayed recognition/treatment complicated by morbidity and mortality

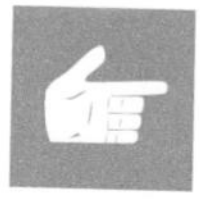

MISCELLANEOUS

ASSOCIATED CONDITIONS
- Systemic infection; infection elsewhere
- Immunodeficiency; immunosuppression
- Rheumatoid arthritis

AGE-RELATED FACTORS
Pediatric: N/A
Geriatric: N/A
Others: N/A

PREGNANCY N/A

SYNONYMS
- Suppurative arthritis
- Septic arthritis

ICD-9-CM
711.00 Pyogenic arthritis, site unspecified

SEE ALSO
Reiter syndrome

OTHER NOTES N/A

ABBREVIATIONS N/A

REFERENCES

- Wilkinson NZ, Kingsley GH, Jones HW, et al. The detection of DNA from a range of bacterial species in the joints of patients with a variety of arthritides using a nested, broad-range polymerase chain reaction. Rheumatol 1999;38:260-266
- Gonzalez-Juanatey C. Rheumatic Manifestations of Infective Endocarditis in Non-Addicts A 12-Year Study. Medicine 2001;80(1);9-19
- Gershwin ME, Robbins DL. Musculoskeletal Diseases of Children, New York, Grune & Stratton, 1983
- Gupta MN, Sturrock RD, Field M. Prospective comparative study of patients with culture proven and high suspicion of adult onset septic arthritis. Ann Rheum Dis 2003;62(4):327-31
- Khachatourians AG, Patzakis MJ, Roidis N, Holtom PD. Laboratory monitoring in pediatric acute osteomyelitis and septic arthritis. Clin Orthop 2003;(409):186-94

Web references: 2 available at www.5mcc.com
Illustrations N/A

Author(s):
Bruce M. Rothschild, MD

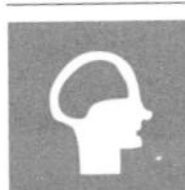

BASICS

DESCRIPTION Invasion of joints by live micro-organisms or their fragments. One of the few curable causes of arthritis. May allow early recognition of systemic infection/disease.

System(s) affected: Musculoskeletal

Genetics: N/A

Incidence/Prevalence in USA:
- One in three million
- Granulomatous arthritis occurs in 1-3% of patients with tuberculosis infections

Predominant age: Diffuse

Predominant sex:
- Male > Female (Brucella and mycobacterial)
- Female > Male (fungal)

SIGNS & SYMPTOMS
- Predominantly monoarticular (90%). Fungal may present as a migratory polyarthritis.
- Joint tenderness
- Limited joint use/motion (especially in children)
- Joint effusion
- Joint warmth - present in less than 50%
- Joint redness - present in less than 50%
- Loss of joint motion
- Tenosynovitis
- Sudden flare of a single joint in a patient with underlying joint disease
- Fever - in 50% at some time during the course of the infection
- Chills
- Malaise
- Cutaneous lesions
- Peripheral neuropathy
- Back pain - especially in tuberculosis and brucellosis
- Hypertrophic osteoarthropathy
- Fretfulness - especially in children
- Doughy swelling, with minimal tenderness
- Dactylitis
- Diaphoresis
- Headache
- Hepatosplenomegaly
- Lymphadenopathy
- Erythema nodosum
- Iritis (with mycobacterial arthritis)

CAUSES
- Hematogenous invasion by microorganisms (80-90%)
- Contiguous spread (10-15%)
- Direct penetration of micro-organisms secondary to trauma

RISK FACTORS
- Concurrent acquired immunodeficiency disease
- Concurrent extra-articular infection
- Prior arthritis in infected joint
- Trauma
- Rheumatoid arthritis
- Joint puncture or surgery
- Prosthetic joint
- Prior antibiotic, corticosteroid, or immunosuppressive therapy
- Serious chronic illness (e.g., diabetes, liver disease, malignancy, primary immunodeficiency)
- Defective phagocytic mechanisms (e.g., chronic granulomatous disease)
- Intravenous drug abuse
- Exposure history (e.g., unpasteurized milk)
- Farmers, butchers, veterinarians
- Travel/habitat history
- Gardening, especially for sporotrichosis

DIAGNOSIS

DIFFERENTIAL DIAGNOSIS
- Gout
- Pseudogout (calcium pyrophosphate deposition disease)
- Spondyloarthropathy (Reiter syndrome, psoriatic arthritis, ankylosing spondylitis, the arthritis of inflammatory bowel disease)
- Juvenile rheumatoid arthritis
- Type IIa hyperlipoproteinemia
- Foreign body synovitis
- Rheumatoid arthritis
- Rheumatic fever
- AIDS
- Cellulitis
- Palindromic rheumatism
- Neuropathic arthropathy
- Lyme arthritis
- Sarcoidosis
- Pyogenic arthritis

LABORATORY
- Synovial fluid usually cloudy with > 20,000 WBC/HPF, but may have fewer white blood cells present or over 100,000. (Caveat - cell count must be performed within 1 hour of obtaining specimen to be valid).
- Synovial fluid white count can be recognized as elevated (in presence of trauma) if RBC:WBC ratio significantly less than 700
- Polymorphonuclear leukocytes usually predominate in synovial fluid. (Granulomatous and viral arthritis may have a mononuclear cell predominance, but polymorphonuclear leukocytes usually predominate).
- Synovial fluid glucose often more than 40 mg/dL (2.22 mmol/L) less than in a simultaneously obtained serum glucose value (in fasting patient). However, arthrocentesis should not be delayed simply to obtain fasting synovial fluid glucose level.
- Synovial fluid eosinophilia may occasionally be seen in the healing phase of an infection, but parasitic (e.g., guinea-worm) infection must also be considered
- Westergren erythrocyte sedimentation - often elevated, but normal in 20%
- Rheumatoid factor positive in 50% - if endocarditis present
- Elevated peripheral white blood cell count
- Cryoglobulins
- Immune complexes
- Febrile agglutinins (to include Brucella and rickettsial related titers)
- Antistreptolysin O (ASO) titer is usually normal
- Depressed synovial fluid and occasionally serum levels of complement
- Presence of crystals in synovial fluid (e.g., urate or calcium pyrophosphate) does not exclude infectious arthritis
- Polymerase chain reaction for specific microorganisms

Drugs that may alter lab results: Insulin, antibiotics

Disorders that may alter lab results: Diabetes

PATHOLOGICAL FINDINGS Synovial biopsy may reveal granulomas and possibly the causative organism

SPECIAL TESTS
- Arthrocentesis - bacterial - for silver and acid fast stain and culture
- Arthrocentesis - mycobacterial - acid fast (positive in 20%); culture (positive in 80%)
- Drug sensitivity testing recommended
- Blood, urine cultures
- Sputum cultures
- Gastric lavage for acid fast - increases yield 7%
- Fungal blood cultures
- All cultures should be held for 2 weeks; acid-fast cultures for 6 weeks
- Polymerase chain reaction (PCR)DNA analysis for tuberculosis

IMAGING
- X-ray
    - ◊ Soft tissue swelling
    - ◊ Osteoporosis
    - ◊ Effacement of the obturator fat pad (with hip involvement) or psoas shadow
    - ◊ X-ray changes are usually a late phenomenon
    - ◊ Rarefaction of subchondral bone
    - ◊ Joint space loss
    - ◊ Erosions
    - ◊ Joint destruction with ankylosis
    - ◊ Subchondral erosion with preservation of joint space is highly suggestive of granulomatous infection
- Other imaging techniques
    - ◊ Technetium joint scans - reveal distribution of inflammation, not just infection
    - ◊ Gallium or Ceretec WBC scan-Indium scans - reveal inflammation as well as infection
    - ◊ Computerized tomography - to identify sequestration
    - ◊ Magnetic resonance imaging - perhaps early cartilage damage, osteomyelitis

DIAGNOSTIC PROCEDURES
- Arthrocentesis with gram, silver and acid fast stain, and culture. Must be done in all patients when possibility of infectious arthritis considered.
- Arthrocentesis approach must avoid contaminated tissue (e.g., overlying cellulitis)
- Biopsy and culture synovial membrane

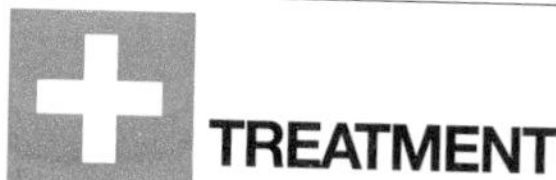

TREATMENT

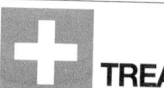

APPROPRIATE HEALTH CARE
- Fungal - initial hospitalization for parenteral therapy
- Mycobacterial - outpatient, once diagnosed
- Brucella - outpatient, once diagnosed

GENERAL MEASURES
- Repeat arthrocentesis to drain the joint, as fluid reaccumulates
- Avoid adding anti-inflammatory therapy so as not to compromise assessment of therapeutic response (to antibiotic)
- Infection associated with prosthetic joints may be difficult to eradicate without removal
- For Brucella or fungal infections, treatment is continued for 1-2 weeks after total resolution of all signs of inflammation, and 6-8 weeks if the joint was previously diseased (e.g., involved by arthritis)
- Anti-granulomatous therapy requires a long program (See Tuberculosis)
- Intra-articular antibiotics are not indicated
- Infectious disease consultation may be helpful

SURGICAL MEASURES
- Arthrotomy indicated only if fluid accumulated is loculated and/or not amenable to needle drainage

ACTIVITY Limit/splint joint initially, while pursuing full passive range of motion. Continuous passive motion is an alternative approach.

DIET As tolerated

PATIENT EDUCATION
- Rothschild, B.M.: Diagnosing and treating infectious arthritis. Geriatric Consultant, 5:14-15, 1986
- Arthritis Foundation

1314 Spring Street, NW
Atlanta, GA 30309
(404) 872-7100

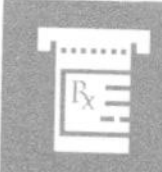

MEDICATIONS

DRUG(S) OF CHOICE
- Medications based on sensitivity of organisms
- Mycobacterial: (use a combination of these three) isoniazid at 5 mg/kg, up to 300 mg po qd, rifampin at 10 mg/kg, up to 600 mg PO qd, and pyrazinamide at 15-30 mg/kg up to 2 gm/d. The latter is replaced after 2 months with ethambutol 15 mg/kg. Continue therapy for 9-24 months. Request infectious disease consultation.
- Brucella: tetracycline plus streptomycin or trimethoprim-sulfamethoxazole or rifampin (for dosage, see manufacturer's literature)
- Fungal infection: amphotericin B, ketoconazole, flucytosine (5-fluorocytosine), dependent upon organism

Contraindications:
- Tetracycline: not for use in pregnancy or children < 8 years.

Precautions:
- Observe for allergic reactions/serum sickness
- Tetracycline: may cause photosensitivity; sunscreen recommended.

Significant possible interactions:
- Tetracycline: avoid concurrent administration with antacids, dairy products, or iron.
- Ketoconazole - multiple drug interactions

ALTERNATIVE DRUGS
- See Tuberculosis

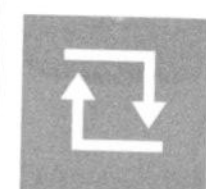

FOLLOWUP

PATIENT MONITORING To verify sterilization of the joint and to verify reversion of inflammatory signs to normal
- Treatment of mycobacterial arthritis requires monthly complete blood count, liver and kidney function and urinalysis assessment
- It is essential to followup frequently after stopping antibiotics to detect relapse
- As dictated by therapy (EG, amphotericin B)

PREVENTION/AVOIDANCE Prophylaxis in presence of predisposing joint condition

POSSIBLE COMPLICATIONS
- Limited joint range of motion
- Flail or fused joint
- Carpal-tunnel syndrome
- Septic necrosis
- Sinus formation
- Ankylosis
- Joint dislocation
- Osteomyelitis
- Shortening of the limb (in children)

EXPECTED COURSE/PROGNOSIS
- Early initiation of treatment should allow cure
- Delayed recognition/treatment complicated by increased morbidity and mortality

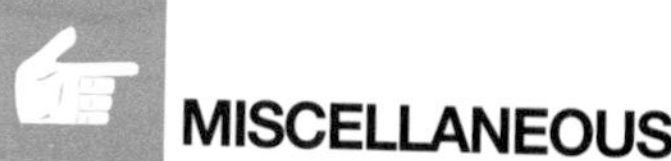

MISCELLANEOUS

ASSOCIATED CONDITIONS
- Systemic infection
- Infection elsewhere
- Immunodeficiency - (medication)
- Immunosuppression

AGE-RELATED FACTORS
Pediatric: Infrequent
Geriatric:
- Grave in elderly
- Tuberculosis much more likely to occur

Others: N/A

PREGNANCY N/A

SYNONYMS
- Fungal arthritis

ICD-9-CM
031.8 Other specified mycobacterial diseases
023.9 Brucellosis, unspecified
115.99 Histoplasmosis, unspecified other

SEE ALSO
Atypical mycobacterial infection
Brucellosis

OTHER NOTES Infectious arthritis may be caused by many other organisms including bacterial (particularly neisseria), rickettsial, parasitic, fungal, and viral agents. Much of the information contained in this profile applies to these other organisms as well as to granulomatous infections.

ABBREVIATIONS
HPF = high power field

REFERENCES

- Gershwin ME, Robbins DL: Musculoskeletal Diseases of Children. New York, Grune & Stratton, 1983
- Rothschild BM, Martin L: Paleopathology: Disease in the Fossil Record. London, CRC Press, 1993
- Kelly WW, Harris ED Jr, Ruddy S, Sledge CB: Textbook of Rheumatology. Philadelphia, W.B. Saunders Co., 1997
- Rothschild BM, Rothschild C: Recognition of hypertrophic osteoarthropathy in skeletal remains. J Rheum 1998;25:2221-2228
- Sawlani V, Chandra T, Mishra RN, Aggarwal A, Jain UK, Gujral RB. MRI features of tuberculosis of peripheral joints. Clin Radiol 2003;58(10):755-62
- Resnick D. Diagnosis of Bone and Joint Disorders. Philadelphia: WB Saunders Co; 2002.p2375-2612

Web references: 1 available at www.5mcc.com
Illustrations N/A

Author(s):
Bruce M. Rothschild, MD

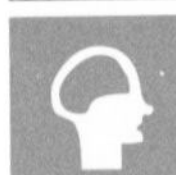

BASICS

DESCRIPTION Juvenile rheumatoid arthritis (JRA) is the most common form of chronic arthritis in children and a major cause of musculoskeletal disability. There are three subtypes of the disease, determined by the clinical characteristics occurring within the first six months of illness.
- Systemic (sys) JRA: occurs in 5-10% of affected children; usually characterized by a febrile onset and evanescent rash with multiple physical and laboratory abnormalities
- Polyarticular (poly) JRA: occurs in 30-40% of affected children; characterized by multiple (> 4) joint involvement and minimal systemic features
- Pauciarticular (pauci) JRA: occurs in 40-50% of affected children; characterized by ≤ 4 joints involved, usually larger joints; a risk for chronic uveitis in young girls and axial skeletal involvement in older boys

System(s) affected: Hemic/Lymphatic/Immunologic, Musculoskeletal
Genetics: HLA-B27 histocompatibility antigen associated with risk of evolving spondyloarthropathy in older boys with pauci JRA. Weaker HLA associations exist for other subtypes (HLA-DR5; HLA-DR8; HLA-DR4).
Incidence/Prevalence in USA: Prevalence approximately 1/1000 children; incidence 1/10,000 children
Predominant age: 1-4 years and 9-14 years
Predominant sex: Female > Male

SIGNS & SYMPTOMS
- Systemic
  - ◊ Arthralgias/arthritis
  - ◊ Chest pain, pericardial friction rub
  - ◊ Dyspnea
  - ◊ Fatigue
  - ◊ Fever
  - ◊ Hepatosplenomegaly
  - ◊ Lymphadenopathy
  - ◊ Myalgias
  - ◊ Rash
  - ◊ Weight loss
- Polyarticular
  - ◊ Arthralgia/arthritis
  - ◊ Cold intolerance
  - ◊ Difficulty writing
  - ◊ Fatigue
  - ◊ Growth retardation
  - ◊ Hand weakness
  - ◊ Limitation of motion
  - ◊ Malaise
  - ◊ Morning stiffness
  - ◊ Rheumatoid nodules
  - ◊ Synovial cysts
  - ◊ Synovial thickening
  - ◊ Weight loss
- Pauciarticular
  - ◊ Abnormal gait
  - ◊ Eye pain, redness
  - ◊ Joint swelling
  - ◊ Leg length abnormality
  - ◊ Morning stiffness
  - ◊ Photophobia

CAUSES Multifactorial including abnormal immune response, genetic predisposition and environmental triggers, possibly infectious

RISK FACTORS
- HLA-B27 in pauci JRA increases risk for development of spondyloarthropathy
- Rheumatoid factor positivity increases risk for severe arthritis in poly JRA
- ANA positivity increases risk for uveitis in pauci and poly JRA

DIAGNOSIS

DIFFERENTIAL DIAGNOSIS Other rheumatic diseases, especially SLE and dermatomyositis; atypical bacterial or viral infections; hemoglobinopathies; malignancy; vasculitis; rheumatic fever; Lyme disease; post-infectious arthritis; musculoskeletal developmental abnormalities; pain syndromes

LABORATORY
- WBC normal or markedly elevated (sys)
- Hb normal or low (especially sys)
- Platelet count normal or elevated
- ANA positive, 40% (poly or pauci)
- RF positive, 10-15% (usually polys)
- HLA-B27 positive, 70% in pauci boys
- Sedimentation rate (ESR) elevated in most patients with active disease; > 100 mL/hr (Westergren) in active systemic disease

Drugs that may alter lab results: Anti-inflammatory therapy may alter CBC and ESR

Disorders that may alter lab results: Hemoglobinopathies (ESR)

PATHOLOGICAL FINDINGS Synovium shows hyperplasia of synovial cells, hyperemia and infiltration of small lymphocytes and mononuclear cells

SPECIAL TESTS
- Echocardiography (pericarditis)
- Radionuclide scans (infection, malignancy)

IMAGING
- Early radiographic changes - soft tissue swelling, periosteal reaction, juxta-articular demineralization; later changes include joint space loss, articular surface erosions, subchondral cyst formation, sclerosis and joint fusion
- CT and MRI very helpful in delineating early erosions

DIAGNOSTIC PROCEDURES
- Joint fluid aspiration and analysis helpful in excluding infection
- Synovial biopsy occasionally indicated in persistent, atypical monoarthritis

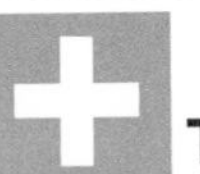

TREATMENT

APPROPRIATE HEALTH CARE
- Outpatient care except for initial diagnostic workup of systemic JRA disease and complications for all subtypes
- Patients require regular (every 4 months in young patients with pauciarticular disease) ophthalmic exams to uncover asymptomatic eye disease, at least for the first 3 years

GENERAL MEASURES Physical therapy including daily home exercise program required for joints with limited motion; moist heat, sleeping bag or electric blanket to relieve morning stiffness

SURGICAL MEASURES Total hip replacement for severe disease may be needed

ACTIVITY
- Full activity as tolerated
- Regular school. May need modified physical education program.

DIET Regular diet with special attention to adequate calcium, iron, protein and caloric intake

PATIENT EDUCATION
- Ongoing education of patients and families needed with special attention to psychosocial needs, behavioral strategies for dealing with pain and noncompliance, and utilization of health care resources
- Printed and audio-visual information available from local Arthritis Foundation

MEDICATIONS

DRUG(S) OF CHOICE

- First-line:
  - ◊ Nonsteroidal anti-inflammatory medications (NSAIDs) adequate in approximately 50% of patients. Average of 2-3 trials needed to determine most effective drug for an individual patient; adequate duration of trial for given NSAID 4-6 weeks (if no adverse reaction). Drugs for children include:
    - Ibuprofen (Motrin, Advil, Nuprin) 30-50 mg/kg/d (usual dose is 40 mg/kg/d)
    - Naproxen (Naprosyn, Aleve) 10-20 mg/kg/d
    - Tolmetin sodium 15-30 mg/kg/d
    - Cox-2 inhibitors
- Second-line:
  - ◊ 30-40% of patients ultimately require addition of disease-modifying antirheumatic drug (DMARD) e.g., antimalarials, sulfasalazine, methotrexate
  - ◊ Other agents - corticosteroids for serious cardiac involvement or unresponsive uveitis; immune globulin IV, etanercept (Enbrel), or cyclosporine (Neoral) in selected patients

Contraindications: Known allergies

Precautions: Most older NSAIDs affect platelet adhesiveness and may worsen a bleeding diathesis. Use caution with all NSAIDs in renal insufficiency and hypovolemic states.

Significant possible interactions: NSAIDs may lower serum levels of digitalis and anticonvulsants, and blunt the effect of loop diuretics. NSAIDs may increase serum methotrexate levels.

ALTERNATIVE DRUGS
Other NSAIDs; analgesics for pain control

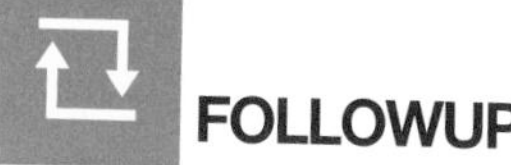

FOLLOWUP

PATIENT MONITORING

- Patients on NSAIDs - CBC, urinalysis, periodically
- Patients on aspirin and/or other salicylates - transaminase and salicylate levels, weekly for first month, then every 3-4 months
- Patient on methotrexate - monthly liver function tests, CBC
- Ophthalmologic monitoring for antimalarials

PREVENTION/AVOIDANCE

- Avoid salicylate therapy during serious viral illness or following varicella exposure due to possible risk for Reye syndrome
- No known preventive measures for JRA

POSSIBLE COMPLICATIONS

- Blindness
- Band keratopathy
- Glaucoma
- Short stature
- Debilitating joint disease
- Patient on NSAIDs
  - ◊ Peptic ulcer
  - ◊ Gastrointestinal hemorrhage
  - ◊ Rashes
  - ◊ CNS reactions
  - ◊ Renal disease
  - ◊ Leukopenia
- Patient on DMARD's
  - ◊ Bone marrow suppression
  - ◊ Hepatitis
  - ◊ Renal disease
  - ◊ Dermatitis
  - ◊ Mouth ulcers
  - ◊ Retinal toxicity (antimalarials) - rare

EXPECTED COURSE/PROGNOSIS

- 50-60% ultimately remit, but functional ability depends on adequacy of long-term therapy (disease control and maintaining muscle and joint function)
- Poorest prognosis in polyarticular patients with positive rheumatoid factor (RF); and in systemic juvenile arthritis

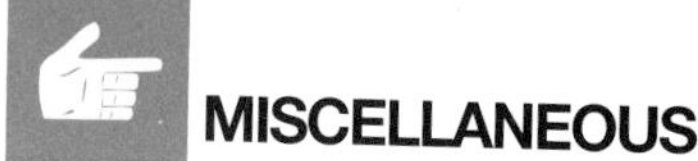

MISCELLANEOUS

ASSOCIATED CONDITIONS
Other autoimmune disorders

AGE-RELATED FACTORS

Pediatric: Behavioral and compliance problems frequent in toddlers and teenagers

Geriatric: N/A

Others: N/A

PREGNANCY
Unpredictable effect on disease activity

SYNONYMS

- Juvenile chronic arthritis
- Juvenile arthritis
- Still disease

ICD-9-CM

714.30 Polyarticular juvenile rheumatoid arthritis, chronic or unspecified
714.31 Polyarticular juvenile rheumatoid arthritis, acute
714.32 Pauciarticular onset JRA
714.33 Monoarticular onset JRA

SEE ALSO

OTHER NOTES
Treatment goal is to control active disease as well as extra-articular manifestations in order to maintain musculoskeletal function as normal as possible

ABBREVIATIONS

JRA = juvenile rheumatoid arthritis
RF = rheumatoid factor
DMARD = disease modifying antirheumatic drug

REFERENCES

- Schaller JG. Juvenile Rheumatoid Arthritis. Pediatrics in Review 1980:2(6);163-174
- Cassidy JT, Petty RE. The Textbook of Pediatric Rheumatology. 4th Ed. Philadelphia: WB Saunders; 2001

Web references: 2 available at www.5mcc.com

Illustrations 1 available

Author(s):

Carol B. Lindsley, MD

BASICS

DESCRIPTION Osteoarthritis (OA) is the most common form of joint disease. Involves progressive loss of articular cartilage and reactive changes at joint margins and in subchondral bone.

- Primary
  - ◊ Idiopathic
  - ◊ Divided into subsets depending on clinical features
- Secondary
  - ◊ Childhood anatomic abnormalities (e.g., congenital hip dysplasia, slipped femoral epiphyses)
  - ◊ Inheritable metabolic disorders (e.g., alkaptonuria, Wilson disease, hemochromatosis)
  - ◊ Neuropathic arthropathy (Charcot's joints)
  - ◊ Hemophilic arthropathy
  - ◊ Acromegalic arthropathy
  - ◊ Paget disease
  - ◊ Hyperparathyroidism
  - ◊ Noninfectious inflammatory arthritis (e.g., rheumatoid arthritis, spondyloarthropathies)
  - ◊ Gout, calcium pyrophosphate deposition disease (pseudogout)
  - ◊ Septic or tuberculous arthritis
  - ◊ Post-traumatic

System(s) affected: Musculoskeletal

Genetics: Genetic transmission is unknown but a woman with distal interphalangeal joint OA is more likely to have a mother or sister with similar joint involvement

Incidence/Prevalence in USA:
- Estimates of radiographic evidence of OA - range from 33% to almost 90% in those people over the age of 65
- Approximately 60 million patients at any one time

Predominant age:
- Over age 40 (for symptomatic disease)
- Leading cause of disability in those over age 65

Predominant sex: Male = Female

SIGNS & SYMPTOMS
- Slowly developing joint pain
- Pain that follows use of a joint
- Stiffness (especially morning and after sitting) of less than 15 minutes duration
- Joint bony enlargement (e.g., Heberden's nodes of distal interphalangeal joints)
- Decreased range of motion
- Tenderness usually absent; may be associated with synovitis, with tenderness along joint margin
- Crepitation as late sign
- Local pain and stiffness with osteoarthritis of spine, with radicular pain (if there is compression of nerve roots)

CAUSES Biomechanical, biochemical, inflammatory, and immunological factors are all implicated in pathogenesis of osteoarthritis

RISK FACTORS
- Age over 50
- Obesity (weight bearing joints)
- Prolonged occupational or sports stress
- Injury to a joint from trauma
- Injury to a joint from pre-existing inflammatory arthritis or infectious arthritis

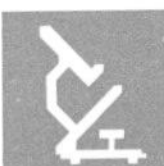

DIAGNOSIS

DIFFERENTIAL DIAGNOSIS
- Distinguish from other types of arthritis by absent systemic findings, minimal articular inflammation, and distribution of involved joints (e.g., distal and proximal interphalangeal joints, not wrist and metacarpophalangeal joints)
- In spine, distinguish from osteoporosis, metastatic disease, multiple myeloma, other bone disease

LABORATORY Not helpful (sedimentation rate not increased) in diagnosis, but may be useful in monitoring treatment with NSAIDs (renal insufficiency and GI bleeding)

Drugs that may alter lab results: N/A

Disorders that may alter lab results: In secondary OA, the underlying disorder may have abnormal lab results, e.g., hemochromatosis - abnormal iron studies

PATHOLOGICAL FINDINGS
- Synovial fluid may have a slightly increased white blood cell count, predominantly mononuclear
- Calcium pyrophosphate dihydrate and/or apatite crystals may occasionally be seen in effusions and require polarized light microscopy or special techniques to see
- Subchondral bone trabecular microfractures
- Degradation response produced by release of proteolytic enzymes, collagenolytic enzymes, prostaglandins, and immune responses

SPECIAL TESTS N/A

IMAGING X-rays usually normal early; later often show narrowed joint space, osteophyte formation, subchondral bony sclerosis, and cyst formation. Erosions may occur on surface of distal interphalangeal (DIP) and proximal interphalangeal (PIP) joints when OA is associated with inflammation (erosive osteoarthritis).

DIAGNOSTIC PROCEDURES
- Joint aspiration
  - ◊ May be helpful to distinguish between OA and chronic inflammatory arthritides
  - ◊ OA - cell count usually < 500 cells/mm3, predominantly mononuclear
  - ◊ Inflammatory - cell count usually > 2000 cells/mm3, predominantly neutrophils

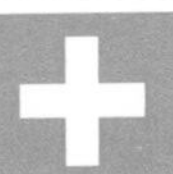

TREATMENT

APPROPRIATE HEALTH CARE Outpatient

GENERAL MEASURES
- Reassurance of absence of generalized systemic disease, with recognition of potential disability from osteoarthritis
- Weight reduction if obese
- General fitness program
- Heat (local, tub baths, etc.)
- Physical therapy to maintain or regain joint motion and muscle strength. Quadriceps strengthening exercises can relieve pain and disability of the knee.
- Protect joints from overuse (e.g., cane, crutches, walker, neck collar, elastic knee support)

SURGICAL MEASURES Surgery may be indicated in advanced disease (e.g., osteotomy, debridement, removal of loose bodies, joint replacement)

ACTIVITY As active as tolerated

DIET No special diet

PATIENT EDUCATION
- For a listing of sources for patient education materials favorably reviewed on this topic, physicians may contact: American Academy of Family Physicians Foundation, P.O. Box 8418, Kansas City, MO 64114, (800)274-2237, ext. 4400
- Arthritis Foundation, PO Box 7669, Atlanta, GA 30357-0669; 800-283-7800

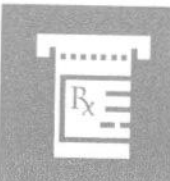

MEDICATIONS

DRUG(S) OF CHOICE

- Acetaminophen for relief of pain. If not effective, non-acetylated salicylates (e.g., salsalate, choline-magnesium salicylate), or low dose ibuprofen ≤ 1600 mg/d.
- Other NSAIDs can be used and have similar efficacy. Their prolonged use is associated with significant side effects, especially in the elderly and includes renal insufficiency, hypertension, leg edema, and GI bleeding. Since pain in osteoarthritis varies from day to day, brief course of a short acting NSAID are preferable.
- Cyclo-oxygenase-2 (COX-2) specific inhibitors are less likely to cause stomach ulcers and they work as well as the nonspecific NSAIDs in reducing arthritis inflammation and pain. They are currently much more expensive than the conventional NSAIDs and should be reserved for those patients who are at a higher risk for stomach ulcers and bleeding.
- Opioid analgesics (e.g., codeine, oxycodone, propoxyphene) should be restricted for treatment of acute episodes of pain

Contraindications: NSAIDs are contraindicated if there is renal disease, congestive heart failure, hypertension, active peptic ulcer disease or previous hypersensitivity to a NSAID or aspirin (asthma, nasal polyps, urticaria/angioedema, hypotension)

Precautions:

- In patients with history of peptic ulcer disease, or risk factors for upper GI bleeding, acetaminophen is recommended. If a NSAID is necessary because of an inadequate response to acetaminophen, it should be given with misoprostol or with a proton pump inhibitor. A COX-2 specific inhibitor NSAID is preferred in patients with a history of upper GI bleeding. Risk factors for upper GI bleeding are a previous history of bleeding or peptic ulcer, age 65, concomitant use of oral corticosteroids or anticoagulants. In these patients, the risk of stomach ulcers can be reduced by such drugs as misoprostol (Cytotec) and the proton pump inhibitors (eg, omeprazole and lansoprazole.
- Oral or parenteral adrenal corticosteroids are contraindicated
- Combinations of 2 or more NSAIDs are contraindicated because of increased risk of adverse reactions without concomitant improved efficacy

Significant possible interactions:

- NSAIDs reduce effectiveness of ACE inhibitors and diuretics
- Aspirin and NSAIDs (except COX-2 inhibitors) may increase effects of anticoagulants
- Increased hypoglycemic effects of oral hypoglycemics with aspirin
- Avoid concomitant use of aspirin with NSAIDs
- Salicylates reduce effectiveness of spironolactone (Aldactone) and uricosurics
- Corticosteroids and some antacids increase salicylate excretion, while ascorbic acid and ammonium chloride reduce salicylate excretion and may cause toxicity

ALTERNATIVE DRUGS

- Judicious use of intra-articular injections of corticosteroids for selected acute flare-ups of joints. No more than 3-4/year intra-articular corticosteroid injections up to a maximal total of 12 injections per joint. Intra-articular corticosteroid injections, if excessive, can accelerate joint deterioration.
- A series of injections of a hyaluronic acid preparation into a painful OA knee may provide relief of pain and improve function
- Capsaicin cream - local application relieves pain - most effective in small joints of the hand. May cause a local burning.

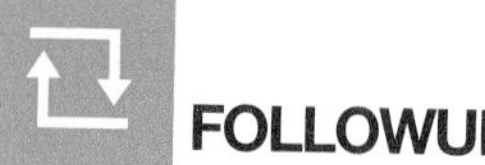

FOLLOWUP

PATIENT MONITORING

- Follow range of motion and functional status at regular intervals
- Watch for GI blood loss and follow cardiac, renal and mental status in older patients on NSAIDs or ASA
- Periodic CBC, renal function tests, stool for occult blood

PREVENTION/AVOIDANCE

Followup of secondary causes

POSSIBLE COMPLICATIONS

- Decompensated CHF, GI bleeding, decreased renal function on NSAIDs or ASA
- Hypoglycemic reactions in diabetic patients taking aspirin (rare)
- Infection or accelerated cartilage loss with intra-articular corticosteroids

EXPECTED COURSE/PROGNOSIS

- Tends to be progressive
- Early in course, pain relieved by rest; later, pain may occur at rest and at night
- Joint effusions may occur, especially in knees
- Joint enlargement occurs later in course due to bony enlargement
- Osteophyte (spur) formation, especially at joint margins, as disease progresses
- Advanced stage with full thickness loss of cartilage down to bone

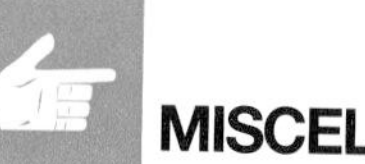

MISCELLANEOUS

ASSOCIATED CONDITIONS

N/A

AGE-RELATED FACTORS

Pediatric: N/A

Geriatric:

- Prevalence increases with age
- Almost universal over 65 (by x-ray but not clinically)

Others: N/A

PREGNANCY

ASA and NSAIDs with some risk to fetus during pregnancy; compatible with breast feeding

SYNONYMS

- Osteoarthrosis
- Degenerative joint disease

ICD-9-CM

715.90 Osteoarthrosis, unspecified whether generalized or localized, site unspecified

SEE ALSO

OTHER NOTES

Surgery may be indicated in advanced disease (for example joint replacement, fusion)

ABBREVIATIONS

N/A

REFERENCES

- Mankin HJ, Brandt KD. Pathogenesis of Osteoarthritis in Kelley's Textbook of Rheumatology, eds. Ruddy S, Harris ED, Sledge CB. 5th Ed, W.B. Saunders, Philadelphia. 2001: 1391-1407.
- Solomon L. Clinical Features of Osteoarthritis in Kelley's Textbook of Rheumatology, eds. Ruddy S, Harris ED, Sledge CB. 5th Ed, W.B. Saunders, Philadelphia. 2001: 1409-1417.
- Brandt KD. Management of Osteoarthritis in Kelly's Textbook of Rheumatology, eds. Ruddy S, Harris ED, Sledge CB. 5th Ed, W.B. Saunders, Philadelphia. 2001: 1419-1432
- Golden BD, Abramson SB. Selective Cyclooxygenase-2 inhibitors. Rheumatic Dis Clin NA 1999;25(2):359-378
- Hochberg MC, Altman RD, Brandt KD. Guidelines for the medical management of osteoarthritis. Part 1. Osteoarthritis of the hip; Part II. Osteoarthritis of the knee: Arthritis Rheum 1995;38:1535-40;1541-46

Web references: 2 available at www.5mcc.com

Illustrations N/A

Author(s):

Bruce C. Gilliland, MD

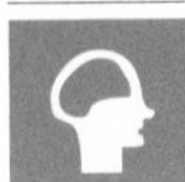

BASICS

DESCRIPTION Arthritis associated with psoriasis. Serologic tests for the rheumatoid factor are usually negative. Patients exhibit sausage-shaped digits and characteristic radiologic changes. Psoriatic arthropathy occurs in about 5% of individuals with psoriasis, especially those with psoriatic nail disease. There are several forms that have been described although the separation into these forms is not distinct. They are called by different descriptive terms by various authors.

- Forms of psoriatic arthropathy:
  - ◊ Psoriatic nail disease and distal interphalangeal involvement (classic psoriatic arthritis). Characteristics - nail pitting, transverse depressions, subungual hyperkeratosis, distal interphalangeal arthritis.
  - ◊ Arthritis mutilans - a destructive, resorptive arthropathy. Produces the so-called opera-glass hand.
  - ◊ Symmetric polyarthropathy resembling rheumatoid arthritis - may be indistinguishable from RA and may represent coincidental rheumatoid arthritis in a patient who has psoriasis
  - ◊ Asymmetric oligoarthropathy - little relationship between joint and skin activity; joints involved may be both large and small
  - ◊ Psoriatic spondylitis - asymmetrical spondylitis and sacroiliitis

System(s) affected: Musculoskeletal, Skin/Exocrine

Genetics: HLA-B27 usually present in patients with spondylitis-type psoriatic arthropathy. Psoriasis itself is associated with HLA-B13, HLA-Bw17, HLA-Cw6, HLA-Bw38, HLA-DR4 and HLA-DR7.

Incidence/Prevalence in USA: Uncommon, approximately 5% of individuals have psoriatic skin disease

Predominant age: Onset age 30-35

Predominant sex: Female > Male (slightly)

SIGNS & SYMPTOMS
- Joint swelling, tenderness, warmth, restricted movement
- Distribution of arthritis dependent upon form of psoriatic arthritis
- Nail changes - pitting, transverse ridging, onycholysis, keratosis, yellowing and destruction of the entire nail
- Fever
- Malaise
- Psoriasis - variable severity
- Other symptoms applying characteristically to the several types of psoriatic arthropathy. See description.

CAUSES
- Unknown
- Probably genetically related

RISK FACTORS
- Psoriasis
- Positive family history

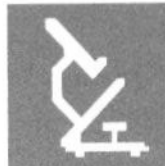

DIAGNOSIS

DIFFERENTIAL DIAGNOSIS
- Psoriasis
- Seropositive inflammatory polyarthritis
- Rheumatoid arthritis
- Osteoarthritis
- Gout
- Reiter syndrome
- Ankylosing spondylitis

LABORATORY
- Serum rheumatoid factor - negative
- Elevated erythrocyte sedimentation rate
- Elevated uric acid
- Anemia
- HLA B27 - spondylitis

Drugs that may alter lab results: N/A

Disorders that may alter lab results: N/A

PATHOLOGICAL FINDINGS Synovitis (resembling rheumatoid arthritis)

SPECIAL TESTS N/A

IMAGING
- X-ray
  - ◊ Gross destructive changes of isolated small joints
  - ◊ Peripheral arthritis mutilans
  - ◊ Erosions, ankylosis
  - ◊ Extensive bone resorption to cause "opera-glass hand"
  - ◊ Fluffy periostitis
  - ◊ Atypical spondylitis with syndesmophyte formation
  - ◊ Acro-osteolysis, "pencil-in-cup" appearance
  - ◊ Asymmetric sacroiliitis
  - ◊ Absence of osteoporosis
- MRI is sensitive in detecting sacroiliitis, joint synovitis, erosions and enthesitis

DIAGNOSTIC PROCEDURES N/A

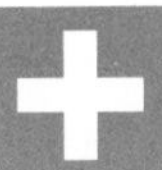

TREATMENT

APPROPRIATE HEALTH CARE Outpatient

GENERAL MEASURES
- Immobilizing splints
- Isometric exercises and swimming later
- Paraffin baths or other heat therapy
- Protect affected joints
- Regular, moderate exposure to sun
- Psoriatic skin care

SURGICAL MEASURES N/A

ACTIVITY Encourage exercise (particularly swimming) to maintain strength and flexibility

DIET No special diet

PATIENT EDUCATION
- Stress non-contagious
- For a listing of sources for patient education materials favorably reviewed on this topic, physicians may contact: American Academy of Family Physicians Foundation, P.O. Box 8418, Kansas City, MO 64114, (800)274-2237, ext. 4400
- Arthritis Foundation, 1314 Spring Street N.W., Atlanta, GA 30309, (404)872-7100

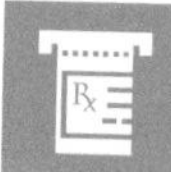

MEDICATIONS

DRUG(S) OF CHOICE
- Several options available depending on involvement of skin and joints:
  - ◊ Non-steroidal anti-inflammatory drugs in usual doses. There is no evidence for superiority of any one NSAID in psoriatic arthritis.
  - ◊ Local corticosteroid injection
  - ◊ Low-dose systemic steroids, if necessary
  - ◊ Topical therapy including steroids for skin
  - ◊ PUVA therapy may be helpful for skin lesions
- Others sometimes useful:
  - ◊ Methotrexate, used only under specific guidelines and by someone experienced with its use.
  - ◊ Gold salts
  - ◊ Antimalarials (controversial)
  - ◊ Sulfasalazine
  - ◊ Immunosuppressives in resistant cases
  - ◊ Cyclosporine (Neoral) in resistant cases
  - ◊ Combination of MTX and Cyclosporine or sulfasalazine under the guidance of a rheumatologist

Contraindications:
- NSAIDs may flare psoriasis
- Methotrexate contraindicated in HIV positive patients

Precautions: Phenylbutazone may cause bone marrow depression. NSAIDs and ASA may cause gastritis and renal failure. Refer to manufacturer's literature.

Significant possible interactions: NSAIDs may impair methotrexate excretion and cause methotrexate toxicity. Refer to manufacturer's literature.

ALTERNATIVE DRUGS
Etretinate 0.5-1.0 mg/kg/day in 2 divided doses

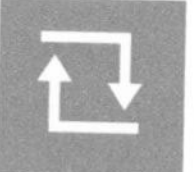

FOLLOWUP

PATIENT MONITORING
Frequent for medication adjustment and encouragement

PREVENTION/AVOIDANCE
N/A

POSSIBLE COMPLICATIONS
- Chronicity
- Severe deforming arthritis (arthritis mutilans)
- Spondylitic form of arthritis with sacroiliitis and spinal involvement
- Corticosteroids may destabilize psoriatic lesions
- Antimalarials can provoke exfoliative dermatitis

EXPECTED COURSE/PROGNOSIS
- Course - acute, intermittent
- More favorable than rheumatoid arthritis (except for arthritis mutilans)
- Treatment of skin lesions can sometime improve arthritic symptoms
- Joint surgery is at least as successful as for rheumatoid arthritis; (RA) infectious complications are more common than RA

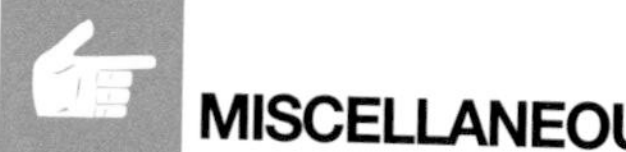

MISCELLANEOUS

ASSOCIATED CONDITIONS
Psoriasis

AGE-RELATED FACTORS
Pediatric: Not commonly seen in this age group
Geriatric: Arthritic symptoms worse
Others: N/A

PREGNANCY
Avoidance of medications (e.g., Methotrexate, gold, antimalarials, sulfasalazine, cyclosporin, etretinate) during pregnancy advised

SYNONYMS
Psoriasis, arthropathic

ICD-9-CM
696.0 Psoriatic arthropathy

SEE ALSO

OTHER NOTES
Pathogenesis: In contrast to the ameliorating affect of AIDS (HIV infection) on rheumatoid arthritis, AIDS is associated with more aggressive joint disease in psoriatic arthritis. Theoretically, then, CD4 cells, which seem to "drive" rheumatoid arthritis, are not involved in the pathogenesis of psoriatic arthritis.

ABBREVIATIONS
N/A

REFERENCES

- Kelley WN, Harris ED, Ruddy S, et al: Textbook of Rheumatology. 5th Ed. Philadelphia, W.B. Saunders, 1997
- Koopman WJ, eds: Arthritis and Allied Disorders. 13th Ed. Philadelphia, Lea & Febiger, 1997
- Salvarini, et al: Psoriatic arthritis. Curr Opin in Rheumatol 1998;10(4):299-305
- Kippel JH, Dippe PA, eds: Rheumatology. St. Louis, Mosby, 1994

Web references: 1 available at www.5mcc.com
Illustrations N/A

Author(s):
Michael Tutt, MD

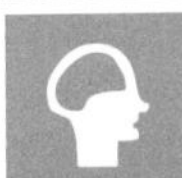

BASICS

DESCRIPTION A chronic systemic inflammatory disease of unknown etiology with a predilection for joint involvement. Articular inflammation may be remitting, but if continued usually results in joint damage and disability. Certain extra-articular manifestations are characteristic, including rheumatoid nodules, arteritis, neuropathy, scleritis, pericarditis, and splenomegaly.

System(s) affected: Cardiovascular, Hemic/Lymphatic/Immunologic, Musculoskeletal, Nervous, Pulmonary

Genetics: Seropositive RA aggregates in families. Genetic factors versus their interaction with environmental facilitators is unclear. HLA-DR4 is found in 70% of Caucasian seropositive patients compared to 25% of controls. Increased relative risk of 4-5 times for the DR4 positive person, although a minority are affected. African Americans tend not to exhibit this predilection.

Incidence/Prevalence in USA:
- 0.3-1.5%; women affected twice as often
- Prevalence in Native Americans is 3.5-5.3%

Predominant age: Third to sixth decades

Predominant sex:
- Female > Male (overall incidence and prevalence of articular manifestations)
- Male > Female (systemic disease)

SIGNS & SYMPTOMS
- Joints: wrists, knees, elbows, shoulders, ankles, and subtalar joints (most often involved) with swelling, heat, deformity, pain on passive motion, morning stiffness. Joint destruction occurs early; 70% show radiologic signs of damage within 3 years of onset.
- Systemic: fatigue, depression, malaise, anorexia, rheumatoid nodules, lymphadenopathy, splenomegaly, ocular disease, entrapment neuropathies
- Patients experience symptoms an average of 36 weeks before diagnosis

CAUSES Antibody-complement complex results in intra-articular inflammation.

RISK FACTORS
- HLA-DR4
- Family history
- Native American ethnicity
- Female gender, age 20-50 years

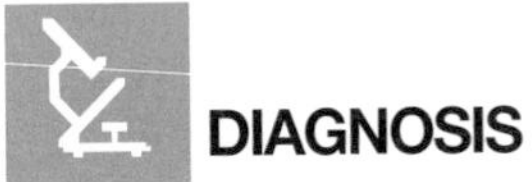

DIAGNOSIS

DIFFERENTIAL DIAGNOSIS
Sjögren syndrome, sarcoidosis, gout, polymyositis, erosive osteoarthritis, seronegative polyarthritis, vasculitis, pseudogout, inflammatory bowel disease, hypersensitivity reactions, Reiter syndrome, Behçet syndrome, psoriatic arthritis, systemic lupus erythematosus, Lyme disease, scleroderma, chronic infection, occult malignancy. Early wrist symptoms not likely in osteoarthritis.

LABORATORY
- Hematocrit - mild anemia common
- ESR: usually elevated
- C-reactive protein (CRP) - direct measure of impact of IL-6 upon liver cells, is linear over a wide range, and is reproducible
- Rheumatoid factor: > 1:80 in 70-80% of patients with RA; 20% negative despite other signs of RA
  - ◊ RF tests are assays for IgM Ab
  - ◊ RF is a poor screening tool with a positive predictive value (PPV) of only 20% in asymptomatic persons. In patients with rheumatologic symptoms, it's PPV = 80%.
  - ◊ Not useful to monitor course of the illness
- ANA: present in 20-30%.
- Electrolytes, Cr, liver function, UA to assess organ comorbid states
- Synovial fluid
  - ◊ Yellowish-white, turbid, poor viscosity
  - ◊ Mucin clot poor due to degradation of hyaluronic acid by lysosomal enzymes
  - ◊ WBC increased (3500-50,000)
  - ◊ Protein: approximately 4.2 g/dL (42 g/L)
  - ◊ Serum-synovial glucose difference ≥ 30 mg/dL (≥ 1.67 mmol/L)

Drugs that may alter lab results: Prior treatment with immunosuppressives may "normalize" results

Disorders that may alter lab results: False positive RF results: Sjögren, mixed cryoglobulinemia, parasitic infections (eg, malaria), liver disease, endocarditis, and acute viral infections (eg, mononucleosis, influenza, rubella)

PATHOLOGICAL FINDINGS
- Synovial infiltration by lymphocytes, plasma cells, and macrophages
- Hypertrophy and hyperplasia of synovial lining cells
- Local production of "self-associating" IgG

SPECIAL TESTS None; biopsy of nodules is not indicated in diagnosis

IMAGING
- X-rays rarely necessary in diagnosis, but useful in following the progression of disease
- Arthrography: to define joint abnormalities or injury to a supporting structure
- Bone scan: if aseptic necrosis is suspected
- CT/MRI: useful in specific situations such as cervical spine symptoms

DIAGNOSTIC PROCEDURES
- American College of Rheumatology criteria: (5 of the 7 must be present. Numbers 1-4 must be continuous > 6 weeks.)

1. Morning stiffness > 1 hour's duration
2. Arthritis of at least three joint groups with soft tissue swelling or fluid
3. Swelling involving at least one of the following joint groups: wrists, proximal interphalangeal, metacarpophalangeal
4. Symmetrical joint swelling
5. Subcutaneous nodules
6. Positive rheumatoid factor test
7. Radiographic changes consistent with RA

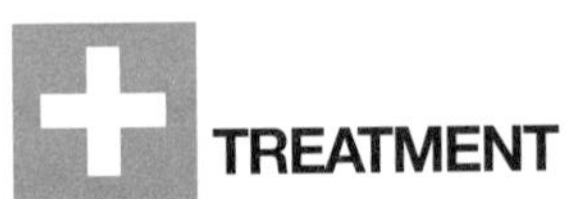

TREATMENT

APPROPRIATE HEALTH CARE
- Primarily outpatient
- Key elements are ongoing evaluation of disease activity and extent of synovitis, structural damage, and psycho/social functional status

GENERAL MEASURES
- Intervene before joint damage occurs
- Emphasis on exercise and mobility; reduction of joint stress; general health care

SURGICAL MEASURES For severe mechanical symptoms

ACTIVITY
- Encourage full activity, but avoid heavy work and vigorous exercise during active phases
- Hydrotherapy or water exercise
- Exercise programs focusing on restoration of function. Isometric exercise with active synovitis.

DIET No special diet. Diets rich in omega-3 fatty acids (25 gm/day) allow some patients to reduce NSAIDs dose.

PATIENT EDUCATION American Rheumatism Association (800)282-7023; Arthritis Foundation, 404-872-7100; www.arthritis.org

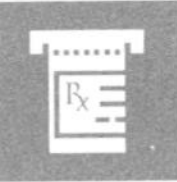

MEDICATIONS

DRUG(S) OF CHOICE
- Pyramid approach has generally been discarded in favor of early treatment with disease modifying agents (DMARDs). Limited evidence from RCTs favors treatment with DMARDs within first year of disease is more effective in limiting disease progression and improving function. No one DMARD is consistently better than another, but methotrexate, hydroxychloroquine, sulfasalazine and leflunomide are preferred over gold, D-Penicillamine, azathioprine and cyclosporine, due to risk/benefit. Combinations of DMARDs may be more effective than using individual drugs, but best combinations for specific circumstances still undetermined.
- Start DMARDs within 2 months if patient has ongoing joint pain/morning stiffness, active synovitis, or persistent increase in ESR/CRP despite appropriate dose NSAIDs
- Early disease or acute/chronic inflammation
  - ◊ Aspirin or other NSAID; try various classes
  - ◊ COX-2 inhibitors - celecoxib (Celebrex) and rofecoxib (Vioxx). Advantages: less risk of GI, renal and platelet injury. Costly.
- Prednisone 5-15 mg q day: Severe disease or to minimize disease activity while awaiting DMARDs to act, decrease activity for a short period of time, or control active disease when NSAIDs/DMARDs have failed. Generally to be used only for short periods. Low dose maintenance therapy (eg, 5 mg qod) controversial.
- Persistent disease activity (chronic synovitis, AM stiffness, increased ESR/CRP, extra-articular disease): add DMARDs; HCQ or SSZ often chosen first. When second line agent's therapeutic level is reached, decrease prednisone slowly.
  - ◊ Minocycline is effective in RA patients compared to placebo and twice as effective compared to hydroxychloroquine in patients also treated with low dose prednisone. Adverse events include GI upset, and dizziness. Serious problems are rare.

◊ Intraarticular steroids - use rarely
◊ Antimalarials: hydroxychloroquine (HCQ, Plaquenil) 400 mg q hs for 2-3 months, then 200 mg/hs; 6 month trial usual
◊ Auranofin (Ridaura) 6-10 mg/d po; reevaluate in 6 months or 1 gram total. Injectable gold (Aurolate): weekly for 22 weeks, then q 2-4 weeks.
◊ Sulfasalazine (SSZ): 500 mg/d, increase to 2 g/d over 1 mo; max: 2-3 g/day; 6 mo trial
◊ Penicillamine (d-penicillamine): 250 mg/d, increase slowly to 750-1000 mg/day; 9 month trial with 8-12 wks at maximum dosage
◊ Azathioprine - due to toxicity, reserve for persons not responsive to other DMARDs
◊ Methotrexate (MTX, Rheumatrex): 5-15 mg/wk po; 3-6 month trial - for steroid dependent disease or after other measures fail. Is DMARD with most predictable benefit. Earlier disease role debated; many recommend MTX in early stage disease. Addition of folate to MTX regimen reduces liver toxicity and discontinuation of methotrexate without lessening effectiveness, although requires a 10-20% increase in dosage of MTX.
◊ Protein A immunoadsorption (Prosorba). For moderate to severe RA in patients failing other DMARDs. Removes antibodies responsible for RA activity. Majority respond in 9-21 weeks. Costly.
◊ Hyaluronate (Hyalgan, Hyalgan G-F20). Hyaluronic acid substitute. Increases the "quality" of joint fluid; exact mechanism unclear. For pain relief. Variable responses. Limited to knee disease at this time. Exact role in RA unclear; expected therapy duration 6-12 mos.
◊ Infliximab (Remicade), adalimumab (Humira) and etanercept (Enbrel). Biologic response modifiers which inhibit tumor necrosis factor (TNF). Administered once monthly IV (infliximab), biweekly (adalimumab) or twice weekly SC (etanercept). Exact role, optimal dosage and duration of treatment unclear. Short term toxicity low, long term toxicity (studies up to 30 months) low as well (7%). Costly.
◊ Leflunomide (Arava). Modifies T-cell function by inhibiting a key enzyme in pyrimidine synthesis, to decrease autoimmune activity. Benefits similar to MTX, but with less side effects. 20 mg qd. For patients not responding to traditional agents or whose use has been limited by side effects.

- Interleukin-1 receptor antagonist (eg, anakinra) new and exciting agent. Dose is 100 mg SC qd. Adverse reactions include rash, pruritus, neutropenia, and severe infections. TNF inhibitors may be more effective. Costly.

Contraindications: Avoid leflunomide in pregnancy

Precautions:
- Consider proton pump inhibitors for patients on NSAIDs chronically, give folic acid (1-2 mg/d) for patients on MTX
- Avoid NSAID combinations

Significant possible interactions:
- NSAIDs:
  ◊ Antacids: reduce absorption
  ◊ Anticoagulants: increase bleeding risk
  ◊ Oral hypoglycemic agents (OHA): Aspirin, phenylbutazone, and oxyphenbutazone may potentiate the activity of OHAs; others currently available do not
  ◊ Antihypertensive/diuretics: NSAIDs may attenuate the effect of diuretics, beta-blockers, hydralazine, prazosin, and ACE inhibitors
  ◊ Lithium: Elevation of plasma lithium levels may occur, especially with indomethacin and diclofenac
  ◊ MTX: Salicylate inhibits the renal clearance of MTX, and toxic levels may occur
  ◊ Phenytoin: Phenylbutazone inhibits metabolism of phenytoin. Salicylates increase the concentration of phenytoin.
  ◊ Probenecid: Inhibits renal clearance of several NSAIDs

ALTERNATIVE DRUGS Combinations of MTX and cyclosporine, gold salts and prednisone, and MTX and hydroxychloroquine all may be useful for resistant disease. Use of MTX and either gold or SSZ is not currently supported by clinical trials.

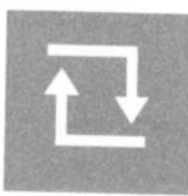

FOLLOWUP

PATIENT MONITORING
- Discuss prognosis, treatment (time and cost), adverse effects, lab and PE monitoring, patient preferences
- Duration of morning stiffness; time of onset of fatigue; NSAID need/day; grip strength; number of joints that are tender or painful on passive range-of-motion; degree of swelling of affected joints
- Functional status assessment
- Progress of established disease on x-ray
- ESR - often best test of disease activity
- Other lab testing, depend on medications and disease progression

PREVENTION/AVOIDANCE Possible decreased risk of RA with oral contraceptive use

POSSIBLE COMPLICATIONS
- Erosive arthritis and joint destruction
- Skin vasculitis
- Pericarditis
- Intracardiac rheumatoid nodules causing valvular, conduction abnormalities
- Pleural, subpleural disease; interstitial fibrosis
- Mononeuritis multiplex, median nerve entrapment
- Sjögren syndrome, scleral rheumatoid nodules
- Felty syndrome

EXPECTED COURSE/PROGNOSIS
- Progressive decline in function, but may be altered significantly with proper medical, surgical, and physiotherapeutic interventions
- Poor prognosis: early age at onset, high RF titer, high ESR, swelling of > 20 joints, extra-articular disease
- Complete remission defined as absence of: 1) symptoms of active inflammatory joint pain. 2) morning stiffness, 3) fatigue, 4) synovitis on physical exam, 5) progression of x-ray damage, 6) elevation of ESR
- Approximately 15-20% of patients have intermittent disease with periods of exacerbation and relatively good prognosis
- Poor prognostic findings:
  ◊ Moderate to severe disease - persistent swelling of the PIP joints, flexor tenosynovitis of the hands, a high ESR, RF or CRP, a large number of swollen joints, extraarticular disease, bone erosions or cartilage loss, SC nodules, and early decline in function
  ◊ Inheritance of shared epitope - RA homozygous for "shared epitope" on DR1 or DR4 HLA class 11 beta chains have poor prognosis. However, it is impractical to assay routinely for these sequences.
  ◊ Early or advanced age at disease onset - onset at advanced age and men before age 50
  ◊ Other factors - concurrent disorders, cigarette smoking, low education, and a lower socioeconomic status

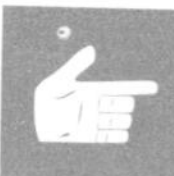

MISCELLANEOUS

ASSOCIATED CONDITIONS Sjögren; Felty, increased incidence of infections, renal impairment, lymphomas and CV disease. Renal disorders include membranous nephropathy d/t gold, pcnNH2, or NSAIDs; secondary amyloidosis d/t chronic inflammation; Focal mesangial proliferative GN; NSAID toxicity.

AGE-RELATED FACTORS
Pediatric: See Juvenile RA

Geriatric:
- Onset uncommon
- Increased contribution/interaction of age-related comorbidities. Pericarditis, septic arthritis, Sjögren syndrome more common.
- Less tolerance to drugs; increased incidence of hydroxychloroquine-associated maculopathy, d-penicillamine rash, and sulfasalazine induced nausea/vomiting. Toxicity from parenteral gold not age-related.

Others: N/A

PREGNANCY
- Use effective contraception when DMARDs given. Modify regimen if pregnancy or breast-feeding desired.
- Labor/delivery pose no serious problems, unless severe mechanical joint disease
- > 75% of RA patients improve during pregnancy, but relapse in 6 months. Occasionally, first episodes occur during pregnancy.
- Fetal abnormalities not increased

SYNONYMS N/A

ICD-9-CM
714.0 Rheumatoid arthritis
714.1 Felty syndrome

SEE ALSO
Arthritis, juvenile rheumatoid (JRA)
Arthritis, osteo
Sjögren syndrome

OTHER NOTES
- Median life expectancy shortened 7 years in males, 3 years in females over 25 years. 50% of patients with RA cannot function in primary job within 10 years of onset
- Functional ability (restriction of normal activities)
  ◊ Class I: None
  ◊ Class II: Moderate
  ◊ Class III: Marked restriction, inability to perform most of the patient's usual occupation or self-care
  ◊ Class IV: Incapacitation or confinement to a bed or wheelchair
- Functional ability tasks (see Pincus, et al)
- A standard measure is Stanford Health Assessment Questionnaire at www.aramis.stanford.edu

ABBREVIATIONS
- DMARD = disease modifying antirheumatic drug

REFERENCES

Web references: 2 available at www.5mcc.com
Illustrations 5 available

Author(s):
Kurt Elward, MD, MPH

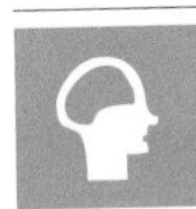

BASICS

DESCRIPTION Artificial insemination is the placement of washed sperm into the female reproductive tract. Placement can be intracervical, intrauterine, intraperitoneal, or intrafollicular. Most common is intrauterine insemination (IUI). Sperm are washed to reduce antigenicity. Insemination can be with partner's sperm or therapeutic insemination with donor sperm (TID).
System(s) affected: Endocrine/Metabolic, Reproductive
Genetics: N/A
Incidence/Prevalence in USA: Varies, depending on etiology of infertility, i.e., male factor is responsible for approximately 35% of cases of infertility, and a cervical factor is responsible for approximately 10% of cases
Predominant age: Reproductive age women (18-45 years of age)
Predominant sex: Female only

SIGNS & SYMPTOMS Inability to conceive

CAUSES
- Indications for IUI include:
  - ◊ Male factor infertility
    - Oligospermia
    - Asthenospermia
    - Hypospadias
    - Retrograde ejaculation
    - Coital dysfunction
  - ◊ Female factors
    - Cervical mucous abnormalities
    - Poor postcoital test
  - ◊ Unexplained infertility

RISK FACTORS
- Male factor 35%
- Cervical factor 10%
- Testicular trauma from vasectomy, prostatitis, a genetic predisposition can predispose to serum antibody production
- Cervical trauma from cryotherapy, LEEP, conization and laser therapy can cause poor sperm-cervical mucous interaction

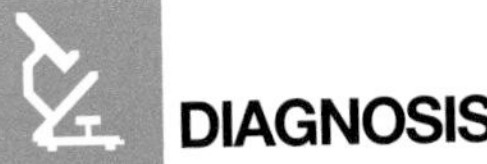

DIAGNOSIS

DIFFERENTIAL DIAGNOSIS
- Primary female cervical factor?
- Primary male factor?

LABORATORY
- Semen analysis
- Postcoital test
- Sperm antibody testing

Drugs that may alter lab results: Clomiphene citrate (Clomid)

Disorders that may alter lab results:
- Abnormal pH of vagina or cervical mucus
- Bacterial infection semen/mucus

PATHOLOGICAL FINDINGS
- Chronic cervicitis
- Chronic prostatitis

SPECIAL TESTS
- Zona free hamster sperm penetration assay
- Bovine cervical mucus sperm penetration test

IMAGING Hysterosalpingogram

DIAGNOSTIC PROCEDURES Postcoital test

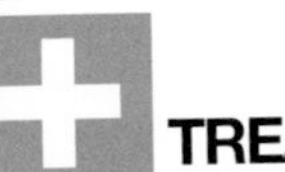

TREATMENT

APPROPRIATE HEALTH CARE Outpatient

GENERAL MEASURES
- Intrauterine insemination should be closely timed with ovulation. Ovulation prediction kits detect the luteinizing hormone (LH) surge which precedes ovulation by 12-36 hours. Intrauterine insemination is performed the day of and/or the day after the LH surge.
- The volume of inseminate that can be transferred into the uterus is 0.25 to 0.5 mL. Small amounts are used to avoid cramping and flushing the oocyte out of the tube. The volume is also limited by space within the uterus.
- Intrauterine insemination is an office procedure. First, the position of the uterus is determined. A speculum is placed in the vagina and the cervix is visualized. The sample of washed sperm is placed into the uppermost portion of the uterine cavity using an insemination catheter with a disposable tuberculin syringe. Avoid touching the uterine fundus with the catheter tip. Occasionally a tenaculum is needed on the anterior lip of the cervix to straighten the endocervical canal. Cervical dilatation or paracervical block is rarely required. The sample is injected slowly over 30-60 seconds.

SURGICAL MEASURES N/A

ACTIVITY No restrictions

DIET No special diet

PATIENT EDUCATION No vaginal lubricants or douching

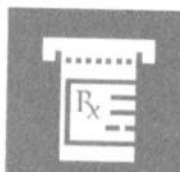

MEDICATIONS

DRUG(S) OF CHOICE
- Clomiphene (Clomid) or human menopausal gonadotropins - menotropins may be used for controlled ovarian hyperstimulation and ovulation may be initiated by the administration of human chorionic gonadotropin (HCG), an LH-like molecule. A recombinant LH product - choriogonadotropin alpha (Ovidrel) may be used subcutaneously for final follicular maturation and ovulation. Intrauterine insemination is performed 24-36 hours after HCG administration. Clomid predisposes to poor cervical mucus, which can adversely alter sperm/mucus interaction.
- Dosages:
  - ◊ Clomiphene: 50 mg daily x 5-7 days to induce ovulation
  - ◊ Menotropins (Pergonal, Repronex, Gonal-F, Follistim) utilized for superovulation induction. Dosage and length of administration depends upon patient response.

Contraindications:
- Uncontrolled thyroid and adrenal dysfunction
- An intracranial lesion
- High follicle-stimulating hormone (FSH) level indicating primary ovarian failure
- Abnormal bleeding of undetermined etiology
- Ovarian cysts of unknown origin
- Hypersensitivity
- Pregnancy

Precautions:
- Multiple births - Clomid 8%, menotropins 25%
- Severe ovarian hyperstimulation (ascites, pleural effusion, dehydration, electrolyte imbalance, pain)
- Ovarian torsion

Significant possible interactions: N/A

ALTERNATIVE DRUGS
Estrogen in follicular phase of cycle to improve mucus (conjugated equine estrogen 1.25-2.5 mg/day cycle days 5-12 or Estraderm patches 0.1-0.2 mg/day cycle days 5-12)

FOLLOWUP

PATIENT MONITORING
- Those patients on Clomid require an ultrasound or a bimanual exam on a monthly basis
- Patients on menotropins require at least serum estradiol measurements and pelvic sonography to monitor ovarian response

PREVENTION/AVOIDANCE
N/A

POSSIBLE COMPLICATIONS
- Uterine cramping
- Mild vasomotor symptoms
- Infection
- Theoretical but unproven risk is development of antisperm antibodies in response to increase exposure of the immune system to sperm antigens

EXPECTED COURSE/PROGNOSIS
- Virtually all pregnancies that result, occur within the first six treatment cycles. A 6 month treatment interval usually represents an adequate therapeutic trial.
- There is a documented increase in efficacy with combination of intrauterine insemination and controlled ovarian hyperstimulation (Pergonal)
- The highest success rates are seen with idiopathic or cervical factor problems
- The poorest outcome is with male factor
- Monthly fecundities of 14% have occurred with therapeutic inseminations utilizing fresh semen

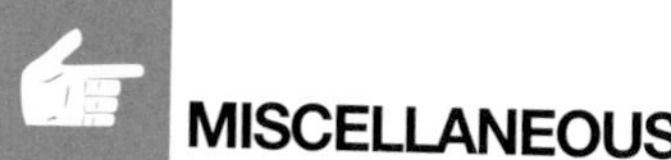

MISCELLANEOUS

ASSOCIATED CONDITIONS
Causes of infertility

AGE-RELATED FACTORS
Pediatric: N/A
Geriatric: N/A
Others:
- Fecundity is inversely related to maternal age
- Contraindications to artificial insemination
  - ◊ Infection (acute cervicitis, endometritis, acute prostatitis, epididymitis, salpingo-oophoritis)
  - ◊ Pregnancy
  - ◊ Unexplained uterine bleeding

PREGNANCY
N/A

SYNONYMS
- Therapeutic insemination
- Intrauterine insemination

ICD-9-CM
628.4 Female infertility of cervical or vaginal origin

SEE ALSO

OTHER NOTES
For donor insemination, only frozen semen is used and only after a 6 month period of "quarantine" to minimize danger of transmission of HIV and other STDs

ABBREVIATIONS
LH = luteinizing hormone
HCG = human chorionic gonadotropin

REFERENCES

- Yen SSC, Jaffe RB, editors. Reproductive Endocrinology. 4th ed. Philadelphia: WB Saunders Co; 1999
- Berek JS, editor. Novak's Gynecology. 13th ed. Baltimore: Williams & Wilkins; 2002
- Khamsi F, Lacanna I. Endman M, Wong J. Recent advances in assisted reproductive technologies. Endocrine 1998;9(1):15-25

Web references: 1 available at www.5mcc.com
Illustrations N/A

Author(s):
Nicholas J. Spirtos, DO

BASICS

DESCRIPTION A chronic non-malignant lung disease caused by inhalation of asbestos, a hazardous dust found in a variety of work places. This disease persists in spite of substantial knowledge about its cause, and effective means of prevention. The disease typically occurs 10-15 years after initial exposure. Asbestosis is a fibrotic interstitial lung disease caused by a cascade of responses to inhaled asbestos fibers. Pleural plaques and mesotheliomas can develop. It increases risk of tuberculosis and lung cancer in cigarette smokers.

System(s) affected: Pulmonary

Genetics: No known genetic pattern

Incidence/Prevalence in USA: There is no uniform surveillance or reporting of asbestosis. In the USA, less than 10 cases per 100,000 people are diagnosed annually; this probably represents an underestimate. 876 deaths reported from 1979 to 1992. Number of cases rising steadily. More than a million people have been exposed to significant levels of asbestos. Peak use was 1940-1975.

Predominant age: Middle age (40-75 years)

Predominant sex: Male > Female, due to exposure pattern

SIGNS & SYMPTOMS
- No unique signs or symptoms
- Insidious onset
- Cough, dry or with sputum production
- Exercise intolerance
- Sexual dysfunction may be associated
- Basilar crackles
- Wheeze with forced exhalation
- Digital clubbing
- Cyanosis
- Right sided heart failure

CAUSES
- Diversity of settings for hazardous exposure
- Asbestos used in more than 3000 commercial products - production peaked in mid-1970s
- Risk to miners and millers of asbestos
- More people at risk in construction sites with unprotected use of asbestos, commonly for insulation
- Maintenance and removal of asbestos-containing material creates high levels
- Office workers, teachers, and students in buildings with asbestos in place have exposure orders of magnitude below those of construction workers. Although societal concern has been high - actual health risk not considered significant.

RISK FACTORS
- Cigarette smoking markedly increases risk
- Asbestos maintenance and removal workers
- Construction workers
- Asbestos miners and millers
- Shipbuilders
- Textile workers
- Railroad workers

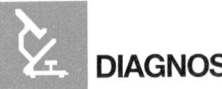

DIAGNOSIS

DIFFERENTIAL DIAGNOSIS Other pneumoconioses (siderosis, stannosis (due to inhalation of tin oxide), baritosis, coal worker pneumoconiosis, silicosis, talcosis, shaver's disease)

LABORATORY
- Hypoxemia
- Bronchoalveolar lavage or biopsy - generally unnecessary in the clinical setting - research tools

Drugs that may alter lab results: N/A

Disorders that may alter lab results: N/A

PATHOLOGICAL FINDINGS
- Lung:
  - ◊ Parietal pleural thickening
  - ◊ Parietal pleural calcification
  - ◊ Interstitial inflammation
  - ◊ Interstitial fibrosis
  - ◊ Alveolar wall fibrosis

SPECIAL TESTS
- Pulmonary function test:
  - ◊ Not diagnostically specific
  - ◊ Useful for following level of impairment
  - ◊ Restrictive, mixed, or obstructive pattern
  - ◊ Reduction in diffusing capacity to carbon monoxide can occur early, even when chest x-ray is normal

IMAGING
- Chest x-ray
  - ◊ Primary diagnostic modality and screening tool - approximately 80% sensitive
  - ◊ Diagnosis based on: credible history of exposure, delay from exposure to detection, and typical radiographic findings
  - ◊ Irregular, linear opacities - start in bases at periphery, and spread upwards
  - ◊ Circumscribed pleural plaques
  - ◊ Rounded atelectasis (pseudotumor)
  - ◊ Pleural thickening
  - ◊ Classification scheme available through International Labour Office
- High resolution CT may increase sensitivity to near 100%
  - ◊ Sub-pleural curvilinear lines

DIAGNOSTIC PROCEDURES Bronchoscopy - research tool

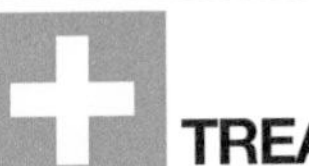

TREATMENT

APPROPRIATE HEALTH CARE Outpatient

GENERAL MEASURES
- No effective treatment to reverse the course
- Early detection essential
- Approach directed at elimination of progression, amelioration of symptoms, reduction of risk of associated disorders
- Withdrawal from exposure
  - ◊ Workers with no symptoms, and only CXR changes may make an informed choice to continue employment, with maximum environmental and personal protection
- Pneumococcal and influenza vaccines
- Chest physiotherapy
- Nutritional advice
- Home oxygen
- Graded exercise
- Stop smoking

SURGICAL MEASURES
- Whole lung lavage to remove retained dust is being investigated
- Lung transplantation for severe advanced cases

ACTIVITY Graded exercise

DIET High calorie, high protein with advanced disease

PATIENT EDUCATION Printed patient information available from: Asbestos Victims of America, P.O. Box 559, Capitola, CA 95010, (408)476-3646 or American Lung Association, 1740 Broadway, New York, NY 10019, (212)315-8700

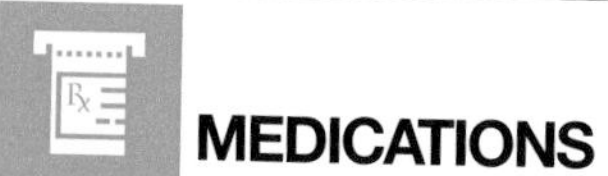

MEDICATIONS

DRUG(S) OF CHOICE
- No specific pharmacologic treatment
- Oxygen
- Bronchodilators for pulmonary toilet

Contraindications: N/A
Precautions: N/A
Significant possible interactions: N/A

ALTERNATIVE DRUGS
- Antibiotics for respiratory infections
- Diuretics
- Treatment of congestive heart failure

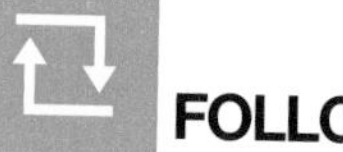

FOLLOWUP

PATIENT MONITORING
- Chest x-rays
- Occasional pulmonary function tests
- Treat infections promptly

PREVENTION/AVOIDANCE
- Primary responsibility of employers
- Exposure control - substitution of safer material or adoption of control technologies
- Monitor workplace exposure
- During high exposure periods such as building repair - use of fit-tested personal respirators for workers
- WHO recommendations for regular health screening of exposed workers
  - ◊ Chest x-ray at baseline
  - ◊ For workers with less than 10 years since first exposure: chest x-ray every 3-5 years
  - ◊ Longer than 10 years: chest x-ray every 1-2 years
  - ◊ Longer than 20 years: chest x-ray annually
  - ◊ All workers: annual respiratory symptom questionnaire, physical exam, and spirometry (alternatively can be done on CXR schedule)
- Reporting of new cases to health authorities

POSSIBLE COMPLICATIONS
- Cancers of the mesothelium of the lung
  - ◊ Unrelated to tobacco use
- Lung cancer
  - ◊ Risk increased in smokers by asbestos workers
- Gastrointestinal cancer risk may be increased
- Exudative pleural effusion
  - ◊ Resolve with residual pleural thickening
- Hyaline plaques on parietal pleura can create pseudotumors
- Increased risk of tuberculosis in smokers

EXPECTED COURSE/PROGNOSIS
- Severity depends on duration of exposure and on intensity of exposure
- Lung disease irreversible
- Further increased lung cancer risk with smoking
- Increased risk for mesotheliomas
- Increased risk for tuberculosis

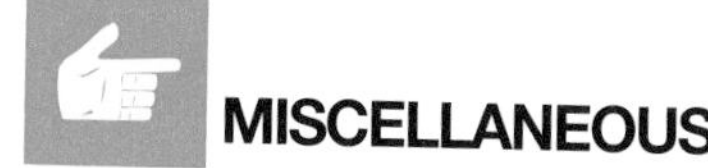

MISCELLANEOUS

ASSOCIATED CONDITIONS N/A

AGE-RELATED FACTORS
Pediatric: N/A
Geriatric: More likely to have terminal respiratory illness
Others: N/A

PREGNANCY N/A

SYNONYMS
- Asbestos pneumoconiosis

ICD-9-CM
501 Asbestosis

SEE ALSO

OTHER NOTES N/A

ABBREVIATIONS
CT = computerized tomography
CXR = chest x-ray
WHO = World Health Organization

REFERENCES

- LaDou J, ed: Occupational Medicine. Norwalk, CT, Appleton and Lange, 1990
- Rosenstock L, Cullen MR: Clinical Occupational Medicine. Philadelphia, W.B. Saunders Co., 1986
- Wagner GR: Asbestosis and silicosis. Lancet 1997;349:1311-1315
- International Labour Office. Guidelines for the use of ILO international classification of radiographs of pneumoconioses, 1980

Web references: 0 available at www.5mcc.com
Illustrations N/A

Author(s):
Nancy N. Dambro, MD

BASICS

DESCRIPTION Effusion and accumulation of fluid in the abdominal cavity. Ascites may occur in any condition that causes generalized edema. In children, nephrotic syndrome and malignancy are the predominant causes. In adults, cirrhosis, heart failure, nephrotic syndrome and chronic peritonitis are most common.
System(s) affected: Cardiovascular, Gastrointestinal, Hemic/Lymphatic/Immunologic, Renal/Urologic
Genetics: N/A
Incidence/Prevalence in USA: Determined by etiology
Predominant age: Determined by etiology
Predominant sex: Determined by etiology

SIGNS & SYMPTOMS
- Abdominal pain
- Abdominal discomfort
- Abdominal distention
- Tight clothing
- Shortness of breath
- Anorexia
- Nausea
- Early satiety
- Pyrosis; heartburn
- Flank pain
- Weight gain
- Orthopnea
- Abdominal fluid wave
- Shifting dullness
- Penile edema; scrotal edema
- Umbilical herniation
- Pleural effusion
- Pedal edema
- Rales
- Tachycardia
- Flatulence

CAUSES
- Peritoneal infection and inflammation:
  - ◊ Tuberculosis
  - ◊ Fungus disease
  - ◊ Chronic bacterial (foreign body, fistula)
  - ◊ Ruptured viscus
  - ◊ Granulomatous peritonitis
  - ◊ Filariasis
- Metabolic diseases
  - ◊ Cirrhosis
  - ◊ Prehepatic and posthepatic portal hypertension
  - ◊ Myxedema
  - ◊ Nephrogenous
  - ◊ Marked hypoalbuminemia (< 2 gm/dL)
- Heart and hepatic congestion
  - ◊ Congestive heart failure
  - ◊ Constrictive pericarditis
  - ◊ Tricuspid stenosis or insufficiency
- Traumatic
  - ◊ Pancreatic fistula
  - ◊ Biliary fistula
  - ◊ Lymphatic fistula (chylous)
  - ◊ Hemoperitoneum (trauma, ectopic pregnancy, tumor)
- Malignancy
  - ◊ Peritoneal seeding - ovarian, colon, pancreas and others
  - ◊ Lymphatic obstruction - leukemia, lymphoma

RISK FACTORS Those associated with possible causes

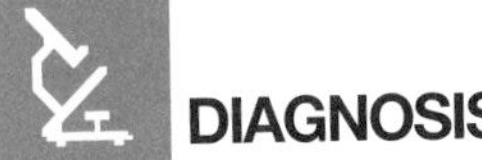

DIAGNOSIS

DIFFERENTIAL DIAGNOSIS
- Obesity
- Air and liquid in distended intestine
- Fluid type:
- Transudate
  - ◊ Likely causes include: Congestive heart failure, constrictive pericarditis, cirrhosis, nephrotic syndrome, hypoalbuminemia
- Exudate
  - ◊ Likely causes include: Neoplasm, tuberculosis, pancreatitis, myxedema, biliary pathology, Budd-Chiari syndrome

LABORATORY
- Ascitic fluid (must be sampled in all new onset, or new to treatment cases; obtain in all:
  - ◊ Culture through inoculating blood culture bottles
  - ◊ Total cell count < 500 mm3
  - ◊ PMN < 200 mm3
  - ◊ Albumin in both serum and ascites calculate. Serum - ascites < 1.1 gm indicates inflammation or exudate, > 1.1 gm indicates portal hypertension. Protein > 2.0 gm (some would suggest 2.5 gm) indicates exudate.
- Of use in specific circumstances
  - ◊ Lactate dehydrogenase < 200 IU/L
  - ◊ Amylase
  - ◊ Acid fast or fungal cultures
  - ◊ Cytology
  - ◊ Triglycerides (with a serum test)
- In blood
  - ◊ Creatinine < 1.4 mg/dL
  - ◊ Electrolytes
- In urine - sodium levels in a single sample:
  - ◊ < 10 mEq/L (< 10 mmol/L) diuretic response unlikely
  - ◊ > 10-70 mEq/L (> 10-70 mmol/L) diuretic response likely
  - ◊ > 70 mEq/L(> 70 mmol/L) diuretics unnecessary

Drugs that may alter lab results: Refer to laboratory test reference

Disorders that may alter lab results: Refer to laboratory test reference

PATHOLOGICAL FINDINGS Peritoneal biopsy when exudative fluid present. May reveal tuberculosis or carcinoma cells. Of no value in other types of fluid.

SPECIAL TESTS Laparoscopy

IMAGING Sonography or CT scan

DIAGNOSTIC PROCEDURES
- Diagnostic paracentesis
- Needle biopsy peritoneum in exudate

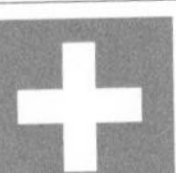

TREATMENT

APPROPRIATE HEALTH CARE May be outpatient or inpatient depending on physical condition

GENERAL MEASURES
- For all patients
  - ◊ Some sodium restriction required, must be most severe when urine sodium is very low
  - ◊ Select a sodium restriction that patient can attain at home; treatment usually required 3-6 months
  - ◊ Water restriction only necessary if sodium < 130 mEq/L
  - ◊ Any persistent elevation of creatinine to > 2.5 mg/dL should lead to decreasing diuretic doses and therapeutic paracentesis
  - ◊ Daily record of weight to monitor gains and losses
- For ascites with edema
  - ◊ Salt restriction and diuretics usually effective
  - ◊ Maximum weight loss of 5 lbs/day
  - ◊ Weekly electrolytes on serum during rapid weight loss
- For ascites without edema
  - ◊ Dietary restrictions and diuretics as above
  - ◊ Maximum loss of 2 lbs/day
- Refractory ascites - ascites that is increasing despite maximal doses of spironolactone (300 mg/day) and furosemide (160-200 mg/day) and dietary sodium restriction OR progressive rise in creatinine to >2.0.
  - ◊ Start paracentesis up to 10 L/session. Replace albumin IV for all removals > 5L at rate of 10 gm albumin for each liter >5 L removed. Continue diuretics at half previous dose.

SURGICAL MEASURES
- TIPS (transjugular intrahepatic portosystemic shunt - a radiological procedure). Effective for refractory ascites.
  - ◊ At the time of placement, the measured portal pressure should drop at least 20 mmHg or to less than 12 mmHg, and the ascites is readily controlled with diuretics. Yearly ultrasonographic study to demonstrate a functional shunt.
  - ◊ Dilation or replacement may be required after 2 or more years. Encephalopathy is a possible complication of TIPS.
- Surgical portacaval shunt. Often an 8-10 mm mesenteric caval shunt is effective in controlling ascites.
  - ◊ Significant operative mortality and morbidity, and some encephalopathy leading most experts to prefer TIPS. When recurrent pleural effusion is present in patient with chronic ascites, fusing of the pleural surfaces is sometimes used. An alternative is placing a TIPS.
  - ◊ Liver transplantation much more difficult and therefore should be considered for non-transplant candidates who have failed TIPS.
- Transplantation. Refractory ascites considered by many as an indication for transplantation.

ACTIVITY Bedrest of benefit in heart failure and when leg edema is prominent, otherwise of limited value.

DIET Sodium restriction needed for several months; regulate on a diet that can be followed outside hospital

PATIENT EDUCATION Diet restrictions

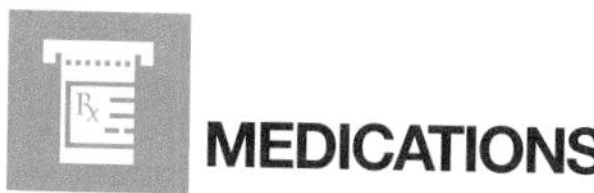

MEDICATIONS

DRUG(S) OF CHOICE

- Diuretics are needed in nearly all patients
  - ◊ Spironolactone 100-300 mg/day orally in one dose best for cirrhotic ascites; furosemide 40-120 mg/day orally best for all other etiologies. May use together.
  - ◊ Dose should be sufficient to obtain net sodium loss in urine
  - ◊ Typical initial dose is 100 or 200 mg of spironolactone and 40 mg furosemide both given in the am.
  - ◊ Discontinue NSAIDs except 80 mg dose of aspirin. Follow body weight daily. If <2 lb loss in next 4 days, increase either spironolactone by 100 mg or furosemide by 40. If 2 lb weight loss/4 days ensues, continue same dose. Emphasize sodium restriction.
  - ◊ Spot sodium in mEq/L x estimated urine output (1 L if no information) should equal estimated dietary sodium. Increase diuretics daily until this is attained. Measure serum electrolytes before each dose change.

Contraindications: See manufacturer's literature

Precautions:

- In hospital, or when rapid diuresis, observe creatinine weekly. NSAIDs may worsen or initiate oliguria or azotemia. Potassium supplements are usually required when diuresis exceeds 1 lb/day.
- Spironolactone or amiloride may increase potassium, monitoring is necessary after the first week of therapy and at least monthly thereafter
- Observe patients closely for signs of volume depletion, encephalopathy and renal insufficiency. NSAIDs may worsen or initiate oliguria or azotemia.

Significant possible interactions: Avoid concomitant use of potassium supplements if spironolactone is used alone

ALTERNATIVE DRUGS

- Only rarely do alternative diuretics lead to success if combinations of spironolactone and furosemide fail or result in azotemia, or creatinine elevations
  - ◊ Most commonly used when there is gastrointestinal intolerance or allergic reactions
  - ◊ Alternatives to spironolactone - amiloride up to 10 mg/day, triamterene up to 200 mg daily in divided dose
  - ◊ Alternatives to furosemide - torsemide up to 100 mg/day, ethacrynic acid 50 mg/IV. May be effective when oral drugs cannot be used.

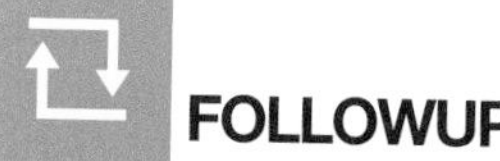

FOLLOWUP

PATIENT MONITORING

- For ascites - changes in body weight and urinary sodium to measure response to therapy
- Monitoring as needed for other therapies
- Measure electrolytes whenever there is appreciable diuresis (>1 lb. loss of weight/day) weekly and at least monthly. Also measure after one week following any change in dose or type of diuretic.

PREVENTION/AVOIDANCE Dependent upon etiology

POSSIBLE COMPLICATIONS

- Overly aggressive diuresis may lead to hypokalemia, worsening hepatic encephalopathy, intravascular volume depletion, azotemia, and possibly to renal failure and death
- Hepatorenal syndrome - urine volume < 300 mL/day, rising blood urea and creatinine. Stop all diuretics. IV fluid challenge of 500 mL 0.9% saline after one day if no improvement.
- Spontaneous peritonitis. Ascites cell count > 250 PMN, may be fever, clinical deterioration. Treat with Cipro or comparable antibiotic.
- Hydrothorax. Always on right side. Cell and lab properties same as ascites. Do not place chest tube. Treat ascites vigorously and if hydrothorax does not disappear, consider TIPS.
- Other complications may be associated with cause of ascites

EXPECTED COURSE/PROGNOSIS

- Ascites is rarely life-threatening. Conservative therapy usually successful.
- Prognosis variable depending upon the underlying cause

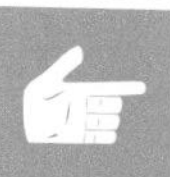

MISCELLANEOUS

ASSOCIATED CONDITIONS Listed in Causes

AGE-RELATED FACTORS

Pediatric: N/A
Geriatric: N/A
Others: N/A

PREGNANCY N/A

SYNONYMS N/A

ICD-9-CM

789.5 Ascites

SEE ALSO

Cirrhosis of the liver
Congestive heart failure
Nephrotic syndrome

OTHER NOTES N/A

ABBREVIATIONS

NSAID = Non-steroidal anti-inflammatory drug

REFERENCES

- Russo MW, Jacques PF, Mauro M, Odell P, Brown RS Jr. Predictors of mortality and stenosis after transjugular intrahepatic portosystemic shunt. Liver Transpl 2002;8(3):271-7
- Runyon, BA. Management of adult patients with ascites due to cirrhosis. Hepatology 2004 ; 39 (3): 841-56
- Gines P,Uriz J, Calahorra B, Garcia-Tsao G, et al. Transjugular intrahepatic portosystemic shunting versus paracentesis plus albumin for refractory ascites in cirrhosis. Gastroenterology 2002 ;123 (6) 139-47

Web references: 1 available at www.5mcc.com
Illustrations N/A

Author(s):
Frank L. Iber, MD

BASICS

DESCRIPTION
Disease caused by a ubiquitous mold that primarily involves the lungs. Disease frequently lethal in neutropenic and bone marrow transplant (BMT) patients. Syndromes include:
- Allergic aspergillosis
  - ◊ Extrinsic allergic alveolitis - hypersensitivity pneumonitis in individuals repeatedly exposed to the fungus
  - ◊ Allergic bronchopulmonary aspergillosis (ABPA) - pulmonary infiltrates, mucous plugging; secondary to allergic reaction to fungus
- Aspergillomas: "fungus ball" saprophytic colonization within pre-existing pulmonary cavities
- Invasive aspergillosis: most common and severe in BMT and neutropenic patients. Also occurs with increased frequency in other immunocompromised persons, such as those with AIDS, solid organ transplant or high dose corticosteroids; commonly fatal.

System(s) affected: Cardiovascular, Gastrointestinal, Musculoskeletal, Nervous, Pulmonary
Genetics: No known genetic pattern
Incidence/Prevalence in USA: Rare
Predominant age: None
Predominant sex: Male = Female

SIGNS & SYMPTOMS
- Allergic - cough, wheezing, constitutional symptoms, plug expectoration
- Aspergillomas - hemoptysis; manifestations of underlying disease
- Invasive - fever, cough, rales, rhonchi; toxicity; CNS signs; GI bleeding

CAUSES
Aspergillus species in decreasing order of frequency: *A. fumigatus, A. flavus, A. niger*

RISK FACTORS
- Allergic - exposure, asthma
- Aspergillomas - COPD, bronchiectasis, TB, malignancy
- Invasive - neutropenia, corticosteroid therapy, graft vs. host disease in recipients of bone marrow transplant, AIDS

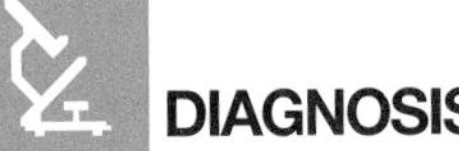

DIAGNOSIS

DIFFERENTIAL DIAGNOSIS
- Allergic - other causes of asthma and hypersensitivity pneumonitis.
- Aspergillomas - neoplasm, TB
- Invasive - bacterial pneumonia, pulmonary hemorrhage, drug toxicity, malignancy; mucor (sinuses).

LABORATORY
- ABPA - eosinophilia, immediate skin reactivity to aspergillus antigen, precipitating-serum antibodies to aspergillus, elevated serum IgE concentrations.
- Invasive - sputum culture, cultures of bronchoalveolar lavage or bronchial washings; biopsy is definitive; blood cultures almost never positive

Drugs that may alter lab results: None

Disorders that may alter lab results: None

PATHOLOGICAL FINDINGS
Necrotizing pneumonia, hemorrhagic infarcts, blood vessel invasion; branching septate hyphae if organism seen microscopically

SPECIAL TESTS
- ABPA - immediate skin reactivity to aspergillus antigen, precipitating serum antibodies (precipitins) against aspergillus antigens, elevated serum IgE concentrations, elevated serum IgE and IgG antibodies specific to *A. fumigatus*.
- Invasive - none

IMAGING
Chest x-ray - fleeting infiltrates (ABPA), round intracavity mass (aspergillomas); nodular or patchy infiltrates progressing to diffuse consolidation and cavitation (invasive); nodular, cavitary or pleural-based wedge-shaped lesions

DIAGNOSTIC PROCEDURES
Bronchoscopy, bronchial washings, bronchoalveolar lavage or transthoracic needle aspiration may be helpful in isolating organism in invasive disease; open lung biopsy is diagnostic but often not possible in severely ill, ventilated patients.

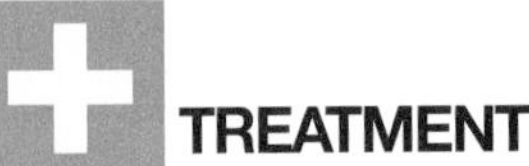

TREATMENT

APPROPRIATE HEALTH CARE
- Allergic - outpatient usually
- Aspergillomas - outpatient usually
- Invasive - inpatient

GENERAL MEASURES
- Allergic
  - ◊ Extrinsic allergic alveolitis - drug therapy, exposure avoidance.
  - ◊ ABPA - corticosteroids
- Aspergillomas - individualized therapy ranging from no therapy to surgical resection of cavities in cases of severe hemoptysis; systemic antifungal therapy is seldom useful
- Invasive - (prognosis tends to be poor) high dose intravenous antifungal therapy; treatment of underlying disease; ?adjunctive cytokine therapy to reverse neutropenia

SURGICAL MEASURES
N/A

ACTIVITY
As tolerated

DIET
No special diet

PATIENT EDUCATION
To specifics of individual circumstances.

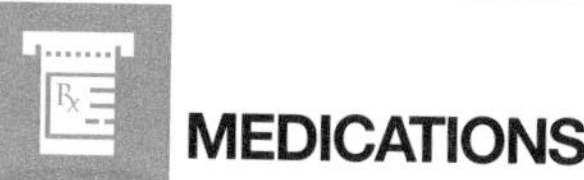

MEDICATIONS

DRUG(S) OF CHOICE

- Allergic
  - ◊ Extrinsic allergic alveolitis - bronchodilators, cromolyn, steroids
  - ◊ ABPA - steroids
- Aspergillomas - none
- Invasive - high dose amphotericin B - up to 1 mg/kg/day. The lipid formulations of amphotericin B (Abelcet, Ambisome) are preferred over standard amphotericin because of the reduced nephrotoxicity in view of the high doses required.
- Caspofungin is approved for patients with aspergillosis unresponsive to other therapy or who have unacceptable toxicity to other agents
- Voriconazole was superior to conventional amphotericin in a large study and is well absorbed orally
- Note: because of the frequent failure of single drug therapy, combination therapy is frequently proposed

Contraindications: Refer to manufacturers literature

Precautions: Amphotericin B can cause significant renal insufficiency and electrolyte abnormalities. Saline infusion at the time of amphotericin B administration may decrease the nephrotoxicity.

Significant possible interactions:

- Amphotericin B - other nephrotoxic drugs (aminoglycosides, cyclosporine, etc): accelerate development of renal insufficiency
- Amphotericin B - diuretics: accelerate electrolyte depletion
- Voriconazole - hepatically metabolized drug; serum levels may be altered
- Itraconazole-hepatically metabolized drugs: serum levels altered
- Itraconazole - gastric pH: normal, low pH is necessary for absorption

ALTERNATIVE DRUGS

Itraconazole is occasionally useful as an alternative agent

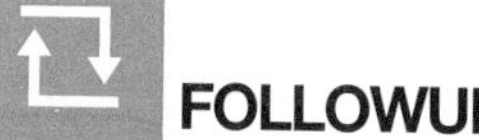

FOLLOWUP

PATIENT MONITORING

- Allergic
  - ◊ Extrinsic allergic, alveolitis - spirometry
  - ◊ ABPA - chest x-ray, IgE levels
- Aspergillomas - chest x-ray, symptoms
- Invasive - chest x-ray, CBC

PREVENTION/AVOIDANCE

- Allergic - avoid exposure
- Aspergillomas - treatment of underlying diseases, eg, COPD, etc.

POSSIBLE COMPLICATIONS

- Allergic - bronchiectasis, pulmonary fibrosis, obstructive lung disease
- Aspergillomas - hemoptyses
- Invasive - metastatic infection of CNS, GI tract and other organs; death

EXPECTED COURSE/PROGNOSIS

- Allergic - with treatment prognosis is good; untreated can progress to severe fibrosis, COPD
- Aspergillomas - prognosis more related to underlying disease
- Invasive - poor prognosis

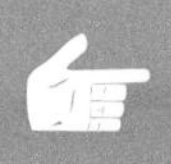

MISCELLANEOUS

ASSOCIATED CONDITIONS

- Allergic - asthma
- Aspergillomas - COPD, TB, pulmonary mycoses, silicosis, sarcoidosis, non-tuberculosis mycobacteria, ankylosing spondylitis, malignancy
- Invasive - neutropenia

AGE-RELATED FACTORS

Pediatric: N/A

Geriatric: N/A

Others:

- Allergic - Tends to occur in younger patients <35.
- Aspergillomas - older patients with chronic lung disease
- Invasive - all ages

PREGNANCY

N/A

SYNONYMS

- Hypersensitivity pneumonitis
- Fungus ball

ICD-9-CM

117.3 Aspergillosis

SEE ALSO

OTHER NOTES

N/A

ABBREVIATIONS

ABPA = allergic bronchopulmonary aspergillosis

REFERENCES

- Soubani AO, Chandrasekar PH. The clinical spectrum of pulmonary aspergillosis. Chest 2002;121(6):1988-99
- Herbrecht R, Denning DW, et al. Invasive Fungal Infections Group of the European Organisation for Research and Treatment of Cancer and the Global Aspergillus Study Group. Voriconazole versus amphotericin B for primary therapy of invasive aspergillosis. N Engl J Med 2002;347(6):408-15
- Petraitis V, Petraitiene R, et al. Combination therapy in treatment of experimental pulmonary aspergillosis: synergistic interaction between an antifungal triazole and an echinocandin. J Infect Dis 2003;187(12):1834-43
- Lin S, Schranz J, Teutsch S. Aspergillosis case-fatality rate: systematic review of the literature. Clin Infect Dis. 2001;32(3):358-66

Web references: 2 available at www.5mcc.com

Illustrations 1 available

Author(s):

Rodney D. Adam, MD

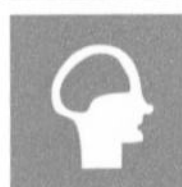

BASICS

DESCRIPTION A disorder of the tracheobronchial tree characterized by mild to severe obstruction to airflow which is at least partially reversible. Symptoms vary, generally episodic or paroxysmal, but may be persistent. The clinical hallmark is wheezing, but cough or chest tightness may be the predominant symptom. Commonly misdiagnosed as recurrent pneumonia or chronic bronchitis.

- Acute symptoms are characterized by narrowing of large and small airways due to spasm of bronchial smooth muscle, edema and inflammation of the bronchial mucosa, and production of mucus
- Occurs in a setting in which asthma is likely and other, rarer conditions have been excluded

System(s) affected: Pulmonary

Genetics: Search for an asthma gene underway; there is a familial association of reactive airway disease (RAD), atopic dermatitis, and allergic rhinitis

Incidence/Prevalence in USA:
- 10 million new cases each year, however, there is confusion due to lack of a uniform definition
- 7-19% of children
- A leading cause of missed school days - 7.5 million/year

Predominant age:
- 50% of cases are children under 10
- Young adult (16-40 years); but may occur at any age

Predominant sex:
- Children under 10: Male > Female
- Puberty: Male = Female
- Adult onset: Female > Male

SIGNS & SYMPTOMS

Variation in pattern of symptoms: paroxysmal, constant, abnormal pulmonary function tests may occur without symptoms

- Wheezing
- Cough
- Chest tightness
- Chest pain
- Periodicity of symptoms
- Exercise-induced wheezing or cough
- Prolonged expiration
- Nocturnal attacks
- Pulsus paradoxus
- Tachycardia
- Hypoxia
- Accessory respiratory muscle use
- Flattened diaphragms
- Nasal polyp; seen in cystic fibrosis and aspirin sensitivity, not in uncomplicated asthma
- Clubbing is not seen in asthma
- Growth is usually normal
- Pectus carinatum

CAUSES

- Allergic factors
  - ◊ Airborne pollens
  - ◊ Molds
  - ◊ House dust (mites)
  - ◊ Cockroaches
  - ◊ Animal dander
  - ◊ Feather pillows
- Other factors
  - ◊ Tobacco smoke and other pollutants
  - ◊ Infections, especially viral
  - ◊ Aspirin
  - ◊ Exercise
  - ◊ Cold air
  - ◊ Sinusitis
  - ◊ Gastroesophageal reflux
  - ◊ Sleep (peak expiratory flow rate [PEFR] lowest at 4 am)
- Current research focuses on inflammatory response (including abnormal release of chemical mediators, eosinophil chemotactic factor, neutrophil chemotactic factor, and leukotrienes, etc.)

RISK FACTORS

- Positive family history of asthma or atopy
- Viral lower respiratory infection during infancy
- Environmental tobacco smoke
- Inner city dwelling

DIAGNOSIS

DIFFERENTIAL DIAGNOSIS Foreign body aspiration - always consider, especially with unilateral wheeze; cystic fibrosis; viral respiratory infections (croup, bronchiolitis); epiglottitis; bronchopulmonary aspergillosis; tuberculosis; hyperventilation syndrome; mitral value prolapse; habit cough; recurrent pulmonary emboli; congestive heart failure; chronic obstructive pulmonary disease; hypersensitivity pneumonitis; vascular anomalies; mediastinal mass; tracheobronchomalacia; vocal cord dysfunction

LABORATORY

- CBC normal
- Nasal eosinophils
- Immunoglobulins
  - ◊ Screen for immunodeficiency (IgA, IgG subclasses)
  - ◊ IgE markedly elevated in allergic bronchopulmonary aspergillosis (ABPA)
- Sweat test in chronic childhood asthmatics
- Arterial blood gases in status asthmaticus
- Theophylline level [therapeutic: 5-15 μg/mL (28-84 μmol/L)]

Drugs that may alter lab results: Antihistamines may alter allergy skin testing

Disorders that may alter lab results: N/A

PATHOLOGICAL FINDINGS Smooth muscle hyperplasia; mucosal edema; thickened basement membrane; inflammatory response; hyperinflated lungs; mucus plugging; bronchiectasis is not seen except in association with ABPA

SPECIAL TESTS

- Pulmonary function tests - reversible airway obstruction (increased airway resistance, decreased airflow rates)
- Allergy testing
- PPD
- Exercise tolerance testing
- Cold air provocation
- Ventilation-perfusion scan
- Methacholine challenge

IMAGING Chest x-ray (hyperinflation, atelectasis, air leak)

DIAGNOSTIC PROCEDURES

- Chest x-ray: do at least one, but not necessary with each exacerbation (right middle lobe atelectasis common)
- Spirometry: decreased FEV1
- Bronchoscopy: rarely indicated
- Laryngoscopy with exercise challenge to diagnose vocal cord dysfunction

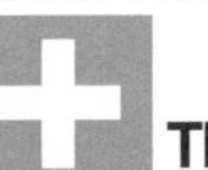

TREATMENT

APPROPRIATE HEALTH CARE

- Outpatient
- Inpatient for bronchospasm not relieved by beta-agonists and steroids

GENERAL MEASURES

- Environmental control of irritants
  - ◊ Molds may grow in vaporizers
  - ◊ Frequent bathing of pets
- Consider hyposensitization - not usually helpful in persistent asthma
- Education essential
- Use spacer device with all metered dose inhalers (MDI)
- Six major classes of drugs are used:
  - ◊ Steroids (budesonide, fluticasone, prednisone, etc)
  - ◊ Mast cell stabilizers (cromolyn and nedocromil)
  - ◊ Beta-agonists (albuterol, bitolterol, salmeterol, etc.); increase in response to symptoms
  - ◊ Methylxanthines (theophylline)
  - ◊ Anticholinergics (atropine, ipratropium)
  - ◊ Leukotriene modifiers
- Prophylactic management with anti-inflammatories (inhaled steroids, cromolyn, leukotriene modifiers)
- Delivery systems
  - ◊ Children < 2 - nebulizer or MDI with valved spacer and mask
  - ◊ Children 2-4 years - MDI and valved spacer
  - ◊ Over 5 years - MDI with spacer or dry powder inhaler
- The following are NOT recommended: mist, large volumes of fluid, breathing exercises, IPPB
- Supplemental oxygen essential for hypoxemia in exacerbations

SURGICAL MEASURES N/A

ACTIVITY Early diagnosis and appropriate treatment facilitate unrestricted activity

DIET No special diet

PATIENT EDUCATION

- American Lung Association, 1740 Broadway, New York, NY 10019, (212)315-8700
- Asthma and Allergy Foundation of America, Suite 305, Washington, DC 20036, (800)7-ASTHMA, (800)727-8462
- Asthma Logbook, Teton NewMedia, (877)306-9793

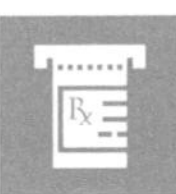

MEDICATIONS

DRUG(S) OF CHOICE

- Mild intermittent asthma: brief wheezing < 2 times a week:
  - ◊ Intermittent beta-agonist (MDI or nebulizer - albuterol, 2 puffs 1.25-5 mg of 0,5% solution (0.25-1.0 mL)
- Mild persistent asthma: symptoms > 2 times a week, but < 1 time a day; affecting activity with PEFR variability < 20%. Medicate daily.
  - ◊ Inhaled steroids (low doses) preferred
  - ◊ Cromolyn qid or nedocromil bid (2 puffs or 2 mL nebulized)
  - ◊ Consider zafirlukast (Accolate) or montelukast (Singulair)

- Moderate persistent asthma: weekly symptoms interfering with sleep or exercise, occasional ER visits, PEFR 60-80% of predicted, PEFR variability >30%. Medicate on regular maintenance schedule.
  - ◊ Inhaled steroids 400-800 μg/day.
  - ◊ If not controlled with moderate dose inhaled steroid (600 μg/day), add long-acting beta agonist
  - ◊ Fluticasone-salmeterol (Advair) (combination drug) helpful with compliance
  - ◊ Consider montelukast
- Severe persistent asthma: frequent symptoms affecting activity, nocturnal symptoms, frequent hospitalizations, PEFR <60% predicted
  - ◊ High dose inhaled steroids; some patients may need alternate day oral steroids
  - ◊ Salmeterol as long-acting bronchodilator
  - ◊ Fluticasone-salmeterol (Advair) helpful with compliance
  - ◊ Theophylline often useful, particularly for nighttime symptoms
  - ◊ Consider montelukast
  - ◊ Consider cromolyn, ipratropium
- Acute exacerbation
  - ◊ Outpatient management
    - Inhaled beta-agonist (albuterol), 1.0 mL/5 mg (dose varies 0.25-1.0 mL with 2 mL NS) to reverse airflow obstruction
    - Levalbuterol (Xopenex) is expensive and of no additional benefit
    - Short course of steroids, 2 mg/kg po qam for 5-7 days
    - IV aminophylline adds toxicity only
    - Observe at least one hour; look for increased work of breathing, air leak syndromes, atelectasis, lowered PEFR
  - ◊ Hospital management
    - Steroids: methylprednisolone (Solu-Medrol) 2 mg/kg IV once, then 1 mg/kg IV q6h
    - Frequent nebulized beta-agonist, even continuous at 5-30 mg/hr
    - Ipratropium neb (250-300 mcg) and/or aminophylline IV drip if not responding well
    - Rarely: isoproterenol or terbutaline IV; magnesium sulfate IV; mechanical ventilation

Contraindications:
- Sedatives, mucolytics
- Antibiotics are usually not necessary
- Avoid beta-adrenergic blocking drugs

Precautions:
- Chronic use of beta agonists may be deleterious; use only when needed (chronic asthma may necessitate chronic use). If beta-agonist used more than twice a week, patient should also be on an anti-inflammatory.
- Do not use salmeterol alone - mortality increased, especially in blacks.

Significant possible interactions: Erythromycin and ciprofloxacin slow theophylline clearance and can increase levels 15-20%

ALTERNATIVE DRUGS
- Ketotifen
- H1-antagonists
- Troleandomycin (TAO)
- Methotrexate
- Immune globulin IV
- Furosemide (Lasix)
- Omalizumab (Xolair), a monoclonal, IgE binding antibody, can be used in patients with moderate to severe persistent asthma, poorly controlled with inhaled steroids and other first-line treatments; administer SC dose q 2-4 weeks; expensive (up to $12,000/year)
  - ◊ Patients should have positive skin test or RAST
  - ◊ Patient IgE should be elevated, but < 700 IU/mL (drug may be ineffective in patients with very high IgE levels)

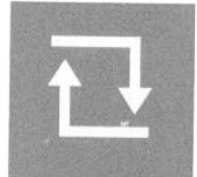

FOLLOWUP

PATIENT MONITORING
- Monitor PEFR at home - record for trend; call if < 70% baseline, ER if < 50% baseline
- pH and arterial blood gases
- Oximetry with status asthmaticus
- Electrolytes - frequent albuterol lowers potassium
- Written and periodically revised action plan is helpful
- Review MDI technique periodically

PREVENTION/AVOIDANCE
- Co-management is essential
  - ◊ Understand medication, inhalers, nebulizers, peak flow meters
  - ◊ Monitor symptoms, possibly peak flows
  - ◊ Pre-arranged action plan for exacerbations
  - ◊ Written guidelines
- Investigate and control triggering factors (pollutants, exercise, house-dust mite, roaches, molds, animal dander) if severe
- Annual influenza immunization
- Avoid aspirin
- Avoid sulfites (food additives)

POSSIBLE COMPLICATIONS
- Respiratory failure; mechanical ventilation
- Atelectasis - most common in right middle lobe
- Flaccid paralysis after exacerbation (self-limited) and rare
- Death
- Air leak syndromes (pneumothorax, etc.)
- SIADH
- Altered theophylline metabolism
- Steroid myopathy
- Inhaled steroid safety has been established

EXPECTED COURSE/PROGNOSIS
- Excellent, with attention to general health and use of medications to control symptoms
- In childhood asthma, < 50% "outgrow it"
- Mortality risk increases with:
  - ◊ Greater than 3 emergency room visits/yr
  - ◊ Nocturnal symptoms
  - ◊ History of ICU admission
  - ◊ Mechanical ventilation
  - ◊ Greater than 2 hospitalizations/yr
  - ◊ Systemic steroid dependence
  - ◊ History of syncope with asthma
  - ◊ History of noncompliance
- Mortality rates are increasing
- If responsive to treatment is poor, review diagnosis and compliance prior to adding more potent therapy

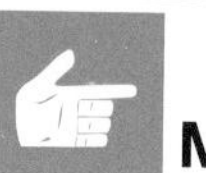

MISCELLANEOUS

ASSOCIATED CONDITIONS
- Reflux esophagitis
- Sinusitis

AGE-RELATED FACTORS
Pediatric: 50% of new cases of asthma occur in children below 10 years
Geriatric: Unusual for initial episode to occur
Others: N/A

PREGNANCY
- About 50% of asthma patients have no changes, 25% seem to improve and 25% have worse symptoms
- Stress prevention
- Avoid medications with contraindications

SYNONYMS
- Bronchial asthma
- Reactive airway disease

ICD-9-CM
493.00 Extrinsic asthma, unspecified
493.10 Intrinsic asthma, unspecified
493.90 Asthma, unspecified

SEE ALSO
Bronchiolitis
Bronchitis, acute
Chronic obstructive pulmonary disease & emphysema
Congestive heart failure
Cystic fibrosis
Epiglottitis
Hypersensitivity pneumonitis
Immunodeficiency diseases
Laryngotracheobronchitis
Tuberculosis

OTHER NOTES Antihistamines are not contraindicated in asthma

ABBREVIATIONS
ABPA = allergic bronchopulmonary aspergillosis
PFT = pulmonary function test
RAD = reactive airway disease
PEFR = peak expiratory flow rate
MDI = metered dose inhaler
NS = normal saline

REFERENCES

- Gwaltney JM JR. Acute bronchitis. In: Mandell Gl, Bennett JE, Dolin R, eds. Principles and Practices of Infectious Disease. 4th ed. New York: Churchill Livingstone; 1995. p606-8
- Seaton A, Seaton D, Leitch AG:.Crofton and Douglas's Respiratory Diseases. Boston, Blackwell Scientific Publications, 1989
- Heuston WJ, Mainous AG III. Acute bronchitis. Am Fam Physician 1998;57(6):1270-6
- Kemper KJ. Chronic asthma: an update. Pediatr Rev 1996;17(4):111-8
- Expert Panel Report. Guidelines for the diagnosis and management of asthma. NHLBI; NIH Publ. No. 97-4051A, 2002

Web references: 10 available at www.5mcc.com
Illustrations N/A

Author(s):
Nancy N. Dambro, MD

BASICS

DESCRIPTION Atelectasis (lung collapse) is a portion of lung which is non-aerated, but otherwise normal. May be an asymptomatic finding on CXR or associated with symptoms. Pulmonary blood flow to area of atelectasis is usually reduced, thereby limiting shunting and hypoxia. Diagnosis and therapy are directed at basic cause.
System(s) affected: Cardiovascular, Pulmonary
Genetics: Depends on basic condition e.g., cystic fibrosis, COPD, asthma, congenital heart disease, congestive heart failure, etc.
Incidence/Prevalence in USA: Common in general anesthesia and in intensive care with high inspired oxygen concentrations
Predominant age: All ages
Predominant sex: Male = Female

SIGNS & SYMPTOMS
- Small atelectasis
  - ◊ Commonly asymptomatic
  - ◊ Produces no change in the overall clinical presentation
- Large atelectasis:
  - ◊ Tachypnea
  - ◊ Cough
  - ◊ Hypoxia which resolves in some cases over 24-48 hours - due to ventilation - perfusion mismatch
  - ◊ Dullness to percussion
  - ◊ Absent breath sounds if airway is occluded
  - ◊ Bronchial breathing if airway is patent
  - ◊ Diminished chest expansion
  - ◊ Tracheal or precordial impulse displacement
  - ◊ Wheezing may be heard with focal obstruction

CAUSES
- Increased alveolar surface tension due to cardiogenic or non-cardiogenic pulmonary edema, primary surfactant deficiency, or infection
- Resorptive atelectasis due to airway obstruction from lumenal blockage (mucus, tumor, foreign body), airway wall abnormality (edema, tumor, bronchomalacia, deformation), or extrinsic airway compression (cardiac, vascular, tumor, adenopathy)
- Compression of the lung (lobar emphysema, cardiomegaly, tumor)
- Increased pleural pressure due to fluid or air in the pleural space (pneumothorax, effusion, empyema, hemothorax, chylothorax)
- Chest wall restriction due to skeletal deformity and/or muscular weakness (scoliosis, neuromuscular disease, phrenic nerve paralysis, anesthesia)

RISK FACTORS
- Varies with condition producing atelectasis
- Atelectasis following anesthesia is increased in smokers, obese individuals, and individuals with short, wide thoraces
- Asthma - right middle lobe most common

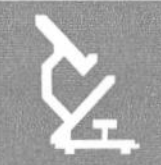

DIAGNOSIS

DIFFERENTIAL DIAGNOSIS
- Atelectasis is not a specific diagnosis, but rather a result of disease or distorted anatomy. The differential is thus found under Causes.
- The roentgenographic differential includes pneumonia, fluid accumulation, lung hypoplasia, or tumor

LABORATORY N/A

Drugs that may alter lab results: N/A

Disorders that may alter lab results: N/A

PATHOLOGICAL FINDINGS
- Pathology varies with cause
- Obstructive atelectasis - non-aerated lung without inflammation or infiltration

SPECIAL TESTS N/A

IMAGING
- CXR
  - ◊ May demonstrate linear, round, or wedge shaped densities
  - ◊ Right middle lobe and lingular atelectasis will obscure the ipsilateral heart border
  - ◊ Lower lobe atelectasis will obscure the diaphragm
  - ◊ Air bronchograms are usually absent in obstructive atelectasis
  - ◊ Evidence of possible airway compression, pleural fluid or air should be sought
  - ◊ Diffuse microatelectasis in surfactant deficiency may lead to a ground-glass appearance with striking air bronchograms
  - ◊ Mediastinal structures and the diaphragm move toward the atelectatic region
  - ◊ Adjacent lung may show compensatory hyperinflation

DIAGNOSTIC PROCEDURES
- Bronchoscopy to assess airway patency. (Bronchoscopy as therapy is controversial with the exception of foreign body or other structural causes).
- Echocardiography to assess cardiac status in cardiomegaly
- Chest CT or MRI to visualize airway and mediastinal structures
- Barium swallow to assess mediastinal vascular compression
- Other procedures vary with potential cause

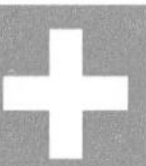

TREATMENT

APPROPRIATE HEALTH CARE Varies with severity

GENERAL MEASURES
- Varies with severity and cause of atelectasis
- Maximize patient mobility
- Ensure adequate oxygenation and humidification
- Chest physiotherapy with percussion and postural drainage. Consider adding treatments using new airway clearance techniques such as Positive Expiratory Pressure (PEP) mask.
- Incentive spirometry
- Positive pressure ventilation or continuous positive airway pressure in subjects with neuromuscular weakness. In-exsufflator may also be helpful here.

SURGICAL MEASURES N/A

ACTIVITY Encourage activity, mobilization as tolerated

DIET No special diet

PATIENT EDUCATION Encourage activity as appropriate. Instruct in basic cause and its therapy.

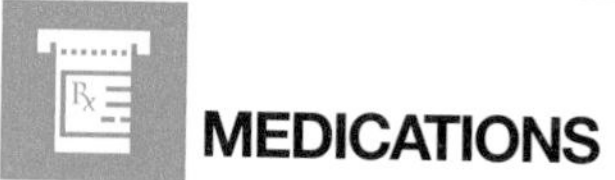

MEDICATIONS

DRUG(S) OF CHOICE

- Bronchodilator therapy (beta-agonist aerosol); efficacy controversial
- Other therapies directed at basic cause - antibiotics, foreign body removal, tumor therapy, cardiac medication, steroids in asthma

Contraindications: Refer to manufacturer's literature
Precautions: Refer to manufacturer's literature
Significant possible interactions: Refer to manufacturer's literature

ALTERNATIVE DRUGS N/A

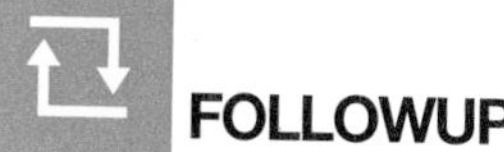

FOLLOWUP

PATIENT MONITORING

- Varies with cause and patient status
- In simple atelectasis associated with asthma or infection, monthly visits are adequate

PREVENTION/AVOIDANCE

- Avoidance of 100% inspired oxygen (which can rapidly absorb causing atelectasis)
- Foreign body/aspiration precautions
- Postoperative mobilization and/or rotation
- Institute therapies such as chest physiotherapy and incentive spirometry as preventive maneuvers in at-risk patients

POSSIBLE COMPLICATIONS

- Infection with chronic lung damage is an unlikely, but unfortunate complication
- Atelectasis is rarely life-threatening and usually spontaneously resolves

EXPECTED COURSE/PROGNOSIS

- Resolution with medical therapy
- Surgical therapy needed only for certain causes, or if chronic infection and bronchiectasis supervene

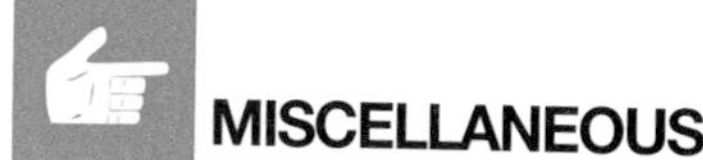

MISCELLANEOUS

ASSOCIATED CONDITIONS N/A

AGE-RELATED FACTORS Very young and very old patients with limited mobility at greater risk

Pediatric: Congenital airway obstruction due to mediastinal cysts, tumor, or vascular rings; foreign body aspiration
Geriatric: Primary and secondary lung tumors sometimes associated
Others: Asthma

PREGNANCY Management is similar to non-pregnant and varies with cause

SYNONYMS Lung collapse

ICD-9-CM

518.0 Pulmonary collapse

SEE ALSO

Asthma
Pneumonia, bacterial
Pneumonia, mycoplasma
Pneumonia, viral

OTHER NOTES

- Round atelectasis:
  - ◊ A pleural based round density on CXR with a comet tail of vessel and airway
  - ◊ More common in patients with asbestos exposure
  - ◊ May mimic tumor, but can usually be definitively diagnosed with imaging studies thereby avoiding surgery

ABBREVIATIONS N/A

REFERENCES

- Hazinski TH. Atelectasis. In: Chernick V, ed. Kendig's Disorders of the Respiratory Tract in Children. 5th Ed. Philadelphia: W.B. Saunders Co.; 1990
- Marini JJ, Pierson DJ, Hudson LD. Acute lobar atelectasis: a prospective comparison of fiberoptic bronchoscopy and respiratory therapy. Am Rev Respir Dis 1971;119:971
- Rickstenste, Sventrik, et al: Effects of periodic positive airway pressure by mask on postoperative pulmonary function. Chest 1986;6:774-81
- Crystal RG, West JB, Barnes PJ, Weibel ER, eds. The Lung. Philadelphia: Lippincott Williams & Wilkins; 1997

Web references: 0 available at www.5mcc.com
Illustrations N/A

Author(s):
Nancy N. Dambro, MD

BASICS

DESCRIPTION The common form of arteriosclerosis in which deposits of yellowish plaques (atheromas) containing cholesterol, lipoid material, and lipophages are formed within the intima and inner media of large and medium sized arteries.
System(s) affected: Cardiovascular
Genetics: Probable genetic link; many risk factors for atherosclerosis (lipid metabolism, hypertension, and diabetes) are clearly inheritable
Incidence/Prevalence in USA:
- Common, but declining steadily. The effects upon the brain, heart, kidneys, extremities and other vital organs form the leading cause of morbidity and mortality in the USA and most Western countries.
- Complications of atherosclerosis account for 1/2 of all deaths, and 1/3 of deaths in persons between ages 35-65

Predominant age: 35 and older
Predominant sex: Male > Female

SIGNS & SYMPTOMS
- Characteristically silent until atheromas produce:
  - ◊ Stenosis
  - ◊ Thrombosis
  - ◊ Aneurysm
  - ◊ Embolus
- For lists of possible symptoms see the following titles elsewhere in this book:
  - ◊ Essential hypertension
  - ◊ Coronary arteriosclerosis
  - ◊ Congestive heart failure
  - ◊ Cerebrovascular accident
  - ◊ Atrial arrhythmias
  - ◊ Ventricular arrhythmias
  - ◊ Renal failure, chronic
  - ◊ Dissecting aneurysm
  - ◊ Thrombosis and embolism, arterial

CAUSES
- Biochemical, physiologic, environmental factors that lead to thickening and occlusion of the lumen of arteries
- Aging (some degree of atherosclerosis is universal)
- One or more of the risk factors listed below

RISK FACTORS
- Modifiable
  - ◊ Hypertension
  - ◊ Tobacco smoking
  - ◊ Diabetes mellitus
  - ◊ Obesity
  - ◊ Physical inactivity
  - ◊ Decreased high-density lipoprotein (HDL) cholesterol
  - ◊ Increased low-density lipoprotein (LDL) cholesterol
- Non-modifiable
  - ◊ Male gender
  - ◊ Increasing age
  - ◊ Family history of premature atherosclerosis

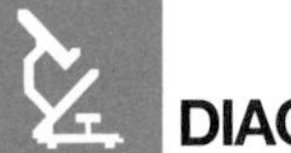

DIAGNOSIS

DIFFERENTIAL DIAGNOSIS N/A

LABORATORY Associated with elevated serum cholesterol; elevated LDL and low HDL

Drugs that may alter lab results: N/A

Disorders that may alter lab results: N/A

PATHOLOGICAL FINDINGS
- Early changes (simple) potentially reversible
  - ◊ Accumulation of lipid-laden cells in the intimal layer of the artery (usually monocytes/macrophages from circulating blood)
  - ◊ Lipid streaks in aortas and coronary arteries
- Late changes (complicated) usually reversible
  - ◊ Atheromatous plaques with necrosis, fibrosis, calcification
  - ◊ Weakening of elastic lamellae
  - ◊ Neovascularization
  - ◊ Arterial obstruction
  - ◊ Thrombosis
- Oxidized LDL induces vascular smooth muscle cell apoptosis and cell death
- Alteration of endothelial function involving mostly nitrous oxide pathways promotes platelet adhesion and aggregation, local clotting, vascular growth and alters vascular tone
- Decrease in elastin with aging along with collagen degeneration and increased intima-media thickness of arterial wall

SPECIAL TESTS N/A

IMAGING Extensively calcified atherosclerotic plaques may be identified in major blood vessels on x-ray

DIAGNOSTIC PROCEDURES
- X-ray (often incidental finding)
- Associated with hypercholesterolemia; elevated LDL and low HDL
- Arterial doppler studies (carotid, renal)
- Angiography
- Ankle-brachial index (ABI)

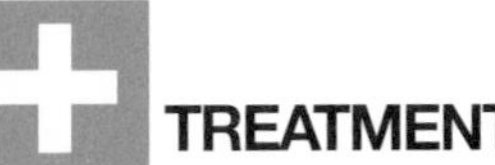

TREATMENT

APPROPRIATE HEALTH CARE Outpatient until complications occur; emphasis on prevention

GENERAL MEASURES
- For details see the following titles:
  - ◊ Essential hypertension
  - ◊ Congestive heart failure
  - ◊ Cerebrovascular accident
  - ◊ Renal failure, chronic
  - ◊ Dissecting aneurysm
  - ◊ Thrombosis & embolism, arterial
  - ◊ Diabetes
  - ◊ Hyperlipidemia

SURGICAL MEASURES N/A

ACTIVITY Encourage physical fitness

DIET
Recommended daily intake
- Initial diet; Step 1
  - ◊ Total fat - < 30% of total calories; saturated fat < 10%
  - ◊ Carbohydrates - 50-60% of total calories
  - ◊ Protein - 10-20% of total calories
  - ◊ Cholesterol - < 300 mg a day
  - ◊ Total calories - amount required to achieve and maintain desirable weight
  - ◊ Sodium - 1650-2400 mg
  - ◊ Alcohol - < 30 g
- Initial diet; Step 2
  - ◊ Total fat - < 30% of total calories; saturated fat < 7%
  - ◊ Carbohydrates - 50-60% of total calories
  - ◊ Protein - 10-20% of total calories
  - ◊ Cholesterol - < 200 mg a day
  - ◊ Total calories - amount required to achieve and maintain desirable weight
  - ◊ Sodium - 1650-2400 mg
  - ◊ Alcohol - < 30 g
  - ◊ Anti-oxidants (vitamin A, E, C)
  - ◊ HMG-CoA inhibitors (statins)

PATIENT EDUCATION
- Crucial parts of preventing and treating atheroscleroses involve nutrition, fitness, and smoking cessation
- Extensive educational materials available from many agencies (e.g., American Heart Association, U.S. Government Printing Office, National Cholesterol Education Program). Use these to help teach patients how to avoid or eliminate risk factors.

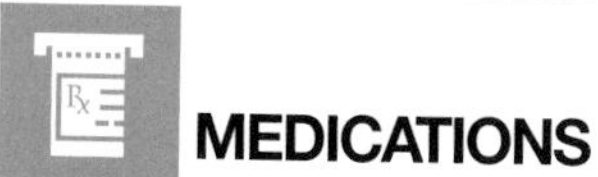

MEDICATIONS

DRUG(S) OF CHOICE
- For details see the following titles:
  - ◊ Essential hypertension
  - ◊ Coronary arteriosclerosis
  - ◊ Congestive heart failure
  - ◊ Stroke
  - ◊ Atrial arrhythmias
  - ◊ Ventricular arrhythmias
  - ◊ Renal failure, chronic
  - ◊ Dissecting aneurysm
  - ◊ Thrombosis and embolism, arterial
  - ◊ Angina
  - ◊ Myocardial infarction
  - ◊ Arteriosclerotic heart disease
  - ◊ Atherosclerotic occlusive disease

Contraindications: Refer to manufacturer's literature
Precautions: Refer to manufacturer's literature
Significant possible interactions: Refer to manufacturer's literature

ALTERNATIVE DRUGS
See specific titles

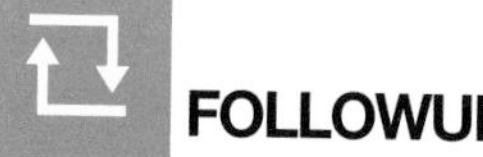

FOLLOWUP

PATIENT MONITORING
See specific titles

PREVENTION/AVOIDANCE
- Treat or control modifiable risk factors
- Hormone replacement therapy in postmenopausal women

POSSIBLE COMPLICATIONS
- Coronary artery disease
- Renal failure
- Cerebrovascular accidents
- Dissecting or ruptured aneurysms
- Congestive heart failure
- Arterial thrombosis
- Gangrene
- Cardiac arrhythmias
- Sudden death

EXPECTED COURSE/PROGNOSIS
Avoiding risk factors has greatly decreased mortality rates in the past decade

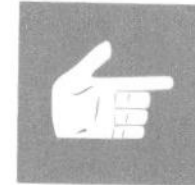

MISCELLANEOUS

ASSOCIATED CONDITIONS
- Essential hypertension
- Coronary arteriosclerosis
- Congestive heart failure
- Cerebrovascular accident
- Atrial arrhythmias
- Ventricular arrhythmias
- Renal failure, chronic
- Aortic dissection
- Thrombosis and embolism, arterial
- Atherosclerotic occlusive disease

AGE-RELATED FACTORS
Pediatric: Fatty streaks and deposits in the intima of the aortas of all children begin as early as age 3 years
Geriatric: Atherosclerosis happens to all who live long enough. Its effects and complications can be minimized and/or delayed by avoiding all risk factors possible.
Others: N/A

PREGNANCY
N/A

SYNONYMS
N/A

ICD-9-CM
414.00 Coronary atherosclerosis of unspecified type of vessel, native or graft

SEE ALSO
Aortic dissection
Arterial embolus & thrombosis
Atherosclerotic occlusive disease
Congestive heart failure
Hypertension, essential
Renal failure, chronic
Stroke (Brain attack)

OTHER NOTES
N/A

ABBREVIATIONS
N/A

REFERENCES

- Hurst JW, et al: The Heart. 8th Ed. New York, McGraw-Hill, 1994
- Hunninghake D, ed: Lipid disorders. Medical Clinics of North America. Vol. 78, No. 1, Jan., 1994
- Guidelines for cardiopulmonary resuscitation and emergency cardiac care. JAMA 1992;268(16)28
- Fauci AS, ed: Harrison's Principles of Internal medicine. 14th ed. New York, McGraw-Hill, 1998

Web references: 2 available at www.5mcc.com
Illustrations 4 available

Author(s):
Chandramohan Batra, MD

BASICS

DESCRIPTION A peripheral arterial disease can be acute or chronic. There is obstruction or narrowing of the lumen of the aorta and its major branches causing interruption of blood flow, usually to feet and legs. Involved arteries may include mesenteric and celiac arteries. Occlusions cause ischemia, discomfort, skin ulceration and gangrene.
System(s) affected: Cardiovascular
Genetics: Family history of early complications of atherosclerosis
Incidence/Prevalence in USA: Increases with age (parallels atherosclerosis)
Predominant age: Older adults
Predominant sex: Male > Female (2:1)

SIGNS & SYMPTOMS
- Intermittent claudication - exercise induced pain that is relieved by rest is pathognomonic
- Site of occlusion determines site of pain
- Occlusion of abdominal aorta and/or iliac vessels produce claudication in the back, buttocks and hips
- Femoral obstruction causes pain in the calf
- The degree of occlusion determines the exercise tolerance and if severe enough produces pain at rest
- Pulses are diminished or absent
- The limb is cold and pale and typically develops dependent rubor
- Atrophic skin changes often result in shiny hairless skin

CAUSES
- Almost always a complication of atherosclerosis
- Mechanism of occlusion - embolus, thrombosis, fracture, or trauma

RISK FACTORS
- Smoking
- Hyperlipidemia
- Diabetes
- Hypertension
- Physical stress

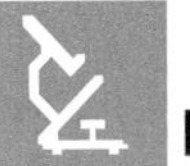

DIAGNOSIS

DIFFERENTIAL DIAGNOSIS
- Thromboangiitis obliterans (inflammatory disease primarily affecting young male smokers)
- Fibromuscular dysplasia of the peripheral vessels (rare)

LABORATORY N/A

Drugs that may alter lab results: N/A

Disorders that may alter lab results: N/A

PATHOLOGICAL FINDINGS
- Occluding mass in lumen of thrombosed artery
- Calcareous deposits in occluded vessel in medial coat with atheromas

SPECIAL TESTS Doppler ultrasound to compare systolic pressure in upper and lower limbs (ankle: brachial ratio should be higher than 0.95 at rest)

IMAGING Angiography for an individual who may be a candidate for surgery

DIAGNOSTIC PROCEDURES History and physical

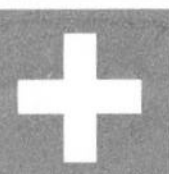

TREATMENT

APPROPRIATE HEALTH CARE Outpatient for conservative management. Inpatient for surgery or more severe cases.

GENERAL MEASURES
- Smoking cessation
- Foot and limb care
- Graduated exercise program
- Weight control
- Pain management
- Cholesterol management
- Appropriate treatment of coexisting disease, i.e., diabetes
- Infection control
- Lifestyle modification

SURGICAL MEASURES
- Indications for surgery are ischemic pain at rest, or changes likely to lead to amputation, or intolerable symptoms
- The procedure depends upon site of lesion. Includes endarterectomy, bypass procedures, transluminal angioplasty, and amputation.
- Patients with aorto-iliac disease tend to have good surgical results to a disabling disorder
- Surgery should not be performed for femoral popliteal disease unless symptoms are very severe or disabling
- Bypass surgery for vessels distal to popliteal artery has little success
- Patch grafting
- Atherectomy
- Laser angioplasty
- Stents (wire plastic mesh to stretch and mold to the arterial wall to prevent re-occlusion)
- Amputation with failure of arterial reconstructive surgery or with development of gangrene, persistent infection, or intractable pain

ACTIVITY To the degree that symptoms permit

DIET
- Good diet control
- Lose weight, if overweight

PATIENT EDUCATION
- Educate patient regarding symptoms or signs that require early assessment by physician
- Teach careful foot care
- Avoid elevating or applying heat to affected parts
- Urge early ambulation after surgery
- Assist patient with a stop smoking program

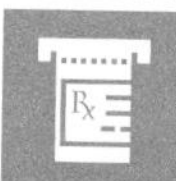

MEDICATIONS

DRUG(S) OF CHOICE
- Vasodilator drugs are ineffective
- Aspirin to decrease platelet aggregation
- Newer antiplatelet agents such as clopidogrel look promising

Contraindications: In patients sensitive to xanthines
Precautions: Most adverse effects are gastrointestinal. Dizziness and headache are also common.
Significant possible interactions: Use cautiously in patients on oral coagulants. Monitor closely for bleeding complications.

ALTERNATIVE DRUGS
Anticoagulants

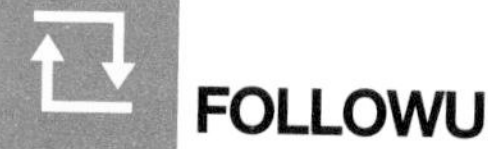

FOLLOWUP

PATIENT MONITORING
- For acute phase with surgery, closely follow all aspects of postoperative recovery
- For mild chronic cases, follow patient at regular intervals, frequency dependent upon severity of symptoms
- Management/modification of risk factors

PREVENTION/AVOIDANCE
- Periodic health maintenance measures
- Healthy lifestyle including appropriate diet and adequate exercise
- Avoidance of smoking

POSSIBLE COMPLICATIONS
- Necrosis
- Gangrene
- Limb amputation

EXPECTED COURSE/PROGNOSIS
Course varies from slow progression with easily controlled symptoms to rapid deterioration with severe symptoms requiring surgical intervention

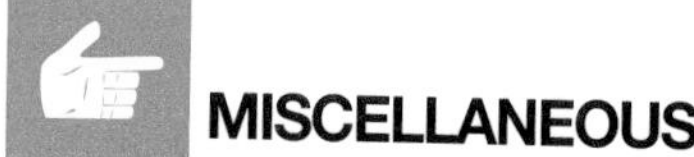

MISCELLANEOUS

ASSOCIATED CONDITIONS
- Atherosclerosis
- Arteriosclerosis obliterans
- Fibromuscular dysplasia
- Thromboangiitis obliterans
- Takayasu arteritis
- Abdominal aortic coarctation
- Radiation injury
- Popliteal artery entrapment syndrome
- Popliteal cystic degeneration
- Arteritis

AGE-RELATED FACTORS
Pediatric: N/A
Geriatric: N/A
Others: N/A

PREGNANCY
N/A

SYNONYMS
- Peripheral arterial disease
- Occlusive arterial disease

ICD-9-CM
444.22 Arterial embolism and thrombosis of arteries of lower extremity
444.21 Arterial embolism and thrombosis of arteries of upper extremity

SEE ALSO
Arteriosclerosis obliterans
Atherosclerosis

OTHER NOTES
N/A

ABBREVIATIONS
N/A

REFERENCES
- Marcus ML. The Coronary Circulation in Health and Disease. New York, McGraw-Hill, 1983
- Hurst JW, et al. The Heart. 8th Ed. New York, McGraw-Hill, 1994
- Braunwald E, ed. Heart Disease: A Textbook of Cardiovascular Medicine. 5th Ed. Philadelphia, W.B. Saunders Co., 1996

Web references: 1 available at www.5mcc.com
Illustrations N/A

Author(s):
Stanley G. Smith, MA, MB

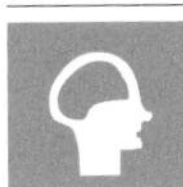

BASICS

DESCRIPTION Atrial fibrillation (AF) is a chronic or paroxysmal arrhythmia characterized by chaotic atrial electrical activity. The electrophysiologic mechanism is most likely multiple reentrant wavelets within the atria. In some patients, triggering premature atrial beats and/or bursts of tachycardia emanate from the pulmonary venous ostia or other sites. Because the AV node is bombarded with nearly continuous atrial electrical impulses, the ventricular response is irregular and usually rapid (up to or exceeding 160 beats per minute). Symptoms vary from none to mild (palpitations, lightheadedness, fatigue, poor exercise capacity) to severe (angina, dyspnea, syncope), and are frequently more serious in patients with significant structural heart disease. In some patients with Wolff-Parkinson-White syndrome, AF may be extremely rapid and degenerate into ventricular fibrillation.
System(s) affected: Cardiovascular, Nervous
Genetics: No specific genetic pattern in most patients
Incidence/Prevalence in USA: Estimated at 1 per 1000 adults per year; estimated at 2-4% of adult population
Predominant age:
Prevalence increases with age:

Age	AF cases/1000
25-35	2-3
55-64	30-40
62-90	50-90

Predominant sex: Male > Female

SIGNS & SYMPTOMS
- Irregular pulse
- Tachycardia
- Heart failure
- Hypotension
- Palpitations
- Lightheadedness
- Poor exercise capacity
- Fatigue
- Dyspnea
- Angina
- Near syncope/syncope
- Stroke
- Arterial embolization

CAUSES
- Hypertensive heart disease
- Valvular/rheumatic heart disease
- Coronary artery disease
- Acute myocardial infarction
- Pulmonary embolus
- Cardiomyopathy
- Congestive heart failure
- Infiltrative heart disease
- Pericarditis
- Intoxication/ingestion (e.g., ethanol in "Holiday Heart")
- Hyperthyroidism
- Postoperative state (especially cardiothoracic surgery)
- Sick sinus syndrome (tachycardia-bradycardia syndrome)
- Idiopathic (including "lone" atrial fibrillation)

RISK FACTORS
- Hypertension
- Diabetes mellitus
- Left ventricular hypertrophy
- Coronary artery disease
- Congestive heart failure
- Rheumatic heart disease

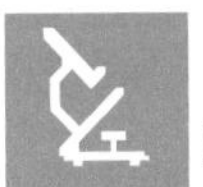

DIAGNOSIS

DIFFERENTIAL DIAGNOSIS
- Multifocal atrial tachycardia (MAT)
- Sinus tachycardia with frequent atrial premature beats
- Atrial flutter (see below)

LABORATORY
- ECG is diagnostic; low amplitude fibrillatory waves without discrete P waves; irregularly irregular pattern of QRS complexes
- Holter monitor and event monitor helpful in diagnosing paroxysmal atrial fibrillation (PAF)
- Echocardiogram to assess for structural heart disease
- Thyroid function tests

Drugs that may alter lab results: N/A

Disorders that may alter lab results: N/A

PATHOLOGICAL FINDINGS
- Atrial dilatation
- Atrial injury (chronic or acute)
- Atrial thrombus, especially in atrial appendage
- Sclerosis/fibrosis of SA node
- Coronary artery disease, valvular/rheumatic disease, cardiomyopathy, pulmonary embolus, etc.

SPECIAL TESTS
- Ventilation-perfusion scan or pulmonary angiography if pulmonary embolus suspected
- Transesophageal echocardiography may be useful in detecting left atrial appendage thrombus and therefore risk of stroke with cardioversion

IMAGING
- Chest x-ray to screen for cardiopulmonary abnormalities
- Echocardiogram to assess for structural heart disease

DIAGNOSTIC PROCEDURES As above

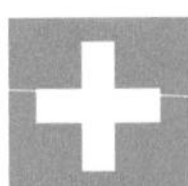

TREATMENT

APPROPRIATE HEALTH CARE
- Inpatient if significant symptoms, extremely rapid ventricular rate, initiating antiarrhythmic therapy, if AF triggered by acute process (acute myocardial infarction, congestive heart failure, pulmonary embolus, etc.), or high risk for stroke (rheumatic heart disease, prior TIA/stroke, etc.)
- Outpatient management appropriate for many patients

GENERAL MEASURES
- Avoidance of potential triggers
  - ◊ Avoid ethanol, caffeine, nicotine
  - ◊ Management of underlying structural heart disease
- Prevention of complications
  - ◊ Anticoagulation to reduce the risk of embolic complications
  - ◊ Antibiotic prophylaxis if AF is due to valvular heart disease
- Therapy strategies
  - ◊ Ventricular rate control with AV nodal blocking agents
  - ◊ Restore and maintain sinus rhythm with antiarrhythmic drugs
  - ◊ Nonpharmacologic therapies

SURGICAL MEASURES
Nonpharmacological therapies
- Cardiac surgery (e.g., the "maze procedure") may be considered in severely symptomatic, medically refractory patients
- Permanent dual chamber pacing may reduce incidence of AF in patients with sick sinus syndrome
- Radiofrequency catheter ablation of AV node with permanent pacemaker implantation is a reasonable alternative in symptomatic medically refractory patients
- Radiofrequency catheter ablation procedures to prevent AF recurrence are becoming more effective
- Implantable atrial defibrillators to detect and cardiovert paroxysms of AF may be considered in highly selected patients

ACTIVITY
- As tolerated
- With medical management, minimal functional impairment in many patients

DIET As appropriate for underlying heart disease and other comorbidities

PATIENT EDUCATION
Printed material available from:
- Du Pont Pharmaceuticals, Wilmington, DE 19880-0026, (800)341-4004
- Krames Communications, 11100 Grundy Lane, San Bruno, CA 94066-9821; tel 800-333-3022
- Health Trend Publishing, PO Box 7390, Menlo Park, CA 94026; 800-747-1606

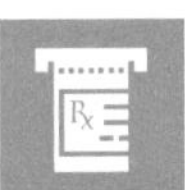

MEDICATIONS

DRUG(S) OF CHOICE
Note: Clinical risk factors for stroke include age > 65, diabetes, hypertension, history of prior stroke or transient ischemic attack (TIA), and prior history of congestive heart failure. Echocardiographic risk factors for stroke include left atrial enlargement, mitral regurgitation, and left ventricular dysfunction.
- Anticoagulation:
  - ◊ Unless contraindications to anticoagulants exist, patients with AF with any of these risk factors should receive warfarin to

maintain an international normalized ratio (INR) of 2.0-3.0

  - ◊ Patients in whom warfarin is contraindicated should receive aspirin 325 mg/day. Aspirin 325 mg/day, is appropriate in low risk patients (e.g., age < 65 years with no risk factors for stroke). Data are fewer with paroxysmal AF, though treatment guidelines are the same for chronic AF.
- Routine use of antiarrhythmic drugs in attempts to maintain sinus rhythm was not beneficial in the AFFIRM trial. Antiarrhythmic drugs may be used when a specific indication for sinus rhythm maintenance (eg, symptoms, hemodynamic embarrasment, etc.) exists.
- Control of ventricular rate
  - ◊ Beta-blockers (propranolol, metoprolol, atenolol, nadolol, etc.)
  - ◊ Non-dihydropyridine calcium channel blockers (diltiazem and verapamil). For example, diltiazem 10 mg IV push, followed by 10 mg/hr IV to control rate to approximately 100.
  - ◊ Cardiac glycosides (digoxin). May be less effective than other agents in controlling ventricular response, particularly in active patients.
- Conversion to/maintenance of sinus rhythm:
  - ◊ Direct current (DC) cardioversion
  - ◊ Antiarrhythmic therapy for chemical cardioversion and maintenance of sinus rhythm following cardioversion carries a risk of pro-arrhythmia
  - ◊ Ibutilide, an intravenous type III agent, has been approved for chemical cardioversion of atrial fibrillation and flutter of short duration (less than 90 days)
  - ◊ If the duration of AF is more than 24-48 hours or is unknown, patients should be treated with warfarin for at least 3 weeks before and 4 weeks after cardioversion. Alternatively, once therapeutic anticoagulation is established, transesophageal echocardiography may be performed. If there is no evidence of atrial thrombus, cardioversion may then be performed. Anticoagulation should be continued for at least 4 weeks following cardioversion. Long-term, and perhaps indefinite, anticoagulation should be considered.
  - ◊ Chronic oral antiarrhythmic therapy to suppress AF recurrences
    - Type IA (procainamide, disopyramide, quinidine)
    - Type IC (flecainide, propafenone) in patients with structurally normal hearts or mild hypertensive heart disease
    - Type III (sotalol, amiodarone, dofetilide)
- Acute therapy for hemodynamically compromised patients:
  - ◊ Heparin for anticoagulation
  - ◊ IV beta or calcium channel blocker for control of ventricular rate
  - ◊ Pharmacologic and/or DC cardioversion

Contraindications:

- Active bleeding precludes anticoagulation; risk of bleeding is a relative contraindication to long-term anticoagulation
- Warfarin is contraindicated in patients with prior history of warfarin skin necrosis
- Type IC drugs are contraindicated in patients with coronary artery disease and cardiomyopathy
- Type IA drugs, sotalol, ibutilide and dofetilide should not be used in patients with torsade de pointes history

Precautions:

- With type IA drugs, ibutilide, dofetilide and sotalol, the risk of torsade de pointes increases with the extent of QT interval prolongation (i.e., the QTc). Avoid other drugs that prolong the QT interval (phenothiazines, tricyclic antidepressants, terfenadine, astemizole, erythromycin, etc.). Avoid hypokalemia and hypomagnesemia. Torsade de pointes due to drug induced long QT syndrome is said to be "pause dependent" as the risk increases with bradycardia, heart block, and sinus pauses.
- With type IC drugs, stress testing is helpful to exclude exercise induced pro-arrhythmia or QRS widening
- With amiodarone, careful surveillance for hepatic, thyroid, pulmonary, skin and ophthalmologic adverse effects is necessary
- In many patients, adequate medical therapy of AF will cause bradycardia necessitating a permanent pacemaker.

Significant possible interactions:

- Quinidine increases digoxin levels
- Amiodarone increases digoxin levels and enhances effects of warfarin

ALTERNATIVE DRUGS N/A

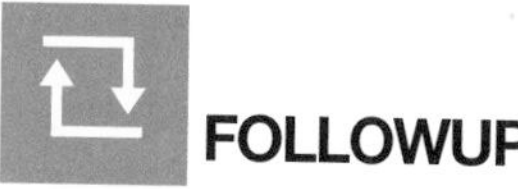

FOLLOWUP

PATIENT MONITORING

- ECG/Holter monitor to assess maintenance of sinus rhythm, control of ventricular rate during AF
- Frequent blood tests to maintain INR at 2.0-3.0
- ECG to monitor QTc interval in patients on antiarrhythmic therapy
- Careful followup of antiarrhythmic drug therapy is mandatory.

PREVENTION/AVOIDANCE

- Ethanol may trigger AF in some patients
- In cardiomyopathy/heart failure, hemodynamic decompensation may trigger AF

POSSIBLE COMPLICATIONS

- Embolic stroke
- Peripheral arterial embolization
- Significant complications of pharmacologic therapy (bradyarrhythmias and torsade de pointes)
- Bleeding with anticoagulation

EXPECTED COURSE/PROGNOSIS

- Stroke risk low with long-term anticoagulation
- AF increases the risk of cardiovascular morbidity and mortality, but long-term prognosis may be a function of underlying structural heart disease

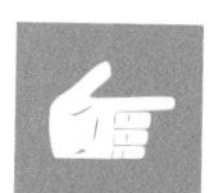

MISCELLANEOUS

ASSOCIATED CONDITIONS

- Wolff-Parkinson-White syndrome
- Sick sinus syndrome
- Atrial flutter:
  - ◊ A related arrhythmia with regular atrial electrical activity, typically at a rate of 250-350, manifested as sawtooth "flutter" waves on the ECG. 2:1 or 4:1 conduction through the AV node to the ventricle is usual, so the pulse is frequently regular.
  - ◊ Many patients have both AF and atrial flutter
  - ◊ Management for these closely related arrhythmias is similar, though atrial flutter is more difficult to control pharmacologically but more easily electrically cardioverted than AF
  - ◊ Although atrial flutter alone may pose a lower a risk of thromboembolism than AF, guidelines for anticoagulation of atrial flutter and AF are the same
  - ◊ Radiofrequency catheter ablation to cure atrial flutter is becoming more widely applied

AGE-RELATED FACTORS

Pediatric: Though extremely uncommon in children with structurally normal hearts, AF may be seen in the setting of congenital heart disease and following surgical repair

Geriatric: Both the incidence of AF and the risk of stroke increase with age

Others: Risk of stroke is extremely low in young patients without structural heart disease, so called "lone atrial fibrillation."

PREGNANCY

- AF is unusual during pregnancy in the absence of structural heart disease (e.g., rheumatic mitral stenosis)
- Digoxin is safe during pregnancy; beta-blockers, procainamide, and quinidine are probably safe. There is limited information regarding calcium blockers.
- Risk of fetal hemorrhage makes anticoagulation problematic; moreover, warfarin causes fetal anomalies. SC heparin is probably the best choice if long-term anticoagulation is necessary.
- DC cardioversion does not seem to adversely affect the fetus

SYNONYMS

- AF
- A Fib

ICD-9-CM

427.31 Atrial fibrillation
427.32 Atrial flutter

SEE ALSO

Atrial flutter
Wolff-Parkinson-White syndrome

OTHER NOTES N/A

ABBREVIATIONS

- AF = atrial fibrillation
- CAF = chronic atrial fibrillation
- PAF = paroxysmal atrial fibrillation
- PT = prothrombin time
- INR = international normalized ratio

REFERENCES

- Prystowsky EN, Benson DW, Fuster V, et al. Management of patients with atrial fibrillation. Circulation 1996;93:1262-77
- Riley RD, Pritchell ELC. Pharmacologic management of atrial fibrillation. J Cardiovasc Electrophys 1997;8:818-29
- Falk RH. Atrial Fibrillation. New Engl J Med 2001;344:1067-78
- ACC/AHA/ESC. Guidelines on the management of patients with atrial fibrillation. J Am Coll Cardiol 2001;38:1231-65

Web references: 5 available at www.5mcc.com
Illustrations 1 available

Author(s):
Leonard Ganz, MD
Leonard S. Lilly, MD

Atrial septal defect (ASD)

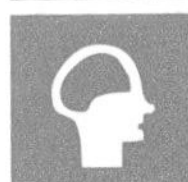

BASICS

DESCRIPTION A defect or opening in the atrial septum allowing flow of blood between the two chambers. Shunting is typically left to right and occurs late in ventricular systole and early diastole. The degree of shunting depends on 1) the size of the defect, and 2) the relative compliance of the two ventricles. There can be minimal right to left shunting in early ventricular systole, especially during inspiration. Symptoms typically occur due to right ventricular and pulmonary vascular volume overload sometimes with resultant pulmonary hypertension.

Types:

- Ostium secundum - occurs in the region of the fossa ovalis (most common)
- Sinus venosus - occurs in the superior-posterior septum
- Ostium primum - occurs in the inferior portion of the septum (often involves mitral valve)

System(s) affected: Cardiovascular, Pulmonary
Genetics: Congenital, associated with multiple syndromes. rarely familial.
Incidence/Prevalence in USA: Accounts for 10% of congenital heart defects
Predominant age: Newborn, but may be diagnosed at any age
Predominant sex: Female > Male (2:1)

SIGNS & SYMPTOMS

- Childhood symptoms - usually minimal. Can include failure to thrive and frequent pulmonary infections
- Adult symptoms - easy fatigability, dyspnea on exertion, heart failure (late)
- Signs vary according to extent of shunting and include:
  - ◊ Prominent precordial bulge
  - ◊ Right ventricular lift
  - ◊ Palpable pulmonary artery pulse
  - ◊ Fixed, widely-split S2
  - ◊ Pulmonic flow murmur
  - ◊ Low pitched diastolic murmur at left lower sternal border
  - ◊ Cyanosis and clubbing (with severe pulmonary hypertension - Eisenmenger syndrome)
  - ◊ Stroke due to paradoxical emboli

CAUSES Unknown

RISK FACTORS Congenital heart disease family history

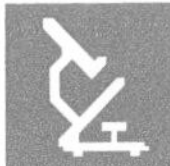

DIAGNOSIS

DIFFERENTIAL DIAGNOSIS Other congenital heart disease, right bundle branch block (for widely split S2)

LABORATORY N/A

Drugs that may alter lab results: N/A

Disorders that may alter lab results: N/A

PATHOLOGICAL FINDINGS

- Gross defect in atrial septum
- Dilated right atrium, right ventricle
- Enlarged pulmonary artery

SPECIAL TESTS

- ECG findings:
  - ◊ Ostium secundum - rightward axis, right ventricular hypertrophy, rSR' pattern in V
  - ◊ Sinus venosus - leftward axis, inverted P wave in lead III
  - ◊ Ostium primum - leftward axis

Note: All may be associated with PR prolongation

IMAGING

- X-ray - varying degrees of cardiac enlargement, increased pulmonary vascular workings
- Cardiac MRI
- Cardiac catheterization (indicated in select patients) demonstrates right ventricle enlargement and location of the shunt
- Echocardiography

DIAGNOSTIC PROCEDURES

- Cardiac MRI
- Cardiac angiography
- Echo and Doppler
- Transesophageal echo in adults

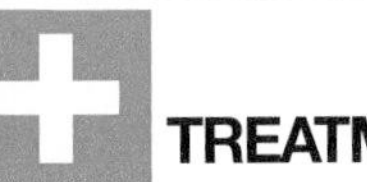

TREATMENT

APPROPRIATE HEALTH CARE Referral/evaluation by a cardiologist

GENERAL MEASURES N/A

SURGICAL MEASURES

- Surgical repair (particularly when the pulmonary systemic flow ratio is ≥ 1.5:1)
- Surgical repair delayed until preschool age (2-4) except for large defects to be repaired earlier
- Small ASD - primary closure with umbrella-like patch via cardiac catheter is experimental
- Surgery if paradoxical emboli result in stroke

ACTIVITY As tolerated

DIET No special diet

PATIENT EDUCATION For patient education materials on this topic, contact: American Heart Association, 7320 Greenville Avenue, Dallas, TX 75231, (214)373-6300

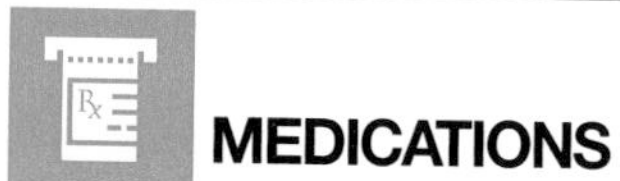

MEDICATIONS

DRUG(S) OF CHOICE
- Antibiotic prophylaxis (not for secundum ASD)
- Anticoagulation if paradoxical emboli

Contraindications: N/A
Precautions: N/A
Significant possible interactions: N/A

ALTERNATIVE DRUGS N/A

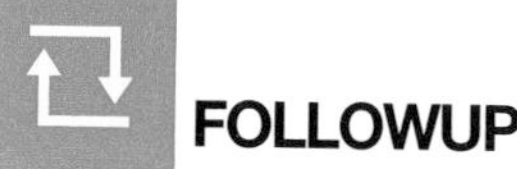

FOLLOWUP

PATIENT MONITORING
- Until defect has closed
- Routine echocardiography followup

PREVENTION/AVOIDANCE
- Evaluation prior to pregnancy

POSSIBLE COMPLICATIONS
- Congestive heart failure
- Cyanosis
- Late-onset arrhythmias 10-20 years after surgery (5%)
- Stroke
- Pulmonary hypertension
- Eisenmenger syndrome
- Infective endocarditis

EXPECTED COURSE/PROGNOSIS
- Course - chronic
- 50% mortality by age 50 in untreated patients with large defects
- Favorable in surgically treated symptomatic patients

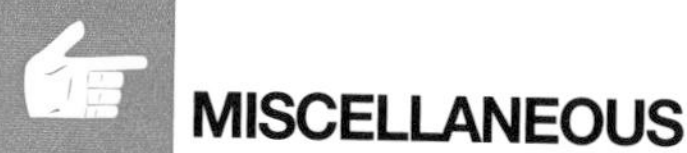

MISCELLANEOUS

ASSOCIATED CONDITIONS
- Mitral stenosis
- Mitral regurgitation
- Anomalous pulmonary venous return
- Multiple congenital syndromes

AGE-RELATED FACTORS
Pediatric: Most frequently appears in this age group
Geriatric: Defects in older persons may still be closed surgically
Others: N/A

PREGNANCY
- Evaluation prior to pregnancy, since condition may worsen

SYNONYMS N/A

ICD-9-CM
429.71 Acquired cardiac septal defect

SEE ALSO
Aortic valvular stenosis
Coarctation of the aorta
Complete atrioventricular (AV) canal
Patent ductus arteriosus
Pulmonic valvular stenosis
Tetralogy of Fallot
Transposition of the great vessels
Tricuspid atresia
Truncus arteriosus
Ventricular septal defect (VSD)

OTHER NOTES N/A

ABBREVIATIONS N/A

REFERENCES

- Friedman WF, Perloff JK: Congenital heart disease in infancy and childhood. In: Braunwald E, ed. Heart Disease. 4th Ed. Philadelphia, W.B. Saunders Co., 1992
- Hillis DL, Lange RA, Winniford MD, Page RL: Manual of Clinical Problems in Cardiology. New York, Little, Brown and Co., 1995

Web references: 0 available at www.5mcc.com
Illustrations N/A

Author(s):
Ricardo Samson, MD

Attention deficit/Hyperactivity disorder

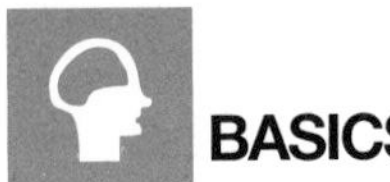

BASICS

DESCRIPTION A behavior problem characterized by a short attention span, low frustration tolerance, impulsivity, distractibility, and usually, hyperactivity. This can result in poor school performance, difficulty in peer relationships, and parent/child conflict.
System(s) affected: Nervous
Genetics: Familial pattern
Incidence/Prevalence in USA: 5% of school aged children
Predominant age:
- Onset < 7 years old
- Lasts into adolescence and adulthood
- 50% meet diagnostic criteria by age 4

Predominant sex: Males > Females (5:1)

SIGNS & SYMPTOMS
DSM-IV-R Criteria - 6 or more inattention criteria and/or 6 or more hyperactivity/impulsivity criteria. Symptoms must begin by age 7, be present for > 6 months and be noticed in 2 settings (eg, home and school).
- Inattention
  - ◊ Careless mistakes in tasks
  - ◊ Difficulty sustaining attention
  - ◊ Doesn't seem to listen
  - ◊ Doesn't follow through or finish tasks
  - ◊ Difficulty organizing tasks
  - ◊ Avoids tasks which require sustained mental effort
  - ◊ Loses things
  - ◊ Easily distracted
  - ◊ Forgetful
- Hyperactivity/Impulsivity
  - ◊ Fidgets
  - ◊ Difficulty remaining seated
  - ◊ Runs or climbs excessively
  - ◊ Difficulty playing quietly
  - ◊ Acts as if "driven by a motor"
  - ◊ Talks excessively
  - ◊ Blurts out answers before question is complete
  - ◊ Has difficulty awaiting turn
  - ◊ Interrupts others

CAUSES Multifactorial

RISK FACTORS
- Family history
- Co-morbid conditions (associated with, but not caused by)
  - ◊ Learning disabilities
  - ◊ Mood disorders
  - ◊ Oppositional defiant disorder
  - ◊ Conduct disorder

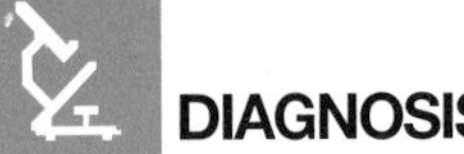

DIAGNOSIS

DIFFERENTIAL DIAGNOSIS
- Refer to DSM IV-R (see References)
- Activity level appropriate for age
- Dysfunctional family situation
- Learning disability (dyslexia, etc.)
- Hearing/vision disorder
- Oppositional/defiant disorder (see DSM IV-R)
- Conduct disorder (see DSM IV-R)
- Lead poisoning
- Medication reaction (decongestant, antihistamine, theophylline, phenobarbital)
- Tourette
- Pervasive developmental delay (autism)
- Absence seizures (attention deficit only)

LABORATORY Rarely needed, can check lead level

Drugs that may alter lab results: N/A

Disorders that may alter lab results: N/A

PATHOLOGICAL FINDINGS
- "Soft" neurological signs - nonspecific (Romberg, mixed hand preference, etc.)
- Motor tics can be present (cough, noises, twitching)

SPECIAL TESTS
- Behavior rating scales should be completed by parents and teachers. They are repeated after therapy is started to gauge differences (DSM-IV criteria can be used for this).
- Testing for learning disability (eg, dyslexia) through the school
- Good psychosocial evaluation of home environment
- See References

IMAGING Not needed

DIAGNOSTIC PROCEDURES Diagnosis is by DSM-IV criteria. EEG not needed unless symptoms are highly suggestive of seizure disorder (eg, absence seizures).

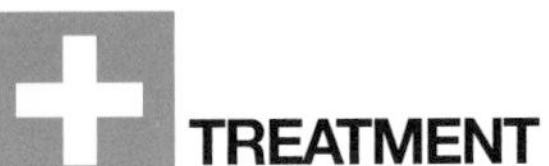

TREATMENT

APPROPRIATE HEALTH CARE Outpatient

GENERAL MEASURES
- Parent/school/patient education
- Work closely with teacher
- Avoid unproved therapies

SURGICAL MEASURES N/A

ACTIVITY N/A

DIET No dietary changes have been proven to help ADHD. Parents can experiment with non-harmful diets by eliminating sugar, dyes, additives

PATIENT EDUCATION
- Key points for parents:
  - ◊ 50% of ADHD children have one parent with ADHD; modify education sessions with parents accordingly
  - ◊ Strong emphasis on behavior therapy such as token systems
  - ◊ Reinforce good behavior (with rewards and attention)
  - ◊ Make eye contact with each request
  - ◊ Give one task at a time
  - ◊ Time out (brief) for problems
  - ◊ Stop behavior before it escalates
  - ◊ Find things child is good at and emphasize these
  - ◊ Some families benefit from "anger training," "social training" and family therapy
  - ◊ Educate parents to realistic expectations
  - ◊ Refer to advocacy and support groups
  - ◊ Help family and child deal with negative feelings
- Key points for teachers:
  - ◊ Short work sessions
  - ◊ Clear rules
  - ◊ Immediate consequences
  - ◊ Reinforce good behavior
  - ◊ Coordinate homework with parents using daily assignment notebook
  - ◊ Have second set of books at home
- Support groups
  - ◊ CHADD - Children and Adults with ADD, 8181 Professional Pl. Suite 201, Landover, MD 20785; 800-233-4050
  - ◊ ADD Warehouse 300 NW 70th Ave, Suite 102, Plantation, FL 33317; 800-233-9273
  - ◊ AD-IN - ADD Information Network, 475 Hillside Ave, Needham, MA 02174; 781-455-9895
  - ◊ LDA - Learning Disabilities Association, 4156 Library Rd, Pittsburgh, PA 15234
  - ◊ National Information Center for Children & Youth with Disabilities www.nichcy.org

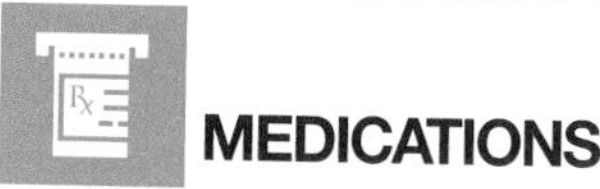

MEDICATIONS

DRUG(S) OF CHOICE
- Nonstimulant:
  - ◊ Atomoxetine (Strattera); selective norepinephrine reuptake inhibitor; 0.5-2 mg/kg/d every AM. Slower onset of efficacy; GI side effects and sedation.
- Stimulant:
  - ◊ Methylphenidate (Ritalin, Concerta, Metadate CD, Ritalin LA)
    - Short-acting - Ritalin 5-20 mg q am, noon and 4 pm; maximum dose 60 mg
    - Long-acting - Concerta 18, 36, 54 mg q am; Metadate CD 40 mg q am; Ritalin LA 20, 30, 40 q am
  - ◊ Several newer stimulant drugs have been developed which have no advantage over older, established drugs

Contraindications: N/A

Precautions:
- If not responding, check compliance and consider another diagnosis
- Methylphenidate has become a drug of abuse and should be monitored carefully - 20 mg nongeneric have highest street value
- Drug holidays should only be given if family/peer relationships aren't harmed
- Some children experience withdrawal (tearfulness, agitation) after a missed dose

Significant possible interactions:
- Atomoxetine interacts with Paxil, Prozac, quinidine
- Stimulants may increase levels of seizure drugs, SSRIs, tricyclics and warfarin

ALTERNATIVE DRUGS
- Amphetamine
  - ◊ Adderall 2.5-20 mg every 4-6 hours
  - ◊ Adderall XR 5-30 mg every am; age 6 and above.
  - ◊ Amphetamines have a higher addiction potential.
- Pemoline (Cylert) 18.75-112.5 mg/day; long-acting, chewable tablet available. Often less effective than methylphenidate.
- Nonstimulant drugs - due to the mixed efficacy and high side effects of these drugs, they are not recommended for use without a consultant. Examples - clonidine, tricyclic antidepressants, selective serotonin reuptake inhibitors (SSRIs).

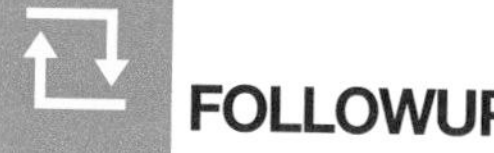

FOLLOWUP

PATIENT MONITORING
- Parent/teacher rating scales initially, in 2 weeks, and regularly
- Office visits to monitor side effects and efficacy. End point is - improved grades, improved rating scales, acceptable family interactions, and improved peer interactions.
  - ◊ Monitor growth and BP
  - ◊ Methylphenidate (Ritalin, Concerta), monitor CBC
  - ◊ Pemoline (Cylert), monitor ALT
  - ◊ Dexmethylphenidate (Focalin), monitor CBC

PREVENTION/AVOIDANCE
- Children are at risk for: abuse, depression, social isolation
- Parents need regular support and advice
- Establish contact with teacher each school year

POSSIBLE COMPLICATIONS
- Untreated ADHD can lead to: failing school, parental abuse, social isolation, poor self esteem
- If appetite poor, offer food morning and evening
- Some children experience withdrawal (tearfulness, agitation) after a missed dose

EXPECTED COURSE/PROGNOSIS
- May last through school years and into adulthood
- It becomes easier to control with increasing age
- Encourage career choices which allow autonomy and mobility
- There is no increased incidence of delinquency unless other co-morbid features exist (eg, conduct disorder)
- Encourage parents to subtract 2 years from their child's chronological age when allowing privileges (eg, treat a 16 year old like a 14 year old; delay driving until age 18)

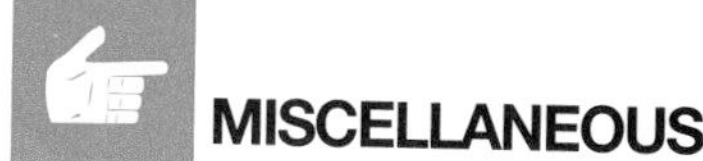

MISCELLANEOUS

ASSOCIATED CONDITIONS
See Risk Factors

AGE-RELATED FACTORS
Pediatric: N/A
Geriatric: N/A
Others: N/A

PREGNANCY
Avoid stimulant medications in pregnancy

SYNONYMS
- Attention deficit disorder
- Hyperactivity

ICD-9-CM
314.00 Attention deficit disorder without mention of hyperactivity
314.01 ADD with hyperactivity

SEE ALSO

OTHER NOTES
N/A

ABBREVIATIONS
ADD = Attention Deficit Disorder
LFT = liver function test

REFERENCES

- Barkley RA. ADHD - A Handbook for Diagnosis and Treatment. 2nd Ed. New York, Guilford Press, 1998
- Behrman RE, Kliegman M, eds. Nelson Textbook of Pediatrics. 16th ed. Philadelphia, W.B. Saunders Co., 2000
- American Psychiatric Association. Diagnostic and Statistical Manual of Mental Disorders. 4th Ed, Revised. Washington, DC, American Psychiatric Association, 1994
- The Parents Guide to Attention Deficit Disorders, Hawthorne Education Services, Columbia, Missouri 65205, 1-314-874-1710
- Barkley RA. Defiant Children. 2nd Ed. New York, Guilford Press, 1997
- Barkley RA. Taking Charge of ADHD. New York, Guilford Press, 1995

Web references: 3 available at www.5mcc.com
Illustrations N/A

Author(s):
Laura L. Novak, MD

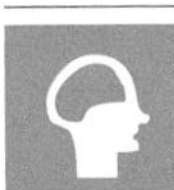

BASICS

DESCRIPTION Autism is a pervasive developmental disorder of early childhood characterized by severe impairment in:
- Effective social skills
- Absent or impaired language development
- Repetitive and/or stereotyped activities and interests, especially inanimate objects

System(s) affected: Nervous
Genetics: High concordance in monozygotic twins, increased prevalence in siblings
Incidence/Prevalence in USA: About 7 in10,000 persons
Predominant age: Onset prior to age 3, but generally abnormal development is apparent well before
Predominant sex: Male > Female (2-4:1)

SIGNS & SYMPTOMS
- Impairment in social interaction:
  - ◊ Inadequate or lack of use of multiple non-verbal behaviors, such as postures and facial expression
  - ◊ Failure to develop appropriate peer relationships
  - ◊ Lack of sharing interests and achievements
  - ◊ Lack of social and/or emotional reciprocity
- Communication impairment:
  - ◊ Delay or lack of development of spoken language without accompanying alternative modes of communication
  - ◊ Impairment in initiating and sustaining conversation
  - ◊ Idiosyncratic language with stereotyped or repetitive usage
  - ◊ Lack of developmentally appropriate play, especially imitative
- Repetitive and stereotyped patterns of behavior:
  - ◊ Abnormal preoccupations either in intensity or focus
  - ◊ Inflexibility to non-functional activities
  - ◊ Stereotyped or repetitive motor mannerisms
  - ◊ Preoccupation with inanimate objects and their parts

CAUSES No single cause has been identified. It is generally believed that it is caused by abnormalities in brain structure or function. Research continues to investigate the link between heredity, genetics and medical problems. Questions regarding immunizations causing autism and associated pervasive developmental disorders are being investigated but not yet substantiated.

RISK FACTORS
- Certain medical conditions, including fragile X syndrome, tuberous sclerosis, congenital rubella syndrome, and untreated phenylketonuria (PKU)
- Sibling with autism

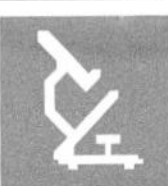

DIAGNOSIS

DIFFERENTIAL DIAGNOSIS
- Other mental and CNS disorders including:
  - ◊ Schizophrenia
  - ◊ Elective mutism
  - ◊ Language disorder
  - ◊ Mental retardation
  - ◊ Stereotyped movement disorder
- Other pervasive developmental disorders including:
  - ◊ Rett disorder
  - ◊ Childhood disintegrative disorder
  - ◊ Asperger disorder

LABORATORY N/A (other than to rule-out associated conditions)

Drugs that may alter lab results: N/A

Disorders that may alter lab results: N/A

PATHOLOGICAL FINDINGS N/A

SPECIAL TESTS
- Parents' Evaluation of Developmental Status (PEDS)
- Pervasive Developmental Disorders Screening Test-Stage I (PDDST).
- Childhood Autism Rating Scale (CARS) rating system
- Checklist for Autism in Toddlers (CHAT) is used to screen for autism at 18 months of age
- Autism Screening Questionnaire has been used with children four and older
- Intellectual level needs to be established and monitored, as it is one of the best measures of prognosis
- EEG as autistic children have a markedly higher incidence of epilepsy which increases with age

IMAGING Could be useful in ruling out associated conditions

DIAGNOSTIC PROCEDURES
- Developmental history
- Psychiatric examination
- Psychological testing
- Comprehensive language assessment

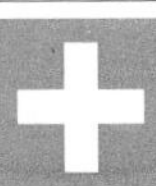

TREATMENT

APPROPRIATE HEALTH CARE Comprehensive structured educational programming of a sustained and intensive design

GENERAL MEASURES
- There is currently no cure for autism. Early diagnosis and initiation of multiple disciplinary intervention will help enhance functioning in later life.

Treatment goals: to improve language and social skills, decrease problem behaviors, foster independence and provide support for parents
- Consider consults: ophthalmology, otolaryngology, lead screening and metabolic testing, genetic screening, skin testing (for tuberous sclerosis) and others as needed
- Parent support groups and respite programs

SURGICAL MEASURES N/A

ACTIVITY
- As tolerated by the child
- Educational specialized programs developed through local school system

DIET No special diet

PATIENT EDUCATION
- The Autism Society of America, 7910 Woodmont Ave., Bethesda, MD 20814-3007; 800-autism; website autism-society.org.
- Atwood T, Wing L. Asperger Syndrome: A Guide for Parents and Professionals, Jessica Kingsley Publisher, 1997
- Siegel B. The world of the autistic child: understanding and treating autistic spectrum disorders. Oxford, England, Oxford University Press

MEDICATIONS

DRUG(S) OF CHOICE None
Contraindications: N/A
Precautions: Risperidone may be associated with hyperglycemia and ketoacidosis
Significant possible interactions: N/A

ALTERNATIVE DRUGS
- Stimulant medications may be used to address concomitant symptoms of attention deficit disorder, such as impulsiveness, hyperactivity and inattention
- SSRI antidepressants, such as fluoxetine and sertraline have shown some help in reducing ritualistic behavior and improving moods
- Clomipramine (Anafranil), a tricyclic antidepressant, has been reported to decrease some forms of self-injurious behavior, obsessive/compulsive symptoms and compulsive, aggressive behavior
- Buspirone (BuSpar) has in some individuals reduced hyperactivity and stereotyped behavior
- Neuroleptics have been used with limited effectiveness
- Risperidone (Risperdal) in low doses has helped socialization in some case reports
- Gabapentin (Neurontin) is being used but no studies exist

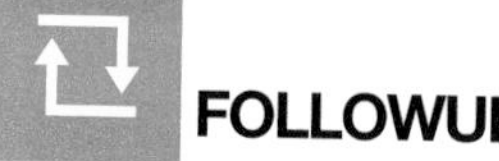

FOLLOWUP

PATIENT MONITORING
- Constant by caregivers. As indicated by physician, prescribed medical management.
- Intellectual and language testing every two years in childhood

PREVENTION/AVOIDANCE None known

POSSIBLE COMPLICATIONS
- Increasing incidents of seizure disorders
- Increased risk for physical and sexual abuse in autistic children

EXPECTED COURSE/PROGNOSIS
- Those who begin treatment at a young age have significantly better outcomes
- Prognosis is closely related to initial intellectual abilities with only 20% functioning above the mentally retarded level
- Communicative language development before age five is also associated with a better outcome
- The general expected course is for a life-long need of supervised structured care. Only 1-2% become independent.

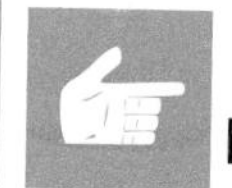

MISCELLANEOUS

ASSOCIATED CONDITIONS
- Mental retardation
- Attention deficit/hyperactivity disorder
- Phenylketonuria, tuberous sclerosis, and fragile X syndrome
- Anxiety
- Depression
- Obsessional behavior
- Seizures

AGE-RELATED FACTORS
Pediatric: Onset seen only in children under three
Geriatric: N/A
Others: N/A

PREGNANCY May be increased risk of autism in complications of pregnancy, labor and delivery

SYNONYMS
- Early infantile autism
- Childhood autism
- Kanner autism
- Pervasive developmental disorder

ICD-9-CM
299.0 Infantile autism

SEE ALSO
Anxiety
Attention deficit/Hyperactivity disorder
Depression
Fragile X syndrome
Mental retardation
Schizophrenia
Seizure disorders

OTHER NOTES
Refer also to Asperger syndrome

ABBREVIATIONS N/A

REFERENCES

- Chakrabarti S, Fombonne E. Pervasive developmental disorders in preschool children. JAMA 2001;285:3093-9
- Prater CD, Zylstra RG. Autism: a medical primer. Am Fam Physician 2002 Nov 1;66(9):1667-74
- Siegel B. Early screening and diagnosis in autism spectrum disorders: the pervasive developmental disorders screening test (PDDST). NIH State of the Science in Autism: Screening and Diagnosis Working Conference, Bethesda, Md., June 15-17, 1998
- Volkmar F, Cook EH Jr, Pomeroy J, Realmuto G, Tanguay P. Practice parameters for the assessment and treatment of children, adolescents, and adults with autism and other pervasive developmental disorders. J Am Acad Child Adolesc Psychiatry 1999;38(12 suppl):32S-54S
- Volkmar FR: Autism and the Pervasive Developmental Disorders. In: Lewis M, ed. Child and Adolescent Psychiatry; A Comprehensive Textbook. Baltimore, Williams and Wilkins, 1991
- Diagnostic and Statistical Manual of Mental Disorders. 4th ed. American Psychiatric Association, Washington, D.C., 1994
- Findling RL, Maxwell K, Wiznitzer M. An open clinical trial of risperidone monotherapy in young children with autistic disorder. Psychopharmacol Bull 1997;33(1):155-9
- Holmes DL. Autism Through the Lifespan: the Eden Model. Woodbine House, 1998
- McDougle CJ, Posey D. Genetics of childhood disorders: XLIV. autism, part 3: psychopharmacology of autism. J Am Acad Child Adolesc Psychiatry 2002;41(11):1380-3

Web references: 3 available at www.5mcc.com
Illustrations N/A

Author(s):
Mark R. Dambro, MD

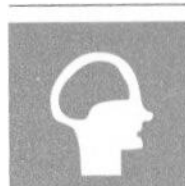

BASICS

DESCRIPTION

- Babesiosis is a worldwide tick-borne hemolytic disease that is caused by intraerythrocytic protozoan parasites of the genus Babesia
- Babesiosis has rarely been reported outside the US. Sporadic cases have been reported from a number of countries including France, Italy, the former Yugoslavia, United Kingdom, Ireland, the former Soviet Union and Mexico. In the US, infections have been reported from many states but the most endemic areas are the islands off the coast of Massachusetts (including Nantucket and Martha's Vineyard) and New York (including eastern and south central Long Island, Shelter Island and Fire Island) and in Connecticut. In these areas, asymptomatic human infection seems to be common.
- After a recognized tick bite, the incubation period of babesiosis varies from 5-33 days. However, most patients do not recall recent tick exposure. After an infected blood transfusion, the incubation period can be up to nine weeks.

System(s) affected: Cardiovascular, Gastrointestinal, Hemic/Lymphatic/Immunologic, Musculoskeletal, Nervous, Pulmonary, Renal/Urologic

Genetics: N/A

Incidence/Prevalence in USA:

- Between 1968 and 1993, > 450 Babesia infections were confirmed in the US by blood smears or serologic testing. Prevalence is difficult to estimate because of lack of surveillance, and because infections are often asymptomatic.
- A recent study evaluated the seroprevalence and seroconversion for tick-borne diseases in a high-risk population in the northeast United States. In this one-year seroconversion study of patients in New York state who were at high risk for tick-borne diseases, antibodies to *B. microti* were seen in seven of 671 participants (1 percent).

Predominant age: All ages; most patients present in their 40s or 50s

Predominant sex: N/A

SIGNS & SYMPTOMS

- Asymptomatic
- High fever (up to 40°C [104°F])
- Chills
- Diaphoresis
- Gastrointestinal (anorexia, nausea, abdominal pain, vomiting, diarrhea)
- Generalized weakness
- Fatigue
- Myalgia
- Respiratory (cough, shortness of breath)
- Headache
- Hepatomegaly and splenomegaly or evidence of shock
- Rash (uncommon)
- Central nervous system involvement includes headache, photophobia, neck and back stiffness, altered sensorium and emotional lability
- Jaundice and dark urine may develop later in course of illness

CAUSES

- *Babesia microti* (in the US) and *Babesia divergens* and *Babesia bovis* (in Europe) cause most infections in humans. Recently, one case of *B. divergens* was reported in the U.S.
- A previously unknown species of Babesia (WA-1) was isolated from an immunocompetent man in Washington state who had clinical babesiosis. Researchers also described another probable new babesial species (MO1) associated with the first reported case of babesiosis acquired in the state of Missouri. MO1 is probably distinct from *B. divergens* but the two share morphologic, antigenic and genetic characteristics.
- Ixodid (or hard-bodied) ticks, in particular *Ixodes dammini* (*Ixodes scapularis*) and *Ixodes ricinus*, are the vectors of the parasite

RISK FACTORS

- Exposure to endemic areas
- Transfusion-associated babesiosis and transplacental/perinatal transmission have been reported

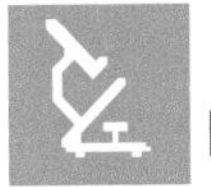

DIAGNOSIS

DIFFERENTIAL DIAGNOSIS

- Bacterial sepsis
- Hepatitis
- Lyme disease
- Ehrlichiosis
- Leishmaniasis
- Malaria

LABORATORY

- Mild to severe hemolytic anemia (common nonspecific finding)
- Normal to slightly depressed leukocyte count (common nonspecific finding)
- Typical morphologic picture on the blood smear
- A Wright- or Giemsa-stained peripheral blood smear is most commonly used to demonstrate the presence of intraerythrocytic parasites
- Rarely, tetrads of merozoites are visible
- Serologic evaluation with the indirect immunofluorescent antibody test with use of *B. microti* antigen is available in a few laboratories. The cutoff titer for determination of a positive result varies with the particular laboratory protocol used, but in most laboratories, titers of more than 1:64 are considered consistent with *B. microti* infection. Tenfold to 20-fold higher titers can be observed in the acute setting, with a gradual decline over weeks to months. The correlation between the level of the titer and the severity of symptoms is poor.
- Detection of *B. microti* by polymerase chain reaction (PCR) is more sensitive and equally specific for the diagnosis of acute cases, in comparison with direct smear examination and hamster inoculation. PCR-based methods may also be indicated for monitoring of the infection.

Drugs that may alter lab results: N/A

Disorders that may alter lab results: N/A

PATHOLOGICAL FINDINGS N/A

SPECIAL TESTS N/A

IMAGING N/A

DIAGNOSTIC PROCEDURES Based on typical morphologic picture on the blood smear in conjunction with epidemiologic information

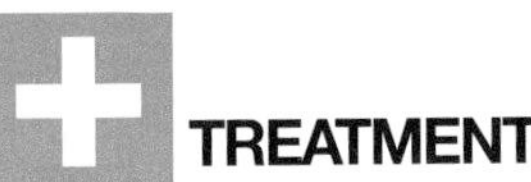

TREATMENT

APPROPRIATE HEALTH CARE Outpatient or inpatient depending on symptoms

GENERAL MEASURES Supportive care

SURGICAL MEASURES N/A

ACTIVITY N/A

DIET N/A

PATIENT EDUCATION AAFP - patient handout - www.aafp.org/afp/20010515/1976ph.html

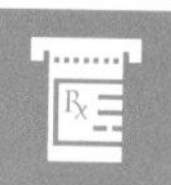

MEDICATIONS

DRUG(S) OF CHOICE

- Atovaquone (Mepron) suspension 750 mg twice daily plus azithromycin (Zithromax) 500-1,000 mg per day
- Combination of quinine (Quinamm) 650 mg of salt orally, three times daily and clindamycin (Cleocin) 600 mg orally, three times daily, or 1.2 g parenterally, twice daily for 7-10 days is the most commonly used treatment. The pediatric dosage is 20-40 mg/kg per day for quinine and 25 mg/kg per day for clindamycin.
- In areas endemic for Lyme disease and ehrlichiosis - may be advisable to add doxycycline (Vibramycin) 100 mg twice a day by mouth in the management of patients with babesiosis until serologic testing is completed
- Exchange transfusion, together with antibabesial chemotherapy, may be necessary in critically ill patients. This treatment is usually reserved for patients who are extremely ill - with blood parasitemia of more than 10 percent, massive hemolysis and asplenia.

Contraindications: N/A
Precautions: Clindamycin can lead to *C. difficile* associated diarrhea
Significant possible interactions: N/A

ALTERNATIVE DRUGS

- Several other drugs have been evaluated, including tetracycline, primaquine, sulfadiazine (Microsulfon) and pyrimethamine (Fansidar). Results have varied. Pentamidine (Pentam) has proved to be moderately effective in diminishing symptoms and decreasing parasitemia.

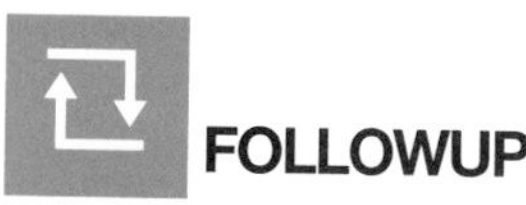

FOLLOWUP

PATIENT MONITORING Monitor for complications (congestive heart failure, etc.) and follow parasitemia as needed

PREVENTION/AVOIDANCE

- Avoid endemic regions during the peak transmission months of May through September (especially relevant for asplenic or immunocompromised persons in whom babesiosis can be a devastating illness).
- Using insect repellant is advised during outdoor activities, especially in wooded or grassy areas. Products with 10 to 35 percent DEET will provide adequate protection under most conditions.
- Early removal of ticks is important; the tick must remain attached for at least 24 hours before the transmission of *B. microti* occurs. Daily self-examination is recommended for persons who engage in outdoor activities in endemic areas.
- Pets must be examined for ticks because they may carry ticks into the home

POSSIBLE COMPLICATIONS

- Congestive heart failure
- Disseminated intravascular coagulation
- Acute respiratory distress syndrome (that can occur even a few days after the onset of effective antimicrobial treatment)
- Renal failure and myocardial infarction also have been associated with severe babesiosis

EXPECTED COURSE/PROGNOSIS

- When left untreated, silent babesial infection may persist for months or even years
- 139 hospitalized cases in New York state between 1982 and 1993
  - ◊ Nine patients (6.5 percent) died
  - ◊ One fourth of the patients were admitted to the intensive care unit
  - ◊ One fourth of the patients required hospitalization for more than 14 days
- Alkaline phosphatase levels greater than 125 U per L, white blood cell counts greater than 5 X 109 per L, history of cardiac abnormality, history of splenectomy, presence of heart murmur and parasitemia values of 4 percent or higher were associated with disease severity

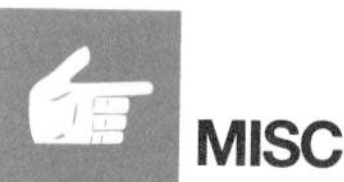

MISCELLANEOUS

ASSOCIATED CONDITIONS

- Co-infection with *Borrelia burgdorferi* and *B. microti* is relatively common in endemic areas
- Co-infection with Ehrlichia species may also be seen. Three species of Ehrlichia have been described that infect humans, *Ehrlichia chaffeensis*, *Ehrlichia phagocytophila* and *Ehrlichia ewingii*. Typically, patients have a nonspecific febrile illness. Rash is uncommon with human granulocytic ehrlichiosis but common with human monocytic ehrlichiosis. Laboratory findings often include leukopenia, thrombocytopenia and increases in serum hepatic enzyme activities.

AGE-RELATED FACTORS

Pediatric: N/A
Geriatric: The morbidity and mortality is higher in patients older than 65
Others: High-level parasitemia is more common in asplenic patients. Such patients have been treated successfully with exchange transfusion in addition to drugs.

PREGNANCY N/A

SYNONYMS N/A

ICD-9-CM

088.82 Babesiosis

SEE ALSO

Lyme disease

OTHER NOTES N/A

ABBREVIATIONS N/A

REFERENCES

- Beattie JF, Michelson ML, Holman PJ. Acute babesiosis caused by Babesia divergens in a resident of Kentucky. N Engl J Med 2002;29;347(9):697-8
- Gelfand JA. Babesia. In: Mandell GL, Douglas RG, Bennett JE, Dolin R, eds. Mandell, Douglas, and Bennett's Principles and practice of infectious diseases. 5th ed. New York: Churchill Livingstone, 2000. p. 2899-902
- Boustani MR, Gelfand JA. Babesiosis. Clin Infect Dis 1996. p. 22:611-5
- Mylonakis E. When to suspect and how to monitor babesiosis. Am Fam Phys 2001;63:1969-74
- Pruthi RK, Marshall WF, Wiltsie JC, Persing DH. Human babesiosis. Mayo Clin Proc 1995;70:853-62
- Persing DH, Herwaldt BL, Glaser C, Lane RS, Thomford JW, Mathiesen D, et al. Infection with a babesia-like organism in northern California. N Engl J Med 1995;332:298-303
- Quick RE, Herwaldt BL, Thomford JW, Garnett ME, Eberhard ML, Wilson M, et al. Babesiosis in Washington State: a new species of Babesia? Ann Intern Med 1993;119:284-90
- White DJ, Talarico J, Chang HG, et al. Human babesiosis in New York State: a review of 139 hospitalized cases and analysis of prognostic factors. Arch Int Med 1998;158:2149-54
- Gutman JD, Kotton CN, Kratz A. Case records of the Massachusetts General Hospital. Weekly clinicopathological exercises. Case 29-2003. A 60-year-old man with fever, rigors, and sweats. N Engl J Med 2003;349(12):1168-75

Web references: 0 available at www.5mcc.com
Illustrations N/A

Author(s):

Eleftherios Mylonakis, MD
Vassiliki Syriopoulou, MD

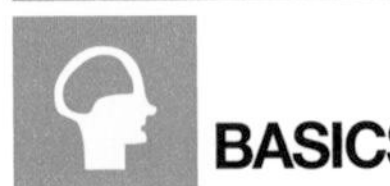

BASICS

DESCRIPTION
Balanitis: inflammation of glans penis
Posthitis: inflammation of the foreskin
System(s) affected: Reproductive, Skin/Exocrine
Genetics: N/A
Incidence/Prevalence in USA: N/A
Predominant age: Adult
Predominant sex: Male only

SIGNS & SYMPTOMS
- Pain, penile
- Dysuria
- Drainage, site of infection
- Erythema
- Prepuce swelling
- Ulceration
- Plaques

CAUSES
- Allergic reaction (condom latex, contraceptive jelly)
- Fungal (*Candida albicans*) and bacterial infections (*Borrelia vincentii*, *Streptococci*)
- Fixed drug eruption (sulfa, tetracycline, barbital)
- Plasma cell infiltration (Zoon balanitis)
- Autodigestion by activated transplant exocrine enzymes

RISK FACTORS
- Presence of foreskin
- Oral antibiotics in male infants can predispose to Candida balanitis

DIAGNOSIS

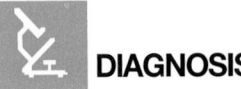

DIFFERENTIAL DIAGNOSIS
- Leukoplakia
- Lichen planus
- Psoriasis
- Reiter syndrome
- Lichen sclerosus et atrophicus
- Erythroplasia of Queyrat
- Balanitis xerotica obliterans

LABORATORY
- Microbiology culture
- Wet mount
- Serology for syphilis
- Serum glucose

Drugs that may alter lab results: None

Disorders that may alter lab results: None

PATHOLOGICAL FINDINGS Plasma cells infiltration with Zoon balanitis

SPECIAL TESTS N/A

IMAGING N/A

DIAGNOSTIC PROCEDURES Biopsy, if persistent

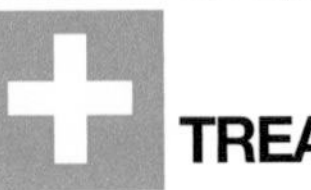

TREATMENT

APPROPRIATE HEALTH CARE Outpatient

GENERAL MEASURES
- Warm compresses or sitz baths
- Local hygiene

SURGICAL MEASURES Consider circumcision as preventative measure

ACTIVITY No limitations

DIET No special diet

PATIENT EDUCATION
- Need for appropriate hygiene
- Avoidance of known allergens

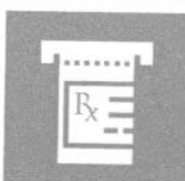

MEDICATIONS

DRUG(S) OF CHOICE

- Fungal - clotrimazole (Lotrimin) 1% bid to affected area or nystatin (Mycostatin) bid to qid to affected area
- Bacterial - bacitracin qid to affected area or neomycin-polymyxin B-bacitracin (Neosporin) qid to affected area. If infection, cephalosporin or sulfa drug by mouth or injection.
- Dermatitis - topical steroids qid to affected area
- Zoon balanitis - topical steroids qid

Contraindications: Refer to manufacturer's profile of each drug

Precautions: Refer to manufacturer's profile of each drug

Significant possible interactions: Refer to manufacturer's profile of each drug

ALTERNATIVE DRUGS N/A

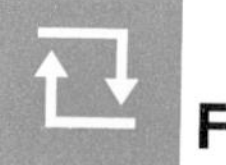

FOLLOWUP

PATIENT MONITORING Every 1-2 weeks until etiology has been established. Persistent balanitis may require biopsy to rule out malignancy.

PREVENTION/AVOIDANCE

- Proper hygiene and avoidance of allergens
- Circumcision

POSSIBLE COMPLICATIONS

- Meatal stenosis
- Premalignant changes from chronic irritations
- Urinary tract infections

EXPECTED COURSE/PROGNOSIS

With appropriate treatment it should resolve

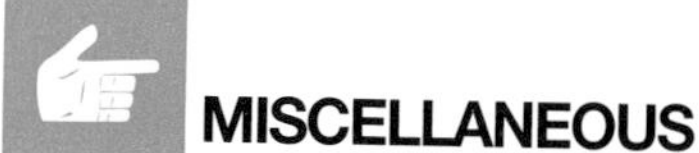

MISCELLANEOUS

ASSOCIATED CONDITIONS Diabetes mellitus

AGE-RELATED FACTORS

Pediatric: Oral antibiotics predispose infants to Candida balanitis

Geriatric: Condom catheters can predispose to balanitis

Others: N/A

PREGNANCY N/A

SYNONYMS N/A

ICD-9-CM

607.1 Balanitis
112.2 Candidiasis of other urogenital sites
099.8 Other specified venereal diseases

SEE ALSO

Reiter syndrome

OTHER NOTES N/A

ABBREVIATIONS N/A

REFERENCES

- Gillenwater JY, Grayhack JT, Howard SS, Duckett JW: Adult and Pediatric Urology. 2nd Ed. Mosby Year Book, Philadelphia, 1991
- Zoon JJ: Balanoposthite chronique cireonscrite benigne à plasmacytes (contra èrythroplasie de Queyrat). Dermatologica 1952;105:1
- Tom WW, Munda R, First MR, et al: Autodigestion of the glans, penis and urethra by activated transplant pancreatic exocrine enzymes. Surgery 1987;102:99-101

Web references: 1 available at www.5mcc.com

Illustrations 2 available

Author(s):

James P. Miller, MD
Timothy L. Black, MD

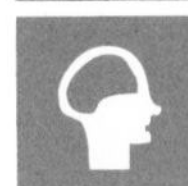

BASICS

DESCRIPTION Acute or chronic traumatic inflammation of the middle ear space secondary to the rapid development of a negative (or less commonly a positive) pressure differential between the surrounding atmosphere of the external canal and the middle ear compartments (tympanic cavity, eustachian tube, and mastoid air cells)
This situation is brought about by the inability of the eustachian tube to adequately equilibrate the middle ear air pressure with the moment-to-moment changes in the environmental atmospheric pressures while descending or ascending in air (flight) and/or especially in water (diving). This causes the retraction or protraction of the tympanic membrane with subsequent inflammation and/or rupture. This also may cause asymmetric pressure stimulation of the inner ear and vestibular end-organ.
System(s) affected: Nervous
Genetics: N/A
Incidence/Prevalence in USA: The most common medical disorder experienced by SCUBA divers. Also highly prevalent among aircraft flight personnel (especially high-performance jet aircraft), passengers, and sky divers.
Predominant age: All ages
Predominant sex: Male = Female

SIGNS & SYMPTOMS
- Abrupt in onset
- Otalgia (ear pain)
- Feeling of fullness in ear
- Conductive hearing loss
- Dizziness
- Tinnitus
- Vertigo
- Nausea and vomiting
- Transient facial paralysis
- With tympanic membrane rupture the ability to blow air and/or fluid out one's ear while performing a Valsalva maneuver or when sneezing
- Crying in children (which is their only means of autoinflation)

CAUSES
- Rapid descent or ascent with eustachian tube obstruction
  - ◊ Eustachian tube lock
  - ◊ Upper respiratory infections - sinusitis, rhinitis, tonsillitis, and adenoiditis
  - ◊ Overzealous forceful Valsalva maneuver (in ascent with vestibular stimulation)
  - ◊ Allergic rhinitis
  - ◊ Non-allergic rhinitis with eosinophilia
  - ◊ Obstructing nasal polyps
  - ◊ Deviated nasal septum
  - ◊ Congenital abnormalities of inner/middle ear (cleft palate)
  - ◊ Nasopharyngeal tumors
- Rapid descent or ascent with external ear canal occlusion
  - ◊ Otitis externa (swimmer's ear)
  - ◊ Impacted cerumen
  - ◊ Ear plugs
- Trauma to external and middle ear
  - ◊ Activities involving external ear trauma - boxing, soccer, water skiing, accidents, etc.
  - ◊ Overzealous use of cotton swab in cleaning ear canals

RISK FACTORS
- Participating in high risk activities without adequate eustachian tube autoinflation (Valsalva maneuver, swallowing) and/or with any of the listed causes of eustachian tube and external ear canal dysfunction:
- SCUBA diving
- Airplane flight
- Sky diving
- High altitude mountain travelers
- High altitude elevator rides
- Hyperbaric oxygen chamber therapy
- High impact sports
- Infants and young otologically healthy children have difficulty in dilating the eustachian tube (by swallowing) even at small pressure changes and therefore are at higher risk (especially with upper respiratory infection)

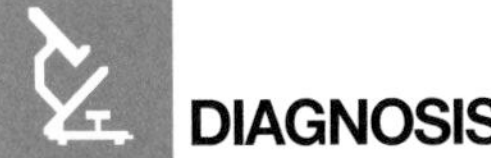

DIAGNOSIS

DIFFERENTIAL DIAGNOSIS
- Serous otitis media
- Acute and chronic otitis media
- External otitis
- Myringitis bullosa

LABORATORY N/A

Drugs that may alter lab results: N/A

Disorders that may alter lab results: N/A

PATHOLOGICAL FINDINGS
- Tympanic membrane retraction or protraction with hemotympanum or rupture
- Edema of mucosal lining and capillary engorgement with transudation of middle ear effusion
- Inner ear involvement with rupture of the round or oval windows and leakage of perilymph into the middle ear and perilymphatic fistula development

SPECIAL TESTS N/A

IMAGING Only to rule out suspected nasopharyngeal tumor or sinusitis

DIAGNOSTIC PROCEDURES
- Otoscopic exam
- Audiogram - conductive (middle ear) versus mixed (inner ear) loss
- Surgical exploration to rule out inner ear involvement if suspected

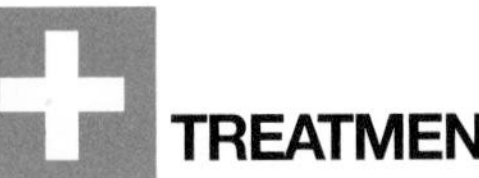

TREATMENT

APPROPRIATE HEALTH CARE
- Outpatient generally
- Inpatient for complicating emergencies,

e.g., incapacitating pain requiring myringotomy, large tympanic perforation requiring tympanoplasty

GENERAL MEASURES
- Perform Valsalva method of eustachian tube autoinflation (patient inhales then closes nose with thumb and index finger on nasal alae, then exhales with mouth closed). This will equalize pressures, relieve pain, and restore hearing. This usually needs to be repeated several times during descent or ascent.
- Nasal decongestant spray with repeated applications
- Antihistamines
- If the suggested maneuvers are unsuccessful return to higher altitude if possible and repeat Valsalva
- If ear block occurs, then outpatient politzerization must be performed followed by systemic and oral decongestants
- If associated infection, treat with appropriate antibiotics

SURGICAL MEASURES N/A

ACTIVITY
- No flying or diving until complete resolution of all signs and symptoms and Valsalva maneuver can be performed
- In severe cases, bedrest

DIET Avoid food allergens that cause rhinitis

PATIENT EDUCATION
- Teach Valsalva maneuver
- Educate on how to create allergy-free environment
- Divers Alert Network of Duke University Medical Center, information line,

(919) 684-2948

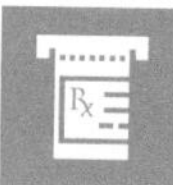

MEDICATIONS

DRUG(S) OF CHOICE
- Decongestants:
  - ◊ 0.05% oxymetazoline (Afrin, Afrin 12-Hour) two initial sprays 5 minutes apart then q12h
  - ◊ 0.05% phenylephrine (Neo-Synephrine) two initial sprays 5 minutes apart then q12h
  - ◊ Pseudoephedrine (Sudafed 12-hour, Afrinol) 120 mg q12h po
- Antihistamines for allergic component:
  - ◊ Diphenhydramine (Benadryl) 25-50 mg q6h
  - ◊ Loratadine (Claritin) 10 mg qday
  - ◊ Fexofenadine (Allegra) 60 mg bid (60 mg qday in patients with decreased renal function)

Contraindications:
- Previous allergic reactions
- Hypertension
- Drowsiness
- Erythromycin and terfenadine or astemizole; cardiac toxicity.

Precautions:
- All medications must be used on the ground to rule out idiosyncratic reactions that could incapacitate in an airplane or underwater environment
- Elderly are more susceptible to drug side effects, especially with diphenhydramine

Significant possible interactions: Refer to manufacturer's profile of each drug. Terfenadine and astemizole have many possible interactions. Avoid with macrolide antibiotics, ketoconazole.

ALTERNATIVE DRUGS
Cetirizine (Zyrtec)

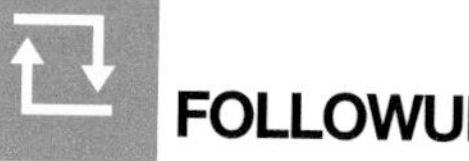

FOLLOWUP

PATIENT MONITORING
- Otoscopic until symptoms clear
- In severe cases, audiograms

PREVENTION/AVOIDANCE
- Avoid altitude changes with any risk factors for eustachian tube dysfunction
- Chewing gum while flying especially for children
- Use of recommended medications before the activity

POSSIBLE COMPLICATIONS
- Permanent hearing loss
- Ruptured tympanic membranes
- Serous otitis media

EXPECTED COURSE/PROGNOSIS
- Ear block - hours to days with complete resolution and return to flight or diving in days to weeks
- Tympanic rupture - weeks to months

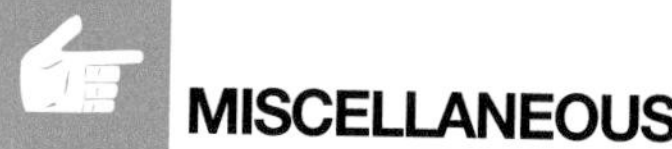

MISCELLANEOUS

ASSOCIATED CONDITIONS
- Aerosinusitis
- Aerodontalgia
- Face mask squeeze
- Epistaxis
- Alternobaric vertigo
- Unequal caloric stimulation vertigo
- Anxiety - leading to panic attack
- Temporomandibular joint syndrome
- Inner ear cochlear damage and/or perilymph fistula

AGE-RELATED FACTORS
Pediatric: Healthy children have difficulty in dilating the eustachian tube (by swallowing) even at small pressure changes and therefore are at higher risk (especially with upper respiratory infection)
Geriatric: Drug side effects
Others: N/A

PREGNANCY
Increased nasal congestion

SYNONYMS
- Aerotitis
- Otitic barotrauma
- Middle ear barotrauma
- Middle ear squeeze

ICD-9-CM
993.0 Barotrauma, otitic
993.1 Barotrauma, sinus

SEE ALSO

OTHER NOTES
N/A

ABBREVIATIONS
SCUBA = self-contained underwater breathing apparatus

REFERENCES

- Paparella MM, Shumrick DA, et al, eds. Otolaryngology. 4th Ed. Philadelphia, W.B. Saunders Co., 1991
- Dehart R, ed. Fundamentals of Aerospace Medicine. Philadelphia, Lea & Febiger, 1985

Web references: 0 available at www.5mcc.com
Illustrations N/A

Author(s):
Smith L. Johnston, III, MD, MS

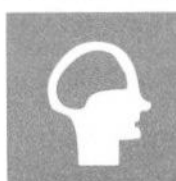

BASICS

DESCRIPTION Bartonella infections cause manifestations in two broad categories:
- Localized skin lesions and prominent regional lymphadenitis, i.e., typical cat scratch disease (CSD). Atypical CSD manifestations often represent disseminated infection.
- Primary bacteremia, potential for persistent disseminated infection with localized inflammatory (and neovascular) lesions in a variety of organ systems and/or ongoing bacteremia.

System(s) affected: Cardiovascular, Gastrointestinal, Hemic/Lymphatic/Immunologic, Musculoskeletal, Nervous, Pulmonary, Skin/Exocrine
Genetics: No defined genetic predisposition
Incidence/Prevalence in USA:
- Non-B. bacilliformis infections:
  - ◊ CSD: estimated 9.3/100,000 people (approximately 25,000 cases annually)
- Others, no incidence estimates

Predominant age:
- B. henselae infections:
  - ◊ CSD: 55% in persons < 18 years old
  - ◊ BA/BP, bacteremia, endocarditis, other syndromes: predominantly adults

Predominant sex: Non-B. bacilliformis infections: Male > Female

SIGNS & SYMPTOMS
- Carrión disease (the spectrum of *B. bacilliformis* infection)
  - ◊ Oroya fever (acute bacteremia): abrupt onset 3 weeks after inoculation, morbid course; severe anemia due to bacterial invasion of erythrocytes, many complications
  - ◊ Asymptomatic persistent bacteremia: <15% of Oroya fever survivors not treated with antibiotics
  - ◊ Verruga peruana: crops of nodular angiomatous skin lesions months after Oroya fever; mucosal and internal lesions also; involute in months to years
- Typical CSD (89% of cases)
  - ◊ 4-6 days after inoculation: 50-75% develop 2-3 mm macule at the trauma site; progresses to a papule or pustule
  - ◊ Regional adenopathy 1-8 weeks post-inoculation; sole manifestation in up to 50%
  - ◊ Nodes involved: 80% upper extremities, neck, head
  - ◊ Suppuration of involved nodes: 15%.
  - ◊ Malaise and/or fever: 30% of patients
  - ◊ Spontaneous resolution: 2-4 months for majority
- Atypical CSD (11% of cases)
  - ◊ Parinaud oculoglandular syndrome: granulomatous conjunctivitis and ipsilateral preauricular lymphadenitis
  - ◊ Neuroretinitis: usually unilateral; macular star exudate, papilledema, retinal nodules, angiomatous subretinal changes; self-limited, with return of visual acuity to near-baseline; concurrent *B. henselae* bacteremia found in some
  - ◊ Encephalopathy: mild-profound changes of higher cortical functions; seizures; neurologic sequelae rare
  - ◊ Other manifestations self-limited, sequelae rare: granulomatous hepatitis/splenitis, osteolysis, atypical pneumonitis, fever of undetermined origin (FUO), mononucleosis-type syndrome, others
- Bacteremia due to non-B. bacilliformis species: short-term fatality uncommon
  - ◊ *B. quintana*: (Eponyms: Trench fever, Wolhynia fever, shin-bone fever, quintan fever) Incubation days-weeks; sudden onset of fever, non-specific symptoms/signs; self-limited illness may be brief (4-5 days), prolonged (2-6 weeks), most commonly paroxysmal (3-5 episodes of 5 days duration).
  - ◊ *B. henselae*: HIV-infected: insidious onset of fatigue, malaise, aches, weight loss, recurring fevers, headache; localizing findings uncommon. HIV-uninfected: abrupt onset of fever, may persist or become relapsing; myalgias, arthralgias, headache; localizing findings unusual; asymptomatic persistence can evolve.
- Endocarditis: fever, new or changed heart murmur
- Bacillary angiomatosis/peliosis (BA/BP): neovascular proliferation disorders
  - ◊ BA: mostly immunocompromised hosts, e.g., HIV-infected; involves skin (crops of subcutaneous or dermal nodules, and/or skin-colored to purple papules; may ulcerate with serous or bloody drainage, and crusting), regional lymph nodes, internal organs; *B. henselae* and *B. quintana* both inculpated
  - ◊ BP involves liver and spleen in HIV-infected and other immunosuppressed persons; can involve lymph nodes as well; nonspecific clinical manifestations
- Neurologic in HIV-infected: cognitive dysfunction, behavioral disturbances; may be mistaken for HIV-related or other dementia, psychiatric disease

CAUSES
- *B. bacilliformis*: Carrión disease (limited to the Andes mountains)
- *B. quintana*: Trench fever, BA/BP, endocarditis
- *B. henselae*: Acute and persistent bacteremia, BA/BP complex, non-neovascular inflammation including endocarditis and CSD, neurologic manifestations
- *B. elizabethae*: Bacteremia with endocarditis (1 reported case)
- *B. clarridgeiae*: CSD (1 reported case)
- *B. vinsonii*: bacteremia (1 reported case)

RISK FACTORS
- Vector exposure with cutaneous inoculation
  - ◊ *B. bacilliformis*: Sandflies of the genus Lutzomyia (formerly Phlebotomus)
  - ◊ *B. quintana*: Human body louse, possibly others as yet unidentified
  - ◊ *B. henselae*: Domestic cat (especially scratch/bite from kitten < 1 year old), possibly cat fleas, possibly ticks
  - ◊ *B. elizabethae, B. vinsonii*: unknown
- Cell-mediated immune dysfunction (a role in BA/BP, possibly endocarditis)
  - ◊ HIV infection, especially with CD4+ lymphocyte count < 100/μL
  - ◊ Chronic corticosteroid, azathioprine, cyclophosphamide, cyclosporine, ethanol

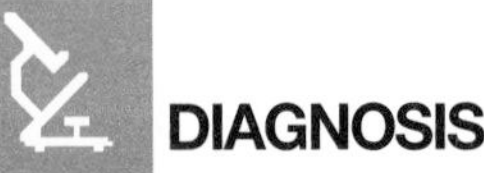

DIAGNOSIS

DIFFERENTIAL DIAGNOSIS
- Typical CSD: other causes of unilateral lymphadenopathy: *Sporothrix schenckii*, *Pasteurella* species, *Yersinia pestis*, *Francisella tularensis*, *Mycobacteria*, *Erysipelothrix rhusiopathiae*, *Staphylococci*, *Streptococci*, other agents associated injection drug use, lymphoma, metastatic malignancy
- Atypical CSD: other agents causing similar syndromes
- Non-bacilliformis *Bartonella* species bacteremia syndromes
  - ◊ In immunocompromised, especially HIV-infected: *Cryptococcus neoformans*, *Histoplasma capsulatum*, *Coccidioides immitis*, Mycobacterium avium-complex
  - ◊ After recent arthropod exposure: rickettsial infections, tularemia, plague, babesiosis, borreliosis (location-dependent).
  - ◊ After cat/dog scratch/bite: *Pasteurella* species infection
  - ◊ Viral illnesses: influenza, infectious mononucleosis, acute hepatitis, etc.
- Endocarditis: other fastidious/slow-growing bacteria associated with endocarditis, e.g. species of *Haemophilus*, *Actinobacillus*, *Cardiobacterium*, *Eikenella*, *Kingella*, *Coxiella*
- BA/BP: Kaposi sarcoma; pyogenic granuloma
- Neurologic in HIV-infected: other causes of encephalopathy, e.g., primary HIV-related, tertiary syphilis, cryptococcal meningitis, toxoplasmosis of brain, progressive multifocal leukoencephalopathy, alcohol or drug abuse

LABORATORY
- Non-bacilliformis *Bartonella spp*
  - ◊ Blood cultures: lysis-centrifugation (Isolator) cultures plated on blood or chocolate agar, incubated at 35-37°C in 5% CO_2 > 2 weeks; enriched broth media, e.g. BACTER, incubated at 35-37°C in 5% CO_2 >2 weeks and subculture to agar if bacilli detected by periodic acridine orange staining.
  - ◊ Tissue cultures: recovery from tissue homogenate plated on blood or chocolate agar may require >4 weeks
  - ◊ 1st generation serologic tests available in reference labs

Drugs that may alter lab results: Antibiotics: cultures falsely negative

Disorders that may alter lab results: N/A

PATHOLOGICAL FINDINGS
- Verruga peruana: neovascular proliferation, bacteria uncommonly identified
- CSD: stellate abscesses, mixed inflammatory infiltrates, granulomata, follicular hyperplasia of lymph nodes; bacilli in tissue demonstrable by silver impregnation stains (Warthin-Starry or Steiner) in about 1/3 cases
- Endocarditis: Warthin-Starry stained bacilli may be seen in vegetations

- BA/BP
  - ◊ BA lesions: lobular proliferations of small blood vessels containing cuboidal endothelial cells interspersed with inflammatory cells, mostly neutrophils. Fibrillar- or granular-appearing amphophilic material often seen in interstitium hematoxylin and eosin stain. Warthin-Starry stain or electron microscopy demonstrate these to be clusters of bacilli.
  - ◊ BP: involved organs contain blood-filled, partially endothelial cell-lined cystic structures and surrounding clumps of bacilli (identified by Warthin-Starry stain) in the midst of inflammatory cells.
- Neurologic in HIV-infected: little information

SPECIAL TESTS
- Skin testing reagents: not commercially available or standardized; use is not recommended
- Co-incubation of tissue homogenates with cell culture lines to enhance culture recovery; PCR and immunohistochemical labeling for non-culture detection in tissue: currently remain research tools

IMAGING Ultrasonography or CT as indicated

DIAGNOSTIC PROCEDURES
- Biopsies for histology/culture of cutaneous nodules, lymph nodes, or internal organs as necessary
- Typical CSD; traditionally, diagnosis required 3 of 4 criteria fulfilled:

(1) Animal contact (usually cat or dog) resulting in a scratch, abrasion or ocular lesion
(2) Positive serologic test (replaces positive skin test)
(3) Characteristic lymph node pathology
(4) Absence of evidence of other causes of lymphadenopathy

- Atypical CSD: compatible syndrome, absence of other evident cause; positive skin or serologic testing
- Bacteremia: clinical suspicion; use of appropriate culture methods
- Endocarditis: compatible clinical syndrome, evidence of valve lesion (ultrasonographic or tissue), positive culture of blood or valve (or non-culture demonstration, e.g., immunohistochemistry, polymerase chain reaction [PCR])
- BA/BP: biopsy for definitive diagnosis; presumptive diagnosis by response to appropriate antibiotics
- Neurologic in HIV-infected: (1) compatible clinical syndrome plus elevated antibodies in CSF or detection in CSF by culture or PCR, (2) no other cause

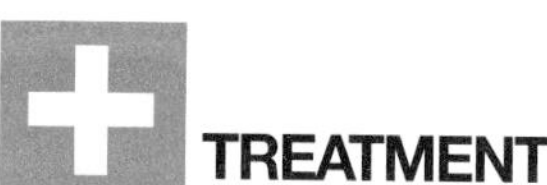

TREATMENT

APPROPRIATE HEALTH CARE
- Outpatient for uncomplicated infection
- Initial hospitalization may be necessary for complications

GENERAL MEASURES
- CSD: symptom-specific supportive therapy, e.g., aspiration of suppurative lymph nodes to alleviate pain
- Other syndromes (including CSD-associated neuroretinitis and encephalopathy): antibiotic therapy

SURGICAL MEASURES N/A

ACTIVITY Fully active if uncomplicated

DIET No special diet

PATIENT EDUCATION N/A

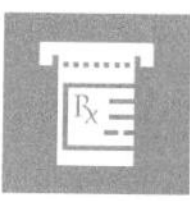

MEDICATIONS

DRUG(S) OF CHOICE
- *B. bacilliformis* infection: chloramphenicol 500 mg po qid for 1 week
- For typical CSD: no proven response to many agents including erythromycin, doxycycline, penicillin, cephalosporins; anecdotal reports of efficacy of rifampin > ciprofloxacin > gentamicin > trimethoprim-sulfamethoxazole. One placebo-controlled trial of oral azithromycin found some efficacy for 5 day course.
  - ◊ Azithromycin dose:
    - Adults and children > 45 kg: 500 mg on day 1, 250 mg daily on days 2-5
    - Children ≤ 45 kg: 10 mg/kg on day 1; 5 mg/kg daily on days 2-5
- Non-bacilliformis Bartonella infections including bacteremia without endocarditis, cutaneous BA + local lymph node involvement, CSD-associated neuroretinitis and encephalopathy, *B. henselae*-related neuro-psychiatric disorders in HIV-infected:
  - ◊ Erythromycin 500-1000 mg po bid or doxycycline 100 mg po bid for 4 weeks in immunocompetent; 8-12 weeks in immunocompromised (rifampin may play adjunctive role); azithromycin 250 mg qd for comparable duration should be effective as well
- Endocarditis, visceral or bony involvement with BA/BP: Erythromycin 500-1000 mg qid or doxycycline 100 mg bid x 2-4 weeks parenteral; complete 8-12 weeks po; azithromycin 250 mg qd for comparable duration should be effective as well

Contraindications: N/A
Precautions: N/A
Significant possible interactions: N/A

ALTERNATIVE DRUGS
- *B. bacilliformis* infection: tetracyclines
- Non-bacilliformis Bartonella infections: other tetracyclines, azithromycin, clarithromycin, chloramphenicol, ofloxacin, ciprofloxacin

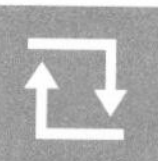

FOLLOWUP

PATIENT MONITORING Relapse may occur in non-CSD syndromes if therapy is too brief, close follow-up after completion of antibiotics is warranted

PREVENTION/AVOIDANCE Avoid contact with potential vectors, especially young cats. If cat scratch or bite occurs, wash the wound promptly and thoroughly.

POSSIBLE COMPLICATIONS Relapse, especially in HIV infection

EXPECTED COURSE/PROGNOSIS
- CSD - spontaneous resolution usually in 2-4 months without specific therapy
- Other syndromes - with proper treatment, full resolution; if relapse, consider long-term suppressive antibiotics after retreatment

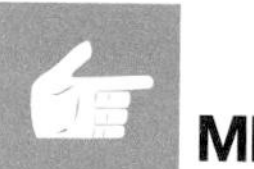

MISCELLANEOUS

ASSOCIATED CONDITIONS In advanced HIV infection, other opportunistic infections may be present

AGE-RELATED FACTORS
Pediatric: N/A
Geriatric: N/A
Others: N/A

PREGNANCY N/A

SYNONYMS
- Bartonellosis

ICD-9-CM
078.3 Cat-scratch disease
083.1 Trench fever
083.8 Other Bartonella-related diagnoses, including BA/BP
088.0 Bartonellosis

SEE ALSO

OTHER NOTES N/A

ABBREVIATIONS
CSD = Cat Scratch Disease
BA = Bacillary angiomatosis
BP = Bacillary peliosis
HIV = Human immunodeficiency virus

REFERENCES

- Bass LN, Vincent JM, Person DA. The expanding spectrum of Bartonella infections. Pediatr Infect Dis 1997;16:2-10, 163-179
- Spach DH, Koehler JE. Bartonella-associated infections. Infect Dis Clinics North Am 1998;12:137-155
- Slater LN, Welch DF. Bartonella species including cat-scratch disease. In: Mandell GL, Bennett JE, Dolin R, eds. Principles and Practices of Infectious diseases. 5th ed. Philadelphia: Churchill Livingstone; 2000

Web references: 0 available at www.5mcc.com
Illustrations 2 available

Author(s):
Leonard N. Slater, MD

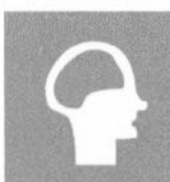

BASICS

DESCRIPTION Malignant tumor of the skin originating from the basal cells of the epidermis and its appendages. Rarely metastasizes but capable of local tissue destruction.
System(s) affected: Skin/Exocrine
Genetics: More common in fair-skin blondes and redheads
Incidence/Prevalence in USA: Approximately 900,000 cases/year
Predominant age: Generally > 40 but incidence is increasing in younger populations
Predominant sex: Males > Female (although incidence is increasing in females)

SIGNS & SYMPTOMS
- Begins as a small, smooth surfaced, well defined nodule
- Color pink to red
- "Pearly" translucent border
- Telangiectatic vessels overlying
- May have varying degrees of melanin pigment
- As nodule enlarges, central ulceration and crusting occurs

CAUSES
- Sun exposure
- Inorganic arsenic exposure
- X-ray exposure

RISK FACTORS
- Chronic sun exposure
- Light complexion
- Tendency to sunburn
- Male sex although increasing risk in women due to lifestyle changes e.g., suntan parlors, etc.
- Family history of skin cancer

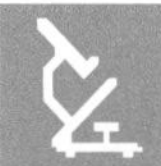

DIAGNOSIS

DIFFERENTIAL DIAGNOSIS Sebaceous hyperplasia, intradermal nevi (pigmented and non-pigmented), molluscum contagiosum

LABORATORY Pathologic examination required to confirm diagnosis

Drugs that may alter lab results: N/A

Disorders that may alter lab results: N/A

PATHOLOGICAL FINDINGS Nidus of basal cells extending into dermis. Characteristic cells resemble normal basal cells with large basophilic, oval nuclei. Rare mitoses. Tumor cells arranged in palisades at periphery.

SPECIAL TESTS N/A

IMAGING N/A

DIAGNOSTIC PROCEDURES Biopsy mandatory to confirm diagnosis

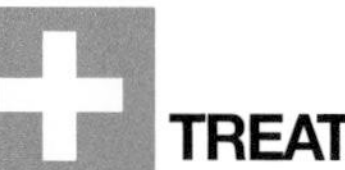

TREATMENT

APPROPRIATE HEALTH CARE Outpatient unless extensive lesion

GENERAL MEASURES N/A

SURGICAL MEASURES
- Treatment selection varies with extent and location of lesion, tumor border distinctiveness
- High risk areas - inner canthus, nasolabial sulcus, philtrum, preauricular area, retroauricular sulcus, lip, temple
- Curettage and electrodesiccation - nodular lesion < l cm, in low risk area, if not deeply invasive. Requires specialized training and experience in surgical technique.
- Excision - useful for lesions in high risk areas, not as dependent on lesion size. Poor choice if multiple lesions. Requires appropriate training.
- Cryosurgery - reserved for small lesions in low risk area. Requires specialized training and equipment. May want pre- and post-treatment biopsies.
- Moh's surgery - the preferred microsurgically- controlled surgical treatment for lesions in high risk area, for recurrent lesion, if there is an aggressive growth pattern. Requires referral to appropriately trained dermatologic surgeon.
- Radiation - useful for patients who could not tolerate minor surgical procedures (e.g., elderly patients). Also may be used when preservation of local tissue important such as near lips and eyelids.

ACTIVITY No restrictions except to avoid overexposure to sun

DIET No special diet

PATIENT EDUCATION
- Teach patient appropriate sun avoidance techniques, sunscreens, etc.
- Skin self exam

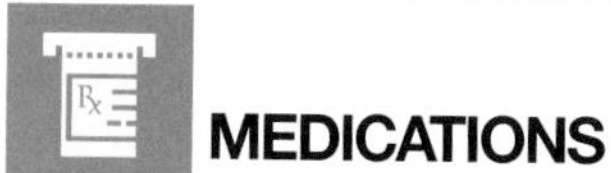

MEDICATIONS

DRUG(S) OF CHOICE Topical antibiotics after excision for 24 to 48 hours (optional)
Contraindications: N/A
Precautions: N/A
Significant possible interactions: N/A

ALTERNATIVE DRUGS N/A

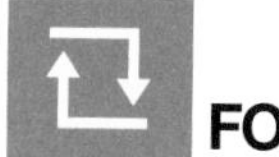

FOLLOWUP

PATIENT MONITORING Every month for 3 months, then twice yearly for 5 years, yearly thereafter

PREVENTION/AVOIDANCE
- Sunscreens
- Hats, long-sleeve shirts
- Avoid tanning and sunburn, especially during childhood

POSSIBLE COMPLICATIONS
- Local recurrence and spread. Usually recurrences will appear within 5 years.
- Metastasis (rare)

EXPECTED COURSE/PROGNOSIS
- Proper treatment yields 90-95% cure
- Most recurrences happen within 5 years
- Development of new basal cell carcinomas. 36% of patients will develop a new lesion within 5 years.

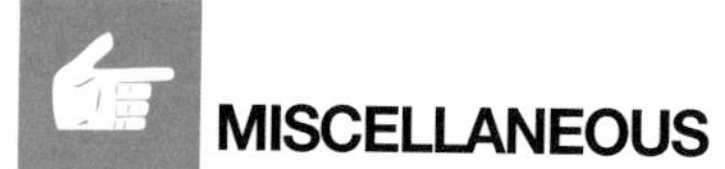

MISCELLANEOUS

ASSOCIATED CONDITIONS
- Xeroderma pigmentosum
- Nevoid basal cell carcinoma syndrome

AGE-RELATED FACTORS
Pediatric: Rare in children
Geriatric: Greater frequency in geriatric patients
Others: N/A

PREGNANCY N/A

SYNONYMS
- Basal cell epithelioma
- Rodent ulcer

ICD-9-CM
173.3 Other malignant neoplasm of skin of other and unspecified parts of face
173.4 Other malignant neoplasm of scalp and skin of neck
173.5 Other malignant neoplasm of skin of trunk, except scrotum
173.6 Other malignant neoplasm of skin of upper limb, including shoulder
173.7 Other malignant neoplasm of skin of lower limb, including hip
173.9 Other malignant neoplasm of skin, site unspecified

SEE ALSO

OTHER NOTES N/A

ABBREVIATIONS N/A

REFERENCES

- Fitzpatrick TN, et al: Dermatology in General Medicine. New York, McGraw-Hill, 1999
- Friedman RJ, et al: Cancer of the Skin. Philadelphia, W.B. Saunders Co., 1991
- Lever WF, et al. Histopathology of the Skin. Philadelphia, JB Lippincott, 1990
- Odom RB, et al. Andrews Diseases of the Skin: Clinical Dermatology. Philadelphia, WB Saunders Co, 2000

Web references: 1 available at www.5mcc.com
Illustrations 10 available

Author(s):
Tim DeBlieck, MD

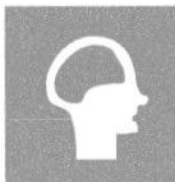

BASICS

DESCRIPTION Rare multisystem, chronic disease characterized by oral and genital mucocutaneous ulcerations, skin rashes, arthritis, thrombophlebitis, uveitis, colitis, and neurologic symptoms.
- Endemic in Japan and Northeastern Mediterranean region.

System(s) affected: Musculoskeletal, Nervous, Renal/Urologic, Reproductive, Skin/Exocrine
Genetics: One report in a mother and newborn (A. Fam, Ann Rheumatic Dis 1981;40:509-512). Very rarely familial.
Incidence/Prevalence in USA:
- 1/100,000 prevalence
- In other countries, per 100,000
  - ◊ Japan: 10
  - ◊ Iran: 16-100
  - ◊ Germany: 2
  - ◊ Saudi Arabia: 20

Predominant age: 3rd to 4th decades
Predominant sex: Male > Female; frequently twice as often. Some studies suggest equal frequency.

SIGNS & SYMPTOMS
- Aphthous stomatitis
- Genital ulcers - painful in the male, usually painless in the female
- Dermal - papulovesicular, erythema nodosum, pathergy, erythema multiforme, vasculitis, pyoderma
- Ocular - iritis, iridocyclitis, chorioretinitis, hypopyon, hemorrhage, papilledema, optic atrophy
- Morning stiffness - in 1/3
- Polyarthritis - self-limited and predominantly affecting lower extremities
- Thrombophlebitis - peripheral, pulmonary, cerebral, Budd Chiari syndrome
- Neurologic - cranial nerve palsy, hemiplegia, intracranial hypertension, meningomyelitis and recurrent meningitis, confusional state
- GI - aphthous ulcers, colitis, melena
- Pulmonary infiltrates - possibly related to thrombosis
- Myopathy/myositis - rare
- Peripheral gangrene - rare
- Epididymitis
- Glomerulonephritis - rare

CAUSES
- Unknown
  - ◊ Classified as vasculopathy or autoimmune
  - ◊ HLA-B5 alloantigen relationship
  - ◊ Possible environmental toxin - heavy metals, pesticides
  - ◊ Possibly English walnuts or Ginkgo nuts
  - ◊ Fibrinolysis abnormality
  - ◊ One report associated with HIV infection (C. Stein, J Rheumatol 1991;18,1427-8)

RISK FACTORS See Causes

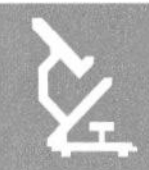

DIAGNOSIS

DIFFERENTIAL DIAGNOSIS
- Reiter syndrome and other forms of spondyloarthropathy
- Inflammatory bowel disease (Crohn disease and ulcerative colitis)
- Syphilis
- Erythema nodosum
- Aphthous stomatitis
- Herpes simplex
- Stevens-Johnson syndrome
- Vasculitis
- Multisystem disease
- Thrombophlebitis related to coagulation factor deficiency
- Mollaret meningitis

LABORATORY
- Erythrocyte sedimentation rate elevation, but can be normal
- Immune complexes detected by Raji cell and C1q solid phase assays, but not clinically useful
- Cryoglobulin
- Hypergammaglobulinemia
- Circulating anticoagulation (rare)
- Anti-cardiolipin antibody (rare)
- Pathergy

Drugs that may alter lab results: N/A

Disorders that may alter lab results: N/A

PATHOLOGICAL FINDINGS
- May be no recognizable changes
- Mononuclear perivascular infiltration
- Mononuclear infiltrate in synovium
- Endothelial cell swelling
- Partial obliteration of vascular lumen
- Neutrophilic dermatitis (Sweet syndrome) rarely

SPECIAL TESTS
- None specific for Behçet, but helpful in following disease course:
  - ◊ Depression of plasma antithrombin III levels with active disease
  - ◊ Increased fibrinolytic activity during attacks
  - ◊ Anti-neutrophil cytoplasmic antigen antibodies, perinuclear variety
  - ◊ Demyelinating antibodies in neuro-Behçet syndrome
  - ◊ Anti-cardiolipin antibodies, lupus anticoagulants
  - ◊ Anti-endothelial antibodies
  - ◊ Pathergy

IMAGING N/A

DIAGNOSTIC PROCEDURES
- Careful history and physical and frequent reevaluation
- Synovial fluid - inflammatory effusion
- Arteriography - for aneurysms or thrombosis

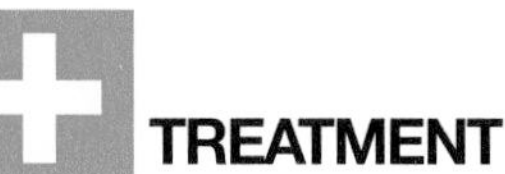

TREATMENT

APPROPRIATE HEALTH CARE Usually outpatient. Inpatient usually required for neurologic complications

GENERAL MEASURES According to body system involved

SURGICAL MEASURES N/A

ACTIVITY As tolerated

DIET No special diet

PATIENT EDUCATION
- American Behçet Association, 421 21st Avenue SW, Rochester, MN 55902, (507)281-3059

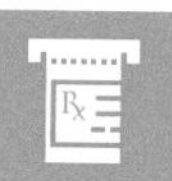

MEDICATIONS

DRUG(S) OF CHOICE
- Colchicine: 0.6 mg bid
- Topical ocular steroids
- Prednisone: 1 mg/kg for severe involvement, especially CNS
- Azathioprine: 2-3 mg/kg/day po
- Methotrexate: Use the lowest possible dose; perhaps 7.5 mg/week
- Cyclosporine: 1-4 mg/kg; but monitor LFT, creatinine, magnesium, lipids q2 wks x 3 mo, then q mo
- Resistant cases may require
  - ◊ Tacrolimus (FK 506) 0.09-0.15 mg/kg/day
  - ◊ Thalidomide 300 mg/day
  - ◊ Interferon alpha
  - ◊ Anti-coagulants for patients with anticardiolipin antibodies - warfarin (Coumadin) to establish PT-INR 3.0-3.5

Contraindications:
- Thalidomide contraindicated in pregnancy
- Refer to manufacturer's literature

Precautions:
- Refer to manufacturer's literature
- Absorption of drugs such as amitriptyline, diazepam, carbamazepine, phenytoin, and acetaminophen may be reduced in Behçet syndrome

Significant possible interactions: Refer to manufacturer's literature

ALTERNATIVE DRUGS
- Levamisole - 100-150 mg two days per week
- Chlorambucil - but concern with respect to toxicity, especially its malignant potential
- Cyclophosphamide: 50-100 mg/day q am. Patient should drink 8-10 glasses of water/day and report any blood in the urine.
- Tumor necrosis factor inhibitors
- Stem cell transplantation
- Anti-CD52 antibody

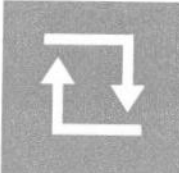

FOLLOWUP

PATIENT MONITORING Dependent on severity of system involvement and medication monitoring

PREVENTION/AVOIDANCE Avoid English walnuts

POSSIBLE COMPLICATIONS
- Death
- Blindness
- Paralysis
- Embolism/thrombosis - pulmonary, vena cava, peripheral
- Aneurysms
- Amyloidosis
- Thrombotic events, especially when anticardiolipin antibodies present

EXPECTED COURSE/PROGNOSIS
- Normal life expectancy, except with neurologic involvement
- Possible vision impairment

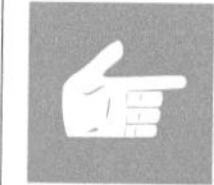

MISCELLANEOUS

ASSOCIATED CONDITIONS
- Amyloid
- Sweet syndrome

AGE-RELATED FACTORS
Pediatric: Rare
Geriatric: Rare
Others: N/A

PREGNANCY
- Thalidomide contraindicated in pregnancy
- Possible increase in thrombosis and fetal demise

SYNONYMS
- Mucocutaneous ocular syndrome
- Franceschetti-Valero syndrome

ICD-9-CM
136.1 Behçet syndrome

SEE ALSO

OTHER NOTES N/A

ABBREVIATIONS N/A

REFERENCES

- International diagnostic study group for Behçet's disease. Evaluation of ('classification') criteria in Behçet's disease - Towards internationally agreed criteria. Brit J Rheumatol 1992;31:299-308
- Shimizu T, et al: Behcet disease. Semin Arthritis Rheum 1979; 8:223-260
- Chaleby K: Clin Chem 1987;33:1679-1681
- O'Duffy JD: Behcet's disease. Curr Opin Rheumatol 1994;6:39-43 (note: this is better than the more recent Curr Opin Rheumatol reviews)
- Hamuryudan V, et al: Systemic interferon alpha-2b treatment in Behcet syndrome. J Rheumatol 1994;21:1098-1100
- Kaklamni VG, Vaiopoulos G, Koklomonis PG. Behcet's disease. Semin in Arthritis Rheum 1998;27:197-217
- Pacor ML, et al: Cyclosporin in Behcet's disease. J Rheumatol 1994;13:224-227
- Huong DL, et al: Arterial lesions in Behcet's disease. J Rheumatol 1995;22:2103-2113
- Akman-Demir G, et al: Seven year follow-up of neurologic involvement in Behcet syndrome. Arch Neurol 1996;53:691-768
- Gerber S, et al: Long-term MR follow-up of cerebral lesions in neuro-Behcet's disease. Neuroradiol 1996;38:761-768
- Kaklamani VG, et al: Behcet's disease. Semin in Arthritis Rheum 1998;27:197-217
- Lockwood CM, Hale G, Waldman H, Jayne DR. Remission induction in Behcet's disease following lymphocyte depletion by the anti-CD52 antibody CAMPATH 1-H. Rheumatology (Oxford) 2003;42(12):1539-44
- Hassard PV, Binder SW, Nelson V, Vasiliauskas EA. Anti-tumor necrosis factor monoclonal antibody therapy for gastrointestinal Behcet's disease: a case report. Gastroenterology 2001;120(4):995-9
- Sakane T, Takeno M, Suzuki N, Inaba G. Behcet's disease. N Engl J Med 1999;341(17):1284-91
- Zouboulis CC, Vaiopoulos G, Marcomichelakis N, Palimeris G, Markidou I, Thouas B, Kaklamanis P. Onset signs, clinical course, prognosis, treatment and outcome of adult patients with Adamantiades-Behcet's disease in Greece. Clin Exp Rheumatol 2003;21(4 Suppl 30):S19-26

Web references: 1 available at www.5mcc.com
Illustrations 1 available

Author(s):
Bruce M. Rothschild, MD

BASICS

DESCRIPTION Paralysis or weakness of the muscles supplied by the facial nerve, typically unilaterally, due to inflammation and swelling of the facial nerve within the facial canal
- Bell palsy: Idiopathic
- Ramsay Hunt syndrome: Bell palsy associated with vesicles within the outer ear canal or behind the ear, due to herpes zoster infection
- Facial diplegia: The simultaneous development of bilateral Bell palsy is highly unusual and conditions such as Guillain-Barré syndrome and chronic meningitis should be considered as possible explanations.

System(s) affected: Nervous
Genetics: There is a familial tendency toward Bell palsy
Incidence/Prevalence in USA: Incidence 16 in 100,000
Predominant age: Affects all ages. Most common in individuals over 30 years of age.
Predominant sex: Male = Female

SIGNS & SYMPTOMS
- Sudden onset or onset over days
- Unilateral total or partial paralysis of the facial muscles
- Mild "numbness" on the affected side
- Ipsilateral inadequate tear production; ipsilateral tearing
- Ipsilateral loss of taste
- Ipsilateral ear ache
- Ipsilateral exaggerated sound
- Ipsilateral loss of corneal reflex

CAUSES
- Bell palsy
  - ◊ Inflammation of the facial nerve within the facial canal
  - ◊ Exposure to cold
  - ◊ Probably viral
- Ramsay Hunt syndrome
  - ◊ Herpes zoster
  - ◊ Rarely Herpes simplex
- Diabetes mellitus

RISK FACTORS
- Age over 30
- Exposure to cold
- Diabetes
- Pregnancy
- Upper respiratory infection (coryza, influenza)

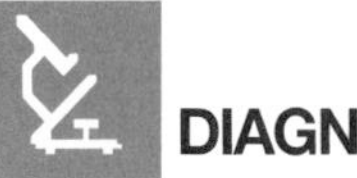

DIAGNOSIS

DIFFERENTIAL DIAGNOSIS
- Neoplastic
  - ◊ Carcinomatous meningitis
  - ◊ Leukemic meningitis
  - ◊ Tumors of the parotid gland
  - ◊ Tumors of the base of the skull
- Infectious
  - ◊ Lyme disease
  - ◊ Chronic meningitis
  - ◊ Bacterial meningitis
  - ◊ Osteomyelitis of the base of the skull
  - ◊ Otitis media
  - ◊ Leprosy
- Other
  - ◊ Sarcoidosis
  - ◊ Melkersson-Rosenthal syndrome (facial paralysis with scrotal tongue)
  - ◊ Head injury with fracture of the temporal bone
  - ◊ Brainstem stroke (anteroinferior cerebellar artery)
  - ◊ Multiple sclerosis
  - ◊ Guillain-Barré syndrome (can initially present as a very typical Bell palsy)
  - ◊ Multifocal acquired demyelinating sensory and motor neuropathy (a variant of CIDP)

LABORATORY
- CSF protein - mildly elevated in 1/3 of cases
- CSF cells - mildly elevated in 10% of cases, with a mononuclear cell predominance

Drugs that may alter lab results: N/A

Disorders that may alter lab results: N/A

PATHOLOGICAL FINDINGS
- Edema of the facial nerve
- Occasional hemorrhagic streaks
- Dilatation of the vasa nervorum
- Infiltration of mononuclear cells in some cases
- Atrophy of the facial nerve

SPECIAL TESTS
- Electromyography in the first three weeks after onset of the condition manifests a decreased or absent interference pattern on the affected side, which reflects a reduction or absence of function of the facial motor units. After three weeks, denervation potentials (fibrillations) are typically seen. Eventually, with recovery, low-amplitude, short-duration, polyphasic (nascent) motor units may appear in previously denervated areas. Recovery may be incomplete.
- Nerve conduction velocities may reveal absence or attenuation of the evoked potential, slowing of the conduction velocity or a normal conduction velocity and amplitude (variable due to varying severity and duration of condition)
- Blink reflex - the electrophysiological equivalent of the corneal reflex, should be abnormal in all cases

IMAGING MRI to rule out posterior fossa lesions and intracanalicular 8th nerve tumors if clinical suspicion is high. Bell palsy can be mimicked by small brainstem strokes.

DIAGNOSTIC PROCEDURES Spinal tap may reveal an elevated protein or cell count, however, it is usually not necessary

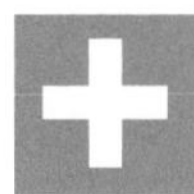

TREATMENT

APPROPRIATE HEALTH CARE
Outpatient except for surgical decompression (very controversial and largely abandoned)

GENERAL MEASURES
- Close and patch ipsilateral eye
- Methylcellulose eye drops

SURGICAL MEASURES Total failure of recovery can be treated by anastomosing the dental VII cranial nerve to the proximal end of another cranial nerve

ACTIVITY Fully active. Due to patching, use caution in activities requiring keen depth perception.

DIET No special diet

PATIENT EDUCATION Explanation and reassurance when appropriate

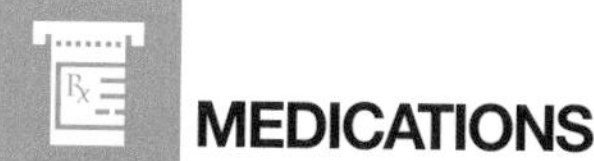

MEDICATIONS

DRUG(S) OF CHOICE
- Corticosteroids: Prednisone 80 mg po qd for three days, then 60 mg po qd for three days, then 40 mg po qd for three days, then 20 mg po qd for three days, then discontinue use. Course of treatment to begin immediately after onset of Bell palsy. There is little benefit in starting steroids after four days. Use of corticosteroids is controversial.
- Antiviral agents with activity against herpes group of viruses in Ramsay Hunt syndrome and idiopathic Bell palsy

Contraindications: Pre-existing infections including tuberculosis and systemic mycosis
Precautions: Use with discretion in pregnancy, peptic ulcer disease, and diabetes
Significant possible interactions: MMR, OPV, and other live vaccines

ALTERNATIVE DRUGS N/A

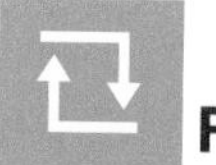

FOLLOWUP

PATIENT MONITORING
- Recheck monthly for six to twelve months
- Look for evidence of corneal abrasions. Expect early recovery.

PREVENTION/AVOIDANCE N/A

POSSIBLE COMPLICATIONS
- Unmasking of subclinical infection (such as tuberculosis) by steroid usage
- Steroid-induced psychological disturbances
- Steroid-induced avascular necrosis of hips, knees and/or shoulders
- Corneal abrasion and ulceration

EXPECTED COURSE/PROGNOSIS
- Complete, partial or no recovery of function. Patients with partial denervation typically fully recover. Patients with total denervation usually partially recover, but may exhibit aberrant regeneration (e.g., crocodile tears) or hemifacial spasm as long term complications.
- May recur on the same or opposite side

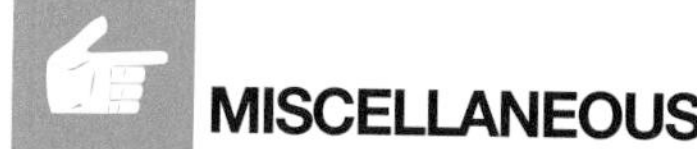

MISCELLANEOUS

ASSOCIATED CONDITIONS N/A

AGE-RELATED FACTORS
Pediatric: N/A
Geriatric: N/A
Others: N/A

PREGNANCY
Use steroids cautiously in pregnancy. Consult with obstetrician.

SYNONYMS
- Idiopathic facial paralysis

ICD-9-CM
351.0 Bell palsy

SEE ALSO
Herpes simplex
Herpes zoster

OTHER NOTES N/A

ABBREVIATIONS N/A

REFERENCES

- Dyck PJ, Thomas PK, et al, eds: Peripheral Neuropathy. 3rd Ed. Philadelphia, W.B. Saunders Co., 1993
- Murakemi S, et al. Bell palsy and herpes simplex virus: identification of viral DNA in endoneurial fluid and muscle.
- Ann Intern Med. 1996 Jan 1;124(1 Pt 1):27-30

Web references: 0 available at www.5mcc.com
Illustrations N/A

Author(s):
Colin R. Bamford, MD

BASICS

DESCRIPTION Due to its well protected location, bladder rupture is unusual. Injury most often secondary to penetrating or blunt trauma and classified as contusion, intraperitoneal or extraperitoneal rupture.
System(s) affected: Renal/Urologic
Genetics: N/A
Incidence/Prevalence in USA: N/A
Predominant age: N/A
Predominant sex: N/A

SIGNS & SYMPTOMS
- Suprapubic pain
- Urinary retention
- Hematuria (94%)
- Muscle rigidity over lower abdomen
- No peritonitis

CAUSES
- Forceful blunt or penetrating blow to lower abdomen, particularly with a full bladder

RISK FACTORS
- Distended bladder at the time of trauma
- Congenital malformation of bladder
- Prior pelvic or bladder surgery
- Frequently associated with pelvic fractures

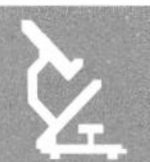

DIAGNOSIS

DIFFERENTIAL DIAGNOSIS
- Rupture of the urethra
- Rupture of abdominal viscus
- Pelvic fracture with hematoma

LABORATORY Hematuria on urinalysis

Drugs that may alter lab results: None

Disorders that may alter lab results: None

PATHOLOGICAL FINDINGS
- Jagged irregular tear in the bladder
- Perforation at the dome of bladder near urachus (blunt trauma)
- Extensive perivesical hematoma

SPECIAL TESTS None

IMAGING
- Cystogram with drain out film
- Urethrogram
- CT - cystogram

DIAGNOSTIC PROCEDURES
- Rarely is cystoscopy indicated

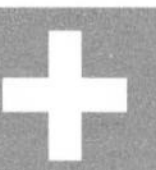

TREATMENT

APPROPRIATE HEALTH CARE Inpatient

GENERAL MEASURES
- Extraperitoneal rupture, insert foley, admit, conservative care
- Antibacterial coverage, broad spectrum
- Anticholinergics for spasm
- Pain medication as required
- Catheter removal in 10-14 days

SURGICAL MEASURES
- Intraperitoneal rupture, immediate surgical repair
- Blunt trauma, contusion, comfort care
- Penetrating injury, exploration, surgical repair

ACTIVITY Full activity when associated injuries permit

DIET No special diet

PATIENT EDUCATION Printed material available from multiple sources

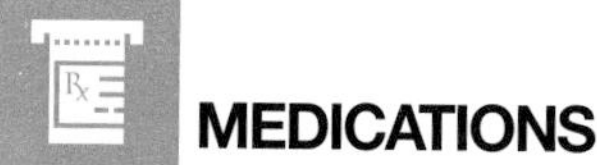

MEDICATIONS

DRUG(S) OF CHOICE
- Broad spectrum coverage, ciprofloxacin (Cipro) 500 mg bid
- Opium and belladonna suppositories q 6-8 hr prn spasms
- Oxybutynin (Ditropan) 5-10 mg tid for spasms
- Adequate pain control as required

Contraindications: Refer to manufacturer's profile of each drug
Precautions: Avoid quinolones (e.g., ciprofloxacin) in children
Significant possible interactions: Refer to manufacturer's profile of each drug

ALTERNATIVE DRUGS
- Other quinolones
- Other antispasmodics; e.g., flavoxate

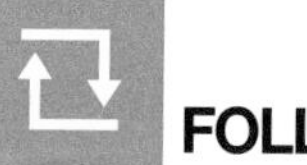

FOLLOWUP

PATIENT MONITORING
- Cystogram repeat in 7-10 days
- Remove catheter when bladder sealed
- Periodic check for infection and stricture formation

PREVENTION/AVOIDANCE
- Use seat belts
- Auto air bag

POSSIBLE COMPLICATIONS
- Infection
- Fistula formation (rare)
- Peritonitis (rare)

EXPECTED COURSE/PROGNOSIS
- Complete recovery
- Stricture (uncommon) - only long term complication

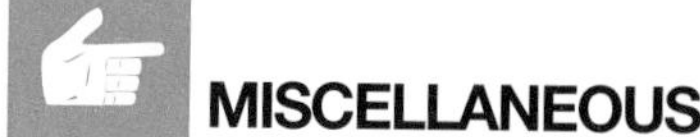

MISCELLANEOUS

ASSOCIATED CONDITIONS Frequently associated with pelvic fractures

AGE-RELATED FACTORS
Pediatric: Position of bladder makes intraperitoneal rupture more common
Geriatric: N/A
Others: N/A

PREGNANCY N/A

SYNONYMS N/A

ICD-9-CM
596.9 Unspecified disorder of bladder

SEE ALSO

OTHER NOTES N/A

ABBREVIATIONS N/A

REFERENCES

- Walsh PC, Gittes RF, Perlmutter AD. Campbell's Urology. 6th Ed. Philadelphia, W.B. Saunders Co., 1992

Web references: 0 available at www.5mcc.com
Illustrations N/A

Author(s):
Kevin Spear, MD

BASICS

DESCRIPTION An uncommon, systemic, fungal infection with a broad range of manifestations including pulmonary, skin, bone and genitourinary involvement

System(s) affected: Endocrine/Metabolic, Musculoskeletal, Pulmonary, Renal/Urologic, Skin/Exocrine

Genetics: N/A

Incidence/Prevalence in USA: Ranges from 0.4-4 cases per 100,000 population per year. Higher prevalence in states bordering the Mississippi and Ohio Rivers. Sporadic cases occurring in other areas.

Predominant age: Adults, but 10-20% of cases occur in children

Predominant sex: Male > Female

SIGNS & SYMPTOMS

- Acute infection
  - ◊ Onset may be abrupt or insidious
  - ◊ May be asymptomatic and self-limiting
  - ◊ Incubation period 30-45 days
  - ◊ Fever, chills, myalgias, arthralgias
  - ◊ Cough initially nonproductive, then productive
  - ◊ Hemoptysis (common)
  - ◊ Erythema nodosum
- Pulmonary blastomycosis
  - ◊ Three forms - acute, chronic, asymptomatic
  - ◊ Acute form presents as nonspecific, flu-like illness
  - ◊ Chronic pneumonia in 60-90% of patients with proven disease
  - ◊ Cough - nonproductive to productive
  - ◊ Hemoptysis
  - ◊ Weight loss
  - ◊ Pleuritic chest pain
  - ◊ Pleural effusions - 10%
  - ◊ Respiratory failure in small percentage
  - ◊ Upper lobe fibronodular infiltrates - 50%
  - ◊ Mass lesion - 30%
  - ◊ Cavitary lesions, nodular infiltrates, mass-like lesions are frequent in chronic pulmonary disease
  - ◊ Pleural thickening
- Cutaneous blastomycosis
  - ◊ Most common extrapulmonary manifestation - 40-80%
  - ◊ May occur with or without pulmonary disease
  - ◊ Two types of lesions
  - ◊ Verrucous lesions begin as small papulopustular lesions, slowly spread, become crusted, have sharp borders; central clearing with scar formation and depigmentation; microabscesses noted at periphery of lesion
  - ◊ Ulcerative lesions (initially pustules) form shallow ulcers with raised edges and granulating base
  - ◊ May be mistaken for pyoderma gangrenosum or squamous cell carcinoma
  - ◊ Mucosal lesions may occur
  - ◊ Regional adenopathy (uncommon)
  - ◊ Subcutaneous nodules - cold abscesses
- Skeletal blastomycosis
  - ◊ Occurs 25-50% of extrapulmonary cases
  - ◊ Long bones, vertebrae, ribs most commonly involved
  - ◊ Well circumscribed osteolytic lesions
  - ◊ May present with contiguous soft tissue abscesses and/or sinus tracts
  - ◊ Paraspinous abscess may occur in vertebral disease
  - ◊ Acute or chronic arthritis may result from extension of contiguous osteomyelitis
  - ◊ Joint involvement (usually large joints) - knees, ankles, hips
- Genitourinary blastomycosis
  - ◊ Occurs in 10-30% of cases
  - ◊ Involves prostate most commonly but also epididymis and testes
  - ◊ Outflow obstruction
  - ◊ Enlarged tender prostate
  - ◊ Involvement of female genitalia uncommon and usually acquired through sexual contact
- Other
  - ◊ Central nervous system involvement with acute or chronic meningitis, epidural or cerebral abscesses: more common in AIDS
  - ◊ Liver, spleen, pericardium, thyroid, gastrointestinal tract, adrenal gland may each be involved

CAUSES

- Inhalation of spores of *Blastomyces dermatitidis* into lung with spread to other organ systems by lymphohematogenous dissemination
- Primary inoculation of skin may rarely occur
- Female genital infection may result from sexual transmission
- Reactivation of previous infection may occur in immunocompromised patients including those with AIDS

RISK FACTORS

- Occupational or recreational exposure to soil containing spores of *B. dermatitidis*
- Residence in areas of increased disease prevalence
- Rarely associated with AIDS
- Long-term corticosteroids, hematologic malignancies

DIAGNOSIS

DIFFERENTIAL DIAGNOSIS

- Pulmonary - acute bacterial pneumonia, tuberculosis, other fungal diseases, bacterial lung abscess, empyema, bronchogenic carcinoma
- Cutaneous - bacterial pyoderma, cutaneous mycobacterial infection, other cutaneous fungal infections (sporotrichosis, histoplasmosis, cryptococcosis), squamous cell carcinoma
- Bone - bacterial osteomyelitis, tuberculosis, neoplastic disease
- Genitourinary - bacterial prostatitis, prostate cancer, other fungal infections, tuberculosis

LABORATORY

- Culture of *B. dermatitidis* from tissue or body secretions on Sabouraud's or other enriched media
- Demonstration of yeast forms (5-15 micrometers in diameter, with refractile cell wall, broad-based budding and no capsule) in tissue or body secretions by wet mount or special stains
- In pulmonary disease, KOH prep of sputum reveals organism 50-70% of time
- Serologic tests include complement fixation, enzyme-linked immunoassay, immunodiffusion precipitin antibody tests. All have variable sensitivity and low specificity and are not helpful in diagnosis.
- Delayed hypersensitivity skin testing with blastomycin also has low sensitivity and specificity and not useful in diagnosis

Drugs that may alter lab results: N/A

Disorders that may alter lab results: Histoplasma cross-reacts with serologic tests for blastomycosis

PATHOLOGICAL FINDINGS

- Early inflammatory response with polymorphonuclear leukocytes followed by granuloma formation with lymphocytes and macrophages
- Granulomas do not show caseation necrosis
- Yeast is often found attached to or inside monocytes, macrophages and giant cells

SPECIAL TESTS

- Special staining of tissue with Gomori methenamine silver stain
- Periodic acid-Schiff's stain colors cell wall pink or red
- Mucicarmine stain helps differentiate from encapsulated Cryptococcus

IMAGING

- CT scan of head for CNS lesions
- CT scan of spine for vertebral lesions
- Bone scan for skeletal lesions
- Chest x-ray may show upper lobe fibronodular infiltrates, consolidation, diffuse alveolar infiltrates, mass lesions or pleural thickening

DIAGNOSTIC PROCEDURES

- Aspiration of abscess contents for wet mount and culture
- Needle or surgical biopsy of involved tissue

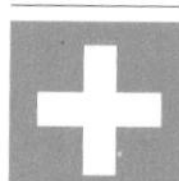

TREATMENT

APPROPRIATE HEALTH CARE
- Acute non-life-threatening pulmonary infection may be treated with oral itraconazole as an outpatient
- Severe life threatening infection, central nervous system disease or disease in immunocompromised host should be treated initially with intravenous amphotericin B in the hospital

GENERAL MEASURES
- Systemic antifungal therapy is indicated for all cases of extrapulmonary blastomycosis
- Systemic antifungal therapy is indicated for all but the very mild or asymptomatic pulmonary cases in which a trial of observation may be appropriate

SURGICAL MEASURES
- Surgical débridement of bone lesions if there are areas of devitalized bone
- Surgical drainage of large cutaneous abscesses or pleural empyemas

ACTIVITY No restrictions, once patient is released from hospital

DIET No special dietary requirement

PATIENT EDUCATION Counsel patient and family on potential adverse effects associated with antifungal therapy, duration of therapy required and potential for relapse or chronic infection

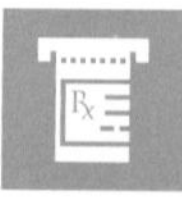

MEDICATIONS

DRUG(S) OF CHOICE
- Milder forms
  - ◊ Itraconazole (Sporanox) 200 mg po twice a day for at least 6 months
    - Bioavailability enhanced when taken with food
    - Antacids or H2 blockers result in lower serum level
    - Very little drug excreted in urine; GU disease more resistant to therapy
- Severe forms
  - ◊ Amphotericin B (Fungizone): 0.5-0.8 mg/kg IV over 4-6 hours daily for a cumulative dose of 1.5-2 gm
    - First dose of amphotericin B is given as a test dose of 1 mg in 200 mL dextrose 5% in sterile water intravenously over 2-4 hours
    - Dose is increased by 10 mg daily until a maintenance dose of 0.5 mg-0.8 mg per kg per day is reached. Slow escalation is not appropriate for severe blastomycosis. Full dose can be given on 1st or 2nd day of treatment.
    - Rigors can be prevented by pre-infusion dose of meperidine 50 mg
    - To reduce infusion-related fever, pre-infusion acetaminophen and diphenhydramine

Contraindications:
- Life threatening intolerance to amphotericin such as anaphylaxis
- CNS disease
  - ◊ Amphotericin B: total dose 2 gm
  - ◊ Alternative to amphotericin B - fluconazole 800 mg/d because of good CNS penetration

Precautions:
- Monitor for hypotension during the infusion
- Monitor renal function, serum sodium, potassium and magnesium, and CBC twice weekly during therapy
- Replace potassium and magnesium as indicated
- When serum creatinine rises to 1.6 mg/dL (141 μmol/L) or greater, dosage interval should be changed to 48 hours
- Watch for phlebitis at infusion site
- Consider peripherally inserted central catheter (PICC) for infusion

Significant possible interactions:
- Avoid use of potentially nephrotoxic drugs such as aminoglycosides which may potentiate nephrotoxicity of amphotericin B
- Itraconazole - concurrent use of rifampin, phenytoin or carbamazepine may increase hepatic metabolism resulting in lower serum drug levels and treatment failure

ALTERNATIVE DRUGS
Efficacy of alternate regimens not well established by controlled studies
- Fluconazole 400 mg daily for 6 months for non-life-threatening blastomycosis
- Ketoconazole (Nizoral): 400-800 mg po daily for 6 months
- Lipid preparations of amphotericin B have not been adequately evaluated in human blastomycosis; they may provide an alternative for selected patients unable to tolerate standard amphotericin B

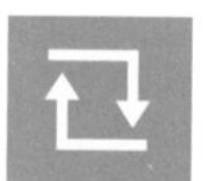

FOLLOWUP

PATIENT MONITORING
- Monitor closely during early therapy
- Frequency of followup depends on severity of disease
- Monitor serum electrolytes, creatinine and CBC twice weekly during amphotericin B therapy
- Post-therapy followup every 3 months for 2 years then twice yearly

PREVENTION/AVOIDANCE
- Unknown
- Condoms for sexual encounters

POSSIBLE COMPLICATIONS Treatment-induced nephrotoxicity, electrolyte imbalance, anemia

EXPECTED COURSE/PROGNOSIS
- Cure in over 90% with appropriate therapy
- Relapse in less than 10% of cases
- Relapse rate higher with ketoconazole therapy
- Adverse reactions with amphotericin B are frequent and significant

MISCELLANEOUS

ASSOCIATED CONDITIONS N/A

AGE-RELATED FACTORS
Pediatric: Uncommon in children
Geriatric: Prognosis is worse in elderly patients with significant underlying pulmonary or renal disease
Others: N/A

PREGNANCY
- Amphotericin B is drug of choice
- Azoles should not be used in pregnancy

SYNONYMS North American blastomycosis

ICD-9-CM
116.0 Blastomycosis

SEE ALSO

OTHER NOTES N/A

ABBREVIATIONS N/A

REFERENCES

- Mandell GL, editor. Principles and Practice of Infectious Diseases. 5th ed. New York: Churchill Livingstone; 2000
- Patel RG, et al. Clinical presentation, radiographic findings, and diagnostic methods of pulmonary blastomycosis: A Review of 100 consecutive cases. South Med J 1999;92:289-95
- Chapman SW, et al. Practice guidelines for the management of patients with blastomycosis. Clinical Infect Dis 2000;30:679-83

Web references: 0 available at www.5mcc.com
Illustrations N/A

Author(s):
William G. Gardner, MD

BASICS

DESCRIPTION An inflammatory reaction of the eyelid margin. It usually occurs as seborrheic (non-ulcerative) or as staphylococcal (ulcerative) blepharitis. Both types may coexist.
System(s) affected: Skin/Exocrine
Genetics: N/A
Incidence/Prevalence in USA: Common (the most frequent ocular disease)
Predominant age: Adult
Predominant sex: Male = Female

SIGNS & SYMPTOMS
- *Staphylococcus aureus* blepharitis
  - ◊ Itching
  - ◊ Lacrimation; tearing
  - ◊ Burning
  - ◊ Photophobia (light sensitivity)
  - ◊ Usually worse in morning
  - ◊ Recurrent stye (external hordeolum, or internal hordeolum)
  - ◊ Recurrent chalazia (chronic inflammation of meibomian glands)
  - ◊ Fine, epithelial keratitis, lower half of cornea
  - ◊ Ulcerations at base of eyelashes
  - ◊ Broken, sparse, misdirected eyelashes(trichiasis)
- Seborrheic blepharitis
  - ◊ Lid margin erythema
  - ◊ Dry flakes, oily secretions on lid margins and/or lashes
  - ◊ Associated dandruff of scalp, eyebrows
  - ◊ Sometimes nasolabial erythema, scaling
- Mixed blepharitis (seborrheic with associated Staph aureus)
  - ◊ Most common type of blepharitis
  - ◊ Symptoms and signs of both staph and seborrheic present

CAUSES
- Seborrheic
  - ◊ Accelerated shedding of skin cells with associated sebaceous gland dysfunction
  - ◊ P. ovale and P. orbiculare yeasts often colonize
  - ◊ Oil and skin cells foster staph growth
- Staphylococcus
  - ◊ Usually part of mixed blepharitis
  - ◊ Colonization of Zeis glands of lid margin and meibomian glands posterior to lashes, with Staphylococcus aureus
  - ◊ Impetigo contagiosa-staphylococcus
  - ◊ Infectious eczematoid dermatitis-Staphylococcus is the hapten
  - ◊ Staphylococcus scalded skin syndrome - entire body involved (in young children)
  - ◊ Angular blepharitis staph - most frequent bacteria involved
- Other types of blepharitis
  - ◊ Contact dermatitis with or without secondary Staphylococcus infection
  - ◊ Meibomian gland dysfunction

RISK FACTORS
- Candida
- Seborrheic dermatitis
- Acne rosacea
- Diabetes mellitus
- Immunocompromised state (AIDS, chemotherapy, etc.)

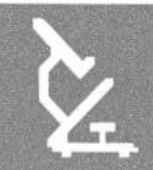

DIAGNOSIS

DIFFERENTIAL DIAGNOSIS
- Masquerade syndrome:
  - ◊ Persistent inflammation and thickening of eyelid margin may indicate squamous cell, basal cell, or sebaceous cell carcinoma masquerading as "blepharitis"
  - ◊ These carcinomas may also mimic styes or chalazions
  - ◊ Sebaceous cell carcinoma has a 23% fatality rate (found in one study of eyelid sebaceous cell carcinomas). Up to one half of potentially fatal sebaceous cell carcinomas may resemble benign inflammatory diseases, particularly chalazions and chronic blepharoconjunctivitis.
  - ◊ Any swelling or inflammation of eyelid which does not resolve promptly (within one month) with treatment, is suspect as a possible underlying carcinoma

LABORATORY N/A

Drugs that may alter lab results: N/A

Disorders that may alter lab results: N/A

PATHOLOGICAL FINDINGS
Acute or chronic inflammatory cell types

SPECIAL TESTS
- Cultures in atypical blepharitis
- Biopsy in atypical cases that are suspect for carcinoma

IMAGING N/A

DIAGNOSTIC PROCEDURES
See Special Tests

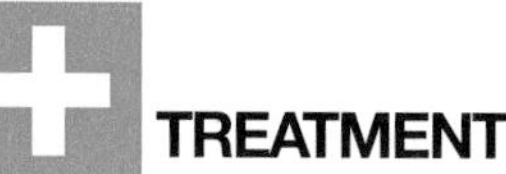

TREATMENT

APPROPRIATE HEALTH CARE
Outpatient

GENERAL MEASURES
- Mild seborrheic blepharitis (dry flakes, minimal inflammation) - apply eyelid margin scrubs with eyelid cleanser at least once daily
- If Staphylococcus likely, follow lid scrubs with application of bacitracin, or (second choice), erythromycin ophthalmic ointment, to eyelid margins, using cotton tipped applicator
- Clean lids and apply ointment nightly in mild cases, up to four times daily in severe cases
- Discontinue soft contact lenses until condition cleared
- Chronic recurrent blepharitis requires referral to ophthalmologist for evaluation as to whether patient should continue in lenses

SURGICAL MEASURES N/A

ACTIVITY
No restrictions

DIET
No restrictions

PATIENT EDUCATION
- Blepharitis "Fact Sheet" from American Academy of Ophthalmology (see References for ordering information)
- Advise patient that blepharitis is a chronic condition, prone to recurrence if hygiene (lid scrubs) are not maintained after antibiotic treatment is discontinued

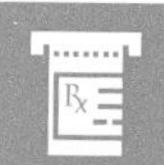

MEDICATIONS

DRUG(S) OF CHOICE

- Topical treatment, if Staphylococcus likely, application of bacitracin, or (second choice), erythromycin ophthalmic ointment
- In some cases of Staphylococcus blepharitis (e.g., rosacea), systemic tetracycline 250 mg qid x several weeks, tapering to 250 mg daily for one to three months, or doxycycline 100 mg bid po. Alternative is oxacillin 250 mg qid for 1-2 weeks. Used for persistent (despite topical treatment) lid inflammation or recurrent meibomian styes.

Contraindications:

- Allergy to medication
- Tetracycline: not for use in pregnancy or children < 8 years

Precautions:

- Avoid medication containing neomycin, as it is sensitizing
- Tetracycline: may cause photosensitivity; sunscreen recommended

Significant possible interactions:

- Tetracycline: avoid concurrent administration with antacids, dairy products, or iron
- Broad-spectrum antibiotics: may reduce the effectiveness of oral contraceptives; barrier method recommended

ALTERNATIVE DRUGS

Quinolones may be helpful for persistent or recurrent Staphylococcal blepharitis

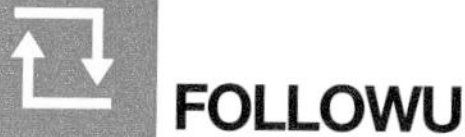

FOLLOWUP

PATIENT MONITORING Every 2 months

PREVENTION/AVOIDANCE Follow treatment guidelines

POSSIBLE COMPLICATIONS

- Hordeolum (stye)
- Scarring of eyelid margin
- Misdirection of eyelashes (trichiasis)
- Corneal infection

EXPECTED COURSE/PROGNOSIS

Long-term eyelid hygiene required to control

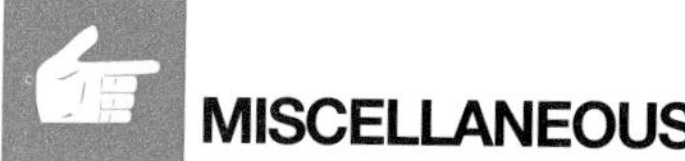

MISCELLANEOUS

ASSOCIATED CONDITIONS See diagnosis section above regarding blepharitis masquerade syndromes

AGE-RELATED FACTORS

Pediatric: N/A
Geriatric: N/A
Others: N/A

PREGNANCY N/A

SYNONYMS N/A

ICD-9-CM

373.00 Blepharitis, unspecified

SEE ALSO

OTHER NOTES N/A

ABBREVIATIONS N/A

REFERENCES

- Tasman W, ed. Duane's Clinical Ophthalmology. Philadelphia, J.B. Lippincott Co., 2002
- Boniuk M, Zimmerman LE. Sebaceous carcinoma of the eyelid, eyebrow, caruncle, and orbit. Trans Am Acad Ophthalmol Otolaryngol 1968;72:619
- Rao NA, McLean IW, Zimmerman LE. Sebaceous carcinoma of the eyelids and caruncles: Correlation of clinicopathological features of prognosis. In: Jakobic FA, ed. Ocular and Adnexal Tumors. Birmingham, Aesculapius 1978:461
- American Academy of Ophthalmology, Department of Patient Education. Blepharitis Fact Sheet. San Francisco, American Academy of Ophthalmology. Available for order as tear-off pads, phone (415)-561-8500 to order or write AAO, P.O. Box 7424, San Francisco, CA 94120-7424

Web references: 1 available at www.5mcc.com
Illustrations N/A

Author(s):
T. Glendon Moody, MD

BASICS

DESCRIPTION Primary malignant bone tumors are rare. Four types make up the majority.
- Malignant fibrous histiocytoma (MFH) - a pleomorphic sarcoma of storiform pattern without differentiation
- Osteosarcoma - similar to malignant fibrous histiocytoma with differentiation to osteoid production
- Osteosarcoma - cellular cartilaginous lesion with abundant binucleate cells, myxoid areas, and pushing borders
- Ewing sarcoma - small, blue-round cell neoplasm

System(s) affected: Musculoskeletal

Genetics:
- Ewing sarcoma has 11/22 chromosomal translocation and EW5-FLI-1 fusion protein
- Osteosarcomas shows loss of retinoblastoma and p53 suppressor genes and amplification of the genes C-myc, mdm-2, SAS, and cyclin-dependent kinase

Incidence/Prevalence in USA:
Rare: 5000 bone and soft tissue sarcomas per year, a practicing orthopedic surgeon may see one primary malignant tumor of bone in every five years of practice. Ewing sarcoma is less common in blacks.

Predominant age:
- MFH - teens and elderly
- Osteogenic sarcoma - teens and early twenties
- Chondrosarcoma - very young and very old
- Ewing sarcoma - children, teens, and early twenties

Predominant sex: Male = Female

SIGNS & SYMPTOMS
- Pain with weight bearing, at rest and at night
- Swelling
- Tenderness
- Fracture with minor trauma
- Minor injury may bring attention to lesion

CAUSES
- Generally unknown
- MFH often follows irradiation or arises in old bone infarct
- Osteosarcoma has association with loss of suppressor retinoblastoma and p53 genes
- Chondrosarcoma may arise in pre-existing enchondroma or exostosis

RISK FACTORS
- Multiple enchondromatosis (Ollier's disease) - chondrosarcoma
- Multiple hereditary exostosis - chondrosarcoma
- Previous irradiation, risk factor for MFH
- Previous history of bilateral retinoblastoma - osteosarcoma

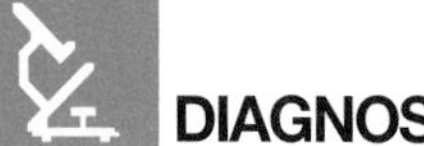

DIAGNOSIS

DIFFERENTIAL DIAGNOSIS
- Solitary metastatic lesion or myeloma especially in the patient over age 40
- Lymphoma at any age
- Benign bone tumors and benign bone tumors that look aggressive (aneurysmal bone cyst, giant cell tumor, eosinophilic granuloma)
- Infection (osteomyelitis)
- Metabolic bone disease (osteopenia, Paget, hyperparathyroidism)
- Synovial diseases (pigmented villonodular synovitis, synovial chondromatosis, degenerative or inflammatory synovitis)
- Myositis ossificans and repair reaction to trauma
- Avascular necrosis

LABORATORY
- 50% of osteosarcomas have an elevated alkaline phosphatase
- Ewing sarcoma may be associated with an elevated ESR and LDH
- Acid phosphatase, prostatic specific antigen to exclude prostatic carcinoma
- Calcium, phosphate, alkaline phosphatase
- Thyroid function tests to exclude thyroid carcinoma
- Elevated ESR and WBC in osteomyelitis
- Serum protein electrophoresis and urine electrophoresis to exclude myeloma

Drugs that may alter lab results: N/A

Disorders that may alter lab results: N/A

PATHOLOGICAL FINDINGS
- Histology and special studies in combination with radiographic findings confirms the diagnosis
- Ewing sarcoma expresses MIC-2 protein (CD99)
- Electron microscopy: glycogen granules in Ewing sarcoma; neurosecretory granules in neuroectodermal tumors; Birbeck bodies in histiocytosis-X
- Osteosarcoma may express Her-2/neu indicating, if present a more aggressive tumor, but one which may respond more favorably to trastuzumab (Herceptin)

SPECIAL TESTS
- Open biopsy or needle biopsy. Needle biopsies may not provide enough tissue for frozen section, touch prep, permanent section, snap freezing, electron microscopy, cytogenetic and molecular studies, DNA indices, immunoperoxidase staining and immunophenotyping (lymphoma).
- Biopsy of associated soft tissue mass may lessen the risk of pathologic fracture
- Biopsy tract should to be excised in continuity with the tumor at the time of resection.

IMAGING
- Plain films provide the most important information regarding the nature of the lesion and guide further testing
- Bone scan - prior to biopsy, looking for other lesions
- CT scan for cortical destruction and internal calcification or ossification. Abdominal CT, MRI or renal ultrasound to exclude hypernephroma.
- MRI scan determines the extent of marrow involvement and associated soft tissue mass
- Chest x-ray and chest CT for metastatic disease.
- Mammogram to exclude breast carcinoma

DIAGNOSTIC PROCEDURES
- Rectal exam for prostatic nodules
- Laboratory studies for metabolic bone disease

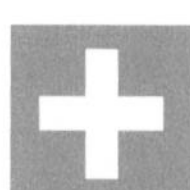

TREATMENT

APPROPRIATE HEALTH CARE Inpatient surgery

GENERAL MEASURES N/A

SURGICAL MEASURES
- Resection with adequate margin is required to minimize risk of local persistence
- For MFH and osteosarcoma, pre-resection neo-adjuvant chemotherapy treats micrometastatic disease immediately, allows time for ordering replacement prosthesis and bone graft, allows for an in vivo assessment of the chemotherapy responsiveness of the tumor, and may facilitate limb salvage by allowing a "safer" close margin
- Chondrosarcoma in the extremities should be treated exclusively by surgery unless it is of the mesenchymal or de-differentiated high grade variety
- Ewing sarcoma was traditionally treated with chemotherapy and surgery was limited to those lesions that were extremely large, associated with pathologic fracture, or involved an expendable bone. Most Ewing sarcoma lesions were irradiated. However, despite irradiation, local recurrence is common up to 25% in pelvic lesions. Therefore, surgery with limb salvage is increasingly accepted. A dramatic decrease in size in Ewing sarcoma occurs after initial chemotherapy and a decision can then be made after restaging as to whether to irradiate or to resect the primary lesion.
- The treatment goal is to minimize local recurrence while preserving function. Limb salvage is employed whenever a safe margin can be obtained.

ACTIVITY Varies with stage of disease and treatment

DIET No special diet

PATIENT EDUCATION Refer to local branch of American Cancer Society for information and support groups

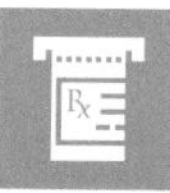

MEDICATIONS

DRUG(S) OF CHOICE

These drugs are administered according to specific protocols. Other protocols may be appropriate.

- MFH and osteosarcoma:
  - ◊ Doxorubicin (Adriamycin)
  - ◊ Intra-arterial and intravenous cisplatin
  - ◊ High dose methotrexate with leucovorin rescue
  - ◊ Ifosfamide [with mesna to protect against hemorrhagic cystitis]
  - ◊ Cyclophosphamide (Cytoxan)
  - ◊ Dactinomycin (actinomycin-D)
  - ◊ Bleomycin
- Liposome-encapsulated muramyl tripeptide phosphatidylethanolamine (liposomal MTP-PE) immune modulating agent for osteosarcoma (under trial in CCSG and POG)
- Ewing sarcoma:
  - ◊ Cyclophosphamide
  - ◊ Vincristine
  - ◊ Actinomycin D
  - ◊ Doxorubicin (Adriamycin)
  - ◊ Ifosfamide
  - ◊ Etoposide

Contraindications: Refer to manufacturer's literature

Precautions:

- Left ventricular dysfunction with Adriamycin. Cumulative dose > 450 mg/m2 increases risk. Follow with serial echocardiograms and/or MUGA scans when cumulative dose > 250 mg/m2.
- With high dose methotrexate, hydration, alkalinization of the urine, and close monitoring of plasma levels are needed

Significant possible interactions:

- Myelosuppression
- Renal tubular dysfunction with ifosfamide
- Renal and hepatic dysfunction and GI mucositis with methotrexate
- Nephrotoxicity and ototoxicity with cisplatin

ALTERNATIVE DRUGS

- Ondansetron (Zofran), dronabinol (Marinol), metoclopramide (Reglan), and others for nausea control

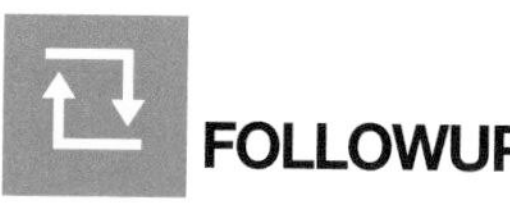

FOLLOWUP

PATIENT MONITORING

- Patients who require adjuvant chemotherapy are treated after resection of the tumor with maintenance chemotherapy
- Blood counts for myelosuppression
- Serial echocardiograms when Adriamycin is being used. G-CSF often used to minimize neutropenia.
- Chest x-rays obtained every two months for the first year, every three months for the second year, and every four months in the third year
- CT scans of the lungs are initially repeated every six months during first two years
- Ewing sarcoma may recur > 5 years after diagnosis

PREVENTION/AVOIDANCE

None identified

POSSIBLE COMPLICATIONS

- Limb salvage with any primary malignant bone tumor is fraught with potential complications
- Micrometastatic disease may have occurred at the time of presentation and can appear at any time during the course of treatment or followup
- Local recurrence risk for osteosarcoma with limb salvage is about 10%
- There can be leg length discrepancy, infection, wound dehiscence, skin coverage problems, arterial and nerve injury, non-union of bone grafts, and mechanical loosening of prosthetic implants
- Thoracotomy and continued chemotherapy is often recommended for metastatic disease to the lung
- Ewing sarcoma, metastatic to the lung, is quite diffuse and is less amenable to thoracotomy

EXPECTED COURSE/PROGNOSIS

- With amputation alone, 80% of patients with osteosarcoma had pulmonary metastatic disease by two years. With chemotherapy, the five year disease-free survival rate is 50-85%.
- Favorable prognostic factors for MFH and osteosarcoma include responsiveness to chemotherapy, distal portions of the extremities, small size, age over ten
- Most chondrosarcomas are of lower grade and have a low risk of metastatic spread and low incidence of local recurrence after adequate surgery
- MFH, osteosarcoma, and Ewing sarcoma have an overall 50% survival with combined treatment modalities

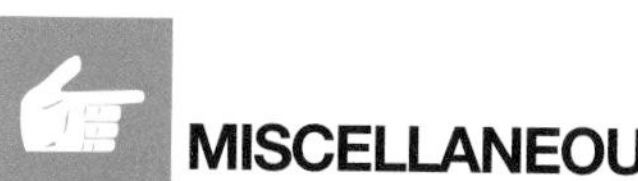

MISCELLANEOUS

ASSOCIATED CONDITIONS

- A higher incidence of chondrosarcoma is seen in patients with multiple hereditary exostosis, multiple enchondromatosis (Ollier disease) and patients with enchondromatosis and hemangiomatosis (Maffucci syndrome)
- Patients with enchondromatosis more often die of GI malignancies than metastatic chondrosarcoma

AGE-RELATED FACTORS

Pediatric: N/A
Geriatric: N/A
Others: N/A

PREGNANCY

- Increased growth of musculoskeletal malignancies during pregnancy
- Soft tissue desmoid tumors have estrogen and progesterone receptors

SYNONYMS

N/A

ICD-9-CM

170.9 Malignant neoplasm of bone and articular cartilage, site unspecified

SEE ALSO

Osteitis deformans

OTHER NOTES

- Osteosarcoma variants like parosteal, periosteal, and intraosseous osteosarcoma are lower grade lesions with a more favorable prognosis, often not requiring chemotherapy. Other variants, post irradiation, and post-Paget osteosarcoma metastasize early.
- Chordoma - rare malignant bone tumor that develops from the remnants of the primitive notochord. May be located in the sacrum or near the base of the skull. Usual course - slowly progressive; recurrent; cure possible.

ABBREVIATIONS

ESR = erythrocyte sedimentation rate
MUGA = nuclear multiple gated acquisition ventriculogram

REFERENCES

- Enneking WF: Musculoskeletal Tumor Surgery, Volumes I and II. New York, Churchill Livingstone, 1983
- Schajowicz F, McGuire MH: Diagnostic difficulties in skeletal pathology. Clinical orthopedics and Related Research 1991;240:281-310
- Womer RB: The cellular biology of bone tumors. Clinical orthopedics and Related Research 1991;262:12-21
- Simon MA: Limb salvage for osteosarcoma in the 1980's. Clinical orthopedics and Related Research 1991;270:264-270
- Velez-Yanguas, Warrier RP: The evolution of chemotherapeutic agents for the treatment of pediatric musculoskeletal malignancies, Orthopedic Clin NA 1996;27:545-549
- Mendelsohn J. Jeremiah Metzger Lecture. Targeted cancer therapy. Trans Am Clin Climatol Assoc. 2000;111:95-110

Web references: 3 available at www.5mcc.com
Illustrations N/A

Author(s):
Mark R. Dambro, MD

BASICS

DESCRIPTION An intoxication producing paralytic disease caused by neurotoxins of Clostridium botulism and is the most toxic substances known to science. The toxin prevents acetylcholine release at presynaptic membranes, blocking neuromuscular transmission in cholinergic nerve fibers.

- Four forms exist:
  - ◊ Foodborne botulism
  - ◊ Infantile botulism
  - ◊ Wound botulism
  - ◊ Classification undetermined

System(s) affected: Endocrine/Metabolic, Gastrointestinal, Nervous

Genetics: N/A

Incidence/Prevalence in USA:
- Rare 0.34/100,000 with 75% the infantile form
- Foodborne - 24 cases/year
- Infantile - 71 cases/year
- Wound botulism - less than 100 cases in literature
- Indeterminate - very rare but incidence unknown

Predominant age:
- Foodborne - all ages
- Infantile - 2 to 4 months (rare after 6 months)
- Wound - usually younger adult
- Undetermined - older than one year

Predominant sex:
- Foodborne, infantile and undetermined - Male=Female
- Wound - Male > Female

SIGNS & SYMPTOMS
- Foodborne
  - ◊ Onset 12-48 hours after ingestion, as long as 14 days
  - ◊ Nonspecific findings early (nausea, vomiting, malaise, dizziness, abdominal distension)
  - ◊ Dry mouth
  - ◊ Constipation, urinary retention
  - ◊ Symmetric descending weakness or paralysis of motor and autonomic nerves, usually beginning with the cranial nerves
  - ◊ Cranial nerve paralysis (ptosis; extraocular muscle paresis; fixed, dilated pupils; dysphagia)
  - ◊ Postural hypotension
  - ◊ Muscle weakness, respiratory paralysis (no sensory deficits)
  - ◊ Afebrile
  - ◊ Progression over several days
- Infantile
  - ◊ Constipation - early sign
  - ◊ Loss of head control
  - ◊ Loss of suck
  - ◊ Loss of facial expression and verbalization
  - ◊ Symmetric descending weakness and cranial nerve paresis similar to foodborne form
  - ◊ Diminished or absent deep tendon reflexes
  - ◊ Autonomic dysfunction
  - ◊ Afebrile
  - ◊ Usual progression over 2-5 days, can be short as few hours
- Wound
  - ◊ Onset 4-14 days post injury
  - ◊ Findings similar to foodborne botulism, but GI symptoms less common
  - ◊ May be febrile
- Undetermined
  - ◊ Possible adult variant of infant botulism
  - ◊ Findings similar to infant botulism

CAUSES
- Ingestions of C. botulinum neurotoxins (A, B, and E most common)
- Foodborne usually from home-canned vegetables, prepared foods or foods incubated in anaerobic conditions
- Infantile from ingestion of spores in environment or occasionally in honey
- Wound due to contamination with toxin-producing C. botulinum
- Undetermined - cause unknown

RISK FACTORS
- Foodborne - ingestion of home-canned or prepared foods
- Infantile from ingestion of honey. Breast feeding (controversial)
- Wound - IV drug use (e.g., black tar heroin) or "skin popping"

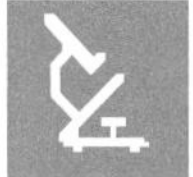

DIAGNOSIS

DIFFERENTIAL DIAGNOSIS
- Guillian-Barre syndrome
- Encephalitis
- Tick paralysis
- Myasthenia gravis
- Eaton Lambert myasthenic syndrome
- Basilar artery stroke
- Congenital neuropathy or myopathy
- Sepsis
- Hypokalemic periodic paralysis
- Polio
- Other poisonings (organophosphate, shellfish, Amanita mushrooms, atropine, aminoglycoside)

LABORATORY
- Routine tests - check for hypokalemia
- CSF testing - normal helps differentiate from Guillian-Barre
- Toxin detected in gastric contents, blood, feces, suspected food and containers
- Confirmation available at CDC and some state laboratories
- Pulmonary function testing

Drugs that may alter lab results: N/A

Disorders that may alter lab results: Underlying myoneural disease

PATHOLOGICAL FINDINGS
- Nonspecific

SPECIAL TESTS
- Stool contains organism and toxin
- Serum toxin present in foodborne form

IMAGING N/A

DIAGNOSTIC PROCEDURES Electromyogram (EMG) shows characteristic brief, low voltage compound motor-unit, small amplitude, overly abundant action potentials (BSAPs), incremental response to repetitive stimulation. Findings not definitive for botulism.

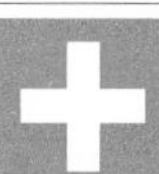

TREATMENT

APPROPRIATE HEALTH CARE
Inpatient, with maximal monitoring capabilities, especially for respiratory failure

GENERAL MEASURES
- Meticulous airway management
- Monitor pulmonary function
- Physical therapy with range of motion exercise and assisted ambulation as tolerated
- Prevention of decubiti

SURGICAL MEASURES Wound excision debridement

ACTIVITY Bedrest initially

DIET
- Nasogastric feedings, if needed
- Fluid restriction if inappropriate antidiuretic hormone (ADH) syndrome

PATIENT EDUCATION
- When preserving food at home, kill Clostridium botulism spores by pressure cooking at 250°F (120°C) for 30 minutes
- Toxin can be destroyed by boiling for 10 minutes or cooking at 175°F (80°C) for 30 minutes
- Avoid honey in first year of life

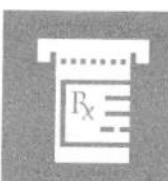

MEDICATIONS

DRUG(S) OF CHOICE
- Antitoxin therapy with trivalent A-B-E antitoxin (available at CDC (404) 639-3670 or 639-2888), one vial IV and one vial IM, repeat IV in 2-4 hours if symptoms persist
- Penicillin therapy of unclear value
- Infantile
  - ◊ Antitoxin therapy not needed
  - ◊ Penicillin therapy of unclear value
  - ◊ Enemas may assist in removal of toxin
- Wound
  - ◊ Antitoxin therapy with trivalent A-B-E antitoxin, one vial IV and one vial IM, repeat in 2-4 hours if persistent symptoms
  - ◊ Penicillin therapy of unclear value
  - ◊ Contradictions: Aminoglycosides - may potentiate paralysis
  - ◊ Precautions: Serum sickness or hypersensitivity reactions in 20% of antitoxin recipients. Test before treating.

Contraindications: N/A
Precautions: N/A
Significant possible interactions: N/A

ALTERNATIVE DRUGS N/A

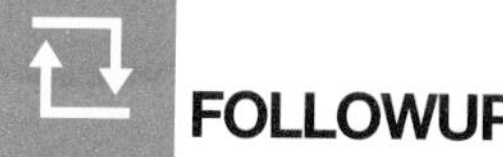

FOLLOWUP

PATIENT MONITORING Cardiorespiratory monitoring during illness

PREVENTION/AVOIDANCE
- Avoid giving honey to infants
- Do not eat or taste food from bulging cans, or if food is off smelling

POSSIBLE COMPLICATIONS
- Aspiration pneumonia
- Nosocomial infection
- Hypoxic tissue damage
- Death

EXPECTED COURSE/PROGNOSIS
- Foodborne and wound
  - ◊ Mortality 25% (<10% under 20 years of age), usually due to delayed diagnosis and respiratory failure
  - ◊ Full recovery may require months
  - ◊ Sequelae due to hypoxic insults
- Infantile
  - ◊ Mortality < 10%
  - ◊ Extended recovery period and sequelae as above

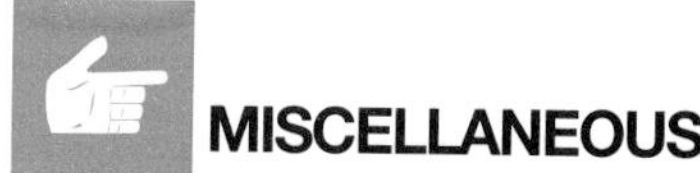

MISCELLANEOUS

ASSOCIATED CONDITIONS N/A

AGE-RELATED FACTORS
Pediatric: Avoid honey first year
Geriatric: N/A
Others: N/A

PREGNANCY N/A

SYNONYMS
- Sausage poisoning
- Kerner's disease

ICD-9-CM
005.1 Botulism

SEE ALSO
Food poisoning, bacterial
Tick paralysis

OTHER NOTES Organism present in stools of 1-2% of healthy individuals. Release of toxins in the gut may worsen symptoms of infantile botulism by bacterial lysis.

ABBREVIATIONS N/A

REFERENCES

- Shapiro RL, Hatheway C, Swerdlow DL. Botulism in the United States: a clinical epidemiologic review. Ann Intern Med 1998;129(3):221-8
- Mandell G, Douglas R, Bennett J. Principles and Practice of Infectious Diseases. 4th Ed. New York, Churchill Livingstone, 1995
- Oski F, DeAngelis C, Feigin R, Warshaw J. Principles and Practice of Pediatrics. Philadelphia, J.B. Lippincott, 1990
- Wigginton JM, Thill P. Infant botulism: A review of the literature. Clin Pediatr 1993:32(11):669-674
- Hatheway CL. Botulism: The present status of the disease. Curr Top Microbiol Immunol 1995; 195:55-75
- Haddad LM, Shannon MW, Winchester JF, eds. Clinical Management of Poisoning and Drug Overdose. 3rd ed. Philadelphia: W.B. Saunders, 1998
- Zajtchuk R, Bellamy RF, eds. Textbook of military medicine, Part 1, Office of the Surgeon General, 1997

Web references: 1 available at www.5mcc.com
Illustrations N/A

Author(s):
Jack Bradford, DO

BASICS

DESCRIPTION Single or multiple abscesses within the brain, usually occurring secondary to a focus of infection outside the central nervous system. May mimic brain tumor but evolves more rapidly (days to a few weeks). It starts as a cerebritis, becomes necrotic, and subsequently becomes encapsulated.
System(s) affected: Nervous
Genetics: No known genetic pattern
Incidence/Prevalence in USA: Infrequent
Predominant age: Median age 30-40
Predominant sex: Male > Female (2:1)

SIGNS & SYMPTOMS
- Recent onset of headache becoming severe
- Nausea and vomiting
- Mental changes progressing to stupor and coma
- Afebrile or low-grade fever
- Neck stiffness
- Seizures
- Papilledema
- Focal neurological signs depending on location

CAUSES
- Direct extension from otitis, mastoiditis, sinusitis or dental infection
- Cranial osteomyelitis
- Penetrating skull trauma
- Prior craniotomy
- Bacteremia from lung abscess, pneumonia
- Bacterial endocarditis
- Fungal infection of the nasopharynx
- Toxoplasma gondii (in AIDS patients)
- Cyanotic congenital heart disease
- Intravenous drug use
- No source found in 20%
- Most common infective organisms - streptococci, staphylococci, enteric gram-negative bacilli and anaerobes (usually same as source of infection), Nocardia

RISK FACTORS
- AIDS
- Immunocompromised
- IV drug abuse

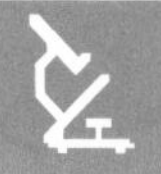

DIAGNOSIS

DIFFERENTIAL DIAGNOSIS
- Brain tumors
- Stroke
- Resolving intracranial hemorrhage
- Subdural empyema
- Extradural abscess
- Encephalitis

LABORATORY
- WBC may be normal or mildly elevated
- Culture of abscess contents, predominant organisms include Toxoplasma (AIDS), Staphylococcus (trauma), aerobic or anaerobic bacteria, fungi (rare)
- Blood studies - mild polymorphonuclear leukocytosis, elevated sedimentation rate

Drugs that may alter lab results: Prior administration of antibiotics

Disorders that may alter lab results: N/A

PATHOLOGICAL FINDINGS
- Suppuration, liquefaction, encapsulation, depending on stage of evolution
- Fibrosis

SPECIAL TESTS Surgical burr hole with aspiration to make a specific bacteriologic diagnosis

IMAGING
- CT or MRI are diagnostic methods of choice - findings are dependent on stages of the abscess
- Radionuclide 117 IN-labeled leukocytes may distinguish abscess from neoplasm

DIAGNOSTIC PROCEDURES
- History, physical exam
- Lumbar puncture often contraindicated
- Search for primary source of infection (chest x-ray, skull film for fracture, sinus films, etc.)

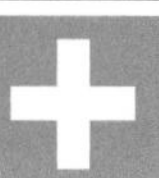

TREATMENT

APPROPRIATE HEALTH CARE Inpatient for close observation, diagnostic evaluation, and specialty consultation (neurology, neurosurgery, infectious disease)

GENERAL MEASURES
- Palliative and supportive
- Medical therapy
  - ◊ For surgical inaccessible, multiple abscesses
  - ◊ For abscesses in early cerebritis stage
  - ◊ Small (< 2.5 cm) abscess
  - ◊ Therapy directed toward most likely organism

SURGICAL MEASURES
- Surgical therapy
  - ◊ Mandatory when neurologic deficits are severe or progressive
  - ◊ Used when the abscess is in the posterior fossa
  - ◊ Abscess drainage - (via needle) under stereotactic CT guidance through a burr hole under local anesthesia, is most rapid and effective method. May be repeated if needed.
  - ◊ Craniotomy - if abscess is large or multilocular
  - ◊ Abscess resulting from trauma

ACTIVITY Bedrest until infection controlled and abscess evacuated or resolving, then up as tolerated

DIET IV fluids if nausea and vomiting present

PATIENT EDUCATION For patient education materials favorably reviewed on this topic, contact: Brain Research Foundation, 208 S. LaSalle Street, Suite 1426, Chicago, IL 60604, (312)782-4311

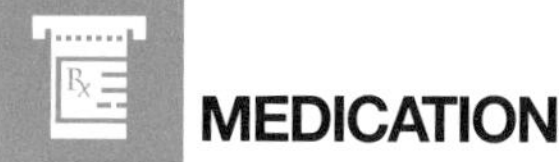

MEDICATIONS

DRUG(S) OF CHOICE
- Antibiotics according to organism if known
- If organism unknown, begin with penicillin G and metronidazole, or chloramphenicol (Chloromycetin), if metronidazole cannot be used
- Add oxacillin or nafcillin if trauma or IV drug user (use vancomycin in penicillin-sensitive patients)
- If gram-negative organism suspected (otic, GI, GU organ) add third-generation cephalosporin
- Abscess associated with HIV infection assumed to be due to Toxoplasma gondii - daily doses of sulfadiazine and pyrimethamine. Therapy will be life-long in AIDS patients.
- Anticonvulsants - phenytoin until abscess resolved or perhaps longer. Obtain anticonvulsant levels.
- Following surgical procedure - corticosteroids to reduce edema. Dexamethasone. Taper rapidly. Use usually limited to 1 week. Continue antibiotics for 6-8 weeks.

Contraindications: Sensitivity or allergy to any prescribed medications

Precautions:
- Sulfadiazine poorly water soluble. Patients must maintain adequate hydration or risk developing crystalluria.
- Decrease dosage of penicillins in patients with renal dysfunction
- Monitor serum levels of anticonvulsants
- Dose of pyrimethamine required for treatment of toxoplasmosis may approach toxic levels. Should observe for folic acid deficiency and treat with folinic acid (leucovorin) 5-15 mg (orally, IM, IV) if necessary

Significant possible interactions: Refer to manufacturer's literature

ALTERNATIVE DRUGS N/A

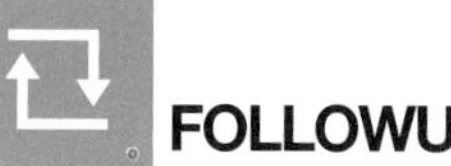

FOLLOWUP

PATIENT MONITORING
- Postsurgical monitoring as needed
- Serial CT or MRI - to confirm progressive resolution, early detection and management of complications

PREVENTION/AVOIDANCE
- Adequate treatment of otitis media, mastoiditis, dental abscess, other predisposing factors
- Prophylactic antibiotics after compound skull fracture or penetrating head wound

POSSIBLE COMPLICATIONS
- Permanent neurological deficits
- Surgical complications
- Recurrent abscess
- Seizures

EXPECTED COURSE/PROGNOSIS
Survival > 80% with early diagnosis and treatment

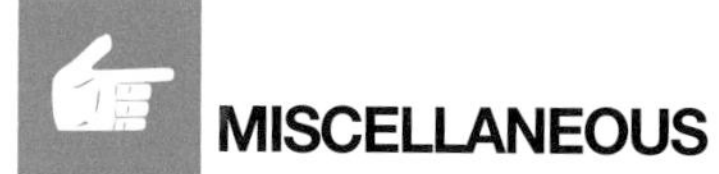

MISCELLANEOUS

ASSOCIATED CONDITIONS
- AIDS
- Congenital heart disease

AGE-RELATED FACTORS
Pediatric:
- About one third of cases in pediatric age group. Rarely found in infants under 1 year of age.
- Cyanotic congenital heart disease frequently associated

Geriatric: Age does not affect outcome as much as abscess size and state of neurological dysfunction at presentation

Others: N/A

PREGNANCY N/A

SYNONYMS Cerebral abscess

ICD-9-CM
324.0 Intracranial abscess

SEE ALSO

OTHER NOTES N/A

ABBREVIATIONS N/A

REFERENCES

- Graham DI, Lantos PL, editors. Greenfield's Neuropathology. 9th ed. London: Arnold; 2002
- Osenbach RK, Loftus CM: Diagnosis and Management of Brain Abscess. Neurosurgery Clinics of North America 1992;3:403-20
- Ropper A, Victor M, editors. Adams and Victor's Principles of Neurology. 7th ed. NewYork: Mcgraw-Hill; 2001
- Rowland LD, editor. Merritt's Textbook of Neurology. 10th ed. Baltimore: Williams & Wilkins; 2000
- Rakel RE, editor. Conn's Current Therapy. Philadelphia: WB Saunders Co; 2003

Web references: 0 available at www.5mcc.com

Illustrations N/A

Author(s):
Peter Kozisek, MD

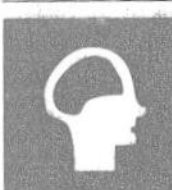

BASICS

DESCRIPTION

Post acute severely brain injured patients with complex injuries, prolonged coma, initial GCS<9 who may have limited responses to environment, are often inconsistently able to communicate their needs and manage personal affairs, and frequently have motor deficits. These patients may reside in a long term care facility or at home with attendant care. Less severely injured individuals may have more evident cognitive and behavioral problems and less physical issues.

Management issues include:

- Changes in level of attention, arousal, cognition and behavior
- Neurogenic bladder and bowel
- Contractures and spasticity
- Heterotopic ossification
- Skin
- Respiratory
- Endocrine

System(s) affected: Endocrine/Metabolic, Musculoskeletal, Nervous, Pulmonary, Renal/Urologic, Reproductive, Skin/Exocrine
Genetics: N/A
Incidence/Prevalence in USA: Brain injury traumatic - 200/100,000; 500,000 hospitalizations and 75,000 deaths per year
Predominant age: Young adults
Predominant sex: Male > Female

SIGNS & SYMPTOMS

- Neurological
  - ◊ Diminished arousal leads to limited responses and may be generalized (eg, decorticate posturing or focal such as eye blink or one limb voluntary movement)
  - ◊ Cognitive impairment
  - ◊ Disinhibited responses and behavior
  - ◊ Impaired memory
  - ◊ Anosognosia (poor self-awareness)
  - ◊ Focal motor deficits, eg, hemiparesis
  - ◊ Cerebellar signs - ataxia, nystagmus, dysmetria, dysdiadochokinesis
  - ◊ Cranial nerve palsies
  - ◊ Hydrocephalus-triad of worse cognition, ataxia, incontinence
  - ◊ Epilepsy - partial or generalized signs
- Urinary frequency and incontinence
- Bowel incontinence
- Spasticity
- Heterotopic ossification - erythema, pain or stiffness in soft tissue around joint
- Decubitus ulcers
- Decreased respiratory strength or poor cough
- Endocrine

CAUSES MVA, assaults, sports injuries, falls

RISK FACTORS See Brain injury, traumatic

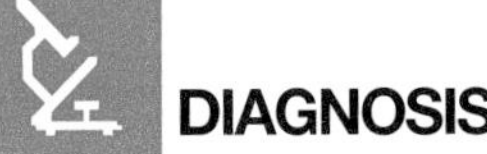

DIAGNOSIS

DIFFERENTIAL DIAGNOSIS

A number of complications can create a change in functional level.

- Chronic infection (e.g., UTI)
- Depression
- Hypothyroidism, other endocrinopathy
- Hydrocephalus, hematoma
- Epilepsy
- Fractures
- Tracheal stricture

LABORATORY

- CBC, electrolytes, BUN, creatinine, calcium, albumin, vitamin B12, folate, TSH, alkaline phosphatase, AST, ALT, morning cortisol level, urine culture
- Culture, ova and parasites for diarrhea
- Skin culture
- Culture tracheal site
- Endocrine workup as indicated

Drugs that may alter lab results: Phenytoin (Dilantin), valproic acid

Disorders that may alter lab results: N/A

PATHOLOGICAL FINDINGS

- Hydrocephalus with periventricular edema
- Joint contractures results in collagen cross linking: decreased range of motion
- Heterotopic ossification: disorganized osteoid calcification in soft tissue

SPECIAL TESTS

- Evoked potentials (auditory, visual and somatosensory)
- Behavioral assessment, neuropsychological testing and vocational assessment in the less severe
- Cognitive testing for orientation and arousal use Western Neuro Sensory Stimulation Profile (WNSS) or Galveston Orientation Amnesia Test (GOAT)
- EEG

IMAGING

- Bone scan: heterotopic ossification
- CT: hydrocephalus, atrophy, hematoma
- Video pharyngeal fluoroscopic swallowing study
- MRI to evaluate diffuse axonal injury

DIAGNOSTIC PROCEDURES

- Altered arousal - visual, auditory and somatosensory evoked potentials
- Neurogenic bladder- check post void residuals 3-4 times. If > 50 cc or 20% of voided volume, urodynamics
- Ultrasound of bladder and kidney: urolithiasis and hydronephrosis
- Endoscopy: cause of dysphagia
- Contractures and spasticity: examination under anesthesia
- Respiratory and neurologic: sleep/oxygen saturation study, bronchoscopy for stricture

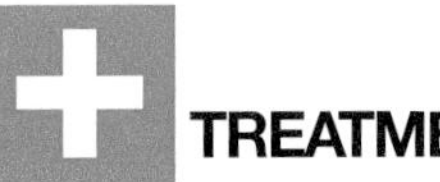

TREATMENT

APPROPRIATE HEALTH CARE

Outpatient; occasional inpatient care

GENERAL MEASURES

- Diminished level of arousal: identify best modality for communication, assess functional skills (proper seating, hand function), behavioral or neuropsychologist. Respiratory therapist (for those with tracheostomy), social work (to assist with family education and long term planning) and nursing
- Reduce sedatives
- Neurogenic bladder - treat UTI
  - ◊ If post void residual < 50 cc then trial of regular voiding routine q2hr
  - ◊ If still incontinent add oxybutynin
  - ◊ If still incontinent try condom catheter during the day; incontinent pads at night.
  - ◊ If raised post void residuals or high pressure bladder or dyssynergic bladder on urodynamics then intermittent catheter q4-6h
- Neurogenic bowel - regular bowel routine
- Contractures and spasticity: stretching
  - ◊ If no progress after 4 weeks consider serial casting or custom made orthotic
  - ◊ Contractures > 45° consider tendon release
- Heterotopic ossification: stretch soft tissue to decrease maturation of osteoid, consider orthotics/splinting. Bone scan at baseline.
- Skin: q2hr turning, avoid seating in position of high shear on buttocks such as in bed at 45 degrees, observe for erythema around tube sites and rule out latex allergy
- Respiratory: night humidification if has a tracheotomy, may require suctioning
- Endocrine- monitor fluid balance
- Dental - assessment and dental x-rays

SURGICAL MEASURES

- Tendons releases; fundoplasty or gastrostomy; tracheostomy; ventriculoperitoneal or ventriculoatrial shunt

ACTIVITY

- As tolerated - outings in wheelchair can be beneficial - skin very sensitive to sun/wind - protect with clothing/golf umbrella clipped to chair
- Age appropriate activities related to premorbid interests yield best attention

DIET

- Consult with dietitian
- Ensure adequate hydration; 2-2.5 L of water/day. More if outside or in hot weather.
- Bolus feeds preferred if fed by gastrostomy
- Upright and quiet activity for half an hour following feeds as aspiration can occur even with a g-tube

PATIENT EDUCATION

- For information and family support groups: http://www.tbinet.org/ or http://www.biausa.org/
- Families need support, advocacy, education, information - verbally and written (audio tape meetings), opportunities to have input regarding priorities, treatment plans and discuss limits of treatment for patient (advance directive)

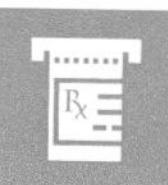

MEDICATIONS

DRUG(S) OF CHOICE
Individualize pharmacotherapy
- Diminished arousal: Consider one of desipramine or amitriptyline 75-150 mg hs, methylphenidate (Ritalin) 20-40 mg/day in 2 divided doses, amantadine 50-200 mg bid, dextroamphetamine, bromocriptine, levodopa
- Agitation: treat epilepsy or depression otherwise, amitriptyline 75-150 mg hs, carbamazepine, valproic acid, lithium, propranolol, serotonin specific re-uptake inhibitor. Minimize use of haloperidol, antipsychotics and benzodiazepines as they worsen cognition. If necessary use antipsychotic with least cognitive side effects, eg, risperidone (Risperdal) or olanzapine (Zyprexa)
- Abulia and lack of initiation: amantadine, bromocriptine, methylphenidate, levodopa
- Epilepsy: if possible avoid phenytoin and phenobarbital - too sedating. Carbamazepine, valproic acid, gabapentin less sedating.
- Neurogenic bladder: oxybutynin 2.5 mg tid to 10 mg qid, if bladder pressures low and/or post void residuals low
- Bowel routine - stool softener such as docusate sodium (daily) combined with laxative (night before suppository), high fiber and suppository (every other day)to induce bowel movement
- Spasticity: all drugs may cause sedation; dantrolene 25-200 mg/day divided tid; or baclofen, benzodiazepines, clonidine. If focal spasticity consider botulinum toxin injection.
- Heterotopic ossification: indomethacin 25-50 mg tid. If severe, progressive or history of GI ulceration then etidronate (Didronel) 20 mg/kg for six months or alendronate 20 mg once a day.

Contraindications: Refer to manufacturer's literature

Precautions:
- Risperidone may be associated with hyperglycemia and ketoacidosis

Significant possible interactions: Refer to manufacturer's literature

ALTERNATIVE DRUGS N/A

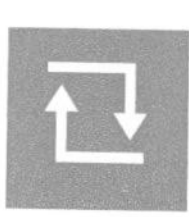

FOLLOWUP

PATIENT MONITORING
- Patients make slow steady gains. Ongoing outcome assessments to determine progress (or not) in abilities and medication efficacy needed. These measures do not need to be sophisticated, for example: length of time able to hold head up or ability to respond to commands written or verbal. Modify program periodically to reflect outcome measures.
- Review medical status monthly

PREVENTION/AVOIDANCE
- Prevent further complications

POSSIBLE COMPLICATIONS
- Major affective disorder (depression, psychosis) in up to 50% of patients
- Family and caregiver burn out
- Substance abuse
- Social isolation
- May be a higher risk of dementia
- Latex allergy to g-tube, catheters
- Dental caries
- Osteoporosis
- Falls
- Aspiration pneumonia
- Pressure ulcers
- Heterotopic ossification
- Dysphagia, esophagitis
- Bladder incontinence
- Contractures/spasticity

EXPECTED COURSE/PROGNOSIS
- Most rapid return of neurological function is during first two years but some patients continue to improve slowly for 5-10 years as long as complications are prevented or managed appropriately.
- Highly variable (80% of individuals with severe injuries become independent in dressing and self-care at 1 year
- Negative prognostic factors:
  - ◊ Age > 40
  - ◊ Abnormal pupillary responses
  - ◊ Prolonged coma i.e., GCS < 9 seven days after injury
  - ◊ Abnormal evoked potentials
  - ◊ Extraocular eye movement abnormalities

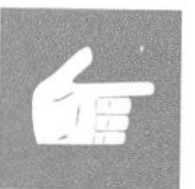

MISCELLANEOUS

ASSOCIATED CONDITIONS
- Psychosis
- Suicide attempts
- Substance abuse
- ADD

AGE-RELATED FACTORS
Pediatric: N/A
Geriatric: N/A
Others: N/A

PREGNANCY N/A

SYNONYMS N/A

ICD-9-CM
530.10 Esophagitis, unspecified
750.6 Congenital hiatus hernia
787.1 Heartburn
733.00 Osteoporosis, unspecified
707.0 Decubitus ulcer
345.3 Epilepsy, grand mal status

SEE ALSO
Brain injury, traumatic
Constipation
Dysphagia
Fecal impaction
Gastroesophageal reflux disease
Hemorrhoids
Osteoporosis
Pressure ulcer
Seizure disorders
Sleep apnea, obstructive
Stomatitis
Stroke (Brain attack)
Stroke rehabilitation

OTHER NOTES
- Paucity of research on this group of patients due to high number of variables, slow progress. However many people are misdiagnosed as being in a persistent vegetative state or locked in syndrome when voluntary responses can be elicited with thorough assessment
- No definitive research on optimum length of time for rehabilitation, slow and steady and over a lifetime appears most effective
- Rehabilitation program guidelines:
  - ◊ Individualized goals: ideally using behavioral approach emphasizing reinforcement of task behavior
  - ◊ Flexible: to account for patient's changing needs (eg, may have an infection that decreased their ability)
  - ◊ Functional (based on practical activities): e.g., helping with self care activities also involves opportunity for range of motion exercises
  - ◊ Consider patient's attention span and best time of day when planning
  - ◊ Allow for as much control and choice as possible (eg, even if can only communicate with eye blinks can participate in choice of clothes to wear, music, preferred activity)
  - ◊ Consistency and familiarity provide opportunities for learning
- Quality of life issues vital, e.g., comfort measures, sensory stimulation as tolerated, attention to spiritual and/or cultural needs, proper positioning
- For agitated behavior, consider consultation with behavioral psychologist to assist in design of program integrating medications and behavior therapy techniques. Minimize use of punishment and reinforce correct behavior. New technique known as Errorless Compliance Training may be helpful.

ABBREVIATIONS
GCS = Glasgow Coma Score

REFERENCES

- Elovic E: Pharmacology and attention and arousal in the low level patient, Neuro Rehabilitation 1996;6:57-67
- Giacino J, Zasler N, Katz D, Kelly J, Rosenberg J, Filley C. Development of practice guidelines for assessment and management of the vegetative and minimally conscious states. Jour of Head Trauma Rehabilitation August 1997;12(4):79-89

Web references: 0 available at www.5mcc.com
Illustrations N/A

Author(s):
Mark R. Dambro, MD

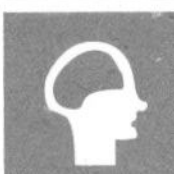

BASICS

DESCRIPTION Frequently related to rapid deceleration such as motor vehicle accidents, diving accidents. May also be due to blunt injury such as with a baseball bat, etc. TBI is a dynamic process with initial bleeding followed by secondary injury due to cerebral edema, continued intracranial bleeding, etc. Predicting outcome initially is difficult and patients may improve for years.

System(s) affected: Cardiovascular, Endocrine/Metabolic, Nervous

Genetics: N/A

Incidence/Prevalence in USA: Incidence: 200/100,000; 500,000 hospitalizations and 75,000 deaths per year

Predominant age: 15-24

Predominant sex: Male > Female

SIGNS & SYMPTOMS

Variable and dependent on degree of injury:

- Loss of consciousness (transient or persistent)
- External signs of head injury
- Headache
- Vomiting
- Amnesia
- Focal signs and symptoms
- Evidence for increased intracranial hypertension (elevated blood pressure, decreased pulse rate, slow or irregular breathing [Cushing triad]) - 30% only have all 3
- Decorticate or decerebrate positioning (both a bad prognostic sign)
- Seizures
- Raccoon eyes, Battle's sign, hemotympanum
- CSF rhinorrhea (see Special tests)
- Unilateral dilated pupil in an alert patient is not consistent with impending herniation since such patients are always unconscious
- Epidural hemorrhage from blunt trauma is generally acute, 30% with a "lucid interval" (initial loss of consciousness followed by recovery of consciousness then loss of consciousness secondary to the intracranial bleed).
- Subdural hemorrhage usually has a slower onset and may present weeks after the initial injury, especially in the elderly.

CAUSES

- Motor vehicle accident (50%), falls, assault
- Child abuse:
  - ◊ Consider if dropped or fell <4 feet (eg, off bed, couch, etc.) and significant injury present
  - ◊ Subdural more likely to be abuse (but epidural could be abuse)
  - ◊ Any retinal hemorrhage (retinal hemorrhage is not caused by seizures or simple head trauma)

RISK FACTORS Alcohol, prior head injury, contact sports, "heading" soccer balls may cause long-term cognitive loss

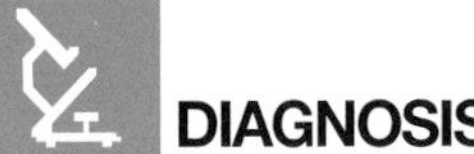

DIAGNOSIS

DIFFERENTIAL DIAGNOSIS Other causes of coma (e.g., drug overdose, infection, metabolic, vascular causes)

LABORATORY

- Patients may rapidly develop DIC; PT/INR, PTT, CBC (for decreased platelets), fibrin degradation products
- Drug and alcohol screening

Drugs that may alter lab results: N/A

Disorders that may alter lab results: N/A

PATHOLOGICAL FINDINGS

- Epidural, subdural or intraparenchymal hemorrhage
- Coup or contra-coup injury
- Evolving, diffuse axonal injury is a principle cause of neurologic sequelae with mild head trauma

SPECIAL TESTS

- Neuropsychometric testing when able
- CSF rhinorrhea contains glucose while nasal mucus does not. Check also for the double-halo sign: put a drop of bloody nasal discharge on filter paper. If it contains both CSF and blood, there will be two rings; a central ring followed by a paler ring.

IMAGING

- CT, C-spine as indicated; use clinical judgment
  - ◊ Absolute require CT scan (adults and children): evidence of basilar skull fracture, CSF rhinorrhea, hemotympanum, Battle's sign, depressed skull fracture; any focal neurologic findings
  - ◊ High risk criteria in adults
    - GCS<15: age >60, 2+ vomiting episodes, seizure; may also include patients with alcohol/drug intoxication, memory deficit and headache
    - GCS=15 (normal): vomiting, severe headache
  - ◊ Moderate risk criteria in adults
    - Amnesia >30 minutes, mechanism of injury (ejection from car, car/pedestrian), fall >3 feet or 5 stairs
  - ◊ Children age <2: loss of consciousness, amnesia, seizure, headache, persistent vomiting, irritability, behavioral changes
  - ◊ Children age >2: any of the above, unusual behavior, large hematoma
  - ◊ Children <3 months: scalp hematoma, significant mechanism
- Skull radiographs are not helpful in most cases, but can be done to document child abuse

DIAGNOSTIC PROCEDURES Placement of intracranial pressure monitor when indicated, serial neurologic exams

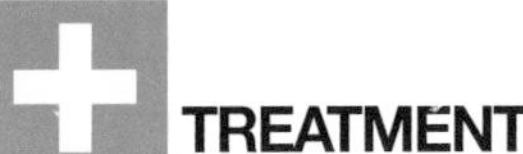

TREATMENT

APPROPRIATE HEALTH CARE

- Outpatient for mild
- Admit: abnormal CT, abnormal GCS, clinical evidence basilar skull fracture, persistent neurological deficits (eg, confusion, somnolence, etc.), patient with no competent adult at home for observation
- Possibly admit: loss of consciousness, amnesia, etc.

GENERAL MEASURES

- Acute management depends on severity of injury. Most patients need no interventions. (Note: There is very little evidence to support or refute the use of most of these measures [including hyperventilation and mannitol]; further studies are in progress.)
- The immediate goal is to determine who needs further therapy, imaging studies (CT) and hospitalization, and to prevent further injury
- All penetrating injury should be evaluated by a neurosurgeon
- C-spine immobilization should be considered in all head trauma. Clear the cervical spine radiographically (AP, lateral showing all 7 cervical vertebrae and the C7/T1 interspace, obliques if indicated).
- ABCs (airway, breathing, circulation) take priority over head injury. Stabilization and prevention of mortality from other injuries is critical to insuring patient survival.
- For the severely injured patient:
  - ◊ Immediate CPR, avoid hypotension or hypoxia. Head injury causes increased ICP secondary to edema and perfusion pressure must be maintained.
  - ◊ Use normal saline for resuscitation fluid. If unable to obtain good IV access, can use 3% or 7% saline for resuscitation fluid (250cc boluses in adults). This does not seem to change mortality, however. Avoid lactated Ringer's which is slightly hypo-osmolar.
  - ◊ Intubate and hyperventilate patients with increased intracranial pressure. Prophylactic hyperventilation for those without signs or symptoms of increased intracranial pressure is contraindicated and may cause additional injury secondary to vasoconstriction. Maintain $PaCO_2$ at 25-30 mm Hg.
  - ◊ Seizure prophylaxis does not change outcomes (death rates, etc.) but may prevent seizures. Consider phenytoin for 1 week post injury.
  - ◊ Manage breakthrough seizures with lorazepam
- Hypothermia is of no benefit

SURGICAL MEASURES Dependent on neurological consult

ACTIVITY See ACTIVITY in topic "Post-concussive syndrome" for sports activity management

DIET As tolerated

PATIENT EDUCATION

- Brain Injury Association help-line: 1-800-444-6443
- Printed patient information: A Chance to Grow, 5034 Oliver Avenue North, Minneapolis, MN 55430, (612)521-2266
- Any patient discharged from your office or the ED should have instructions to watch for symptoms indicating the need for further intervention (changing mental status, worsening headache, focal findings, etc.). Give these instructions to a competent surrogate who will observe the patient. A patient who deteriorates, is not likely to remember or act on any instructions.

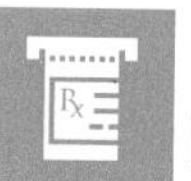

MEDICATIONS

DRUG(S) OF CHOICE
- Acute management (do not hesitate to use morphine or benzodiazepines as indicated, but remember that they may alter the patient's mental status):
  - ◊ Morphine 1-2 mg IV prn for pain control up to 15 mg or more per hour as needed
- Increased intracranial pressure
  - ◊ Mannitol 0.25-2 gm/kg (0.25-1 gm/kg in children) given over 30-60 minutes in patients with adequate renal function. Only one dose should be needed since these patients will require neurosurgical consultation. Mannitol should not be used unless there is evidence of increased ICP; prophylactic use associated with worse outcomes.
  - ◊ Furosemide 20-40 mg IV to promote diuresis
- Seizures
  - ◊ Phenytoin (Dilantin) 15 mg/kg IV (1 mg/kg/min IV not to exceed 50 mg/min). Do not exceed 1 gm in adults. Stop infusion if QT interval increases by > 50% (risk of torsades de pointes).
- Fosphenytoin (Cerebyx) 15 mg/kg IV not to exceed 150 mg/min if phenytoin unavailable or need rapid infusion due to active seizures
  - ◊ Lorazepam (Ativan) 1-2 mg (0.1 mg/kg in children) IV. Higher doses may be needed and are okay as long as the patient is ventilated. Preferred over diazepam.
  - ◊ Phenobarbital 15 mg/kg IV at 25-50 mg/min. May give IM.
- For paralysis
  - ◊ Vecuronium: 10 mg adults, followed by 2-5 mg IV as needed
  - ◊ Pancuronium: 4 mg adults, and hourly as needed. Patient should be immediately intubated or airway should otherwise be controlled.
  - ◊ Avoid succinylcholine which will increase ICP
- To prevent secondary injury from CNS arterial spasm:
  - ◊ Nimodipine: after acute injury generally in consultation with neurosurgery or neurology
- Spinal cord injury
  - ◊ Corticosteroids. Detrimental in acute head injury alone

Contraindications: Allergy

Precautions:
- Mannitol will initially raise the blood pressure by increasing intravascular volume, but will cause hypotension when diuresis begins
- Neither furosemide or mannitol should be given to the hypotensive patient
- Make sure you can manage the airway before paralyzing the patient
- Do not use morphine, benzodiazepines or phenobarbital unless you are prepared to manage the patient's airway

Significant possible interactions: Phenobarbital, morphine and the benzodiazepines can have additive respiratory depression

ALTERNATIVE DRUGS
Diuretics and IV beta-blockers (e.g. esmolol or labetalol) can be used to maintain mean arterial pressure between 130 mm Hg and 70 mm Hg (American Heart Association guideline for blood pressure in intracranial bleeding). No good controlled trials of blood pressure management in traumatic bleeding. Use labetalol 5-10 mg IV until blood pressure is controlled. Nitroprusside may be helpful. However, nitrates may increase intracranial pressure. Antibiotics (e.g., cefazolin) should be given if penetrating trauma is present. Prophylactic antibiotics are not useful in basilar skull fractures.

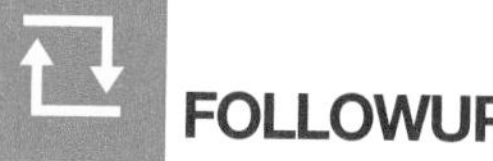

FOLLOWUP

PATIENT MONITORING
- Schedule regular followup
- Gradual return to work or school, even after mild to moderate head injury
- The post-concussion syndrome can follow mild head injury without loss of consciousness and includes headaches, dizziness, fatigue and subtle cognitive or affective changes. Most of these improve within 3 months.
- Most important element of mild TBI management is recognizing the genuine organic basis for patient's symptoms
- Proper counseling, symptomatic management and gradual return to normal activities is essential to prevent a post-traumatic neurosis which can become refractory to treatment

PREVENTION/AVOIDANCE
- Safety education
- Seat belts, bicycle and motorcycle helmets
- Protective headgear for contact sports

POSSIBLE COMPLICATIONS
- Delayed hematomas
- Chronic subdural hematoma, which may follow even "mild" head injury, especially in the elderly. Often present with headache, decreased mentation.
- Delayed hydrocephalus
- Emotional disturbances and psychiatric disorders resulting from head injury may be refractory to treatment
- Seizure disorders - in about 50% of penetrating head injuries, in about 20% of severe closed head injuries, and in < 5% of head injuries overall. Hematomas significantly increase risk of epilepsy.
- Second impact syndrome occurs when the CNS loses autoregulation. Generally, an individual with a minor head injury is returned to a contact sport. Following even minor trauma (eg, whiplash), the patient will lose consciousness and herniate within 1-2 minutes with a 50% mortality. A similar syndrome of "malignant edema" can occur in children with even a single injury.

EXPECTED COURSE/PROGNOSIS
- Gradual improvement for many
- 30-50% of severe head injuries may be fatal
- Prolonged coma may be followed by satisfactory outcome
- Rehabilitation indicated following a significant acute injury. Involve the family in decision making and setting realistic goals.

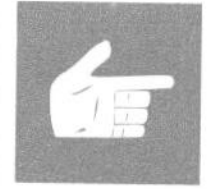

MISCELLANEOUS

ASSOCIATED CONDITIONS
Alcohol and drug abuse

AGE-RELATED FACTORS
Pediatric: Outcome for children more positive, except in severe TBI

Geriatric:
- Poorer prognosis with increasing age
- Subdural hematomas are common after fall or blow; symptoms may be subtle

Others: None

PREGNANCY
N/A

SYNONYMS
- Head injury

ICD-9-CM
800.00 Fracture of vault of skull, closed without mention of intracranial injury, unspecified state of consciousness
850.9 Concussion, unspecified
851.xx Cerebral laceration or contusion
852.00 Subarchnoid hemorrhage following injury without mention of open intracranial wound, unspecified state of consciousness
854.00 Intracranial injury of other and unspecified nature, without mention of intracranial wound, unspecified state of consciousness

SEE ALSO
Brain injury - post acute care issues
Post-concussive syndrome
Seizure disorders

OTHER NOTES
The GCS is not a linear scale; a score of 14 (normal being 15) represents a moderately severe injury category

ABBREVIATIONS
GCS = Glasgow Coma Score
ICP = intracranial pressure

REFERENCES

- McNaughton H, Harwood M. Traumatic brain injury: assessment and management. Hosp Med 2002;63(1):8-11
- Society of Critical Care Medicine. Guidelines for the acute medical management of severe traumatic brain injury in infants, children, and adolescents. Critical Care Medicine 2003;31(6suppl):s407-91
- Haydel MJ . Indications for computed tomography in patients with minor head injury. N Engl J Med 2000;343(2):100-5
- Roberts I, Schierhout G, Alderson P. Absence of evidence for the effectiveness of five interventions routinely used in the intensive care management of severe head injury: a systematic review. J Neurol Neurosurg Psychiatry 1998;65(5):729-33
- Skippen P, Seear M, Poskitt K, et al. Effect of hyperventilation on regional cerebral blood flow in head-injured children. Crit Care Med 1997;25(8):1402-9
- Graber MA. Emergency medicine. In: Graber MA, et al, editors. The Family Practice Handbook. St Louis: Mosby-Yearbook; 1997
- Concussive Guidelines. 226 MMWR March 14, 1997
- Schierhout G, et al. Prophylactic antiepileptic agents after head injury: A systematic review. J Neurol Neurosurg Psych 1998;64(1):108-12
- Skippen P, et al. Effect of hyperventilation on regional cerebral blood flow in head-injured children. Crit Care Med 1997;25(8):1402-9
- Stiell IG, Wells GA, Vandemheen K, Clement C, et al. The Canadian CT Head Rule for patients with minor head injury. Lancet 2001;357(9266):1391-6
- Schutzman SA, Greenes DS. Pediatric minor head trauma. Ann Emerg Med 2001;37(1):65-74
- Batchelor J, McGuiness A. A Meta-analysis of GCS 15 head injured patients with loss of consciousness or post-traumatic amnesia. Emerg Med J. 2002;19(6):515-9

Web references: 0 available at www.5mcc.com

Illustrations N/A

Author(s):
Dana Collaguazo, MD
Hans House, MD

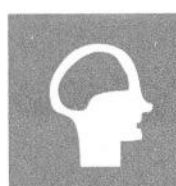

BASICS

DESCRIPTION A congenital, abnormal tract connecting the skin of neck with an internal structure, resulting from failure of closure of a branchial cleft.
- May involve branchial clefts I-IV, which develop in the 4th gestational week

System(s) affected: Skin/Exocrine
Genetics: 10% have family history
Incidence/Prevalence in USA: Unknown
Predominant age: By definition are all present at birth although may remain unnoticed for some time. (Branchial cleft cysts may not present until later childhood.)
Predominant sex: Unknown

SIGNS & SYMPTOMS
- Presence of tiny external opening usually on lower neck along anterior border of sternocleidomastoid muscle
- Spontaneous mucoid drainage
- External openings may also be marked by a skin tag or cartilage
- Infection may rarely be the presenting sign with erythema, swelling, pain, fever
- 10% are bilateral

CAUSES
- The 1st branchial cleft contributes to the tympanic cavity and eustachian tube. Related fistulae are very rare and tend to be infra- or retroauricular. (Preauricular cysts and sinuses are not thought to be of branchial cleft origin.)
- The 2nd branchial cleft forms the hyoid bone and tonsillar fossa. Related fistulae (most common variant) course between the internal and external carotid arteries. Internal opening usually at level of tonsillar fossa. External opening along anterior border of sternocleidomastoid muscle.
- 3rd and 4th branchial clefts form parathyroid glands, thymus and portions of thyroid (parafollicular cells). Fistulae are rare, those from 3rd cleft course lateral to carotid artery, both should have external ostia on lower anterior neck.

RISK FACTORS Positive family history

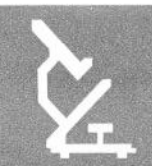

DIAGNOSIS

DIFFERENTIAL DIAGNOSIS
- External sinuses
- Cystic hygroma
- Dermoid cysts
- Lymphadenopathy

LABORATORY Culture only if signs of infection

Drugs that may alter lab results: N/A

Disorders that may alter lab results: N/A

PATHOLOGICAL FINDINGS Lined by stratified squamous epithelium, may contain hair follicles, sweat glands, sebaceous glands, cartilage. Some are lined by ciliated columnar epithelium.

SPECIAL TESTS N/A

IMAGING N/A

DIAGNOSTIC PROCEDURES Sinogram or fistulogram may be done but is of little value

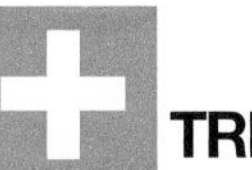

TREATMENT

APPROPRIATE HEALTH CARE
- Surgical excision
- Outpatient status usually appropriate

GENERAL MEASURES N/A

SURGICAL MEASURES
- Small transverse incision at external ostium with careful dissection of fistula
- Stepladder incisions may be needed
- End of fistula ligated flush with pharyngeal mucosa
- Drains are not used
- Antibiotics only for infection

ACTIVITY N/A

DIET N/A

PATIENT EDUCATION

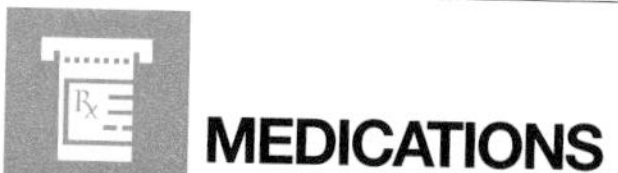

MEDICATIONS

DRUG(S) OF CHOICE N/A
Contraindications: N/A
Precautions: N/A
Significant possible interactions: N/A

ALTERNATIVE DRUGS N/A

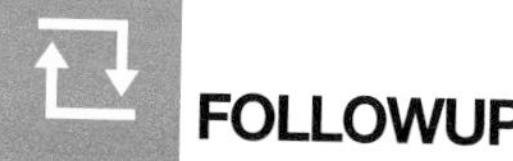

FOLLOWUP

PATIENT MONITORING
- Follow at weekly intervals, if infected, until resolution, than excision
- Postoperative visit at 2 weeks

PREVENTION/AVOIDANCE N/A

POSSIBLE COMPLICATIONS
- Facial nerve injury
- Infection
- Carotid artery injury
- Possible recurrence if any epithelium remains
- Neoplastic degeneration of branchial remnants (about 250 reported cases) if not resected

EXPECTED COURSE/PROGNOSIS
Good

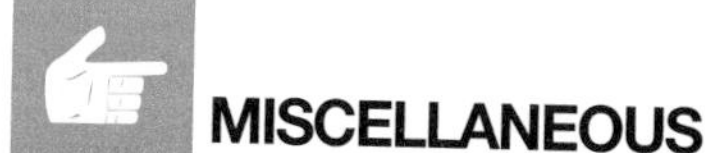

MISCELLANEOUS

ASSOCIATED CONDITIONS Microtia and aural atresia occur with failure of development of 1st branchial cleft.

AGE-RELATED FACTORS
Pediatric: Almost all occur in pediatric age group
Geriatric: N/A
Others: N/A

PREGNANCY N/A

SYNONYMS N/A

ICD-9-CM
744.41 Branchial cleft sinus or fistula

SEE ALSO

OTHER NOTES Branchial cleft remnants, sinuses, cysts are also the result of failure of branchial cleft to complete its normal development

ABBREVIATIONS N/A

REFERENCES

- Ashcraft KW, Murphy JP, Sharp RJ, editors. Pediatric Surgery. 3rd ed. Philadelphia: WB Saunders Co; 2000
- O'Neill JA, Rowe MI, Grosfeld JL, et al. Pediatric Surgery. 5th ed. St Louis: Mosby; 1998
- Ziegler M, Azizkhan R, Weber T, et al, editors. Operative Pediatric Surgery. New York: McGraw-Hill Companies; 2003.

Web references: 0 available at www.5mcc.com
Illustrations N/A

Author(s):
Timothy L. Black, MD

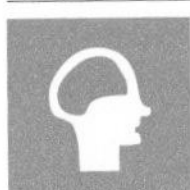

BASICS

DESCRIPTION Collection of pus usually localized. Can be associated with lactation or fistulous tracts secondary to squamous epithelial neoplasm or duct occlusion.
System(s) affected: Skin/Exocrine
Genetics: N/A
Incidence/Prevalence in USA: Common
Predominant age:
- Subareolar abscess - postmenopausal
- Puerperal abscess - premenopausal

Predominant sex: Female

SIGNS & SYMPTOMS
- Tender breast lump, fluctuant, usually unilateral
- Erythema
- Draining pus
- Local edema
- Systemic malaise
- Fever
- Nipple and skin retraction
- Proximal lymphadenopathy

CAUSES
- Puerperal abscesses - blocked lactiferous duct
- Subareolar abscess - squamous epithelial neoplasm with keratin plugs or ductal extension with associated inflammation
- Peripheral abscess - stasis of the duct

RISK FACTORS
- Puerperal mastitis 5-11% go on to abscess
- Diabetes
- Rheumatoid arthritis
- Steroids
- Silicone/paraffin implants
- Lumpectomy with radiation
- Heavy cigarette smoking
- Nipple retraction

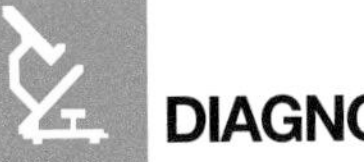

DIAGNOSIS

DIFFERENTIAL DIAGNOSIS
- Carcinoma (inflammatory)
- Tuberculosis (may be associated with HIV infection)
- Actinomycosis
- Typhoid
- Sarcoid
- Syphilis
- Hydatid cyst
- Sebaceous cyst

LABORATORY
- Leukocytosis
- Elevated sedimentation rate
- Culture and sensitivity of drainage to identify pathogen, usually staphylococci or streptococcus. Non-lactational abscess associated with anaerobic bacteria.

Drugs that may alter lab results: None

Disorders that may alter lab results: None

PATHOLOGICAL FINDINGS
- Squamous metaplasia of the ducts
- Intraductal hyperplasia
- Epithelial overgrowth
- Fat necrosis
- Duct ectasia

SPECIAL TESTS None

IMAGING
- Ultrasound
- Mammogram - cannot exclude carcinoma

DIAGNOSTIC PROCEDURES
- Aspiration for culture
- Fine needle aspiration (FNA) not accurate to exclude carcinoma

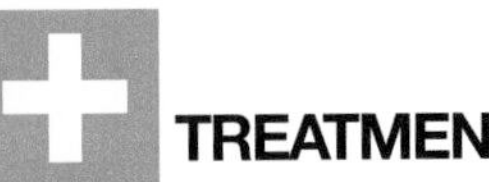

TREATMENT

APPROPRIATE HEALTH CARE Outpatient, unless systemically immunocompromised

GENERAL MEASURES
- Cold compresses
- Expression of milk

SURGICAL MEASURES
- Aspiration possibly under ultrasound guidance
- Incision and drainage with removal of loculations and biopsy of all non-puerperal abscesses to rule out carcinoma
- Open all fistulous tracts, especially in nonlactating abscesses

ACTIVITY No restrictions

DIET No restrictions

PATIENT EDUCATION
- Care of wound
- Breast feeding precautions

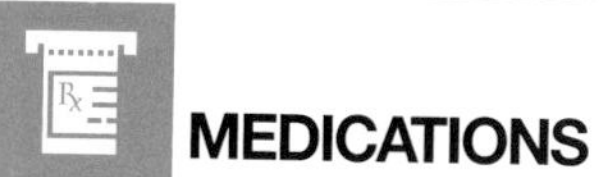

MEDICATIONS

DRUG(S) OF CHOICE
- Non-steroidal anti-inflammatory agents
- Erythromycin 250-500 mg qid
- First generation, oral cephalosporin
  - ◊ Cephalexin 500 mg bid
  - ◊ Cefaclor 250 mg tid
- Amoxicillin-clavulanate (Augmentin) 250 mg tid
- Clindamycin 300 mg tid if anaerobes suspected

Contraindications: Allergy to antibiotic
Precautions: Refer to manufacturer's profile of each drug
Significant possible interactions: Refer to manufacturer's profile of each drug

ALTERNATIVE DRUGS N/A

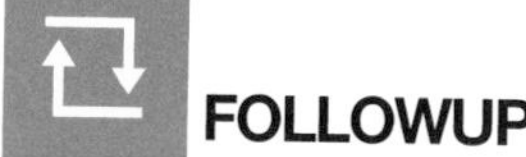

FOLLOWUP

PATIENT MONITORING Assure resolution to exclude carcinoma

PREVENTION/AVOIDANCE
- Early treatment of mastitis with milk expression and cold compresses
- Early treatment with antibiotics

POSSIBLE COMPLICATIONS Fistula

EXPECTED COURSE/PROGNOSIS
Good. Complete healing expected in 8 to 10 days, particularly if abscess can be incised and drained.

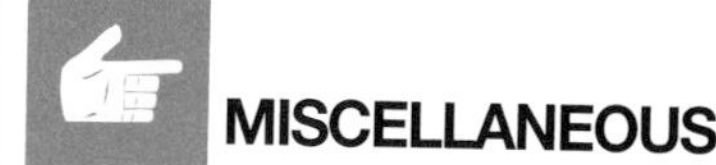

MISCELLANEOUS

ASSOCIATED CONDITIONS N/A

AGE-RELATED FACTORS
Pediatric: N/A
Geriatric: N/A
Others: N/A

PREGNANCY Most commonly associated with postpartum lactation

SYNONYMS
- Mammary abscess
- Peripheral breast abscess
- Subareolar abscess
- Puerperal abscess

ICD-9-CM
611.0 Inflammatory disease of breast
675.1 Puerperal, postpartum

SEE ALSO

OTHER NOTES N/A

ABBREVIATIONS N/A

REFERENCES

- Benson EA: Management of breast abscesses. World J Surg 1989;13:753-756
- Dixon JM: Periductal mastitis/duct ectasia. World J Surg 1989;13:715-720
- Ferrara JJ, et al: Non surgical management of breast infections in non-lactating women. Am Surg 1990;56:668-671
- Olsen CG, Gordon RE: Breast disorders in nursing mothers. Am Fam Physician 1990;41:1509-1515
- Smallwood JA: Benign breast disease. Baltimore, Urban & Schwarzenberg, 1990
- Maier WP, et al: Nonlactational breast infection. Amer Surg 1994;60:247-250
- Bundred NJ, Dover MS, et al: Breast abscess and cigarette smoking. Br Jour Surg 1992;79(1):58-59
- Karstoup S, et al: Acute puerperal breast abscess: US-guided drainage. Radiology 1993;188(3):807-809

Web references: 0 available at www.5mcc.com
Illustrations N/A

Author(s):
Thomas R. Strigle, MD

BASICS

DESCRIPTION Malignant neoplasm in the breast. Breast cancers are classified as noninvasive (in situ) or invasive (infiltrating) with approximately 70% of all breast cancers possessing a component of invasion.

System(s) affected: Gastrointestinal, Musculoskeletal, Nervous, Pulmonary, Skin/Exocrine

Genetics:
- Only 20% of patients have a significant family history of breast cancer. This predisposition tends to be autosomal dominant with maternal lineage.
- Recent studies have revealed families with breast cancer susceptibility genes including BRCA1 and BRCA2. Family history suggestive of breast cancer susceptibility genes include multiple first and second degree relatives with early breast cancer diagnosis and the presence of ovarian cancer. Approximately 1 in 400 U.S. women will carry a germ-line mutation for BRCA1. BRCA1 and BRCA2 carriers have a 50 - 85 % lifetime risk of breast cancer, ovarian cancer, or both. BRCA2 carriers have a higher risk of male breast cancer.

Incidence/Prevalence in USA:
- 1 in 8 women will develop breast cancer within a lifetime
- The American Cancer Society estimates that 217,440 new cases will be diagnosed in 2004 with 40,580 deaths (including 470 men)

Predominant age: 30-80 with peak age 45-65; 77% of cases occur in women > age 50

Predominant sex: Female > Male (1% occurs in male)

SIGNS & SYMPTOMS
- Palpable mass (55%)
- Abnormal mammogram without a palpable mass (35%)
- Color changes
- Lymphedema (peau d'orange)
- Dimpling
- Nipple retraction
- Breast enlargement
- Axillary mass
- Bone pain (rare)
- Discharge (bloody discharge is more ominous)

CAUSES Unknown

RISK FACTORS
- Increased breast cancer risk occurs in first degree relatives (relative risk [RR] = 2.3), with bilateral disease in premenopausal relatives (RR = 10.5), or bilateral disease in postmenopausal relatives (RR = 5.0)
- Increased hormone risks include early menarche, late menopause, nulliparity or first full term pregnancy after age 30
- Women with a prior history of breast cancer or previous breast biopsies revealing atypical changes are at increased risk (5-10 times) for subsequent cancer
- Exogenous estrogen use, especially in conjunction with progestins increase the risk of breast cancer

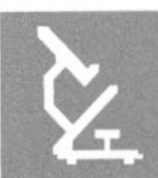

DIAGNOSIS

DIFFERENTIAL DIAGNOSIS
- Differential diagnosis is extensive
- Benign breast disorders such as abscesses, hematomas, or fibroadenomas
- Proliferative breast diseases such as fibrocystic changes, ductal and lobular hyperplasia, or sclerosing adenosis
- Malignant breast diseases including sarcomas, lymphomas, or metastatic disease to breast

LABORATORY Initial lab tests include CBC, LFTs, CXR, bilateral mammography +/- ultrasound, pathologic review of biopsy, estrogen and progesterone receptor determination, and S phase determination

Drugs that may alter lab results: N/A

Disorders that may alter lab results: N/A

PATHOLOGICAL FINDINGS
- Noninvasive cancers (carcinoma in situ)
  - ◊ The percentage of non-invasive cancers diagnosed is increasing due to increased mammography screening
  - ◊ Usually detected by abnormal mammogram
  - ◊ Noninvasive cancers are of two types: Intraductal or intralobular. Intraductal cancers are subdivided by growth patterns: Micropapillary, cribriform, solid, or comedo. The comedo growth pattern is considered more aggressive.
- Invasive cancers
  - ◊ Tend to present with a breast lump
  - ◊ Subdivided into - not-otherwise-specified (50%), lobular (5%), Paget disease (2%), and miscellaneous (metaplastic, neuroendocrine, or squamous cell carcinomas [1%])
  - ◊ Patients with invasive histologies with medullary 6%, colloid 7%, tubular, papillary, and adenoid cystic carcinomas 2%, have improved survival

SPECIAL TESTS
- Bone scan should be performed if symptoms suggest bony metastasis, if alkaline phosphatase is elevated, or if widespread disease is suspected
- CT or US of the abdomen may be indicated if widespread or recurrent disease is suspected

IMAGING
- Mammography
  - ◊ Detects 80% of breast cancers, is the best technique for the detection of minimal (< 0.5 cm) breast cancer. The most common abnormality representing cancer is an irregular mass.
  - ◊ Microcalcifications can occur as the only sign of malignancy in 35% of breast cancers
  - ◊ 10-20% of palpable cancers have normal mammograms. Do not fail to biopsy a mass because of a "normal" mammogram.
- Ultrasound may confirm whether a suspicious lump is solid or cystic and help define its size and extent

DIAGNOSTIC PROCEDURES
- Tissue confirmation of the suspicious mass or abnormal mammogram is essential. Biopsy may be excisional or incisional depending upon the size and location of the abnormality.
- Biopsy of non-palpable lesions is achieved with needle localization
- Cytologic confirmation of a palpable abnormality may be obtained by fine needle aspiration or core needle biopsy

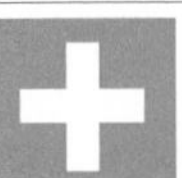

TREATMENT

APPROPRIATE HEALTH CARE Patients are usually treated by a team consisting of a medical oncologist, a surgeon, and a radiation oncologist

GENERAL MEASURES
- Early breast cancer treatment (Stage I/II)
  - ◊ Lumpectomy (wide excision with breast conservation) and radiotherapy is the treatment of choice for early primary breast cancer.
  - ◊ Axillary node dissection is indicated with all invasive tumors and large noninvasive ones. Identification and biopsy of sentinel nodes may be preferred over axillary dissection because of its lower morbidity rate, but is only appropriate in women with tumors <5cm and who have not had radiation or chemotherapy
  - ◊ Most women with primary breast cancer have subclinical metastases and many will have recurrence of disease despite apparently curative surgery and the use of radiotherapy. Combination chemotherapy is indicated for most patients with early breast cancer.
- Treatment of locally advanced breast cancer (Stage III)
  - ◊ Usually multidisciplinary treatment consisting of mastectomy, axillary dissection, radiation, and chemotherapy +/- tamoxifen
  - ◊ Preoperative chemotherapy or hormonal therapy often converts inoperable tumors to operable ones
- Treatment of advanced or recurrent disease (Stage IV)
  - ◊ Surgical resection if possible; chemotherapy, radiation, hormonal therapy.

SURGICAL MEASURES
- Breast conserving surgery is appropriate for most breast cancers
- Studies comparing mastectomy to breast conserving procedures show no difference in long-term survival
- If any axillary nodes are positive, 60-70% risk of relapse within 5 years
- If all axillary nodes are negative, there is 70-80% chance of long-term cure

ACTIVITY Minimal activity restrictions exist during treatment

DIET No proven relationship exists between breast cancer and diet

PATIENT EDUCATION
- Patients should be reminded of the importance of regular mammography in the early detection of breast cancer. Physicians may choose to recommend self breast examination (SBE).
- For a listing of sources for patient education materials, physicians may contact: American Cancer Society and the National Cancer Institute

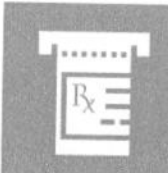

MEDICATIONS

DRUG(S) OF CHOICE

- Metastatic disease is considered incurable, but treatable with remissions occurring in 30-40% of patients
- Chemotherapy reduces the risk of recurrence 22-37% and death 14-27%
- Combination chemotherapy is preferred over single agents
- High dose chemotherapy with bone marrow transplant doesn't appear to improve survival
- Tamoxifen reduces the risk of recurrence and death for women of all ages; treatment should be continued for five years. It probably is not of benefit to women with estrogen receptor negative tumors.

Contraindications: Strict hematologic, renal, hepatic, and cardiac guidelines need to be followed for the administration of cytotoxic chemotherapy

Precautions: Monitoring for infection is important for patients receiving chemotherapy. Tamoxifen increases the patient's risk of developing endometrial cancer and interacts with warfarin, erythromycin, cyclosporin, nifedipine, and diltiazem.

Significant possible interactions: Drug interactions are common and depend on combinations used. Refer to manufacturer's literature.

ALTERNATIVE DRUGS N/A

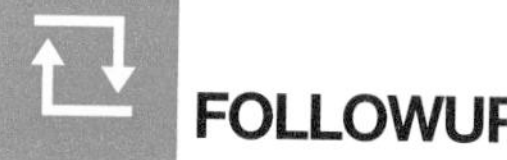

FOLLOWUP

PATIENT MONITORING

- Up to 60% of patients with invasive disease will relapse within five years despite initial therapy
- The status of the axillary lymph nodes is the most important indicator for disease relapse
- Surveillance for recurrent disease should include physical examination every 4 months for 2 years, every six months for 3 years, then yearly. Mammography and routine chemistries should be done annually. Women on tamoxifen should have annual pelvic exams.
- Workup of suspected recurrence should include CBC, LFTs, CXR, bone scan, CT of affected area, +/- biopsy

PREVENTION/AVOIDANCE

- Estrogen use and alcohol consumption increase risk
- Decreasing dietary fat has not been shown to alter breast cancer risk
- The synthetic antiestrogen, tamoxifen, may be a useful prophylactic agent in high risk women
- The selective estrogen receptor modulator, raloxifene (Evista), reduced the risk of breast cancer in short term studies and may play a role in prevention in the future
- Mammography
  - ◊ Screening for disease: US Preventive Services Task Force recommends mammography with or without clinical breast examination every 1-2 years for women over 40. American Cancer Society recommends mammography and a clinical breast examination every year after age 40. They also recommend clinical breast examination every 3 years for ages 20-39. ACOG and AMA recommend mammogram every 1-2 years and annual clinical breast examination starting at age 40 and then annual mammograms at age 50.
  - ◊ Diagnostic mammography should be performed at the advice of the patient's physician
  - ◊ In women ages 50-69, mammography screening can reduce mortality by 30%; the reduction in mortality is less impressive for women younger than 50 or older than 70

POSSIBLE COMPLICATIONS

- Postoperative: lymphedema (< 5% in modified radical mastectomy), seromas, wound infection, and limited shoulder motion
- Chemotherapy: nausea, vomiting, alopecia, leukopenia, bladder irritation, stomatitis, fatigue, and menstrual abnormalities
- Tamoxifen: hot flushes, menstrual irregularities including menopause, vaginal discharge, hypercalcemia, skin rashes, and possible endometrial carcinoma
- Irradiation: skin reaction, fibrosis (1%), brachial plexopathy (1%), rib fracture (1%), arm edema, pulmonary fibrosis (1%), and rarely second breast malignancy.

EXPECTED COURSE/PROGNOSIS

- 5 year survival
  - ◊ Stage 0 (noninvasive) 100%
  - ◊ Stage I (2 cm, no spread) 98%
  - ◊ Stage II (>2 cm, or spread to axillary lymph nodes) 76-88%
  - ◊ Stage III (>5 cm or fixed nodes, metastatic disease to the skin, inflammatory changes, chest wall extension, or supraclavicular lymph nodes) 49-56%
  - ◊ Stage IV (distant metastatic disease) 16%

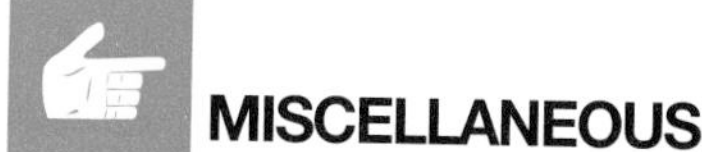

MISCELLANEOUS

ASSOCIATED CONDITIONS Organ disease at metastatic sites

AGE-RELATED FACTORS Age-specific incidence of breast cancer increases sharply until menopause and continues to increase at a slower rate in the geriatric population

Pediatric: Breast cancer occurs rarely in children with the most common pathology being secretory carcinoma

Geriatric: There is a higher percentage of ER positive tumors (80%) in the geriatric population. This correlates with improved disease-free survival.

Others: N/A

PREGNANCY Breast cancer occurs infrequently during pregnancy (2.8%). Delay in diagnosis is common, and most series report poorer survival related to advanced stage at diagnosis.

SYNONYMS N/A

ICD-9-CM

174.9 Malignant neoplasm of female breast, unspecified

175.9 Malignant neoplasm of male breast, other and unspecified sites

SEE ALSO

OTHER NOTES N/A

ABBREVIATIONS

ER = estrogen receptor

PgR = progesterone receptor

REFERENCES

- Morrow M. The evaluation of common breast problems. Am Fam Physician 2000;61(8):2371-8, 2385
- Margolese RG. Surgical considerations for invasive breast cancer. Surg Clin No Amer 1999;79(5):1031-46
- Smith RA, Mettlin C, Johnson-Davis K, et al. American Cancer Society guidelines for the early detection of cancer. CA Cancer J Clin 2004;54:41-52
- Schairer C, Lubin J, Troisi R, et al. Menopausal estrogen and estrogen-progestin replacement therapy and breast cancer risk. JAMA 2000;283(4):485-91
- Hortobagyi G. Treatment of breast cancer. N Engl J Med 1998;339(14):974-84
- Krag D, Weaver D, et al. The sentinel node in breast cancer. N Engl J Med 1998;339(14):941-946
- Osborne C Tamoxifen in the treatment of breast cancer. N Engl J Med 1998;339(22):1609-18.
- National Comprehensive Cancer Network (NCCN) Practice Guidelines, 2004

Web references: 4 available at www.5mcc.com

Illustrations 1 available

Author(s):

Stephen M. Adams, MD

BASICS

DESCRIPTION
- Advantages
  - ◊ Fewer respiratory, gastrointestinal and otitis media infections
  - ◊ Ideal food - easily digestible, nutrients well absorbed, less constipation
  - ◊ Increased contact between mother and baby and, perhaps, added self-esteem for mother
  - ◊ Economical, portable, easy to meet needs quickly
  - ◊ Decreased incidence of allergies in childhood
  - ◊ Decreased incidence of breast cancer in mother
  - ◊ More rapid and complete reversion of mother's pelvis and uterus to pre-puerperal state
- Contraindications
  - ◊ HIV infection
  - ◊ Active TB
  - ◊ Hepatitis is not a contraindication
  - ◊ Substances of abuse will pass into human milk; please see Reference on drugs in lactation
- Physiology
  - ◊ Stimulation of areola causes secretion of oxytocin
  - ◊ Oxytocin is responsible for let-down reflex when milk is ejected from cells into milk ducts
  - ◊ Sucking stimulates secretion of prolactin which triggers milk production. Thus milk is made in response to nursing and increases supply.
- Technique
  - ◊ Get in comfortable position, usually sitting or reclining with baby's head in crook of mother's arm (side-lying position often useful following C-section delivery)
  - ◊ Bring baby to mother to decrease stress on back
  - ◊ Baby's belly and mother's belly should face each other or touch (belly-to-belly)
  - ◊ Initiate the rooting reflex by tickling baby's lips with nipple or finger. As baby's mouth opens wide, mother guides her nipple to back of her baby's mouth while pulling the baby closer. This will ensure that the baby's gums are sucking on the areola, not the nipple.

System(s) affected: Endocrine/Metabolic, Skin/Exocrine
Genetics: N/A
Incidence/Prevalence in USA: According to the 2001 National Immunization Survey, 65% of new mothers initiated breast feeding and 27% were doing at least some breast feeding at six months of age. The national goal is 75% and 50% respectively.
Predominant age: 16-45
Predominant sex: Female only

SIGNS & SYMPTOMS N/A

CAUSES N/A

RISK FACTORS N/A

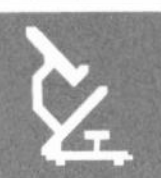

DIAGNOSIS

DIFFERENTIAL DIAGNOSIS N/A

LABORATORY N/A

Drugs that may alter lab results: N/A

Disorders that may alter lab results: N/A

PATHOLOGICAL FINDINGS N/A

SPECIAL TESTS N/A

IMAGING N/A

DIAGNOSTIC PROCEDURES N/A

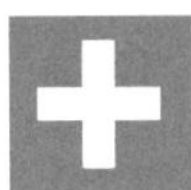

TREATMENT

APPROPRIATE HEALTH CARE Outpatient

GENERAL MEASURES See Patient Education

SURGICAL MEASURES N/A

ACTIVITY No restrictions

DIET
- Adequate calorie and protein intake while nursing. Drinking cow's milk is not necessary.
- Drink plenty of fluids
- Continue prenatal vitamins
- Fluoride supplement unnecessary
- New National Academy of Science guidelines recommend that children get at least 200 IU/day of vitamin D beginning in the newborn period to prevent rickets. For exclusively breastfed babies, this will require taking a vitamin supplement such as PolyViSol or Vi-Daylin vitamin drops, 1/2 cc/day.

PATIENT EDUCATION
- Antepartum
  - ◊ Regular promotion of advantages of breast-feeding
  - ◊ Discuss woman's postpartum plans, i.e., if going to work. Emphasize possibility of nursing part-time after returning to work or nursing until weaning the week before returning to work
  - ◊ Emphasize importance of only breast-feeding for first 3 weeks of life to allow adequate build up of sufficient milk supply. Substitution of a bottle feed can occur after this time and still allow for continued nursing.
  - ◊ Counsel women on technique
- Natural history
  - ◊ Colostrum present in breast at birth but may not be seen
  - ◊ Milk will not come in before 3rd day postpartum
  - ◊ Frequent nursing (at least 9 or more times/24 hours) will lead to milk coming in sooner and in greater quantities
  - ◊ Allow baby to determine duration of each nursing; baby will lose weight the first few days and may not get back to birth weight until

day 10
- Postpartum
  - ◊ Immediate breast-feeding after the birth
  - ◊ Rooming-in to encourage on-demand feeding
  - ◊ Observation of a nursing session by experienced physician, nurse or lactation consultant
  - ◊ Avoid formula or water supplementation
  - ◊ Review expectations, techniques. Be very encouraging.
  - ◊ See in office within a few days of discharge, especially if first-time nursing
- Signs of adequate nursing
  - ◊ Breasts become hard before and soft after feeding
  - ◊ 6 or more wet diapers in 24 hours
  - ◊ Baby satisfied; appropriate weight gain (average one ounce/day in first few months)
  - ◊ Growth spurts - anticipate these around 10 days, 6 weeks, 3 months, and 4-6 months. Baby will nurse more often at these times for several days. This will increase milk production to allow for further adequate growth.
  - ◊ Supplemental baby vitamins are unnecessary unless the baby has very limited exposure to sun (then needs vitamin D)
- Weaning
  - ◊ Breast milk alone is adequate food for first 6 months
  - ◊ Solids may be introduced at 4-6 months
  - ◊ For mothers going to work, start switching the baby to bottle feeding during the hours mother will be gone about a week ahead of time. Do this by dropping a breast-feed every few days and substituting pumped breast milk or formula, preferably given by another caregiver.
  - ◊ To increase the likelihood that baby will take a bottle occasionally, introduce it at 3-4 weeks and give once or twice a week

- Family planning
  - ◊ Frequent nursing increases the duration of postpartum amenorrhea; however, breast-feeding is not a completely reliable form of contraception. Options include barrier methods, implants, Depo-Provera, oral contraceptions, IUDs and the lactational amenorrhea method. There is some disagreement on estrogen's effect on milk supply, so some providers use progesterone-only birth control pills in the early postpartum period.

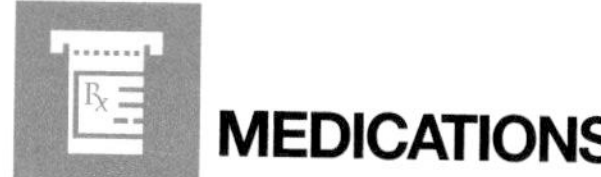

MEDICATIONS

DRUG(S) OF CHOICE N/A
Contraindications: N/A
Precautions: N/A
Significant possible interactions: N/A

ALTERNATIVE DRUGS N/A

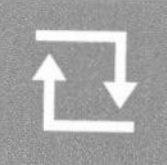

FOLLOWUP

PATIENT MONITORING See mother and baby within a few days of hospital discharge if she is a first-time breast-feeder

PREVENTION/AVOIDANCE N/A

POSSIBLE COMPLICATIONS
- Plugged ducts (mother is well except for)
  - ◊ Sore lump in one or both breasts without fever
  - ◊ Use moist hot packs on lump prior to and during nursing; more frequent nursing on affected side; ensure good technique
- Mastitis
  - ◊ Sore lump in one or both breasts plus fever and/or redness on skin overlying lump
  - ◊ Use moist hot packs on lump prior to and during nursing; more frequent nursing on affected side; antibiotics covering for Staph. aureus (the most common organism) for at least 7 days
  - ◊ Patients can be quite ill with mastitis
  - ◊ Other possible sources of fever should be ruled out - endometritis, pyelonephritis in particular. Mother should get increased rest, use acetaminophen (Tylenol) as necessary. Fever should resolve within 48 hours or consider changing antibiotics. Lump should also resolve. If it continues, an abscess may be present requiring surgical drainage.
- Milk supply inadequate
  - ◊ Check weight gain
  - ◊ Review signs of adequate supply; review technique, frequency and duration of nursing
  - ◊ Check to see if mother has been supplementing, thereby decreasing her own milk production
- Sore nipples
  - ◊ Check technique
  - ◊ Baby should be taken off the breast by breaking the suction with a finger in the mouth
  - ◊ Air-dry nipples after each nursing; no breast creams and do not wash nipples with soap and water; check for signs of thrush in baby and mother
- Engorgement
  - ◊ Usually develops after milk first comes in (day 3 or 4)
  - ◊ Signs are warm, hard, sore breasts
  - ◊ To resolve, offer baby more frequent nursing; may have to hand express a little milk to soften areola enough to let baby latch on; nurse long enough to empty breasts; generally resolves within a day or two
- Flat or inverted nipples
  - ◊ When stimulated, inverted nipples will retract inward, flat nipples remain flat; should check for this on initial prenatal physical
  - ◊ Nipple shells, a doughnut-shaped insert, can be worn inside the bra during the last month of pregnancy to gently force the nipple through the center opening of the shell
  - ◊ Babies can nurse successfully even if the shell does not correct the problem before birth. A lactation consultant or La Leche League member may be a good resource in this situation. Another source: J Human Lactation. 9(1):27-29, 1993.

EXPECTED COURSE/PROGNOSIS
Healthy baby

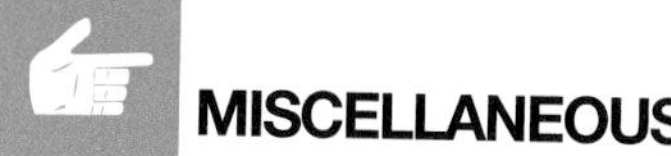

MISCELLANEOUS

ASSOCIATED CONDITIONS N/A

AGE-RELATED FACTORS N/A
Pediatric: N/A
Geriatric: N/A
Others: N/A

PREGNANCY N/A

SYNONYMS N/A

ICD-9-CM

SEE ALSO

OTHER NOTES N/A

ABBREVIATIONS N/A

REFERENCES

- Briggs GG, et al. Drugs in Pregnancy and lactation. 6th ed. Baltimore: Williams & Wilkins; 2001
- Riordan J, Auerback K. Pocket Guide to Breast-feeding and Human Lactation. 2nd ed. Spira-bound. Boston: Jones and Bartlett; 2000
- Moreland J, Coombs J. Promoting and supporting breast-feeding. Am Fam Physician 2000;61(7):2093-100, 2103-4
- Sinusas K, Gagliardi A. Initial management of breast-feeding. Am Fam Physician 2001;15;64(6):981-8
- Mortensen EL, Michaelsen KF, et al. The association between duration of breastfeeding and adult intelligence. JAMA 2002;287(18):2365-71

Web references: 1 available at www.5mcc.com
Illustrations N/A

Author(s):
Eric Henley, MD, MPH

BASICS

DESCRIPTION At the time of delivery the fetal buttocks are the presenting part in the maternal pelvis
- Frank breech presentation - the fetal hips are flexed and the knees extended with the feet near the shoulders, accounting for 60-65% of breech presentations at term
- Incomplete breech presentation - one or both of the fetal hips are incompletely flexed, resulting in some part of the fetal lower extremity as the presenting part. Thus the terms single footling, double footling, knee presentation. Accounts for 25-35% of breech presentations.
- Complete breech - similar to frank breech except knees are flexed rather than extended. Accounts for 5% of breech presentations.

System(s) affected: Reproductive
Genetics: Fetal anomalies including anencephaly, hydrocephalus, trisomy 21 and 18 have higher incidence of breech birth
Incidence/Prevalence in USA: 3-4% of singleton term deliveries and up to 15-30% of low birth weight infants (< 2500 grams). Breech presentation is common in early pregnancy. At 25-26 week about 20-30% of singleton fetus are in breech position but this decreases near term.
Predominant age: N/A
Predominant sex: Female only

SIGNS & SYMPTOMS
- Anus palpable on digital vaginal exam
- Leopold's maneuver reveals ballottable head in fundal region
- Mom reports kicking in lower abdomen
- Presenting part not palpable in pelvis near term

CAUSES Probably a combination of one or more of the risk factors listed below

RISK FACTORS
- Fetal anomalies including anencephaly, hydrocephalus, trisomy 21, fetal alcohol syndrome, Potter's syndrome, myotomic dystrophy
- Uterine anomalies including bicornate uterus
- Uterine relaxation associated with great parity
- Uterine overdistension as in polyhydramnios or multiple gestation
- Placenta previa
- Placental implantation in cornual-fundal region
- Low birth weight or premature infant
- Macrosomia
- Pelvic contractions or irregularly shaped pelvis - such as android or platypelloid pelvis
- Pelvic tumors
- Nulliparity
- Previous history of breech birth

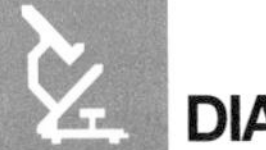

DIAGNOSIS

DIFFERENTIAL DIAGNOSIS
- In labor, diagnosis is made by vaginal exam and confirmed by ultrasound. Can be confused with face presentation on digital vaginal exam.
- In breech greater trochanter and anus form a straight line. In face presentation mouth and malar bones form a triangle.

LABORATORY None

Drugs that may alter lab results: N/A

Disorders that may alter lab results: N/A

PATHOLOGICAL FINDINGS
- Congenital malformation among term breech infants: Overall incidence 6-9%
- There is a higher incidence of congenital hip dislocation in infants with breech presentation at term

SPECIAL TESTS N/A

IMAGING
- Ultrasound - confirms presenting part
- X-ray - flat plate of abdomen and pelvimetry to determine extent of head flexion and pelvic measurements (rarely done)

DIAGNOSTIC PROCEDURES Near term women should be examined to determine presenting part. If breech is suspected on ultrasound should be done to confirm presenting part. When breech presentation confirmed, the option for external version or elective C-section should be discussed with the patient.

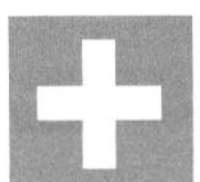

TREATMENT

APPROPRIATE HEALTH CARE Inpatient for labor and delivery

GENERAL MEASURES
- Continuous electronic fetal monitoring during labor
- Breech presentation may be converted by external version (see Prevention/Avoidance) but this is not always successful and has risks
- Currently ACOG recommends external version at term and planned cesarean delivery for persistent breech presentation. This recommendation is based on large randomized clinical trial showing decreased perinatal and neonatal morbidity and mortality in planned breech cesarean delivery vs. planned breech vaginal delivery. There was no difference in maternal morbidity or mortality.

SURGICAL MEASURES
- Breech delivery is accomplished either vaginally or by cesarean section
- Most physicians and patients opt for elective cesarean delivery for breech presentation near term, which is usually scheduled after patient is 39 weeks.
- When a patient presents in labor with the fetus in breech position, a decision about a trial of labor or immediate cesarean section must be made. Preferably this decision is made prior to onset of labor.
- Obtain ultrasound to document fetal presentation, to check for fetal abnormalities, and to estimate fetal weight in deciding candidacy for vaginal delivery
- The selection criteria for vaginal delivery are fairly strict to reduce morbidity and mortality for both mother and infant (rarely done)
- Cesarean section is recommended in the following circumstances unless the fetus is too immature to survive:
  - ◊ Large (> 3500 grams) or small (< 2500 grams) fetus, estimated by ultrasound or skilled observer
  - ◊ Pelvic contraction or unfavorable pelvic shape (platypelloid and android)
  - ◊ Hyperextended head
  - ◊ Significant fetal heart rate abnormality
  - ◊ Footling breech
  - ◊ Severe fetal growth retardation
  - ◊ Premature fetus greater than 26 weeks with mother in active labor
  - ◊ Previous cesarean section (sometimes)
  - ◊ Abnormal labor including failure to dilate, prolonged second stage, and failure of descent
  - ◊ Mother primipara
  - ◊ Mother unable or unwilling to cooperate
- Cesarean section procedure:
  - ◊ Prepare for cesarean section by starting IV fluids and obtaining blood type and screen, in all patients, in case needed for emergency
  - ◊ A low transverse cesarean section may need to be extended vertically if there is difficulty with head entrapment (this extension produces a weak scar)
  - ◊ General anesthesia with isoflurane can rapidly relax the uterus and allow delivery of an entrapped after-coming head
  - ◊ Delivery usually accomplished with spinal anesthesia
  - ◊ Cord blood gases should be obtained following delivery
- Vaginal delivery procedures:
  - ◊ Currently not recommended but may be an option in limited circumstances. (Patient presenting in advanced labor or second twin.)
  - ◊ The candidate for vaginal delivery needs to be attended by a birth attendant skilled in breech delivery, a scrubbed assistant, an anesthesiologist capable of rapid induction of general anesthesia, and an individual skilled in neonatal resuscitation.
  - ◊ Epidural is preferred anesthesia
  - ◊ Leave membranes intact as long as possible to prevent possible cord prolapse
  - ◊ The patient should not push until fully dilated due to risk of partial delivery through a cervix that is not fully dilated which can lead to head entrapment
  - ◊ Consider cutting a large episiotomy to allow sufficient room for delivery
  - ◊ Use abdominal guidance of fetal head to keep it flexed as it descends into pelvis
  - ◊ The infant should not be touched before the umbilicus crosses the maternal perineum
  - ◊ Traction prior to this point constitutes a complete breech extraction and is associated with higher risk of perinatal morbidity and mortality
  - ◊ With the fetal back anterior, maintain downward traction while grasping the fetal hips until the scapula becomes visible
  - ◊ Check for nuchal arm
  - ◊ As one axilla becomes visible rotate the infant until the shoulders are oriented anteriorly and posteriorly allowing their delivery
  - ◊ The fetal head is delivered in a face down position with either piper forceps or manual flexion of the head
  - ◊ Cord blood gases should be obtained following delivery

ACTIVITY Bedrest during labor

DIET Nothing by mouth until delivery accomplished

PATIENT EDUCATION
- Educate patient about increased risk of fetal distress, and fetal trauma in both cesarean and vaginal breech delivery compared to vaginal vertex delivery
- Vaginal breech delivery is associated with increased risk of prolapsed cord and/or cord compression; fetal hypoxia; nuchal arm, with attendant risk of trauma including humerus fracture, clavicle fracture, and nerve palsies; and entrapment of fetal head
- External version may allow for vaginal vertex delivery with decreased risk of infant and maternal morbidity. (see prevention/avoidance)
- When planned elective cesarean breech delivery is chosen mode of delivery, the patient should be instructed to go to the hospital at the first signs of labor, if she goes into labor prior to scheduled cesarean section which is usually scheduled at 39-40 week gestation
- Risk of cesarean delivery including infection, bleeding, possible damage to maternal bladder or bowel. Slight increased risk maternal morbidity and mortality compared to vaginal vertex delivery.

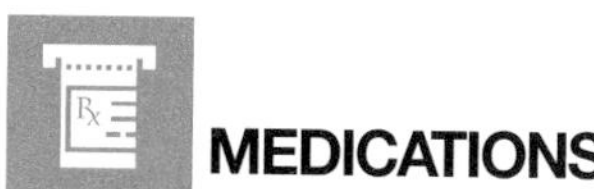

MEDICATIONS

DRUG(S) OF CHOICE None
Contraindications: N/A
Precautions: N/A
Significant possible interactions: N/A

ALTERNATIVE DRUGS N/A

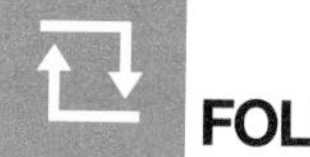

FOLLOWUP

PATIENT MONITORING
- Continuous fetal heart rate monitoring should be done during labor and delivery
- Six weeks postpartum care is done as with other deliveries

PREVENTION/AVOIDANCE
- External cephalic version (ECV)
  - ◊ Conversion of breech to vertex can be attempted after 36 week gestation and if successful allows for vaginal vertex delivery. Success rates 48-78% with reversion rates back to breech of 2%.
  - ◊ ECV associated with risk (1-2%) of umbilical cord entanglement, abruptio placenta, preterm labor, premature rupture of membranes (PROM), fetal brachycardia, fetal-maternal hemorrhage, and severe maternal discomfort
  - ◊ Prior to procedure tocolytics are usually administered and RhoGAM is given to Rh negative mothers
  - ◊ ECV should only be attempted with continuous fetal heart monitoring in the delivery suite where immediate cesarean delivery can be done
  - ◊ ECV requires two operators, one to monitor fetal cardiac activity via ultrasound and holding fetal position while the second person lifts buttocks out of pelvis by abdominal manipulation and then guides the fetal head into pelvis
  - ◊ Contraindications to ECV include multiple pregnancy, non-reassuring fetal monitoring, placenta previa, PROM, abruption, previous uterine surgery, uterine malformation, oligohydramnios, maternal cardiac disease, or major fetal anomalies
  - ◊ Successful ECV factors include - multiparity, relaxed abdominal wall, adequate amniotic fluid, nonfrank breech, floating presenting part, posterior placenta, and average maternal body weight
  - ◊ Failure of ECV associated with maternal obesity, nulliparity, anteriorly located placenta, large fetus, decrease amniotic fluid, frank breech that is engaged in pelvis
- Prevention of fetal anomalies by tight glucose control in diabetics. Antenatal folate therapy to decrease risk of neural tube detects.

POSSIBLE COMPLICATIONS
- Trauma to the head, soft tissue, brachial plexus and spinal cord - not always prevented by cesarean
- Asphyxia secondary to cord compression or prolapse
- Congenital hip dislocation

EXPECTED COURSE/PROGNOSIS
- Perinatal morbidity and mortality are much higher in breech births. A large proportion of the deaths are related to congenital abnormalities.
- In patients properly selected for vaginal delivery, potentially perinatal morbidity and mortality, and maternal morbidity are reduced
- For infants 750 -1500 grams or less than 32 weeks gestational age, there is a much higher rate of cerebral hemorrhage and perinatal death associated with vaginal compared to cesarean delivery

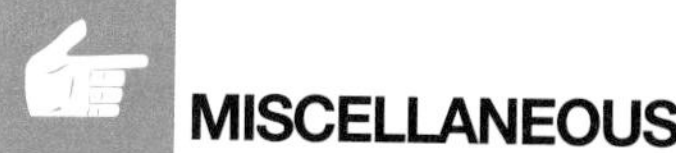

MISCELLANEOUS

ASSOCIATED CONDITIONS
- See Risk Factors
- Congenital hip dislocation is more common in first born females

AGE-RELATED FACTORS
Pediatric: N/A
Geriatric: N/A
Others: N/A

PREGNANCY A problem of pregnancy

SYNONYMS N/A

ICD-9-CM
652.20 Breech presentation without mention of version, unspecified
763.0 Breech delivery and extraction
763.4 Cesarean delivery

SEE ALSO
Placenta previa
Premature labor

OTHER NOTES Maneuvers of cesarean breech delivery are similar to vaginal breech extraction and can be associated with severe trauma to the infant

ABBREVIATIONS N/A

REFERENCES

- Cunningham FG, Gant NF, eds. Williams' Obstetrics. 21st ed. New York, NY: McGraw-Hill; 2001
- Scorza W. Intrapartum management of breech presentation. Clinics in Pernat 1996;23(1):31-49
- Erkkola R: Controversies: Selective vaginal delivery for breech presentation, J Perinat Med 1996;24:553-61
- Committee on Obstetric Practice. ACOG committee opinion. Mode of term singleton breech delivery. Number 265, December 2001. American College of Obstetricians and Gynecologists. Int J Gynaecol Obstet 2002;77(1):65-6

Web references: 2 available at www.5mcc.com
Illustrations N/A

Author(s):
Kimberle Vore, MD

BASICS

DESCRIPTION Chronic irreversible, abnormal dilatation of the bronchi, usually accompanied by infection and productive cough
System(s) affected: Pulmonary
Genetics: Associated with many conditions including some that are congenital or hereditary
Incidence/Prevalence in USA:
- No reliable figures available
- Less common than it once was, probably due to more effective treatment of childhood respiratory infections

Predominant age: Begins most often in early childhood, but symptoms may not appear until later in life
Predominant sex: Male = Female

SIGNS & SYMPTOMS
- Cough
- Sputum - copious and purulent
- Hemoptysis
- Wheezing
- Coarse or moist crackles
- Cyanosis
- Digital clubbing
- Dyspnea
- Barrel chest
- Emaciation
- Fatigue
- Fever
- Recurrent pneumonia
- Tachycardia
- Tachypnea

CAUSES
- Alpha-1-antitrypsin deficiency
- Allergic bronchopulmonary aspergillosis
- Bronchial obstruction
- Cystic fibrosis
- Dyskinetic cilia syndromes
- Hypogammaglobulinemia
- Inhaling noxious chemicals
- Kartagener syndrome (situs inversus, sinusitis, immotile spermatozoa, bronchiectasis)
- Necrotizing pulmonary infections
- Pulmonary abscess
- Severe lung infection in childhood (measles, adenovirus, influenza, pertussis, or bronchiolitis)
- Tuberculosis
- Congenital immunodeficiency syndromes
- Chronic aspiration
- Rheumatic diseases
- Transplant graft rejection

RISK FACTORS
- Repeated bouts of pneumonia
- Any chronic respiratory illness
- Retained foreign body
- Immunodeficiency
- Gastroesophageal reflux
- Sinusitis

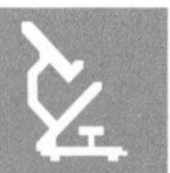

DIAGNOSIS

DIFFERENTIAL DIAGNOSIS
- Chronic bronchitis
- Chronic obstructive pulmonary disease
- Cystic fibrosis
- Pulmonary tuberculosis
- Allergic bronchopulmonary aspergillosis

LABORATORY
- Positive sputum culture (yields H. influenzae, Streptococcus pneumoniae, staphylococcal, klebsiella, pseudomonas, or anaerobes)
- Hypoxemia
- Leukocytosis, usually
- Serum immunoglobulins - check for hypogammaglobulinemia, IgE level helpful

Drugs that may alter lab results: N/A

Disorders that may alter lab results: N/A

PATHOLOGICAL FINDINGS
- Bronchial dilation
- Inflamed bronchi
- Purulent bronchorrhea
- Necrosis of bronchial mucosa
- Peribronchial scarring

SPECIAL TESTS
- Sweat test
- Skin test for aspergillus
- Bronchoscopy useful in locating bleeding site and to exclude adenoma or foreign body
- Ciliary biopsy with electron microscopy (EM)
- Pulmonary function tests show variable obstruction and restriction; include test for reversible component
- Sputum culture/sensitivity, AFB, fungus

IMAGING
- CT scan
  - ◊ Shows dilation and truncation of airways with signet rings prominent in lower lobes
  - ◊ High resolution CT is best to establish diagnosis and extent of disease
  - ◊ Spiral CT helpful for questionable findings
- Bronchography has limited role
- Chest x-ray
  - ◊ Can be normal
  - ◊ Coarse lung markings - honeycomb/tram tracks
  - ◊ Air-fluid level
  - ◊ Cystic lesions
  - ◊ Atelectasis

DIAGNOSTIC PROCEDURES
- Fiberoptic bronchoscopy
  - ◊ Recommended when disease is of recent onset or is unilateral
  - ◊ May be combined with bronchography
  - ◊ Obtain culture

TREATMENT

APPROPRIATE HEALTH CARE Outpatient except for possible surgery

GENERAL MEASURES
- Airway clearance techniques
  - ◊ Chest physical therapy
  - ◊ Percussion (mechanical)
  - ◊ Postural drainage
  - ◊ Hydration
  - ◊ Nebulized saline
  - ◊ Pulmonary rehabilitation with inspiratory muscle training
  - ◊ Noninvasive positive pressure ventilation, nocturnal or chronic
- Bronchoscopy may be required for extraction of mucus or mycelial plugs, or if physiotherapy has failed
- Pulmonary rehabilitation to improve functional status
- Bronchial artery embolization may be lifesaving for massive pulmonary hemorrhage
- Avoid cigarette smoking
- Treat acid reflux if needed

SURGICAL MEASURES Segmental pulmonary resection for localized disease or refractory hemoptysis

ACTIVITY As fully active as possible

DIET No restrictions

PATIENT EDUCATION Printed patient information available from: American Lung Association, 1740 Broadway, New York, NY 10019, (212)315-8700

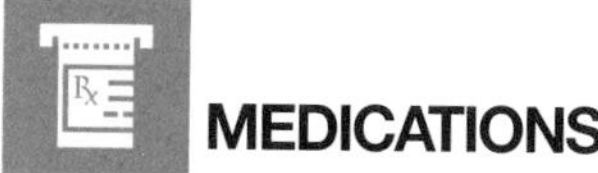

MEDICATIONS

DRUG(S) OF CHOICE
- Bronchodilators
  - ◊ Use chronically to enhance sputum clearance; particularly beneficial with asthma or aspergillosis
  - ◊ Beta-adrenergic agonists (e.g., albuterol) given by metered dose inhaler with use of a spacer (reservoir device)
- Inhaled corticosteroids
  - ◊ Use chronically to enhance sputum clearance
  - ◊ Beclomethasone, fluticasone, etc., given by metered dose inhaler
- Antibiotics
  - ◊ Use early for exacerbations. Continue minimum of 7-10 days. May use culture to guide choice. Chronic prophylaxis not recommended.
  - ◊ Ciprofloxacin
  - ◊ Levofloxacin
  - ◊ Ampicillin: 250-500 mg orally q 6 hours (50 mg/kg/day in divided doses q 6-8 hours in children less than 20 kg)

or
  - ◊ Trimethoprim-sulfamethoxazole: DS q12h
  - ◊ Tetracycline: 250-500 mg orally q 6 hours
  - ◊ Nebulized aminoglycosides - tobramycin 300 mg by aerosol bid
- Steroids
  - ◊ Consider for patients with bronchopulmonary aspergillosis. IgE level guides steroid dosing.

Contraindications:
- Tetracycline: not for use in pregnancy or children < 8 years.

Precautions:
- Tetracycline: may cause photosensitivity; sunscreen recommended.

Significant possible interactions:
- Tetracycline: avoid concurrent administration with antacids, dairy products, or iron.
- Broad-spectrum antibiotics: may reduce the effectiveness of oral contraceptives; barrier method recommended.

ALTERNATIVE DRUGS
- For chronic persistent infection, long-term high dose of amoxicillin 3 g every 12 hours may be useful. It does not provide relief for everyone and has more side effects.
- Other broad-spectrum antimicrobials including anti-pseudomonals if required. Choice would depend on pathogen and susceptibility.
- Inhaled corticosteroids if reversible obstruction present
- Oxygen - if PO2 < 60 mm Hg
- Nicotine replacement, consider to aid smoking cessation

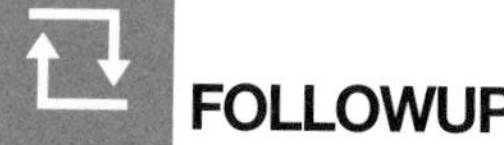

FOLLOWUP

PATIENT MONITORING
- Frequent followup for progress of illness, prevention of infection, smoking cessation, and to check on physiotherapy
- Pulmonary function and C-reactive protein may be monitored to assess inflammation and disease progression
- At some point in followup, need to discuss with patient the possibility of mechanical ventilation and cardiopulmonary resuscitation in the future. The patient, family and provider should determine if this type of treatment is appropriate.

PREVENTION/AVOIDANCE
- Treat all pneumonias adequately
- Immunizations for viral illnesses (e.g., influenza)
- Immunization for pneumococcal pneumonia
- Routine childhood immunizations (e.g., pertussis, measles, Hib)
- Genetic counseling if inherited etiology

POSSIBLE COMPLICATIONS
- Recurrent pulmonary infections
- Pulmonary hypertension
- Secondary amyloidosis
- Cor pulmonale
- Brain abscess
- Massive hemoptysis
- Atelectasis
- Lung abscess

EXPECTED COURSE/PROGNOSIS
- Chronic. Surgery may be curative if disease localized.
- Average life expectancy - 55 years
- 10% of patients have a rapidly progressive course

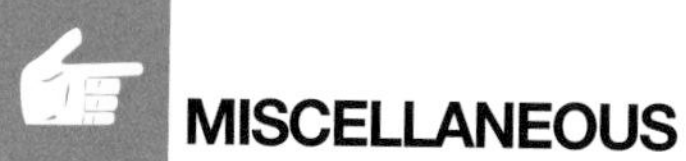

MISCELLANEOUS

ASSOCIATED CONDITIONS
- Sinusitis
- Cor pulmonale
- Kartagener syndrome
- Cystic fibrosis
- Ulcerative colitis
- Marfan syndrome
- Ehlers-Danlos syndrome
- Yellow nail syndrome

AGE-RELATED FACTORS
Pediatric: Cystic fibrosis and other congenital disorders
Geriatric: Elderly more likely to need hospitalization for treatment
Others: N/A

PREGNANCY N/A

SYNONYMS N/A

ICD-9-CM
494.0 Bronchiectasis without acute exacerbation
494.1 Bronchiectasis with acute exacerbation

SEE ALSO
Aspergillosis
Bronchiolitis obliterans & organizing pneumonia
Cystic fibrosis
Kartagener syndrome
Lung abscess

OTHER NOTES Conditions that may lead to bronchiectasis include severe pneumonia (especially measles, pertussis, adenoviral infections in children), necrotizing infections due to Klebsiella, staphylococci, influenza virus, fungi, mycobacteria, mycoplasma, bronchial obstruction from any cause (foreign body, carcinoma, enlarged mediastinal lymph nodes

ABBREVIATIONS N/A

REFERENCES
- Hardy KA. A review of airway clearance: New techniques, indications and recommendations. Respir Care 1994;39(5):440-5
- Lewiston NJ. Bronchiectasis in childhood. Pediatr Clin North Am 1984;31(4):865-78
- Marwah OS. Bronchiectasis: How to identify, treat and prevent. Postgrad Med 1995;97:149-59
- Barker AF. Bronchiectasis. N Engl J Med 2002;346(18):1383-93

Web references: 1 available at www.5mcc.com
Illustrations N/A

Author(s):
Gregory Snyder, MD

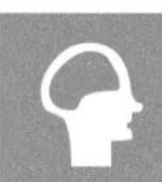

BASICS

DESCRIPTION Inflammation of the bronchioles, usually seen in young children, occasionally in high-risk adults. May be seasonal (winter and spring) and often occurs in epidemics. Usual course: insidious; acute; progressive.
System(s) affected: Pulmonary
Genetics: N/A
Incidence/Prevalence in USA: Medical care provided to 1000-1500/100,000 annually. Estimated incidence is higher. Annual winter-spring epidemics.
Predominant age: newborn-2 years (peak age 2-6 months)
Predominant sex: Male > Female

SIGNS & SYMPTOMS
- Anorexia
- Cough
- Cyanosis
- Expiratory wheezing
- Apnea
- Fever
- Grunting
- Inspiratory crackles
- Intercostal retractions
- Irritability
- Noisy breathing
- Otitis media
- Pharyngitis
- Tachycardia
- Tachypnea
- Vomiting

CAUSES
- Respiratory syncytial virus - most prevalent
- Parainfluenza
- Adenovirus
- Rhinovirus
- Influenza virus
- Chlamydia
- Eye, nose, mouth inoculation
- Exposure to adult with URI
- Day care exposure (significant)
- Idiopathic (many adult cases)

RISK FACTORS
- Contact with infected person
- Children in day care environment
- Heart-lung transplantation patient
- Adults - exposure to toxic fumes, connective tissue disease

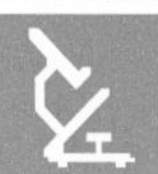

DIAGNOSIS

DIFFERENTIAL DIAGNOSIS
- Asthma
- Vascular ring
- Lobar emphysema
- Foreign body
- Heart disease
- Pneumonia
- Reflux
- Aspiration
- Cystic fibrosis

LABORATORY
- Arterial blood gas - hypoxemia, hypercarbia, acidemia
- Respiratory viral culture
- Respiratory viral antigens

Drugs that may alter lab results: N/A

Disorders that may alter lab results: N/A

PATHOLOGICAL FINDINGS
- Abundant mucous exudate
- Mucosal - hyperemia, edema
- Submucosal lymphocytic infiltrate, monocytic infiltrate, plasmacytic infiltrate
- Small airway debris, fibrin, inflammatory exudate, fibrosis
- Peribronchiolar mononuclear infiltrate

SPECIAL TESTS
Infant pulmonary function studies - research tool

IMAGING
- Chest x-ray
  - ◊ Focal atelectasis - RUL common
  - ◊ Air trapping
  - ◊ Flattened diaphragm
  - ◊ Increased anteroposterior diameter
  - ◊ Peribronchial cuffing

DIAGNOSTIC PROCEDURES N/A

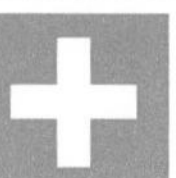

TREATMENT

APPROPRIATE HEALTH CARE
- Most patients can be treated at home
- Inpatient indicated for patient with increased respiratory distress, cyanosis, and dehydration or inability to feed

GENERAL MEASURES
- Most critical phase is first 48-72 hours after onset. Treatment is usually symptomatic.
- Fluid at maintenance
- Mechanical ventilation in respiratory failure
- Isolation: contact; handwashing most important
- Antiviral agents for selected high-risk patients
- Cardio-respiratory monitoring
- Inhaled bronchodilators are commonly used, although efficacy has been hard to demonstrate in controlled studies
- Steroids may not change course - except in patients with reactive airway disease

SURGICAL MEASURES N/A

ACTIVITY
- Avoid exposure to crowds, viral illness for 2 months
- Avoid smoke

DIET
- Frequent small feedings of clear liquids
- If hospitalized, may require intravenous fluids

PATIENT EDUCATION
- Griffith: Instructions for Patients; Philadelphia, Elsevier
- American Academy of Pediatrics; website www.aap.org

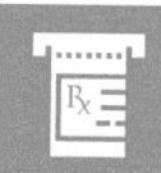

MEDICATIONS

DRUG(S) OF CHOICE
- Oxygen
- Albuterol: may be effective for acute symptoms
- Epinephrine aerosols may be of more benefit
- Ribavirin: For infants and children, an inhaled antiviral agent active against RSV, may be indicated in patients with underlying cardio-pulmonary disease, young age (< 6 weeks), or with severe RSV (elevated pCO2; require mechanical ventilation - use with caution via ventilator). Nebulize via small particle aerosol generator (SPAG). Use of ribavirin has decreased in recent years, secondary to lack of significant clinical efficacy.

Contraindications: Refer to manufacturer's literature

Precautions: None

Significant possible interactions: None

ALTERNATIVE DRUGS
- Antibiotics only if secondary bacterial infection present (rare)
- Corticosteroids do not change course, unless infant has reactive airway disease. In adults corticosteroids may be helpful.

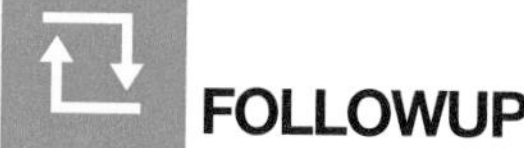

FOLLOWUP

PATIENT MONITORING
- If patient is receiving home care, follow daily by telephone for 2-4 days
- For hospitalized patient, monitor as needed depending on severity of infection. Bronchiolitis can be associated with apnea.

PREVENTION/AVOIDANCE
- Hand washing
- Contact isolation of infected babies
- Persons with colds should keep contacts with infants to a minimum
- Palivizumab (Synagis), a monoclonal product, administered monthly, November thru March, 15 mg/kg IM. Available in single use vials of 100mg and 50mg. Used for RSV prevention in high risk patients:
    - ◊ 28-32 weeks gestation and less than 6 months old in November
    - ◊ Less than 28 weeks gestation and less than 12 months old
    - ◊ Moderately severe BPD and up to two years old
    - ◊ Hemodynamically significant congenital heart disease (until age 6 months)
- RSV immune globulin, a human blood product, can also be used in at-risk patients. Monthly infusions of 750 mg/kg, November thru March, in a controlled setting. Avoid fluid overload. Vial is 50 mg/mL; infuse at 1.5-6 mL/kg/hr; monitor oximeter and vital signs.
- Both of these medications are quite expensive.

POSSIBLE COMPLICATIONS
- Bacterial superinfection
- Bronchiolitis obliterans
- Apnea
- Respiratory failure
- Death
- Increased incidence of RAD

EXPECTED COURSE/PROGNOSIS
- In most cases, recovery is complete within 7-10 days
- Mortality statistics differ, but probably under 1%
- High-risk infants (BPD, CHD) may have prolonged course

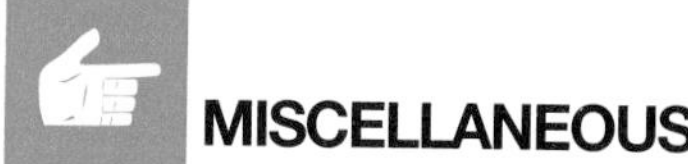

MISCELLANEOUS

ASSOCIATED CONDITIONS
- Common cold
- Conjunctivitis
- Pharyngitis
- Otitis media
- Diarrhea

AGE-RELATED FACTORS
Pediatric: Most common in infants

Geriatric: N/A

Others: N/A

PREGNANCY N/A

SYNONYMS N/A

ICD-9-CM
466.11 Acute bronchiolitis due to respiratory syncytial virus

466.19 Acute bronchiolitis due to other infectious organisms

SEE ALSO

OTHER NOTES N/A

ABBREVIATIONS
BPD = bronchopulmonary dysplasia

CHD = congenital heart disease

RAD = reactive airway disease

SPAG = small particle aerosol generator

REFERENCES

- Mandell GL, ed. Principles and Practice of Infectious Diseases. 4th Ed. New York: Churchill Livingstone; 1995
- Fields BN, et al, eds. Virology. 2nd Ed. New York: Raven Press; 1990
- Red Book: 2003 Report of the Committee on Infectious Diseases. 26th ed. Elk Grove Village, IL: American Academy of Pediatrics; 2003.p.523-27

Web references: 1 available at www.5mcc.com

Illustrations N/A

Author(s):
Nancy N. Dambro, MD

BASICS

DESCRIPTION This is a specific reaction of lung tissue to a variety of injuries. The lungs show a pattern of multiple patchy pneumonia. These are seen on chest x-ray as patchy alveolar or ground glass opacifications with or without interstitial infiltrates and may have air bronchograms as well.
System(s) affected: Pulmonary
Genetics: N/A
Incidence/Prevalence in USA: Uncommon
Predominant age: Reported cases range age 0-70, mean age 50's
Predominant sex: N/A

SIGNS & SYMPTOMS
- Most cases present with a flu-like illness that lasts 4-10 weeks or longer. Most have been treated with antibiotics without success.
- Fever
- Dry cough
- Weight loss
- Dyspnea may be severe
- Crackles and perhaps squeaks over involved area
- Fatigue

CAUSES Idiopathic. A complex response to a variety of injuries, such as toxic inhalation; post mycoplasma, viral and bacterial infection; aspiration; immunologic factors.

RISK FACTORS
- AIDS
- Immunocompromised patients, including transplant patients

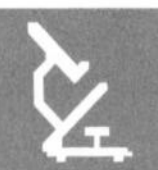

DIAGNOSIS

DIFFERENTIAL DIAGNOSIS
- Usual interstitial pneumonitis (UIP)
- Noninfectious diseases
- Tuberculosis
- Sarcoidosis
- Histoplasmosis
- Berylliosis
- Goodpasture syndrome
- Neoplasm
- Polyarteritis nodosa
- Systemic lupus erythematosus
- Wegener granulomatosis
- Sjögren syndrome
- Chronic eosinophilic pneumonia
- Cryptogenic bronchiolitis

LABORATORY
- Leukocytosis with a normal differential
- Elevated ESR, usually quite elevated
- Negative cultures
- Negative serology for mycoplasma, Coxiella, Legionella, psittacosis, and fungus
- Negative viral studies

Drugs that may alter lab results: N/A

Disorders that may alter lab results: N/A

PATHOLOGICAL FINDINGS
- Intraluminal fibrosis of distal airspaces is the major pathologic feature
- Fibroblasts and plugs of inflammatory cells and loose connective tissue fill these distal airways
- The inflammatory cells are mainly lymphocytes and plasma cells
- Interstitial fibrosis is present
- The plugs of edematous granulation tissue in the terminal and respiratory bronchioles and alveolar ducts do not cause permanent damage

SPECIAL TESTS
- Pulmonary function shows a restrictive/obstructive pattern
- Flow-volume loop shows terminal airway obstruction
- Chest x-ray may show patchy alveolar opacities often in the mid or upper lung area. A ground glass pattern that may have air bronchograms.
- V/Q scan: matched patchy defects

IMAGING
- Chest x-ray - often appears more normal than the physical examination
- CT scans more accurately define the distribution and extent of the patchy alveolar opacities with areas of hyperlucency

DIAGNOSTIC PROCEDURES
- Open lung biopsy
- Transbronchial biopsy
- It may be well to use a trial of steroids as a diagnostic trial, though not all would agree
- If a diagnostic trial is successful, be prepared to treat the patient for at least a year

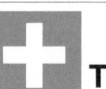

TREATMENT

APPROPRIATE HEALTH CARE Inpatient

GENERAL MEASURES
- Monitor blood gases or pulse oximetry
- Oxygen as necessary

SURGICAL MEASURES N/A

ACTIVITY As tolerated

DIET No special diet

PATIENT EDUCATION Followup is especially important. Relapse is common. Treatment is prolonged. If medication tapered too rapidly, relapse may well occur.

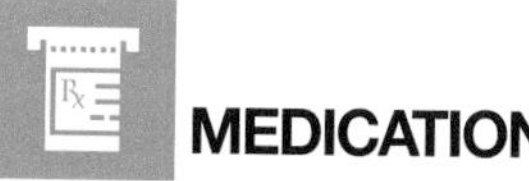

MEDICATIONS

DRUG(S) OF CHOICE
- Prednisone
  - ◊ 60 mg daily for 1-3 months
  - ◊ Then tapered over a few weeks to 20 mg (this dose may later be given as alternate day therapy). Increase length of taper for patients on long-term therapy to avoid precipitating Addisonian crisis.
  - ◊ Treatment may be needed for one year or more

Contraindications: Refer to manufacturer's literature

Precautions: Be aware of the patient's Mantoux status and history of peptic ulcer disease. Long-term steroid associated with significant adverse effects including Cushing syndrome, fluid retention, osteoporosis, hyperkalemia, poor wound healing.

Significant possible interactions: Refer to manufacturer's literature

ALTERNATIVE DRUGS
- Steroids other than prednisone may be used
- One paper reported the use of erythromycin 600 mg/ day for 3-4 months after initial control with prednisone
- Antimicrobials if original infection is persistent. Choice depends on the pathogen.

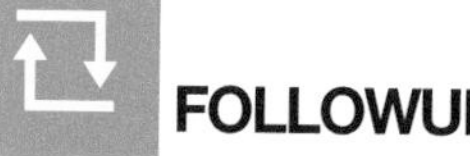

FOLLOWUP

PATIENT MONITORING
- Frequent visits, weekly initially
- Emphasize the need to continue the prednisone because of the chance of relapse
- Monitor the lung disease and the side effects of prednisone therapy (Mantoux, monthly CBC, funduscopic exam every 3-6 months)

PREVENTION/AVOIDANCE
Except for prevention of relapse, none known

POSSIBLE COMPLICATIONS
- Bronchiectasis
- Death, but with proper treatment, recovery is usually complete without permanent sequelae

EXPECTED COURSE/PROGNOSIS
Complete recovery but individual case management is mandatory

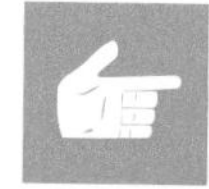

MISCELLANEOUS

ASSOCIATED CONDITIONS
- Drug-induced pneumonitis
  - ◊ Paraquat poisoning
  - ◊ Amiodarone toxicity
  - ◊ Acebutolol toxicity
  - ◊ Freebase cocaine pulmonary toxicity
  - ◊ Overdose of L-tryptophan
  - ◊ Though most were treated with antibiotics only penicillamine and sulfasalazine have been implicated
- Infections
  - ◊ Chronic infectious pneumonia
  - ◊ Malaria
- Immuno-compromise
  - ◊ Bone marrow transplantation
- Connective tissue diseases
  - ◊ Rheumatic lung
  - ◊ Sjogren syndrome
  - ◊ Polymyositis
  - ◊ Scleroderma
  - ◊ Essential mixed cryoglobulinemia
- Miscellaneous
  - ◊ Cystic fibrosis
  - ◊ Bronchopulmonary dysplasia
  - ◊ Renal failure
  - ◊ Congestive heart failure
  - ◊ Adult respiratory distress syndrome
  - ◊ Chronic eosinophilic pneumonia
  - ◊ Hypersensitivity pneumonitis
  - ◊ Histiocytosis X
  - ◊ Sarcoidosis
  - ◊ Pneumoconioses
  - ◊ Radiation pneumonitis

AGE-RELATED FACTORS
Pediatric: Rare, but has been reported after viral pneumonia (adenovirus influenza). Characteristics include delayed recovery, persistent cough, crackles or wheezing after pneumonia. The laboratory findings are generally not helpful. Imaging shows: V/Qm matched defects; HRCT, bronchiectasis, bronchogram, pruned tree appearance. Diagnosis confirmed by biopsy. Treatment includes steroids - 1 mg/kg/24 hrs for one month, followed by weaning over several months.

Geriatric: Not common

Others: Apparently only seen in adults

PREGNANCY
N/A

SYNONYMS
- Intraluminal fibrosis of distal airways
- Idiopathic BOOP
- Cryptogenic organizing pneumonia (COP)
- Obliterative bronchiolitis

ICD-9-CM
491.8 Other chronic bronchitis

SEE ALSO
Sjögren syndrome

OTHER NOTES
This disease behaves differently than bronchiolitis obliterans (BO). BOOP is a restrictive problem, BO is an obstructive problem. BO causes permanent lung damage and BOOP is completely reversible.

ABBREVIATIONS
V/Q = ventilation-perfusion ratio

HRCT = high resolution computerized tomography

REFERENCES

- Cordier JF, Loire R, Brune J: Idiopathic Bronchiolitis Obliterans Organizing Pneumonia. Chest 1989;96:999-1004
- Mueller NL, Staples CA, Miller RR: Bronchiolitis Obliterans Organizing Pneumonia: CT features in 14 patients. AJR 1990;154:983-987
- Epler GR, Colby TV, et al: Bronchiolitis Obliterans Organizing Pneumonia. N Eng J Med 1985;312:152-158
- Hardy KA, Schidlow D, Zaeri N: Obliterative Bronchiolitis in Children. CHEST 1988;93:460-466
- St John RC, Dorinsky PM: Cryptogenic bronchiolitis. Clin Chest Med 1993;14(4): 667-75
- Lynch DA: Imaging of small airways diseases. Clin Chest Med 1993;14(4):623-34

Web references: 1 available at www.5mcc.com

Illustrations N/A

Author(s):
David A. Pope, MD

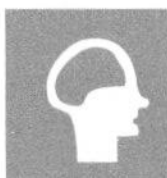

BASICS

DESCRIPTION Inflammation of trachea, bronchi and bronchioles resulting from a respiratory tract infection or chemical irritant. Generally self-limited with complete healing and full return of function. Most infections are viral.

System(s) affected: Pulmonary
Genetics: No known genetic pattern
Incidence/Prevalence in USA: Common
Predominant age: All ages
Predominant sex: Male = Female

SIGNS & SYMPTOMS
- Preceding respiratory tract infection, such as a common cold with coryza, malaise, chills, slight fever, sore throat, back and muscle pain
- Cough, initially dry and unproductive, then productive. Later, mucopurulent sputum.
- Fever
- Fatigue, aching
- Hemoptysis
- Chest burning
- Dyspnea (sometimes)
- Rales, rhonchi, wheezing
- No evidence of pulmonary consolidation
- Pharynx injected

CAUSES
- *Adenovirus*
- *Influenza* A and B
- *Parainfluenza*
- *Chlamydia pneumoniae* (TWAR agent)
- *Bordetella pertussis*
- *Respiratory syncytial virus*
- *Coxsackievirus*
- *Herpes simplex*
- *Haemophilus influenzae*
- Possibly fungi
- *Mycoplasma*
- Secondary bacterial infection as part of an acute upper respiratory infection
- *Streptococcus pneumoniae*
- *Moraxella catarrhalis*
- *Mycobacterium tuberculosis*
- *Rhinovirus*
- *Coronovirus* (types 1-3)

RISK FACTORS
- Chronic bronchopulmonary diseases
- Chronic sinusitis
- Bronchopulmonary allergy
- Hypertrophied tonsils and adenoids in children
- Immunosuppression
- Air pollutants
- Elderly
- Infants
- Smoking
- Second-hand smoke
- Alcoholism
- Gastroesophageal reflux disease (GERD)
- Tracheostomy
- Environmental changes
- Immunoglobulin deficiency

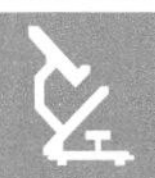

DIAGNOSIS

DIFFERENTIAL DIAGNOSIS
- Asthma
- Influenza
- Bronchopneumonia
- Bronchiectasis
- Acute sinusitis
- Aspiration
- Cystic fibrosis
- Reactive airways dysfunction syndrome (RADS)
- Bacterial tracheitis
- Retained foreign body
- Inhalation injury
- Heart failure
- Bronchogenic carcinoma
- GERD (Gastroesophageal Reflux Disease)

LABORATORY
- Arterial blood gases - hypoxemia (rarely)
- Leukocytosis
- Sputum culture/gram stain
- Viral titers
- Mycoplasma titers

Drugs that may alter lab results: N/A

Disorders that may alter lab results: N/A

PATHOLOGICAL FINDINGS
- Mucosal hyperemia and inflammation
- Desquamation of columnar epithelium
- Mucopurulent exudate

SPECIAL TESTS Pulmonary function tests (seldom needed during acute stages) - increased residual volume, decreased maximal expiratory rate

IMAGING Chest x-ray - lungs normal if uncomplicated. Helps rule out other diseases or complications.

DIAGNOSTIC PROCEDURES Symptoms and signs

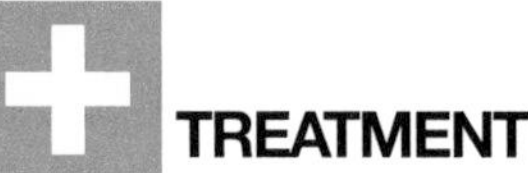

TREATMENT

APPROPRIATE HEALTH CARE
Outpatient unless elderly or complicated by severe underlying disease

GENERAL MEASURES
- Rest
- Steam inhalations
- Vaporizers
- Antibiotics if bacterial etiology suspected
- Adequate hydration
- Stop smoking
- Treat associated illnesses (e.g., GERD)
- Antitussives

SURGICAL MEASURES N/A

ACTIVITY Rest until fever subsides

DIET Increased fluids (up to 3-4 L/day) while febrile

PATIENT EDUCATION For patient education materials favorably reviewed on this topic, contact: American Lung Association, 1740 Broadway, New York, NY 10019, (212)315-8700

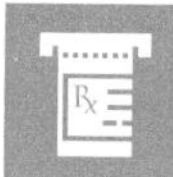

MEDICATIONS

DRUG(S) OF CHOICE
- Amantadine or rimantadine therapy if influenza A suspected; most effective if started within 24-48 hours of development of symptoms
- Decongestants if accompanied by sinus condition
- Antipyretic analgesic such as aspirin or ibuprofen
- Antibiotics - for more severe symptoms (high fever persists, concomitant COPD, purulent discharge).
  - ◊ amoxicillin 500 mg q8hrs or trimethoprim-sulfa-methoxazole DS q12hrs for routine infection
  - ◊ Macrolide - clarithromycin (Biaxin) 500 mg q12hr or azithromycin (Zithromax) Z-pack for PCN or sulfa allergy or mycoplasma infection
  - ◊ Doxycycline 100 mg qd for 10 days if *Moraxella*, *Chlamydia* or *Mycoplasma* suspected
  - ◊ Quinolone for more serious infection or other antibiotic failure
- Cough suppressant for troublesome cough (not with COPD); guaifenesin with codeine or dextromethorphan
- Bronchodilators (aerosols/steroids)
- Consider steroids for bronchospasm

Contraindications:
- Doxycycline should not be used during pregnancy or in children
- Avoid using clarithromycin (Biaxin) if using oral contraceptives

Precautions: Refer to manufacturer's literature. Watch for theophylline toxicity with macrolides and quinolones. Macrolides also interfere with oral contraceptives.

Significant possible interactions: Refer to manufacturer's literature

ALTERNATIVE DRUGS
- Other antibiotics if indicated by sputum culture (*Moraxella* needs different set of antibiotics)
- Antivirals
- Other macrolides or quinolones according to pathogen and sensitivity

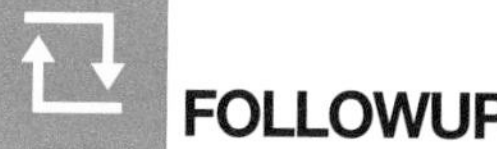

FOLLOWUP

PATIENT MONITORING
- Oximetry until no longer hypoxemic
- Recheck for chronicity

PREVENTION/AVOIDANCE
- Avoid smoking
- Control underlying risk factors (asthma, sinusitis, reflux)
- Avoid exposure
- Vaccinations

POSSIBLE COMPLICATIONS
- Bronchopneumonia
- Acute respiratory failure
- Bronchiectasis
- Chronic cough
- Hemoptysis
- Superinfection

EXPECTED COURSE/PROGNOSIS
- Usual - complete healing with good return of function
- Can be serious in elderly or debilitated patients
- Cough may persist for several weeks after initial improvement
- Post-bronchitic reactive airways disease (rare)
- Bronchiolitis obliterans and organizing pneumonia (BOOP) (rare)

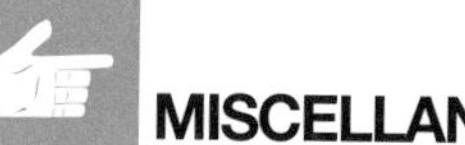

MISCELLANEOUS

ASSOCIATED CONDITIONS
- Asthma
- Epiglottitis
- Coryza
- Pharyngitis
- Croup
- Influenza
- Smoking
- Pneumonia
- Emphysema
- Sinusitis
- Bronchial obstruction
- Gastroesophageal reflux disease

AGE-RELATED FACTORS
Pediatric:
- Occurrence in this age group usually is in association with other conditions of upper and lower respiratory tract (trachea usually involved)
- Some children seem to be more susceptible than others (if repeated attacks, child should be evaluated for anomalies of the respiratory tract including immune deficiencies)
- If acute bronchitis is caused by respiratory syncytial virus, may be fatal

Geriatric: Can be a serious illness in this age group, particularly if part of influenza

Others: N/A

PREGNANCY N/A

SYNONYMS Tracheobronchitis

ICD-9-CM
466.0 Acute bronchitis

SEE ALSO
Asthma

Chronic obstructive pulmonary disease & emphysema

OTHER NOTES N/A

ABBREVIATIONS
GERD = gastroesophageal reflux disease

RADS = reactive airways dysfunction syndrome

REFERENCES

- Baum GL, Wolinsky E, editors. Textbook of Pulmonary Diseases. 4th ed. Boston: Little, Brown & Co.; 1989
- Gwaltney JM JR. Acute bronchitis. In: Mandell Gl, Bennett JE, Dolin R (eds): Principles and Practices of Infectious Disease. 4th ed. New York, Churchill Livingstone, 1995:606-08
- Seaton A, Seaton D, Leitch AG: Crofton and Douglas's Respiratory Diseases. Boston, Blackwell Scientific Publications, 1989
- Heuston WJ, Mainous AG III. Acute bronchitis. Am Fam Phys 1998;57(6):1270-76

Web references: 0 available at www.5mcc.com

Illustrations N/A

Author(s):
Alan J. Cropp, MD

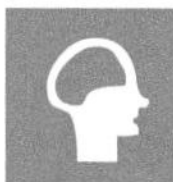

BASICS

DESCRIPTION Systemic bacterial infection caused by Brucella species in infected animal products, or vaccine. Incubation period usually 5-60 days, but highly variable and may be several months. Characterized by intermittent or irregular fevers, with symptoms ranging from subclinical disease to infection of almost any organ system. Bone and joint involvement common. May be chronic or recurrent. Case fatality untreated less than 2%.

System(s) affected: Cardiovascular, Endocrine/Metabolic, Gastrointestinal, Musculoskeletal, Nervous, Pulmonary, Renal/Urologic, Skin/Exocrine

Genetics: None; some evidence for intrauterine transmission

Incidence/Prevalence in USA:
- About 100/year (105 cases in 1992; 0.34/100,000), but probably underreported
- Common in developing countries; consider in immigrants
- Highest rates in Hispanic population, along US-Mexico border
- Considered a potential biological terror agent in aerosolized form
- Reportable in all states except Nevada

Predominant age: All ages, but especially 20-60 (occupational exposure), sometimes children (milk-related outbreaks)

Predominant sex:
- Male > Female (occupational exposure)
- Female ≥ Male (milk exposure)

SIGNS & SYMPTOMS
- Fever (may be undulant, increased in afternoon and evening, maximum 101-104° daily); weakness; headache; sweating; chills; generalized aching; arthralgia (90%)
- Also common - weight loss, depression, irritability, hepatosplenomegaly (20-30%)
- Hepatic dysfunction (abnormal liver function test) 30-60%
- Gastrointestinal symptoms (unusual)
- Lymphadenopathy, especially cervical, inguinal (12-21%)
- Orchitis, epididymitis (normal urinalysis) (2-40%)
- Nephritis, prostatitis (rare)
- Cystitis
- Pulmonary - cough or other pulmonary symptoms, x-ray may be normal (15-25%)
- Cutaneous - many transient, non-specific rashes have been described; also, purpura from thrombopenia (5%)
- Visual disturbances, eye pain
- Chronic fatigue syndrome and various neuro-psychiatric symptoms described. Unclear relationship.
- Also localized suppurative infections (see Complications)

CAUSES
- Brucella ingestion from tissue or milk
- Worst disease: *B. melitensis, B. suis*; also *B. canis, B. abortus*. Enter through mucous membrane, broken skin, occasionally inhaled. Facultative intracellular parasite, releases endotoxin when destroyed.
- Person-to-person transmission rare; sexual, vertical, possibly breast milk. Case report of neonatal brucellosis from a blood transfusion

RISK FACTORS
- In US, from occupational exposure to infected animals (especially cattle, sheep). Veterinarians, meat processors, farm workers; who may experience accidental exposure to vaccine. 18 case outbreak in pork processing plant, 1992.
- Consumer exposure to unpasteurized milk products, cheese
- Exposure while traveling in countries where endemic (Mediterranean, Middle East, N. and E. Africa, central Asia, India, Mexico, Central and South America)
- Worse in chronically ill, immunosuppressed, malnourished
- Iron deficiency increases susceptibility

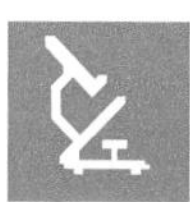

DIAGNOSIS

DIFFERENTIAL DIAGNOSIS
- Many non-specific systemic febrile illnesses; a great mimic
- Tularemia
- Psittacosis
- Rickettsial disease
- Tuberculosis
- Visceral leishmaniasis
- Other disease of infected organs
- HIV infection

LABORATORY
- Isolation of organism from blood, discharge, bone or other tissue. Fastidious and slow-growing. Watch 3-4 weeks, with periodic subcultures. Automated systems shorten time, but not all recognize brucellosis. PCR accurate including non-blood samples, but not available in most clinical labs. Skin tests not standardized, not recommended for diagnosis.
- Acute illness: Blood culture is positive 70%, bone marrow 90%
- May have thrombopenia, disseminated intravascular coagulation; granulopenia, lymphopenia, lymphocytosis. 30-60% with abnormal liver function test. Up to 70% may have normal labs.
- Serology: Brucella standard tube agglutination (STA) paired sera, > 1:160 or 4 x rise (cheapest). Easy, accurate, rapid dipstick for IgM now exists for developing countries.
- More effective ELISA, indirect fluorescent antibody test (IFAT), Coombs tests, immunocapture-agglutination (Brucellacapt). With ELISA, IgM, IgG or IGA may be present at low levels > 1 year even if treated.
- IgM increased initially for several weeks, declines by 3 months
- IgG begins rise 2 weeks, may stay up (low levels) > 1 yr if treated or not treated (though IgM increase may be lower or gone by 6 months if treated, can also persist > 1 year at low levels). IgG titer rises again with reinfection or reactivation. IgG and IGA titer > 1:160 at 1 year implies ongoing disease.
- New research: gene cloning and amplification for discriminatory markers detection and strain differences; PCR-ELISA

Drugs that may alter lab results: None

Disorders that may alter lab results: Serologic cross-reaction with *F. tularensis, Yersinia enterocolitica, V. cholerae*, or vaccinated patients. It has been misdiagnosed in culture as *Moraxella phenylpyruvica*.

PATHOLOGICAL FINDINGS
- Facultative intracellular gram negative *coccobacillus*; can survive inside phagocytic cells, circulate to regional lymph nodes, and into circulation. (Cell-mediated immunity necessary to kill intracellular organism.)
- Macrophages kill, releasing endotoxin that may cause symptoms of acute disease
- Variable tissue reaction depending on site, organisms. Causes local microabscesses; noncaseating granulomas; possibly some immune reaction in arthritis, including elevated C3, C4; ANA, RF.

SPECIAL TESTS Echocardiogram depending on location

IMAGING
- Bone scan, CT, depending on location
- Chest x-ray - pleural effusion, lung cavitation
- Joint x-rays frequently normal, requiring scan or MRI

DIAGNOSTIC PROCEDURES Biopsy, aspiration depending on location

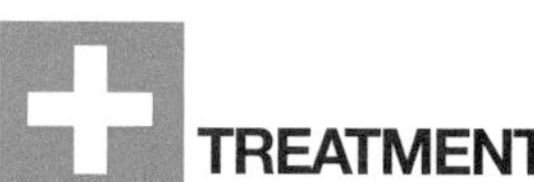

TREATMENT

APPROPRIATE HEALTH CARE Outpatient in mild cases, hospitalization in severe illness. Cardiac care unit in patients with complicating cardiac disease.

GENERAL MEASURES
- Supportive care
- In milk-related or occupational outbreak, look for other cases

SURGICAL MEASURES Specific complications may require surgical drainage, or valve replacement in endocarditis

ACTIVITY Bedrest during febrile periods and restricted activity in acute cases

DIET No special diet. May need to provide supplemental foods, e.g., milk shakes, to counter weight loss.

PATIENT EDUCATION Food Safety and Inspection Service, Office of Public Awareness, Department of Agriculture, Room 1165-S, Washington, DC 20205, (202)447-9351

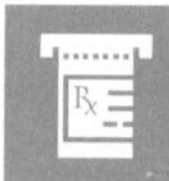

MEDICATIONS

DRUG(S) OF CHOICE
- Optimal therapy includes two drugs, at least one with good intracellular penetration. In some cases, 3 drugs may give a better long-term cure. Longer courses (months) may improve relapse rate in complicated disease.
  - ◊ Rifampin 600-900 mg and doxycycline 200 mg given together every day for at least 6 weeks (possible for several months with severe complications). 5% relapse rate, not related to drug resistance - use same drugs for relapse. Usual cause is localized sequestration of organisms, or noncompliance with medication.
  - ◊ Steroids in Herxheimer's reaction, severe illness, pancytopenia

Contraindications: Avoid doxycycline in children, pregnant women

Precautions: May get Herxheimer's reaction when therapy initiated

Significant possible interactions:
- Rifampin is a potent inducer for the hepatic P450 enzyme system, and may increase metabolism of many drugs metabolized by the liver
- Doxycycline: Antacids, anticoagulants, barbiturates, carbamazepine, hydantoins, cimetidine, digoxin, insulin, iron salts, lithium, methoxyflurane, oral contraceptives, penicillins, sodium bicarbonate

ALTERNATIVE DRUGS
- In recent studies, ciprofloxacin 1 gm/qd and rifampin 600 mg/day for 30 days as effective as rifampin/doxycycline for 45 days
- Doxycycline orally bid and streptomycin by injection - very effective. (Streptomycin currently not available in the USA except by special request from CDC in Atlanta.) Slightly more effective than doxycycline/rifampin, especially with spondylitis, but more toxic and less convenient.
- In children, trimethoprim-sulfamethoxazole (cotrimoxazole) plus rifampin 15 mg/kg (don't use alone) - higher relapse rate
- In children and pregnant women, rifampin 15 mg/kg for 45 weeks plus: cotrimoxazole for 6 weeks or gentamicin for 7 days or netilmicin 5-6 mg/kg IM. Significant cotrimoxazole resistance in some countries.
- Ofloxacin plus rifampin effective in recent study
- No single drug is effective alone

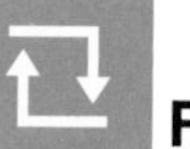

FOLLOWUP

PATIENT MONITORING Check serology at 6 months and 1 year for chronic disease (difficult to evaluate if continuing exposure). Investigate any evidence of complication, recurrence. PCR recently shown sensitive and specific for monitoring treatment relapse.

PREVENTION/AVOIDANCE
- Avoid infected dairy products
- For occupational exposure - caution, animal vaccination, use of protective goggles, protective gloves. Possible future human vaccine.
- Post-exposure prophylaxis same as treatment in large scale exposure such as bioterrorism
- Susceptible to heat, disinfectant but can survive in dust, soil or water for weeks

POSSIBLE COMPLICATIONS
- Relapse (5% overall)
- Localized suppurative infections - osteo-articular (20-85%). Includes arthritis (possibly also immune effect), bursitis, tenosynovitis, osteomyelitis, sacroiliitis, vertebral or paraspinous abscess.
- Endocarditis - rare, but main cause of death in brucellosis
- Thrombophlebitis
- Neuro-brucellosis - most are meningeal. Also peripheral neuritis (usually single, bilateral is possible), encephalitis, myelitis, radiculopathy. Possibly neuro-psychiatric symptoms; a chronic fatigue type syndrome may exist.
- Intrinsic ocular lesions - uveitis, retinal thrombophlebitis, nummular keratitis
- Pneumonitis with pleural effusion
- Hepatitis
- Cholecystitis
- Chronic infection. Persistent (> 1 year) signs of infection, elevated titers, occasional bacteria in blood or tissue. Chronic fatigue syndrome with everything negative is controversial.

EXPECTED COURSE/PROGNOSIS
- Untreated case fatality < 2%
- Most cases resolve with treatment. 2-3 weeks for acute uncomplicated cases, but at least 6 weeks treatment recommended
- Relapse rate overall, 5%

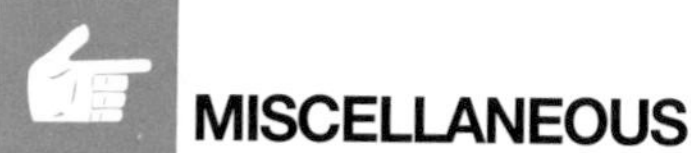

MISCELLANEOUS

ASSOCIATED CONDITIONS N/A

AGE-RELATED FACTORS
Pediatric: May be mild, subclinical
Geriatric: N/A
Others: Worse in chronically ill, immunosuppressed

PREGNANCY High rates of miscarriage or abortion (can occur in subclinical cases). Early antibiotic treatment is preventive.

SYNONYMS
- Undulant fever
- Malta fever

ICD-9-CM
023.9 Brucellosis, unspecified

SEE ALSO
Abortion, spontaneous
Chronic fatigue syndrome
Thrombosis, deep vein (DVT)

OTHER NOTES N/A

ABBREVIATIONS N/A

REFERENCES

- Young E. An overview of human brucellosis. Clin Infect Dis 1995;21:283-90
- Corbel MJ. Brucellosis: an overview. Emerg Infect Dis 1997;3(2)213-21
- Berenson AS, editor. Control of Communicable Diseases Manual. 17th ed. Washington, DC: American Public Health Association; 2000
- Montejo JM, et al. Open randomized therapeutic trial of six antimicrobial regimens in brucellosis. Clin Inf Dis 1993;16:671-76
- Trujillo IZ, Zavala AN, Caceres JG, Miranda CQ. Brucellosis. Infect Dis Clin of NA 1994;8(1)
- Mandell GL, editor. Principles and Practice of Infectious Diseases. 5th ed. New York: Churchill Livingstone; 1999
- Smit S, Henk L. Development and evaluation of a rapid dipstick assay for serodiagnosis of acute human brucellosis. J Clin Microbiol 1999;12:4179-82
- Sauret J, Vilissova N. Human Brucellosis. J Am Board Fam Pract 2002;15(5);401-6
- Al Dahouk S, Tomaso H, et al. Laboratory-based diagnosis of brucellosis--a review of the literature. Part I: Techniques for direct detection and identification of Brucella spp. Clin Lab 2003;49(9-10):487-505
- Al Dahouk S, Tomaso H, et al. Laboratory-based diagnosis of brucellosis--a review of the literature. Part II: serological tests for brucellosis. Clin Lab 2003;49(11-12):577-89

Web references: 0 available at www.5mcc.com
Illustrations N/A

Author(s):
Nancy Snapp, MD, MPH

BASICS

DESCRIPTION Classified in purging and non-purging subtypes. Purging often by self-induced vomiting, laxatives, diuretics. Non-purging type consists of - binges followed by sharply restricted diet and/or vigorous exercise.
System(s) affected: Cardiovascular, Endocrine/Metabolic, Gastrointestinal, Nervous
Genetics: Genetic component
Incidence/Prevalence in USA: Approximately 2% of females; higher among university women. True incidence is not known as this is a secretive disease.
Predominant age: Adolescents and young adults; can occur at any age
Predominant sex: Female > Male (5:1)

SIGNS & SYMPTOMS
- Patients may switch back and forth between purging and non-purging bulimia
- Onset may be stress related
- May be average weight or even somewhat obese; most are slightly below average weight
- Frequent fluctuations in weight
- Deny that there is a problem
- Gobble high calorie foods during binge
- Preoccupation with weight control
- Food collection and hoarding
- Diet pill, diuretic, laxative, ipecac and thyroid medication abuse
- Prefers vigorous exercise, especially running, aerobics
- Diabetic patients often withhold insulin
- Depressed mood and self-depreciation following the binges
- Relief and increased ability to concentrate following the purges
- Vomiting (may be effortless)
- Abdominal pain
- Parotid swelling
- Eroded teeth
- Scarred hands or abrasions on back of hands
- Cardiomyopathy and muscle weakness due to ipecac abuse

CAUSES
- Thought to be largely emotional
- Moderate genetic influence

RISK FACTORS
- Depression, obsessionality, impulsivity
- Low self-esteem
- Achievement pressure; high self-expectations; social anxiety
- Acceptance of the culturally condoned ideal of slimness
- Ambivalence about dependence/independence
- Stress due to multiple responsibilities, tight schedules, competition
- Weight dissatisfaction; perceived overweight
- Environment that stresses thinness or physical fitness (eg, armed forces)
- Family history of substance abuse, eating disorder, obesity, depression
- Poor impulse control, ETOH misuse
- Difficulty resolving conflict, expressing negative emotions

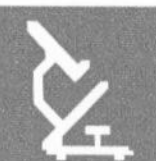

DIAGNOSIS

DIFFERENTIAL DIAGNOSIS
- Major depressive disorder
- Anorexia, binge eating/purging type
- Psychogenic vomiting
- Hypothalamic brain tumor
- Epileptic equivalent seizures
- Kluver-Bucy-like syndromes
- Kleine-Levin syndrome
- Body dysmorphic disorder

LABORATORY
- All results may be within normal limits
- Elevated BUN
- Hypokalemia, hypochloremia
- Hypomagnesemia
- Elevated basal serum prolactin
- Mild elevation serum amylase
- Positive dexamethasone suppression test
- Low CD4/CD8 ratio
- Reduced serotonin activity
- Blunted prolactin response to serotonin agonists

Drugs that may alter lab results: N/A

Disorders that may alter lab results: N/A

PATHOLOGICAL FINDINGS
- Eroded tooth enamel
- Esophagitis, Mallory-Weiss tears
- Asymptomatic, non-inflammatory parotid enlargement
- Gastric dilatation
- Infarction and perforation of the stomach
- Acute pancreatitis
- Spontaneous pneumomediastinum

SPECIAL TESTS
- ECG
- Gastric motility
- Thyroid, liver, renal function
- Drug screen

IMAGING Not indicated

DIAGNOSTIC PROCEDURES Psychological screening: Eating Attitudes Test, BULIT, SCANS, EDI

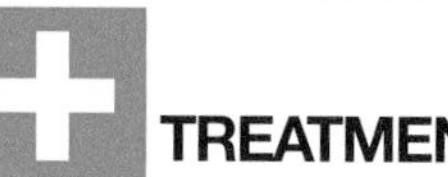

TREATMENT

APPROPRIATE HEALTH CARE
- Most patients can be treated as outpatients
- Hospitalize if patient is suicidal; if there is lab or ECG evidence of marked electrolyte imbalance; marked dehydration; or if there has been no response to outpatient therapy

GENERAL MEASURES
- Inpatient:
  - ◊ If possible, admit to eating disorders unit or unit with structured eating disorders program
  - ◊ Supervised meals and bathroom privileges
  - ◊ No access to the bathroom for 2 hours after meals
  - ◊ Monitor weight and physical activity
  - ◊ Assess psychological state and nutritional status
  - ◊ Identify precipitants to bingeing
  - ◊ Develop alternatives to purging
  - ◊ Monitor electrolytes
  - ◊ Focal individual and cognitive behavioral therapy. Frequent visits by physician.
  - ◊ Gradually shift control to patient as she demonstrates responsibility
- Outpatient:
  - ◊ Build trust, treatment alliance
  - ◊ Assess psychological state and nutritional status
  - ◊ Involve patient in establishing target goals
  - ◊ Use self-monitoring techniques such as food diary
  - ◊ Identify prodromal states, precipitants
  - ◊ Address ruminations about calories, weight, purging
  - ◊ Focus on overall well-being, developing gratifying relationships
  - ◊ Challenge fear of loss of control
  - ◊ Cognitive-behavioral therapy and interpersonal therapy
  - ◊ Family therapy for adolescents
  - ◊ Nutritional education, relaxation techniques, couples therapy, self-help group may also be helpful.

SURGICAL MEASURES N/A

ACTIVITY
- Monitor excess activity
- Stress importance of playful, pleasurable activities

DIET
- Goal is a balanced diet with adequate calories and a normal eating pattern
- Reintroduce feared foods

PATIENT EDUCATION
- Seriousness and consequences of bulimic behavior including cognitive impairment
- Information on nutrition, metabolic balance
- Tools for self monitoring when appropriate

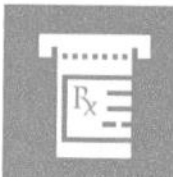

MEDICATIONS

DRUG(S) OF CHOICE

- SSRIs - fluoxetine (Prozac) 10-80 mg or fluvoxamine (Luvox) 50-300 mg/day are effective in reducing symptoms with relatively few side effects. High dose treatment often needed.
- MAO inhibitors - phenelzine (Nardil) 60-90 mg/day. Patients with atypical depression may respond to MAO inhibitors and not SSRIs.
- Augment with buspirone (BuSpar) if desired. To prevent relapse, maintain antidepressant medication at full therapeutic dose for at least one year.
- Note: Dishonesty and noncompliance are common

Contraindications: Refer to manufacturer's literature

Precautions:

- Serious toxicity following overdose is common
- Patients often vomit medications

Significant possible interactions:

- Lithium and tricyclic medication can be lethal when administered to hypokalemic patients
- SSRIs may increase tricyclic levels
- Because of danger of food related hypertensive crises, use irreversible MAO inhibitors only with fully cooperative patients
- To avoid the serotonin syndrome, allow 5 weeks between discontinuing fluoxetine and beginning MAO inhibitor
- Avoid co-administration of bupropion (Wellbutrin, Zyban) as this may precipitate seizures

ALTERNATIVE DRUGS

- Inositol (a nutrient) 10-18 g/day; controlled trial indicated effects comparable to SSRIs
- Domperidone (Motilium) 10 mg before meals relieves bloating, abdominal pain; favorable safety profile
- Sibutramine (Meridia) 13 mg in AM is of theorized interest; research is lacking
- If there is an underlying bipolar disorder, patients may benefit from lithium (Eskalith), 300 mg bid, increase gradually to therapeutic blood level of 0.6-1.2 mEq/L (0.6-1.2 mmol/L)
- Ondansetron (Zofran) 4-8 mg tid between meals can help prevent vomiting
- Psyllium (Metamucil) preparations 1 tbsp hs with glass of water, can prevent constipation during laxative withdrawal

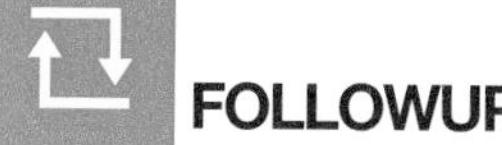

FOLLOWUP

PATIENT MONITORING

- Binge-purge activity
- Level of exercise activity
- Self-esteem, comfort with body and self
- Ruminations and depression
- Repeat any abnormal lab values weekly or monthly until stable

PREVENTION/AVOIDANCE

- Encourage rational attitude about weight
- Moderate overly high self-expectations
- Enhance self-esteem
- Diminish stress

POSSIBLE COMPLICATIONS

- Suicide
- Drug and alcohol abuse
- Potassium depletion; cardiac arrhythmia; cardiac arrest
- Maternal and fetal problems if pregnant

EXPECTED COURSE/PROGNOSIS

- Highly variable, tends to wax and wane
- May spontaneously remit
- Most patients continue to binge/purge, but do so less often
- Patients who do not establish trust likely to drop out of therapy, be lost to follow-up
- Those who stay in therapy tend to improve
- Patients with personality disorders have a generally poor prognosis
- 30-50% relapse rate per year for several years
- Impulsive patients may engage in stealing, suicide gestures, substance abuse, promiscuity

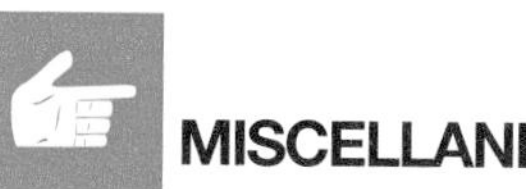

MISCELLANEOUS

ASSOCIATED CONDITIONS

- Major depression and dysthymia
- Bipolar disorder
- Obsessive-compulsive disorder
- Social phobia and other anxiety disorders
- Schizophrenic disorder
- Substance abuse disorder
- Borderline personality disorder
- Compulsive shoplifting (kleptomania)

AGE-RELATED FACTORS

Pediatric: N/A

Geriatric: N/A

Others: Less frequently diagnosed in men or in older women

PREGNANCY

- Poor nutritional status may affect fetus
- Binge-purge may increase or decrease during pregnancy

SYNONYMS N/A

ICD-9-CM

307.51 Bulimia

SEE ALSO

Hyperkalemia
Laxative abuse
Salivary gland tumors

OTHER NOTES

- Anorexic patients may deal with the frustration of chronic food deprivation by converting to bulimia
- High risk
  - ◊ Ballet dancers, models, cheerleaders
  - ◊ Athletes, especially runners, gymnasts, weight lifters, body builders, jockeys, divers, wrestlers, figure skaters, field hockey players
- Sub-clinical eating disorders are common in university populations
- Sexual abuse is not causally related to bulimia
- Chronic, extreme hypokalemia can occur without physical symptoms

ABBREVIATIONS

MAO = monoamine oxidase
SRI = serotonin reuptake inhibitors

REFERENCES

- Lewinsohn PM, Striegel-Moore RH, Seeley JR. Epidemiology and natural course of eating disorders in young women from adolescence to young adulthood. J Am Acad Child Adolesc Psychiatry 2000;39(10):1284-92
- Davis C. Eating disorders and hyperactivity: a psychobiological perspective. Can J Psychiatr 1997;42:168-75
- Mitchell JE, Peterson CB, Myers T, Wonderlich S. Combining pharmacotherapy and psychotherapy in the treatment of patients with eating disorders. Psychiatr Clin North Am. 2001;24(2):315-23
- Ben-Tovin. Eating disorders: outcome, prevention and treatment. Curr Opin Psychiatry 2003;16:65-9
- Fairburn CG, Harrison PJ. Eating disorders. Lancet 2003;361(9355):407-16
- Striegel-Moore R, Smolak L. Eating Disorders: Innovative Directions in Research and Practice. Washington DC: Am Psychiatry Assn: 2001

Web references: 3 available at www.5mcc.com

Illustrations N/A

Author(s):

Alayne Yates, MD

BASICS

DESCRIPTION Burns are tissue injuries caused by application of heat, chemicals, electricity, or irradiation to the tissue. Extent of injury (depth of burn) is result of intensity of heat (or other exposure) and the duration of exposure.
- Partial thickness: First degree involves superficial layers of epidermis. Second degree involves varying degrees of epidermis (with blister formation) and part of the dermis.
- Full thickness: Third degree involves destruction of all skin elements with coagulation of subdermal plexus

System(s) affected: Endocrine/Metabolic, Skin/Exocrine
Genetics: N/A
Incidence/Prevalence in USA:
- Per year in USA (1999 data):
  - ◊ Total population: 1.25-2 million burns, 600,000 emergency room admissions, 45,000 hospitalizations, 4,500 deaths
  - ◊ In children: 250,000 are burned, 15,000 hospitalizations, 1,100 deaths

Predominant age: All ages
Predominant sex: Male = Female

SIGNS & SYMPTOMS
- First degree
  - ◊ Erythema of involved tissue
  - ◊ Skin blanches with pressure
  - ◊ Skin may be tender
- Second degree
  - ◊ Skin is red and blistered
  - ◊ Skin is very tender
- Third degree
  - ◊ Burned skin is tough and leathery
  - ◊ Skin is not tender

CAUSES
- Open flame and hot liquid are most common (heat usually 15-45°C or greater)
- Caustic chemicals or acids (may show little signs or symptoms for the first few days)
- Electricity (may have significant injury with very little damage to overlying skin)
- Excess sun exposure

RISK FACTORS
- Hot water heaters set too high
- Work place exposure to chemicals, electricity or irradiation
- Young children and elderly adults with thin skin are more susceptible to injury
- Carelessness with burning cigarettes
- Inadequate or faulty electrical wiring

DIAGNOSIS

DIFFERENTIAL DIAGNOSIS
- Toxic epidermal necrolysis
- Scalded skin syndrome

LABORATORY
- Hematocrit
- Type and cross
- Electrolytes
- Blood urea nitrogen
- Urinalysis

Drugs that may alter lab results: N/A

Disorders that may alter lab results: Pre-existing cardiac disease

PATHOLOGICAL FINDINGS
- First degree: devitalization of superficial layers of epidermis, congestion of intradermal vessels
- Second degree: coagulation necrosis of varying depths of epidermis, clefting of epidermis (blister), coagulation of subdermal plexus, skin appendages intact
- Third degree: necrosis of all skin elements, coagulation of subdermal plexus

SPECIAL TESTS
- Children - glucose (hypoglycemia may occur in children because of limited glycogen storage)
- Smoke inhalation - arterial blood gas, carboxyhemoglobin
- Electric burns - electrocardiogram, urine myoglobin, creatine kinase (CK) isoenzymes

IMAGING
- Chest x-ray
- Xenon scan may be useful in suspected smoke inhalation

DIAGNOSTIC PROCEDURES Bronchoscopy may be necessary in smoke inhalation to evaluate lower respiratory tract

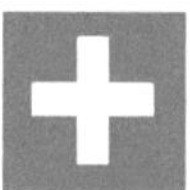

TREATMENT

APPROPRIATE HEALTH CARE
- Hospitalization for all serious burns
  - ◊ Second degree burns over 10% body surface area (BSA), any 3rd degree burn
  - ◊ Burns of hands, feet, face or perineum
  - ◊ Electrical/lightning burns
  - ◊ Inhalation injury
  - ◊ Chemical burns
  - ◊ Circumferential burn
- Transfer to burn center for:
  - ◊ 2nd and 3rd degree burns over 10% BSA in patients under 10 years and over 50 years of age
  - ◊ 2nd and 3rd degree burns over 20% BSA in any age range
  - ◊ Burns of hands, feet, face or perineum
  - ◊ Electrical/lightning burns
  - ◊ Inhalation injury
  - ◊ Chemical burns
  - ◊ Circumferential burn
  - ◊ Chemical burns with threat of functional impairment

GENERAL MEASURES
Based on depth of burns and accurate estimate of total body surface area (BSA) involved (Rule of nines)
- Rule of nines
  - ◊ Each upper extremity - adult and child 9%
  - ◊ Each lower extremity - adult 18%; child 14%
  - ◊ Anterior trunk - adult and child 18%
  - ◊ Posterior trunk - adult and child 18%
  - ◊ Head and neck - adult 10%; child 18%
- Quick estimate (for smaller burns)
  - ◊ The surface area of the patient's hand is approximately 1% of their BSA.
- Tetanus prophylaxis (if not current)
- Remove all rings, watches, etc., from injured extremities to avoid tourniquet effect
- Remove clothing and cover all burned areas with dry sheet
- Flush area of chemical burn (for approximately 2 hours)
- 100% oxygen administration in all major burns, consider early intubation
- Do not apply ice to burn site
- Nasogastric tube (high risk of paralytic ileus)
- Foley catheter
- Pain relief
  - ◊ IV Demerol, morphine or methadone for severe pain
  - ◊ Oral analgesics eg, Tylenol with codeine, Percocet, Lortab) for moderate pain
- ECG monitoring in first 24 hours following electrical burn
- Whirlpool hydrotherapy followed by silver sulfadiazine (Silvadene) occlusive dressings in severe burns
- Once or twice a day cleansing with dressing changes
- Epilock or Elasto-Gel may be used as dressing in selected patients (especially useful for outpatient treatment of minor burns)
- Burn fluid resuscitation

Calculate fluid resuscitation from time of burn, not from time treatment begins.
  - ◊ 2-4 mL Ringer's lactate x body weight (kg) x % BSA burn (1/2 given in first eight hours, 1/4 in second eight hours and 1/4 in third eight hours). In children, this is given in addition to maintenance fluids and is adjusted according to urine output and vital signs.
  - ◊ Colloid solutions are not recommended during the first 12-24 hours of resuscitation
- Other
  - ◊ Use of biological membranes or skin substitutes may be indicated for burn coverage

SURGICAL MEASURES
- Escharotomy may be necessary in constricting circumferential burns of extremities or chest
- Tangential excision with split thickness skin grafts

ACTIVITY Early mobilization is the goal

DIET High protein, high calorie diet when bowel function resumes; nasogastric tube feedings may be required in early post-burn period. TPN if NPO expected for > 5 days.

PATIENT EDUCATION
- Use of sunscreen
- Access to electrical cords/outlets
- Isolate household chemicals
- Use low temperature setting for hot water heater
- Household smoke detectors with special emphasis on maintenance
- Family/household evacuation plan
- Proper storage and use of flammable substances

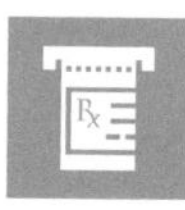

MEDICATIONS

DRUG(S) OF CHOICE
- Morphine small frequent IV doses (0.1 mg/kg/dose in children; 2.5-20 mg q 2-6 hours in adults)
- Silver sulfadiazine (Silvadene) topically to burn site (can cause leukopenia)
- Electrical burn with myoglobinuria will require alkalinization of urine and mannitol
- No indication for prophylactic antibiotics
- Consider H2 blockers: cimetidine, ranitidine, famotidine, or nizatidine for stress ulcer prophylaxis in severely burned patients

Contraindications: Specific drug allergies
Precautions: Be alert for respiratory depression with narcotics
Significant possible interactions: Refer to manufacturer's profile of each drug

ALTERNATIVE DRUGS
- Mafenide (Sulfamylon) - full thickness burn (caution: metabolic acidosis)
- Silver nitrate 0.5% (messy, leaches electrolytes from burn and causes water toxicity)
- Povidone-iodine (Betadine) may result in Iodine absorption from burn, "tan eschar". Makes débridement more difficult.
- Travase-enzymatic débridement

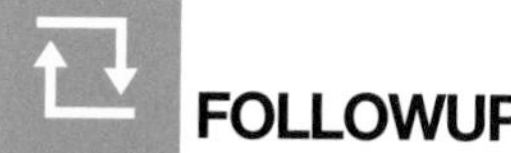

FOLLOWUP

PATIENT MONITORING According to extent of burn and treatment

PREVENTION/AVOIDANCE Skin grafts or newly epithelialized skin is highly sensitive to sun exposure and thermal extremes

POSSIBLE COMPLICATIONS
- Gastroduodenal ulceration (Curling ulcer)
- Marjolin ulcer - squamous cell carcinoma developing in old burn site
- Burn wound sepsis-usually gram negative organisms
- Pneumonia
- Decreased mobility with possibility of future flexion contractures

EXPECTED COURSE/PROGNOSIS
- First degree burn: complete resolution
- Second degree burn: epithelialization in 10-14 days (deep second degree burns will probably require skin graft)
- Third degree burn: no potential for re-epithelialization, skin graft required
- Length of hospital stay and need for ICU care depends on extent of burn, smoke inhalation and age
- A 50% survival can be expected with a 62% burn in ages 0-14 years, 63% burn in ages 15-40 years, 38% burn in age 40-65 years, 25% burn in patients over 65 years
- 90% of survivors can be expected to return to an occupation as remunerative as their pre-burn employment

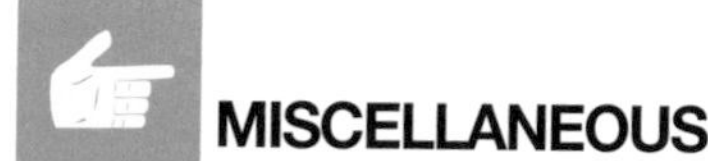

MISCELLANEOUS

ASSOCIATED CONDITIONS
- Smoke inhalation syndrome
  - ◊ Occurs within 72 hours of burn
  - ◊ Suspected in burns occurring in an enclosed space
  - ◊ Intubation, ventilation with positive end-expiratory pressure (PEEP) assistance

AGE-RELATED FACTORS
Pediatric:
- Consider child abuse when dealing with hot water burns in children
  - ◊ Observe distribution of burns
  - ◊ Pay attention to straight lines, especially if bilateral

Geriatric: Prognosis poorer for severe burns
Others: N/A

PREGNANCY N/A

SYNONYMS N/A

ICD-9-CM
940.9 Unspecified burn of eye and adnexa
941.00 Unspecified degree burn of face and head, unspecified site
942.00 Unspecified degree burn of trunk, unspecified site
948.0 Burn, any degree <10% of BSA (fifth digit can indicate BSA involved in 3rd degree burn)
949.0 Unspecified burn, unspecified degree
949.1 Unspecified burn, erythema [first degree]
949.2 Unspecified burn, blisters, epidermal loss [second degree]
949.3 Unspecified burn, full thickness skin loss [third degree NOS]

SEE ALSO

OTHER NOTES N/A

ABBREVIATIONS
BSA = body surface area
PEEP = positive end expiratory pressure
TPN = total parenteral nutrition

REFERENCES

- Gillespie RW, Dimik AR, Hallberg PW. Advanced Burn Life Support Course Provider's Manual. Lincoln, Nebraska Burn Institute; 1990
- Eichelberger MR. Pediatric Trauma: Prevention, Acute Care, Rehabilitation, St Louis: Mosby year Book; 1993
- Schwartz SI, Shires GT, Spencer FC, et al, editors. Principles of Surgery. 7th ed. New York: McGraw-Hill Book Co; 1999
- Touloukian RJ. Pediatric Trauma. 2nd ed. St. Louis: Mosby Year Book;1990
- Ziegler MM, Azizkhan RG, Weber TR, eds. Operative Pediatric Surgery. New York: McGraw-Hill; 2003

Web references: 4 available at www.5mcc.com
Illustrations 3 available

Author(s):
Timothy L. Black, MD
James P. Miller, MD

BASICS

DESCRIPTION A bursa is a sac that is formed or found in areas subject to friction, such as locations where tendons pass over bony landmarks. Most common sites are subdeltoid, olecranon, prepatellar, trochanteric, radiohumeral. They essentially lubricate the region with synovial fluid. Large bursae usually communicate with joints and are responsible for retaining the synovial fluid in place. Bursae are fluid-filled sacs that serve as a cushion between tendons and bones. Bywaters, an English rheumatologist, found at least 78 bursae symmetrically placed on each side of the body.

System(s) affected: Musculoskeletal
Genetics: N/A
Incidence/Prevalence in USA: Common. Traumatic bursitis more likely in patients less than 35 years of age.
Predominant age: 15-50 years (most common in skeletally mature)
Predominant sex: Males > Females

SIGNS & SYMPTOMS
- Includes pain/tenderness
- Decreased range of motion of affected region (rare except at shoulder)
- Erythema if infection present
- Swelling
- Crepitus sometimes found

CAUSES
- Bursitis may be acute or chronic, and its etiology is often unknown
- There are many types of bursitis, including infectious, traumatic, inflammatory or gouty
- Less often rheumatoid disease or TB as well as gout and pseudogout

RISK FACTORS Individuals who engage in repetitive and vigorous training or others who suddenly increase their level of activity (e.g., "weekend warriors"). Also, improper or over-zealous stretching may lead to injury.

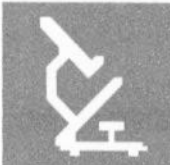

DIAGNOSIS

DIFFERENTIAL DIAGNOSIS
- Tendinitis, strains and sprains
- Joint pains may be caused by gout, pseudogout, rheumatoid arthritis, osteoarthritis
- Arthritis. Many elderly patients think it is the cause of their pain. (Lars Goran-Larsson, a rheumatologist from Sweden, and John Barn, M.D., reviewed their referrals for a 26-month period and found that 108 of 600 (18%) patients had some form of soft tissue problem rather than arthritis).

LABORATORY
Following will all help in differentiating soft tissue disease from rheumatic and connective tissue disease:
- CBC
- ESR
- Serum protein electrophoresis
- Rheumatoid factor (RF)
- Serum uric acid
- Calcium
- Phosphorus
- Alkaline phosphatase
- VDRL
- Joint fluid analysis (when available)

Drugs that may alter lab results:
- ESR may be increased with coexistent use of dextran, methyldopa, methysergide, penicillamine, theophylline, vitamin A
- ESR may be decreased with coexistent use of quinine, salicylates, and drugs which cause a high glucose level

Disorders that may alter lab results: N/A

PATHOLOGICAL FINDINGS
- Acute - with early inflammation, bursa is distended with watery or mucoid fluid
- Chronic - bursal wall is thickened and inner surface is shaggy and trabeculated. The space is filled with granular, brown, inspissated blood admixed with gritty, calcific precipitations. Upper extremity tendonitis and bursitis are usually the result of repetitive microtrauma, probably resulting in disruption of fibers leading to pain, spasm and disability.

SPECIAL TESTS ECG (if shoulder pain mimics cardiac pain)

IMAGING
- CT or MRI
- Calcific deposits may be seen on plain x-ray

DIAGNOSTIC PROCEDURES
- Aspiration of swollen bursa and evaluation of synovial fluid
- The clinician must differentiate infected from inflammatory bursitis. Fluid analysis and culture help make the diagnosis. If the gram stain and culture yield an infective cause, treat with appropriate antibiotics. If the etiology is inflammatory, give local care.

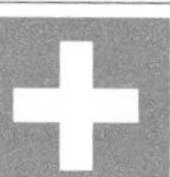

TREATMENT

APPROPRIATE HEALTH CARE Outpatient; refer only difficult cases

GENERAL MEASURES
- Conservative therapy consists of rest, ice and local care, elevation, gentle compression (often referred to as RICE therapy [rest-ice-compression-elevation])
- Physical therapy/hydrocollator treatments
- Invasive therapy would include aspiration of the bursa, injection of steroids
- Have patient wear a sling to protect arm and support shoulder
- Treatment of any underlying infection

SURGICAL MEASURES In severe cases, possibly surgical excision

ACTIVITY Rest and elevation of affected extremity

DIET Consider changes if bursitis directly related to obesity/crystalline deposition

PATIENT EDUCATION
- Advice concerning prevention via appropriate warm-up and stretching and avoidance of repetitive injury
- Possible life-style changes to prevent recurrent joint irritation

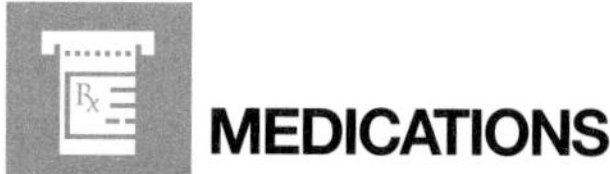

MEDICATIONS

DRUG(S) OF CHOICE
- Non-steroidal anti-inflammatories (NSAIDs) or aspirin. Injectable steroids and stronger analgesics if needed.
- Antibiotic therapy if infection present

Contraindications: Refer to manufacturer's profile of each drug
Precautions: Refer to manufacturer's profile of each drug
Significant possible interactions: Refer to manufacturer's profile of each drug

ALTERNATIVE DRUGS
- Application of local analgesic balms, capsaicin cream, injection of a corticosteroid along with lidocaine
- Systemic steroids (if not contraindicated)

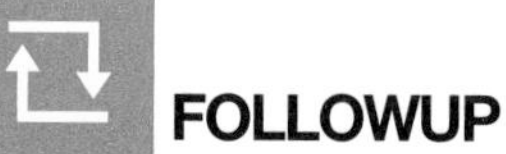

FOLLOWUP

PATIENT MONITORING
- Discontinue NSAIDs as soon as possible to avoid side effects
- Some patients may require repeated injections (usually no more than three) of a corticosteroid and lidocaine (Xylocaine)

PREVENTION/AVOIDANCE
- Appropriate warm-up and cool-down maneuvers, avoidance of overuse or inadequate rest between workouts
- Range of motion exercises
- Maintain high level of fitness and general good health

POSSIBLE COMPLICATIONS
- Acute bursitis may progress to chronic
- Severe long-range limitation of motion

EXPECTED COURSE/PROGNOSIS
- Most bouts of bursitis heal without sequelae
- Repetitive acute bouts may lead to chronic bursitis necessitating repeated joint/bursal aspirations or eventually surgical excision of involved bursa

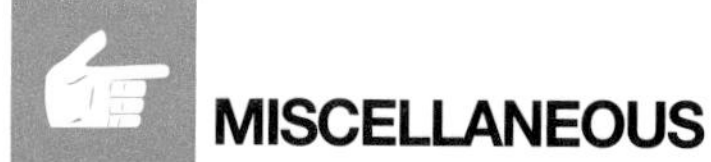

MISCELLANEOUS

ASSOCIATED CONDITIONS
- Tendinitis
- Sprains, strains
- Associated stress fractures

AGE-RELATED FACTORS
Pediatric: Look for other causes
Geriatric: More common
Others: N/A

PREGNANCY N/A

SYNONYMS N/A

ICD-9-CM
727.3 Other bursitis

SEE ALSO
Tendinitis

OTHER NOTES N/A

ABBREVIATIONS N/A

REFERENCES

- Robbins SL, Cotran RS: Pathological Basis of Disease. 2nd Ed. Philadelphia, W.B. Saunders Co., 1989
- Rotstein BR: Soft tissue rheumatism of the upper extremities: diagnosis and management. MEDLINE Professional, Sept, 1991

Web references: 0 available at www.5mcc.com
Illustrations N/A

Author(s):
Timothy Robinson, DO
Brenda Oshea-Robinson, RPAC

BASICS

DESCRIPTION *Candida albicans* and related species cause a variety of infections. Cutaneous candidiasis syndromes include erosio interdigitalis blastomycetica, folliculitis, balanitis, intertrigo, paronychia, onychomycosis, diaper rash, perianal candidiasis, and the syndromes of chronic mucocutaneous candidiasis. Mucous membrane infections include oral candidiasis (thrush), esophagitis, and vaginitis. The most serious manifestation of candidiasis is hematogenously disseminated invasive candidiasis (sometimes referred to as acute systemic candidiasis).
System(s) affected: Gastrointestinal, Pulmonary, Renal/Urologic, Reproductive, Skin/Exocrine
Genetics: N/A
Incidence/Prevalence in USA: Approximately 50/100,000. Hematogenously disseminated candidiasis affects at least 120,000 patients annually in the USA.
Predominant age: All ages are susceptible to hematogenously disseminated candidiasis. Premature neonates are at particularly high risk.
Predominant sex: Male = Female (hematogenously disseminated candidiasis)

SIGNS & SYMPTOMS
- Fever
- Malaise
- Tachycardia
- Hypotension
- Altered mental status
- Hepatosplenomegaly
- Maculopapular or nodular skin rash

CAUSES
- *Candida albicans* is the most frequent pathogen. However, other important human pathogens include *C. tropicalis*, *C. krusei*, *C. stellatoidea*, *C. pseudotropicalis*, *C. guilliermondi*, *C. parapsilosis*, *C. lusitaniae*, *C. rugosa*, *C. lambica*, and *Candida glabrata*.
- Candida species colonize human mucocutaneous surfaces, and most infections are endogenously acquired from this reservoir
- Human-to-human transmission of Candida occurs in some settings

RISK FACTORS
- For hematogenously disseminated invasive candidiasis:
  - ◊ Neutropenia
  - ◊ Antibacterial chemotherapy
  - ◊ Indwelling intravascular access devices
  - ◊ Prior hemodialysis
  - ◊ Mucocutaneous candidiasis
  - ◊ Cardiothoracic or abdominal surgery
  - ◊ Diabetes
  - ◊ Hyperalimentation (TPN)
- Non-*albicans* species are more prevalent in those with leukemia, neutropenia, and on fluconazole prophylaxis

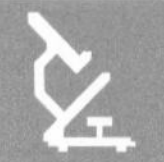

DIAGNOSIS

DIFFERENTIAL DIAGNOSIS Includes a variety of cryptic bacterial infections and, in the neutropenic host, multiple opportunistic infections

LABORATORY N/A

Drugs that may alter lab results: N/A

Disorders that may alter lab results: N/A

PATHOLOGICAL FINDINGS The characteristic histopathology of lesions of Candida invasion of visceral organs is microabscess formation

SPECIAL TESTS
- The diagnosis is established by isolating the causative organism from blood cultures (lysis/centrifugation blood cultures are superior to broth culture techniques for this purpose) or other normally sterile body sites, or by demonstration of organisms in histopathologic specimens of normally sterile tissues
- Isolation of Candida from multiple sites should raise the diagnostic suspicion of hematogenously disseminated invasive candidiasis
- Candida species isolated from a normally sterile site should be identified to the species level
- Fungal sensitivity testing should be employed in cases of persistent or recurrent Candida infections
- Azole resistant *C. albicans* species are reported with increasing frequency
- Fungal sensitivity testing should be employed for all cases of fungemia with Candida spp.

IMAGING Imaging techniques are generally not specifically useful in the diagnosis of hematogenously invasive disseminated candidiasis. However, in the syndrome of hepatosplenic candidiasis (chronic systemic candidiasis) imaging of the liver and spleen by liver scan, ultrasound, or CT (the most sensitive) may be useful in suggesting this syndrome as the cause of persistent fever and liver dysfunction in patients who have recently recovered from neutropenia.

DIAGNOSTIC PROCEDURES
- If blood cultures remain consistently negative, excisional biopsy may be useful in diagnosis
- Aspiration and biopsy of skin lesions occasionally seen with hematogenously disseminated candidiasis is also useful
- Endoscopy with brushings and biopsy is useful in esophageal candidiasis

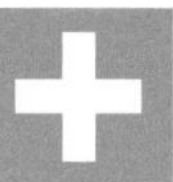

TREATMENT

APPROPRIATE HEALTH CARE Inpatient for hematogenously invasive disseminated candidiasis

GENERAL MEASURES
- Fluid and electrolyte therapy is often required
- Hemodynamic and respiratory support may be required in seriously ill patients
- Removal of potentially infected intravascular access devices is imperative

SURGICAL MEASURES N/A

ACTIVITY As tolerated

DIET No special diet

PATIENT EDUCATION Patients should be advised of the nature of the infection and the toxicities associated with therapy

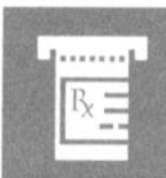

MEDICATIONS

DRUG(S) OF CHOICE

- Caspofungin (Cancidas)
  - ◊ Useful as preferred therapy for candidemia in patients with prior azole therapy, immune compromised, neutropenia
  - ◊ Initial therapy of choice for any patient with candidemia
  - ◊ 70 mg IV load over 1 hour on day one followed by 50 mg IV daily
  - ◊ Modify dose for severe hepatic insufficiency
- Fluconazole
  - ◊ 400-800 mg IV daily for first week, followed by additional IV or oral therapy at the same dose for at least 2 weeks after last positive blood culture or last evidence of infection. Higher doses of fluconazole may be required if non-albicans species are known or suspected.
  - ◊ Has been shown to be as effective as amphotericin B therapy and less toxic for treatment of candidemia in patients who are not neutropenic, do not have AIDS, and are not severely immunosuppressed by therapy after organ transplantation
- Amphotericin B
  - ◊ Is an initial therapy of choice for any patient with candidemia and the preferred therapy for patients with neutropenia, severe immune compromise prior azole therapy
  - ◊ Administer first in a test dose of 1 mg and then in incrementally increasing doses to 0.3-0.7 mg/kg/day. (Some authorities administer full dose after the test dose. In a critically ill patient, slow increase in dose is not warranted). Depending on host status and form of hematogenously invasive disseminated candidiasis, total dose requirement ranges from 200 mg to 2.0 gm over a therapeutic duration of 2-10 weeks.

Contraindications:

- The safety of amphotericin B therapy in pregnant patients has not been established
- Caspofungin is category C

Precautions:

- Amphotericin B
  - ◊ Toxicity is formidable. Acute reactions occur commonly during initiation of therapy, including fever, rigors, and hypotension. These can be ameliorated or eliminated by premedication with acetaminophen, ibuprofen or hydrocortisone, and tend to decline over time with continuing daily therapy. Use meperidine if needed to abort rigors.
  - ◊ Azotemia is a common complication and may be an indication for reducing therapy in some patients (to reduce toxicity, not because of renal elimination of drug). Generally recommended to hold drug if BUN > 40 mg/dL (14.3 mmol/L) or creatinine > 3.0 mg/dL (266 μmol). Hold until above levels decline, then administer drug every other day. Maintenance of optimal fluid status and prevention of dehydration help minimize risk of azotemia. "Sodium loading" with 77 mEq (77 mmol) sodium daily (= 1 L 1/2 normal saline) has been suggested by some authorities to decrease renal toxicity.
  - ◊ Significant hypokalemia (often requires therapy) and renal tubular acidosis (rarely requires therapy) may develop. Significant hypomagnesemia may worsen hypokalemia.
  - ◊ Anemia commonly develops in patients on protracted therapy but is almost always reversible
  - ◊ Headache and phlebitis are common
  - ◊ Leukopenia, thrombocytopenia, and liver function abnormalities are rarely encountered
- Itraconazole, voriconazole and caspofungin do not enter the urinary stream in sufficient concentrations to treat urinary tract infections

Significant possible interactions:

- Caspofungin - potentially important interactions with carbamazepine, phenytoin, cyclosporine, tacrolimus, sirolimus, NNRTIs, and rifampin
- Amphotericin B - concomitant therapy with cyclosporine or other nephrotoxic agents such as aminoglycoside or vancomycin may increase risk of amphotericin-induced nephrotoxicity
- Fluconazole - potentially important drug-drug interactions may occur in patients receiving oral hypoglycemics, coumarin-type anticoagulants, phenytoin, cyclosporine, rifampin, theophylline or terfenadine or astemizole, Drug-drug interactions are more likely with itraconazole and voriconazole

ALTERNATIVE DRUGS

- Liposomal preparations of amphotericin B appear to be less nephrotoxic
- Fluconazole therapy may be preferred for infections with *C. lusitaniae*, which may be resistant to amphotericin B
- Caspofungin or amphotericin B is preferred for infections with *C. krusei* which is likely resistant to fluconazole, as may be *C. glabrata*
- Other azole antifungals depending on activity and safety (itraconazole and voriconazole)
- Flucytosine may be used as adjunctive therapy with fluconazole for peritonitis
- Caspofungin in candidiasis. Data suggest that caspofungin is as effective as conventional amphotericin B for treatment of candidemia and is less frequently associated with adverse effects.

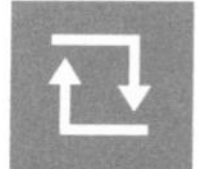

FOLLOWUP

PATIENT MONITORING Complete blood count, serum electrolytes, and serum creatinine should be measured at least twice weekly in patients on daily amphotericin B therapy. If blood cultures are positive, they should be repeated until negative.

PREVENTION/AVOIDANCE Fluconazole, liposomal amphotericin B and voriconazole reduce the incidence of candidiasis in patients undergoing induction therapy for acute leukemia or bone marrow transplantation

POSSIBLE COMPLICATIONS

- Of hematogenously disseminated candidiasis
  - ◊ Pyelonephritis
  - ◊ Endophthalmitis
  - ◊ Endocarditis, myocarditis, pericarditis
  - ◊ Arthritis, chondritis, osteomyelitis
  - ◊ Pneumonitis
  - ◊ Central nervous system infection

EXPECTED COURSE/PROGNOSIS

Overall mortality for patients with hematogenously disseminated candidiasis is 40-75%, with mortality attributable to candidemia being 15-37%

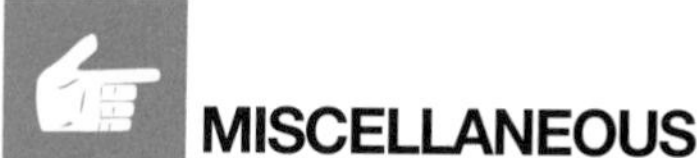

MISCELLANEOUS

ASSOCIATED CONDITIONS See Risk Factors

AGE-RELATED FACTORS

Pediatric: N/A
Geriatric: N/A
Others: N/A

PREGNANCY N/A

SYNONYMS N/A

ICD-9-CM

112.5 Candidiasis, disseminated
112.9 Candidiasis of unspecified site

SEE ALSO

Candidiasis, mucocutaneous
Vulvovaginitis, candidal

OTHER NOTES Other candidal infections: Intraperitoneal infection in patients with major abdominal surgery, biliary tract candidiasis, isolated lower urinary tract infection

ABBREVIATIONS N/A

REFERENCES

- Rex JH, Walsh TJ, Sobel JD, et al. Practice guidelines for the treatment of candidemia. Clin Infec Dis 2000;30:662-78
- Blumberg HM, Jarvis WR, Soucie JM, et al. NEMIS Study Group: Risk factors for candidal bloodstream infetions in surgical intensive care unit patients. The NEMIS prospective multicenter study. Clin Infect Dis 2001;33:177-86
- Uzon D, Anaissie EJ. Predictors in outcome in cancer patients with candidemia. Am Oncol 2000;11:1517-21
- Lundstrom T, Sobel J. Nosocomial candiduria: A review. Clin Infect Dis 2001;32:1602-7
- Kontoyiannis DP, Luna MA, Samuels BI, Bodey GP. Hepatosplenic candidiasis. A manifestation of chronic disseminated candidiasis. Infect Dis Clin North Am 2000;14(3):721-39
- Vincent JL, Anaissie E, Bruining H, Demajo W, et al. Epidemiology, diagnosis and treatment of systemic Candida infection in surgical patients under intensive care. Intensive Care Med 1998;24(3):206-16

Web references: 0 available at www.5mcc.com
Illustrations 8 available

Author(s):

Brock D. Lutz, MD
Ronald A. Greenfield, MD

BASICS

DESCRIPTION A mucocutaneous disorder caused by infection with various species of *Candida*. *Candida* is normally present, in very small amounts, in the oral cavity, gastrointestinal tract, and female genital tract.

- *Candida* vulvovaginitis - infection on the vaginal mucosa, often associated with cutaneous vulvar involvement
- Oropharyngeal candidiasis - infection of the oral cavity ("thrush") and/or pharynx.
- *Candida* esophagitis - usually associated with an immunosuppressed host
- Gastrointestinal candidiasis - gastritis, sometimes with ulcers, usually associated with thrush. The small and large bowel can also be affected.
- Angular cheilitis - fissures formed by *Candida* infection at the corners of the mouth.

System(s) affected: Gastrointestinal, Skin/Exocrine

Genetics: Chronic mucocutaneous candidiiasis is a heterogeneous clinical syndrome that usually presents in childhood and can have an autosomal recessive, dominant or sporadic mode of inheritance. Sera from HIV-infected patients with thrush have been screened for *C. albicans* genomic expression. Identified genes include some encoding immunogenic antigens. Notably, when disrupted, genes can confer defects in morphogenesis, adherence, and mortality. Additionally, family analysis has identified an isolated form of mucocutaneous candidiasis that affects nails only, and its chromosomal region. This and multiple other studies suggest that there are distinct phenotypes that respond in varying degrees to *Candida* replication in their host.

Incidence/Prevalence in USA: More common, particularly vaginal. Very common in persons with immunodeficiency.

Predominant age:
- Infants and older geriatrics predominate for thrush and cutaneous infections
- Women during their child bearing years predominate for vaginitis

Predominant sex: Female > Male (due to the entity of *Candida* vaginitis)

SIGNS & SYMPTOMS
- In pediatrics
  - ◊ Oral lesions - white, raised, painless, distinct patches within oral cavity
  - ◊ Perineal - erythematous maculopapular rash with white "satellite" pustules
- In adults (whether or not immunocompromised)
  - ◊ Vulvovaginal lesions - thin to thick whitish, "cottage cheese"-like discharge; erythematous patches in vagina or on perineum. Range from asymptomatic to intense pruritus with "burning" irritation
- In immunocompromised hosts
  - ◊ Oral lesions - white, raised, painless, distinct patches; erythematous slightly raised patches; thick dark brownish coating; deep fissures
  - ◊ Esophagitis - dysphagia, odynophagia, retrosternal pain. Usually associated with thrush.
  - ◊ Gastrointestinal - ulcerations, pain
  - ◊ Balanitis - erythema, linear erosions and scaling

CAUSES Species of *Candida albicans* and, less frequently, *Candida tropicalis*

RISK FACTORS
- Immunosuppression
- Antibacterial therapy
- Douching, chemical irritants, other vaginitides predispose some women to yeast vaginitis
- Dentures
- Chronic steroids (oral or inhaled)
- Birth control pills
- Hyperglycemia

DIAGNOSIS

DIFFERENTIAL DIAGNOSIS
- Baby formula can mimic thrush
- Hairy leukoplakia can mimic thrush but does not rub off to an erythematous base and is usually on the lateral sides of the tongue.
- Other yeasts may present like *Candida*
- Some of the symptoms of *Trichomonas vaginalis* (TV) can mimic those of *Candida* vulvovaginitis (CV). Specific symptom overlaps include: Both may have 1) initial symptoms post-menstrually, 2) marked vulvar irritation, 3) labial erythema, 4) external dysuria, and 5) vaginal tenderness.

LABORATORY
- Potassium hydroxide 10% microscopic slide preparation ("KOH prep"). Breaks down epithelial cell walls allowing yeast forms to be more easily identified. Best if heated. Lack of slide identification does not rule out and, conversely, one may identify a scant number of fungal forms without symptoms or pathogenesis.
- Gram stain reveals gram positive yeast forms
- Culture - blood or Sabouraud's agar. A positive may be result of normal flora.

Drugs that may alter lab results:
- Douches and spermicides
- Inadequately dosed antifungal medication

Disorders that may alter lab results: Other vaginitides (may obscure vaginal slide findings)

PATHOLOGICAL FINDINGS Slide prep - Mycelia (hyphae) or pseudomycelia (pseudohyphae) yeast forms. A polymorphonuclear leukocyte response is not usually seen.

SPECIAL TESTS N/A

IMAGING Esophageal candidiasis will sometimes reveal a "cobblestone" appearance with a barium swallow and, less commonly, fistulas or esophageal dilatation (from denervation)

DIAGNOSTIC PROCEDURES
- For KOH prep, will need sample of discharge or "coating" of infected area or ulcer
- Esophagitis may need endoscopic biopsy
- HIV seropositivity plus thrush with dysphagia relieved by antifungal treatment is consistent with diagnosis of *Candida* esophagitis

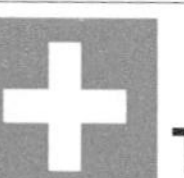

TREATMENT

APPROPRIATE HEALTH CARE Outpatient

GENERAL MEASURES Screen both well infants and patients with severe immunodeficiency using appropriate history and physical at all routine visits

SURGICAL MEASURES N/A

ACTIVITY N/A

DIET A few authorities say rectal colonization may be decreased with active culture yogurt or other live lactobacillus, but no clear correlation

PATIENT EDUCATION
- Advise patients at risk for recurrence about antibacterial therapy overgrowth
- Inform appropriate patients of over-the-counter vaginitis medications
- Cotton underwear may allow for better perineal ventilation and, thus, a less suitable environment for yeast

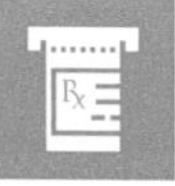

MEDICATIONS

DRUG(S) OF CHOICE
- Vaginal (choose one):
  - ◊ Miconazole (Monistat) 2% cream: one applicator or 100 mg suppositories, intravaginally q hs x 7 days
  - ◊ Clotrimazole (Gyne-Lotrimin, Mycelex): intravaginal suppositories 100 mg q hs x 6-7 days or 200 mg q hs x 3 days. 1% cream one applicator intravaginally q hs x 6-7 days.
  - ◊ Nystatin (Mycostatin, Nilstat) 100,000 U/gram cream (one applicator) or 100,000 U tablets (one) intravaginally bid x 7 days
  - ◊ Fluconazole (Diflucan) 150 mg tablet once
- Oropharyngeal:
  - ◊ Clotrimazole (Mycelex) 10 mg troche, slowly dissolve in mouth 5 times per day, preferably over 20 minutes for 7-14 days (2 days after disappearance of thrush) (first choice in most literature)
  - ◊ Nystatin pastilles - 1 or 2, qid for 7-14 days (48 hours after disappearance of thrush)
  - ◊ Nystatin oral suspension (100,000 units/mL): Children apply 5-10 mL qid x10 days directly to oral lesions. Adults swish and swallow 5-10 mL over 20 minutes qid x14 days. Prophylaxis for relapses consists of above dosages 2-5 times per day.
  - ◊ Amphotericin B (Fungizone) oral suspension (100 mg/mL): 1 mL qid, swish "for as long as reasonable" before swallowing. Use between meals if possible.
- Esophagitis:
  - ◊ Ketoconazole (Nizoral) 200-400 mg tablets - one po qd x14-21 days

or

  - ◊ Fluconazole (Diflucan) 200 mg, then 100 mg po qd x10-21 days

- Gastrointestinal (therapy not well defined)
  - ◊ Fluconazole 200 mg tablets - one po qd x14-21 days

or

  - ◊ Amphotericin B (Fungizone) IV
- Note: Resistant candidiasis is common in severely immunocompromised hosts. Some patients with otherwise resistant oropharyngeal and/or esophageal infection benefit from amphotericin B, 50 mg 3 times a week or from itraconazole (Sporanox) 200 mg bid for the same number of days described under fluconazole dosing for the various sites of infection mentioned above.

Contraindications:
- Any drug is contraindicated if it causes severe allergic response or a severe adverse reaction
- Ketoconazole, itraconazole or nystatin (if swallowed) - severe hepatotoxicity
- Amphotericin B - renal failure

Precautions:
- Vaginal - miconazole is usually drug of choice in pregnancy
- Ketoconazole - rarely, men may have difficulty achieving erections secondary to this drug. May cause light sensitivity. Teratogen in pregnancy and probably excreted in milk. Not well studied in children. Anaphylaxis is reported. Hepatic toxicity has been noted, predominantly with long-term therapy.
- Fluconazole - adjust dose with renal compromise. Hepatotoxicity is rare. Very expensive relative to most other oral agents. Resistance has often been noted.
- Amphotericin B - renal toxicity and hypokalemia common. Careful monitoring is mandatory. Ketotic diabetics should have well controlled blood sugars prior to administration. Safety during pregnancy is not established.
- Itraconazole - doubling the Itraconazole dose results in approximately a three-fold increase in the Itraconazole plasma concentrations

Significant possible interactions:
- Rarely seen with creams, lotions or suppositories
- Ketoconazole
  - ◊ Antacids, H2 blockers (achlorhydria) - reduce ketoconazole concentration
  - ◊ Amphotericin - drug antagonism; do not give together
  - ◊ Antiretrovirals - many have problematic interactions with ketoconazole; check drug reference
  - ◊ Coumadin - potentiates anticoagulation
  - ◊ Hypoglycemics - enhanced hypoglycemia
  - ◊ INH/rifampin - reduce ketoconazole concentration
  - ◊ Cyclosporine - increased cyclosporine concentration
  - ◊ Phenytoin - metabolism altered; check levels
  - ◊ Alcohol - disulfiram reaction possible
  - ◊ Others - check drug interaction reference
- Amphotericin
  - ◊ Nephrotoxic drugs - enhanced toxicity
  - ◊ Corticosteroids - potentiates hypokalemia
  - ◊ Ketoconazole - drug antagonism; do not give together
- Fluconazole
  - ◊ Rifampin - decreased fluconazole concentrations
  - ◊ Tolbutamide - decreased tolbutamide concentrations
  - ◊ Warfarin, phenytoin, cyclosporine - metabolism altered; check levels
- Itraconazole - this potent cytochrome P450 3A4 isoenzyme system (CYP3A4) inhibitor may increase plasma concentrations of the many drugs metabolized by that pathway and cause serious cardiovascular events. Carefully assess all co-administered medications.

ALTERNATIVE DRUGS
- Vaginal
  - ◊ Terconazole (Terazol) particularly for recurrent cases that may involve imidazole resistance. 0.4% cream - one applicator intravaginally q hs x 7 days; 0.8% cream/80 mg suppositories - one applicator or one suppository intravaginally q hs x 3 days
  - ◊ Any of the antifungal creams or suppositories can be tried every month for a few days near menses to help curb recurrent infections
- Oropharyngeal
  - ◊ Ketoconazole 200-400 mg po qd x 14-21 days
  - ◊ Fluconazole 50-200 mg tablets - one po qd x 14-21 days, although a majority of fungal strains found in the oropharynx are likely to be resistant
- Esophagitis
  - ◊ Amphotericin B (variable dosing)

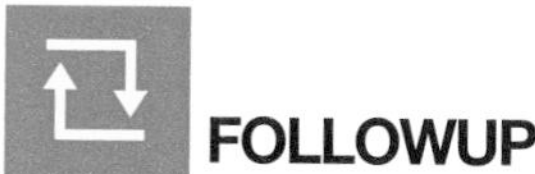

FOLLOWUP

PATIENT MONITORING
Immunocompromised persons may need to monitor themselves regularly. Use symptoms to monitor as well as "routine" KOH preps and or visual investigations during vaginal or oral exams.

PREVENTION/AVOIDANCE
- Antibiotics can potentiate candidiasis
- *Candida* overgrowth is more likely with pH changes from douching, chemicals (such as spermicides) or other vaginitides
- Moist environments are conducive to overgrowth of *Candida*. Cotton underwear may help deter some *Candida* infections.

POSSIBLE COMPLICATIONS
- Rarely develops major complications in immunocompetent persons
- With immunocompromised, generally depends on severity of immune status (CD4 count is the most common marker). Moderate immunodepression (CD4 200-500) may be associated with chronic candidiasis. With severe immunodepression (CD4 < 100) thrush can lead to esophagitis and, later, a full systemic infection can involve every organ system, particularly the kidney (candiduria).

EXPECTED COURSE/PROGNOSIS
- For immunocompetent individuals, a benign course and excellent prognosis is the norm
- In immunosuppressed persons, *Candida* may become an "AIDS defining illness" by CDC criteria and chronicity can cause much morbidity and, less commonly, mortality

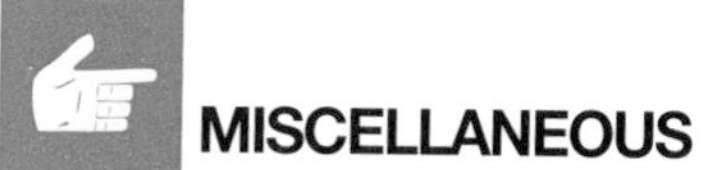

MISCELLANEOUS

ASSOCIATED CONDITIONS
- Human immunodeficiency virus
- Other leukopenias
- Diabetes mellitus
- Cancer
- Other immunosuppressive disorders
- Those disorders that call for steroids (oral or intranasal)

AGE-RELATED FACTORS
Pediatric: Newborn thrush may be acquired in the birth canal
Geriatric: Thrush is common
Others: Vaginitis is common in women of childbearing age. Uncommon to see prepubertal or post-menopausal yeast vaginitis due to hormonal induced changes in the vaginal wall.

PREGNANCY
- No known fetal complications of maternal *Candida*
- See specific "medication precautions" above
- Miconazole is usually drug of choice in pregnancy

SYNONYMS
- Monilia
- Thrush
- Yeast

ICD-9-CM
112.0 Candidiasis of mouth
112.1 Candidiasis of vulva and vagina
112.9 Candidiasis of unspecified site

SEE ALSO
Candidiasis
HIV infection & AIDS
Vulvovaginitis, candidal

OTHER NOTES
- Most *Candida* infections are associated with endogenous flora
- Transmission from person to person is rare
- Occasionally *Candida* vaginitis may be sexually transmitted
- Rarely, oral *Candida* leukoplakia can be precancerous
- Skin testing, often used to diagnose or exclude anergy, is positive in 70-85% of individuals randomly checked in studies

ABBREVIATIONS N/A

REFERENCES

- Betts RF, Chapman SW, Penn RL. Reese and Betts' a Practical Approach to Infectious Diseases. Boston: Littlr, Brown and Co; 2002
- Vazquez JA, Sobel JD. Mucosal candidiasis. Infect Dis Clin North AM 2002;16(4):793-820

Web references: 0 available at www.5mcc.com
Illustrations N/A

Author(s):
Susan Louisa Montauk, MD

BASICS

DESCRIPTION Carbon monoxide (CO) is produced by incomplete combustion of carbon containing compounds such as wood. Inhalation of CO leads to displacement of oxygen from binding sites on hemoglobin. CO has about 250 times the affinity for hemoglobin than oxygen.

Detrimental effects are related to tissue hypoxia from decreased oxygen content and a shift of the oxyhemoglobin dissociation curve to the left. CO also binds to cytochrome oxidase impairing mitochondrial function. Muscle activity is affected by CO by binding to myoglobin.

System(s) affected: Cardiovascular, Musculoskeletal, Nervous

Genetics: N/A

Incidence/Prevalence in USA: Approximately 3800 deaths annually

Additional 10,000 individuals miss one or more days of work

Predominant age: N/A

Predominant sex: N/A

SIGNS & SYMPTOMS
- Headaches
- Tinnitus
- Nausea
- Dizziness
- Weakness
- Confusion
- CNS depression
- Syncope
- Angina
- Tachycardia
- Cardiac dysrhythmias
- Nystagmus
- Ataxia
- Seizures
- Coma
- Cardiopulmonary arrest

CAUSES Carbon monoxide inhalation

RISK FACTORS
- Cigarette smokers
- Smoke inhalation
- Closed space with faulty furnaces or stoves
- Coal miners
- Mechanics (inhalation of car exhaust)
- Paint strippers
- Solvent manufacturing

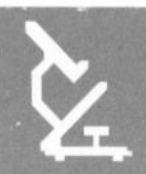

DIAGNOSIS

DIFFERENTIAL DIAGNOSIS Cyanide toxicity

LABORATORY Measurement of carboxyhemoglobin

Drugs that may alter lab results: N/A

Disorders that may alter lab results: N/A

PATHOLOGICAL FINDINGS N/A

SPECIAL TESTS N/A

IMAGING N/A

DIAGNOSTIC PROCEDURES N/A

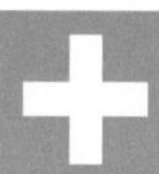

TREATMENT

APPROPRIATE HEALTH CARE
- Emergency room for mild poisoning
- Inpatient for moderate or severe poisoning

GENERAL MEASURES
- Removal from offending source
- Rapid reduction in tissue hypoxia with 100% oxygen to reduce the half-time of elimination of carbon monoxide to 40 minutes
- Supportive care as necessary
- Intubation and mechanical ventilation may be necessary for severe intoxication
- Volume resuscitation

SURGICAL MEASURES N/A

ACTIVITY Rest until carboxyhemoglobin reduced and symptoms abate

DIET N/A

PATIENT EDUCATION N/A

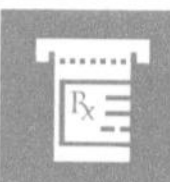

MEDICATIONS

DRUG(S) OF CHOICE
- 100% Oxygen by tight fitting non-rebreathing mask
- Hyperbaric oxygen for severe poisoning
- Mild poisoning: carboxyhemoglobin levels < 30%
  - ◊ No signs or symptoms of cardiovascular or neurologic dysfunction
  - ◊ Treatment - admission if carboxyhemoglobin > 25%
  - ◊ Symptomatic medication - acetaminophen for headache etc.
  - ◊ 100% Oxygen by nonrebreather until carboxyhemoglobin < 5%
  - ◊ Patients with underlying heart disease should be admitted regardless of level of carboxyhemoglobin
- Moderate poisoning: carboxyhemoglobin 30-40%
  - ◊ No signs or symptoms of cardiovascular or neurologic dysfunction
  - ◊ Treatment - admission
  - ◊ Cardiovascular status should be followed closely even in the absence of clear cardiac effects
  - ◊ Determination of acid-base status - corrected by oxygen
  - ◊ 100% Oxygen by nonrebreather until carboxyhemoglobin < 5%
- Severe poisoning: carboxyhemoglobin > 40%
  - ◊ Cardiovascular or neurologic functional impairment at any carboxyhemoglobin
  - ◊ Treatment - admission
  - ◊ Cardiovascular function monitoring
  - ◊ Acid-base status monitoring
  - ◊ 100% Oxygen by nonrebreather until carboxyhemoglobin < 5%
  - ◊ Hyperbaric oxygen immediately if available, if unavailable then treat as in moderate poisoning
  - ◊ No improvement in cardiovascular or neurologic function within 4 hours - transport to nearest facility with hyperbaric oxygen, regardless of distance

Contraindications: N/A
Precautions: N/A
Significant possible interactions: N/A

ALTERNATIVE DRUGS N/A

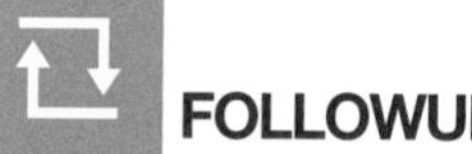

FOLLOWUP

PATIENT MONITORING
- Measurement of carboxyhemoglobin levels
- Arterial blood gases
- Psychiatric evaluation and follow up for intentional exposure

PREVENTION/AVOIDANCE
- Maintenance of furnaces and stoves to avoid faulty combustion
- Adequate ventilation in high risk occupations

POSSIBLE COMPLICATIONS
- Myocardial infarction
- Long term neuropsychiatric complications
  - ◊ Intellectual deterioration
  - ◊ Memory impairment
- Personality changes
  - ◊ Irritability
  - ◊ Aggressiveness
  - ◊ Violence
  - ◊ Moodiness

EXPECTED COURSE/PROGNOSIS
Most survivors recover completely with only a minority developing chronic neuropsychiatric impairment

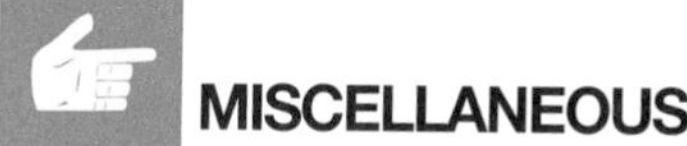

MISCELLANEOUS

ASSOCIATED CONDITIONS N/A

AGE-RELATED FACTORS
Pediatric: N/A
Geriatric: Higher incidence of cardiovascular and neurologic disease increasing complications
Others: N/A

PREGNANCY
Tissue hypoxia includes the fetus. Can cause significant fetal abnormalities depending on the developmental stage.

SYNONYMS N/A

ICD-9-CM
986 Toxic effect of carbon monoxide

SEE ALSO

OTHER NOTES N/A

ABBREVIATIONS
CO = Carbon monoxide
CNS = Central nervous system

REFERENCES

- Murray JF, Nadel JA, eds: Textbook of Respiratory Medicine. Philadelphia, W.B. Saunders Co., 1988
- Ingbar DH, ed: Clinics in Chest Medicine: Respiratory Emergencies I. Philadelphia, W.B. Saunders Co., March, 1994
- Shoemaker WC, Ayers S, et al, eds: Textbook of Critical Care. Philadelphia, W.B. Saunders Co., 1989
- Ilano AL, Raffin TA: Management of Carbon Monoxide Poisoning. Chest 1990;91:165-169

Web references: 1 available at www.5mcc.com
Illustrations N/A

Author(s):
Robert DeMarco, MD

BASICS

DESCRIPTION Absence of effective mechanical cardiac activity.
- This section is not a substitute for an American Heart Association approved ACLS course and is intended only as a quick reference

System(s) affected: Cardiovascular
Genetics: N/A
Incidence/Prevalence in USA: 200:100,000
Predominant age: Increases with age
Predominant sex: Male > Female

SIGNS & SYMPTOMS
- Unconscious secondary to CNS hypoperfusion
- No pulses in large arteries
- Apnea or agonal breathing
- Cyanosis or pallor

CAUSES
- Asystole (confirm in 2 leads; 11% actually fine V-fib)
- Ventricular fibrillation (V-fib)
- Pulseless ventricular tachycardia (V-tach)
- Pulseless electrical activity (PEA, previously known as electrical mechanical dissociation [EMD])

RISK FACTORS
- Male
- Increasing age
- Hypercholesterolemia
- Hypertension
- Cigarette smoking
- Positive family history of atherosclerosis

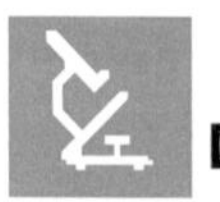

DIAGNOSIS

DIFFERENTIAL DIAGNOSIS
- Drugs: barbiturates, narcotics, calcium channel blockers, beta blockers, tricyclics
- Shock: septic or blood loss induced
- Hypothermia
- Pulmonary embolism
- Cardiac tamponade
- Pneumothorax
- Acidosis
- Electrolyte abnormality
- Carbon monoxide

LABORATORY
- Arterial blood gas
- Electrolytes
- CBC
- Drug levels
- PT (international normalized ratio [INR]), PTT, type and cross, if indicated

Drugs that may alter lab results: Digoxin toxicity may cause hyperkalemia

Disorders that may alter lab results:
- Hypo- or hyperventilation will change pO_2 and pCO_2
- Acidosis increases serum potassium

PATHOLOGICAL FINDINGS Based on underlying cause

SPECIAL TESTS ECG

IMAGING Chest x-ray for endotracheal (ET) tube placement, pneumothorax. Consider echocardiogram for pericardial effusion.

DIAGNOSTIC PROCEDURES N/A

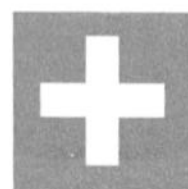

TREATMENT

APPROPRIATE HEALTH CARE
Pre-hospital emergency medical service (EMS) personnel, emergency department, "cardiac arrest team", intensive care setting

GENERAL MEASURES
- Defibrillation first
  - ◊ Adult: 200, 300, or 360J
  - ◊ Children: Use largest paddles that will fit on child even adult size if can get good contact. Defibrillate at 2J/kg once. Increase to 4J/kg twice.
- 100% oxygen by bag-valve-mask or endotracheal tube (preferred)
- Start 2 IV's as close to the heart as possible (central line OK but don't waste time). Large bore peripheral lines can deliver fluid more quickly than a central line. This is especially important in PEA secondary to hypovolemia.
- Perform CPR including closed chest compression. Intermittent abdominal compression and active compression /decompression show no survival advantage.
- Keep patient warm if possible, especially in children
- Monitor:
  - ◊ Pulse after three initial defibrillations
  - ◊ Check monitor between each defibrillation and after any intervention
  - ◊ Use end-tidal CO_2 monitor to assess gas exchange, if available. Esophageal intubation will produce a very low end-tidal CO_2.

SURGICAL MEASURES
If indicated:
- Pericardiocentesis to treat cardiac tamponade
- Needle decompression (second intercostal space midclavicular line), then chest tube insertion to treat tension pneumothorax

ACTIVITY N/A

DIET N/A

PATIENT EDUCATION Suggest basic life support (BLS) training to all patients in your practice, especially those who have family members at risk for cardiac arrest

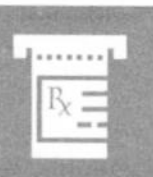

MEDICATIONS

DRUG(S) OF CHOICE
- Lidocaine, atropine, naloxone, and epinephrine [LANE] can all be given by endotracheal tube. Follow by 10 cc of NS or sterile water followed by bagging.
- Epinephrine:
  - ◊ 1 mL = 1 mg (1:1000)
  - ◊ 1 mL = 0.1 mg (1:10,000)

ADULT: Ventricular tachycardia and pulseless ventricular tachycardia.
Use in order listed below:
- Defibrillate x3 at 200J, 300J, 360J
  - ◊ Check monitor rhythm
  - ◊ Follow each drug administration by repeated defibrillation at 360J
  - ◊ Check monitor and pulses after each subsequent intervention
- Epinephrine: 1 mg IV every 3-5 minutes or vasopressin 40U IV single dose, one time only. May choose to resume epinephrine if no response after a single dose of vasopressin. High dose epinephrine is permissible but discouraged and may actually worsen outcomes.
- Amiodarone 300 mg IV push may be used prior to lidocaine
- Lidocaine: 1.5 mg/kg IV, repeat in 5 minutes to total dose of 3 mg/kg
- Magnesium sulfate: 1-2 mg IV in suspected Torsades de pointes or refractory V-fib/V-tach
- Procainamide 30 mg/min IV in refractory V-fib/V-tach (maximum dose of 17 mg/kg) is permissible. However, since the time to a useful level by infusion is so long, it is discouraged and is unlikely to be of any benefit. No improvement in survival to discharge.
- Bicarbonate: 1 mEq/kg IV only in known preexisting bicarbonate responsive acidosis, tricyclic overdose, to alkalinize the urine in known overdose

ADULT: asystole
- CPR
- Confirm in 2 leads
- Consider possible causes including hypoxia, hyperkalemia, hypokalemia, preexisting acidosis, drug overdose, hypothermia
- Consider defibrillation as per V-tach/V-fib since V-fib may be mistaken for asystole
- Consider immediate transcutaneous pacing
- Epinephrine: 1 mg IV push repeated every 3-5 minutes
  - ◊ May use intermediate dose or high dose epinephrine (2-5 mg IV or 0.1 mg/kg IV) every 3-5 minutes
- Atropine: 1 mg IV push every 3-5 minutes to total dose of 0.04 mg/kg
  - ◊ Shorter atropine dosing intervals are acceptable (every 1-2 minutes)
- Consider termination of efforts if no reversible underlying cause is found

For pulseless electrical activity (PEA)
- Includes EMD, idioventricular rhythms, ventricular escape rhythms, bradyasystole rhythms, post-defibrillation idioventricular rhythms
- Assess blood flow by Doppler ultrasound if available
- Consider possible reversible causes: cardiogenic shock (weak pump), cardiac tamponade, tension pneumothorax, severe hypovolemia, pulmonary embolism (consider thrombolytics), hypothermia, hypoxia, acidosis, hyperkalemia, drug overdose such as beta-blockers, calcium channel blockers, tricyclics, digoxin
- Epinephrine: 1 mg IV push. Repeat every 3-5 minutes. Can use intermediate or high dose epinephrine (2-5 mg IV or 0.1 mg/kg IV respectively) every 3-5 minutes, but this shows no proven improvement in survival.
- Atropine: 1 mg IV every 3-5 minutes to total dose of 0.04 mg/kg: if absolute bradycardia (< 60 beats per minute) or relative bradycardia. May decrease interval to 1-2 minutes if desired.

CHILDREN:
(in alphabetical order)
- Amiodarone for pulseless VF/VT 5 mg/kg IV or IO rapid bolus. For perfusing tachyarrhythmias loading 5 mg/kg IV or IO over 20-60 minutes, maximum dose 15 mg/kg/d.
- Atropine 0.01-0.02 mg/kg/dose; minimum dose is 0.1 mg, maximum single dose is 0.5 mg in child, 1.0 mg in adolescent
- Epinephrine
  - ◊ Bradycardia: 0.01 mg/kg IV/IO or 0.1 mg/kg ET (1:1000)
  - ◊ Asystolic or pulseless arrest: First dose is 0.01-0.03 mg/kg IV/IO. Doses as high as 0.2 mg/kg may be effective.
  - ◊ Infusion: 0.1 μg/kg/min. Titrate to desired effect (0.1 μg/kg/min-1.0 μg/kg/min)
- Lidocaine
  - ◊ Bolus: 1 mg/kg/dose (maximum 3 mg/kg)
  - ◊ Infusion: 20-50 μg/kg/min
- Sodium bicarbonate 1 mEq/kg/dose or 0.3 x kg x base deficit. Infuse slowly and only if ventilation adequate.

Contraindications: None during an arrest

Precautions:
- Calcium can be used if known (pre-existing) hyperkalemia precipitated arrhythmia. Calcium is contraindicated in hyperkalemia secondary to digoxin.
- Magnesium is relatively contraindicated in renal failure but given consequences of not terminating rhythm, this is only a relative contraindication in this setting

Significant possible interactions: N/A

ALTERNATIVE DRUGS Asystole: Aminophylline 250 mg IV bolus has been effective in uncontrolled trials, but should be used only when conventional therapy has failed

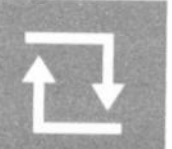

FOLLOWUP

PATIENT MONITORING Intensive care setting on continuous monitor, look for precipitating cause including serial EKG's and enzymes to rule out myocardial infarction

PREVENTION/AVOIDANCE Treat underlying disease

POSSIBLE COMPLICATIONS
- Can have significant neurologic, hepatic, renal, and cardiac ischemic injury
- May have rib fractures or pneumothorax from CPR

EXPECTED COURSE/PROGNOSIS
- Outcome related to underlying disease, age, duration of arrest, etc.
- Outcome poor if
  - ◊ > 4 minutes to CPR or > 8 minutes to ACLS
  - ◊ Arrest in field
  - ◊ Resuscitation effort > 30 minutes
- About 14% survive in-hospital arrest; fewer after field arrest.

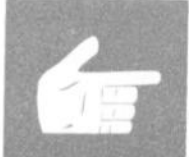

MISCELLANEOUS

ASSOCIATED CONDITIONS
- Coronary artery disease (cardiac arrest may be first presenting symptom)
- Valvular heart disease
- Hypertension

AGE-RELATED FACTORS
Pediatric: Bradycardia is most common initial form of cardiac arrest. Most frequently is primarily a response to underlying pulmonary disease and hypoxia. Adequate oxygenation and ventilation is especially important.
Geriatric: Poor risk for survival and long-term outcome
Others: N/A

PREGNANCY
- Displace uterus either manually or by placing a rolled towel or pad under right hip. If not able to resuscitate within 5-15 minutes, consider emergency C-section to relieve uterine obstruction and increase blood return to the heart. This may also be done to save the fetus if at a viable age.
- Consider amniotic fluid embolism or eclampsia related seizures as precipitating factors

SYNONYMS
- Code Blue

ICD-9-CM
427.5 Cardiac arrest

SEE ALSO

OTHER NOTES N/A

ABBREVIATIONS
ACLS = Advanced Cardiac Life Support
EMD = electro-mechanical dissociation
ET = endotracheal
IO = intraosseous
PEA = pulseless electrical activity

REFERENCES

- Guidelines 2000 for Cardiopulmonary Resuscitation and Emergency Cardiovascular Care. Part 6: advanced cardiovascular life support: section 3: adjuncts for oxygenation, ventilation and airway control. The American Heart Association in collaboration with the International Liaison Committee on Resuscitation. Circulation 2000; 102(8Suppl):95-104
- Graber MA. Emergency Medicine. In: Graber MA, et al, eds. The Family Practice Handbook. St. Louis: Mosby-Yearbook; 1997

Web references: 2 available at www.5mcc.com
Illustrations N/A

Author(s):
Bobby Peters, MD

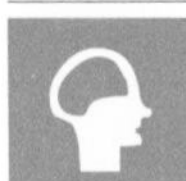

BASICS

DESCRIPTION Compression of cardiac chambers by acute pressure on the heart from increased volume and pressure of the pericardial fluid
- As fluid accumulates, pressure primarily affects the compliant cardiac wall and transmits the pressure transmurally, resulting in increased ventricular pressure. This decreases ventricular filling and reduces cardiac output by reducing stroke volume.
- The compensatory mechanisms for tamponade are: Increased peripheral resistance, increased CVP and increased heart rate. All three increase myocardial oxygen denied the heart at a time when perfusion is limited.
- In some patients, pulsus paradoxus and equalization of pressures may not occur
- In patients with elevated left ventricular diastolic pressures (as with chronic hypertension), resistance to left ventricle (LV) filling is constant. Throughout the cardiac cycle, equalization of pressures in these patients may only be noted in the right heart chambers with LV pressures being higher than right ventricle (RV) pressures.
- The absence of pulsus paradoxus and classic hemodynamic finding does not rule out tamponade

System(s) affected: Cardiovascular
Genetics: N/A
Incidence/Prevalence in USA: N/A
Predominant age: N/A
Predominant sex: N/A

SIGNS & SYMPTOMS
- Beck's triad - distant heart sounds, hypotension, distended neck veins
- Most common complaints are of intolerance to minimal activity and dyspnea. Later may develop agitation, CNS depression, coma and cardiac arrest.
- Decreased systolic blood pressure
- Narrow pulse pressure
- Pulsus paradoxus - greater than 15 mm Hg drop in systolic blood pressure between inspiration and expiration
- Neck veins may be distended and reveal a rapid systolic (X) descent and attenuated or absent diastolic (Y) descent
- Tachycardia - a compensatory mechanism to maintain output
- Right upper quadrant tenderness due to hepatic engorgement
- Increased area of cardiac dullness outside the apical point of maximum impulse

CAUSES
- Physiology of tamponade depends on size and rapidity of development
- Uremia
- Neoplasm - breast, lung, lymphoma, leukemia
- Postmyocardial infarction (Dressler's)
- Postoperative - as high as 30% post pericardiotomy
- HIV - particularly symptomatic
- Other viruses - Coxsackie group B, influenza, echo, herpes
- Bacterial infection - S. aureus, M. tuberculosis, S. pneumoniae (rare)
- Fungal infection - M. capsulatum
- Lupus and rheumatologic disease
- Trauma
- Placement of central venous catheter, pacer wires
- Hypothyroidism
- Drug induced

RISK FACTORS
- Cardiac tamponade should be suspected in the hemodynamically unstable patient:
  - ◊ With known pericarditis
  - ◊ Following blunt or penetrating chest trauma
  - ◊ Following open heart surgery or cardiac catheterization
  - ◊ With known or suspected intrathoracic neoplasm
  - ◊ With suspected dissecting aortic aneurysm
  - ◊ Renal failure on dialysis

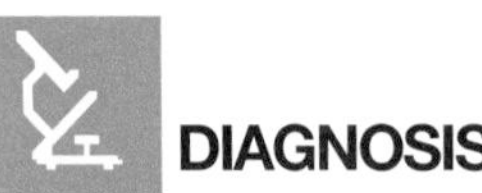

DIAGNOSIS

DIFFERENTIAL DIAGNOSIS
- Tension pneumothorax
- Acute RV failure
- Chronic obstructive pulmonary disease
- Constrictive pericarditis
- Acute acceleration of chronic bronchitis
- Acute pulmonary emboli
- Fat emboli
- Excessive or rapid administration of fluids
- Abdominal distention from ascites or ileus
- Increased intrathoracic pressure from pneumothorax, hemothorax, airway obstruction, or mechanical ventilation
- Administration of vasopressors

LABORATORY
- CBC
- Sed rate
- Cardiac enzymes to rule out acute myocardial infarction
- Antinuclear antibodies (ANA)
- Rheumatoid factor
- BUN/creatinine
- Pericardial fluid for - culture of bacteria, fungus, mycobacteria, Gram stain, hematocrit, cell count, cytology, glucose, protein, rheumatoid factors, complement levels

Drugs that may alter lab results: N/A

Disorders that may alter lab results: N/A

PATHOLOGICAL FINDINGS Pericardial blood usually does not clot, but occasionally will

SPECIAL TESTS
- ECG
  - ◊ May show sinus tachycardia, low voltage QRS complexes, diffuse ST segment elevation and PR segment depression of pericarditis
  - ◊ Electrical alternans (R wave variation from beat to beat)
  - ◊ Electrical alternans is seen in 10-20% of cases of tamponade and 50-60% of these are neoplastic in origin
- Right heart catheterization
  - ◊ Equalization (within 2-3 mm) of right atrial, pulmonary artery diastolic pressure, pulmonary capillary wedge pressure, left atrial and left ventricular diastolic pressure
  - ◊ The intracardiac diastolic pressure will approximate the intrapericardial pressure
  - ◊ The dip and plateau pattern of constriction or restriction pericardial disease is absent
  - ◊ Loss of Y descent on atrial wave form

IMAGING
- Chest x-ray:
  - ◊ May or may not show enlargement of cardiac shadow (if > 250 cc fluid present)
- Echocardiography:
  - ◊ Diagnostic cardiac compression
  - ◊ Doppler - right sided transvalvular flow greatly exaggerated; left sided flows greatly reduced with inspiration

DIAGNOSTIC PROCEDURES N/A

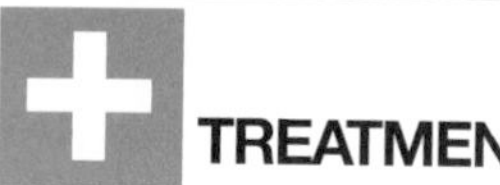

TREATMENT

APPROPRIATE HEALTH CARE Inpatient

GENERAL MEASURES
- Maintain hemodynamic stability until definitive correction of the pericardial tamponade
- All patients should have q 15 minute blood pressures, heart rate and at a minimum CVP measurement. Strong consideration should be given to placement of a Swan-Ganz catheter if time allows.
- Fluids may be of temporary benefit, but rising filling pressures may further compromise coronary perfusion

SURGICAL MEASURES
- Pericardiocentesis surgical treatment:
  - ◊ Indications - when there is rapid deterioration of hemodynamic function, when there is delay in operation for traumatic effusion and for diagnostic reasons
  - ◊ If rapid re-accumulation is anticipated (as in malignancy) it may be helpful to insert a long term drainage catheter. Also consider instillation of sclerosing agents.
  - ◊ Surgery should be performed under the most optimal circumstances available to the operation as the patient's condition allows
  - ◊ Blind pericardiocentesis should be performed only in life threatening emergencies
  - ◊ Ideally echocardiography can be brought to the bedside to assist in needle placement and progress of fluid removal
  - ◊ Invasive monitoring is also helpful to follow decrease in pericardial pressures
  - ◊ Fluoroscopy can also be used
  - ◊ EKG guidance using the "V" lead to avoid contact with the epicardium may be useful
  - ◊ 20% of patients with tamponade will have a negative tap because the pericardial sac contains coagulated material. Hemorrhagic pericardial effusions usually do not clot.

ACTIVITY Bedrest

DIET As tolerated

PATIENT EDUCATION N/A

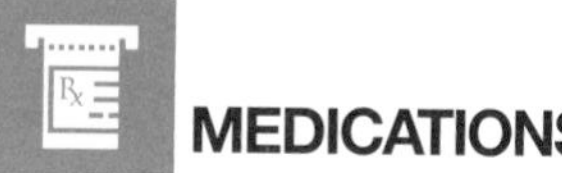

MEDICATIONS

DRUG(S) OF CHOICE Isoproterenol may temporarily increase cardiac output
Contraindications: Refer to manufacturer's literature
Precautions: Refer to manufacturer's literature
Significant possible interactions: Refer to manufacturer's literature

ALTERNATIVE DRUGS N/A

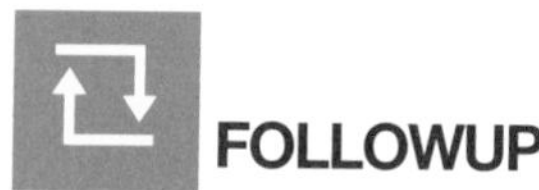

FOLLOWUP

PATIENT MONITORING Close monitoring until stable

PREVENTION/AVOIDANCE None

POSSIBLE COMPLICATIONS
- Cardiac perforation and/or laceration at time of pericardiocentesis
- Pneumothorax at time of pericardiocentesis
- Constriction of pericardium

EXPECTED COURSE/PROGNOSIS
Good results expected with appropriate treatment

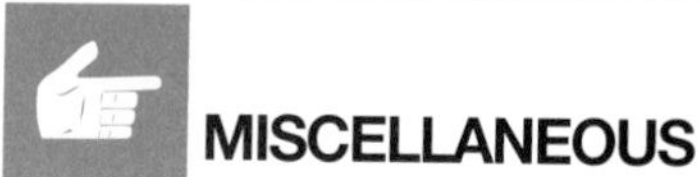

MISCELLANEOUS

ASSOCIATED CONDITIONS
- Myocardial infarction
- Aortic aneurysm

AGE-RELATED FACTORS
Pediatric: N/A
Geriatric: N/A
Others: N/A

PREGNANCY N/A

SYNONYMS N/A

ICD-9-CM
423.9 Unspecified disease of pericardium

SEE ALSO

OTHER NOTES N/A

ABBREVIATIONS N/A

REFERENCES

- Silva-Cardoso J, Moura B, Martins L, Mota-Miranda A, Roche-Goncalves F, LeCour H. Pericardial involvement in human immunodeficiency virus infection. Chest 1999, Feb;115(2):418-22
- Heger JW, et al: Cardiology for the House Officer. Baltimore, Williams & Wilkins, 1982
- Civettee JM, Taylor RW, Kirby RR: Critical Care. Philadelphia, J.B. Lippincott, 1988
- Rippie JM, et al: Intensive Care Medicine. Boston, Little, Brown and Company, 1991
- Shoemaker WC, et al: Textbook of Critical Care. Philadelphia, W.B. Saunders Co., 1989

Web references: 1 available at www.5mcc.com
Illustrations N/A

Author(s):
Todd S. Carran, MD

Cardiomyopathy, end stage

BASICS

DESCRIPTION In 1988, WHO defined cardiomyopathy as "heart muscle diseases of unknown causes," but now have expanded to include diseases with dominant pathophysiology as well as etiology and pathologic factors.

- Classification of cardiomyopathy (each of which can be caused by many disorders):
  - ◊ Dilated
  - ◊ Hypertrophic
  - ◊ Restrictive
  - ◊ Arrhythmogenic
  - ◊ Unclassified
- Types of cardiomyopathy:
  - ◊ Systolic failure: low cardiac output, decreased left ventricular ejection, tendency to accumulate salt and water causing increased intravascular volume, peripheral edema, and left and right heart failure symptoms. Etiologies include idiopathic, viral, postpartum, alcoholic, and many ischemic cardiomyopathies. An neurohormonal imbalance in norepinephrine causes fluid retention, peripheral vasoconstriction, and overstimulation of cardiac beta-receptors. These changes initially allow the heart to maintain a normal blood flow, but later cause progressive heart enlargement, pulmonary congestion, and right heart failure. The recognition of this imbalance has led to changes in medical therapy; angiotensin converting enzyme (ACE) inhibitors are an important part of therapy.
  - ◊ Diastolic failure: normal or super normal systolic function, non-compliant (stiff) left ventricle with increased filling pressures. Scarring (eg, post MI), amyloidosis, and hypertrophic cardiomyopathy may result in diastolic failure. Generally, the heart is not as enlarged as in the systolic failure group.

System(s) affected: Cardiovascular

Genetics: Idiopathic hypertrophic subaortic stenosis has a familial distribution

Incidence/Prevalence in USA:
- 60,000 patients, under 65, die each year with end-stage heart disease.
- 35,000 to 70,000 of the population might benefit from cardiac replacement or chronic support
- Most rapidly growing form of heart disease

Predominant age:
- Ischemic cardiomyopathy is seen mostly in age > 50
- Idiopathic and familial cardiomyopathies are seen at an earlier age, as are those related to congenital heart disease, viral cardiomyopathy, alcoholic cardiomyopathy and post partum cardiomyopathy

Predominant sex: Male > Female (ischemic cardiomyopathy)

SIGNS & SYMPTOMS
- Shortness of breath at rest
- Dyspnea on minimal exertion
- Paroxysmal nocturnal dyspnea/orthopnea
- Postprandial dyspnea
- Fatigue
- Syncope
- Tachypnea
- Cyanosis, pallor
- Cool vasoconstricted extremities
- Diaphoresis
- Jugular venous distention
- Bi-basilar inspiratory rales
- S3 cardiac gallop
- Liver and spleen enlargement
- Ascites, edema
- Chest pain

CAUSES
- Infectious
  - ◊ Viral (e.g., Coxsackie virus)
  - ◊ Poliomyelitis
  - ◊ Diphtheria
  - ◊ Toxoplasmosis
  - ◊ Trichinosis
  - ◊ Trypanosomiasis
  - ◊ Acute rheumatic fever
- Congenital
  - ◊ Congenital heart disease
  - ◊ Glycogen storage disease
  - ◊ Pompe disease
  - ◊ Hurler syndrome
  - ◊ Hunter syndrome
  - ◊ Fabry disease
  - ◊ Duchenne muscular dystrophy
  - ◊ Friedreich ataxia
  - ◊ Familial cardiomyopathies, such as "asymmetric septal hypertrophy"
- Toxic/metabolic
  - ◊ Alcoholism
  - ◊ Radiation
  - ◊ Beriberi
  - ◊ Kwashiorkor
  - ◊ Potassium deficiency
  - ◊ Cobalt
  - ◊ Hemosiderosis
- Drugs
  - ◊ Adriamycin
- Inflammatory
  - ◊ Giant cell myocarditis
  - ◊ Loeffler eosinophilia
  - ◊ Sarcoidosis
- Idiopathic
- Others
  - ◊ Coronary artery disease
  - ◊ Peripartum and postpartum
  - ◊ Amyloidosis
  - ◊ Idiopathic hypertrophic subaortic stenosis
  - ◊ Endomyocardial fibrosis

RISK FACTORS
- Hypertension
- Hyperlipidemia
- Obesity
- Diabetes mellitus
- Smoking
- Stress
- Sedentary lifestyle
- Cardiac surgery

DIAGNOSIS

DIFFERENTIAL DIAGNOSIS
- Severe pulmonary disease
- Primary pulmonary hypertension
- Recurrent pulmonary embolism
- Hypothyroidism
- Some advanced forms of malignancy

LABORATORY
- Hyponatremia
- Pre-renal azotemia
- Mild hyperbilirubinemia
- ECG: left ventricular hypertrophy, left bundle branch block (LBBB) ventricular strain pattern, left and right atrial enlargement are often seen. In ischemic cardiomyopathies evidence of previous myocardial infarctions (Q-waves and poor R-wave progression in the precordial leads).

Drugs that may alter lab results: Digoxin, furosemide, ACE inhibitors (by improving cardiac function)

Disorders that may alter lab results: N/A

PATHOLOGICAL FINDINGS N/A

SPECIAL TESTS
- Cardiac catheterization. Helps differentiate between ischemic and other types of cardiomyopathy, elucidates intracavitary pressures, cardiac output, left ventricular function and coronary anatomy. Also provides an opportunity to measure pulmonary artery pressures and pulmonary vascular resistance (mean pulmonary artery pressure minus the mean left atrial [wedge] pressure divided by the cardiac output [normal 1.2])
- Maximal oxygen consumption. This treadmill exercise study provides the most prognostic information. Max-oxygen consumption <10 cc/kg/mm correlates with >50% one year mortality, and >18 cc/kg/mm correlates with >90% one year survival.
- For transplant candidates, the following are recommended: CT scans of the chest and abdomen; 24 hour creatinine clearance; routine pulmonary function studies (including blood gas determination); serologies for hepatitis A, B, C, HIV, Toxoplasma, CMV and EB virus; full panels of renal and liver function; complete blood count with differential; and Panorex dental x-ray. Additional studies indicated if any findings are suspicious for disease which would be a contraindication to transplantation. For instance, any undiagnosed roentgenographic abnormality of the lungs is a contraindication to transplantation.

IMAGING
- Chest x-ray
  - ◊ Cardiac enlargement (four chamber) in the dilated cardiomyopathies
  - ◊ Increased vascular markings to the upper lobes: elevated pulmonary venous pressure
  - ◊ Hazy diffuse densities in the hilar areas: pulmonary edema
  - ◊ Pleural effusions and curly B-lines in the lung periphery: engorged pulmonary lymphatics
  - ◊ In hypertrophic cardiomyopathies and cardiomyopathies with normal cardiac size, usually see pulmonary signs of cardiac failure
- Echocardiogram:
  - ◊ In the dilated cardiomyopathies, demonstrates four chamber enlargement and global hypokinesias
  - ◊ In hypertrophic cardiomyopathies, severe left ventricular hypertrophy
  - ◊ In ischemic cardiomyopathy, the heart may be normal or enlarged
  - ◊ Usually segmental abnormalities in contraction of the left ventricle can be detected, indicative of previous localized myocardial infarction
- Multiple-gated acquisition scan (MUGA): Best study to quantitate ejection fraction, often < 25%

DIAGNOSTIC PROCEDURES N/A

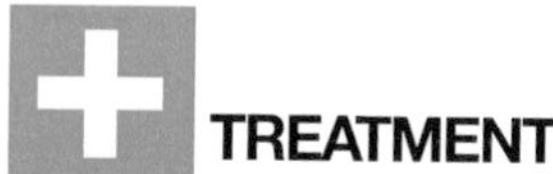

TREATMENT

APPROPRIATE HEALTH CARE Outpatient until time for myocardial transplant or for treatment of severe heart failure

GENERAL MEASURES
- Treatment of heart failure
- Treatment of electrolyte disturbances

SURGICAL MEASURES Myocardial transplant

ACTIVITY Limited by varying degrees. Bedrest may be necessary.

DIET Low fat, low salt, fluid restriction

PATIENT EDUCATION Careful instructions and precautions for all medications

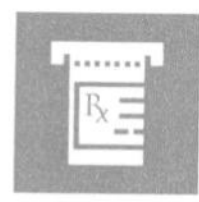

MEDICATIONS

DRUG(S) OF CHOICE
- Systolic failure syndromes, ACE inhibitors, diuretic, and digitalis are the current treatments of choice.
  - ◊ Digoxin (Lanoxin) 0.125-0.25 mg/day
  - ◊ Furosemide 40-120 mg bid to qid
  - ◊ Potassium chloride 20 mEq for each 40 mg of furosemide
  - ◊ ACE inhibitors: captopril (Capoten) 6.25-50 mg tid or enalapril (Vasotec) 2.5-25 mg/day
  - ◊ Isosorbide dinitrate 20-100 mg qid
  - ◊ Hydralazine 5-25 mg qid (maximum of 300 mg/day divided)
  - ◊ Oxygen: 2-4 liters/minute by nasal cannula at bedtime
  - ◊ Metolazone 2.5-5 mg/day; use only in Lasix-resistant patients
  - ◊ Carvedilol or metoprolol; these beta-blockers must be started at very low dosage and increased carefully
  - ◊ Angiotensin II receptor blocker, eg, losartan) 25 mg/day
- Diastolic failure
  - ◊ Beta blockers (eg metoprolol)
  - ◊ Calcium channel bockers, especially verapamil and diltiazem
  - ◊ ACE inhibitors
  - ◊ Antihypertensive therapy

Contraindications:
- Digoxin - 1st or 2nd degree heart block
- Furosemide - oliguria, anuria, renal dysfunction
- Metolazone - hypokalemia

Precautions:
- Digoxin - in patients with renal dysfunction requiring quinidine therapy, the digoxin dosage should be 0.125 mg/day and levels followed carefully. Serum potassium must also be monitored.
- Furosemide - careful titration of patients with end stage heart disease is necessary. Over diuresis may result in dehydration and hyponatremia. Potassium chloride should accompany furosemide therapy to prevent hypokalemia and hypochloremic alkalosis. Furosemide plus aminoglycosides is nephrotoxic and/or ototoxic.
- ACE inhibitors - must be used with extreme care. If blood pressure is already low, begin with captopril at a very low dose such as 6.25 mg tid.
- Metolazone - this powerful adjunct to Lasix therapy can cause hypovolemia and hypokalemia and is most often used for short durations or on alternate days
- Carvedilol and metoprolol should not be given to "wet" congestive failure patients since they may depress systolic function
- Beta adrenergic drugs are contraindicated for long term use since they increase mortality

Significant possible interactions: Digoxin has many interactions including antibiotics, amiodarone, verapamil, cholestyramine. Digoxin levels increase in patients on quinidine.

ALTERNATIVE DRUGS
- IV continuous infusion of dobutamine. It may be applicable in an outpatient setting.
- Other ACE inhibitors at appropriate doses
- IV infusion of amrinone or milrinone
- Beta blockers such as carvedilol; with cardiologist supervision

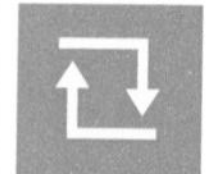

FOLLOWUP

PATIENT MONITORING Monthly followup is usually adequate

PREVENTION/AVOIDANCE Reduce salt and water intake, home blood pressure measurement, daily weight check are helpful

POSSIBLE COMPLICATIONS Worsening congestive heart failure, syncope, arrhythmias, sudden death

EXPECTED COURSE/PROGNOSIS
- 20-40% of patients in New York functional class IV die within one year. With transplant, one year survival as high as 94%. Patients on ACE inhibitors have a longer survival due to afterload reduction and subsequent reduction in cardiac size and improved cardiac efficiency.
- Expert medical therapy can significantly improve outcomes

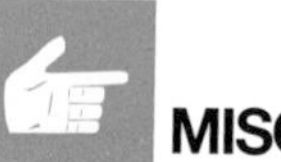

MISCELLANEOUS

ASSOCIATED CONDITIONS N/A

AGE-RELATED FACTORS
Pediatric: Idiopathic, viral, congenital heart disease, and familial cardiomyopathies more likely in children
Geriatric: N/A
Others: N/A

PREGNANCY May occur postpartum

SYNONYMS N/A

ICD-9-CM
425.4 Other primary cardiomyopathies
425.5 Alcoholic cardiomyopathy

SEE ALSO
Alcohol use disorders
Amyloidosis
Diabetes mellitus, Type 1
Diabetes mellitus, Type 2
Diphtheria
Hypertension, essential
Hypothyroidism, adult
Idiopathic hypertrophic subaortic stenosis (IHSS)
Malnutrition, protein-calorie
Poliomyelitis
Rheumatic fever
Sarcoidosis
Toxoplasmosis
Trichinosis
Trypanosomiasis, East African
Trypanosomiasis, West African

OTHER NOTES N/A

ABBREVIATIONS
CMV = cytomegalovirus
EBV = Epstein-Barr virus
MUGA = Multiple-gated acquisition scan

REFERENCES

- Copeland JG: Cardiac Transplantation. Curr Probl Surg 1988;25(9):607-72
- Emery RW, et al: The cardiac donor: A six-year experience. Ann Thorac Surg 1986;41:356-362
- Wahlers T, et al: Donor heart related variables and early mortality after heart transplantation. J. Heart Transplant 1991;10:22-27
- Pickering JG, et al: Fibrosis in the transplanted heart and its relation to donor ischemic time. Circulation 1990;81:949-958
- Hosenpud JO, et al: Relation between recipient: Donor body size match and hemodynamics three months after heart transplantation. J. Heart Transplant 1989;8:241-243

Web references: 0 available at www.5mcc.com
Illustrations N/A

Author(s):
David G. Pocock, MBBS
William J. Moran, DO

BASICS

DESCRIPTION In carotid sinus syndrome (CSS), stimulation of one or both of the hypersensitive carotid sinuses at the bifurcation of the common carotid arteries produces brief episodes of faintness or loss of consciousness. Four types are described:
- Cardioinhibitory: vagally mediated causing bradycardia, sinus arrest or atrioventricular block for > 3 seconds
- Vasodepressor: a sudden drop of peripheral vascular resistance leads to > 50 mm Hg decrease in systolic BP without change in heart rate, or to > 30 mm Hg symptomatic drop in systolic BP
- Mixed: combined cardioinhibitory and vasodepressor changes
- Cerebral: extremely rare, carotid sinus hypersensitivity occurs without bradycardia or hypotension

System(s) affected: Cardiovascular, Nervous
Genetics: N/A
Incidence/Prevalence in USA: 64 out of 132 consecutive patients (48.5%) older than 65, evaluated for dizziness, falls or syncope were found to have carotid sinus type sensitivity
Predominant age: Elderly
Predominant sex: Male > Female

SIGNS & SYMPTOMS
- Dizziness
- Syncope
- Falls
- Blurred vision
- Vertigo
- Tinnitus
- Bradycardia
- Hypotension
- Pallor
- Sweating
- Tachypnea
- No postictal symptoms

CAUSES
- Unknown etiology
- Stimulation of the hypersensitive baroreceptors in the carotid sinus affects vagus and sympathetic nerve outflow
- Carotid body tumors
- Inflammatory and malignant lymph nodes in the neck
- Metastatic cancer
- Coronary artery disease

RISK FACTORS
- Diffuse atherosclerosis
- Wearing tight collars
- Shaving over region of carotid sinus
- Emotional upheaval
- Head movement

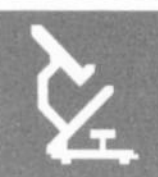

DIAGNOSIS

DIFFERENTIAL DIAGNOSIS
- Vasovagal syncope
- Postural hypotension
- Primary autonomic insufficiency
- Hypovolemia
- Arrhythmias
- Sick sinus syndrome
- Syncope secondary to reduced cardiac output
- Cerebrovascular insufficiency
- Emotional disturbances
- Other causes of syncope

LABORATORY N/A

Drugs that may alter lab results: N/A

Disorders that may alter lab results: N/A

PATHOLOGICAL FINDINGS N/A

SPECIAL TESTS With the patient in the supine position and while the ECG is monitored, manual massage of the carotid sinus causes asystole of more than 3 seconds (cardioinhibitory) and/or a drop in systolic BP as described in Description.

IMAGING N/A

DIAGNOSTIC PROCEDURES
- Carotid sinus massage (check for potential contraindications before performing massage including carotid bruits, known carotid hypersensitivity, demonstrated carotid artery disease)
- Electrophysiologic studies
- Electrocardiogram
- Carotid duplex scan

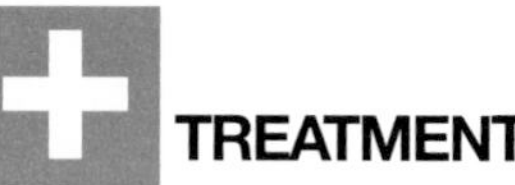

TREATMENT

APPROPRIATE HEALTH CARE
Outpatient. No treatment is required for asymptomatic individuals.

GENERAL MEASURES Cardiac pacing (dual chamber) is the treatment of choice

SURGICAL MEASURES
- Carotid sinus denervation (CSD) by surgery or radiation therapy for selected patients
- Implantation of a permanent pacemaker helps in preventing recurrent symptoms in patients with cardioinhibitory component
- Surgery for selected patients with atheromata

ACTIVITY No restrictions

DIET No special diet

PATIENT EDUCATION Avoidance of exacerbating factors that might stimulate the carotid sinus - tight neck collar, shaving, turning of the head to one side, straining at stool

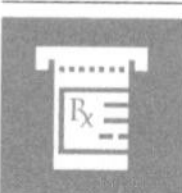

MEDICATIONS

DRUG(S) OF CHOICE

- Anticholinergics - atropine for the cardioinhibitory type
- Sympathomimetics - ephedrine
- Theophylline
- In one recent study, SSRIs were successful in controlling symptoms

Contraindications: Refer to manufacturer's instructions
Precautions: Concomitant usage of digitalis, beta-blockers, clonidine and alpha-methyldopa may accentuate response to carotid sinus massage
Significant possible interactions: Refer to manufacturer's instructions

ALTERNATIVE DRUGS

- Fludrocortisone has been used in clinical trials for patients with vasopressor CSS

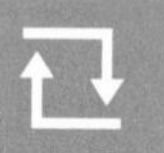

FOLLOWUP

PATIENT MONITORING Follow as an outpatient

PREVENTION/AVOIDANCE

- Avoidance of pressure on the neck
- Support hose may be helpful for some patients with vasodepressor type

POSSIBLE COMPLICATIONS

- Prolonged confusion
- Frequent falls leading to injuries and fractures

EXPECTED COURSE/PROGNOSIS

Serious if syncope associated with atheromatous narrowing of sinus artery or basilar artery

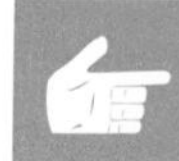

MISCELLANEOUS

ASSOCIATED CONDITIONS

- Sick sinus syndrome
- Atrioventricular block
- Coronary artery disease

AGE-RELATED FACTORS

Pediatric: N/A
Geriatric: More likely to occur in elderly. Associated with atheromata secondary to coronary artery disease. Should be considered in elderly patients with frequent falls.
Others: N/A

PREGNANCY N/A

SYNONYMS

- Hypersensitive carotid sinus syndrome
- Carotid sinus syncope
- Carotid sinus hypersensitivity

ICD-9-CM

337.0 Idiopathic peripheral autonomic neuropathy

SEE ALSO

Atherosclerosis

OTHER NOTES It is clinically important to distinguish CSS from sick sinus syndrome

ABBREVIATIONS

CSS = carotid sinus syndrome

REFERENCES

- McIntoch SJ, Lawson J, Kenny RA. Clinical characteristics of vasopressor, cardioinhibitory, and mixed carotid sinus syndrome in the elderly. Amer J of Med 1993;95(2):203-8
- Isselbacher KJ, et al, eds. Harrison's Principles of Internal Medicine. 14th Ed. New York, McGraw-Hill, 1998
- Braunwald E, ed. Heart Disease: A Textbook of Cardiovascular Medicine. 6th Ed. Philadelphia, W.B. Saunders Co., 2001

Web references: 0 available at www.5mcc.com
Illustrations N/A

Author(s):

George E. Kikano, MD

BASICS

DESCRIPTION This is the most common cause of peripheral nerve compression. The median nerve is compressed as it traverses the carpal tunnel in the wrist and hand. The tunnel is composed of the carpal bones dorsally and the transverse carpal ligament ventrally. It contains flexor tendons and the median nerve. Symptoms tend to affect the dominant hand but over half the patients experience bilateral symptoms.
System(s) affected: Musculoskeletal, Nervous
Genetics: Unknown, however a familial type has been reported
Incidence/Prevalence in USA: Most common entrapment neuropathy. Most recent estimates of prevalence indicate that the disorder occurs in 346/100,000 population.
Predominant age: 40 to 60
Predominant sex: Female > Male (3-10:1)

SIGNS & SYMPTOMS

The symptoms characteristically are relieved by shaking or rubbing the hands. During waking hours symptoms occur when driving the car, reading the newspaper and occasionally when using the hands for repetitive maneuvers. The altered sensation is characteristically confined to the thumb, index and middle finger but many patients do not distinguish this localization and feel the entire hand is affected

- Tingling or prickling sensations in the fingers
- Burning pain in the fingers particularly at night (acroparesthesias)
- Arm pain
- Finger sensory loss
- Positive Tinel's sign
- Positive Phalen's sign
- Wasting of the thenar and hypothenar muscles is a late sign
- Weakness of the hand, however, for such tasks as opening jars is often noted by the patient early in the disorder

CAUSES

- Disorders affecting the musculoskeletal system in the region of the wrist including trauma or Colles' fracture, degenerative joint disease, rheumatoid arthritis, ganglion cyst, scleroderma
- Hypothyroidism and diabetes are frequently associated with this condition which also occurs with increased frequency during pregnancy
- Other miscellaneous causes include acromegaly, lupus erythematosus, leukemia, pyogenic infections, sarcoidosis, primary amyloidosis and Paget disease
- Hyperparathyroidism, hypocalcemia

RISK FACTORS Repetitive flexion and extension of the wrist may influence the development of carpal tunnel syndrome. Occupation as a seamstress or computer operator may aggravate carpal tunnel syndrome. There is, however, no universal agreement that carpal tunnel syndrome is job related.

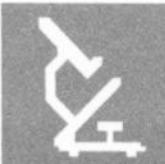

DIAGNOSIS

DIFFERENTIAL DIAGNOSIS

- Cervical spondylosis
- Generalized peripheral neuropathy
- Brachial plexus lesion

LABORATORY

- No one laboratory test is diagnostic
- Normal thyroid function studies and normal glucose metabolism studies may be helpful in excluding these conditions which may be associated with CTS

Drugs that may alter lab results: N/A

Disorders that may alter lab results: N/A

PATHOLOGICAL FINDINGS N/A

SPECIAL TESTS

- Electromyography
  - ◊ Will be abnormal in more than 85% of cases
  - ◊ Prolonged distal latency of the median motor nerves may be seen
  - ◊ The most sensitive indicator is the median sensory distal latency which is prolonged. Furthermore the sensory nerve action potential may be reduced or unobtainable.
- Stimulation of the ulnar nerve should be done as well to exclude generalized polyneuropathy

IMAGING

- Special x-ray views of the carpal tunnel may be obtained. These are of limited usefulness unless heterotopic calcification can be identified.
- Magnetic resonance (MR) neurography may be used to confirm compression of the median nerve in the carpal tunnel and to assess the success of surgical decompression

DIAGNOSTIC PROCEDURES

- Tinel's sign - tapping of the wrist proximal to the carpal tunnel may produce electric sensation perceived by the patient, a sign of nerve compression
- Phalen's sign - holding the wrist flexed for 60 seconds may precipitate the paresthesias experienced by the patient
- A blood pressure tourniquet to cut off circulation to the arm may precipitate symptoms promptly

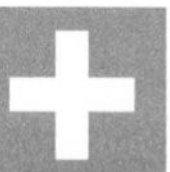

TREATMENT

APPROPRIATE HEALTH CARE

- Outpatient
- Outpatient surgery

GENERAL MEASURES

- Splinting of the wrist in extension may provide significant relief of symptoms. Prolonged use of splinting if possible may allow some symptoms to resolve.
- Injection of the carpal tunnel with hydrocortisone (Medrol 40 mg/mL). 1 mL + 1% lidocaine (1 mL) may provide significant temporary relief. This is particularly useful during pregnancy.

SURGICAL MEASURES

- Surgical decompression of the carpal tunnel by dividing the transverse carpal ligament completely provides almost complete relief of symptoms in over 95% of patients
- Surgical decompression is usually done as an outpatient under local anesthesia
- Healing of the incision generally takes two weeks; an additional two weeks of recuperation may be required before the hand can be fully utilized for tasks requiring strength
- Recent randomized, controlled studies indicate that surgery is more effective than splinting at 18 months

ACTIVITY As tolerated

DIET No special diet

PATIENT EDUCATION Carpal Tunnel Syndrome Foundation. For patient education materials favorably reviewed on this topic, contact: American Academy of Family Physicians Foundation, P.O. Box 8418, Kansas City, MO 64114, (800)274-2237, ext.4400

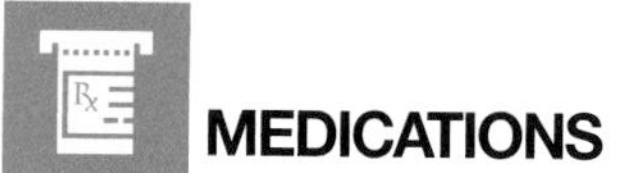

MEDICATIONS

DRUG(S) OF CHOICE There is no medication at present to prevent or slow the progression of cataracts

Contraindications: N/A

Precautions: N/A

Significant possible interactions: N/A

ALTERNATIVE DRUGS N/A

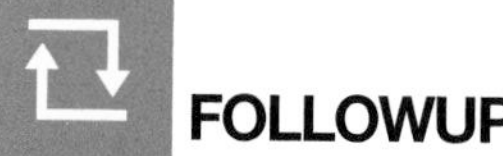

FOLLOWUP

PATIENT MONITORING

- As cataract progresses, the ophthalmologist may change spectacle correction to maintain vision. When this is no longer practical or successful, surgery is recommended.
- Following surgery, spectacle correction may be required to maximize visual acuity for the patient's need. Usually measured several weeks after surgery.

PREVENTION/AVOIDANCE

- Use of ultraviolet protecting glasses in sunny climates may slow progression of cataract, but this is not proven by controlled studies to date
- Antioxidants (vitamins C, E, etc.) theoretically beneficial, but not proven

POSSIBLE COMPLICATIONS Blindness

EXPECTED COURSE/PROGNOSIS

- Ocular prognosis good after cataract removal if no prior ocular disease.
- In congenital cataracts prognosis is often poor because of the high risk of amblyopia.

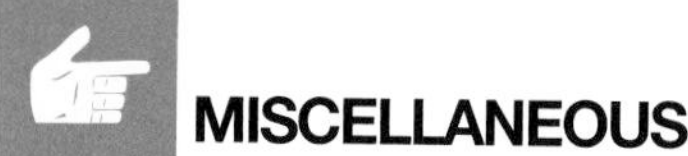

MISCELLANEOUS

ASSOCIATED CONDITIONS

- Diabetes
- Ocular diseases

AGE-RELATED FACTORS

Pediatric: See information on congenital cataracts

Geriatric: 92% of people over age 75 have cataracts

Others: N/A

PREGNANCY See information on congenital cataracts (e.g., rubella syndrome)

SYNONYMS N/A

ICD-9-CM

366.19 Other and combined forms of senile cataract

743.30 Congenital cataract, unspecified

SEE ALSO

OTHER NOTES If patient has cataract and symptoms do not seem to support recommended surgery, a second opinion by another ophthalmologist may be indicated

ABBREVIATIONS N/A

REFERENCES

- Tasman W, ed. Duane's Ophthalmology. Philadelphia: J.B. Lippincott Co; 2002

Web references: 1 available at www.5mcc.com

Illustrations N/A

Author(s):

T. Glendon Moody, MD

BASICS

DESCRIPTION A chronic diarrheal disease characterized by intestinal malabsorption of virtually all nutrients and precipitated by eating gluten-containing foods.
System(s) affected: Gastrointestinal
Genetics: See Risk factors
Incidence/Prevalence in USA: 1 in 120-300 persons in North America. Prevalence - Irish, Italians reportedly 1/250.
Predominant age: Two incidence peaks - age 1 (80%) and adult (20%).
Predominant sex: Female > Male (3:2)

SIGNS & SYMPTOMS
- Diarrhea
- Steatorrhea
- Muscle cramps
- Iron deficiency anemia
- Nervousness
- Weight loss
- Failure to thrive (slowing velocity of weight gain)
- Weakness
- Lassitude
- Fatigue
- Large appetite
- Abdominal distention
- Explosive flatulence
- Abdominal pain, nausea, vomiting are rare
- Recurrent aphthous stomatitis
- Elevated LFTs

CAUSES Sensitivity to gluten, specifically gliadin fraction

RISK FACTORS
- First order relatives - 10% incidence
- 71% in monozygotic twins

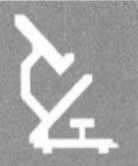

DIAGNOSIS

DIFFERENTIAL DIAGNOSIS Rule out short bowel syndrome, pancreatic insufficiency, Crohn disease, Whipple disease, hypogammaglobulinemia, tropical sprue, lymphoma, acquired immune deficiency syndrome, acute enteritis, giardiasis, eosinophilic gastroenteritis, pancreatic disease

LABORATORY
- Positive anti-gliadin IgA and IgG
- Positive anti-endomysial antibodies and IgA tissue transglutaminase
- IgA deficient patients have "false-negative" IgA antiendomysial and IgA antitransglutaminase antibodies
- 72 hour fecal fat showing greater than 7% fat malabsorption
- D-Xylose test showing malabsorption of this sugar
- Decreased calcium
- Decreased prothrombin time
- Decreased neutral fats
- Decreased cholesterol
- Decreased vitamin A
- Decreased vitamin B12 (rare)
- Decreased vitamin D
- Decreased vitamin C
- Decreased folic acid
- Decreased iron
- Decreased total protein
- Anemia

Drugs that may alter lab results: N/A

Disorders that may alter lab results: N/A

PATHOLOGICAL FINDINGS Small bowel biopsy - flattened villi, hyperplasia and lengthening of crypts, infiltration of plasma cells and lymphocytes in lamina propria

SPECIAL TESTS Endoscopy

IMAGING Upper GI series showing flocculation of barium, edema and flattening of mucosal folds

DIAGNOSTIC PROCEDURES Biopsy of the duodenal mucosa with repeat endoscopy and normal biopsy on a gluten-free diet is necessary before a firm diagnosis can be made.

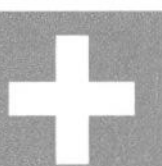

TREATMENT

APPROPRIATE HEALTH CARE Outpatient

GENERAL MEASURES Removal of gluten from the diet. Rice, corn and soybean flour are safe, palatable substitutes. Levels of IgA antigliadin normalize with gluten abstinence.

SURGICAL MEASURES N/A

ACTIVITY No restrictions

DIET Removal of gluten - wheat, rye, barley and those with gluten additives

PATIENT EDUCATION
- Clinical dietitian
- Copy of gluten-free diet
- Possible lay self-help group
- American Celiac Society, 45 Gifford Avenue, Jersey City, NJ 07304,
(201)432-1207
- Gluten Intolerance Group (206) 325-6980

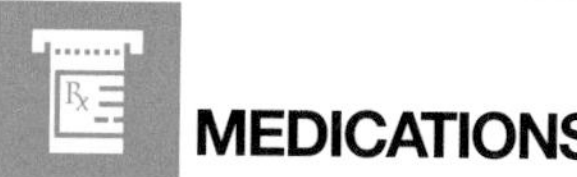

MEDICATIONS

DRUG(S) OF CHOICE
- Usually none
- Prednisone, 40-60 mg/day po in cases of refractory sprue
- Refractory disease
  - ◊ Steroids
  - ◊ Azathioprine
  - ◊ Cyclosporine
  - ◊ Possible future role of infliximab (Remicade)

Contraindications: History of tuberculosis, fungus or herpes infections
Precautions: Use with caution in congestive heart failure, diabetes, peptic ulcer, myasthenia gravis
Significant possible interactions: Diuretics taken concomitantly may lead to potassium depletion

ALTERNATIVE DRUGS May require supplemental calcium, calcium carbonate, 500 mg po bid, and vitamin D (ergocalciferol) 10-100 mcg/day; in severe malabsorption, up to 2.5 mg/day may be required

FOLLOWUP

PATIENT MONITORING Repeat endoscopy after 6-8 weeks on a gluten-free diet (in selected cases)

PREVENTION/AVOIDANCE Avoid all gluten containing products

POSSIBLE COMPLICATIONS
- Malignancy - less than 10% of patients (50% of which are small bowel lymphoma)
- Refractory sprue - may respond to prednisone 40-60 mg/day po. Refractory sprue unresponsive to corticosteroid therapy raises the specter of adult-onset autoimmune enteropathy or cryptic T-cell lymphoma. In this circumstance, screening for antienterocyte autoantibodies and careful scrutiny of the small intestine, including retroperitoneal lymph node biopsy with full thickness small bowel biopsy may be needed.
- Chronic ulcerative jejunoileitis - associated with multiple ulcers, intestinal bleeding, strictures, perforation, obstruction, peritonitis - 7% mortality
- Osteoporosis secondary to decreased vitamin D and calcium absorption
- Dehydration
- Electrolyte depletion
- refractory cases may need total parenteral nutrition
- Death (rare)

EXPECTED COURSE/PROGNOSIS
Good with correct diagnosis and adherence to gluten free diet. Feel better in seven days. All symptoms usually disappear in four to six weeks. It is unknown whether strict dietary adherence decreases cancer risk.

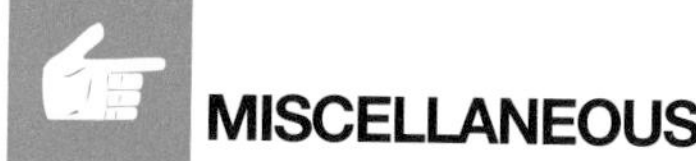

MISCELLANEOUS

ASSOCIATED CONDITIONS
- May have secondary lactase deficiency
- Extraintestinal manifestation may include marked decrease in bone density
- Dermatitis herpetiformis
- Autoimmune thyroiditis
- Diabetes, type 1 (prevalence of celiac disease in type 1 diabetes is 3-8%)
- Hypertransaminasemia

AGE-RELATED FACTORS
Pediatric: Children reaching adolescence may outgrow intolerance to wheat but should be cautioned to watch for signs of recurrence in middle age
Geriatric: N/A
Others: N/A

PREGNANCY Consider celiac disease in pregnant women with severe anemia

SYNONYMS
- Sprue
- Gluten enteropathy
- Celiac sprue

ICD-9-CM
579.0 Celiac disease

SEE ALSO

OTHER NOTES The most common cause of refractory diarrhea is noncompliance with a gluten-free diet

ABBREVIATIONS N/A

REFERENCES

- McClave S. Celiac and Tropical Sprue. In: Chobanian SJ, Van Ness MM, eds. A Manual of Clinical Problems in Gastroenterology. 2nd ed. Boston: Little-Brown; 1993
- Ryan BM, Kelleher D. Refractory celiac sprue. Gastro 2000;119:243-51
- Carroccio A, Soresi M, Di Prima L, Montalto G. Screening for celiac disease in patients with chronic liver disease. Gastroenterology 2003;125(4):1289
- Kaukinen K, Halme L, et al. Celiac disease in patients with severe liver disease: gluten-free diet may reverse hepatic failure. Gastroenterology 2002;122(4):881-8

Web references: 0 available at www.5mcc.com
Illustrations N/A

Author(s):
Michael M. Van Ness, MD

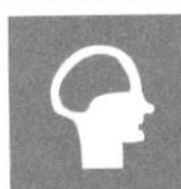

BASICS

DESCRIPTION An acute, spreading infection of the dermis and subcutaneous tissue. Several entities are recognized:
- Cellulitis of the extremities - characterized by an expanding, red, swollen, tender or painful plaque with an indefinite border that may cover a wide area
- Recurrent cellulitis of the leg after saphenous venectomy - patients have an acute onset of swelling, erythema of the legs arising months to years after coronary artery bypass. (Surgery using lower extremity veins for bypass grafts.)
- Dissecting cellulitis of the scalp - recurrent painful, fluctuant dermal and subcutaneous nodules
- Facial cellulitis in adults - a rare event. Patients usually develop pharyngitis, followed by high fever, rapidly progressive anterior neck swelling, tenderness and erythema associated with dysphagia.
- Facial cellulitis in children - potentially serious. Swelling and erythema of the cheek develop rapidly, usually unilateral.
- Perianal cellulitis - bright perianal erythema extending from the anal verge approximately 2 to 3 cm onto the surrounding perianal skin
- Pseudomonas cellulitis - may be a localized phenomenon or it may occur during pseudomonas septicemia

System(s) affected: Skin/Exocrine
Genetics: No known genetic pattern
Incidence/Prevalence in USA: Unknown
Predominant age:
- Perianal cellulitis - principally in children
- Facial cellulitis - in adults, usually older than 50 years. In children, between 6 months and three years.

Predominant sex: Male = Female (perianal cellulitis more common in boys)

SIGNS & SYMPTOMS
- General
  - ◊ Local tenderness
  - ◊ Pain
  - ◊ Erythema
  - ◊ Malaise
  - ◊ Fever, chills
  - ◊ Involved area is red, hot, and swollen
  - ◊ Borders of the area are not elevated and not demarcated
  - ◊ Regional lymphadenopathy is common
- Recurrent cellulitis
  - ◊ Same as above
  - ◊ Edema
  - ◊ High fever, chills and toxicity
- Dissecting cellulitis of the scalp
  - ◊ Purulent drainage from burrowing interconnecting abscesses
- Facial cellulitis in adults
  - ◊ Malaise
  - ◊ Anorexia
  - ◊ Vomiting
  - ◊ Itching
  - ◊ Burning
  - ◊ Dysplasia
  - ◊ Anterior neck swelling
- Facial cellulitis in children
  - ◊ Irritability
  - ◊ Upper respiratory tract infection symptoms
- Perianal cellulitis
  - ◊ Intense perianal erythema
  - ◊ Pain on defecation
  - ◊ Blood streaked stools
  - ◊ Perianal pruritus

CAUSES
- By site
  - ◊ Cellulitis of the extremities: *Group A streptococcus, Staphylococcus aureus*
  - ◊ Recurrent cellulitis of the leg: Non-group A beta hemolytic Streptococci (group C,G,B)
  - ◊ Dissecting cellulitis of the scalp: *Staphylococcus aureus*
  - ◊ Facial cellulitis in adults: *H. influenzae* type B
  - ◊ Facial cellulitis in children: *H. influenzae* type B, over 3 years with portal of entry: staphylococcal and streptococcal
  - ◊ Synergetic necrotizing cellulitis: Mixed aerobic-anaerobic flora
  - ◊ Intravenous drug use: *Staphylococcus aureus*, Streptococci, Enterobacteriaceae, Pseudomonas, Fungi
  - ◊ Synergetic necrotizing cellulitis: Mixed aerobic-anaerobic flora
- Specific diseases
  - ◊ Diabetes mellitus: *Staphylococcus aureus*, Streptococci, Enterobacteriaceae, Anaerobes
  - ◊ Human bites: Eikenella corrodens
  - ◊ Animal bites (cat and dog): Staphylococci, *Pasteurella multocida*
- Patient groups
  - ◊ Neonates: *Group B streptococcus*
  - ◊ Immunocompromised
    - Bacteria (Serratia, Proteus and other Enterobacteriaceae)
    - Fungi (*Cryptococcus neoformans*)
    - Atypical mycobacterium
  - ◊ Children with nephrotic syndrome: *E. coli*
  - ◊ Environmental and occupational exposures
    - *Erysipelothrix rhusiopathiae*
    - *Vibrio species*
    - *Aeromonas hydrophilia*
- Rare causes
  - ◊ Anaerobic
  - ◊ *Clostridium perfringens* (gas forming cellulitis)
  - ◊ Tuberculosis
  - ◊ Syphilitic gumma
  - ◊ Fungal: Mucormycosis, Aspergillosis

RISK FACTORS
- General
  - ◊ Previous trauma (laceration, puncture, human or animal bite)
  - ◊ Underlying skin lesion (furuncle, ulcer)
  - ◊ Surgical wound
  - ◊ Recurrent cellulitis
  - ◊ Post coronary artery bypass in patients whose saphenous veins have been removed
  - ◊ Lower extremity lymphedema secondary to a) radical pelvic surgery b) radiation therapy c) neoplastic involvement of pelvic lymph nodes
  - ◊ Mastectomy
  - ◊ Diabetes mellitus
  - ◊ Intravenous drug use
  - ◊ Immunocompromised host
  - ◊ Burns
  - ◊ Environmental and occupational factors

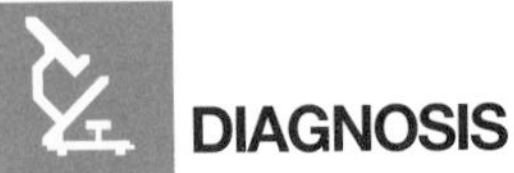

DIAGNOSIS

DIFFERENTIAL DIAGNOSIS
- Perianal cellulitis
  - ◊ Candida intertrigo
  - ◊ Psoriasis
  - ◊ Pin worm infection
  - ◊ Inflammatory bowel disease
  - ◊ Behavioral problem
  - ◊ Child abuse
- Others
  - ◊ Acute gout
  - ◊ Fasciitis/myositis
  - ◊ Mycotic aneurysm
  - ◊ Ruptured Baker's cyst
  - ◊ Thrombophlebitis
  - ◊ Osteomyelitis
  - ◊ Herpetic whitlow
  - ◊ Cutaneous diphtheria
  - ◊ Pseudogout

LABORATORY
- Aspirates from the point of maximum inflammation. Yield a 45% positive culture rate as compared to a 5% from leading edge culture.
- Blood cultures - potential pathogens isolated in 25% of patients
- Mild leucocytosis with a left shift
- A mildly elevated sedimentation rate
- CBC

Drugs that may alter lab results: Previous antibiotic therapy may alter the results

Disorders that may alter lab results: N/A

PATHOLOGICAL FINDINGS Biopsy of skin shows marked infiltration of the dermis with eosinophils and inflammatory changes

SPECIAL TESTS
- Serial serological testing with antistreptolysin O, anti-deoxyribonuclease B, and anti-hyaluronidase tests may be successful in diagnosing cellulitis caused by group A, C, or G hemolytic streptococci
- Sinus drainage and culture of aspirate

IMAGING
- Gas forming cellulitis
  - ◊ Plain x-rays show gas bubbles in the soft tissue
  - ◊ CT shows gas and myonecrosis

DIAGNOSTIC PROCEDURES
- Skin biopsy
- Lumbar puncture should be considered for all children with H. influenzae type B cellulitis

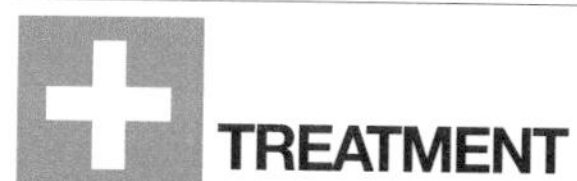

TREATMENT

APPROPRIATE HEALTH CARE Outpatient for mild cases, inpatient for severe infections

GENERAL MEASURES
- Immobilization and elevation of the involved limb to reduce swelling may be needed in *H. influenzae type B*
- Sterile saline dressings to decrease local pain
- Moist heat to localize the infection
- Cool aluminum acetate (Burow's solution) compresses for pain relief

SURGICAL MEASURES
- Debridement for gas/purulent collections
- Intubation or tracheotomy may be needed for cellulitis of the head or neck
- Hand infections - wide filleting incision in necrotizing cellulitis

ACTIVITY Ambulatory in mild infection; bedrest in severe infection

DIET Regular diet

PATIENT EDUCATION
- Good skin hygiene
- Avoid skin traumas
- Report early skin changes to physician

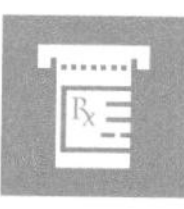

MEDICATIONS

DRUG(S) OF CHOICE
Treat 10-30 days. Guided by culture results whenever possible.
- Mild early suspected streptococcal etiology: Aqueous penicillin G, 600,000 U, then IM procaine penicillin at 600,000 U q8-12 hrs
- Staphylococcal infection or no clues to etiology: penicillinase-resistant penicillin (e.g., oxacillin 0.5-1.0 g po q6 hrs)
- Severe infection: penicillinase-resistant penicillin (e.g., nafcillin 1.0-1.5 g IV q4 hrs)
- Gram negative bacillus as possible etiology: aminoglycoside (gentamicin) plus a semisynthetic penicillin
- Rapidly progressive cellulitis after a fresh water injury: penicillinase-resistant penicillin plus gentamicin or chloramphenicol
- Human bites: amoxicillin-clavulanate (Augmentin)
- Animal bites (cellulitis at the saphenous site): penicillin or nafcillin, in high dosage, IV for 7 days before switching to oral therapy
- Facial cellulitis in adults and children: (H. influenza B) cefotaxime IV
- Gas forming cellulitis: Aqueous penicillin G 10-20 million U/day IV
- Diabetes mellitus: Cefoxitin or if toxic, clindamycin and gentamicin
- Intravenous drug abuse: Vancomycin and gentamicin
- Compromised hosts: clindamycin and gentamicin
- Burn patients: vancomycin and gentamicin

Contraindications:
- Allergies to the antibiotic

Precautions: Renal failure, other organ failure
Significant possible interactions: Refer to manufacturer's literature

ALTERNATIVE DRUGS
- Mild infection
  - ◊ Penicillin allergy: erythromycin, 500 mg po q6 hrs
- Severe infection
  - ◊ Vancomycin 1.0-1.5 g/day IV
  - ◊ Human bite and animal bites: IV cefoxitin
- Gas forming cellulitis
  - ◊ Metronidazole 500 mg IV q6h
  - ◊ Clindamycin 600 mg IV q8h
- Fluoroquinolones (adults)

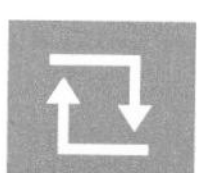

FOLLOWUP

PATIENT MONITORING
- A blood culture at the end of treatment to ensure cure
- Repeat needle aspirate culture
- Repeat blood count if patient was toxic
- Repeat lumbar puncture in case of meningitis

PREVENTION/AVOIDANCE
- Treatment of tinea pedis with antifungal (such as clotrimazole) will prevent recurrent cellulitis of the legs in patients who have had coronary bypass
- Avoid trauma
- Avoid swimming in fresh water or salt water in the presence of skin abrasion
- Avoid human or animal bite
- Support stocking with peripheral edema
- Good skin hygiene
- For recurrent cellulitis - prophylactic penicillin G (250-500 mg po bid)
- H. influenzae cellulitis - rifampin prophylaxis for entire family of index case or in day-care classroom in which one or two children exposed. Dosage: 20 mg/kg/day (maximum: 600 mg/day) for 4 days.

POSSIBLE COMPLICATIONS
- Bacteremia
- Local abscesses
- Super infection with gram negative organisms
- Lymphangitis especially in recurrent cellulitis
- Thrombophlebitis of lower extremities in older patients
- Dissecting cellulitis of the scalp - scarring; alopecia
- Facial cellulitis in children - meningitis in 8% of patients
- Gas forming cellulitis - gangrene; amputation; 25% mortality

EXPECTED COURSE/PROGNOSIS
With adequate antibiotic treatment, outlook is good

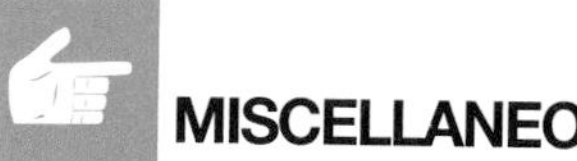

MISCELLANEOUS

ASSOCIATED CONDITIONS
- Facial cellulitis in children
  - ◊ Upper respiratory tract infection
  - ◊ Unilateral or bilateral otitis media in 68% of patients
  - ◊ Meningitis in 8% of patients
- Perianal cellulitis
  - ◊ Pharyngitis may precede the infection
- Frontal sinus in adult
  - ◊ Subacute bacterial endocarditis
  - ◊ Scarlet fever
  - ◊ Vaccinia
  - ◊ Herpes simplex
  - ◊ Herpes zoster

AGE-RELATED FACTORS
Pediatric: N/A
Geriatric: In cellulitis of lower extremities, patients are more prone to develop thrombophlebitis
Others: N/A

PREGNANCY N/A

SYNONYMS N/A

ICD-9-CM
682.9 Cellulitis and abscess at unspecified site

SEE ALSO
Animal bites
Cellulitis, periorbital & orbital
Erysipelas
Thrombophlebitis, superficial

OTHER NOTES N/A

ABBREVIATIONS N/A

REFERENCES

- Habif T. Clinical Dermatology. 4th Ed. St. Louis, CV Mosby, 2004
- Mandell GL, ed. Principles and Practice of Infectious Diseases. 5th ed. New York: Churchill Livingstone; 2000

Web references: 1 available at www.5mcc.com
Illustrations 18 available

Author(s):
Abdulrazak Abyad, MD, MPH

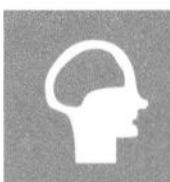

BASICS

DESCRIPTION An acute, spreading infection of the dermis and subcutaneous tissue. Several entities are recognized.
Cellulitis around the eyes is a potentially dangerous periorbital and orbital infection.
System(s) affected: Nervous, Skin/Exocrine
Genetics: No known genetic pattern
Incidence/Prevalence in USA: Unknown
Predominant age: N/A
Predominant sex: Male = Female

SIGNS & SYMPTOMS
- Lid edema
- Rhinorrhea
- Orbital pain, tenderness
- Headache
- Conjunctival hyperemia
- Chemosis
- Ptosis
- Limitation to ocular motion
- Increase intraocular pressure
- Disease in corneal sensation
- Congestion of retinal veins
- Chorioretinal stria
- Gangrene and sloughing of lids

CAUSES
- Cellulitis around the eye in adult
  - ◊ *Staphylococcus aureus* most common
  - ◊ *Streptococcus pyogenes*
  - ◊ *Streptococcus pneumonia*
  - ◊ Mixed infection
- Cellulitis around the eye in children less than five years
  - ◊ *H. influenzae* most common

RISK FACTORS
- Trauma
- Chronic sinusitis (anaerobic)
- Acute sinusitis (aerobic)
- Retained orbital foreign bodies
- Puncture wound
- Surgical procedure: Exploration of orbital tumor, retinal detachment procedure, strabismus operation
- Acute dacryocystitis
- Dental or intracranial infection
- Bacteremia

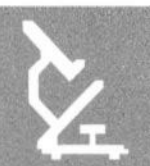

DIAGNOSIS

DIFFERENTIAL DIAGNOSIS
- Retro-orbital cellulitis/abscess

LABORATORY
- Aspiration of fluid from the orbit is contraindicated
- Blood culture more likely to be positive in children < 5 years
- Culture of discharge from nasal mucosa, nasopharynx and conjunctiva

Drugs that may alter lab results: Previous antibiotic therapy

Disorders that may alter lab results: N/A

PATHOLOGICAL FINDINGS N/A

SPECIAL TESTS Serial serological testing with antistreptolysin O, anti-deoxyribonuclease B, and anti-hyaluronidase tests may be successful in diagnosing cellulitis caused by group A, C, or G hemolytic streptococci

IMAGING
- B-scan ultrasound
- Plain orbital and sinus films
- Computerized tomography (CT) is the most accurate and provides the most important information
- Magnetic resonance imaging is the imaging modality of choice in diagnosing suspected cases of cavernous sinus thrombosis

DIAGNOSTIC PROCEDURES
- Skin biopsy
- Lumbar puncture should be considered for all children with H. influenzae type B cellulitis

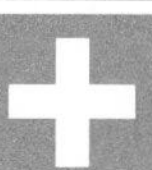

TREATMENT

APPROPRIATE HEALTH CARE Outpatient for mild cases, inpatient for severe infections

GENERAL MEASURES N/A

SURGICAL MEASURES
- Surgical debridement and/or drainage is needed if abscess develops or if clinical situation deteriorates despite adequate therapy in 24-48 hours or if visual acuity decreases
- In orbital mucormycosis, surgical debridement of devitalized tissue is extremely important

ACTIVITY
- Ambulatory in mild infection
- Bedrest in severe infection

DIET Regular diet

PATIENT EDUCATION
- Good skin hygiene
- Avoid skin traumas
- Report early skin changes to health professional

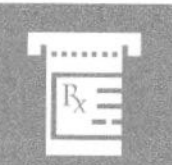

MEDICATIONS

DRUG(S) OF CHOICE
- In adults, nafcillin or oxacillin 1.5 g every 4 hours
- In children, ampicillin 200 mg/kg/day in divided doses intravenously plus nafcillin or oxacillin (100 mg/kg/day)
- Sinus decongestion - nasal sprays, oral decongestants, oral antihistamines

Contraindications:
- Allergies to the antibiotic
- Previous history of allergy to the drug

Precautions: Renal failure, other organ failure
Significant possible interactions: Refer to manufacturer's literature

ALTERNATIVE DRUGS
- In adults, cefotaxime or clindamycin or chloramphenicol or vancomycin
- In children, if *H. influenzae* resistant to ampicillin - third generation cephalosporin, cefotaxime or chloramphenicol
- In immunocompromised - piperacillin and gentamicin
- Fluoroquinolones (adults)
- Linezolid (Zyvox)

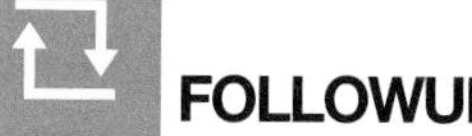

FOLLOWUP

PATIENT MONITORING Repeat imaging in patients with orbital cellulitis

PREVENTION/AVOIDANCE
- Avoid trauma
- Avoid swimming in fresh water or salt water in the presence of skin abrasion
- In *H. influenzae* cellulitis - rifampin prophylaxis for the entire family of an index case. Rifampin prophylaxis in day-care classroom in which one or two children exposed. Dosage - 20 mg/kg/24 h (maximum of 600 mg a day) for 4 days.

POSSIBLE COMPLICATIONS
- Osteomyelitis
- Strabismus
- Afferent pupillary defect
- Chronic draining sinus
- Scarred upper eyelid
- Profound visual loss
- Blindness
- Ophthalmoplegia
- Cavernous sinus thrombosis
- Meningitis
- Intracranial abscess
- Acute infarction of retina and choroid

EXPECTED COURSE/PROGNOSIS
With adequate antibiotic treatment, outlook is good

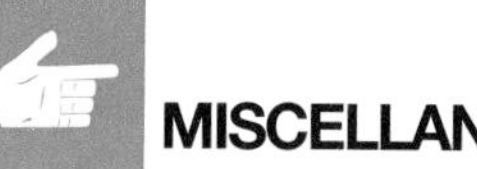

MISCELLANEOUS

ASSOCIATED CONDITIONS Sinusitis ethmoiditis in children in 84% of patients

AGE-RELATED FACTORS
Pediatric: Newborn may acquire orbital cellulitis secondary to intrauterine infection
Geriatric: N/A
Others: N/A

PREGNANCY N/A

SYNONYMS N/A

ICD-9-CM
376.01 Orbital cellulitis

SEE ALSO
Animal bites
Cellulitis
Erysipelas
Thrombophlebitis, superficial

OTHER NOTES N/A

ABBREVIATIONS N/A

REFERENCES

- Habif T. Clinical Dermatology. 4th Ed. St. Louis, CV Mosby, 2004
- Mandell GL, ed. Principles and Practice of Infectious Diseases. 5th ed. New York: Churchill Livingstone; 2000
- Morgan SJ. Purulent orbital cellulitis. Eye 2002;16(2):215

Web references: 0 available at www.5mcc.com
Illustrations N/A

Author(s):
Abdulrazak Abyad, MD, MPH

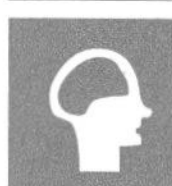

BASICS

DESCRIPTION A term used to describe a group of patients with a non-progressive but not unchanging disorder of movement or posture that is a result of a central nervous system insult that occurred prenatally, perinatally, or during the first three years of life

System(s) affected: Musculoskeletal, Nervous

Genetics: Rarely inherited. Small percentage of cases with symmetric signs are associated with autosomal recessive transmission. Symmetric and idiopathic spastic CP (4% of cases) has 1:8 recurrence risk.

Incidence/Prevalence in USA: 1 to 2 per 1,000 live births. Up to 10% of infants with birthweight less than 1500 grams.

Predominant age: Causative CNS insult during period of rapid brain growth but effects are life long and evolve with time.

Predominant sex: Male > Female (1.3:1)

SIGNS & SYMPTOMS

By classification

- Spastic 40%
  - ◊ Spasticity
  - ◊ Hemiplegia, quadriplegia or diplegia
  - ◊ Triplegia, monoplegia are rare
  - ◊ Contractures
  - ◊ Mental retardation with quadriplegia and mixed forms
  - ◊ Normal intelligence with hemiplegia or paraplegia
  - ◊ Scissors gate, toe walking
  - ◊ Tremors with hemiplegia
  - ◊ Aphonia with quadriplegia
  - ◊ Seizures
- Athetotic (dyskinetic) 30%
  - ◊ Usually normal intelligence
  - ◊ Choreoathetoid type is the most common with jerky motions of proximal muscle groups and slow writhing of extremities face neck and trunk
  - ◊ Dystonic type due to simultaneous contraction of opposing muscle groups
  - ◊ Speech difficulties
  - ◊ Muscular hypertrophy
  - ◊ Deafness common with athetosis caused by kernicterus
- Ataxic 10%
  - ◊ Normal intelligence
  - ◊ Clumsy disposition with wide based gate and difficulty with fine

movements.

  - ◊ Best prognosis for functional improvement
- Mixed 20%
  - ◊ Spasticity and choreoathetosis most common
  - ◊ Athetosis and ataxia can occur
  - ◊ Mental retardation common.

CAUSES

- 70% of the time, neither causes nor risk factors can be identified
- In utero bacterial infections (chorioamnionitis), viral infections (e.g. rubella), CNS malformations, chromosomal abnormalities, coagulation disorders, kernicterus, CNS trauma and intraventricular hemorrhage
- While most cases are due to prenatal events and prematurity, 10% or less of cases are due to intrapartum events. Such cases are almost always of spastic quadriplegic type or dyskinetic type and are associated with evidence of severe metabolic acidosis at birth (pH ≤ 7.00) and early onset neonatal encephalopathy at birth. Criteria which individually are nonspecific but which together suggest intrapartum cause include a sentinel hypoxic event immediately before or during labor (e.g. cord prolapse, abruption or uterine rupture); sudden, rapid and sustained deterioration of the fetal heart rate pattern which was previously normal; Apgar scores of ≤ 6 for greater than five minutes; early evidence of multisystem involvement and early imaging showing acute cerebral abnormality.

RISK FACTORS

- Prematurity
- Hypoxic ischemia
- Encephalopathy in the perinatal period
- Seizures in the perinatal period
- Germinal matrix and interventricular hemorrhage in the perinatal period
- In utero infections
- Meningitis/encephalitis postnatally
- Child abuse
- Intrauterine growth restriction
- Breech
- Multiple gestation

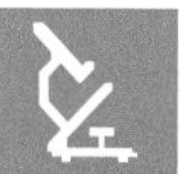

DIAGNOSIS

DIFFERENTIAL DIAGNOSIS Cerebral palsy is a descriptive term based on clinical observation. Chromosomal and metabolic abnormalities must be excluded. Early diagnosis made at 12 months of life may be wrong more than half the time. Evidence of disease progression excludes cerebral palsy. early warning signs include delay in motor milestones, toe walking, persistent fisting, seizures, irritability, poor suck, established handedness before 2 years of age, and abnormal limb posture.

LABORATORY

- Laboratory data is not required to make the diagnosis.
- Other tests may help exclude Tay-Sachs metachromatic leukodystrophy, mucopolysaccharidosis

Drugs that may alter lab results: None

Disorders that may alter lab results: None

PATHOLOGICAL FINDINGS Central nervous system abnormalities: CT and MRI might show abnormalities of the brain including cysts, cerebral atrophy, calcification, tumors, malformation, strokes, etc.

SPECIAL TESTS

- Urine amino acid screening
- High resolution karyotype

IMAGING N/A

DIAGNOSTIC PROCEDURES

- History and careful physical exam
- Pedigree
- EEG, MRI, CT

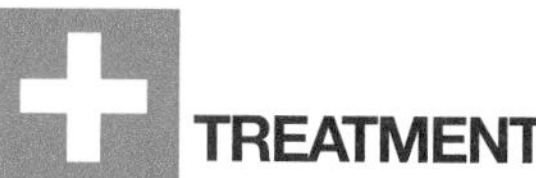

TREATMENT

APPROPRIATE HEALTH CARE The goal of therapy is to improve function

GENERAL MEASURES

- Early intervention services
- Physical therapy, occupational therapy, orthosis, adaptive equipment
- Oral medications should be carefully titrated upward to avoid side effects
- Alter muscle tone, assuming that the abnormal tone is adversely affecting function, by:
  - ◊ Injection of botulinum toxin into the abnormal muscles
  - ◊ Rhizotomy
  - ◊ Continuous infusion of intrathecal baclofen
- Strabismus, refractive errors and visual field defects are common and should be addressed early to prevent deterioration
- Anti-convulsants for seizures
- Alternative therapies
  - ◊ Hyperbaric oxygen therapy and therapeutic electrical stimulation were shown to have no benefit in randomized clinical trials
  - ◊ Conductive Education (The Peto Method) was as good as, but not better than standard care in a randomized trial
  - ◊ Constraint-induced movement or forced use therapy may be effective, but there are no large controlled studies
  - ◊ Adeli Suit which is based on a design for Soviet cosmonauts is available only in Poland as part of intensive physio-therapy program. Little information is available.

SURGICAL MEASURES

- Tendon transfers and contracture release to prevent bone deformation
- Open reduction of hip subluxation and dislocation
- Dorsal rhizotomy to decrease spasticity
- Implantation of reservoir for intrathecal baclofen
- Spinal fusion and rods for scoliosis

ACTIVITY Full activity depending upon the patient's dysfunction

DIET

- Normal diet, although constipation is frequent and stool softeners might be considered
- Poor suck, dysphagia and reflux often lead to nutritional difficulties. Nasogastric tube (short term) or gastrostomy tube (long term) may be necessary.

PATIENT EDUCATION

- It is very important to educate the patient and parents about the child's disabilities as well as prognosis; mental retardation seen in 20-25% of patients with cerebral palsy.
- United Cerebral Palsy, 1660 L Street, NW, Suite 700, Washington, DC 20036, (800)872-5827/(202)776-0406; TTY (202)973-7197; Fax (202)776-0414
- Disabled children are at higher risk of physical abuse, neglect and sexual abuse. The usual adolescent issues such as sexuality must be addressed.
- Patients and their families should be made aware of their rights under the Americans with Disabilities Act

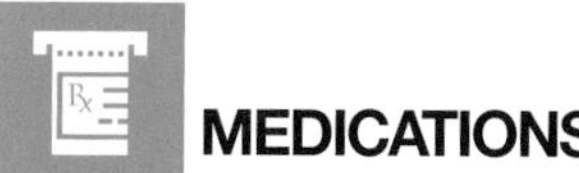

MEDICATIONS

DRUG(S) OF CHOICE

- Drugs to decrease spasticity:
  - ◊ Baclofen is most commonly used
  - ◊ Diazepam, clonazepam and clorazepate also are used and may also help with sleep disturbances and irritability
  - ◊ Dantrolene sodium is sometimes used, but can be hepatoxic
  - ◊ Tizanidine and clonidine , also available as transdermal patch, are alpha-2 adrenergic agents
- Intrathecal baclofen via an implantable reservoir minimizes systemic side effects
- Anti-seizure medications as needed

Contraindications: Refer to manufacturer's literature
Precautions: Refer to manufacturer's literature
Significant possible interactions: Refer to manufacturer's literature

ALTERNATIVE DRUGS Other centrally acting muscle relaxants

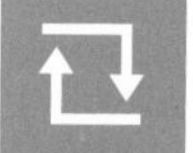

FOLLOWUP

PATIENT MONITORING Followup visits are important to determine the development of contractures and the presence of associated problems (e.g., epilepsy, learning disabilities, strabismus, hearing loss and mental retardation).

PREVENTION/AVOIDANCE In theory measures which decrease premature birth and fetal growth restriction would be of benefit. These include good prenatal care, smoking cessation, avoidance of substance abuse and care in infertility treatment to decrease the risk of multiple pregnancies. Antenatal corticosteroids (betamethasone or dexamethasone) should be given to the mother when premature birth is anticipated between 24 and 34 weeks gestation. While given mainly to decrease the risk of respiratory distress syndrome, their use has been associated with a decreased incidence of neonatal intraventricular hemorrhage.

POSSIBLE COMPLICATIONS

- Chronicity with permanent disability
- Bladder dysfunction may lead to frequent urinary tract infections

EXPECTED COURSE/PROGNOSIS

- The patient should improve in function with time
- Muscle tone may change for the worse during adolescence (does not mean that the disease is progressive)

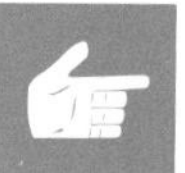

MISCELLANEOUS

ASSOCIATED CONDITIONS

- Epilepsy
- Learning disabilities
- Mental retardation
- Behavioral problems
- Strabismus
- Hearing loss

AGE-RELATED FACTORS

Pediatric: Contractures will increase as a result of growth associated with asymmetrical muscle tone and strength. Scoliosis may develop as a result.
Geriatric: N/A
Others: N/A

PREGNANCY

- Reproductive function should not be affected. Contractures may make positioning for vaginal delivery difficult but cesarean is usually reserved for usual obstetric indications
- For patients with seizures the risks of poor seizure control outweigh the teratogenic potential of almost all anticonvulsants. Periconceptional folate supplementation (1 to 4 mg per day) may decrease the risk of anticonvulsant teratogenesis.
- There is little information on baclofen and dantrolene use in pregnancy although no adverse fetal or newborn effects have been reported

SYNONYMS

- Little disease
- Cerebral diplegia
- Infantile cerebral paralysis

ICD-9-CM

343.9 Infantile cerebral palsy, unspecified

SEE ALSO

OTHER NOTES N/A

ABBREVIATIONS N/A

REFERENCES

- Murphy N, Such-Neibar T. Cerebral palsy diagnosis and management: the state of the art. Curr Probl Pediatr Adolesc Health Care. 2003;33(5):146-69
- Kuban KCK, Leviton A. Cerebral Palsy. N Engl J Med 1994;330(3):188-95
- Neonatal Encephalopathy and Cerebral Palsy: Defining the Pathogenesis and Pathophysiology. American College of Obstetricians and Gynecologists; American Academy of Pediatrics, Washington, DC 2003

Web references: 2 available at www.5mcc.com
Illustrations N/A

Author(s):
Michael Krew, MD

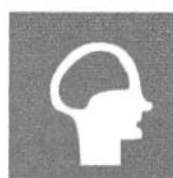

BASICS

DESCRIPTION Pre-invasive neoplastic epithelial changes in the transformation zone of the uterine cervix often associate with human papilloma virus infections

- Mild dysplasia (CIN I or SIL low grade) - cellular changes are limited to the lower one-third of the squamous epithelium
- Moderate dysplasia (CIN II or SIL high grade) - cellular changes are limited to the lower two-thirds of the squamous epithelium
- Severe dysplasia (CIN III or SIL high grade or carcinoma in situ) - cellular changes involves the full thickness of the squamous epithelium

System(s) affected: Reproductive
Genetics: N/A
Incidence/Prevalence in USA: Difficult to assess due to wide variability in false negative Pap smear reporting and uneven distribution of qualified colposcopy practitioners. Prevalence 3,600/100,000 at age 27-28.
Predominant age: The median age for carcinoma in situ is 28 years. Earlier lesions can be expected at younger ages
Predominant sex: Female only

SIGNS & SYMPTOMS

- Frequently none
- Occasionally associated with condyloma acuminata in the vulva, vagina, or anus
- Occasionally there are co-existing sexually transmitted diseases in the lower reproductive tract, e.g., chlamydia, gonorrhea

CAUSES Strong linkage with infections by human papilloma viruses types 16, 18, 31, 33, and 35. Other types of the same virus have also been implicated.

RISK FACTORS

- Multiparity and pregnancy before age 20 years
- Multiple sexual partners
- Early age in first sexual intercourse
- Condyloma acuminatum infection elsewhere in the body
- Cigarette smoking
- Prostitution
- Lower socioeconomic status

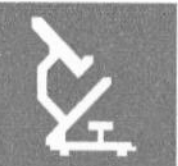

DIAGNOSIS

DIFFERENTIAL DIAGNOSIS

- Invasive carcinoma of the cervix
- Condyloma acuminatum

LABORATORY

- Pap smear

Drugs that may alter lab results:

- Surgical lubricants e.g., K-Y Jelly

Disorders that may alter lab results: N/A

PATHOLOGICAL FINDINGS

- Clumping of the nuclear chromatin material
- Reversal of the nuclear/cytoplasmic ratio
- Koilocytosis
- Hyperchromasia

SPECIAL TESTS

- Viral DNA hybridization (Virapap) and others
- Colposcopy
- PAPNET system to review negative Pap smears
- CYTYC 2000 thin prep Pap test (replacement of current Pap preparations)

IMAGING N/A

DIAGNOSTIC PROCEDURES

- Papanicolaou smear
- Colposcopy and directed cervical biopsies
- Cone biopsy (by cold knife, laser, or loop excision)
- Endocervical curettage
- Loop electrosurgical excision procedure (LEEP)
- Cervicography
- Speculum examination
- Use of HPV DNA typing to select certain cases with borderline abnormalities, e.g., atypical squamous cells of undetermined significance (ASCUS), for closer followup and colposcopy

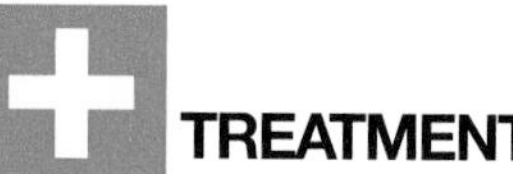

TREATMENT

APPROPRIATE HEALTH CARE Outpatient

GENERAL MEASURES Office evaluation and observation

SURGICAL MEASURES Outpatient surgery - cryotherapy, laser ablative or excisional cone, cold knife cone, electrosurgical loop excision of transformation zone

ACTIVITY Four weeks of pelvic rest after cone biopsy

DIET No restriction

PATIENT EDUCATION See Followup section

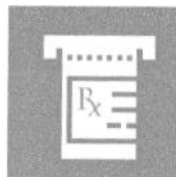

MEDICATIONS

DRUG(S) OF CHOICE
- Treatment is primarily surgical
- Fluorouracil (Efudex) once or twice daily as 5% vaginal cream supplemental therapy

Contraindications: Hypersensitivity to 5-fluorouracil

Precautions:
- If hand is used in application of 5-fluorouracil, wash hand immediately afterwards
- Avoid contact of 5-fluorouracil with eyes, nose, or mouth

Significant possible interactions: N/A

ALTERNATIVE DRUGS N/A

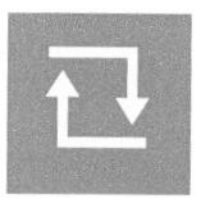

FOLLOWUP

PATIENT MONITORING
Repeat Pap smears every 4 months during the first year after cone excision for severe dysplasia, every 6 months thereafter. For lesser lesions, repeat Pap smear yearly. Probe endocervical canal to assure patency.

PREVENTION/AVOIDANCE
- Monogamy of both sexual partners
- Use of condom during coitus if unable to practice monogamy
- Abstain from smoking
- Emphasize importance of yearly Pap smears for patients
- Ability to obtain skilled colposcopy service as needed
- Patient education (individually or by community services) to emphasize the need for Pap smear
- Educate medical care providers to make patient referrals for the screening service unless they provide it themselves

POSSIBLE COMPLICATIONS
- Some severe dysplasia will progress to invasive carcinoma of the cervix
- Possible complications following cone biopsy of the cervix:
  - ◊ Hemorrhage
  - ◊ Infection
  - ◊ Cervical stenosis
  - ◊ Cervical incompetence
  - ◊ Infertility
  - ◊ Incomplete excision of dysplastic tissue
  - ◊ Recurrence

EXPECTED COURSE/PROGNOSIS
- Generally excellent
- Persistence of dysplasia can occur due to incomplete excision
- Recurrence of dysplasia can occur due to inability to eradicate the human papilloma virus in the patient's body or prevent new infections

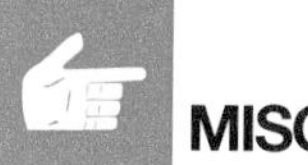

MISCELLANEOUS

ASSOCIATED CONDITIONS
- Condyloma acuminatum
- Carcinoma of the cervix

AGE-RELATED FACTORS
Pediatric: Very rare

Geriatric: Less frequent

Others: This is usually a problem for the women in the reproductive age group. The median age is 28 years for severe dysplasia. For lesser lesions, the median ages tend to be much lower.

PREGNANCY
- Dysplasia may progress during pregnancy
- It is important to determine the severity of dysplasia and to exclude the presence of invasive carcinoma during pregnancy
- Dysplasia does not require definitive treatment during pregnancy
- Dysplasia by itself is not an indication for cesarean section

SYNONYMS N/A

ICD-9-CM
622.1 Dysplasia of cervix (uteri)

SEE ALSO
Abnormal Pap smear
Cervical malignancy
Condyloma acuminata

OTHER NOTES
Squamous intraepithelial lesion (SIL) is in reference to Pap smear only

ABBREVIATIONS
CIN = cervical intraepithelial neoplasia
SIL = squamous intraepithelial lesion

REFERENCES

- Koss LG. Reducing the error rate in Papanicolaou smears. The Female Patient 1994;19:6
- Sherman ME, et al. PAPNET analysis of reportedly negative smears preceding the diagnosis of high grade intraepithelial lesion or carcinoma. Modern Pathol 19947(5):578-581
- Disaia PJ, Creasman WT. Clinical Gynecologic Oncology. 4th Ed. St. Louis, The C.V. Mosby Co., 1993
- Wright TC, Richart RM, Ferencz A. Electrosurgery for HPV-related diseases of the lower genital tract. New York, Arthur Vision, Inc. & Biovision, Inc., 1992
- Kurman RJ, ed. Blaustein's Pathology Of The Female Genital Tract. 3rd Ed. New York, Springer-Verlag, 1987
- Novak ER, Woodruff JD. Novak's Gynecologic and Obstetric Pathology With Clinical and Endocrine Relations. 8th Ed. Philadelphia, W.B. Saunders Company, 1979
- Herbst AL, Mishell DR, Stenchever MA, Droegemueller W. Comprehensive Gynecology. 2nd Ed. St. Louis, C.V. Mosby Co., 1992
- Richart R, Jones HW III, Reid R. Classification and Interpretation of Pap smears. ACOG Update 1993;18;10:1-10
- Korn AP. Management of abnormal cervical/vaginal Pap smears. Medscape Women's Health 1996;1(3)
- Update: National Breast and Cervical Cancer Early Detection Program MMWR 1996;45(23):484-487
- Block BB, Branham RA. Efforts to improve the follow-up of abnormal Papanicolaou test results. J of Am Board of Fam Prac 1998;11:1
- Manos M, Kinney W, Hurley L, Sherman M, Shich-Ngai J, Kurman R. Identifying women with cervical neoplasia, using human papilloma virus DNA testing for equivocal Papanicolaou results. JAMA 1999;281(17):1605-10

Web references: 1 available at www.5mcc.com

Illustrations N/A

Author(s):
Albert T. Shiu, MD

BASICS

DESCRIPTION Result from upward or backward injury to frontal head, jaw, and face. May involve:
- Soft tissue injury around cervical spine - "whiplash" or acute cervical musculoligamentous strain/sprain
- Vertebral structures - fractures, dislocations, ligamentous tears, and disc disruption
- Spinal cord - acute central cord syndrome (CCS) secondary to cord compression or vascular insult

System(s) affected: Musculoskeletal, Nervous
Genetics: Related to predisposing factors like ankylosing spondylitis associated with HLA-B27
Incidence/Prevalence in USA: About 1/4 of spinal injuries caused by hyperextension
Predominant age: Trauma and sports injuries most common in young adults, average age 29.4 years; CCS most common among elderly, average age 53 years
Predominant sex: Male > Female

SIGNS & SYMPTOMS
- Neck pain, stiffness and tenderness
- Headaches
- Paresthesia
- Numbness
- Shoulder pain, spasms and tenderness; range of motion limitation; radicular signs
- Classically, with forehead, face, or jaw abrasion, laceration, or contusion
- CCS
  - ◊ Typically distal upper extremity (UE) weakness or paralysis worse than proximal UE, worse than lower extremity
  - ◊ Variable sensory changes below level of lesion and sphincter dysfunction (including urinary retention)
  - ◊ Horner syndrome if C8-T11 involved
  - ◊ Lhermitte's sign (7% of cases)

CAUSES
- Trauma
  - ◊ Mostly vehicular accidents
  - ◊ Sports injuries
  - ◊ Falls
  - ◊ Assaults

RISK FACTORS
Present in 65% of CCS
- Spinal stenosis
  - ◊ Congenital
  - ◊ Acquired - prior trauma, spondylosis
- Spinal rigidity
  - ◊ Klippel-Feil syndrome
  - ◊ Ankylosing spondylitis

DIAGNOSIS

DIFFERENTIAL DIAGNOSIS
- Herniated discs
- Arthritis
- Radiculopathy
- Myelopathy
- For CCS
  - ◊ Bell cruciate palsy
  - ◊ Bilateral brachial plexus injuries

LABORATORY N/A

Drugs that may alter lab results: N/A

Disorders that may alter lab results: N/A

PATHOLOGICAL FINDINGS
- Acute cervical strain/sprain - based on animal, cadaver and postmortem studies
- Muscle tears of the sternocleidomastoid or partial avulsion of the longus colli
- Stretching or rupture of anterior longitudinal ligament
- Injuries to Intervertebral discs and facet joint capsules
- Rarely, retropharyngeal hematoma.
- Vertebral fractures: See General Measures
- CCS - secondary to cord compression or vascular insult
- Traditionally reported as central gray matter injury with hemorrhage
- Central hemorrhage is seen with more severe injuries
- It is currently thought that there is predominately white matter injury with involvement of the lateral column, particularly, corticospinal tracts
- Pathological hallmark - diffuse axonal disruption

SPECIAL TESTS See Imaging

IMAGING
- Plain c-spine films still main initial diagnostic tool
  - ◊ Static - c-spine series with minimum of two views, lateral view reveals post-trauma abnormalities in 70-83% of cases, addition of anteroposterior and open mouth increases sensitivity; may show prevertebral soft-tissue swelling without other radiological signs in

CCS, craniocervical soft tissue swelling in C2 fractures or bony abnormalities
  - ◊ Dynamic - flexion/extension, only if asymptomatic neck and no neurological deficits or mental impairment, evaluates ligamentous integrity in acute setting, also evaluates spine stability and union, by amount of movement, in fractures during or after treatment
- CT scan or tomograms - better delineation of fractures, spinal canal status
- CT myelogram - alternative to MRI, delineates neural impingement
- MRI - diagnostic procedure of choice in CCS with direct visualization of traumatic cord lesions (edema or hematomyelia), soft tissue compressing cord and stenosis of canal. It also detects a high percentage of occult disc, ligament or soft tissue abnormalities, but is poor with fractures.

DIAGNOSTIC PROCEDURES Discussed in other sections; care needs to be taken to avoid overlooking subtle hyperextension injuries

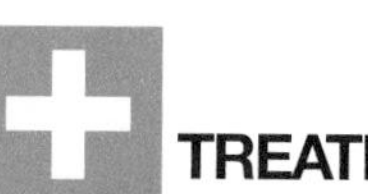

TREATMENT

APPROPRIATE HEALTH CARE Outpatient or inpatients as required by injury

GENERAL MEASURES
- Whiplash; depending on severity
  - ◊ Activity restriction with increases after patient improvement
  - ◊ Soft to rigid collar
  - ◊ Medicines - analgesics, muscle relaxants, anti-inflammatory
  - ◊ Post resolution of spasms, repeat flexion/extension lateral c-spine to confirm stability
- CCS
  - ◊ See Medications
  - ◊ If no instability, bed rest with soft collar for 4-6 weeks followed by mobilization with collar for another 4-6 weeks
- Fractures; stability determined by usual radiologic criteria; surgical decompression and stabilization is indicated:
  - ◊ In patients with incomplete spinal cord injuries and spinal canal compromise from bone, disc, subluxation, or hematoma
  - ◊ In those who deteriorate or do not improve on conservative therapy
- Hangman's fracture - traumatic spondylolisthesis of the axis with bilateral fractures through the C2 pedicles, often with anterior subluxation of C2 over C3
  - ◊ Usually stable, managed with orthosis, SOMI (sternal-occipital-mental orthosis)
  - ◊ Unstable if C2 subluxation over C3 is greater than 50% of vertebral body of C3 in anterioposterior diameter
  - ◊ Unstable if excessive angulation of C2 over C3
  - ◊ Then treated with halo vest immobilization for 8-14 weeks until repeat flexion/extension films
  - ◊ If stable, rigid collar for additional 8-12 weeks
- Odontoid fracture - treated according to type
  - ◊ I - through apex, may be unstable and require surgical fusion
  - ◊ II - most common type, at base of dens, usually unstable; nonunion rates of about 30% with immobilization alone, especially with increased dens displacement more than 6 mm in patients more than 7 years old
  - ◊ III - through C2 body, usually stable; immobilized in halo for 8-14 weeks, rigid collar for 8-14 weeks, then mobilization
- C3-C7 hyperextension fractures
  - ◊ If stable, rigid collar for 8-14 weeks then mobilization
  - ◊ If unstable, halo brace; serial lateral c-spine films from supine to upright; if still unstable, surgical stabilization
  - ◊ Post-op, followup x-rays until trabeculation across fracture site or interbody fusion achieved

SURGICAL MEASURES

- CCS
  - ◊ In acute cases, surgery is associated with deterioration and increased complications, and therefore contraindicated
  - ◊ Surgery may be indicated in patient who is improving and then deteriorates
  - ◊ Otherwise, surgical decompression and stabilization performed only when neurologic function has reached a plateau or maximum recovery
  - ◊ Fractures: See General Measures

ACTIVITY Rest and immobilization until pain is controlled; followed by gradual mobilization, and rehabilitation exercises if needed

DIET No special diet

PATIENT EDUCATION For patient instruction on prevention: THINK FIRST Foundation, 22 S. Washington St., Park Ridge, IL 60068, (708)692-2740

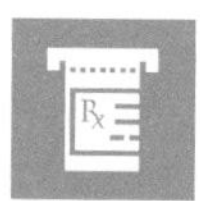

MEDICATIONS

DRUG(S) OF CHOICE CCS - methylprednisolone 30 mg/kg IV over one hour followed by 5.4 mg/kg IV per hour for 23 hours (continue for 47 hours if started more than eight hours after injury). It improves neurological outcome, motor and sensory function at 6 weeks, 6 months, and l year after incomplete spinal cord injury.

Contraindications: N/A

Precautions: N/A

Significant possible interactions: N/A

ALTERNATIVE DRUGS N/A

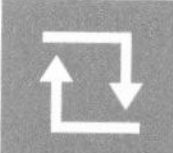

FOLLOWUP

PATIENT MONITORING

- Patients seen and checked with x-rays every 3-4 weeks for about 3 months, when bone healing is usually adequate
- Halo then replaced with rigid collar for next 3 months or rigid collar replaced with soft collar for comfort

PREVENTION/AVOIDANCE Wearing seat belts; using proper equipment when participating in sports activities

POSSIBLE COMPLICATIONS

- Persistent symptoms
- Nonunion of fractures
- Persistent instability requiring another procedure
- Reactions and infection related to orthosis

EXPECTED COURSE/PROGNOSIS

Most important prognostic factor is the initial neurologic status

- Whiplash - most patients recover well, mild symptoms resolving within 6 months
  - ◊ On the average, more severe injuries without disc involvement resolve in 21 months
  - ◊ 30 months for those with degenerative changes
  - ◊ At 2 years, 42% complete recovery, 15% mild discomfort, 43% significant discomfort affecting work
- CCS
  - ◊ Most patients recover motor strength within 2 weeks
  - ◊ Younger patients have better prognosis
  - ◊ Leg, bowel, and bladder function return first
  - ◊ Return of arm strength follows, then that of hand
  - ◊ However, upper extremities recover less well, and fine finger movements is usually not regained completely
  - ◊ With cord contusion but no hematomyelia, 50% recover enough strength and sensation to ambulate independently although usually with spasticity
- Fracture-dislocation
  - ◊ Hangman's fracture - 93-100% fusion rate after 8-14 weeks external immobilization
  - ◊ Odontoid fracture - type III, 90% fusion with immobilization

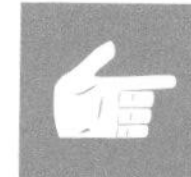

MISCELLANEOUS

ASSOCIATED CONDITIONS N/A

AGE-RELATED FACTORS

Pediatric: Consider spinal cord injury without radiographic abnormality (SCIWORA), which has a high incidence at < 9 years. MRI may help detect the injury.

Geriatric: Degenerative disease of cervical spine may be confused with acute traumatic change on imaging

Others: N/A

PREGNANCY N/A

SYNONYMS N/A

ICD-9-CM

952.00 Cervical spinal cord injury without evidence of spinal bone injury, C1-C4 level with unspecified spinal cord injury

SEE ALSO

OTHER NOTES N/A

ABBREVIATIONS

CCS = central cord syndrome

REFERENCES

- Eichler ME, Vollmer DG. Cervical spine trauma. In: Youmans JR, ed. Neurological surgery. 4th ed. Philadelphia, W.B. Saunders, 1996,1939-6
- Greenberg MS. Handbook of neurosurgery. 4th ed. Florida, Greenberg Graphics, 1997
- McDowell GS, Cammisa FP, Eismont FJ. Hyperextension injuries of the cervical spine. In: Levine AM, Eismont FJ, Garfin SR, Zigler JE, eds. Spine trauma. Philadelphia, W.B. Saunders, 1998,367-86
- Sonntag VKH, Francis PM. Controversies in spinal cord syndromes. In: Garfin SR, Northup BE. eds. Surgery for Spinal Cord Injuries. New York, Raven Press, 1993,15-31
- Travis RL. Hyperextension and hyperflexion injuries of the cervical spine. In: Youmans JR, ed. Neurological Surgery. 4th Ed. Philadelphia, W.B. Saunders, 1996,2037-42
- Wong WB, Parjabi MM, White AA. Mechanisms of injury in the cervical spine. In: Clark CR, editor. The Cervical Spine. 3rd Ed. Philadelphia, Lippincott-Raven, 1998,79

Web references: 5 available at www.5mcc.com

Illustrations N/A

Author(s):

Oren N. Gottfried, MD

Martin E. Weinand, MD

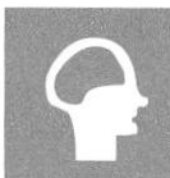

BASICS

DESCRIPTION Invasive cancer of the uterine cervix commonly involves the vagina, parametria and the pelvic side-walls. In advanced cases, the cancer may invade the bladder, rectum, or other pelvic sites.
System(s) affected: Reproductive
Genetics: Not an inherited disease
Incidence/Prevalence in USA: In 1997, there were 14,500 new cases, and 4,800 deaths due to the disease
Predominant age: Greater than 25% of all cervical cancer cases occur in women 65 years or older. 40-50% of women dying from cervical cancer are over 65 years of age.
Predominant sex: Female only

SIGNS & SYMPTOMS
- Abnormal vaginal bleeding
- Post-coital vaginal bleeding
- Pelvic pain, leg pain, back pain
- Dyspareunia
- Hematuria
- Rectal bleeding
- Foul vaginal discharge
- Cervical ulcer, crater, or fungating mass
- Extension of the cervical mass into upper vagina and/or parametria, with induration, nodularity, and fixation to surrounding tissue

CAUSES Unknown. There is a strong association with genital infection by the oncogenic strains of human papilloma virus (HPV) in 90% of cases.

RISK FACTORS
- Multiple sexual partners
- Male partner with multiple sexual partners
- Male partner who has had a partner with cervical carcinoma
- Early onset of first sexual intercourse
- Current or previous HPV infections, eg, condyloma acuminatum, cervical intraepithelial neoplasia (CIN)
- History of sexually transmitted diseases
- Smoker
- Immunosuppression from drugs or HIV infection
- Diethylstilbestrol (DES) offspring

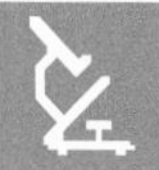

DIAGNOSIS

DIFFERENTIAL DIAGNOSIS
- Marked cervicitis and erosion
- Cervical polyp
- Cervical condyloma
- Metastasis from endometrial carcinoma or gestational trophoblastic disease
- Cervical pregnancy

LABORATORY
- For initial diagnosis: Papanicolaou smear and cervical biopsies
- Complete blood count
- BUN, creatinine

Drugs that may alter lab results: Vaginal lubricants may obscure Pap smears

Disorders that may alter lab results: Vaginitis or excessive vaginal bleeding may obscure Pap smears

PATHOLOGICAL FINDINGS
- Invasive squamous cell carcinoma is the major cell type
- Invasive adenocarcinoma is becoming increasingly evident
- Other cell types are also present in the minority

SPECIAL TESTS
- Colposcopy, if indicated
- Endocervical curettage
- Cervical conization, if indicated
- Liver function tests
- Cystoscopy
- Sigmoidoscopy

IMAGING
- Computed tomographic scans of the abdomen and pelvis, if needed, for detection of lymph node metastasis, and for evaluation of planned radiation therapy
- Lymphangiography, if needed, for detection of pelvic and para-aortic lymph node metastasis
- Chest x-ray
- Excretory pyelogram

DIAGNOSTIC PROCEDURES Cervical conization can resolve the question of early invasion, and if present, can determine the depth of invasion, and the presence of lymphatic and vascular involvement

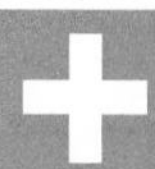

TREATMENT

APPROPRIATE HEALTH CARE According to the depth of invasion and clinical staging

GENERAL MEASURES
- Improve the patient's nutritional state, correct any anemia and treat any vaginal and/or pelvic infections
- Chemotherapy has been used extensively as adjuvant therapy to metastatic disease and more recently as neoadjuvant therapy

SURGICAL MEASURES
- Stage 1a1 (lesions with less than 3 mm invasion from basement membrane): cervical conization with total hysterectomy later when patient's family is completed; otherwise total hysterectomy by either the abdominal or vaginal route.
- Stage 1a2 (lesions with greater than 3 mm but less than 5 mm invasion from the basement membrane) and for stages 1b1, 1b2, 2a: patient has the option of radical hysterectomy, bilateral pelvic lymphadenectomy, and para-aortic nodes sampling; or primary radiation with brachytherapy and teletherapy
- Stage 4A (lesions limited to central metastasis to the bladder and/or rectum): pelvic exenteration may be feasible
- Radiation measures
  - ◊ Stages 1a2 or higher, the following techniques have been used:
    - Brachytherapy with intracavitary radium or cesium or interstitial cesium needles to treat the central tumor sites, and
    - Teletherapy with external megavoltage radiation to treat tumor metastasis in the pelvic walls
- For localized persistent or recurrent disease, radiation therapy or pelvic exenteration as appropriate

ACTIVITY As tolerated

DIET As appropriate

PATIENT EDUCATION American Cancer Society, 1599 Clifton Rd., Atlanta, GA 30329, (404)320-3333

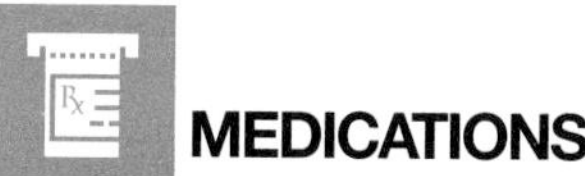

MEDICATIONS

DRUG(S) OF CHOICE

- Cisplatin, hydroxyurea, and fluorouracil have been used as adjuvant sensitizer to radiation therapy
- Cisplatin/carboplatin, etoposide (VP-16), ifosfamide, bleomycin have been used as adjuvant therapy for recurrent, metastatic disease

Contraindications: Refer to manufacturer's profile of each drug.

Precautions: Refer to manufacturer's profile of each drug

Significant possible interactions: Refer to manufacturer's profile of each drug

ALTERNATIVE DRUGS

- Ondansetron (Zofran), dronabinol (Marinol), metoclopramide (Reglan), and others for nausea control

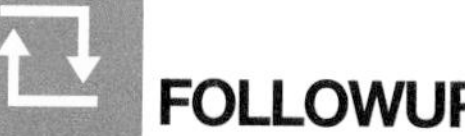

FOLLOWUP

PATIENT MONITORING

- With completion of definitive therapy. each patient is evaluated with physical/pelvic examinations and Pap smear at the following intervals:
  - ◊ Every 3 months for 1-2 years
  - ◊ Every 6 months until the 5th year
  - ◊ Yearly thereafter
- The three most common signs of cancer recurrence are: unexplained weight loss, leg edema, and pelvic or thigh pain

PREVENTION/AVOIDANCE

- Stop smoking
- Avoid sexually transmitted diseases
- Regular Pap smears and pelvic exams; appropriate interval for Pap smear (reference: 1988 American College of Obstetricians and Gynecologists and American Cancer Society):
  - ◊ All women who are or who have been sexually active, or who have reached age 18, should undergo an annual Pap test and pelvic examination.
  - ◊ After a woman has had three or more consecutive satisfactory annual examinations with normal findings, the Pap smear may be performed less frequently at the discretion of her physician

POSSIBLE COMPLICATIONS

- Hemorrhage
- Pelvic infection
- Bladder dysfunction
- Genitourinary fistula
- Ureteral obstruction with renal failure
- Bowel obstruction
- Lymphocyst
- Pulmonary embolism
- Loss of ovarian function from radiotherapy or indication for bilateral oophorectomy

EXPECTED COURSE/PROGNOSIS

After commonly accepted surgical and radiation treatments.

Five year survival after accepted surgical and radiation management of cervical malignancy:

Stage	5 yr survival
1	80%
2	65%
3	30%
4	15%

MISCELLANEOUS

ASSOCIATED CONDITIONS

- Condyloma acuminatum
- Preinvasive/invasive lesions of the vulva and vagina

AGE-RELATED FACTORS

Pediatric: N/A

Geriatric: Since more than half the invasive cancer cases are seen in the over 65 age group, efforts should be concentrated in expanding the availability of Pap smear screening to the geriatric population

Others: Selection of surgical therapy in younger women with early stages of cancer provides ovarian conservation

PREGNANCY Generally, the choice of treatment is dependent on the length of gestation, the patient's wish to continue pregnancy to attainment of fetal lung maturity, and the treating physician's comfort level in delaying definitive therapy. If treatment is delayed, the patient must receive close follow-up care with its frequency dependent upon the severity of the disease. Selection of the mode of therapy is based upon clinical staging as noted previously.

SYNONYMS

- Cancer of the uterine cervix
- Cervical cancer
- Cervical carcinoma

ICD-9-CM

180.0 Malignant neoplasm of body of cervix uteri, endocervix

SEE ALSO

OTHER NOTES N/A

ABBREVIATIONS N/A

REFERENCES

- McMeekin DS, McGonigle KH, Vasilev SA. Cervical cancer prevention: towards cost effective screening. Medscape Women's Health 12-2-1997
- Parke SL, Tong T, Bolden S, et al. Cancer statistics, 1997. Ca-A cancer Jour for Clinicians 1997;47(1):5-27
- National Cancer Institute: Cancer Statistics Review 1973-1987. Bethesda, NCI Publication No. (NIH)90-2789, 1990
- Nanda K, McCrory D, Myers E, Bastian L, Hasselblad V, Hickey J.
- Accuracy of the Papanicolaou test in screening for and follow-up of cervical cytological abnormalities: A systematic review. Ann Intern Med 2000;132:810-819

Web references: 0 available at www.5mcc.com

Illustrations N/A

Author(s):
Albert T. Shiu, MD

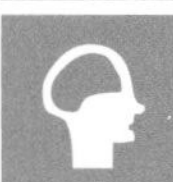

BASICS

DESCRIPTION Pedunculated masses, usually single, which vary in size from a few millimeters to 3 centimeters and protrude from the cervix; may bleed
System(s) affected: Reproductive
Genetics: N/A
Incidence/Prevalence in USA: Common
Predominant age: Most often ages 40-60
Predominant sex: Female only

SIGNS & SYMPTOMS
- Painless
- Intermenstrual bleeding (spotting)
- May cause post-coital or postmenopausal bleeding
- Leukorrhea

CAUSES
- Unknown for most
- Secondary reaction to cervical inflammatory or hormonal stimulation

RISK FACTORS None known

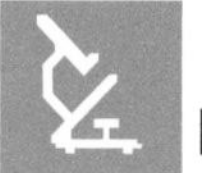

DIAGNOSIS

DIFFERENTIAL DIAGNOSIS
- Prolapsed submucous myoma or endometrial polyp
- Other causes of intermenstrual bleeding
- Decidualized endometrium

LABORATORY N/A

Drugs that may alter lab results: N/A

Disorders that may alter lab results: N/A

PATHOLOGICAL FINDINGS Benign hyperplastic endocervical epithelium often with a large number of blood vessels

SPECIAL TESTS
- Diagnosis usually made by pelvic examination
- Perform Pap smear prior to treatment
- Send to pathology for analysis

IMAGING N/A

DIAGNOSTIC PROCEDURES Characteristic appearance noted at time of pelvic examination

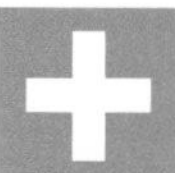

TREATMENT

APPROPRIATE HEALTH CARE Outpatient usually. Very large polyps may require removal in the operating room.

GENERAL MEASURES N/A

SURGICAL MEASURES Simple surgical excision in office with traction or electrocautery, control bleeding with silver nitrate, Monsels solution or cautery. Larger polyps may require ligature.

ACTIVITY Avoid sexual intercourse, tampons, and douching for 2 weeks

DIET General diet

PATIENT EDUCATION Routine care instructions

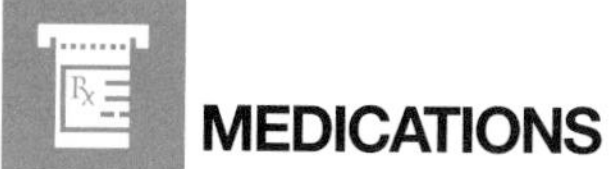

MEDICATIONS

DRUG(S) OF CHOICE None
Contraindications: N/A
Precautions: N/A
Significant possible interactions: N/A

ALTERNATIVE DRUGS N/A

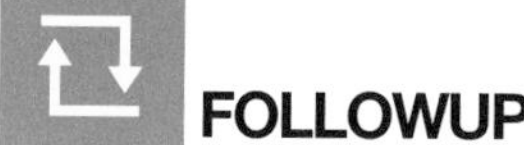

FOLLOWUP

PATIENT MONITORING Recheck at routine appointments or as needed

PREVENTION/AVOIDANCE None known

POSSIBLE COMPLICATIONS
- Bleeding and mild pain with removal
- Spotting for 1 or 2 days

EXPECTED COURSE/PROGNOSIS
Almost always benign. Very rare incidence of dysplasia in polyp. Very rare possibility of malignancy arising.

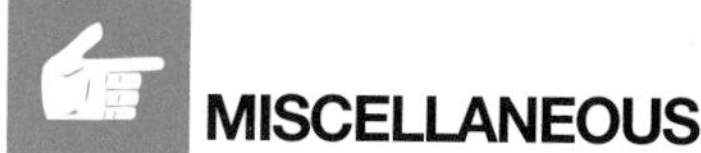

MISCELLANEOUS

ASSOCIATED CONDITIONS None

AGE-RELATED FACTORS
Pediatric: Very rare
Geriatric: Rare
Others: N/A

PREGNANCY Delay removal until postpartum unless causing significant bleeding or cervical dilation

SYNONYMS N/A

ICD-9-CM
622.7 Mucous polyp of cervix

SEE ALSO

OTHER NOTES N/A

ABBREVIATIONS N/A

REFERENCES

- Blaustein A, et al, eds. Blaustein's Pathology of the Female Genital Tract. 5th ed. New York: Springer-Verlag; 2002
- Novak ER, et al, eds: Novak's Gynecology. 13th ed. Baltimore: Lippincott Williams & Wilkins; 2002

Web references: 0 available at www.5mcc.com
Illustrations N/A

Author(s):
Nicole Pilevsky, MD

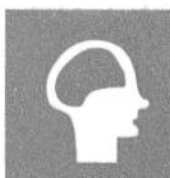

BASICS

DESCRIPTION Though an over-simplification, it is best to classify injuries as flexion, extension, compression, or unknown

- Flexion injuries
  - ◊ Anterior subluxation - best seen on lateral view of cervical spine as a kyphotic angulation at the point of ligamentous injury. Widening of spinous process at the point of injury may occur.
  - ◊ Facet dislocation - unstable injury, especially when bilateral. Anterior displacement of vertebra (50% of its width) usually indicates bilateral facet dislocation.
  - ◊ Compression fractures - usually associated with disruption of the posterior ligament complex and therefore unstable
  - ◊ Clay-shoveler's fracture - avulsion fracture of C7-C6 or T1 spinous process with intact posterior ligaments and therefore stable
- Extension injuries
  - ◊ Hangman's fracture - fracture of the pars interarticularis of the axis. It accounts for 10-15% of fractures.
  - ◊ Laminar fracture - difficult to see. Usually in older people who have spondylosis.
  - ◊ Fracture posterior arch atlas - usually stable when an isolated injury
  - ◊ Fracture dislocations - may resemble a flexion injury since the vertebral body is propelled forward and therefore appears as a flexion subluxation
- Compression
  - ◊ Jefferson's fracture - a fracture of the arches of C1, best seen on the open mouth view as displacement of C1 lateral masses
  - ◊ Burst fracture - seen on the AP radiograph as a vertical fracture of the body and on the lateral as a commutation of the body with varying degrees of retropulsion of the body
- Unknown mechanisms
  - ◊ Odontoid fractures - best seen on the AP view, but lateral views may show a tilt or displacement

System(s) affected: Musculoskeletal, Nervous
Genetics: N/A
Incidence/Prevalence in USA: Cervical injuries account for twelve thousand deaths in the U.S. each year. One-half of these are from motor vehicular accidents.
Predominant age: Most common in ages 16-25
Predominant sex: Male > Female

SIGNS & SYMPTOMS

- Pain, stiffness, and/or tenderness in an alert patient. If none of these are present the incidence of cervical spine injury is only 1-2%, provided the patient is alert and without alcohol or drug intake. (A lateral cervical spine x-ray should be taken routinely in all severe trauma).
- Head and/or facial trauma/lacerations in patients with altered consciousness

CAUSES Trauma

RISK FACTORS

- Motor vehicle accidents
- Diving accidents

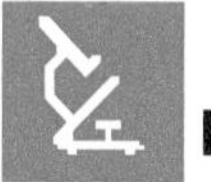

DIAGNOSIS

DIFFERENTIAL DIAGNOSIS

- Joint, muscle or ligament inflammation
- Paresthesias
- Arthritis
- Cervical disk protrusion
- Cervical spondylosis

LABORATORY N/A

Drugs that may alter lab results: N/A

Disorders that may alter lab results: N/A

PATHOLOGICAL FINDINGS N/A

SPECIAL TESTS Tomograms may be obtained to visualize otherwise obscure fractures, but even these are usually inferior to imaging by CT. MRI is superior in evaluating soft tissue injury.

IMAGING

- The use of CT and MRI scanning has greatly facilitated diagnosis of obscure cervical injuries. The CT may be a little better in some bone injuries, especially in the foramen, while the MRI has the edge with soft tissue evaluation. Both are superior to any previous method.
- X-ray - a lateral view of the cervical spine is only 80-85% accurate in picking up abnormalities. Adding an AP and open mouth odontoid view will increase the accuracy of screening to 90-95%. However, in the presence of pain, tenderness, and/or stiffness, the use of a CT or MRI scan should be considered since 5-10% of cases will have normal radiographs even with a significant cervical injury.
- X-rays vary with the type of injury, but a few salient features to be observed are:
  - ◊ Soft-tissue swelling on the lateral view of greater than 5 mm when measured from the inferior border of C3 to the trachea indicates a severe injury (except children)
  - ◊ Widely divergent spinous processes on the lateral view indicates rupture of ligaments
  - ◊ Abnormal widening of either a complete interspace or a portion of the anterior or posterior interspace on lateral view (compare with interspaces above and below)
  - ◊ Malrotation of the spinous processes on the AP view (they should form a straight line)
  - ◊ Inequality of the space on either side of the odontoid on open mouth views

DIAGNOSTIC PROCEDURES N/A

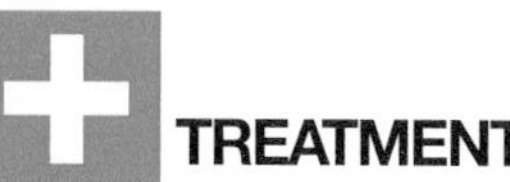

TREATMENT

APPROPRIATE HEALTH CARE

- Transportation
  - ◊ A carefully applied rigid collar supplemented by sand bags on either side of the head on a rigid backboard is probably the safest method
  - ◊ Oxygen should be given to all patients with injury to the spinal cord. (Patients with high cord lesions die of asphyxiation so assisted ventilation may be needed).
  - ◊ 50% of serious cervical injuries will have associated head, chest, abdominal or major extremity injuries in association. Give first aid to these patients maintaining the "ABC" principle of airway, breathing, and circulation.
  - ◊ Military antishock garment (MASG) can be used in cases of shock
  - ◊ Start an intravenous line if it can be done rapidly. Otherwise, this should not be done as valuable time may be wasted. The principle of "load and go" in cases of ambulance or "swoop and scoop" in the case of helicopters is a good one if an acute care center is close at hand.
- Hospital
  - ◊ Prior to dealing with the cervical injury, attention should be directed towards the ABC's (airway, breathing, circulation)
  - ◊ Arterial oxygen should be measured immediately since oxygenation of an injured spinal cord helps prevent further damage and aids in recovery. If the oxygen partial pressure (pO2) is less than 70 mm of mercury, or the cervical lesion is above C5, intubation is indicated. If the patient is breathing, blind nasal intubation can be tried; otherwise the oral approach with a laryngoscope is necessary. Both require careful technique with avoidance of neck extension. If this cannot be done with ease or if there are severe facial injuries, a cricothyroidotomy should be done.
  - ◊ A nasogastric (NG) tube should always be inserted to prevent vomiting, aspiration. It also prevents gastric dilatation with lung compression and difficult breathing.
  - ◊ In most cases, volume replacement is best accomplished through the femoral route. The subclavian approach risks pneumothorax and further oxygenation problems.
  - ◊ If a pneumothorax is present, a chest tube should always be inserted (first confirmed by x-ray). Needle aspiration is indicated only as a temporary measure to relieve symptoms in a tension pneumothorax prior to insertion of the tube.
  - ◊ In all cord injuries, abdominal and chest CT scan should be done to rule out a severe intra-abdominal injury. This procedure is highly accurate while all physical findings and symptoms are unreliable. (The NG tube and an indwelling Foley catheter should be done prior to the scans.)

GENERAL MEASURES

- Spinal shock occurs in 25-40% of spinal cord injuries. It is characterized by systolic hypotension and bradycardia. The cause is loss of distal sympathetic tone.
- Head injuries alone do not cause hypotension but can cause hypertension
- Because patients with cervical trauma may sustain other significant injuries, systolic hypotension may be from blood loss and/or spinal shock. Remember that several liters of blood can be lost from a head or perineal wound.
- Shock other than from volume loss or spinal shock can come from pericardial tamponade, tension pneumothorax, or cardiac contusion

SURGICAL MEASURES Surgical management as needed for type of injury

ACTIVITY N/A

DIET N/A

PATIENT EDUCATION N/A

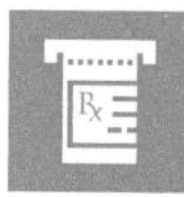

MEDICATIONS

DRUG(S) OF CHOICE

- Methylprednisolone
    - ◊ If given within 8 hours after the injury, has been shown to not only minimize further injury, but to improve both motor function and sensation for up to six months. This steroid apparently prevents lipid hydrolysis and subsequent destruction of the cell membrane.
    - ◊ Initial dose: 30 mg/kg over a 15 minute period. Then 45 minutes later, 5.4 mg/kg/hr for the next 23 hours. See Bracken 1990, N Engl J Med 322:1405-1411.

Contraindications: None

Precautions: Intravenous cimetidine (Tagamet) 300 mg q6h or ranitidine (Zantac) 50 mg q8h can be given if a history of ulcer is present. In cases of multiple injuries this is a good way to prevent stress ulcer.

Significant possible interactions: None

ALTERNATIVE DRUGS

- Naloxone, nimodipine and thyrotropin releasing hormones have been tried with equivocal results. Tests are underway using chemotherapeutic drugs, but these await the outcome of several studies.
- Other H2 receptor antagonists

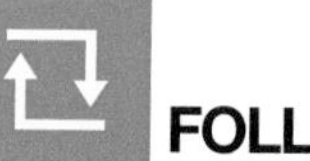

FOLLOWUP

PATIENT MONITORING Critical care facilities must be available initially and later physical and occupational therapy units with special skills in spinal cord injuries

PREVENTION/AVOIDANCE N/A

POSSIBLE COMPLICATIONS

- Paresthesia
- Muscle weakness
- Reflex loss
- Sensory loss
- Radiculopathy

EXPECTED COURSE/PROGNOSIS

In cases of significant cord injuries, the prognosis is guarded. Development of newer orthopedic devices can stabilize the spine and allow early mobilization, but do not help to reverse neurological damage if present.

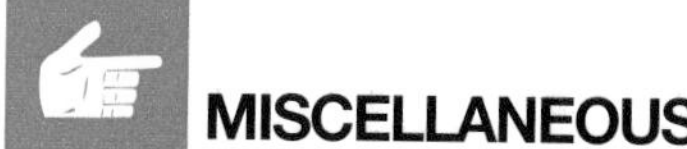

MISCELLANEOUS

ASSOCIATED CONDITIONS N/A

AGE-RELATED FACTORS

Pediatric: N/A
Geriatric: N/A
Others: N/A

PREGNANCY N/A

SYNONYMS Cervical fracture, dislocation

ICD-9-CM

952.00 Cervical spinal cord injury without evidence of spinal bone injury, C1-C4 level with unspecified spinal cord injury

SEE ALSO

OTHER NOTES N/A

ABBREVIATIONS N/A

REFERENCES

- Torg JS, Sennett B, et al: Axial loading injuries to middle cervical spine segment. An analysis and classification of 25 cases. American Journal of Sports Medicine 1991:19(1):6-20
- Soderstrom CA, Brumback RJ: Orthopedic Clinics of North America 1986;17(1):3-13
- Bracken MB, et al: Efficacy of methylprednisolone in acute spinal cord Injury; JAMA 1984;251:45-52
- Bracken MB, et al: A randomized control trial of methylprednisolone or naloxone in the treatment of acute spinal cord injury. Results of the second acute spinal cord Injury study. N Engl J Med 1990;322:1405-1411
- Jacobs B: Cervical Fractures and Dislocations, Clinical Orthopedics 1975;109:18

Web references: 1 available at www.5mcc.com
Illustrations N/A

Author(s):
R. Bruce Hall, MD

Cervical spondylosis

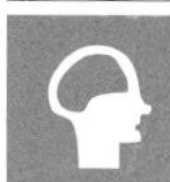

BASICS

DESCRIPTION Degenerative changes in the cervical vertebra and/or disk with spur formation and subsequent impingement of neural elements in a narrow cervical canal
System(s) affected: Musculoskeletal
Genetics: N/A
Incidence/Prevalence in USA: 30-40% of the population above age 40 years
Predominant age: Above 40 the incidence increases with each passing decade
Predominant sex: Male > Female (3:2)

SIGNS & SYMPTOMS
- Pain in the posterior neck often associated with radiation into the arms
- Scapular pain
- Pain in the arms is almost always on the outer aspect of the arm at least to elbow level (coronary heart pain is almost always on the inner aspect of the arm)
- Radicular pain into the arms or scapular area may be present without neck pain
- Dysphagia may develop with large anterior osteophytes
- Weakness of extremities - upper and/or lower
- Bladder or bowel incontinence in severe cases
- If an osteophyte develops on a neurocentral joint and extends laterally, it can encroach on the vertebral artery and may cause dizziness, vertigo, tinnitus or interorbital blurring of vision. Symptoms are exacerbated by extremes of movement and even minor neck trauma.
- Loss of neck extension (common)
- Lateral flexion of the cervical spine is limited in the erect position, but greatly increased on lying down. (Functional disorders are not improved by lying down.)
- Long tract signs may develop in severe cases with positive Babinski
- Tenderness of biceps and pectoralis major in C5-6 segment disease
- Triceps tenderness in C6-7 segment disease

CAUSES Degenerative changes with osteophytes and disk space narrowing

RISK FACTORS N/A

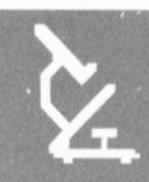

DIAGNOSIS

DIFFERENTIAL DIAGNOSIS
- Cervical disk disease (the two often co-exist)
- Pancoast tumor of lung
- Rheumatoid arthritis
- Neurological disorders such as multiple sclerosis

LABORATORY N/A

Drugs that may alter lab results: N/A

Disorders that may alter lab results: N/A

PATHOLOGICAL FINDINGS N/A

SPECIAL TESTS N/A

IMAGING
- X-rays of cervical spine, AP, lateral open mouth odontoid and both oblique views should be obtained. Osteophytes and/or joint space narrowing will be evident.
- CT or MRI scans are quite valuable in cases where surgery is contemplated or the diagnosis is in doubt. It is not indicated in the great majority of cases as a careful history and physical examination coupled with routine cervical spine x-rays will make the diagnosis. The decision as to which is better, the CT scan or MRI, is controversial. The MRI depicts cord changes, enlargement, compression, or atrophy better. While the CT, especially in conjunction with myelography, shows the bony changes, especially in foramina involvement. MRI has the obvious advantage of not requiring a myelogram. Postoperatively, the MRI is excellent in evaluation of patients who have failed to obtain relief from surgery or have developed new symptoms. If this does not demonstrate a cause, then a CT scan with contrast can be obtained.

DIAGNOSTIC PROCEDURES N/A

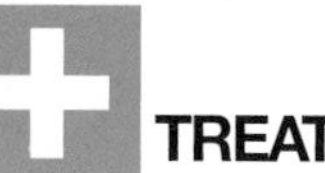

TREATMENT

APPROPRIATE HEALTH CARE Outpatient for conservative treatment, inpatient if surgery indicated

GENERAL MEASURES
- Acute phase - moist heat, gentle massage and temporary immobilization with a cervical collar that holds the neck in slight flexion. Intermittent cervical traction may be helpful, but the line of pull should be such that the neck is slightly flexed. Ultrasonic treatments, especially combined with gentle muscle stimulation (US-MS) for 15-20 minutes daily or bid may be helpful in the acute phase.
- Chronic - no treatment necessary except for non-narcotic analgesics for symptoms. Any type of activity or work which causes strain of the neck should be avoided.

SURGICAL MEASURES
- Indications: Severe pain unresponsive to conservative measures, significant or progression of neurologic deficits, long tract signs, vertebral artery syndrome
- Most common surgery is anterior interbody fusion with excision of disk and any accessible osteophytes

ACTIVITY Any activity which does not cause symptoms should be encouraged as the disease is chronic. Needless restrictions can make the patient a medical invalid.

DIET No special diet

PATIENT EDUCATION
- Personally instruct (or have a therapist instruct) in the proper use of orthopedic appliances. Cervical collars should produce a slight flexion of the neck as should traction. Avoid extension in all situations.
- Instruct patient in home traction to relieve symptoms; instruct patient in home exercise routine to relieve spasm and discomfort
- Instruct patients to report any weaknesses, eye symptoms, bladder or bowel incontinence immediately

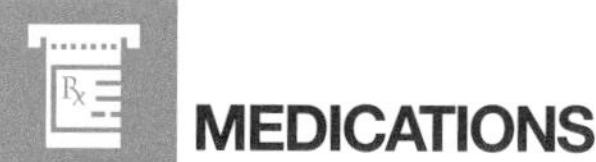

MEDICATIONS

DRUG(S) OF CHOICE

- Acetaminophen (Tylenol) 500 mg qid is the safest regimen. Studies have shown it to be at least as effective as NSAIDs.
- NSAIDs - aspirin 1.0 gm qid is effective in many cases. If this fails, any of the other NSAIDs are used with all having about the same success rate. Piroxicam 10 mg daily, tolmetin 600 mg tid are some examples. If aspirin therapy is used, salicylate levels should be obtained; therapeutic range is 10-30 mg/dL (0.724-2.17 mmol/L). Enteric coated aspirin may be helpful to minimize GI upset.
- Cortisone should not be used in long term management. Occasional injections of trigger zones with 40 mg methylprednisolone (Depo-Medrol) may be used, but this should be saved for severe exacerbations.
- Trigger point injection of lidocaine 1%, injected into the "hot areas", especially in the scapular area. Often as effective in relieving symptoms alone as when combined with methylprednisolone

Contraindications: NSAIDs, except aspirin, should not be used in patients with chronic liver disease. Use with caution in cases of ulcers. If NSAIDs are used, misoprostol (Cytotec) 200 μg qid should be given concomitantly.

Precautions: Patients on long term NSAIDs should be monitored with liver studies 6-8 weeks after initial treatment and then every 3-4 months

Significant possible interactions: Refer to manufacturer's profile of each drug

ALTERNATIVE DRUGS N/A

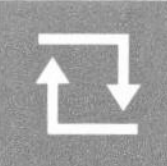

FOLLOWUP

PATIENT MONITORING Patients should be seen in 3-4 weeks for evaluation of neurologic status. If this has not changed follow at intervals of 3-6 months, depending on severity of symptoms.

PREVENTION/AVOIDANCE The midcervical spine is the area usually involved in spondylosis. This portion will develop a flexion deformity causing extension of the upper spine as the body tries to keep the head erect. Avoid any extension strain such as a "spinal manipulation," extension during intubation for a general anesthesia, or cervical strain from auto accidents, especially rear-end collisions. These can cause a basilar artery thrombosis or thrombosis of the posterior inferior cerebellar artery with a subsequent Wallenberg syndrome. Dysphagia, pain and temperature loss to the same side of the face and opposite side of the body, nystagmus and Horner syndrome are present in Wallenberg syndrome.

POSSIBLE COMPLICATIONS Loss of motion, especially extension, may require adjustments to certain occupations to prevent uncommonly significant muscle loss and instability of gait, bladder or bowel function

EXPECTED COURSE/PROGNOSIS

Fortunately, the prognosis is for a benign course in the overwhelming majority of cases, though for most of their lives patients will be plagued by pain which exacerbates often with no known cause

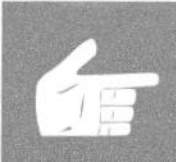

MISCELLANEOUS

ASSOCIATED CONDITIONS Cervical disk disease

AGE-RELATED FACTORS

Pediatric: N/A
Geriatric: N/A
Others: N/A

PREGNANCY As in the case of rheumatoid arthritis, the symptoms often improve but occasionally are made worse

SYNONYMS

- Cervical arthritis
- Cervical myelopathy
- Cervical osteophyte

ICD-9-CM

722.4 Degeneration of cervical intervertebral disc
721.0 Cervical spondylosis without myelopathy
721.1 Cervical spondylosis with myelopathy

SEE ALSO

OTHER NOTES N/A

ABBREVIATIONS

US-MS = ultrasonic treatment with muscle stimulation

REFERENCES

- McNab I: Cervical Spondylosis: Clinical Orthopedics 1975;109:69-77
- Clifton AG, et al: Identifiable causes for poor outcome in surgery for cervical spondylosis. Neuroradiology 1990;177(2):313-325
- Karnaze MG, et al: Comparison of MR and CT myelography in imaging the cervical and thoracic spine. American Journal of Roentgenography 1988;150(2);397-403

Web references: 0 available at www.5mcc.com
Illustrations N/A

Author(s):
R. Bruce Hall, MD

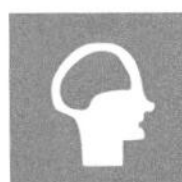

BASICS

DESCRIPTION An inflammation of the uterine cervix. Infectious cervicitis may be caused by Chlamydia trachomatis, Neisseria gonorrhoeae, herpes simplex or Trichomonas vaginalis.
- Chronic cervicitis is characterized by inflammation of the cervix without an identified pathogen

System(s) affected: Reproductive
Genetics: N/A
Incidence/Prevalence in USA:
- Gonorrhea 166/100,000
- Chlamydia 290/100,000 women
- Trichomonas 1200/100,000
- Gonorrhea 2% of sexually active women under age 30
- Chlamydia 5-35% of women
- Trichomonas 5-25%

Predominant age: Infectious cervicitis is most common in adolescents, but can be seen in women of any age
Predominant sex: Female only

SIGNS & SYMPTOMS
- Mucopurulent (yellow) discharge from the cervix
- Cervical erosion or erythema
- Easily induced endocervical mucosal bleeding
- Tenderness of cervix
- Postcoital bleeding
- Frequently asymptomatic

CAUSES
- Chlamydia trachomatis
- Neisseria gonorrhoeae
- Herpes simplex virus
- Trichomonas vaginalis
- Cause of chronic cervicitis unknown

RISK FACTORS
- Multiple sexual partners
- History of sexually transmitted disease
- Postpartum period

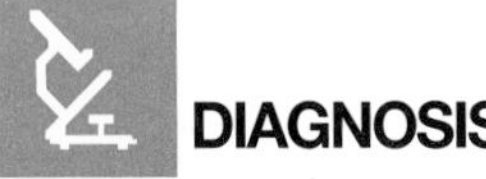

DIAGNOSIS

DIFFERENTIAL DIAGNOSIS
- Vaginal infections with Candida albicans or Trichomonas vaginalis extending onto the cervix
- Carcinoma of the cervix

LABORATORY
- Endocervical gram stain, more than 10 WBC's per high power field (hpf) suggests cervicitis
- Cervical cultures for *C. trachomatis, N. gonorrhoeae*
- Polymerase chain reaction (PCR) and ligase chain reaction (LCR) more sensitive than cultures for chlamydia. LCR can be used with urine.
- Enzyme immunoassays (EIAs) of endocervical swabs for chlamydia and gonorrhea
- Nucleic acid amplification tests (NAATs) are more sensitive and can also be used on urine specimens
- Wet mount for Trichomonas vaginalis
- If ulcerations present, culture for herpes simplex virus
- Venereal Disease Research Laboratory (VDRL) or rapid plasma reagin (RPR) to rule out concurrent syphilis

Drugs that may alter lab results: Recent antibiotic treatment

Disorders that may alter lab results: N/A

PATHOLOGICAL FINDINGS Inflammatory changes on Pap smear

SPECIAL TESTS N/A

IMAGING N/A

DIAGNOSTIC PROCEDURES Colposcopy is indicated in chronic inflammation, with biopsy of suspicious areas

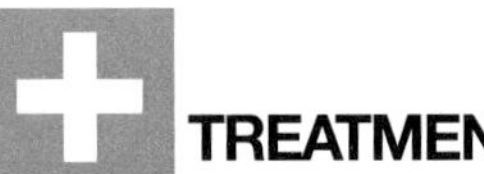

TREATMENT

APPROPRIATE HEALTH CARE Outpatient treatment

GENERAL MEASURES Chronic cervicitis with negative cultures and biopsies may be treated with cryosurgery

SURGICAL MEASURES N/A

ACTIVITY Full activity

DIET No special diet

PATIENT EDUCATION
- Advise patient to use condoms consistently
- If infectious etiology, advise patient to inform her partners

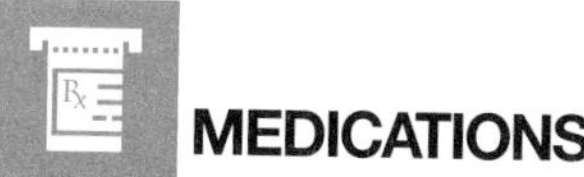

MEDICATIONS

DRUG(S) OF CHOICE

- If infectious cervicitis suspected, treat without awaiting culture results. Ceftriaxone (Rocephin) 125 mg IM single dose; followed by either doxycycline (Vibramycin) 100 mg po bid for 7 days or azithromycin (Zithromax) 1 g single dose.
- For Trichomonas, metronidazole (Flagyl) 2 g single dose
- For herpes, acyclovir (Zovirax) 200 mg po 5 times daily (or 400 mg tid) for 7 days
- Chronic cervicitis associated with postmenopausal vaginal atrophic changes may respond to topical estrogen creams

Contraindications:

- Doxycycline should not be used in pregnant or nursing mothers
- Metronidazole contraindicated in first trimester of pregnancy

Precautions: Doxycycline should not be taken with milk, antacids, or iron containing preparations

Significant possible interactions: Doxycycline - warfarin (Coumadin) and oral contraceptives may have their effectiveness reduced

ALTERNATIVE DRUGS

- Any of the following can be substituted for ceftriaxone (quinolones should not be used for gonorrhea in patients who have traveled to Hawaii, California, or Viet Nam because of high levels of resistance):
  ◊ Ofloxacin (Floxin) 400 mg po single dose
  ◊ Ciprofloxacin (Cipro) 500 mg po single dose
  ◊ Levofloxacin (Levaquin) 250 mg single dose
- Erythromycin base or stearate 500 mg po qid, or erythromycin ethylsuccinate 800 mg po qid can be substituted for doxycycline

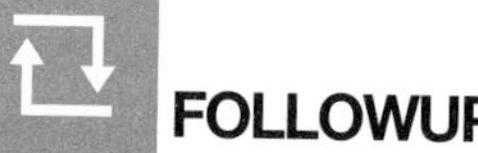

FOLLOWUP

PATIENT MONITORING

- Repeat cultures after treatment for chlamydia or gonorrhea are indicated in pregnant or high risk patients
- Annual Pap smears in sexually active patients screen for chronic cervicitis

PREVENTION/AVOIDANCE Patients with more than one sexual partner should be advised to use condoms at every encounter

POSSIBLE COMPLICATIONS

- Cervicitis with C. trachomatis or N. gonorrhoeae is associated with an 8-10% risk of subsequent pelvic inflammatory disease
- Moderate to severe inflammation is associated with condyloma acuminatum and cervical carcinoma

EXPECTED COURSE/PROGNOSIS

- Infectious cervicitis usually responds to systemic antibiotics
- Chronic cervicitis may be resistant to treatment, and should be monitored closely for cervical dysplasia

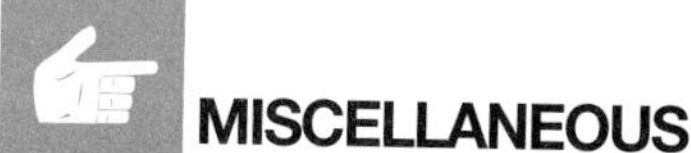

MISCELLANEOUS

ASSOCIATED CONDITIONS Patients with infectious cervicitis should be screened for other sexually transmitted diseases, syphilis, trichomonas, and possibly human immunodeficiency virus (HIV)

AGE-RELATED FACTORS

Pediatric: Infectious cervicitis in children should lead to investigation for possible sexual abuse

Geriatric:

- Chronic cervicitis in postmenopausal women may be related to lack of estrogen
- The possibility of infectious cervicitis should not be overlooked, as many geriatric patients remain sexually active

Others: Adolescents remain a high-risk group for sexually transmitted diseases

PREGNANCY Screen all pregnant women for infectious cervicitis because of the risk of transmission to the fetus

SYNONYMS Mucopurulent cervicitis

ICD-9-CM

616.0 Cervicitis and endocervicitis
098.15 Acute gonococcal cervicitis
079.88 Chlamydia infection
099.53 Other venereal diseases due to Chlamydia trachomatis, lower genitourinary sites

SEE ALSO

Cervical dysplasia
Cervicitis, ectropion & true erosion
Chlamydial sexually transmitted diseases
Gonococcal infections
Trichomoniasis

OTHER NOTES The presence of Trichomonas does not rule out other concurrent infection

ABBREVIATIONS N/A

REFERENCES

- Sexually Transmitted Diseases - Treatment Guidelines 2002: MMWR:51(No. RR-6):32-42
- Miller KE, Graves JC. Update on the prevention and treatment of sexually transmitted diseases. Am Fam Phys 2000;61(2):379-86
- Drug treatment of genital chlamydial infection. Drug & Therapeutics Bulletin 2001;39(4):27-30
- Screening Tests To Detect Chlamydia trachomatis and Neisseria gonorrhoeae Infections 2002;MMWR:51(No. RR-15):1-38
- Hollier LM, Workowski K. Treatment of sexually transmitted diseases in women. Obstet Gynecol Clin North Am 2003;30(4):751-5

Web references: 1 available at www.5mcc.com

Illustrations N/A

Author(s):
Barbara A. Majeroni, MD

BASICS

DESCRIPTION
- Cervicitis - inflammatory changes due to infections
- Ectropion - eversion of the cervix in pregnancy
- True erosion - loss of overlying vaginal epithelium due to trauma, e.g., forceful insertion of vaginal speculum in patient with atrophic mucosa

System(s) affected: Reproductive
Genetics: N/A
Incidence/Prevalence in USA:
- Cervicitis - very common in sexually active women
- Ectropion - with oral contraceptive use; very common in pregnant women
- True erosion - occasionally seen in postmenopausal women

Predominant age: Sexually active women
Predominant sex: Female only

SIGNS & SYMPTOMS
- Cervicitis - metrorrhagia, post-coital bleeding, vaginal discharge
- Ectropion - red cervix due to color of the columnar epithelium
- True erosion - vaginal bleeding, sharply defined ulcers of cervix

CAUSES
- Cervicitis - Chlamydia trachomatis, Trichomonas vaginalis
- Ectropion - hormonal changes with oral contraceptive use (especially with progesterone) or during pregnancy,
- True erosion - injury to atrophic epithelium due to estrogen deficiency in menopause

RISK FACTORS
- Cervicitis - sexual contact with infected partner(s), recurrence due to inadequate therapy
- Ectropion - pregnancy
- True erosion - estrogen deficiency, trauma

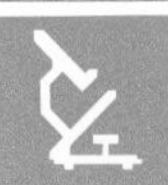

DIAGNOSIS

DIFFERENTIAL DIAGNOSIS
- Cervical dysplasia
- Carcinoma of the cervix

LABORATORY
- Saline and potassium hydroxide preparation of cervical/vaginal smears
- Chlamydiazyme or chlamydia cell culture, gonorrhea culture
- Papanicolaou (Pap) smear of the cervix
- Chlamydia DNA probe
- Gonorrhea DNA probe

Drugs that may alter lab results: N/A

Disorders that may alter lab results: N/A

PATHOLOGICAL FINDINGS
- Cervicitis - acute and chronic inflammatory changes, presence of infective organisms
- Ectropion - none/squamous metaplasia
- True erosion - sharply defined ulcer borders, loss of epithelium

SPECIAL TESTS None

IMAGING None

DIAGNOSTIC PROCEDURES Colposcopy

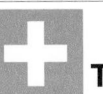

TREATMENT

APPROPRIATE HEALTH CARE Outpatient

GENERAL MEASURES N/A

SURGICAL MEASURES N/A

ACTIVITY No restrictions

DIET No special diet

PATIENT EDUCATION Provide printed material about sexually transmitted diseases and about estrogen deficiency and estrogen replacement therapy

MEDICATIONS

DRUG(S) OF CHOICE
- Trichomoniasis - metronidazole 500 mg bid for 7 days or 2 g once or 1 g bid for 2 doses
- Chlamydial infection - for non-pregnant women, doxycycline 100 mg bid po for 7 days; for pregnant women, erythromycin base 500 mg qid po for 7 days, or erythromycin ethylsuccinate 800 mg qid for 7 days
- Ectropion - none
- True erosion - estrogen, conjugated vaginal cream daily for 2 weeks, follow by estrogen replacement therapy

Contraindications:
- Metronidazole - first trimester of pregnancy
- Doxycycline - pregnancy or lactation
- Estrogen - see extended list of contraindications to estrogen use in standard texts

Precautions:
- Metronidazole - possible fetal harm if used in first trimester of pregnancy, disulfiram reaction with alcohol
- Doxycycline - possible fetal harm if used during pregnancy, staining of the infant's teeth if used during breast-feeding, allergy, photosensitization
- Erythromycin - nausea or vomiting
- Estrogens - history of estrogen dependent neoplasms, history of thromboembolic diseases, see extended list of contraindications to estrogen therapy in standard texts

Significant possible interactions:
- Metronidazole and alcohol
- Doxycycline and dairy products, iron preparations, warfarin, and oral contraceptives (use backup contraceptive method)
- Erythromycin with astemizole - may increase latter's levels with subsequent ECG changes
- Erythromycin and theophylline (elevated theophylline level)
- Estrogen - N/A

ALTERNATIVE DRUGS
- Metronidazole - sulfanilamide-aminacrine-allantoin cream (AVC cream)
- Doxycycline - erythromycin or azithromycin
- Erythromycin - clindamycin
- Estrogen - lubricant, same as that used for vaginal speculum
- Azithromycin 1 g for one dose only (pregnancy category B)
- Ofloxacin 300 mg bid x 7 days
- Amoxicillin-clavulanate (Augmentin) 250 mg po q8h for 7 days

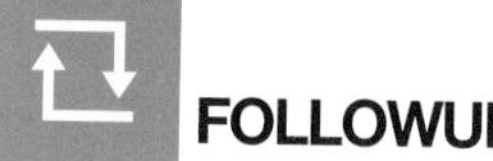

FOLLOWUP

PATIENT MONITORING
- Trichomoniasis - repeat vaginal smear until infection is cleared
- Chlamydial infection - repeat chlamydial culture post antibiotic therapy
- Estrogen deficiency - re-examine in one month to confirm healing

PREVENTION/AVOIDANCE
- Trichomoniasis or chlamydial infection - treatment of sexual partners and use of condom during coitus
- Estrogen deficiency - estrogen replacement therapy

POSSIBLE COMPLICATIONS N/A

EXPECTED COURSE/PROGNOSIS
- Cervicitis - excellent healing once infection is eradicated
- Ectropion - spontaneous regression postpartum, cessation or oral contraceptive use
- True erosion - spontaneous healing

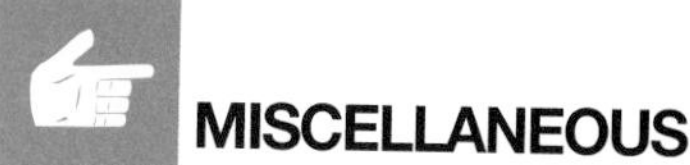

MISCELLANEOUS

ASSOCIATED CONDITIONS
- Gonorrhea
- Bacterial vaginosis

AGE-RELATED FACTORS
Pediatric: N/A
Geriatric: Menopause
Others: N/A

PREGNANCY
- Ectropion
- Azithromycin should be used with caution
- Doxycycline should not be used in pregnancy

SYNONYMS N/A

ICD-9-CM
616.0 Cervicitis and endocervicitis

SEE ALSO

OTHER NOTES N/A

ABBREVIATIONS N/A

REFERENCES

- Disaia PJ, Creasman WT: Clinical Gynecologic Oncology. 3rd Ed. St. Louis, The C.V. Mosby Company, 1989
- Herbst AL, Mishell DR, Stenchever MA, Droegemueller W: Comprehensive Gynecology. 2nd Ed. St. Louis, The C.V. Mosby Co., 1992
- Kurman RJ, ed: Blaustein's Pathology Of The Female Genital Tract. 3rd Ed. New York, Springer-Verlag, 1987
- Novak ER, Woodruff JD: Novak's Gynecologic and Obstetric Pathology With Clinical and Endocrine Relations. 8th Ed. Philadelphia, W.B. Saunders Company, 1979
- Lebhere TB: In: Hacker NF, Moore JG, eds. Essentials Obstetrics and Gynecology. 2nd Ed. Philadelphia, W.B. Saunders Co., 1992
- Iglesias E, Alderman E, Fox A. Use of wet smear to screen for sexually transmitted disease. Infections In Medicine 2000;17(3):175-85

Web references: 1 available at www.5mcc.com
Illustrations N/A

Author(s):
Albert T. Shiu, MD

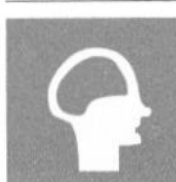

BASICS

DESCRIPTION A sexually transmitted disease characterized by painful genital ulcerations and inflammatory inguinal adenopathy. It is uncommon in the United States but found worldwide. Chancroid is endemic in developing countries and a cofactor for HIV transmission.
System(s) affected: Reproductive, Skin/Exocrine
Genetics: N/A
Incidence/Prevalence in USA: Fewer than 100 cases reported to the CDC in 2000-2002. Actual numbers felt to be greater due to underreporting of cases.
Predominant age: Teenagers and adults
Predominant sex: Male > Female

SIGNS & SYMPTOMS
- Tender genital papule that ulcerates after 24 hours
- Irregular edged, painful ulcer(s)
- Ulcers may be 1 mm to 5 cm in size
- Ulcers may occur on the shaft of the penis, glans and meatus in men
- Ulcers in women most commonly occur in labia majora but also seen in labia minora, perineum, thigh, and cervix
- Painful inguinal adenopathy with abscess (bubo) formation in 30% of patients
- Atypical presentations include folliculitis and foreskin abscess

CAUSES *Haemophilus ducreyi* (gram negative bacterium)

RISK FACTORS
- Multiple sexual partners
- Uncircumcised males
- Prostitutes often are carriers

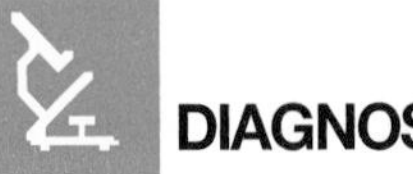

DIAGNOSIS

DIFFERENTIAL DIAGNOSIS
- Syphilis
- Herpes simplex virus (HSV 1 and 2)
- Lymphogranuloma venereum (LGV)
- Granuloma inguinale

LABORATORY Serologic testing for antibody with ELISA technique. Gram stain; culture of organism on Mueller-Hinton agar with incorporated vancomycin. Polymerase chain reaction (PCR) where available.

Drugs that may alter lab results: Previous antibiotics

Disorders that may alter lab results: None expected

PATHOLOGICAL FINDINGS "School of fish" pattern on gram stain

SPECIAL TESTS N/A

IMAGING N/A

DIAGNOSTIC PROCEDURES
- Gram stain and culture of ulcer exudate
- Aspiration of inguinal bubo (lymph node)
- PCR testing of ulcer exudate for *H. Ducreyi* DNA
- Dark-field examinations of exudate to rule out Treponema pallidum
- Culture or PCR testing for HSV

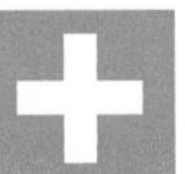

TREATMENT

APPROPRIATE HEALTH CARE Outpatient treatment

GENERAL MEASURES
- Saline or Burow's solution soaks to ulcers
- Aspiration of buboes if greater than 5 cm; done through adjacent uninvolved skin

SURGICAL MEASURES N/A

ACTIVITY Refrain from sexual intercourse until genital lesions fully resolved

DIET N/A

PATIENT EDUCATION
- Sexual counseling
- Use of condoms
- Local wound care
- Treatment of all sexual partners with same regimen as index case
- HIV testing

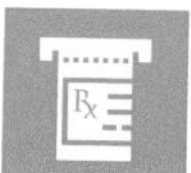

MEDICATIONS

DRUG(S) OF CHOICE

- Azithromycin 1 gm po single dose (more expensive than other treatments)
- Ceftriaxone 250 mg IM single dose
- Ciprofloxacin 500 mg po bid for 3 days or other quinolone
- Erythromycin base 500 mg qid x 7 days

Contraindications:

- Allergy to the medication
- Ciprofloxacin in pregnancy and lactation, and patients less than age 18

Precautions: Refer to manufacturer's profile of each drug

Significant possible interactions: Refer to manufacturer's profile of each drug

ALTERNATIVE DRUGS N/A

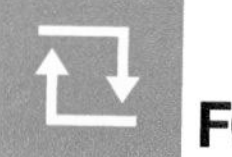

FOLLOWUP

PATIENT MONITORING

- Patient followed until all clinical signs of infection resolved
- Should see symptomatic improvement within 3 days and objective improvement by day 7
- Baseline syphilis serology and at 3 months
- HIV testing at baseline and at 3 months post-treatment

PREVENTION/AVOIDANCE

Avoidance of sexual activity until ulcers resolved

POSSIBLE COMPLICATIONS

- Phimosis
- Balanoposthitis
- Rupture of buboes with fistula formation and scarring

EXPECTED COURSE/PROGNOSIS

- Full clinical resolution with appropriate treatment
- 5% relapse after treatment
- Primary infection is not believed to provide immunity

MISCELLANEOUS

ASSOCIATED CONDITIONS

- Syphilis - concurrently in 10% of patients (per new CDC data)
- HSV or HIV infection

AGE-RELATED FACTORS N/A

Pediatric: N/A

Geriatric: N/A

Others: HIV disease may affect treatment response

PREGNANCY

Maternal to infant transmission has not been reported

SYNONYMS

- Soft chancre
- Ulcus molle

ICD-9-CM

099.0 Chancroid

SEE ALSO

Syphilis

OTHER NOTES

Chancroid has been shown to be an established risk factor for acquisition of HIV infection

ABBREVIATIONS N/A

REFERENCES

- Centers for Disease Control and Prevention. Sexually Transmitted Diseases Treatment Guidelines - 2002. MMWR 2002 / 51(RR06);1-80]
- Montero JA. Chancroid: An update. Infect Med 2002;191:174-8
- Schulte JM, Schmid G. Recommendations for treatment of chancroid. Clin Infect Dis 1995;20(Suppl 1):539-46
- Trees DL, Morse SA. Chancroid and haemophilus ducreyi: an update. Clin Microbiol Rev 1995;8(3):357-75

Web references: 0 available at www.5mcc.com

Illustrations N/A

Author(s):

Jeffery T. Kirchner, DO

BASICS

DESCRIPTION A common, highly contagious, childhood exanthem characterized by the development of typical crops of vesicles on the skin and mucous membranes.

- The virus is spread by respiratory droplets or direct contact with vesicles or indirectly through freshly soiled articles
- Outbreaks tend to occur from January to May
- The usual incubation period is 14-16 days (range 11-21). Patients are infectious from approximately 48 hours before appearance of the rash until the final lesions have crusted. Most people acquire chickenpox during childhood and develop long immunity.

System(s) affected: Nervous, Skin/Exocrine
Genetics: No known genetic pattern
Incidence/Prevalence in USA: Common
Predominant age: Peak incidence 5-9 years, but may occur at any age
Predominant sex: Male = Female

SIGNS & SYMPTOMS

- Prodromal symptoms - fever, malaise, anorexia, mild headache
- Characteristic rash - crops of "teardrop" vesicles on erythematous bases
- Lesions erupt in successive crops
- Progress from macule to papule to vesicle, then begin to crust
- Rash present in various stages of development
- Pruritic
- Usually begins on trunk, then spreads to face and scalp
- Minimal involvement of the extremities
- Lesions may be present on mucous membranes, oral and vaginal

CAUSES

- Human (alpha) herpesvirus 3 (varicella-zoster virus, V-Z virus), a member of the Herpesvirus group; a double-stranded DNA virus. (Reservoir: humans.)

RISK FACTORS

- No prior history of varicella
- Immunosuppressed (especially children with leukemia/lymphoma in remission or on high-dose corticosteroids)

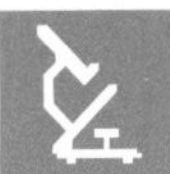

DIAGNOSIS

DIFFERENTIAL DIAGNOSIS

- Herpes simplex
- Herpes zoster
- Impetigo
- Coxsackievirus infection
- Papular urticaria
- Scabies
- Dermatitis herpetiformis
- Drug rash
- Rickettsialpox

LABORATORY

- Leukocyte count may be normal, low, or mildly increased
- Marked leukocytosis is suggestive of secondary infection
- Multinucleated giant cells on Tzanck smear from scrapings of vesicles
- Isolated virus from human tissue culture

Drugs that may alter lab results: N/A

Disorders that may alter lab results:

- Herpes zoster
- Herpes simplex

PATHOLOGICAL FINDINGS

- Skin lesions histologically identical to herpes simplex virus
- In fatal cases intranuclear inclusions can be found in the endothelium of blood vessels and most organs

SPECIAL TESTS

For complicated cases and epidemiologic studies:

- Visualization of the virus by EM
- Serologic testing by FAMA or ELISA
- Detection of viral DNA by PCR

IMAGING N/A

DIAGNOSTIC PROCEDURES N/A

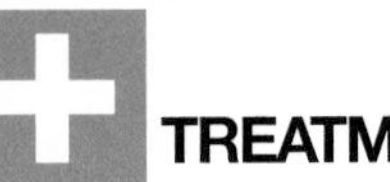

TREATMENT

APPROPRIATE HEALTH CARE Outpatient except for complicating emergencies

GENERAL MEASURES

- Supportive/symptomatic treatment
- Good hygiene to avoid secondary infection

SURGICAL MEASURES N/A

ACTIVITY As tolerated. Children may return to school when lesions have scabbed over, temperature is normal and sense of well-being has returned.

DIET No special diet

PATIENT EDUCATION Griffith: Instructions for Patients; Philadelphia, Elsevier

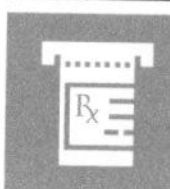

MEDICATIONS

DRUG(S) OF CHOICE
- Antipyretics for fever
- Avoid aspirin because of its link to Reye syndrome
- Local and/or systemic antipruritic agents for itching
- In immunocompromised host - varicella-zoster immune globulin (VZIG) available for passive immunization. VZIG must be given within 96 hours after exposure to be beneficial. After 4th day postexposure, wait for rash to develop then give acyclovir 500 mg/m2/day intravenously every 8 hours for 7 days.
- Acyclovir - decreases duration of fever and shortens time of viral shedding. Recommended for adolescents, adults and high-risk patients. Most beneficial if initiated early in the disease (≤ 24 hours).
  - ◊ 2-16 yr: 20 mg/kg/dose (max. 800 mg/dose), qid for 5 days
  - ◊ Adults: 800 mg, 5 times daily.

Contraindications: Hypersensitivity to the drug
Precautions: Possible renal insufficiency with acyclovir
Significant possible interactions: Concurrent administration of probenecid increases half-life. Increased effect with zidovudine (drowsiness, lethargy)

ALTERNATIVE DRUGS
- Famciclovir 500 mg tid x 7-10 days
- Valacyclovir 1 gm tid x 7-10 days
- Vidarabine
- Interferon

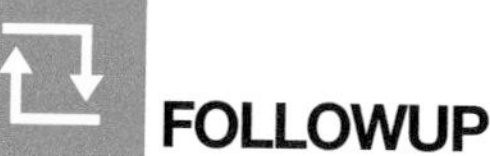

FOLLOWUP

PATIENT MONITORING Usually none in mild cases. If complications occur, intensive supportive care may be required.

PREVENTION/AVOIDANCE
- Exposed, susceptible individuals considered infectious for 21 days
- Isolation of hospitalized patients
- Passive immunization with ZIG, VZIG, or the intravenous formulation of ZIP. Both ZIG and VZIG should be given within 96 hours (preferably within 72 hours) of exposure to ensure efficacy. ZIP can be given somewhat later. Recommended for persons exposed to chickenpox or shingles within 96 hours who are immunocompromised, ≥15 years old without prior history of chickenpox, newborns of mothers with onset of chickenpox < 5 days before delivery or < 2 days after delivery. Exposure criteria: continued household contact, prolonged face-to-face contact (same room), or indoor playmate > 1 hour.
- Varicella vaccine effectiveness decreases significantly after 1 year (most cases of breakthrough disease are mild). If administered at younger than 15 months, the vaccine's effectiveness was lower in the first year after vaccination, but the difference in effectiveness was not statistically significant for subsequent years.
- Varicella-Virus vaccine (Varivax) - a live attenuated vaccine approved by the FDA and recommended by ACIP for immunization of healthy individuals, 12 months and above, who have not had chickenpox
  - ◊ 12m-12y: single dose 0.5 mL SC. Cumulative efficacy 70-90%.
  - ◊ 13y and above: two 0.5 mL SC doses 4-8 weeks apart. Efficacy 70%.
  - ◊ Has been shown to prevent or significantly reduce the severity of varicella if given within 72 hours and possibly up to 5 days, postexposure in several studies
  - ◊ Maybe considered for a subset of HIV positive children in CDC Class I with CD4 > 25%
- Vaccine recipients should avoid contact with immunocompromised people, and pregnant women who have never had chickenpox and their newborns, for up to 6 weeks after vaccination

POSSIBLE COMPLICATIONS
- Secondary bacterial infection - cellulitis, abscess, erysipelas, sepsis, septic arthritis/osteomyelitis, staphylococcal pyomyositis
- Pneumonia (20-30% of adults with chickenpox have lung involvement)
- Encephalitis (the most common CNS complication)
- Reye syndrome
- Purpura
- Lymphadenitis
- Nephritis

EXPECTED COURSE/PROGNOSIS
- In the healthy child, chickenpox is rarely a serious disease and recovery is complete
- Confers long immunity
- Second attack rare, but subclinical infection common
- Infection latent and may recur years later as herpes zoster in adults (and sometimes in children)
- Fatalities rarely occur from complications

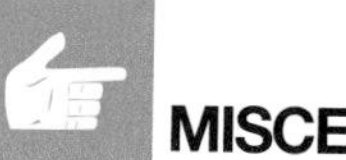

MISCELLANEOUS

ASSOCIATED CONDITIONS N/A

AGE-RELATED FACTORS
Pediatric:
- Neonates born to mothers who develop chickenpox 5 days before or 2 days after delivery are at risk for serious disease. Must give VZIG.
- Varicella bullosa seen mainly in children under two. Lesions appear as bullae instead of vesicles. Clinical course unchanged.
- Case-fatality (in USA) 2/100,000
- Most common cause of death: septic complications and encephalitis

Geriatric:
- Infection more severe than in children
- Latent varicella infection may reactivate and cause the exanthem shingles or zoster
- Case-fatality 30/100,000
- Most common cause of death: primary viral pneumonia

Others: N/A

PREGNANCY Risk of transplacental infection following maternal infection is 25%. Congenital malformations are seen in 5% when the fetus is infected during the 1st or 2nd trimester. There is an increased morbidity for women infected during pregnancy (e.g., pneumonia).

SYNONYMS
- Varicella

ICD-9-CM
052.9 Varicella without mention of complication

SEE ALSO
Herpes zoster
Immunizations

OTHER NOTES N/A

ABBREVIATIONS
ACIP = Advisory Committee on Immunization Practices
FAMA = fluorescent antibody to membrane antigen
ZIG = zoster immune globulin
ZIP = zoster immune plasma
DNA = deoxyribonucleic acid
EM = electron microscopy
PCR = polymerase chain reaction
VZIG = varicella-zoster immune globulin

REFERENCES

- Mandell GL, editor. Principles and Practice of Infectious Diseases. 5th ed. New York: Churchill Livingstone; 2000
- Benenson, AS, editor. Control of Communicable Diseases Manual. 16th ed. Baltimore, United Book Press, Inc, 1995
- Fauci AS, editor. Harrison's Principles of Internal medicine. 15th ed. New York: McGraw-Hill; 2001
- Vazquez M, LaRussa PS, et al. Effectiveness over time of varicella vaccine. JAMA 2004;291(7):851-5

Web references: 2 available at www.5mcc.com
Illustrations 6 available

Author(s):
Kathryn Reilly, MD, MPH

BASICS

DESCRIPTION

- Emotional abuse: sustained, repetitive, inappropriate emotional response to the child's experience of emotion and its accompanying expressive behavior
- Psychological abuse: sustained, repetitive, inappropriate behavior which damages or substantially reduces the creative and developmental potential of crucially important mental faculties and mental processes of a child
- Physical abuse: injury to a child caused by a caretaker for no apparent reason including reaction to unwanted behavior. The use of an instrument on any part of the body is abuse, i.e., belt.
- Sexual abuse: any contact or interaction between a child and another person in which the child is sexually exploited for the gratification or profit of the perpetrator. Offenders can be juveniles.
- Neglect: occurs when those responsible for meeting the basic needs of a child fail to do so, either acute or chronic

System(s) affected: Endocrine/Metabolic, Gastrointestinal, Musculoskeletal, Nervous, Reproductive, Skin/Exocrine

Genetics: N/A

Incidence/Prevalence in USA: More than 1.4 million per year (1 in 2000 die); extremely difficult to estimate

Predominant age: 7 years old

Predominant sex: Male = Female

SIGNS & SYMPTOMS

- Non-specific symptoms of abuse
  - ◊ Behavior regression
  - ◊ Anxiety, depression
  - ◊ Sleep disturbances, night terrors
  - ◊ Increased sex play
  - ◊ School problems
  - ◊ Self-destructive behaviors
- Physical abuse
  - ◊ Children do not suffer life-threatening injuries in household falls
  - ◊ May be no physical signs
  - ◊ Skin markings (lacerations, burns, ecchymoses, linear contusions)
  - ◊ Contusions with definite shapes (coat hangers, belt buckles)
  - ◊ Circular contusions on trunks or limbs (finger pressure points)
  - ◊ Bites
  - ◊ Cigarette burns on palms, extremities
  - ◊ Immersion injuries with clearly demarcated lines
  - ◊ Oral trauma (torn frenulum, loose teeth)
  - ◊ Ear trauma (ear pulling)
  - ◊ Eye trauma (hyphema, hemorrhage)
  - ◊ Abdominal blunt trauma
  - ◊ Fractures
  - ◊ Head trauma
- Sexual abuse
  - ◊ Unequivocal abnormalities are found in a small number of children (2-8%)
  - ◊ Abuse often consists of fondling, rubbing and other contacts not likely to produce detectable injuries
  - ◊ Unexplained vaginal injuries or bleeding
  - ◊ Pregnancy
  - ◊ Sexually transmitted diseases
  - ◊ Sexual promiscuity/prostitution
  - ◊ Erythema and increased vascularity of the perihymenal tissues
  - ◊ Increased friability of the posterior fourchette
  - ◊ Hymenal attenuation and asymmetry, lacerations, especially if hymenal margin is altered
  - ◊ Perianal lacerations, scars and fissures, circumferential edema (Tyre sign), delta-shaped abrasion
  - ◊ May be no physical signs
- Neglect
  - ◊ May be small, thin, dirty, with rashes
  - ◊ Fearful or too trusting
  - ◊ Clinging to or avoiding mother
  - ◊ Flat or balding occiput
  - ◊ Abnormal development or growth parameters

CAUSES
Not well-defined

RISK FACTORS
May be many, but poverty (5 times greater risk), parental substance abuse, lower educational status, maternal history of abuse and negative maternal attitude toward pregnancy appear to be strongly associated, history of parent(s) having been abused, mentally ill parent, parental isolation, presence of domestic violence, family history

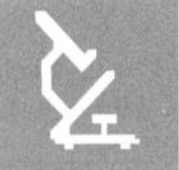

DIAGNOSIS

DIFFERENTIAL DIAGNOSIS

- Physical trauma
  - ◊ Accidental injury
  - ◊ Bleeding disorders (e.g., classic hemophilia)
  - ◊ Metabolic diseases (e.g., vitamin K deficiency)
  - ◊ Congenital (type I Ehlers-Danlos syndrome)
  - ◊ Salicylate toxicity
  - ◊ Conditions with skin manifestations: Mongolian spots, Henoch-Schönlein purpura, purpura fulminans of meningococcemia, erythema multiforme, hypersensitivity vasculitis, platelet aggregation disorders, disseminated intravascular coagulation (DIC), phytophotodermatitis, car seat burns, staphylococcal scalded skin syndrome, chicken pox, impetigo, osteogenesis imperfecta, congenital syphilis
- Neglect
  - ◊ Endocrinopathies (e.g., diabetes mellitus, diabetes insipidus, thyroid disorders, adrenal problems, pituitary problems)
  - ◊ Constitutional
  - ◊ GI (clefts, chalasia, gastroesophageal reflux, celiac disease, inflammatory bowel disease)
  - ◊ Cystic fibrosis
  - ◊ Liver disease
  - ◊ Renal tubular acidosis
  - ◊ CNS abnormalities
- Skeletal trauma
  - ◊ Obstetrical trauma
  - ◊ Prematurity
  - ◊ Nutritional - metabolic defects (scurvy, rickets, mucolipidosis II, secondary hyperparathyroidism)
  - ◊ Infection (congenital syphilis, osteomyelitis)
  - ◊ Osteogenesis imperfecta
  - ◊ Infantile cortical hyperostosis
  - ◊ Leukemia
  - ◊ Histiocytosis X
  - ◊ Metastatic neuroblastoma

LABORATORY

- Urinalysis, urine culture and sensitivity
- CBC
- Electrolytes, creatinine, BUN, glucose
- May add PT, PTT, bleeding time, platelet count, factor XIII, urine toxicology screen

Drugs that may alter lab results: N/A

Disorders that may alter lab results: See Differential Diagnosis

PATHOLOGICAL FINDINGS

- Spiral fractures in non-ambulatory patients
- Chip fractures or bucket-handle fractures (classic for abuse)
- Epiphyseal - metaphyseal rib fractures in infants
- Rupture of liver and spleen in abdominal blunt trauma
- Retinal hemorrhages in shaken baby syndrome
- Abnormalities strongly suggesting sexual abuse include: Recent or healed lacerations of the hymen and vaginal mucosa, proctoepisiotomy, bite marks
- The presence of sperm is a definitive finding of child abuse

SPECIAL TESTS

- Sexual abuse
  - ◊ Wet mount for motile sperm and one fixed for cytopathology exam for sperm
  - ◊ Tests for gonorrhea, chlamydia
  - ◊ Serum pregnancy tests
  - ◊ Rapid plasma reagin (RPR)
  - ◊ Consider HIV testing (repeat in 6 months)
  - ◊ Acid phosphatase test of secretions for sperm
  - ◊ If the assault occurred within 72 hours of the examination, samples should be collected for the forensic laboratory (contact police investigator for proper protocol)
- Neglect
  - ◊ Stool exam
  - ◊ Calorie count
  - ◊ Purified protein derivative (PPD) and anergy panel
  - ◊ Sweat test
  - ◊ Lead and zinc protoporphyrin levels

IMAGING

- Photographs
- Chest x-ray, skeletal survey (skull frontal and lateral, lateral thoracolumbar spine, frontal upper extremities to include shoulder girdle and hands, frontal lower extremities to include lower lumbar spine, pelvis and feet)
- In some hospitals a standard set of x-rays called a SNAT (suspected non-accidental trauma) series is defined
- Possible bone scan

DIAGNOSTIC PROCEDURES
Consider photocolposcopy in sexual abuse

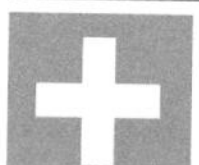

TREATMENT

APPROPRIATE HEALTH CARE
- Acute episodes, especially of sexual abuse, are often best managed in an emergency room equipped for collecting forensic specimens and maintaining "chain of evidence"
- Hospital admission for children with moderate to severe injuries, unstable neurologic or cardiovascular exams and those with acute psychological trauma
- If not hospitalized, a child should be sent to another relative or arrange for foster care if the suspected abuser lives with the child
- Counseling is imperative
- Mandatory reporting to Child Protective Authorities
- Counseling for entire family
- Consultation with local child abuse specialist advisable

GENERAL MEASURES
- After initial evaluation, consider referral to sexual assault center
- Always explain what the physical exam will involve and why certain procedures are necessary
- Examine child in a quiet, comfortable setting and allow child to choose who will be in the room
- To examine female genitalia, use dorsolithotomy position for older girls and the "frog leg" position for younger girls
- Examine anus of all young children in prone knee-chest position

SURGICAL MEASURES As clinically indicated

ACTIVITY As clinically indicated

DIET As clinically indicated

PATIENT EDUCATION Counsel family not to use negative terms such as "ruined," "violated," or "dirty" in reference to the child. The child's emotional reaction to abuse will be profoundly influenced by the responses of adult caretakers.

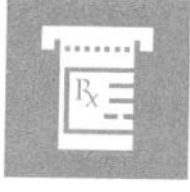

MEDICATIONS

DRUG(S) OF CHOICE Antibiotics as indicated for treatment of documented sexually-transmitted disease
Contraindications: Refer to manufacturer's profile of each drug
Precautions: Refer to manufacturer's profile of each drug
Significant possible interactions: Refer to manufacturer's profile of each drug

ALTERNATIVE DRUGS Other postcoital contraceptive drugs

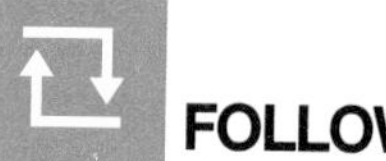

FOLLOWUP

PATIENT MONITORING Patient must be referred to the appropriate state protective services and followed as closely as clinically and psychologically indicated

PREVENTION/AVOIDANCE Early detection of and intervention in dysfunctional families whenever possible

POSSIBLE COMPLICATIONS Long-term physical and psychological damage

EXPECTED COURSE/PROGNOSIS Without intervention, child abuse is a recurrent and escalating phenomenon

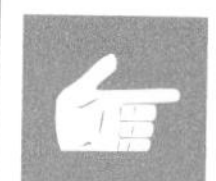

MISCELLANEOUS

ASSOCIATED CONDITIONS
- Failure-to-thrive
- Shortfalls in development
- Poor school performance
- Poor social skills
- Psychological illnesses

AGE-RELATED FACTORS
Pediatric: N/A
Geriatric: N/A
Others: N/A

PREGNANCY Use of ethinyl estradiol and norgestrel (Ovral) reduces rate of pregnancy after rape to under 2% which is one-third the rate that would be expected without intervention. It is thought to work by making the uterine lining inhospitable to implantation and must be considered an abortifacient in this setting.

SYNONYMS
- Battered child syndrome
- SNAT
- Child maltreatment

ICD-9-CM
995.50 Child abuse, unspecified

SEE ALSO

OTHER NOTES When documenting an examination on an allegedly or suspected abused child, especially in cases of possible sexual abuse, never record "findings not consistent with abuse" or "no evidence of abuse." Simply record findings and note that the findings neither exclude nor confirm allegations of abuse. The absence of physical findings does not indicate the child's history is incorrect.

ABBREVIATIONS
SNAT = suspected non-accidental trauma

REFERENCES

- Reece RM, ed. Pediatric Clinics of North America, Vol 37, No. 4. Philadelphia, W.B. Saunders Co, August 1990
- Rosenstein BJ, Fosarelli PD. Pediatric Pearls. Yearbook Medical Publishers, Inc, 1989:330-4
- Flaherty EG, Weiss H. Medical Evaluation of Abused and Neglected Children. American Journal of Diseases of Children 1990;144
- Muram D. Child Sexual Abuse. Obstetrics and Gynecology Clinics of North America 1992;19(1)
- Child Abuse and Neglect Statistical Fact Sheet. National Clearinghouse on Child Abuse Information, 1996
- Gibbons M, Vincent EC. Childhood Sexual Abuse. Amer Fam Phys 1994;49:125-36
- O'Hagan KP: Emotional and psychological abuse: Problems of definition. Child Abuse and Neglect 1995;19:4
- Mcintosh BJ. Child abuse. AAFP Home Study Audio 2000;273:9-15

Web references: 0 available at www.5mcc.com
Illustrations 3 available

Author(s):
Sumner T. McAllister, MD
Hugh S. Smith, MD

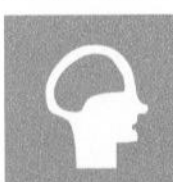

BASICS

DESCRIPTION *Chlamydia pneumoniae*, an obligate intracellular bacteria, has been established as an important cause of adult respiratory disease including pneumonia, bronchitis, sinusitis and pharyngitis. There is no animal reservoir.
System(s) affected: Pulmonary
Genetics: No known genetic predisposition
Incidence/Prevalence in USA: Estimated incidence of 100 to 200 cases of pneumonia/100,000/year. Accounts for 6 to 12% of pneumonias and 3 to 6% of bronchitis cases. Numbers do not necessarily apply to all areas. Incidence of subclinical infection much greater.
Predominant age: Less common in children under 5 years. Pneumonia more common in elderly.
Predominant sex: Male > Female (10-25% more)

SIGNS & SYMPTOMS
- 70% to 90% of infections are mild or subclinical
- Onset often gradual with delayed presentation
- Sore throat and hoarseness may precede cough by a week or more, giving biphasic appearance to illness
- Cough (often prominent with scant sputum)
- Fever (usually early in illness)
- Sore throat
- Rhinitis
- Headache
- Malaise
- Hoarseness
- Sinus congestion
- Rales, rhonchi or wheezing
- Pharyngeal erythema
- Retropharyngeal lymphoid granulation

CAUSES Infection with *C. pneumoniae*

RISK FACTORS
- Outbreaks have occurred among groups of military recruits, university students, students and nursing home residents. Incubation period is approximately 30 days. Sporadic cases often have no apparent source of exposure. No known animal hosts.
- Serologic evidence of acute and chronic *C. pneumoniae* infection found in approximately 1/3 of patients admitted to hospital with acute COPD exacerbation, often together with other concurrent bacterial infection
- Associated with acute respiratory exacerbation in children with cystic fibrosis

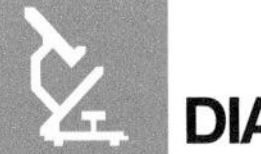

DIAGNOSIS

DIFFERENTIAL DIAGNOSIS Consider other common bacterial respiratory pathogens, including *Streptococcus*, *Bordetella*, *Haemophilus*, *Klebsiella*, *Mycoplasma* and *Legionella* species

LABORATORY
- Leukocyte count usually normal or low
- Sedimentation rate often moderately elevated
- Sputum usually negative by gram stain and routine culture

Drugs that may alter lab results: Early treatment with tetracycline may blunt IgG antibody response

Disorders that may alter lab results: None known

PATHOLOGICAL FINDINGS Not usually available

SPECIAL TESTS
- *C. pneumoniae* can be identified from clinical specimens (not sputum) by culture in HL or HEp2 and by polymerase chain reaction (PCR). Both culture and PCR require a sophisticated laboratory and are not widely available.
- Serologic testing with microimmunofluorescence (MIF) antibody and enzyme immunoassay (EIA) antibody are both commercially available. Testing with MIF is recommended by the CDC. EIA is less specific. Testing acute and convalescent (at least 3 weeks after disease onset) sera is preferable.

IMAGING
- Chest radiograph may be abnormal even in clinically mild disease
- Variable radiographic abnormalities include unilateral and bilateral infiltrates and pleural effusions. Single, subsegmental infiltrate is common.

DIAGNOSTIC PROCEDURES Definite diagnosis of acute infection requires a positive culture or PCR or a four-fold rise in antibody titer. Very high antibody titer or antibody in the IGM fraction suggest a recent infection.

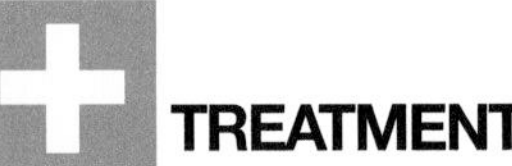

TREATMENT

APPROPRIATE HEALTH CARE
- Usually outpatient
- Patients with severe pneumonia or coexisting illness may require hospitalization

GENERAL MEASURES No specific general measures

SURGICAL MEASURES N/A

ACTIVITY Usually reduced during illness

DIET No special diet

PATIENT EDUCATION
- Griffith HW: Instructions for Patients; Philadelphia, W.B. Saunders Co.
- For a listing of sources for patient education materials favorably reviewed on this topic, physicians may contact: American Academy of Family Physicians Foundation, P.O. Box 8418, Kansas City, MO 64114, (800)274-2237, ext. 4400

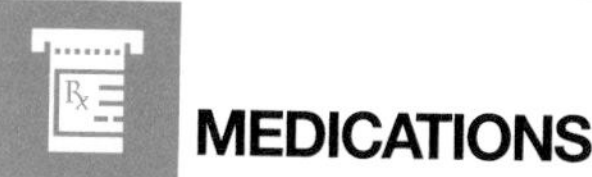

MEDICATIONS

DRUG(S) OF CHOICE
- Azithromycin (Zithromax) 500 mg on day 1, then 250 mg a day on days 2 through 5

or
- Clarithromycin (Biaxin) 500 mg po every 12 hours for 10-14 days

or
- Tetracycline 500 mg po qid for at least 14 days

or
- Doxycycline 100 mg po q 12 hours for at least 14 days

Contraindications:
- Tetracycline not for use in pregnancy or children < 8 years.

Precautions: Tetracycline may cause photosensitivity; sunscreen recommended.

Significant possible interactions:
- Tetracyclines may increase the anticoagulant effect of warfarin
- Broad-spectrum antibiotics may reduce the effectiveness of oral contraceptives; barrier method recommended.

ALTERNATIVE DRUGS
- Erythromycin base 250-500 mg qid for 14-21 days
- Levofloxacin 250-500 mg qd PO or IV
- Beta-lactam (penicillin based) antibiotics and sulfisoxazole not effective

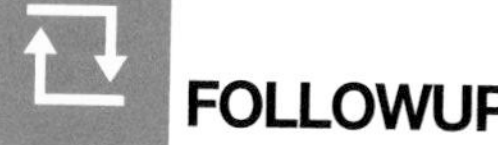

FOLLOWUP

PATIENT MONITORING Weekly until well, for response to treatment and resolution of radiographic abnormalities

PREVENTION/AVOIDANCE
- Transmission presumably via respiratory secretions. Avoid infected persons.
- Hand washing

POSSIBLE COMPLICATIONS
- Reactive airway disease
- Erythema nodosum
- Otitis media
- Endocarditis
- Myocarditis
- Pericarditis
- Sarcoidosis
- Meningitis/encephalitis
- Reactive arthritis
- Acute chest syndrome in sickle cell disease
- Associated with atherosclerotic disease - effect of treatment unknown

EXPECTED COURSE/PROGNOSIS
- Resolution of cough and malaise often requires several weeks or longer
- Chronic bronchospastic disease has been reported following acute infection
- Persistent or relapsed symptoms may respond to second course of antibiotics

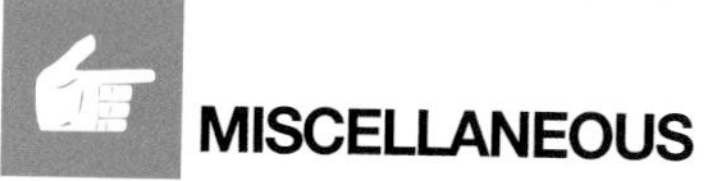

MISCELLANEOUS

ASSOCIATED CONDITIONS
- Chronic obstructive pulmonary disease
- HIV infection
- Cystic fibrosis

AGE-RELATED FACTORS
Pediatric: Usually milder disease in children
Geriatric: Usually more severe in older adults
Others: None known

PREGNANCY
- No known special risks
- Tetracyclines contraindicated

SYNONYMS
- TWAR

ICD-9-CM
078.88 Other specified diseases due to Chlamydiae

SEE ALSO
Pneumonia, mycoplasma
Psittacosis

OTHER NOTES
- No significant seasonal variation
- Most cases occur sporadically, though intrafamilial spread also occurs
- Infection in debilitated or hospitalized patients can be severe
- Reinfection is possible
- Individuals have been reported who are persistently culture positive despite antibiotic treatment
- Country-wide epidemics of *C. pneumoniae* infections have been documented in the Scandinavian countries
- Found in atherosclerotic plaque in coronary arteries, carotid arteries and the aorta. Also associated with MI and stroke in seroepidemiologic studies. Role in atherogenesis in humans not established. Clinical significance not known.

ABBREVIATIONS N/A

REFERENCES

- Kauppinen M, Saikku P. Pneumonia due to Chlamydia pneumoniae: prevalence, clinical features, diagnosis and treatment. Clin Infect Dis 1995;21:s244-252
- Jackson LA, Grayston JT. Chlamydia pneumoniae (TWAR). In: Mandell GI, Bennett JE, Dolin R, editors. Principles and Practices of Infectious Disease. 5th ed. New York: Churchill Livingstone; 2000. p.2007-10
- Miyashita N, Fukano H, Okimoto N, et al. Clinical presentation of community-acquired Chlamydia pneumoniae pneumonia in adults. Chest 2002;121(6):1776-81

Web references: 1 available at www.5mcc.com
Illustrations N/A

Author(s):
David H. Thom, MD, PhD
J. Thomas Grayston, MD

BASICS

DESCRIPTION An obligate intracellular membrane-bound prokaryotic organism, chlamydia trachomatis causes an estimated 3 million new sexually transmitted infections in the US each year. The estimated cost of chlamydia STDs in 1994 was $2 billion per year in the U.S., largely due to costly complications such as PID, infertility, and ectopic pregnancy. Studies indicate that 75-90% of women and 50-90% of men with chlamydial STD are asymptomatic. Persons with asymptomatic infection can remain infectious for years. Currently many more women than men are screened, leaving a large male reservoir of infection.
System(s) affected: Reproductive
Genetics: Unknown
Incidence/Prevalence in USA: 3-5% general medical population, 5-15% of teens and young adults, 10-20% STD clinics
Predominant age: 15-25
Predominant sex: Male = Female

SIGNS & SYMPTOMS A substantial majority of cases are asymptomatic. Of those with symptoms, the following are most common:
- Males
  - ◊ Urethritis
  - ◊ Epididymitis
  - ◊ Proctitis
  - ◊ Reiter syndrome
- Females
  - ◊ Cervicitis - typically mucopurulent
  - ◊ Urethral syndrome
  - ◊ Bartholinitis
  - ◊ Endometritis
  - ◊ Salpingitis/pelvic inflammatory disease (PID)
  - ◊ Fitz-Hugh-Curtis perihepatitis syndrome
- Infants
  - ◊ Conjunctivitis
  - ◊ Pneumonitis
  - ◊ Carriage-pharynx/GI tract
- Symptoms most strongly associated with chlamydia include urethral or cervical discharge, and pelvic or testicular pain. Persons with such symptoms, or with rectal pain, discharge, or tenesmus, should be tested for chlamydia.
- While chlamydia (and gonorrhea) can cause mucopurulent cervicitis (MPC), these organisms cannot be isolated from most cases of MPC, and most women who have these organisms do not have MPC. Therefore, neither women with mucopurulent cervicitis nor their partners should be treated empirically for chlamydia in the absence of other evidence supporting such treatment.

CAUSES Chlamydia trachomatis serovars D-K

RISK FACTORS
- Risk correlates with number of sexual partners
- Risk correlates inversely with age

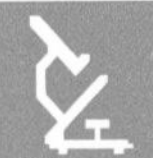

DIAGNOSIS

DIFFERENTIAL DIAGNOSIS
- Neisseria gonorrhea
  - ◊ Urethritis
  - ◊ Proctitis
  - ◊ Epididymitis
  - ◊ Cervicitis
  - ◊ PID
  - ◊ Bartholin's abscess
  - ◊ Perihepatitis
- Ureaplasma urealyticum
  - ◊ Urethritis, epididymitis
  - ◊ Reiter disease
  - ◊ PID
- Chlamydia trachomatis (Serovars LI-3)
  - ◊ Lymphogranuloma venereum
  - ◊ Proctitis

LABORATORY
- Chlamydial cell culture - sensitivity 50-70%, specificity 100%, takes up to 7 days
- Antigen detection and enzyme immunoassay - sensitivity 50-90%
- Direct fluorescent antibody detection (DFA) - sensitivity ≈75% in an experienced lab technician's hands; specificity > 99%
- Amplified molecular testing (e.g., PCR, LCR, SDA, HCS, TMA) - sensitivity ≈ 95%, specificity ≈ 99%, rapid turnaround times, urine or swab specimens, relatively expensive

Drugs that may alter lab results: Amplified molecular tests may remain positive for as long as three weeks after successful treatment

Disorders that may alter lab results: Many amplified molecular tests are not approved for rectal or pharyngeal chlamydia

PATHOLOGICAL FINDINGS N/A

SPECIAL TESTS N/A

IMAGING N/A

DIAGNOSTIC PROCEDURES Specimens should contain cell scrapings rather than inflammatory discharge, since the organism lives only inside the epithelial cells

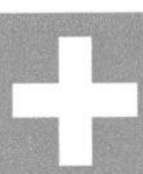

TREATMENT

APPROPRIATE HEALTH CARE Outpatient, unless moderately or severely ill with PID or other complications

GENERAL MEASURES
- All patients with known or suspected chlamydia should be tested for gonorrhea, syphilis, and HIV (the latter requires individual counseling and consent)
- Some experts recommend that all patients treated for chlamydia should be treated empirically for gonorrhea simultaneously, unless they are known to be negative for gonorrhea by sensitive lab testing
- All partners of patients treated for chlamydia should be tested if possible but treated empirically regardless, rather than waiting for test results
- Some experts recommend treating partners of men being treated for non-specific urethritis, others recommend testing partners and waiting for test results
- Neither women with mucopurulent cervicitis nor their partners should be treated empirically for chlamydia in the absence of other evidence supporting such treatment

SURGICAL MEASURES N/A

ACTIVITY Abstain from sexual contact until diagnosis and treatment complete for patient and all partners

DIET N/A

PATIENT EDUCATION
- Risk-reduction counseling
- Safe sex practices, such as barrier protection
- Serious sequelae of chlamydial disease such as tubal infertility, chronic pelvic pain
- Stress need to finish entire course of antibiotics
- For a listing of sources for patient education materials favorably reviewed on this topic, physicians may contact: American Academy of Family Physicians Foundation, P.O. Box 8418, Kansas City, MO 64114, (800)274-2237, ext. 4400

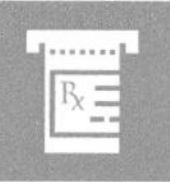

MEDICATIONS

DRUG(S) OF CHOICE

- Urethritis, cervicitis, sexual partners of infected persons
  - ◊ Doxycycline - 100 mg po bid x 7 days
  - ◊ Azithromycin - 1 gm orally in a single dose
  - ◊ Pregnant women - erythromycin base, 250 mg po qid x 14 days
- Other chlamydial syndromes
  - ◊ Epididymitis - tetracycline, doxycycline, erythromycin for 10-14 days as above.
  - ◊ Pelvic inflammatory disease - doxycycline for 10-14 days to cover the chlamydial component of PID (gonorrhea and anaerobic organisms must be treated as well; see CDC recommendations: ceftriaxone 250 mg IM once, cefoxitin, other 3rd generation cephalosporin, or a quinolone), erythromycin for 10-14 days may be needed in pregnant or tetracycline intolerant females to treat chlamydial component.

Contraindications: Tetracyclines (e.g., doxycycline) and quinolones (e.g., ofloxacin, levofloxacin) contraindicated in children and pregnant women

Precautions: Tetracyclines: may cause photosensitivity; sunscreen recommended

Significant possible interactions:

- Tetracyclines: avoid concurrent administration with antacids, dairy products, or iron
- Broad-spectrum antibiotics: may reduce the effectiveness of oral contraceptives; barrier method recommended

ALTERNATIVE DRUGS

- Erythromycin base 500 mg po qid x 7 days
- Erythromycin ethylsuccinate 800 mg po qid x 7 days
- Ofloxacin 300 mg po bid x 7 days
- Levofloxacin 500 mg po daily x 7 days

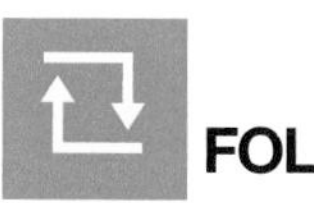

FOLLOWUP

PATIENT MONITORING

- Test of cure is not routine, although it is reasonable to retest persons treated with erythromycin one to two months after treatment
- Sexual partners need to be evaluated and treated empirically if necessary, to prevent passing the disease back and forth between partners. Partnerships with community health departments should be fostered to assist with partner tracing.
- Lack of resolution or recurrence of symptoms must be immediately reported to the physician
- Severe cases of urethritis/cervicitis as well as the chlamydial syndromes should be seen in followup after completion of therapy
- Up to 25% of asymptomatic patients screened for chlamydia may not return for treatment post-chlamydia culture results. Strategies must be developed to insure treatment can be instituted.

PREVENTION/AVOIDANCE

- Populations with prevalence >5% should be screened at least annually. These include:
  - ◊ New or more than one sex partner in last 6 months
  - ◊ Attending adolescent or family planning clinic
  - ◊ Attending an STD or abortion clinic
  - ◊ Attending a jail or other detention center or clinic
  - ◊ Rectal pain, discharge, or tenesmus
  - ◊ Testicular pain
  - ◊ All sexually active woman <25 years old
  - ◊ Consider for all sexually active men <25 years old (studies are pending)
- Only sure way to avoid infection is abstinence, which is not a viable option for many patients. Risk reduction counseling is an effective prevention measure, emphasizing using barrier protection (e.g., condoms) and minimizing the number of different sex partners. Modifiable risk behaviors related to number of sex partners include alcohol or drug use.

POSSIBLE COMPLICATIONS

- Enhances transmission of and susceptibility to HIV in both sexes
- Males
  - ◊ Transient oligospermia
  - ◊ Post epididymitis urethral stricture (rare)
- Females
  - ◊ Tubal infertility
  - ◊ Tubal pregnancy
  - ◊ Chronic pelvic pain

EXPECTED COURSE/PROGNOSIS

Prognosis good with early and compliant therapy. However, due to the asymptomatic nature of early disease and the population affected, symptomatic PID still accounts annually for 2.5 million outpatient visits and more than one quarter million hospitalizations.

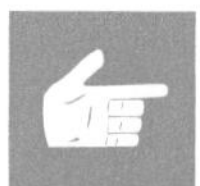

MISCELLANEOUS

ASSOCIATED CONDITIONS

- Pelvic inflammatory disease, epididymitis, cervicitis, urethritis
- Other diseases caused by other chlamydial species:
  - ◊ Psittacosis - Chlamydia psittaci
  - ◊ Pneumonia - Chlamydia pneumoniae - Chlamydia trachomatis (infants)
  - ◊ Lymphogranuloma venereum - Chlamydia trachomatis serovars L1-L3
  - ◊ Trachoma - Chlamydia trachomatis serovars A-C

AGE-RELATED FACTORS

Pediatric: N/A

Geriatric: N/A

Others: Prevalence inversely proportional to age (after onset of sexual activity)

PREGNANCY Perinatal acquisition may result in neonatal pneumonia and/or conjunctivitis. Tetracycline and ofloxacin contraindicated in pregnancy; erythromycin or azithromycin should be used in this situation.

SYNONYMS N/A

ICD-9-CM

615.9 Unspecified inflammatory disease of uterus, except cervix

616.0 Cervicitis and endocervicitis

616.10 Vaginitis and vulvovaginitis, unspecified

SEE ALSO

Cervicitis
Epididymitis
Gonococcal infections
HIV infection & AIDS
Pelvic inflammatory disease (PID)
Syphilis
Urethritis

OTHER NOTES N/A

ABBREVIATIONS

- STD = sexually transmitted disease
- PID = pelvic inflammatory disease
- HIV = human immunodeficiency virus
- MPC = mucopurulent cervicitis

REFERENCES

- Stamm WE, Holmes K, et al. Chlamydia trachomatis Infections in the Adult. In: Sexually Transmitted Diseases. 2nd ed. New York: McGraw-Hill; 1990
- Centers for Disease Control and Prevention: Sexually Transmitted Disease Treatment Guidelines 2002. MMWR 2002;51(RR-6):32-6
- Hook EW III, et al. Use of cell culture and a rapid diagnostic assay for Chlamydia trachomatis screening. JAMA 1995;272(11):867
- Heath C, Heath J. Chlamydia trachomatis infection update. Am Fam Phys 1995;52:1455-61
- Stamm WE. Chlamydia trachomatis - The persistent pathogen. Sexually Transmitted Diseases 2001;28(12):684-9
- US Preventive Services Task Force: Screening for Chlamydial Infection: Recommendations and Rationale. American Journal of Preventive Medicine 2001;20(3S):90-4
- Turner CF, Rogers SM, et al. Untreated gonococcal and chlamydial infection in a probability sample of adults. JAMA 2002;287(6):726-33
- Swain GR, McDonald RA, et al. Decision analysis: point-of-care chlamydia testing vs. laboratory-based methods. Clinical Medicine & Research 2004;2(1):29-35

Web references: 0 available at www.5mcc.com

Illustrations N/A

Author(s):

Geoffrey R. Swain, MD, MPH

Cholangitis (acute)

BASICS

DESCRIPTION Bacterial infection of the bile duct system that is associated with obstructive biliary duct pathology
System(s) affected: Gastrointestinal
Genetics: N/A
Incidence/Prevalence in USA: N/A
Predominant age: 55-70 years, rare in children, more common in adults
Predominant sex: Female > Male

SIGNS & SYMPTOMS
May have only one or two symptoms, and the abdominal exam may be unrevealing
- Right upper quadrant pain (RUQ), not severe
- Jaundice
- Chills and fever
- Shock
- CNS depression

CAUSES
- Biliary tract obstruction from:
  - ◊ Stones
  - ◊ Tumor (pancreatic, CBD, ampulla, metastatic)
  - ◊ Benign strictures (postsurgical, PSC)
  - ◊ Parasites (Ascaris)
  - ◊ Pancreatitis
  - ◊ Blood clots
- Reflux of small bowel bacteria
  - ◊ Choledochoenterostomy
  - ◊ "Sump syndrome"
- Other
  - ◊ Cholecystitis
  - ◊ Bacteriemia
  - ◊ Surgical, radiographic, endoscopic manipulation
  - ◊ Biliary stent

RISK FACTORS
- Cholelithiasis
- Endoscopic or surgical manipulation
- Foreign bodies, such as parasites, biliary stent

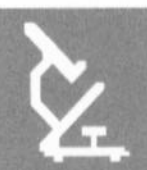

DIAGNOSIS

DIFFERENTIAL DIAGNOSIS
- Acute cholecystitis - pain and tenderness are invariably present. (May be very difficult to distinguish between cholangitis and acute cholecystitis).
- Pyogenic liver abscess
- Hepatitis
- Acute pancreatitis
- Perforated duodenal ulcer
- Pelvic inflammatory disease with peritonitis
- Kidney stones
- Pancreatitis

LABORATORY
- Increasing WBC with left shift
- Hyperbilirubinemia - in 90%
- Alkaline phosphatase - increasing in 90%
- Positive blood culture - in 50% (gram negative aerobes, and some anaerobes)

Drugs that may alter lab results: N/A

Disorders that may alter lab results: N/A

PATHOLOGICAL FINDINGS In acute toxic disease, pus under pressure in the common bile duct

SPECIAL TESTS
- Need to delineate underlying biliary tract abnormality
- Cholangiography is definitive test
- Percutaneous transhepatic cholangiography (PTC) or endoscopic retrograde cholangiopancreatography (ERCP)

IMAGING Ultrasound will diagnose gallbladder stones and common bile duct size, but will demonstrate common bile duct calculi in less than 15%

DIAGNOSTIC PROCEDURES Cholangiography as described above

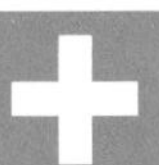

TREATMENT

APPROPRIATE HEALTH CARE Inpatient

GENERAL MEASURES Control sepsis, then evaluate with cholangiography and treat underlying biliary tract pathology. Urgent bile duct decompression may be necessary.

SURGICAL MEASURES
- Patients who do not respond to antibiotics and supportive care require emergency decompression of the biliary duct system. This may be accomplished by surgery, endoscopy, or transhepatic cholangiography.
- In case of obstruction secondary to stones, endoscopic papillotomy and stone extraction will drain the duct and may be definitive treatment of the underlying cause and is shown to reduce mortality

ACTIVITY As tolerated

DIET Nothing by mouth until acute phase is terminated

PATIENT EDUCATION For patient education materials favorably reviewed on this topic, contact: National Digestive Diseases Information Clearinghouse, Box NDDIC, Bethesda, MD 20892, (301)468-6344

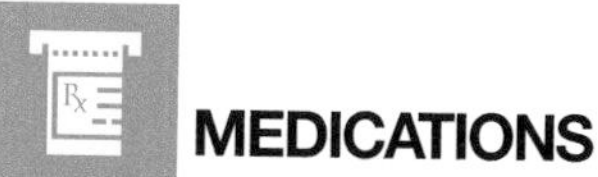

MEDICATIONS

DRUG(S) OF CHOICE
- Antibiotic regimen should cover gram negative aerobes, enterococci, and anaerobes.
  - ◊ Ampicillin 1 gm q6h IV (substitute ciprofloxacin or levofloxacin in penicillin allergic patient) +
  - ◊ Aminoglycoside (e.g., tobramycin, amikacin is an alternative but is expensive) +
  - ◊ Metronidazole 500 mg q8h IV

Contraindications: Refer to manufacturer's profile of each drug
Precautions: Renal toxicity of aminoglycoside therapy; check peak and trough levels
Significant possible interactions: Refer to manufacturer's profile of each drug

ALTERNATIVE DRUGS
- Piperacillin-tazobactam (Zosyn) OR
- Ampicillin-sulbactam (Unasyn) OR
- Ticarcillin-clavulanate (Timentin)

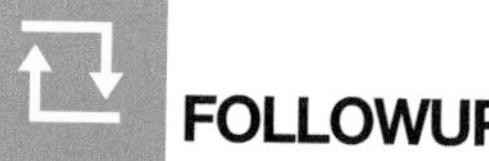

FOLLOWUP

PATIENT MONITORING Requires careful monitoring of hemodynamic parameters

PREVENTION/AVOIDANCE Cholangiography when indicated at time of cholecystectomy with endoscopic, radiographic, or surgical clearance of retained CBD stones

POSSIBLE COMPLICATIONS
- Hepatic abscess
- Sepsis
- Hepatic dysfunction

EXPECTED COURSE/PROGNOSIS
- Acute cholangitis - good
- Acute toxic cholangitis - mortality high

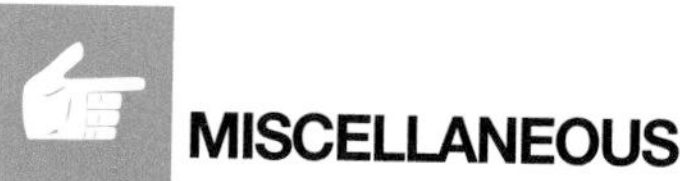

MISCELLANEOUS

ASSOCIATED CONDITIONS
- Choledocholithiasis
- Malignant tumors
- Benign strictures
- Biliary-enteric anastomosis
- Invasive procedures
- Foreign bodies
- Parasites
- Secondary sclerosing cholangitis

AGE-RELATED FACTORS
Pediatric: N/A
Geriatric: N/A
Others: N/A

PREGNANCY N/A

SYNONYMS N/A

ICD-9-CM
576.1 Cholangitis

SEE ALSO
Cholelithiasis

OTHER NOTES N/A

ABBREVIATIONS N/A

REFERENCES

- Nahrwold DL: Cholangitis. In: Sabiston DC, ed. Textbook of Surgery. 15th Ed. Philadelphia, W.B. Saunders Co., 1996
- Boeg JH, Way LW: Acute Cholangitis. Ann Surg 1980;191:264
- Pitt HA, Longmire WP Jr: Suppurative Cholangitis. In: Hardy JM, ed. Critical Surgical Illness. 2nd Ed. Philadelphia, W.B. Saunders Co., 1980

Web references: 0 available at www.5mcc.com
Illustrations N/A

Author(s):
Mark Horattas, MD

BASICS

DESCRIPTION
Inflammation of the gallbladder occurring acutely or chronically, often secondary to previously asymptomatic gallstones.

System(s) affected: Gastrointestinal

Genetics: Increased prevalence in Native Americans and Caucasians, less prevalent in African Americans

Incidence/Prevalence in USA:
- Increases with age, body mass index. Prevalence by ultrasound surveys:
  - ◊ By age 30, 30% of Native Americans
  - ◊ By age 60, 80% of Native Americans
  - ◊ By age 60, 30% of Caucasians
  - ◊ By age 60, 20% of African Americans

Predominant age: 5th and 6th decade

Predominant sex: Female > Male (2:1)

SIGNS & SYMPTOMS
- Asymptomatic. 5-10% become symptomatic each year.
- Acute cholecystitis
  - ◊ Abdominal pain - sudden onset, intense, in epigastrium or right upper quadrant, radiates to shoulder or back. Pathognomonic feature is "biliary colic" a pain rising over 2-3 minutes to a plateau of intensity that is maintained for > 20 minutes.
  - ◊ Nausea and vomiting
  - ◊ Recurrent attacks following meals by 1-6 hours, lasting > 12 hours until recovered, usually < 3 days
  - ◊ Elevated temperature - mild to moderate
  - ◊ Local tenderness, rarely diffuse
  - ◊ Murphy's sign - inspiratory arrest elicited when palpating right upper quadrant while asking the patient for deep inhalation
  - ◊ Palpable gall bladder - 5% of cases
- Common duct stone
  - ◊ Jaundice in 50%
  - ◊ Biliary colic 60%
  - ◊ Fever and chills 30%
  - ◊ Pruritus 10%
  - ◊ Loose bowel movements, light color
  - ◊ Mild to marked hepatomegaly > 80%
  - ◊ Tenderness infrequent
  - ◊ Palpable gall bladder 10%
  - ◊ Gallstone ileus (rare)
  - ◊ Gallstone > 3 cm fistulizes into bowel and obstructs at ileocecal area
  - ◊ Antecedent pain, often over weeks with non-biliary colic
  - ◊ Abdominal distension, mild tenderness
  - ◊ Air in biliary passages on plain x-ray
  - ◊ Intestinal obstruction at level of terminal ileum
- Pancreatitis
  - ◊ Pain over upper abdomen
  - ◊ Nausea and vomiting
- Empyema
  - ◊ Phlegmon of obstructed gall bladder
  - ◊ Insidious weight loss, mild wasting
  - ◊ Gradual onset of occult infection signs, fever, anorexia
  - ◊ Mass usually present
  - ◊ Tenderness usually absent
- Chronic cholecystitis
  - ◊ Associated with gallstones, often asymptomatic; 20% become symptomatic over 15-20 years
  - ◊ Mild dyspepsia following fatty meals

CAUSES
- Gallstones in 90-95% of cases. May obstruct the cystic duct, leading to acute cholecystitis; obstruction of the common bile duct, causing jaundice, or obstruction of the pancreatic duct, causing pancreatitis.
- Gallbladder sludge, a viscous material, insoluble in bile, that layers on sonogram, and occasionally produces cholecystitis, common duct obstruction or pancreatitis. Occurs in most pregnant women, most total parenteral nutrition, and most patients with rapid weight loss
- Acalculous cholecystitis in 5% of cases. Associated with severe stressful situations including cardiac surgery, multiple trauma. May be associated with ischemic damage to the gallbladder wall.
- Bacteria. Usually do not initiate the inflammation but important in the complications of empyema and ascending cholangitis. In emphysematous cholecystitis, Clostridia are probably responsible for both initiation and complications.
- Neoplasms and strictures of common bile duct. Usually associated with cholangitis and pancreatitis.

RISK FACTORS
- Cardiac surgery
- Trauma
- Biliary parasites
- Gallstones (see topic Cholelithiasis)
- Rapid weight loss
- Prolonged parenteral alimentation
- Pregnancy

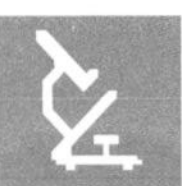

DIAGNOSIS

DIFFERENTIAL DIAGNOSIS
Acute pancreatitis, ulcer, diverticulitis, pyelonephritis, pneumonitis, hepatic abscess, hepatic tumors, Irritable bowel disease, non-ulcer dyspepsia

LABORATORY
- Acute cholecystitis
  - ◊ Leukocytosis - 12,000-15,000
  - ◊ Liver tests usually abnormal; ALT, AST slightly elevated, alkaline phosphatase, GGT elevated with common duct obstruction
- Common duct stone
  - ◊ High bilirubin in 50%, in 100% after 10 days
  - ◊ Elevated alkaline phosphatase and gamma glutamyl transpeptidase (GGT) in 85%
  - ◊ Positive blood culture in 15%
  - ◊ Barely abnormal ALT, AST
  - ◊ Elevated fasting bile salts
  - ◊ Elevated WBC if infection
  - ◊ Serum amylase may be elevated. If > 1000 units, concomitant pancreatitis should be considered.

Drugs that may alter lab results:
- Steroids
- Immunosuppressive drugs. These may mask leukocytosis and early signs of inflammation.

Disorders that may alter lab results:
- Old age, malnutrition
- Lymphoma, other immunocompromised states

PATHOLOGICAL FINDINGS
N/A

SPECIAL TESTS
99mTc Imino diacetic acid (HIDA) scan - highly sensitive (97%) for diagnosis of acute cholecystitis. HIDA derivatives are taken up by hepatocytes and excreted in bile and concentrated in gallbladder. Failure to see gallbladder in 1 hour is highly suspicious for acute cholecystitis. Usually abnormal in acalculous cholecystitis.

IMAGING
- Plain radiographs (upright)
  - ◊ 20% of gallstones are radiopaque
  - ◊ Air cholangiogram if there is gallbladder-gut fistula
  - ◊ Emphysematous cholecystitis - air in the gallbladder wall or in lumen
- Ultrasonography
  - ◊ Best technique to diagnose gallstones (high sensitivity - 95%, and specificity - 98%)
  - ◊ Best noninvasive imaging technique to diagnose acute cholecystitis. Findings include thick gall bladder wall (> 3 mm), gallbladder distension, sludge in lumen, pericholecystic fluid.
- CT scan
  - ◊ No advantage over ultrasonography in gallstone/acute cholecystitis diagnosis
  - ◊ Better than ultrasonography to detect enlargement of pancreas. Helpful in the diagnosis of abscess formation. Shows thickened gall bladder wall in cancer.
  - ◊ Better than US for dilated common bile duct

DIAGNOSTIC PROCEDURES
- Ultrasound or CT scan often diagnostic
- Tc HIDA test during acute pain
- Endoscopic retrograde cholangiopancreatography (ERCP) - to see status of biliary and pancreatic ducts
- Percutaneous transhepatic cholangiography test (PTC) - gives more information about intrahepatic biliary system
- Magnetic resonance almost as sensitive as ERCP to detect common bile duct stones. Endoscopic ultrasound is superior to ERCP in detecting common duct stones and has fewer complications.
- Laparotomy - if unable to make diagnosis by less invasive means

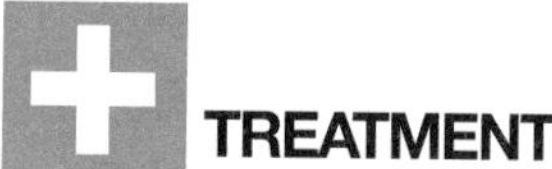

TREATMENT

APPROPRIATE HEALTH CARE
- Outpatient for patients with mild symptoms
- Inpatient - patients with biliary colic lasting for more than 6 hours and showing toxicity, jaundice, rigors, or requiring narcotics for pain
- Ascending cholangitis is a surgical emergency. If laparotomy is inappropriate, drainage can be obtained by ERCP or transhepatic cholangiography.
- Direct drainage of gallbladder by invasive radiologist occasionally required

GENERAL MEASURES
NPO, IV fluids, nasogastric suction

SURGICAL MEASURES
- Surgery (cholecystectomy) is the appropriate treatment for symptomatic cholecystitis
  - ◊ Best performed by laparoscopy, but a standard laparotomy is acceptable
  - ◊ Mortality rate - 0.1% in age <50 years and 0.8% age >50
  - ◊ Early cholecystectomy is the general practice rather than delayed interval cholecystectomy (delay only if surgery is contraindicated).
- If there is jaundice, evaluation of the common bile duct is essential by intraoperative cholangiogram, or by a separate ERCP
- Laparoscopic cholecystostomy
  - ◊ Rapidly replacing alternative surgical drainage procedure
  - ◊ If the patient is a poor risk, drainage of the gallbladder or biliary passages can be achieved by radiological or endoscopic techniques. This will allow control of infection and jaundice for several weeks or months.
- Dissolution therapy - rarely used if laparoscopic cholecystectomy can be performed
  - ◊ Ursodeoxycholic acid (Actigall) in 10 mg/kg is the drug of choice
  - ◊ To be effective there must be a functioning gallbladder on oral cholecystography
  - ◊ Stones must be free of calcium. Few small stones have best prognosis to dissolve. An alternative drug is chenodeoxycholic acid (Chenodiol) 12-15 mg/kg/day.
- Other indications for emergency surgery include - toxic patient, doubtful diagnosis, perforation or abscess

ACTIVITY
As tolerated by the patient

DIET
- NPO during acute cholecystitis
- Fatty meals precipitate mild attacks. Avoid if possible.

PATIENT EDUCATION
National Digestive Diseases Information Clearinghouse, Box NDDIC, Bethesda, MD 20892, (301) 468-6344

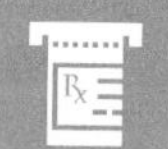

MEDICATIONS

DRUG(S) OF CHOICE
- Mild attack
  - ◊ Diclofenac 75 mg IV may abort early attack
  - ◊ Ampicillin 4-6 gm/day or cefazolin (Ancef) 2-4 gm/day
- Severe attack - gentamicin 3-5 mg/kg/day and clindamycin 1.8-2.7 gm/day. A penicillin could be added if needed.
- The formation of gallstones during rapid weight loss after bariatric surgery or severe diets is prevented by ursodiol (ursodeoxycholic acid) 10 mg/kg/day
- Formation of gallstones in prolonged parenteral alimentation is prevented by daily feeding of 100 kcal or daily injection of cholecystokinin

Contraindications: Hypersensitivity reactions

Precautions:
- Nephrotoxicity, ototoxicity with aminoglycosides
- Adjust the dose according to creatinine clearance

Significant possible interactions: Refer to manufacturer's profile of each drug

ALTERNATIVE DRUGS
For acute cholecystitis - 3rd generation cephalosporins

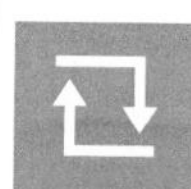

FOLLOWUP

PATIENT MONITORING
Post cholecystectomy - follow through postoperative period

PREVENTION/AVOIDANCE
- Avoid risk factors when possible
- During rapid weight loss following bariatric surgery or very low calorie diets, ursodeoxycholic acid (ursodiol)10 mg/kg/day
- During total parenteral alimentation for more than one month, daily ingestion of 100 kcal, or injection of cholecystokinin

POSSIBLE COMPLICATIONS
Occur in about 5% cases of acute cholecystitis and include - perforation, abscess formation, fistula formation (intestine, colon, cutaneous), gangrene, empyema, cholangitis, hepatitis, pancreatitis, gallstone ileus, carcinoma

EXPECTED COURSE/PROGNOSIS
- In general the prognosis is good for gallbladder disease. Those who die during acute episodes are mainly due to other conditions, especially coronary artery disease.
- Symptomatic gallstones usually have recurrent symptoms in 3 to 6 months indicating need for future action
- After cholecystectomy, stones may recur in bile ducts

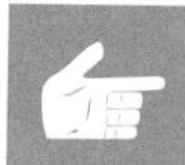

MISCELLANEOUS

ASSOCIATED CONDITIONS
- Pancreatitis
- Hemolytic anemias such as sickle cell disease, spherocytosis
- Cirrhosis, hypersplenism

AGE-RELATED FACTORS
Pediatric: N/A
Geriatric: Sometimes difficult to diagnose; complications more likely; cholecystectomy mortality rate higher
Others: N/A

PREGNANCY
N/A

SYNONYMS
N/A

ICD-9-CM
574.00 Calculus of gallbladder with acute cholecystitis, without mention of obstruction
574.11 Calculus of gallbladder with other cholecystitis, with obstruction
575.0 Acute cholecystitis
575.10 Cholecystitis, unspecified
574.01 Calculus of gallbladder with acute cholecystitis, with obstruction

SEE ALSO
Adenocarcinoma of the gallbladder
Cholangitis (acute)
Choledocholithiasis
Cholelithiasis
Jaundice

OTHER NOTES
Lithotripsy - can be used in patients with chronic cholecystitis. Contraindications - stones greater than 25 mm, more than 3 stones, calcified stones, bile duct stones, poor general condition. Largely replaced by laparoscopic cholecystectomy.

ABBREVIATIONS
N/A

REFERENCES

- Trowbridge RL, Rutkowski NK, Shojania KG. Does this patient have acute cholecystitis? JAMA 2003;289(1):80-6
- Puc MM, Tran HS, Wry PW, Ross SE. Ultrasound is not a useful screening tool for acute acalculous cholecystitis in critically ill trauma patients. Am Surg 2002;68(1):65-9
- Indar AA, Beckingham IJ. Acute cholecystitis. BMJ 2002;21;325(7365):639-43
- Cameron IC, Chadwick C, Phillips J, Johnson AG. Acute cholecystitis--room for improvement? Ann R Coll Surg Engl 2002;84(1):10-3
- Chopra S, Dodd GD 3rd, Mumbower AL, et al. Treatment of acute cholecystitis in non-critically ill patients at high surgical risk: comparison of clinical outcomes after gallbladder aspiration and after percutaneous cholecystostomy. AJR Am J Roentgenol 2001;176(4):1025-31
- Soto JA. Bile duct stones: diagnosis with MR cholangiography and helical CT. Seminars in Ultrasound, CT & RM 1999;20:304-16

Web references: 1 available at www.5mcc.com
Illustrations N/A

Author(s):
Frank L. Iber, MD

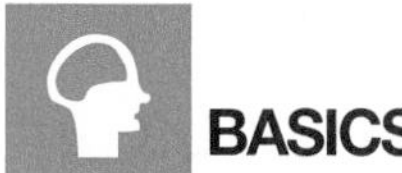

BASICS

DESCRIPTION Stones in common bile duct that migrate from the gallbladder. Calcium bilirubinate stones may form de novo.
System(s) affected: Gastrointestinal
Genetics: N/A
Incidence/Prevalence in USA: Up to 10% of patients with gallbladder stones discovered at time of cholecystectomy
Predominant age: Incidence increases with age
Predominant sex: Female > Male

SIGNS & SYMPTOMS
- May be asymptomatic
- Biliary colic
- Common bile duct obstruction
- Cholangitis
- Pancreatitis
- Pain can't be differentiated from pain arising from gallbladder
- Epigastric pain
- Abdominal tenderness
- Pain unrelieved by antacids
- Anorexia, vomiting
- Dark urine
- Light colored feces
- Right upper quadrant tenderness
- Palpable gallbladder
- Jaundice

CAUSES
- Chronic hemolytic states
- Hepatobiliary parasitism
- Duct stricture
- Gallbladder disease

RISK FACTORS
- Cholelithiasis
- Obesity
- Chronic hemolysis
- Prior cholecystectomy

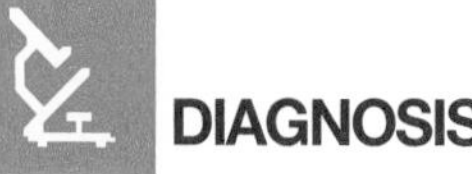

DIAGNOSIS

DIFFERENTIAL DIAGNOSIS
- Biliary stricture
- Narrowed biliary - enteric anastomosis
- Sclerosing cholangitis
- Sphincter of Oddi dysfunction
- Biliary parasites
- Papillary stenosis
- Blood clots

LABORATORY
- Increasing WBC
- Increasing alkaline phosphatase
- Hypercholesterolemia (when associated with chronic cholestasis)
- Increased transaminases
- Hyperbilirubinemia

Drugs that may alter lab results: N/A

Disorders that may alter lab results: N/A

PATHOLOGICAL FINDINGS
- Dilated bile ducts
- Bile plugging
- Small bile duct proliferation
- Cholesterol gallstones

SPECIAL TESTS
- Nuclear medicine (PIPIDA)
- Endoscopic retrograde cholangiopancreatography (ERCP),
- Percutaneous transhepatic cholangiography (PTC)
- Endoscopic ultrasound (EUS)
- Magnetic resonance cholangiopancreatography (MRCP)

IMAGING
- Intraoperative cholangiography - common bile duct filling defects
- Nuclear medicine cholescintigraphy
- Endoscopic cholangiography or PTC - common bile duct filling defects
- Endoscopic ultrasonography - can likely detect stones, but no therapeutic capability

DIAGNOSTIC PROCEDURES
- Ultrasound will reveal gallbladder stones - not reliable for common bile duct stones, but may reveal ductal dilatation over 75% of the time
- ERCP will visualize the common bile duct and other portions of the upper gastrointestinal tract and will allow for papillotomy plus stone extraction in majority of cases.

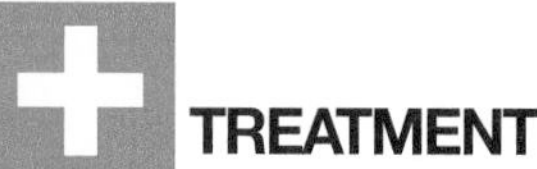

TREATMENT

APPROPRIATE HEALTH CARE Inpatient

GENERAL MEASURES N/A

SURGICAL MEASURES
- In the elderly, ERCP and papillotomy with stone removal may prevent or delay the need for cholecystectomy
- Identification and removal of stones in the course of cholecystectomy
- If the gallbladder has been previously removed, ERCP, papillotomy plus stone extraction

ACTIVITY As tolerated

DIET Low fat may be helpful

PATIENT EDUCATION National Digestive Diseases Information Clearinghouse, Box NDDIC, Bethesda, MD 20892, (301)468-6344

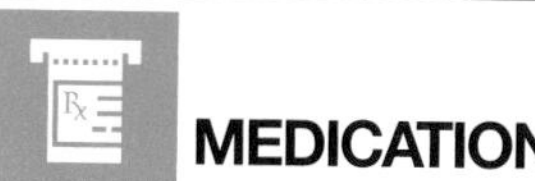

MEDICATIONS

DRUG(S) OF CHOICE
- Antibiotic regimen should cover gram negative aerobes, enterococci, and anaerobes if infection is present
  - ◊ Ampicillin 1 gm q6h IV (substitute ciprofloxacin or levofloxacin in penicillin allergic patient) +
  - ◊ Aminoglycoside (e.g., tobramycin, amikacin is an alternative but is expensive) +
  - ◊ Metronidazole 500 mg q8h IV

Contraindications: Refer to manufacturer's profile of each drug
Precautions: Refer to manufacturer's profile of each drug
Significant possible interactions: Refer to manufacturer's profile of each drug

ALTERNATIVE DRUGS
- Piperacillin-tazobactam (Zosyn) OR
- Ampicillin-sulbactam (Unasyn) OR
- Ticarcillin-clavulanate (Timentin)

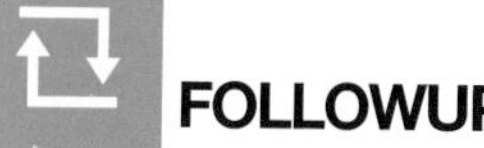

FOLLOWUP

PATIENT MONITORING Routine postoperative care. Liver function tests and bilirubin levels may be beneficial.

PREVENTION/AVOIDANCE
- Operative cholangiography at time of cholecystectomy to identify common bile duct stones and then duct exploration or endoscopic sphincterotomy for their removal
- T-tube cholangiogram before removal of tube after operative bile duct exploration

POSSIBLE COMPLICATIONS
- Cholangitis - most frequent (60%)
- Bile duct obstruction
- Pancreatitis
- Biliary enteric fistula
- Hemobilia
- Liver dysfunction

EXPECTED COURSE/PROGNOSIS
Good prognosis if treated

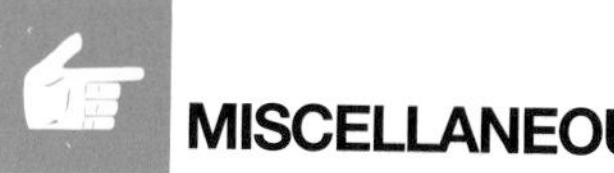

MISCELLANEOUS

ASSOCIATED CONDITIONS
- Cholecystitis
- Cholangitis
- Periampullary diverticula
- Stricture tumor

AGE-RELATED FACTORS
Pediatric: N/A
Geriatric: Prognosis guarded
Others: N/A

PREGNANCY Cholestasis of pregnancy may lead to choledocholithiasis

SYNONYMS
- Common bile duct stone
- Common bile duct calculi

ICD-9-CM
574.30 Calculus of bile duct with acute cholecystitis, without mention of obstruction
574.50 Calculus of bile duct without mention of cholecystitis, without mention of obstruction

SEE ALSO
Adenocarcinoma of the gallbladder
Cholangitis (acute)
Cholecystitis
Cholelithiasis
Jaundice

OTHER NOTES N/A

ABBREVIATIONS
- ERCP = endoscopic retrograde cholangiopancreatography
- PTC = percutaneous transhepatic cholangiography

REFERENCES
- Nahrwold DL: The Biliary System. In: Sabisto DC, ed. Textbook of Surgery. Philadelphia, W.B. Saunders, 1996
- Jordan GL Jr: Choledocholithiasis. Curr Prob Surg 1982;19:723

Web references: 0 available at www.5mcc.com
Illustrations N/A

Author(s):
Mark Horattas, MD

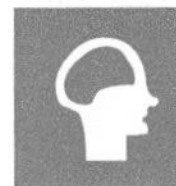

BASICS

DESCRIPTION Cholesterol or pigmented stones formed and contained in the gallbladder
System(s) affected: Gastrointestinal
Genetics: N/A
Incidence/Prevalence in USA: 8-10% of population. Increased incidence in American Indians and Hispanics.
Predominant age: Increases with age - peak at sixth decade
Predominant sex: Female > Male (2:1)

SIGNS & SYMPTOMS
- Mostly asymptomatic. 5-10% become symptomatic each year. Over lifetime, less than half of patients with gallstones develop symptoms.
- Episodic right upper quadrant or epigastric pain radiating to back (biliary colic)
- Nausea
- Vomiting
- Fatty food intolerance (not proven)
- Indigestion

CAUSES
- Production of bile supersaturated with cholesterol
- Decrease in bile content of either phospholipids or bile acids
- Biliary stasis
- Hemolytic diseases
- Biliary infection

RISK FACTORS
- Short gut syndrome
- Inflammatory bowel disease
- Multiparity
- Long term total parenteral nutrition
- Cirrhosis (for pigment stones)
- Hemolytic disorders - hereditary spherocytosis, sickle cell anemia
- Prosthetic cardiac valves
- Biliary parasites
- Rapid weight loss
- Childhood malignancy
- Native American descent
- Diabetes (for complications)
- Female gender

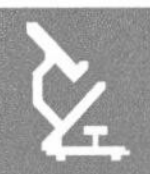

DIAGNOSIS

DIFFERENTIAL DIAGNOSIS
- Peptic ulcer
- Hepatitis, pancreatitis
- Coronary artery disease
- Appendicitis
- Pneumonia
- Gallbladder cancer
- Renal stones
- Blood clots
- Stricture
- Gallbladder polyps
- Biliary sludge

LABORATORY None

Drugs that may alter lab results: N/A

Disorders that may alter lab results: N/A

PATHOLOGICAL FINDINGS Gallstones

SPECIAL TESTS Hepatobiliary radionuclide scan

IMAGING
- Ultrasound (best technique to diagnose gallstones)
- Oral cholecystogram
- CT scan (no advantage over ultrasound)

DIAGNOSTIC PROCEDURES N/A

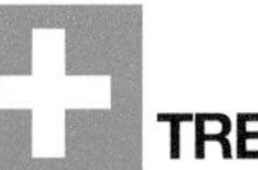

TREATMENT

APPROPRIATE HEALTH CARE Inpatient for surgical procedures

GENERAL MEASURES
- Treat only symptomatic gallstones
- Advise patient of presence of stones
- Observe asymptomatic stones
- Oral dissolution - only if surgery option not available (less than 25% of all patients eligible)

SURGICAL MEASURES
- Laparoscopic cholecystectomy
- Open cholecystectomy
- Direct contact dissolution - only for a small subset of patients - high recurrence rate
- Extracorporeal shock wave lithotripsy - role of this modality unclear and currently under study - not FDA approved
- Percutaneous cholecystostomy in high risk patients

ACTIVITY N/A

DIET Low fat diet may be helpful

PATIENT EDUCATION
- National Digestive Diseases Information Clearinghouse, Box NDDIC, Bethesda, MD 20892, (301)468-6344

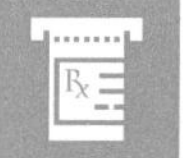

MEDICATIONS

DRUG(S) OF CHOICE
- Analgesic for symptom relief
- Ursodiol (ursodeoxycholic acid, Actigall) 8-10 mg/kg/day bid-tid - for up to two years - oral dissolution
- Chenodiol (Chenix) 250 mg bid for 2 weeks; then increase by 250 mg increments until a dose of 13-16 mg/kg daily is reached or intolerance develops - oral dissolution
- Methyl tert-butyl ether - contact dissolution

Contraindications:
- Known allergy
- Acute cholecystitis - dissolution agents
- Severe abnormal liver function tests
- Non-functioning gallbladder
- Calcified (radiopaque) stones - relative
- Multiple stones
- Stones greater than 2 cm
- Stones that don't float on oral cholecystogram

Precautions:
- Monitor liver enzymes - may rise in up to 30% of patients
- Monitor serum cholesterol
- Methyl tert-butyl ether should only be used by one experienced with this contact dissolution method
- Observe for severe diarrhea

Significant possible interactions: N/A

ALTERNATIVE DRUGS
NSAIDs may have a role in pain relief since prostaglandins are important in the development of pain

Note:
- Oral dissolution only effective for radiolucent (cholesterol) stones
- Ursodiol probably preferred over chenodiol as it has a lower incidence of adverse effects

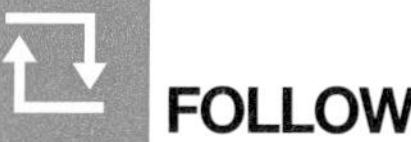

FOLLOWUP

PATIENT MONITORING
- Medical attention if asymptomatic stones become symptomatic
- Patients on oral dissolution agents should be followed with liver enzymes, serum cholesterol and imaging studies

PREVENTION/AVOIDANCE
Use of ursodiol (Actigall) with rapid weight loss prevents stone formation

POSSIBLE COMPLICATIONS
- Acute cholecystitis (90-95% secondary to gallstones)
- Gallstone pancreatitis
- Acute cholangitis
- Common bile duct stones with obstructive jaundice
- Gallstone ileus
- Liver abscess
- Biliary-enteric fistula
- Peritonitis
- Gallbladder cancer

EXPECTED COURSE/PROGNOSIS
- Less than half of patients with gallstones will become symptomatic
- Cholecystectomy - mortality 0.5% elective, 3-5% emergency, morbidity less than 10% elective, 30-40% emergency
- 10-15% will have associated choledocholithiasis
- After cholecystostomy, stones may recur in bile duct

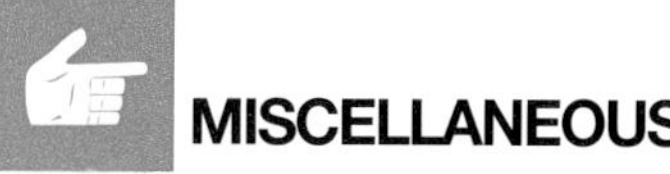

MISCELLANEOUS

ASSOCIATED CONDITIONS
90% of gallbladder carcinomas have gallstones

AGE-RELATED FACTORS
Pediatric:
- Uncommon before 10 years of age
- Associated with blood dyscrasia

Geriatric:
- Incidence increases with age
- Age alone should not alter therapy plan

Others: N/A

PREGNANCY
Attempt conservative therapy but surgery if indicated

SYNONYMS
Gallstones

ICD-9-CM
574.00 Calculus of gallbladder with acute cholecystitis, without mention of obstruction
574.10 Calculus of gallbladder with other cholecystitis, without mention of obstruction
574.20 Calculus of gallbladder without mention of cholecystitis, without mention of obstruction
575.0 Acute cholecystitis
575.10 Cholecystitis, unspecified
574.01 Calculus of gallbladder with acute cholecystitis, with obstruction

SEE ALSO
Adenocarcinoma of the gallbladder
Cholangitis (acute)
Cholecystitis
Choledocholithiasis
Jaundice

OTHER NOTES
Laparoscopic cholecystectomy has become most frequently used procedure. (Lithotripsy can be considered in rare circumstances.)

ABBREVIATIONS
N/A

REFERENCES

- Hardy JD, ed: Hardy's Textbook of Surgery. 2nd Ed. Philadelphia, J.B. Lippincott, 1988
- Pitt HA, ed: The Surgical Clinics of North America. Vol. 70, No. 6. Philadelphia, W.B. Saunders, Dec, 1990

Web references: 0 available at www.5mcc.com
Illustrations N/A

Author(s):
Gary B. Williams, MD

BASICS

DESCRIPTION An acute infectious disease caused by Vibrio cholerae (El Tor type is responsible for current epidemic, the other type, classic, is found only in Bangladesh). (New serotype now in Bangladesh, India (0139). Important because of lack of efficacy of standard vaccine.) Characteristics include severe diarrhea with extreme fluid and electrolyte depletion, and vomiting, muscle cramps and prostration. Usual course: acute; chronic; relapsing.

- Clinical course is 3-5 days, and in the early stages a severely affected patient can lose one liter of fluid per hour
- Endemic areas: India; Southeast Asia; Africa; Middle East; Southern Europe; Oceania; South and Central America

System(s) affected: Gastrointestinal
Genetics: N/A
Incidence/Prevalence in USA: 0.01 cases/100,000. The few cases in the U.S. have been in returning travelers or associated with food brought into the country illicitly.
Predominant age: All ages
Predominant sex: Male = Female

SIGNS & SYMPTOMS

- Abdominal discomfort
- Anorexia
- Anuria
- Apathy
- Cholera gravis
- Cyanosis
- Decreased skin turgor
- Dehydration
- Diarrhea, painless
- Distant heart sounds
- Diuresis, sudden
- Dysrhythmias
- Fever
- Hypotension
- Hypothermia
- Hypovolemic shock
- Increased or decreased bowel sounds
- Lethargy
- Listlessness
- Malaise
- Non-tender abdomen
- Oliguria
- Rice-water diarrhea
- Seizures
- Sunken eyes
- Tachycardia
- Thirst
- Vomiting
- Washerwoman's fingers
- Weak peripheral pulses
- Weakness

CAUSES

- Enterotoxin elaborated by gram-negative
- Vibrio cholera (O-group 1)
- Human host
- Contaminated food
- Contaminated water
- Contaminated shellfish

RISK FACTORS

- Traveling or living in epidemic areas
- Exposure to contaminated food or water
- Person-to-person transmission (rare)
- In endemic areas, children under age 5
- Attack more severe in blood group O as compared to AB
- Individual with low gastric acid secretion
- Gastrectomy
- Individuals on acid-suppressing medications

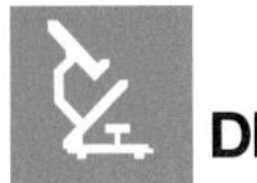

DIAGNOSIS

DIFFERENTIAL DIAGNOSIS Other causes of severe diarrhea and dehydration (e.g., Shigella, E. coli, viruses)

LABORATORY

- Stool culture - on selective media (thiosulfate citrate bile salts sucrose [TCBS])
- Typed antisera specific agglutination
- Dark field microscopy - characteristic vibrio motility in stool
- Increased vibriocidal antibodies in unimmunized individual
- Laboratory abnormalities of severe dehydration:
  - ◊ Acidemia
  - ◊ Acidosis
  - ◊ Hypokalemia
  - ◊ Hyponatremia
  - ◊ Hypochloremia
  - ◊ Hypoglycemia
  - ◊ Increased specific gravity
  - ◊ Polycythemia
  - ◊ Mild neutrophilic leukocytosis

Drugs that may alter lab results: N/A

Disorders that may alter lab results: N/A

PATHOLOGICAL FINDINGS

- Electron microscopy - organism adherent to mucosa
- Intact mucosa
- Increased cellularity of lamina propria
- Increased cellularity of mucosa
- Vascular congestion
- Lymphoid hyperplasia of Peyer's patches
- Lymphoid hyperplasia of mesenteric lymph nodes
- Lymphoid hyperplasia of spleen
- Cerebral edema
- Acute tubular necrosis
- Vacuolar hypokalemic nephropathy
- Pulmonary edema
- Hyaline membranes
- Bronchopneumonia
- Focal myocardial damage
- Lipid-depleted adrenals
- Tubularization of zona fasciculata

SPECIAL TESTS N/A

IMAGING

- Abdominal film - ileus
- Chest x-ray - microcardia

DIAGNOSTIC PROCEDURES Physical examination and medical history that includes recent travel

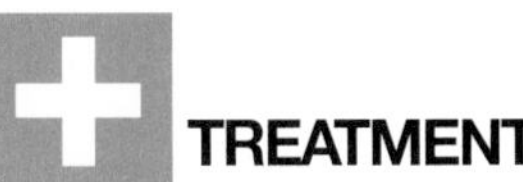

TREATMENT

APPROPRIATE HEALTH CARE Outpatient for mild cases, inpatient for moderate or severe cases

GENERAL MEASURES

- Determination of the amount of fluid loss (may compare patient's previous weight to current weight)
- Rehydration therapy. Oral for mild to moderate cases. Patients with severe dehydration may require intravenous replacement.

SURGICAL MEASURES N/A

ACTIVITY Bedrest until symptoms resolved and strength returns

DIET Small, frequent meals when vomiting stops and appetite returns

PATIENT EDUCATION

- Centers for Disease Control. Traveler's Information Hotline: (404)332-4559 (available 24 hours via a touch-tone telephone).
- International Association for Medical Assistance to Travelers, 417 Center St., Lewiston, NY 14092, (716)754-4883

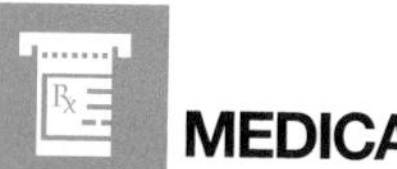

MEDICATIONS

DRUG(S) OF CHOICE
- Oral rehydration therapy

For mild disease:
- ◊ Oral rehydration solution (ORS) commercial brands available (Pedialyte, Rehydralyte, Resol, Rice-Lyte) or
- ◊ ORS formula from World Health Organization (WHO) - per liter:
  - Sodium chloride 3.5 grams
  - Potassium chloride 1.5 grams
  - Glucose 20 grams
  - Trisodium citrate 2.9 grams
- Parenteral rehydration

Severely dehydrated patients
- ◊ IV rehydration (Ringer's lactate) is followed by oral or nasogastric administration of glucose or sucrose-electrolyte solution
- Antibiotics
  - ◊ For older children and adults - doxycycline (Vibramycin) - 300 mg once or 100 mg bid for 3 days or tetracycline 50 mg/kg/day for 3 days
  - ◊ For young children - trimethoprim-sulfamethoxazole (SMX-TMP, Bactrim, Septra) 8 mg/kg trimethoprim plus 40 mg/kg sulfamethoxazole per day, divided q12h. This dosage is equivalent to 1 mL/kg of SMX/TMP suspension. Alternatively, furazolidone (Furoxone) 5-10 mg/kg/day divided q6h for 3 days.
  - ◊ In pregnancy - furazolidone 100 mg qid x 7-10 days.

Contraindications:
- Tetracycline: not for use in pregnancy or children < 8 years.
- Furazolidone and alcohol may cause disulfiram-like reaction.

Precautions:
- Tetracycline: may cause photosensitivity; sunscreen recommended.

Significant possible interactions:
- Tetracycline: avoid concurrent administration with antacids, dairy products, or iron.

ALTERNATIVE DRUGS N/A

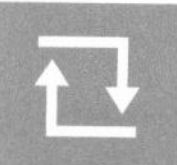

FOLLOWUP

PATIENT MONITORING Follow patient until symptoms resolved

PREVENTION/AVOIDANCE
- Water purification
- Careful food selection, e.g., no unpeeled raw fruits or vegetables, no raw or undercooked seafood
- Enteric precautions
- Tetracycline for contacts
- Natural infection confers long-lasting immunity
- Prophylactic vaccine
  - ◊ 50% effective for 3 to 6 months
  - ◊ Not recommended unless required by destination country, and if so, a single dose is sufficient
  - ◊ Concomitant administration with yellow fever vaccine may result in reduced vaccine response to yellow fever
  - ◊ Invariably associated with local side effects
  - ◊ Systemic side effects of fever and malaise
  - ◊ A new vaccine shows promise, but still in the testing stage

POSSIBLE COMPLICATIONS
- Hypovolemic shock
- Chronic biliary infection
- Up to 50% mortality with untreated shock
- Intermittent stool shedding

EXPECTED COURSE/PROGNOSIS
- Prompt oral or IV treatment can be lifesaving
- Appropriate disposal of human waste
- Antibiotic treatment reduces duration and infectivity of disease
- Mortality less than 1% with appropriate supportive care
- Increased mortality with untreated hypovolemic shock

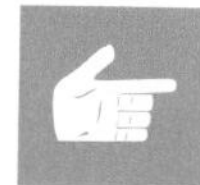

MISCELLANEOUS

ASSOCIATED CONDITIONS Increased risk of disease with gastric achlorhydria

AGE-RELATED FACTORS
Pediatric:
- Breast-feeding is protective against cholera
- Vaccine not recommended for children less than 6 months

Geriatric: N/A
Others: N/A

PREGNANCY N/A

SYNONYMS
- Asiatic cholera
- Epidemic cholera
- Rice water diarrhea
- Cholera gravis

ICD-9-CM
001.9 Cholera, unspecified

SEE ALSO
Diarrhea, acute
Oral rehydration

OTHER NOTES Centers for Disease Control does not expect a major outbreak of cholera in the U.S., but it has issued a "Cholera Preparedness Plan," outlining steps for proper surveillance, treatment, laboratory diagnosis, investigation of outbreaks, and public education

ABBREVIATIONS N/A

REFERENCES

- Mandell GL, ed. Principles and Practice of Infectious Diseases. 4th Ed. New York, Churchill Livingstone, 1995
- Warren KS, Mahmoud AA, eds. Tropical and Geographical Medicine. New York, McGraw-Hill, 1990
- Dhiman BR, Greenough CB III, eds. Cholera. New York, Plenum Medical Book Co., 1992
- Shears P. Recent developments in cholera. Curr Opin Infect Dis 2001;14(5):553-8

Web references: 1 available at www.5mcc.com
Illustrations N/A

Author(s):
Abdulrazak Abyad, MD, MPH

BASICS

DESCRIPTION Chronic cough is defined as cough of >3 weeks duration. Patients present for fear of underlying pathology (eg, cancer), annoyance, self-consciousness, hoarseness. Patients with stress urinary incontinence may find cough particularly troubling. COPD and smoking-related cough are most common etiologies at the primary care level.
System(s) affected: Gastrointestinal, Pulmonary
Genetics: N/A
Incidence/Prevalence in USA: Prevalence of 14-23% in nonsmokers
Predominant age: All age groups
Predominant sex: Male = Female

SIGNS & SYMPTOMS
- Variable and related to the underlying cause
- Usually nonproductive cough with no other signs or symptoms. May persist up to 6 weeks after resolution of viral illness.
- Possible signs and symptoms of allergic diathesis, rhinitis, sinusitis, GERD, CHF, connective tissue disorders

CAUSES
- Often multiple etiologies, but most are related to bronchial irritation. Up to 42% of patients have more than one cause. Most frequent (account for 94% of cases):
  - ◊ Postnasal drip (PND)
  - ◊ Asthma
  - ◊ Gastroesophageal reflex disease (GERD)
  - ◊ Chronic bronchitis
- Other causes:
  - ◊ Aberrant innominate artery
  - ◊ ACE inhibitor therapy
  - ◊ Aspiration
  - ◊ Bronchiectasis
  - ◊ Congestive heart failure
  - ◊ Cystic fibrosis
  - ◊ Eosinophilic lung disease
  - ◊ External auditory canal irritation
  - ◊ Laryngeal cancer
  - ◊ Laryngotracheomalacia
  - ◊ Lung neoplasm (e.g.,, bronchogenic carcinoma)
  - ◊ Pertussis
  - ◊ Post-viral bronchial hyperresponsiveness
  - ◊ Psychogenic (habit cough)
  - ◊ Restrictive lung disease
  - ◊ TB, atypical mycobacterium, and other chronic lung infections

RISK FACTORS
- Smoking
- Stress (particularly school stress in children)

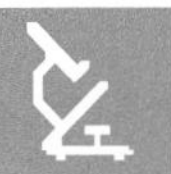

DIAGNOSIS

DIFFERENTIAL DIAGNOSIS N/A

LABORATORY N/A

Drugs that may alter lab results: N/A

Disorders that may alter lab results: N/A

PATHOLOGICAL FINDINGS Specific to underlying etiology

SPECIAL TESTS
- Sputum for eosinophils and cytology
- Purified protein derivative (PPD) skin testing
- Pulmonary function testing with beta-2 agonist
- Sweat chloride testing

IMAGING
- Chest x-ray
- Chest CT if needed
- Upper GI series
- Sinus series or sinus CT

DIAGNOSTIC PROCEDURES
- History and physical
  - ◊ Age of the patient, presence of associated signs/symptoms, medical history, medication (ACE inhibitor), environmental exposures, smoking history may make some causes more likely
  - ◊ Absence of additional signs/symptoms of a particular condition not necessarily helpful (eg, 75% of GERD patients have no other signs or symptoms)
  - ◊ Character of cough is rarely helpful
- 24 hour pH probe
- Rarely bronchoscopy
- Extensive testing only if indicated by the history and physical. Simple testing (chest x-ray, sinus studies) followed by empiric therapy directed at likely underlying etiology.

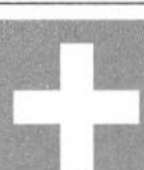

TREATMENT

APPROPRIATE HEALTH CARE Outpatient

GENERAL MEASURES
- Directed at most likely etiology
- Eliminate smoking and ACE inhibitors
- Often empiric treatment of PND and GERD
- Attempt maximal therapy for single most likely cause for several weeks, then search for coexistent etiologies

SURGICAL MEASURES
- Fundoplication is often effective for cough secondary to refractory GERD
- Cough secondary to chronic sinusitis may improve post-surgically

ACTIVITY GERD patients may benefit from elevation of head of the bed and elimination of pre-bedtime meals

DIET GERD patients may benefit from avoidance of EtOH, caffeine, nicotine, citrus, fatty foods

PATIENT EDUCATION
- Reassurance that vast majority of causes are not life threatening, and they can be managed effectively
- Counsel - that several weeks-months may be required for significant reduction or elimination of cough
- Prepare for the possibility of multiple diagnostic tests and therapeutic regimens as treatment is often empiric

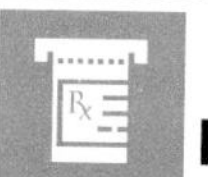

MEDICATIONS

DRUG(S) OF CHOICE
- Antitussives
  - ◊ Dextromethorphan (Delsym) 30mg bid, age > 6 years
  - ◊ Narcotics: codeine 15-30 mg q6h, hydrocodone (Vicodin) 5mg q6h
- Other treatments (antacids, bronchodilators, antibiotics, etc.) directed at etiology of cough

Contraindications: N/A
Precautions: N/A
Significant possible interactions: N/A

ALTERNATIVE DRUGS N/A

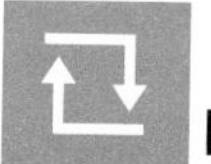

FOLLOWUP

PATIENT MONITORING
- Frequent followup to assess effectiveness of treatment and addition of other medications as needed
- Consider stepwise withdrawal of medications after resolution of cough

PREVENTION/AVOIDANCE N/A

POSSIBLE COMPLICATIONS
- Tussive syncope
- Tussive headache
- Stress urinary incontinence
- Abdominal and intercostal muscle strain
- Inguinal hernia
- Pneumothorax
- Medication side-effects

EXPECTED COURSE/PROGNOSIS
- Most patients (>90%) can be effectively diagnosed and treated with a systematic approach
- Cough from any cause may take weeks to months until resolution, and resolution is highly dependent on efficacy of treatment directed at underlying etiology

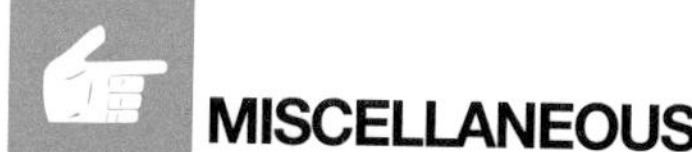

MISCELLANEOUS

ASSOCIATED CONDITIONS N/A

AGE-RELATED FACTORS
Pediatric: Habit cough more likely in school-aged children
Geriatric: N/A
Others: N/A

PREGNANCY N/A

SYNONYMS N/A

ICD-9-CM
786.2 Cough
306.1 Physiological malfunction arising from mental factors, respiratory
491.0 Simple chronic bronchitis

SEE ALSO
Asthma
Bronchiectasis
Congestive heart failure
Eosinophilic pneumonias
Gastroesophageal reflux disease
Laryngeal cancer
Lung, primary malignancies
Pertussis
Pulmonary edema
Rhinitis, allergic
Sinusitis
Tuberculosis

OTHER NOTES
Algorithms for diagnosis and treatment can be found in references

ABBREVIATIONS
GERD = Gastroesophageal reflux disease
PPI = Proton pump inhibitor
MAI = mycobacterium avium-intracellulare
PND = Postnasal drip

REFERENCES

- Chung KF, Lalloo UG. Diagnosis and management of chronic persistent dry cough. Postgrad Med J 1996;72:594-8
- Irwin RS. Silencing chronic cough. Hosp Pract (Off Ed) 1999;34(4):53-9
- Irwin RS, et al. Clinical consensus statement: Managing cough as a defense mechanism and a symptom, ACCP. Chest 1998;114(2 Suppl):133S-181S
- Lawler WR. An office approach to the diagnosis of chronic cough. Am Fam Physician 1998;58(9):2015-22
- Parvez L, et al. Evaluation of antitussive agents. Man Pulm Pharm 1996;9:299-308

Web references: 0 available at www.5mcc.com
Illustrations N/A

Author(s):
Jon C. Seager, MD

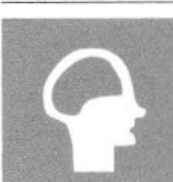

BASICS

DESCRIPTION Chronic fatigue syndrome (CFS) is characterized primarily by profound fatigue, in association with multiple systemic and neuropsychiatric symptoms, lasting at least 6 months. The fatigue must have a new or definite onset (i.e., not lifelong), is not relieved by rest, and results in a substantial reduction in previous activities (occupation, education, social, and personal).

System(s) affected: Endocrine/Metabolic, Musculoskeletal

Genetics: N/A

Incidence/Prevalence in USA: 10/100,000

Predominant age: Young adult

Predominant sex: Female > Male (slightly)

SIGNS & SYMPTOMS

- Fatigue (100%)
- Ability to date onset of illness (100%)
- Unexplained general muscle weakness (90%)
- Arthralgias (90%)
- Forgetfulness (90%)
- Inability to concentrate (90%)
- Emotional lability (90%)
- Myalgias (90%)
- Confusion (90%)
- Mood swings (90%)
- Low-grade fever (37.5-38.6°C) (85%)
- Irritability (85%)
- Prolonged fatigue lasting 24 hours after exercise (80%)
- Depression (80%)
- Headaches (76%)
- Photophobia (76%)
- Difficulty sleeping (76%)
- Allergies (70%)
- Vertigo (40%)
- Adenopathy (40%)
- Shortness of breath (33%)
- Chest pain (33%)
- Nausea (33%)
- Weight loss (30%)
- Hot flushes (30%)
- Palpitations (30%)
- Painful lymph nodes (30%)
- Gastrointestinal complaints (30%)
- Night sweats (25%)
- Weight gain (15%)
- Rash (15%)

CAUSES Unknown. Multiple immunologic abnormalities suggestive of viral reactivation syndrome have been reported. Attention has been to viruses (EBV, HHV-6, enteroviruses), possibly in concert, possibly with environmental factors. No infectious agent has been implicated in the syndrome.

RISK FACTORS Some studies have found an increased risk of developing chronic fatigue syndrome in patients who had a history of childhood abuse or tauma

DIAGNOSIS

DIFFERENTIAL DIAGNOSIS

- Malignancies
- Autoimmune disease
- Localized infection (occult abscess, etc.)
- Chronic or subacute bacterial disease (endocarditis)
- Lyme disease
- Fungal disease (histoplasmosis, coccidioidomycosis)
- Parasitic disease (amebiasis, giardiasis, helminths)
- HIV related disease
- Psychiatric disorders
    - ◊ Drug dependency or abuse (including prescription drugs)
    - ◊ Depression
    - ◊ Hypochondriasis
    - ◊ Anxiety disorders
    - ◊ Somatization disorder
- Chronic inflammatory disease (sarcoidosis, Wegener granulomatosis)
- Known chronic viral disease (chronic hepatitis)
- Neuromuscular disease (multiple sclerosis, myasthenia gravis)
- Endocrine disorder (hypothyroidism, Addison, Cushing, diabetes mellitus)
- Iatrogenic (as from medication side effects)
- Toxic agent exposure
- Other known or defined systemic disease (chronic pulmonary, cardiac, hepatic, renal, or hematologic disease)
- Physiologic (inadequate or disrupted sleep, menopause, etc.)

LABORATORY

- Initial lab studies
    - ◊ Chemistry panel
    - ◊ CBC
    - ◊ Urinalysis
    - ◊ Thyroid function
- Additional studies
    - ◊ ESR
    - ◊ ANA
    - ◊ VDRL
    - ◊ Rheumatoid factor
    - ◊ Purified protein derivative
    - ◊ Serum cortisol
    - ◊ HIV
    - ◊ Immunoglobulin
    - ◊ Epstein-Barr serology

Drugs that may alter lab results: N/A

Disorders that may alter lab results: N/A

PATHOLOGICAL FINDINGS N/A

SPECIAL TESTS None. Diagnosis of exclusion. History, physical exam normal.

IMAGING Experimental at present

DIAGNOSTIC PROCEDURES

To establish the diagnosis - 2 major criteria and at least 6 symptoms plus at least 2 physical signs; or at least 8 symptoms

- Major criteria:
    - ◊ New onset fatigue lasting longer than 6 months with a 50% reduction in activity
    - ◊ No other medical or psychiatric conditions that could cause symptoms
- Symptoms:
    - ◊ Low grade fever
    - ◊ Sore throat
    - ◊ Painful cervical or axillary adenopathy
    - ◊ Generalized muscle weakness
    - ◊ Myalgias
    - ◊ Headaches
    - ◊ Migratory arthralgias
    - ◊ Sleep disturbances (hypersomnia or insomnia)
    - ◊ Neuropsychological complaints (one or more of: photophobia, visual scotomas, forgetfulness, irritability, confusion, difficulty concentrating, depression)
- Physical signs:
    - ◊ Low grade fever (37.5-38.6°C)
    - ◊ Pharyngitis (nonexudative)
    - ◊ Cervical or axillary adenopathy

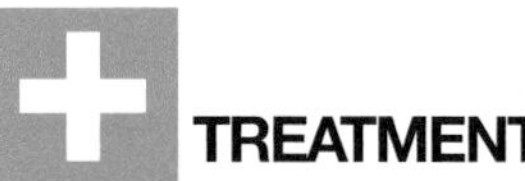

TREATMENT

APPROPRIATE HEALTH CARE Outpatient

GENERAL MEASURES

- Because the cause of CFS is unknown and no specific therapy has shown consistent results, mainstay of therapy is supportive care
- A program of moderate exercise (with rest periods during exacerbations of the disease), a healthy diet, stress reduction, and support groups or counseling is likely to be beneficial and while not necessarily curative will help the patient cope with their disease
- Alternative therapies (chiropractic, homeopathy, acupuncture, enforced rest, guided image hypnosis) helpful for some; may be worth trying
- Psychiatric symptoms often prominent but generally felt secondary rather than causative, but symptom treatment beneficial

SURGICAL MEASURES N/A

ACTIVITY As tolerated, but strenuous exercise tends to exacerbate symptoms in most

DIET Rich in vitamins and minerals

PATIENT EDUCATION

- Support groups available. Contact CFS Association, 3521 Broadway, Suite 222, Kansas City, MO 64111, (816)931-4777
- CFIDS Association. P.O. Box 220398, Charlotte, NC 28222-0398
- International Chronic Fatigue Syndrome Society. P.O. Box 230108, Portland, OR 97223

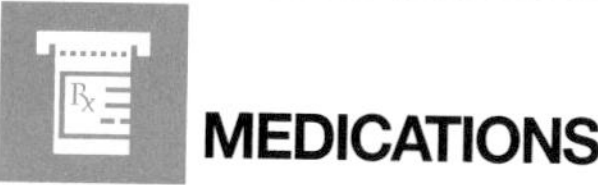

MEDICATIONS

DRUG(S) OF CHOICE
- None
- Poly1:polyC12U (Ampligen), essential fatty acid therapy, immune globulin IV, vitamin B12, and bovine liver extract (LEFAC) are used experimentally
- Supportive therapy directed toward symptoms with NSAIDs, antidepressants including fluoxetine, buspirone, and others

Contraindications: Refer to manufacturer's literature
Precautions: Refer to manufacturer's literature
Significant possible interactions: Refer to manufacturer's literature

ALTERNATIVE DRUGS N/A

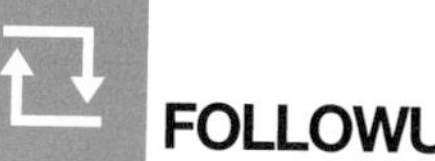

FOLLOWUP

PATIENT MONITORING No consensus. Periodic re-evaluation appropriate for support, symptom relief, assessment for other cause.

PREVENTION/AVOIDANCE Unknown

POSSIBLE COMPLICATIONS
- Depression
- Socioeconomic problems

EXPECTED COURSE/PROGNOSIS
- Indolent; waxes and wanes
- Generally very slow improvement over months or years

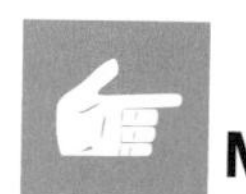

MISCELLANEOUS

ASSOCIATED CONDITIONS
- Fibromyalgia (70% reported to meet criteria)
- Depression
- Hypochondriasis

AGE-RELATED FACTORS
Pediatric: Reported in children
Geriatric: Reported in elderly
Others: N/A

PREGNANCY No information

SYNONYMS
- CFS
- Chronic Epstein-Barr syndrome
- Yuppie flu

ICD-9-CM
300.5 Neurasthenia
780.71 Chronic fatigue syndrome

SEE ALSO
Depression
Epstein-Barr virus infections
Fibromyalgia

OTHER NOTES Controversial topic, data often conflicting

ABBREVIATIONS
CFS = chronic fatigue syndrome

REFERENCES

- Afari N, Buchwald D. Chronic fatigue syndrome: a review. Am J Psychiatry 2003;160(2):221-36
- Cleare AJ. The neuroendocrinology of chronic fatigue syndrome. Endocr Rev 2003;24(2):236-52
- Aktan NM. Chronic fatigue syndrome. An overview of current concepts. Adv Nurse Pract 2003;11(12):64-6
- Craig T, Kahumanu S. Chronic fatigue syndrome. Amer Fam Phys 2002:65(6):1083-90
- Taylor RR, Jason LA. Sexual abuse, physical abuse, chronic fatigue and chronic fatigue syndrome, A community based study. J Nerv Ment Dis 2001;189(10):709-15
- Baschetti R. Cognitive behavior therapy for chronic fatigue syndrome. Lancet 2001;359(9259)841-7
- Holmes GP, Kaplan JE, et al: Chronic Fatigue Syndrome: A Working Case Definition. Annals of Internal Medicine 1988;108, 387-389
- Klimas NG, et al: Immunologic Abnormalities in Chronic Fatigue Syndrome. J. Clinical Microbiology 1990;28(6),1403-1410
- English T: Skeptical of Skeptics. JAMA 1991;265(8):964,
- An information packet, for health care providers, is available from the CDC's Viral Diseases Division (404)639-1338
- Deale A, Chalder T, Wessely S. Illness beliefs and treatment outcome in chronic fatigue syndrome. J Psychsom Res 1998;45:77-83
- Jason LA, Melrose H, et al. Managing chronic fatigue syndrome: Overview and case study. AAOHN J 1999;47:(1)17-21
- Wessely S. The epidemiology of chronic fatigue syndrome. Epidemiol Psychiatr Soc 1998;7(1):10-24
- Friedberg F, Jason LA. Understanding chronic fatigue syndrome: An empirical guide to assessment and treatment. Am Psychological Assoc 1998 - Washington, DC
- Richards J. Chronic fatigue syndrome in children and adolescents: A review article. Clinical Child Psychology & Psychiatry 2000;5(1):31-51
- Cohn S. Taking time to smell the roses: Accounts of people with chronic fatigue syndrome and their struggle for legitimization. J Anthropology and Medicine 1999;6(2):195-215
- Soderberg S, Evengard B. Short-term group therapy for patients with chronic fatigue syndrome. Psychother Psychosom 2001 Mar-Apr;70(2):108-11.
- Ridsdale L, Godfrey E, Chalder T, Seed P, King M, Wallace P, Wessely S. Chronic fatigue in general practice: is counselling as good as cognitive behaviour therapy? A UK randomised trial. Br J Gen Pract. 2001 Jan;51(462):19-24.
- Friedman TC, Echeverry D, Poland RE. Orthostatic hypotension and chronic fatigue syndrome. JAMA 2001 Mar 21;285(11):1441-43
- Kenny RA, Graham LA. Chronic fatigue syndrome symptoms common in patient with vasovagal syncope. Am J Med 2001 Feb 15;110(3):242-3

Web references: 1 available at www.5mcc.com
Illustrations N/A

Author(s):
Moshe S. Torem, MD

Chronic obstructive pulmonary disease & emphysema

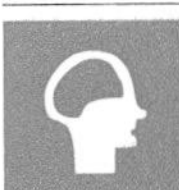

BASICS

DESCRIPTION Chronic obstructive pulmonary disease (COPD) encompasses several diffuse pulmonary diseases including chronic bronchitis, asthma, cystic fibrosis, bronchiectasis, and emphysema. The term usually refers to a mixture of chronic bronchitis and emphysema. COPD is characterized by airflow limitation that is not fully reversible.
- Chronic bronchitis is defined clinically by increased mucus production and recurrent cough present on most days for at least three months during at least two consecutive years.
- Emphysema is the destruction of interalveolar septa. The disease occurs in the distal or terminal airways and involves both airways and lung parenchyma.

System(s) affected: Pulmonary

Genetics:
- Chronic bronchitis is not a genetic disorder although some studies have hinted at a predisposition for development of this condition.
- A rare form of emphysema, antiprotease deficiency (due to alpha 1-antitrypsin deficiency), is an inherited disorder that is an expression of two autosomal codominant alleles.

Incidence/Prevalence in USA:
- 10-20% of adults; more than 100,000 deaths/year (4th most common cause of death)
- 14 million people have chronic bronchitis; 2 million people have emphysema
- Fourth leading cause of death in the United States

Predominant age: Over 40 years

Predominant sex: Male > Female

SIGNS & SYMPTOMS
- Chronic bronchitis
  - ◊ Cough
  - ◊ Sputum production
  - ◊ Frequent infections
  - ◊ Intermittent dyspnea
  - ◊ Hemoptysis
  - ◊ Morning headache
  - ◊ Pedal edema
  - ◊ Plethora
  - ◊ Cyanosis
  - ◊ Wheezing
  - ◊ Weight gain
  - ◊ Diminished breath sounds
  - ◊ Distant heart sounds
- Emphysema
  - ◊ Minimal cough
  - ◊ Scant sputum
  - ◊ Dyspnea
  - ◊ Often significant weight loss
  - ◊ Occasional infections
  - ◊ Barrel chest
  - ◊ Minimal wheezing
  - ◊ Use of accessory muscles of respiration
  - ◊ Pursed lip breathing
  - ◊ Cyanosis is slight or absent
  - ◊ Breath sounds very diminished
  - ◊ Weight loss

CAUSES
- Cigarette smoking
- Air pollution
- Antiprotease deficiency (alpha-1 antitrypsin)
- Occupational exposure (i.e., firefighters, dusty jobs)
- Infection possibly (viral)
- Occupational pollutants (cadmium, silica)

RISK FACTORS
- Passive smoking (especially adults whose parents smoked)
- Severe viral pneumonia early in life
- Aging
- Ethyl alcohol (EtOH) consumption
- Airway hyperactivity

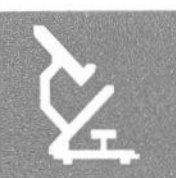

DIAGNOSIS

DIFFERENTIAL DIAGNOSIS Acute bronchitis, asthma, bronchiectasis, bronchogenic carcinoma, acute viral infection, normal aging of lungs, occupational asthma, chronic pulmonary embolism, sleep apnea, primary alveolar hypoventilation, chronic sinusitis, reactive airways dysfunction syndrome (RADS), congestive heart failure

LABORATORY
- Chronic bronchitis
  - ◊ Hypercapnia
  - ◊ Polycythemia
  - ◊ Hypoxia can be moderate to severe
- Emphysema
  - ◊ Normal serum hemoglobin or polycythemia
  - ◊ Normal $PaCO_2$; unless FEV1 < 1 L, then can be elevated
  - ◊ Mild hypoxia - especially at night

Drugs that may alter lab results: Sedatives including alcohol

Disorders that may alter lab results: Obesity, concurrent restrictive lung dysfunction, primary pulmonary hypertension, acute infections, anemia, pulmonary embolism, sleep apnea, congestive heart failure

PATHOLOGICAL FINDINGS
- Chronic bronchitis
  - ◊ Bronchial mucous gland enlargement
  - ◊ Increased number of secretory cells in surface epithelium
  - ◊ Thickened small airways from edema and inflammation
  - ◊ Smooth muscle hyperplasia
  - ◊ Mucus plugging
  - ◊ Bacterial colonization of airways
- Emphysema
  - ◊ Entire lung affected
  - ◊ Bronchi usually clear of secretions
  - ◊ Anthracotic pigment
  - ◊ Alveoli enlarged with loss of septa
  - ◊ Cartilage atrophy
  - ◊ Bullae

SPECIAL TESTS
- Pulmonary function testing
  - ◊ Decreased FEV1 with concomitant reduction in FEV1/FVC ratio
  - ◊ Poor or absent reversibility to bronchodilators
  - ◊ FVC may be normal or reduced
  - ◊ Normal or increased total lung capacity
  - ◊ Increased residual volume
  - ◊ Diffusing capacity is normal or reduced
- Nocturnal oximetry

IMAGING
- Chronic bronchitis chest x-ray shows increased bronchovascular markings and cardiomegaly
- Emphysema chest x-ray shows small heart, hyperinflation, flat diaphragms and possibly bullous changes
- CAT scan may show bullous changes, especially if it is high resolution

DIAGNOSTIC PROCEDURES
- Pulmonary function tests
- ABGs
- Chest x-ray

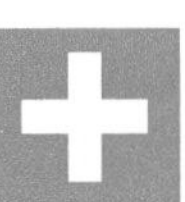

TREATMENT

APPROPRIATE HEALTH CARE
- Outpatient treatment is usually adequate. However, hospitalization may be required for exacerbation, infection, or diagnostic procedures (i.e., transbronchial lung biopsy).
- Acute respiratory failure may require an intensive care unit and possibly a mechanical ventilator to support the patient

GENERAL MEASURES
- Smoking cessation
- Aggressive treatment of infections
- Treat any reversible bronchospasm
- Reduction of secretions through good pulmonary hygiene
- Cor pulmonale may necessitate use of home oxygen
- Pulmonary rehabilitation
- Appropriate vaccinations
- Adequate hydration

SURGICAL MEASURES
- Lung reduction surgery (selected cases)
- Lung transplantation (selected cases)

ACTIVITY As tolerated. Full activity should be encouraged.

DIET A well balanced, high protein diet is suggested. Low carbohydrates may benefit those with hypercarbia.

PATIENT EDUCATION
- Printed material is available from the National Jewish Hospital in Denver, Colorado. The local branch of the American Lung Association also has educational material.
- Coach patients in pulmonary rehabilitation

MEDICATIONS

DRUG(S) OF CHOICE
- Theophylline (Theo-Dur, Unidur, Uniphyl) 400 mg/day. Increase by 100-200 mg in one to two weeks if necessary.
- Sympathomimetics - e.g., metaproterenol (Alupent), albuterol (Proventil, Ventolin), pirbuterol (Maxair), 1-2 puffs from the metered dose inhaler every 4-6 hrs. May be increased to every 3 hrs. Use of spacer device (AeroChamber, Inspirease) may be beneficial. (Up to 4 puffs recommended by some.) Long acting sympathomimetics - salmeterol (Serevent) or formoterol (Foradil) to be considered.
- Anticholinergics
  - ◊ Ipratropium (Atrovent) two puffs (36 μg) 4 times daily. May take additional inhalations not to exceed 12 in 24 hrs.
  - ◊ Tiotropium (Spiriva), one puff daily
- Corticosteroids - prednisone (Deltasone). Given orally 7.5-15 mg/day. Most useful in bronchitis with some reversibility. Inhaled corticosteroids also may be beneficial with less side effects.
- Purified human alpha1-antitrypsin for patients with this deficiency - 60 mg/kg weekly to maintain level more than 80 mg/dL
- Mucolytic agents may improve secretion management

Contraindications:
- Theophylline - hypersensitivity
- Sympathomimetics - cardiac arrhythmias associated with tachycardia; hypersensitivity
- Anticholinergics - hypersensitivity to atropine or its derivatives
- Corticosteroids - systemic fungal infections; hypersensitivity

Precautions:
- Theophylline - reduce dosage in patients with impaired renal or liver function; age over 55; CHF. Therapeutic drug level is 5-15 μg/mL (55.5-111 μmol).
- Rifampin - may cause a decrease in theophylline levels by increasing theophylline metabolism. Monitor serum theophylline level.
- Sympathomimetics - excessive use may be dangerous. May need to reduce dose in patients with cardiovascular disease, hypertension, hyperthyroidism, diabetes or convulsive disorders.
- Anticholinergics - narrow angle glaucoma, prostatic hypertrophy, bladder-neck obstruction
- Corticosteroids - may mask infection or predispose to infection, especially fungal; subcapsular cataracts; glaucoma; adrenocortical insufficiency; psychic derangements; gastrointestinal bleeding; diabetes mellitus, reactivation of tuberculosis

Significant possible interactions:
- Theophylline - lithium carbonate; propranolol; erythromycin; cimetidine; ranitidine; rifampin; ciprofloxacin

Addition of cimetidine, ciprofloxacin, or erythromycin will decrease theophylline clearance causing theophylline levels to rise. Careful monitoring of serum theophylline levels is warranted. (Note: cimetidine is now an OTC drug.)
- Sympathomimetics - other sympathomimetics, monoamine oxidase inhibitors or tricyclic antidepressants
- Anticholinergics - refer to manufacturer's profile
- Corticosteroids - NSAIDs (indomethacin), aspirin, synthetic thyroid hormone

ALTERNATIVE DRUGS
- Theophylline may be given orally, intravenously or by rectal suppository
- Sympathomimetics may be given as aerosolized solution (albuterol, metaproterenol [Metaprel], levalbuterol, isoetharine) when mixed with saline; orally (Alupent, Proventil, Brethine, Ventolin) or subcutaneously (terbutaline)
- Anticholinergics - atropine sulfate, glycopyrrolate. Ipratropium (Atrovent) now available in aerosolized solution and may be mixed with albuterol.
- Corticosteroids may be given intravenously (hydrocortisone, methylprednisolone) or inhaled (beclomethasone, flunisolide, triamcinolone acetonide)
- Home oxygen

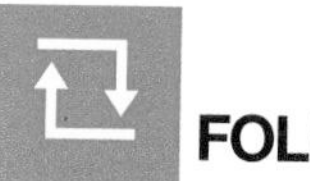

FOLLOWUP

PATIENT MONITORING
- Severe or unstable patients should be seen monthly
- When stable, may be seen biannually
- Check theophylline level with each dose adjustment until the desired level (or result) is achieved, then check every 6-12 months
- With home oxygen, check arterial blood gasses yearly or with any change in condition. Monitor oxygen saturation (pulse oximetry) more frequently.
- Some patients only desaturate at night thereby only needing nocturnal oxygen
- Avoid travel at high altitude. Air travel with oxygen requires pre-arrangement.
- Discuss advanced directive in severe cases

PREVENTION/AVOIDANCE
Avoidance of smoking is the most important preventive measure. Passive smoke also has been shown to be harmful. Early detection may be useful in preserving remaining lung function.

POSSIBLE COMPLICATIONS
- Infection is common
- Cor pulmonale, secondary polycythemia, bullous lung disease, acute or chronic respiratory failure, pulmonary hypertension, malnutrition, pneumothorax, poor sleep quality, arrhythmias, acute respiratory failure

EXPECTED COURSE/PROGNOSIS
- The patient's age and post-bronchodilator forced expiratory volume (FEV1) are the most important predictors of prognosis. Young age and FEV1 > 50% predicted have a good prognosis. Older patients with more severe lung disease do worse.
- Supplemental oxygen, when indicated, has been shown to increase survival
- Smoking cessation is also important for an improved prognosis
- Malnutrition, cor pulmonale, hypercapnia and pulse > 100 indicate a poor prognosis

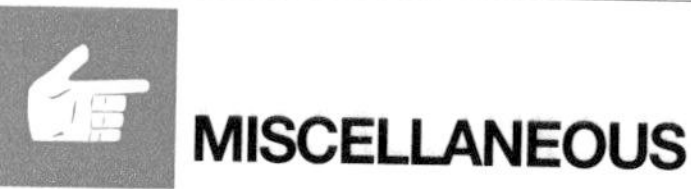

MISCELLANEOUS

ASSOCIATED CONDITIONS
- Lung cancer
- Coronary artery disease
- Peptic ulcer disease
- Chronic sinusitis
- Malnutrition
- Laryngeal carcinoma
- Acute bronchitis

AGE-RELATED FACTORS
Pediatric: Repeated childhood respiratory illnesses make COPD a greater risk

Geriatric: Relative risk is 1.2 to 2.3 times greater than in younger person

Others: Unusual under age 25 unless antiprotease deficiency is present. Incidence increases as age approaches 60.

PREGNANCY N/A

SYNONYMS
- Bronchitis
- COLD (Chronic obstructive lung disease)
- OAD (Obstructive airways disease)
- COPD

ICD-9-CM
496 Chronic airway obstruction, NEC

492.8 Other emphysema

SEE ALSO
Asthma

Bronchitis, acute

OTHER NOTES
- Albuterol is also known as salbutamol
- Other important considerations for treatment include adequate hydration, supplemental oxygen, antibiotics when indicated, mucolytic agents, pulmonary rehabilitation, good pulmonary hygiene

ABBREVIATIONS
FVC = forced vital capacity

FEV1 = forced expiratory volume at 1 second

COPD = chronic obstructive pulmonary disease

ABG = arterial blood gases

REFERENCES

- Pauwels RA. Global strategy for the diagnosis, management, and prevention of chronic obstructive pulmonary disease. NHLBI/WHO Global Initiative for Chronic Obstructive Lung Disease (GOLD) Workshop summary. Am J Respir Crit Care Med 2001;163(5):1256-76
- Chodosh S. Treatment of chronic bronchitis: state of the art. Am J Med 1991;91(6A):875
- Rochester CL. Clinics in Chest Medicine. Philadelphia: WB Saunders Co; 2000. p.21-4

Web references: 1 available at www.5mcc.com

Illustrations N/A

Author(s):
Alan J. Cropp, MD

BASICS

DESCRIPTION Cirrhosis refers to the pathological changes in the liver of extensive fibrosis and regenerative nodules and the clinical syndromes associated with this pathological state. Although often clinically silent, suspected only by altered biochemistry or liver imaging, it is characteristically associated with jaundice, fluid retention, wasting, coagulopathy, altered mental status, and fulminant gastrointestinal bleeding.
System(s) affected: Cardiovascular, Endocrine/ Metabolic, Gastrointestinal
Genetics: Minority of cases clearly inherited (hemachromatosis, hepatolenticular degeneration [Wilson disease] and alpha-antitrypsin deficiency in adults, many other very rare inherited diseases in the first few years of life). Glycogen storage disease is a common one.
Incidence/Prevalence in USA: 6th or 7th leading cause of death age 30 to 50, approximately 30,000 deaths/year
Predominant age: Etiology dependent, but peak in 40-50
Predominant sex: Male > Female

SIGNS & SYMPTOMS

- Asymptomatic cirrhosis:
  - ◊ May be skin changes including spider angioma, xanthomas, increased pigmentation, ecchymoses or bruising
  - ◊ May be abdominal collateral circulation
  - ◊ Hepatic firmness, hepatomegaly, splenomegaly
- Diffuse liver failure
  - ◊ Fatigue after minimal exertion
  - ◊ Anorexia , loss of weight
  - ◊ Weakness, malaise
  - ◊ Heaviness or tenderness in right upper quadrant
  - ◊ Absent or irregular menses
  - ◊ Diminished sexual interest and impaired performance
  - ◊ Jaundice, tea colored urine
  - ◊ Leg edema and/or abdominal swelling
  - ◊ Bruising, abnormal bleeding
  - ◊ Hepatomegaly
  - ◊ Episodic confusion, asterixis
  - ◊ Hematemesis or melena
  - ◊ Spider angioma
  - ◊ Palmar erythema
- Alcoholic etiology
  - ◊ Cheilosis
  - ◊ Parotid enlargement
  - ◊ Night blindness
- Biliary cirrhosis
  - ◊ Xanthelasma
  - ◊ Scratch marks
- Nonalcoholic steatohepatitis
  - ◊ Obesity - BMI >30
- Age difference - under age 15 rarely see confusion and asterixis, extremely common after age 50 Jaundice infrequent under age 8, more common with increasing age

CAUSES Chronic damage to the liver from toxins, viruses, cholestasis, or metabolic disorders. Scar tissue slowly replaces normal functioning liver tissue, progressively diminishing blood flow through the liver and preventing normal function.

RISK FACTORS

- Alcoholism and hepatitis C cause 60%
- Hepatitis B
- Progressive fatty liver
- Nonalcoholic steatohepatitis
- Biliary cirrhosis
- Hemachromatosis
- Less frequent causes
  - ◊ Wilson disease, alpha-1-antitrypsin deficiency
  - ◊ Hepatotoxic drugs
  - ◊ Chronic and recurrent heart failure
  - ◊ Chronic biliary obstruction
  - ◊ Sclerosing cholangitis
  - ◊ Cystic fibrosis
  - ◊ Polycystic or multiple telangiectasis diseases
  - ◊ Veno-occlusive disease
  - ◊ Granulomatous liver disease
  - ◊ Idiopathic portal fibrosis
  - ◊ Shared intravenous needles
  - ◊ Multiple transfusions before 1994

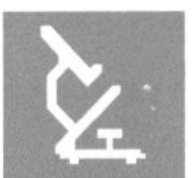

DIAGNOSIS

DIFFERENTIAL DIAGNOSIS

- Diffuse liver disease without cirrhosis vs with cirrhosis
- Cirrhosis vs metastatic or multifocal cancer in the liver
- Cirrhosis vs vascular congestion of the liver
- Temporary and reversible liver disease vs cirrhosis
- Hepatic encephalopathy
- Bleeding esophageal varices
- Ascites
- Jaundice
- Liver biochemical abnormalities

LABORATORY

- Changes of hepatic cell injury
  - ◊ ALT, AST most commonly elevated
  - ◊ Globulin increased if chronic
  - ◊ Protein electrophoresis shows broad band elevation
- Changes of cholestasis
  - ◊ Alkaline phosphatase elevated
  - ◊ GGTP elevated
  - ◊ 5'-nucleotidase, is liver specific alkaline phosphatase
  - ◊ Bile acids elevated
  - ◊ Cholesterol elevated (when condition chronic)
- Changes of impaired amount of functioning liver
  - ◊ Reduced albumin
  - ◊ Prolonged INR for prothrombin time
  - ◊ Elevated bilirubin
- Changes suggesting portal hypertension and large spleen
  - ◊ Diminished platelet count
- Specific tests to determine etiology
  - ◊ Hepatitis
    - Hepatitis B surface antigen, hepatitis B DNA viral load
    - Anti-hepatitis C antibody, hepatitis C RNA viral load
  - ◊ Alcoholism - alcohol in serum in patient who claims to be abstinent
    - Carbohydrate deficient transferrin
    - Elevated GGTP (gamma glutamyl transpeptidase) with normal alkaline phosphatase and decreased K, Mg, Zn or phosphate
  - ◊ Biliary cirrhosis - antimitochondrial antibody
  - ◊ Chronic active hepatitis - anti-smooth muscle, or anti-nuclear antibody
  - ◊ Hemachromatosis - iron saturation >50%, increased ferritin, gene
  - ◊ Hepatolenticular degeneration (Wilson disease) ceruloplasmin, copper excretion
  - ◊ Hepatocellular carcinoma - alpha fetoprotein

Drugs that may alter lab results: N/A

Disorders that may alter lab results: N/A

PATHOLOGICAL FINDINGS

- Fibrous scars, regenerative nodules a feature of all types of cirrhosis. Alcoholic cirrhosis has large nodules, necrotic cells surrounded by PMNs.
  - ◊ Mallory bodies, usually increased fat. May have giant mitochondria.
- Nonalcoholic steatohepatitis may have all of the features of alcoholic but usually more fat
- Biliary cirrhosis. PMN infiltration in the wall of bile ducts, inflammation markedly increased in portal spaces. Progressive loss of bile ducts in portal spaces.
- Hemachromatosis - marked increase in iron
- Chronic active hepatitis - great increase in lymphocytes and cells damaged immediately adjacent to lymphocytes
- Alpha-1-antitrypsin deficiency - PAS positive bodies in hepatocytes
- Hepatitis B and C. Periportal lymphocytic inflammation but damage in central vein region or throughout the lobule.

SPECIAL TESTS

- Endoscopy: identifies esophageal varices or portal hypertensive gastropathy, other bleeding lesions, and to effect emergency treatment of the bleeding lesion if necessary
- Electroencephalography may be required to clarify etiology of confusion
- Diagnostic paracentesis to clarify etiology of ascites and possible complications
- Liver biopsy is the gold standard of diagnosis. Can be conducted safely in a percutaneous fashion if INR < 1. 5 and there is no bleeding tendency and modest or no ascites. Otherwise transjugular biopsy must be performed by an experienced radiologist, infrequently available.

IMAGING

- Ultrasound sometimes required to verify ascites
- Doppler ultrasound used to indicate patency of hepatic and portal veins
- Ultrasound to identify status of biliary passages and presence of gall bladder stones, shows scars in liver. Usually done just before liver biopsy to determine optimal needle insertion site.
- If status of the extrahepatic biliary passages uncertain, CT scan or magnetic resonance exam. If stones likely or biopsy required ERCP is then performed.
- Abdomen CT scan may clarify scars of cirrhosis vs. metastatic disease or fatty liver
- MRI performed to clarify patency of blood vessels and collaterals as in Budd-Chiari syndrome, thrombosis of portal vein, varices or periumbilical collaterals. It also clearly identifies the extrahepatic biliary passages.
- Endoscopic ultrasound useful to identify dilated common duct or masses in the pancreas. Guided needle biopsy can determine histology.

DIAGNOSTIC PROCEDURES

- History, examination, biochemistry and imaging provide diagnosis more than half the time
- Liver biopsy performed 80% of time to verify probable diagnosis or establish uncertain one and to clarify prognosis

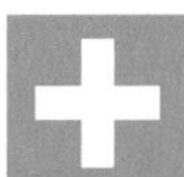

TREATMENT

APPROPRIATE HEALTH CARE Outpatient care except for emergencies (major gastrointestinal bleeding, hepatic encephalopathy, systemic bacteria) infection, unexplained rapidly progressing hepatic decompensation, renal failure

GENERAL MEASURES
- Remove/treat the underlying cause when possible
- Patients must abstain from alcohol, drugs and supplements with no benefit
- Immunize for pneumococcal disease, hepatitis A and B, and influenza
- Review, alcohol, prescription medications, OTC medications and health food items
- Nutritious diet including 1-1.5 gm protein/kg body wt, from all food groups. Weight changes adjusted toward ideal body weight. Daily multivitamin recommended.
- Specific measures:
  - ◊ Hemachromatosis - phlebotomy until iron stores depleted as judged by the ferritin and production of a mild iron deficiency anemia. Usually 25-150 units of blood must be removed.
  - ◊ Fatty liver syndromes - weight reduction, control of abnormal lipids, tight control of diabetes

SURGICAL MEASURES
- Bleeding varices - endoscopic ligation; 4-6 treatments required (may also need propranolol). If bleeding occurs, consider TIPS (transjugular intrahepatic shunt). Rarely a surgically placed side to side portacaval shunt is performed (should be the basis for listing for transplantation).
- Ascites - may require paracentesis each 2 weeks, or more often, despite sodium restriction and diuretic therapy. TIPS may render the ascites easier to control.
- Transplantation - either cadaver liver (average wait time 18 months, 10% on waiting list die annually) or partial transplant from living donor (rapidly growing segment of liver transplants)
- Hepatocellular carcinoma. Cure with partial resection of liver in well compensated cirrhosis. Treat < 5cm nodules with direct ethanol injection, or intra-arterial chemoembolism.

ACTIVITY Conditioning will overcome fatigue

DIET Nutritious diet 1-1.5 gm protein unless liver encephalopathy. Low sodium useful in all patients, essential when there is ascites.

PATIENT EDUCATION
- Educate patient and family and/or care givers on possible complications and a course of action to be taken for each
- Avoid crowds particularly during flu season
- Should not use NSAIDs or gentamicin

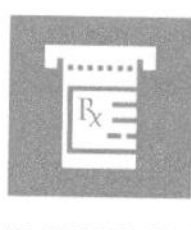

MEDICATIONS

DRUG(S) OF CHOICE
- Hepatitis C - PEG-alpha-interferon weekly and ribavirin bid for 6 months (eliminates virus permanently in about 50% of patients). Patients <age 69 with grade 3 or 4 fibrosis on biopsy, and no history of depression should be treated. Most patients without fibrosis or persistently normal ALT, AST are not treated, but this may be individualized.
- Hepatitis B - lamivudine 100 mg daily for 1 to 2 years. Alternatively PEG-alpha interferon for one year.
- Biliary cirrhosis - ursodeoxycholic acid 10 mg/kg daily for patients life
- Wilson disease - penicillamine 1-3 gm/day as tolerated or tetrathiomolybdate from 100-400 mg/day. After one year zinc acetate alone 250 mg bid is used for maintenance.
- Autoimmune chronic active hepatitis - prednisone 5-20 mg/day as needed with azathioprine (Imuran) 0.5-1 mg/kg for at least 2 years, repeat with relapses
- Complications of cirrhosis
  - ◊ Esophageal varices - propranolol long acting 40-160 mg/day sufficient to lower portal pressure by 20 mm of Hg or lower pulse rate by 25%. May add long acting nitrates, spironolactone or losartan if pressure is not lowered.
  - ◊ Ascites - sodium restricted diet and spironolactone 100-400 mg/day with furosemide 40-160. Torsemide may substitute for furosemide.
- Encephalopathy - lactulose 15 mL of 50% solution 3 times daily, titrate up until 3 loose bowel movements daily. If fail to control, add oral neomycin 250 mg tid.
- Renal insufficiency - stop diuretics, nephrotoxic drugs, normalize serum electrolytes. Hospitalization with plasma expansion or temporary dialysis may be necessary.

Contraindications: Refer to manufacturer's literature
Precautions: Refer to manufacturer's literature
Significant possible interactions: Refer to manufacturer's literature

ALTERNATIVE DRUGS
- Milkweed thistle taken according to the manufacturer's recommendation improves symptoms and is without harm. It is widely used by patients for whom no specific treatment exists.
- Recombinant factor VIIa rapidly corrects bleeding associated with hepatic coagulopathy

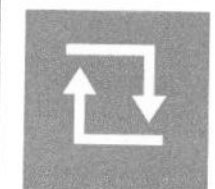

FOLLOWUP

PATIENT MONITORING
- Yearly, if etiology of liver disease corrected and free of complications
- If varices recur, repeat endoscopy each 2-3 years to identify and treat
- Patients with cirrhosis develop hepatocellular carcinoma at the rate of 5% yearly. Those over 55, with hepatitis B or C, decreased INR (prothrombin), or decreased platelets are at highest risk. Many recommend obtaining a serum alpha-fetoprotein, a marker of hepatoma each 6-12 months and a yearly ultrasound. If a new mass appears it should be biopsied. If alpha fetoprotein has become elevated and the US is negative, then CT scan is appropriate. These should only be done if the patient is a candidate for definitive treatment with alcohol injection or surgery.
- Yearly vaccination for influenza. Review that Pneumovax, hepatitis A, B immunization are current.

PREVENTION/AVOIDANCE
- Prophylactic antibiotics recommended for invasive procedures and when there is a gastrointestinal bleed
- Patients with esophageal varices requiring banding should be maintained on a proton pump inhibitor of gastric acid

POSSIBLE COMPLICATIONS
- Ascites
- Edema
- Hepatic encephalopathy
- Bleeding esophageal varices
- Hepatocellular carcinoma
- Susceptibility to bacterial infections
- Spontaneous bacterial peritonitis
- Renal failure
- Liver failure
- Coagulopathy
- Jaundice

EXPECTED COURSE/PROGNOSIS
- If the etiology is removed, variable course
- Life is shortened due to portal hypertension and its complications
- Course after diagnosis of cirrhosis 5-20 years of asymptomatic disease. Once complications start, death within 5 years without transplantation. If etiology cannot be removed, course is more rapid. With transplantation, approximately 15% die in first year, then about 5% a year.
- Transplantation: < 25% of cirrhotics have one due to organ shortage. Obtaining a portion of a living donors liver is the fastest growing group of liver transplantations.

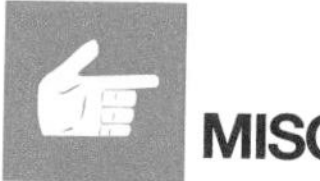

MISCELLANEOUS

ASSOCIATED CONDITIONS N/A

AGE-RELATED FACTORS
Pediatric:
- Jaundice and encephalopathy less frequent indicate more severe liver damage
- Many rare inborn errors of metabolism known, some treatable with diet, surgery

Geriatric: Jaundice and encephalopathy much more common
Others: N/A

PREGNANCY
- Rare in cirrhosis but does not harm the disease
- Feasible after transplantation

SYNONYMS N/A

ICD-9-CM
571.2 Alcoholic cirrhosis of liver
571.5 Cirrhosis of liver without mention of alcohol

SEE ALSO
Alcohol use disorders
Ascites
Esophageal varices
Hemochromatosis
Hepatic encephalopathy
Hepatitis A
Hepatitis B
Hepatitis C
Hepatoma

OTHER NOTES N/A

ABBREVIATIONS N/A

REFERENCES

- Giallourakis CC, Rosenberg, Friedman LS. The liver in heart failure. Clini in Liver Dis 2002;6:947-67
- Ayata G, Gordon FD, Lewis WD, et al. Cryptogenic cirrhosis: clinicopathologic findings at and after liver transplantation. Human Pathol 2002;33:1098-104
- Mathurin P, Mendenhall CL, Carithers RL Jr, et al. Corticosteroids improve short-term survival in patients with severe alcohollic hepatitis: individual data analysis of the last three randomized placebo controlled double blind trials of corticosteroids in severe alcoholic hepatitis. J of Hepatol 2002;36:480-7

Web references: 0 available at www.5mcc.com
Illustrations N/A

Author(s):
Frank L. Iber, MD
Mark C. Iber, PA

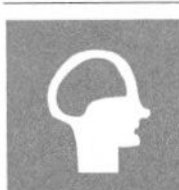

BASICS

DESCRIPTION A sensation of functionally impairing muscle fatigue, cramps and/or pain of the lower extremities brought on by exertion and relieved with rest. Less than 10% of patients with known lower extremity atherosclerosis develop claudication. Approximately 90% of all patients with claudication are cigarette smokers.

System(s) affected: Cardiovascular, Musculoskeletal

Genetics: Geni loci unidentified

Incidence/Prevalence in USA:
- Biennial incidence (Framingham study): .07% in men aged 35-44 years and 1.4% in men older than 65 years; diabetic patients 4-6 times that of nondiabetics
- Prevalence: approximately 1.7-2.2% among older patients

Predominant age: Common in males > 55, females > 60

Predominant sex: Male > Female (by a less than 2:1 ratio)

SIGNS & SYMPTOMS
- Cold feet are an early warning symptom
- Sudden or gradual onset
- Restricted walking distance due to symptom onset
- Symptom continuum from calf muscle fatigue to severe cramps/pain
- Dependent rubor
- Hairless lower extremities
- Leg color may be normal when horizontal, but may appear dusky crimson hue when in lowered position
- Marked blanching on evaluation
- Poorly palpable or absent lower extremity pulses (may not be true for patients with blood vessel calcifications i.e. diabetic patients)
- Paresthesias or numbness are later symptoms
- Symptoms of pain may not be detected in a diabetic patient
- Nonhealing ulcer associated with poor circulation

CAUSES
- Sites affected depends on involved vasculature:
- Aortoiliac disease - pain may extend from buttocks to thigh
- Femoropoliteal disease - pain may extend from calves to feet
- Superficial femoral artery occlusion accounts for most cases of lower extremity claudication symptoms.
- Subclavian, axillary and/or brachial artery blockages may lead to upper extremity claudication symptoms.
- Other causes of arterial occlusion to consider: emboli, popliteal entrapment, adventitious cystic disease of the popliteal arteries, and thromboangiitis obliterans (Buerger disease)

RISK FACTORS
(Cigarette smoking and hypertension are most closely linked with worsening claudication symptoms)
- Smoking
- Diabetes mellitus
- Hypertension
- Hypercholesterolemia
- Family history
- Obesity
- Preexisting heart disease

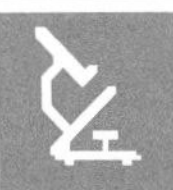

DIAGNOSIS

DIFFERENTIAL DIAGNOSIS
[Neither pseudoclaudication nor osteoarthritis affects ankle brachial indices (see below)]
- Pseudoclaudication: attributed to spinal cord impingement or spinal stenosis. Sitting or squatting helps relieve symptoms.
- Osteoarthritis: pain made worse by weight bearing

LABORATORY N/A

Drugs that may alter lab results: None

Disorders that may alter lab results: Calcified, non-compressible vessels would affect ankle brachial indices (see below).

PATHOLOGICAL FINDINGS N/A

SPECIAL TESTS
- The ankle brachial index (ABI) is the systolic blood pressure at the ankle divided by that of the brachial artery. Normal indices are minimally greater than or equal to 1. The ABI provides information on proximal arterial disease extent and a general idea concerning functional compromise. For example, an ABI greater than 0.5 suggests stenosis of a single arterial segment. An ABI less than 0.5 suggests multisegmental arterial stenoses. Claudicants tend to have ABIs ranging from 0.5 to 0.8. Probable tissue death and rest pain is usually found at ABIs less than 0.3.
- Since calcified vasculature impairs compressibility and ABIs cannot be conventionally measured, photoplethysmography is another option to evaluate toe pressures. Normal toe pressures are 80-90% of brachial artery systolic blood pressures.
- Two claudication screening tools are the Rose and Edinburgh questionnaires.
  - ◊ The Rose queries if calf pain while walking is relieved by 10 minutes of rest or if pain exacerbated by an increased pace (or walking uphill) is relieved by tapering or stopping the activity. Other items include persistent pain if walking continues and absence of calf pain while sedentary. If physicians' diagnosis of claudication is the gold standard, the Rose questionnaire has a specificity of approximately 99% and a sensitivity of 66%.
  - ◊ The Edinburgh is a modified Rose questionnaire taking into account that some patients might continue to walk through calf pain. This questionnaire has a sensitivity of approximately 91% for the detection of claudicants.

IMAGING
- Duplex ultrasound
- Angiography
- Role of computed tomographic angiography (CTA) and magnetic resonance angiography (MRA) in comparison to conventional angiography remains to be determined.

DIAGNOSTIC PROCEDURES
- Arteriography - when surgical correction is anticipated
- Noninvasive vascular tests

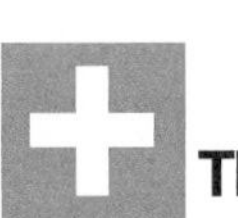

TREATMENT

APPROPRIATE HEALTH CARE
Outpatient. An exception is those patients with severe disease who may require inpatient evaluation

GENERAL MEASURES
- Medical treatment
- Elimination of risk factors whenever possible
- Smoking cessation
- Dietary optimization (low fat and low cholesterol diet)
- Exercise (however, approximately 70% of claudicants will require medication for symptom control)

SURGICAL MEASURES
(Note: Most patients do not require surgical management.)
- Angioplasty
- Arterial bypass surgery

ACTIVITY Ambulatory

DIET Low fat, low cholesterol diet for avoidance and control of hyperlipidemia

PATIENT EDUCATION
- Primary prevention: Encourage an exercise program, no smoking, healthy dietary choices, management of blood glucose in diabetic patients, hypertension control
- Secondary prevention: As above. Emphasize smoking cessation and hypertension control.

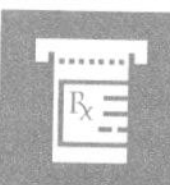

MEDICATIONS

DRUG(S) OF CHOICE
- Aspirin - 80 mg qd to reduce platelet aggregation
- Pentoxifylline (Trental) - to decrease internal configuration of red cells - 400-800 mg bid-tid. Administer for at least 6-8 weeks to determine if therapy is effective.
- Cilostazol (Pletal) 50-100 mg bid

Contraindications:
- Cilostazol is contraindicated in patient's with congestive heart failure
- Pentoxifylline is contraindicated in patient's with recent cerebral and/or retinal hemorrhage

Precautions:
- Headache occurs frequently (>30%) in patients taking cilostazol

Significant possible interactions:
- Cilostazol: Metabolized via the cytochrome P-450 isoenzymes. Use caution during coadministration of other inhibitors of CYP3A4 (e.g., grapefruit juice, ketoconazole, itraconazole, erythromycin and diltiazem), and during coadministration of inhibitors of CYP2C19 (e.g. omeprazole).
- Pentoxifylline: theophylline levels may rise
- Concurrent use of beta blockers in patients with coexisting cardiovascular disease does not appear to worsen claudication symptoms in affected patients

ALTERNATIVE DRUGS
- Ticlopidine (Ticlid)
- Vasodilators
- Calcium channel blockers
- Anticoagulants
- Role of PGE1 and PGI2 analogues and stimulants (i.e., AS-103, iloprost, beraprost, defibrotide) continues to be investigated

FOLLOWUP

PATIENT MONITORING Peripheral non-invasive vascular studies every 6 months. If worsening, would be indication for surgery.

PREVENTION/AVOIDANCE
- Walking program
- Avoid smoking

POSSIBLE COMPLICATIONS
- Tissue/ limb loss- predominantly affects diabetic patients as disease progresses
- Complications of reperfusion
  - ◊ Compartmental syndrome
  - ◊ Venous thrombosis induced by low flow state which may flush to right side of heart to pulmonary circulation

EXPECTED COURSE/PROGNOSIS
- Gradual improvement with use of medical therapy/walking program and diminution/elimination of risk factors. Some patients may require revascularization. Disease progression may include rest pain, tissue loss and gangrene.
- Chronic intermittent ischemia may cause lasting defects in muscle function resulting in weakness which could be an early sign of peripheral arterial disease

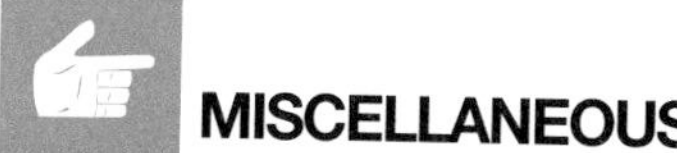

MISCELLANEOUS

ASSOCIATED CONDITIONS Other manifestations of arteriosclerotic vascular disease - myocardial infarction(s), carotid artery occlusive disease, renovascular occlusive disease, and hypertension

AGE-RELATED FACTORS
Pediatric: N/A
Geriatric: More common with advancing age
Others: N/A

PREGNANCY N/A

SYNONYMS N/A

ICD-9-CM
443.9 Peripheral vascular disease, unspecified

SEE ALSO
Thromboangiitis obliterans (Buerger disease)

OTHER NOTES N/A

ABBREVIATIONS N/A

REFERENCES

- Lennihan, Porter, et al. When chronic ischemia worsens. Patient Care 1988;22:77-89
- Flannery DP, Schuler FF, et al. Risk factors affecting natural history of intermittant claudication. Arch Surg 1988;123:867-70
- Rutherford RB, ed: Vascular Surgery. 4th Ed. Philadelphia, WB Saunders Co, 1995
- Cooke JA, Ma AO. Medical therapy of peripheral arterial occlusive disease. Surgical Clinics of North America 1995;75(4):569-79
- Velazquez AC, Baum RA, Carpenter JP. Magnetic resonance angiography of lower extremity arterial disease. Surg Clin NA 1998;78(4):519-35
- McNamara DB, Champion HC, Kadowitz PJ. Pharmacologic management of peripheral vascular disease. Surg Clin NA 1998;78(3):447-64
- Bassiouny HS. Noninvasive evaluation of the lower extremity arterial tree and graft surveillance. Surg Clin NA 1995;75(4):593-606
- Rubin GA, Zarins CK. MR and spiral/helical CT imaging of lower extremity occlusive disease. Surg Clin NA 1995;75(4):607-19

Web references: 0 available at www.5mcc.com
Illustrations N/A

Author(s):
J. C. Chava-Zimmerman, MD

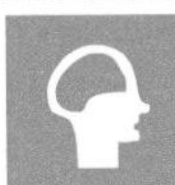

BASICS

DESCRIPTION A constriction (discrete or of varying lengths) of the aorta usually located just distal to the left subclavian artery at the junction of the ligamentum arteriosum

System(s) affected: Cardiovascular

Genetics: No Mendelian inheritance, but common in Turner syndrome

Incidence/Prevalence in USA: 64/100,000 under 1 year of age

Predominant age: Usually diagnosed in infancy

Predominant sex: Male > Female (1.7:1)

SIGNS & SYMPTOMS
- Headaches
- Exertional leg fatigue and pain
- Prominent neck pulsations
- Epistaxis
- Hypertension
- Pulse disparity: radial - femoral pulse delay and increased amplitude in brachial verses femoral pulse
- Fundoscopy: corkscrew tortuosity of retinal arterioles
- Delayed, weak, or absent pulse
- Prominent left ventricular impulse
- Murmur (aortic stenosis or insufficiency, ventricular septal defect, rarely mitral valve)
- S4 systolic ejection click
- Bruit (coarctation, collaterals, patent ductus arteriosus)
- Cyanosis, rarely
- In infancy may also have heart failure, failure to thrive, irritability, tachypnea, and dyspnea
- Extensive collaterals develop from branches of the subclavian, internal mammary, superior intercostal, and axillary arteries

CAUSES Congenital: Takayasu arteritis, Turner syndrome, multiple left-sided obstruction

RISK FACTORS
- Turner syndrome
- Congenital left heart abnormalities

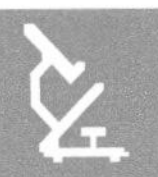

DIAGNOSIS

DIFFERENTIAL DIAGNOSIS
- Takayasu arteritis
- Neurofibromatosis
- Pseudocoarctation (with or without hypertension, peripheral vascular disease)

LABORATORY N/A

Drugs that may alter lab results: N/A

Disorders that may alter lab results: N/A

PATHOLOGICAL FINDINGS
- Segmental tubular hypoplasia
- Discrete obstruction with medial thickening
- Distal aneurysm

SPECIAL TESTS
- Doppler examination of pulses reveals disparity
- Electrocardiogram may show left ventricular hypertrophy
- Blood pressures - all 4 extremities: upper limb systemic hypertension and differential of > 10mmHg

IMAGING
- Chest x-ray may show rib notching, "3" sign, rarely cardiomegaly
- Echocardiography for coarctation and coexisting cardiac anomalies
- Transesophageal echocardiography
- Magnetic resonance imaging (MRI)

DIAGNOSTIC PROCEDURES Cardiac catheterization and angiography: post-stenotic dilation

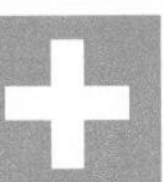

TREATMENT

APPROPRIATE HEALTH CARE Inpatient surgery

GENERAL MEASURES N/A

SURGICAL MEASURES
- Surgical correction or balloon angioplasty can be done in infancy if urgently needed. Best results when performed age 1-2 years.
- Surgery should be done in childhood and adulthood as soon as coarctation diagnosed to prevent late complications
- Three common surgical procedures for correction of coarctation include (1) end-to-end anastomosis, (2) patch aortoplasty (insertion of Dacron patch), and, (3) subclavian flap procedure
- Balloon angioplasty of coarctation offers good results for primary treatment and for postoperative re-stenosis
- Stent placement
  - ◊ May prevent unnecessary dilation of coarctation during angioplasty
  - ◊ May further prevent late recoarctation than angioplasty alone

ACTIVITY Exercise may exacerbate hypertension, but normal activity recommended after correction

DIET No special diet

PATIENT EDUCATION
- Discuss post-coarctation syndrome
- For patient education materials favorably reviewed on this topic, contact: American Heart Association, 7320 Greenville Avenue, Dallas, TX 75231, (214)373-6300

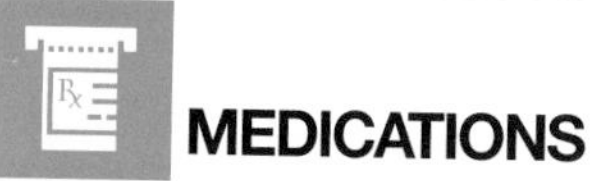

MEDICATIONS

DRUG(S) OF CHOICE

- Alprostadil (prostaglandin E1), patency of ductus arteriosus
- Antibiotic prophylaxis (for dental and/or invasive procedures) for life (even after correction)
- Antihypertensives if needed
- Preload and afterload reduction if heart failure develops

Contraindications: Refer to manufacturer's profile of each drug

Precautions:

- Lowering upper extremity blood pressure may cause hypoperfusion of lower extremities
- Lowering blood pressure not advised in pregnancy unless emergency

Significant possible interactions: Refer to manufacturer's profile of each drug

ALTERNATIVE DRUGS N/A

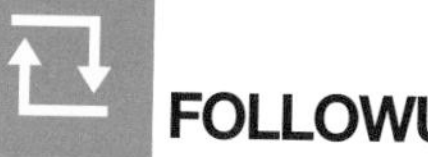

FOLLOWUP

PATIENT MONITORING Frequent postoperative followup for evidence of re-stenosis (check for hypertension and pulse disparities) and late complications

PREVENTION/AVOIDANCE Patients should be encouraged to have normal lifestyles and activities after coarctation correction

POSSIBLE COMPLICATIONS

- Most common with late or no correction
- Heart failure
- Aneurysm of circle of Willis, rupture possible
- Hypertension
- Rupture or dissection of aortic aneurysm
- Endarteritis or endocarditis (need antibiotic prophylaxis)
- Aortic valve disease (stenosis or insufficiency)
- Post coarctectomy syndrome: recurrence, hypertension, atherosclerotic heart disease, aneurysm at site of coarctectomy, progressive aortic stenosis and/or regurgitation
- Fistula formation between aorta and airways leading to hemoptysis

EXPECTED COURSE/PROGNOSIS

- Depends on age of repair and presence of other cardiac abnormalities
- Residual or restenosis (6-33%)
- Subsequent cardiac surgery (11%)
- Hypertension (25%)
- Survival after surgery: 10 years (91%), 20 years (84%), 30 years (72%)
- Uncorrected, 80% mortality before age 50

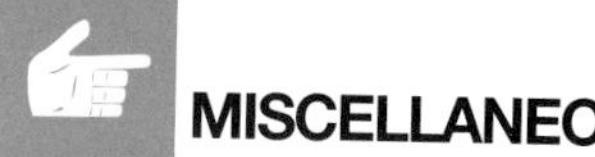

MISCELLANEOUS

ASSOCIATED CONDITIONS

- Bicuspid aortic valve (85%)
- Patent ductus arteriosus (65%)
- Ventricular septal defect (30-35%)
- Aortic stenosis and/or insufficiency
- Subvalvular aortic stenosis
- Mitral valve abnormalities (common)
- Transposition of great vessels or double outlet right ventricle
- Aneurysm of circle of Willis
- Neurofibromatosis I
- Acquired intercostal aneurysms

AGE-RELATED FACTORS Greater risk of complications if correction is delayed beyond early childhood. Often diagnosis is delayed.

Pediatric: N/A

Geriatric: N/A

Others: N/A

PREGNANCY Uncorrected (or restenosis) coarctation carries high risk of aortic rupture or dissection and cerebral hemorrhage (aneurysm of circle of Willis rupture), but lower risk of pre-eclampsia than other forms of hypertension

SYNONYMS N/A

ICD-9-CM

747.1 Coarctation of aorta

SEE ALSO

OTHER NOTES N/A

ABBREVIATIONS N/A

REFERENCES

- Fuster V, ed. Hurst's The Heart. 10th ed. New York: McGraw-Hill; 2001
- Chizer MA. Classic Teachings in Cardiology. New Jersey: Laennec Publishing Inc; 1996
- Braunwald E, et al. Heart Disease. 6th ed. Philadelphia: WB Saunders Co; 2001
- Rosenthal E. Stent Implantation of Aortic coarctation: The treatment of choice in adults?: Journal of American Cardiology 2001;38 (5):1524-7
- Ledesma M, et al. Results of Stenting for Aortic Coarcatation: American Journal of Cardiology 2001;88(4):460-2
- Manganas C, et al. Reoperation and Coarctation of the Aorta: the need for lifelong surveillance: Ann Thorac Surg 2001;7(4):1222-4
- Heikkinen LO, et al. Aortopulmonary fistula after coarctation repair: Ann Thorac Surg 2002;73(5):1634-6

Web references: 0 available at www.5mcc.com

Illustrations N/A

Author(s):
Timothy McCurry, MD
Vernan Atienza, MD
Ejaz Khan, MD

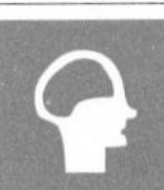

BASICS

DESCRIPTION Pulmonary fungal infection endemic to the Southwest USA. Can become progressive and involve extrapulmonary sites, including bone, CNS, and skin. Known as the "great imitator." Incubation period is 1 to 4 weeks after exposure.
System(s) affected: Endocrine/Metabolic, Musculoskeletal, Nervous, Pulmonary, Skin/Exocrine
Genetics: Unknown
Incidence/Prevalence in USA: 100,000 cases per year. (0.5% extrapulmonary)
Predominant age: All ages
Predominant sex: Male = Female

SIGNS & SYMPTOMS
- Anorexia
- Arthralgias
- Chest pain
- Chills
- Confusion
- Cough, dry or productive
- Cyanosis
- Dyspnea
- Erythema nodosum
- Fatigue
- Fever
- Headache
- Hepatomegaly
- Hydrocephalus
- Hyperreflexia
- Malaise
- Night sweats
- Pleural friction rub
- Rash
- Sore throat
- Splenomegaly
- Tachycardia
- Tenosynovitis
- Toxic erythema
- Weight loss
- Note: Over half of cases are subclinical

CAUSES Coccidioides immitis, a soil fungus especially adapted to arid conditions. Liberated spores are inhaled when soil is disturbed: digging, construction sites, archaeological sites, dust storms, spelunking (exploring caves). Soil that lines rodent burrows is worst.

RISK FACTORS
- Certain groups are more prone to dissemination: immunocompromised hosts, pregnant women, African-Americans, Filipinos.
- CNS involvement more common in young white males
- Immunosuppression. Previously infected patients can experience relapse years later through the mechanism of cell-mediated immune deficiency.
- Diabetes mellitus
- AIDS
- Chronic steroid use

DIAGNOSIS

DIFFERENTIAL DIAGNOSIS
- Pneumonia, all etiologies
- Lung carcinoma
- Sarcoidosis
- Histoplasmosis, other fungi
- Lung abscess
- TB
- Lymphoma
- Meningitis
- Plus all other causes of cough, fever, fatigue
- Old granulomas can be mistaken for tumors

LABORATORY
- Skin test turns positive at 3 weeks to 3 months; may remain positive indefinitely; applying skin test will not interfere with serologies. Skin test is currently not being manufactured and it is unclear when it will be available again.
- Serology - immunodiffusion measures precipitin antibodies (IgM) rise within 2 weeks and fall after 2 months; complement fixation antibodies (IgG) rise at 1-3 months; patients with mild symptoms may never develop detectable serology
- May have elevated sedimentation rate and peripheral eosinophilia
- Culture of sputum, wound exudate, joint aspirate; unlikely to grow fungus in urine, blood, pleural fluid

Drugs that may alter lab results: Steroids may alter ability to react to skin testing

Disorders that may alter lab results: N/A

PATHOLOGICAL FINDINGS Fungal elements, spherules

SPECIAL TESTS Biopsy of affected tissue, e.g., lung nodule, skin lesion

IMAGING Chest x-ray findings include - normal, infiltrate(s), nodule(s), cavity, adenopathy mediastinal or hilar, pleural effusion

DIAGNOSTIC PROCEDURES If unable to establish diagnosis from skin testing and serologies - bronchoscopy, fine-needle biopsy, open lung biopsy, pleural biopsy, bone/skin/node biopsy, CSF stain, serology, culture

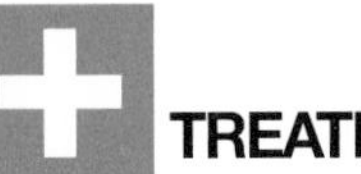

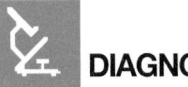

TREATMENT

APPROPRIATE HEALTH CARE
- Outpatient except in very severe cases
- Recommend referral to pulmonary or infectious disease specialist if drug treatment becomes imperative. Consider such treatment if IgG titers > 1:16, if disease persists without improvement over 6 weeks, or if skin test remains negative in the face of positive serology.

GENERAL MEASURES
- Cool mist humidifier for dry cough or sore throat
- Rest
- Supportive therapy

SURGICAL MEASURES N/A

ACTIVITY As tolerated

DIET No special diet

PATIENT EDUCATION For patient education materials favorably reviewed on this topic, contact: American Lung Association, 1740 Broadway, New York, NY 10019, (212)315-8700

MEDICATIONS

DRUG(S) OF CHOICE

- In mild cases, treat for symptomatic relief of cough with antitussives plus treat pleuritic pain with non-steroidal anti-inflammatory agents
- For persistent, progressive, or disseminated disease the following drugs are indicated. However, dosing, whom to treat, and length of treatment is controversial.
  - ◊ Amphotericin B: 0.5-1.0 mg/kg with a total cumulative dose of 2-4 gm
  - ◊ Ketoconazole: 400 mg/day
  - ◊ Fluconazole: 400 mg/day. Fluconazole is also the treatment of choice for coccidioidomeningitis with a usual dose of 800 mg/day.
- Itraconazole: 200 mg bid

Contraindications: Avoid steroids

Precautions: Amphotericin is highly nephrotoxic.

Significant possible interactions:

- Ketoconazole-H2 blockers: decrease absorption of ketoconazole (ketoconazole requires an acidic pH for absorption).
- Azole antifungals - QT prolongation and ventricular arrhythmias

ALTERNATIVE DRUGS N/A

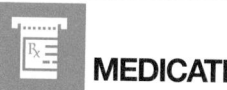

FOLLOWUP

PATIENT MONITORING

- If serology negative but index of suspicion is high, repeat every 2 weeks (skin test currently not available). With positive serologies, follow titers every 2 weeks until titers are dropping and patient has clinical improvement or resolution.
- Follow abnormal chest x-rays until findings are resolved or scarring process is complete

PREVENTION/AVOIDANCE

- Not contagious between host and contacts
- Cultures in lab are highly contagious via inhalation and lab personnel must be very cautious when handling specimens
- High risk populations (see Risk factors) should consider avoiding high risk activities, such as construction, archaeological digs, etc.

POSSIBLE COMPLICATIONS

- Severe cases are fatal, especially if associated with meningitis. Can cause destruction of pulmonary tissue due to scarring, cavities, etc.
- Hemoptysis

EXPECTED COURSE/PROGNOSIS

- Most cases are self-limited, resolve within a few months. Progressive and disseminated disease can be difficult to eradicate.
- Prognosis poor if weak cell mediated immunity response or high IgG
- Relapse of extrapulmonary or disseminated disease is common.

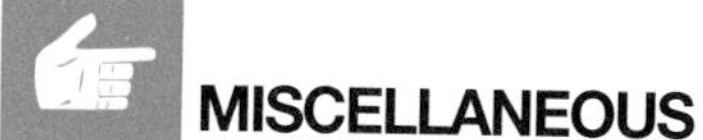

MISCELLANEOUS

ASSOCIATED CONDITIONS N/A

AGE-RELATED FACTORS

Pediatric: N/A
Geriatric: N/A
Others: N/A

PREGNANCY Increased risk for dissemination, especially if contracted late in gestation

SYNONYMS

- Cocci
- Desert fever
- Posada-Wernicke disease
- Valley fever
- San Joaquin fever

ICD-9-CM

114.9 Coccidioidomycosis, unspecified

SEE ALSO

OTHER NOTES Travel history is essential when working up any pulmonary infection not responding to normal measures

ABBREVIATIONS N/A

REFERENCES

- Galgiani JN. Primary coccidioidal infection. UpToDate Online 2002. UpToDate Clinical Reference. Available at: http://www.uptodate.com
- Isselbacher KJ, et al, editors. Harrison's Principles of Internal Medicine. 13th Ed. New York: McGraw-Hill; 1994
- Hedges E, Miller S. Coccidioidomycosis: Office diagnosis and treatment. Amer Fam Phys 1990;(5):1499-506

Web references: 0 available at www.5mcc.com
Illustrations N/A

Author(s):
Sandra Miller, MD

BASICS

DESCRIPTION Colic is an incompletely understood state of excessive crying seen in young infants who are otherwise well. A working definition - abnormal crying that lasts > 3 hours/day for at least 3 times/week.
System(s) affected: Gastrointestinal, Nervous
Genetics: N/A
Incidence/Prevalence in USA: Common. 10,000/100,000 in some reports, as high as 25,000/100,000 in others
Predominant age: 3 weeks of age to 3 months of age
Predominant sex: Male = Female

SIGNS & SYMPTOMS
- Rhythmic crying, paroxysmal
- Inconsolability
- Fist clenching
- Back arching
- Drawing up of infant's legs
- Excessive flatus

CAUSES
- The cause is unknown. Factors that may play a role include:
  - ◊ Swallowing air during the process of crying, feeding, or sucking on hands or fingers
  - ◊ Overfeeding with large amounts of formula or breast milk
  - ◊ Family tension
  - ◊ Parental anxiety
  - ◊ Allergies to cow's milk
  - ◊ Esophageal reflux
  - ◊ Baby's inability to console itself when dealing with stimuli

RISK FACTORS Physiologic predisposition in infant

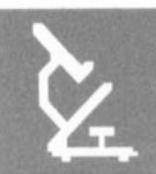

DIAGNOSIS

DIFFERENTIAL DIAGNOSIS
- Any organic cause for excessive crying in infants (e.g., meningitis, sepsis, strangulated hernia, occult fracture)
- Entirely a clinical diagnosis

LABORATORY N/A

Drugs that may alter lab results: N/A

Disorders that may alter lab results: N/A

PATHOLOGICAL FINDINGS N/A

SPECIAL TESTS N/A

IMAGING N/A

DIAGNOSTIC PROCEDURES Physical examination may be performed to rule out other causes

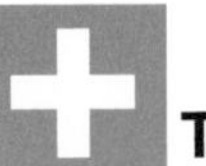

TREATMENT

APPROPRIATE HEALTH CARE Outpatient management

GENERAL MEASURES
- Handling of the colicky infant in a calm and non-stimulating manner should be demonstrated
- Use of pacifier
- Use of gentle rhythmic motion (e.g., car rides)
- Use of music

SURGICAL MEASURES N/A

ACTIVITY N/A

DIET Removal of cow's milk from diet for a one week trial

PATIENT EDUCATION
- Explain normal crying behavior. Reassure parents that colic is not the result of bad parenting.
- American Academy of Pediatrics, 141 Northwest Point Blvd., P.O. Box 927, Elk Grove Village, IL 60009-0927, (800)433-9016

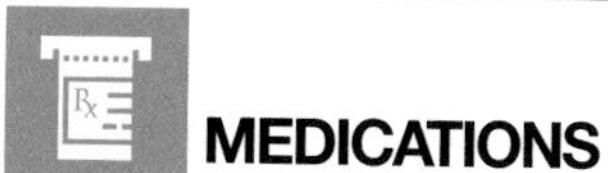

MEDICATIONS

DRUG(S) OF CHOICE N/A
Contraindications: N/A
Precautions: N/A
Significant possible interactions: N/A

ALTERNATIVE DRUGS N/A

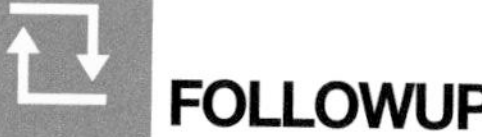

FOLLOWUP

PATIENT MONITORING Frequent outpatient visits as needed for parental reassurance and education

PREVENTION/AVOIDANCE Colic is normally not preventable

POSSIBLE COMPLICATIONS None expected

EXPECTED COURSE/PROGNOSIS
- Usually subsides by 3 months of age
- In spite of apparent abdominal pain, colicky infants eat well and gain weight normally
- Colic has no bearing on the baby's intelligence or future development

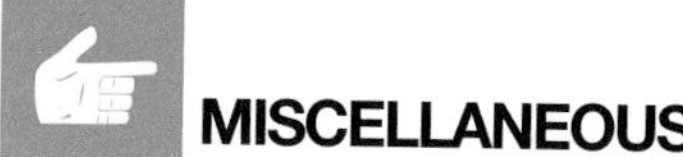

MISCELLANEOUS

ASSOCIATED CONDITIONS N/A

AGE-RELATED FACTORS
Pediatric: A problem of infancy
Geriatric: N/A
Others: N/A

PREGNANCY N/A

SYNONYMS N/A

ICD-9-CM
789.0 Abdominal pain

SEE ALSO

OTHER NOTES N/A

ABBREVIATIONS N/A

REFERENCES

- McCollough M. Common complaints in the first 30 days of life. Emerg Med Clin North Am 2002; 20(1): 27-48
- Clemons RM. Issues in newborn care. Prim Care 2000; 27(1):251-67
- Garrison MM. A systematic review of treatments for infant colic. Pediatrics 2000;106(1 Pt 2):184-90
- Behrman RE, Kliegman RM. Nelson Textbook of Pediatrics. 17th ed. Philadelphia: WB Saunders Co; 2003

Web references: 0 available at www.5mcc.com
Illustrations N/A

Author(s):
Mark R. Dambro, MD

BASICS

DESCRIPTION A malignant neoplasm arising from the luminal surface of the colon, rectum or anus. The fourth most common malignancy in the U.S. and the second most common cause of cancer-related deaths.
- Adenocarcinoma - by far, most common histologic form, usually arising from benign adenoma. Unequally distributed, with 38% in proximal colon and 62% in distal colon or rectum.
- Carcinoid - uncommon, arising from enterochromaffin cells. Usually located in appendix or rectum; not likely to metastasize unless larger than 2 cm in diameter.
- Squamous cell carcinoma - uncommon form; located in the anal canal. Also called epidermoid or cloacogenic.
- Melanoma - rare; usually presents as pigmented lesion adjacent to dentate line

System(s) affected: Gastrointestinal
Genetics:
- Hereditary colon and rectal cancer accounts for approximately 15-20% of colorectal cancer
- Ras oncogene mutations seen in 40-50% of adenocarcinoma; alterations of suppressor genes also seen in 75%, especially involving chromosomes 17,18

Incidence/Prevalence in USA: 155,000 new cases/year
Predominant age: Adenocarcinoma usually occurs in individuals > age 50 years with peak incidence in the seventh decade
Predominant sex: Male = Female

SIGNS & SYMPTOMS
- Vary with location
- Early lesions are frequently asymptomatic
- Right-sided adenocarcinoma
  ◊ Anemia
  ◊ Pain and/or mass in right lower quadrant
  ◊ Occult blood in stool
  ◊ Change in appearance of stool (infrequent)
- Left-sided adenocarcinoma
  ◊ Change in bowel habits (may be constipation or diarrhea)
  ◊ Reduced caliber of stool
  ◊ Red blood mixed in stool
- Rectal adenocarcinoma
  ◊ Bright red rectal bleeding
  ◊ Tenesmus
  ◊ Mass on digital exam
- Carcinoid
  ◊ Often incidental finding
  ◊ Appendicitis-like if located in appendix
  ◊ Rectal bleeding
  ◊ Cramping abdominal pain
  ◊ Carcinoid syndrome; occurs with metastases to liver; includes facial flushing, abdominal cramps, diarrhea
- Squamous cell carcinoma
  ◊ Painful defecation
  ◊ Rectal bleeding
  ◊ Mass or ulcer in anal canal
  ◊ Non-healing anal fissure

CAUSES
- Undetermined; both genetic and environmental factors may contribute
- Environmental - high dietary animal fat, low dietary fiber

RISK FACTORS
- Adenocarcinoma
  ◊ Two-thirds of patients are over 50 years old
  ◊ Pancolonic ulcerative colitis, (2% per year after 10 years active disease)
  ◊ Familial polyposis (100%)
  ◊ Hereditary nonpolyposis colorectal cancer (family history)
  ◊ Benign adenomas (tubular 3%; villous 9-12%)
  ◊ Coexisting (synchronous) colon cancer (5%)
  ◊ Previous (metachronous) colon cancer (2-5%)
- Carcinoid
  ◊ Multiple endocrine adenopathy (MEA), rare
  ◊ Other organs with carcinoid (small bowel, bronchial)
- Squamous cell carcinoma
  ◊ Bowen disease
  ◊ Paget disease

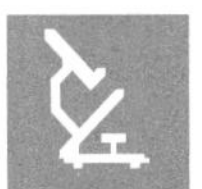

DIAGNOSIS

DIFFERENTIAL DIAGNOSIS
- Strictures (ischemic, Crohn, diverticulosis)
- Other neoplasms (prostatic carcinoma, lipoma, leiomyoma, sarcoma, others)
- Infectious/inflammatory lesions (ameboma, tuberculoma, hemorrhoids)
- Extrinsic masses (abscesses, cysts/pseudocysts, phlegmons)

LABORATORY
- Positive fecal occult blood test
- Anemia
- Urinary 5-hydroxyindoleacetic acid (5-HIAA); elevated in carcinoid
- Elevated plasma carcinoembryonic antigen (CEA)

Drugs that may alter lab results:
- Aspirin-containing medications and non-steroidal anti-inflammatory drugs - positive fecal occult blood test
- Smoking - increased carcinoembryonic antigen

Disorders that may alter lab results:
- Peptic ulcer disease, ulcerative colitis, hemorrhoids, benign polyps - positive fecal occult blood test
- Renal failure - increased carcinoembryonic antigen

PATHOLOGICAL FINDINGS
- Adenocarcinoma
  ◊ May appear as ulcerated, polypoid, or fungating mass. May extend to local structures or metastasize by blood, lymphatics; staging of tumor reflects level of penetration.
  ◊ TNM staging

Stage I - invades to muscularis propria
Stage II - into serosa or adjacent organs
Stage III - regional nodes involved
Stage IV - distant metastases
- Carcinoid
  ◊ Tend to be multicentric
  ◊ Metastasize by blood, lymphatics
- Squamous cell carcinoma
  ◊ Most are ulcerative but may vary greatly in size
  ◊ Metastasize to inguinal lymphatics

SPECIAL TESTS Carcinoembryonic antigen - usually elevated with bulky tumor or metastases, useful in postoperative assessment

IMAGING
- Computerized tomography - used to determine extent of pelvic involvement in rectal cancer; not usually necessary in colon cancer
- Transrectal ultrasound - useful in defining extent of involvement by rectal lesions
- Virtual colonography - using CT scanning technology the entire colon can be visualized. This does not replace the colonoscope as a means of visualizing the colon and rectum.

DIAGNOSTIC PROCEDURES
- Anoscopy - useful for anal canal visualization, biopsies
- Proctoscopy/flexible sigmoidoscopy with biopsy - used for distal lesions when complementary barium enema available for proximal colon
- Colonoscopy with biopsy - for primary diagnosis, screening of high-risk patients and post-resection surveillance; consider as screening modality of choice in all patients

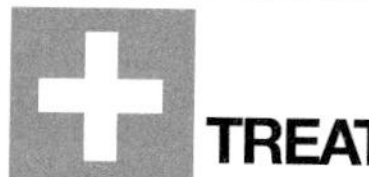

TREATMENT

APPROPRIATE HEALTH CARE Inpatient

GENERAL MEASURES N/A

SURGICAL MEASURES
- Surgical procedures - radical resection of tumor with wide margins; includes segments of normal colon, mesentery, lymph nodes
- Right hemicolectomy for proximal tumors
- Left hemicolectomy for descending colon cancers
- Sigmoid colectomy for sigmoid cancers
- Abdominoperineal resection with colostomy for cancers of distal rectum (within 5-7 cm of dentate line)
- Preoperative or postoperative radiotherapy and chemotherapy: May improve outcome when used for rectal carcinoma
- For carcinoma of anus - combined chemotherapy (5-fluorouracil and mitomycin C) and radiotherapy. Convert to abdominoperineal resection for residual or recurrent tumor or consider salvage chemotherapy (5-FU + cisplatin).

ACTIVITY Usually normal; may be slightly modified for patient with stoma

DIET Usually normal; avoidance of gas-producing foods may be helpful in ostomates (cabbage, beans, onions, alcoholic beverages)

PATIENT EDUCATION
- American Cancer Society
- National Cancer Institute, Department of Health And Human Services, Public Inquiries Section, Office of Cancer Communications, Building 31, Room 101-18, 9000 Rockville Pike, Bethesda, MD 20892, (301)496-5583,

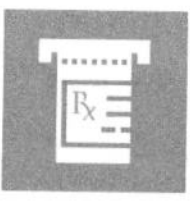

MEDICATIONS

DRUG(S) OF CHOICE
- Steroids, somatostatin or methysergide may ameliorate symptoms of carcinoid syndrome
- Stage III colon adenocarcinoma - fluorouracil (5-FU) plus leucovorin
- Stage II and III rectal - 5-FU + radiation

Contraindications: Peptic ulcer disease (steroids)
Precautions: Refer to manufacturer's literature
Significant possible interactions: Refer to manufacturer's literature

ALTERNATIVE DRUGS N/A

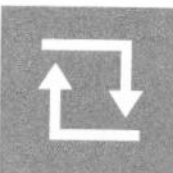

FOLLOWUP

PATIENT MONITORING
- Adenocarcinoma (after remainder of colon is cleared of all lesions)
  - ◊ Colonoscopy - repeat in 1 year; then every 3 years
  - ◊ Carcinoembryonic antigen test, liver chemistries, fecal occult blood test - every 3 months for 2 years; then every 4 months for year 3; then every 6 months for year 4; then annually
- Carcinoid:
  - ◊ 5-HIAA every 6 months x 2 years, then annually
- Squamous cell carcinoma:
  - ◊ Clinical evaluation every 4 months x 1 year, then annually
  - ◊ Biopsy suspicious areas in anus, groin

PREVENTION/AVOIDANCE
- Colonic polyps should be removed, examined microscopically. If benign, surveillance colonoscopy should be performed after 3 years, and if normal, every 5 years
- Screening - asymptomatic population
  - ◊ Average risk (ie > 50 years)
    - Flexible sigmoidoscopy every 5 years
    - Colonoscopy every 10 years
    - Barium enema every 5 years
  - ◊ High risk (history of polyps, personal history of colorectal cancer, family history of colorectal cancer, history of IBD, FAP [familial adenomnononppatous polyposis], hereditary non-polyposis colon cancer)
    - Colonoscopy
    - Schedules vary depending upon underlying risk

POSSIBLE COMPLICATIONS
- Following resections:
  - ◊ Mortality 5-10%
  - ◊ Wound infection 5-15%
  - ◊ Anastomotic stricture/leak/abscess 2-5%
  - ◊ Pneumonia 5-10%
  - ◊ Urinary tract infection 5-20%
- During chemotherapy or radiation therapy:
  - ◊ Stomatitis
  - ◊ Proctitis/diarrhea
  - ◊ Temporary loss of hair

EXPECTED COURSE/PROGNOSIS
- Adenocarcinoma: Overall 5-year survival is 55% but relates to tumor stage in individual patients

Five year survival for colorectal adenocarcinoma by initial stage:

Stage	5-year Survival
I	92%
II	70%
III	50%
IV	5%

- Carcinoid:
  - ◊ Overall 5-year survival is 65%
  - ◊ Relates to tumor stage as in adenocarcinoma
- Squamous cell carcinoma:
  - ◊ Overall 5-year survival is 79%

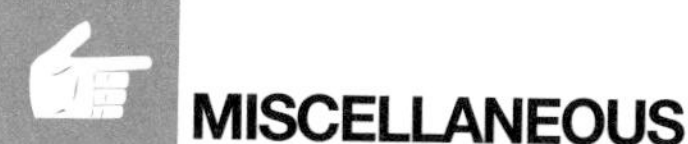

MISCELLANEOUS

ASSOCIATED CONDITIONS Colonic carcinoid - multiple endocrine neoplasia types I, II

AGE-RELATED FACTORS
Pediatric: Adenocarcinoma of colon occurs rarely in children; prognosis is very poor
Geriatric: Coexistence of medical illness may complicate postoperative course
Others: N/A

PREGNANCY N/A

SYNONYMS N/A

ICD-9-CM
154.0 Malignant neoplasm of rectosigmoid junction

SEE ALSO

OTHER NOTES N/A

ABBREVIATIONS N/A

REFERENCES

- Benson AB, Choti MA, Cohen AM, et al. NCCN Practice guidelines for colorectal cancer. Oncology 2000;14:203-12
- Burke CA, Van Stolk R. Colorectal screening: making sense of the different guidelines. Clev Clin J Med 1999;66:303-11
- Lynch HT, Smyrk R. Hereditary colorectal cancer. Semin Oncol 1999;26:478-84

Web references: 1 available at www.5mcc.com
Illustrations N/A

Author(s):
Wayne H. Schwesinger, MD
Morton S. Kahlenberg, MD

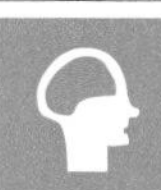

BASICS

DESCRIPTION Inflammation of the nasal passages due to any number of respiratory viruses. Usually not serious; vast majority are self-treated.
System(s) affected: Pulmonary
Genetics: American Indians and Eskimos at higher risk than other ethnic groups and have more frequent complications such as otitis media; individuals with certain alpha-1-antitrypsin genotypes may be unusually susceptible to the common cold.
Incidence/Prevalence in USA: Preschool children 6-10 colds/yr; kindergarten 12/yr; schoolchildren 7/yr; adolescents/adults 2-4/yr. National Ambulatory Survey: 31 episodes/100 persons/year (counting only colds that lead to medical attention or at least one day of restricted activity).
Predominant age: Children > adults
Predominant sex: Male = Female

SIGNS & SYMPTOMS
- Nasal stuffiness and/or obstruction (80-100%)
- Sneezing (50-70%)
- Scratchy throat (50%)
- Cough (40%)
- Hoarseness (30%)
- Malaise (20-25%)
- Headache (25%)
- Fever > 100°F/37.7°C (0-1%)

CAUSES
- Usually due to one of 200 virus strains from six virus families; many strains present within the same geographic region or family
  - ◊ Rhinovirus (> 200 serotypes)
  - ◊ Influenza A, B, C viruses
  - ◊ Parainfluenza viruses
  - ◊ Respiratory syncytial viruses
  - ◊ Coronaviruses
  - ◊ Adenoviruses
  - ◊ Certain ECHO viruses
- In 40% cases, no agent can be identified

RISK FACTORS
- Exposure to infected individuals
- Touching one's nose or conjunctiva with contaminated fingers
- Allergic disorders

DIAGNOSIS

DIFFERENTIAL DIAGNOSIS
- Allergic rhinitis
- Mumps
- Rubeola
- Cytomegalovirus
- Epstein-Barr virus
- Mycoplasma pneumonia
- Influenza - systemic symptoms including myalgias, malaise, severe headache and ocular symptoms overshadow the respiratory complaints

LABORATORY
- CBC if symptoms persist for more than 10 days or with fever > 100°F (37.8°C)
- Nasal smear for eosinophilia may be useful in select individuals

Drugs that may alter lab results: N/A

Disorders that may alter lab results: N/A

PATHOLOGICAL FINDINGS
- Rhinovirus infects the ciliated epithelium lining the nose. Edema and hyperemia of nasal mucous membranes results.
- Exudation of serous and mucinous fluid containing immunoglobulins
- Histology: edema of subepithelial connective tissue, and a scanty cellular infiltrate containing neutrophils, plasma cells, lymphocytes, and eosinophils
- Rhinovirus causes a "non-destructive" inflammation of the mucous membranes, in contrast to influenza and parainfluenza which denude epithelium to the basement membrane

SPECIAL TESTS In some centers, rapid antigen tests for various respiratory viruses are available for patients requiring hospitalization or for research purposes

IMAGING Not indicated unless there is concern for bacterial superinfection of the sinuses, supraglottic region, trachea, or lungs

DIAGNOSTIC PROCEDURES In rare cases, may want to attempt to culture virus from nasal washings or identify by ELISA or RIA methods

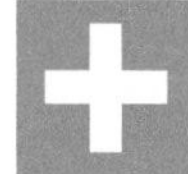

TREATMENT

APPROPRIATE HEALTH CARE Outpatient self-care

GENERAL MEASURES
- Rest, fluids, and symptomatic measures
- Reassure that usual course is 6-10 days
- Humidify inspired air
- Discontinue tobacco and alcohol products (if not already done)
- In infants, clear nasal passages with a bulb syringe, position mattress at 45°, use saline nasal drops

SURGICAL MEASURES N/A

ACTIVITY Up as tolerated with increased rest in the first few days

DIET Encourage fluids

PATIENT EDUCATION
- Reassure that colds are ubiquitous and a normal part of human existence
- Spread is primarily via hand-to-hand transmission of virus contaminated nasal secretions; persons with colds touch their nose and eyes and then touch others
- Small-particle aerosols released in talking, coughing, and sneezing do not travel very far and contain only a low concentration of rhinovirus
- Rhinovirus survives for hours on the hands and hard surfaces, but does not survive long on porous surfaces such as tissues
- Individual susceptibility to colds, depends in large part, on pre-existing antibody levels
- Serum immunity lasts for years, but most individuals gain little protection against future colds due, in part, to the large number of viral serotypes and the antigenic drift that occurs over time in some viral types (rhinovirus, influenza)
- Educate about the expected course and symptomatic measures
- Advise patients to contact you if they develop dyspnea, productive cough, temperature > 102°F (38.9°C), or shaking chills
- Patient information at www.niaid.nih.gov/factsheets/cold.htm

MEDICATIONS

DRUG(S) OF CHOICE
No cure or practical preventive measure documented. Medications targeting a particular symptom reduce the likelihood of adverse systemic effects
- Topical decongestants (sympathomimetics) reduce edema and swelling of the nasal mucosa, promote drainage, and reduce nasal airflow resistance. Preferred over oral because of minimal systemic effects. Sprays preferred over drops in ages > 6.
  - ◊ Oxymetazoline
    - Adults and children ages 6-12: 0.05% solution, 2 or 3 sprays in each nostril bid
    - Children ages 2-6: 0.025% solution, 2 or 3 drops in each nostril bid
    - Rebound congestion (rhinitis medicamentosa) unlikely if used < 5 days
- Topical anticholinergics. Control rhinorrhea but do not relieve nasal congestion or sneezing
  - ◊ Ipratropium: Adults and children >11: 0.06% solution, 2 sprays to each nostril TID for 4 days
- Oral decongestants (sympathomimetics)

Advantages over topical decongestants: longer duration of action, lack of local irritation and no risk of rhinitis medicamentosa
  - ◊ Pseudoephedrine
    - Adults: 60 mg q4-6h (120 mg sustained release q12h)
    - Children ages 6-12: 30 mg q4-6h
    - Children 2-5: 15 mg q4-6h
- Antihistamines. Histamine does not play a significant role in the common cold, but are safe and effective in alleviating sneezing and rhinorrhea. Their perceived benefit may come from anticholinergic effects, drying nasal and pharyngeal secretions and sedative effects promoting rest.
- Chlorpheniramine
  - ◊ Adults: 4 mg q4-6h (or 8 mg tid, 12 mg bid)
  - ◊ Children ages 6-12: 2 mg q4-6h
  - ◊ Children ages 2-6: 1 mg q4-6h
- Cough suppressants. Cough most likely due to irritation of tracheobronchial receptors by post-nasal drip and may therefore benefit from decongestants. If nonproductive or interferes with sleep or normal activities, a cough suppressant is indicated. Codeine and dextromethorphan exhibit comparable efficacy. Adverse effects: drowsiness and GI upset.
  - ◊ Codeine
    - Adults: 10-20 mg q4-6h
    - Children ages 6-12: 5-10 mg q4-6h
    - Children ages 2-6: 2.5-5 mg q4-6h
  - ◊ Dextromethorphan
    - Adults: 10-30 mg q4-8h
    - Children ages 6-12: 15 mg q6-8h
    - Children ages 2-6: 2.5-7.5 mg q4-8h
- Expectorants. Though commonly employed, efficacy not proven
  - ◊ Guaifenesin
    - Adults: 100-400 mg q4h
    - Children ages 6-12: 100-200 mg q4h
    - Children ages 2-5: 50-100 mg q4h

Contraindications:
- Oral decongestants - monoamine oxidase inhibitors or selegiline

Precautions:
- Oral decongestants
  - ◊ Affect all vascular beds and may increase blood pressure. They are cardiac stimulants and may result in arrhythmias. They may increase glucose levels in individuals with glucose intolerance or diabetes mellitus.
  - ◊ Other adverse effects include headache, nervousness, sleeplessness, and dizziness
  - ◊ Should be used with caution in patients taking guanethidine
- Antihistamines
  - ◊ Nasal blockage and sinus congestion may worsen
- Cough suppressants
  - ◊ Misuse and dependence can occur with codeine, but dextromethorphan abuse by adolescents is reported
- Expectorants
  - ◊ Liquid preparations may contain high concentrations of alcohol
  - ◊ Nausea, vomiting or abdominal pain are common adverse effects

Significant possible interactions: See manufacturer's literature

ALTERNATIVE DRUGS
- Many mouthwashes, gargles and lozenges are promoted to relieve the pain of sore throat. The demulcent effects of hard candy, gargling with warm saline, and products with anesthetics (e.g., benzocaine or phenol), may provide pain relief.
- Aromatic oils (e.g., menthol, camphor, eucalyptus), when applied topically or taken in a lozenge, produce a sensation of increased airflow in the absence of a significant change in airflow resistance.
- Antibacterials are of no value
- Antivirals
  - ◊ Interferon. Prevents viral invasion of mucosa to prevent colds; side effects include nasal irritation or bleeding in about 10% of patients; may be useful in groups that have close contact
  - ◊ Zinc chloride. Prevents viral replication in vitro, but efficacy of lozenges unproven
- Vitamin C (ascorbic acid)
  - ◊ No preventative effects and only a modest (average 23%) reduction in the severity and duration of symptoms.
  - ◊ Precipitation of urate, oxalate, or cystine stones has been seen, and urine glucose monitoring may be inaccurate in individuals taking large doses
  - ◊ Interferes with stool guaiac testing

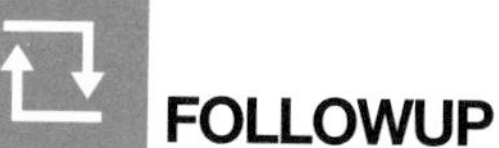

FOLLOWUP

PATIENT MONITORING Patients should contact their physician if they develop fever associated with systemic symptoms, difficulty breathing, dyspnea, and/or purulent drainage

PREVENTION/AVOIDANCE Frequent hand washing and avoiding touching the face may help prevent colds

POSSIBLE COMPLICATIONS
- Lower respiratory tract infection
- Bronchial hyperreactivity
- May lead to decompensation in patients with asthma and chronic lung disease
- Otitis media (2% of colds)
- Acute sinusitis (0.5% of colds)
- Pneumonia
- Rhinitis medicamentosa

EXPECTED COURSE/PROGNOSIS
Complete recovery expected within 3-10 days

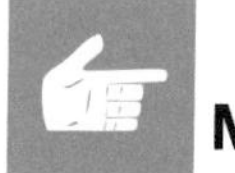

MISCELLANEOUS

ASSOCIATED CONDITIONS
- Pharyngitis
- Sinusitis
- Bronchitis
- Bronchiolitis
- Pneumonia
- Croup
- Asthma

AGE-RELATED FACTORS
Pediatric:
- Medications are likely to produce adverse effects or toxicity in young children
- Incidence of colds is highest

Geriatric: Medications commonly produce adverse effects in the elderly

Others: N/A

PREGNANCY
- Decongestants: no clear association between drug use and congenital defects
- Antihistamines: no clear association between drug use and congenital defects
- Codeine: indiscriminate use during pregnancy may pose a risk to the fetus

SYNONYMS
- URI
- Upper respiratory infection

ICD-9-CM
460 Acute nasopharyngitis (common cold)

SEE ALSO
Cytomegalovirus inclusion disease
Epstein-Barr virus infections
Influenza
Measles, rubeola
Mumps
Pharyngitis
Pneumonia, mycoplasma
Rhinitis, allergic

OTHER NOTES N/A

ABBREVIATIONS
- ELISA = enzyme linked immunosorbent assay
- RIA = radioimmunoassay
- URI = upper respiratory infection

REFERENCES

- Bryant BG, Lombardi TP. Cold, cough and allergy products. In: Covington CR, Lawson LC, Young LL, eds. Handbook of Nonprescription Drugs.10th Ed. Washington, D.C.:American Pharmaceutical Association; 1993:89-115
- Gadomski A. Rational use of over-the-counter medications in young children. JAMA 1994;272:1063-4
- Hemila H. Does vitamin C alleviate the symptoms of the common cold?-a review of current evidence. Scandinavian Journal of Infectious Diseases 1994;26(1):1-6
- Hendeles L. Efficacy and safety of antihistamines and expectorants in nonprescription cough and cold preparations. Pharmacotherapy 1993;13(2):154-8
- Hendeles L. Selecting a decongestant. Pharmacotherapy 1993;13(6 Pt2):129S-134S
- Hendley JO, Gwaltney JM Jr. Mechanisms of transmission of rhinovirus infections. Epidemiologic Reviews 1988;10:243-58
- Lowenstein SR, Parrino TA. Management of the common cold. Advances in Internal Medicine 1987;32:207-33
- Saroea HG. Common colds: Causes, potential cures, and treatment. Canadian Family Physician 1993;39:2215-16, 2219-20
- Smith MB, Feldman W. Over-the-counter cold medications. A critical review of clinical trials between 1950 and 1991. JAMA 1993;269(17):2258-63
- Tyrrell DA. A view from the common cold unit. Antiviral Research 1992;18(2):105-25

Web references: 0 available at www.5mcc.com

Illustrations N/A

Author(s):
Lisa M. Schroeder, MD

Complete atrioventricular (AV) canal

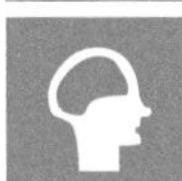

BASICS

DESCRIPTION The central atrioventricular (AV) portion of the cardiac septum and the contiguous mitral and tricuspid valves are abnormal, allowing for an unobstructed atrioventricular canal. Children with Down syndrome and this anomaly rapidly progress to pulmonary vascular obstructive disease (within 3 to 6 months).

- Rastelli classification:
  - ◊ Type A: Common anterior AV valve leaflet is divided and attached to the crest of the ventricular septum by chordae
  - ◊ Type B: Common anterior AV valve leaflet is divided and chordae tendineae from the midportions of the divided anterior leaflet are attached to the right ventricular medial papillary muscle
  - ◊ Type C: Common anterior AV valve leaflet is undivided and not attached to the ventricular septum (free-floating leaflet)

System(s) affected: Cardiovascular
Genetics: No known genetic pattern
Incidence/Prevalence in USA: 1 in 250,000 live births; type A being the most common
Predominant age: Congenital, present at birth
Predominant sex: Female > Male

SIGNS & SYMPTOMS
- Pulmonary congestion
- Congestive heart failure
- Low systemic arterial blood oxygen saturation
- Tachycardia
- Poor feeding
- Growth failure
- Mitral regurgitation
- Pulmonary vascular obstructive disease, and cyanosis (30% in the first 2-3 years)

CAUSES Defective development of the endocardial cushions

RISK FACTORS Unknown

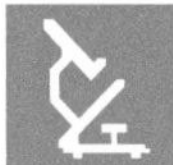

DIAGNOSIS

DIFFERENTIAL DIAGNOSIS
- Atrial septal defect
- Ventricular septal defect
- Incomplete or intermediate AV canal
- Patent ductus arteriosus
- Mitral valve prolapse
- Secondary mitral regurgitation
- Pulmonary vascular obstructive disease
- Anomalous pulmonary venous return

LABORATORY Arterial blood gas

Drugs that may alter lab results: N/A

Disorders that may alter lab results: N/A

PATHOLOGICAL FINDINGS Low oxygen saturation in the arterial blood gas

SPECIAL TESTS
- Cardiac 2-D echo-Doppler showing anatomic defect, increased pulmonary pressures, mitral regurgitation, tricuspid regurgitation, right and left atrial and ventricular enlargements
- ECG - superior QRS axis, right ventricular hypertrophy (RVH), left ventricular hypertrophy (LVH), possibly peaked P waves

IMAGING
- Cardiac angiogram demonstrating AV canal and mitral and tricuspid regurgitation, left and right atrial and ventricular enlargement
- Chest x-ray showing increased pulmonary vasculature, left and right atrial and ventricular enlargement
- MRI offers excellent imaging of crux

DIAGNOSTIC PROCEDURES
- Pulmonary artery catheter showing prominent "V" waves, elevated pulmonary capillary wedge pressures, right atrial "step-up" in oxygen saturations
- Angiography

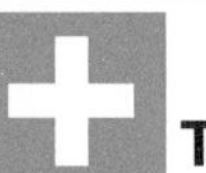

TREATMENT

APPROPRIATE HEALTH CARE Medical management (digoxin, diuretics, afterload reducers) either as an inpatient or an outpatient, dependent upon the patient's condition

GENERAL MEASURES Provide general treatment for congestive heart failure

SURGICAL MEASURES If pulmonary edema, growth failure and congestive heart failure is refractive in spite of optimal medical therapy, reparative surgery should be pursued as early as possible. Repair should be especially early in children with Down syndrome (approximately 3 months). Repair should be performed before 2 years of age to avoid the continued progression of pulmonary vascular obstructive disease. Patients more than 2 years of age can undergo repair if the pulmonary vascular resistance (PVR) does not exceed 8-10 units-meters squared. At a minimum, surgical correction includes closure of the interatrial and interventricular septal defects and suspension of the medial aspects of the left and right AV valve leaflets. Pulmonary artery banding might still be a possibility.

ACTIVITY As tolerated

DIET High calorie, low salt

PATIENT EDUCATION Instruct regarding travel to altitudes and plane travel causing potential hypoxia

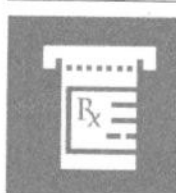

MEDICATIONS

DRUG(S) OF CHOICE Digoxin, ACE inhibitors or isosorbide dinitrate plus hydralazine, furosemide, potassium supplementation

- Doses for term infants
  - ◊ Digoxin - oral 30 μg/kg (digitalizing), then 10 μg/kg/24 hrs. Adjust to maintain levels within therapeutic range - 0.5-2.0 ng/mL (0.64-2.6 nmol/L)
  - ◊ Captopril - 0.05-0.1 mg/kg/dose tid-qid
  - ◊ Isosorbide dinitrate - refer to manufacturer's literature
  - ◊ Hydralazine - 0.75-3.0 mg/kg/dose, increase as needed to maximum of 6 mg/kg/dose
  - ◊ Furosemide - oral 2 mg/kg, increase as needed to maximum of 6 mg/kg
  - ◊ Potassium - supplement patients who require furosemide. Maintenance dose is 2-3 mEq/kg/24 hours.

Contraindications: Profound systemic hypotension, worsening hypoxia and V/Q mismatch with treatment

Precautions: Refer to manufacturer's literature

Significant possible interactions: Refer to manufacturer's literature

ALTERNATIVE DRUGS Dobutamine or amrinone drips

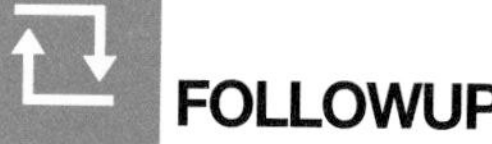

FOLLOWUP

PATIENT MONITORING

- As indicated by clinical intervention and disease progression
- Serial measurements of arterial oxygen content
- Serial measurements of pulmonary vascular resistance

PREVENTION/AVOIDANCE Avoid hypoxic embarrassment in environments of low oxygen tension

POSSIBLE COMPLICATIONS

- Refractive hypoxia secondary to progressive pulmonary vascular obstructive disease
- Cyanosis
- Polycythemia
- Growth failure
- Congestive heart failure/pulmonary edema
- Complications of surgery:
  - ◊ Residual ventricular septal defect
  - ◊ Residual left ventricular to right atrial shunting
  - ◊ Complete AV block

EXPECTED COURSE/PROGNOSIS

- PVR less than 5:
  - ◊ If undergoing reparative surgery, are at risk for an approximate 10% surgical mortality
  - ◊ The majority of those surviving realize complete relief of their symptoms and will need no further treatment
- PVR between 5-13 undergoing surgery:
  - ◊ Perioperative mortality approaches 33%
  - ◊ Survivors realize functional class I or II (New York Heart Association [NYHA] classification)
- PVR greater than 5 who do not or can not undergo surgical intervention:
  - ◊ Deterioration is progressive with death ranging from 2-16 years of age

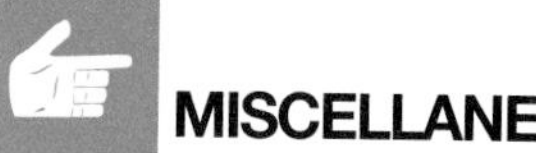

MISCELLANEOUS

ASSOCIATED CONDITIONS

- Down syndrome. Very high percentage have complete atrioventricular canal lesions.
- Tetralogy of Fallot
- Unbalanced canal with left or right dominance

AGE-RELATED FACTORS

Pediatric: Surgical intervention before age 2 or before marked increase in PVR occurs

Geriatric: N/A

Others: N/A

PREGNANCY N/A

SYNONYMS N/A

ICD-9-CM

745.69 Endocardial cushion defects, other

SEE ALSO

Atrial septal defect (ASD)

OTHER NOTES N/A

ABBREVIATIONS

AVC = atrioventricular canal
PVR = pulmonary vascular resistance
V/Q = ventilation-perfusion ratio

REFERENCES

- Brandenburg RO, Fuster V, Giuliani ER, McGoon DC. Cardiology: Fundamentals and Practice. Chicago, Year Book Medical Publishers, 1987
- Braunwald E, ed. Heart Disease: A Textbook of Cardiovascular Medicine. 5th Ed. Philadelphia, W.B. Saunders Co., 1996

Web references: 0 available at www.5mcc.com

Illustrations N/A

Author(s):

David J. Framm, MD

Complex regional pain syndrome

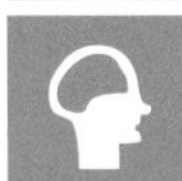

BASICS

DESCRIPTION Pain syndrome following injury to bone and soft tissue. Pathogenesis is obscure. Evidence suggests that these syndromes involve areas of the brain and nervous system.
- Type I - no nerve injury (reflex sympathetic dystrophy [RSD])
- Type II - associated with a demonstrable nerve injury (causalgia)

System(s) affected: Nervous
Genetics: No known genetic pattern
Incidence/Prevalence in USA: Unknown
Predominant age: No predominant age
Predominant sex: Male > Female

SIGNS & SYMPTOMS
- Type I
  - ◊ Hypersensitivity to light touch
  - ◊ Thermal hypersensitivity
  - ◊ Osteoporosis
  - ◊ Hair loss
  - ◊ Mottled skin
  - ◊ Muscle spasms
  - ◊ Nail brittleness
- Type II
  - ◊ Burning pain
  - ◊ Paroxysms of pain
  - ◊ Partial motor paralysis
  - ◊ Worse with emotional stress

CAUSES Other than known nerve injury (type II or causalgia), there is no known definitive pathogenesis

RISK FACTORS
- Minor or severe trauma
  - ◊ Surgery
  - ◊ Lacerations
  - ◊ Burns
  - ◊ Frostbite
  - ◊ Casting
  - ◊ Penetrating injury

DIAGNOSIS

DIFFERENTIAL DIAGNOSIS Infection, hypertrophic scar, bone fragments, neuroma, central nervous system tumor or syrinx

LABORATORY N/A

Drugs that may alter lab results: N/A

Disorders that may alter lab results: N/A

PATHOLOGICAL FINDINGS
- Partial or complete damage to afferent nerve pathways and probably reorganized central pain pathways
- Most common nerves involved are median and sciatic
- Atrophy in affected muscles
- Incomplete nerve plexus lesion

SPECIAL TESTS EMG/NCV to evaluate peripheral nerve function

IMAGING Bone scan to delineate presence of demineralization or occult osteomyelitis

DIAGNOSTIC PROCEDURES May use drop of acetone on skin of involved limbs to evaluate thermal hypersensitivity

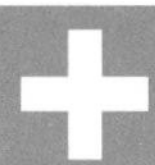

TREATMENT

APPROPRIATE HEALTH CARE Outpatient, except for operative procedures or intravenous sympathetic nerve blockade

GENERAL MEASURES
- Available information about treatment is based on small studies or treatment reports, therefore remains largely empiric
- Treatment response can be predicted by diagnosis (type I vs type II)
- Type I
  - ◊ Physical therapy
  - ◊ Transcutaneous nerve stimulation
  - ◊ Biofeedback
  - ◊ Psychotherapy
- Type II
  - ◊ Sympathetic blocks
  - ◊ Sympathectomy
- Anesthetic blockade (chemical or surgical) of sympathetic nerve function (transient relief suggests that chemical or surgical sympathectomy will be helpful)
- Intravenous regional sympathetic block with guanethidine or reserpine by pain specialist or anesthetist
- Physical therapy (essential during all phases of treatment)
- Transcutaneous electric nerve stimulation (controversial)
- Inject myofacial painful trigger points
- Briskly rub the affected part several times per day
- Acupuncture can be tried
- Hypnosis
- Relaxation training (alternate muscle relaxing and contracting)
- Biofeedback
- Discourage maladaptive behaviors
- Refer the patient to a specialty pain clinic in difficult cases

SURGICAL MEASURES Sympathectomy sometimes necessary

ACTIVITY Maintain as high a level of physical and intellectual activity as possible

DIET No special diet

PATIENT EDUCATION
- Stress staying active physically
- Careful instructions about any prescribed medications
- Internet: Reflex Sympathetic Dystrophy Syndrome Association (RSDSA) www.rsds.org; 203-877-3790 or American RSD Hope Group www.rsdhope.org; 207-583-4589

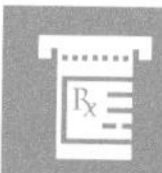

MEDICATIONS

DRUG(S) OF CHOICE

No single drug or combination of drugs has produced consistent results; early therapy is beneficial

- Alpha-adrenergic blockers
  - ◊ Phenoxybenzamine 40-120 mg daily, orally in divided doses. The initial dose should not exceed 10 mg.
- Miscellaneous
  - ◊ Prednisone 60-80 mg/day orally, tapered over 2-4 weeks
- Tricyclic antidepressants
  - ◊ Amitriptyline (Elavil) 25-100 mg/day qHS
  - ◊ Nortriptyline (Pamelor) 25-100 mg/day
- Anticonvulsants (serum drug level monitoring may be needed, except for clonazepam; Individualize doses):
  - ◊ Carbamazepine (Tegretol) 200-1000 mg/day orally
  - ◊ Phenytoin (Dilantin) 100-300 mg/day orally
  - ◊ Clonazepam (Klonopin) 1-10 mg/day orally
  - ◊ Valproic acid (Depakene) 750-2250 mg/day orally, maximum of 60 mg/kg
  - ◊ Gabapentin 100 mg q hs up to 600-1200 mg tid
- Skeletal muscle relaxant:
  - ◊ Baclofen 10-40 mg/day orally - may act synergistically with carbamazepine and phenytoin

Contraindications: Refer to manufacturer's literature

Precautions: Refer to manufacturer's literature

Significant possible interactions: There are many with this group of drugs. Refer to manufacturer's literature.

ALTERNATIVE DRUGS

Narcotics - only after all non-opioid therapies are exhausted. May be necessary to use to allow patient to engage in physical therapy.

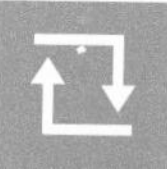

FOLLOWUP

PATIENT MONITORING

- Watch carefully for adverse reactions to medications
- Several different forms of therapy may need to be tried

PREVENTION/AVOIDANCE

- Mobilization following injury
- Avoidance of nerve damage during surgical procedures
- Splinting of an injured extremity for adequate period of time
- Adequate analgesics during recovery from injuries

POSSIBLE COMPLICATIONS

- Drug mishaps
- Joint contractures
- Contralateral spread of symptoms

EXPECTED COURSE/PROGNOSIS

- Course - variable; chronic; remitting
- Outlook only satisfactory, may need attempts at several treatment modalities. No one form of therapy is superior to others. Failure to respond to one form does not mitigate against success with another.
- Those patients receiving work compensation for an injury or secondary gain from family or friends are in a separate category and may never get well

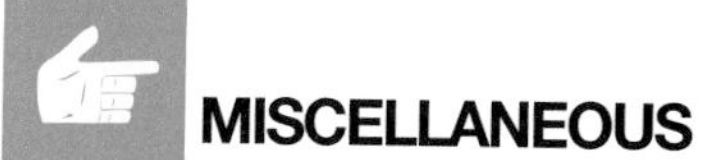

MISCELLANEOUS

ASSOCIATED CONDITIONS

- Serious injury to bone and soft tissue
- Herpes zoster

AGE-RELATED FACTORS

Pediatric: N/A

Geriatric: Painful perception is frequently worse in older patients. Start with smaller than usual doses of drugs.

Others: N/A

PREGNANCY

Many of the useful drugs are contraindicated in pregnancy

SYNONYMS

- Traumatic erythromelalgia
- Weir-Mitchell causalgia
- Causalgia
- Reflex sympathetic dystrophy
- Post-traumatic neuralgia
- Sympathetically maintained pain

ICD-9-CM

337.21 Reflex sympathetic dystrophy of the upper limb
337.22 Reflex sympathetic dystrophy of the lower limb
354.4 Causalgia of upper limb
355.71 Causalgia of lower limb

SEE ALSO

Arterial embolus & thrombosis
Herpes zoster

OTHER NOTES

- Postherpetic neuralgia is a result of partial or complete damage to afferent nerve pathways
- Pain occurring in dermatomes as a sequela of herpes zoster

ABBREVIATIONS

N/A

REFERENCES

- Atkins RM. Complex regional pain syndrome. J Bone Joint Surg Br 2003;85(8):1100-6
- Hendler NH. Complex regional pain syndrome, types I and II. In: Weiner RS, ed. Pain Management: A Practical Guide for Clinicians. 6th Ed. Boca Raton, CRC Press; 2002
- Rho RH, Brewer RP, Lamer TJ, Wilson PR. Complex regional pain syndrome. Mayo Clin Proc 2002;77(2):174-80

Web references: 2 available at www.5mcc.com

Illustrations N/A

Author(s):
Dennis E. Hughes, DO

Condyloma acuminata

BASICS

DESCRIPTION Condyloma acuminata are soft, skin colored, fleshy warts that are caused by the HPV (human papilloma virus). There are now > 100 known types of HPV and types 6, 11, 16, 18, 31, 33, 35 have been associated with condyloma acuminata. The disease is highly contagious, can appear singly or in groups, small or large. They appear in the vagina, on the cervix, around the external genitalia and rectum, in the urethra, anus, also conjunctival, nasal, oral and laryngeal warts and occasionally, the throat. The incubation period may be from 1-6 months.

System(s) affected: Reproductive, Skin/Exocrine

Genetics: N/A

Incidence/Prevalence in USA:

- Most common viral sexually transmitted disease in the U.S.
- ≈ 1% of sexually active population in U.S. has genital warts
- 26% transmission after single encounter
- Minimum of 10-20% of sexually active women may be infected with HPV. Studies in men suggest a similar prevalence.
- 750,000 new cases per year; rates are increasing
- Peak prevalence is in ages 17-33

Predominant age: 15-30 years of age

Predominant sex: Male = Female

SIGNS & SYMPTOMS

- Tumors, soft, sessile
- Surface smooth to very rough
- Multiple fingerlike projections
- Perianal condylomata acuminatum usually rough and cauliflower-like
- Penile lesions often smooth and papular
- Penile lesions often occur in groups of three or four
- Male sites - frenulum, corona, glans, prepuce, meatus, shaft, scrotum
- Female sites - labia, clitoris, periurethral area, perineum, vagina, cervix (flat lesions)
- Pruritus
- Irritation
- Bleeding (result of trauma)
- Perianal area (both sexes)
- Subclinical HPV infection
- May be detected by Pap test

CAUSES Human papillomaviruses. These are circular double-stranded DNA molecules. There are over 70 HPV subtypes. The cause of common venereal warts is types 6 and 11. Cervical dysplasia and carcinoma in situ are likely caused by types 16, 18, 31, 33, and 35.

RISK FACTORS

- Young adult
- Sexually active
- Not using condoms
- Possibly subclinical infection
- Young age of commencing sexual activity
- Cigarette smoking
- Poor hygiene
- Pregnancy
- Caucasian
- History of genital warts

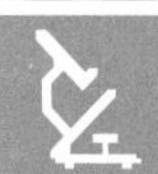

DIAGNOSIS

DIFFERENTIAL DIAGNOSIS

- Condyloma lata (flat warts of syphilis)
- Lichen planus
- Normal sebaceous glands
- Seborrheic keratosis
- Molluscum contagiosum
- Keratomas
- Scabies
- Crohn disease
- Skin tags
- Melanocytic nevi
- Vulvar intraepithelial neoplasia
- Buschke-Lowenstein tumor

LABORATORY Serologic test for syphilis - negative

Drugs that may alter lab results: N/A

Disorders that may alter lab results: N/A

PATHOLOGICAL FINDINGS

- Possible cervical dysplasia in females
- Benign
- Well organized basal layer
- Underlying infiltration of lymphocytes
- Plasma cells
- Hyperplastic epithelial changes
- Basement membrane intact
- Sometimes difficult to differentiate from squamous cell carcinoma

SPECIAL TESTS Aceto-whitening: Subclinical lesions can be visualized by wrapping the penis with gauze soaked with 5% acetic acid for 5 minutes. Using a ten X hand lens or colposcope, warts appear as tiny white papules. A shiny white appearance of the skin represents foci of epithelial hyperplasia (subclinical infection). Not highly specific, low positive predictive value.

IMAGING N/A

DIAGNOSTIC PROCEDURES

- Biopsy with highly specialized identification techniques (not clinically useful). HPV DNA detection is done by PCR on biopsy tissue.
- Colposcopy, antroscopy, anoscopy, Pap smear

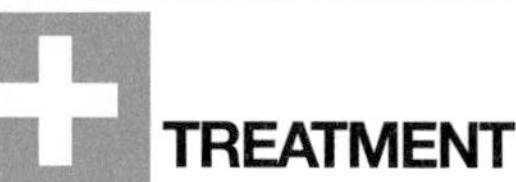

TREATMENT

APPROPRIATE HEALTH CARE Outpatient

GENERAL MEASURES

- May resolve on their own
- Treatment determined by location and size of warts
- Small warts may be treated with topical applications
- Cryotherapy
- Change therapy if no improvement after 3 treatments, no complete clearance after 6 treatments, or therapy exceeding manufacturer's recommendations
- Appropriate screening and counseling of partners

SURGICAL MEASURES

- Larger warts require laser treatment or electrocoagulation
- Surgical excision for large warts

ACTIVITY No restrictions

DIET No special diet

PATIENT EDUCATION

- Explain preventive measures and chronic nature of the infection
- Numerous pamphlets on HPV, STD prevention, condom use
- Emphasize need for women to get regular Pap smears

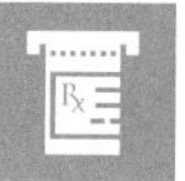

MEDICATIONS

DRUG(S) OF CHOICE

- Imiquimod (Aldara) 5% cream applied overnight 3 times weekly until warts clear for up to 16 weeks
- Cryotherapy - liquid nitrogen is applied to warts in 5-10 second bursts. Usually requires 2-3 weekly sessions.
- Podophyllin in tincture of Benzoin. Apply directly to warts. Leave on for 1-4 hours, then wash off. Repeat treatment every 7 days until gone (in office procedure)

or

- Podofilox (Condylox) - for external warts. Apply to external warts every 12 hours (allowing to dry) for 3 consecutive days. May repeat after 4 days (home application).
- Trichloroacetic acid - 25-85%. Apply only to warts. Use powder/talc to remove un-reacted acid. Repeat in office at weekly intervals.
- Topical cidofovir gel - undergoing trials; applied once daily for 5 days every other week for maximum of 6 cycles

Contraindications:

- Podophyllin - do not use during pregnancy or on oral, cervical, urethral or perianal warts. Can use on small number of vaginal warts with careful drying after application.
- Cryotherapy - cryoglobulinemia

Precautions:

- Podophyllin - to minimize local and systemic reactions, wash treated areas 1-4 hours after application and use ointments to protect surrounding skin from contact with podophyllin
- Cryotherapy - none
- Electrocautery - don't use in patient with pacemaker

Significant possible interactions: N/A

ALTERNATIVE DRUGS

- External (penile and perianal)
  - ◊ Podophyllin
  - ◊ Podofilox (Condylox) self-treatment
  - ◊ Electrocautery, laser, intralesional interferon
  - ◊ Small study of topical BCG use for penile lesions
- Urethral meatus
  - ◊ Laser
  - ◊ Podophyllin
  - ◊ Topical fluorouracil
- Anal
  - ◊ Trichloroacetic acid (TCA) - apply weekly
  - ◊ Topical fluorouracil
- Oral
  - ◊ Electrocautery
  - ◊ Surgery
  - ◊ Laser
- Trichloroacetic acid is ideal for isolated lesions in pregnant women
- Oral cimetidine 30-40 mg/kg divided tid for 3 months in children with genital and perigenital condyloma. Used as a primary and adjunctive therapy.

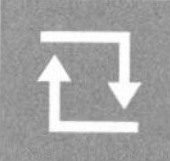

FOLLOWUP

PATIENT MONITORING

- Every 2 weeks for treatment until clear
- Pap test every 1 year for indefinite period
- Biopsy for persistent warts
- Monitor sex partners
- Treatment does not decrease infectivity

PREVENTION/AVOIDANCE

- Use of condoms by male sexual partners of individuals who have been treated for HPV infection
- Use of condoms by infected men (preventive effects not adequately evaluated; 40% of infected men have scrotal warts)
- Abstinence by women until treatment completed
- Circumcision may prevent recurrence in some men
- HPV vaccine - phase II trial in progress, appears encouraging

POSSIBLE COMPLICATIONS

- Cervical dysplasia
- Malignant change: Progression to cancer rarely, if ever occurs
- Male urethral obstruction
- The prevalence of high grade dysplasia (HGD) and cancer in anal canal is higher in HIV-positive than in HIV-negative patients, probably because of HPV activity

EXPECTED COURSE/PROGNOSIS

- Warts clear with treatment or spontaneous regression
- Recurrences: Frequent and may necessitate repeated treatment
- Some studies identified 3 independent risk factors for condyloma relapse: Positive HIV, male sex, and Langerhans' cells - LCs/mm anal tissue (15 vs. 30)
- Without treatment: May remain stable, worsen, or resolve completely
- Asymptomatic infection persists indefinitely

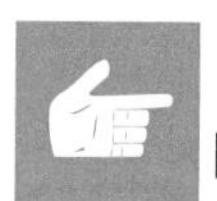

MISCELLANEOUS

ASSOCIATED CONDITIONS

- 90% of cervical cancer contains evidence of HPV infection
- Gonorrhea
- Syphilis
- AIDS
- Chlamydia
- Other sexually transmitted disease

AGE-RELATED FACTORS

Young adults, infants and children

Pediatric: Consider sexual abuse if seen in children; although can acquire by other means (eg, transfer from wart on child's hand)

Geriatric: N/A

Others:

- Venereal warts are increasing in an ever younger population. A recent study of 487 college women showed an infection rate of 48%.
- Increased size and number in immunocompromised states

PREGNANCY

- Warts often grow larger in pregnancy and regress spontaneously after delivery. Use cryotherapy.
- Virus does not cross the placenta. Treatment during pregnancy is somewhat controversial. C-section is not indicated.
- HPV can be transmitted to infant at time of delivery and cause laryngeal papillomas, a rare and life threatening condition

SYNONYMS

- Genital warts
- Venereal warts
- Papilloma acuminatum

ICD-9-CM

078.11 Condyloma acuminata

SEE ALSO

Abnormal Pap smear

OTHER NOTES

N/A

ABBREVIATIONS

N/A

REFERENCES

- Franco I. Oral cimetidine for the management of genital and perigenital warts in children. J Urol 2000;164(3 Pt 2):1074-5
- Bohle A, Buttner H, Jocham D. Primary treatment of condylomata acuminata with viable bacillus Calmette-Guerin. J Urol 2001;165(3):834-6
- Fitzpatrick TB, et al: Color Atlas and Synopsis of Clinical Dermatology. New York, McGraw-Hill, 1992
- Beutner KR, Wiley DJ, et al: Genital warts and their treatment. Clin Infect Dis 1999;28(suppl1):537-56
- Edwards L: Imiquimod in clinical practice. Australia J Dermatol 1998;39(suppl1)s14-16
- Sobhani I, Vuagnat A, Walker F, et al. Prevalence of high-grade dysplasia and cancer in the anal canal in human papillomavirus-infected individuals. Gastroenterology 2001;120(4):857-66

Web references: 4 available at www.5mcc.com

Illustrations 2 available

Author(s):

Carrie A. Jaworski, MD
Shefali K. Shah, MD

Congenital megacolon

BASICS

DESCRIPTION Congenital disease of the colon, characterized by functional obstruction and accumulation of feces and massive dilatation of colon

System(s) affected: Gastrointestinal, Nervous

Genetics: Familial 50 times base rate. Sometimes associated with Down syndrome.

Incidence/Prevalence in USA: 1 in 2000 to 5000 births (Caucasians 91%, Blacks 8%, Oriental 0.5%)

Predominant age: Infancy

Predominant sex:
- Males > Females for short segment (8:2)
- Males > Females for long segment (5:4)

SIGNS & SYMPTOMS
- Early infancy:
  - ◊ Onset early in infancy, newborn fails to pass meconium in 24 to 48 hours after birth
  - ◊ Obstipation
  - ◊ May have diarrhea
  - ◊ Marked enlargement and distention of abdomen
  - ◊ Colonic peristalsis visible
  - ◊ Vomiting
  - ◊ Palpable fecal mass
  - ◊ Growth retardation (possible)
- Older infants:
  - ◊ Failure to thrive
  - ◊ Anorexia
  - ◊ Lack of physiologic urge to defecate
  - ◊ Empty rectum on digital examination
  - ◊ Palpable colon
  - ◊ Visible peristalsis
  - ◊ Hypoalbuminemia

CAUSES Congenital absence of Auerbach's and Meissner's autonomic plexuses in bowel wall - usually limited to the colon

RISK FACTORS
- Family history of Hirschsprung disease
- Offspring risk if parent has short segment - 2%; if parent has long segment - up to 50%
- Sibling risk if male affected - female has 0.6% risk (short segment)
- Sibling risk if female affected - male has 18% risk (long segment)

DIAGNOSIS

DIFFERENTIAL DIAGNOSIS
- Megacolon, secondary (to Chagas disease)
- Megacolon, acquired, functional
- Functional constipation
- Hypoganglionosis
- Meconium plug syndrome
- Small left colon syndrome
- Meconium ileus

LABORATORY Electrolytes, albumin, CBC, urinalysis, thyroid function

Drugs that may alter lab results: N/A

Disorders that may alter lab results: N/A

PATHOLOGICAL FINDINGS
- Congenital absence of Auerbach's and Meissner's autonomic plexuses in myenteric plexus of colon wall
- Obstruction may begin at anus, and may extend proximally to involve varying portions of the colon or terminal ileum (rarely may involve entire small bowel)
- Enormous dilatation and hypertrophy of all layers of involved colon
- Aganglionosis of involved bowel
- Submucosal hypertrophied nerve bundles

SPECIAL TESTS
- Proctoscopy: Ampulla empty of feces
- Biopsy: Absence of ganglia in wall of narrowed rectum
- Anorectal manometry

IMAGING
- X-ray - barium enema shows:
  - ◊ Large ovoid mass mottled by small, irregular gas shadows
  - ◊ Dilatation of sigmoid colon above narrowed distal sigmoid or rectum
  - ◊ Narrowed portion rippled or segmented
  - ◊ Fluid levels within bowel
  - ◊ Diaphragm elevated

DIAGNOSTIC PROCEDURES
- Suction aspiration biopsy of bowel wall
- Barium enema
- Proctosigmoidoscopy
- Large bowel wall biopsy
- Laparoscopy: Normal proximal colon dilatation
- Anorectal manometry: Internal sphincter relaxation failure

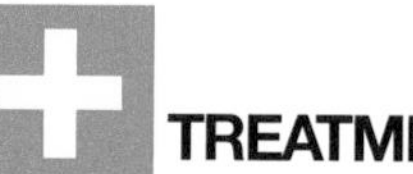

TREATMENT

APPROPRIATE HEALTH CARE Early work-up (ambulatory or hospital). Inpatient for surgery.

GENERAL MEASURES
- Treatment may be symptomatic or definitive
- May need emergency correction of fluid and electrolyte imbalance
- Removal of fecal accumulation - retention enemas of 3-4 ounces (90-120 mL) of mineral oil followed by repeated colonic irrigations with isotonic saline solution. Avoid use of other solutions, e.g., water, soapsuds enemas.

SURGICAL MEASURES
- Inpatient surgery
  - ◊ Proximal colostomy and resection of agangliononic bowel is gold standard (and necessary when there is significant proximal dilation)
  - ◊ Definitive pull-through procedure (Duhamel, Soave, or Swenson) when dilation has resolved (usually 2-4 months)
  - ◊ Single stage procedure may be possible in infants
  - ◊ Transanal pull-through in infants
  - ◊ Laparoscopic technique may be used
- Confirmation of normal ganglion cells mandatory at colostomy site and proximal resection site prior to anastomosis

ACTIVITY No restrictions

DIET
- Diet will not control the obstipation of Hirschsprung
- Postoperative diet - standard for age when bowel function returns

PATIENT EDUCATION
- After surgery instruct parents to detect and report dehydration, decreased urinary output, sunken eyes, poor skin turgor, vomiting, fever
- Encourage bonding with parents by having parents participate in child's care as much as possible
- Request enterotomy therapist to teach family

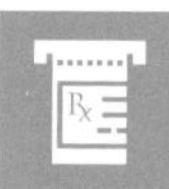

MEDICATIONS

DRUG(S) OF CHOICE
- None recommended for treatment
- Preliminary to surgery: Bowel prep with neomycin or nystatin

Contraindications: N/A
Precautions: N/A
Significant possible interactions: N/A

ALTERNATIVE DRUGS
- Metronidazole (Flagyl) for bowel preparation

FOLLOWUP

PATIENT MONITORING Closely until recuperated fully from surgical intervention

PREVENTION/AVOIDANCE N/A

POSSIBLE COMPLICATIONS
- Toxic enterocolitis, possibly fatal
- Bleeding and/or perforation

EXPECTED COURSE/PROGNOSIS
- Favorable
- Requires long-term followup
- Requires aggressive management of any suspected Hirschsprung enterocolitis with:
  - ◊ Rectal irrigation
  - ◊ IV antibiotics
  - ◊ Nasogastric decompression

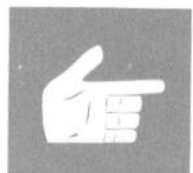

MISCELLANEOUS

ASSOCIATED CONDITIONS
- Chagas disease (secondary aganglionic megacolon may be a late complication of Chagas)
- Megacolon, acquired, functional usually begins in 3rd or 4th year of life
- Down syndrome
- Septal defects
- Tetralogy of Fallot
- Dandy-Walker syndrome
- Associated with anomalies 22% of the time, especially neurological, cardiovascular, urological, gastrointestinal

AGE-RELATED FACTORS
Pediatric: Occasionally infants have only mild or intermittent constipation with intervening bouts of diarrhea. These cases may not be diagnosed until later in infancy.
Geriatric: N/A
Others: N/A

PREGNANCY N/A

SYNONYMS
- Aganglionic megacolon
- Hirschsprung disease
- Zuelzer-Wilson disease (total colonic aganglionosis)

ICD-9-CM
751.3 Hirschsprung disease and other congenital functional disorders of colon

SEE ALSO
Constipation

OTHER NOTES Diagnosis must be made as early as possible to prevent toxic enterocolitis

ABBREVIATIONS N/A

REFERENCES

- Ryan ET, et al: J Ped Surg 1992;1:76-81
- Walsh K, et al, eds. Pediatric Surgery. New York: Yearbook Medical Publishers; 1986
- Eastwood GL, Avunduk C, eds. Manual of Gastroenterology. Boston: Little, Brown; 1988
- Barakat AY, ed. Renal Disease in Children: Clinical Evaluation & Diagnosis. New York: Springer-Verlag; 1990
- O'Neill J, Rowe M, Fonkalsrud E, et al, eds. Pediatric Surgery, 5th ed. St. Louis: Mosby; 1998

Web references: 0 available at www.5mcc.com
Illustrations N/A

Author(s):
Timothy L. Black, MD

BASICS

DESCRIPTION Congestive heart failure (CHF) is the principal complication of heart disease. It is a pathophysiologic state produced by an abnormality in cardiac pump function (either transient or prolonged). The heart is unable to transport blood in a sufficient flow to meet metabolic needs. CHF occurs at some time in most cases of severe heart disease.

- This produces a variety of clinical circumstances from acute left ventricular dysfunction (due to tachyarrhythmia, bradyarrhythmia, and acute myocardial infarction) to chronic left ventricular dysfunction (due to chronic volume/pressure overload as seen in valvular heart disease)
- Two physiologic components explain most of the clinical findings of CHF - most patients have findings consistent with both mechanisms:
  - ◊ an inotropic abnormality resulting in diminished systolic emptying (systolic failure)
  - ◊ a compliance abnormality in which the ability of the ventricles to accept blood is impaired (diastolic dysfunction).

System(s) affected: Cardiovascular, Pulmonary
Genetics: N/A
Incidence/Prevalence in USA: Most common inpatient diagnosis for patients over 65
Predominant age: Varies by etiology of heart disease
Predominant sex:

- Male > Female - ages 40-75
- Male = Female - ages 75 and over

SIGNS & SYMPTOMS

- Early and mild impairment:
  - ◊ Dyspnea on exertion-cardinal sign of left heart failure
  - ◊ Deteriorating exercise capacity
  - ◊ Easy fatigue
  - ◊ Difficulty breathing
  - ◊ Weakness
  - ◊ Tachypnea with mild exertion
  - ◊ Basilar rales
  - ◊ Positive hepatojugular reflux
  - ◊ Faint S3 gallop
  - ◊ Nocturia
- Moderate impairment:
  - ◊ Nocturnal nonproductive cough
  - ◊ Orthopnea
  - ◊ Paroxysmal nocturnal dyspnea
  - ◊ Wheezing, especially nocturnal in absence of history of asthma or infection (cardiac asthma)
  - ◊ Anorexia
  - ◊ Fullness or dull pain in RUQ
  - ◊ Tachypnea at rest
  - ◊ Anxiety
  - ◊ Hepatomegaly with tenderness to palpation
  - ◊ Cool extremities due to peripheral vasoconstriction
  - ◊ Prominent rales over bases
  - ◊ Right pleural effusion
  - ◊ Edema
  - ◊ Gallop rhythm
  - ◊ Diastolic hypertension
  - ◊ Elevated jugular venous pressure
  - ◊ Cardiomegaly
- Severe impairment:
  - ◊ Cerebral dysfunction
  - ◊ Abdominal bloating (ascites)
  - ◊ Cyanosis
  - ◊ Hypotension
  - ◊ Pulsus alternans
  - ◊ Anasarca
  - ◊ Frothy and/or pink sputum
  - ◊ Increased P2
  - ◊ Cardiac cachexia
  - ◊ Cheyne-Stokes respirations

CAUSES

- Coronary artery disease
- Myocardial infarction
- Cardiomyopathy
  - ◊ Alcoholic
  - ◊ Viral
  - ◊ Long-standing hypertension
  - ◊ Drugs (e.g., chemotherapeutic agents)
  - ◊ Muscular dystrophy
  - ◊ Amyloidosis
  - ◊ Postpartum state
- Valvular abnormalities
  - ◊ Aortic stenosis or regurgitation
  - ◊ Rheumatic heart disease (mitral and aortic valvular disease)
- Renal artery stenosis, usually bilateral, may cause recurrent "flash" pulmonary edema
- Volume overload
- Cardiac depressants; negative inotropes (e.g., beta blockers, IV amiodarone)
- Arrhythmias, eg, atrial fibrillation
- High output states
  - ◊ Hyperthyroidism
  - ◊ Beriberi heart disease
- HIV

RISK FACTORS

- Iatrogenic reduction of intensity of therapy
- Inappropriate sodium and/or fluid excess
- Patient non-compliance
- Intercurrent arrhythmia, eg, atrial fibrillation
- Administration of drug with negative inotropic effects
- Excessive physical, emotional, or environmental stress
- Thyrotoxicosis, pregnancy, or any condition associated with increased metabolic demand
- Recent pregnancy (postpartum cardiomyopathy)

DIAGNOSIS

DIFFERENTIAL DIAGNOSIS

- Simple dependent edema
- Exertional asthma
- Severe diffuse CAD
- Occult COPD
- Nephrotic syndrome: excluded by absence of history of asymptomatic edema, proteinuria in nephrotic range, and history of renal disease
- Cirrhosis: excluded by absence of stigmata of liver disease, and history of liver disease and its risk factors
- Left heart failure: findings of pulmonary congestion and diminished cardiac output appearing in patients with myocardial infarction, aortic and mitral valve disease, and hypertensive disease
- Right heart failure: findings of systemic vascular congestion (edema, ascites) appear in patients with cor pulmonale, tricuspid insufficiency, and most commonly in patients with uncorrected prolonged left heart failure
- Venous occlusive disease with subsequent peripheral edema

LABORATORY

- B-type natriuretic peptide (BNP) is a marker of ventricular dysfunction; >100 is consistent with CHF. May be helpful in:
  - ◊ Evaluating treatment since its value changes rapidly
  - ◊ The emergency setting to help differentiate the cause of dyspnea
- Lab findings in early and mild to moderately severe CHF
  - ◊ Respiratory alkalosis
  - ◊ Mild azotemia
  - ◊ Decreased erythrocyte sedimentation rate
  - ◊ Proteinuria (usually less than 1 gm/24 h that clears with treatment)
- Lab findings in severe CHF
  - ◊ Increased creatinine
  - ◊ Hyperbilirubinemia in severe cases
  - ◊ Dilutional hyponatremia

Drugs that may alter lab results: N/A

Disorders that may alter lab results: Renal failure may elevate BNP

PATHOLOGICAL FINDINGS

- Early and acute
  - ◊ Firm lungs with microscopic revealing engorged capillaries with thickening of the alveolar septa with extravasation of red cells and edema fluid
  - ◊ Liver is engorged, firm, and fluid-filled. Microscopic - reveals dilated central hepatic veins and sinusoids.
- Late and chronic
  - ◊ Hemosiderin deposits in lungs
  - ◊ "Nutmeg" liver with centrilobular necrosis
  - ◊ Occasionally hemorrhagic nonbacterial enterocolitis with hemorrhagic necrosis secondary to mesenteric vasoconstriction

SPECIAL TESTS N/A

IMAGING

- X-ray - mild changes: pulmonary artery wedge pressure = 18-23 mm Hg (2.4-3.1 kPa)
  - ◊ Increased heart size
  - ◊ Increased blood flow to the upper lobes
  - ◊ Equalization of flow between the upper and lower lobes
- X-ray - moderate severe pulmonary artery wedge pressure = 20-25 mm Hg (2.7-3.3 kPa)
  - ◊ Interstitial edema
  - ◊ Kerley's B lines
  - ◊ Perivascular edema
  - ◊ Subpleural effusions
- X-ray - severe changes: pulmonary artery wedge pressure > 25 mm Hg (> 3.3 kPa)
  - ◊ Alveolar edema
  - ◊ Butterfly pattern of pulmonary edema

DIAGNOSTIC PROCEDURES

- Echocardiographic studies are the most useful tests
- Cardiac catheterization, both right and left, for full diagnosis and prognosis
- B-type natriuretic peptide (BNP) is a useful marker of ventricular dysfunction. It is a cardiac neuro-hormone secreted from the ventricles in an increasing amount in response to abnormal pressure overload and increasing volume. The levels of BNP have been shown to increase in patients in correlation with progressive worsening of NYHA class of congestive heart failure (CHF). B-type natriuretic peptide has been shown to better predict the presence or absence of CHF than any set of clinical or lab measures of the cause of dyspnea. A level of over 100 is consistent with CHF. The level changes rapidly in response to treatment or worsening of the situation, so may be helpful not only in diagnosis but in following the benefit of treatment. It is helpful in the emergency room to differentiate the cause of dyspnea.
- Complete PFTs
- Nuclear imaging to evaluate LV and RV size and systolic function

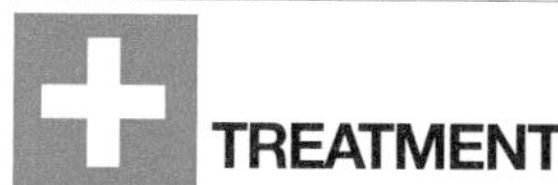

TREATMENT

APPROPRIATE HEALTH CARE Inpatient when severe

GENERAL MEASURES
- Immediate treatment of the heart failure
- Search for underlying correctable conditions
- Eliminate contributing factors when possible
- Supplemental oxygen
- Antiembolism stockings
- Fluid and sodium restriction. Education about this is imperative for long term control. Daily weights guide overall therapy.
- Identify and control underlying correctable conditions (e.g., acute MI, valvular disease, hyperthyroidism, but most commonly inadvertent salt and/or fluid overload)

SURGICAL MEASURES
- Heart valve surgery - possibly, if defective heart valve is responsible; mitral valve repair especially helpful if mitral regurgitation is aggravating CHF
- Cardiac transplantation - to be considered in patients (age < 55) without other disqualifying medical problems, who are developing CHF unresponsive to other therapeutic maneuvers, and who are felt to have a life expectancy of less than a year
- Biventricular pacing

ACTIVITY
- During severe stage, bed rest with elevation of head of bed and anti-embolism stockings to help control leg edema
- Gradual increase in activity with walking will help increase strength

DIET
- Sodium restriction (initially 4 gm sodium qd)
- Weight reduction diet if appropriate
- Low fat diet to retard coronary artery disease
- Appropriate fluid restriction

PATIENT EDUCATION
- Printed patient information available from:
  - ◊ American Heart Association, 7320 Greenville Avenue, Dallas, TX 75231, (214)373-6300
  - ◊ American College of Cardiology, 911 Old Georgetown Road, Bethesda, MD 20814, (301) 897-5400

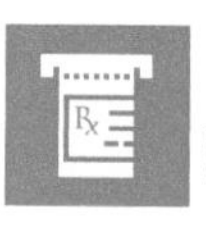

MEDICATIONS

DRUG(S) OF CHOICE
- Diuretics, usually in combination with digitalis are used to initiate therapy. ACE inhibitors have become a mainstay of therapy. For acute pulmonary edema, IV morphine remains cornerstone of therapy.
- Digoxin
  - ◊ Improves contractility, slows ventricular rate in atrial fibrillation
  - ◊ May be harmful in acute MI, hypertrophic cardiomyopathy, or aortic stenosis
  - ◊ Loading dose should be sufficient to have early beneficial effect, especially in atrial fibrillation with a rapid rate, e.g., 0.5-1.0 mg IV/PO, then another 1.0-1.5 mg in divided doses q4-6h
- Diuretics
  - ◊ Furosemide (Lasix): IV or PO, depending on severity of pulmonary congestion. May require continuous drip.
  - ◊ Metolazone (Zaroxolyn): excellent addition when furosemide does not seem to be sufficient
  - ◊ Spironolactone: when used carefully, to avoid hyperkalemia. An important addition to difficult chronic cases.
- ACE Inhibitors
  - ◊ Used to decrease afterload - shown to increase survival
  - ◊ Improve general symptomatology and overall exercise capacity
- Beta-blockers
  - ◊ Carvedilol (Coreg) 3.125 mg po bid for 2 weeks, then 6.25 mg bid for 2 weeks, increased to maximum 25 mg bid for class I to III CHF
  - ◊ Bisoprolol (Zebeta) 5-20 mg/day: in CIBIS-II study significantly decreases all-cause mortality and sudden death ("treatment effects were independent of the severity or cause of heart failure")
- Vasodilators
  - ◊ IV nitroglycerin may be of short-term benefit to decrease preload, afterload, and systemic resistance.
  - ◊ Oral medications, e.g., hydralazine, prazosin, and Isosorbide dinitrate demonstrate tachyphylaxis

Contraindications: Refer to manufacturer's literature

Precautions: ACE inhibitors may produce hypotension on first use in volume depleted patients. Beta-blockers may produce profound hypotension.

Significant possible interactions: Calcium channel blockers may impair LV function especially when used with beta blockers. Amlodipine seems less likely to be a problem.

ALTERNATIVE DRUGS
- Sympathomimetic amines. Can be used in severe CHF unresponsive to above measures
  - ◊ Dopamine and dobutamine have been successful for short periods in treatment
  - ◊ Dobutamine can be used on an intermittent outpatient basis with intermittent infusion. However, in spite of possibly improving quality of life, reduces long-term survival.

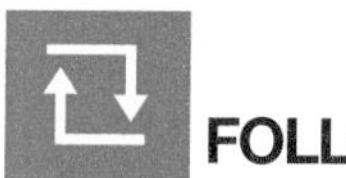

FOLLOWUP

PATIENT MONITORING
- Variable depending on clinical circumstances. Initially every 2-3 weeks after patient stabilized.
- Closely follow - history and physical findings, chest x-ray, electrolytes, BUN, and creatinine

PREVENTION/AVOIDANCE Treatment of underlying disorders when possible

POSSIBLE COMPLICATIONS
- Electrolyte disturbance
- Atrial and ventricular arrhythmias
- Mesenteric insufficiency
- Protein enteropathy
- Digitalis intoxication

EXPECTED COURSE/PROGNOSIS
- Result of initial treatment is usually good, whatever the cause
- Long-term prognosis variable. Mortality rates range from 10% with mild symptoms to 50% with advanced, progressive symptoms.

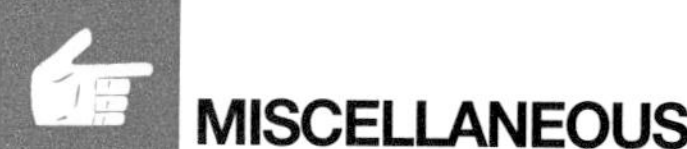

MISCELLANEOUS

ASSOCIATED CONDITIONS See Causes

AGE-RELATED FACTORS

Pediatric: Usually associated with congenital heart disease

Geriatric:
- Medications may need dosage adjustment
- Age-related cardiomyopathy is an increasing problem. It should be considered when the elderly complain of unusual dyspnea or easy fatigue. Beta-blockers may be of help.

Others: N/A

PREGNANCY If occurs, will require special care

SYNONYMS
- Heart failure
- Dropsy
- Circulatory failure
- Cardiac failure

ICD-9-CM
428.0 Congestive heart failure, unspecified

SEE ALSO

OTHER NOTES N/A

ABBREVIATIONS
CCF = congestive cardiac failure

REFERENCES

- Maisel AS, Krishnaswamy P, Nowak RM, McCord J, et al. Rapid measurement of B-type natriuretic peptide in the emergency diagnosis of heart failure. N Engl J Med 2002;18;347(3):161-7
- Topol E, ed. Textbook of Cardiovascular Medicine. Philadelphia: Lippincott-Raven; 1997
- Consensus recommendations for the management of chronic heart failure. On behalf of the membership of the advisory council to improve outcomes nationwide in heart failure. Am J Cardiol 1999;83(2A):1A-38A
- The Cardiac Insufficiency Bisoprolol Study II. Lancet 1999;353:9-13

Web references: 0 available at www.5mcc.com

Illustrations 8 available

Author(s):
Phil Lobstein, MD

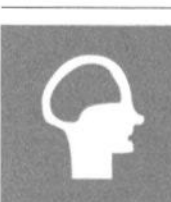

BASICS

DESCRIPTION Iinflammation of the bulbar and/ or palpebral conjunctiva of less than 4 weeks duration
System(s) affected: Nervous, Skin/Exocrine
Genetics: N/A
Incidence/Prevalence in USA: Variable, but accounts for 1-2% of all ambulatory office visits
Predominant age: Depends on cause
Predominant sex: Male = Female

SIGNS & SYMPTOMS
- General: for viral, bacterial, allergic, atopic and nonspecific
  - ◊ Red eye, conjunctival injection
  - ◊ Discharge
  - ◊ Foreign body sensation
  - ◊ Eyelid sticking or crusting
  - ◊ Normal visual acuity and papillary reactivity, otherwise, see Differential Diagnosis
- Viral, adenoviral or enteroviral most common sporadically in children, or may be associated with influenza, measles or mumps
  - ◊ History of upper respiratory infection or systemic viral symptoms
  - ◊ May start with 1 eye, then progresses to both eyes in 1-2 days
  - ◊ Watery mucous discharge
  - ◊ Inferior palpebral conjunctival follicles
  - ◊ Palpable preauricular lymphadenopathy
- Viral, herpes simplex or zoster
  - ◊ May have history of recurrent ocular herpes simplex
  - ◊ Burning sensation, rarely itching
  - ◊ Unilateral, with concurrent herpetic skin vesicles on eyelid or in distribution of ophthalmic branch of trigeminal nerve if herpes zoster
  - ◊ Palpable preauricular node
- Bacterial, gonococcal hyperacute infection
  - ◊ Rapid onset 12-24 hours
  - ◊ Severe purulent discharge
  - ◊ Chemosis-conjunctival edema
  - ◊ May have rapid growth of superior corneal ulceration
  - ◊ Eyelid swelling
  - ◊ Preauricular adenopathy
  - ◊ ? History or signs of other sexually transmitted diseases (chlamydia, HIV, etc.)
- Bacterial, nongonococcal: may be epidemic
  - ◊ Mild pruritus
  - ◊ Mild purulent discharge
  - ◊ Conjunctival chemosis- edema
  - ◊ No preauricular adenopathy
  - ◊ If contact lens user, must rule out pseudomonal keratitis
- Allergic
  - ◊ Itching most dominant symptom
  - ◊ Watery discharge
  - ◊ History of seasonal or dander allergies
  - ◊ Chemosis-conjunctival edema
  - ◊ Eyelids edematous and red
  - ◊ No preauricular adenopathy
- Atopic/vernal recurrent
  - ◊ History of atopy
  - ◊ Itching
  - ◊ Thick sticky discharge
  - ◊ Seasonal recurrences
  - ◊ Large conjunctival papillae (bumps) under upper eyelid
  - ◊ Sometimes superior corneal "shield" ulcer (sterile, gray-white infiltrate)
  - ◊ Sometimes raised white dots on inner lids or limbus
  - ◊ Sometimes superficial punctate keratopathy on fluorescein staining
- Nonspecific irritative
  - ◊ Dry eyes with intermittent redness and mucus
  - ◊ Irritation after a chemical exposure or drug reaction
  - ◊ Foreign body: may still have redness and discharge 24 hours after removal

CAUSES
- Viral
  - ◊ Adenovirus (common cold)
  - ◊ Coxsackie
  - ◊ Enterovirus (acute hemorrhagic conjunctivitis)
  - ◊ *Herpes simplex*, primary and recurrent
  - ◊ *Herpes zoster* or varicella
  - ◊ Molluscum contagiosum
  - ◊ Measles, mumps or influenza
- Bacterial
  - ◊ *Staphylococcus aureus*
  - ◊ *S. epidermidis*
  - ◊ *Streptococcus pneumoniae*
  - ◊ *Haemophilus influenzae* (especially in children)
  - ◊ Pseudomonas species (must rule out in contact lens users; frequently progresses to corneal ulcers)
  - ◊ *Neisseria gonorrhoeae*
  - ◊ *Neisseria meningitidis*
  - ◊ *Chlamydia trachomatis* causes a chronic conjunctivitis - gradual onset over 4 weeks
- Allergic
  - ◊ Hay fever, seasonal allergies
  - ◊ Vernal conjunctivitis/atopy
- Nonspecific
  - ◊ Irritative: topical medications, wind, or dry eye, ultraviolet light exposure, smoke
  - ◊ Autoimmune: Sjogren's, pemphigoid, Wegener granulomatosis
  - ◊ Rare: Rickettsial, fungal, parasitic, tuberculosis, syphilis, Kawasaki disease, Grave disease, gout, carcinoid, sarcoid, psoriasis, Stevens-Johnson, Reiter syndrome

RISK FACTORS
- History of contact with infected persons; epidemic bacterial or viral conjunctivitis
- Sexually transmitted disease contact: gonococcal, chlamydial, syphilis, herpes
- Use of contact lenses: pseudomonal

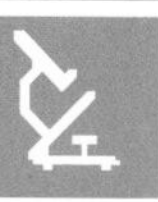

DIAGNOSIS

DIFFERENTIAL DIAGNOSIS
- Uveitis (iritis, iridocyclitis, choroiditis): limbal flush (red band at corneal margin, less on other areas of conjunctiva) hazy anterior chamber, decreased visual acuity
- Penetrating ocular trauma: ophthalmologic emergency; hospitalize
- Acute glaucoma (ophthalmologic emergency) headache, corneal clouding, decreased visual acuity
- Corneal ulcer(s) or foreign body: abnormal fluorescein exam
- Dacryocystitis: tenderness and swelling over tear sac (near nasal bridge)
- Scleritis and episcleritis: red injected vessels are radially oriented, sectoral (pie wedge) inflammation, sometimes with nodularity of sclera
- Ophthalmia neonatorum: neonates in first 2 day of life - gonococcal; 5-12 days of life - chlamydial, consider HSV if maternal cultures were positive for herpes simplex. Consider specialty consultation. All of these require systemic therapy as well as topical.

LABORATORY
- Usually not needed initially for the most common causes of conjunctivitis
- Culture swab if thought to be bacterial or if contact lens user
- Gram stain of discharge if thought to be gonococcal

Drugs that may alter lab results: N/A

Disorders that may alter lab results: N/A

PATHOLOGICAL FINDINGS N/A

SPECIAL TESTS
- Pap stain for giant cells of herpes simplex.
- Viral culture or immunofluorescence for herpes simplex

IMAGING N/A

DIAGNOSTIC PROCEDURES
- Document visual acuity/Snellen Chart
- Fluorescein staining to detect foreign bodies, corneal ulcers or punctate keratitis, and look for dendritic lesions of herpes simplex or zoster
- Examine eyelid skin also for herpetic vesicles, lice or nits, blepharitis or styes

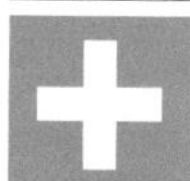

TREATMENT

APPROPRIATE HEALTH CARE Outpatient

GENERAL MEASURES
- Cool compresses and eyelid cleansing with wet cloth up to 4 times per day
- Discontinue use of contact lenses for duration of inflammation
- Patching of eye not beneficial
- Try to avoid irritants such as smoke, dry wind, prolonged sun exposure

SURGICAL MEASURES N/A

ACTIVITY No restrictions

DIET No restrictions

PATIENT EDUCATION
- Discuss handwashing techniques to decrease transmission of disease
- Do not re-use eye cosmetics after an infection. They should be discarded.
- Demonstrate eye dropper techniques: while eye is closed, and head tipped back, drop several drops in a lake at nasal margin then patient can open eyes to allow liquid to enter. Never touch tip of applicator to skin or eye.
- Demonstrate ointment techniques; apply 1/2 inch to edge of lower lid

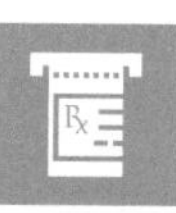

MEDICATIONS

DRUG(S) OF CHOICE
- Viral - nonherpetic
  - ◊ Artificial tears for symptomatic relief
  - ◊ Vasoconstrictor/antihistamine (e.g. naphazoline/pheniramine) qid for severe itching
  - ◊ Consider bland, inexpensive, topical antibiotic ointments in an empiric approach "in case" a viral infection is complicated by skin flora:
    - Erythromycin ophthalmic ointment inch twice a day for 5 days, or
    - 10% sodium sulfacetamide ophthalmic drops 2 gtts every 4 hours for 5 days.
- Viral - herpetic
  - ◊ Trifluorothymidine 1% drops one drop 5 times a day, or vidarabine 3% ointment 5 times per day.
  - ◊ Acyclovir oral, consult drug reference
  - ◊ If corneal lesions seen, consider ophthalmologist referral
- Bacterial - gonorrheal
  - ◊ If ulceration visible, or can not be ruled out consider emergent ophthalmologic consultation and hospitalization for IV ceftriaxone
  - ◊ If no corneal lesions, ceftriaxone 1 gm IM, as single dose and topical bacitracin ophthalmic ointment 1/2 inch, 4 times per day.
- Bacterial - nongonococcal
  - ◊ Bacitracin ophthalmic 1/2 inch 2-4 times per day for 5 days or
  - ◊ Erythromycin ophthalmic ointment, 1/2 inch 2-4 times per day for 5 days, or
  - ◊ Sodium sulfacetamide 10% solution, 2 drops every 4 hours (while awake) for 5 days
  - ◊ Fluoroquinolone eye drops (such as ciprofloxacin) are more expensive but also are acceptable
  - ◊ Avoid aminoglycoside drops and neomycin ointments as they can cause a reactive keratoconjunctivitis after a few days of use
- Allergic and atopic
  - ◊ Artificial tears 4 to 8 times per day
  - ◊ Vasoconstrictor/antihistamine 4 times per day
  - ◊ Ketorolac (Acular) 0.5% or levocabastine (Livostin) anti-inflammatory ophthalmic, 4 times per day or olopatadine (Patanol) 2-3 times per day to relieve itching
  - ◊ Topical cromolyn (Opticrom) 4%, 4 times per day
  - ◊ Oral antihistamine (e.g., diphenhydramine 25 mg 3-4 times per day) in severe cases
  - ◊ Avoid topical steroids in nonophthalmologic setting as patients must be monitored for development of steroid related cataracts and glaucoma. If superior shield ulcer of vernal conjunctivitis is present, refer to ophthalmology for steroids.

Contraindications: Avoid use of topical steroids unless in ophthalmologic setting and able to monitor intraocular pressure

Precautions:
- Do not allow dropper to touch eye or skin to avoid contamination. Do not re-use same eye cosmetics after an infection - they should be discarded
- Vasoconstrictor/antihistamine - rebound vasodilation after prolonged use

Significant possible interactions: N/A

ALTERNATIVE DRUGS
- Viral - numerous over-the-counter and prescription topical vasoconstrictors and antihistamines
- Bacterial
  - ◊ Polymyxin-gramicidin
  - ◊ Neomycin-polymyxin b-bacitracin (Neosporin) (15% of people have reaction to neomycin)
  - ◊ Ciprofloxacin
  - ◊ Norfloxacin
  - ◊ Chloramphenicol (warning: slight hematological adverse effect risk)
  - ◊ Oral erythromycin for chlamydia in neonate (see drug reference for dosing)
- Allergic
  - ◊ Numerous topical vasoconstrictors and antihistamines
  - ◊ Numerous oral antihistamines

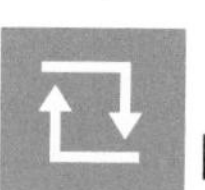

FOLLOWUP

PATIENT MONITORING Referral if worse in 24 hours. Bacterial: expect improvement in 24 hours and resolution in 2-5 days.

PREVENTION/AVOIDANCE
- Avoid listed causes when possible
- Wash hands frequently

POSSIBLE COMPLICATIONS
- Viral
  - ◊ Corneal scars with herpes simplex
  - ◊ Neonatal herpes simplex could include encephalitis
  - ◊ Lid scars or entropion with Varicella zoster
  - ◊ Bacterial superinfection
- Bacterial
  - ◊ Chronic marginal blepharitis
  - ◊ Conjunctival scar if membrane develops.
  - ◊ Corneal ulcers or perforation, very rapid with gonococcal
  - ◊ Hypopyon: pus in anterior chamber
  - ◊ Chlamydial neonatal ophthalmia: could have concomitant pneumonia
- Allergic, chemical or nonspecific
  - ◊ Bacterial superinfection

EXPECTED COURSE/PROGNOSIS
- Viral
  - ◊ 10 days for pharyngitis with conjunctivitis
  - ◊ Several weeks for epidemic keratoconjunctivitis
  - ◊ 2-3 weeks for herpes simplex
- Bacterial
  - ◊ 2-4 days with treatment
  - ◊ 10-14 days if untreated

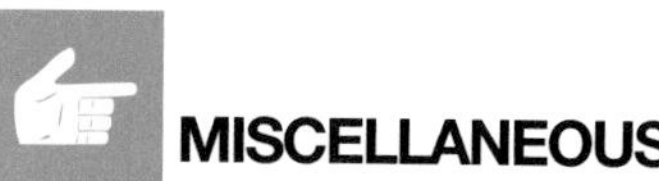

MISCELLANEOUS

ASSOCIATED CONDITIONS
- Viral infection (e.g., common cold)
- Sexually transmitted diseases

AGE-RELATED FACTORS
Pediatric: Neonatal conjunctivitis may be gonococcal, chlamydial, irritative or related to dacryocystitis. Gonococcal ophthalmia neonatorum is an emergency.
Geriatric: More likely to have autoimmune, systemic or irritative conditions
Others: Epidemic bacterial (streptococcal) conjunctivitis reported on college campuses

PREGNANCY N/A

SYNONYMS Pink eye

ICD-9-CM
077.99 Unspecified diseases of conjunctiva due to viruses
372.50 Conjunctival degeneration, unspecified
372.14 Other chronic allergic conjunctivitis

SEE ALSO
Rhinitis, allergic
Sjögren syndrome
Vernal keratoconjunctivitis

OTHER NOTES N/A

ABBREVIATIONS N/A

REFERENCES

- Rhee D, Pyfer M. The Will's Eye Manual. 3rd ed. Baltimore: Lippincott Williams & Wilkins; 1999
- David SP. Should we prescribe antibiotics for acute conjunctivitis? Am Fam Physician 2002;66(9):1649-50
- Martin M, Turco JH, Zegans ME, et al. An outbreak of conjunctivitis due to atypical Streptococcus pneumoniae. N Engl J Med 2003;348(12):1112-21
- Vaughan D, Asbury T, et al. General Ophthalmology. 13th Ed. Stamford: Appleton & Lange;1992
- Greenberg MF, Pollard ZF. The red eye in childhood. Pediatr Clin North Am 2003;50(1):105-2

Web references: 1 available at www.5mcc.com
Illustrations 1 available

Author(s):
Frances Y. Wu, MD

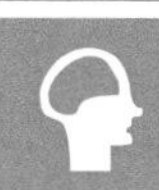

BASICS

DESCRIPTION A combination of changes in the frequency, size, consistency, and ease of stool passage, which leads to an overall decrease in volume of bowel movements. Very subjective, each individual has their own threshold level.
System(s) affected: Gastrointestinal
Genetics: Unknown (the condition may be familial)
Incidence/Prevalence in USA:
- Higher at extremes of life, i.e., among infants/children and the elderly
- Common; affects a majority of persons during their lifetimes

Predominant age: All ages can be affected; more frequent at the extremes of life (infancy and old age)
Predominant sex: Female > Male

SIGNS & SYMPTOMS
- Less frequency of stooling than the patient perceives as "normal" (normal is 3-5 times/week)
- Harder stool than "normal"
- Smaller stools than normal (average < 35 grams/day is abnormal)
- Impaction of stool secondary to hardness
- Inspissated stool
- Lack of consistent urgency to stool
- Difficulty expelling feces from the rectum
- Painful evacuation of feces
- Lingering sense of incomplete emptying of the bowel
- Abdominal fullness or a feeling of malaise secondary to inadequate bowel evacuation
- Tenesmus

CAUSES
- Electrolyte abnormalities
  - ◊ Hypercalcemia
  - ◊ Hypokalemia
- Hormonal abnormalities
  - ◊ Hypothyroidism
  - ◊ Diabetes
- Congenital impediments, e.g., aganglionic megacolon (Hirschsprung disease) or excessively elongate, redundant, capacious bowel (dolichocolon)
- Congenital or acquired neuromuscular bowel impairment ("pseudo-obstruction")
- Concomitant illness, injury, or debility
- Mechanical bowel impediment (obstruction or ileus, due to any cause)
- Inadequate fluid intake
- Side-effect of drugs (e.g., anticholinergic agents, opiates)
- Chronic abuse of laxatives or cathartics
- Psychiatric, cultural, emotional, environmental factors
- Painful fecal evacuation from anal disease (e.g., fissures)

RISK FACTORS
- Extremes of life (very young and very old)
- Neurosis
- Polypharmacy
- Sedentary life style or condition
- Diet and fluid intake

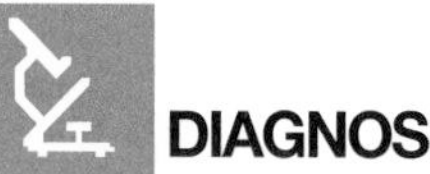

DIAGNOSIS

DIFFERENTIAL DIAGNOSIS
- Congenital
  - ◊ Hirschsprung
  - ◊ Hypoganglionosis
  - ◊ Congenital dilation of the colon
  - ◊ Small left colon syndrome
- Meconium ileus
- "Normal" stooling with anxious patient or parent
- Illnesses predisposing to constipation
  - ◊ Dehydration
  - ◊ Hypothyroidism
  - ◊ Hypokalemia
  - ◊ Hypercalcemia
- Other causes of abdominal pain

LABORATORY
- Only necessary when other disorders are being considered
  - ◊ CBC to detect anemia that may indicate colorectal neoplasm
  - ◊ Thyroid functions
  - ◊ Electrolytes, glucose, calcium

Drugs that may alter lab results: N/A

Disorders that may alter lab results: N/A

PATHOLOGICAL FINDINGS
- None in common, "functional" constipation
- Paucity or absence of intramural enteric ganglia in certain cases of congenital or acquired megacolon
- Neuromuscular abnormalities in certain cases of "pseudo-obstruction"

SPECIAL TESTS
- Endoscopic evaluation
  - ◊ Flexible sigmoidoscopy
  - ◊ Colonoscopy
- In selected cases of long-standing constipation, timed measure of passage of ingested stool markers may help discern differing impediments
- Anorectal motility in patients with suspected Hirschsprung or anorectal motility disorders

IMAGING
- Plain (KUB) film of the abdomen may help to discern the extent and nature of the problem
- Barium enema or barium swallow with small bowel follow through looking for anatomical defects (mass lesions, ileus)
- Cineradiography of passage of barium, instilled in, then expelled from the rectosigmoid segment ("defecography"), may help define evacuation disorders in selected cases

DIAGNOSTIC PROCEDURES
- Digital rectal exam to rule out a rectal mass, check for blood in the stool, and define stool consistency
- Sigmoidoscopy or colonoscopy is seldom required, unless needed to define an abnormality discovered by barium enema or when there is evidence of iron deficiency anemia or blood in the stool

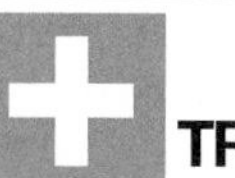

TREATMENT

APPROPRIATE HEALTH CARE Outpatient usually, except when investigation discloses an underlying lesion or obstruction that requires hospitalization

GENERAL MEASURES
- Attempt to eliminate medications that may cause or worsen constipation
- Increase fluid intake
- Modify diet
- Enemas if other methods fail

SURGICAL MEASURES N/A

ACTIVITY Encourage exercise

DIET
- If no anatomic abnormalities, increase fiber to approximately 15 gm/day (bran, fruit, green vegetables, and whole grain cereals and breads)
- Encourage liberal intake of fluids

PATIENT EDUCATION
- Define constipation and normal variations
- Occasional mild constipation is normal
- Instruction in consistent "bowel training" i.e., allowing adequate time for bowel evacuation in a quiet, unhurried environment; instruction in facilitating posture on commode, e.g., thighs flexed toward abdomen
- Parents sometimes needs more treatment/advice than the constipated child

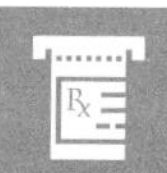

MEDICATIONS

DRUG(S) OF CHOICE

- Hydrophilic colloids (bulk-forming agents; not really drugs)
  - ◊ Psyllium (Konsyl, Metamucil, Perdiem)
  - ◊ Methylcellulose (Citrucel)
  - ◊ Polycarbophil (Mitrolan, FiberCon)
- Osmotic laxatives - appropriate for short-term use. The usual dose is 15 mL to 30 mL once or twice a day.
  - ◊ Milk of magnesia 15-30 mL bid
  - ◊ Magnesium citrate 15-30 mL bid
  - ◊ Phosphate of soda 15-30 mL bid
  - ◊ Lactulose (Chronulac) 15-30 mL bid
  - ◊ Sorbitol 15-30 mL bid
  - ◊ Alumina-magnesium (Maalox, Mylanta)
  - ◊ Polyethylene glycol (MiraLax) 17 g in 8 oz of water q day
- Stool softeners
  - ◊ Docusate sodium (Colace) 100 mg bid

Contraindications:

- Any impediment to bowel transit, such as an obstructing lesion or ileus. Osmotic laxatives may result in overdistension or bowel perforation
- Any acute intra-abdominal inflammatory condition
- Renal and heart failure are relative contraindications

Precautions: Advise patient against chronic use of irritant and osmotic laxatives

Significant possible interactions:

- Magnesium containing laxatives
  - ◊ Bind tetracyclines preventing their absorption
  - ◊ Reduce the effectiveness of digitalis and phenothiazines
  - ◊ Sodium polystyrene sulfonate (Kayexalate) bind and prevent neutralization of bicarbonate, leading to systemic alkalosis, which may be severe

ALTERNATIVE DRUGS

- Lubricants (e.g., mineral oil) are unpalatable to many patients, subject to leakage, and impose the risk of aspiration
- Emollient suppositories are useful, if at all, in allaying anorectal soreness
- Irritant cathartics (stimulants)
  - ◊ Ricinoleic acid or castor oil (Neoloid); 30-60 mL/day
  - ◊ Phenolphthalein (Ex-Lax, Modane)
  - ◊ Bisacodyl (Dulcolax); 2-3 tabs swallowed whole or 1 suppository bid
- Motor and secretory properties
  - ◊ Anthraquinones: senna (Senokot); 1-2 cap or 15-30 mL qhs
- Enemas (avoid soap suds - may lead to colitis)
  - ◊ Sodium phosphate (Fleet enema)
- Suppositories
  - ◊ Osmotic: sodium phosphate
  - ◊ Lubricant: glycerin
  - ◊ Stimulatory: bisacodyl
- Prokinetic agents

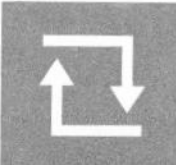

FOLLOWUP

PATIENT MONITORING What seems to be simple, "functional" constipation, if it persists, should be further investigated for a possible "organic" cause

PREVENTION/AVOIDANCE Because for some patients a tendency to constipation is habitual, instruction in proper diet, bowel training, and use of bulk-forming supplements must be reinforced

POSSIBLE COMPLICATIONS

- Volvulus
- Cancer risk
- Acquired megacolon: in severe, long-standing cases
- Cathartic colon: repeated laxative abuse
- Fluid and electrolyte depletion: laxative abuse
- Rectal ulceration ("stercoral ulcer") related to recurrent fecal impaction
- Anal fissures

EXPECTED COURSE/PROGNOSIS

Constipation that is only occasional, brief, and responsive to simple measures is harmless. That which is habitual can be a lifelong nuisance.

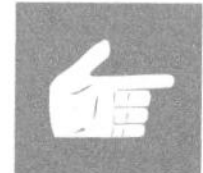

MISCELLANEOUS

ASSOCIATED CONDITIONS Debility, either general, as in the aged, or that imposed by specific, underlying illness

AGE-RELATED FACTORS

Pediatric: Consider Hirschsprung disease

Geriatric:

- Elderly persons, who have enjoyed regular bowel action throughout their lives, seldom suffer constipation due to age alone
- Persons with a lifelong tendency to constipation often encounter increasing difficulty with advancing age
- There is an increased incidence of colorectal neoplasms with age that may be associated with constipation.

Others: N/A

PREGNANCY Women with a tendency to constipation may find the condition more troublesome in the third trimester and require dietary adjustment and supplements

SYNONYMS

- Costive bowel
- Locked bowels

ICD-9-CM

564.00 Constipation, unspecified
564.7 Megacolon, other than Hirschsprung
564.89 Other functional disorders of intestine
751.3 Hirschsprung disease and other congenital functional disorders of colon

SEE ALSO

Congenital megacolon
Encopresis

OTHER NOTES

Obstipation refers to intractable constipation

ABBREVIATIONS N/A

REFERENCES

- Rogers AI: Constipation In: Berk JE, Haubrich WS, eds. Gastrointestinal Symptoms: Clinical Interpretation. Philadelphia, B.C. Decker Inc., 1991
- Haubrich WS: Constipation. In: Berk JE, et al, eds. Bockus Gastroenterology. 4th Ed. Philadelphia, W.B. Saunders Co., 1985
- Devroede G: Constipation. In: Sleisenger MH, Fordtran JS, eds. Gastrointestinal Disease. 4th Ed. Philadelphia, W.B. Saunders Co., 1989
- Wald A: Approach to the patient with constipation. In: Yamada T, ed. Textbook of Gastroenterology. Vol. I. Philadelphia, J.B. Lippincott Co., 1991
- Nunez M, Robinson B: Management of Constipation in the Older Patient. J Florida MA 1991;78:12, 829-831
- Leonard-Jones JE: Clinical Management of Constipation, Pharmacology 1993;47(suppl1):216-223
- Goroll AH, May LA, Mulley AG: Approach to the Patient with Constipation. In Primary Care Medicine, Lippincott, 1987
- Abyad A, Murad F. Constipation common sense care of the older patient. Geriatrics 1996; 51(12):28-36

Web references: 0 available at www.5mcc.com

Illustrations N/A

Author(s):
Abdulrazak Abyad, MD, MPH

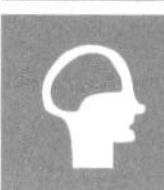

BASICS

DESCRIPTION Variety of methods used to prevent pregnancy. This may be done by preventing implantation, ovulation, or entry of sperm into uterus. Natural family planning's objective is to limit coitus around the time of suspected ovulation. The most effective method of contraception, aside from abstinence, is permanent sterilization. While these methods may be reversible under certain circumstances, patients should consider them irreversible.

Failure rates for reversible contraceptive methods:

Method	--Failure Rates (%)-- Theoretical	Actual
Chance	85	85
Female condom	5	21
Spermicides	6	21
Fertility awareness†	1-9	20
Withdrawal	4	19
Cervical cap	9	18
Sponge	6-9	18-28
Diaphragm	6	18
Male condom	2	12
Combined pill	0.1	3
Minipill	0.5	3
Tubal ligation	0.4	0.4
Depo-Provera	0.3	0.3
Vasectomy	0.1	0.15
IUD	0.1-0.5	0.1-2.0
Norplant	0.09	0.09
EC	2	2

† BBT, calendar, & cervical mucus

System(s) affected: Reproductive
Genetics: N/A
Incidence/Prevalence in USA:
- About two-thirds of women at risk for unwanted pregnancies use contraception
- Among individuals of reproductive age having regular coitus:
  - ◊ Tubal sterilization 27%
  - ◊ Vasectomy 12%
  - ◊ Oral contraceptives 27%
  - ◊ Condoms 21%
  - ◊ Diaphragms 3.5%
  - ◊ IUD 1.2%
  - ◊ Natural family planning 2%
  - ◊ Foam 0.6%
  - ◊ Injectable contraceptive 2.5%

Predominant age:
- Female - 11-52 years
- Male - any age after puberty

Predominant sex: Female. However, condom or vasectomy are methods most commonly used by males.

SIGNS & SYMPTOMS N/A

CAUSES N/A

RISK FACTORS
- For pregnancy
  - ◊ Any ovulating woman who engages in intercourse with a fertile male
  - ◊ Young adolescents
  - ◊ Those who are from a lower socioeconomic status, or have limited knowledge about reproduction

DIAGNOSIS

DIFFERENTIAL DIAGNOSIS N/A

LABORATORY
- Female
  - ◊ Cervical cytology
  - ◊ Cultures for gonorrhea and Chlamydia
  - ◊ Blood lipids, blood sugar
  - ◊ Pregnancy test (if hormonal contraception is not initiated at time of menses)
- Male
  - ◊ None except routine pre-operative studies prior to vasectomy
  - ◊ Semen analysis after vasectomy; aspermia will require up to 15 ejaculations

Drugs that may alter lab results: N/A

Disorders that may alter lab results: N/A

PATHOLOGICAL FINDINGS N/A

SPECIAL TESTS N/A

IMAGING N/A

DIAGNOSTIC PROCEDURES N/A

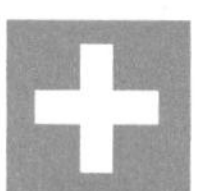

TREATMENT

APPROPRIATE HEALTH CARE
- Outpatient

GENERAL MEASURES
Non-drug methods
- Latex condom
- IUD. Insert during menses (assures patient is not pregnant), but may be inserted any time. Contraindications: pregnancy, history of PID, undiagnosed genital bleeding, uterine anomalies(woman with two uterine cavities may use two IUDs), large fibroids.
- Diaphragm
- Periodic abstinence
  - ◊ Mucus method: abstain from intercourse while cervix builds up its mucus to a peak level. Between four days after noticing the cervix is becoming drier (mucus is decreasing) and until mucus is again detected is the period during which intercourse is allowed.
  - ◊ Calendar method: calculate fertile period as shortest cycle minus 18 days to longest cycle minus 11 days after recording length of menstrual cycles over a year
  - ◊ Symptothermal method: involves calculate the first day of abstinence by subtracting 21 from the length of the shortest menstrual cycle in the previous six months, or the first day cervical mucus is detected, whichever comes first. End calculated as 3 days after the woman's body temperature rises 1°C.

SURGICAL MEASURES
- Permanent sterilization
  - ◊ Tubal sterilization in the female
  - ◊ Vasectomy in the male

ACTIVITY N/A

DIET N/A

PATIENT EDUCATION
- Condoms. Water-based lubricants reduce the risk of breakage. More effective if pre-lubricated with spermicide. Leave space at tip to act as reservoir. Withdraw from vagina before penis becomes flaccid.
- IUD. Check string periodically
- Diaphragm
  - ◊ Refit after childbirth or if weight change by more than 10%
  - ◊ Before inserting, one tablespoon of water-soluble spermicidal jelly or cream should be placed in the dome
  - ◊ Check for proper placement once inserted
  - ◊ Leave in at least 6 hours after coitus
  - ◊ If coitus is repeated before 6 hours, insert another teaspoon of spermicidal cream or jelly into the vagina without removing the diaphragm
- Female condom
  - ◊ New condom required for each sex act
  - ◊ Insert properly so that inner ring is well into vagina and outer ring lies against vulva. Make sure that penis enters inside the sheath.
  - ◊ Remove condom after intercourse being careful not to spill any semen
- Oral contraception
  - ◊ Pill should be taken same time each day
  - ◊ If a pill is missed, take two the following day, but use a barrier method, until next period
  - ◊ If two periods are missed, check a pregnancy test. Do not stop pills if period is missed.
- Norplant: replace after 5 years
- Printed materials available from ACOG (1.800.673.8444)
- Emergency contraception (EC) prevents pregnancy via several proposed mechanisms including: inhibition of sperm motility, alterations in tubal transport, unfavorable uterine receptivity, and/or fertilization inhibition. EC does not affect an established pregnancy. EC includes three methods: progestin only pills, combination estrogen-progestin pills, and the copper bearing IUD. Safety of these methods is excellent, but should not be utilized in a known, established pregnancy. (Telephone information available at 888-NOT-2-LATE.)

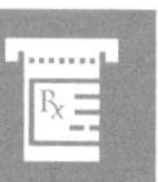

MEDICATIONS

DRUG(S) OF CHOICE
- Oral contraceptives (OC)
  - ◊ Side effects minimized with sub-50 microgram estrogen dose pills. OCs with 35 μg of ethinyl estradiol provide the same blood hormone levels as 50 μg of mestranol.
  - ◊ Triphasics contain less total progestogen; less likely to affect lipid profile adversely
  - ◊ The progesterone (derivatives of testosterone) varies between manufacturers. Newer progestogens are less androgenic and therefore should have less adverse effects on lipoproteins. However, there is concern about an increased risk of stroke with pills containing desogestrel.

◊ Generics should be avoided because of fluctuating dosage in each pill batch
◊ If side effects occur, pill may be changed in a trial and error fashion
- Spermicides
◊ All contain nonoxynol-9
- Levonorgestrel (Norplant)
◊ 6 silastic tubes implanted by physician
◊ Effective up to 5 years
- Medroxyprogesterone (Depo-Provera)
◊ 150 mg IM q 3 months
◊ Contraceptive levels of hormone persist for up to 4 months (2-4 week margin of safety)
- Emergency contraception. Start hormones as soon as possible after unprotected intercourse, but before 72 hours for maximum effectiveness.
◊ Estradiol-levonorgestrel (Preven, Ovral, Ogestrel) 50mg/0.25 mg. 2 tabs q12h (4 tabs total). [Anti-nausea medication (e.g., Phenergan) should be prescribed in conjunction with this method, to be given 1-2 hours before the EC doses.]
◊ Levonorgestrel (Plan B) 0.75mg. 1 tab q12h (2 tabs total). Less nausea than with estrogen containing products and slightly more effective.
◊ Copper bearing IUD. May be inserted up to the time of implantation (5-7 days after ovulation or generally 5 days after intercourse); over 99% effective in preventing pregnancy and continues to provide contraception for up to 10 years.

Contraindications:
- Implantable or injectable contraceptives
◊ Active liver disease
◊ Thrombophlebitis
◊ Pregnancy
◊ Unexplained, abnormal uterine bleeding
◊ Cholestatic jaundice
◊ Hyperlipidemia
- Oral contraceptives
◊ Same as implantable contraception plus noncompliance and estrogen dependent malignancies
◊ Relative contraindications are uterine leiomyomata, hypertension, insulin-requiring diabetes mellitus, and migraine headaches

Precautions: N/A

Significant possible interactions:
- When these drugs needed, add a barrier method (or rarely, use a 50 mcg estrogen pill)
◊ Phenytoin (Dilantin) - induces microsomal liver enzymes causing accelerated metabolism of hormones with subsequent reduced blood levels. The same effect occurs in implantable contraception.
◊ Antibiotics - decreased enterohepatic circulation. Rifampin may also increase metabolism of oral contraceptives.

ALTERNATIVE DRUGS N/A

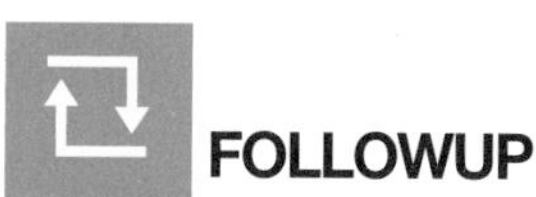

FOLLOWUP

PATIENT MONITORING
- Annual pelvic exam and Pap smear
- Whenever side effects or problems occur
- Check for presence of IUD 1 month after insertion. If string is nor found, use pelvic ultrasound to locate.
- Oral contraceptive users: 3 months after starting for hypertension; then annually

PREVENTION/AVOIDANCE N/A

POSSIBLE COMPLICATIONS
- Oral contraceptives, serious
◊ Thromboembolism - stop method and treat the disorder. Do not resume oral contraception.
◊ Hypertension - stop method; do not resume
◊ M I - main risk is in smokers beyond age 35. Do not use in these patients.
- Oral contraceptives, minor
◊ Nausea and vomiting - advise patient to take after eating
◊ Breakthrough bleeding - usually self-limiting after 3 months; if persists, change pill
◊ Amenorrhea - pregnancy must be ruled out, then either change to a different pill or add conjugated estrogen 0.3 mg for the first 10 days of pill package
◊ Cyclic weight gain - use smallest dose of estrogen available
◊ Breast tenderness - rare with low dose pill
◊ Depression - rare with low dose pill
◊ Chloasma - stop pill or cover with makeup
◊ Acne or hirsutism - change to a less androgenic progesterone
◊ Cholestatic jaundice - stop pill; do not restart
◊ Weight gain throughout cycle - use triphasic pill to minimize dose of progesterone or use newer progesterone
- Implantable contraceptive (Norplant)
◊ Amenorrhea - about 33% (if it persists for 2 months, must rule out pregnancy)
◊ Irregular bleeding - about 33%

Note: Both are self limited and last about 1 year and the patient should be informed of side effects before choosing this method
- Injectable contraceptive (Depo-Provera)
◊ Irregular bleeding during first few months
◊ Not readily reversible
◊ Amenorrhea - common after 1 year of use
- IUD
◊ PID or salpingitis - remove IUD and start antibiotics
◊ Heavy bleeding and cramps - remove IUD

EXPECTED COURSE/PROGNOSIS
- Pregnancy may occur with any method
◊ After permanent sterilization - pregnancy indicates failure of the procedure and the need for reoperation; must evaluate for tubal implantation
◊ With an IUD, remove the device if string is visible. If string is not seen, leave in position since there is only a slightly increased risk of spontaneous abortion.
◊ With oral contraceptives - stop pill. Only very slight chance of virilization of female fetus.
◊ With implantable contraceptive - remove implants

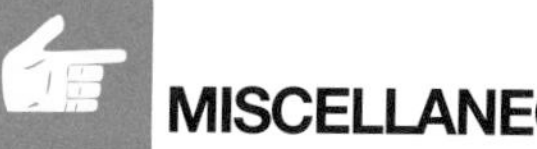

MISCELLANEOUS

ASSOCIATED CONDITIONS N/A

AGE-RELATED FACTORS
Pediatric: Use of estrogen prior to pubertal growth spurt may lead to a reduction in ultimate height due to epiphyseal closure
Geriatric: High dose oral contraceptives should be avoided for estrogen replacement therapy
Others: Healthy non-smokers may use oral contraceptives until age >= 50. When stopped, observe for menopause signs. Use other contraceptive method during this period.

PREGNANCY
Relationship to breast cancer is uncertain; some suggest a slight increase in risk in certain groups

SYNONYMS
- Birth control
- Family planning

ICD-9-CM

SEE ALSO

OTHER NOTES
- Other benefits of oral contraception
◊ Clearly established benefits: reductions in ovarian cancers, endometrial cancers, ectopic pregnancies and pelvic inflammatory disease; less dysmenorrhea and anemia; reduced functional ovarian cysts and a regular menstrual cycle
◊ Benefits not clearly established: less osteopenia, endometriosis and atherosclerosis; fewer new cases of rheumatoid arthritis

ABBREVIATIONS
EC = emergency contraception
PID = pelvic inflammatory disease

REFERENCES

- Speroff L, Glass RH, Kase NG. Clinical Gynecologic Endocrinology and Infertility. 5th Ed. Baltimore, Williams & Wilkins, 1994
- Berek, Jonathan S, et al. Novak's Gynecology. 12th Ed. Baltimore, Williams & Wilkins, 1996
- Nordenberg T. Protecting against unintended pregnancy: A guide to contraceptive choices. FDA Consumer, June 2000
- Ellertson C, Trussell J, et al. Emergency Contraception. Semin Reprod Med 19(4):323-330, 2001.

Web references: 0 available at www.5mcc.com
Illustrations N/A

Author(s):
William Dobak, DO
Nicholas J. Spirtos, DO

BASICS

DESCRIPTION Right ventricular enlargement/dysfunction and failure caused by pulmonary hypertension (increased right ventricular afterload) secondary to diseases of the lung, thorax, and pulmonary vasculature.
- Acute cor pulmonale: acute dilatation or overload of the right ventricle secondary to massive pulmonary embolism
- Chronic cor pulmonale: hypertrophy and dilatation of the right ventricle resulting from diseases of the pulmonary parenchyma and/or pulmonary vasculature (most commonly COPD)

System(s) affected: Cardiovascular, Pulmonary, Renal/Urologic
Genetics: No known genetic pattern
Incidence/Prevalence in USA: 5-10% of adult heart diseases
Predominant age: >45
Predominant sex: Male > Female

SIGNS & SYMPTOMS
- Acute cor pulmonale:
  - ◊ Severe dyspnea
  - ◊ Pallor
  - ◊ Diaphoresis
  - ◊ Jugular venous distention with inspiration (Kussmaul's sign)
  - ◊ Systolic murmur loudest at left sternal border (tricuspid regurgitation)
  - ◊ Distended, tender, pulsatile liver
  - ◊ S3 gallop
  - ◊ Hypoxemia
  - ◊ Cardiovascular collapse because of right ventricle's low output state
- Chronic cor pulmonale:
  - ◊ Tachypnea/shortness of breath not relieved by sitting upright
  - ◊ Hoarseness secondary to compression of the left recurrent laryngeal nerve by enlarged pulmonary vessels (Ortner syndrome)
  - ◊ Productive or nonproductive cough
  - ◊ Chest pain secondary to pulmonary artery root dilatation and right ventricular ischemia
  - ◊ Hepatomegaly
  - ◊ Peripheral edema
  - ◊ Cyanosis
  - ◊ Right ventricular systolic heave
  - ◊ Pulmonary ejection click
  - ◊ S3 gallop that increases with inspiration
  - ◊ Jugular venous distention with prominent a- and v-waves
  - ◊ Systolic murmur of tricuspid regurgitation
  - ◊ Diastolic murmur of pulmonary regurgitation
  - ◊ Right ventricular failure (indicated by increased venous pressure, edema, hepatojugular reflux, worsening tricuspid regurgitation, right ventricular pulsus alternans, development of S3 and S4).

CAUSES
- Disease affecting pulmonary air spaces
  - ◊ Diffuse interstitial lung diseases: idiopathic pulmonary fibrosis, radiation induced fibrosis
  - ◊ Pulmonary resection
  - ◊ Chronic obstructive pulmonary diseases (chronic bronchitis, emphysema, asthma)
  - ◊ Granulomatous and connective tissue diseases: sarcoidosis, rheumatoid arthritis, systemic lupus erythematosus, eosinophilic granuloma, mixed connective tissue disease
  - ◊ Bronchiectasis
  - ◊ Cystic fibrosis
  - ◊ Malignant infiltration
  - ◊ Chronic hypoxia at high altitude
  - ◊ Congenital structural defects
- Diseases affecting the pulmonary vasculature
  - ◊ Primary pulmonary hypertension
  - ◊ Pulmonary embolism
  - ◊ CREST
  - ◊ Tumor embolism
  - ◊ Amniotic fluid embolism
  - ◊ Schistosomiasis
  - ◊ Sickle cell disease
  - ◊ Pulmonary vascular disease secondary to systemic illness
  - ◊ Human immunodeficiency virus
  - ◊ Granulomatous pulmonary arteritis
  - ◊ Chronic liver disease
  - ◊ Intravenous drug abuse
- Diseases affecting thoracic cage function
  - ◊ Obesity
  - ◊ Kyphoscoliosis
  - ◊ Neuromuscular diseases
  - ◊ Sleep apnea
  - ◊ Pleural fibrosis
  - ◊ Idiopathic hypoventilation
- Pharmacologic induction
  - ◊ Appetite suppressants, including aminorex, fenfluramine, dexfenfluramine

RISK FACTORS
- Tobacco abuse
- Living at high altitudes
- Industrial exposures

DIAGNOSIS

DIFFERENTIAL DIAGNOSIS
- Primary disease of the left side of the heart
- Congenital heart disease with left-to-right shunting

LABORATORY
- Acute cor pulmonale: ventilation/perfusion mismatch with hypoxia and hypocarbia
- Chronic cor pulmonale: pulmonary function testing shows airflow obstruction with reduced pO_2 and possibly elevated hematocrit

Drugs that may alter lab results: N/A

Disorders that may alter lab results: N/A

PATHOLOGICAL FINDINGS
- Evidence of underlying etiology
- Dilated, hypertrophic right ventricle

SPECIAL TESTS
ECG: often normal, but findings can include:
- RVH: most common in primary pulmonary hypertension. Indicated by clockwise rotation of electrical axis, right axis deviation, and P pulmonale (increased P wave amplitude in II, III, and AVF)
- Right-sided heart failure suggested by:
  - ◊ R/S in V1>1
  - ◊ R/S in V6<1
  - ◊ R wave in V1>5mm
  - ◊ P wave in II>2.5 mm, consistent with right atrial enlargement
- Transient changes with hypoxia (arterial O_2 saturation <85% and mean pulmonary arterial pressure >25 mm Hg) which may include:
  - ◊ Rightward mean QRS axis (shift of 30° or more from former position)
  - ◊ Biphasic, flattened, or inverted T waves in the precordial leads
  - ◊ ST segment depression in II, III and aVF
  - ◊ Incomplete or complete (rare) right bundle-branch block

IMAGING
- Chest x-ray:
  - ◊ Heart size may be normal in mild to moderate disease
  - ◊ There may be counter-clockwise cardiac rotation and loss of aortic knob prominence with severe disease
  - ◊ In the PA view, the left heart border is mostly comprised of the right ventricle
  - ◊ Pulmonary hypertension gives rise to dilatation of the pulmonary trunk and hilar vessels
- Echocardiography estimates right ventricular dimensions, right atrial pressure, systolic pulmonary artery pressure, and the severity of tricuspid regurgitation. In patients with chronic cor pulmonale secondary to COPD, there may also be late diastolic LV filling secondary to RV pressure/volume overload-induced structural distortion of the left ventricle.
- Thallium-201 myocardial scintigraphy and MRI can be used to diagnose right ventricular hypertrophy
- MRI can be used more specifically to characterize right ventricular ejection fraction and ventricular volume, including end-systolic and end-diastolic wall sizes

DIAGNOSTIC PROCEDURES
Right heart catheterization for quantitation of ventricular and pulmonary pressures and exclusion of congenital heart disease as etiology of right heart failure. Lung biopsy also helpful in discriminating among granulomatous and collagen-vascular diseases.

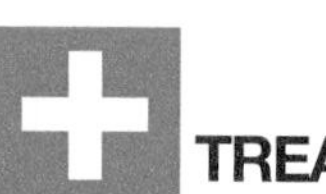

TREATMENT

APPROPRIATE HEALTH CARE
- Acute cor pulmonale: ICU setting
- Chronic cor pulmonale: outpatient

GENERAL MEASURES
- Vigorous antibiotic treatment of acute respiratory tract infections
- Avoidance of airway irritants (eg, tobacco smoke), sedatives and tranquilizers
- Treatment of underlying pulmonary disease, for example:
  - ◊ Chronic obstructive pulmonary disease
    - Bronchodilators to relieve obstruction
    - Supplemental oxygen to correct hypoxia and acidemia
    - Vasodilators, diuretics and phlebotomy (when HCT 55-60%) are possibly useful
    - Digoxin with concomitant left ventricular failure
  - ◊ Ventilatory abnormalities, eg, sleep apnea
    - CPAP (continuous positive airway pressure) or BiPAP (biphasic positive airway pressure)
    - Progestins
    - Tracheostomy
- Acute or chronic thromboembolic disease
  - ◊ Appropriate anticoagulation and hemodynamic support

SURGICAL MEASURES N/A

ACTIVITY As tolerated

DIET Moderate salt restriction

PATIENT EDUCATION
- Signs of COPD exacerbation
- Sudden unilateral swelling of lower extremity in patient with hypercoagulability
- Diet restrictions
- Signs of edema to watch for
- Stress the need for adequate rest
- Referral to social service agency for home care help (oxygen, suctioning, etc)
- Report any signs of infections to physician
- Avoid use of nonprescription medications, especially sedatives

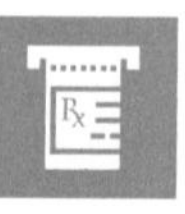

MEDICATIONS

DRUG(S) OF CHOICE
- Oxygen: Maintain arterial oxygen over 60 mm Hg (>8.0 kPa), if possible, to reduce pulmonary vascular resistance and improve myocardial dynamics. Excess oxygen depresses respiratory drive in patients with carbon dioxide retention.
- Theophylline: Bronchodilator, increases right ventricular ejection fraction (RVEF), and decreases pulmonary and systemic vascular resistance.
- Beta-adrenergic agonists: During acute, short-term administration, terbutaline beneficial probably by increasing RVEF and lowering pulmonary vascular resistance.
- Bronchodilators: (e.g., ipratropium, metaproterenol, albuterol) used every six hours and more often if necessary in order to maintain airway patency and arterial oxygen saturation
- Diuretics: (e.g., furosemide) for the relief of peripheral edema, combinations of furosemide and spironolactone (Aldactone) for ascites.
- Vasodilators: (e.g., hydralazine, nifedipine, diltiazem, prazosin) may be tried if conventional measures (oxygen and bronchodilators) fail. Success with these agents can only be accurately assessed with invasive monitoring. Benefit is obtained if the following criteria are met:
  - ◊ Pulmonary vascular resistance reduced by 20%
  - ◊ Cardiac output increases or remains unchanged
  - ◊ Pulmonary artery pressure decreases or remains unchanged
  - ◊ Systemic vascular resistance does not drop significantly. Consistent with the latter, monitor for systemic hypotension during initiation of therapy.
- In patients with primary pulmonary hypertension, calcium channel blockers (diltiazem, nifedipine) are a therapeutic mainstay as long as left ventricular dysfunction is not exacerbated. Patients at high-risk for thromboembolic phenomena should be anticoagulated with warfarin. Warfarin provides symptomatic improvement and decreases mortality in patients with primary pulmonary hypertension.
- Preliminary data with oral sildenafil shows it is an effective and selective pulmonary vasodilator that increases cardiac output without increasing wedge pressure in patients with pulmonary hypertension. Additional studies will be needed to determine the drug's effect on outcomes in these patients.
- In patients with pulmonary arterial hypertension and WHO class III or IV symptom severity, bosentan (Tracleer) administered at 125mg po bid has been shown to improve exertional tolerance and walking distance. Tracleer has also been shown to improve cardiac function and reduce pulmonary vascular resistance, pulmonary arterial pressure, and mean right atrial pressure. Tracleer is an endothelin-1 receptor antagonist. Liver function tests must be monitored while patients are on this medication as it has been associated with liver toxicity. If ALT or AST levels exceed three times the upper limit of normal on therapy, it must be discontinued. The use of Tracleer is absolutely contraindicated in pregnant patients because of the high likelihood of inducing teratogenic effects.

Contraindications: Avoid sedatives and respiratory depressants

Precautions: Diuretics - monitor electrolytes as excessive loss of potassium and chloride may result in metabolic alkalosis, further impairing respiratory drive.

Significant possible interactions: Refer to manufacturer's literature

ALTERNATIVE DRUGS
- Digoxin: Controversial; increases right heart contractility, but also induces pulmonary vasoconstriction, which may exacerbate right heart failure. Digoxin should be used in patients with cor pulmonale and concomitant left ventricular failure. Because of hypoxia and diuretic use, dangerous arrhythmias may develop.
- Other therapies being tested: inhalational nitric oxide, intravenous epoprostenol, and endothelin receptor blockers

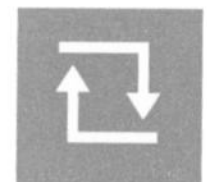

FOLLOWUP

PATIENT MONITORING
- Dependent on severity of underlying disease(s), extent of right heart failure, and medications in use
- Appropriate patients with advancing disease should be referred to centers specializing in lung and heart-lung transplantation. Right ventricular geometry and function tends to normalize subsequent to lung transplantation.

PREVENTION/AVOIDANCE Discontinue tobacco use, limit exposure to inhalational irritants and allergens

POSSIBLE COMPLICATIONS N/A

EXPECTED COURSE/PROGNOSIS
- Depends on underlying disease and degree of pulmonary hypertension. 50,000 deaths per year in US from acute pulmonary embolism. In more chronic forms of cor pulmonale, there is a 10-50% 5 year mortality which improves with supplemental oxygen. In COPD with cor pulmonale, 3 year mortality is 60%.
- S1S2S3 on EKG, alveolar-arterial gradient >48 mm Hg during oxygen therapy, and right atrial overload indicate a poor prognosis when chronic cor pulmonale is secondary to COPD

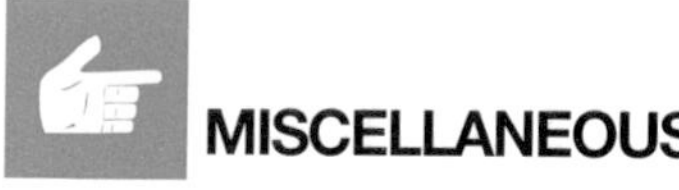

MISCELLANEOUS

ASSOCIATED CONDITIONS
- Left heart failure

AGE-RELATED FACTORS
Pediatric: N/A

Geriatric: Metabolism of sedatives and narcotics slowed, thus the respiratory drive of these patients may be affected for prolonged periods

Others: N/A

PREGNANCY Increased demand for placental perfusion may be severe

SYNONYMS N/A

ICD-9-CM
416.9 Chronic pulmonary heart disease, unspecified
415.0 Acute cor pulmonale

SEE ALSO
Alveolar proteinosis of the lung
Congestive heart failure
Cystic fibrosis
Obesity

OTHER NOTES N/A

ABBREVIATIONS N/A

REFERENCES

- Restrepo CI, Tapson VF. Pulmonary hypertension and cor pulmonale. In Topol EJ, ed. Textbook of Cardiovascular Medicine. Philadelphia, Lippincott-Raven, 1997:707-25
- Braunwald E. Cor Pulmonale. In: Fauci AS, et al, eds: Harrison's Principles of Internal Medicine.14th ed. new York, McGraw Hill, 1998:1324-8
- Wiedemann HP, Matthay RA. Cor Pulmonale. In: Braunwald E, ed: Heart Disease: A Textbook of Cardiovascular Disease. 5th ed. Philadelphia, WB Saunders Co, 1997:1604-25
- Incalzi RA, et al. Electrocardiographic chronic cor pulmonale: a negative prognostic finding in chronic obstructive pulmonary disease. Circulation 1999;99:1600-5
- Tutar E, et al. Echocardiographic evaluation of left ventricular diastolic function in chronic cor pulmonale. Am J Cardiol 1999;83:1414-7

Web references: 0 available at www.5mcc.com

Illustrations N/A

Author(s):
Peter P. Toth, MD, PhD

BASICS

DESCRIPTION Corneal ulcers represent an infection of the cornea by bacteria, virus or fungi as a result of breakdown in the protective epithelial barrier. If left untreated, corneal ulcers can result in blindness. Ulcerations may be central or marginal.
System(s) affected: Nervous
Genetics: None
Incidence/Prevalence in USA: Common
Predominant age: None
Predominant sex: Male = Female

SIGNS & SYMPTOMS
- Eyelid and conjunctiva become inflamed
- Mucopurulent discharge
- The corneal epithelium will be absent with underlying ulceration and infiltration of the corneal stroma with leukocytes
- Foreign body sensation
- Blurred vision
- Light sensitivity
- Pain

CAUSES
- Corneal ulcers are predisposed by the presence of an entry to the external eye. Dry eye, burns, abrasion, contact lenses, inappropriate use of topical anesthetics, antibiotics, or antiviral drops, immunosuppressant drugs, diabetes, immunodeficiency.
- Causative agents for foreign entry:
  - ◊ Gram positive organisms (staphylococci, streptococci, and bacilli)
  - ◊ Anaerobes (cocci, bacilli)
  - ◊ Gram negative organisms (diplococcus, rods, and anaerobes)
  - ◊ Pseudomonas
  - ◊ Viruses such as herpes

RISK FACTORS
- Any abrasive injury
- Contact lenses (especially soft lenses)
- Chronic topical steroid use

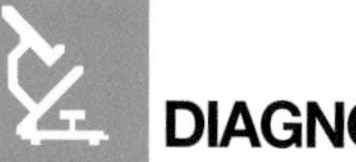

DIAGNOSIS

DIFFERENTIAL DIAGNOSIS Identify infecting organisms

LABORATORY Culture the ulcer

Drugs that may alter lab results: Pretreatment with topical antibiotics or corticosteroids may delay diagnosis

Disorders that may alter lab results: N/A

PATHOLOGICAL FINDINGS Scrapings for Gram's and Giemsa's stain may demonstrate bacteria, yeast, or intranuclear inclusions which may aid in the diagnosis

SPECIAL TESTS N/A

IMAGING N/A

DIAGNOSTIC PROCEDURES Scrapings of the corneal ulcer may be necessary to identify the underlying organism. The sample should be plated onto the culture media directly.

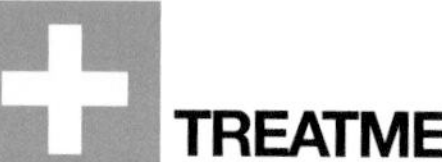

TREATMENT

APPROPRIATE HEALTH CARE
- Outpatient or inpatient for severe ulcer or noncompliant patient
- All cases of corneal ulceration should be promptly referred to an ophthalmologist

GENERAL MEASURES
- Aggressive topical antibiotic treatment directed toward the causative agent should be instituted immediately while culture studies are pending
- Supplemental topical cycloplegia reduces the inflammation and aids in patient comfort
- Bandaging the eye should be avoided and topical steroids should never be used. Daily evaluation is necessary and prompt consultation with an ophthalmologist or corneal specialist is advised.

SURGICAL MEASURES N/A

ACTIVITY Reduced, until vision returns to normal and healing is complete

DIET No special diet

PATIENT EDUCATION Prevention of abrasions and proper handling of contact lenses can prevent recurrence of corneal ulcers

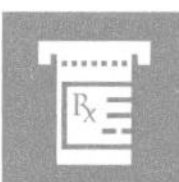

MEDICATIONS

DRUG(S) OF CHOICE

- Sulfacetamide 10% suspension (bacteriostatic) is only good for low grade conjunctival infections
- Topical gentamicin and tobramycin are effective against Pseudomonas, Enterobacter, Klebsiella, and aerobic gram negative organisms, while cephalosporins (e.g., cefazolin 50 mg/mL) may be effective against many gram negative organisms. The combination aminoglycoside and cephalosporin may be the most appropriate initial therapy.
- Topical quinolones, e.g., ciprofloxacin (Ciloxan) 0.3%, also ofloxacin (Ocuflox) 0.3%. These may be treatment of choice for Pseudomonas infections.
- Fungal keratitis needs to be treated with parenteral amphotericin B for candida and aspergillus; clotrimazole, miconazole, econazole, and ketoconazole may also be required

Contraindications: Refer to manufacturer's profile of each drug
Precautions: Refer to manufacturer's profile of each drug
Significant possible interactions: Refer to manufacturer's profile of each drug

ALTERNATIVE DRUGS N/A

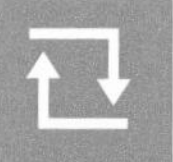

FOLLOWUP

PATIENT MONITORING The patient should be monitored at least daily

PREVENTION/AVOIDANCE Avoid corneal abrasion or injury and improper contact lens handling

POSSIBLE COMPLICATIONS Scarring of the cornea and loss of vision

EXPECTED COURSE/PROGNOSIS

- Corneal ulcerations should improve daily and heal with appropriate therapy
- If healing does not occur or the ulcer extends, then consideration should be given to an alternative diagnosis and treatment

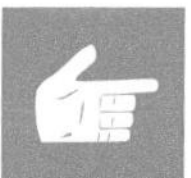

MISCELLANEOUS

ASSOCIATED CONDITIONS Chronic ulcerations may be associated with neurotrophic keratitis due to lack of fifth nerve innervation of the cornea. Individuals with thyroid disease, diabetes, immunosuppressive conditions are particularly at risk.

AGE-RELATED FACTORS

Pediatric: N/A
Geriatric: Ring ulceration more common
Others: N/A

PREGNANCY N/A

SYNONYMS N/A

ICD-9-CM

370.00 Corneal ulcer, unspecified

SEE ALSO

OTHER NOTES N/A

ABBREVIATIONS N/A

REFERENCES

Web references: 0 available at www.5mcc.com
Illustrations N/A

Author(s):
Robert M. Kershner, MD

BASICS

DESCRIPTION Anterior chest wall pain associated with pain and tenderness of the costochondral and costosternal regions.
System(s) affected: Musculoskeletal
Genetics: Unknown
Incidence/Prevalence in USA: 10% of chest pain complaints. 15-20% of teenagers with chest pain.
Predominant age: 20-40
Predominant sex: Female

SIGNS & SYMPTOMS
- Insidious onset
- Pain usually sharp in nature, sometimes pleuritic
- Pain involves multiple locations, the second through fifth costal cartilage most often involved
- Pain worse with movement and breathing
- Heat often provides relief of pain
- Chest tightness is often associated with the pain
- Pain sometimes radiates into arm
- Non-suppurative edema and tenderness at rib articulations
- Redness and warmth at sites of tenderness

CAUSES
- Not fully understood
- Trauma
- Overuse

RISK FACTORS
- Unusual physical activity or overuse
- Recent upper respiratory infection

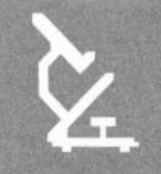

DIAGNOSIS

DIFFERENTIAL DIAGNOSIS
- Cardiac
  - ◊ Coronary artery disease
  - ◊ Aortic aneurysm
  - ◊ Mitral valve prolapse
  - ◊ Pericarditis
  - ◊ Myocarditis
- Gastrointestinal
  - ◊ Gastroesophageal reflux
  - ◊ Peptic esophagitis
  - ◊ Esophageal spasm
  - ◊ Gastritis
- Musculoskeletal
  - ◊ Fibromyalgia
  - ◊ Slipping rib syndrome - involves the lower ribs
  - ◊ Costovertebral arthritis
  - ◊ Painful xiphoid syndrome
  - ◊ Rib trauma with swelling
  - ◊ Thoracic disk compression
  - ◊ Ankylosing spondylitis
  - ◊ Epidemic myalgia
  - ◊ Precordial catch syndrome
- Psychogenic
  - ◊ Anxiety disorder
  - ◊ Panic attacks
  - ◊ Hyperventilation
- Respiratory
  - ◊ Asthma
  - ◊ Pneumonia
  - ◊ Chronic cough
  - ◊ Pneumothorax
- Other
  - ◊ Herpes zoster
  - ◊ Spinal tumor
  - ◊ Metastatic cancer
  - ◊ Substance abuse (cocaine)

LABORATORY The diagnosis of costochondritis is based on a complete and thorough history and physical examination. Laboratory exams should only be utilized if there is concern regarding other elements of the differential diagnosis. Erythrocyte sedimentation rate inconsistently elevated.

Drugs that may alter lab results: N/A

Disorders that may alter lab results: N/A

PATHOLOGICAL FINDINGS Costochondral joint inflammation

SPECIAL TESTS None indicated for the diagnosis of costochondritis

IMAGING No imaging is indicated for the diagnosis of costochondritis. Chest x-ray normal.

DIAGNOSTIC PROCEDURES None

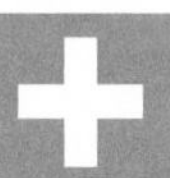

TREATMENT

APPROPRIATE HEALTH CARE Outpatient therapy

GENERAL MEASURES Patient reassurance. Rest and heat.

SURGICAL MEASURES N/A

ACTIVITY As tolerated

DIET Regular

PATIENT EDUCATION Educate the patient in regards to the self-limited nature of the illness. Instruct patient on proper physical activity regimens to avoid overuse syndromes. Also stress the importance of avoiding sudden, significant changes in activity.

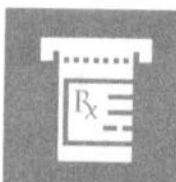

MEDICATIONS

DRUG(S) OF CHOICE Non-steroidal anti-inflammatory drugs (NSAIDs) such as aspirin, ibuprofen (Advil, Motrin), naproxen (Anaprox, Naprosyn, Aleve) or diclofenac (Voltaren). Other analgesics may be used as needed.

Contraindications:
- History of anaphylaxis to aspirin
- Peptic ulcer disease
- Renal insufficiency

Precautions:
- Peptic ulcers may occur with chronic use of non-steroidal anti-inflammatory drugs
- Acute interstitial nephritis
- Drug accumulation with renal insufficiency
- Liver function abnormalities in up to 15% of patients

Significant possible interactions:
- NSAIDs
  - ◊ Albumin-bound drugs - displacement of either drug
  - ◊ Warfarin - increased prothrombin time. Monitor prothrombin times closely and adjust warfarin dosage as needed. Monitor lithium levels and adjust lithium dosage as needed. May need to increase lithium dosage when non-steroidal anti-inflammatory drugs have been discontinued.
  - ◊ Lithium - increased lithium plasma level
  - ◊ Furosemide - decreased natriuretic effect and increased risk of acute renal failure secondary to decreased renal blood flow
  - ◊ Propranolol - decreased antihypertensive effect

ALTERNATIVE DRUGS Acetaminophen

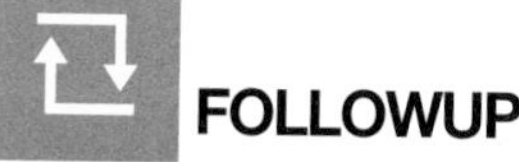

FOLLOWUP

PATIENT MONITORING Followup in one week

PREVENTION/AVOIDANCE Avoid activity which increases the pain

POSSIBLE COMPLICATIONS Incomplete attention to differential diagnosis or inappropriate interventions in a desire to ensure that a more life-threatening diagnosis is not missed

EXPECTED COURSE/PROGNOSIS
- Self-limited illness, although sometimes chronic
- Often recurs

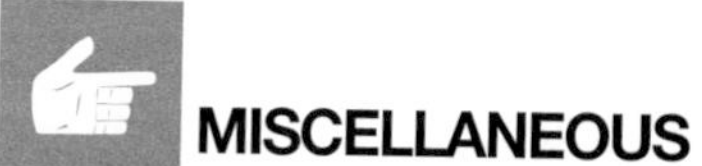

MISCELLANEOUS

ASSOCIATED CONDITIONS Upper respiratory infections

AGE-RELATED FACTORS
Pediatric: Special attention should be paid to psychogenic chest pain with children who perceive family discord
Geriatric: Often present with multiple problems capable of causing chest pain, making a thorough history and physical exam imperative.
Others: N/A

PREGNANCY Unknown

SYNONYMS
- Costosternal syndrome
- Parasternal chondrodynia
- Anterior chest wall syndrome
- Tietze disease
- Tietze syndrome
- Chondrocostal junction syndrome

ICD-9-CM
733.6 Tietze disease

SEE ALSO

OTHER NOTES N/A

ABBREVIATIONS N/A

REFERENCES

- Gregory PL, Biswas AC, Batt ME. Musculoskeletal problems of the chest wall in athletes. Sports Med 2002;32(4):235-50¥ A report from ASPN: An exploratory report of chest pain in primary care. J Am Board Fam Prac 1990, 3:143-150
- Klinkman MS, Stevens D, Gorenflow DW. Episodes of care for chest pain: A preliminary report. From MIRNET, J Fam Practice 1994;38(4):345-52
- Disla E, Rhim HR, Reddy A, Karten I, Taranta A. Costochondritis. a prospective analysis in an emergency department setting. Archives Int Med 1994:154(21):2466-2469
- Mukamel M, Kornreich L, Horev G, Zaharia A, Mimoun M. Tietze's syndrome in children. J Ped 1997;131(5):774-775
- Klinkman MS, Stevens D, Gorenflow DU. Episodes of cure for chest pain: a preliminary report from MIRNET. Michigan Research Network. J Fam Prac 1994;38(4):345-352
- Jenson S. Musculoskeletal causes of chest pain. Australian Fam Physician 2001;30(9):534-9

Web references: 1 available at www.5mcc.com
Illustrations N/A

Author(s):
Scott A. Fields, MD

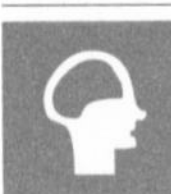

BASICS

DESCRIPTION An idiopathic inflammatory disease of the small intestine (60%), the colon (20%) or both; involving all of the layers of the bowel, but most commonly involving the terminal ileum. It is a slowly progressive and recurrent disease with prominent involvement of multiple regions of the intestine with normal sections in between.

System(s) affected: Gastrointestinal

Genetics: 15% of patients have first-degree relatives with inflammatory bowel disease. Family members develop the disease with similar patterns and similar age of onset.

Incidence/Prevalence in USA:
- More common in Caucasians than African-Americans or Asians
- More common in Jews
- 20-100/100,000 prevalence

Predominant age:
- Most cases 15-25 age of onset
- Second smaller peak in ages 55-65

Predominant sex: Female > Male (slightly)

SIGNS & SYMPTOMS
- All forms of Crohn
  - ◊ Diarrhea occurs in most patients
  - ◊ Abdominal pain in two-thirds
  - ◊ Weight loss
  - ◊ Abdominal tenderness often less than expected, in view of symptoms
  - ◊ Abdominal mass (occasionally)
  - ◊ Fistula - perirectal, bladder, skin, vagina
  - ◊ Extraluminal disease (10%) skin, iritis, arthritis, sclerosing cholangitis
- Small bowel disease only
  - ◊ Diarrhea prominent, including nocturnal
  - ◊ Vague abdominal pain frequent. Only half of patients with abdominal pain have associated tenderness, not relieved with evacuation and often aggravated by food.
  - ◊ Intestinal obstruction in 1/3. Cramping abdominal pain precedes for months.
  - ◊ Bleeding in 20%, rarely massive
  - ◊ Perianal disease, including fistulae
  - ◊ Internal fistulae
- Colon disease only
  - ◊ Diarrhea prominent, including nocturnal
  - ◊ Hematochezia
  - ◊ Abdominal pain in 1/2, often relieved by stooling
  - ◊ Perianal disease in 40%, fistulae
  - ◊ Weight loss prominent
  - ◊ Megacolon occurs in about 10%
  - ◊ Intestinal obstruction occasional
- Colon and small bowel disease
  - ◊ Intestinal obstruction much more common

CAUSES
- Idiopathic
- Aggravated by bacterial infection
- Aggravated by inflammatory cascade
- Aggravated by smoking cessation

RISK FACTORS
- More cigarette smokers than expected

DIAGNOSIS

DIFFERENTIAL DIAGNOSIS
- Colon disease
  - ◊ Ulcerative colitis
  - ◊ Ischemic colitis (older age group)
  - ◊ Enteric pathogens: Amebiasis, Tuberculosis, Yersinia, Campylobacter, Gonorrhea, Clostridium difficile toxin, Shigella, Salmonella, LGV and non-LGV Chlamydia, Fungi(e.g., actinomycosis)
  - ◊ Malignancy: Lymphoma, adenocarcinoma
  - ◊ Caustic enemas (e.g., H2O2)
- Small bowel disease
  - ◊ Enteric pathogens: Tuberculosis, Yersinia, Campylobacter, LGV and non-LGV Chlamydia, Fungi (e.g., actinomycosis), Chlamydial pelvic inflammation in women
  - ◊ Lymphoma
  - ◊ Drugs (e.g., NSAIDs)
  - ◊ Eosinophilic gastroenteritis

LABORATORY
- Elevated sedimentation rate
- Anemia common
- Albumin decreased in severe cases
- Serum electrolytes imbalance
- Specific nutrient deficiency: B12, fat soluble vitamins, folate
- C reactive protein elevated
- pANCA (perinuclear antineutrophil cytoplasmic antibody) is elevated in 85% ulcerative colitis, 15% Crohn disease. Antiglycan antibody is elevated in 75% Crohn disease, 5% ulcerative colitis. This pair of markers helps distinguish which disease is present in obscure cases.

Drugs that may alter lab results: Sulfa drugs may lower folate after years of administration

Disorders that may alter lab results: All tests are non-specific, similar degrees of disease from other causes produce similar changes

PATHOLOGICAL FINDINGS
- Involvement of all layers of gut wall with inflammation in > 95% cases at least focal areas
- Skip areas in 80% (a normal segment between two involved segments)
- Granuloma in 15%
- Fat hypertrophy following mesenteric vessels in 50% of small bowel disease

SPECIAL TESTS Colonoscopy is most helpful. The colon is not uniformly involved. The typical lesion is nodular with undermined pus filled mucosal ulcers. Strictures commonly present, occasionally preventing passage of the endoscope. The terminal ileum often has aphthous ulcers and may have nodularity. Small bowel proximal to an anastomosis is a very common site of recurrence.

IMAGING
- Barium x-rays - enema and small bowel
  - ◊ Loss of smooth mucosa, undermined ulcers prominent
  - ◊ Narrowed lumen in most involved segments of small bowel
  - ◊ Fistulae from involved segment to other bowel loops, bladder, vagina or external
  - ◊ Skip areas, multiple lesions common
  - ◊ Failure to reflux into ileum on barium enema (not specific)
  - ◊ Ulcers undermining mucosa
  - ◊ Small bowel ulcerated wall
  - ◊ Narrowed lumen
  - ◊ Fistula to other parts of intestine
- Plain x-rays
  - ◊ Intestinal obstruction
  - ◊ Toxic patient with colon disease, toxic megacolon
  - ◊ Evaluation of arthritis
  - ◊ Sacroiliitis
- CT Scans
  - ◊ Defines thickening of bowel wall, strictures and dilatation
  - ◊ Define abscess cavities and fistulae
  - ◊ Identify extensive perirectal disease

DIAGNOSTIC PROCEDURES
- Ileoscopy and enteroscopy
- The constellation of barium-identified distribution of lesions, endoscopic findings, and biopsies usually establish the diagnosis
- Biopsies of mucosa in involved areas usually compatible with diagnosis, but not diagnostic. Helps rule out other causes.

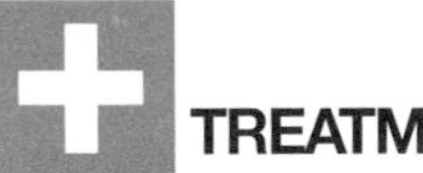

TREATMENT

APPROPRIATE HEALTH CARE
- Outpatient customary, inpatient for complications or special treatments
- Progressive disease - average patient requires surgery each 4-7 years

GENERAL MEASURES
- Attention to maintaining weight and nutrition
- Monitor severe cases for fat malabsorption
- Perirectal disease, sitz baths, soap and water after stooling, surgical drainage of perirectal abscesses, surgical treatment of recurrent fistulae if medical management fails
- Extracolonic disease (uveitis, arthritis, dermatitis, sclerosing cholangitis) managed as other diseases in that special area
- Folate supplements often needed

SURGICAL MEASURES
- Indications for surgery:
  - ◊ Severe recurrent hemorrhage
  - ◊ Inability to thrive
  - ◊ Abscess
  - ◊ Total or recurrent intestinal obstruction
  - ◊ Toxic megacolon or extensive disease
  - ◊ Symptomatic fistulae other than rectal
  - ◊ Failure of ostomy to function after ≥1 year

ACTIVITY Full activity as tolerated

DIET
- Usually no restrictions
- If fat malabsorption, diminish fat in diet
- If strictures or recurrent obstruction, avoid highly fibrous substances
- If diarrhea prominent, increase dietary fiber (sometimes recommended), decrease fat

PATIENT EDUCATION
- An important part of management
- Crohn and Colitis Foundation of America Inc, 11th floor, Park Ave South, NY 10016, Phone (800)343-3637. Joining local chapters recommended.

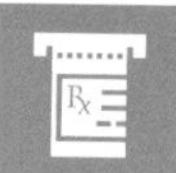

MEDICATIONS

DRUG(S) OF CHOICE

- Naive patient, relapse, major symptoms
  - ◊ Prednisone orally 20-60 mg/day. Response 1-3 weeks. Start tapering after 4-6 weeks.
  - ◊ Start mesalamine (5-aminosalicylic acid, Asacol, Claversal, Rowasa) at same time. Use minimal dose bid or tid, increase each 4 days to reach maximum recommended dose.
  - ◊ If tenesmus or bleeding prominent - mesalamine enema or hydrocortisone enema bid
- Maintenance therapy
  - ◊ Usually with mesalamine, methotrexate, or azathioprine (Imuran) prolongs remission and delays additional surgery
  - ◊ Several delivery forms of mesalamine exist; each targets a different portion of the intestine. Select form appropriate to patient.
- Predominantly perirectal disease with fistulae
  - ◊ Metronidazole (Flagyl) 250 mg tid for max of 8 weeks
- Patients who relapse with prednisone tapering or fail to respond
  - ◊ Add azathioprine (Imuran) 2-2.5 mg/kg/day or mercaptopurine (6-MP) 1-1.5 mg/kg/day. After 6-12 weeks, expect maximum benefit. If good response, taper steroid.
  - ◊ If inadequate response, maintain patient on immunosuppressant and start a course of infliximab (Remicade) 5 mg/kg at 0, 2 and 6 weeks. May repeat as clinically indicated at 8 week intervals.
- Patients with symptomatic fistula failing to heal with conservative therapy
  - ◊ Infliximab used as above permits more than half to heal
- Patients with joint, eye, and skin extra-intestinal manifestations
  - ◊ Unresponsive to mesalamine, occasionally responsive to prednisone
  - ◊ Usually responsive to infliximab
- For all well-controlled patients, supply loperamide (Imodium) 2 mg to control diarrhea on those occasions it would interfere with social life

Contraindications: Allergy to prescribed drugs

Precautions:

- Allergies common
- Male sterility problem with chronic use of mesalamine
- Watch for thrombocytopenia and pancytopenia
- Azathioprine (Imuran) or 6-
  - ◊ A small number of patients have genetically determined altered levels of the enzyme thiopurine methyltransferase (TPMT). 1/300 have none of this enzyme and exhibit severe marrow toxicity to low doses of either azathioprine or 6-MP. 1/10 have increased sensitivity. Determining the TPMT level before initiating treatment allows dose adjustment.
  - ◊ In all patients, careful monitoring of the WBC is required. It is now known that treatment efficacy correlates with the level of 6-thioguanine nucleotides reached in erythrocytes. In patients who have not had a remission with azathioprine or 6-MP, obtaining these levels after 12 weeks indicates whether a therapeutic level of drug has been given and permits dose adjustment.

Significant possible interactions: Folic acid supplements needed with mesalamine. Refer to manufacturer's profile of each drug.

ALTERNATIVE DRUGS

- Budesonide - a steroid almost totally removed by the liver; use instead of prednisone in patients requiring long term steroid; partially avoids steroid complications
- Methotrexate 25 mg IM weekly may be used instead of 6-MP or azathioprine
- Cyclosporine has assisted in closing fistulae when other measures fail
- Etanercept, a newly released agent similar to infliximab is being increasingly used
- Natalizumab an integrin blocking agent has benefit, appropriate use not yet defined

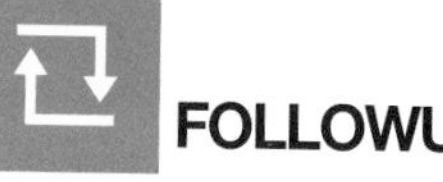

FOLLOWUP

PATIENT MONITORING

- Regular assessment (each 3-6 months if patient is stable) of symptoms, particularly status of weight, pain, diarrhea, hemoglobin and sedimentation rate
- Regular calculation of an activity index based upon:

1) loose stools/day, 2) pain, 3) general well being, 4) systemic manifestations, 5) use of antidiarrheal, 6) presence of abdominal mass, 7) hematocrit, 8) change in body weight. Highly useful in following patients and making decisions to increase or diminish medications and/or hospitalize.

- Endoscopy and further images if there are changes in symptoms and signs
- Check liver tests yearly
- Check vitamin B12 level in those with ileal disease or ileal resection
- Check folate level in all on 5-aminosalicylate, use supplements in all

PREVENTION/AVOIDANCE

- Ongoing care with available physician
- Consultant for review; long term advice

POSSIBLE COMPLICATIONS

- Progression nearly certain - both expansion of old lesions and new lesions occur
- Recurrence after operation nearly certain, usually occurs in gut segment most proximal to anastomoses
- Fistulae occur about 15% of patients; perirectal, cutaneous, enterovaginal, enterovesicular are all seen
- Extraluminal disease occurs in 10% with skin, uveal tract, joint, and biliary tract disease most common. All fairly specific in pattern; do not parallel activity of the luminal disease.
- Extensive colon disease associated with increased risk of adenocarcinoma
- Colon perforation and massive bleeding
- Toxic megacolon
- Gall stones occur in > 25%
- Osteoporosis commonly occurs; more frequent and severe when chronic use of steroids

EXPECTED COURSE/PROGNOSIS

- Average patient has surgery each 7 years; >4 surgeries, expect short-bowel syndrome
- Expect disease to recur
- Majority will have normal life (work, children, full activities); overall life is shortened

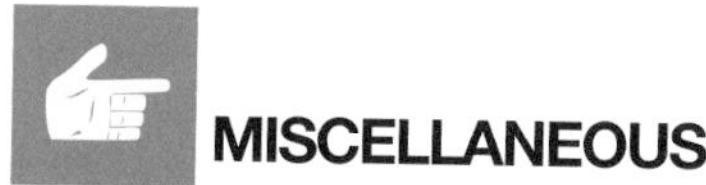

MISCELLANEOUS

ASSOCIATED CONDITIONS

- Viral gastroenteritis may be more devastating
- Arthritis of two types - similar to rheumatoid and spondylitis
- Variety of skin lesions, erythema nodosum, non-specific rashes, pyoderma gangrenosum
- Uveal tract disease rare but related
- Sclerosing cholangitis in about 10%, manifest from mild liver test abnormalities including pericholangitis on biopsy to full syndrome
- Pigment gallstones are increased with ileal disease

AGE-RELATED FACTORS

Pediatric: Rare
Geriatric: N/A
Others: Occurs at any age

PREGNANCY

- Reversible male sterility after long time on sulfasalazine - folate defers
- No contraindications to pregnancy

SYNONYMS

- Granulomatous colitis
- Regional enteritis
- Regional ileitis
- Regional colitis
- Regional ileocolitis

ICD-9-CM

555.0 Regional enteritis of small intestine
555.1 Regional enteritis of large intestine
555.9 Regional enteritis of unspecified site

SEE ALSO

Celiac disease
Diarrhea, acute
Diarrhea, chronic
Intestinal parasites
Short-bowel syndrome
Ulcerative colitis

OTHER NOTES N/A

ABBREVIATIONS N/A

REFERENCES

- Baert F, Noman M, Vermeire S,et al. Influence of immunogenicity on the long-term efficacy of infliximab in Crohn's disease. N Engl J Med 2003;348(7):601-8
- Ljung T, Staun M, Grove O, et al. Pyoderma gangrenosum associated with Crohn disease: effect of TNF-alpha blockade with infliximab. Scand J Gastroenterol 2002;37(9):1108-10
- Harrison J, Hanauer SB. Medical treatment of Crohn's disease. Gastroenterol Clin North Am 2002;31(1):167-84
- Poggioli G, Pierangeli F, Laureti S, Ugolini F. Review article: indication and type of surgery in Crohn's disease. Aliment Pharmacol Ther 2002;16 Suppl 4:59-64
- Berg DF, Bahadursingh AM, Kaminski DL, Longo WE. Acute surgical emergencies in inflammatory bowel disease. Am J Surg 2002;184(1):45-51
- Fraser AG, Orchard TR, Jewell DP. The efficacy of azathioprine for the treatment of inflammatory bowel disease: a 30 year review. Gut 2002;50(4):485-9
- Hanauer SB, Feagan BG, Lichtenstein GR et al. Maintenance infliximab for Crohn's disease: the ACCENT 1 randomized trial. Lancet 2002;359:1541-9

Web references: 3 available at www.5mcc.com
Illustrations 5 available

Author(s):
Frank L. Iber, MD

BASICS

DESCRIPTION Cryptococcus neoformans is a fungus which rarely causes disease in hosts with normal immune function. Cryptococcal meningitis is one of the more common AIDS-defining infections in HIV seropositive persons.
System(s) affected: Endocrine/Metabolic, Nervous, Pulmonary, Skin/Exocrine
Genetics: N/A
Incidence/Prevalence in USA: Accounts for 5-8% of opportunistic infections in AIDS patients. Incidence has been decreasing in recent years.
Predominant age: Generally adults
Predominant sex: Male > Female (reflects HIV prevalence)

SIGNS & SYMPTOMS
- Cryptococcal meningitis
  - ◊ Often insidious onset with subtle findings
  - ◊ Frontal or temporal headache (80-95% of patients)
  - ◊ Fever (60-80% of patients)
  - ◊ Impaired mentation
  - ◊ Seizures or focal neurologic signs (less common)
  - ◊ Meningismus may be absent (80% of patients)
  - ◊ Deaths within first few weeks of diagnosis is often related to increased intracranial pressure
- Pulmonary cryptococcus
  - ◊ May be asymptomatic
  - ◊ Cough
  - ◊ Shortness of breath
  - ◊ Fever
  - ◊ Hemoptysis
  - ◊ Frequently disseminates in immunosuppressed patients
- Disseminated cryptococcus
  - ◊ Painless skin nodules (5-10% of patients). May occur as erythematous papules, vesicles, macules, or ulcers.
  - ◊ The heart, bone, kidney, adrenals, eyes, prostate and lymph nodes may harbor infection with symptoms referable to affected organ

CAUSES The cryptococcus fungus is ubiquitous. Person to person transmission is rare.

RISK FACTORS Immunosuppression which results in reactivation of latent infection (usually foci in lungs). Rarely, invasive infection may occur in normal hosts.

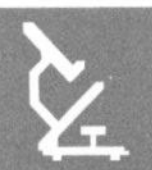

DIAGNOSIS

DIFFERENTIAL DIAGNOSIS
- In CNS disease - toxoplasmosis, lymphoma, AIDS dementia complex, progressive multifocal leukoencephalopathy, herpes encephalitis, other fungal disease
- In pulmonary disease - tuberculosis, Pneumocystis, histoplasmosis, coccidioidomycosis, Kaposi sarcoma, lymphoma
- In disseminated disease - tuberculosis, histoplasmosis, lymphoma, coccidioidomycosis

LABORATORY
- Serum cryptococcal antigen (if positive, search for dissemination, perform L.P.)
- CSF cryptococcal antigen (positive in 95% of culture-proven positive cases)
- India ink preparation of CSF (50% positive in non-AIDS patients; 80% (bronchoalveolar lavage) positive in AIDS patients)
- Culture of CSF, sputum, blood, urine

Drugs that may alter lab results: N/A

Disorders that may alter lab results: In presence of rheumatoid factor, false positive latex agglutination tests have occurred

PATHOLOGICAL FINDINGS Inflammation, granuloma formation (may caseate and cavitate), basilar meningitis with mucoid exudate

SPECIAL TESTS Lumbar puncture in cryptococcal meningitis: Imperative to check opening pressure initially (may repeat if clinical deterioration) significantly increased intracranial pressure associated with poor prognosis. In non-AIDS patients - elevated opening pressure, elevated CSF protein, decreased glucose and lymphocytic pleocytosis. In AIDS patients - abnormal CSF findings in 40% of patients. high opening pressure > 200 mm water in 70% of patients.

IMAGING
- In cryptococcal meningitis - CT of brain is negative unless focal cryptococcomas present
- In pulmonary cryptococcosis - chest x-ray may show infiltrates, nodules, mass lesions (with rare cavitation), miliary spread, hilar adenopathy (10%), pleural effusions (less than 5%)

DIAGNOSTIC PROCEDURES Biopsies of skin lesions may be diagnostic

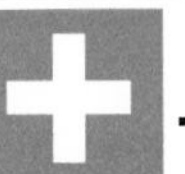

TREATMENT

APPROPRIATE HEALTH CARE Inpatient; outpatient for mild cases

GENERAL MEASURES N/A

SURGICAL MEASURES N/A

ACTIVITY As tolerated

DIET As tolerated

PATIENT EDUCATION Life-long antifungal medication generally required for suppression. In severely immune deficient patients, consider prophylaxis with fluconazole.

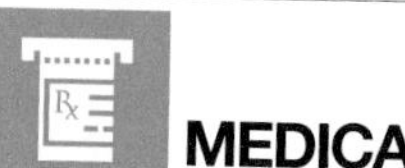

MEDICATIONS

DRUG(S) OF CHOICE

- Amphotericin B at 0.7 mg/kg/day IV plus flucytosine 100 mg/kg/day until patient is clinically improving (2-3 weeks); followed by
- Fluconazole (Diflucan) 400 mg/day (oral or intravenous) until a total of 8 weeks of primary therapy has been completed

Contraindications: Refer to manufacturer's profile of each drug

Precautions: With amphotericin B - permanent renal impairment may occur, hypokalemia, hypomagnesemia; during infusion - fever, chills, headache - pretreat with diphenhydramine, acetaminophen to decrease fever and chill. Add heparin 500 U and hydrocortisone 50 mg to IV amphotericin B to decrease phlebitis.

Significant possible interactions: Refer to manufacturer's literature

ALTERNATIVE DRUGS

- For patients with elevated intracranial pressure - aggressive management with daily lumbar punctures; lumbar drains or acetazolamide is indicated
- Combination fluconazole 400-800 mg/day po plus flucytosine 100 mg/kg/day po is being studied (may be useful in patients intolerant or non-responsive to amphotericin B)
- Liposomal amphotericin (AmBisome) 4 mg/kg/day IV for 14 days followed by fluconazole

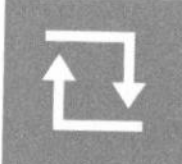

FOLLOWUP

PATIENT MONITORING

- Monitor clinical status and repeat LP if indicated
- Foci in the prostate may be difficult to eliminate

PREVENTION/AVOIDANCE

- Without suppression, relapse is common (50% in AIDS patients within one year)
- Suppress with fluconazole 200 mg po daily
- May consider discontinuing suppressive fluconazole when CD4 cells > 100-200 for over 6 months. When patients respond to antiretroviral therapy.
- Avoid bird roosts
- Primary prophylaxis with fluconazole (100-200 mg/day or tiw) or 400mg/wk in selected patients with CD4 < 50-100 decreases the incidence of cryptococcosis. Cost; possible drug resistance; and drug interactions should be considered.

POSSIBLE COMPLICATIONS

- Cryptococcal infections are fatal unless treated
- Increased intracranial pressure

EXPECTED COURSE/PROGNOSIS

- Fatal without treatment
- No statistics available on survival

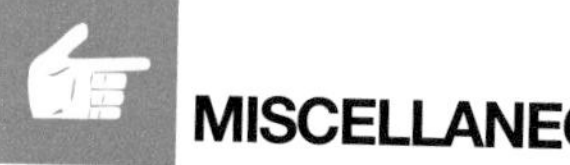

MISCELLANEOUS

ASSOCIATED CONDITIONS

- HIV infection
- AIDS

AGE-RELATED FACTORS

Pediatric: N/A
Geriatric: N/A
Others: N/A

PREGNANCY Amphotericin contraindicated in pregnancy except when treating cryptococcal meningitis

SYNONYMS Torulosis

ICD-9-CM

117.5 Cryptococcosis

SEE ALSO

HIV infection & AIDS

OTHER NOTES N/A

ABBREVIATIONS

CSF = cerebrospinal fluid
AIDS = acquired immunodeficiency syndrome

REFERENCES

- Mitchell TG, Perfect JR. Cryptococcosis in the era of AIDS - 100 years after the discovery of Cryptococcus neoformans. Clin Microbiol Rev 1998;8:51-548
- Aberg JA, Powderly WG. Cryptococcosis. In: Cohen PT, Sande MA, Volberding PA (eds). AIDS Knowledge Base. On the Internet
- Van der Horst CM, Saag MS, Cloud GA, et al. Treatment of cryptococcal meningitis associated with the acquired immunodeficiency syndrome. NEJM 1997;337:15-21
- Haubrich RM, et al. High dose fluconazole for treatment of cryptococcal disease in patients with human immunodeficiency virus infection. J Infect Dis 1994;170:238-44
- Park MK, Hospenthal DR, Bennett JE. Treatment of hydrocephalus secondary to cryptococcal meningitis by use of shunting. Clin Infect Dis 1999;28(3):629-33
- 2001 USPHS/IDSA Guidelines for the Prevention of Opportunistic Infections in Persons Infected with Human Immunodeficiency Virus;July, 2001 (Draft Revisions to MMWR 1999;48:NoRR10
- Chetchotisakd P, Sungkanuparph S, Thinkhamrop B, et al.A multicentre, randomized, double-blind, placebo-controlled trial of primary cryptococcal meningitis prophylaxis in HIV-infected patients with severe immune deficiency. HIV Med. 2004;5(3):140-3.

Web references: 1 available at www.5mcc.com
Illustrations 2 available

Author(s):

Cynthia Gail Carmichael, MD

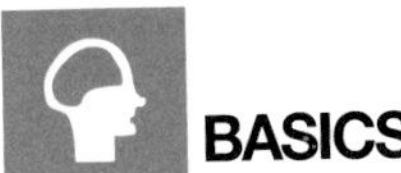

BASICS

DESCRIPTION Incomplete or improper descent of one or both testicles. Normally, descent is in the 7th to 8th month of gestation. The cryptorchid testis may be palpable or non-palpable.
1. Abdominal - located inside the internal ring
2. Canalicular - located between the internal and external ring
3. Ectopic - located outside the normal path of testicular descent from abdominal cavity to scrotum - may be ectopic to perineum, femoral canal, superficial inguinal pouch (most common), suprapubic area and opposite hemiscrotum
4. Retractile - fully descended testis that moves freely between the scrotum and the groin
5. Iatrogenic - previously descended testis becomes undescended secondary to scar tissue after inguinal surgery, such as an inguinal hernia repair or hydrocelectomy

System(s) affected: Reproductive
Genetics: Occurrence of undescended testes in siblings as well as fathers suggests a genetic etiology
Incidence/Prevalence in USA: 3% of full-term and 33% of premature newborn males. Spontaneous testicular descent occurs by age 1 to 3 months in 50-70% of full term males with cryptorchidism. Descent at 6 to 9 months of age is rare.
Predominant age: Premature newborns
Predominant sex: Male only

SIGNS & SYMPTOMS One or both testicles in a site other than the scrotum. May be an isolated defect or associated with other congenital anomalies.

CAUSES
- Not fully known
- May involve alterations in mechanical factors (gubernaculum, length of vas deferens and testicular vessels, groin anatomy, epididymis, cremasteric muscles, and abdominal pressure), hormonal factors (gonadotropin, testosterone, dihydrotestosterone, and Müllerian inhibiting substance), and neural factors (ilioinguinal nerve and genitofemoral nerve)

RISK FACTORS Family history of cryptorchidism. Some have noted the following to be associated with an increased risk of cryptorchidism: firstborn child, c-section delivery, toxemia of pregnancy, hypospadias, congenital subluxation of hip, low birth weight and prematurity.

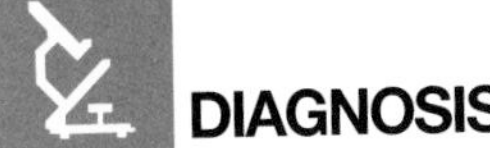

DIAGNOSIS

DIFFERENTIAL DIAGNOSIS
- Retractile testis (hypermobile testis): A normally descended testis that ascends into the inguinal canal because of an active cremasteric reflex
- Atrophic testis: May occur as a result of neonatal torsion

LABORATORY If bilateral nonpalpable undescended testes, check basal gonadotropin levels (FSH), if increased in boys < 9 years of age no further workup necessary to diagnose bilateral anorchia. If FSH not increased, HCG stimulation test to determine presence/absence of testicular tissue - HCG 2000 IU daily for 3 days and check testosterone pre- and post stimulation.

Drugs that may alter lab results: N/A

Disorders that may alter lab results: N/A

PATHOLOGICAL FINDINGS
- Higher incidence of carcinoma in undescended testis and alterations in spermatogenesis
- Histologic changes occur by 1.5 years of age and include smaller seminiferous tubules, fewer spermatogonia and more peritubular tissue

SPECIAL TESTS N/A

IMAGING Ultrasonography is able to detect testicles in the inguinal canal and pubic region in 70% of cases, but is only able to detect 20% of intra-abdominal testicles. CT scan findings in children are inconsistent.

DIAGNOSTIC PROCEDURES
- Physical exam
  - ◊ Performed with child in sitting, standing and squatting positions with warm hands
  - ◊ A Valsalva maneuver and applied pressure to lower abdomen may help identify the testes, especially a gliding testis
  - ◊ Failure to palpate a testis after repeated exams suggests an intra-abdominal or atrophic testis
  - ◊ An enlarged contralateral testis in the presence of a non-palpable testis suggests testicular atrophy/absence
  - ◊ Laparoscopy is useful in the child with impalpable cryptorchidism to accurately confirm testicular absence or presence and to determine the feasibility of performing a standard orchiopexy

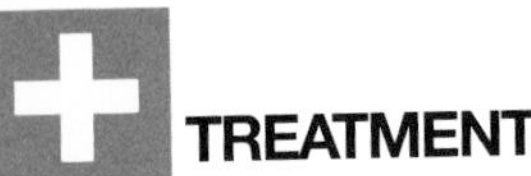

TREATMENT

APPROPRIATE HEALTH CARE
Outpatient until surgery performed

GENERAL MEASURES
- Rule out retractile testis
- Administration of chorionic gonadotropin - may cause testicular descent in some boys. Reports of efficacy are inconsistent.

SURGICAL MEASURES
- Reasons to consider: Avoids torsion, averts trauma, decreases but does not eliminate risk of malignancy, and prevents further alterations in spermatogenesis
- Orchiopexy should be performed by age 1. Alterations in germ cell count in the cryptorchid testis have been identified by age 2.

ACTIVITY No restrictions

DIET No special diet

PATIENT EDUCATION Discuss with parents about causes, available treatments, and possible effects on patient's reproductive potential; also increased risk for testicular cancer and need for self-examination

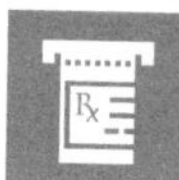

MEDICATIONS

DRUG(S) OF CHOICE The International Health Foundation recommendations for HCG therapy is biweekly injections of 250 IU for infants, 500 IU for children up to 6 years of age and 1000 IU for those 6 years of age and older, for a total of 5 weeks
Contraindications: Contraindicated in patients with a clinically apparent inguinal hernia, those with a history of previous ipsilateral groin surgery or in ectopic testicles. Also refer to manufacturer's literature.
Precautions: May induce precocious puberty - discontinue drug, effects should reverse in 4 weeks. Premature epiphyseal closure.
Significant possible interactions: Refer to manufacturer's literature

ALTERNATIVE DRUGS N/A

FOLLOWUP

PATIENT MONITORING
- Patients should be followed after surgery to evaluate testicular growth
- Testicular tumors occur mainly at puberty or after and thus these children should be taught self-examination when older

PREVENTION/AVOIDANCE No preventive measures known

POSSIBLE COMPLICATIONS
- Progressive failure of spermatogenesis, if left untreated. Even with orchiopexy, the fertility rate is still reduced, especially with bilateral undescended testicles. Spermatogenesis related to duration of cryptorchidism and the location of the testis. Abnormalities have also been identified in the contralateral descended testis, although less severe
- Higher risk (20-46 times) of testicular cancer (risk may remain despite orchiopexy)
- Hernia development (25%)

EXPECTED COURSE/PROGNOSIS
- Disorder usually corrected with medical or surgical therapy, however; possible lifelong consequences
- If testicle is absent or orchiectomy required, may consider placement of testicular prosthesis

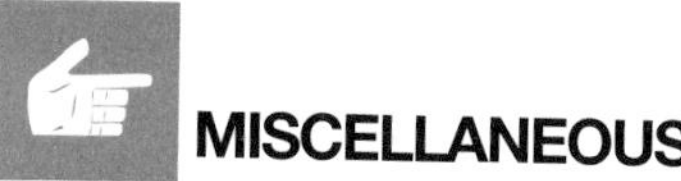

MISCELLANEOUS

ASSOCIATED CONDITIONS
- Inguinal hernia
- Hemiscrotum
- Hydrocele
- Abnormalities of vas deferens and epididymis
- Klinefelter syndrome
- Hypogonadotropic hypogonadism
- Germinal cell aplasia
- Mullerian inhibiting factor deficiency
- 5 alpha-reductase deficiency
- True hermaphrodite
- Prune belly syndrome
- Meningomyelocele
- Hypospadias
- Wilm tumor
- Kallmann syndrome
- Prader Willi syndrome
- Cystic fibrosis

AGE-RELATED FACTORS
Pediatric: This problem is usually detectable at birth or soon thereafter. If surgery is to be the treatment, it should be performed during the first year of life.
Geriatric: N/A
Others: Puberty: If unilateral cryptorchidism is discovered at or after puberty, usual treatment is orchiectomy

PREGNANCY N/A

SYNONYMS
- Undescended testes

ICD-9-CM
752.51 Undescended testis

SEE ALSO
Hydrocele
Meningomyelocele
Wilms tumor

OTHER NOTES N/A

ABBREVIATIONS
IU = international units

REFERENCES

- Leissner J, Filipas D, Wolf HK, Fisch M. The undescended testis: considerations and impact on fertility. BJU Int 1999;83(8):885-91
- Docimo SG, Silver RI, Cromie W. The undescended testicle: diagnosis and management. Am Fam Physician 2000;62(9):2037-44, 2047-8
- Callaghan P. Undescended testis. Pediatr Rev 2000;21(11):395
- Oh J, Landman J, Evers A, Yan Y, Kibel AS. Management of the postpubertal patient with cryptorchidism: an updated analysis. J Urol 2002;167(3):1329-33
- Cortes D, Thorup JM, Visfeldt J. Cryptorchidism: aspects of fertility and neoplasms. A study including data of 1,335 consecutive boys who underwent testicular biopsy simultaneously with surgery for cryptorchidism. Horm Res 2001;55(1):21-7
- Giannopoulos MF, Vlachakis IG, Charissis GC. 13 Years' experience with the combined hormonal therapy of cryptorchidism. Horm Res 2001;55(1):33-7
- Merguerian PA, Mevorach RA, et al. Laparoscopy for the evaluation and management of the nonpalpable testis. Urology 1998;51(5A suppl):3-6
- Cryptorchidism: a prospective study of 7500 consecutive male births, 1984-8. John Radcliffe Hospital Cryptorchidism Study Group. Arch Dis Child. 1992;67(7):892-9

Web references: 1 available at www.5mcc.com
Illustrations N/A

Author(s):
Pamela I. Ellsworth, MD
William A. Primack, MD

BASICS

DESCRIPTION Clinical abnormalities associated with chronic exposure to excessive amounts of cortisol (the major adrenocorticoid). The most frequent cause is prolonged use of exogenous glucocorticoids.
System(s) affected: Cardiovascular, Endocrine/Metabolic, Musculoskeletal, Skin/Exocrine
Genetics:
- Multiple endocrine neoplasia type I
- Carney complex

Incidence/Prevalence in USA: Uncommon
Predominant age: All ages
Predominant sex: Females > Males

SIGNS & SYMPTOMS
- Moon face (facial adiposity)
- Increased adipose tissue in neck and trunk
- Central weight gain
- Emotional lability
- Hypertension
- Osteoporosis
- Purple striae on the skin
- Diabetes or glucose intolerance with fasting hyperglycemia and/or glycosuria
- Muscle weakness due to loss of muscle mass from increased catabolism
- Skeletal growth retardation in children
- Easy bruising
- Hirsutism

CAUSES
- Exogenous glucocorticoids and/or ACTH
- Endogenous ACTH-dependent hypercortisolism
  - ◊ ACTH-secreting pituitary tumor
  - ◊ Ectopic ACTH production (e.g., small-cell carcinoma of lung, bronchial carcinoid)
- Endogenous ACTH-independent hypercortisolism
  - ◊ Adrenal adenoma
  - ◊ Adrenal carcinoma
  - ◊ Macro/micro nodular hyperplasia

RISK FACTORS
- Any medical problem requiring prolonged use of corticosteroids
- Pituitary tumor
- Adrenal mass
- Neuroendocrine tumor (e.g., bronchial carcinoid)

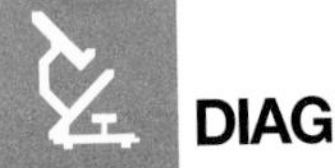

DIAGNOSIS

DIFFERENTIAL DIAGNOSIS
- Obesity, diabetes mellitus, hypertension
- Hypercortisolism secondary to alcoholism (pseudo-Cushing)

LABORATORY
- 24 hour urinary cortisol
- Plasma cortisol (am and pm)
- Plasma ACTH concentration
- Glycosuria (possible)
- Neutrophilia
- Lymphopenia
- Hyperglycemia
- Hyperlipidemia
- Hypokalemia
- Dynamic endocrine testing (e.g., dexamethasone suppression test)

Drugs that may alter lab results: Refer to lab test or drug reference

Disorders that may alter lab results: Refer to lab test reference

PATHOLOGICAL FINDINGS
- Hyalinization of basophilic cells (anterior pituitary) - Crooke's cell changes
- Muscular atrophy
- Nephrosclerosis
- Corticotroph pituitary tumor
- Ectopic ACTH-secreting tumor
- Adrenal adenoma or carcinoma
- Micro- or macronodular hyperplasia

SPECIAL TESTS If ACTH-dependent, inferior petrosal sinus sampling for ACTH

IMAGING
- Chest films
- X-rays of the lumbar spine - osteoporosis is common
- If pituitary tumor suspected - pituitary MRI scan
- If adrenal disease suspected - abdominal CT scan
- If ectopic ACTH-secretion suspected - chest CT scan

DIAGNOSTIC PROCEDURES Not all tests indicated for every case. Choice of diagnostic procedure dependent on circumstances and judgment.

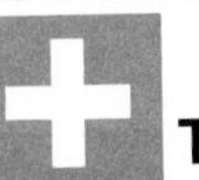

TREATMENT

APPROPRIATE HEALTH CARE Inpatient for surgical procedures

GENERAL MEASURES
- Depends on etiology. Surgery is the treatment of choice; persistent disease may require - radiation, drug therapy, or surgery
- Medical treatment with adrenocortical inhibitors
  - ◊ Has not been too successful
  - ◊ Should be used when other methods fail
  - ◊ In consultation with a clinician having experience in their use

SURGICAL MEASURES
- Primary hypersecretion of ACTH
  - ◊ Transsphenoidal microsurgery. Bilateral adrenalectomy as an adjunct for patients not cured.
- Adrenocortical tumors
  - ◊ Surgical removal when possible
  - ◊ If adrenocortical carcinoma, prognosis is poor
- Ectopic ACTH production
  - ◊ Removal of the neoplastic tissue
  - ◊ Metastatic spread makes surgical cure unlikely/impossible
  - ◊ Bilateral adrenalectomy

ACTIVITY Determined by patient's symptoms and form of treatment used

DIET
- Potassium supplements
- High protein diet

PATIENT EDUCATION
- National Adrenal Disease Foundation (NADF), 505 Northern Blvd, Great Neck, NY 11021; 516-407-4992; e-mail: nadf@aol.com
- Instructions on drug therapy, diet, activity
- Early treatment of infections
- Monitor weight daily
- Emotional lability prevention

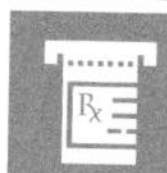

MEDICATIONS

DRUG(S) OF CHOICE
- Medications in treatment should be used in consultation with an endocrinologist
- Adjunctive management considerations
  - ◊ Inhibit cortisol production - ketoconazole 400-600 mg twice daily (dosages higher than conventionally recommended)
  - ◊ Glucocorticoid replacement following pituitary surgery. In most cases, can be discontinued by 3-12 months.

Contraindications: Refer to manufacturer's literature

Precautions: Refer to manufacturer's literature

Significant possible interactions: Refer to manufacturer's literature

ALTERNATIVE DRUGS
- Mitotane
- Aminoglutethimide
- Metyrapone

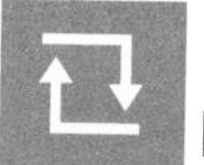

FOLLOWUP

PATIENT MONITORING
- Individualize depending on therapy
- Check regularly for signs of adrenal hypofunction

PREVENTION/AVOIDANCE
- Avoid excessive corticosteroid treatment when possible
- Comprehensive teaching to help patient cope with lifelong treatment (if needed)

POSSIBLE COMPLICATIONS
- Osteoporosis
- Increased susceptibility to infections
- Hirsutism
- Metastases of malignant tumors

EXPECTED COURSE/PROGNOSIS
- Usual course - chronic with cyclic exacerbations and rare remissions
- Guardedly favorable prognosis with surgery

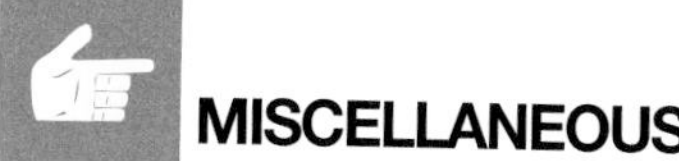

MISCELLANEOUS

ASSOCIATED CONDITIONS Tumors of the pituitary; multiple endocrine neoplasia Type I, Carney complex

AGE-RELATED FACTORS
Pediatric: Rare in infancy and childhood. Most cases (under age 8) are due to malignant adrenal tumors.

Geriatric: N/A

Others: N/A

PREGNANCY Can cause exacerbation of Cushing disease

SYNONYMS N/A

ICD-9-CM
255.0 Cushing syndrome

SEE ALSO

OTHER NOTES Pituitary ACTH excess due to a pituitary tumor causes what is called Cushing disease

ABBREVIATIONS
CRH = corticotropin releasing hormone

REFERENCES

- Kaye TB, Crapo L: The Cushing syndrome. An update in diagnostic tests. Ann Intern Med 1990;112:434
- Flack MR, Oldfield EH, Cutle GB Jr, et al: Urine free cortisol in the high dose dexamethasone suppression test for the differential diagnosis of the Cushing syndrome. Ann Intern Med 1992;116:211
- Miller JW, Crapo L: The medical treatment of Cushing's syndrome. Endocrine Reviews 1993;14:443
- Young WF Jr: Cushing's syndrome. In: Rakel RE, ed. Conn's Current Therapy. New York, NY, W.B. Saunders Co., 2002

Web references: 1 available at www.5mcc.com

Illustrations 4 available

Author(s):
William F. Young, Jr, MD

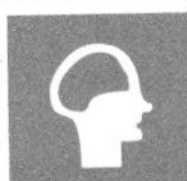

BASICS

DESCRIPTION Cutaneous or mucocutaneous eruptions are the most common adverse reactions to oral or parenteral drug therapy. Reactions may be immunologically mediated (either IgE dependent or immune complex dependent).
- Non-immunologic reactions occur more commonly. The majority of reactions occur within one week of initiation of drug therapy but make occur up to 4 weeks after initiation of therapy.
- Maculopapular and urticarial eruptions are the most common but multiple morphologic types of reactions may occur

System(s) affected: Hemic/Lymphatic/Immunologic, Skin/Exocrine
Genetics: No known genetic inheritance pattern
Incidence/Prevalence in USA:
- Three reactions per 1000 drug courses
- Approximately 120 million inpatient drug courses annually in the USA, therefore approximately 144/100,000
- Approximately 125 million Americans regularly use prescription drugs as outpatients; overall prevalence in this group is unknown

Predominant age: All ages affected
Predominant sex: Female > Male (specific ratio unknown)

SIGNS & SYMPTOMS
(note: in order of frequency)
- Maculopapular eruptions (exanthems):
  - ◊ Most frequent cutaneous reaction
  - ◊ Maybe indistinguishable from viral exanthem
  - ◊ Erythematous macules and papules
  - ◊ Often confluent and symmetrical
  - ◊ Pruritus common
  - ◊ Mucous membranes, palms and soles may be involved
  - ◊ Onset typically 7-21 (average 10) days after initiation of drug
- Urticaria:
  - ◊ Pruritic red wheals distributed anywhere on the body including mucous membranes
  - ◊ Individual lesions fade within 24 hours but new urticaria may develop
  - ◊ May be mediated by anaphylactic or accelerated IgE reactions, serum sickness or non-immunologic histamine reactions
  - ◊ Deep dermal and subcutaneous swelling constitute angioedema and when mucous membranes are involved, may be life-threatening
- Acneform eruptions
  - ◊ Pustular lesions but unlike true acne, no comedones
- Eczematous reactions
  - ◊ Pruritic scale-like erythematous lesions typically on flexor surfaces of arms or legs
- Erythema multiforme
  - ◊ Target lesions
  - ◊ Bullous lesions
  - ◊ Mucous membrane involvement (Stevens-Johnson syndrome)
- Exfoliative erythroderma
  - ◊ Generalized erythema and scaling
  - ◊ Potentially life-threatening
- Fixed drug eruptions
  - ◊ Single or multiple round sharply defined dark red plaques
  - ◊ Appear shortly after drug exposure and reappear in the same location after drug ingestion. Lesions can occur anywhere: glans penis common in men (especially with tetracycline)
  - ◊ Onset usually 2 hours after ingestion of drug
  - ◊ Some patients have a refractory period during which the drug fails to activate lesions
- Lichen planus like eruptions
  - ◊ Violaceous papules extensor wrist surfaces
  - ◊ Reticular pattern, buccal mucosa
- Lupus erythematosus-like reactions
  - ◊ Malar erythema
- Photosensitivity reaction
  - ◊ Phototoxic reactions within 24 hours of light exposure
  - ◊ Photoallergic reactions; less common
- Vasculitis
  - ◊ Petechiae or purpura concentrated on lower legs
- Vesiculobullous eruptions
  - ◊ Small isolated bullae, erythema multiforme, toxic epidermal necrolysis (potentially fatal)

CAUSES
- Acneform: OCP's, corticosteroids, iodinated compounds, hydantoins, lithium
- Erythema multiforme: sulfonamides, penicillins, barbiturates, hydantoins, NSAIDs, tetracycline, cefaclor, terbinafine
- Erythema nodosum: OCP's, sulfonamides, penicillins
- Fixed drug eruptions: OCP's, barbiturates, salicylates barbiturates, tetracycline, sulfonamides, sulfonylureas
- Lichenoid: gold, antimalarials, tetracycline
- Photosensitivity: phenothiazines, griseofulvin, sulfonamides, tetracycline
- Vasculitis: thiazides, gold, sulfonamides, NSAIDs, tetracycline
- Bullous: NSAIDs, thiazides, barbiturates, captopril
- Skin necrosis: warfarin

RISK FACTORS Drug therapy, especially with sulfonamides, penicillins

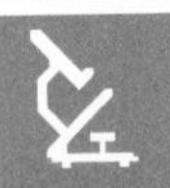

DIAGNOSIS

DIFFERENTIAL DIAGNOSIS
- Viral exanthem: since maculopapular eruptions are the most common form of drug reaction these are often difficult to distinguish from viral exanthems. Presence of fever, lymphocytosis, and other systemic findings may help differentiate.
- Drug eruptions manifest as many types of dermatosis as previously listed; consider a primary dermatosis in the differential diagnosis. Resolution of the eruption upon withdrawal of a drug will help to clarify. The histopathology of skin biopsy can also be helpful in persistent cases.
- Skin reactions in young children - may be due to the dye in the liquid antibiotic

LABORATORY
- Routine laboratory tests generally nonspecific and usually not helpful
- Eosinophilia: Possible in certain allergic reactions but generally of little value clinically

Drugs that may alter lab results: Procainamide, hydralazine - positive ANA

Disorders that may alter lab results: N/A

PATHOLOGICAL FINDINGS
- Pathological findings dependent upon type of reaction; may be nonspecific
- Punch biopsy sometimes helpful for fixed drug eruptions which show certain characteristic histological features, e.g., lichen planus-like or erythema multiforme

SPECIAL TESTS
- Skin testing (useful in IgE mediated reactions)
- IgG and IgM: hemagglutination assays can detect drug-specific antibodies, but not routinely useful

IMAGING N/A

DIAGNOSTIC PROCEDURES
- Detailed drug-use history including all OTC medicines, duration of therapy, medications used within the last four weeks
- Withdrawal of suspected offending agent and observation for resolution of rash
- Selective special testing for suspected IgE mediated reactions

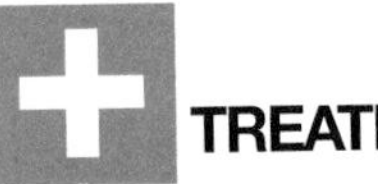

TREATMENT

APPROPRIATE HEALTH CARE
- Urticaria, angioedema, or bullous lesions are all potentially more serious than other types of reactions therefore these patients should be seen as soon as possible for evaluation
- Consider inpatient treatment for anaphylactic reactions, Stevens-Johnson syndrome, extensive bullous reactions, or toxic epidermal (TEN) necrolysis

GENERAL MEASURES
- Discontinue suspected offending agent. In patients with multiple medications, the decision to discontinue each medication should be based on the likelihood of each individual medication causing the reaction (e.g., 7% for penicillins, sulfonamides) and the risk/benefit ratio of continuing each medication.
- Re-challenge with specific medications thought to have caused urticaria, angioedema, anaphylaxis, erythema multiforme, or other bullous lesions is potentially dangerous

SURGICAL MEASURES N/A

ACTIVITY
- No specific restrictions in general
- For acute eczematous or urticarial reactions with intense pruritus, tepid bathing and avoidance of activities resulting in perspiration may be helpful
- For toxic epidermal necrolysis, admit to burn unit

DIET No dietary restrictions

PATIENT EDUCATION Printed patient information is available from American Academy of Dermatology, 930 N. Meacham Rd., P.O. Box 4014, Schaumberg, IL 60168-4014; (708)330-0230

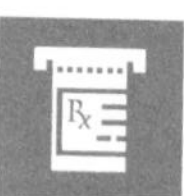

MEDICATIONS

DRUG(S) OF CHOICE
- Specific therapy depends on the type of drug eruption. Most require no specific therapy.
- Symptomatic therapy helpful for pruritus, xeroses, urticaria and angioedema
- For pruritus - antihistamines, e.g., diphenhydramine (Benadryl) 25-50 mg q6h, hydroxyzine (Atarax) 10-25 mg q6-8h)
- Anaphylaxis or widespread urticaria - epinephrine 1:1000, 0.01 mL per kilogram (0.3 mL maximum) subcutaneous
- For anaphylaxis, severe urticaria, erythema multiforme - corticosteroids parenterally as indicated by patient's condition; or on tapering po schedule (10-14 days). Therapy of toxic epidermal necrolysis controversial; majority do not favor use of systemic corticosteroids; intravenous IgG therapy can be life saving.
- Topical lubricants, emollients for eczematous reactions
- Topical corticosteroids (Group I-III) for limited eczematous type eruptions, or for lichenoid eruptions
- Systemic corticosteroids (for urticaria, angioedema, and anaphylaxis) - prednisone 40-60 mg/d for 5-10 days. Also useful in severe diffuse eczematous reactions.

Contraindications: Refer to manufacturer's information
Precautions: Refer to manufacturer's information
Significant possible interactions: Refer to manufacturer's information

ALTERNATIVE DRUGS N/A

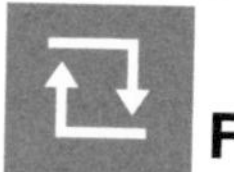

FOLLOWUP

PATIENT MONITORING
- For urticarial, bullous, or erythema multiforme-like lesions, close patient followup is indicated to insure there is no progression
- Patients with systemic anaphylaxis or wide spread bullous lesions, including toxic epidermal necrolysis, should be admitted to hospital until condition improves
- Maintain at least telephone follow-up until eruption has completely cleared
- Label patient's chart with the suspected agent and the specific type of reaction

PREVENTION/AVOIDANCE
- Future avoidance of specific drugs and any analogs
- Be aware of any potential cross over reactions (i.e., 8-10% incidence of reactions of cephalosporins in patients sensitized to penicillins and the cross-over for the anticonvulsive drugs hydantoin, barbiturates, and carbamazepine [Tegretol])
- Always question patients about prior drug reactions, specific type of reaction, and use of OTC medicines

POSSIBLE COMPLICATIONS
- Anaphylaxis
- Laryngeal edema
- Possible associated bone marrow suppression
- Hepatitis and hematologic changes (dapsone, hydantoin)
- Possible cross reaction to chemically similar agents with future exposure

EXPECTED COURSE/PROGNOSIS
- Eruptions generally fade within days after removing offending agent
- Urticaria, angioedema, bullous reactions, are potentially more serious, even life-threatening

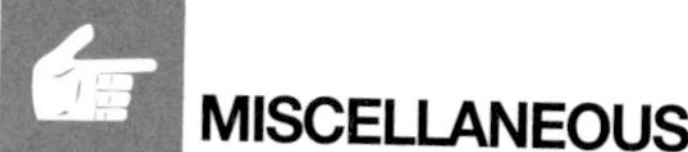

MISCELLANEOUS

ASSOCIATED CONDITIONS N/A

AGE-RELATED FACTORS
Pediatric: May occur in this age group
Geriatric:
- Possibly more likely in this age group due to greater number of medications
- Severe systemic reactions less well tolerated

Others: N/A

PREGNANCY N/A

SYNONYMS
- Drug eruptions
- Dermatitis medicamentosa

ICD-9-CM
693.0 Dermatitis due to drugs or medicines taken internally

SEE ALSO

OTHER NOTES N/A

ABBREVIATIONS
TEN = toxic epidermal necrolysis

REFERENCES

- Habif T. Clinical Dermatology. 4th ed. St. Louis: CV Mosby; 2004
- Lazarou J, et al. Incidence of adverse drug reactions in hospitalized patients. JAMA 1998;279:1200-05
- Daoud MS, et al. Recognizing cutaneous drug eruptions. Post Grad Med 1998;104(1):101-15
- Roujeau JC. Treatment of severe drug eruptions. J Dermatol 1999;26(11):718-22
- Heller HM. Adverse cutaneous drug reactions in patients with human immunodeficiency virus-1 infection. Clin Dermatol 2000;18(4):485-9
- Bigby M. Rates of cutaneous reactions to drugs. Arch Dermatol 2001;137(6):765-70
- Yates AB, deShazo RD. Allergic and nonallergic drug reactions. South Med J 2003;96(11):1080-7

Web references: 0 available at www.5mcc.com
Illustrations 37 available

Author(s):
J. Randall Richard, MD

Cutaneous squamous cell carcinoma

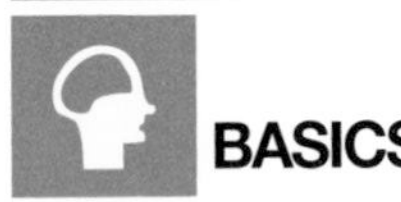

BASICS

DESCRIPTION Malignant epithelial tumor arising from keratinocytes
System(s) affected: Skin/Exocrine
Genetics: N/A
Incidence/Prevalence in USA: Varies within geographic U.S. From 30/100,000 for white males in Detroit to 154/100,000 for white males in New Orleans
Predominant age: Elderly population
Predominant sex: Male > Female

SIGNS & SYMPTOMS
- Occurs most commonly in chronically sun-exposed areas in light-skinned people e.g., scalp, neck, upper extremities, back of hands, superior surface of pinna
- Often develops in previously damaged skin, e.g., solar keratoses, actinic cheilitis
- In African Americans - equal frequency in sun-exposed and unexposed
- Tumors present often as small, firm nodules with indistinct margins or as plaques
- Surface may be smooth, verrucous or papillomatous
- Varying degrees of ulceration, erosion, crust, scale
- Color often red to red-brown to tan
- May appear white in areas of moisture
- May arise in chronic skin ulcers, e.g., venous stasis ulcers
- May arise in scars
- Can arise in skin damaged by radiation, x-rays, etc.
- Varies from slowly growing, locally invasive to aggressive tumor with propensity to metastasis
- On lip, often arises in patch of leukoplakia

CAUSES
- Exact mechanism not established, epidemiologic and experimental evidence suggests the following as causative agents
- Sunlight (solar radiation)
- Radiation exposure
- Inorganic arsenic exposure
- Exposure to coal tar, other oil and tar derivatives
- Immunosuppression by medications or disease

RISK FACTORS
- Older age - risk may be ten times higher in the elderly
- Male - 2-3 times the risk for females
- Sunlight exposure
- Irish-Scottish-British descent
- Fair complexion, fair hair
- Light blue or green eyes
- Poor tanning ability with tendency to burn

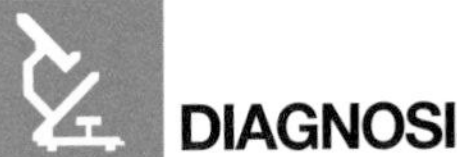

DIAGNOSIS

DIFFERENTIAL DIAGNOSIS Keratoacanthoma, basal cell carcinoma, actinic keratosis, malignant melanoma

LABORATORY Requires biopsy for precise pathologic diagnosis

Drugs that may alter lab results: N/A

Disorders that may alter lab results: N/A

PATHOLOGICAL FINDINGS Abnormal epithelial cells extending into the dermis from the epidermis. Varying degrees of atypical appearance can be noted.

SPECIAL TESTS N/A

IMAGING N/A

DIAGNOSTIC PROCEDURES Surgical biopsy mandatory to ensure proper and precise diagnosis

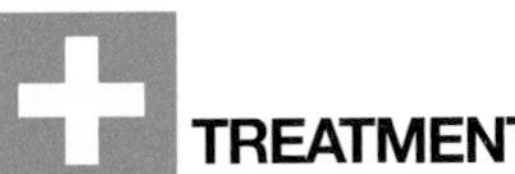

TREATMENT

APPROPRIATE HEALTH CARE All outpatient unless extensive lesion

GENERAL MEASURES N/A

SURGICAL MEASURES
- Excisional surgery - appropriate for almost all squamous cell lesions
- Electrodesiccation and curettage - used for small lesions (generally < 1.0 cm) on flat surfaces, e.g., forehead, cheek. Requires training and expertise in electrosurgery.
- Indications for Moh's micrographic surgery include: Recurrent tumor; larger, ill-defined lesions; presence of bone or cartilage invasion; multiple carcinomas; lesion in area of late radiation change. Requires referral to appropriately trained dermatologic surgeon.
- Radiation therapy - suitable for larger advanced lesions. Requires specialized training.

ACTIVITY Full activity

DIET No restrictions

PATIENT EDUCATION
- Instruct patient in skin self exam
- Appropriate sun avoidance measures, e.g., sunscreens, protective clothing
- Patient education materials available from American Cancer Society

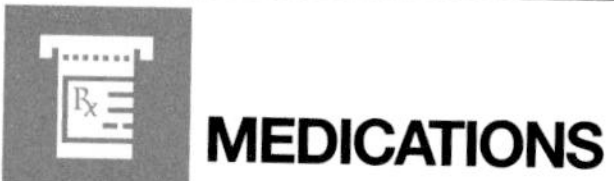

MEDICATIONS

DRUG(S) OF CHOICE N/A
Contraindications: N/A
Precautions: N/A
Significant possible interactions: N/A

ALTERNATIVE DRUGS N/A

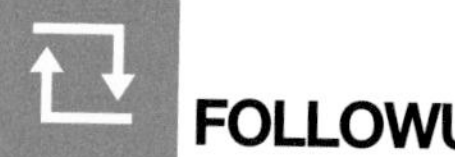

FOLLOWUP

PATIENT MONITORING After therapy, skin exam every month for 3 months, 6 months post-treatment, then yearly

PREVENTION/AVOIDANCE
- Sun-avoidance measures - sunscreens, hats, etc.
- Avoid contact with known carcinogenic compounds

POSSIBLE COMPLICATIONS
- Recurrence locally
- Metastatic disease

EXPECTED COURSE/PROGNOSIS
- About 90-95% cure rate with appropriate treatment
- Lesion equal to or greater than 2 cm more prone to recur
- Head and neck lesions have better prognosis

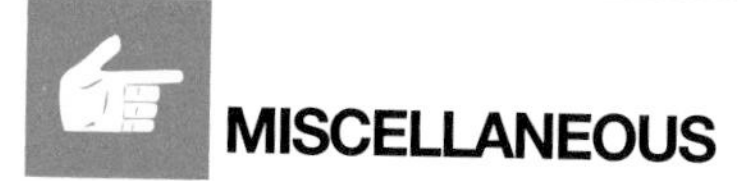

MISCELLANEOUS

ASSOCIATED CONDITIONS
- Xeroderma pigmentosum
- Albinism
- Chronic skin ulcers of the leg
- Chronic thermal burns
- Actinic keratosis (cutaneous horn)
- Bowen disease

AGE-RELATED FACTORS
Pediatric: N/A
Geriatric: N/A
Others: N/A

PREGNANCY N/A

SYNONYMS
- Squamous cell carcinoma of the skin
- Epidermoid carcinoma
- Prickle cell carcinoma

ICD-9-CM
173.3 Other malignant neoplasm of skin of other and unspecified parts of face
173.4 Other malignant neoplasm of scalp and skin of neck
173.5 Other malignant neoplasm of skin of trunk, except scrotum
173.6 Other malignant neoplasm of skin of upper limb, including shoulder
173.7 Other malignant neoplasm of skin of lower limb, including hip
173.9 Other malignant neoplasm of skin, site unspecified

SEE ALSO

OTHER NOTES N/A

ABBREVIATIONS N/A

REFERENCES

- Fitzpatrick TN, et al: Dermatology in General Medicine. New York, McGraw-Hill Book Company, 1999
- Friedman RJ, et al: Cancer of the Skin. Philadelphia, WB Saunders Co, 1991
- Alam M, Ratner D. Cutaneous squamous cell carcinoma. N Engl J Med. 2001;344(13):975-83

Web references: 1 available at www.5mcc.com
Illustrations 4 available

Author(s):
Tim DeBlieck, MD

Cutaneous T cell lymphoma

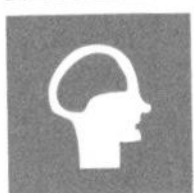

BASICS

DESCRIPTION Cutaneous T cell lymphoma (mycosis fungoides) is an uncommon chronic lymphoma characterized by a malignant proliferation of T helper cells in the skin. In the late stage, the lymph nodes and viscera are affected.
System(s) affected: Hemic/Lymphatic/Immunologic, Skin/Exocrine
Genetics: Evidence suggests increased frequency of HLA antigens Aw31 and Aw32
Incidence/Prevalence in USA: 0.29 cases per 100,000 per year
Predominant age: Most cases occur in fifth and sixth decades, incidence increases with age
Predominant sex: Male > Female

SIGNS & SYMPTOMS
- Skin eruption
  - ◊ Patches (eczema-like rash)
  - ◊ Plaques
  - ◊ Tumors
  - ◊ Pruritus
  - ◊ Exfoliative erythroderma
  - ◊ Ulcers of the skin
- Lymphadenopathy
- Hepatomegaly (late)
- Splenomegaly (late)
- Central nervous system (late)

CAUSES Unknown

RISK FACTORS
- HTLV-I
- Exposure to petrochemicals, metals and solvents
- Association with lymphomatoid papulosis

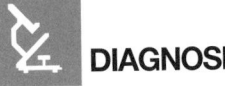

DIAGNOSIS

DIFFERENTIAL DIAGNOSIS
- Patches:
  - ◊ Parapsoriasis
  - ◊ Atopic eczema
  - ◊ Nummular eczema
- Plaques:
  - ◊ Parapsoriasis
  - ◊ Psoriasis
- Tumors:
  - ◊ Other primary skin cancers
  - ◊ Internal malignancies metastatic to skin
  - ◊ Histiocytosis X
- Exfoliative erythroderma:
  - ◊ Psoriasis
  - ◊ Atopic dermatitis
  - ◊ Drug eruption

LABORATORY
- CBC with differential and platelets
- Total lymphocyte count
- Automated chemical profile

Drugs that may alter lab results: N/A

Disorders that may alter lab results: N/A

PATHOLOGICAL FINDINGS
- Skin biopsy:
  - ◊ Epidermotropism of lymphocytes
  - ◊ Sentinel lymphocytes in epidermis
  - ◊ Pautrier's microabscesses of lymphocytes
  - ◊ Widened, fibrotic papillary dermis
  - ◊ Superficial band-like dermal infiltrate
  - ◊ Occasionally granulomatous component

SPECIAL TESTS
- Sézary cell preparation
- Electron microscopy
- HTLV-I serology
- Enzyme histochemistry
- DNA flow cytometry
- Immunophenotyping
- Immunogenotyping
- Molecular cytogenetics
- Polymerase chain reaction

IMAGING
- Chest x-ray
- CT scan of abdomen

DIAGNOSTIC PROCEDURES
- Skin biopsy - diagnostic procedure of choice
- Lymph node biopsy
- Bone marrow biopsy
- Liver biopsy

TREATMENT

APPROPRIATE HEALTH CARE The majority of patients can be managed on an outpatient basis

GENERAL MEASURES
- No disease-specific special measures
- Treatment should be individualized for each patient as in most cases this is a chronic slowly progressive disease.

SURGICAL MEASURES N/A

ACTIVITY Fully active

DIET No special diet

PATIENT EDUCATION
- By physician on individual basis
- Mycosis Fungoides Foundation, PO Box 374, Birmingham, MI 48012-0374; 248-644-9014; web site mffoundation.org

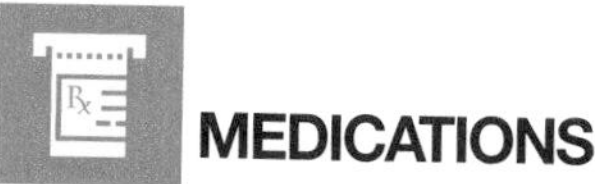

MEDICATIONS

DRUG(S) OF CHOICE

- Therapy must be individualized. There is no universally accepted standard approach to treatment of this disease. The extent and the rapidity of progression of the disease (stage of disease) dictates the aggressiveness of therapy.
- For early and less aggressive disease:
  - ◊ Topical potent corticosteroids
  - ◊ Topical mechlorethamine (nitrogen mustard, Mustargen)
  - ◊ PUVA or RePUVA (retinoids plus PUVA)
  - ◊ Topical carmustine (BCNU)
- For more resistant disease:
  - ◊ Electron beam therapy
  - ◊ Combination therapy - interferon or retinoids plus phototherapy (UVA or UVB)
  - ◊ Methotrexate
  - ◊ Extracorporeal photochemotherapy (especially Sézary syndrome)
- For advanced and resistant disease:
  - ◊ Systemic chemotherapy
  - ◊ Interleukin-2
- Bexarotene (Targretin)
- Topical mechlorethamine (nitrogen mustard, Mustargen) for early disease, in aqueous or ointment preparation applied once daily to entire skin surface avoiding genitalia

Contraindications: See manufacturer's profile of each drug

Precautions:

- Delayed hypersensitivity occurs in 50%
- Radiomimetic - patients should practice prudent sun avoidance
- Maintenance treatment required after clearing

Significant possible interactions: See manufacturer's profile of each drug

ALTERNATIVE DRUGS

- Narrow band or broad band UVB
- PUVA (psoralen and ultraviolet A light)
- Topical carmustine (BCNU)
- Total body electron beam therapy
- Localized orthovoltage x-ray therapy
- Interferon
- Retinoids (e.g., etretinate)
- Extracorporeal photochemotherapy
- Denileukin diftitox (Ontak)
- Purine analogues (deoxycoformycin, fludarabine, and 2-chlorodeoxyadenosine)
- Bone marrow transplantation

FOLLOWUP

PATIENT MONITORING Must be individualized

PREVENTION/AVOIDANCE N/A

POSSIBLE COMPLICATIONS Metastatic spread to organs other than skin

EXPECTED COURSE/PROGNOSIS

- The development of lymphadenopathy, tumors or cutaneous ulcerations during the course of the disease is associated with a median survival of 4 years
- The appearance of the third sign (irrespective of the order developed) is associated with a median survival of 1 year

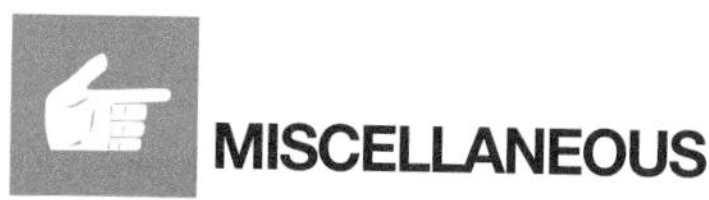

MISCELLANEOUS

ASSOCIATED CONDITIONS N/A

AGE-RELATED FACTORS

Pediatric: N/A
Geriatric: N/A
Others: N/A

PREGNANCY N/A

SYNONYMS

- Mycosis fungoides
- Sézary syndrome

ICD-9-CM

202.80 Other malignant lymphomas, unspecified site, extranodal and solid organ sites

SEE ALSO

HIV infection & AIDS

OTHER NOTES Sézary syndrome is the leukemic variant of cutaneous T cell lymphoma. Characteristics include erythroderma, pruritus, adenopathy and circulating atypical cells with cerebriform nuclei.

ABBREVIATIONS

HTLV = Human T-lymphotropic virus

REFERENCES

- Kempf W, Kettelhack N, Duvic M, Burg G. Topical and systemic retinoid therapy for cutaneous T-cell lymphoma. Hematol Oncol Clin North Am 2003;17(6):1405-19
- Rook AH, Kuzel TM, Olsen EA. Cytokine therapy of cutaneous T-cell lymphoma: interferons, interleukin-12, and interleukin-2. Hematol Oncol Clin North Am 2003;17(6):1435-48
- Seo N, Furukawa F, Tokura Y, Takigawa M. Vaccine therapy for cutaneous T-cell lymphoma. Hematol Oncol Clin North Am 2003;17(6):1467-74
- Oyama Y, Guitart J, Kuzel TM, Burt RK, Rosen ST. High-dose therapy and bone marrow transplantation in cutaneous T-cell lymphoma. Hematol Oncol Clin North Am 2003;17(6):1475-83
- Brecher A. Mycosis fungoides. Dermatol Online J 2003;9(4):23
- Nguyen NQ. Subcutaneous T-cell lymphoma. Dermatol Online J 2003;9(4):4
- Wollina U, Dummer R, Brockmeyer NH, Konrad H, Busch JO, Kaatz M, et al. Multicenter study of pegylated liposomal doxorubicin in patients with cutaneous T-cell lymphoma. Cancer 2003;98(5):993-1001
- Herbert CR, McBurney EI. Cutaneous T-cell lymphoma in a patient with neurofibromatosis type 1. Cutis 2003;72(1):27-30
- McGinnis KS, Shapiro M, Vittorio CC, Rook AH, Junkins-Hopkins JM. Psoralen plus long-wave UV-A (PUVA) and bexarotene therapy: An effective and synergistic combined adjunct to therapy for patients with advanced cutaneous T-cell lymphoma. Arch Dermatol 2003;139(6):771-5
- Demierre MF, Vachon L, Ho V, Sutton L, Cato A, Leyland-Jones B. Phase 1/2 pilot study of methotrexate-laurocapram topical gel for the treatment of patients with early-stage mycosis fungoides. Arch Dermatol 2003;139(5):624-8
- Kim YH, Martinez G, Varghese A, Hoppe RT. Topical nitrogen mustard in the management of mycosis fungoides: update of the Stanford experience. Arch Dermatol 2003;139(2):165-73
- Guitart J, Wickless SC, Oyama Y, Kuzel TM, Rosen ST, Traynor A, Burt R. Long-term remission after allogeneic hematopoietic stem cell transplantation for refractory cutaneous T-cell lymphoma. Arch Dermatol 2002;138(10):1359-65
- Muche JM, Sterry W. Vaccination therapy for cutaneous T-cell lymphoma. Clin Exp Dermatol 2002;27(7):602-7
- Suchin KR, Junkins-Hopkins JM, Rook AH. Treatment of stage IA cutaneous T-Cell lymphoma with topical application of the immune response modifier imiquimod. Arch Dermatol 2002;138(9):1137-9
- Leman JA, Dick DC, Morton CA. Topical 5-ALA photodynamic therapy for the treatment of cutaneous T-cell lymphoma. Clin Exp Dermatol 2002;27(6):516-8
- Suchin KR, Cucchiara AJ, Gottleib SL, Wolfe JT, DeNardo BJ, et al. Treatment of cutaneous T-cell lymphoma with combined immunomodulatory therapy: a 14-year experience at a single institution. Arch Dermatol 2002;138(8):1054-60
- Sarris AH, Phan A, Duvic M, Romaguera J, McLaughlin P, Mesina O, et al. Trimetrexate in relapsed T-cell lymphoma with skin involvement. J Clin Oncol 2002;20(12):2876-80

Web references: 0 available at www.5mcc.com
Illustrations 6 available

Author(s):

Vera Y. Soong, MD

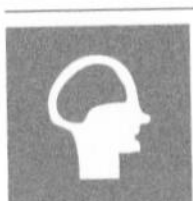

BASICS

DESCRIPTION Generalized, autosomal recessive disorder of infants, children and young adults with widespread dysfunction of the exocrine glands. Characteristics include chronic pulmonary disease, pancreatic insufficiency, abnormally high levels of electrolytes in the sweat, pansinusitis, digital clubbing and less frequently biliary cirrhosis, diabetes mellitus.
System(s) affected: Endocrine/Metabolic, Gastrointestinal, Pulmonary, Reproductive
Genetics: Autosomal recessive mutation of gene on chromosome 7. Linkage detection in families with known disease. Probes for direct detection available.
Incidence/Prevalence in USA: The most common lethal genetic disease. Caucasians: 1 in 2500 births, 1 in 17,000 African-Americans, and low in Native Americans and Asians.
Predominant age: Infants, children and young adults (oldest patient at time of diagnosis was 65)
Predominant sex: Male = Female

SIGNS & SYMPTOMS
- Sweat gland secretions:
  - ◊ Increased concentrations of sodium, potassium and chloride leading to hyponatremia, hypochloremia, metabolic alkalosis, arrhythmias
  - ◊ Dehydration with heat and infections
- Respiratory:
  - ◊ Wheezing, chronic cough, dyspnea, barrel chest, tachypnea
  - ◊ Cyanosis, digital clubbing
  - ◊ Nasal polyposis, pansinusitis
  - ◊ Recurrent bronchitis and pneumonia leading to bronchiectasis
  - ◊ Predominant flora - *Staphylococcus aureus* and *Pseudomonas aeruginosa*. *Burkholderia cepacia* carries a poorer prognosis.
- Gastrointestinal:
  - ◊ Characteristically frequent, bulky, foul - smelling, pale stool with a high fat content due to fat malabsorption
  - ◊ Failure to thrive
  - ◊ Meconium ileus in newborns
  - ◊ Distal intestinal obstruction syndrome (DIOS)
  - ◊ Colonic strictures possible with high-dose enzyme replacement (>15,000 U lipase /kg/day)
  - ◊ Chronic, recurrent abdominal pain
  - ◊ Gastroesophageal reflux
  - ◊ Voracious appetite prior to treatment
  - ◊ Abdominal distension
  - ◊ Hypoelectrolytemia and alkalosis
  - ◊ Vitamin deficiencies (A,D,E,K)
  - ◊ Rectal prolapse
- Others:
  - ◊ Delayed weight gain during growth and development
  - ◊ Retarded bone growth
  - ◊ Delayed sexual development
  - ◊ Males ≈95% infertile
  - ◊ Decreased female fertility

CAUSES Autosomal recessive genetic defect

RISK FACTORS Positive family history (rarely seen due to recessive nature)

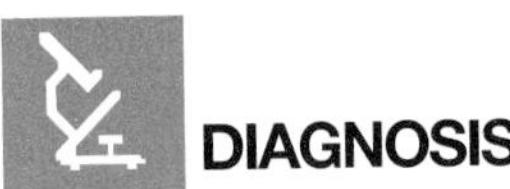

DIAGNOSIS

DIFFERENTIAL DIAGNOSIS
- Immunodeficiency
- Recurrent pneumonias
- Bronchiectasis
- Infertility
- Dyskinetic cilia
- Asthma

LABORATORY
- Elevation of sodium and chloride concentrations in sweat (quantitative pilocarpine iontophoresis sweat test)
- Genetic screening if sweat test inadequate (see Special Tests below)
- Stool trypsin and chymotrypsin absent or diminished
- 72 hour fecal fat excretion - increased fat in stool
- Decreased albumin, fat soluble vitamin levels
- CF gene probe (reference lab)
- Mucoid *Pseudomonas* in respiratory secretions. Also *S. aureus*.

Drugs that may alter lab results: Systemic steroids

Disorders that may alter lab results:
- Edema
- Hypoproteinemia
- Inadequate quantities of sweat to study
- Adrenal insufficiency

PATHOLOGICAL FINDINGS
- Lungs (major problem) - chronic inflammation, inspissated mucus, bronchiectasis with areas of fibrosis and atelectasis
- Pancreas - obstructed ducts, acini replaced by fibrotic tissue, cysts, amorphous eosinophilic concretions and thick mucus
- Liver - secretions obstruct biliary ducts; fatty infiltration; focal biliary cirrhosis
- Intestine - hypertrophied mucous glands
- Males - hypoplasia or atrophy of vas deferens

SPECIAL TESTS
- Pulmonary function studies (3-4 times a year)
- Sputum culture and sensitivity yearly or more frequently
- Atypical mycobacterium smear and culture (surveillance and before starting azithromycin [Zithromax] protocol)
- Exercise testing
- Response to bronchodilators - may show paradoxical drop
- In newborns - serum concentration of immunoreactive trypsin elevated, and can be used in newborn screening. Radioimmunoassay developed for use with dried blood spots that are routinely collected for newborn metabolic screening.
- Genetic testing to identify patient defect and analyze family for carrier status or prenatal diagnosis
- Echocardiogram
- Hearing testing if aminoglycosides given
- Careful monitoring of nutritional status; skin-fold thickness annually
- Aggressive monitoring of glucose metabolism
- INR and vitamin A and E levels annually

IMAGING
- Chest x-ray - hyperaeration, hilar adenopathy, occasional pneumothorax, bronchiectasis, blebs, increased involvement in right upper lobe
- High resolution CT of chest to localize bronchiectasis

DIAGNOSTIC PROCEDURES Diagnosis made in presence of clinical symptoms and positive sweat test or gene probe

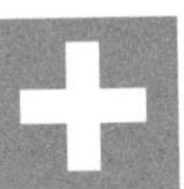

TREATMENT

APPROPRIATE HEALTH CARE
- Outpatient usually
- Inpatient during infections or other crisis
- Home care for IV antibiotics

GENERAL MEASURES
- Care by experienced physician and team (respiratory therapist, nurse, nutritionist, physical therapist, counselor, social worker)
- Goals are to prevent and treat respiratory failure and pulmonary complications
- Postural drainage and chest physiotherapy - adjuncts include flutter valve and CPT vest (expensive)
- Pancreatic enzyme replacement; H2 receptor blockers can increase utilization of enteric coated enzymes
- Regular exercises for fitness
- Press for adequate growth through good nutrition - supplements may be needed
- Aerosol B2 agonists; consider ipratropium
- Antibiotics - especially to target *Pseudomonas*, *Staphylococcus*
- DNase: aerosolized mucolytic, 2.5 mg neb q day. Use pari-plus nebulizer cup.
- Oxygen: when needed
- Monitor sleeping O2 saturation
- Hypaque or diatrizoate (Gastrografin) enemas or surgery for unrelieved meconium ileus (newborn)
- For fecal accumulation and intussusception in older children or adults - enemas of diatrizoate (Gastrografin) or polyethylene glycol (Golytely) per NG
- Early identification of diabetes, and treatment with insulin
- Assisted ventilation with BiPAP is acceptable and temporary. May be used nightly as a bridge to lung transplant.

SURGICAL MEASURES
- Surgery may be indicated for some complications
- Organ transplants possible for lung, liver, pancreas

ACTIVITY Physical conditioning to the extent possible for cardiorespiratory fitness (does not improve pulmonary function)

DIET
- Allow liberal salting of foods per patient preference
- High protein
- High calories (1.5 x recommended for general population)
- High fat (previously not recommended)
- Vitamin supplements (double RDA)
- May need supplemental feeds, oral or by gastrostomy

PATIENT EDUCATION Written information and support: Cystic Fibrosis Foundation, 6931 Arlington Road, Ste. 2000, Bethesda, MD 20814, (800)344-4823; website www.cff.org

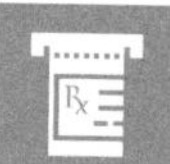

MEDICATIONS

DRUG(S) OF CHOICE
- Oral antibiotics
  - ◊ Ciprofloxacin for exacerbations
  - ◊ Cephalexin (Keflex) for *Staphylococcus aureus*
- Aerosolized antibiotics
  - ◊ Tobramycin 300 mg bid. 28 day on/28 day off rotating schedule for patients colonized with Pseudomonas
- IV antibiotics
  - ◊ According to culture and sensitivity studies when ill with respiratory infections
  - ◊ For *Pseudomonas* infections - IV tobramycin, start with 10 mg/kg/24 hrs; peak 8-12 μg/mL (17-26 μmol/L); trough 1-2 μg/mL (2-4 μmol/L) plus IV ceftazidime or antipseudomonal penicillin.
  - ◊ For staphylococcal infections - IV oxacillin or ticarcillin-clavulanate (Timentin). Vancomycin if resistant.
- Other therapies
  - ◊ Pancreatic enzyme replacements - dose 500-2500 units lipase/kg/meal. Distal colonic strictures possible with high doses.
  - ◊ Bronchodilators, if response demonstrated
  - ◊ Dornase alfa (DNase) nebulized daily 2.5 mg
  - ◊ Azithromycin, by anti-inflammatory protocol; if < 40 kg, 250 mg po q MWF; if > 40 kg, 500 mg po q MWF. Patient should not be colonized with atypical TB (could suppress).
  - ◊ Ibuprofen, regular use, may retard lung disease, but levels must be monitored
  - ◊ Oxygen therapy for severe pulmonary insufficiency or hypoxemia, pulmonary hypertension
  - ◊ Night-time mask BiPap effective with significant respiratory insufficiency
  - ◊ Occasional assisted ventilation, controversial
  - ◊ IPPB contraindicated
  - ◊ Routine administration of annual influenza vaccine

Contraindications: Refer to manufacturer's literature

Precautions: Refer to manufacturer's literature. Higher dosages or shorter administration intervals usually required.

Significant possible interactions: Refer to manufacturer's literature

ALTERNATIVE DRUGS
- Other antipseudomonal antibiotic
- Cephalexin for staphylococcal prophylaxis in infants not indicated

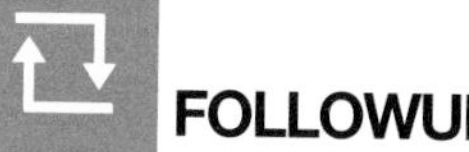

FOLLOWUP

PATIENT MONITORING At least 3 times a year; Cystic Fibrosis Center recommended

PREVENTION/AVOIDANCE
- In prenatal situations
  - ◊ Genetic counseling
  - ◊ Prenatal diagnosis for future pregnancies
- For complications
  - ◊ For respiratory infections - maintain pertussis and measles immunity; annual influenza immunization
  - ◊ Avoid general anesthetics. Consider epidural, spinal, or local.
  - ◊ Good medical teamwork in the management of the multifaceted problems of the disease

POSSIBLE COMPLICATIONS
- Diabetes: affects growth, lung function
- Atelectasis
- Pneumothorax
- Hemoptysis
- Right heart failure
- Pulmonary hypertension
- Pulmonary emphysema
- Digital clubbing
- Hypertrophic pulmonary osteoarthropathy
- Metabolic alkalosis
- Volume depletion
- Bleeding esophageal varices
- Symptomatic biliary cirrhosis
- Intestinal obstruction
- Female fertility rate about 80% of normal
- Numerous psychosocial aspects
- Malnutrition
- Retarded growth
- Hypovitaminosis A (increased ICP)
- Hypovitaminosis E (hemolytic anemia)
- Hypovitaminosis K (bleeding tendency)

EXPECTED COURSE/PROGNOSIS
- Largely dependent on pulmonary involvement
- Prognosis improving due to early detection and aggressive treatment
- Median survival is to age 33

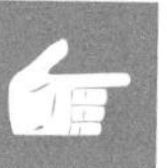

MISCELLANEOUS

ASSOCIATED CONDITIONS
- Pansinusitis
- Nasal polyposis

AGE-RELATED FACTORS
Pediatric: Diagnosis usually confirmed in infancy or early childhood but some go undetected until adolescence. Newborn screening methods are in development. Psychosocial considerations.

Geriatric: N/A

Others: N/A

PREGNANCY If cystic fibrosis patient's condition (pulmonary and nutrition) good at start of pregnancy, usually returns to that level following birth. If these conditions are compromised before pregnancy, they may deteriorate following birth.

SYNONYMS
- CF

ICD-9-CM
277.00 Cystic fibrosis without mention of meconium ileus

277.01 Cystic fibrosis with meconium ileus

SEE ALSO
Asthma

Bronchiectasis

OTHER NOTES
- Advise genetic counseling for at-risk individuals
- Encoded protein on long arm of chromosome 7 contains 1480 amino acids
- Multiple types of gene defects are possible (>500 defined). Most common mutation (70%) is DeltaF 508.

ABBREVIATIONS
CF = cystic fibrosis

IPPB = intermittent positive pressure breathing

ICP = intracranial pressure

RDA = recommended daily allowance

REFERENCES

- Tizzano F, Buchwald M. Cystic fibrosis: Beyond the gene to therapy. Jour of Pediatrics 1992;120;337-43
- Tizzano F, Buchwald M. Recent advances in cystic fibrosis research. Jour of Pediatrics 1993;122:985-88
- Schidlow DV, Taussig LM, Knowles MR. Cystic Fibrosis Foundation Conference Report on Pulmonary Complications of Cystic Fibrosis; Pediatric Pulmonology 1993;15:187-98
- Taussig LM:.Cystic Fibrosis. New York: Thieme-Stratton Inc.,;1984
- Orenstein DM, Stern RC, Rosenstein BJ. Cystic Fibrosis: Medical Care. Philadelphia: Lippincott Williams & Wilkins; 2000
- Consensus Conferences - Concepts in CF Care. Cystic Fibrosis Foundation; 2004

Web references: 0 available at www.5mcc.com

Illustrations N/A

Author(s):

Nancy N. Dambro, MD

BASICS

DESCRIPTION Cytomegalovirus (CMV) is a beta herpesvirus. CMV may remain latent throughout a person's life and rarely reactivates. CMV cannot be propagated in laboratory animals or in most cell cultures.

- The disease occurs world-wide and almost two thirds of the U.S. population is seropositive from prior exposure during childhood or early adulthood. In most of these, the disease is mild and overlooked. Populations at risk for active disease include neonates, transplant recipients, and AIDS patients.
- CMV infection during pregnancy can be hazardous to the fetus and may lead to stillbirth, brain damage, birth defects or to severe neonatal illness
- The name derives from the infected cells that are large and bear intranuclear inclusions
- Infection may be in almost any organ, but the salivary glands are the most common site in children and the lungs in adults. This infection can occur congenitally, postnatally, or at any age.
- Categories of CMV infections include:
  - ◊ Congenital: These infections vary greatly from mild cytomegaloviremia in a normal infant to the cause of abortion, stillbirth, postnatal death from hemorrhage, anemia, liver or CNS damage.
  - ◊ Acute infection in a normal host
  - ◊ Infections in bone marrow transplant patients - usually pneumonia
  - ◊ Infection in patients with AIDS - usually retinitis or colitis
  - ◊ Infections in other immunocompromised patients - pulmonary, gastrointestinal, or renal disease

System(s) affected: Nervous, Pulmonary, Skin/Exocrine

Genetics: May be passed from mother to fetus

Incidence/Prevalence in USA:
- Common, but frequently asymptomatic
- Up to 70% of adults have been infected, almost all with inapparent disease. CMV infection is even more prevalent in populations at higher risk for HIV infection (IV drug users 75%, homosexual males 90%)

Predominant age: All ages, peaks at < 3 months; 16-40 years, and 40-75 years

Predominant sex: Male > Female

SIGNS & SYMPTOMS
- Congenital:
  - ◊ Abortion
  - ◊ Asymptomatic cytomegaloviremia
  - ◊ Hemorrhage
  - ◊ Anemia
  - ◊ Jaundice
  - ◊ Signs of CNS damage
- Acquired: (acute infection in a normal or immunocompromised host)
  - ◊ May be asymptomatic
  - ◊ Fatigue
  - ◊ Nausea
  - ◊ Vomiting
  - ◊ Bone pain
  - ◊ Chills
  - ◊ Fever
  - ◊ Diarrhea
  - ◊ Jaundice
  - ◊ Hepatomegaly
  - ◊ Splenomegaly
  - ◊ Dyspnea
- Infections in transplant patients:
  - ◊ Pneumonitis with cough, fever, chills, chest pain
- Infections in AIDS patients:
  - ◊ Retinitis
  - ◊ Esophageal, gastric, small bowel and colonic ulcerations
  - ◊ Pneumonitis
  - ◊ CNS with radiculopathy or encephalitis

CAUSES
- Infection with cytomegalovirus
- Reactivation of a latent process in patients who are immunosuppressed

RISK FACTORS
- HIV infection
- AIDS
- Organ transplantation (50% attack rate, depending on serologic status)
- Blood transfusion. A postperfusion syndrome may develop in 2 to 4 weeks in patients having fresh blood transfusions. Characteristics include fever lasting 2 to 3 weeks, hepatitis, with or without jaundice, atypical lymphocytosis similar to that of infectious mononucleosis, and a skin rash.
- Immunocompromised host
- Living in closed population
- Corticosteroid therapy
- Day care environment - infant or geriatric
- For congenital infection - maternal infection during pregnancy

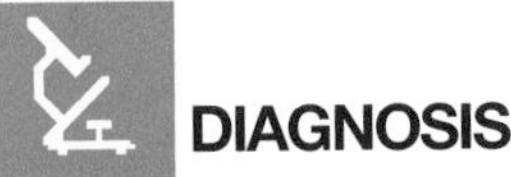

DIAGNOSIS

DIFFERENTIAL DIAGNOSIS
- Congenital: Bacterial, viral, and protozoan infections, such as toxoplasmosis, rubella, syphilis
- Acquired: Viral hepatitis, infectious mononucleosis

LABORATORY
- Human fibroblastic cell culture inoculation may isolate the virus from urine, blood, other body fluids, or tissues
- Leukopenia
- Thrombocytopenia
- Increased lymphocytes
- Demonstration of CMV in secretions or tissues by immunofluorescence with commercially available monoclonal antibodies or by in situ hybridization

Drugs that may alter lab results: N/A

Disorders that may alter lab results: N/A

PATHOLOGICAL FINDINGS Giant cells with basophilic inclusion bodies

SPECIAL TESTS
- Human fibroblastic tissue cultures to isolate the virus
- Immunofluorescence techniques for virus demonstrations

IMAGING Skull film - intracranial calcifications

DIAGNOSTIC PROCEDURES
- Bronchoscopy in bone marrow transplant patients if suspicious of CMV pneumonia
- Buffy coat culture
- Endoscopic biopsy of gastrointestinal tract

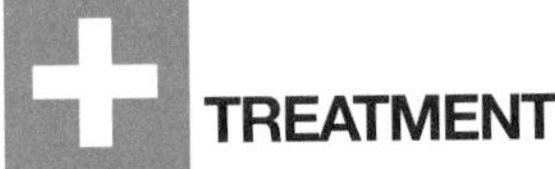

TREATMENT

APPROPRIATE HEALTH CARE Inpatient for disseminated infection or CMV reactivation syndrome

GENERAL MEASURES Isolation

SURGICAL MEASURES N/A

ACTIVITY Bedrest

DIET No special diet

PATIENT EDUCATION N/A

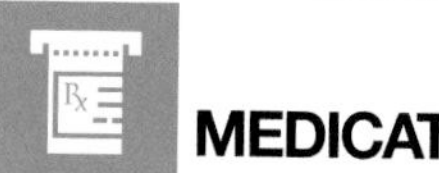

MEDICATIONS

DRUG(S) OF CHOICE
- Valacyclovir - oral prophylaxis in adult bone marrow transplant recipients (neutropenia)
- Ganciclovir - nucleoside analog that is virostatic; useful in all ages; IV or oral
- Foscarnet - adult CMV illnesses (renal toxicity)
- Cidofovir - adult CMV illnesses (nephrotoxicity)

Contraindications: Refer to manufacturer's literature
Precautions: Refer to manufacturer's literature
Significant possible interactions: Refer to manufacturer's literature

ALTERNATIVE DRUGS
Future - ganciclovir implants for control of CMV retinitis; vaccines?

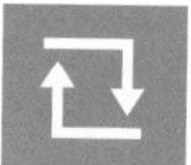

FOLLOWUP

PATIENT MONITORING
Close followup in ICU (isolated) during infection with disseminated form

PREVENTION/AVOIDANCE
Avoid immunosuppression (when possible)

POSSIBLE COMPLICATIONS
- Chorioretinitis
- Encephalitis
- Mononucleosis
- Colitis
- Deafness
- Mental retardation

EXPECTED COURSE/PROGNOSIS
Disseminated form often fatal

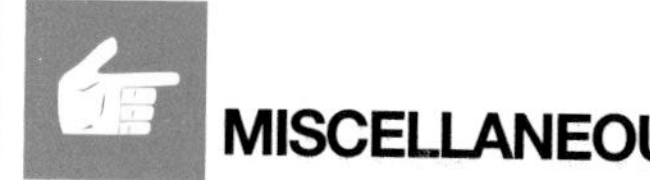

MISCELLANEOUS

ASSOCIATED CONDITIONS
- Acquired immune deficiency syndrome (AIDS)
- Corticosteroid therapy
- Leukemia
- Lymphoma

AGE-RELATED FACTORS
Pediatric: May occur congenitally or postnatally
Geriatric: N/A
Others: N/A

PREGNANCY
N/A

SYNONYMS
- Giant cell inclusion disease
- CID
- CMV
- Salivary gland virus disease

ICD-9-CM
078.5 Cytomegaloviral disease

SEE ALSO

OTHER NOTES
N/A

ABBREVIATIONS
N/A

REFERENCES

- Winston DJ, Yeager AM, Chandrasekar PH, et al. Valacyclovir Cytomegalovirus Study Group. Randomized comparison of oral valacyclovir and intravenous ganciclovir for prevention of cytomegalovirus disease after allogeneic bone marrow transplantation. Clin Infect Dis 2003;36(6):749-58
- Mandell GL, editor. Principles and Practice of Infectious Diseases. 5th Ed. New York: Churchill Livingstone; 2000
- Onorato IM, et al. Epidemiology of Cytomegaloviral Infection: Recommendations for Prevention & Control. Rev Infect Dis 1985;7:479
- Cohen JI, Corey GR. Cytomegalovirus Infection in the Normal Host. Medicine 1985;64:100-114
- Drew WL, et al. Cytomegalovirus: disease syndrome and treatment. Curr Clin Top Infect Dis 1999;19:16-29

Web references: 2 available at www.5mcc.com
Illustrations 1 available

Author(s):
Kathi Clement, MD

Expanded Topics

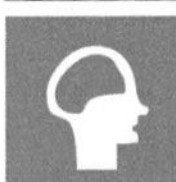

BASICS

DESCRIPTION Metastatic dissolution of gas bubbles (usually nitrogen) into tissues caused by a relatively rapid decrease in the environmental pressure. Five types based on symptomatology:
- Limb bends - gas deposition in tissues causes a poorly-localized "pain-only" syndrome; may herald more serious disease (shoulder most common).
- Cerebral bends - stroke-like picture due to paradoxical arterial gas embolism (via A-V or intracardiac shunt), de novo arterial gas formation, and/or cerebral edema.
- Spinal cord bends - transverse paresis caused by retrograde venous thrombosis with patchy necrosis and edema of the spinal cord; predilection for high lumbar nerve roots due to lack of collateral circulation.
- Inner ear bends - development of bubble formation and hemorrhage in labyrinthine fluid spaces and vasculature.
- Lung bends ("chokes") - excessive venous bubbles develop and release vasoactive substances causing pulmonary irritation and bronchoconstriction. The primary symptoms are substernal chest pain (worse with inspiration), dyspnea, and cough. Decompression sickness (DCS) - type I (mild) - mild pain, rash; type II - (serious) pulmonary, shock, nervous system; AGE - arterial gas embolism

System(s) affected: Cardiovascular, Musculoskeletal, Nervous, Pulmonary
Genetics: N/A
Incidence/Prevalence in USA: Uncommon, < 1% even in high-density diving areas and areas of caisson work; 13.4 per 100,000 dives
Predominant age: 20-29
Predominant sex: 95% males, although there is no evidence to suggest increased susceptibility based on sex.

SIGNS & SYMPTOMS
- 95% present in 3-4 hours, but may be delayed for 24 hours or more
- Burning blebs (skin bends), lymphedema
- Painful pruritic red rash ("cutis marmorata")
- Vague, poorly localized pain
- Headache, visual field deficits
- Ataxia, nystagmus
- Delirium
- Coma
- Convulsions
- Confusion
- Patchy numbness
- Respiratory "chokes" in 2%
- Coughing paroxysm's (Behnke's sign)
- Arrhythmia
- Bradycardia or tachycardia
- Hypotension
- Tachypnea, hemoptysis
- Subcutaneous emphysema along tendon sheaths (rare)
- Rapidly ascending paraplegia
- Negative or positive scotomata
- Sharply defined area of pallor on tongue (Liebermeister sign)
- Air in retinal vessels

CAUSES
- Rapid ascent from scuba diving (depth > 33 feet)
- Rapid ascent/decompression in an airplane
- Tunnel work = caisson disease
- Inadequate pressurization/denitrogenation when flying
- Flying to high altitude too soon after scuba diving

RISK FACTORS
- Prolonged dive at depth over 33 feet
- Obesity
- Multiple, repetitive scuba dives
- Cold water diving
- Poor physical conditioning
- Vigorous physical activity
- Dehydration
- Local injury
- Patent foramen ovale (for neurologic symptoms) - routine screening not recommended

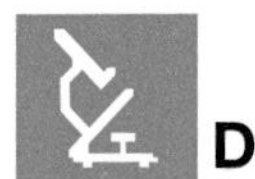

DIAGNOSIS

DIFFERENTIAL DIAGNOSIS
- Arterial gas embolism
- Traumatic injury to extremity
- Cerebrovascular accident
- Musculoskeletal strains
- Urticaria
- Malingering

LABORATORY
- ABGs - may show decreased pO2, decreased pCO2, and metabolic acidosis.
- CBC - increased hematocrit in severe cases due to dehydration. Thrombocytopenia.
- Coagulation tests - may see increased fibrin split products and increased prothrombin time

Drugs that may alter lab results: N/A

Disorders that may alter lab results: N/A

PATHOLOGICAL FINDINGS
- Skin lesions: painful, pruritic, blotchy red rash on torso, burning blebs on skin, lymphedema
- Joints: erythema and edema on the periarticular surfaces

SPECIAL TESTS EEG - irregular slowing with cerebral bends

IMAGING
- Chest x-ray - pneumothorax, mediastinal emphysema; +/- right heart enlargement. Plain x-ray or ultrasound - gas bubbles in joints, tendons, bursae, muscles.
- CT scan - should be performed on all patients with history of trauma or neurologic signs

DIAGNOSTIC PROCEDURES "Test of pressure" = trial of recompression to 2.8 ATA/100% oxygen/10'

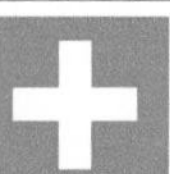

TREATMENT

APPROPRIATE HEALTH CARE Referral through Divers' Alert Network [DAN (919)684-8111] to nearest hyperbaric facility for recompression test. The specific treatment may vary from institution to institution, but is based on the procedures first established in the Armed Services (e.g., US Navy Table 6). Patients may be sent home when cutaneous symptoms only are present, if the appropriate response to therapy is observed in the emergency department.

GENERAL MEASURES
- 100% oxygen via tight nonbreathing mask
- Fluid resuscitation (avoid D5W or hypotonic IV solutions with cord injury). Despite the theoretical advantages of volume expanders (dextran, albumin, etc.), no experimental or clinical studies support their use since they are not without risk.
- Rapid referral to hyperbaric chamber facility
- Position recumbent - not Trendelenburg
- Transport via ground, low-altitude airplane, or aircraft pressurized to sea level

SURGICAL MEASURES N/A

ACTIVITY Bedrest when neurologic involvement present

DIET As tolerated

PATIENT EDUCATION Anyone who desires to perform scuba diving should be certified by an appropriate diving agency: NAUI, PADI, SSI, or YMCA. Sport divers who have not been diving for > 6 months should review diving principles/skills via a refresher course.

MEDICATIONS

DRUG(S) OF CHOICE 100% oxygen; diazepam 5-15 mg IV (IM absorption unpredictable) for inner ear decompression sickness. Symptoms of vertigo, nausea and vomiting may get significant relief. The use of steroids has been advocated by some for the assumed vasogenic edema seen in decompression sickness. This form of therapy remains controversial and not proven in controlled clinical trials. If steroids are prescribed, they should not be used for more than 4-5 days for neurological symptoms.
Contraindications: Hypersensitivity to benzodiazepines and acute narrow-angle glaucoma
Precautions: Administration of diazepam requires monitoring of the respiratory status, blood pressure and heart rate. Dosage reductions are required in the elderly and patients with hepatic dysfunction.
Significant possible interactions: Benzodiazepines potentiate the effects of other CNS depressants.

ALTERNATIVE DRUGS
- Adjunctive therapy:
  - ◊ Digitalization for CHF/tachycardia
  - ◊ Aminophylline NOT useful for "chokes"
  - ◊ Roles of steroids and heparin not determined

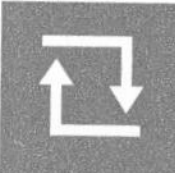

FOLLOWUP

PATIENT MONITORING Symptomatic assessment for relapse/progression which occurs in 25%

PREVENTION/AVOIDANCE
- Follow decompression tables (Navy, NAUI, PADI) for diving to depth (> 33 feet) or use dive computers that calculate nitrogen content of various tissues
- Allow adequate time between diving and flying to altitude (24 hours)

POSSIBLE COMPLICATIONS
- Oxygen toxicity with seizures (infrequent and unpredictable)
- Neurologic sequelae for non-responders
- Long-term risk of aseptic necrosis

EXPECTED COURSE/PROGNOSIS
- Excellent for early symptomatic presentation, referral and treatment
- Related to duration and severity of symptoms prior to treatment
- Although recompression therapy is best administered early as possible, some patients may still benefit even at six to nine days after the incident, referral is critical, even if symptoms resolve, since 25% of patients will relapse

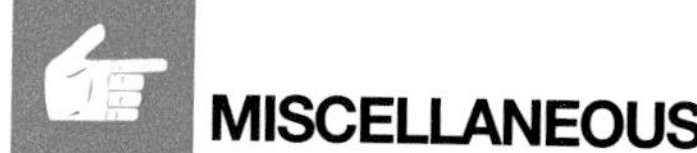

MISCELLANEOUS

ASSOCIATED CONDITIONS N/A

AGE-RELATED FACTORS
Pediatric: N/A
Geriatric: N/A
Others: N/A

PREGNANCY Pregnant patient with decompression sickness a priority as fetus may also be affected; no contraindication to recompression

SYNONYMS
- Bends
- Paretic bends
- Caisson disease

ICD-9-CM
993.3 Caisson disease

SEE ALSO

OTHER NOTES
- The diagnosis may be difficult due to the variable clinical manifestations. The most important clue is recent decompression.
- 71% of nervous system decompression sickness present as skin or limb bends
- Limb bends with musculoskeletal complaints frequently diagnosed as malingering due to vague nature
- Only way to exclude the diagnosis in patient at risk is a negative test of pressure

ABBREVIATIONS
DCS = decompression sickness
NAUI = National Association for Underwater Instructors
PADI = Professional Association for Diving Instructors
SSI = Sport SCUBA Instructors
YMCA = Young Men's Christian Association
ATA = atmospheres absolute

REFERENCES

- Bove A, Davis JC. Diving Medicine. 2nd Ed. Philadelphia, W.B. Saunders Co., 1990
- Catron PW, Flynn ET. Adjuvant drug therapy for decompression sickness: A review. Undersea Biomed Res 1982;9:161-73

Web references: 0 available at www.5mcc.com
Illustrations N/A

Author(s):
Darell E. Heiselman, DO

BASICS

DESCRIPTION Delirium is a neurologic complication of illness and/or medication use that is especially common in older patients. The key diagnostic features are an acute change in mental status that fluctuates, abnormal attention, and either disorganized thinking or altered level of consciousness. Delirium is a medical emergency requiring immediate evaluation in order to decrease morbidity, mortality, and health-care costs. The Confusion Assessment Method (CAM), which focuses on diagnostically important issues, is an easily used and well-validated tool for delirium screening. The CAM has been adapted for use in the ICU setting.
While the neuropathophysiology of delirium is not clearly defined, a multi-component approach addressing multiple potential contributing factors can reduce its incidence and complications.
System(s) affected: Nervous
Genetics: None known
Incidence/Prevalence in USA: The prevalence of delirium in hospitalized older patients ranges from 10-40%, with and incidence of 25-60%. In high-risk older patients such as those with hip fracture, >50% experience delirium. Since about 1/3 of adults age > 65 are hospitalized annually in the United States, and assuming a conservative delirium rate of 20%, each year 7% of all persons age 65 or older develop delirium.
Predominant age: Older persons
Predominant sex: Male = female

SIGNS & SYMPTOMS

Diagnostic criteria
- CAM: Five features indicate the presence of delirium
- First 3 along with either of the last 2 are present
  - ◊ Acute onset
  - ◊ Fluctuating course
  - ◊ Abnormal attention and inability to sustain focus
  - ◊ Disorganized thinking; problems with planning/reasoning/insight
  - ◊ Abnormal level of consciousness
- Any of the following may also be present in the delirious patient, but are not diagnostically specific to delirium:
  - ◊ Short- and long-term memory problems
  - ◊ Sleep-wake cycle disturbances
  - ◊ Misperceptions, hallucinations, and/or delusions
  - ◊ Emotional lability
  - ◊ Tremors and asterixis

Delirium subtypes
- Four subtypes based on level of consciousness
  - ◊ Hyperactive delirium (15%): Patients are loud, rambunctious, and disruptive.
  - ◊ Hypoactive delirium (20%): Patients are quietly confused, and may sit in bed without eating, drinking, or moving.
  - ◊ Mixed delirium (50%): Features of both hyper- and hypoactive delirium
  - ◊ Normal consciousness delirium (15%): Patients have an apparently normal level of consciousness, but still display disorganized thinking (confused, irrelevant, rambling speech), along with the acute onset, inattention, and fluctuating mental state

CAUSES

- Usually multifactorial; often an interaction between predisposing and precipitating risk factors. With more predisposing factors (i.e. the frailer the patients), the less severe the precipitating factors must be to produce delirium. Conversely, those with few predisposing factors (i.e. very robust patients) require a greater illness-related insult to manifest delirium.
- Consider medications strongly in searching for a cause

RISK FACTORS

- Predisposing risk factors: Advanced age, prior cognitive impairment, functional impairment, high BUN/Cr ratio, dehydration, malnutrition, hearing or vision impairment, or any underlying medical condition that produces frailty
- Precipitating risk factors: Severe illness in any organ system(s), need for a urinary catheter, more than three medications, pain, any adverse iatrogenic event. Medications deserve special attention - the most important include sedative-hypnotics (especially long-acting benzodiazepines, e.g., diazepam and flurazepam), narcotics (especially meperidine), and anticholinergics (especially diphenhydramine, which should not be used to treat insomnia in older persons)

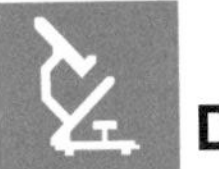

DIAGNOSIS

DIFFERENTIAL DIAGNOSIS

- Depression (slower onset, primarily a disturbance of mood, a normal level of consciousness and fluctuates over weeks to months)
- Dementia (insidious onset, memory problems, normal level of consciousness and fluctuates over days to weeks)
- Psychosis

LABORATORY

- Initially: CBC, electrolytes, BUN/Cr, urinalysis, and chest X-ray
- If needed: ECG, ABGs, drug screen, and liver function tests

Drugs that may alter lab results: N/A

Disorders that may alter lab results: N/A

PATHOLOGICAL FINDINGS N/A

SPECIAL TESTS N/A

IMAGING

- Non-contrast head CT scan if diagnosis unclear, recent fall, receiving anticoagulants or new focal neurologic signs; or to rule out increased intracranial pressure prior to lumbar puncture

DIAGNOSTIC PROCEDURES

- Lumbar puncture, rarely, but perform if clinical suspicion of a CNS bleed or infection is high

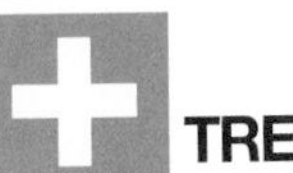

TREATMENT

APPROPRIATE HEALTH CARE New delirium is a medical emergency usually deserving of evaluation in the inpatient setting

GENERAL MEASURES

- There is little evidence to suggest that restraints decrease the risk of falls or injury and should be used only in the most difficult to manage patients, for as brief a time as possible
- Post-operative patients should be monitored and treated for:
  - ◊ Myocardial infarction/ischemia
  - ◊ Arrhythmias
  - ◊ Pulmonary complications/pneumonia (especially if COPD present)
  - ◊ Pulmonary embolism
  - ◊ Urinary or stool retention (attempt urinary catheter removal by postoperative day 2)
- The route of anesthesia (general versus epidural) does not effect the risk of delirium
- Treatment is multifactorial, involving identification of contributing factors and preemptive care to avoid iatrogenic problems. Several areas of care deserve special attention in all patients:
  - ◊ CNS oxygen delivery (attempt to attain the following)
    - SaO2 > 90% with goal of SaO2>95%
    - Systolic BP > 2/3 baseline or > 90 mmHg
    - Hematocrit > 30%
  - ◊ Fluid/electrolyte balance
    - Sodium, potassium, and glucose normal (glucose < 300 mg/dl in diabetics)
    - Treat fluid overload or dehydration
  - ◊ Treat pain
    - Scheduled acetaminophen at 1 gram QID if daily pain
    - Morphine or oxycodone for breakthrough pain if acetaminophen ineffective
    - Avoid meperidine (Demerol)
  - ◊ Eliminate unnecessary medications
    - Discontinue or minimize benzodiazepines, anticholinergics, and antihistamines
    - Eliminate medication redundancies
    - Investigate new patient symptoms as potential manifestation of medication side effect
  - ◊ Regulate bowel/bladder function
    - Bowel movement at least every 48 hours
    - Screen for urinary retention or incontinence, especially after catheter removal
  - ◊ Nutrition
    - Dentures used properly
    - Proper positioning for meals
    - Assistance with meals when necessary
    - Nutritional supplements (1-3 cans daily) if intake is poor
    - Temporary nasogastric tube if unable to take food orally and bowels working
  - ◊ Mobilization
    - Out of bed on hospital day 2 (or postoperative day 1) if no contraindications
    - Out of bed several hours daily if no contraindications
    - Daily physical therapy if not ambulating independently
    - Daily occupational therapy if not functionally independent

◊ Prevention of major hospital-acquired problems
  - 6-inch thick foam mattress overlay if not on a special pressure reducing bed
  - Avoid urinary catheter.
  - Institute skin care program for patients with established incontinence
  - Incentive spirometry if bed-bound
  - Subcutaneous heparin 5000 units BID if bed-bound

◊ Environmental stimulation
  - Glasses and hearing aids if used prior to illness
  - Clock and calendar
  - Soft lighting
  - Radio, tapes, television if desired

◊ Sleep
  - Quiet environment
  - Soft music
  - Therapeutic massage
  - Medication if required: trazodone 25 mg qhs prn sleep; zolpidem (Ambien) 5 mg qhs prn sleep; no diphenhydramine, no benzodiazepines

SURGICAL MEASURES N/A

ACTIVITY As tolerated. Early physical therapy consultation may help prevent deconditioning.

DIET N/A

PATIENT EDUCATION N/A

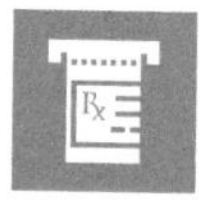

MEDICATIONS

DRUG(S) OF CHOICE

Nonpharmacological approaches are preferred for initial treatment. Medications often only treat the symptoms of delirium and do not address the underlying cause.

- Neuroleptics are the preferred medications
  ◊ Haloperidol (Haldol). Initially, 0.25-0.5mg PO/IM/IV unless urgent sedation is required such as with an intubated patient
  ◊ Quetiapine (Seroquel). 25mg q/day bid
- Short acting benzodiazepines, if neuroleptics don't work or should be avoided
  ◊ Lorazepam (Ativan). Initially, 0.25-0.5mg PO/IM/IV.

Contraindications: Avoid neuroleptics in patients with parkinsonism or Parkinson disease

Precautions:

- Neuroleptics may cause significant extrapyramidal problems and benzodiazepines may lead to sedation. Both may increase the risk of falls.
- Risperidone may be associated with hyperglycemia and ketoacidosis

Significant possible interactions: N/A

ALTERNATIVE DRUGS

- Risperidone (Risperdal) 0.25-0.5mg
- Olanzapine (Zyprexa) 2.5-5.0mg

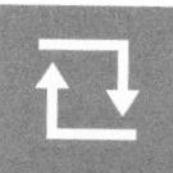

FOLLOWUP

PATIENT MONITORING Patients should be monitored and mental status reassessed at least daily. Other monitoring depends upon the specific medical conditions present.

PREVENTION/AVOIDANCE In patients at high risk for delirium due to age and/or frailty the approach to prevention is the same as for treatment of delirium.

POSSIBLE COMPLICATIONS Falls, pressure ulcers, malnutrition, functional decline, oversedation, polypharmacy.

EXPECTED COURSE/PROGNOSIS Delirium is usually thought of as acute and hence usually improves with treatment of the underlying condition. However, it is not unusual for delirium to become chronic. In one study, only 42% of patients had resolution of their symptoms 6 months after discharge.

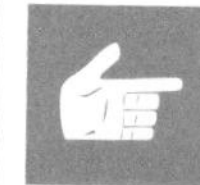

MISCELLANEOUS

ASSOCIATED CONDITIONS

- New medicine or medicine changes
- Infections (especially lung and urine)
- Heart attack
- Stroke
- Alcohol or drug withdrawal

AGE-RELATED FACTORS

Pediatric: N/A

Geriatric: Older patients are at the highest risk of delirium

Others: N/A

PREGNANCY N/A

SYNONYMS

- Acute confusional state
- Altered mental status
- Organic brain syndrome
- Acute mental status change

ICD-9-CM

780.09 Alterations of consciousness, other
293.0 Acute delirium
293.1 Subacute delirium
293.89 Other specified transient organic mental disorders, other
292.81 Drug-induced delirium
290.11 Presenile dementia with delirium
290.3 Senile dementia with delirium
291.0 Alcohol withdrawal delirium
291.1 Alcohol amnestic syndrome
292.0 Drug withdrawal syndrome

SEE ALSO

Alcohol use disorders
Dementia
Depression
Restlessness

OTHER NOTES

ABBREVIATIONS

CAM = Confusion Assessment Method

REFERENCES

- Inouye SK, van Dyck CH, Alessi CA, et al. Clarifying confusion: the confusion assessment method. Ann Intern Med 1990;113:941-948
- Inouye SK, Bogardus ST, Charpentier PA, et al. A Multicomponent Intervention to Prevent Delirium in Hospitalized Older Patients. NEJM 1999;340(9):669-676
- Marcantonio ER, Flacker JM, Wright RJ, Resnick NM. Reducing Delirium After Hip Fracture: A Randomized Trial. J of the Amer Geriatr Soc 2001;49(5):516-522
- Ely EW, Margolin R, Francis J, et al. Evaluation of delirium in critically ill patients: Validation of the Confusion Assessment Method for the Intensive Care Unit (CAM-ICU). Crit Care Med 2001;29(7):1370-1379
- Anonymous. Practice Guidelines for the treatment of patients with delirium. Amer J Psych 1994;156:(5 supp):1-20

Web references: 0 available at www.5mcc.com

Illustrations N/A

Author(s):
Jonathan M. Flacker, MD

Dementia

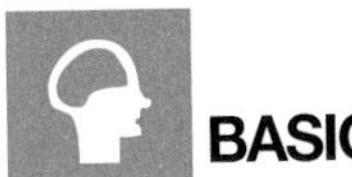

BASICS

DESCRIPTION A pathologic process defined as a persistent impairment of a prior level of intellectual functioning

- Alzheimer dementia (AD) is the most common form and characterized by a relentless deterioration of higher cortical functioning. The rate of deterioration is variable.
- Ischemic vascular dementia (IVD) formerly multi-infarct dementia, occurs as a result of clinical or subclinical cerebral infarcts secondary to atherosclerosis. Deterioration is stepwise with periods of clinical plateaus.
- Frontotemporal dementia (FTD) - insidious change in personality with cognitive dysfunction. Onset usually prior to age 65.
- Secondary dementias - also referred to as "reversible dementias" because the cognitive impairment may reverse with treatment of the primary disorder
- Dementia with Lewy bodies (DLB) - early onset dementia with associated psychosis, depression

System(s) affected: Nervous

Genetics:

- At least 15% of patients with AD will report a positive family history
- Persons with Trisomy 21 (Down syndrome) who survive into their 20's and 30's will inevitably develop a progressive dementia

Incidence/Prevalence in USA:

- 0.5% between ages 60 and 64; 3.2% between ages 80-90
- 1480/100,000
- 1.2 million people in the U.S. have severe dementia and another 2.5 million have moderate illness; 10% of all persons over the age of 65 have clinically important dementia

Predominant age: Increasing incidence with increasing age. Can occur in younger persons secondary to trisomy 21 or AIDS.

Predominant sex: Male = Female

SIGNS & SYMPTOMS

- Impaired short- and long-term memory
- Impaired abstract thinking
- Impaired judgment
- Aphasia
- Apraxia
- Agnosia
- Anomia
- Personality change, emotional outbursts, wandering, restlessness, hyperactivity, especially with FTD
- Sleep disturbances
- Mood disturbances
- Urinary incontinence (usually late in DAT or normal pressure hydrocephalus)
- Fecal incontinence (late)
- Rigidity
- Tremor (especially with DLB)
- Hallucinations (especially with DLB)
- Delusions
- Overt paranoid behavior
- Weight loss
- Seizures

CAUSES

- AD - genetic predisposition in > 15%
- IVD - due to cerebral atherosclerosis or emboli with clinical or subclinical infarcts
- Secondary dementias - causes include hypothyroidism, vitamin B deficiency, normal pressure hydrocephalus, AIDS, syphilis, and various medications. The dementia will be accompanied by the other signs and symptoms characteristic of the primary disorder.

RISK FACTORS

- Increasing age
- Prevalence of atherosclerotic disease (IVD)
- Trisomy 21 (Down syndrome)
- History of head trauma
- History of CNS infection
- Midlife depression

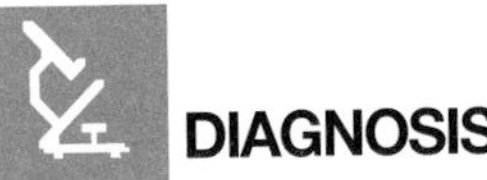

DIAGNOSIS

DIFFERENTIAL DIAGNOSIS

- Delirium
- Normal aging (age-associated memory impairment)
- Depression
- Schizophrenia
- Sensory deprivation states
- Chronic alcoholism
- Heat stroke
- Postsurgical and/or postanesthesia state

LABORATORY

Done primarily to rule out potentially reversible causes

- Thyroid function tests
- Syphilis serology
- Serum B12 and folate
- Complete blood count and screening metabolic profile

Drugs that may alter lab results: Thyroid hormone replacement and iodine preparations may affect thyroid function tests

Disorders that may alter lab results: False positive syphilis serology with acute infections, leprosy, subacute bacterial endocarditis, and autoimmune disorders

PATHOLOGICAL FINDINGS

- AD - granulovesicular degeneration, neurofibrillary tangles, senile neuritic plaques, microvascular amyloid
- Old infarcts, atherosclerotic disease

SPECIAL TESTS

- Mental status testing
- Neuropsychologic testing
- Electroencephalogram for patients with altered consciousness or associated seizures

IMAGING

- Head computerized tomography (CT) if history suggestive of a mass, or focal neurologic signs or in patient with dementia of brief duration
- Magnetic resonance imaging (MRI) is more sensitive than computerized tomography (CT) for detection of soft tissue lesions (small infarcts, mass lesions, atrophy of the brainstem, and other subcortical structures). MRI may also clarify ambiguous computed tomography findings.
- Isotope cisternography if suspicious of normal pressure hydrocephalus
- Positive emission tomography (PET) shows cortical hypometabolism

DIAGNOSTIC PROCEDURES N/A

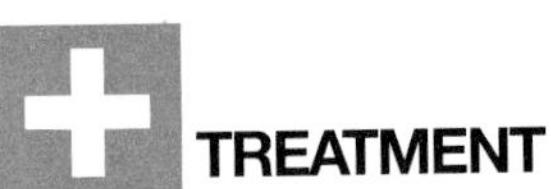

TREATMENT

APPROPRIATE HEALTH CARE

- Outpatient except when complications warrant hospitalization
- Nursing home - if disease progresses to the point that long-term care becomes necessary

GENERAL MEASURES

- Daily schedules and written directions
- Support and education of caregivers
- Emphasis on nutrition, personal hygiene, personal safety (accident-proofing the home) and supervision
- Discussions with the family concerning advanced directives
- Socialization (adult day care)
- Sensory stimulation (prominent displays of clocks and calendars)
- Improvement in sleep hygiene
- Pharmacotherapy should be reserved for specific behavioral symptoms after nonpharmacologic therapy has failed

SURGICAL MEASURES N/A

ACTIVITY Fully active with direction and supervision

DIET No special diet

PATIENT EDUCATION

- The 36-Hour Day by Mace and Rabins
- Printed material available from the Alzheimer Association, (800)621-0379

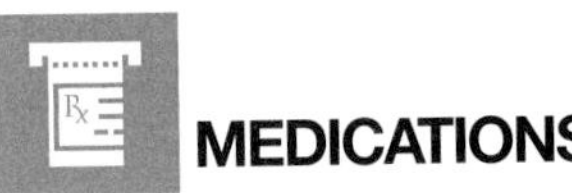

MEDICATIONS

DRUG(S) OF CHOICE

- Appropriately treat secondary causes, such as hypothyroidism or vitamin B12 deficiency
- With other causes, drugs are used to treat behavioral symptoms after nonpharmacologic therapy has failed

- Sun-downing, aggressive behavior: antipsychotics such as haloperidol (Haldol) or risperidone (Risperdal) 0.5-1.0 mg at bedtime are reasonable choices in a non-emergency situation
- Depression: nortriptyline (Pamelor) 20-50 mg or desipramine (Norpramin) 25 mg bid or the serotonin reuptake inhibitors - sertraline (Zoloft), fluoxetine (Prozac), paroxetine (Paxil), or citalopram (Celexa), escitalopram (Lexapro)
- Sleep disturbance: Intermittent use of temazepam (Restoril) 15 mg, zolpidem (Ambien) 5 mg, trazodone (Desyrel) 25-50 mg, mirtazapine (Remeron) 15 mg, or chloral hydrate 500 mg at bedtime is occasionally warranted
- Cognitive dysfunction: donepezil (Aricept) 5-10 mg every AM, rivastigmine (Exelon) 1.5-6 mg bid, galantamine (Reminyl) 4-12 mg bid, vitamin E 500-1000 IU per day, memantine (Namenda) 5-20 mg daily

Contraindications:
- Antipsychotics (haloperidol, risperidone, thioridazine) - severe depression; Lewy body dementia, Parkinson disease; hypo- or hypertension
- Tricyclic antidepressants (nortriptyline, desipramine) - acute recovery phase following myocardial infarction, acute narrow-angle glaucoma
- Acute active liver disease, active untreated peptic ulcers

Precautions:
- Hypnotics should not be used on a regular basis
- In the elderly, begin with small doses and increase slowly
- Lorazepam (Ativan) may produce paradoxical excitation or daytime drowsiness
- Triazolam (Halcion) can produce confusion and psychotic reactions in the elderly
- Antipsychotics
  - ◊ Risperidone may be associated with hyperglycemia and ketoacidosis
  - ◊ Use with caution in patients with severe cardiovascular disorders because of the possibility of severe hypotension
  - ◊ Tardive dyskinesia
  - ◊ Neuroleptic malignant syndrome
  - ◊ Lowered seizure threshold
  - ◊ Monitor bone marrow function with CBC
- Tricyclic antidepressants (TCA)
  - ◊ Anticholinergic effects
  - ◊ Sedation, increased confusion
  - ◊ May produce arrhythmia, sinus tachycardia, and prolong conduction time
  - ◊ Lowered seizure threshold
- Benzodiazepines
  - ◊ Dependence
  - ◊ Sedation, increased confusion
  - ◊ Respiratory depression
  - ◊ Withdrawal symptoms
- Tacrine (Cognex)
  - ◊ Use with caution in persons with a history of elevated liver function tests, neuromuscular disease, seizures or asthma
- Donepezil (Aricept) use with caution:
  - ◊ If at risk for gastrointestinal ulcers
  - ◊ In persons with sick sinus syndrome or other supraventricular cardiac conduction conditions
- Serotonin reuptake inhibitors
  - ◊ Weight loss
  - ◊ Might decrease seizure threshold
  - ◊ Dry mouth
  - ◊ Tremor
  - ◊ Nausea, vomiting, diarrhea
- Galantamine (Reminyl)
  - ◊ Bradycardia
  - ◊ Nausea, vomiting
  - ◊ Urinary retention
- Rivastigmine (Exelon) use with caution:
  - ◊ Bradycardia/sick sinus
  - ◊ Cardiovascular disease
  - ◊ Asthma/COPD
  - ◊ PUD
- Memantine (Namenda)
  - ◊ Agitation
  - ◊ Urinary incontinence
  - ◊ Diarrhea

Significant possible interactions:
- Antipsychotics: lithium may induce extrapyramidal symptoms and disorientation
- Tricyclic antidepressants (TCA): monoamine oxidase inhibitors should not be administered with TCA. Antipsychotic administration, cimetidine and estrogens may increase the TCA concentration.
- Benzodiazepines: increased serum phenytoin concentration. Cimetidine may increase the benzodiazepine concentration.
- Tacrine (Cognex): decrease theophylline dose by 50%. Use with caution with anticholinergic medications and NSAIDs.
- Serotonin reuptake inhibitors: do not use in combination with monoamine oxidase inhibitors; allow 6 weeks between stopping SSRI and starting MAO-I. May increase warfarin effect. Monitor lithium levels closely in those patients on lithium when a serotonin reuptake inhibitor is added.

ALTERNATIVE DRUGS
- Lithium carbonate
- Carbamazepine (Tegretol)
- Selegiline (Eldepryl)
- Divalproex (Depakote)

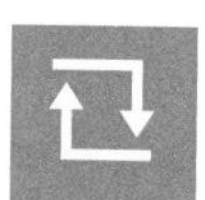

FOLLOWUP

PATIENT MONITORING
- Periodic mental status testing to assess progression and predict prognosis
- Periodic monitoring of nutritional status
- Periodic monitoring of the caregiver status to assess for caregiver stress
- Periodic assessment of the environment for safety
- Liver function tests with tacrine therapy

PREVENTION/AVOIDANCE N/A

POSSIBLE COMPLICATIONS
- Antipsychotic-induced extrapyramidal effects
- Falls
- Pressure sores
- Malnutrition
- Constipation
- Various infections

EXPECTED COURSE/PROGNOSIS
- AD - a progressive disease with variable rates of progression, but inevitably leading to profound cognitive impairment
- IVD - less likely to be progressive but cognitive improvement is unlikely
- Secondary dementias - treatment of the underlying condition may lead to improvement

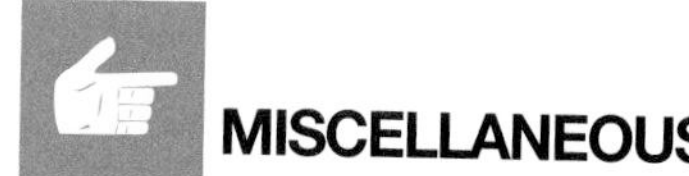

ASSOCIATED CONDITIONS
- Depression
- Insomnia

AGE-RELATED FACTORS
Pediatric: N/A

Geriatric:
- In the elderly, begin drugs with small doses and increase slowly
- Drugs with a long half-life (fluoxetine, lorazepam, etc.) require closer monitoring in the elderly; it may be better to choose a drug with a shorter half-life (sertraline, paroxetine, temazepam)

Others: N/A

PREGNANCY N/A

SYNONYMS Senility

ICD-9-CM
290.0 Senile dementia, uncomplicated
290.10 Presenile dementia, uncomplicated
290.40 Arteriosclerotic dementia, uncomplicated
331.0 Alzheimer disease

SEE ALSO
Alcohol use disorders
Alzheimer disease
Creutzfeldt-Jakob disease
Down syndrome
Huntington disease
Hypothyroidism, adult
Juvenile amaurotic familial idiocy
Parkinson disease
Pellagra
Pick disease
Stroke (Brain attack)
Syphilis
Wilson disease

OTHER NOTES N/A

ABBREVIATIONS
AD = Alzheimer dementia
IVD = ischemic vascular dementia
FTD = frontotemporal dementia
DLB = dementia with Lewy bodies

REFERENCES

- Diagnostic and Statistical Manual of Mental Disorders. 4th Ed., Washington, D.C., American Psychiatric Association, 1994
- Small GW, et al: Diagnosis and treatment of Alzheimer disease and related disorders: consensus statement of the American Association for Geriatric Psychiatry, the Alzheimer's Association, and the American Geriatrics Society. JAMA 1997;278(16):1363-1371

Web references: 8 available at www.5mcc.com

Illustrations N/A

Author(s):
Aubrey L. Knight, MD

BASICS

DESCRIPTION Depression is a primary mood disorder that is characterized by a depressed mood and/or a decrease in interest in things that used to give pleasure (anhedonia). It may have several accompanying symptoms and signs. It may accompany several different somatic and psychological illnesses. The etiology is multifactorial, but it is thought that depression is associated with changes in receptor-neurotransmitter relationship in the limbic system. Serotonin and norepinephrine are the primary neurotransmitters involved, but dopamine also has been related to depression. A family history of depression is a common finding.
- Bipolar disorder has a prominent depressive phase, but is a different clinical entity that is treated differently from depression

System(s) affected: Nervous
Genetics: Possible defect on chromosome II or X
Incidence/Prevalence in USA: Estimated that 5-20% of population will experience a significant depression at some time
Predominant age:
- Bipolar - mean, 30 years
- Unipolar - mean, 40 years

Predominant sex: Female > Male

SIGNS & SYMPTOMS
- Depressed mood
- Anhedonia
- Depression is probable when at least four of the following exist in addition to depressed mood or anhedonia:
  - ◊ Poor appetite - either weight gain or loss (may eat or drink out of boredom or reasons other than appetite)
  - ◊ Sleep disorder - either insomnia or hypersomnia
  - ◊ Fatigue - tiredness is out of proportion to the amount of energy expended
  - ◊ Psychomotor retardation or agitation (restlessness, irritability or withdrawal)
  - ◊ Poor self image - self reproach, excessive guilt
  - ◊ Difficulty in concentrating, poor memory, unable to make decisions
  - ◊ Suicidal ideation. Sometimes when people begin to recover they gain enough energy to think about and sometimes to attempt suicide.

CAUSES
- Impaired synthesis of the neurotransmitters
- Increased breakdown or metabolism of the neurotransmitters
- Increased pump uptake of the neurotransmitters. The action potential is passed on from neuron to neuron. Following this the neurotransmitter is (1) reabsorbed into the neuron where it is either destroyed by an enzyme or actively removed by a reuptake pump and stored until needed or (2) destroyed by monoamine oxidase (MAO) located in the mitochondria.
- Lack of these neurotransmitters causes certain types of depression, e.g., decreased norepinephrine causes dullness and lethargy, while decreased serotonin causes irritability, hostility and suicide ideation
- Environmental factors and learned behavior may effect neurotransmitters and/or have independent influence on depression
- Many life stresses and losses

RISK FACTORS
- Females more likely to develop depressive illness than males
- Strong family history (depression, suicide, alcoholism, other substance abuse)
- Presence of chronic disease, especially multiple diseases
- Migraine headaches
- Back pain
- Chronic pain
- Recent myocardial infarction
- Peptic ulcer disease
- Insomnia
- Stressful situations
- Adolescence
- Advancing age
- Retirement
- Children with behavioral disorders, especially hyperactivity
- Substance abuse
- Menopause
- Losses

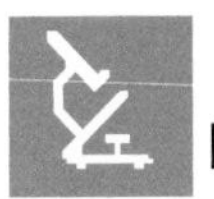

DIAGNOSIS

DIFFERENTIAL DIAGNOSIS
- Organic brain diseases
- Endocrine diseases, such as hypothyroid and hyperthyroid diseases
- Diabetes mellitus
- Liver failure
- Renal failure
- Malignancy
- Chronic fatigue syndrome
- Vitamin deficiency (pernicious anemia, pellagra)
- Medication side effects (many drugs cause or worsen depression)
- Medication overdose
- Medication abuse
- Withdrawal from medication
- Alcohol abuse
- Substance abuse
- Withdrawal from abused substance (alcohol, cocaine, marijuana)

LABORATORY Depression is a clinical diagnosis. Laboratory tests are used primarily to rule out other diagnoses.

Drugs that may alter lab results: All psychoactive drugs

Disorders that may alter lab results: Thyroid disease

PATHOLOGICAL FINDINGS N/A

SPECIAL TESTS
- ECG (diagnosis of arrhythmia, especially heart block)
- EEG (only if organic brain disease is suspected)

IMAGING CT or MRI of brain, if organic brain syndrome (OBS) included in differential

DIAGNOSTIC PROCEDURES
- Depression is primarily a clinical diagnosis that depends on skillfully eliciting family, social and psychosocial factors
- Validated standard rating scales can assist in identifying and following depressed patients
  - ◊ Zung Self-rating Depression Scale
  - ◊ BDI - Beck's Depression Inventory
  - ◊ CES-D Scale - Criteria for Epidemiologic Studies - Depression Scale
  - ◊ CDI - Children's Depression Inventory
  - ◊ Yesavage's Geriatric Depression Scale

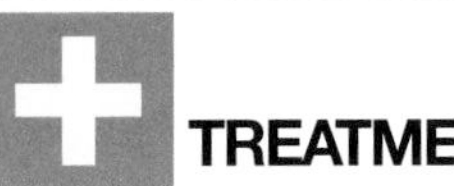

TREATMENT

APPROPRIATE HEALTH CARE Outpatient; inpatient care is indicated for seriously depressed or suicidal patients

GENERAL MEASURES
- Psychotherapeutic interventions act synergistically with pharmacologic therapy
- Psychotherapy alone is effective and appropriate for milder forms of depression
- Use the correct medication
- Use the correct dosage
- Use the correct medication long enough
- ECT can be very effective in refractory cases

SURGICAL MEASURES N/A

ACTIVITY No restrictions

DIET No special diet

PATIENT EDUCATION
- Carefully teach about medications
- Consider referral to support groups
- Stress need for long-term treatment and followup
- Recommend reading for patients, e.g., How to Cope With Depression by DePaulo and Ablow; Depression is a Treatable Illness: A Patient's Guide, AHCPR Publications Clearinghouse
- Contact local support groups through National Depression Manic Depression Association (DMDA) (800)82-MDMDA

MEDICATIONS

DRUG(S) OF CHOICE
All of the below listed medications are equally efficacious for depression. Selection is based on side effects profile.
- Polycyclic (mostly tricyclic [TCAs]) antidepressants with sedating properties (also have anticholinergic properties, potential for fatal overdose):
  - ◊ Amoxapine (Asendin) 50-400 mg/day in divided doses. Maximum hs dose 300 mg
  - ◊ Amitriptyline (Elavil, Endep) 150-300 mg/day qhs
  - ◊ Maprotiline (Ludiomil) 75-225 mg/day. Useful with associated anxiety.
  - ◊ Mirtazapine (Remeron) 15-45 mg/day at hs
  - ◊ Nortriptyline (Pamelor, Aventyl) 75-150 mg/day qhs (a metabolite of amitriptyline)
  - ◊ Doxepin (Adapin, Sinequan) 150-300 mg/day qhs
  - ◊ Trimipramine (Surmontil) 75-250 mg/day qhs
  - ◊ Trazodone (Desyrel) 150-300 mg/day qhs
- Polycyclic antidepressants with activating properties (also have anticholinergic properties, insomnia, anxiety, potentially fatal overdose):
  - ◊ Imipramine (Tofranil) 150-300 mg/day
  - ◊ Desipramine (Norpramin, Pertofrane) 150-300 mg/day
  - ◊ Protriptyline (Vivactil) 30-60 mg/day
- Selective serotonin reuptake inhibitors (can cause insomnia, anxiety, appetite suppression, sexual dysfunction [a common reason why patients discontinue their use]; overdose less likely to be fatal):
  - ◊ Fluoxetine (Prozac) 20 mg/day q am
  - ◊ Sertraline (Zoloft) 50-100 mg/day q am
  - ◊ Paroxetine (Paxil) 10-30 mg/day q am
  - ◊ Citalopram (Celexa) 20-40 mg q am
  - ◊ Escitalopram (Lexapro) 10-20 mg q am (metabolite of citalopram)
- Others:
  - ◊ Venlafaxine (Effexor) 75-100 mg/day in divided doses. Increases effective serotonin and norepinephrine; can cause insomnia, anxiety, anorexia).
  - ◊ Bupropion (Wellbutrin) 100-450 mg/day in divided doses (catecholamine reuptake inhibitor); seizure risk in higher doses, minimal risk of sexual dysfunction

Contraindications: Refer to manufacturer's profile of each drug

Precautions:
- Decrease beginning dose by half for children and elderly
- Fluoxetine, sertraline, paroxetine best given in the morning
- Polycyclic antidepressant prescriptions should initially be written for small total amounts to prevent suicide (TCAs fatal with doses > 1-1.5 gm in adults)
- TCAs may produce arrhythmias and lower seizure threshold
- Venlafaxine - allow approximately two weeks washout of other medications before instituting therapy with venlafaxine
- SSRIs - abrupt discontinuation may result in withdrawal symptoms

Significant possible interactions:
- Refer to manufacturer's profile of each drug
- Avoid nonprescription drugs containing pseudoephedrine, or phenylephrine (cold medicines)
- MAOI - serious hypertension a risk if prior use of SSRIs

ALTERNATIVE DRUGS
- Clomipramine (Anafranil) 100-250 mg/day (although primarily used to treat obsessive-compulsive disorder)
- Fluvoxamine (Luvox) 100-300 mg/day in divided doses. Indicated for obsessive-compulsive disorder.
- MAO inhibitors - significant drug and food interactions limit their use, but can be useful in refractory cases
- Hypericum perforatum (St. John's Wort) maybe useful in mild depression, avoid simultaneous use of SSRIs or MAO inhibitors

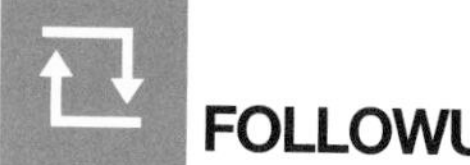

FOLLOWUP

PATIENT MONITORING
- See patient within 2 weeks after starting medication. The patient will probably not feel greatly improved at this visit.
- During followup visits evaluate side effects, dosage and effectiveness of the medication
- Follow about every 2 weeks until improvement begins. If treatment is adequate, the depression should improve within 4 weeks of initiating treatment.
- Follow every 3 months thereafter
- Explain to the patient that the treatment must continue even after improvement
- Plan to treat at least 6 months to 2 years. Longer in patients with family history of depression and the very young.
- The quality of the relationship (therapeutic alliance) between the patient and the health care professional is important in the overall success of treatment of depression

PREVENTION/AVOIDANCE
See Causes and Risk factors

POSSIBLE COMPLICATIONS
- Suicide
- Failure to improve

EXPECTED COURSE/PROGNOSIS
- This is one of the most rewarding conditions to treat because once you find the right drug, the right dose, and have a positive relationship with the patient, improvement is likely
- Anticipate recurrences

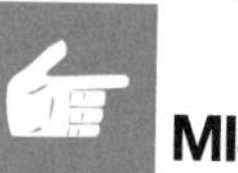

MISCELLANEOUS

ASSOCIATED CONDITIONS
- Manic depression (bipolar)
- Schizophrenia
- Schizo-affective disorders
- Psycho-physiological disorders
- Physical disorders
- Cyclothymic and grief reactions
- Alcoholism

AGE-RELATED FACTORS
Pediatric: Depression occurs in children
Geriatric: More common in elderly and difficult to precisely diagnose. Depression frequently coexists with dementia or delirium.
Others: N/A

PREGNANCY
Caution in using psychoactive medications in pregnancy. Rely on psychotherapy and support groups until pregnancy is completed.

SYNONYMS
Unipolar affective disorder

ICD-9-CM
311 Depressive disorder, not elsewhere classified
296.20 Major depressive disorder, single episode, unspecified
296.30 Major depressive disorder, recurrent episode, unspecified

SEE ALSO
Obsessive compulsive disorder
Postpartum depression

OTHER NOTES
- Depression is the fourth most common reason to visit the family physician
- Like so many other medical illnesses with psychological symptoms, family, doctors and patients tend to try to overlook this condition because they feel they should be able to control it themselves
- Attention deficit syndromes are being treated with antidepressants. They may be more effective than methylphenidate (Ritalin) or amphetamines.
- Bipolar disorder may first present as an episode of depression

ABBREVIATIONS
OBS = organic brain syndrome
TCA = tricyclic antidepressant
TSH = thyroid stimulating hormone

REFERENCES

- Diagnosis and Treatment (Quick Reference Guide for Clinicians; AHCPR publication 93-0552). Agency for Health Care Policy and Research Publications Clearinghouse, PO Box 8547, Silver Spring, MD
- Shearer SL, Adams GK. Nonpharmacologic aids in the treatment of depression. Am Fam Physician 1993;47(2):435-43

Web references: 3 available at www.5mcc.com
Illustrations N/A

Author(s):
Dannen D. Mannschreck, MD

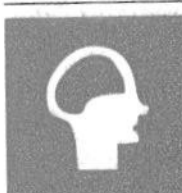

BASICS

DESCRIPTION Chronic pruritic eczematous condition affecting characteristic sites. Associated with family history of atopy (asthma, allergic rhinitis, atopic dermatitis).

System(s) affected: Skin/Exocrine

Genetics: Genetic predisposition - family history positive in two-thirds of cases

Incidence/Prevalence in USA: Common; increased since 1970

Predominant age: Mainly childhood disease. Affects 10% of all children, usually appearing in the first year of life and gradually subsiding over subsequent years.

Predominant sex: Male = Female (females tend to have somewhat worse prognosis)

SIGNS & SYMPTOMS

- Pruritus is the most common symptom
- Distribution of lesions
  - ◊ Infants - trunk, face, and extensor surfaces
  - ◊ Children - antecubital and popliteal fossae
  - ◊ Adults - face, neck, upper chest, and genital areas
  - ◊ In adults with limited distribution of lesions a history of childhood eczema is a clue to diagnosis
- Morphology of lesions
  - ◊ Infants - erythema and papules; may develop oozing, crusting vesicles
  - ◊ Children and adults - lichenification and scaling are typical with chronic eczema
  - ◊ Family history of atopic dermatitis may be more useful than morphology in making the diagnosis
- Associated features
  - ◊ Facial erythema, mild to moderate
  - ◊ Perioral pallor
  - ◊ Infraorbital fold (Dennie sign/Morgan line)
  - ◊ Dry skin
  - ◊ Increased palmar linear markings
  - ◊ Pityriasis alba (hypopigmented asymptomatic areas on face and shoulders)
  - ◊ Keratosis pilaris

CAUSES Unknown. Genetically determined, non-allergic disease.

RISK FACTORS

- Skin infections
- Emotional stress
- Irritating clothes and chemicals
- Excessively hot or cold climate
- Food allergy in children (controversial)
- Exposure to tobacco smoke

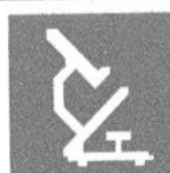

DIAGNOSIS

DIFFERENTIAL DIAGNOSIS

- Photosensitivity rashes
- Contact dermatitis (especially if only the face is involved)
- Scabies
- Seborrheic dermatitis (especially in infants)
- Psoriasis or lichen simplex chronicus if only localized disease is present in adults
- Rare conditions of infancy: histiocytosis X, Wiskott-Aldrich syndrome, ataxia-telangiectasia syndrome
- Ichthyosis vulgaris

LABORATORY Serum IgE levels are frequently elevated

Drugs that may alter lab results: N/A

Disorders that may alter lab results: N/A

PATHOLOGICAL FINDINGS Epidermis is thickened and hyperkeratotic. Dermis shows perivascular inflammation.

SPECIAL TESTS None

IMAGING None

DIAGNOSTIC PROCEDURES Skin biopsy shows nonspecific eczematous changes. (Biopsy is rarely required since diagnosis is made on clinical grounds.)

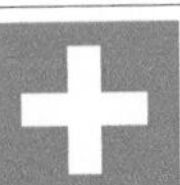

TREATMENT

APPROPRIATE HEALTH CARE Generally outpatient, using topical corticosteroids

GENERAL MEASURES

- Decrease stress if possible
- Avoid agents that may cause irritation (e.g., wool, perfumes)
- Minimize sweating
- Lukewarm (not hot) baths
- Minimize use of soap (superfatted soaps best)
- Frequent systemic lubrication with thick emollient creams (eg, Eucerin) over moist skin
- Sun exposure may be helpful
- Humidify the house
- Avoid excessive contact with water
- Avoid lotions that contain alcohol

SURGICAL MEASURES N/A

ACTIVITY No restrictions

DIET There is controversy regarding the role of food allergies and exacerbations of atopic dermatitis. The most common suspicious foods are eggs, milk, wheat and peanuts. Consider elimination diets (e.g., for 3-4 weeks) and food challenges. Also consider delaying introduction of the common suspicious foods until an infant is 6 months old.

PATIENT EDUCATION

- Goal is control, not cure (although many patients will outgrow their disease)
- See: www.niams.nih.gov/hi/topics/dermatitis

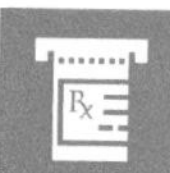

MEDICATIONS

DRUG(S) OF CHOICE

- Topical steroids achieve good control in 90% of patients
- In infants and children, use 0.5-1% topical hydrocortisone creams or ointments
- In adults, may use higher potency (over 1%) topical corticosteroids in areas other than face and skin folds
- Use short courses of higher potency corticosteroids for flares, then return to the lowest potency (creams preferred) that will control dermatitis

Contraindications: None

Precautions: Beware that chronic potent fluorinated corticosteroids use may cause striae or atrophy, especially in children. High potency topical corticosteroids may produce systemic effects if used for prolonged periods.

Significant possible interactions: None

ALTERNATIVE DRUGS

- Topical immunomodulators (tacrolimus or pimecrolimus) are 2nd line agents for episodic use for children over age 2
- Antihistamines for pruritus (e.g., hydroxyzine, 10-25 mg at bedtime and prn)
- Plastic occlusion - in combination with topical medication, this promotes absorption
- For severe atopic dermatitis, consider systemic steroids for 1-2 weeks, e.g., prednisone 2 mg/kg/day po (max 80 mg) initially, tapered over 7-14 days.
- Topical tricyclic doxepin as a 5% cream may decrease pruritus
- Evening primrose oil, includes high content of fatty acids, believed to decrease prostaglandin synthesis, believed to promote conversion of linoleic acid to omega-6 fatty acid
- Modified Goeckerman regimen (tar + UV light)
- Immune modifiers (methotrexate, azathioprine, cyclosporine)

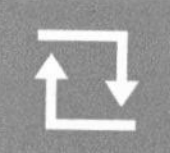

FOLLOWUP

PATIENT MONITORING Individualize, depending on severity of disease

PREVENTION/AVOIDANCE

- Smallpox vaccine should be avoided because of risk of eczema herpeticum (see Possible Complications)

POSSIBLE COMPLICATIONS

- Cataracts are more common in patients with atopic dermatitis
- Skin infections (usually *Staphylococcus aureus*); sometimes subclinical
- Eczema herpeticum - generalized vesiculopustular eruption caused by infection with herpes simplex or vaccinia virus. Patients are acutely ill and require hospitalization.
- Atrophy and/or striae if fluorinated corticosteroids are used on face or skin folds
- Systemic absorption may occur if large areas of skin are treated, particularly if high-potency medications and occlusion are combined

EXPECTED COURSE/PROGNOSIS

- Chronic disease that tends to burn out with age. 90% of patients have spontaneous resolution by puberty.
- Some adults may continue to have localized eczema, e.g., chronic hand or foot dermatitis, eyelid dermatitis, or lichen simplex chronicus

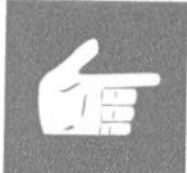

MISCELLANEOUS

ASSOCIATED CONDITIONS

- Asthma
- Allergic rhinitis
- Hyper-IgE syndrome (Job syndrome) which is characterized by atopic dermatitis, elevated IgE, recurrent pyodermas, and decreased chemotaxis of mononuclear cells

AGE-RELATED FACTORS

Pediatric: More frequent
Geriatric: Relatively rare
Others: N/A

PREGNANCY N/A

SYNONYMS

- Eczema
- Disseminated neurodermatitis
- Atopic eczema
- Atopic neurodermatitis
- Constitutional dermatitis
- Besnier prurigo

ICD-9-CM

691.8 Other atopic dermatitis and related conditions

SEE ALSO

OTHER NOTES If very resistant to treatment, search for a coexisting contact dermatitis

ABBREVIATIONS N/A

REFERENCES

- Duarte AM, Schachner LA. Atopic dermatitis. In: Hoekelam RA, ed. Primary Pediatric Care. 4th ed. St. Louis: Mosby; 2001
- Tofte SJ, Hanifin JM. Current management and therapy of atopic dermatitis. J Am Acad Dermatol 2001;44(1 Suppl):S13-6
- Eichenfield LF, Hanifin JM, Luger TA, et al. Consensus conference on pediatric atopic dermatitis. J Am Acad Dermatol 2003;49(6):1088-95

Web references: 2 available at www.5mcc.com
Illustrations 19 available

Author(s):
Dennis E. Hughes, DO

BASICS

DESCRIPTION The cutaneous reaction to an external substance
- Primary irritant dermatitis (80%) is due to direct injury of the skin. It affects individuals exposed to specific irritants and generally produces discomfort immediately after exposure.
- Allergic contact dermatitis (ACD) (20%) affects only individuals previously sensitized to the contactant. It represents a delayed hypersensitivity reaction, requiring several hours for the cascade of cellular immunity to be completed to manifest itself.

System(s) affected: Skin/Exocrine
Genetics: Increased frequency of ACD in families with allergies
Incidence/Prevalence in USA: Contact dermatitis represents > 90% of all occupational skin disorders
Predominant age: All ages
Predominant sex: Male = Female. Variations due to differences in exposure to offending agents as well as normal cutaneous variations between male and female (eccrine and sebaceous gland function and hair distribution).

SIGNS & SYMPTOMS
- Acute
  - ◊ Papules, vesicles, bullae with surrounding erythema
  - ◊ Crusting and oozing may be present
  - ◊ Pruritus
- Chronic
  - ◊ Erythematous base
  - ◊ Thickening with lichenification
  - ◊ Scaling
  - ◊ Fissuring
- Distribution
  - ◊ Where epidermis is thinner (eyelids, genitalia)
  - ◊ Areas of contact with offending agent (e.g., nail polish)
  - ◊ Palms and soles more resistant
  - ◊ Deeper skin-folds spared
  - ◊ Linear arrays of lesions
  - ◊ Lesions with sharp borders and sharp angles - pathognomonic

CAUSES
- Plants
  - ◊ Rhus-urushiol (poison ivy, oak, sumac)
  - ◊ Primary contact - plant (roots/stems/leaves)
  - ◊ Secondary contact - clothes/fingernails (not blister fluid)
- Chemicals
  - ◊ Nickel - jewelry, zippers, hooks, watches
  - ◊ Potassium dichromate - tanning agent in leather
  - ◊ Paraphenylenediamine - hair dyes, fur dyes, industrial chemicals
  - ◊ Turpentine - cleaning agents, polishes, waxes
  - ◊ Soaps, detergents
- Topical medicines
  - ◊ Neomycin - topical antibiotics
  - ◊ Thimerosal (Merthiolate) - preservative in topical medications
  - ◊ Anesthetics - benzocaine
  - ◊ Parabens - preservative in topical medications
  - ◊ Formalin - cosmetics, shampoos, nail enamel

RISK FACTORS
- Occupation
- Hobbies
- Travel
- Cosmetics
- Jewelry

DIAGNOSIS

DIFFERENTIAL DIAGNOSIS
- Based on clinical impression - appearance, periodicity, localization
- Groups of vesicles - herpes simplex
- Diffuse bullous or vesicular lesions - bullous pemphigoid
- Photo-distribution - phototoxic/allergic reaction to systemic allergen
- Eyelids - seborrheic dermatitis
- Scaly eczematous lesions - atopic dermatitis, nummular eczema, lichen simplex chronicus, stasis dermatitis, xerosis

LABORATORY N/A

Drugs that may alter lab results: N/A

Disorders that may alter lab results: N/A

PATHOLOGICAL FINDINGS
- Intercellular edema
- Bullae

SPECIAL TESTS Patch tests for allergic contact dermatitis (systemic corticosteroids or recent, aggressive use of topical steroids may alter results)

IMAGING N/A

DIAGNOSTIC PROCEDURES Patch test

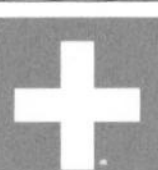

TREATMENT

APPROPRIATE HEALTH CARE Outpatient

GENERAL MEASURES
- Removal of offending agent
- Topical soaks with cool tap water, Burow's solution (1:40 dilution), or saline (1 tsp/pint water), or silver nitrate solution
- Lukewarm water baths - antipruritic
- Aveeno (oatmeal) baths
- Chronic - emollients (white petrolatum, Eucerin)

SURGICAL MEASURES N/A

ACTIVITY Stay active, but avoid overheating

DIET No special diet

PATIENT EDUCATION
- Avoidance of irritating substance
- Cleaning of secondary sources (nails, clothes)
- Fallacy of blister fluid spreading disease

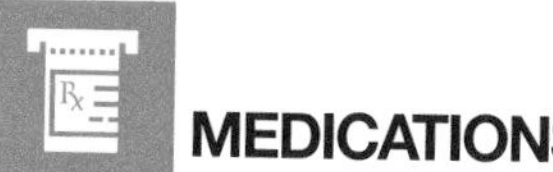

MEDICATIONS

DRUG(S) OF CHOICE

- Topical
  - ◊ Shake lotion of zinc oxide, talc, menthol 0.25%, phenol 0.5%
  - ◊ Corticosteroids: high potency steroids, fluocinonide (Lidex) 0.05% ointment 3-4 times daily. Caution regarding face/skinfolds - use lower potency steroids and avoid prolonged usage. Switch to lower potency topical steroid once acute phase resolved. Avoid prolonged use.
  - ◊ Calamine lotion
  - ◊ Topical antibiotics for secondary infection (bacitracin, gentamicin, erythromycin)
- Systemic
  - ◊ Antihistamine: hydroxyzine 25-50 mg qid, diphenhydramine 25-50 mg qid
  - ◊ Corticosteroids: prednisone. Taper starting at 60-80 mg/d, tapered over 10-14 days.
  - ◊ Antibiotics: erythromycin 250 mg qid if secondarily infected
  - ◊ Dicloxacillin 250 mg po qid for 7-10 days or amoxicillin-clavulanate (Augmentin) 500 mg po bid for 7-10 days for secondary bacterial infection

Contraindications: N/A

Precautions:

- Drowsiness from antihistamines
- Local skin effects: atrophy, stria, telangiectasia from prolonged use of potent topical steroids

Significant possible interactions: N/A

ALTERNATIVE DRUGS

Other topical antibiotics depending on organisms and sensitivity

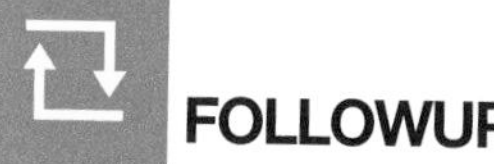

FOLLOWUP

PATIENT MONITORING

- As necessary for recurrence
- Patch testing for etiology after resolved

PREVENTION/AVOIDANCE

Avoid causative agents. Use of protective gloves (with cotton lining) may be helpful.

POSSIBLE COMPLICATIONS

- Generalized eruption secondary to autosensitization
- Secondary bacterial infection

EXPECTED COURSE/PROGNOSIS

Self-limited, benign

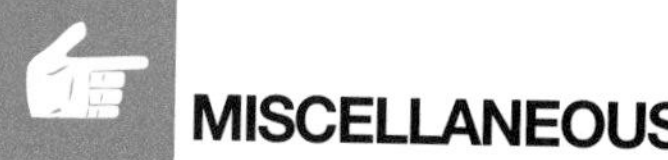

MISCELLANEOUS

ASSOCIATED CONDITIONS

N/A

AGE-RELATED FACTORS

Pediatric: Younger individuals - increased incidence of positive patch testing due to better delayed hypersensitivity reactions

Geriatric: Increased incidence of irritant dermatitis secondary to skin dryness

Others: N/A

PREGNANCY

Usual cautions with medications

SYNONYMS

Dermatitis venenata

ICD-9-CM

692.0 Contact dermatitis and other eczema due to detergents

692.9 Contact dermatitis and other eczema due to unspecified cause

SEE ALSO

OTHER NOTES

N/A

ABBREVIATIONS

ACD = allergic contact dermatitis

REFERENCES

- Bondi E, Jegasothy B, Lazarus G. Dermatology, Diagnosis and Therapy. Norwalk, CT: Appleton & Lange; 1992
- Abel E, Farber E. Scientific American Inc., New York, 1985

Web references: 3 available at www.5mcc.com

Illustrations 32 available

Author(s):

Aamir Siddiqi, MD

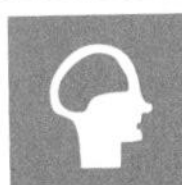

BASICS

DESCRIPTION Diaper dermatitis is a rash occurring under the covered area of a diaper. The rash may be an irritant contact dermatitis, candidiasis, atopic dermatitis or seborrheic dermatitis.
System(s) affected: Skin/Exocrine
Genetics: N/A
Incidence/Prevalence in USA: Common
Predominant age: Infants; highest incidence 9-12 months
Predominant sex: Male = Female

SIGNS & SYMPTOMS
- Irritant contact diaper dermatitis
  - ◊ Prominent rash on buttocks and pubic skin
  - ◊ Creases of skin are relatively spared
  - ◊ Rash is dusky red and shiny
  - ◊ Skin seems chapped
  - ◊ Weeping, crusting, and excoriations are not prominent
- Candidiasis diaper rash
  - ◊ Initial involvement of creases with rapid extension
  - ◊ Color: bright red
  - ◊ Accompanying edema
  - ◊ Isolated satellite papules and pustules at margins of inflammatory plaques
  - ◊ Excoriations are prominent
  - ◊ Positive KOH preparation
  - ◊ Positive cultures
- Atopic diaper dermatitis
  - ◊ Distribution spares creases
  - ◊ Genitalia frequently involved
  - ◊ Itch-scratch cycle with excoriations are prominent
  - ◊ Child scratches vigorously at night
  - ◊ Weeping, crusting, excoriations sometimes present; secondary bacterial infection can occur
- Seborrheic diaper dermatitis
  - ◊ Dusky-red patches and plaques deep within skin creases
  - ◊ Non-intertriginous skin is relatively spared
  - ◊ Weeping, crusting, excoriations - not prominent
  - ◊ Other sites of seborrheic dermatitis are frequently present: retroauricular, axillary folds, scalp

CAUSES Irritation to skin from prolonged contact with urine or feces

RISK FACTORS
- Infrequent diaper changes
- Waterproof diapers
- Improper laundering
- Family history of dermatitis
- Hot, humid weather
- Recent treatment with oral antibiotics
- Diarrhea

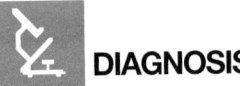

DIAGNOSIS

DIFFERENTIAL DIAGNOSIS
- Contact dermatitis
- Seborrheic dermatitis
- Candidiasis
- Atopic dermatitis
- Scabies
- Acrodermatitis enteropathica
- Letterer-Siwe disease
- Congenital syphilis
- Child abuse
- Streptococcal infection
- Kawasaki disease
- Biotin deficiency
- Psoriasis

LABORATORY Culture will reveal candida, if present

Drugs that may alter lab results: N/A

Disorders that may alter lab results: N/A

PATHOLOGICAL FINDINGS Varying inflammation is the most prominent finding

SPECIAL TESTS
- KOH preparation
- Culture pustules if present

IMAGING N/A

DIAGNOSTIC PROCEDURES
- Culture lesions
- KOH preparation

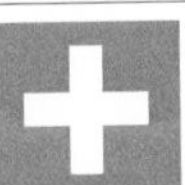

TREATMENT

APPROPRIATE HEALTH CARE Outpatient

GENERAL MEASURES
- Expose the buttocks to air as much as possible
- Don't use waterproof pants during treatment - day or night. They keep skin wet and subject to rash or infection.
- Change diapers frequently - even at night if the rash is extensive
- Super absorbable diapers beneficial
- Discontinue using baby lotion, powder, ointment or baby oil (except zinc oxide)
- Zinc oxide ointment or other barrier cream to the rash at the earliest sign of diaper rash, and 2 or 3 times a day thereafter (apply to clean, thoroughly dry skin)
- Use mild soap and pat dry

SURGICAL MEASURES N/A

ACTIVITY Protect from overheating

DIET No special diet

PATIENT EDUCATION N/A

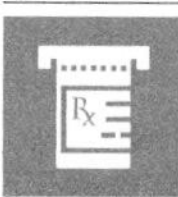

MEDICATIONS

DRUG(S) OF CHOICE

- If candidiasis suspected or diaper rash persistent, use antifungal such as miconazole nitrate 2% cream, miconazole powder, econazole (Spectazole), clotrimazole (Lotrimin), or ketoconazole (Nizoral) cream, at each diaper change.
- If inflammation is prominent, consider very low potency steroid cream, such as hydrocortisone 0.5-1% tid along with an antifungal cream or and combination product such as clioquinol-hydrocortisone (Vioform-Hydrocortisone) cream
- If a secondary bacterial infection is suspected, use an anti-Staphylococcal oral antibiotic or mupirocin (Bactroban) ointment topically

Contraindications: N/A

Precautions: Avoid high or moderate potency steroids often found in combination steroid-antifungal mixtures

Significant possible interactions: N/A

ALTERNATIVE DRUGS
Sucralfate paste for resistant cases

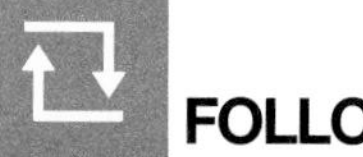

FOLLOWUP

PATIENT MONITORING
Recheck weekly until clear, then at times of recurrence

PREVENTION/AVOIDANCE
See General Measures

POSSIBLE COMPLICATIONS

- Secondary bacterial infection
- Secondary yeast infection

EXPECTED COURSE/PROGNOSIS
Quick complete clearing with appropriate treatment

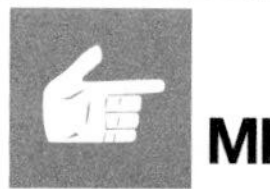

MISCELLANEOUS

ASSOCIATED CONDITIONS

- Contact (allergic or irritant) dermatitis
- Seborrheic dermatitis
- Psoriasis
- Candidiasis
- Atopic dermatitis

AGE-RELATED FACTORS
Pediatric: Problem most common in this age group

Geriatric: Incontinence

Others: N/A

PREGNANCY
N/A

SYNONYMS

- Diaper rash

ICD-9-CM
691.0 Diaper or napkin rash

SEE ALSO
Candidiasis

Dermatitis, atopic

Dermatitis, contact

Psoriasis

OTHER NOTES
Two or more types of diaper dermatitis can exist concomitantly. If so, treat each accordingly.

ABBREVIATIONS
N/A

REFERENCES

- Dershewitz R, editor. Ambulatory Pediatric Care. 3rd ed. Philadelphia: Lippincott-Raven; 1999
- Liptak GS. Diaper rash. In: Hoekelam RA, editor. Primary Pediatric Care. 4th ed. St. Louis: Mosby; 2001
- Kazaks EL, Lane AT. Diaper dermatitis. Pediatr Clin North Am 2000;47(4):909-19

Web references: 1 available at www.5mcc.com

Illustrations N/A

Author(s):
Dennis E. Hughes, DO

BASICS

DESCRIPTION A generalized scaling eruption of the skin, either idiopathic in nature or secondary to underlying cutaneous or systemic disease
System(s) affected: Skin/Exocrine
Genetics: No known genetic pattern
Incidence/Prevalence in USA: Rare; estimated 1% of hospitalizations for skin disease
Predominant age: 75% of patients are over age 40
Predominant sex: Male > Female (2:1)

SIGNS & SYMPTOMS
- Fine generalized scales with mild erythema and lichenification of skin
- With acute onset and in early stages of exudative dermatitis, may have thin epidermis, erythema, and exudation with subsequent development of crusting
- Initial distribution is that of any underlying cutaneous disease, Subsequently, as exfoliative dermatitis further develops, this distribution is lost and the scaling is generalized.
- With no underlying cutaneous disease, the distribution initially favors the genital region, trunk, and head before generalizing
- Sensation of skin tightness
- Nail dystrophy
- Hair loss, with alopecia in up to 25%
- Pruritus
- Fever in 40-50%
- Chills
- Malaise/weakness
- Mucous membranes spared
- Anemia (both microcytic and macrocytic) in up to 65%
- Eosinophilia (30%)
- Nontender generalized lymphadenopathy
- Steatorrhea
- Hepatomegaly in 20-35%
- Splenomegaly when underlying lymphoma/leukemia present
- Gynecomastia
- Hypoproteinemia
- Dehydration
- High output cardiac failure
- Tachycardia
- Lymphadenopathy in 60% or more
- Hyper/hypopigmented areas of the skin

CAUSES
- Idiopathic in up to 20% or more of cases
- Up to 80% may occur in response to one of the following:
  - ◊ Atopic dermatitis
  - ◊ Colon carcinoma
  - ◊ Contact dermatitis (5-10%)
  - ◊ Drug eruptions (14%)
  - ◊ Fungal disease with id reaction
  - ◊ HIV infection
  - ◊ Ichthyosiform dermatoses
  - ◊ Leukemia
  - ◊ Lichen planus
  - ◊ Lung carcinoma
  - ◊ Lymphoma - 15% of cases overall and 35-50% of patients over age 40
  - ◊ Medications - sulfonamides and sulfones, penicillins, cephalosporins, anticonvulsants, NSAIDs, codeine, heavy metals, INH, quinidine, captopril, iodine, antimalarials, Phenothiazines, methotrexate
  - ◊ Multiple myeloma
  - ◊ Mycosis fungoides
  - ◊ Pemphigus foliaceus
  - ◊ Photosensitivity reaction
  - ◊ Pityriasis rosea
  - ◊ Pityriasis rubra pilaris
  - ◊ Psoriasis
  - ◊ Pyoderma with id reaction
  - ◊ Reiter syndrome
  - ◊ Scabies
  - ◊ Seborrheic dermatitis
  - ◊ Sézary syndrome
  - ◊ Staphylococcal scalded skin syndrome
  - ◊ Stasis dermatitis
  - ◊ Systemic lupus erythematosus
  - ◊ Toxic epidermal necrolysis

RISK FACTORS
- Underlying diseases as noted above
- Male sex
- Age greater than 40

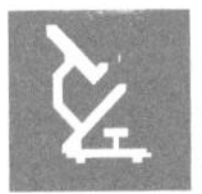

DIAGNOSIS

DIFFERENTIAL DIAGNOSIS Acutely eczematous dermatoses such as contact dermatitis and drug eruptions should be considered

LABORATORY None diagnostic. May have elevated WBC with eosinophilia, anemia, elevated ESR, decreased albumin and electrolyte abnormalities

Drugs that may alter lab results: N/A

Disorders that may alter lab results: N/A

PATHOLOGICAL FINDINGS May have characteristics of the underlying cutaneous disease. Other changes are nonspecific: Hyperkeratosis, parakeratosis, acanthosis in the epidermis; and edema, vasodilation, perivascular infiltrates with lymphocytes, histiocytes, and eosinophils in the dermis.

SPECIAL TESTS None

IMAGING Chest x-ray and other imaging procedures as indicated to investigate any underlying disease process

DIAGNOSTIC PROCEDURES
- Careful history and physical exam
- Skin biopsy; lymph node biopsy and bone marrow biopsy as indicated to investigate an underlying disease process

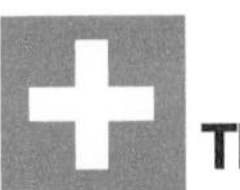

TREATMENT

APPROPRIATE HEALTH CARE Outpatient except in those cases with complications of secondary infection, dehydration, or heart failure

GENERAL MEASURES
- Withdrawal of any implicated medications or treatment of any identified underlying infection/disease
- Protection from development of hypothermia
- Cool colloid baths with oatmeal (Aveeno) - 1 cup in 10 inches (25.4 cm) water
- Local moisturizing ointments/lotions

SURGICAL MEASURES N/A

ACTIVITY As tolerated

DIET
- High protein. Increased fluid intake should be encouraged in those with more extensive skin involvement.
- Watch for folate iron deficiency in chronic cases

PATIENT EDUCATION
- Patients should avoid any identified etiologic agents
- Patients with underlying diseases that have caused exfoliative dermatitis can be educated regarding symptomatic treatment of the dermatitis and be advised that successful treatment of the underlying disease will usually also be successful for the exfoliative dermatitis
- Protection against hypothermia and dehydration and identification of signs of infection should be part of the education process
- Advise those patients, without an identified cause for the exfoliative dermatitis, that many cases spontaneously remit (exact number uncertain) and that medical therapy to control symptoms can be provided
- American Academy of Dermatology (708)330-0230

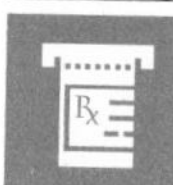

MEDICATIONS

DRUG(S) OF CHOICE
- Systemic corticosteroids initial dosage equivalent to prednisone 40 mg/day with increases in dosage by 20 mg/day if there is no response after 3-4 days at a given dose. Subsequently, dosage should be tapered to control symptoms.
- In addition, treatment specific to any underlying infection or disease should be provided

Contraindications: Psoriasis as the underlying cause of the exfoliative dermatitis
Precautions:
- Atopic dermatitis and seborrheic dermatitis as underlying causes
- Avoid coal tar treatment except with psoriasis, and then only use after 24-48 hours of hydration therapy

Significant possible interactions: Refer to manufacturer's literature

ALTERNATIVE DRUGS
- Antihistamines can be useful for pruritus and topical steroids can be used for more localized disease
- When psoriasis is the underlying cause, cyclosporine, methotrexate, etretinate, phototherapy, or other treatments specific to this disease should be provided
- Photochemotherapy may be useful therapy for treating exfoliative dermatitis associated with mycosis fungoides
- Isotretinoin has been used when pityriasis rubra pilaris is the underlying cause
- Antibiotic or antifungal therapy as indicated for superinfection

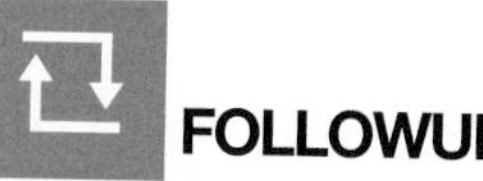

FOLLOWUP

PATIENT MONITORING Patients should be monitored for response to therapy, development of complications, and for adverse effects related to therapy

PREVENTION/AVOIDANCE Known or suspected etiologic agents should be avoided

POSSIBLE COMPLICATIONS
- Infection
- Hypothermia
- Dehydration/electrolyte disturbances
- Heart failure
- Bacterial/fungal superinfection

EXPECTED COURSE/PROGNOSIS
- In patients with an identified underlying cause, the course and prognosis will parallel the primary disease
- For patients with idiopathic exfoliative dermatitis, the prognosis is poor with frequent recurrences or chronic symptoms requiring chronic steroid therapy

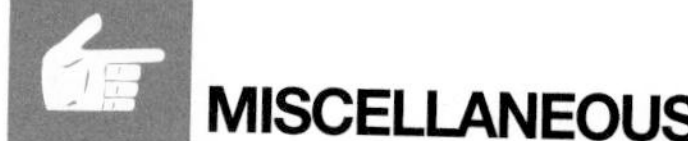

MISCELLANEOUS

ASSOCIATED CONDITIONS Any of the infections or diseases listed under causes

AGE-RELATED FACTORS
Pediatric: Less common, but may occur, associated with atopic dermatitis medications or the inherited dermatoses
Geriatric: N/A
Others: N/A

PREGNANCY N/A

SYNONYMS
- Erythroderma
- Pityriasis rubra

ICD-9-CM
695.89 Other specified erythematous conditions, other

SEE ALSO

OTHER NOTES N/A

ABBREVIATIONS N/A

REFERENCES

- Fitzpatrick TB, et al, editors. Dermatology In General Medicine. 5th ed. New York: McGraw-Hill; 1999
- Rothe MJ, Bialy TL, Grant-Kels JM. Erythroderma. Dermatol Clin 2000;18(3):405-15
- Domonkos AN, Arnold HL, Odom RB. Andrews' Diseases of the Skin. 9th ed. Philadelphia: WB Saunders Co; 2000
- Sauer GC. Manual of Skin Diseases. 8th ed. Philadelphia: JB Lippincott Co; 2000

Web references: 1 available at www.5mcc.com
Illustrations 4 available

Author(s):
Mitchell S. King, MD

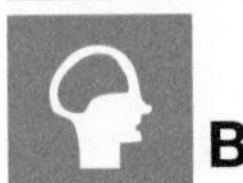

BASICS

DESCRIPTION Dermatitis herpetiformis is an intensely pruritic papulovesicular disease on extensor skin surfaces
System(s) affected: Skin/Exocrine
Genetics: High incidence of HLA B8/Dw3
Incidence/Prevalence in USA: Uncommon. Prevalence not known and most likely varies with the race and ethnicity of the population studied.
Predominant age: 15-60, mean age of onset is in the fourth decade
Predominant sex: Male > Female (1.5:1)

SIGNS & SYMPTOMS
- Symmetrical intensely pruritic, papulovesicular eruption
- Elbows and extensor forearms are the most common site of involvement
- Buttocks, knees, upper back, posterior neck and scalp also frequent
- Oral lesions infrequent
- Secondary excoriations may be prominent
- Burning or stinging feeling may be prominent

CAUSES Unknown

RISK FACTORS
- Gluten-sensitive enteropathy
- Family history of dermatitis herpetiformis

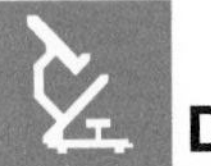

DIAGNOSIS

DIFFERENTIAL DIAGNOSIS
- Scabies
- Erythema multiforme
- Bullous pemphigoid
- Linear IgA disease
- Transient acantholytic dermatosis
- Subcorneal pustular dermatosis
- Erythema elevatum diutinum
- Papular urticaria
- Eczema
- Tinea corporis
- Excoriations

LABORATORY Abnormal thyroid function tests may occur

Drugs that may alter lab results:
- Thyroid
- Steroids

Disorders that may alter lab results: N/A

PATHOLOGICAL FINDINGS
- Papillary dermal neutrophilic microabscesses
- Subepidermal vesicles

SPECIAL TESTS Direct immunofluorescence reveals granular IgA deposition in the dermal papilla

IMAGING Thyroid scan if indicated by physical exam

DIAGNOSTIC PROCEDURES
- Skin biopsy
- IgA anti-endomysial antibodies

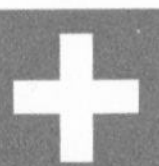

TREATMENT

APPROPRIATE HEALTH CARE Outpatient

GENERAL MEASURES No special measures

SURGICAL MEASURES N/A

ACTIVITY Fully active

DIET Clinical improvement occurs with gluten-free diet

PATIENT EDUCATION
- Contact American Academy of Dermatology, 930 N. Meacham Rd., P.O. Box 4014, Schaumberg, IL 60168-4014, (708)330-0230
- Gluten Intolerance Group of North America, 15110 10th Av. SW, Suite A, Seattle, WA 98166-1820; 206-246-6652, fax 206-246-6531; website www.gluten.net

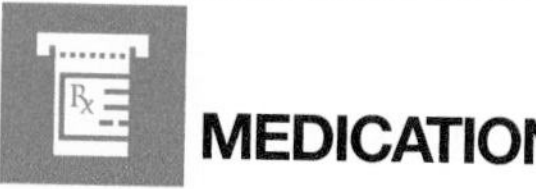

MEDICATIONS

DRUG(S) OF CHOICE Dapsone 50 mg per day will usually improve symptoms within 24 to 48 hours in adults. Average maintenance dose is 25 to 200 mg per day.

Contraindications: See manufacturer's profile of each drug

Precautions:

- Side effects of dapsone include:
  - ◊ Hemolytic anemia
  - ◊ Methemoglobinemia
  - ◊ Toxic hepatitis
  - ◊ Cholestatic jaundice
  - ◊ Hypoalbuminemia
  - ◊ Sensory and motor neuropathy
  - ◊ Psychosis
  - ◊ Infectious mononucleosis syndrome with fever and lymphadenopathy
  - ◊ Agranulocytosis
  - ◊ Aplastic anemia
  - ◊ Exfoliative dermatitis
  - ◊ Erythema multiforme
  - ◊ Erythema nodosum
  - ◊ Urticaria
  - ◊ Dapsone is secreted in breast milk and will produce hemolytic anemia in infants
  - ◊ Dapsone will produce a severe hemolytic anemia in patients with glucose-6-phosphate dehydrogenase (G6PD) deficiency

Significant possible interactions: See manufacturer's profile of each drug

ALTERNATIVE DRUGS Sulfapyridine, colchicine, prednisone, tetracycline plus nicotinamide, cyclosporin, systemic steroids, topical steroids

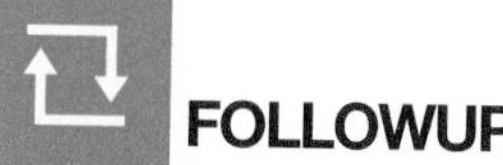

FOLLOWUP

PATIENT MONITORING

- Baseline CBC and liver function studies should be obtained
- G6PD should be quantified in Asians, blacks and those of southern Mediterranean descent
- CBC should be checked weekly for first month, monthly for the next five months and semi-annually thereafter
- Chemistry profile should be checked every six months
- Patient should be made aware of potential hemolytic anemia and the blue-gray discoloration associated with methemoglobinemia

PREVENTION/AVOIDANCE N/A

POSSIBLE COMPLICATIONS N/A

EXPECTED COURSE/PROGNOSIS

- Patients respond dramatically to dapsone
- Strict adherence to a gluten-free diet will produce improvement of clinical symptoms and a decrease in dapsone requirement in the majority of patients
- Occasional new lesions (2-3 per week) are to be expected and are not an indication for altering daily dosage

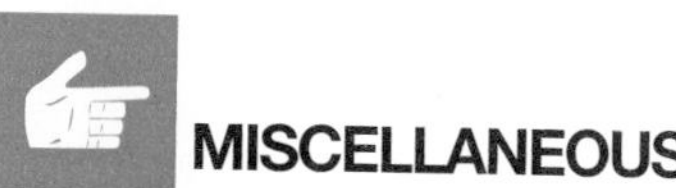

MISCELLANEOUS

ASSOCIATED CONDITIONS

- Gluten-sensitive enteropathy
- Hyperthyroidism
- Hypothyroidism
- Thyroid nodules
- Multi-nodular goiter
- Thyroid carcinoma
- Pernicious anemia
- Gastrointestinal lymphoma
- Glomerulopathy
- Immunologic disorders including systemic lupus erythematosus, Addison disease, rheumatoid arthritis, ulcerative colitis, Raynaud phenomenon, atopy, Sjögren syndrome, vitiligo, and dermatomyositis have been reported to be associated with dermatitis herpetiformis

AGE-RELATED FACTORS

Pediatric: Dapsone dose must be adjusted
Geriatric: N/A
Others: N/A

PREGNANCY Data is inconclusive but suggests that dapsone is safe during pregnancy. It is recommended that adherence to a strict gluten-free diet, preferably for 6-12 months before conception be instituted in the hope of eliminating the need for dapsone during pregnancy.

SYNONYMS Duhring disease

ICD-9-CM

694.0 Dermatitis herpetiformis

SEE ALSO

Sjögren syndrome

OTHER NOTES N/A

ABBREVIATIONS N/A

REFERENCES

- Leonard J. Management of dermatitis herpetiformis. Clin & Exp Dermatol 2002;27(4)328
- Enta T, Adams SP. Dermacase. Dermatitis herpetiformis. Can Fam Physician 2000;46:2199, 2211
- Kosann MK. Dermatitis herpetiformis. Dermatol Online J 2003;9(4):8
- Lovett W. Dermatitis herpetiformis and a gluten-free diet. Am Fam Physician 2003;67(3):470
- McCleskey PE, Erickson QL, David-Bajar KM, Elston DM. Palmar petechiae in dermatitis herpetiformis: a case report and clinical review. Cutis 2002;70(4):217-23
- Bickle K, Roark TR, Hsu S. Autoimmune bullous dermatoses: a review. Am Fam Physician 2002;65(9):1861-70
- Porter WM, Dawe SA, Bunker CB. Dermatitis herpetiformis and cutaneous T-cell lymphoma. Clin & Exp Dermatol 2001;26(3)305-6
- Varma S, Lanigan SW. Management difficulties due to concurrent dermatitis herpetiformis and variegate porphyria. Br J Dermatol 2000;143(3)654-5
- Shah SA, Ormerod AD. Dermatitis herpetiformis effectively treated with heparin, tetracycine and nicotinamide. Clin & Exp Dermatol 2000;25(3)204-5
- Woollons A, Darley, et al. Childhood dermatitis herpetiformis: an unusual presentation. Clin & Exp Dermatol 1999;24(4)283-5
- Collin P, Pukkala E, Reunala T. Malignancy and survival in dermatitis herpetiformis: a comparison with coeliac disease. Gut 1996;38(4):528-30
- Isaac M, McNeely MC. Dermatitis herpetiformis associated with lichen planopilaris. J Am Acad Dermatol 1995;33(6):1050-1
- Zaenglein AL, Hafer L, Helm KF. Diagnosis of dermatitis herpetiformis by an avidin-biotin-peroxidase method. Arch Dermatol 1995;131(5):571-3
- Sigurgeirsson B, Agnarsson BA, Lindelof B. Risk of lymphoma in patients with dermatitis herpetiformis. BMJ 1994;308(6920):13-5

Web references: 1 available at www.5mcc.com
Illustrations N/A

Author(s):

Vera Y. Soong, MD

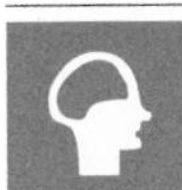

BASICS

DESCRIPTION Chronic, superficial, inflammatory condition affecting hairy regions of the body, especially scalp, eyebrows, and face. Mechanism of disease unknown.

System(s) affected: Skin/Exocrine
Genetics: Positive family history common
Incidence/Prevalence in USA: Common
Predominant age: Infancy, adolescence, and adulthood
Predominant sex: Male > Female

SIGNS & SYMPTOMS
- Infants
  - ◊ Cradle cap - greasy scaling of scalp, sometimes with associated mild erythema
  - ◊ Diaper and/or axillary rash
  - ◊ Onset typically about age one month
  - ◊ Usually resolves by age 8-12 months
- Adults
  - ◊ Red, greasy, scaling rash in most locations, consisting of patches and plaques with indistinct margins
  - ◊ Red, smooth, glazed appearance in skin folds
  - ◊ Minimal pruritus
  - ◊ Chronic waxing and waning course
  - ◊ Bilateral and symmetrical
  - ◊ Most commonly located in hairy skin areas with numerous sebaceous glands, e.g., scalp and scalp margins, eyebrows and eyelid margins, nasolabial folds, ears and retroauricular folds, presternal area and mid-upper back

CAUSES
- Skin surface yeasts (Pityrosporum ovale) may be a contributing factor
- Genetic and environmental factors also contribute to disease, i.e., disease flares are common with any stress or illness
- Disease also seems to parallel increased sebaceous gland activity in infancy and adolescence or as a result of some acnegenic drugs

RISK FACTORS
- Parkinson disease
- AIDS (disease severity correlated with progression of immune deficiency)
- Emotional stress

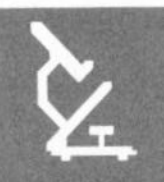

DIAGNOSIS

DIFFERENTIAL DIAGNOSIS
- Atopic dermatitis - (distinction may be difficult in infants)
- Psoriasis - usually knees, elbows, nails will be involved. Scalp psoriasis will be more sharply demarcated than seborrhea, with crusted, infiltrated plaques rather than mild scaling and erythema.
- Candida
- Tinea cruris or capitis - suspect these when usual medications fail, or if there is hair loss
- Eczema of auricle or otitis externa
- Rosacea
- Discoid lupus erythematosus
- Histiocytosis X - may appear as seborrheic type eruption. Consider biopsy if usual therapies fail and especially if petechiae are noted.
- Dandruff (scalp only, noninflammatory)

LABORATORY N/A

Drugs that may alter lab results: N/A

Disorders that may alter lab results: N/A

PATHOLOGICAL FINDINGS Nonspecific changes of eczematous dermatitis. (Biopsy unnecessary unless there is a suspicion of histiocytosis X).

SPECIAL TESTS N/A

IMAGING N/A

DIAGNOSTIC PROCEDURES N/A

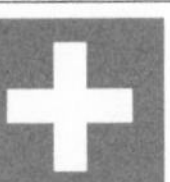

TREATMENT

APPROPRIATE HEALTH CARE Outpatient

GENERAL MEASURES
- Increase frequency of shampooing
- Sunlight in moderate doses may be helpful

SURGICAL MEASURES N/A

ACTIVITY Full activity

DIET No special diet

PATIENT EDUCATION Goal of treatment is control, rather than cure, of disease. Seborrheic dermatitis does not cause hair loss.

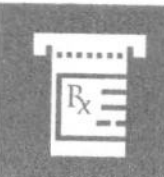

MEDICATIONS

DRUG(S) OF CHOICE
- Cradle cap:
  - ◊ Frequent shampooing with a mild, non-medicated shampoo
  - ◊ Remove thick scale by applying warm olive or mineral oil and then wash off several hours later with Dawn dishwashing detergent and a soft bristle toothbrush
  - ◊ May use a coal tar shampoo or ketoconazole (Nizoral) shampoo if the non-medicated shampoo is ineffective
- Adults:
  - ◊ Wash off all affected areas with antiseborrheic shampoos. Start with over-the-counter brands (Tegrin, Selsun Blue) and increase to more potent preparations (containing coal tar, sulfur, selenium or salicylic acid) if no improvement is noted.
  - ◊ For dense scalp scaling, 10% Liquor Carbonic Detergens (LCD) in Nivea Oil may be used at bedtime, covering the head with a shower cap. This should be done nightly for 1-3 weeks.
  - ◊ Ketoconazole (Nizoral) cream may be used to clear scales in other areas, followed by application of steroids to reduce inflammation. Begin with 1% hydrocortisone and advance to more potent (fluorinated) steroid preparations as needed. Avoid continuous use of the more potent steroids to reduce the risk of skin atrophy or systemic absorption (especially in infants and children).
  - ◊ Once controlled, washing with zinc soaps or selenium lotion with periodic use of steroid cream will help maintain remission
- For secondary infections: Short course of erythromycin or dicloxacillin

Contraindications: None
Precautions: Fluorinated corticosteroids and higher concentrations of hydrocortisone (e.g., 2.5%) may cause atrophy or striae if used on the face or on skin folds
Significant possible interactions: None

ALTERNATIVE DRUGS In severe seborrhea nonresponsive to topical therapy - isotretinoin (0.1-0.3 mg/kg/day) may be helpful. This agent should be used cautiously.

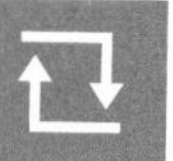

FOLLOWUP

PATIENT MONITORING Every 2 to 12 weeks as necessary, depending on disease severity and degree of patient sophistication

PREVENTION/AVOIDANCE N/A

POSSIBLE COMPLICATIONS
- Skin atrophy or striae possible from fluorinated corticosteroids, especially if used on the face
- Glaucoma - can result from use of fluorinated steroids around the eyes
- Photosensitivity - occasionally caused by tars
- Herpes keratitis - rare complication of herpes simplex. Instruct patient to stop eyelid steroids if herpes simplex develops.

EXPECTED COURSE/PROGNOSIS
- In infants, seborrheic dermatitis usually remits after 6 to 8 months
- In adults, seborrheic dermatitis is usually chronic and unpredictable, with exacerbations and remissions. Disease is usually easily controlled with shampoos and topical steroids.

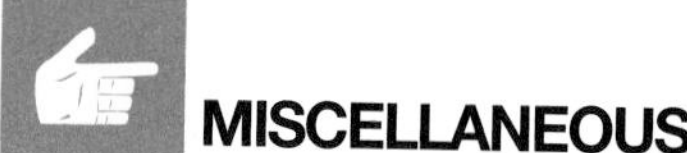

MISCELLANEOUS

ASSOCIATED CONDITIONS Parkinson disease, AIDS (disease severity correlated with progression of immune deficiency)

AGE-RELATED FACTORS
Pediatric: Common in infants
Geriatric: N/A
Others: N/A

PREGNANCY N/A

SYNONYMS
- Seborrhea
- Cradle cap

ICD-9-CM
690.10 Seborrheic dermatitis, unspecified

SEE ALSO
Dermatitis, atopic
Tinea capitis
Tinea cruris

OTHER NOTES N/A

ABBREVIATIONS N/A

REFERENCES

- Habif T. Clinical Dermatology. 4th ed. St. Louis: CV Mosby; 2004
- Dershewitz R, ed. Ambulatory Pediatric Care. 3rd ed. Philadelphia: Lippincott-Raven; 1999
- Johnson BA, Nunley JR. Treatment of seborrheic dermatitis. Am Fam Physician. 2000;61(9):2703-10, 2713-4

Web references: 1 available at www.5mcc.com
Illustrations 3 available

Author(s):
Dennis E. Hughes, DO

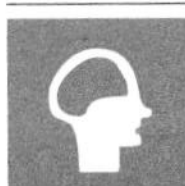

BASICS

DESCRIPTION Chronic, noninflammatory edema of the lower leg accompanied by cycle of scratching, excoriations, weeping, crusting, and inflammation; venous stasis

System(s) affected: Skin/Exocrine

Genetics: Familial link probable

Incidence/Prevalence in USA: Common in patients over 50 years of age (6-7% of patients > 50 yr)

Predominant age: Adult, geriatric

Predominant sex: Female > Male

SIGNS & SYMPTOMS

- Insidious onset
- Usually bilateral
- Scaly, eczematous patches
- Violaceous (sometimes brown), erythematous colored lesions - due to deoxygenation of venous blood (postinflammatory hyperpigmentation and hemosiderin deposition within the cutaneous tissue)
- Distribution - medial aspect of ankle with frequent extension onto the foot and lower leg
- Noninflammatory edema precedes the skin eruption and ulceration
- Brawny induration
- Stasis ulcers (frequently accompanies stasis dermatitis) secondary to cuts, bruises, excoriations to the weakened skin around the ankle
- Mild pruritus, pain (if ulcer present)
- Varicosities are often associated with ulcers

CAUSES

- Incompetence of perforating veins causing blood to backflow to the superficial venous system leading to venous hypertension and cutaneous inflammation
- Continuous presence of edema in ankles, usually present because of venous valve incompetency (varicose veins)
- Weakness of venous walls in lower extremities
- Trauma to edematous, eczematized skin

RISK FACTORS

- Atopy
- Superimposition of itch-scratch cycle
- Trauma
- Previous deep vein thrombosis
- Previous pregnancy
- Prolonged medical illness
- Obesity
- Secondary infection
- Low-protein diet
- Old age
- Deposition of fibrin around capillaries
- Microvascular abnormalities
- Ischemia
- Genetic propensity
- Edema
- Wearing of tight garments that constrict the thigh
- Vein stripping
- Vein harvesting in patients requiring coronary artery bypass grafting

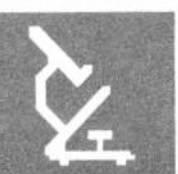

DIAGNOSIS

DIFFERENTIAL DIAGNOSIS

- Other eczematous diseases such as:
  - ◊ Atopic dermatitis
  - ◊ Contact dermatitis (due to topical agents used to self-treat)
  - ◊ Neurodermatitis
  - ◊ Arterial insufficiency
  - ◊ Sickle cell disease causing skin ulceration
  - ◊ Cellulitis
- Tinea dermatophyte infection
- Pretibial myxedema
- Nummular eczema
- Lichen simplex chronicus
- Xerosis
- Asteatotic eczema

LABORATORY Culture stasis ulcers if you decide to use antibiotics (use of antibiotics topically or systemically is controversial)

Drugs that may alter lab results: N/A

Disorders that may alter lab results: N/A

PATHOLOGICAL FINDINGS Chronic inflammation, characterized histologically by proliferation of small blood vessels in the papillary dermis

SPECIAL TESTS Culture ulcer base or prurient crusted areas to determine whether secondary infection is present

IMAGING venous Doppler studies should be considered if DVT is suspected

DIAGNOSTIC PROCEDURES Rule out arterial insufficiency

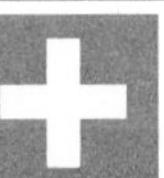

TREATMENT

APPROPRIATE HEALTH CARE

- Outpatient
- Inpatient for vein stripping, sclerotherapy or skin grafts
- Venous ulcer treatment includes autolytic, chemical, mechanical, surgical and biologic
  - ◊ Autolytic - hydrogels, alginates, hydrocolloids, foams and films
  - ◊ Biologic - topical application of granulocyte macrophage colony stimulating factor promotes healing of ulcers
  - ◊ Chemical - enzyme débriding agents
  - ◊ Mechanical - wet to dry dressings, hydrotherapy, irrigation
  - ◊ Surgical modifying cause of venous hypertension, treat ulcer by graft

GENERAL MEASURES

- Primary role of treatment is to reverse effects of venous hypertension
- Reduce edema:
  - ◊ Leg elevation - heels higher than knees, knees higher than hips
  - ◊ Compression therapy: elastic bandage wraps - Ace bandages or Unna's paste boot (zinc gelatin) if lesions are dry or compression stockings (Jobst or non-fitted type)
  - ◊ Pneumatic compression devices
  - ◊ Diuretic therapy
- Treat infection:
- Debride the ulcer base of necrotic tissue
- Improvement of lipodermatosclerosis

SURGICAL MEASURES

- Sclerotherapy and surgery may be required

ACTIVITY

- Avoid standing still
- Stay active, exercise regularly
- Elevate foot of bed unless contraindicated

DIET No special diet. Lose weight, if overweight.

PATIENT EDUCATION

- Stress staying active to keep circulation and leg muscles in good condition. Walking is ideal.
- Keeping legs elevated while sitting or lying
- Don't wear girdles, garters, or pantyhose with tight elastic tops
- Don't scratch
- Elevate foot of bed with 2-4 inch blocks

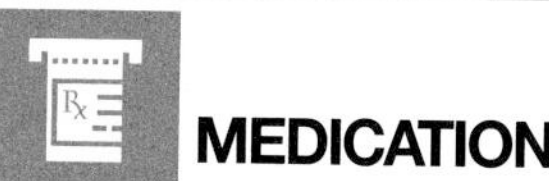

MEDICATIONS

DRUG(S) OF CHOICE
- If secondary infection, treat with oral antibiotics for staphylococcus or streptococcus organisms (eg, dicloxacillin 250 mg qid; cephalexin 250 mg qid or levofloxacin 250 mg qd)
- S. aureus or beta-hemolytic streptococcus, treat with oral antibiotics
- Gram-negative colonization, treat with topical antimicrobial agents (e.g., benzoyl peroxide, acetic acid, silver nitrate, or Hibiclens) or broad-spectrum topical antibiotics (eg neomycin or bacitracin-polymyxin b [Polysporin])
- 5% aluminum acetate (Burow's solution) wet dressings and cooling pastes
- Topical triamcinolone 0.1% (Kenalog, Aristocort) cream/ointment tid or topical betamethasone
- Betamethasone valerate (Valisone) 0.1% cream/ointment/solution tid
- Topical antipruritic - pramoxine, camphor, menthol, doxepin
- Systemic steroids for severe cases
- Calcium dobesilate has been shown to be an effective adjuvant therapy

Contraindications: N/A
Precautions: Refer to manufacturer's literature
Significant possible interactions: N/A

ALTERNATIVE DRUGS
- Consider antibiotics on basis of culture results of exudate from ulcer craters
- Lubricants when dermatitis is quiescent
- Chronic stasis dermatitis can be treated with topical emollients (eg, white petroleum, lanolin, Eucerin)
- Antipruritic medications (eg, diphenhydramine, cetirizine hydrochloride, desloratadine)

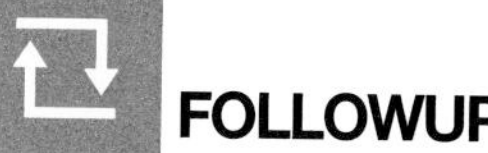

FOLLOWUP

PATIENT MONITORING
If Unna's boot is used - cut off and reapply boot once a week (restricts edema and prevents scratching)

PREVENTION/AVOIDANCE
- Avoid recurrence of edema with compression stockings
- Topical lubricants twice daily to prevent fissuring and itching

POSSIBLE COMPLICATIONS
- Secondary bacterial infection
- Deep vein thrombus
- Bleeding at dermatitis sites
- Squamous cell carcinoma in edges of long standing stasis ulcers
- Scarring, which in turn leads to further compromise to blood flow and increased likelihood of minor trauma

EXPECTED COURSE/PROGNOSIS
- Chronic course with intermittent exacerbations and remissions
- The healing process for ulceration is often prolonged and may take months

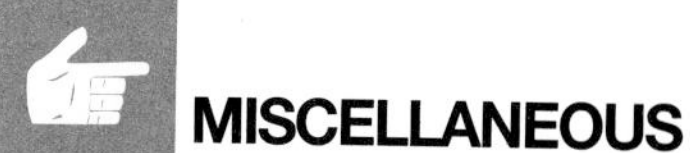

MISCELLANEOUS

ASSOCIATED CONDITIONS
- Varicose veins
- Other eczematous disease

AGE-RELATED FACTORS
Pediatric: N/A
Geriatric: Common in this age group. It is estimated to affect 15-20 million patients over the age of 50 years in the United States.
Others: N/A

PREGNANCY N/A

SYNONYMS
- Gravitational eczema
- Varicose eczema
- Venous dermatitis

ICD-9-CM
454.1 Varicose veins of lower extremities with inflammation
459.81 Venous (peripheral) insufficiency, unspecified

SEE ALSO
Varicose veins

OTHER NOTES N/A

ABBREVIATIONS N/A

REFERENCES

- Petropoulos P. Stasis dermatitis. In: Ferri F, ed. Ferri's Clinical Advisor: Instant Diagnosis and Treatment. 6th ed. New York: Mosby, Inc; 2004. p805-6
- Theodosat A. Skin diseases of the lower extremities in the elderly. Dermatol Clin 2004;22(1):13-21
- Sams WM Jr, Lynch PR, eds. Principles and Practices of Dermatology. New York, Churchill Livingstone, 1996
- Fitzpatrick TB, et al, eds. Dermatology in General Medicine. 5th Ed. New York, McGraw-Hill, 1999
- Sauer GC: Manual of Skin Diseases. 8th Ed. Philadelphia, J.B. Lippincott, 1999
- Valencia IC, Falabella A, Kirsner RS, Eaglstein WH. Chronic venous insufficiency and venous leg ulceration. J Am Acad Dermatol 2001;44(3):401-21

Web references: 1 available at www.5mcc.com
Illustrations 9 available

Author(s):
Joseph A. Florence, MD

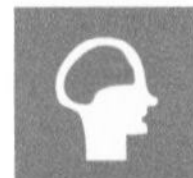

BASICS

DESCRIPTION Defective regulation of water balance secondary to decreased secretion of, or failure of response to, vasopressin

- Inadequate secretion of vasopressin may be due to loss of or malfunction of the neurosecretory neurons that make up the neurohypophysis (posterior pituitary) and the pituitary stalk
- Insensitivity to vasopressin - a disorder of renal tubular function resulting in inability to respond to vasopressin in absorption of water
- Excessive water intake - (primary polydipsia) usually of functional origin

System(s) affected: Endocrine/Metabolic

Genetics:

- Familial cases of vasopressin deficiency have been reported (commonly autosomal dominant; more than 20 mutations have been identified), but the disease is usually isolated, and often secondary to other disorders
- Nephrogenic diabetes insipidus (insensitivity to vasopressin) - usually inherited (sex linked recessive), expressed in males, rarely in females. Two gene defects involving response elements to arginine vasopressin (AVP) have been defined.

Incidence/Prevalence in USA: N/A

Predominant age:

- Vasopressin deficiency may occur at any age including infancy and childhood
- Nephrogenic diabetes insipidus is usually manifest in infancy

Predominant sex: Nephrogenic diabetes insipidus is encountered in males with rare exception, reflecting its X-linked recessive mode of inheritance

SIGNS & SYMPTOMS

- Thirst/polydipsia (with a particular preference for cold or iced drinks)
- Polyuria
- Nocturia
- Dehydration
- Headache
- Visual disturbance

CAUSES

- Inadequate secretion of vasopressin: a variety of pathological lesions may produce damage including tumors (craniopharyngioma, lymphoma, metastasis); infections (meningitis, encephalitis); trauma, granulomas (sarcoid, histiocytosis); or vascular disorders. Some are idiopathic or familial.
- Excessive water intake (psychogenic)
- Insensitivity to vasopressin: genetic defect in resorption of water in renal tubule (collecting ducts)
- Drugs: Lithium, demeclocycline, vincristine, amphotericin B and methoxyflurane may produce nephrogenic diabetes insipidus
- Hypercalcemia
- Hypokalemia

RISK FACTORS N/A

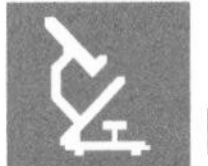

DIAGNOSIS

DIFFERENTIAL DIAGNOSIS

- Diabetes mellitus and other causes of polydipsia and polyuria
- Increased solute load for excretion as occurs with high salt intake
- Psychogenic polydipsia (ultimately impairs vasopressin secretion)
- Nephrogenic diabetes insipidus (differentiate from vasopressin deficiency by clinical trial of desmopressin [DDAVP])

LABORATORY

- Hypernatremia (presenting manifestation, particularly in infants and children)
- Inability to concentrate urine (measure by osmolality, rather than specific gravity)
- Urinary glucose (to rule out diabetes mellitus)
- Plasma vasopressin or urinary vasopressin following osmotic stimulus, such as fluid restriction or administration of hypertonic saline

Drugs that may alter lab results: Lithium, demeclocycline and methoxyflurane may produce vasopressin insensitivity

Disorders that may alter lab results: Hypokalemia and hypercalcemia alter ability to concentrate urine

PATHOLOGICAL FINDINGS Degeneration and death of neurosecretory neurons in the neurohypophysis

SPECIAL TESTS

- Testing ability to concentrate urine in face of water deprivation should be done by measuring urine and plasma osmolality before and after a six hour period of thirst. This should be done during the day. It is not wise to do overnight thirst tests, particularly in children.
- The most valuable measurements are the urine/plasma osmolal ratio and plasma vasopressin concentrations. The results are sometimes difficult to interpret since low ratios may be found in patients with primary polydipsia. If results support the diagnosis, desmopressin should be administered to test renal concentrating ability.

IMAGING If the diagnosis of diabetes insipidus is made, appropriate studies for cause including imaging of the brain must be performed

DIAGNOSTIC PROCEDURES Fluid deprivation to concentrate urine

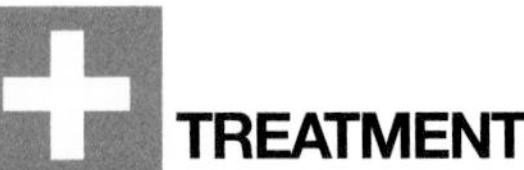

TREATMENT

APPROPRIATE HEALTH CARE Initial diagnosis and management may require hospitalization. Continuing care is provided on an outpatient basis with self-medication.

GENERAL MEASURES

- Control fluid balance and prevent dehydration
- Check weight daily
- Provide good skin and mouth care

SURGICAL MEASURES N/A

ACTIVITY Not restricted

DIET Normal with free access to fluids except that young infants with nephrogenic diabetes insipidus may benefit from low solute formula

PATIENT EDUCATION

- Administration and dosage of intranasal desmopressin
- Importance of having access to fluids as thirst dictates
- Wear a medical identification neck tag or bracelet

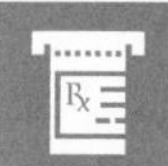

MEDICATIONS

DRUG(S) OF CHOICE
- Central (vasopressin deficient) diabetes insipidus
  - desmopressin (DDAVP) (a derivative of vasopressin) given intranasally two times daily in dosage necessary to control polyuria or polydipsia usually (10-25 μg) or 2-4 μg parenterally in 2 divided doses
- Nephrogenic diabetes insipidus - thiazide diuretics combined with amiloride

Contraindications: Desmopressin should be used with caution in the immediate postoperative period for intracranial lesions because of possible cerebral edema

Precautions: Overdose of desmopressin may produce water intoxication in patients with excessive water intake

Significant possible interactions: See manufacturer's profile of each drug

ALTERNATIVE DRUGS
- Chlorpropamide (Diabinese) 250-500 mg/day reduces polyuria and polydipsia
- Clofibrate (Atromid-S) at a maximum dose of 1 gm tid also has an antidiuretic effect
- Hydrochlorothiazide 50 mg/day

Note: The effects of these alternate drugs are not as predictable as desmopressin

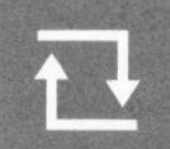

FOLLOWUP

PATIENT MONITORING
- Requires regular followup at intervals of 2-3 weeks initially and 3-4 months later
- Adjustment of treatment based on the urine and electrolyte concentrations and patient's symptoms

PREVENTION/AVOIDANCE
Avoid situations of marked increase in water loss. Take fluids as dictated by thirst with no water restriction.

POSSIBLE COMPLICATIONS
- Dilatation of urinary tract has been observed (probably secondary to large volume of urine)
- Complications of primary disease (tumor histiocytosis, etc.) should be anticipated
- In nephrogenic diabetes, there is an associated retardation of mental development in some patients (cause undetermined)
- Subnormal growth rate

EXPECTED COURSE/PROGNOSIS
- Condition is usually permanent, although an occasional case following trauma or tumor goes into permanent remission
- Prognosis of diabetes insipidus per se is good depending on underlying disorder
- Without treatment, dehydration can lead to confusion, stupor and coma

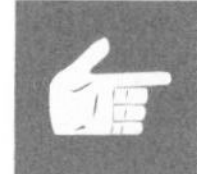

MISCELLANEOUS

ASSOCIATED CONDITIONS
- Infection (e.g., encephalitis, tuberculosis, syphilis)
- Tumors
- Xanthomatosis
- Pyelonephritis
- Renal amyloidosis
- Potassium depletion
- Sjögren syndrome
- Sickle cell anemia
- Chronic hypercalcemia
- Wolfram syndrome (DIDMOAD)

AGE-RELATED FACTORS
Pediatric: Nephrogenic diabetes insipidus is usually manifest in infancy

Geriatric: N/A

Others: N/A

PREGNANCY
N/A

SYNONYMS
N/A

ICD-9-CM
253.5 Diabetes insipidus

SEE ALSO
Sjögren syndrome

OTHER NOTES
N/A

ABBREVIATIONS
DI = diabetes insipidus

DIDMOAD = diabetes insipidus, diabetes mellitus, optic atrophy and deafness

REFERENCES

- Robertson G. Posterior pituitary hormones. In: Felig P, Baxter JD, Broadus AE, Frohman LA, editors. Endocrinology and Metabolism. New York: McGraw-Hill; 1995. p. 385
- Reeves WB, et al. Posterior pituitary and water metabolism. In: Wilson JD, editor. William's Textbook of Endocrinology. 9th ed. Philadelphia: WB Saunders; 1998. p. 341-388

Web references: 0 available at www.5mcc.com

Illustrations N/A

Author(s):
William W. Cleveland, MD

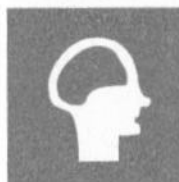

BASICS

DESCRIPTION A chronic disease caused by pancreatic insufficiency (deficiency) of insulin production, resulting in hyperglycemia and end-organ complications such as accelerated atherosclerosis, neuropathy, nephropathy, and retinopathy. Features include:
- Patients insulinopenic and require insulin
- Prone to ketosis
- Usually of rapid onset
- Nutritional status - normal or thin
- Disease lability
- Response to oral drugs uncommon
- Seasonable: January-April are peak onset periods (children < 6 years old have greater degree of seasonal risk)

System(s) affected: Endocrine/Metabolic

Genetics:
- Mode of genetic expression not clear
- Genes located on major histocompatibility complex on chromosome 6
- HLA DR3 and DR4 are individually associated with increased risk factor of 4; if carrying both susceptibility genes, relative risk factor increases to 12
- HLA B8 and B15 also associated with increased risk

Incidence/Prevalence in USA: Incidence of 15/100,000/ year. Racial predilection for Caucasian. African-Americans have lowest overall incidence.

Predominant age: Mean age of onset 8-12 years, peaking in adolescence; onset about 1.5 years earlier in girls than boys. Rapid decline in incidence after adolescence.

Predominant sex: Male = Female

SIGNS & SYMPTOMS
- Polyuria and polydipsia
- Polyphagia is classic, but not common
- Anorexia is commonly observed
- Weight loss (usually from 10-30%, and often almost devoid of body fat at time of diagnosis)
- Increased fatigue
- Decreased energy levels and lethargy
- Muscle cramps
- Irritability and emotional lability
- Vision changes, such as blurriness
- Altered school and work performance
- Headaches
- Anxiety attacks
- Chest pain and occasional difficult breathing
- Abdominal discomfort and pain
- Nausea
- Diarrhea or constipation

CAUSES
- The inherited defect causes an alteration in immunologic integrity, placing the beta cell at special risk for inflammatory damage. The mechanism of damage is autoimmune.
- Environmental factors include:
  - ◊ Viruses (such as mumps, Coxsackie, CMV, and hepatitis viruses)
  - ◊ Dietary factors - breast feeding may provide a degree of protection against the disease while diets high in dairy products are associated with increased risk
  - ◊ Possible risk in diets high in nitrosamines
  - ◊ Environmental toxins
  - ◊ Emotional and physical stress

RISK FACTORS
- Certain HLA types (see above)
- Presence of a specific 64K protein which may be responsible for antibody formation
- Increased risk when either insulin-dependent or non-insulin dependent diabetes present in any first-degree relatives
- Slightly greater risk of a child developing diabetes especially if the father has type 1 diabetes

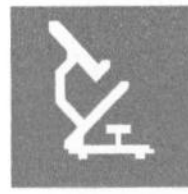

DIAGNOSIS

DIFFERENTIAL DIAGNOSIS
- Benign renal glycosuria
- Glucose intolerance
- Type II (non-insulin-dependent) diabetes mellitus - children might have MODY (maturity-onset diabetes of the young) - becoming more frequent
- Infantile-onset diabetes mellitus
- Secondary diabetes
  - ◊ Pancreatic disease (pancreatitis, cystic fibrosis)
  - ◊ Hormonal disorders (pheochromocytoma, multiple endocrine adenomatosis)
  - ◊ Inborn errors of metabolism (glycogen storage disease, Type I)
  - ◊ Genetic disorders with insulin resistance (acanthosis nigricans)
  - ◊ Hereditary neuromuscular disease
  - ◊ Progeroid syndromes
  - ◊ Obesity (Prader-Willi syndrome)
  - ◊ Cytogenetic syndromes (trisomy 21, Klinefelter and Turner syndromes)
  - ◊ Drug or chemical-induced glucose intolerance (see list below)
  - ◊ Acute poisonings (salicylate poisoning can be associated with hyperglycemia and glycosuria, and may mimic diabetic ketoacidosis)

LABORATORY
- Blood glucose
- Electrolytes
- Venous pH
- U/A for glucose and ketones
- CBC (WBC may be elevated)
- Hemoglobin A1C level
- C-peptide insulin level
- Islet-cell antibodies
- T4 and thyroid antibodies
- GAD antibodies

Drugs that may alter lab results:
- The following may cause hyperglycemia (particularly in patients prone to diabetes)
  - ◊ Hormones: glucagon, glucocorticoids, growth hormone, epinephrine, estrogen and progesterone (oral contraceptives), thyroid preparations
  - ◊ Drugs: thiazide diuretics, furosemide, acetazolamide, diazoxide, beta-blockers, alpha-agonists, calcium channel blockers, phenytoin, phenobarbital sodium, nicotinic acid, cyclophosphamide, l-asparaginase, epinephrine-like drugs (decongestants and diet pills), non-steroidal anti-inflammatory agents, nicotine, caffeine, sugar-containing syrups, fish oils

Disorders that may alter lab results: See Differential Diagnosis

PATHOLOGICAL FINDINGS Inflammatory changes with lymphocytic infiltration around the Islets of Langerhans, or islet cell destruction

SPECIAL TESTS
- Oral glucose tolerance test (possibly with insulin levels, if diagnosis is questionable)
- Intravenous glucose test (for possible early detection of subclinical diabetes)
- Consider HLA-typing

IMAGING None indicated

DIAGNOSTIC PROCEDURES N/A

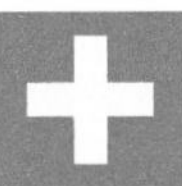

TREATMENT

APPROPRIATE HEALTH CARE
- Initial care: inpatient stabilization versus outpatient management, preferably in a diabetes unit where a team approach is used
- If in diabetic ketoacidosis (DKA): initially IV fluids and IV insulin until stable, then restore electrolyte and acid-base balance, correct hyperglycemia, prevent hypoglycemia and hypokalemia, risk of cerebral edema
- Remaining health care is done by the family at home. Encourage the child to do as much self-care as possible.

GENERAL MEASURES
- Overall "control" of carbohydrate metabolism for the very young child:
  - ◊ Normoglycemia (adjusted for age) "tight" control with striving for blood glucose levels in range of 80-150 mg/dL (4.4-8.3 mmol/L) all the time, might be dangerous (risk of repeated hypoglycemia)
  - ◊ Hemoglobin A1C level as close to the normal (non-diabetic) range as possible
- Overall good health
  - ◊ Asymptomatic
  - ◊ Normal appearance
  - ◊ Try to keep lipid profile normal
- Normal growth and development
  - ◊ Reach optimal height for genetic potential
  - ◊ Appropriate and timely pubertal maturation
  - ◊ Coping psychosocial development: Normal school or work attendance and performance. Normal future goals and career plans.
- Prevent acute complications
  - ◊ Hypoglycemic insulin reactions
  - ◊ Ketoacidosis
- Delay or prevent chronic complications

SURGICAL MEASURES N/A

ACTIVITY
- All normal activities, including full participation in sports activities
- Regular, rather than periodic, aerobic exercise is preferable

DIET Appropriate diabetes exchange (ADA) diet for age (carbohydrate-50%, protein-20%, fat-30%)

PATIENT EDUCATION
- Complete initial education and ongoing education for patient and family. Team approach is ideal, if available
- For a listing of sources, physicians may contact: American Academy of Family Physicians Foundation, P.O. Box 8418, Kansas City, MO 64114, (800)274-2237, ext. 4400

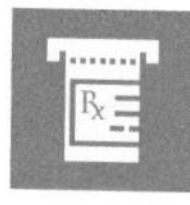

MEDICATIONS

DRUG(S) OF CHOICE
- Insulin
  - ◊ Source: Human (Humulin or Novolin)
  - ◊ Types: NPH, Lente, Regular, Ultralente, 70/30 premixture, (not used much in children) Humalog and Novolog (used much more than regular insulin, and can be given immediately before or after eating); insulin glargine (Lantus)
- Insulin regimens (given subcutaneously by syringe or various pen devices, some disposable))
  - ◊ 2 doses: NPH/Lente and Regular/Humalog/Novolog in a 2:1 ratio typically given before breakfast and before supper. AM dose usually 1/2 to 2/3 of total daily dose (other than for newly-onset diabetics, this 2 dose regimen will not achieve optimal glycemic control)
  - ◊ 3 doses: NPH/Lente and Regular/Humalog/Novolog at supper; and a bedtime dose of NPH/Lente (this regimen may prevent nighttime hypoglycemia and the dawn or Somogyi phenomenon)
  - ◊ 4 doses (a common regimen in recent years): Humalog or Novolog insulin at breakfast, lunch, and supper, and NPH/Lente at bedtime
- Newest insulin regimen using insulin glargine (Lantus): Humalog or Novolog at breakfast, lunch, and supper and before snacks as well - dosage based on a determined insulin/carbohydrate ratio and correction factor for elevated blood sugar, plus Lantus insulin (a 24 hour nearly "peakless" insulin, providing basal insulin throughout the day). This insulin regimen is very physiologic and gives similar insulin profiles as the insulin pump (without having to wear a pump).
  - ◊ Insulin pump (external) therapy: used more commonly in diabetic patients these days (adults and children); basal insulin is given continuously (rates preset); and bolus doses given pre-meals and snacks. based on insulin/carbohydrate ratios; ALL insulin is Humalog or Novolog.

Contraindications: None
Precautions: Avoid hypoglycemia, the dawn phenomenon, and Somogyi syndrome (rebound hyperglycemia)
Significant possible interactions:
- Beta-blockers may mask symptoms of hypoglycemia and delay return to normoglycemia

ALTERNATIVE DRUGS
- Oral hypoglycemics usually not indicated in Type I diabetes (unless an obese patient, who may have MODY; or a combination of Type 1 and Type 2) - metformin (Glucophage)
- Immunosuppressants
  - ◊ Cyclosporine: reduces rate of autoimmune beta cell destruction, must be started in initial weeks after the diagnosis of diabetes is made (studies: at 1 year, 20% of cyclosporine - treated patients on no insulin, compared to 12-15% of placebo controls; after 1 year, progressive decline in beta cell function and loss of remission. Toxic side effects include renal disease, hypertension, lymphoma formation.
  - ◊ Other interventional drugs being studied - azathioprine, steroids, nicotinamide

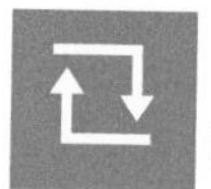

FOLLOWUP

PATIENT MONITORING
- Initially, frequent outpatient followup visits till stable; every 2-3 months thereafter. Monitor height, weight, sexual maturation.
- Daily home blood glucose monitoring with home blood glucose meter: One-Touch (Profile, Fasttake and Ultra); Accuchek (Advantage, Complete, Active); Precision (X-tra or QID); Glucometer Elite XL; Freestyle; In Duo (combination meter and insulin pen). Blood tests should be done at least 4-6 times daily for optimal monitoring, with adjustment and supplementation of insulin doses based on blood glucose levels-regardless of which insulin regimen.
- Periodic (about every 3 months) measurement of hemoglobin A1c to assess overall glycemic control
- Yearly measurement of serum lipids and thyroid function
- Regular review and update of dietary management. Adjust for increased caloric needs for age, level of physical activity, pubertal growth spurt, changes in weight.

PREVENTION/AVOIDANCE None known

POSSIBLE COMPLICATIONS
- Microvascular disease (retinopathy, nephropathy, neuropathy)
- Hyperlipidemia
- Macrovascular disease (coronary and cerebral artery disease)
- Foot problems
- Hypoglycemia
- Diabetic ketoacidosis
- Excessive weight gain
- Psychologic problems related to chronic disease

EXPECTED COURSE/PROGNOSIS
- Initial remission or "honeymoon" phase with decreased insulin needs and easier overall control, usually lasts 3-6 months and rarely beyond a year
- Progression to "total diabetes" when endogenous insulin is insignificant; usually is gradual, but a major stress or illness may bring it on more acutely
- Current prognosis
  - ◊ Increasing longevity and "quality of life" with careful blood glucose monitoring and improvement in insulin delivery regimens and systems
  - ◊ At this time, probable reduced life expectancy, but this has improved dramatically over the past 20 years
  - ◊ Continue to be optimistic about advances in understanding diabetes that may prevent or minimize complications

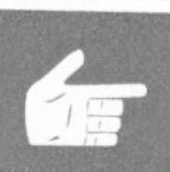

MISCELLANEOUS

ASSOCIATED CONDITIONS
- Other autoimmune diseases such as hypothyroidism and Addison Disease (screening regularly for hypothyroidism particularly important in females, who have a much higher incidence of this already)
- Diabetes mellitus can also be seen as part of multiple endocrine adenomatosis

AGE-RELATED FACTORS
Pediatric: More prevalent in this age. Over the past 10 years, a larger percentage of very young children (less than 5 years of age) present with diabetes.
Geriatric: N/A
Others: N/A

PREGNANCY
- At the time of embryogenesis, hyperglycemia increases the incidence of congenital malformations. Hence, tight control of blood sugar before conception is important.
- Safe pregnancy possible, with vaginal delivery of a term baby.

SYNONYMS
- Childhood diabetes
- Brittle diabetes

ICD-9-CM
250.00 Diabetes mellitus without mention of complication, type 2 or unspecified type, not stated as uncontrolled
250.01 Diabetes mellitus without mention of complication, type 1, not stated as uncontrolled

SEE ALSO
Diabetes mellitus, Type 2
Diabetic ketoacidosis (DKA)

OTHER NOTES N/A

ABBREVIATIONS
MODY = maturity-onset diabetes of the young

REFERENCES

- Travis L, et al: Diabetes Mellitus in Children and Adolescents. Philadelphia, WB Saunders Co, 1987
- Pediatric and Adolescent Endocrinology. Pediatric Clinics of North America, Volume 34, Number 4, W.B. Saunders Co., August 1987
- Lebovitz HE, ed: Therapy for Diabetes Mellitus and Related Disorders. American Diabetes Association, Inc., 1991
- Clark CM, et al: Prevention and treatment of the complications of diabetes mellitus. New Engl J Med 1995;332(18):1210-1217

Web references: 4 available at www.5mcc.com
Illustrations 16 available

Author(s):
Robert M. Schultz, MD

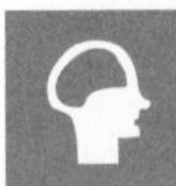

BASICS

DESCRIPTION Non-ketosis prone hyperglycemia and glucose intolerance due to defects in insulin secretion and peripheral insulin action. Accounts for 80% of diabetic cases.
System(s) affected: Cardiovascular, Endocrine/Metabolic, Nervous, Renal/Urologic
Genetics: Strong polygenic familial susceptibility. Concordance is nearly complete in identical twins.
Incidence/Prevalence in USA:
- Incidence:
  - ◊ 300/100,000 (males 230/100,000, females 340/100,000)
- Prevalence:
  - ◊ 5,000/100,000
  - ◊ More common in some groups such as Pima Indians with 35% prevalence

Predominant age: Typically occurs after age 40
Predominant sex: Female > Male in Caucasian populations

SIGNS & SYMPTOMS
- Related to hyperglycemia and complications including nephropathy, neuropathy, and retinopathy
- Polyuria
- Polydipsia
- Polyphagia
- Weight loss
- Weakness
- Fatigue
- Frequent infections

CAUSES Genetic factors and obesity are important

RISK FACTORS
- Family history
- Gestational diabetes
- Obesity

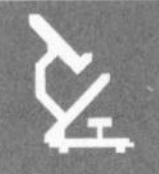

DIAGNOSIS

DIFFERENTIAL DIAGNOSIS
- Type 1 diabetes mellitus
- Other specific types of diabetes mellitus
  - ◊ Genetic defects of ß-cell function
  - ◊ Genetic defects in insulin action
  - ◊ Diseases of exocrine pancreas
  - ◊ Endocrinopathies
  - ◊ Drug or chemical induced (see below)
  - ◊ Infections
  - ◊ Immune mediated
  - ◊ Genetic syndromes sometimes associated with diabetes
  - ◊ Hemochromatosis
- Gestational diabetes mellitus

LABORATORY
Criteria for diagnosis
- Symptoms of diabetes (polyuria, polydipsia, weight loss) plus casual (random) plasma glucose ≥ 200 mg/dL (11.1 mmol/L)

or
- Fasting plasma glucose ≥ 126 mg/dL (7.0 mmol/L) on 2 occasions

or
- 2 hour plasma glucose ≥ 200 mg/dL (11.1 mmol/L) during OGTT with 75 g glucose load

Drugs that may alter lab results:
- Pentamidine
- Nicotinic acid
- Glucocorticoids
- Thyroid hormone
- Diazoxide
- Beta adrenergic agonists
- Thiazides
- Dilantin
- Alpha-interferon
- Some fluoroquinolones
- Some second generation (atypical) antipsychotics

Disorders that may alter lab results: See Differential Diagnosis

PATHOLOGICAL FINDINGS N/A

SPECIAL TESTS
- Glucose tolerance test usually not necessary, except when diagnosing gestational diabetes
- Hemoglobin A1C not recommended for diagnosis, but helpful in management

IMAGING N/A

DIAGNOSTIC PROCEDURES N/A

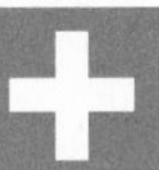

TREATMENT

APPROPRIATE HEALTH CARE Regular outpatient follow-up except for complicating emergencies such as severe hyperglycemia, hyperosmolar coma, and severe infections

GENERAL MEASURES
- Home monitoring of blood glucose
- Regular examination for complications: retinopathy, neuropathy, nephropathy
- Diabetes is a high risk factor for coronary heart disease. NCEP Adult Treatment Panel III recommends an LDL-cholesterol goal of < 100 mg/dL.
- Strict control of hypertension (goal BP <130/80) reduces the risk of complications and death related to diabetes and decreases progression of diabetic retinopathy and deterioration in vision

SURGICAL MEASURES N/A

ACTIVITY Regular aerobic exercise can improve glucose tolerance and decrease medication requirements

DIET
- American Diabetes Association (ADA) provides dietary recommendations for NIDDM. The emphasis is on achieving glucose, lipid, and blood pressure goals. Mild caloric restriction is recommended to achieve mild to moderate weight loss (5-10 kg).
- Food choices are similar to Dietary Guidelines for Americans and the Food Guide Pyramid:
  - ◊ 10-20% of calories from protein
  - ◊ < 10% of calories each from saturated and polyunsaturated fat
  - ◊ Remainder of calories from monounsaturated fat and carbohydrates, depending on individual patient factors
  - ◊ Sugar is not specifically prohibited

PATIENT EDUCATION
- Education is critical for patients with NIDDM. Include information on the disease, medication treatment, self-monitoring, foot care, physical activity and diet management
- Support groups and classes certified by the ADA are recommended
- The ADA has prepared numerous patient education materials (430 North Michigan Ave. Chicago, IL 60611 or contact local ADA affiliate listed in white pages of telephone directory)

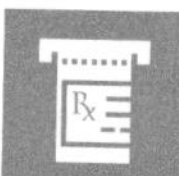

MEDICATIONS

DRUG(S) OF CHOICE

The following classes of agents may be used alone or in combination. Sulfonylureas are generally used as initial treatment, but recent data suggest that metformin may be the preferred first medication in obese patients. If one drug does not produce adequate control, a drug from a different class should be added. If two agents are not adequate, insulin might be the next best addition.

- Biguanides
  - ◊ Metformin (Glucophage) 500-850 mg bid-tid
- Sulfonylureas
  - ◊ Glimepiride (Amaryl) 1-8 mg/d in 1 dose
  - ◊ Glipizide (Glucotrol) 2.5-40 mg/d in 1-2 doses (1st 20 mg in AM)
  - ◊ Glipizide extended release tablets 5-20 mg/d in 1 dose
  - ◊ Glyburide (DiaBeta, Micronase) 1.25-20 mg/d in 1-2 doses (1st 10 mg in AM)
  - ◊ Note: sulfonylureas may be taken with meals except glipizide which should be taken 30 min before meals
- Thiazolidinediones
  - ◊ Pioglitazone (Actos) 15-45 mg qd
  - ◊ Rosiglitazone (Avandia) 2-4 mg bid. Monitor serum transaminase q 2 mo for 1st year.
- a-Glucosidase inhibitors
  - ◊ Acarbose(Precose)25-100 mg tid
  - ◊ Miglitol (Glyset) 25-100 mg tid
  - ◊ Taken at beginning of meals to decrease postprandial glucose peaks. Avoid use in renal insufficiency, inflammatory bowel disease, colonic ulceration or partial bowel obstruction.
- Insulin (NPH, Lente, Regular, Ultralente, 70/30, Humalog, Novolog); insulin glargine (Lantus)
- Combinations
  - ◊ Fixed dose combinations of metformin with glipizide, glyburide, and rosiglitazone are available

Contraindications:

- To oral agents: type I (insulin dependent) diabetes mellitus, ketotic patient, pregnancy, history of specific drug allergy
- Use caution in liver or renal disease and acute infection or stress

Precautions:

- Warn patients of signs of hypo- and hyperglycemia
- Home glucose monitoring (1-4 times/d) recommended for most patients taking insulin
- Avoid metformin in situations which increase risk for lactic acidosis: renal insufficiency, radiocontrast agents, surgery or acute illnesses such as liver disease, cardiogenic shock, pancreatitis or hypoxia. Use caution in CHF, alcohol abuse, elderly or with tetracycline.

Significant possible interactions:

- Drugs which may potentiate sulfonylureas include: salicylates, clofibrate, warfarin (Coumadin), chloramphenicol, ethanol, and ACE inhibitors
- Beta-blockers may mask symptoms of hypoglycemia and delay return to normoglycemia
- Thiazolidinedione pioglitazone may decrease effectiveness of oral contraceptives
- Drugs which bind others in the intestine, such as cholestyramine resin, should be taken at least 2 hours apart from a-glucosidase inhibitors
- Gatifloxacin

ALTERNATIVE DRUGS

- Aspirin recommended for diabetics with known macrovascular disease and those over 40 years old with another risk factor for vascular disease
- First generation sulfonylureas
  - ◊ Chlorpropamide (Diabinese) 100-500 mg/d in 1 dose
  - ◊ Tolazamide (Tolinase) 100-1000 mg/d in 1-2 doses
  - ◊ Tolbutamide (Orinase) 500-3000 mg/d in 2-3 doses
- Insulin - lispro, aspart, regular insulin, NPH, Lente, Ultralente, insulin glargine in 1 or preferably 2-3 injections per day. Insulin may be used in combination with oral agents. Most often required in late stages of type 2 diabetes mellitus when oral agents fail to control blood glucose. Insulin can be started as 10 units combination intermediate/short acting with evening meal or intermediate (NPH) or insulin glargine at bedtime.
- Meglitinides
  - ◊ Repaglinide (Prandin) 0.5-4 mg before meals tid. May be useful in patients with sulfa allergy or renal impairment who are not candidates for sulfonylureas.
  - ◊ Nateglinide (Starlix) 60-120 mg before meals tid

FOLLOWUP

PATIENT MONITORING

- Frequency of followup depends on compliance and degree of metabolic control. Every two to four months is typical.
- Review of symptoms and home blood glucose levels
- Hemoglobin A1c
- Funduscopy
- Cardiopulmonary exam
- Foot exam for ulcers, arterial insufficiency, neuropathy
- After five years, perform yearly: Ophthalmologist exam, monitor for proteinuria and renal insufficiency

PREVENTION/AVOIDANCE

Avoidance of weight gain and obesity and maintenance of regular physical activity may prevent or delay NIDDM

POSSIBLE COMPLICATIONS

- Appear to be due to effects of diabetes mellitus on arterial walls in one form or another
- Peripheral neuropathy
- Proliferative retinopathy
- Nephropathy and chronic renal failure
- Atherosclerotic cardiovascular and peripheral vascular disease
- Hyperosmolar coma
- Gangrene of extremities
- Blindness
- Glaucoma
- Cataracts
- Skin ulceration
- Charcot joints

EXPECTED COURSE/PROGNOSIS

- Maintenance of normal blood sugar levels may delay or prevent complications of diabetes
- In susceptible individuals, complications begin to appear 10-15 years after onset, but can be present at time of diagnosis since disease may go undetected for years

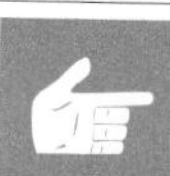

MISCELLANEOUS

ASSOCIATED CONDITIONS

- Hypertension is common (see treatment above)
- Hyperlipidemia
- Impotence

AGE-RELATED FACTORS

Pediatric: The incidence of type 2 diabetes mellitus in children is increasing dramatically, possibly related to increases in childhood obesity

Geriatric: Common in the elderly and is a significant contributing factor to blindness, renal failure, and lower limb amputations

Others: Generally diagnosed after age 40

PREGNANCY

Diabetes can cause significant maternal complications and fetal wasting. Intensive management has improved the outcome dramatically.

SYNONYMS

- Adult onset diabetes mellitus
- Nonketotic diabetes mellitus
- NIDDM

ICD-9-CM

250.00 Diabetes mellitus without mention of complication, type 2 or unspecified type, not stated as uncontrolled

250.02 Diabetes mellitus without mention of complication, type 2 or unspecified type, uncontrolled

SEE ALSO

Diabetes mellitus, Type 1

Diabetic ketoacidosis (DKA)

Hypertension, essential

OTHER NOTES

N/A

ABBREVIATIONS

NIDDM = Non-insulin dependent diabetes mellitus

ADA = American Diabetic Association

REFERENCES

- Report of the Expert Committee on the diagnosis and classification of diabetes mellitus. Diabetes 1997;20:1183-97
- Holmboe ES. Oral antihyperglycemic therapy for type 2 diabetes: clinical applications. JAMA 2002;287(3):373-6
- Inzucchi SE. Oral antihyperglycemic therapy for type 2 diabetes: scientific review. JAMA 2002;287(3):360-72
- Clinical Practice Recommendations 2004. Diabetes Care 2004; 27:S1-S137
- UK Prospective Diabetes Study Group. Tight blood pressure control and risk of macrovascular and microvascular complications in type 2 diabetes: UKPDS 38. Br Med J 1998; 317: 703-13
- UK Prospective Diabetes Study Group. Efficacy of atenolol and captopril in reducing risk of macrovascular and microvascular complications in type 2 diabetes: UKPDS 39. Br Med J 1998; 317: 713-20
- UK Prospective Diabetes Study Group. Intensive blood-glucose control with sulphonylureas or insulin comopared with conventional treatment and risk of complications in patients with type 2 diabetes (UKPDS 33). Lancet 1998; 352: 837-53

Web references: 4 available at www.5mcc.com

Illustrations 16 available

Author(s):

David S. Gray, MD

Diabetic ketoacidosis (DKA)

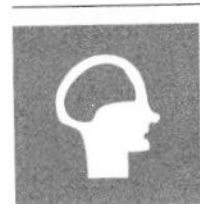

BASICS

DESCRIPTION A true medical emergency secondary to absolute or relative insulin deficiency characterized by hyperglycemia, ketonemia, metabolic acidosis, and electrolyte depletion
System(s) affected: Endocrine/Metabolic
Genetics: N/A
Incidence/Prevalence in USA: 46 episodes/10,000 diabetic patients; 2 per 100 patient years of type 1 DM
Predominant age: 0-19 years of age
Predominant sex: Male = Female

SIGNS & SYMPTOMS
- Polyuria
- Polydipsia
- Generalized weakness
- Malaise/lethargy
- Nocturia
- Nausea/vomiting
- Abdominal pain and tenderness
- Decreased bowel sounds
- Decreased perspiration
- Hypotension
- Hypothermia
- Decreased reflexes
- Coma
- Confusion
- Tachycardia
- Tachypnea
- Fever +/-
- Breath fruity, with acetone smell
- Dry mucous membranes
- Anorexia or increased appetite

CAUSES
- Insulin dependent diabetes mellitus (20-30% in newly diagnosed diabetics)
- Infarction (myocardial) 5-7%
- Infection (30-40%) usually respiratory or urinary
- Idiopathic (20-30%)
- Medication non-compliance
- CVA
- Trauma
- Surgery
- Emotional stress

RISK FACTORS
- Any condition that leads to an absolute or relative insulin deficiency
- History of corticosteroid therapy

DIAGNOSIS

DIFFERENTIAL DIAGNOSIS
- Hyperosmolar non-ketotic coma
- Alcoholic ketoacidosis
- Lactic acidosis
- Acute hypoglycemic coma
- Uremia

LABORATORY
- Blood sugar elevated (usually 250-800 mg/dL [13.88-44.4 mmol/L] range)
- Serum ketosis
- Urine ketosis
- Glycosuria
- Hyponatremia
- Hyperamylasemia
- Hypertriglyceridemia
- Hypercholesterolemia
- Increased BUN
- $HCO_3 < 15$ (< 15 mmol/L)
- Decreased calculated total body K^+
- Metabolic acidosis on ABGs
- Increased serum osmolality
- Increased anion gap

Drugs that may alter lab results: N/A

Disorders that may alter lab results:
- With concomitant lactic acidosis, acetoacetate production may be inhibited in presence of high levels of beta hydroxybutyrate. The nitroprusside reaction, which measures only acetoacetate, may not be strongly positive.
- A very low serum sodium (< 110 mmol/L) suggests an artifact due to severe hypertriglyceridemia
- Severe acidosis gives artificially high K^+ level
- Markedly increased serum ketones may cross react and cause a falsely high serum creatinine

PATHOLOGICAL FINDINGS N/A

SPECIAL TESTS
- ECG (especially if MI suspected). May also assist in evaluation of K^+ status. Usually shows sinus tachycardia.
- Urine and blood cultures

IMAGING Chest x-ray to rule out pulmonary infection

DIAGNOSTIC PROCEDURES N/A

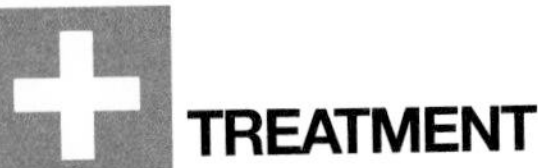

TREATMENT

APPROPRIATE HEALTH CARE
- Inpatient intensive care. This is a life threatening emergency.
- Goals are to increase rate of glucose utilization by insulin-dependent tissues, to reverse ketonemia and acidosis, and to correct the depletion of water and electrolytes.

GENERAL MEASURES
- IV Fluids adults: 1000 mL over first hour, then 500 mL/hr (approximately 7 mL/kg/hr) x 4 hrs or until dehydration improves, then 250 mL/hour (3.5 mL/kg/hr). Switch to D5 in 1/2 NS when serum glucose < 300 mg/dL (16.65 mmol/l). Expect to give 4-8 L/ first 24 hrs. (Some do not recommend initial IV bolus).
- Pediatric maintenance requirements: 100 mL/kg for first 10 kg, 50 mL/kg for second 10 kg and 20 mL/kg thereafter. Fluid deficit: (Multiply patient's body weight by percentage dehydration). Replace maintenance and deficit evenly over 48 hours.

SURGICAL MEASURES N/A

ACTIVITY Bedrest

DIET Nothing by mouth initially. Advance to pre-ketotic diet when nausea and vomiting are controlled.

PATIENT EDUCATION
- For prevention, careful control of blood glucose (usually HgbA1c $\leq 7\%$)
- Monitor glucose carefully during periods of stress, infection, trauma etc.

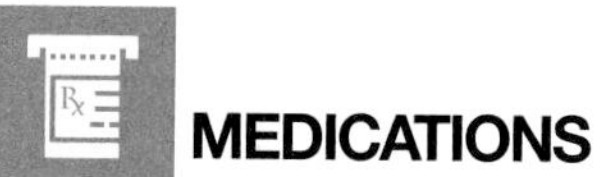

MEDICATIONS

DRUG(S) OF CHOICE
- Insulin - initiate infusion at 0.1U/kg/hr
- Potassium phosphate or Potassium chloride
- Sodium bicarbonate, rarely

Contraindications:
- No demonstrable clinical benefit from bicarbonate with a pH > 7.0.
- Hold K+ if > 5.5 (> 5.5 mmol/L)

Precautions:
- Double insulin if no response in serum glucose over first 2 hours
- Must continue insulin until serum bicarbonate and anion gap normalize
- Add dextrose to IV fluid when blood sugar < 300 mg/dL (16.65 mmol/L)
- If using bicarbonate, add 50 mg NaHCO3 to 1L 1/2 NS and give over 2 hours
- Delay K+ administration in patients with inadequate urine output or evidence of diabetic nephropathy
- If blood sugar does not fall by approximately 75 mg % q2h, increase insulin rate
- Taper IV insulin and start NPH/Reg insulin after acidosis clears and patient is eating

Significant possible interactions: For each 0.1 unit of pH, serum K+ will change by approximately 0.6 mEq (0.6 mmol/L) K in the opposite direction

ALTERNATIVE DRUGS N/A

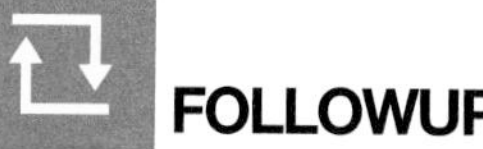

FOLLOWUP

PATIENT MONITORING
- Monitor mental status, vital signs, urine output q 30-60 minutes until improved, then q2-4 h x 24 hrs
- Blood sugar q 1 hr until < 300 mg/dL (16.65 mmol/L), then q2-6h
- Potassium, bicarbonate, sodium, anion gap; q 2 hrs
- Phosphate, calcium, magnesium; q4-6h

PREVENTION/AVOIDANCE
- Monitor glucose closely during stressful situations
- Careful insulin control
- Educational program for sick-day management instructions

POSSIBLE COMPLICATIONS
- Cerebral edema
- Pulmonary edema
- Venous thrombosis
- Hypokalemia
- Myocardial infarction
- Acute gastric dilatation
- Late hypoglycemia
- Erosive gastritis
- Infection
- Respiratory distress
- Hypophosphatemia
- Mucormycosis

EXPECTED COURSE/PROGNOSIS
- DKA accounts for 14% of all hospital admissions for diabetes and for 16% of all diabetic related fatalities
- Mortality of 1-2%
- In children < 10 years old, DKA causes 70% diabetes related fatalities

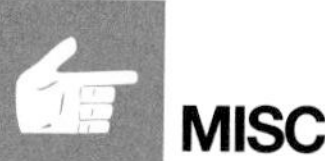

MISCELLANEOUS

ASSOCIATED CONDITIONS Look for complications of chronic diabetes (nephropathy, neuropathy, retinopathy, etc.)

AGE-RELATED FACTORS
Pediatric:
- Occasionally children or adolescents with DKA exhibit marked mental deterioration, including development of coma 4-6 hrs after therapy has begun. Mortality is high.
  - ◊ Diagnose by CT scan (cerebral edema)
  - ◊ Treat with IV bolus of 1 gram mannitol/kg in 20% solution
  - ◊ If no response, hyperventilation to a pCO2 of 28 mm Hg

Geriatric: Must be careful with renal status or congestive heart failure

Others: N/A

PREGNANCY Risk of fetal death with DKA during pregnancy is nearly 50%

SYNONYMS N/A

ICD-9-CM
250.12 Diabetes with ketoacidosis, type 2 or unspecified type, uncontrolled

SEE ALSO
Diabetes mellitus, Type 1

OTHER NOTES N/A

ABBREVIATIONS
NS = normal saline
ABG = arterial blood gases
D5 = 5% dextrose

REFERENCES

- Isselbacher KJ, et al, eds: Harrison's Principles of Internal Medicine. 13th Ed. New York, McGraw-Hill, 1994
- Bennett JC, Plum F, eds: Cecil Textbook of Medicine. 20th Ed. Philadelphia, W.B. Saunders Co., 1996
- Bell DS, et al: Diabetic ketoacidosis: Why early detection and aggressive treatment are crucial. Postgrad Med 1997;101(9):193-200

Web references: 2 available at www.5mcc.com
Illustrations N/A

Author(s):
Stoney A. Abercrombie, MD

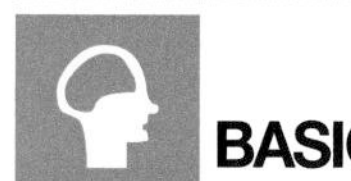

BASICS

DESCRIPTION Diarrhea of abrupt onset in a healthy individual is most often related to an infectious process. A variety of symptoms are often observed, including frequent passage of loose or watery stools, fever, chills, anorexia, vomiting and malaise.

- Acute viral diarrhea - the most common form, usually occurs for 1-3 days, and is self-limited. It causes changes in the small intestine cell morphology such as villous shortening and an increase in the number of crypt cells.
- Bacterial diarrhea - may be suspected if there is a history of a similar and simultaneous illness in individuals who have shared contaminated food with the patient. Diarrhea developing within 12 hours of the meal is most likely due to ingestion of a preformed toxin.
- Protozoal infections - such as *Giardia lamblia* cause prolonged, watery diarrhea that often afflicts travelers returning from endemic areas where the water supply has been contaminated.
- Traveler's diarrhea - typically begins three to seven days after arrival in a foreign location and is generally quite acute

System(s) affected: Endocrine/Metabolic, Gastrointestinal
Genetics: N/A
Incidence/Prevalence in USA: N/A
Predominant age: All ages
Predominant sex: N/A

SIGNS & SYMPTOMS
- Loose liquid stools +/- blood or mucus
- Fever
- Abdominal pain and distension
- Headache
- Anorexia
- Malaise
- Vomiting
- Myalgia
- With Giardia - cramping, pale-greasy stools, fatigue, weight loss, chronicity

CAUSES
- Bacterial
  - ◊ E. coli
  - ◊ Salmonella
  - ◊ Shigella
  - ◊ Campylobacter jejuni
  - ◊ Vibrio parahaemolyticus
  - ◊ Vibrio cholerae
  - ◊ Yersinia enterocolitica
- Viral
  - ◊ Rotavirus
  - ◊ Norwalk virus
- Parasitic
  - ◊ Giardia lamblia
  - ◊ Cryptosporidium
  - ◊ Entamoeba histolytica

RISK FACTORS
- Individual from an industrialized country visiting a developing country
- Immunocompromised host

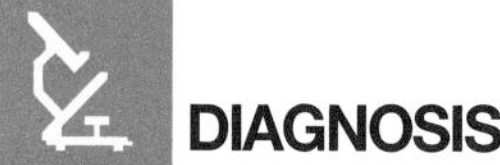

DIAGNOSIS

DIFFERENTIAL DIAGNOSIS
- Ulcerative colitis
- Crohn disease
- Drugs (cholinergic agents, magnesium-containing antacids)
- Pseudomembranous colitis secondary to antibiotic use
- Diverticulitis
- Spastic (irritable) colon
- Fecal impaction
- Malabsorption
- Zollinger-Ellison syndrome
- Ischemic bowel
- Gastrinoma

LABORATORY
- CBC - increased WBC with a left shift may indicate an infectious process; decreased hemoglobin/hematocrit may indicate anemia from blood loss
- Serum electrolytes - increased sodium from dehydration, decreased potassium from diarrhea
- BUN, creatinine - elevated in dehydration
- pH - hyperchloremic acidosis
- Stool sample - occult blood (present in IBD, bowel ischemia, bacterial infections), fecal leukocytes (present in diarrhea caused by Salmonella, Campylobacter, Yersinia), bacterial culture and sensitivity (for Salmonella, Yersinia, Shigella, Campylobacter), ova and parasites, C. difficile toxin, Ziehl-Neelsen stain (for Cryptosporidium)

Drugs that may alter lab results: N/A

Disorders that may alter lab results: N/A

PATHOLOGICAL FINDINGS
- Viral diarrhea - changes in small intestine cell morphology that include villous shortening, increased number of crypt cells and increased cellularity of the lamina propria
- Bacterial diarrhea - bacterial invasion of colonic wall leads to mucosal hyperemia, edema and leukocytic infiltration

SPECIAL TESTS N/A

IMAGING Abdominal x-rays (flat plate and upright) are indicated in patients with abdominal pain or evidence of obstruction to rule out toxic megacolon and bowel ischemia

DIAGNOSTIC PROCEDURES Sigmoidoscopy indicated in patients with bloody diarrhea or suspected pseudomembranous or ulcerative colitis

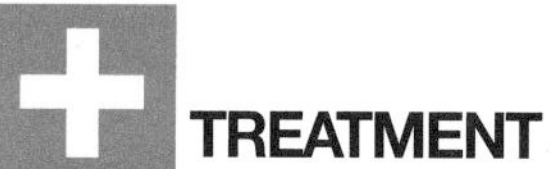

TREATMENT

APPROPRIATE HEALTH CARE Outpatient except for complicating emergencies (dehydration)

GENERAL MEASURES
- Replacement of lost fluid and electrolytes
- Clear liquids such as tea, broth, carbonated beverages (without caffeine) and rehydration fluids (e.g., Gatorade) to replace lost fluid
- Packets of rehydration salts (one packet to be diluted in one quart of water); drink until thirst is quenched; will help in replacing lost electrolytes. Treatment of choice for pediatric patients.

SURGICAL MEASURES N/A

ACTIVITY Bedrest

DIET
- During periods of active diarrhea, avoid coffee, alcohol, dairy products, most fruits, vegetables, red meats, and heavily seasoned foods
- After 12 hours with no diarrhea, begin by eating clear soup, salted crackers, dry toast or bread, and sherbet
- As stooling rate decreases, slowly add to diet, rice, baked potato, and chicken soup with rice or noodles
- As stool begins to retain shape, add to diet baked fish, poultry, applesauce, and bananas

PATIENT EDUCATION See guidelines in Prevention/Avoidance

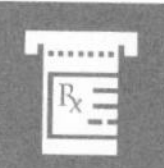

MEDICATIONS

DRUG(S) OF CHOICE
- Loperamide, 4 mg followed by 2 mg capsule after each unformed stool, or bismuth subsalicylate, 30 mL every half hour until 8 doses, may be helpful in mild diarrhea
- If diarrhea persists and a bacterial or parasitic organism is identified, antibiotic therapy should be started:
  - ◊ Giardia: metronidazole 250 mg tid for 5 days
  - ◊ E. histolytica: metronidazole 750 mg tid for 10 days
  - ◊ Shigella: trimethoprim-sulfamethoxazole 160 mg and 800 mg, respectively, bid for five days, or ciprofloxacin (Cipro) 500 mg bid for 3 days
  - ◊ Campylobacter: erythromycin 500 mg qid for 5 days or ciprofloxacin (Cipro) 500 mg bid for 3 days
  - ◊ C. difficile: metronidazole 500 mg tid for 10-14 days
  - ◊ Traveler's diarrhea: Ciprofloxacin (Cipro) 750 mg one dose or if severe, 500 mg divided PO bid for 3 days

Contraindications:
- Antibiotics are contraindicated in Salmonella infections unless caused by S. typhosa or the patient is septic
- Avoid alcoholic beverages with metronidazole due to possibility of disulfiram reaction

Precautions:
- Antiperistaltic agents (e.g., loperamide) should be used with caution in patients suspected of having infectious diarrhea or antibiotic associated colitis
- Doxycycline, sulfamethoxazole-trimethoprim, ciprofloxacin - may cause photosensitivity. Use sunscreen.

Significant possible interactions:
- Salicylate absorption from bismuth subsalicylate can cause toxicity in patients already taking aspirin containing compounds and may alter anticoagulation control in patients taking coumadin
- Ciprofloxacin and erythromycin increase theophylline levels

ALTERNATIVE DRUGS
- Doxycycline 100 mg bid for 3 days
- Diphenoxylate-atropine in nonpregnant adults
- Tinidazole or secnidazole for E. histolytica
- Vancomycin for C. difficile infections
- Alosetron in IBS

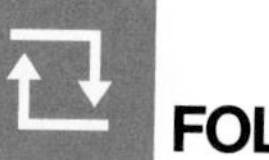

FOLLOWUP

PATIENT MONITORING If diarrhea continues for three to five days with or without blood or mucus then consult physician

PREVENTION/AVOIDANCE
- Frequent oversights during foreign travel include brushing teeth with contaminated water, ingesting ice cubes, or eating cold salads or meats
- Avoid uncooked or undercooked seafood or meat, buffet meals left out for several hours, or food served by street vendors

POSSIBLE COMPLICATIONS
- Dehydration
- Sepsis
- Shock
- Anemia

EXPECTED COURSE/PROGNOSIS A common problem that is rarely life-threatening if attention is given to maintaining adequate hydration

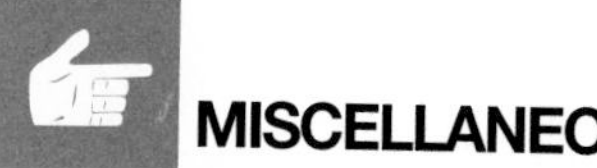

MISCELLANEOUS

ASSOCIATED CONDITIONS
- Diabetes mellitus
- Ileal resection
- Gastrectomy
- Hyperthyroidism

AGE-RELATED FACTORS
Pediatric:
- Rotavirus is a common cause of viral diarrhea in the winter months and is accompanied with vomiting
- Other etiologies include overfeeding, medications, cystic fibrosis and malabsorption

Geriatric: Watery diarrhea in elderly patient with chronic constipation may be caused by fecal impaction or obstructing neoplasm

Others: N/A

PREGNANCY Avoid dehydration since this may lead to preterm labor

SYNONYMS N/A

ICD-9-CM
005.9 Food poisoning, unspecified
558.2 Toxic gastroenteritis and colitis
558.9 Other and unspecified noninfectious gastroenteritis and colitis
787.91 Diarrhea

SEE ALSO
Botulism
Cholera
Food poisoning, bacterial

OTHER NOTES N/A

ABBREVIATIONS
IBD = inflammatory bowel disease

REFERENCES

- Hirschhorn N, Greenough WB: Progress in oral rehydration therapy. Scientific American 1991;264:5
- Dupont HL, Edelman R: Infectious diarrhea: From E. coli to Vibrio. Patient Care, May 30,1991

Web references: 1 available at www.5mcc.com
Illustrations N/A

Author(s):
Tejal Parikh, MD

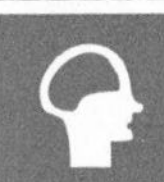

BASICS

DESCRIPTION Healthy adults have daily stool weights < 200 grams (7 oz). Stool weights in excess are abnormal and if > 3 weeks are considered chronic. Causes include: inflammatory diarrhea, osmotic diarrhea (malabsorption), secretory diarrhea (endogenous and exogenous), and intestinal dysmotility.
System(s) affected: Gastrointestinal
Genetics:
- Celiac sprue and inflammatory bowel disease may be familial
- Lactose intolerance - increased incidence in certain geographic regions

Incidence/Prevalence in USA:
- Unknown, but felt to be underdiagnosed, especially in celiac sprue
- Inflammatory bowel disease probably underdiagnosed because many patients don't seek therapy

Predominant age: Determined by certain illnesses
Predominant sex: Female > Male

SIGNS & SYMPTOMS
- Frequent loose stools, fever, abdominal pain, weight loss, tenesmus, flatus, bulky stools plus
  - ◊ Inflammatory: blood (must rule out colonic neoplasm), anemia, abdominal pain
  - ◊ Osmotic: steatorrhea, azotorrhea, weight loss, improves with fasting
  - ◊ Secretory: large volumes, persists with fasting
  - ◊ Altered intestinal motility: alternating diarrhea and constipation, passage of mucus and incomplete evacuation, bloating, anxiety, depression (not nocturnal)
  - ◊ Factitious: peripheral edema, weakness, nausea, nocturnal, hypokalemia

CAUSES
- Inflammatory diarrhea
  - ◊ Inflammatory bowel disease (ulcerative colitis and Crohn disease)
  - ◊ Radiation enterocolitis
  - ◊ Eosinophilic gastroenteritis
  - ◊ Hypersensitivity, e.g., food allergy
  - ◊ AIDS - mucosal and submucosal inflammation with possible impairment in absorption and excessive secretion
- Infectious
  - ◊ Parasites (e.g., *Giardia lamblia*, *Isospora*)
  - ◊ Helminths (e.g., *Strongyloides*)
  - ◊ Bacterial (e.g., *Mycobacterium avium intracellulare*, *Clostridium difficile*)
- Osmotic diarrhea
  - ◊ Pancreatic insufficiency (e.g., alcohol-induced, cystic fibrosis)
  - ◊ Bacterial overgrowth
  - ◊ Celiac disease
  - ◊ Thyrotoxicosis
  - ◊ Lactase deficiency
  - ◊ Whipple disease
  - ◊ Abetalipoproteinemia
  - ◊ Post-surgical (short gut, PUD surgery)
  - ◊ Drugs: colchicine, neomycin, and para-aminosalicylic acid, antacids with magnesium, nondigestible intraluminal solute that exerts an osmotic force increasing the intraluminal fluid overwhelming the colonic mucosal absorptive capacities
- Secretory diarrhea (endogenous)
  - ◊ Carcinoid syndrome
  - ◊ Zollinger-Ellison syndrome
  - ◊ Vasoactive intestinal peptide-secreting pancreatic adenomas
  - ◊ Medullary carcinoma of thyroid
  - ◊ Villous adenoma of rectum
  - ◊ Microscopic colitis
  - ◊ Choleraic diarrhea - excessive secretion of electrolytes
  - ◊ Diabetic
  - ◊ Alcohol-induced
- Secretory (exogenous)
  - ◊ Factitious
  - ◊ Laxatives (phenolphthalein, cascara , senna, aloe)
  - ◊ Medications (cholinergics, ACE inhibitors, colchicine, theophyllines, thyroid)
  - ◊ Toxins (arsenic, mushrooms, insecticides, alcohol)
- Altered intestinal motility (most common in clinical practice)
  - ◊ Irritable bowel syndrome (most common in young females)
  - ◊ Fecal impaction
  - ◊ Neurologic diseases
  - ◊ Diabetes - increased transit and possible bacterial overgrowth

RISK FACTORS
- Inflammatory: AIDS, infections, radiation, family history
- Osmotic: infectious, abdominal surgery including cholecystectomy, resection gastric and small bowel, vagotomy, chronic alcohol abuse, Sorbitol, fructose, gluten
- Secretory: distal ileal surgery
- Altered intestinal motility: diabetes, fecal impaction or neurological diseases
- Factitious: laxative use

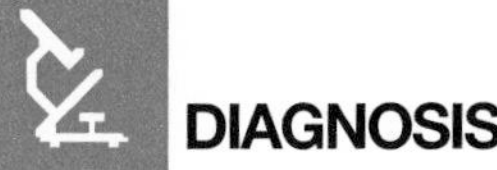

DIAGNOSIS

DIFFERENTIAL DIAGNOSIS
- Functional disorder
- Inflammatory bowel disease: look for systemic illness or extra-intestinal manifestations (arthritis, pyoderma gangrenosum, erythema nodosum, uveitis or vasculitis); consider Crohn or ulcerative colitis
- Factitious: psychiatric disease or history of
- Irritable bowel syndrome: alternating diarrhea and constipation, psychiatric overtones
- Tropical sprue
- TB enteritis
- Chronic radiation enterocolitis
- Colonic neoplasm
- Diverticular disease

LABORATORY
- Stool ova and parasites
- Stool leukocytes
- Stool fat, osmolality, and occult blood
- Stool for *C. difficile* toxin
- Serum electrolytes and CBC
- Serum iron studies, vitamin B12, folate, vitamin D, PT, blood chemistry for albumin and cholesterol, serum carotene
- D-Xylose absorption test
- Inflammatory diarrhea: blood or leukocytes in stool, hypoproteinemia (hypoalbuminemia and hypoglobulinemia)
- Factitious: hypokalemia

Drugs that may alter lab results: Screen for laxative abuse, e.g., phenolphthalein

Disorders that may alter lab results: Unspecified noninfectious gastroenteritis; psychiatric behavior in factitious diarrhea may contaminate stool study

PATHOLOGICAL FINDINGS
- When present, findings are those of the associated or underlying disease
- None seen in functional disorder

SPECIAL TESTS
- Inflammatory: colonic biopsies
- Biopsies with esophagogastroduodenoscopy (EGD) or colonoscopy when performed
- Fecal fat stool collections: 48-72 hours
- Breath test for labeled CO_2 to assess fat, carbohydrate, and bile salt malabsorption
- Blood and urine hormone levels in endocrine diseases
- Malabsorption - small bowel biopsies
- Capsule endoscopy - small bowel visualization

IMAGING Barium enema, KUB

DIAGNOSTIC PROCEDURES
- Thorough history and physical exam helpful
- Colonoscopy for inflammatory lesions and associated occult blood in stool or with iron deficiency
- If barium enema is negative and diarrhea persists, biopsies are required (to rule out microscopic colitis in which the mucosa may appear normal). UGI evaluation with small bowel biopsies for malabsorption evaluation
- Melanosis coli suggests cathartic abuse

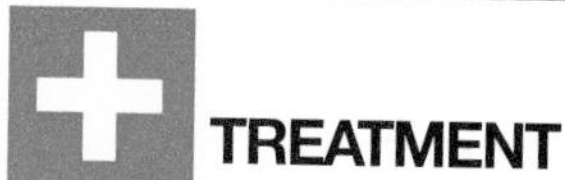

TREATMENT

APPROPRIATE HEALTH CARE Unless electrolyte abnormality, deconditioning or hypotensive, outpatient therapy is adequate

GENERAL MEASURES Fluids with electrolyte supplementation

SURGICAL MEASURES
- For villous adenomas, hormone producing tumors, and refractory ulcerative colitis

ACTIVITY Restricted only for the debilitated patient

DIET
- Abstain from gluten products, sorbitol, lactose-containing products, food allergens
- In IBS, may need to add dietary fiber (bulking agents) (e.g. 20-30 grams of supplemental fiber per day)

PATIENT EDUCATION
- Explain in simple terms of bowel physiology
- Reassure that normal frequency varies widely
- Dietary consult when appropriate
- Restrict colon stimulants

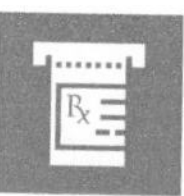

MEDICATIONS

DRUG(S) OF CHOICE
- Efforts to increase stool consistency may be undertaken using psyllium or other hydrophilic agents
- In secretory diarrhea, opiates may help
- Diphenoxylate-atropine (Lomotil) 5-20 mg daily or loperamide (Imodium) 4-16 mg daily; given in doses calculated and timed according to the patient's individual needs. These agents may be contraindicated in infectious diarrheas because of possible organism enhancement of tissue. also avoid in ulcerative colitis toxic megacolon.
- Kaolin-pectin (Kapectolin, Donnagel) 2-16 tablespoons daily, divided and timed according to individual need
- Specific agents include:
  - ◊ Octreotide (Sandostatin) a analogue of somatostatin used in carcinoid syndrome and severe fluid loss in AIDs patients
  - ◊ Omeprazole: an H-K-ATPase inhibitor for use in Zollinger-Ellison syndrome
  - ◊ Indomethacin: prostaglandin inhibitor used in medullary carcinoma of the thyroid and villous adenomas (rare)
  - ◊ H1 and H2 receptor antagonists combination for systemic mastocytosis
  - ◊ Cholestyramine (Questran) for bile salt malabsorption and certain post-surgical patients
  - ◊ Lactase (Lactaid, Lactrase) for lactose intolerance
  - ◊ Alosetron (Lotronex) - restricted use for diarrhea predominant IBS

Contraindications: Any impediment to bowel transit, obstruction, ileus
Precautions: Excessive treatment may lead to obstipation
Significant possible interactions: N/A

ALTERNATIVE DRUGS
- Anti-cholinergics, antispasmodics, and alosetron (Lotronex) which has restricted use in irritable bowel syndrome
- Steroids and sulfasalazine derivatives in inflammatory bowel disease
- Clonidine in diabetes mellitus diarrhea

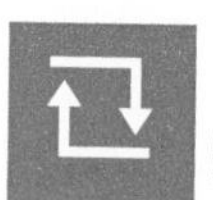

FOLLOWUP

PATIENT MONITORING If diarrhea persists, further evaluation recommended

PREVENTION/AVOIDANCE Refrain from dietary or pharmacological agents that may precipitate a diarrhea event

POSSIBLE COMPLICATIONS
- Fluid and electrolyte abnormalities
- Malnutrition
- Anemia
- Sepsis
- Cachexia

EXPECTED COURSE/PROGNOSIS
Variable, from a short (factitious and altered intestinal motility) and treatable course, to a chronic illness (e.g., Crohn, ulcerative colitis, etc.)

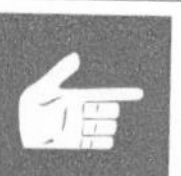

MISCELLANEOUS

ASSOCIATED CONDITIONS
- Immune-complex mediated extra-intestinal complications of inflammatory bowel disease
  - ◊ Arthritis
  - ◊ Uveitis
  - ◊ Pyoderma gangrenosum
  - ◊ Nephritis

AGE-RELATED FACTORS
Pediatric: Diarrhea secondary to dietary products, e.g., fructose and apple juice
Geriatric: Patients with life-long diarrhea may suffer increasing difficulty with advanced age
Others: N/A

PREGNANCY N/A

SYNONYMS
- Loose bowels
- The runs

ICD-9-CM
005.9 Food poisoning, unspecified
558.2 Toxic gastroenteritis and colitis
558.9 Other and unspecified noninfectious gastroenteritis and colitis
787.91 Diarrhea

SEE ALSO
Crohn disease
Cryptococcosis
Diarrhea, acute
Giardiasis
Irritable bowel syndrome
Ulcerative colitis
Uveitis

OTHER NOTES N/A

ABBREVIATIONS
IBD = inflammatory bowel disease
IBS = irritable bowel syndrome

REFERENCES
- Spiro HM. Diarrhea Diseases. In: Spiro HM, ed. Clinical Gastroenterology. 4th ed. New York: McGraw-Hill, Inc; 1993: p356-358
- Krejs GJ. Diarrhea. In: Wyngaarden JB, Smith HL, eds. Cecil Textbook of Medicine. 19th ed. Philadelphia: WB Saunders Co; 1992: p680-687
- Freidman LS, Isselbacher KJ. Chronic Diarrhea. In: Braunwald E, Isselbacher KJ, et al, eds. Harrison's Principles of Internal Medicine. 13th ed. New York: McGraw-Hill, 1994: p216-219.
- Fine KD, Krejs GJ, Fo;dtran JS. Diarrhea. In: Sleisenger MH, Fordtran JS, eds. Gastrointestinal Disease. 5th ed. Philadelphia: WB Saunders Co; 1994: p1043-1072
- Powell D. Approach to the patient with diarrhea. In: Yamada T, et al, eds. Textbook of Gastroenterology. 3rd ed. Baltimore: Lippincott Williams & Wilkins; 1998

Web references: 1 available at www.5mcc.com
Illustrations N/A

Author(s):
Robert Burgos, MD

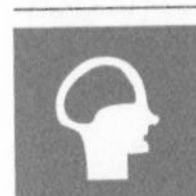

BASICS

DESCRIPTION A condition that may result from digitalis overdosage, hypokalemia, advanced degenerative heart disease with conduction disturbances, or a combination of factors. Toxicity may develop even when serum levels are within normal range. Usual course - acute; chronic.
System(s) affected: Cardiovascular, Gastrointestinal, Nervous
Genetics: No known genetic pattern
Incidence/Prevalence in USA: Occurs in 5-23% of patients sometime during therapy
Predominant age: Middle age to elderly (40-75 years)
Predominant sex: Male = Female

SIGNS & SYMPTOMS
- Abdominal pain
- Anorexia
- Bilateral central scotomata
- Bizarre mental symptoms in elderly patients
- Blurred vision
- Bradycardia
- Confusion
- Delirium
- Depression
- Diarrhea
- Disorientation
- Drowsiness
- Fatigue
- Hallucinations
- Halos around lights
- Headache
- Hypotension
- Impaired color vision
- Irregular pulse
- Lethargy
- Loss of visual acuity
- Mydriasis
- Nausea
- Neuralgia
- Nightmares
- Personality changes
- Photophobia
- Restlessness
- Vertigo
- Vomiting
- Weakness

CAUSES
- Alkalosis
- Amiodarone
- Broad spectrum antibiotics
- Cor pulmonale
- Diltiazem
- Hemodialysis
- Hypernatremia
- Hypokalemia
- Hypomagnesemia
- Hypothyroidism
- Macrolides
- Myocarditis
- Overdosage
- Poisoning with plants containing cardiac glycosides, such as oleander, foxglove
- Procaine
- Quinidine
- Reserpine
- Spironolactone
- Steroids

RISK FACTORS
- Anoxia
- Catecholamines
- Decompensating heart failure
- Diuretics
- Hypercalcemia
- Myocardial infarction
- Recent cardiac surgery
- Renal failure
- Suicide attempt

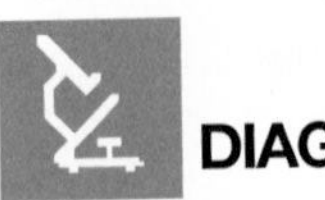

DIAGNOSIS

DIFFERENTIAL DIAGNOSIS
- Heart block
- Renal disease
- Other causes of life-threatening arrhythmia

LABORATORY
- Eosinophilia
- Increased digitalis level, especially if ≥ 4 ng/mL (≥ 5.1 nmol/L). Digoxin levels may not correlate with amount taken in acute ingestion.
- Potassium - hyperkalemia with acute ingestion; hypokalemia with chronic ingestion of excess or chronic renal failure

Drugs that may alter lab results: Any digitalis drug

Disorders that may alter lab results: Many cardiac abnormalities

PATHOLOGICAL FINDINGS N/A

SPECIAL TESTS
- EKG (Note that no arrhythmia is unique to digitalis toxicity, thus any sudden change in cardiac rhythm suggests possible toxicity)
  - ◊ Accelerated junctional rhythms
  - ◊ Atrial flutter
  - ◊ Atrial premature contractions
  - ◊ Atrial tachycardia with AV block
  - ◊ Bidirectional tachycardia
  - ◊ Bundle branch block
  - ◊ Junctional premature beats
  - ◊ Sinus bradycardia
  - ◊ Sinus bradycardia with junctional tachycardia
  - ◊ Ventricular fibrillation
  - ◊ Ventricular premature contractions
  - ◊ Wenckebach's block with junctional premature beats
  - ◊ P-R changes
  - ◊ Q-T changes

IMAGING N/A

DIAGNOSTIC PROCEDURES N/A

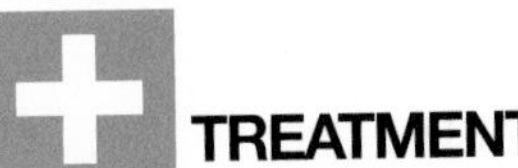

TREATMENT

APPROPRIATE HEALTH CARE
Inpatient - coronary care unit

GENERAL MEASURES
- Maintain airways
- Continuous cardiac monitoring
- Discontinue digitalis
- Check serum electrolytes; maintain potassium in high-normal range. Treat hyperkalemia (K >5.5) with NaHCO3 (1 mEq/kg) glucose (0.5 g/kg), and insulin 0.1 U/kg. Do not use calcium as it may worsen ventricular arrhythmias.
- Correct calcium and magnesium abnormalities
- Avoid quinidine, which may increase serum digoxin levels by displacing digoxin from its binding sites and by decreasing renal and nonrenal excretion
- Avoid beta-adrenergic blocking drugs and isoproterenol
- Procainamide may be used
- If the patient is hemodynamically stable with primarily enhanced vagal activity (1st or 2nd degree AV block) and if the peak digitalis effect has been reached, no acute therapy is required
- Must monitor for 24 hours after ingestion

SURGICAL MEASURES N/A

ACTIVITY
Bedrest with monitoring

DIET
Low salt, low fat

PATIENT EDUCATION
Griffith, H.W.: Instructions for Patients; Philadelphia, W.B. Saunders Co.

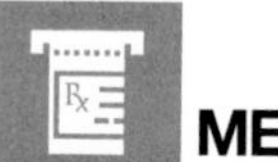

MEDICATIONS

DRUG(S) OF CHOICE
- Fluid plus electrolyte therapy
- Correct acidosis
- Digoxin Immune Fab (Digibind)
  - ◊ Indicated for treatment of severe, life-threatening arrhythmias due to digoxin or digitoxin overdosage
  - ◊ Obtain a digoxin level before administration - be aware that the digoxin level may be falsely high if measured < 6 hours after ingestion
  - ◊ Do not draw another digoxin level for 4 days after digoxin antibody (Digibind) administration since drug's half-life is up to 20 hours in patients with normal renal function
  - ◊ For adults and children ingesting an unknown amount of digoxin, administer 10 vials of digoxin Immune Fab in 50 mL of NS IV over 30 minutes. However, if there is a life-threatening arrhythmia, give as bolus. Observe response and administer an additional 10 vials if clinically indicated. Watch for volume overload in children.
  - ◊ For toxicity during chronic therapy: Adults, 15 vials digoxin Immune Fab in 50 mL NSS IV over 30 minutes; children, < 20 kg, 1 vial should suffice
- For ventricular arrhythmias use
  - ◊ Lidocaine 50 to 100 mg IV (for ventricular arrhythmias), repeated in 3-5 minutes if needed, up to a total of 300 mg. Give no more than 300 mg in 1 hour. One protocol calls for an initial bolus of lidocaine followed by 20-50 mcg/kg/min infusion for maintenance.
  - ◊ Phenytoin - 100 mg q 3-5 minutes up to 1000 mg
  - ◊ Magnesium
  - ◊ Digoxin Immune Fab (Digibind)
- Treat bradycardia and heart block with atropine 0.5-2 mg IV. There is a controversy as to whether pacing should be done as it is associated with a high complication rate in digoxin intoxicated patients and should be used for those to whom Fab is ineffective.

Contraindications: Refer to manufacturer's literature
Precautions: Refer to manufacturer's literature
Significant possible interactions: Refer to manufacturer's literature

ALTERNATIVE DRUGS
Consider atropine, cholestyramine

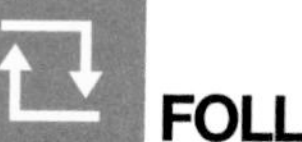

FOLLOWUP

PATIENT MONITORING
- Close EKG monitoring, potassium and digitalis levels throughout total treatment
- Monitor kidney function

PREVENTION/AVOIDANCE
- Store digitalis safely
- Monitor for toxicity
- Fluid plus electrolyte therapy according to need as determined by periodic studies, particularly of potassium level
- If there is a documentable recent exposure, consider gastric decontamination by lavage and administer activated charcoal
- Symptomatic overdose patients might best be managed by a poison control center or toxicologist
- Educate regarding potential for drug interactions
- Onset of vague symptoms should raise suspicion of toxicity
- Be aware of illnesses that predispose to toxicity such as heart failure and dehydration

POSSIBLE COMPLICATIONS
- Death
- Conduction defects
- Life threatening rhythm disturbances

EXPECTED COURSE/PROGNOSIS
Recovery likely if patient survives 24 hours

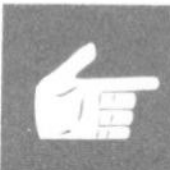

MISCELLANEOUS

ASSOCIATED CONDITIONS
- Chronic heart failure
- Acute pulmonary edema

AGE-RELATED FACTORS
Pediatric: N/A
Geriatric: Morbidity and mortality greater
Others: N/A

PREGNANCY N/A

SYNONYMS N/A

ICD-9-CM
972.1 Poisoning by cardiotonic glycosides and drugs of similar action

SEE ALSO
Ventricular tachycardia (VT)

OTHER NOTES N/A

ABBREVIATIONS
NS = normal saline

REFERENCES

- Carter BL, et al: Monitoring digoxin therapy in two long-term facilities. J Am Geriatr Soc 1981;29:263
- Beller GA, et al: Digitalis intoxication: a prospective clinical study with serum level correlations. N Engl J Med 1971;284:989
- Duhme DW, et al: Reduction of digoxin toxicity associated with measurement of serum levels. Ann Int Med 1974;80:516
- Marcus FI: Diagnosing digitalis intoxication. Hospital Med 1990;7:75
- Burroughs Wellcome Co: Digibind product information. Research Triangle Park, NC., 1991
- Borron SW, et al: Advances in the management of digoxin toxicity in the older patient. Drugs and Aging 1997;10:18-33
- Cauffield JS, et al: The serum digoxin concentration. 10 questions to ask. Amer Fam Phys 1997;56(2):495-503
- Olson K, et al: Poisoning and Drug Overdose. Norwalk, CT, Appleton & Lange, 1994:124-125

Web references: 1 available at www.5mcc.com
Illustrations N/A

Author(s):
Lisa Vantrease, MD
Bruce T. Vanderhoff, MD

BASICS

DESCRIPTION Acute respiratory tract infection caused by *Corynebacterium diphtheriae*, usually producing a membranous pharyngitis
- Incubation period 2 to 5 days. Infection usually occurs in fall and winter in temperate regions. In the tropics, seasonal trends are less distinct.
- Transmission by respiratory route from infected person or carrier. Humans are the only reservoir.
- Several forms occur:
  - ◊ Membranous pharyngotonsillar diphtheria - the membrane is gray, adheres to the pharynx and is surrounded by erythema. The underlying mucosa bleeds when the membrane is removed.
  - ◊ Nasal diphtheria - unilateral discharge
  - ◊ Obstructive laryngotracheitis - complication when membrane descends into larynx or bronchial tree. When it breaks up in young children, total obstruction of the airway may occur.
  - ◊ Cutaneous diphtheria - punched-out ulcer covered by gray membrane (particularly in tropics and among homeless). Peaks August to October in southern United States.

System(s) affected: Cardiovascular, Nervous, Pulmonary, Skin/Exocrine
Genetics: N/A
Incidence/Prevalence in USA: 1.6 in 100,000,000 for non-cutaneous form
Predominant age: Children less than 15 and poorly immunized adults. Diphtheria is a rare condition in the U.S. today. Recent outbreaks have occurred in the new independent states of the former Soviet Union.
Predominant sex: Male = Female

SIGNS & SYMPTOMS
- Membranous pharyngotonsillar diphtheria:
  - ◊ Initially, white to yellow membrane which is easily removed
  - ◊ Adherent, whitish-gray, leathery membrane on tonsils or pharynx
  - ◊ Removing membrane causes bleeding of mucosa
  - ◊ Injected pharynx
  - ◊ Membrane may become black due to hemorrhage
  - ◊ Sore throat
  - ◊ Cervical adenopathy with swelling
  - ◊ Malaise and prostration
  - ◊ Enlarged, tender cervical and submandibular lymph nodes
  - ◊ May progress to edematous, swollen neck (bull neck)
  - ◊ Paralysis of soft palate
  - ◊ Low grade fever of 37.8-38.8°C (100-100.9°F)
  - ◊ Thrombocytopenia and purpura
- Nasal diphtheria:
  - ◊ Serosanguineous or seropurulent discharge and excoriations
  - ◊ Often discharge is unilateral
  - ◊ Often chronic, mild course
- Obstructive laryngotracheitis:
  - ◊ Hoarseness
  - ◊ Croupy cough
  - ◊ Progresses to dyspnea and stridor
  - ◊ Labored breathing
  - ◊ Thick speech
- Cutaneous diphtheria:
  - ◊ On skin, conjunctiva, vulva, vagina, penis
  - ◊ Primary cutaneous diphtheria - starts as tender pustule on lower extremity and becomes deep, round, punched-out ulcer covered by grayish membrane
  - ◊ Secondary infection of preexisting wound - purulent exudate, partial membrane

CAUSES *Corynebacterium diphtheriae*

RISK FACTORS
- Crowded living conditions
- Inadequate immunization. In the USA, 22-62% of people age 18 to 39 years and 41-84% of people over 60 years of age lack protective levels of antibody.
- Lower socioeconomic status
- Native Americans
- Alcoholism
- Travelers - outbreaks have occurred in the Ukraine and Russia

DIAGNOSIS

DIFFERENTIAL DIAGNOSIS
- Bacterial pharyngitis including group A streptococcus
- Viral pharyngitis
- Mononucleosis
- Oral syphilis
- Candidiasis
- Vincent's angina
- Acute epiglottitis

LABORATORY
- Gram-positive rods in the pathognomonic Chinese character configuration
- Moderate leukocytosis
- Thrombocytopenia
- Transient albuminuria
- Methylene-blue stains can assist in a presumptive diagnosis in experienced hands
- Culture from nose and throat beneath membrane and have plated on special media; inform lab that diphtheria is suspected
- Should test for toxigenicity of strain

Drugs that may alter lab results: If an antibiotic was used, then 5 or more days may be required for the culture to grow on Loeffler's medium

Disorders that may alter lab results: N/A

PATHOLOGICAL FINDINGS
- Pleomorphic gram-positive rods
- Necrotic epithelium
- Hyaline degeneration

SPECIAL TESTS
- Serial ECG's and cardiac enzymes to detect myocarditis
- Delayed peripheral nerve conduction velocities
- Culture on Loeffler's or tellurite medium is positive in 8 to 12 hours if not previously treated with an antibiotic. Laboratory must be alerted to use one of the special media.

IMAGING N/A

DIAGNOSTIC PROCEDURES
- Culture throat or lesions
- Smear of exudate for gram stain

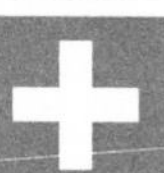

TREATMENT

APPROPRIATE HEALTH CARE
- Inpatient, initially hospitalized in unit which can monitor cardiac and respiratory status. (Must act on presumptive diagnosis because therapy cannot wait for culture confirmation).
- Isolation until cultures on two consecutive days are negative. The first culture must be taken at least 24 hours after the cessation of antibiotic therapy.

GENERAL MEASURES
- Have intubation or tracheostomy readily available. For laryngeal disease, laryngoscopy is desirable. Intubation or tracheostomy should be considered early for laryngeal disease.
- Avoid hypnotics and sedatives while monitoring respiratory status
- Physical therapy in convalescence for range of motion exercises to prevent contractions

SURGICAL MEASURES N/A

ACTIVITY Rest (for at least 3 weeks until risk of developing myocarditis has passed)

DIET Liquid to soft as tolerated

PATIENT EDUCATION Explain aspects of illness and complications

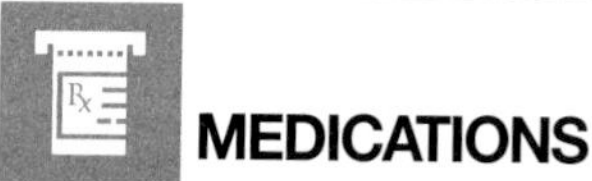

MEDICATIONS

DRUG(S) OF CHOICE

Both antitoxin and antibiotics are needed for non-cutaneous diphtheria

- Diphtheria antitoxin, equine: Use 20,000 to 40,000 units of antitoxin for laryngeal or pharyngeal disease of less than 48 hours duration, 40,000 to 60,000 units for nasopharyngeal lesions, 80,000 to 120,000 units for extensive disease of 3 or more days duration or swelling of the neck (bull neck). Administer antitoxin by IV infusion over 60 minutes and/or by intramuscular injection. Some experts recommend treating cutaneous disease with 20,000 to 40,000 units of antitoxin while others doubt its value when there are no signs of systemic disease. Antitoxin is obtained from the CDC.
- Erythromycin parenterally or orally, 40-50 mg/kg/day; maximum of 2 grams/day for 14 days

Contraindications: See Precautions

Precautions:

- Equine antitoxin: 7% of patients are sensitive to equine antitoxin and need desensitization. Always test for hypersensitivity to antitoxin prior to its administration.
  - ◊ First, a drop of 1:100 dilution of antitoxin is placed on a scratch on the forearm. If negative, an intradermal skin test is done with 1:1000 dilution (0.02 mL).
  - ◊ A positive reaction is the development of urticaria within 20 minutes of injection
  - ◊ If no reaction to first intradermal, then repeat test with a 1:100 dilution. If the person has a negative history for animal allergy, has not previously received animal serum and had a negative scratch test, then 1:100 dilution may be used initially.

Significant possible interactions: N/A

ALTERNATIVE DRUGS

- Penicillin G intramuscularly, 100,000 to 150,000 units/kg/day in four divided doses up to 600,000 units per day
- DL-carnitine 100 mg/kg/day given bid po in children for 4 days in myocarditis (experimental)

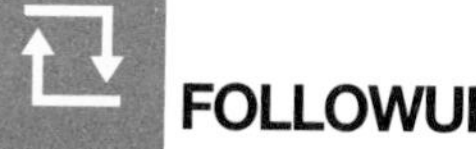

FOLLOWUP

PATIENT MONITORING

- ECG, cardiac enzymes and respiratory status. Serial ECG 2-3 times per week for 4-6 weeks to detect myocarditis.
- Elimination of the organism should be documented by three negative cultures at least 24 hours apart. The first culture should be at least 24 hours after the completion of antimicrobial therapy.
- During convalescence, patients should be immunized against diphtheria because infection does not necessarily confer immunity

PREVENTION/AVOIDANCE

- Prevention is by immunization:
  - ◊ Children 6 weeks up to 7 years of age should receive doses at 2, 4, 6 and 15-18 months and 4-6 years of age with 0.5 mL of DTaP vaccine IM If the pertussis component is contraindicated then pediatric DT should be used. A booster dose of adult Td should be given at age 11-12 years.
  - ◊ Unimmunized persons 7 years of age or older should receive two doses of Adult Td 4-8 weeks apart with a third dose 6-12 months later. 0.5 mL of Td should be given IM.
  - ◊ Subsequently, booster doses with Td should be given every 10 years to all individuals without a contraindication. An alternative strategy after the booster at age 11-12 years is a single adult booster at 50 years of age, in addition to following the recommendations for Td boosters in the event of an injury or wound.
  - ◊ Immunized individuals may develop diphtheria but their course is milder; immunization protects against the toxin, not infection or microbial carriage in the nose, pharynx or skin
  - ◊ Disinfect all articles in contact with patient
  - ◊ Close contacts should be cultured and given antibiotic prophylaxis regardless of immunization status. Previously immunized contacts should receive a booster of diphtheria toxoid unless vaccinated within last 5 years. Unimmunized contacts should begin the series. Erythromycin prophylaxis for 7 days.

POSSIBLE COMPLICATIONS

- Myocarditis (in 10-25%) may occur early
- Cranial and peripheral neuropathy (2-6 weeks after onset)
- ECG abnormalities in two-thirds of patients, including: bundle branch block, tachycardia, atrial or ventricular fibrillation, extrasystoles
- Right sided heart failure
- Local paralysis of soft palate and posterior pharynx demonstrated by regurgitation of fluids through the nares
- Peripheral and cranial neuropathy affecting primarily motor nerve functions. Motor dysfunction starts proximally and extends distally. Usually slowly resolves.
- Syndrome like Guillain-Barré

EXPECTED COURSE/PROGNOSIS

- < 5% mortality rate
- Prognosis guarded until recovery
- 5-10% persistence in nasopharynx in convalescing patients

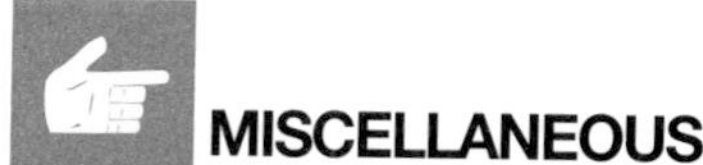

MISCELLANEOUS

ASSOCIATED CONDITIONS N/A

AGE-RELATED FACTORS

Pediatric: N/A
Geriatric: N/A
Others: N/A

PREGNANCY N/A

SYNONYMS N/A

ICD-9-CM

032.0 Faucial diphtheria
032.1 Nasopharyngeal diphtheria
032.2 Anterior nasal diphtheria
032.3 Laryngeal diphtheria
032.81 Conjunctival diphtheria
032.82 Diphtheritic myocarditis
032.83 Diphtheritic peritonitis
032.84 Diphtheritic cystitis
032.85 Cutaneous diphtheria
032.89 Other specified diphtheria, other
032.9 Diphtheria, unspecified

SEE ALSO

OTHER NOTES N/A

ABBREVIATIONS N/A

REFERENCES

- Red Book Report of the Committee on Infectious Diseases, 2003. Elk Grove Village, American Academy of Pediatrics, 2003
- Advisory Committee on Immunization Practices
- Centers for Disease Control and Prevention. Atkinson W, Hamborsky J, Wolfe S, eds Epidemiology and Prevention of Vaccine-Preventable Diseases (Pink Book). 8th ed. Washington DC: Public Health Foundation; 2004

Web references: 3 available at www.5mcc.com
Illustrations N/A

Author(s):

Richard Kent Zimmerman, MD, MPH
Gregory A. Poland, MD

Disseminated intravascular coagulation (DIC)

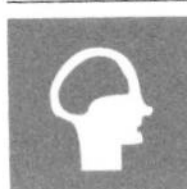

BASICS

DESCRIPTION Generation of fibrin in the blood and consumption of pro-coagulants and platelets occurring in complications of obstetrics, (e.g., abruptio placenta), infection (especially gram-negative), malignancy and other severe illnesses
System(s) affected: Hemic/Lymphatic/Immunologic
Genetics: Homozygous protein C or protein S deficiency
Incidence/Prevalence in USA: Unknown
Predominant age: None
Predominant sex: Male = Female

SIGNS & SYMPTOMS
- Epistaxis
- Gingival bleeding
- Mucosal bleeding
- Hemoptysis
- Hematemesis
- Metrorrhagia
- Cough
- Dyspnea
- Confusion
- Disorientation
- Stool blood
- Hematuria
- Oliguria
- Fever
- Skin petechiae
- Purpura
- Ecchymosis
- Skin hemorrhagic necrosis
- Localized rales
- Tachypnea
- Pleural friction rub
- Retinal hemorrhages
- Anuria
- Thrombosis
- Stupor
- Peripheral cyanosis

CAUSES
- Coagulation disorder due to widespread activation of clotting mechanism
- Obstetric complications
- Infection
- Neoplasms
- Intravascular hemolysis
- Vascular disorders; thrombosis
- Snake bite
- Massive tissue injury
- Trauma
- Hypoxia
- Liver disease
- Infant and adult RDS
- Purpura fulminans
- Thermal injury

RISK FACTORS
- Pregnancy
- Prostatic surgery
- Head injury
- Inflammatory states

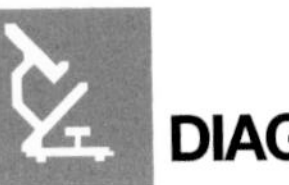

DIAGNOSIS

DIFFERENTIAL DIAGNOSIS
- Massive hepatic necrosis
- Vitamin K deficiency
- Thrombocytopenic purpura
- Hemolytic-uremic syndrome
- Primary fibrinolysis

LABORATORY
- Thrombocytopenia
- Increased partial thromboplastin time
- Increased prothrombin time
- Increased thrombin time
- Decreased fibrinogen
- Increased fibrin degradation product (FDP)
- Decreased antithrombin III
- Positive D-Dimer assay
- Increased bleeding time
- Schizocytosis
- Anemia
- Leukocytosis
- Increased lactate dehydrogenase (LDH)
- Increased BUN
- Decreased factor V
- Decreased or increased factor VIII
- Decreased factor X
- Decreased factor XIII
- Hemoglobinemia
- Hematuria
- Guaiac-positive stools
- Decreased protein C

Drugs that may alter lab results: N/A

Disorders that may alter lab results: N/A

PATHOLOGICAL FINDINGS N/A

SPECIAL TESTS N/A

IMAGING Chest x-ray: Bilateral perihilar soft density

DIAGNOSTIC PROCEDURES N/A

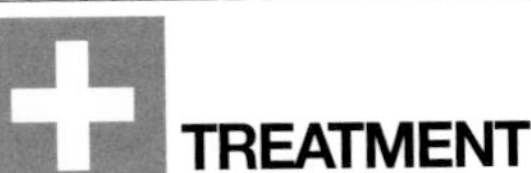

TREATMENT

APPROPRIATE HEALTH CARE Inpatient

GENERAL MEASURES
- Treat underlying condition e.g., evacuation of uterus in abruptio placenta. Broad-spectrum antibiotics for gram-negative sepsis.
- Replacement of blood loss
- Platelet concentrates
- Fresh frozen plasma
- Cryoprecipitate
- Antithrombin III concentrate
- Anticoagulants

SURGICAL MEASURES N/A

ACTIVITY As tolerated

DIET No special diet

PATIENT EDUCATION Griffith, H.W.: Instructions for Patients; Philadelphia, W.B. Saunders Co.

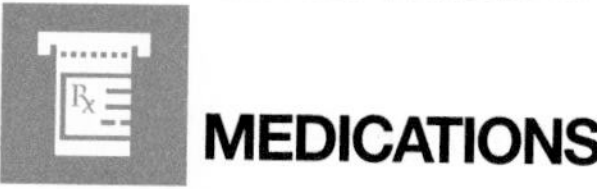

MEDICATIONS

DRUG(S) OF CHOICE

- Anticoagulants (heparin) if clinical findings suggest developing thrombotic complications, but never after head injury
- Broad-spectrum antibiotics for sepsis

Contraindications:

- Head injury
- Hemorrhagic stroke

Precautions: Refer to manufacturer's literature

Significant possible interactions: Refer to manufacturer's literature

ALTERNATIVE DRUGS For DIC associated with metastatic prostatic carcinoma, consider heparin, aminocaproic acid (Amicar). Do not use fibrinolytic inhibitors (Amicar) unless severe fibrinolysis is documented.

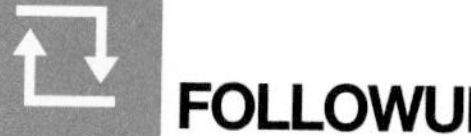

FOLLOWUP

PATIENT MONITORING Closely until much improved

PREVENTION/AVOIDANCE No preventive measures known

POSSIBLE COMPLICATIONS

- Acute renal failure
- Shock
- Cardiac tamponade
- Hemothorax
- Intracerebral hematoma
- Gangrene and loss of digits

EXPECTED COURSE/PROGNOSIS

Related to severity of cause of DIC

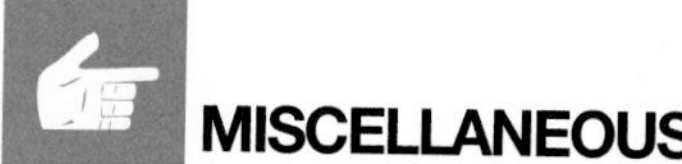

MISCELLANEOUS

ASSOCIATED CONDITIONS Thromboembolic phenomena associated with venous thrombosis, thrombotic vegetations on the aortic heart valve, arterial emboli, neonatal purpura fulminans (homozygous protein C or protein S deficiency)

AGE-RELATED FACTORS

Pediatric: Neonatal purpura fulminans associated with DIC and protein C or protein S deficiency (homozygous)

Geriatric: N/A

Others: N/A

PREGNANCY N/A

SYNONYMS

- Consumptive coagulopathy
- Defibrination syndrome
- DIC

ICD-9-CM

286.6 Defibrination syndrome

SEE ALSO

OTHER NOTES N/A

ABBREVIATIONS

RDS = respiratory distress syndrome

FDP = fibrin degradation products

REFERENCES

- Isselbacher KJ, et al, eds: Harrison's Principles of Internal Medicine. 13th Ed. New York, McGraw-Hill, 1994
- Stites DP, Stobo JD, Wells JV, eds: Basic and Clinical Immunology. 8th Ed. New York, Appleton & Lange, 1994

Web references: 1 available at www.5mcc.com

Illustrations 2 available

Author(s):

Stanley G. Smith, MA, MB

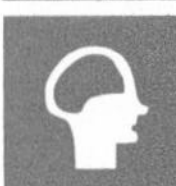

BASICS

DESCRIPTION A sudden change in state of consciousness, identity, motor behavior, thoughts, feelings and perception of external reality to such an extent that these functions do not operate congruently. Many pathologic symptoms can be found, but the patient experiences dysphoria, suffering, and maladaptive functioning. Disorders include:
- Dissociative amnesia
- Dissociative fugue
- Dissociative identity disorder
- Depersonalization disorder
- Dissociative disorder not otherwise specified (NOS). Authors may include somnambulism (sleep-walking disorder), conversion reactions, pseudo-epilepsy and (in some cultures) a variety of possession syndromes.

System(s) affected: Nervous
Genetics: N/A
Incidence/Prevalence in USA: 8-10% of the general psychiatrically ill. As many as 70% of young adults report short periods of dissociative experiences that are self-limiting and resolve spontaneously.
Predominant age: Adolescents and young to middle age adults; rare as a new illness in elderly. If untreated, may linger from childhood into adult and old age.
Predominant sex: Female > Male (2:1)

SIGNS & SYMPTOMS
All disorders share:
- Symptoms cause significant distress or impairment in social, occupational, or other important areas of functioning
- Symptoms are not due to the direct physiological effects of a substance (e.g., drug of abuse, a medication) or a general medical condition (e.g., temporal lobe epilepsy)
- Dissociative amnesia:
  - ◊ One or more episodes of inability to recall important personal information that is too extensive to be explained by ordinary forgetfulness
  - ◊ Not occurring during another psychiatric illness and not due to effects of chemical substance (drug abuse or medication)
  - ◊ Not due to a neurological or other medical condition (e.g., head trauma)
- Dissociative fugue:
  - ◊ Sudden unexpected travel away from home or one's customary place of work with an inability to recall one's past
  - ◊ Confusion about personal identity or assumption of a new identity (partial or complete)
  - ◊ Above symptoms do not occur exclusively during course of dissociative identity disorder
  - ◊ Symptoms cause significant distress or impairment in social, occupational, or other important areas of functioning with activities of daily living
- Dissociative identity disorder:
  - ◊ Presence of two or more distinct identities or personality states (each with its own relatively enduring pattern of perceiving, relating to, and thinking about environment and self).
  - ◊ At least two of these identities or personality states recurrently take control of the person's behavior
  - ◊ Inability to recall important personal information (too extensive to be explained by ordinary forgetfulness)
  - ◊ Reports of time distortion, lapses and discontinuities
  - ◊ Experiencing voices from inside one's head
  - ◊ Chronic headaches
  - ◊ History of severe emotional or physical abuse as a child
  - ◊ Referring to self as "he/she," "we," "us"
  - ◊ Eating disorders
  - ◊ Flashbacks
  - ◊ Feelings of derealization
  - ◊ Feelings of depersonalization
  - ◊ Amnesia about important childhood events
  - ◊ Personal objects and belongings that cannot be accounted for
  - ◊ Disowning unrecalled behaviors
  - ◊ Different handwriting styles
  - ◊ Different signatures and names found in personal diary
  - ◊ Sudden mood changes
  - ◊ Sudden behavioral changes, i.e., from adult to young child
  - ◊ Episodes of déjà vu
  - ◊ Feeling controlled by "another person" from within
  - ◊ Self-inflicted violence such as wrist cutting
- Depersonalization disorder:
  - ◊ Persistent or recurrent experiences of feeling detached from, and as if one is an outside observer of one's mental processes or body (e.g., feeling like one is in a dream)
  - ◊ During the depersonalization experience, reality testing remains intact
  - ◊ The depersonalization experience does not occur exclusively during the course of another mental disorder, such as schizophrenia, panic disorder, acute stress disorder or another dissociative disorder
- Dissociative disorder NOS: Predominant feature is a dissociative symptom (i.e., a disruption in the usually integrated functions of consciousness, memory, identity, or perception of the environment) that does not meet the criteria for any specific dissociative disorder. Examples:
  - ◊ Clinical presentations similar to dissociative identity disorder that fail to meet the full criteria for this disorder. Examples include a) there are not two or more distinct personality states or b) amnesia for important personal information does not occur
  - ◊ Derealization unaccompanied by depersonalization in adults
  - ◊ States of dissociation that occur in individuals who have been subjected to periods of prolonged and intense coercive persuasion (e.g., brainwashing, thought reform, or indoctrination while captive)
  - ◊ Dissociative trance disorder: Single or episodic disturbances in the state of consciousness, identity, or memory that are indigenous to particular locations and cultures. Dissociative trance involves narrowing of awareness of immediate surroundings or stereotyped behaviors or movements that are experienced as being beyond one's control.
  - ◊ Possession trance: Involves replacement of the customary sense of personality identity, attributed to the influence of a spirit, power, and associated with stereotyped "involuntary" movements or amnesia.
  - ◊ Loss of consciousness, stupor, or coma not attributed to a general medical condition
  - ◊ Ganser syndrome: The giving of approximate answers to questions (e.g., "2 plus 2 equals 5") when not associated with dissociative amnesia or dissociative fugue

CAUSES
- Physical, emotional, verbal, or sexual abuse in childhood
- Sudden and severe trauma or threat to one's psychological or physical integrity
- Sudden and unexpected exposure to watching others being killed or severely injured (as in an industrial or car accident)
- A preponderance of coping with trauma and internal or inter-personal conflicts by the use of dissociation
- Psychological/social support to cope with the trauma/abuse was not available

RISK FACTORS
- Exposure to neglect, abuse and trauma in one's childhood
- Tendency to cope with life stresses by excessively using an escape mechanism of day dreaming and/or dissociation

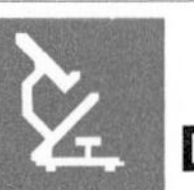

DIAGNOSIS

DIFFERENTIAL DIAGNOSIS
- Other mental/CNS disorder: Schizophrenia, depression, anxiety disorder, mania, obsessive/compulsive disorder, identity disorder, phobic disorders, eating disorders
- Other: Extreme sensory deprivation, epilepsy; early phases of dementia, encephalitis, head trauma, migraine, cerebral vascular disease, brain tumors
- Endocrinopathy: Hypoglycemia, hypothyroidism, hyperthyroidism
- Miscellaneous: Huntington disease, carbon monoxide poisoning, mescaline intoxication, botulism, hyperventilation
- Obstructive sleep apnea, nocturnal myoclonus

LABORATORY Toxicology screening may be helpful

Drugs that may alter lab results: Lithium carbonate may produce hypothyroidism

Disorders that may alter lab results:
Patients (especially those with dissociative identity disorder) may present with medical oddities such as fast healing of broken bones, radiographs resembling brain atrophy, brain infarcts, lupus, or abnormal pulmonary function tests.
A variety of symptoms (including blurred vision, nausea and vomiting, rapid heart beat, palpitation, extreme bradycardia, urinary frequency and urgency, extreme changes in levels of blood glucose) may lead to erroneous diagnosis

PATHOLOGICAL FINDINGS N/A

SPECIAL TESTS EEG to rule out epilepsy and sleep disorders. Polysomnogram to rule out sleep apnea.

IMAGING CT scan and MRI of the head to rule out multiple infarct dementia, brain tumors, and some forms of encephalopathy

DIAGNOSTIC PROCEDURES
- Neuro-psychological testing is helpful in ruling out learning disabilities and cognitive deficits due to early dementia or borderline mental retardation
- Psychological testing helps identify specific psychiatric disorders, personality structure and dynamics
- Dissociation scales help assess the tendency to dissociate in daily living activities
- Amobarbital (Amytal) interviews (narcoanalysis) and special interviews under hypnosis are useful in selected cases
- Clinician reviews patient's diary for handwriting and signature changes.

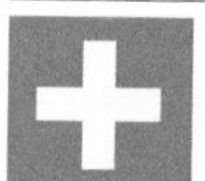

TREATMENT

APPROPRIATE HEALTH CARE
- Outpatient, individual psychotherapy
- At times of crisis: intensive hospital-based treatment (as a protection for patients with suicidal or homicidal impulses, and/or self-inflicted violence)
- Use inpatient care to verify diagnosis with special tests and begin treatment program that continues on outpatient basis
- Note: Treatment emphasis on progress in the adaptive functions with daily living activities, symptom alleviation, ego strengthening, prevent regressions

GENERAL MEASURES
- Individual psychotherapy plus behavior modification, narcoanalysis and narcosynthesis, hypnoanalysis and hypnotherapy
- Adjuncts: support groups, group therapy, expressive art therapy, occupational and recreational therapy
- Bibliotherapy and grapho-therapy are useful

SURGICAL MEASURES N/A

ACTIVITY Based on patient's condition

DIET N/A

PATIENT EDUCATION
- Self-hypnosis, relaxation exercises and guided imagery
- Encourage patients to read about their condition and be inspired by others who have been diagnosed, treated, and recovered, e.g., "A Mind of My Own" by Chris Sizemore, published by W. Morrow, New York, 1989

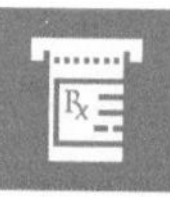

MEDICATIONS

DRUG(S) OF CHOICE
No medications are specifically curative. The following have been helpful:
- Antidepressants: depression
- Benzodiazepines: anxiety and insomnia
- Propranolol 80-400 mg/day: flashbacks and other dissociative symptoms
- Neuroleptics (in low doses): self-abusive behavior. Thioridazine 10-200 mg/day; haloperidol 2-10 mg/day; chlorprothixene 3-200 mg/day, and perphenazine 4-22 mg/day or risperidone 1-4 mg/day.
- Severe agitation, droperidol 1-5 mg IM (effective in producing calm sleep/stopping agitation)
- Mood swings, in dissociative disorders, do not respond to the use of lithium carbonate, carbamazepine or valproic acid unless patient has co-morbid bipolar disorder

Contraindications: N/A

Precautions:
- Short-acting benzodiazepines abuse potential
- Overdose/suicide potential with TCAs
- Very low doses of neuroleptics can be used without producing tardive dyskinesia (try to avoid higher doses)
- Risperidone may be associated with hyperglycemia and ketoacidosis

Significant possible interactions: Avoid MAO inhibitors with TCAs or SSRIs

ALTERNATIVE DRUGS
- Buspirone for anxiety 30-80 mg/day
- Clomipramine, 75-200 mg/day or fluvoxamine 100-300 mg/day for obsessive-compulsive symptoms
- Recently the use of alternative neuroleptic medicines have been found useful for the control of self-inflicted violence
  - ◊ Risperidone (Risperdal) 0.5-4 mg per day
  - ◊ Olanzapine (Zyprexa) 2.5-10 mg per day
  - ◊ Quetiapine (Seroquel) 25-200 mg per day

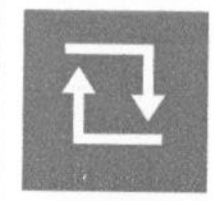

FOLLOWUP

PATIENT MONITORING
- Outpatients: 1-4 hrs of psychotherapy per week to avoid hospitalization
- Inpatients: more intensive treatment, e.g. daily psychotherapy

PREVENTION/AVOIDANCE
- Child abuse prevention via parent education and community agency intervention
- Crisis intervention following individual trauma or disasters for prevention of chronic morbidity/disability

POSSIBLE COMPLICATIONS Self-inflicted violence; suicide attempts; substance abuse and chemical dependency

EXPECTED COURSE/PROGNOSIS
Ranges from spontaneous improvement, in cases of dissociative amnesia, dissociative fugue, and depersonalization disorder, to acute and chronic morbidity in others
- Without treatment, dissociative identity disorder patient may have a healthy functioning facade, with episodes of depression, confusion, mood swings, etc. With age, intensity/frequency of dissociative experiences may decrease and crystallize around 1-2 major personality states.
- Effective treatment produces partial or full recovery for many patients

MISCELLANEOUS

ASSOCIATED CONDITIONS See Causes

AGE-RELATED FACTORS
Pediatric: Suspect abuse or neglect
Geriatric: Decrease in dissociative disorders. Medication side effects more likely.
Others: N/A

PREGNANCY N/A

SYNONYMS
- Hysterical neurosis, dissociative type
- Ganser syndrome

ICD-9-CM
300.15 Dissociative disorder or reaction, unspecified
301.50 Histrionic personality disorder, unspecified

SEE ALSO

OTHER NOTES N/A

ABBREVIATIONS N/A

REFERENCES

- Moskowitz A. Dissociation and violence: a review of the literature. Trauma Violence Abuse 2004;5(1):21-46
- Markowitsch HJ. Psychogenic amnesia. Neuroimage 2003;20 Suppl 1:S132-8
- Chefetz, RA. Reassociating Psychoanalysis and dissociation: A review of Dissociation of Trauma: Theory, Phenomenology, and Technique. Contemporary Psychoanalysis 2004;40(1):123-33
- Maldonado JR, Butler LD, Spiegal D. Treatment for dissociative disorders. In: Natham P, Gorman JM, eds. A Guide to Treatments That Work. 2nd Ed. London, England, Oxford University; 2002; p463-496
- Dell PF. Dissociative phenomenology of dissociative identity disorder. J Nerv Ment Dis.2002;190(1):1-15
- Torem MS. Medications in the treatment of dissociative identity disorder. Spira JL, ed. In: Treating Dissociative Identity Disorder. San Francisco, CA, Jossey-Bass, 1996:99-132
- Steinberg M. Handbook for the assessment of dissociation, a clinical guide. American Psychiatric Press, 1995
- Kirsh I, Lynn SJ. Dissociation theories of hypnosis. Psychological Bulletin, 1998;123:100-15
- Spiegel D. Trauma, dissociation, and memory. Annals New York Academy of Sciences, 1997;821:225-237
- Chu JA, et al. Memories of childhood abuse; dissociation, amnesia, and corroboration. Am J Psychiatry 1999;156:749-55
- Spitzer C, et al. Dissociative experiences and psychopathology in conversion disorders. J of Psychosomatic Research 1999;46:291-294
- Lipsanen T, et al. Visual distortions and dissociation. J of Nerv and Ment Disease 1999;187:109-12
- Meares R. The contribution of Hughlings Jackson to an understanding of dissociation. Am J Psychiatr 1999;156(12):1850-55
- American Psychiatric Association: Diagnostic and Statistical Manual of Mental Disorders. 4th Ed. Washington, DC, American Psychiatric Association, 1994:477-491
- Putnam FW: Diagnosis & Treatment of Multiple Personality Disorder. NY, Guilford Press, 1989
- Kluft RP, Fine CG: Clinical Perspectives on Multiple Personality Disorder. Washington, DC, American Psychiatric Press, Inc., 1993
- Spiegel D, ed: Dissociative Disorders: A clinical review. Lutherville, MD, Sidran Press, 1993
- Michelson LK, Ray WJ, eds. Handbook of Dissociation. New York, Plenum Press, 1996
- Merckelbach H, Muris P. The causal link between self-reported trauma and dissociation: a critical review. Behav Res Ther 2001 Mar;39(3):245-54
- Fine CG, Berkowitz AS. The wreathing protocol: the imbrication of hypnosis and EMDR in the treatment of dissociative identity disorder and other dissociative responses. Am J Clin Hypn 2001 Jan-Apr;43(3-4):275-90
- Steinberg M. Hughlings Jackson and dissociation. Am J Psychiatry. 2001 Jan;158(1):145-6
- Nijenhuis ER. Somatoform dissociation: Major symptoms of dissociative disorders. Jour Trauma and Dissociation 2000;1(4):7-29
- Steinberg M. Updating diagnostic criteria for dissociative disorders: Learning from scientific advances. 2001;2(1):59-63

Web references: 3 available at www.5mcc.com
Illustrations N/A

Author(s):
Moshe S. Torem, MD

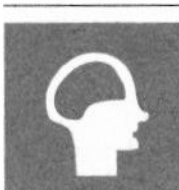

BASICS

DESCRIPTION Diverticulosis of the colon and its varied clinical consequences. Diverticula develop in people in countries eating a low fiber diet and are much more prevalent in western societies.

- Diverticula of colon: Herniation of the colon mucosa through the muscular layer, usually at the site of a perforating artery, lying between two layers of serosa in the mesentery. They are more common in the sigmoid and distal colon and increase in numbers with age.
- Diverticulitis: An abscess or peridiverticular inflammation initiated by the rupture of a mucosal microscopic abscess into the mesentery. Such infection may progress, fistulize into the genitourinary system, obstruct, or spontaneously resolve. Develops in about 5% of subjects with diverticulosis each year. Over a lifetime about half of patients with diverticulosis develop inflammation.

System(s) affected: Gastrointestinal

Genetics: No known genetic pattern

Incidence/Prevalence in USA:

- 2200-3000/100,000 (diverticulitis)
- Diverticuli in up to 20% in general population but increases progressively with age reaching up to 40%-50% in 6th-8th decade

Predominant age: Rare below 40 years, most common in 6th-8th decade

Predominant sex: Male = Female

SIGNS & SYMPTOMS

- Diverticulosis
  - ◊ Only 10-25% of subjects harboring diverticula will develop symptoms (possibly related to coexistent irritable bowel disease)
  - ◊ Pain - due to tension in colonic wall, mostly in left lower quadrant, worse after eating, some relief following bowel movement or passage of flatus
  - ◊ Diarrhea or constipation
  - ◊ Palpable mass in left iliac fossa - firm, tender
  - ◊ Abdomen may be distended and tympanitic
  - ◊ Absent signs of peritoneal inflammation
  - ◊ Melena, hematochezia if diverticula bleed
- Diverticulitis
  - ◊ Pain - acute onset, mostly localized in left lower quadrant. Prominently associated with tenderness in same region.
  - ◊ Fever with chills as severity increases
  - ◊ Anorexia, nausea, vomiting
  - ◊ Constipation or diarrhea
  - ◊ Rebound tenderness, involuntary guarding, board-like rigidity
  - ◊ Palpable mass - tender, firm, fixed
  - ◊ Abdomen distended and tympanitic
  - ◊ Bowel sounds depressed or could be exaggerated if obstruction ensues
  - ◊ Dysuria, frequency if bladder involved
  - ◊ Pneumaturia, fecaluria if colovesical fistula develops
  - ◊ Rectal exam may reveal tenderness, induration, mass in the cul-de-sac
  - ◊ Enterocutaneous, enterovaginal, and perirectal fistulae may be initial manifestation

CAUSES

- Causes are speculative/not clearly proven
- Defects in colonic motility and increased intraluminal pressure, partially brought about by too little fecal volume
- Colonic segmentation - nonpropulsive contractions producing isolated segments or little chambers with high pressure in them
- Low fiber diet - increases segmentation and causes higher intraluminal pressure
- Defects in colonic wall strength
- Cause of bleeding unclear, not related to diverticulitis. Right sided diverticula, though less common, account for 50% of all bleeding from diverticula.

RISK FACTORS

- Age over 40
- Low residue diet
- Previous diverticulitis
- Number of diverticula in the colon

DIAGNOSIS

DIFFERENTIAL DIAGNOSIS

- Irritable bowel syndrome
- Lactose intolerance
- Carcinoma of distal colon
- Ulcerative colitis, Crohn disease
- Angiodysplasia (for rectal bleed)
- Ischemic or infectious colitis
- Appendicitis
- Other gynecologic and urologic disorders

LABORATORY

- WBC count normal in diverticulosis, elevated with immature polymorphs in diverticulitis
- Hemoglobin low if bleeding is a symptom
- Sedimentation rate elevated in diverticulitis
- Urine analysis may reveal WBC's, RBC's, pus cells in fistula formation
- Urine culture - persistent infection in colovesical fistula
- Blood culture - positive in diverticulitis with generalized peritonitis

Drugs that may alter lab results:

- Steroids
- Other immunosuppressive drugs

Disorders that may alter lab results: Severe malnutrition

PATHOLOGICAL FINDINGS

- Prediverticular state - myochosis (thickening of circular layer of muscle, shortening of tenia, restriction of lumen)
- Multiple diverticula - spastic colon diverticulosis, simple massed diverticulosis, right sided diverticulosis
- Solitary diverticulum - giant sigmoid diverticulum
- Diverticulitis - inflammation, necrosis, perforation
- Diverticulitis - earliest stage, rupture of a mucosal abscess into mesentery. Does not start with obstruction of the neck as does appendicitis.

SPECIAL TESTS

- 99mTc labeled RBC scan for bleeding (rarely used) and/or angiography
- Gallium or indium labeled leukocytes to localize abscess (rarely used)

IMAGING

- Plain film abdomen supine and upright - useful in peritonitis and perforation
- Barium enema - best means for diagnosis of diverticulosis. Less useful in diagnosis of diverticulitis.
- Diverticula may be seen on endoscopy, but less sensitive than Barium enema.
- CT scan with or without rectal contrast - diagnostic for abscess, fistula, size and location of inflammatory mass
- Angiography - diagnostic as well as therapeutic in diverticular bleeding
- Fistulograms
- Spiral CT scan with bolus of IV contrast dye may demonstrate bleeding

DIAGNOSTIC PROCEDURES

- Colonoscopy and flexible sigmoidoscopy - helpful in diagnosis of diverticulosis and extremely valuable in differential diagnosis to prove or rule out cancer. Ulcerative or ischemic colitis can uniformly be diagnosed by these modalities.
- Cystoscopy - in colovesical fistula

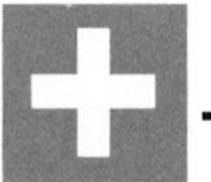

TREATMENT

APPROPRIATE HEALTH CARE

- Diverticulosis - outpatient with fiber supplements to soften stools
- Outpatient diverticulitis (pain, tenderness, leukocytosis, but no toxicity or peritoneal signs)
- About 2% subjects require hospitalization for toxicity, septicemia, peritonitis or failure to resolve in a few days. About half of these will require surgery.
- Toxic patients require hospitalization and intravenous antibiotics at least until response

GENERAL MEASURES

- IV fluids, analgesics, nasogastric suction
- Indications for surgery - severe diverticulitis, perforation, abscess, fistula, severe diverticular bleeding (requiring more than 2,000 mL of blood in 24 hours), recurrent episodes

SURGICAL MEASURES

- Usual indication related to diverticulitis. Multiple attacks in 2 years, unhealing fistulae, abscess or toxicity may lead to surgery.
- Large pus collections are usually drained radiologically and when resolved, the most involved segment of the colon resected

ACTIVITY Fully active in diverticulosis, restricted activity in diverticulitis

DIET
- NPO during acute diverticulitis, progress to fluids, then to high fiber as normal bowel function returns
- All patients with diverticula should increase dietary fiber to high level through foods, and/or fiber supplement if appropriate

PATIENT EDUCATION
- Importance of high fiber diet and recognizing the symptoms of complications at early stage
- Additional material from:

National Digestive Diseases Information Clearinghouse, Box NDDIC, Bethesda, MD 20892, (301)468-6344

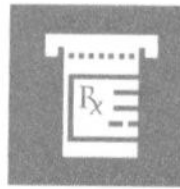

MEDICATIONS

DRUG(S) OF CHOICE
- Diverticulosis
  - ◊ Pain syndromes may be treated with antispasmodics - hyoscyamine (Levsin) 0.125 mg or 2 each 4 hours; buspirone (BuSpar) 15-30 mg/day; or meperidine (Demerol) 100-150 mg/day along with high fiber diet
  - ◊ Constipation and diarrhea, manage as indicated for irritable bowel disease
- Diverticulitis
  - ◊ Oral treatment for mild disease - metronidazole (Flagyl) 250-500 mg q 8 hours and amoxicillin 500 mg q 8 hours combination, or ciprofloxacin 500 mg bid. Expect response within 3 days. Continue oral therapy for one week.
  - ◊ More severe cases in hospital - gentamicin 3-5 mg/kg/day plus clindamycin 1.8-2.7 gm/day along with analgesic. Aminoglycoside dose varies with creatinine clearance.
- Diverticular bleeding
  - ◊ Vasopressin 0.2-0.3 units/minute through selective intra-arterial catheter. Used when bleeding demonstrated at angiography.

Contraindications: Hypersensitivity reaction

Precautions:
- Avoid morphine and other opiates except for Demerol
- Watch for renal toxicity and ototoxicity with aminoglycosides

Significant possible interactions: Refer to manufacturer's profile of each drug

ALTERNATIVE DRUGS
Tobramycin and metronidazole, 3rd generation cephalosporins

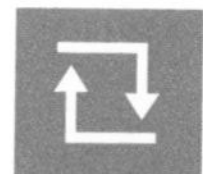

FOLLOWUP

PATIENT MONITORING
- Some physicians would not do any invasive studies; others have recommended repeat barium enema every 3 years if symptoms infrequent or absent, or following corrective surgery
- Colonoscopy, if needed based on above results

PREVENTION/AVOIDANCE
High fiber diet, psyllium, agar, methylcellulose

POSSIBLE COMPLICATIONS
- Hemorrhage
- Perforation
- Peritonitis
- Bowel obstruction
- Abscess - paracolic, subhepatic, subphrenic
- Fistula - colovesical, colovaginal, colocutaneous

EXPECTED COURSE/PROGNOSIS
- Prognosis is good with early detection and treatment of the complications
- Of those with a first episode of diverticulitis who are successfully managed medically, up to 67% will not have subsequent attacks requiring hospitalization; 33% will recur. Two or three recurrences in 1-2 years is an indication to electively remove the involved segment of colon.
- Of those with diverticular bleeding, up to 20% will rebleed in a period of months to years

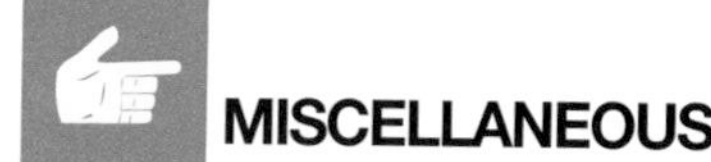

MISCELLANEOUS

ASSOCIATED CONDITIONS
Often occurs in conjunction with spastic colon

AGE-RELATED FACTORS
Pediatric: Very rare

Geriatric:
- More common
- May sometimes be difficult to diagnose

Others: N/A

PREGNANCY
Differentiate from ectopic pregnancy

SYNONYMS
N/A

ICD-9-CM
562.10 Diverticulosis of colon (without mention of hemorrhage)

562.11 Diverticulitis of colon (without mention of hemorrhage)

SEE ALSO
Irritable bowel syndrome

OTHER NOTES
N/A

ABBREVIATIONS
N/A

REFERENCES

- Morris CR, Harvey IM, Stebbings WS, et al. Epidemiology of perforated colonic diverticular disease. Postgrad Med J 2002;78(925):654-8
- Schweitzer J, Casillas RA, Collins JC. Acute diverticulitis in the young adult is not 'virulent'. Am Surg 2002;68(12):1044-7
- Biondo S, Pares D, Marti Rague J, et al. Acute colonic diverticulitis in patients under 50 years of age. Br J Surg 2002;89(9):1137-41
- Ambrosetti P, Becker C, Terrier F. Colonic diverticulitis: impact of imaging on surgical management - a prospective study of 542 patients. Eur Radiol 2002;12(5):1145-9
- Horgan AF, McConnell EJ, Wolff BG, et al. Atypical diverticular disease: surgical results. Dis Colon Rectum 2001;44(9):1315-8

Web references: 1 available at www.5mcc.com

Illustrations N/A

Author(s):
Frank L. Iber, MD

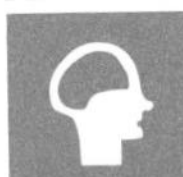

BASICS

DESCRIPTION A common form of mental retardation whose cause is unknown. All patients have extra chromosome 21 material; chromosome non-disjunction usually occurs in female meiosis. The syndrome occurs in all races with equal frequency.
- Trisomy 21: 90% of patients, an extra chromosome 21 is found in all cells
- Translocation 21: 5% of patients, extra chromosome 21q material is translocated to another chromosome, usually 13 or 15. For the 5% of translocation trisomies, 2/3 are new, 1/3 have a parental carrier.
- Mosaic 21: 5% of patients, 2 or more cell populations found, usually normal and trisomy 21. Clinical manifestations milder.

System(s) affected: Cardiovascular, Nervous, Skin/Exocrine
Genetics: As above. Extra chromosome comes from mother in > 90% of the cases.
Incidence/Prevalence in USA: 1 in 1000 births
Predominant age: Most identified at birth. Lifespan shortened.
Predominant sex: Male = Female

SIGNS & SYMPTOMS
- Infants and children
  - ◊ Brachycephaly (100%)
  - ◊ Hypotonia (80%)
  - ◊ Posterior 3rd fontanel
  - ◊ Small ears, +/- superior ear folds, +/- low set ears
  - ◊ Mongoloid slant, eyes (90%)
  - ◊ Epicanthic folds (90%)
  - ◊ Brushfield's (speckled) spots of iris (50%)
  - ◊ Esotropia (50%)
  - ◊ Depressed nasal bridge
  - ◊ Enlarged tongue (75%)
  - ◊ Small chin
  - ◊ Short neck
  - ◊ Cardiac murmur (50%)
  - ◊ Abnormal dermatoglyphics, including single palmar crease, distal palmar triradius, and absence of plantar whorl (ball of foot)
  - ◊ Developmental delay, which may not be apparent in 1st year
  - ◊ Thyroid defects; low or high (5%)
  - ◊ Mild-moderate instability of neck at C1-C2
- Adults
  - ◊ Most findings milder, but brachycephaly remains
  - ◊ Patients are retarded (IQ = 40-45) but usually personable and cooperative
  - ◊ Most adults can care for their personal needs. Some have jobs, but all require a sheltered environment.
  - ◊ A small percent of patients have some autistic features. A small percent of patients are non-verbal.
  - ◊ A small percent of patients have breathing problems and tracheomalacia

CAUSES
- Genetic - unequal chromosome division
- Genetic - translocation (5% of cases)

RISK FACTORS
- Increases with mother's age:
  - ◊ 1/2000, age 20
  - ◊ 1/200, age 35
  - ◊ 1/100, age 37
  - ◊ 1/20, age 45

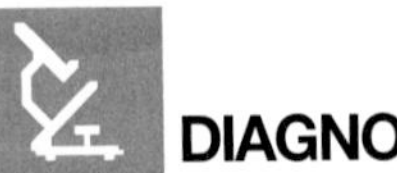

DIAGNOSIS

DIFFERENTIAL DIAGNOSIS
- Minor familial anomalies such as Mongoloid slant, epicanthic folds and depressed nasal bridge, particularly in a child with hypotonia
- The presence of a whorl on the ball of the foot usually indicates a normal child

LABORATORY A chromosome test is definitive and should always be done because of the chance of translocation

Drugs that may alter lab results: N/A

Disorders that may alter lab results: N/A

PATHOLOGICAL FINDINGS Alzheimer plaques found in 100% of brains after age 20

SPECIAL TESTS N/A

IMAGING Abdominal ultrasound for urinary tract anomalies in children with pyuria or fevers of unknown origin

DIAGNOSTIC PROCEDURES
- Echocardiography in all children. A VSD/endocardial cushion defect may not be apparent at birth.
- X-ray of neck for minor trauma, or there is neck pain, long tract symptoms or breathing problems
- Thyroid testing for children with poor weight gain, constipation
- Thyroid testing annually until age 5, then as indicated

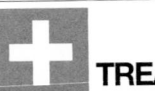

TREATMENT

APPROPRIATE HEALTH CARE
- Genetic evaluation and counseling
- Cardiac evaluation and ECG
- Appropriate pediatric health care
- Thyroid testing for any reasons (slowing of growth or weight gain, constipation) and thyroid treatment

GENERAL MEASURES
- Parents can usually adapt to a special child
- Most important is to address parental fears and treat the infant normally
- Infant stimulation programs recommended, but definitive proof of effectiveness is lacking

SURGICAL MEASURES N/A

ACTIVITY
- Fully active unless heart disease
- A controlled environment is needed for older children and adults

DIET No special diet. Programs suggesting megavitamin therapy have been disproved.

PATIENT EDUCATION
- National Down Syndrome Congress (800)232-NDSC
- Down syndrome Usenet list serv: listserv@vm1.nodak.edu
- Down syndrome information and counseling is available: http://www.nas.com/downsyn
- Frank discussion of health issues including piracetam is available - www.ds-health.com/

MEDICATIONS

DRUG(S) OF CHOICE N/A
Contraindications: N/A
Precautions: N/A
Significant possible interactions: N/A

ALTERNATIVE DRUGS
- Current enthusiasm for "neural enhancers", e.g., piracetam, a GABA analog, not proven, but under study
- Experimental evidence that Vitamin E prolongs the life of DS neurons in tissue culture

FOLLOWUP

PATIENT MONITORING
- 1 or 2 subsequent genetic visits to complete counseling and a visit at 1-2 years
- Follow cardiac status carefully
- Thyroid and possibly cardiac investigation if growth rate decreased

PREVENTION/AVOIDANCE
- Prenatal chorion villus biopsy at 9-10 weeks and amniocentesis at 13-15 weeks
- A low screening maternal serum alpha-fetoprotein (MSAFP, and abdominal triple screen at 14-16 weeks gestation finds 50-60% of cases
- Prenatal testing recommended for all pregnant females over 35, but this only impacts 25% of cases
- Recurrence:
  - ◊ 1% for trisomy 21 if child has trisomy 21
  - ◊ Is one-fifth to one-sixth for parents with a balanced translocation
  - ◊ If the parental translocation is 21:21 (45,t (21:21)), the recurrence is 100%
  - ◊ Increased recurrence in families with mosaic Down syndrome is not clear, but prenatal testing is recommended

POSSIBLE COMPLICATIONS
- Bowel obstruction (fistula, intestinal anomalies [10%])
- Hirschsprung's disease (3%)
- Thyroid disease (hypo-and hyperthyroidism 5-8%)
- Leukemia (0.5%)
- Congenital heart disease (50%) especially endocardial cushion defect, ventricular septal defect
- Alzheimer disease
- Seizures (3-4%)

EXPECTED COURSE/PROGNOSIS
- Development is normal in the first year in about one-third of cases and mildly delayed in the rest
- Development slows after age 1 and language and cognition are moderately delayed
- The outcome and longevity may be dependent on congenital heart disease
- Some adult individuals can work in protected situations; a few largely independent
- Intestinal complications and congenital heart disease may be of immediate concern
- Hypothyroid disease occurs after 6 months when found, and diminished growth is the principal sign
- Clinical Alzheimer disease in 1/3 of patients after age 35
- There is premature aging. Most patients die at 50-60, earlier if there is heart disease.

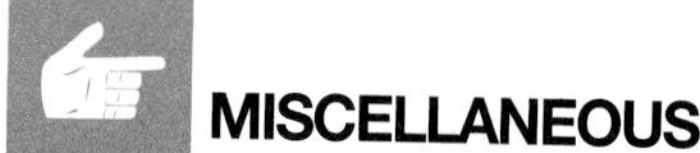

MISCELLANEOUS

ASSOCIATED CONDITIONS N/A

AGE-RELATED FACTORS
Pediatric: N/A
Geriatric: Seldom survive to geriatric age
Others: N/A

PREGNANCY Pregnancy is possible in patients with Down syndrome. The risk for Down syndrome in an infant is 50%.

SYNONYMS
- Trisomy 21
- Trisomy G
- Down syndrome

ICD-9-CM
758.0 Down syndrome

SEE ALSO

OTHER NOTES Mongolism is a term no longer used

ABBREVIATIONS N/A

REFERENCES

- Behrman RE, Kliegman RM, eds: Nelson Textbook of Pediatrics. 14th Ed. Philadelphia, W.B. Saunders Co., 1992
- Smith D: Recognizable Patterns of Human Malformation. 4th Ed. Philadelphia, W.B. Saunders Co., 1988

Web references: 2 available at www.5mcc.com
Illustrations N/A

Author(s):
Paul J. Benke, MD, PhD

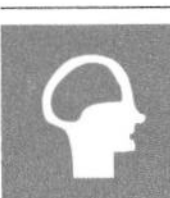

BASICS

DESCRIPTION Gastrointestinal symptoms resulting from rapid gastric emptying. Usually occurs following gastric surgery (gastrectomy, vagotomy, pyloroplasty).
System(s) affected: Gastrointestinal
Genetics: N/A
Incidence/Prevalence in USA: After vagotomy: 0.9% of proximal gastric vagotomy; 10-22% truncal vagotomy
Predominant age: Middle age to elderly
Predominant sex: Male = Female

SIGNS & SYMPTOMS
Most common to least common:
- Abdominal discomfort, pain
- Diarrhea (postprandial)
- Bloating
- Nausea
- Palpitations
- Diaphoresis
- Weight loss
- Flushing
- Lightheadedness
- Confusion and syncope

CAUSES Multifactorial including:
- Rapid delivery of hyperosmolar material into intestine
- Supraphysiologic release of various peptides/vasoactive mediators
- Reactive hypoglycemia

RISK FACTORS Surgical drainage procedures, particularly gastrectomy; anti-ulcer surgery

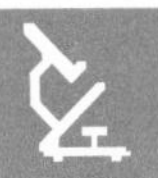

DIAGNOSIS

DIFFERENTIAL DIAGNOSIS
- Mechanical obstruction
- Gastroenteric fistula
- Celiac sprue
- Crohn disease
- Pancreatic exocrine insufficiency
- Neuroendocrine tumors (e.g., carcinoid)
- Irritable bowel syndrome

LABORATORY
- Postprandial hypoglycemia
- Anemia
- Hypoalbuminemia

Drugs that may alter lab results: Insulin

Disorders that may alter lab results: Diabetes mellitus

PATHOLOGICAL FINDINGS N/A

SPECIAL TESTS N/A

IMAGING
- Upper GI series - barium rapidly emptying from stomach
- Nuclear medicine gastric emptying study
- Endoscopy (exclude mechanical obstruction)

DIAGNOSTIC PROCEDURES N/A

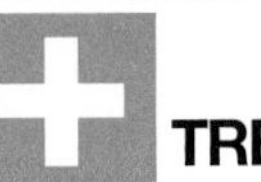

TREATMENT

APPROPRIATE HEALTH CARE Outpatient except in rare circumstances

GENERAL MEASURES Dietary and medical management

SURGICAL MEASURES Surgery only if dietary and medical management unsuccessful and symptoms debilitating; variable results

ACTIVITY
- No restrictions
- Lying down after eating or when symptoms occur

DIET
- Low carbohydrate
- Frequent small meals with minimal liquid
- Drink fluids between meals only
- High protein diet
- Adequate caloric intake

PATIENT EDUCATION National Digestive Diseases Information Clearinghouse, Box NDDIC, Bethesda, MD 20892, (301)468-6344

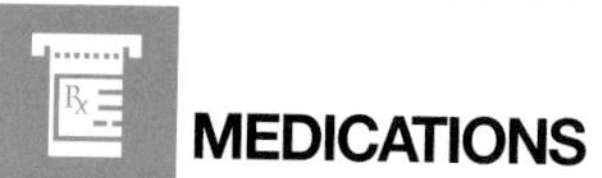

MEDICATIONS

DRUG(S) OF CHOICE
- Octreotide (Sandostatin) 200-400 mcg/day subcutaneous, given in divided doses q8h. Can be very expensive.
- Pectin/guar gum

Contraindications:
- Hypersensitivity

Precautions: N/A

Significant possible interactions: Refer to manufacturer's literature

ALTERNATIVE DRUGS Anticholinergics. Results generally disappointing.

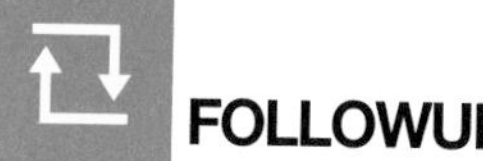

FOLLOWUP

PATIENT MONITORING Follow to be sure of adequate nutrition

PREVENTION/AVOIDANCE
- Eating frequent, small, dry meals that contain no refined carbohydrates
- Restrict fluids to between meals

POSSIBLE COMPLICATIONS
- Hypoglycemia
- Malnutrition
- Electrolyte disturbances including hypokalemia

EXPECTED COURSE/PROGNOSIS
Favorable

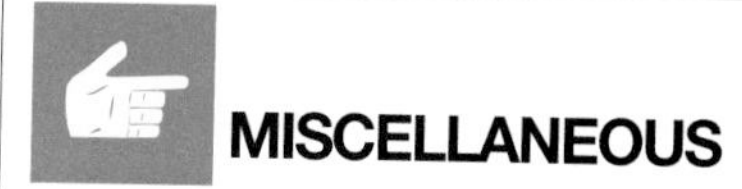

MISCELLANEOUS

ASSOCIATED CONDITIONS
- Peptic ulcer disease
- Reactive hypoglycemia
- Gastrectomy/vagotomy

AGE-RELATED FACTORS
Pediatric: N/A
Geriatric: N/A
Others: N/A

PREGNANCY N/A

SYNONYMS Early postgastrectomy syndrome

ICD-9-CM
564.2 Postgastric surgery syndromes

SEE ALSO
Diarrhea, chronic
Hypoglycemia, nondiabetic
Peptic ulcer disease

OTHER NOTES N/A

ABBREVIATIONS N/A

REFERENCES
- Vecht J, Masclee AA, Lamers CB. The dumping syndrome. Current insights into pathophysiology, diagnosis and treatment. J Gastroenterol Suppl 1997; 223:21-7
- Mallory G, MacGregor A, Nand C. The influence of dumping on weight loss after gastric surgery for obesity. Obes Surg 1996;6:474-8
- Sleisenger MH, Fordtran JS, editors. Gastrointestinal Disease: Pathophysiology, Diagnosis, Management. 5th ed. Philadelphia: W.B. Saunders Co.; 1994
- Spiro HW, editor. Clinical Gastroenterology. 4th ed. New York: McGraw-Hill; 1993

Web references: 3 available at www.5mcc.com
Illustrations N/A

Author(s):
Philip E. Jaffe, MD

BASICS

DESCRIPTION Contracture of the palmar fascia due to fibrous proliferation resulting in flexion deformities and loss of function. Similar change may rarely occur in plantar fascia. It usually appears simultaneously.
System(s) affected: Musculoskeletal
Genetics:
- Autosomal dominant with variable penetrance
- 10% of patients have a positive family history

Incidence/Prevalence in USA:
- Unknown
- Norway - 9% males and 3% females

Predominant age: 50 for males; 60 for females
Predominant sex: Male > Female (ranges from 2:1 to 10:1)

SIGNS & SYMPTOMS
- Typical
  - ◊ Caucasian male 50-60
  - ◊ Bilateral with one hand more involved
  - ◊ Family history
  - ◊ Unilateral or bilateral (50%)
  - ◊ Right hand more frequent
  - ◊ Ring finger more frequent
  - ◊ Ulnar digits more affected than radial
  - ◊ Mild pain early
  - ◊ Later painless plaques or nodules in palmar fascia
  - ◊ Extends into a cord-like band in the palmar fascia
  - ◊ Skin adheres to fascia and becomes puckered
  - ◊ Nodules can be palpated under the skin
  - ◊ Digital fascia becomes involved as disease progresses
  - ◊ Web space contractures
  - ◊ Dupuytren diathesis can involve plantar (Ledderhose's - 10%) and penile (Peyronie - 2%) fascia
  - ◊ Knuckle pads
- Atypical
  - ◊ No age, gender differences
  - ◊ No family history
  - ◊ May have systemic disease (see Risk Factors)
  - ◊ May have a history of trauma
  - ◊ More common unilateral
  - ◊ No ectopic manifestations (Ledderhose's or Peyronie)
  - ◊ Nonprogressive

CAUSES
- Unknown
- Ischemia to the fascia with oxygen free radical formation
- Possibly related to release of angiogenic basic fibroblast growth factor
- Related to microhemorrhage and release of growth factors

RISK FACTORS
- Smoking (mean 16 pack-years, odds ratio 2.8)
- Increasing age
- Male/Caucasian
- Diabetes mellitus (one-third affected, increases with time, usually mild; middle and ring finger involved)
- Epilepsy
- Chronic illness (e.g., pulmonary tuberculosis, liver disease)
- Hypercholesterolemia
- Liver disease
- HIV infection

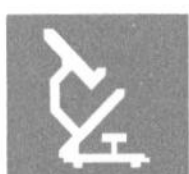

DIAGNOSIS

DIFFERENTIAL DIAGNOSIS
- Early for callosity
- Tendon abnormalities
- Camptodactyly - early teens tight facial bands ulnar side of small finger

LABORATORY N/A

Drugs that may alter lab results: N/A

Disorders that may alter lab results: N/A

PATHOLOGICAL FINDINGS
- Myofibroblasts
- First stage (proliferative) - increased myofibroblasts
- Second stage (residual) - dense fibroblast network
- Third stage (involutional) - myofibroblasts disappear

SPECIAL TESTS N/A

IMAGING MR can assess cellularity of lesions which correlate with higher recurrence after surgery

DIAGNOSTIC PROCEDURES N/A

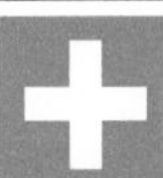

TREATMENT

APPROPRIATE HEALTH CARE
- Outpatient monitoring and physical therapy
- Inpatient if surgery indicated

GENERAL MEASURES
- Steroid injection for acute tender nodule
- Physiotherapy is ineffective alone
- Isolated involvement of palmar fascia can be followed
- Metacarpophalangeal (MP) joint involvement can be followed if flexion contracture is < 30 degrees
- Clostridial collagenase injections in phase 2 trial looks promising

SURGICAL MEASURES
- Surgery - selective fascial ray release
  - ◊ Indications: Any involvement of the proximal interphalangeal (PIP) joints or metacarpophalangeal (MCP) joints are contracted at least 30 degrees. Hueston's table-top test, if positive, consider surgery (when the palm is placed on a flat surface, the digits can not be simultaneously placed fully on the same surface as the palm because of flexion contractures).
  - ◊ May require skin grafts for wound closure with severe cutaneous shrinkage
  - ◊ 80% have full range of movement if operated on early
  - ◊ Continuous elongation technique is useful to prepare a severely contracted PIP joint for surgery. The digit can frequently be completely extended, however, will relapse if surgery not performed.
  - ◊ Amputation of little finger, if severe and deforming
  - ◊ MCP joints respond better than PIP joints, especially if > 45°

ACTIVITY
- No restrictions
- Physical therapy after surgery - started 3-5 days after surgery (passive and active exercises, posterior dynamic extension splints)

DIET No special diet

PATIENT EDUCATION
- Avoid risk factors especially with a strong family history
- Regular follow-up by physician every 6 months-1 year

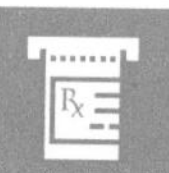

MEDICATIONS

DRUG(S) OF CHOICE
- Steroid injection for an acute tender nodule, painful knuckle pad
- Clostridial collagenase injections may also be effective

Contraindications: N/A
Precautions: N/A
Significant possible interactions: N/A

ALTERNATIVE DRUGS
Topical high-potency steroids - case report of improvement with clobetasol 0.1% bid and hs for 2-4 weeks

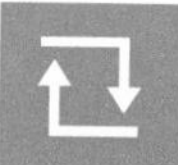

FOLLOWUP

PATIENT MONITORING
Follow patient in early stages of disease

PREVENTION/AVOIDANCE
None known. Avoid risk factors when possible.

POSSIBLE COMPLICATIONS
- Post-surgery development of reflex sympathetic dystrophy
- Postoperative recurrence or extension 46-80%
- Postoperative hand edema and skin necrosis
- Digital infarction

EXPECTED COURSE/PROGNOSIS
- Typical
  - ◊ Unpredictable, but usually slowly progressive
  - ◊ Patients likely to have aggressive disease (one or more) < 40 at onset, knuckle pads, positive family history, bilateral disease involving radial side of hand
  - ◊ Reports of clinical regression with continuous passive skeletal traction in extension and under a skin graft
  - ◊ Recurrence rate after surgery is 10-34%
  - ◊ Prognosis better for MP joint vs PIP joint after surgery
- Atypical
  - ◊ Nonprogressive
  - ◊ Surgery rarely needed
  - ◊ Recurrence unlikely if surgery performed

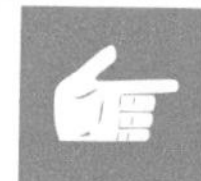

MISCELLANEOUS

ASSOCIATED CONDITIONS
- Alcoholism
- Epilepsy
- Diabetes mellitus
- Chronic lung disease
- Occupational hand trauma (vibration white finger)
- Shoulder-hand syndrome
- Status post myocardial infarction
- Hypercholesterolemia

AGE-RELATED FACTORS
Pediatric: N/A
Geriatric: Primarily in this age group
Others: N/A

PREGNANCY
N/A

SYNONYMS
N/A

ICD-9-CM
728.6 Contracture of palmar fascia

SEE ALSO

OTHER NOTES
N/A

ABBREVIATIONS
MP = metacarpophalangeal
PIP = proximal interphalangeal

REFERENCES

- Attali P, Ink O, et al. Dupuytren's contracture, alcohol consumption and chronic liver disease. Arch Intern Med 1987;147:1065-67
- Hill N, Hurst L. Dupuytren's contracture. Hand Clinics 1989;5(3):349-57
- Way LW. Current Surgical Diagnosis & Treatment. 8th Ed. Los Altos, CA, Lange, 1989
- Hueston JT. Repression of Dupuytren's contracture. J of Hand Surg 1992;17(4):453-57
- McFarlane RM. The current status of Dupuytren's disease. J of Hand Surg 1995;8(3):181-4
- Rayan G. Clinical presentation of Dupuytren's disease. Hand Clinics 1999;15(1):87-96
- Hunt TR 3rd. What is the appropriate treatment for Dupuytren contracture? Cleve Clin J Med 2003;70(2):96-7

Web references: 0 available at www.5mcc.com
Illustrations N/A

Author(s):
Jeffrey F. Minteer, MD

Dysfunctional uterine bleeding (DUB)

BASICS

DESCRIPTION Abnormal uterine bleeding, usually associated with anovulatory cycles, in the absence of other detectable organic lesions. This unit will deal only with women of reproductive age. Three major categories are:
- Estrogen breakthrough bleeding
- Estrogen withdrawal bleeding
- Progestin breakthrough bleeding

System(s) affected: Endocrine/Metabolic, Reproductive
Genetics: Unclear; tendency to have familial characteristics
Incidence/Prevalence in USA: Exact numbers not available, widespread prevalence, without specific geographic variation
Predominant age: 12-45
Predominant sex: Female only

SIGNS & SYMPTOMS
- Uterine bleeding:
  - ◊ Unrelated to menses
  - ◊ In excess of normal menstrual flow
  - ◊ Occurring in an irregular pattern
  - ◊ Rarely painful
- Absence of:
  - ◊ Other systemic symptoms
  - ◊ Unusual bleeding from other areas
  - ◊ Urinary or gastrointestinal irregularities
  - ◊ Sustained aspirin or anticoagulant use
  - ◊ Use of hormonal preparations
  - ◊ Evidence of thyroid disease
  - ◊ Galactorrhea
  - ◊ Pregnancy (especially ectopic)
  - ◊ Evidence for reproductive tract malignancy

CAUSES
- After Eisenberg:
  - ◊ Midcycle spotting - caused by a decrease in estrogen at midcycle following ovulation
  - ◊ Frequent menses - due to short follicular phase as a result of inappropriate feedback at pituitary/hypothalamic level
  - ◊ Deficiency of luteal phase - associated with premenstrual spotting or polymenorrhea when luteal phase is suddenly shortened by prematurely decreased progesterone; due to corpus luteum insufficiency
  - ◊ Prolonged corpus luteum activity - caused by persistent progesterone production - results in prolonged cycles or protracted episodes of bleeding
  - ◊ Anovulation - production of estrogen unaccompanied by cyclic surges of luteinizing hormone (LH) or secretion of progesterone from the corpus luteum. 90% of all DUB is anovulatory. Usually seen at extremes of reproductive life.
  - ◊ Other - uterine lesions, leiomyomata, polyps, carcinoma, vaginal infection, foreign body, ectopic pregnancy, hydatid mole, endocrine dysfunction (especially thyroid), blood dyscrasias

RISK FACTORS Listed with Causes

DIAGNOSIS

DIFFERENTIAL DIAGNOSIS
- Advanced liver disease
- Anabolic steroids
- Hematological disease (von Willebrand, leukemia, thrombocytopenia)
- Hormonal imbalance
- Iatrogenic causes
- Intrauterine devices
- Medications (oral contraceptives, corticosteroids, hypothalamic depressants, anticholinergics, digitalis, anticoagulants)
- Pregnancy (ectopic, incomplete miscarriage)
- Thyroid disease
- Trauma
- Uterine cancer
- Uterine leiomyomas

LABORATORY
- Rarely necessary unless clinical picture suggests other endocrine or hematological disease, or if patient is perimenopausal
- Consider thyroid function tests, CBC, PT, PTT, workup for hirsutism, HCG (to rule out pregnancy and/or hydatid mole), prolactin (pituitary dysfunction)

Drugs that may alter lab results: N/A

Disorders that may alter lab results: N/A

PATHOLOGICAL FINDINGS Variable, depending on the disease process present. Pathological review of endometrial sampling specimens is mandatory in all patients.

SPECIAL TESTS
- Determination of ovulatory status:
  - ◊ a) menstrual cycle charting
  - ◊ b) basal body temperature monitoring
  - ◊ c) measurement of the serum progesterone concentration in the mid-luteal phase 18-24 days after the onset of menses. Normal mid-luteal phase progesterone levels are between 6-25 ng/mL. A single low value does not reliably indicate an abnormal luteal phase due to LH pulses. A single level > 6 ng/mL usually indicates a normal luteal phase.
- An endometrial biopsy (EMB) should be performed in all women > age 35 with menorrhagia to rule out endometrial cancer or a premalignant lesion. EMB also should be considered in women 18-35 with AUB with risk factors for endometrial cancer, including obesity, chronic anovulation, history of breast cancer; tamoxifen use; family history of endometrial, ovarian, breast, or colon cancer. EMB is performed at or beyond day 18. Secretory endometrium confirms ovulation occurred in that cycle. EMB will not diagnose leiomyosarcoma or leiomyoma, since these lesions are deep to the endometrial lining.

IMAGING
- Ultrasound may be helpful in identifying ovarian cysts and uterine tumors
- Transvaginal ultrasound (TVS) to measure endometrial thickness may be considered in addition to endometrial biopsy. Consider TVS if you suspect pregnancy, anatomic problems, polycystic ovarian syndrome. The ultrasonographer should have a great deal of experience with the technique.

DIAGNOSTIC PROCEDURES
- Careful history of bleeding, with graphic display of cycles often helpful
- Pelvic examination
- Pap smear
- Endometrial biopsy in selected patients:
  - ◊ All patients over 35 years of age
  - ◊ Obese patients
  - ◊ Patients with diabetes mellitus
  - ◊ Patients with hypertension
  - ◊ Patients with suspected polycystic ovary syndrome
- Dilatation and curettage in those who have higher risk for endometrial hyperplasia and carcinoma (consider D&C more strongly over endometrial biopsy if the suspected diagnosis is endometritis, atypical hyperplasia, or carcinoma):
  - ◊ Heavy, uncontrolled bleeding
  - ◊ Histological examination is necessary, but biopsy is contraindicated
  - ◊ Medical curettage fails

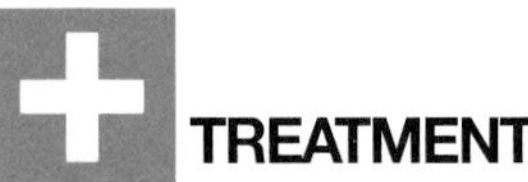

TREATMENT

APPROPRIATE HEALTH CARE Almost always outpatient; may need hospitalization for profuse bleeding and hemodynamic instability

GENERAL MEASURES See Medications

SURGICAL MEASURES
- Acute (profuse bleeding, hemodynamic instability):
  - ◊ Dilatation and curettage
  - ◊ Hysterectomy in selected (rare) cases
- Non-acute:
  - ◊ Hysterectomy in selected patients if medical therapy fails
  - ◊ Endometrial ablation in selected patients if medical therapy fails

ACTIVITY As tolerated

DIET Normal; include adequate iron

PATIENT EDUCATION
- Thorough yet easily comprehended explanation of diagnostic approach and plan of treatment is important. Many questions regarding fertility, cancer, and infectious disease.
- Discuss ways for patient to avoid prolonged stress or emotional turmoil
- American College of Obstetricians & Gynecologists (ACOG), 409 12th St., SW, Washington, DC 20024-2188, (800)762-ACOG

MEDICATIONS

DRUG(S) OF CHOICE

- Acute (heavy bleeding, unstable):
  - ◊ Conjugated equine estrogens (25 mg intravenously) every 4 hours for a maximum of six doses
  - ◊ When bleeding has stopped, induce shedding of the endometrium with 10 mg medroxyprogesterone (Provera) qd for 10-13 days, or with oral contraceptive medication containing 35 mcg of ethinyl estradiol or equivalent
  - ◊ Correct anemia with supplemental iron therapy
- Nonacute:
  - ◊ Progestin: Medroxyprogesterone 10 mg each day for 10-13 days
  - ◊ Estrogen and progesterone (if bleeding when seen or bleeding continues with progesterone or with OCP's): Add 1.25 mg conjugated estrogens daily for days 1-25
  - ◊ Oral contraceptives: Any preparation is usually adequate; initial therapy is one pill qid for 5-7 days. After withdrawal bleeding, may begin normal regimen, usually for at least 3 months or give medroxyprogesterone, 10 mg every day for 10 days every 30 days to regulate menses. Can add estrogen, conjugated (Premarin), 1.25 mg daily for 7 days during and in addition to regimen in order to stop intermenstrual bleeding.
  - ◊ Prostaglandin synthetase inhibitors (e.g., naproxen sodium, mefenamic acid): Can decrease amount of blood loss
  - ◊ GnRH agonists - create a hypogonadotropic state; provide only short-term benefits (6-9 months) and are expensive. Common side effects include hot flashes, vaginal dryness, decreased libido, insomnia, breast tenderness, depression, headaches, and transient menstruation. GnRH analog treatment for six months or more causes loss in bone density.
  - ◊ Correct anemia with supplemental iron therapy
  - ◊ Special considerations in perimenopausal women. Administration of a low dose oral contraceptive in women who do not smoke and are free of other contraindications to oral contraceptive therapy. There are also noncontraceptive benefits of oral contraceptives in this age group, including protection against endometrial and ovarian cancer, prevention of benign breast disease, and prevention of bone loss. Oral contraceptives can be continued until the onset of menopause.

Contraindications: Therapy should not be instituted until a reasonable attempt at diagnosis has been made, and other causes of uterine bleeding have been considered. "Blind" hormonal therapy is ill-advised and potentially dangerous.

Precautions: Absence of withdrawal bleeding requires workup. Estrogens should not be administered to perimenopausal women or those at risk for endometrial cancer until endometrial hyperplasia and carcinoma have been excluded. Failure of a particular regimen should prompt thorough review of the diagnostic pathway before further steps are taken.

Significant possible interactions: Refer to manufacturer's profile of each drug

ALTERNATIVE DRUGS

- Progesterone:
  - ◊ 100 mg IM progesterone in oil (an alternate to oral medroxyprogesterone). This works well for active bleeding. Not appropriate for cyclic therapy.
  - ◊ Vaginal suppositories due to leakage and uncertain amount of effective medication should not be used
  - ◊ "Natural" progesterone lozenges (sublingual/oral) have not be adequately studied for use with DUB and have questionable safety.
- Danazol (Danocrine) [unlabeled use]: 200-400 mg/day. Much more expensive and may cause masculinization. Usually reserved for women planning to undergo endometrial ablation soon.

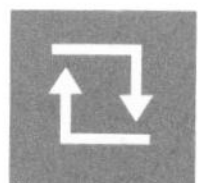

FOLLOWUP

PATIENT MONITORING All women treated for DUB with estrogens should maintain a menstrual calendar to document the pattern of bleeding abnormalities and their relation to therapy

PREVENTION/AVOIDANCE N/A

POSSIBLE COMPLICATIONS

- Anemia
- Adenocarcinoma of the uterus if prolonged unopposed estrogen stimulation in women with intact uterus
- Significant side effects of individual preparations. See manufacturer's printed information.

EXPECTED COURSE/PROGNOSIS

- Varies with pathophysiologic process
- In young women, most anovulatory cycles can be treated confidently and successfully with physiologically sound therapeutic regimens, without surgical intervention

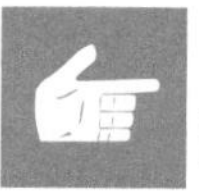

MISCELLANEOUS

ASSOCIATED CONDITIONS Listed with Causes

AGE-RELATED FACTORS

Pediatric: N/A

Geriatric: Uterine bleeding in a postmenopausal female must be pursued as if there were carcinoma or other significant pathology present

Others: Early postpubertal females and those in their later reproductive years most often affected

PREGNANCY May confuse with ectopic pregnancy, hydatidiform mole

SYNONYMS N/A

ICD-9-CM

626.8 Disorders of menstruation and other abnormal bleeding from female genital tract, other

SEE ALSO

Dysmenorrhea
Ectopic pregnancy
Menorrhagia

OTHER NOTES If DUB cannot be controlled with medical treatment, options besides hysterectomy are available. Among these are the ND:YAG laser or electrocautery of the endometrium with a ball-end resectoscope.

ABBREVIATIONS N/A

REFERENCES

- Ash SJ, Farrell SA, Flowerdew G. Eadometrial biopsy in DUB. J Reprod Med 1996;41:892-6.
- Granberg S, Ylostalo P, Wrikland M, Karlsson R. Endometrial sonographic and histologic findings in women with and without hormonal replacement therapy suffering from postmenopausal bleeding. Maturitas 1997;1:35-40
- Munro MG. Abnormal uterine bleeding in the reproductive years. Part II-medical management. J Am Assoc Gynecol Laparosc 2000;7:17-35
- Colacurci N, De Placido G, Mollo A, et al. Short-term use of Goserelin depot in the treatment of dysfunctional uterine bleeding. Clin Exp Obstet Gynecol 1995;22(3):212-9
- Casper RF, Senoz S, Ben-Chetrit A. The use of oral contraceptives in women over age 35. Reprod Med Rev 1995;4:115-20
- Anderson ABM, Haynes PJ, Guilleband J, Turnbull AC. Reduction of menstrual blood loss by prostaglandin synthetase inhibitors. Lancet 1976;1:774
- DeVore GR, Owens O, Kase N. Use of intravenous Premarin in the treatment of dysfunctional uterine bleeding - a double-blind randomized control study. Obstet Gynecol 1982;59:285
- Speroff L, Glass RH, Kase NG, eds. Clinical Gynecologic Endocrinology and Infertility. 6th ed. Baltimore: Williams and Wilkins; 1999
- Cowan BD, Morrison JC. Management of abnormal genital bleeding in girls and women. N Engl J Med 1991;324:1710
- Apgar BS. Dysmenorrhea and dysfunctional uterine bleeding. Primary Care; Clinics in Office Practice 1997:24:161-78
- Goldfarb HA: A review of 35 endometrial ablations using ND:YASG laser for recurrent menorrhagia. Obstet Gynecol Clin 1990;79(5pt1):833-5

Web references: 0 available at www.5mcc.com

Illustrations N/A

Author(s):
Kurt Elward, MD, MPH

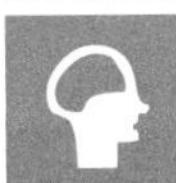

BASICS

DESCRIPTION
- Dyshidrotic eczema: Recurrent, non-erythematous, vesicular eruption primarily of the palms, soles and interdigital areas. The term pompholyx (Greek "bubble") is generally reserved for the cases of deep-seated pruritic vesicles (the so-called "sago grain" appearance). Generally associated with, but not caused by, hyperhidrosis.
- Lamellar dyshidrosis: A fine spreading exfoliation of the superficial epidermis in the same distribution as described above. Hyperhidrosis may or may not be associated.

System(s) affected: Skin/Exocrine
Genetics: N/A
Incidence/Prevalence in USA: 20/100,000
Predominant age: Usually < age 40
Predominant sex: Male = Female

SIGNS & SYMPTOMS
- Dyshidrotic eczema
  - ◊ Small superficial vesicles of the palms and soles and between the fingers and toes
  - ◊ Scaling, fissures and lichenification may follow vesicle formation
  - ◊ Burning and itching are common
  - ◊ Bilateral and frequently symmetrical lesions
  - ◊ Vesicles may sometimes coalesce to form larger vesicles or even bullae
  - ◊ Vesicles may rupture leading to a fine scaling similar to tinea
- Lamellar dyshidrosis
  - ◊ Small white macules which spread peripherally
  - ◊ Central area begins to scale
  - ◊ Desquamation of the horny layer of the skin that continues to spread

CAUSES
- Exact cause is not known
- May represent an id reaction especially to a dermatophyte infection, atopic reaction, reaction to allergens
- Stress may play a role since dyshidrosis is more frequent in anxious individuals, and those with psychosocial stress
- Hyperhidrosis is not a cause, but is often associated with the disease

RISK FACTORS
- Atopic dermatitis
- Contact dermatitis
- Dermatophytosis
- Bacterial infections
- Foods
- Drugs, such as aspirin or other salicylates

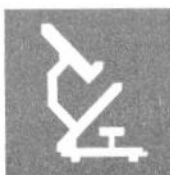

DIAGNOSIS

DIFFERENTIAL DIAGNOSIS
- Tinea manuum or pedis
- Id reaction
- Contact dermatitis
- Atopic dermatitis
- Drug reaction
- Dermatophytid
- Pustular psoriasis
- Seborrheic dermatitis
- Acrodermatitis continua
- Pustular bacterid

LABORATORY N/A

Drugs that may alter lab results: N/A

Disorders that may alter lab results: N/A

PATHOLOGICAL FINDINGS
- Dyshidrotic eczema: Reveals fine 1-2 mm spongiotic vesicles intraepidermally. Sweat ducts are not involved.
- Lamellar dyshidrosis: Exfoliation of the horny layer of the epidermis

SPECIAL TESTS N/A

IMAGING N/A

DIAGNOSTIC PROCEDURES
- Diagnosis is usually based on clinical exam
- Skin biopsy

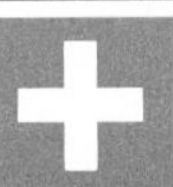

TREATMENT

APPROPRIATE HEALTH CARE Outpatient

GENERAL MEASURES
- Avoidance of possible causative factors (see Risk factors)
- Though hyperhidrosis is not a cause, excessive sweating may increase pruritus and burning
- Moisturizers will give symptomatic relief of dry scaly lesions
- If feet involved:
  - ◊ Wear shoes with leather soles rather than rubber (e.g., sneakers)
  - ◊ Wear socks made of cotton instead of synthetic materials
  - ◊ Remove shoes and socks whenever possible to allow sweat evaporation and to apply lubricants

SURGICAL MEASURES N/A

ACTIVITY
- Avoid, when possible, stress or excessive sweating (may be psychological or thermal sweating)
- Avoid excess detergents and water

DIET No restrictions

PATIENT EDUCATION
- Instructions on self-care, complications and avoidance
- Explain the association between stress and dyshidrosis and suggest counseling if appropriate

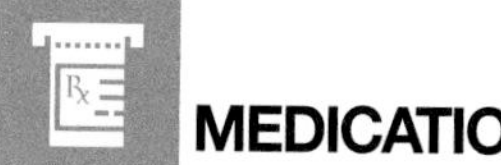

MEDICATIONS

DRUG(S) OF CHOICE
- Dyshidrotic eczema-mild cases
  - ◊ Topical steroids (medium to high potency), or
  - ◊ 5% salicylate in alcohol (provided salicylates are not a cause), or aluminum acetate (Burow's solution) compresses
  - ◊ Moisturizers for symptomatic relief
- Dyshidrotic eczema-moderate to severe cases
  - ◊ A systemic corticosteroid such as short course of oral prednisone
  - ◊ Intramuscular ACTH or triamcinolone acetonide 40 mg
  - ◊ PUVA (psoralens and ultraviolet A) therapy is effective therapy (including mild cases)
  - ◊ Tap water iontophoresis and low dose methotrexate have also been shown to be helpful in recalcitrant cases
  - ◊ UV-B has also shown benefit
- Lamellar dyshidrosis
  - ◊ Application of coal tar (Estar) preparations
  - ◊ Intramuscular corticosteroids
  - ◊ Keratolytics and moisturizers are sometimes helpful

Contraindications: Refer to manufacturer's profile of each drug

Precautions: Refer to manufacturer's profile of each drug

Significant possible interactions: Refer to manufacturer's profile of each drug

ALTERNATIVE DRUGS N/A

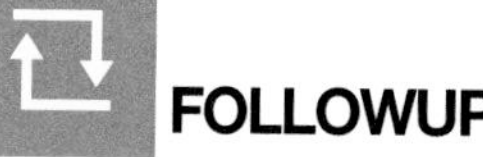

FOLLOWUP

PATIENT MONITORING As needed

PREVENTION/AVOIDANCE
- Control of emotional stress, avoid sweating
- Treatment for psychological factors, if appropriate

POSSIBLE COMPLICATIONS Bacterial secondary infections

EXPECTED COURSE/PROGNOSIS
- Benign and without scarring
- Lesions will often resolve spontaneously, though faster with appropriate treatment
- Recurrence is the rule rather than the exception

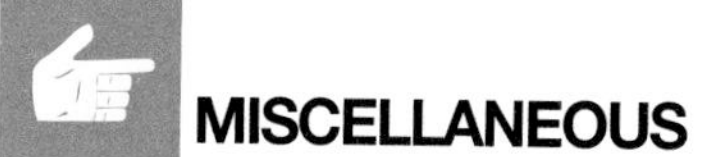

MISCELLANEOUS

ASSOCIATED CONDITIONS N/A

AGE-RELATED FACTORS
Pediatric: N/A

Geriatric: N/A

Others: N/A

PREGNANCY N/A

SYNONYMS
- Pompholyx
- Cheiropompholyx
- Keratolysis exfoliativa

ICD-9-CM
705.81 Dyshidrosis

SEE ALSO

OTHER NOTES N/A

ABBREVIATIONS N/A

REFERENCES

- Domonkos AN, Arnold HL, Odom RB: Andrew's Diseases of the Skin. 8th Ed. Philadelphia, W.B. Saunders Co., 1990
- Fitzpatrick TB, et al, eds. Dermatology in General Medicine. 5th Ed. New York, McGraw-Hill, 1999
- Fitzpatrick TB: Color Atlas and Synopsis of Clinical Dermatology. 2nd Ed. New York, McGraw-Hill, 1992
- Sauer R: Manual of Skin Diseases. 6th Ed. Philadelphia, J.B. Lippincott, 1991

Web references: 0 available at www.5mcc.com

Illustrations 2 available

Author(s):
Scott A. Kincaid, MD

BASICS

DESCRIPTION Pelvic pain occurring at or around the time of menses. A leading cause of absenteeism for women under age 30.
- Primary dysmenorrhea - without pathological physical findings
- Secondary dysmenorrhea - often more severe than primary, having a secondary pathologic (structural) cause

System(s) affected: Reproductive
Genetics: Not well studied
Incidence/Prevalence in USA:
- >50% of adult females have menstrual pain
- 10% are incapacitated for 1-3 days each cycle

Predominant age:
- Primary - teens to early 20's
- Secondary - 20's to 30's

Predominant sex: Female only

SIGNS & SYMPTOMS
- Mild - pelvic discomfort or cramping or heaviness on first day of bleeding with no associated symptoms
- Moderate - discomfort occurring on first 2-3 days of menses and accompanied by mild malaise, diarrhea and headache
- Severe - intense, cramp-like pain lasting 2-7 days; often with nausea, diarrhea, back pain, thigh pain, and headache

CAUSES
- Primary:
  - ◊ Elevated production (2-7 times normal) of prostaglandins and other mediators in the uterus which produce uterine ischemia through:
    - Platelet aggregation
    - Vasoconstriction
    - Dysrhythmic contractions with pressures higher than the systemic blood pressure
- Secondary:
  - ◊ Congenital abnormalities of uterine or vaginal anatomy
  - ◊ Cervical stenosis
  - ◊ Pelvic infection
  - ◊ Adenomyosis
  - ◊ Endometriosis
  - ◊ Pelvic tumors - especially leiomyomata
  - ◊ Uterine polyps
  - ◊ Intrauterine device

RISK FACTORS
- Primary:
  - ◊ Nulliparity
  - ◊ Obesity
  - ◊ Cigarette smoking
  - ◊ Positive family history
- Secondary:
  - ◊ Pelvic infection
  - ◊ Sexually transmitted diseases
  - ◊ Endometriosis

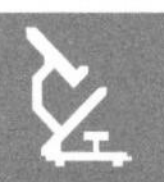

DIAGNOSIS

DIFFERENTIAL DIAGNOSIS
- Primary:
  - ◊ History is characteristic
- Secondary:
  - ◊ Pelvic or genital infection
  - ◊ Complication of pregnancy
  - ◊ Missed or incomplete abortion
  - ◊ Ectopic pregnancy
  - ◊ Uterine or ovarian neoplasm
  - ◊ Endometriosis
  - ◊ Urinary tract infection
  - ◊ Complication of uterine device

LABORATORY Noncontributory except in case of acute infection, in which case white blood cell count may be elevated and blood or cervical cultures positive

Drugs that may alter lab results: Antibiotics

Disorders that may alter lab results: N/A

PATHOLOGICAL FINDINGS
- Primary:
  - ◊ None
- Secondary:
  - ◊ Uterine enlargement
  - ◊ Leiomyomata
  - ◊ Ligamentous thickening
  - ◊ Fixation of pelvic structures
  - ◊ Endometritis
  - ◊ Salpingitis

SPECIAL TESTS N/A

IMAGING N/A
- Primary - consider ultrasound to rule out secondary abnormalities if history not characteristic
- Secondary - ultrasound or laparoscopy to define anatomy

DIAGNOSTIC PROCEDURES
- Primary:
  - ◊ History is characteristic
  - ◊ Physical examination should be normal
  - ◊ Response to NSAIDs helps confirm diagnosis
- Secondary:
  - ◊ History of onset at least 18-24 months after menarche
  - ◊ Physical examination may reveal anatomic abnormalities or tenderness
  - ◊ Laparoscopy (rarely needed)

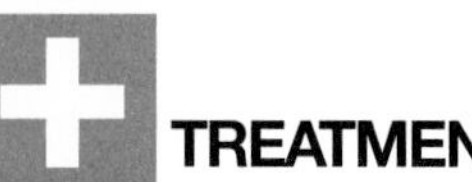

TREATMENT

APPROPRIATE HEALTH CARE
- Primary - outpatient
- Secondary - usually outpatient

GENERAL MEASURES
- General physical conditioning, exercise to raise endorphins
- Transcutaneous electrical nerve stimulator (TENS)
- Secondary dysmenorrhea - treatment of infections. Suppression of endometrium if endometriosis is suspected.
- Acupuncture may be effective

SURGICAL MEASURES Adenomyosis may require hysterectomy

ACTIVITY Normal

DIET
- Dietary supplementation with vitamin B1 (thiamine) 100 mg po daily has been found effective when used for at least 90 days
- Dietary supplementation with fish oil capsule daily found effective when used for 2 months
- Low fat vegetarian diet significantly decreases pain

PATIENT EDUCATION
- Reassure patient that primary dysmenorrhea is treatable with use of non-steroidal anti-inflammatory agents prior to menses and/or oral contraceptives, and will usually abate with age and parity
- Refer to web site: www.5mcc for resources for patient education material
- Vitamin E 500 IU daily 2 days prior to menses and 3 days after onset, found effective in teens with primary dysmenorrhea

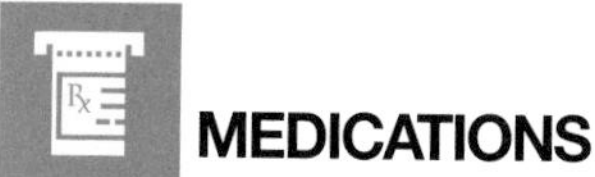

MEDICATIONS

DRUG(S) OF CHOICE
- Ibuprofen 400-600 mg every 4-6 hours,

or
- Naproxen sodium 550 mg every 12 hours,

or
- Aspirin 650 mg every 4-6 hours,

or
- Valdecoxib 20 mg every 12 hours or celecoxib 400 mg day one, 200 mg every 12 hours or rofecoxib 50 mg daily (not FDA approved for this use)

or
- Other nonsteroidal anti-inflammatory drugs
- Oral contraceptives in monthly or 3 monthly cycles

Contraindications:
- Platelet disorders
- Gastric ulceration or gastritis
- Thromboembolic disorders
- Vascular disease
- Contraindications to oral contraceptives

Precautions:
- GI irritation
- Lactation
- Coagulation disorders
- Impaired renal function
- Congestive heart failure
- Liver dysfunction

Significant possible interactions:
- Coumarin-type anticoagulants
- Aspirin with other NSAID's
- Methotrexate
- Furosemide
- Lithium

ALTERNATIVE DRUGS
- Mefenamic acid 500 mg at once, then 250 mg every 6 hours may be tried if other NSAIDs are ineffective, as it blocks both production of prostaglandins as well as already-formed prostaglandins
- Hydrocodone or tramadol (Ultram) for management of severe symptoms
- Calcium channel blockers (nifedipine, others) in low doses; efficacy reported, but not FDA approved for this use
- Transdermal nitroglycerin (not FDA approved for this use)
- Nafarelin acetate 200-400 mg/day for endometriosis (will simulate menopause)
- Progestin-containing intrauterine device (IUD) in suitable candidates

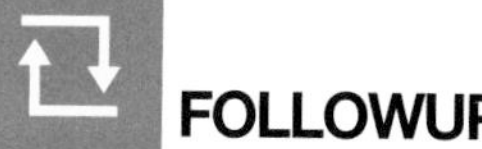

FOLLOWUP

PATIENT MONITORING N/A

PREVENTION/AVOIDANCE
- Primary - choose a diet low in animal fats, dairy products and eggs. Increase vegetables, raw seeds and nuts to increase production of beneficial prostaglandins.
- Secondary - reduce risk of sexually-transmitted diseases

POSSIBLE COMPLICATIONS
- Primary - anxiety and/or depression
- Secondary - infertility from underlying pathology

EXPECTED COURSE/PROGNOSIS
- Primary - improves with age and parity
- Secondary - likely to require therapy based on underlying cause

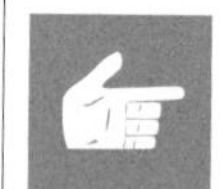

MISCELLANEOUS

ASSOCIATED CONDITIONS N/A

AGE-RELATED FACTORS N/A
Pediatric: Onset with first menses raises probability of genital tract anatomic abnormality such as transverse vaginal septum, uterine anomalies
Geriatric: N/A
Others: N/A

PREGNANCY
Consider ectopic pregnancy in differential diagnosis of pelvic pain with vaginal bleeding

SYNONYMS
Menstrual cramps

ICD-9-CM
625.3 Dysmenorrhea

SEE ALSO
Endometriosis

OTHER NOTES N/A

ABBREVIATIONS N/A

REFERENCES

- Harel Z, Biro FM, et al. Supplementation with omega-3 polyunsaturated fatty acids in the management of dysmenorrhea in adolescents. Am J Ob Gyn 1996;174(4):1335-8
- Transdermal nitroglycerin in the management of pain associated with primary dysmenorrhea: a multinational study. J Int Med Res 1997;25(1):41-4
- Milson I, Hedner N, Mannheimer C. A comparative study of the effect of high-intensity transcutaneous nerve stimulation and oral naproxen on intrauterine pressure and menstrual pain in patients with primary dysmenorrhea. Am J Obstet Gynecol 1994;170(1 Pt 1):123-9
- Nigam S, Benedetto C, et al. Increased concentrations of eicosanoids and platelet-activating factor in menstrual blood from women with primary dysmenorrhea. Eicosanoids 1991;4(3):137-31
- Smith RP. Cyclic pelvic pain and dysmenorrhea. Obstet Gynecol Clin North Am 1993;20(4):753-64
- Ziaei S, Faghihzadeh S, Sohrabvand F, Lamyian M, Emamgholy T. A randomised placebo-controlled trial to determine the effect of vitamin E in treatment of primary dysmenorrhoea. BJOG 2001;108(11):1181-3
- Chavez ML, DeKorte CJ. Valdecoxib: a review. Clin Ther 2003 Mar;25(3):817-51
- Coco AS. Primary dysmenorrhea. Am Fam Physician 1999;60(2):489-96
- Lethaby A, Augood C, Duckitt K. Nonsteroidal anti-inflammatory drugs for heavy menstrual bleeding (Cochrane Review). In: The Cochrane Library, Issue4, 2003, Chichester, UK: John Wiley & Sons. Ltd.
- Marjoribanks J, Proctor ML, Farquhar C. Nonsteroidal anti-inflammatory drugs for primary dysmenorrhoea (Cochrane Review). In: The Cochrane Library, Issue4, 2003, Chichester, UK: John Wiley & Sons. Ltd.
- Morgan PJ, Kung R, Tarshis J. Nitroglycerin as a uterine relaxant: a systematic review. J Obstet Gynaecol Can 2002;24(5):403-9
- Proctor ML, Roberts H, Farquhar CM. Combined oral contraceptive pill (OCP) as treatment for primary dysmenorrhoea (Cochrane Review). In: The Cochrane Library, Issue4, 2003, Chichester, UK: John Wiley & Sons. Ltd.
- Proctor ML, Smith CA, Farquhar CM, Stones RW. Transcutaneous electrical nerve stimulation and acupuncture for primary dysmenorrhoea (Cochrane Review). In: The Cochrane Library, Issue4, 2003, Chichester, UK: John Wiley & Sons. Ltd.
- Stones RW, Mountfield J. Interventions for treating chronic pelvic pain in women (Cochrane Review). In: The Cochrane Library, Issue4, 2003, Chichester, UK: John Wiley & Sons. Ltd.
- White AR. A review of controlled trials of acupuncture for women's reproductive health care. J Fam Plann Reprod Health Care 2003;29(4):233-6

Web references: 6 available at www.5mcc.com
Illustrations N/A

Author(s):
Janice E. Daugherty, MD

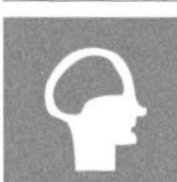

BASICS

DESCRIPTION Recurrent and persistent genital pain associated with sexual activity, in either the male or female. Dyspareunia may be due to organic, emotional or psychogenic causes.
- Primary: Present throughout one's sexual history
- Secondary: Arising from some specific event or condition, e.g., menopause, drugs
- Superficial: Difficulty or pain at or near the introitus or vaginal barrel associated with penetration
- Deep: Pain after penetration located at the cervix or lower abdominal area
- Complete: Present under all circumstances
- Situational: Occurring selectively with specific situations

System(s) affected: Reproductive
Genetics: N/A
Incidence/Prevalence in USA:
- Most women who are sexually active will experience dyspareunia at some time in their lives. Approximately 15% (4-40%) of adult women will have dyspareunia on a few occasions during a year. About 1-2% of women will have painful intercourse on a more than occasional basis.
- Male prevalence unknown

Predominant age: All ages
Predominant sex: Female > Male

SIGNS & SYMPTOMS Varying degrees of pelvic/genital pressure, aching, tearing and/or burning

CAUSES
- Disorders of vaginal outlet
  - ◊ Hymenal ring abnormalities
  - ◊ Postmenopausal atrophy
  - ◊ Decreased lubrication
  - ◊ Episiotomy scars
  - ◊ Vulvar vestibulitis/vulvodynia
  - ◊ Infections
  - ◊ Trauma
  - ◊ Adhesions
  - ◊ Clitoral irritation
  - ◊ Vulvar papillomatosis
- Disorders of vagina
  - ◊ Infections
  - ◊ Masses or tumors
  - ◊ Decreased lubrication
  - ◊ Pelvic relaxation resulting in rectocele, uterine prolapse or cystocele
  - ◊ Inflammatory or allergic response to foreign substance
  - ◊ Abnormality of vault due to surgery or radiation
  - ◊ Congenital malformations
- Disorders of pelvic structures
  - ◊ Pelvic inflammatory disease
  - ◊ Endometriosis
  - ◊ Malignant or benign tumors of the uterus
  - ◊ Ovarian pathology
  - ◊ Pelvic adhesions
  - ◊ Prior pelvic fracture
  - ◊ Levator ani myalgia
  - ◊ Pelvic venous congestion
- Disorders of the gastrointestinal tract
  - ◊ Inflammatory bowel disease
  - ◊ Crohn disease
  - ◊ Diverticular disease
  - ◊ Constipation
  - ◊ Hemorrhoids
  - ◊ Fistulas
- Disorders of the urinary tract
  - ◊ Interstitial cystitis
  - ◊ Ureteral or vesical lesions
- Male
  - ◊ Genital muscle spasm
  - ◊ Infection and irritation of penile skin
  - ◊ Cancer of penis
  - ◊ Phimosis
  - ◊ Penile anatomy disorders
  - ◊ Prostate infections and enlargement
  - ◊ Infection of seminal vesicles
  - ◊ Testicular disease
  - ◊ Torsion of spermatic cord
  - ◊ Musculoskeletal disorders of pelvis and lower back
  - ◊ Urethritis
- Psychologic disorders
  - ◊ Fear
  - ◊ Depression
  - ◊ Anxiety
  - ◊ Phobic reactions
  - ◊ Conversion reactions
  - ◊ Hostility towards partner
  - ◊ Psychological trauma

RISK FACTORS
- Diabetes
- Estrogen deficiency
- Alcohol/marijuana consumption
- Menopause
- Medroxyprogesterone use
- Stress
- Fatigue or overwork
- Lactation
- Vaginal surgery
- Medication side effects (antihistamines, tamoxifen, bromocriptine, low estrogen oral contraceptives, depo-medroxyprogesterone, desipramine)

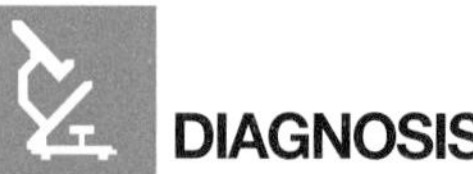

DIAGNOSIS

DIFFERENTIAL DIAGNOSIS
- Vaginismus

LABORATORY
- Gonorrhea culture
- Wet mount
- Chlamydia culture
- Herpes culture
- Urine analysis
- Urine culture
- Pap smear to assess estrogen status

Drugs that may alter lab results: N/A

Disorders that may alter lab results: N/A

PATHOLOGICAL FINDINGS Dependent on etiology

SPECIAL TESTS N/A

IMAGING
- Voiding cystourethrogram if urinary tract involvement
- Gastrointestinal contrast studies if GI symptoms
- US and CT of limited value; perform if clinically indicated

DIAGNOSTIC PROCEDURES
- Colposcopy and biopsy if vaginal/vulvar lesions
- Laparoscopy if complex deep penetration pain
- Cystoscopy if urinary tract involvement
- Sigmoidoscopy if GI involvement

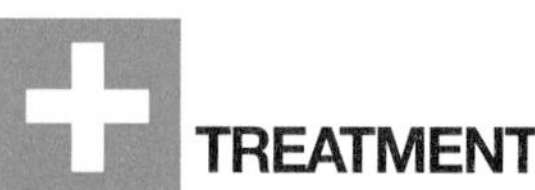

TREATMENT

APPROPRIATE HEALTH CARE Outpatient

GENERAL MEASURES
- The first step in treatment is to educate the patient and partner as to the nature of the problem and reassure them the problem can be solved
- Organic causes can generally be identified during the initial evaluation and specific treatment initiated
- Once organic causes have been ruled out, individual and/or couple behavioral therapy should be initiated
- Behavioral therapy
  - ◊ Designed to systemically desensitize to intercourse through a series of interventions over a period of weeks
  - ◊ Interventions range from muscle relaxation and mutual body massage to sexual fantasies and erotic massage, with the ultimate goal of intercourse and sexual responsiveness
- Individual therapy
  - ◊ Indicated to help the patient deal with intrapsychic issues and assess the role of the partner
- Couple therapy
  - ◊ Indicated to help resolve interpersonal problems
  - ◊ May involve short-term structured intervention or sexual counseling
  - ◊ Referral for long-term therapy may be necessary

SURGICAL MEASURES
- Should be avoided
- Surgical vestibulectomy can be considered when conservative measures fail with vulvar-vestibulitis

ACTIVITY Routine; sitz baths may relieve painful inflammation

DIET Regular; a high-fiber diet may help if constipation is the cause

PATIENT EDUCATION
- Patient education models, information on sexual arousal techniques, Kegel exercise information (Instructions for Patients, Griffith, H.W., W.B. Saunders Co., Philadelphia; Our Bodies, Ourselves for the New Century: A book by and for women, Boston Women's Health Collective, Simon & Schuster, New York)
- www.dyspareunia.org

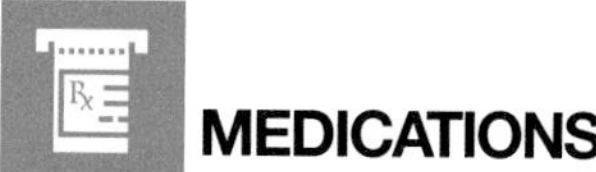

MEDICATIONS

DRUG(S) OF CHOICE
- ◊ Dependent on the etiology. May include antibiotics, antifungals and antivirals for infection; estrogen for vaginal atrophy; analgesics and topical anesthetics for pain; and lubricants for dryness.
- ◊ Vulvar vsetibulitis/vulvodynia may respond to tricyclic antidepressants or gabapentin.

Contraindications: Refer to manufacturer's profile on each drug
Precautions: Refer to manufacturer's profile on each drug
Significant possible interactions: Refer to manufacturer's profile on each drug

ALTERNATIVE DRUGS N/A

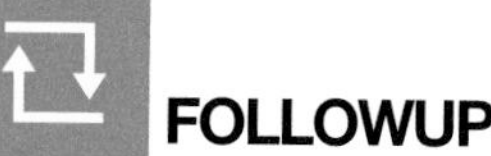

FOLLOWUP

PATIENT MONITORING Dependent on therapy. Every 6-12 months once resolved.

PREVENTION/AVOIDANCE Avoidance of alcohol and tobacco products

POSSIBLE COMPLICATIONS N/A

EXPECTED COURSE/PROGNOSIS
The majority of cases will respond to treatment

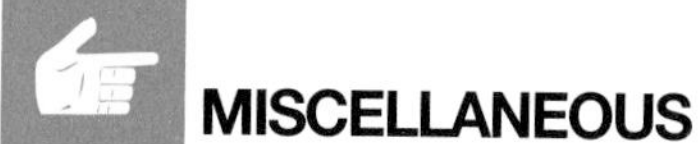

MISCELLANEOUS

ASSOCIATED CONDITIONS Vaginismus

AGE-RELATED FACTORS
Pediatric: N/A
Geriatric: The incidence increases dramatically in the postmenopausal woman who is not receiving HRT primarily because of vaginal atrophy. Over half of all sexually active women will report dyspareunia.
Others: N/A

PREGNANCY
- Pregnancy is a potent influence on sexuality; dyspareunia is common
- Episiotomies have been associated with dyspareunia. Mediolateral episiotomies have greater incidence when compared to midline.

SYNONYMS N/A

ICD-9-CM
302.76 Psychosexual dysfunction with functional dyspareunia
625.0 Dyspareunia
608.89 Other specified disorders of male genital organs, other

SEE ALSO
Balanitis
Endometriosis
Pelvic inflammatory disease (PID)
Peyronie disease
Sexual dysfunction in women
Vaginismus
Vulvovaginitis, bacterial
Vulvovaginitis, candidal
Vulvovaginitis, estrogen deficient

OTHER NOTES N/A

ABBREVIATIONS N/A

REFERENCES

- Canavan TP, Heckman CD. Dyspareunia in women. Breaking the silence is the first step toward treatment. Postgrad Med 2000;108(2):149-52, 157-60, 164-6
- Butcher J. ABC of sexual health: female sexual problems II: sexual pain and sexual fears. BMJ 1999:318(7176):110-112
- Heim LJ. Evaluation and differential diagnosis of dyspareunia. Am Fam Physician 2001;63(8):1535-44

Web references: 0 available at www.5mcc.com
Illustrations N/A

Author(s):
Scott T. Henderson, MD

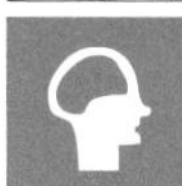

BASICS

DESCRIPTION An ill-defined condition characterized by the presence of chronic intermittent symptoms of epigastric pain and fullness, early satiety, nausea and/or vomiting without mucosal lesions or other structural abnormalities of the gastrointestinal tract

System(s) affected: Gastrointestinal

Genetics: N/A

Incidence/Prevalence in USA: Common, affecting 15-20% of patients referred to gastroenterologists

Predominant age: Adults, but can be seen in children

Predominant sex: Females > Males

SIGNS & SYMPTOMS
- Belching
- Aerophagia, gaseousness, abdominal distension
- Borborygmus
- Epigastric pain, gnawing or burning; eating may improve or worsen symptoms
- Substernal pain, gnawing or burning
- Anorexia, nausea, or vomiting
- Change in bowel habits
- Abdominal tenderness
- No anatomic abnormalities

CAUSES
- Often unknown, may be of several different etiologies
- Evanescent ulcers (20-30% go on to develop ulcers)
- Gastric motility disorder
- Adverse drug effects
- Doubtful relationship to helicobacter pylori

RISK FACTORS
- Other functional disorders
- Anxiety
- Depression

DIAGNOSIS

DIFFERENTIAL DIAGNOSIS
- Gastroesophageal reflux
- Cholecystitis
- Peptic ulcer disease
- Gastric cancer
- Esophageal spasm
- Malabsorption syndromes
- Pancreatic disease
- Irritable bowel syndrome
- Aerophagia
- Ischemia heart disease
- Diabetes mellitus
- Thyroid disease
- Connective tissue disorders
- Conversion disorder

LABORATORY
- CBC
- Chemistry panel
- Stool for occult blood

Drugs that may alter lab results: Too many to list

Disorders that may alter lab results: N/A

PATHOLOGICAL FINDINGS None (by definition)

SPECIAL TESTS
- Esophageal manometry (rarely needed)
- 24-hour intra-esophageal pH monitoring (rarely needed)

IMAGING
- Recommended in:
  - ◊ Patients over 45 years of age at onset of symptoms
  - ◊ Patients with symptoms and signs suggesting more serious disease
  - ◊ Patients who need added reassurance
  - ◊ Younger patients who do not respond rapidly to empiric treatment
- Usual:
  - ◊ Endoscopy, or
  - ◊ Upper GI series
- Sometimes:
  - ◊ Barium enema
  - ◊ Gallbladder studies (e.g., ultrasound or oral cholecystogram)
  - ◊ Nuclear medicine gastric emptying study (in selected cases)

DIAGNOSTIC PROCEDURES
- Careful history and physical
- Normal studies of esophagus, stomach and duodenum (particularly in patients over 45)

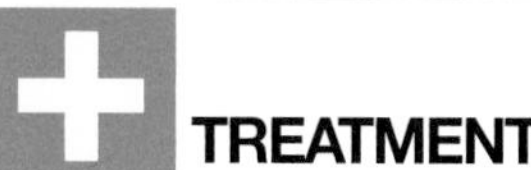

TREATMENT

APPROPRIATE HEALTH CARE Outpatient

GENERAL MEASURES
- Supportive measures
  - ◊ Reassurance
  - ◊ Do not investigate excessively
  - ◊ Dietary changes (see below)
  - ◊ Elevate head of bed (where applicable)
  - ◊ Maintain ideal body weight
  - ◊ Explore psychological issues

SURGICAL MEASURES N/A

ACTIVITY
- Stress reduction
  - ◊ Relaxation techniques
  - ◊ Physical exercise
  - ◊ Reflux precautions where applicable

DIET
- Avoid foods known to exacerbate symptoms
- Frequent small meals
- Avoid regular and decaffeinated coffee
- Avoid tea, cocoa, chocolate
- Avoid heavy alcohol use
- Avoid cigarette smoking
- Avoid aspirin containing compounds and NSAIDs

PATIENT EDUCATION See Web site

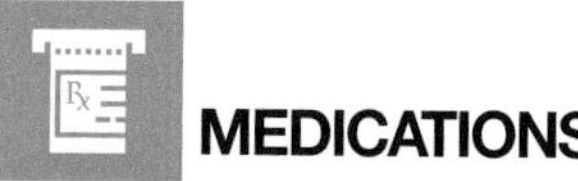

MEDICATIONS

DRUG(S) OF CHOICE
- 60% of patients improve with placebo
- Acid reduction drugs
  - ◊ H2 antagonists
  - ◊ Proton pump inhibitors (PPI)
  - ◊ Antacids

Contraindications:
- Magnesium containing antacids should be avoided in patients with significant renal dysfunction

Precautions:
- H2 antagonist and PPI dosages should be adjusted in patients with renal disease
- Calcium containing antacids may precipitate the formation of kidney stones

Significant possible interactions:
- H2 blockers interact with drugs metabolized by, and affecting the liver
- Antacids compete with digoxin, iron salts, tetracycline, fluoroquinolones, and other drugs for absorption from the stomach

ALTERNATIVE DRUGS
- Gastric motility drugs
  - ◊ Metoclopramide (Reglan); although side effects are significant
  - ◊ Erythromycin
- Amitriptyline 50mg qHS

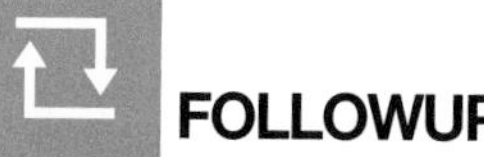

FOLLOWUP

PATIENT MONITORING
- Usual duration of medication is 4 weeks, then 2 weeks intermittently for exacerbations. If chronic medication use is needed, should do imaging to rule out serious pathology.
- Continuing observation to provide support and reassurance
- Minimize diagnostic studies unless disabling symptoms persist or new problems arise

PREVENTION/AVOIDANCE Continued health habits suggested under Treatment (i.e., avoid activities known to exacerbate problems, maintain healthy lifestyle, continue stress reduction techniques)

POSSIBLE COMPLICATIONS Undiagnosed serious pathology

EXPECTED COURSE/PROGNOSIS
Long-term or chronic symptoms with periods that are symptom free

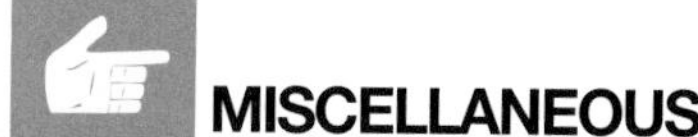

MISCELLANEOUS

ASSOCIATED CONDITIONS Other functional bowel disorders

AGE-RELATED FACTORS
Pediatric: Look for family system dysfunction
Geriatric: Cancer risk is higher
Others: N/A

PREGNANCY May exacerbate

SYNONYMS
- Non-ulcer dyspepsia
- Moynihan dyspepsia
- Pseudo-ulcer dyspepsia
- Phantom ulcer
- Non-organic dyspepsia
- Nervous dyspepsia

ICD-9-CM
536.8 Dyspepsia and other specified disorders of function of stomach

SEE ALSO
Gastritis
Irritable bowel syndrome

OTHER NOTES N/A

ABBREVIATIONS N/A

REFERENCES

- Talley NJ. Non-ulcer dyspepsia: Current approaches to diagnosis and management. Am Fam Phys 1993;47:1407-1416
- Veldhuyzen van Zanten SJ. Drug treatment of functional dyspepsia: a systematic analysis of trial methodology with recommendations for design of future trials. Am J Gastroenterol 1996;91(4):660-73
- Fisher RS, Parkman HP. Management of nonulcer dyspepsia. N Engl J Med. 1998;339(19):1376-81

Web references: 2 available at www.5mcc.com
Illustrations N/A

Author(s):
K. Patricia McGann, MD, MSPH

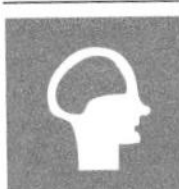

BASICS

DESCRIPTION The sensation of difficulty swallowing. This is a disorder of esophageal transfer or transport and is a symptom of an underlying process. The problem is commonly divided into oropharyngeal and esophageal types.
System(s) affected: Gastrointestinal, Nervous
Genetics: N/A
Incidence/Prevalence in USA: 7% incidence lifetime; increasing prevalence with age
Predominant age: All ages
Predominant sex: Male = Female

SIGNS & SYMPTOMS
- Oropharyngeal type
  - ◊ Choking with swallowing
  - ◊ Coughing with swallowing
  - ◊ Weak voice
  - ◊ Aspiration pneumonia
  - ◊ Weight loss
- Esophageal type
  - ◊ Pressure sensation in mid-chest (patient may localize pathology to correct anatomic site)
  - ◊ Symptoms should distinguish whether dysphagia is for solids or liquids or both
  - ◊ Aspiration pneumonia
  - ◊ Weight loss
  - ◊ Symptoms of GERD
  - ◊ Longer time required to eat meals (patient unconsciously chews food more thoroughly)

CAUSES
- In children
  - ◊ Malformations - congenital (esophageal atresia, choanal atresia)
  - ◊ Malformations - acquired (corrosive or herpetic esophagitis)
  - ◊ Neuromuscular/neurologic - delayed maturation, cerebral palsy, muscular dystrophy
  - ◊ Gastroesophageal reflux disease
- In adults - esophageal
  - ◊ Structural - tumors (cancer or benign), strictures (peptic, chemical, trauma, radiation), rings & webs, extrinsic compression, vascular anomaly (goiter)
  - ◊ Gastroesophageal reflux disease
  - ◊ Neuromuscular - achalasia, diffuse esophageal spasm, scleroderma, myasthenia gravis
- In adults - oropharyngeal
  - ◊ CVA
  - ◊ Parkinson
  - ◊ Multiple sclerosis
  - ◊ Zenker's diverticulum
  - ◊ Myasthenia gravis

RISK FACTORS
- Children - hereditary and/or congenital malformations
- Adults - age > 50 years, when cancer of the esophagus is more likely
- Smoking
- Long history of gastroesophageal reflux disease
- Medications (quinine, potassium chloride, vitamin C, tetracycline, non-steroidal anti-inflammatory drugs, and others)

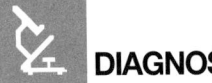

DIAGNOSIS

DIFFERENTIAL DIAGNOSIS
- Cardiac chest pain
- Globus hystericus

LABORATORY N/A

Drugs that may alter lab results: N/A

Disorders that may alter lab results: N/A

PATHOLOGICAL FINDINGS
- Squamous cell or adenocarcinoma
- Barrett's metaplasia
- Fibrous tissue of a ring, web or stricture
- Acute or chronic inflammatory change
- Heterotopic gastric mucosa (inlet patch)
- Oropharyngeal lesions

SPECIAL TESTS
- In infants/children
  - ◊ Observe sucking/eating
  - ◊ Attempt to pass nasogastric tube to assess esophageal patency
  - ◊ X-ray neck and chest
  - ◊ Contrast x-ray
  - ◊ Endoscopy
- In adults
  - ◊ X-ray of neck and chest
  - ◊ Endoscopy
  - ◊ Barium cine/video esophagogram
  - ◊ Ambulatory, 24 hour pH testing
  - ◊ Esophageal manometry

IMAGING
- X-ray: chest, neck, abdomen
- Contrast x-ray: esophagram, cine-esophagram, modified cine-esophagram (cookie swallow)
- CT scan of chest

DIAGNOSTIC PROCEDURES
- Endoscopy with biopsy
- Esophageal manometry (altered by anticholinergics [propantheline], calcium channel blockers [nifedipine], nitrates [nitroglycerin], prokinetic [metoclopramide], sedatives [diazepam])
- Esophageal pH monitoring (altered by anticholinergics [propantheline], H2 receptor antagonists [cimetidine], proton pump inhibitors [omeprazole], prokinetic [metoclopramide])

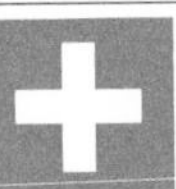

TREATMENT

APPROPRIATE HEALTH CARE
- Outpatient for those conditions where the patient is able to maintain nutrition and where there is little risk of complication
- Hospitalization may be required for either infants or adults where dysphagia is associated with total or near total obstruction of the esophageal lumen
- Endoscopy and/or esophageal dilatation may be needed for stenoses
- Surgery may be needed in either benign or malignant processes

GENERAL MEASURES
- Exclude cardiac disease
- Determine esophageal patency to exclude inflammation
- Ensure airway and pulmonary function
- Assess nutritional status

SURGICAL MEASURES
- Esophageal dilatation (pneumatic or bougie)
- Esophageal stent; laser for late cancer
- treatment for underlying problem (eg, thyroid goiter, esophageal atresia)
- Photodynamic therapy (cancer)

ACTIVITY No restriction

DIET
Varies from nothing by mouth to near normal, depending on the degree of obstruction.

PATIENT EDUCATION
- Counsel on avoiding irritating drugs
- Counsel on chewing, consistency of food
- In infants/children - discuss underlying problem and therapy for recurrent aspiration
- In adults - discuss etiology and therapy (need for repeat dilatations). Speech therapy may be helpful in teaching swallowing techniques.

MEDICATIONS

DRUG(S) OF CHOICE
- For spasms:
  - ◊ Nitrates
  - ◊ Calcium channel blockers (nifedipine [Procardia]10-30 mg tid)
- For esophagitis:
  - ◊ Antacids
  - ◊ H2-blockers (cimetidine [Tagamet], ranitidine [Zantac], nizatidine [Axid], famotidine [Pepcid])
  - ◊ Proton pump inhibitors (omeprazole [Prilosec], lansoprazole [Prevacid]), rabeprazole (Aciphex), esomeprazole (Nexium), pantoprazole (Protonix)
  - ◊ Prokinetic agents - metoclopramide (Reglan)

Contraindications:
- Anticholinergics - obstructive uropathy, glaucoma, myasthenia gravis, achalasia
- Nitrates - early myocardial infarction, severe anemia, increased intracranial pressure

Precautions: May need to use liquid forms of medications

Significant possible interactions: Refer to manufacturer's profile of each drug

ALTERNATIVE DRUGS N/A

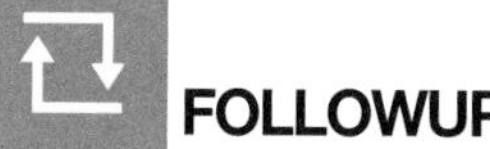

FOLLOWUP

PATIENT MONITORING The type of reassessment and frequency of follow-up is related to the specific etiology of the dysphagia

PREVENTION/AVOIDANCE
- Very hot or very cold foods may worsen.
- Observe feeding of infants closely for aspirations - have suction available
- Advise for correction of poorly fitting dentures in adults or elderly
- Avoid drinking alcohol with meals
- Avoid soft breads, solid meats

POSSIBLE COMPLICATIONS
- Aspiration
- Esophageal "asthma"
- Pneumonia
- Barrett's esophagus
- Death

EXPECTED COURSE/PROGNOSIS
Course and prognosis varies with the specific diagnosis (cancer - poor; esophageal peptic stricture - good)

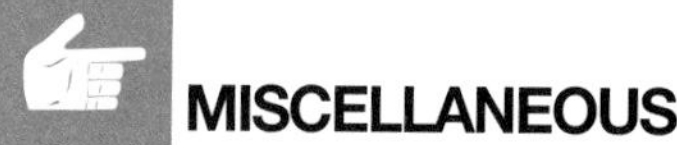

MISCELLANEOUS

ASSOCIATED CONDITIONS
- Esophageal carcinoma
- Gastroesophageal reflux disease
- Dysphagia lusoria
- Achalasia
- Symptomatic diffuse esophageal spasm
- Scleroderma
- Myasthenia gravis
- CVA

AGE-RELATED FACTORS
Pediatric: Congenital malformations

Geriatric:
- Poor dentition and/or dentures
- Drug induced

Others: N/A

PREGNANCY N/A

SYNONYMS N/A

ICD-9-CM
787.2 Dysphagia

SEE ALSO
Esophageal tumors
Gastroesophageal reflux disease
Schatzki ring

OTHER NOTES This is a symptom of an abnormal process. A search for the etiology is of great importance.

ABBREVIATIONS
GERD = gastroesophageal reflux disease

REFERENCES

- Clouse RE. Approach to the patient with dysphagia or odynophagia. In: Yamada T, et al, eds. Textbook of Gastroenterology. 4th ed. Philadelphia: Lippincott Williams & Wilkins; 2003
- Domenech E, Kelly J. Swallowing disorders. Med Clin North Am 1999;83(1):97-113
- Kosko JR, Moser JD, Erhart N, Tunkel DE. Differential diagnosis of dysphagia in children. Otolaryngol Clin North Am 1998;31(3):435
- Trate DM, Parkman HP, Fisher RS. Dysphagia - evaluation, diagnosis and treatment. Primary Care 1996;23(3)417-32
- Rothstein RD. A systematic approach to the patient with dysphagia. Hosp Pract 1997;32(3):169-175

Web references: 1 available at www.5mcc.com

Illustrations N/A

Author(s):
Duane C. Roe, MD

BASICS

DESCRIPTION The presence of seizure activity in an obstetric patient with the syndrome of hypertension, edema, and proteinuria (pre-eclampsia), in a patient without underlying neurological disease. Nearly all postpartum cases occur within 24 hours of delivery.
System(s) affected: Hemic/Lymphatic/Immunologic, Nervous, Reproductive
Genetics: There does seem to be some genetic predisposition. The single-gene model best explains the frequency of about 25%, but multifactorial inheritance is also possible.
Incidence/Prevalence in USA: Incidence of pregnancy-induced hypertension affects approximately 6% of pregnancies, with preeclampsia complicating 2-4%. Of preeclamptic patients, eclampsia develops in l/2000 deliveries in developed countries. In developing countries, estimates range from l/100 to 1/1700.
Predominant age: Most of the cases occur in younger women because of the higher incidence of preeclampsia in younger (nulliparous) women. However, older (> 40 years), preeclamptic patients have 4 times the incidence of seizures compared with patients in their 20's.
Predominant sex: Female only

SIGNS & SYMPTOMS
- Tonic-clonic seizure activity (focal or generalized)
- Headache, visual disturbance and epigastric or right upper quadrant pain often precedes seizure
- Seizures may occur once or repeatedly
- Postictal coma, cyanosis (variable)
- Temperatures > 39°C consistent with CNS hemorrhage
- Disseminated intravascular coagulation (DIC), thrombocytopenia, liver dysfunction, renal failure associated
- Proteinuria
- Up to 30% may not have edema, 20% may not have proteinuria
- Normal blood pressure - however, normal blood pressure, even in "response" to treatment, does not rule out potential for seizures
- Hemoconcentration - predisposition to pulmonary and or cerebral edema with fluid therapy. There is actually an excess of extracellular fluid that is inappropriately distributed to the extracellular spaces.

CAUSES
- Exact cause of seizures remains unclear
- Trophoblastic tissue seems to be required, and somehow results in widespread vasospasm
- Severe cerebral vasoconstriction; hemorrhages occur due to failure of the constriction to limit perfusion pressure in the capillaries, with consequent rupture and vasogenic cerebral edema and ring hemorrhages
- Now considered to be primarily an endothelial disorder

RISK FACTORS
- Nulliparity 5-1
- Age > 40 3:1
- African American 1.5.1
- Family history of PIH 5:1
- Chronic HTN 10:1
- Chronic renal disease 20:1
- Antiphospholipid syndrome 10-1
- Diabetes 2:1
- Twins 4:1
- High BMI 3:1

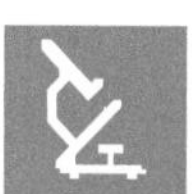

DIAGNOSIS

DIFFERENTIAL DIAGNOSIS
- Epilepsy
- Cerebral tumors
- Ruptured cerebral aneurysm
- Until other causes are proven, however, all pregnant women with convulsions should be considered to have eclampsia

LABORATORY
- CBC/platelets
- 24 hour urine for protein/creatinine clearance
- Creatinine
- Serum transaminase
- Serum albumin
- LDH, uric acid
- Coagulation profiles - abnormalities suggest severe disease
- Serum markers such as hCG, leptin, and inhibin A have not proven to be useful as screening tests

Drugs that may alter lab results: Concurrent treatment with Dilantin, barbiturates (not with magnesium)

Disorders that may alter lab results: N/A

PATHOLOGICAL FINDINGS Cerebral edema, hyperemia, focal anemia, thrombosis, and hemorrhage; cerebral lesions account for 40% of eclamptic deaths

SPECIAL TESTS
- Fetal monitoring - dependent on other clinical factors. Consider nonstress testing weekly to twice weekly when diagnosis is established, and if clinical condition/laboratory testing indicates progressive disease.
- Ultrasound - used to monitor growth, cord blood now, Bishop score. Perform as indicated based on clinical stability and laboratory findings.

IMAGING Computerized tomography can evaluate for mass lesions, infarct, hemorrhages, but is rarely used when usual clinical picture is present. Should be considered if focal findings persist or uncharacteristic signs/symptoms present.

DIAGNOSTIC PROCEDURES
- No additional procedures generally applicable
- EEG may vary from posterior slow waves to status epilepticus, but is rarely useful
- Cerebral spinal fluid studies are of no value unless other causes (e.g., meningitis) are seriously considered in differential diagnosis

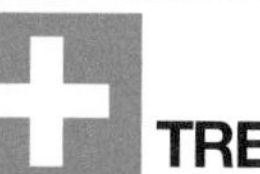

TREATMENT

APPROPRIATE HEALTH CARE
- Inpatient management for severe/deteriorating disease
- Outpatient management with close (days to weekly) follow up for stable mild to moderate disease. Consider home blood pressure and urine protein monitoring.

GENERAL MEASURES
- Control of convulsions, correction of hypoxia and acidosis, lowering blood pressure, steps to effect delivery as soon as convulsions are controlled
- See Medications
- Indications for delivery
  - ◊ Gestational age > 38 weeks
  - ◊ Platelet count < 100,000
  - ◊ Progressive deterioration in liver/renal function
  - ◊ Suspected abruption
  - ◊ Persistent severe neurological symptoms
  - ◊ Severe growth retardation
  - ◊ Nonreassuring fetal testing results
  - ◊ Oligohydramnios
- Women with severe disease and between 32 and 37 weeks and worsening clinical/fetal status merit delivery, preferably after an attempt to demonstrate/promote fetal lung maturity

SURGICAL MEASURES If fetal distress is evident or maternal condition at high risk of deterioration in spite of medical therapy, Cesarean section may be indicated. Patient is still at some risk for post partum eclampsia, however.

ACTIVITY Bedrest

DIET Nothing by mouth until stable, then usual seizure precautions; low salt diet commonly recommended

PATIENT EDUCATION
- Explain to the patient and partner/family what has happened and the need for the prompt actions necessary to ensure the safety of the mother and infant
- Additional materials from: American College of Obstetricians & Gynecologists, 409 12th St., SW, Washington, DC 20024-2188, (800)762-ACOG

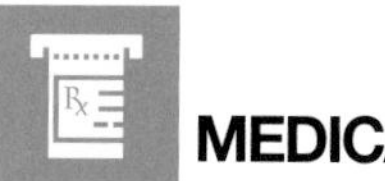

MEDICATIONS

DRUG(S) OF CHOICE

Recent randomized trials: magnesium sulfate superior to phenytoin in treatment and prevention of eclampsia and probably more effective and safer than diazepam

- Magnesium sulfate
  - ◊ 2-4 g IV, repeated every 15 minutes to a maximum of 6 g to achieve resolution of an ongoing convulsion
  - ◊ Magnesium then is continued at 1-3 g/hour with the amount given based on the neurological exam and patellar reflex
  - ◊ Levels of 6-8 mEq/mL are considered therapeutic, but clinical status is most important
  - ◊ May be given safely even in presence of renal insufficiency
  - ◊ As magnesium is continued, must ensure that
    - a) patellar reflex is present
    - b) respirations are not depressed
    - c) urine output is at least 25 cc/hr
- Fluid therapy:
  - ◊ Ringer's lactate with 5% dextrose at 60-120 mL/hr, with careful attention to fluid-volume status
  - ◊ Invasive monitoring may be needed
  - ◊ Earlier transfusion may be considered due to attenuated intravascular volume and hemoconcentration
- Hypertension, if present and severe (eg, greater than 160/110) should also be treated
  - ◊ IV hydralazine - 5 mg IV, then 5-10 mg boluses prn q 20 minutes

or

  - ◊ Labetalol - 10 or 20 mg intravenously, then double dose q 10 minute intervals up to 80 mg; maximum total cumulative dose of 220 -230 mg (eg, 20-40-80-80 or 10-20-40-80)

Contraindications:

- Previous sensitivity/intolerance to a specific drug
- Avoid diuretics which can decrease the already lowered intravascular volume
- Hyperosmotic agents are dangerous due to capillary leakage

Precautions: Careful monitoring of neurological status, urine output, respirations, and fetal status

Significant possible interactions: Combinations of medications may cause respiratory depression. Calcium carbonate (1 gram administered slowly IV) can reverse magnesium-induced respiratory depression.

ALTERNATIVE DRUGS

- Benzodiazepines, eg, diazepam 2 mg/min until resolution or 20 mg given, or lorazepam 1-2 mg/min up to total of 10 mg, or phenytoin 18-20 mg/kg at a rate of 20-40 mg/min, or phenobarbital 100 mg/min to a total of 20 mg/kg given
- Nifedipine may be added to magnesium sulfate, but is not yet standard therapy (Austral N Zeal J OBstet Gynecol 1994;34: 144-48)

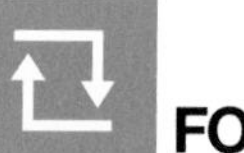

FOLLOWUP

PATIENT MONITORING Blood pressure, neurological examination, condition of fetus

PREVENTION/AVOIDANCE

- Adequate prenatal care
- Good control of preexisting hypertension
- Recognition and treatment of preeclampsia
- Aspirin has been suggested to lower fetal death; recent evidence in a large RCT showed no benefit
- Calcium supplementation has been shown to reduce the risk of preeclampsia by 30% (9 RCTs)
- There is some evidence for vitamin C (1000/mg/d) plus E (400U/d) in reducing risk for preeclampsia

POSSIBLE COMPLICATIONS

- 56% have transient deficits including cortical blindness
- Most women do not have long-term sequelae from eclampsia
- Death from toxemia or its complications
- Death of fetus

EXPECTED COURSE/PROGNOSIS

- 25% of eclamptic women will have hypertension in subsequent pregnancies, but only 5% of these will be severe, and only 2% will be eclamptic again
- Eclamptic, multiparous women may be at higher risk for subsequent essential hypertension
- Multiparous women with eclampsia have higher mortality in subsequent pregnancies than primiparous women
- Racial factors are unclear, since the higher incidence of essential hypertension in blacks may predispose them to higher rates of hypertension postpartum, rather than a history of eclampsia

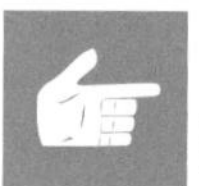

MISCELLANEOUS

ASSOCIATED CONDITIONS None

AGE-RELATED FACTORS

Pediatric: Essential for adequate neonatal care/facilities

Geriatric: N/A

Others: Younger patients have highest incidence, but most likely related to the fact that younger patients represent largest numbers of primigravidas

PREGNANCY By definition, a complication of pregnancy

SYNONYMS

- Pregnancy-associated seizures
- Toxemic seizures

ICD-9-CM

642.40 Mild or unspecified pre-eclampsia, unspecified
642.50 Severe pre-eclampsia, unspecified
642.60 Eclampsia, unspecified
642.90 Unspecified hypertension complicating pregnancy, childbirth, or the puerperium, unspecified
780.39 Other convulsions

SEE ALSO

Preeclampsia

OTHER NOTES N/A

ABBREVIATIONS N/A

REFERENCES

- Cunningham FG, MacDonald PC, Gant NF, eds. Williams' Obstetrics. 19th ed. Norwalk, CT: Appleton and Lange; 1993
- Chesley LC, Annitto JE, Cosgrove RA. Long-term follow-up study of eclamptic women: sixth periodic report. Am J Obst Gyneco 1976;124:446
- American College of Obstetrics and Gynecology. Technical bulletin, Number 91, 1986
- Lucas MJ, Leveno KJ, Cunningham FG. A comparison of magnesium sulfate with phenytoin for the prevention of preeclampsia. N Engl J Med 1995;333:201-5
- Lindheimer MD. Preeclampsia-eclampsia 1996: preventable? Have disputes on its treatment been resolved? Current Opinion in Nephrology and Hypertension 1996;5:452-8
- Knight M, Duley L. The effectiveness and safety of antiplatelet agents for prevention and treatment of preeclampsia. In Cochrane Library, Issue 3. Oxford: Update software, 2000
- Atallah AN, Hofineyr GJ, Duley L. Calcium supplementation during pregnancy to prevent hypertensive disorders. In Cochrane Library, Issue 3. Oxford: Update software, 2000
- Chappell LD, Seed PT, Briley AL. Effect of antioxidants on the occurrence of preeclampsia in women at increased risk. Lancet 1999;354:810-16.
- Duley L. Magnesium sulphate versus phenytoin for preeclampsia: In Cochrane Library, Issue 3. Oxford: Update software, 2000
- Cards S, et al. Low dose aspirin to prevent preeclampsia in women at high risk. N Engl J Med 1998;338:701-5
- National High Blood Pressure Education Program Working Group on High Blood Pressure in Pregnancy. Am J Obstet Gynecol 2000;183(I)S1-22

Web references: 0 available at www.5mcc.com

Illustrations N/A

Author(s):

Kurt Elward, MD, MPH

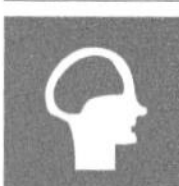

BASICS

DESCRIPTION Extrauterine pregnancy - any pregnancy existing outside the confines of the uterine cavity
- Tubal pregnancy - pregnancy existing within the different portions of the fallopian tubes, i.e., ampullary (55%), isthmic (25%), fimbrial (17%), interstitial (cornual) (2%)
- Ovarian pregnancy - pregnancy existing within the confines of an ovary
- Abdominal pregnancy - pregnancy existing in the abdominal (peritoneal) cavity, most commonly within the cul-de-sac. Occasionally it may implant on the intestines, pelvic side-walls, omentum, or even on the surfaces of the liver or spleen.
- Cervical pregnancy - pregnancy is implanted in the substance of the cervix below the level of the internal os
- Intraligamentary pregnancy - after a tubal pregnancy ruptures, the surviving embryo secondarily implants within the confines of the anterior and posterior leaves of the broad ligament

System(s) affected: Reproductive
Genetics: N/A
Incidence/Prevalence in USA:
- 88,000 cases in 1987
- 16.8 per 1000 pregnancies (live birth, legally induced abortions, and ectopic pregnancies)

Predominant age: Over 40% occurred in women between ages 20 and 29
Predominant sex: Female only

SIGNS & SYMPTOMS
- Tubal pregnancy:
  - ◊ Pelvic pain
  - ◊ Amenorrhea followed by irregular vaginal bleeding
  - ◊ Abdominal tenderness
  - ◊ Adnexal tenderness or mass
  - ◊ Tenesmus
  - ◊ Shoulder pain
  - ◊ Syncope
  - ◊ Passage of decidual cast
- Ovarian pregnancy:
  - ◊ Pain and cramps
  - ◊ Pelvic mass
  - ◊ Vaginal bleeding after a period of amenorrhea
  - ◊ Clinical shock after rupture
- Abdominal pregnancy:
  - ◊ History suggestive of tubal abortion or rupture
  - ◊ Pregnancy complicated by unusual gastrointestinal symptoms
  - ◊ Fetal movements very marked or painful
  - ◊ Easy palpation of the fetal parts or movements
  - ◊ Pregnancy described by a multipara as "different"
  - ◊ False labor near term
  - ◊ High lying fetus in abnormal presentation, often transverse
  - ◊ Displacement of a firm, long cervix
  - ◊ Palpation of the fetal parts through the vaginal fornix
  - ◊ Unusually loud vascular souffle
- Cervical pregnancy:
  - ◊ A soft and disproportionately enlarged cervix equal to or greater than the uterine corpus (hourglass effect)
  - ◊ Extrusion of dark tissue through the external os
  - ◊ Continuous vaginal bleeding after amenorrhea
- Intraligamentary pregnancy:
  - ◊ History suggestive of tubal abortion or rupture
  - ◊ Unilateral pelvic mass associated with pain

CAUSES
- Tubal pregnancy:
  - ◊ Previous tubal pregnancy
  - ◊ Pelvic inflammatory disease
  - ◊ Endometriosis
  - ◊ Previous tubal surgery
  - ◊ Salpingitis isthmica nodosa
  - ◊ Pelvic adhesions
  - ◊ Pelvic tumors
- Ovarian pregnancy:
  - ◊ Implantation of the fertilized ovum on the ovarian surface
  - ◊ Tubal abortion with secondary implantation of the embryo on the tubal surface
- Abdominal pregnancy:
  - ◊ Tubal abortion with secondary implantation
  - ◊ Uteroperitoneal fistula following rupture of cesarean section or myomectomy scars
  - ◊ External transmigration theory
  - ◊ Menstrual regurgitation of a fertilized ovum theory
- Cervical pregnancy:
  - ◊ Unreceptive endometrium to implantation due to infection
  - ◊ Uterine myomas
  - ◊ Atrophic endometrium
  - ◊ Septate uterus
  - ◊ Presence of intrauterine device (IUD)
  - ◊ Scarring of the endometrium
  - ◊ Oral contraceptive use
- Intraligamentary pregnancy:
  - ◊ Rupture of a tubal pregnancy and secondary implantation between the anterior and posterior leaves of the broad ligament

RISK FACTORS
- Previous tubal surgery
- Previous pelvic inflammatory disease
- Pelvic adhesions
- Previous tubal pregnancy
- Previous uterine surgery
- Use of an intrauterine device
- History of endometritis
- Recipients of assisted reproductive technologies, e.g., in-vitro fertilization and embryo transfer

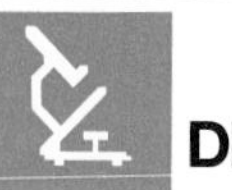

DIAGNOSIS

DIFFERENTIAL DIAGNOSIS
- Uterine abortion
- Appendicitis
- Salpingitis
- Ruptured corpus luteum cyst
- Cornual myoma or abscess
- Ovarian tumor
- Endometrioma
- Cervical cancer
- Cervical phase of uterine abortion
- Placenta previa

LABORATORY
- Urine pregnancy test
- Human chorionic gonadotropin (HCG) - serial quantitative serum beta
- Serial blood counts to quantify blood loss
- Serum progesterone level

Drugs that may alter lab results: N/A

Disorders that may alter lab results: N/A

PATHOLOGICAL FINDINGS
- Tubal pregnancy:
  - ◊ Presence of chorionic villi within the tubal wall
- Ovarian pregnancy (Spiegelberg's criteria):
  - ◊ The pregnancy must occupy the position of the ovary
  - ◊ The pregnancy must be connected to the uterus by the utero-ovarian ligament
  - ◊ The ipsilateral oviduct must be normal
  - ◊ The pregnancy sac must show the presence of ovarian tissue
- Abdominal pregnancy - primary form:
  - ◊ Both ovaries and oviducts must be normal
  - ◊ There is no uteroperitoneal fistula
  - ◊ Attachment of the conceptus is exclusively to the peritoneal surface
- Abdominal pregnancy - secondary form:
  - ◊ Fetal or placental tissue is found within the abdominal cavity beyond the ovaries or oviducts
- Cervical pregnancy:
  - ◊ Chorionic villi are implanted within the substance of the uterine cervix below the level of the internal os
  - ◊ The uterine cavity above the internal os is free of the products of conception
- Intraligamentary pregnancy:
  - ◊ The products of conception are within the confines of the broad ligament

SPECIAL TESTS
- Culdocentesis
- Endometrial biopsy and/or dilatation and curettage

IMAGING
- Vaginal and abdominal ultrasonography
- CT scan
- MRI
- Endovaginal color Doppler flow imaging

DIAGNOSTIC PROCEDURES
- Laparoscopy
- Laparotomy

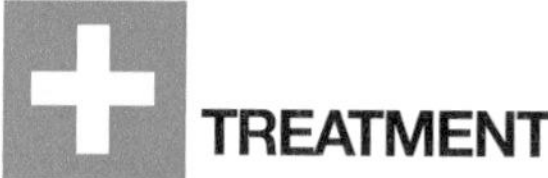

TREATMENT

APPROPRIATE HEALTH CARE
- Outpatient for most evaluation and treatment
- Outpatient surgery for unruptured tubal pregnancy
- Inpatient surgery for unstable hemodynamic conditions after resuscitation

GENERAL MEASURES N/A

SURGICAL MEASURES
- Laparotomy is often required for ovarian, abdominal, and intraligamentary pregnancy
- Careful curettage, packing of the cervix and uterine cavity, bilateral internal iliac artery ligations, or even hysterectomy may be necessary as treatment for cervical pregnancy
- Unruptured tubal pregnancy may be treated by salpingostomy
- Unruptured tubal pregnancy of less than 4 cm. diameter may be treated through laparoscopy. With methotrexate, best results obtainable when unruptured tubal pregnancy is less than 2 cm diameter or HCG less than 10000 mIU/mL, and before ultrasound evidence of fetal heart beats.

ACTIVITY Variable

DIET Variable

PATIENT EDUCATION American College of Obstetricians & Gynecologists (ACOG), 409 12th St., SW, Washington, DC 20024-2188, (800)762-ACOG

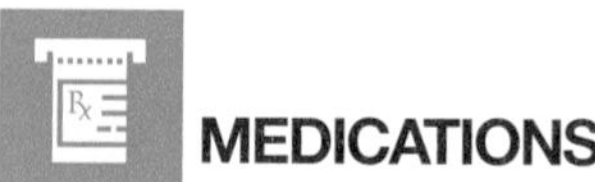

MEDICATIONS

DRUG(S) OF CHOICE
- Methotrexate as primary treatment for unruptured tubal pregnancy and for persistent disease after salpingostomy
- Methotrexate as supplementary treatment for retained placenta after delivery of the fetus in abdominal pregnancy
- Dosage: Methotrexate 1 mg/kg IM every other day with leucovorin 0.1 mg/kg IM in between. Maximum of 4 doses of methotrexate or methotrexate x 1 without leucovorin, at 50 mgm per square meter of body surface area; may repeat once if unsatisfactory response.

Contraindications: Pregnant women with psoriasis
Precautions: Methotrexate has toxic effects on the hematologic, renal, gastrointestinal, pulmonary, and neurologic systems
Significant possible interactions: Refer to manufacturer's profile of each drug

ALTERNATIVE DRUGS Dactinomycin

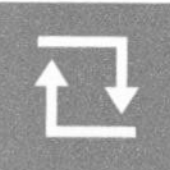

FOLLOWUP

PATIENT MONITORING
- Serial serum quantitative ß-HCG until level drops to near zero
- Followup pelvic ultrasonogram for persistent or recurrent masses
- Followup imaging studies for retained placenta in abdominal pregnancy, e.g., ultrasonography, CT scan, and MRI

PREVENTION/AVOIDANCE
- Reliable contraception
- Repeat tubal pregnancies occur in about 12%. For patient who becomes pregnant again, use ultrasound to verify intrauterine pregnancy.

POSSIBLE COMPLICATIONS
- Hemorrhage and hypovolemic shock
- Infection
- Loss of reproductive organs after complicated surgery
- Infertility
- Urinary and/or intestinal fistulas after complicated surgery
- Need for blood transfusions with its hazards
- Disseminated intravascular coagulation

EXPECTED COURSE/PROGNOSIS
With early diagnosis and treatment, rupture unlikely to occur

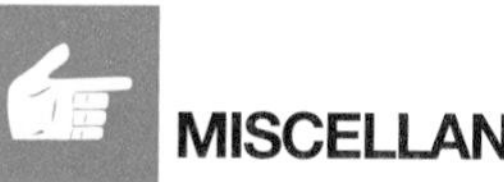

MISCELLANEOUS

ASSOCIATED CONDITIONS N/A

AGE-RELATED FACTORS
Pediatric: N/A
Geriatric: N/A
Others: N/A

PREGNANCY N/A

SYNONYMS
- Extrauterine pregnancy
- Tubal pregnancy
- Ovarian pregnancy
- Abdominal pregnancy
- Cervical pregnancy
- Intraligamentary pregnancy

ICD-9-CM
633.90 Unspecified ectopic pregnancy without intrauterine pregnancy

SEE ALSO
Abortion, spontaneous

OTHER NOTES N/A

ABBREVIATIONS N/A

REFERENCES

- Herbst AL, Mishell DR, Stenchever MA, Droegemueller W. Comprehensive Gynecology. 2nd ed. St. Louis: The C.V. Mosby Co.; 1992
- Durfee RB, Pernoll ML. Early pregnancy risks In: Pernoll M, Benson RC, eds. Current Obstetric and Gynecologic Diagnosis and Treatment. 7th ed. Norwalk, CT: Appleton and Lange; 1991
- Kurman RJ, ed: Blaustein's Pathology of the Female Genital Tract. 3rd ed. New York: Springer-Verlag; 1987
- Novak ER, Woodruff JD. Novak's Gynecologic and Obstetric Pathology With Clinical and Endocrine Relations. 8th ed. Philadelphia: W.B. Saunders Co.; 1979
- Stovall TG, Ling FW. Single dose methotrexate, an expanded clinical trial. Am J OB-GYN 1993;168:1759-1765
- Stovall TG, Ling FW. Gonadotrophin in screening for ectopic pregnancy. Human Repro 1992;7:723-725
- Wolf GC, et al. Completely non-surgical management of ectopic pregnancies. Gynecol-Obstet Invest 1994;37:232-235
- Kadar N, et al. The discriminatory HCG zone for endovaginal sonography, a prospective randomized study. Fertil Steril 1994;61:1016-1020
- Emerson DS, et al. Diagnostic efficacy of endovaginal color Doppler flow imaging in an ectopic pregnancy screening. Radiology 1992;183:413-420
- Pellerito JS, et al. Ectopic pregnancy: Evaluation with endovaginal color flow imaging. Radiology 1992;183:407-411
- Tay J, Moore J, Walker J, Ectopic Pregnancy: Regular Review. Brit Med Jour 2000;1 April:916-19
- Medical Management of Tubal Pregnancy. ACOG Practice Bulletin. Clinical Management Guidelines For Obstetricians & Gynecologists, Number 3, December 1998:973-79

Web references: 2 available at www.5mcc.com
Illustrations N/A

Author(s):
Albert T. Shiu, MD

BASICS

DESCRIPTION Premature ejaculation: Inability to constantly control the ejaculatory reflex is a common sexual disorder affecting all age groups. Definition criteria vary, e.g., inability to maintain an erection of sufficient duration to satisfy a partner, or ejaculation that occurs before individual wants it to. Natural biological response is to ejaculate within 2 minutes after vaginal penetration. Ejaculatory control is an acquired behavior that increases with experience.

- Retarded ejaculation: A condition in which erection is normal, or prolonged, but ejaculation does not occur
- Retrograde ejaculation: The valve at the base of the bladder fails to close during ejaculation and the ejaculate is forced backward into the bladder. Erection and sexual pleasure are usually not diminished.

System(s) affected: Nervous, Reproductive
Genetics: No known genetic pattern
Incidence/Prevalence in USA: Premature ejaculation is common (particularly in the adolescent)
Predominant age: All age groups
Predominant sex: Male only

SIGNS & SYMPTOMS
- Ejaculation occurring before individual wishes
- Ejaculation does not occur following normal erection (including masturbation)

CAUSES
- Never any ejaculate
  - ◊ Congenital structural disorder (Müllerian duct cyst, Wolffian abnormality)
  - ◊ Acquired (radical prostatectomy, postinfectious, posttraumatic, T10-12 neuropathy)
- Retrograde ejaculation
  - ◊ TURP (25%)
  - ◊ Surgery on the neck of the bladder
  - ◊ Extensive pelvic surgery
  - ◊ Retroperitoneal lymph node dissection for testicular cancer (also can produce failure of emission)
  - ◊ Neurologic disorders, eg, multiple sclerosis
  - ◊ Drugs, eg, amoxapine, desipramine, imipramine
- Retarded ejaculation
  - ◊ Rarely may be due to underlying painful disorder, eg, prostatitis, seminal vesiculitis
  - ◊ May be psychogenic as part of erectile dysfunction
  - ◊ Sympathectomy, eg, spinal cord injury, diabetes mellitus
  - ◊ Some drugs may impair ejaculation, eg, certain MAO inhibitors, SSRIs, alpha-blockers, antipsychotics, tricyclic antidepressants
- Premature ejaculation
  - ◊ Sexual inexperience
  - ◊ High level of sexual arousal
  - ◊ Fear of sexually transmitted disease
  - ◊ Anxiety
  - ◊ Guilty feelings about sex
  - ◊ Interpersonal maladaptation (marital problems, unresponsiveness of mate)
  - ◊ Lack of privacy

RISK FACTORS
Listed with Causes

DIAGNOSIS

DIFFERENTIAL DIAGNOSIS N/A

LABORATORY
- Laboratory test results are usually normal
- Post-ejaculate urinalysis will confirm retrograde ejaculation when infertility is a concern

Drugs that may alter lab results: N/A

Disorders that may alter lab results: N/A

PATHOLOGICAL FINDINGS N/A

SPECIAL TESTS Look for diabetes, multiple sclerosis, spinal cord injury

IMAGING N/A

DIAGNOSTIC PROCEDURES Detailed sexual history

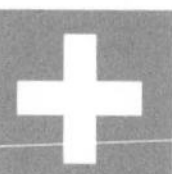

TREATMENT

APPROPRIATE HEALTH CARE Outpatient

GENERAL MEASURES
- Identification of any medical cause (even if not reversible) helps patient accept condition
- Improve partner communication
- Reduce performance pressure through reassurance
- Use sensate focus therapy
- Techniques to learn ejaculatory control, e.g., coronal squeeze technique or start-and-stop technique
- Use of a variety of resources may be necessary, e.g., psychiatrists, psychologists, sex therapists, vascular surgeons, urologists, endocrinologists, neurologists
- If drugs are a possible cause, consider discontinuing or changing dosage
- Retrograde ejaculation may be helped if intercourse occurs when bladder is full

SURGICAL MEASURES N/A

ACTIVITY No restrictions

DIET No special diet except for diabetics

PATIENT EDUCATION See General Measures

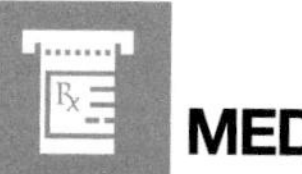

MEDICATIONS

DRUG(S) OF CHOICE
- Premature ejaculation may respond to topical anesthesia gel applied under a condom for 30 minutes prior to intercourse. Clomipramine or sertraline have been shown to delay ejaculation for 4-6 minutes.
- Switching antidepressants to bupropion, nefazodone, or mirtazapine or possibly trazodone often eliminates drug-induced ejaculatory disturbance
- Retarded orgasm and ejaculation in patients who must continue SSRI drugs may respond to sildenafil

Contraindications: N/A
Precautions: N/A
Significant possible interactions: N/A

ALTERNATIVE DRUGS N/A

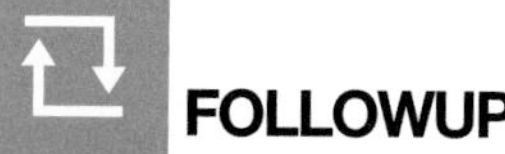

FOLLOWUP

PATIENT MONITORING As needed depending on type of therapy

PREVENTION/AVOIDANCE Better sexuality education may reduce problems

POSSIBLE COMPLICATIONS Psychological impact on some males - signs of severe inadequacy, self-doubt, additional anxiety and guilt

EXPECTED COURSE/PROGNOSIS
Often improves with therapy and counseling

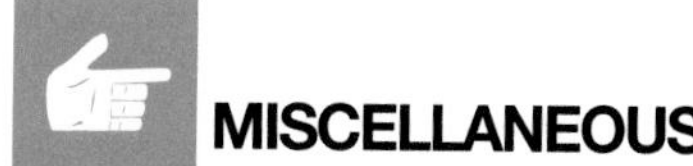

MISCELLANEOUS

ASSOCIATED CONDITIONS
- Neurological disorders, e.g., multiple sclerosis
- Prostatitis
- Psychological disorders
- Interpersonal disorders

AGE-RELATED FACTORS
Pediatric: N/A
Geriatric: Age alone does not cause ejaculation problems
Others: N/A

PREGNANCY N/A

SYNONYMS
- Premature ejaculation
- Retarded ejaculation
- Retrograde ejaculation
- Inhibited orgasm in males

ICD-9-CM
608.89 Other specified disorders of male genital organs, other
306.59 Physiological malfunction arising from mental factors, genitourinary, other
302.75 Psychosexual dysfunction with premature ejaculation

SEE ALSO

OTHER NOTES N/A

ABBREVIATIONS N/A

REFERENCES

- Hendry WF. Disorders of ejaculation: congenital, acquired and functional. Brit J Urol 1998;82(3):331-41
- Antidepressants and sexual dysfunction: a patient-centered approach. J Clin Psychiatry (Monograph Series) 1999;17(1)
- Vale J. Ejaculatory dysfunction. BJU Int 1999;83(5):557-563
- Yaffe M, Fenwick E. Sexual Happiness: A Practical Approach. New York, H. Holt & Co., 1988
- Stine CC, Collins M. Male sexual dysfunction. Prim Care 1989;16:1031
- Walsh PC, Gittes RF, Perlmutter AD, eds. Campbell's Urology. 6th Ed. Philadelphia, W.B. Saunders Co., 1992
- Segraves RT. Effects of psychotropic drugs on human erection and ejaculation. Arch Gen Psych 1989;46:275-284
- Kamischke A, Nieschlag E. Update in medical treatment of ejaculatory disorders. International Journal of Andrology.□vol 25(6), Dec 2002, pp. 333-344

Web references: 1 available at www.5mcc.com
Illustrations N/A

Author(s):
Bruce Block, MD

BASICS

DESCRIPTION Acute inflammation of the brain caused by viral invasion or by a viral-mediated inflammatory response in the brain following an acute, systemic infection. Meningeal, spinal cord, and peripheral nerve involvement may accompany encephalitis. Most cases of viral encephalitis are rare complications of common systemic viral infections. Post-viral encephalitis usually occurs via immune-mediated mechanisms and has onset 2-12 days after the primary viral infection.
System(s) affected: Nervous
Genetics: N/A
Incidence/Prevalence in USA: Uncommon; total of 117 cases reported to Centers for Disease Control and Prevention in 2000. Estimated 20,000 cases per year overall, most of which are mild. HSV encephalitis (most common) estimated incidence 1 in 250,000 per year. Seasonal variation:
- Arthropod-borne diseases (e.g., arboviruses) are predominantly spring and summer
- Enteroviruses peak in late summer, early fall (most common cause of viral meningitis in the U.S. and are responsible for up to 20% of viral encephalitis)
- Mumps and varicella prevalent in spring
- Most others (e.g., herpes simplex virus) are not seasonal

Predominant age: Age extremes at highest risk, especially for *Herpes simplex* encephalitis
Predominant sex: None

SIGNS & SYMPTOMS
- Nonspecific symptoms (malaise, skin rash, fever, myalgia) may precede neurologic symptoms
- Meningeal involvement is signified by stiff neck and headache
- Photophobia, lethargy progressing to coma, seizures, and focal neurologic deficits may be observed
- Progression is variable; may be rapid or follow a more indolent course
- Temporal lobe involvement by *Herpes simplex* leads to temporal lobe seizures, aphasia, and anosmia

CAUSES
- Endemic
  - ◊ *Herpes simplex* virus types 1 and 2
  - ◊ *Epstein-Barr* virus
  - ◊ *Varicella-zoster* virus
  - ◊ *Adenovirus*
  - ◊ Rabies
  - ◊ Dengue
  - ◊ Benign lymphocytic choriomeningitis V
  - ◊ Infectious mononucleosis
  - ◊ California encephalitis (CE) virus
  - ◊ St. Louis encephalitis (SLE) virus
  - ◊ Russian spring-summer encephalitis
  - ◊ Murray Valley
  - ◊ LaCrosse encephalitis
  - ◊ Powassan encephalitis
- Epidemic
  - ◊ Arboviruses (e.g., St. Louis encephalitis, Japanese encephalitis (JE), eastern equine encephalitis, western equine encephalitis, Venezuelan equine encephalitis, West Nile fever)
  - ◊ Enteroviruses (most commonly Coxsackie B viruses, but also includes poliovirus, echovirus)
  - ◊ *Nipah virus*
  - ◊ Mumps
  - ◊ Varicella-zoster
  - ◊ Influenza
  - ◊ HTLV III (HIV)

RISK FACTORS
- Many of the agents produce more severe disease in newborns and the elderly
- Travel to endemic areas; contact with animals
- Exposure to vectors (e.g., culicine mosquitoes)
- Poor hygiene (principal mode of transmission of enteroviruses is fecal-oral although respiratory transmission is important for some EVs)
- HIV positivity
- Immunosuppression

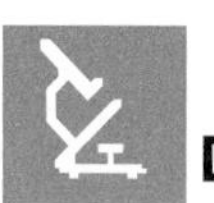

DIAGNOSIS

DIFFERENTIAL DIAGNOSIS
- Bacterial infection
  - ◊ Meningitis
  - ◊ Brain abscess
  - ◊ Tuberculosis
  - ◊ Cat-scratch disease
- Rickettsial infection
  - ◊ Rocky Mountain spotted fever
  - ◊ Ehrlichiosis
- Spirochetal infection
  - ◊ Syphilis
  - ◊ Lyme disease
  - ◊ Leptospirosis
  - ◊ Tick-borne relapsing fever
- Other infectious agents
  - ◊ Free-living amoeba (Naegleria, Acanthamoeba)
  - ◊ Toxoplasmosis
- Intracranial hemorrhage
- Intracranial tumor
- Trauma
- Thromboembolism
- Systemic lupus erythematosus
- Toxic ingestion
- Hypoglycemia

LABORATORY
- Standard laboratory studies (CBC, serum chemistries) are usually normal or nonspecifically abnormal
- Cerebrospinal fluid examination is essential
  - ◊ White cell count usually increased (10-2000 cells/mm3) but may be normal, especially in immunocompromised host; neutrophils predominate early, then see shift to mononuclear cells
  - ◊ Red cell count usually normal (more likely elevated in herpes simplex infections)
  - ◊ Protein may be normal or mildly elevated
  - ◊ Glucose may be normal or mildly decreased
  - ◊ ELISA detection of IgM helpful retrospectively to determine causative agent
  - ◊ Polymerase chain reaction (PCR) to amplify viral DNA is the diagnostic choice for HSV (particularly in neonatal HSV), CMV, human herpesvirus 6 (HHV-6), and enterovirus infections. However, local unavailability of this test limits its application.

Drugs that may alter lab results: Steroid therapy may mask CSF inflammatory findings

Disorders that may alter lab results: Immunocompromised patients may have normal CSF findings

PATHOLOGICAL FINDINGS
- Varies according to etiology
- Usually have prominent perivascular inflammation
- Swelling and degenerative changes of neural elements
- Negri bodies may be seen in brain, conjunctiva, and skin from the base of the neck in rabies patients

SPECIAL TESTS
- Electroencephalographic findings are usually abnormal, with slowing or epileptiform activity present. Temporal lobe abnormalities, particularly periodic lateralized epileptic form discharges (PLEDS), should suggest a diagnosis of HSV encephalitis.
- Most viral encephalitis cases have specific diagnosis made by measurement of acute and convalescent (2-3 weeks) serum antibody concentrations for the specific pathogen. A four-fold change in titer is suggestive of the diagnosis.
- CSF antibody index can be used to ascertain specific central nervous system production of antibody against the infecting agent: Serum and CSF IgG antibody and serum and CSF albumin concentrations are determined. Infection may be suggested by a higher specific antibody: albumin ratio in CSF than in serum.
- Antigen detection in CSF by polymerase chain reaction has been useful in cases of HSV and enteroviral disease, but is available only in some centers
- Enteroviruses may be recovered from CSF viral culture about 60% of cases, but most other viral agents are present in too low quantities to be detected by these techniques

IMAGING Imaging studies (CT scan, MRI, brain scan) may be normal early; later, nonspecific abnormalities are seen. Temporal lobe pathology suggests the diagnosis of HSV. MRI more sensitive than CT in viral encephalidities

DIAGNOSTIC PROCEDURES Brain biopsy, coupled with immunohistochemistry, may be useful in certain cases, particularly to identify treatable causes

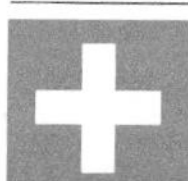

TREATMENT

APPROPRIATE HEALTH CARE Inpatient with symptomatic and supportive therapy as needed

GENERAL MEASURES
- Maintenance of adequately respiratory and circulatory support
- Control cerebral edema if necessary (hyperventilation, osmotic diuresis)
- Anticonvulsant as needed
- Monitor for SIADH
- Prevent bed sores

SURGICAL MEASURES N/A

ACTIVITY As indicated by clinical condition

DIET As indicated by clinical condition. May need fluid restriction for SIADH or cerebral edema.

PATIENT EDUCATION Advice to travelers to specific areas (e.g., Asia for Japanese encephalitis, Australia for many arthropod-borne infections). Vaccine availability.

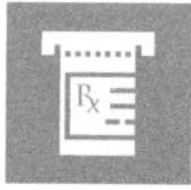

MEDICATIONS

DRUG(S) OF CHOICE
- Acyclovir 10 mg/kg IV q8h for 2-3 weeks for HSV infections. Resistance may be seen in immunocompromised patients.
- Foscarnet (Foscavir) is an effective option in patients with acyclovir resistant HSV
- Immunocompromised patients with VZV should be treated the same as for HSV infection.
- No specific antiviral therapy for other etiologies

Contraindications: None
Precautions:
- Not approved for pregnant women, but benefits probably outweigh risks to fetus
- Adjust dose of acyclovir in patients with renal insufficiency

Significant possible interactions:
- Acyclovir and famciclovir must be phosphorylated by viral enzymes before they are active. Patients previously treated with these antiviral drugs may have mutant virus lacking viral thymidine kinase activity and hence are resistant to these antivirals. These mutant virus are significant is producing cutaneous infection, but probably don't cause encephalitis.

ALTERNATIVE DRUGS
- Vidarabine (adenine arabinoside) for acyclovir-resistant HSV; has been used in combination with acyclovir
- Pleconaril (Picovir), an orally active inhibitor of enteroviruses (EV) and rhinoviruses, has been administered to patients with life threatening EV CNS infections on a compassionate use basis; preliminary results are encouraging.

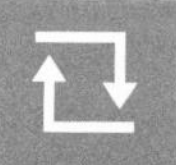

FOLLOWUP

PATIENT MONITORING Intracranial pressure monitoring may be needed for severe cases

PREVENTION/AVOIDANCE
- Use of appropriate insect repellants, protective clothing, avoidance and removal of ticks
- Vaccines:
  - ◊ Japanese encephalitis (3 doses of 1 mL each administered SC on days 0, 7, and 30; vaccinees should be observed for 30 minutes after vaccination and should remain in areas with ready access to medical care for the next 10 days)
  - ◊ Eastern equine - vaccine only available for horses

POSSIBLE COMPLICATIONS
- Varies with etiologic agent
- HSV encephalitis has highest morbidity and mortality of the common viral encephalitides (untreated mortality 70%; < 5% of survivors have normal neurologic function)

EXPECTED COURSE/PROGNOSIS
- Prognosis generally difficult to predict; somewhat based on infecting agent (e.g., HSV-2 severe, varicella mild)
- With disseminated neonatal HSV, antiviral therapy, initiated early reduces mortality rate to 60% (85% without therapy), but subsequent neurologic impairment is approximately 40%.
- With CNS neonatal HSV disease only, mortality is approximately 15% (50% without therapy). Unfortunately, antiviral therapy has had no impact on the morbidity of survivors; 65% have neurologic impairment

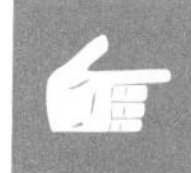

MISCELLANEOUS

ASSOCIATED CONDITIONS N/A

AGE-RELATED FACTORS
Pediatric:
- Children more commonly symptomatic from arboviral infection than are adults
- Neonatal - newborns at higher risk for severe HSV and enteroviral CNS disease

Geriatric: May also be at risk for severe disease
Others: N/A

PREGNANCY Risk of HSV infection in an infant delivered vaginally to a mother with a primary genital infection is approximately 40%; drops to 3-5% in reactivation genital lesions. Enteroviruses may be transmitted transplacentally to fetus; cause of neonatal disease if mother infected just prior to delivery.

SYNONYMS
- Meningoencephalitis

ICD-9-CM
047.9 Unspecified viral meningitis
049.9 Unspecified non-arthropod-borne viral diseases of central nervous system

SEE ALSO
Adenovirus infections
Ehrlichiosis
Encephalitis, Saint Louis
Epstein-Barr virus infections
Herpes simplex
Herpes zoster
HIV infection & AIDS
Meningitis, viral
Rabies
West Nile fever

OTHER NOTES N/A

ABBREVIATIONS
EV = enterovirus
HSV = herpes simplex virus
SIADH = syndrome of inappropriate antidiuretic hormone secretion
VZV = varicella-zoster virus

REFERENCES

- Whitley RJ. Viral encephalitis. New Engl J Med 1990;323:242
- Whitley RJ. Viral encephalitis. Pediatr Rev. 1999 Jun 20(6):192-8
- Griffin DE, Johnson RT. Encephalitis, myelitis, and neuritis. In: Mandell GL, et al, eds. Principles and Practice of Infectious Diseases. 4th Ed. New York, Churchill Livingstone, 1995
- Read SJ. Laboratory diagnosis of common viral infections of the central nervous system by using a single multiplex PCR screening assay. J Clin Microbiol 1999 May;37(5):1352-5
- Hinson VK, Tyou WR. Update on viral encephalitis. Curr Opin Neurol 2001 Jun 14(3):369-374
- Redington J, Tyler KL. Viral infections of the nervous system. Arch Neurol 2002 May 59(5):712
- Romero JR, Newland JG. Viral meningitis and encephalitis: Traditional and emerging viral agents. Sem Ped Inf Dis 2003 14(3):72-82

Web references: 1 available at www.5mcc.com
Illustrations N/A

Author(s):
Mary Cataletto, MD

BASICS

DESCRIPTION The regular passage of fecal material into clothes or other inappropriate places by a child older than four years of age
System(s) affected: Gastrointestinal
Genetics: None known
Incidence/Prevalence in USA: 1.3% of all children > 4 years of age
Predominant age: 70% have onset before 5 years of age
Predominant sex: Males > Females 1.5:1.

SIGNS & SYMPTOMS
- Constipation (retentive encopresis) usually accompanies encopresis (there is a subgroup of children who do not have constipation - nonretentive 20%)
- Unrecognized constipation and/or stool retention often precedes the symptom presented to the care provider
- Large amount of fecal material on abdominal, pelvic or rectal exam
- Pasty stool found on underclothes
- Fecal or foul odor surrounds the child
- Often intermittent periumbilical pain
- Occasional passage of a voluminous stool
- History of painful bowel movements
- Some children seem shy and withdrawn
- Some children may act out or display aggressive behavior
- Some have had recurrent urinary tract infections

CAUSES
- Psychologic
  - ◊ Difficulty with toilet training
  - ◊ Resistance to using toilet facilities, such as school bathrooms or outdoor toilets during camping trips
  - ◊ Association with sexual abuse in boys
- Anatomic
  - ◊ Anal fissure
  - ◊ Painful defecation of any kind
  - ◊ Muscle hypotonia
  - ◊ Slow intestinal motility
  - ◊ Aganglionic megacolon or Hirschsprung disease
  - ◊ Spinal cord defects
  - ◊ Anal stenosis
  - ◊ Anterior displacement of the anus: anogenital index - the distance from the posterior aspect of the vagina or scrotum to the anus divided by the full distance to the tip of the coccyx) > 0.34 females/> 0.45 males
  - ◊ Post surgical stricture of anus or rectum
  - ◊ Pelvic mass
  - ◊ Neurofibromatosis
- Dietary or metabolic
  - ◊ Lack of fiber
  - ◊ Excessive protein or milk intake
  - ◊ Inadequate water intake
  - ◊ Hypothyroidism

RISK FACTORS
- Boys are more often affected
- Difficulty with bowel training
- Unresolved fecal retention and impaction

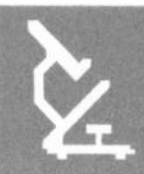

DIAGNOSIS

DIFFERENTIAL DIAGNOSIS
- Not difficult when brought to provider's attention
- Suspect when exam detects soiling of underclothes
- Must look for underlying treatable causes of constipation

LABORATORY
- Urinalysis and urine culture may be indicated
- Thyroid function studies

Drugs that may alter lab results: N/A

Disorders that may alter lab results: N/A

PATHOLOGICAL FINDINGS N/A

SPECIAL TESTS N/A

IMAGING Abdominal plain films are occasionally necessary if an impaction is suspected but not detected by abdominal or rectal examination

DIAGNOSTIC PROCEDURES
- Detailed history and complete physical exam
  - ◊ Neurological examination of lower extremities
  - ◊ Genital area
  - ◊ Digital rectal
  - ◊ Abdominal radiograph
- History of constipation prior to one month of age is almost always present with aganglionic megacolon and that history would warrant a barium enema and/or rectal biopsy

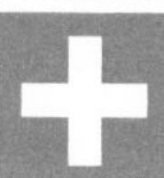

TREATMENT

APPROPRIATE HEALTH CARE Hospital admission and abdominal x-ray may be necessary to insure complete removal of impaction

GENERAL MEASURES
- Anticipatory guidance relative to toilet training beginning at 18 months
- The impaction must be eliminated before starting maintenance treatment
- Avoid redevelopment of an impaction
- Avoid frequent and repeated digital examinations, enemas, and suppositories
- Biofeedback training has be used in conjunction with standard treatment, but results are disappointing
- Child to sit on toilet twice a day at the same time each day for 10-15 minutes and 10-15 minutes after meals

SURGICAL MEASURES N/A

ACTIVITY Unrestricted

DIET
- Avoid excessive milk, bananas, apples, gelatin
- Increased fiber

PATIENT EDUCATION
- Education and demystifying the process
- Careful and full explanation of the treatment plan
- Allay the guilt and avoid punishment for soiling

MEDICATIONS

DRUG(S) OF CHOICE
- Remove stool impaction: (before starting maintenance treatment program)
- Give 1 ounce of mineral oil the first day
- On the next day, give 1-3 enemas till clear; this may need to be repeated on 1-2 subsequent days
  - ◊ First give an oil retention enema
  - ◊ Follow the oil retention enema with hypophosphate enemas, e.g., sodium phosphate (Fleet's) 1 ounce (28.4 gm) per 20 pounds (9.1 kg) of body weight, or
  - ◊ Normal saline enemas - 2 tsp table salt per quart (946 mL) of warm water and give 2 ounces (60 mL) per year of age to a maximum of 16 ounces (480 mL)
  - ◊ A bisacodyl (Dulcolax) suppository can be inserted to assist the evacuation
- Alternative: give an oral solution of polyethylene glycol (Colyte, Nulytely) at 20 mL/kg/hr for 4 hours on 2 consecutive days
- Maintenance treatment
  - ◊ Up to 6 months or more to keep stool soft and mobile
  - ◊ Give mineral oil (may mix with orange juice to make palatable)
  - ◊ Fiber or other hydrophilic agents may be used to soften the stool - lactulose, methylcellulose, psyllium, polycarbophil, malt soup extract
  - ◊ Multivitamins must be given between doses of mineral oil to ensure absorption of fat soluble vitamins (A, D, E, K)

Contraindications: Refer to manufacturer's profile of each drug
Precautions: Avoid bedtime doses of mineral oil to decrease risk of aspiration
Significant possible interactions: Refer to manufacturer's profile of each drug

ALTERNATIVE DRUGS N/A

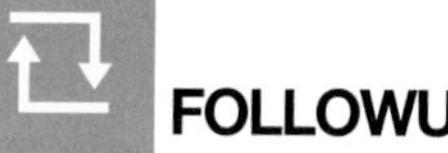

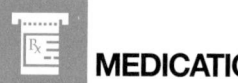

FOLLOWUP

PATIENT MONITORING
- Continue the maintenance treatment program for at least 6 months and maybe for as long as 1-2 years
- Visits every 4-10 weeks for support and to ensure compliance
- Telephone availability to prevent problems and adjust doses
- Redevelopment of impaction must be removed as above
- Counseling and/or referral for associated psychosocial issues

PREVENTION/AVOIDANCE
- Optimal feeding practices
- Normal bowel function and recommendations for bowel training
- Early detection of problems
- Avoid Karo syrup
- Prompt treatment of perianal dermatitis to avoid painful defecation
- Look for signs of relapse which include large caliber stools, decrease in frequency of defecation, soiling

POSSIBLE COMPLICATIONS
- Excessive enemas or suppositories may cause colitis
- Perianal dermatitis
- Anal fissure

EXPECTED COURSE/PROGNOSIS
- Usually responds well though relapses may occur
- Children with psychosocial or emotional problems which preceded the encopresis are more recalcitrant to treatment

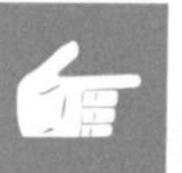

MISCELLANEOUS

ASSOCIATED CONDITIONS
- Perianal dermatitis
- Urinary tract infections
- Sexual abuse in boys

AGE-RELATED FACTORS
Pediatric: N/A
Geriatric: N/A
Others: N/A

PREGNANCY N/A

SYNONYMS
Soiling

ICD-9-CM
787.6 Incontinence of feces

SEE ALSO

OTHER NOTES N/A

ABBREVIATIONS N/A

REFERENCES

- Hatch TF. Encopresis and constipation in children. Pediatric Clinics of N Am 1988;35(2):257-78
- Kuhn BR, Marcus BA, Pitner SL. Treatment guidelines for primary nonretentive encopresis and stool toileting refusal. Amer Fam Physician 1999;59(8):2172-8

Web references: 0 available at www.5mcc.com
Illustrations N/A

Author(s):
James F. Broomfield, MD

BASICS

DESCRIPTION A disease resulting from infection primarily of the valvular endocardium and occasionally the mural endocardium
System(s) affected: Cardiovascular, Endocrine/Metabolic, Hemic/Lymphatic/Immunologic, Pulmonary, Renal/Urologic, Skin/Exocrine
Genetics: Unknown
Incidence/Prevalence in USA: 1.7-4.2/100,000; 0.32-1.3/1000 hospital admissions
Predominant age: All ages
Predominant sex: Male > Female (slightly)

SIGNS & SYMPTOMS
- Fever, may be high, low or absent. May be only symptom in prosthetic valve endocarditis.
- Night sweats, chilly sensation
- Malaise, myalgia, joint pain
- Back pain, may be severe
- Anorexia, weight loss
- Delirium, headache
- Paralysis, hemiparesis, aphasia
- Numbness, muscle weakness
- Cold extremity with pain
- Bloody urine, may be gross or microscopic
- Bloody sputum, from septic pulmonary emboli
- Petechiae
- Conjunctival hemorrhage
- Hemorrhagic or necrotic pustule
- Pain of finger tip, or toe tip (subjective symptom of Osler node)
- Chest pain, shortness of breath, cough
- Roth spot
- Osler node
- Janeway lesion
- Heart murmur, may be absent
- Pericardial rub
- Pleural friction rub
- Splenomegaly

CAUSES
- Acute endocarditis (often an aggrressive course and may not be associated with an underlying valve lesion)
  - ◊ *Staphylococcus aureus*
  - ◊ Streptococcus groups A, B, C, G
  - ◊ *Haemophilus influenzae* or *parainfluenzae*
  - ◊ *Streptococcus pneumoniae*
  - ◊ *Staphylococcus lugdunensis*
  - ◊ Enterococcus spp (*E. faecalis*, *E. faecium*, *E. durans*)
  - ◊ *Neisseria gonorrhoeae*
- Subacute endocarditis (indolent course, often is setting of structural valve disease)
  - ◊ *Alpha-hemolytic streptococci*
  - ◊ *Streptococcus bovis*
  - ◊ Enterococcus spp
  - ◊ *Haemophilus aphrophilus* or *paraphrophilus*
  - ◊ *Actinobacillus actinomycetemcomitans*
  - ◊ *Cardiobacterium hominis*
  - ◊ *Eikenella corrodens*
  - ◊ *Kingella kingae*
  - ◊ *Staphylococcus aureus*
- Endocarditis in intravenous drug-abusers (often involves the tricuspid valve)
  - ◊ *Staphylococcus aureus*
  - ◊ *Pseudomonas aeruginosa*
  - ◊ *Burkholderia cepacia*
  - ◊ Other gram-negative bacilli
  - ◊ Enterococcus spp
  - ◊ Candida spp
- Early prosthetic valve endocarditis (<60 days after valve implantation)
  - ◊ *Staphylococcus aureus*
  - ◊ *Staphylococcus epidermidis*
  - ◊ Gram-negative bacilli
  - ◊ Candida spp
  - ◊ Aspergillus spp
- Late prosthetic valve endocarditis (>60 days after valve implantation)
  - ◊ *Alpha-hemolytic streptococci*
  - ◊ Enterococcus spp
  - ◊ *Staphylococcus epidermidis*
  - ◊ Candida spp
  - ◊ Aspergillus spp
- Culture-negative endocarditis (5-10%)
  - ◊ Patients on antibiotics
  - ◊ *Bartonella quintana* (homeless people)
  - ◊ *Bartonella henselae* (cat owners)
  - ◊ Fastidious organism: Brucella spp, fungi, *Coxiella burnetii* (Q fever), *Chlamydia trachomatis*, *Chlamydia psittaci*, HACEK organisms (*Haemophilus species, Actinobacillus actinomycetemcomitans, Cardiobacterium hominis, Eikenella corrodens*, Kingella spp)

RISK FACTORS
- Underlying conditions
  - ◊ Prosthetic cardiac valves, including bioprosthetic and homograft valves
  - ◊ Previous bacterial endocarditis, even in the absence of heart disease
  - ◊ Most congenital cardiac malformations
  - ◊ Rheumatic and other acquired valvular dysfunction, even after valvular surgery
  - ◊ Hypertrophic cardiomyopathy
  - ◊ Mitral valve prolapse with valvular regurgitation
  - ◊ Indwelling intravascular devices
- Associated with transient bacteremia
  - ◊ Gingival irritation, including professional cleaning
  - ◊ Tonsillectomy and/or adenoidectomy
  - ◊ Procedures on intestinal or respiratory mucosa
  - ◊ Rigid bronchoscopy
  - ◊ Sclerotherapy of esophageal varices
  - ◊ Esophageal dilatation
  - ◊ Gallbladder surgery
  - ◊ Cystoscopy
  - ◊ Urethral dilatation
  - ◊ Urethral catheterization in the presence of infection
  - ◊ Urinary tract surgery in the presence of infection
  - ◊ Prostatic surgery
  - ◊ Incision and drainage of infected tissue
  - ◊ Vaginal hysterectomy
  - ◊ Vaginal delivery in the presence of infection

DIAGNOSIS

DIFFERENTIAL DIAGNOSIS
- Connective tissue diseases
- Fever of unknown origin
- Intra-abdominal infections
- Rheumatic fever
- Salmonellosis
- Tuberculosis

LABORATORY
- Positive blood cultures taken at different times
- 2-dimensional echocardiography, not always positive for vegetations (transesophageal echocardiography has high sensitivity)
- Leukocytosis in acute endocarditis
- Anemia in subacute endocarditis
- Elevated ESR
- Decreased C3, C4, CH50 in subacute endocarditis
- Hematuria, microscopic or macroscopic
- Rheumatoid factor in subacute endocarditis
- Serologies for Chlamydia, Q fever (Coxiella) and Bartonella may be useful in "culture-negative" endocarditis

Drugs that may alter lab results: Antibiotics may make blood cultures falsely negative

Disorders that may alter lab results: N/A

PATHOLOGICAL FINDINGS
- Vegetations are composed of platelets, fibrin and colonies of micro-organisms. Destruction of valvular endocardium, perforation of valve leaflets, rupture of chordae tendineae, abscesses of myocardium, rupture of sinus of Valsalva, pericarditis may occur.
- Emboli, infarction, abscesses and/or infarction may be found in any organ.
- Immune-complex glomerulonephritis possible

SPECIAL TESTS N/A

IMAGING
- Pulmonary ventilation perfusion scan may be useful in right-sided endocarditis
- CT scan may be useful in locating abscesses

DIAGNOSTIC PROCEDURES
- Transesophageal echocardiography
- Cardiac catheterization may be indicated to ascertain the degree of valvular damage
- Aortic root injection may be useful when aortic root abscess or rupture of sinus of Valsalva is suspected

Duke criteria for diagnosis of infective endocarditis (2 major criteria, OR 1 major and 3 minor criteria, OR 5 minor criteria)
- Major criteria
  - ◊ Positive blood culture
    - Typical microorganism for infective endocarditis from 2 separate blood cultures, or
    - Persistently positive blood culture. Defined as recovery of a microorganism consistent with infective endocarditis from: blood cultures drawn more than 12 hours apart, or all of 3 or a majority of 4 or more separate blood cultures, with first and last drawn at least 1 hour apart
  - ◊ Positive echocardiogram: (a) oscillating intracardiac mass, on valve or supporting structures, or in the path of regurgitant jets, or on implanted material, in the absence of an alternative anatomic explanation, or (b) abscess, or (c) new partial dehiscence of prosthetic valve
  - ◊ New valvular regurgitation (increase or change in pre-existing murmur not sufficient)
- Minor criteria
  - ◊ Predisposing heart condition or IV drug use
  - ◊ Fever ≥ 38.0°C (100.4°F)
  - ◊ Vascular phenomena: major arterial emboli, septic pulmonary infarcts, mycotic aneurysm, intracranial hemorrhage, conjunctival hemorrhage, Janeway lesions
  - ◊ Immunologic phenomena: glomerulonephritis, Osler's nodes, Roth spots, rheumatoid factor
  - ◊ Microbiologic evidence: positive blood culture, but not meeting major criterion (excluding single positive cultures for coagulase-negative staphylococci and organisms that do not cause endocarditis) or serologic evidence of active infection with organism consistent with infective endocarditis
  - ◊ Echocardiogram: consistent with infective endocarditis but not meeting major criterion

TREATMENT

APPROPRIATE HEALTH CARE
- Initial hospitalized care
- Intensive care for critically ill patients
- Outpatient home IV antibiotic therapy in selected stable and reliable patients

GENERAL MEASURES
- Treat CHF if it occurs
- Oxygen treatment as needed
- Consider hemodialysis

SURGICAL MEASURES
- Valve replacement may be performed before antibiotic treatment course is completed when any of the following are present:
  - ◊ CHF due to valve incompetence
  - ◊ Multiple major systemic emboli
  - ◊ Infection is caused by resistant organisms, e.g., fungus, Pseudomonas aeruginosa
  - ◊ Dehiscence of infected prosthetic valve
  - ◊ Relapse of prosthetic valve endocarditis
  - ◊ Persistent bacteremia despite antibiotics

ACTIVITY
- Bedrest is indicated initially
- Ambulation when clinically improved

DIET No special diet

PATIENT EDUCATION
- Importance of dental hygiene
- Antibiotic prophylaxis when undergoing certain dental/surgical procedures
- Give patient an AHA wallet card listing antibiotic regimens for prophylaxis. Obtain the AHA wallet card, 78-1005 (CP), from local chapters of American Heart Association.

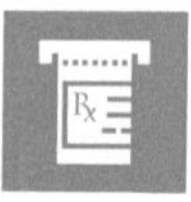

MEDICATIONS

DRUG(S) OF CHOICE
- Penicillin-susceptible streptococci: Penicillin 2-4 million UIV q4h, plus gentamicin for 2 weeks (6 weeks for prosthetic valve endocarditis). In patients with native valve endocarditis: patient > 65 years of age, those with impairment of the eighth nerve or of renal function, or those with central nervous system involvement, use penicillin only, in the same dosage alone for 4 weeks.
- Enterococci: Penicillin 5-10 million U q4h, plus gentamicin or streptomycin for 4-6 weeks (6 weeks for prosthetic valve endocarditis). Test the enterococcal strain in vitro for high-level resistance to gentamicin and streptomycin (minimal inhibitory concentration [MIC] > 2000 μg/mL). Use streptomycin, 1 gm IM q24h, instead of gentamicin if there is high-level resistance to gentamicin and not to streptomycin.
- Staphylococcus of native valve: Oxacillin or nafcillin 2 g IV q4h for 6 weeks. For the first 3-5 days, add gentamicin.
- Staphylococcus of prosthetic valve: Vancomycin 15 mg/kg (usual dose 1 g) IV infused over 1 h q12h, plus rifampin 300 mg po q8h, both for 6 weeks, plus gentamicin for the first 2 weeks
- HACEK organisms: ceftriaxone 2 gm IM or IV q24h for 4 weeks

Contraindications: For patients who are allergic to penicillin, use alternative drugs

Precautions:
- In patients with renal impairment, dosage adjustment should be made for penicillin G, gentamicin, cefazolin, vancomycin
- Rapid infusion of vancomycin (less than one hour) may cause "red-neck syndrome". This is due to histamine release and not an allergic reaction. It will disappear when the rate of infusion is reduced.

Significant possible interactions:
- Vancomycin plus gentamicin increases renal toxicity
- Rifampin increases the requirement for coumarin and oral hypoglycemic agents

ALTERNATIVE DRUGS
- For patients allergic to penicillin
  - ◊ Penicillin-susceptible streptococci: ceftriaxone 2 g IM or IV qday for 4 weeks or ceftriaxone 2 g IV plus gentamicin 3 mg/kg qday for 2 weeks (not to be used in patients with immediate type hypersensitivity to penicillin), or vancomycin 15 mg/kg (usual dose 1 g) IV over 1 hr q12h for 4 weeks (6 weeks for prosthetic valve endocarditis)
  - ◊ Enterococci: Desensitization to penicillin should be considered. Vancomycin 15 mg/kg (usual dose 1 g) IV infused over 1 hr q12h, plus gentamicin (see Other Notes) for 4-6 weeks (6 weeks for prosthetic valve endocarditis).
  - ◊ Staphlococcus of native valve: Cefazolin 2 gm IV q8h (not to be used in patients with immediate-type hypersensitivity to penicillin), or vancomycin 15 mg/kg (usual dose 1 g) IV infused over 1 hr q12h, for 6 weeks

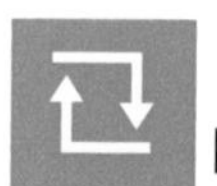

FOLLOWUP

PATIENT MONITORING
- Check gentamicin peak (approx 3 μg/mL) and trough (<1 μg/mL) levels if used for more than 5 days, and in patients with renal dysfunction.
- Check vancomycin peak (30-45 μg/mL) and trough (<10 μg/mL) levels in patients with renal dysfunction.
- Perform twice weekly BUN and serum creatinine while the patient is receiving gentamicin
- Consider audiometry baseline and follow-up during long-term aminoglycoside therapy

PREVENTION/AVOIDANCE
- Treat dental caries while the patient is being treated for endocarditis
- Maintain good oral hygiene
- Give antibiotic prophylaxis to patients undergoing procedures that may cause transient bacteremia
- Antibiotic regimen for dental/oral/upper respiratory tract procedures: (may be used in patients with prosthetic valves)
  - ◊ Amoxicillin 2 g po (or for penicillin allergic patients, clindamycin 600 mg po) 1 hr before procedure
  - ◊ Alternative: Ampicillin 2.0 g IV (or IM) (or for penicillin allergic patients clindamycin 600 mg IV) 30 minutes before procedure
- Antibiotic regimen for GU/GI procedures
  - ◊ Ampicillin 2 g IV (or IM) plus gentamicin 1.5 mg/kg IV (or IM) (not to exceed 120 mg) 30 minutes before procedure
  - ◊ For patients allergic to penicillin: vancomycin 1.0 g IV infused over 1 hr plus gentamicin 1.5 mg/kg IV (or IM) (not to exceed 120 mg); complete infusion 30 minutes before procedure
- Alternate oral regimen for moderate-risk patients undergoing GU/GI procedures
  - ◊ Amoxicillin 2.0 g po 1 hr before or ampicillin 2 g IV (or IM) 30 minutes before procedure
  - ◊ For patients who are allergic to penicillin: vancomycin 1.0 g IV infused over 1 hr; complete infusion 30 minutes before procedure

POSSIBLE COMPLICATIONS
- Arterial emboli and infarcts (e.g., MI, mesenteric, splenic, cerebral infarct)
- Infectious emboli (e.g., abscesses of heart, lung, brain, meninges, bone, pericardium)
- Inflammatory/immune disorders (e.g., arthritis, myositis, glomerulonephritis)
- Miscellanous complications (e.g., congestive heart failure, ruptured valve cusp, sinus of Valsalva aneurysm, cardiac arrhythmia, ruptured mycotic aneurysm)

EXPECTED COURSE/PROGNOSIS
- Staphylococcal endocarditis, fever and positive blood cultures may persist up to 10 days after appropriate treatment started
- Streptococcal endocarditis, clinical response expected within 48 hours of antibiotic treatment and blood cultures negative soon after antibiotics
- Prognosis depends largely on complications

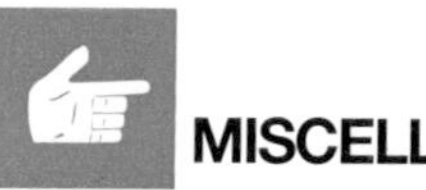

MISCELLANEOUS

ASSOCIATED CONDITIONS
- Substance abuse
- Central vascular access

AGE-RELATED FACTORS
Pediatric: N/A
Geriatric: Prognosis is worse in elderly
Others: N/A

PREGNANCY Use gentamicin with caution

SYNONYMS
- Bacterial endocarditis
- Subacute bacterial endocarditis
- Acute bacterial endocarditis

ICD-9-CM
421.0 Acute and subacute bacterial endocarditis
421.9 Acute endocarditis, unspecified
996.61 Infection and inflammatory reaction due to cardiac device, implant, and graft

SEE ALSO
Bartonella infections
Brucellosis

OTHER NOTES N/A

ABBREVIATIONS
IE = Infective endocarditis
ABE = Acute bacterial endocarditis
SBE = Subacute bacterial endocarditis

REFERENCES

- Watanakunakorn C, Burkert T: Infective endocarditis at a large community teaching hospital, 1980-1990. A review of 210 episodes. Medicine 1993;72:90-102

Web references: 0 available at www.5mcc.com
Illustrations 2 available

Author(s):
Mark R. Dambro, MD

BASICS

DESCRIPTION Heterotopic islands of uterine mucosa (endometrium) found in many locations.
- Pelvic sites - peritoneal surfaces (bladder, cul-de-sac, pelvic side walls, broad ligaments, uterosacral ligaments, fallopian tubes, and uterus), lymph nodes, ovaries, bowel
- Distant sites - vagina, cervix, abdominal wall, arm, leg, pleura, lung, diaphragm, kidneys, spleen, gallbladder, nasal mucous membranes, spinal canal, stomach, breast

System(s) affected: Reproductive
Genetics: N/A
Incidence/Prevalence in USA: May be as high as 25% in women of reproductive age
Predominant age: Women of reproductive age and possibly in menopausal women with signs and symptoms aggravated by hormone replacement therapy
Predominant sex: Female only

SIGNS & SYMPTOMS
- Infertility (30-40% of patients with endometriosis)
- Dyspareunia
- Dysmenorrhea
- Dyschezia
- Chronic pelvic pain
- Premenstrual spotting
- Spontaneous abortion (theoretical)
- Luteinized unruptured follicle syndrome

CAUSES
- Retrograde menstruation (Sampson's theory)
- Lymphatic/vascular metastases (Halban's theory)
- Direct implantation
- Coelomic metaplasia (coelomic epithelium undergoes metaplasia forming functioning endometrium)

RISK FACTORS
- Hereditary/genetic predisposition
- Delayed childbearing
- Luteinized unruptured follicle syndrome (granulosa/theca cells undergo luteinization but actual follicular rupture fails to occur, thereby predisposing to limited progesterone secretion into peritoneal cavity thus allowing refluxed endometrial cells to implant and proliferate)

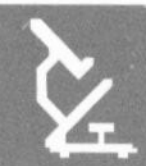

DIAGNOSIS

DIFFERENTIAL DIAGNOSIS Differential diagnosis of pelvic pain include all causes of acute abdomen including complications of intrauterine and extrauterine pregnancy, urinary tract infection, irritable bowel syndrome, ulcerative colitis, Crohn disease, pelvic adhesions, acute salpingitis, ruptured ovarian cyst, intussusception, malignancies, and other conditions

LABORATORY No special value, but CA-125 levels may be elevated

Drugs that may alter lab results: N/A

Disorders that may alter lab results: N/A

PATHOLOGICAL FINDINGS Biopsy of endometriotic lesions usually demonstrate both endometrial glands and stroma

SPECIAL TESTS CA-125

IMAGING
- Vaginal/abdominal ultrasound (identify only endometriomas of ovaries)
- MRI for pelvic masses (endometriomas)
- Hysterosalpingography for tubal occlusion proximally or distally and periadnexal adhesions

DIAGNOSTIC PROCEDURES Laparoscopy

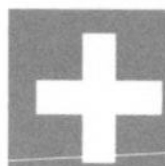

TREATMENT

APPROPRIATE HEALTH CARE Diagnose and treat "early" to prevent sequelae such as infertility and pelvic pain

GENERAL MEASURES N/A

SURGICAL MEASURES
- At the time of laparoscopy, attempt laser vaporization or fulguration of implants, drainage/resection of ovarian endometriomas, and lysis of pelvic adhesions
- Consider uterosacral ligament laser vaporization/fulguration for presacral neurectomy for severe pelvic pain or dysmenorrhea. Microsurgery or in-vitro fertilization (IVF) or gamete intrafallopian tube transfer (GIFT) may be necessary when laparoscopic surgery followed by superovulation induction with human menopausal gonadotropins, pure follicle-stimulating hormone and artificial intrauterine insemination have failed to achieve pregnancy.

ACTIVITY Activity may be limited depending upon severity of pelvic pain

DIET No special diet

PATIENT EDUCATION
- Prevention of disease difficult but may be maintained in quiescent state with oral contraceptive agents
- Printed materials available from The American Fertility Society, 2140 11th Ave South, Suite 200, Birmingham, AL 35205-2800, (205)933-8494

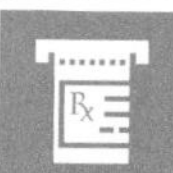

MEDICATIONS

DRUG(S) OF CHOICE

- Gonadotropin-releasing hormone (GnRH) agonists such as
  - ◊ Nafarelin (Synarel) intranasal 400 μg/day divided as 2 inhalations/day, one in each nostril. If patient continues with menses after 2 months of treatment, dose may be increased to 800 μg
  - ◊ Leuprolide acetate (Lupron, Lupron Depot) 0.5-1.0 mg/day or 3.75-7.5 mg/month, respectively
  - ◊ Goserelin (Zoladex) implant 3.6 mg subcutaneously every 4 weeks for 6 months
- Maintenance:
  - ◊ 6-9 months of therapy followed by "active" attempts at pregnancy or maintenance therapy with oral contraceptive agents
  - ◊ Calcium supplementation 1000-1500 mg/day is recommended when using GnRH analog therapy to prevent calcium loss as women become severely hypoestrogenic

Contraindications: Any contraindication to the drug itself or of hypoestrogenemia

Precautions:

- Calcium loss secondary to hypoestrogenemia
- Hot flashes secondary to hypoestrogenemia
- Paresthesias of face and upper extremities
- Contraception measures should be used by sexually active women since ovulation may not be suppressed even if menses cease

Significant possible interactions: Refer to manufacturer's literature

ALTERNATIVE DRUGS

- Danazol (Danocrine) 400-800 mg/day for 6-9 months
- Medroxyprogesterone (Provera) 30 mg/day for 6-9 months
- Megestrol (Megace) 40 mg/day for 6-9 months
- "Continuous" oral contraceptives, e.g., ethinyl estradiol-norgestrel (Lo/Ovral, Ovral) until childbearing is desired

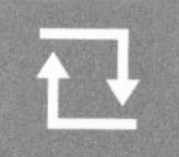

FOLLOWUP

PATIENT MONITORING

- Monitor serum estradiol levels until less than 10 pg/mL (37 pmol/L) when using GnRH analogs
- Monitor patient's pain response with history and physical exams every 8-12 weeks
- Monitor size of ovarian endometriomas with ultrasound every 8-12 weeks
- May need additional surgery depending upon patient's fertility and/or pelvic pain

PREVENTION/AVOIDANCE

- Pregnancy seems to have a temporary ameliorating effect upon the course of the disease
- Endometriosis is generally a recurring disorder that may persist even into early menopause

POSSIBLE COMPLICATIONS

- Infertility/subfertility
- Sterility
- Chronic pelvic pain
- Total abdominal hysterectomy and bilateral salpingo-oophorectomy
- Intussusception

EXPECTED COURSE/PROGNOSIS

- Pregnancy should occur, but depends upon the severity of the disease
- Signs and symptoms generally regress with the onset of the menopause, but can usually be controlled during the reproductive years

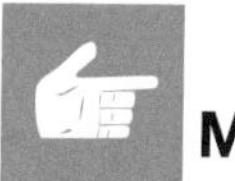

MISCELLANEOUS

ASSOCIATED CONDITIONS

- Pelvic endometriosis is rarely associated with endometrioid carcinoma of the ovary
- Hematuria with bladder involvement
- Rectal bleeding with bowel involvement
- Hemoptysis with lung involvement

AGE-RELATED FACTORS

Pediatric: N/A

Geriatric: Endometriosis may persist even during early menopause and may be exacerbated with estrogen replacement therapy

Others:

- Endometriosis of the intramural portion of the fallopian tube may cause isthmic proximal tubal obstruction and infertility
- Infertility may not only be related to anatomical disruption of pelvic structures but to liberation of peritoneal macrophages which can predispose to gamete phagocytosis
- Immune disorders such as production of anti-endometrial antibodies can also be associated with reproductive dysfunction

PREGNANCY Refer to board certified reproductive endocrinologist or gynecologist with expertise in infertility

SYNONYMS Endometriosis externa

ICD-9-CM

617.0 Endometriosis of uterus
617.3 Endometriosis of pelvic peritoneum

SEE ALSO

Appendicitis, acute
Ectopic pregnancy

OTHER NOTES Educate female patients of reproductive age as to the signs and symptoms of pelvic endometriosis, especially teenagers complaining of dysmenorrhea and/or dyspareunia

ABBREVIATIONS N/A

REFERENCES

- Speroff L, Glass RH, Kase NG: Endometriosis and Infertility. In: Brown CL, ed. Clinical Gynecologic Endocrinology and Infertility. 5th Ed. Baltimore, Williams & Wilkins, 1994
- Berger DL, Mohammadkhani MS. Weekly Clinicopathological Exercises: Case 13-2000: A 26-Year-Old Women with Bouts of Abdominal Pain, Vomiting, and Diarrhea. NEJM 4/27/2000;Vol 342

Web references: 0 available at www.5mcc.com

Illustrations N/A

Author(s):
Nicholas J. Spirtos, DO

BASICS

DESCRIPTION Involuntary loss of urine. Nocturnal enuresis (NE) or bedwetting is the term used in children. Diurnal/daytime enuresis is loss of urine while awake. Two general classifications:
- Persistent primary NE (1% of adult population; 87.4% of all cases of enuresis)
  - ◊ Child/adult who has never been continent for an extended period (up to 1 year)
  - ◊ May have subtle diurnal symptoms: mild urgency, frequency, and urge incontinence (UI)
  - ◊ Incidence of organic disease in adults with NE similar to that in children with NE
- Adult onset or secondary NE (11.6% of all cases of enuresis)
  - ◊ Return of involuntary loss of urine after an extended period of urinary control; most adults with secondary NE have organic disease
  - ◊ Consider sexual abuse in children
  - ◊ Not uncommon particularly in the elderly
  - ◊ Adult onset NE with absent daytime incontinence is a serious symptom; usually heralds significant urethral obstruction, and a high incidence of bladder diverticulum, hydronephrosis and vesicoureteral reflux. Complete urologic evaluation and aggressive therapy warranted. UDS needed to assess for lower urinary tract dysfunction (anatomic or neurologic).
  - ◊ Usually associated with diurnal symptoms, voiding dysfunction and UI

System(s) affected: Nervous, Renal/Urologic

Genetics:
- Genetics important in nocturnal enuresis; somatic, and psychosocial and environmental factors have a major modulatory effect
- Nocturnal bladder control is more heritable in boys (33%) than girls (10%) • Most commonly, nocturnal enuresis is an autosomal dominant inheritance pattern with high penetrance (90%). 1/3 of all cases are sporadic. Four loci associated with nocturnal enuresis identified. 75% of children with enuresis have a first degree relative with the condition; if both parents had enuresis, 77% will also have enuresis; if one parent had enuresis, 44% of children affected; 15% of children have enuresis if neither parent had enuresis.

Incidence/Prevalence in USA: 5-7 million children have primary nocturnal enuresis

Predominant age: Most children obtain bladder control by 2-4 years. Enuresis is seen as follows: 5 years 3% females, 7% males; 10 years 2% females, 3% males; > 18 years 1%.

Predominant sex: Male > Female (2:1)

SIGNS & SYMPTOMS
- Voiding pattern (intermittently continent or wet all the time)
- Inability to keep from urinating while asleep at least once per month
- Diurnal enuresis may be associated with frequency, dysuria, or activities that cause an increase in intra-abdominal pressure
- Some children may be withdrawn and shy and some may show aggressive behaviors; both may be secondary to the enuresis and not primary behaviors
- Stress factors such as intrafamilial discord, significant life events, psychosocial or emotional problems may be present

CAUSES
- Many theories, none confirmed; both functional and organic causes
- Current research suggests nocturnal enuresis is caused by a mismatch in nocturnal urine production, small functional bladder capacity and arousability
- Organic urologic causes 1-4% enuresis in children
  - ◊ UTI, occult spina bifida, ectopic ureters, lazy bladder syndrome, irritable bladder with wide bladder neck
- Organic nonurologic causes:
  - ◊ Epilepsy, diabetes mellitus, sleep apnea, food allergies, sleep apnea; there is an increased release of atrial natriuretic factor which may increase urine output and contribute to enuresis
- Deficiency of nocturnal production of arginine vasopressin, antidiuretic hormone, by the anterior pituitary is seen in majority of enuretic patients
- CNS maturational delay has been implicated as a cause
- Sleep disorders or alteration in sleep pattern - no evidence. Nocturnal enuresis occurs in all stages of sleep.

RISK FACTORS
- Emotional and psychological problems in children
- An increased incidence of family and social problems (death in the family, temporary separation of mother, moving, accidents or surgery)
- Family history
- Any reason that increases overall risk of incontinence
- Increased age with increased incidence of medical and urologic disease
- Altered mental status or impaired mobility

DIAGNOSIS

DIFFERENTIAL DIAGNOSIS
- Persistent nocturnal enuresis
  - ◊ Delayed physiologic urinary control
  - ◊ UTI
  - ◊ Spina bifida occulta
  - ◊ Obstructive sleep apnea
  - ◊ Idiopathic detrusor instability
  - ◊ Previously unrecognized myelopathy or neuropathy (Multiple sclerosis, tethered cord, epilepsy)
  - ◊ Anatomic urinary tract abnormally (ectopic ureter, etc)
- Secondary NE
  - ◊ Bladder outlet obstruction
  - ◊ UTI
  - ◊ Neurologic disease
  - ◊ Neurogenic bladder (spinal cord compression/injury, etc)

LABORATORY
- Not usually needed for children
- Urinalysis and urine culture: UTI, pyuria, hematuria, proteinuria, glycosuria, and poor concentrating ability (low specific gravity) may suggest an organic etiology, especially in adults
- BUN and creatinine - suspected renal insufficiency
- Urine cytology if carcinoma/CIS suspected

Drugs that may alter lab results: Diuretics may cause low urinary specific gravity

Disorders that may alter lab results: Anatomic abnormalities may predispose to UTI

PATHOLOGICAL FINDINGS N/A

SPECIAL TESTS Urodynamic testing may be beneficial in adults. More UDS findings than children (28-70%). Detrusor instability and/or reduced bladder capacity most common finding.

IMAGING
- Rule out anatomic abnormalities
- IVP, renal ultrasound, voiding cystourethrogram, or retrograde pyelogram as clinically indicated. Duplication and ureteral ectopia, urethral strictures or diverticula may be detected.
- Spine x-rays detect spina bifida occulta

DIAGNOSTIC PROCEDURES
- See Special Tests
- General medical history
- Diagnosis criteria:
  - ◊ In a child greater than 5 years of age, who has nocturnal enuresis at least twice per week for more than 3 months (DSM-IV, American Psychiatric Association, 1994)
  - ◊ In an adult, any evidence of wetting at night, with or without daytime leakage

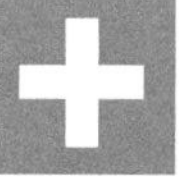

TREATMENT

APPROPRIATE HEALTH CARE Outpatient

GENERAL MEASURES
- Pharmacotherapy, psychotherapy and behavioral modifications
- First address any obvious correctable cause (eg, diabetes mellitus, bladder outlet obstruction)
- Psychotherapy requires participation of child along with the entire family
- Behavioral modifications. These include:
  - ◊ Self monitoring and record keeping is primary technique to improve enuresis
  - ◊ Motivation and responsibility training. Child made responsible for changing/laundering bed linen.
  - ◊ Calendar with "star" rewards for dry nights and some reward system
  - ◊ Efficacy of 25% with 5% relapse rate
  - ◊ Penalties for wet beds is counter-productive
- Bladder training. Exercises to increase bladder capacity. May include biofeedback. Effectiveness in nocturnal enuresis is variable.
- Enuresis alarms - 70% success with 30% relapse. Alarms appear more effective than desmopressin or tricyclics by the end of treatment, and subsequently in most studies.
- Acupuncture (traditional and laser) may be beneficial in the treatment of NE by increasing nocturnal bladder capacity. A promising alternative to conventional therapies for monosymptomatic NE.

SURGICAL MEASURES Only necessary if enuresis is secondary to other surgically correctable cause (eg, tethered cord, ectopic ureter, benign prostatitic hypertrophy)

ACTIVITY No restrictions

DIET
- Restricting liquids after 6 PM may help
- Avoid caffeinated beverages entirely due to diuretic effect
- Avoid foods that appear to cause urinary problems (eg, spicy foods, certain fruits)

PATIENT EDUCATION Explain to parents that most cases of childhood enuresis resolve spontaneously

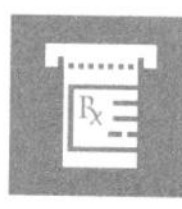

MEDICATIONS

DRUG(S) OF CHOICE
- Oxybutynin (Ditropan, Ditropan XL, Oxytrol patch) - anticholinergic: increases functional bladder capacity and aids in timed voiding
  - ◊ Ditropan - adults and peds > 5 years - 5 mg po tid-qid; peds 1-5 years - 0.02 mg/kg/dose bid-qid (syrup 5 mg/5 mL)
  - ◊ Ditropan XL - adults 5 mg po qd; increase to 30 mg/d po (5 and 10 mg/tab)
  - ◊ Oxytrol patch, apply one patch every 3-4 days (3.9 mg/patch)
  - ◊ Periodic drug holidays recommended
  - ◊ Ditropan 5 mg single night time dose - success rate of 30-50% with 50% relapse with stopping drug. Best in children with frequency, urgency, concomitant day time wetting, and urodynamic evidence of uninhibited detrusor contractions (success rate of 85-91%).
- Imipramine (Tofranil) - tricyclic antidepressant with anticholinergic effects
  - ◊ Dose - adults 25-75 mg po qhs; peds: > 6 y: 10-25 mg po hs
  - ◊ Increase by 10-25 mg at 1-2 wk intervals, treat for 2-3 mo, then taper, success rate of 25-30% when used > 3 months
- Desmopressin (DDAVP) - synthetic analogue of vasopressin, a naturally occurring human ADH decreases nocturnal urine output. Intranasally 10-40 mcg.
  - ◊ Peds > 6 years 20 mcg intranasally hs. Success rate 10-60%. Safe even when used for more than 12 months. Desmopressin reduces the number of nights of primary nocturnal enuresis by at least 1 per week, and increases the likelihood of "cure" (defined as 14 consecutive dry nights) while treatment is continued.
- Tolterodine (Detrol, Detrol LA) - anticholinergic
  - ◊ Detrol 1-2 mg po bid
  - ◊ Detrol LA 2-4 mg/d; no extensive experience in children

Contraindications: Imipramine - do not use with MAOI

Precautions:
- Oxybutynin - glaucoma, myasthenia gravis, GI or GU obstruction, ulcerative colitis, megacolon. Decrease dose in elderly.
- Tolterodine - urinary retention, gastric retention, or uncontrolled narrow-angle glaucoma; significant drug interactions with CYP2D6, CYP3A3/4 substrates
- DDAVP - should be used judiciously or avoided in patient at risk for electrolyte changes or fluid retention (congestive heart failure, renal insufficiency, and cystic fibrosis)

Significant possible interactions: Refer to manufacturer's profile of each drug

ALTERNATIVE DRUGS N/A

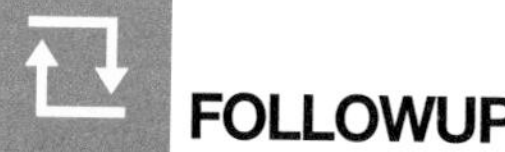

FOLLOWUP

PATIENT MONITORING Follow until enuresis resolved or to monitor therapy

PREVENTION/AVOIDANCE No preventive measures known.

POSSIBLE COMPLICATIONS
- Urinary tract infection
- Perineal excoriation
- Psychologic problems (especially in children)

EXPECTED COURSE/PROGNOSIS
- In children, nocturnal enuresis is generally self limiting
- 1% will persist as adult nocturnal enuresis; requires detailed evaluation for organic causes

MISCELLANEOUS

ASSOCIATED CONDITIONS
- Bronchial asthma
- Verified food allergy
- Spina bifida
- Ectopic ureter
- Attention-deficit hyperactivity disorder

AGE-RELATED FACTORS
Pediatric: Common
Geriatric: Infrequent, often associated with diurnal enuresis
Others: N/A

PREGNANCY Voiding pattern changes common and usually resolve after delivery

SYNONYMS
- Bedwetting
- Sleep enuresis
- Nocturnal incontinence
- Primary nocturnal enuresis

ICD-9-CM
307.6 Enuresis
788.30 Urinary incontinence, unspecified

SEE ALSO
Urinary incontinence

OTHER NOTES Self-concept and self-esteem are adversely effected by enuresis in children, therefore early successful treatment is advocated

ABBREVIATIONS
NE = nocturnal enuresis
UDS = urodynamic studies
UI = urinary incontinence

REFERENCES

- Diehr S, Bercaw D. How effective is desmopressin for primary nocturnal enuresis? Fam Pract 2003;52(7):568-9
- Djurhuus JC, Rittig S. Nocturnal enuresis. Curr Opin Urol 2002;12(4):317-20
- Glazener CM, Evans JH, Peto RE. Alarm interventions for nocturnal enuresis in children. Cochrane Database Syst Rev 2003;(2):CD002911
- Hvistendahl GM, Rawashdeh YF, et al. The relationship between desmopressin treatment and voiding pattern in children. BJU Int 2002;89(9):917-22
- Rawashdeh YF, Hvistendahl GM, Kamperis K, et al. Demographics of enuresis patients attending a referral centre. Scand J Urol Nephrol 2002;36(5):348-53
- Sakamoto K, Blaivas JG. Adult onset nocturnal enuresis. Urol 2001;165(6 Pt 1):1914-7

Web references: 2 available at www.5mcc.com
Illustrations N/A

Author(s):
Leonard G. Gomella, MD

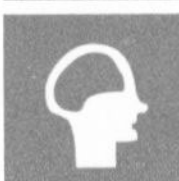

BASICS

DESCRIPTION Eosinophilic pneumonias are characterized by eosinophilic lung infiltrates with or without peripheral blood eosinophilia. They are classified as acute or chronic and can be either idiopathic or secondary to other causes.

- Included are:
  - ◊ Löffler's syndrome (simple pulmonary eosinophilia)
  - ◊ Allergic bronchopulmonary aspergillosis (ABPA)
  - ◊ Drug-induced pulmonary eosinophilia
  - ◊ Tropical pulmonary eosinophilia
  - ◊ Chronic or prolonged pulmonary eosinophilia
  - ◊ The hypereosinophilic syndrome
  - ◊ Churg-Strauss syndrome (polyarteritis nodosa) or allergic angiitis

System(s) affected: Pulmonary
Genetics: No known genetic pattern
Incidence/Prevalence in USA: Rare
Predominant age: Any age
Predominant sex: Male = Female (male in 4th decade; female in 6th decade)

SIGNS & SYMPTOMS

- Dyspnea
- Fever in acute cases
- Cough with sputum
- Chills
- Hypoxia
- Wheezing in some patients
- Anorexia
- Decreased localized breath sounds
- Tachycardia
- Malaise
- Symptoms may be mild or life-threatening

CAUSES

- Idiopathic (though hypersensitivity suspected) in one third of cases
- Drugs/toxins (penicillin, nitrofurantoin, isoniazid, chlorpropamide, sulfonamides, antituberculous therapy (PAS), gold, aspirin, hydralazine)
- Tropical
  - ◊ Parasites
  - ◊ Toxocara larvae
  - ◊ Filariae
  - ◊ Nematodes (Strongyloides, Ascaris, Ancylostoma
- Aspergillus fumigatus (asthmatic pulmonary eosinophilia)
- Systemic vasculitis

RISK FACTORS

- Patients with chronic disorders, e.g., asthma, cystic fibrosis
- Living or traveling in certain geographical areas, e.g., India, Ceylon, Burma, Malaysia, Indonesia, tropical Africa, South America, South Pacific
- Cigarette smoking has recently been suggested

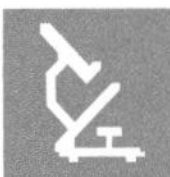

DIAGNOSIS

DIFFERENTIAL DIAGNOSIS

- Tuberculosis
- Sarcoidosis
- Hodgkin disease
- Other lymphoproliferative disorders
- Eosinophilic granuloma of the lung
- Desquamative interstitial pneumonitis
- Hypereosinophilic syndrome
- Wegener granulomatosis
- Interstitial lung disease

LABORATORY

- Findings determined by etiology
- Leukocytosis
- Eosinophilia in peripheral blood and lungs
- A. fumigatus found in sputum
- Positive filarial complement fixation
- Elevated IgE levels
- Increased WBC
- Elevated ESR
- Stool examination for parasites

Drugs that may alter lab results: N/A

Disorders that may alter lab results: N/A

PATHOLOGICAL FINDINGS

- Lung
  - ◊ Alveolar eosinophilic filling
  - ◊ Septal eosinophilic infiltration

SPECIAL TESTS

- Bronchoscopy with broncho alveolar lavage
- Lung biopsy when diagnosis uncertain or clinical course is severe (rare)
- Pulmonary function studies

IMAGING High resolution CT (HRCT), chest x-ray - migratory infiltrates, small pleural effusion; transient infiltrates; interstitial opacities

DIAGNOSTIC PROCEDURES

- History and physical exam with particular emphasis on drug intake, recent travel to tropical areas, and systemic symptoms
- Bronchoscopy with broncho-alveolar lavage (BAL)

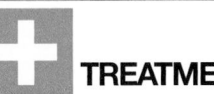

TREATMENT

APPROPRIATE HEALTH CARE Outpatient for milder cases. More severe cases may require inpatient care.

GENERAL MEASURES

- Evaluate for secondary causes
- Mild cases may require no specific therapy
- Coughing and deep breathing exercises to clear secretions
- Discontinuing offending drug
- Treatment of underlying parasite infestation

SURGICAL MEASURES N/A

ACTIVITY As tolerated.

DIET High calorie, high protein, soft diet

PATIENT EDUCATION Information about activity, diet, symptoms of recurrence

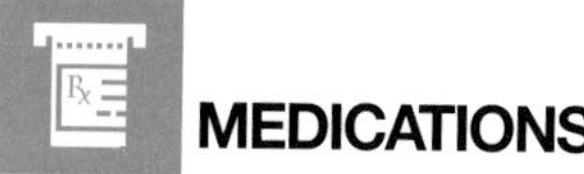

MEDICATIONS

DRUG(S) OF CHOICE

- Corticosteroid therapy. In chronic pulmonary eosinophilia, 20-40 mg prednisone daily. In Churg-Strauss syndrome may require large doses e.g., 40-60 mg of prednisone daily. Withdrawal should be possible after recovery. In chronic conditions, treatment should continue for 6-12 months.
- Treat asthma, if present
- Piperazine for Ascaris infestation
- Diethylcarbamazine [available only from the manufacturer] 6-8 mg/kg orally in 3 divided doses a day for 10-14 days for tropical pulmonary eosinophilia
- Appropriate vermifuges for helminthic infections

Contraindications: Refer to manufacturer's literature

Precautions: Refer to manufacturer's literature

Significant possible interactions: Refer to manufacturer's literature

ALTERNATIVE DRUGS

- In Churg-Strauss syndrome, cases resistant to corticosteroid therapy, adding azathioprine or cyclophosphamide may be helpful
- Some patients may require oxygen therapy

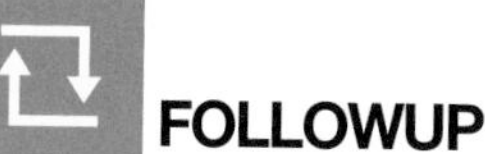

FOLLOWUP

PATIENT MONITORING Physical examinations and chest x-rays until resolved

PREVENTION/AVOIDANCE Avoid exposure to offending agent

POSSIBLE COMPLICATIONS

- Some patients may show evidence of small airways dysfunction
- Delay in treatment of tropical pulmonary eosinophilia may result in irreversible pulmonary fibrosis

EXPECTED COURSE/PROGNOSIS

- Excellent in the milder forms
- Corticosteroid therapy is dramatically effective in more severe cases

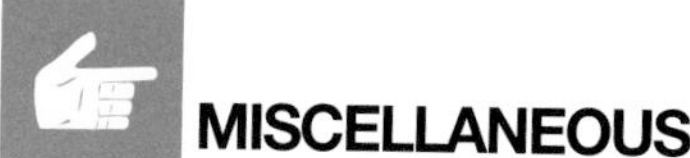

MISCELLANEOUS

ASSOCIATED CONDITIONS

- Asthma
- Hypersensitivity pneumonitis
- Wegener granulomatosis

AGE-RELATED FACTORS

Pediatric: N/A

Geriatric: More morbidity, probably due to decreased lung capacity and likelihood of concomitant diseases

Others: N/A

PREGNANCY N/A

SYNONYMS

- Löffler syndrome
- Pulmonary infiltrates with eosinophilia syndrome (PIE)

ICD-9-CM

518.3 Pulmonary eosinophilia

SEE ALSO

Aspergillosis
Hodgkin disease
Roundworms, tissue
Sarcoidosis
Tuberculosis
Wegener granulomatosis

OTHER NOTES N/A

ABBREVIATIONS N/A

REFERENCES

- Murray JF, Nadel JA, editors. Textbook of Respiratory Medicine. 3rd ed. Philadelphia: W.B. Saunders Co; 2000

Web references: 0 available at www.5mcc.com

Illustrations N/A

Author(s):
George E. Kikano, MD

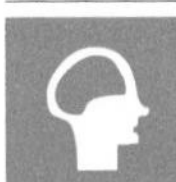

BASICS

DESCRIPTION Inflammation of the epididymis resulting in scrotal pain, swelling and induration of the posterior-lying epididymis, and eventual scrotal wall edema, involvement of the adjacent testicle, and hydrocele formation
System(s) affected: Reproductive
Genetics: N/A
Incidence/Prevalence in USA: Common
Predominant age: Usually younger sexually active men or older men with urinary infection, but may also rarely occur in prepubertal boys
Predominant sex: Male only

SIGNS & SYMPTOMS
- Scrotal pain, sometimes extending to the groin region, may begin relatively acutely over several hours
- Urethral discharge or symptoms of urinary tract infection, such as frequency of urination, dysuria, cloudy urine, or hematuria
- Initially, only the posterior-lying epididymis, usually the lowermost tail section, will be very tender and indurated
- Elevation of the testes/epididymis improves the discomfort
- Entire hemiscrotum becomes swollen, the testis becomes indistinguishable from the epididymis, the scrotal wall becomes thick and indurated, and reactive hydrocele may occur
- Fever and chills occur with severe infection and abscess formation

CAUSES
- Younger than age 35
  - ◊ Usually chlamydia or *Neisseria gonorrhea*
  - ◊ Look for serous urethral discharge (chlamydia) or purulent discharge (gonorrhea)
- Older than age 35
  - ◊ Coliform bacteria usually, but sometimes Staphylococcus aureus or epidermidis
  - ◊ Often associated with distal urinary tract obstruction
  - ◊ Tuberculosis, if sterile pyuria and nodularity of vas deferens
  - ◊ Sterile urine reflux after transurethral prostatectomy
  - ◊ Granulomatous reaction following bacillus Calmette-Guerin (BCG) intravesical therapy for superficial bladder cancer
- Prepubertal boys
  - ◊ Usually coliform bacteria
  - ◊ Evaluate for underlying congenital abnormalities, such as vesicoureteral reflux, ectopic ureter, or anorectal malformation (rectourethral fistula)
- At any age
  - ◊ Amiodarone, an antiarrhythmic agent, may cause a non-infectious epididymitis, that resolves with decreasing the drug dose

RISK FACTORS
- Urinary tract infection, particularly prostatitis
- Indwelling urethral catheter
- Urethral instrumentation or transurethral surgery
- Urethral stricture
- Transrectal prostate biopsy
- Prostate brachytherapy (seeds) for prostate cancer
- Anal intercourse
- HIV immunosuppressed patient
- Severe Behçet disease

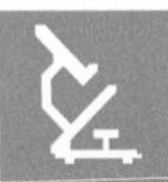

DIAGNOSIS

DIFFERENTIAL DIAGNOSIS
- Epididymal congestion following vasectomy
- Testicular torsion
- Torsion of appendix testis
- Mumps orchitis
- Testicular tumor
- Testicular trauma
- Epididymal cyst
- Spermatocele
- Hydrocele
- Varicocele
- Epididymal adenomatoid tumor
- Epididymal rhabdomyosarcoma

LABORATORY Pyuria on urinalysis, leukocytosis, gram stain urethral discharge

Drugs that may alter lab results: N/A

Disorders that may alter lab results: N/A

PATHOLOGICAL FINDINGS
- Gross and microabscesses
- Organisms reach the epididymis through the lumen of the vas deferens
- Interstitial congestion
- Fibrous scarring

SPECIAL TESTS N/A

IMAGING Ultrasound of scrotum, radionuclide scan

DIAGNOSTIC PROCEDURES Scrotal exploration or aspiration of epididymis (rarely performed)

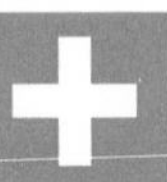

TREATMENT

APPROPRIATE HEALTH CARE
- Outpatient, usually
- Inpatient, if septic or if surgery is scheduled

GENERAL MEASURES
- Scrotal elevation
- Ice pack
- Spermatic cord block with local anesthesia in severe cases

SURGICAL MEASURES
- Aspiration of hydrocele to assist examination of scrotal contents and relieve discomfort
- Vasostomy to drain infected material
- Scrotal exploration, if uncertain whether this is epididymitis or testicular torsion
- Drainage of abscesses, epididymectomy, or epididymo-orchiectomy in severe cases not responding to antibiotics

ACTIVITY Bedrest for minimum of 1-2 days

DIET No restrictions, but force fluids

PATIENT EDUCATION
- Limit activity, immobilize scrotal contents
- Stress completing course of antibiotics, even when asymptomatic

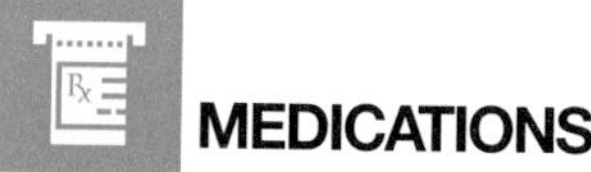

MEDICATIONS

DRUG(S) OF CHOICE
- Younger than age 35 for chlamydia
  - ◊ Doxycycline 100 mg po bid for 10 days and ceftriaxone 250 mg IM
- Older men with bacteriuria
  - ◊ Trimethoprim-sulfamethoxazole (Bactrim, Septra) double strength po bid for 10-14 days
  - ◊ Ciprofloxacin (Cipro) 500 mg po bid x 10-14 days
  - ◊ Levofloxacin (Levaquin) 250 mg po q day x 10-14 days
  - ◊ Norfloxacin (Noroxin) 400 mg po bid x 10-14 days
- Analgesia
  - ◊ Non-steroidal anti-inflammatory drug (e.g., naproxen or ibuprofen) for mild to moderate pain
  - ◊ Acetaminophen-codeine or acetaminophen-oxycodone for moderate to severe pain
- Septic or toxic patient
  - ◊ Third generation cephalosporin (ceftriaxone 1-2 gm IV/IM every 24 hours)
  - ◊ Aminoglycoside (gentamicin 1 mg/kg IV/IM every 8 hours, adjusted for renal function) after a loading dose of 2 mg/kg

Contraindications: None
Precautions: Refer to manufacturer's profile of each drug
Significant possible interactions: Refer to manufacturer's profile of each drug

ALTERNATIVE DRUGS
- Other aminoglycosides or third generation cephalosporin depending on specific pathogen
- Add rifampin (rifampicin) or vancomycin as required

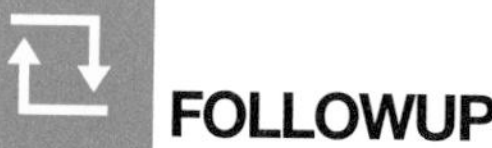

FOLLOWUP

PATIENT MONITORING Office visits until all signs of infection have cleared

PREVENTION/AVOIDANCE
- Vasectomy or vasoligation during transurethral surgery
- Antibiotic prophylaxis for urethral manipulation
- Early treatment of prostatitis
- Avoid vigorous rectal examination with acute prostatitis

POSSIBLE COMPLICATIONS
- Recurrent epididymitis
- Infertility
- Fournier's gangrene (necrotizing synergistic infection)

EXPECTED COURSE/PROGNOSIS
- Pain improves within 1-3 days, but induration may take several weeks/months to completely resolve
- If bilateral involvement, sterility may result

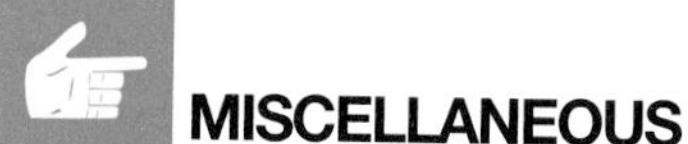

MISCELLANEOUS

ASSOCIATED CONDITIONS
- Prostatitis
- Urethritis

AGE-RELATED FACTORS
Pediatric:
- In prepubertal, may be post-infectious inflammatory condition, treated with analgesics and usually no antibiotics
- Bacteremia from Haemophilus influenzae infection may produce acute epididymitis
- In adolescent males, must rule out acute testicular torsion

Geriatric: Diabetic patients with sensory neuropathy may have little pain despite severe infection/abscess
Others: N/A

PREGNANCY N/A

SYNONYMS
Epididymo-orchitis

ICD-9-CM
604.90 Orchitis and epididymitis, unspecified

SEE ALSO

OTHER NOTES
- Syphilis, brucellosis, blastomycosis, coccidioidomycosis, and cryptococcosis are rare causes of epididymitis
- Nonbacterial epididymitis and epididymo-orchitis are not rare. Cause is not clear, but may be secondary to retrograde extravasation.

ABBREVIATIONS N/A

REFERENCES

- Berger RE. Acute epididymitis. Semin Urol 1991;9:28
- Donzella JG, Merrick GS, Lindert DJ, et al. Epididymitis after transrectal ultrasound-guided needle biopsy of prostate gland. Urology 2004;63(2):306-8
- Somekh E, Gorenstein A, Serour F. Acute epididymitis in boys: evidence of a post-infectious etiology. J Urol 2004;171(1):391-4

Web references: 0 available at www.5mcc.com
Illustrations N/A

Author(s):
Peter T. Nieh, MD

BASICS

DESCRIPTION An illness with acute onset characterized by inflammation and edema of the supraglottic structures, epiglottis, vallecula, arytenoepiglottic folds and arytenoids

System(s) affected: Pulmonary

Genetics: N/A

Incidence/Prevalence in USA:
- Incidence has decreased dramatically since the introduction of the *Haemophilus influenzae type b* (Hib) vaccine
- Incidence in adults 1-3/100,000

Predominant age:
- In the pre-vaccine era the most commonly affected group were children 2-6 years old
- With increasing use of Hib vaccine the predominant age is shifting to older children (median age, 7 years).

Predominant sex: Male > Female: 1.5 : 1

SIGNS & SYMPTOMS
- Sudden onset and fulminant course
- Fever
- Sore throat
- Dysphagia, drooling
- Cervical adenopathy
- Airway obstruction resulting in respiratory distress
- "Tripod" position (sitting propped up on hands with head forward and tongue out)
- Muffled voice/cry (vs. hoarseness in croup)
- Minimal cough (vs. barking cough in croup)
- Toxic appearance/shock (occasionally, due to associated septicemia)
- Stridor softer and less prominent than croup
- Usually no history of prodromal upper respiratory infection (vs. positive history in croup)
- In adults, presentation more indolent (sore throat the predominate symptom)

CAUSES
- Bacterial
  - ◊ *Haemophilus influenzae type b*
  - ◊ *Streptococcus pyogenes*
  - ◊ *Streptococcus pneumoniae*
  - ◊ *Staphylococcus aureus*
- Fungal
- Viral
- Traumatic
  - ◊ Caustic ingestion
- Allergic reactions

RISK FACTORS N/A

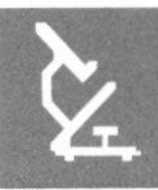

DIAGNOSIS

DIFFERENTIAL DIAGNOSIS
- Viral croup (laryngotracheobronchitis)
- Acute angioneurotic edema (no fever)
- Aspirated foreign body
- Bacterial tracheitis (pseudomembranous croup)
- Retropharyngeal or peritonsillar abscess
- Diphtheria in an unimmunized patient (often an adult)
- Sepsis of other cause

LABORATORY
- Blood culture (positive in over 75-90% of children with Hib acute epiglottitis). See under Diagnostic Procedures - should not visualize/swab epiglottis except in controlled environment, i.e., operating room. Blood tests also contraindicated until airway secured.
- Epiglottic swab culture (positive in 70%)
- CBC. Leukocytosis with left shift
- Hib antigen test in blood/urine useful in children with previous antibiotic treatment
- Hypoxia, usually not present until airway obstructed

Drugs that may alter lab results: N/A

Disorders that may alter lab results: N/A

PATHOLOGICAL FINDINGS N/A

SPECIAL TESTS N/A

IMAGING
- Neck radiographs are contraindicated if epiglottitis is suspected, due to danger of sudden complete airway obstruction although lateral neck films are often obtained (insure adequate staff present if complete airway obstruction occurs)
- CXR, after intubation, to check position of endotracheal tube and to rule out pneumonia which can occur as a complication up to 25% of cases.

DIAGNOSTIC PROCEDURES
- Visualization of epiglottis with tongue depressor is contraindicated due to danger of sudden complete airway obstruction
- Controlled visualization of epiglottis at intubation in operating room is diagnostic ("cherry red", edematous epiglottis)
- Lumbar puncture is indicated if there is clinical suspicion of meningitis
- In adult, indirect laryngoscopy is generally safe

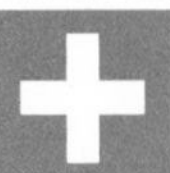

TREATMENT

APPROPRIATE HEALTH CARE Acute epiglottitis is a medical emergency. Hospitalize during acute illness in ICU.

GENERAL MEASURES
- Each institution should have emergency protocol involving a team of emergency room physicians, pediatricians, anesthesiologists, surgeons, pediatric intensivists, and pediatric ICU nurses (principles are similar for pediatric and adult patients)
- Call anesthesiologist to bedside
- Have equipment for intubation and needle cricothyrotomy or percutaneous tracheostomy at bedside
- Notify OR
- Notify pediatric surgery or ENT for standby in OR in case tracheostomy becomes necessary
- Keep patient quiet, calm, sitting up (in parent's arms)
- Avoid venipuncture, blood gases, oxygen masks, intravenous lines, injections, monitors, and radiographs
- Judicious use of sedation that does not depress respirations may be appropriate
- Racemic epinephrine is without benefit
- Avoid examining the pharynx
- Transport patient and parent together to OR in a wheelchair
- Intubate all patients, preferably in OR under controlled circumstances by experienced anesthesiologist with surgery or ENT on standby for emergency tracheostomy
- Tracheostomy not indicated unless intubation unsuccessful
- Tape airway securely in place and use a bite block if indicated
- Splint elbows and restrain arms to avoid self-extubation
- Use humidity in a tent and avoid T-piece (traction increases risk of accidental extubation)
- CPAP, mechanical ventilation, and sedation usually unnecessary
- Pay attention to supervision and pulmonary toilet/suctioning to minimize risk of endotracheal tube plugs

SURGICAL MEASURES Emergency tracheotomy may be necessary

ACTIVITY N/A

DIET IV fluid initially, then nasogastric feedings while intubated

PATIENT EDUCATION Reassurance about treatment and outcome

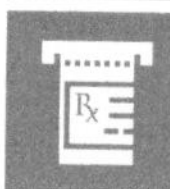

MEDICATIONS

DRUG(S) OF CHOICE
- Begin empiric antibiotic promptly after blood and epiglottic cultures are obtained. Antibiotics guided by cultures thereafter. Duration of antimicrobial: 7 days
- Cefotaxime (Claforan) 100-200 mg/kg/day q 8 hours IV
- Ceftriaxone (Rocephin) 50-100 mg/kg/day q 12 hours IV
- Ampicillin-sulbactam (Unasyn) 150 mg/kg/day q 6 h IV
- Amoxicillin-clavulanate 100 mg/kg/day q 8 h IV

Contraindications: Refer to manufacturer's profile
Precautions: Refer to manufacturer's profile
Significant possible interactions: Refer to manufacturer's profile

ALTERNATIVE DRUGS
- Ampicillin 100 mg/kg/day divided q 6 hours IV and chloramphenicol 100 mg/kg/day divided q 6 hours. Follow levels. May stop chloramphenicol only if *H. influenzae* b sensitive to ampicillin.
- Steroids and racemic epinephrine of no benefit
- Antipyretics if necessary

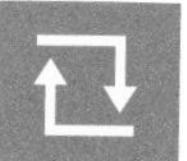

FOLLOWUP

PATIENT MONITORING
- Rule out secondary foci of infection
- Follow swallowing ability and presence of an air leak around endo/nasotracheal tube
- Followup laryngoscopy prior to extubation (advocated by some)
- Observe in ICU for 24 hours following extubation

PREVENTION/AVOIDANCE
- *H. influenzae* vaccine is effective though not 100% protective
- Rifampin prophylaxis (20 mg/kg once daily for 4 days, maximum daily dose 600 mg) for all household and day care contacts. Family and close contacts may be asymptomatic carriers of *H. influenzae*.

POSSIBLE COMPLICATIONS
- Pneumonia, meningitis, cervical adenitis, septic arthritis, pericarditis, cellulitis (rare)
- Epiglottic abscess
- Septic shock (in about 1%)
- Pneumothorax, pneumomediastinum (very rare)
- Death from asphyxia

EXPECTED COURSE/PROGNOSIS
- Most can be extubated after 24 to 48 hours
- Morbidity and mortality is low with appropriate intervention

MISCELLANEOUS

ASSOCIATED CONDITIONS N/A

AGE-RELATED FACTORS
Pediatric: Rare since introduction of Hib vaccine
Geriatric: Rare
Others: N/A

PREGNANCY N/A

SYNONYMS Supraglottitis

ICD-9-CM
464.30 Acute epiglottitis without mention of obstruction
464.31 Acute epiglottitis with obstruction

SEE ALSO
Immunizations

OTHER NOTES N/A

ABBREVIATIONS
Hib = Hemophilus influenza type b

REFERENCES

- Gerber AC, Pfenninger J. Acute epiglottitis: Management during intubation and hospitalization. Intensive Care Med 1986;12:407-411
- Vernon DD, Ashok PS. Acute epiglottitis in children: A conservative approach to diagnosis and management. Crit Care Med 1986;14:23-25
- Blanc VF, Duquenne P, Charest J: Acute epiglottitis: An overview. Acta Anaesthesial Belg 1986;37:171-178
- Chery JD. Epiglottitis (Supraglottitis) in Feigin RD, Chery JD, Demmer GJ, Kaplan SL; eds. Textbook of Pediatric Infectious Diseases 5th edition. W. B. Saunders Company, Philadelphia. 2004:241-51
- Shepherd M, Kidney E. Adult epiglottitis. Accid Emerg Nurs. 2004;12:28-30
- Berger G, Landau T, Berger S, Finkelstein Y, Bernheim J, Ophir D. The rising incidence of adult acute epiglottitis and epiglottic abscess. Am J Otolaryngol 2003;24(6):374-83
- Low YM, Leong JL, Tan HK. Paediatric acute epiglottitis re-visited. Singapore Med J 2003;44(10):539-41
- Mathur KK, Mortelliti AJ. Candida epiglottitis. Ear Noe Throat J 2004;83(1):13
- Shah RK, Roberson DW, Jones DT. Epiglottitis in the hemophilus type B vaccine era: changing trends. Laryngoscope 2004 Mar;114(3):557-60
- McEwan J, Giridharan W, Clarke RW, Shears P. Peadiatric acute epiglottitis: not a disappearing entity. J Pediatr Otorhinolaryngol 2003;67:317-21

Web references: 0 available at www.5mcc.com
Illustrations N/A

Author(s):
Vassiliki Syriopoulou, MD

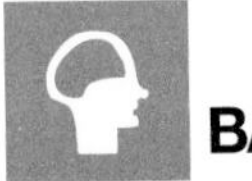

BASICS

DESCRIPTION Hemorrhage from nostril, nasal cavity or nasopharynx
- Anterior bleed: Originates from anterior nasal cavity, usually Little's area (Kiesselbach's plexus) on septum just above posterior end of nasal vestibule. Second most common is anterior end of inferior turbinate.
- Posterior bleed: Originates from posterior nasal cavity or nasopharynx usually under the posterior half of the inferior turbinate or the roof of the nasal cavity

System(s) affected: Pulmonary
Genetics: N/A
Incidence/Prevalence in USA: Common
Predominant age: Less than 10 years and over 50 years
Predominant sex: Male = Female

SIGNS & SYMPTOMS Usually nostril hemorrhage, however cases of posterior bleed may be asymptomatic or present with hemoptysis, nausea, hematemesis or melena

CAUSES
- Idiopathic (most common)
- Traumatic/blunt - nose picking (epistaxis digitorum), low humidity, foreign body
- Infection - upper respiratory, acute/chronic rhinitis, acute/chronic sinusitis
- Vascular abnormalities - sclerotic vessels of age, hereditary hemorrhagic telangiectasia, arteriovenous malformation
- Neoplasm (especially when unilateral)
- Hypertension (usually in combination with another cause)
- Coagulopathy - hereditary (e.g., hemophilia), therapeutic or adverse effect of drugs, blood dyscrasias, leukemias, thrombocytopenia or platelet dysfunction
- Septal perforation
- Septal deviation (one side is overexposed to dry air)
- Bleeding originating in a sinus (fracture, tumor)
- Endometriosis (nasal ectopic endometrium)

RISK FACTORS N/A

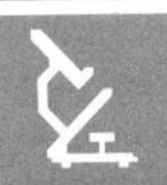

DIAGNOSIS

DIFFERENTIAL DIAGNOSIS Epistaxis is a symptom or a sign, not a disease. Less than 10% are caused by neoplasm or coagulopathy.

LABORATORY CBC, crossmatch for hypovolemic shock or anemia

Drugs that may alter lab results: N/A

Disorders that may alter lab results: N/A

PATHOLOGICAL FINDINGS N/A

SPECIAL TESTS As indicated for unusual causes

IMAGING CT scan if neoplasm is suspected

DIAGNOSTIC PROCEDURES
- Angiography (rarely)
- Nasal endoscopy to locate and cauterize bleeding vessel

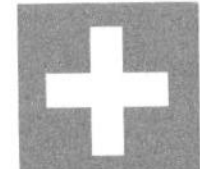

TREATMENT

APPROPRIATE HEALTH CARE
- Outpatient (usually). Inpatient for severe hemorrhage.
- Elderly patient with posterior bleeds and balloon or packing usually requires inpatient management

GENERAL MEASURES
- Resuscitation as indicated
- Sedation, analgesic, antihypertensive or anticoagulant reversal as needed
- Patient should be gowned and sitting, if stable. Gown, gloves, and eye protection for examiner.
- Attempt to locate bleeding site using headlamp, suction, nasal speculum and assistant. Clear nasal cavity of blood with suction, forceps withdrawal of clot or patient blowing nose. If bleeding has stopped, rub suspicious areas with wet cotton tipped applicator to identify site. Diffuse ooze or multiple sites suggests systemic cause. In cases of posterior bleed try to identify as either roof or low posterior site since each has different arterial supply (will be important if arterial ligation is necessary).
- Locating the site may be difficult with bilateral bleeding. Usually there is only one bleeding site and the blood appears on the other side because of (1) septal perforation, (2) obstruction of the affected side by pinching or packing or (3) there is a posterior bleed and blood passes behind the nasal septum. Clues are the side on which bleeding started and a careful examination using suction, headlamp and speculum.
- Anterior bleed:
  - ◊ Place pledget soaked in vasoconstrictor and local anesthetic in cavity and pinch nostril for several minutes to stop bleeding by direct pressure
  - ◊ Remove pledget and visualize vessel. Cauterize with silver nitrate stick directly on vessel with firm pressure for 30 seconds.
  - ◊ Alternative chemical cautery includes bead of chromic acid or 25% trichloroacetic acid. Larger vessels respond better to thermal cautery or bipolar electrocautery. Avoid indiscriminate cauterization of a large area.
  - ◊ If unsuccessful, apply second dose of anesthetic and place anterior pack using 1/2 x 72 inch ribbon gauze impregnated with petroleum jelly (Vaseline) or nasal tampons may be used. Use bayonet forceps and nasal speculum to insert in folding layers as far back as possible. Press each layer firmly down on the last in one continuous strip with the folded ends alternating front and back. The average nasal cavity will accommodate the full length if properly placed. Tape 2x2 gauze over nostril as drip catch and to prevent packing end from falling out of nostril.
- Posterior bleed:
  - ◊ Traditional posterior packing has been replaced by various balloon systems. However it is very effective if balloon systems fail to control bleeding.
  - ◊ Balloon systems include single large balloon with or without central tube for airway. They usually come in 3 or 4 sizes and right or left. Other systems provide a small (10 cc) posterior balloon and larger (30 cc) anterior balloon. After local anesthesia, the tube is placed in the affected nostril and is passed to the nasopharynx as one would a nasogastric tube. Then inflate the posterior balloon with air or water (see manufacturer's directions) and pull forward to press upon the posterior area. Then inflate the anterior balloon (see note under Complications) . A very effective method uses a 10 to 14 Fr Foley catheter. Place tip of Foley through the nostril to nasopharynx or upper oropharynx. Visualize through mouth avoiding placement in hypopharynx. Inflate balloon 7 to 15 cc. Pull forward until balloon wedges in posterior passage. Assistant maintains gentle traction while catheter is placed along mid-section of lateral wall of nasal cavity. Insert anterior pack described above. Maintain catheter traction and stretch slightly. Place umbilical cord clamp on catheter across nostril against anterior pack so that elasticity of catheter compresses balloon against anterior pack. Protect facial skin from clamp by padding with 2x2 gauze. Drape rest of catheter over ear and tape in place.
- Intractable bleed:
  - ◊ Bilateral packing is sometimes required (admission required)
  - ◊ Bleeding from roof may be controlled by placing double balloon system with small anterior pack placed above anterior balloon. Inflation then raises pack to place pressure on roof.
  - ◊ Intractable bleed requires surgical cauterization or arterial ligation (ideally after visual identification of bleeding site to define appropriate arterial supply). This can usually be achieved through transnasal endoscopy. Alternative is angiographic selective arterial embolization.

SURGICAL MEASURES
- Arterial ligation for intractable bleeding

ACTIVITY Bedrest with head at 45 to 90 degrees

DIET No alcohol or hot liquids

PATIENT EDUCATION Demonstrate proper pinching pressure techniques

MEDICATIONS

DRUG(S) OF CHOICE
- Vasoconstrictors
  - ◊ Cocaine 4%
  - ◊ Phenylephrine 0.25%,
  - ◊ Xylometazoline 0.1%
  - ◊ Epinephrine 1:1000
- Anesthetics
  - ◊ Cocaine 4%
  - ◊ Tetracaine (Pontocaine) 2%
  - ◊ Lidocaine laryngeal spray, jelly 2%, solution 4%, viscous 2%
- Systemic antibiotics and decongestants to prevent sinusitis with packs or balloon use
- Iron supplementation for patients with considerable blood loss

Contraindications: Allergy to any component

Precautions:
- Hypertension, coronary artery disease with epinephrine
- Large doses of cocaine in children

Significant possible interactions: Refer to manufacturer's profile of each drug

ALTERNATIVE DRUGS Numerous other topical anesthetics and vasoconstrictors

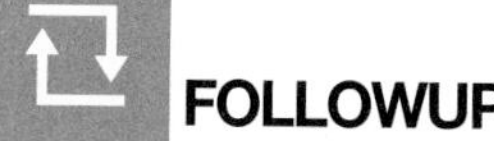

FOLLOWUP

PATIENT MONITORING Hemodynamics and blood loss as indicated. Packs or balloons removed in 24 to 36 hours.

PREVENTION/AVOIDANCE Liberal application of petroleum jelly (Vaseline) to nostril to prevent drying and picking. Humidification at night. Cut fingernails.

POSSIBLE COMPLICATIONS
- Sinusitis
- Double balloon systems tend to migrate posteriorly, if anterior balloon breaks, patient may obstruct airway with migrated posterior balloon. Prevent by placing umbilical cord clamp across end of tubing at nostril after inflation.
- Septal hematoma or abscess from excessive trauma during packing
- Septal perforation secondary to aggressive cauterization
- External nasal deformity secondary to pressure necrosis from the anterior component of posterior packing
- Mucosal pressure necrosis secondary to high balloon inflation pressures
- Cocaine, lidocaine toxicity
- Vasovagal episode during packing

EXPECTED COURSE/PROGNOSIS
Good results with proper treatment

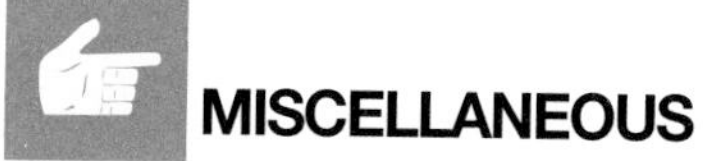

MISCELLANEOUS

ASSOCIATED CONDITIONS In the elderly - hypertension, atherosclerosis and conditions that decrease platelets and clotting functions

AGE-RELATED FACTORS
Pediatric: More likely anterior bleed
Geriatric: More likely posterior bleed
Others: N/A

PREGNANCY N/A

SYNONYMS Nosebleed

ICD-9-CM
784.7 Epistaxis

SEE ALSO

OTHER NOTES N/A

ABBREVIATIONS N/A

REFERENCES

- Votey R, Dudley JP: Emergency ear, nose and throat procedures. Emerg. Clin. NA 1989;7(1)117-154
- Perretta LJ, et al: Emergency evaluation and management of epistaxis. Emerg. Clin. NA 1987;5(2)265-277
- Wong, Jafek: Pediatric Otorhinolaryngology. Appleton-Century-Crofts,1989

Web references: 0 available at www.5mcc.com
Illustrations N/A

Author(s):
Mark R. Dambro, MD

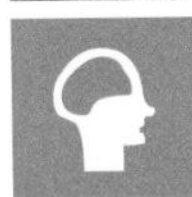

BASICS

DESCRIPTION Epstein-Barr virus (EBV) is tropic for B lymphocytes which apparently are infected in the oropharynx through salivary exchange; infected B cells then circulate in the blood and are distributed to the bone marrow and lymphoreticular system. The virus can also be found in infected epithelial cells of the buccal mucosa, salivary glands, tongue and endocervix. This suggests that chronic epithelial replication brings about continuous reinfection of B lymphoid cells. Immune T cell responses to latently infected B cells account for the clinical findings. All seropositive persons actively shed virus in the saliva.

System(s) affected: Hemic/Lymphatic/Immunologic

Genetics: N/A

Incidence/Prevalence in USA:
- Infects over 90% of humans
- Military and college student groups have most active infection rate
- Worldwide in distribution, but clinical IM is observed predominantly in countries with advanced sociohygienic conditions

Predominant age:
- Older children, adolescents and young adults
- By young adult life, 60-90% of persons are antibody positive

Predominant sex: Male = Female

SIGNS & SYMPTOMS
- May begin abruptly or insidiously
- In adults, the temperature may rise to 103°F (39.4°C) and gradually falls over a variable period of 7-10 days; in severe cases temperature elevations of 104-105° F (40.0-40.6°C) may persist for 2 weeks
- Children usually have a low-grade fever or may be afebrile
- Diffuse hyperemia and hyperplasia of oropharyngeal lymphoid tissue
- Gelatinous, grayish-white exudative tonsillitis persists for 7-10 days in 50%
- Petechiae develop at the border of the hard and soft palates in 60%
- Tender lymphadenopathy (cervical nodes are most commonly enlarged)
- Axillary, epitrochlear, popliteal, inguinal, mediastinal and mesenteric nodes may also be affected
- Lymph node enlargement subsides over days or weeks
- Splenomegaly in 50%
- Abnormal hepatic enzymes in 80% of patients for several weeks after onset. Hepatomegaly in 15-20%.
- Pneumonitis
- Chest pain (myocarditis and pericarditis)
- Hilar adenopathy may be observed in IM cases having extensive lymphoid hyperplasia
- Neurologic (rare)
  - ◊ Aseptic meningitis
  - ◊ Bell palsy
  - ◊ Meningoencephalitis
  - ◊ Guillain-Barré syndrome
  - ◊ Transverse myelitis
  - ◊ Cerebellar ataxia
  - ◊ Acute psychosis
- Hematologic (rare)
  - ◊ Thrombocytopenia, slight to moderate, early in illness
  - ◊ Hemolytic anemia with marked neutropenia during early weeks of disease
  - ◊ Aplastic anemia
  - ◊ Agammaglobulinemia
- Skin manifestations (3-16%)
  - ◊ Erythematous macular or maculopapular rash
  - ◊ Petechial and purpuric exanthems have been reported
  - ◊ Rash location - trunk and upper arms; occasionally the face and forearms involved
  - ◊ Urticarial lesions on the abdomen, arms, legs

CAUSES The Epstein-Barr virus, a member of the herpesvirus (DNA virus) group.

RISK FACTORS
- Age
- Sociohygienic level
- Geographic location
- Close, intimate contact

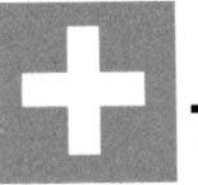

DIAGNOSIS

DIFFERENTIAL DIAGNOSIS
- Streptococcal pharyngitis and tonsillitis
- Diphtheria
- Blood dyscrasias
- Rubella
- Measles
- Viral hepatitis
- Cytomegalovirus
- Toxoplasmosis

LABORATORY
- Lymphocytes and atypical lymphocytes
  - ◊ Increased numbers of lymphocytes and atypical lymphocytes (may be up to 70% of leukocytes) in peripheral blood.
  - ◊ In the first week after onset of illness, the white blood cell count is normal or moderately decreased. By the second week, lymphocytosis develops with more than 10% atypical lymphocytes. Such cells vary in size and shape with indented, oval or horseshoe-shaped nuclei and basophilic, vacuolated, foamy cytoplasm.
  - ◊ During early illness, atypical lymphocytes are B cells transformed by EBV; later, the atypical cells are primarily T cells having immunoregulatory function
- Antibodies
  - ◊ Heterophil antibodies in 80-90% of adults.
  - ◊ The responsible heterophile antibody is an IgM response which appears during the first or second week of illness and persists for 3-6 months. Sheep cell agglutinins are not specific for IM and may occur in other conditions including serum sickness, infectious hepatitis, rubella, leukemia and Hodgkin disease; low titers may also be found in normal healthy individuals.
  - ◊ Differential absorption techniques distinguish these agglutinins from IM-associated heterophile antibodies. In general, the agglutinin titer is higher in IM than in other disorders; an unabsorbed heterophile titer greater than 1:128 and 1:40 or higher after absorption is significant.
- Specific antibodies to EBV-associated antigens
  - ◊ Develop regularly in IM
  - ◊ Viral capsid (VCA)-specific IgM and IgG are present early in illness; VCA-IgM responses disappear after several months whereas VCA-IgG antibodies persist for life.
  - ◊ Antibodies to EBV early antigen (EA) complexes, associated with viral replication, are present in 70-80% of patients during acute disease and usually disappear after 6 months
  - ◊ Antibodies to the EBV nuclear antigen complex (EBNA) appear slowly and develop 1-6 months after onset of illness

Drugs that may alter lab results: N/A

Disorders that may alter lab results: Atypical lymphocytes are not specific for Epstein-Barr infections and may be present in other clinical conditions including rubella, infectious hepatitis, allergic rhinitis, asthma and primary atypical pneumonia. In IM, increased numbers of atypical forms are present in peripheral blood whereas in other disorders the quantitative percentage is usually less.

PATHOLOGICAL FINDINGS
- Widespread focal and perivascular aggregates of mononuclear cells are found throughout the body
- Mononuclear infiltrations involve lymph nodes, tonsils, spleen, lungs, liver, heart, kidneys, adrenal glands, skin and central nervous system
- Bone marrow hyperplasia develops regularly and small granulomas may be present; these are non-specific and have no prognostic significance
- A polyclonal B cell proliferative response is characteristic of IM. Relatively few circulating lymphocytes are infected by EBV and represent less than 0.1% of circulating mononuclear cells in acute illness.

SPECIAL TESTS N/A

IMAGING Ultrasound, splenomegaly

DIAGNOSTIC PROCEDURES See under Laboratory

TREATMENT

APPROPRIATE HEALTH CARE Outpatient usually

GENERAL MEASURES
- The treatment is chiefly supportive
- During acute stage, rest in bed

SURGICAL MEASURES
- With profound thrombocytopenia, refractory to corticosteroid therapy, splenectomy may be necessary.

ACTIVITY
- Decided on an individual basis during convalescence
- Excess exertion, heavy lifting and participation in contact sports are prohibited during acute illness and also in the presence of splenomegaly. Rupture of the spleen may be fatal if not recognized and requires blood transfusions, treatment for shock, and splenectomy.

DIET
- Maintain adequate fluid intake
- Low fat, high carbohydrate diet
- Avoid alcohol for 6-8 months

PATIENT EDUCATION Reassurance and support

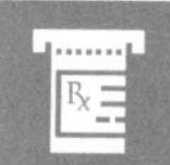

MEDICATIONS

DRUG(S) OF CHOICE

- Antimicrobial agents (usually a penicillin) if throat culture is positive for Group A, beta-hemolytic streptococci. Avoid ampicillin because of rash that occurs with ampicillin in mononucleosis.
- Aspirin and warm saline gargles for the pain of pharyngeal involvement and enlarged lymph nodes
- Codeine or meperidine, for unrelieved pain
- Corticosteroids
  - ◊ With severe pharyngotonsillitis with oropharyngeal edema and airway encroachment, a short course of corticosteroids may be utilized. Prednisone or its equivalent is used. Start with an initial dosage of 10-15 mg qid for 2 days. Decrease by 5 mg daily so that steroid treatment is discontinued in approximately 10 days.
  - ◊ Considered for patients with marked toxicity or major complications (e.g., hemolytic anemia, thrombocytopenic purpura, neurologic sequelae, myocarditis, pericarditis and severe generalized dermatologic lesions).

Contraindications: Steroids not recommended for mild, uncomplicated IM

Precautions: Refer to manufacturer's literature

Significant possible interactions: Refer to manufacturer's literature

ALTERNATIVE DRUGS N/A

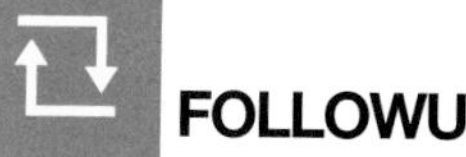

FOLLOWUP

PATIENT MONITORING

- Avoid contact sports, heavy lifting, and excess exertion until the spleen and liver have returned to normal size.
- Eliminate alcohol or exposure to other hepatotoxic drugs until liver function studies return to normal
- Monitor patients closely during the first 2-3 weeks after onset of symptoms. Thereafter follow until symptoms subside.
- Rarely, laboratory results resolve more slowly and symptoms (malaise, fatigue, intermittent sore throat, lymphadenopathy) may persist for several months

PREVENTION/AVOIDANCE N/A

POSSIBLE COMPLICATIONS

- Airway obstruction
- Hematologic or neurologic complications
- Toxemia
- Splenic rupture (rare); greatest risk is during the 2nd-3rd week of illness
- Hypersensitivity rash
  - ◊ Develops 7-10 days after initiation of ampicillin (or its analogues and other penicillins like methicillin) treatment; this generalized erythematous maculopapular eruption occurs mainly over the trunk and extremities, including palms and soles. Rash persists for a week; desquamation may continue for several days

EXPECTED COURSE/PROGNOSIS

- IM usually mild or moderate severity
- Acute symptoms 2-3 weeks with full recovery in 4-8 weeks

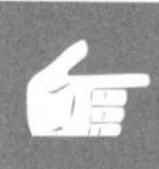

MISCELLANEOUS

ASSOCIATED CONDITIONS

- Infectious mononucleosis (IM): the symptomatic primary EBV infection seen in otherwise healthy older children, adolescents and young adults. Clinical features are variable in severity and duration; in children the disease is generally mild, whereas in adults it is more severe and protracted. The incubation period is 30-50 days.
- X-linked lymphoproliferative syndrome (Duncan disease)
- Lymphoproliferative syndromes due to EBV infections in transplant patients
- Lymphomas (B cell lymphoblastic, T cell)
- Lymphocytic interstitial pneumonitis
- Hairy leukoplakia of the tongue and central nervous system lymphomas in AIDS patients
- Burkitt lymphoma
- Nasopharyngeal carcinoma
- Parotid carcinoma
- Hodgkin disease

AGE-RELATED FACTORS

Pediatric:

- Infection during infancy and childhood usually subclinical and inapparent
- Clinical IM more common in older children and young adults

Geriatric: Heterophile positive IM has been reported in an elderly patient 5 weeks following blood transfusion

Others: N/A

PREGNANCY One large prospective study of pregnant women failed to demonstrate evidence of any intrauterine EBV infection. However, rare birth defects considered to be due to congenital EBV infection have been reported; such defects include cataracts, hypotonia, cryptorchidism and micrognathia.

SYNONYMS N/A

ICD-9-CM

075 Infectious mononucleosis

SEE ALSO

OTHER NOTES N/A

ABBREVIATIONS

IM = infectious mononucleosis

EBNA = Epstein-Barr nuclear antigen

REFERENCES

- Halstead ME, Bernhardt DT. Common infections in the young athlete. Pediatr Ann 2002;31(1):42-8
- Schooley R. Epstein-Barr Infections. In: Mandell GL. Bennett JE. Dolin R, editors. Principles and Practices of Infectious Diseases. 5th ed. Philadelphia: Churchill Livingston; 2000
- Cohen J. Epstein-Barr virus infection. New Engl J Med 2000;343:481-92

Web references: 0 available at www.5mcc.com

Illustrations N/A

Author(s):

Dennis E. Hughes, DO

BASICS

DESCRIPTION Dissatisfaction with size, rigidity, or duration of erection. Male sexual dysfunction encompasses an even larger group of complaints and disorders of arousal, desire, orgasm, sensation, and relationship. Transient periods of impotence occur in about half of adult males and are not considered dysfunctional.

System(s) affected: Cardiovascular, Nervous, Renal/Urologic, Reproductive

Genetics: Rarely related to chromosomal disorders

Incidence/Prevalence in USA: Erectile failure involves about 10% of men, but is underreported by patients

Predominant age:

- Patients with psychologic, gender, and primary organic problems often present themselves for help between adolescence and the third decade
- Patients with relationship problems, but concerned mainly about physical problems, tend to seek care in the sixth decade
- Most patients with physical problems are in the seventh and eighth decade, but rarely seek help

Predominant sex: Male only

SIGNS & SYMPTOMS

- Reduction of erectile size and rigidity
- Inability to maintain erection
- Inability to achieve erection
- Reduced body hair
- Thyromegaly
- Gynecomastia
- Testicular atrophy or absence
- Deformed penis
- Peripheral vascular disease
- Neuropathy

CAUSES

- Endocrine
- Neurologic
- Vascular
- Medication(s)
- Psychological
- Structural

RISK FACTORS

- Prior pelvic surgery
- Medication use
- Risk factors for disorders listed in Causes

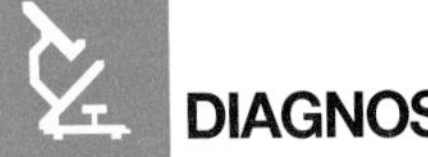

DIAGNOSIS

DIFFERENTIAL DIAGNOSIS

- Endocrine
  - ◊ Low or high thyroxine
  - ◊ Low testosterone
  - ◊ High prolactin
  - ◊ Diabetes
  - ◊ High estrogen effect
  - ◊ Renal failure
  - ◊ Zinc deficiency
- Neurological
  - ◊ Central
  - ◊ Spinal
  - ◊ Peripheral
- Vascular
  - ◊ Arterial insufficiency
  - ◊ Cavernosal insufficiency
  - ◊ Venous insufficiency
- Medication
  - ◊ Many types, e.g., beta-blockers, thiazides
- Psychological
  - ◊ Depression
  - ◊ Schizophrenia
  - ◊ Relationship disorders
  - ◊ Personality disorders
  - ◊ Anxiety
- Structural
  - ◊ Microphallus
  - ◊ Chordee and Peyronie disease
  - ◊ Cavernosal scarring
  - ◊ Phimosis
  - ◊ Hypospadias
  - ◊ Postsurgical sequelae

LABORATORY

- CBC
- BMP (glucose, K+, Na+, BUN, Cr)
- Albumin
- TSH
- Prolactin
- Free testosterone (morning sample)

Drugs that may alter lab results: N/A

Disorders that may alter lab results: N/A

PATHOLOGICAL FINDINGS Most men over age 55 will have some test abnormality or risk factor, but it is not necessarily the cause of the patient's erectile dysfunction

SPECIAL TESTS

- 24 hour urine zinc
- Dorsal nerve somatosensory evoked potentials
- Sacral evoked response
- Penile-brachial blood pressures
- Aortogram
- Selective pudendal angiogram
- Dynamic cavernosography
- Nocturnal penile tumescence (NPT) testing
- Penile blood pressure

IMAGING Doppler, angiogram, cavernosogram

DIAGNOSTIC PROCEDURES Response to papaverine or alprostadil injection

TREATMENT

APPROPRIATE HEALTH CARE Since erectile dysfunction is multifactorial, evaluation by a generalist in an outpatient setting

GENERAL MEASURES

- Early use of penile implants is now discouraged because of success with vacuum erectile devices, sensate focus therapy, injection therapy and oral therapy
- Improve partner communication
- Reduce performance pressure
- Use sensate focus therapy
- Try vacuum erectile device or oral therapy (and can be used in conjunction with intracavernous injections)
- Use of psychiatrists, psychologists, sex therapists, vascular surgeons, urologists, endocrinologists, neurologists, plastic surgeons, etc., often necessary for refractory cases

SURGICAL MEASURES N/A

ACTIVITY No restrictions

DIET Control diabetes if present

PATIENT EDUCATION The New Male Sexuality by Bernie Zilbergeld, PhD., Bantam Books, 1992; and problem-specific handouts

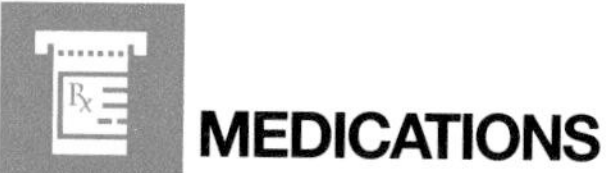

MEDICATIONS

DRUG(S) OF CHOICE
- Erection induction: Prostaglandins
  - ◊ Intracavernous injection (1/2", 30 gauge needle), starting with 0.1 mL

Compounded intracavernousal solution:

Drug	Amt	Conc/mL
PGE-1(500mcg/mL)	50mcg	6.6mcg
Papaverine(300mg/10mL)	150mg	20mg
Phentolamine	5mg	0.67mg
Bacteriostatic NaCl	QS 7.5mL	

Compounds 7.5mL; usual dose 0.1-0.5mL

or
  - ◊ Alprostadil (Caverject) 10-20 µg/mL; inject into the dorsolateral aspect of proximal third of the penis. Do not exceed 60 mg dose. Do not use more than 3 times a week or more than once in 24 hours. Patient to notify physician if erection lasts > 6 hours for immediate attention.
  - ◊ Alprostadil (Muse) urethral suppository 125 mg, 250 mg, 500 mg, and 1000 mg pellets. Maximum of 2 uses in 24 hrs.
- Erection induction: Phosphodiesterase type 5 (PDE-5) inhibitors
  - ◊ Sildenafil (Viagra) 25 mg, 50 mg, or 100 mg tablets. Usual dose, 50 mg 1 hr prior to sexual activity. Duration up to 4 hrs.
  - ◊ Vardenafil (Levitra) 2.5 mg, 5 mg, 10 mg, 20 mg tablets. Usual dose, 10 mg 1 hr prior to sexual activity. Duration up to 4 hrs.
  - ◊ Tadalafil (Cialis) 5mg, 10 mg, 20 mg tablets. Usual dose, 10 mg 1 hr prior to sexual activity. Duration up to 36 hrs.
- Miscellaneous
  - ◊ Testosterone cypionate 200 mg IM every two weeks when hypogonadism is present. Testosterone patch or gel also available.
  - ◊ Bromocriptine 2.5 mg bid up to 40 mg/day when hyperprolactinemia is present

Contraindications:
- Injections should be avoided in patients with bleeding disorders, patients with sickle cell disease or trait, and in patients with penile deformities.
- Avoid use in patients with known allergies to constituents
- Nitroglycerin (or other nitrates) & phosphodiesterase inhibitors - potential for severe, potentially fatal, hypotension

Precautions:
- Testosterone: urinary retention, acne, sodium retention and gynecomastia
- Bromocriptine: self-limited nausea, vomiting
- Injection therapy: priapism, fibrosis, hypotension and nausea
- Urethral suppositories: penile pain and irritation, as well as testicular pain. No reports yet of priapism.
- Sildenafil: hypotension
- PDE-5 inhibitors: use caution with congential prolonged QT syndrome, class Ia or II antiarrhythmics, NTG, alpha-blockers (e.g., terazosin, tamsulosin), retinal disease, unstable cardiac disease, liver and renal failure.

Significant possible interactions:
- PDE-5 inhibitor concentration is affected by CYP3A4 inhibitors (e.g., erythromycin, indinavir, ketoconazole, and ritonavir, amiodarone, cimetidine, clarithromycin, delavirdine, diltiazem, fluoxetine, fluvoxamine, grapefruit juice, itraconazole, nefazodone, nevirapine, ritonavir, saquinavir, and verapamil). Serum concentrations and/or toxicity may be increased. When used with these drugs reduce the dose of PDE-5 inhibitor (1/2 of the usual initial dose q 3 days).
- PDE-5 inhibitor concentration may be reduced by rifampin and phenytoin

ALTERNATIVE DRUGS N/A

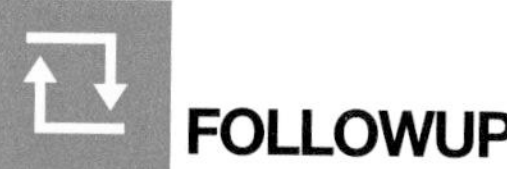

FOLLOWUP

PATIENT MONITORING Meet with patient and, if possible, his partner, as required by cause, therapy, and response

PREVENTION/AVOIDANCE Since erectile dysfunction is multifactorial, referral to a sex therapist or couples therapist may help to speed recovery and prevent future problems

POSSIBLE COMPLICATIONS Specific to therapy

EXPECTED COURSE/PROGNOSIS
- Given that the majority of patients have unspecified causes of their erectile disorders, vacuum erection device, injection or suppository therapy with alprostadil, oral sildenafil and penile implant have improved the outlook greatly
- Expect 20% failure rate of vacuum erection device, high drop-out rate from injection therapy, and a 10-30% non-use rate for penile implants
- Spontaneous cure rate is about 15%
- Studies indicate a response rate of 40-60% for urethral alprostadil compared to 85-90% for the injection
- Sildenafil and other PDE-5 inhibitors are effective in 70% of men at maximum dose, but are less effective in patients with diabetes and those who have had a prostatectomy for cancer

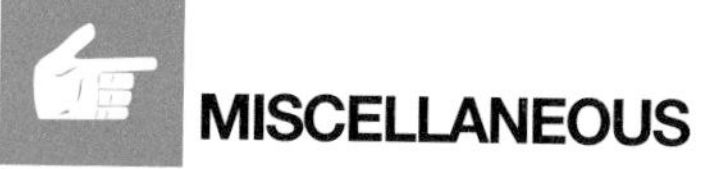

MISCELLANEOUS

ASSOCIATED CONDITIONS N/A

AGE-RELATED FACTORS
Pediatric: N/A
Geriatric: Aging alone is not a cause of impotence
Others: N/A

PREGNANCY N/A

SYNONYMS Impotence

ICD-9-CM
302.70 Psychosexual dysfunction, unspecified
302.71 Psychosexual dysfunction with inhibited sexual desire
302.72 Psychosexual dysfunction with inhibited sexual excitement
302.9 Unspecified psychosexual disorder
V41.7 Problems with sexual function
607.84 Impotence of organic origin

SEE ALSO
Priapism

OTHER NOTES N/A

ABBREVIATIONS N/A

REFERENCES

- Montague D. Disorders of Male Sexual Dysfunction. Boca Raton, Year Book Medical Publishers, 1988
- Wagner G, Green R. Impotence. New York, Plenum Press, 1981
- Segraves RT, Schoenberg HW: Diagnosis and Treatment of Erectile Disturbances. New York, Plenum Medical Book Company, 1985
- Evans C. The use of penile prostheses in the treatment of impotence. [Review] [25 refs]. Brit J of Urology 1998:81(4):591-8
- Gingell JC. New developments in self-injection therapy for erectile dysfunction. [Review] [33 refs]. Brit J of Urology 1998:81(4):599-603
- Lue TF. Erectile dysfunction. New Engl J Med 2000;342(24):1802-1813
- Gholami SS, Gonzalez-Cadavid NF, et al. Peyronie's disease: a review. J Urol 2003;169(4):1234-41
- Schover LR, Fouladi RT, Warneke CL, et al. The use of treatments for erectile dysfunction among survivors of prostate carcinoma. Cancer 2002;95(11):2397-407

Web references: 0 available at www.5mcc.com
Illustrations 1 available

Author(s):
Bruce Block, MD

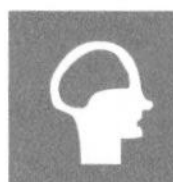

BASICS

DESCRIPTION Bacterial cellulitis involving the superficial skin and lymphatics usually due to group A streptococcus. Usually acute, but a chronic recurrent form also exists.
System(s) affected: Skin/Exocrine
Genetics: N/A
Incidence/Prevalence in USA: Unknown
Predominant age: Usually infants and adults over 40. Greatest in elderly (> 75 years).
Predominant sex: Male = Female

SIGNS & SYMPTOMS
- Prodrome of malaise, fever and chills
- Headache, vomiting are prominent
- Arthralgias
- Pruritus
- Skin discomfort
- Vesicles
- Facial redness
- Acute onset of erythema
- Begins as erythematous patch
- Sharply demarcated raised border
- Center of lesion clears as periphery spreads
- Desquamation and vesicle formation can occur
- Face is the most common area involved, especially nose and ears
- Chronic form may recur hours to years after initial episode
- Chronic form usually recurs at site of the previous infection
- Fever is usually the differentiating factor among similar skin manifestations

CAUSES Group A beta-hemolytic streptococcus primarily; occasionally other strep groups or staph

RISK FACTORS
- Operative wounds
- Fissured skin (especially at the nose and ears)
- Any inflamed skin
- Traumatic wounds/abrasions
- Leg ulcers/stasis dermatitis
- Chronic diseases (diabetes, malnutrition, nephrotic syndrome)
- Immunocompromised or debilitated individual

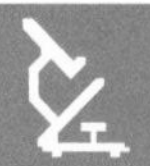

DIAGNOSIS

DIFFERENTIAL DIAGNOSIS
- Erysipeloid (little toxicity)
- Contact dermatitis (no fever)
- Angioneurotic edema (no fever)
- Scarlet fever (usually more widespread without edema)
- Lupus (of the face, less fever, positive antinuclear antibodies)
- Polychondritis (of the ear)
- Dermatophytid
- Tuberculoid leprosy

LABORATORY
- Leukocytosis (usually > 15,000)
- Strep may be cultured from exudate or from non-involved sites
- Antistreptolysin (ASO), streptozyme, anti-DNase may be helpful
- Blood culture (< 5% positive)

Drugs that may alter lab results: N/A

Disorders that may alter lab results: N/A

PATHOLOGICAL FINDINGS
- Edema
- Vasodilation and enlarged lymphatics
- Infiltration of polymorphonuclear leukocytes, lymphocytes and other inflammatory cells
- Endothelial cell swelling
- Gram positive cocci

SPECIAL TESTS N/A

IMAGING N/A

DIAGNOSTIC PROCEDURES None

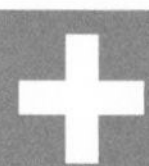

TREATMENT

APPROPRIATE HEALTH CARE Outpatient

GENERAL MEASURES
- Symptomatic treatment of aches and fever
- Adequate fluid intake
- Local treatment with cold compresses

SURGICAL MEASURES N/A

ACTIVITY Bedrest with activity based on severity of illness

DIET No special diet

PATIENT EDUCATION Importance of completing medication regimen prescribed

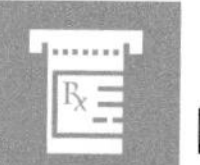

MEDICATIONS

DRUG(S) OF CHOICE
- Penicillin V (Pen VK) for at least ten days (improvement in 24-48 hours). Children: 90 mg/kg/day divided q6h; adults: 500 mg/dose q6h (approximately 1000 mg bid).
- Parenteral antibiotics are recommended for severe or complicated cases (1-2 million units every 4-6 hours)
- In chronic recurrent infections some authors recommend lower dose daily maintenance/prophylactic treatment after the acute infection resolves

Contraindications: Penicillin allergy
Precautions: Refer to manufacturer's profile of each drug
Significant possible interactions: Refer to manufacturer's profile of each drug

ALTERNATIVE DRUGS
- Erythromycin. Children: 30-40 mg/kg/day divided q6h; adults: 250 mg/dose q6h.
- Clarithromycin total 1000 mg/day
- Azithromycin
- Cephalosporins
- Consider penicillinase-resistant penicillin such as dicloxacillin 500 mg q6h in facial involvement due to possible staph

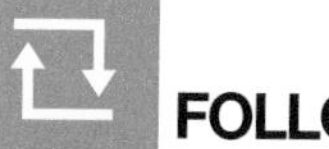

FOLLOWUP

PATIENT MONITORING
Patients should be treated until all symptoms and skin manifestations have resolved

PREVENTION/AVOIDANCE
- Maintenance antibiotics for chronic recurrent cases
- Men who shave within five days of facial erysipelas are more likely to have a recurrence
- In recurrent cases, search for other possible source of streptococcal infection (e.g., tonsils, sinuses, teeth, toenails, etc.)

POSSIBLE COMPLICATIONS
- Bacteremia
- Scarlet fever
- Pneumonia
- Abscess
- Embolism
- Gangrene
- Meningitis
- Sepsis
- Death

EXPECTED COURSE/PROGNOSIS
- Adequate treatment results in full recovery
- Chronic edema/scarring can result from chronic recurrent cases
- Rarely elephantiasis may result from chronic recurrent cases
- Untreated cases sometimes will resolve spontaneously

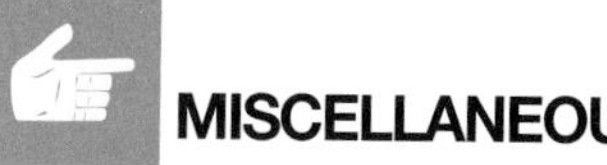

MISCELLANEOUS

ASSOCIATED CONDITIONS
N/A

AGE-RELATED FACTORS
Pediatric:
- Group B strep may be a cause in neonates/infants
- Abdominal involvement more common in infants
- Face, scalp, and leg common in older children

Geriatric:
- Fever may not be as prominent
- More prone to complications
- High output cardiac failure may occur in debilitated patients with underlying cardiac disease
- Face and lower extremity most common areas

Others: N/A

PREGNANCY
N/A

SYNONYMS
- Saint Anthony fire
- Ignis sacer

ICD-9-CM
035 Erysipelas

SEE ALSO

OTHER NOTES
Patients on systemic steroids may be more difficult to diagnose since signs and symptoms of the infection may be masked by anti-inflammatory action of the steroids

ABBREVIATIONS
N/A

REFERENCES

- Fitzpatrick TB, et al: Color Atlas and Synopsis of Clinical Dermatology. 2nd Ed. New York, McGraw-Hill, 1992
- Sauer R: Manual of Skin Diseases. Philadelphia, J.B. Lippincott, 1985
- Domonkos AN, Arnold HL, Odom RB: Andrew's Diseases of the Skin. 8th Ed. Philadelphia, W.B. Saunders Co., 1990
- Wherle PF, Tops FH Sr: Communicable and Infectious Diseases. St. Louis, C.V. Mosby, 1981
- Fitzpatrick TB, et al, eds: Dermatology in General Medicine. 3rd Ed. New York, McGraw-Hill, 1987
- Bratton RL, Nesse RE. St. Anthony's Fire: diagnosis and management of erysipelas. Am Fam Physician 1995;51(2):401-4
- Gilbert D, et al. The Sanford Guide to Antimicrobial Therapy 2003. Hyde Park, New York: Antimicrobial Therapy, Inc; 2003

Web references: 1 available at www.5mcc.com
Illustrations N/A

Author(s):
Scott A. Kincaid, MD

BASICS

DESCRIPTION
Erythema multiforme (EM) is an acute self limited hypersensitivity reaction involving the skin and sometimes the mucus membranes. Erythema multiforme minor- also called the erythema multiforme - Hebra, is a mild form appearing as a pleomorphic rash which includes target lesions, but not large vesicles or petechia, affecting the skin with or without involving one mucus membrane site. Erythema multiforme major is a more severe form, involving more than one mucus membrane site. While many authors consider this to be the same as Stevens-Johnson syndrome, there appears to be a growing consensus that EM and SJS are unrelated.

System(s) affected: Skin/exocrine
Genetics: Possibly associated with HLA-B15
Incidence/Prevalence in USA: Not known. In Germany the incidence of erythema multiforme major, Stevens Johnson syndrome and toxic epidermal necrolysis combined appears to be 0.189/100,000 persons per year.
Predominant age: Peak incidence in 20's and 30's; rare under 3 and over age 50
Predominant sex: Male > Female (3:2)

SIGNS & SYMPTOMS
- The typical pleomorphic eruption is a mixture of macules of various sizes and target lesions. These consist of a central inflamed and superficially necrotic area, surrounded by a halo of less inflamed skin, enclosed within an outer erythematous rim. Purpuric lesions are uncommon, and vesicles may be related to antecedent herpes 1 infections. The rash occurs on the palms, soles, dorsum of the hands and extensor surface of the extremities and the face. It is often recurrent, following a viral infection.
- Involvement of the mucus membranes is quite common, which caused confusion with Stevens Johnson syndrome. In EM mucus membrane involvement consists of target lesions of the lips or herpetic lesions without extensive necrosis.
- Pruritus is usually absent
- The skin may feel normal, or there may be a mild burning sensation.
- If corneal ulceration occurs it is a serious complication

CAUSES
- Most cases appear to be due to a preceding infection. Drugs seem to be an infrequent cause.
- Viral infections - particularly herpes simplex; also Epstein-Barr, Coxsackie, echovirus, varicella, mumps and poliovirus
- Bacterial infections- including Brucellosis, diphtheria (etc.), borreliosis. Mycoplasma appears to more often precede Stevens-Johnson syndrome.
- Protozoan infections
- Fungal infection, including *Trichophyton rubrum*
- Collagen vascular diseases
- Malignancy
- Pregnancy
- Premenstrual hormone changes
- Consumption of beer
- Reiter syndrome
- Sarcoidosis
- Vaccines- tetanus/diphtheria (Td), bacillus Calmette-Guerin (BCG), oral polio vaccine (OPV)
- Medications- the accepted list includes sulfonamides, penicillins, anticonvulsants, salicylates, but many of these were actually associated with Stevens Johnson syndrome when it was considered to be a type of erythema nodosum major
- Radiotherapy

RISK FACTORS
- Previous history of erythema multiforme
- Male sex

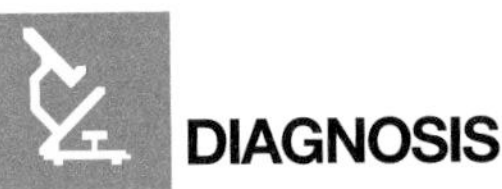

DIAGNOSIS

DIFFERENTIAL DIAGNOSIS
- Stevens Johnson syndrome
- Urticaria
- Necrotizing vasculitis
- Drug eruptions
- Contact dermatitis
- Pityriasis rosea
- Secondary syphilis
- Ringworm
- Pemphigus vulgaris
- Pemphigoid
- Dermatitis herpetiformis
- Herpes gestationis
- Septicemia
- Serum sickness
- Viral exanthems
- Rocky Mountain spotted fever
- Collagen vascular diseases
- Mucocutaneous lymph node syndrome
- Meningococcemia
- Lichen planus
- Behçet syndrome
- Recurrent aphthous ulcers
- Herpetic gingivostomatitis
- Granuloma annulare

LABORATORY None

Drugs that may alter lab results: N/A

Disorders that may alter lab results: N/A

PATHOLOGICAL FINDINGS
A predominantly inflammatory pattern characterized by a lichenoid infiltrate which is of high density and rich in T-lymphocytes, and epidermal necrosis that mainly affects the basal layer

SPECIAL TESTS N/A

IMAGING N/A

DIAGNOSTIC PROCEDURES Skin biopsy

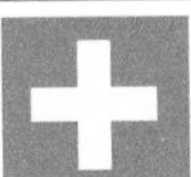

TREATMENT

APPROPRIATE HEALTH CARE
Care at home, unless mouth herpes precludes oral intake.

GENERAL MEASURES
- Treatment of any underlying or causative disease
- Withdrawal of any causative drugs
- For mild cases, symptomatic treatment is sufficient. For more severe cases, meticulous wound care and use of Burow's solution or Domeboro solution dressings.
- Oral lesions can be treated with mouthwashes with warm saline, or a solution of diphenhydramine, lidocaine (Xylocaine), and Kaopectate to provide symptomatic relief and oral hygiene, and to facilitate oral intake

SURGICAL MEASURES N/A

ACTIVITY As tolerated

DIET As tolerated with increased fluid intake

PATIENT EDUCATION
Patients should be reassured that the disease is self-limited. Recurrences are possible. Encourage avoidance of any identified etiologic agent.

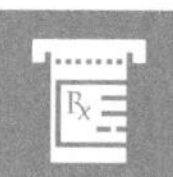

MEDICATIONS

DRUG(S) OF CHOICE The use of steroids is controversial. Patients who have recurrent herpes-induced EM may benefit from acyclovir, by reducing the number of herpetic episodes. Other causative infections should be treated appropriately.
Contraindications: Some underlying infections or health problems such as diabetes may contraindicate the use of steroids
Precautions: Refer to manufacturer's profile of each drug
Significant possible interactions: Refer to manufacturer's profile of each drug

ALTERNATIVE DRUGS None have been shown to be useful

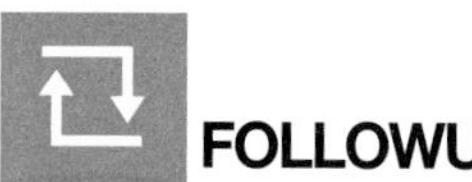

FOLLOWUP

PATIENT MONITORING The disease is self-limiting. Complications are rare with no mortality.

PREVENTION/AVOIDANCE
- Known or suspected etiologic agents should be avoided
- Acyclovir may help prevent herpes-related erythema multiforme
- Tamoxifen has been shown to prevent premenstrual related disease

POSSIBLE COMPLICATIONS Corneal ulceration is a serious complication of Stevens-Johnson syndrome. It is not clear whether this can occur in true EM. While there may be complications of the underlying disease, there are no other complications of EM.

EXPECTED COURSE/PROGNOSIS
- Rash evolves over 1-2 weeks and subsequently resolves within 2-3 weeks, generally without scarring or sequelae
- Following resolution there may be some post-inflammatory hyperpigmentation
- Risk of recurrence may be as high as 37%

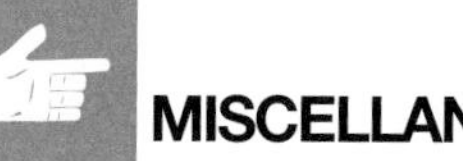

MISCELLANEOUS

ASSOCIATED CONDITIONS
Any of the infections or diseases listed under causes.

AGE-RELATED FACTORS
Pediatric: More severe forms of the disease tend to occur in younger males. Rare under age 3 years.
Geriatric: Rare over age 50 years
Others: N/A

PREGNANCY Reported as a possible etiologic condition

SYNONYMS Erythema exudativum multiforme

ICD-9-CM
695.1 Erythema multiforme

SEE ALSO
Dermatitis, contact
Dermatitis, herpetiformis
Herpes gestationis
Pemphigus vulgaris
Pityriasis rosea
Serum sickness
Stevens-Johnson syndrome
Tinea corporis
Urticaria

OTHER NOTES Because it is an immunologic reaction, drug-related erythema multiforme will not occur until 7-14 days after exposure to the offending agent, unless the patient has had the medication previously

ABBREVIATIONS N/A

REFERENCES

- Saunders Electronic Atlas of Dermatology. Philadelphia, WB Saunders Co, 1996
- Rzany B, et al: Epidemiology of erythema exudativum multiforme majus, Stevens-Johnson syndrome, and toxic epidermal necrolysis in Germany (1991-1992): structure and results of a population-based registry. Journal of Clinical Epidemiology 1996;49(7):769-773
- Weston WL, et al: Target lesions on the lips: childhood herpes simplex associated with erythema multiforme mimics Stevens-Johnson syndrome. Journal of the American Academy of Dermatology 1997;37(5 pt2):848-850
- Assier H, et al: Erythema multiforme with mucous membrane involvement and Stevens-Johnson syndrome are clinically different disorders with distinct causes. Archives of Dermatology 1995;131(5):539-543
- Tay YK, et al: Mycoplasma pneumonia infection is associated with Stevens-Johnson syndrome, not erythema multiforme (von Hebra) Journal of the American Academy of Dermatology 1996;35(5pt1):757-760
- Rahman SA, et al: Erythema multiforme associated with superficial fungal disease. Cutis. 1995 ;55(4):329-351
- Vaness MJ, Dwyer PK: Erythema multiforme-like reaction associated with radiotherapy. Australian Radiology 1996;40(3):334-347
- Cote B, et al: Clinicopathological correlation in erythema multiforme and Stevens-Johnson syndrome. Archives of Dermatology 1995;131(11):1268-1272
- Paquet P, Pierard GE: Erythema multiforme and toxic epidermal necrolysis: a comparative study. American Journal of Dermatopathology 1997;19(2):127-132
- Kakourou T, et al: Corticosteroid treatment of erythema multiforme major (Stevens-Johnson syndrome) in children. European Journal of Pediatrics 1997;156(2):90-93
- Revuz JE, Roujeau JC: Advances in toxic epidermal necrolysis. Seminars in Cutaneous Medicine & Surgery 1966;15(4):258-266

Web references: 1 available at www.5mcc.com
Illustrations 4 available

Author(s):
Lewis C. Rose, MD

BASICS

DESCRIPTION Clinical pattern of multiple, bilateral, cutaneous, inflammatory, non-ulcerating, non-scarring eruptions that undergo characteristic color changes ending in temporary bruise-like areas. Occurs most commonly on the extensor surface of the shins, less common on thighs and forearms. It is often idiopathic, but may be seen as a response to a variety of clinical entities. Will usually subside in 3 to 6 weeks without scarring or atrophy.
System(s) affected: Skin/Exocrine
Genetics: N/A
Incidence/Prevalence in USA: Unknown
Predominant age: 20-30 years
Predominant sex: Female > Male (3:1)

SIGNS & SYMPTOMS
- Initially raised, warm, tender, brightly erythematous nodules on anterior shins. Lesions become bluish and fluctuant, gradually fading to yellowish resembling a bruise
- Can also occur on any area with subcutaneous fat
- Diameter 1-15 cm
- Fever, malaise, chills
- Hilar adenopathy
- Episcleral lesions
- Eruptions often preceded by URI symptoms
- Headache
- Arthralgias (rare)

CAUSES
- Idiopathic (37-60%)
- Bacterial - streptococcal infections (most common cause in children), tuberculosis, leprosy, Yersinia enterocolitica, tularemia, Campylobacter, salmonella, Shigella, gonorrhea
- Sarcoid
- Drugs - sulfonamides, oral contraceptives, bromides
- Pregnancy
- Deep fungal - dermatophytes, coccidioidomycosis, histoplasmosis, blastomycosis
- Viral/chlamydial - infectious mononucleosis, lymphogranuloma venereum, paravaccinia
- Enteropathies - ulcerative colitis, Crohn disease
- Malignancies - lymphoma/leukemia, sarcoma, post radiation therapy

RISK FACTORS Listed with Causes

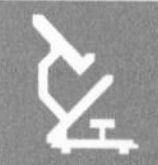

DIAGNOSIS

DIFFERENTIAL DIAGNOSIS
- Superficial thrombophlebitis
- Cellulitis
- Septic emboli
- Erythema induratum (cold, ulcerating nodules on calves)
- Nodular vasculitis (warm, ulcerating nodules)
- Weber-Christian disease (violaceous, scarring nodules)
- Lupus panniculitis
- Cutaneous polyarteritis nodosa
- Sarcoidosis granulomata
- Cutaneous T cell lymphoma
- Erythema nodosum leprosum

LABORATORY
- Elevated erythrocyte sedimentation rate
- CBC: mild leukocytosis
- Throat culture, ASO titers (throat culture usually not positive because infection typically resolves before lesions appear)
- Stool culture and leukocytes if indicated
- Skin testing for mycobacteria if indicated

Drugs that may alter lab results: Antecedent antibiotics may affect cultures

Disorders that may alter lab results: N/A

PATHOLOGICAL FINDINGS
- Septal panniculitis
- Neutrophilic infiltrate in septa of fat tissue, early in course
- Fibrosis, periseptal granulation tissue, lymphocytes and multinucleated giant cells predominate late in course
- Lower dermis/subcutis involvement and septal fibrosis may occur

SPECIAL TESTS N/A

IMAGING Chest x-ray for hilar adenopathy or infiltrates

DIAGNOSTIC PROCEDURES Deep skin excisional biopsy including subcutaneous fat. Usually not necessary.

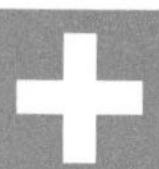

TREATMENT

APPROPRIATE HEALTH CARE Outpatient

GENERAL MEASURES
- Wet dressings (hot soaks and topical medications are not useful)
- Discontinue potentially causative drugs
- Treat underlying disease

SURGICAL MEASURES N/A

ACTIVITY
- Bedrest, keep legs elevated
- Elastic wraps or support stockings may be helpful if patients want to be up and around

DIET No restrictions

PATIENT EDUCATION
- Lesions will resolve over a few months
- No scarring is anticipated
- Joint aches and pains may persist
- Less than 20% recur

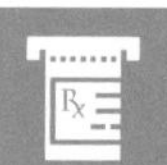

MEDICATIONS

DRUG(S) OF CHOICE
- Medication usually more effective after initial onset versus with chronic disease
- Condition often self-limited
- Nonsteroidal anti-inflammatory drugs (NSAIDs):
  - ◊ Indomethacin: 75-150 mg per day, divided tid
  - ◊ Naproxen (Naprosyn): 500-1000 mg per day, divided bid
  - ◊ Aspirin: 325 mg 8-12 per day; use enteric coated to decrease GI upset. Titrate to blood levels.

Contraindications:
- Active or recent peptic ulcer disease
- History of NSAIDs hypersensitivity

Precautions:
- Gastrointestinal upset/bleeding
- Fluid retention
- Dose reduction in elderly, especially those with renal disease, diabetes, heart failure
- May mask fever
- NSAIDs may elevate liver function tests

Significant possible interactions:
- May blunt antihypertensive effects of diuretics and beta-blockers
- NSAIDs can elevate plasma lithium levels
- Caution advised with naproxen or any highly protein-bound drug since it may compete for albumin binding and elevate levels
- NSAIDs can cause significant elevation and prolongation of methotrexate levels

ALTERNATIVE DRUGS
- Potassium iodide 400-900 mg daily, divided bid-tid for 3-4 weeks (for persistent lesions)
- Corticosteroids only in very severe, refractory cases
- Other NSAIDs
- Recent reports of improvement with colchicine 0.6-1.2 mg bid

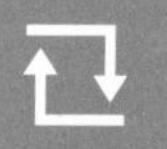

FOLLOWUP

PATIENT MONITORING Monthly followup or as dictated by underlying disorder

PREVENTION/AVOIDANCE N/A

POSSIBLE COMPLICATIONS Vary according to underlying disease. None expected from lesions of erythema nodosum.

EXPECTED COURSE/PROGNOSIS
- Individual lesions resolve over 3-6 week course
- Total time course of 6-12 weeks, but may vary with etiologic disease if present
- Joint aches and pains may persist for years
- Lesions do not scar
- One or more recurrences in 12-14% of cases; these occur over variable periods, averaging several years, seen most often with sarcoid, streptococcal infection, pregnancy, and oral contraceptives

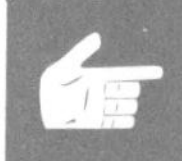

MISCELLANEOUS

ASSOCIATED CONDITIONS See Causes

AGE-RELATED FACTORS
Pediatric: Incidence equal male and female
Geriatric: N/A
Others: N/A

PREGNANCY May have repeat outbreaks during pregnancy

SYNONYMS Dermatitis contusiformis

ICD-9-CM
695.2 Erythema nodosum

SEE ALSO

OTHER NOTES
- Lofgren syndrome (erythema nodosum and hilar adenopathy) is seen with multiple etiologies and does not exclusively indicate sarcoid
- Clinical variant of erythema nodosum migrans (subacute nodular migratory panniculitis) is often unilateral with nodules fewer in number, smaller in size and longer lasting, often extending radially by division into smaller nodules
- In patients with a history of Hodgkin disease, erythema nodosum is a warning of impending recurrence

ABBREVIATIONS N/A

REFERENCES

- Fitzpatrick TB, Eisen AZ, et al, editors. Dermatology in General Medicine. 5th ed. New York: McGraw-Hill; 1999
- Habif T. Clinical Dermatology. 4th Ed. St. Louis, CV Mosby, 2004
- Hannuksela M. Erythema nodosum. Clin Dermatol 1986;4(4):88-95
- Gonzalez-Gay MA, Garcia-Porrua C, Pujol RM, Salvarani C. Erythema nodosum: a clinical approach. Clin Exp Rheumatol 2001;19(4):365-8
- Requena L, Requena C. Erythema nodosum. Dermatol Online J 2002;8(1):4

Web references: 1 available at www.5mcc.com
Illustrations 3 available

Author(s):
Bruce T. Vanderhoff, MD
Matthew Hintz, MD

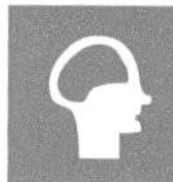

BASICS

DESCRIPTION Hemolytic anemia of the fetus or newborn caused by transplacental transmission of maternal antibody. When severe, the anemia can result in extramedullary hematopoiesis, secondary organ dysfunction, heart failure, hydrops, and death. The name erythroblastosis refers to the presence of immature erythrocytes in the peripheral blood from accelerated hematopoiesis.
System(s) affected: Cardiovascular, Hemic/Lymphatic/Immunologic, Nervous
Genetics: Can occur when the fetus inherits a paternal blood group antigen lacking in the mother. The Rh D antigen is most frequently implicated. (For more on inheritance of Rh antigens, see Rh incompatibility.)
Incidence/Prevalence in USA:
- Uncommon
- About 9% of pregnancies have an Rh-negative mother with an Rh-positive fetus
- With Rho(D) immune globulin prophylaxis, risk of sensitization is reduced to less than 1% of susceptible pregnancies

Predominant age: Fetus and newborn
Predominant sex: Male = Female

SIGNS & SYMPTOMS
- Pallor
- Respiratory distress
- Hepatomegaly
- Splenomegaly
- Ascites
- Hypotension/shock
- Edema/anasarca/hydrops
- Jaundice of newborn
- Purpura/bleeding problems
- Fetal death in utero

CAUSES
- Maternal isoimmunization to Rh antigen by transfusion of Rh-positive blood
- Maternal isoimmunization from exposure to fetal Rh antigens in prior pregnancy or current pregnancy
- Maternal isoimmunization to other blood group antigens (Kell, Duffy, Kidd, M, S, Diego, etc.) is unusual but may cause serious disease

RISK FACTORS
- Prior transfusion with incompatible blood
- Any Rh-positive pregnancy in Rh-negative woman
- Without prophylactic immunotherapy (Rh immune globulin), risk of Rh sensitization is up to 16% during or after term pregnancy, about 3% for spontaneous abortion and 5-6% for surgical abortion
- Sensitization by exposure to fetal blood can occur also with ectopic pregnancy, amniocentesis, chorionic villus sampling, placental trauma or manipulation, placental abruption
- Prophylaxis with Rh immune globulin greatly reduces but does not eliminate the risk

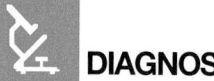

DIAGNOSIS

DIFFERENTIAL DIAGNOSIS
- Fetal blood loss anemia
- Twin-to-twin transfusion
- Arteriovenous or cardiac malformations
- Hereditary hemolytic anemias
- Drug-induced hemolytic anemia
- Nonimmune fetal hydrops
- Hemolysis from intrauterine infection (syphilis, toxoplasmosis, CMV, others)

LABORATORY
- Positive indirect Coombs test (antibody screen) during pregnancy
- Positive direct Coombs test in fetus or newborn
- Anemia in fetus or newborn
- Reticulocytosis
- Nucleated RBC's on differential count
- Hyperbilirubinemia (indirect bilirubin)
- Thrombocytopenia

Drugs that may alter lab results: Prior administration of Rho(D) immune globulin may lead to weakly (false) positive indirect Coombs test in mother and direct Coombs test in infant

Disorders that may alter lab results: N/A

PATHOLOGICAL FINDINGS
- Erythroid hyperplasia of bone marrow
- Extramedullary hematopoiesis
- Hepatomegaly
- Splenomegaly
- Cardiac enlargement
- Pulmonary hemorrhages
- Enlargement, edema of placenta

SPECIAL TESTS
- Elevated amniotic fluid bilirubin (delta OD 450)
- Paternal blood typing may exclude pregnancy from being at risk

IMAGING
- Ultrasonography can demonstrate hepatomegaly, abdominal enlargement, ascites, or signs of hydrops
- Doppler flow studies of fetus are experimental in assessing degree of anemia
- Fetus may be severely affected without hydrops; ultrasound poor at predicting need for intervention

DIAGNOSTIC PROCEDURES
- Amniocentesis
- Umbilical cord blood sampling

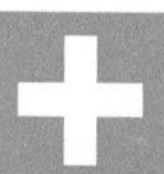

TREATMENT

APPROPRIATE HEALTH CARE
- Affected pregnancies usually managed at the tertiary care level because of the specialized, somewhat hazardous treatment measures involved
- Delivery should occur in an institution capable of performing exchange transfusion even if only mild involvement of infant is expected
- Infants with moderate or severe disease require neonatal intensive care

GENERAL MEASURES
- See Patient Monitoring
- Depending on severity of involvement, treatment of infant may include:
  - ◊ Phototherapy
  - ◊ Transfusion after delivery
  - ◊ Exchange transfusion
  - ◊ Diuretics and digoxin for hydrops
  - ◊ Early delivery
  - ◊ Intrauterine transfusion. Intravascular approach via the umbilical vein is becoming preferred over the intraperitoneal approach and appears to be more effective.

SURGICAL MEASURES N/A

ACTIVITY N/A

DIET N/A

PATIENT EDUCATION Griffith: Instructions for Patients, 5th Ed. Philadelphia, W.B. Saunders Co., to photocopy for patient

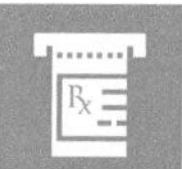

MEDICATIONS

DRUG(S) OF CHOICE N/A
Contraindications: N/A
Precautions: N/A
Significant possible interactions: N/A

ALTERNATIVE DRUGS
- Diuretics, inotropic agents, etc., may be used in addition to transfusion to manage heart failure in the newborn
- Promethazine, immune serum globulin, corticosteroids, and plasmapheresis have been tried as alternatives to invasive treatments but have not been effective

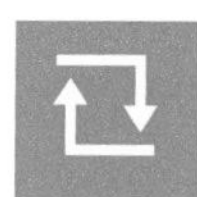

FOLLOWUP

PATIENT MONITORING
- Antibody titer measured every few weeks during pregnancy. A titer of 1:16 or greater indicates need for further testing.
- Periodic amniocentesis for photometric determination of amniotic fluid bilirubin levels in pregnancies with elevated antibody titers. Results estimate the extent of fetal hemolysis and the need for cord blood sampling.
- Percutaneous umbilical blood sampling (PUBS, cordocentesis) for fetal blood type, hematocrit, reticulocyte count, presence of erythroblasts
- Fetal heart rate testing/ultrasonography to assess fetal status
- Amniocentesis for fetal lung maturity

PREVENTION/AVOIDANCE
- Rho(D) Immune Globulin (RhIG, RhoGAM, Gamulin Rh) given prophylactically to unsensitized, Rh-negative pregnant women at risk. Usually at 28-32 weeks gestation and at birth if infant is Rh positive (see Rh incompatibility topic).
- Artificial insemination with sperm from antigen-negative donor for isoimmunized woman whose partner is antigen positive

POSSIBLE COMPLICATIONS
- Fetal distress requiring emergent delivery
- Fetal death in utero
- Disseminated intravascular coagulation (DIC)
- Pregnancy loss from umbilical blood sampling
- Pregnancy loss from intrauterine transfusion
- Asphyxia
- Neonatal hemolytic anemia, mild to severe
- Neonatal anemia from hematopoietic suppression after intrauterine transfusion
- Pulmonary edema
- Congestive heart failure
- Shock
- Neonatal jaundice, mild to severe
- Kernicterus

EXPECTED COURSE/PROGNOSIS
- 50% of affected infants have mild disease and require no treatment (or treatment of anemia and jaundice only after delivery), and can be delivered at or near term
- 30% have moderate disease with anemia and hepatomegaly. They require close followup of the pregnancy for signs of deterioration which may require early delivery after 32-34 weeks or intrauterine transfusion prior to that age. After delivery exchange transfusion is likely to treat anemia and hyperbilirubinemia.
- 20% have fetal hydrops, require intrauterine transfusion and delivery as early as 32-34 weeks
- Disease severity tends to worsen in successive affected pregnancies
- Hydrops is associated with poorer prognosis
- Without treatment overall perinatal mortality is 30%
- With appropriate monitoring and treatment most infants do well, even those requiring intrauterine transfusion
- Fortunately, with universal screening for Rh sensitization and widespread use of Rh immune globulin in 3rd trimester and/or birth have made disease relatively rare

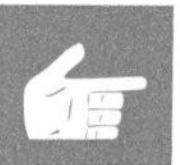

MISCELLANEOUS

ASSOCIATED CONDITIONS N/A

AGE-RELATED FACTORS
Pediatric: Exclusively affects fetus and neonate
Geriatric: N/A
Others: N/A

PREGNANCY N/A

SYNONYMS
- Erythroblastosis neonatorum
- Hemolytic disease of the newborn
- Congenital anemia of the newborn
- Immune hydrops fetalis
- Icterus gravis neonatorum

ICD-9-CM
773.0 Rh hemolytic disease in fetus or newborn
773.1 ABO hemolytic disease in fetus or newborn
773.2 Other hemolytic disease in fetus or newborn
773.3 Isoimmune hydrops fetalis
773.4 Kernicterus due to isoimmunization
773.5 Isoimmune late anemia

SEE ALSO
Rh incompatibility

OTHER NOTES N/A

ABBREVIATIONS N/A

REFERENCES

- Grab D, Paulus WE, Bommer A, Buck G, Terinde R. Treatment of fetal erythroblastosis by intravascular transfusions: outcome at 6 years, Obstet Gyenol 1999;93:165-8
- Cunningham FG, MacDonald PC, Gant NF, eds. Williams' Obstetrics. 19th ed. Norwalk, CT: Appleton and Lange; 1993
- Scott JR, et al, eds. Danforth's Obstetrics and Gynecology. 7th ed. Philadelphia: J.B. Lippincott; 1994
- Duerbeck NB, Seeds JW. Rhesus immunization in pregnancy: A Review. Obstetrical and Gynecological Survey 1993;48(12):801-10

Web references: 2 available at www.5mcc.com
Illustrations N/A

Author(s):
Donald A. F. Nelson, MD

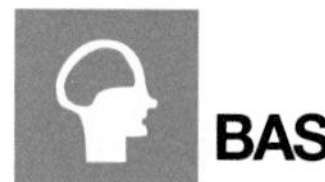

BASICS

DESCRIPTION
- Carcinomas - begin in the esophagus (primary) and usually occur in the lower third. Types: Squamous cell carcinoma; adenocarcinoma (may now account for more than 25% of esophageal cancer). At the time of diagnosis, 80% have metastases to the lymph nodes.
- Benign neoplasms - rare. Types: Leiomyoma (most common), papilloma, and fibrovascular polyps.

System(s) affected: Gastrointestinal
Genetics: No known genetic pattern
Incidence/Prevalence in USA:
- Squamous cell: 3-15/100,000 males; 3-4/100,000 females (highest incidence in Blacks)
- Adenocarcinoma: Rising incidence (vast majority have Barrett's esophagus)

Predominant age: > 50 years (peak incidence 50-60)
Predominant sex: Male > Female (2.6:1)

SIGNS & SYMPTOMS
- Progressive dysphagia for solids over weeks to months
- Progressive weight loss
- Regurgitation and aspiration are common (especially at night)
- Cachexia
- Supraclavicular lymphadenopathy
- Esophageal obstruction
- Hiccups
- Cough
- Hoarseness
- Gastrointestinal blood loss

CAUSES Unknown. Most esophagus cancers are primary, but some spread from other body parts.

RISK FACTORS
- Smoking
- Excess alcohol consumption
- Head and neck tumors
- Nitrates in foods
- Lye stricture
- Achalasia
- Tylosis
- Plummer-Vinson syndrome (anemia and esophageal web)
- Coexisting primary oro-pharyngeal carcinoma
- Barrett's metaplasia (develops in 10-40% of patients with chronic gastroesophageal reflux)
- Gastroesophageal reflux

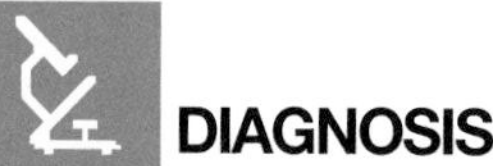

DIAGNOSIS

DIFFERENTIAL DIAGNOSIS
- Benign causes of dysphagia, achalasia
- Motility disorders of the esophagus
- Extrinsic esophageal compression secondary to mediastinal/pulmonary disease

LABORATORY
- Esophageal biopsy/brushing
- Anemia

Drugs that may alter lab results: N/A

Disorders that may alter lab results: N/A

PATHOLOGICAL FINDINGS
- Location - 20% in upper third, 30% in middle third, 50% in lower third
- Elevated plaques
- Ulceration
- Strictures

SPECIAL TESTS Esophagoscopy

IMAGING
- Barium swallow - stenosing lesion
- CT scan - valuable for looking for metastases
- X-ray of the upper-intestinal tract may show pneumonitis, pleural effusion, lung abscess
- Endoscopic ultrasound - staging (most accurate)

DIAGNOSTIC PROCEDURES
- Esophagoscopy with biopsy
- Brush cytology (> 95% positive)
- Bronchoscopy - distortion of the bronchial lumen, blunting of the carina, or intrabronchial tumor
- Once tumor is identified, liver function studies and ultrasonography and/or CT scan for evidence of liver metastases
- Endoscopic ultrasound is most sensitive and specific test to determine local spread

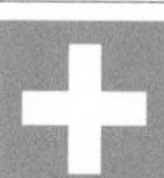

TREATMENT

APPROPRIATE HEALTH CARE
- Inpatient occasionally
- Home care or extended-care facility following definitive treatment

GENERAL MEASURES
- Palliative therapeutic options include: surgery, radiotherapy, chemotherapy, laser photocoagulation, photodynamic therapy, dilation, placement of endoluminal prosthesis (stent) or combination of these methods. The specific choice will depend on the extent of the tumor and symptoms and the individual patient's state of health.

SURGICAL MEASURES
- Majority of tumors are not resectable for cure at time of presentation
- Important to stage the lesion before determining treatment plan
- Strictures may be dilated for temporary relief
- Prior to surgery - average patient requires nutritional and pulmonary preparation, e.g., feeding tube with formula diet and respiratory therapy
- Endoluminal prosthesis may be attempted for patients who have failed other methods of palliation

ACTIVITY Adjusted to patient's ability

DIET
- Soft to liquid
- High calorie supplements (usually liquid)

PATIENT EDUCATION For patient education materials favorably reviewed on this topic, contact: National Cancer Institute, Department of Health And Human Services, Public Inquiries Section, Office of Cancer Communications, Building 31, Room 101-18, 9000 Rockville Pike, Bethesda, MD 20892, (301)496-5583

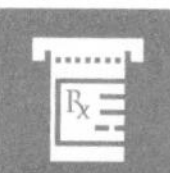

MEDICATIONS

DRUG(S) OF CHOICE
- Chemotherapy in selected patients
- Analgesics
- Antacids, H2 receptor antagonist, or proton pump inhibitors when gastroesophageal reflux symptoms co-exist
- Metoclopramide if gastric emptying problems coexist (frequently paraneoplastic)

Contraindications: Refer to manufacturer's literature
Precautions: Refer to manufacturer's literature
Significant possible interactions: Refer to manufacturer's literature

ALTERNATIVE DRUGS
- Cisapride if gastric emptying problems coexist (frequently paraneoplastic) (not generally recommended)

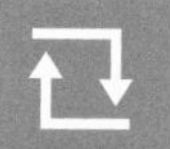

FOLLOWUP

PATIENT MONITORING Individualized to follow results of preoperative and postoperative treatment

PREVENTION/AVOIDANCE
- Avoid tobacco, excess alcohol, corrosive chemicals
- Endoscopic surveillance of those at high risk (Barrett's, esophagus, head and neck cancer)

POSSIBLE COMPLICATIONS
- Metastases to anterior jugular, supraclavicular, subdiaphragmatic lymph nodes, liver, lungs
- Complications from surgical procedures (anastomotic leak or stricture, fistula formation, empyema, malnutrition)
- Radiation can cause esophageal perforation, stricture, fistula, esophagitis, pneumonitis, myelitis, and pulmonary fibrosis
- Toxicities of chemotherapy - nausea, vomiting, hair loss, gastroenteritis, hematopoietic and immune depression
- Tubes can become blocked or dislodged
- Aspiration from esophageal obstruction

EXPECTED COURSE/PROGNOSIS
- Overall 5-year survival 5%; in squamous cell carcinoma with uninvolved lymph nodes 15-20%
- Death rate following resection or bypass is 10-15%

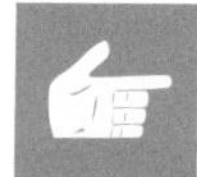

MISCELLANEOUS

ASSOCIATED CONDITIONS
- Barrett metaplasia
- Head and neck cancer
- Achalasia

AGE-RELATED FACTORS
Pediatric: N/A
Geriatric: Most common in males over 60
Others:
- Uncommon under age 50
- Definitive treatment is standard regardless of age
- Symptomatic therapy requires dose adjustment for very old and very young

PREGNANCY N/A

SYNONYMS
- Esophagus squamous cell carcinoma
- Esophagus adenocarcinoma

ICD-9-CM
150.9 Malignant neoplasm of esophagus, unspecified

SEE ALSO
Gastroesophageal reflux disease

OTHER NOTES N/A

ABBREVIATIONS N/A

REFERENCES

- Chabner BA, Collins JM. Cancer Chemotherapy: Principles and Practice. Philadelphia: J.B. Lippincott Co.; 1990
- Livstone EM. General considerations of tumors of the esophagus. In: Berk JE, ed. Bockus' Gastroenterology. 4th ed. Philadelphia: W.B. Saunders Co.; 1985
- Fox JR, Kuwada SK. Today's approach to esophageal cancer. What is the role of the primary care physician? Postgrad Med 2000;107(5):109-14
- Lambert R. treatment of esophagogastric tumors. Endoscopy 2000;32:322-30
- Jenkins T, Friedman L. Adenocarcinoma of the esophagogastric junction. Dig Dis 1999;17:153-62

Web references: 3 available at www.5mcc.com
Illustrations N/A

Author(s):
Philip E. Jaffe, MD

BASICS

DESCRIPTION Large collateral veins located in the submucosa of the esophagus and stomach, most prominent in the distal esophagus, connecting the portal vein with the superior vena cava. These veins result from chronic high pressure in the portal vein and are particularly prone to rupture with associated gastrointestinal bleeding and often exsanguination and death. Bleeding from varices is the single most common cause of death in cirrhosis of the liver.
System(s) affected: Cardiovascular, Gastrointestinal
Genetics: No known pattern
Incidence/Prevalence in USA: Present in 85% of cases of cirrhosis of the liver. Causes 5-11% of upper gastrointestinal bleeding.
Predominant age: Parallels the ages of cirrhosis with most cases 40-60 years, but can occur at any age
Predominant sex: Male > Female

SIGNS & SYMPTOMS
- Intestinal bleeding only symptoms
  - ◊ Upper GI, 75% of time, painless hematemesis
  - ◊ Occult GI with anemia 25%
- Abdominal periumbilical collateral circulation
- Signs of cirrhosis
  - ◊ Large, hard liver
  - ◊ Splenomegaly
  - ◊ Ascites

CAUSES
- Cirrhosis accounts for > 90% of cases. Alcoholic and hepatitis C most common causes of cirrhosis, but hemochromatosis, hepatitis B, nonalcoholic steatonecrosis, biliary cirrhosis, autoimmune cirrhosis account for some.
- Extrahepatic portal vein occlusion from umbilical vein infection, trauma, chronic pancreatitis, thrombotic conditions, polycythemia cause a few
- Noncirrhotic portal hypertension common in patients from Asian continents
- Malignant invasion of liver sinusoids or portal vein. Seen in lymphoma, leukemia, hepatocellular carcinoma, pancreatic carcinoma.
- Metabolic diseases altering liver sinusoids - amyloid, Gaucher disease, fatty liver
- Budd-Chiari syndrome, veno-occlusive disease due to senecio, thrombotic conditions

RISK FACTORS
- Cirrhosis of the liver
- Inherited thrombotic conditions such as anti-thrombin III, substance S or R deficiencies
- Prolonged use of estrogen-progesterone

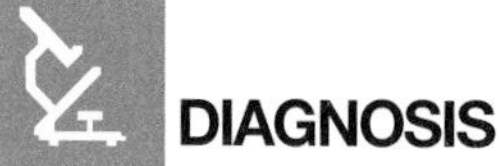

DIAGNOSIS

DIFFERENTIAL DIAGNOSIS
- Upper GI bleeding
  - ◊ Pulmonary bleeding; hemoptysis
  - ◊ Peptic ulcer disease
  - ◊ Gastric malignancy
- Lower GI bleeding
  - ◊ Hemorrhoids
  - ◊ Colon malignancy
  - ◊ Colonic polyp
  - ◊ Diverticulitis

LABORATORY Reflects only the anemia of bleeding, or the abnormalities related to the cirrhosis or other cause

Drugs that may alter lab results: N/A

Disorders that may alter lab results: N/A

PATHOLOGICAL FINDINGS Extensive collateral circulation in the mediastinum and in the abdomen in addition to large vessels in the submucosa of the esophagus. When bleeding occurs, these large veins explode into the submucosa of esophagus and rupture in turn into the lumen.

SPECIAL TESTS N/A

IMAGING
- Esophagram following barium swallow with adherent barium demonstrates very advanced varices, but is insensitive to small ones. Is not used when bleeding present for it precludes possible urgent angiography.
- MRI demonstrates large vascular channels intra-abdominally, and in the mediastinum. Demonstrates patency of the intrahepatic portal vein and splenic vein if this is required.
- Doppler sonography demonstrates patency, diameter, and flow in portal vein, and splenic vein, and large collaterals intra-abdominally
- Venous phase celiac arteriography demonstrates portal vein and its collaterals

DIAGNOSTIC PROCEDURES
- Esophagoscopy as part of EGD endoscopy can identify and treat. Large, protruding, lumenal veins in the distal 1/3 of the esophagus are diagnostic. If recent bleeding, they may be seen to be bleeding in 5%. Useful when active bleeding is present, to identify early varices, and to follow course of treatment.

Grading endoscopic findings and risk of variceal bleeding:

```
-Findings-
1  2  3  4    Grade  Risk
------------------------------
A  A  A  A      1    Rare
B  A  A  A      2    Unlikely
C  B  A  B      3    Possible
C  C  C  C      4    Likely
------------------------------
Endoscopic Findings==========
1.Size of varices
  A. Small B. Medium C. Large
2.Number of columns of varices
  A. 1-2    B. 2-3    C. >3
3.Red wale markings
  A. None  B. Mild    C. Severe
4.Cherry red spots
  A. None  B. Mild    C. Severe
==============================
```

- Gastric varices may be identified. Fundic varices are large and tortuous. Other regions are more discrete, harder to identify and treat. Diffuse telangiectatic lesion called portal hypertension gastropathy also seen. All of these may bleed.
- Doppler sonography to demonstrate patency of:
  - ◊ Portal and splenic veins
  - ◊ Porta-caval shunts
- Venous phase angiography
  - ◊ Diagnose hepatic vein occlusion
- Endoscopic ultrasound particularly sensitive to gastric varices
- Portal pressure measure
  - ◊ Radiologist introduces a catheter retrograde into the hepatic veins in a wedged position to occlude flow
  - ◊ Catheter is withdrawn to a free position and pressure again measured. Difference between wedged and free is portal pressure. If under 12 mm Hg, bleeding is extremely unlikely. Progressive increases above 12 correlate with likelihood of hemorrhage.
  - ◊ This is sometimes used to monitor successful treatment with beta adrenergic blocking agents

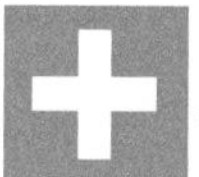

TREATMENT

APPROPRIATE HEALTH CARE
Inpatient for acute bleeding

GENERAL MEASURES
- As related to cirrhosis
- Hospital management of bleeding varices
  - ◊ Appropriate resuscitation and maintenance of blood volume
  - ◊ Urgent upper endoscopy for diagnosis and treatment. Injections of somatostatin or octreotide to control bleeding permit endoscopic treatment of varices. If bleeding not controlled with these drugs, vasopressin and spironolactone have been added with additional benefit.
  - ◊ Variceal ligation or sclerosant injection for bleeding varices
  - ◊ Repeat ligation or sclerosant injection if bleeding recurs
  - ◊ If ligation or sclerosant injection fails to stop bleeding or cannot be accomplished, consider TIPS (transjugular intrahepatic portacaval shunt)

- Management of non-bleeding varices
  - ◊ If ligation or sclerotherapy started, complete the sequence at intervals of 1-4 weeks. 4-6 treatments usually required to eradicate varices.
  - ◊ If no bleeding has occurred, and varices are rated grade 2 or more severe, by endoscopy, treat with propranolol - 10 mg q 12h initially titrated up each few days until pulse rate slowed by 25%, average dose 80 mg bid. Remain on this dose for life or until transplant or some form of portacaval shunt.
- If bleeding recurs, or pressure measurement shows portal pressure still above 12 mm Hg, isosorbide mononitrate is usually added. Some limited successful experience with losartan or spironolactone has been reported.
- Gastric varices
  - ◊ Injection of prominent fundic varices with sclerosant or methacrylate has been effective. Retrograde sclerosis in the balloon occluded varices has also been used.
  - ◊ Propranolol sufficient to normalize the portal pressure (less than 12 mm Hg) or lower resting pulse by 15%, often in conjunction with long acting nitrate or losartan should be used in all patients with abnormal gastric vessels.
  - ◊ TIPS effectively lowers portal pressure and prevents bleeding. Though no better than regularly used drugs, occasionally patients are noncompliant.

SURGICAL MEASURES
- Portocaval shunt
- Esophageal transection
- Liver transplantation

ACTIVITY
No restrictions

DIET
Appropriate to cirrhosis or other conditions present

PATIENT EDUCATION
- Appropriate to cirrhosis
- National Digestive Information Clearinghouse, 2 Information Way, Bethesda, MD 20892 or American Liver Foundation, 1425 Pompton Way, Cedar Grove, NJ 07009

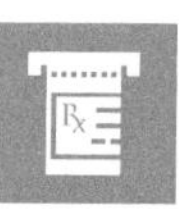

MEDICATIONS

DRUG(S) OF CHOICE
- For varices grade 2 or worse:
  - ◊ propranolol 80 mg bid. Increase until pulse rate decreased by 25% from basal
  - ◊ Other nonspecific beta blockers probably effective. Nadolol proven effective.
  - ◊ Isosorbide mononitrate further reduces portal pressure and is often used in conjunction with beta adrenergic blocking agents. Spironolactone or losartan in conjunction with beta blockers are reported to achieve the same thing (with more limited experience, but fewer side effects).
- During banding or sclerotherapy: proton pump blocker such as lansoprazole 30 mg q d for one month
- During bleeding: antibiotic prophylaxis for spontaneous peritonitis. Norfloxacin 400 mg q12h for 7 days.

Contraindications: Severe asthma with beta blockers
Precautions: Symptomatic hypotension
Significant possible interactions: N/A

ALTERNATIVE DRUGS
N/A

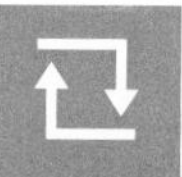

FOLLOWUP

PATIENT MONITORING
- Varix ligation or sclerotherapy, repeated every 1-4 weeks until varices eradicated
- If varices grade 1 or 2 on endoscopy (do not hemorrhage), repeat endoscopy each year. If eradicated, repeat endoscopy each 2 years.
- If TIPS or other portacaval shunt, repeat endoscopy only if clinically bleeding
- If TIPS present, followup as recommended by radiologist, usually Doppler sonogram each 6 months

PREVENTION/AVOIDANCE
- Endoscope esophagus each 2 years in cirrhosis
  - ◊ If grade 3, propranolol, 40-120 mg bd
  - ◊ If grade 4, prophylactic endoscopic ligation

POSSIBLE COMPLICATIONS
- Bleeding. Gastric or other uncommon varices may occur following successful eradication of esophageal varices.
- Educate patient to plan of action if bleeding occurs, particularly if traveling

EXPECTED COURSE/PROGNOSIS
- Bleeding diminished and survival prolonged
- Recurrent bleeding is an indication for transplantation listing
- In progressive worsening, grade changes are one grade in 2 years

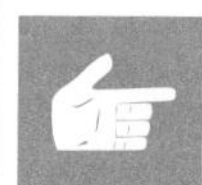

MISCELLANEOUS

ASSOCIATED CONDITIONS
- Infections associated with underlying cirrhosis: e.g., influenza and pneumococcal
- Gastric varices often occur after eradication
- Portal hypertensive gastropathy can also bleed. Recognized by endoscopy, and responds to beta blockade and TIPS.
- Collateral circulation may occur with thrombosis of the superior or inferior vena cava
- Hemorrhoids

AGE-RELATED FACTORS
Pediatric: N/A
Geriatric: N/A
Others: Can occur in all age groups

PREGNANCY
N/A

SYNONYMS
N/A

ICD-9-CM
456.0 Esophageal varices with bleeding
456.1 Esophageal varices without mention of bleeding

SEE ALSO
Cirrhosis of the liver
Hemorrhoids
Portal hypertension
Portal vein thrombosis

OTHER NOTES
N/A

ABBREVIATIONS
N/A

REFERENCES

- Matsuo M, Kanematsu M, Kim T, et al. Esophageal varices: diagnosis with gadolinium-enhanced MR imaging of the liver for patients with chronic liver damage. AJR Am J Roentgenol 2003;180(2):461-6
- Zhou Y, Qiao L, Wu J, Hu H, Xu C. Comparison of the efficacy of octreotide, vasopressin, and omeprazole in the control of acute bleeding in patients with portal hypertensive gastropathy: a controlled study. J Gastroenterol Hepatol 2002;17(9):973-9
- Shimizu T, Onda M, Tajiri T, Yoshida H, Mamada Y, Taniai N, Aramaki T, Kumazaki T. Bleeding portal-hypertensive gastropathy managed successfully by partial splenic embolization. Hepatogastroenterology 2002;49(46):947-9
- Jensen DM. Endoscopic screening for varices in cirrhosis: findings, implications, and outcomes. Gastroenterology 2002;122(6):1620-30
- Lo GH, Chen WC, Chen MH, Hsu PI, Lin CK, Tsai WL, Lai KH.
- Banding ligation versus nadolol and isosorbide mononitrate for the prevention of esophageal variceal rebleeding. Gastroenterology 2002;123(3):728-34
- Lui HF, Stanley AJ, Forrest EH, et al. Primary prophylaxis of variceal hemorrhage: a randomized controlled trial comparing band ligation, propranolol, and isosorbide mononitrate. Gastroenterology 2002;123(3):735-44

Web references: 2 available at www.5mcc.com
Illustrations N/A

Author(s):
Frank L. Iber, MD

BASICS

DESCRIPTION Factor V Leiden is a genetic disease that is the most common congenital cause of venous thrombosis. It leads to resistance to activated protein C.
System(s) affected: Cardiovascular, Gastrointestinal, Hemic/Lymphatic/Immunologic, Nervous, Pulmonary, Reproductive
Genetics: Autosomal dominant. Deep and superficial thrombosis of the venous system occurs with an odds ratio of 50 to 100 for homozygotes. The odds ratio is closer to 2.5 for heterozygotes.
Incidence/Prevalence in USA: Approximately 3-12% of Caucasians are affected. The mutation is rare in other ethnic groups. Approximately 15-20% of patients who present with thrombosis have factor V Leiden.
Predominant age: Thrombosis typically occurs after the second decade
Predominant sex: Male = Female

SIGNS & SYMPTOMS
- Arterial thrombosis is rare in adults with factor V Leiden
- Thrombosis in unusual locations such as the saggital sinus, mesentery and portal systems is less common in patients with factor V Leiden than in patients with deficiency of protein C or S.
- Obstetrical complications are increased in patients with factor V Leiden and factor V Leiden increases the risk of venous thrombosis in patients who are pregnant or taking oral contraceptives.

CAUSES Point mutation causing substitution of arginine for glycine in residue 506 of factor V gene rendering it less susceptible to inactivation by activated protein C. Activated protein C is generated when protein C binds to its endothelial receptor, thrombomodulin. Activated protein C and its cofactor, protein S, lead to inactivation of factors V and VIII. Factor V Leiden is the most common cause of resistance to activated protein C.

RISK FACTORS
- Oral contraceptives increase the risk of thrombosis. In homozygotes the risk increases approximately 100-fold; in heterozygotes approximately 35-fold. The risk is halved when the patient uses a desogestrel-containing OC.
- Hormone replacement therapy (HRT) and selective estrogen receptor modulators (SERM) both increase the risk of thrombosis and in patients with factor V Leiden that risk is increased substantially
- Pregnancy and factor V Leiden increase the risk of thrombosis 7 to 16-fold during pregnancy and the puerperium. Other complications of pregnancy may be increased in patients with factor V Leiden.

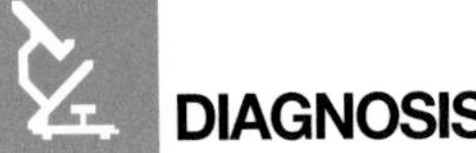

DIAGNOSIS

DIFFERENTIAL DIAGNOSIS
- Protein C deficiency
- Protein S deficiency
- Antithrombin deficiency
- Other causes of activated protein C resistance (e.g., antiphospholipid antibodies)
- Dysfibrinogenemia
- Dysplasminogenemia
- Homocysteinemia
- Prothrombin 20210 mutation
- Elevated factor VIII levels

LABORATORY
- Factor V Leiden Mutation Analysis

Drugs that may alter lab results: N/A

Disorders that may alter lab results: N/A

PATHOLOGICAL FINDINGS N/A

SPECIAL TESTS
- DNA-based test for factor V mutation
- Plasma-based coagulation assay using factor V deficient plasma to which patient plasma is added along with purified activated protein C. The relative prolongation of the activated partial thromboplastin time (aPTT) is used to assay for the defect.

IMAGING Magnetic resonance angiography (MRA), venography, arteriography to detect thrombosis

DIAGNOSTIC PROCEDURES N/A

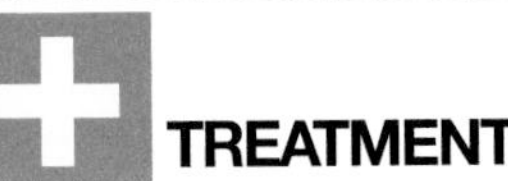

TREATMENT

APPROPRIATE HEALTH CARE Outpatient

GENERAL MEASURES
- Patients with factor V Leiden and a first thrombosis should be anticoagulated initially with heparin or low molecular weight heparin followed by oral anticoagulation with warfarin. Patients should be maintained on warfarin with an INR of 2 to 3 for at least 6 months. Recurrent thrombosis requires indefinite anticoagulation.

SURGICAL MEASURES N/A

ACTIVITY No restrictions

DIET No restrictions

PATIENT EDUCATION
- Patients should be educated about use or oral anticoagulant therapy if taking such
- Avoid NSAIDs while on warfarin
- The role of family screening is unclear since most patients with this mutation do not have thrombosis. In a patient with a family history of Factor V Leiden, consider screening during pregnancy or if considering oral contraceptive use.

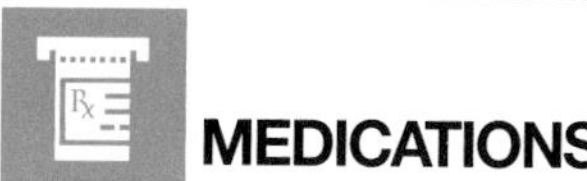

MEDICATIONS

DRUG(S) OF CHOICE
- Low molecular weight heparin (LMWH)
  - ◊ Enoxaparin (Lovenox) 1mg/kg SC bid initially for at least 5 days or until INR is 2-3 at which time it can be stopped
  - ◊ Tinzaparin (Innohep) 175 anti Xa IU/kg SC qd
  - ◊ Dalteparin (Fragmin) 200 IU/kg SC qd
- Oral anticoagulant
  - ◊ Warfarin (Coumadin) 5 mg qd initially and adjusted to an INR of 2-3

Contraindications:
- Active bleeding precludes anticoagulation; risk of bleeding is a relative contraindication to long-term anticoagulation
- Warfarin is contraindicated in patients with prior history of warfarin skin necrosis

Precautions:
- Observe patient for signs of embolization, further thrombosis or bleeding
- Avoid IM injections. Periodically check stool and urine for occult blood, monitor complete blood counts including platelets.
- Heparin - thrombocytopenia and/or paradoxical thrombosis with thrombocytopenia
- Warfarin - necrotic skin lesions (typically breasts, thighs, buttocks)
- LMWH - adjust dosage in renal insufficiency

Significant possible interactions:
- Agents that intensify the response to oral anticoagulants: Alcohol, allopurinol, amiodarone, anabolic steroids, androgens, many antimicrobials, cimetidine chloral hydrate, disulfiram, all NSAIDs, sulfinpyrazone, tamoxifen, thyroid hormone, vitamin E, ranitidine, salicylates, acetaminophen
- Agents that diminish the response to anticoagulants: Aminoglutethimide, antacids, barbiturates, carbamazepine, cholestyramine, diuretics, griseofulvin, rifampin, oral contraceptives

ALTERNATIVE DRUGS
- Heparin 80 mg/kg IV bolus followed by 18 mcg/kg/hr. Adjust dose depending on aPTT.

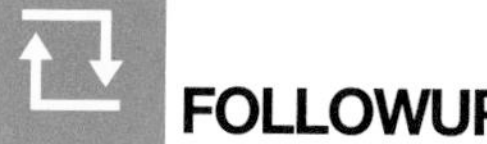

FOLLOWUP

PATIENT MONITORING
- Warfarin use requires periodic (approximately monthly after initial stabilization) INR measurements with a goal of 2-3

PREVENTION/AVOIDANCE
- Patients with factor V Leiden without thrombosis do not require prophylactic treatment

POSSIBLE COMPLICATIONS
- Venous or arterial thrombosis
- Bleeding in anticoagulated patients

EXPECTED COURSE/PROGNOSIS
Most patients heterozygous for factor V Leiden do not have thrombosis. Homozygotes have about a 50% incidence of thrombosis. Recurrence rates after a first thrombosis are not clear with some investigators finding rates as high as 5% and others finding rates similar to the general population. Despite the increased risk for thrombosis, factor V Leiden does not increase overall mortality.

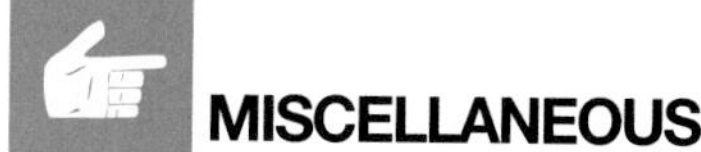

MISCELLANEOUS

ASSOCIATED CONDITIONS N/A

AGE-RELATED FACTORS
Pediatric: Thrombosis rare in this group, but has been described
Geriatric: N/A
Others: N/A

PREGNANCY
Increases thrombosis risk in patients with factor V Leiden

SYNONYMS
- Factor V Leiden thrombophilia
- Factor V Leiden mutation

ICD-9-CM
289.81 Primary hypercoagulable state

SEE ALSO
Thrombosis, deep vein (DVT)

OTHER NOTES

ABBREVIATIONS
LMWH = low molecular weight heparin

REFERENCES

- Greengard JS, Eichinger S, Griffin JH, Bauer KA. Variability of thrombosis among heterozygous siblings with resistance to activated protein C due to Arg -> Gln mutation in the gene for factor V. N Engl J Med 1994;331:1559
- Dahlback B. Resistance to activated protein C as risk factor for thrombosis; molecular mechanisms, laboratory investigation, and clinical management. Seminhematol 1997;34:217
- Kim RJ, Becker RC. Association between factor V Leiden, prothrombin G20210A, and methylenetetrahydrofolate reductase C677T mutations and events of the arterial circulatory system: a meta-analysis of published studies. Am Heart J. 2003;146:948

Web references: 1 available at www.5mcc.com
Illustrations 1 available

Author(s):
Marc Jeffrey Kahn, MD

Failure to thrive (FTT)

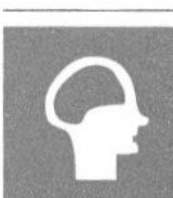

BASICS

DESCRIPTION Failure to thrive is a symptom (rather than a disease) characterized by disproportionate failure to gain weight in comparison to height due to caloric insufficiency (or under utilization of ingested food) without obvious etiology.
System(s) affected: Endocrine/Metabolic, Musculoskeletal, Nervous
Genetics: No consistent genetic pattern
Incidence/Prevalence in USA:
- Not known
- 2-4% of pediatric in-patient admissions are for evaluation of failure to thrive (FTT). It is a common and difficult diagnostic problem.

Predominant age: Usually 6-12 months; almost all are under 3-5 years
Predominant sex: Male = Female

SIGNS & SYMPTOMS
- Weight low for age and height
- Growth chart shows significant deceleration of weight gain
- Difficult personality, feeding and sleep problems
- Apathetic and withdrawn, or watchful and alert
- Poor hygiene
- Signs of inflicted trauma
- Primary caretaker characteristics - psychosocial problems, often depressed
- Family characteristics - unstable, disturbed

CAUSES
- Organic etiology: less than 20%, usually gastrointestinal or neurologic. Includes some infants who were profoundly premature. Less commonly - chronic infection, malignancies, cardiac and renal
- Environmental deprivation: about 70%, of which one-third are simple educational problems, such as incorrect feeding
- Normal, small children (about 10%) not truly FTT

RISK FACTORS
- Parent with psychosocial problems
- Premature or sick newborn
- Infant with physical deformity
- Unstable, disturbed family

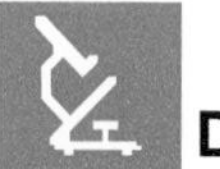

DIAGNOSIS

DIFFERENTIAL DIAGNOSIS Any condition of sufficient severity to cause failure to gain weight adequately, including child abuse and/or neglect

LABORATORY
- Routine laboratory work-up should be kept to a minimum
  - ◊ CBC
  - ◊ Sedimentation rate
  - ◊ Urinalysis
  - ◊ Urine culture
  - ◊ Chemical profile, including BUN, calcium, phosphorus: electrolytes, total protein, albumin and bicarbonate
- Other studies dictated by results of history and physical examination, such as thyroid profile, pituitary studies

Drugs that may alter lab results: NA

Disorders that may alter lab results: Various blood chemistries may be altered by malnutrition regardless of cause

PATHOLOGICAL FINDINGS N/A

SPECIAL TESTS N/A

IMAGING
- Skeletal survey if there is suspicion or evidence of physical abuse
- X-rays for bone age (wrist film)

DIAGNOSTIC PROCEDURES
- Careful, detailed history and physical examination are most important
- Observation of infant and his or her interaction with caretakers and environment essential
- If suspicious of Turner syndrome, a karyotype is indicated. Buccal smears were previously the test of choice but are no longer considered appropriate.
- Carefully plotted growth curves, including weight, height, and head circumference
- Evaluation may require involvement of many disciplines, including endocrine, behavioral, social service, nursing, dietetics
- Consider sleep study and/or nasopharyngoscopy if upper airway obstruction is likely (eg, snoring, sweating during sleep)

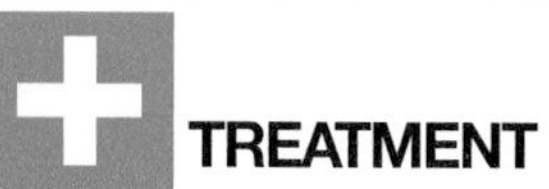

TREATMENT

APPROPRIATE HEALTH CARE Outpatient, except inpatient when all other attempts to improve have failed

GENERAL MEASURES
- Admission to inpatient setting
- Use of few sympathetic primary caretakers in hospital
- Provision of stimulation, cuddling, affection as inpatient or outpatient

SURGICAL MEASURES N/A

ACTIVITY No restrictions

DIET Provision of balanced, high caloric diet on both a scheduled and ad lib basis, 150-200 kcal/kg/day

PATIENT EDUCATION Depends on etiology of FTT. When environmental deprivation is established, attempts to re-educate in a non-punitive way is essential.

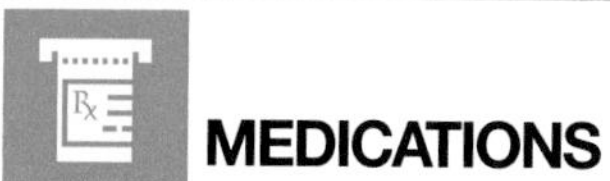

MEDICATIONS

DRUG(S) OF CHOICE None; routine vitamin supplementation
Contraindications: N/A
Precautions: N/A
Significant possible interactions: N/A

ALTERNATIVE DRUGS N/A

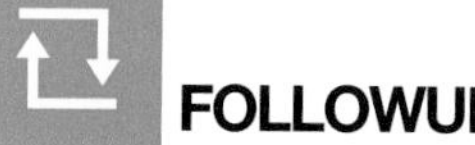

FOLLOWUP

PATIENT MONITORING
- When etiology is organic, followup depends on particular disease involved
- When environmental deprivation is established, extremely close followup, both at home and in office is essential. If family fails to comply, child protection authorities must be notified and foster care may be necessary.

PREVENTION/AVOIDANCE Stable home life with caring parents

POSSIBLE COMPLICATIONS N/A

EXPECTED COURSE/PROGNOSIS
Long-term prognosis of children with FTT due to environmental deprivation is not encouraging. Many children remain small, most demonstrate developmental and educational deficiencies and personality disorders. Only one-third are ultimately normal.

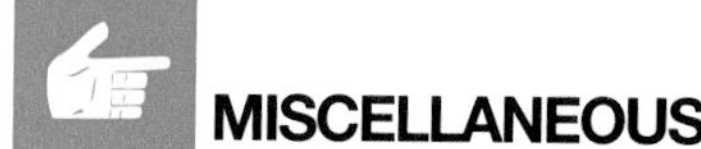

MISCELLANEOUS

ASSOCIATED CONDITIONS N/A

AGE-RELATED FACTORS N/A
Pediatric: N/A
Geriatric: N/A
Others: N/A

PREGNANCY N/A

SYNONYMS N/A

ICD-9-CM
783.40 Lack of normal physiological development, unspecified

SEE ALSO
Down syndrome
Turner syndrome

OTHER NOTES N/A

ABBREVIATIONS FTT = failure to thrive

REFERENCES

- Sills RH. Failure to Thrive. In: Stockman JA, editor. Difficult Diagnosis in Pediatrics. Philadelphia: W.B. Saunders Co.; 1990
- Gartner, Zitelli. Common and Chronic Symptoms in Pediatrics. CV Mosby, 1997
- Gartner B, Zitelli BJ, Carlton J Jr. Common & Chronic Symptoms in Pediatrics: A Companion to the Atlas of Pediatric Physical Diagnosis. St. Louis: Mosby Year Book; 1997
- Stallings VA: Nutrition. In: FD Burg (ed): Gellis and Kagan's Current Pediatric Therapy. Philadelphia, WB Saunders, 1999

Web references: 1 available at www.5mcc.com
Illustrations N/A

Author(s):
Kurt J. Wegner, MD

BASICS

DESCRIPTION
- Fatty liver - a liver biopsy diagnosis showing fatty deposits in greater than 30% of liver cells. There is no necrosis, no fibrosis, and the ALT and AST enzymes are normal. This syndrome is asymptomatic, is a non-progressive condition and has essentially no adverse health consequences.
- Non-alcoholic steatohepatitis (NASH) - a liver biopsy diagnosis of fatty deposits in greater than 50% of liver cells associated with acute and chronic inflammation and increased fibrosis. Though asymptomatic in most patients, the ALT and AST enzymes are elevated. This disease progresses to cirrhosis.

System(s) affected: Endocrine/Metabolic, Gastrointestinal, Reproductive

Genetics: Largely unknown. All types of obesity and diabetes, and carriers of hemochromatosis gene are more likely to be affected.

Incidence/Prevalence in USA:
- Account for 10% of outpatient referrals to hepatologist
- Present in 20-25% of obese (body mass index >30)
- Present in 5-10% type 2 diabetics
- Reason for liver transplantation in 1% transplants

Predominant age: 50's, but occurs at any age

Predominant sex: Male = Female

SIGNS & SYMPTOMS
- Vast majority of patients are asymptomatic, disease is suspected by:
  - ◊ Hepatomegaly Incidentally observed enlarged liver or spleen on image
  - ◊ Unsuspected elevation of ALT or AST enzymes on screening biochemistry
- Commonest signs and symptoms
  - ◊ Liver pain or tenderness
  - ◊ Mild to marked hepatomegaly
  - ◊ Splenomegaly
  - ◊ Fatigue
- Infrequent - limited to advanced cases
  - ◊ Abdominal collateral veins
  - ◊ Variceal hemorrhage
  - ◊ Ascites
  - ◊ Edema

CAUSES
- Fatty liver - most commonly impaired ability of the liver to remove fatty acids
- In hyperinsulinemia, alcoholism, and a few other conditions, there is an increased production of fatty acids for the liver to store and dispose of
- Non-alcoholic steatohepatitis - almost always 2 factors occur simultaneously. There is a peripheral insulin resistance and increased hepatic oxidative stress from at least one of many different causes. Mitochondrial damage leading to impaired restoration of ATP stores, lipid peroxidation, and increased iron stores have each been found in 25-40% of NASH cases.

RISK FACTORS
- Protein-calorie malnutrition
- Total parenteral nutrition > 6 weeks
- Bariatric surgery
- Hepatitis C
- Alcohol intake exceeding 50 gm/day
- HIV infection
- Organic solvents (chlorinated hydrocarbons, toluene)
- Obesity; BMI > 30
- Diabetes type 2
- Gene for hemochromatosis or other conditions with increased iron stores
- Small intestinal bacterial overgrowth
- Pituitary insufficiency
- Hyperlipidemia, particularly hypertriglyceridemia
- Drugs - tetracycline, glucocorticoids, tamoxifen, methotrexate, valproic acid, zidovudine, didanosine, fialuridine, most chemotherapy regimes

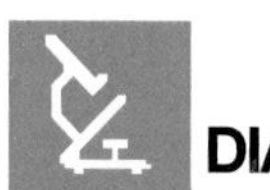

DIAGNOSIS

DIFFERENTIAL DIAGNOSIS
- Viral hepatitis
- Drug induced hepatitis
- Occupational exposure
- Metabolic liver disease

LABORATORY
- CBC is normal
- Sedimentation rate normal
- Liver tests (albumin, bilirubin, prothrombin time, alkaline phosphatase, GGPT) normal but both ALT and AST enzymes elevated with ALT>AST
- Lipids almost always abnormal. Cholesterol elevated 60%. 45% decreased HDL, 58% increased LDL. 50 to 80% elevated triglycerides.
- 30-100 % are diabetic with elevated insulin
- Leptin elevated more than expected for obesity

Drugs that may alter lab results: None

Disorders that may alter lab results:
- Obesity associated with many of these abnormalities
- Uncontrolled diabetes

PATHOLOGICAL FINDINGS
- Anatomic pathology
  - ◊ Liver biopsy the gold standard to differentiate fatty liver with good prognosis from NASH
  - ◊ In NASH, inflammation in the lobule with both acute and chronic cellular response, and fibrosis starting in the pericentral region are the major markers of poor future prognosis. Staging based largely on the extent of fibrosis. Mallory hyaline may be present.
  - ◊ Biopsy is required in those patients with abnormal ALT, AST, symptoms or marked hepatomegaly

SPECIAL TESTS N/A

IMAGING
- Ultrasound often detects hepatomegaly with "bright irregularities" which is usual finding in fat
- CT scan can be diagnostic of fat for it has decreased density in Hounsfield Units compared to all other conditions of the liver. Focal fat deposits usually represents a transient change when marked weight loss occurs and is not related.

DIAGNOSTIC PROCEDURES
- Liver biopsy
  - ◊ Patients with unexplained hepatomegaly and elevation of the ALT, AST enzymes persisting for at least 3 months
  - ◊ Liver biopsy separates benign fatty liver from NASH, thereby helping to establish prognosis

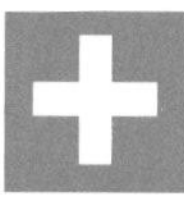

TREATMENT

APPROPRIATE HEALTH CARE Outpatient

GENERAL MEASURES
- Obesity; when body mass index (BMI) greater than 30, should be treated. Weight loss to ideal body weight is the single most evaluated and effective treatment. Fully half of obese NASH patients will normalize the ALT, AST enzymes and loose fat on CT scan.
- Diabetes should be tightly regulated
- Other identified risk factors should be corrected if possible
- All alcohol use should be discontinued permanently

SURGICAL MEASURES
- Weight reduction operations such as gastric bypass are frequently utilized with reduction of obesity and improvement in NASH

ACTIVITY
- No restrictions
- Daily regimen of physical activity recommended

DIET
- Weight, diabetes, and blood lipid control are the goals
- Regular visits to a dietitian are useful
- Usually restriction of both total energy (calories), simple carbohydrates, and alcohol are required to control diabetes, weight and lipids

PATIENT EDUCATION Planning for lifelong change in eating, exercise, and alcohol use is required. As such, regular education and motivation sessions are of value.

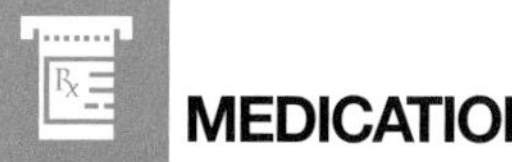

MEDICATIONS

DRUG(S) OF CHOICE
- General:
  - ◊ Drugs to control diabetes and elevated lipid levels are required if those conditions are present
  - ◊ Drugs to facilitate weight loss may be used on a temporary basis
- Specific, used only in biopsy proven NASH when weight reduction, diabetes and lipid control have failed. These treatments are considered experimental but have normalized ALT and AST and reduced fat in the liver in pilot studies:
  - ◊ Troglitazone
  - ◊ Metformin
  - ◊ Pioglitazone

Contraindications: N/A
Precautions: N/A
Significant possible interactions: N/A

ALTERNATIVE DRUGS N/A

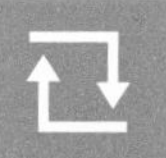

FOLLOWUP

PATIENT MONITORING
- Repeat liver tests (ALT, AST) each 2 to 4 months
- Yearly US or CT scan to show diminution in fat
- Changes toward normal provide major motivation to continue life style changes

PREVENTION/AVOIDANCE
- Avoid alcohol
- Avoid unessential medications including health food and OTC agents
- Obtain hepatitis A and B vaccination if not immune
- Obtain Pneumovax and yearly influenza vaccination

POSSIBLE COMPLICATIONS
- Limited to patients with NASH:
  - ◊ Progression of liver fibrosis to cirrhosis. Believed to be the major cause of cryptogenic cirrhosis.
  - ◊ Liver failure with ascites, encephalopathy, and bleeding varices
  - ◊ Hepatocellular carcinoma
  - ◊ Consideration of transplantation

EXPECTED COURSE/PROGNOSIS
- Goals of treatment:
  - ◊ Fatty liver without NASH (no fibrosis, no hepatitis): non-progressive disease, treat to control symptoms
  - ◊ Fatty liver with NASH: progressive disease, treat to normalize ALT, AST and to diminish fat in liver as verified by yearly ultrasounds
- NASH form of fatty liver
  - ◊ Slowly progressive
  - ◊ Normalization of AST, ALT with treatment slows progression but does not stop it
  - ◊ Diminution of fat on serial images or biopsy slows progression but does not stop it
  - ◊ Cirrhosis develops in about 25% of patients after 20-30 years
  - ◊ Liver failure from cirrhosis occurs in 1-5%. Transplantation is effective. NASH has infrequently recurred after transplantation.

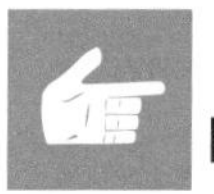

MISCELLANEOUS

ASSOCIATED CONDITIONS
Preeclampsia, in pregnancy-related disease

AGE-RELATED FACTORS
Pediatric: N/A
Geriatric: N/A
Others: Usually identified in the 40s and 50s, may occur at any age

PREGNANCY
A severe complication of 3rd trimester is acute fatty liver of pregnancy. Abrupt onset of confusion and restlessness. ALT and AST always elevated. Emergency liver biopsy confirms. Prompt delivery corrects the liver disease. In most cases fetus has an inborn error of lipid metabolism blocking same in mother.

SYNONYMS
- Steatosis
- Steatonecrosis
- Steatohepatitis
- Non-alcoholic steatohepatitis

ICD-9-CM
646.70 Liver disorders in pregnancy, unspecified
571.0 Alcoholic fatty liver
571.8 Other chronic nonalcoholic liver disease

SEE ALSO
Alcohol use disorders
Cirrhosis of the liver
Diabetes mellitus, Type 1
Diabetes mellitus, Type 2

OTHER NOTES N/A

ABBREVIATIONS
NASH = non-alcoholic steatohepatitis

REFERENCES

- Farrell GC. Drugs and steatohepatitis. Seminars in Liver Disease 2002;22:185-94
- Yu AS, Keeffe EB. Nonalcoholic fatty liver disease. Reviews in Gastroenterological Disorders 2002;2:11-19
- Clark JM, Diehl AM. Defining nonalcoholic fatty liver disease- implications for epidemiologic studies. Gastroenterology 2003;124:248-50
- Talwalkar JA All patients with NASH need to have a liver biopsy: arguments for the motion. Canadian J of Gastroenterology 2002;16--718-21
- Laurin J. All patients with Nash need to have a liver biopsy: arguments against the motion. Canadian J of Gastroenterology 2002;16:722-6
- Yang Z, Yamada J, Zhao Y, et al. Prospective screening for pediatric mitochondrial trifunctional protein defects in pregnancies complicated by liver disease. JAMA 2002;288:2163-6
- Li Z, Clark J, Diehl AM. The liver in obesity and type 2 diabetes mellitus. Clinics in Liver Disease 2002;6:867-77
- Marrero A Fontana RJ, Su GL. NAFLD may be a common underlying liver disease in patients with hepatocellular carcinoma in the United States. Hepatology 2002;36:1349-54
- Youssef W, McCullough AJ. Diabetes mellitus, obesity and hepatic steatosis. Seminars in Gastrointestinal Disease 2002;13:17-30
- Brunt EM, Janney CG, Di Bisceglie AM, et al. Non-alcoholic steatohepatitis: a proposal for grading and staging the histological lesions. Am J Gastroenterol 1999;94(9):2467-74
- Promrat K, Lutchman G, Uwaifo GI, et al. A pilot study of pioglitazone treatment for nonalcoholic steatohepatitis. Hepatology 2004; 39 (1) :188-96
- Neuschwander-Terri BA, Brunt EM, Wehmeier KR et al. Improved nonalcoholic steatohepatitis after 48 weeks of treatment with the PPAR-gamma ligand rosiglitazone. Hepatology 2003;38:1008-17
- Harrison SA, Torgerson S, Hayashi P et al. Vitamin E and vitamin C treatment improves fibrsois in patients with nonalcoholic steatohepatitis. Am J Gastroenterol 2003;98 (11): 2485-90
- Wang RT, Koretz RL, Jee HF Jr. Is weight reduction an effective therapy for nonalcoholic fatty liver? A systematic review. Am J Med 2003;115 (7): 554-9

Web references: 0 available at www.5mcc.com
Illustrations N/A

Author(s):
Frank L. Iber, MD

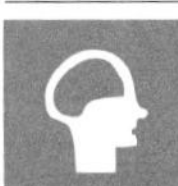

BASICS

DESCRIPTION Incomplete evacuation of feces, leading to formation of a large, firm, immovable mass of stool in the rectum (70%), sigmoid flexure (20%) or proximal colon (10%). The rectosigmoid colon dilates to accommodate the mass, which, in turn, is not pliable enough to pass through the disproportionately small anal canal by the patient's weak defecation effort. Impacted stool may exist as a single mass (stercolith) or as a composite of small, rounded fecal particles (scybalum).

System(s) affected: Gastrointestinal

Genetics: Fecal impaction of the cecum may be seen in cystic fibrosis

Incidence/Prevalence in USA:
- General population - 1% (1000/100,000)
- Children - 1.5%
- Nursing home residents - 30%

Predominant age: Over age 60

Predominant sex: No sex preponderance in adults. Among children, 75% are boys.

SIGNS & SYMPTOMS
- Fecal incontinence, interpreted as "diarrhea"
- Postprandial abdominal pain
- Tenesmus
- Colic
- Nausea, vomiting
- Anorexia, weight loss
- Dehydration
- Headache
- General malaise
- Agitation; confusion
- Fever to 39.4°C (103°F)
- Tachycardia
- Tachypnea
- Urinary frequency, incontinence
- Large mass of stool palpable in lower left quadrant and rectal vault

CAUSES
- Diet lacking in fiber
- Drugs (stimulant laxatives, opiates, benzodiazepines, tricyclic antidepressants, phenothiazines, antihypertensives, sucralfate, iron)
- Local or generalized neurogenic bowel disorders (e.g., stroke, parkinsonism, spinal cord lesions)
- Painful rectal conditions inhibiting voluntary defecation, (e.g., anal fissure, hemorrhoids)
- Neoplastic or inflammatory obstructing lesions (e.g., rectal bezoars)
- Hypothyroidism
- Hypokalemia
- Hypercalcemia
- Excess of gastrointestinal inhibitory hormones (prolactin, endorphins, glucagon, secretin)

RISK FACTORS
- Institutionalization
- Psychogenic illness
- Immobility, inactivity
- Pica
- Chronic renal failure; renal transplant recipients
- Urinary incontinence
- Cognitive decline

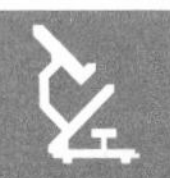

DIAGNOSIS

DIFFERENTIAL DIAGNOSIS
- Irritable bowel syndrome
- Gastroenteritis, colitis
- Diverticulitis
- Appendicitis
- Carcinoma of the colon

LABORATORY
- Leukocytosis to 15,000 WBC/cu.mm
- Hyponatremia
- Hypokalemia
- Stool may be positive for occult blood
- Anemia, due to blood loss

Drugs that may alter lab results: N/A

Disorders that may alter lab results: N/A

PATHOLOGICAL FINDINGS N/A

SPECIAL TESTS Sigmoidoscopy may be used to clarify the nature of a rectosigmoid mass beyond digital reach

IMAGING
- Plain abdominal radiography identifies masses of stool or signs of obstruction if digital exam unrevealing
- Barium enema can differentiate feces from tumor

DIAGNOSTIC PROCEDURES N/A

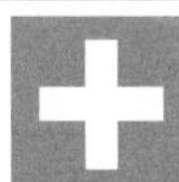

TREATMENT

APPROPRIATE HEALTH CARE Outpatient

GENERAL MEASURES
- Manual fragmentation and extraction of fecal mass (after lubrication with lidocaine jelly) by physician or nurse
- More proximal masses can be disimpacted with water jet directed through fiberoptic sigmoidoscope
- Enemas - containing 20% water soluble contrast material (Gastrografin, Hypaque) may further fragment stool bolus
- For complete evacuation after partial fragmentation - bisacodyl suppositories or enemas with mineral oil, tap water or sodium phosphate
- Ensure minimum fluid intake of 1.5-2.0 liters/day

SURGICAL MEASURES Laparotomy - necessary only in extreme cases

ACTIVITY Increased activity important

DIET
- High fiber
- Home remedy: mix 2 cups bran, 2 cups applesauce and 1 cup unsweetened prune juice. Refrigerate. Take 2 to 3 tablespoons bid.

PATIENT EDUCATION
- Avoid catharsis
- No hot water, soap or hydrogen peroxide enemas! They may burn or irritate rectal mucosa, causing bleeding.

MEDICATIONS

DRUG(S) OF CHOICE

- A daily one-liter bolus of polyethylene glycol-electrolyte (GoLYTELY, Colyte) solution given over 4-6 hours for up to 3 days is reported to be highly effective and acceptable oral therapy in adults
- For disimpaction in children, consider one of the following:
  - ◊ Combination (enema, suppository, oral laxative)
    - Day 1: 1-2 enemas, 1 oz/10 kg to 4.5 oz maximum
    - Day 2: Bisacodyl suppository per rectum every day or twice daily
    - Day 3: Bisacodyl tablet orally every day or twice daily
    - Repeat 3-day cycle if needed 1-2 times
  - ◊ High-dose mineral oil
    - 15-30 mL orally per year of age per day to 8 oz maximum, once or twice daily for 3 days
  - ◊ Enemas
    - 1-2 oz/10 kg to 4.5 oz maximum, once or twice daily for 1-2 days
  - ◊ Polyethylene glycol 3350 (GoLYTELY) is safe and effective in children at doses of 1.0-1.5 g/kg per day for 3 days

Contraindications: N/A

Precautions:

- Use magnesium citrate with caution in patients with renal insufficiency
- Be careful with lactulose; colonic distention can result from its bacterial fermentation

Significant possible interactions: N/A

ALTERNATIVE DRUGS N/A

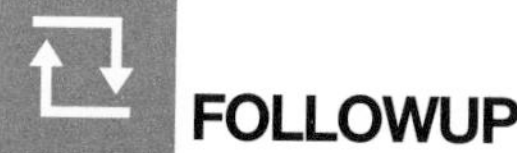

FOLLOWUP

PATIENT MONITORING

- Less than one bowel movement every other day suggests impaction
- Periodic rectal exam

PREVENTION/AVOIDANCE

- Establish regular, consistent toilet time by evoking gastrocolic reflex
- Maintain high fiber diet
- Reinforce exercise
- Install user-friendly commodes
- Use hydrophilic mucilloids (Metamucil) or stool-wetting agents (Colace) as needed
- Consider biofeedback; bowel training
- Periodic enemas, if indicated
- Periodic polyethylene glycol powder (MiraLax), 1 heaping teaspoon in 8 oz water daily for 2 weeks

POSSIBLE COMPLICATIONS

- Complications of impaction
  - ◊ Urinary tract obstruction
  - ◊ Recurrent urinary tract infections
  - ◊ Intestinal obstruction
  - ◊ Spontaneous perforation of colon
  - ◊ Stercoral ulceration
  - ◊ Hernia
  - ◊ Volvulus
  - ◊ Megacolon
  - ◊ Rectal prolapse
  - ◊ Pneumothorax
  - ◊ Hypoxia
  - ◊ Hypovolemic shock
  - ◊ Iliac occlusion
- Complications of disimpaction
  - ◊ Sepsis
  - ◊ Hypotension
  - ◊ Instrumental perforation
  - ◊ Bleeding
  - ◊ Postoperative obstruction

EXPECTED COURSE/PROGNOSIS

- Reimpaction likely, if bowel program not followed
- Prognosis poor for perforation with peritonitis
- Mortality with impaction and obstruction highest in very young and very old (up to 16%)

MISCELLANEOUS

ASSOCIATED CONDITIONS Pulmonary aspiration

AGE-RELATED FACTORS

Pediatric:

- Habitual neglect of defecation urge, because of interference with play, may promote impaction
- Fecal impaction has been reported to occur in over half of all children with chronic constipation

Geriatric:

- Measure thyroid function, electrolyte activity and urea nitrogen levels in elderly patients presenting with impaction
- Much more likely to occur in patients over 80

Others: N/A

PREGNANCY Impaction can produce dysfunctional labor, dystocia

SYNONYMS Terminal reservoir syndrome

ICD-9-CM

560.39 Impaction of intestine, other

SEE ALSO

Constipation
Diarrhea, chronic
Encopresis

OTHER NOTES Electrohydraulic lithotripsy has been used to safely remove large calcified fecaliths

ABBREVIATIONS N/A

REFERENCES

- Feldman M, Friedman LS, Sleisenger MH, editors. Sleisenger & Fordtran's Gastrointestinal and Liver disease. 7th ed. Philadelphia: W.B. Saunders Co; 2002
- Chassagne P, Landrin I, Neveu C, Czernichow P, et al. Fecal incontinence in the institutionalized elderly: incidence, risk factors, and prognosis. Am J Med 1999;106(2):185-190
- Felt B, Wise CG, Olson A, Kochhar P, et al. Guideline for the management of pediatric idiopathic constipation and soiling. Arch Pediatr Adolesc Med 1999;153:380-85
- Whitehead WE, Wald A, Norton NJ. Treatment options for fecal incontinence. Dis Colon Rectum 2001;44:131-144
- Youssef NN, Peters JM, Henderson W, et al. Dose response of PEG 3350 for the treatment of childhood fecal impaction. J Pediatr 2002;141(3):410-4

Web references: 0 available at www.5mcc.com

Illustrations N/A

Author(s):

Richard Viken, MD

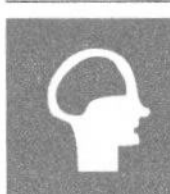

BASICS

DESCRIPTION Failure to conceive after one year of unprotected intercourse
System(s) affected: Endocrine/Metabolic, Reproductive
Genetics: PCO; clusters in families. Possibly genetic defects - insulin gene polymorphism, Klinefelter syndrome (XXY), Y chromosomal defects, Turner syndrome (mosaics).
Incidence/Prevalence in USA: 10-15% of all couples. Incidence increasing as 20% of women are delaying childbearing until after age 35.
Predominant age: Increases with age, e.g., ages 30-34: 14% infertile, ages 35-39: 20% infertile, ages 40-45: 25% infertile
Predominant sex: N/A

SIGNS & SYMPTOMS
- Thorough history and physical should be performed on each partner
- Genital/pelvic infection (e.g., pelvic inflammatory disease often associated with an obstruction of reproductive tract)
- Endocrine dysfunction (e.g., hypothyroidism, hypogonadism, abnormal puberty) often associated with abnormalities of ovulation or spermatogenesis
- Sexual dysfunction (e.g., premature ejaculation) may contribute to the problem
- Anovulatory cycles are frequently irregular, without premenstrual symptoms or dysmenorrhea. Some patients may have features (e.g., hirsutism, obesity, acne) suggestive of polycystic ovarian disease.
- Endometriosis is often associated with cyclic premenstrual pain, secondary dysmenorrhea and dyspareunia

CAUSES
Most couples have more than one factor
- Male factors 30-40%
- Ovulation factors 15%
- Cervical/uterine factors 10%
- Tubal/peritoneal factors including endometriosis 40%
- Immunologic factors 5%
- Psychogenic/nutritional/metabolic factors 5%
- Unexplained infertility 10-20%

RISK FACTORS Multiple - see under Causes

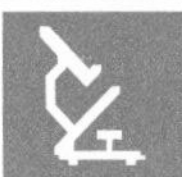

DIAGNOSIS

DIFFERENTIAL DIAGNOSIS N/A

LABORATORY
Only basic elements of evaluation and diagnosis will be discussed here. Most of the tests of spermatogenesis and ovulation should be repeated at least once if abnormal.
- Semen analysis, normal values are (modified strict Krueger):
  - ◊ Volume 2-6 mL
  - ◊ pH 7-8
  - ◊ Viscosity - liquefies within one hour
  - ◊ Count - 20 million/cc or greater
  - ◊ Motility - 50% or more
  - ◊ Morphology - 14% or more normal morphology
- Basal body temperature charting
  - ◊ Assesses ovulation and adequacy of the luteal phase
  - ◊ Morning temperature should rise about one degree Fahrenheit at the time of ovulation and remain elevated for 13-14 days (less than 11 is abnormal)
- Serum progesterone
  - ◊ Assesses ovulation and corpus luteum function
  - ◊ A level of 10mg/mL or greater correlates with ovulation
  - ◊ Should be obtained on approximately day 21-23 of a 28 day menstrual cycle
  - ◊ Assessment of ovarian reserve-day 3 FSH <15mlu/mL
- Endometrial biopsy (short luteal phase) (day 13 progesterone <10)
  - ◊ Obtain on day 25-27 of a 28 day cycle or 11-14 days after the LH surge
  - ◊ Assesses ovulation, function of the corpus luteum, and normalcy of the endometrium (luteal phase defect - out of phase endometrium > 2 days in at least 2 cycles)
- The following tests are useful to evaluate underlying causes of anovulation or low sperm counts:
  - ◊ Thyroid stimulating hormone
  - ◊ Prolactin >20mg/mL
  - ◊ Testosterone - decreased in primary male gonadal failure; increased in female hyperandrogenism, PCO
  - ◊ Follicle stimulating hormone (FSH) and luteinizing hormone (LH) (elevated in primary gonadal failure, decreased in hypopituitarism); LH/FSH ratio > 2.5 consistent with PCO
  - ◊ Karyotype (elevated FSH/LH), e.g., Klinefelter syndrome, Turner syndrome (mosaic)
  - ◊ Glucose intolerance - glucose tolerance test, fasting glucose/insulin ratio < 4.5, fasting insulin > 20mU/cc - insulin resistance, PCO (some diagnose insulin resistance by clinical picture)
  - ◊ Late onset congenital adrenal hyperplasia - 17 OH progesterone
  - ◊ Adrenal disease - DHEAS
- Post coital test (not that useful - historical value)
  - ◊ Evaluates sperm/cervical mucus interaction
  - ◊ Cervical mucus is aspirated with a nasal polyps forceps or a tuberculin syringe from the os after intercourse during the mid cycle (ferning, elasticity of mucus)
  - ◊ If 20 or more sperm with directional movement are seen per high-power field of a microscope, the result is good. Sperm with shaking motion suggest sperm antibody.

Drugs that may alter lab results:
- Semen abnormalities can be caused by:
  - ◊ Cimetidine
  - ◊ Spironolactone
  - ◊ Nitrofurantoin
  - ◊ Sulfasalazine
  - ◊ Marijuana
  - ◊ Chemotherapeutic agents
  - ◊ Cocaine
  - ◊ Excessive alcohol
  - ◊ Occupational/environmental hazards/toxins

Disorders that may alter lab results:
- Polycystic ovarian disease
- Endometriosis
- Severe hypospadias
- Retrograde ejaculation (often associated with diabetes)
- Varicocele (controversial)
- Testicular injury (e.g., surgery, mumps, trauma)
- Occupational/environmental hazards/toxins
- Loop electrosurgical excision procedure (LEEP) - no cervical mucus

PATHOLOGICAL FINDINGS N/A

SPECIAL TESTS Multiple tests (e.g., hamster egg penetration assay - to assess sperm's ability to fertilize) are available to study specific aspects of reproduction, but are used only by fertility specialists, and available in only specialized labs. Also hemizona assay, immunobead binding test. Tests now bypassed by intracytoplasmic sperm injection (ICSI).

IMAGING
- Hysterosalpingogram (HSG) - evaluates tubal patency and uterine contour. This procedure may have some therapeutic benefit. Avoid if history suggests an infection.
- Pelvic ultrasound - fibroids, ovarian pathology, endometriomas, subcortical ovarian cysts (PCO), Müllerian defects
- MRI - Müllerian defects

DIAGNOSTIC PROCEDURES Laparoscopy - should be deferred until basic evaluation is complete. Can be diagnostic and therapeutic (eg, chromotubation, simultaneous hysteroscopy and operative laparoscopy). May be bypassed for intrauterine insemination/clomiphene trial. Ovarian drilling in clomiphene resistant PCO decreases testosterone load (can cause adhesions).

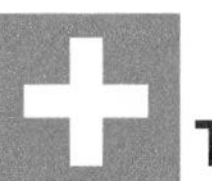

TREATMENT

APPROPRIATE HEALTH CARE Outpatient evaluation, with attention to the emotional support of the couple

GENERAL MEASURES
- Dispel myths and provide accurate information
- Simultaneously evaluate and counsel both partners without blame!
- Find and correct causes of infertility
- Provide information on adoption when appropriate, early in work-up
- Consider donor insemination or intrauterine insemination for refractory abnormalities of semen analysis. Intracytoplasmic sperm injection (ICSI) available for oligospermia, antisperm antibodies, poor cervical mucus, or poor capacitation.
- Discontinue smoking, excessive alcohol, and/or illicit drugs, limit toxin exposure
- IVF-severe tubal disease: need for donor eggs, sperm manipulation. IVF indicated after 2 years of unexplained infertility, after 1 year of treatment for a particular defect, or after 1 year of donor insemination or ovulation induction.
- Unexplained infertility - IUI (intrauterine insemination) and clomiphene trial increases fertility rate 3x compared to placebo

SURGICAL MEASURES
- Laparoscopy if workup suspicious for tubal blockage/ endometriosis. Destruction of endometriosis in mild-moderate disease helpful
- Consider laparoscopy for endometriosis tubal factor, lysis of adhesions, and correction of tubal obstruction
- Correction of Müllerian defects
- Removal of polyps, fibroids (only after other factors ruled out) - if large, prevents implantation/blocks tubes
- Vasovasostomy
- Vasoepididymostomy
- Testicular sperm extraction procedure
- Consider varicocele repair for abnormal semen analysis (controversial, refuted by scientific trials)

ACTIVITY
- Males with low sperm counts should avoid hot tubs/saunas (decreased spermatogenesis with elevated scrotal temperature)
- If the male has low sperm counts, intercourse should be timed to occur approximately every 24-36 hours during the fertile period. Start 5-6 days prior to expected ovulation and continue for 2 days afterwards.
- Regular intercourse 2-3 times a week for most couples
- Abstaining to "save up" - not proven

DIET N/A

PATIENT EDUCATION
- RESOLVE, 5 Water St, Arlington, MA 02174
- Fertility Research Foundation, 1430 Second Avenue, Suite 103, New York, NY 10021, (212)744-5500
- American College of Obstetricians & Gynecologists, 409 12th St, SW, Washington, DC 20024-2188, (800)762-ACOG
- Endometriosis Association 8585 N. 76th Pl., Milwaukee, WI 53223

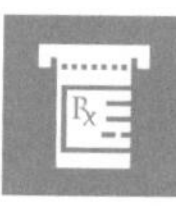

MEDICATIONS

DRUG(S) OF CHOICE
- Clomiphene (Clomid): Indicated for induction of ovulation. Typical dose - 25-50 mg daily x 5 days on days 3-7 of cycle. Increase monthly by 50 mg increments until ovulation (BBT, progesterone) and continue for 3-4 months. Maximum 150-200 mg. This estrogen antagonist binds to receptors in the hypothalamus and stimulates increased release of gonadotropin releasing hormone (GnRH), leading to increased secretion of follicle stimulating hormone (FSH) and luteinizing hormone (LH) from the pituitary.
- Bromocriptine/cabergoline: Indicated for treatment of anovulation associated with galactorrhea, hyperprolactinemia or pituitary microadenomas

Contraindications: N/A

Precautions:
- Clomiphene - hyperstimulation syndrome, multiple pregnancy, hot flashes. Pelvic exams are useful to rule out ovarian enlargement. Cervical mucus may be scant and require estrogen supplementation.
- Bromocriptine/cabergoline - headaches, nausea, lightheadedness

Significant possible interactions: N/A

ALTERNATIVE DRUGS
- Fertility specialists with access to specialized lab
  - ◊ Human menopausal gonadotropin (FSH, LH) or urofollitropin (FSH)
  - ◊ GnRH analogs - hypogonadotrophic hypogonadism - pulsatile
- Treatment of insulin resistance
  - ◊ Metformin (Glucophage) - gradually increase from 500 mg qd x 5 days to 500 mg bid x 5 days, and finally 500 mg tid. This minimizes side effects. No reports of hypoglycemia. Repeat abnormal hormones in 1 month. Restart clomiphene at lower level.
- Intrauterine insemination - oligospermia, cervical factors (LEEP), coital problems
- Inadequate luteal phase - clomiphene, supplemental progesterone
- Adrenal component - glucocorticoids

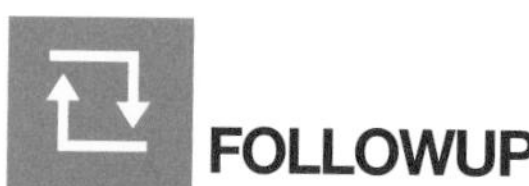

FOLLOWUP

PATIENT MONITORING See under Diagnosis

PREVENTION/AVOIDANCE
- Maintain normal BMI; even loss of 5-10% helps
- Prevention of sexually transmitted disease and subsequent pelvic inflammatory disease
- Treat endometriosis when diagnosis is made - chronic condition. Birth control pills until fertility desired controls disease progression.

POSSIBLE COMPLICATIONS
- Plural gestation with ovulation induction
- Ectopic pregnancy following tubal re-anastomosis - 15% risk
- Risk of ovarian cancer with 11 cycles or more of clomiphene has recently been discounted

EXPECTED COURSE/PROGNOSIS
- About half of couples conceive during the second year of unprotected intercourse
- If the couple has been infertile for four or more years, the prognosis tends to be poor
- Encourage initiation of adoption process

MISCELLANEOUS

ASSOCIATED CONDITIONS IUD use and non-monogamous sex increases risk of infection. Also small risk at insertion.

AGE-RELATED FACTORS
Pediatric: N/A

Geriatric: N/A

Others:
- Increasing anovulation with increasing age
- Increased disease burden with age from diseases like endometriosis, and cumulative exposure to environmental/occupational hazards
- Decreased ovarian reserve - menstrual day 3 FSH. If > 10, poor reserve (newer assays). If < 10, adequate reserve. Good IVF candidate.
- Clomiphene challenge test: clomiphene 100 mg/day days 5-9. FSH > 26 on day 10, poor prognosis
- Consider oocyte donation with older couples, or poor ovarian reserve
- Unruptured luteinized follicle - avoid NSAIDs

PREGNANCY N/A

SYNONYMS N/A

ICD-9-CM
606.9 Male infertility, unspecified

628.9 Female infertility of unspecified origin

SEE ALSO
Erectile dysfunction

Hypothyroidism, adult

Klinefelter syndrome

Pelvic inflammatory disease (PID)

Polycystic ovarian disease

Turner syndrome

OTHER NOTES N/A

ABBREVIATIONS
PCO = polycystic ovarian disease

LEEP = loop electrosurgical excision procedure

REFERENCES

- ACOG Practice Bulletin. Number 34, February 2002. Management of infertility caused by ovulatory dysfunction. American College of Obstetricians and Gynecologists. Obstet Gynecol 2002;99(2):347-58
- ACOG Practice Bulletin. Number 41, Dec 2002. Clinical Management Guidelines for Obstetrician-Gynecologists. American College of Obstetricians and Gynecologists. Obstet Gynecol 2002;100(6):1389-402
- Barbieri RL. Metformin for the treatment of polycystic ovary syndrome. Obstet Gynecol 2003;101(4):785-93
- Forti G, Krausz C. Evaluation and treatment of the infertile couple. J Clin Endocrinol & Metab 1998;83:4177-88
- Futterweit W. Polycystic ovary syndrome: clinical perspectives and management. Obstet Gynecol Surv 1999;54(6):403-13
- Guzick DS, et al. Efficacy of superovulation and intrauterine insemination in the treatment of infertility. NEJM 1999;340:117-83
- Hull MGR, Cahill DJ. Female infertility. Endocrinol Metab Clin North Am 1998;27:851-76
- Hunter MH, Sterrett JJ. Polycystic ovary syndrome: it's not just infertility. Am Fam Physician 2000;62(5):1079-88,1090
- Legro RS. Polycystic ovary syndrome: current and future treatment paradigms. Am J Obstet Gynecol 1998;179(6 Pt 2):S101-S108
- Nestler JE, et al. Effects of metformin on spontaneous and clomiphene induced ovulation in the polycystic ovary syndrome. NEJM 1998;338:1876-80
- Precis, reproductive endocrinology: an update in obstetrics and gynecology. Washington DC, ACOG, 1998
- Speroff L, Glass R, Kase N. Clinical Gynecologic Endocrinology and Infertility. 6th ed. Baltimore: Williams & Wilkins; 1999
- Stanford JB, White GL, Hatasaka H. Timing intercourse to achieve pregnancy: current evidence. Obstet Gynecol 2002;100(6):1333-41
- Taylor A. Polycystic ovary syndrome. Endocrinol Metab Clin North Am 1998;27:877-902
- Velasquez E, Acosta A, Mendoza S. Menstrual cyclicity after metformin therapy in polycystic ovary syndrome. Obstet & Gynecol 1997;90:392-5
- Marcoux S, Maheux R, Berube S, The Canadian Collaborative Group on Endometriosis. Laparoscopic Surgery in Infertile Women with Minimal or Mild Endometriosis. N Engl J Med 1997; 337:217-222

Web references: 1 available at www.5mcc.com

Illustrations N/A

Author(s):
Eric S. Miller, MD

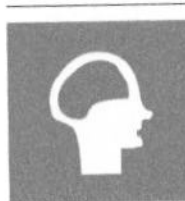

BASICS

DESCRIPTION Current criteria:
- Fever greater than 38.3°C (101°F) on at least four occasions over a 14 day period
- Illness of 14 days duration without an obvious cause

System(s) affected: Endocrine/Metabolic
Genetics: N/A
Incidence/Prevalence in USA: No data on actual incidence
Predominant age: All ages
Predominant sex: Dependent on etiology

SIGNS & SYMPTOMS
- Fever does not present as the only manifestation of a disease. The type and pattern of fever is of little help in making the diagnosis.
- Constitutional symptoms that almost always accompany a fever: headache, myalgia, malaise

CAUSES
- Over 200 causes; each with a prevalence of 5% or less
- Infection
  - ◊ Abdominal abscesses
  - ◊ Mycobacterial infection
  - ◊ Cytomegalovirus
  - ◊ Endocarditis/pericarditis
  - ◊ Sinusitis
  - ◊ HIV (late stage)
  - ◊ Renal
  - ◊ Osteomyelitis
  - ◊ Catheter infections
  - ◊ Amebic hepatitis
  - ◊ Wound infections
  - ◊ Other miscellaneous infections
- Neoplasms
  - ◊ Lymphoma
  - ◊ Leukemia
  - ◊ Solid tumors (hypernephroma)
  - ◊ Hepatoma
  - ◊ Atrial myxoma
  - ◊ Colon cancer
- Collagen vascular disease
  - ◊ Giant cell arteritis
  - ◊ Polyarteritis nodosa
  - ◊ Rheumatic fever
  - ◊ Systemic lupus erythematosus
  - ◊ Rheumatoid arthritis
  - ◊ Polymyalgia rheumatica
- Other causes
  - ◊ Granulomatous diseases
  - ◊ Pulmonary emboli/deep vein thrombosis
  - ◊ Drug fever
  - ◊ Thermoregulatory disorders
  - ◊ Endocrinologic diseases
  - ◊ Occupational causes
  - ◊ Periodic fever
  - ◊ Factitious/fraudulent fever
  - ◊ Cerebrovascular accident
  - ◊ Cirrhosis
  - ◊ Alcoholic hepatitis
  - ◊ Other

RISK FACTORS
- Recent travel
- Exposure to biologic or chemical agents
- Persons in AIDS risk group
- Elderly persons
- Drug abuse
- Immigrants

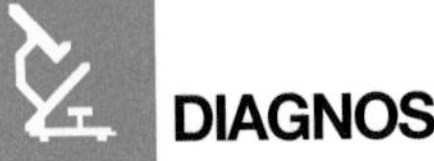

DIAGNOSIS

DIFFERENTIAL DIAGNOSIS See Causes

LABORATORY
- CBC - leukopenia, anemia, thrombocytopenia/thrombocytosis
- C-reactive protein
- Sedimentation rate - elevated
- Liver function tests (especially alkaline phosphatase) - evidence of inflammation, obstruction or infiltrative disease
- Blood cultures (not to exceed 6)
- Urinalysis and urine culture

Drugs that may alter lab results: N/A

Disorders that may alter lab results: N/A

PATHOLOGICAL FINDINGS Dependent on etiology

SPECIAL TESTS
- Tuberculin skin test - may not be helpful if anergic or acute infection. If test negative, repeat in 2 weeks.
- Sputum and urine cultures for tuberculosis
- Gastric washing for tuberculosis
- Serologic tests - Epstein-Barr, hepatitis, syphilis, Lyme disease, Q fever, cytomegalovirus, amebiasis/coccidioidomycosis
- HIV antibody test
- Serum protein electrophoresis - if immunologic etiology suspected
- Thyroid function tests - if thyroiditis suspected
- Rheumatoid factor and antinuclear antibody test - if collagen vascular disease suspected

IMAGING
- Chest x-ray
- Abdominal films
- Sinus x-rays - if clinically indicated
- Bone scan - if osteomyelitis or metastatic disease suspected
- CT scan or MRI of abdomen and pelvis (plus directed biopsy, if indicated) - if infectious process or mass lesions suspected
- 67-gallium or Tc-sulfur colloid scan - if infectious process or tumor suspected
- FDG PET (positron emission tomography using the radiolabeled glucose analogue 18 F-fluorodeoxyglucose scan) - if infectious process, inflammatory process, or tumor suspected
- Ultrasound of abdomen and pelvis (plus directed biopsy, if indicated) - if mass lesions, renal obstruction or gallbladder/biliary tree pathology suspected
- Leg Doppler - if DVT/PE suspected
- Echocardiogram - if cardiac valve lesions, atrial myxomas or pericardial effusion suspected (transthoracic vs transesophageal)
- Ventilation/perfusion scan - if pulmonary emboli suspected
- Indium-labeled leukocyte scanning - if inflammatory process suspected

DIAGNOSTIC PROCEDURES
- Bone marrow - if granulomatous disease, infection or malignancy suspected
- Liver biopsy - if granulomatous disease suspected
- Temporal artery biopsy - if giant cell arteritis suspected
- Lymph node, muscle or skin biopsy - if clinically indicated
- Spinal tap - if clinically indicated
- Exploratory laparotomy - if otherwise unsuccessful in determining etiology

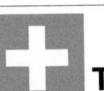

TREATMENT

APPROPRIATE HEALTH CARE
- Outpatient
- Hospitalization reserved for ill and debilitated and also in those in which factitious fever has been ruled out or an invasive procedure is indicated

GENERAL MEASURES
- Attempt to determine etiology before initiating therapy
- Avoid therapeutic trials unless as a last resort and only if therapy is reasonably specific
- "Shotgun" approaches are condemned since they do not solve the problem, obscure the clinical picture and have effects

SURGICAL MEASURES N/A

ACTIVITY Ambulatory primarily

DIET With temperature elevations, patients will have increased caloric and fluid demands

PATIENT EDUCATION Maintain an open line of communication between physician and patient/family as the workup progresses; the extended time required in establishing a diagnosis can be frustrating for all parties

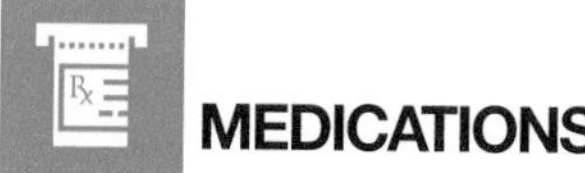

MEDICATIONS

DRUG(S) OF CHOICE

- Dependent on diagnosis. In up to a fifth of patients, the cause of the fever will not be identified in spite of a thorough work up. If the patient has symptoms with the fever or continues to decline, a therapeutic trial may be indicated.
  - ◊ Antipyretics such as acetaminophen or aspirin
  - ◊ Non-steroidal anti-inflammatory drugs such as indomethacin or naproxen
  - ◊ Steroid trial based on patient's history
  - ◊ Antibiotic trial based on patient's history
  - ◊ Antituberculous therapy if at high risk for granulomatous disease pending culture results

Contraindications: Aspirin should be avoided in children because of the risk of Reye syndrome
Precautions: If a steroid trial is initiated, the physician must be aware the patient may have a relapse after treatment or if certain conditions (such as tuberculosis) have been undiagnosed, the therapy may have deleterious effects
Significant possible interactions: Refer to manufacturer's literature

ALTERNATIVE DRUGS N/A

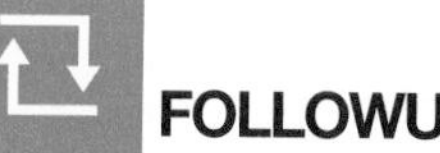

FOLLOWUP

PATIENT MONITORING If the etiology of the fever continues to elude the physician, a history and physical examination along with screening laboratory studies should be repeated. Special attention should be paid to travel, occupational, sexual, and drug exposure.

PREVENTION/AVOIDANCE N/A

POSSIBLE COMPLICATIONS Dependent on etiology

EXPECTED COURSE/PROGNOSIS

- Dependent on etiology and age
  - ◊ HIV infected patients have highest mortality
  - ◊ One year survival rates reflecting deaths due to all causes:

91% < 35 year olds
82% 35-64 year olds
67% > 64 year olds

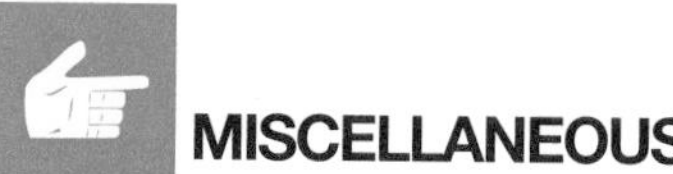

MISCELLANEOUS

ASSOCIATED CONDITIONS N/A

AGE-RELATED FACTORS

Pediatric:

- Infections and collagen-vascular diseases most likely etiology
- Inflammatory bowel disease common etiology in older children and adolescents
- Has a better prognosis than in non-pediatric cases

Geriatric:

- Most common causes are acute leukemia, Hodgkin lymphoma, intra-abdominal infections, tuberculosis and temporal arteritis
- Signs and symptoms in the elderly are much more nonspecific
- Co-existing diseases and numerous medications may cloud features
- Mortality rates are higher in the elderly

Others: Consider factitious fever in young female health care workers. In HIV infected patients, FUO usually occurs with advanced disease. Mycobacterium is the most common cause.

PREGNANCY Fever is known to increase the risk of neural tube defects and trigger preterm labor

SYNONYMS N/A

ICD-9-CM

780.6 Fever
778.4 Other disturbances of temperature regulation of newborn
659.20 Pyrexia of unknown origin during labor
672.0 Pyrexia of unknown origin during puerperium

SEE ALSO

Arthritis, juvenile rheumatoid (JRA)
Atrial myxoma
Colorectal malignancy
Cytomegalovirus inclusion disease
Endocarditis, infective
Giant cell arteritis
Granulomatous disease of childhood, chronic
Hepatitis, alcoholic
Hepatoma
HIV infection & AIDS
Leukemia
Osteomyelitis
Polyarteritis nodosa
Polymyalgia rheumatica
Pulmonary embolism
Rheumatic fever
Sinusitis
Stroke (Brain attack)
Systemic lupus erythematosus (SLE)

OTHER NOTES N/A

ABBREVIATIONS

PUO = pyrexia of unknown origin

REFERENCES

- Davies GR, Finch RG. Fever of unknown origin. Clin Med 2001;1(3):177-9
- Mourad O, Palda V, Detsky AS. A comprehensive evidence-based approach to fever of unknown origin. Arch Intern Med 2003;163(5):545-51
- Roth AR, Basello GM. Approach to the adult patient with fever of unknown origin. Am Fam Physician 2003;68(11):2223-8

Web references: 0 available at www.5mcc.com
Illustrations N/A

Author(s):

Scott T. Henderson, MD

BASICS

DESCRIPTION Fibrocystic breast disease is a generalized term for benign breast disorders such as lumps and pain. The term benign breast disease is preferred. Benign lumps are usually smooth, regular, and mobile. The following classifications are useful:
- Lumps:
  - ◊ Physiologic nodularity - lumps vary with the phase of the menstrual cycle, common in young women
  - ◊ Mastoplasia - a ropy, thickening of the breast tissue, most common in the upper outer quadrant, persists throughout the menstrual cycle
  - ◊ Cysts - distended, fluid filled masses caused by an imbalance between secretion and absorption in the breast lobule, common in the decade preceding menopause
  - ◊ Fibroadenoma - benign solid tumor, smooth margins, mobile, most common tumor in teenagers and young women, may occur at any age after thelarche
  - ◊ Phyllodes tumors - painless, solid, smooth, lobular, bulky; stromal hyperplasia; 10% are malignant
- Nipple discharge
  - ◊ Although considered one of the warning signs for breast cancer, 90% of patients with nipple discharge have benign disease
  - ◊ Bilateral duct ectasia - most common cause of nipple discharge; benign inflammatory condition; bilateral, sticky, multicolored discharge; usually has to be expressed
  - ◊ Bilateral galactorrhea-prolactin-secreting pituitary tumors - usually in association with amenorrhea; drugs (isoniazid, methyldopa, thiazides, reserpine, tricyclic antidepressants, BCP's); trauma; hypothyroidism
  - ◊ Unilateral intraductal papilloma - spontaneous discharge from one duct. Carcinoma must be excluded.
- Pain
  - ◊ Cyclical mastodynia - hormonal, an exaggeration of the normal premenstrual tenderness
  - ◊ Non-cyclical - sclerosing adenosis, cysts, chest wall muscle spasm, costochondritis, fibromyalgia, neuritis, stress, referred pain
- Inflammatory conditions
  - ◊ Fat necrosis - a solid lump with or without pain that can mimic carcinoma
  - ◊ Superficial phlebitis of the thoracoepigastric vein (Mondor disease) - local tenderness and induration
  - ◊ Mastitis/abscess - exquisite pain and tenderness, erythema (common), not always a definite mass, common with lactation and squamous metaplasia of lactiferous ducts (Zuska disease), usually caused by staphylococcal organisms
- Growth disorders
  - ◊ Accessory nipples (polythelia)
  - ◊ Absence of the breast (amastia)
  - ◊ Absence of the nipple (athelia)
  - ◊ Hypoplasia (often associated with hypoplasia of the thorax and pectoral muscles, and abnormalities of the hand, i.e., Poland syndrome)
  - ◊ Gigantomastia: occurs during puberty and pregnancy
  - ◊ Gynecomastia: occurs in men in association with puberty, senescence, liver disease, and testicular tumors, and medications such as digoxin and cimetidine

System(s) affected: Skin/Exocrine
Genetics: Family history of cysts common
Incidence/Prevalence in USA: Unknown. It is estimated that at least 50% of women have benign breast symptoms during their lifetime.
Predominant age:
- Symptoms tend to occur in menstruating women
- Mastoplasia - most common in women from mid 20's to 55 years of age
- Cysts - usually seen in women in their 40's
- Cyclical mastodynia - common in menstruating women
- Non-cyclical pain - can occur at any age after breast development

Predominant sex: Female > Male (almost exclusively)

SIGNS & SYMPTOMS
- Asymptomatic
- Breast pain
- Breast tenderness
- Pain subsides after menses
- Smooth masses
- Tense masses
- Fluctuant masses
- Bilateral masses
- Breast engorgement
- Breast thickening
- Nipple discharge

CAUSES
- The etiology of benign breast disease is unknown
- Possible causes:
  - ◊ Luteal phase defect in progesterone
  - ◊ Increased estrogen (17 beta estradiol)
  - ◊ Hyperprolactinemia
  - ◊ End organ hypersensitivity to estrogen
  - ◊ Sensitivity to methylxanthines
  - ◊ Dietary fat intake

RISK FACTORS
- Unknown
- The effect of consumption of methylxanthine-containing substances, e.g., coffee, tea, cola, and chocolate is controversial

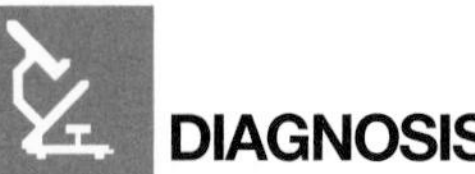

DIAGNOSIS

DIFFERENTIAL DIAGNOSIS
- Lumps - breast cancer, sebaceous cyst
- Skin changes - breast cancer, eczema
- Pain - costochondritis, chest wall muscle spasm, neuralgia, anxiety, depression, breast cancer, angina pectoris, gastroesophageal reflux, Pancoast tumor

LABORATORY Prolactin, TSH (if galactorrhea), aspiration cytology or biopsy of discrete mass

Drugs that may alter lab results: N/A

Disorders that may alter lab results: N/A

PATHOLOGICAL FINDINGS Hyperplasia of breast epithelium or stroma, adenosis, microcysts, macrocysts, duct ectasia (plasma cell mastitis), apocrine metaplasia

SPECIAL TESTS N/A

IMAGING
- Mammography
  - ◊ Signs of malignancy include irregular mass, clustered masses, calcifications, architectural distortion, dilated duct
  - ◊ May be normal in presence of malignancy; mammograms are difficult to interpret in women less than age 35 due to dense breast tissue
- Ultrasonography
  - ◊ Useful for differentiating cystic from solid lesions
- Thermography (available at a few institutions)

DIAGNOSTIC PROCEDURES
- Fine needle aspiration and biopsy - allows differentiation of cystic and solid lesion. Cells sent for cytology can diagnose cancer with a relatively high degree of accuracy. Low morbidity. If mass disappears, no further evaluation is necessary.
- Core needle biopsy - usually not indicated for fibrocystic disease. Useful in diagnosis of a large cancer.
- Excisional biopsy - indicated for all solid lumps that are not clearly benign

TREATMENT

APPROPRIATE HEALTH CARE Outpatient. May be inpatient for biopsy or surgery.

GENERAL MEASURES
- Evaluate to be certain there is no malignancy by means of imaging and diagnostic procedures
- Pain rarely severe or disabling
- Frequently resolves spontaneously
- Reassure patient there is no malignancy
- Cold compresses may be helpful
- Well fitting, supportive brassiere (worn night and day)

SURGICAL MEASURES Possibly excision (under local anesthesia) of benign fibroadenoma or phyllode tumors, and fat necrosis lesions

ACTIVITY No restrictions. Avoid activities that may cause trauma to the breasts.

DIET Abstention from methylxanthines (coffee, tea, caffeine-containing soda and chocolate)

PATIENT EDUCATION
- American College of Obstetricians & Gynecologists, 409 12th St., SW, Washington, DC 20024-2188, (800)762-ACOG
- Booklet on Breast Self Examination from Primary care and Care and Cancer, 17 Prospect St., Huntington, NY 11743, (516)424-8900
- National Cancer Institute, (800)4-CANCER
- American Cancer Society; http://www3.cancer.org/cancerinfo/documents/bbreast.asp?ct=5

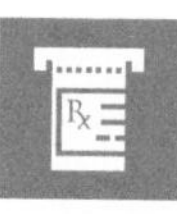

MEDICATIONS

DRUG(S) OF CHOICE
- For cyclical pain and swelling unresponsive to general measures - oral contraceptives have been shown to decrease the risk of fibrocystic breast disease; spironolactone (Aldactone) 10 mg bid premenstrually may be helpful or vitamin A 150,000 IU daily for 3 months; vitamin E 300-600 IU a day for 3 months
- For more severe disease - danazol (Danocrine) 100-200 mg per day or bromocriptine 2.5 mg bid for 3 months may be useful, but side effects and expense limit their usefulness

Contraindications: Refer to manufacturer's literature
Precautions: Refer to manufacturer's literature
Significant possible interactions: Refer to manufacturer's literature

ALTERNATIVE DRUGS N/A

FOLLOWUP

PATIENT MONITORING
- Patients with fibrocystic change may have an increased risk of malignancy
- If there is no atypia on biopsy the risk is only minimally increased
- Patients need to be assessed with clinical examination, radiological studies, and, sometimes, biopsy to be certain a given lump is not malignant
- Followup times are variable depending on the clinical situation. A young patient in whom physiological nodularity is suspected should be observed through one menstrual cycle.
- Mammograms should be obtained at age 35, at least every 1-2 years after age 40, and yearly after age 50
- Ultrasound is useful to differentiate cysts from solid lesions, but is not used for screening
- Aspiration cytology is useful for diagnosis of cysts and solid lesions. The false positive rate ranges from 0-5.8%, and the false negative rate from 1.7-22%.
- When physical examination, mammography, and needle aspiration are used in combination, detection rates for breast cancer range from 93-100%

PREVENTION/AVOIDANCE Avoiding caffeine may reduce breast pain

POSSIBLE COMPLICATIONS
- Fibrocystic change can make physical examination and mammograms difficult to interpret
- Atypical hyperplasia may lead to cancer

EXPECTED COURSE/PROGNOSIS
Benign, chronic, recurring, intermittent

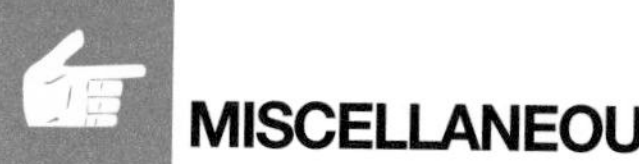

MISCELLANEOUS

ASSOCIATED CONDITIONS Breast carcinoma

AGE-RELATED FACTORS
Pediatric: Biopsy in children should be avoided since a developing breast bud may be inadvertently removed
Geriatric: Not as common in this age group
Others: Prophylactic mastectomy for pain is rarely indicated since many patients have underlying psychiatric problems

PREGNANCY N/A

SYNONYMS
- Chronic cystic mastitis
- Adenosis
- Benign breast disease
- Mammary dysplasia
- Fibrocystic disease

ICD-9-CM
610.1 Diffuse cystic mastopathy

SEE ALSO

OTHER NOTES N/A

ABBREVIATIONS N/A

REFERENCES

- Rohan TE, Miller AB: A cohort study of oral contraceptive use and risk of benign breast disease. Int J Cancer 1999;82(2):191-6
- Smith BL. The Breast. In: Ryan KJ, editor. Kistner's Gynecology & Women's Health. 7th ed. St Louis: Mosby; 1999

Web references: 0 available at www.5mcc.com
Illustrations N/A

Author(s):
Cathryn Heath, MD
John C. Smulian, MD, MPH

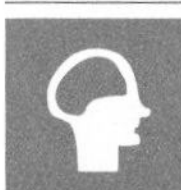

BASICS

DESCRIPTION Extremely common pain phenomenon occurring in a defined pattern, reproduced by pressure on "trigger points".
System(s) affected: Musculoskeletal, Nervous
Genetics: N/A
Incidence/Prevalence in USA: Prevalence: 7-10%
Predominant age: 18-70
Predominant sex: Female > Male

SIGNS & SYMPTOMS
- Pressure manually applied to specific sites, referred to as "trigger points" reproduce the patient's symptoms:
  - ◊ Temporalis - above the ear
  - ◊ Anterior to tragus of ear
  - ◊ Scalenus capitis
  - ◊ Sternocleidomastoid
  - ◊ Low anterior neck
  - ◊ Pectoralis minor
  - ◊ Manubriosternal
  - ◊ Anterior and posterior axillary folds
  - ◊ Trapezius ridge
  - ◊ Upper rhomboids
  - ◊ Lower rhomboids
  - ◊ Iliac crest
  - ◊ Mid-buttocks
  - ◊ Mid-rectus femoris
  - ◊ Mid-vastus lateralis
  - ◊ Quadriceps insertion - at the patella
  - ◊ Humeral epicondyles (many investigators would diagnose fibromyalgia, while some prefer epicondylitis) and negative tenderness at "neutral sites" (e.g., scapula, glabella)
  - ◊ Absence of neutral point tenderness
- Other signs and symptoms often of a chronic nature
  - ◊ Non-restorative sleep, with early morning awakening in an unrefreshed state
  - ◊ Typically insidious in onset
  - ◊ Pain is increased in the morning, with weather changes, anxiety, stress
  - ◊ Pain improved by mild physical activity or vacations (stress-relieving situations)
  - ◊ Abnormal non-rapid eye movement (non-REM) stage IV sleep
  - ◊ Generalized fatigue or tiredness
  - ◊ Anxiety
  - ◊ Chronic headache
  - ◊ Irritable bowel syndrome
  - ◊ Subjective, non-confirmable complaints of swelling or numbness, not associated with objective neurologic findings
  - ◊ Depression
  - ◊ Reduced physical endurance
  - ◊ Decreased social interaction

CAUSES
- Loss of non-REM stage IV sleep
- Stress
- Trauma

RISK FACTORS
- Sleep disturbance (e.g., sleep apnea)
- Trauma
- Depression
- Weather changes

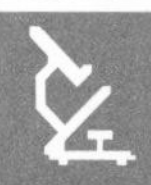

DIAGNOSIS

DIFFERENTIAL DIAGNOSIS
- Hypothyroidism
- Psychogenic rheumatism
- Muscle strain/sprain
- Muscle disease (e.g., polymyositis)
- Polymyalgia rheumatica
- Temporal arteritis

LABORATORY
- Normal Westergren erythrocyte sedimentation rate
- Normal creatine phosphokinase and aldolase
- Normal TSH, T3 resin uptake and T4
- Normal complete blood count, renal and liver function

Drugs that may alter lab results: Steroids

Disorders that may alter lab results: N/A

PATHOLOGICAL FINDINGS None

SPECIAL TESTS
- Sleep study; rarely indicated, but consider if obstructive sleep apnea a consideration or patient fails initial sleep hygiene measures
- Thermography of trigger point areas

IMAGING N/A

DIAGNOSTIC PROCEDURES The clinical history and physical examination

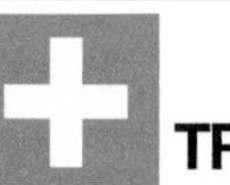

TREATMENT

APPROPRIATE HEALTH CARE Outpatient

GENERAL MEASURES
- Electroprobe. A direct current technique utilizing 500-1000 mA in 30 second intervals repeated over 15 minutes, 4 times per week for several weeks to break the cycle of pain.
- Electrical stimulation pads. Used as an adjunctive therapy to the electroprobe for fibromyalgia. They provide inferential stimulation (alternating current) at 80-150 Hz in 15 second sweeps for 15 minutes.
- Ultrasound, hot packs, conditioning, increasing social interactions and general conditioning exercises (the last is supplemental only)
- Stress management
- TENS and the variant called MENS has not proven effective in treating fibromyalgia

SURGICAL MEASURES N/A

ACTIVITY
- Fully active. However, the pain of fibrositis may be so distracting as to reduce attentiveness, predisposing to error and accident.
- Conditioning exercises as tolerated

DIET No restrictions

PATIENT EDUCATION
- Printed material: Rothschild, B.: Diagnosing and treating fibrositis and fibromyalgia. Geriatric Consultant, 9(5/6):26-28, 1990
- Your personal guide to living with fibromyalgia. Arthritis Foundation, Atlanta, 1997

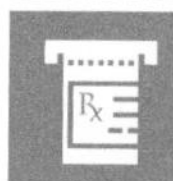

MEDICATIONS

DRUG(S) OF CHOICE
- Sleep restorative without interfering with stage IV sleep:
  - ◊ Zolpidem (Ambien) 5-10 mg hs prn
  - ◊ Temazepam (Restoril) 15-30 mg hs prn
- Local injection of trigger points
  - ◊ Lidocaine 1% injectable 1/2 cc

Contraindications: Drug allergy, suicide potential

Precautions:
- NSAIDs - refer to manufacturer's literature
- Consider discontinuation of sleep restoratives if grogginess, aberrant behavior, memory loss, or thought process changes.
- Psychological and/or physical dependence may occur. However, if the patient is nonfunctional without them, long-term use is reasonable.

Significant possible interactions:
- NSAIDs - refer to manufacturer's literature
- Others - digoxin, phenytoin, MAO inhibitors

ALTERNATIVE DRUGS
- Trazodone (Desyrel) 50 mg po hs prn
- Flurazepam (Dalmane) 15-30 mg hs prn (note: Significant "hangover" potential secondary to long half-life)
- Triazolam (Halcion) 0.125 mg po hs prn increased gradually to 0.5 mg (use is controversial)
- Cyclobenzaprine (Flexeril) 10 mg tid prn (of lesser efficacy)
- Amitriptyline (Elavil) 20-50 mg hs prn (of lesser efficacy)
- NSAIDs may provide non-narcotic symptomatic pain relief (of lesser efficacy)

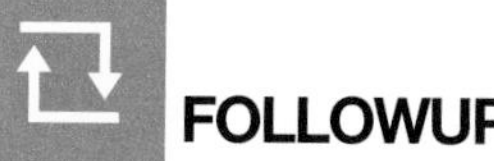

FOLLOWUP

PATIENT MONITORING
- For efficacy at 2-4 weeks
- For medication side effects every 3-6 months

PREVENTION/AVOIDANCE
- Adequate sleep
- General conditioning exercises

POSSIBLE COMPLICATIONS
- Chronic pain, chronic loss of work
- Fibromyalgia is allegedly a greater source of work loss and dysfunction than rheumatoid arthritis

EXPECTED COURSE/PROGNOSIS
- With resolution of sleep disturbance, may resolve totally
- Aggressive physical therapy is critical in those who do not respond
- Approximately 5% do not respond to any form of therapeutic intervention. Hypnosis may be attempted in that group.

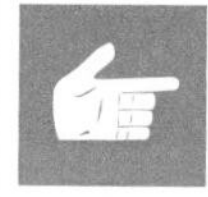

MISCELLANEOUS

ASSOCIATED CONDITIONS
- Restless legs syndrome
- Leg cramps
- Obesity

AGE-RELATED FACTORS
Pediatric: Uncommon

Geriatric: Common; polypharmacy may be part of the problem

Others: N/A

PREGNANCY Limits therapeutic approach to physical therapy modalities

SYNONYMS
- Fibrositis
- Myofascial pain syndrome

ICD-9-CM
729.1 Myalgia and myositis, unspecified

SEE ALSO
Chronic fatigue syndrome
Insomnia
Irritable bowel syndrome
Restless legs syndrome

OTHER NOTES Perhaps the most common cause of neck or back pain in this patient population and most common rheumatologic problem in general

ABBREVIATIONS
TENS = transcutaneous electrical neural stimulation
EMS = electronic muscle stimulation
IF = interferential stimulation
NSAID = non-steroidal anti-inflammatory drug

REFERENCES

- Wallace DJ, Linker-Israel M, Hallegua D, et al. Cytokines play an aetiopathogenetic role in fibromyalgia: A hypothesis and pilot study. Rheumatol 2001;40:743-9
- Rothschild BM. Fibromyalgia: An explanation for the aches and pains of the 90's. Comprehensive Therapy 1991;17(6):9-14
- Vu J, Rothschild BM. Retrospective assessment of fibromyalgia therapeusis. Comprehensive Therapy 1994;20:545-49
- Wolfe F, Smythe HA, Yunus MB, Bennett RM, et al. The American College of Rheumatology criteria for the classification of fibromyalgia. Arthritis Rheum 1990;33:160-72
- Siceloff E, et al. Variability of fibromyalgia-like symptoms. Comp Ther, Cin Press
- Inanici F, Yunus MB. Fibromyalgia syndrome: Diagnosis and management. Hospital Physician 2002;8:53-66
- Wallace DJ, et al. Cytokines play an aetiopathogenetic role in fibromyalgia: A hypothesis and pilot study. Rheumatol 2001;40:743-9
- Thieme K, Gromnica-Ihle E, Flor H. Operant behavioral treatment of fibromyalgia: a controlled study. Arthritis Rheum 2003;49(3):314-20
- Desmeules JA, Cedraschi C, et al. Neurophysiologic evidence for a central sensitization in patients with fibromyalgia. Arthritis Rheum 2003;48(5):1420-9
- Hsu ES. Myofascial pain syndrome and fibromyalgia. Semin Anesthesia 2003;22:152-8
- Sayar K, Aksu G, Ak I, Tosun M. Venlafaxine treatment of fibromyalgia. Ann Pharmacother 2003;37(11):1561-5
- Efficacy of electroprobe/electroanalgesia (Cheng and Pomeranz, 1979; Dai et al, 2001; Ledergerber, 1979; Lehmann et al, 1983; Leo, 1983; Sola, 1981)
- Lack of efficacy of TENS (Graff-Radford et al, 1989; Lehmann et al, 1983; Milne et al, 2001; Sluka and Walsh, 2003). The latter indicates that the low voltage TENS approach is no better than placebo.
- Cheng RS, Pomeranz B. Electroacupuncture anlgesia could be mediated by at least two pain-relieving mechanisms: Endorphin and non-endorphin systems. Life Sciences 1979;25:1957-1962.
- Dai Y, Kondo E, Fukuoka T, Tokunaga A, Miki K, Noguchi K. The effect of electroacupuncture on pain behaviors and noxious stimulus-evoked Fos expression in a rat model of neuropathic pain. J Pain 2:151-159.
- Graff-Radford SB, Reeves JL, Baker RL, Chiu D. Effects of transcutaneous electrical stimulation on myofascial pain and trigger point sensitivity. Pain 1989;37:1-5.
- Ledergerber CP. Transcutaneous electroacupuncture and electroanalgesia. Amer J Acupuncture 1979;2:127-136.
- Lehmann TR, Russell DW, Spratt KF. The impact of patients with nonorganic physical findings on a controlled trial of transcutaneous electrical nerve stimulation and electroacupuncture. Spine 1983;6:625-634.
- Leo KC. Use of electrical stimulatin at acupuncture points for the treatment of reflex sympathetic dystrophy in a child. Physical Therapy 1983;63:957-959.
- Milne S, Welch V, Brosseau L. Transcutaneous electrical stimulation (TENS) for chronic low back pain. Cochrane Database Syst Rev 2001;(2)CD003008.
- Sluka KA, Walsh D. Transcutaneous electric nerve stimulation: Basic science mechanisms and clinical effectiveness. J Pain 2003;4:109-121.
- Sola AE. Myofascial trigger point therapy. Resident & Staff Physician 1981;(8):38-46.

Web references: 4 available at www.5mcc.com

Illustrations N/A

Author(s):
Bruce M. Rothschild, MD

BASICS

DESCRIPTION Inflammation of hair follicles, often in clusters, often due to local infection or chemical irritation or associated with underlying disease. May be superficial or deep.
System(s) affected: Skin/Exocrine
Genetics: No known genetic pattern
Incidence/Prevalence in USA: Common (no statistics available)
Predominant age: All ages
Predominant sex: Male > Female

SIGNS & SYMPTOMS
- Characteristic lesions are small yellow or gray pustules surrounded by erythema and pierced by a hair. Common folliculitis can appear on any part of the body. Sycosis barbae is folliculitis of the beard area of the shaved face, particularly common in black men. Hot tub folliculitis occurs in the bathing suit area. Eosinophilic pustular folliculitis (EPF) occurs mainly on the trunk of HIV positive patients, but can occur in atopic children sensitive to skin fungi, and as Ofuji disease in non-HIV patients, especially in Japan.
- Lesions are commonly grouped
- Eosinophilic folliculitis is often very pruritic, but other types of folliculitis are only mildly pruritic, or not at all
- Patients who are not HIV positive are usually afebrile and without systemic symptoms

CAUSES
- Staphylococcus aureus
- Pseudomonas aeruginosa in hot-tub folliculitis
- Gram negative bacteria in patients on long term antibiotics
- Candida albicans in patients on immunosuppressants or long term antibiotic therapy
- Dermatophyte fungi - uncommon
- Occasionally herpes simplex 1, herpes zoster, molluscum contagiosum virus
- Plastic occlusive dressings

RISK FACTORS
- Abrasion
- Injury
- Nearby surgical wounds or draining abscesses
- Tight clothing (jeans folliculitis)
- Poor hygiene
- Exposure to hydrocarbons
- Use of hot tubs or saunas
- Immunodeficiency
- Diabetes mellitus
- Lithium therapy
- Wax epilation

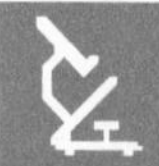

DIAGNOSIS

DIFFERENTIAL DIAGNOSIS
- Keratosis pilaris (follicular papules on the extensor surfaces of extremities in atopic individuals)
- Contact dermatitis
- Tinea
- Acne
- Pustular miliaria (10)
- Flat warts
- Molluscum contagiosum
- Scabies
- Perioral dermatitis
- Diaper dermatitis

LABORATORY
- Gram stain - look for bacteria or eosinophils
- KOH preparation - looking for budding yeast or hyphae
- Culture of pus
- Fasting blood sugar
- HIV status

Drugs that may alter lab results: N/A

Disorders that may alter lab results: N/A

PATHOLOGICAL FINDINGS
- For common or hot tub folliculitis - suppurative inflammation of hair follicles
- For eosinophilic pustular folliculitis there is a perifollicular and perivascular infiltrate in which eosinophils exceed the numbers of neutrophils

SPECIAL TESTS N/A

IMAGING N/A

DIAGNOSTIC PROCEDURES Biopsy if diagnosis is in doubt or in cases resistant to treatment

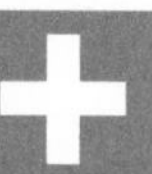

TREATMENT

APPROPRIATE HEALTH CARE Outpatient

GENERAL MEASURES
- Cleanse areas bid with antibacterial soap (e.g. Dial)
- Shampoo daily with Selsun Blue for scalp lesions
- Apply moist heat to pustules to encourage them to drain
- For shaved areas:
  - ◊ Try electric razor instead of blade, and sterilize electric razor cutting parts with alcohol for 30 minutes daily.
  - ◊ Or change blade of sharp razor daily
  - ◊ Allow hair to grow.
- Avoid wax epilatories if they cause a rash.
- Avoid skin oils or greasy ointments
- Avoid topical oils

SURGICAL MEASURES N/A

ACTIVITY Full

DIET No special diet

PATIENT EDUCATION As listed above under General measures

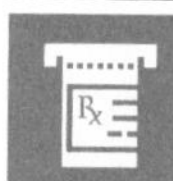

MEDICATIONS

DRUG(S) OF CHOICE
- Staphylococcal folliculitis,
  - ◊ Dicloxacillin 250 mg qid
  - ◊ Erythromycin 250 mg qid
  - ◊ Cephalosporin
- Pseudomonas folliculitis
  - ◊ Usually self limited, no antibiotic indicated
  - ◊ If severe or persistent adults can use ciprofloxacin 500 mg or ofloxacin 400 mg bid for 10 days
- Eosinophilic pustular folliculitis
  - ◊ No local causative organism, no specific antibiotic
  - ◊ Non-HIV related EPF often responds to oral indomethacin
  - ◊ For EPF in HIV positive patients isotretinoin therapy appears to be promising

Contraindications:
- History of hypersensitivity to the drug
- Quinolone antibiotics are contraindicated in pregnancy and for children
- Indomethacin is contraindicated in patients who have had a peptic ulcer

Precautions: Refer to manufacturers literature

Significant possible interactions:
- Ciprofloxacin and ofloxacin - antacids, sucralfate, oral anticoagulants, theophylline, caffeine, probenecid
- Erythromycin - theophylline, oral anticoagulants, carbamazepine, corticosteroids, digoxin, ergot alkaloids, cyclosporine, phenytoin, terfenadine, astemizole

ALTERNATIVE DRUGS
- Mupirocin (Bactroban) topical therapy to affected area tid
- First generation cephalosporins for Staph. aureus
- For pseudomonas, third generation cephalosporins, aminoglycosides, or ticarcillin

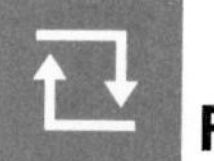

FOLLOWUP

PATIENT MONITORING
- One return visit in two weeks if symptoms abate
- Resistant cases should be followed every two weeks until cleared

PREVENTION/AVOIDANCE
- Good personal hygiene; avoid sharing a towel or washcloth
- Discard any dressings carefully
- Avoid causative factors
- Find and treat family members or friends who may be a source of reinfection

POSSIBLE COMPLICATIONS
May progress to become furuncles or abscesses

EXPECTED COURSE/PROGNOSIS
- Usually resolves with treatment
- May recur in staph carriers. Mupirocin may be required on nares of patient to treat carrier state. Family carriers may also require treatment.
- Resistant or severe cases may warrant testing for diabetes mellitus or immunodeficiency

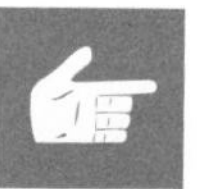

MISCELLANEOUS

ASSOCIATED CONDITIONS
- Diabetes mellitus
- Immunodeficiency

AGE-RELATED FACTORS
Pediatric: N/A
Geriatric: N/A
Others: N/A

PREGNANCY
Pruritic folliculitis of pregnancy is a rare disorder that resolves spontaneously after delivery

SYNONYMS
Sycosis

ICD-9-CM
704.8 Other specified diseases of hair and hair follicles

SEE ALSO

OTHER NOTES
N/A

ABBREVIATIONS
EPF = eosinophilic pustular folliculitis

REFERENCES

- Fitzpatrick TB, et al: Color Atlas & Synopsis of Clinical Dermatology. 2nd Ed. New York, McGraw Hill, 1992
- Majors MJ, et al: HIV-related eosinophilic folliculitis: a panel discussion Seminars in Cutaneous Medicine and Surgery 1997;16(3):219-223
- Saunders Electronic Atlas of Dermatology. Philadelphia, WB Saunders Co, 1996
- Schmidt A: Malassezia furfur; a fungus belonging to the physiological skin flora and its relevance in skin disorders. Cutis 1997;59(1):21-24
- Abdel-Razek M, et al: Pityrosporon, (Malassezia) folliculitis in Saudi Arabia - diagnosis and therapeutic trials. Clinical & Experimental Dermatology 1995;20(5):406-409
- Wakelin SH, et al: Lithium-induced follicular hyperkeratosis. Clinical & Experimental Dermatology 1996;21(4):296-298
- Mimouni-Bloch A, et al: Severe folliculitis with keloid scars induced by wax epilation in adolescents. Cutis 1997;59(1):41-42
- Fushimi M, et al: Eosinophilic pustular folliculitis effectively treated with recombinant interferon-gamma: suppression of mRNA expression of interleukin 5 in peripheral blood mononuclear cells British Journal of Dermatology 1996;134(4):766-772
- Callen J, et al: Color Atlas of Dermatology. Philadelphia, WB Saunders Co, 1993
- Teraki Y: Ofuji's disease and cytokines: Remission of eosinophilic pustular folliculitis associated with increase serum concentrations of interferon gamma. Dermatology. 192(1): 16-18
- Otley CC, et al: Isotretinoin treatment of human immunodeficiency virus-associated eosinophilic folliculitis. Results of an open pilot trial. Archives of Dermatology 1995;131(9):1047-1050

Web references: 0 available at www.5mcc.com
Illustrations N/A

Author(s):
Lewis C. Rose, MD

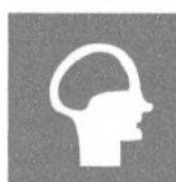

BASICS

DESCRIPTION Food allergy is a hypersensitivity reaction which is caused by certain foods. Adverse reactions after food ingestion may be caused by immunologic mechanisms, such as the classic IgE allergic response, or by non-immunologic mediated mechanisms.

System(s) affected: Gastrointestinal, Hemic/Lymphatic/Immunologic, Nervous, Pulmonary, Skin/Exocrine

Genetics: In family members with a history of food hypersensitivity, the probability of food allergy in subsequent siblings may be as high as 50%

Incidence/Prevalence in USA:
- The incidence of IgE mediated food allergy has been estimated to range from 1-7% of the population
- In children up to 4 years of age the incidence is between 8-16%
- Only about 3-4% of children over 4 years of age have persisting food allergy. Therefore, it is frequently a transient phenomena.

Predominant age: All ages, but more common in infants and children

Predominant sex: Male > Female (2:1)

SIGNS & SYMPTOMS
- Gastrointestinal (system usually affected)
  - ◊ More common: Nausea, vomiting, diarrhea, abdominal pain, occult bleeding, flatulence, bloating
  - ◊ Less common: Malabsorption, protein losing enteropathy, eosinophil-gastroenteritis, and colitis
- Dermatologic
  - ◊ More common: Urticaria/angioedema, atopic dermatitis, pallor or flushing
  - ◊ Less common: Contact rashes
- Respiratory
  - ◊ More common: Allergic rhinitis, asthma and bronchospasm, cough, serous otitis media
  - ◊ Less common: Pulmonary infiltrates (Heiner syndrome), pulmonary hemosiderosis
- Neurologic
  - ◊ Less common: Hyperkinesis, tension-fatigue syndrome, migraine headaches, syncope
- Other symptoms:
  - ◊ Systemic anaphylaxis, vasculitis
  - ◊ Suspected manifestations include enuresis, proteinuria and arthropathy
  - ◊ Growth retardation

CAUSES
- Any food or ingested substance can cause allergic reactions. Most commonly implicated foods include cow's milk, egg whites, wheat, soy, peanut, fish, tree nuts (walnut and pecan), shellfish, melons, sesame seeds, sunflower seeds.
- Several food dyes and additives can elicit allergic-like reactions

RISK FACTORS
- Persons with allergic or atopic predisposition are at increased risk of hypersensitivity reaction to foods
- Family members with a history of food hypersensitivity

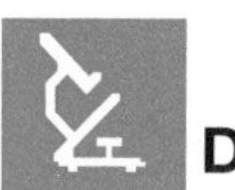

DIAGNOSIS

DIFFERENTIAL DIAGNOSIS
- A careful history is necessary to document a temporal relationship with the manifestations of suspected food hypersensitivity
- The gastrointestinal, dermatologic, respiratory, neurologic or other systemic manifestations may mimic a variety of clinical entities

LABORATORY
- Eosinophilia in either blood or tissue suggests atopy
- Epicutaneous (prick or puncture) allergy skin tests are useful in documenting IgE mediated immunologic hypersensitivity. In most clinical situations, the allergy skin tests are good for screening. Skin testing using the suspect food may be helpful. An oral challenge may be completed to accurately determine the clinical hypersensitivity. The overall agreement between allergy skin testing and oral food challenge is approximately 60% (i.e., a positive skin test showing a positive challenge reaction to a particular food).
- Radioallergosorbent (RAST) test can also detect specific IgE antibodies to offending foods. In certain laboratories, the RAST test was almost as accurate as a skin test in predicting positive oral challenges.
- Leukocyte histamine release and assays for circulating immune complexes are predominantly research procedures and are of limited use in clinical practices. Assays for IgG and IgG 4 subclass antibodies are commercially available. There are no convincing data that these tests are reliable for the diagnosis of food allergy.
- The provocative injection and sublingual provocative tests are both highly controversial and have been proven to be useless for the diagnosis of food allergy
- The leukocytotoxic assay is an unproven diagnostic procedure and is not useful for the diagnosis of allergy

Drugs that may alter lab results: N/A

Disorders that may alter lab results: N/A

PATHOLOGICAL FINDINGS
Pathologic findings are not common in food allergies however, inflammatory changes can be seen in the gastrointestinal tract.

SPECIAL TESTS
Stool exam, mucus, eosinophilia

IMAGING
Upper GI series for gastric antral inflammation, in rare cases

DIAGNOSTIC PROCEDURES
- Elimination and challenge test
  - ◊ The best procedure for confirming food allergy
  - ◊ First, the suspected food is eliminated from the diet for 1-2 weeks
  - ◊ The patient's symptoms are monitored. If the patient's symptoms disappear or substantially improve, an oral challenge with the suspected food should be performed under medical supervision.
  - ◊ Optimally, this challenge should be performed in a double-blind, placebo controlled manner
  - ◊ Patients with a history of anaphylaxis should not generally have an oral challenge
  - ◊ Most allergic reactions will occur within 30 minutes to 2 hours after the challenge, although late reactions have also been described, which may occur from 12-24 hours

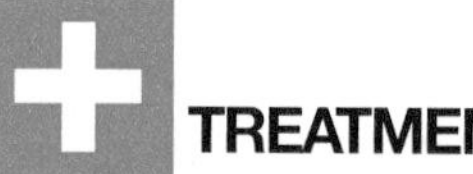

TREATMENT

APPROPRIATE HEALTH CARE
Outpatient

GENERAL MEASURES
- Avoidance of the offending food is the most effective mode of treatment for patients with food allergies
- Those patients with exquisite and severe allergy hypersensitivity to a food should be more cautious in their avoidance of that food. They should carry epinephrine for self-administration in the event that the offending food is ingested unknowingly, and a subsequent immediate reaction develops.
- Immunotherapy or hyposensitization with food extracts by various routes, including subcutaneous immunotherapy or sublingual neutralization are not recommended since the success with these methods have not been proven in controlled scientific studies

SURGICAL MEASURES
N/A

ACTIVITY
No restrictions

DIET
As determined by tests

PATIENT EDUCATION
- Patients should be counseled by a dietitian to be sure that they maintain a nutritionally sound diet, in spite of avoiding those foods to which patient is sensitive
- Patient support - Food Allergy Network, 4744 Holly Ave., Fairfax, VA 22030-5647, 703-691-3179; website www.foodallergy.org

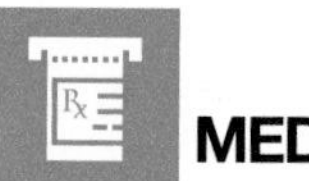

MEDICATIONS

DRUG(S) OF CHOICE
- Symptomatic treatment, e.g., antihistamine
- The use of cromolyn has been suggested, but is not practical for use in most patients with food allergy
- Recent studies have suggested the use of ketotifen, which is a mast cell stabilizer. This drug is not available in the United States.

Contraindications: N/A
Precautions: N/A
Significant possible interactions: N/A

ALTERNATIVE DRUGS N/A

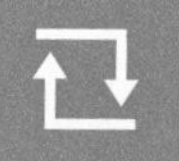

FOLLOWUP

PATIENT MONITORING As needed

PREVENTION/AVOIDANCE Avoidance of offending food

POSSIBLE COMPLICATIONS
- Anaphylaxis
- Angioedema
- Bronchial asthma
- Enterocolitis
- Eczematoid lesions

EXPECTED COURSE/PROGNOSIS
- Most infants will outgrow their food hypersensitivity by 2-4 years. It may be possible to reintroduce the offending food cautiously into the diet (particularly helpful when the food is one that is difficult to avoid).
- Adults with food hypersensitivity (particularly to milk, fish, shellfish or nuts) tend to maintain their allergy for many years

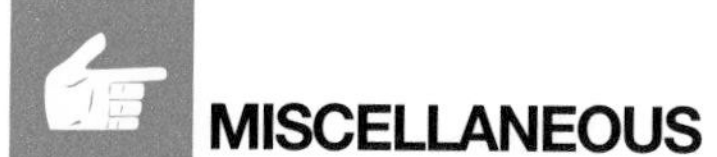

MISCELLANEOUS

ASSOCIATED CONDITIONS N/A

AGE-RELATED FACTORS
Pediatric: N/A
Geriatric: N/A
Others: N/A

PREGNANCY N/A

SYNONYMS
- Allergic bowel disease
- Dietary protein sensitivity syndrome

ICD-9-CM
693.1 Dermatitis due to food taken internally
692.5 Contact dermatitis and other eczema due to food in contact with skin
995.60 Anaphylactic shock or reaction due to unspecified food

SEE ALSO
Celiac disease
Epiglottitis
Irritable bowel syndrome
Pyloric stenosis

OTHER NOTES N/A

ABBREVIATIONS N/A

REFERENCES

- Sampson HA. Food allergy. J Allergy Clin Immunol 2003;111(2Suppl):S540-7
- Chandra RK, ed. Food Allergy. Clin Rev Allergy/Immu 1995;13:291-376
- Sampson HA. Food Allergy. Part 1: Immunopathogenesis and clinical disorders. J Allergy Clin Immunol 1999;103:717-23
- Sampson HA. Food Allergy. Part 2: Diagnosis and management. J Allergy Clin Immunol 1999;103:981-89

Web references: 6 available at www.5mcc.com
Illustrations N/A

Author(s):
Stanley Fineman, MD

BASICS

DESCRIPTION A variety of related illnesses resulting from ingestion of food contaminated with bacteria capable of causing disease. The illness may be produced by bacterial infection itself (salmonellosis, shigellosis) or by toxins produced by the bacteria (*Staphylococcus aureus*, *Clostridium perfringens*, *Bacillus cereus*). Usually involves the large bowel, whereas viral etiologies generally involve the small intestine.
System(s) affected: Gastrointestinal
Genetics: N/A
Incidence/Prevalence in USA: Poor reporting overall. Estimated 6 million cases/year. 1 in 10 Americans with food-borne diarrhea/year. Approximate incidence is 2,500/100,000. Most commonly reported cause in the US are *C. jejuni*, Salmonella, *C. perfringens, S. aureus* - accounting for 90% of cases, totaling approximately 45,000 hospitalizations and 2,700 deaths in U.S.
Predominant age: All ages
Predominant sex: Male = Female

SIGNS & SYMPTOMS

Most cases of gastroenteritis have a viral etiology, some of which (Norwalk-like virus) can be foodborne. Suspect bacterial food poisoning when multiple persons become ill after eating the same meal. Timing and type of clinical presentation can aid in establishing etiology.

- Fever more suggestive of invasive organisms (Shigella, Salmonella, Campylobacter)
- Nausea, vomiting 1-6 hours after meal (*S. aureus*, *B. cereus*)
- Cramps, diarrhea 8-16 hours after meal (*C. perfringens*, *B. cereus*)
- Fever, cramps, diarrhea 18-72 hours after meal (*Campylobacter jejuni*, *Yersinia enterocolitica*, *E. coli*, *Vibrio parahaemolyticus*, Shigella and Salmonella species)
- Bloody diarrhea without fever 3-5 days after meal (verotoxigenic *E. coli*, occasionally *C. jejuni*)
- Pseudoappendicitis (*Y. enterocolitica*)
- Sepsis, meningitis (*Listeria monocytogenes*, *Shigella* and *Salmonella* species)
- Occasional metastatic foci of infection, ie, arthritis (*L. monocytogenes*, *Salmonella*)
- HUS/TTP (HUS = hemolytic-uremic syndrome, TTP = thrombotic thrombocytopenic purpura) in 10-15% of *E. coli*) 0157:H7 infections

CAUSES

- *S. aureus* (preformed enterotoxin)
- *B. cereus* (preformed enterotoxin)
- *C. perfringens* (enterotoxin elaborated in gut)
- *C. jejuni* (tissue invasion)
- *Y. enterocolitica* (tissue invasion)
- *E. coli* (enterotoxigenic, verotoxigenic [hemorrhagic], and tissue invasive forms), including *E. coli* 0157:H7
- *V. parahaemolyticus* (toxin elaboration, possibly invasion)
- *Shigella species* (tissue invasion)
- *Salmonella species* (tissue invasion), including *Salmonella* serotype Typhimurium definitive type 104
- *L. monocytogenes* (tissue invasion)

RISK FACTORS

Ingestion of:

- High protein foods: egg salad, cream-filled pastries, poultry, ham - *S. aureus*
- Cereals, fried rice, dried foods and herbs, meats, vegetables - *B. cereus*
- Meats, gravies, dried foods, vegetables - *C. perfringens*
- Under-cooked poultry, meat, raw dairy products, contaminated water, mushrooms - *C. jejuni*
- Under-cooked pork, other meat and dairy products - *Y. enterocolitica*
- Raw vegetables (especially sprouts), meats tainted fruit and juices, contaminated water and milk - *E. coli*
- Raw and cooked seafood - *V. parahaemolyticus*
- Raw vegetables, egg salads, contaminated water - *Shigella*
- Raw or under-cooked eggs, poultry, dairy products, meat - *Salmonella*
- Under-cooked meat, dairy products, and many other foods - *L. monocytogenes*
- Daycare contacts
- Travel to developing regions
- Exposure to asymptomatic animals harboring infections and spreading them through feces and milk - *E. coli*, *Listeria*, *Salmonella*

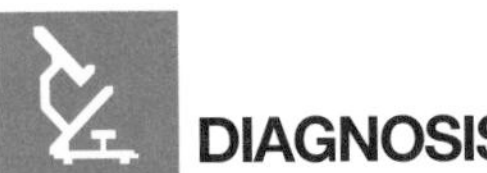

DIAGNOSIS

DIFFERENTIAL DIAGNOSIS

- Infectious gastroenteritis of any kind
- Inflammatory bowel disease
- Appendicitis and other acute surgical abdominal processes
- Hepatitis

LABORATORY Culture of stool most reliable. Routine cultures detect Shigella, Salmonella, Campylobacter and *E. coli* 0157:H7. Vibrio and most *E. coli* species require specific media and orders to laboratory.

Drugs that may alter lab results: Prior or concomitant antibiotic therapy may eliminate pathogen from stool

Disorders that may alter lab results: N/A

PATHOLOGICAL FINDINGS Only present in invasive or colitic syndromes

SPECIAL TESTS Sigmoidoscopy in persistent and unresponsive cases

IMAGING N/A

DIAGNOSTIC PROCEDURES

- Stool culture - obtain if diarrhea is severe (patient is bedfast), temperature > 101.5°F (38.5°C), persistently bloody stools, presence of fecal leukocytes
- Epidemiologic investigation
- Culture of suspected food source if available

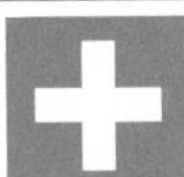

TREATMENT

APPROPRIATE HEALTH CARE Usually outpatient management sufficient with attention to dehydration and electrolyte imbalances. Hospitalization for septicemias or focal infections, severe electrolyte imbalance or dehydration.

GENERAL MEASURES

- Most are self-limited syndromes and do not require specific therapy
- Oral solutions for rehydration. Sport drinks and diluted fruit juices with broth and crackers sufficient in mild cases.
- For moderate cases, consider 8 oz orange or apple juice plus 1/2 teaspoon honey and a pinch of salt followed by 8 oz water with 1/4 teaspoon baking soda
- Intravenous fluid or oral rehydration solutions containing 50-100 mEq Na/L and electrolyte replacement if necessary for more severe dehydration (particularly in the elderly)
- For infants, rehydration products (e.g., Pedialyte) provides adequate fluid and electrolyte replacement. Don't use for more than 1 to 2 days without clinical reassessment of nutritional needs.

SURGICAL MEASURES N/A

ACTIVITY Bedrest for comfort if needed during the acute phase

DIET Eliminate contaminated food. Reintroduction of bland or normal age-appropriate diets as soon as hydrated and able. Generally, no dietary restrictions are broadly recommended.

PATIENT EDUCATION

- Avoidance of raw or under-cooked foods
- Proper food storage and preparation techniques such as refrigeration
- Instruction on prevention if patient traveling to foreign countries
- Avoid antidiarrheal drugs in most cases; they may prolong the carrier state

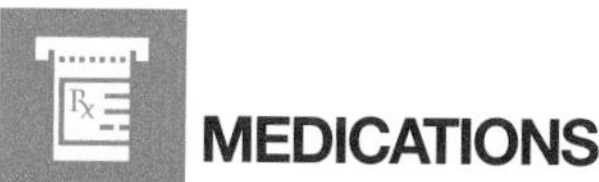

MEDICATIONS

DRUG(S) OF CHOICE

- Antibiotic use is controversial and often of limited benefit
- For septicemias and focal infections, systemic antibiotic therapy may be indicated
- Consider antibiotics in prolonged febrile state with fecal blood and/or leukocytes or moderate to severe traveler's diarrhea
- Shigella or salmonella: trimethoprim-sulfamethoxazole 160 mg and 800 mg, respectively, bid for five days, or ciprofloxacin (Cipro) 500 mg bid for 10 days if acquired outside the U.S.
- Campylobacter: erythromycin 250 mg qid for 5 days or ciprofloxacin (Cipro) 500 mg bid for 7 days
- Yersinia: Ceftriaxone 1 g IV qd
- Listeriosis: ampicillin plus aminoglycoside
- Traveler's diarrhea: trimethoprim-sulfamethoxazole one double strength tablet bid for 3 days or ciprofloxacin (Cipro) 500 mg bid for 3 days
- Bismuth subsalicylate may have anti-inflammatory and bactericidal activity

Contraindications:

- Avoid antiperistaltic agents in colitic (bloody diarrhea) syndromes since they may increase the chance of systemic dissemination
- Antiemetics may be given but are usually unnecessary

Precautions: N/A

Significant possible interactions:

- Certain antibiotics have recognized drug-drug interactions
- Anticholinergics may have side effects in elderly or cardiac patients

ALTERNATIVE DRUGS N/A

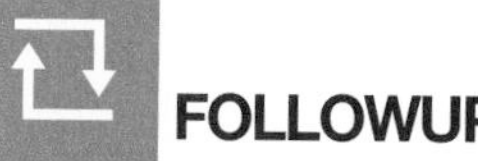

FOLLOWUP

PATIENT MONITORING

- Individualized based on degree of dehydration and electrolyte imbalance, or signs of sepsis
- Close medical follow up and evaluation should be considered for persistence of symptoms unabated > 48 hours, and in infants, elderly, and immunocompromised
- Serious disturbances require hospitalization, frequent vital signs, strict recording of input and output with appropriate fluid replacement

PREVENTION/AVOIDANCE

- No ingestion of raw or undercooked seafood, meats, or poultry
- Avoid any unpasteurized dairy products; juices or eggs
- Clean thoroughly any food preparation area in contact with causative items
- Ensure proper cold storage of any prepared foods not immediately consumed
- Wash hands frequently and thoroughly when handling or preparing foods
- Be wary of frozen fruit products from developing nations

POSSIBLE COMPLICATIONS

- Cardiovascular collapse
- Arrhythmias from electrolyte disturbance
- Septicemias or other metastatic infections
- Hypoglycemic seizures or coma

EXPECTED COURSE/PROGNOSIS

- Resolution of signs and symptoms over a few days in most cases
- Chronic sequelae include Guillain-Barre syndrome, reactive arthritis

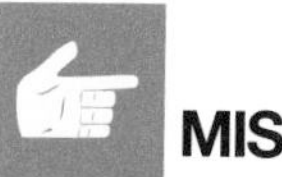

MISCELLANEOUS

ASSOCIATED CONDITIONS N/A

AGE-RELATED FACTORS

Pediatric:

- Day care center outbreaks may occur. Perhaps at higher risk of complications from antiperistaltic drugs.
- Newborns and infants are a high risk for mortality and complications
- Shigellosis is a rare cause of chronic vaginal discharge in young girls

Geriatric:

- Nursing home outbreaks may occur
- Significant cause of mortality

Others: N/A

PREGNANCY Perinatal salmonellosis, listeriosis, and campylobacteriosis may secondarily infect newborn with severe consequences of sepsis and meningitis

SYNONYMS N/A

ICD-9-CM

003.0 Salmonella gastroenteritis
004.0 Shigella dysenteriae
004.9 Shigellosis, unspecified
005.0 Staphylococcal food poisoning
005.1 Botulism
005.9 Food poisoning, unspecified
008.00 Intestinal infection due to Escherichia coli, unspecified

SEE ALSO

Appendicitis, acute
Botulism
Brucellosis
Dehydration
Diarrhea, acute
Eosinophilic gastroenteritis
Guillain-Barré syndrome
Hypokalemia
Intestinal parasites
Salmonella infection
Typhoid fever

OTHER NOTES

- *C. jejuni* antimicrobial therapy resistance is increasing

ABBREVIATIONS N/A

REFERENCES

- Diagnosis and management of foodborne illnesses: a primer for physicians. MMWR Recomm Rep. 2001;50(RR-2):1-69
- Mandell GL, Douglas RG Jr, Bennett JE. Principles and Practice of Infectious Diseases. 4th Ed. New York, Churchill Livingstone, 1995
- Mead P. Food related illness and death in the United States. Emerg Infect Dis 1999;5(5):607-25
- Dupont H. American College of Gastroenterology: Guidelines on acute infectious diarrhea in adults. J of Gastroenterol 1997;92(11):1962-74

Web references: 2 available at www.5mcc.com
Illustrations N/A

Author(s):

Karl M. Schmitt, MD

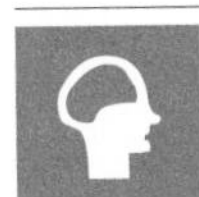

BASICS

DESCRIPTION The fragile X mutation that produces the fragile X syndrome is the most common known heritable cause of mental retardation. As a result, it is the most common form of familial mental retardation. This condition received its name from the cytogenetic "fragile site" which is seen on the long arm of the X chromosome (Xq27.3). It is associated with abnormal increase in CGG repeats in the untranslated region of the FMR-1 gene in both carriers and affected individuals. Affected individuals also exhibit hypermethylation at the fragile site.

System(s) affected: Musculoskeletal, Nervous, Reproductive

Genetics:

- The pattern of inheritance is X-linked, however, this condition is seen in both sexes. Males usually more severely affected than females.
- The specific factors controlling the expression of genes at the fragile X site are not fully understood
- 80% of males with the fragile X chromosome will be affected with moderate to severe mental retardation, with 20% unaffected and defined as transmitting males
- Only one third of the female carriers will have mental retardation, and their degree of handicap usually is less severe. Females may demonstrate emotional problems.
- Females with the permutation appear to be at increased risk of premature ovarian failure, while males with the permutation appear to be at risk for early onset of ataxia in middle age

Incidence/Prevalence in USA: Recent epidemiological studies indicate that the prevalence of fully mutated FRAXA males is 1:4,000. This would suggest the prevalence of affected females is 1:12,000. Overall prevalence would be 1:6,000 individuals. Other studies report approximately 1:300 females may be premutation carriers.

Predominant age: Life-long condition

Predominant sex: Males usually more severely affected, but females demonstrate a higher carrier rate

SIGNS & SYMPTOMS

- The signs and symptoms seen in the "classic" case of fragile X syndrome may be diagnostic; however, the clinical presentation is extremely varied, is age-dependent, and sex-influenced. African-Americans are also less likely to show the characteristic features.
- Early childhood:
  - ◊ Global developmental delay with speech and language severely affected
  - ◊ Overgrowth
  - ◊ Autistic-like behaviors
- Postpubertal males (affected)
  - ◊ Mental retardation (100%)
  - ◊ Connective tissue dysplasia
  - ◊ Characteristic physical features
    - Macroorchidism (95%)
    - Long, thin face (60-65%)
    - Prominent jaw (60-65%)
    - Large ears (> 7.0 cm) (60-65%)
    - Midface hypoplasia (50-60%)
    - Prominent forehead (40%)
    - Large, fleshy hands (30%)
    - Unusual dermatoglyphics

CAUSES Transmission of affected X chromosome

RISK FACTORS

- Transmitting males are intellectually normal and pass the affected chromosome to all of their daughters, the latter who may have affected sons
- Affected females transmit the affected chromosome to their offspring on a 50/50 chance basis

DIAGNOSIS

DIFFERENTIAL DIAGNOSIS

- Fragile X syndrome should be considered in patients (male or female) with mental retardation of unknown etiology
- Many male children will present primarily with speech delay or overgrowth and may have been misdiagnosed as having cerebral gigantism (Soto) syndrome
- Males or females with significant learning disabilities with speech and language deficits
- Familial pattern of MR
- Pervasive developmental disorder
- Significant learning disability
- FRAXE - cytogenetically positive/DNA negative
- Autism
- William syndrome

LABORATORY Molecular genetic testing (DNA) is the diagnostic test of choice. Molecular studies can identify full mutations, mosaic patterns, and permutations thereby identifying affected carriers among normal relatives.

Drugs that may alter lab results: N/A

Disorders that may alter lab results: N/A

PATHOLOGICAL FINDINGS N/A

SPECIAL TESTS Affected patients are in need of educational and psychological evaluation for the development of learning programs

IMAGING N/A

DIAGNOSTIC PROCEDURES N/A

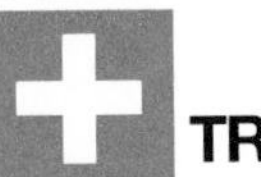

TREATMENT

APPROPRIATE HEALTH CARE Affected individuals will usually require life-long adult supervision and should be referred to the local mental retardation board for case management

GENERAL MEASURES Early detection allows initiation of pre-school intervention programs

SURGICAL MEASURES N/A

ACTIVITY Full activity

DIET No special diet

PATIENT EDUCATION

- The patient and the family should receive genetic evaluation and counseling
- Patient and family could contact: The National Fragile X Foundation (800)688-8765
- FRAXA Research Foundation www.fraxa.org

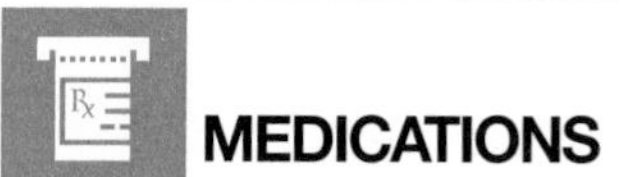

MEDICATIONS

DRUG(S) OF CHOICE Folic acid 20 mg qd, has been reported anecdotally to improve behavior and attention span in prepubertal males. No statistically significantly benefit has been observed in children or adults during double-blind studies.
Contraindications: N/A
Precautions: N/A
Significant possible interactions: N/A

ALTERNATIVE DRUGS N/A

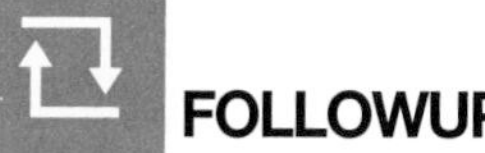

FOLLOWUP

PATIENT MONITORING General health maintenance

PREVENTION/AVOIDANCE Genetic counseling and evaluation of at-risk family members and pregnancies. Prenatal diagnosis is available.

POSSIBLE COMPLICATIONS Severe learning and/or behavioral problems; the latter of which are more frequent among female patients

EXPECTED COURSE/PROGNOSIS
- Males with a full mutation may require life-long adult supervision
- Among affected males and females, life-span is generally not affected
- Among males, intellect manifests early plateauing which causes a decline in IQ scores
- Females are less affected but may have mild to moderate mental retardation
- Approximately 1/3 of affected females manifest learning disabilities

MISCELLANEOUS

ASSOCIATED CONDITIONS
- Speech and language problems
- Developmental delay
- Mental retardation
- Maladaptive behavior
- Attention deficit disorder/hyperactivity disorder (ADHD)
  - ◊ Is found with greater frequency among individuals with neuropsychological dysfunction
  - ◊ Treatment for ADHD among the mentally retarded is not unlike that for the general population
  - ◊ Data indicate overuse of psychoactive substances to aid caretakers

AGE-RELATED FACTORS
Pediatric: N/A
Geriatric: N/A
Others: N/A

PREGNANCY Patient and family should receive genetic evaluation and counseling as prenatal diagnosis is available

SYNONYMS
- Martin-Bell syndrome
- Marker X syndrome
- X-linked mental retardation
- FRAXA

ICD-9-CM
758.9 Conditions due to anomaly of unspecified chromosome

SEE ALSO
Attention deficit/Hyperactivity disorder
Autism
Down syndrome
Mental retardation

OTHER NOTES Extensive family history is mandatory

ABBREVIATIONS ADHD = attention deficit disorder/hyperactivity disorder

REFERENCES

- Fisch GS, editor. Genetics and Genomics of Neurobehavioral Disorders. Totowa, NJ: Humana Press; 2003
- Simensen RJ, Rogers RC: Fragile X Syndrome. Amer Fam Phys 1989;39(5):185-193
- Special Issue: X-Linked Mental Retardation. American Journal of Medical Genetics 1996;64:1&2
- Hagerman RJ, Hagerman PJ. Fragile X Syndrome: Diagnosis, Treatment and Research. 3rd ed. Baltimore: Johns Hopkins University; 2002

Web references: 5 available at www.5mcc.com
Illustrations N/A

Author(s):
Richard J. Simensen, PhD
Gene S. Fisch, PhD

BASICS

DESCRIPTION A localized complication of exposure to cold, resulting in diminished blood flow to the affected part (especially hands, face or feet). Dehydration, enzymatic destruction and ultimately cell death occurs. In severe cases, deep tissue freezing may occur with damage to underlying blood vessels, muscles and nerve tissue.
System(s) affected: Endocrine/Metabolic, Skin/Exocrine
Genetics: N/A
Incidence/Prevalence in USA: N/A
Predominant age: All ages
Predominant sex: Male = Female

SIGNS & SYMPTOMS
- Injured area first appears cold, hard, white and is anesthetic to touch. Progresses to blotchy-red, swollen and painful regions after rewarming.
- Loss of cutaneous sensation
- Numbness
- Throbbing pain
- Paresthesia
- Excessive sweating
- Joint pain
- Pallor
- Subcutaneous edema
- Hyperemia
- Blistering
- Blue discoloration
- Skin necrosis
- Gangrene

CAUSES
- Prolonged exposure to cold
- Refreezing thawed extremities

RISK FACTORS
- Impaired cerebral function
- Under the effects of alcohol or drug abuse
- Underlying psychiatric disturbance
- Ambient temperature less than 0°F (-17.8°C)
- Smoker
- Elderly
- Raynaud phenomenon

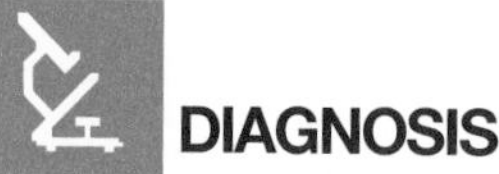

DIAGNOSIS

DIFFERENTIAL DIAGNOSIS Frostnip - superficial damp cold injury

LABORATORY
- Hemoconcentration
- Decreased hepatic function

Drugs that may alter lab results: N/A

Disorders that may alter lab results: N/A

PATHOLOGICAL FINDINGS
- Ice crystallization in the intravascular extracellular space
- Atrophy
- Fibroblastic proliferation
- Skin necrosis

SPECIAL TESTS ECG - bradycardia, atrial fibrillation, atrial flutter, ventricular fibrillation, diffuse T wave inversion

IMAGING N/A

DIAGNOSTIC PROCEDURES Various imaging techniques such as thermography, angiography, digital plethysmography and radioisotope vascular and bone scanning have been used to assess degree of vascular injury. Helps surgeons make decisions - but no technique is entirely reliable during vascular instability which lasts 2-3 weeks.

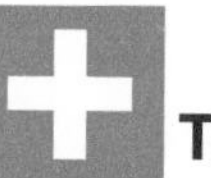

TREATMENT

APPROPRIATE HEALTH CARE Outpatient or inpatient, depending on severity

GENERAL MEASURES
- Emergency measures for patient without pulse or respiration. Such measures may include CPR and internal warming with warm IV's and warm oxygen (see hypothermia)
- Prevent refreezing. May be necessary to keep frostbitten part frozen until patient can be transported to a care facility.
- Treat for hypothermia
- Treat for pain, NSAIDs, and/or narcotics if needed
- Cautious rewarming. May immerse frozen body part for several minutes in water no hotter than 40-42°C (104-107°F).
- After rewarming, injured parts should be covered with nonadhesive dressings, splinted, and elevated.
- Application of aloe vera, administration of non-steroidal anti-inflammatory drugs are considered helpful in removal and inhibition of deleterious prostaglandins (eg ibuprofen 400-800 mg orally bid or a systemic anti-inflammatory given as early as possible)
- Keep patient dry. If conscious, give warm fluids with high sugar content.
- Amputation not to be considered until it is definite that tissues are dead. May take about 3 weeks to know if the tissue is permanently injured.
- Prevention of infection, once treatment begins
- Ongoing whirlpool therapy for cleansing and debridement
- Prevention of damage to other body parts

SURGICAL MEASURES N/A

ACTIVITY
- As tolerated, protect injured body parts
- Initiate physical therapy once healing progresses sufficiently

DIET
- As tolerated
- Warm oral fluids

PATIENT EDUCATION
- Local library
- Exposure protection
- Early signs and symptoms of frostbite

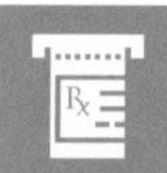

MEDICATIONS

DRUG(S) OF CHOICE
- Warm IV fluids via central venous pressure (CVP) line
- Heated oxygen
- For myxedema coma - Levothyroxine 500 μg IV plus 300 mg hydrocortisone IV diluted in D5W or NS
- Tetanus toxoid
- For severe pain - analgesics or narcotics
- Antibiotics may be required for infection
- Maintenance - gastric lavage, peritoneal dialysis, hemodialysis, and mediastinal lavage if needed (using warmed fluids)

Contraindications: Refer to manufacturer's profile of each drug
Precautions: Refer to manufacturer's profile of each drug
Significant possible interactions: Refer to manufacturer's profile of each drug

ALTERNATIVE DRUGS
Consider nifedipine 10 mg po tid 30 mg XL po qd or pentoxifylline 400 mg po tid

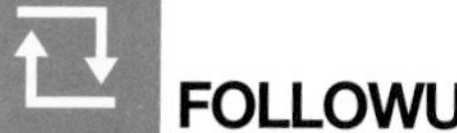

FOLLOWUP

PATIENT MONITORING
- Preferably electronic probe for temperature monitoring (rectal or vascular)
- Followup for physical therapy progress, infection, other complications

PREVENTION/AVOIDANCE
- Dress in layers with appropriate cold weather gear. Cover exposed areas and extremities appropriately.
- Proper preparation for trips to cold climates. Avoid alcohol.

POSSIBLE COMPLICATIONS
- Hyperglycemia
- Acidosis
- Refractory arrhythmias
- Tissue loss. Distal parts of an extremity may undergo spontaneous amputation.
- Gangrene
- Death

EXPECTED COURSE/PROGNOSIS
- Anesthesia and bullae may occur
- The affected areas will heal or mummify without surgery. The process may take 6-12 months for healing. Patient may be sensitive to cold and experience burning and tingling.

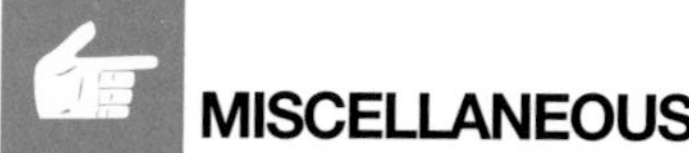

MISCELLANEOUS

ASSOCIATED CONDITIONS
Alcohol and/or drug abuse

AGE-RELATED FACTORS
Pediatric: Loss of epithelial growth centers
Geriatric:
- Associated disease states increase mortality
- Periarticular osteoporosis complicates
- More prone to hypothermia

Others: N/A

PREGNANCY
Acidosis

SYNONYMS
- Dermatitis congelationis
- Frostnip
- Environmental injuries

ICD-9-CM
991.0 Frostbite of face
991.1 Frostbite of hand
991.2 Frostbite of foot
991.3 Frostbite of other and unspecified sites

SEE ALSO
Hypothermia

OTHER NOTES
N/A

ABBREVIATIONS
N/A

REFERENCES

- Rakel RE, ed: Textbook of Family Practice. 5th Ed. Philadelphia, W.B. Saunders Co., 1995
- Berkow R, et al, eds: Merck Manual. 16th Ed. Rahway, NJ, Merck Sharp & Dohme, 1992
- Kelly KJ, Glaeser P, Rice TB, Wendelberger KJ: Profound accidental hypothermia and freeze injury of the extremities in a child. In Critical Care Medicine. Baltimore, Williams & Wilkins, 1990
- Urschel JD: Frostbite: Predisposing factors and predictors of poor outcome. In Trauma. Baltimore, Williams & Wilkins, 1990
- Mills WF, et al: Cold Injury: A Collection of Papers. Alaska Med 1993;35(1)

Web references: 0 available at www.5mcc.com
Illustrations N/A

Author(s):
Timothy Robinson, DO
Brenda Oshea-Robinson, RPAC

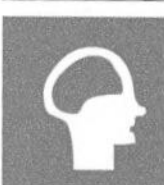

BASICS

DESCRIPTION Syndrome of painful restriction of active and passive range of motion in one or both shoulders. Idiopathic adhesive capsulitis has 3 stages: painful, adhesive, and recovery.
System(s) affected: Musculoskeletal
Genetics: N/A
Incidence/Prevalence in USA: Primary (idiopathic) 2-3%
Predominant age: 40-70, rare in children
Predominant sex: Female > Male

SIGNS & SYMPTOMS
- General signs and symptoms
  - ◊ Pain aggravated with movement and alleviated with rest
  - ◊ Pain and tenderness over the shoulder area with pressure - may interrupt sleep
  - ◊ Preceding injury, illness, or immobilization (sometimes)
  - ◊ Loss of active and passive range of motion in all planes
  - ◊ Loss of natural arm swing with gait
  - ◊ Because of compensatory scapular elevation (to lift the arm) muscles may be painful and spastic
  - ◊ Muscle atrophy and weakness with time
  - ◊ Inability to reach into a back pocket or fasten the back of a garment
- Stages of adhesive capsulitis
  - ◊ Painful stage (weeks to months)
    - Pain with movement
    - Generalized shoulder ache that is difficult to pinpoint
    - Muscle spasm
    - Increasing pain at night and at rest
  - ◊ Adhesive stage (up to 1 year)
    - Less pain
    - Increasing stiffness and restriction of movement
    - Decreasing pain at night and at rest
    - Discomfort felt at extreme ranges of movement
  - ◊ Recovery stage (weeks to months)
    - Decreased pain
    - Marked restriction with slow gradual increase in range of motion
    - Recovery is spontaneous; frequently incomplete

CAUSES
- Idiopathic (primary)
- Diseases and conditions associated with secondary adhesive capsulitis
  - ◊ Trauma
  - ◊ Diabetes
  - ◊ Post-inflammatory
  - ◊ Post CVA, post-MI, post-mastectomy (immobilization is the speculated cause)
  - ◊ Hypo/hyper-thyroidism
  - ◊ Avascular necrosis
  - ◊ Tuberculosis
  - ◊ Scleroderma
  - ◊ Rheumatoid arthritis
  - ◊ Lung cancer or chronic lung disease

RISK FACTORS
- Systemic diseases (see above: causes - secondary adhesive capsulitis)
- Prolonged immobilization
- Age (more common in elderly)
- Diabetes

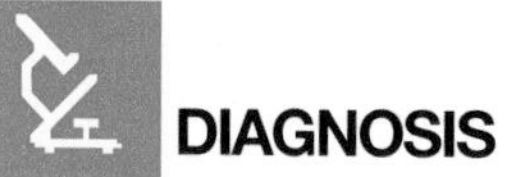

DIAGNOSIS

DIFFERENTIAL DIAGNOSIS
- Rotator cuff strain/tear
- Bicipital/rotator/calcific tendinitis
- Septic arthritis
- Bursitis
- Glenohumeral or AC joint osteoarthritis
- Rheumatoid arthritis
- Bony neoplasm/metastases
- Dislocation
- Fracture (distal clavicle, proximal humerus)

LABORATORY Rule out systemic/autoimmune disease: TSH, ESR, ANA, CBC, glucose

Drugs that may alter lab results: N/A

Disorders that may alter lab results: SLE, RA

PATHOLOGICAL FINDINGS Fibrous bands traversing the glenohumeral joint space (occasional). Surgical findings of adherence of capsule to humeral head.

SPECIAL TESTS N/A

IMAGING
- Plain x-ray (AP, axillary, supraspinatus outlet views) to rule out osteoarthritis, calcific tendinitis, AVN, osteomyelitis, fracture, dislocation, and tumor
  - ◊ AP - check osteopenia, fractures, dislocations, superior migration of humeral head
  - ◊ Axillary - check subluxation or articular head damage
  - ◊ Supraspinatus outlet views - check supraspinatus outlet narrowing to rule out acromial impingement
- Arthrography - joint volume is reduced to 5-10 mL (normal 20-30 mL). Since this is invasive, arthrography is reserved for patients with uncertain diagnosis.
- Consider MRI to evaluate rotator cuff

DIAGNOSTIC PROCEDURES
- Joint aspiration if septic joint is suspected (rarely necessary)
- Arthroscopy to visualize fibrous bands in the joint space (rarely necessary)

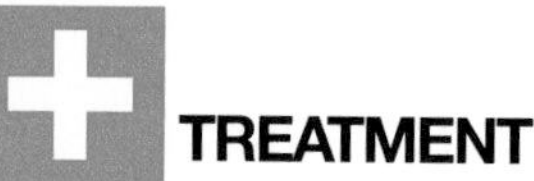

TREATMENT

APPROPRIATE HEALTH CARE
- Outpatient

GENERAL MEASURES
- Control of pain and preservation of mobility
- Avoid prolonged immobilization
- Heat and/or ice
- Address underlying causes of secondary adhesive capsulitis (see Causes and Differential Diagnosis)
- Physical therapy

SURGICAL MEASURES Arthroscopic lysis of adhesions and manipulation under anesthesia are reserved for refractory cases (controversial).

ACTIVITY
- Encourage shoulder range of motion
- Forceful shoulder exercises not recommended

DIET
- No restrictions

PATIENT EDUCATION
- Stretching exercises qd or bid - during and after improvement
  - ◊ Codman exercises: sit sideways in a straight chair. Rest armpit on the back of the chair. Swing the arm slowly in circles. Start with smaller circles and then bigger circles (clockwise and counterclockwise).
  - ◊ Climbing the wall: Put the hand flat on a wall in front of you. Use the fingers to "climb" the wall. Pause 30 seconds every few inches.
  - ◊ Reaching: Put everyday objects on a high shelf so that reaching is done more often

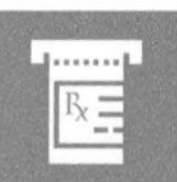

MEDICATIONS

DRUG(S) OF CHOICE
- NSAIDs during painful stage
- Opioid analgesics (with physical therapy) if NSAID contraindicated
- Oral corticosteroids for a taper of 3-4 weeks (40 mg, 30, 20, 10, then discontinue)

Contraindications:
- NSAIDS: GI ulcer disease/bleeding,
- Renal disease (see manufacturer's literature)

Precautions: See manufacturer's literature
Significant possible interactions: See manufacturer's literature

ALTERNATIVE DRUGS
- Low-dose tricyclic antidepressants (e.g. amitriptyline) may help with pain and sleep
- Intra-articular steroids (e.g. triamcinolone, betamethasone): do not shorten recovery but may aid in decreasing discomfort with mobility exercises (controversial). Systemic steroids not indicated.

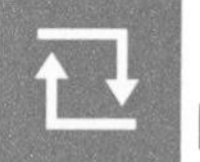

FOLLOWUP

PATIENT MONITORING Close monitoring and frequent encouragement usually needed for successful recovery

PREVENTION/AVOIDANCE
- Early range of motion exercises after injury
- Stretching, frequent physical activity

POSSIBLE COMPLICATIONS
- Long term loss of some mobility (7-30%) or function (rare); residual pain and stiffness

EXPECTED COURSE/PROGNOSIS
- Adhesive capsulitis may last from 6 to 9 months to as long as 1 to 3 years
  - ◊ Painful stage: 2-6 months
  - ◊ Adhesive stage: 4-6 months
  - ◊ Recovery stage: 1-3 months

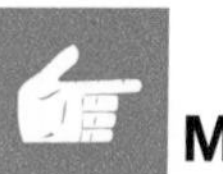

MISCELLANEOUS

ASSOCIATED CONDITIONS Above - see causes

AGE-RELATED FACTORS
Pediatric: Rare, but reported
Geriatric: Common
Others: N/A

PREGNANCY N/A

SYNONYMS
- Peri-capsulitis
- Adherent bursitis
- Obliterative bursitis
- Adhesive capsulitis

ICD-9-CM
726.0 Adhesive capsulitis of shoulder

SEE ALSO

OTHER NOTES
- Iontophoresis (electromotive drug administration) generally not recommended in this condition

ABBREVIATIONS N/A

REFERENCES

- Siegel LB, Cohen NJ, Gall EP. Adhesive capsulitis: A sticky issue. Am Fam Phys 1999;59(7):1843-1851
- Daigneault J, Cooney LM Jr. Shoulder pain in older people. J Am Geriatr Soc 1998;46(9):1145-1151
- Woodward T, Best T. The painful shoulder: Part II. Acute and chronic disorders. Am Fam Phys 2000;61(11):3291-3300
- Pearsall AW, Speer KP. Frozen shoulder syndrome: diagnostic and treatment strategies in the primary care setting. Med Sci Sports Exerc 1998;30(4 Suppl):S33-9

Web references: 0 available at www.5mcc.com
Illustrations N/A

Author(s):

Frances Biagioli, MD
Jonathan Vinson, MD

BASICS

DESCRIPTION Acute abscess of a hair follicle due to infection by Staphylococcus aureus. Spreads away from hair follicle into surrounding dermis.
System(s) affected: Skin/Exocrine
Genetics: Unknown
Incidence/Prevalence in USA:
- Uncommon in children unless immunodeficiency state present (i.e., can appear in young girls with hyperimmunoglobulin E-Staphylococcal syndrome [Job's syndrome])
- Increase in frequency after puberty

Predominant age: Adolescents and young adults. Uncommon in young children unless immunodeficiency state present (i.e., can appear in young girls with hyperimmunoglobulin E-staphylococcal syndrome [Job syndrome]).
Predominant sex: Males = Females

SIGNS & SYMPTOMS
- Painful erythematous papules/nodules (1-5 cm) with central pustulation
- Located only in hirsute sites of body, especially areas prone to friction or minor trauma (i.e., underneath belt, anterior thighs)
- May be singular or multiple
- No fever or systemic symptoms
- Tender red perifollicular swelling, terminating in discharge of pus and necrotic plug
- Pus usually drains spontaneously

CAUSES Pathogenic strain of Staphylococcus aureus

RISK FACTORS
- Carriage of pathogenic strain of Staphylococcus in nares, skin, axilla, and perineum
- Rarely, polymorphonuclear leukocyte defect or hyperimmunoglobulin-E/Staphylococcus abscess syndrome
- Diabetes mellitus, malnutrition, alcoholism
- Primary immunodeficiency disease (chronic granulomatous disease, Chediak-Higashi syndrome, C3 deficiency, C3 hypercatabolism, transient hypogammaglobulinemia of infancy, immunodeficiency with thymoma, Wiskott-Aldrich syndrome)
- Secondary immunodeficiency (leukemia, leukopenia, neutropenia, therapeutic immunosuppression)
- Medication use that impairs neutrophil function (eg, omeprazole)

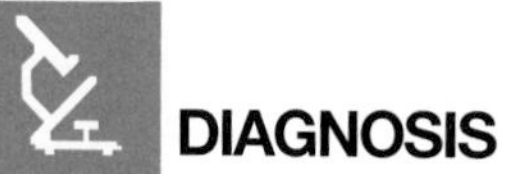

DIAGNOSIS

DIFFERENTIAL DIAGNOSIS
- Folliculitis
- Pseudofolliculitis
- Carbuncles
- Ruptured epidermal cyst
- Hidradenitis suppurativa

LABORATORY Culture of abscess material

Drugs that may alter lab results: Antibiotics

Disorders that may alter lab results: N/A

PATHOLOGICAL FINDINGS Histopathologically - perifollicular necrosis containing fibrinoid material and neutrophils. At deep end of necrotic plug, in subcutaneous tissue, is a large abscess with a gram stain positive for small collections of staph aureus.

SPECIAL TESTS None except for immunoglobulin levels in rare cases

IMAGING N/A

DIAGNOSTIC PROCEDURES Culture of abscess material

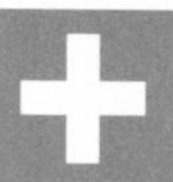

TREATMENT

APPROPRIATE HEALTH CARE Outpatient

GENERAL MEASURES
- Moist, warm compresses (provides comfort, encourages localization/pointing/drainage) 30 minutes, 4 times a day
- If pointing or large, incise and drain
- Consider packing to promote drainage
- Routine culture not necessary for localized abscess in non-diabetic patients with normal immune system
- Systemic antibiotics usually unnecessary, unless extensive surrounding cellulitis or fever
- If recurrent, problem usually related to chronic skin carriage of particular strain of Staphylococcus in nares or on skin. Treatment goals are to 1) decrease or eliminate pathogenic strain or 2) in very difficult cases, implant less aggressive strain.
- Suppression of pathogenic strain
  - ◊ Culture nares, skin, axilla, perineum
  - ◊ Begin therapeutic antibiotic doses
  - ◊ Wash entire body and fingernails (with nailbrush) daily for 1-3 weeks with povidone-iodine (Betadine), hexachlorophene (Hibiclens), or pHisoHex soap (all can cause dry skin)
  - ◊ After shower ointments
  - ◊ Sanitary practices - change towels, washcloths and sheets daily; clean shaving instruments; avoid nose-picking; change wound dressings frequently
- Replacement of pathogenic strain with nonpathogenic strain (502A bacterial interference)
  - ◊ Culture nose and lesions to document pathogenic strain
  - ◊ Culture family members if disease involves them
  - ◊ Treat patient and infected household members with antibiotics
  - ◊ Discontinue topical/oral antibiotics 48 hours then inoculate anterior nares with Staphylococcus aureus 502A (stock bacteria) (tilt head back, swab each anterior nares with 2 soaked cotton swabs of culture while patient sniffs material into nares and nasopharynx)
  - ◊ Followup 1 month later; repeat process if abscesses not controlled

SURGICAL MEASURES N/A

ACTIVITY Avoid contact sports (i.e., wrestling) if active lesions. Otherwise no restrictions.

DIET Unrestricted

PATIENT EDUCATION Refer to: Habif T: Clinical Dermatology. 3rd Ed. St. Louis, CV Mosby, 1996

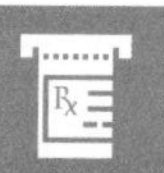

MEDICATIONS

DRUG(S) OF CHOICE
- If abscesses multiple, if lesions have marked surrounding inflammation, or if immunocompromised
  - ◊ Obtain culture and place on antibiotics for at least 14 days
  - ◊ Cloxacillin (Tegopen) or dicloxacillin (Dynapen, Pathocil) 250 mg qid, or
  - ◊ Erythromycin (E-mycin, PCE) 250-500 tid
- Suppression of pathogenic strain
  - ◊ Dicloxacillin or cloxacillin 250 mg qid x 21 days
  - ◊ Erythromycin 250-500 mg tid (if penicillin allergic) x 21 days
  - ◊ If above fails - begin 1-3 month course of antibiotics. May need to add rifampin 600 mg q day x 10 days
  - ◊ After showering - bacitracin ointment or mupirocin to both anterior nares with cotton swab tid-qid x > 14 days
- Replacement of pathogenic strain
  - ◊ Treat patient and infected household members with dicloxacillin 250 mg qid or if child/infant with 50 mg/kg/day qid x 7-10 days

Contraindications:
- Cloxacillin and dicloxacillin - penicillin allergy
- Erythromycin, mupirocin - hypersensitivity

Precautions:
- Cloxacillin and dicloxacillin - anaphylactic reaction
- Erythromycin - cautious use in patients with impaired hepatic function; GI side effects especially abdominal cramping; pregnancy category B. Increased cardiac toxicity with astemizole

Significant possible interactions: Erythromycin - increases theophylline and carbamazepine levels; decreases warfarin clearance

ALTERNATIVE DRUGS
- Resistant strains of Staph. aureus: first generation cephalosporins, clindamycin, ciprofloxacin + rifampin (rifampicin), Trimethoprim-sulfamethoxazole (cotrimoxazole) + rifampicin
- If known or suspected impaired neutrophil function (i.e., impaired chemotaxis, phagocytosis, superoxide generation), add vitamin C 1000 mg/day for 4-6 weeks (prevents oxidation of neutrophils)
- If fail with antibiotic regimens
  - ◊ May try oral pentoxifylline 400 mg tid for 2-6 months
  - ◊ Contraindications - recent cerebral and/or retinal hemorrhage; intolerance to methylxanthines (i.e., caffeine, theophylline)
  - ◊ Precautions - prolonged prothrombin time and/or bleeding; if on warfarin, frequent monitoring of prothrombin time

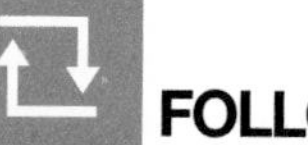

FOLLOWUP

PATIENT MONITORING Instruct patient to see physician if compresses unsuccessful

PREVENTION/AVOIDANCE Patient education regarding self care (see General Measures section. Treatment and prevention are interrelated.)

POSSIBLE COMPLICATIONS
- Scarring
- Bacteremia
- Metastatic seeding (i.e., septal/valve defect, arthritic joint)

EXPECTED COURSE/PROGNOSIS
- Self-limited (usually drains pus spontaneously and will heal with or without scarring within several days)
- Recurrent/chronic lasting for months or years

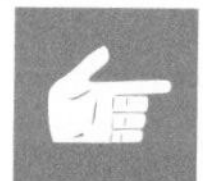

MISCELLANEOUS

ASSOCIATED CONDITIONS
- Usually normal immune system
- Diabetes mellitus
- Polymorphonuclear leukocyte defect (rare)
- Hyperimmunoglobulin-E/staphylococcal abscess syndrome (rare)
- See Risk Factors for others

AGE-RELATED FACTORS
Pediatric: N/A
Geriatric: N/A
Others: Most common after puberty. Clusters have been reported in teenagers living in crowded quarters.

PREGNANCY N/A

SYNONYMS
- Boils

ICD-9-CM
680.9 Carbuncle and furuncle, unspecified site

SEE ALSO
Folliculitis
Hidradenitis suppurativa

OTHER NOTES
- If abscess culture grows gram negative bacteria or fungus then consider polymorphonuclear neutrophil (PMN) leukocyte function defect
- Hydradenitis suppurativa is a particular form of furunculosis
- Can order Staphylococcus aureus 502A from American Type Culture Collection, Rockville, Md.

ABBREVIATIONS N/A

REFERENCES

- Sams WM Jr, Lynch P: Principles and Practice of Dermatology. New York, Churchill Livingstone, 1990
- du Vivier A: Dermatology in Practice. Philadelphia, J.B. Lippincott Co., 1990
- Habif T. Clinical Dermatology. 4th Ed. St. Louis, CV Mosby, 2004
- Wahba-Yahav AV: Intractable chronic furunculosis: Prevention of recurrence with pentoxifylline. Acta Dermato-Venereologica 1992;72(6):461-462
- West BC, et al. Furunculosis associated with repeated courses of omeprazole therapy. Clin Infec Dis 1998;26:1234-5
- Levy R, Shriker O, et al. Vitamin C for the treatment of recurrent furunculosis in patients with impaired neutrophil function. J Infect Dis 1996;173:1502

Web references: 0 available at www.5mcc.com
Illustrations 4 available

Author(s):
W. Paul Slomiany, MD

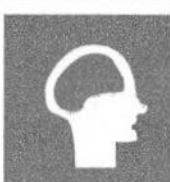

BASICS

DESCRIPTION Milky nipple discharge not associated with gestation. Galactorrhea does not include serous, purulent or bloody nipple discharge. Disorders of lactation are associated with hyperprolactinemia either from over production or loss of inhibitory regulation by dopamine.
System(s) affected: Endocrine/Metabolic, Nervous, Reproductive
Genetics: N/A
Incidence/Prevalence in USA: 1-50% of non-pregnant reproductive age women
Predominant age: 15-50 (reproductive)
Predominant sex: Males are rarely affected

SIGNS & SYMPTOMS
Bilateral milky nipple discharge, other findings vary with causes
- Hypogonadism from hyperprolactinemia
  - ◊ Oligomenorrhea, amenorrhea
  - ◊ Inadequate luteal phase, anovulation, infertility
  - ◊ Decreased libido (especially in affected males)
- Mass effects from pituitary enlargement
  - ◊ Headache, cranial neuropathies
  - ◊ Bitemporal hemianopsia, amaurosis, scotomata
- Signs/symptoms of associated conditions
  - ◊ Adrenal insufficiency, acromegaly, hypothyroidism, chest wall conditions

CAUSES
- Pituitary gland overproduction
  - ◊ Prolactinoma, acromegaly, empty sella, lymphocytic hypophysitis
- Hypothalamic region dysregulation
  - ◊ Craniopharyngiomas, meningiomas, dysgerminomas, tumors, sarcoid, irradiation, vascular insult, stalk disruption or dissection
- Medications that suppress dopamine
  - ◊ Phenothiazines, SSRIs, TCAs, butyrophenones, cimetidine, ranitidine, reserpine, alpha methyl-dopa, verapamil, estrogens, isoniazid, opioids, stimulants, neuroleptics, metoclopramide
- Chest wall conditions
  - ◊ Zoster, fibrocystic breast disease, surgical or other trauma
- Post surgical condition especially oophorectomy
- Other causes
  - ◊ Primary hypothyroidism, cirrhosis, Cushing disease, ectopic prolactin secretion, renal failure, sarcoid, lupus, multiple sclerosis, polycystic ovary syndrome
- Physiologic with pregnancy or up to 6 month after stopping lactation
  - ◊ Chiari-Frommel - idiopathic galactorrhea more than six month postpartum
- Idiopathic - normal prolactin levels

RISK FACTORS N/A

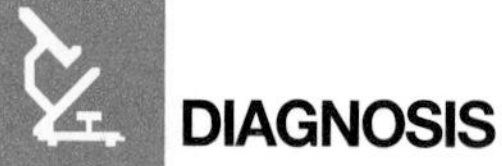

DIAGNOSIS

DIFFERENTIAL DIAGNOSIS
- Primary hypothyroidism
- Non-milky nipple discharge
  - ◊ Intraductal papilloma, fibrocystic disease
- Purulent breast discharge
  - ◊ Mastitis, breast abscess, impetigo, eczema
- Bloody breast discharge - think malignancy

LABORATORY
- Confirm microscopic of secretions is lipoid
- Check prolactin level and thyroid functions
- Check pregnancy test, liver and renal functions
- Consider FSH/LH if amenorrheic
- Consider growth hormone levels if acromegaly suspected
- Check adrenal steroids if signs of Cushing disease

Drugs that may alter lab results: See medications that can cause hyperprolactinemia

Disorders that may alter lab results: See disorders listed under Causes

PATHOLOGICAL FINDINGS None unless pituitary resection required, gland can have woody fibrosis if patient took bromocriptine (Parlodel) for very long

SPECIAL TESTS
- Formal visual field testing if pituitary adenoma suspected
- Progesterone withdrawal bleed if amenorrheic

IMAGING Pituitary MRI (CT, coned-down views or tomograms are substandard)

DIAGNOSTIC PROCEDURES No additional

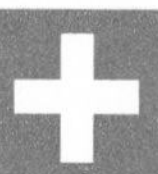

TREATMENT

APPROPRIATE HEALTH CARE
- Out patient care unless pituitary resection required
- Bromocriptine patients need good hydration

GENERAL MEASURES
- Treat underlying cause if possible
- Treat to manage symptoms, reduce patient anxiety, restore fertility
- Reduce tumor size or prevent progression to prevent neurologic sequelae
- If microadenoma "watchful waiting" can be appropriate as 95% to do not enlarge
- Treat asymptomatic tumors if >10 mm
- Discontinue offending medications

SURGICAL MEASURES
- Macroadenomas need surgery if medical management does not halt growth, if any

neurologic symptoms, if >10 mm, or patient cannot tolerate medications
  - ◊ Transsphenoidal pituitary resection
  - ◊ 50% recurrence after surgery
- Radiation is an alternate therapy
  - ◊ 20-30% success rate
  - ◊ 50% risk of panhypopituitarism after radiation
- In some research centers gamma knife is being tried

ACTIVITY No restrictions

DIET No restrictions

PATIENT EDUCATION
- Warn about symptoms of mass enlargement in pituitary
- Discuss treatment rationale and risks of treating or not
- Patient education material available from: Pituitary Tumor Network Assoc., 16350 Ventura Blvd. #231, Encino, CA 91436: (805) 499-9973

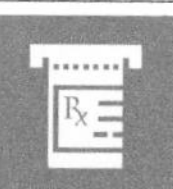

MEDICATIONS

DRUG(S) OF CHOICE The dopamine antagonist bromocriptine (Parlodel) works to reduce prolactin levels and shrink tumor size. Therapy is suppressive not curative. Start low 1.25 mg at night with a snack and increase to 2.5 mg tid. Doses as high as 30 mg/day may be required for tumor regression. 10 -15% are resistant so try alternates.

Contraindications: Uncontrolled hypertension, sensitivity to ergot alkaloids, preeclampsia

Precautions:

- Nausea, vomiting, drowsiness are common
- Orthostasis, lightheadedness or syncope
- Hypertension, seizures, acute psychosis, digital vasospasm are rare
- Long term treatment can cause woody fibrosis of the pituitary gland

Significant possible interactions: Phenothiazines, butyrophenones, other drugs listed under Causes

ALTERNATIVE DRUGS

- Other forms of bromocriptine - intravaginal, sustained release, intramuscular
- Pergolide (Permax) 0.05 - 0.15 mg once daily; fewer side effects than bromocriptine
- Cabergoline (Dostinex) 0.25 - 1.0 mg weekly; convenient dosing
- Quinagolide, Metergoline marketed in Europe

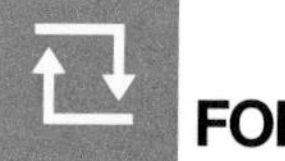

FOLLOWUP

PATIENT MONITORING

- Varies with cause, check prolactin levels every six weeks until normalized, then every 6-12 months
- Monitor visual fields and MRI at least yearly, if clinical course is stable, then every 2-5 years

PREVENTION/AVOIDANCE Keep medication causes in mind

POSSIBLE COMPLICATIONS

- Depends on underlying cause
- If enlarging pituitary adenoma risk of permanent visual field loss
- Panhypopituitarism can complication radiation or surgical therapy.
- Osteoporosis if amenorrhea persists without estrogen replacement

EXPECTED COURSE/PROGNOSIS

- Depends on underlying cause
- Symptoms recur after discontinuation of medication
- Surgery can have 50% recurrence
- Prolactinomas less than 10 mm can resolve spontaneously

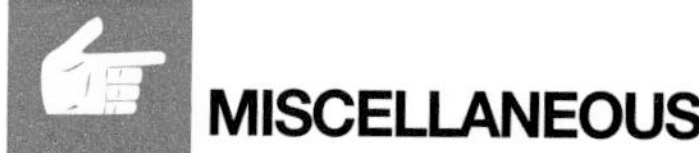

MISCELLANEOUS

ASSOCIATED CONDITIONS See Causes

AGE-RELATED FACTORS

Pediatric: N/A

Geriatric: N/A

Others: N/A

PREGNANCY Adenomas can grow rapidly during pregnancy. The majority of galactorrhea during pregnancy is physiologic.

SYNONYMS

- Disordered lactation
- Nipple discharge

ICD-9-CM

676.60 Galactorrhea associated with childbirth, unspecified

SEE ALSO

Hyperprolactinemia
Pituitary basophilic adenoma
Pituitary chromophobe adenoma

OTHER NOTES Can occur in males, 20% of patients with MEN-1 have prolactinomas

ABBREVIATIONS

SSRI = selective serotonin reuptake inhibitor
MAOI = monoamine oxidase inhibitor
TCA = tricyclic antidepressant
FSH = follicle stimulating hormone
LH = luteinizing hormone

REFERENCES

- Cho DY, Liau WR. Comparison of endonasal endoscopic surgery and sublabial microsurgery for prolactinomas. Surg Neurol 2002;58(6):371-5; discussion 375-6
- Biller BM, Luciano A, Crosignani PG, et al. Guidelines for the diagnosis and treatment of hyperprolactinemia. J Reprod Med 1999;44(12 Suppl):1075-84
- Pena KS, Rosenfeld JA. Evaluation and Treatment of Galactorrhea. Am Fam Physician 2001;63(9):1763-70
- Freda PU. Long-term treatment of prolactin-secreting macroadenomas with pergolide. J Clin Endocrinol Metab 2000;85(1):8-13
- Nomikos P, Buchfelder M, Fahlbusch R. Current management of prolactinomas. J Neurooncol 2001;54(2):139-50
- Tansey MJ, Schlechte JA. Pituitary production of prolactin and prolactin-suppressing drugs. Lupus 2001;10(10):660-4

Web references: 5 available at www.5mcc.com
Illustrations N/A

Author(s):
Patricia Borman, MD

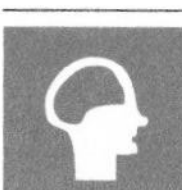

BASICS

DESCRIPTION Gastric malignancy may occur anywhere in the stomach. Over the last 20 years the incidence of adenocarcinoma of the proximal stomach and the gastroesophageal junction has risen while the incidence of distal cancers has remained unchanged or decreased slightly. Infiltration to lymph nodes, omentum, lungs and liver is rapid. Uncommon in U.S. natives.

System(s) affected: Gastrointestinal

Genetics:
- 2 to 4 times more common in first degree relatives
- More common in people with blood group A

Incidence/Prevalence in USA: 7/100,000; 22,400 new cases per year

Predominant age: Over 55 (2/3 over age 65)

Predominant sex: Male > Female (1.7:1)

SIGNS & SYMPTOMS
- Chronic non-colicky abdominal pain (especially in epigastrium) ranging from postprandial fullness to severe steady pain
- Anorexia
- Pain unrelieved by antacids
- Pain exacerbated by food
- Pain relieved by fasting
- Dysphagia
- Hematemesis
- Melena
- Cachexia
- Hepatomegaly
- Nausea and vomiting
- Constipation
- Early satiety
- Weight loss

CAUSES Unknown. Probably arises from a non-specific mucosal injury. H. pylori may trigger carcinogenesis by causing chronic atrophic gastritis and intestinal metaplasia. Probable association with food preservatives (e.g., nitrates, sulfites).

RISK FACTORS
- Helicobacter pylori infection
- Diet rich in additives (smoked, pickled or salted foods; highly spiced oriental foods)
- Achlorhydria
- Atrophic gastritis/intestinal metaplasia
- Pernicious anemia
- Prior gastric resection
- Smoking/tobacco abuse
- Ethnic background: Hispanic, Japanese, Chilean, Costa Rican. First or second generation Japanese, Chilean or Costa Rican in the United States.
- Polyps or dysplasia anywhere in alimentary canal
- Familial polyposis
- Barrett's esophagus
- Low consumption of fruits and vegetables
- Individuals with blood group A

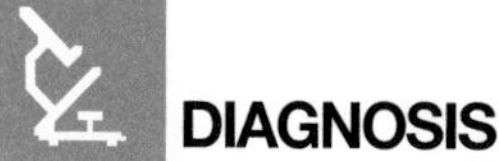

DIAGNOSIS

DIFFERENTIAL DIAGNOSIS
- Gastric lymphoma
- Peptic ulcer with or without hemorrhage
- Eosinophilic gastroenteritis
- Giant hypertrophic gastritis (Ménétrier's disease)
- Carcinoma of the colon
- Functional dyspepsia
- Carcinoma of body or tail of the pancreas
- Angiodysplasia of the colon
- GI sarcoidosis
- Small intestinal lymphoma
- Crohn disease

LABORATORY
- Positive stool guaiac for blood
- Hemoglobin less than 12 g/dL (1.86 mmol/L)
- Hematocrit less than 35 (0.35)
- Albumin less than 3 g/dL (30 g/L)

Drugs that may alter lab results: N/A

Disorders that may alter lab results: Pernicious anemia may cause a false positive pentagastrin test

PATHOLOGICAL FINDINGS
- Adenocarcinomas 90% (types: intestinal and diffuse [linitis plastica])
- Gastric lymphomas, sarcomas, and other rare types 10%

SPECIAL TESTS Pentagastrin test - stomach pH less than 6

IMAGING Double contrast upper GI study - barium filling defect, endoscopy, endoscopic ultrasound, CT scan

DIAGNOSTIC PROCEDURES Upper endoscopy for direct visualization, cytology and biopsy, endoscopic ultrasound is most accurate preoperative staging tool

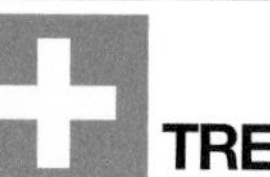

TREATMENT

APPROPRIATE HEALTH CARE Inpatient

GENERAL MEASURES
- Surgical excision of the tumor with resection of the local lymph nodes offers the only chance for cure. Even patients who are not felt to have a curable lesion should be offered an attempt at surgical reduction of the tumor since it offers the best form of palliation and improves the likelihood of benefit if chemotherapy and/or radiation therapy is administered. Exception is early (superficial) gastric cancer where nonsurgical ablation (usually endoscopic) may be curative. Gastric cardia tumors may be effectively palliated by nonsurgical means.
- Radiation therapy is of little benefit due to the radioresistancy of gastric tumors and the high doses of radiation required. It does have use in the palliation of pain, bleeding and obstruction
- Preoperative chemotherapy particularly in patients with locally advanced disease may be of benefit

SURGICAL MEASURES
- Radical subtotal gastrectomy with gastrojejunostomy or gastroduodenostomy is the usual treatment of choice. A large part of the stomach along with the greater and lesser omentum is removed en bloc. At times a splenectomy and distal pancreatectomy are also performed. Direct extensions are also excised.
- Total gastrectomy is indicated only if necessary to remove the local lesion
- Local excision or endoscopic laser therapy or electrocautery for palliation of incurable lesion by resection of bleeding area or area of obstruction

ACTIVITY Adjusted to patient's ability

DIET Dependent on the surgical procedure. Supplemental feedings or total parenteral nutrition (TPN) may be necessary to ensure adequate caloric intake.

PATIENT EDUCATION
- Contact local American Cancer Society
- Cancer Research Institute Helpbook: What to Do If Cancer Strikes. FDR Station, Box 5199, New York, NY 10150-5199

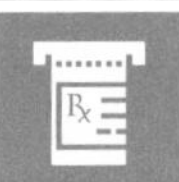

MEDICATIONS

DRUG(S) OF CHOICE

- Chemotherapy has little activity in the treatment of gastric malignancy. Multiple combinations have been tried. The following combinations may offer some palliation or possible prolongation of life:
  - ◊ Fluorouracil
  - ◊ Fluorouracil + leucovorin
  - ◊ Fluorouracil + doxorubicin ± methotrexate
  - ◊ Fluorouracil + doxorubicin + mitomycin
  - ◊ Etoposide + fluorouracil + cisplatin
  - ◊ Etoposide + cisplatin ± doxorubicin
  - ◊ Etoposide + leucovorin + fluorouracil
  - ◊ Fluorouracil + epirubicin + carmustine

Note: Dosing of these agents is patient specific; refer to Drug Evaluations Annual. American Medical Association or other sources

Contraindications:

- 5-fluorouracil: Poor nutritional state, depressed bone marrow function, serious infections, major surgery in last month
- Doxorubicin: Preexisting myelosuppression, impaired cardiac function
- Mitomycin-C: Platelet count less than 75,000/mm3, leukocyte count less than 3000/mm3, serum creatinine greater than 1.7 mg/dL (150 μmol/L), coagulation disorders, serious infections

Precautions:

- Myelosuppression can occur with any of these agents
- Fluorouracil: Stomatitis, gastrointestinal injury, alopecia
- Doxorubicin: Stomatitis, gastrointestinal injury, alopecia, cardiac toxicity
- Mitomycin-C: Renal toxicity, hypercalcemia, gastrointestinal injury, cardiac toxicity
- Etoposide: Peripheral neuropathy, mucositis, hepatic damage
- Methotrexate: Stomatitis, mucositis, gastrointestinal damage, pulmonary infiltrates and fibrosis
- Epirubicin: cardiac toxicity
- Cisplatin: Ototoxicity, renal tubular damage, hypomagnesemia, hypokalemia, hypocalcemia, hemorrhagic cystitis

Significant possible interactions:

- Cisplatin: Aminoglycosides may potentiate nephrotoxicity and ototoxicity
- Loop diuretics may potentiate ototoxicity

ALTERNATIVE DRUGS

- Ondansetron (Zofran), dronabinol (Marinol), metoclopramide (Reglan), and others for nausea control

FOLLOWUP

PATIENT MONITORING Routine, frequent followup is necessary to monitor disease state, assess treatments, monitor for recurrence/metastasis, and assess nutritional status

PREVENTION/AVOIDANCE

- Insufficient data to establish that screening would decrease mortality in US population
- Screening may be of benefit in high prevalence areas
- Diets including 5-20 servings of both fruits and vegetables each week reduce the risk of gastric malignancy by about half

POSSIBLE COMPLICATIONS

- Metastatic disease (especially hepatic, cerebral and pulmonary)
- Anemia (especially pernicious)
- Pyloric stenosis

EXPECTED COURSE/PROGNOSIS

- The prognosis for gastric carcinoma is not optimistic. Since most lesions do not produce symptoms until late in their course, gastric carcinomas are usually advanced at the time of diagnosis. Surgery offers the only chance for a cure.
- Overall 5 year relative survival rate 19% (if local disease 57%, regional spread 19%, distant spread 2%)
- Early gastric cancers are usually detected as incidental findings or when screening endoscopy is performed in endemic areas. Five year survival rate is > 40% depending on specific staging and tumor differentiation.
- Primary gastric lymphoma more treatable than adenocarcinoma of the stomach. 5 year survival rate of 40% - 60% with subtotal gastrectomy followed by combination chemotherapy.

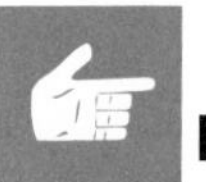

MISCELLANEOUS

ASSOCIATED CONDITIONS

- Predisposed by giant hypertrophic gastritis (Ménétrier's disease)
- Predisposed by intestinal metaplasia of the stomach
- Atrophic gastritis
- H. pylori

AGE-RELATED FACTORS

Pediatric: Rare
Geriatric: Prevalence greater
Others: N/A

PREGNANCY Gastric cancer is rarely diagnosed in pregnancy. Prognosis is poor if diagnosed.

SYNONYMS Linitis plastica

ICD-9-CM

151.0 Malignant neoplasm of stomach, cardia
151.1 Malignant neoplasm of stomach, pylorus
151.2 Malignant neoplasm of stomach, pyloric antrum
151.3 Malignant neoplasm of fundus of stomach
151.4 Malignant neoplasm of body of stomach
151.5 Malignant neoplasm of lesser curvature of stomach, unspecified
151.6 Malignant neoplasm of greater curvature of stomach, unspecified
151.8 Malignant neoplasm of other specified sites of stomach
151.9 Malignant neoplasm of stomach, unspecified

SEE ALSO

Esophageal tumors
Multiple endocrine neoplasia (MEN)

OTHER NOTES

- Patients in lower socioeconomic classes are at greater risk of developing gastric tumors
- Migrants from high incidence areas (such as Iceland, Chile or Japan) to low incidence areas maintain an increased risk while their offspring have an occurrence rate that corresponds to the new location

ABBREVIATIONS N/A

REFERENCES

- Ellis KK, Fennerty MB. Gastric malignancy. Gastrointest Endosc Clin N Am 1996;6(3):545-63
- Bowles MJ, Benjamin IS. ABC of the upper gastrointestinal tract: Cancer of the stomach and pancreas. BMJ 2001;323(7326):1413-6
- Layke JC, Lopez PP. Gastric cancer: diagnosis and treatment options. Am Fam Physician 2004;69(5):1133-40, 1145-6

Web references: 1 available at www.5mcc.com
Illustrations N/A

Author(s):

Scott T. Henderson, MD

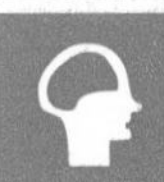

BASICS

DESCRIPTION Inflammatory reaction in the stomach; typically involves the mucosa, seldom the full thickness of the stomach wall

- Patchy erythema of gastric mucosa: a common endoscopic finding; usually insignificant
- Erosive gastritis: a reaction to mucosal injury by a noxious chemical agent, e.g., drugs (especially NSAID's) or alcohol
- Reflux gastritis: a reaction to protracted reflux exposure to bile and pancreatic juice, usually associated with a defective pylorus; typically limited to the prepyloric antrum
- Hemorrhagic gastritis (stress ulceration): a reaction to hemodynamic disorder, eg, hypovolemia or hypoxia (as in shock). Also, very common in intensive care units (ICU).
- Infectious gastritis: commonly associated with Helicobacter pylori (possibly causative, maybe opportunistic); viral infection, usually as a component of systemic infection, is common; significant infection by other specific microbes is rare
- Gastric mucosal atrophy, sometimes called atrophic gastritis: frequent, in varying degrees, in the elderly; invariable in primary (pernicious) anemia

System(s) affected: Gastrointestinal
Genetics: Unknown (except, probably, for gastric mucosa atrophy)
Incidence/Prevalence in USA: N/A
Predominant age: All ages; an estimated 60% of persons older than 60 years harbor H. pylori in their gastric mucosa, but in only a small fraction is this significant
Predominant sex: Male = Female

SIGNS & SYMPTOMS

- Nondescript epigastric distress, often aggravated by eating
- Anorexia
- Nausea, with or without vomiting
- Significant bleeding is unusual except in hemorrhagic gastritis
- Hiccups

CAUSES

- Alcohol
- Aspirin and other non-steroidal anti-inflammatory drugs
- Bile reflux
- Pancreatic enzyme reflux
- Stress (hypovolemia or hypoxia)
- Radiation
- Staphylococcus aureus exotoxins
- Bacterial infection (eg: Helicobacter pylori)
- Viral infection
- Pernicious anemia
- Gastric mucosal atrophy
- Portal hypertension gastropathy
- Emotional stress

RISK FACTORS

- Age over 60
- Exposure to potentially noxious drugs or chemical agents
- Hypovolemia, hypoxia (shock)
- Candidal autoimmune

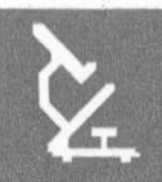

DIAGNOSIS

DIFFERENTIAL DIAGNOSIS

- Functional gastrointestinal disorder
- Peptic ulcer disease
- Linitis plastica
- Viral gastroenteritis
- Pancreatic disease
- Gastric cancer (elderly)

LABORATORY Usually unremarkable, except when blood loss results in anemia

Drugs that may alter lab results: Antibiotics or omeprazole may affect urea breath test for H. pylori

Disorders that may alter lab results: N/A

PATHOLOGICAL FINDINGS Acute or chronic inflammatory infiltrate in gastric mucosa, often with distortion or erosion of adjacent epithelium. Presence of H. pylori may be confirmed.

SPECIAL TESTS

- 13C-urea breath test for H. pylori (not widely available)
- Serologic test available for H. pylori (office and clinical laboratory), inexpensive
- Gastric acid analysis may be abnormal, but is not a reliable indicator of gastritis

IMAGING Nuclear scintigraphy not done clinically

DIAGNOSTIC PROCEDURES Gastroscopy, usually with biopsy, is essential for a precise diagnosis. (Recommend if poor response to initial treatment.)

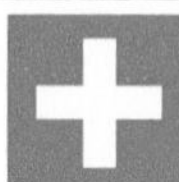

TREATMENT

APPROPRIATE HEALTH CARE Outpatient, except for severe hemorrhagic gastritis

GENERAL MEASURES

- No specific therapy for gastritis (with the exception of H. pylori infection)
- Parenteral fluid and electrolyte supplements required if vomiting prevents food intake
- Consider discontinuing NSAIDs or adding misoprostol

SURGICAL MEASURES N/A

ACTIVITY Usually no restriction

DIET Restriction, if any, depends on severity of symptoms (e.g., light, soft diet); avoid caffeine and spicy foods.

PATIENT EDUCATION

- Explanation, reassurance
- Smoking cessation
- Dietary changes
- Relaxation therapy

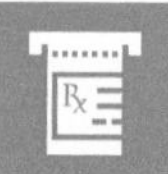

MEDICATIONS

DRUG(S) OF CHOICE
- Antacids - best given in liquid form, 30 mL 1 hour after meals and at bedtime; useful mainly as an emollient
- H2 receptor antagonists e.g., cimetidine (Tagamet) - "priming" dose of 300 mg IV, then a steady infusion of 37.5-75 mg per hour, dissolved in the running fluid. Patients less severely ill - oral cimetidine 300 mg q6h (or ranitidine [Zantac] or famotidine [Pepcid] or nizatidine [Axid]). Not shown to be clearly superior to antacids.
- Sucralfate (Carafate) 1 g q4-6h on an empty stomach. Rationale uncertain, but empirically helpful.
- Prostaglandins, e.g., misoprostol (Cytotec), can help allay gastric mucosal injury, suggested dosage of 100-200 μg qid
- To eradicate H. pylori:
  - ◊ "Triple therapy" is advised - bismuth (as Pepto-Bismol) 30 mL liquid or 2 tablets qid for 4 weeks plus metronidazole 250 mg qid for the first week, plus tetracycline 250 mg qid or amoxicillin 250 mg tid for 2-4 weeks

or
  - ◊ "Dual therapy" with omeprazole 20 mg bid plus amoxicillin 500 mg qid for 2 weeks
  - ◊ Short course therapy with 1 week of metronidazole, omeprazole, and clarithromycin bid - 90% effective

Contraindications: Hypersensitivity to the drug(s)
Precautions:
- If bismuth is prescribed, warn patient of black stools
- Refer to manufacturer's profile of each drug

Significant possible interactions: Refer to manufacturer's profile of each drug

ALTERNATIVE DRUGS N/A

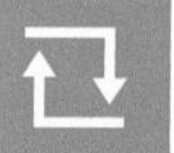

FOLLOWUP

PATIENT MONITORING Gastroscopy should be repeated after 6 weeks if gastritis has been severe or if symptomatic response to treatment has not been achieved

PREVENTION/AVOIDANCE
- Patients should be warned of known or potentially injurious drugs or chemical agents
- Patients liable to hypovolemia or hypoxia (especially patients confined to an intensive care ward) should receive prophylactic therapy

POSSIBLE COMPLICATIONS Bleeding from extensive mucosal erosion or ulceration

EXPECTED COURSE/PROGNOSIS
- Most cases clear spontaneously when the cause has been identified and allayed
- Recurrence of H. pylori infection may require a repeated course of treatment

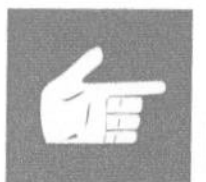

MISCELLANEOUS

ASSOCIATED CONDITIONS
- Gastric or duodenal peptic ulcer
- Primary (pernicious) anemia
- Portal hypertension

AGE-RELATED FACTORS
Pediatric: Gastritis rarely occurs in infants or children
Geriatric: Persons over 60 often harbor apparently harmless H. pylori infection
Others: N/A

PREGNANCY N/A

SYNONYMS
- Erosive gastritis
- Reflux gastritis
- Hemorrhagic gastritis
- Acute gastritis

ICD-9-CM
535.50 Unspecified gastritis and gastroduodenitis without mention of hemorrhage

SEE ALSO

OTHER NOTES N/A

ABBREVIATIONS
NSAID = non-steroidal anti-inflammatory drug

REFERENCES

- Richardson CT: Gastritis. In: Wyngaarden JB, Smith LH Jr, eds. Cecil Textbook of Medicine. Philadelphia, W.B. Saunders Co., 1988:689-692
- Graham DY, Malaty HM, Evans G, et al: Epidemiology of Helicobacter pylori in an asymptomatic population in the US. Gastroenterology 1991;100:1495-1501
- Zinner MJ, Rypins EB, Martin LR, et al: Misoprostol versus antacid titration for preventing stress ulcers in postoperative surgical ICU patients. Ann Surg 1989;210:590-595
- Cutler AP: Testing for Helicobacter pylori in clinical practice. Am J Med 1996;100:355-415
- Ofman JJ, et al: Management strategies for Helicobacter pylori seropositive patients with dyspepsia: clinical and economic consequences. Ann Inter Med 1997;126:280-291

Web references: 0 available at www.5mcc.com
Illustrations N/A

Author(s):
Douglas M. Hoy, MD

BASICS

DESCRIPTION Reflux of gastroduodenal contents into the esophagus, larynx or lungs with or without esophageal inflammation
System(s) affected: Gastrointestinal
Genetics: N/A
Incidence/Prevalence in USA: 65% of adults have suffered heartburn; 24% have had symptoms for > 10 years. 17% of adults use indigestion aids at least once weekly, only 24% of sufferers have consulted a physician. Children affected 1/300-1000. 30-80% of pregnant women report heartburn.
Predominant age: All ages
Predominant sex: Male = Female

SIGNS & SYMPTOMS
- Heartburn (pyrosis) 70-85%
- Regurgitation 60%
- Dysphagia (possible stricture) 15-20%
- Angina-like chest pain 33%
- Bronchospasm (asthma) 15-20%
- Laryngitis (dysphonia)
- Chronic cough
- Globus sensation
- Loss of dental enamel
- In infants: Recurrent emesis, failure to thrive, apnea syndrome

CAUSES
- Inappropriate relaxation of lower esophageal sphincter (LES) (idiopathic, food- or drug-related)
- Chronic eructation (belching), aerophagia
- Pregnancy (progestational hormones cause decreased LES pressure)
- Scleroderma (reduced esophageal motility and incompetent LES)
- Chalasia of infancy
- Delayed gastric emptying (impaired acid clearance)
- Acid hypersecretion (e.g., Zollinger-Ellison syndrome)
- Heller's myotomy for achalasia

RISK FACTORS
- Foods that lower LES pressure (high-fat content, yellow onions, chocolate, peppermint)
- Foods that irritate esophageal mucosa (citrus fruits, spicy tomato drinks)
- Hiatal hernia - acid trapping
- Chronic belching, aerophagia
- Medications that lower LES pressure (e.g., theophylline, anticholinergics, progesterone, calcium channel blockers (nifedipine, verapamil), alpha adrenergic agents, diazepam, meperidine
- Indwelling nasogastric tube
- Chest trauma
- In children: Down syndrome, mental retardation, cerebral palsy, repaired tracheoesophageal fistula
- Eradication of H. pylori infection (resulting in increased acid production, loss of acid buffering, etc.)
- Risks for erosive esophagitis: male, caucasian, hiatal hernia, basal metabolic index (BMI) >30 and NSAIDs

DIAGNOSIS

DIFFERENTIAL DIAGNOSIS
- Infectious esophagitis (candida, herpes, HIV, cytomegalovirus)
- Chemical esophagitis (lye ingestion)
- Radiation injury
- Crohn disease of esophagus
- Angina pectoris
- Esophageal carcinoma
- Pill-induced esophagitis (e.g., doxycycline, ascorbic acid, quinidine, potassium chloride, bisphosphonates, etc.)
- Achalasia
- Ulcer disease
- Alkaline reflux

LABORATORY N/A

Drugs that may alter lab results: N/A

Disorders that may alter lab results: N/A

PATHOLOGICAL FINDINGS
- Acute inflammation (especially eosinophils)
- Hyperplasia (thickening) of the basal zone of the epithelium seen in 85%
- Lengthening of vascular channels within vascular papillae so that they approach the luminal surface
- Barrett's epithelial change - gastric columnar epithelium (intestinal metaplasia) migrates upward into the distal esophagus; may be associated with strictures and peptic ulceration; dysplasia and malignant transformation

SPECIAL TESTS
- Esophageal pH monitoring (antacids, H2 blockers, proton pump inhibitors and other antisecretory agents can give false negative pH monitoring)
- Esophageal manometry (anticholinergics, theophylline, calcium channel blockers, meperidine, diazepam may give falsely low LES pressure on manometry)

IMAGING
- Barium swallow: Presence of a sliding hiatal hernia appears to be a predictor of reflux esophagitis; mucosal irregularity due to inflammation and edema; prominent longitudinal folds, erosions, ulcers; smoothly tapered strictures; pseudodiverticula
- Radionuclide scintigraphy

DIAGNOSTIC PROCEDURES
- "Once in a lifetime" endoscopy in chronic GERD patients to exclude Barrett's and adenocarcinoma is becoming an accepted practice
- Endoscopy (or upper GI series), pH monitoring to evaluate patients with warning symptoms (dysphagia, hematemesis, unexplained weight loss, chest pain, etc.)
- 50-70% of patients with heartburn have negative findings on endoscopy (nonerosive or endoscopy-negative reflux disease [ENRD])
- Patients with esophagitis are graded according to the LA (Los Angeles) Classification as follows:
  - ◊ Grade A: one or more mucosal breaks < 5 mm in maximal length (30-35% of patients)
  - ◊ Grade B: one or more mucosal break > 5 mm in length but not continuous between the tops of two mucosal folds (40% of patients)
  - ◊ Grade C: mucosal breaks continuous between the tops of two or more mucosal folds but involving < 75% of the esophageal circumference (20% of patients)
  - ◊ Grade D: mucosal breaks involving > 75% of the esophageal circumference (5-7% of patients)
- Barrett's change suspected when salmon colored mucosa extends > 2 cm above normal squamocolumnar junction (in up to 10%).
- Mucosal biopsy
- Cytology for Barrett's dysplasia (flow cytometry useful adjunct when available)
- Metoclopramide or cisapride may give falsely negative gastric emptying results
- Empiric trial of proton pump inhibitor compares well to pH monitoring as a diagnostic tool in diagnosing reflux in patients without alarm symptoms

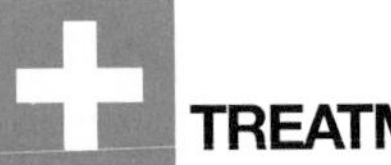

TREATMENT

APPROPRIATE HEALTH CARE Outpatient (typical heartburn history has a positive predictive value of > 80%; warrants empiric therapy in absence of alarm symptoms)

GENERAL MEASURES
- Elevate head of bed, avoid lying down directly after meals; avoid stooping, bending, tight-fitting garments
- Avoid drugs that decrease LES pressure
- Weight loss
- Avoid voluntary eructation
- Stepped therapy
  - ◊ Phase I: lifestyle and diet modifications plus antacids or OTC H2 blockers
  - ◊ Phase II: H2 blockers in prescription doses; proton pump inhibitors
  - ◊ Phase III: (1) proton pump inhibitor or high-dose H2 blocker or (2) H2 blockers or proton pump inhibitor plus promotility agent
  - ◊ Phase IV: surgery
- Endoscopic therapy - designed to increase pressure and/or improve the antireflux barrier
  - ◊ Radiofrequency energy delivered to LES area (Stretta procedure) improved symptoms, but did not reduce acid exposure or need for medications when compared to a sham procedure
  - ◊ Plication of the LES by endoscopic suturing system
  - ◊ Injection of microspheres into the LES

SURGICAL MEASURES Open or laparoscopic Nissen ot Toupet fundoplication. Good-excellent response: if abnormal 24 hr pH score, typical primary symptom and poor prior response to medical treatment; poor response: if normal 24 hr pH score, poor esophageal motility, aerophagia

ACTIVITY Full activity

DIET Avoid chocolate, peppermint, onions, high-fat foods, alcohol, tobacco, coffee, citrus

PATIENT EDUCATION Digestive Diseases Clearinghouse, Suite 600, 1555 Wilson Blvd., Rosslyn, VA 22209, (212)685-3440

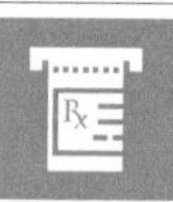

MEDICATIONS

DRUG(S) OF CHOICE
- Mild to moderate disease: H2 blockers in equipotent oral doses, eg, cimetidine (Tagamet) 800 mg bid or 400 mg qid or ranitidine (Zantac) 150 bid or famotidine (Pepcid) 20 mg bid or nizatidine (Axid) 150 mg bid. Proton pump inhibitors (eg, omeprazole (Prilosec) 20 mg/d, lansoprazole (Prevacid) 30 mg/d, pantoprazole (Protonix) 40 mg/d, rabeprazole (Aciphex) 20 mg/d, esomeprazole (Nexium) 40 mg/d may be used as initial therapy for symptomatic GERD.
- Erosive esophagitis: Proton pump inhibitors are significantly more effective than the H2 blockers in ulcer healing doses
- Severe disease (refractory to initial therapy): Proton pump inhibitor given once or twice daily or higher
- Extraesophageal symptoms (eg laryngitis, asthma) often require higher doses of proton pump inhibitors (PPI) for prolonged duration
- Nonerosive reflux disease (NERD): PPIs more effective than H2 blockers
- Pantoprazole available in intravenous formulation for patients who cannot take po

Contraindications: Known hypersensitivity to H2 blockers, omeprazole, lansoprazole, cisapride

Precautions:
- Dose reduction of H2 blockers for renal failure
- Avoid cimetidine when potentially interacting drugs are co-administered (or closely monitor prothrombin time or serum theophylline levels, etc.)

Significant possible interactions:
- Cimetidine interacts with > 60 drugs (e.g., theophylline, warfarin, phenytoin, lidocaine). Refer to manufacturer's profile.
- Omeprazole
  - ◊ May prolong the elimination of diazepam, warfarin and phenytoin
  - ◊ Prolonged PPI use associated with hypergastrinemia and potential for vitamin B12 deficiency

ALTERNATIVE DRUGS
- Antacids; alginates e.g., alumina-magnesium (Gaviscon)
- Metoclopramide (Reglan) 5-10 mg before meals used adjunctively with H2 blockers (neuropsychiatric side effects in 30% limits its usefulness)
- Cisapride (Propulsid) 10-20 mg qid (before meals and at bedtime) available only for investigational limited access program through the manufacturer
- Baclofen 40 mg/d has reduced acid reflux episodes and belching

FOLLOWUP

PATIENT MONITORING Follow symptomatically; repeat endoscopy at 4-8 weeks for poor symptomatic response; endoscopy and biopsy for Barrett's esophagus (to detect dysplasia) every 1-2 years

PREVENTION/AVOIDANCE
- Nocturnal breakthrough of heartburn treated with hs dose of H2 blocker or bid PPI
- Long-term maintenance therapy with H2 blockers or proton pump inhibitors along with lifestyle and diet modifications to prevent symptomatic relapse
- Peptic strictures may require periodic dilatation (although frequency of dilatation is reduced by PPI maintenance)
- Proton pump inhibitors are most effective in acute healing doses for chronic maintenance in severe GERD
- Consider antireflux surgery (laparoscopic approach increasingly being used) in patients with severe disease in lieu of chronic drug therapy
- Annual or every other year endoscopy, biopsy and cytology to detect dysplasia in Barrett's epithelium (more frequently if dysplasia present)
- Photodynamic therapy for Barrett esophagus with dysplasia

POSSIBLE COMPLICATIONS
- Peptic stricture (10-15%)
- Hemorrhage (3%)
- Barrett's esophagus (10%)
- Pulmonary or ear, nose, throat complications (5-10%)
- Noncardiac chest pain
- Adenocarcinoma from Barrett's epithelium

EXPECTED COURSE/PROGNOSIS
- Majority of patients respond well to antisecretory therapy. Overall healing rate at $\le$ 12 weeks for PPIs = 84% vs H2 blockers 52%. Speed of healing is 12% per week for PPI vs 6% per week for H2 blockers. Complete freedom from heartburn is 77% for PPI vs 48% for H2 blockers.
- Symptoms and esophageal inflammation often return promptly when treatment withdrawn
- Relapse prevention therapy with H2 blockers/proton pump inhibitor often requires the full healing dose be maintained
- Antireflux surgery (e.g., fundoplication) for complications or "refractory" disease; excellent short-term results. But long-term follow up shows many patients eventually require medical therapy for acid suppression; doses of 40 mg/d omeprazole or equivalent yield similar long-term results compared to surgery.
- Regression of Barrett's epithelium does not routinely occur despite aggressive medical or surgical therapy
- Cost effectiveness of long-term maintenance therapy has been shown for PPIs and H2 blockers (PPI more cost effective than high dose H2 blockers)
- Successful eradication of Helicobacter pylori associated with worsening of GERD in some patients
- Long-term safety of omeprazole (up to 11 years) recently demonstrated

MISCELLANEOUS

ASSOCIATED CONDITIONS
- Extraesophageal reflux
- Reflux-induced asthma
- Pulmonary aspiration
- Chronic cough/throat clearing
- Loss of dental enamel
- Halitosis
- Laryngitis, laryngeal carcinoma
- Globus sensation
- Vocal cord granulomas

AGE-RELATED FACTORS
Pediatric:
- Reflux symptoms usually resolve by 18 mo
- Vomiting, weight loss, failure to thrive more common than heartburn
- Positional treatment = use of infant seat for 2-3 hours after meals; thickened feedings
- Drug treatment = antacids or liquid H2 blockers (e.g., Zantac syrup); omeprazole
- Surgery for severe symptoms (apnea, choking, persistent vomiting) successful in 85-95%

Geriatric: Complications more likely

Others: N/A

PREGNANCY
- Heartburn (when first experienced): 52% 1st trimester, 24% 2nd trimester, 9% 3rd trimester
- Tends to recur in subsequent pregnancies
- Symptomatic therapy includes multiple small meals, avoid lying down for 2-3 hours after meals, elevating the head of the bed at night
- Antacids, alginates, sucralfate appear safe in all trimesters
- Ranitidine, cimetidine, and omeprazole also appear safe in early as well as late pregnancy

SYNONYMS
- Reflux esophagitis
- Peptic esophagitis
- Barrett esophagus
- Symptomatic hiatal hernia
- Nonerosive reflux disease
- Supraesophageal reflux disease

ICD-9-CM
530.10 Esophagitis, unspecified
750.6 Congenital hiatus hernia
787.1 Heartburn

SEE ALSO
Esophageal tumors
Peptic ulcer disease

OTHER NOTES Alkaline (bile) reflux accounts for up to 15% of Barrett's esophagus and severe esophagitis; promotility agent or surgery may be required in this setting

ABBREVIATIONS
LES = lower esophageal sphincter
GER = gastroesophageal reflux
GERD = gastroesophageal reflux disease
PPI = proton pump inhibitor
NERD = nonerosive reflux disease

REFERENCES

- Corley DA, Katz P, Wo JM, et al. Improvement of gastroesophageal reflux symptoms after radiofrequency energy: a randomized, sham-controlled trial. Gastroenterology. 2003;125(3):668-76¥ Inadomi JM, Sampliner R, Lagergren J, et al. Screening and surveillance for Barrett esophagus in high-risk groups: a cost-utility analysis. Ann Intern Med 2003;138(3):176-86
- Zhang Q, Lehmann A, Rigda R, Dent J, Holloway RH. Control of transient lower oesophageal sphincter relaxations and reflux by the GABA(B) agonist baclofen in patients with gastro-oesophageal reflux disease. Gut 2002;50(1):19-24
- Cange L, Johnsson E, Rydholm H, et al. Baclofen-mediated gastro-oesophageal acid reflux control in patients with established reflux disease. Aliment Pharmacol Ther 2002;16(5):869-73

Web references: 1 available at www.5mcc.com
Illustrations N/A

Author(s):
James H. Lewis, MD

Giant cell arteritis

BASICS

DESCRIPTION A systemic granulomatous, predominantly large vessel arteritis, most commonly affecting the branches of the cranial arteries, (but may involve other aortic branches), seen primarily in the elderly. Frequently associated with polymyalgia rheumatica (PMR).
System(s) affected: Cardiovascular, Hemic/Lymphatic/Immunologic, Musculoskeletal, Nervous
Genetics: May be important, several family clusters have been identified
Incidence/Prevalence in USA: More common in northern latitudes (15-30/ 100,000 person over 50/year) vs. southern latitudes (less than 2/100,000 in some series). Primarily Caucasian, Northern European descent.
Predominant age: 60 years or older (very rare under 50). Incidence increases with age.
Predominant sex: Female > Male (2:1)

SIGNS & SYMPTOMS
- Onset may be abrupt or insidious over months
- Local
  - ◊ Headache (usually unilateral temporal, may be generalized or occipital) seen in 2/3 of patients
  - ◊ Jaw/tongue "claudication" upon mastication (fairly specific)
  - ◊ Visual disturbances early - amaurosis fugax, scotoma, diplopia); late - ischemic optic neuritis, blindness
  - ◊ Scalp tenderness
  - ◊ Swollen, red temporal artery (rare)
  - ◊ Decreased temporal artery pulse (may be increased early)
  - ◊ Sore throat, cough (10%)
  - ◊ Neurologic manifestations - TIA, stroke
- Systemic
  - ◊ Polymyalgia rheumatica - seen in 40-60%
  - ◊ Fever (low grade) - 15% with FUO
  - ◊ Fatigue/malaise
  - ◊ Weight loss/anorexia
  - ◊ Arthralgias, myalgias, arthritis

CAUSES
- Etiology unknown
- Possibly immunologic mechanism

RISK FACTORS
- Age over 50
- Presence of polymyalgia rheumatica

DIAGNOSIS

DIFFERENTIAL DIAGNOSIS
- Cerebral vasculitides
- Other causes of headache (tumor, sinusitis, cervical or temporomandibular joint arthritis)
- Cerebral vascular insufficiency
- Other connective tissue disease
- Retinal detachment or other causes of loss of vision
- Septic arteritis
- Embolic disease

LABORATORY
- ESR (Westergren) usually greater than 50 (may be over 100)
- ESR may be normal in < 10% of patients
- Elevated alkaline phosphatase over 1.5 x normal (unusual)
- Elevated aspartate aminotransferase (AST) over 1.5 x normal (unusual)
- Anemia - mild to moderate, normochromic/normocytic
- Mild leukocytosis
- Mild thrombocytosis

Drugs that may alter lab results: Prednisone, methotrexate, other immunosuppressives

Disorders that may alter lab results:
- Tumor, infection, serum protein abnormalities all raise the ESR
- Congestive heart failure, microcytic anemia, and hemoglobinopathy may lower ESR

PATHOLOGICAL FINDINGS
- Inflammatory infiltrate (either mononuclear cells or granulomas with giant multinucleated cells) seen in the intima and media of large vessels with resultant disruption of the internal elastic lamina. Lesions may be isolated (i.e., skip lesions)
- Biopsy may not show evidence of active arteritis. However, changes of healing arteritis or vasculitis supports the diagnosis of GCA. If clinically active disease (headache, jaw claudication, elevated ESR), treat as GCA and use high dose steroids.

SPECIAL TESTS Temporal artery biopsy - need serial section in specimen of adequate size (at least 1 inch). Bilateral biopsy may be necessary.

IMAGING Temporal arteriography (in selected cases)

DIAGNOSTIC PROCEDURES
- Temporal artery biopsy
  - ◊ Minimum 2.5 cm segment of vessel with serial sections
  - ◊ Within 96 hours of starting steroids
  - ◊ If negative, must consider biopsy of contralateral artery (may increase yield up to 10-14%)

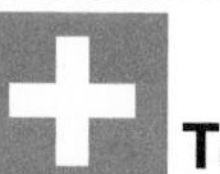

TREATMENT

APPROPRIATE HEALTH CARE
- Outpatient surgery (initially for temporal artery biopsy)
- With reasonable suspicion, immediately institute high dose corticosteroid therapy while arranging temporal artery biopsy

GENERAL MEASURES Institute surveillance for corticosteroid side effects, including osteoporosis screening

SURGICAL MEASURES
- Temporal artery biopsy

ACTIVITY Ambulatory ad lib

DIET
- Appropriate salt restriction
- Adequate calcium intake (1500 mg/day)
- Watch serum glucose

PATIENT EDUCATION
- Precautions regarding steroid use, especially osteoporosis
- Exacerbation of disease with medication dose adjustment
- Adrenal suppression - patients should get medical alert bracelet or neck tag
- With CNS symptoms or headache, call physician immediately for adjustment of steroid dose
- Excellent material available from Arthritis Foundation, http://www.arthritis.org

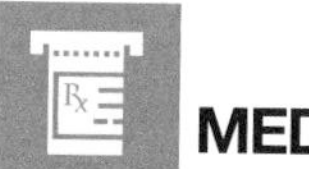

MEDICATIONS

DRUG(S) OF CHOICE

- Prednisone - early:
  - ◊ 60 mg prednisone/d; single morning dose (never use every other day steroids)
  - ◊ Begin slow taper after 6-8 weeks if asymptomatic and ESR decreased (occasionally patient may not normalize ESR)
- Prednisone - taper:
  - ◊ Taper initially by 5 mg every 2 weeks to dose of 25 mg. Then slow taper by 2.5 mg decrements every 2-4 weeks to a dose of 10-15 mg if above guidelines are met. (Must be individualized).
  - ◊ Continue 10-15 mg daily for several months-year, with periodic attempts to taper (i.e., every 3-6 months) by 1 or 2 mg
  - ◊ Use symptoms and ESR to help guide taper
  - ◊ Average time to disease remission 3-4 years, range 1-10 years

Contraindications:

- Systemic fungal infections, although physician must evaluate risks and benefits.
- Relative contraindications: Avoid, if possible, in patients with congestive heart failure, diabetes mellitus, systemic fungal or bacterial infection (must treat infection concurrently if steroids are necessary).

Precautions:

- Long term steroid use
  - ◊ Associated with several potentially severe adverse effects, including: Increased susceptibility to infection, glucose intolerance, adrenal suppression, muscle wasting, osteoporosis, peptic ulcer disease, sodium and water retention, cataracts, avascular necrosis, GI bleeding, psychosis, weight gain
  - ◊ Use lowest possible dose
  - ◊ Upon discontinuing, if the patient has received long-term therapy, taper slowly to avoid Addisonian crisis. May need temporary stress dose steroids for surgical procedures, accidents or severe infections.

Significant possible interactions: Refer to manufacturer's literature

ALTERNATIVE DRUGS

Methotrexate only if patient cannot use steroids (brittle diabetes mellitus, severe osteoporosis, congestive heart failure, etc.) or fails to respond to steroids

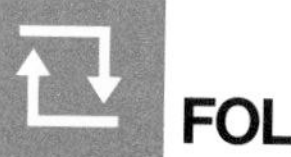

FOLLOWUP

PATIENT MONITORING

- ESR - repeat at monthly intervals initially and while tapering, then every 3 months
- Follow visual/constitutional symptoms monthly initially, then as needed

PREVENTION/AVOIDANCE

N/A

POSSIBLE COMPLICATIONS

- Complications related to steroids
- Exacerbation of disease during therapy or taper
- Blindness, stroke

EXPECTED COURSE/PROGNOSIS

- With early treatment, resolution of symptoms and preservation of vision
- Average length of disease 3-4 years
- With no treatment, high risks of blindness and stroke
- Occasionally ESR elevation not related to GCA activity and cannot be used to monitor and/or adjust treatment

MISCELLANEOUS

ASSOCIATED CONDITIONS

Polymyalgia rheumatica

AGE-RELATED FACTORS

Pediatric: Does not occur in this age group
Geriatric: Incidence increases with age (twice as common in patients over 80 as it is in 50-59 age group)
Others: N/A

PREGNANCY

N/A

SYNONYMS

- Temporal arteritis
- Horton's headache

ICD-9-CM

446.5 Giant cell arteritis

SEE ALSO

Depression
Fibromyalgia
Headache, cluster
Headache, tension
Polymyalgia rheumatica
Polymyositis/dermatomyositis

OTHER NOTES

Westergren ESR is preferable. If other ESR used (e.g., Wintrobe) then cannot use the listed guidelines for abnormalities.

ABBREVIATIONS

GCA = Giant cell arteritis
TA = temporal arteritis

REFERENCES

- Hunder GG. Giant Cell Arteritis and Polymyalgia Rheumatica. In: Kelly WN, Harris ED, Ruddy S, Sledge CB, eds. Textbook of Rheumatology. 6th Ed. p1155-64, Philadelphia, W.B. Saunders Co., 2001
- Hunder GG, et al. The American College of Rheumatology 1990 Criteria for the Classification of Giant Cell Arteritis. In Arthritis Rheum 1990;33:1122-8
- Wayland CM, Goronzy JJ. Polymyalgia rheumatica and giant cell arteritis. In: Koopman WJ, ed. Arthritis and Allied Conditions. 14th Ed. Philadelphia, Lippincott Williams & Wilkins, 2001
- Hazelman BL. Polymyalgia rheumatica and giant cell arteritis. In: Hochberg MC, Silman AJ, Smolen JS, Weinblatt ME, Weisman MH. Rheumatology. 3rd ed. Edinburgh: Mosby; 2003. p. 1623-1633

Web references: 2 available at www.5mcc.com
Illustrations N/A

Author(s):
Eric P. Gall, MD

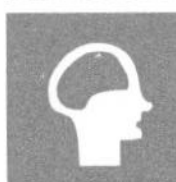

BASICS

DESCRIPTION Intestinal infection caused by the protozoan parasite, *Giardia lamblia*. Infection results from ingestion of the cysts that excyst into trophozoites which colonize the small intestine and cause the symptoms. The cycle is continued when the trophozoites encyst in the small intestine and water, food, or hands are contaminated by feces of the infected person. Most infections result from fecal-oral transmission or ingestion of contaminated water, less commonly from contaminated food.
System(s) affected: Gastrointestinal
Genetics: N/A
Incidence/Prevalence in USA: 5% of patients with stools submitted for ova and parasite exams. Overall prevalence is lower and variable.
Predominant age: All ages, but most common in early childhood
Predominant sex: Slightly more common in males

SIGNS & SYMPTOMS
- Approximately 25-50% of infected persons are symptomatic
- Chronic diarrhea (lasting more than 5-7 days and frequently weeks)
- Abdominal bloating
- Flatulence
- Loose, greasy, foul-smelling stools
- Weight loss
- Nausea
- Lactose intolerance

CAUSES Protozoan parasite (*Giardia lamblia*) infection acquired through fecal-oral transmission or ingestion of contaminated water, less commonly from contaminated food

RISK FACTORS
- Day care centers
- Male homosexuality
- Wilderness camping

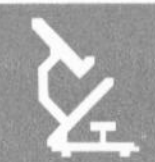

DIAGNOSIS

DIFFERENTIAL DIAGNOSIS
- Includes other etiologies of small intestinal diarrhea
- Infectious causes include cryptosporidiosis, isosporiasis, cyclosporiasis
- Other causes of malabsorption includes celiac sprue, tropical sprue, bacterial overgrowth syndromes, Crohn ileitis
- Irritable bowel is suspected when diarrhea is not accompanied by weight loss

LABORATORY
- Stool for ova and parasites, repeated 3 times if necessary. Cysts are seen in fixed or fresh stools and occasionally, trophozoites are found in fresh diarrheal stools.
- Fluorescent antibody and ELISA tests of fecal specimens are available

Drugs that may alter lab results: A number of drugs interfere with stool exams

Disorders that may alter lab results: N/A

PATHOLOGICAL FINDINGS Intestinal biopsy shows flattened, mild lymphocytic infiltration and trophozoites on the surface.

SPECIAL TESTS String test (Entero-Test). A gelatin capsule on a string is swallowed and left in the duodenum for several hours or overnight.

IMAGING N/A

DIAGNOSTIC PROCEDURES Esophagogastroduodenoscopy with biopsy and sample of small intestinal fluid.

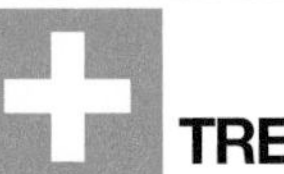

TREATMENT

APPROPRIATE HEALTH CARE Outpatient for mild cases, inpatient if symptoms are severe

GENERAL MEASURES
- Medical therapy for all infected individuals
- Fluid replacement if dehydrated

SURGICAL MEASURES N/A

ACTIVITY As tolerated

DIET Good nutrition, low lactose, low fat

PATIENT EDUCATION Avoidance of risk factors

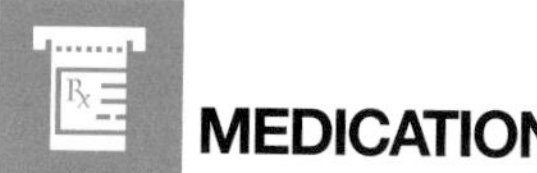

MEDICATIONS

DRUG(S) OF CHOICE

- Metronidazole (Flagyl) 250 mg tid for 5-7 days

Contraindications: Relatively contraindicated in pregnancy, especially first trimester

Precautions:

- Rare toxic psychosis with quinacrine
- Theoretical risk of carcinogenesis with metronidazole

Significant possible interactions: Occasional disulfiram reaction with metronidazole

ALTERNATIVE DRUGS

- Furazolidone 8 mg/kg/day tid for 10 days (slightly less effective, but commonly used in pediatrics because it is well tolerated)
- Paromomycin (Humatin), a nonabsorbable aminoglycoside which is probably less effective, but commonly recommended in pregnancy because of theoretical risk of teratogenicity of other agents
- Tinidazole is effective when given as a single dose. It is the treatment of choice in many other countries, but is not available in the US.
- Quinacrine 100 mg tid for 5-7 days. Was the treatment of choice for giardiasis, but is not available from most pharmacies in the US.
- Albendazole 400 mg daily for 5 days. Antihelminthic drug which may be as effective as metronidazole and better tolerated.
- Nitazoxanide suspension was approved by the FDA in 2003 for treatment of giardiasis in children ages 1-11. Children ages 1-4 receive 100 mg bid, and ages 5-11 receive 200 mg bid for 3 days.

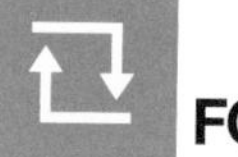

FOLLOWUP

PATIENT MONITORING Symptoms, weight, stool exams

PREVENTION/AVOIDANCE Good hand washing when caring for diapered children, water purification when camping

POSSIBLE COMPLICATIONS Those of malabsorption and weight loss

EXPECTED COURSE/PROGNOSIS

Untreated giardiasis lasts for weeks. Patients usually (90%) respond to treatment within a few days and most of the non-responders or relapses respond to a second course with the same or a different agent.

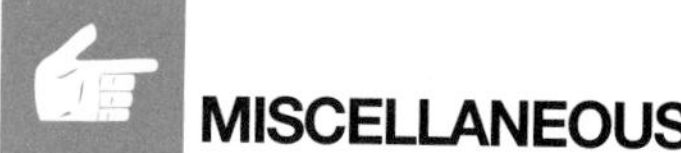

MISCELLANEOUS

ASSOCIATED CONDITIONS Hypogammaglobulinemia and possibly IgA deficiency. The diarrhea is more severe and prolonged in these patients.

AGE-RELATED FACTORS

Pediatric: Most common in early childhood
Geriatric: N/A
Others: N/A

PREGNANCY Concern for potential teratogenicity of medications. Consult infectious disease specialist or gastroenterologist for symptomatic disease.

SYNONYMS N/A

ICD-9-CM

007.1 Giardiasis

SEE ALSO

OTHER NOTES *G. lamblia* is also called *G. duodenalis*, *G. intestinalis*

ABBREVIATIONS N/A

REFERENCES

- Adam R.D. The Biology of Giardia spp. Microbiol Rev 1991;55:706-732
- Hill DR. <I>Giardia lamblia</I>. In: Mandell GL, Bennett JE, Dolin R, eds. Principles and Practice of Infectious Diseases. 5th Ed. New York, Churchill Livingstone, 2000
- Ortega I, Adam RD. Giardia: overview and update. Clin Infec Dis 1997;25:545-549
- Adam RD. The biology of <I>Giardia lamblia</I>. Clin Infec Dis 2001;14:447-475
- Gardner TB, Hill DR. Treatment of giardiasis. Clin Microbiol Rev 2001;14(1):114-28

Web references: 1 available at www.5mcc.com
Illustrations N/A

Author(s):
Rodney D. Adam, MD

BASICS

DESCRIPTION Mild chronic or intermittent unconjugated hyperbilirubinemia (not due to hemolysis) with otherwise normal liver function
System(s) affected: Hemic/Lymphatic/Immunologic
Genetics: A gene defect resulting in reduced bilirubin UDP-glucuronosyltransferase-1 appears to be necessary but not sufficient for Gilbert syndrome.
Incidence/Prevalence in USA: About 7% of the population
Predominant age: Present from birth, but most often presents in the second or third decade of life; heterozygous for single abnormal gene
Predominant sex: Male > Female (2-7:1)

SIGNS & SYMPTOMS No significant symptoms have been attributed to this disorder, although a variety of nonspecific symptoms have been described. There are no abnormal physical findings other than occasional mild jaundice

CAUSES The hyperbilirubinemia results from impaired hepatic bilirubin clearance (approximately 30% of normal). Hepatic bilirubin conjugation (glucuronidation) is reduced, though this is likely not the only defect.

RISK FACTORS None

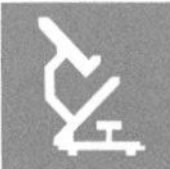

DIAGNOSIS

DIFFERENTIAL DIAGNOSIS Hemolysis, ineffective erythropoiesis (megaloblastic anemias, certain porphyrias, thalassemia major, sideroblastic anemia, severe lead poisoning, congenital dyserythropoietic anemias), cirrhosis, chronic persistent hepatitis, pancreatitis or biliary tract disease

LABORATORY
- Bilirubin: less than 6 mg/dL (103 μmol/L) and usually less than 3 mg/dL (51 μmol/L), virtually all unconjugated (indirect)
- CBC with peripheral smear is normal
- Reticulocyte count is normal
- Liver function tests (SGOT, SGPT, alkaline phosphatase, GGT) are normal
- Fasting and postprandial serum bile acids are normal
- Up to 60% of patients have clinically insignificant mild hemolysis which frequently can only be detected with sophisticated red cell survival studies

Drugs that may alter lab results: Bilirubin level may be raised by nicotinic acid and lowered by phenobarbital

Disorders that may alter lab results: Bilirubin levels increase during fasting, and may increase during a febrile illness

PATHOLOGICAL FINDINGS None

SPECIAL TESTS None

IMAGING N/A

DIAGNOSTIC PROCEDURES
- A liver biopsy is not usually needed to exclude other diagnoses
- Some clinicians recommend confirming the diagnosis by reducing daily caloric intake to 400 kcal for 48 hours, which results in a two to threefold increase in unconjugated bilirubin

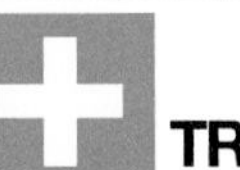

TREATMENT

APPROPRIATE HEALTH CARE Outpatient. The most important treatment is to make a positive diagnosis of Gilbert disease to reassure the patient and prevent further unnecessary procedures

GENERAL MEASURES None

SURGICAL MEASURES N/A

ACTIVITY Full activity

DIET Normal

PATIENT EDUCATION Reassure the patient that the condition is benign with no known sequelae

MEDICATIONS

DRUG(S) OF CHOICE N/A
Contraindications: N/A
Precautions: N/A
Significant possible interactions: N/A

ALTERNATIVE DRUGS N/A

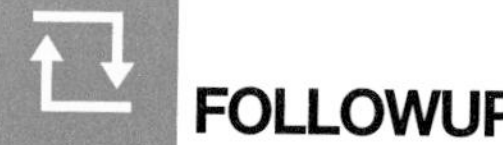

FOLLOWUP

PATIENT MONITORING If history, physical examination, and laboratory tests are normal, see the patient on two or three further occasions during the ensuing 12 to 18 months. If the patient develops no symptoms, reticulocytosis or new liver function abnormalities, make the diagnosis of Gilbert disease.

PREVENTION/AVOIDANCE N/A

POSSIBLE COMPLICATIONS No known complications

EXPECTED COURSE/PROGNOSIS
The disorder is benign with an excellent prognosis

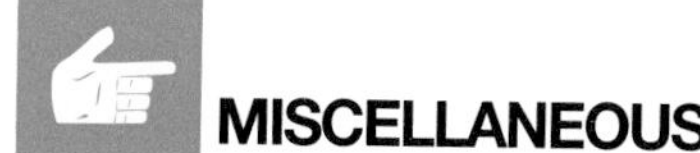

MISCELLANEOUS

ASSOCIATED CONDITIONS Gilbert disease may be part of a spectrum of hereditary disorders which includes types I and II Crigler-Najjar syndrome

AGE-RELATED FACTORS
Pediatric: It is rare for the disorder to be diagnosed before puberty
Geriatric: N/A
Others: N/A

PREGNANCY The relative fasting that may occur with morning sickness can elevate the bilirubin level

SYNONYMS Gilbert syndrome

ICD-9-CM
277.4 Disorders of bilirubin excretion

SEE ALSO
Crigler-Najjar syndrome

OTHER NOTES N/A

ABBREVIATIONS N/A

REFERENCES

- Okolicsanyi L, Fevery J, Billing B, et al: How should mild, isolated unconjugated hyperbilirubinemia be investigated? Sem Liver Dis 1983;3(1):36-41
- Watson KJR, Gollan JL: Gilbert's syndrome. Bailliere's Clin Gastroenterol 1989;3(2):337-55
- Bosma PJ, Choudhury JR, Bakker C, et al: The genetic basis of the reduced expression of bilirubin UDP-glucuronosyltransferase-1 in Gilbert's syndrome. NEJM 1995;333:1171-5

Web references: 0 available at www.5mcc.com
Illustrations N/A

Author(s):
Robert A. Marlow, MD, MA

BASICS

DESCRIPTION Inflammation of the gingiva, one of the forms of significant oral infections
- Others forms of oral infection:
  - ◊ Periodontitis - progression of gingivitis to connective tissue and alveolar bone
  - ◊ Vincent's angina (trench mouth, necrotizing ulcerative gingivitis, fusospirochetosis) - fusiform bacillus or spirochete infection
  - ◊ Glossitis - inflammation of the tongue (see separate title on this subject)

System(s) affected: Gastrointestinal
Genetics: No known genetic pattern
Incidence/Prevalence in USA: Pandemic, 90% of the population affected
Predominant age: Mostly adult
Predominant sex: Male = Female

SIGNS & SYMPTOMS
- Mouth odor (bad breath)
- Gum swelling (painless)
- Gum redness
- Change of normal gum contours
- Gum bleeding when flossing or brushing
- Edema of interdental papillae
- Narrow band of bright red inflamed gum surrounding neck of tooth
- Vincent's angina - ulcers, fever, malaise, regional lymphadenopathy, pain

CAUSES
- Noncontagious
- Inadequate plaque removal
- Blood dyscrasias
- Reaction to oral contraceptives
- Vincent's - fusiform bacillus or spirochete infection
- Allergic reactions
- Endocrine disturbances, i.e., pregnancy, menses
- Chronic debilitating disease

RISK FACTORS
- Diabetes mellitus
- Malocclusion
- Poor dental hygiene
- Mouth breathing
- Faulty dental restoration
- HIV positive
- Pregnancy

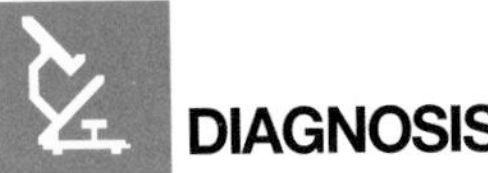

DIAGNOSIS

DIFFERENTIAL DIAGNOSIS
- Acute necrotizing ulcerative gingivitis (Vincent's disease)
- Afunctional gingivitis
- Chronic desquamative gingivitis
- Diabetic gingivitis
- Diphenylhydantoin gingivitis
- Hormonal gingivitis
- Leukemic gingivitis
- Pregnancy gingivitis
- Pericoronitis
- HIV

LABORATORY Smear to identify causative agent

Drugs that may alter lab results: N/A

Disorders that may alter lab results: N/A

PATHOLOGICAL FINDINGS
- Acute or chronic inflammation
- Broken crepuscular epithelium
- Hyperemic capillaries
- Polymorphonuclear infiltration
- Papillary projections in subepithelial tissue
- Fibroblasts

SPECIAL TESTS N/A

IMAGING N/A

DIAGNOSTIC PROCEDURES N/A

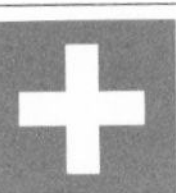

TREATMENT

APPROPRIATE HEALTH CARE Outpatient

GENERAL MEASURES
- Remove irritating factors (plaque, calculus, faulty dentures)
- Good oral hygiene
- Regular dental check-ups
- No smoking
- Warm saline rinses twice daily
- Prophylaxis by dental hygienist

SURGICAL MEASURES N/A

ACTIVITY No restrictions

DIET Assure adequate vitamins and minerals

PATIENT EDUCATION Printed patient information available from: American Dental Association, 211 E. Chicago Avenue, Chicago, IL 60611, (800)621-8099

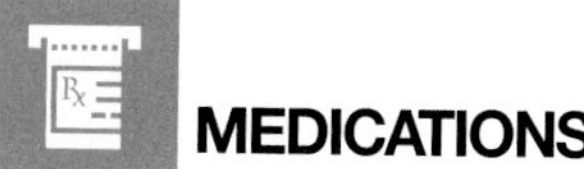

MEDICATIONS

DRUG(S) OF CHOICE
- Antibiotics indicated only for acute necrotizing ulcerative gingivitis (Vincent's angina)
- Antibiotics, e.g., penicillin V, pediatric dose 25-50 mg/kg/day divided q6h; adult dose 250-500 mg q6h, or
- Erythromycin - pediatric dose 30-40 mg/kg/day divided q6h; adult dose 250 mg q6h
- Topical corticosteroids e.g., triamcinolone in Orabase)

Contraindications: Allergy to antibiotics
Precautions: Erythromycin frequently causes significant gastrointestinal upsets
Significant possible interactions: Refer to manufacturer's literature

ALTERNATIVE DRUGS Other antibiotics according to culture or smear

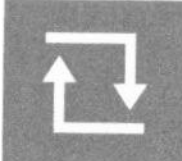

FOLLOWUP

PATIENT MONITORING Until clear

PREVENTION/AVOIDANCE
- Good oral hygiene, daily brushing and flossing
- Cleaning by a dentist or hygienist every 6 months or sooner

POSSIBLE COMPLICATIONS Severe periodontal disease

EXPECTED COURSE/PROGNOSIS
- Usual course - acute; relapsing; intermittent; chronic
- Prognosis - generally favorable, responds well to appropriate treatment

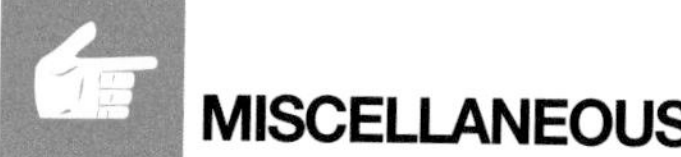

MISCELLANEOUS

ASSOCIATED CONDITIONS
- Periodontitis
- Glossitis

AGE-RELATED FACTORS
Pediatric: Mild cases common in children and usually requires no treatment
Geriatric: More frequent in this age group (due more to lifelong accumulation, rather than increased susceptibility)
Others: N/A

PREGNANCY Characteristics - hyperplasia, pedunculated gingival growths, pyogenic granuloma

SYNONYMS Denture sore mouth

ICD-9-CM
523.1 Chronic gingivitis

SEE ALSO
Glossitis

OTHER NOTES N/A

ABBREVIATIONS N/A

REFERENCES

- Berkow, R., et al. (eds.): Merck Manual, 16th Ed. Rahway, NJ, Merck Sharp & Dohme, 1992

Web references: 1 available at www.5mcc.com
Illustrations 1 available

Author(s):
David deVlaming, DDS

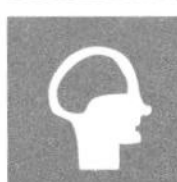

BASICS

DESCRIPTION Primary angle-closure glaucoma results from obstruction of aqueous humor outflow through the trabecular meshwork by peripheral iris apposition to the cornea which causes a consequent elevation in intraocular pressure (IOP). The underlying mechanism is pupillary block, in which aqueous egress through the pupil is limited causing forward iris displacement. Angle-closure glaucoma can occur in subacute, acute, and chronic forms and is associated with an anatomically narrow anterior chamber angle; the angle comprises the peripheral iris, anterior ciliary body, trabecular meshwork, and peripheral cornea and can only be observed with a special examination technique called gonioscopy. In its acute form, primary angle-closure glaucoma is an ophthalmic emergency with a natural history of severe visual loss.

System(s) affected: Nervous

Genetics: Polygenic inheritance; first degree relatives have a 2-5% lifetime risk

Incidence/Prevalence in USA:
- 100 cases/100,000 population
- 500/100,000 (Blacks and Asians more common than Caucasians)

Predominant age: 55-70

Predominant sex: Female > Male

SIGNS & SYMPTOMS
- Subacute
  - ◊ Dull ache in or around one eye
  - ◊ Mildly blurred vision
  - ◊ Symptoms occur when watching TV or movies in dark room, reading, or when fatigued. Relieved by sleep or rest.
  - ◊ Normal intraocular pressure (10-23 mmHg)
  - ◊ Shallow anterior chamber
  - ◊ Iris bombé
  - ◊ Intermittent peripheral anterior synechiae
  - ◊ Enlarged pupil
- Acute
  - ◊ Ocular pain
  - ◊ Blurred vision
  - ◊ Lacrimation
  - ◊ Halos around lights
  - ◊ Frontal headache
  - ◊ Nausea and vomiting
  - ◊ Symptoms likely to occur with times of emotional stress and with activities as for subacute form
  - ◊ Elevated intraocular pressure (usually 40-80 mm Hg)
  - ◊ Corneal microcystic edema
  - ◊ Lid edema, conjunctival hyperemia, and circumcorneal injection
  - ◊ Fixed mid-dilated pupil, often oval
  - ◊ Shallow anterior chamber often with inflammatory reaction
- Chronic
  - ◊ May have symptoms of subacute form or may be asymptomatic
  - ◊ Multiple peripheral anterior synechiae
  - ◊ Normal or elevated intraocular pressure
  - ◊ Increased cup to disc ratio
  - ◊ Normal pupil

CAUSES Predisposing ocular anatomy

RISK FACTORS
- Small cornea
- Hyperopia
- Shallow anterior chamber
- Eskimo ancestry
- Female sex
- Use of antidepressants or other drugs with cholinergic inhibition
- Cataract
- Iris and ciliary body cysts

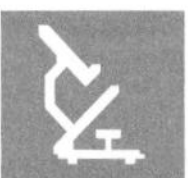

DIAGNOSIS

DIFFERENTIAL DIAGNOSIS
- Neovascular glaucoma
- Absolute glaucoma
- Malignant glaucoma
- Plateau iris syndrome
- Miotic induced glaucoma
- Phacomorphic glaucoma
- Anterior uveitis

LABORATORY None

Drugs that may alter lab results: N/A

Disorders that may alter lab results: N/A

PATHOLOGICAL FINDINGS
- Corneal stromal and epithelial edema
- Endothelial cell loss
- Iris stromal necrosis
- Anterior subcapsular cataract (glaukomflecken)
- Optic disc congestion, cupping
- Optic nerve atrophy

SPECIAL TESTS Gonioscopy

IMAGING N/A

DIAGNOSTIC PROCEDURES Careful ophthalmic examination including indentation gonioscopy and tonometry

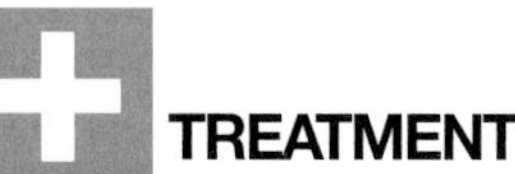

TREATMENT

APPROPRIATE HEALTH CARE
- For acute form - inpatient admission from office or emergency room
- Other forms - outpatient
- Ophthalmology consultation

GENERAL MEASURES
- For acute form
  - ◊ Intravenous access for administering medications is helpful, antiemetics may be necessary
  - ◊ Definitive treatment is laser iridotomy once the attack is broken, intraocular pressure has normalized, and intraocular inflammation has subsided

SURGICAL MEASURES
- Peripheral iridectomy
- Argon or Nd:YAG laser iridotomy (procedure of choice for subacute and chronic forms)
- Argon laser gonioplasty

ACTIVITY For acute form - bedrest until attack subsides

DIET Usual for patient

PATIENT EDUCATION
- Usually patients need bilateral treatment since second eye is at risk for same disease process
- For patient education materials favorably reviewed on this topic, contact:
  - ◊ Foundation for Glaucoma Research, 490 Post Street, Suite 830, San Francisco, CA 94102, (415)986-3162
  - ◊ American Academy of Ophthalmology,

655 Beach Street, San Francisco, CA 94109, (415)561-8500; www.eyenet.org

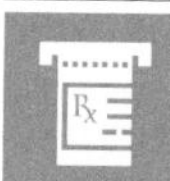

MEDICATIONS

DRUG(S) OF CHOICE

- For acute form: (a combination of the following)
  - ◊ Hyperosmotic agents - oral 50% glycerin 0.1-1.5 g/kg or oral isosorbide dinitrate 1.5-2.0 g/kg, and/or intravenous mannitol 20% 1-2 g/kg over 45 minutes
  - ◊ Carbonic anhydrase inhibition - acetazolamide (Diamox) 500 mg IV plus 500 mg po, then 250 mg po q6h prn; dorzolamide 2% eyedrops q8h.

Note: Use of the intravenous and oral agents above is sometimes necessary prior to the use of eye drops in order to lower the IOP enough to permit intraocular penetration.
  - ◊ Beta-blockers - timolol (Timoptic) 0.5% q12h or levobunolol (Betagan) 0.5% q12h or betaxolol (Betoptic) 0.5% q12h
  - ◊ Miotics - pilocarpine 2-4% one dose. In complicated cases with multiple mechanisms, miotics may paradoxically worsen the condition. Hence, they must be used with caution. See Contraindications.
  - ◊ Corticosteroid - prednisolone acetate (Pred Forte) 1% q4-6h
  - ◊ Other - apraclonidine (Iopidine) 0.5% or 1% q8h; also, latanoprost (Xalatan) 0.005% q24h
- For subacute and chronic forms:
  - ◊ Treatment is surgical

Contraindications: With history of recent intraocular surgery, possibility of malignant glaucoma is increased and miotics may be contraindicated

Precautions:
- Timolol, levobunolol, and betaxolol, use with caution in patients with chronic heart failure or chronic obstructive pulmonary disease
- Mannitol, use with caution in patients with chronic heart failure or renal failure
- Acetazolamide, use with caution in patients with history of nephrolithiasis or metabolic acidosis

Significant possible interactions: Acetazolamide may accelerate potassium loss and metabolic acidosis in patients on other diuretics

ALTERNATIVE DRUGS
As above

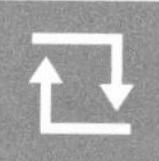

FOLLOWUP

PATIENT MONITORING
- Subacute and chronic forms, check tonometry and gonioscopy initially every 3 months after laser iridotomy, follow visual fields every 6-12 months
- Acute form, discharge after laser iridotomy and intraocular pressure are controlled and follow as with the chronic form
- Consider frequent serum electrolytes while on mannitol
- Semi-annual CBC while on acetazolamide

PREVENTION/AVOIDANCE
Prophylactic laser treatment of second eye

POSSIBLE COMPLICATIONS
- Chronic corneal edema
- Corneal fibrosis and vascularization
- Iris atrophy
- Cataract
- Lens subluxation
- Optic atrophy
- Malignant glaucoma
- Central retinal vein occlusion

EXPECTED COURSE/PROGNOSIS
- Varies with delay of patient presentation and severity of attack
- Preceding chronic angle-closure may have caused optic atrophy
- Recurrence is quite rare following peripheral iridotomy or iridectomy and implies a rare variant known as the iris plateau syndrome

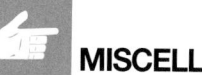

MISCELLANEOUS

ASSOCIATED CONDITIONS
- Cataract
- Microphthalmos
- Hyperopia

AGE-RELATED FACTORS
Pediatric: Rare

Geriatric: Secondary angle closure glaucoma can be caused by many common eye conditions in the elderly including cataract, ocular surgery and diabetes

Others: N/A

PREGNANCY
N/A

SYNONYMS
- Acute glaucoma
- Narrow angle glaucoma

ICD-9-CM
365.20 Primary angle-closure glaucoma, unspecified
365.02 Borderline glaucoma, anatomical narrow angle

SEE ALSO
Glaucoma, primary open-angle

OTHER NOTES
- Medications (higher risk) that may exacerbate angle-closure glaucoma:
  - ◊ Systemic or topical anticholinergics
  - ◊ Topical sympathomimetics
  - ◊ Antihistamines
  - ◊ Phenothiazines
  - ◊ Antidepressants
- Medications (lower risk) that may exacerbate angle-closure glaucoma:
  - ◊ Benzodiazepine
  - ◊ Carbonic anhydrase inhibitors
  - ◊ CNS stimulants (including cocaine)
  - ◊ MAO inhibitors
  - ◊ Systemic sympathomimetics
  - ◊ Theophylline
  - ◊ Vasodilators

ABBREVIATIONS
NAG = narrow angle glaucoma

REFERENCES

- Ritch R, Shields MB, Krupin T: The Glaucomas. St. Louis, C.V. Mosby, 1995
- Fraunfelder FT, Roy FH: Current Ocular Therapy 3. 5th Ed. Philadelphia, W.B. Saunders Co., 1999

Web references: 2 available at www.5mcc.com

Illustrations N/A

Author(s):
Robert G. Fante, MD

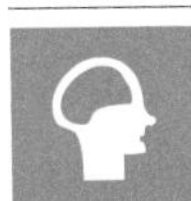

BASICS

DESCRIPTION An optic neuropathy resulting in visual field loss, frequently associated with increased intraocular pressure. Normal intraocular pressure (IOP) is 10-22 mm Hg. However, glaucomatous optic nerve damage can also occur in the setting of normal IOP and can also occur as a secondary manifestation of other disorders, such as corticosteroid-induced glaucoma. Aqueous is produced by the ciliary epithelium of the ciliary body and is secreted into the posterior chamber of the eye. Aqueous then flows through the pupil and enters the anterior chamber to be drained by the trabecular meshwork in the iridocorneal angle of the eye, into Schlemm's canal and into the venous system of the episclera. 5 to 10 % of the total aqueous outflow leaves via the uveoscleral pathway.

System(s) affected: Nervous

Genetics: A family history of glaucoma increases one's risk for developing glaucoma

Incidence/Prevalence in USA: At least 2.25 million persons, over 45 years of age, have primary open-angle glaucoma (POAG), and half of them may be unaware that they have the disease. Prevalence of POAG in persons > age 40 is about 1.8%.

Predominant age: Incidence increases with age. Primary open-angle glaucoma usually occurs after 40 years of age.

Predominant sex: Male = Female

SIGNS & SYMPTOMS

- Painless, slowly progressive visual loss. Patients are generally unaware of the visual loss until late in the disease, because central visual acuity generally remains unaffected until late in the disease.
- Increased IOP
- Cup-to-disk ratio (C/D) > 0.5
- Earliest visual field defects are paracentral scotomas and peripheral nasal steps

CAUSES

- Impaired aqueous outflow through the trabecular meshwork
- Increased resistance within the aqueous drainage system

RISK FACTORS

- Increased IOP
- African American
- Elderly
- Positive family history
- Myopia
- Diabetes mellitus
- Central corneal thinness < 555 microns
- Larger vertical cup-disc ratio
- Larger horizontal cup-disc ratio
- Disc hemorrhage
- Prolonged use of topical, periocular, inhaled or systemic corticosteroids

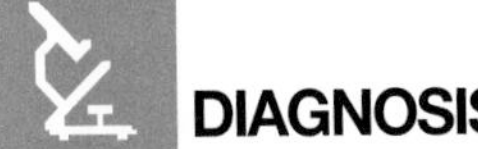

DIAGNOSIS

DIFFERENTIAL DIAGNOSIS

- Normal-tension glaucoma
- Optic nerve pits
- Anterior ischemic optic neuropathy
- Compressive lesions of the optic nerve or chiasm
- Posthemorrhagic (shock optic neuropathy)

LABORATORY N/A

Drugs that may alter lab results: N/A

Disorders that may alter lab results: N/A

PATHOLOGICAL FINDINGS

- Atrophy and cupping of the optic nerve
- Loss of retinal ganglion cells and their axons produces defects in the retinal nerve fiber layer

SPECIAL TESTS

- Visual field testing
- Gonioscopy
- Tonometry - the measurement of the intraocular pressure

IMAGING

- Optical coherence tomography (OCT) can be useful in the detection of early glaucoma by measuring the thickness of the nerve fiber layer (NFL). The NFL is thinner in patients with glaucoma.
- Confocal scanning laser ophthalmoscope may provide objective measurements of the optic disc

DIAGNOSTIC PROCEDURES

- Tonometry to measure IOP
- Perimetry to assess visual fields
- Ophthalmoscopy to assess the optic nerve for glaucomatous damage

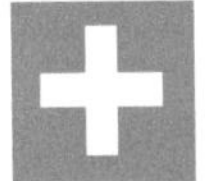

TREATMENT

APPROPRIATE HEALTH CARE Outpatient

GENERAL MEASURES

- The Early Manifest Glaucoma Trial (EMGT) showed:
  - ◊ Early treatment of POAG significantly delays disease progression
  - ◊ The magnitude of initial IOP reduction was a major factor influencing disease progression
- The Ocular Hypertension Treatment Study (OHTS) showed:
  - ◊ Patients who only had increased IOP, in the range of 24 to 32 mm Hg, were treated with topical ocular hypotensive medication
  - ◊ Treatment produced approximately a 20% reduction in IOP
  - ◊ At 5 years, treatment reduced the incidence of POAG by more than 50%, that is 9.5% in the observation group vs 4.4% in the medication treated group
- The Collaborative Normal-Tension Glaucoma Study Group showed:
  - ◊ Therapeutic intervention which resulted in a 30% decrease in IOP helped prevent progression of visual field loss
- The Advanced Glaucoma Intervention Study (AGIS) showed:
  - ◊ Eyes were randomized to laser trabeculoplasty or filtering surgery when medical therapy failed
  - ◊ In follow-up, if the IOP was always < 18 mm Hg then the visual fields tended to stabilize. When IOP > 17 mm Hg more than half the time patients tended to worsen their visual fields.
  - ◊ Caucasians did best with trabeculectomy first, whereas African Americans did better with argon laser trabeculoplasty as initial procedure
- The Collaborative Initial Glaucoma Treatment Study (CIGTS) showed:
  - ◊ Both initial medical and surgical treatment achieved significant IOP reduction and both groups had little visual field loss over a long period of time

SURGICAL MEASURES

- Argon laser trabeculoplasty (ALT)
  - ◊ Applied to 180 degrees of the trabecular meshwork
  - ◊ Improves aqueous outflow
  - ◊ The Glaucoma Laser Trial (GLT) Research Group showed, in newly diagnosed, previously untreated POAG patients that ALT was as effective as topical glaucoma medication within the first 2 years of follow-up
  - ◊ Usually reserved for patients needing better IOP control while taking topical glaucoma drops
- Trabeculectomy (glaucoma filtering surgery)
  - ◊ Usually reserved for patients needing better IOP control after maximal medical therapy and who may have also previously undergone an ALT
  - ◊ A superficial flap of sclera is dissected anteriorly to the trabecular meshwork, and a segment of the trabecular meshwork is removed underneath the scleral flap
  - ◊ Mitomycin C can be applied at the time of surgery to increase the chances of a surgical success
- Shunt surgery
  - ◊ E.g., Molteno and Ahmed devices
  - ◊ Generally reserved for difficult glaucoma cases in which conventional filtering surgery has failed or is likely to fail
  - ◊ A tube is place into the anterior chamber or through the pars plana that allows aqueous to flow to an extraocular reservoir, which is placed in the equatorial region on the sclera
- Ciliary body ablation
  - ◊ Indicated to lower IOP in patients with poor visual potential or poor candidates for filtering or shunt procedures

ACTIVITY No limitations

DIET No restrictions

PATIENT EDUCATION

- Importance of follow-up to monitor disease progression
- POAG is a silent robber of vision, and patients may not appreciate the significance of their disease until much of their visual field is lost
- American Academy of Ophthalmology, 655 Beach Street, San Francisco, CA 94109-1336

MEDICATIONS

DRUG(S) OF CHOICE
More than one medication, with different mechanisms of action, may be needed. When 3 or more medications required, compliance is difficult and surgical therapy may be needed to lower the IOP further.

Ocular hypotensive agent categories:
- Beta-adrenergic antagonists (nonselective and selective); decrease aqueous formation
  - ◊ Timolol
- Parasympathomimetics (miotic), including cholinergic (direct-acting) and anticholinesterase agents (indirect-acting parasympathomimetic); increase aqueous outflow
  - ◊ Pilocarpine; cholinergic
  - ◊ Echothiophate, anticholinesterase
- Carbonic anhydrase inhibitors (oral, topical); decrease aqueous formation
  - ◊ Acetazolamide
- Adrenergic agonists (nonselective and selective alpha 2 agonists)
  - ◊ Epinephrine and dipivefrin. Nonselective agents which increase aqueous outflow through the trabecular meshwork and also uveoscleral outflow
  - ◊ Brimonidine tartrate, alpha 2-adrenergic agonist, decreases aqueous formation and increases uveoscleral outflow
- Prostaglandin analogues; enhance uveoscleral outflow
  - ◊ Latanoprost
- Hyperosmotic agents; increase blood osmolality, drawing water from the vitreous cavity
  - ◊ Mannitol
  - ◊ Glycerin

Contraindications:
- Nonselective beta-adrenergic antagonists: avoid in asthma, chronic obstructive pulmonary disease, second- and third-degree AV block, and in decompensated heart failure. Betaxolol is a selective beta-antagonist and is safer in pulmonary disease.
- Parasympathomimetics (miotic)
  - ◊ Indirect-acting parasympathomimetic agents have the potential for significant ocular and systemic side effects and are rarely used today. Systemically absorbed anticholinesterase eye drops reduce serum pseudocholinesterase levels. If succinylcholine is used for induction of general anesthesia, prolonged apnea may result.
  - ◊ Anticholinesterase agents (indirect-acting parasympathomimetics) are cataractogenic
- Carbonic anhydrase inhibitors
  - ◊ Do not use in patients with sulfa drug allergies
  - ◊ Do not use in patients with cirrhosis - risk of hepatic encephalopathy
- Adrenergic agonists: Caution recommended when using brimonidine and monoamine oxidase inhibitor or tricyclic antidepressant and in patients with vascular insufficiency
- Prostaglandin analogues: Caution in patients with uveitis and should be avoided during pregnancy
- Hyperosmotic agents
  - ◊ Glycerin can produce hyperglycemia or ketoacidosis in diabetic patients
  - ◊ Can cause congestive heart failure
  - ◊ Do not use in patients with anuria

Precautions:
- Beta-adrenergic antagonists: Caution with obstructive pulmonary disease, heart failure, and diabetes
- Parasympathomimetics (miotic) cause pupillary constriction and may cause decreased vision in patients with a cataract. May also cause an eye ache or myopia due to increased accommodation. All miotics break down the blood-aqueous barrier and may induce chronic iridocyclitis.
- Adrenergic agonists (e.g., brimonidine): Caution with vascular insufficiency
- Prostaglandin analogues may cause increased pigmentation of the iris and periorbital tissue (eyelid). Increased pigmentation and growth of eyelashes. Should be used with caution in patients with active intraocular inflammation (iritis/uveitis). Caution is advised in the use of prostaglandin analogues in eyes with risk factors for *Herpes simplex*, iritis, and cystoid macular edema. Macular edema may be a complication associated with treatment.
- Hyperosmotic agents: Caution in diabetics, dehydrated patients, and in patients with cardiac, renal and hepatic disease

Significant possible interactions:
- Beta-adrenergic antagonists: Caution in patients taking calcium antagonists because of possible atrioventricular conduction disturbances, left ventricular failure or hypotension. Catecholamine-depleting drugs such as reserpine may cause hypotension and/or bradycardia. Quinidine can potentiate the systemic beta-blockade.
- Parasympathomimetics (miotic): indirect-acting parasympathomimetic agents, anticholinesterase eye drops, can reduce serum pseudocholinesterase levels. If succinylcholine is used for induction of general anesthesia, prolonged apnea may result.

ALTERNATIVE DRUGS N/A

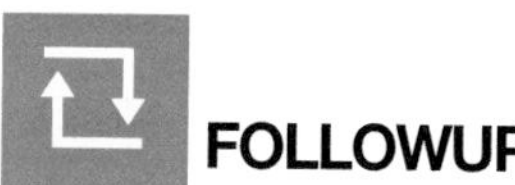

FOLLOWUP

PATIENT MONITORING
- Monitor vision and IOP every 3-6 months
- Visual field testing every 6-18 months
- Optic nerve evaluated every 3-18 months, depending on how well controlled the POAG

PREVENTION/AVOIDANCE
Genetic testing is being evaluated to help screen for POAG

POSSIBLE COMPLICATIONS
Blindness

EXPECTED COURSE/PROGNOSIS
- With standard glaucoma therapy, the rate of visual field loss in POAG is slow
- Patients may still lose vision and develop blindness, even when treated appropriately. In one study the rate of legal blindness from POAG over a follow-up of 22 years was 19%.

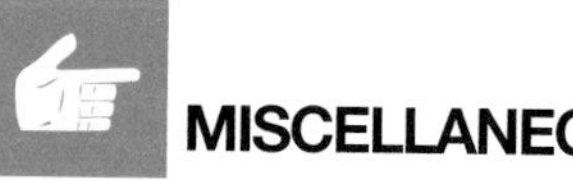

MISCELLANEOUS

ASSOCIATED CONDITIONS
Diabetes mellitus

AGE-RELATED FACTORS
Pediatric: N/A

Geriatric: Increasing prevalence with increasing age

Others: N/A

PREGNANCY
Prostaglandins should be avoided in pregnancy in the treatment of POAG

SYNONYMS
Chronic open-angle glaucoma

ICD-9-CM
365.11 Primary open angle glaucoma
377.14 Glaucomatous atrophy (cupping) of optic disc
365.12 Low tension glaucoma
365.00 Preglaucoma, unspecified

SEE ALSO

OTHER NOTES N/A

ABBREVIATIONS
POAG = primary open-angle glaucoma
COAG = chronic open-angle glaucoma
IOP = intraocular pressure

REFERENCES

- Kwon YH, Kim CS, Zimmerman MB, Alward WL, Hayreh SS. Rate of visual field loss and long-term visual outcome in primary open-angle glaucoma. Am J Ophthalmol 2001;132(1):47-56
- American Academy of Ophthalmology. Preferred Practice Pattern: Primary Open-Angle Glaucoma 2000; 1-36
- Heijl A, Leske MC, Bengtsson B, Hyman L, et al. Early Manifest Glaucoma Trial Group. Reduction of intraocular pressure and glaucoma progression: results from the Early Manifest Glaucoma Trial. Arch Ophthalmo 2002;120(10):1268-79
- Gordon MO, Beiser JA, Brandt JD, et al. The Ocular Hypertension Treatment Study: baseline factors that predict the onset of primary open-angle glaucoma. Arch Ophthalmol 2002;120(6):714-20
- The Advanced Glaucoma Intervention Study (AGIS): 4. Comparison of treatment outcomes within race. Seven-year results. Ophthalmology 1998;105(7):1146-64
- The Advanced Glaucoma Intervention Study (AGIS): 7. The relationship between control of intraocular pressure and visual field deterioration.The AGIS Investigators. Am J Ophthalmol 2000;130(4):429-40
- Kass MA, Heuer DK, Higginbotham EJ, et al. The Ocular Hypertension Treatment Study: a randomized trial determines that topical ocular hypotensive medication delays or prevents the onset of primary open-angle glaucoma. Arch Ophthalmol 2002;120(6):701-13
- Comparison of glaucomatous progression between untreated patients with normal-tension glaucoma and patients with therapeutically reduced intraocular pressures. Collaborative Normal-Tension Glaucoma Study Group. Am J Ophthalmol 1998;126(4):487-97
- Lichter PR, Musch DC, Gillespie BW, et al, CIGTS Study Group. Interim clinical outcomes in the Collaborative Initial Glaucoma Treatment Study comparing initial treatment randomized to medications or surgery Ophthalmology. 2001;108(11):1943-53
- Medeiros FA, Sample PA, Zangwill LM, et al. Corneal thickness as a risk factor for visual field loss in patients with preperimetric glaucomatous optic neuropathy. Am J Ophthalmol 2003;136(5):805-13

Web references: 0 available at www.5mcc.com

Illustrations N/A

Author(s):
Richard W. Allinson, MD

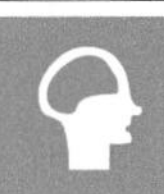

BASICS

DESCRIPTION An immunologic response to an infection (usually streptococcal) which damages the renal glomeruli. It can be initiated by other bacterial and viral infections. This is an immune complex, hypocomplementemic glomerulonephritis. Most common in children. Characterized by diffuse inflammatory changes in the glomeruli and clinically by the abrupt onset of hematuria with red blood cell casts, and mild proteinuria. Accompanied in many cases by hypertension, edema, and azotemia.

System(s) affected: Renal/Urologic
Genetics: No known genetic pattern
Incidence/Prevalence in USA: 20/100,000/ year (1-2% of pyodermas and 8% of streptococcal infections in children; occurs with impetigo in the late summer and with streptococcal pharyngitis in the winter)
Predominant age:
- 60% of cases in children 2-12 years old
- Only 10% older than 40 years of age

Predominant sex: Male > Female (60:40)

SIGNS & SYMPTOMS
- Classic findings of acute nephritis
  - ◊ Hematuria (100%)
  - ◊ Oliguria or anuria (52%)
  - ◊ Edema (85%)
  - ◊ Hypertension (82%)
  - ◊ Hypocomplementemia (C3) (83%)
  - ◊ Gross hematuria (30%), tea-colored urine
  - ◊ Edema of face and eyes in the am and feet and ankles in the afternoons and evenings
  - ◊ Fever (rare)
- Other signs and symptoms
  - ◊ Pharyngitis
  - ◊ Respiratory infection
  - ◊ Scarlet fever
  - ◊ Dark urine
  - ◊ Weight gain
  - ◊ Abdominal pain
  - ◊ Anorexia
  - ◊ Back pain
  - ◊ Pallor
  - ◊ Impetigo

CAUSES
- Follows group A beta-hemolytic streptococcus infection
- "Nephritogenic" strains of strep - groups 1, 4, 11, 12, 49 "Red Lake", 55, 60
- Unusual to have a second attack - protective immunity to nephritogenic antigen
- Cases of "postinfective" glomerulonephritis have also been reported from pneumococcus, staphylococcus, meningococcus, chickenpox, and hepatitis
- Streptococcal infection precedes renal lesions by 1-3 weeks
- Pharyngitis precedes renal lesions by 1-2 weeks (types 1, 2, 4, 12)
- Impetigo - (types 49, 55, 57) usually precedes throat or otitis media infection by 2-4 weeks

RISK FACTORS
- 15% occurrence rate after infection with nephritogenic strain
- Endemic with cyclic epidemics
- Subclinical cases 20 times more common
- Streptococcal infection (e.g., scarlet fever or erysipelas) can be associated with rheumatic fever or acute glomerulonephritis, rarely both

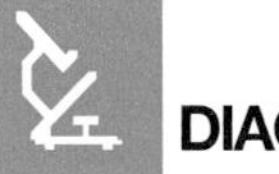

DIAGNOSIS

DIFFERENTIAL DIAGNOSIS
- Membranoproliferative glomerulonephritis
- Other postinfective glomerulonephritis
- Systemic lupus erythematosus
- IgA nephropathy
- Anaphylactoid purpura
- Rapidly progressive glomerulonephritis

LABORATORY
- Streptococcal tests (Streptozyme) that include many antigens are most sensitive (+ or -) for screening but not quantitative
- Antistreptolysin O (ASO) - quantitative titer. Increased in 60-80% of cases. Increase begins 1-3 weeks, is highest 3-5 weeks, normal in 6 months. ASO titer is unrelated to severity, duration or prognosis of renal disease.
- Red blood cells casts on urinalysis:
  - ◊ destroyed by centrifugation
  - ◊ disintegrate in urine, particularly alkaline urine
- Characteristically, red blood cells from glomerular bleeding are distorted while those from lower urinary tract have normal morphology
- U/P creatinine > 40, decreased renin
- Culture throat and skin lesions for streptococcus
- C3 and C4 complements are best for evaluation
- Streptozyme
- Hypertriglyceridemia
- Proteinuria
- Decreased glomerular filtration rate
- Uremia
- Increased serum creatinine
- Anemia
- ANA to rule out systemic lupus erythematosus

Drugs that may alter lab results: N/A

Disorders that may alter lab results: N/A

PATHOLOGICAL FINDINGS
- On renal biopsy
  - ◊ Diffuse proliferative and exudative glomerulonephritis
  - ◊ Electron microscopy - subepithelial deposits
  - ◊ Immunofluorescence - C3 in almost all cases, some with IgG and IgM

SPECIAL TESTS N/A

IMAGING
X-rays and/or ultrasound are not necessary to make the diagnosis

DIAGNOSTIC PROCEDURES
- If progressive, consider renal biopsy. Biopsy usually not indicated.

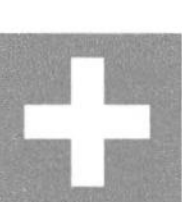

TREATMENT

APPROPRIATE HEALTH CARE
- Most patients can be safely followed as outpatients
- Inpatient usually until blood pressure and creatinine normalized and edema begins to recede

GENERAL MEASURES
- Decrease salt: no-added salt diet until edema and hypertension clear
- Decrease fluids to insensible losses plus 2/3 of the urine output until diuresis
- Control hypertension with diuretics
- Dialysis: peritoneal dialysis or hemodialysis for symptomatic azotemia, unresponsive hyperkalemia, intractable acidosis, diuretic resistant pulmonary edema

SURGICAL MEASURES N/A

ACTIVITY
Can return to full activity after clinically improved. May have increased hematuria after exercise for up to two years.

DIET
- "No-added" salt diet until edema, hypertension, and azotemia clear
- Restrict protein in presence of azotemia and metabolic acidosis
- Avoid high potassium foods

PATIENT EDUCATION
- National Kidney Foundation, 30 E. 33rd Street, Suite 1100, New York, NY 10016, (212)889-2210
- Web site - www.healthanswers.com

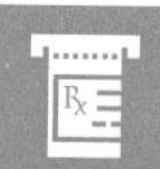

MEDICATIONS

DRUG(S) OF CHOICE

- Hyperkalemia
  - ◊ No potassium in IV fluids until hyperkalemia resolves
  - ◊ Sodium polystyrene sulfonate (Kayexalate) resin: 1 gm/kg in 10% sorbitol, pr or po
  - ◊ If acidosis present, treat as indicated below
  - ◊ Hypocalcemia with symptomatic hyperkalemia: 0.5 cc/kg 10% calcium gluconate IV over 30 minutes
  - ◊ Hypocalcemia with asymptomatic hyperkalemia: oral calcium carbonate (Tums) 1-2 gm calcium/day. (Tums have 650 mg calcium/tablet)
- Pulmonary edema
  - ◊ Oxygen
  - ◊ Furosemide (Lasix)
  - ◊ Digitalization is not effective
- Peripheral edema
  - ◊ Furosemide 1-2 mg/kg/dose given bid-tid po or IV
  - ◊ Treatment with diuretics decreases the duration and severity of edema and hypertension
- Acidosis
  - ◊ Sodium bicarbonate 1-2 mEq/kg/dose (1-2 mmol/kg/dose) IV over 30 minutes to correct acidosis
- Strep infection
  - ◊ Give penicillin for 10 days (po if possible)
  - ◊ Erythromycin in penicillin allergic patients
- Hypertension
  - ◊ Control with diuretics (furosemide 0.5-1 mg/kg IV or 2 mg/kg po bid or tid) and vasodilators (hydralazine [Apresoline] 0.25-1.0 mg/kg qid or nifedipine 0.25 mg/kg po prn or qid)

Contraindications: Refer to manufacturer's literature
Precautions: Refer to manufacturer's literature
Significant possible interactions: Refer to manufacturer's literature

ALTERNATIVE DRUGS N/A

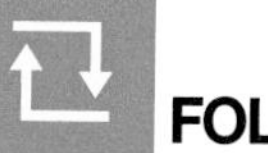

FOLLOWUP

PATIENT MONITORING

- Depends on severity of disease
- Urinalysis at 2, 4 and 8 weeks and 4, 6 and 12 months
- Stop followup when urinalysis is normal
- Monitor blood pressure each visit
- Monitor serum creatinine at 2, 6, and 12 months
- C3 complement should be normal by 6 weeks

PREVENTION/AVOIDANCE Treat streptococcal infections aggressively

POSSIBLE COMPLICATIONS

- Hypertensive retinopathy
- Hypertensive encephalopathy
- Rapidly progressive glomerulonephritis
- Abnormal urinalysis may persist for years (microhematuria)
- Chronic renal failure (rare)
- Nephrotic syndrome (approximately 10%)
- Marked decline in glomerular filtration rate (rare)

EXPECTED COURSE/PROGNOSIS

- Usually self-limited to 2-3 weeks
- Immediate mortality < 0.5%
- Long-term: excellent in children; almost all patients recover completely.
- May have more morbidity in adults or in those with pre-existing renal lesions
- Microscopic hematuria may persist for 24 months (or longer with complete recovery)
- Proteinuria persists for up to 3 months
- Symptoms can be exacerbated by a intercurrent illness but rarely after 12 months
- Urine may be darker (microscopic hematuria) after strenuous exercise

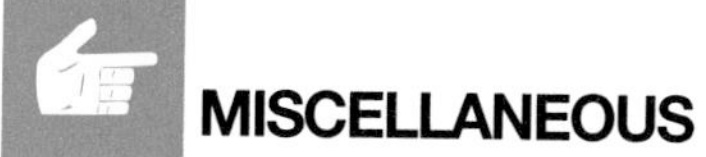

MISCELLANEOUS

ASSOCIATED CONDITIONS N/A

AGE-RELATED FACTORS

Pediatric: Common in children ages 2-16
Geriatric: N/A
Others: N/A

PREGNANCY N/A

SYNONYMS

- Acute nephritic syndrome
- Postinfectious glomerulonephritis
- Acute post-streptococcal glomerulonephritis

ICD-9-CM

580.9 Acute glomerulonephritis with unspecified pathological lesion in kidney

SEE ALSO

Glomerulonephritis, membranous
Hyperkalemia
Hypertensive emergencies
Hypocalcemia
Renal failure, acute (ARF)

OTHER NOTES N/A

ABBREVIATIONS N/A

REFERENCES

- Brenner B, Rector F, editors. The Kidney. 6th Ed. Philadelphia: W.B. Saunders Co.; 2000
- Barratt T, Avner E, W. Harmon, editors. Pediatric Nephrology. 4th ed. Baltimore: Williams & Wilkins; 2000

Web references: 2 available at www.5mcc.com
Illustrations N/A

Author(s):

Watson C. Arnold, MD

BASICS

DESCRIPTION Acute or chronic inflammation of the tongue either as a primary disease or symptom of systemic disease
System(s) affected: Gastrointestinal
Genetics: N/A
Incidence/Prevalence in USA: Common
Predominant age: All ages
Predominant sex: Male > Female

SIGNS & SYMPTOMS
- Reddened tip and edges of tongue (with pellagra, anemia, excess smoking)
- Fiery red, swollen, ulcerated tongue (pellagra)
- Tongue smooth and pale (anemias)
- Ulcers (herpetic or aphthous lesions, streptococcal infection, erythema multiforme, pemphigus)
- White patches (candidiasis, syphilis, leukoplakia, lichen planus, mouth breathing)
- Denuded smooth areas (geographic tongue)
- Painful tongue (anemia, pellagra, viral)
- Hairy tongue (follows antibiotic therapy, fever or excessive use of mouthwashes with peroxide)
- Tenderness, pain, swelling of the tongue (infections or trauma)
- Burning, painful tongue (candidiasis, anemia, diabetes, malignancies)
- Non-painful solitary ulcerations (malignancy)
- Painful combination of ulcers, nodules, linear fissures (herpetic geometric glossitis in HIV)
- Malignancy - painless red and/or white lesions
- Verrucous plaque, lateral aspect (EBV-oral hairy leukoplakia, in HIV patients)

CAUSES
- Systemic:
  - ◊ Malnutrition with avitaminosis (e.g., B group)
  - ◊ Anemia (pernicious, iron deficiency)
  - ◊ Skin diseases (e.g., lichen planus, erythema multiforme, aphthous lesions, Behçet syndrome, pemphigus vulgaris, syphilis)
  - ◊ HIV (candidiasis, HSV, loss of papillae)
  - ◊ Lansoprazole plus clarithromycin, amoxicillin, metronidazole (for treatment of H. Pylori in PUD)
- Local:
  - ◊ Infections (HSV, EBV, candidiasis, tuberculosis, streptococcal)
  - ◊ Trauma (ill-fitting dentures, burns, convulsive seizures)
  - ◊ Primary irritants (alcohol, tobacco, hot foods, spices, excessive peppermint, citrus)
  - ◊ Sensitization (chemical irritants, e.g., dyes, mouth wash, toothpaste, systemic drugs)
  - ◊ Malignancy

RISK FACTORS
- Low socioeconomic status
- Poor nutrition
- Dentures
- Smoking, smokeless tobacco
- Alcoholism
- Anxiety, stress
- Depression
- Advancing age
- Immunocompromised state

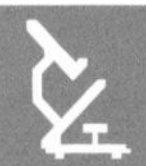

DIAGNOSIS

DIFFERENTIAL DIAGNOSIS
- Systemic:
  - ◊ Avitaminosis (particularly B group, e.g., pellagra)
  - ◊ Anemia (pernicious, iron deficiency)
  - ◊ Skin diseases (e.g., lichen planus, erythema multiforme, aphthous lesions, Behçet syndrome, pemphigus vulgaris, syphilis)
  - ◊ HIV
- Local:
  - ◊ Infections (herpes simplex virus [HSV], Epstein-Barr virus [EBV], candidiasis, tuberculosis, streptococcal)
  - ◊ Trauma (ill-fitting dentures, burns, convulsive seizures)
  - ◊ Primary irritants: alcohol, tobacco, hot foods, spices
  - ◊ Sensitization (chemical irritants, e.g., dyes, mouth wash, toothpaste, systemic drugs)
  - ◊ Malignancy (95% are squamous cell)
  - ◊ Geographic tongue (also known as migratory glossitis) - benign, but recurrent

LABORATORY
- CBC
- Serologic tests for syphilis
- Chemical profile
- Tests for vitamin B12 deficiency
- Postprandial glucose
- Smear and culture lesions when indicated

Drugs that may alter lab results: N/A

Disorders that may alter lab results: N/A

PATHOLOGICAL FINDINGS Varies according to underlying causes

SPECIAL TESTS
- Biopsy solitary lesions that do not respond to treatment in one week
- 10% KOH scrapings for suspected candidiasis

IMAGING N/A

DIAGNOSTIC PROCEDURES
- Biopsy
- KOH scrapings

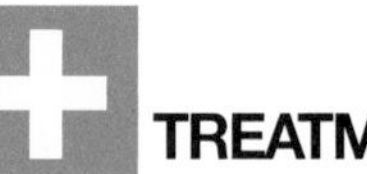

TREATMENT

APPROPRIATE HEALTH CARE Outpatient

GENERAL MEASURES
- Avoid any possible sensitizing irritants or agents
- Specific therapy for oral infections (see Medications)
- Local treatment (see Medications)
- Analgesics when needed
- Request dental evaluation
- Scrupulous oral hygiene

SURGICAL MEASURES N/A

ACTIVITY No restrictions unless there is a systemic infection

DIET Bland or liquid diet

PATIENT EDUCATION Griffith: Instructions for Patients; 7th ed. Philadelphia, Elsevier, 2004

MEDICATIONS

DRUG(S) OF CHOICE
- For candidiasis:
  - ◊ Nystatin oral suspension 400,000 units (4 mL) to 600,000 units qid for 10 days as an oral rinse, then swallowed
- For oral infections:
  - ◊ Oral penicillin V
  - ◊ Multivitamins (vitamin B-complex, vitamin E)
  - ◊ Iron (if deficient)
- Local treatment:
  - ◊ Mouth rinse with 2% lidocaine viscous, 1 tablespoon before each meal and every 3 hours if needed for pain
  - ◊ Mouth wash of 1/2 teaspoon sodium bicarbonate in 8 oz (240 mL) warm water qid
  - ◊ Mouth rinse with carbamide peroxide (Gly-Oxide) 10% 0.5 mL or 10 drops qid (expectorate after use) for irritation, aphthous ulcers
  - ◊ Triamcinolone (Kenalog) in dental paste (Orabase): Compound triamcinolone 0.1% in emollient dental paste applied to specific lesions, especially aphthous ulcers
  - ◊ 50/50 mixture of kaolin-pectin and diphenhydramine (Benadryl) as mouth rinse (coats and topically anesthetizes)

Contraindications: Refer to manufacturer's literature
Precautions: Depressed gag reflex with lidocaine viscous. Decreased sensitivity to hot/cold liquids.
Significant possible interactions: Refer to manufacturer's literature

ALTERNATIVE DRUGS
- For candidiasis:
  - ◊ Clotrimazole - 10 mg oral lozenges 5 times a day for 10 days

or
  - ◊ Ketoconazole - one 200 mg tablet (for children 1/4 tablet) orally once a day

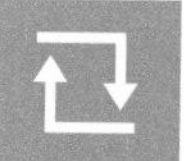

FOLLOWUP

PATIENT MONITORING
- Re-visits periodically when needed until healing occurs
- If lesions do not heal, biopsy is indicated

PREVENTION/AVOIDANCE
- Evaluation of nutritional status including B-vitamin deficiencies, anemias
- Cessation of tobacco use (including "smokeless")
- Assess for irritation from teeth, dentures

POSSIBLE COMPLICATIONS
- Lymphadenopathy
- Chronicity

EXPECTED COURSE/PROGNOSIS
- Prompt improvement when cause can be identified and treated
- Aphthous ulcers, erythema multiforme and hairy tongue often recur

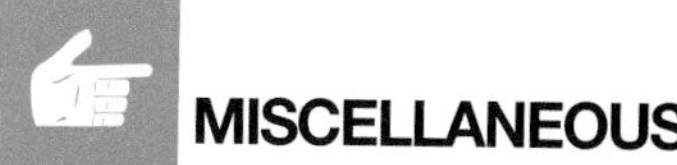

MISCELLANEOUS

ASSOCIATED CONDITIONS
- Diabetes mellitus
- HIV infection

AGE-RELATED FACTORS
Pediatric: Median rhomboid glossitis is a developmental lesion causing a rhomboid-shaped, smooth, reddish, nodular area on the dorsal surface of the back portion of the middle third of the tongue. This type of glossitis is innocuous and requires no treatment.
Geriatric: Many patients with glossitis are postmenopausal or elderly
Others: N/A

PREGNANCY N/A

SYNONYMS N/A

ICD-9-CM
529.0 Glossitis

SEE ALSO
Candidiasis
HIV infection & AIDS
Vitamin deficiency

OTHER NOTES
Some symptoms of glossitis have no organic cause. Treat symptoms and reassure regarding malignancy.

ABBREVIATIONS
EBV = Epstein-Barr virus
HSV = herpes simplex virus

REFERENCES

- Itin PH, Lautenschlager S. Viral lesions of the mouth in HIV-infected patients. Dermatol 1997;194(1):1-7
- Kretzschmar JL, Kretzschmar DP. Common oral conditions. Amer Fam Phys 1996;54(1):225-34
- Drezner DA, Schaffer SR. Geographic tongue: Otolaryngology-Head and Neck Surgery 1997;117(3):291
- Porter SR, Scully C. Adverse drug reactions in the mouth. Clin Dermatol 2000;18(5):525-32
- Byrd JA, Bruce AJ, Rogers RS 3rd. Glossitis and other tongue disorders. Dermatol Clin 2003;21(1):123-34
- Assimakopoulos D, Patrikakos G, Fotika C, Elisaf M. Benign migratory glossitis or geographic tongue: an enigmatic oral lesion. Am J Med 2002;113(9):751-5

Web references: 0 available at www.5mcc.com
Illustrations 1 available

Author(s):
J. Randall Richard, MD

BASICS

DESCRIPTION Gonorrhea is a purulent inflammation of mucous membrane surfaces caused by a sexually transmitted microorganism, Neisseria gonorrhoeae. Virtually any mucous membrane can be infected. Occasionally the organism may become blood-borne causing a syndrome comprised of combinations of any of the following features: Fever, skin lesions, arthralgias/tenosynovitis, and septic arthritis.
- Hematogenous dissemination may also lead to endocarditis, or rarely, meningitis
- In women, salpingitis, local extension from the endocervical canal to the fallopian tubes is common. The ovaries may be involved with abscess formation. The entire complex of upper genital tract infection in women is referred to as pelvic inflammatory disease (PID).
- In men, the epididymis may become infected with extension to the testicle
- An asymptomatic carrier state can occur in both sexes

System(s) affected: Cardiovascular, Musculoskeletal, Nervous, Reproductive, Skin/Exocrine
Genetics: Individuals with congenital deficiency of the late components of the complement cascade (C 7,8,9) are prone to develop dissemination of local gonococcal infections
Incidence/Prevalence in USA: 358,995 cases reported to CDC in 2000, resulting in a rate of 132/100,000 population
Predominant age: 15-24
Predominant sex: Male > Female (symptomatic disease)

SIGNS & SYMPTOMS
- Adolescent and adult males:
  - ◊ Scant to copious purulent urethral discharge (98%)
  - ◊ Dysuria (98%)
  - ◊ Testicular pain (1%)
  - ◊ Asymptomatic urethral infection (incidence of about 1%)
  - ◊ Urethral stricture
- Adolescent and adult females without PID:
  - ◊ Asymptomatic cervical infection (approximately 20%)
  - ◊ Endocervical discharge (on pelvic exam) (96%)
  - ◊ Vaginal discharge
  - ◊ Dysuria
  - ◊ Bartholin's gland abscess
- Adolescent and adult females with PID:
  - ◊ Dysmenorrhea
  - ◊ Metromenorrhagia
  - ◊ Lower abdominal pain and tenderness
  - ◊ Fever
  - ◊ Cervical traction tenderness
  - ◊ Palpable, tender fallopian tubes and/or ovaries
  - ◊ Abdominal rebound tenderness
  - ◊ Infertility
  - ◊ Chronic pelvic pain
- Either sex, if receptive partner in anal intromission:
  - ◊ Rectal discharge: purulent or bloody
  - ◊ Tenesmus
  - ◊ Rectal burning or itching
  - ◊ Asymptomatic rectal infection
- Either sex, other syndromes:
  - ◊ Pharyngeal infection - asymptomatic infection (98%), sore throat, exudative pharyngitis (< 1%)
  - ◊ Eye infection (rare) - purulent discharge, conjunctivitis, chemosis, eyelid edema, corneal ulceration
  - ◊ Disseminated syndromes - fever; chills; arthralgias (small joints); synovial sheath tenderness and swelling (hands and/or feet); painful skin lesions (pustular, red, tender); septic arthritis (usually asymmetric, polyarticular, and mainly involving elbows, knees and more distal joints; manifested by joint pain, swelling, erythema, and induration)
  - ◊ Endocarditis - rapid cardiac valve destruction, high fevers
  - ◊ Meningitis - meningeal signs, headache, skin lesions, fever, altered mental status
- Infants and children
  - ◊ Eye infection (rare - because of routine ocular prophylaxis in the USA)
  - ◊ Pneumonia (of the newborn) - fever, infiltrate on chest x-ray
  - ◊ Vulvovaginitis - vaginal discharge
  - ◊ Rectal infection
  - ◊ Pharyngeal infection
  - ◊ Meningitis
  - ◊ Other forms of disseminated infection - fever, chills, arthralgias, synovial sheath tenderness and swelling, skin lesions, septic arthritis, endocarditis

CAUSES Neisseria gonorrhoeae (gonococcus)

RISK FACTORS
- Sexual exposure to an infected individual without barrier protection (condom)
- Multiple sexual partners
- Infant - passage through the infected birth canal of the mother
- Children - sexual abuse by infected individual
- Auto-inoculation (finger to eye)
- For PID - use of intrauterine devices

DIAGNOSIS

DIFFERENTIAL DIAGNOSIS
- Chlamydia infections (may mimic all aspects of gonococcal infections except disseminated syndromes)
- Urinary tract infections
- Vaginitis caused by other infectious agents (yeast, trichomonas, bacterial vaginosis)

LABORATORY
- Gram stain of exudate from infected mucosal surface
- Demonstration of pairs or clumps of Gram-negative kidney-shaped diplococci associated with the cytoplasm of polymorphonuclear leukocytes. The adjacent surfaces are slightly concave.
- Sensitivity of urethral smear in symptomatic male ≥95%
- Sensitivity of endocervical smear in infected woman = 40-60%
- DNA probes and PCR: sensitivity 92->99% dependent upon population; specificity >97%: can replace culture confirmation in most cases of adult infection
- Culture of exudate on selective medium (Thayer-Martin or Martin-Lewis, containing antibiotics to inhibit other microorganisms). Demonstration of typical organisms by Gram-stain morphology and growth on selective media constitutes a "presumptive" diagnosis of gonococcal infection. Culture should always be done in suspected cases of infection in children.
- Sensitivity of blood culture in disseminated disease - 50%
- Sensitivity of joint fluid culture in septic arthritis - 50%

Drugs that may alter lab results: Prior administration of even small amounts of many antibiotics may render a culture falsely negative; PCR or DNA probe may remain positive

Disorders that may alter lab results: N/A

PATHOLOGICAL FINDINGS
- Exudate of polymorphonuclear leukocytes is typical
- In PID - loss of ciliated columnar epithelium from the fallopian tubes. Tubes, pelvic mesentery, and ovaries may be bound together with dense fibrosis and abscess formation.

SPECIAL TESTS
- Confirmation of the isolate as the gonococcus by standard sugar fermentation tests, enzymatic tests or DNA probes. Important in medicolegal situations such as rape or child abuse since other Neisseria, which are normal inhabitants of mucosal surfaces, may look like gonococcus on Gram-stained smear.
- Testing for antimicrobial susceptibility. ß-lactamase production and chromosomally mediated resistance to penicillin and/or tetracycline are becoming more common. Although routine ß-lactamase testing of N. gonorrhoeae has been recommended by the U.S. Public Health Service, the need for such testing is questionable if current therapy guidelines are observed. However, in face of rising fluoroquinolone resistance as well, all cases of apparent therapy failure should have cultures and susceptibility studies performed.

IMAGING Pelvic ultrasound or CT scan may demonstrate thick, dilated fallopian tubes or abscess formation

DIAGNOSTIC PROCEDURES
- Culdocentesis may demonstrate free purulent exudate, and provide material for gram staining and culture
- Gram staining material from unroofed skin lesions may show typical organisms

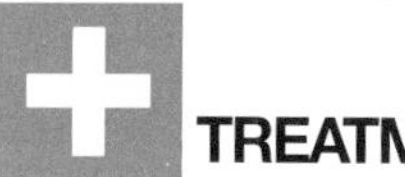

TREATMENT

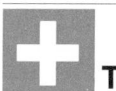

APPROPRIATE HEALTH CARE
- Outpatient for uncomplicated infection, with contact notification and contact treatment
- Hospitalize for:
  - ◊ Hematogenously disseminated infection
  - ◊ Pneumonia or eye infection in infants
  - ◊ PID: if unable to take oral medications, significant tubo-ovarian abscess, or patient is pregnant

GENERAL MEASURES
- Abstain from sexual activity until after full treatment, plus testing and treatment of partner(s)
- DNA probe or PCR testing for chlamydia
- Serologic test for syphilis
- Encourage testing for HIV infection

SURGICAL MEASURES N/A

ACTIVITY Fully active for uncomplicated disease

DIET No special diet

PATIENT EDUCATION
- Discuss sexually transmitted diseases and methods of prevention
- Discuss HIV infection and risks; encourage patient and partner(s) to be tested

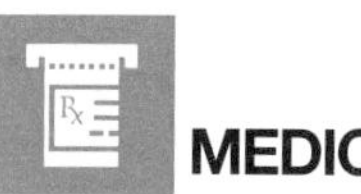

MEDICATIONS

DRUG(S) OF CHOICE
- Treatment of adults:
  - ◊ Uncomplicated N. gonorrhoeae infection of urethra, cervix, rectum: Initial single dose of ceftriaxone 125 mg IM or cefixime 400 mg po or ofloxacin 400 mg po or ciprofloxacin 500 mg po or levofloxacin 250 mg po plus an agent with activity against chlamydia, e.g., doxycycline 100 mg po bid x 7 days or azithromycin 1.0 g po as a single dose

Note: In pregnancy, ceftriaxone is the treatment of choice. Erythromycin 500 mg po qid x 7 days is an alternative antichlamydia agent for use in pregnancy. In the absence of pregnancy, ofloxacin 300 mg po bid x 7 days is another alternative antichlamydia therapy. Alternative parenteral agents for therapy of gonococcal infections include other 3rd generation cephalosporins and spectinomycin.

  - ◊ Uncomplicated infection of the rectum: ceftriaxone 125 mg IM or ciprofloxacin 500 mg po (plus an agent with activity against chlamydia - see above)
  - ◊ Conjunctivitis: ceftriaxone 1 g IM
  - ◊ PID: outpatient regimens (see citations for treatment of hospitalized patients)
    - Regimen A: Ofloxacin 400 mg po bid x 14 days plus clindamycin 450 mg po qid x 14 days or metronidazole 500 mg po bid x 14 days
    - Regimen B: Cefoxitin 2g IM + probenecid 1g po or ceftriaxone 250 mg IM; plus doxycycline 100 mg po bid x 14 days
- Disseminated infections in adults
  - ◊ Bacteremia and dermatitis-arthritis complex: ceftriaxone 1g IV daily. With clinical improvement, complete 7-10 days of therapy with cefixime 400 mg po bid, ciprofloxacin 500 mg po bid, levofloxacin 500 mg po qd, or other agents to which the infecting organism has been proven fully susceptible.
  - ◊ Meningitis: Ceftriaxone 1-2g IV q 12 hours for 10-14 days
  - ◊ Endocarditis: Ceftriaxone 1-2g IV q 12 hours for 4 weeks

Note: Parenteral penicillin G can be used to treat disseminated infection if full susceptibility is documented. Other third generation cephalosporins also can be substituted for ceftriaxone for parenteral therapy; spectinomycin 2 g IM q12hr is an alternative to initial ß-lactam; ofloxacin, levofloxacin, or ciprofloxacin are also alternatives.

- Treatment of infants and children < 45 kg:

(patients >45 kg should receive full adult dose)
  - ◊ Uncomplicated genital, pharyngeal, rectal, or conjunctival infection and infants born to mothers with untreated gonorrhea
    - Ceftriaxone 125 mg IM in single dose. Alternative is spectinomycin 40 mg/kg up to 2 g as single IM dose.
  - ◊ Disseminated infections: ceftriaxone 25-50 mg/kg IV or IM daily or cefotaxime 25 mg/kg IV or IM q12h
    - 7 days for bacteremia or dermatitis/arthritis complex
    - 10-14 days for meningitis
    - 28 days for endocarditis
  - ◊ Ophthalmic neonatorum prophylaxis: single application of:
    - 1% silver nitrate aqueous solution, or
    - 0.5% erythromycin ophthalmic ointment, or
    - 1% tetracycline ophthalmic ointment

Contraindications: Fluoroquinolones and tetracyclines such as doxycycline are contraindicated in pregnancy

Precautions: Refer to manufacturer's profile of each drug

Significant possible interactions: Refer to manufacturer's profile of each drug

ALTERNATIVE DRUGS If organisms not penicillin-resistant, use IV penicillin G. Note: Some penicillin resistance is now due to penicillinase production. Oral ampicillin or amoxicillin plus probenecid may be substituted for cephalosporins in uncomplicated disease, also after lab confirms absence of penicillin-resistance. Spectinomycin is an alternative if ß-lactam agents or fluoroquinolones cannot be used. Fluoroquinolone resistance is rising. Drug susceptibility testing after culture must be performed in the event of apparent fluoroquinolone therapy failure.

FOLLOWUP

PATIENT MONITORING Retesting to document cure is not necessary if one of the recommended regimens is used unless symptoms persist or there is concern about poor compliance with therapy

PREVENTION/AVOIDANCE
- Condoms offer partial protection
- Sexual contacts should be treated

POSSIBLE COMPLICATIONS
- Urethral stricture in men
- Infertility in women
- Corneal scarring after eye infections
- Destruction of joint articular surfaces
- Destruction of cardiac valves
- Death from CHF or meningitis

EXPECTED COURSE/PROGNOSIS
With adequate, early therapy complete cure and return to normal function is the rule

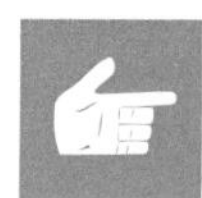

MISCELLANEOUS

ASSOCIATED CONDITIONS Other sexually transmitted infections (chlamydia, syphilis, HIV, hepatitis B, herpes) and vaginal infections

AGE-RELATED FACTORS
Pediatric: N/A
Geriatric: N/A
Others: N/A

PREGNANCY PID may lead to fetal loss, or premature labor and delivery

SYNONYMS
- GC
- Clap

ICD-9-CM
098.0 Acute gonoccal infection of lower genitourinary tract
614.9 Unspecified inflammatory disease of female pelvic organs and tissue

SEE ALSO
Chlamydial sexually transmitted diseases
Pelvic inflammatory disease (PID)
Syphilis

OTHER NOTES N/A

ABBREVIATIONS
GC = gonococcal
PID = pelvic inflammatory disease

REFERENCES

- Centers for Disease Control and Prevention (CDC). Sexually transmitted diseases treatmetn guidelines 2002. Morbidity Mortality Weekly report 2002;51(RR06):1-80
- Sparling PF, Handsfield HH. Neisseria gonorrhoeae. In: Mandell GL, Bennett JE, Dolin R, eds. Principles and Practices of Infectious Diseases. 5th ed. Philadelphia: Churchill Livingstone; 2000.p. 2242-2258

Web references: 2 available at www.5mcc.com
Illustrations 1 available

Author(s):
Leonard N. Slater, MD

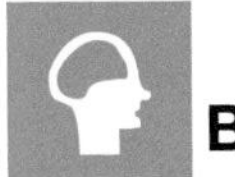

BASICS

DESCRIPTION Inflammatory reaction to urate crystals in joints, bones and subcutaneous structures. Initially, a hyperacute arthritis which may progress to a chronic arthritis. Rarely it may present as a chronic arthritis. Recognition of the crystals in fluid is pathognomonic.

- Primary gout - the most common: underexcretion or overproduction of uric acid
- Secondary gout - related to myeloproliferative diseases or their treatment, therapeutic regimens producing hyperuricemia, renal failure, renal tubular disorders, lead poisoning, hyperproliferative skin disorders, enzymatic defects (e.g., deficient hypoxanthine guanine phosphoribosyltransferase, glycogen storage diseases)

System(s) affected: Endocrine/Metabolic, Musculoskeletal, Renal/Urologic
Genetics: N/A
Incidence/Prevalence in USA: 100/100,000 prevalence. Under age 18: rare; age 18-44: 3; age 45-64: 21; age over 65: 35
Predominant age: 30-60
Predominant sex: Male > Female (20:1)

SIGNS & SYMPTOMS

- Hyperacute onset (within 24 hours) of severe pain, swelling, redness, and warmth in one or two joints (75% are monoarticular)
- Soft tissue redness, swelling, warmth
- Exquisite tenderness
- Propensity for first MTP joint, symptomatic in 50% of initial attacks; eventually in 75%
- Acute untreated attacks last 2-21 days
- Attack may be isolated, more often repetitive, 2nd attack may not occur for years
- Recurrent attacks last longer and occur more frequently with each recurrence
- Between critical periods - absence of inflammation (until the chronic or tophaceous phase occurs)
- Rarely polyarticular - proximal interphalangeal, distal interphalangeal, metacarpal phalangeal, wrist, knee, ankle, midtarsal joints, heel
- Migratory polyarthritis is a rare presentation
- 50% of untreated patients develop a chronic arthritis within 3-42 years
- Inflammatory synovial effusion
- Subcutaneous or intraosseous nodules (20%), referred to as tophi - may affect ears (antihelix), extensor aspects of peripheral joints (e.g., olecranon), rarely fingertips, cornea, aorta, spine or even intracranial
- Subcutaneous nodules may have a creamy (urate) discharge
- Fever, chills
- Carpal tunnel syndrome
- Kidney stones

CAUSES

- Hyperuricemia
- Dietary excess (e.g., anchovies, sardines, sweetbreads, kidney, liver and meat extracts)
- Inborn errors of metabolism
- Lead poisoning (Saturnine gout from moonshine)
- Kidney disease
- Hemoproliferative disorders
- Dehydration
- Low dose aspirin

RISK FACTORS

- Ethanol ingestion
- Family history
- Polynesian extraction (e.g., Samoan gout)
- Medications - aminophylline, caffeine, corticosteroids, cytotoxic drugs (cyclosporine), diazepam, diphenhydramine, diuretics, L-dopa, dopamine, epinephrine, ethambutol, methaqualone, alpha-methyl dopa, nicotinic acid, probenecid (low dose), pyrazinamide, salicylates (< 10/dL blood levels), sulfinpyrazone (low dose), vitamins B12 and C.
- Diuretics may be responsible for 20% of secondary gout
- Ketosis
- Surgery or trauma
- Obesity (50%)
- Hypertension (50%)
- Vascular disease
- Diabetes
- Renal failure
- Hypothyroidism
- Hyperparathyroidism; hypoparathyroidism
- Hyperlipidemia types II, IV, V
- Paget disease
- Hyperproliferative skin disorders (e.g., psoriasis)
- Lymphoproliferative disorders
- Calcium pyrophosphate deposition disease
- Sarcoidosis
- Hemolytic anemia
- Hemoglobinopathies
- Pernicious anemia
- Radiation treatment
- Type I glycogen storage disease
- Down syndrome
- Gut sterilization by antibiotics

DIAGNOSIS

DIFFERENTIAL DIAGNOSIS Infectious arthritis, pseudogout (calcium pyrophosphate deposition disease), type IIa hyperproteinemia, amyloidosis, multicentric reticulohistiocytosis, hyperparathyroidism, spondyloarthropathy, rheumatoid arthritis (rarely)

LABORATORY

- WBC usually elevated with left shift during acute attacks
- ESR usually elevated during acute attacks
- Hyperuricemia may be present, although not diagnostic

Drugs that may alter lab results:

- Intra-articular steroids - many have inherent birefringence, which will cause confusion on synovial fluid analysis
- Hyperuricemia - induced by drugs that reduce effective circulating blood volume (induced by low dose aspirin, probenecid or sulfinpyrazone)
- Cyclosporine - induced renal insufficiency

Disorders that may alter lab results:

Alcoholism, sarcoidosis, lead poisoning, kidney failure, psoriasis, hemoglobinopathy

PATHOLOGICAL FINDINGS

- Urate crystals in synovial membrane (98% of specimens processed entirely anhydrously [urate is water soluble])
- Tophus in 29% of individuals with untreated gout of 5 years duration, in 74% of individuals with untreated gout of 40 years duration

SPECIAL TESTS

- Synovial fluid white blood cell count is usually inflammatory (10,000-70,000 cells/dL), but may have as few as 1,000 WBC/dL
- Wet mounts of synovial fluid reveal strongly negatively birefringent urate crystals on polarizing exam
- Gout crystals may be identified in asymptomatic joints

IMAGING

- X-ray is usually normal in the first year of uncontrolled disease.
- X-ray in chronic gout reveals "punched-out" erosions (lytic areas) often with periosteum overgrowing the erosion ("overhanging edge" sign). This is highly suggestive, but may also be caused by amyloidosis, type IIa hyperlipoproteinemia, and by multicentric reticulohistiocytosis.
- X-ray erosions with preservation of joint space is similarly characteristic. X-ray rarely reveals intraosseous lytic areas (tophi).
- Bone scan reveals increased nuclide concentration at affected sites

DIAGNOSTIC PROCEDURES

- Arthrocentesis with polarizing optical examination
- Biopsy of synovial membrane or subcutaneous nodule, processing the specimen anhydrously (urate is water soluble) and examining with polarizing optics

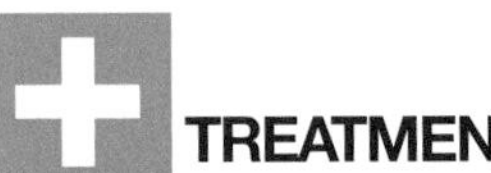

TREATMENT

APPROPRIATE HEALTH CARE Outpatient, except for consideration of associated joint infection or for therapeutic unresponsiveness

GENERAL MEASURES

- Control the acute attack of gout
- Addressing the underlying cause

SURGICAL MEASURES N/A

ACTIVITY Affected joint(s) at rest until hyperacute phase is controlled

DIET Reduce ingestion of fat, alcoholic beverages, sardines, anchovies, liver, sweetbreads

PATIENT EDUCATION

- Arthritis Foundation pamphlet on gout
- Rothschild, BM.: Hyperuricemia in the elderly. Geriatric Consultant, 4:14-16, 31, 1985.

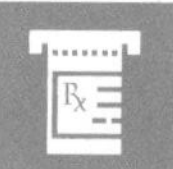

MEDICATIONS

DRUG(S) OF CHOICE

- Acute attack
  - ◊ A NSAID at full dosage for 2-5 days
  - ◊ When acute attack is controlled, reduce dose by 1/4-1/2
- Chronic treatment
  - ◊ Initiate when acute attack controlled (unless kidneys at risk because of unusual uric acid load)
  - ◊ Generally not pursued unless recurrent attacks or evidence of tophaceous or renal disease
  - ◊ Any contributing medication regimens are first altered and any predisposing medical conditions/habits addressed
  - ◊ Patient is tested for uric acid excretion (<600 mg/day while on purine free diet or <800 mg/day on unrestricted diet implies hypoexcretor)
    - Hypoexcretor: probenecid is initiated at 500 mg qd and increased by 500 mg at monthly intervals, until the uric acid is lowered to normal range or at least 2 mg/dL (0.12 mmol/L) less than the levels during which attacks are noted. (Maximum dose 2-3 g/day.) Urinary alkalinization and recommendation of ingestion of copious amounts of fluid are adjunctive.
    - Hyperexcretor, tophaceous or renal disease are present: allopurinol, initiated at 100 mg qd and increased by 100 mg weekly, to a maximum of 600 mg per day.

Contraindications:

- NSAIDs:
  - ◊ Peptic ulcer disease
  - ◊ Psychosis
  - ◊ Severe headache
  - ◊ Pregnancy
  - ◊ Concomitant anticoagulant use
  - ◊ Presence of a blood dyscrasia
  - ◊ Use with caution when renal insufficiency present
- Probenecid:
  - ◊ Uric acid overproduction
  - ◊ Uric acid stones
  - ◊ Renal impairment
  - ◊ Concomitant salicylates
  - ◊ Tophi (relative)
- Allopurinol:
  - ◊ Bone marrow suppression
  - ◊ Liver disease
  - ◊ Concomitant cytotoxic drugs
  - ◊ Diuretics may require increased amount of allopurinol

Precautions:

- Probenecid and allopurinol may predispose to acute gouty attacks. Use low dose NSAID for 6-24 mos to reduce risk.
- Reduce NSAID dosage in presence of renal or liver disease
- Reduce cytotoxic drug dose in presence of allopurinol
- With allopurinol risk of skin rash

Significant possible interactions:

- NSAIDs:
  - ◊ Anticoagulants
  - ◊ Antidiabetic agents
  - ◊ Anticonvulsants
  - ◊ Lithium
- Probenecid:
  - ◊ Antibiotics
  - ◊ Antidiabetic agents
  - ◊ Thiopental
  - ◊ Ketamine
  - ◊ NSAIDs
  - ◊ Lorazepam
  - ◊ Rifampin
  - ◊ Antagonized by pyrazinamide, salicylates
- Allopurinol:
  - ◊ Mercaptopurine (requires reduction of chemotherapy dose to 1/3 of usual dose)
  - ◊ Azathioprine (requires reduction of chemotherapy dose to 1/3 of usual dose)
  - ◊ Methotrexate
  - ◊ Possibly cyclophosphamide
  - ◊ Anticoagulants
  - ◊ Antidiabetic agents

ALTERNATIVE DRUGS

- Related to control of the acute attack:
  - ◊ Colchicine, a controversial toxic agent which must be taken within 24 hours of onset of the acute attack to be effective; IV preferred 2 mg, followed by 1 mg q6h for 2 doses; do not repeat in less than 3 days
  - ◊ Intra-articular long-acting (depot) corticosteroid (if infection definitely ruled out)
  - ◊ ACTH 40-80 IU IM
- Related to control of the underlying hyperuricemia in the hypoexcretor:
  - ◊ Sulfinpyrazone, initiated at 400 mg qd
  - ◊ Oxypurinol 200-800 mg/day on compassionate use or research protocol only
  - ◊ Fenofibrate 160 mg qd; augments renal urate clearance

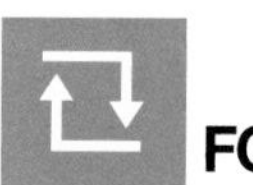

FOLLOWUP

PATIENT MONITORING

- Related to medicinal control of the acute attack and suppressing attacks:
  - ◊ Adjusting therapeutic regimen if no significant clinical response to therapy within 3 days of its initiation.
  - ◊ CBC, renal and hepatic blood testing and urinalysis at 1 wk, 6 wks and every 3 months
- Related to control of the underlying hyperuricemia:
  - ◊ CBC, uric acid level, renal and hepatic blood testing, and urinalysis at monthly intervals (with dosage/regimen modification) until desired serum uric acid level achieved

PREVENTION/AVOIDANCE

- Avoidance of exacerbating medications/diets/habits
- Maintain serum uric acid <7

POSSIBLE COMPLICATIONS

- Increased susceptibility to infection
- Urate nephropathy
- Uric acid nephropathy
- Renal stones
- Nerve/spinal cord impingement
- Recognition of urate crystals does not preclude concomitant infectious arthritis

EXPECTED COURSE/PROGNOSIS

- With early treatment, total control
- If recurrent attacks, successful uric acid adjustment (requiring lifelong use of uricosuric or allopurinol medication) usually effective
- During the first 6-24 months of uricosuric or allopurinol therapy, acute gout may occur

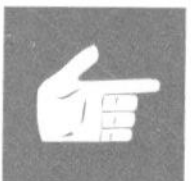

MISCELLANEOUS

ASSOCIATED CONDITIONS

- Myeloproliferative disorders
- Lymphoproliferative disorders
- Alcoholism
- Hyperlipidemia
- Obesity
- Hypertension
- Diabetes
- Lesch-Nyhan syndrome - chorea, spasticity, self-mutilation in childhood

AGE-RELATED FACTORS

Pediatric: Onset in this age group identifies gout secondary to an inborn error of metabolism or underlying disease process
Geriatric: Usually related to medications
Others: N/A

PREGNANCY Usual pregnancy precautions

SYNONYMS N/A

ICD-9-CM

274.0 Gouty arthropathy
274.10 Gouty nephropathy, unspecified
274.11 Uric acid nephrolithiasis
274.81 Gouty tophi of ear
984.9 Toxic effect of unspecified lead compound (including fumes)

SEE ALSO

Alcohol use disorders
Anemia, sickle cell

OTHER NOTES N/A

ABBREVIATIONS

MP = metatarsal phalangeal
NSAID = non-steroidal anti-inflammatory drug

REFERENCES

- Yu TF. Gout. In: Katz W, editor. Diagnosis and Management of Rheumatic Diseases. Philadelphia: JB Lippincott; 1988
- Kelley WN, Harris ED Jr, Ruddy S, Sledge CB. Textbook of Rheumatology. Philadelphia: WB Saunders Co; 1997
- Rothschild BM, Heathcote GM. Characterization of gout in a skeletal population sample. Amer J Phys Anthrol 1995;98(4):519-25
- Vazquez-Mellado J, et al. Intradermal tophi in gout. J Rheum 1997;26:136-40
- Hepburn AL, Kaye SA, Feher MD. Long-term remission from gout associated with fenofibrate therapy. Clin Rheumatol 2003;22:73-6
- Yu KH, Luo SF, Liou LB, Wu YJ, Tsai WP, Chen JY, Ho HH. Concomitant septic and gouty arthritis--an analysis of 30 cases. Rheumatology (Oxford) 2003;42(9):1062-6
- Weniger FG, Davison SP, Risin M, Salyapongse AN, Manders EK. Gouty flexor tenosynovitis of the digits: report of three cases. J Hand Surg [Am] 2003;28(4):669-72
- Takahashi S, Moriwaki Y, Yamamoto T, Tsutsumi Z, Ka T, Fukuchi M. Effects of combination treatment using anti-hyperuricaemic agents with fenofibrate and/or losartan on uric acid metabolism. Ann Rheum Dis 2003;62(6):572-5

Web references: 3 available at www.5mcc.com
Illustrations 1 available

Author(s):

Bruce M. Rothschild, MD

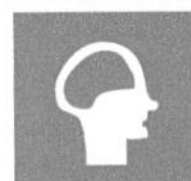

BASICS

DESCRIPTION Chronic, self-limited inflammation of the skin exhibited by annularly arranged papules

- Localized granuloma annulare: the most common form consists of a solitary group of flesh colored papules that gradually involute centrally to form circles or semicircles
- Disseminated granuloma annulare: occurs less often (approximately 15%) and usually consists of widespread lesions with the same characteristics as the localized type as well as infiltrated papules
- Generalized perforating granuloma annulare: characterized by pinpoint umbilicated papules on the extremities
- Subcutaneous granuloma annulare: usually seen as a painless subcutaneous nodule

System(s) affected: Skin/Exocrine
Genetics: Not specified, although a familial incidence has been noted among siblings, twins, and successive generations
Incidence/Prevalence in USA: N/A
Predominant age:

- Localized granuloma annulare: young adults
- Disseminated granuloma annulare: younger than age 10 or older than 40 years
- Generalized perforating granuloma annulare: children and young adults
- Subcutaneous granuloma annulare: children

Predominant sex: Females > Males (2:1)

SIGNS & SYMPTOMS

- Papular, flesh-colored or slightly pink, circular or semicircular lesions
- Papules usually found on dorsal surface of hands, fingers, feet, extensor aspects of arms and legs, trunk
- Subcutaneous nodules seen on palms, legs, buttocks, scalp (usually the occiput)
- Papules can perforate
- Lesions may be pruritic on rare occasions, but usually asymptomatic

CAUSES Unknown

RISK FACTORS

- Diabetes mellitus
- Positive family history
- Rheumatoid arthritis
- HIV
- Herpes zoster

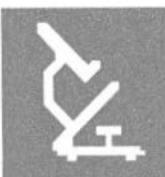

DIAGNOSIS

DIFFERENTIAL DIAGNOSIS

- Papular lesions
  - ◊ Necrobiosis lipoidica
  - ◊ Cutaneous amyloidosis
  - ◊ Annular elastolytic granuloma
  - ◊ Papular sarcoid
  - ◊ Lichen planus
  - ◊ Tinea
  - ◊ Tuberculoid (TT) or borderline tuberculoid (BT) leprosy
  - ◊ Erythema migrans
  - ◊ Verruca plana
  - ◊ Majocchi granuloma
  - ◊ Appendageal hamartomas, e.g., eruptive syringomata
- Subcutaneous nodules
  - ◊ Rheumatoid nodules

LABORATORY If disseminated form, check blood sugar. Also rheumatoid factor if symptoms of RA present.

Drugs that may alter lab results: N/A

Disorders that may alter lab results: N/A

PATHOLOGICAL FINDINGS Palisading granuloma with histiocytes and epithelial cells surrounding a central zone of altered collagen in the mid to upper dermis

SPECIAL TESTS N/A

IMAGING N/A

DIAGNOSTIC PROCEDURES

- Inspection of skin usually reveals diagnosis
- Skin scraping to rule out fungi can be done
- If diagnosis is in doubt, skin biopsy can be performed

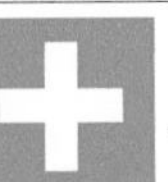

TREATMENT

APPROPRIATE HEALTH CARE Outpatient

GENERAL MEASURES Treatment is not always satisfactory.

SURGICAL MEASURES N/A

ACTIVITY Full activity

DIET American Diabetic Association guidelines when associated with diabetes

PATIENT EDUCATION If patient has disseminated form, papules may be accentuated by sun exposure

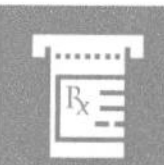

MEDICATIONS

DRUG(S) OF CHOICE
- Localized form - intralesional triamcinolone acetonide, 5-10 mg/mL injected into the elevated border only. A 30 gauge needle is used. May be repeated at monthly intervals.
- Topical steroids with occlusion or incorporated in tape are occasionally useful for localized form
- Superficial lesions of the localized form respond to cryotherapy with liquid nitrogen, but atrophy is possible
- Disseminated form - dapsone 100 mg qd or bid; PUVA or RePUVA

Contraindications: Dapsone should not be given to patients with G6PD deficiency
Precautions: See manufacturer's profile of each drug
Significant possible interactions: See manufacturer's profile of each drug

ALTERNATIVE DRUGS
- For disseminated form isotretinoin 80 mg qd
- For disseminated form, PUVA therapy is used in more refractive cases
- Niacin 1.5 gm qd, potassium iodide or topical vitamin E have all been reported to be effective

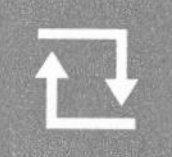

FOLLOWUP

PATIENT MONITORING Depends on nature of treatment; generally two week intervals while undergoing treatment

PREVENTION/AVOIDANCE Avoid sun-exposure in patients with disseminated form if association with light

POSSIBLE COMPLICATIONS Rarely granuloma annulare may involve fascia and tendons leading to sclerosis and deformity

EXPECTED COURSE/PROGNOSIS
- Lesions disappear without scarring in 75% of patients in two years
- 40% of patients experience recurrences, often at the original site

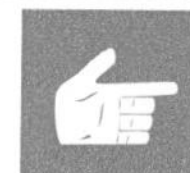

MISCELLANEOUS

ASSOCIATED CONDITIONS
- Diabetes mellitus is mainly associated with disseminated granuloma annulare up to 20% of the time. Likewise, some patients with rheumatoid arthritis have developed granuloma annulare.
- Can be associated with other granulomatous disease, such as, necrobiosis lipoidica, rheumatoid nodules and sarcoidosis
- No definite relationship has been uncovered between granuloma annulare and the presence of occult malignancies. However, in older patients with skin lesions that histologically resemble classic granuloma annulare, investigation for lymphoma or other malignancy should be considered.

AGE-RELATED FACTORS
Pediatric: N/A
Geriatric: Disseminated form is more common in older patients
Others: N/A

PREGNANCY N/A

SYNONYMS N/A

ICD-9-CM
695.89 Other specified erythematous conditions, other

SEE ALSO
Arthritis, rheumatoid (RA)
Diabetes mellitus, Type 1
Diabetes mellitus, Type 2
Sarcoidosis

OTHER NOTES N/A

ABBREVIATIONS N/A

REFERENCES

- Odom RB, James WD, Berger TG. Andrews' Diseases of the Skin. 9th ed. Philadelphia: WB Saunders; 2000
- Habif TP. Clinical Dermatology. 4th ed. New York: Mosby; 2004
- Lebwohl MG, et al, eds. Treatment of Skin Disease. 1st ed. New York: Mosby; 2002
- Li A, Hogan DJ, Sanusi ID, Smoller BR. Granuloma annulare and malignant neoplasms. Am J Dermatopathol 2003;25(2):113-6

Web references: 1 available at www.5mcc.com
Illustrations 6 available

Author(s):
Gary J. Silko, MD, MS

BASICS

DESCRIPTION Benign, solitary mass that involves exposed areas such as distal extremities and face as well as the oral cavity (most frequently the gingiva)
System(s) affected: Gastrointestinal, Skin/Exocrine
Genetics: N/A
Incidence/Prevalence in USA: Unknown
Predominant age: Any, most frequently children and second to fifth decades
Predominant sex: Slight predilection for females

SIGNS & SYMPTOMS
- Sessile or pedunculated
- Granular, smooth or slightly nodular
- Soft
- May be ulcerated, bleeding easily
- Red, purple, or brown in color
- Ranges from a few millimeters to 2-3 centimeters in diameter

CAUSES
- Thought to be an over-reaction to minor trauma
- May be related to hormonal changes in pregnancy

RISK FACTORS
- Pregnancy
- Intraoral trauma or surgery

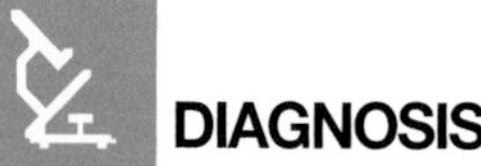

DIAGNOSIS

DIFFERENTIAL DIAGNOSIS
- Peripheral ossifying granuloma
- Giant cell granuloma
- Odontogenic fibroma
- Kaposi sarcoma
- Malignant melanoma
- Angiolymphoid hyperplasia with eosinophilia
- Metastatic carcinoma
- IN AIDS patients, bacillary angiomatosis, deep mycoses

LABORATORY N/A

Drugs that may alter lab results: N/A

Disorders that may alter lab results: N/A

PATHOLOGICAL FINDINGS
- Micro-small, endothelial lined vascular spaces
- Micro- loose or dense connective tissue stroma
- Micro- acute and chronic inflammatory cells
- Micro- no true granuloma formation
- Micro- abundant mitotic activity

SPECIAL TESTS N/A

IMAGING N/A

DIAGNOSTIC PROCEDURES Excisional biopsy

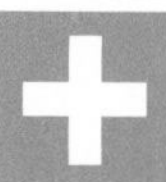

TREATMENT

APPROPRIATE HEALTH CARE Outpatient

GENERAL MEASURES
- Occasional spontaneous resolution
- Good oral hygiene

SURGICAL MEASURES
- Electrosurgery (electrodesiccation and curettage)
- CO2 laser destruction
- Surgical excision of lesion (with cleaning of adjacent teeth if lesion is gingival)
- May recur if inadequately excised

ACTIVITY As tolerated

DIET As tolerated

PATIENT EDUCATION Patient should avoid trauma to the area following excision

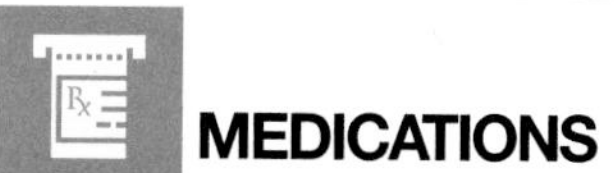

MEDICATIONS

DRUG(S) OF CHOICE None
Contraindications: N/A
Precautions: N/A
Significant possible interactions: N/A

ALTERNATIVE DRUGS N/A

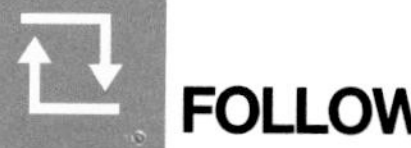

FOLLOWUP

PATIENT MONITORING As needed

PREVENTION/AVOIDANCE Good oral hygiene

POSSIBLE COMPLICATIONS Recurrence. After removal or destruction of a solitary lesion, multiple satellite lesions can form around the original treatment site.

EXPECTED COURSE/PROGNOSIS
Complete resolution expected with adequate excision.

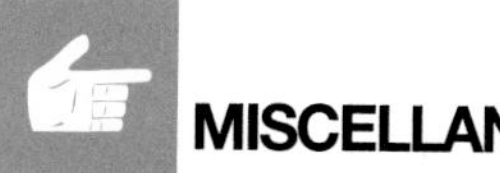

MISCELLANEOUS

ASSOCIATED CONDITIONS N/A

AGE-RELATED FACTORS N/A
Pediatric: N/A
Geriatric: N/A
Others: N/A

PREGNANCY Lesion also occurs in pregnant women, and is known as "pregnancy tumor"

SYNONYMS
- Pregnancy tumor
- Granuloma gravidum

ICD-9-CM
686.1 Pyogenic granuloma
522.6 Chronic apical periodontitis
528.9 Other and unspecified diseases of the oral soft tissues

SEE ALSO

OTHER NOTES N/A

ABBREVIATIONS N/A

REFERENCES

- Wood NK, Goaz PW: Differential Diagnosis of Oral Lesions. St. Louis, C.V. Mosby, 1985
- Ash MM: Oral Pathology. Philadelphia, Lea & Febiger, 1986

Web references: 0 available at www.5mcc.com
Illustrations 3 available

Author(s):
Gregg W. Suits, MD

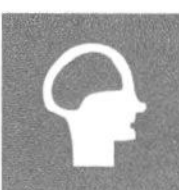

BASICS

DESCRIPTION A group of predominately demyelinating diseases of the peripheral nerves causing acute progressive weakness, usually an ascending paralysis. 30% have respiratory paralysis requiring mechanical ventilation, but complete or substantial recovery is the rule.

- GBS divided into two disease forms:
  - ◊ Demyelinating
    - AIDP (acute inflammatory demyelinating polyradiculoneuropathy): more than 90% cases in western countries, 30% patients have non-specific elevated anti-GM I antibodies
    - Miller-Fisher syndrome: ophthalmoplegia, areflexia, and ataxia of limbs with relatively preserved muscle strength; 90% patients have elevated anti-GQ1b antibodies
  - ◊ Axonal loss (poor prognosis)
    - AMAN (acute motor axonal neuropathy): 5% cases in western countries, more than 50% in northern China. Predominant motor involvement, recent Campylobacter jejuni gastroenteritis.
    - AMSAN (acute motor-sensory axonal neuropathy): occurs mostly in adults

System(s) affected: Nervous
Genetics: Not directly genetically inherited. presumed to be individual's idiosyncratic response to preceding infection, which may have a genetic basis
Incidence/Prevalence in USA: 1-8/100,000 incidence, non-seasonal, non-epidemic
Predominant age: All ages
Predominant sex: Male > Female (1.5:1)

SIGNS & SYMPTOMS
- Dysesthesias, paresthesias of feet and hands are usually the earliest symptoms
- Acute, symmetric, and usually ascending weakness of limbs was notable within days after onset of dysesthesias
- Areflexia associated with muscle weakness, decreased position and vibratory sensation often present
- Gait disorder common in all age groups; the most common presentation in children
- Pain common, especially back, legs; may be severe
- Autonomic neuropathy (50%) with labile blood pressure, cardiac arrhythmias, ileus, and/or urinary retention
- Respiratory muscle paralysis 30% in untreated cases. Neck muscle weakness, dysphagia, and dysarthria were predictors of impending respiratory failure.
- Cranial nerve involvement less than 50%; usually facial weakness, 10-20% ophthalmoparesis

CAUSES
- Autoimmune destruction of myelin and/or axon by antiganglioside antibodies. Activated T-cells, macrophages, and increased matrix metalloproteinases may also play a role.
- Upper respiratory or diarrheal illness within previous 1-3 weeks in 50-70%, including Campylobacter jejuni (30-40%), CMV (13%), EBV (10%), Mycoplasma pneumoniae (5%), HIV
- Vaccinations: swine flu (but not other influenza vaccine) and rabies
- Malignancies (lymphoma, especially Hodgkin)
- Surgery
- Drugs: gold, penicillamine, streptokinase, captopril, danazol, IV heroin, IV gangliosides

RISK FACTORS
- Antecedent infection, especially *C. jejuni*, which has more severe course and higher residual disability. Recent CMV predicts delay in early recovery.
- Diabetes mellitus, recent surgery, organ transplantation

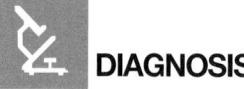

DIAGNOSIS

DIFFERENTIAL DIAGNOSIS
- Brain: acute cerebral vascular strokes, encephalitis
- Spinal cord syndromes: transverse myelitis may have identical presentation in the beginning of the course as GBS, cord compression, cauda equina syndrome, B12 deficiency, HIV, Lyme disease, sarcoid, carcinomatous meningoradiculitis
- Motor neuron: polio
- Peripheral nerve: neuropathy caused by or associated with vasculitis (PAN, Wegner's, Churg-Strauss, nonsystemic vasculitis limited to peripheral nerve), connective tissue disorder, metabolic (diabetes mellitus, alcoholic, hypophosphatemia), disimmune process (paraneoplastic syndrome, POEMS, angiofollicular lymphoma, monoclonal gammopathy, sarcoidosis, multifocal motor neuropathy with conduction block), acute ICU neuromyopathy, amyloidosis, toxin (arsenic or thallium poisoning, Vitamin B6 overdose, glue sniffing, chemotherapeutics), infectious disease (tick paralysis, diphtheria, Lyme disease), flaring of hereditary/congenital neuropathy (porphyria, hereditary neuropathy with liability to pressure palsy, Fabry disease, mitochondria cytopathy), AIDP as initial presentation of 2% of CIDP patients
- Neuromuscular junction: myasthenia gravis, Eaton-Lambert, toxins (botulism, organophosphates), hypermagnesemia
- Muscle: polymyositis, periodic paralysis, toxic myopathy
- Psychiatric: hysteria

LABORATORY
- CSF: elevated protein with normal white cell count (albuminocytological dissociation) is characteristic, except that in patients with HIV aseptic meningitis cell counts may be high. Protein normal in 50% cases in first week of illness.
- Blood:
  - ◊ a) Routine: CBC/eosinophil, TSH/T4, B12/folate, liver and renal function, electrolytes, CK, ESR, hemoglobin A1C, anti-DNA antibodies
  - ◊ b) Others: when appropriate, RF, ANCA, SS-A, SS-B, ACE level, hepatitis B or C antigens, cryoglobulinemia, IPEP, delta-aminolevulinic acid, and Lyme titer
- Urine: 24-hour urine for light chain for disimmune or amyloidosis
- Optional: drug/toxin and heavy metal screen, HIV testing. In children, may check arylsulfatase A activity.

Drugs that may alter lab results: N/A

Disorders that may alter lab results: Demyelinating neuropathy associated with diabetes mellitus may have similar CSF profile as GBS; however GBS usually has higher CSF protein (>0.4g/dL)

PATHOLOGICAL FINDINGS Primary autoimmune attack predominantly involved in motor nerve roots and proximal nerve segments. Sural nerve biopsy not indicated/ considered unless it is necessary to rule out vasculitis or amyloidosis; multifocal inflammatory cell infiltration with demyelination and/or axonal degeneration can be seen.

SPECIAL TESTS Serum anti-GM1 antibody titer in axonal variant

IMAGING
- MRI spinal cord if myelopathy or cord lesion suspected
- Chest X-ray

DIAGNOSTIC PROCEDURES
- Nerve conduction studies: most sensitive test. At the beginning of disease, it may only show prolonged F-wave latency. Conduction block is common in GBS, and characteristic of acquired demyelinating neuropathy (excepting that it can be seen in HNPP uncommonly). Prolonged distal latency and slowing of conduction velocity in at least two nerves each in arms or legs confirms the diagnosis. Very low CMAP amplitude reflects severe axonal loss and portends a prolonged recovery phase in adults.
- Lumbar puncture: elevated protein with normal cell counts

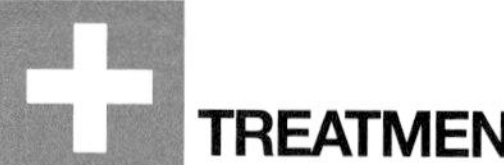

TREATMENT

APPROPRIATE HEALTH CARE
- Hospitalization with monitoring of respiratory function and elective intubation for impending respiratory failure
- IVIG/plasmapheresis for all patients too weak to walk, rapid progression, or poor prognostic indicators
- Intensive care monitoring for dysautonomia and arrhythmias as indicated
- In university hospitals, about 60% GBS patients were admitted into ICU, 50% of those need mechanical ventilation; 10-20% patients have mild disease without the need for intervention by IVIG or plasmapheresis

GENERAL MEASURES
- Serial measurements FVC and oximetry with intubation for respiratory distress or FVC<20 mL/kg (<1L in adults). FVC best measurement (oximetry/ABGs normal until respiratory failure has occurred; peak flow measures air flow resistance not respiratory muscle strength).
- Intubation for difficulty swallowing/aspiration from bulbar palsy
- Cardiac monitoring for arrhythmias: tachyarrhythmias usually do not require treatment; bradyarrhythmias - atropine; sinus arrest and complete heart block - temporary pacemaker
- Hypertension: often does not need treatment. Avoid use beta-blockers or vasodilators, both could precipitate hypotension. In severe HTN, use morphine bolus to prevent congestive heart failure.
- Hypotension: Trendelenburg position and volume expansion (IV fluids)
- Pain common, can be severe and recalcitrant: analgesics including opioids; TCAs, carbamazepine, TENS helpful adjuncts
- Constipation/ileus from autonomic neuropathy: laxatives, enemas
- Urinary retention from autonomic neuropathy: catheterization
- Prevent complications of immobilization, e.g. pneumonia, decubitus ulcers, DVT/PE, contractures
- Depression: frequent reminders that recovery is the rule; antidepressants

SURGICAL MEASURES Tracheostomy for prolonged intubation

ACTIVITY No limitation. Prevent contractures and assist with weakness.

DIET No special diet. Enteral feedings if intubated.

PATIENT EDUCATION Important to stress expectation of full/significant recovery

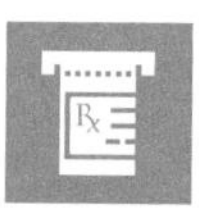

MEDICATIONS

DRUG(S) OF CHOICE
- Immune globulin IV (IVIG) and plasma exchange equally effective, shorten duration and severity of disease. IVIG more available with fewer side effects, but more expensive.
  - ◊ IVIG: 2 g/kg x 2-4 days OR 400 mg/kg/day x 5 consecutive days
  - ◊ Plasmapheresis/plasma exchange: 200-250 mL/kg in 3-5 sessions over 8-13 d
  - ◊ Headache and aseptic meningitis were the frequent side effects of IVIG. Slowing the infusion rate will mitigate such events.
- Steroids not effective and possibly deleterious
- Analgesics for pain

Contraindications: IVIG in IgA deficiency

Precautions:
- IVIG: risk of anaphylaxis (IgA deficiency), acute renal failure in elderly diabetics or pre-existing renal disease, and hepatitis C
- Plasmapheresis: hypotension, autonomic instability, sepsis

Significant possible interactions: N/A

ALTERNATIVE DRUGS
- No advantage to using both IVIG and plasmapheresis over using either one by itself
- Intravenous infusion of monoclonal antibodies to adhesion molecules (eg, integrin), is under investigation and appears to be a promising therapy

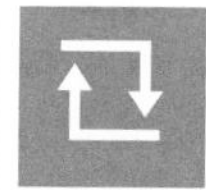

FOLLOWUP

PATIENT MONITORING Physical rehabilitation to regain muscle strength

PREVENTION/AVOIDANCE Avoid influenza vaccination unless clearly indicated

POSSIBLE COMPLICATIONS
- Paralysis, permanent residual weakness
- Respiratory failure, mechanical ventilation
- Hypotension, hypertension, labile BP
- Cardiac arrhythmias
- Ileus
- Urinary retention
- Aspiration, pneumonia, sepsis
- DVT, PE
- Psychiatric problems including depression

EXPECTED COURSE/PROGNOSIS
- Untreated: 3 phases of illness - initial progression phase 24 hours-3 weeks, more than 50% patients reach nadir before 14 days, highest risk of death and complications during this phase. Plateau phase same approximate duration as initial phase. Recovery phase 1-6 months. In adults, no discernible improvement after 2 years.
- 2-5% mortality (most often from dysautonomia or complications), 50% complete recovery, 45% some residual disability, 5% severe permanent disability. Relapses may occur both before and after recovery.
- Poor prognostic signs:
  - ◊ Rapid progression to severe disease (<7d)
  - ◊ Mechanical ventilation
  - ◊ Nerve conduction studies: CMAP <10% or mean distal motor amplitude <20%
  - ◊ AMAN (see Differential Diagnosis)
  - ◊ Preceding *C. jejuni* infection
  - ◊ Age over 60 years

MISCELLANEOUS

ASSOCIATED CONDITIONS Chronic inflammatory demyelinating polyneuropathy (CIDP)

AGE-RELATED FACTORS
Pediatric: Disease tends to be milder
Geriatric: Worse prognosis >60 years
Others: N/A

PREGNANCY No data

SYNONYMS
- Acute inflammatory demyelinating polyradiculopathy
- GBS
- Landry-Guillain-Barre-Strohl syndrome
- Acute inflammatory neuropathy
- Acute idiopathic polyneuritis
- Acute immune mediated polyneuritis (AIMP)
- Landry ascending paralysis
- Acute segmentally demyelinating polyradiculoneuropathy

ICD-9-CM
357.0 Acute infective polyneuritis

SEE ALSO
Amyotrophic lateral sclerosis
Arsenic poisoning
Botulism
Diphtheria
Lead poisoning
Poliomyelitis
Spinal cord compression
Thallium poisoning

OTHER NOTES N/A

ABBREVIATIONS
GBS = Guillain-Barre syndrome
AIDP = acute inflammatory demyelinating polyradiculopathy
AMAN = acute motor axonal neuropathy
AMSAN = acute motor-sensory axonal neuropathy
CMAP = compound muscle action potential
CIDP = chronic inflammatory demyelinating polyneuropathy
DVT = deep vein thrombosis
PE = pulmonary embolism
IVIG = intravenous immunoglobulin
IgA = immunoglobulin A
SLE = systemic lupus erythematosus
PAN = polyarteritis nodosa
CMV = cytomegalovirus
EBV = Epstein-Barr virus
HIV = human immunodeficiency virus

REFERENCES

- Barisic N, et al. Long-term follow-up of children with chronic relapsing polyneuropathy. Pediatric Neurol 2002;26:293-7
- Inaba A, et al. Electrophysiological evaluation of conduction in the most proximal motor root segment. Muscle Nerve 2002;25:608-11
- Bella I, Chad D. Neuromuscular disorders and acute respiratory failure. Neurol Clinics 1998; 6(2):391-417
- Wijdicks EFM. The Clinical Practice of Critical Care Neurology, Chapter 23 Guillain-Barré Syndrome: 290-306. Lippincott-Raven; 1997
- Van Doorn PA, Garssen MP. Treatment of immune neuropathies. Curr Opin Neurol 2002;15(5):623-31
- Green DM, Ropper AH. Mild Guillain-Barré syndrome. Arch Neurol 2001;58(7):1098

Web references: 5 available at www.5mcc.com
Illustrations N/A

Author(s):
Mian Li, MD, PhD
David A. Griesemer, MD

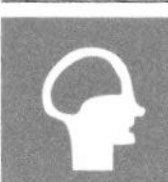

BASICS

DESCRIPTION A benign glandular enlargement of the male breast that is generally bilateral (may be asymmetric or unilateral)
- Type I: Benign adolescent hypertrophy
  - ◊ Physiologic discoid subacute mass
  - ◊ Resolves spontaneously
- Type II: Physiologic gynecomastia
  - ◊ Generalized enlargement to greater degree
- Type III:
  - ◊ Obesity simulates gynecomastia
- Type IV:
  - ◊ Pectoral muscle hypertrophy

System(s) affected: Endocrine/Metabolic, Skin/Exocrine
Genetics: Some instance of familial gynecomastia may be inherited as a male-limited autosomal trait
Incidence/Prevalence in USA:
- 38-64% of pubertal males may have mild form
- Non-pubertal forms are rare except when drug induced

Predominant age: Puberty; and over the age of 65 (especially with a weight gain)
Predominant sex: Male only

SIGNS & SYMPTOMS
- Usually asymptomatic
- May be painful and tender if it has developed rapidly (drug-induced, refeeding gynecomastia)

CAUSES
- Physiologic - transient in neonatal boys and at puberty
- Exposure to a high level of estrogen compared to testosterone concentration
- Tumors - estrogen secreting, gonadotropin secreting and prolactin secreting pituitary adenomas
- Drug-induced (hormones, marijuana, digitalis, spironolactone, cimetidine, ketoconazole, phenytoin, furosemide, verapamil, cytotoxic drugs, antihypertensives, sedatives, antidepressants, amphetamine)
- Systemic disorders - cirrhosis, thyrotoxicosis, renal failure
- Androgen production deficiency
- Androgen resistant syndromes
- Trauma
- Idiopathic

RISK FACTORS
- Klinefelter syndrome
- Obesity
- Testicular failure
- Recovery from prolonged severe illness associated with malnutrition and weight loss (refeeding gynecomastia)
- Family history
- Peutz-Jeghers syndrome
- Male pseudohermaphroditism
- Hyperthyroidism
- Hypothyroidism
- Hepatic disease

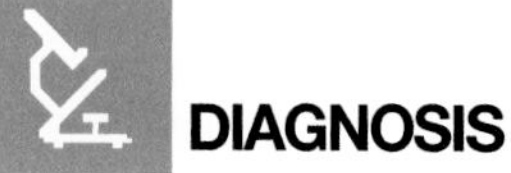

DIAGNOSIS

DIFFERENTIAL DIAGNOSIS
- Obesity with increase in adipose tissue
- Carcinoma of the male breast
- Lipomas
- Neurofibromas

LABORATORY
- Laboratory evaluation rarely indicated
- Human chorionic gonadotropin levels - high levels may lead to finding a choriocarcinoma or other hCG-secreting tumor
- Plasma testosterone and luteinizing hormone measurements - help diagnose hypogonadism
- Serum estradiol
- Serum prolactin
- Liver function
- Others if clinically indicated e.g., thyroid function, chromosomal analysis

Drugs that may alter lab results: N/A

Disorders that may alter lab results:
- Cirrhosis
- Thyrotoxicosis
- Renal failure

PATHOLOGICAL FINDINGS
- Dense, periductal hyaline, collagenous connective tissue
- Hyperplastic ductal lining
- Plasma cell infiltrate

SPECIAL TESTS Full endocrine investigations may be indicated

IMAGING CT, ultrasonography (rarely indicated)

DIAGNOSTIC PROCEDURES
- History and physical exam to determine possible etiology
- Biopsy, if suspicious

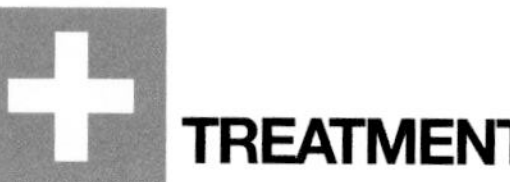

TREATMENT

APPROPRIATE HEALTH CARE Outpatient

GENERAL MEASURES
- Correct underlying disorder
- Withdrawal of causative drug if feasible
- Observation with reassurance that problem is transient
- Danazol and tamoxifen have been used (side effects may be significant)

SURGICAL MEASURES
- Biopsy if suspicious for cancer
- Subcutaneous mastectomy for severe, persistent cases or those with psychological concerns

ACTIVITY No restrictions

DIET
- No special diet
- If obesity a problem, weight loss diet

PATIENT EDUCATION N/A

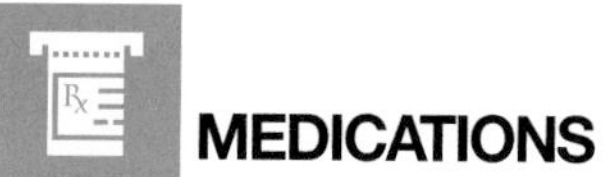

MEDICATIONS

DRUG(S) OF CHOICE None
Contraindications: N/A
Precautions: N/A
Significant possible interactions: N/A

ALTERNATIVE DRUGS N/A

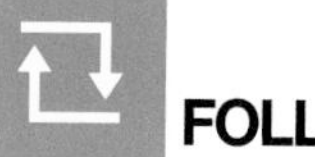

FOLLOWUP

PATIENT MONITORING
- Every 3-6 months for physiologic gynecomastia
- Until well for non-physiologic gynecomastia

PREVENTION/AVOIDANCE In men taking estrogen for prostate cancer - low dose radiation prior to institution of diethylstilbestrol

POSSIBLE COMPLICATIONS
- Nipple inversion may occur following subcutaneous mastectomy
- Asymmetry of breasts
- Postoperative fluid collection
- Withdrawal behavior
- Depression

EXPECTED COURSE/PROGNOSIS
- Physiologic gynecomastia clears without treatment (may take up to 2 years)
- Drug withdrawal cures
- Other causes - outcome depends on etiology
- Little change in Type III without substantial weight loss
- Good results with subcutaneous mastectomy

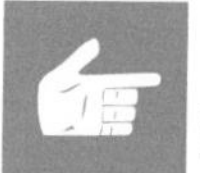

MISCELLANEOUS

ASSOCIATED CONDITIONS Listed with Causes

AGE-RELATED FACTORS
Pediatric:
- Transient gynecomastia seen in neonatal boys
- At puberty, may be observed in 38-64% of boys

Geriatric: Drug induced form more common
Others: N/A

PREGNANCY N/A

SYNONYMS Male breast hypertrophy

ICD-9-CM
611.1 Hypertrophy of breast

SEE ALSO
Klinefelter syndrome

OTHER NOTES N/A

ABBREVIATIONS N/A

REFERENCES

- Becker KL, editor. Principles and Practice of Endocrinology and Metabolism. Philadelphia: J.B. Lippincott Co; 1990
- Ashcraft KW, Murphy JP, Sharp RJ, editors. Pediatric Surgery. 3rd ed. Philadelphia: W.B. Saunders Co; 2000
- Mahoney CP. Adolescent gynecomastia. Differential diagnosis and management. Pediatr Clin North Am 1990;37:1389
- Schwartz SI, Shires GT, Spencer FC, et al, editors. Principles of Surgery. 7th ed. New York: McGraw-Hill Book Co; 1999

Web references: 0 available at www.5mcc.com
Illustrations N/A

Author(s):
Timothy L. Black, MD

BASICS

DESCRIPTION Attacks of severe, unilateral headache typically localized in periorbital area and temple associated with ipsilateral lacrimation, rhinorrhea, ptosis, miosis, and nasal congestion. Individual attacks last 30-180 minutes and occur 1-6 times per day. Two forms exist: episodic with attack phases lasting 4-16 weeks, followed by a cluster-free interval of generally 6 months to years duration; and chronic, with a cluster-free interval of less than 1 week in a 12 month period of time.

System(s) affected: Nervous

Genetics: Unknown

Incidence/Prevalence in USA: 0.5-1% of adult population

Predominant age: Mean age of onset: 30 years in men, later in women

Predominant sex: Male > Female (6:1)

SIGNS & SYMPTOMS

- Sudden onset of severe headache
- Headache reaches crescendo within 15 minutes, lasts < 3 hours
- Pain is unilateral, oculotemporal or oculofrontal; rare in other locations
- Severe, piercing, boring, exploding, penetrating (occasionally throbbing) pain
- Ipsilateral partial Horner syndrome (ptosis and miosis)
- Lacrimation (84%)
- Injected conjunctiva (58%)
- Ptosis (57%)
- Nasal stuffiness (48%)
- Rhinorrhea (43%)
- Bradycardia (43%)
- Nausea (40%)
- Perspiration (26%)
- Restlessness and agitation during attacks
- Attacks may occur at same time for consecutive days; frequently an attack occurs within 90 minutes of falling to sleep (corresponding to first REM sleep)

CAUSES

- Unknown, perhaps:
  - ◊ Disruption of circadian rhythm based on hypothalamus
  - ◊ Disturbed autoregulation of cerebral arteries
  - ◊ Disorder of serotonin metabolism or transmission in CNS
  - ◊ Disorder of histamine concentrations or receptors

RISK FACTORS

- Male gender
- Age > 30 years
- Small amounts of vasodilators, such as, alcohol or nitroglycerin
- Occasional relationship to previous head trauma or surgery

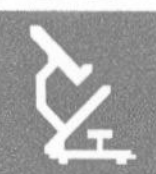

DIAGNOSIS

DIFFERENTIAL DIAGNOSIS Diagnosis generally made through careful history. Differential includes other head and neck pathology, migraine, trigeminal and other facial neuralgias, chronic paroxysmal hemicrania (probably a cluster variant), temporal arteritis, pheochromocytoma.

LABORATORY Not useful except to rule out differential diagnosis

Drugs that may alter lab results: N/A

Disorders that may alter lab results: N/A

PATHOLOGICAL FINDINGS N/A

SPECIAL TESTS N/A

IMAGING Generally of little value except in atypical presentations or those unresponsive to therapy

DIAGNOSTIC PROCEDURES N/A

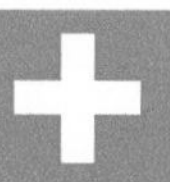

TREATMENT

APPROPRIATE HEALTH CARE Outpatient except in patient at suicidal risk

GENERAL MEASURES

- During cluster periods, avoid alcohol, bright lights and glare, excessive emotion and stress as these may precipitate attacks
- Avoid narcotic analgesics, especially oral preparations
- Tobacco (high predilection for tobacco abuse in this population) may make patients more refractory to therapy

SURGICAL MEASURES Radiofrequency trigeminal gangliolysis in carefully selected refractory patients with strictly unilateral attacks

ACTIVITY

- Avoid self-injury during bouts of excruciating pain
- Vigorous physical activity at first symptom may abort attack in some
- Compression of ipsilateral carotid or temporal artery may reduce pain in some. Caution exercised in recommending carotid massage in patient at risk for occult carotid disease.

DIET

- During cluster phase, alcohol even in small amounts frequently precipitates attacks
- Rarely, specific foods may trigger attacks

PATIENT EDUCATION

- Focus on the validity, natural history, and pathology of the condition
- Advise patient to avoid known precipitants
- Assist patient with learning self-treatment methods
- Provide supportive relationship and follow-up
- Avoid high altitudes

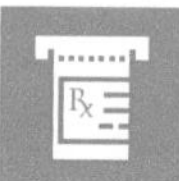

MEDICATIONS

DRUG(S) OF CHOICE

- General information
  - ◊ Prophylactic therapy is paramount
  - ◊ Avoid pain therapy for acute attacks, especially narcotic analgesics
  - ◊ Assess cardiovascular risk before instituting vasoactive drugs, such as, ergotamine or sumatriptan
- Acute attacks
  - ◊ Oxygen 100% at 7-10 liters for 10-15 minutes administered through a tight-fitting face mask with patient in sitting position and breathing at normal respiratory rate
  - ◊ Sumatriptan (Imitrex) 6 mg subcutaneous, maximum of 12 mg per 24 hours with at least 1 hour between injections
  - ◊ Dihydroergotamine mesylate (DHE 45) 1 mg IM or IV. May teach self-administration with SC.
- Prophylaxis (to shorten cluster period or prevent expected attacks):
  - ◊ Verapamil up to 80 mg PO qid spaced evenly through waking hours
  - ◊ Lithium carbonate (Eskalith) 300 mg 2-4 times a day
  - ◊ Ergotamine timed to be at peak serum level during anticipated attack, e.g., 2 mg rectal or 1-2 mg oral 2 hours before. This is especially useful to prevent nocturnal attacks.
  - ◊ Prednisone, various schedules, e.g., 60-80 mg PO for 7 days followed by rapid tapering over 6 days or 40 mg/day for 5 days tapered over 3 weeks. This therapy is initiated while other long-term agent is being employed, such as, verapamil or lithium.

Contraindications: Refer to manufacturer's literature

Precautions: Refer to manufacturer's literature

Significant possible interactions: Refer to manufacturer's literature

ALTERNATIVE DRUGS

- Acute attack:
  - ◊ Lidocaine intranasal instillation of 1 mL of 4% topical solution slowly on same side as symptoms. Position patient supine with head extended 45 degrees and rotated 40 degrees to the side of pain. May need to premedicate with 1-2 drops of intranasal 0.5% phenylephrine for nasal stuffiness.
- Prophylaxis
  - ◊ Indomethacin up to 150 mg per day in divided doses. Absolute responsiveness in chronic paroxysmal hemicrania (CPH) and useful in female cluster patients.
  - ◊ Nifedipine 40-120 mg/day
  - ◊ Nimodipine up to 240 mg/day
  - ◊ Combinations of verapamil and lithium with or without ergotamine may be useful when single drug therapy is ineffective
  - ◊ Histamine desensitization done at certain major headache centers

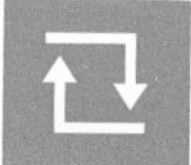

FOLLOWUP

PATIENT MONITORING

- To anticipate cluster bouts and initiate early prophylaxis
- Monitor for adverse medication response and side-effects
- Monitor for unmasking of underlying cardiovascular disorder
- Education for patient and family

PREVENTION/AVOIDANCE

- Alcohol, nitroglycerine, and some foods can induce cluster attack
- Disturbances in sleep cycle can induce attacks (sleep cycle disruption common due to anticipation and occurrence of nocturnal attacks)
- Strong emotions, anger, excessive physical activity may induce attacks
- Tobacco may slow responsiveness to medication
- Narcotics may expedite transformation of episodic cluster to chronic cluster

POSSIBLE COMPLICATIONS

- Self-injury during attack
- Side-effects of medication including unmasking of coronary heart disease
- Potential for drug abuse
- High flow oxygen may be problematic in patients with COPD or who smoke

EXPECTED COURSE/PROGNOSIS

- Recurrent attacks
- Prolonged remissions
- Possibility of transformation of episodic cluster to chronic cluster and occasionally chronic cluster to episodic cluster

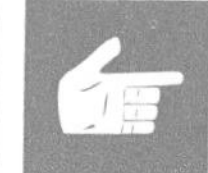

MISCELLANEOUS

ASSOCIATED CONDITIONS

- Significantly higher incidence of peptic ulcer and coronary heart disease (males)
- Prior history of migraine frequently in female patients
- Increased risk of suicide

AGE-RELATED FACTORS

Pediatric: Very rare cases reported

Geriatric: N/A

Others:

- With age - more likely to begin in women, often in peri- or post-menopausal years
- Characteristic appearance - "leonine" face, thickened skin, above average height, more likely to have hazel eye color, and be heavy smokers. No evidence of specific psychologic type.

PREGNANCY Very rare in pregnancy

SYNONYMS

- Migrainous neuralgia
- Sphenopalatine neuralgia
- Histamine cephalalgia
- Horton headache

ICD-9-CM

346.20 Variants of migraine without mention of intractable migraine

346.21 Variants of migraine with intractable migraine, so stated

784.0 Headache

SEE ALSO

Headache, tension

OTHER NOTES N/A

ABBREVIATIONS N/A

REFERENCES

- Cady RK, Fox AW, editors. Treating the Headache Patient. New York: Marcel Dekker; 1995
- Dechant KC, Clissol SP. Sumatriptan (review). Drugs 1992;43:776-98
- Dalessio DJ, Silberstein SD. Wolff's Headache and Other Head Pain. 6th ed. New York: Oxford University Press; 1993
- Raskin NH. Headache. 2nd ed. New York: Churchill Livingstone; 1988

Web references: 2 available at www.5mcc.com

Illustrations N/A

Author(s):

Roger Cady, MD

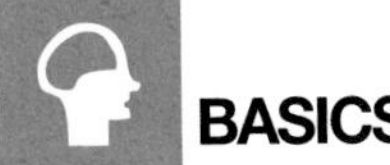

BASICS

DESCRIPTION Tension headache can be divided into two types:
- Episodic - usually associated with some stressful event, is of moderate intensity, self-limited, and usually responds to nonprescription preparations
- Chronic - often recurring daily, bilateral location, usually occipitofrontal and associated with contracted muscles of the neck and scalp

System(s) affected: Musculoskeletal
Genetics: 40% have a positive family history for headache
Incidence/Prevalence in USA: Common
Predominant age: 60% have onset after age 20 (unusual to begin after age 50)
Predominant sex: Female > Male

SIGNS & SYMPTOMS
- Bilateral headache in 90%
- Located fronto-occipital or generalized
- Dull, pressing or band-like
- Intensity varies throughout the day
- Often present upon arising or shortly thereafter
- Chronic headaches have a duration greater than 5 years in 75% of patients
- Insomnia
- Teeth grinding
- Not aggravated by physical activity
- Difficulty concentrating
- Muscular tightness or stiffness in neck, occipital and frontal regions

CAUSES
- Poor posture
- Stress and/or anxiety
- Depression (found in 70% of those with daily headache)
- Low platelet serotonin
- Cervical osteoarthritis
- Intramuscular vasoconstriction

RISK FACTORS
- Obstructive sleep apnea
- Medications
- Excess caffeine

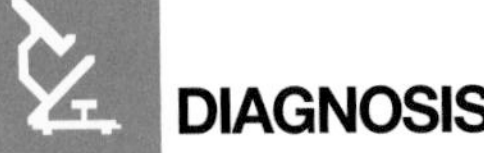

DIAGNOSIS

DIFFERENTIAL DIAGNOSIS
- Cervical spondylosis
- TMJ syndrome
- Caffeine-dependency
- Non-prescription analgesic dependency
- Depression
- Head injury
- Severe anemia or polycythemia
- Uremia and hepatic disorders
- Toxic effects from drugs or fumes
- Dental disease
- Paget disease of bone
- Chronic sinusitis
- Refractive error
- Hypertension
- Hypoxia
- Temporal arteritis
- Migraine
- Lesions of the eye or middle ear
- Lesions of the oral cavity

LABORATORY
- CBC
- SMAC-20
- Thyroid studies
- ESR in anyone over 50 years of age

Drugs that may alter lab results: N/A

Disorders that may alter lab results: Chronic hepatitis, renal and thyroid conditions

PATHOLOGICAL FINDINGS Normal neurological examination, furrowed brow, tense masseter muscle, tight muscles in the scalp and neck

SPECIAL TESTS N/A

IMAGING
- X-rays of cervical spine
- Head CT or MRI necessary only when headache pattern has recently changed or there is a positive finding on neurological exam

DIAGNOSTIC PROCEDURES NA

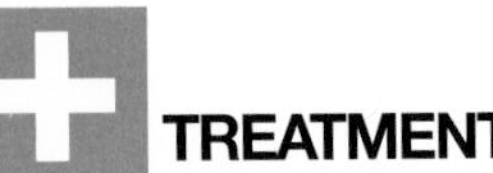

TREATMENT

APPROPRIATE HEALTH CARE Outpatient setting

GENERAL MEASURES
- Relief measures - use relaxation routines; rest in quiet, dark room with cold washcloth over eyes; hot bath or shower; massaging back of neck and temples
- Biofeedback training offers a nonpharmacologic alternative which is often beneficial

SURGICAL MEASURES N/A

ACTIVITY Encourage physical fitness, range of motion and strengthening exercises for the neck

DIET No demonstrated link between diet and tension headache

PATIENT EDUCATION
- Life style changes to minimize stress. Suggest patient seek counseling, if appropriate.
- Encourage relaxation techniques, aerobic exercise, assertiveness training
- Patient information available from the National Headache Foundation, 5252 N. Western Ave., Chicago, IL 60625, (800)843-2256

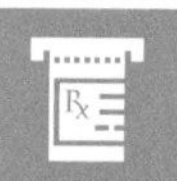

MEDICATIONS

DRUG(S) OF CHOICE
- Acute attack: non-steroidal anti-inflammatory drugs (NSAIDs):
  - ◊ Naproxen sodium (Naprosyn, Aleve) 500 mg/bid
  - ◊ Fenoprofen calcium (Nalfon) 600 mg/day (200 mg q 4-6 hours)
  - ◊ Ibuprofen (Motrin, Advil) 400 mg/tid
  - ◊ Ketoprofen (Orudis) 50 mg/tid
- Prophylaxis for chronic tension headache - antidepressants
  - ◊ Amitriptyline (Elavil) 50-100 mg/day
  - ◊ Desipramine (Norpramin) 50-100 mg/day
  - ◊ Imipramine (Tofranil) 50-100 mg/day
  - ◊ Nortriptyline (Pamelor) 25-50 mg/day

Contraindications:
- NSAIDs and antidepressants, in general, not suitable for use in children
- Antidepressants should not be used concomitantly with MAO inhibitors

Precautions:
- Do not use antidepressants in presence of acute myocardial infarction
- Avoid over dependence on nonprescription caffeine-containing preparations
- Use NSAIDs with precaution in patients with history of previous peptic disease

Significant possible interactions: Antidepressants and alcohol create accentuated depression

ALTERNATIVE DRUGS
- Beta blockers - prophylaxis (select one):
  - ◊ Propranolol (Inderal LA) 80 mg/daily
  - ◊ Nadolol (Corgard) 40 mg/daily
  - ◊ Atenolol (Tenormin) 50-100 mg/daily
- Combination agent - prophylaxis
  - ◊ Isometheptene - dichloralphenazone - acetaminophen (Midrin) one capsule tid
- Other NSAIDs

FOLLOWUP

PATIENT MONITORING A warm, nonjudgmental, understanding relationship with the physician is the best predictor for a successful treatment program

PREVENTION/AVOIDANCE
- Physical therapy
- Biofeedback and relaxation therapy
- Cervical traction
- Injection of trigger points

POSSIBLE COMPLICATIONS
- Undue reliance on non-prescription caffeine-containing analgesics
- Dependence/addiction to narcotic analgesics
- GI bleed from NSAID use
- Risk of addiction to analgesics
- Risk of epilepsy is four times that of the general population

EXPECTED COURSE/PROGNOSIS
- Usually follows a chronic course when life stressors are not changed
- Most cases are intermittent and should not interfere with work or normal life span

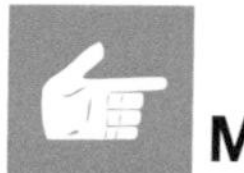

MISCELLANEOUS

ASSOCIATED CONDITIONS 10% of patients with tension headache also have migraine headache

AGE-RELATED FACTORS
Pediatric: 15% will have onset at age less than 10 years
Geriatric: Onset of new headache in the elderly is always worrisome and cause for careful study
Others: Unusual for tension-type headaches to begin after age 50

PREGNANCY No documented relationship

SYNONYMS
- Muscle contraction headache
- Cephalgia

ICD-9-CM
307.81 Tension headache

SEE ALSO

OTHER NOTES N/A

ABBREVIATIONS N/A

REFERENCES

- Coutin IB, Glass SF Recognizing uncommon headache syndromes. Am Fam Phys 1996;54(7):2247-52
- Maizels M: The clinician's approach to the management of headache. West J Med, March 1998;168:203-12
- Smith R. Chronic headaches in family practice. J Am Board Fam Pract 1992;5(6):589-99
- Holroyd KA, O'Donnell FJ, Stensland M, et al. Management of chronic tension-type headache with tricyclic antidepressant medication, stress management therapy, and their combination: a randomized controlled trial. JAMA 2001;285(17):2208-15
- Clinch CR. Evaluation of acute headaches in adults. Am Fam Phys 2001;63(4):685-92
- Lewis DW. Headaches in children and adolescents. Am Fam Phys 2002;65(4):625-32

Web references: 1 available at www.5mcc.com
Illustrations N/A

Author(s):
Don McHard, MD

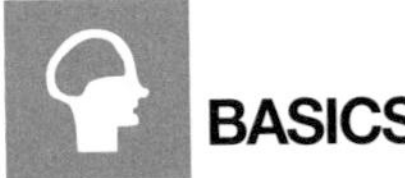

BASICS

DESCRIPTION Complete or partial hearing loss that may involve the middle ear (mechanical, conductive) or the inner ear (nerve, sensorineural)
System(s) affected: Nervous
Genetics: Both types may be on a genetic basis
Incidence/Prevalence in USA:
- 140/100,000/year (134 adults, 6 school age children)
- 3,494 (cases/100,000), with 3,333 for adults and 161 for school age children

Predominant age: All ages, but more common in elderly
Predominant sex: Male = Female

SIGNS & SYMPTOMS Obvious difficulty hearing, with possible association of other symptoms such as tinnitus, dizziness, pain, and fullness

CAUSES
- Conductive
  - ◊ Cerumen impaction
  - ◊ Perforation of tympanica membrane
  - ◊ Middle ear fluid (serous otitis media)
  - ◊ Acute otitis media
  - ◊ Adhesive otitis media
  - ◊ Damage to ossicles (trauma, infection, etc.)
  - ◊ Tympanosclerosis (thickening of drum that may produce fixation)
  - ◊ Otosclerosis (new bone growth that produces stapes fixation)
  - ◊ Cholesteatoma (growth of skin into middle ear)
  - ◊ Middle ear tumor (glomus, etc.)
  - ◊ Congenital problems (atresia, ossicular fixation, etc.)
  - ◊ Temporal bone fracture, injuries
- Sensorineural
  - ◊ Acoustic tumor
  - ◊ Ménière disease
  - ◊ Noise induced (industrial, recreational, occupational)
  - ◊ Hereditary
  - ◊ Congenital
  - ◊ Viral (relatively common, especially mumps)
  - ◊ Ototoxicity (ASA, quinine, gentamicin, kanamycin, etc.)
  - ◊ Syphilis - hearing loss, tinnitus, dizzy
  - ◊ Presbycusis (hearing loss related to aging)
  - ◊ Temporal bone injury, fracture
  - ◊ Metabolic (hypothyroid, etc.)
  - ◊ Perilymphatic (inner ear) fistula (usually secondary to pressure changes or trauma)
  - ◊ Autoimmune disease

RISK FACTORS Nasal allergy and other causes of eustachian tube obstruction; exposure to loud noise levels; use of ototoxic antibiotics; prematurity; heredity (otosclerosis)

DIAGNOSIS

DIFFERENTIAL DIAGNOSIS
- In conductive loss, must rule out cholesteatoma
- In sensorineural loss, must rule out acoustic tumor

LABORATORY N/A

Drugs that may alter lab results: N/A

Disorders that may alter lab results: N/A

PATHOLOGICAL FINDINGS N/A

SPECIAL TESTS
- Audiometry including pure tone and speech testing, and impedance (middle ear pressure) testing. Both types of hearing loss may fluctuate, making audiometric results variable from test to test. Marked conductive loss in one ear may be difficult to exclude (mask) when testing opposite ear.
- Otoscopy with operating microscope (sometimes necessary to see small superior, attic perforation, indicating a cholesteatoma)

IMAGING
- CT scan (not routinely needed) is useful to demonstrate tumors and cholesteatoma of the temporal bone
- MRI scan is more useful to show acoustic and other cerebellopontine angle tumors (usually produce a sensorineural hearing loss)

DIAGNOSTIC PROCEDURES
- Exploratory tympanotomy sometimes necessary to confirm presence of middle ear fluid, tumor, etc.
- Underlying conditions are identified primarily on basis of history of hearing loss, otoscopy, and hearing test (audiometry)
- FTA or equivalent
- Sed rate for autoimmune disease

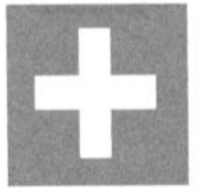

TREATMENT

APPROPRIATE HEALTH CARE Outpatient

GENERAL MEASURES
- Conductive (mechanical)
  - ◊ Cerumen: Remove with suction and irrigation (not if perforation is present). Don't direct water against drum but against canal wall. Manipulation with wire curette may help.
  - ◊ Tympanic membrane perforation: Surgical correction
  - ◊ Serous otitis (primarily in children). Treat underlying conditions. Use decongestants, antibiotics. Urge inflation of eustachian tube (hold nose and blow).
  - ◊ Adhesive otitis: Looks like perforation. Treat eustachian tube problem. May need surgery.
  - ◊ Damage to ossicles: Don't manipulate. Refer to otolaryngologist.
  - ◊ Tympanosclerosis: Drum has white plaques. Treat only if hearing loss is present.
  - ◊ Otosclerosis: Suspect on basis of history of onset, early in life, that is progressive, with positive family history of hearing loss. Consider surgery. Refer to otolaryngologist.
  - ◊ Cholesteatoma: Identify by perforation that is located near margin of drum. Refer to otolaryngologist.
  - ◊ Middle ear tumor: May see through drum. Most commonly will be glomus tumor, which has red color and may cause pulsation. Significant problem, needs prompt referral to otolaryngologist.
  - ◊ Congenital deformity: Don't attribute all hearing loss in children to infections and middle ear fluid. Refer to otolaryngologist.
  - ◊ Temporal bone injury: If limited, may only involve middle ear. Drum likely to appear blue. Refer to otolaryngologist.
- Sensorineural (nerve)
  - ◊ Acoustic tumor: Most significant type of hearing loss. Very important to diagnose promptly. Suspect when unilateral hearing loss and tinnitus (with or without dizziness) are present. Needs much higher degree of suspicion on part of primary care physician. Refer to otolaryngologist.
  - ◊ See topic on Ménière disease
  - ◊ Noise damage: The most common cause of hearing loss in this country. Very frequent on occupational basis, and has the attention of federal government (OSHA regulations). Also occurs secondary to sports and recreation (hunting, use of guns, loud music, chain saws, shop tools). Needs much greater level of recognition at primary care level. Refer to otolaryngologist.
  - ◊ Hereditary/congenital: Needs immediate recognition early in life, so that if significant, hearing aids can be placed. For total or near total hearing loss, cochlear implantation may be suitable with placement of electronic device into mastoid and cochlea.
  - ◊ Viral: A relatively common cause of permanent hearing loss, frequently unilateral, e.g., mumps
  - ◊ Ototoxic (medication): Needs much more recognition at primary care level. Suspect when hearing loss, and perhaps dizziness and tinnitus come on during course of treatment with certain antibiotics (and many other medications). See Medications.
  - ◊ Syphilis: Treat with high dose penicillin given intravenously, as well as steroids
  - ◊ Presbycusis: No specific treatment available, but important to provide hearing rehabilitation. This includes counseling patient to avoid factors that may cause further loss (noise exposure, ototoxic drugs). Emphasize development of lip reading skills, and counseling family to pronounce words clearly, face patient when speaking, etc. Offer hearing aid trial when patient is a suitable candidate.
  - ◊ Temporal bone injury: No treatment available specifically for hearing loss unless middle ear is involved
  - ◊ Metabolic: Treatment of specific problem (e.g. hyperlipidemia, hypothyroid)
  - ◊ Perilymphatic fistula: Diagnosis based on history of injury to ear including barotrauma during diving. Treatment is early exploration to confirm fistula in round or oval window of middle ear, with repair of fistula. Refer to otolaryngologist.

◊ Total or near total sensorineural hearing loss: Cochlear implant (electronic device inserted into mastoid and inner ear)
◊ Autoimmune sensorineural hearing loss: Steroids and chemotherapy. Refer to otolaryngologist.

SURGICAL MEASURES
See General Measures

ACTIVITY
- Patients having perforation of the ear drum or ventilation tube in place should be advised not to swim or allow water to enter the ear
- Patients having hearing loss secondary to noise exposure should be advised to avoid loud noise, or to use suitable protection (ear plugs or ear muffs)

DIET Patients whose hearing loss is due to Ménière disease should avoid excessive use of salt

PATIENT EDUCATION See information under other headings

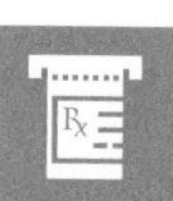

MEDICATIONS

DRUG(S) OF CHOICE
- Cerumen impaction - it is frequently helpful to soften the wax prior to removing it. triethanolamine polypeptide oleate-condensate (Cerumenex) is popular, but should not be used in the presence of a perforation, and may produce a skin reaction. A good alternative is simply to place, or have the patient place mineral oil in the ear canal overnight prior to wax removal. Hexachlorophene (pHisoHex) and topical docusate sodium (Colace) are also useful to soften very hard wax.
- Acute otitis media - erythromycin or amoxicillin
- Chronic otitis media with purulent drainage - neomycin-polymyxin B-hydrocortisone (Cortisporin) otic drops (or an equivalent) placed into the ear canal (3-6 drops bid)
- Serous otitis media - decongestant, e.g., pseudoephedrine - guaifenesin (Entex PSE) and erythromycin
- Sudden sensorineural hearing loss with no apparent cause - steroid therapy in high dosage form (80 mg/day of prednisone, or equivalent steroid) may be helpful

Contraindications: History of sensitivity to any of the antibiotics referred to above
Precautions: Avoid the temptation of over-diagnosing "red ear" and using antibiotics without a well thought out diagnosis
Significant possible interactions: Refer to manufacturer's literature

ALTERNATIVE DRUGS
- Acute otitis media - cefaclor
- Chronic ear infection with drainage - ear drops and powder containing ciprofloxacin. Gentamicin drops is another alternative.

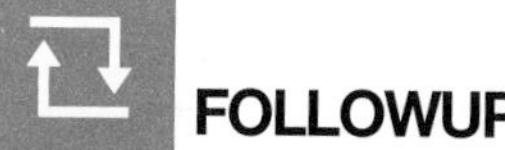

FOLLOWUP

PATIENT MONITORING Hearing testing (audiometry) is the primary means of monitoring patient progress

PREVENTION/AVOIDANCE
- Impaired eustachian tube function (serous otitis media, acute otitis media) - improve tubal function with treatment of allergic and sinus disease. Treat upper respiratory infections (URI) promptly and aggressively if ear problems are frequent.
- Sensorineural hearing loss due to noise exposure (or any type of nerve deafness) - advise against excessive noise exposure; recommend ear plugs/ear muffs
- Nerve deafness due to ototoxic medications may be prevented by the avoidance, or careful use of drugs known to be ototoxic (consider audiometric monitoring if used). The most frequently implicated antibiotics are gentamicin, kanamycin, neomycin, vancomycin, and streptomycin. Other implicated drugs include lidocaine, morphine, digitalis, quinidine, and furosemide. Use of these drugs cannot always be avoided. Be more suspicious of the possibility that a given medication might be ototoxic, and when hearing loss is a problem, to prescribe with care.
- Serious nerve deafness resulting from CNS disease (meningitis, lues) may be prevented by thorough treatment of the primary problem
- If URI present, avoid flying or diving

POSSIBLE COMPLICATIONS
- Middle ear problems may progress to chronic ear problems (perforations, cholesteatoma)
- Cholesteatoma is capable of producing major complications including permanent loss of hearing, balance problems, facial nerve paralysis, meningitis, lateral sinus thrombosis, and brain abscess. Glomus tumors and acoustic tumors must be identified, or major CNS complications may result.
- Ménière disease may proceed to total and permanent hearing loss if not treated, and may occur in spite of treatment
- Severe nerve deafness, particularly associated with tinnitus may produce such an emotional impact on the patient that suicide may occur. Treat the patient with empathy and understanding, offer help even if it seems limited. Encouragement and followup care are extremely helpful in managing these patients.

EXPECTED COURSE/PROGNOSIS
Sensorineural hearing loss is usually permanent, but in a few instances, may be stabilized, improved, or even cured

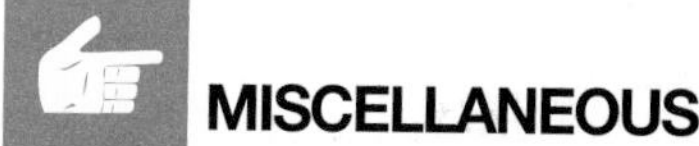

MISCELLANEOUS

ASSOCIATED CONDITIONS Noise, allergy, sinus disease, trauma, heredity, ototoxicity, CNS infections (meningitis, lues), age, hyperlipidemia, hypothyroid, barotrauma and autoimmune disease

AGE-RELATED FACTORS
Pediatric: Eustachian tube problems and secondary middle ear problems are more common in infants and small children, usually becoming less frequent by approximately age 10
Geriatric: Presbycusis is common and is made worse by noise exposure and other factors
Others: N/A

PREGNANCY Otosclerosis may become active during pregnancy

SYNONYMS N/A

ICD-9-CM
380.4 Impacted cerumen
385.00 Tympanosclerosis, unspecified as to involvement
387.9 Otosclerosis, unspecified
382.00 Acute suppurative otitis media without spontaneous rupture of ear drum
382.01 Acute suppurative otitis media with spontaneous rupture of ear drum

SEE ALSO
Ménière disease

OTHER NOTES N/A

ABBREVIATIONS SNHL = sensorineural hearing loss

REFERENCES

- Lucente FE, Gady HE. Essentials of Otolaryngology. 4th ed. Philadelphia, Lippincott Williams & Wilkins, 1999:63-76

Web references: 3 available at www.5mcc.com
Illustrations N/A

Author(s):
Gale Gardner, MD

Heat exhaustion & heat stroke

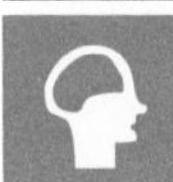

BASICS

DESCRIPTION A continuum of increasingly severe heat illnesses caused by dehydration, electrolyte losses, and failure of the body's thermoregulatory mechanisms
- Heat exhaustion is an acute heat injury with hyperthermia due to dehydration
- Heat stroke is extreme hyperthermia with thermoregulatory failure and profound central nervous system dysfunction

System(s) affected: Endocrine/Metabolic, Nervous
Genetics: N/A
Incidence/Prevalence in USA: Dependent on predisposing conditions in combination with environmental factors
Predominant age: More likely in children or elderly
Predominant sex: Male = Female

SIGNS & SYMPTOMS
- Heat Exhaustion
  - ◊ Fatigue and lethargy
  - ◊ Weakness
  - ◊ Dizziness
  - ◊ Nausea, vomiting
  - ◊ Myalgias
  - ◊ Headache
  - ◊ Profuse sweating
  - ◊ Tachycardia
  - ◊ Hypotension
  - ◊ Lack of coordination
  - ◊ Agitation
  - ◊ Intense thirst
  - ◊ Hyperventilation
  - ◊ Paresthesias
  - ◊ Core temperature elevated but < 103°F (< 39.4°C)
- Heat Stroke
  - ◊ Exhaustion
  - ◊ Confusion, disorientation
  - ◊ Coma
  - ◊ Hot, flushed, dry skin
  - ◊ Core temperature > 105°F (> 40.5°C)

CAUSES Failure of heat-dissipating mechanisms or an overwhelming heat stress leading to a rise in core temperature, dehydration and salt depletion

RISK FACTORS
- Poor acclimatization to heat or poor physical conditioning
- Salt or water depletion
- Obesity
- Acute febrile or gastrointestinal illnesses
- Chronic illnesses - uncontrolled diabetes or hypertension, cardiac disease
- Alcohol and other substance abuse
- High heat and humidity, poor air circulation in environment
- Heavy, restrictive clothing
- Nutritional supplementation that includes ephedra

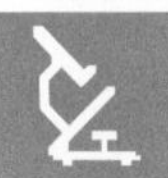

DIAGNOSIS

DIFFERENTIAL DIAGNOSIS
- Other causes of elevated temperature, dehydration or circulatory collapse
  - ◊ Febrile illnesses, sepsis
  - ◊ Drug-induced fluid loss
  - ◊ Cardiac arrhythmia or infarction
  - ◊ Acute cocaine intoxication
  - ◊ Malignant hyperthermia (an autosomally inherited disorder of skeletal and cardiac muscle in which patients have abnormal muscle metabolism on exposure to halothane or skeletal muscle reactants)

LABORATORY
- Used primarily to detect end-organ damage
- Electrolytes, urinalysis
- Creatinine, blood urea nitrogen
- Liver enzymes
- Complete blood count
- Increased urine specific gravity
- Results of above studies yield hypernatremia, hyperchloremia, hemoconcentration

Drugs that may alter lab results: Diuretics

Disorders that may alter lab results: N/A

PATHOLOGICAL FINDINGS Only those associated with major organ system failure

SPECIAL TESTS N/A

IMAGING N/A

DIAGNOSTIC PROCEDURES Rectal temperature monitoring

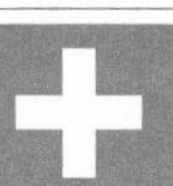

TREATMENT

APPROPRIATE HEALTH CARE Emergency treatment - best in a hospital setting

GENERAL MEASURES
- Rapid cooling - remove clothing, wet patient down, ice packs
- Fluid and electrolyte replacement with hypotonic oral fluids or IV 0.5-1.0 liter normal saline
- Consider central venous pressure monitoring

SURGICAL MEASURES N/A

ACTIVITY Rest with legs elevated

DIET
- Cool or cold clear liquids only (non-carbonated)
- Avoid caffeine
- Unrestricted sodium

PATIENT EDUCATION
- Stress the importance of proper conditioning and acclimatization
- Instruct patients to recognize heat stress signs and symptoms
- Maintain as much skin exposure as possible in hot, humid conditions, while using proper sun block protection
- Avoid dehydration with proper fluids during activity or exercise - 8 oz fluid intake for every 15 minutes of moderate exercise
- Never leave children unattended in cars during hot weather
- Try to gain access to air conditioned environment during hot weather

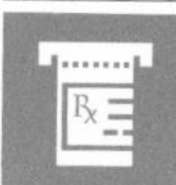

MEDICATIONS

DRUG(S) OF CHOICE No medications are required in the initial management. Use isotonic saline solution to rehydrate.
Contraindications: N/A
Precautions: N/A
Significant possible interactions: N/A

ALTERNATIVE DRUGS
- Consider immunomodulators such as corticosteroids
- In disseminated intravascular coagulation, consider appropriate replacement therapy

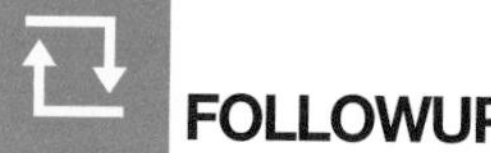

FOLLOWUP

PATIENT MONITORING
- Rectal temperature monitoring - cooling may be discontinued when the core temperature drops to 102°F (38.9°C) and stabilizes
- Heat stroke patients may require airway management, hemodynamic monitoring and careful fluid and electrolyte administration and monitoring
- Consider central venous pressure monitoring

PREVENTION/AVOIDANCE Most important factor in preventing heat stress is adequate fluid replacement. Allow acclimatization to hot weather through proper conditioning and activity modification. Dress appropriately with loose-fitting, open weave, light-colored clothing.

POSSIBLE COMPLICATIONS
- May involve failure of any major organ system
- Cardiac arrhythmias or infarction
- Pulmonary edema, adult respiratory distress syndrome
- Coma, seizures
- Acute renal failure
- Rhabdomyolysis
- Disseminated intravascular coagulation
- Hepatocellular necrosis

EXPECTED COURSE/PROGNOSIS
- Good when mental function is not altered and when serum enzymes are not elevated. Recovery is within 24-48 hours in most cases.
- The mortality rate for heat stroke (10-80%) is directly related to the duration and intensity of hyperthermia as well as to the speed and effectiveness of diagnosis and treatment

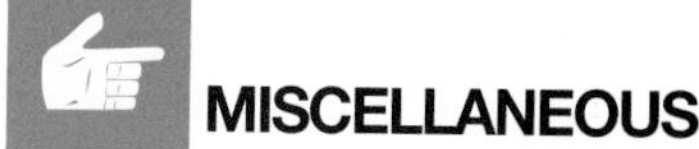

MISCELLANEOUS

ASSOCIATED CONDITIONS N/A

AGE-RELATED FACTORS
Pediatric: Children are more susceptible
Geriatric: Elderly are more susceptible
Others: N/A

PREGNANCY May be more prone to volume depletion with heat stress

SYNONYMS
- Heat illness
- Heat injury
- Hyperthermia
- Heat collapse
- Heat prostration

ICD-9-CM
992.5 Heat exhaustion, unspecified
992.0 Heat stroke and sun stroke

SEE ALSO
Hyperthermia, malignant

OTHER NOTES N/A

ABBREVIATIONS N/A

REFERENCES

- Graham BS. Features and outcomes of classic heat stroke. Annals of Int Med 1999;130(7):613-14
- Griffin SL, Gardner JW, Flinn SD. Cooling methods for heat stroke victims. Annuls Int Med 2000;132(8):678
- Khosla R; Guntupalli KK. Heat related illnesses. Crit Care Clin 1999;15(2):251-63
- Brouchama A. Heat stroke: a new look at an ancient disease. Int Care Med 1995;21(8):623-25
- Bross MH, Nash BT, Carlton F. Heat emergencies. Am Fam Phys 1994;50(2):389-96
- Keatinge WR, Donaldson GC, Cordioli E, et al. Heat related mortality in warm and cold regions of Europe: observational study. BMJ 2000;321(7262):670-3
- Bouchama A, Knochel JP. Heat stroke. N Engl J Med 2002;346(25):1978-88
- Charaton F. Ephedra supplement may have contributed to sportsman's death. BMJ 2003;326(7387):464

Web references: 2 available at www.5mcc.com
Illustrations N/A

Author(s):
Scott A. Fields, MD

BASICS

DESCRIPTION Can be gross or microscopic. Symptomatic or asymptomatic. It can be at the beginning (initial), end (terminal) or throughout (total) the urine stream.
System(s) affected: Renal/Urologic
Genetics: N/A
Incidence/Prevalence in USA: Up to 15% of general population, though typically <1%
Predominant age: All ages
Predominant sex: Female>Male

SIGNS & SYMPTOMS
- Generally none
- Red or rose-colored urine with gross hematuria

CAUSES
- Trauma
  - ◊ Exercise-induced (resolves with rest)
  - ◊ Abdominal trauma with renal or ureteral injury
  - ◊ Pelvic fracture with bladder or urethral injury
  - ◊ Iatrogenic trauma after catheterization, abdominal, or pelvic surgery
  - ◊ Foreign body, physical/sexual abuse
- Neoplasms
  - ◊ Malignancies of prostate, urethra, bladder, ureter, kidney may present with hematuria (30% of patients with gross hematuria will have a malignancy, 5% of patients with microscopic hematuria)
  - ◊ Benign tumors
  - ◊ Endometriosis of the urinary tract (suspect in females with cyclic hematuria)
- Inflammatory
  - ◊ UTI: probably the most common cause of hematuria in adults
  - ◊ Renal diseases: glomerulonephritis, radiation nephritis, radiation cystitis, pyelonephritis
  - ◊ Endocarditis
- Metabolic
  - ◊ Calculus disease (85% of patients have hematuria)
  - ◊ Hypercalciuria with microcalculi or nephrocalcinosis; most common cause of hematuria in children without UTI or glomerulonephritis
- Congenital
  - ◊ Cystic disease: polycystic kidney disease, solitary renal cyst
  - ◊ Benign familial hematuria or thin basement membrane nephropathy
  - ◊ Alport syndrome (hematuria, proteinuria, hearing loss)
  - ◊ Renal tubular acidosis type 1, cystinuria, oxalosis
- Hematologic
  - ◊ Bleeding dyscrasias: e.g., hemophilia
  - ◊ Henoch-Schönlein purpura
  - ◊ Sickle-cell anemia
- Vascular
  - ◊ Hemangioma
  - ◊ A-V malformations (rare)
  - ◊ "Nutcracker syndrome". Compression of left renal vein and subsequent renal parenchymal congestion
  - ◊ Renal vein thrombosis
  - ◊ Arterial emboli to kidney
- Chemical
  - ◊ Nephrotoxins: aminoglycosides, cyclosporine
- Obstruction
  - ◊ Hydronephrosis, from any cause
  - ◊ BPH - rule out other causes of hematuria
- Idiopathic
  - ◊ Loin pain hematuria (most often young women on oral contraceptives)

RISK FACTORS
- Smoking
- Occupation exposures, e.g., organic chemical exposure
- Analgesic abuse (eg, phenacetin)
- Medications (eg. cyclophosphamide)
- Pelvic irradiation
- Chronic infection, especially with calculi
- Recent upper respiratory tract infection
- Positive family history of renal diseases (stones, glomerulonephritis)

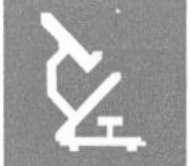

DIAGNOSIS

DIFFERENTIAL DIAGNOSIS
- Artifactual discoloration of the urine (pseudohematuria)
  - ◊ Dehydration
  - ◊ Dyes, e.g., phenazopyridine (Pyridium), rifampin, food colorings
  - ◊ Precipitated urate crystals cause a pink or red urine color (e.g., in neonates)
- Vaginal bleeding (e.g., menses, dysfunctional uterine bleeding, vaginal trauma)
- Genital/perineal trauma
- Malingering/other secondary gain (urine obtained by catheterization will be helpful)

LABORATORY
- Urine dipstick
  - ◊ False negatives: high-dose Vitamin C; low urine pH (<5)
  - ◊ False positives: oxidizers (povidone, bacterial peroxidases, bleach), myoglobin
- Urinalysis; confirm dipstick findings and quantify RBCs (normal urine contains ≤ 5 RBCs/high power field on any single specimen and ≤ 3 RBCs/high power field on any 2 successive specimens on centrifuged specimens). Red cell casts pathognomonic of glomerular bleeding. Proteinuria (large) suggests glomerular leak. Dysmorphic RBCs most often from glomerular origin.
- Urine culture if pyuria is present
- Renal function tests: BUN and creatinine
- PT for patients on warfarin or suspected of abusing warfarin
- CBC may show elevated WBC, anemia unlikely from hematuria although gross hematuria can produce significant blood loss. Anemia and microscopic hematuria usually secondary to chronic disease
- Urine cytology, although "atypical" cells can be seen with benign conditions. Good for high grade transitional cell carcinoma

Drugs that may alter lab results:
- Vitamin C; false negative dipstick
- Phenazopyridine may discolor the dipstick making interpretation difficult

Disorders that may alter lab results: N/A

PATHOLOGICAL FINDINGS
- Glomerulonephritis

SPECIAL TESTS
- Renal biopsy may be necessary to diagnosis glomerulonephritis and with gross hematuria and crescentic nephritis, urgent immunosuppressive therapy may be needed
- Retrograde pyelogram can be considered in patients with documented allergy to IV contrast
  - ◊ Sensitive for small lesions of supravesical collecting system
  - ◊ Valuable for patients with allergy or contraindication to iodine contrast because contrast is not absorbed in this test
  - ◊ Requires cystoscopy
- Cystoscopy
  - ◊ Best for evaluation of bladder pathology especially small transitional carcinomas
  - ◊ Flexible cystoscopy is less painful and may have increased sensitivity
- Ureteroscopy/pyeloscopy
  - ◊ Best for visualization of suspected supravesical collecting system lesions
  - ◊ Biopsy, excision, fulguration, or extraction of lesions/stones possible
  - ◊ Requires anesthesia
  - ◊ Requires cystoscopy
  - ◊ Risk of injury to collecting system

IMAGING
- Intravenous pyelogram (IVP)
  - ◊ Overall best study, widely available, cost efficient
  - ◊ Limited sensitivity for small renal masses, and differentiating cystic from solid masses
  - ◊ Addition of tomography increases sensitivity
  - ◊ Potential reactions to intravenous iodine contrast media (especially with dehydration, diabetic, on metformin, and in pre-existent renal insufficiency)
- Renal ultrasonography
  - ◊ Best for differentiating cystic from solid masses and finding radiolucent stones
  - ◊ Sensitive for hydronephrosis
  - ◊ No radiation or iodinated contrast exposure
  - ◊ Cost efficient
  - ◊ Poor sensitivity for small renal masses
- CT
  - ◊ Most sensitive for evaluating renal masses, and perirenal pathology
  - ◊ Visualizes major renal vasculature
  - ◊ Satisfactory for stone detection but can misinterpret non-urologic calcifications
  - ◊ Visualization of ureters is discontinuous
  - ◊ Less cost efficient
  - ◊ Potential reactions to intravenous iodine contrast media identical to IVP
  - ◊ Need for oral contrast media to opacify bowel
- MRI
  - ◊ Similar to CT in sensitivity for renal masses
  - ◊ No radiation exposure
  - ◊ Least cost efficient

DIAGNOSTIC PROCEDURES

- Urine dipsticks are not adequately reliable because specificity is only 65% (high sensitivity however).
- Criterion is based on midstream fresh clean catch voided urine sample. More than 3 RBC per high power field on 2 of 3 successive urine specimens or more than 5 RBC per high power field on any single specimen is considered abnormal. (See OTHER NOTES for urine preparation.)
- Casts are best observed in fresh urine and may only be observed near the edges of the slide; delays in performing the urinalysis will decrease its usefulness as a diagnostic test, particularly for nephritis
- Exclude benign, factitious, or non-urinary causes such as menstruation, mild trauma, exercise-induced, poor collection technique, chemical/drug causes, infection and hematologic
- Differentiate intrinsic renal parenchymal disease from other causes. Indicators of renal disease are significant proteinuria, red cell casts, increased creatinine in absence of obstruction
- Consider nephrology evaluation to determine etiology of primary renal disease
- Non-intrinsic renal parenchyma] disease requires urologic evaluation. Depth of evaluation depends on high- or low-risk status for presence of pathology:
  - ◊ Upper urinary tract imaging adequate to determine presence or absence of abnormalities
  - ◊ Cystoscopy to evaluate lower urinary tract
  - ◊ Urine cytology for high risk of transitional cell carcinoma
  - ◊ Other modalities as needed to obtain detailed enough view of entire urinary system

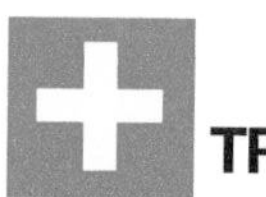

TREATMENT

APPROPRIATE HEALTH CARE Outpatient

GENERAL MEASURES N/A

SURGICAL MEASURES

- Gross hematuria: Clots may require continuous bladder irrigation with a large bore Foley catheter (2 or 3-way catheter may be helpful) to prevent clot retention
- In trauma, the degree of hematuria is not well related to the degree of injury and additional imaging and surgical intervention may be required

ACTIVITY Not restricted although trauma may necessitate inpatient care

DIET Not restricted; consider dye/drug ingestion in artifactual urine discoloration

PATIENT EDUCATION N/A

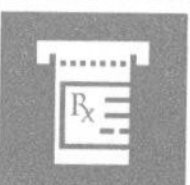

MEDICATIONS

DRUG(S) OF CHOICE

- None indicated for undiagnosed hematuria

Contraindications: N/A
Precautions: N/A
Significant possible interactions: N/A

ALTERNATIVE DRUGS N/A

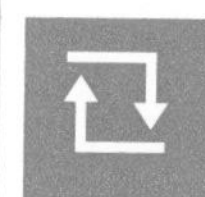

FOLLOWUP

PATIENT MONITORING

- After initial workup, 35% of patients remain without a diagnosis
- Followup of hematuria is unclear; some experts recommend "periodic" urinalysis and cytology while others suggest only symptomatic patients be re-evaluated
- Re-evaluation indicated for recurrence of gross hematuria, positive cytology, or significant symptoms, increasing proteinuria, presence of red cell casts, worsening renal function

PREVENTION/AVOIDANCE

- Minimize indwelling catheterization; attempt to remove post-operative urinary catheters by post-op day 3

POSSIBLE COMPLICATIONS N/A

EXPECTED COURSE/PROGNOSIS

- Generally excellent for common causes of hematuria
- Malignant tumors and certain types of nephritis have a poorer prognosis

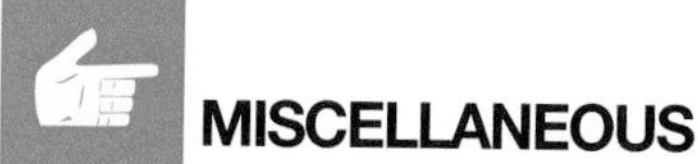

MISCELLANEOUS

ASSOCIATED CONDITIONS

- Hypertension
- Nephrotic syndrome

AGE-RELATED FACTORS

Pediatric: Consider glomerulonephritis, child abuse. Cystoscopy rarely needed, voiding cystourethrogram may be helpful
Geriatric: Suspect UTI, sometimes occult
Others: N/A

PREGNANCY Consider vaginal source of bleeding

SYNONYMS N/A

ICD-9-CM

599.7 Hematuria

SEE ALSO

Endocarditis, infective
Hemophilia
Renal calculi
Renal cell carcinoma
Urinary tract infection in females
Urinary tract infection in males

OTHER NOTES

- Preparation for routine urinalysis
  - ◊ Centrifuge approximated 10 mL of fresh, midstream, clean-catch voided urine
  - ◊ Discard the supranatant
  - ◊ Place the spun sediment on a glass slide and cover with a cover slip
  - ◊ Observe with the 40 power microscope lens

ABBREVIATIONS

REFERENCES

- Grossfeld GD, Litwin MS, Wolf JS, et al. Evaluation of asymptomatic microscopic hematuria in adults: the American Urological Association best practice policy--part I: definition, detection, prevalence, and etiology. Urology 2001;57(4):599-603
- Walsh PC, ed. Campbell's Urology. 7th Ed. Philadelphia: Saunders: 1998
- Sutton JM. Evaluation of hematuia in adults. JAMA 1990;263:2475-80

Web references: 0 available at www.5mcc.com
Illustrations N/A

Author(s):
Ira N. Hollander, MD

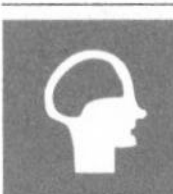

BASICS

DESCRIPTION A hereditary disorder in which the small intestine absorbs excessive iron. Since the body lacks any way to excrete iron, the excess is stored in glands and muscle, such as the liver, pancreas, and heart. Over the years, the involved organs begin to fail.
System(s) affected: Endocrine/Metabolic
Genetics: Autosomal recessive; acquired; mutation in HFE gene. The stereotypic expression of the mutation is variable. A small proportion of homozygotes have no evidence of iron overload, indicating other influences such as environmental factors.
Incidence/Prevalence in USA: 3 cases/1000 people (heterozygote frequency 1 in 10) - the most common abnormal gene in the US population
Predominant age: Present from birth, but symptoms usually present in the fifth and sixth decades
Predominant sex: Male = Female (clinical signs are more frequent in men [8:1 male to female ratio])

SIGNS & SYMPTOMS

- Weakness (83%)
- Abdominal pain (58%)
- Arthralgia (43%)
- Loss of libido or potency (38%)
- Amenorrhea (22%)
- Dyspnea on exertion (15%)
- Neurologic symptoms (6%)
- Hepatomegaly (83%)
- Increased skin pigmentation (75%)
- Loss of body hair (20%)
- Splenomegaly (13%)
- Peripheral edema (12%)
- Jaundice (10%)
- Gynecomastia (8%)
- Ascites (6%)
- Testicular atrophy
- Hepatic tenderness
- Diabetes mellitus symptoms

CAUSES

- The mechanism for increased iron absorption in the face of excessive iron stores is unknown. Iron metabolism appears normal in this disease except for a higher level of circulating iron.
- Iron overload may be due to thalassemia, sideroblastic anemia, liver disease, excess iron intake, chronic transfusion

RISK FACTORS

- The disease is a genetic disorder. Some variables influence the age of onset and severity of symptoms.
- Intake of iron, especially from vitamin supplements. These may contain large amounts of iron as well as vitamin C, which enhances iron absorption.
- Alcohol increases the absorption of iron (as high as 41% of patients with symptomatic disease are alcoholic)
- Loss of blood delays the onset of symptoms, such as blood loss in women because of menstruation and pregnancy.

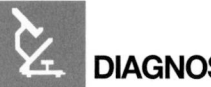

DIAGNOSIS

DIFFERENTIAL DIAGNOSIS

- Repeated transfusions
- Hereditary anemias with ineffective erythropoiesis
- Alcoholic cirrhosis
- Porphyria cutanea tarda
- Atransferrinemia
- Excessive ingestion of iron (rare)

LABORATORY

- Transferrin saturation (serum iron concentration divided by total iron-binding capacity x 100): greater than 70% is virtually diagnostic of iron overload; 45% or higher warrants further evaluation
- Serum ferritin: greater than 300 μg/L for men and postmenopausal women and 200 μg/L for pre-menopausal women
- Urinary iron
- Increased urine hemosiderin
- Hyperglycemia
- Decreased FSH
- Decreased LH
- Decreased testosterone
- Increased SGOT
- Hypoalbuminemia

Drugs that may alter lab results: Iron supplements, transfusions may elevate serum iron

Disorders that may alter lab results: Inflammatory reactions, other forms of liver disease, certain tumors (e.g., acute granulocytic leukemia), rheumatoid arthritis may elevate serum ferritin

PATHOLOGICAL FINDINGS

- Increased hepatic parenchymal iron stores
- Hepatic fibrosis and cirrhosis with hepatomegaly
- Pancreatic enlargement
- Excess hemosiderin in liver, pancreas, myocardium, thyroid, parathyroid, joints, skin
- Cardiomegaly
- Joint deposition of iron

SPECIAL TESTS After diagnosis established, consider oral glucose tolerance test to rule out diabetes and echocardiogram to rule out cardiomyopathy

IMAGING Not indicated unless used to evaluate suspected liver disease

DIAGNOSTIC PROCEDURES

- Liver biopsy for stainable iron is the standard for diagnosis. Presence or absence of cirrhosis can also be ascertained.
- DNA PCR testing for HFE gene mutations C282Y and H63D - present in 85-90% of patients
- Homozygosity for the C282Y mutation with biochemical evidence for iron overload can confirm the diagnosis

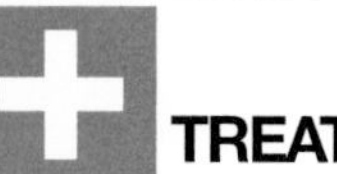

TREATMENT

APPROPRIATE HEALTH CARE Outpatient

GENERAL MEASURES

- Removal of excess iron by repeated phlebotomy once or twice weekly to establish and maintain a mild anemia (hematocrit of 37-39%)
- When the patient finally becomes iron deficient, a lifelong maintenance program of 4-6 phlebotomies a year to keep storage iron normal - maintain serum ferritin ≤ 50 μg/L

SURGICAL MEASURES N/A

ACTIVITY Full activity unless significant heart disease

DIET

- An iron-poor diet is not of significant benefit
- Avoid alcohol, iron-fortified foods, iron-containing supplements, and uncooked shellfish
- Restrict vitamin C to small doses between meals
- Tea chelates iron and may be drunk with meals

PATIENT EDUCATION

- Iron Overload Diseases Association, Inc., 433 Westwind Dr., North Palm Beach, FL 33408
- American Hemochromatosis Society, Inc., 4044 W. Lake Mary Blvd., Unit #104, Lake Mary, FL 32746-2012

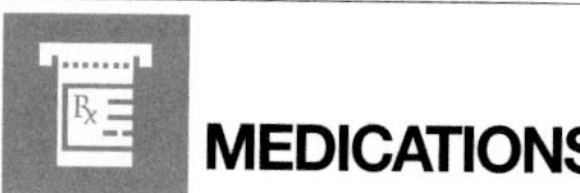

MEDICATIONS

DRUG(S) OF CHOICE None. Only when phlebotomy is not feasible or in the presence of severe heart disease should the iron-chelating agent deferoxamine (Desferal) be considered.
Contraindications: N/A
Precautions: N/A
Significant possible interactions: N/A

ALTERNATIVE DRUGS None

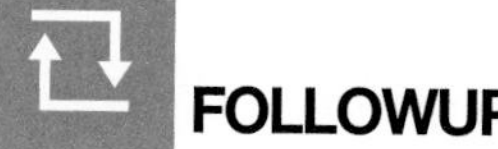

FOLLOWUP

PATIENT MONITORING
- Measure hematocrit before each phlebotomy - skip phlebotomy if hematocrit is less than 36%
- Schedule an additional phlebotomy when hematocrit is greater than 40%
- When anemia becomes refractory, repeat transferrin saturation and serum ferritin to confirm depletion of iron stores
- When iron stores are depleted, 4 to 6 phlebotomies a year should keep iron stores normal - maintain serum ferritin ≤ 50 μg/L
- During maintenance therapy, measure transferrin saturation and serum ferritin yearly
- Liver biopsy to assess iron stores when serum iron transferrin and ferritin results have not normalized

PREVENTION/AVOIDANCE Family members should be screened

POSSIBLE COMPLICATIONS
- Cirrhosis
- Hepatoma (only in patients with cirrhosis)
- Diabetes mellitus
- Cardiomyopathy
- Arthritis
- Hypogonadism

EXPECTED COURSE/PROGNOSIS
- Patients diagnosed before cirrhosis develops and treated with phlebotomy have a normal life expectancy
- Life expectancy is reduced in patients with cirrhosis, diabetes mellitus, and patients that require longer than 18 months of phlebotomy therapy to return iron stores to normal

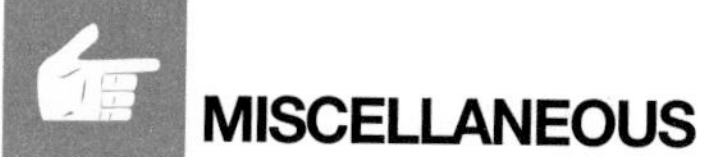

MISCELLANEOUS

ASSOCIATED CONDITIONS See Possible complications

AGE-RELATED FACTORS
Pediatric: Although rare, iron overload can occur even as early as 2 years of age. The disorder can be diagnosed before iron overload is clinically apparent.
Geriatric: N/A
Others: N/A

PREGNANCY Avoid iron supplements

SYNONYMS
- Bronze diabetes
- Troisier-Hanot-Chauffard syndrome

ICD-9-CM
275.0 Disorders of iron metabolism

SEE ALSO

OTHER NOTES Most patients with hemochromatosis go undiagnosed. Since treatment with phlebotomy will prevent all complications when begun early, the diagnosis of hemochromatosis should be considered much more frequently by physicians.

ABBREVIATIONS N/A

REFERENCES

- Brandhagen DJ, Fairbanks VF, Baldus W. Recognition and management of hereditary hemochromatosis. Am Fam Physician 2002;1;65(5):853-60
- Powell LW, George DK, et al. Diagnosis of hemochromatosis. Ann Intern Med 1998;129:925-31
- Barton JC, McDonnel SM, et al. Management of hemochromatosis. Ann Intern Med 1998;129:932-9

Web references: 2 available at www.5mcc.com
Illustrations 1 available

Author(s):
Robert A. Marlow, MD, MA

BASICS

DESCRIPTION
- Hemophilia A and hemophilia B are clinically indistinguishable, inherited bleeding disorders due to a deficiency of coagulant factor VIII (hemophilia A) or factor IX (hemophilia B)
- Disease severity is determined by percent of coagulant factor present
  - ◊ Severe; < 2%
  - ◊ Moderate; 2-5%
  - ◊ Mild; > 6%. Patients with greater than 25% factor activity rarely bleed, however bleeding after major surgery can occur in patients or carriers with factor VIII levels in the range of 25-35%.

System(s) affected: Hemic/Lymphatic/Immunologic

Genetics: Both hemophilia A and hemophilia B are X-linked, recessive

Incidence/Prevalence in USA:
- Hemophilia A - 10 in 100,000 males
- Hemophilia B - 2 in 100,000 males

Predominant age:
- Both are congenital conditions
- Severe disease generally noted at birth or in first year
- Mild disease may not be diagnosed until young adulthood

Predominant sex: Females are generally asymptomatic carriers unless their factor level is < 40%. Rare exceptions occur from consanguinity within families, concomitant Turner syndrome, or extremely disproportionate lyonization resulting in the preponderance of cells in the carrier female containing the X chromosome with the hemophilic gene.

SIGNS & SYMPTOMS
- Bleeding into soft tissues, muscles, and weight-bearing joints
- Bleeding occurs hours to days after injury, can involve any organ, and can continue for hours to days
- Compartment syndromes and ischemic nerve damage from large hematomas
- Repeated bleeding into a joint causes osteoarthritis, articular fibrosis, and joint ankylosis
- Hematuria
- CNS bleeding, usually post-traumatic

CAUSES Congenital

RISK FACTORS Positive family history. Can predict risk to offspring using simple Mendelian genetics for an X-linked recessive disorder.

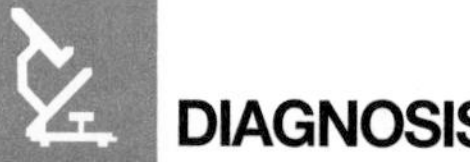

DIAGNOSIS

DIFFERENTIAL DIAGNOSIS
- Von Willebrand disease
- Vitamin K deficiency (factor IX is vitamin K dependent)
- Other factor deficiencies, afibrinogenemia, dysfibrinogenemia, fibrinolytic defects, platelet disorders

LABORATORY
- Activated partial thromboplastin time (PTT) is prolonged while platelet count, and prothrombin time are normal
- Bleeding time is prolonged in 15-20% of patients with hemophilia A
- PTT is corrected when mixed with normal plasma
- Hemophilia A - diagnostic test is low factor VIII.
- Hemophilia B - diagnostic test is low factor IX

Drugs that may alter lab results: Recent aspirin use will increase bleeding time, leading to confusion with Von Willebrand disease

Disorders that may alter lab results: N/A

PATHOLOGICAL FINDINGS
- Synovial hemosiderosis
- Articular cartilage degeneration
- Thickening of periarticular tissues
- Bony hypertrophy

SPECIAL TESTS Hemophilia A - carrier detection compares the ratio of factor VIII to von Willebrand factor protein and is predictive in up to 95% of cases. Molecular diagnosis is preferred for carrier testing.

IMAGING N/A

DIAGNOSTIC PROCEDURES N/A

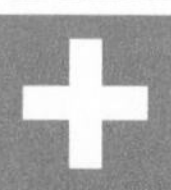

TREATMENT

APPROPRIATE HEALTH CARE
- Outpatient
- Home infusion therapy
- Inpatient for infusions following significant bleeding episodes

GENERAL MEASURES
- Avoid aspirin or aspirin-containing drugs
- Treat early. Symptoms often precede obvious bleeding.
- An uncomplicated, soft tissue bleeding or an early hemarthrosis requires a single infusion to 20-30% activity
- More extensive hemarthrosis or retroperitoneal bleeding requires bid infusions for 72 or more hours to 25-50% activity
- Life-threatening bleeding into the CNS requires maintaining levels greater than 50% activity for 2 weeks
- Major surgery requires greater than 50% activity preoperatively, continued for 1-2 weeks postoperatively
- Orthopedic care and physical therapy to prevent contractures and maintain joint mobility
- Vaccinate against hepatitis B at time of diagnosis
- Maintain good dental care
- Annual evaluation in a comprehensive hemophilia center
- Consideration for three times weekly prophylaxis in severe factor VIII deficiency

SURGICAL MEASURES
- Surgical or radionucleotide synovectomy, in selected patients
- Joint replacement, in selected patients

ACTIVITY
- Attempt to lead as normal a life as possible
- Restrict activities in proportion to the degree of factor deficiency, but maintaining a trim physical condition is important

DIET No special diet

PATIENT EDUCATION
- Teach patient and family about signs and symptoms to watch for
- Genetic counseling
- Home care with self administered replacement therapy is often used
- Printed patient information available from: National Hemophilia Foundation, 110 Green Street, Room 406, New York, NY, 10012, (212)219-8180

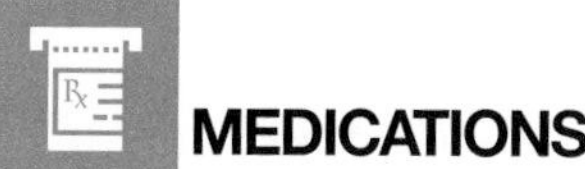

MEDICATIONS

DRUG(S) OF CHOICE

- Hemophilia A: Recombinant or monoclonal factor VIII is treatment of choice for hemophilia A patients who are HIV negative and who have had minimal prior concentrate exposure. Less optimal are plasma products enriched in factor VIII [cryoprecipitate, factor VIII concentrate]
  - ◊ 1 unit of factor VIII (the amount in 1 mL of plasma) per kg of body weight will raise the plasma level of the recipient by 2%
  - ◊ Number units = [(desired percent activity - current percent activity) times (body weight in kilograms)] divided by 2
  - ◊ For example: 70 kg patient with 5% activity needs to be taken to 25% activity. Units needed: [(25% - 5%) x (70 kg)] / 2 = [(25 - 5) x (70)] / 2 = 700 units of factor VIII needed
  - ◊ Half-life of factor VIII is 8-12 hours, therefore need to infuse at least bid to maintain a chosen factor VIII level, and tid when tight control of the level is needed
- Hemophilia B: Recombinant factor IX became available in mid 1997 and is treatment of choice for hemophilia B patients who are HIV negative and who have had minimal prior concentrate exposure. Monoclonal antibody purified factor IX is an effective and apparently safe plasma derived product
  - ◊ For mild patients: Desmopressin (DDAVP); 0.3 mcg/kg diluted in 10-20 mL of saline IV over 20 minutes. An intranasal preparation is also available.
  - ◊ Factor IX concentrate for moderate to severe hemorrhage and patients to undergo surgery. One unit/kg will raise levels 1%
  - ◊ Number units = [(desired percent activity - current percent activity) times (body weight in kilograms)] divided by 1
  - ◊ For example: 70 kg patient with 5% activity needs to be taken to 25% activity. Units needed: [(25% - 5%) x (70 kg)] / 2 = [(25 - 5) x (70)] / 1 = 1400 units of factor IX needed

Contraindications: None

Precautions: Hemophilia B - some factor IX concentrates contain trace amounts of activated vitamin K-dependent factors and therefore are thrombogenic and carry a risk for thromboembolism

Significant possible interactions: N/A

ALTERNATIVE DRUGS

- Aminocaproic acid (epsilon-aminocaproic acid, EACA) can be used for minor dental work following a single factor VIII infusion. Aminocaproic acid greatly enhances the risk of thromboembolism and should be used with caution with factor IX concentrates.
- Patients with inhibitors to factor VIII may require intensive plasmapheresis, large doses of concentrate, infusion of prothrombin complex concentrates (bypassing products), porcine factor VIII, or recombinant factor VIIA.

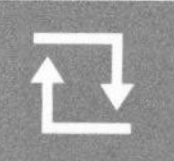

FOLLOWUP

PATIENT MONITORING Regular evaluations every 6 to 12 months include a musculoskeletal evaluation, an inhibitor screen, liver tests, and tests for antibodies to hepatitis viruses and human immunodeficiency virus (HIV)

PREVENTION/AVOIDANCE Genetic counseling

POSSIBLE COMPLICATIONS

- Factor VIII and IX preparations and transfusions may result in viral hepatitis, chronic liver disease, and acquired immunodeficiency syndrome (AIDS). However, recent advances in factor VIII concentrate preparation should prevent future HIV infection and hepatitis B and C.
- Hemophilia A - 10-20% of patients develop inhibitors to factor VIII, typically those with severe disease receiving multiple transfusions. Type I (high responders) inhibitors to factor VIII rapidly neutralize factor VIII and prevent effective transfusion therapy. Type II (low responders) inhibitors are low-titer and may respond to higher than normal doses of factor VIII.

EXPECTED COURSE/PROGNOSIS

- Repeated hemarthroses result in eventual deformity and crippling
- Survival is normal for those with mild disease, and mortality is increased 2 to 6 fold in those with moderate to severe disease, primarily due to complications of infection
- Median life expectancy with this condition peaked in late 1970's at 68 years, and is now declining due to the AIDS epidemic
- Up to 70% are HIV seropositive, especially those with severe disease, and 4% with severe disease develop AIDS. Younger patients whose treatment began since the mid-late 80's are largely HIV negative and are not expected to be exposed by modern replacement products. The proportion of HIV positive hemophiliacs is therefore declining.

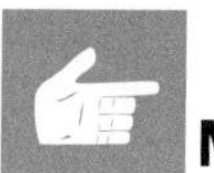

MISCELLANEOUS

ASSOCIATED CONDITIONS None

AGE-RELATED FACTORS

Pediatric: Mean age of onset of symptoms is 1.5 years for severe disease (often noted in first year), 3 years for moderate disease, and 5 years or later for mild disease

Geriatric: N/A

Others: N/A

PREGNANCY

- The vast majority of females are asymptomatic carriers, although an occasional carrier will bleed at time of surgery. They require no specific treatment during pregnancy or delivery.
- Prenatal diagnosis previously required sampling fetal blood for coagulant activity. Newer prenatal detection schemes detect an identifiable restriction fragment length polymorphism or a gene deletion or rearrangement in a sample of chorionic villus or from fluid obtained at amniocentesis.

SYNONYMS

- Hemophilia A
- Factor VIII deficiency
- Classic hemophilia
- Hemophilia B
- Factor IX deficiency
- Christmas disease

ICD-9-CM

286.0 Congenital factor VIII disorder
286.1 Congenital factor IX disorder

SEE ALSO

OTHER NOTES Recombinant factor VIII is available. It has biologic activity and clinical efficacy comparable to plasma factor VIII, while posing no risk of transmitting hepatitis viruses or HIV. There are factor VIII and factor IX concentrates prepared from human plasma using a monoclonal antibody method plus either heat or detergent treatment of the concentrate. These monoclonal-prepared concentrates have the lowest risk for hepatitis B and essentially no risk for HIV infection. (Recombinant factor IX became available in mid 1997, and has no risk of viral infection.)

ABBREVIATIONS N/A

REFERENCES

- Jones PK, Ratnoff OD. The changing prognosis of classic hemophilia (factor VIII 'deficiency'). Ann Int Med 1991;114(8):641-8
- Schwartz RS, et al. Human Recombinant DNA-Derived Antihemophilic Factor (Factor VIII) in the Treatment of Hemophilia A. N Engl J Med 1990;323(26):1800-5

Web references: 0 available at www.5mcc.com

Illustrations N/A

Author(s):

Mark R. Dambro, MD

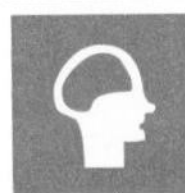

BASICS

DESCRIPTION Varicosities of the hemorrhoidal venous plexus. Usual course - acute; chronic; relapsing.
- External hemorrhoids are located below the dentate line and covered by squamous epithelium
- Internal hemorrhoids are located above the dentate line

System(s) affected: Cardiovascular, Gastrointestinal
Genetics: No known genetic pattern
Incidence/Prevalence in USA: Common
Predominant age: Adults, although may occur at any age
Predominant sex: Male = Female

SIGNS & SYMPTOMS
- All cases:
  - ◊ Constipation or diarrhea
  - ◊ Straining with defecation
- Small or minimal
  - ◊ Episodic bleeding on stool
- Extensive internal
  - ◊ Feeling of incomplete evacuation
- Small or minimal external
  - ◊ Pruritus
- Protruding but can be reduced
  - ◊ Mass
  - ◊ Prominent bleeding
  - ◊ Pruritus
  - ◊ Thrombosis with severe acute pain
- Protruding, not reducible
  - ◊ Mass
  - ◊ Inability to clean after stool
  - ◊ Thrombosis common
  - ◊ Strangulation possible
  - ◊ Ulceration

CAUSES
- Dilated veins of hemorrhoidal plexus
- Tight internal anal sphincter

RISK FACTORS
- Pregnancy
- Colon malignancy
- Liver disease
- Portal hypertension
- Constipation
- Occupations that require prolonged sitting
- Loss of muscle tone in old age, rectal surgery, episiotomy, anal intercourse
- Obesity
- Chronic diarrhea

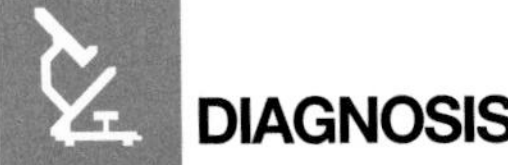

DIAGNOSIS

DIFFERENTIAL DIAGNOSIS
- Rectal or anal neoplasia
- Condyloma

LABORATORY N/A

Drugs that may alter lab results: N/A

Disorders that may alter lab results: N/A

PATHOLOGICAL FINDINGS N/A

SPECIAL TESTS N/A

IMAGING N/A

DIAGNOSTIC PROCEDURES
- Anorectal examination including anoscopy
- Sigmoidoscopy
- Inspection following straining at stool

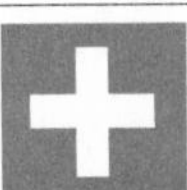

TREATMENT

APPROPRIATE HEALTH CARE
All of these treatments, except surgical, are outpatient with recovery and freedom from symptoms within 48 hours

GENERAL MEASURES
- Hemorrhoids are a recurrent disease, even after surgical excision; measures for prevention should be taken
- Mild symptoms or prevention:
  - ◊ Avoid prolonged sitting at stool
  - ◊ Avoid straining
  - ◊ Avoid constipation through stool softeners, and high fiber intake in diet or with supplements
  - ◊ Use soap and water for cleanup after stool
- For pain, sitz baths with soapy water, or hypertonic epsom salts (cup per 2 quarts of water)
- Mild and minimal hemorrhoids respond to changed diet, relief of constipation, soap and water cleanup and brief stooling
- Pruritus or mild discomfort after stooling responds to hydrocortisone ointment, anesthetic ointments or sprays
- Mild bleeding with external hemorrhoids responds to sitz baths and ointments or suppositories
- Hemorrhoids often progress from itching bleeding stage, to protrusion with easy reduction, then difficult reduction, and finally rectal prolapse. Thrombosis may occur at any protrusion stage. Constipation relief, anal hygiene, local ointments, and soaks are effective through the stage of easy reduction, but the more severe stages require rubber band ligation or rectal surgery.

SURGICAL MEASURES
- Indications
  - ◊ Persisting and soiling bleeding
  - ◊ Prolapsed internal hemorrhoids
  - ◊ Poor anal hygiene due to prolapsed hemorrhoids
  - ◊ Persistent pain
- Treatments
  - ◊ For severe pain:
    - Incision of thrombosed hemorrhoid
  - ◊ Severe protruding hemorrhoids:
    - Rubber band ligation (internal hemorrhoids only)
    - Injection therapy (suitable for one or two)
    - Cryosurgery, infrared or laser surgery for external hemorrhoids
  - ◊ Prolapsed rectum
    - Requires surgical correction
  - ◊ Surgical resection - for major external or internal hemorrhoids

ACTIVITY
- No restrictions
- Encourage physical fitness
- Avoid prolonged sitting and straining on the toilet

DIET High fiber

PATIENT EDUCATION Explain recurrence benignity, need for good diet, exercise and stooling health

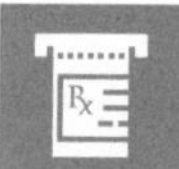

MEDICATIONS

DRUG(S) OF CHOICE
- Prevention:
  - ◊ Fiber supplements
  - ◊ Stool softeners
- Pain:
  - ◊ Analgesic sprays or ointments - benzocaine, dibucaine (Nupercainal). Use sprays with caution as they may contain alcohol that can cause burning sensation when applied.
- Pruritus:
  - ◊ Hydrocortisone (Anusol-HC, Cortifoam) ointment
- Bleeding:
  - ◊ Astringent suppositories (Preparation H)
  - ◊ Hydrocortisone (Anusol; Cortifoam) ointment

Contraindications: Refer to manufacturer's literature
Precautions: Refer to manufacturer's literature
Significant possible interactions: Refer to manufacturer's literature

ALTERNATIVE DRUGS N/A

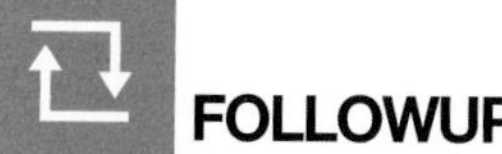

FOLLOWUP

PATIENT MONITORING
As needed, depending on treatment

PREVENTION/AVOIDANCE
- Avoid constipation
- Lose weight, if overweight
- Avoid prolonged sitting on the toilet
- Avoid prolonged sitting at work. Get up and move around periodically.

POSSIBLE COMPLICATIONS
- Thrombosis
- Secondary infection
- Ulceration
- Anemia (rare)
- Incontinence

EXPECTED COURSE/PROGNOSIS
- Spontaneous resolution
- Recurrence

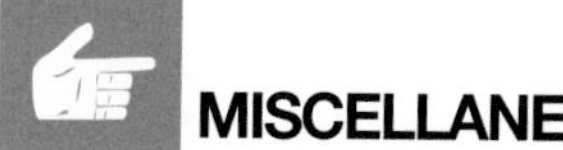

MISCELLANEOUS

ASSOCIATED CONDITIONS
- Liver disease
- Pregnancy
- Portal hypertension
- Constipation

AGE-RELATED FACTORS
Pediatric:
- Uncommon in infants and children. Look for underlying cause, e.g., venacaval or mesenteric obstruction, cirrhosis, portal hypertension.
- Occasionally, as in adults, hemorrhoids may result from chronic constipation, fecal impaction and straining at stool. Surgery is rarely required.

Geriatric: Common in elderly along with rectal prolapse
Others: N/A

PREGNANCY
Common in pregnancy. Usually resolves after pregnancy. No treatment required, unless extremely painful.

SYNONYMS
Piles

ICD-9-CM
455.6 Unspecified hemorrhoids without mention of complication

SEE ALSO
Colorectal malignancy
Portal hypertension
Portal vein thrombosis

OTHER NOTES N/A

ABBREVIATIONS N/A

REFERENCES

- Sardinha TC, Corman ML. Hemorrhoids. Surg Clin North Am 2002;82(6):1153-67
- Nonsurgical treatment of hemorrhoids. J Gastrointest Surg 2002;6(3):290-4
- Senagore AJ. Surgical management of hemorrhoids. J Gastrointest Surg 2002;6(3):295-8
- Hetzer FH, Demartines N, Handschin AE, Clavien PA. Stapled vs excision hemorrhoidectomy: long-term results of a prospective randomized trial. Arch Surg 2002;137(3):337-40
- Sohn N, Aronoff JS, Cohen FS, Weinstein MA. Transanal hemorrhoidal dearterialization is an alternative to operative hemorrhoidectomy. Am J Surg 2001;182(5):515-9
- Hulme-Moir M, Bartolo DC. Hemorrhoids. Gastroenterol Clin North Am 2001;30(1):183-97
- Komborozos VA, Skrekas GJ, Pissiotis CA. Rubber band ligation of symptomatic internal hemorrhoids: results of 500 cases. Dig Surg 2000;17(1):71-6

Web references: 1 available at www.5mcc.com
Illustrations N/A

Author(s):
Frank L. Iber, MD

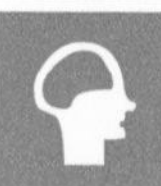

BASICS

DESCRIPTION Rare multisystem disease characterized by pleomorphic, but predominantly purpuric skin and mucous membrane lesions, gastrointestinal symptoms, and joint pain. Nephritis may occur. Epidemiology - it is the most common acute vasculitis affecting children.

System(s) affected: Endocrine/Metabolic, Gastrointestinal, Hemic/Lymphatic/Immunologic, Musculoskeletal, Nervous, Pulmonary, Renal/Urologic, Reproductive, Skin/Exocrine

Genetics: One case report in a father and son

Incidence/Prevalence in USA:
- Rare; seasonal, especially in spring and autumn
- 0.5/10,000 to 2.9/10,000 in geographically focal outbreaks in children
- 22.1/100,000 under age 14; 70.3/100,000 between ages 4 and 6

Predominant age:
- 75% between age of 2 and 11 years (but reported from 6 months to 86 years)
- < age 2 - milder renal and gastrointestinal manifestations
- Adults - extremely rare

Predominant sex: Male > Female (1.5-2:1)

SIGNS & SYMPTOMS
- Dermal
  - ◊ Purpura, petechiae, urticaria, erythematous, maculopapules, ecchymoses, rarely vesicular, livedo reticularis, ulceration and necrosis
  - ◊ Nonpitting angioedema - scalp - 20%, extremities - 46%; especially under age 3; present in 100%; presenting feature in 50%
- GI - 35-85
  - ◊ Precedes rash in 14%
  - ◊ Vomiting, colicky abdominal pain, gastrointestinal hemorrhage, ileus, intussusception (1-5%, especially ileoileal, related to submucosal hematomas), pancreatitis, gallbladder hydrops, protein losing enteropathy, ischemic necrosis of bile ducts
- Joint pain - 68-82%
  - ◊ Presenting sign in 25%
  - ◊ Periarticular tenderness and swelling especially of knees and ankles, with hand/wrist and elbow involvement less common
  - ◊ Additive pattern of arthritis, transient intramuscular hemorrhage
- Renal
  - ◊ May be transient hematuria or progress to glomerulonephritis and renal failure or death in 41-68% of children. If it occurs, does so within 3 months of rash onset.
  - ◊ 3% precedes purpura
  - ◊ Oliguria, edema, hypertension, renal failure
  - ◊ Nephrotic syndrome is rare
  - ◊ Hematuria alone - no progression
  - ◊ Hematuria and proteinuria - 15% develop renal failure
  - ◊ Nephrotic syndrome - 50% develop end stage renal disease within 10 years
  - ◊ 2-4% have rapidly progressive renal failure
  - ◊ Persistent nephropathy - 1%
- Neurologic (uncommon) - seizures, paresis, chorea, peripheral neuropathy, Guillain-Barré syndrome, uveitis
  - ◊ Lethargy, stupor, hyperactivity, irritability, rarely convulsions, chorea, headache, cortical blindness, paralysis, mononeuropathy
- Pulmonary - 6%
  - ◊ Hemorrhage, pleural effusion
- Scrotal swelling
  - ◊ 2-35% of cases from scrotal vessel vasculitis
- Cardiac - myocardial infarction, pericarditis
- Gastrointestinal - intussusception, pancreatitis, cholecystitis, perforation
- Constitutional - fever
- Anemia
- Thrombophlebitis perhaps from the thrombocytosis seen in 67%

CAUSES
- Probably an IgA-mediated small vessel vasculitis
- Preceding streptococcal infection
- *Salmonella*
- *Shigella*
- *Yersinia*
- *Legionella*
- Parvovirus
- Adenovirus
- *Mycoplasma*
- Epstein-Barr virus
- Varicella
- Vaccination against typhoid, paratyphoid A and B, yellow fever and cholera
- *Toxocara canis*
- Penicillin, ampicillin
- Erythromycin
- Tetracycline
- Vancomycin
- Quinidine and quinine
- Lisinopril
- Enalapril
- Losartan
- Diphenhydramine
- Tetramethylthiuram disulfide
- Insect bites

RISK FACTORS
- Hypertriglyceridemia
- Hyperuricemia

DIAGNOSIS

DIFFERENTIAL DIAGNOSIS
- Vasculitis
- Allergic angiitis
- Polyarteritis nodosum
- Erythema multiforme
- Inflammatory bowel disease (Crohn disease and ulcerative colitis)
- Systemic lupus erythematosus
- Syphilis
- Multisystem disease
- Thrombophlebitis related to coagulation factor deficiency
- Acute abdomen
- Coagulopathies
- Testicular torsion
- Thrombocytopenic purpura
- Sepsis
- Acute glomerulonephritis
- Acute hemorrhagic edema of infancy

LABORATORY
- Erythrocyte sedimentation rate elevation - 75%
- ASO titer - 30%
- CH50 - low in 30-40%
- Properdin depression -30%
- Cellular casts indicate significant renal disease
- Prothrombin deficiency
- IgA immune complexes
- Vitamin K deficiency
- Factor VIII deficiency
- Amylase, if pancreatitis
- Stool guaiac in 49%
- IgD elevation
- IgA1 O-linked oligosaccharide abnormalities, diminished galactose content

Drugs that may alter lab results: N/A

Disorders that may alter lab results: Higher frequency of HLA-DRB1*01 phenotype and anticardiolipin antibodies

PATHOLOGICAL FINDINGS
- Subserosal hemorrhages
- Swollen vascular endothelium
- Leukocytoclastic vasculitis
- Esophageal, gastric and small bowel ulcerations and intramural edema
- Pericapillary and periarteriolar neutrophilic infiltrates
- Occasional fibrinoid necrosis of vascular wall
- Glomerulonephritis with hypercellularity, focal necrotizing, crescent formation, and perivascular mononuclear or polymorphonuclear infiltrate, IgA, IgM, C3, fibrin, IgG and properdin deposition
- Necrotizing vasculitis
- IgA deposition and IgA nephropathy
- Submucosal and intramural fluid/blood intestinal wall extravasation

SPECIAL TESTS
- Immunofluorescent examination of involved tissue reveals IgA deposition
- Anti-cardiolipin antibodies should probably be sought
- Ultrasound - for intussusception
- Pulmonary function tests - reduced diffusing capacity, but unclear that it is clinically significant

IMAGING
- X-ray
  - ◊ Uniform small bowel wall fold thickening - may even produce 'coin stack' pattern
  - ◊ Edema and thumbprinting or filling defects of bowel walls
  - ◊ Intussusception

DIAGNOSTIC PROCEDURES
- Careful history and physical and frequent reevaluation

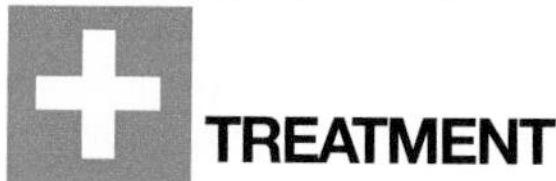

TREATMENT

APPROPRIATE HEALTH CARE Supportive measures

GENERAL MEASURES
- Sudden increase in abdominal pain may be caused by bowel infarction or perforation, gall bladder hydrops, intussusception or pancreatitis
- Treatment of the underlying/associated infection
- Discontinuation of unnecessary drugs
- Closely monitor blood pressure, urinalysis and renal function

SURGICAL MEASURES N/A

ACTIVITY As tolerated

DIET N/A

PATIENT EDUCATION Vigilance for recurrence of symptoms

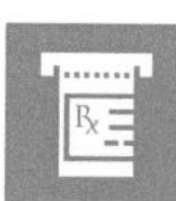

MEDICATIONS

DRUG(S) OF CHOICE
- Nonsteroidal anti-inflammatory drugs at intermediate doses
- Avoid prednisone for rash or abdominal pain, as aggravates systemic aspects of the disease
- Prednisone - 1-2.5 mg/kg for renal disease (not just hematuria) or possible pulmonary hemorrhage

Contraindications:
- Refer to manufacturer's literature
- Steroids contraindicated for solely dermal/GI/joint manifestations

Precautions:
- Refer to manufacturer's literature

Significant possible interactions: Refer to manufacturer's literature

ALTERNATIVE DRUGS
- Full anticoagulation (PTT 60-80 seconds; PT INR 2.5-3.5)
- Antiplatelet drugs - e.g., dipyridamole - 3 mg/kg to 6 mg/kg
- The above two in combination with prednisone and cyclophosphamide
- High dose immune globulin IV - 1 gm/kg/day in 12 hour infusions
- Cyclosporine - 5 mg/kg/day
- Cyclophosphamide - 2 mg/day in adults
- Danazol 400-600 mg/day
- Plasmapheresis
- Recombinant Factor VIII infusion

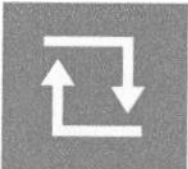

FOLLOWUP

PATIENT MONITORING
- Dependent on severity of system involvement
- Long-term followup required if renal involvement, as progression may not be noted for years

PREVENTION/AVOIDANCE N/A

POSSIBLE COMPLICATIONS
- Death
- Renal failure
- Bowel infarction or perforation
- Gall bladder hydrops
- Pancreatitis
- Stenosing ureteritis
- Isolated reports as presenting sign of cancer
- Recurrence in renal transplant - 75% in living related donors; 0 in cadaver donors
- Antiphospholipid syndrome

EXPECTED COURSE/PROGNOSIS
- Typically lasts 4-6 weeks
- 50% have recurrences
- Significant proteinuria, altered renal function, hypertension are adverse prognostic indicators
- Rarely fatal

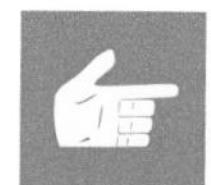

MISCELLANEOUS

ASSOCIATED CONDITIONS
- Polychondritis
- Antiphospholipid antibody syndrome
- Familial Mediterranean fever
- Thyroiditis

AGE-RELATED FACTORS
Pediatric: < age 2 - milder renal and gastrointestinal manifestations
Geriatric: N/A
Others: N/A

PREGNANCY No evidence of fetal damage in one report

SYNONYMS
- Schönlein-Henoch purpura
- Anaphylactoid purpura
- Allergic purpura
- Peliosis rheumatica
- Hemorrhagic capillary toxicosis
- IgA nephropathy
- Leukocytoclastic vasculitis
- Allergic vasculitis
- Berger disease

ICD-9-CM
287.0 Allergic purpura

SEE ALSO

OTHER NOTES N/A

ABBREVIATIONS N/A

REFERENCES

- Hasegawa, et al. Fate of renal grafts with recurrent Henoch-Schönlein purpura nephritis in children. Transplant Proc 1989;21:2130-2133
- Iijima K, et al. Multiple combined therapy for severe Henoch-Schönlein nephritis in children. Pediatr Nephrol 1998;12:244-248
- Lanzkowsky S, Lanzkowsky L, Lanzkowsky P. Henoch-Schönlein purpura. Pediatrics in Review 1992;13:130-137
- Saulsbury FT. Corticosteroid therapy does not prevent nephritis in Henoch-Schönlein purpura. Pediatr Nephrol 1993;7:69-71
- Saulsbury FT. Henoch-Schönlein purpura in children. Medicine 1999;78:395-409
- Szer IS. Henoch-Schönlein purpura: When and how to treat. J Rheumatol 1996;23:1661-1665
- Saulsbury FT. Henoch-Schönlein purpura. Curr Opin Rheumatol 2001;13(1):35-40
- Singh S, et al. Severe Henoch-Schoenlein nephritis: Resolution with azathioprine and steroids. Rheumatol Intl 2002;22:133-137
- Donadio JV, Grande JP. IgA nephropathy. N Engl J Med 2002;347:738-48.
- Yang, Y-H, et al. Increasing transforming growth factor-=beta (TGF-B)-secreting T cells and IgA anticardiolipin antibody levels during acute stage of childhood Henoch-Schoenlein purpura. Clin Exp Immun 2000;122:285-90

Web references: 0 available at www.5mcc.com
Illustrations N/A

Author(s):
Bruce M. Rothschild, MD

BASICS

DESCRIPTION Altered mental and neuromotor functioning associated with acute or chronic liver disease and/or portal systemic shunting of blood. The prominent features are mild to marked forgetfulness, impaired arousability, and a "flapping tremor" (asterixis).

System(s) affected: Gastrointestinal, Nervous

Genetics: Unknown

Incidence/Prevalence in USA:
- Occurs in 1/3 cases of cirrhosis
- Occurs in all cases of fulminant hepatic failure
- Present in nearly half of patients who reach the stage of liver disease requiring transplantation

Predominant age: Parallels that of fulminant liver disease with peak in the 40's, and cirrhosis with peak in late 50's. May occur at any age.

Predominant sex: Male = Female (reflecting the underlying liver disease)

SIGNS & SYMPTOMS
- Ages 10-60
  - ◊ Prominent signs of underlying liver disease (50%), jaundice most common, ascites second most common
  - ◊ Gastrointestinal hemorrhage with hematemesis or melena (20%)
  - ◊ Systemic infection, urinary tract or pulmonary (20%)
  - ◊ Four stages of confusion and obtundity described. (1) forgetfulness, disturbance in nocturnal sleep, daytime drowsiness, (2) mild confusion but can be aroused, (3) can be aroused, but markedly confused, limited orientation and thought content, (4) unable to be aroused.
  - ◊ Asterixis prominent in stages 2, 3
  - ◊ Handwriting and hand coordination deteriorated in stages 1, 2
  - ◊ Tremor prominent in stage 2
  - ◊ Psychotic thoughts infrequent
  - ◊ Reflexes symmetrically hyperactive
  - ◊ Tremor and asterixis not observed in ocular muscles
  - ◊ Mental and neurological signs change rapidly (over 6 to 12 hours)
- Age over 60
  - ◊ Signs of underlying liver disease diminished (25%)
  - ◊ Confusion more prominent
  - ◊ Precipitating gastrointestinal hemorrhage or infection less often identified
  - ◊ Remains in stage 1 or 2 for many days
  - ◊ Progression slower
- Age under 10
  - ◊ Signs of underlying liver disease prominent, usually fulminant hepatic failure or extremely advanced cirrhosis
  - ◊ Progression through the stages very rapid, often 6 to 12 hours
  - ◊ Precipitating cause frequently not identified

CAUSES
- Shunting of intestinal blood through the severely diseased liver without the intervention of viable liver cells. TIPS (transjugular intrahepatic portacaval shunt), a widely used radiologically inserted shunt to lower portal pressure, produces liver encephalopathy.
- Shunting of such blood through collateral circulation or surgically constructed portacaval shunts
- Most common in long standing cirrhosis of the liver with spontaneous shunting of intestinal blood through collaterals.
- Failure of liver to detoxify agents noxious to CNS, eg, ammonia, mercaptans, fatty acids
- Increased aromatic and reduced branched chain amino acids in blood
- Precipitation of acute event, search for:
  - ◊ New overt or occult infection including spontaneous peritonitis
  - ◊ Potassium, magnesium or other electrolyte depletion
  - ◊ Use of opiate, sedative, tranquilizer, drugs
  - ◊ Gastrointestinal bleeding

RISK FACTORS
- Infection
- Sedative or opiate drugs
- Electrolyte disturbance
- Anemia
- Gastrointestinal hemorrhage

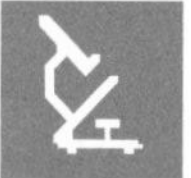

DIAGNOSIS

DIFFERENTIAL DIAGNOSIS
- Head trauma, concussion, subdural hematoma
- Alcohol withdrawal syndrome
- Toxic confusion due to medication
- Toxic confusion due to illicit drug use
- Meningitis
- Metabolic encephalopathy related to anoxia, hypoglycemia, hypokalemia, hypo- or hypercalcemia, uremia

LABORATORY
- Screening blood, sputum and urine cultures to identify infection
- Hematology to identify anemia and signs of infection
- Standard biochemistry profile to identify hypokalemia, bilirubinemia, altered calcium status, hypomagnesemia, urea, hypoglycemia
- Arterial blood gases
- Liver tests to evaluate severity of underlying liver disease
- Prothrombin and partial thromboplastin time
- Toxicology screen for illicit drugs
- Elevated ammonia often present

Drugs that may alter lab results:
- Infusion of amino acid solutions may affect ammonia level
- Opiate administration - producing severe constipation may affect ammonia level

Disorders that may alter lab results:
- Uremia may affect ammonia level
- Rapid and severe tissue breakdown, massive burns, trauma or infection may affect ammonia level

PATHOLOGICAL FINDINGS
- Brain edema in 100% of fatal cases
- Glial hypertrophy in chronic encephalopathy

SPECIAL TESTS
- Electroencephalogram shows symmetrical slowing of basic (alpha) rhythm in common with other forms of metabolic encephalopathy
- Visually-evoked potential specific in stages 2, 3 and 4

IMAGING
- Useful only to rule out other diagnoses
- CT scan of head most useful
- Brain MRI shows increased glutamine in basal ganglia

DIAGNOSTIC PROCEDURES
- Clinical setting and findings adequate in 80% of cases
- Venous ammonia of great aid in patients with chronic liver disease when the clinical findings are confusing
- EEG is useful to a limited extent, but findings are similar in other forms of metabolic encephalopathy
- Treatment response often confirms diagnosis
- Trail marking test and other psychometric tests of value in alert, ambulatory patients with slight slowing down or changed behavior

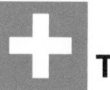

TREATMENT

APPROPRIATE HEALTH CARE
- Outpatient for stages 1 and 2 when diagnosis is clear and if recurrent can be managed satisfactorily
- Stage 3 or 4 requires inpatient management
- Stage 3 or 4 in fulminant hepatic failure is a strong indication for evaluation for liver transplantation. Transfer to a transplant center should be considered.

GENERAL MEASURES
- Identify and treat vigorously precipitating causes - gastrointestinal bleed, infection, sedative drugs, or electrolyte imbalance are most common
- Stage 2 or higher - attention to adequate fluid intake, and at least 1000 kcal (4.19 MJ) of food daily
- Give Fleet's enema to all patients without diarrhea
- Clumsiness and poor judgment prominent. Be sure patient has the care needed to avoid falls, cuts on broken glass, smoking burns, machinery or auto accidents.
- Avoid sedative or opiate medications. Benzodiazepine sedatives and opiate derivatives such as Lomotil have caused liver coma.
- In stage 4 patients - must protect the airway as aspiration is common. Tracheal intubation often used. Feeding IV or with endoscope introduced jejunal feeding tube.

SURGICAL MEASURES Artificial liver perfusion devices have proven useful in fulminant hepatic failure to bridge the patient until a donor liver is available for transplantation

ACTIVITY
- As tolerated
- Avoid driving and machinery

DIET
- Integrate with needs of underlying liver disease
- Lower total protein. Stage 1 - avoid protein gluttony. Stage 2 - limit red meat and consume small portions of all other protein foods, total protein for day 50-60 grams. Stage 3 - consume 40 gram protein or vegetable protein diet (about 20 grams). Stage 4 - consume 10 or fewer grams of protein. Feeding IV or endoscope introduced jejunal feeding tube to avoid aspiration. For all stages at least 1000 kcal (4.19 MJ) ingested daily.
- As coma improves, increase dietary protein as tolerated

PATIENT EDUCATION
- Include family in education
- Dietitian instruction in eating lower protein diets, avoid protein bingeing
- Avoid unnecessary sedative or antianxiety medications and opiates
- Recognition of early signs and to get treatment promptly
- Pamphlets (quite good for family) - American Association for the Study of Liver Diseases, 6900 Grove Road, Thorofare, NJ 08086, (609)848-1000)

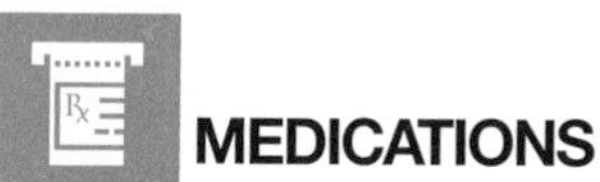

MEDICATIONS

DRUG(S) OF CHOICE
- Lactulose (Cephulac) syrup 30 mL of 50% solution four times daily. Diminish to bid when 3 or more bowel movements a day occur daily.
- If stage 4 is present, worsening occurs, or no improvement in 2 days, add antibiotics. Amoxicillin 4 gm/day is suitable. Neomycin 1-4 gm/day in 4 divided doses may be used if renal status is good.
- Antacids as needed

Contraindications:
- Total ileus
- Hypersensitivity reaction

Precautions:
- Potassium depletion
- Electrolyte imbalance
- Renal failure

Significant possible interactions: Refer to manufacturer's profile of each drug

ALTERNATIVE DRUGS
- Any antibiotic affecting intestinal flora such as:
  - ◊ Metronidazole or vancomycin in refractory cases
  - ◊ Dopamine agonists, e.g., bromocriptine have been tried
  - ◊ Branched-chain amino acids IV
  - ◊ Flumazenil

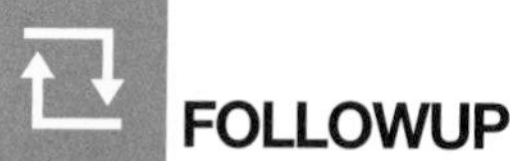

FOLLOWUP

PATIENT MONITORING
- To optimize treatment a trail-making test should be followed (provided by Cephulac makers). Apply to Stage 1 and 2 patients to determine how much maintenance treatment and diet needed. Should be run daily at first and then at each visit when changes in drugs and diet are made.
- Patients with changed findings should be seen twice weekly
- Stable patients should be seen monthly
- Trail-making test performed at each office visit
- In cirrhosis, evaluate for transplantation for death likely in

24 months

PREVENTION/AVOIDANCE
- Avoid unessential medications, particularly opiates, sedatives
- Avoid protein binges

POSSIBLE COMPLICATIONS
- Recurrence
- Stable, chronic, impaired status
- With many recurrences, permanent basal ganglion injury (non-Wilsonian hepatolenticular degeneration)
- Hepatorenal syndrome
- Acute tubular necrosis
- Bleeding
- Disseminated intravascular coagulation
- Bacteremia
- Shock

EXPECTED COURSE/PROGNOSIS
- In acute or fulminant
  - ◊ With adequate aggressive treatment, disappears without residue or recurrence
- In chronic liver disease
  - ◊ Coma returns
  - ◊ With each recurrence it becomes more and more difficult to treat
  - ◊ Plateau of maximum improvement shows a decrement over several years, such that the degree of improvement with treatment is less and less. Eventual 80% mortality.

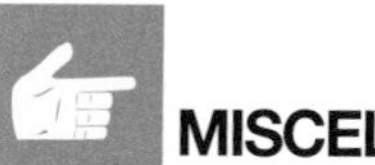

MISCELLANEOUS

ASSOCIATED CONDITIONS
- Liver disease
- Rarely with portacaval shunt with normal liver function

AGE-RELATED FACTORS See under Signs and symptoms
Pediatric: N/A
Geriatric: N/A
Others: N/A

PREGNANCY May occur as a complication of pregnancy

SYNONYMS
- Hepatic coma
- Liver coma

ICD-9-CM
572.2 Hepatic coma

SEE ALSO

OTHER NOTES N/A

ABBREVIATIONS N/A

REFERENCES

- Sorkine P, Ben Abraham R, Szold O, et al. Role of the molecular adsorbent recycling system (MARS) in the treatment of patients with acute exacerbation of chronic liver failure. Crit Care Med 2001;29(7):1332-6.
- Blei AT, Cordoba J; Practice Parameters Committee of the American College of Gastroenterology. Hepatic Encephalopathy. Am J Gastroenterol 2001;96(7):1968-76
- Ong JP, Aggarwal A, Krieger D, et al. Correlation between ammonia levels and the severity of hepatic encephalopathy. Am J Med 2003;15;114(3):188-93
- Saxena N, Bhatia M, Joshi YK, et al. Electrophysiological and neuropsychological tests for the diagnosis of subclinical hepatic encephalopathy and prediction of overt encephalopathy. Liver 2002;22(3):190-7
- McDougall AJ, Davies L, McCaughan GW. Rapid improvement of autonomic and peripheral neuropathy after liver transplantation: a single case report. Liver Transpl 2002;8(2):164-6
- Lee SS, Mathiasen RA, Lipkin CA, et al. Endoscopically placed nasogastrojejunal feeding tubes: a safe route for enteral nutrition in patients with hepatic encephalopathy. Am Surg 2002;68(2):196-200
- Cadranel JF, Lebiez E, Di Martino V, et al. Focal neurological signs in hepatic encephalopathy in cirrhotic patients: an underestimated entity? Am J Gastroenterol 2001;96(2):515-8
- Amodio P, Caregaro L, Patteno E, et al. Vegetarian diets in hepatic encephalopathy: facts or fantasies? Dig Liver Dis 2001;33(6):492-500
- Als-Nielsen B, Kjaergard LL, Gluud C. Benzodiazepine receptor antagonists for acute and chronic hepatic encephalopathy. Cochrane Database Syst Rev. 2001;(4): CD002798
- Das A, Dhiman RK, Saraswat VA, Verma M, Naik SR. Prevalence and natural history of subclinical hepatic encephalopathy in cirrhosis. J Gastroenterol Hepatol 2001;16(5):531-5
- Als-Nielsen B, Koretz RL, Kjaergard LL et al. Branched-chain amino acids for hepatic encephalopathy. Cochrane Database Syst Rev 2003; (2)pp CD001939

Web references: 1 available at www.5mcc.com
Illustrations N/A

Author(s):
Frank L. Iber, MD

BASICS

DESCRIPTION A systemic viral infection primarily involving the liver
System(s) affected: Gastrointestinal
Genetics: Some predisposition to immunologic manifestations; DR4 - positive increase with concurrent immunologic disease
Incidence/Prevalence in USA: 33% of Americans have antibodies; 125,000-200,000 infections/yr; 70% symptomatic; declining incidence with vaccination
Predominant age: HAV rare in infants; susceptibility increases with age.
Predominant sex: Male = Female

SIGNS & SYMPTOMS
- Fever (60%)
- Malaise (67%)
- Nausea and vomiting
- Anorexia (54%)
- Jaundice (in adults, 62%)
- Hepatomegaly
- Dark urine (84%)
- Pale stools, usually transient
- Abdominal/RUQ pain
- Fatigue
- Meningismus (occasional)
- Vast majority are minimally symptomatic or asymptomatic, especially children

CAUSES
- Multiple viruses possible as coinfection
- HAV and HEV transmitted enterically (fecal-oral); parenteral route rare
- Maximum infectivity 2 weeks before jaundice
- May be endemic in institutions; day care centers - vaccinate for HBV
- No chronicity in HAV

RISK FACTORS
- Health care workers/other occupational risks
- Household exposure
- Intimate exposure
- Recent body piercing; tattoos less likely, role controversial
- Transmission rare through blood exposure

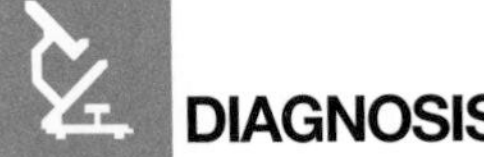

DIAGNOSIS

DIFFERENTIAL DIAGNOSIS
- Other hepatitis viruses
- Infectious mononucleosis
- Primary or secondary hepatic malignancy
- Ischemic hepatitis
- Drug-induced hepatitis
- Alcoholic hepatitis
- Autoimmune hepatitis
- Wilson disease
- Rheumatic and skin manifestation may suggest immunologic disorder

LABORATORY
- Marked elevation of AST/ALT (acute hepatitis, particularly ALT, 400-several thousand U/L)
- Mild elevation of alkaline phosphatase
- Bilirubin from normal to markedly elevated; with elevation, conjugated and unconjugated fractions usually increased

Positive serum markers in hepatitis A:

Status	Marker
A, R	Anti-HAV (total) and IgM both positive
P	Anti-HAV total positive, Anti-HAV IgM negative

Infection status:
A=acute
R=recent
P=previous

- For severe hepatitis, measure PT and PTT, albumin, electrolytes, glucose and CBC

Drugs that may alter lab results: Corticosteroids, other immunosuppressive drugs

Disorders that may alter lab results: Leukopenia may exacerbate viral replication

PATHOLOGICAL FINDINGS Features of acute hepatocellular injury with variable inflammation and necrosis. Lymphoid aggregates are uncommon. Chronic liver disease or cirrhosis does not occur.

SPECIAL TESTS Liver biopsy usually not needed

IMAGING Usually not needed

DIAGNOSTIC PROCEDURES
- History; exposure source; exclude drugs; both prescription, over the counter and herbs
- Tenderness over the liver; may be hepatomegaly
- Jaundice often not present
- Serum "liver function tests" often elevated before bilirubin increases; measure aminotransferases in acute illnesses when there is no evident cause
- Serum biochemical markers for each virus, diagnostic in 90% of patients

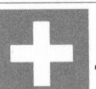

TREATMENT

APPROPRIATE HEALTH CARE
- Outpatient care usual; severe cases need to be admitted
- Segregation helpful for food handlers with HAV

GENERAL MEASURES
- Monitor: coagulation defects, fluid and electrolytes, acid-base imbalance, hypoglycemia, impairment of renal function
- Report acute cases to public health department

SURGICAL MEASURES N/A

ACTIVITY As tolerated

DIET Adequate calories; balanced nutrition

PATIENT EDUCATION
- Proper hygiene
- Handwashing - particularly patients, food handlers and day care workers
- Vaccinate against HAV
- Blood exposure rare
- Wash and cover cuts and bruises

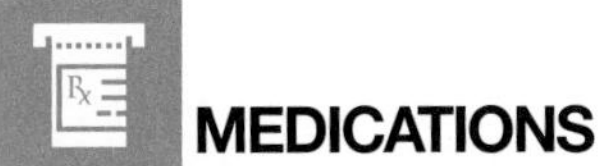

MEDICATIONS

DRUG(S) OF CHOICE Antiviral therapy not indicated in acute HAV infections as spontaneous resolution occurs in almost all patients
Contraindications: Corticosteroids may add to morbidity/increased mortality.
Precautions: N/A
Significant possible interactions: Refer to manufacturer's profile of each drug

ALTERNATIVE DRUGS N/A

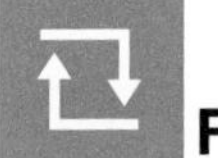

FOLLOWUP

PATIENT MONITORING
- Serial measurement of serum AST/ALT
- Appropriate serum viral markers useful for evaluation of recovery or progression
- Liver biopsies in acute cases if diagnosis remains in doubt
- Monitor for metabolic complications

PREVENTION/AVOIDANCE
- Good sanitation, hygiene
- Immune globulin (passive immunization): 0.02 mL/kg IM (given 1-2 weeks after exposure prevents illness in 80-90%). With prolonged exposure give q 5 months. Also use for close contacts, day care staff/children (if case occurs), institutions with multiple cases, travelers to areas of high prevalence (with 3 week lead time, use vaccine).
- Hepatitis A vaccine (Havrix, Vaqta): 0.5 mL dose IM in children > 2 yrs; 1 mL in adults IM; 2nd dose 6-12 mo later for >8 yrs. Separate syringe site from immune globulin. Use for travelers, day-care staff/children, custodial facility employees, sewage workers, military, homosexual men, food handlers, Native Americans, Alaskan natives.

POSSIBLE COMPLICATIONS
- Icteric disease
- 3 rare variants: relapsing, cholestatic, fulminant

EXPECTED COURSE/PROGNOSIS
- Mild disease usual, often no jaundice
- No chronic liver disease
- Mortality < 1%
- Lifetime immunity usual with recovery

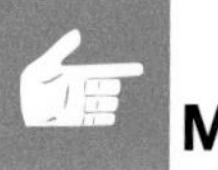

MISCELLANEOUS

ASSOCIATED CONDITIONS
- Arthritis
- Urticaria
- Immune complex nephritis (particularly membranous glomerulopathy)
- Anemias (including aplastic anemia)

AGE-RELATED FACTORS
Pediatric: Milder; usually anicteric; may be unrecognized
Geriatric: N/A
Others: N/A

PREGNANCY N/A

SYNONYMS N/A

ICD-9-CM
070 Viral hepatitis

SEE ALSO
Hepatitis B
Hepatitis C
Immunizations

OTHER NOTES N/A

ABBREVIATIONS N/A

REFERENCES

Web references: 1 available at www.5mcc.com
Illustrations N/A

Author(s):
Rajiv R. Varma, MD

BASICS

DESCRIPTION A systemic viral infection primarily involving the liver
System(s) affected: Gastrointestinal
Genetics: Some predisposition to immunologic manifestations; DR4 - positive increase with concurrent immunologic disease
Incidence/Prevalence in USA:
- 140,000 - 320,000 infections/year
- 1-1.25 million chronically infected
- Post-transfusion hepatitis B (rare)

Predominant age: All ages
Predominant sex: Fulminant HBV: Male > Female (2:1)

SIGNS & SYMPTOMS
- Fever (60%)
- Malaise (67%)
- Nausea and vomiting
- Anorexia (54%)
- Jaundice (in adults, 62%)
- Hepatomegaly
- Dark urine (84%)
- Pale stools, usually transient
- Abdominal/RUQ pain
- Fatigue
- Meningismus (occasional)
- Arthralgia/arthritis
- Vast majority are minimally symptomatic or asymptomatic

CAUSES Hepatitis B virus

RISK FACTORS
- Health care workers/other occupational risks
- Hemodialysis
- Recipients of blood and/or blood products (esp. prior to 1992)
- IV drug users 60-70% of new infections
- Sexually active homosexual males
- Household exposure
- Intimate exposure
- Positive needlestick
- Transplanted organs
- Snorting cocaine
- Recent body piercing; tattoos less likely, role controversial
- Perinatal transmission of neonate of hepatitis B infected mother rare with HCV unless HIV positive

DIAGNOSIS

DIFFERENTIAL DIAGNOSIS Infectious mononucleosis, primary or secondary hepatic malignancy, ischemic hepatitis, drug-induced hepatitis, alcoholic hepatitis, autoimmune hepatitis, Wilson disease, rheumatic and skin manifestation may suggest immunologic disorder

LABORATORY
- Marked elevation of AST/ALT (acute hepatitis, particularly ALT, 400-several thousand U/L)
- Mild elevation of alkaline phosphatase
- Bilirubin from normal to markedly elevated; with elevation, conjugated and unconjugated fractions usually increased

Positive serum markers in hepatitis B:

```
Status    Marker
-----------------------------------------
 HBV      HBsAg & Anti-HBs &
  panel   (Anti-HBc IgM, window period)
 A, E     HbsAg & ±
           (Anti-HBC IgM, window period)
 Rcv      Anti-HBe, -HBs, & -HBc IgG
 C        HbsAg, HbeAg
           Markers of replications:
              HBeAg & Anti-HBe & HBV-DNA
 V        Anti-HBs, ±Anti-HBc
---------------------------
Infection status:
   A=acute        R=recent
   C=chronic      P=previous
   Rcv=recovered  V=vaccinated
   E=early/carrier state
```

- For severe hepatitis, measure PT and PTT, albumin, electrolytes, glucose and CBC
- If HBV chronic, test HBV DNA titer
- Patients with severe HBV infection should be tested for coinfection or superinfection with HDV. Testing for HDV also indicated in sexually active gay men, and those with history of IV drug abuse.
- HBeAg indicates high infectivity (horizontal and vertical transmission)
- Persistence > 6 months indicates probable chronic liver disease

Drugs that may alter lab results: Corticosteroids, other immunosuppressive drugs

Disorders that may alter lab results: Leucopenia may exacerbate viral replication

PATHOLOGICAL FINDINGS
- Liver biopsy in persistent or chronic disease shows wide range of histologic changes (variable inflammation and/or necrosis, cholestasis, fibrosis, cirrhosis or chronic active hepatitis)
- Clinical course may not predict severity of histopathologic changes
- Microvesicular steatosis and lymphoid aggregates suggest hepatitis C infection

SPECIAL TESTS Liver biopsy usually needed for determining type and extent of liver injury in persistent disease and to exclude other diseases. Also, usually necessary prior to start of antiviral treatment such as interferon alfa.

IMAGING
- Usually helpful
- Ultrasound may demonstrate ascites or exclude obstruction. Helpful when cancer is suspected.
- CT with IV contrast and MRI in selected cases
- Early cirrhosis usually not detected by imaging studies - need liver biopsy

DIAGNOSTIC PROCEDURES
- History; exposure source; exclude drugs; both prescription, over the counter and herbs
- Tenderness over the liver; may be hepatomegaly
- Jaundice may not be present in most
- Serum "liver function tests" often elevated before bilirubin increases; measure aminotransferases in acute illnesses when there is no evident cause
- Serum biochemical markers, diagnosis in 90% of patients

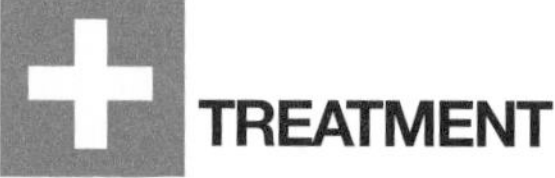

TREATMENT

APPROPRIATE HEALTH CARE
- Outpatient care usual; severe cases need inpatient care

GENERAL MEASURES
- Monitor: coagulation defects, fluid and electrolytes, acid-base imbalance, hypoglycemia, impairment of renal function
- Report acute cases to public health department
- Need multidisciplinary approach, especially in those with cirrhosis. Familiarity with risks, side effects and monitoring for liver cancer and mutations of hepatitis B is essential.

SURGICAL MEASURES Consider liver transplantation in fulminant acute hepatitis/end-stage liver disease (HCV) and in early stages of primary liver cancer. Refer to a tertiary care center with liver and other organ transplant facilities.

ACTIVITY As tolerated

DIET Adequate calories; balanced nutrition

PATIENT EDUCATION
- Avoid sharing razors, tooth brushes and nail clippers
- Wash and cover cuts and bruises
- Proper use and disposal of needles
- Proper hygiene, particularly food handlers
- HBV sexually transmitted
- HBV present in saliva, vaginal secretions, vaccinate sexual partner, household contacts against HAV, HBV

MEDICATIONS

DRUG(S) OF CHOICE

- Acute hepatitis B: Antiviral therapy not indicated as spontaneous resolution occurs in about 95%; others need close monitoring for chronicity or fulminant hepatic failure.
- Chronic hepatitis B: persistent hepatitis B surface antigenemia > 6 months
  - ◊ Interferon-alpha (IFN-a) and lamivudine (LAM) are equally effective.
  - ◊ Goals of therapy: Decrease in HBV DNA to undetectable level; loss of hepatitis Be antigen and appearance of anti -Hbe; loss of HBsAg from serum is seldom achieved but will be ideal.

Chronic hepatitis B therapy:

HBeAg	HBV-DNA	ALT†	Rx
+	+	+	IFN, ADV or LAM
-	-	N	Monitor
+/-	+	CC	LAM or ADV
+/-	+	DC	LAM or ADV; Liver transplant
+/-	-	CC	Monitor
+/-	-	DC	Liver transplant

† ALT + when >2x normal
CC: compensated cirrhosis
DC: decompensated cirrhosis

Contraindications: Interferon: platelet count < 50,000. Mouse immunoglobulin, egg protein or neomycin allergy. Corticosteroids may add to morbidity/increased mortality.

Precautions:

- Other disorders of coagulation, myelosuppression, seizures, depression (esp. suicide ideation), pregnancy, fertile age group, lactation
- Increased serum triglycerides may occur during IFN therapy; may cause abnormal ALT
- Psychiatric evaluation may be prudent prior to IFN treatment
- Lamivudine resistant mutations

Significant possible interactions: Refer to manufacturer's profile of each drug

ALTERNATIVE DRUGS

Adefovir 10 mg qid, Famciclovir (Famvir) 500 mg tid for chronic hepatitis B

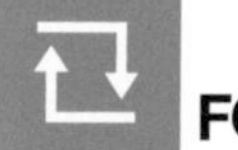

FOLLOWUP

PATIENT MONITORING

- Serial measurement of serum AST/ALT
- Appropriate serum viral markers useful for evaluation of recovery or progression
- Liver biopsies in chronic disease; in acute cases if diagnosis remains in doubt
- Monitor for metabolic complications
- WBC, platelets with interferon alfa therapy
- Chronic HBV, HBV-DNA valuable for prediction of favorable response to IFN. High pretreatment ALT and low pretreatment HBV-DNA associated with favorable response.
- Monitor for hepatic decompensation (ascites, hepatic encephalopathy, spontaneous bacterial peritonitis, etc) in cirrhotics

PREVENTION/AVOIDANCE

- General
  - ◊ Screen blood products
  - ◊ Proper disposal of needles
  - ◊ Good sanitation, hygiene
  - ◊ Maximum infectivity 2 weeks before jaundice
  - ◊ May be endemic in institutions; day care centers - vaccinate for HBV
  - ◊ HBV transmitted sexually, perinatally, occupationally, and via parenteral drug use (e.g., shared needles); also enterically.
- Specific
  - ◊ Hepatitis B vaccine. A new hepatitis B vaccine to include pres, and S2 antigens will be available soon; more effective especially in nonresponders.
  - ◊ High risk groups: hepatitis B human immune globulin within 24 hr of exposure (0.06 mL/kg IM)
  - ◊ HBV screening in pregnant women; vaccinate all infants at birth.

POSSIBLE COMPLICATIONS

Acute or subacute necrosis, chronic active or chronic hepatitis, cirrhosis, hepatic failure; hepatocellular carcinoma (HBV, HCV)

EXPECTED COURSE/PROGNOSIS

- Recovery from acute infection in 95% of patients
- Severity of hepatic encephalopathy best predictor of poor survival in hepatic failure
- HBV (mortality 1%) and HDV (with icterus, mortality 2-20%) more severe symptoms; often leads to persistent/chronic liver disease, cirrhosis, liver failure, hepatocellular carcinoma; more severe problems if impaired immune function. Follow treatment with HBV-DNA levels.

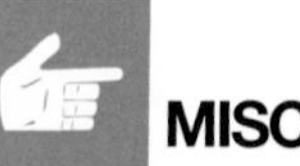

MISCELLANEOUS

ASSOCIATED CONDITIONS

- Arthritis, urticaria, immune complex nephritis (particularly membranous glomerulopathy), anemias (including aplastic anemia), dermatitis and cardiomyopathy (usually with HBV, rare with HCV).

AGE-RELATED FACTORS

Pediatric: HBV more acute, less prolonged, less complications, but may become chronic.
Geriatric: N/A
Others: Alcohol abuse a major factor for chronic liver disease. Measure viral biochemical markers in patients with alcoholic liver disease (especially anti-HCV).

PREGNANCY

- Test, in later gestation, for HBsAg
- HBV transmitted vertically (< 10%) as well as perinatally and produces carrier state in 30%. Give infant HBIg 0.5 mL and HBV vaccine (Recombivax HB; separate sites) within 12 hrs of birth followed by HBV vaccine, 0.5 mL IM at ages 1 and 6 months. Check HBsAg and HBsAb at age 12 months
- Vertical transmission increased in HIV

SYNONYMS

N/A

ICD-9-CM

070 Viral hepatitis

SEE ALSO

Hepatitis A
Hepatitis C
Immunizations

OTHER NOTES

N/A

ABBREVIATIONS

HBsAg = hepatitis B surface antigen
HBeAg = hepatitis Be antigen

REFERENCES

- Lok ASF, McMahon BJ. Chronic hepatitis B. Practice guidelines on chronic hepatitis B. Hepatology 2004;39:857-61

Web references: 1 available at www.5mcc.com
Illustrations N/A

Author(s):

Rajiv R. Varma, MD
Kia Saeian, MD

Hepatitis C

BASICS

DESCRIPTION A systemic viral infection primarily involving the liver
System(s) affected: Gastrointestinal
Genetics: Some predisposition to immunologic manifestations; DR4 - positive increase with concurrent immunologic disease
Incidence/Prevalence in USA:
- 16% of sporadic hepatitis; 40,000 new cases year ; 3 million chronically infected (85% of infected); donor blood screening has reduced risk

Predominant age: All ages
Predominant sex: Male = Female

SIGNS & SYMPTOMS
- Fever (60%)
- Malaise (67%)
- Nausea and vomiting
- Anorexia (54%)
- Jaundice (34%)
- Hepatomegaly
- Dark urine (84%)
- Pale stools, usually transient
- Abdominal/RUQ pain
- Fatigue (major complaint)
- Meningismus (occasional)
- Arthralgia/arthritis
- Vast majority are minimally symptomatic or asymptomatic

CAUSES
- Hepatitis C virus

RISK FACTORS
- Health care workers/other occupational risks
- HCV transmitted through blood or its products; in 40%, mode unknown
- Hemodialysis
- Recipients of blood and/or blood products (esp. prior to 1992)
- IV drug users 60-70% of new infections
- Sexually active homosexual males (much more likely with hepatitis B than with C
- Household exposure
- Intimate exposure
- Positive needlestick
- Transplanted organs
- Snorting cocaine
- Recent body piercing; tattoos less likely, role controversial
- HIV positivity increases risk of hepatitis C or C virus infection in coinfected patients
- Perinatal transmission of neonate of hepatitis B infected mother rare with HCV unless HIV positive

DIAGNOSIS

DIFFERENTIAL DIAGNOSIS Infectious mononucleosis, primary or secondary hepatic malignancy, ischemic hepatitis, drug-induced hepatitis, alcoholic hepatitis, autoimmune hepatitis, Wilson disease, rheumatic and skin manifestation may suggest immunologic disorder

LABORATORY
- Marked elevation of AST/ALT (acute hepatitis, particularly ALT, 400-several thousand U/L); HCV may have normal ALT; AST/ALT ratio =>1 associated with cirrhosis in chronic HCV
- Mild elevation of alkaline phosphatase
- Bilirubin from normal to markedly elevated; with elevation, conjugated and unconjugated fractions usually increased

Positive serum markers in hepatitis C:

Status	Marker
A, C	Anti-HCV ELISA III or RIBA HCV RNA: (qual. & quan.) Genotypes I-IV

Infection status:
A=acute
C=chronic

- For severe hepatitis, measure PT and PTT, albumin, electrolytes, glucose and CBC
- Persistence > 6 months indicates probable chronic liver disease
- Acute, ongoing HCV, confirm by other markers, RIBA, HCV-RNA (for chronic HCV); >viral counts, genotypes 1, 2, 3 & 4
- In early acute HCV infection, anti-HCV may be negative; may need retest in 3-6 weeks
- HCV-RNA becomes positive early in acute cases
- HCV genotypes may be useful. Genotypes with favorable prognosis - 2a, 2b, 3a; less favorable 1a, 1b

Drugs that may alter lab results: Corticosteroids, other immunosuppressive drugs

Disorders that may alter lab results: Leucopenia may exacerbate viral replication

PATHOLOGICAL FINDINGS Liver biopsy in persistent or chronic disease shows wide range of histologic changes (variable inflammation and/or necrosis, cholestasis, lymphoid aggregate, steatosis, fibrosis, cirrhosis or chronic active hepatitis. Clinical course may not predict severity of histopathologic changes. Microvesicular steatosis and lymphoid aggregates suggest hepatitis C infection.

SPECIAL TESTS Liver biopsy usually needed for determining type and extent of liver injury in persistent disease and to exclude other diseases. Also, usually necessary prior to start of antiviral treatment such as interferon-alfa.

IMAGING Usually helpful. Ultrasound may demonstrate ascites or exclude obstruction. Helpful when cancer is suspected. CT with IV contrast and MRI in selected cases. Early cirrhosis usually not detected by imaging studies - need liver biopsy.

DIAGNOSTIC PROCEDURES
- History; exposure source; exclude drugs; both prescription, over the counter and herbs
- Tenderness over the liver; may be hepatomegaly
- Jaundice may not be present in most
- Serum "liver function tests" often elevated before bilirubin increases; measure aminotransferases in acute illnesses when there is no evident cause
- Serum biochemical markers for each virus, diagnosis in 90% of patients

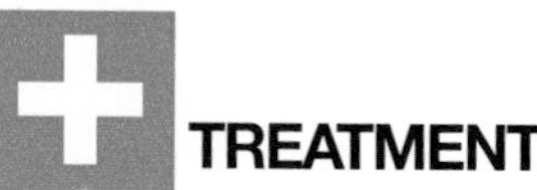

TREATMENT

APPROPRIATE HEALTH CARE
- Outpatient care usual; severe cases need inpatient care

GENERAL MEASURES
- Monitor: coagulation defects, fluid and electrolytes, acid-base imbalance, hypoglycemia, impairment of renal function
- Report acute cases to public health department
- Need multidisciplinary approach monitored by experienced physician-led-team
- Careful patient selection essential

SURGICAL MEASURES Consider liver transplantation in fulminant acute hepatitis/end-stage liver disease and in early stages of primary liver cancer. Refer to a tertiary care center with liver and other organ transplant facilities.

ACTIVITY As tolerated

DIET Adequate calories; balanced nutrition

PATIENT EDUCATION
- Avoid sharing razors, tooth brushes and nail clippers
- Wash and cover cuts and bruises
- Proper use and disposal of needles
- Proper hygiene, particularly food handlers
- Sexual transmission low, but does occur

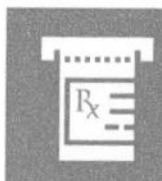

MEDICATIONS

DRUG(S) OF CHOICE

- Acute hepatitis C: Antiviral therapy is highly effective for acute infections. Interferon-alfa 5 mg SC or IM daily for HCV-RNA for 4 weeks followed by 3 times per week for 20 weeks.
- Chronic hepatitis C: pegylated interferon + ribavirin
  - ◊ Pegylated interferon-alpha 2b 1.5 mcg/kg/week
  - ◊ Pegylated interferon-alpha 2a 180 mcg/week
  - ◊ Ribavirin 800-1200 mg po bid in combination with pegylated interferon

Contraindications: Interferon: platelet count < 50,000. Mouse immunoglobulin, egg protein or neomycin allergy. Corticosteroids may add to morbidity/increased mortality.

Precautions:

- Other disorders of coagulation, myelosuppression, seizures, depression (esp suicide ideation), pregnancy, fertile age group, lactation
- Ribavirin may induce hemolytic anemia (hemoglobin 2 gm/dL below pretreatment) is common. Avoid in pregnancy.
- Increased serum triglycerides may occur during IFN therapy; may cause abnormal ALT. Measure HCV-RNA to assess response in such patients.
- Psychiatric evaluation may be prudent prior to IFN treatment

Significant possible interactions: Refer to manufacturer's profile of each drug

ALTERNATIVE DRUGS N/A

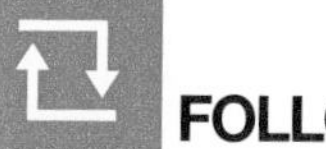

FOLLOWUP

PATIENT MONITORING

- Serial measurement of serum AST/ALT
- Appropriate serum viral markers useful for evaluation of recovery or progression
- Liver biopsies in chronic disease; in acute cases if diagnosis remains in doubt
- Monitor for metabolic complications
- WBC, platelets with interferon-alfa therapy
- Lower viral load, genotypes 2 and 3 and absence of cirrhosis are predictors of favorable therapeutic response. Undetectable HCV-RNA (quantitative serum HCV-RNA) at 12 weeks is associated with sustained response. Persistently positive HCV-RNA at 24 weeks indicates lack of response; prolonged course is unlikely to be beneficial.
- Monitor for hepatic decompensation (ascites, hepatic encephalopathy, spontaneous bacterial peritonitis, etc) in cirrhotics
- Goal of therapy is eradication of hepatitis C virus; HCV-RNA test should become persistently undetectable
- Early virologic response is defined as ≥2 log decrease in HCV-RNA level after 12 weeks of treatment
- In patients with cirrhosis the risk of hepatic cellular carcinoma is high (20% life-time risk). Monitor for hypervascular lesions by imaging (ultrasound, helical CT) every 6 months.

PREVENTION/AVOIDANCE

- No specifics on prevention/avoidance
- Maximum infectivity 2 weeks before jaundice

POSSIBLE COMPLICATIONS

- Acute or subacute necrosis, chronic hepatitis, hepatic failure
- Primary liver cancer risk
- HCV-associated cirrhosis: 1-3% per year, lifetime risk 20%. Cirrhosis patients need surveillance for hepatocellular carcinoma.

EXPECTED COURSE/PROGNOSIS

- Severity of hepatic encephalopathy best predictor of poor survival in hepatic failure
- In HCV, regardless of severity:
  - ◊ >80% progress to chronic hepatitis
  - ◊ 20-50% to cirrhosis, and some, liver failure
  - ◊ Typically slow progression 10-30 years
  - ◊ May progress to HCC, but IFN may decrease HCC risk
  - ◊ Associated with type II AI
  - ◊ Chronic HCV unlikely to clear HCV-RNA spontaneously
  - ◊ HCV after needlestick, usually sustained IFN response
  - ◊ Final phase HCV rare cause of fulminant hepatic failure
- Alcohol increases severity of chronic HCV

MISCELLANEOUS

ASSOCIATED CONDITIONS

- Arthritis, urticaria, immune complex nephritis (particularly membranous glomerulopathy), anemias (including aplastic anemia), dermatitis and cardiomyopathy (rare with HCV). HCV implicated in sporadic form of idiopathic mixed cryoglobulinemia, porphyria cutaneous tarda, polyarteritis nodosa.
- HIV-HCV: more severe course

AGE-RELATED FACTORS

Pediatric: Uncommon
Geriatric: N/A
Others: Alcohol abuse a major factor for chronic liver disease from HCV. Measure viral biochemical markers in patients with alcoholic liver disease (especially anti-HCV).

PREGNANCY

- Vertical transmission increased in HIV

SYNONYMS N/A

ICD-9-CM

070 Viral hepatitis

SEE ALSO

Hepatitis A
Hepatitis B
Immunizations

OTHER NOTES N/A

ABBREVIATIONS

PCR = polymerase chain reaction
IFN = interferon
HCC = hepatocellular carcinoma
AI = autoimmune hepatitis

REFERENCES

- Alter MJ, Kruszan-Moran D, Naiman OV, et al. The prevalence of hepatitis C virus infection in the United States. N Engl J Med 1999;341:556-62
- Seeff LP. Emerging and reemerging issues, infections diseases: Hepatitis C: A meeting ground for the generalist and the specialist. Amer J Med 1999;107(6B): ls-100s.
- Jaeckel E, Comberg M, Wedemeyer H, et al. Treatment of acute hepatitis C interferon alfa 2b. N Engl J Med 2001;345:1452-7
- Manns MP, McHutchison JG, Gordon SC, et al. Peg-interferon alfa 2b plus ribavirin compared with interferon alfa 2b plus ribavirin for initial treatment of chronic hepatitis C: a randomized controlled trial. Lancet 2001;358:958-65
- Lauer GM, Walker BD. Hepatitis C virus infection. Medical Progress. N Engl J Med 2001;345:41-52
- Gane E, Portmann B, Naouniov N, et al: Long-term outcome of Hepatitis C infection after liver transplantation. N Engl J Med 1996:334;815-820

Web references: 1 available at www.5mcc.com
Illustrations N/A

Author(s):

Rajiv R. Varma, MD
Kia Saeian, MD

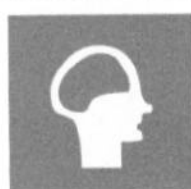

BASICS

DESCRIPTION Primary malignant tumor of liver arising from hepatic parenchymal cells (hepatocytes), blood vessels or cholangioles within the liver, excluding gallbladder and biliary passages. With the exception of fibrolamellar type, 85% associated with an underlying liver disease, usually cirrhosis.

System(s) affected: Gastrointestinal

Genetics: No known genetic pattern

Incidence/Prevalence in USA:
- 1-5 new cases per 100,000 of population per year
- Among known cirrhotics, 2-5 cases/100/year
- Asians > caucasians > blacks > hispanics > native americans

Predominant age:
- 6th-8th decade (mean age 55-62 years) in USA and western countries
- Among immigrants from Asia and Africa occurs 2-3 decades earlier
- Under age 5, hepatoma presents in noncirrhotic livers, 70% cured by surgical resection

Predominant sex: Male > Female (3-4:1)

SIGNS & SYMPTOMS
- Early curable stage
  - ◊ Paraneoplastic syndrome - feminization, precocious puberty
  - ◊ Palpable nodule on liver
  - ◊ Age 2 to 6 years - abdominal mass in liver, abdominal pain, irregular hepatomegaly
- Usual adult manifestations
  - ◊ Known cirrhosis or prominent clinical signs of cirrhosis - 80%
  - ◊ Abdominal pain - 80%, right upper quadrant, dull ache to severe, aggravated by jolting
  - ◊ Hepatomegaly - 80-90%, irregular, nodular, firm to hard, tender
  - ◊ Weight loss, 30%
  - ◊ Hepatic arterial bruit, 20%
  - ◊ Friction rub - rare, more common in metastatic liver disease
  - ◊ Nausea, vomiting
  - ◊ Fever - 10-50%, low grade, intermittent
  - ◊ Paraneoplastic manifestations - hypertrophic osteoarthropathy, carcinoid syndrome, feminization, polycythemia
  - ◊ Hemoperitoneum, most common tumor cause
  - ◊ Unexplained deterioration of stable cirrhosis
  - ◊ Budd-Chiari syndrome
  - ◊ Blockage of portal vein, inferior vena cava, renal veins

CAUSES
- Cirrhosis - accounts for 60 to 80% of cases. Alcoholic cirrhosis most important in western world. Reported risk of hepatoma in alcoholic cirrhosis is 3-10% with micronodular pattern.
- Hepatitis B virus infection - associated with > 70% of cases worldwide. Most important factor in Africa and Asia but less important in western countries. In USA, HBsAg is positive in 20% cases of this tumor.
- Hepatitis C virus infection - 50-70% of HBsAg negative patients are positive for anti-HCV antibody, an important factor in hepatoma patients not due to HBV infection.
- Mycotoxins (aflatoxins) - metabolite of fungus Aspergillus flavus that contaminates foods. Two series, B1 and derivatives and G1 and derivatives. B1 being the most potent carcinogen, important in Sub-Saharan Africa and Southeast Asia, no significant role in USA.
- Vinyl polymer, but not the finished product, produces angiosarcoma

RISK FACTORS
- For hepatocellular carcinoma
  - ◊ All forms of cirrhosis
    - Hepatitis B and C
    - Alcoholism
    - Hemachromatosis
    - NASH (nonalcoholic steatohepatitis)
    - Alpha-1-antitrypsin deficiency
    - Biliary cirrhosis
  - ◊ Long term use of oral contraceptives
  - ◊ Repeated use of fungus-infected food
- For cholangiocarcinoma
  - ◊ Gallstones
  - ◊ Sclerosing cholangitis
  - ◊ Choledochal cysts
  - ◊ Clonorchiasis
- For fibrolamellar type
  - ◊ Risk factors unknown
- For angiosarcoma
  - ◊ Vinyl polymer

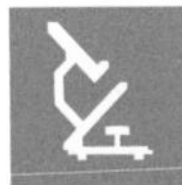

DIAGNOSIS

DIFFERENTIAL DIAGNOSIS
- Early asymptomatic tumor - underlying liver conditions, e.g., cirrhosis, chronic hepatitis; benign liver nodules, hamartoma, hemangioma, metastatic adenocarcinoma, gallstones, or gallbladder polyp
- Late symptomatic tumor with hepatomegaly - hepatic cyst, adenoma, hemangioma, abscess, metastatic malignancy of liver, cirrhosis with activity, infarction of liver, fatty infiltration, thrombosis of hepatic veins, portal vein, inferior vena cava, active viral hepatitis, alcoholic hepatitis
- Ruptured tumor - all causes of acute abdomen, traumatic hemoperitoneum

LABORATORY
- Erythrocytosis, elevated Ca, low glucose
- Liver function test abnormalities
- Tumor markers
  - ◊ Alpha-fetoprotein (AFP) - single most important lab test for screening and diagnosis of hepatoma - 70%. Negative in angiosarcoma, cholangiocarcinoma and fibrolamellar carcinoma. Level > 400 ng/mL (> 400 μg/L) is diagnostic, level does not correlate with prognosis.
  - ◊ Other markers - des-gamma-carboxyprothrombin, gamma glutamyl transferase, carcinoembryonic antigen (CEA), variant alkaline phosphatase, isoferritins

Drugs that may alter lab results: Hypoglycemic agents, calcitonin, vitamin D

Disorders that may alter lab results: Acute or chronic hepatitis, germ cell tumors, pregnancy. All cause slight elevation of AFP.

PATHOLOGICAL FINDINGS
- Tumors up to 2 cm (and often 3-4 cm) are not metastatic. Most common metastatic site is the liver.
- Nodular - 75%, usually in cirrhotic liver
- Massive - common in children and non-cirrhotic livers, more prone to rupture
- Diffuse - rare, a large part of liver is involved
- Hepatocellular origin - most commonly multicentric, well differentiated, usually superimposed on underlying cirrhosis. Anaplastic form often difficult to be certain of cell of origin or differentiate from metastatic malignancy.
- Fibrolamellar - single nodule, non-cirrhotic, extensive fibrous stroma
- Cholangiocarcinoma - multicentric, most often mixed with hepatocellular elements
- Angiosarcoma

SPECIAL TESTS N/A

IMAGING
- Plain x-ray - useful to demonstrate metastatic involvement to lung and bone
- Ultrasound - best diagnostic imaging technique, capable of detecting tumor > 1 cm, and may be positive when AFP is normal. Has been useful in serially following cases of cirrhosis to identify hepatocellular cancer when under 2 cm and curable.
- CT scan - valuable in determining extrahepatic spread of the disease; diagnostic of fibrolamellar
- MRI - helpful in delineating the details of tumor, and invasion of vessels
- Hepatic arteriography - mostly done to see the anatomy of hepatic vessels and extent of tumor while considering resection, embolization, dearterialization or intra-arterial infusion of cytotoxic agents. Most useful in detecting angiosarcoma, separating benign vs. malignant.
- Lipoidal angiography and CT - lipoidal is readily taken up by tumor cells, this technique can detect even millimeter sized lesions. Lipoidal also serves as a vehicle to deliver chemotherapeutic or radioactive agents to the tumor.

DIAGNOSTIC PROCEDURES
- Tissue diagnosis must be made for appropriate treatment
- Liver biopsy - usually US or CT guided when nodules not palpable
- Laparoscopic occasionally used to evaluate extent in cirrhosis

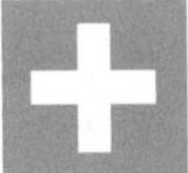

TREATMENT

APPROPRIATE HEALTH CARE Inpatient initially

GENERAL MEASURES Precautions to avoid falls, attention to nutrition

SURGICAL MEASURES
- Surgical resection is the only cure. Surgical removal should be considered in Child's A (and some B) patients and may include up to a lobe of the liver.
- Surgical resection has a high cure rate when 3 or fewer nodules each <5 cm.
- X-ray guided radiofrequency ablation (or the less effective alcohol injection) is effective palliation and may make surgery possible.
- Embolization of the tumor supplying artery with chemotherapy, under x-ray guidance is effective palliation and may make surgery possible.
- The presence of small (no more than 3 tumors, less than 5 cm.) increases the priority for transplantation if it is otherwise indicated

ACTIVITY As tolerated

DIET High calorie, low protein diet

PATIENT EDUCATION Important for prevention; abstinence from alcohol and IV drugs, vaccination against HBV

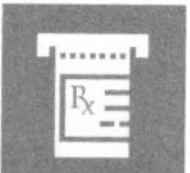

MEDICATIONS

DRUG(S) OF CHOICE
- Chemotherapy has no survival benefit
- Treatment of hepatoma in patients with hepatitis C with PEG-alpha- interferon and ribavirin prolongs survival and improves quality of life

Contraindications: N/A
Precautions: N/A
Significant possible interactions: N/A

ALTERNATIVE DRUGS : N/A

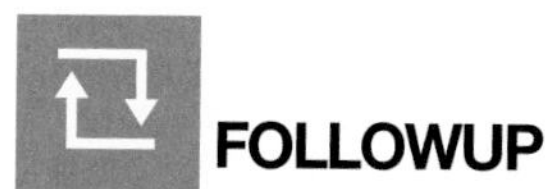

FOLLOWUP

PATIENT MONITORING
- After successful resection there is high risk for recurrence
- Check AFP every 3 months
- Ultrasound every 4-6 months

PREVENTION/AVOIDANCE
- Prevention against HBV infection/cirrhosis
  - ◊ General education regarding risks of exposure to HBV and precautions to avoid this
  - ◊ Vaccination in high risk individuals - nurses, doctors, dialysis unit staff, lab technicians
  - ◊ Vaccination of all children
  - ◊ Abstinence from alcohol, IV drugs, homosexual behavior
  - ◊ Persistent HBV and HCV infections eradicated with alpha interferon, lamivudine
- Screening and early diagnosis
  - ◊ Early diagnosis to detect asymptomatic tumor (< 3 cm) at a potentially curable stage has been emphasized. The only screening test available so far is AFP testing which can detect 70-80% of tumors < 3 cm when used in conjunction with serial high resolution sonography - each 6-12 months.
  - ◊ AFP should be done every 6 months in high risk individuals (cirrhosis, chronic active hepatitis) along with annual ultrasound. In moderate risk subjects (HBsAg positive but asymptomatic), AFP should be done yearly followed by ultrasound if it is abnormal with prompt biopsy of any new nodules.
  - ◊ Patients exposed to 10 or more years of vinyl chloride polymerization should have q 6 months sonography. New nodules should be promptly biopsied.

POSSIBLE COMPLICATIONS
Rupture; hemoperitoneum; liver failure; cachexia; metastases to other organs; thrombosis of portal, hepatic, renal veins

EXPECTED COURSE/PROGNOSIS
- Unresectable symptomatic tumors: grave prognosis patients seldom live more than 6 months
- Resectable asymptomatic tumors
  - ◊ Surgery is curative in > 70% of children. 40% of adults
  - ◊ Surgery curative in >80% of tumors <3 cm in cirrhosis
- Transplantation has same survival as tumor-free patients when hepatoma is incidentally discovered or is less than 2 cm in diameter. Only slight reduction in survival with up to 3 tumor nodules <5 cm

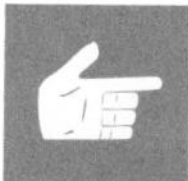

MISCELLANEOUS

ASSOCIATED CONDITIONS
- Infections - chronic hepatitis B, hepatitis C, Delta hepatitis, clonorchiasis and schistosomiasis
- Primary liver diseases - alcoholic cirrhosis, primary biliary cirrhosis
- Metabolic diseases - Alpha1-antitrypsin deficiency, hemochromatosis, tyrosinemia

AGE-RELATED FACTORS
Can occur in all age groups

Pediatric: Second most common tumor in first year of life following Wilms' tumor. High cure rate.
Geriatric: N/A
Others: N/A

PREGNANCY N/A

SYNONYMS
- Hepatocellular carcinoma
- Liver cancer
- Fibrolamellar carcinoma
- Cholangiocarcinoma

ICD-9-CM
155.0 Malignant neoplasm of liver, primary

SEE ALSO

OTHER NOTES
- In Africa and Southeast Asia:
  - ◊ Incidence of hepatoma is high - 15-20 cases/100,000/year
  - ◊ Age group is younger - 3rd and 4th decade
  - ◊ Male to female ratio is high - 6:1 to 7:1
  - ◊ Aflatoxin and HBV are the major factors and cirrhosis is less important
  - ◊ Course is more progressive and fulminant
  - ◊ Tumors are mostly at unresectable stage at first presentation

ABBREVIATIONS
HBsAg = hepatitis B surface antigen
HCV = hepatitis C virus
HBV = hepatitis B virus
AFP = alpha-fetoprotein

REFERENCES

- Velazquez RF, Rodriguez M, Navascues CA, et al. Prospective analysis of risk factors for hepatocellular carcinoma in patients with liver cirrhosis. Hepatology 2003;37:520-7
- Shiratori Y, Shiina S, Teratani T, et al. Interferon therapy after tumor ablation improves prognosis in patients with hepatocellular carcinoma associated with hepatitis C virus. Ann Internal Medicine 2003;138:299-306
- Ebied OM, Federle MP, Carr BI, et al. Evaluation of responses to chemoembolization in patients with unresectable hepatocellular carcinoma. Cancer 2003;97:1042-50
- Iwamoto S, Sanefuji H, Okuda K. Angiographic subsegmentectomy for the treatment of patients with small hepatocellular carcinoma. Cancer 2003;97:1051-6
- Leung TW, Yu S, Johnson PJ, et al. Phase 11 study of the efficacy and safety of cisplatin-epinephrine injectable gel administered to patients with unresectable hepatocellular carcinoma. J of Clinical Oncology 2003;21:652-8
- Lau WY, Leung TW, Yu SC, Ho SK. Percutaneous local ablative therapy for hepatocellular carcinoma: a review and look into the future. Ann Surgery 2003;237:171-9
- Llovet JM, Bruix J. Systematic review of randomized trials for unresectable hepatocellular carcinoma: Chemoembolization improves survival. Hepatology 2003;37:429-42
- Befeler AS, Di Bisceglie AM. Hepatocellular carcinoma: diagnosis and treatment. Gastroenterology 2002;122:1609-19
- Poon RT, Fan ST, Wong J. Selection criteria for the hepatic resection in patients with large hepatocellular carcinoma larger than 10 cm in diameter. J of the Amer College of Surgeons 2002;194:592-602
- Llovet JM, Burroughs, A, Bruix J. Hepatocellular carcinoma. Lancet 2003;362:1907-17
- Lam CM, Ng KK, Poon RT et al. Impact of radiofrequency ablation on the management of patients with hepatocellular carcinoma in a specialized center. Brit J Surg 2004;91(3):334-8
- Yoshida H, Tateishi R, Arakawa Y et al. Benefit of interferon therapy in hepatocellular carcinoma prevention for individual patients with chronic hepatitis C. Gut 2004;53 (3):425-30
- Lang BH, Poon RT, Fan ST et al. Perioperative and long-term outcome of major hepatic resection for small solitary hepatocellular carcinoma in patients with cirrhosis. Arch Surg 2003;138 (11): 1207-13
- Cha C, Fong Y, Jarnagin WR, et al. Predictors and patterns of recurrence after resection of hepatocellular carcinoma. J Am Coll Surg 2003;197 (5): 753-8
- Harrison LE, Koneru B, Baramipour P et al. Locoregional recurrences are frequent after radiofrequency ablation for hepatocellular carcinoma. J Am Colll Surg 2003;197 (5): 759-64
- Adam R, Azoulay D, Castaing D et al. Liver resection as a bridge to transplantation for hepatocellular carcinoma on cirrhosis: a reasonable strategy? Ann Surg 2003;238 (4): 508-19
- De Baere T, Risse O, Kuoch V et al. Adverse evetnts during radiofrequency treatments of 582 hepatic tumors. Am J Roentgenol 2003;181 (3):695-700
- O'Suilleabhain CB, Poon RT, Yong JL et al. Factors predictive of 5 year survival after transarterial chemoembolization for inoperable hepatocellular carcinoma. Br J Surg 2003;90 (3): 325-31
- Ebied OM, Federle MP, Carr BI et al. Evaluation of responses to chemoembolization in patients with unresectable hepatocellular carcinoma. Cancer 2003;97 (4):1042-50

Web references: 1 available at www.5mcc.com
Illustrations 1 available

Author(s):
Frank L. Iber, MD

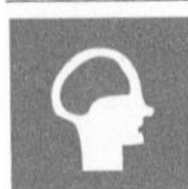

BASICS

DESCRIPTION An acute, functional and progressive reduction in renal blood flow and glomerular filtration rate (GFR) secondary to intense renal cortical vasoconstriction in the setting of decompensated cirrhosis. Other etiologies for renal failure in cirrhosis must be absent to diagnose hepatorenal syndrome (HRS). HRS may be classified as (1) type 1 HRS with a rapidly progressive decline in GFR (< 2 weeks); or (2) type II HRS which is not as rapidly progressive (> 2 weeks).

System(s) affected: Endocrine/Metabolic, Gastrointestinal, Hemic/Lymphatic/Immunologic, Nervous, Renal/Urologic

Genetics: Not important except as risk for liver disease (e.g., infantile or autosomal recessive polycystic kidney disease or alpha-1-antitrypsin deficiency, etc.)

Incidence/Prevalence in USA: Unknown (clear cut differentiation between hepatorenal syndrome and acute tubular necrosis [ATN] or pre-renal state not always made). Estimate: 32-41/100 admitted to the hospital for cirrhosis with ascites develop HRS at 2 and 5 years. One other study in patients with cirrhosis and ascites: 18% and 39% (of HRS) at 1 and 5 years.

Predominant age: Usually > 4th decade (increased incidence of alcoholic cirrhosis) but may occur at any age

Predominant sex: Male > Female (increased incidence and prevalence of alcoholic cirrhosis)

SIGNS & SYMPTOMS

- Oliguria in the setting of cirrhosis
- Jaundice, ascites, encephalopathy
- GI bleeding
- Poor nutritional status
- Splenomegaly
- Spider angioma
- Peripheral vasodilatation
- Tachycardia and bounding pulse often present with HRS. Almost always develops during a hospitalization, not on admission.

CAUSES End stage liver disease from alcohol or toxins, viral hepatitis, fulminant hepatic failure, malignancy or any other injury which leads to cirrhosis (e.g., Schistosoma) with accompanying risk factors

RISK FACTORS

- Any reduction of effective blood volume in cirrhosis including:
  - ◊ Excessive diuresis and gastrointestinal blood loss (e.g., variceal bleeding)
  - ◊ Excessive diarrhea (lactulose-induced)
  - ◊ Bacteremia
  - ◊ Reduction in venous return with tense ascites
  - ◊ Vomiting; GI bleeding
  - ◊ Protein-calorie malnutrition, especially with alcoholic cirrhosis

DIAGNOSIS

DIFFERENTIAL DIAGNOSIS

- For abrupt onset of oliguria in cirrhosis
  - ◊ Volume contraction
  - ◊ Cardiac failure (possibly alcoholic cardiomyopathy)
  - ◊ Acute vasomotor nephropathy
  - ◊ Obstruction
  - ◊ Interstitial nephritis (drug-induced)

LABORATORY

- Azotemia in the setting of cirrhosis with appropriate spot urine values (consistent with tubular function):
  - ◊ Na+ < 10 mEq/L (10 mmol/L)
  - ◊ Fractional excretion of sodium < 1%
  - ◊ Urine/plasma creatinine > 30:1
  - ◊ Osmolality mild to moderate reduction in concentrating ability (400-600 mOsm/kg/water)
  - ◊ All reversible causes should be ruled out (e.g., pre-renal; obstruction).
- Urinalysis - absence of ATN casts; < 500 mg/dL protein
- Lack of improvement in renal function following diuretic withdrawal and expansion of plasma volume with 1.5 L of normal saline
- Minor criteria: urine volume < 500 cc/day; urine red cells < 50 hpf; serum sodium < 130 mcg/L
- Other: prolonged prothrombin time, decreased serum albumin concentration, elevated bilirubin

Drugs that may alter lab results: N/A

Disorders that may alter lab results: N/A

PATHOLOGICAL FINDINGS

- Liver: cirrhosis or acute fulminant failure
- Kidneys: would function if transplanted into hosts without liver disease, a functional renal derangement only

SPECIAL TESTS Xenon 133 washout curves show a profound reduction in renal cortical perfusion (historic interest)

IMAGING Renal ultrasound shows normal kidneys without obstruction

DIAGNOSTIC PROCEDURES Though experimental presently, renal duplex Doppler ultrasonography appears to have predictive value in separating cirrhotics who will develop HRS from those who won't based on resistive index

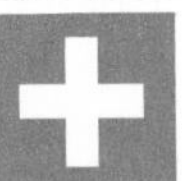

TREATMENT

APPROPRIATE HEALTH CARE Maintenance of volume status in cirrhosis

GENERAL MEASURES

- Supportive
  - ◊ Avoid iatrogenic events that precipitate HRS
  - ◊ Diagnose and treat correctable causes of azotemia in cirrhosis: volume expanders (100 gm albumin in 500 cc normal saline) should always be tried if possible, left ventricular function maximized if possible, relief of urinary obstruction when present
- Other
  - ◊ Large volume paracentesis
  - ◊ Dialysis is only indicated as ancillary support for patients awaiting liver transplant or in patients with acute potentially reversible liver failure
  - ◊ Head-out water immersion and LaVeen shunts of dubious value
  - ◊ Acute liver failure with HRS may reverse if the liver regenerates

SURGICAL MEASURES Liver transplantation when feasible is the only curative treatment. The observed 3 month to estimated 6 months to 1 year survival in patients with transjugular intrahepatic portosystemic stent-shunts is improved. LeVeen shunt may provide similar benefit.

ACTIVITY Bedrest

DIET N/A

PATIENT EDUCATION In alcoholic cirrhosis, abstention from alcohol is essential and may prevent further deterioration of cirrhosis

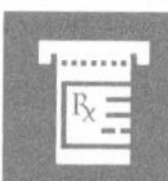

MEDICATIONS

DRUG(S) OF CHOICE Low dose dopamine may provide temporary benefit. Not curative.

Contraindications: N/A

Precautions:
- Avoid NSAIDs, demeclocycline, aminoglycosides or other nephrotoxins
- Judicious use of loop diuretics
- Avoid iatrogenic volume contraction in cirrhotic inpatients

Significant possible interactions: Refer to manufacturer's literature

ALTERNATIVE DRUGS Vasopressin analogues (terlipressin and ornipressin) combined with plasma volume expansion demonstrate some effect on the short-term reversibility of renal dysfunction. May act as a bridge to liver transplant. Questions of efficacy persist, however.

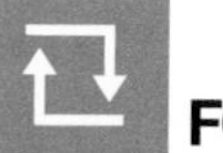

FOLLOWUP

PATIENT MONITORING N/A

PREVENTION/AVOIDANCE See Risk Factors

POSSIBLE COMPLICATIONS Death

EXPECTED COURSE/PROGNOSIS
- Grave without liver transplant in chronic cirrhosis or without regeneration of the liver in acute fulminant failure
- If a liver transplant is performed, actuarial patient survival after transplant is less in patients with preceding hepatorenal syndrome
- The patient may be supported with hemodialysis, continuous arteriovenous hemofiltration (CAVH) or continuous arteriovenous hemodialysis (CAVHD) and transjugular portosystemic stent-shunt prior to organ availability for transplant

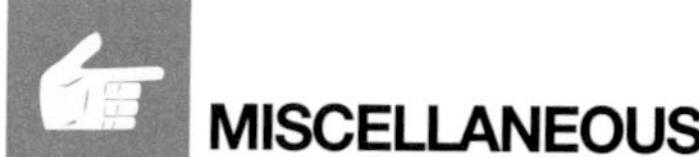

MISCELLANEOUS

ASSOCIATED CONDITIONS See Causes and Differential Diagnosis

AGE-RELATED FACTORS
Pediatric: See Genetics
Geriatric: N/A
Others: N/A

PREGNANCY May be associated with HRS if liver failure occurs during pregnancy

SYNONYMS
- Renal failure of cirrhosis
- Functional renal failure of cirrhosis
- Hepatic nephropathy
- Heyd syndrome
- Oliguric renal failure of cirrhosis
- Hemodynamic renal failure of cirrhosis

ICD-9-CM
572.4 Hepatorenal syndrome
997.4 Digestive system complications, NEC

SEE ALSO
Acetaminophen poisoning
Cirrhosis of the liver
Hepatitis A
Hepatitis B
Hepatitis C
Renal failure, acute (ARF)
Schistosomiasis of the liver, chronic

OTHER NOTES N/A

ABBREVIATIONS
HRS = hepatorenal syndrome

REFERENCES

- Celeb H, Dondy E, Celikes H: Renal blood flow detection with Doppler ultrasonography in patients with hepatic cirrhosis. Arch Int Med 1997;157:564-566
- Arroyo V, Gines P, Gerbes AL et al: Definition and diagnostic criteria of refractory ascites and hepatorenal syndrome in cirrhosis. Hepatology 1996;23:164-176
- Roberts LR, Kamath PS: Ascites and hepatorenal syndrome; pathophysiology and management. Mayo Clin Proc 1996;71:874881
- Van Roey G, Moore K: The hepatorenal syndrome. Pediatr Nephrol 1996;10:100-107
- Brensing KA, Textor J, Strunk H, et al: Transjugular intrahepatic portosystemic stent-shunt for hepatorenal syndrome. Lancet 1997;349:697-698
- Sussman NL, Lake JR: Treatment of hepatic failure-1996: current concepts and progress toward liver dialysis. Am J Kid Dis 1996;27:605-621
- Gines P. Arroyo V, Rodes J: Ascites and hepatorenal syndrome: pathogenesis and treatment strategies. Advances In Internal Med 1998;43:99-143
- Bateller R, Sort P, Gines P, Arroyo V: Hepatorenal syndrome: definition, pathophysiology, clinical features and management. Kidney Intl 1998;53(suppl 66):S47-S53
- Epstein M: Hepatorenal syndrome: emerging perspectives. Seminars in Nephrology 1997;17(6):563-575

Web references: 1 available at www.5mcc.com
Illustrations N/A

Author(s):
Michael M. Van Ness, MD

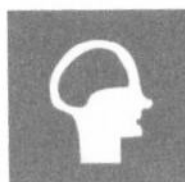

BASICS

DESCRIPTION Infectious disease caused by Coxsackievirus group A. Characteristics - fever of short duration, typical vesicular or ulcerated lesions in the post pharynx or on the soft palate. Usual course - acute.
System(s) affected: Endocrine/Metabolic, Gastrointestinal
Genetics: N/A
Incidence/Prevalence in USA: Year around in tropical climate and in summer and fall in temperate climate
Predominant age: 3 months-16 years
Predominant sex: Male = Female

SIGNS & SYMPTOMS
- Anorexia
- Drooling
- Sore throat
- Fever
- Malaise
- Irritability
- Listlessness
- Local pain
- Emesis
- Backache
- Headache
- Coryza
- Diarrhea
- Bilateral discrete vesicles, gray base
- Erythematous patches
- Vesicles may rupture to form ulcers
- Posterior pharynx location - pharynx, tonsils, soft palate, little involvement of anterior 2/3 of mouth

CAUSES
- Common
  - ◊ Coxsackievirus A - types 1-10, 16 and 22
- Infrequent
  - ◊ Coxsackievirus B - types 1-5
  - ◊ Echovirus - types 6, 9, 11, 17, 22, 25
  - ◊ Other enterovirus

RISK FACTORS Contact with infected person

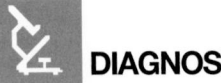

DIAGNOSIS

DIFFERENTIAL DIAGNOSIS
- Herpes simplex - multiple ulcers on lips and anterior mouth. Diagnose with Herpes culture.
- Drug reactions - cutaneous lesions often present (urticaria, erythema multiforme)
- Recurrent aphthous stomatitis
  - ◊ Buccal, labial, alveolar, mucosal ulcers
  - ◊ Recurrent crops
  - ◊ Few systemic symptoms
- Lichen planus - painful ulcer, white "lacy" pattern on mucosa or may have cutaneous lesions which are purple and pruritic
- Hand, foot and mouth disease - classic distribution of vesicular rash on hands, buttocks, feet and mouth

LABORATORY
- Slight leukocytosis (< 50%)
- Positive viral culture - mouth washings, stool

Drugs that may alter lab results: N/A

Disorders that may alter lab results: N/A

PATHOLOGICAL FINDINGS N/A

SPECIAL TESTS
- Complement fixation
- Hemagglutinin inhibition tests
- Serum antibodies to coxsackievirus - titers should show a fourfold rise in serial samples

IMAGING N/A

DIAGNOSTIC PROCEDURES N/A

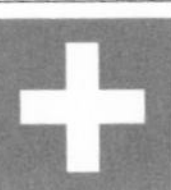

TREATMENT

APPROPRIATE HEALTH CARE
Outpatient

GENERAL MEASURES
- Self-limited
- Palliative and supportive
- Hydration

SURGICAL MEASURES N/A

ACTIVITY No restrictions

DIET Clear liquids

PATIENT EDUCATION N/A

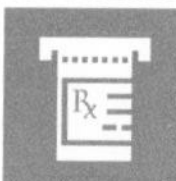

MEDICATIONS

DRUG(S) OF CHOICE
- Analgesics - acetaminophen, NSAIDs
- Topical anesthetics
- Mouthwash - aqueous solution of 1% dyclonine and 1% diphenhydramine (Benadryl) in 50% attapulgite (Kaopectate)
- 2% viscous lidocaine solution

Contraindications: N/A
Precautions: N/A
Significant possible interactions: N/A

ALTERNATIVE DRUGS N/A

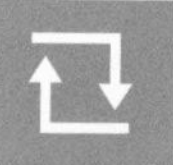

FOLLOWUP

PATIENT MONITORING Hydration

PREVENTION/AVOIDANCE Avoid contact with infected individual

POSSIBLE COMPLICATIONS
- Complications are rare
  - ◊ Exanthem
  - ◊ Aseptic meningitis
  - ◊ Myocarditis
  - ◊ Encephalitis

EXPECTED COURSE/PROGNOSIS
Complete recovery

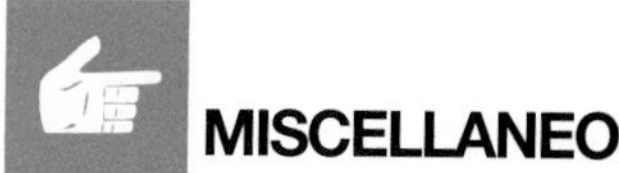

MISCELLANEOUS

ASSOCIATED CONDITIONS N/A

AGE-RELATED FACTORS
Pediatric: N/A
Geriatric: N/A
Others: N/A

PREGNANCY N/A

SYNONYMS N/A

ICD-9-CM
074.0 Herpangina

SEE ALSO
Hand-foot-and-mouth disease
Herpes simplex

OTHER NOTES N/A

ABBREVIATIONS N/A

REFERENCES

- Bondi J, Jegasothy B, Lazarus G. Dermatology, Diagnosis and Therapy. Norwalk, CT: McGraw-Hill/Appleton & Lange; 1992
- Ho M, Chen ER, Hsu KH, et al. An epidemic of enterovirus 71 infection in Taiwan. Taiwan Enterovirus Epidemic Working Group. N Engl J Med 1999;341(13):929-35

Web references: 2 available at www.5mcc.com
Illustrations N/A

Author(s):
Aamir Siddiqi, MD

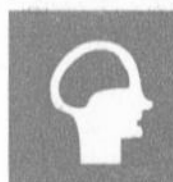

BASICS

DESCRIPTION Infections of the eye caused by one of the herpes viruses. Herpes simplex (HSV) types 1 and 2 or varicella-zoster virus. These infections may affect the eyelids and surrounding skin and may also cause conjunctivitis, keratitis, uveitis, as well as retinitis or optic neuritis. These viruses establish latent infections and eye involvement is most often from reactivation of latent viruses. Epstein-Barr virus may cause conjunctivitis or keratitis in infectious mononucleosis. Cytomegalovirus, which is also a herpesvirus, can cause a severe retinitis in immunocompromised patients with AIDS.

System(s) affected: Nervous, Skin/Exocrine

Genetics: No genetic pattern

Incidence/Prevalence in USA:
- HSV - 500,000 cases per year; 1/10,000 infants born with neonatal HSV
- Zoster - 300,000 new cases per year

Predominant age:
- HSV may affect any age
- Zoster usually affects older people

Predominant sex: Male = Female

SIGNS & SYMPTOMS

Varies according to the virus and the ocular structures involved
- Eye pain
- Red eye (usually unilateral)
- Photophobia
- Tearing
- Decreased vision
- Skin/eyelid rash and pain
- Fever (varicella-zoster or infectious mononucleosis)
- Malaise (varicella-zoster or infectious mononucleosis)

CAUSES
- Primary infections:
  - ◊ Neonatal HSV, usually HSV-2
  - ◊ Primary ocular HSV, usually HSV-1
- Recurrent infections:
  - ◊ Reactivation of HSV or herpes zoster virus (HZV) from trigeminal ganglion
- Reactivating factors:
  - ◊ Fever
  - ◊ Ultraviolet light
  - ◊ Cold wind
  - ◊ Systemic illness
  - ◊ Menstruation
  - ◊ Emotional stress
  - ◊ Local trauma
  - ◊ Immunosuppression

RISK FACTORS
- Family members/close contact with HSV
- History of varicella infection

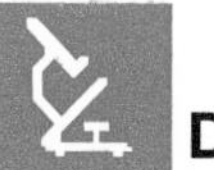

DIAGNOSIS

DIFFERENTIAL DIAGNOSIS
- Viral conjunctivitis of other cause
- Bacterial keratoconjunctivitis
- Adult inclusion (chlamydial) conjunctivitis
- Allergic conjunctivitis
- Corneal abrasion
- Recurrent corneal erosion
- Toxic conjunctivitis
- Fungal keratitis
- Iritis/uveitis
- Scleritis

LABORATORY
- Laboratory tests are usually not required unless diagnosis in doubt
- Viral culture from cornea, conjunctiva, or skin; fluorescent antibody; polymerase chain reaction (PCR)
- Giemsa stain of corneal or skin lesion scrapings for multinucleated giant cells

Drugs that may alter lab results: N/A

Disorders that may alter lab results: N/A

PATHOLOGICAL FINDINGS
- Vesicular skin rash
- Zoster rash follows dermatome, does not cross midline and involves upper eyelid
- Dendritic keratitis
- HSV dendrites stain with fluorescein
- Large geographic corneal ulcers may occur
- Corneal stromal inflammation, opacity and neovascularization may occur
- Decreased corneal sensation
- Uveitis
- Secondary glaucoma

SPECIAL TESTS
- Fluorescein staining of the cornea - positive staining with HSV
- Rose bengal staining of cornea - positive with zoster and HSV
- Corneal sensation - usually decreased
- Slit-lamp exam
- Measure intraocular pressure
- Dilated funduscope exam
- Evaluate zoster patients under age 40 for immunodeficiency

IMAGING N/A

DIAGNOSTIC PROCEDURES As above

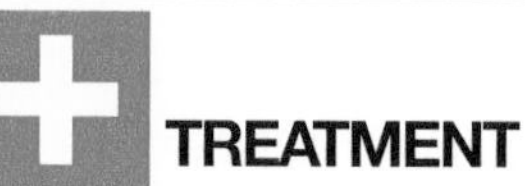

TREATMENT

APPROPRIATE HEALTH CARE
- Outpatient
- Hospitalize if severe systemic spread for IV therapy

GENERAL MEASURES
- Warm compresses to skin lesions
- Gentle debridement of corneal epithelial lesions

SURGICAL MEASURES Occasionally, débridement of involved epithelium

ACTIVITY As tolerated

DIET Regular

PATIENT EDUCATION American Academy of Ophthalmology

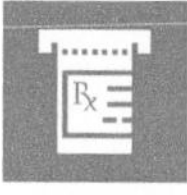

MEDICATIONS

DRUG(S) OF CHOICE
- Skin and eyelid lesions:
  - ◊ Prophylactic topical antibiotic ointment, such as bacitracin or erythromycin bid for 1-2 weeks
  - ◊ Trifluorothymidine (Viroptic) 1% drops or vidarabine 3% ointment 5 times per day if eyelid margin involved
  - ◊ Zoster - acyclovir 800 mg po 5 times per day for 10 days or famciclovir 500 mg po tid for 7 days; useful if started within 7 days of onset and active lesions are present
  - ◊ Severe or persistent zoster - hospitalize; acyclovir 5-10 mg/kg IV q 8 hours for 5-10 days
  - ◊ For postherpetic neuralgia in herpes zoster:
    - Consider prednisone 60 mg po for 3-7 days and taper off over the next 1-2 weeks
    - Cimetidine 400 mg po bid during prednisone treatment
    - Consider antidepressant such as amitriptyline 25 mg po tid
- Corneal disease:
  - ◊ HSV epithelial disease:
    - Trifluorothymidine 1% drops 9 times per day or vidarabine 3% ointment 5 times per day; taper over 10-21 days based on response
    - Cycloplegia with scopolamine 0.25% or cyclopentolate 1% drops tid
  - ◊ Stromal keratitis or uveitis (without epithelial disease):
    - Cycloplegia with scopolamine 0.25% or cyclopentolate 1% drops tid
    - Topical steroid such as prednisolone acetate 1% drops qid
    - Trifluorothymidine 1% drops qid for prophylaxis while on topical steroids
- Optic neuritis, chorioretinitis, or cranial nerve involvement with zoster:
  - ◊ Acyclovir 5-10 mg/kg IV q 8 hours for 1 week
  - ◊ Prednisone 60 mg po for 3-7 days and taper over the next 1-2 weeks
- Secondary glaucoma
  - ◊ Aqueous humor suppressant such as timolol 0.5% drops bid or methazolamide 50 mg po bid or tid
- Neurotrophic ulcer or persistent epithelial disease:
  - ◊ Consider reducing or discontinuing topical antivirals to avoid toxicity
  - ◊ Preservative-free lubricant ointment
  - ◊ Erythromycin 3% ophthalmic ointment q hs or bid
  - ◊ Consider patching or tarsorrhaphy

Contraindications:
- Topical steroids are contraindicated with active corneal epithelial disease
- Acyclovir is contraindicated in pregnancy
- Prednisone should not be used in immunocompromised patients

Precautions:
- Topical antiviral agents are toxic and may cause an allergic reaction; substitution with another agent may be tried
- Topical steroids can raise intraocular pressure
- Acyclovir dosage should be reduced in renal insufficiency
- See manufacturer's literature for additional precautions

Significant possible interactions: See manufacturer's literature

ALTERNATIVE DRUGS
- Idoxuridine 0.5% ointment or 0.1% drops 5 times per day is more toxic than the other antivirals, but may be substituted if allergic reaction develops to others
- Topical acyclovir ointment to skin lesions - effectiveness uncertain
- Medroxyprogesterone 1% drops in place of other steroids if corneal thinning
- Capsaicin 0.025% cream tid to 6 times per day for months to years for post-herpetic neuralgia
- Non-steroidal anti-inflammatory agents po for scleritis associated with zoster
- Amitriptyline may also be helpful for postherpetic neuralgia
- Oral acyclovir 2 gm/day in divided doses x 10 days may be used in patients intolerant of topical antivirals
- Oral valacyclovir 500-1000mg bid has been used as an alternative to acyclovir

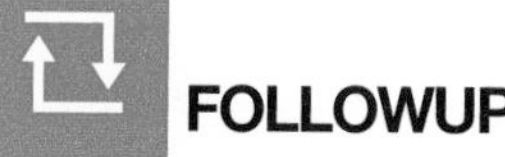

FOLLOWUP

PATIENT MONITORING
- Size of epithelial defect
- Vision
- Corneal opacity
- Anterior chamber inflammation
- Intraocular pressure

PREVENTION/AVOIDANCE
- Avoid close contact with patients with active lesions
- Herpes zoster virus can be spread to individuals who have not had chicken pox
- Avoid known precipitating factors for recurrent HSV
- Topical steroids alone do not reactivate the virus, but may exacerbate spontaneous recurrences
- Very slow taper of topical steroids over many months for corneal epithelial disease
- Antiviral prophylaxis while on topical steroids
- Varicella vaccination prior to infection
- Oral acyclovir 400 mg bid reduces recurrence rate of HSV keratitis by 50%

POSSIBLE COMPLICATIONS
- Corneal neovascularization and scarring resulting in poor vision
- Neurotrophic ulcer with perforation
- Secondary bacterial or fungal infection
- Secondary glaucoma from uveitis or steroid treatment
- Necrotizing interstitial keratitis
- Corneal transplant may be required
- Post-herpetic neuralgia with zoster
- Vision loss from optic neuritis or chorioretinitis
- Systemic involvement

EXPECTED COURSE/PROGNOSIS
- Neonatal primary HSV often disseminated with high mortality rate, 37% have vision worse than 20/200
- Primary HSV in children and adults often asymptomatic; overt disease usually self-limited
- Recurrent ocular HSV:
  - ◊ Skin lesions in clusters last for 5-7 days
  - ◊ HSV epithelial disease - without treatment, 40% resolve without sequelae; with treatment, 90-95% resolve without complication
  - ◊ HSV stromal keratitis usually resolves in weeks to months with some scarring; neovascularization increases risk for severe scarring
- Ocular varicella - may produce a keratitis; usually self-limited, but with occasional complications
- Herpes zoster ophthalmicus
  - ◊ Dermatitis 8-14 days acute phase with subsequent scarring possible
  - ◊ Conjunctivitis, episcleritis and scleritis may occur
  - ◊ Two-thirds of patients develop keratitis and decreased corneal sensation
  - ◊ Uveitis occurs in about 40%
  - ◊ Neurotrophic keratitis occurs in one-half; most recover sensation in 2-3 months
  - ◊ Secondary glaucoma occurs in 10%
  - ◊ Post-herpetic neuralgia in 20-40%; usually longer lasting in older patients
- Recurrence common for HSV and HZO

MISCELLANEOUS

ASSOCIATED CONDITIONS
- Immunosuppression
- AIDS
- Malignancy

AGE-RELATED FACTORS
Pediatric: Neonatal HSV often systemic and life-threatening
Geriatric: Zoster more common in older age groups
Others: Consider immunodeficiency in zoster patients under age 40

PREGNANCY
- May increase recurrence
- Avoid systemic steroids, acyclovir and other medications contraindicated in pregnancy
- Pregnant women who have not had chicken pox should especially avoid contact with patients with active zoster

SYNONYMS
- Herpes simplex keratitis
- Herpes zoster ophthalmicus
- Herpetic keratitis or keratouveitis

ICD-9-CM
054.40 Herpes simplex with unspecified ophthalmic complication
053.29 Herpes zoster (HZV) with ophthalmic complications, other

SEE ALSO
Conjunctivitis, acute

OTHER NOTES N/A

ABBREVIATIONS
HSV = herpes simplex virus
HZV = herpes zoster virus
HZO = herpes zoster ophthalmicus
VZV = varicella-zoster virus

REFERENCES

- Albert DM, Jakobiec FA, eds. Principles and Practice of Ophthalmology. Philadelphia, W.B. Saunders Co., 1994
- Rhee DJ, Pyfer MF, eds. The Wills Eye Manual - Office and Emergency Room Diagnosis and Treatment of Eye Diseases. 3rd Ed. Philadelphia, Lippincott Williams & Wilkins, 1999
- Pepose JS, Holland GN, Wilhelmus KR. Ocular Infection and Immunity. St. Louis, Mosby, 1996

Web references: 1 available at www.5mcc.com
Illustrations N/A

Author(s):
Thomas W. Hejkal, MD, PhD

BASICS

DESCRIPTION Herpes (from Greek "to creep or crawl") simplex virus (usually HSV-2) infection involving the genitals

- Primary genital herpes: genital herpes due to HSV-1 or HSV-2 with absence of antibody to HSV-1 or HSV-2 at time of infection
- Non-primary first episode genital herpes: genital herpes due to HSV-2 with existing antibody to HSV-1 or genital herpes due to HSV-1 with existing antibody to HSV-2
- Recurrent genital herpes: reactivation of latent genital herpes with existing antibody to the same HSV type recovered from the lesion

System(s) affected: Nervous, Reproductive, Skin/Exocrine

Genetics: N/A

Incidence/Prevalence in USA:

- 50-200/100,000 (300,000 - 700,000 cases/year)
- 10,000-30,000/100,000 people (45 million)

Predominant age: 18-40

Predominant sex: Female > Male

SIGNS & SYMPTOMS

- It is difficult to differentiate primary, 1st episode non-primary, and recurrent disease on the basis of symptoms and clinical findings
- 60-70% of patients infected with HSV-2 are asymptomatic or do not recognize clinical manifestations of disease
- Presence of multiple, shallow, tender ulcers has 94% specificity for diagnosis of genital HSV in males
- Primary genital herpes
  - ◊ Fever; headache; malaise; myalgia
  - ◊ Burning genital pain
  - ◊ Dysuria (female)
  - ◊ Dyspareunia
  - ◊ Sacral paresthesia
  - ◊ Inguinal adenopathy
  - ◊ Aseptic meningitis in 30%
  - ◊ Occasional urinary retention
  - ◊ Vesicles, on an erythematous base, which ulcerate, crust over, and resolve spontaneously within 21 days. Vesicles persist longer on dry skin.
  - ◊ Bilateral lesions, primarily affecting the external genitalia: female - labia majora/minora, inner thighs, vaginal mucosa, cervix, perianal skin; male - penile glans, penile shaft, urethra
- Non-primary: first episode
  - ◊ Burning genital pain
  - ◊ Vesicles, on an erythematous base, which ulcerate, crust over, and resolve spontaneously within 14-17 days
- Non-primary: recurrent
  - ◊ Prodromal symptoms - burning, numbness, tingling, paresthesia of genitals at site of previous lesions which occur approximately 24 hours prior to the eruption of new vesicles
  - ◊ Burning genital pain
  - ◊ Vesicles, on an erythematous base, which ulcerate, crust over, and resolve spontaneously within 7-10 days
  - ◊ Unilateral lesions
  - ◊ Endometritis, salpingitis, urethritis, prostatitis may be associated with recurrent HSV-2 infection

CAUSES

- Herpes simplex virus; a double stranded DNA, Alphaherpesvirinae virus subfamily
  - ◊ HSV-1: 10-30% (increasing incidence); is now greater than HSV-2 in some clinical settings; falling incidence of childhood HSV-1; oral sex
  - ◊ HSV-2: 70-90% (99% with HSV-2 antibodies have genital lesions)

RISK FACTORS

- Primary inoculation
  - ◊ Increasing age, lower socioeconomic status, African-American
  - ◊ Sexual activity - number of lifetime partners, duration of sexual activity, and past history of STD's
  - ◊ Fomites - wet towels (rare)
- Transmission:
  - ◊ Incubation period: 1-45 days (mean 5.8)
  - ◊ Annual risk for susceptible female acquiring disease from an infected male partner is 10-30%; for susceptible male from infected female approximately 5%
  - ◊ Patients without HSV-1 antibody are at greater risk for acquiring HSV-2 infection than those with HSV-1 antibody
  - ◊ Over 70% of new cases result from transmission during asymptomatic or clinically unrecognized shedding
  - ◊ Risk of asymptomatic shedding is highest within 1 year of occurrence of first episode of genital herpes, occurs 2-3% of days, in HSV-2 infection, and in women with frequent symptomatic episodes
  - ◊ Oral acyclovir daily suppresses shedding of HSV-2 (80-90% reduction)
  - ◊ Valacyclovir, given once daily, reduces transmission of HSV-2 to uninfected partners by 77%
- Triggers (recurrent): genital trauma, menses, intercurrent infection, emotional stress, ultraviolet light; recurrences more common in men

DIAGNOSIS

DIFFERENTIAL DIAGNOSIS

- Primary syphilis, chancroid, lymphogranuloma venereum, atypical genital warts, molluscum contagiosum, candidiasis, herpes zoster, folliculitis, scabies, allergic contact dermatitis, trauma, inflammatory bowel disease, Behçet syndrome, Stevens-Johnson syndrome, psoriasis, lichen planus, ulcerative balanitis, granuloma inguinale, neoplasia

LABORATORY

- Viral detection from lesion: swab vesicle fluid or ulcer; viral culture, EIA, DNA detection by PCR (2-3x more sensitive than culture)
- Tzanck prep: sensitivity = 40-50% compared to culture; multinucleated giant cells.
- Pap smear - sensitivity = 60-70%
- Serology: ELISA, direct fluorescent assay (DFA), radioimmunoassay (RIA) and complement fixation. Do not reliably discriminate between HSV-1 and HSV-2. Sensitivity = 80% compared to culture. Primary herpes - 4 x increase acute/convalescent titer; recurrent herpes - no increase in acute/convalescent titer. Seroconversion usually occurs within 4-6 weeks after onset of symptoms.
- Type specific serologic assays: Immunodot, Western Blot (gold standard) and monoclonal antibody (glycoprotein-G) blocking RIA - discriminate between HSV-1 and HSV-2. Commercially available tests include HerpesSelect-1 & 2 (ELISA), HerpesSelect 1/2 (immunoblot), and POCkit-HSV-2 (point of care test).
- Potential indications for obtaining type specific herpes virus serology:
  - ◊ Evaluation of asymptomatic long-term sexual partner of infected individual
  - ◊ Recurrent undiagnosed genital ulcers
  - ◊ Screening of pregnant women with infected partners
  - ◊ Differentiation between primary and non-primary genital infection
- Screening of following groups - STD clinic attendees, semen donors, candidates for immunosuppression, individuals at high risk for HIV infection

Drugs that may alter lab results: Calcium agglutinate swabs may be toxic to HSV and are not recommended for culture; use Dacron tipped swabs

Disorders that may alter lab results: Varicella-zoster will give identical Tzanck prep results

PATHOLOGICAL FINDINGS

- Histopathologic-cytopathic changes
  - ◊ Intracellular edema of epithelial cells
  - ◊ Nuclear margination of chromatin
  - ◊ Formation of Cowdry type A intranuclear inclusions
  - ◊ Cell fusion into multinucleated giant cells
- Pathologic stages:
  - ◊ Primary mucocutaneous infection
  - ◊ Acute sacral ganglionic infection
  - ◊ Establishment of latency
  - ◊ Ganglionic reactivation
  - ◊ Recurrent infection

SPECIAL TESTS

Herpes simplex serology:

Lesion†	Serology††	Stage†††
HSV1	Negative	P HSV1
HSV2	Negative	P HSV2
HSV1	HSV2	NP HSV1
HSV2	HSV1	NP HSV2
HSV1	HSV1 ± HSV2	R HSV1
HSV2	HSV2 ± HSV1	R HSV2

† culture, EIA or PCR
†† type-specific antibody
††† P=primary; R=recurrent; NP=non-primary first episode

IMAGING N/A

DIAGNOSTIC PROCEDURES N/A

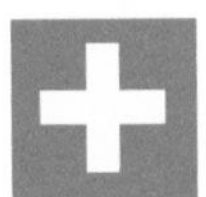

TREATMENT

APPROPRIATE HEALTH CARE Outpatient, self-care

GENERAL MEASURES Cool compresses of aluminum acetate (Burow's solution) 4-6 times a day), ice packs to perineum, sitz baths, local perineal hygiene, topical anesthetic, analgesics (NSAIDs)

SURGICAL MEASURES N/A

ACTIVITY
- Avoid intercourse in the presence of symptomatic genital lesions
- Appropriate rest if systemic manifestations (primary) are present

DIET N/A

PATIENT EDUCATION
Herpes Resource Center Hotline (919)361-8488

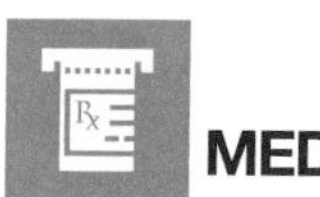

MEDICATIONS

DRUG(S) OF CHOICE
- Acyclovir (Zovirax)
  - ◊ Primary episode: 400 mg tid x10 days or 200 mg po 5 q day x7-10 days
  - ◊ Severe local or disseminated disease: 5 mg/kg IV q 8 hrs x7 days
  - ◊ Encephalitis: 10 mg/kg IV, q 8 hrs x10 days
  - ◊ Recurrent: 200 mg po 5 q day x5 days (or 400 mg tid x5 days, or 800 mg bid x5 days or 800 mg tid x2 days)
  - ◊ Chronic suppression: recommended for frequent (≥ 6/year) or clinical/psychological disabling recurrences: 400 mg po bid (or 200 mg po 3-5 times/day) - appears safe and efficacious for at least 10 years of therapy. Patients prefer suppression over episodic treatment of recurrences.
  - ◊ HIV infection: 400 mg po 3-5 q day until clinical resolution attained

Contraindications: Allergy to acyclovir

Precautions:
- Acyclovir
  - ◊ Pregnancy: Not FDA approved for routine use (category C), studies have demonstrated safety when used, appropriate use is advocated by ACOG
  - ◊ Drug is excreted in breast milk
  - ◊ Modify dose in patients with significant renal insufficiency
  - ◊ Acyclovir resistance (also famciclovir and valacyclovir resistance): mostly in HIV infected patients (5-10%)

Significant possible interactions:
- Acyclovir
  - ◊ Methotrexate - use with caution in patients who have had a neurologic reaction to intrathecal methotrexate
  - ◊ Interferon - acyclovir is synergistic in vitro with interferon. Clinical significance is unknown. Use with caution in patients with prior neurological reactions to interferon.
  - ◊ Probenecid - will decrease renal excretion, increase serum concentration
  - ◊ Use with caution in combination with nephrotoxic agents

ALTERNATIVE DRUGS
- Acyclovir topical ointment - less effective; use is discouraged
- Valacyclovir (Valtrex)
  - ◊ Metabolized to acyclovir and valine; greater bioavailability than acyclovir
  - ◊ May cause thrombotic thrombocytopenia purpura/hemolytic uremic syndrome in small % of immunocompromised patients
  - ◊ Pregnancy category B
  - ◊ First episode: 1 g po bid x 7-10 days
  - ◊ Recurrent: 500 mg bid x 3-5 days
  - ◊ Chronic suppression: 250 mg po bid or 500 mg po daily (< 9 episodes/yr) or 1000 mg po daily (> 9 episodes/yr)
- Famciclovir (Famvir)
  - ◊ Metabolized to penciclovir, inhibits viral replication
  - ◊ Activity/side effects similar to acyclovir; greater bioavailability than acyclovir
  - ◊ Pregnancy category B
  - ◊ First episode: 250 mg po tid x 7-10 days
  - ◊ Recurrent: 125 mg po bid x 5 days
  - ◊ Chronic suppression: 250 mg po bid
- Foscarnet: 40 mg/kg IV every 8 hours in severe disease with proven or suspected acyclovir resistant strains
- Vidarabine: 10 mg/kg/d infused over 10 hrs; benefits HIV patients with HSV-1 infection failing acyclovir and foscarnet therapy
- Cidofovir (Vistide) topical 0.1-0.3% gel x 5 days, for progressive/resistant lesions
- Trifluridine (Viroptic) ophthalmic solution used for mucocutaneous lesions resistant to acyclovir

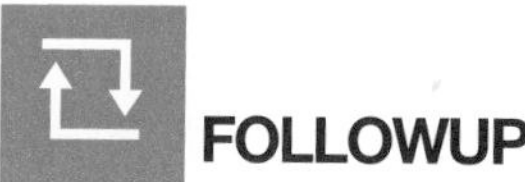

FOLLOWUP

PATIENT MONITORING
- Acute episode - followup if complications
- Latent infection - annual pap smear; check pregnant women at prenatal visits and onset of labor
- Reassess chronic suppression therapy after 1 year

PREVENTION/AVOIDANCE
- Condoms/spermicide in sexual activity
- Avoid multiple sexual partners
- Avoid stress when possible
- Avoid sex if lesions or prodromal symptoms present and for 2 days after resolved
- Pregnant women without evidence of HSV antibody should avoid unprotected sex in late pregnancy
- Screening for asymptomatic HSV infection is not recommended by USPSTF

POSSIBLE COMPLICATIONS
- Vaginal discharge
- Secondary bacterial infection
- Urinary retention
- Aseptic meningitis
- Transmission to neonate; spontaneous abortion, preterm birth, low birthweight infants
- Increased risk for HIV infection (2-3 times)
- Emotional impact - lowered self esteem, guilt, anger, depression, fear of rejection

EXPECTED COURSE/PROGNOSIS
- Resolution of signs/symptoms: Primary in 14-21 days; first episode - non-primary 14-17 days; recurrent 7-10 days
- Latent infection - recurrences in 80% of patients within 1 year of initial HSV-2 infection; immunocompetent average 3-4/year
- HSV infection in immunocompromised (AIDS) patient - more severe, difficult to treat
- Monthly recurrence rates - HSV-1 = 0.02-0.08, HSV-2 = 0.33 - 0.35

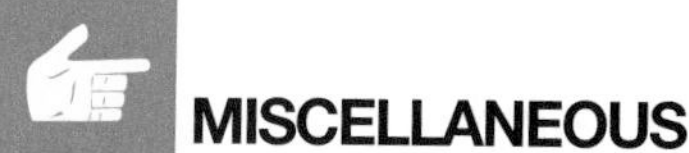

MISCELLANEOUS

ASSOCIATED CONDITIONS
- Herpes labialis
- Syphilis
- Gonorrhea
- Non-gonococcal urethritis/cervicitis
- Genital warts (HPV)
- AIDS (HIV)
- Trichomoniasis

AGE-RELATED FACTORS
Pediatric:
- Genital lesions in prepubertal child suggests sexual abuse
- Neonatal infection occurs in 10-20/100,000 live births. Most result from maternal asymptomatic viral shedding.
- Neonatal infection survival rates-localized - > 95%; CNS - 85%; systemic - 30%
- High risk infant: acyclovir 30 mg/kg/day IV q8h for 10-14 days
- Low risk infant: asymptomatic, culture eyes, nasopharynx, mouth at 24-36 hrs old and observe

Geriatric: N/A

Others: N/A

PREGNANCY
- Primary/1st episode - spontaneous abortion (45%); preterm labor (35%)
- Greatest risk for neonatal infection occurs with primary (50% transmission rate) or non-primary first episode (30% transmission rate) infected mother at delivery; enhanced by prolonged rupture of membranes, use of fetal scalp electrode, presence of lesions on cervix, and prematurity
- Low risk - recurrent asymptomatic HSV shedding in mother (3%); mothers with high titer of neutralizing antibodies
- Cesarean section is indicated if herpetic genital lesions are present during labor
- Culture suspicious lesions during pregnancy
- ACOG Clinical Management Guidelines:
  - ◊ Women with primary HSV during pregnancy, or active genital herpes infection near term or at delivery, should receive antiviral therapy
  - ◊ Women with 1st episode non-primary genital herpes or at risk for recurrent genital herpes at or beyond 36 weeks gestation should be considered for anti-viral therapy; can reduce C-section rate, clinical HSV and HSV shedding at delivery, should continue until delivery, acyclovir 400mg tid or valacyclovir 500mg bid
  - ◊ Pregnant women on acyclovir: report to CDC/ Wellcome 800-722-9292, x38465

SYNONYMS
Herpes genitalis

ICD-9-CM
054.10 Genital herpes, unspecified

SEE ALSO
Herpes simplex

OTHER NOTES N/A

ABBREVIATIONS N/A

REFERENCES

- Bernstein DI: Effects of prior HSV-1 infection on genital HSV-2 infection. Prog Med Virol 1991;38:109-127

Web references: 2 available at www.5mcc.com

Illustrations N/A

Author(s):
Gary Levine, MD

BASICS

DESCRIPTION Often called pemphigoid gestationis, a rare dermatopathic, immune-mediated and self-limited eruption most often occurring during mid-pregnancy
- Onset is in second trimester of pregnancy with remission after delivery except for some postpartum flares. May recur in subsequent pregnancies.
- Characterized by pruritic polymorphous vesicles, papules, and/or bullae often located in periumbilical or other truncal areas. May affect the buttocks, forearms, palms, or soles; less frequently scalp and face may be involved. Clustered vesicles may coalesce to form bullae, rupture to form crusts, then heal with hyperpigmentation.
- Mucous membranes are spared but intestinal mucosa may have celiac-like lesions without significant clinical malabsorption

System(s) affected: Reproductive, Skin/Exocrine
Genetics: Genetic predisposition possible, suggested by increased HLA-A1, -B8, and -DR3 antigens in affected women
Incidence/Prevalence in USA: Rare; 1 per 50,000 pregnancies; mainly whites
Predominant age: Child-bearing years
Predominant sex: Female only

SIGNS & SYMPTOMS Intensely pruritic papules and/or vesicles, occurring first in periumbilical area and spreading more generally

CAUSES
- Unknown but immune alterations suspected
- Higher association with HLA-DR3 and HLA-DR4
- Possibly role of major histocompatibility complexes (MHC) class II antigen
- Not caused by herpes virus

RISK FACTORS
- Episode in prior pregnancy
- Herpes simplex does not increase risk

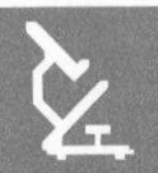

DIAGNOSIS

DIFFERENTIAL DIAGNOSIS
- Other pruritic conditions of pregnancy
  - ◊ Besnier's prurigo gestationis with excoriated papules and no vesicles; usually limited to extensor surface of extremities
  - ◊ Papular urticarial papules and plaques of pregnancy (PUPPP syndrome) which has urticarial plaques and small papules with a narrow, pale halo and no vesicles; usually in primagravidas near term
  - ◊ Impetigo herpetiformis has sterile pustules, not vesicles, and may involve mucous membranes, groin, and inner thighs
  - ◊ Papular dermatitis of pregnancy
- Non-pregnancy conditions to consider
  - ◊ Dermatitis herpetiformis (much more chronic and more often in middle-aged males)
  - ◊ Bullous pemphigoid
  - ◊ Toxic drug eruption including erythema multiforme

LABORATORY
- Tzanck smear negative
- Herpes simplex virus culture negative
- Peripheral eosinophilia may be present

Drugs that may alter lab results: N/A

Disorders that may alter lab results: N/A

PATHOLOGICAL FINDINGS
- Subepidermal vesicle often with eosinophils and edema of dermal papillae
- Acantholysis is rare
- Inflammation surrounds superficial and deep dermal vessels

SPECIAL TESTS Biopsy with direct immunofluorescence shows intense deposition of C3 (100%) and IgG (25-30%) along basement membrane. Serum may have circulating IgG antibasement membrane autoantibodies (10-20%) by indirect immunofluorescence; if not, half have herpes gestationis (HG) factor (a protein that fixes complement to basement membrane in-vitro human skin preparations).

IMAGING N/A

DIAGNOSTIC PROCEDURES Biopsy

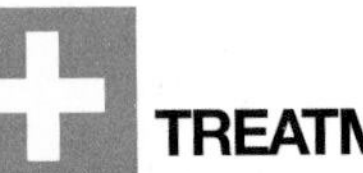

TREATMENT

APPROPRIATE HEALTH CARE Outpatient

GENERAL MEASURES
- Differentiate from herpes virus infection
- Relieve pruritus
- Prevent secondary infection
- Soothing compresses such as with aluminum acetate (Burow's solution, Domeboro) may help relieve itching

SURGICAL MEASURES N/A

ACTIVITY As tolerated

DIET No special diet

PATIENT EDUCATION
- Educate about difference between this and herpes virus infection
- Inform of possible fetal risks and possibility of limited disease in newborn

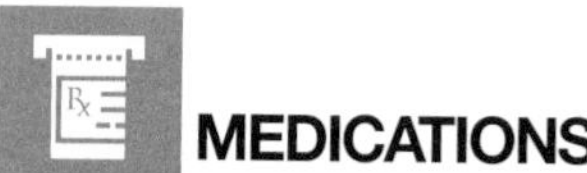

MEDICATIONS

DRUG(S) OF CHOICE

- Topical steroids and oral antihistamines for mild pruritus
- Most will require systemic corticosteroids in doses of 20-40 mg/day (at the minimum effective dose) through first month postpartum. Often able to taper off before delivery, and then increase in the postpartum period as needed.

Contraindications: Weigh risk of aggravating hyperglycemia, potential effects on maternal and fetal bone, increased susceptibility to infections versus benefit of relieving pruritus, and resolving the lesions

Precautions:

- Use prednisone cautiously in patients with immune impairment, diabetes, or thrombophlebitis
- If prednisone has been used over several weeks, taper when discontinuing to prevent cortisol deficiency

Significant possible interactions: Methylprednisolone may enhance toxicity of erythromycin

ALTERNATIVE DRUGS

Pyridoxine

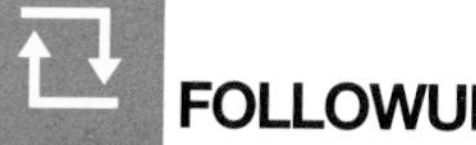

FOLLOWUP

PATIENT MONITORING

Watch for secondary bacterial infection

PREVENTION/AVOIDANCE

- Avoid other people with infections, since there is susceptibility of open skin lesions and decreased resistance secondary to corticosteroids
- Some authorities recommend cesarean section when mother is known to be infected
- Avoid scalp monitors if disease involves maternal genitalia
- Use of estrogens or progesterone may trigger flare-up

POSSIBLE COMPLICATIONS

- Secondary bacterial infection
- Excess systemic medication in pregnancy
- Fetal deaths
- Premature births
- Fetal growth retardation
- Conjunctivitis
- Keratitis
- Cataracts
- Shock
- Transient herpes gestationis in the neonate

EXPECTED COURSE/PROGNOSIS

- Spreads during 2nd-3rd trimester
- Remits after delivery within weeks
- Often flares in puerperium, especially with oral contraceptives
- Tends to recur in subsequent pregnancies and when recurs, it is likely to begin earlier and be more severe
- Systemic steroids may suppress new lesions, relieve pruritus, and dampen course; fetal outcome may be worsened
- Duration observed less in breast-feeding women

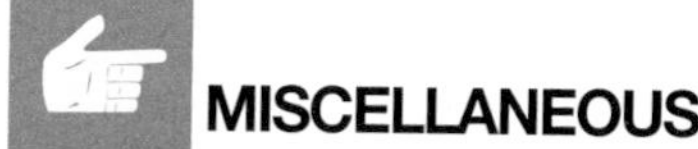

MISCELLANEOUS

ASSOCIATED CONDITIONS

- Pregnancy
- Hydatidiform mole
- Choriocarcinoma

AGE-RELATED FACTORS

Pediatric:

- Has been associated with preterm birth (22%) and still birth (< 10%)
- Rare cases of transient neonatal herpes gestationis are usually mild and resolve spontaneously; these are probably from passive transfer of antibasement membrane antibodies and HG factor

Geriatric: N/A

Others: N/A

PREGNANCY

By definition, a condition of pregnancy and puerperium. Rarely seen also with hydatiform moles and choriocarcinoma.

SYNONYMS

- Dermatitis gestationis
- Pemphigoid gestationis

ICD-9-CM

646.80 Other specified complications of pregnancy, unspecified

646.83 Other specified complications of pregnancy, antepartum condition or complication

SEE ALSO

OTHER NOTES

Uncommon intrauterine infections are associated with microcephaly intracranial calcification and chorioretinitis

ABBREVIATIONS

N/A

REFERENCES

- Engineau L. Pemphigoid gestationis: a review. Am J Obstet Gynecol 2000;183(2):483-91
- Roger D, et al. Specific pruritic diseases of pregnancy. Arch Dermatol 1994:130:734-9
- Borradori L, Saura J. Specific dermatoses of pregnancy. Arch Dermatol 1994;130:778-80

Web references: 0 available at www.5mcc.com

Illustrations N/A

Author(s):

Arthur R. Slaughter, MD

BASICS

DESCRIPTION Viral disease with many manifestations, usually seen as painful vesicles that often occur in clusters on skin, cornea, or mucous membranes; may occur as encephalitis, pneumonia, or disseminated infection.
Usual course of primary disease is 2 weeks; duration of recurrences varies; viral shedding in recurrence is briefer than with primary disease. Newborns or individuals with immune compromise are at risk for major morbidity or mortality.
System(s) affected: Nervous, Skin/Exocrine
Genetics: N/A
Incidence/Prevalence in USA:
- 29.2/100,000 office visits/year
- Widespread; 0.65-20% of adults may be excreting HSV1 or HSV2 at any given time
- Prevalence of antibodies varies from 30% in higher socioeconomic strata to 100% in lower socioeconomic strata; 20,000-70,000/100,000

Predominant age: All ages
Predominant sex: Male = Female

SIGNS & SYMPTOMS
- Vesicles - usually cluster and open as painful ulcerated lesions, often with erythematous base
- Primary disease classic variations include:
  - ◊ Herpetic whitlow: localized primary infection on a finger with intense itching and pain, followed by vesicles that may coalesce with swelling, erythema, and may mimic pyogenic paronychia; neuralgia and axillary adenopathy sometimes; heals over 2-3 weeks without incision. Primary inoculation of other abraded skin can occur (e.g., herpes gladiatorum in wrestlers).
  - ◊ Primary herpetic gingivostomatitis and pharyngitis: first infection with HSV1 usually in early childhood; incubation from 2-12 days, then fever, sore throat, pharyngeal edema and erythema; small vesicles develop on pharyngeal and oral mucosa, rapidly ulcerate and increase in number to involve soft palate, buccal mucosa, tongue, floor of mouth, and often lips and cheeks; tender gums may bleed; fetid breath, cervical adenopathy; fever, general toxicity, poor oral intake, and drooling contribute to dehydration; autoinoculation of other sites may occur; resolves in 10-14 days with slower resolution of adenopathy
  - ◊ Primary genital herpes: see Herpes, genital topic
  - ◊ Primary herpes keratoconjunctivitis: by HSV1 usually; can present as unilateral conjunctivitis with regional adenopathy, as blepharitis with vesicles on lid margin, as keratitis with dendritic lesions or with punctate opacities; lasts 2-3 weeks but systemic involvement prolongs process
  - ◊ Eczema herpeticum: diffuse pox-like eruption complicating atopic dermatitis; one cause of Kaposi varicelliform eruption; sudden appearance of lesions in typical atopic areas (upper trunk, neck, head); high fever, local edema, adenopathy, umbilicated vesicles develop hemorrhagic crust or become pustular; appear in crops for up to a week; significant fluid or blood loss and secondary bacterial infections can cause fatality; similar serious inoculations can occur with severe burn patients and go unrecognized under the eschar.
  - ◊ Neonatal herpes simplex: perinatal primary infection is life-threatening and usually acquired by vaginal birth of infected mother; fetal risk and neonatal risk are greater in mothers with primary genital herpes infection since shedding is more prolonged and the inoculum is greater; incubation from 5-7 days usually (rarely 4 weeks); cutaneous, mucous membrane, or ocular signs in only 70%; congenital infection via prenatal transplacental virus transfer may present with jaundice, hepatosplenomegaly, DIC, encephalitis, seizures, temperature instability, chorioretinitis, and/or conjunctivitis with or without skin vesicles; neurologic morbidity worse with HSV2 than with HSV1 in neonates; fatal hepatic or adrenal necrosis may occur
- Recurrent diseases from endogenous reactivation include:
  - ◊ Herpes labialis: recurrent lesions on lips with HSV1, usually less than one recurrence per six months, but 5-25% may have more than one attack per month; precipitating events may be sunlight, fever, trauma, menses, stress; prodrome of pain, burning, itching may last 6-48 hrs before vesicles appear, often at vermilion border with increased pain; will ulcerate and crust within 48 hrs; heals within 8-10 days generally; may have local adenopathy
  - ◊ Ocular herpes: may recur as keratitis, blepharitis, or keratoconjunctivitis; may have dendritic ulcers, decreased corneal sensation, less visual acuity; uveitis may cause permanent visual loss
  - ◊ Recurrent genital herpes (herpes progenitalis): see Herpes, genital topic

CAUSES Herpes simplex virus, a DNA virus of two major types: HSV1 and HSV2; most often HSV1 is associated with oral lesions and HSV2 with genital lesions but reverse occurs also

RISK FACTORS
- Immune compromise (brief as with occurrence of other illness or stress, or more chronic as with chemotherapy, malignancy, or AIDS)
- Newborns - if exposed to actively infected mother via birth canal or if exposed to case in nursery (insufficient maternal passive antibody transfer); risk greatest for neonate of mother with active primary H. simplex infection
- Prior HSV infection
- Sexual intercourse with infected person (condoms can help prevent but location of some lesions may permit spread even with condoms)
- Occupational exposure (medical/dental risk more for HSV1 whitlow and general community to HSV2 whitlow)

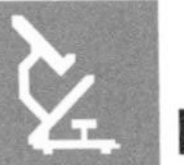

DIAGNOSIS

DIFFERENTIAL DIAGNOSIS
- Impetigo - straw-colored vesicles that crust
- Aphthous stomatitis - grayish, shallow erosions with ring of hyperemia, usually only anterior in mouth and lips
- Herpes zoster - unilateral dermatome distribution
- Syphilitic chancre - usually painless ulcer
- Herpangina - vesicles predominate on anterior tonsillar pillars, soft palate, uvula and oropharynx but not more anteriorly on lips or gums (usually caused by group A Coxsackievirus)
- Stevens-Johnson syndrome
- Other causes of Kaposi varicelliform eruption are varicella and Coxsackievirus A16

LABORATORY
- Tzanck smear shows multinucleated giant cells often with intranuclear inclusions (scrape material from lesion onto slide, fix with ethanol or methanol, stain with Giemsa or Wright preparation; alternatively spray slide with cytological fixative and stain as for Pap smear)
- Herpes simplex virus culture - only half of true positives available in 2 days; rest may take 6 days or longer to be positive; not considered as reasonable means to follow activity of recurrent disease near labor and delivery

Drugs that may alter lab results: N/A

Disorders that may alter lab results: Varicella (herpes zoster) has identical findings on Tzanck smear

PATHOLOGICAL FINDINGS Multinucleated giant cells with 2-15 nuclei per cell with eosinophilic inclusion bodies within nuclei; intraepithelial edema (ballooning degeneration) and intracellular edema; brain biopsy (in encephalitis) has hemorrhagic necrosis of gray and white matter with acute and chronic inflammation, thrombosis and fibrinoid necrosis of parenchymal vessels, and intranuclear inclusions in astrocytes, oligodendroglia, and neurons

SPECIAL TESTS
- Clinically available antibody tests do not reliably distinguish between HSV-1 and HSV-2, but initially high titers or less than a fourfold rise of titers between acute and convalescent sera may help rule-out a primary infection
- IgM HSV antibodies may appear in first 4 weeks of life in infected infants

IMAGING N/A

DIAGNOSTIC PROCEDURES
- Occasionally biopsy is needed
- Screen for other sexually transmitted diseases with primary genital herpes

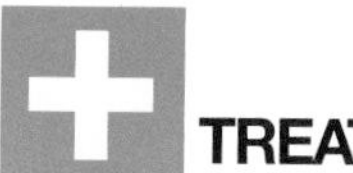

TREATMENT

APPROPRIATE HEALTH CARE Outpatient

GENERAL MEASURES
- Limited skin lesions (as in recurrent herpes labialis) may benefit from early unroofing of vesicles and application of Campho-Phenique
- Intermittent cool moist dressings with Domeboro or Burow's solution
- Inability to void from severe periurethral lesions may be remedied by pouring a cup of warm water over genitals while urinating or sitting in a warm bath to urinate
- Children with gingivostomatitis may require IV hydration
- Extensive skin disease (as with neonates or with eczema herpeticum) may require vigorous volume replacement

SURGICAL MEASURES N/A

ACTIVITY No restrictions

DIET Avoid acidic foods with gingivostomatitis

PATIENT EDUCATION
- Avoid contact with immunocompromised
- Wash hands often
- Genital herpes: avoid sexual contact while disease is active; discuss condom benefits and limits and reinforce benefits of mutually monogamous sexual relations.
- Reassure and reduce stigma

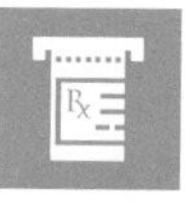

MEDICATIONS

DRUG(S) OF CHOICE
- Acyclovir
  - ◊ Primary herpes labialis: 15 mg/kg (up to 200 mg) po x 5 doses daily for days
  - ◊ Primary genital herpes: 400 mg po tid or 200 mg po x 5 doses daily for 7-10 days
  - ◊ Recurrent genital herpes: 800 mg bid or 200 mg po x 5 doses daily for 5 days; for chronic suppression in persons with frequent recurrences - 400 mg bid
  - ◊ Neonatal herpes simplex or encephalitis: 20 mg/kg IV over 1 hour q8h x 14-21 days
  - ◊ Primary herpes gingivostomatitis, recurrent herpes labialis and other HSV skin infections: 200 mg po q4h x 5 doses daily for 10 days
- Penciclovir (Denavir)
  - ◊ Oroherpes recurrence: 1% cream q2h while awake for 4 days
- Valacyclovir (Valtrex): better bioavailability orally than acyclovir, is converted to acyclovir
  - ◊ Primary genital herpes: 1 gm po bid for 10 days
  - ◊ Recurrent genital herpes: 500 mg po bid for 3 days; chronic suppression 1 g po q/day (10 or more recurrences per year) or 500 mg po q/day (9 or less recurrences per year)
- Famciclovir (Famvir): is converted to penciclovir, with longer intracellular half-life and higher levels than acyclovir
  - ◊ Primary genital herpes: 250 mg po tid for 7-10 days
  - ◊ Recurrent genital herpes: 125 mg po bid for 5 days; chronic suppression 250 mg po bid

Contraindications: Acyclovir, valacyclovir, or famciclovir: Hypersensitivity or intolerance

Precautions:
- Reduce dosage in renal insufficiency for acyclovir, valacyclovir and famciclovir
- Acyclovir may produce encephalopathic reactions, particularly in the elderly
- Valacyclovir: Thrombotic thrombocytopenia purpura/hemolytic uremic syndrome (TTP/HUS) reported in some immunocompromised persons in trials on high doses (8 grams daily) for CMV suppression
- Pregnancy - see Miscellaneous section

Significant possible interactions: Probenecid with IV acyclovir, possibly probenecid with valacyclovir can reduce renal clearance and elevate antiviral drug levels

ALTERNATIVE DRUGS
- Foscarnet: Drug of choice for acyclovir-resistance in immunocompromised persons with systemic HSV; 40 mg/kg IV q8h (assume valacyclovir and famciclovir resistance also if acyclovir resistance occurs)
- Other topicals:
  - ◊ Ophthalmic preparations for herpes keratoconjunctivitis: Acyclovir, vidarabine (Vira-A), idoxuridine and trifluorothymidine; refer to ophthalmologist

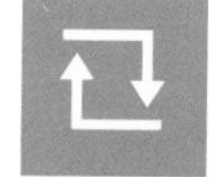

FOLLOWUP

PATIENT MONITORING Observe for disappearance of lesions and resolution of systemic manifestations

PREVENTION/AVOIDANCE See Patient Education

POSSIBLE COMPLICATIONS Herpes encephalitis - brain biopsy may be needed for diagnosis; herpes pneumonia; aseptic meningitis; herpes viremia

EXPECTED COURSE/PROGNOSIS Good for treatment of recurrent episodes. Expect frequent recurrences.

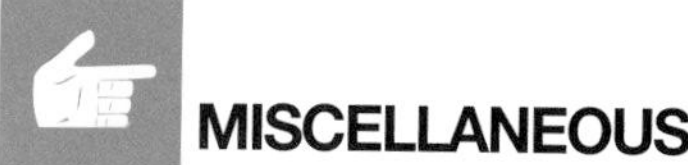

MISCELLANEOUS

ASSOCIATED CONDITIONS Erythema multiforme

AGE-RELATED FACTORS
Pediatric: Previously described
Geriatric: Decreased immunological competence of old age may increase risk
Others: N/A

PREGNANCY
- May give acyclovir orally for first episode genital herpes or severe recurrent herpes. Give IV for severe or complicated disease.
- Risk of viral shedding at delivery from asymptomatic recurrent genital HSV low (≈1.6%); not predicted by monitoring cultures
- Attack rate for neonatal HSV is 30-50% if primary maternal genital HSV present at time of delivery and < 1% for recurrent genital HSV at time of delivery. Avoid fetal scalp electrodes if maternal history of genital HSV.
- C-section and/or acyclovir indicated if any active genital lesions (or prodrome) present at time of delivery; consider if primary genital herpes occurred within 4 wks of expected delivery
- Obtain HSV cultures (urine, stool, CSF, eyes, throat) of neonates exposed to primary maternal genital HSV at delivery; treat with acyclovir if clinically ill, cultures positive, CSF abnormal
- Neonates with possible exposure to HSV with signs of infection: lethargy, poor feeding, fever, or lesions; admit, culture; treat immediately with IV acyclovir if HSV illness suspected

SYNONYMS N/A

ICD-9-CM
054.0 Eczema herpeticum
054.9 Herpes simplex without mention of complication
771.2 Other congenital infections

SEE ALSO
Herpes, genital

OTHER NOTES N/A

ABBREVIATIONS N/A

REFERENCES

- Dwyer DE, Cunningham AL. Herpes simplex virus infection in pregnancy. Bailliere's Clin Obstet Gynecol 1993;7:75-105
- Hirsch MS: Herpes simples virus. In: Mandell GL, et al, eds. Principles and Practice of Infectious Diseases. New York: Churchill Livingstone; 1990
- CDC Sexually Transmitted Diseases Treatment Guidelines 2002. MMWR 2002;51(RR6):12-17
- Amir J, Harel L, Smetana Z, Varsano I. Treatment of herpes simplex gingivostomatitis with acyclovir in children: a randomised double blind placebo controlled study. BMJ 1997;314(7097):1800-3

Web references: 0 available at www.5mcc.com
Illustrations 18 available

Author(s):
Arthur R. Slaughter, MD

BASICS

DESCRIPTION Herpes zoster usually presents as a painful unilateral dermatomal eruption. Zoster results from reactivation of varicella-zoster (chickenpox) virus that has been dormant.
- Postherpetic neuralgia (PHN) is usually defined as pain persisting at least one month after rash has healed. Due to variable definitions of PHN used in research, the term zoster associated pain (ZAP) may be more useful clinically.

System(s) affected: Nervous, Skin/Exocrine
Genetics: N/A
Incidence/Prevalence in USA:
- 215/100,000/year; incidence is increasing as population ages
- Occurs in 10-20% of the population at some time
- Active herpes zoster 23.9/100,000
- Postherpetic neuralgia 86/100,000

Predominant age:
- Herpes zoster incidence increases with age. 80% of cases occur in persons over age 20 years (2-3 per 1000 age 20 to 50; 10 per 1000 > 80 years).
- Postherpetic neuralgia incidence increases dramatically with age (4% age 30-50; 50% over age 80 years)

Predominant sex: Male = Female

SIGNS & SYMPTOMS
- Prodromal phase (sensations over involved dermatome prior to rash)
  - ◊ Tingling
  - ◊ Itching
  - ◊ Boring or knifelike pain
- Acute phase
  - ◊ Constitutional symptoms variable (fatigue, malaise, headache, low-grade fever)
  - ◊ Dermatomal rash
  - ◊ Weakness (1% may have weakness in distribution of rash)
  - ◊ Initially erythematous and maculopapular that evolves rapidly to grouped vesicles
  - ◊ Vesicles become pustular and/or hemorrhagic in 3 to 4 days
  - ◊ Resolution of rash with crusts separating by 14 to 21 days
- Possible sine herpete (zoster without rash) and other chronic disorders associated with varicella-zoster virus without the typical rash
- Chronic phase
  - ◊ Postherpetic neuralgia (15% overall; increases dramatically with age)
  - ◊ A small percentage (1-5%) may affect the motor nerves causing weakness (called zoster motoricus), e.g., facial nerve (Ramsay Hunt syndrome), spinal motor radiculopathies

CAUSES Reactivation of dormant varicella-zoster (chickenpox) virus in dorsal root ganglia or gasserian ganglia

RISK FACTORS
- The vast majority of persons affected have no underlying illness
- Increasing age
- Compromised cell-mediated immunity in immunosuppressed patients or patients with malignancy (especially leukemia and lymphoma)
- Spinal surgery
- Spinal cord radiation
- History of chickenpox

DIAGNOSIS

DIFFERENTIAL DIAGNOSIS
- Rash - herpes simplex virus, Coxsackievirus, contact dermatitis, superficial pyoderma
- Pain - cholecystitis, pleuritis, myocardial infarction, diabetic neuropathy

LABORATORY
- Rarely necessary
- Viral culture
- Tzanck smear (does not distinguish from herpes simplex and false negatives occur)
- PCR analysis and antibody testing of CSF may be valuable for diagnostic challenges and research

Drugs that may alter lab results: N/A

Disorders that may alter lab results: N/A

PATHOLOGICAL FINDINGS
- Multinucleated giant cells with intralesional inclusion
- Lymphatic infiltration of sensory ganglia with focal hemorrhage and nerve cell destruction

SPECIAL TESTS N/A

IMAGING N/A

DIAGNOSTIC PROCEDURES Biopsy for direct immunofluorescence testing (rarely done)

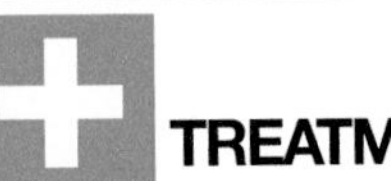

TREATMENT

APPROPRIATE HEALTH CARE Outpatient unless disseminated or occurring as complication of serious underlying disease requiring hospitalization

GENERAL MEASURES
- Wet dressings with tap water or 5% aluminum acetate (Burow's) applied 30 to 60 minutes 4-6 times per day
- Lotions such as calamine

SURGICAL MEASURES N/A

ACTIVITY No restrictions

DIET No special diet

PATIENT EDUCATION
- Duration of rash is 2-3 weeks
- Potential for dissemination (dissemination must be suspected with constitutional illness signs and/or spreading rash)
- Potential postherpetic neuralgia
- Potential risk of transmitting illness (chickenpox) to susceptible persons

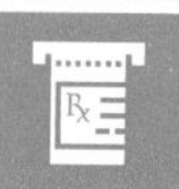

MEDICATIONS

DRUG(S) OF CHOICE

- Acute treatment
  - ◊ Antiviral agents initiated within 72 hours of rash may relieve symptoms, speed resolution of rash and perhaps modify postherpetic neuralgia. These agents are indicated for immunocompromised patients, ophthalmic zoster and disseminating zoster.
    - Valacyclovir 1000 mg tid for 7 days
    - Famciclovir 500 mg tid for 7 days
    - Acyclovir 800 mg every 4 hours (5 doses daily) for 7 days
  - ◊ Analgesics (acetaminophen, codeine, NSAIDs) prn
  - ◊ Corticosteroids may help acute symptoms, but theoretically increase risk of dissemination
- Treatment of complications
  - ◊ Secondary bacterial skin infections
    - Silver sulfadiazine topically and/or systemic antibiotics
- Postherpetic neuralgia and zoster-associated pain
  - Tricyclic antidepressants (amitriptyline 25 mg qhs and other low dose TCAs) relieve pain acutely and may reduce pain duration
  - Lidocaine (Lidoderm) patch 5% applied after skin rash closure over painful areas (limit 3 patches simultaneously or trim single patch) for up to 12 hours is reported effective in one limited trial
  - Gabapentin 100-600 mg tid for pain and other quality of life indicators, but is limited by adverse effects
  - Opioids and other analgesics may be useful adjuncts
  - Pregabalin 50-100 mg tid reduces pain, but usefulness limited by side effects
  - Capsaicin (Zostrix) cream, percutaneous nerve stimulation, and over 40 other medications and treatments have been advocated in the literature without good quality evidence
- Prevention of postherpetic neuralgia and zoster-associated pain (these treatments should be limited to patients over age 50 years)
  - Antiviral therapy with valacyclovir, famciclovir or acyclovir given during acute skin eruption may be effective in limiting duration of pain
  - Low dose amitriptyline (in the same dosage as for treatment of postherpetic neuralgia) but started within 72 hours of rash onset and continued for 90 days may reduce postherpetic neuralgia incidence or duration
  - Corticosteroids do not reduce incidence, severity or duration of postherpetic neuralgia

Contraindications: Refer to manufacturer's profile of each drug

Precautions:

- Assess renal function prior to using valacyclovir, famciclovir or acyclovir
- Valacyclovir, famciclovir, acyclovir - pregnancy category B
- Refer to manufacturer's profile of each drug

Significant possible interactions: Refer to manufacturer's profile of each drug

ALTERNATIVE DRUGS

Over 40 have been advocated (but no good supporting evidence is published)

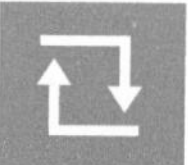

FOLLOWUP

PATIENT MONITORING

Symptom dependent

PREVENTION/AVOIDANCE

- Varicella vaccines currently available will theoretically reduce zoster incidence in the future
- Vaccines are being tested for prevention of herpes zoster in individuals previously infected with wild VZ virus
- Zoster patients may transmit virus causing varicella (chickenpox) to susceptible persons

POSSIBLE COMPLICATIONS

- Postherpetic neuralgia
- Ocular involvement with facial zoster. Corneal ulceration (classically a "dendritic" ulcer).
- Superinfection of skin lesions
- Meningoencephalitis
- Cutaneous dissemination
- Hepatitis
- Pneumonitis
- Peripheral motor weakness
- Segmental myelitis
- Cranial nerve syndromes especially ophthalmic and facial (Ramsay Hunt syndrome)
- Guillain-Barré syndrome
- Arteritis, large vessel
- Encephalitis, small vessel

EXPECTED COURSE/PROGNOSIS

- Resolution of acute rash within 14 to 21 days
- Postherpetic neuralgia may occur in patients over age 50

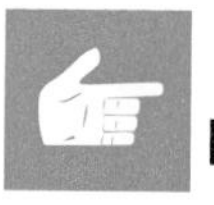

MISCELLANEOUS

ASSOCIATED CONDITIONS

Immunocompromise including HIV infection, transplant recipients, and malignancies. Most people with zoster are immunocompetent.

AGE-RELATED FACTORS

Pediatric:

- Occurs less frequently in children
- Has been reported in newborns primarily infected in utero

Geriatric:

- Increased incidence
- Increased incidence of postherpetic neuralgia

Others: N/A

PREGNANCY

Can occur during pregnancy

SYNONYMS

Shingles

ICD-9-CM

053.9 Herpes zoster without mention of complication

SEE ALSO

Bell palsy
Chickenpox
Herpes eye infections
Herpes simplex
Ramsay Hunt syndrome, Type 1

OTHER NOTES

N/A

ABBREVIATIONS

N/A

REFERENCES

- Helgason S, Sigurdsson JA, Gudmundsson S. The clinical course of herpes zoster: a prospective study in primary care. Eur J GM Pract 1996;2:12-6
- Stankus SJ, Dlugopolski M, Packer D. Management of herpes zoster (shingles) and postherpetic neuralgia. Am Fam Phys 2000;61:2437-44, 2447-8
- Gilden DH, Kleinschmidt-DeMasters BK, LaGuardia JJ, Mahalingam R, Cohrs RJ. Neurologic complications of the reactivation of varicella-zoster virus. N Engl J Med 2000;342:634-45
- Alper BS, Lewis PR. Does treatment of acute herpes zoster prevent or shorten postherpetic neuralgia? J Fam Pract 2000;49:255-264

Web references: 0 available at www.5mcc.com

Illustrations 8 available

Author(s):

Larry W. Halverson, MD

BASICS

DESCRIPTION Sudden, involuntary, contraction of the inspiratory muscles (predominantly the diaphragm) terminated by abrupt closure of the glottis stopping the inflow of air and producing the characteristic sound.
System(s) affected: nervous, Pulmonary
Genetics: N/A
Incidence/Prevalence in USA: Self limited hiccups are extremely common; intractable hiccups are rare
Predominant age: All ages (including fetus)
Predominant sex: Male > Female (4:1)

SIGNS & SYMPTOMS Hiccup attacks usually occur at brief intervals and last only a few seconds or minutes. Bouts lasting more than 48 hours often imply an underlying physical or metabolic disorder. Intractable hiccups may occur continuously for months or years. Hiccups usually occur with a frequency of 4 to 60 per minute.

CAUSES
- Pathophysiologic significance is unknown; hiccups have been associated with more than 100 underlying disorders.
- Results from stimulation of one or more limbs of the hiccup reflux arc (vagus and phrenic nerves) with a "hiccup center" located in the upper spinal cord
- In men greater than 90% have an organic basis while in women a psychogenic cause is more likely
- Specific underlying causes include:
  - ◊ Alcoholism
  - ◊ CNS lesions (brainstem tumors, vascular lesions, Parkinson disease)
  - ◊ Diaphragmatic irritation (tumors, pericarditis, eventration, splenomegaly, hepatomegaly, peritonitis)
  - ◊ Hair, insect or foreign body irritating tympanic membrane
  - ◊ Pharyngitis, laryngitis
  - ◊ Mediastinal and other thoracic lesions (pneumonia, aortic aneurysm, tuberculosis, myocardial infarction, lung cancer)
  - ◊ Esophageal lesions (reflux esophagitis, achalasia, Candida esophagitis, carcinoma, obstruction)
  - ◊ Gastric lesions (ulcer, distention, cancer)
  - ◊ Hepatic lesions (hepatitis, hepatoma)
  - ◊ Pancreatic lesions (pancreatitis, pseudocysts, cancer)
  - ◊ Inflammatory bowel disease
  - ◊ Cholelithiasis, cholecystitis
  - ◊ Prostatic disorders
  - ◊ Appendicitis
  - ◊ Postoperative, abdominal procedures
  - ◊ Toxic metabolic causes (uremia, hyponatremia, gout, diabetes)
  - ◊ Drug induced (dexamethasone, methylprednisolone, anabolic steroids, benzodiazepines, alpha methyldopa)
  - ◊ Psychogenic causes (hysterical neurosis, grief, malingering)
  - ◊ Idiopathic

RISK FACTORS
- General anesthesia
- Postoperative state
- Irritation of the vagus nerve branches
- Structural, vascular, infectious or traumatic CNS lesions

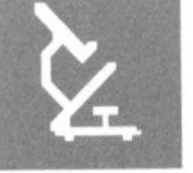

DIAGNOSIS

DIFFERENTIAL DIAGNOSIS See Causes (burping [eructation] may be confused with hiccups)

LABORATORY N/A

Drugs that may alter lab results: N/A

Disorders that may alter lab results: N/A

PATHOLOGICAL FINDINGS N/A

SPECIAL TESTS N/A

IMAGING Fluoroscopy is useful to determine if one hemidiaphragm is dominant

DIAGNOSTIC PROCEDURES N/A

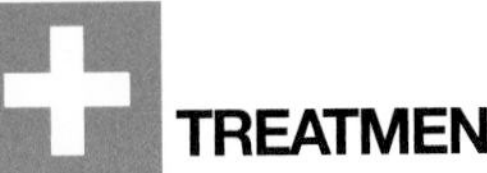

TREATMENT

APPROPRIATE HEALTH CARE
- Outpatient (usually)
- Inpatient (if elderly, debilitated or intractable hiccups)

GENERAL MEASURES
- Treat any specific underlying cause when identified.
  - ◊ Dilate esophageal stricture or obstruction
  - ◊ Remove hair or foreign body from ear canal
  - ◊ Angostura bitters for alcohol induced hiccups
  - ◊ Catheter stimulation of pharynx for operative and postoperative hiccups
  - ◊ Antifungal treatment for Candida esophagitis
  - ◊ Correct electrolyte imbalance
- Simple home remedies
  - ◊ Swallowing a spoonful of sugar
  - ◊ Sucking on a hard candy or swallowing peanut butter
  - ◊ Holding breath and increasing pressure on diaphragm (Valsalva maneuver)
  - ◊ Tongue traction
  - ◊ Lifting the uvula with a cold spoon
  - ◊ Drinking from the far side of a glass
  - ◊ Inducing fright
  - ◊ Smelling salts
  - ◊ Rebreathing into a paper (not plastic) bag
  - ◊ Sipping ice water
- Medical measures
  - ◊ Relief of gastric distention (gastric lavage, nasogastric aspiration, induced vomiting)
  - ◊ Counterirritation of the vagus nerve (supraorbital pressure, carotid sinus massage, digital rectal massage), to be used with caution
  - ◊ Respiratory center stimulants (breathing 5% carbon dioxide)
  - ◊ Phrenic nerve block or electrical stimulation of dominant hemidiaphragm
  - ◊ Psychiatric (hypnosis, behavioral modification)
  - ◊ Miscellaneous (cardioversion, acupuncture)

SURGICAL MEASURES Phrenic nerve crush or transection

ACTIVITY As tolerated

DIET Avoid gastric distension from overeating, carbonated beverages, aerophagia

PATIENT EDUCATION See General Measures

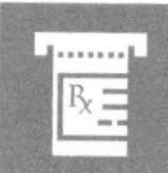

MEDICATIONS

DRUG(S) OF CHOICE

Possible drug remedies:

- Baclofen, a GABA analog, 5-10 mg tid (best choice)
- Chlorpromazine 25-50 mg IV
- Haloperidol 2-12 mg IM
- Phenytoin 200 mg IV then 100 mg qid
- Metoclopramide 5-10 mg qid
- Nifedipine 10-20 mg qd-tid
- Amitriptyline 10 mg tid
- Lidocaine 1.5 mg/kg IV infusion followed by 0.75 mg/kg on subsequent days
- Gabapentin (Neurontin) up to 1800 mg/d in divided doses

Contraindications: Refer to manufacturer's literature (baclofen is not recommended in patients with stroke or other cerebral lesions)
Precautions: Refer to manufacturer's literature (abrupt withdrawal of baclofen should be avoided)
Significant possible interactions: Refer to manufacturer's literature

ALTERNATIVE DRUGS

- Amantadine, carbidopa-levodopa in Parkinson disease
- Steroid replacement in Addison disease
- Antifungal agent in Candida esophagitis
- Ondansetron in carcinomatosis with vomiting
- Nefopam (a nonopiod analgesic with anti-shivering properties related to antihistamines and antiparkinsonian drugs) is available outside the US in both IV and oral formulations

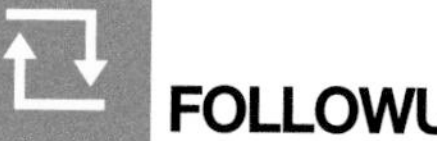

FOLLOWUP

PATIENT MONITORING Until hiccups cease

PREVENTION/AVOIDANCE

- Correct underlying cause
- Maintenance drug therapy (e.g., baclofen 5-10 mg tid; phenytoin 100 mg qid; valproic acid 15 mg/kg undivided doses; nifedipine 10-20 mg qd-tid; metoclopramide 10 mg qid)

POSSIBLE COMPLICATIONS

- Inability to eat
- Weight loss
- Exhaustion, debility
- Insomnia
- Cardiac arrhythmias
- Wound dehiscence
- Death (rare)

EXPECTED COURSE/PROGNOSIS

- Hiccups often cease during sleep
- Most acute benign hiccups resolve with home remedies or spontaneously
- Intractable hiccups may last for years and decades
- Hiccups have persisted despite bilateral phrenic nerve transection

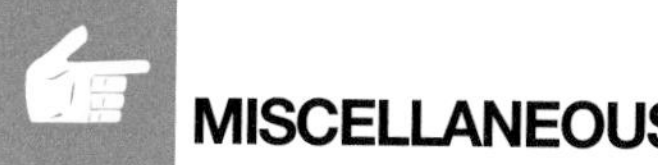

MISCELLANEOUS

ASSOCIATED CONDITIONS See Causes

AGE-RELATED FACTORS

Pediatric: May persist from fetal state
Geriatric: Can be a serious problem among the elderly
Others: N/A

PREGNANCY Fetal hiccups noted as rhythmic fetal movements (confirmed sonographically), fetal hiccups often recur in subsequent pregnancies

SYNONYMS

- Hiccoughs
- Singultus

ICD-9-CM

786.8 Hiccough

SEE ALSO

OTHER NOTES N/A

ABBREVIATIONS

- GABA = gamma amino butyric acid

REFERENCES

- Lewis JH: Hiccups: Reasons and remedies. In: Lewis JH, ed. A Pharmacologic Approach to Gastrointestinal Disorders. Baltimore, Williams & Wilkins, 1994
- Lewis JH: Hiccups and their cures. Clin Perspectives in Gastroenterol 2000;3(5):277-283
- Ramirez FC; Graham DY. Treatment of intractable hiccup with baclofen: results of a double-blind randomized, controlled, cross-over study. Am J Gastroenterol 1992 Dec;87(12):1789-91
- Schlager A. Korean hand acupuncture in the treatment of chronic hiccups. Am J Gastroenterol 1998 Nov;93(11):2312-3
- Okuda Y. Use of a nerve stimulator for phrenic nerve block in treatment of hiccups. Anesthesiology 1998 Feb;88(2):525-7
- Bilotta F; Rosa G. Nefopam for severe hiccups. N Engl J Med 2000;343(26):1973-4
- Dickerman RD, Jaikumar S. The hiccup reflex arc and persistent hiccups with high-dose anabolic steroids: is the brainstem the steroid-responsive locus? Clin Neuropharmacol 2001;24(1):62-4
- Cohen SP, Lubin E, Stojanovic M. Intravenous lidocaine in the treatment of hiccup.South Med;94(11):1124-5
- Schiff E, River Y, Oliven A, Odeh M. Acupuncture therapy for persistent hiccups.Am J Med Sci 2002;323(3):166-8
- Moretti R, Torre P, Antonello RM, et al. Gabapentin as a drug therapy of intractable hiccup because of vascular lesion: A three-year follow up. Neurologist 2004;10(2):102-106
- Porzio G, Aielli F, Narducci F, et al. Hiccup in patients with advanced cancer successfully treated with gabapentin: report of three cases. N Z Med J 2003;116(1182): U605

Web references: 0 available at www.5mcc.com
Illustrations N/A

Author(s):

James H. Lewis, MD

BASICS

DESCRIPTION Acute, tender, cyst-like abscesses in apocrine gland bearing skin (axillae, anogenital area, pubes, areolae, also apocrine glands scattered around umbilicus, scalp, trunk and face). In chronic cases, fibrotic sinus tracts develop with intermittent drainage and periodic acute abscesses.
System(s) affected: Skin/Exocrine
Genetics: Unknown, possibly single gene transmission (autosomal dominant), possibly polygenic
Incidence/Prevalence in USA: 0.3-4%
Predominant age: Peak onset age 11-30, commonly 30-40; rare before puberty
Predominant sex: Female (perianal) > Male (axillary)

SIGNS & SYMPTOMS
- Early signs of pruritus, erythema, and local hyperhidrosis
- Comedones may be present
- Distribution - area of apocrine glands with axillae and groin most common
- Papules (dome-shaped) 1-3 cm in size
- Nodules (dome-shaped) 1-3 cm in size
- Larger lesions fluctuant
- Multiple recurrences at the same site
- Healing sites accompanied by scarring and sinus tracts
- Associated arthritis (rare)

CAUSES
- Traditionally considered a disorder of apocrine glands but now felt to be due to occlusion of terminal follicular epithelium within apocrine gland-bearing skin. Bacteria involvement is not a primary pathogenic event, but secondary.
- Historically part of "follicular occlusive triad"; acne conglobata, dissecting cellulitis of scalp, hidradenitis suppurativa. Pilonidal sinus later added to form a tetrad.
- Smoking may be a major triggering factor

RISK FACTORS
- Obesity
- African American
- Female
- Acne
- Diabetes mellitus
- Hypercholesterolemia
- Low basal metabolic rate
- Smoking possibly

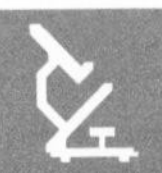

DIAGNOSIS

DIFFERENTIAL DIAGNOSIS
- Furunculosis. Differentiate by specific culture and also by the response to specific antibiotics.
- Carbuncles, granulomatous disease, infected epidermoid cysts, tuberculosis cutis, actinomycosis, tularemia and carcinoma. With inguinal involvement: granuloma inguinale and lymphogranuloma venereum.
- Inflammatory bowel disease with anogenital fistula (may also coexist with hidradenitis suppurativa or be mistaken for it)

LABORATORY
- Culture of exudate from lesion: Staphylococci, Streptococci, E. Coli, Proteus with chronic condition, usually not anaerobes. Increasing antibiotic resistance.
- Possibly increased ESR, leukocytosis, decreased serum iron, normocytic anemia, and changes in serum electrophoresis pattern - probably due to chronic inflammatory process

Drugs that may alter lab results: N/A

Disorders that may alter lab results: N/A

PATHOLOGICAL FINDINGS Acute and chronic inflammation, multiple comedones, sinus tracts when recurrent

SPECIAL TESTS Culture discharge from lesion(s)

IMAGING N/A

DIAGNOSTIC PROCEDURES
- Incision and drainage of lesion(s) with biopsy
- Clinical criteria for early diagnosis (proposed by Mortimer)
  - ◊ Recurrent deep boils > 6 months in flexural sites
  - ◊ Onset after puberty
  - ◊ Poor response to conventional antibiotics
  - ◊ Strong tendency toward relapse or recurrence
  - ◊ Comedones in apocrine gland-bearing skin
  - ◊ Routine culture of pus from boils - no pathogens
  - ◊ Personal or family history of acne or pilonidal sinuses and exacerbation of boils premenstrually in women

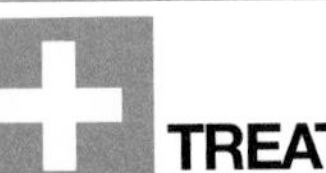

TREATMENT

APPROPRIATE HEALTH CARE Generally outpatient

GENERAL MEASURES
- Symptomatic treatment acute lesions
- Prevent new lesions
- Local cleansing (germicidal soap)
- Improve environmental factors that cause follicular blockage

SURGICAL MEASURES
- Wide excision with healing by granulation (considered more efficacious then drug treatment); but medical treatment tried first because of extensive nature of surgery treatment
- Incision and drainage of lesions
  - ◊ Remove sinus tracts
  - ◊ Exteriorization with curettage and electrodesiccation
- Treatment for severe, intractable cases: excision and skin graft
- CO2 laser stripping with healing by secondary intention

ACTIVITY Fully active

DIET No restrictions

PATIENT EDUCATION
- Minimize heat exposure and sweating
- Reduce weight if obese
- Avoid constrictive clothing
- Medication precautions

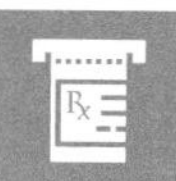

MEDICATIONS

DRUG(S) OF CHOICE
- Antibiotics (not curative, relapse almost always inevitable); treatment sometimes for 2 or more months:
  - ◊ Clindamycin 2% lotion or neomycin cream topically to control odor. Topical clindamycin as effective as systemic tetracyclines for stage 1 or 2 disease. Oral clindamycin also effective.
  - ◊ Tetracycline 250 mg qid or 500 mg tid
  - ◊ Minocycline (Minocin) 100 mg bid po
  - ◊ Erythromycin 1-1.5 gm qd po
  - ◊ Doxycycline 100 mg bid 7-14 days
  - ◊ Other antibiotics depending on culture
- Consider oral retinoids
  - ◊ Isotretinoin (Accutane) 40-80 mg/day po for 4 months. No Accutane during pregnancy (highly teratogenic). Equivocal results, still frequent recurrences.
- Birth control pills (female only), if antibiotic therapy fails. Low-dose progesterone BCPs (e.g., Norinyl, Ortho-Novum, Enovid).
- Consider steroids
  - ◊ Injection of lesions with depot-type steroids (e.g., triamcinolone)
  - ◊ Consider brief course of systemic corticosteroids
  - ◊ Anti-androgen therapy - controversial

Contraindications: Tetracycline - pregnancy, children < 8 years

Precautions:
- Tetracycline - use sunscreen (SPF 15 or better) to avoid phototoxicity.
- Review professional literature before prescribing birth control pills or Accutane

Significant possible interactions:
- Tetracycline - do not take dairy products, antacids, or iron preparations within 2 hours of tetracycline dose.

ALTERNATIVE DRUGS N/A

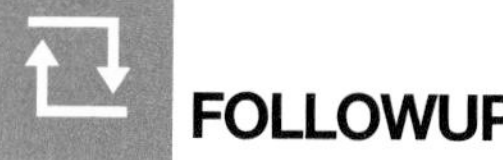

FOLLOWUP

PATIENT MONITORING
Revisits monthly, or more often if needed

PREVENTION/AVOIDANCE
- Minimize heat exposure and sweating
- Lose weight if overweight
- Avoid constrictive clothing/frictional trauma
- Avoid underarm antiperspirants and deodorants

POSSIBLE COMPLICATIONS
- Contracture formation at the sites of lesions
- Restricted limb mobility
- Squamous cell carcinoma may develop in indolent sinus tracts (usually anogenital)
- Disseminated infection septicemia- unusual
- Lymphedema
- Urethral/rectal fistula
- Anemia
- Arthritis (asymmetrical pauciarticular to symmetrical polyarthritis/polyarthralgia. Typically larger joints of upper or lower extremities, particularly the knee)
- Amyloidosis
- Renal failure
- Interstitial keratitis

EXPECTED COURSE/PROGNOSIS
- Individual lesions (with or without drainage) heal slowly in 10-30 days
- Recurrences may last for several years
- Rare spontaneous resolution
- Relentlessly progressive scarring and sinus tracts

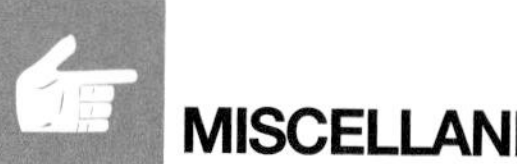

MISCELLANEOUS

ASSOCIATED CONDITIONS
- Acne
- Perifolliculitis capitis abscedens et suffodiens (dissecting cellulitis of scalp)
- Obesity with associated diabetes mellitus, atopy, acanthosis nigricans

AGE-RELATED FACTORS
Pediatric: Rarely occurs before puberty (1 case reported in a 2 year old)

Geriatric: Rare after menopause

Others: Common late puberty through age 40

PREGNANCY
No Accutane treatment during pregnancy

SYNONYMS
- Apocrinitis
- Hidradenitis axillaris
- Acne inversa

ICD-9-CM
705.83 Hidradenitis

SEE ALSO
Folliculitis
Furunculosis

OTHER NOTES
- Some patients develop only two or three papules per year. Others develop new lesions and drain as rapidly as old ones resolve.
- Although 50% of patients receiving Accutane, in doses similar to those for acne, obtain appreciable improvement, relapse occurs quickly upon discontinuing

ABBREVIATIONS N/A

REFERENCES

- Konig A. Cigarette smoking as a triggering factor of hydradenitis suppurativa. Dermatol 1999;198(3):261-4
- Brown TJ, Rosen T: Hydradenitis Suppurativa. Southern Med J 1998;91(12):1107-1114
- Moschella SL, Hurley HJ: Dermatology. 3rd Ed. Philadelphia, W.B. Saunders, 1992
- Lynch PJ: Dermatology for the House Officer. 3rd Ed. Baltimore, Williams & Wilkins, 1994
- Bell BA, Ellis H: Hydradenitis Suppurativa. Journal of the Royal Society of Medicine 1978;71:511-515
- Sauer GC: Manual of Skin Diseases. 6th Ed. Philadelphia, J.B. Lippincott, 1991
- Orkin M, ed: Dermatology. Los Altos, CA, Lange Medical Publishers, 1991
- Lapins J, Marcusson JA, Emtestam L: Surgical treatment of chronic hidradenitis suppurativa: CO2 laser stripping-secondary intention technique. British J of Dermatol 1994 131:551-556

Web references: 0 available at www.5mcc.com

Illustrations N/A

Author(s):
Sean Herrington, MD

BASICS

DESCRIPTION Fracture of the head or neck of the femur, usually as the result of a fall. The following classification derives from the vascular anatomy of the head and neck of the femur.
- Intracapsular
  - ◊ Femoral neck, subcapital or transcervical
  - ◊ Intracapsular femoral neck fractures may disrupt the blood supply to the femoral head, resulting in avascular necrosis
- Extracapsular
  - ◊ Intertrochanteric
  - ◊ Subtrochanteric

System(s) affected: Musculoskeletal
Genetics: No known genetic factor
Incidence/Prevalence in USA:
- 200,000 patients per year over the age of 65 have fracture of hips
- In women over age 75, there is a 1% incidence per year

Predominant age: 80% occur in those over age 60
Predominant sex: Female > Male (3:1)

SIGNS & SYMPTOMS
- Pain in hip. If severe, it usually indicates a displaced fracture. Mild pain usually occurs in non-displaced fractures.
- Pain in knee. Pain is referred from hip and may occur in absence of hip pain.
- External rotation of leg
- Shortening of leg

CAUSES
- Osteoporosis
- Direct blunt trauma
- Spontaneous in pathologic conditions

RISK FACTORS
- Bone mineral density
- Metastatic cancer
- Neurological disease with gait impairment
- Severe renal disease with secondary hyperparathyroidism
- Use of long-acting sedatives and hypnotics in the elderly
- Age
- Propensity to fall
- History of previous fracture
- Weight loss
- Frailty
- Impaired vision
- Osteoarthritis
- Hyperthyroidism
- Deconditioning
- Cigarette smoking
- Alcohol use

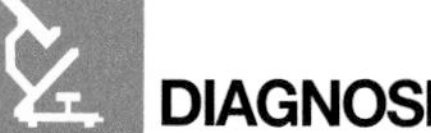

DIAGNOSIS

DIFFERENTIAL DIAGNOSIS Rule out primary or metastatic malignancy, pelvic fracture

LABORATORY Routine pre-operative laboratory including CBC, chemical profile, electrolytes

Drugs that may alter lab results: N/A

Disorders that may alter lab results: N/A

PATHOLOGICAL FINDINGS Osteoporosis

SPECIAL TESTS N/A

IMAGING
- X-rays - AP and "frog leg" lateral of hip
- X-ray AP pelvis to rule out pelvis fracture as cause of pain. Also provides information regarding appearance of opposite side.
- X-ray remainder of femur to include knee
- X-ray any other tender or painful area as other fractures are common and symptoms may be ignored with severe pain of hip fracture
- CT or MRI scans are not routinely indicated as the diagnosis is usually obvious from plain radiographs

DIAGNOSTIC PROCEDURES N/A

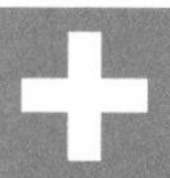

TREATMENT

APPROPRIATE HEALTH CARE
- Treat emergently
- During transportation to hospital, gentle traction of the leg may help relieve discomfort. This can be maintained in bed, but requires close observation of circulation and skin changes.
- Pain control (may need narcotic analgesics)

GENERAL MEASURES
- Medical evaluation to have patient in best possible condition before surgery
- Surgery is almost always indicated. Older patients do not tolerate long periods of bed confinement.
- Protect pressure points to avoid decubitus ulcers, especially on the sacrum, heels and malleoli
- Oxygen therapy as needed per oxymetry assessment
- Pressure gradient stockings
- Situations where non-operative treatment may be appropriate include:
  - ◊ Immediately preterminal
  - ◊ Nonambulatory, demented
    - Bed bound
    - Unable to transfer independently
- Compression-type fatigue fracture of the femoral neck
  - ◊ Occurs in normal bone exposed to excessive loads, e.g., young athlete
  - ◊ Patients must be compliant with 6-8 weeks of sharply restricted activity

SURGICAL MEASURES
- Displaced intracapsular fractures have no clearly superior treatment. Options are internal fixation or arthroplasty. Internal fixation is associated with a higher risk of implant failure than hemiarthroplasty (femoral head replacement). At present, the choice of treatment is determined by patient factors, e.g., age, presence of arthritis, availability and cost of different types of treatment, surgeon experience, and surgeon preference.
- Undisplaced intracapsular fractures should have internal fixation with a widely used method that is familiar to the surgeon, e.g., cancellous screws or compression screw and plate
- Extracapsular (trochanteric) fractures should be treated surgically. A compression hip screw and plate has less chance of failure, leading to reoperation, compared with a fixed device. And it may prove to be more cost-effective in the long term.
- For subtrochanteric fractures, the Medoff sliding plate has been associated with fewer failures of fixation when compared with other screw plates and is recommended for this fracture

ACTIVITY
- Patients should be up (for toilet, and prevention of deep vein thrombosis and decubiti) as soon as possible after surgery, usually the next day
- Ambulate as soon as possible after surgery, e.g., with use of a walker. Close supervision by an experienced therapist necessary.

DIET No special diet

PATIENT EDUCATION Refer to physical therapy for walking instructions; usually non-weight bearing for several weeks at least

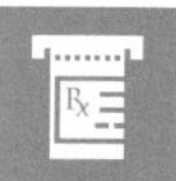

MEDICATIONS

DRUG(S) OF CHOICE
- Analgesics, as indicated. Drug of choice might be morphine sulfate 2-10 mg q3h prn with change to oral opioids as soon as possible.
- Prophylactic anticoagulation with unfractionated low dose heparin, 5000 u SC q8-12 hours or low molecular weight heparin (Lovenox) 30 mg SC q 12h
- Prophylactic antibiotics at induction of anesthesia: ceftriaxone 2 gm IV or IM x 1 dose

Contraindications: Associated head injury or severe respiratory disease
Precautions: Dosage should be lower in older people to avoid respiratory problems
Significant possible interactions: Refer to manufacturer's literature

ALTERNATIVE DRUGS N/A

FOLLOWUP

PATIENT MONITORING
- X-rays of the hip taken prior to discharge from the hospital and every 8-12 weeks afterward until healed
- Monitor postoperative physical therapy for full recovery

PREVENTION/AVOIDANCE
- Prophylactic treatment for osteoporosis
- Calcium supplementation, 1,000-1,500 mg PO daily
- Vitamin D supplementation 400-800 IU PO daily
- Bisphosphonates
  - ◊ Alendronate (Fosamax), 35-70 mg PO weekly
  - ◊ Risedronate (Actonel), 35 mg PO weekly
- Salmon calcitonin
  - ◊ Nasal spray (Miacalcin), one spray daily in alternate nostrils
  - ◊ Injectable (Calcimar), 100 IU SC/IM daily
- Avoid long-acting sedatives and hypnotics in the elderly
- Use walking canes or walkers if patient has unsteady gait
- Have older people use proper chair for sitting. Should not allow hip flexion greater than 90 degrees since rising from this position requires external rotation of the extremity with subsequent torsional forces which can cause fracture.
- Use sturdy rails in showers, bathrooms, stairs, or ramps

POSSIBLE COMPLICATIONS
- Mental deterioration. Present in 90% of older patients for varying periods of time after surgery. Usually subsides, but may persist due to pre-existing arteriosclerosis.
- Infection. More common in comminuted fractures and patients with diabetes. Surgical implants should be left in place and antibiotics given as indicated by culture and sensitivity. Some require the wound to be opened and drained.
- Aseptic necrosis of femoral head. Occurs in 25-30% of femoral neck fractures. Treatment requires a prosthetic replacement in older patients.
- Phlebitis. Prophylaxis with warfarin (Coumadin) to keep INR 2.0-2.5 or pro-time 15-18 scc - for at least 4 weeks; or enoxaparin (Lovenox) 30 mg SQ q12h beginning 12 hours after surgery and continuing until patient is mobile
- Nonunion
  - ◊ In case of neck fractures, a prosthetic replacement is indicated
  - ◊ In the intertrochanteric fracture, a bone graft, usually with replacement of the nail and plate, is indicated

EXPECTED COURSE/PROGNOSIS
- Hip fractures remain a serious injury in older people. There is a 15-20% three month mortality in trochanteric fractures and 10% in neck fractures.
- Sixty-five percent of patients can be expected to return to their former state of health

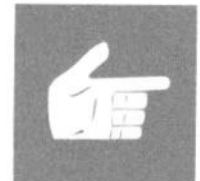

MISCELLANEOUS

ASSOCIATED CONDITIONS
- Osteoporosis
- Metastatic malignancy

AGE-RELATED FACTORS
Pediatric: N/A
Geriatric: Hip fractures common in geriatric age group
Others: N/A

PREGNANCY N/A

SYNONYMS
- Subcapital fracture
- Trochanteric fracture
- Femoral neck fracture

ICD-9-CM
820. Fracture of neck of femur (use appropriate modifier)

SEE ALSO
Osteoporosis

OTHER NOTES None

ABBREVIATIONS N/A

REFERENCES

- Chilov MN, Cameron ID, March LM; Australian National Health and Medical Research Council. Evidence-based guidelines for fixing broken hips: an update. Med J Aust 2003;179(9):489-93x
- Marx JA, editor. Rosen's emergency medicine: concepts and clinical practice.5th ed. St. Louis: Mosby, Inc.; 2002.
- Bruyere O, Edwards J, Reginster JY. Fracture prevention in postmenopausal women. Clin Evid Concise 2003;10:249-251
- Brunner LC, Eshilian-Oates L, Kuo TY. Hip fractures in adults. Am Fam Physician 2003;67(3):537-542
- Wehren LE. The epidemiology of osteoporosis and fractures in geriatric medicine. Clin Geriatr Med 2003;19:245-258
- Teasdall RD, Webb LX. Innovations in the management of hip fractures. Orthopedics 2003 Aug;26(8 suppl): s843-s849

Web references: 0 available at www.5mcc.com
Illustrations N/A

Author(s):
Richard Viken, MD

BASICS

DESCRIPTION Presence of excessive body and facial hair, in a male pattern, especially in women; may be present in normal adults as an ethnic characteristic or may develop as a result of androgen excess due to tumor or drugs

- Often accompanied by menstrual irregularities

System(s) affected: Endocrine/Metabolic, Reproductive
Genetics: Multifactorial
Incidence/Prevalence in USA: 8% of adult women
Predominant age: Postpubertal females
Predominant sex: Postpubertal females

SIGNS & SYMPTOMS

- Hair thickens and darkens in "male" pattern - beard, moustache, chest hair
- Often accompanied by irregular menses and anovulation
- Often accompanied by acne
- May be accompanied by infertility
- Onset is usually gradual
- Extreme androgenic effects (deep voice, clitorimegaly, balding) is known as virilization

CAUSES Most hirsutism is idiopathic and no etiology is found. The underlying process appears to be increased binding of androgenic (male) hormones at the skin level. These hormones may be from the ovary or adrenal gland. Anovulation, obesity and insulin resistance can also contribute and is then called polycystic ovary syndrome.

RISK FACTORS

- Family history
- Anovulation

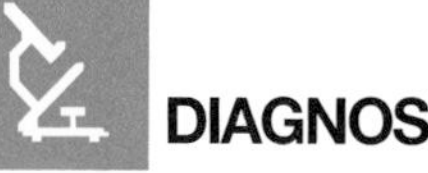

DIAGNOSIS

DIFFERENTIAL DIAGNOSIS

- Normal variant, ethnic trait
- Idiopathic - probably due to peripheral binding
- Polycystic ovary disease - a syndrome of cystic ovaries with decreased ovulation, insulin resistance and hirsutism
- Excessive androgen production from the ovary (measured by testosterone), the adrenal (measured by DHEAS [dehydroepiandrosterone sulfate]), or late onset congenital adrenal hyperplasia (measured by 17-OHP [17 hydroxyprogesterone])
- Ovarian tumor (testosterone > 200) - rare
- Adrenal tumor (DHEAS > 700) - rare
- Hypothyroidism
- Hyperprolactinemia
- Supplements in performance athletes
- Cushing disease - rare

LABORATORY

- Lab testing is performed to r/o underlying tumor and pituitary disease which are rare. Empiric treatment without lab workup is an acceptable option.
- Basic workup - total testosterone, DHEAS, 17-OHP, TSH, prolactin, ± LH/FSH
- If testosterone > 200, do ovarian tumor workup
- If DHEAS > 700, do adrenal tumor workup
- LH/FSH ratio is elevated (>2) in 75% of polycystic ovarian disease
- If testosterone, DHEAS or 17 OHP are elevated, but not in tumor range, treat as described below
- Fasting glucose/insulin ratio to rule out insulin resistance in polycystic ovary syndrome (> 4.5 is normal)

Drugs that may alter lab results: N/A

Disorders that may alter lab results: N/A

PATHOLOGICAL FINDINGS N/A

SPECIAL TESTS

- If 17-OHP is 300-800, do ACTH (Cortrosyn) test (ACTH 0.25 mg IV and check 17-OHP at 0 and 1 hour) to confirm congenital adrenal hyperplasia
- If DHEAS is high, but not in tumor range, can do low dose dexamethasone test (0.5 mg dexamethasone qid x 5 days, then recheck DHEAS and testosterone - they will decrease if androgens are adrenal and won't if they are ovarian)
- If dysfunctional uterine bleeding is present, consider endometrial biopsy

IMAGING

- If testosterone > 200 or DHEAS > 700, get CT of ovaries or adrenals
- Ovarian ultrasound can help in the diagnosis of polycystic ovary syndrome

DIAGNOSTIC PROCEDURES N/A

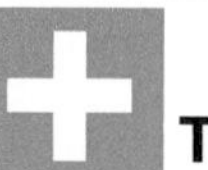

TREATMENT

APPROPRIATE HEALTH CARE Outpatient

GENERAL MEASURES

- Treatment is slow and often lifelong
- If patient desires pregnancy, induction of ovulation may be necessary
- Provide contraception as needed
- Encourage patient to maintain ideal weight
- Treat accompanying acne

SURGICAL MEASURES N/A

ACTIVITY No special activity

DIET No special diet

PATIENT EDUCATION

- Hormonal treatment stops further hair growth but will not usually reverse present hair
- Treatment takes 6-24 months and may be life long
- Cosmetic measures include - plucking, bleaching, shaving, electrolysis, laser hair removal and cover up cosmetics
- Electrolysis should be by a licensed professional

MEDICATIONS

DRUG(S) OF CHOICE
After tumor has been ruled out:
- Oral contraceptives:
  - ◊ Any brand is effective
  - ◊ Estrogen and progesterone can be given separately
  - ◊ Medroxyprogesterone (Depo-Provera) IM every 3 months; less effective
- Metformin: decreases insulin secretion which decreases androgen production in polycystic ovaries
- Chronic dexamethasone therapy can be used in late onset congenital adrenal hyperplasia (0.5 mg qhs), but oral contraception is also effective
- Eflornithine (Vaniqa) HCL cream - apply bid; reduces facial hair in 40% of women (with long term use)

Contraindications: Avoid giving medications in pregnancy
Precautions: N/A
Significant possible interactions: N/A

ALTERNATIVE DRUGS
- Antiandrogenic drugs (often used when workup is negative and oral contraceptives are not helping. They have low efficacy and many side effects):
  - ◊ Spironolactone: up to 200 mg/day - onset of action is slow; side effects include menorrhagia; contraindicated in pregnancy
  - ◊ Cyproterone: orphan drug not routinely available - usually combined with estrogen - contraindicated in pregnancy. Monitor LFTs.
  - ◊ Flutamide: 250 mg tid - nonsteroidal antiandrogen. Monitor LFTs. Need concurrent oral contraceptives.
  - ◊ Ketoconazole: 400 mg day - avoid with astemizole, triazolam, cisapride
  - ◊ Leuprolide (Lupron): lowers LH. Side effects of menopause.
  - ◊ Danazol: lowers LH. Side effects of menopause
  - ◊ Serenoa repens (saw palmetto) - in small studies decreases hair growth via blocking 5-alpha-reductase activity in the skin

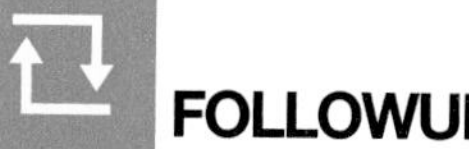

FOLLOWUP

PATIENT MONITORING Monitor for known side effects of medications

PREVENTION/AVOIDANCE
- As hormone balance improves, fertility may increase - provide contraception as needed
- Patients desiring pregnancy may need fertility intervention such as ovulation induction
- Prolonged amenorrhea may, over time, put the patient at risk for endometrial hyperplasia or carcinoma
- There is an increased incidence of diabetes and insulin resistance in polycystic ovarian disease which can increase risk of heart disease
- Women with late onset congenital adrenal hyperplasia may be carriers for the severe early onset childhood disease - counsel
- Avoid quackery and unlicensed electrolysis

POSSIBLE COMPLICATIONS
- Dysfunctional uterine bleeding and anemia
- Androgenic excess may adversely affect lipid status, cardiac risk and bone density
- Poor self image/shame

EXPECTED COURSE/PROGNOSIS
- Good (with long term therapy) for halting further hair growth
- Moderate to poor for reversing current hair growth

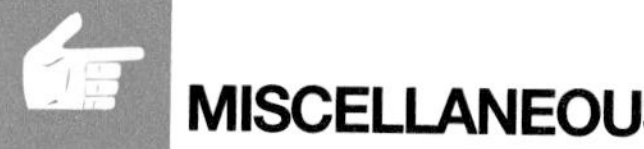

MISCELLANEOUS

ASSOCIATED CONDITIONS
- Acne
- Infertility
- Obesity
- Hyperinsulinemia

AGE-RELATED FACTORS
Pediatric: N/A
Geriatric: Can occur after menopause if peripheral conversion of estrogen is poor
Others: N/A

PREGNANCY
- May have related infertility
- If pregnancy occurs, must discontinue known contraindicated drugs
- Pregnancy outcome is related to underlying cause of hirsutism

SYNONYMS
- Excessive hair

ICD-9-CM
704.1 Hirsutism

SEE ALSO
Acne vulgaris
Fertility problems
Hyperprolactinemia
Hypothyroidism, adult
Obesity
Polycystic ovarian disease

OTHER NOTES N/A

ABBREVIATIONS
LFT = liver function test

REFERENCES
- Speroff L, Glass R, Kase N. Clinical Gynecologic Endocrinology and Infertility. 6th Ed. Williams & Wilkins, Baltimore, 1999
- Franks S. Polycystic ovarian disease. NEJM 1995;333(13):853-868
- Kalve E, Klein JF. Evaluation of women with hirsutism. Am Fam Phys 1996;54)1):117-124
- Hirsutism and polycystic ovarian syndrome. Society for Reproductive Medicine, 1995

Web references: 0 available at www.5mcc.com
Illustrations 1 available

Author(s):
Laura L. Novak, MD

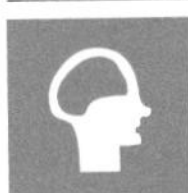

BASICS

DESCRIPTION Fungal infection with Histoplasma capsulatum, a dimorphic soil-dwelling saprophyte that has multiple clinical manifestations. Initial infection in the normal host is often asymptomatic. Other manifestations include a self-limited flu-like syndrome, mediastinal fibrosis, scar tissue residual, chronic cavitary disease in those with obstructive lung disease and disseminated histoplasmosis which is more frequent in the immunocompromised host and infants.

- H. capsulatum has worldwide distribution; the most endemic region in North America is the central U.S. The fungus exists in mycelial form in nature and in yeast phase when exposed to mammalian temperatures. Spores may remain active for up to ten years. Exposure to bird or bat excrement promotes growth of the fungus for unexplained reasons.
- Chronic pulmonary histoplasmosis - usually occurs in white males with obstructive lung disease and apical bullous lung pathology. These patients exhibit evidence of an indolent infectious process.
- Disseminated histoplasmosis infection in the immunocompromised is a rare opportunistic infection which may mimic sepsis syndrome and progress to multiple organ system failure

System(s) affected: Gastrointestinal, Hemic/Lymphatic/Immunologic, Pulmonary, Skin/Exocrine

Genetics: None known

Incidence/Prevalence in USA:
- Infection in endemic areas is virtually 100%; few patients develop active disease; approximately 500,000 new infections in the U.S./yr
- Occurrence in AIDS patients is 2%-5%
- Disseminated histoplasmosis occurs in

< 0.05% of infections, one-third of these are infants < 1 year old, in adults there is an increased prevalence with age > 60 years

Predominant age:
- None in acute histoplasmosis
- Infants < 1 year old are at higher risk for disseminated histoplasmosis

Predominant sex:
- Acute histoplasmosis - Male = Female
- Disseminated histoplasmosis -

Male > Female (5-10:1)

SIGNS & SYMPTOMS
- Primary infection in the normal host is usually asymptomatic
- 1% immunocompetent individuals with low-level exposure develop symptoms
- 99% subclinical infection
- Arthralgia-erythema nodosum-erythema multiforme is associated with acute infection
- Low grade fever, anorexia, weight loss, night sweats, and productive cough are associated with chronic infections

CAUSES Dimorphic fungus Histoplasma capsulatum

RISK FACTORS
- Spelunking
- Cleaning chicken coops
- Excavation near bird roosts
- Demolition or remodeling of old buildings
- Exposure to decayed wood or dead trees
- Performing routine activities in areas with high accumulation of bird droppings
- Immunosuppression

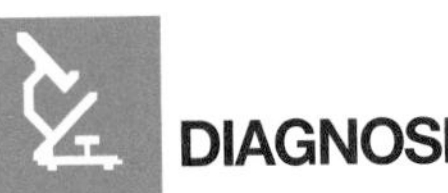

DIAGNOSIS

DIFFERENTIAL DIAGNOSIS
- Atypical pneumonia and viral pneumonitis
- Other fungal diseases such as blastomycosis, coccidioidomycosis
- Other granulomatous diseases such as M. tuberculosis and sarcoidosis
- Pneumoconiosis
- Lymphoma
- Malignancies associated with hilar lymphadenopathy

LABORATORY
- For disseminated histoplasma antigen in AIDS patients, urinary and blood histoplasmosis
- Polysaccharide antigen detection is a rapid test for diagnosis and for monitoring relapse
- Complement fixation may be negative approximately 30% in acute histoplasmosis and 50% in disseminated histoplasmosis
- Immunodiffusion test may be negative in approximately 50% of patients with acute histoplasmosis. Maximum positivity of test occurs 4-6 weeks after exposure.
- Complement fixation antibodies at titers 1:8 or 1:16 are presumptive for diagnosis, > 1:32 is strongly supportive as is an acute 4-fold titer rise. Determining the presence of H and M bands may be helpful.
- For chronic histoplasmosis and disseminated disease, cultures of sputum, bronchoalveolar lavage, bone marrow, lymph nodes, blood, liver and cerebrospinal fluid may be positive. Demonstration of characteristic organisms by silver stain on biopsy and bronchoalveolar lavage and bronchial washing specimens is diagnostic.

Drugs that may alter lab results: N/A

Disorders that may alter lab results:
- Serologic tests may be falsely negative early in infection or in the immunocompromised
- False positive results may occur with tuberculosis and other fungal diseases
- Slow clearance of antibodies may identify patients with past Histoplasmosis infection who now present with a different disease
- False positive complement fixation titers may occur after histoplasmin skin antigen testing
- False positive H. capsulatum polysaccharide antigen test may occur with patients with disseminated blastomycosis and coccidioidomycosis

PATHOLOGICAL FINDINGS Poorly formed caseating granulomas on biopsy or bronchoscopy specimens with identification of characteristic yeast forms by methenamine silver stain

SPECIAL TESTS
- Determine the presence of urinary H. capsulatum antigen
- Bronchoscopy
- Liver and bone marrow biopsies

IMAGING
- Routine CXR may reveal focal mid-lung field infiltrates (27%), hilar or mediastinal adenopathy (25%) or both (30%). May see miliary or diffuse pattern with disseminated disease following large antigen load.
- If indicated, chest CT scan to differentiate mediastinal fibrosis from mediastinal granuloma

DIAGNOSTIC PROCEDURES
- Serologic blood work
- Bronchoscopy with bronchoalveolar lavage and transbronchial biopsy
- Liver and bone marrow biopsies for suspected disseminated disease
- Mediastinoscopy for lymph node biopsy

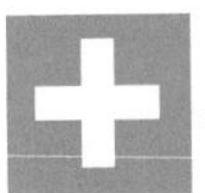

TREATMENT

APPROPRIATE HEALTH CARE
- Usually outpatient
- Disseminated histoplasmosis requires hospitalization for initial treatment

GENERAL MEASURES 99% of acute primary histoplasmosis resolve spontaneously; symptomatic treatment only

SURGICAL MEASURES N/A

ACTIVITY Avoid high risk exposures

DIET No restrictions

PATIENT EDUCATION Extended treatment needs in chronic cavitary histoplasmosis; maintenance therapy in AIDS

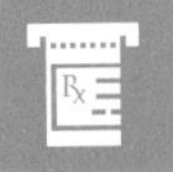

MEDICATIONS

DRUG(S) OF CHOICE
- Disseminated histoplasmosis
  - ◊ Amphotericin B - test dose is 1 mg followed by 0.25 mg/kg/dose, which may be slowly increased to 0.5 mg/kg/dose. Cumulative dose to 1-2 gm (at least 35 mg/kg is indicated).
  - ◊ Ketoconazole or itraconazole for mild disease
    - Ketoconazole: Induction therapy with 400 mg/day for 3 days, then maintenance therapy 200 mg or 400 mg a day
    - Itraconazole: Induction therapy with 200 mg twice a day for 3 days, then 200 mg once or twice daily

- AIDS patients
  - ◊ Itraconazole for mild disease: Induction therapy with 600 mg/day for 3 days, then 400 mg/day. Drug of choice for primary and maintenance therapy is itraconazole. Ketoconazole is not effective in AIDS-related histoplasmosis. Maintenance therapy with itraconazole 400 mg/day or amphotericin-B 50-100 mg weekly (1 mg/kg).
- Chronic cavitary histoplasmosis
  - ◊ Amphotericin-B for severe or moderately severe disease, 2.0-2.5 g cumulative
  - ◊ Ketoconazole or itraconazole for mild disease
    - Ketoconazole: Induction therapy with 400 mg/day for 3 days, then maintenance therapy 200 mg or 400 mg/day
    - Itraconazole: Induction therapy with 200 mg twice daily for 3 days, then 200 mg once or twice daily
- Acute pulmonary histoplasmosis
  - ◊ Amphotericin B for severe or moderately severe disease; test dose is 1 mg followed by 0.25 mg/kg/dose which may be slowly increased to 0.5 mg/kg/dose. Cumulative dose at least 35 mg/kg.
  - ◊ Ketoconazole or itraconazole for mild disease
    - Ketoconazole: Induction therapy with 400 mg/day for 3 days, then maintenance therapy 200 mg or 400 mg/day
    - Itraconazole: Induction therapy with 200 mg twice daily for 3 days, then 200 mg once or twice daily
- Duration of treatment
  - ◊ Optimal duration of treatment with antifungals has not been established
  - ◊ Disseminated histoplasmosis - 6 months course
  - ◊ Chronic cavitary histoplasmosis - at least 12 months course with stable CXR findings over 3-6 months
  - ◊ Acute pulmonary histoplasmosis - 2-3 month course
  - ◊ AIDS-related or relapsed - chronic, lifelong, maintenance therapy
- Mediastinal granuloma
  - ◊ Can mimic fibrosing mediastinitis, may respond to treatment with amphotericin B
- Fibrosing mediastinitis
  - ◊ Has no active infection present and is not treatable

Contraindications: No contraindications to treatment in patients with progressive cavitary disease or disseminated histoplasmosis. The latter has a mortality rate of 80% if untreated.

Precautions:
- Amphotericin B
  - ◊ Dosage probably does not need to be adjusted for creatinine clearance
  - ◊ It is nephrotoxic. Renal function must be monitored closely. Monitor electrolytes, especially potassium and magnesium.
  - ◊ Rigors can be prevented by pre-infusion meperidine. Fever and chills can be diminished by pre-infusion dose of acetaminophen plus diphenhydramine.
- Ketoconazole
  - ◊ Is associated with gastrointestinal upset
  - ◊ May inhibit testosterone synthesis and should be used with caution in patients with underlying hepatic dysfunction

Significant possible interactions:
- Expected benefits outweigh possible risks.
- Ketoconazole
  - ◊ Requires an acid environment for dissolution. If the patient requires antacid or H2 blockade, administer at least 2 hours after dose of ketoconazole
  - ◊ May increase cyclosporine levels
  - ◊ May decrease Rifampin and INH levels as well as ketoconazole levels
  - ◊ May increase phenytoin levels
- Itraconazole
  - ◊ Rifampin levels may decrease itraconazole to undetectable levels
  - ◊ May increase digoxin levels
  - ◊ Questionable effect on cyclosporine levels
- Fluconazole
  - ◊ May increase cyclosporine levels
  - ◊ May increase warfarin effect
  - ◊ Questionable effect of rifampin on fluconazole

ALTERNATIVE DRUGS
- Fluconazole has not been approved for histoplasmosis therapy. Fluconazole is undergoing investigational studies in its use for chronic pulmonary and disseminated histoplasmosis. Preliminarily, fluconazole doses of 400 mg/day or higher may be necessary for therapeutic outcome.
- Liposomal amphotericin may be used if amphotericin nephrotoxicity encountered

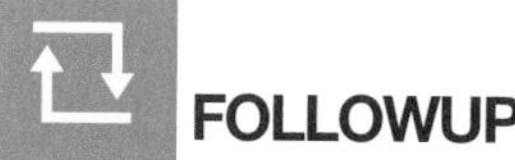

FOLLOWUP

PATIENT MONITORING Renal function and liver chemistries every 1-2 months for chronic therapy patients; chest x-ray to evaluate therapy response at regular intervals

PREVENTION/AVOIDANCE Maintenance therapy is required in AIDS

POSSIBLE COMPLICATIONS
- Bronchial, tracheal or esophageal obstruction secondary to adenopathy, broncholithiasis
- Pulmonary, splenic and hepatic calcifications, rarely pericarditis, pleurisy or effusion
- CNS histoplasmosis (rare): Chronic meningitis or intracranial histoplasmosis
- Endocarditis involving aortic or mitral valves
- Pericardial effusions (sterile exudates) not thought to be secondary to hematogenous spread
- Fibrosing mediastinitis can cause stenosis of vascular and bronchial structures within the mediastinum causing pulmonary hypertension, superior vena cava syndrome and bronchial obstruction
- Acute renal failure and hepatic dysfunction secondary to medications
- Amphotericin induced hypokalemia
- Relapse occurring in the immunocompromised or inadequately treated patient with disseminated histoplasmosis

EXPECTED COURSE/PROGNOSIS
- Primary histoplasmosis - 99% resolve spontaneously
- The prognosis for chronic cavitary pulmonary histoplasmosis is determined by the loss of lung parenchyma and pulmonary function
- Treatment of disseminated disease in AIDS/non-AIDS cases does improve outcome with ketoconazole having > 80% success rate and amphotericin B being 60-100% successful. Despite maintenance therapy, AIDS patients, have 10-50% relapse rate.

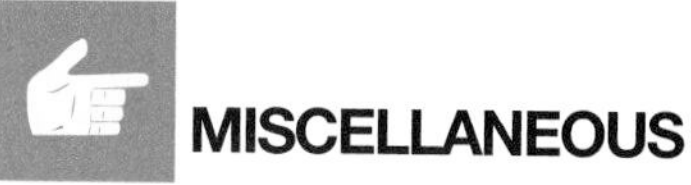

MISCELLANEOUS

ASSOCIATED CONDITIONS
- Disseminated histoplasmosis is an opportunistic infection in the immunocompromised host
- HIV infection

AGE-RELATED FACTORS
Pediatric: 1/3 of cases of disseminated histoplasmosis occur in infants < 1 year old
Geriatric: Increased incidence of disseminated histoplasmosis in males during 6th and 7th decades
Others: N/A

PREGNANCY No increased incidence

SYNONYMS N/A

ICD-9-CM
115.90 Histoplasmosis, unspecified without mention of manifestation
115.99 Histoplasmosis, unspecified other

SEE ALSO

OTHER NOTES N/A

ABBREVIATIONS N/A

REFERENCES

- Dismukes WE, Cloud G, Bowles C, et al: Treatment of blastomycosis and histoplasmosis with ketoconazole. Ann Intern Med 1985;103:861-872
- Como JA, Dismukes WE: Oral azole drugs as systemic antifungal therapy. N Engl J Med 1994;330:263-272
- Wheat JL, Connolly-Stringfield P, Kohler RB, et al: Histoplasma capsulatum polysaccharide antigen detection in diagnosis and management of disseminated histoplasmosis in patients with acquired immunodeficiency syndrome. Am J Med 1989;87:396-400
- Wheat JL, Connolly-Stringfield PA, Baker RL, et al: Histoplasmosis in the acquired immune deficiency syndrome: clinical findings diagnosis and treatment, and review of the literature. In Medicine 1990;69:361-374
- Wheat J: Histoplasmosis: recognition and treatment. Clin Infect Dis. (suppl) 1994;1:S19-27

Web references: 1 available at www.5mcc.com
Illustrations 2 available

Author(s):
Robert P. Baughman, MD

BASICS

DESCRIPTION A chronic infection with variable course (requiring about 10 years from the time of infection for 50% of persons to develop AIDS). HIV infects cells with CD4 receptors, most notably the CD4 lymphocytes. Infection results in cell death and a decline in immune function resulting in opportunistic infections (O.I.), malignancies, and neurologic problems. These opportunistic conditions define the acquired immunodeficiency syndrome (AIDS). As of 1/1/93 all HIV infected persons with <200 CD4 cells are categorized as AIDS. HIV also has direct effects on the central nervous system, GI tract and other systems.
System(s) affected: Gastrointestinal, Hemic/Lymphatic/Immunologic, Nervous, Pulmonary
Genetics: Unclear, some genotypes may be protective
Incidence/Prevalence in USA: > 800,000 AIDS cases; > 450,000 deaths
Predominant age: Young adults - 25-44
Predominant sex: Male > Female

SIGNS & SYMPTOMS

- Acute infection: Mononucleosis-like syndrome with fever, rash, myalgia, and malaise a self-limited syndrome occurring about 6-8 weeks postinfection, associated with the development of HIV antibody
- Asymptomatic infection: Follows initial infection; variable duration
- Persistent generalized lymphadenopathy: Characteristics - lymph node enlargement 1 cm or greater in 2 or more extra-inguinal sites. Adenopathy persists longer than 3 mos.
- Other diseases:
  - ◊ Constitutional: Fever lasting more than one month, involuntary weight loss of more than ten percent baseline weight, persistent diarrhea, skin rash, severe chronic fatigue
  - ◊ Neurologic disease: Dementia, myelopathy or peripheral neuropathy not explained by other illness
  - ◊ Secondary infectious disease:
    - AIDS-defining opportunistic infections: Pneumocystis carinii pneumonia; chronic cryptosporidial diarrhea; cerebral toxoplasmosis; extra-intestinal Strongyloides; isosporiasis; esophageal, bronchial/pulmonary candidiasis; cryptococcosis; histoplasmosis; coccidioidomycosis; disseminated mycobacterial disease; cytomegalovirus disease; chronic mucocutaneous or disseminated herpes simplex; progressive multifocal leukoencephalopathy.
    - Other specified infections: Oral hairy leukoplakia, dermatomal zoster, nocardioses, tuberculosis (pulmonary), recurrent salmonella bacteremia, oral candidiasis.
  - ◊ Secondary cancers: Kaposi sarcoma, Hodgkin and non-Hodgkin lymphoma, and primary brain lymphoma, invasive cervical cancer
  - ◊ Cardiac myopathy, pericarditis
  - ◊ Renal - HIV nephropathy
  - ◊ Other conditions not classified above that may be attributed to HIV infection: idiopathic thrombocytopenic purpura, seborrheic dermatitis, chronic lymphoid interstitial pneumonitis
- 1993 revised classification: For HIV infection and expanded surveillance case definition for AIDS among adolescents and adults (from MMWR)
- Categories:

A	B	C
Asymptomatic or persistent general lymphadenopathy	Symptomatic; not category A or C conditions	AIDS indicator conditions

(includes acute [primary] infection)

- CD4 cell categories:

1	2	3
≥ 500/μg	200-499/μg	< 200/μg
A1, B1, C1†	A2, B2, C2†	A3†, B3†, C3†

(† = expanded AIDS surveillance case definition)

- Conditions: Included in the AIDS surveillance case definition
  - ◊ Candidiasis of bronchi, trachea, or lungs
  - ◊ Candidiasis, esophageal
  - ◊ Cervical cancer, invasive
  - ◊ Coccidioidomycosis, disseminated or extrapulmonary
  - ◊ Cryptococcosis, extrapulmonary
  - ◊ Cryptosporidiosis, chronic intestinal (> 1 month duration)
  - ◊ Cytomegalovirus disease (other than liver, spleen or nodes)
  - ◊ HIV encephalopathy
  - ◊ Herpes simplex: chronic ulcer(s) (> than 1 month duration) or bronchitis, pneumonitis, or esophagitis
  - ◊ Histoplasmosis, disseminated or extrapulmonary
  - ◊ Isosporiasis, chronic intestinal (> 1 month duration)
  - ◊ Kaposi sarcoma
  - ◊ Lymphoma, Burkitt (or equivalent term)
  - ◊ Lymphoma, immunoblastic (or equivalent term)
  - ◊ Lymphoma, primary in brain
  - ◊ Mycobacterium avium complex or M. kansasii, disseminated or extrapulmonary
  - ◊ Mycobacterium tuberculosis, any site (pulmonary or extrapulmonary)
  - ◊ Mycobacterium, other species or unidentified species, disseminated or extrapulmonary
  - ◊ Pneumocystis carinii pneumonia
  - ◊ Progressive multifocal leukoencephalopathy
  - ◊ Salmonella septicemia, recurrent
  - ◊ Toxoplasmosis of brain
  - ◊ Wasting syndrome resulting from HIV infection

CAUSES Human immunodeficiency virus (HIV); a retrovirus

RISK FACTORS

- Sexual activity
  - ◊ Post-sexual exposure prophylaxis is under investigation
- Injection drug use
- Recipients of blood products: Highest risk 1975 to 3/1985
- Hemophiliacs who received pooled plasma
- Children of HIV-infected women:
  - ◊ 30% of the these children during pregnancy will be infected without treatment
  - ◊ Breast feeding is a possible route of transmission
  - ◊ Prenatal, intrapartum and postpartum zidovudine significantly decreases the risk of HIV transmission from mother to child (from 29% to 8%)
- Occupational exposure
  - ◊ Postexposure treatment (in conjunction with expert consultation) with 2 or 3 antiretrovirals for significant exposures

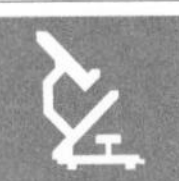

DIAGNOSIS

DIFFERENTIAL DIAGNOSIS Screen for HIV infection when there is prolonged illness without ready explanation.

LABORATORY

- ELISA
  - ◊ Sensitivity and specificity > 98%
  - ◊ Reported as reactive or non-reactive. Reactive tests should be repeated. Confirm repeatedly reactive tests by another test (most commonly the Western Blot).
- Western blot
  - ◊ Test results are positive, negative, or indeterminate (indeterminate tests result from non-specific reactions of HIV-negative sera with some HIV proteins)
  - ◊ The CDC recommends reaction with two of the following three bands as criteria for positivity: P24; gp41, and gp 120/160. If the test is indeterminate, repeat test in 3-6 months.

Drugs that may alter lab results: N/A

Disorders that may alter lab results: Collagen vascular disease, pregnancy, syphilis, recent immunization

PATHOLOGICAL FINDINGS N/A

SPECIAL TESTS As indicated by suspicion of opportunistic infection or HIV-associated condition.

IMAGING N/A

DIAGNOSTIC PROCEDURES N/A

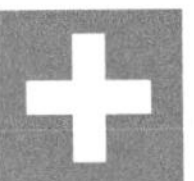

TREATMENT

APPROPRIATE HEALTH CARE Outpatient setting. Consultation with an experienced HIV expert is strongly encouraged.

GENERAL MEASURES

- The initial visit:
  - ◊ Past medical history including STDs and TB with dates and treatment
  - ◊ Review of systems to include fever, chills, diarrhea, weight loss, fatigue, adenopathy, oral sores, cough, shortness of breath, dyspnea on exertion, visual changes, headaches, skin rash, neurologic changes, sinusitis, odynophagia
  - ◊ Social history
  - ◊ Physical examination, with Pap smear
  - ◊ Immunization review (pneumococcal, influenza, and Td recommended in adults. OPV contraindicated in children [use IPV]). Hepatitis A and B if not immune.
  - ◊ Studies: CBC with differential and platelets; SMAC; RPR; CD4 absolute count and %lymphocytes CD4; Hep A IgG, Hep B sAg and sAb; Hep C antibody; chest x-ray; PPD with control; HIV-1 RNA viral quantitation (viral load); toxoplasmosis IgG, CMV IgG, Pap smears in females
- Patients with CD4<350 or CD4 >350 and viral burden >50,000 copies/mL may benefit from antiretroviral treatment
- Patients with CD4<200 or with oral candidiasis or other signs of significant immune suppression should receive Pneumocystis carinii prophylaxis

- Patients with CD4<100 and toxoplasmosis IgG should receive toxoplasmosis prophylaxis and regular screening for CMV retinitis
- Patients with CD4<50 should receive prophylaxis against Mycobacterium avium complex (MAC)
- When antiretroviral treatment results in significant increase in CD4#, then certain O.I. prophylaxis may be discontinued

SURGICAL MEASURES N/A

ACTIVITY Encourage regular exercise.

DIET
- Encourage good nutrition
- Avoid raw eggs, unpasteurized milk and other potentially contaminated foods
- May require vitamin supplementation

PATIENT EDUCATION
- Provide frank, complete, non-judgmental information on the routes of transmission (primarily sexual and needle sharing). Teach HIV infected how to minimize risk to others.
- Pre-printed and additional information material is available from a wide variety of sources including: National AIDS Hotline -

(800)342-2437 [Spanish (800)342-7432]
- National Institute of Health AIDS Clinical Trials Group (800)874-2572. Information on AIDS/HIV clinical trials.
- American Foundation for AIDS Research: (212)719-0033; new treatments and research

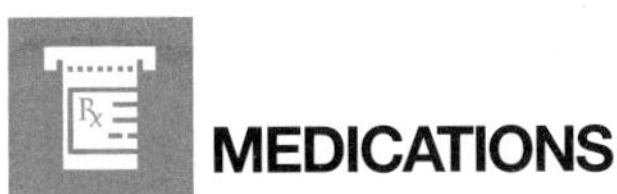

MEDICATIONS

DRUG(S) OF CHOICE
- Nucleoside reverse transcriptase inhibitors:
  - ◊ Abacavir (ABC, Ziagen)
  - ◊ Didanosine (ddI, Videx)
  - ◊ Emtricitabine (FTC, Emtriva)
  - ◊ Lamivudine (3TC, Epivir)
  - ◊ Stavudine (d4T, Zerit)
  - ◊ Zalcitabine (ddC, Hivid)
  - ◊ Zidovudine (AZT, Retrovir)
- Protease inhibitors:
  - ◊ Amprenavir (Agenerase)
  - ◊ Atazanavir (Reyataz)
  - ◊ Indinavir (Crixivan)
  - ◊ Lopinavir-ritonavir (Kaletra)
  - ◊ Nelfinavir (Viracept)
  - ◊ Ritonavir (Norvir)
  - ◊ Saquinavir (Fortovase)
- Non-nucleoside reverse transcriptase inhibitors:
  - ◊ Delavirdine (Rescriptor)
  - ◊ Efavirenz (Sustiva)
  - ◊ Nevirapine (Viramune)
- Nucleotide reverse transcriptase inhibitors:
  - ◊ Tenofovir (Viread)
- Fusion inhibitors
  - ◊ Enfuviritide (Fuzeon)
- Current standard of care requires the use of 3 drugs to attempt to prevent the emergence of resistance. Goal of therapy is to reduce viral load as much as possible and delay or reverse immunodeterioration.

Contraindications: Significant drug interactions
Precautions: Antiretroviral drugs have significant toxicities; refer to specific drug information
Significant possible interactions: Antiretroviral drugs, especially the protease inhibitors have potentially life-threatening interactions; refer to specific drug information

ALTERNATIVE DRUGS N/A

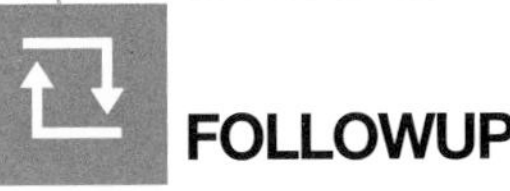

FOLLOWUP

PATIENT MONITORING
- Frequency determined largely by the patient's clinical and psychological status and by the need to monitor drug toxicity and immune function
- Recheck CD4 counts and viral load at least every 3-6 months depending on stage of illness and medical regimen
- Check at subsequent visits:
  - ◊ Complete, careful physical exam
  - ◊ Complete review of systems especially focused on neurologic symptoms (CNS infection, malignancy, or dementia), visual changes (CMV retinitis), diarrhea, fever, night sweats, shortness of breath, dyspnea on exertion (early P. carinii pneumonia), and odynophagia (esophageal candidiasis)
- Genotypic and phenotypic tests for resistance to antiretrovirals are available and appear to improve clinical outcome

PREVENTION/AVOIDANCE When possible: avoid unscreened blood products; avoid unprotected sexual intercourse; use condoms; avoid injection drug abuse; needle exchange for active IDUs

POSSIBLE COMPLICATIONS
- Immunodeficiency
- Opportunistic infections
- Neuropsychiatric symptoms
- HIV-associated malignancies

EXPECTED COURSE/PROGNOSIS
When untreated HIV infection leads to AIDS, life expectancy is two to three years. AIDS defining opportunistic infections usually do not develop until CD4<200. In HIV untreated infection, CD4 counts decline at a rate of 50-80/year with more rapid decline as counts drop below 200. Potent antiretroviral regimens may delay or reverse immune dysfunction.

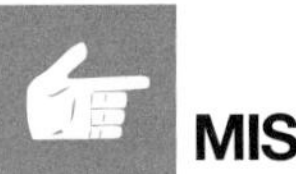

MISCELLANEOUS

ASSOCIATED CONDITIONS
- Syphilis: May be more aggressive in HIV-infected persons. Definitive treatment for syphilis in HIV infected persons is controversial; consult with an STD specialist.
- Tuberculosis is co-epidemic with HIV. HIV infection changes the management of TB; should test all persons with TB for HIV, or if not tested, should treat with multiple drugs as if HIV-infected.
- Hepatitis C co-infected patients have more rapid progression to cirrhosis

AGE-RELATED FACTORS
Pediatric: Progresses more rapidly in infants
Geriatric: Progresses more rapidly in age >50
Others: N/A

PREGNANCY Antiretroviral therapy has been demonstrated to decrease the risk of HIV transmission to infants. Pregnant women should be treated based on their HIV disease status. Current guidelines are cited below.

SYNONYMS
- Acquired immune deficiency syndrome

ICD-9-CM
042 Human immunodeficiency virus (HIV) disease

SEE ALSO
Candidiasis
Candidiasis, mucocutaneous
Cryptococcosis
Cytomegalovirus inclusion disease
Idiopathic thrombocytopenic purpura (ITP)
Kaposi sarcoma
Pneumonia, Pneumocystis (PCP)
Rhodococcus infections
Tuberculosis

OTHER NOTES Increased risk of cervical cancer in HIV-infected women. Perform PAP smears every 6 months.

ABBREVIATIONS N/A

REFERENCES

- CDC. Guidelines for the use of Antiretroviral Agents in HIV-1-Infected Adults and Adolescents. (last updated Mar 2004; see www.aidsinfo.nih.gov for latest version of the 'living document')
- Yeni PG, Hammer SM, Hirsch MS, Saag MS, Schechter M, Carpenter CC, et. al. Treatment for adult HIV infection: 2004 recommendations of the International AIDS Society-USA Panel. JAMA. 2004;292(2):251-65
- CDC. Guidelines for Preventing Opportunistic Infections Among HIV-Infected Persons-2002. MMWR 2002;51(No. RR-8)
- U.S. Public Health Service Task Force Recommendations for Use of Antiretroviral Drugs During Pregnancy for Maternal Health and Reduction of Perinatal Transmission of HIV Type 1 in the US. Fed Reg, 12-97
- CDC. Updated U.S. Public Health Guidelines for the Management of Occupational Exposures to HBV, HCV, and HIV and Recommendations for Postexposure Prophylaxis. MMWR 2001;50(No.RR-1)

Web references: 7 available at www.5mcc.com
Illustrations 39 available

Author(s):
Kevin Carmichael, MD

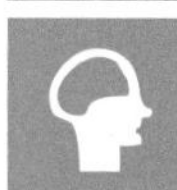

BASICS

DESCRIPTION A malignant disease of lymphoid tissue. Probable clonal proliferation of transformed B cells in majority; rarely may involve T cells. Reed-Sternberg cells are pathognomonic. Disease spreads to contiguous lymphoid tissue and eventually to non-lymphoid tissue.

- Rye classification-based on pathologic findings (frequency by percent):
  - ◊ Lymphocyte predominant (2-10)
  - ◊ Mixed cellularity (20-40)
  - ◊ Lymphocyte depleted (2-15)
  - ◊ Nodular sclerosis (40-80)

System(s) affected: Hemic/Lymphatic/Immunologic

Genetics:
- First degree relatives - 3 times risk
- Siblings of younger patients - 7 times risk

Incidence/Prevalence in USA:
- 3.1/100000
- About 7000 new cases expected yearly
- Incidence is lower in underdeveloped countries

Predominant age:
- Bimodal age distribution
  - ◊ Early peak in mid to late 20s
  - ◊ Later peak around 60-70
- Rare under age 5

Predominant sex: Male > Female (1.4:1)

SIGNS & SYMPTOMS
- Asymptomatic lymphadenopathy (usually cervical or supraclavicular)
- Fever (Pel-Epstein pattern)
- Night sweats
- Weight loss
- Fatigue
- Anorexia
- Unexplained itching
- Alcohol-induced pain

CAUSES
- Unknown; EB virus may play a role

RISK FACTORS
- Immunodeficiency (inherited or acquired)
- Autoimmune disorders
- HIV infection

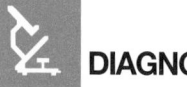

DIAGNOSIS

DIFFERENTIAL DIAGNOSIS
- Non-Hodgkin lymphoma
- Infectious lymphadenopathy
- Other solid tumor metastases
- Sarcoidosis
- Autoimmune disease
- AIDS/HIV infection
- Drug reaction

LABORATORY
- CBC
- Chemistry profile
- ESR
- Liver function tests
- Renal function tests
- HIV (if risk factors present)
- Hepatitis serology (if risk factors present)

Drugs that may alter lab results: Phenytoin may produce pseudolymphoma

Disorders that may alter lab results: N/A

PATHOLOGICAL FINDINGS
- Reed-Sternberg (RS) cell
  - ◊ Abundant cytoplasm
  - ◊ Two or more nuclei or nuclear lobes, each with a prominent nucleoli
- Background infiltrate of lymphocytes, histiocytes, granulocytes, plasma cells and fibroblasts

SPECIAL TESTS N/A

IMAGING
- Chest X-ray
- Thoracic CT scan
- Abdominal and pelvic CT scan (or possibly MR scan)
- PET scan (exact role is under investigation)
- Lymphangiography
- Bone scan, gallium scan, abdominal ultrasound (used infrequently)

DIAGNOSTIC PROCEDURES
- Excisional lymph node biopsy (needle biopsy not sufficient)
- Exploratory laparotomy with splenectomy - becoming uncommon
- Bone marrow biopsy-especially with systemic symptoms
- Liver biopsy (in selected cases)

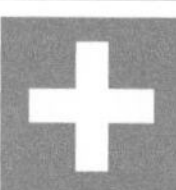

TREATMENT

APPROPRIATE HEALTH CARE
- Initial staging is critical to therapy
- Cotswold classification
  - ◊ Stage I - single lymph node group
  - ◊ Stage II - two or more node groups on same side of diaphragm
  - ◊ Stage III - Node groups on both sides of diaphragm
  - ◊ Stage IV - dissemination involving extra-nodal organs (not the spleen which is considered lymphoid tissue)
  - ◊ Subclass designations: A = no symptoms; B = systemic symptoms (fever, night sweats, weight loss >10% body weight); X = bulky disease (widened mediastinum > 1/3 intrathoracic diameter or > 10 cm nodal mass); E = single extra-nodal site involvement in proximity with known nodal site

GENERAL MEASURES
- Treatment aimed for cure with minimum toxicity, including treatment-induced late mortality
- Treatment can be radiation therapy (RT), chemotherapy, or combined radiation and chemotherapy (CMT), based on stage and tumor burden
  - ◊ Early stages - favorable prognosis - low amount (2-3 cycles) chemotherapy plus involved field RT; or extended field RT
  - ◊ Early stages - unfavorable prognosis - moderate chemotherapy (≈4 cycles) plus RT
  - ◊ Advanced stages - extensive chemotherapy (≈8 cycles) with or without RT
- Autologous bone marrow transplant for selected patients who fail conventional therapy

SURGICAL MEASURES N/A

ACTIVITY As tolerated

DIET No restrictions

PATIENT EDUCATION
- Reproductive impact
  - ◊ Spermatogenesis often impaired prior to therapy
  - ◊ Gonadal side effects of therapy
  - ◊ Sperm banking option for males
  - ◊ Oophoropexy in premenopausal female if pelvic RT contemplated
- Risks of secondary malignancy
- Careful oral and dental care during therapy
- Patient education material
  - ◊ Leukemia Society of America, 733 3rd Avenue, New York, NY 10017

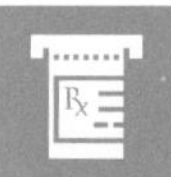

MEDICATIONS

DRUG(S) OF CHOICE
- Note: Must be monitored by experienced oncologist
- ABVD chemotherapy - 4 week cycles
  - ◊ Doxorubicin (Adriamycin) - 25 mg/m2 IV days 1 and 15
  - ◊ Bleomycin 10 mg/m2 IV days 1 and 15
  - ◊ Vinblastine 6.0 mg/m2 IV days 1 and 15
  - ◊ Dacarbazine 375 mg/m2 IV days 1 and 15

Contraindications: As in general for chemotherapy

Precautions: Chemotherapy toxicity, bone marrow suppression

Significant possible interactions: Refer to manufacturer's literature

ALTERNATIVE DRUGS
- MOPP chemotherapy - 4 week cycles
  - ◊ Mechlorethamine (nitrogen mustard) 6.0 mg/m2 IV days 1 and 8
  - ◊ Vincristine (Oncovin) 1.4 mg/m2 IV days 1 and 8
  - ◊ Procarbazine 100 mg/m2 po days 1 through 14 (avoid vanilla, cheese and wine)
  - ◊ Prednisone 40 mg/m2 po days 1 through 14 during cycles 1 and 4
- Alternate cycles with MOPP/ABVD to minimize toxicity
- BEACOPP (bleomycin, etoposide, doxorubicin, cyclophosphamide, vincristine, procarbazine, prednisone)
- Stanford V regimen (nitrogen mustard, doxorubicin, vinblastine, vincristine, bleomycin, etoposide, prednisone)

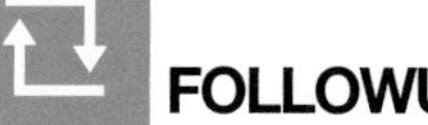

FOLLOWUP

PATIENT MONITORING
- CBC, nutrition and hydration during therapy
- Post-treatment monitoring (at least yearly)
  - ◊ CBC, ESR
  - ◊ TSH, if RT to the neck
  - ◊ Chest x-ray

PREVENTION/AVOIDANCE
- Pneumococcal vaccine, if splenectomy is planned for staging
- Consider vaccines for Haemophilus and Neisseria species as well

POSSIBLE COMPLICATIONS
- Secondary malignancies following therapy
- Sterility, gonadal dysfunction
- Hypothyroidism
- Bone marrow suppression
- Immunosuppressed infections, including herpes zoster
- Anemia
- ITP, TTP
- Coronary artery disease, cardiomyopathy
- Radiation pneumonitis, pulmonary fibrosis
- Transient radiation myelopathy (Lhermitte's sign)

EXPECTED COURSE/PROGNOSIS
- Overall 5 year survival 83%
- 75% long term survival
- 10 year survival rates correlate with stage at diagnosis
  - ◊ Stage IA, IB, IIA non-bulky 85-95%
  - ◊ Stage IIA bulky, IIB 80-85%
  - ◊ Stage IIIA 75-90%
  - ◊ Stage IIIB 60-65%
  - ◊ Stage IV 55-60%
- Unfavorable prognostic factors in advanced disease
  - ◊ Sed rate > 70
  - ◊ Age > 45
  - ◊ Male gender
  - ◊ Albumin < 4g/dL
  - ◊ Hemoglobin < 10.5 g/dL
  - ◊ Lymphopenia < 600 cells/μL
  - ◊ Leukocyte count ≥ 15,000 cells/μL

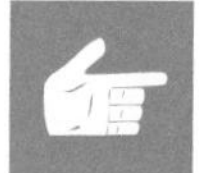

MISCELLANEOUS

ASSOCIATED CONDITIONS
- T lymphocyte defects, which persist after successful treatment
- Patients with HIV tend to present with more advanced disease

AGE-RELATED FACTORS
Pediatric:
- Increased risk for males
- Young females (< 20) who have treatment with thoracic radiation are at high risk for breast cancer

Geriatric: Usually presents in more advance stage and shows unfavorable histology

Others: N/A

PREGNANCY
- Pregnancy not known to affect course of disease
- Hodgkin disease not known to affect pregnancy or fetus IF therapy can be postponed until delivery
- Normal pregnancy can occur after treatment, if fertility is maintained
- Risk of disease progression during pregnancy is variable. Management must be individualized

SYNONYMS
Malignant lymphoma

ICD-9-CM
201.90 Hodgkin disease, unspecified, unspecified site, extranodal and solid organ sites

SEE ALSO
Lymphoma, non-Hodgkin

OTHER NOTES
N/A

ABBREVIATIONS
N/A

REFERENCES

- Fung HC, Nademanee AP. Approach to Hodgkin's lymphoma in the new millennium. Hematol Oncol 2002;20(1):1-15
- Horwitz SM, Horning SJ. Advances in the treatment of Hodgkin's lymphoma. Curr Opin Hematol 2000;7(4):235-40
- Tesch H, Sieber M, Diehl V. Treatment of advanced stage Hodgkin's disease. Oncology 2001;60(2):101-9
- National Comprehensive Cancer Network. NCCN practice guidelines for Hodgkin's disease. Oncology (Huntingt) 1999 May;13(5A):78-110
- Urba WJ, Longo DL. Hodgkin's disease. NEJM 1992;326(10):678-87

Web references: 0 available at www.5mcc.com

Illustrations N/A

Author(s):
Rich Londo, MD

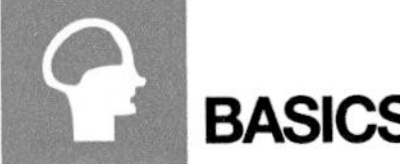

BASICS

DESCRIPTION The common term "stye" refers to any inflammation or infection of the eyelid margin involving the hair follicles of the eyelashes (external hordeolum), meibomian glands (internal hordeolum), or granulomatous infection of the meibomian glands (chalazion)
System(s) affected: Skin/Exocrine
Genetics: No known genetic pattern
Incidence/Prevalence in USA: Extremely common
Predominant age: None
Predominant sex: Male = Female

SIGNS & SYMPTOMS
- Redness of the margin of the eyelid with scaling, collection of discharge
- Localized inflammation of the eyelashes
- Patients may experience itching or scaling of the eyelids, chronic redness, eye irritation leading to localized tenderness and pain

CAUSES
- The most common causes of eyelid infections are staphylococcal, although other organisms may also be involved
- Seborrhea can predispose to infections of the eyelid

RISK FACTORS
- Predisposing blepharitis (low grade infections of the eyelid margin)
- Poor eyelid hygiene
- Contact lens wearers
- Application of make-up

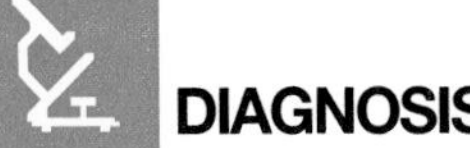

DIAGNOSIS

DIFFERENTIAL DIAGNOSIS
- Blepharitis
- Eyelid neoplasms

LABORATORY Culture of the eyelid margins is usually not necessary

Drugs that may alter lab results: None

Disorders that may alter lab results: None

PATHOLOGICAL FINDINGS Bacterial contamination and white cells in eyelid discharge

SPECIAL TESTS None

IMAGING None

DIAGNOSTIC PROCEDURES History and eye examination

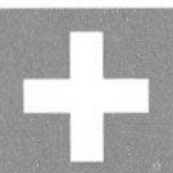

TREATMENT

APPROPRIATE HEALTH CARE Outpatient

GENERAL MEASURES
- Warm compresses to the area of inflammation can help increase blood supply and potentiate spontaneous drainage
- Good personal hygiene with attention to cleansing the eyelids on a daily basis to prevent recurrent infections
- Application of an antibiotic ointment (such as erythromycin) to the margin of the eyelid after proper cleansing. (Except children under 12, where there is a risk of blurred vision and amblyopia.) Helps reduce bacterial proliferation.

SURGICAL MEASURES If the infection becomes localized to a single gland, incision, drainage, and curettage is sometimes necessary. This is an in-office procedure with a local anesthetic.

ACTIVITY No restrictions

DIET No special diet

PATIENT EDUCATION
- The patient should be instructed in proper cleansing of the eyelids using a solution of tap water and baby shampoo or a commercially prepared hypoallergenic cleanser
- The stye should not be squeezed

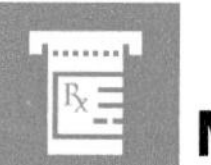

MEDICATIONS

DRUG(S) OF CHOICE
- Erythromycin ophthalmic ointment
- Occasionally use of an aminoglycoside ophthalmic ointment such as gentamicin may be necessary if refractory to simpler treatment
- Oral dicloxacillin for 2 weeks if refractory to topical ointment
- Treat underlying dry eye with artificial tears

Contraindications: None
Precautions: None
Significant possible interactions: None

ALTERNATIVE DRUGS None

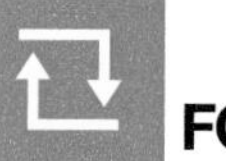

FOLLOWUP

PATIENT MONITORING The patient should be seen within several weeks to assess the effectiveness of therapy

PREVENTION/AVOIDANCE Eyelid hygiene

POSSIBLE COMPLICATIONS None expected. An internal hordeolum, if untreated, may lead to generalized cellulitis of the lid.

EXPECTED COURSE/PROGNOSIS
Responds well to treatment, but tends to recur in some patients

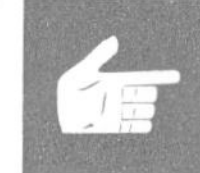

MISCELLANEOUS

ASSOCIATED CONDITIONS
- Acne
- Seborrhea

AGE-RELATED FACTORS
Pediatric: N/A
Geriatric: N/A
Others: N/A

PREGNANCY N/A

SYNONYMS
- Internal hordeolum
- External hordeolum
- Chalazion hordeolum
- Zeisian sty
- Meibomian sty

ICD-9-CM
373.11 Hordeolum externum
373.2 Chalazion
373.00 Blepharitis, unspecified

SEE ALSO

OTHER NOTES N/A

ABBREVIATIONS N/A

REFERENCES

Web references: 0 available at www.5mcc.com
Illustrations N/A

Author(s):
Robert M. Kershner, MD

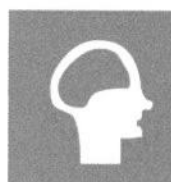

BASICS

DESCRIPTION Horner syndrome is caused by interruptions of the sympathetic nerve supply to the eye and results in miosis, ptosis, enophthalmos (sometimes), and absence of sweating of the ipsilateral face and neck
- Peripheral lesion (complete syndrome) - distal to superior cervical ganglion
- Central lesion (incomplete syndrome) - proximal to superior cervical ganglion

System(s) affected: Nervous, Skin/Exocrine
Genetics: Some autosomal dominant familial incidence
Incidence/Prevalence in USA: Unknown
Predominant age: May occur at any age
Predominant sex: Male = Female

SIGNS & SYMPTOMS
- Ptosis (drooping of the eyelid)
- Miosis (narrowing of the pupil of the eye)
- Anhidrosis
- Enophthalmos is sometimes found
- In congenital Horner, iris reduced - pigmentation, blue-gray, mottling of the affected eye (heterochromia iridis)
- Loss of ciliospinal reflex. Pinching skin of neck normally produces ipsolateral pupil dilation

CAUSES
- Interruption of the sympathetic nerve fibers that originate in the hypothalamus and travel down to the lateral part of the brain stem to exit in the thoracic area. These fibers synapse in the cervical sympathetic ganglia and the postganglionic fibers travel to the eye along the wall of the carotid and ophthalmic arteries.
- Idiopathic

RISK FACTORS
- Apical bronchogenic carcinoma (Pancoast tumor)
- Aneurysm of the carotid or subclavian artery
- Injuries to the carotid artery high in the neck
- Congenital Horner syndrome
- Dissection of the carotid arteries
- Cluster headaches, approximately 20% of which have an accompanying ipsilateral Horner syndrome. The syndrome may outlast the headaches.
- Carotid artery occlusion, approximately 15% of patients with carotid artery occlusion develop ipsilateral Horner syndrome - may occur without evidence of cerebral ischemia, neck injuries or operative procedures
- Syringomyelia
- Inflammatory process
- Cervical nerve root avulsion

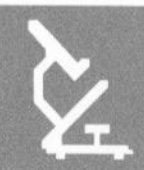

DIAGNOSIS

DIFFERENTIAL DIAGNOSIS Neurological diseases

LABORATORY N/A

Drugs that may alter lab results: N/A

Disorders that may alter lab results: N/A

PATHOLOGICAL FINDINGS
- Brainstem lesion
- Massive hemisphere lesion
- Cervical cord lesion
- Root lesion
- Sympathetic chain lesion

SPECIAL TESTS A normal pupil will dilate in response to installation of 10% cocaine.
- The miotic pupil in Horner won't dilate, or will dilate poorly, because of the absence of norepinephrine at the nerve endings.
- To distinguish a third order neuron disorder from a first and second neurone disorder 1% hydroxyamphetamine (Paredrine) or 4-hydroxyamphetamine 5% Pholedrine can be instilled 48 hours later. In a first or second neuron lesion, dilation will take place. Failure of the Horner pupil to dilate, or poor dilatation indicates a third-order neuron lesion.

IMAGING CT/MRI of the brain, chest, spinal cord

DIAGNOSTIC PROCEDURES Spinal tap - occasionally indicated in addition to above

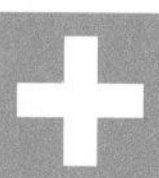

TREATMENT

APPROPRIATE HEALTH CARE Inpatient or outpatient, depending upon cause

GENERAL MEASURES
- Search for tumor or other compressive lesion is indicated for any patient who develops Horner syndrome
- Horner syndrome in itself does not produce any disability or require treatment
- Treatment is management of the underlying condition

SURGICAL MEASURES N/A

ACTIVITY Disease dependent

DIET Disease dependent

PATIENT EDUCATION N/A

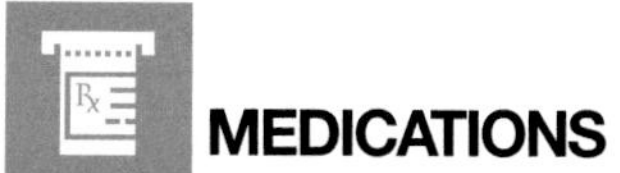

MEDICATIONS

DRUG(S) OF CHOICE Therapy appropriate for the underlying disease
Contraindications: N/A
Precautions: N/A
Significant possible interactions: N/A

ALTERNATIVE DRUGS N/A

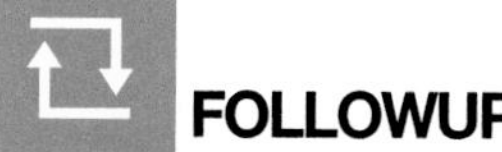

FOLLOWUP

PATIENT MONITORING Disease dependent

PREVENTION/AVOIDANCE None known

POSSIBLE COMPLICATIONS Chronic pupillary constriction

EXPECTED COURSE/PROGNOSIS
Variable with cause

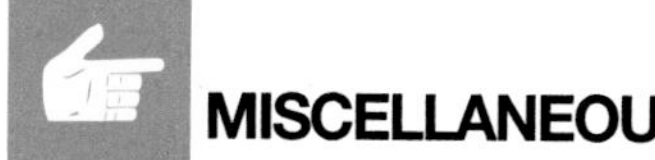

MISCELLANEOUS

ASSOCIATED CONDITIONS
- Wallenberg syndrome
- Pancoast's tumor
- C8 radiculopathy

AGE-RELATED FACTORS
Pediatric: N/A
Geriatric: N/A
Others: N/A

PREGNANCY N/A

SYNONYMS
- Bernard-Horner syndrome
- Bernard syndrome
- Cervical sympathetic syndrome
- Oculosympathetic syndrome

ICD-9-CM
337.9 Unspecified disorder of autonomic nervous system

SEE ALSO

OTHER NOTES N/A

ABBREVIATIONS N/A

REFERENCES

- Pryce-Phillips W, Murray TJ. Essential Neurology. New York: Scientific American Medicine,;1991
- Rhee DJ, Pyfer MF, eds. The Wills Eye Manual - Office and Emergency Room Diagnosis and Treatment of Eye Diseases. 3rd Ed. Philadelphia: Lippincott Williams & Wilkins; 1999

Web references: 1 available at www.5mcc.com
Illustrations N/A

Author(s):
Stanley G. Smith, MA, MB

BASICS

DESCRIPTION An inherited disease characterized by dementia and chorea that has a gradual onset and slow progression. Symptoms usually don't develop until after 30 years of age. By the time of diagnosis the patient has usually reproduced and passed the disease to another generation.

System(s) affected: Nervous

Genetics: Autosomal dominant; genetic marker on chromosome 4

Incidence/Prevalence in USA: 4-8 cases/100,000 people in the U.S.

Predominant age: Young adult (16-40); middle age (40-75)

Predominant sex: Male = Female

SIGNS & SYMPTOMS

- Early
  - ◊ Anxiety
  - ◊ Emotional lability
  - ◊ Impaired problem solving
  - ◊ Depression
  - ◊ Hypotonia
  - ◊ Abnormal eye movements
  - ◊ Facial twitching
  - ◊ Bradykinesia
  - ◊ Impulsiveness
  - ◊ Hostility
  - ◊ Agitation
  - ◊ Impaired odor recognition and discriminability
- Late
  - ◊ Chorea
  - ◊ Dysphagia
  - ◊ Dysarthria
  - ◊ Bladder and bowel incontinence
  - ◊ Gait disturbance
  - ◊ Postural instability
  - ◊ Hyperkinesia
  - ◊ Dementia
  - ◊ Rigidity
  - ◊ Hypertonia
  - ◊ Clonus
  - ◊ Primitive reflexes
- Variable
  - ◊ Weight loss
  - ◊ Aggressiveness, including sexual
  - ◊ Mania
  - ◊ Hallucinations
  - ◊ Paranoia

CAUSES HD is associated with a cytosine-adenine-guanine (CAG) trinucleotide repeat expansion in a large gene on the short arm of chromosome 4. The gene encodes the protein Huntingtin, which selectively accumulates in clumps within brain cells. These cells appear sensitive to damage by the aggregated, toxic levels of huntingtin.

RISK FACTORS Family history is a definite risk factor. Although a small percent of patients with DNA-proven Huntington disease will have a negative family history.

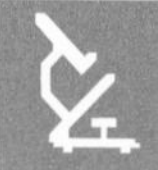

DIAGNOSIS

DIFFERENTIAL DIAGNOSIS

- Movement disorder - hereditary
  - ◊ Huntington disease
  - ◊ Hereditary nonprogressive chorea
  - ◊ Neuroacanthocytosis
  - ◊ Wilson disease
  - ◊ Ataxia-telangiectasia
  - ◊ Lesch-Nyhan syndrome
  - ◊ Hallervorden-Spatz disease
  - ◊ Fahr disease
- Movement disorder - secondary
  - ◊ Infections/immunologic
    - Sydenham chorea
    - Encephalitis
    - Systemic lupus erythematosus
    - Tertiary syphilis
  - ◊ Drug induced
    - Levodopa
    - Anticonvulsants
    - Anticholinergics
    - Cimetidine
    - Isoniazid
  - ◊ Metabolic and endocrine
    - Chorea gravidarum
    - Hyperthyroidism
    - Birth control pills
    - Hyperglycemic nonketotic encephalopathy
  - ◊ Vascular
    - Hemichorea/hemiballism with subthalamic nucleus lesion
    - Periarteritis nodosa
- Movement disorder - unknown etiology
  - ◊ Senile chorea
  - ◊ Essential chorea
  - ◊ Parkinson disease
- Dementia
  - ◊ Alzheimer disease
  - ◊ Creutzfeldt-Jakob
  - ◊ Pick disease
- Emotional and perceptual disorders
  - ◊ Bipolar disorder
  - ◊ Schizophrenia
- Abnormal behavior
  - ◊ Alcoholism
  - ◊ Antisocial personality disorder

LABORATORY

- Decreased endogenous gamma-aminobutyric acid (GABA)
- Decreased glutamic acid decarboxylase
- Decreased choline-acetyltransferase

Drugs that may alter lab results: N/A

Disorders that may alter lab results: N/A

PATHOLOGICAL FINDINGS

- Gross - cerebral atrophy
- Gross - atrophic caudate nucleus
- Gross - atrophic putamen
- Gross - ventricular enlargement
- Gross - atrophic globus pallidus
- Gross - atrophic frontal lobes
- Gross - atrophic parietal lobes
- Gross - cortical atrophy
- Micro - loss of small neurons of striatum with fibrillary gliosis
- Micro - loss of small neurons with fibrillary gliosis in ventrolateral thalamic nucleus
- Micro - loss of small neurons with fibrillary gliosis in substantia nigra
- Electron microscopy - membranous whorls
- Electron microscopy - increased numbers of dense synaptic vesicles in presynaptic nerve terminals

SPECIAL TESTS Presymptomatic detection of the disease via genetic linkage analysis is possible; but widespread testing awaits the resolution of social and ethical considerations

IMAGING

- CT or MRI - cerebral atrophy and atrophy of basal ganglia
- Positron emission tomography (PET) - reduced glucose utilization, lowered dopamine receptor binding
- Head CT - enlarged lateral ventricle

DIAGNOSTIC PROCEDURES Neuropsychological testing measures may capture early striatal neuron loss by demonstrating impairment 2 years before development of motor disease

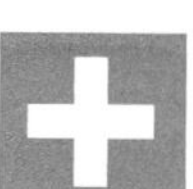

TREATMENT

APPROPRIATE HEALTH CARE

- Outpatient
- About 7% to 8% of HD patients are in nursing homes. Women outnumber men, with the most robust predictor of placement being advanced motor impairment (marked chorea, bradykinesia, impaired gait and balance).

GENERAL MEASURES

- Genetic counseling
- Symptomatic treatment (dopamine receptor blocking drugs), such as phenothiazines or haloperidol
- Consider electroconvulsive therapy (ECT) for drug-resistant depression
- Speech and occupational therapy

SURGICAL MEASURES N/A

ACTIVITY Full activity as long as possible

DIET No special diet, but soft diet with liquid supplements may be needed. Coenzyme Q10 (Ubiquinone), a popular vitamin supplement, shows promise in reversing the generalized energy defect in HD.

PATIENT EDUCATION

- Counseling for offspring
- Newsletter and printed information available from: Huntington Disease Society of America, 140 W. 22nd St, 6th Floor, New York, NY 10011-2420, phone (212)242-1968; fax (212)243-2443; www.hdsa.org
- www.stanford.edu/group/hopes

MEDICATIONS

DRUG(S) OF CHOICE
- For dyskinesia and/or behavioral problems: Haloperidol (Haldol) 1 mg bid and increased every 3 or 4 days until satisfactory response. Suggested daily maximum 10 mg.
- For choreoathetosis: clonazepam (Klonopin), start at 0.5 mg q hs, increasing over several months to 9 mg maximum in a divided daily dose; reserpine, start at 0.1 mg/day, increase at 7-10 day intervals to 3 mg/day maximum; tetrabenazine, start at 12.5 mg/day, increase by 12.5 mg every 7 days to 25 mg qid maximum
- For rigidity: baclofen (Lioresal), start at 10 mg/day, increase slowly to 120 mg maximum in a divided dose. May combine with clonazepam.
- For depression: fluoxetine (Prozac), start at 10 mg/day, increase by 10 mg increments to 60 mg/day maximum

Contraindications: Refer to manufacturer's literature

Precautions: Extrapyramidal reactions, tardive dyskinesia may occur. Can be treated with anticholinergic medication.

Significant possible interactions: Do not administer haloperidol with meperidine due to possibility of serotonin syndrome.

ALTERNATIVE DRUGS
- Presynaptic dopamine-depleting agents
- Postsynaptic dopamine antagonists
- Tricyclic antidepressants
- Antipsychotics

FOLLOWUP

PATIENT MONITORING
Periodically for behavioral changes

PREVENTION/AVOIDANCE
- Genetic counseling
- Smoking cessation in late (choreiform) stage

POSSIBLE COMPLICATIONS
- Choking
- Subdural hematoma
- Personality changes
- Suicide

EXPECTED COURSE/PROGNOSIS
Poor, progressive impairment, fatal outcome within 20 years, usually from pneumonia

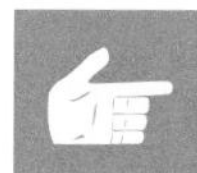

MISCELLANEOUS

ASSOCIATED CONDITIONS
- A lower incidence of cancer among patients with Huntington disease seems to be related to intrinsic biologic factors
- An autosomal dominant disorder arising from a different CAG expansion mutation, termed "Huntington disease-like 2", has clinical and MRI features indistinguishable from HD. Further genetic investigation may yield insight into the pathogenesis of HD.

AGE-RELATED FACTORS
Pediatric: Juvenile form, defined by onset before age 21, occurs in 7% of HD cases. Characteristics are: 1) transmission from an HD affected father, 2) large numbers of CAG repeats, 3) more severe neuropathological involvement, including rigidity and seizures.

Geriatric: Usually fatal before geriatric age group; but onset is after age 50 in 20%

Others: About 20% of relatives at 1-in-2 risk of inheriting Huntington disease from an affected parent now accept the offer of presymptomatic testing

PREGNANCY
N/A

SYNONYMS
- Chronic progressive hereditary chorea
- Huntington chorea

ICD-9-CM
333.4 Huntington disease

SEE ALSO
Wilson disease

OTHER NOTES
- Experiments using a mouse model of HD suggest that intracerebroventricular administration of a caspase inhibitor delays disease progression and activity. The caspases are a family of proteases, active in the brains of mice and humans with HD, which regulate apoptosis.
- Medical historians may be interested in the following article: Innes Am, Chudley AE. Genetic landmarks through philately: Woodrow Wilson 'Woody' Guthrie and Huntington disease. Clin Genet 2002;61:263-267

ABBREVIATIONS
N/A

REFERENCES

- Victor M, Ropper AH. Adams & Victor's Prinicples of Neurology. 7th ed. New York: McGraw-Hill Publishing Co; 2000
- Wusthoff C. The dilemma of confidentiality in Huntington disease. JAMA 2003;290:1219-20
- Wleelock VL, Tempkin T, Marder K, Nance M, et al. Predictors of nursing home placement in Huntington disease. Neurology 2003;60(6):998-1001
- Bonelli RM, Wenning GK, Kapfhammer HP. Huntington's disease: present treatments and future therapeutic modalities. Int Clin Psychopharmacol 2004 Mar;19(2):51-62
- Gilroy J. Basic Neurology. 3rd ed. New York: McGraw-Hill; 2000
- Higgins DS. Chorea and its disorders. Neurologic Clinics 2001;19(3):707-22
- Paulson JS, Zhao H, Stout JC, Brinkman RR, et al. Clinical markers of early disease in persons near onset of Huntington's disease. Neurology 2001;57(4):658-662
- Nance MA, Myers RH. Juvenile onset Huntington's disease-clinical and research perspectives. Ment Retard Dev Disabil Res Rev 2001;7(3):153-7

Web references: 3 available at www.5mcc.com

Illustrations N/A

Author(s):
Richard Viken, MD

BASICS

DESCRIPTION Hydrocele is a collection of fluid within the scrotum.
- Communicating hydrocele: Associated with a patent processus vaginalis, has associated indirect inguinal hernia
- Non-communicating hydrocele: Infantile type - no communication, frequent spontaneous resolution. Adult type - no communication, infrequent resolution.
- Hydrocele of the cord: Distal portion of processus vaginalis has closed, mid-portion patent and fluid filled, proximal portion may be open or closed
- Acute hydrocele: Acute fluid collection resulting from an acute process within the tunica vaginalis

System(s) affected: Reproductive
Genetics: Unknown
Incidence/Prevalence in USA: Estimated to be 1% of adult males; prevalence 1000/100,000
Predominant age: Childhood
Predominant sex: Male only

SIGNS & SYMPTOMS
- Swelling in scrotum or inguinal canal
- Demonstrated fluctuation in size (communicating hydrocele)
- Usually not painful
- Sensation of heaviness in scrotum
- Pain radiating to back (occasionally)
- Fluid collection in scrotum that transilluminates

CAUSES
- Closure of processus vaginalis trapping peritoneal fluid (non-communicating)
- Closure of distal processus, trapping fluid in mid portion of processus vaginalis (hydrocele of cord)
- Failure of closure of processus vaginalis (communicating hydrocele)
- Infection
- Tumors
- Trauma
- Ipsilateral renal transplantation

RISK FACTORS
- Ventriculoperitoneal shunt
- Exstrophy of the bladder
- Ehlers-Danlos syndrome
- Peritoneal dialysis

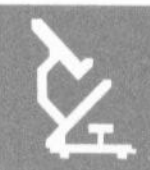

DIAGNOSIS

DIFFERENTIAL DIAGNOSIS
- Indirect inguinal hernia
- Orchitis
- Epididymitis
- Traumatic injury to testicle
- Torsion of testicle or torsion of appendix testes

LABORATORY N/A

Drugs that may alter lab results: N/A

Disorders that may alter lab results: N/A

PATHOLOGICAL FINDINGS Patent processus vaginalis in communicating hydroceles

SPECIAL TESTS N/A

IMAGING
- Abdominal x-ray - may be useful to distinguish incarcerated hernias from hydrocele (rarely needed)
- Inguinoscrotal ultrasound - should be able to demonstrate presence of bowel, e.g., distinguish incarcerated hernia in child from a hydrocele of the cord
- Testicular nuclear scan or doppler ultrasound - to distinguish testicular torsion

DIAGNOSTIC PROCEDURES N/A

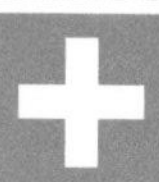

TREATMENT

APPROPRIATE HEALTH CARE
- Outpatient surgery
- Observation in early infancy until definite communication demonstrated or until 1-2 years of age

GENERAL MEASURES N/A

SURGICAL MEASURES
- Inguinal approach with ligation of processus vaginalis and drainage of hydrocele sac in children. (In hydrocele of cord, sac can be completely removed.)
- Scrotal approach with drainage of hydrocele and resection of tunica vaginalis in adults
- In adults no therapy is needed unless hydrocele causes discomfort or unless there is a significant underlying cause such as tumor
- Jaboulay-Winkelmann procedure (for thick hydrocele sac) - hydrocele sac wrapped posteriorly around cord structures
- Lord procedure (for thin hydrocele sac) - radial sutures used to gather hydrocele sac posterior to testis and epididymis
- Aspiration of hydrocele should not be done (with possible exception of postoperative hydrocele)

ACTIVITY Full activity after surgery

DIET For age

PATIENT EDUCATION N/A

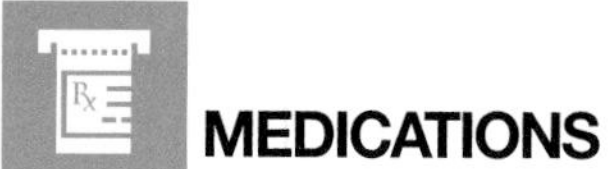

MEDICATIONS

DRUG(S) OF CHOICE N/A
Contraindications: N/A
Precautions: N/A
Significant possible interactions: N/A

ALTERNATIVE DRUGS N/A

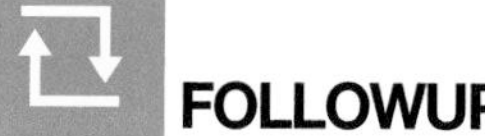

FOLLOWUP

PATIENT MONITORING
- Follow at 3 month intervals until decision for/against surgery made
- Postoperative, follow up at 2-4 weeks and then at 2-3 month intervals until resolution of any postoperative (traumatic) hydrocele

PREVENTION/AVOIDANCE N/A

POSSIBLE COMPLICATIONS
- Postoperative traumatic hydrocele common. Usually resolves spontaneously.
- Injury to vas deferens or spermatic vessels
- Suture granuloma
- Hematoma
- Wound infection

EXPECTED COURSE/PROGNOSIS
Recovery should be rapid and complete

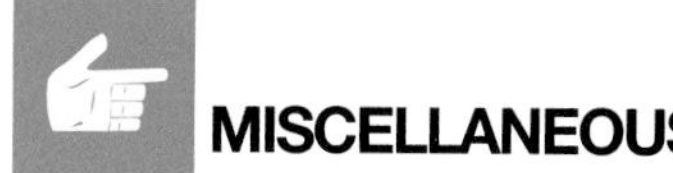

MISCELLANEOUS

ASSOCIATED CONDITIONS
- Ehlers-Danlos syndrome
- Exstrophy of bladder
- Indirect inguinal hernia
- Hydrocephalus with ventriculoperitoneal shunt
- Peritoneal dialysis

AGE-RELATED FACTORS
Pediatric: In communicating hydrocele consider contralateral inguinal exploration
Geriatric: N/A
Others: N/A

PREGNANCY N/A

SYNONYMS N/A

ICD-9-CM
603.9 Hydrocele, unspecified

SEE ALSO
Hernias, external

OTHER NOTES N/A

ABBREVIATIONS N/A

REFERENCES

- Gillenwater JY, Grayhack JT, Howards SS, Duckett J. Adult & Pediatric Urology. 2nd Ed. Philadelphia, Marby Year Book, 1991
- Ashcraft KW, Murphy JP, Sharp RJ, eds. Pediatric Surgery. 3rd Ed. Philadelphia, W.B. Saunders Co., 2000
- Kelalis PP, King LR, Belman AB. Pediatric Urology. 3rd Ed. Philadelphia, W.B. Saunders Co., 1992
- Resnick MI, Kursh ED. Current Therapy in GenitoUrinary Surgery. 2nd Ed. St. Louis, Mosby-Year Book, 1992

Web references: 1 available at www.5mcc.com
Illustrations N/A

Author(s):
Timothy L. Black, MD
James P. Miller, MD

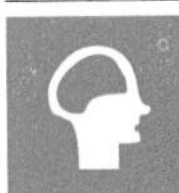

BASICS

DESCRIPTION

Unilateral or bilateral dilatation of the renal pelvis and calyces secondary to intrinsic and/or extrinsic obstruction to urine flow. May also be functional.

System(s) affected: Renal/Urologic

Genetics: Unknown

Incidence/Prevalence in USA:
- Children 2 in 100
- Adults 3.8 in 100

Predominant age: All ages. Bimodal peaks: congenital and over age 60.

Predominant sex:
- Age 0 - 20 years: Male = Female
- Age 20 to 60 years: Female > Male
- Age greater than 60 years: Male > Female

SIGNS & SYMPTOMS
- Varies with acute or chronic presentation
- Chronic may be completely asymptomatic
- "Colic" referred to vulva or to testicle (lithiasis) with acute obstruction
- Change in urine output (anuria, polyuria, intermittent variation in urine volume)
- Hesitancy, frequency, urgency
- Dribbling
- Urinary tract infections
- Decreased force of urine or interrupted stream
- Nocturia
- Abdominal mass
- Thirst
- Hypertension (may be accelerated)
- Edema
- After relief - post obstructive diuresis
- Epididymitis
- Acute or chronic urinary retention

CAUSES
- Intrinsic, congenital
  - ◊ Stenosis (ureteral, urethral and meatal)
  - ◊ Adynamic ureter
  - ◊ Spinal cord defects, e.g., spina bifida
  - ◊ Bladder neck obstruction
  - ◊ Duplication of the ureter
  - ◊ Ureterocele
- Intrinsic, acquired
  - ◊ Prostate hyperplasia, carcinoma
  - ◊ Renal lithiasis (most common)
  - ◊ Neoplasm (renal, ureteral or bladder)
  - ◊ Papillary necrosis with sloughed papilla
  - ◊ Ureterocele
  - ◊ Trauma
  - ◊ Blood clot
  - ◊ Fungus ball
  - ◊ Granuloma (tuberculosis)
  - ◊ Neurogenic bladder
  - ◊ Other nervous system diseases - tabes dorsalis, multiple sclerosis, diabetic neuropathy, traumatic spinal cord injury
  - ◊ Anticholinergics
  - ◊ Phimosis, ureteral valve, polyp or stricture
  - ◊ Schistosomiasis (hematobium)
  - ◊ Wegener granulomatosis
  - ◊ Psychogenic polydipsia
  - ◊ Imperforate hymen
- Extrinsic
  - ◊ Retroperitoneal-neoplasm, blood, abscess, fibrosis, aneurysm
  - ◊ Crohn disease
  - ◊ Lymphocele, hydrocele
  - ◊ Fecaloma
  - ◊ Gynecologic - gravid uterus, endometriosis, pelvic inflammatory disease, abscess, cyst, gynecologic malignancy, uterine prolapse, uterine leiomyomata
  - ◊ Sjögren syndrome (pseudolymphoma)
- Functional or non-mechanical - congenital
  - ◊ Mega-ureter
  - ◊ Prune belly syndrome
  - ◊ Extra-renal pelvis
- Functional or non-mechanical - other
  - ◊ Accidental surgical ligation
  - ◊ Diabetes insipidus
  - ◊ Diuretics
  - ◊ Vesicoureteral reflux
  - ◊ Postobstructive residual
  - ◊ Postsurgical: post ureteral anastomosis, adhesions
  - ◊ Progestational agents

RISK FACTORS
- Any of the disorders listed in causes
- Radiation
- Prostatic hypertrophy and/or malignancy
- Renal lithiasis
- Methysergide
- Analgesic abuse (papillary necrosis, transitional cell carcinoma)
- Sickle cell anemia (papillary necrosis)
- Diabetes mellitus (papillary necrosis)
- Bleeding diathesis
- Anticholinergics

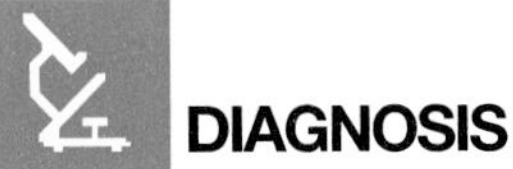

DIAGNOSIS

DIFFERENTIAL DIAGNOSIS See Causes

LABORATORY
- May be normal
- Azotemia
- Hyperkalemia
- Metabolic acidosis (with and without anion gap)
- Hypernatremia (nephrogenic diabetes insipidus)
- Urine analysis - hematuria, crystals, bacteriuria
- Decreased urine concentrating ability
- Polycythemia (rare)
- Anemia of chronic renal disease

Drugs that may alter lab results: Nephrotoxins may aggravate azotemia (non-steroidal anti-inflammatory drugs, immunosuppressants, aminoglycosides, iodinated contrast, anticholinergics)

Disorders that may alter lab results: N/A

PATHOLOGICAL FINDINGS
- Thin renal cortex
- Renal tubular atrophy
- Medullary destruction

SPECIAL TESTS
- Voiding cystourethrogram
- Post void residual
- Ultrasound prostate with biopsy if nodule found
- Prostatic specific antigen (malignancy); controversial - yes (American Cancer Society), no (National Cancer Institute)
- Prenatal sonography
- Rectal examination in males age > 50

IMAGING
- Kidney ureter bladder (KUB) plain film
- Unenhanced helical CT for lithiasis
- Ultrasound - abnormal renal function, cortical thinning, ureteral dilatation
- IVP with tomograms (normal renal function): Renal pelvis dilatation
- Renal flow scan, diuretic renogram
- CT scan; MRI
- Pulsed and color Doppler
- Diuretic enhanced duplex Doppler sonography

DIAGNOSTIC PROCEDURES
- To determine location and etiology:
  - ◊ Cystoscopy/retrograde pyelography
  - ◊ Antegrade pyelography
  - ◊ Loopography (obstruction with ureteral diversion)

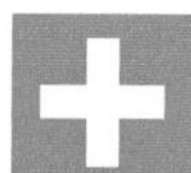

TREATMENT

APPROPRIATE HEALTH CARE Outpatient

GENERAL MEASURES
- Females: Pelvic exam and pap smear for potential gynecologic malignancy. Appropriate work-up for recurrent urinary tract infections.
- Males: Anatomic study of the urinary tract for any urinary tract infection, appropriate review of systems and digital rectal exam for prostatic hypertrophy. Prostatic specific antigen, acid phosphatase, rectal transducer ultrasound of prostate for enlargement.
- Relief of obstruction
  - ◊ Foley catheter for prostatic hypertrophy
  - ◊ Transurethral resection of the prostate gland for prostatic hypertrophy
  - ◊ Nephrostomy tube
  - ◊ Pyeloplasty
  - ◊ Surgical diversion of ureters
  - ◊ Ureteral stents
  - ◊ Urolithiasis - extra corporeal shock wave lithotripsy, percutaneous nephrolithotomy, ureteroscopic stone removal or surgical removal. Treatment depends on stone size.
  - ◊ Nephrectomy
- Neurogenic hydronephrosis
  - ◊ Frequent voiding
  - ◊ Double voiding
  - ◊ Suprapubic pressure
  - ◊ Intermittent catheterization
  - ◊ Cholinergics
  - ◊ Surgical reimplantation of ureters
  - ◊ Antibiotics, when needed for infection
- Uremia
  - ◊ Dialysis
  - ◊ Treat hyperkalemia
  - ◊ Treat acidosis (1-2 teaspoons sodium bicarbonate tid or Shohl's solution)
  - ◊ Treat hypocalcemia (calcium acetate, vitamin D - dihydrotachysterol

SURGICAL MEASURES N/A

ACTIVITY As tolerated

DIET
- If not uremic, no restriction
- When uremic - protein, salt, potassium restriction as needed
- For stone-formers, increased oral fluids

PATIENT EDUCATION
Printed material available from National Kidney Foundation, 30 East 33rd, St., Ste. 1100, New York, New York, 10016 (800)622-9010. "What Everyone Should Know About Kidneys and Kidney Disease" (Order #01-01 BP English, #01-02 BP Spanish); also Urinary Tract Obstructions. How they Can Affect You.

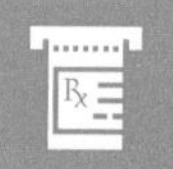

MEDICATIONS

DRUG(S) OF CHOICE
- Lithiasis - treatment is stone-specific:
  - ◊ Hypercalciuric calcium oxalate - hydrochlorothiazide 25-50 mg po every day to decrease urine calcium excretion
  - ◊ Uric acid - acutely alkalinize urine to pH ≥ 6.5 with sodium bicarbonate, chronic allopurinol 100-300 mg po every day
- Prostatic hypertrophy
  - ◊ Terazosin, doxazosin, tamsulosin, finasteride

Contraindications: Allergy to drug
Precautions: N/A
Significant possible interactions: N/A

ALTERNATIVE DRUGS N/A

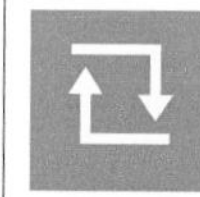

FOLLOWUP

PATIENT MONITORING
- Imaging procedure of choice depending on etiology and anatomic location (IVP, renal scan, cysto-retrogrades, ultrasound)
- Metabolic studies for nephrolithiasis
- Appropriate cancer screening if applicable

PREVENTION/AVOIDANCE
- Avoid anticholinergics when obstruction present
- Avoid dehydration with lithiasis
- Drug therapy appropriate to prevent future calculi

POSSIBLE COMPLICATIONS
- Urinary tract infection from instrumentation
- Fibrosis from radiation for pelvic malignancy
- Obstruction from stone fragments on lithotripsy
- Postoperative bleeding

EXPECTED COURSE/PROGNOSIS
- Contingent on relief of obstruction and residual renal function
- Excellent course and prognosis with relief of obstruction and restoration of normal renal function
- Nonmechanical ureteropelvic junction (UPJ) obstruction has a good prognosis
- Reflux with pyelonephritis worsens prognosis significantly
- Poor if obstruction secondary to advanced malignancy

MISCELLANEOUS

ASSOCIATED CONDITIONS See causes

AGE-RELATED FACTORS
Pediatric: Hydronephrosis most often congenital
Geriatric: In males, most often due to prostatic enlargement
Others: N/A

PREGNANCY Frequent temporary cause of hydronephrosis

SYNONYMS
- Urinary tract obstruction
- Obstructive uropathy
- Obstructive nephropathy
- Postrenal insufficiency
- Caliectasis
- Pyelectasis
- Ureterectasis

ICD-9-CM
753.20 Unspecified obstructive defect of renal pelvis and ureter
591 Hydronephrosis

SEE ALSO
Prostatic hyperplasia, benign (BPH)
Renal failure, acute (ARF)
Renal failure, chronic
Sjögren syndrome

OTHER NOTES N/A

ABBREVIATIONS N/A

REFERENCES

- Chen MYM, Zagoria RJ. Can noncontrast helical CT replace IVP for evaluation of patients with acute urinary tract colic? J Emerg Med 1999;17:299-303
- Chevalier RL, Klahr S. Therapeutic approaches in obstructive uropathy. Semin in Nephrol 1998;18:652-8
- Heilburg IP. Update on dietary recommendations and medical treatment of renal stone disease. Nephrol Dial Transplant 2000;15:117-23
- Knobel B, Rosman P, Gewurtz G. Bilateral hydronephrosis due to fecaloma in an elderly woman. J Clin Gastroenterol 2000;30(3):311-3
- Reznicek SB. Common urologic problems in the elderly. Prostate cancer, outlet obstruction and incontinence require special management. Postgrad Med 2000;107:163-4,167-70,177-78

Web references: 3 available at www.5mcc.com
Illustrations N/A

Author(s):
Neal S. Gold, MD

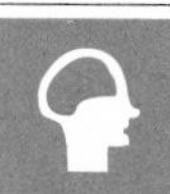

BASICS

DESCRIPTION The most common cause of hypercalcemia diagnosed in a hospital setting is malignancy, often heralding the patient's demise. Because of the extremely poor prognosis, it must be differentiated from other, more treatable, entities.
System(s) affected: Endocrine/Metabolic, Gastrointestinal, Musculoskeletal, Nervous
Genetics: N/A
Incidence/Prevalence in USA: Occurs in 5-10% of cancer patients
Predominant age: N/A
Predominant sex: N/A

SIGNS & SYMPTOMS
- Severity of symptoms depends on calcium level, rapidity of onset of hypercalcemia, state of hydration, and underlying malignancy
- Anorexia, nausea
- Polyuria, dehydration
- Lethargy, stupor, coma

CAUSES
- Solid tumors:
  - ◊ 80% have increased levels of nephrogenous cyclic AMP, reflecting activity of ectopic parathormone-related peptide(s). True ectopic PTH production is exceedingly rare.
  - ◊ PTH-related protein has been found to be a major mediator of hypercalcemia in malignancy, and appears to influence bone metastases, especially in breast cancer
  - ◊ Lung cancer (25% of cases usually squamous, less common are adenocarcinoma and large cell, rarely small cell)
  - ◊ Squamous carcinoma of head, neck, esophagus, female genital tract (20% of cases)
  - ◊ Renal cell carcinoma (8% of cases)
- Myeloma, lymphoma, breast cancer with osseous metastases, and others. Tumors may induce hypercalcemia by one or more of the following mechanisms:
  - ◊ Nephrogenous cyclic AMP is reduced, reflecting suppression of PTH by nonparathyroid hypercalcemia
  - ◊ Factors implicated include interleukin-1, interleukin-6, tumor necrosis factor, macrophage colony stimulating factor, prostaglandin (E series), lymphotoxin, vascular cell adhesion molecule-1, hepatocyte growth factor, and others
  - ◊ Direct resorption of bone by metastatic tumor (controversial)
  - ◊ 1-alpha hydroxylase activity of some lymphomas, causing tumoral production of 1,25-dihydroxyvitamin D

RISK FACTORS
- Dehydration
- Immobilization

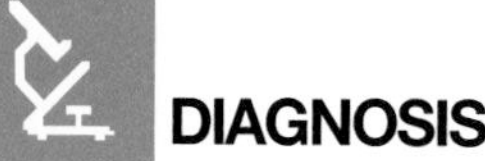

DIAGNOSIS

DIFFERENTIAL DIAGNOSIS
(not including benign familial hypercalcemia)
- Vitamins A and D
- Immobilization
- Thyrotoxicosis
- Addison disease
- Milk-alkali syndrome
- Inflammatory disorders
- Neoplastic-related disorders
- Sarcoidosis, TB, and other granulomatous diseases
- Thiazides, lithium; theophylline and aspirin toxicity
- Rhabdomyolysis
- AIDS
- Paget disease
- Parenteral nutrition
- Hyperparathyroidism

LABORATORY
- Serum calcium: Total calcium level depends on binding proteins. Adjusted calcium can be estimated by:

Ca(adj) = Ca(tot) - 0.8 x (albumin - 4)
- Ionized calcium: Physiologically most important, affected by pH. May be measured directly if specimen is collected under anaerobic conditions and analyzed promptly.
- PTH assay: "Intact" molecule (especially two-site, noncompetitive) methods have greatest specificity, almost always suppressed, in malignancy. If elevated in a cancer patient, suspect concomitant hyperparathyroidism.
- PTH-related peptide: Assays now are clinically available; often elevated in hypercalcemia of malignancy (see above)
- 25-hydroxyvitamin D: May be elevated in vitamin D intoxication
- 1,25-dihydroxyvitamin D: Elevated in up to 50% of hypercalcemic patients with lymphoma

Drugs that may alter lab results:
- Lithium, thiazide diuretics, vitamin D preparations can all increase serum calcium
- Bisphosphonates can lower serum phosphate

Disorders that may alter lab results: N/A

PATHOLOGICAL FINDINGS N/A

SPECIAL TESTS Staging techniques as necessary to determine extent of malignancy

IMAGING If there is laboratory evidence of primary hyperparathyroidism, imaging (such as ultrasound, CT, MRI, or nuclear parathyroid scans) may be required in patients with previous neck surgery, prior to re-exploration

DIAGNOSTIC PROCEDURES N/A

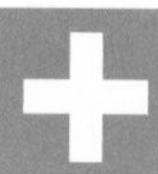

TREATMENT

APPROPRIATE HEALTH CARE Inpatient

GENERAL MEASURES
- Treatment of underlying malignancy
- Maintain hydration, encourage oral fluids; intravenous saline diuresis
- Hemodialysis can be utilized when saline diuresis and medications fail

SURGICAL MEASURES N/A

ACTIVITY Avoid bed rest or immobilization as much as possible

DIET No special diet

PATIENT EDUCATION N/A

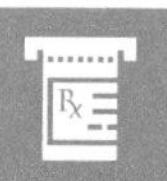

MEDICATIONS

DRUG(S) OF CHOICE

- Volume expansion. IV saline increases urinary calcium excretion. Adjust to maintain urine output of 100-150 mL/hr. Requires close monitoring to avoid over-hydration in critical patients.
- Loop diuretics. Use only after adequate hydration.
- Calcitonin. Decreases osteoclast maturation and inhibits bone resorption. 4-8 IU/kg SC or IM q 8-12 hours. IM route preferred if patient is dehydrated. Nontoxic, acts in 12-24 hours, lowers calcium 1-2 mg/dL. Minor but uncomfortable side effects include nausea, flushing, and cramps. Steroids may antagonize "Escape" phenomenon.
- Bisphosphonates. Analogs of inorganic pyrophosphate adsorb to bone hydroxyapatite and interfere with osteoclast maturation and function.
  - ◊ Zoledronic acid (Zometa). Agent of choice. 4mg IV over 15 minutes. Normalizes serum calcium in 80-90% of patients. Duration of control over 30 days. Nephrotoxic potential, especially in myeloma patients receiving thalidomide. Can be given for many years if needed.
  - ◊ Pamidronate (Aredia). 60 mg IV over 4 hours. Normalizes calcium up to 3 weeks or more. May repeat dose. 70% effective.
- Glucocorticoids: (40-60 mg/day prednisone or equivalent). Most effective in vitamin D intoxication, may be helpful in myeloma, lymphoma and other granulomatous disorders. Usually not effective in solid tumors.
- Gallium nitrate. Inhibits bone resorption by inhibiting ATPase dependent proton pump on osteoclast membrane. Dose is 200 mg IV diluted in 1000 mL 5% dextrose and infused over 24 hours, repeat for 5 days. Nephrotoxic potential.

Contraindications: Refer to manufacturer's literature

Precautions:

- Be aware that hypocalcemia and hypophosphatemia may rarely occur with bisphosphonate therapy
- Check magnesium, creatinine, phosphate and calcium prior to bisphosphonate use
- Exercise caution in patients with renal insufficiency
- Zoledronic acid: increased risk of renal impairment with rapid (<15 min) IV infusions; also use caution in patients with active upper GI symptoms.
- Gallium nitrate: use caution when co-administered with amphotericin B or aminoglycosides.

Significant possible interactions:

- NSAIDs may enhance the nephrotoxicity of some therapies

ALTERNATIVE DRUGS

- Plicamycin (mithramycin). Second-line agent. 25 μg/kg IV over several hours. Onset < 12 hours, peak effect 48-72 hours, duration 3-9 days. Toxicity: nausea, thrombocytopenia, hepatic and renal.
- Etidronate (Didronel) and clodronate are weaker agents with limited use
- Risedronate (Actonel) can be given orally - investigational
- Phosphates. Not first-line drugs.
  - ◊ Oral: 1-2 gm/day neutral phosphates, 4 divided doses. Modest hypocalcemic effect, but significant GI distress.
  - ◊ IV: should be avoided because of calcium-phosphate precipitation in tissues, risk of severe hypotension
- Calcitriol analogs (22-oxacalcitriol) may reduce release of PTH-RP
- Immunization with synthetic PTH peptides may lower serum calcium by inducing blocking antibodies to PTH-RP

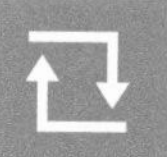

FOLLOWUP

PATIENT MONITORING Frequent serum calcium and electrolyte determinations, expect relapse

PREVENTION/AVOIDANCE Encourage adequate hydration and activity, especially in multiple myeloma

POSSIBLE COMPLICATIONS N/A

EXPECTED COURSE/PROGNOSIS

Median survival after diagnosis of tumoral hypercalcemia depends on the type and extent of the malignancy, but usually indicates a poor prognosis

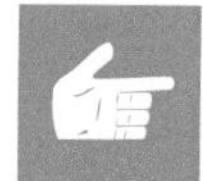

MISCELLANEOUS

ASSOCIATED CONDITIONS N/A

AGE-RELATED FACTORS N/A

Pediatric: N/A
Geriatric: N/A
Others: N/A

PREGNANCY Careful consideration of treatment options during pregnancy

SYNONYMS Tumoral hypercalcemia

ICD-9-CM

275.40 Unspecified disorder of calcium metabolism
275.42 Hypercalcemia

SEE ALSO

Addison disease
HIV infection & AIDS
Hyperparathyroidism
Hyperthyroidism
Milk-alkali syndrome
Rhabdomyolysis
Sarcoidosis
Tuberculosis

OTHER NOTES

- Future approaches to therapy
  - ◊ Calcitriol analogs (22-oxacalcitriol) may reduce release of PTH-RP
  - ◊ Immunization with synthetic PTH peptides may lower serum calcium by inducing blocking antibodies to PTH-RP

ABBREVIATIONS N/A

REFERENCES

- Marcus R, ed. Endocrinology and Metabol Clin of NA 1989;18(3):778-828
- Mundy GR, Guise TA. Hypercalcemia of malignancy. (81 refs) [Review] Amer J of Med 1997;103:134-45
- Deftos LJ. Hypercalcemia in malignant and inflammatory diseases. Endocrinol Metab Clin North Am 2002;31(1):141-58
- Kyle RA. The role of biphosphonates in multiple myeloma. Ann Int Med 2000;132(9):734-6
- Powles T, el al. Randomized, placebo-controlled trial of clodronate in patients with primary operable breast cancer. J of Clin Oncol 2002;20(15):3219-24

Web references: 1 available at www.5mcc.com
Illustrations N/A

Author(s):

James H. Rudick, MD

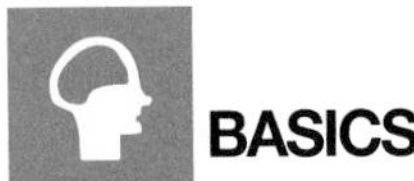

BASICS

DESCRIPTION
- Serum cholesterol > 200 mg/dL (5.18 mmol/L)
- High density lipoprotein fraction of cholesterol (HDL) - protective
- Low density lipoprotein (LDL) - atherogenic

System(s) affected: Cardiovascular, Endocrine/ Metabolic

Genetics: Heterozygous familial. Hypercholesterolemia, 1 in 500 cases. Autosomal dominant hypercholesterolemia 1 in 1 million.

Incidence/Prevalence in USA: 120 million people with cholesterol 200 mg/dL (5.18 mmol/L) or more, 60 million with 240 mg/dL (6.22 mmol/L) or more

Predominant age: Prevalence increases with age

Predominant sex: Male > Female

SIGNS & SYMPTOMS
- Corneal arcus before 50
- Xanthomata
- Xanthelasma
- Arterial bruits
- Claudication
- Angina pectoris
- Stroke
- Myocardial infarction

CAUSES
- Primary
  - ◊ Diet
  - ◊ Heredity
  - ◊ Obesity
  - ◊ Sedentary life-style
- Secondary
  - ◊ Hypothyroidism
  - ◊ Diabetes mellitus
  - ◊ Nephrotic syndrome
  - ◊ Obstructive liver disease
  - ◊ Progestins
  - ◊ Anabolic steroids
  - ◊ Corticosteroids
  - ◊ Diuretics except indapamide (Lozol)
  - ◊ Beta blockers except those with intrinsic sympathomimetic activity (ISA)
  - ◊ Some immunosuppressants

RISK FACTORS
- Obesity
- Heredity
- Physical inactivity

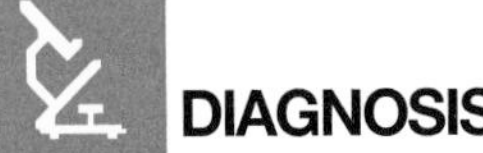

DIAGNOSIS

DIFFERENTIAL DIAGNOSIS N/A

LABORATORY
- Lipoprotein panel; total cholesterol, HDL, LDL, triglycerides must be checked fasting
- Cholesterol is considered elevated if > than 200 mg/dL (5.18 mmol/L)
- TSH initially because hypothyroidism may cause hypercholesterolemia

Drugs that may alter lab results: Caffeine may increase cholesterol

Disorders that may alter lab results:
- Hypothyroidism
- Nephrotic syndrome
- Obstructive liver disease

PATHOLOGICAL FINDINGS N/A

SPECIAL TESTS N/A

IMAGING N/A

DIAGNOSTIC PROCEDURES N/A

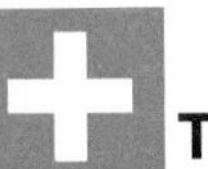

TREATMENT

APPROPRIATE HEALTH CARE
Outpatient, except for complicating emergencies, e.g., myocardial infarction

GENERAL MEASURES
- Requires intervention: HDL less than 40 mg/dL (0.78 mmol/L), LDL greater than 160 mg/dL (4.14 mmol/L), coronary heart disease (CHD) or CHD risk equivalent
- Treatment depends on LDH, HDL, and triglyceride levels as modified by the number of following risk factors:
  - ◊ Smoking
  - ◊ Male over 45
  - ◊ Female over 55
  - ◊ HDL less than 40
  - ◊ Hypertension
  - ◊ MI or stroke in first degree relative (male under 55 and female under 65)
- CHD risk equivalent = diabetes mellitus; carotid, aortic or peripheral vascular disease; or a risk for major coronary events ≥ 20% per 10 years per the Framingham point scale derived from the above risk factors

SURGICAL MEASURES N/A

ACTIVITY
Walking or other sustained cardiovascular exercise for 2.5 hours per week or more. Important for increasing HDL, lowering total cholesterol, and losing weight.

DIET
- Reduce all dietary fats to approximately 30% of total calories. Olive oil should be preferentially used.
- Increase fiber, increase intake of fruits, vegetables, whole grains, and garlic
- Emphasize, vegetarian, meatless, eggless, cheese-less meals, with poultry, fish, and nonfat milk or yogurt
- Minimal daily alcohol use may increase HDL
- Dietary adherence to low fat and cholesterol generally may be expected to result in a 10% LDL reduction
- Intake of too many carbohydrates with a high glycemic index, eg, bread rice, pasta, potatoes, may make weight loss and cholesterol reduction more difficult

PATIENT EDUCATION
American Heart Association publications

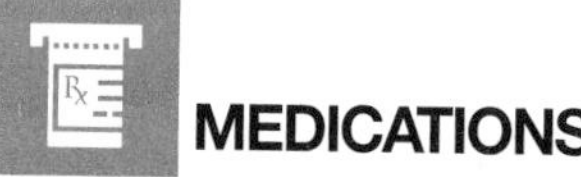

MEDICATIONS

DRUG(S) OF CHOICE

- Indications for initiating medications:
  - ◊ No coronary heart disease (CHD) and fewer than 2 risk factors: if after 3 months of diet, exercise, LDL ≥ 190
  - ◊ No CHD, but 2 or more risk factors: if after 3 months diet, exercise, LDL ≥ 160
  - ◊ CHD or CHD risk equivalents if after 6-12 week diet, exercise, LDL ≥ 100
- HMG-CoA reductase inhibitors (statins):
  - ◊ Fluvastatin (Lescol), lovastatin (Mevacor), or pravastatin (Pravachol), 20-80 mg per day. Effects: 20-40% LDL decrease, increase HDL and lower triglycerides.
  - ◊ Simvastatin (Zocor) 10-80 mg may decrease LDL 50%, increase HDL, and lower triglycerides
  - ◊ Atorvastatin (Lipitor)10-80 mg may be taken any time of day, may decrease LDL 60% and lowers triglycerides
  - ◊ Rosuvastatin (Crestor) 10-40mg may decrease LDL 60%, lower triglycerides and increases HDL

Contraindications:

- Cholestyramine - complete biliary obstruction, triglycerides > 200
- Nicotinic acid - hepatic dysfunction, acute peptic ulcer, diabetes mellitus, hyperuricemia
- HMG-CoA reductase inhibitors - active liver disease, pregnancy

Precautions:

- HMG-CoA reductase inhibitors - liver function tests 6-12 weeks after initiation of therapy, then every 6 months for one year, then periodically. Myositis with markedly elevated creatine kinase (CK) may occur.
- Cholestyramine - gradually increase dose on weekly basis to minimize GI side effects (particularly constipation, flatulence)

Significant possible interactions:

- Cholestyramine - other drugs taken less than one hour before or within six hours after may be bound and not absorbed as well. Fat soluble vitamins A, D, E and K absorption may be impeded.
- Nicotinic acid and HMG-CoA reductase inhibitors - concomitant gemfibrozil, niacin, or immunosuppressives increase possibility of myositis

ALTERNATIVE DRUGS

- Cholestyramine (Questran) or colestipol (Colestid) bile acid binding resins. One to six packets per day taken qd, bid, or tid or colesevelam (Welchol) 6 tablets daily. Effect: 15-30% fall in LDL.
- Niacin (nicotinic acid): 500 mg to 3 gm taken one to three times daily with meals in timed release formulation to minimize side effects, or Niaspan at bedtime. Effect: 15-30% LDL lowering, decreases triglycerides. Hepatic dysfunction more common in patients who take sustained release niacin than in those who take immediate release form. Best to start with low doses and increase as tolerated.
- Ezetimibe (Zetia) - selectively inhibits intestinal absorption of cholesterol and related phytosterols. 10 mg/day. Effect: 18-25% LDL lowering either when used primarily or added to a statin.

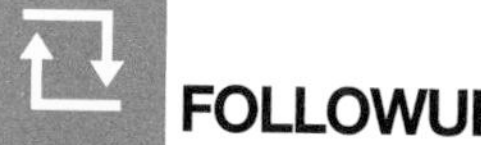

FOLLOWUP

PATIENT MONITORING

- While on medication, monitor cholesterol, HDL, LDL, triglycerides, liver enzymes (on statins, niacin) every 6-12 weeks until goal LDL reached, then every 6-12 months
- All adults 20 and over - lipoprotein panel every 5 years

PREVENTION/AVOIDANCE Prudent diet, frequent exercise and weight control for all

POSSIBLE COMPLICATIONS Coronary heart disease, cerebrovascular disease, generalized arteriosclerosis

EXPECTED COURSE/PROGNOSIS

- 1% decrease in cholesterol results in 2% decreased risk of CHD
- Goals:
  - ◊ LDL < 160 if 0-1 risk factors
  - ◊ LDL < 130 if 2 or more risk factors
  - ◊ LDL < 80 if CHD or CHD risk equivalent
  - ◊ Risk factors
    - Smoking
    - Male over 45
    - Female over 55
    - HDL less than 40
    - Hypertension
    - MI or stroke in first degree relative under (male under 55 and female under 65)

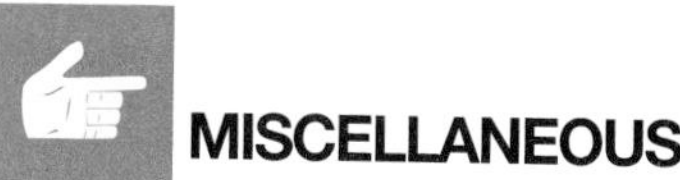

MISCELLANEOUS

ASSOCIATED CONDITIONS

- Hypertension
- Obesity
- Diabetes mellitus
- Hypothyroidism
- Coronary artery disease
- Cerebrovascular disease
- Peripheral vascular disease

AGE-RELATED FACTORS

Pediatric:

- Screening every five years beginning as early as 12. (Childhood screening is controversial because no studies have shown a clear link between hypercholesterolemia in childhood and hypercholesterolemia in adulthood. Furthermore, the risks of reducing cholesterol in childhood are not known.)
- If total cholesterol greater than 170 mg/dL (4.40 mmol/L), check HDL and LDL levels. If LDL is 110-125 mg/dL (2.85-3.24 mmol/L) = moderate risk, if LDL is greater than 125 mg/dL (3.24 mmol/L) = high risk.

Geriatric: The benefit of cholesterol reduction in preventing coronary disease persists in the elderly, though very low cholesterol readings are associated with higher mortality in the elderly without coronary artery disease

Others: N/A

PREGNANCY Fetal nutritional demands may alter diet and drug treatment; statins contraindicated

SYNONYMS N/A

ICD-9-CM

272.0 Pure hypercholesterolemia

SEE ALSO

Hypothyroidism, adult

OTHER NOTES N/A

ABBREVIATIONS N/A

REFERENCES

- Kwiterovich PO Jr. State-of-the-art update and review: clinical trials of lipid-lowering agents. Am J Cardiol 1998;82(12A):3U-17U
- Havel RJ, Rapaport E. Management of primary hyperlipidemia. New Engl J Med 1995;332(22):1491-98
- Shepherd J. Prevention of CHD with pravastatin in men with hypercholesterolemia, NEJM 1995;220:1302-07
- Scandinavian simvastatin study group. Randomized trial of cholesterol lowering in 4,444 patients with CHD. Lancet 1994;344:1383-89
- Brown WV. Epidemiology and treatment of hypercholesteremia; where we are today. Am J of Med 1997;102(2A)
- Hebert P, Henneker C, et al. Cholesterol lowering with statin drugs. Risk of stroke, and total mortality. JAMA 1997;278:313-21
- Amsterdam, Ezra, et al. Managing dyslipidemia. Supplement to Patient Care. 1999:2-28
- Downs JR, et al. Results of AFCAPS, TexCAPS. JAMA 1998;29:1615-1622
- Medical Letter. Choice of lipid lowering drugs. 1998;40:12-18
- Executive Summary of The Third Report of The National Cholesterol Education Program (NCEP) Expert Panel on Detection, Evaluation, And Treatment of High Blood Cholesterol In Adults (Adult Treatment Panel III). JAMA 2001;285(19):2486-97
- Heart Protection Study Collaborative Group. MRC/BHF Heart Protection Study of cholesterol lowering with simvastatin in 20,536 high-risk individuals: a randomised placebo-controlled trial. Lancet 2002;360(9326):7-22
- Cannon CP, Braunwald E, McCabe CH, et al. Comparison of intensive and moderate lipid lowering with statins after acute coronary syndromes. NEJM 2004; 350:1495-1504

Web references: 0 available at www.5mcc.com
Illustrations 5 available

Author(s):

John Z. Carter, MD

Hyperemesis gravidarum

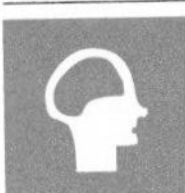

BASICS

DESCRIPTION Persistent vomiting in a pregnant woman that interferes with fluid and electrolyte balance, as well as nutrition. Usually associated with the first 8 to 20 weeks of pregnancy. Believed to have biomedical and behavioral aspects. Associated with high estrogen levels. Symptoms usually begin about 2 weeks after first missed period.

System(s) affected: Endocrine/Metabolic, Gastrointestinal, Reproductive

Genetics: Unknown

Incidence/Prevalence in USA:
- 2% of pregnancies have electrolyte disturbances
- 50% of pregnancies have at least some gastrointestinal disturbance

Predominant age: 21-31

Predominant sex: Female only

SIGNS & SYMPTOMS
- Hypersensitivity to smell
- Alteration in taste
- Nausea
- Vomiting with retching
- Acidosis
- Decreased urine output
- Volume depletion
- Fatigue
- Starvation

CAUSES
- Unknown
- May be psychological factors
- Hyperthyroidism
- Hyperparathyroidism
- Gestational hormones
- Liver dysfunction
- Autonomic nervous system dysfunction

RISK FACTORS
- Trophoblastic activity
- Gonadotropin production stimulated
- Altered gastrointestinal function
- Various odors
- Taste or sight of food
- Hyperthyroidism
- Hyperparathyroidism
- Obesity
- Multiple gestations
- Nulliparity
- Liver dysfunction

DIAGNOSIS

DIFFERENTIAL DIAGNOSIS
- Other common causes of vomiting must be considered:
  - ◊ Gastroenteritis
  - ◊ Gastritis
  - ◊ Reflux esophagitis
  - ◊ Peptic ulcer disease
  - ◊ Cholelithiasis
  - ◊ Cholecystitis
  - ◊ Pyelonephritis
  - ◊ Anxiety

LABORATORY
- Electrolytes decreased
- Urinalysis - glucosuria, albuminuria, granular casts and hematuria (rare)
- Increased uric acid
- Reduced protein

Drugs that may alter lab results: None likely

Disorders that may alter lab results: N/A

PATHOLOGICAL FINDINGS Fatty degeneration of the liver; renal tubular damage; heart damage; petechial brain hemorrhages

SPECIAL TESTS None indicated for the diagnosis of hyperemesis gravidarum

IMAGING No imaging is indicated for the diagnosis of hyperemesis gravidarum

DIAGNOSTIC PROCEDURES Only indicated if it is necessary to rule out other diagnoses

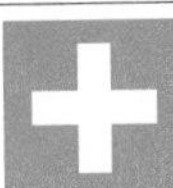

TREATMENT

APPROPRIATE HEALTH CARE
- Outpatient therapy
- In some severe cases, inpatient parenteral or enteral volume and nutrition repletion may be indicated

GENERAL MEASURES
- Patient reassurance
- Bedrest
- If dehydrated, IV fluids. Repeat if there is a recurrence of symptoms following initial improvement.

SURGICAL MEASURES N/A

ACTIVITY As tolerated after improvement

DIET
- Nothing by mouth for first 24 hours if patient is ill enough to require hospitalization
- For outpatient: A diet rich in carbohydrates and protein, such as fruit, cheese, cottage cheese, eggs, beef, poultry, vegetables, toast, crackers, rice. Limit intake of butter. Patients should avoid spicy meals and high fat foods.

PATIENT EDUCATION
- Attention should be given to psychosocial issues such as possible ambivalence about the pregnancy
- Patients should be instructed to take small amounts of fluid frequently to avoid volume depletion

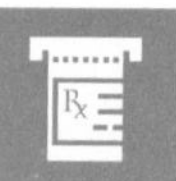

MEDICATIONS

DRUG(S) OF CHOICE

- Pyridoxine 10-30 mg daily IV. Not always effective, but not harmful.
- Antihistamines (e.g., diphenhydramine [25-50 mg q4-6h] or dimenhydrinate, or doxylamine)
- Phenothiazines (e.g., promethazine or prochlorperazine)
- Meclizine 25 mg q6h
- Methylprednisolone 16 mg po qd x 3 days then taper over 2 weeks

Contraindications: All medications taken during pregnancy should balance the risks and benefits both to the mother and the fetus

Precautions:

- Phenothiazines - associated with prolonged jaundice, extrapyramidal effects, hyper- or hyporeflexia in newborns

Significant possible interactions: Refer to manufacturer's profile of each drug

ALTERNATIVE DRUGS

Avoid all drugs if possible

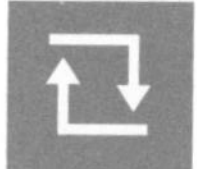

FOLLOWUP

PATIENT MONITORING

- Follow up on a daily basis for weight monitoring in severe cases
- Special attention should be given to monitoring for ketosis, hypokalemia, or acid-base disturbances due to hyperemesis

PREVENTION/AVOIDANCE

Anticipatory guidance in first and second trimester regarding dietary habits in hopes of avoiding volume and nutritional depletion

POSSIBLE COMPLICATIONS

- Patients with greater than a 5% weight loss are associated with intrauterine growth retardation and fetal anomalies
- Hemorrhagic retinitis
- Liver damage
- CNS deterioration, sometimes to coma

EXPECTED COURSE/PROGNOSIS

- Self-limited illness with good prognosis if patient's weight is maintained at greater than 95% of the pre-pregnancy weight
- With complication of hemorrhagic retinitis, mortality rate is 50%

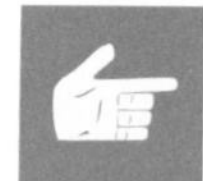

MISCELLANEOUS

ASSOCIATED CONDITIONS

Hyperthyroidism

AGE-RELATED FACTORS

N/A

Pediatric: N/A

Geriatric: N/A

Others: N/A

PREGNANCY

Problem is confined to early pregnancy

SYNONYMS

Morning sickness

ICD-9-CM

643.00 Mild hyperemesis gravidarum, unspecified

643.1 Hyperemesis gravidarum with metabolic disturbance, unspecified

SEE ALSO

OTHER NOTES

N/A

ABBREVIATIONS

N/A

REFERENCES

- Cowan MJ. Hyperemesis gravidarum: implications for home cure and infusion therapies. J Intraven Nurs 1996;19)1):46-58
- Strong TH Jr. Alternative therapies of morning sickness. Clin Obstet Gynecol 2001;44(4):653-60
- Goodwin TM. Hyperemesis gravidarum. Clin Ob/Gyn 1998;41(3):597-605
- Eliakim R, Abulafia O, Sherer DM. Hyperemesis gravidarum: a current review. Am J Perinatol 2000;17(4):207-18
- Yost NP, McIntire DD, Wians FH, Ramin SM, Balko JA, Leveno KJ. A randomized, placebo-controlled trial of corticosteroids for hyperemesis due to pregnancy. Obstet Gynecol. Dec 2003;102(6):1250-1254

Web references: 0 available at www.5mcc.com

Illustrations N/A

Author(s):

Scott A. Fields, MD

BASICS

DESCRIPTION A common electrolyte disorder with plasma potassium concentration > 5.0 mEq/L (> 5.0 mmol/L). Four major causes:
- Increased load - either endogenous from tissue release or exogenous from a high intake which is usually in association with impaired excretion
- Decreased excretion - due to decreased glomerular filtration rate
- Cellular redistribution - shifting of intracellular (which is the major store of potassium) to extracellular space
- Factitious - related to improper collection or transport of blood sample

System(s) affected: Cardiovascular, Endocrine/Metabolic, Nervous
Genetics: Rare, autosomal dominant skeletal muscle sodium channel defect causing hyperkalemic paralysis
Incidence/Prevalence in USA: Common
Predominant age: N/A
Predominant sex: Male = Female

SIGNS & SYMPTOMS
- Cardiac - most important, dominating, and frequent symptoms
  - ◊ Peaked T wave
  - ◊ Flattened p wave
  - ◊ Prolonged p-Q interval
  - ◊ Widened QRS complex
  - ◊ Sine wave
  - ◊ Ventricular fibrillation
  - ◊ Cardiac arrest
- Neuromuscular
  - ◊ Numbness
  - ◊ Weakness
  - ◊ Flaccid paralysis

CAUSES
- Spurious
  - ◊ Hemolysis (most common)
  - ◊ Thrombolysis
  - ◊ Leukocytosis
  - ◊ Infectious mononucleosis
  - ◊ Familial
  - ◊ Pseudohyperkalemia
  - ◊ Procedural technical error (ischemic blood draw due to tight, prolonged tourniquet application)
- Redistribution
  - ◊ Acidosis
  - ◊ Insulin deficiency
  - ◊ Beta blockade due to beta blocking drugs
  - ◊ Digitalis intoxication
  - ◊ Succinylcholine
  - ◊ Arginine hydrochloride/lysine hydrochloride
  - ◊ Periodic paralysis
  - ◊ Fluoride intoxication
  - ◊ Exercise with heavy sweating
- Excessive endogenous potassium load
  - ◊ Hemolysis
  - ◊ Rhabdomyolysis
  - ◊ Internal bleeding
- Excessive exogenous potassium load
  - ◊ Parenteral administration
  - ◊ Excess in diet
  - ◊ Overdose of potassium supplements
- Diminished potassium excretion
  - ◊ Decreased glomerular filtration rate (acute or far-advanced chronic renal failure)
  - ◊ Decreased mineral corticoid activity
  - ◊ Defect in tubular secretion (renal tubular acidosis II and IV)
  - ◊ Drugs: non-steroidal anti-inflammatory agents, cyclosporine, potassium sparing diuretics, ACE inhibitors

RISK FACTORS
- Impaired urinary excretion
- Acidemia
- Massive cell breakdown
- Use of potassium sparing diuretics
- Excess potassium supplementation

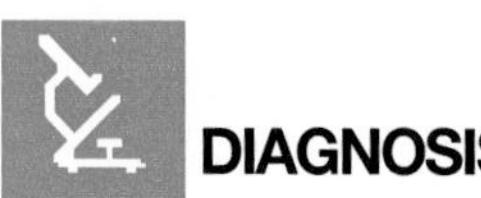

DIAGNOSIS

DIFFERENTIAL DIAGNOSIS
- Cardiac arrhythmias
- Hypocalcemia

LABORATORY Potassium greater than 5.0 mEq/L (5.0 mmol/L)

Drugs that may alter lab results: N/A

Disorders that may alter lab results:
- Acidemia - potassium shifts from intracellular to extracellular space in effort to buffer acid load. Once acidemia is corrected, the potassium may return to normal or even become decreased.
- Insulin deficiency

PATHOLOGICAL FINDINGS N/A

SPECIAL TESTS
- Cortisol and aldosterone levels to check for mineralocorticoid deficiency when other causes are ruled out
- ECG changes usually evolve as potassium rises above 6.0 mEq/L

IMAGING N/A

DIAGNOSTIC PROCEDURES N/A

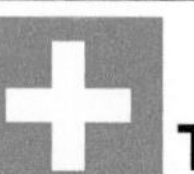

TREATMENT

APPROPRIATE HEALTH CARE Inpatient with cardiac monitoring if ECG changes are present or potassium is greater than 6.0 mEq/L (6.0 mmol/L)

GENERAL MEASURES
- Discontinue any K-sparing drugs or dietary K
- Major goal is to find the cause of hyperkalemia
- If hyperkalemia is severe, treat first, then do diagnostic investigations

SURGICAL MEASURES N/A

ACTIVITY Bedrest

DIET 80 mEq (80 mmol) or less of potassium per 24 hours

PATIENT EDUCATION Consult with dietitian

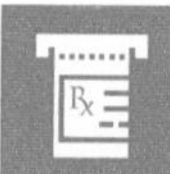

MEDICATIONS

DRUG(S) OF CHOICE
- Dextrose (1 ampule of D50) and insulin, 10 units of regular subcutaneous). Temporary shift of potassium intracellularly taking effect in the first 30 minutes but only lasting a short time.
- Sodium bicarbonate, 50-100 mEq [50-100 mmol], in conjunction with the pH. Especially recommended if serum bicarbonate is ≤ 10 mmol/L. Effects are temporary.
- Sodium polystyrene sulfonate (Kayexalate) 30-60 grams by mouth or by rectum. Effective in 1-4 hours and is a definitive treatment. May repeat q6h if necessary.
- Calcium gluconate, 1 ampule, is cardio-protective only and should only be used when ECG changes are present
- Hemodialysis when other measures are not effective

Contraindications: None

Precautions: Sodium bicarbonate and Kayexalate provide a sodium load that may exacerbate fluid overload in cardiac or renal failure patients

Significant possible interactions: See manufacturer's profile of each drug

ALTERNATIVE DRUGS N/A

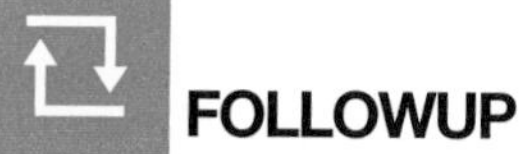

FOLLOWUP

PATIENT MONITORING Serial renal panels until correction complete

PREVENTION/AVOIDANCE Diet and oral supplement compliance

POSSIBLE COMPLICATIONS
- Life threatening cardiac arrhythmias
- Hypokalemia

EXPECTED COURSE/PROGNOSIS Full resolution with correction of the underlying etiology. Reduction of plasma potassium should begin within the first hour of initiation of treatment.

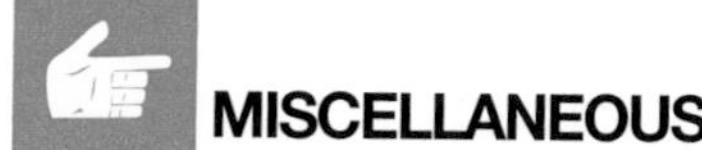

MISCELLANEOUS

ASSOCIATED CONDITIONS
- Renal failure
- Mineralocorticoid deficiency

AGE-RELATED FACTORS
Pediatric: Rare in this group

Geriatric: Increased risk for hyperkalemia in this age group due to decreases in renin and aldosterone

Others: N/A

PREGNANCY N/A

SYNONYMS
- Hyperpotassemia

ICD-9-CM
276.7 Hyperpotassemia

SEE ALSO
Addison disease

Hypokalemia

OTHER NOTES

ABBREVIATIONS N/A

REFERENCES

- Isselbacher KJ, et al, editors: Harrison's Principles of Internal Medicine. 15th Ed. New York: McGraw-Hill; 2001
- Mandal AK, Nahman NS Jr, eds: Kidney Diseases in Primary Care. Baltimore: Lippincott Williams & Wilkins; 1998
- Perazella, MA. Drug-induced hyperkalemia: old culprits and new offenders. Amer J of Med 2000;109(4):307-314

Web references: 0 available at www.5mcc.com

Illustrations N/A

Author(s):
Mark D. Darrow, MD

BASICS

DESCRIPTION Water content of body fluid is deficient compared to sodium content (serum Na > 150 mEq/L [150 mmol/L])
- Significant hypernatremia (serum Na > 160 mEq/L [160 mmol/L]) - may not indicate total body sodium content
- Hypertonicity - increased solutes in extracellular fluid (ECF) which do not cross cell membranes, e.g., sodium, mannitol or glucose. Shifts water from intracellular fluid (ICF) to ECF.
- Hyperosmolality - increased solutes e.g., urea or alcohol, which freely cross all membranes or glucose which does not cross cell membranes. May be present without hypertonicity.

System(s) affected: Endocrine/Metabolic
Genetics: No known genetic pattern. Some diabetes insipidus (DI) may be hereditary.
Incidence/Prevalence in USA: Common in the elderly (e.g., 1% of hospitalized patients over age 65); also may occur with diarrhea in infants
Predominant age: N/A
Predominant sex: Male = Female

SIGNS & SYMPTOMS
- Severity of symptoms usually correlate with the extent of hyperosmolality
- Primary neurological - thirst, restlessness, irritability, disorientation, delirium, coma, convulsions
- Dry mouth and mucous membranes
- Lack of tears and decreased salivation
- Flushed skin
- Fever
- Oliguria or anuria
- Hyperventilation
- Hyperreflexia
- Brain hemorrhage
- Thirst is the primary protection against hypertonicity

CAUSES
- Sodium excess - total body sodium increased
  - ◊ Oral - improperly mixed infant formula, salt given as "punishment" or as a prank, sea water ingestion
  - ◊ IV - NaCl or $NaHCO_3$ during cardiopulmonary resuscitation, intrauterine NaCl for abortion
- Water deficit - total body sodium normal
  - ◊ Decreased intake: e.g., thirst, decreased access to water
  - ◊ Increased urine water loss, e.g., diabetes insipidus
  - ◊ Increased insensible water loss, e.g., fever, hyperventilation, hypermetabolic state
- Hypotonic fluid loss - total body sodium decreased
  - ◊ Loss of fluid containing sodium - without adequate water replacement
- Urinary loss
  - ◊ Osmotic diuretics
  - ◊ Diabetes mellitus
  - ◊ Diuresis from acute tubular necrosis (ATN) or from relief of acute urinary obstruction
- GI loss
  - ◊ Diarrhea, especially in children
- Insensible loss
  - ◊ Sweat
  - ◊ Newborns under radiant warmers

RISK FACTORS
- Children
- Elderly
- Comatose patients

DIAGNOSIS

DIFFERENTIAL DIAGNOSIS
- Diabetes insipidus
- Hyperosmotic coma
- Salt ingestion
- Hypertonic dehydration

LABORATORY
- Serum Na > 150 to 170 mEq/L (> 150-170 mmol/L) - usually dehydration
- Serum Na > 170 mEq/L (> 170 mmol/L) - usually diabetes insipidus
- Serum Na > 190 mEq/L (> 190 mmol/L) - usually chronic salt ingestion
- Diabetes insipidus
  - ◊ Urine osmolality less than serum osmolality
  - ◊ Urine sodium usually low
  - ◊ Polyuria
  - ◊ Neurogenic vs. nephrogenic diabetes insipidus
- Hyperosmolar coma
  - ◊ Blood sugar elevated
  - ◊ Decreased urine output
  - ◊ Increased urine osmolality
- Salt ingestion
  - ◊ Increased urine Na
  - ◊ Increased urine osmolality
- Hypertonic dehydration
  - ◊ Decreased urine sodium
  - ◊ Increased urine osmolality

Drugs that may alter lab results: A variety of medications may raise or lower sodium levels. Refer to a laboratory test reference.

Disorders that may alter lab results: N/A

PATHOLOGICAL FINDINGS N/A

SPECIAL TESTS
- Water deprivation (with diabetes insipidus urine osmolality does not increase when hypernatremic)
- Antidiuretic hormone (ADH) stimulation (with nephrogenic diabetes insipidus urine osmolality does not increase after ADH or DDAVP)

IMAGING CAT scan or MRI in diabetes insipidus - to rule out craniopharyngioma, tumor or median cleft syndrome

DIAGNOSTIC PROCEDURES History, physical, laboratory studies, family history for NDI

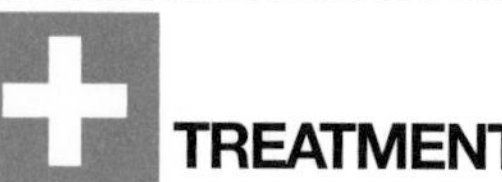

TREATMENT

APPROPRIATE HEALTH CARE Inpatient (many patients are already hospitalized and hypernatremia develops after admission)

GENERAL MEASURES
- Water replacement orally, if patient conscious
- Treat hypovolemia first, then treat hypernatremia
- Calculated water deficit (liters) =

$$[(0.6 \times wt) \times (Na - 140)] \div 140$$

wt = weight in kilograms
Na = current serum sodium

- Dialysis - especially with serum Na > 200 mEq/L (200 mmol/L)

SURGICAL MEASURES N/A

ACTIVITY Bedrest until stable or underlying condition resolved or controlled

DIET
- Assure proper nutrition during acute phase
- After resolution of acute phase, may want to consider sodium restricted diet for patient
- Severe salt restriction in nephrogenic diabetes insipidus

PATIENT EDUCATION
- Patients with nephrogenic diabetes insipidus must avoid salt and drink large amounts of water
- www. healthanswers.com
- www.hometown.aol.com

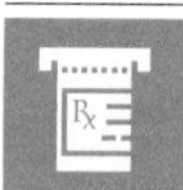

MEDICATIONS

DRUG(S) OF CHOICE

- Hypovolemia
  - ◊ Isotonic saline (normal saline or Ringer's lactate) 10-20 mL/kg IV over 1-2 hrs. May repeat if 10% or greater dehydration.
  - ◊ Isotonic fluids: 5% dextrose with half-normal saline until urine output established
- Hypernatremia
  - ◊ Hypotonic fluids (NaCl or dextrose 5% in water)
  - ◊ Decrease serum sodium by 0.5 mEq/L/hour (0.5 mmol/L/hour) or by no more than 20 mEq/L/day (20 mmol/L/day). Allows idiogenic osmoles to resolve (mostly taurine in brain cell water).
  - ◊ Hypocalcemia may occur during correction of hypernatremia. Add calcium (50 mg/kg 10% calcium gluconate) to IV fluids.
  - ◊ Acidosis is often present in severely dehydrated patients. Add sodium bicarbonate, 50 mEq/L, to IV fluids. If both acidosis and hypocalcemia are present simultaneously, correct the calcium deficit first.
  - ◊ Potassium and phosphate, if needed
- Neurogenic diabetes insipidus (DI)
  - ◊ Desmopressin (DDAVP) acetate: adults 10-40 μg intranasally in 1-3 divided doses; children 5-30 μg in a single evening dose or in 2 divided doses. Oral DDAVP now available - dosage varies.
  - ◊ May use 2.5 dextrose in water if giving large volumes of water in DI or NDI to avoid glycosuria
- Nephrogenic diabetes insipidus (NDI)
  - ◊ Chlorothiazide: 10 mg/kg/dose given bid
  - ◊ Chlorpropamide: 100-250 mg each morning

Contraindications: Refer to manufacturer's literature

Precautions:

- Rapid correction of hypernatremia can cause pulmonary edema. Hypocalcemia often occurs during correction.
- In diabetes insipidus - high rates of dextrose 5% in water can cause hyperglycemia and glucose induced diuresis

Significant possible interactions: Refer to manufacturer's literature

ALTERNATIVE DRUGS

Consider non-steroidal anti-inflammatories in nephrogenic diabetes insipidus

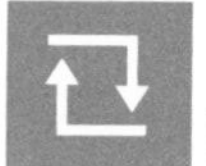

FOLLOWUP

PATIENT MONITORING

- For patient in an acute setting, frequent re-examinations
- Electrolytes frequently
- Urine osmolality and urine output in DI
- Ensure adequate calories are ingested. Patients may ingest so much water that they feel full and do not eat.
- Daily weights

PREVENTION/AVOIDANCE

- Treatment or prevention of underlying cause
- Avoid preparing infant formula at home, and never add salt to any commercial infant formula

POSSIBLE COMPLICATIONS

- CNS thrombosis or hemorrhage
- Seizures
- Mental retardation
- Hyperactivity
- Chronic hypernatremia - over two days duration has higher mortality
- Serum sodium > 180 mEq/L (> 180 mmol/L) - often have residual CNS damage

EXPECTED COURSE/PROGNOSIS

Most recover but rate of neurological impairment is high

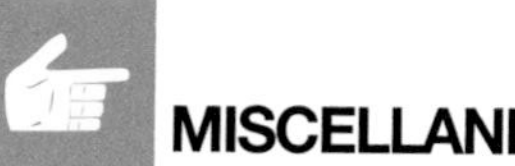

MISCELLANEOUS

ASSOCIATED CONDITIONS

- Sodium excess - total body sodium increased
- Water deficit - total body sodium normal
- Hypotonic fluid loss - total body sodium decreased
- Urinary loss

AGE-RELATED FACTORS N/A

Pediatric:

- May occur in low birth weight newborns
- May result from incorrect preparation of infant formula

Geriatric:

- More common in the elderly hospitalized patient, resulting in a higher morbidity or mortality
- Hypernatremia may be caused by administration of loop diuretics

Others: N/A

PREGNANCY N/A

SYNONYMS N/A

ICD-9-CM

270.6 Disorders of urea cycle metabolism

SEE ALSO

Diabetes insipidus

OTHER NOTES N/A

ABBREVIATIONS

DI = diabetes insipidus

REFERENCES

- Brenner B, Rector F, editors. The Kidney. 6th Ed. Philadelphia: W.B. Saunders Co.; 2000
- Barratt T, Avner E, W. Harmon, editors. Pediatric Nephrology. 4th ed. Baltimore: Williams & Wilkins; 2000
- Kokko J, Tannen R, editors. Fluid and Electrolytes. 3rd ed. Philadelphia: W.B. Saunders Co.; 1996

Web references: 0 available at www.5mcc.com

Illustrations N/A

Author(s):

Watson C. Arnold, MD

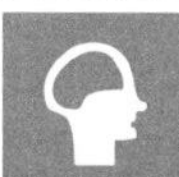

BASICS

DESCRIPTION Hyperparathyroidism represents a loss in control of the body's normal regulatory feedback mechanism on the parathyroid glands and their ability to maintain a normal serum calcium

- Primary hyperparathyroidism - direct hyperfunction of the parathyroid glands due to either glandular hyperplasia or adenoma
- Secondary hyperparathyroidism - usually found in chronic renal disease or vitamin D deficient states which cause hyperplasia of all four glands and associated increase in activity
- Multiple endocrine neoplasia (MEN syndromes) - disease states with associated endocrine malfunctions with parathyroid gland hyperplasia leading to a hyperparathyroid state
- Parathyroid carcinoma - extremely rare

System(s) affected: Endocrine/Metabolic
Genetics: N/A
Incidence/Prevalence in USA:

- Rare in children
- Male adults 60 years or older - 100 cases/100,000
- Female adults 60 years or older - 300-400 cases/100,000
- All-age adjusted incidence - 42 cases/100,000
- Prevalence all ages - 250 cases/100,000 population

Predominant age: Age greater than 50
Predominant sex: Females > Males (4:1)

SIGNS & SYMPTOMS

- "Painful bones, renal stones, abdominal groans and psychic moans." You must think of it to diagnose it.
- Renal:
  - ◊ Nephrolithiasis
  - ◊ Nephrocalcinosis
  - ◊ Reduced glomerular filtration rate
  - ◊ Thirst
  - ◊ Polydipsia
  - ◊ Polyuria
- Gastrointestinal:
  - ◊ Abdominal distress
  - ◊ Gastroduodenal ulcer
  - ◊ Pancreatitis
  - ◊ Pancreatic calcification
  - ◊ Constipation
  - ◊ Vomiting
  - ◊ Anorexia
  - ◊ Weight loss
- Skeletal:
  - ◊ Bone pain and tenderness
  - ◊ Cystic bone lesions
  - ◊ Skeletal demineralization
  - ◊ Spontaneous fracture
  - ◊ Vertebral collapse
  - ◊ Osteoporosis
- Mental:
  - ◊ Fatigue
  - ◊ Apathy
  - ◊ Anxiety
  - ◊ Depression
  - ◊ Psychosis
- Neurologic:
  - ◊ Somnolence
  - ◊ Coma
  - ◊ Diffuse EEG abnormalities
- Neuromuscular:
  - ◊ Muscle fatigue
  - ◊ Weakness
  - ◊ Hypotonia
- Cardiovascular:
  - ◊ Hypertension
  - ◊ Short QT interval
- Articular/periarticular:
  - ◊ Arthralgia
  - ◊ Gout
  - ◊ Pseudogout
  - ◊ Periarticular calcification
- Ocular:
  - ◊ Band keratopathy
  - ◊ Conjunctivitis
  - ◊ Conjunctival calcium deposits

CAUSES

- Primary hyperparathyroidism
  - ◊ Caused by usually one but sometimes multiple parathyroid gland hyperplasia or adenomatous changes which cause an unregulated increase of parathyroid hormone (PTH) production and release, causing increase in serum calcium
- Secondary hyperparathyroidism
  - ◊ Seen most often in chronic renal failure because of adaptive parathyroid gland hyperplasia and hyperfunction
  - ◊ Renal parenchymal loss resulting in hyperphosphatemia
  - ◊ Impaired calcitriol production leading to hypocalcemia
  - ◊ General skeletal and renal resistance to PTH for reasons unknown

RISK FACTORS

- Age greater than 50
- Female
- Occurs more frequently in temperate than tropical climates
- Higher incidence in people exposed to therapeutic low dose radiation

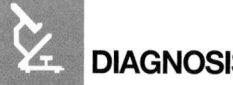

DIAGNOSIS

DIFFERENTIAL DIAGNOSIS

- Other causes of elevated serum calcium level must be excluded
- Due to increased PTH:
  - ◊ Ectopic hyperparathyroidism
  - ◊ Bronchogenic carcinoma
  - ◊ Carcinoma of the kidney
- Nonparathyroid causes:
  - ◊ Malignancy - breast carcinoma, multiple myeloma, lymphoma, leukemia, prostate cancer, Paget disease
  - ◊ Granulomatous disease - sarcoidosis, tuberculosis, berylliosis, histoplasmosis, coccidioidomycosis
  - ◊ Drugs - thiazide diuretics, furosemide, vitamin D intoxication, vitamin A excess, lithium, milk alkali syndrome, exogenous calcium intake
  - ◊ Endocrine - hyperthyroidism, hypothyroidism, acute adrenal insufficiency, vipoma, pheochromocytoma
  - ◊ Familial hypocalciuric hypercalcemia
  - ◊ Immobilization

LABORATORY

- Elevated serum calcium greater than 10.2 mg/dL (2.55 mmol/L) on 3 successive measurements
- Elevated serum immunoreactive parathyroid hormone (iPTH) levels
- Low serum phosphate levels, less than 2.5 mg/dL (0.81 mmol/L)
- Elevated serum chloride levels
- Decreased serum CO2
- Hyperchloremic metabolic acidosis
- Increase in urinary cyclic AMP

Drugs that may alter lab results: N/A

Disorders that may alter lab results: N/A

PATHOLOGICAL FINDINGS

- Parathyroid hyperplasia - all parathyroid glands with cellular changes
- Parathyroid adenoma - only one gland usually with cellular changes
- Parathyroid carcinoma - cellular changes consistent with malignancy, i.e., cellular atypia, lymph node changes

SPECIAL TESTS Immunoassay directed against intact PTH molecule

IMAGING

- Neck ultrasonography
- Thallium technetium scanning
- Magnetic resonance imaging
- CT scanning with and without contrast
- Sestamibi scan for neck

DIAGNOSTIC PROCEDURES

- Percutaneous needle biopsy aspiration for cytology and PTH determination
- Open surgical removal with frozen section diagnosis

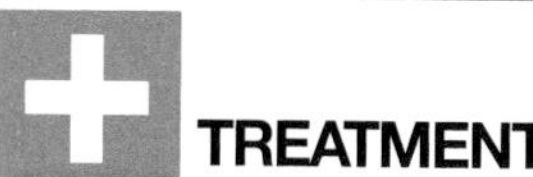

TREATMENT

APPROPRIATE HEALTH CARE Outpatient usually. Inpatient for surgery or for treatment of underlying cause.

GENERAL MEASURES
- A few patients with mild asymptomatic hypercalcemia due to hyperparathyroidism may not be candidates for surgery and may be managed conservatively. Avoiding dehydration is the most important treatment.

SURGICAL MEASURES
- Surgical removal of diseased gland is only proven curative therapy for hyperparathyroidism (subtotal resection)
- In preoperative and immediately postoperative patients, large fluid intake is indicated to help prevent formation of renal stones
- Open neck surgical exploration advocated approach
- Removal of obviously diseased gland with biopsies of other glands to make sure physiologically viable
- Total resection of all four glands with transplantation of normal gland to forearm advocated by some
- Special attention must be made during exploration and removal of parathyroid glands for ectopic gland in the neck area
- Postoperative course needs special attention paid to airway and risk of airway compromise
- Monitoring renal functions closely

ACTIVITY As tolerated

DIET As indicated by condition of patient

PATIENT EDUCATION
- Educate about medications
- Importance of periodic lab exams

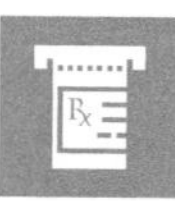

MEDICATIONS

DRUG(S) OF CHOICE
- Furosemide (Lasix) may be helpful in well hydrated individuals who are hypercalcemic
- Estrogens, e.g., conjugated estrogens (Premarin), estradiol (Estrace, Estraderm) are indicated in postmenopausal females with hyperparathyroidism

Contraindications: Avoid diuretics in individuals who are hypercalcemic
Precautions: Refer to manufacturer's literature
Significant possible interactions: Refer to manufacturer's literature

ALTERNATIVE DRUGS N/A

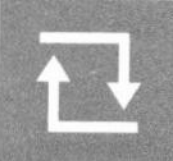

FOLLOWUP

PATIENT MONITORING
- Postoperatively
  - ◊ Monitor renal function closely
  - ◊ Potential precipitous fall in serum calcium resulting in development of transient tetany

PREVENTION/AVOIDANCE N/A

POSSIBLE COMPLICATIONS
- Skeletal damage (pathologic fractures)
- Renal damage
- Urinary tract infections
- "Parathyroid poisoning"
- Hypertension
- From surgery:
  - ◊ Hypoparathyroidism
  - ◊ Recurrent laryngeal nerve damage
  - ◊ Bleeding
  - ◊ Infection
  - ◊ Unsuccessful surgery (5%)

EXPECTED COURSE/PROGNOSIS
- Postoperative course requires following of serum calcium to make sure hyperparathyroid state does not redevelop
- Prognosis is excellent in primary hyperparathyroidism with resolution of many of the preoperative symptoms
- Secondary hyperparathyroidism carries a poor prognosis because of the primary disease state of chronic renal failure

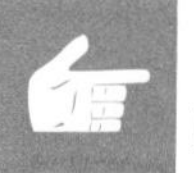

MISCELLANEOUS

ASSOCIATED CONDITIONS Multiple endocrine neoplasia (MEN) syndromes

AGE-RELATED FACTORS
Pediatric: N/A
Geriatric:
- Common in the elderly
- More likely to have a secondary disease
- May cause confusion and be interpreted as senile dementia

Others: N/A

PREGNANCY Rarely occurs during pregnancy

SYNONYMS N/A

ICD-9-CM
252.0 Hyperparathyroidism
259.3 Ectopic hormone secretion, NEC
588.8 Other specified disorder resulting from impaired renal function

SEE ALSO
Multiple endocrine neoplasia (MEN)

OTHER NOTES N/A

ABBREVIATIONS PTH = parathyroid hormone

REFERENCES

- Arnaud CD: The parathyroid glands, hypercalcemia, and hypocalcemia. In: Wyngaarden JB, Smith LH, eds. Cecil Textbook of Medicine. 18th Ed. Philadelphia, W.B. Saunders Co., 1988
- Clark O, Quan-Yank D: Primary hyperparathyroidism: a surgical perspective. In Endocrinology and Metabolism Clinics of North America 1989;18(3):701-715

Web references: 0 available at www.5mcc.com
Illustrations 3 available

Author(s):
Mark R. Dambro, MD

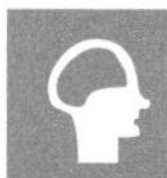

BASICS

DESCRIPTION An abnormal elevation in the serum prolactin level.
System(s) affected: Endocrine/Metabolic, Nervous, Reproductive
Genetics: N/A
Incidence/Prevalence in USA: 1% to 50% of non-pregnant, reproductive-aged women (studies vary widely). Less common in men.
Predominant age: Reproductive age
Predominant sex: Female > Male

SIGNS & SYMPTOMS
- Galactorrhea (milky nipple discharge)
- Amenorrhea (usually secondary amenorrhea)
- Menstrual disorders
- Infertility
- Osteoporosis/osteopenia
- Decreased libido
- Impotence in males
- May also have signs and symptoms of pituitary enlargement
  - ◊ Headache
  - ◊ Visual field impairment
  - ◊ Hypopituitarism (secondary to tumor pressure on surrounding structures)
- May also have signs and symptoms of associated conditions.
  - ◊ Hypothyroidism
  - ◊ Cushing disease
  - ◊ Acromegaly

CAUSES
- Physiologic
  - ◊ Pregnancy
  - ◊ Puerperium
  - ◊ Up to 6 months after weaning
- Prolactin producing pituitary adenoma
- Medications
  - ◊ Phenothiazines
  - ◊ Tricyclics
  - ◊ Opioids
  - ◊ Metoclopramide
  - ◊ Verapamil
  - ◊ Alpha-methyldopa
  - ◊ Isoniazid
  - ◊ Estrogen
  - ◊ Oral contraceptive pills
  - ◊ Reserpine
  - ◊ Butyrophenones
- Hypothyroidism (due to elevated TRH)
- Chest wall conditions
  - ◊ Herpes zoster
  - ◊ Post thoracotomy
  - ◊ Fibrocystic changes
- Postoperative stress
- Pituitary stalk compression
  - ◊ Craniopharyngioma
  - ◊ Pinealoma
  - ◊ Meningioma
  - ◊ Astrocytoma
  - ◊ Metastases
  - ◊ Head trauma
- Miscellaneous causes
  - ◊ Renal failure
  - ◊ Cirrhosis
  - ◊ Sarcoid
  - ◊ Lupus
  - ◊ Carcinoma of lung or kidneys
  - ◊ Ovarian teratoma
  - ◊ Myoma
  - ◊ Eosinophilic granuloma
  - ◊ Other pituitary or hypothalamic disease

RISK FACTORS Listed with Causes.

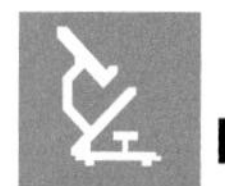

DIAGNOSIS

DIFFERENTIAL DIAGNOSIS As hyperprolactinemia is defined by an abnormal laboratory result, the differential is limited to lab error

LABORATORY
- Prolactin level
- Pregnancy test
- Thyroid function tests
- LH/FSH if amenorrheic
- Blood chemistries, liver and kidney function tests if indicated.

Drugs that may alter lab results: See medications listed under Causes.

Disorders that may alter lab results: See disorders listed under Causes.

PATHOLOGICAL FINDINGS None, unless pituitary resection needed.

SPECIAL TESTS Formal visual field testing if pituitary adenoma suspected.

IMAGING
- MRI (even if prolactin minimally elevated, to rule out hypothalamic tumors which may compress the pituitary stalk thereby decreasing delivery of prolactin inhibitory hormone with subsequent rise in prolactin)
- CT if MRI not available.
- Avoid "coned-down" or plain tomograms of the pituitary as they are relatively insensitive and will not rule out the presence of hypothalamic lesions compressing the pituitary stalk.

DIAGNOSTIC PROCEDURES Usually limited to history, physical exam, blood work, and imaging as described above

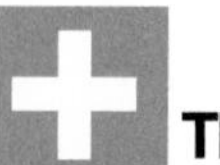

TREATMENT

APPROPRIATE HEALTH CARE Out patient unless pituitary resection needed

GENERAL MEASURES
- Discontinue offending medications, if any
- Treat underlying causes.
- Symptom management
  - ◊ Galactorrhea causing patient anxiety
  - ◊ Fertility restoration
  - ◊ Pituitary adenoma
  - ◊ Prevention of osteoporosis
- "Watchful waiting" is appropriate but pituitary macroadenomas (tumors >10 mm) warrant treatment even if asymptomatic.
- Radiation therapy is usually limited to patients not responding satisfactorily to medical or surgical therapy or sometimes given after surgery to prevent recurrence. The risk is pituitary insufficiency. Long term follow up is needed.

SURGICAL MEASURES
- Indications:
  - ◊ Intolerance or resistance to medical treatment for macroadenomas
- Risks:
  - ◊ High recurrence rate (up to 40%)
  - ◊ Transient DI
  - ◊ CSF leakage
  - ◊ Meningitis
  - ◊ Pituitary insufficiency

ACTIVITY No restrictions

DIET No restrictions

PATIENT EDUCATION
- Discussion of risks of untreated hyperprolactinemia
  - ◊ Headache
  - ◊ Visual field loss
  - ◊ Decreased bone density
  - ◊ Infertility
  - ◊ Patient education material available from: Pituitary Tumor Network Assn, 16350 Ventura Blvd. #231, Encino, CA 91436: (805)499-9973

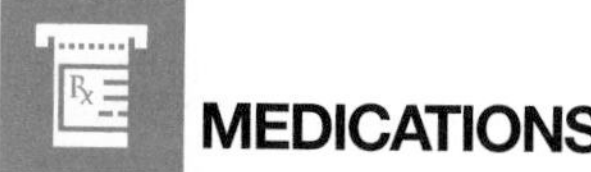

MEDICATIONS

DRUG(S) OF CHOICE
- Bromocriptine (Parlodel). Start with low dose of 1.25 mg or 2.5 mg daily, then increase as tolerated over several weeks to 2.5 mg tid. Doses up to 30 mg daily are occasionally required for prolactinoma regression, after which lower doses can be used for maintenance. First dose should be taken with evening meal.

Contraindications: Uncontrolled hypertension, sensitivity to any ergot alkaloids.

Precautions:
Adverse effects (decreased with gradual increase in dosage):
- Nausea/vomiting
- Headache
- Dizziness
- Fatigue
- Lightheadedness
- Vomiting
- Abdominal cramps
- Nasal congestion
- Drowsiness
- Postural hypotension

Significant possible interactions:
Phenothiazines, butyrophenones, other drugs listed under Causes.

ALTERNATIVE DRUGS
- Intravaginal bromocriptine
- Sustained release bromocriptine (Parlodel SRO)
- Intramuscular bromocriptine (Parlodel LAR)
- New dopamine agonists:
  - ◊ Quinagolide - administered daily
  - ◊ Pergolide (Permax) - 0.05 mg QD
  - ◊ Cabergoline (Dostinex) - 0.25 mg twice weekly; may increase monthly as needed up to 1.0 mg twice weekly

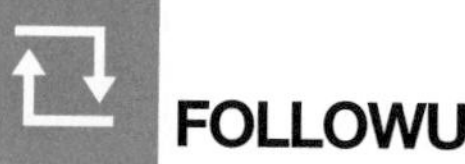

FOLLOWUP

PATIENT MONITORING
- Depends on etiology. Consider:
  - ◊ Prolactin level every 6 to 12 months.
  - ◊ Formal visual field testing yearly.
  - ◊ MRI in one year and then every 2 to 5 years, depending on clinical course.

PREVENTION/AVOIDANCE N/A

POSSIBLE COMPLICATIONS
- Depends on underlying cause.
- If pituitary adenoma, risk of permanent visual field loss.

EXPECTED COURSE/PROGNOSIS
- Depends on underlying cause.
- Tends to recur after discontinuation of medical therapy.
- Microadenomas sometimes regress without intervention.

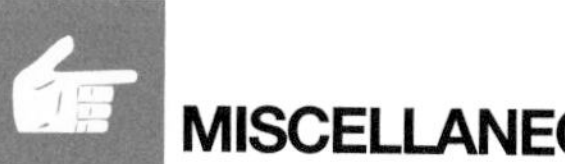

MISCELLANEOUS

ASSOCIATED CONDITIONS See Causes.

AGE-RELATED FACTORS
Pediatric: N/A
Geriatric: N/A
Others: N/A

PREGNANCY
- Hyperestrogenic environment during pregnancy causes pituitary enlargement due to lactotroph hyperplasia.
  - ◊ Microadenomas - 1% risk of enlargement - medical treatment controversial due to low risk of enlargement and possible teratogenic effects.
  - ◊ Macroadenomas - 10% risk of tumor expansion - medical therapy may be discontinued once pregnancy is confirmed and restarted if close observation reveals headaches or visual impairment.

SYNONYMS N/A

ICD-9-CM
611.6 Galactorrhea not associated with childbirth
259.9 Unspecified endocrine disorder

SEE ALSO
Galactorrhea
Pituitary basophilic adenoma
Pituitary chromophobe adenoma
Prolactinoma

OTHER NOTES
- Symptomatic hyperprolactinemia rarely occurs in males. Males require very high levels of prolactin in order to develop symptoms.

ABBREVIATIONS N/A

REFERENCES

- Jones TH: The management of hyperprolactinemia. Brit J of Hosp Med 1995;53(8):374-378
- Conner P, Gabriel F: Hyperprolactinemia; etiology, diagnosis and treatment alternatives. Acta Obstet Gynecol Scand 1998;77:249-262
- Kleinberg DL, Noel GH, Frantz G: Galactorrhea: A study of 235 cases including 48 with pituitary tumors. N Engl J Med 1977;296:589
- Schlechte JA: Clinical impact of hyperprolactinemia. Bailliere's Clinical Endocrinology and Metabolism 1995;9(2):359-366
- Kaye TB: Hyperprolactinemia - Causes, consequences, and treatment options. Postgrad Med 1996;99(5):265-268
- Molitch ME: Pathologic hyperprolactinemia. Endocrinology and Metabolism clinics of North America 1992;21(4):877-901
- New drugs for hyperprolactinemia. Drug and Therapeutics Bulletin 1995;33(9):65-67

Web references: 4 available at www.5mcc.com
Illustrations N/A

Author(s):
Doreen L. Hock, MD

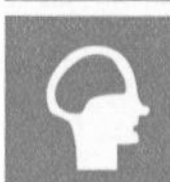

BASICS

DESCRIPTION Hypersensitivity pneumonitis (extrinsic allergic alveolitis) is a diffuse inflammatory disease of the lung caused by repeated inhalation of dust constituted of animal proteins, plant proteins or reactive inorganic compounds. Regardless of the etiologic inhalant, most forms share common features:
- Involvement of peripheral airways, alveoli and interstitium
- Mononuclear cell infiltration of interstitium with granuloma formation and increased alveolar macrophage activity
- Precipitating antibodies against offending dust without complement activation
- Normal IgE and eosinophil levels in chronic form. May present as either acute or sub-acute to chronic progressive pneumonitis.

System(s) affected: Pulmonary
Genetics:
- Not related to:
  - ◊ Atopic predisposition
  - ◊ Blood type
  - ◊ HLA type

Incidence/Prevalence in USA:
- National prevalence unknown
- 1-8% of farmers and 6-15% of pigeon breeders develop related pneumonitis

Predominant age: All ages, but tends to occur in adults because of occupation related exposure
Predominant sex: Male = Female

SIGNS & SYMPTOMS
- Acute hypersensitivity pneumonitis - the following occur within 6 hours of exposure to the offending antigen and may mimic an acute infectious pneumonia:
  - ◊ Fever up to 40°C
  - ◊ Cough
  - ◊ Dyspnea
  - ◊ Malaise
  - ◊ Body aches
  - ◊ Rare hemoptysis or sputum production
  - ◊ Hypoxia
  - ◊ Fine, mid- to end-inspiratory crackles in chest
- Chronic hypersensitivity pneumonitis - chronic progressive condition without acute exacerbation:
  - ◊ Chronic cough
  - ◊ Dyspnea and exercise limitation
  - ◊ Anorexia and weight loss
  - ◊ Fatigue
  - ◊ Progressive hypoxia and cyanosis
  - ◊ Clubbing
  - ◊ Fine, mid- to end-inspiratory crackles in chest
  - ◊ Cor pulmonale with right heart failure

CAUSES
- Exposure to dust capable of inciting immune response, for example:
  - ◊ Farmer's lung (Thermophilic actinomycetes)
  - ◊ Air conditioner lung (Thermophilic actinomycetes)
  - ◊ Bagassosis (Thermophilic actinomycetes)
  - ◊ Bird breeder's lung (avian protein and blood)
  - ◊ Rat handler's lung (rat urine and protein)
  - ◊ Isocyanate lung (toluene diisocyanate [TDI], methylene diisocyanate [MDI] exposure)
  - ◊ Washing powder lung (Bacillus subtilis enzymes)

RISK FACTORS
- Intensity of exposure
- Size (1-5 micron particles reach deep into lung)
- Smokers at lower risk than non-smokers

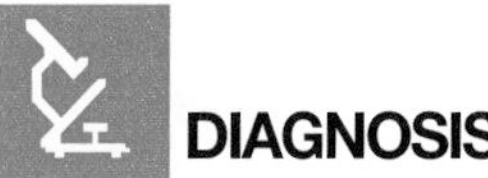

DIAGNOSIS

DIFFERENTIAL DIAGNOSIS
- Acute hypersensitivity pneumonia:
  - ◊ Acute infectious pneumonia
  - ◊ Influenza
  - ◊ Adenovirus
  - ◊ Mycoplasma
  - ◊ Pyogenic bacteria
  - ◊ Pneumocystis carinii
  - ◊ Fungus
- Chronic hypersensitivity pneumonia:
  - ◊ Tuberculosis
  - ◊ Sarcoidosis
  - ◊ Pneumoconiosis
  - ◊ Scleroderma
  - ◊ Rheumatoid lung
  - ◊ Lupus erythematosus
  - ◊ Eosinophilic granuloma
  - ◊ Lymphangitic carcinomatosis
  - ◊ Fungal infections
  - ◊ Pneumocystis carinii pneumonia
  - ◊ Drug reactions
  - ◊ Hemosiderosis
  - ◊ Idiopathic pulmonary fibrosis

LABORATORY
- Leukocytosis with polymorphonuclear predominance in acute form
- Non-specific elevation of immunoglobulins and erythrocyte sedimentation rate
- Positive rheumatoid test and mononucleosis spot test
- Negative blood, sputum, throat cultures

Drugs that may alter lab results: Bronchodilators alter lung function

Disorders that may alter lab results: Asthma or atopy may lead to eosinophilia or increased IgE levels and confuse picture

PATHOLOGICAL FINDINGS
- Acute hypersensitivity pneumonitis:
  - ◊ Alveolar walls infiltrated by polymorphs, lymphocytes, macrophages, plasma cells
  - ◊ Eosinophils are rare
  - ◊ Alveolar space contains proteinaceous exudate and edema
  - ◊ Alveolar capillaries with fibrin/platelet thrombi, but no vasculitis
- Chronic hypersensitivity pneumonitis:
  - ◊ Alveolitis and interstitial inflammation with lymphocytes, plasma cells and histiocytes with non-caseating granulomas
  - ◊ Focal granulomatous inflammation of bronchioles
  - ◊ Interstitial fibrosis and honeycombing in severe cases

SPECIAL TESTS
- Serum IgG precipitating antibodies to offending agent. Note: 40-50% of non-hypersensitive individuals with high exposure have positive precipitating antibodies.
- Skin testing: Standardized agents poorly available and of limited use
- Inhalation challenge testing can cause severe reactions and therefore is usually not performed except in specialized, in-hospital units
- Pulmonary function studies demonstrate:
  - ◊ Reduced lung volume
  - ◊ Impaired gas transfer
  - ◊ Forced expiratory volume (FEV) 1, forced vital capacity (FVC) and FEV1/FVC ratio may be normal early on and then drop with the development of chronic airway obstruction
  - ◊ Forced expiratory flow (FEF) 25-75 and flows near residual volume may be reduced
  - ◊ Decreased lung compliance
- Bronchoalveolar lavage
  - ◊ Acute form with neutrophils and lymphocytes
  - ◊ Chronic form with high lymphocytes (60%) mostly T-cells of CD-8 type
  - ◊ Differentiate from sarcoid which has mostly T-cells of CD-4 type
- Lung biopsy
  - ◊ Rarely needed if treatment and avoidance of exposure results in improvement (see Pathological Findings)

IMAGING
- Acute hypersensitivity pneumonitis on CXR:
  - ◊ 30-40% abnormal CXR
  - ◊ Diffuse interstitial infiltrate with hazy background
  - ◊ Fine nodular shadows from 1-3 mm in size
  - ◊ Linear striated shadows
  - ◊ Occasional lower lobe consolidation
  - ◊ Resolution between attacks
- Chronic hypersensitivity pneumonitis on CXR:
  - ◊ Reticulonodular pattern
  - ◊ Linear shadows and nodules change from fine to coarse pattern with progression of disease
  - ◊ No hilar adenopathy, pleural effusion, or pneumothorax
  - ◊ Upper lobe predominance in 40-50% of cases with ring shadows and bronchiectasis

DIAGNOSTIC PROCEDURES
- Lung biopsy rarely needed for diagnosis
- Role of CT scan is unclear

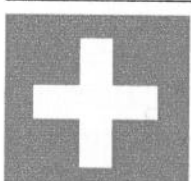

TREATMENT

APPROPRIATE HEALTH CARE Outpatient except for acute pneumonitis cases and admission for workup (bronchial alveolar lavage [BAL], lung biopsy, challenge studies)

GENERAL MEASURES Avoidance of offending antigen

SURGICAL MEASURES N/A

ACTIVITY Full activity, unless advanced disease

DIET Normal

PATIENT EDUCATION
- Stress pathogenesis and critical importance of avoidance of allergen
- Stress risk of irreversible lung damage with continued exposure
- Note that chronic exposure may lead to a loss of acute symptoms with exposure, i.e., patient may lose awareness of exposure-symptom relationship
- Printed patient information available from: American Lung Association, 1740 Broadway, New York, NY 10019, (212)315-8700

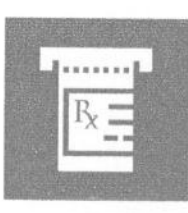

MEDICATIONS

DRUG(S) OF CHOICE
- Avoidance is primary therapy
- Corticosteroids: Prednisone, 2 mg/kg/day or 60 mg/m2/day, or other comparable corticosteroid. Initial course of one to two weeks with progressive withdrawal of medication. Alternate day therapy if exposure cannot be discontinued may help, but may not prevent progression.

Contraindications: Refer to manufacturer's literature

Precautions:
- Observation for side effects:
  - ◊ Immunosuppression
  - ◊ Salt and water retention
  - ◊ Osteoporosis
  - ◊ Acne
  - ◊ Hirsutism
  - ◊ Behavioral changes
  - ◊ Weight gain/appetite increase

Significant possible interactions: In patients with renal or cardiovascular disease a corticosteroid with minimal sodium retention should be chosen

ALTERNATIVE DRUGS
- Bronchodilators may symptomatically improve patients
- Oxygen may be needed in advanced cases

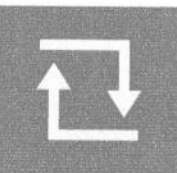

FOLLOWUP

PATIENT MONITORING Initial followup should be weekly to monthly depending upon severity and course

PREVENTION/AVOIDANCE Antigens must be avoided to stop process

POSSIBLE COMPLICATIONS
- Progressive interstitial fibrosis with end-stage lung disease
- Cor pulmonale and right heart failure

EXPECTED COURSE/PROGNOSIS
- Excellent prognosis with reversal of pathologic findings with effective treatment of early disease
- Stabilization of severe, advanced disease with avoidance and anti-inflammatory medication

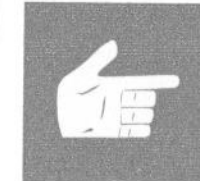

MISCELLANEOUS

ASSOCIATED CONDITIONS N/A

AGE-RELATED FACTORS
Pediatric: N/A
Geriatric: N/A
Others: N/A

PREGNANCY Avoidance of antigen in early pregnancy. Avoidance and medication in later pregnancy.

SYNONYMS
- Extrinsic allergic alveolitis
- Allergic interstitial pneumonitis

ICD-9-CM
495.9 Unspecified allergic alveolitis and pneumonitis

SEE ALSO

OTHER NOTES In acute form, consider other toxic, non-hypersensitivity related conditions such as silo-filler's lung

ABBREVIATIONS N/A

REFERENCES

- Sharma OP: Hypersensitivity pneumonitis. Disease-a-Month 1991;37(7):409-71
- Krumpe PE, Lum CCQ, Cross CE: Approach to the patient with diffuse lung disease. Med Clin North Am 1988;72(5):1225-1246

Web references: 0 available at www.5mcc.com
Illustrations N/A

Author(s):
Nancy N. Dambro, MD

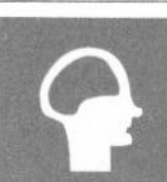

BASICS

DESCRIPTION Hypertension is defined as a sustained elevated blood pressure (systolic blood pressure of 140 mm Hg or greater and/or diastolic blood pressure of 90 mm Hg or greater). Also conceptually includes the blood pressure level at which the benefits of action exceed those of inaction. Prehypertension is defined as systolic pressure 120-139 mm Hg or diastolic 80-89 mm Hg. Hypertension is a strong risk factor for cardiovascular disease.

System(s) affected: Cardiovascular

Genetics: Blood pressure levels are strongly familial but no clear genetic pattern has been discerned. The strong familial risk for cardiovascular diseases should be concomitantly considered.

Incidence/Prevalence in USA: 50 million (1988-1991 NHANES III); 20% of the U.S. population

Predominant age: Essential (primary, benign, idiopathic) hypertension usually has its onset in the 20's to 30's

Predominant sex: Males > Females (males tend to run higher pressures than females but more importantly have a significantly higher risk of cardiovascular disease at any given blood pressure)

SIGNS & SYMPTOMS
- Hypertension should be considered asymptomatic except in extremes or after related cardiovascular complications develop
- Headache can be seen especially with higher blood pressures. This is often present on awakening and occipital in nature.
- Retinopathy - narrowed arteries, AV nicking, copper or silver wiring of retinal arterioles
- Increased A2 heart sound

CAUSES
Over 90% of hypertension has no identified cause. These can be labeled essential or primary hypertension. Secondary causes of hypertension include five areas:
- Renal parenchymal
  - ◊ Glomerulonephritis
  - ◊ Pyelonephritis
  - ◊ Polycystic kidneys
- Endocrine
  - ◊ Primary hyperaldosteronism
  - ◊ Pheochromocytoma
  - ◊ Hyperthyroidism
  - ◊ Cushing syndrome
- Vascular
  - ◊ Coarctation
  - ◊ Renal artery stenosis
- Chemical
  - ◊ Oral contraceptives
  - ◊ NSAIDs
  - ◊ Decongestants
  - ◊ Antidepressants
  - ◊ Sympathomimetics
  - ◊ Many industrial chemicals
  - ◊ Corticosteroids
  - ◊ Ergotamine alkaloids
  - ◊ Lithium
  - ◊ Cyclosporine
- Sleep apnea

RISK FACTORS
- Family history
- Obesity
- Alcohol
- Excess dietary sodium
- Stress
- Physical inactivity

DIAGNOSIS

DIFFERENTIAL DIAGNOSIS Secondary hypertension (because of the low incidence of reversible secondary hypertension, special tests should be considered only if the history, physical, or basic laboratory evaluation indicates the possibility)

LABORATORY
- Hemoglobin and hematocrit or CBC
- Complete urinalysis (sometimes reveals proteinuria)
- Potassium, calcium and creatinine
- Cholesterol (total and HDL)
- Fasting blood glucose
- Uric acid

Drugs that may alter lab results: Numerous drugs and foods interfere with catecholamine measurements in considering pheochromocytoma

Disorders that may alter lab results: N/A

PATHOLOGICAL FINDINGS
- Late complications include
  - ◊ Stroke
  - ◊ Retinal vascular narrowing, hemorrhages, exudates, papilledema
  - ◊ Left ventricular hypertrophy
  - ◊ Congestive heart failure
  - ◊ Ischemic heart disease
  - ◊ Proteinuria and nephrosclerosis

SPECIAL TESTS
- Only if history, physical or lab indicates
  - ◊ IVP and renal arteriogram
  - ◊ Plasma catecholamines, urinary metanephrines/vanillylmandelic acid
  - ◊ Plasma renin
  - ◊ Aortogram
  - ◊ ECG

IMAGING
- If history or physical indicate
  - ◊ Chest x-ray
  - ◊ Ultrasonography
  - ◊ IVP
  - ◊ Provocative renal nuclear scans (e.g., captopril renogram)
  - ◊ Digital subtraction arteriography
  - ◊ Angiogram

DIAGNOSTIC PROCEDURES
- Renal biopsy if renal parenchymal disease is suspected
- A presumptive diagnosis of hypertension can be made if the average of at least two blood pressure measurements exceeds either 90 mm Hg diastolic or 140 mm Hg systolic, assuming proper resting conditions, cuff size and application are maintained
- The Joint National Committee on Detection, Evaluation, and Treatment of High Blood Pressure (JNC): Recommends a good history and physical exam with emphasis on:
  - ◊ Family history of hypertension and cardiovascular disease
  - ◊ Personal past history of cardiovascular, cerebrovascular and renal disease as well as diabetes
  - ◊ Previous elevated blood pressures
  - ◊ Previous treatments
  - ◊ History of weight gain, exercise activities, sodium intake, fat intake and alcohol use
  - ◊ Symptoms suggesting secondary hypertension
  - ◊ Psychosocial and environmental factors affecting blood pressure and risk for cardiovascular disease
  - ◊ Other cardiovascular risk factors such as obesity, smoking, hyperlipidemia, and diabetes
  - ◊ Funduscopic exam for arteriolar narrowing, arteriovenous compression, hemorrhages, exudates, and papilledema
  - ◊ Body mass index
  - ◊ Waist circumference
  - ◊ Blood pressure in both arms
  - ◊ Complete cardiac and peripheral pulse exam. Compare radial and femoral pulse for differences in volume and timing, auscultation for carotid abdominal and femoral bruits.
  - ◊ Abdominal exam for masses and bruits. Listen high in the flanks over the kidneys.
  - ◊ Neurological assessment

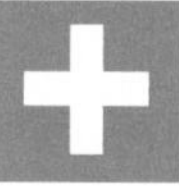

TREATMENT

APPROPRIATE HEALTH CARE Outpatient

GENERAL MEASURES
- Individualize goal blood pressures based on risk factors but generally treat to diastolic < 90 mm Hg (< 12 kPa) and systolic < 140 mm Hg (< 21.3 kPa)
- Weight reduction for obese patients may lower blood pressures
- Smoking cessation is an important part of a cardiovascular risk reduction program
- Biofeedback and relaxation exercises reduce blood pressure
- Risk stratification affects treatment
  - ◊ Prehypertension (120-129/80-89) - drug therapy for chronic renal disease or diabetic patients
  - ◊ Stage 1 hypertension (140-159/90-99) - begin thiazide diuretics for most patients
  - ◊ Stage 2 hypertension (>160/>100) - consider starting 2 drugs or a thiazide-containing combination
- Primary focus is achieving systolic BP goal

SURGICAL MEASURES N/A

ACTIVITY Encourage regular aerobic activity; 30 minutes/day

DIET
- Some patients will respond to a reduced salt diet (<100 mmol/day; < 6gm NaCl or <2.4gm sodium)
- Limit alcohol consumption to < 1 oz/day
- Decrease saturated fats and increase monounsaturated fats
- Consider potassium and calcium, although absolute effect uncertain

PATIENT EDUCATION
- Emphasize asymptomatic nature of hypertension and importance of lifetime treatment
- Review risk factors for cardiovascular disease with emphasis on comprehensive preventive program
- Printed Aids for High Blood Pressure Education, NIH Publication 03-5232; http://nhlbi.nih.gov/health/public/heart/hbp/hbp_low/index.htm

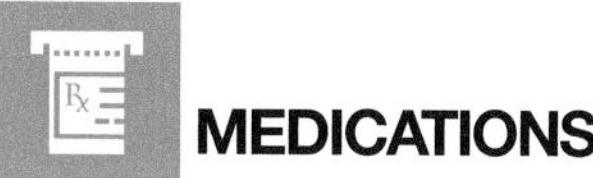

MEDICATIONS

DRUG(S) OF CHOICE
Diuretics and beta blockers have the most documented benefits. ACE inhibitors should be used in patients with diabetes or CHF. Alpha adrenergic agents might benefit males with BPH. Beta blockers might benefit patients with ischemic heart disease, congestive heart failure or migraine. Calcium channel blockers could be considered in patients with migraine or asthma. Combination products are available and may improve compliance with multi-drug regimens.
First line choices include the following categories and their representatives:
- Diuretics
  - ◊ Hydrochlorothiazide 6.25-50 mg qd; chlorthalidone 12.5-50 mg qd; indapamide 1.25-5 mg qd
- ACE inhibitors
  - ◊ Captopril 25-450 mg bid; enalapril 2.5-40 mg qd; fosinopril 10-80 mg qd; lisinopril 5-40 mg qd; ramipril 2.5-20 mg qd; quinapril 10-80 mg qd; benazepril 10-40 mg qd
- Angiotensin II receptor blocker
  - ◊ Losartan 25-100 mg in 1 or 2 doses; valsartan 80-320 mg qd; irbesartan 75-300 mg qd; candesartan 4-32 mg qd; telmisartan 40-80 mg qd
- Calcium channel blockers
  - ◊ Diltiazem CD, 180-360 mg qd; felodipine 5-20 mg qd; nicardipine 20-40 mg tid; nifedipine SR, 30-120 mg qd; verapamil SR, 120-480 mg qd; amlodipine 2.5-10 mg qd
- Beta blockers
  - ◊ Acebutolol 400-800 mg qd; atenolol 25-100 mg qd; metoprolol 50-200 mg qd; nadolol 40-320 mg qd; pindolol 5-30 mg bid; propranolol 20-120 mg bid; timolol 5-20 mg bid; betaxolol 5-40 mg qd; bisoprolol 2.5-20 mg qd

Contraindications:
- Diuretics may worsen gout and diabetes
- Beta blockers are relatively contraindicated in reactive airway disease, and heart block. Diabetes and peripheral vascular disease are relative contraindications.
- Diltiazem or verapamil: caution with heart failure or block
- Bilateral renovascular disease can be worsened by ACE inhibitors

Precautions: See manufacturer's profile of each drug
Significant possible interactions: See manufacturer's profile of each drug

ALTERNATIVE DRUGS
Many may be added to the above for combination therapy
- Centrally acting adrenergic inhibitors
  - ◊ Clonidine 0.1-1.2 mg bid or weekly patch 0.1 mg/day to 0.3 mg/day; guanabenz 4-32 mg bid; guanfacine 1-3 mg qd; methyldopa 250-2000 mg bid
- Alpha adrenergic agents
  - ◊ Prazosin 1-10 mg bid; terazosin 1-20 mg qd; doxazosin 1-16 mg qd
- Peripherally acting adrenergic inhibitors
  - ◊ Guanadrel 2.5-37.5 mg bid; guanethidine 10-50 mg qd; reserpine 0.1-0.25 mg qd; labetalol 100-900 mg bid
- Vasodilators
  - ◊ Hydralazine 25-150 mg bid; minoxidil, rarely used due to adverse effects
- Loop diuretics (for patients with volume overload)
  - ◊ Furosemide 20-320 mg qd; bumetanide 0.5-2 mg qd; ethacrynic acid 25-100 mg qd
- Potassium sparing diuretics, in patients with hypokalemia while taking thiazides
  - ◊ Amiloride 5-10 mg qd; spironolactone 25-100 mg qd; triamterene 50-150 mg qd

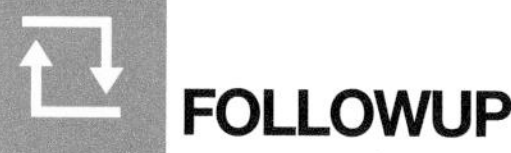

FOLLOWUP

PATIENT MONITORING
- Once stable, patients should be reevaluated at least every 3 to 6 months
- Review compliance, effectiveness and adverse reactions
- Quality of life issues should be considered, including sexual function
- At least annual evaluation of urinalysis, creatinine and potassium are appropriate, generally as part of a screening laboratory panel

PREVENTION/AVOIDANCE Diet, exercise, reduce stress, stop smoking, little or no alcohol, compliance in taking medications

POSSIBLE COMPLICATIONS
- Congestive heart failure
- Renal failure
- Myocardial infarction
- Stroke
- Hypertensive heart disease

EXPECTED COURSE/PROGNOSIS
Good with adequate control

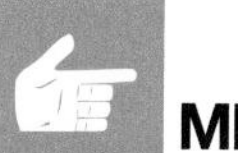

MISCELLANEOUS

ASSOCIATED CONDITIONS See list in Causes

AGE-RELATED FACTORS
Pediatric:
- Blood pressure should be measured during routine examinations
- Hypertension can accompany a wide variety of acute and chronic illnesses in this age group

Geriatric: Isolated systolic hypertension more common in this group. Therapy has been shown to be effective although adverse reactions to medications are more frequent.
Others: N/A

PREGNANCY Elevated blood pressures during pregnancy may be either chronic hypertension or pregnancy induced preeclampsia. Maternal and fetal mortality benefit from treatment. See topic on preeclampsia. Some medications may adversely affect the fetus.

SYNONYMS
- Benign hypertension
- Idiopathic hypertension
- Familial hypertension
- High blood pressure
- Chronic hypertension
- Genetic hypertension

ICD-9-CM
401.1 Essential hypertension, benign

SEE ALSO
Hypertensive emergencies
Polycystic kidney disease

OTHER NOTES
Normal saline (0.9% NaCl) contains 154 mmol/L of sodium (1 liter contains 1.5 times the recommended sodium per day for salt restricted patients)

ABBREVIATIONS
SR = sustained release

REFERENCES

- Kaplan NM. Clinical Hypertension. 8th ed. Baltimore: Lippincott Williams & Wilkins; 2002
- The Fourth Report on the Diagnosis, Evaluation, and Treatment of High Blood Pressure in Children and Adolescents. Pediatrics 2004;114(2):555-76
- The Seventh Report of the Joint National Committee on Prevention, Detection, Evaluation, and Treatment of High Blood Pressure. JAMA 2003;289(19):2560-72

Web references: 1 available at www.5mcc.com
Illustrations 5 available

Author(s):
David E. Burtner, MD

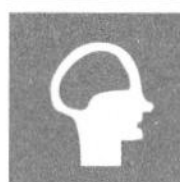

BASICS

DESCRIPTION Terminology describing hypertensive emergencies can be confusing. Terms such as "hypertensive crisis," "malignant hypertension," "hypertensive urgency," "accelerated hypertension" and "severe hypertension" are all used in the literature and often overlap. Some definitions include a specific diastolic or systolic blood pressure reading, while others emphasize an acute change in the blood pressure or the presence of specific clinical syndromes.
- Severe hypertension is defined as a diastolic blood pressure of 115 mm Hg (15.3 kPa) or greater. Patients with severe hypertension may or may not have a hypertensive emergency.
- A hypertensive emergency occurs when an acute elevation of blood pressure causes rapid and progressive end-organ damage, particularly in the cardiovascular, renal and central nervous systems.

System(s) affected: Cardiovascular, Nervous, Pulmonary, Renal/Urologic
Genetics: N/A
Incidence/Prevalence in USA: Less than 1% of patients with hypertension
Predominant age: Young or middle-aged patients with known hypertensive disease
Predominant sex: Male > Female

SIGNS & SYMPTOMS
- Hypertension
- Headache
- Nausea, vomiting
- Seizure
- Retinopathy
- Visual disturbances
- Chest pain
- Shortness of breath, dyspnea, orthopnea
- Focal neurologic deficits
- Stupor, coma
- Pulmonary edema
- Hemorrhage
- Thrombosis
- Embolus
- Acute renal failure
- Abdominal pain

CAUSES
- Medications including: SSRIs, decongestants, appetite suppressants, steroids (including oral contraceptives), MAO inhibitors in combination with certain foods or drugs, and drugs of abuse such as cocaine or amphetamine
- Withdrawal from antihypertensives, especially clonidine (Catapres)
- Withdrawal from CNS depressants
- Eclampsia/preeclampsia
- Thrombotic thrombocytopenic purpura (TTP)
- Pheochromocytoma
- Idiopathic hypertension
- Renal disease
- Severe burns
- Postoperative hypertension

RISK FACTORS
- History of hypertension
- Drug abuse
- Non-compliance with medications

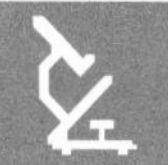

DIAGNOSIS

DIFFERENTIAL DIAGNOSIS Other CNS pathology

LABORATORY
- Urinalysis and renal function tests (red cell casts, hematuria, proteinuria are all common)
- Urine drug screen in selected patients
- Blood count and smear may indicate microangiopathic hemolytic anemia, thrombocytopenia
- Serum electrolytes (may indicate hypokalemic alkalosis)
- Calcium, glucose, uric acid and lipid profiles
- Subsequent work-up for renal artery stenosis or pheochromocytoma in selected patients

Drugs that may alter lab results: N/A

Disorders that may alter lab results: N/A

PATHOLOGICAL FINDINGS Extreme blood pressure elevations can overwhelm the autoregulatory mechanisms for organ blood flow resulting in damage to the arteriolar and capillary beds. This process produces organ hemorrhages and edema from the leakage of blood and fluid.

SPECIAL TESTS
- Electrocardiography may reveal ischemia or left ventricular hypertrophy
- Funduscopic examination may reveal papilledema, exudates or hemorrhages

IMAGING
- Chest radiographs:
  - ◊ May show pulmonary edema and cardiomegaly due to congestive heart failure
  - ◊ Mediastinal widening and blunting of the aortic knob consistent with a dissecting aneurysm
- Head CT
  - ◊ Assess the patient with CNS symptoms for intracranial bleed

DIAGNOSTIC PROCEDURES
- Blood pressure - measured with an appropriately sized cuff, and two or more readings from both arms should be averaged before the blood pressure is accepted as elevated
- Sphygmomanometer is recommended

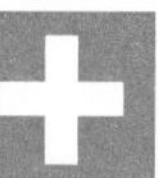

TREATMENT

APPROPRIATE HEALTH CARE
Intensive care unit

GENERAL MEASURES
- Comfortable environment, which may lower the blood pressure
- General goal is to lower the mean arterial pressure by approximately 20-25% or reduce diastolic pressure to 100-110 mm Hg (13.3-14.6 kPa) over one hour
- If ongoing end-organ damage is thought to be secondary to the hypertensive state, prompt treatment with intravenous medication is indicated. Monitor patient closely so that a rapid fall in blood pressure can be avoided.
- Optimally, an arterial catheter is used to monitor blood pressure
- Intravenous infusion pump
- Mean arterial pressure is approximately one-third of the sum of twice the diastolic pressure plus the systolic pressure

SURGICAL MEASURES N/A

ACTIVITY Bedrest

DIET Low sodium when tolerated

PATIENT EDUCATION
- Importance of medication compliance
- Lack of symptoms with hypertension until organ damage occurs

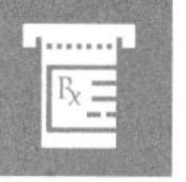

MEDICATIONS

DRUG(S) OF CHOICE The drug(s) used depends on the end organs affected and the patient's clinical status. All medications are IV unless otherwise indicated.
- DRUGS:
  - ◊ Nitroprusside (Nipride, Nitropress) infusion 0.5-10 μg/kg/min; contraindicated in pregnancy
  - ◊ Hydralazine bolus 5-15 mg; preferred in pregnancy
  - ◊ Diazoxide (Hyperstat) infusion 7.5-30 mg/min
  - ◊ Labetalol (Normodyne, Trandate) bolus 20-80 mg q10-15 minutes; infusion 0.5-2.0 mg/min
  - ◊ Nitroglycerin (NTG) infusion 5-100 μg/min
  - ◊ NTG 0.4 mg SL tablet. Repeat q5min if needed. Consider IV infusion after 3 doses.
  - ◊ Trimethaphan (Arfonad) infusion 0.5-5 mg/min
  - ◊ Propranolol (Inderal) 2-4 mg/hr
  - ◊ Phentolamine (Regitine) bolus 5-10 mg q5-15 minutes
  - ◊ Oral clonidine: oral loading dose of 0.2 mg followed by 0.1 mg per hour until blood pressure has been lowered or a total dose of 0.8 mg has been administered
  - ◊ Esmolol 0.05-0.3 mg/kg/min
  - ◊ Enalaprilat 0.625-1.25 mg
  - ◊ Nicardipine 4-15 mg/hr

- DISEASE STATES:
  - ◊ Hypertensive encephalopathy
    - Nitroprusside infusion or
    - Diazoxide infusion or
    - Labetalol or enalaprilat
  - ◊ Central nervous system events
    - Nitroprusside infusion (treat only if diastolic pressure > 130 mm Hg [> 17.3 kPa])
  - ◊ Myocardial ischemia
    - Nitroglycerin infusion or
    - Labetalol or esmolol or enalaprilat
  - ◊ Congestive heart failure
    - Nitroprusside infusion or
    - Nitroglycerin infusion or enalaprilat or nicardipine
  - ◊ Aortic dissection
    - Nitroprusside and propranolol infusions or
    - Trimethaphan and propranolol infusions
  - ◊ Renal failure
    - Nitroprusside infusion or
    - Labetalol
  - ◊ Pheochromocytoma
    - Phentolamine or
    - Labetalol or
    - Nitroprusside infusion
  - ◊ Antihypertensive withdrawal
    - Labetalol or
    - Phentolamine
  - ◊ Interactions between MAO inhibitors and foods or drugs
    - Phentolamine or
    - Labetalol
  - ◊ Eclampsia/preeclampsia
    - Hydralazine
  - ◊ Severe hypertension (hypertensive urgencies) without evidence of acute end-organ damage. Treatment is controversial. No emergent treatment recommended.

Contraindications:

- Diazoxide: not recommended for patients with suspected myocardial ischemia, congestive heart failure or aortic dissection
- Labetalol: not recommended for patients with asthma, chronic obstructive lung disease, congestive heart failure, heart block, cardiogenic shock or severe bradycardia (due to its beta-blockade property)
- Nitroprusside: not recommended in pregnancy

Precautions:

- Nitroprusside: when IV nitroprusside is continued for more than 48-72 hours, or the patient has compromised renal function, plasma thiocyanate levels should be monitored. Use with clonidine has caused myocardial infarction.
- Diazoxide and hydralazine: may produce reflex tachycardia with increased myocardial oxygen consumption (can be prevented by pretreatment with intravenous propranolol). Use with caution in suspected myocardial infarction.
- Topical clonidine has a slow onset of action and is generally not useful in hypertensive emergencies
- Oral/SL nifedipine (Adalat, Procardia) may cause serious adverse effects such as cerebral vascular ischemia, stroke, or severe hypotension and should probably not be used for hypertensive emergencies

Significant possible interactions: N/A

ALTERNATIVE DRUGS Dopamine-1 receptor agonists (investigational) may preserve renal function better than other agents.

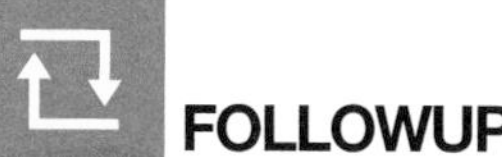

FOLLOWUP

PATIENT MONITORING

- Monitor closely to avoid a rapid fall in blood pressure
- Begin oral therapy as soon as possible after control achieved with IV medications

PREVENTION/AVOIDANCE Counsel patient on importance of compliance with antihypertensive treatment and dangers of abrupt stoppage of medication

POSSIBLE COMPLICATIONS

- Abrupt lowering of the blood pressure may result in inadequate cerebral or cardiac blood flow, leading to stroke or myocardial ischemia
- Authorities have questioned whether the benefits of aggressive treatment outweigh the risks in patients with severe hypertension but no end-organ damage. No studies have proven that aggressive treatment reduces the risk of long-term morbidity or mortality from hypertensive urgencies.

EXPECTED COURSE/PROGNOSIS

- The blood pressure should return to normal levels within 24 hours

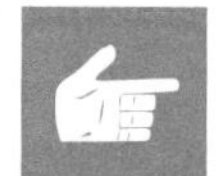

MISCELLANEOUS

ASSOCIATED CONDITIONS

- Chronic renal failure
- Renovascular hypertension
- Acute glomerulonephritis
- Renal vasculitis

AGE-RELATED FACTORS

Pediatric: Usually associated with renal disease. May present with abdominal pain.
Geriatric: N/A
Others: N/A

PREGNANCY Hydralazine is drug of choice since nitroprusside decreases placental blood flow and cyanide metabolite crosses the placenta and is therefore relatively contraindicated in pregnancy. Treat eclampsia.

SYNONYMS

- Hypertensive crisis
- Severe hypertension
- Malignant hypertension
- Accelerated hypertension

ICD-9-CM

401.0 Essential hypertension, malignant
405.01 Secondary malignant renovascular hypertension
437.2 Hypertensive encephalopathy
642.90 Unspecified hypertension complicating pregnancy, childbirth, or the puerperium, unspecified

SEE ALSO

Aortic dissection
Eclampsia (toxemia of pregnancy)
Hypertension, essential
Pheochromocytoma
Preeclampsia

OTHER NOTES N/A

ABBREVIATIONS

MAO = monoamine oxidase
SSRI = selective serotonin reuptake inhibitor

REFERENCES

- Gifford R. Management of Hypertensive Crisis. J Amer Med Soc 1991;226:829-835
- Calhoun DA, Oparil S. Treatment of hypertensive crisis. N Engl J Med 1990;323:1177-83
- The sixth report of the Joint National Committee on Detection, Evaluation, and Treatment of High Blood pressure. Arch Intern Med 1997;157:2413-2445
- Haber E, Slater E. Hypertensive Emergencies in High Blood Pressure. In: Rubenstein E, Federman DD, editors. Scientific American Medicine, Scientific American Inc., 1978-1992
- Graber MA. Emergency Medicine. In: Graber MR, et al, editors. The Family Practice Handbook. St Louis: Mosby-Yearbook; 1994
- Abdelwahab W, Frishman W, Landau A. Management of hypertensive urgencies and emergencies. J Clin Pharmacol 1995;35:747-62
- Murphy C. Hypertensive emergencies. Advances and Updates in Cardiovascular Emergencies 1995;13:973-1007
- Grossman E, Messerli FH, Grodzicki T, et al. Should a moratorium be placed on sublingual nifedipine capsules given for hypertensive emergencies and pseudoemergencies? JAMA 1996; 276:1328-31
- Shayne PH, Pitts SR. Severely increased blood pressure in the emergency department. Ann Emerg Med 2003;41(4):513-29

Web references: 0 available at www.5mcc.com
Illustrations N/A

Author(s):

John Guisto, MD
Arthur Sanders, MD

BASICS

DESCRIPTION The reaction to excess thyroid hormone. Types of hyperthyroidism include:

- Graves' disease (GD) - the most common form - an autoimmune disease. Thyroid stimulating immunoglobulins (TSI's) of the IgG class are produced and bind to thyrotropin (TSH) receptors on the thyroid gland. The TSI's mimic the action of TSH and cause excess secretion of thyroxine (T4) and triiodothyronine (T3). Goiter and ophthalmopathy are common characteristics. Pretibial myxedema is rare.
- Toxic multinodular goiter - occurs later in life. Nodules are insidious and almost never malignant. No ophthalmopathy or localized myxedema present.
- Toxic uninodular goiter - solitary nodule with autonomous function. Almost always benign.
- Other causes are rare and include TSH-secreting pituitary tumors, surreptitious ingestion of T4 or T3, functioning trophoblastic tumors, and iodine-induced hyperthyroidism, especially from the cardiac drug amiodarone

System(s) affected: Endocrine/Metabolic
Genetics: Unknown
Incidence/Prevalence in USA: 1:1000 in women, 1:3000 in men
Predominant age: Any age, peaks in 3rd and 4th decades
Predominant sex: Female > Male

SIGNS & SYMPTOMS

- In adults
  - ◊ Nervousness (85%)
  - ◊ Increased sweating (70%)
  - ◊ Heat intolerance (70%)
  - ◊ Palpitations and tachycardia (75%)
  - ◊ Dyspnea (75%)
  - ◊ Fatigue and weakness (60%)
  - ◊ Weight loss (52%)
  - ◊ Increased appetite (40%)
  - ◊ Exophthalmos (34%)
  - ◊ Goiter (87%)
  - ◊ Tremor (65%)
  - ◊ Warm and moist skin (72%)
  - ◊ Emotional lability
  - ◊ Subclinical; may present with atrial fibrillation, cardiomegaly, skeletal demineralization with a low TSH
- In children
  - ◊ Linear growth acceleration
  - ◊ Ophthalmic abnormalities more common

CAUSES

- Graves' disease - autoimmune disease
- Toxic multinodular goiter - iodine deprivation followed by iodine repletion
- Toxic uninodular goiter - unknown
- Hashimoto's thyroiditis - "hashitoxicosis"

RISK FACTORS

- Positive family history
- Female sex
- Other autoimmune disorders
- Iodide repletion after iodide deprivation

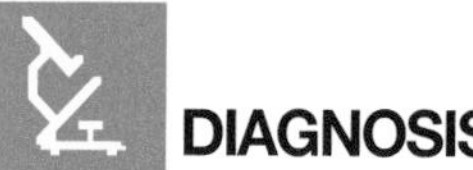

DIAGNOSIS

DIFFERENTIAL DIAGNOSIS

- Anxiety
- Malignancy
- Diabetes
- Pregnancy
- Menopause
- Pheochromocytoma

LABORATORY

- T3 - Total T3 by immunometric assay > 200 ng/mL
- T4 - by immunometric assay >12.5 μg/dL (161 nmol/L)
- Free thyroxine index (FTI) >12
- Free thyroxine > 1.5 ng/dL
- TSH - below normal, often undetectable
- Radioiodine uptake (RIU) - high in Graves' disease, high or normal in toxic nodules

Drugs that may alter lab results:

- Anabolic steroids
- Androgens
- Estrogens
- Heparin
- Iodine containing compounds (especially amiodarone)
- Phenytoin
- Rifampin
- Salicylates
- Thyroxine
- Triiodothyronine

Disorders that may alter lab results:

- A variety of non-thyroidal illnesses can alter T4 and T3 with little effect on TSH
- FTI permits correction of misleading results caused by pregnancy and estrogens

PATHOLOGICAL FINDINGS

- Graves' disease - hyperplasia
- Toxic nodules - nodule formation

SPECIAL TESTS N/A

IMAGING

- Thyroid scans using radioiodine: diffuse in GD, focal in toxic nodules
- Ultrasonography with fine needle aspiration to investigate nodules

DIAGNOSTIC PROCEDURES N/A

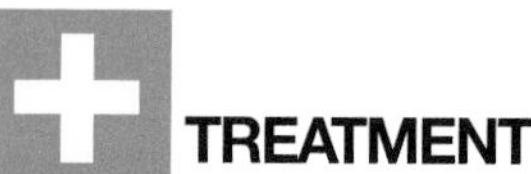

TREATMENT

APPROPRIATE HEALTH CARE

- Outpatient except for treatment of thyroid storm, a rare life-threatening condition, which may cause heart failure, fever, and mania

GENERAL MEASURES Antithyroid drugs, therapeutic radioiodine, beta blockers for tachycardia and tremor

SURGICAL MEASURES Rarely, subtotal thyroidectomy

ACTIVITY Modify activity according to disease severity

DIET Sufficient calories to prevent weight loss

PATIENT EDUCATION Importance of compliance with drug therapy and surveillance for hypothyroidism

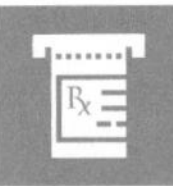

MEDICATIONS

DRUG(S) OF CHOICE
- Initial treatment
  - ◊ Methimazole (Tapazole)
    - Adults: 15-60 mg/day po given once daily.
    - Children: 6-10, 0.4 mg/kg/day po once daily
  - ◊ Propylthiouracil (PTU)
    - Adults (preferred in elderly, those with cardiac disease, thyroid storm, and pregnant and lactating women) 100-900 mg/day po given tid. No more than 300 mg/day during pregnancy. Radioiodine often first choice.
    - Children age > 10, 150-300 mg/day po given tid or 5-7 mg/kg/day
    - Children age 6-10, 50-150 mg/day po given tid or 5-7 mg/kg/day
- Maintenance with antithyroids
  - ◊ Methimazole
    - Adults: 5-30 mg/day po given daily. No more than 20 mg/day during pregnancy.
    - Children 0.2 mg/kg/day po given daily
  - ◊ PTU
    - Adults: 50-600 mg/day given bid po
    - Children: 50 mg bid po (or 1/2-2/3 of initial dose)
- Thyrotoxic crisis
  - ◊ PTU
    - Adults 15-20 mg po q4h during the first day (as an adjunct to other therapies)
    - Neonates 10 mg/kg/day po given q4h
    - Dosage adjustments by following clinical status, free T4 (or FTI) and, when appropriate, TSH
- Saturated solution of potassium iodide (SSKI) 5 drops every 6 hours for 24-72 hours until improvement
- Additional drugs:
  - ◊ Radioiodine therapy: sodium iodide I-131 (Iodotope). Dosage calculation: estimated thyroid weight multiplied by 120 μCi/g divided by 24 hour radioiodine uptake.
  - ◊ Beta blocker: propranolol (Inderal) 40-240 mg daily po

Contraindications:
- Radioiodine therapy - pregnancy and nursing
- Propranolol - congestive heart failure, asthma, chronic bronchitis, pregnancy, hypoglycemia

Precautions:
- PTU and MMI - may cause dermatitis, agranulocytosis or hepatotoxicity
- Radioiodine therapy often causes permanent hypothyroidism and may cause fetal hypothyroidism or malformation if administered during pregnancy

Significant possible interactions: Oral anticoagulants may be potentiated by PTU

ALTERNATIVE DRUGS
Ipodate sodium (Oragrafin) - 0.5 g qid po

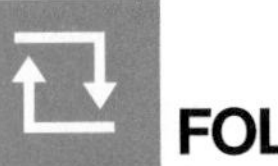

FOLLOWUP

PATIENT MONITORING
- Repeat thyroid tests once a year
- CBC and liver function tests when appropriate
- Therapy with antithyroids continues 3-12 months
- After radioiodine therapy, thyroid function tests at 6 weeks, 12 weeks, 6 months and annually thereafter if euthyroid

PREVENTION/AVOIDANCE
N/A

POSSIBLE COMPLICATIONS
- Hypoparathyroidism, recurrent laryngeal nerve damage, and hypothyroidism with subtotal thyroidectomy
- Development of hypothyroidism after radioiodine treatment
- Visual loss or diplopia due to severe ophthalmopathy
- Localized pretibial myxedema at any time
- Cardiac failure in the elderly with underlying heart disease
- Muscle wasting; proximal muscle weakness

EXPECTED COURSE/PROGNOSIS
With precise diagnosis and adequate treatment, prognosis is good

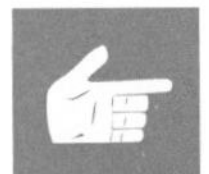

MISCELLANEOUS

ASSOCIATED CONDITIONS
Other autoimmune diseases and Down syndrome

AGE-RELATED FACTORS
Pediatric: Neonates treated with antithyroids 2-3 months. Most children treated with antithyroids.

Geriatric:
- Characteristic symptoms and signs may be absent in elderly
- Harder to diagnose
- Cardiac failure more likely

Others: N/A

PREGNANCY
- Treat with small doses of PTU or MMI due to increased risk of spontaneous abortion and premature delivery in hyperthyroid pregnant women
- Avoid treatment induced hypothyroidism
- Symptoms may be confusing
- Thyrotoxicosis often improves during pregnancy and relapses postpartum
- Radioiodine therapy absolutely contraindicated

SYNONYMS
Thyrotoxicosis

ICD-9-CM
242.00 Toxic diffuse goiter without mention of thyrotoxic crisis or storm

242.01 Toxic diffuse goiter with mention of thyrotoxic crisis or storm

242.90 Thyrotoxicosis without mention of goiter or other cause without mention of thyrotoxic crisis or storm

242.91 Thytotoxicosis without mention of goiter or other cause with mention of thyrotoxic crisis or storm

SEE ALSO

OTHER NOTES
N/A

ABBREVIATIONS
TSI = thyroid stimulating immunoglobulins
TSH = thyroid stimulating hormone
T4 = thyroxine
T3 = triiodothyronine
FTI = free thyroxine index
RIU = radioiodine uptake
PTU = propylthiouracil
MMI = methimazole

REFERENCES

- Ross DS. Hyperthyroidism. Wellesley, MA: UpToDate: 2004
- Federman DD. Scientific American Medicine, revised August 1997;3(I):6-12
- Greenspan FS, Strewler GJ. Basic and Clinical Endocrinology. 5th ed. Stamford CT: Appleton & Lange; 1997. p.233-247
- Mestman JH. Hyperthyroidism in pregnancy. Endocrinol Metab Clin North Am 1998;27(I):127-49
- Attia J, Margetts P, Guyatt G. Diagnosis of thyroid disease in hospitalized patients: a systematic review. Arch Intern Med 1999;159(7):658-65
- Woeber KA. Update on the management of hyperthyroidism and hypothyroidism. Arch Fam Med 2000;9(8):743-7
- Surks MI, Ortiz E, Daniels GH, et al. Subclinical thyroid disease: scientific review and guidelines for diagnosis and management. JAMA. 2004;291(2):228-38

Web references: 0 available at www.5mcc.com
Illustrations 2 available

Author(s):
Richard P. Levy, MD

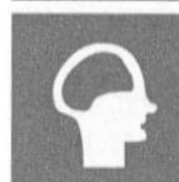

BASICS

DESCRIPTION Triglycerides (TG) are fatty molecules of long-chain fatty acids and glycerol. The hypertriglyceridemias are a heterogeneous family of disorders due to disturbances in synthesis and/or degradation of triglycerides rich plasma lipoprotein.
- Normal triglycerides is less than 100 mg/dL (1.13 mmol/L) in children and less than 150 mg/dL (1.70 mmol/L) in adults.
- Abnormal hypertriglyceridemia: 150-500 mg/dL (1.7-5.65 mmol/L)
- Distinct hypertriglyceridemia: More than 500 mg/dL (5.65 mmol/L)
- Physiology: The major triglycerides containing lipoproteins are:
  - ◊ Chylomicron: In post prandial state from absorption of dietary fat from the gut.
  - ◊ Very low density lipoprotein (VLDL): In fasting state endogenous synthesis from carbohydrates and fatty acid in the liver.
  - ◊ Intermediate density lipoprotein (IDL): From degradation of chylomicron and VLDL
- Classification: Hypertriglyceridemia falls into one of the following groups based on the lipoprotein pattern
  - ◊ Type I: Markedly elevated chylomicron. Presents with high triglyceridemia and minimally elevated cholesterol. Usually present in childhood. Clinically associated with abdominal pain due to pancreatitis, eruptive xanthoma, hepatosplenomegaly and lipemia retinalis. The risk for atherosclerosis is not increased. The causes are either primary (autosomal recessive due to lipoprotein lipase or apo-C deficiency) or secondary, i.e., SLE and dysgammaglobulinemia.
  - ◊ Type II-A: Elevated LDL. Presenting with high cholesterol
  - ◊ Type II-B: Elevated LDL and VLDL. Presents with high cholesterol and high triglycerides. The risk for atherosclerosis is strong. The primary disorder includes several genetic disorders. Secondary causes include hypothyroidism, liver and kidney disease, porphyria, multiple myeloma.
  - ◊ Type III: Elevated IDL (dysbetalipoproteinemia). Presents with high cholesterol and triglycerides. Majority of patients with primary disorder are homozygous for apoprotein E2. Secondary causes are hypothyroidism and dysgammaglobulinemia.
  - ◊ Type IV: Elevated VLDL. Presents with high triglycerides and minimally elevated cholesterol. In some, the risk for atherosclerosis is increased.
  - ◊ Type V: Elevated chylomicrons and VLDL. Presents with very high triglycerides and high cholesterol. Genetic form is autosomal recessive due to LPL or apo-C deficiency. There is increased risk of atherosclerosis.

Note: Above classification is only descriptive and provides little insight into the genetic and mechanism of the disorder. The plasma lipoprotein change with time in any individual, a phenomenon to be expected because of the precursor-product relationship in the metabolism of VLDL and LDL and effect of diet on VLDL. A single disease state can lead to several different lipoprotein patterns and a single lipoprotein phenotype can be caused by multiple disease states.

System(s) affected: Cardiovascular, Endocrine/Metabolic, Gastrointestinal

Genetics:
- Familial hypercholesterolemia: autosomal dominant
- Polygenic hypercholesterolemia: polygenic
- Familial hypertriglyceridemia: autosomal dominant
- Familial combined hyperlipidemia: autosomal dominant
- Familial dysbetalipoproteinemia: autosomal recessive
- LPL and apo-C deficiency: autosomal recessive

Incidence/Prevalence in USA:
- Familial combined hyperlipidemia - 1-2%
- Familial hypertriglyceridemia - 1-2%
- Familial dyslipoproteinemia - 1/10,000

Predominant age: N/A

Predominant sex: Male > Female

SIGNS & SYMPTOMS
- Pancreatitis (TG over 1000)
- Chylomicronemia syndrome (TG over 2,000)
  - ◊ Memory loss/dementia
  - ◊ Dyspnea
  - ◊ Headache/vertigo
  - ◊ Eruptive xanthoma
  - ◊ Lipemia retinalis
  - ◊ Hepatosplenomegaly
  - ◊ Lymphadenopathy
  - ◊ Peripheral neuropathy/paresthesia
- Atherosclerosis

CAUSES
- Primary
  - ◊ Sporadic
  - ◊ Genetic
- Secondary
  - ◊ Condition associated with hypertriglyceridemia: Obesity, metabolic syndrome, diabetes mellitus, pregnancy, uremia/dialysis, hypothyroidism, nephrotic syndrome, acromegaly, Cushing syndrome, systemic lupus erythematosus, dysgammaglobulinemias, glycogen storage Type I, lipodystrophy
  - ◊ Drugs associated with hypertriglyceridemia: Alcohol, estrogen, tamoxifen, birth control pill, beta blockers, diuretics, glucocorticoid, isotretinoin/retinoid, bile acid binding resins cause a modest (<10%) elevation in some patients with Type II hyperlipidemia, HIV antiretroviral and protease inhibitors.

RISK FACTORS
- Genetic susceptibility
- Obesity
- Diabetes
- Alcoholism
- Exacerbated by medical illness and/or drug (see secondary causes)

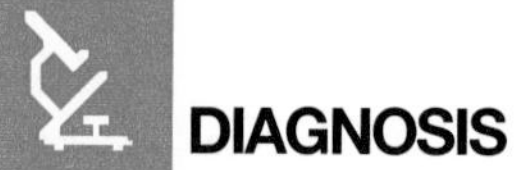

DIAGNOSIS

DIFFERENTIAL DIAGNOSIS Primary versus secondary

LABORATORY
- Turbid and milky serum
- Measurement of fasting plasma lipids

Drugs that may alter lab results: N/A

Disorders that may alter lab results:
- In TG induced pancreatitis, both serum and urinary amylase concentration may be normal due to interference of the plasma lipids or some other inhibitor with the assay
- TG may interfere with hemoglobin measurement, while bilirubin may be artificially elevated
- Pseudohyponatremia may result from very high TG

PATHOLOGICAL FINDINGS
- Atherosclerosis
- Pancreatitis
- In chylomicronemia syndrome - lipid laden macrophage (foam cell) infiltration of visceral organs, bone marrow and skin.

SPECIAL TESTS
- HDL cholesterol measurement (inversely related to TG)
- Apoprotein B measurement (may define a subset of mild hypertriglyceridemia patients at excess risk for CHD)
- LDL fractionation (type B or dense LDL is seen with atherogenic hypertriglyceridemia)
- Genetic testing for apoprotein E2

IMAGING
- Pancreatitis - CT of pancreas
- Atherosclerosis - doppler, angiography, ultra-fast CT of heart

DIAGNOSTIC PROCEDURES
- TG measured after a fast of 12-14 hours in:
  - ◊ Any individual with total cholesterol level of ≥ 240 mg/dL (6.22 mmol/L)
  - ◊ Men with HDL-C < 40 mg/dL and women with HDL-C < 50 mg/dL
  - ◊ Patients with acute pancreatitis, signs and symptoms of chylomicronemia syndrome and lactescence plasma
  - ◊ Individuals with past and present history of atherosclerosis, family history of premature arteriosclerosis
  - ◊ Individuals with 2 or more CHD risk factors; a disease or medications which raise triglycerides
  - ◊ Diabetic patients - impaired fasting glucose
  - ◊ Hypertensive (BP ≥ 130/85 mmHg) patients
  - ◊ Patients with abdominal obesity waist circumference: men > 40 in; women > 35 in

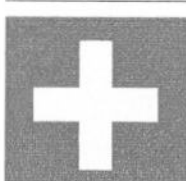

TREATMENT

APPROPRIATE HEALTH CARE Outpatient usually. Inpatient, if underlying disorder warrants.

GENERAL MEASURES
- A thorough search for correctable secondary causes and treating an underlying illness or removing an incriminated drug
- In case of primary hypertriglyceridemia, screening the other family members
- Treatment is indicated in distinct hypertriglyceridemia to prevent acute pancreatitis and in mild hypertriglyceridemia to prevent CAD in patients with high risk, strong family or personal history of atherosclerosis.
- Treatment of severe hypertriglyceridemia associated with pancreatitis - hospitalization, elimination of dietary fat; if diabetic, continuous IV infusion of insulin

SURGICAL MEASURES N/A

ACTIVITY Usually no restrictions. Exercise is important.

DIET Weight reduction to ideal body weight with AHA Step I Diet (50-55% carbohydrate, less than 30% fat)

PATIENT EDUCATION
- Smoking cessation
- Elimination of alcohol

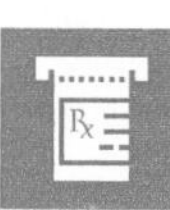

MEDICATIONS

DRUG(S) OF CHOICE
- Fibrates: reduce triglycerides 20-70%, decrease hepatic VLDL synthesis and increase VLDL metabolism
  - ◊ Fenofibrate (Tricor) 54-160 mg/day
  - ◊ Gemfibrozil (Lopid) 600 mg bid
- Niacin (Niaspan) 1-3 g/day
  - ◊ Reduces triglycerides by 20-50%
  - ◊ Inhibit hepatic VLDL synthesis

Contraindications: Refer to manufacturer's literature

Precautions:
- Gemfibrozil and fenofibrate
  - ◊ Side effects - upper and lower GI side effects (usually mild and are the most frequent adverse effects), cholelithiasis, myalgia, hepatotoxicity
  - ◊ May increase the incidence of myopathy/rhabdomyolysis if given with HMG-CoA reductase inhibitors
- Nicotinic acid
  - ◊ Side effects - flushing and pruritus (prostaglandin mediated and alleviated by ASA)
  - ◊ Upper GI discomfort and peptic ulcer disease (PUD)
  - ◊ Hepatotoxicity (more with sustained release preparation)
  - ◊ Hyperuricemia and gout, hyperglycemia, toxic amblyopia
  - ◊ Flushing less with extended release forms
  - ◊ Fulminant hepatic necrosis reported with extended release forms

Significant possible interactions: Gemfibrozil with warfarin - enhanced anticoagulation effect; monitor PT closely following addition or withdrawal of gemfibrozil

ALTERNATIVE DRUGS
- HMG-CoA reductase inhibitors [lovastatin (Mevacor, Altocor), pravastatin (Pravachol), simvastatin (Zocor), fluvastatin (Lescol), atorvastatin (Lipitor), rosuvastatin (Crestor)] lower triglycerides 10-30%
- Fish oil
- Glitazones - pioglitazone and rosiglitazone
- Clofibrate (Atromid-S)

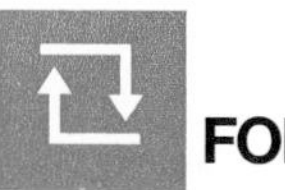

FOLLOWUP

PATIENT MONITORING
- Fasting lipid profile
- Liver function test, CPK, CBC diff
- Target goals
  - ◊ For pancreatitis - TG < 500 mg/dL (< 5.65 mmol/L)
  - ◊ For CHD: patients with CHD, diabetes, and 2 or more risk factors TG<150 mg/dL (<1.7 mmol/L)

PREVENTION/AVOIDANCE Covered in other headings

POSSIBLE COMPLICATIONS
- Acute pancreatitis
- Atherosclerosis

EXPECTED COURSE/PROGNOSIS
- Good in secondary disorder if the underlying causes are eliminated
- In primary, may need life-long treatment

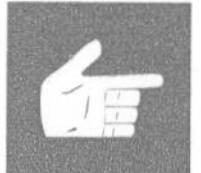

MISCELLANEOUS

ASSOCIATED CONDITIONS
- Mostly associated with low HDL cholesterol
- Mostly associated with dense LDL particle (type B)
- May be associated with hypercholesterolemia
- Metabolic syndrome (3 out of the following)
  - ◊ Abdominal obesity (male waist > 40 in; female waist > 35 in)
  - ◊ Triglycerides > 150 mg/dL
  - ◊ HDL cholesterol (male < 40; female < 50)
  - ◊ Blood pressure > 130/85
  - ◊ Fasting glucose > 100-125 mg/dL

AGE-RELATED FACTORS
Pediatric: In severe cases only, diet is recommended
Geriatric: N/A
Others: N/A

PREGNANCY All drugs are contraindicated during pregnancy

SYNONYMS
- Hyperlipidemia
- Chylomicronemia syndrome

ICD-9-CM
272.4 Other and unspecified hyperlipidemia
272.3 Hyperchylomicronemia
272.1 Pure hypertriglyceridemia
272.2 Mixed hyperlipidemia
272.0 Pure hypercholesterolemia

SEE ALSO
Hypercholesterolemia

OTHER NOTES N/A

ABBREVIATIONS
AHA = American Heart Association
CAD = coronary artery disease
HDL = high density lipoprotein
IDL = intermediate density lipoprotein
LDL = low density lipoprotein
LPL = lipoprotein lipase
PUD = peptic ulcer disease
TG = triglycerides
VLDL = very low density lipoprotein

REFERENCES

- The National Cholesterol Education Program (NCEP) expert panel on detection, evaluation, and treatment of high blood cholesterol in adults (Adult Treatment Panel III). JAMA 2001;285(19):2486-97
- Grundy SM. Hypertriglyceridemia, insulin resistance, and the metabolic syndrome. Am J Cardiol 1999;83(9B):25F-29F
- Miller M. Current perspectives on the management of hypertriglyceridemia. Am Heart J 2000;140(2):232-40

Web references: 0 available at www.5mcc.com
Illustrations 5 available

Author(s):
Reza Moattari, MD

BASICS

DESCRIPTION Hypochondriasis is a mental disorder associated with an excessive worry about one's health and a preoccupation with a variety of symptoms whereby the person is convinced he/she is suffering from some sort of disease. Patients suffering from this condition mostly seek medical attention searching for the physician that will diagnose them with a physical illness to explain their symptoms. This often leads to a variety of excessive work-ups, including many repetitive and expensive lab tests and diagnostic procedures. Even though these are necessary to rule out some serious physical disease, this diagnosis should not be made by exclusion alone, but should also be made by using inclusive criteria as mentioned below.

System(s) affected: Nervous

Genetics: Some studies show an increase prevalence of hypochondriasis in families, especially among identical twins and first degree relatives.

Incidence/Prevalence in USA:
- Some studies point out that hypochondriasis is present in 3-14% of patients seen by primary care physicians.
- Some surveys show that 10-20% of the general population worry about illness from time to time. About 45% of patients seen by mental health professional worry about illness from time to time.

Predominant age: The peak incidence is believed to happen during the fourth or fifth decade of life, although all age groups can be affected, including children, adolescents, and the elderly.

Predominant sex: It is found equally in men and women; however, women tend to seek help more often than men

SIGNS & SYMPTOMS
- Preoccupation with fears of having, or the idea that one has, a serious disease based on the person's misinterpretation of bodily symptoms
- The preoccupation persists despite appropriate medical evaluation and reassurance
- The belief is not of delusional intensity (as in delusional disorder, somatic type) and is not restricted to a circumscribed concern about appearance (as in body dysmorphic disorder).
- The preoccupation causes clinically significant distress impairment in social, occupational, or other important areas of functioning.
- The duration of the disturbance is at least 6 months
- The preoccupation is not better accounted for by generalized anxiety disorder, obsessive-compulsive disorder, panic disorder, a major depressive episode, separation anxiety, or another somatoform disorder.

CAUSES
- Biological: There is some evidence suggesting that patients with hypochondriasis may be born with a tendency to amplify somatic sensations and that they have lower threshold and a lower tolerance of physical discomfort
- Life events: Medical diseases may predispose a patient to hypochondriasis, such as certain patients being highly sensitive to certain physical symptoms following an acute stroke, myocardial infarction, intensive treatment following malignant illness, organ transplantation, etc. These may be experienced by the patient or by a close family member or friend.
- Childhood events: The experience of numerous or serious actual medical illnesses during one's childhood may predispose the individual to hypochondriasis later on in life.
- Psychological: Many authors view hypochondriasis as the patient's psychodynamic defense against guilt, shame, low self-esteem, and a narcissistic over-indulgence with one's self. Other authors view it as the patient's way of seeking attention by overly identifying with the sick role which offers the patient a way to alleviate symptoms of anxiety and seek reassurance.
- Sociocultural: Some societies and cultures view mental symptoms in a pejorative and stigmatized way, blaming the patient for his/her illness, however, if the patient has physical symptoms and a bona fide medical diagnosis, he/she are treated with greater empathy, dignity, and respect and are not blamed for causing their illness.

RISK FACTORS Exposure to life-threatening medical conditions and procedures in one's childhood, adolescence, or in adult life

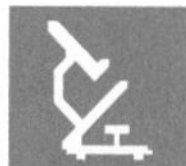

DIAGNOSIS

DIFFERENTIAL DIAGNOSIS
- Any patient suffering from hypochondriasis, as with any other psychiatric disorder is not immune from developing a medical/organic disease. Such organic diseases as those affecting many organ systems like connective tissue diseases, autoimmune diseases, as well as more focused single-organ type diseases must always be considered as a possibility in these patients.
- Underlying depressive disorders
- Schizophrenia
- Delusional disorders
- Conversion disorder
- Anxiety disorder
- Panic disorder
- Obsessive-compulsive disorder
- Factitious disorder with physical symptoms
- Somatization disorder
- Chronic pain disorder
- Body Dysmorphic disorder
- Malingering
- Munchausen syndrome

LABORATORY
- Lab tests are used to rule out organic diseases

Drugs that may alter lab results: N/A

Disorders that may alter lab results: N/A

PATHOLOGICAL FINDINGS N/A

SPECIAL TESTS N/A

IMAGING N/A

DIAGNOSTIC PROCEDURES
- Thorough mental status examination
- Psychological testing is used to rule out other psychiatric disorders and specifically confirm the diagnosis of hypochondriasis

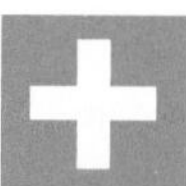

TREATMENT

APPROPRIATE HEALTH CARE Outpatient

GENERAL MEASURES
- Treatment of choice is individual psychotherapy delivered on an outpatient basis
- Many patients do better with supportive psychotherapy and behavior modification focused on the alleviation of their symptoms
- Group therapy: Some patients do better in a group setting where they get social support and interaction with others
- Reassuring the patient by repeating lab tests is only short-lived and does not solve the underlying problem

SURGICAL MEASURES N/A

ACTIVITY Regular exercise in moderation

DIET Good nutrition

PATIENT EDUCATION Providing cognitive knowledge about the condition strengthens the patient's intellectual capacities and provides a structure for better response to somatic symptoms, cognitive behavioral and other psychotherapeutic interventions.

MEDICATIONS

DRUG(S) OF CHOICE
- No specific drug is known to cure hypochondriasis
- Antidepressants and antianxiety medications are most successful in patients who have a preponderance of anxiety and depressive symptoms
- The SSRI group (selective serotonin reuptake inhibitors) are most helpful and have to be used selectively based on patient's tolerance to side effects
- Select patients with a preponderance of obsessive-compulsive symptoms have responded to such drugs as clomipramine 50-150 mg/day or fluoxetine 20-80 mg/day or fluvoxamine 100-300 mg/day
- Sertraline 50-100 mg/day
- Citalopram 20-60 mg/day
- Escitalopram 10-20 mg/day
- Paroxetine 10-60 mg/day
- Paroxetine CR 12.5-25 mg/day

Contraindications:
- Avoid medications that patient is allergic to
- Avoid medications with many side effects
- Avoid medications with known drug interactions

Precautions: Avoid long term use of narcotics and other addictive medication

Significant possible interactions: N/A

ALTERNATIVE DRUGS
- Lithium carbonate: 300-900 mg/day with an optimal blood level of 0.5-0.9 mEq/L
- Valproic acid: 500-2000 mg/day or 15-60 mg/kg/day with an optimal plasma level of 50-100 μg/mL

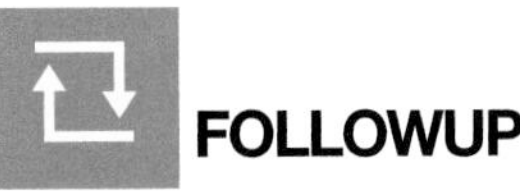

FOLLOWUP

PATIENT MONITORING
- Patients should be seen on a regular basis in the primary care physician's office or with a psychotherapist
- Appointments should be scheduled regardless of whether the patient has new symptoms or not
- Avoid the use of long hospitalizations and unnecessary lab work-ups
- Avoid statements such as, "Call me if you have a problem" or "Make an appointment only if you have a problem"
- Provide reassurance by careful listening to the patient's concerns. Allow the patient to talk about psychosocial issues.
- Provide a safe environment for empathic listening and understanding

PREVENTION/AVOIDANCE N/A

POSSIBLE COMPLICATIONS
- Risks of repeated and unnecessary lab and diagnostic procedures
- Narcotic and other drug addictions

EXPECTED COURSE/PROGNOSIS
- The natural history of this condition is usually chronic
- It has fluctuations in the intensity with periods of relative remission and exacerbation of acuity that may create destruction in the patient's life
- Prognosis varies depending on the patient's personality structure, education, social support system, intelligence, and motivation for change
- Many psychiatrists consider this condition to have a poor prognosis for psychoanalytic treatment

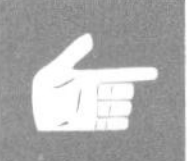

MISCELLANEOUS

ASSOCIATED CONDITIONS
Somatization disorder, conversion disorder, depressive disorder NOS, anxiety disorder NOS

AGE-RELATED FACTORS
Pediatric: Early childhood exposure to serious medical illness and diagnostic procedures predisposes these patients to develop hypochondriasis in adult life

Geriatric: Elderly patients usually have a higher frequency for chronic medical illness which may co-exist with hypochondriasis and complicates the treatment of hypochondriasis

Others: N/A

PREGNANCY N/A

SYNONYMS
- Hypochondriacal neurosis
- Hypochondria

ICD-9-CM
300.7 Hypochondriasis

SEE ALSO

OTHER NOTES N/A

ABBREVIATIONS N/A

REFERENCES

- Creed F, Barsky A. A systematic review of the epidemiology of somatisation disorder and hypochondriasis. J Psychosom Res 2004;56(4):391-408
- Magarinos M, Zafar U, Nissenson K, Blanco C. Epidemiology and treatment of hypochondriasis. CNS Drugs 2002;16(1):9-22
- Phillips KA. Somatoform and factitious disorders. Rev of Psychiatr 2001:20(3):27-65
- Noyes R Jr. The relationship of hypochondriasis to anxiety disorders. General Hosp Psychiatry 1999;21:8-17
- Clark DM, et al. Two psychological treatments for hypochondriasis. A randomized controlled trial. British J of psychiatry 1999;173:218-225
- Rief W, et al. Cognitive aspects of hypochondriasis and the somatization syndrome. J of Abnormal psychiatry 1998;107:587-595
- Bouman TK, Visser S. Cognitive and behavioral treatment of hypochondriasis. Psychotherapy and Psychosomatics 1998;67:214-221
- Ferguson E. Hypochondriacal concerns symptoms reporting and secondary gain mechanism. British J of Medical Psychology 1998;71:281-295
- Marcus DK. The cognitive-behavioral model of hypochondriasis: Misinformation and triggers. J of Psychosomatic Research 1999;47(1):79-91
- Barsky AJ, Cleary PD, Sarnie MD, Klerman GL: The course of transient hypochondriasis. Psychiatry 1993;150:484-488
- Diagnostic and Statistical Manual of Mental Disorders (DSM-IV). 4th Ed. Washington, DC, American Psychiatric Association, 445-469, 1994
- Ford CV: Dimensions of somatization & hypochondriasis. Neurol Clin 1995;13:241-253
- Ford CV: The Somatizing Disorders. Psychosomatic 1986;27:327-337
- Kellner R: Hypochondriasis and somatization. JAMA 1987;258:2718-2722
- Smith GR: Somatization disorder: In the Medical Setting. Washington, DC, National Institute of Mental Health, 1990
- Fallon BA, Schneier FR, Marxhal R, Campeas R, Vermes D, Goetz D, Liebowitz MR: The pharmacotherapy of hypochondriasis. Psychopharmacology Bulletin 1996;32(4);607-11
- Mabe PA, Riley WT, Jones LR, Hobson DP: The medical context of hypochondriacal traits. International Journal of Psychiatry in Medicine, 1996;26(4):443-459
- Gureje O, Ustun TB, Simon GE: The syndrome of hypochondriasis: a cross-national study in primary care. Psychological Medicine 1997;27(5):1001-1010
- Fallon BA. Pharmacologic strategies for hypochondriasis. In: Hypochondriasis: Modern Perspectives on an Ancient Malady. Starcevic V, Lipsitt Dr, editors. New York; Oxford University Press:2001:p329-351
- Visser S, Bouman TK. The treatment of hypochondriasis: exposure plus response prevention vs cognitive therapy. Behav Res Ther. 2001 Apr;39(4):423-42
- Barsky AJ, Cleary PD, Sarnie MD, Klerman GL: The course of transient hypochondriasis. Psychiatry 1993;150:484-488
- Diagnostic and Statistical Manual of Mental Disorders (DSM-IV). 4th Ed. Washington, DC, American Psychiatric Association, 445-469, 1994
- Ford CV: Dimensions of somatization & hypochondriasis. Neurol Clin 1995;13:241-253
- Ford CV: The Somatizing Disorders. Psychosomatic 1986;27:327-337

Web references: 0 available at www.5mcc.com

Illustrations N/A

Author(s):
Moshe S. Torem, MD

BASICS

DESCRIPTION An abnormally low concentration of glucose in the circulating blood of a diabetic. A side effect of insulin and/or sulfonylurea treatment in the course of normal treatment of diabetes mellitus. Hypoglycemia may also occur as a condition in itself or in association with other disorders. Often referred to as an "insulin reaction".

System(s) affected: Endocrine/Metabolic

Genetics: No known genetic pattern

Incidence/Prevalence in USA:
- Most type 1 diabetics experience hypoglycemia. Tightly controlled type 1 often experience hypoglycemia weekly.
- Type 2 diabetics experience hypoglycemia much less frequently than type 1 diabetics
- Most common in type 1 diabetics
- Common in type 2 diabetic patients treated with insulin and/or insulin secretagogues
- Apha-glucosidase inhibitors, biguanides and thiazolidinediones do not cause hypoglycemia when used as monotherapy, but may enhance the risk of hypoglycemia when used in combination with insulin and/or sulfonylureas or meglitinides.
- Uncommon in diabetics treated with diet and exercise alone
- Studies comparing insulin lispro (human analog) with human regular insulin did not demonstrate a difference in frequency of hypoglycemia
- Hypoglycemia is the most common immediate health problem for students with diabetes

Predominant age: All ages

Predominant sex: Male = Female

SIGNS & SYMPTOMS
- Adrenergic hypoglycemia signs and symptoms include:
  - ◊ Pallor
  - ◊ Tremulousness
  - ◊ Nervous anxiety
  - ◊ Irritability
  - ◊ Tachycardia
  - ◊ Diaphoresis
  - ◊ Weakness
- Neuroglycopenic hypoglycemia signs and symptoms include:
  - ◊ Diplopia
  - ◊ Lethargy
  - ◊ Inability to concentrate or remember
  - ◊ Confusion
  - ◊ Behavior change
  - ◊ Paresthesias
  - ◊ Hunger
  - ◊ Stupor
  - ◊ Seizure
  - ◊ Coma
- Glycemic threshold/response
  - ◊ ≈80 mg/dL - decreased insulin secretion
  - ◊ ≈65 mg/dL - increased glucagon, epinephrine, cortisol, and growth hormone secretion
  - ◊ ≈55 mg/dL - symptoms
  - ◊ ≈45 mg/dL - cognitive dysfunction

CAUSES
- Loss of the hormonal counter-regulatory mechanism in glucose metabolism
- Diet - too little food (skipping a meal)
- Medication - too much insulin or oral hypoglycemic agent (improper dose or timing)
- Erratic absorption of insulin or oral hypoglycemics
- Adverse reaction from other medications
- Exercise - unplanned or excessive exercise
- Alcohol consumption
- Vomiting or diarrhea
- Gastroparesis

RISK FACTORS
- 2-3 times more common in the "tight control" patient (according to data from the Diabetes Control and Complications Trial).
- Most type 1 diabetics experience hypoglycemia. Type 2 diabetics experience hypoglycemia much less frequently unless insulin is used. Uncommon in those treated with diet and exercise alone.
- Nearly 3/4 of severe hypoglycemic episodes occur during sleep
- Autonomic neuropathy
- Illness, stress and unplanned life events
- Greater than 5 years duration of diabetes
- Elderly patient
- Renal disease
- Liver disease
- Congestive heart failure
- Hypothyroidism
- Hypoadrenalism
- Gastroenteritis
- Starvation or prolonged fasting
- Alcoholism
- Oral hypoglycemics with long duration and high potency have greater hypoglycemic risks

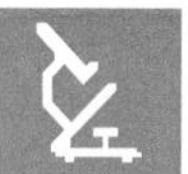

DIAGNOSIS

DIFFERENTIAL DIAGNOSIS
- Aspirin induces hypoglycemia in some children
- Drinking alcohol can cause blood sugar to drop in sensitive individuals
- Hypoglycemia is well documented in chronic alcoholics and binge drinkers
- Eating unripe ackee fruit from Jamaica is a rare cause of low blood sugar
- Gastrointestinal dysfunction causing postprandial hypoglycemia or alimentary reactive hypoglycemia
- Hormonal deficiency states (hormonal reactive hypoglycemia)
- Idiopathic reactive hypoglycemia
- Hypoglycemia of sepsis
- Islet cell tumors
- Factitious hypoglycemia from surreptitious injection of insulin
- Hypoglycemia may be found in nondiabetics under certain conditions such as early pregnancy, prolonged fasting, and long periods of strenuous exercise
- Reactive hypoglycemia a popular diagnosis 20 years ago, is actually quite rare

LABORATORY
- Plasma glucose ≤ 45 mg/dL (≤ 2.5 mmol/L) or less
- Suspect low when plasma glucose is 45-60 mg/dL (2.5 and 3.33 mmol/L)
- In children plasma glucose ≤ 40 mg/dL (≤ 2.22 mmol/L)
- Suspect hypoglycemic unawareness in asymptomatic type 1 diabetes with low or normal HgbA1c

Drugs that may alter lab results: N/A

Disorders that may alter lab results: Hemoglobinopathies may alter HgbA1c results

PATHOLOGICAL FINDINGS N/A

SPECIAL TESTS
Chronic hypoglycemia is evidenced by a low glycohemoglobin level

IMAGING N/A

DIAGNOSTIC PROCEDURES
- History and physical exam
- Plasma, or whole blood glucose
- Severe hypoglycemia episodes are defined as those in which the patient has incapacity sufficient to require the assistance of another person

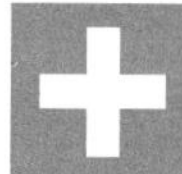

TREATMENT

APPROPRIATE HEALTH CARE
- Outpatient except for complicating emergencies (coma, inapparent cause, long acting oral hypoglycemic)
- Admit the patient if:
  - ◊ There is any doubt of the cause
  - ◊ Expectation of prolonged hypoglycemia (eg, caused by a sulfonylurea drug)
  - ◊ Inability of the patient to drink
  - ◊ The treatment has not resulted in prompt recovery of sensorium
  - ◊ Seizures, coma, or altered behavior (eg, ataxia, disorientation, unstable motor coordination, dysphasia) secondary to documented or suspected hypoglycemia

GENERAL MEASURES
- Glucose is the preferred treatment for hypoglycemia, however, any form of carbohydrate that contains glucose should be effective
- Education is the mainstay of prevention
- Blood glucose targets should be individualized
- Any sugar-containing food or beverage which can be rapidly absorbed, eg, juice (4-6 ounces), candy (5-6 pieces of hard candy) or non-diet soda
- OTC glucose tablets or gels
- Hypoglycemic unawareness (most commonly found in patients with long-standing type 1 DM) is a major risk factor for severe hypoglycemic reactions
- Intensive therapy for diabetes should be adjusted to minimize the occurrence of severe hypoglycemia
- Meticulous prevention of hypoglycemia can reverse hypoglycemia unawareness
- Hypoglycemia unawareness can be reversed by avoidance of iatrogenic hypoglycemia
- In younger children, blood glucose profiles should include early morning measurements

SURGICAL MEASURES N/A

ACTIVITY
- Rest until glucose is normal
- For patients taking insulin
  - ◊ For planned exercise, consider a reduced insulin dosage to prevent hypoglycemia
  - ◊ Additional carbohydrates may be needed for unplanned exercise
- Moderate intensity exercise increases glucose uptake by 2-3 mg/kg/min above usual requirements (a 70 kg person needs ≈10-15 g carbohydrates per hour of moderate physical activity)

DIET
- Avoid extra calories without changing the source of the problem - excess insulin or oral hypoglycemic
- If alcohol is consumed, it should be with food to reduce the risk of hypoglycemia
- Protein does not slow the absorption of carbohydrates
- Fats may slow the absorption of carbohydrates

PATIENT EDUCATION
- Most important measure is prevention
- Educate patients, their relatives and close friends, teachers and supervisors
- Teach self-monitoring of blood glucose (SMBG) and self-adjustment for insulin therapy, diet control, and exercise regimen
- Emergency medical assistance may be needed if the person does not recover within a few minutes
- Carry an ID tag
- Always keep some type of quick-acting carbohydrate close by

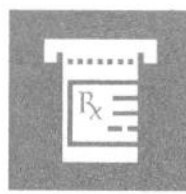

MEDICATIONS

DRUG(S) OF CHOICE
- General
  - ◊ Oral administration of small molecule sugars (saccharose/glucose) - glucose is preferred
  - ◊ Approximately 60-90 calories (15-20 g of glucose) repeated every 15 minutes until blood sugar is 100 mg/dL (5.55 mmol/L) or more
  - ◊ It takes about 15 minutes for the carbohydrates to be digested and to enter the blood stream as glucose
- In patients with loss of consciousness at home
  - ◊ Administer glucagon IM or subcutaneous in the deltoid or anterior thigh:
  - ◊ If under 5 years old, give 0.25 to 0.50 mg
  - ◊ Older child (5-10 years old) give 0.50 to 1 mg
  - ◊ Over 10 years old, give 1 mg
- If emergency medical personnel are present or patient hospitalized
  - ◊ Give one-half amp 50% dextrose every 5-10 minutes until the patient awakens
  - ◊ Then feed orally and/or administer 5% dextrose intravenously at a level that will maintain the blood glucose at a level above 100 mg/dL.
  - ◊ Patients with hypoglycemia secondary to oral hypoglycemics should be monitored for 24-48 hours since hypoglycemia may recur after apparent clinical recovery

Contraindications: None
Precautions: Refer to manufacturer's literature
Significant possible interactions:
- Treatment may cause hyperglycemia (called Somogyi phenomenon)
- Clearance of certain oral hypoglycemics from plasma may be prolonged in persons with liver disease

ALTERNATIVE DRUGS Acarbose, a potent alpha-glucosidase inhibitor slows the absorption kinetics of dietary carbohydrates by reversible competitive inhibition of alpha-glucosidase activity, and so reduces the post-prandial blood glucose increment and insulin response

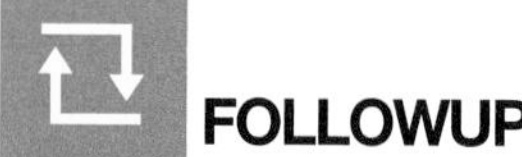

FOLLOWUP

PATIENT MONITORING Self-monitoring of blood glucose

PREVENTION/AVOIDANCE
- Educating patients, family, teachers and close friends
- Maintaining a routine schedule of diet, medication and exercise
- Regular blood glucose testing
- Continuous subcutaneous glucose monitoring
- Wearing a medical alert identification bracelet or necklace
- Those patients who experience recurrent hypoglycemic episodes should be individually evaluated and when appropriate, the employment position should be modified
- Information should be given to the school or daycare setting so that personnel are aware of the diagnosis of diabetes in a student and the signs, symptoms and treatment of hypoglycemia
- Blood glucose testing should be available at school or workplace

POSSIBLE COMPLICATIONS
- Coma
- Seizure
- Prolonged or severe hypoglycemia may cause permanent neurological damage and/or cognitive impairment
- Evaluation of neuropsychological functioning of DCCT participants shows no evidence of significant cognitive deterioration associated with repeated episodes of severe hypoglycemia. Repeated episodes of severe hypoglycemia are not necessarily associated with cognitive dysfunction.
- Significant differences have been documented between adults and children in the incidence of hypoglycemia
- Myocardial infarction, stroke, especially in the elderly

EXPECTED COURSE/PROGNOSIS
Full recovery is usual depending on the rapidity of diagnosis and treatment

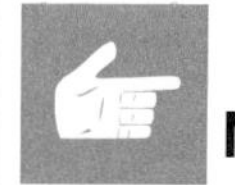

MISCELLANEOUS

ASSOCIATED CONDITIONS
- Autonomic dysfunction
- Neuropathies
- Cardiomyopathies

AGE-RELATED FACTORS
Pediatric: Significance of hypoglycemia in infants of diabetic mothers remains to be defined
Geriatric: Often not diagnosed in the elderly
Others: N/A

PREGNANCY With hypoglycemic reactions during pregnancy the fetus is less likely to be hypoglycemic because of active transport of glucose across the placenta

SYNONYMS
- Low blood sugar
- Insulin reaction
- Insulin shock
- Reactive hypoglycemia

ICD-9-CM
250.82 Diabetes with other specified manifestations, type 2 or unspecified type, uncontrolled
300.19 Other and unspecified factitious illness
579.3 Other and unspecified postsurgical nonabsorption
775.0 Syndrome of "infant of a diabetic mother"
775.6 Neonatal hypoglycemia
962.3 Poisoning by insulins and antidiabetic agents

SEE ALSO
Diabetes mellitus, Type 1
Diabetes mellitus, Type 2

OTHER NOTES
- The tighter the diabetic control the greater the importance of home glucose monitoring to avoid hypoglycemia
- In patients receiving beta blockers, the drug will mask tachycardia, but not the sweating

ABBREVIATIONS N/A

REFERENCES

- American Diabetes Association Clinical Practice recommendations. Diabetes Care 2003:26(s1)
- Diabetes Control and Complications Trial (DCCT). Adverse events and their association with treatment regimens in the Diabetes Control and Complications Trial. Diabetes Care 1995;18(11):1415-27
- National Diabetes Information Clearinghouse (NDIC) a service of the National Institute of Diabetes and Digestive and Kidney Diseases (NIDDK)
- American Diabetes Association
- Herbel G, Boyle PJ. Hypoglycemia. Pathophysiology and treatment. Endocrinol Metab Clin North Am 2000;29(4):725-43

Web references: 2 available at www.5mcc.com
Illustrations N/A

Author(s):
Joseph A. Florence, MD

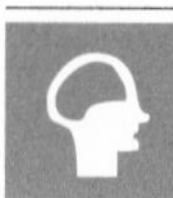

BASICS

DESCRIPTION Hypoglycemia is defined by Whipple triad: 1) low plasma glucose level, 2) symptoms (see list below), 3) symptoms are relieved with correction of low blood sugar. It occurs often in diabetic patients (covered under a separate topic) and has a less common appearance in nondiabetic patients.
- Reactive hypoglycemia - in response to a meal, specific nutrients, or drugs. May occur within 2-3 hours after a meal, or later. Also seen after gastrointestinal surgery (in association with dumping syndrome in some patients).
- Spontaneous (fasting) hypoglycemia - may be associated with a primary condition, e.g., hypopituitarism, Addison disease, myxedema, or in disorders related to liver malfunction, and renal failure. If hypoglycemia presents as a primary manifestation, other disorders to consider include hyperinsulinism and extrapancreatic tumors.

System(s) affected: Endocrine/Metabolic
Genetics: Some aspects may involve genetics (e.g., hereditary fructose intolerance)
Incidence/Prevalence in USA: Unknown
Predominant age: Older adult
Predominant sex: Female > Male

SIGNS & SYMPTOMS
- Central nervous system (CNS); these symptoms predominate if glucose dropping gradually:
  - ◊ Headache
  - ◊ Confusion
  - ◊ Visual disturbances
  - ◊ Changes in personality
  - ◊ Convulsions
  - ◊ Coma
- Heart
  - ◊ Palpitations
  - ◊ Hypotension
- Gastrointestinal
  - ◊ Hunger
  - ◊ Nausea
  - ◊ Belching
- Adrenergic; these symptoms are more prominent in acute drop in glucose (as in insulin reaction)
  - ◊ Sweating
  - ◊ Anxiety
  - ◊ Tremulousness
  - ◊ Dizziness
  - ◊ Diaphoresis
  - ◊ Nervousness

CAUSES
- Reactive: Post-prandial hypoglycemia
  - ◊ Alimentary hyperinsulinism
  - ◊ Meals (high in refined carbohydrates)
  - ◊ Certain nutrients, e.g., fructose, galactose, leucine
  - ◊ Glucose intolerance (prediabetic)
  - ◊ Pseudohypoglycemia - patients with symptoms of hypoglycemia or self-diagnosis in whom low blood sugars may not be detectable and who may be impossible to convince that they do not suffer from hypoglycemia after all tests are found to be normal
  - ◊ Gastrointestinal surgery
  - ◊ Idiopathic (unknown)
- Spontaneous: Fasting hypoglycemia
  - ◊ Drugs or alcohol (insulin or sulfonylureas, propranolol, salicylates, quinine, disopyramide, or pentamidine
  - ◊ Surreptitious drug use (self-injection of insulin or taking oral hypoglycemic in nondiabetic patients
  - ◊ Hepatic disease
  - ◊ Islet cell hyperplasia or tumor
  - ◊ Catecholamine deficiency
  - ◊ Glucagon deficiency
  - ◊ Extrapancreatic tumor
  - ◊ Exercise
  - ◊ Fever
  - ◊ Pregnancy
  - ◊ Renal glycosuria
  - ◊ Large tumor
  - ◊ Ketotic hypoglycemia of childhood
  - ◊ Adrenal insufficiency
  - ◊ Hypopituitarism
  - ◊ Enzyme deficiencies or defects
  - ◊ Severe malnutrition
  - ◊ Sepsis

RISK FACTORS Listed with Causes

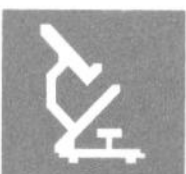

DIAGNOSIS

DIFFERENTIAL DIAGNOSIS
- CNS disorders
- Psychogenic

LABORATORY
- Lab studies best done when patient is symptomatic
- Measurement of blood and plasma glucose
- C-peptide measurement
- Check liver studies, serum insulin, cortisol

Drugs that may alter lab results: Many drugs can affect levels. Refer to a drug or laboratory reference.

Disorders that may alter lab results: N/A

PATHOLOGICAL FINDINGS N/A

SPECIAL TESTS
- Plasma glucose overnight fasting - < 60 mg/dL (< 3.33 mmol/L)
- Plasma glucose 72-hour fasting - < 45 mg/dL (< 2.5 mmol/L) for females and < 55 mg/dL (< 3.05 mmol/L) for males
- Oral glucose tolerance - < 50 mg/dL (< 2.78 mmol/L)
- IV tolbutamide test - normal
- Insulin radioimmunoassay - elevated insulin levels if islet cell tumor present

IMAGING Abdominal CT to rule out abdominal tumor

DIAGNOSTIC PROCEDURES
- Misinterpretation of glucose tolerance tests may lead to an misdiagnosis of hypoglycemia. More than 1/3 of normal patients have hypoglycemia with or without symptoms during a 4 hour glucose tolerance test. However, these individuals may be at risk for developing type II diabetes mellitus.
- For definitive diagnosis - patient should have(1) documented occurrence of low blood glucose levels(2) symptoms that occur when the blood glucose is low(3) evidence that the symptoms are relieved specifically by the ingestion of sugar or other food(4) identification of the particular type of hypoglycemia

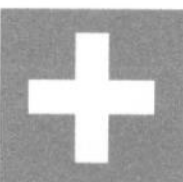

TREATMENT

APPROPRIATE HEALTH CARE Outpatient except for severe cases. May also be inpatient for testing.

GENERAL MEASURES
- Oral carbohydrate for alert patient without drug overdose (2-3 tablespoons of sugar in glass of water or fruit juice, 1-2 cups of milk, a piece of fruit, soda cracker)
- If patient unable to swallow, glucagon IM or subcutaneously
- In hypoglycemia caused by drugs or certain nutrients, avoid or control the causative agents
- In hypoglycemia following meals - try high protein diet with restricted carbohydrates
- Avoid stress
- "Nonhypoglycemic hypoglycemia" or "pseudohypoglycemia"
  - ◊ Many patients (often females, ages 20-45) present with the diagnosis of reactive hypoglycemia (self-diagnosed or misinterpretation of tests)
  - ◊ Symptoms usually pertain to chronic fatigue and somatic complaints (stress often has a role in these symptoms)
  - ◊ Management is difficult. Listening is important. Dietary changes, e.g., 120 gm carbohydrate diet, low in simple sugars can be recommended.
  - ◊ Counseling - for stress or other problems may be useful

SURGICAL MEASURES If islet cell tumor (insulinoma) - surgery is the treatment of choice. If it is inoperable, drug therapy may relieve symptoms.

ACTIVITY May need to revise exercise routine

DIET
- High protein, low carbohydrate
- Frequent small feedings (6) instead of 2-3 larger meals
- Avoid fasting

PATIENT EDUCATION
- Instructions about fasting tests and interpretations of results
- Dietary instruction
- Counseling for stress, if appropriate
- Recognition of early symptoms of hypoglycemia and how to take corrective action

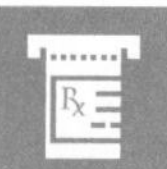

MEDICATIONS

DRUG(S) OF CHOICE
- Once an established diagnosis is made, drug therapy appropriate to the underlying disorder
- In patient unable to swallow - glucagon IM or subcutaneously. If no response, give IV glucose. For serious hypoglycemia, give IV bolus of 25-50 g of 50% glucose solution followed by a constant infusion of glucose until the patient can take by mouth.
- Insulinoma - see separate topic in book
- Postsurgical gastrectomy patients unresponsive to diet changes may benefit from propantheline which delays gastric emptying

Contraindications: Refer to manufacturer's literature
Precautions: Refer to manufacturer's literature
Significant possible interactions: Refer to manufacturer's literature

ALTERNATIVE DRUGS N/A

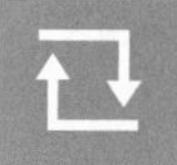

FOLLOWUP

PATIENT MONITORING
- Dependent on type and severity of symptoms, and treatment of underlying cause
- Hypoglycemia from sulfonylurea can last for days

PREVENTION/AVOIDANCE
- Follow dietary and exercise guidelines
- Patient recognition of early symptoms and taking corrective action

POSSIBLE COMPLICATIONS If tumor removed (insulinoma), some surgical risk involved

EXPECTED COURSE/PROGNOSIS
Favorable, with recognition and appropriate treatment

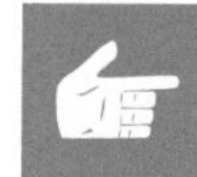

MISCELLANEOUS

ASSOCIATED CONDITIONS
- Insulinoma
- Severe liver disease
- Alcoholism
- Adrenocortical insufficiency
- Myxedema
- Malnutrition (patients with renal failure)
- Gastrointestinal surgery
- Panhypopituitarism
- Addison disease

AGE-RELATED FACTORS
Pediatric: Usually divided into 2 syndromes
(1) transient neonatal hypoglycemia and
(2) hypoglycemia of infancy and childhood
Geriatric: More likely to have underlying disorders or be using causative drugs
Others: N/A

PREGNANCY N/A

SYNONYMS
- Postprandial hypoglycemia
- Functional hypoglycemia
- Idiopathic hypoglycemia
- Alimentary hypoglycemia
- Postgastrectomy hypoglycemia
- Alcohol-induced hypoglycemia
- Factitious hypoglycemia
- Iatrogenic hypoglycemia
- Exogenous hypoglycemia

ICD-9-CM
251.2 Hypoglycemia, unspecified
251.0 Hypoglycemic coma
251.1 Other specified hypoglycemia

SEE ALSO
Hypoglycemia, diabetic
Insulinoma

OTHER NOTES N/A

ABBREVIATIONS N/A

REFERENCES

- Service FJ. Classification of hypoglycemic disorders. Endocrinol & Metabol Clin of NA 1999;28(3):501-17
- Cryer PE. Hypoglycemia. In: Braunwald E, Fauci AS, et al, eds. Harrison's Principles of Internal Medicine. 15th ed. New York, McGraw-Hill, 2001: p2138-43

Web references: 3 available at www.5mcc.com
Illustrations N/A

Author(s):
F. David Schneider, MD, MSPH

BASICS

DESCRIPTION Hypokalemia occurs when serum potassium (K+) concentration is below the normal range, commonly 3.5-5.0 mEq/L (3.5-5.0 mmol/L).
System(s) affected: Endocrine/Metabolic, Musculoskeletal, Nervous, Renal/Urologic
Genetics:
- Some familial disorders are rare causes of hypokalemia
  - ◊ Familial hypokalemic periodic paralysis
  - ◊ Congenital adrenogenital syndromes
  - ◊ Liddle syndrome
  - ◊ Familial interstitial nephritis

Incidence/Prevalence in USA: Common
Predominant age: N/A
Predominant sex: Male = Female

SIGNS & SYMPTOMS
- Neuromuscular (most prominent manifestations) - skeletal muscle weakness (may range from mild weakness to total paralysis, including respiratory muscles); may lead to rhabdomyolysis in severe cases. Smooth muscle involvement may lead to gastrointestinal hypomotility producing ileus and constipation.
- Cardiovascular - ventricular arrhythmias, hypotension, cardiac arrest
- Renal - polyuria, nocturia due to impaired concentrating ability
- Metabolic - hyperglycemia

CAUSES
- General causes
  - ◊ Decreased intake (uncommon): anorexia nervosa, deficient diet in alcoholics
  - ◊ Gastrointestinal loss: vomiting, diarrhea, laxative abuse, fistulas, villous adenoma, ureterosigmoidostomy
  - ◊ Intracellular shift of K: metabolic alkalosis, insulin excess, beta adrenergic catecholamine excess (acute stress, intake of B2 agonists), hypokalemic periodic paralysis, intoxications (theophylline, barium, toluene)
- Renal potassium loss
  - ◊ Drugs: diuretics, penicillin antibiotics, aminoglycosides
  - ◊ Mineralocorticoid excess states: primary hyperaldosteronism, secondary hyperaldosteronism (congestive heart failure, cirrhosis, nephrotic syndrome, malignant hypertension, renin-producing tumors), Bartter syndrome, congenital adrenogenital syndromes, exogenous mineralocorticoids (glycyrrhizic acid in licorice, carbenoxolone, steroids in nasal sprays), Liddle syndrome
  - ◊ Glucocorticoid excess states: Cushing syndrome, exogenous steroids, ectopic ACTH production, II ß hydroxysteroid dehydrogenase deficiency
  - ◊ Renal tubular acidosis (RTA)
  - ◊ Leukemia
  - ◊ Magnesium depletion
  - ◊ Thyrotoxic hypokalemic paralysis

RISK FACTORS Any disorder or medication regimen requiring potassium supplementation

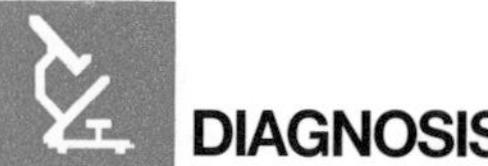

DIAGNOSIS

DIFFERENTIAL DIAGNOSIS Spurious hypokalemia which occurs when blood with a high WBC count (> 100,000/mm3) is allowed to stand at room temperature (WBC's extract K from plasma), thyrotoxicosis

LABORATORY Serum potassium < 3.5 mEq/L (< 3.5 mmol/L)

Drugs that may alter lab results: Diuretics

Disorders that may alter lab results: Leukemia and other conditions with high WBC

PATHOLOGICAL FINDINGS
- Vacuolization of proximal and distal renal tubular cells
- In severe hypokalemia, necrosis of cardiac and skeletal muscle

SPECIAL TESTS
- ECG - flattening or inversion of T waves, increased prominence of U waves, depression of ST segment, ventricular ectopia
- Work-up for etiology - excessive renal K loss is present when urinary K is in excess of 20 mEq/day in the presence of hypokalemia. In the patient with excessive renal K loss and hypertension (HTN), plasma renin and aldosterone levels should be determined to differentiate adrenal from non-adrenal causes of hyperaldosteronism. If HTN is absent and the patient is acidotic, RTA should be considered. If HTN is absent and serum pH is normal to alkalotic, a high urine chloride (> 10 mEq/day) (> 10 mmol/day) suggests hypokalemia secondary to diuretics or Bartter syndrome and a low urine chloride (< 10 mEq/day) (< 10 mmol/day) suggests vomiting as the probable cause.

IMAGING If there is evidence of mineralocorticoid excess (see Special tests), proceed with CT scan of adrenal glands

DIAGNOSTIC PROCEDURES N/A

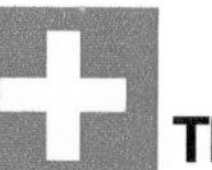

TREATMENT

APPROPRIATE HEALTH CARE
- Hypokalemia is usually not an emergency. For asymptomatic patients being treated with oral replacement, outpatient followup is sufficient.
- Patients with cardiac manifestations will require intravenous replacement with cardiac monitoring in an intensive care setting

GENERAL MEASURES
- Treatment of the underlying cause, if hypokalemia is mild
- When hypokalemia is severe, potassium replacement is necessary

SURGICAL MEASURES N/A

ACTIVITY No restrictions

DIET In mild hypokalemia (K = 3.0-3.5 mEq/L) (K = 3.0-3.5 mmol/L) not caused by GI losses, dietary supplementation may be sufficient. Potassium-rich foods include oranges, bananas, cantaloupes, prunes, raisins, dried beans, dried apricots, and squash.

PATIENT EDUCATION
- Instructions for diet
- If potassium supplementation is necessary, stress need for compliance

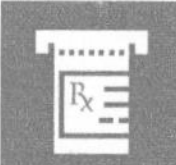

MEDICATIONS

DRUG(S) OF CHOICE

- For non-emergent conditions (serum K > 2.5 mEq/L [K > 2.5 mmol/L], no cardiac manifestations), oral therapy is preferred and doses of 40-120 mEq/day (40-120 mmol/day) are usually adequate. Potassium chloride is suitable for all forms of hypokalemia. Other K salts may be indicated if there is a coexisting disorder: Potassium bicarbonate or bicarbonate precursor (gluconate, acetate, or citrate) in metabolic acidosis or phosphate in phosphate deficiency.
- For emergent situations (serum K < 2.5 mEq/L [< 2.5 mmol/L], arrhythmias), intravenous replacement is indicated. The rate of administration should not exceed 20 mEq/hour (20 mmol/hour) and maximum recommended concentration is 60 mEq/L (60 mmol/L) of saline for peripheral administration. Central may give higher concentration.
- In non-emergent situations, intravenous K should be given only when oral administration is not feasible (e.g., vomiting, postoperative state). In this setting, rate should not exceed 10 mEq/hour and concentration should not exceed 40 mEq/L.

Contraindications: None

Precautions:

- Any form of K replacement carries the risk of hyperkalemia
- Serum K should be checked more frequently in groups at higher risk: Elderly, diabetics, and patients with renal insufficiency
- Patients receiving digitalis and patients with diabetic ketoacidosis in whom intracellular shift in K is expected after insulin therapy is initiated must have more aggressive replacement

Significant possible interactions: Concomitant administration of K sparing diuretics (spironolactone, triamterene, amiloride ACE inhibitors) magnify the risk of hyperkalemia

ALTERNATIVE DRUGS None

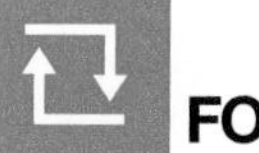

FOLLOWUP

PATIENT MONITORING

- Patients receiving intravenous therapy should have their serum K level checked frequently (q4-6 h)
- Patients requiring potassium supplements should have serum potassium studied at intervals dictated by calculation of patient compliance

PREVENTION/AVOIDANCE Patients being started on diuretics should be advised to increase their dietary K intake (see Diet)

POSSIBLE COMPLICATIONS Hyperkalemia

EXPECTED COURSE/PROGNOSIS

The ease of correction of hypokalemia and the need for prolonged treatment rests on the primary cause. If this can be eliminated (e.g., resolution of diarrhea, discontinuation of diuretics, removal of adrenal tumor), hypokalemia is expected to resolve and no further treatment is indicated.

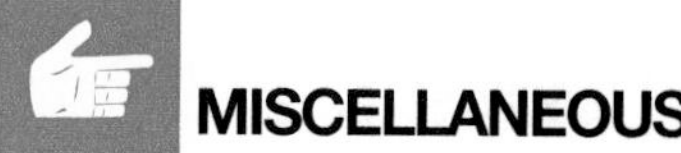

MISCELLANEOUS

ASSOCIATED CONDITIONS N/A

AGE-RELATED FACTORS N/A

Pediatric: Not common in this age group, but may occur in chronic gastrointestinal loss or secondary to hyperadrenalism

Geriatric:

- Diuretic therapy, diarrhea and chronic laxative abuse are most common causes for hypokalemia in this age group
- May need to correct magnesium depletion

Others: Acute GI illnesses with severe vomiting or diarrhea

PREGNANCY Treatment is same

SYNONYMS N/A

ICD-9-CM

276.8 Hypopotassemia

SEE ALSO

Hyperkalemia
Liddle syndrome

OTHER NOTES N/A

ABBREVIATIONS

RTA = renal tubular acidosis
K+ = potassium

REFERENCES

- Peterson LN, Moshe L. Disorders in potassium metabolism. In: Schrier RW, ed: Renal and Electrolyte Disorders. Philadelphia, Lippincott-raven, 1997:192-240
- Mandal A. Hypokalemia and hyperkalemia. Med Clin of North Amer 1997;81(3):611-639
- Isselbacher KJ, et al, Harrison's Principles of Internal Medicine. 15th Ed. New York, McGraw-Hill, 2001
- Cohn J, et al, New Principles for Potassium Replacement in Clinical Practice: A contemporary Review by the National Council on Potassium in Clinic Practice. Arch of Intern Med 2000;160 (16): 2429-2436
- Mandal AK, Nahman HS Jr, eds: Kidney Diseases In: Primary Care, Baltimore. Lippincott Williams and Wilkins, 1998

Web references: 0 available at www.5mcc.com

Illustrations N/A

Author(s):

Mark D. Darrow, MD

Hypokalemic periodic paralysis

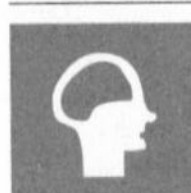

BASICS

DESCRIPTION Episodic weakness associated with low serum potassium (K+) levels.

- Two forms exist:
  - ◊ Familial hypokalemic periodic paralysis; the more common form (FHPP) is usually inherited as an autosomal dominant trait
  - ◊ Hypokalemic periodic paralysis with thyrotoxicosis (thyrotoxic hypokalemic periodic paralysis or THPP); rarer, usually affects Asian males

System(s) affected: Endocrine/Metabolic, Musculoskeletal, Nervous

Genetics: Autosomal dominant (FHPP)

Incidence/Prevalence in USA: 1:100,000 (estimated)

Predominant age: Onset of disease in late childhood or adolescence (FHPP), early adulthood (THPP). Onset of disease after age 35 extremely rare. Age of onset with FHPP depends on type of genetic mutation.

Predominant sex:

- Male > Female (3:1) (FHPP)
- Male > Female (20:1) (THPP)

SIGNS & SYMPTOMS

- Episodic attacks of limb muscle weakness which last from a few hours to several days
- Typical attack comes on during sleep which was preceded by strenuous exercise
- Attacks also provoked by high carbohydrate or high sodium (Na+) meals
- Cold, stress, alcohol, diuretics, insulin, or epinephrine may also exacerbate attack
- Strength between attacks usually normal
- After years of prolonged, frequent attacks patient may develop persistent proximal weakness
- Myalgias
- Proximal weakness greater than distal weakness
- Muscles of the eyes, face, tongue, pharynx, larynx, diaphragm, and sphincters rarely involved
- Deep tendon reflexes hypoactive
- Sensation preserved
- Patients with THPP may manifest signs of hyperthyroidism (especially systolic hypertension and tachycardia)

CAUSES

- Exact pathogenesis unknown
- Abnormality is in the muscle membrane
- Hypokalemia due to intracellular shift of potassium
- Total body potassium is normal (i.e., hypokalemia is not due to potassium loss)
- Muscle fibers chronically depolarized by 10-15 mV, but membrane conductance normal between attacks
- Several mutations in either calcium (type 1 FHPP) or sodium (type 2 FHPP) have been identified (alpha-1 subunit of ion channel protein)
- Very rare form of FHPP due to potassium channel mutation recently reported
- Calcium channel mutation may induce FHPP by changing behavior or expression of other ion channels in muscle
- Contractile apparatus normal
- Pathogenesis of FHPP and THPP may be different since thyroid hormone doesn't worsen FHPP
- Acetazolamide may precipitate attacks in patients with type 2 FHPP caused by sodium channel mutation

RISK FACTORS

- Male
- Age under 35
- Family history (FHPP)
- Asian (THPP)

DIAGNOSIS

DIFFERENTIAL DIAGNOSIS

- Hyperkalemic periodic paralysis (adynamia episodica)
- Myotonia congenita
- Paramyotonia congenita
- Normokalemic periodic paralysis
- Barium poisoning
- Hyperventilation
- Secondary hypokalemia (laxative or diuretic use, diarrhea, vomiting, renal or adrenal disease, clay ingestion)
- Myasthenia gravis
- Guillain-Barré syndrome
- Tick paralysis
- Cataplexy
- Sleep paralysis
- Presyncope
- "Drop attacks"
- Akinetic epilepsy
- Andersen's syndrome (episodic paralysis, ventricular dysthymias, and dysmorphic features)
- Episodic ataxia

LABORATORY

- Hallmark is low serum K+ (as low as 1.3 mEq/L [1.3 mmol/L])
- Low serum phosphorous and low serum magnesium also found
- Urine K+ normal
- Elevated T3, T4, free thyroid index, and decreased TSH (THPP only)
- Serum CK level normal or slightly increased
- Acid-base balance normal
- Urine potassium/creatinine ratio low (<2)

Drugs that may alter lab results: N/A

Disorders that may alter lab results: N/A

PATHOLOGICAL FINDINGS

- Muscle biopsy may show atrophy, centrally placed vacuoles of sarcoplasm
- Electromicroscopy studies show vacuoles are due to progressive dilatation of sarcoplasmic reticulum

SPECIAL TESTS

- With mild hypokalemia electrocardiogram (ECG) may show S-T depression, flattened T waves, presence of U waves
- With severe hypokalemia ECG may show peaked P waves, prolonged P-R interval, widened QRS
- Electromyography not helpful (usually normal between attacks)
- Genetic testing (DNA sequencing) to differentiate type 1 FHPP from type 2 FHPP (calcium vs sodium channel mutations)

IMAGING Thyroid scans using radioiodine (THPP only)

DIAGNOSTIC PROCEDURES Provocative testing (50 to 100 g oral glucose with 2 to 4 g oral sodium followed by exercise, or 50 to 100 g oral glucose with 10-20 IU subcutaneous insulin) may be required. Patient should have cardiac monitoring during testing.

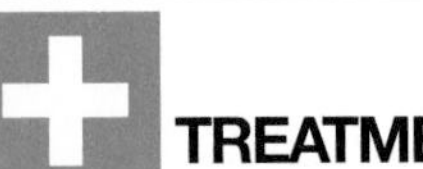

TREATMENT

APPROPRIATE HEALTH CARE

- Severe hypokalemia or weakness - inpatient with cardiac monitoring
- Mild hypokalemia or weakness - outpatient with close follow up

GENERAL MEASURES May rarely need respiratory support

SURGICAL MEASURES N/A

ACTIVITY As tolerated

DIET

- Avoid high carbohydrate, high sodium foods
- K+ rich fruit of dubious benefit

PATIENT EDUCATION Genetic counseling (FHPP) as there is a 50% risk of transmitting abnormal gene to offspring and a ≈50% chance of affected siblings

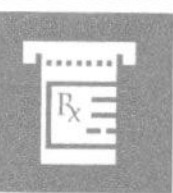

MEDICATIONS

DRUG(S) OF CHOICE
- Acute attack
  - ◊ Oral potassium chloride, 0.2 to 0.4 mEq/kg (0.2-0.4 mmol/kg), repeated every 15 to 30 min depending on response of ECG, serum K+, muscle strength (usual dose: 40 mEq [40 mmol])
  - ◊ In life-threatening situation or if vomiting give intravenous KCl in mannitol (5% glucose or normal saline IV may worsen situation). Bolus 0.1 mEq/kg (0.1 mmol/kg) every 5 to 10 min; monitor ECG, serum K+. (Usual dose: 15 mEq [15 mmol] over 15 minutes then 10 mEq/hr [10 mmol/hr] if peripheral IV, up to 60 mEq/hr [60 mmol/hr] if central IV and cardiac monitoring.)
  - ◊ IV propranolol (THPP only)
- Prevention of attacks in FHPP
  - ◊ Oral KCl
  - ◊ Acetazolamide (Diamox), 125 to 1000 mg/d divided qd to bid (type 1 FHPP only)
- Prevention of attacks in THPP
  - ◊ Treat underlying thyrotoxicosis with beta-adrenergic blocking agents (propranolol [Inderal] and others)
  - ◊ Acetazolamide contraindicated

Contraindications:
- Acetazolamide - marked hepatic or renal dysfunction, hypersensitivity, adrenal failure, hyperchloremic acidosis, low serum Na+, K+ (type 2 FHPP, THPP)
- Propranolol - cardiogenic shock, sinus bradycardia, 2nd or 3rd degree AV block, congestive heart failure, bronchial asthma

Precautions:
- Infusion of IV KCl must be monitored to avoid inadvertent infusion of large and potentially fatal doses
- Peripheral intravenous KCl infusion rates greater than 10 mEq/h (10 mmol/h) may be painful
- Rebound hyperkalemia may occur in patients who receive more than 90 mEq KCl in 24 hours and in patients with THPP who receive KCl and propranolol
- Acetazolamide - drowsiness or paresthesias at high doses. May precipitate or worsen paralysis in patients with type 2 FHPP.
- Propranolol - impaired hepatic or renal function

Significant possible interactions:
- Acetazolamide - high dose aspirin
- Propranolol - reserpine, verapamil, aluminum hydroxide, phenytoin, rifampin, chlorpromazine, cimetidine, theophylline

ALTERNATIVE DRUGS
- Acute attack
  - ◊ None
- Prevention of attacks in FHPP
  - ◊ Triamterene (Dyrenium) 25 to 100 mg/d
  - ◊ Spironolactone (Aldactone) 25 to 100 200 mg/d
- Prevention of attacks in THPP
  - ◊ Propylthiouracil, radioactive ablation of the thyroid

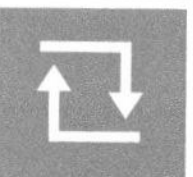

FOLLOWUP

PATIENT MONITORING
- Follow serum K+, electrolytes (if on acetazolamide)
- Follow thyroid function tests (if on propranolol or propylthiouracil)

PREVENTION/AVOIDANCE See Medication (prevention of attacks) and Diet

POSSIBLE COMPLICATIONS Cardiac arrhythmias, respiratory collapse

EXPECTED COURSE/PROGNOSIS
- Frequency of attacks usually lessens with age
- After years of prolonged, frequent attacks patient may develop persistent proximal weakness

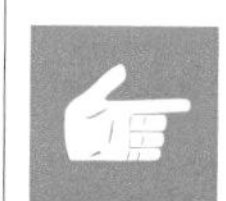

MISCELLANEOUS

ASSOCIATED CONDITIONS Hyperthyroidism with THPP

AGE-RELATED FACTORS
Pediatric: Onset of disease in late childhood or adolescence

Geriatric: Onset of disease after age 25-35 extremely rare; frequency of attacks usually lessens with age

Others: N/A

PREGNANCY N/A

SYNONYMS
- Paroxysmal myoplegia

ICD-9-CM
359.3 Familial periodic paralysis

SEE ALSO
Guillain-Barré syndrome
Hyperthyroidism
Hypokalemia
Myasthenia gravis
Tick paralysis

OTHER NOTES N/A

ABBREVIATIONS
K+ = potassium
Na+ = sodium
FHPP = hypokalemic periodic paralysis (familial)
THPP = thyrotoxic (hypokalemic) periodic paralysis

REFERENCES

- Antes LM, Kujuba DA, Fernandez PC. Hypokalemia and the pathology of ion transport molecules. Semin Nephrol 1998;18:31-45
- Cannon SC. An expanding view for the molecular basis of familial periodic paralysis. Neuromuscul Disord 2002;12(6):533-43
- Dias da Silva MR, Cerutti JM, Tengan CH, et al. Mutations linked to familial hypokalaemic periodic paralysis in the calcium channel alpha1 subunit gene (Cav1.1) are not associated with thyrotoxic hypokalaemic periodic paralysis. Clin Endocrinol (Oxf) 2002;56(3):367-75
- Gutmann L. Periodic paralyses. Neurologic Clin 2000;18:195-202
- Hoffman EP. Voltage-gated ion channelopathies: inherited disorders caused by abnormal sodium, chloride, and calcium regulation in skeletal muscle. Annual Review of Medicine 1995;46:431-41
- Ko GTC, Chow CC, Yeung HHL, et al. Thyrotoxic periodic paralysis in a Chinese population. QJ Med 1996;89:463-8
- Lehmann-Horn F, Jurkat-Rott K, Rüdel R. Periodic paralysis: understanding channelopathies. Curr Neurol Neurosci Rep 2002;2(1):61-9
- Lehmann-Horn F, Rüdel R. Channelopathies: the nondystrophic myotonias and periodic paralyses. Seminars in Pediatric Neurology 1996;3(2):122-39
- Lin S, Chiu J, Hsu C, et al. A simple and rapid approache to hypokalemic paralysis. Am J Emerg Med 2003;21:487-91
- Lin S, Lin Y. Propranolol rapidly reverses paralysis, hypokalemia, and hypophosphatemia in thyrotoxic periodic paralysis. Am J Kid Dis 2001;37:620-3
- Lin Y, Wu C, Pei D, et al. Diangosing thyrotoxic periodic paralysis in the ED. Am J Emerg Med 2003;21:339-42
- Magsino CH, Ryan AJ. Thyrotoxic periodic paralysis. South Med J 2000;93:996-1003
- Manoukian MA, Foote JA, Crapo LM. Clinical and metabolic features of thyrotoxic periodic paralysis in 24 episodes. Arch Int Med 1999;159:601-6
- Ober KP. Thyrotoxic periodic paralysis in the United States: Report of 7 cases and review of the literature. Medicine 1992;71(3):109-20
- Ptacek L. The familial periodic paralyses and nondystrophic myotonias. Am J Med 1998;104:58-70
- Renner DR, Ptacek LJ. Periodic paralyses and nondystrophic myotonias. Adv Neurol 2002;88:235-52
- Ruff RL. Insulin acts in hypokalemic periodic paralysis by reducing inward rectifier K+ current. Neurol 1999;53:1556-63
- Ruff RL. Skeletal muscle sodium current is reduced in hypokalemic periodic paralysis. Proc Natl Acad Sci 2000;97(18):9832-3
- Stedwell R, Allen KM, Binder LS. Hypokalemic paralysis: A review of the etiologies, pathophysiology, presentation, and therapy. Am J Emerg Med 1992;10:143-8
- Starnberg D, Maisonobe T, Jurkat-Rott K. Hypokalemic periodic paralysis type 2 caused by mutations at codon 672 in the muscle sodium channel gene SCN4A. Brain 2001;124:1091-9
- Tassone H, Moulin A, Henderson S. The pitfalls of potassium replacement in thyrotoxic periodic paralysis: A case report and review of the literature. J Emerg Med 2004;2:157-61

Web references: 3 available at www.5mcc.com
Illustrations N/A

Author(s):
Chris Vincent, MD

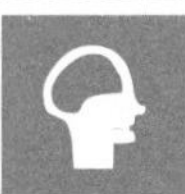

BASICS

DESCRIPTION Defined as a plasma sodium concentration < 135 mEq/L (< 135 mmol/L)
- Hypovolemic hyponatremia - there is a decrease in total body water (TBW) and a greater decrease in total body sodium. The extracellular fluid (ECF) volume is decreased. Orthostatic hypotension and other changes consistent with hypovolemia are present.
- Euvolemic hyponatremia - there is an increase in TBW with a normal total body sodium. The ECF volume is minimally to moderately increased but there is no edema.
- Hypervolemic hyponatremia - there is an increase in total body sodium and a greater increase in TBW. The ECF is increased markedly and there is edema.
- Redistributive hyponatremia - there is a shift of water from the intracellular compartment to the extracellular compartment with a resultant dilution of sodium. TBW and total body sodium are unchanged. This occurs with hyperglycemia.
- Pseudohyponatremia - there is a dilution of the aqueous phase by excessive proteins or lipids. TBW and total body sodium are unchanged. This occurs in hypertriglyceridemia or multiple myeloma.

System(s) affected: Endocrine/Metabolic
Genetics: N/A
Incidence/Prevalence in USA: Described as the most common electrolyte disorder seen in a general hospital population. A recent study of hospitalized patients found an incidence of 1% and a prevalence of 2.5%.
Predominant age: All ages
Predominant sex: Male = Female

SIGNS & SYMPTOMS
- Lethargy
- Disorientation
- Generalized weakness
- Muscle cramps
- Anorexia
- Hiccups
- Nausea and vomiting
- Agitation or delirium
- Stupor
- Coma
- Depressed deep tendon reflexes
- Hypothermia
- Positive Babinski responses
- Cheyne-Stokes respiration
- Pseudobulbar palsy
- Seizures
- Orthostatic hypotension
- Cranial nerve palsies

CAUSES
- Hypovolemic hyponatremia (extrarenal loss of sodium)
  - ◊ Gastrointestinal loss - vomiting, diarrhea
  - ◊ Third spacing - peritonitis, pancreatitis, burns, rhabdomyolysis
  - ◊ Skin loss - burns, sweating, cystic fibrosis
  - ◊ Lung loss - bronchorrhea
- Hypovolemic hyponatremia (renal loss of sodium)
  - ◊ Salt losing nephritis
  - ◊ Mineralocorticoid deficiency
  - ◊ Diuretic
  - ◊ Bicarbonaturia - renal tubular acidosis, metabolic alkalosis
  - ◊ Ketonuria or anion gap acidosis
  - ◊ Partial urinary tract obstruction
  - ◊ Osmotic diuresis
- Euvolemic hyponatremia
  - ◊ Hypothyroidism
  - ◊ Pure glucocorticoid deficiency
  - ◊ Drugs
  - ◊ Stress
  - ◊ Syndrome of inappropriate antidiuretic hormone release (SIADH). Causes include pulmonary and central nervous system disorders.
- Hypervolemic hyponatremia
  - ◊ Nephrotic syndrome
  - ◊ Cirrhosis
  - ◊ Congestive heart failure
  - ◊ Renal failure
- Redistributive hyponatremia
  - ◊ Hyperglycemia
  - ◊ Mannitol infusion
- Pseudohyponatremia
  - ◊ Hypertriglyceridemia
  - ◊ Multiple myeloma

RISK FACTORS
Excessive fluid intake

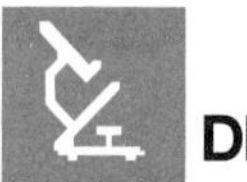

DIAGNOSIS

DIFFERENTIAL DIAGNOSIS See Causes

LABORATORY
- Serum sodium less than 135 mEq/L (135 mmol/L)
- Plasma osmolality
- Urine sodium
- BUN
- Creatinine
- Hypovolemic hyponatremia
  - ◊ Plasma osmolality low
  - ◊ BUN/creatinine ratio greater than 20/1
  - ◊ Urine sodium > 20 mEq/L (> 20 mmol/L) - renal loss
  - ◊ Urine sodium < 10 mEq/L (< 10 mmol/L) - extrarenal loss
  - ◊ Serum potassium > 5.0 mEq/L (> 5 mmol/L) - consider mineralocorticoid deficiency
- Euvolemic hyponatremia
  - ◊ Plasma osmolality low
  - ◊ BUN/creatinine ratio less than 20/1
  - ◊ Urine sodium > 20 mEq/L (> 20 mmol/L)
- Hypervolemic hyponatremia
  - ◊ Plasma osmolality low
  - ◊ Urine sodium < 10 mEq/L (< 10 mmol/L) in nephrotic syndrome, CHF, cirrhosis
  - ◊ Urine sodium > 20 mEq/L (> 20 mmol/L) in acute and chronic renal failure
- Redistributive hyponatremia
  - ◊ Plasma osmolality normal or high
  - ◊ Glucose or mannitol levels elevated
- Pseudohyponatremia
  - ◊ Plasma osmolality normal
  - ◊ Triglyceride or protein levels elevated

Drugs that may alter lab results: N/A

Disorders that may alter lab results: N/A

PATHOLOGICAL FINDINGS N/A

SPECIAL TESTS For euvolemic hyponatremia a thyroid stimulating hormone (TSH) to rule out hypothyroidism and a one-hour cosyntropin stimulation test to rule out adrenal insufficiency

IMAGING
- CT of head if pituitary problem suspected or if SIADH from CNS problem suspected
- Chest x-ray to rule out pulmonary pathology if SIADH diagnosed

DIAGNOSTIC PROCEDURES N/A

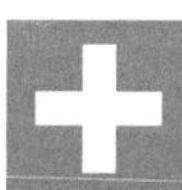

TREATMENT

APPROPRIATE HEALTH CARE
- Inpatient treatment mandatory if acute hyponatremia or symptomatic
- Inpatient treatment advised if asymptomatic and serum sodium less than 125 mEq/dL

GENERAL MEASURES
- Assess all medications patient is taking
- Institute seizure precautions

SURGICAL MEASURES N/A

ACTIVITY Varies according to patient mental status

DIET
- Euvolemic hyponatremia - water restriction to 1000 cc/day
- Hypervolemic hyponatremia - water and sodium restriction
- Hypovolemic hyponatremia - isotonic saline
- Redistributive or pseudohyponatremia - treat underlying cause

PATIENT EDUCATION N/A

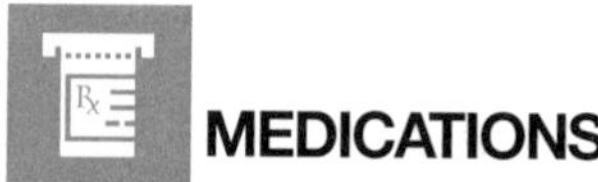

MEDICATIONS

DRUG(S) OF CHOICE

- Severe symptomatic hyponatremia: The use of hypertonic saline (3%) is clearly indicated only in patients who are both severely symptomatic and have sodium concentrations less than 120 mEq/L (120 mmol/L). Three percent saline should be used at a rate of 1 cc/kg/hr. This will raise the serum sodium level by approximately 1 mEq/L/hr (1 mmol/L/hr). The hypertonic saline infusion should only continue until a serum sodium of 120 mEq/L (120 mmol/L) is reached or the patient becomes asymptomatic. Avoid correction by more than 12 mEq/L/day (12 mmol/day).
- Chronic hyponatremia: If hyponatremia does not improve with fluid restriction or other appropriate treatment, consider using demeclocycline. In doses of 600-1200 milligrams per day, the drug produces a nephrogenic diabetes insipidus.
- Maintenance: Clinical judgment

Contraindications: Demeclocycline can cause nephrotoxicity in patients with liver disease

Precautions:

- Demeclocycline - photosensitivity and nausea can occur
- Three percent saline-rapid correction of severe symptomatic hyponatremia has been associated with central pontine myelinolysis (CPM). This neurologic disorder induces loss of myelin and supportive structures in the pons and occasionally in other areas of the brain. CPM is seen one to several days after rapid correction of serum sodium and is characterized by gradual neurologic deterioration.

Significant possible interactions: Demeclocycline - oral anticoagulants, oral contraceptives, penicillin

ALTERNATIVE DRUGS N/A

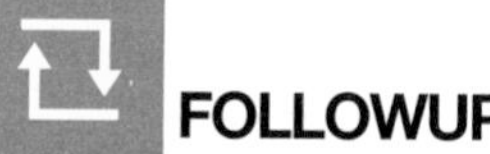

FOLLOWUP

PATIENT MONITORING

- Serum sodium level should be monitored when clinically indicated. If three percent saline is used the sodium level should be checked hourly.
- Volume status should be monitored if 3% or 0.9% saline is used

PREVENTION/AVOIDANCE

Dependent on underlying condition

POSSIBLE COMPLICATIONS

- Occult tumor may present with SIADH
- Hypervolemia if saline used
- Central pontine myelinolysis

EXPECTED COURSE/PROGNOSIS

With recognition and proper treatment a return to normal serum sodium and resolution of neurologic symptoms is expected. Prognosis is dependent on underlying condition.

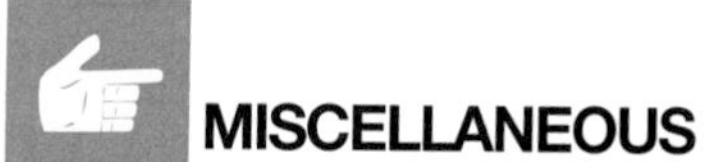

MISCELLANEOUS

ASSOCIATED CONDITIONS

- Hypothyroidism
- Hypopituitarism
- Adrenocortical hormone deficiency

AGE-RELATED FACTORS N/A

Pediatric: N/A
Geriatric: N/A
Others: N/A

PREGNANCY N/A

SYNONYMS N/A

ICD-9-CM

276.1 Hyposmolality and/or hyponatremia

SEE ALSO

OTHER NOTES N/A

ABBREVIATIONS

TBW = total body water
ECF = extracellular fluid
SIADH = syndrome of inappropriate antidiuretic hormone secretion

REFERENCES

- Schrier RW. Renal and Electrolyte Disorders. 4th ed. Boston, Little Brown and Co; 1997
- Rose BD, Post TW. Clinical Physiology of Acid-Base and Electrolyte Disorders. 5th ed. NewYork: McGraw-Hill; 2001

Web references: 0 available at www.5mcc.com
Illustrations N/A

Author(s):

Peter Kozisek, MD

BASICS

DESCRIPTION Deficiency of parathyroid hormone (PTH) from disease, injury or congenital absence or malfunction of the parathyroid glands. Manifested as hypocalcemia producing neuromuscular symptoms ranging from paresthesia to tetany.
- Classifications:
  - ◊ Hypoparathyroidism (follows accidental removal or damage to parathyroid glands during surgery; may be transient or permanent)
  - ◊ Idiopathic (parathyroids absent or atrophied)
  - ◊ Pseudohypoparathyroidism (no PTH deficiency, but target organs do not respond to its action)

System(s) affected: Endocrine/Metabolic, Musculoskeletal, Nervous
Genetics: Idiopathic hypoparathyroidism may have a genetic component
Incidence/Prevalence in USA: All forms are rare
Predominant age: All ages
Predominant sex: Male = Female

SIGNS & SYMPTOMS
- Chronic hypocalcemia may be asymptomatic
- Neuromuscular excitability as carpopedal spasm
- Increased deep tendon reflexes
- Chvostek's sign: hyperirritability of the facial nerve when tapped
- Trousseau's sign: carpopedal spasm within 2 minutes of inflating a blood pressure cuff over systolic pressure
- Dysphagia
- Organic brain syndrome
- Psychosis
- Mental deficiency (children)
- Tetany (paresthesias, pain, difficulty walking, laryngospasm, stridor, cyanosis, seizures)
- Dry hair
- Brittle fingernails
- Dry, scaly skin
- Cataracts
- Cardiac arrhythmias

CAUSES
- Idiopathic
  - ◊ DiGeorge syndrome
  - ◊ Congenital absence
  - ◊ Late onset, autoimmune
- Postsurgical (may be transient)
- Infiltrative - metastatic carcinoma and others
- Irradiation
- Hypomagnesemia
- Alcohol

RISK FACTORS
- Neck surgery, especially thyroid
- Neck trauma
- Head and neck malignancies

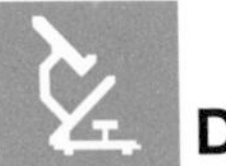

DIAGNOSIS

DIFFERENTIAL DIAGNOSIS
- Rickets and osteomalacia
- Candidiasis
- Pseudohypoparathyroidism
- Addison disease
- Pernicious anemia
- Hypocalcemia of severe illness

LABORATORY
- Serum total and ionized calcium - decreased
- Serum phosphorus - increased (> 5.4 mg/dL [> 1.74 mmol/L])
- Immunometric assay for parathyroid hormone - decreased

Drugs that may alter lab results: Corticosteroids

Disorders that may alter lab results: Other hormonal disorders; hypoalbuminuria

PATHOLOGICAL FINDINGS
- Complete or almost complete replacement of parathyroid gland parenchymal tissue by fat
- Brain blood vessels calcified

SPECIAL TESTS
- ECG - increased Q-T and S-T intervals (due to hypocalcemia)
- Serum beta-carotene (normal)
- D-Xylose absorption
- 72 hour stool fat
- Slit-lamp - may show early posterior lenticular cataract formation

IMAGING
- X-ray:
  - ◊ Increased bone density
  - ◊ Tooth roots absent
  - ◊ Calcification of cerebellum, choroid plexus, cerebral basal ganglia

DIAGNOSTIC PROCEDURES N/A

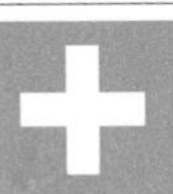

TREATMENT

APPROPRIATE HEALTH CARE
- Outpatient unless severe
- Inpatient for tetany
- Outpatient followup

GENERAL MEASURES
- Transient forms of hypoparathyroidism may not require treatment
- Acute attack hypoparathyroid tetany
  - ◊ Is life-threatening and requires immediate IV calcium treatment to raise calcium levels
  - ◊ Verify adequate airway is present
  - ◊ If patient is awake, breathing into paper bag can help raise serum ionized calcium levels also
  - ◊ Seizure prevention
  - ◊ May require tracheostomy
- Maintenance
  - ◊ Lifelong calcitriol and calcium
  - ◊ Maintain serum calcium in the low normal range 8.5-9 mg/dL (2.12-2.25 mmol/L)
  - ◊ Skin softeners for scaly skin
  - ◊ Adequate control requires careful attention to avoid overtreatment or undertreatment

SURGICAL MEASURES N/A

ACTIVITY As tolerated

DIET No special diet

PATIENT EDUCATION
- Careful and detailed instructions about maintenance therapy
- Importance of periodic blood chemical evaluations
- Signs and symptoms of overtreatment and undertreatment to watch for

MEDICATIONS

DRUG(S) OF CHOICE
- For tetany:
  - ◊ Immediate IV calcium gluconate 10-20 mL of 10% solution given slowly until tetany ceases
  - ◊ Calcium salts orally as soon as possible, 1-2 g daily
  - ◊ Oral vitamin D (ergocalciferol) 500 IU/day

or
  - ◊ Calcitriol - pediatric dose: 0.04-0.08 μg/kg/24 hr. Adult dose: 0.25 μg/24 hr. Then 0.25 μg qod. Adjust based on calcium and phosphorus levels.
- Maintenance:
  - ◊ Calcium - 1-2 g daily in divided doses
  - ◊ Oral vitamin D or calcitriol
  - ◊ If associated endocrinopathies - appropriate hormone replacement
  - ◊ Thiazide diuretic - for some patients to increase phosphate excretion and decrease calcium excretion

Contraindications: Refer to manufacturer's literature
Precautions: Refer to manufacturer's literature
Significant possible interactions: Refer to manufacturer's literature

ALTERNATIVE DRUGS N/A

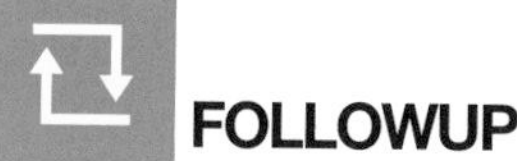

FOLLOWUP

PATIENT MONITORING
- Outpatient after tetany corrected
- Periodic blood chemical evaluations

PREVENTION/AVOIDANCE
Care in surgical procedure that may cause damage to parathyroid glands

POSSIBLE COMPLICATIONS
- Neuromuscular symptoms (reversible)
- Cataracts
- Basal ganglia calcifications
- If condition starts early in childhood - stunting of growth, malformation of teeth, mental retardation
- Hypothyroidism
- Parkinsonian symptoms
- Ossification of the paravertebral ligaments
- Complications of overtreatment or undertreatment
- Institutionalized due to permanent mental damage

EXPECTED COURSE/PROGNOSIS
- Course - acute, chronic
- Transient hypoparathyroidism following neck surgery
- Good outlook with diagnosis and treatment

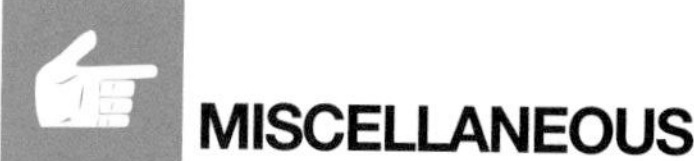

MISCELLANEOUS

ASSOCIATED CONDITIONS
- DiGeorge syndrome
- Addison disease
- Mucocutaneous candidiasis

AGE-RELATED FACTORS
Pediatric:
- May occur in premature infants
- Congenital absence of parathyroids
- May appear later in childhood as idiopathic

Geriatric: Hypocalcemia fairly common in the elderly and may be due to multiple abnormalities
Others: N/A

PREGNANCY N/A

SYNONYMS Parathyroid tetany

ICD-9-CM
252.1 Hypoparathyroidism

SEE ALSO

OTHER NOTES N/A

ABBREVIATIONS N/A

REFERENCES

- Agus ZS. Etiology of hypocalcemia in adults. Wellesley, MA: UpToDate: 2004
- Obermayer-Straub P, et al. Autoimmune polyglandular syndromes. Bailliere's Clin Gastroenterol 1998;12(2):293-315
- Mestman JH. Parathyroid disorders of pregnancy. Semin Perinatol 1998;22(6):485-96
- Federman DD. Scientific American Medicine New York: WebMD; 1998 3Vi;9-11
- Becker KL, editor. Principles and Practice of Endocrinology and Metabolism. 3rd ed. Philadelphia: Lippincott Williams & Wilkins; 2001. p. 588-597

Web references: 0 available at www.5mcc.com
Illustrations N/A

Author(s):
Richard P. Levy, MD

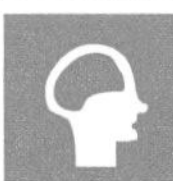

BASICS

DESCRIPTION Generalized condition caused by partial or total failure of the pituitary gland's vital hormones - ACTH, TSH, LH, FSH, GH, prolactin (PRL)
System(s) affected: Endocrine/Metabolic, Gastrointestinal, Musculoskeletal, Nervous, Reproductive, Skin/Exocrine
Genetics: Some pituitary defects are congenital
Incidence/Prevalence in USA: Relatively rare
Predominant age: Occurs in adults and children. In children it causes dwarfism and pubertal delay.
Predominant sex: Male = Female

SIGNS & SYMPTOMS
- Usually starts with hypogonadism or gonadotropin failure (decreased FSH and LH)
- Signs of hypofunction of target glands
- Secondary amenorrhea
- Impotence
- Infertility
- Decreased libido
- Diabetes insipidus (rare)
- Lethargy
- Tiredness
- Sensitivity to cold
- Anorexia
- Nausea
- Abdominal pain
- Lactation failure
- Retarded growth
- Failure of secondary sexual characteristics to develop
- Mental aberrations
- Headache
- Visual field defects
- Blindness

CAUSES
- Lesions or tumors of the anterior pituitary gland (intrasellar or extrasellar)
- Congenital defects
- Pituitary apoplexy
- Hypophysectomy
- Infiltrative diseases (e.g., sarcoidosis, histiocytosis X)
- Sometimes idiopathic
- Lymphocytic hypophysitis
- Irradiation
- Accidental or surgical trauma
- Hypothalamic disease

RISK FACTORS
- Trauma
- Pregnancy and delivery

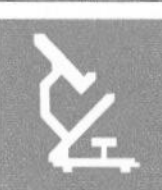

DIAGNOSIS

DIFFERENTIAL DIAGNOSIS
- Primary hypothyroidism
- Anorexia nervosa
- Chronic liver disease
- Myotonia dystrophica
- Addison disease
- Primary psychosis
- Primary hypogonadism

LABORATORY
- Confirms hormonal deficiencies
- Radioimmunoassay of pituitary and target gland hormones
- Provocative tests

Drugs that may alter lab results: Any hormone

Disorders that may alter lab results:
- Cushing syndrome
- Addison disease
- Hyperthyroidism
- Hypothyroidism

PATHOLOGICAL FINDINGS
- Destruction of anterior pituitary
- Atrophy of adrenal cortex, thyroid, gonads

SPECIAL TESTS
- Careful testing for smell
- Visual field examination by quantitative perimetry

IMAGING
- X-rays - chest, skull, hands, wrists (for bone age)
- Pituitary CT or MRI

DIAGNOSTIC PROCEDURES N/A

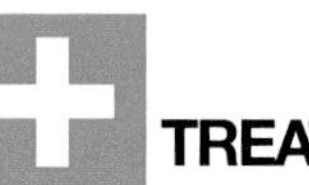

TREATMENT

APPROPRIATE HEALTH CARE
- Outpatient
- Inpatient for surgery when hypopituitarism is due to a pituitary tumor

GENERAL MEASURES
- Hormonal replacement
- Exercise program to rehabilitate
- Wear medical identification

SURGICAL MEASURES
- Surgery for pituitary tumor

ACTIVITY Encourage active physical exercise program

DIET High calorie, high protein

PATIENT EDUCATION
- Wear medical identification bracelet or necklace
- In patient with documented ACTH deficiency, stress need for additional cortisone at time of any major physical stress (e.g., fever above 101°F [38.3°C]; acute illness)

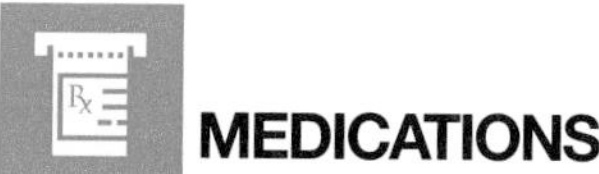

MEDICATIONS

DRUG(S) OF CHOICE
- Replacement of hormones secreted by the target glands:
  - ◊ Hydrocortisone
  - ◊ Thyroxine
  - ◊ Androgen or cyclic estrogen
  - ◊ Human growth hormone (for treating dwarfism and in selected adult patients)
  - ◊ Dosages and administration schedule vary according to age and sex, refer to manufacturer's literature

Contraindications: Refer to manufacturer's literature
Precautions: Refer to manufacturer's literature
Significant possible interactions: Refer to manufacturer's literature

ALTERNATIVE DRUGS N/A

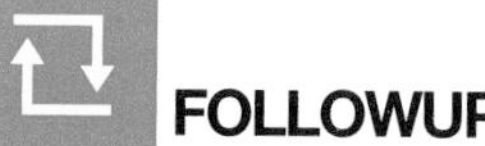

FOLLOWUP

PATIENT MONITORING 3 and 12 month evaluations for post-treatment hormonal status. For patients with pituitary tumors include visual fields, thyroid and adrenal function, sellar computerized imaging.

PREVENTION/AVOIDANCE None

POSSIBLE COMPLICATIONS
- Blindness
- Adrenal crisis
- Long-term medications

EXPECTED COURSE/PROGNOSIS
- Course - acute, chronic
- Variable, but guardedly favorable with replacement therapy
- If due to postpartum necrosis, may have complete or partial recovery

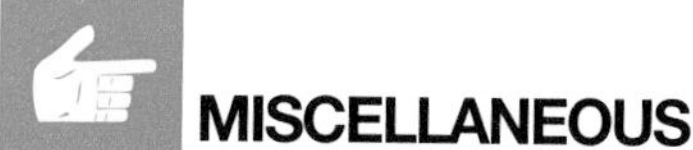

MISCELLANEOUS

ASSOCIATED CONDITIONS
- Childhood hypopituitarism
- Sheehan syndrome
- Hypothyroidism
- Kallman syndrome

AGE-RELATED FACTORS
Pediatric: Hypopituitarism in this age group leads to dwarfism due to lack of growth hormone
Geriatric: More difficult to diagnose
Others: N/A

PREGNANCY
- Severe postpartum hemorrhage can lead to hypopituitarism
- Lymphocytic hypophysitis may be triggered by pregnancy

SYNONYMS
- Pituitary cachexia
- Hypopituitarism syndrome
- Simmonds syndrome
- Panhypopituitarism

ICD-9-CM
253.2 Panhypopituitarism

SEE ALSO

OTHER NOTES N/A

ABBREVIATIONS N/A

REFERENCES

- Sheehan H, Summers VK: The syndrome of hypopituitarism. Q.J. Med 1949;42:319
- Vance M: Hypopituitarism. N Eng J Med 1994;330:1651

Web references: 0 available at www.5mcc.com
Illustrations N/A

Author(s):
William F. Young, Jr, MD

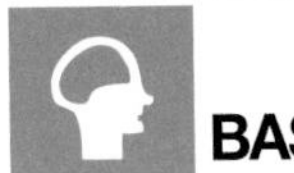

BASICS

DESCRIPTION Hypothermia occurs when a core (rectal, tympanic or esophageal) temperature falls below 35°C (95°F). It may take several hours or several days to develop. As the body temperature falls, all organ system are affected; cerebral blood flow decreases and the metabolic rate declines rapidly. Patients who have been immersed for as long as 45 minutes in very cold water and appear to be dead have still been resuscitated.
System(s) affected: Cardiovascular, Endocrine/Metabolic, Nervous, Skin/Exocrine
Genetics: N/A
Incidence/Prevalence in USA: Estimates vary widely due to lack of pathological evidence, and that hypothermia is usually considered a secondary cause in diagnosing disorders
Predominant age: Very young and the elderly
Predominant sex: Male > Female

SIGNS & SYMPTOMS
- Mild (34-35°C)
  - ◊ Lethargy
  - ◊ Mild confusion
  - ◊ Shivering
  - ◊ Tachypnea
  - ◊ Loss of fine motor coordination
  - ◊ Increased pulse and blood pressure
  - ◊ Peripheral vasoconstriction
- Moderate (30-34°C)
  - ◊ Delirium
  - ◊ Bradycardia
  - ◊ Hypotension
  - ◊ Hypoventilation
  - ◊ Cyanosis
  - ◊ Arrhythmias
  - ◊ Semicoma and coma
  - ◊ Muscular rigidity
  - ◊ Generalized edema
  - ◊ Slowed reflexes
- Severe (< 30°C)
  - ◊ Very cold skin
  - ◊ Rigidity
  - ◊ Apnea
  - ◊ No pulse - ventricular fibrillation or asystole
  - ◊ Areflexia
  - ◊ Unresponsive
  - ◊ Fixed pupils

CAUSES
- Decreased heat production
- Increased heat loss
- Impaired thermoregulation

RISK FACTORS
- Malnutrition
- Cold water immersion
- Exposure to high winds
- Homeless
- Vehicle breakdown
- Outdoor workers
- Trauma victims (especially head)
- Alcohol consumption
- Mental illness; Alzheimer disease
- Drug intoxication (barbiturates, phenothiazines, cyclic antidepressants, parasympatholytics, benzodiazepines, narcotics)
- Endocrinopathies (hypothyroidism, hypopituitarism, hypoadrenalism, hypoglycemia)
- Hypothalamic and CNS dysfunction
- Sepsis
- Cardiovascular disease
- Bronchopneumonia
- Hepatic failure
- Uremia
- Extensive skin disease (psoriasis dermatitis)
- Excessive fluid loss

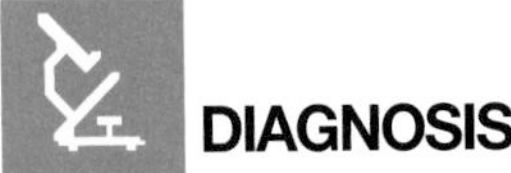

DIAGNOSIS

DIFFERENTIAL DIAGNOSIS
- Cerebrovascular accidents
- Intoxication
- Drug overdose
- Complications of diabetes, hypothyroidism, hypopituitarism

LABORATORY
- Arterial blood gases (reported in the uncorrected form)
- Complete blood and platelet counts
- Toxicology screen
- Serum electrolytes
- Urinalysis
- Prothrombin time
- Partial thromboplastin time
- Fibrinogen levels
- Blood culture
- BUN/creatinine
- Glucose
- Amylase
- Liver function studies
- Thyroid function tests
- Serum cortisol
- Cardiac enzymes

Drugs that may alter lab results: Refer to laboratory test reference

Disorders that may alter lab results: Refer to laboratory test reference

PATHOLOGICAL FINDINGS
- Moderate dilation of right heart
- Pulmonary edema

SPECIAL TESTS
- Temperature measure - with special thermometers that can record low temperatures and measure core temperatures. Oral temperatures are of no value.
- Electrocardiogram - slowing of sinus rate with T-wave inversion, QT-interval prolongation, hypothermic J waves (Osborn waves) characterized by a notching of the QRS complex and ST segment
- Thyroid and pituitary function tests

IMAGING X-rays of the cervical spine, chest, abdomen, if appropriate

DIAGNOSTIC PROCEDURES History of prolonged exposure to cold may make the diagnosis obvious, but hypothermia may be overlooked, especially if patient is comatose

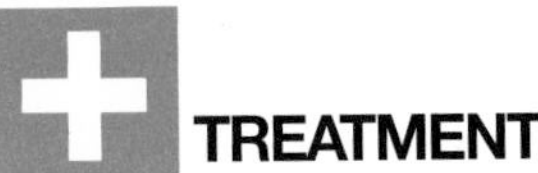

TREATMENT

APPROPRIATE HEALTH CARE Inpatient (emergency room or intensive care)

GENERAL MEASURES
- Establish ABC's of basic life support; establish airway, intubate if necessary. Give warm humidified oxygen (42-46°C). Correct metabolic acidosis.
- Evaluate for frostbite and other trauma
- Rewarming
  - ◊ Dependent on severity of hypothermia
  - ◊ Warm center of body first
  - ◊ Rate of rewarming should be 0.5-2°C/hour. More rapid rewarming can cause ventricular fibrillation and hypovolemic shock.
- With all patients
  - ◊ Remove wet garments
  - ◊ Protect against heat loss and wind chill
  - ◊ Maintain horizontal position
  - ◊ Monitor core temperature and cardiac rhythm
- Mild hypothermia
  - ◊ Passive rewarming (wrap in heated blanket or clothing)
  - ◊ Administration of heated (43°C) IV solutions (D5NS)
  - ◊ Warm fluids may be given if fully alert
- Moderate hypothermia
  - ◊ Active external rewarming
  - ◊ Heated blankets; heating pads
  - ◊ Radiant heat sources
  - ◊ Alcohol-circulating blankets
- Severe hypothermia
  - ◊ Active internal (core) rewarming
  - ◊ Peritoneal dialysis
  - ◊ Gastrointestinal, colonic, or bladder lavage with warm fluids (43°)
  - ◊ Heated intravenous fluids
  - ◊ Heated humidified oxygen
  - ◊ Thoracic cavity lavage (43°)
  - ◊ Extracorporeal blood rewarming
- Cardiac arrhythmias
  - ◊ Atrial fibrillation and sinus bradycardia are common, but patients usually convert to normal sinus rhythm with rewarming
  - ◊ Transient type ventricular arrhythmias should not be treated. If treatment is required, bretylium is recommended.
  - ◊ If cardiac pacing required, preferable to use external noninvasive pacemaker
- Sepsis bacterial infections
  - ◊ In infants - signs may not be evident, initiate treatment with broad-spectrum antibiotic until culture results are available
  - ◊ Older children and adults - if no signs, can usually wait for culture results
  - ◊ Diabetic adults - consider prophylactic antibiotic coverage

SURGICAL MEASURES N/A

ACTIVITY Bedrest. Because of the cold, heart is irritable and susceptible to arrhythmias. Take special care in moving and transporting.

DIET Warm fluids only, if alert and able to swallow

PATIENT EDUCATION
- Preventive measures to avoid recurrence
- If due to inadequate clothing or housing, refer patient to a social service agency
- Urge persons with cardiovascular disease to avoid outdoor exercise in cold weather
- Accidental hypothermia, NIH publication, No. 93-1464

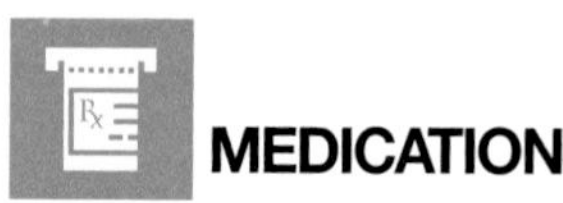

MEDICATIONS

DRUG(S) OF CHOICE
- For sepsis or bacterial infections - antibiotics based on site and etiology. Prophylactic antibiotics are not indicated.
- If ventricular fibrillation requires treatment, bretylium, 5 mg/kg, may be helpful. Magnesium sulfate, 100 mg/kg, is also effective.
- For hypoglycemia, D50W at a dose of 1 mg/kg IV
- Thiamine, 100 mg IV, should be given to any alcoholic or cachectic patient
- Naloxone, 2.0 mg IV, should be given to any patient with a depressed level of consciousness
- Levothyroxine 150-500 μg IV for hypothermic myxedema
- For severe acidosis - sodium bicarbonate

Contraindications:
- Medications, including epinephrine, lidocaine and procainamide can accumulate to toxic levels if used repeatedly in severely hypothermic patients
- Routine use of steroids, barbiturates or antibiotics have not been shown to increase survival or decrease postresuscitative damage

Precautions:
- If the patient fails to respond to the initial three defibrillation attempts or initial drug therapy, subsequent defibrillations or additional boluses of medication should be avoided until core temperature > 30°C. When temperature > 30°C, IV medications are indicated, but at longer than the standard intervals.
- Avoid vasopressors because of arrhythmogenic potential and delayed metabolism
- To prevent fluid overload, IV fluids should be slowly administered because of the decreased cardiac output
- Avoid lactated Ringer's solution because of decreased lactate metabolism

Significant possible interactions: Use all drugs cautiously because metabolism and renal elimination are impaired and once rewarming has occurred, there is mobilization of depot stores

ALTERNATIVE DRUGS N/A

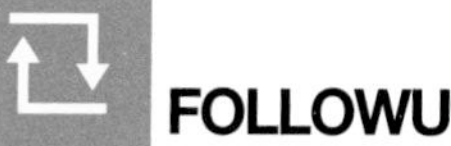

FOLLOWUP

PATIENT MONITORING
- During acute episode
  - ◊ Lab work repeated frequently (with particular attention to electrolytes and glucose)
  - ◊ Continuous cardiac monitoring
  - ◊ Urinary output monitoring
  - ◊ Temperature monitoring
  - ◊ Follow blood gases, both corrected and uncorrected
- Following acute episode
  - ◊ Continued therapy for any underlying disorder

PREVENTION/AVOIDANCE
- Appropriate clothing for cold weather, with particular attention to head, feet and hand coverings
- If walking or climbing in cold climate, carry survival bags lined with space blankets for use if stranded or injured
- Avoid alcohol, especially if anticipating exposure to cold weather
- Alertness to early symptoms and initiating preventive steps, e.g., drinking warm fluids
- Adequate heat in the home
- Review patient's medications that may predispose to hypothermia (e.g., neuroleptics, sedatives, hypnotics, tranquilizers) and decrease dosage or discontinue if appropriate and feasible
- Referral of patient to social service agency for help with adequate housing, heat or clothing

POSSIBLE COMPLICATIONS
- Cardiac arrhythmias
- Hypotension secondary to marked vasodilatation of rewarming
- Hyperkalemia
- Hypoglycemia
- Rhabdomyolysis
- Bladder atony
- Pneumonia (aspiration and broncho)
- Pulmonary edema
- Pancreatitis
- Peritonitis
- Gastrointestinal bleeding
- Acute tubular necrosis
- Intravascular thromboses
- Metabolic acidosis
- Gangrene of extremities
- Compartment syndromes

EXPECTED COURSE/PROGNOSIS
- Mortality rates are decreasing for hypothermia due to increased recognition and advanced therapy. Mortality usually dependent upon the severity of underlying cause of hypothermia.
- In previously healthy individuals, recovery is usually complete
- Mortality rate in healthy patients < 5%
- Mortality rate in patients with co-existing illness > 50%

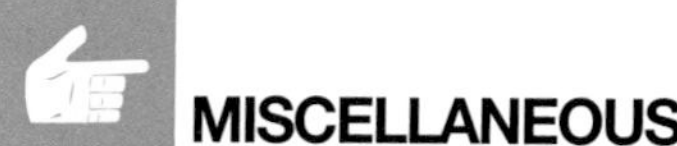

MISCELLANEOUS

ASSOCIATED CONDITIONS
- Congestive heart failure
- Hypothyroidism
- Hypopituitarism
- Uremia
- Addison disease
- Ketoacidosis
- Pulmonary infection
- Sepsis
- Brain injury, tumor
- Diabetes

AGE-RELATED FACTORS
Pediatric:
- All infants are at increased risk of hypothermia because of their limited ability to produce heat when placed in a cold environment. This is particularly true during the first 12 hours of life and in asphyxiated infants. Newborns should be placed under a radiant heat source and the amniotic fluid dried off.
- A child's body temperature drops faster than an adult's when immersed in cold water. This may increase tolerance of the heart's arrhythmias.

Geriatric:
- Mortality rates increase with increasing age
- Older adults have a lower metabolic rate and it is more difficult for them to maintain normal body temperature when environment drops below 18°C
- Aging also impairs the ability to detect temperature changes
- This population also has increased incidence of diseases that decrease heat production, increase or impair thermoregulation

Others: N/A

PREGNANCY Controlled hypothermia in the operating suite is safe during pregnancy, especially with cerebrovascular surgery

SYNONYMS Accidental hypothermia

ICD-9-CM
991.6 Hypothermia
995.89 Other specified adverse effects, NEC, Other
778.2 Cold injury syndrome of newborn
780.99 Hypothermia not associated with low environmental temperature
778.3 Other hypothermia of newborn

SEE ALSO
Frostbite
Near drowning

OTHER NOTES N/A

ABBREVIATIONS N/A

REFERENCES

- Weinberg AD. Hypothermia. Annual of Emergency Medicine 1993; 22(part 2):370-377
- Danzl DT, Pozos R. Accidental hypothermia. New Engl J Med 1994;331:1756-1760
- Hanania NA, Zimmerman JL. Accidental hypothermia. Crit Care Clin 1999;15(2):235-49
- Biem J, Koehncke N, Dosman J. Out of the cold: Management of hypothermia and frostbite. CMAJ 2003;Feb 4;168(3):305-11. Review.

Web references: 1 available at www.5mcc.com
Illustrations N/A

Author(s):
Scott T. Henderson, MD

Hypothyroidism, adult

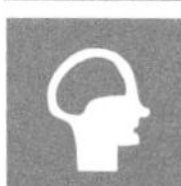

BASICS

DESCRIPTION A clinical state resulting from decreased circulating levels of free thyroid hormone or from resistance to hormone action. Myxedema connotes severe hypothyroidism.

System(s) affected: Endocrine/Metabolic

Genetics:
- No known genetic pattern for idiopathic primary hypothyroidism
- Hypothyroidism may be associated with Type II autoimmune polyglandular syndrome, which is associated with HLA-DR3, DR4
- Secondary hypothyroidism frequently results from treatment for Graves disease, which may be familial

Incidence/Prevalence in USA:
- 5-10/1000 in general population
- Over age 65, increases to 6-10% of women, 2-3% of men

Predominant age: Over 40

Predominant sex: Female > Male, 5-10:1

SIGNS & SYMPTOMS
- Symptoms
  - ◊ Onset may be insidious, subtle
  - ◊ Weakness, fatigue, lethargy
  - ◊ Cold intolerance
  - ◊ Decreased memory
  - ◊ Hearing impairment
  - ◊ Constipation
  - ◊ Muscle cramps
  - ◊ Arthralgias
  - ◊ Paresthesias
  - ◊ Modest weight gain (10 pounds [4.5 kg])
  - ◊ Decreased sweating
  - ◊ Menorrhagia
  - ◊ Depression
  - ◊ Hoarseness
  - ◊ Carpal tunnel syndrome
- Signs
  - ◊ Dry, coarse skin
  - ◊ Dull facial expression
  - ◊ Coarsening or huskiness of voice
  - ◊ Periorbital puffiness
  - ◊ Swelling of hands and feet
  - ◊ Bradycardia
  - ◊ Hypothermia
  - ◊ Reduced systolic blood pressure
  - ◊ Increased diastolic blood pressure
  - ◊ Reduced body and scalp hair
  - ◊ Delayed relaxation of deep tendon reflexes
  - ◊ Macroglossia
  - ◊ Dilutional hyponatremia
  - ◊ Anemia (usually normochromic, normocytic)
  - ◊ Enlarged heart on chest x-ray (often due to pericardial effusion)

CAUSES
- Post-ablative follows radioactive iodine therapy or thyroid surgery. Delayed hypothyroidism may develop in patients treated with thioamide drugs (propylthiouracil, methimazole) 4 to 25 years later.
- Primary hypothyroidism may develop as a result of autoimmune thyroiditis, or be idiopathic
- With goiter, most commonly due to autoimmune disease, such as Hashimoto thyroiditis; or heritable biosynthetic defects, iodine deficiency (rare in the US), or drug induced (iodides, lithium, phenylbutazone, aminosalicylic acid, amiodarone, aminoglutethimide and interferon a)
- Central hypothyroidism, may be due to deficiency of thyrotropin-releasing hormone (TRH) from the hypothalamus or thyroid-stimulating hormone (TSH) from the pituitary
- Transient hypothyroidism may result from silent thyroiditis (most common in post partum period) and subacute granulomatous thyroiditis

RISK FACTORS
- Risk increases with increasing age
- Autoimmune diseases
- Previous postpartum thyroiditis
- Previous head or neck irradiation

DIAGNOSIS

DIFFERENTIAL DIAGNOSIS
- Nephrotic syndrome
- Chronic nephritis
- Neurasthenia
- Depression
- Euthyroid sick syndrome
- Congestive heart failure
- Primary amyloidosis
- Dementia from other causes

LABORATORY
- TSH (radioimmunoassay) - elevated
- Total serum thyroxine (T4) - decreased
- T3 resin uptake - increased
- Free T4 index (= T3 resin uptake x total serum T4) - low
- In severe hypothyroidism, anemia, elevated cholesterol, CPK, LDH, AST, hyponatremia

Drugs that may alter lab results:
- Thyroid supplement
- Cortisone
- Dopamine
- Phenytoin
- Estrogen or androgen therapy in excess of replacement
- Amiodarone
- Salicylates

Disorders that may alter lab results:
- Any severe illness
- Pregnancy
- Chronic protein malnutrition
- Hepatic failure
- Nephrotic syndrome

PATHOLOGICAL FINDINGS Thyroid may be small, atrophic or enlarged

SPECIAL TESTS Radioimmunoassay

IMAGING None necessary

DIAGNOSTIC PROCEDURES Elevated TSH (greater than 20 μU/mL [3-20 mIU/L]) is diagnostic of primary thyroid failure

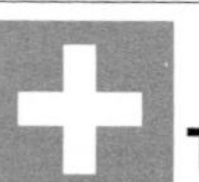

TREATMENT

APPROPRIATE HEALTH CARE Outpatient except for complicating emergencies (coma, hypothermia)

GENERAL MEASURES Goals of treatment are to restore and maintain a euthyroid state

SURGICAL MEASURES N/A

ACTIVITY As tolerated

DIET
- High-bulk diet may be helpful to avoid constipation
- Low fat diet for obese patients

PATIENT EDUCATION
- Importance of compliance with thyroid replacement therapy
- Need for lifelong treatment
- Report to physician any signs of infection, heart problems
- Signs of thyrotoxicity

MEDICATIONS

DRUG(S) OF CHOICE
- Levothyroxine (Synthroid, Levothroid)
  - ◊ 50-100 µg/day. Increase by 25 µg/day every 4-6 weeks until TSH is in normal range.
  - ◊ Dosage requirements may vary with age, sex, residual secretory capacity of thyroid gland, other drugs being taken by patient, intestinal function
  - ◊ Elderly patients may require lower dose because clearance is decreased

Contraindications:
- Thyrotoxic heart disease
- Uncorrected adrenocorticoid insufficiency

Precautions:
- Start with lower doses in the elderly and patients with heart disease
- Diabetic patients may need readjustment of hypoglycemic agents with institution of thyroxine
- Dosage of oral anticoagulants may need adjustment; monitor prothrombin time while initiating treatment

Significant possible interactions:
- Oral anticoagulants
- Insulin
- Oral hypoglycemics
- Estrogen
- Oral contraceptives
- Cholestyramine
- Ferrous sulfate may decrease absorption when taken concomitantly

ALTERNATIVE DRUGS
None currently recommended

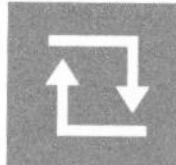

FOLLOWUP

PATIENT MONITORING
- Every 6 weeks until stabilized, then every 6 months
- Follow cardiac status closely in older patients

PREVENTION/AVOIDANCE
N/A

POSSIBLE COMPLICATIONS
- Treatment induced congestive heart failure in people with coronary artery disease
- Myxedema coma - life threatening complication of hypothyroidism
- Increased susceptibility to infection
- Megacolon
- Organic psychosis with paranoia
- Adrenal crisis with vigorous treatment of hypothyroidism
- Infertility
- Hypersensitivity to opiates
- Overtreatment over long periods can lead to bone demineralization

EXPECTED COURSE/PROGNOSIS
- With early treatment, striking transformations in approved appearance and mental function. Return to normal state is the rule.
- Relapses will occur if treatment is interrupted
- If untreated, may progress to myxedema coma

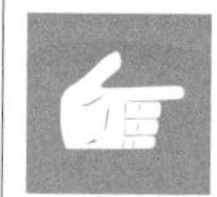

MISCELLANEOUS

ASSOCIATED CONDITIONS
- Hyponatremia
- Anemia
- Idiopathic adrenocorticoid deficiency
- Diabetes mellitus
- Hypoparathyroidism
- Myasthenia gravis
- Vitiligo
- Hypercholesterolemia
- Mitral valve prolapse
- Depression
- Rapid cycling bipolar disorder

AGE-RELATED FACTORS
Pediatric: N/A

Geriatric:
- Characteristic signs and symptoms frequently changed or absent. Hypothyroidism is common in elderly. Diagnosis based on laboratory criteria.
- Replacement therapy is usually about two thirds of the dose used in young adults.

Others: N/A

PREGNANCY
- Replacement therapy may need adjustment. TSH levels should be monitored monthly during first trimester.
- Postpartum - check TSH levels at about 6 weeks
- Painless subacute thyroiditis may occur in the post partum period leading to transient hypothyroidism lasting about 3 months. Treatment with replacement therapy may be warranted. Up to 30% of these individuals develop permanent hypothyroidism.

SYNONYMS
Myxedema

ICD-9-CM
244.0 Postsurgical hypothyroidism
244.2 Iodine hypothyroidism
244.8 Other specified acquired hypothyroidism
244.9 Unspecified hypothyroidism

SEE ALSO
Hyperthyroidism
Thyroiditis

OTHER NOTES
- Surgical procedures
  - ◊ Hypothyroid patients (mild to moderate) tolerate surgery with mortality and complications similar to euthyroid patients
  - ◊ If surgery is elective, render patient euthyroid prior to procedure
  - ◊ If surgery is urgent, proceed with the procedure with individualized replacement therapy preoperatively and postoperatively

ABBREVIATIONS
N/A

REFERENCES

- Barzel US. Hypothyroidism: diagnosis and management. Clin Geriatric Med 1995;11(2):239-49
- Hueston WJ. Treatment of hypothyroidism. Am Fam Phys 2001;64(10):1717-24
- Woeber KA. Update on the management of hypothyroidism and hyperthyroidism. Arch Int Med 2000; 160(8):1067-71
- Guha B, Krishnaswamy G, Peiris A. The diagnosis and management of hypothyroidism. South Med J 2002;95(5):475-80
- Roberts CG, Ladenson PW. Hypothyroidism. Lancet 2004;363(9411):793-803

Web references: 1 available at www.5mcc.com

Illustrations N/A

Author(s):
Barbara A. Majeroni, MD

BASICS

DESCRIPTION A cutaneous eruption associated with, but distant to, the main lesion of the disease.
Id is a word termination often combined with a root reflecting the causative factor. For example, bacterid, syphilid, and tuberculid. The dermatophytid is the most frequently referenced id reaction in dermatology. A dermatophytid is an autosensitization reaction where a secondary cutaneous reaction occurs at a site distant to a primary fungal infection. The distant eruption is due to circulating fungal antigen from the primary site reacting with antibodies at sensitized areas of the skin.
System(s) affected: Skin/Exocrine
Genetics: N/A
Incidence/Prevalence in USA: Not infrequent
Predominant age: All affect all ages
Predominant sex: Male = Female

SIGNS & SYMPTOMS
- Usual
  - ◊ Pruritic vesicles on the hands
  - ◊ Tinea infection on the feet
  - ◊ Generalized reactions can occur
- Less common
  - ◊ Papules
  - ◊ Lichenoid eruption
  - ◊ Eczematoid eruption

CAUSES Circulating antigens react with antibodies at sensitized areas of the skin

RISK FACTORS
- Fungal infection of the skin

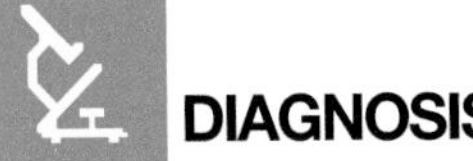

DIAGNOSIS

DIFFERENTIAL DIAGNOSIS
- Pompholyx
- Contact dermatitis
- Drug eruptions
- Pustular psoriasis

LABORATORY
- Fungal infection at the primary site proven by potassium hydroxide (KOH) or fungal culture
- No fungal demonstrable at the site of the presumed id reaction

Drugs that may alter lab results: N/A

Disorders that may alter lab results: N/A

PATHOLOGICAL FINDINGS
- Vesicles in the upper dermis
- Moderate acanthosis
- Increased granular cell layer
- Lack of inflammation

SPECIAL TESTS Skin shows a positive trichophytin reaction

IMAGING N/A

DIAGNOSTIC PROCEDURES
- Potassium hydroxide (KOH) prep
- Fungal culture

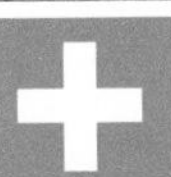

TREATMENT

APPROPRIATE HEALTH CARE Outpatient

GENERAL MEASURES
- treatment of the underlying fungal infection
- Symptomatic treatment of pruritus with antihistamines and/or topical steroids if needed
- Treatment for secondary bacterial infection

SURGICAL MEASURES N/A

ACTIVITY As tolerated

DIET No special diet

PATIENT EDUCATION
- Avoidance of hot humid conditions which promote fungal growth
- Aeration of susceptible body areas, eg, wear sandals or open foot wear
- If possible, wearing boxer shorts or loose fitting clothing, drying off wet skin after bathing, using powders and antiperspirants to make the environment less conducive to fungal growth

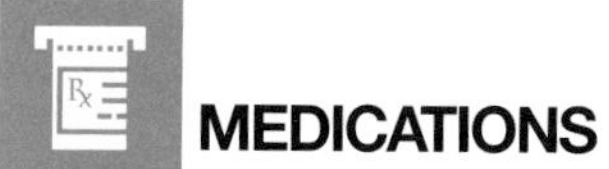

MEDICATIONS

DRUG(S) OF CHOICE Antifungals - topical and/or systemic

Contraindications: Refer to manufacturer's profile of each drug

Precautions: Refer to manufacturer's profile of each drug

Significant possible interactions: Refer to manufacturer's profile of each drug

ALTERNATIVE DRUGS
- Topical or systemic antibiotics for any secondary infection
- Antihistamines for any pruritus
- Topical steroids for pruritus
- Systemic steroids only if reaction is florid or generalized nature

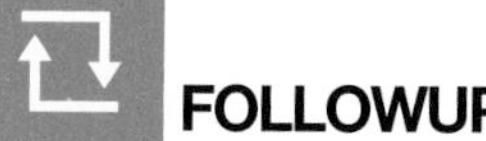

FOLLOWUP

PATIENT MONITORING Followup in a few days or a week pending clinical course

PREVENTION/AVOIDANCE
- Minimize factors for developing fungal infections
- Prompt treatment of any developing fungal infection

POSSIBLE COMPLICATIONS
- Secondary bacterial infection (cellulitis)

EXPECTED COURSE/PROGNOSIS After appropriate treatment, virtual resolution in a few days to two weeks

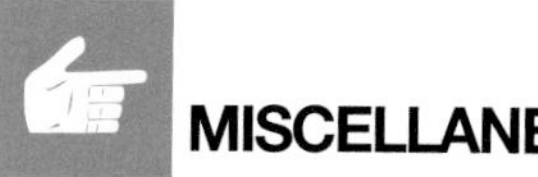

MISCELLANEOUS

ASSOCIATED CONDITIONS Primary fungal infection

AGE-RELATED FACTORS
Pediatric: N/A
Geriatric: N/A
Others: N/A

PREGNANCY N/A

SYNONYMS
- Dermatophytid
- Trichophytid

ICD-9-CM
692.89 Contact dermatitis and other eczema due to other specified agents, other

SEE ALSO
Tinea corporis
Tinea pedis

OTHER NOTES N/A

ABBREVIATIONS N/A

REFERENCES

- Habif T. Clinical Dermatology. 4th Ed. St. Louis, CV Mosby, 2004

Web references: 1 available at www.5mcc.com
Illustrations 1 available

Author(s):
Joseph Shrum, MD

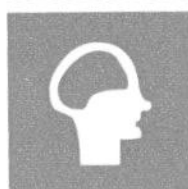

BASICS

DESCRIPTION This entity was the first known form of the hypertrophic cardiomyopathies (HCM) with the characteristic finding of inappropriate (disproportionate to the hemodynamic load) myocardial hypertrophy
- IHSS is characterized by a dynamic pressure gradient in the subaortic area leading clinically to both:
  - ◊ Diastolic dysfunction with impaired ventricular filling and elevated atrial filling pressures producing dyspnea
  - ◊ Systolic dysfunction with limitation of cardiac output response to exercise, exertional syncope, and secondary left ventricular hypertrophy
- Diagnosis usually is made by recognition of signs associated with outflow obstruction, but symptoms are predominantly characterized by diastolic dysfunction

System(s) affected: Cardiovascular
Genetics:
- Autosomal dominant with > 50% penetrance
- Evidence of disease (usually milder) is found in 25% of first degree relatives. Relatives usually do not have outflow obstruction, exhibit only localized hypertrophy, and are asymptomatic.

Incidence/Prevalence in USA: Uncommon
Predominant age: Most commonly presents in third decade (disease of young adulthood), but occurs from newborns to elderly
Predominant sex: Male = Female

SIGNS & SYMPTOMS
- Dyspnea: mainly a result of diastolic dysfunction and initially exertional in onset (50-90%)
- Angina pectoris (50-90%)
- Syncope: exertional (50-90%)
- Presyncope: exertional (50-90%)
- Fatigue (50-90%)
- Palpitations (50-90%)
- Paroxysmal nocturnal dyspnea (50%)
- Double apical impulse due to prominent atrial system
- PMI displaced laterally
- Rapidly rising bifid carotid pulse
- Prominent S4
- S2 variable splitting (depending on degree of outflow obstruction)
- Harsh systolic crescendo-decrescendo murmur best heard between apex and left sternal border
- Murmur: increases and lengthens with Valsalva, standing, amyl nitrite; decreases with sudden squatting, lying down, passive leg raising, isometric handgrip

CAUSES Thickened septum impinging on the anterior mitral valve leaflet during systole causing outflow obstruction

RISK FACTORS Family history of HCM

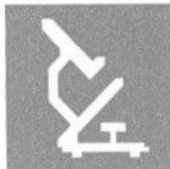

DIAGNOSIS

DIFFERENTIAL DIAGNOSIS
- Fixed outflow obstruction such as aortic stenosis (AS). In AS the carotid pulse is slow-rising and reduced in volume versus the rapid-rising bifid pulse of IHSS. Bedside hemodynamic maneuvers (Valsalva, etc.) also help to differentiate.

LABORATORY N/A

Drugs that may alter lab results: N/A

Disorders that may alter lab results: N/A

PATHOLOGICAL FINDINGS
- Distinctive pattern of left ventricular (LV) hypertrophy - localized disproportionate hypertrophy of the LV septum with the ratio of septal to free wall thickness > 1.3:1 without anatomic evidence of pressure overload
- Dilated atria
- Increased LV mass and small chamber sizes
- Mural plaque of LV outflow tract
- Mitral valve thickening
- Anatomic variants:
  - ◊ Apical form; not associated with intraventricular gradients
  - ◊ Localized mid-ventricular obstructive form
- Disorganization and disarray septal muscle bundles
- Abnormal intramural coronary arteries

SPECIAL TESTS
- Electrocardiogram: Common findings (50-90%)
  - ◊ Non-specific ST-T wave abnormalities
  - ◊ Left ventricular hypertrophy
- Electrocardiogram: Less common findings (< 50%)
  - ◊ Prominent and abnormal Q waves in anterior precordial and lateral limbs lead, simulating myocardial infarction
  - ◊ P-wave abnormalities indicating left atrial enlargement
  - ◊ Short PR interval with QRS morphology suggestive of pre-excitation without clear evidence of pre-excitation (rare in IHSS)
  - ◊ Holter findings - frequent ventricular arrhythmias with up to 25% revealing ventricular tachycardia
  - ◊ Atrial fibrillation - late finding and poor prognostic sign

IMAGING Chest x-ray - variable findings from normal cardiac size to cardiomegaly, none of which is pathognomonic

DIAGNOSTIC PROCEDURES
- Echocardiography
  - ◊ Asymmetric septal hypertrophy with septal to free wall ratio > 1.3:1
  - ◊ Abnormal systolic anterior leaflet motion of the mitral valve
  - ◊ Left ventricular hypertrophy
  - ◊ Left atrial enlargement
  - ◊ Small ventricular chamber size with increased contractility
  - ◊ Partial systolic closure of aortic valve in mid-systole
  - ◊ Mitral valve prolapse
  - ◊ Mitral regurgitation by Doppler
  - ◊ Decreased mid-aortic flow coincident with systolic anterior leaflet motion of mitral valve by Doppler
- Radionuclide
  - ◊ Thallium scintigraphy with stress at times reveals positive defects in setting of arteriographically normal coronary arteries
- Cardiac catheterization and angiocardiography
  - ◊ Hemodynamic measurement documents degree and lability of outflow obstruction, and diastolic characteristics of left ventricle
  - ◊ Angiocardiography documents left and right ventricular anatomy and coronary arterial anatomy

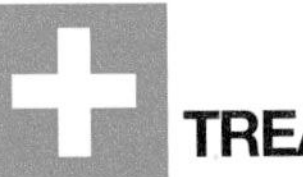

TREATMENT

APPROPRIATE HEALTH CARE Outpatient usually. Inpatient for studies and/or surgery.

GENERAL MEASURES
- Therapy based on pathophysiology, namely interventions to reduce ventricular contractility or increase ventricular volume, ventricular compliance, and outflow tract dimensions
- Digitalis glycosides are contraindicated except for atrial fibrillation with uncontrolled response
- Nitrates and sympathomimetic amines (e.g., isoproterenol) are contraindicated except with concomitant coronary heart disease
- Diuretics are relatively contraindicated because of their effect on ventricular volume and left ventricular myotomy
- Pacemaker therapy - AV sequential pacing is frequently helpful in symptomatic patients with an outflow obstruction who do not respond to medical therapy

SURGICAL MEASURES Left ventricular myomectomy - done only in setting of severe symptoms refractory to medical therapy or sequential pacing in those patients with outflow gradient >50 mm Hg (<6.65 kPa), either at rest or with provocation. 95% successful in abolishing gradient with 70% of patients having a marked symptomatic improvement for at least 5 years.

ACTIVITY
- Strenuous exercise, especially competitive sports, should not be undertaken because of high risk of sudden death. Younger patients with little or no functional impairment have the greatest risk of sudden death.
- Sports participation by patients with IHSS is not permitted if any of the following are present: Marked left ventricle hypertrophy, significant outflow gradient, significant supraventricular and/or ventricular arrhythmias, or history of sudden death in relatives with hypertrophic cardiomyopathy

DIET No special diet, but may need to reduce caloric intake, due to reduced activity

PATIENT EDUCATION
- Activity restrictions
- Refer for psychosocial counseling if appropriate (patient and family may suffer from restricted life-style and chronic disease problems)
- Recommend family learn cardiopulmonary resuscitation methods

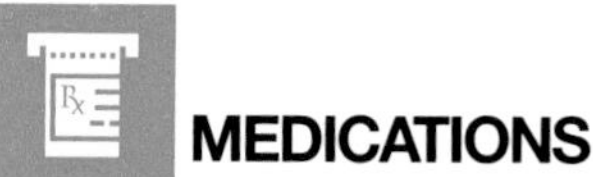

MEDICATIONS

DRUG(S) OF CHOICE
- Beta blockers (propranolol, metoprolol, etc)
  - ◊ May decrease outflow obstruction: Some evidence suggests that it may increase ventricular compliance. No clear evidence that it reduces incidence of sudden death.
  - ◊ 1/3 to 2/3 of patients experience symptomatic improvement
  - ◊ May titrate up to 320 mg/day of propranolol equivalent to obtain clinical effect provided patient tolerates dose
- Calcium channel blockers (primarily verapamil)
  - ◊ Alternative to therapy with propranolol
  - ◊ May have better effect on exercise performance
  - ◊ Decrease in outflow gradient due to depression of cardiac contractility
  - ◊ Improves diastolic filling by improved diastolic relaxation
- Amiodarone (Cordarone)
  - ◊ Limited use in treating ventricular arrhythmias because of documented pro-arrhythmic effects in HCM
  - ◊ Only to be used in patients with ventricular tachycardia associated with hemodynamic compromise. Use of drug is to be guided by initial and followup electrophysiological studies.

Contraindications:
- Verapamil:
  - ◊ Major side effects include depression of impulse formation and A-V block, negative inotropism, and vasodilatation - all of which can result in hypotension, shock, pulmonary edema, and death
  - ◊ Therefore, relatively contraindicated for use in patients with increased left ventricle end diastolic pressure (LVEDP), paroxysmal nocturnal dyspnea (PND), orthopnea, and/or in patients with sinus node disease and A-V block (unless there is an appropriate pacing device)

Precautions: See manufacturer's profile of each drug

Significant possible interactions: See manufacturer's profile of each drug

ALTERNATIVE DRUGS
- Diltiazem
- Disopyramide

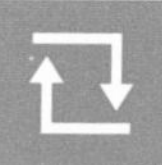

FOLLOWUP

PATIENT MONITORING Yearly when symptoms and pharmacologic regimens become stable

PREVENTION/AVOIDANCE
- Avoid strenuous exercise, especially competitive sports
- Avoid rapid standing
- Avoid inotropic drugs and diuretics
- Use antitussives for infections that are accompanied by a cough

POSSIBLE COMPLICATIONS
- Sudden death
- Congestive heart failure
- Arrhythmia
- Atrial fibrillation with mural thrombosis formation
- Infective mitral endocarditis

EXPECTED COURSE/PROGNOSIS
- Annual mortality rate - 4% a year (sudden death most common reason)
- Chronic illness with restricted life-style

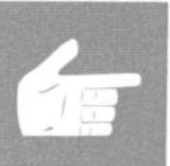

MISCELLANEOUS

ASSOCIATED CONDITIONS
- Mitral regurgitation
- Essential hypertension
- Mitral valve prolapse
- Angina pectoris

AGE-RELATED FACTORS
Pediatric:
- IHSS being recognized with increasing frequency
- Children may be asymptomatic. Evaluation of a heart murmur may disclose IHSS.

Geriatric: Occurrence is more frequent with increasing age. Female prevalence is greater in this age group.

Others: N/A

PREGNANCY N/A

SYNONYMS
- Hypertrophic obstructive cardiomyopathy (HOCM)
- Muscular subaortic stenosis

ICD-9-CM
425.1 Hypertrophic obstructive cardiomyopathy

SEE ALSO

OTHER NOTES Genetic counseling may be appropriate

ABBREVIATIONS
- HCM = hypertrophic cardiomyopathy
- AS = aortic stenosis
- LV = left ventricle
- PMI = Point of maximal impulse

REFERENCES

- Braunwald E, editor Heart Disease: A Textbook of Cardiovascular Medicine. 6th ed. Philadelphia: WB Saunders Co; 2001
- Maron BJ, et al. Sudden death in hypertrophic cardiomyopathy. A profile of 78 patients. Circulation 1982;65:1388
- Goldman L, Braunwald E, editors. Primary Cardiology. 2nd ed. Philadelphia: WB Saunders Co; 2003

Web references: 0 available at www.5mcc.com

Illustrations N/A

Author(s):
Peter Kozisek, MD

Idiopathic thrombocytopenic purpura (ITP)

BASICS

DESCRIPTION A decrease in the circulating number of platelets (< 100,000 per microliter) in absence of toxic exposure or a disease associated with a low platelet count. It occurs as a secondary effect of peripheral platelet destruction as well as decreased platelet production. It is a diagnosis of exclusion.
- Acute ITP - a disease of childhood which often follows an acute infection and has spontaneous resolution within 2 months. Platelet counts < 20,000. This is a common disorder.
- Chronic ITP - a disease which persists after 6 months without a specific cause. Usually seen in adults and persists for months to years. Platelet count typically 30,000-80,000.

System(s) affected: Hemic/Lymphatic/Immunologic
Genetics: No known genetic pattern
Incidence/Prevalence in USA: 1 in 10,000
Predominant age:
- Acute ITP - children ages 2-6 years old
- Chronic ITP - >50 years

Predominant sex:
- Acute ITP - Male = Female
- Chronic ITP - Female > Male (2:1)

SIGNS & SYMPTOMS
- Post traumatic bleeding at 40,000-60,000 platelet count
- Petechial hemorrhages
- Purpura
- Bruising tendency
- Gingival bleeding
- Gastrointestinal bleeding
- Mucocutaneous hemorrhages
- Menometrorrhagia
- Menorrhagia
- Recurrent epistaxis
- Neurological symptoms secondary to intracerebral bleeding
- Non-palpable spleen (absence of splenomegaly is an essential diagnostic criterion)
- Spontaneous bleeding < 20,000 platelet count

CAUSES IgG autoantibodies on platelet surface which are bound to and destroyed by reticuloendothelial (RE) phagocytes

RISK FACTORS
- Acute infection
- Age
- Cardiopulmonary bypass
- Hypersplenism
- Antiphospholipid antibody syndrome
- Preeclampsia
- HIV infection

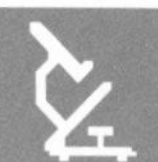

DIAGNOSIS

DIFFERENTIAL DIAGNOSIS
- Drug induced immune thrombocytopenia. Over 150 drugs have been implicated.
- Infections
- Acute leukemia
- Thrombotic thrombocytopenia purpura (TTP)
- Hemolytic uremic syndrome
- Factitious: "platelet clumping on the peripheral smear"
- Thrombocytopenia secondary to sepsis
- Myelodysplastic syndrome, particularly in the older patient
- Decreased production in marrow: malignancy, drugs, viruses, megaloblastic anemia
- Post transfusion
- Isoimmune neonatal purpura
- Disseminated intravascular coagulation (DIC)
- Alcohol induced

LABORATORY
- Decreased platelet count: 5,000-75,000
- Relative lymphocytosis and slight eosinophilia
- Prolonged bleeding time (not useful in the presence of thrombocytopenia)
- Anemia
- PT, PTT normal

Drugs that may alter lab results: N/A

Disorders that may alter lab results: N/A

PATHOLOGICAL FINDINGS
- Peripheral smear shows normal red and white cells with diminished but large platelets; smear helps to rule out pseudothrombocytopenia
- Marrow reveals abundant megakaryocytes with normal erythroid and myeloid precursors

SPECIAL TESTS
- Peripheral smear - routinely recommended
- Platelet associated antibody (PA-IgG) - optional bound and unbound test available; bound is superior with sensitivity of 49-66% and specificity of 78-92%

IMAGING CT of head to rule out intracranial bleeding if clinically indicated

DIAGNOSTIC PROCEDURES
- Bone marrow aspiration/biopsy (consider in refractory cases)
  - ◊ Does not need to be done before giving gamma globulin
  - ◊ Not needed in patients < 60 who have typical clinical and lab presentation
  - ◊ Rarely indicated in children, but preferred by some hematologists if steroids will be used in treatment

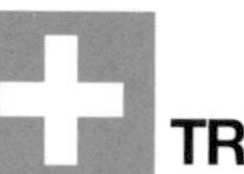

TREATMENT

APPROPRIATE HEALTH CARE
- Outpatient management unless patient at risk for bleeding (platelet count < 20,000)
- Admit patients with active bleeding

GENERAL MEASURES
- Children with platelet counts > 30,000 do not require treatment if they are asymptomatic or those with minor purpura do not need treatment
- Treatment for adults if platelet < 20,000, or platelets < 50,000 with symptoms or risks for bleeding such as HTN or peptic ulcers
- Specific treatment usually not necessary unless count is < 100,000; possibly < 30,000 with chronic ITP
- Platelet transfusions for significant bleeding

SURGICAL MEASURES
- Splenectomy
  - ◊ In patients who fail medical therapy
  - ◊ Consider Hib and meningococcal vaccine
  - ◊ Be sure to administer pneumococcal vaccine at least 2 weeks prior to splenectomy
  - ◊ Criteria remain not well-defined. Decision based on response, severity. and patient preference regarding risks/benefits of surgery.
  - ◊ Splenectomy considered if after 3-6 months, patient needs > 10-20 mg prednisone/day to keep platelets above 30,000/mm3

ACTIVITY Minimal activity to prevent injury or bruising. Avoid contact sports.

DIET No special diet

PATIENT EDUCATION Avoidance of ASA and other platelet inhibiting drugs. No data on immunizations-strictly recommendations.

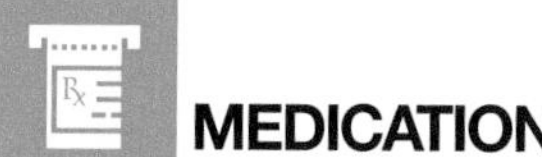

MEDICATIONS

DRUG(S) OF CHOICE

- Acute ITP: prednisone 1-2 mg/kg/day for 2-4 weeks, then taper.
- Chronic ITP: oral prednisone 1-2 mg/kg/day with tapers over 4-6 weeks; most responses occur within first week of treatment. For patients who do not respond, consider IV immune globulin (IVIG) 0.4g/kg per day for 5 days, or anti-D, 50 μg/kg once (repeat as necessary) or dexamethasone 20-40 mg/d for 4 days. If no response to these therapies, then consider splenectomy. Also limited data to screen for and eradicate *H. pylori*.
- Emergency treatment of patients with internal or mucocutaneous bleeding or who need emergent surgery treatment should include:
  - ◊ IV immune globulin 1g/kg/d for 2 days
  - ◊ IV methylprednisolone 1g/d for 3 days
  - ◊ Platelet transfusions (5U every 4-6 hours or 2 U/h)

Contraindications: Do not administer gamma globulin if patient has IgA deficiency

Precautions: Refer to manufacturer's literature

Significant possible interactions: Anaphylaxis in patients with IgA deficiency who have IgA auto-antibodies

ALTERNATIVE DRUGS

- Acute ITP: immune globulin (IVIG, gamma globulin) 1-2 gm/kg single dose or 400 mg/kg/day for 5 days. Minor adverse reactions - chills, nausea, headache, joint pains in 2-7%. If this occurs, slow the rate of infusion. Gamma globulin may be effective alone or as a pretreatment to facilitate platelet transfusion. May delay need for splenectomy.
- Chronic ITP: high doses of intravenous gamma globulin in emergencies
- Anti-Rho(D) immune globulin 250 IU (50-75 μg/kg) as a single dose or in two divided doses given over 2 days; indications for use:
  - ◊ Children with acute or chronic ITP
  - ◊ Adults with chronic ITP who are RhD positive
  - ◊ ITP secondary to HIV infection
- Azathioprine 1-4mg/kg/d modified according to WBC
- Cyclophosphamide 1 to 2 mg/kg/day
- Vincristine or vinblastine
- Danazol 400-800 mg/d
- Cyclosporin A 3m/kg/d
- Rituximab, campath-1H, mycophenolate mofetil
- Plasmapheresis
- Autologous hematopoietic stem cell transplantation
- Investigational or experimental therapies
  - ◊ Monoclonal antibodies against CD20 and CD154
  - ◊ Autologous bone marrow transplant
  - ◊ Immune globulin IV 1g/kg for 2-3 days if platelets <5,000 despite several days of steroids
  - ◊ Thrombopoietin
  - ◊ Etanercept
  - ◊ Monoclonal antibody to FcγRI receptor
  - ◊ Monoclonal antibody to CD40 ligand

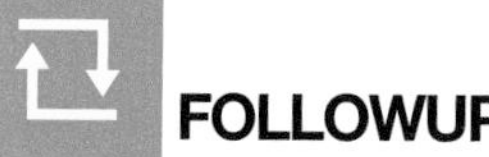

FOLLOWUP

PATIENT MONITORING

- Frequent platelet counts, daily to weekly, depending on severity and treatment
- Follow clinical status of hemostasis

PREVENTION/AVOIDANCE

Avoid medications (when feasible) that inhibit platelet function (such as aspirin), or those that suppress bone marrow

POSSIBLE COMPLICATIONS

- 1% mortality due to intracranial hemorrhage
- Severe blood loss
- Corticosteroid adverse effects
- Pneumococcal infections if patient must have splenectomy. Use pneumococcal vaccine.

EXPECTED COURSE/PROGNOSIS

- Acute ITP:
  - ◊ 80-85% completely recover within 2 months
  - ◊ 15% proceed to chronic ITP
- Chronic ITP:
  - ◊ 10-20% recover spontaneously
  - ◊ Remainder with diminished platelets for months to years
  - ◊ May see spontaneous remissions (5%) and relapses

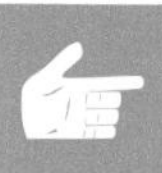

MISCELLANEOUS

ASSOCIATED CONDITIONS

- Acute ITP:
  - ◊ Varicella
  - ◊ Other viral infections
- Chronic ITP:
  - ◊ HIV
  - ◊ H. Pylori
  - ◊ Graves' disease
  - ◊ Hashimoto thyroiditis
  - ◊ Sarcoidosis
  - ◊ Systemic lupus erythematosus
  - ◊ Autoimmune hemolytic anemia (Evans' syndrome)

AGE-RELATED FACTORS

Pediatric:

- The acute form is primarily a childhood disease
- Better prognosis than adults

Geriatric: ITP is uncommon in this age group; look for other cause of low platelet count

Others: N/A

PREGNANCY

- Only if < 50,000 platelet count, may consider C-section
- Patient in labor should receive intravenous gamma globulin due to risk to the infant
- Platelet autoantibodies cross the placenta and may cause neonatal thrombocytopenia. Consider prednisone 10-20 mg/day for 10-14 days prior to delivery.
- Preeclampsia or gestational thrombocytopenia may cause thrombocytopenia unrelated to ITP

SYNONYMS

- Postinfectious thrombocytopenia
- Immune thrombocytopenic purpura
- Werlhof disease

ICD-9-CM

287.3 Primary thrombocytopenia

SEE ALSO

OTHER NOTES N/A

ABBREVIATIONS N/A

REFERENCES

- Di Paola JA, Buchanan GR. Immune thrombocytopenic purpura. Pediatr Clin North Am 2002;49(5):911-28
- McMillan R. Classical management of refractory adult immune (idiopathic) thrombocytopenic purpura. Blood Rev 2002;16(1):51-5
- Cines DB. Thrombocytopenic purpura. N Engl J Med 2002;346:995-1008
- George JN. Treatment options for chronic idiopathic thrombocytopenia purpura. Semin Hematol 2000;37(suppl2):31-4
- Stasi R, Provan R. Management of ITP in adults. Mayo Clin Proc 2004; 79:504-22

Web references: 0 available at www.5mcc.com

Illustrations N/A

Author(s):

Jeffery T. Kirchner, DO

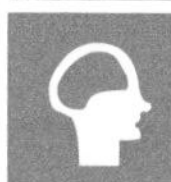

BASICS

DESCRIPTION For the prevention of certain diseases.
Specific indications include:
- Hepatitis B
  - ◊ Infants
  - ◊ Healthcare workers
  - ◊ Laboratory personnel who might be exposed to the virus
  - ◊ Intravenous drug users
  - ◊ Male homosexuals
  - ◊ Patients with a sexually transmitted disease
- Pneumococcal polysaccharide
  - ◊ All persons age 65 and over (once)
  - ◊ All patients prior to splenectomy
  - ◊ Patients with chronic liver, heart, lung or renal disease
  - ◊ Patients with diabetes mellitus, HIV, asplenia
- Influenza inactivated (annually)
  - ◊ All persons age 50 and older
  - ◊ Healthcare workers
  - ◊ Patients with chronic heart, lung or renal disease (may begin at 6 months of age)
  - ◊ Patients with diabetes mellitus, HIV
  - ◊ Healthy children age 6-23 months
  - ◊ Contacts of high-risk persons
- Live, attenuated influenza vaccine (LAIV)for healthy persons 5-49 years old who wish to be vaccinated
- Diphtheria, tetanus, acellular pertussis (DTaP)
  - ◊ All children starting at age 2 months
  - ◊ May be given up to the 7th birthday
- Diphtheria and tetanus (pediatric) toxoids
  - ◊ Children < 7 years who cannot take DTaP
- Tetanus and diphtheria (adult) toxoids
  - ◊ Booster at ages 11-12 or 14-16 and either every 10 years thereafter or a single booster dose at age 50
- Measles, mumps and rubella (MMR)
  - ◊ Children at age 12 to 15 months and again between 4 and 6 years
  - ◊ Adults (especially medical personnel and daycare workers) without prior immunization or uncertain immunizations born after 1956
  - ◊ International travelers
  - ◊ College students - 2 doses total if not previously vaccinated
- Varicella
  - ◊ Children at age 12 to 18 months (1 dose)
  - ◊ Catch-up vaccination for children 18 months to 12 years (1 dose) without history of chickenpox
  - ◊ Susceptible persons ≥ 13 years without history of chickenpox (2 doses)
  - ◊ Health care workers without a previous history of chickenpox
  - ◊ Varicella vaccine may be given within 3-5 days for postexposure prophylaxis
- Polio - all IPV schedule
  - ◊ All children starting at 2 months of age
  - ◊ Adults previously immunized who will travel to areas where polio is prevalent
  - ◊ 4 doses of IPV now recommended
  - ◊ For school entry, 4 doses of polio vaccine (IPV and/or OPV) needed
- Haemophilus influenzae type b
  - ◊ All children starting at 2 months of age
- Hepatitis A
  - ◊ Travelers to higher risk countries
  - ◊ Patients with chronic liver disease
  - ◊ Certain high-risk communities, states, and ethnic groups, e.g., Native American/Alaskan
  - ◊ Homosexual males
  - ◊ Street drug users
  - ◊ Laboratory personnel who might be exposed
- Pneumococcal conjugate vaccine
  - ◊ Infants at 2, 4, 6, 12-15 months
  - ◊ Special catch-up schedule
  - ◊ Catch-up all children through 23 months
  - ◊ Catch-up children 24-59 months who are high-risk, including chronic illness, African American, Native American, sickle cell disease

System(s) affected: Hemic/Lymphatic/Immunologic
Genetics: N/A
Incidence/Prevalence in USA: N/A
Predominant age: N/A
Predominant sex: N/A

SIGNS & SYMPTOMS N/A

CAUSES N/A

RISK FACTORS N/A

DIAGNOSIS

DIFFERENTIAL DIAGNOSIS N/A

LABORATORY N/A

Drugs that may alter lab results: N/A

Disorders that may alter lab results: N/A

PATHOLOGICAL FINDINGS N/A

SPECIAL TESTS N/A

IMAGING N/A

DIAGNOSTIC PROCEDURES N/A

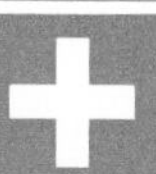

TREATMENT

APPROPRIATE HEALTH CARE N/A

GENERAL MEASURES
- Informed patient consent should discuss consequences of specific diseases and risks of immunizations - Vaccine Information Statements should be given prior to vaccination
- Antipyretics (eg, acetaminophen) are useful for the fever which may accompany certain immunizations

SURGICAL MEASURES N/A

ACTIVITY No restrictions after immunization

DIET No specific restrictions after immunization

PATIENT EDUCATION Report adverse events promptly. Minor redness, swelling, and or soreness at the site of injections can be expected; ice packs and acetaminophen may be helpful. Report serious reactions to VAERS at 800-822-7967.

IMMUNIZATION SCHEDULE #1:

```
       <--------- months ---------->
       0  1  2  4  6  12  15  18  23
------------------------------------
Hep B† 1----->
Hep B†    2------->3----------->
DTaP         1  2  3        4--->
Hib          1  2  3   4--->
IPV          1  2  3----------->
PCV-7        1  2  3   4--->
MMR                    1--->
Var                    1------->
INFL††             1--------------->
------------------------------------
Dash (-->) indicate range of acceptable
    ages for vaccination
R = Review immunizations/administer
    needed dose(s)
 †Start hep B series at birth for
    children of HBsAg+ mothers
††Influenza vaccine encouraged for
    children 6-23 months
```

IMMUNIZATION SCHEDULE #2:

```
       <-------- years --------->
       4-6  11-12  14-16  50  65+
--------------------------------------
Hep B       R
DTaP    5
Td          1-----> and q 10 yrs
IPV     4
MMR     2   R
Var         R
INFL                      1--> yrly
PNEU                         1 once
--------------------------------------
R = Review immunizations/administer
    needed dose(s)
```

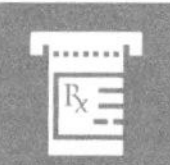

MEDICATIONS

DRUG(S) OF CHOICE

Immunization administration guide:

Agent	Dose (mL)	Route
DTaP	0.5	IM
MMR	0.5	SC
Polio (IPV)	0.5	SC
PCV-7	0.5	IM
HBv†	††	IM
Hib	0.5	IM
Influenza Inactivated	0.5†††	IM
Td and DT	0.5	IM
Pneumococcal Polysaccharide	0.5	IM or SC
Varicella	0.5	SC
LAIV	-	Nasal

†Newborns of HBsAg-positive mothers also receive HBIG
††Variable - see manufacturer instructions
†††0.25mL for children 6-35 months old

Wounds and immunization recommendations
- Tetanus immune globulin (TIG)
  - ◊ 3+ doses of Td given in past: TIG not needed
  - ◊ <3 doses of Td given in past: Give TIG, except in patients with a clean (minor) wound.
- Tetanus toxoid (Td)
  - ◊ Give Td if patient not immunized within 10 yrs
  - ◊ Give Td if patient not immunized within 5 yrs and wound is dirty (contaminated with dirt, feces, or saliva), puncture (penetration beyond epidermis), or major (burn, frostbite, crush injury)

Contraindications:
- Anaphylaxis to thimerosal: See manufacturer's insert. Thimerosal has been removed from almost all childhood vaccines.
- Anaphylaxis to neomycin: MMR, DTP, Hib, IPV, varicella contraindicated
- Anaphylaxis to streptomycin: IPV contraindicated
- Anaphylaxis to previous dose
- Encephalopathy within 7 days after DTP: Give DT for next dose(s)
- Pregnancy: MMR, varicella
- Known, active, untreated tuberculosis: varicella contraindicated
- Anaphylaxis to eggs: influenza (inactivated and LAIV)
- Immunocompromised patients should, in general, not receive live viral vaccines (MMR, LAIV and varicella), although patients with HIV may receive MMR if not severely immunocompromised. Varicella vaccine is generally contraindicated but may be given to some specified groups - see ACIP recommendations for details (i.e., certain HIV infected children and humoral immunodeficiencies).

Precautions:
- DTaP
  - ◊ Suspected neurologic disease: Delay immunization until clarified
  - ◊ Fever of ≥ 40.5°C (105°F) within 48 hours after previous DTP/DTaP
  - ◊ Collapse or shock-like state (hypotonic-hyporesponsive episode) within 48 hours after DTP/DTaP
  - ◊ Seizure within 3 days after DTP/DTaP
  - ◊ Persistent, inconsolable crying lasting ≥ 3 hrs within 48 hours after DTP/DTaP
  - ◊ The following are NOT contraindications and DTaP may be given if present:
    - Family history of convulsions: Pre-treat with acetaminophen and after DTaP q4h for 24 hrs
    - Family history of SIDS
    - Family history of adverse event following DTaP/DTP
    - Temperature < 40.5°C (105°F) following a prior DTaP/DTP
- Varicella, LAIV
  - ◊ Avoid salicylates for 6 weeks

Significant possible interactions:
- Avoid MMR and varicella vaccine within 3-11 months after gamma globulin (see ACIP)
- Give MMR and varicella either together or separated by 1 month

ALTERNATIVE DRUGS None

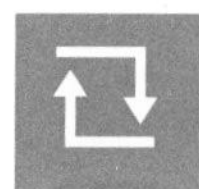

FOLLOWUP

PATIENT MONITORING
- None routinely needed
- Hepatitis: Measure antibody (anti-HBs) response after HBv for healthcare workers, immunocompromised persons and offspring of hepatitis B carriers

PREVENTION/AVOIDANCE N/A

POSSIBLE COMPLICATIONS
- Fever, malaise, local reactions (redness, pain) are most common
- Rarely, allergic reactions
- Febrile seizures rarely occur after DTaP

EXPECTED COURSE/PROGNOSIS
Most patients develop antibodies

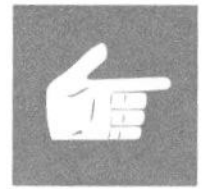

MISCELLANEOUS

ASSOCIATED CONDITIONS N/A

AGE-RELATED FACTORS
Pediatric:
- Most vaccines are given before entry into school
- Do not delay DTaP immunization of the preterm infant unless specific contraindications exist

Geriatric: Pneumococcal polysaccharide, influenza, and Td are needed in older age groups

Others: N/A

PREGNANCY
MMR and varicella should not be routinely given to pregnant women or women who are planning pregnancy within 28 days

SYNONYMS
- Vaccinations
- Inoculations

ICD-9-CM
V05.9 Need for prophylactic vaccination and inoculation against unspecified single disease

SEE ALSO
Chickenpox
Diphtheria
Hepatitis A
Hepatitis B
Influenza
Measles, rubella
Measles, rubeola
Mumps
Pertussis
Pneumonia, bacterial
Poliomyelitis
Tetanus

OTHER NOTES
- PPD may be given at same time as MMR or wait 4 weeks after immunization to do skin test
- Culture-proven pertussis provides immunity; use DT instead of DTaP
- Haemophilus disease: Immunity not provided when child under 2 years; administer Hib as if no disease has occurred
- Combination vaccines are available

ABBREVIATIONS
DTaP = pediatric diphtheria and tetanus toxoids, and acellular pertussis vaccine
DT = pediatric diphtheria and tetanus toxoids
Td = adult diphtheria and tetanus toxoids
TIG = tetanus immune globulin
HBv = hepatitis B vaccine
HBIG = hepatitis B immune globulin
OPV = trivalent oral poliovirus vaccine
IPV = enhanced inactivated poliovirus vaccine
HbOC = Hib vaccine (HibTITER)
PRP-OMP = Hib vaccine (PedvaxHIB)
PRP-T = Hib vaccine (ActHIB, OmniHIB)
MMR = measles, mumps, and rubella vaccine
Hib = conjugated Haemophilus influenzae type b vaccine inactivated
LAIV = live attenuated influenza vaccine
INFL = influenza vaccine
PCV-7 = pneumococcal conjugate vaccine
PNEU = pneumococcal polysaccharide vaccine
PPD = purified protein derivative
VZIG = varicella-zoster immune globulin
Var = varicella zoster vaccine

REFERENCES
- Advisory Committee on Immunization Practices (ACIP)
- Red Book 2003 Report of the Committee on Infectious Diseases. American Academy of Pediatrics, 2003
- American Academy of Family Physicians
- 2003 Immunization Supplement to Journal of Family Practice
- Shots 2004 PDA software free from www.immunizationed.org

Web references: 5 available at www.5mcc.com
Illustrations N/A

Author(s):
Richard Kent Zimmerman, MD, MPH
Richard D. Clover, MD

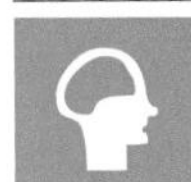

BASICS

DESCRIPTION Disorders associated with disruption of the integrity of the immune system resulting in a wide spectrum of illnesses
- May be primary or secondary and involve any or all of the system's cells and their products (T cells, B cells, monocytes, macrophages, etc.) their receptors, metabolic pathways and products which are normally involved in health maintenance and protection
- Primary
  - ◊ Combined immunodeficiencies, e.g., severe combined immunodeficiency (SCID), adenosine deaminase (ADA) deficiency, and reticular dysgenesis
  - ◊ Antibody deficiencies, e.g., X-linked agammaglobulinemia, IgA deficiency, Ig deficiency with increased IgM (hyper-IgM syndrome), common variable immunodeficiency (CVID) and transient hypogammaglobulinemia of infancy
  - ◊ Other well-defined syndromes, e.g., Wiskott-Aldrich syndrome (eczema, thrombocytopenia and repeated infections), ataxia telangiectasia (cerebellar ataxia, oculocutaneous telangiectasia and immunodeficiency) and DiGeorge syndrome (isolated T cell deficiency)
  - ◊ Associated syndromes e.g., Down syndrome, chronic mucocutaneous candidiasis, hyper-IgE syndrome, chronic granulomatous disease, partial albinism and WHIM syndrome (warts, hypogammaglobulinemia, infection, myelokathexis [retention of leukocytes in a hypercellular marrow]), phagocytic defects with early onset of periodontal disease.
  - ◊ Complement deficiencies
- Secondary
  - ◊ AIDS
  - ◊ Other infections, malignancies, malnutrition, protein-losing enteropathy, drugs, and chronic stress

System(s) affected: Hemic/Lymphatic/Immunologic

Genetics: Included in Description

Incidence/Prevalence in USA:
- 1 in every 500 (including IgA deficiency) born with an immune system defect
- Many more will acquire a defect which may be transient or permanent

Predominant age:
- All ages. Children most likely to present with primary or inherited deficiencies.
- Number of newborns with AIDS increasing. In part associated with: (1) increased premature infant survival, (2) improved treatment and care of other primary diseases, (3) use of immunosuppressive agents.

Predominant sex: Male > Female

SIGNS & SYMPTOMS
- Common features
  - ◊ Unusual susceptibility to infection. Frequency and severity vary with type of defect.
  - ◊ Malignancies, especially lymphoreticular
  - ◊ Increased tendency toward autoimmune disorders
  - ◊ Weight loss
  - ◊ Fever
- More specific features
  - ◊ Combined T and B cell deficiencies associated with severe fungal, bacterial and viral infections. Enzyme deficiencies may be involved.
  - ◊ T cell deficiencies may be acquired (as with the human immunodeficiency virus) or congenital with wide spectrum manifestations. Children with DiGeorge syndrome show cardiac defects, micrognathia, hypertelorism and hypocalcemic tetany.
  - ◊ B cell or immunoglobulin deficiency syndromes may be associated with chronic sinusitis, recurrent respiratory infection, chronic diarrheal disease, rheumatoid arthritis, systemic lupus erythematosus (SLE), atopy, splenomegaly, anemia, recurrent pneumococcal pneumonia and meningococcal meningitis
  - ◊ Chronic giardiasis, fever of unknown origin and malabsorption should cause suspicion of immunodeficiency
  - ◊ Miscellaneous syndromes include chronic mucocutaneous candidiasis, fatal Epstein-Barr virus infection, and complement component deficiencies

CAUSES
- Primary immunodeficiency diseases
  - ◊ Faulty genes and gene products resulting in inherited defects of the immune system including: antibody, cellular, phagocytic cytokine production, and complement deficiencies
  - ◊ Manifested by infections soon after birth but may not be expressed clinically until later in life
- Secondary immunodeficiency diseases
  - ◊ Treatment with immunosuppressive agents
  - ◊ Nutritional deficiencies
  - ◊ Use of drugs and exposure to chemicals should be considered
  - ◊ X-ray treatment
  - ◊ IgA deficiency associated with phenytoin or penicillamine
  - ◊ Thymoma associated with hypogammaglobulinemia
  - ◊ Viruses e.g., HIV-1 and HIV-2

RISK FACTORS
- Family history
- Almost anything less than good health practices
- Drug abuse and parenteral blood exposure
- Sexual lifestyle
- Aging

DIAGNOSIS

DIFFERENTIAL DIAGNOSIS
- Must consider all immunodeficiency disorders
- Careful history and physical will direct proper search

LABORATORY
- High percentage of immunodeficiencies will be discovered by a CBC with a differential smear and immunoglobulin levels including: IgG, IgA, IgM and IgE. IgG subclasses should be included.
- Further assays include mononuclear cell populations which may be quantified
- Total lymphocyte a good screen
- Functional evaluation by skin testing (anergy battery) and antibody levels to common viruses and bacterial toxins
- Complement levels
- Phagocyte function
- Specific cytokine function
- Additional specific tests for suspected acquired causes for immunodeficiencies (AIDS, chronic diarrhea, malignancy, drugs, etc.)

Drugs that may alter lab results: N/A

Disorders that may alter lab results: N/A

PATHOLOGICAL FINDINGS Vary with type of deficiency and resultant disease(s)

SPECIAL TESTS N/A

IMAGING
- MRI helpful in evaluation of CNS lesions associated with toxoplasmosis
- Techniques and technology continue to improve dramatically

DIAGNOSTIC PROCEDURES
- Careful history and physical
- Try to deduce whether infections associated with T cell response inadequacies (fungal and other opportunistic infections) or lack of B cell (antibodies) response or both

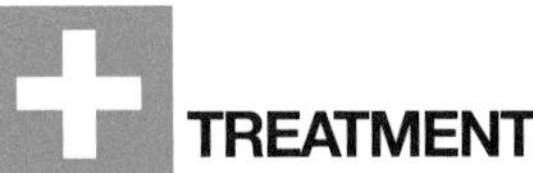

TREATMENT

APPROPRIATE HEALTH CARE
- Outpatient or inpatient management appropriate to clinical problem

GENERAL MEASURES
- Depends mainly on complexity of the immune deficiency
- Bone marrow transplant with donor T cell engraftment in severe abnormalities of T cell function. Best done at referral research centers.
- Intravenous immunoglobulin - for patients deficient in IgG. Not appropriate for treatment for Ig deficiency other than IgG, but may be helpful in the hyper-IgM syndrome.

SURGICAL MEASURES N/A

ACTIVITY As appropriate

DIET Severe immunodeficiencies require sterile conditions

PATIENT EDUCATION Printed patient information available from: Immune Deficiency Foundation, 25 West Chesapeake Ave. Room 206, Rowson, MD 21204

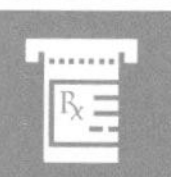

MEDICATIONS

DRUG(S) OF CHOICE
- Antibiotics with appropriate spectra for infecting organism(s). Ketoconazole reported to be effective in some chronic fungal infections.
- Enzyme replacement therapy for ADA deficiency
- Autologous genetically corrected T cells with normal ADA gene
- Zidovudine (AZT) reduces rate of maternal transmission of HIV
- Combination drug therapy in HIV
- Recombinant interleukin-2 conjugated with polyethylene glycol (PEG), promising

Contraindications: Refer to manufacturer's literature

Precautions:
- Multidisciplinary input in order
- Refer to manufacturer's literature

Significant possible interactions: Refer to manufacturer's literature

ALTERNATIVE DRUGS N/A

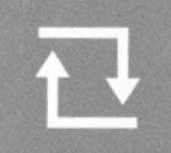

FOLLOWUP

PATIENT MONITORING
- Children with SCID must remain in controlled environment, exposure to any pathogen may result in death
- IgG levels monitored and maintained in common variable hypogammaglobulinemia
- Meticulous instruction and checks for infections

PREVENTION/AVOIDANCE
Genetic counseling for primary cases

POSSIBLE COMPLICATIONS
- Autoimmune disorders
- Serum sickness reactions to gamma globulin treatment
- Malignancies
- Overwhelming infection
- Fatal graft-versus-host disease following blood transfusions in SCID patients

EXPECTED COURSE/PROGNOSIS
Related closely to type and degree of immunodeficiency

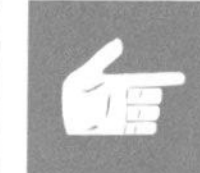

MISCELLANEOUS

ASSOCIATED CONDITIONS N/A

AGE-RELATED FACTORS
Pediatric: Depends on specific immunodeficiency disorder
Geriatric: Depends on specific immunodeficiency disorder
Others: N/A

PREGNANCY
AIDS transmission

SYNONYMS N/A

ICD-9-CM
279.3 Unspecified immunity deficiency

SEE ALSO
HIV infection & AIDS
Wiskott-Aldrich syndrome

OTHER NOTES
- Research opportunities:
  - ◊ Continue studies at the cellular, cytokine, and molecular level
  - ◊ Continue to develop techniques of replacing gene and gene products where deficiencies are either inherited or acquired
  - ◊ Expand acquired immunodeficiency research and the addressing of clinical and social problems
  - ◊ AIDS vaccine evaluation group

ABBREVIATIONS N/A

REFERENCES

- NIAID Task Force on Immunology and Allergy
- Isselbacher KJ, et al, eds: Harrison's Principles of Internal Medicine. 13th Ed. New York, McGraw-Hill, 1994
- Lichtenstein L, Fauci A: Current Therapy in Allergy, Immunology and Rheumatology. Toronto, B.C. Decker, Inc., 1988
- Stiehm ER, Blaese RM: Pediatric Research. Vol. 33, No. 1 (suppl)/Jan, 1993
- Immune Deficiency Foundation Clinical Updates, Littleton, CO
- Cunningham-Rundles C, et al: Brief Report - Enhanced Humoral Immunity in Common Variable Immune-Deficiency with Polyethylene glycol-conjugated interleukin-2. NEJM 1995;331(14):918-921

Web references: 0 available at www.5mcc.com
Illustrations N/A

Author(s):
Mark R. Dambro, MD

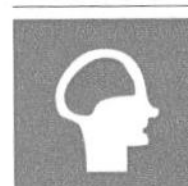

BASICS

DESCRIPTION A superficial, intraepidermal, unilocular, vesiculopustular infection. Typically begins as erythematous tender papule that rapidly progresses through a vesicular to a honey-crusted stage. Cultures now give over 80% with Staphylococcus aureus alone or combined with group A beta-hemolytic streptococci. Change over past 20 years to predominately Staph. aureus.

- Bullous impetigo: Staphylococci impetigo that progress rapidly to small to large flaccid bulla. No lymphadenopathy; < 30% of cases.
- Folliculitis: Considered by some to be Staph aureus impetigo of hair follicle
- Ecthyma: A deeper, ulcerated, impetigo infection often with lymphadenitis

System(s) affected: Skin/Exocrine
Genetics: N/A
Incidence/Prevalence in USA: Unreported
Predominant age: 2-5 years
Predominant sex: Male = Female

SIGNS & SYMPTOMS
- May be slow and indolent or rapidly spreading
- Tender red macule or papule as early lesion
- Thin roofed vesicle to bullae - usually nontender
- Pustules
- Weeping shallow red ulcer
- Honey-colored crusts
- Most frequent on face around mouth and nose, or at site of trauma
- Satellite lesions
- Often multiple sites
- Bullae on buttocks, trunk, face

CAUSES
- Coagulase positive staphylococci - pure culture about 50-90%. More contagious via contact.
- Beta-hemolytic streptococci - pure culture only about 10% of the time
- Mixed infections of streptococci and staphylococci common. Data suggest increasing importance of staphylococci over past 20 years.
- Direct contact or insect vector
- Can be contamination at trauma site
- Regional lymphadenopathy

RISK FACTORS
- Warm, humid environment
- Tropical or subtropical climate
- Summer or fall season
- Minor trauma, insect bites, etc.
- Poor hygiene, epidemics, during war, etc.
- Familial spread
- Poor health with anemia and malnutrition
- Complication to pediculosis, scabies, chickenpox, eczema
- Contact dermatitis (Rhus)
- Burns
- Atopic dermatitis
- Contact sports
- Children in day care

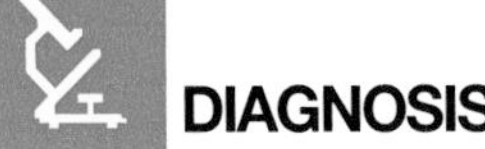

DIAGNOSIS

DIFFERENTIAL DIAGNOSIS
- Nonbullous:
  - ◊ Chickenpox
  - ◊ Herpes
  - ◊ Folliculitis
  - ◊ Erysipelas
  - ◊ Insect bites
  - ◊ Severe eczematous dermatitis
  - ◊ Scabies
  - ◊ Tinea corporis
- Bullous:
  - ◊ Burns
  - ◊ Pemphigus vulgaris
  - ◊ Bullous pemphigoid
  - ◊ Stevens-Johnson syndrome

LABORATORY
None usually required
- Culture - taken from the base of lesion after removal of crust. Blood agar grows both staphylococci and group A streptococci
- ASO titer - can be weak positive for streptococci (not usually done)
- Streptozyme - positive for streptococci (not usually done)

Drugs that may alter lab results: N/A

Disorders that may alter lab results: Streptococci pharyngitis will alter streptococci enzyme tests

PATHOLOGICAL FINDINGS N/A

SPECIAL TESTS Cultures as listed under Laboratory

IMAGING N/A

DIAGNOSTIC PROCEDURES N/A

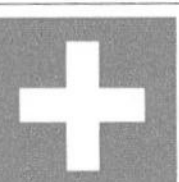

TREATMENT

APPROPRIATE HEALTH CARE Outpatient

GENERAL MEASURES Removal of crusts, cleanliness with gentle washing 2-3 times daily. Clean with antibacterial soap, chlorhexidine or betadine.

SURGICAL MEASURES N/A

ACTIVITY
- Athletes restricted from contact sports
- School and daycare contagious restrictions

DIET No special diet

PATIENT EDUCATION Good hygiene important to prevent possible spread

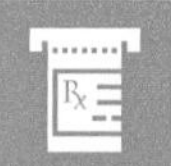

MEDICATIONS

DRUG(S) OF CHOICE

Note: Increasing incidence of Staphylococcus resistant to erythromycin may make the following suggestions inaccurate in your community.

- Nonbullous (minor spread, treat 7 days; widespread, treat 10 days); bullous (treat 10 days)
  - ◊ Erythromycin base - adults 1 gm/day divided doses q6h in adults. Pediatric 30-40 mg/kg/d q6h.
  - ◊ Mupirocin (Bactroban) topical ointment apply tid, 7-10 days (nonbullous only). Not as effective on scalp as around mouth.
  - ◊ Dicloxacillin - adult 250 mg qid. Pediatric 12-25 mg/kg/d divided q6h.

Contraindications: Drug allergy

Precautions: Refer to manufacturer's profile of each drug

Significant possible interactions:

- Erythromycin with theophyllines, astemizole, and other drugs
- Refer to manufacturer's profile of each drug

ALTERNATIVE DRUGS

Oral doses:

- 1st generation cephalosporins - children
  - ◊ Cephalexin: 25-50 mg/kg/24 h divided q6h
  - ◊ Cefaclor: 20-40 mg/kg/24 h divided q8h
  - ◊ Cephradine: 25-50 mg/kg/24 h divided q6-12h
  - ◊ Cefadroxil: 30 mg/kg/24 h divided bid
- 1st generation cephalosporins - adults
  - ◊ Cephalexin: 250 mg qid
  - ◊ Cefaclor: 250 mg tid
  - ◊ Cephradine: 500 mg bid
  - ◊ Cefadroxil: 1 gm/day in divided doses
- Amoxicillin-clavulanate acid
  - ◊ Adult: 250 mg tid
  - ◊ Pediatric: 20-40 mg/kg/day of amoxicillin divided q8h
- Azithromycin
  - ◊ Adult 500 mg on day 1 followed by 250 mg daily for days 2-5
  - ◊ Pediatric 10 mg/kg on day 1 followed by 5 mg/kg days 2-5
- Clarithromycin
  - ◊ Adult 250 mg bid
  - ◊ Pediatric 15 mg/kg/d bid
- Vancomycin
- Clindamycin
- Ciprofloxacin plus rifampin (rifampicin)
- Severe bullous disease may require IV therapy such as nafcillin or cefazolin

FOLLOWUP

PATIENT MONITORING If not clear within 7-10 days, culture the lesions

PREVENTION/AVOIDANCE Close attention to family hygiene, particularly hand washing. Avoid crowding. Treat atopic dermatitis.

POSSIBLE COMPLICATIONS

- Ecthyma
- Erysipelas
- Post-streptococcal acute glomerulonephritis
- Deep cellulitis
- Bacteremia
- Osteomyelitis
- Septic arthritis
- Pneumonia
- Lymphadenitis

EXPECTED COURSE/PROGNOSIS

- Complete resolution in 7-10 days with treatment
- Antibiotic treatment will not prevent or halt glomerulonephritis as it will with rheumatic fever
- If not clear within 7-10 days, culture is necessary to find resistant organism

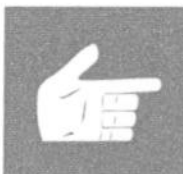

MISCELLANEOUS

ASSOCIATED CONDITIONS

- Malnutrition and anemia
- Crowded living conditions
- Poor hygiene
- Neglected minor trauma
- Any chronic dermatitis

AGE-RELATED FACTORS

Pediatric: Impetigo neonatorum may occur by nursery contamination

Geriatric: N/A

Others: N/A

PREGNANCY N/A

SYNONYMS

- Pyoderma
- Impetigo contagiosa
- Impetigo vulgaris
- Fox impetigo

ICD-9-CM

684 Impetigo

SEE ALSO

OTHER NOTES N/A

ABBREVIATIONS N/A

REFERENCES

- Isselbacher KJ, et al, editors. Harrison's Principles of Internal Medicine. 13th Ed. New York: McGraw-Hill; 1994
- Dagan R. Impetigo in childhood: changing epidemiology and new treatments. Pediatric Annuals 1993;22(4):235-240
- Peters G, editor. Red Book. New York: American Academy of Pediatrics; 1997
- Rakel RE, editor. 1997 Conn's Current Therapy. Philadelphia: WB Saunders Co; 1997
- Rhody C. Bacterial infections of the skin. Prim Care 2000;27(2):459-73
- Ko WT, Adal KA, Tomecki KJ. Infectious diseases. Med Clin North Am 1998;82(5):1001-31

Web references: 1 available at www.5mcc.com

Illustrations 7 available

Author(s):

William H. Billica, MD

BASICS

DESCRIPTION A form of hyponatremia with inappropriately elevated urine osmolality. The resulting abnormal urinary water retention and normal sodium excretion leads to dilutional hyponatremia. Total body sodium levels may be normal or near normal. Total body water is usually increased. Associated with an underlying disorder, e.g., neoplasm, pulmonary disorder, or central nervous system disease.
System(s) affected: Endocrine/Metabolic
Genetics: No known genetic pattern
Incidence/Prevalence in USA: Usually found in the hospital setting where incidence can be as high as 35%
Predominant age: Common in the elderly
Predominant sex: N/A

SIGNS & SYMPTOMS
- Usually neurological
- Lethargy
- Restlessness
- Confusion
- Edema (rare)
- Anorexia
- Nausea/vomiting
- Headache
- Irritability
- Decreasing reflexes
- Seizures
- Coma
- Asymptomatic

CAUSES
- Drugs (vincristine, narcotics, thiazide diuretics, cyclophosphamide, carbamazepine, barbiturates, morphine, chlorpropamide, nicotine, beta-adrenergic agents, general anesthetics, oxytocin, bromocriptine)
- Neoplasms
  - ◊ Ectopic ADH production
  - ◊ Oat cell carcinoma of the lung
  - ◊ Hodgkin disease
  - ◊ Pancreatic carcinoma
  - ◊ Bronchogenic carcinoma
- Infectious diseases
  - ◊ Meningitis
  - ◊ Pneumonia
  - ◊ Pulmonary tuberculosis
  - ◊ Rocky Mountain spotted fever
  - ◊ HIV
- Miscellaneous cardiopulmonary conditions
  - ◊ Asthma
  - ◊ Atelectasis
  - ◊ Myocardial infarction
  - ◊ Positive-pressure breathing
  - ◊ Vascular diseases
- Other
  - ◊ Chronic pain
  - ◊ Multiple sclerosis
  - ◊ Guillain-Barre syndrome
  - ◊ Lupus erythematosus
  - ◊ Porphyria
  - ◊ Hypothyroidism, myxedema
  - ◊ Idiopathic

RISK FACTORS
- Patient with causative disorder
- Use of predisposing drugs
- Elderly patient
- Postoperative
- Institutionalized patient

DIAGNOSIS

DIFFERENTIAL DIAGNOSIS
- Postoperative:
  - ◊ caused by non-osmotic release of ADH
  - ◊ affects women more than men
  - ◊ ADH increased by pain and narcotics
- Postprostatectomy syndrome:
  - ◊ irrigating solution must be non-conducting (i.e., electrolyte free)
  - ◊ D5W absorbed
- Psychotic polydipsia:
  - ◊ active therapy rarely needed
  - ◊ diuresis occurs when intake stopped
  - ◊ intake usually over 10 L/day
  - ◊ interaction with other psychotropic drugs
- Acute (usually in children):
  - ◊ swallowing water during swimming
  - ◊ diluted formula
  - ◊ tap water enemas
- Drug induced:
  - ◊ oxytocin infusion - given in D5W during labor (oxytocin has antidiuretic effect)
  - ◊ cyclophosphamide - usually with IV administration
  - ◊ chlorpropamide (oral hypoglycemic agent)
  - ◊ carbamazepine - central ADH release
  - ◊ vincristine - central SIADH
  - ◊ non-steroidal anti-inflammatory drugs (NSAIDs) - decreased renal prostaglandins
- Diuretic drug induced:
  - ◊ usually thiazide
  - ◊ vasopressin increased by decreasing EABV
  - ◊ usually elderly patients or in bulimia
  - ◊ correct slowly
- Tumor induced
  - ◊ bronchogenic carcinoma (secretes ADH-like substance)
  - ◊ unexplained persistent hyponatremia may indicate a tumor
- Pulmonary:
  - ◊ tuberculosis - secretes ADH
  - ◊ mechanical ventilation - increased intrathoracic pressure, decreased cardiac output, causes decreased EABV, causes increased ADH
  - ◊ asthma, acute respiratory failure, pneumonia
- CNS/hypothalamic irritation:
  - ◊ meningitis
  - ◊ Rocky Mountain spotted fever
  - ◊ encephalitis
  - ◊ trauma - especially after CNS surgery
- Endocrine:
  - ◊ Addison disease
  - ◊ hypothyroidism
- Factitious hyponatremia
  - ◊ caused by increased serum glucose, cholesterol or proteins
- Other:
  - ◊ "Appropriate" ADH secretion and hyponatremia with decreased effective arterial blood volume, e.g., congestive heart failure, nephrotic syndrome, cirrhosis

LABORATORY
- BUN low or normal
- Creatinine low or normal
- Urine osmolality 200+ mOsm/kg
- Urinary Na concentration > 20 mEq/L (> 20 mmol/L)
- Elevated serum concentration ADH
- Normal adrenal and renal function
- Uric acid low

Drugs that may alter lab results: N/A

Disorders that may alter lab results: N/A

PATHOLOGICAL FINDINGS N/A

SPECIAL TESTS Oral water-loading test may be helpful in diagnosis in some patients. Response to water-load will be impaired in SIADH. May be unsafe and often not necessary to establish diagnosis

IMAGING Not usually require for diagnosis

DIAGNOSTIC PROCEDURES N/A

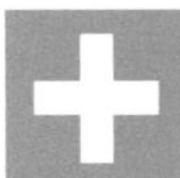

TREATMENT

APPROPRIATE HEALTH CARE Outpatient or inpatient depending on severity of symptoms or underlying cause

GENERAL MEASURES
- Mildly symptomatic
  - ◊ Patient has serum Na > 125 mEq/L (> 125 mmol/L)
  - ◊ Restrict fluid to 800-1000 mL/day
- Acute (less than 48 hours duration)
  - ◊ Hypertonic saline
  - ◊ Water diuresis (loop diuretics, e.g. furosemide)
- Symptomatic (seizure, coma)
  - ◊ High mortality due to cerebral edema if serum Na < 120 mEq/L (< 120 mmol/L)
  - ◊ Decrease oral free water to 2/3 maintenance
  - ◊ Increase oral salt
  - ◊ Correct serum Na deficit. (mEq sodium deficit = desired sodium minus actual sodium times 0.5 times weight [kg])
  - ◊ Increase serum sodium slowly with hypertonic saline by 0.5 mEq/L /hour until it reaches 120 mEq/L

SURGICAL MEASURES N/A

ACTIVITY As tolerated

DIET May need increased salt or decreased water intake depending on cause

PATIENT EDUCATION Diet and fluid restrictions

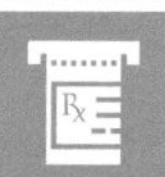

MEDICATIONS

DRUG(S) OF CHOICE
- Water diuresis - furosemide (Lasix) plus hourly sodium chloride and potassium chloride replacement - requires frequent monitoring. Treatment of choice for acute management.
- Demeclocycline - blocks ADH at renal tubule - produces nephrogenic diabetes insipidus. (Dosage for long term management: 600-1200 mg/day. Onset of action is within one week, therefore not best for acute management).
- Lithium - blocks ADH at renal tubule - has the problem of lithium toxicity, anti-anabolic effects especially in cirrhosis and congestive heart failure
- Hypertonic (3%) saline
  - ◊ Increase serum Na by 10-12 mEq/L (10-12 mmol/L) every 24 hrs
  - ◊ Increase serum Na 5% over first few hours
  - ◊ Increase serum Na to only 120 mEq/L (120 mmol/L), acutely
  - ◊ Increase serum Na by 0.5 mEq/hr (0.5 mmol/hr)

Contraindications: Avoid fluids in congestive heart failure, nephrotic syndrome or cirrhosis

Precautions:
- Too rapid correction can cause:
  - ◊ Congestive heart failure
  - ◊ Subdural and intracerebral hemorrhage
  - ◊ Permanent CNS damage, especially with serum Na < 120 mEq/L (< 120 mmol/L)
  - ◊ Demyelination syndrome

Significant possible interactions: Refer to manufacturer's literature

ALTERNATIVE DRUGS N/A

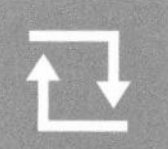

FOLLOWUP

PATIENT MONITORING
- Careful, continuous, clinical and laboratory monitoring of the hyponatremic state during acute phase
- For chronic management, monitor underlying cause as needed

PREVENTION/AVOIDANCE
- Search for cause of SIADH, if unknown
- Monitor electrolytes in postoperative patients to determine if fluid intake needs restriction
- Reducing or changing medications, if a drug is the cause
- Life-long restriction of fluid intake

POSSIBLE COMPLICATIONS
- Central pontine myelinolysis:
  - ◊ Chronic hyponatremia - usually < 120 mEq/L (< 120 mmol/L)
  - ◊ Too rapid correction - > 12 mEq/L/day (> 12 mmol/day)

EXPECTED COURSE/PROGNOSIS
Dependent on underlying cause

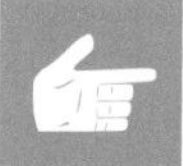

MISCELLANEOUS

ASSOCIATED CONDITIONS Listed with Causes

AGE-RELATED FACTORS
Pediatric: N/A
Geriatric: Most common in this age group
Others: N/A

PREGNANCY N/A

SYNONYMS
- SIADH
- Syndrome of inappropriate secretion of ADH

ICD-9-CM
276.9 Electrolyte and fluid disorders NEC
253.6 Syndrome of inappropriate secretion of antidiuretic hormone

SEE ALSO
Hyponatremia

OTHER NOTES N/A

ABBREVIATIONS N/A

REFERENCES

- Brenner B, Rector F, editors. The Kidney. 6th Ed. Philadelphia: W.B. Saunders Co.; 2000
- Kokko J, Tannen R, editors. Fluid and Electrolytes. 3rd ed. Philadelphia: W.B. Saunders Co.; 1996

Web references: 1 available at www.5mcc.com
Illustrations N/A

Author(s):
Deogracias R. Pe□a, MD

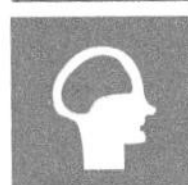

BASICS

DESCRIPTION An acute, usually self-limited, viral, febrile, infection caused by influenza virus types A and B. It is marked by inflammation of the nasal mucosa, pharynx, conjunctiva, and respiratory tract. Outbreaks occur almost every winter with varying degrees of severity.
- The influenza virus displays antigenic shift (variation) which leads to strains of the virus to which there is little immunologic resistance in the population and may result in pandemics. The influenza virus displays minor antigenic variation called drift.

System(s) affected: Pulmonary
Genetics: N/A
Incidence/Prevalence in USA: 95 million cases/year. Attack rates in healthy children are 10-40% each year. Morbidity is also high in young children.
Predominant age:
- Incidence: highest in school-aged children (3 months-16 years); young adult (16-40 years)
- Morbidity: highest in elderly (> 75 years) and concurrent medical illnesses, such as lung disease
- Hospitalization rates also higher in infants

Predominant sex: Male = Female

SIGNS & SYMPTOMS
Sudden onset of:
- High Fever
- Myalgia (sometimes severe and lasting for days)
- Sore throat/pharyngitis
- Nonproductive cough
- Headache
- Cervical lymphadenopathy
- Chills
- Nasal congestion
- Malaise
- Rhinorrhea
- Sinusitis
- Sneezing
- Conjunctivitis

CAUSES Orthomyxovirus (influenza antigenic types A and B) that are transmitted person-to-person, often by the airborne route

RISK FACTORS
- For contracting disease:
  - ◊ Patients in semi-closed environments such as nursing homes
  - ◊ Students, prisoners
  - ◊ Crowded, close environments during times of epidemics
- For complications
  - ◊ Chronic pulmonary diseases
  - ◊ Cardiovascular diseases including valvular problems and congestive heart failure
  - ◊ Metabolic diseases
  - ◊ Hemoglobinopathies
  - ◊ Malignancies
  - ◊ Pregnancy, especially in the 3rd trimester
  - ◊ Neonates, infants, elderly
  - ◊ Immunosuppression

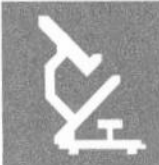

DIAGNOSIS

DIFFERENTIAL DIAGNOSIS
- Respiratory viral infections including RSV, parainfluenza, adenovirus, enterovirus
- Atypical Mycoplasma pneumonia
- Q fever
- Viral or streptococcal tonsillitis
- Infectious mononucleosis
- Coxsackievirus infections
- Chlamydia pneumoniae

LABORATORY
- Rapid antigen test
- Culture of nasopharyngeal swab or aspirate
- Lymphopenia
- Leukocytosis may signal complications

Drugs that may alter lab results: N/A

Disorders that may alter lab results: N/A

PATHOLOGICAL FINDINGS Inflammation of respiratory tract

SPECIAL TESTS N/A

IMAGING
- Chest x-ray
  - ◊ Usually normal unless secondary infection
  - ◊ Basilar streaking
  - ◊ Patchy infiltrate - mild disease

DIAGNOSTIC PROCEDURES
- Tissue culture of nasopharyngeal swab or aspirate
- Rapid ELISA antigen test. Some rapid tests diagnose influenza A, while others diagnose influenza A+B.
- History and physical examination - close attention to epidemiology (e.g., current outbreak in community). Contact CDC at (404)332-4555 or health department to determine type or do rapid testing.

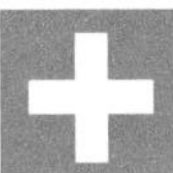

TREATMENT

APPROPRIATE HEALTH CARE Outpatient except for treatment of severe complications or treatment of those in high risk groups

GENERAL MEASURES
- Symptomatic treatment (saline nasal spray, analgesic gargle)
- Cool-mist, ultrasonic humidifier to increase moisture of inspired air
- Modified respiratory isolation techniques
- Hospitalized patients may require oxygen or ventilatory support
- Avoid smoking

SURGICAL MEASURES N/A

ACTIVITY As tolerated. Strict hand washing procedures.

DIET Increase fluid intake

PATIENT EDUCATION
- For a listing of sources for patient education materials favorably reviewed on this topic, physicians may contact: American Academy of Family Physicians Foundation, P.O. Box 8418, Kansas City, MO 64114, (800)274-2237, ext. 4400
- Educate high-risk patients about prevention

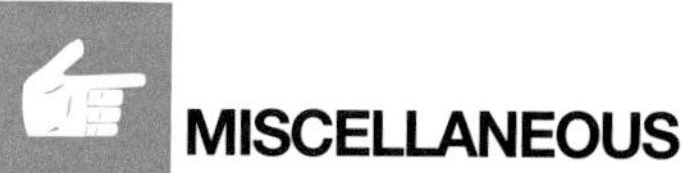

MEDICATIONS

DRUG(S) OF CHOICE
Antivirals effective if administered within the first 48 hours
- Rimantadine is effective only for influenza A
  - ◊ Rimantadine is now preferred over amantadine due to fewer side effects
  - ◊ 100 mg twice per day orally for 3-5 days. It shortens duration of fever, systemic and respiratory symptoms by about one day. Effective if taken within the first 48 hours.
  - ◊ The rimantadine dose should be decreased to 100 mg/d for elderly nursing home residents and those with either liver or severe renal impairment.
  - ◊ See manufacturer's guidelines for children's dosages
- Zanamivir and oseltamivir are effective for influenza types A and B; shortens duration by 1 day
  - ◊ Oseltamivir also reduces complications of influenza
  - ◊ Zanamivir dose is 2 inhalations twice per day for 5 days (persons 7 years and older)
  - ◊ Oseltamivir dose is 75 mg po twice per day for 5 days (persons 13 years and older). If severe renal impairment, 75 mg po once per day. 2 mg/kg/day in two divided doses for children (up to 150 mg).
- Antipyretics
  - ◊ Acetaminophen - fever control in children.
  - ◊ Aspirin should not be used in children under 16 years due to risk of Reye syndrome

Contraindications: Rimantadine - nursing mothers

Precautions:
- Rimantadine:
  - ◊ May cause mild CNS symptoms (e.g., lightheadedness, insomnia, anxiety) which are dose related and clear when stopped
  - ◊ May potentiate underlying seizure disorders and exacerbate epilepsy; EEG abnormalities are increased
  - ◊ Cautious use if uncontrolled psychosis or severe psychoneurosis
  - ◊ Those being treated with rimantadine should avoid contact with unaffected individuals taking a drug for prophylaxis
- Zanamivir may cause bronchospasm; have bronchodilator available
- Oseltamivir:
  - ◊ May cause nausea and vomiting; this may be less severe if taken with food
  - ◊ Dose should be decreased if renal failure creatinine clearance < 30 mL/min

Significant possible interactions: N/A

ALTERNATIVE DRUGS
Ibuprofen or other NSAIDs for symptomatic relief (no aspirin in children)

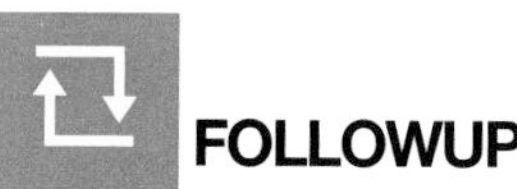

FOLLOWUP

PATIENT MONITORING
In mild cases, usually no follow-up required. Follow moderate or severe cases until symptoms resolved and any complications are treated effectively.

PREVENTION/AVOIDANCE
- Incubation - 1 to 4 days; infected persons most contagious during peak symptoms
- Trivalent influenza vaccine
  - ◊ Recommended for all adults age 50 and older
  - ◊ Recommended for high risk individuals: chronic pulmonary disease, cardiovascular disease, immunosuppression, hemoglobinopathies, renal diseases, metabolic disease, diabetes, HIV, long term aspirin therapy, asplenia, alcoholism
  - ◊ Recommended for health care providers, home care providers, staff and residents of nursing homes and other chronic care facilities, homeless, public safety workers and close contacts of high risk individuals
  - ◊ In 2004, vaccination of healthy 6-23 month-olds is recommended
  - ◊ Should be administered in the Fall prior to influenza season
  - ◊ Some side effects possible, e.g., fever and mild, local reaction at vaccination site.
  - ◊ Dose is 0.5 IM except for children < 3 years old. Children 6 through 35 months old should receive 0.25 mL.
  - ◊ Single dose/year except for children < 9 years old who should receive 2 doses the first year that they receive influenza vaccine (1 month apart)
    - Vaccine contraindications: Anaphylaxis to eggs (do skin testing first)
    - 1-2 weeks after immunization before protection occurs
- Live attenuated influenza vaccine (LAIV)
  - ◊ For healthy persons 5-49 years old
  - ◊ Persons who should not be vaccinated: anaphylaxis to eggs, immunocompromising conditions, pregnant women, persons with high-risk conditions, persons with a history of Guillain-Barre syndrome
- Amantadine, rimantadine and oseltamivir:
  - ◊ May be used prophylactically in high risk groups (that have not been vaccinated or need additional control measures) during epidemics of influenza. It should not be considered as a substitute for vaccination unless vaccine contraindicated.
  - ◊ Take for duration of outbreak, if no vaccine given. Discontinue after 14 days if used in addition to vaccine.
  - ◊ Prophylactically during influenza season for those with contraindications to vaccine
  - ◊ Prophylactically for staff and residents in nursing home outbreaks of influenza
  - ◊ Prophylactically for immune deficient persons who are expected not to respond to vaccination
  - ◊ Oseltamivir at 75 mg qd can be used for influenza types A and B, whereas rimantadine is effective for only type A

POSSIBLE COMPLICATIONS
- Otitis media
- Pneumonia
- Reye syndrome
- Rhabdomyolysis
- Post-influenza asthenia
- Acute sinusitis
- Croup
- Apnea in neonates
- Bronchitis
- Death
- Exacerbation of CHF

EXPECTED COURSE/PROGNOSIS
Favorable

MISCELLANEOUS

ASSOCIATED CONDITIONS
Bacterial pneumonia

AGE-RELATED FACTORS
Pediatric:
- Reye syndrome is a rare and severe complication associated with aspirin use. Avoid aspirin in children with influenza.
- Vaccinate 6-23 month-olds with inactivated vaccine

Geriatric:
- Elderly more likely to have complications
- Immunization recommended age 50 and older

Others: N/A

PREGNANCY
- Women at risk from influenza complications should receive influenza vaccine regardless of trimester
- ACIP recommends vaccinating all women who will be pregnant during influenza season
- Amantadine is contraindicated in pregnant women

SYNONYMS
- Flu
- Grip
- Acute catarrhal fever

ICD-9-CM
487.0 Influenza with pneumonia
487.1 Influenza with other respiratory manifestations

SEE ALSO

OTHER NOTES
Persons with HIV infection should get annual influenza vaccination, however the antibody response to the vaccine may be low in persons with advanced HIV-related illnesses

ABBREVIATIONS
N/A

REFERENCES
- Report of the Committee on Infectious Diseases, 2003 Elk Grove Village: American Academy of Pediatrics; 2003
- Prevention and control of influenza. Recommendations of the Immunization Practices Advisory Committee (ACIP). MMWR; 2004
- Mandell GL, ed. Principles and Practice of Infectious Diseases. 5th ed. New York: Churchill Livingstone; 2000

Web references: 3 available at www.5mcc.com

Illustrations N/A

Author(s):
Richard Kent Zimmerman, MD, MPH

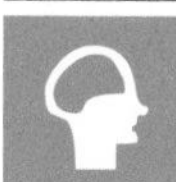

BASICS

DESCRIPTION Arthropods affect man by being pests, inoculating poison, invading tissue, or transmitting disease. Inoculation of poison may occur as either a bite or a sting. This discussion is limited to the irritative, poisonous, allergic effects of these pests.
- Harmful arthropods of the U.S. include:
  - ◊ Bees: Bumblebees, sweat bees, honeybees
  - ◊ Wasps: Hornets, wasps
  - ◊ Ants: Fire ants, harvester ants
  - ◊ Brown recluse spider
  - ◊ Black widow spider
  - ◊ Hobo spiders
  - ◊ Scorpions
  - ◊ Mosquitoes
  - ◊ Flies: Deer, horse, black, stable, and biting midges
  - ◊ Lice: Body, head, pubic
  - ◊ Bugs: Kissing, bed, wheel
  - ◊ Fleas: Human, cat, dog
  - ◊ Mites: Itch mite (scabies), red bugs (chiggers)
  - ◊ Ticks
  - ◊ Caterpillars: Puss, browntail, buck, moth saddleback
  - ◊ Centipedes
- Characteristic reactions include:
  - ◊ Local tissue irritation, inflammation and destruction
  - ◊ Systemic effects related to inoculated poisons
  - ◊ Allergic reactions: Immediate or delayed

System(s) affected: Skin/Exocrine
Genetics: N/A
Incidence/Prevalence in USA: Widespread (seasonal and regional variance)
Predominant age: All ages
Predominant sex: Male = Female

SIGNS & SYMPTOMS
- Local reactions:
  - ◊ Erythema
  - ◊ Pain
  - ◊ Heat
  - ◊ Swelling
  - ◊ Itching
  - ◊ Blisters
  - ◊ Secondary infection - cellulitis, abscess
  - ◊ Necrosis
  - ◊ Ulceration
  - ◊ Drainage
- Toxic reactions: Non-antigenic
  - ◊ Nausea
  - ◊ Vomiting
  - ◊ Headache
  - ◊ Fever
  - ◊ Diarrhea
  - ◊ Lightheadedness
  - ◊ Syncope
  - ◊ Drowsiness
  - ◊ Muscles spasms
  - ◊ Edema
  - ◊ Convulsions
- Systemic reactions: Allergic
  - ◊ Itching eyes
  - ◊ Facial flushing
  - ◊ Generalized urticaria
  - ◊ Dry cough
  - ◊ Chest/throat constriction
  - ◊ Wheezing
  - ◊ Dyspnea
  - ◊ Cyanosis
  - ◊ Abdominal cramps
  - ◊ Diarrhea
  - ◊ Nausea
  - ◊ Vomiting
  - ◊ Vertigo
  - ◊ Chills/fever
  - ◊ Stridor
  - ◊ Shock
  - ◊ Loss of consciousness
  - ◊ Involuntary bowel/bladder action
  - ◊ Frothy sputum
  - ◊ Respiratory failure
  - ◊ Cardiovascular collapse
  - ◊ Death
- Delayed reaction:
  - ◊ Serum-sickness-like reactions
  - ◊ Fever
  - ◊ Malaise
  - ◊ Headache
  - ◊ Urticaria
  - ◊ Lymphadenopathy
  - ◊ Polyarthritis
- Unusual reactions:
  - ◊ Encephalopathy
  - ◊ Neuritis
  - ◊ Vasculitis
  - ◊ Nephrosis
  - ◊ Extreme fear/anxiety

CAUSES
- Local tissue inflammation and destruction from poison
- Allergic reaction from previous sensitization
- Toxic reaction from large inoculation of poison

RISK FACTORS
- Living environment
- Climate
- Season
- Clothing
- Lack of protective measures
- Perfumes, colognes
- Previous sensitization
- Young or elderly at more risk

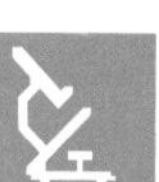

DIAGNOSIS

DIFFERENTIAL DIAGNOSIS
- Local reaction: Infection, cellulitis, dermatoses, punctures, foreign bodies
- Toxic reaction: Chemical exposure/ingestion, medications, IV drug abuse, environmental, plants
- Allergic reaction: Medications, illicit drugs, foods, topical products, environmental, plants, chemicals

LABORATORY Leukocytosis, thrombocytopenia, hypofibrinogenemia, abnormal coagulation, DIC, proteinuria, hemoglobinemia, hemoglobinuria, myoglobinemia, myoglobinuria, and azotemia are uncommon but possible manifestations in severe reactions

Drugs that may alter lab results: N/A

Disorders that may alter lab results: N/A

PATHOLOGICAL FINDINGS Inflammation, ulceration, vesiculation, pustulation, rupture, eschar, swelling

SPECIAL TESTS N/A

IMAGING N/A

DIAGNOSTIC PROCEDURES N/A

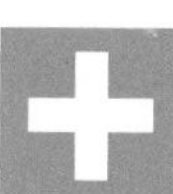

TREATMENT

APPROPRIATE HEALTH CARE
- Outpatient or inpatient, depending on individual response to injury
- Hospitalize for severe systemic reactions with threatened airway obstruction, bronchospasm, hypotension, severe angiodermatitis or pain

GENERAL MEASURES
- First aid measures, local treatment, activate emergency services in severe reactions. If history of allergy or large envenomations, don't wait to seek emergency care.
- Use ANA kit and over-the-counter antihistamines, if available and required
- Local (depending on severity)
  - ◊ Remove stinger (scrape it out - don't squeeze with tweezer)
  - ◊ Cleanse wound
  - ◊ Ice packs to bite or sting site (alternate 10 minutes on/10 minutes off)
  - ◊ Elevation of affected part
  - ◊ Rest the affected area
  - ◊ Debride ulcers
  - ◊ Drain abscesses
- Systemic (depending on severity, and type of reaction); home use - Epi-Pen
  - ◊ Adequate airway (intubation, tracheostomy) - if needed to bypass obstruction
  - ◊ Oxygen (4-6 L/min) - if needed for respiratory distress
  - ◊ Hospitalize and observe 24-48 hours

SURGICAL MEASURES Optimal treatment of necrotic spider bites is not well defined. Surgical repair may be required of severe ulcerative lesions, but not until primary necrotizing process is complete.

ACTIVITY Rest to limit spread of poison

DIET No special diet; nothing by mouth if severe systemic reaction

PATIENT EDUCATION
- Protective measures, ANA kit use, risks
- Individuals with known sensitivity should wear medical identification (bracelet, tag) or carry a card

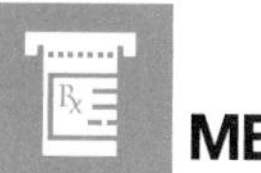

MEDICATIONS

DRUG(S) OF CHOICE

- Local (depending on severity)
  - ◊ Analgesics
  - ◊ Antihistamines - diphenhydramine (Benadryl) 25-50 mg qid
  - ◊ Steroids topical or oral - prednisone 20-40 mg/day
  - ◊ Antibiotics
- Systemic (depending on severity and reaction type)
  - ◊ Epinephrine [1:1000] subcutaneous: to combat urticaria, wheezing, angioedema - child 0.01 mL/kg, adult 0.3-0.5 mL
  - ◊ Diphenhydramine: 25-50 mg IV or IM, to combat urticaria, wheezing, angioedema
  - ◊ Aminophylline: adult 500 mg IV over 20-30 minutes, child 7.5 mg/kg, if needed for bronchospasm
  - ◊ IV fluids (Ringer's lactate): if needed for hypotension, hypovolemia
  - ◊ Dopamine: 200 mg in 250 mL at 5 mcg/kg/min - to correct vascular collapse. Titrate to maintain systemic blood pressure over 90 mm Hg.
  - ◊ Hydrocortisone: 100-250 mg IV, if needed for severe urticaria or spider bite
  - ◊ Tetanus prophylaxis and antibiotics: if indicated
  - ◊ Diazepam (Valium): 5-10 mg, if needed for severe muscle spasms
  - ◊ Morphine or meperidine (Demerol): if needed for pain
- Antivenins (e.g., Black Widow spider, scorpion) are available and appropriate in certain cases based on availability and identification of organism
- Topical insecticides
  - ◊ Lice: 1% permethrin (Nix, Elimite) is drug of choice, but 1% lindane (Kwell) or pyrethrin (Rid) are effective.
  - ◊ Scabies: 5% permethrin is drug of choice, but 10% crotamiton (Eurax) or lindane are effective

Contraindications: Refer to manufacturer's literature

Precautions:

- Dosing appropriate to age
- If severe reaction, don't delay treatment
- Severe vascular collapse may require central pressure monitor

Significant possible interactions: Refer to manufacturer's literature

ALTERNATIVE DRUGS

- Other antihistamines, e.g., loratadine (Claritin), fexofenadine (Allegra), etc.
- Oral ivermectin (Mectizan) appears effective for lice and scabies, but is not FDA approved for this purpose

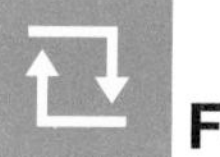

FOLLOWUP

PATIENT MONITORING Followup wound care

PREVENTION/AVOIDANCE

- Avoid re-exposure in known hypersensitive individuals
- Prescribe anaphylactic (ANA kit) or Epi-Pen, if indicated
- Educate on risks of increasing anamnestic responses in future
- Consider desensitization with immunotherapy in severe cases
- DEET or other proven insect repellants
- Permethrin applied to clothes is better against ticks than DEET

POSSIBLE COMPLICATIONS

- Infection
  - ◊ Bacterial
  - ◊ Arthropod associated diseases with tick, fly, bug and mosquito bites, e.g., lyme borreliosis, rickettsial disease (Rocky Mountain spotted fever), arboviral encephalitis, malaria, leishmaniasis, trypanosomiasis, dengue
- Scarring
- Drug reactions
- Multisystem failure
- Death

EXPECTED COURSE/PROGNOSIS

- Minor reactions - excellent
- Severe reactions - excellent with early, appropriate treatment

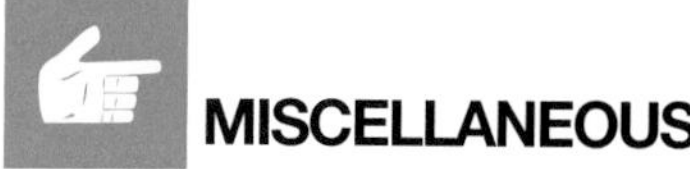

MISCELLANEOUS

ASSOCIATED CONDITIONS N/A

AGE-RELATED FACTORS

Pediatric: More at risk
Geriatric: More at risk
Others: N/A

PREGNANCY Not a contraindication to appropriate management

SYNONYMS N/A

ICD-9-CM

989.5 Toxic effect of venom
910.8 Other and unspecified superficial injury of face, neck, and scalp except eye, without mention of infection

SEE ALSO

Pediculosis
Scabies

OTHER NOTES

- Imported fire ants and Africanized bees in endemic areas of the Southern United States pose increased risks to persons living in these areas

ABBREVIATIONS N/A

REFERENCES

- Tintinalli JE, Krome RL, eds: Emergency Medicine. New York, McGraw-Hill, 1988
- Schroeder SA, Krupp MA, Tierne, LM, McPhee SJ, eds: Current Medical Diagnosis and Treatment. Norwalk, CT, Appleton & Lange, 1989
- MMWR: Necrotic arachnidism-Pacific Northwest, 1988-1996. 1996;Vol45:No 21
- Isselbacher KJ, et al, eds: Harrison's Principles of Internal Medicine. 13th Ed. New York, McGraw-Hill, 1994
- The Medical Letter. Vol 40 (Issue 1017) Jan 2, 1998
- Mosquitoes and mosquito repellants: A clinician's guide. Annals of Internal Medicine 1198;Jun 1:128(11):931-940

Web references: 0 available at www.5mcc.com
Illustrations 11 available

Author(s):

Gregory G. Gaar, MD

BASICS

DESCRIPTION Difficulty in falling asleep or maintaining sleep, intermittent wakefulness, early morning awakening or a combination of these. Can be:
- Transient - due to a life crisis, bereavement, change in environment or concomitant illness
- Chronic - associated with medical and psychiatric conditions or drug intake.

System(s) affected: Nervous
Genetics: N/A
Incidence/Prevalence in USA: Affects an estimated 35% of the adult population. One of the most frequent complaints in primary care practice.
Predominant age: Elderly
Predominant sex: Male = Female

SIGNS & SYMPTOMS
- Perceived reduction in sleeping time
- Initial insomnia - difficulty initiating sleep at usual time
- Middle insomnia - wakefulness during the usual sleep cycle, "tossing and turning"
- Terminal insomnia - early awakening
- Daytime sleepiness and napping
- Tiredness
- Anticipatory anxiety

CAUSES
- Medical illnesses - arthritis, fibromyalgia, hyperthyroidism, gastroesophageal reflux disease, duodenal ulcer, Alzheimer disease and other dementias, restless leg syndrome, sleep apnea, respiratory diseases, and all painful conditions (e.g., muscle cramps)
- Psychiatric illnesses - mostly depression, classically associated with early morning awakening, but can also be manifested by initial or middle insomnia
- Anxiety
- Schizophrenia
- Manic disorders
- Drug induced insomnia - alcohol, caffeine, nicotine
- Nonprescription drugs - diet aids, decongestants, cough preparations
- Prescribed drugs - steroids, theophylline, phenytoin (Dilantin), levodopa (Sinemet, Dopar)
- Obstructive sleep apnea
- Jet lag (transient)
- Heavy smoking

RISK FACTORS
- Chronic illnesses
- Age over 50
- Multiple drug intake
- Obesity

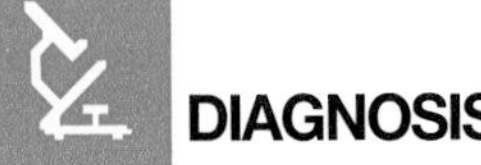

DIAGNOSIS

DIFFERENTIAL DIAGNOSIS N/A

LABORATORY N/A

Drugs that may alter lab results: N/A

Disorders that may alter lab results: N/A

PATHOLOGICAL FINDINGS N/A

SPECIAL TESTS Diagnosis can be confirmed by the use of polysomnography, particularly if sleep apnea is suspected. This is generally not necessary or practical.

IMAGING N/A

DIAGNOSTIC PROCEDURES Insomnia is a self-reported condition

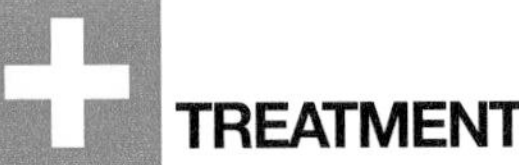

TREATMENT

APPROPRIATE HEALTH CARE Outpatient

GENERAL MEASURES
- Transient insomnia
  - ◊ Lasts less than three to four weeks
  - ◊ Reassurance and supportive counseling are appropriate treatment modalities
- Chronic insomnia
  - ◊ Address the underlying cause: Pain, drugs, depression
  - ◊ Avoid alcohol after 5 PM or within 6 hours of retiring because of secondary rebound stimulation
  - ◊ Patient should be encouraged to avoid daytime napping and to develop bedtime rituals conducive to sleep
  - ◊ A thorough review of the patient's habits, drug intake, diet, and exercise pattern may uncover correctable causes of insomnia
  - ◊ Prescribe hypnotics only if the above strategies fail

SURGICAL MEASURES N/A

ACTIVITY
- No restriction
- A daily exercise routine is helpful. Avoid exercise close to bedtime.

DIET
- Avoid caffeine
- Avoid heavy, late night snacks (sometimes a light snack before bedtime may help)
- Avoid alcohol after 5 PM or within 6 hours of retiring, because of secondary rebound stimulation

PATIENT EDUCATION
- Explain sleep patterns and sleep hygiene
- Show limitations and noxious effects of drugs used for insomnia
- Incorporation of appropriate dietary and exercise protocol

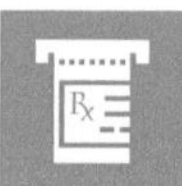

MEDICATIONS

DRUG(S) OF CHOICE
- Analgesics as indicated for pain
- Benzodiazepines
  - ◊ Flurazepam (Dalmane), 15-30 mg, long half-life, elderly might benefit from smaller dose
  - ◊ Temazepam (Restoril), 15 mg one to two hours before bedtime
  - ◊ Triazolam (Halcion), shortest half-life, 0.125 mg to 0.25 mg, smaller dose recommended for the elderly. Useful as part of treatment regimen for jet lag.
- Non-benzodiazepines
  - ◊ Zolpidem (Ambien), 10 mg for adults and 5 mg for the elderly/debilitated
  - ◊ Zaleplon (Sonata) 5, 10 or 20 mg. Short-acting.
- Tricyclic antidepressants
  - ◊ Widely used for insomnia associated with depression
  - ◊ Preferred agent is amitriptyline (Elavil) because of its marked sedative effect. A typical starting dose is 50-100 mg at bedtime.

Contraindications:
- Pregnancy and lactation
- Psychoses
- Acute narrow angle glaucoma
- Significant liver disease
- Depressed patient who may be suicide risk

Precautions:
- All benzodiazepines can cause paradoxical, agitated states, anterograde amnesia, and rebound insomnia
- Flurazepam may cause incoordination ataxia and impairment of intellectual functions
- Triazolam has been associated with withdrawal psychosis and seizures in some patients after abrupt cessation, psychological dependence, physical dependence
- Amitriptyline can cause constipation and orthostatic hypotension
- Zolpidem, although generally well tolerated, should be used with the same precautions taken with other sedative hypnotics. Most common reported side effects are drowsiness, dizziness, headache.
- Zaleplon appears to be a good choice for elderly patients since it does not cause residual sedation or affect psychomotor function. However, clinical experience is limited.

Significant possible interactions:
- Alcohol may potentiate the CNS effects of the benzodiazepines
- Digoxin serum concentrations may be increased
- Levodopa efficacy may be reduced

ALTERNATIVE DRUGS
- Diphenhydramine (Benadryl) has been used to induce sleep in the elderly, but it may also cause confusion and "hangover"
- Chloral hydrate (Noctec), 250-500 mg, is favored by some clinicians since it does not cause tolerance or withdrawal. The nightly dose is 250-500 mg.
- Melatonin, a pineal hormone. Marketed as a dietary supplement. There is some evidence that controlled-release melatonin improves sleep quality in a selected elderly population. Not FDA approved. Appears useful for jet lag. Has mild hypnotic effect. No adverse effects have been reported, but controlled studies are lacking.

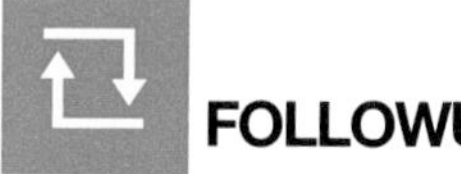

FOLLOWUP

PATIENT MONITORING
- Need for benzodiazepines to be reassessed periodically. Avoid standing prescriptions.
- Followup as needed depending on individual patient. Refer for psychosocial counseling, if appropriate.

PREVENTION/AVOIDANCE Avoidance, when possible, of all possible causes

POSSIBLE COMPLICATIONS
- Transient insomnia becomes chronic
- Increased daytime sleepiness

EXPECTED COURSE/PROGNOSIS
Should resolve with time. Treatment of underlying symptoms helpful.

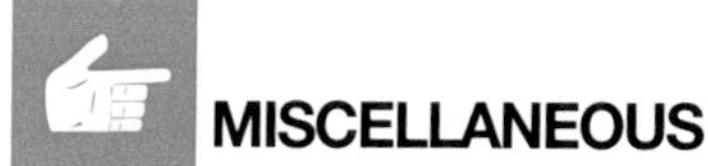

MISCELLANEOUS

ASSOCIATED CONDITIONS
- Obstructive sleep apnea
- Drug or alcohol addiction and dependence

AGE-RELATED FACTORS
Pediatric: N/A

Geriatric:
- Exert caution when prescribing benzodiazepines or other sedative-hypnotics to the elderly
- Educate older patients about age-related sleep changes

Others: N/A

PREGNANCY Transient insomnia occurs due to discomfort in sleeping positions

SYNONYMS Sleeplessness

ICD-9-CM
780.50 Sleep disturbance, unspecified
780.51 Insomnia with sleep apnea
780.52 Other insomnia

SEE ALSO
Anxiety
Depression
Fibromyalgia
Jet lag
Prion diseases
Sleep apnea, obstructive

OTHER NOTES L-Tryptophan: formerly widely used - no longer available as a single ingredient

ABBREVIATIONS N/A

REFERENCES

- Rakel R, editor. Textbook of Family Practice. 5th ed. Philadelphia: W.B. Saunders Co.; 1995
- Goldman HH: Review of General Psychiatry. 4th ed. Norwalk, CT: Appleton & Lange; 1995
- Bahrat RS, Nakra MD, et al. Insomnia in the Elderly. Amer Fam Phys 1991;477-483
- The Medical Letter on Drugs and Therapeutics. Vol 35, Issue 895, April 30, 1993
- The Medical Letter on Drugs and Therapeutics. Vol 37, Issue 962, November 24, 1995
- Maczaj M. Pharmacological treatment of insomnia. Drugs 1993;45(1):44-55
- Garfinkel D, Laudon M, Nof D, Zisapel N. Improvement of sleep quality in elderly people by controlled-release melatonin. Lancet 1995;346(8974):541-544
- Dockhorn RJ, Dockhorn DW. Zolpidem in the treatment of short-term insomnia: a randomized placebo-controlled trial. Clin Neuropharmacol 1996;19(4):333-340
- Ancoli-Israel S. Insomnia in the elderly: a review for the primary care
- practitioner. Sleep 2000 Feb 1;23 Suppl1: S23-30

Web references: 1 available at www.5mcc.com

Illustrations N/A

Author(s):
Michel J. Dodard, MD

BASICS

DESCRIPTION Insulinomas are tumors of the pancreatic beta cells of the islets of Langerhans. They are usually very small with 70% measuring less than 1.5 cm. They are usually single and benign with only 10-15% being malignant and only 10% being multiple tumors. Their malignant potential is not as clinically important as their functional ability to secrete insulin, which leads to symptomatic hypoglycemia.

- The symptomatic hypoglycemia is secondary to persistent, absolute, or relative hyperinsulinemia that is unresponsive to normal feedback mechanisms
- The hypoglycemic episodes are irregular, recurrent, and tend to increase in frequency and severity over time
- Hypoglycemic episodes are especially likely to occur when fasting or after exercise
- Pancreatic beta cells secrete both insulin and C-peptide
- Whipple triad is the basis for the clinical diagnosis of insulinomas.
  - ◊ Symptomatic fasting or postexercise hypoglycemia
  - ◊ Low blood glucose levels less than 50 mg/dL (2.78 mmol/L) during symptoms.
  - ◊ Resolution of symptoms when treated with oral or IV glucose
- Laboratory diagnosis is based on inappropriately high serum insulin and C-peptides during periods of low blood glucose (shows over-secretion and endogenous origin)
- Awareness is the key to early diagnosis

System(s) affected: Cardiovascular, Endocrine/Metabolic, Gastrointestinal, Nervous

Genetics: No known genetic pattern unless part of MEN 1 syndrome

Incidence/Prevalence in USA: Annual incidence of 1 in 1.25 million persons

Predominant age:
- Rare less than 20 years old
- 20% of cases in adults under 40 years old
- 40% of cases in adults between 40 and 60 years old
- 40% or cases in adults over 60 years old

Predominant sex: 60% of new cases occur in females

SIGNS & SYMPTOMS
Due to hypoglycemia or catecholamine compensatory release
- Neurological
  - ◊ Apathy
  - ◊ Irritability
  - ◊ Confusion
  - ◊ Disorientation
  - ◊ Delirium
  - ◊ Coma
  - ◊ Convulsions
  - ◊ Diplopia
  - ◊ Blurred vision
  - ◊ Vertigo
  - ◊ Inarticulate speech
  - ◊ Tremor
  - ◊ Dizziness
  - ◊ Hallucinations
- Cardiovascular
  - ◊ Palpitations
  - ◊ Tachycardia
  - ◊ Angina
  - ◊ Sweating
- Gastrointestinal
  - ◊ Hunger
  - ◊ Abdominal discomfort
  - ◊ Nausea
  - ◊ Vomiting
  - ◊ Weight gain

CAUSES Etiology unknown

RISK FACTORS
- Older than 40
- MEN 1 syndrome

DIAGNOSIS

DIFFERENTIAL DIAGNOSIS
- Medications
  - ◊ Inappropriate insulin
  - ◊ Sulfonylureas
  - ◊ Beta-blockers
  - ◊ Salicylates
  - ◊ Quinine
- Very rare causes
  - ◊ Nesidioblastosis
  - ◊ Large sarcomas
  - ◊ Hepatocellular carcinoma
- Reactive hypoglycemia

LABORATORY
- Document low blood sugar during symptoms
- RIA of serum insulin and C-peptide (inappropriately elevated during symptoms)
- Malignant tumors may secrete ß-HCG

Drugs that may alter lab results: N/A

Disorders that may alter lab results: N/A

PATHOLOGICAL FINDINGS
- Usually small and single
- Malignant tumors tend to be larger and multiple
- Metastases are found in the liver or regional lymph nodes (distant metastases rare)
- Tumors evenly distributed throughout the pancreas (1/3 in head, 1/3 in body, 1/3 in tail)

SPECIAL TESTS
- Fast for 72 hours or until symptoms develop. When symptomatic, determine insulin, C-peptide, and glucose levels.
- Provocative testing
  - ◊ IV calcium gluconate (15 mg/kg of elemental calcium) over 4 hours determining insulin and glucose levels
  - ◊ Tolbutamide bolus (1 gram after an overnight fast) and determine insulin and glucose levels at 150 minutes
  - ◊ C-peptide suppression with 0.1 unit/kg of insulin and determine C-peptide and glucose levels

IMAGING
- Selective mesenteric angiography (detects 52-85%)
- Preoperative CT (detects 70%)
- Endoscopic ultrasound
- Preoperative ultrasound (detects 22-63%)
- Intraoperative ultrasound (detects 86%)
- Somatostatin analogue I123 labeled TyR 3-octreotide

DIAGNOSTIC PROCEDURES
- Document high insulin/glucose ratio during symptoms
- 72 hour fast
- Portal venous sampling
- Intraoperative ultrasound
- Intraoperative palpation

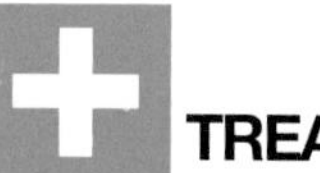

TREATMENT

APPROPRIATE HEALTH CARE Treatment is primarily surgical; medical treatment for surgically incurable lesions

GENERAL MEASURES
- Closely observe for severe hypoglycemic symptoms
- Attempt to increase glucose levels
- Attempt to decrease insulin levels
- Keep a ready glucose source available

SURGICAL MEASURES
- Enucleation if tumor is superficial
- Partial pancreatectomy if tumor is deep-seated or invasive
- Mechanical ablative techniques (hepatic arterial embolization for refractory metastases)

ACTIVITY Avoid exercise

DIET Frequent high carbohydrate meals and snacks

PATIENT EDUCATION N/A

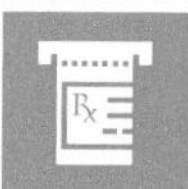

MEDICATIONS

DRUG(S) OF CHOICE

- To decrease insulin secretion
  - ◊ Diazoxide 100-150 mg po q8h (3-8 mg/kg daily in 2 or 3 divided doses)
  - ◊ Octreotide acetate (long acting analog of somatostatin); 50-100 mcg SQ bid, increase as needed to control symptoms
- To increase glucose levels
  - ◊ Oral or IV glucose
  - ◊ IM or SQ glucagon
- For metastatic disease
  - ◊ Streptozocin plus doxorubicin
  - ◊ Fluorouracil

Contraindications: Refer to manufacturer's literature

Precautions:

- Strenuous exercise
- Prolonged fasts
- May need diuretic to counteract the sodium and fluid retention of diazoxide

Significant possible interactions: Refer to manufacturer's literature

ALTERNATIVE DRUGS

- Octreotide acetate. Continue treatment until surgery or lifelong if tumor is unresectable.
- Dacarbazine (DTIC, 5-dimethyltriazenoimidazole-4-carboxamine) for metastatic disease
- To increase glucose levels
  - ◊ Corticosteroids
  - ◊ Propranolol
  - ◊ Phenytoin

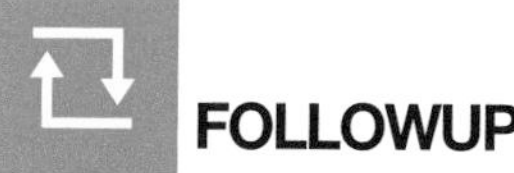

FOLLOWUP

PATIENT MONITORING Watch for recurrence of hypoglycemic symptoms

PREVENTION/AVOIDANCE N/A

POSSIBLE COMPLICATIONS

- From surgery
  - ◊ Pancreatitis
  - ◊ Pancreatic leaks
  - ◊ Fistulae
  - ◊ Peritonitis
  - ◊ Abscess
  - ◊ Pseudocysts

EXPECTED COURSE/PROGNOSIS

Excellent if tumor solitary, benign, and completely resected

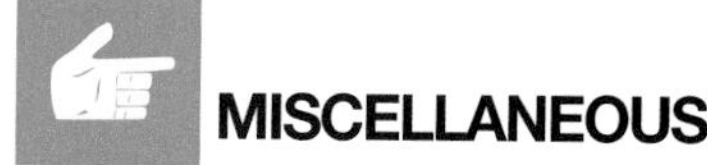

MISCELLANEOUS

ASSOCIATED CONDITIONS MEN 1 syndrome

AGE-RELATED FACTORS

Pediatric: N/A
Geriatric: N/A
Others: N/A

PREGNANCY N/A

SYNONYMS

- Beta cell tumor
- Beta cell adenoma
- Nesidioblastoma

ICD-9-CM

157.4 Malignant neoplasm of Islets of Langerhans
211.7 Benign neoplasm of Islets of Langerhans

SEE ALSO

Multiple endocrine neoplasia (MEN)

OTHER NOTES

- 8% of patients with MEN 1 syndrome have insulinomas
- Insulinomas associated with MEN 1 syndrome tend to be multiple tumors and present at an earlier age

ABBREVIATIONS N/A

REFERENCES

- Proyle CA. Endocrine tumors of the pancreas: an update. Aust NZ J Surg 1998;68:90-100
- Modlin IM, Lewis JJ, Ahlman H, Bilchik AJ, Kumar RR. Management of unresectable malignant endocrine tumors of the pancreas. Surg Gynecol & Obstet 1993;176:507-18
- Grant CS. Insulinoma. Surg Oncol Clin of NA 1998;7:819-44
- Brentjens R, Saltz L. Islet cell tumors of the pancreas: the medical oncologist's perspective. Surg Clin North Am 2001;81(3):527-42
- Pereira PL, Wiskirchen J. Morphological and functional investigations of neuroendocrine tumors of the pancreas. Eur Radiol 2003;13(9):2133-46
- Burns AR, Dackiw AP. Insulinoma. Curr Treat Options Oncol 2003;4(4):309-17

Web references: 2 available at www.5mcc.com
Illustrations N/A

Author(s):

Rick Ricer, MD

BASICS

DESCRIPTION A disease of unknown cause probably representing a final common pathway from several etiologies. At least four types can be separated for treatment purposes. Likely pathogenesis is loss of elasticity of bladder muscular wall with adherence of mucosal layer.

- Classic type: Normal bladder capacity under anesthesia. Ulceration, cracking, or glomerulation of mucosa with bladder distention under anesthesia. No incontinence. Symptoms wax and wane. Non-progressive. A bladder sensory problem.
- Type 2: Same as classic type, except no bladder mucosa changes on cystoscopy with bladder distention.
- Type 3: Progressive bladder fibrosis. Small true bladder capacity under anesthesia. Poor bladder wall compliance. Often ulcer present at cystoscopy. Sometimes incontinence present if bladder fills beyond capacity.
- Type 4: Same as type 3, but with chronic bacteriuria that is unresponsive to antibiotics.

System(s) affected: Renal/Urologic
Genetics: Probably not an inherited disease
Incidence/Prevalence in USA: Up to 500,000 affected. Many cases likely unreported.
Predominant age: 20's to 40's for types 1 and 2. 20's to 70's for types 3 and 4.
Predominant sex: Female > Male (10:1)

SIGNS & SYMPTOMS

- Frequent, urgent, relentless urination day and night
- Pain with full bladder that resolves with bladder emptying (except if bacteriuria present)
- Urge urinary incontinence if bladder capacity is small
- Dyspareunia especially with full bladder
- Secondary symptoms from chronic pain and sleeplessness

CAUSES

- Unknown. Not primarily psychosomatic, though many secondary effects present
- Possible causes:
  - ◊ Subclinical urinary infection
  - ◊ Increased bladder wall permeability to irritants such as urea
  - ◊ Autoimmune

RISK FACTORS Unknown

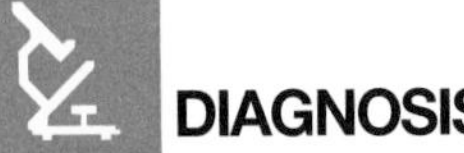

DIAGNOSIS

DIFFERENTIAL DIAGNOSIS

- Uninhibited bladder (urgency, frequency, urge incontinence, less pain, symptoms usually decrease when asleep)
- Urinary infection: Cystitis, prostatitis
- Bladder neoplasm
- Bladder stone
- Neurologic bladder disease
- Non-urinary pelvic disease (sexually transmitted diseases, endometriosis, pelvic relaxation)

LABORATORY

- Urinalysis: Normal except with chronic bacteriuria (rare)
- Urine culture: Normal except with chronic bacteriuria (rare)
- Urine cytology: Normal

Drugs that may alter lab results: False negative culture if on antibiotics

Disorders that may alter lab results: N/A

PATHOLOGICAL FINDINGS

- Non-specific chronic inflammation on bladder biopsies
- Urine cytology negative for dysplasia and neoplasia

SPECIAL TESTS

- Cystoscopy under anesthesia: Possible bladder ulcer
- Bladder hydraulic distention: Cracking of mucosa after partial emptying with "watershed hemorrhage"
- Bladder biopsies: Chronic inflammation

IMAGING N/A

DIAGNOSTIC PROCEDURES Cystoscopy (as above)

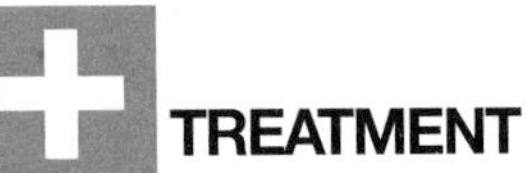

TREATMENT

APPROPRIATE HEALTH CARE Outpatient

GENERAL MEASURES

- Eliminate foods and liquids that exacerbate symptoms on individual basis
- Biofeedback bladder retraining

SURGICAL MEASURES

- Hydraulic distention of bladder under anesthesia
- Cauterization of bladder ulcer
- Augmentation cystoplasty to increase bladder capacity and decrease pressure, with or without partial cystectomy. Expected results in severe cases: 75% much improved, 20% with residual discomfort, 5% unchanged.
- Urinary diversion with total cystectomy

ACTIVITY N/A

DIET

- Variable effects from person to person
- Common irritants include caffeine, spicy foods, acidic foods, alcohol

PATIENT EDUCATION Interstitial Cystitis Association of America, P.O. Box 1553, Madison Square Station, New York, N.Y. 10159-1553. 1-800-ICA-1626

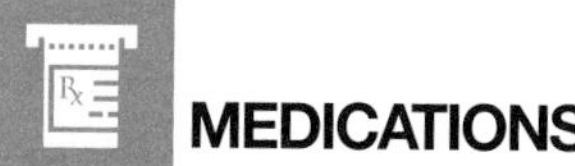

MEDICATIONS

DRUG(S) OF CHOICE

- Oxybutynin, hyoscyamine, and other anticholinergic medications decrease frequency
- Doxepin decreases frequency
- NSAIDs for pain and any inflammatory component
- Pentosan polysulfate (Elmiron) 100 mg three times daily. May take several months to become effective.
- Triple drug therapy - 6 months of pentosan, hydroxyzine, doxepin
- Antibacterials for bacteriuria
- Bladder instillations:
  - ◊ DMSO every 1 to 2 weeks for 3 to 6 weeks, then as needed
  - ◊ Heparin sometimes added to DMSO
  - ◊ Other agents: steroids, lidocaine (Xylocaine), silver nitrate, oxychlorosene (Clorpactin)

Contraindications: No anticholinergics with closed angle glaucoma.
Precautions: N/A
Significant possible interactions: Refer to manufacturer's profile of each drug

ALTERNATIVE DRUGS

- Note that phenazopyridine, a local bladder mucosal anesthetic, is usually not very effective

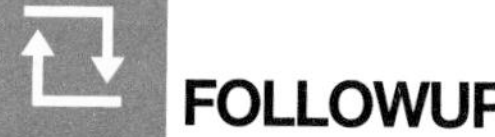

FOLLOWUP

PATIENT MONITORING Not specifically needed unless symptoms unresponsive to treatment

PREVENTION/AVOIDANCE N/A

POSSIBLE COMPLICATIONS Type 3 with long term continuous high bladder pressure could be associated with renal damage

EXPECTED COURSE/PROGNOSIS

- Types 1 and 2: Exacerbations and remissions of symptoms. Generally not progressive. Does not predispose to other diseases.
- Type 3 and 4: Progressive problems that usually require surgery to control symptoms

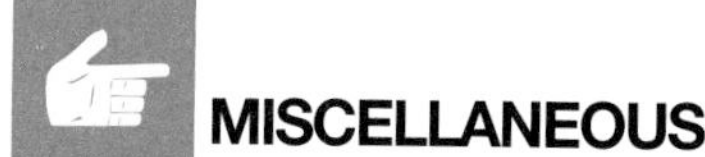

MISCELLANEOUS

ASSOCIATED CONDITIONS N/A

AGE-RELATED FACTORS

Pediatric: N/A
Geriatric: N/A
Others: N/A

PREGNANCY Unpredictable symptom improvement or exacerbation during pregnancy. No known fetal effects from interstitial cystitis. Usual problems of unknown effect on fetus with medications taken during pregnancy.

SYNONYMS

- Urgency frequency syndrome
- Painful bladder syndrome

ICD-9-CM

595.1 Chronic interstitial cystitis

SEE ALSO

Urinary tract infection in females

OTHER NOTES N/A

ABBREVIATIONS

IC = interstitial cystitis
DMSO = dimethyl sulfoxide

REFERENCES

- McGuire, E. J. Urgency Frequency Syndromes, at Voiding Dysfunction and Pelvic Reconstruction, 1996.

Web references: 0 available at www.5mcc.com
Illustrations N/A

Author(s):

Ira N. Hollander, MD

BASICS

DESCRIPTION Intestinal obstruction exists where there is a failure, reversal or impairment of the normal transit of intestinal contents. Obstructions may be partial or complete and are manifested by abdominal pain, emesis and obstipation.
System(s) affected: Gastrointestinal
Genetics: Unknown
Incidence/Prevalence in USA: Accounts, for approximately 20% of all admissions for acute abdominal conditions
Predominant age: N/A
Predominant sex: Male = Female

SIGNS & SYMPTOMS
- Abdominal pain - diffuse, poorly localized abdominal cramping at intervals of 5 to 15 minutes
- Emesis - usually occurs immediately after obstruction of bowel. More frequent in proximal obstruction. Unusual in colon obstruction until small bowel distention occurs.
- Obstipation - common symptom. May pass contents distal to obstruction especially in high intestinal obstruction. Pain followed by explosive diarrhea often seen in partial obstruction.
- Inspection - with or without distention (a late finding), less likely in proximal obstructions
- Auscultation - high pitched bowel sounds, peristaltic rushes
- Palpation - tenderness, mass, presence of peritoneal signs (these suggest strangulation)
- Rectal examination - may reveal fecal impaction. Occult blood may suggest colon malignancy.

CAUSES
- Luminal lesions
  - ◊ Impactions
  - ◊ Gallstones
  - ◊ Meconium in newborns
  - ◊ Intussusception in infants
- Intrinsic lesions
  - ◊ Congenital (e.g., atresia and stenosis, imperforate anus, duplications, Meckel diverticulum)
  - ◊ Trauma
  - ◊ Inflammatory (e.g., Crohn disease, diverticulitis, ulcerative colitis, radiation, toxic [ingestions]
  - ◊ Neoplastic (most common etiology of colon obstruction)
  - ◊ Miscellaneous (e.g., endometriosis)
- Extrinsic lesions
  - ◊ Adhesions (most common etiology of small bowel obstruction)
  - ◊ Hernia and wound dehiscence
  - ◊ Masses (e.g., annular pancreas, anomalous vasculature, abscess and hematoma, neoplasms)
  - ◊ Volvulus
  - ◊ Neuromuscular defect (e.g., megacolon, neuro/myopathic motility disorders)

RISK FACTORS
- Previous abdominal and/or pelvic surgery
- Hernia
- Chronic constipation
- Cholelithiasis
- Inflammatory bowel disease
- Ingested foreign bodies - pica, enteric potassium tablets, etc.
- Diverticular disease

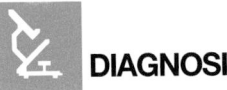

DIAGNOSIS

DIFFERENTIAL DIAGNOSIS Adynamic ileus

LABORATORY
- WBC: Slight rise (15,000/mm3). Significant increases associated with strangulation.
- Hematocrit: Moderate rise associated with extracellular fluid loss
- Renal: Urine specific gravity 1.025-1.030 and rise in BUN and creatinine due to extracellular volume loss
- Amylase: May be elevated. Unreliable as an indicator of obstruction or strangulation.
- Blood gases: May be normal. Late changes are those of acidosis.
- No single or series of laboratory studies are useful in diagnosis of intestinal strangulation

Drugs that may alter lab results: N/A

Disorders that may alter lab results: N/A

PATHOLOGICAL FINDINGS
- Edema of mucosa
- Hypersecretion
- Necrosis

SPECIAL TESTS N/A

IMAGING
- Abdominal and chest radiographs
  - ◊ Distention of small bowel or colon
  - ◊ Air-fluid levels (may be seen in ileus, gastroenteritis, constipation)
  - ◊ Lack of colon gas
  - ◊ Free intraperitoneal air (strangulation with perforation)
  - ◊ "Bird beak" lesion in colonic volvulus
  - ◊ Foreign body visualization
- Contrast studies
  - ◊ Barium enema useful for diagnosis of colonic obstruction and may be therapeutic in intussusception
  - ◊ Barium or Gastrografin orally may differentiate obstruction from ileus
  - ◊ Enteroclysis may identify site of small bowel obstruction

DIAGNOSTIC PROCEDURES
- Rigid proctoscopy. May be therapeutic in sigmoid volvulus.
- Flexible sigmoidoscopy

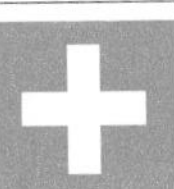

TREATMENT

APPROPRIATE HEALTH CARE
- Inpatient
- Treatment directed at early gastrointestinal decompression, correction of fluid and electrolyte abnormalities, timely operative intervention, surgical/GI consultation required

GENERAL MEASURES
- Nasogastric suction
- Foley catheter
- Swan-Ganz catheter or other central monitor, if required
- Intravenous fluids: Normal saline/Ringer's solution with potassium supplementation as required
- Antibiotic use controversial in absence of sepsis, but prophylactic antibiotics probably appropriate

SURGICAL MEASURES
- Timing of operative intervention critical, must correct electrolytes, volume quickly prior to surgery
- Surgical procedures:
  - ◊ Closed bowel procedures: lysis of adhesions, reduction of intussusception, reduction of volvulus, reduction of incarcerated hernia
  - ◊ Enterotomy for removal of bezoars, foreign bodies, gallstones
  - ◊ Resection of bowel for obstructing lesions, strangulated bowel
  - ◊ Bypasses of intestine around obstruction
  - ◊ Enterocutaneous fistulae proximal to obstruction: colostomy, cecostomy

ACTIVITY Bedrest

DIET NPO

PATIENT EDUCATION N/A

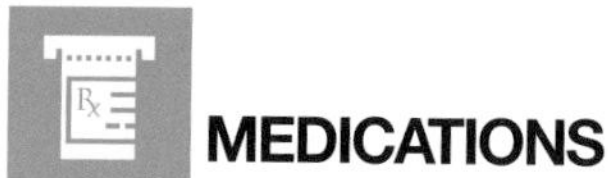

MEDICATIONS

DRUG(S) OF CHOICE Surgeon's choice for prophylaxis
Contraindications: N/A
Precautions: N/A
Significant possible interactions: N/A

ALTERNATIVE DRUGS N/A

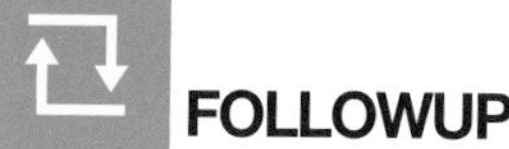

FOLLOWUP

PATIENT MONITORING Follow weekly postoperatively for 2-8 weeks

PREVENTION/AVOIDANCE N/A

POSSIBLE COMPLICATIONS
- Slow return of bowel function
- Higher risk of subsequent obstruction
- Sepsis

EXPECTED COURSE/PROGNOSIS
Usually excellent prognosis. In general, mortality from intestinal obstruction ranges from < 1% to > 20% depending upon etiology, bowel viability, co-morbidities, etc.

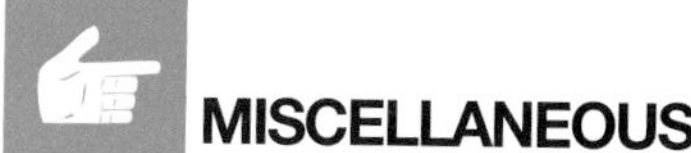

MISCELLANEOUS

ASSOCIATED CONDITIONS N/A

AGE-RELATED FACTORS
Pediatric:
- Different etiologies of obstruction in childhood
  - ◊ Duodenal malformations
  - ◊ Jejunoileal atresia
  - ◊ Malrotation and midgut volvulus
  - ◊ Meconium ileus
  - ◊ Necrotizing enterocolitis
  - ◊ Hirschsprung disease
  - ◊ Intussusception
  - ◊ Duplications
  - ◊ Meckel diverticulum
  - ◊ Imperforate anus

Geriatric:
- Colon neoplasms more common
- Chronic constipation/impactions more common

Others: N/A

PREGNANCY N/A

SYNONYMS N/A

ICD-9-CM
560.0 Intussusception
560.30 Impaction of intestine, unspecified
560.9 Unspecified intestinal obstruction

SEE ALSO

OTHER NOTES Rectal examination showing occult blood may represent colon malignancy as etiology of the obstruction

ABBREVIATIONS N/A

REFERENCES

- Sleisenger MH, Fordtran JS, eds. Gastrointestinal and Liver Disease: Pathophysiology, Diagnosis, Management. 6th Ed. Philadelphia, W.B. Saunders Co., 1998

Web references: 0 available at www.5mcc.com
Illustrations N/A

Author(s):
Abdulrazak Abyad, MD, MPH

Expanded Topics

BASICS

DESCRIPTION

- The class of infectious agents called parasites is divided into two parts:
  - ◊ Protozoa are single cell animals which characteristically divide and multiply within the host, are usually direct fecal-oral in transmission, and do not cause an eosinophilia
  - ◊ Helminths (worms) are multi-cellular animals and with rare exceptions (i.e., *Strongyloides stercoralis*, *Hymenolepis nana*) do not multiply within the host and are often associated with some degree of eosinophilia. The level of eosinophilia is associated with the degree of mucosal invasiveness. The worms have a limited life span within the host and without reinfection would eventually die on their own.
- Not all of the parasites that start out by ingestion in the bowel will remain in the bowel. Some are invasive and some do not release their infective forms into the bowel. This later group, including *Toxoplasma gondii*, *Echinococcus*, *Trichinella spiralis* will not be covered in this topic.
- Most worms require either a prolonged incubation period outside the host before being infectious or need a specific vector for transmission. A notable exception to this rule is *Enterobius vermicularis* (pinworm), the eggs of which are infectious shortly after being passed, so auto-infection occurs readily.
- Direct person-to-person transmission of worms is uncommon
- The likelihood of acquiring an intestinal parasite depends on several factors - the presence of the specific infectious agent, an appropriate "vector" or mode of transmission, and a host who is susceptible to the infectious agent. The world-wide distribution of parasites is determined by geographic factors, socioeconomic factors, age, and crowding with poor food preparation and a break in the standard of water and personal sanitation being the major factors.

System(s) affected: Gastrointestinal

Genetics: Genetic factors play a minor role in the acquisition, pathogenesis and clearance of these infections

Incidence/Prevalence in USA:

- From laboratory statistics: 5-30% general population
- From day care surveys: Asymptomatic 20-30%; symptomatic 50-80%
- Intestinal protozoa account for the majority of parasitological findings in North America (most considered to be non-pathogenic)
- In a random sampling, at least one parasite would be found in the stools of 5-10% of all people. If *Blastocystis hominis* were included in this accounting, 20-30% of specimens examined in parasitology will be positive.
- Helminths are considerably rarer and are highly dependent on population demographics and prior geographic exposure risk factors. In general, less than 10% of all parasitology reports include a helminth.

Predominant age: Pediatric
Predominant sex: Male = Female

SIGNS & SYMPTOMS

- Diarrhea
- Abdominal pain/tenderness
- Excessive gas - bloating, eructation, flatulence, borborygmi
- Nausea or vomiting
- Weight loss and anorexia
- Dysentery, i.e., bleeding (rare, but associated with *Entamoeba histolytica*, *Balantidium coli*)
- Pruritus ani (*E. vermicularis*, *Trichuris trichiura*, *S. stercoralis*, tapeworms)
- Passing a worm or a worm segment
- Increased bowel sounds
- Perirectal or vulvar rash

CAUSES

- Protozoan pathogens:
  - ◊ *Giardia lamblia*
  - ◊ *Entamoeba histolytica*
  - ◊ *Cryptosporidium*
  - ◊ *Isospora belli*
  - ◊ *Balantidium coli*
  - ◊ *Cyclospora cayetanensis*
  - ◊ *Microsporida*
- Possible protozoan pathogens:
  - ◊ *Dientamoeba fragilis*
- Probable non-pathogenic protozoa
  - ◊ All other Entamoeba species
  - ◊ *Endolimax nana*
  - ◊ All other intestinal flagellates
- Helminthic pathogens - nematodes (roundworms):
  - ◊ *Enterobius vermicularis*
  - ◊ *Trichuris trichiura*
  - ◊ *Ascaris lumbricoides*
  - ◊ Hookworm (*Necator americanus*, *Ancylostoma duodenale*)
  - ◊ *Strongyloides stercoralis*
  - ◊ *Capillaria philippinensis*
  - ◊ *Trichostrongylus spp*
- Helminthic pathogens - trematodes (flukes)
  - ◊ *Fasciolopsis buski*
  - ◊ *Clonorchis sinensis*
  - ◊ *Opisthorchis viverrini*
  - ◊ *Heterophyes heterophyes*
  - ◊ *Fasciola hepatica*
  - ◊ *Paragonimus westermani*
  - ◊ *Schistosoma mansoni*
  - ◊ *S. japonicum*
  - ◊ *S. hematobium*
  - ◊ *S. mekongi*
- Helminthic pathogens - cestodes (tapeworms)
  - ◊ *Taenia saginata*
  - ◊ *Taenia solium*
  - ◊ *Diphyllobothrium latum*
  - ◊ *Hymenolepis nana*
  - ◊ *Hymenolepis diminuta*
  - ◊ *Dipylidium caninum*

RISK FACTORS

- Age (children)
- Low socioeconomic status
- Poor sanitation - personal, food, water
- International travel
- Crowding - day care centers, institutional care
- Intercurrent medical conditions, pregnancy, gastric hypoacidity, immunosuppression (AIDS)

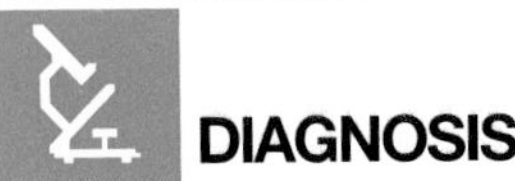

DIAGNOSIS

DIFFERENTIAL DIAGNOSIS

- Other intestinal infections
- Food poisoning
- Malabsorption
- Inflammatory bowel disease
- Hemorrhoids
- Rectal fissures

LABORATORY

- Examination of a single stool specimen collected into a preservative (i.e., sodium acetate formalin [SAF]), well mixed to fix and preserve all elements, will provide an accurate diagnosis in 90% of patients. Additional specimens will need to be examined for greater diagnostic accuracy.
- Newer techniques of lab exam of stool specimens (such as monoclonal antibodies, other antigen detection techniques, DNA detection) are exciting developments but currently provide little advantage over routine techniques and represent additional costs. These techniques are needed to differentiate E. histolytica from E. dispar
- Serology - for specific infections, especially if they do not produce a patent infection in the bowel (i.e., no eggs or parasites released into the stool), or if low numbers of parasites. May be indicated rarely, but are usually available only through referral centers.

Drugs that may alter lab results: Use of antibiotics, oil based laxatives, and the presence of barium in the stool may make a parasitological diagnosis difficult or impossible

Disorders that may alter lab results: N/A

PATHOLOGICAL FINDINGS

- Majority of intestinal parasites are not invasive and produce no or non-specific changes in the histology of the bowel
- Invasive amebiasis of the bowel produces a classical endoscopic and histological picture of ulceration and inflammation in the colon
- Protozoa and helminths may be seen in bowel biopsies

SPECIAL TESTS

- Special techniques for the detection of *Cryptosporidium*, *Isospora belli*, *Cyclospora*, and *microsporidia* often require that the laboratory be informed of the "risk" profile of the patient before these tests will be done
- Pinworm paddles provide a greater diagnostic yield when *Enterobius vermicularis* is being considered. Multiple tests (5) may be needed to exclude the diagnosis of pinworms.
- Parasite culture is possible for a few organisms - *Giardia lamblia*, *Entamoeba histolytica*, *Strongyloides stercoralis*, but are rarely indicated and are usually available only in referral laboratories
- String tests and upper bowel intubations are rarely needed to diagnose the upper intestinal parasites

- Rarely, a biopsy will demonstrate the presence of an invasive helminth on tissue section. Worms can be extremely difficult to diagnose in this manner, usually needing the expertise of a tissue parasite pathologist. The other parasites may be visualized on the mucosa or in the mucous layer.

IMAGING Diagnostic radiology is rarely needed. Exception is for invasive infections such as amebiasis where colitis, amebomas and liver abscesses may be demonstrated by the appropriate techniques.

DIAGNOSTIC PROCEDURES

- Invasive diagnostic procedures are rarely needed or indicated
- With hemorrhagic colitis and a possible diagnosis of invasive amebiasis, sigmoidoscopy will reveal a mucopurulent colitis with ulceration. A scraping from an ulcer, promptly examined by microscopy, will reveal the motile hematophagous trophozoites of *E. histolytica*.
- Upper intestinal endoscopy can yield fluid to be examined for *Giardia lamblia* and *Strongyloides stercoralis*. Impression smears and biopsies obtained with the endoscope can also be examined.

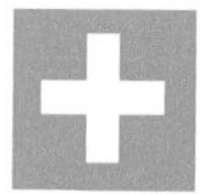

TREATMENT

APPROPRIATE HEALTH CARE Outpatient except for rare surgery or inpatient medical treatment

GENERAL MEASURES

- Therapy must be assessed in the best interest of the patient. Not all patients need to be treated with drugs.
- Symptomatic treatment is indicated for patient comfort once specific therapy has been initiated
- Bowel paralyzing drugs, for diarrhea caused by invasive organisms, are relatively contraindicated

SURGICAL MEASURES

- Surgical procedures play little role in treatment except when amebic liver abscesses need to be drained, e.g., multiple or large abscesses not responding to medical management, or threatened rupture, especially left lobe abscesses. Drainage of such abscesses is often accomplished by directed catheter placement in radiology, with surgical back-up as required.
- Surgery may be required if bowel or other organ obstruction occurs, as can be seen with Ascaris lumbricoides migration

ACTIVITY As tolerated

DIET

- Nutritional support may be required
- Many patients during and following bowel infections, especially when infected with Giardia lamblia, will experience irritable bowel syndrome and/or lactose intolerance. The majority of these patients will respond to a lactose free diet, reduction of caffeine intake, and an increase in dietary fiber.

PATIENT EDUCATION

- Educating the patient is important to reduce the risk of reinfection or transmission
- Education will depend on the parasite, host characteristics and the environment that the two interact in

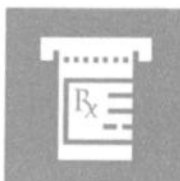

MEDICATIONS

DRUG(S) OF CHOICE

- Protozoa
  - ◊ *Entamoeba histolytica* asymptomatic needs individual assessment
  - ◊ *Entamoeba histolytica* symptomatic intestinal - iodoquinol or diloxanide furoate
  - ◊ *Entamoeba histolytica* invasive disease - iodoquinol or diloxanide furoate. Plus metronidazole, alone or dehydroemetine or emetine plus chloroquine phosphate.
  - ◊ *Giardia lamblia* - metronidazole or tinidazole or furazolidone or quinacrine. Note: albendazole, available in US only from manufacturer, may have activity against *G. lamblia*.
  - ◊ *Cryptosporidium*: none proven effective
  - ◊ *Isospora belli* protozoa: trimethoprim-sulfamethoxazole
  - ◊ *Balantidium coli*: tetracycline or iodoquinol or metronidazole
  - ◊ *Cyclospora*: sulfamethoxazole-trimethoprim
  - ◊ *Microsporidia*: albendazole (some species)
- Helminths
  - ◊ Nematodes (except *Strongyloides* and *Trichostrongylus*): mebendazole or pyrantel pamoate or piperazine citrate or albendazole (available in US only from manufacturer)
  - ◊ *Strongyloides* and *Trichostrongylus*: thiabendazole or albendazole (available in US only from manufacturer)
  - ◊ Cestodes: praziquantel or niclosamide
  - ◊ Trematodes: niclosamide or praziquantel

Contraindications: Refer to manufacturer's profile of each drug

Precautions: Refer to manufacturer's profile of each drug

Significant possible interactions: Refer to manufacturer's profile of each drug

ALTERNATIVE DRUGS N/A

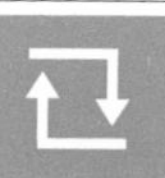

FOLLOWUP

PATIENT MONITORING Repeat examination, to ensure clearance, should be timed taking into account: The life cycle of the parasite (how long would it take to regenerate and become patent) and the risk of reinfection, as well as the specific test likely to find the parasite (stool, pinworm paddle, culture, serology)

PREVENTION/AVOIDANCE The specific nature of the infection often dictates the specific methods needed to avoid reinfection. This usually involves matters of personal, food and/or water sanitation.

POSSIBLE COMPLICATIONS Chronic persistent diarrhea

EXPECTED COURSE/PROGNOSIS See specific text on individual parasite

MISCELLANEOUS

ASSOCIATED CONDITIONS N/A

AGE-RELATED FACTORS

Pediatric: Most common age group affected
Geriatric: Illness may cause more severe debilitation
Others: AIDS - susceptibility to infection, severity of disease

PREGNANCY Some of these infections can be particularly serious in pregnancy. Many of the drugs are contraindicated in pregnancy.

SYNONYMS N/A

ICD-9-CM

129 Intestinal parasitism, unspecified

SEE ALSO

OTHER NOTES N/A

ABBREVIATIONS N/A

REFERENCES

- DuPont HL. Persistent diarrhea in travelers. Clin Infect Dis 1996;22:124-8
- Abramowicz M, editor. Drugs for parasitic infections. In: The Medical Letter. New York, The Medical Letter Inc. 2002;Apr:1-12
- Mandell GL, editor. Principles and Practice of Infectious Diseases. 5th Ed. New York, Churchill Livingstone, 2000

Web references: 3 available at www.5mcc.com
Illustrations N/A

Author(s):
D. W. MacPherson, MD

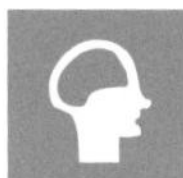

BASICS

DESCRIPTION Invagination of a portion of intestine into itself (may involve any part of small intestine, ileocolic [95%], or colocolic)
System(s) affected: Gastrointestinal
Genetics: N/A
Incidence/Prevalence in USA: 1.5-4/1000 live births
Predominant age: 5-10 months (65% are less than one year of age)
Predominant sex: Male > Female (3:2) - male preponderance is more notable in older infants

SIGNS & SYMPTOMS
- Vomiting (80-100%)
- Blood per rectum - currant-jelly stools (65%-95%) highest percent in infants
- Intermittent, colicky abdominal pain (almost all children)
- Lethargy (22%) (more pronounced with longer duration of illness)
- Palpable mass (16-41%)
- Diarrhea (7%)
- Prolapse of intussusception through anus (3%)
- Fever
- Extreme pallor in some

CAUSES
- Children
  - ◊ Marked hypertrophy of Peyer's patches (92-98%)
  - ◊ Lead point in 2%-8% (polyp, Meckel diverticulum, duplication cyst, ectopic pancreas, lymphoma, Henoch-Schönlein purpura, lipoma, carcinoma)
  - ◊ Allergic reactions, diet changes, changes in intestinal activity may be other causes
  - ◊ Possible adenovirus or rotavirus infection
- Adults
  - ◊ Virtually always associated with lead point

RISK FACTORS
- Henoch-Schönlein purpura
- Leukemia
- Lymphoma
- Cystic fibrosis
- Recent upper respiratory infection (21%)
- Recent operation (1-24 days previously)
- Recent viral gastrointestinal illness

DIAGNOSIS

DIFFERENTIAL DIAGNOSIS
- Adhesive band small bowel obstruction
- Appendicitis
- Gastroenteritis

LABORATORY
- Electrolytes
- CBC
- Urinalysis
- Stool guaiac

Drugs that may alter lab results: N/A

Disorders that may alter lab results: N/A

PATHOLOGICAL FINDINGS
- Hyperplasia of Peyer's lymphatic patches of terminal ileum (92%) with or without mesenteric lymphadenopathy
- Recognizable lead point (see list in Causes) (2-8%)

SPECIAL TESTS N/A

IMAGING
- Ultrasound
- Plain film - flat and upright abdominal films may suggest the diagnosis

DIAGNOSTIC PROCEDURES
- Contrast enema (barium, water soluble contrast or air)
- Abdominal ultrasound

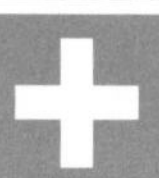

TREATMENT

APPROPRIATE HEALTH CARE Inpatient until resolved

GENERAL MEASURES
- IV fluid resuscitation
- Foley catheter (if child severely dehydrated)
- Nasogastric tube
- Antibiotics useful only if necrotic bowel present
- Non-operative care:
  - ◊ Hydrostatic/pneumatic reduction of intussusception (50-80% success)
  - ◊ Barium column should be 40-42 inches high
  - ◊ Enema continued as long as progress is made. Bowel may be drained and the enema repeated.
  - ◊ Pneumatic reduction pressure should not exceed 120-140 mm Hg (16-18.6 kPa)

SURGICAL MEASURES
- Right lower quadrant incision
- Gentle manipulation by pushing intussusception (not pulling)
- If unable to reduce or non-viable bowel, segmental resection with re-anastomosis
- Enterotomy if lead point suspected
- Incidental appendectomy commonly done

ACTIVITY As tolerated after reduction

DIET Liquids started after abdominal distension resolves and bowel function returns

PATIENT EDUCATION
- Instruct family on possibility of recurrence (5-13%)
- Most recurrences occur in first 24 hours postreduction

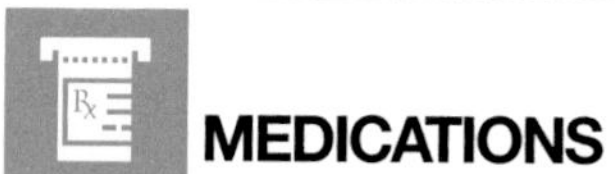

MEDICATIONS

DRUG(S) OF CHOICE N/A
Contraindications: N/A
Precautions: N/A
Significant possible interactions: N/A

ALTERNATIVE DRUGS N/A

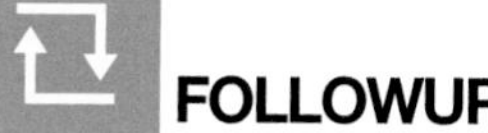

FOLLOWUP

PATIENT MONITORING Office visit one week after discharge

PREVENTION/AVOIDANCE N/A

POSSIBLE COMPLICATIONS
- Bowel perforation during attempted reduction
- Prolonged ileus
- Adhesions with intestinal obstruction
- Incisional hernia
- Ischemic intestine requiring second operation
- Electrolyte abnormality
- Anemia
- Pleural effusion
- Sepsis
- Recurrence

EXPECTED COURSE/PROGNOSIS
- Mortality should not exceed 1-2%
- Possible recurrence (5-13%) after hydrostatic reduction
- Possible recurrence (3%) after operative reduction

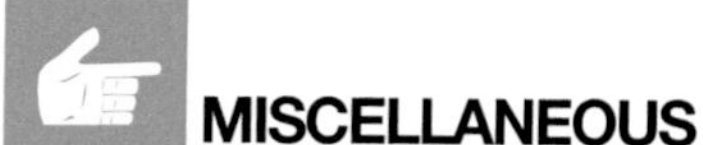

MISCELLANEOUS

ASSOCIATED CONDITIONS
- Henoch-Schönlein purpura
- Cystic fibrosis

AGE-RELATED FACTORS
Pediatric:
- Usually no lead point
- Postoperative intussusception (1-24 days postoperatively) is virtually always in small bowel and only rarely can be reduced hydrostatically

Geriatric: 90% have lead point
Others: N/A

PREGNANCY N/A

SYNONYMS N/A

ICD-9-CM
560.0 Intussusception

SEE ALSO
Cystic fibrosis
Henoch-Schönlein purpura
Intestinal obstruction

OTHER NOTES N/A

ABBREVIATIONS N/A

REFERENCES

- Pang C. Intussusception revisited: Clinicopathologic analysis of 261 cases, with emphasis on pathogenesis. Southern Medical J 1989;82(2):215-228
- Skipper RP, Boeckman R, Klein R. Childhood intussusception. Surg Gynecol Obstet 1990;171(2):151-3
- O'Neill JA, Rowe MI, Grosfeld JL, et al. Pediatric Surgery. 5th ed. St Louis: Mosby; 1998
- West KW, Stephens B, Rescorla FJ, et al. Postoperative intussusception: Experience with 36 cases in children. Surgery 1988;104:781-787

Web references: 1 available at www.5mcc.com
Illustrations N/A

Author(s):
Timothy L. Black, MD
James P. Miller, MD

BASICS

DESCRIPTION Anemia due to decreased iron stores. Poor iron utilization and poor iron re-utilization (e.g., anemia of chronic disease) are also due to iron deficiency, but iron stores are not depleted. Onset may be acute with rapid blood loss, or chronic with poor diet or slow blood loss. This is the most common cause of anemia in the U.S.
System(s) affected: Hemic/Lymphatic/Immunologic
Genetics: No known genetic pattern
Incidence/Prevalence in USA: Affects 7-10% of the adult population, 10-20% of the infants and toddlers, and 15-45% of pregnant patients. Most likely in the poor and in children who are under-immunized.
Predominant age: All ages but especially toddlers and menstruating women
Predominant sex: Female > Male

SIGNS & SYMPTOMS
- Asymptomatic in most cases
- Cheilosis
- Dyspnea on exertion, fatigue, tachycardia, palpitation, vasomotor disturbances
- Effects of underlying GI ulceration, neoplasm, uterine disorders or bleeding varices
- Headache, inability to concentrate, irritability, listlessness
- Neuralgic pain, peripheral paresthesias
- Pica (dirt, paint, ice)
- Spoon-shaped, brittle nails
- Susceptibility to infection

CAUSES
- Blood loss (e.g., menses, GI bleed)
- Poor iron intake
- Poor iron absorption (e.g., postgastrectomy)
- Increased demand for iron (e.g., infancy, adolescence, pregnancy)
- Hookworm infestation
- Gastric carcinoma

RISK FACTORS See Causes

DIAGNOSIS

DIFFERENTIAL DIAGNOSIS
- Defective iron utilization (e.g., thalassemia trait, sideroblastosis, G6PD deficiency)
- Defective iron re-utilization (e.g., infection, inflammation, cancer, other chronic diseases)
- Hypoproliferation (e.g., decreased erythropoietin from hypothyroidism, renal failure, etc.)

LABORATORY
- Stainable iron in bone marrow aspiration is the gold standard
- Low serum ferritin is best non-invasive test in adults, but may miss some deficient patients since ferritin is an acute phase reactant. Fe/TIBC (transferrin ratio) is no longer recommended since it is less sensitive and less specific than ferritin.
- Peripheral smear usually shows hypochromia and microcytosis, but may be normal
- Hemoglobin is usually lower than 12 g/dL, but patients with higher premorbid hemoglobin (such as smokers and patients with chronic hypoxemia) may be anemic at higher Hgb levels. Abnormal values for infants and toddlers, and for pregnant persons, are less than 10.5-11.0 g/dL.
- Low RBC count helps to distinguish thalassemia trait where count is high or high-normal
- Microcytosis with ovalocytosis and anemia unresponsive to iron suggest thalassemia trait
- Low MCV may be absent in mild anemia, or hidden by population of larger cells (e.g., reticulocytes or macrocytes)
- An empiric trial of iron at 3 mg/kg/day may be the best way to diagnose decreased iron stores in infants and children, if reticulocytes elevated in 7-10 days, or Hgb increased > 1.0 g/dL after 4 weeks

Drugs that may alter lab results: Iron supplements or multivitamin-mineral preparations that contain iron

Disorders that may alter lab results:
- Ferritin elevated by acute liver disease, cirrhosis, Hodgkin disease, acute leukemia, solid tumors, fever, acute inflammation, renal dialysis
- Hemoglobin may be elevated by smoking or chronic hypoxemia, thereby hiding anemia if standard anemia limits are used

PATHOLOGICAL FINDINGS
- Absent marrow iron stores
- Marrow - hyperplastic, micronormoblastic

SPECIAL TESTS
- Cause of iron loss - stool guaiac testing, GI endoscopy, stool for O & P, clotting studies
- Rule-out thalassemia - review prior CBC's for persisting mild anemia and marked micro-ovalocytosis, elevated Hgb A2 or Hgb F, family history, and especially high or high normal RBC count
- Rule-out G6PD deficiency - assay at least 6 weeks after last drop in Hgb
- Rule-out poor re-utilization - trial of iron (oral or parenteral), bone marrow aspiration and iron stain
- Rule-out gastric carcinoma, especially in the elderly

IMAGING GI endoscopy to discover occult bleeding sites

DIAGNOSTIC PROCEDURES
- Bone marrow aspiration
- Sigmoidoscopy
- Gastroscopy
- Colonoscopy

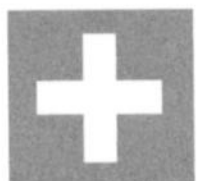

TREATMENT

APPROPRIATE HEALTH CARE Outpatient

GENERAL MEASURES
- Search for cause and correct it. There can be no excuse for not searching for a bleeding site.
- Avoid transfusions except in rare instances

SURGICAL MEASURES N/A

ACTIVITY Patients with hypoxemia, low cardiac output or angina may require reduced activity prescriptions

DIET
- Limit milk to 1 pint a day (adults)
- Emphasize protein- and iron-containing foods (meat, beans, leafy green vegetables)
- Increase dietary fiber to decrease likelihood of constipation during iron replacement therapy
- No milk, other dairy product, antacid, or tetracycline within two hours of drug dosage

PATIENT EDUCATION For patient education materials contact: National Heart, Lung & Blood Institute, Communications & Public Information Branch, National Institutes of Health, Building 31, Room 41-21, 9000 Rockville Pike, Bethesda, MD 20892, (301)251-1222

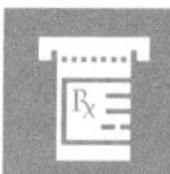

MEDICATIONS

DRUG(S) OF CHOICE

- Ferrous sulfate 300 mg tid on an empty stomach one hour before meals is an ideal dose that provides 180 mg of elemental iron a day. Dose can be reduced as needed for GI symptoms, which affect 15% of patients on standard iron therapy. Or the dose can be taken with meals, which may reduce the delivery of iron by 50%. People with a moderate anemia (Hgb = 10 g/dL) need only 1500-2000 mg of elemental iron replacement. Reducing the amount of iron per dose as much as necessary to abate symptoms will make parenteral iron therapy unnecessary in almost all cases. Special iron formulations and compounds are very expensive and reduce symptoms only to the degree that they reduce delivery of iron.
- Liquid iron preparations are useful for children with a recommended dose of 3 mg/kg/day given in a single dose.
- Consider parenteral iron for patients with malabsorption if higher doses and use of vitamin C fail

Contraindications:

- Antacids concomitantly
- Tetracycline concomitantly

Precautions:

- Iron preparations cause black bowel movements
- Iron overdose is highly toxic. Patients should be instructed to keep tablets and liquids out of the reach of small children.

Significant possible interactions:

- Allopurinol
- Antacids
- Penicillamine
- Tetracyclines
- Vitamin E

ALTERNATIVE DRUGS N/A

FOLLOWUP

PATIENT MONITORING Regularly after return to normal (in order to detect recurrences)

PREVENTION/AVOIDANCE

- Good nutrition with adequate iron intake
- Correction of gynecologic or other problems causing excess blood loss

POSSIBLE COMPLICATIONS Neglecting to identify hidden bleeding points, particularly a bleeding malignancy

EXPECTED COURSE/PROGNOSIS

Curable with iron therapy if the underlying cause can be discovered and cured

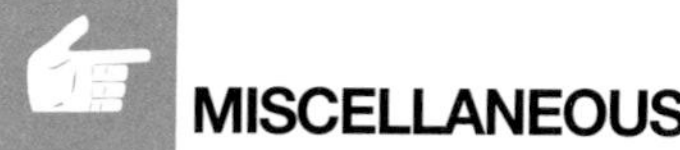

MISCELLANEOUS

ASSOCIATED CONDITIONS N/A

AGE-RELATED FACTORS

Pediatric: Frequent problem in infants whose major source of nutrition is cow's milk and juices
Geriatric: Accounts for 60% of anemias in people over 65
Others: N/A

PREGNANCY Common during pregnancy unless iron supplements are included in the diet

SYNONYMS

- Anemia of chronic blood loss
- Hypochromic, microcytic anemia
- Chlorosis

ICD-9-CM

280.9 Iron deficiency anemia, unspecified

SEE ALSO

OTHER NOTES N/A

ABBREVIATIONS N/A

Hgb = hemoglobin
TIBC = total iron binding capacity

REFERENCES

- Lee RG, Bithell TC, et al. Wintrobe's Clinical Hematology. 9th Ed. Philadelphia, Lea & Febiger, 1993
- Williams WJ, Beutler E, Erslev AJ, et al, eds. Hematology. 4th Ed. New York, McGraw-Hill, 1990
- Van den Broek et al. Iron status in pregnant women: which measurements are valid? Brit J Haem 1998;103(3):817-824
- Farrell R, LaMont JT. Rational approach to iron-deficiency anaemia in premenopausal women. Lancet 1998;352(9145):1953-1954
- Adams WG, et al.Anemia and elevated lead levels in underimmunized inner-city children. Pediatrics 1998;101(3)
- Fireman Z, Kopelman Y, Sternberg A. Endoscopic evaluation of iron deficiency anemia and follow-up in patients older than age 50. J Clin Gastroent 1998;26(1):7- 10
- Waterbury L. Anemia. In Barker LR, Burton JR, Zieve PD. (ed): Principles of Ambulatory Medicine 4th ed. Philadelphia, Lippincott Williams & Wilkins, 1995:593-607

Web references: 0 available at www.5mcc.com
Illustrations N/A

Author(s):
Bruce Block, MD

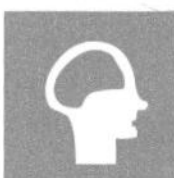

BASICS

DESCRIPTION Acute iron overload due to accidental or intentional ingestion. Accidental ingestion is not uncommon since iron-containing compounds are readily available, brightly colored, and are often sugar coated. Acute symptoms are characterized by vomiting, diarrhea, mild lethargy, upper abdominal pain, pallor, and hyperglycemia with more severe clinical findings including cyanosis, stupor, acidosis, hematemesis, shock, and coma.

System(s) affected: Cardiovascular, Gastrointestinal, Hemic/Lymphatic/Immunologic

Genetics: N/A

Incidence/Prevalence in USA: 3699 cases reported in 1988 along with 15,977 cases of intoxication with iron-fortified vitamins; leading cause of poisoning mortality of children in the US

Predominant age:
- Children most frequently involved (in 1984, 1337 out 1738 iron poisoning cases were reported in children < 6 years of age)
- From 1988-92, approximately 17% of children's deaths reported to poison control centers in the U.S. were iron poisonings

Predominant sex: N/A

SIGNS & SYMPTOMS
- 0.5 to 2 hours - vomiting, hematemesis, abdominal pain, diarrhea, lethargy, shock, acidosis, and coagulopathy
- Apparent recovery may contribute to a false sense of security after initial ingestion, observe patient closely
- 2 to 12 hours - profound shock, severe acidosis, cyanosis and fever
- 12 to 48 hours - symptoms may recur and can include pulmonary edema, shock, acidosis, convulsions, anuria, hyperthermia, and death
- 2 to 6 weeks - if patient survives, pyloric or antral stenosis, hepatic cirrhosis and CNS damage can be seen

The phases listed above do not occur in all patients. For example, in massive overdose, patients may present in shock.

CAUSES
- Excessive iron ingestion - the average human lethal dose is 200 to 250 mg of elemental iron per kg of body weight (equivalent to about 230 ferrous sulfate based on 60 mg of elemental iron per tablet)
- Toxicity is likely following 60 mg/kg of elemental iron ingestion

RISK FACTORS Access to iron products by children resulting in accidental ingestion

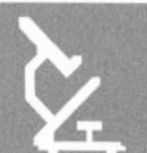

DIAGNOSIS

DIFFERENTIAL DIAGNOSIS
If unknown iron ingestion
- Gastritis
- Small bowel obstruction
- Drug intolerance/overdose
- Alcohol toxicity
- Viral illness
- Diabetic ketoacidosis
- Metabolic acidosis

LABORATORY
- CBC
- Electrolytes and glucose
- Serum iron; total iron binding capacity (TIBC) (may not be available in some hospitals)
- PT/INR (prothrombin time /International Normalized Ratio) and activated partial thromboplastin time (APTT)
- Serum bicarbonate
- Liver function tests in severe overdose

Drugs that may alter lab results: Deferoxamine can falsely lower serum iron unless a reducing agent is added to the specimen. Should obtain a free iron concentration.

Disorders that may alter lab results: TIBC rises factitiously in the presence of high iron levels

PATHOLOGICAL FINDINGS
- None (by definition)

SPECIAL TESTS N/A

IMAGING Abdominal and chest x-ray

DIAGNOSTIC PROCEDURES Abdominal x-ray to evaluate for tablets in the gut

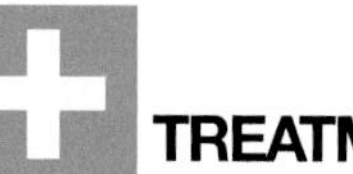

TREATMENT

APPROPRIATE HEALTH CARE
- Emergency room for acute ingestion
- Inpatient for severe ingestion
- Supportive treatment

GENERAL MEASURES
- Maintain proper airway, respiration and circulation
- Assess the amount of iron ingested
- Removal of iron from the gastrointestinal tract
- Hemodialysis, peritoneal dialysis, and exchange transfusion have also be used in lethal overdoses
- Maintain electrolyte balance, treat shock, hypotension, hyperglycemia
- Explore psychological issues if an intentional ingestion

SURGICAL MEASURES N/A

ACTIVITY N/A

DIET N/A

PATIENT EDUCATION
- Prevention counseling on proper storage of iron products out of the reach of children
- Educational material from poison control centers may be available to use
- An informative poster is available, at no charge, from the Department of Health and Human Services, 5600 Fishers Lane (HFI-40), Rockville, MD 20857

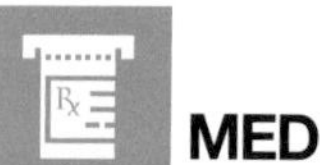

MEDICATIONS

DRUG(S) OF CHOICE

- Decontamination with syrup of ipecac [1-12 years: 15 mL; adult: 30 mL] if a patient has recent iron ingestion and is a candidate for emesis. Contraindications are signs of oral pharyngeal/esophageal irritation, a depressed gag reflex, or CNS excitation/depression. Controversy exists as to whether to give ipecac to children < 6 mo of age.
- Criteria for emesis/lavage:
  - ◊ > 20 mg/kg ingested
  - ◊ Symptomatic
  - ◊ Adults
- Gastric lavage, using tepid water, may be indicated in patients who are comatose or at risk for convulsing. Use if over 20 mg/kg or unknown amount of iron has been ingested.
- Whole bowel irrigation with a solution containing polyethylene glycol (Colyte, Golytely) electrolyte lavage, gives rapid diarrhea with relatively little fluid and electrolyte imbalance; (children: 25 mL/kg/h; adults: 1.5-2 L/h); indicated when radiographic evidence of iron past the pylorus or if tablets persist in the GI tract after other attempts of decontamination. End point: clear rectal effluent, disappearance of radiopacities.
- If large clumps of coalesced iron tablets persist in stomach or duodenum: these can lead to perforation so may need removal by gastroscopy or gastrotomy
- If serum iron exceeds TIBC or peak serum iron is > 300 mcg/dL, administer IV deferoxamine, 15 mg/kg/hr, for not more than 24 hrs to chelate iron and prevent it from entering into chemical reactions. Serum iron levels drop usually within 12 to 48 hours.

Contraindications: Deferoxamine is relatively contraindicated in patients with severe renal disease or anuria, primary hemochromatosis

Precautions: Deferoxamine may cause flushing of skin, urticaria, hypotension and shock with rapid IV injections

Significant possible interactions: N/A

ALTERNATIVE DRUGS N/A

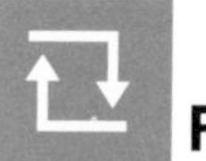

FOLLOWUP

PATIENT MONITORING

- KUB until no pills are seen
- Serum iron concentration
- CBC, electrolytes, serum bicarbonate, blood glucose, serum iron, and TIBC
- Some patients' urine will turn a characteristic vin rose color after treatment with deferoxamine (previously this was used as a diagnostic test of significant iron poisoning)

PREVENTION/AVOIDANCE

- Keep prescription and over-the-counter iron products/ vitamins out of reach of children
- Keep syrup of ipecac on hand in case of accidental acute ingestion

POSSIBLE COMPLICATIONS

2-4 weeks after severe ingestion has resulted in pyloric or antral stenosis, hepatic cirrhosis and CNS damage

EXPECTED COURSE/PROGNOSIS

Depends on amount ingested and length of time patient exposed

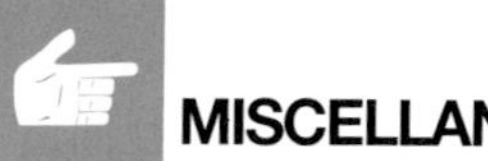

MISCELLANEOUS

ASSOCIATED CONDITIONS N/A

AGE-RELATED FACTORS

Pediatric: For a 2 year old, the average lethal dose of elemental iron is 3 grams

Geriatric: N/A

Others: N/A

PREGNANCY N/A

SYNONYMS Iron poisoning

ICD-9-CM

964.0 Poisoning by iron and its compounds

SEE ALSO

OTHER NOTES N/A

ABBREVIATIONS

TIBC = total iron binding capacity

REFERENCES

- Aisen P, Cohen G, Kang JO. Iron Toxicosis. Int Rev Exp Pathol 1990;31:1-46
- Banner WJ, Tong TG. Iron poisoning. Ped Clin North Am, 1986;33:393-409
- Iron, Poisondex Toxicologic Management, 1974-2002 Micromedex Inc. Vol 00
- FDA Medical Bulletin 1995; 25.3. Washington, DC, Federal Food & Drug Administration, 1995
- Thompson DF. Reassessment of measuring total iron binding capacity in acute iron overdose. Ann Pharmacother 1994;28:63-66
- Chyka PA, Butler AY, Holley JE. Serum iron concentrations and symptoms of acute poisoning in children. Pharmacotherapy 1996;16(6):1053-8

Web references: 0 available at www.5mcc.com

Illustrations N/A

Author(s):

Julienne K. Kirk, PharmD

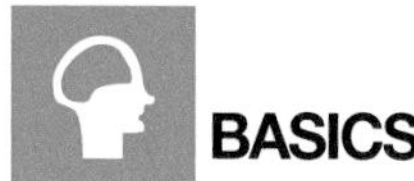

BASICS

DESCRIPTION Altered bowel habits, abdominal pain, gaseousness, in the absence of organic pathology (divided into four types):
- Alternating diarrhea with constipation
- Diarrhea predominant
- Constipation predominant
- Upper abdominal bloating and discomfort

System(s) affected: Gastrointestinal
Genetics: Unknown, but more common in families of patients
Incidence/Prevalence in USA:
- Unknown, but 50% of gastrointestinal visits, and second to upper respiratory infection as cause for lost workdays
- At least 15% of population (uncommon in children and early teens)

Predominant age:
- Late 20's, rarely in late teens
- If over age 40, other disease more likely

Predominant sex:
- Female > Male (2:1) in the US
- In other parts of the world - Male > Female

SIGNS & SYMPTOMS
- All present in most patients but not with every episode
- Abdominal pain, usually lower quadrant, relieved by defecation
- Mucus in stools
- Constipation
- Diarrhea
- Distention
- Upper abdominal discomfort after eating
- Straining for normal consistency stools
- Urgency of defecation
- Feelings of incomplete evacuation
- Scybalous stools
- Nausea, vomiting (rarely)
- Rome II criteria: 12 weeks or more in past 12 months of abdominal bowel pain or discomfort that has 2 out of 3:
  - ◊ Relieved by defecation
  - ◊ Onset associated with change in frequency of stool
  - ◊ Onset associated with change in form of stool

CAUSES Unknown but patients show some gut motility abnormalities with increased response to stress and stimulants, and increase in the 3 cycles/minute smooth muscle contractions. Up to 1/3 of patients develop IBS after an episode of gastroenteritis.

RISK FACTORS
- Other members of the family with the same or similar gastrointestinal disorder
- History of childhood sexual abuse
- Sexual or domestic abuse in women

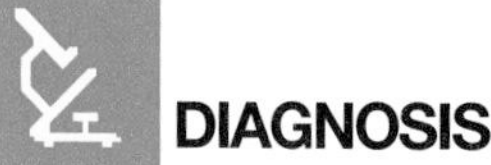

DIAGNOSIS

DIFFERENTIAL DIAGNOSIS
- Inflammatory bowel syndromes
- Lactose intolerance
- Infections (*Giardia lamblia*, *Entamoeba histolytica*, *Salmonella*, *Campylobacter*, *Yersinia*, *Clostridium difficile*)
- Diverticula
- Cathartic use
- Magnesium containing antacids
- Celiac sprue
- Pancreatic insufficiency
- Depression
- Somatization
- Adenocarcinoma of the colon
- Villous adenoma
- Endocrine tumors
- Hypo/hyperthyroidism
- Diabetes mellitus
- Radiation damage to colon or small bowel

LABORATORY
- As needed to rule out other pathology
  - ◊ ESR
  - ◊ CBC
  - ◊ Stool for ova, parasites and culture

Drugs that may alter lab results: N/A

Disorders that may alter lab results: N/A

PATHOLOGICAL FINDINGS All labs normal except for sigmoidoscopy

SPECIAL TESTS Not needed for diagnosis

IMAGING
- Barium enema, if indicated is usually normal
- Small bowel series

DIAGNOSTIC PROCEDURES Sigmoidoscopy (often normal), can show spasm that reproduces pain and increase mucosal folds

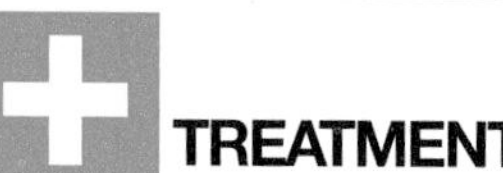

TREATMENT

APPROPRIATE HEALTH CARE Outpatient

GENERAL MEASURES
- Heat to abdomen can help
- Biofeedback may help
- Reduce stress

SURGICAL MEASURES N/A

ACTIVITY As normal

DIET
- Increase fiber - may make some patients worse
- Avoid - large meals; spicy, fried, fatty foods; milk products, carbohydrates

PATIENT EDUCATION
- Many materials available nationally and locally
- Stress the organicity of the disease versus any psychosocial interpretation
- Teach patient to avoid problem stimulants

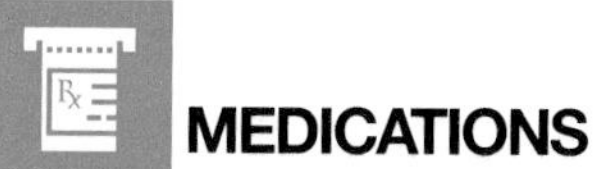

MEDICATIONS

DRUG(S) OF CHOICE
- Use from among this list according to need or response
  - ◊ Bulk producing agents - psyllium (Metamucil) products 1 tbsp bid or tid
  - ◊ Constipating agents (if diarrhea is significant) - loperamide (Imodium) 4 mg initial dose, then 2 mg after each unformed stool or diphenoxylate-atropine (Lomotil) 2.5-5.0 mg (1-2 tablets) after each unformed stool
  - ◊ Antispasmodics/anticholinergics/sedatives
    - dicyclomine (Bentyl) 10-20 mg bid to qid
    - chlordiazepoxide-clidinium (Librax) 1 or 2 ac and qhs
    - hyoscyamine (Levbid) 0.375 mg bid
    - phenobarbital-scopolamine-hyoscyamine-atropine (Donnatal) 1 or 2 tablets ac and hs
    - amitriptyline (Elavil) 25-50 mg qhs
  - ◊ 5-HT4 receptor agonist - tegaserod (Zelnorm) 6 mg bid for 4-6 weeks in patients with prominent constipation, may repeat course once (for women only)
  - ◊ Antiflatulents - simethicone (Mylicon) 2 or 4 tablets pc and hs
  - ◊ Lactose intolerance - lactase (Lactaid) capsules or tablets; 1-2 tablets prior to ingesting milk products

Contraindications: Refer to manufacturer's profile of each drug
Precautions: Refer to manufacturer's profile of each drug
Significant possible interactions: Refer to manufacturer's profile of each drug

ALTERNATIVE DRUGS N/A

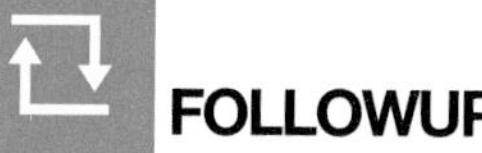

FOLLOWUP

PATIENT MONITORING As needed for symptoms

PREVENTION/AVOIDANCE See Diet

POSSIBLE COMPLICATIONS N/A

EXPECTED COURSE/PROGNOSIS
- No progression to cancer or inflammatory disease
- Expect recurrences, when under stress, throughout life. Frequency lessens as age increases.

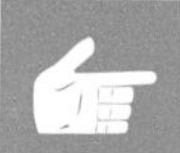

MISCELLANEOUS

ASSOCIATED CONDITIONS
- Migraine
- Bladder frequency
- Nocturia
- Urgency
- Fecal incontinence
- Fibromyalgia
- Dyspareunia
- Depression
- Stress incontinence

AGE-RELATED FACTORS N/A
Pediatric: N/A
Geriatric: N/A
Others: N/A

PREGNANCY Anecdotal information implies that irritable bowel syndrome gets worse in pregnancy. But there are no increased risks to fetus or mother.

SYNONYMS
- Mucous colitis
- Spastic colon
- Irritable colon

ICD-9-CM
564.1 Irritable bowel syndrome

SEE ALSO

OTHER NOTES Must not give patients the impression that this is a psychiatric illness

ABBREVIATIONS
IBS = irritable bowel syndrome

REFERENCES

- Verne GN, Cerda JJ. Irritable bowel syndrome: streamlining the diagnosis. Post Grad Med 1997;102(3):197-208
- Dalton CB, Drossman DA. Diagnosis and treatment of irritable bowel syndrome. Am Fam Phys 1997;55(3):875-85
- Read NW, ed. Irritable Bowel Syndrome. London, Grune and Stratton, 1991
- Rakel R, ed. Textbook of Family Practice. 5th Ed. Philadelphia, W.B. Saunders Co., 1995

Web references: 5 available at www.5mcc.com
Illustrations N/A

Author(s):
S. Shevaun Duiker, MD

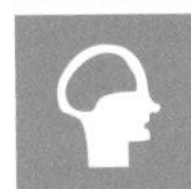

BASICS

DESCRIPTION A neoplasm characterized by vascular tumors of skin and viscera in several different forms:
- Indolent (classic) Kaposi sarcoma (KS)
- African (endemic) KS
- AIDS-related (epidemic) KS
- Form associated with immunosuppressive medications

System(s) affected: Hemic/Lymphatic/Immunologic, Skin/Exocrine
Genetics: Unknown
Incidence/Prevalence in USA:
- Indolent/lymphadenopathic - rare
- In AIDS patients - common

Predominant age: 16-75
Predominant sex: Male > Female

SIGNS & SYMPTOMS
- Indolent Kaposi
  - ◊ Multicentric red-blue violaceous tumors on the skin
  - ◊ Tender skin tumors
  - ◊ Pruritic skin tumors
  - ◊ In older men, lesions appear first on toes or legs
- African (endemic) Kaposi
  - ◊ Usually involves skin, viscera or lymph nodes
- Kaposi associated with HIV infection (epidemic)
  - ◊ Skin lesions widely disseminated, on the face, arms, trunk
  - ◊ Lesions on mucous membranes
  - ◊ Lesions in lymph nodes
  - ◊ Lesions in viscera
- Immunosuppression-associated Kaposi
  - ◊ Tends to be aggressive
  - ◊ High amount of lymph node involvement
  - ◊ Visceral organs involved in one-half

CAUSES
- A herpes virus designated "Kaposi sarcoma herpes virus" (KSHV) or human herpes virus type 8 (HHV8) is required for the development of KS
- Samples from KS lesions have been found to contain DNA sequences identical with HHV8, and HHV8 can be propagated from skin lesions of patients with KS
- Immunosuppression of host is important co-factor in development of KS

RISK FACTORS
- HIV infection
- Living in endemic area (especially Zaire or Uganda)
- Immunosuppressant medications
- Transplantation and chemotherapy
- Sexual activity
- Maternal-fetal transmission
- Maternal-child transmission
- Injection drug use
- Exposure to infectious saliva
- Possible association with trauma in susceptible host
- Many cases transmitted by unknown route

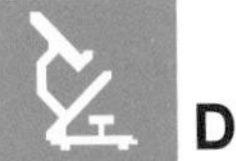

DIAGNOSIS

DIFFERENTIAL DIAGNOSIS Bacillary angiomatosis, granuloma faciale, vascular proliferation and purpuric lesions

LABORATORY
- Specific HHV8 antibodies present in 70-90%
- Southern blot hybridization assay of KS lesions for HHV8
- Polymerase chain reaction (PCR) assay

Drugs that may alter lab results: N/A

Disorders that may alter lab results: N/A

PATHOLOGICAL FINDINGS
- Micro - proliferation of atypical spindle cells
- Micro - proliferation of vascular channels
- Micro - large hyperchromic nuclei
- Micro - spindle-shaped perivascular cells
- Micro - hemosiderin laden macrophages

SPECIAL TESTS Tissue examination

IMAGING CT or MRI scan (chest, abdomen) may assess visceral involvement

DIAGNOSTIC PROCEDURES
- Biopsy of skin or lymph node
- Bronchoscopy with biopsy
- Liver biopsy

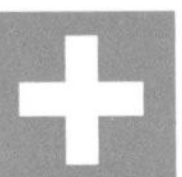

TREATMENT

APPROPRIATE HEALTH CARE
- Outpatient
- Outpatient surgery

GENERAL MEASURES
- If KS due to immunosuppressant medications, eliminate or reduce medication dosage
- If KS is HIV-related, optimize anti-HIV therapy to reduce HIV viral load
- Treatment is otherwise determined by extent and location of the disease
- Observation
- Radiotherapy (electron beam) or x-ray therapy 1000 to 2000 rads
- Systemic chemotherapy, immunotherapy, or antiviral therapy

SURGICAL MEASURES
- Cryotherapy
- Intralesional chemotherapy or immunotherapy
- Surgical excision
- CO_2 laser

ACTIVITY Remain active as long as possible

DIET No special diet

PATIENT EDUCATION
- HIV risk prevention
- Injection drug rehabilitation

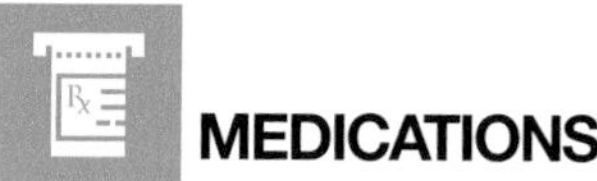

MEDICATIONS

DRUG(S) OF CHOICE
- Chemotherapy
  - ◊ Doxorubicin
  - ◊ Bleomycin
  - ◊ Vinblastine - parenteral or intralesional
  - ◊ Vincristine
  - ◊ Daunorubicin
  - ◊ Paclitaxel
  - ◊ Interleukins
  - ◊ Thalidomide
  - ◊ Interferon - parenteral or intralesional
  - ◊ Alitretinoin gel

Note: Both doxorubicin and daunorubicin are available and approved for use in liposomal forms. These liposomal formulations offer improved outcome with less toxicity.

Contraindications: Refer to manufacturer's literature

Precautions: Refer to manufacturer's literature. Myelosuppression with chemotherapy.

Significant possible interactions: Refer to manufacturer's literature

ALTERNATIVE DRUGS
- Several studies have reported that some individuals have responded to anti-viral medications such as foscarnet (Foscavir), ganciclovir (Cytovene, Vitrasert), and cidofovir (Vistide)
- Photodynamic therapy

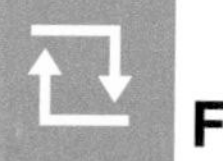

FOLLOWUP

PATIENT MONITORING In HIV patients with KS, other opportunistic infections must be aggressively treated

PREVENTION/AVOIDANCE
- Safe sex practices
- Possible prophylaxis with anti-viral medications
- Avoid needle sharing
- Avoid deep kissing

POSSIBLE COMPLICATIONS
- Extensive pulmonary involvement may lead to hypoxemia
- Extensive lymphatic involvement may lead to severe edema

EXPECTED COURSE/PROGNOSIS
- Improved HIV treatments and anti-viral drugs may result in improved HIV-related KS survival
- Indolent form - 10 year survival

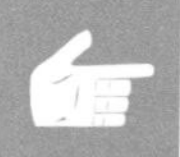

MISCELLANEOUS

ASSOCIATED CONDITIONS
- AIDS
- HIV infection
- Lymphoma

AGE-RELATED FACTORS
Pediatric: In eastern and southern Africa, KS represents 25-50% of all soft tissue sarcomas

Geriatric: Indolent form most likely to occur in men in this age group

Others: N/A

PREGNANCY Maternal-infant HIV transmission may occur

SYNONYMS
- Endotheliosarcoma
- Idiopathic hemorrhagic sarcoma
- Human herpesvirus 8

ICD-9-CM
176.0 Kaposi sarcoma of skin

SEE ALSO
HIV infection & AIDS

OTHER NOTES N/A

ABBREVIATIONS
KS = Kaposi sarcoma

REFERENCES

- Antman K, Chang V. Kaposi's sarcoma. N Engl J Med 2000;342:1027-38
- Cesarman E. Kaposi's sarcoma-associated herpes-like DNA sequences in AIDS-related body cavity-based lymphomas. NEJM 1995;332(18):1186-91
- Moore PS, Chang Y. Detection of a herpesvirus-like DNA sequence in Kaposi's sarcoma in patients with and without HIV infection. NEJM 1995;331:1181-85
- Martin JN, et al. Sexual transmission and the natural history of human herpesvirus 8 infection. NEJM 1997;338:948-954
- Kedes DH, Ganem D. Sensitivity of Kaposi's-associated herpesvirus replication to antiviral drugs: Implications for potential therapy. J Clin Invest 1997;99:2082-6
- Pauk J, et al. Mucosal shedding of human herpesvirus 8 in men. NEJM 2000;343:1369-85
- Cannon MJ, et al. Blood-borne and sexual transmission of human herpesvirus 8 in women with or at risk for human immunodeficiency virus. Infection. NEJM 2001;344:637-43
- Webster-Cyriaque J. Development of Kaposi's sarcoma in a surgical wound. N Engl J Med 2002;346(16):1207-10

Web references: 4 available at www.5mcc.com

Illustrations 9 available

Author(s):
R. Scott Gorman, MD

BASICS

DESCRIPTION An acute, distinct, self-limited, exanthematous febrile disease of young children which is notable for vasculitis of coronary blood vessels with potential dilation and subsequent aneurysms, thrombosis, rupture, or myocardial ischemia. KS should be considered in febrile children with non-tender cervical adenitis(>=1.5 cm) unresponsive to antibiotics and antipyretics, without an alternative diagnosis.

System(s) affected: Cardiovascular, Gastrointestinal, Hemic/Lymphatic/Immunologic, Musculoskeletal, Nervous, Pulmonary, Renal/Urologic, Skin/Exocrine

Genetics: Increased incidence of HLA-Bw 22 in Japanese patients; increased incidence of HLA-Bw 51 in US Caucasians and in Jewish, Israeli patients. Slight increase in siblings of cases.

Incidence/Prevalence in USA:
- Worldwide, affects all races but most prevalent in Japan. In the US, the annual incidence rate among children less than 5 years is 10 cases/100,000 for non-Asians, and 44 cases/100,000 for Asian Americans.
- The incidence in Japan is approximately 95 cases /100,000 children under 5 years
- Highest to lowest prevalence: Asians > Blacks > Caucasians. Seasonal variation - increased in late winter and spring. Increased outbreaks at 2-3 year intervals.

Predominant age:
- 1-5 years (peak age US = 18-24 mo /; Japan = 6-11 mo)
- 80% are < 5 years old; 50% are < 2 years old. Seldom seen after 8 years of age.
- Patients less than 6 mo will present atypically.

Predominant sex: Males > Females (1.6:1 US; 1.35:1 Japan)

SIGNS & SYMPTOMS
- Fever for 5 days or more
  - ◊ Fever is high (103-105°F [39.4-40.5°C]) and unresponsive to antibiotics
  - ◊ May be prolonged (2-3 weeks with average duration of 11 days)
- Polymorphous rash
  - ◊ May be maculopapular, scarlatiniform, morbilliform, erythema multiforme, or rarely vesiculopustular
  - ◊ Frequently confluent in the perineum where it desquamates
- Bilateral conjunctival suffusion
  - ◊ Nonpurulent
- Changes of lips and oral cavity
  - ◊ Reddening of lips in the acute stage which crack, fissure and bleed in the subacute phase
  - ◊ Strawberry or erythematous tongue
  - ◊ Diffuse injection of oral and pharyngeal mucosa without exudate
- Acute, nonpurulent cervical lymphadenopathy
  - ◊ Lymph nodes 1 cm or greater in diameter
  - ◊ Generalized lymphadenopathy usually absent
- Extremity changes
  - ◊ Reddened palms and soles on days 3-5
  - ◊ Indurative edema of hands and feet on days 4-7
  - ◊ Membranous desquamation from fingertips in convalescent phase
- Other organ system involvement:
  - ◊ Cardiovascular
    - Acutely may have tachycardia (disproportionate to fever), gallop rhythms, and ECG changes suggestive of myocarditis
    - Pericarditis, often subclinical
    - Coronary artery and other medium-sized arterial aneurysms
  - ◊ Gastrointestinal
    - Anorexia
    - Vomiting or diarrhea
    - Acute, acalculous cholecystitis may present as a right upper quadrant mass and pain
    - Pancreatitis
  - ◊ Renal
    - Nephritis
    - Urethritis
  - ◊ Pulmonary
    - Pneumonitis, atelectasis, or pleural effusions
  - ◊ Joints
    - Arthritis of wrists, knees, and ankles may appear in third week of illness
  - ◊ Neurologic
    - Irritability
    - Aseptic meningitis
    - Peripheral neuropathies

CAUSES
- Unknown
- Microbial agent is favored because of acute, self-limited course and community-wide outbreaks
  - ◊ Leading theory is that a staphylococcal or streptococcal superantigen, in the appropriate host, stimulates T cell populations which in turn cause activation of immune responses directed against endothelial cell antigens

RISK FACTORS Environmental - exposure to rug shampoo and residing in close proximity to bodies of water have been inconsistently associated risk factors in large epidemics

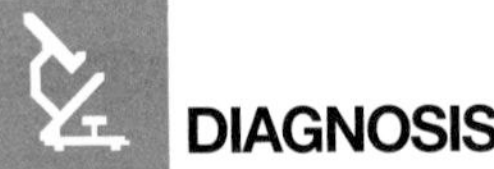

DIAGNOSIS

DIFFERENTIAL DIAGNOSIS
- Staphylococcal scalded skin syndrome
- Toxic shock syndrome
- Stevens-Johnson syndrome
- Reiter syndrome
- Juvenile rheumatoid arthritis
- Scarlet fever
- Measles
- Rubella
- Roseola
- Epstein-Barr virus infections
- Mycoplasma infection
- Leptospirosis
- Lyme disease
- Rocky Mountain spotted fever
- Toxoplasmosis
- Acrodynia
- Drug reactions
- Other vasculitides

LABORATORY
- Anemia (normochromic, normocytic)
- Leukocytosis (12,000-40,000 cells/mm3) with immature forms
- Elevated CRP, ESR, and alpha1-antitrypsin concentrations
- Platelet counts rise in subacute phase and peak in convalescent at 750,000-1,500,000
- Thrombocytopenia associated with severe coronary disease and myocardial infarction
- Mildly elevated serum liver enzymes and bilirubin
- CSF pleocytosis may be seen
- Measles immunoglobulin (IgM) titer helpful in differentiating KS from measles
- Sterile urethral pyuria occurs in 30% of patients

Drugs that may alter lab results: N/A

Disorders that may alter lab results: N/A

PATHOLOGICAL FINDINGS
- During acute stage, neutrophilic infiltrates involving pericardium, myocardium, endocardium, and vascular endothelium may be present
- Necrosis may develop and result in aneurysmal dilatation of medium-sized arteries
- Mononuclear infiltration predominates in the second week of illness, gradually resolving with or without fibrosis
- In addition to cardiac involvement, arteritis may also develop in lungs, kidneys, gastrointestinal tract, and other organs

SPECIAL TESTS
- Quantitative serum immunoglobulins
- ANA, RF, VDRL, immune complexes, complement levels

IMAGING
- Electrocardiogram may show ischemia, arrhythmias
- Echocardiogram may show cardiomyopathy, pericardial effusion, coronary artery dilatation or aneurysms
- Radiography including angiography

DIAGNOSTIC PROCEDURES
- No laboratory study proves diagnosis; diagnosis rests on clinical features and exclusion of other illnesses in differential diagnosis
- Diagnosis of typical syndrome requires fever of at least 5 days' duration, plus 4 of the following 5 criteria:
  - ◊ Mucous membrane changes
  - ◊ Extremity changes
  - ◊ Cervical lymphadenopathy of at least 1 cm in size
  - ◊ Rash
  - ◊ Conjunctival suffusion
- Atypical cases occur with incomplete clinical findings; frequency of coronary artery aneurysms may be higher in this subset of patients

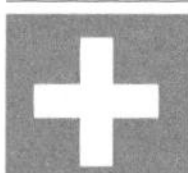

TREATMENT

APPROPRIATE HEALTH CARE When seen acutely, most children are hospitalized for diagnostic evaluation and supportive care. Older children with mild disease may be managed on an outpatient basis.

GENERAL MEASURES
- Antibiotics are given until bacterial etiologies are excluded
- Once KS is suspected, all patients need a cardiac evaluation, including electrocardiogram and echocardiogram
- Diuretics, inotropic agents, and pacemakers may be required for myocarditis

SURGICAL MEASURES Aortocoronary artery bypass surgery for symptomatic patients with severe stenotic lesions (> 75% occluded)

ACTIVITY May be limited if cardiac involvement

DIET IV fluids may be needed if fever and irritability make feeding difficult

PATIENT EDUCATION N/A

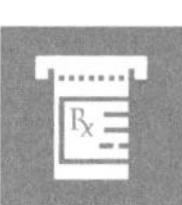

MEDICATIONS

DRUG(S) OF CHOICE
- Aspirin: 80-100 mg/kg/day during the febrile phase. When child is afebrile, continue with low, single dose (5 mg/kg/day, to maximum of 80 mg) therapy for antithrombotic effects until active disease subsides.
- Immune globulin (IVIG) IV 2 gm/kg at the time diagnosis is made (preferably within the first 10 days of illness) lowers the risk of coronary artery aneurysms and may shorten the duration of the acute phase. Retreatment is occasionally considered if clinical response is incomplete, although this has not been well studied.

Contraindications: Corticosteroids may increase the chance of aneurysm formation and should be avoided except in exceptional cases
Precautions: High dose salicylate therapy can cause tinnitus and hepatitis
Significant possible interactions: Aspirin therapy is associated with Reye syndrome in children who develop viral infections, particularly influenza B and varicella. Influenza vaccination is recommended for children requiring aspirin therapy during influenza season, and aspirin should probably be discontinued if influenza or varicella infection occurs.

ALTERNATIVE DRUGS
- Dipyridamole, 4 mg/kg/d, is sometimes administered if coronary artery abnormalities develop
- Fibrinolytic agents (urokinase) for coronary artery thrombosis
- Alprostadil (prostaglandin E1) for peripheral artery ischemia
- Heparin followed by warfarin for large or multiple nonobstructive or obstructive aneurysms

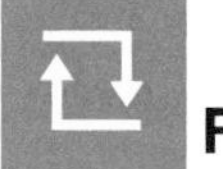

FOLLOWUP

PATIENT MONITORING
- Monitor platelet count and acute phase reactant along with clinical course; when all return to normal, aspirin can be stopped
- Repeat ECG and echocardiogram at 3 and 8 weeks if initial studies are normal; may need further studies (e.g., angiography) if abnormal

PREVENTION/AVOIDANCE N/A

POSSIBLE COMPLICATIONS
- 20% of untreated patients develop coronary artery aneurysms in convalescent phase. Risk factors include:
  - ◊ Male sex
  - ◊ Age < 1 year old
  - ◊ Fever > 2 weeks
  - ◊ Elevated ESR for > 4 weeks
- Ischemic heart disease risk factors include:
  - ◊ Aneurysms > 8 mm
  - ◊ Diffuse or saccular aneurysm
  - ◊ Fever > 21 days
  - ◊ Steroid therapy
  - ◊ Age > 2 years old
- Mortality 0.5%, related to cardiovascular disease

EXPECTED COURSE/PROGNOSIS
- Usually self-limited
- Only potentially permanent sequelae involve cardiovascular system
- Unknown but possible increased risk of atherosclerotic heart disease in adulthood
- Sudden death is possible

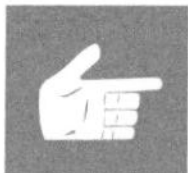

MISCELLANEOUS

ASSOCIATED CONDITIONS N/A

AGE-RELATED FACTORS
Pediatric: See Description
Geriatric: N/A
Others: N/A

PREGNANCY N/A

SYNONYMS
- Mucocutaneous lymph node syndrome
- Infantile periarteritis nodosa

ICD-9-CM
446.1 Acute febrile mucocutaneous lymph node syndrome [MCLS]

SEE ALSO
Polyarteritis nodosa

OTHER NOTES N/A

ABBREVIATIONS
KS = Kawasaki syndrome

REFERENCES

- Feigin RD, et al. Kawasaki disease. In: McMillan JA, et al, editors. Oski's Pediatrics: Principles and Practice. 3rd ed. Philadelphia: Lippincott Williams & Wilkins; 1999
- American Academy of Pediatrics. Kawasaki disease. In: Peter G, editor. 2000 Red Book: Report of the Committee on Infectious Diseases. 25th ed. Elk Grove Village, IL: Academy of Pediatrics; 2000
- Sundel R, Szer I. Vasculitis in childhood. Rheum Dis Clin North Am 2002;28(3):625-54
- Rowley AH. Kawasaki syndrome. Pediatr Clin North Am 1999;46(2):313-29
- Habif T. Clinical Dermatology. 4th Ed. St. Louis, CV Mosby, 2004
- Leung DYM, Schlievert PM, Meissner HC. The immunopathogenesis and management of Kawasaki syndrome. Arthritis and Rheumatism 1998;41(9):1538-47

Web references: 0 available at www.5mcc.com
Illustrations 2 available

Author(s):
Mitchell S. King, MD

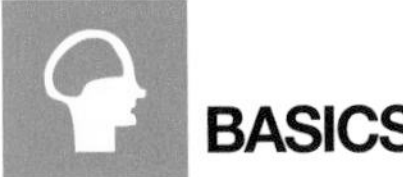

BASICS

DESCRIPTION Abnormally large overgrowth of fibrous tissue (scar) occurring as a result of trauma or irritation that does not subside with time

System(s) affected: Skin/Exocrine

Genetics:
- 5-15 times more common in blacks and Asians than Caucasians. In all races, more darkly pigmented individuals are at higher risk.
- Both autosomal dominant and autosomal recessive familial inheritance have been reported

Incidence/Prevalence in USA: Largely unknown, but does affect 4-16% of the black and Hispanic population

Predominant age: N/A

Predominant sex: Male = Female

SIGNS & SYMPTOMS
- Pain
- Tenderness
- Hyperesthesia
- Pruritus
- Firm, smooth, elevated scar with sharply demarcated borders
- Initially may be pale or mildly erythematous
- Older lesion hypo- or hyperpigmented
- Scar extends beyond margins of the initial wound
- Over period of years, keloids may continue to grow and may develop claw-like projections

CAUSES
- Wounds: traumatic, surgical, body piercing
- Burn injury
- Other injuries
  - ◊ Insect bite
  - ◊ Folliculitis barbae and nuchae
  - ◊ Acne

RISK FACTORS
- Family history of keloids
- Dark skin pigment
- Certain locations on the body, e.g., deltoids, chest, earlobes
- Pregnancy
- Adolescence

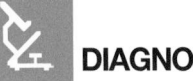

DIAGNOSIS

DIFFERENTIAL DIAGNOSIS
- Hypertrophic scar (usually spontaneously regress; do not cross wound margins)
- Dermatofibroma
- Infiltrating basal cell carcinoma
- Sclerosing metastatic malignancies
- Desmoplastic melanoma
- Other fibronodular skin diseases
- Sarcoidosis

LABORATORY N/A

Drugs that may alter lab results: N/A

Disorders that may alter lab results: N/A

PATHOLOGICAL FINDINGS Histology shows whorl-like arrangements of hyalinized collagen bundles with pressure thinning of papillary dermis and minimal elastic tissue

SPECIAL TESTS N/A

IMAGING N/A

DIAGNOSTIC PROCEDURES
- Biopsy, only if unable to differentiate from carcinoma or infectious disease, since a biopsy may increase the keloid's size. If possible, use a 2 mm punch biopsy to minimize trauma.

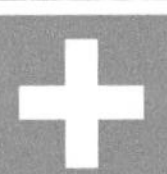

TREATMENT

APPROPRIATE HEALTH CARE Outpatient

GENERAL MEASURES
"Step care" is warranted, adding pressure and then radiation if steroid injections fail.
- Intralesional corticosteroid injections: cause atrophy and are most successful therapy
- Pressure bandages: must maintain 24 mm Hg, and should be worn for 6-12 months. Bandages should not be removed for more than 30 minutes/day. Pressure clips (Zimmer splints) useful for earlobes. Designer splints look like fashion earrings.
- Radiation: no advantage over other methods, therefore use if other methods fail, and then use in conjunction with steroids and pressure
- Topical agents: No evidence to support efficacy; e.g., retinoic acid, vitamin E, antineoplastic agents, silicone gel

SURGICAL MEASURES
- Surgery - high recurrence rate (45-100%), therefore used only for debulking of large keloids or if a lesion is unresponsive to steroid injections or other therapy
- Laser surgery - no definitive evidence of efficacy

ACTIVITY Full activity

DIET No special diet

PATIENT EDUCATION
- Stress possibility of recurrence despite appropriate treatment
- May require many months of treatment with combined modalities

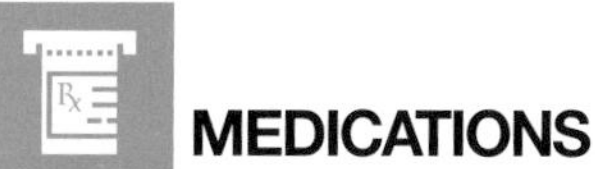

MEDICATIONS

DRUG(S) OF CHOICE
- Triamcinolone (Kenalog) suspension 10 mg/mL
  - ◊ Using 27-30 gauge needle and a TB syringe (total dose 20-30 mg of triamcinolone). May inject 3 lesions at a time, using 10 mg/lesion.
  - ◊ Advance needle while injecting in order to evenly distribute medication
  - ◊ Early keloids are more responsive to this therapy than older lesions
  - ◊ Reinject every 4 weeks until keloid shrinks to near skin surface
  - ◊ If no response to 10 mg/mL triamcinolone suspension, may try 40 mg/mL suspension
  - ◊ May mix dilute triamcinolone (5-10 mg/mL) with local anesthetic for excision of keloids. Postoperative steroid injections at 2-4 weeks and then monthly for 6 months helps prevent recurrences.

Contraindications: None are absolute

Precautions:
- Systemic absorption with adrenal suppression (reversible)
- Local affects - skin atrophy, ulceration, depigmentation, telangiectasias
- Both types of side effects more common with 40 mg/mL triamcinolone suspension

Significant possible interactions: Rare interactions (only with very large doses of corticosteroids and systemic absorption)

ALTERNATIVE DRUGS
- Verapamil locally may be helpful. One study (D'Andrea, 2002) supports repeated intralesional injections of 2.5 mg/mL of verapamil at repeated intervals as an "adjuvant" following excision and topical silicone.
- Interferon-alpha 2b may be helpful after excision
- Imiquimod 5% cream daily for 8 weeks following surgical keloid excision prevented recurrence in small series of 11 patients (Berman and Kaufman 2002)
- Intralesional 5-fluorouracil
- Intralesional bleomycin

FOLLOWUP

PATIENT MONITORING Monthly visits, up to a year, for evaluation and possible steroid re-injections

PREVENTION/AVOIDANCE
- Primary prevention: avoid elective surgery or body piercing in high-risk patients
- When feasible, laparoscopic approaches are preferred in keloid formers
- Compressive pressure dressings may be useful in high risk (e.g., burn) patients. Local steroid injection postoperatively in high risk patients is also effective.

POSSIBLE COMPLICATIONS Skin atrophy, ulceration, depigmentation, telangiectasias can occur as a result of local steroid injections

EXPECTED COURSE/PROGNOSIS
When treatment is successful, lesions gradually diminish with therapy over a 6-18 month period, leaving a flat, shiny scar

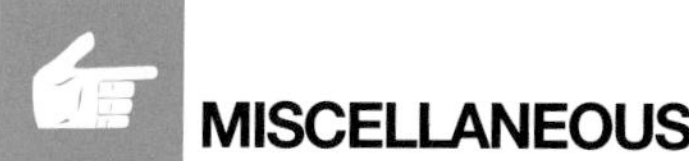

MISCELLANEOUS

ASSOCIATED CONDITIONS None

AGE-RELATED FACTORS
Pediatric: Keloid formation is more common during adolescence

Geriatric: None

Others: N/A

PREGNANCY Keloid formation more likely during pregnancy

SYNONYMS
- Razor bumps

ICD-9-CM
701.4 Keloid scar

SEE ALSO
Animal bites
Burns
Warts

OTHER NOTES N/A

ABBREVIATIONS N/A

REFERENCES

- Marneros AG, Norris JE, Olsen BR, Reichenberger E. Clinical genetics of familial keloids. Arch Dermatol 2001;137(11):1429-34
- Ragoowansi R, Cornes PG, Glees JP, et al. Ear-lobe keloids: treatment by a protocol of surgical excision and immediate postoperative adjuvant radiotherapy. Br J Plast Surg 2001;54(6):504-8
- D'Andrea F, Brongo S, Ferraro G, Baroni A. Prevention and treatment of keloids with intralesional verapamil. Dermatology 2002;204(1):60-2
- Russell R, Horlock N, Gault D. Zimmer splintage: a simple effective treatment for keloids following ear-piercing. Br J Plast Surg 2001;54(6):509-10
- Berman B, Flores F. The treatment of hypertrophic scars and keloids. Eur J Derm 1998;8:591-5
- Poston J. The use of silicone gel sheeting in the management of hypertrophic and keloid scars Jour of Wound Care 2000;9(1):10-6
- Rahban SR, Garner WL. Fibroproliferative scars. Clin Plast Surg 2003;30(1):77-89
- Mustoe TA, Cooter RD, Gold MH, et al. International Advisory Panel on Scar Management. International clinical recommendations on scar management. Plast Reconstr Surg 2002;110(2):560-71
- Gupta S, Kalra A. Efficacy and safety of intralesional 5-fluorouracil in the treatment of keloids. Dermatology 2002;204(2):130-2
- Berman B, Kaufman J. Pilot study of the effect of postoperative imiquimod 5% cream on the recurrence rate of excised keloids. J Am Acad Dermatol 2002;47(4 Suppl):S209-11

Web references: 1 available at www.5mcc.com

Illustrations 4 available

Author(s):
Ronald E. Pust, MD

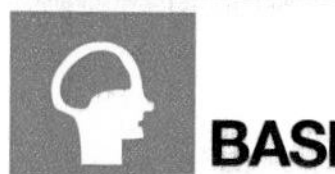

BASICS

DESCRIPTION Common, usually multiple premalignant skin lesions of sun-exposed areas. They are the most common indicator of excessive cumulative ultraviolet light exposure. The risk of transformation to squamous carcinoma is quite low: 1/4% risk of malignant transformation per lesion per year.
System(s) affected: Skin/Exocrine
Genetics: Relates to complexion
Incidence/Prevalence in USA: Common in blondes and redheads; rare in blacks
Predominant age: 40+; progressive with age (if child, look for freckling and other stigmata of xeroderma pigmentosum)
Predominant sex: Male > Female (from occupational sun exposure)

SIGNS & SYMPTOMS
- Lesions usually fairly flat, red, and rough to palpitation; can be lichenoid (ie, resembling lichen - a flat papule or aggregate of papules)
- Mild hyperesthesia common over lesions
- Hypertrophic verrucous lesions (called "cutaneous horns" if extreme) may be impossible to differentiate from squamous cell carcinoma clinically
- A brown, pigmented variant also exists
- Actinic cheilitis usually involves lower lip
- Only photo-exposed areas involved, often with other stigmata of chronic actinic damage: lentigines, actinic elastosis, atrophy

CAUSES
- Short-wave ultraviolet light (UVB)
- Possibly ultraviolet (UVA)
- Bowen disease can be caused by the carcinogenic types of human papilloma virus and arsenic exposure

RISK FACTORS
- Equatorial latitudes
- High elevations
- Outdoor occupation (farmers, sailors, ranchers)
- Outdoor athletics
- Sun worshippers
- Accompanying heat, wind, humidity augment carcinogenic effect
- Occupational exposure, i.e., petroleum products
- Immunosuppression, especially organ transplantation

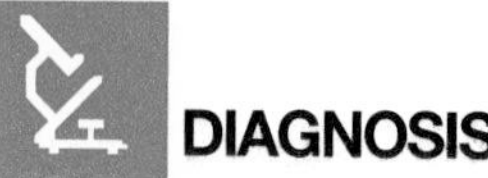

DIAGNOSIS

DIFFERENTIAL DIAGNOSIS
- Squamous cell carcinoma (hypertrophic type)
- Verruca vulgaris (hypertrophic type)
- Seborrheic dermatitis or psoriasis (near hairline)
- Lentigo maligna (pigmented type)
- Lupus erythematosus

LABORATORY N/A

Drugs that may alter lab results: N/A

Disorders that may alter lab results: N/A

PATHOLOGICAL FINDINGS
Diagnosis usually made clinically except where there is a suspicion of carcinoma
- Malignant cells sparse except in Bowenoid variety
- Hyperkeratosis
- Hypertrophic, atrophic, Bowenoid, acantholytic, and pigmented varieties show the corresponding epidermal findings
- Usually a sparse lymphocytic and plasma cell infiltrate

SPECIAL TESTS N/A

IMAGING N/A

DIAGNOSTIC PROCEDURES Biopsy (shave)

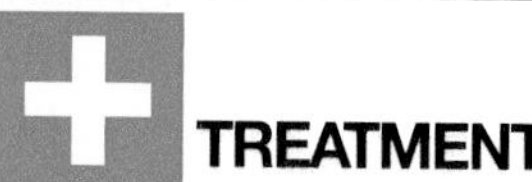

TREATMENT

APPROPRIATE HEALTH CARE Outpatient

GENERAL MEASURES Sun-protective techniques (See Patient Education)

SURGICAL MEASURES
- Cryosurgery for smaller number of lesions
- For extensive lesions (but medical treatment usually preferred)
  - ◊ Skin peels, i.e., 35% trichloroacetic acid
  - ◊ CO2 laser therapy
  - ◊ Dermabrasion

ACTIVITY No restrictions

DIET No special diet

PATIENT EDUCATION
- Teach sun-protective techniques
- Transfer hobbies and other outdoor activities to early morning or late afternoon
- Wear protective clothing and hats
- Daily use of topically applied sunscreens with SPF greater than 15; preferably containing titanium dioxide or avobenzone (Parsol-1789) to afford protection in the UVA range also
- Teach self-examination for cutaneous carcinoma (melanoma, squamous cell, basal cell)

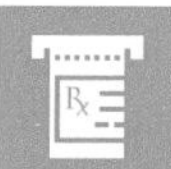

MEDICATIONS

DRUG(S) OF CHOICE Topical fluorouracil (Efudex, Carac, Fluoroplex cream, Fluoroplex solution) destroys even subclinical lesions, also non-scarring; usually applied bid for 3-4 weeks (for larger number of lesions)
Contraindications: N/A
Precautions: Continue treatment to involved skin
Significant possible interactions: N/A

ALTERNATIVE DRUGS
- Topical tretinoin (Retin-A) or tazarotene (Tazorac) may be used to enhance the efficacy of topical fluorouracil
- Photodynamic therapy with aminolevulinic acid and blue light
- 3% diclofenac (Solaraze) gel bid for 3 months
- Topical imiquimod, an interferon-inducer, is an evolving therapy

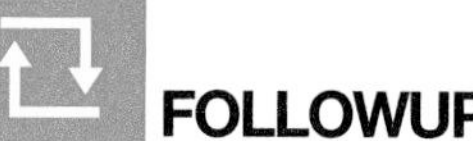

FOLLOWUP

PATIENT MONITORING Dependent on associated malignancy and frequency with which new actinic keratoses appear

PREVENTION/AVOIDANCE Sun protective techniques (See Patient Education)

POSSIBLE COMPLICATIONS Actinic keratosis is a premalignant lesion and may undergo carcinomatous proliferation to become squamous cell carcinoma

EXPECTED COURSE/PROGNOSIS
Excellent, if prevention taken by patient

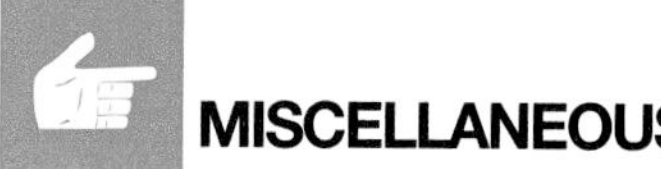

MISCELLANEOUS

ASSOCIATED CONDITIONS
- Squamous cell carcinoma

AGE-RELATED FACTORS
Pediatric: Rare
Geriatric: Frequent problem
Others: N/A

PREGNANCY N/A

SYNONYMS N/A

ICD-9-CM
702.0 Actinic keratosis

SEE ALSO
Dermatitis, seborrheic

OTHER NOTES N/A

ABBREVIATIONS N/A

REFERENCES

- Dodson JM, et al. Malignant potential of actinic keratoses and controversy over treatment. Archives of Dermatology 1991;127:1029
- Lever WF, Schaumburg-Lever G. Histopathology of the Skin. 7th Ed. Philadelphia, J.B. Lippincott, 1990

Web references: 1 available at www.5mcc.com
Illustrations 5 available

Author(s):
John R. Person, MD

BASICS

DESCRIPTION Inflammation of the vestibular labyrinth (a system of intercommunicating cavities and canals in the inner ear). There are many possible causes (see Differential Diagnosis). The most constant and pervasive symptom is vertigo.
System(s) affected: Nervous
Genetics: No known genetic pattern
Incidence/Prevalence in USA: Second most common cause of dizziness due to peripheral vestibular condition (9%) after benign positional vertigo (16%)
Predominant age: All ages beyond infancy
Predominant sex: Male = Female

SIGNS & SYMPTOMS
- Vertigo
- Dizziness
- Hearing loss, fluctuating
- Nausea and vomiting
- Tinnitus
- Perspiration
- Increased salivation
- Generalized malaise
- Hypercapnia
- Nystagmus
- Ataxia

CAUSES
- Physiological - mismatch of vestibular, visual and somatosensory systems triggered by an external stimulus, such as a stop after whirling turns, heights, motion sickness
- Pathological - imbalance in the vestibular system caused by a lesion within vestibular pathways (inner ear to cerebral cortex)
- Infections (especially viral, such as mumps)
- Tumors
- Vasculitis
- Infarction
- Ototoxic drugs, especially aminoglycosides
- Head injury
- Neuronitis

RISK FACTORS
- Trauma
- Stress
- Drug ingestion
- Predisposing virus infection
- Cardiovascular disease
- Cerebrovascular disease

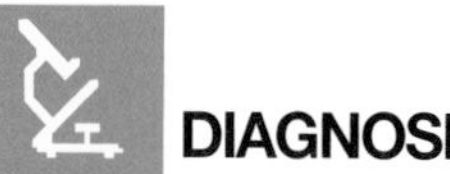

DIAGNOSIS

DIFFERENTIAL DIAGNOSIS
- Acute viral labyrinthitis
- Benign paroxysmal positional vertigo (BPPV)
- Ménière syndrome
- Post-concussive syndrome
- Chronic bacterial otomastoiditis
- Drug-induced damage to vestibular labyrinth
- Vascular insufficiency
- Cerebellopontine-angle tumors, such as acoustic neuroma
- Multiple sclerosis
- Para-infectious encephalomyelitis
- Para-infectious cranial polyneuritis
- Ramsay Hunt syndrome
- Cerebral or systemic vasculitis
- Temporal lobe epilepsy
- HIV infection
- Perilymphatic fistula

LABORATORY Routine laboratory studies not helpful

Drugs that may alter lab results: All drugs with potential ototoxicity

Disorders that may alter lab results: N/A

PATHOLOGICAL FINDINGS N/A

SPECIAL TESTS
- Electronystagmography
- Caloric test
- Doll's eye test
- Forced voluntary hyperventilation for 1 to 3 minutes to mimic symptoms if cause is physiologic or emotional

IMAGING CT or MRI for suspected lesions involving the eighth cranial nerve

DIAGNOSTIC PROCEDURES History and physical

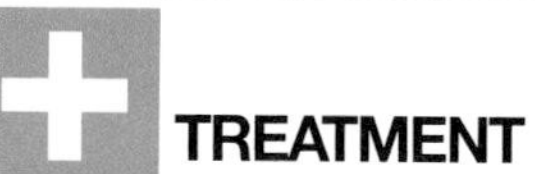

TREATMENT

APPROPRIATE HEALTH CARE Outpatient

GENERAL MEASURES
- Treat underlying disorder when possible
- Symptomatic treatment to accompany specific treatment
- Visual-vestibular exercises for prolonged cases

SURGICAL MEASURES N/A

ACTIVITY
- Lie still with eyes closed in darkened room during acute attacks. Otherwise, activity as tolerated.
- Minimize head movement

DIET Reduced sodium

PATIENT EDUCATION Griffith, H.W.: Instructions for Patients, Philadelphia, W.B. Saunders Co.

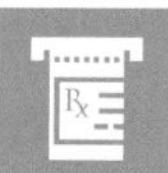

MEDICATIONS

DRUG(S) OF CHOICE
- Meclizine (Antivert) 25 mg qid
- Diazepam (Valium) 5 mg qid
- Promethazine (Phenergan) 25 mg qid
- Prochlorperazine (Compazine) suppositories 25 mg, for vomiting
- Scopolamine transdermal where available

Contraindications: Refer to manufacturer's literature

Precautions: All the listed medications have significant adverse reactions. Use with caution. Avoid scopolamine in the elderly.

Significant possible interactions: Refer to manufacturer's literature

ALTERNATIVE DRUGS N/A

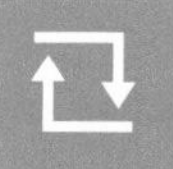

FOLLOWUP

PATIENT MONITORING As needed

PREVENTION/AVOIDANCE No preventive measures

POSSIBLE COMPLICATIONS Permanent hearing loss

EXPECTED COURSE/PROGNOSIS
Depends on cause. Physiological labyrinthitis usually clears completely.

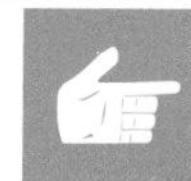

MISCELLANEOUS

ASSOCIATED CONDITIONS
- Ménière disease
- Head injury

AGE-RELATED FACTORS
Pediatric: Unusual in this age group

Geriatric:
- Very common in this age group, especially benign positional vertigo
- Avoid scopolamine or use with extreme caution in this age group

Others: N/A

PREGNANCY Avoid medications

SYNONYMS
- Acute peripheral vestibulopathy
- Vestibular neuronitis
- Vestibular neuritis

ICD-9-CM
386.30 Labyrinthitis, unspecified

SEE ALSO
Ménière disease
Post-concussive syndrome
Ramsay Hunt syndrome, Type 1
Tinnitus

OTHER NOTES N/A

ABBREVIATIONS N/A

REFERENCES

- Baloh RW, Honrobia V. Clinical Neurology of the Vestibular System. 2nd ed. Philadelphia: F.A. Davis Co; 1990
- Rakel RE (ed). Conn's Current therapy. 54th ed. Philadelphia: WB Saunders Co; 2002
- Goetz CG. Textbook of Clinical Neurology. Philadelphia: WB Saunders; 1999
- Noble J. Textbook of Primary Care Medicine. 3rd ed. St. Louis: Mosby, Inc; 2001
- Kroenke K, et al. How common are various causes of dizziness? A critical review. South Med J 2000;93:160-7

Web references: 1 available at www.5mcc.com

Illustrations N/A

Author(s):
Tadao Okada, MD, MPH

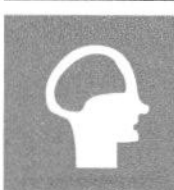

BASICS

DESCRIPTION Lacrimal disorders refer to diseases and abnormalities of tear production and tear film. The most common lacrimal disorder is "dry eye." Lacrimal duct disorders, seen in the pediatric age group, often result in "overflow" tearing.
System(s) affected: Skin/Exocrine
Genetics: None
Incidence/Prevalence in USA: Very common and more often seen in arid climates of the desert Southwest
Predominant age: Dry eye symptoms increase with age. Most common in the elderly.
Predominant sex: Female > Male

SIGNS & SYMPTOMS
- Gritty sensation to the eyes
- Visual blurring
- Redness
- Excessive tearing and mucus production
- Inadequate tears on the ocular surface

CAUSES Poor tear production and/or rapid evaporation of the tears

RISK FACTORS Individuals who live in arid regions, are on diuretics or have a history of collagen vascular diseases such as rheumatoid arthritis, Sjögren syndrome, Bell palsy, eyelid abnormalities and thyroid disease, are most at risk.

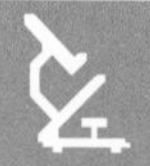

DIAGNOSIS

DIFFERENTIAL DIAGNOSIS Lacrimal disorders need to be differentiated from ocular infections and allergy. Another important consideration is the variety of anticholinergic affecting drugs that decrease tear production.

LABORATORY Tear production can be measured using a Schirmer's filter strip after instillation of topical anesthetic. Wetting of less than 10 mm of the slip after 5 minutes is indicative of insufficient tear production.

Drugs that may alter lab results: N/A

Disorders that may alter lab results: N/A

PATHOLOGICAL FINDINGS In Sjögren syndrome infiltration of the lacrimal gland with inflammatory cells may be evident

SPECIAL TESTS N/A

IMAGING None

DIAGNOSTIC PROCEDURES Staining of the ocular surface with fluorescein will show areas of abnormal uptake and patches of drying. Rose bengal will be taken up by dead or dying epithelial cells and may be a more sensitive test.

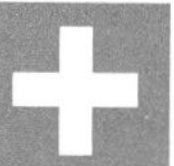

TREATMENT

APPROPRIATE HEALTH CARE Outpatient

GENERAL MEASURES
- Those with systemic illnesses predisposed to dry eye should be informed and instructed in the appropriate use of artificial tear supplements
- Cool mist vaporizer and home humidification is helpful

SURGICAL MEASURES N/A

ACTIVITY No restrictions

DIET No special diet

PATIENT EDUCATION All individuals with systemic illnesses predisposed to dry eye, menopausal women, and those residing in arid climates or over the age of 60 should be instructed in the use of artificial tear supplements to combat dry eye symptoms

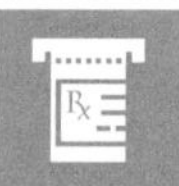

MEDICATIONS

DRUG(S) OF CHOICE
- Artificial tear drops excluding those that have preservatives. The dosage of the drop varies depending on the severity of the symptoms. Usually one drop in each eye several times throughout the day can prevent ocular discomfort.
- The use of a bland ophthalmic ointment at bedtime between the eyelid and the eye can help prevent drying of the eye at night
- Vitamin A supplements

Contraindications: N/A
Precautions: N/A
Significant possible interactions: N/A

ALTERNATIVE DRUGS N/A

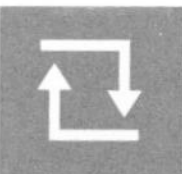

FOLLOWUP

PATIENT MONITORING Monitor early to determine the effectiveness of treatment. Occasionally the use of more viscous drops or increased frequency of tear supplements may be required.

PREVENTION/AVOIDANCE
- Prevent exposure to eye irritants from pollution, cigarette smoke, and sun exposure
- Ensure adequate vitamin A intake in the diet or as a supplement

POSSIBLE COMPLICATIONS Severe dry eye can lead to corneal break-down, secondary invasion by bacteria and eye infections

EXPECTED COURSE/PROGNOSIS
Lacrimal disorders can be adequately managed with artificial tear supplements. Blocked tear ducts can be managed with probing and punctal dilation and/or dacryocystorhinostomy procedures in more severe cases.

MISCELLANEOUS

ASSOCIATED CONDITIONS Sjögren syndrome and age-related factors more commonly seen in the elderly population

AGE-RELATED FACTORS
Pediatric: May find lacrimal duct blockage in infants
Geriatric: Most common in this age group
Others: N/A

PREGNANCY Dry eyes can frequently be associated with pregnancy in an otherwise healthy individual. Vitamin A intake should not exceed 6000 IU a day.

SYNONYMS Epiphora (excessive tearing)

ICD-9-CM
375.11 Dacryops
375.15 Tear film insufficiency, unspecified

SEE ALSO
Sjögren syndrome

OTHER NOTES Symptoms of dry eye are most often overlooked by practitioners when considering conjunctivitis (pink eye) and allergic disorders

ABBREVIATIONS N/A

REFERENCES

- Orbit Eyelids And Lacrimal System, Basic and Clinical Course. San Francisco, American Academy of Ophthalmology

Web references: 0 available at www.5mcc.com
Illustrations N/A

Author(s):
Robert M. Kershner, MD

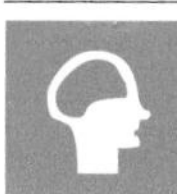

BASICS

DESCRIPTION Inability to digest lactose (the primary sugar in milk) into its constituents, glucose and galactose, due to low levels of lactase enzyme in the brush border of the duodenum
- Congenital lactose intolerance - very rare
- Primary lactose intolerance - common in adults in whom a low level of lactase has developed after childhood. Symptoms are experienced after consumption of milk. Intolerance varies with amount of lactose consumed.
- Secondary lactose intolerance - inability to digest lactose caused by any condition injuring the intestinal mucosa (e.g., diarrhea) or a reduction of available mucosal surface (e.g., resection). This is usually transient, with the duration of the intolerance determined by the nature and course of the primary condition.
- 50% or more of infants with acute or chronic diarrhea have lactose intolerance, especially with rotavirus disease. Also, fairly common with giardiasis and ascariasis, inflammatory bowel disease, and the AIDS malabsorption syndrome.
- Lactose malabsorption - inability to absorb lactose. This does not necessarily parallel lactose intolerance.

System(s) affected: Endocrine/Metabolic, Gastrointestinal
Genetics: Unknown
Incidence/Prevalence in USA:
- Primary lactose intolerance - varies according to race. 75-90% of American Indians, blacks, Asians, Mediterraneans and Jews, less than 5% of descendants of Northern and Central Europeans.
- Secondary lactose intolerance - 50% or more of infants with acute or chronic diarrheal disease have lactose intolerance, especially with rotavirus disease. Also fairly common with giardiasis and ascariasis, inflammatory bowel disease and the AIDS malabsorptive syndrome.

Predominant age:
- Primary - teenage and adult
- Secondary - depends on the underlying condition

Predominant sex: Male = Female. However, 44% of lactose intolerant women will regain the ability to digest lactose during pregnancy.

SIGNS & SYMPTOMS
- Bloating
- Cramping
- Abdominal discomfort
- Diarrhea or loose stools
- Flatulence
- Rumbling (borborygmi)
- Only one-third to one-fifth of people with lactose malabsorption will develop symptoms. Degree of symptoms varies with lactose load and with other foods consumed at the same time.
- In children - vomiting is common; frothy, acid stools; malnutrition can occur

CAUSES
- Primary lactose intolerance - normal decline in the lactase activity in the intestinal mucosa after weaning which is genetically controlled and permanent
- Secondary lactose intolerance - associated with gastroenteritis in children
- Also nontropical and tropical sprue, regional enteritis, abetalipoproteinemia, cystic fibrosis, ulcerative colitis, immunoglobulin deficiencies in both adults and children

RISK FACTORS
- Race
- Age

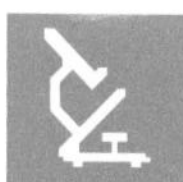

DIAGNOSIS

DIFFERENTIAL DIAGNOSIS
- Sucrase deficiency
- Diseases listed under secondary lactose intolerance
- Irritable bowel syndrome

LABORATORY Low fecal pH and reducing substances only valid when stools are collected fresh and assayed immediately. Fairly insensitive.

Drugs that may alter lab results: None

Disorders that may alter lab results: None

PATHOLOGICAL FINDINGS Lactase deficiency in intestinal mucosa - may be patchy or focal. Rarely used in clinical practice.

SPECIAL TESTS
- Lactose breath hydrogen test - especially in children
- Lactose absorption test - alternative to lactose breath hydrogen test in adults

IMAGING None

DIAGNOSTIC PROCEDURES Small bowel biopsy for assay of lactase activity - may be normal if deficiency is focal or patchy (not readily available and usually not necessary)

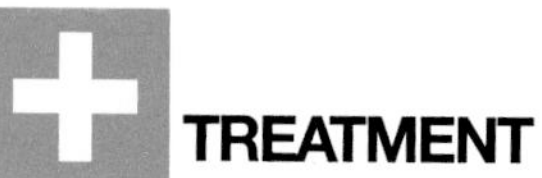

TREATMENT

APPROPRIATE HEALTH CARE Outpatient except severe cases of malnutrition

GENERAL MEASURES No disease specific measures

SURGICAL MEASURES N/A

ACTIVITY Full activity

DIET
- Reduce or restrict dietary lactose to control symptoms
- Yogurt and fermented products such as hard cheeses are tolerated better than milk
- Supplement calcium in the form of calcium carbonate
- Commercially available "lactase" preparations (Lactaid or Lactrase) are effective in reducing symptoms in many people
- Prehydrolyzed milk (Lactaid) is available and effective

PATIENT EDUCATION
- Patients must read labels on commercial products since milk-sugar is used in many products and may cause symptoms
- Lactose intolerant patients may tolerate whole milk or chocolate milk better than skim
- Lactose consumed with other food products is better tolerated than when it is consumed alone
- Primary lactase deficiency is permanent; secondary lactose intolerance is usually temporary, though it may persist for several months after the inciting disease has been cured.
- 20% of prescription drugs and 6% of OTC medicines use lactose as a base

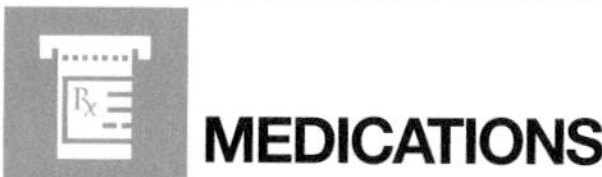

MEDICATIONS

DRUG(S) OF CHOICE
- Lactase (Lactaid, Lactrase) tablets
  - ◊ 1 to 2 capsules or tablets prior to ingesting milk products. These vary in effectiveness at preventing symptoms.
  - ◊ Can add tablets or contents of capsules to milk before drinking
  - ◊ Also available in milk in some areas

Contraindications: None
Precautions: Not effective for all people with lactose intolerance
Significant possible interactions: None

ALTERNATIVE DRUGS
None

FOLLOWUP

PATIENT MONITORING
N/A

PREVENTION/AVOIDANCE
Avoidance of lactose in large quantities will relieve symptoms. Patients can learn what level of lactose is tolerable in their diet.

POSSIBLE COMPLICATIONS
Calcium deficiency

EXPECTED COURSE/PROGNOSIS
- Normal life expectancy
- Symptoms can be controlled

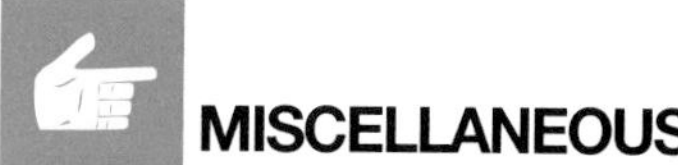

MISCELLANEOUS

ASSOCIATED CONDITIONS
- Tropical or nontropical sprue
- Giardiasis
- Immunoglobulin deficiencies
- Crohn disease
- Cystic fibrosis

AGE-RELATED FACTORS
Pediatric:
- Primary lactose intolerance occurs after weaning - usually beginning in late childhood
- Breast milk contains a large quantity of lactose but does not seem to worsen diarrhea associated with viral or bacterial diseases
- Lactose free formulas are available

Geriatric: No increase in lactose intolerance in this age group
Others: Secondary lactose intolerance can begin at any age

PREGNANCY
44% of lactose intolerant women will be able to tolerate lactose while pregnant

SYNONYMS
Lactase deficiency

ICD-9-CM
271.3 Intestinal disaccharidase deficiencies and disaccharide malabsorption

SEE ALSO

OTHER NOTES
N/A

ABBREVIATIONS
N/A

REFERENCES

- Patel YT, Minocha A. Lactose intolerance: diagnosis and management. Compr Ther 2000;26(4):246-50
- Vesa TH, Marteau P, Korpela R. Lactose intolerance. J Am Coll Nutr 2000;19(2 Suppl):165S-175S

Web references: 2 available at www.5mcc.com
Illustrations N/A

Author(s):
Kathryn Reilly, MD, MPH

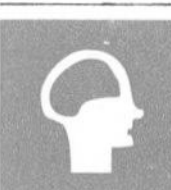

BASICS

DESCRIPTION Most common cancer representing less than 1% of all malignant lesions. Squamous cell carcinomas comprise 5-98% of all malignant neoplasms of the larynx.
- Less than 2% of all carcinomas
- At the time of diagnosis, 62% will have local disease, 26% regional disease and 8% distant disease in the lungs, liver and/or bone
- No racial predilection

System(s) affected: Pulmonary
Genetics: Unknown
Incidence/Prevalence in USA: 5/100,00 (12,500 new cases per year)
Predominant age:
- Median age of occurrence in the 6th and 7th decades
- Less than 1% of laryngeal cancers arise in patients under 30 years of age

Predominant sex: Male > Female (5:1). However, increasing incidence in women who smoke.

SIGNS & SYMPTOMS
- Persistent hoarseness in an elderly or middle aged cigarette smoker
- Dyspnea and stridor
- Ipsilateral otalgia
- Dysphagia
- Odynophagia
- Chronic cough
- Hemoptysis
- Weight loss due to poor nutrition
- Halitosis due to tumor necrosis
- Mass in the neck from metastatic lymph node
- Laryngeal tenderness due to tumor necrosis or suppuration
- Lump in the neck
- Broadening of the larynx on palpation with loss of crepitation
- Tenderness of the larynx
- Fullness of the cricothyroid membrane

CAUSES
- Smoking
- Alcohol abuse

RISK FACTORS Included in Causes

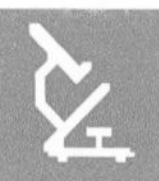

DIAGNOSIS

DIFFERENTIAL DIAGNOSIS
- Acute or chronic laryngitis
- Benign vocal cord lesions such as polyps, nodules, and papillomas
- Tuberculosis or fungal infection of the larynx

LABORATORY Liver function studies to rule out metastatic disease

Drugs that may alter lab results: N/A

Disorders that may alter lab results: N/A

PATHOLOGICAL FINDINGS N/A

SPECIAL TESTS
- Laryngoscopy - fungating, friable tumor with heaped up edges and granular appearance with multiple areas of central necrosis and exudate surrounding areas of hyperemia
- CT or MRI if chest and liver or brain metastasis suspected

IMAGING
- Bone scan if bone metastasis suspected
- Screening chest x-ray to rule out metastatic disease

DIAGNOSTIC PROCEDURES Indirect and/or direct laryngoscopy and biopsy to determine stage of disease as well as histologic confirmation

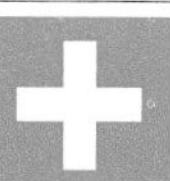

TREATMENT

APPROPRIATE HEALTH CARE Outpatient primarily

GENERAL MEASURES Tracheotomy care, when applicable

SURGICAL MEASURES
- Tracheotomy may be necessary if tumor is large enough to cause upper airway obstruction
- Early disease may be treatable by either radiation therapy or laser cordectomy on an outpatient basis. 90% cure rates are the rule.
- More advanced disease needs inpatient care necessitating partial or total laryngectomy, and postoperative radiation therapy 4-5 weeks after surgery depending on the stage of disease

ACTIVITY Fully active unless the patient is debilitated from more advanced disease and/or greater degree of surgery

DIET
- Nasogastric or gastrostomy feeding may be necessary if tumor involves esophageal inlet
- No special diet otherwise

PATIENT EDUCATION Material is available from local cancer society

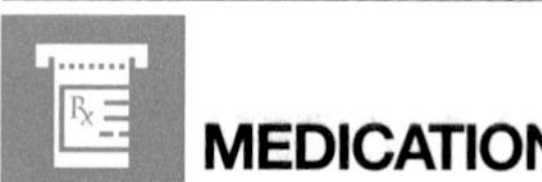

MEDICATIONS

DRUG(S) OF CHOICE
- Narcotics may be necessary for pain control during treatment for mucositis secondary to radiation therapy
- Nystatin mouth rinses for oral thrush

Contraindications: N/A
Precautions: N/A
Significant possible interactions: N/A

ALTERNATIVE DRUGS N/A

FOLLOWUP

PATIENT MONITORING
- Repeat indirect laryngoscopy and complete head and neck examinations for at least five years after treatment to detect early recurrence or second primary
- Yearly chest x-ray and liver function tests
- Patients with dysphagia should undergo barium swallow and/or esophageal endoscopy to rule out second tumor in the esophagus
- Patients with unexplained pain should have appropriate radiological or nuclear medicine, bone scans
- Mental status change indicates CT scan of the brain to rule out brain metastases

PREVENTION/AVOIDANCE
- Indirect laryngoscopy for patients with persistent hoarseness lasting beyond one to two weeks
- Cessation of smoking and/or alcohol abuse

POSSIBLE COMPLICATIONS
- Temporary odynophagia or dysphagia secondary to mucositis and/or thrush during radiation therapy
- Persistent hoarseness despite adequate treatment necessitating further adjunctive procedures and/or speech therapy
- Tracheostomal stenosis requiring stenting with laryngectomy tubes or further surgery
- Dysphagia, secondary to upper esophageal stricture after total laryngectomy necessitating dilatation
- Aspiration, after partial laryngectomy necessitating completion laryngectomy or tracheotomy
- Inability to decannulate after partial laryngectomy due to laryngeal stenosis and/or aspiration
- Radiation induced chondronecrosis which mimics tumor recurrence
- Radiation edema necessitating emergent tracheotomy

EXPECTED COURSE/PROGNOSIS
- Early disease is expected to have greater than 90% cure

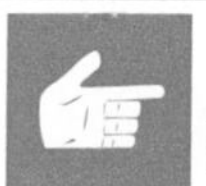

MISCELLANEOUS

ASSOCIATED CONDITIONS
- Less than 10% of patients may have a synchronous squamous cell carcinoma in the lower or upper aerodigestive tract; most notably in the esophagus or lungs

AGE-RELATED FACTORS
Pediatric: N/A
Geriatric: N/A
Others: N/A

PREGNANCY
- Very rare in young patients in general
- Natural history of disease and treatment side effects have to be weighed against the possibilities of continuing on to delivery

SYNONYMS Cancer of larynx

ICD-9-CM
161.9 Malignant neoplasm of larynx, unspecified

SEE ALSO

OTHER NOTES N/A

ABBREVIATIONS N/A

REFERENCES

- Cumming CW, Fredrickson JM, et al, eds. Otolaryngology Head and Neck Surgery, Vol 3. New York, C.V. Mosby Co, 1998
- Suen JY, Myers EN: Cancer of the Head and Neck. 3rd Ed. Philadelphia, WB Saunders Co, 1996
- Ariyan S: Cancer of the Head and Neck. St. Louis, C.V. Mosby, 1987

Web references: 2 available at www.5mcc.com
Illustrations N/A

Author(s):
Roy R. Casiano, MD

BASICS

DESCRIPTION Inflammation of the mucosa of the larynx. Most common during peaks paralleling epidemics of individual viruses, late fall, winter, early spring. In predisposed individuals may also occur intermittently during period of vocal misuse or abuse. Course may be acute or chronic. Includes atrophic, hypertrophic, reflux, catarrhal, sicca, acute infectious, membranous, granulomatous.
System(s) affected: Pulmonary
Genetics: No known genetic pattern
Incidence/Prevalence in USA: Common
Predominant age: All ages
Predominant sex: Male = Female

SIGNS & SYMPTOMS
- Hoarseness
- Abnormal sounding voice
- Aphonia or dysphasia
- Throat tickling
- Feeling of throat rawness
- Constant urge to clear the throat
- Fever
- Malaise
- Dysphagia
- Odynophagia
- Cough
- Regional lymphadenopathy
- Stridor in children
- Referred otalgia

CAUSES
- Virus infections - influenza A, B, parainfluenza, adenovirus, coronavirus, rhinovirus, HPV, CMV, HSV, RSV, Coxsackie
- Bacterial infections - beta-hemolytic streptococcus, Streptococcus pneumoniae, H. influenza, tuberculosis, leprosy, Moraxella catarrhalis
- Misuse or abuse of voice
- Inhaling irritating substances (eg, air pollution)
- Aspiration of caustic chemical
- Aging changes - muscle atrophy, loss of moisture in larynx, bowing of vocal cords
- Esophageal reflux
- Fungal infections: Histoplasmosis, blastomycosis and Candida
- Parasites
- Spirochetes (syphilis)
- Allergic
- Autoimmune
- Idiopathic
- Vocal cord nodules/polyps - "singer's nodes"
- Injury or compression of recurrent laryngeal nerve
- Retropharyngeal abscess
- Tumor
- Trauma - e.g., endotracheal intubation

RISK FACTORS
- Acute
  - ◊ Upper respiratory tract infection
  - ◊ Bronchitis
  - ◊ Pneumonia
  - ◊ Influenza
  - ◊ Pertussis
  - ◊ Measles
  - ◊ Diphtheria
  - ◊ Immunocompromised
- Chronic
  - ◊ Allergy
  - ◊ Chronic rhinitis
  - ◊ Chronic sinusitis
  - ◊ Voice abuse
  - ◊ Reflux of gastric contents
  - ◊ Smoking
  - ◊ Alcohol abuse
  - ◊ Constant exposure to dust or other irritants
  - ◊ Previous endotracheal intubation

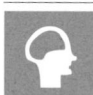

DIAGNOSIS

DIFFERENTIAL DIAGNOSIS
- Croup
- Measles
- Diphtheria
- Vocal nodules or polyps
- Laryngeal malignancy
- Thyroid malignancy
- Gastroesophageal reflux
- Epiglottitis

LABORATORY WBC elevated in bacterial laryngitis

Drugs that may alter lab results: N/A

Disorders that may alter lab results: N/A

PATHOLOGICAL FINDINGS N/A

SPECIAL TESTS Virus culture (seldom necessary)

IMAGING Only if needed for differential diagnosis

DIAGNOSTIC PROCEDURES
- Fiberoptic or indirect laryngoscopy - red, inflamed and occasionally hemorrhagic vocal cords, with rounded edges, and exudate (Reinke's edema)
- Consider otolaryngologic evaluation and biopsy - laryngitis of greater than 2 weeks in adults with history of smoking or alcohol abuse
- Consider 24 hour pH probe - chronic laryngitis in adults with gastroesophageal reflux
- Strobovideo laryngoscopy - for diagnosis of subtle lesions

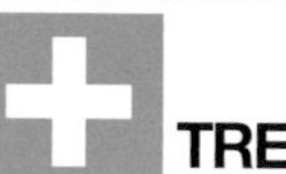

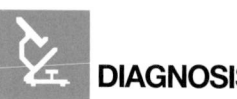

TREATMENT

APPROPRIATE HEALTH CARE Outpatient

GENERAL MEASURES
- Acute
  - ◊ Usually a self-limited illness and not severe
  - ◊ Vocal conservation without excessive voice use
  - ◊ Steam inhalations or cool-mist humidifier
  - ◊ Increase fluid intake
  - ◊ Analgesics
  - ◊ Avoid smoking (or second hand exposure)
- Chronic
  - ◊ Symptomatic treatment as above
  - ◊ Voice therapy (for patients with intermittent dysphagia and vocal abuse)
  - ◊ Stop smoking
  - ◊ Reduce alcohol intake
  - ◊ Occupational change or modification, if exposure
  - ◊ For reflux laryngitis - elevate head of bed, other antireflux management
- Consider otolaryngology consultation for:
  - ◊ Hoarseness > 2-3 weeks
  - ◊ Hoarseness associated with hemoptysis, difficulty swallowing or breathing, or a lump in neck
  - ◊ Loss or severe voice change for more than a few days
  - ◊ Professional singer

SURGICAL MEASURES
- Vocal cord biopsy of hyperplastic mucosa and areas of leukoplakia if cancer or TB is suspected
- Removal of nodules or polyps if voice therapy fails

ACTIVITY Rest until fever subsides then, no restrictions

DIET No special diet

PATIENT EDUCATION
- Provide assistance with smoking cessation
- Help patient with modification of other predisposing habits or occupational hazards

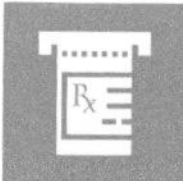

MEDICATIONS

DRUG(S) OF CHOICE
- Usually none
- Analgesics
- Antipyretics
- Cough suppressants
- Penicillin V 250 mg or erythromycin 250 mg - orally q6h for 10-12 days (for streptococcal or pneumococcal infections)
- Antacids or H2 blockers for GERD. Dosage may have to be doubled in cases with symptoms suggestive of pharyngeal or laryngeal reflux disease.
- Consider empiric PPI for chronic laryngitis without obvious reflux symptoms

Contraindications: Refer to manufacturer's literature
Precautions: Refer to manufacturer's literature
Significant possible interactions: Refer to manufacturer's literature

ALTERNATIVE DRUGS N/A

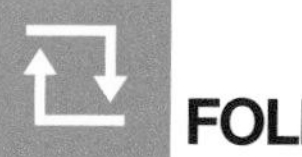

FOLLOWUP

PATIENT MONITORING None needed (usually)

PREVENTION/AVOIDANCE
- Avoid overuse of voice
- Prompt treatment of respiratory infections
- Influenza virus vaccine for high-risk individuals
- Quit smoking
- Avoid alcohol and caffeine
- Maintain proper hydration status

POSSIBLE COMPLICATIONS Chronic hoarseness

EXPECTED COURSE/PROGNOSIS
Complete clearing of the inflammation without sequelae

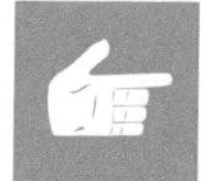

MISCELLANEOUS

ASSOCIATED CONDITIONS
- Viral pharyngitis
- Croup
- Bronchitis
- Pneumonitis

AGE-RELATED FACTORS
Pediatric: Common in this age group
Geriatric: May be sicker and slower to heal
Others: N/A

PREGNANCY Use only safe antibiotics, if antibiotics are essential

SYNONYMS
- Acute laryngitis
- Chronic laryngitis

ICD-9-CM
464.00 Acute laryngitis without mention of obstruction
464.01 Acute laryngitis with obstruction
476.0 Chronic laryngitis

SEE ALSO

OTHER NOTES N/A

ABBREVIATIONS
PPI = proton pump inhibitor

REFERENCES

- Avila MM, Carballal G, Rovaletti H, et al. Viral etiology in acute respiratory infections. Am Rev Respir Dis 1989;140:634
- Adams GL, et al. Fundamentals of Otolaryngology. 6th ed. Philadelphia: W.B. Saunders Co.; 1989
- Ballenger JI, Snow JB, editors. Otorhinolaryngology Head and Neck Surgery. 15 ed. Philadelphia: Williams & Wilkins; 1996
- Banfiels G, Tandon F, Solomons N. Hoarse voice: an early symptom of many conditions. Practitioner 2000;244:267-71
- Rosen CA, Anderson D, Murry T. Evaluating Hoarseness: Keeping Your Patient's Voice Healthy. Am Fam Phys 1998;57(11):2775-82
- Braunwald E, Fauci AS, Kasper DL, Hauser SL, Longo DL, Jameson JL, editors. Harrison's Principles of Internal Medicine, 15th edition, New York, McGraw-Hill; 2001
- Neuenschwander MC, et al. Laryngeal candidiasis. Ear Nose Throat J 2001;80(3):138-9
- El-Serag HB, Hepworth EJ, Lee P, Sonnenberg A. Lansoprazole treatment of patients with chronic idiopathic laryngitis: a placebo-controlled trial. Am J Gastro 2001;96(4):979-83

Web references: 0 available at www.5mcc.com
Illustrations N/A

Author(s):
Bruce T. Vanderhoff, MD
Rohit Uppal, MD

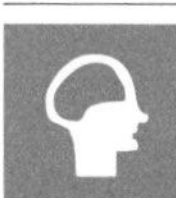

BASICS

DESCRIPTION Subacute viral illness, characterized by barking cough, stridor and fever, often causing upper airway obstruction in children. Most common cause of stridor in children.
System(s) affected: Pulmonary
Genetics: Unknown, though 15% have family history
Incidence/Prevalence in USA: 15,000-40,000/100,000
Predominant age: Childhood
Predominant sex: Male = Female

SIGNS & SYMPTOMS
- Barking, spasmodic cough
- Biphasic stridor
- Low-grade to moderate fever
- Upper respiratory infection prodrome lasting 1-7 days
- Hypoxia/cyanosis
- Fatigue
- Non-toxic appearing child
- Normal voice, no drooling
- No change in stridor with positioning
- Non-tender larynx
- Inflamed subglottic region
- Normal appearing supraglottic region

CAUSES
- Parainfluenza 1
- Paramyxovirus
- Influenza virus type A
- Other parainfluenza and influenza viruses
- Respiratory syncytial virus
- Other viruses - adenovirus, rhinovirus, enterovirus, coxsackievirus, ECHO virus, reovirus, measles virus

RISK FACTORS
- Past history of croup
- Recurrent upper respiratory infections

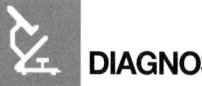

DIAGNOSIS

DIFFERENTIAL DIAGNOSIS
- Epiglottitis
- Foreign body aspiration
- Subglottic stenosis (congenital or acquired)
- Bacterial tracheitis
- Simple upper respiratory infection
- Subglottic hemangioma
- Diphtheria

LABORATORY
- Leukopenia early
- Leukocytosis in severe later stage

Drugs that may alter lab results: N/A

Disorders that may alter lab results: N/A

PATHOLOGICAL FINDINGS
- Inflammatory reaction of respiratory mucosa
- Loss of epithelial cells
- Thick mucoid secretions

SPECIAL TESTS Rapid antigen tests are available in some centers

IMAGING
- PA and lateral neck films show funnel-shaped subglottic region with normal epiglottis - "steeple sign" or "pencil-point sign" (present in 40% of children with LTB)
- Patient should be monitored during imaging - progression of airway obstruction may be rapid

DIAGNOSTIC PROCEDURES
- Direct laryngoscopy - if child is not in acute distress
- Fiberoptic laryngoscopy - procedure of choice where available
- Bronchoscopy

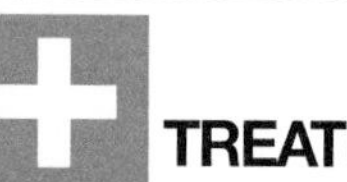

TREATMENT

APPROPRIATE HEALTH CARE
- Outpatient in mild cases only
- Intensive care unit for patients with tachypnea, tachycardia, hypoxia, cyanosis, reactions, pneumonia, or congestive heart failure

GENERAL MEASURES
- Intravenous fluids
- Electrocardiographic monitoring and pulse oximetry

SURGICAL MEASURES
- Intubation required in 6-10% for 3-5 days; use smallest tube possible
- Tracheotomy - rarely

ACTIVITY Must keep patient quiet; crying may exacerbate symptoms

DIET
- NPO with IV fluids for severe cases
- Frequent small feedings with increased fluids for mild cases

PATIENT EDUCATION
- Educate parents about when to seek emergency care if mild cases progress
- Emotional support and reassurance for the patient

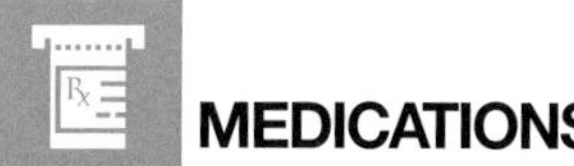

MEDICATIONS

DRUG(S) OF CHOICE
- Dexamethasone: 0.6 mg/kg/day
- Racemic epinephrine (Vaponefrin): 0.2-0.5 mL of 2.25 percent racemic epinephrine delivered in 2-3 mL of normal saline - one dose per 30 minutes, monitoring for side effects and rebound
- Antibiotics controversial in this viral illness
- Oxygen as needed

Contraindications: Refer to manufacturer's literature
Precautions: Avoid over sedation
Significant possible interactions: Refer to manufacturer's literature

ALTERNATIVE DRUGS
- Budesonide 2 mg nebulized; a topical glucocorticoid
- Amantadine for influenza A

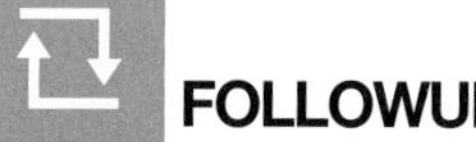

FOLLOWUP

PATIENT MONITORING Severe cases require ICU care with respiratory monitoring for hypoxemia and hypercapnia

PREVENTION/AVOIDANCE N/A

POSSIBLE COMPLICATIONS
- Subglottic stenosis in intubated patients
- Bacterial tracheitis
- Cardiopulmonary arrest
- Pneumonia

EXPECTED COURSE/PROGNOSIS
- Upper respiratory infection prodrome of 1-7 days
- If required, intubation is maintained for 3-5 days
- If required, tracheotomy is maintained for 3-7 days
- Recovery is usually full, without lasting effects

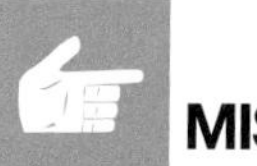

MISCELLANEOUS

ASSOCIATED CONDITIONS If recurrent, search for underlying anatomic abnormality such as subglottic stenosis or consider foreign body

AGE-RELATED FACTORS
Pediatric: Common in children under the age of three
Geriatric: N/A
Others: N/A

PREGNANCY N/A

SYNONYMS
- Croup
- Infectious croup
- Viral croup
- LTB

ICD-9-CM
464.20 Acute laryngotracheitis without mention of obstruction
464.21 Acute laryngotracheitis with obstruction
476.1 Chronic laryngotracheitis

SEE ALSO
Bronchiolitis
Common cold
Epiglottitis
Tracheitis, bacterial

OTHER NOTES Less severe " variant" form, spasmodic croup, consists of croupy cough which becomes worse at night, but has no fever or x-ray changes. Usually resolves with mist therapy at home.

ABBREVIATIONS LTB = laryngotracheobronchitis

REFERENCES

- Ballenger JJ. Diseases of the Nose, Throat and Ear. Philadelphia, Lea & Febiger, 1991
- Gates GA. Current Therapy in Otolaryngology - Head and Neck Surgery. 5th Ed. Philadelphia, B.C. Decker, Inc., 1993

Web references: 0 available at www.5mcc.com
Illustrations N/A

Author(s):
Gregg W. Suits, MD

BASICS

DESCRIPTION Diarrhea caused by self-medication or by a patient simulating diarrhea by the addition of fluid (e.g., urine) to the stool.
System(s) affected: Gastrointestinal, Nervous
Genetics: N/A
Incidence/Prevalence in USA: N/A
Predominant age:
- 18 to 40 years with bulimia nervosa
- 40 to 60 years without bulimia.

Predominant sex: Female > Male

SIGNS & SYMPTOMS
- Diarrhea
- Additional symptoms - abdominal pain, rectal pain, nausea, vomiting, weight loss, muscle weakness, bone pain
- Additional signs - hypokalemia, skin pigmentation, finger clubbing, cyclic edema, kidney stones, melanosis coli
- The signs and symptoms will persist in spite of years of investigation and re-evaluation

CAUSES
- Ingestion of any laxative agent
- Psychological factors
  - ◊ Bulimia nervosa
  - ◊ Secondary gain of attention
  - ◊ Hysterical behavior
  - ◊ Multiple personality disorders
  - ◊ Inappropriate perception of "normal" bowel habits
- Chronic constipation

RISK FACTORS See Causes

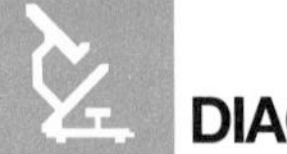

DIAGNOSIS

DIFFERENTIAL DIAGNOSIS Include any source of diarrhea of secretory or osmotic source

LABORATORY
- Serum test - hypokalemia, metabolic alkalosis
- Urinalysis may be abnormal
- Stool Na+, K+
- Stool pH (alkalinization suggests presence of phenolphthalein)
- Stool for laxative titers
- Urine volume and electrolytes

Drugs that may alter lab results: N/A

Disorders that may alter lab results: N/A

PATHOLOGICAL FINDINGS
- Melanosis coli
- "Cathartic colon" - refers to dilation and ahaustral appearance on barium enema

SPECIAL TESTS Hospital room search

IMAGING Barium enema - cathartic colon

DIAGNOSTIC PROCEDURES
- Carefully selected when needed to rule out other diseases
- Try not to repeat prior evaluations
- Sigmoidoscopy
- High index of suspicion

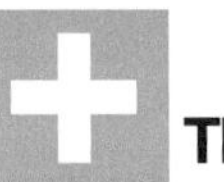

TREATMENT

APPROPRIATE HEALTH CARE Hospitalization may be needed (hypokalemia, malnutrition)

GENERAL MEASURES
- Psychological support is essential
- Confrontation of the patient, gently and with support and understanding
- Discontinue laxative use
- Long term laxative abuse requires weaning
- Treat constipation

SURGICAL MEASURES N/A

ACTIVITY Physical exercise program

DIET
- Ensure good nutritional habits
  - ◊ Increase fiber intake
  - ◊ Adequate calories, especially with bulimia

PATIENT EDUCATION See General Measures

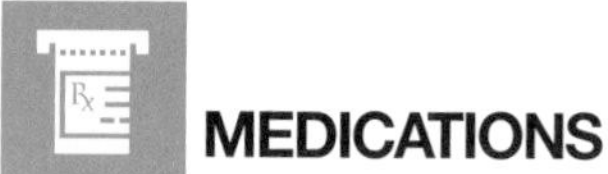

MEDICATIONS

DRUG(S) OF CHOICE
- Based on psychological assessment
- Non-stimulant laxatives if needed
  - ◊ Senna best during pregnancy and lactation
  - ◊ Lactulose
  - ◊ Fiber

Contraindications: Danthron - hepatotoxic
Precautions: Patients will be manipulative in attempts to hide problem, and often large quantities of laxatives
Significant possible interactions:
- Increased rate of intestinal flow may affect rate of absorption of medications: antibiotics, hormones, etc.
- Docusate sodium may potentiate hepatotoxicity of other drugs

ALTERNATIVE DRUGS N/A

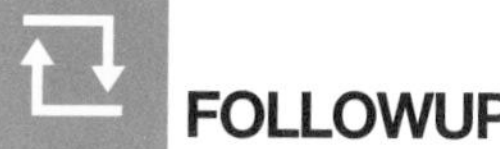

FOLLOWUP

PATIENT MONITORING
- Careful psychological counseling
- Careful medical support. Show concern by frequent visits as needed.
- Assess serum electrolytes

PREVENTION/AVOIDANCE
- Suspicion in patients with unsolved chronic diarrhea
- Monitor "doctor hopping"
- Avoid exploratory surgery
- Avoid repeated testing for diagnosis

POSSIBLE COMPLICATIONS
- Risk of multiple tests and procedures and surgeries
- Malnutrition
- Electrolyte imbalances (hypokalemia)
- Renal failure
- Fatalities especially in children given laxatives by parents
- Renal calculi

EXPECTED COURSE/PROGNOSIS
- Protracted course
- Prognosis related to psychological response

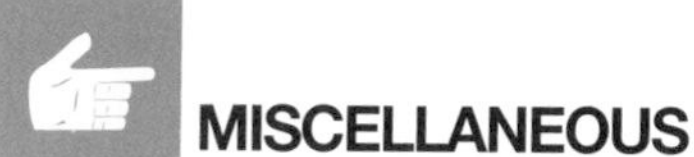

MISCELLANEOUS

ASSOCIATED CONDITIONS N/A

AGE-RELATED FACTORS
Pediatric:
- Death
- Life long laxative dependence

Geriatric:
- Unusual to start beyond age of 60 years
- Rectal incontinence

Others: N/A

PREGNANCY N/A

SYNONYMS
- Factitious diarrhea
- Cathartic colon

ICD-9-CM
305.90 Other, mixed, or unspecified drug abuse, unspecified

SEE ALSO
Bulimia nervosa
Constipation
Hypokalemia
Renal calculi
Renal failure, acute (ARF)
Renal failure, chronic

OTHER NOTES N/A

ABBREVIATIONS N/A

REFERENCES

- Sleisenger MH, Fordtran JS., eds: Gastrointestinal Disease: Pathophysiology, Diagnosis, Management. 6th Ed. Philadelphia, WB Saunders Co, 1998
- Baker EH, Sandle GI: Complications of laxative abuse. Ann Rev of Med 1996;47:127
- Batal H, Johnson M, et al: Bulimia: a primary care approach. J Women's Health 1998;7(2):211

Web references: 2 available at www.5mcc.com
Illustrations N/A

Author(s):
Duane C. Roe, MD

BASICS

DESCRIPTION Consequence of a high body burden of lead, an element with no known physiologic value

System(s) affected: Endocrine/Metabolic, Gastrointestinal, Nervous

Genetics: N/A

Incidence/Prevalence in USA:
- 17% of preschoolers in the US have a blood lead greater than 15 μg/dL (0.72 μmol/L). Sporadic cases in adults.
- Estimated (1990's) in children 6 months to age 5 years (≥ 15 μg/dL [0.72 μmol/L]): 17,000/100,000

Predominant age: 1-5 years old; adult worker

Predominant sex: Male = Female

SIGNS & SYMPTOMS
- Often asymptomatic
- Mild to moderate toxicity
  - ◊ May cause myalgia or paresthesia, fatigue, irritability, lethargy
  - ◊ Abdominal discomfort, arthralgia, difficulty concentrating, headache, tremor, vomiting, weight loss, muscular exhaustibility
- Severe toxicity - leads to 3 major clinical syndromes
  - ◊ Alimentary type - anorexia, metallic taste, constipation, severe abdominal cramps due to intestinal spasm and sometimes associated with rigidity of the abdominal wall
  - ◊ Neuromuscular type (characteristic of adult plumbism) - peripheral neuritis usually painless and limited to extensor muscles
  - ◊ Cerebral type or lead encephalopathy (more common in children) - seizures, coma, long-term sequelae including neurologic defects, retarded mental development, chronic hyperactivity
  - ◊ Chronic exposure may cause renal failure

CAUSES Inhalation of lead dust or fumes, or ingestion of lead

RISK FACTORS
- Children with pica
- Children with iron deficiency anemia
- Residence or frequent visitor in deteriorating, pre-1960 housing with leaded-paint surfaces
- Children with seizures
- Children with hyperkinetic or autistic behavior
- Sibling or playmate with lead poisoning
- Dust from clothing of lead worker
- Lead dissolved in water from lead or lead-soldered plumbing
- Lead glazed ceramics, especially with acidic food or drink
- Food stored in inverted plastic bread bags printed with colored ink
- Colored comics
- Soil/dust near lead industries and roads
- Folk remedies (Mexican - azarcon, greta; Asian - chuifong tokuwan, pay-loo-ah, ghasard, bali goli, kandu; Middle Eastern - alkohl, surma, saoott, cebagin)
- Exposure to litargirio, topical agent from Dominican Republic
- Hobbies - glazed pottery making; target shooting at firing ranges; lead soldering; painting; preparing lead shot, fishing sinkers; stained-glass making; car or boat repair; home remodeling
- Occupational exposure - plumbers, pipe fitters, lead miners, auto repairers, glass manufacturers, shipbuilders, printers, plastic manufacturers, lead smelters and refiners, policemen, steel welders or cutters, construction workers, rubber product manufacturers, gas station attendants, battery manufacturers, bridge reconstruction workers
- Dietary - zinc or calcium deficiency

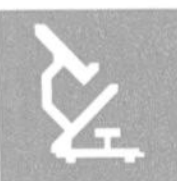

DIAGNOSIS

DIFFERENTIAL DIAGNOSIS
- Elevated erythrocyte protoporphyrin may be due to iron deficiency anemia, less commonly hemolytic anemia. Erythropoietic protoporphyria produces a very high erythrocyte protoporphyrin.
- Alimentary type may be confused with acute abdomen
- Neuromuscular type may be confused with other polyneuropathies
- Cerebral type may be confused with attention deficit disorder, mental retardation, autism, dementia, other causes of seizures

LABORATORY
- Blood lead (Pb) greater than 10 μg/dL (0.48 μmol/L), collected with lead-free container

CDC lead poisoning classification:

Class	Lead (μg/dL)
I	< 10
II	10-19
III	20-44
IV	45-69
V	> 70

1 μg/dL = 0.04826 μmol/L
e.g., 70 μg/dL = 3.38 μmol/dL

- Screening capillary lead levels greater than 10 μg/dL (0.48 μmol/L) should be confirmed with a venous sample
- Asymptomatic patient screening with erythrocyte protoporphyrin level (EP) greater than 35 μg/dL (0.62 μmol/L) indicates need for testing blood Pb
- Hgb and Hct slightly low. Eosinophilia or basophilic stippling on peripheral smear may be seen, but are not diagnostic of lead toxicity.
- Renal function decreased in late stages

Drugs that may alter lab results: N/A

Disorders that may alter lab results: N/A

PATHOLOGICAL FINDINGS N/A

SPECIAL TESTS Calcium ethylenediaminetetraacetic acid (Ca EDTA) mobilization test if blood Pb 25-44 μg/dL (1.21-2.12 μmol/L). This test is not widely used because it is technically difficult to perform and may delay diagnosis and treatment.

IMAGING Abdominal radiograph for lead particles in gut if recent ingestion is suspected. X-ray of long bones may show lines of increased density in the metaphyseal plate resulting from growth arrest, but do not usually alter management.

DIAGNOSTIC PROCEDURES N/A

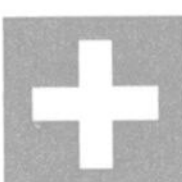

TREATMENT

APPROPRIATE HEALTH CARE Outpatient unless parenteral chelation required. Consider consultation if chelation required.

GENERAL MEASURES
- Case report to local health department for Class III-V. Complete inspection of home or work-place to determine source of lead. Screen all family members.
- Consider oral chelation for Class III or IV. Chelation (preferably parenteral) for Class V or symptomatic Class III or IV.
- Remove from potential source of lead for Class IV or V, until complete inspection is performed

SURGICAL MEASURES N/A

ACTIVITY
- Avoid activity at any site of potential contamination

DIET
- If symptomatic, avoid excessive fluids
- Avoidance of pica
- Consume adequate calcium and iron
- Eat a low fat diet to reduce absorption and retention of lead
- Consume at least 2 servings daily of foods high in vitamin C, such as fruits, vegetables, and juices

PATIENT EDUCATION
- HL Needleman, PJ Landrigan. Raising Children Toxic Free: How to keep your child safe from lead, asbestos, pesticides, and other environmental hazards. New York: Avon Books; 1994
- National Lead Information Center, 801 Roeder Rd., Suite 600, Silver Spring, MD 20910; 800-424-5323; www.epa.gov/lead/nlic.htm
- Alliance to End Childhood Lead Poisoning, 227 Massachusetts Ave, NE, Suite 200, Washington, DC 20002; 202-543-1147; http://www.aeclp.org
- Lead Poisoning Prevention Outreach Program, National Safety Council's Environmental Health Center, 1025 Connecticut Ave, NW, Suite 1200, Washington, DC 20036; (202)293-2270; www.nsc.org/ehc/lead.htm

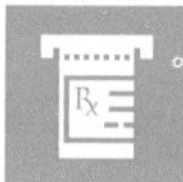

MEDICATIONS

DRUG(S) OF CHOICE
- Oral chelation:
  - ◊ Succimer (Chemet, dimercaptosuccinic acid, DMSA) 10 mg/kg q8h x 5 days, then 10 mg/kg q12h x 2 weeks. May be repeated after 2 weeks off if lead levels are not stabilized below < 15 μg/dL (< 0.72 μmol/L).
- Parenteral chelation (begin after establishment of adequate urine output):
  - ◊ Class V or symptomatic: dimercaprol (British anti-Lewisite, BAL) 75 mg/m2 given deep IM, then BAL 450 mg/m2/d divided q4h x 5 days + Ca EDTA (edetate calcium disodium) 1500 mg/m2/d continuous IV infusion x 5 days. If rebound lead level ≥ 45 μg/dL (≥ 2.17 μmol/L), chelation may be repeated after 2 day interval if symptomatic, after 5 day interval if asymptomatic.
  - ◊ Class IV asymptomatic: Ca EDTA 1000 mg/m2/d x 5 days. May be repeated after 5-7 days.
- Diazepam for initial control of seizures, further control maintained with paraldehyde

Contraindications:
- BAL should not be given to persons allergic to peanuts (the drug solution contains peanut oil)

Precautions:
- Succimer: Gastrointestinal upset, rash, nasal congestion, muscle pains, elevated liver function tests
- Ca EDTA: Renal failure, increased excretion of zinc, copper and iron
- BAL: Nausea, vomiting, fever, headache, transient hypertension, hepatocellular damage

Significant possible interactions:
- Vitamins should not be given concurrently with oral chelation
- BAL may precipitate hemolytic crisis in a patient with G6PD deficiency

ALTERNATIVE DRUGS
- Oral chelation with penicillamine (d-penicillamine, Depen, Cuprimine)
  - ◊ Penicillin allergic patient should not receive D-penicillamine (cross-sensitivity is common)
  - ◊ 10-20 mg/kg bid mixed in apple juice/sauce on empty stomach (not FDA approved)
  - ◊ D-penicillamine may cause gastrointestinal upset, renal failure, granulocytopenia, liver dysfunction, iron deficiency, drug induced lupus-like syndrome

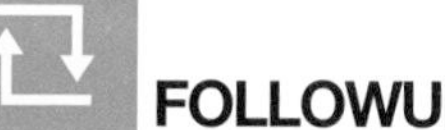

FOLLOWUP

PATIENT MONITORING
- After chelation, check for rebound Pb level in 7-10 days. Follow with regular monitoring, initially biweekly or monthly.
- Correct iron deficiency or any other nutritional deficiencies present
- For Class II or higher, repeat testing every 3 months until Class I level achieved

PREVENTION/AVOIDANCE
- Family should receive counseling on potential sources of lead and methods to decrease lead exposure. Wet mopping and dusting with a high phosphate solution (e.g., powdered automatic dishwasher detergent with 1/4 cup per gallon of water) will help control lead-bearing dust.
- If the source is in the home, the patient must reside elsewhere until the abatement process is completed

POSSIBLE COMPLICATIONS
- CNS toxicity may be long lasting or permanent
- Long-term lead exposure may cause chronic renal failure (Fanconi-like syndrome); gout; lead line (blue-black) on gingival tissue

EXPECTED COURSE/PROGNOSIS
- Symptomatic lead poisoning without encephalopathy generally improves with chelation, but subtle CNS toxicity may be long lasting or permanent
- If encephalopathy occurs, permanent sequelae (mental retardation, seizure disorder, blindness, hemiparesis) in 25-50%

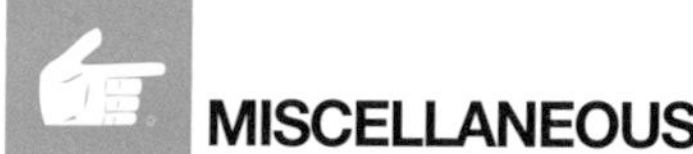

MISCELLANEOUS

ASSOCIATED CONDITIONS Iron deficiency anemia

AGE-RELATED FACTORS
Pediatric:
- Increasing evidence that low lead level exposure (as low as 10 μg/dL [0.48 μmol/L]) may produce neurotoxicity in children
- Children are at increased risk because of incomplete development of the blood-brain barrier before age 3 years allowing more lead into the central nervous system; ingested lead has 40% bioavailability in children compared with 10% in adults
- Common childhood behaviors such as frequent hand-to-mouth activity and pica (repeated ingestion of nonfood products) greatly increase the risk of ingesting lead

Geriatric: N/A

Others: N/A

PREGNANCY
- Lead exposure in pregnancy is associated with reduced birth weight and premature birth
- Lead is an animal teratogen

SYNONYMS Lead poisoning, inorganic

ICD-9-CM
984.9 Toxic effect of unspecified lead compound (including fumes)

SEE ALSO
Iron deficiency anemia

OTHER NOTES Screening is recommended for asymptomatic children during their first 4 years of life living in high risk areas (> 12% elevated). Children in a low risk area should be screened by a questionnaire. Screening EP is not sensitive for blood Pb less than 25 μg/dL (1.20 μmol/L).

ABBREVIATIONS
Pb = lead
EP = erythrocyte protoporphyrin
BAL = British anti-Lewisite

REFERENCES

- Nastoff T, Rush V, Tucker P. Case studies in environmental medicine: lead toxicity. US Department of Health and Human Services, PHS, ATSDR, 2000
- Centers for Disease Control and Prevention. Recommendations for Blood Lead Screening of Young Children Enrolled in Medicaid: Targeting a Group at High Risk. Advisory Committee on Childhood Lead Poisoning Prevention. MMWR 2000;49(No.RR-14):1-13
- Centers for Disease Control and Prevention. Managing Elevated Blood Lead Levels Among Young Children: Recommendations from the Advisory Committee on Childhood Lead Poisoning Prevention. Atlanta, CDC; 2002

Web references: 8 available at www.5mcc.com
Illustrations 1 available

Author(s):
Jason Chao, MD, MS

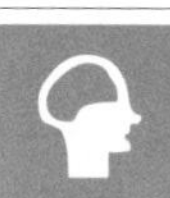

BASICS

DESCRIPTION Idiopathic necrosis of capital femoral epiphysis of the femoral head. 10-20% of cases are bilateral.

System(s) affected: Musculoskeletal

Genetics: No known genetic pattern identified

Incidence/Prevalence in USA: Incidence 15/100,000; prevalence 75/100,000

Predominant age: Susceptible age 2-12 years. However, approximately 80% occur between the ages of 4 and 9 years

Predominant sex: Males > Females (4:1). In bilateral cases males predominate 7:1. However, females seem to have more severe involvement.

SIGNS & SYMPTOMS

- Primarily hip or groin pain although referred pain to the knee and thigh not uncommon
- Range of motion limited, especially in internal rotation and abduction
- Atrophy of thigh musculature due to disuse
- Leg length discrepancy secondary to collapse of the femoral head

CAUSES

- Etiology unclear
- Related to interruption of blood flow to femoral epiphysis

RISK FACTORS

- No genetic risk factors
- Increased incidence in children with low birth weight and delayed physical maturation

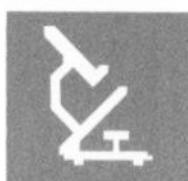

DIAGNOSIS

DIFFERENTIAL DIAGNOSIS

- Unilateral - septic arthritis, toxic synovitis, juvenile rheumatoid arthritis
- Bilateral - spondyloepiphyseal dysplasia, metaphyseal dysplasia, hypothyroidism

LABORATORY

- CBC
- Sedimentation rate (elevated in infection)

Drugs that may alter lab results: N/A

Disorders that may alter lab results: N/A

PATHOLOGICAL FINDINGS

- Early (necrosis, resorption) stage - necrosis of bone with subchondral bone fracture and subsequent collapse of subchondral bone
- Late (healing) stage - revascularization by creeping substitution of necrotic bone

SPECIAL TESTS

IMAGING

- Serial radiographs, AP and frog lateral, of the pelvis are crucial for determining of extent of involvement and progression of healing.
- Full extent of involvement may not be evident for several months as radiographic findings lag symptoms
- MRI - Most sensitive test; facilitates early diagnosis of necrosis and visualization of articular surface
- Dynamic arthrography - used to assess congruency of femoral head
- Technetium 99 bone scan - may be helpful in delineating the extent of avascular changes

DIAGNOSTIC PROCEDURES Hip aspiration to rule out septic arthritis

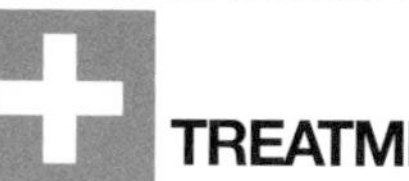

TREATMENT

APPROPRIATE HEALTH CARE

- A pediatric orthopaedic consultation
- Ambulatory treatment is usual, however, some patients may require inpatient traction or surgical procedures

GENERAL MEASURES

- Goals of treatment:
    - ◊ Relieve weight bearing across affected hip, thus reducing irritability of the hip
    - ◊ Obtain and maintain hip range of motion
    - ◊ Maximize regeneration and spherical development of the femoral head by containing the femoral epiphysis within the acetabulum

SURGICAL MEASURES

- Adductor tenotomy to help restore range of motion secondary to adductor contracture
- Femoral and/or pelvic osteotomy to help contain femoral epiphysis within the confines of the acetabulum (in older children or in cases of hip subluxation)

ACTIVITY

- Ambulatory status depends on extent/stage of disease
- Limit weight bearing in cases of hip irritation

DIET No special diet

PATIENT EDUCATION

- Légg-Calvé-Pérthes disease is a self-limited disease with revascularization occurring within 3 years
- Treatment is directed at maintaining an appropriate range of motion and maximizing the containment of the femoral head

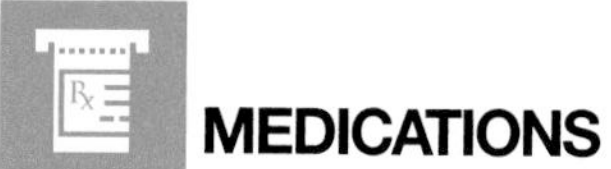

MEDICATIONS

DRUG(S) OF CHOICE
- Ibuprofen 10 mg/kg tid-qid

Contraindications: Allergy to ibuprofen
Precautions: GI irritation
Significant possible interactions: N/A

ALTERNATIVE DRUGS N/A

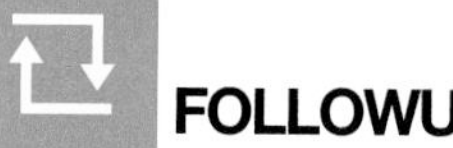

FOLLOWUP

PATIENT MONITORING
- Initially, close followup, with radiographic evaluation, is needed to determine extent of necrosis
- Once healing phase entered, followup can be every 6 months
- Long-term followup necessary to determine final outcome

PREVENTION/AVOIDANCE
Since etiology is not clearly understood, prevention is not possible

POSSIBLE COMPLICATIONS
- Permanent distortion of the femoral head
- Distorted joint susceptible to early degenerative joint disease

EXPECTED COURSE/PROGNOSIS
- Most patients have a favorable outcome
- Outcome is dependent on the patient's age at the time of the diagnosis (the younger the better)
- Prognosis is also related to the degree of involvement of the femoral head (as determined by radiography)

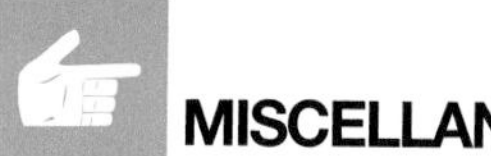

MISCELLANEOUS

ASSOCIATED CONDITIONS N/A

AGE-RELATED FACTORS
Pediatric:
- Physical maturation is delayed
- The younger the patient at the time of diagnosis, the greater the chance for remodeling

Geriatric: N/A
Others: N/A

PREGNANCY N/A

SYNONYMS N/A

ICD-9-CM
732.1 Juvenile osteochondrosis of hip and pelvis

SEE ALSO

OTHER NOTES N/A

ABBREVIATIONS N/A

REFERENCES

- Lovell WW, Morrissy BT, et al (eds). Lovell and Winter's Pediatric Orthopaedics. 5th ed. Philadelphia: Lippincott Williams & Wilkins; 2001
- Thompson GH, Price CT, Roy D, Meehan PL, Richards BS. Legg-Calve-Perthes disease: current concepts. Instr Course Lect 2002;51:367-84
- Herring JA. The treatment of Legg-Calve-Perthes disease. A critical review of the literature. J Bone Joint Surg Am 1998;73A(3):448-58
- Herring JA, ed. Tachdjian's Pediatric Orthopaedics. 3rd ed. Philadelphia: WB Saunders; 2001

Web references: 0 available at www.5mcc.com
Illustrations N/A

Author(s):
Francisco G. Valencia, MD
Patrick C. Henderson, MD

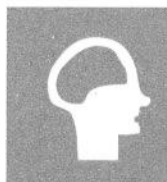

BASICS

DESCRIPTION Legionnaires disease was coined for an epidemic of lower respiratory tract disease occurring in Philadelphia in 1976 in war veterans. The causative bacterium was identified and named Legionella pneumophila and may cause pneumonia or flu-like illness. It ranks among the three most common pneumonias in the clinical setting.

System(s) affected: Gastrointestinal, Pulmonary

Genetics: None known

Incidence/Prevalence in USA:
- The true incidence is not well known. It may increase with the rise in population density in some urban areas, certain travel and leisure activities and more complex infrastructures. Only 2-10% of cases are probably reported.
- Most commonly outbreaks occur at the end of summer and early fall

Predominant age: 15 months-84 years, increased after age 50

Predominant sex: Male > Female

SIGNS & SYMPTOMS
- Range of illness from asymptomatic seroconversion, mild febrile illness, to severe pneumonia
- Incubation 2-10 days
- Fever, chills
- Malaise, weakness, lethargy
- Anorexia
- Myalgia
- Headache
- Watery diarrhea in up to 50%
- Nausea and vomiting in 10-20%
- Dry cough which may become productive
- Pleuritic chest pain in up to 33%
- Relative bradycardia in up to 67% of patients
- Neuropsychiatric symptoms of confusion, disorientation, obtundation, depression, hallucinations, insomnia, seizures in up to 25%
- Blood streaked sputum; gross hemoptysis rare
- Hyponatremia
- Hypophosphatemia
- Elevated serum transaminases
- Elevated creatine kinase
- Approximately 50% of hospitalized patients present with arterial PP < 60 mmHg
- Hypotension (17%)
- Wound infections with Legionella have been reported

CAUSES
- Legionella pneumophila, a weakly gram negative organism is a saprophytic water bacteria, widely distributed in soil and water. Serogroups 1,2, and 6 account for most cases. The optimum temperature for growth is 40-45°C temperatures. It can also be associated with organic material in sediment.
- Mode of transmission:
  - ◊ Aerosolization
  - ◊ Aspiration
  - ◊ Direct instillation into the lungs by equipment (such as respiratory equipment)
  - ◊ Most important mode - aerosolization and airborne dissemination of contaminated water
    - Patients may acquire by inhaling organisms while showering
    - Recently, community outbreaks have been associated with whirlpools, spas, and fountains

RISK FACTORS
- Smoking
- Alcohol abuse
- Immunosuppression/HIV
- Chronic cardiopulmonary disease
- Surgery
- Advanced age
- Renal failure
- Fever > 39°C
- Hyponatremia
- Liver dysfunction
- Creatine kinase elevation

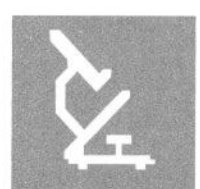

DIAGNOSIS

DIFFERENTIAL DIAGNOSIS Other bacterial pneumonias, atypical pneumonias with mycoplasma and chlamydia, viral pneumonias

LABORATORY

Tests: sensitivity, specificity and time:

Test	Sensitivity %	Specificity %	Time
Sputum culture	10-80	100	3-7day
Serology	40-70	95-99	1-6mo
DFA (sputum)	33-70	95-99	2-4hr
Urinary Ag assay (Elisa)	>90	99-100	2-3hr
Immunochromatography (IC)	>90	99-100	15min†
PCR-serum, urine, resp sample	33-70	98-100	2-4hr

† nonconcentrated urine

Drugs that may alter lab results: N/A

Disorders that may alter lab results: Direct immunofluorescence can cross react with Pseudomonas and Bacteroides species, E. coli, Haemophilus

PATHOLOGICAL FINDINGS
- Multifocal pneumonia with alveolitis and bronchiolitis, with fibrinous pleuritis, and may have serous or serosanguinous pleural effusion. Abscess formation in up to 20%.
- Progression of infiltrates, despite appropriate therapy, may be suggestive of Legionnaires disease. Also, improvement on x-ray may not correlate with clinical findings (longer lag times on x-ray findings).

SPECIAL TESTS Silver and Gimenez stains for lung tissue/specimens

IMAGING
- Chest x-ray
  - ◊ Not specific for Legionella
  - ◊ Commonly with lower lobe patchy alveolar infiltrate with consolidation, usually unilateral
  - ◊ Cavitation or abscess, especially in immunocompromised
  - ◊ Pleural effusion in up to 50%
  - ◊ May take from 1-4 months for the x-ray to return to normal. Progression of infiltrate may be seen despite antibiotic therapy.

DIAGNOSTIC PROCEDURES Transtracheal aspiration or bronchoscopy for sputum/lung samples

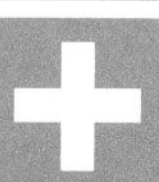

TREATMENT

APPROPRIATE HEALTH CARE Severity of illness and support available in the outpatient setting will dictate the appropriate site for care

GENERAL MEASURES
- Supportive care
- Maintaining oxygenation, hydration, and electrolyte balance while providing antibiotic therapy

SURGICAL MEASURES N/A

ACTIVITY As tolerated

DIET As tolerated

PATIENT EDUCATION
- Can educate patients regarding prevention/avoidance measures, lowering their risk status, and if infected already, about the expected course of the disease
- Disease prevention - elimination of the pathogens from water supplies
- Person-to-person transmission has not been observed

MEDICATIONS

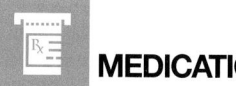

DRUG(S) OF CHOICE
- Azithromycin 500 mg po qd
- Clarithromycin 500 mg po bid
- Levofloxacin 500 mg po or IV every 24 hours
- Ciprofloxacin IV 400 mg every 8 hours or po 750 mg every 12 hours
- Addition of rifampin 600 mg q 12 hours po or IV should be provided along with above in very ill patients

Contraindications: Hypersensitivity reactions
Precautions: Liver disease
Significant possible interactions:
- Erythromycin can increase theophylline, carbamazepine, and digoxin levels and can increase activity of oral anticoagulants
- Rifampin may decrease the effectiveness of oral anticoagulants, steroids, digoxin, quinidine, oral contraceptives and hypoglycemic agents

ALTERNATIVE DRUGS
- Erythromycin 30-60 mg/kg/day po or IV divided into four doses for 10-21 days
- Tetracyclines may be used along with rifampin
  - ◊ Doxycycline IV 200 mg every 12 hours x 2 doses, then 100 mg bid or po 200 mg x 1 dose, then 100 mg bid
  - ◊ Minocycline 100 mg IV or po every 12 hours
- Trimethoprim-sulfamethoxazole IV or po 5 mg/kg TMP every 8 hours

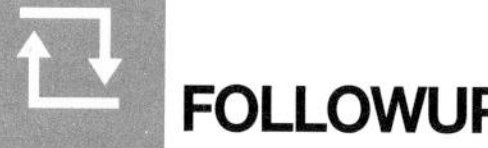

FOLLOWUP

PATIENT MONITORING
- Respiratory status, hydration and electrolyte status should be monitored closely
- Chest x-ray not useful to monitor clinical response

PREVENTION/AVOIDANCE Heating water to 60-70 degrees centigrade may help prevent water contamination. UV light or copper-silver ionization are bactericidal.

POSSIBLE COMPLICATIONS
- Dehydration
- Hyponatremia
- Respiratory insufficiency requiring ventilator support
- Endocarditis
- Disseminated intravascular coagulation
- Renal failure
- Multiple organ dysfunction syndrome (MODS)
- Coma
- Death in 10% of treated non-immunocompromised patients, and in up to 80% of untreated immunocompromised patients
- Bacteremia or abscess formation in immunocompromised

EXPECTED COURSE/PROGNOSIS
- Recovery is variable, some patients experience rapid improvement with defervescence in 3-5 days and recovery in 6-10 days, while others may have a much more protracted course despite treatment
- Mortality rate can approach 50% with nosocomial infections

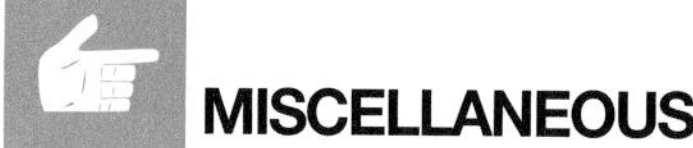

MISCELLANEOUS

ASSOCIATED CONDITIONS Pontiac fever - self limited flu-like illness with pneumonia

AGE-RELATED FACTORS
Pediatric: Less common
Geriatric: Increased incidence in those over age 50
Others: N/A

PREGNANCY N/A

SYNONYMS
- Legionella pneumonia
- Legionellosis

ICD-9-CM
482.83 Pneumonia due to other gram-negative bacteria
482.84 Legionnaires disease

SEE ALSO
Pneumonia, bacterial

OTHER NOTES
- Extrapulmonary disease can occur in the form of:
  - ◊ Encephalitis
  - ◊ Cellulitis
  - ◊ Sinusitis
  - ◊ Pancreatitis
  - ◊ Pyelonephritis
  - ◊ Endocarditis
  - ◊ Pericarditis
  - ◊ Perirectal abscess

ABBREVIATIONS N/A

REFERENCES

- Hoeprich P, Jordan MC. Infectious Diseases. 5th ed. Philadelphia: JB Lippincott; 1994
- Mandell GL, editor. Principles and Practice of Infectious Diseases. 5th ed. New York: Churchill Livingstone; 2000
- Rubenstein E, Federman DD. Scientific American Medicine; 1999
- Edelstein PH. Legionnaire's disease. Clinical Infectious Diseases 1993;16:741-9
- Waterer GW, Baselski VS, Wunderink RG. Legionella and community-acquired pneumonia: a review of current diagnostic tests from a clinician's viewpoint. Am J Med 2001;110:41-8
- Fields BS, Benson RF, Besser RE. Legionella and Legionnaires' disease: 25 years of investigation. Clin Microbiol Rev. 2002;15(3):506-26
- Roig J, Rello J. Legionnaires' disease: a rational approach to therapy. J Antimicrob Chemother 2003;51(5):1119-29
- Sabria M, Campins M. Legionnaires' disease: update on epidemiology and management options. Am J Respir Med 2003;2(3):235-43

Web references: 1 available at www.5mcc.com
Illustrations N/A

Author(s):
Mitchell S. King, MD
Linda Bigi, DO

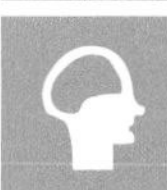

BASICS

DESCRIPTION An infective condition caused by several species of the protozoan *Leishmania*. Currently, about 12 million cases are affected, with 350 million at risk. WHO puts the global burden due to this disease at 2.4 million life years lost and 59,000 deaths in 2001. Four major clinical syndromes are recognized.

- Visceral leishmaniasis (Kala-azar, Black fever) may be endemic, epidemic or sporadic. Different forms are:
  - ◊ African Kala-azar: Found in the eastern half of Africa from the Sahara in the North to the Equator. Disease of older children and young adults (10-25 years); males > females.
  - ◊ Mediterranean or infantile Kala-azar: Seen primarily in the Mediterranean area, China and Latin America. Dogs, jackals, foxes and rats are potential reservoirs. The strains responsible for the Mediterranean and American disease are sometimes referred to as *L. infantum* and *L. chagasi* respectively.
  - ◊ Indian Kala-azar: Age and sex distribution similar to African Kala-azar. Humans are the only known reservoir and transmission is by anthropophilic sandflies.
- Cutaneous leishmaniasis of the old and new worlds. Characterized by one or more localized lesions on exposed areas. These ulcerate centrally and spread centrifugally. Spontaneous healing less common in new world disease. Satellite lesions and lymphadenopathy may or may not occur.
- Mucocutaneous leishmaniasis (espundia). One or more lesions on the legs which may ulcerate. In 2-5% of patients, metastatic lesions appear in the nasopharynx after months or years, and may result in painful mutilating erosions of soft tissue. Lesions may occur rarely in perineum.
- Diffuse cutaneous leishmaniasis. Extensive skin lesions, but no visceral lesions. Clinical picture may be similar to lepromatous leprosy.

System(s) affected: Gastrointestinal, Hemic/Lymphatic/Immunologic, Pulmonary, Skin/Exocrine

Genetics: N/A

Incidence/Prevalence in USA:

- Rare, but reported in states bordering Mexico
- Two confirmed cases of visceral leishmaniasis have been reported in U.S. military personnel who had returned to the United States after serving in Afghanistan during 2002-2004

Predominant age: Children and young adults. (10-25 years). Mediterranean or infantile Kala-azar - usually < 4 years age.

Predominant sex: African Kala-azar, Indian Kala-azar: Male > female

SIGNS & SYMPTOMS

- Incubation period - about 3 months for the visceral form and 2-24 months for others
- Onset - insidious/abrupt
- Malabsorption; failure to thrive in infants and children
- Fever - nocturnal, no signs of toxemia
- Cough
- Diarrhea, GI bleeding
- Lymphadenopathy
- Splenomegaly
- Moderate hepatomegaly
- Cirrhosis, portal hypertension (in 10% of patients)
- Anemia, pancytopenia
- Cutaneous lesions, may ulcerate and heal spontaneously
- Nasal stuffiness
- Epistaxis
- Edema, cachexia and hyperpigmentation in late stages
- Hypoalbuminemia
- Hypergammaglobulinemia

CAUSES

Several species of *Leishmania* including *L. donovani* (Kala-azar), *L. infantum*, *L. chagasi* (Mediterranean and American forms), *L. tropica* (cutaneous form), *L. major* (in Middle East, Afghanistan and India), *L. mexicana*, *L. braziliensis* and others. The organisms are transmitted by female sandflies of the genus phlebotomus in the old world and Lutzomyia in the new world.

RISK FACTORS

- Children > young adults in endemic areas
- Malnutrition
- AIDS
- Incomplete therapy of initial disease

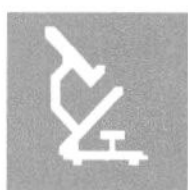

DIAGNOSIS

DIFFERENTIAL DIAGNOSIS

- Malaria
- Brucellosis
- Tuberculosis
- Typhoid
- Hepatic abscess
- Lepromatous leprosy for diffuse leishmaniasis

Post Kala-azar dermal lesion (PKDL) must be differentiated from leprosy, syphilis and yaws

LABORATORY

- Demonstration of parasites in
  - ◊ Splenic aspirate - most sensitive
  - ◊ Bone marrow aspirate
  - ◊ Lymph node aspirate or biopsy
  - ◊ Biopsy material from suspicious skin lesions after cleaning with alcohol to reduce bacterial contamination
  - ◊ The intracellular amastigote form in the macrophages, formerly known as the Leishman-Donovan (LD) body, has a characteristic pear-shaped body with a dark circular nucleus and short rod-shaped kinetoplasts
- Hypergammaglobulinemia
- Direct agglutination test detects IgM antibody which indicates acute disease

Drugs that may alter lab results: N/A

Disorders that may alter lab results: N/A

PATHOLOGICAL FINDINGS

- Marked lymphocytic infiltration
- Ulcerating lesions in the skin and mucosa of nasopharynx

SPECIAL TESTS

- Leishmanin skin test is positive 6-8 weeks after recovery in cutaneous forms, but not in diffuse leishmaniasis. It is negative in visceral leishmaniasis.
- Monoclonal antibodies or hybridization of tissue touch blots with labeled kinetoplast DNA probes used for identification of different strains of Leishmania
- ELISA highly sensitive and specific in visceral disease
- Montenegro skin test is nonstandardized and used only in epidemiological studies. It is negative in visceral leishmaniasis.
- An immunochromatographic strip test for rapid detection of antibodies to leishmania antigen rK39

IMAGING N/A

DIAGNOSTIC PROCEDURES

- Demonstration of the organism by smear or culture from aspirate or biopsy material. Novy-MacNeal-Nicolle medium or other liquid media used for cultures are maintained at 22-28°C for 21 days. Motile promastigotes can be observed microscopically.
- Speciation using monoclonal Ab or labeled DNA probes is unlikely to be cost effective

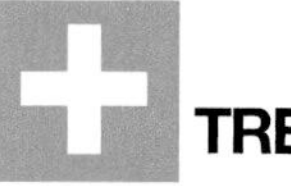

TREATMENT

APPROPRIATE HEALTH CARE Inpatient for blood transfusions and complicating superinfections. Outpatient care once the condition stabilizes.

GENERAL MEASURES

- Bed rest, oral hygiene, and good nutrition are important.
- Transfusions for anemia and antibacterial chemotherapy for bacterial complications must supplement specific therapy.
- Periodic ECG monitoring during prolonged therapy with pentavalent antimonials

SURGICAL MEASURES

- Adjunctive splenectomy
- Reconstructive surgery for tissue damage

ACTIVITY

Bed rest during acute stages. Level of activity dependent on severity of disease and organ systems involved.

DIET

Rich nutritious diet

PATIENT EDUCATION

- Explain prevention measures
- Help for patients: www.cdc.gov/ncidod/dpd/parasites/leishmania

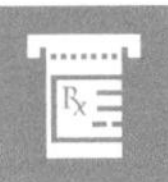

MEDICATIONS

DRUG(S) OF CHOICE

- Sodium antimony gluconate (Pentostam) 100 mg Sb5+/mL IV/IM: single daily dose of 20 mg/kg/day for 20-30 days
- Meglumine antimonate (Glucantime) 85 mg Sb5+/mL, same dose and duration of treatment as above, can also be used

Note: In the U.S., these drugs are available only from the CDC, Atlanta, GA 30333; emergency telephone 404-639-2888 (http://www.cdc.gov)

- Relapses and incomplete responses should be treated with the same regimen for 40-60 days. Addition of oral allopurinol (Zyloprim) 20-30 mg/kg/day in three divided doses has been effective.

Contraindications: Refer to manufacturer's profile of each drug

Precautions: Refer to manufacturer's profile of each drug. Periodic ECG monitoring is recommended during prolonged therapy.

Significant possible interactions: Refer to manufacturer's profile of each drug

ALTERNATIVE DRUGS

- Relapses with drug resistant organisms are usually treated with:
  - ◊ Amphotericin B (Fungizone) IV: 0.5-1 mg/kg on alternate days
  - ◊ Liposomal amphotericin B is excellent for visceral leishmaniasis. It has been administered IV at a total dose of 21 mg/kg given at 3 mg/kg/day on days 1-5, 7 and 14.

  OR
  - ◊ Pentamidine (Pentam): 3-4 mg/kg, 3 times a week for 5-25 weeks
- In patients with concomitant HIV, the disease is resistant to all current drugs
- The new orally effective drug miltefosine is approved in India for visceral leishmaniasis - 2.5 mg/kg (100 mg/day) for 4 weeks (94% cure rate). It has been effective in the cutaneous form at 133 mg and 150 mg daily.
- Paromomycin ointment has been shown to be effective for the cutaneous form

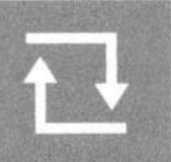

FOLLOWUP

PATIENT MONITORING

- Follow-up at 3 and 12 months to detect relapses
- PKDL should be treated in the same fashion as the initial illness
- Periodic monitoring of ECG, liver function and renal function during prolonged therapy

PREVENTION/AVOIDANCE

- Use of pesticides against sandflies, especially synthetic pyrethroids. Resistance to DDT is high in many areas.
- Insect repellants - for travelers
- Permethrin - coated fine netting for travelers
- Early treatment of human cases
- Elimination of diseased dogs
- Deltamethrin-treated collars fitted to dogs have reduced incidence of the disease in children in the treated areas

POSSIBLE COMPLICATIONS

- Edema, cachexia, hyperpigmentation in late stages
- Superinfections and gastrointestinal bleeding may cause death in untreated patients with visceral disease (Kala-azar)
- 3-10% of the treated cases develop PKDL characterized by depigmented macules and wart-like nodules over the face and extensor surfaces of limbs
- Metastatic lesions in nasopharynx with tissue destruction in patients with mucocutaneous leishmaniasis

EXPECTED COURSE/PROGNOSIS

With early treatment, cure rate is over 90%, though in advanced cases, mortality remains at 15-25%. In untreated cases, death occurs in 3-20 months in up to 95% of adults and 85% of children.

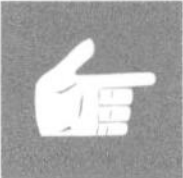

MISCELLANEOUS

ASSOCIATED CONDITIONS Fulminant Kala-azar has been described in association with AIDS and malnutrition

AGE-RELATED FACTORS

Pediatric:

- Pediatric Mediterranean or infantile Kala-azar usually a disease of children under 4 years
- African or Indian Kala-azar: usually a disease of children and young adults (10-25 years)

Geriatric: N/A

Others: N/A

PREGNANCY N/A

SYNONYMS

- Visceral leishmaniasis
- Kala-azar
- Black fever
- Dumdum fever

ICD-9-CM

085.0 Leishmaniasis, visceral (kala-azar)

085.9 Leishmaniasis, unspecified

SEE ALSO

OTHER NOTES N/A

ABBREVIATIONS

PKDL = Post Kala-azar Dermal Leishmaniasis

LD bodies = Leishman-Donovani bodies

REFERENCES

- Davies CR, Kaye P, Croft SL, Sundar S. Leishmaniasis: new approaches to disease control. BMJ 2003;326(7385):377-82
- Jha TK, Sundar S, Thakur CP, et al. Miltefosine, an oral agent, for the treatment of Indian visceral leishmaniasis. N Engl J Med 1999;341(24):1795-800
- Herwaldt BL. Leishmaniasis. In: Fauci AS, et al, editors. Harrison's Principles of Internal Medicine. 15th ed. New York: McGraw-Hill; 2001. p. 1213
- Sundar S. Drug resistance in Indian visceral leishmaniasis. Trop Med Int Health 2001;6(11):849-54. Erratum in: Trop Med Int Health 2002;7(3):293
- CDC. Cutaneous leishmaniasis in U.S. military personnel---Southwest/Central Asia, 2002--2003. MMWR 2003;52:1009-12
- Morbidity and Mortality Weekly Report (MMWR). Two Cases of Visceral Leishmaniasis in U.S. Military Personnel--Afghanistan, 2002-2004. 2004:53(12);265-8
- Jacobs S. An oral drug for leishmaniasis. N Engl J Med. 2002;347(22):1737-8
- Sundar S, Jha TK, et al. Oral miltefosine for Indian visceral leishmaniasis. N Engl J Med 2002;347(22):1739-46

Web references: 3 available at www.5mcc.com

Illustrations N/A

Author(s):

V. Vasudeviah, BSc, MBBS

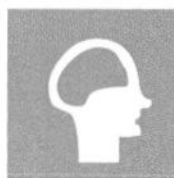

BASICS

DESCRIPTION

A chronic granulomatous infection caused by *Mycobacterium leprae*, an organism which has a high predilection for cooler regions - skin, mucous membrane and peripheral nerves. In the year 2000. 738,284 cases were identified; 70% of which were in India, Nepal and Myanmar. In the recent decade or two, introduction of multidrug therapy (MDT) with the global effort of the WHO in eliminating leprosy has had a great impact on leprosy control. Over 10 million patients have been treated successfully with MDT consisting of rifampicin, ofloxacin and minocycline. Newer drugs with higher activity against *M. leprae* are undergoing trials. Leprosy is classified on a spectrum reflecting degrees of lost immunity (Ridley-Jopling classification).

- Indeterminate leprosy:

Early cutaneous lesions; Findings are very subtle most commonly diagnosed in contacts of known leprosy cases. The lesions tend to heal spontaneously, but may progress to any of the other leprosy types.

- Tuberculoid leprosy (TT):

Characterized by early localized skin lesions and/or nerve lesions. Bacilli are few and difficult to find. Resistance to infection is high, and spontaneous recovery may occur; however peripheral nerves can be destroyed.

- Lepromatous leprosy (LL):

A generalized infection involving skin, oral, nasal, and upper respiratory mucous membrane, the anterior eye, cutaneous and peripheral nerve trunks, the RE system, adrenals, and testes. Numerous bacilli are easily found in tissue specimens. Patient's resistance to infection is low, and untreated disease is progressive.

- Borderline (dimorphous) leprosy:

This has features of both TT and LL poles in various combinations. Usually sub-divided into borderline tuberculoid (BT), mid-borderline (BB) and borderline lepromatous (BL). Borderline forms are unstable and may regress (reversal reaction) toward TT form or progress (downgrading reaction) toward the LL form, depending on the effects of treatment and shifts in immune status.

System(s) affected: Endocrine/Metabolic, Hemic/Lymphatic/Immunologic, Musculoskeletal, Nervous, Pulmonary, Reproductive, Skin/Exocrine

Genetics: Specific HLA-associated genes may be linked to different classes of disease, HLA-DR2 with TT and HLA-MT1 with LL

Incidence/Prevalence in USA: Extremely low; 108 cases in 1999, mostly in immigrants from leprosy-endemic areas. In the USA, leprosy is a reportable disease.

Predominant age: Leprosy can present at any age, although cases in infants under 1 year are extremely rare

Predominant sex:
- Childhood: Male = Female
- Adults: Male > Female (2:1)

SIGNS & SYMPTOMS

- Indeterminate leprosy
  - ◊ One or more hypopigmented or hyperpigmented macules or plaques
  - ◊ Anesthetic patches, though sensation is preserved in early stages
- TT
  - ◊ Initial hypopigmented, hypesthetic macules with sharp demarcations
  - ◊ Fully developed lesions are asymmetric and densely anesthetic with depressed atrophic central areas and elevated margins; loss of sweat glands and hair follicles near the lesion
  - ◊ Nerve involvement occurs early
    - Ulnar, peroneal, and greater auricular nerves may be palpably and visibly enlarged
    - Neuritic pain
    - Muscle atrophy - small muscles of the hand
    - Facial nerve involvement leads to lagophthalmos, keratitis and corneal ulceration
  - ◊ Hand and foot contracture
  - ◊ Hand infection and plantar ulcers secondary to trauma
  - ◊ Resorption and loss of phalanges may supervene
- LL
  - ◊ Extensive cutaneous involvement, usually bilaterally symmetrical
  - ◊ Highly variable cutaneous lesions macules, nodules, papules or plaques
  - ◊ Sites of predilection are face, ears, wrists, elbows, buttocks and knees
  - ◊ Loss of lateral eye brows
  - ◊ Leonine facies
  - ◊ Nasal stuffiness, epistaxis, septal perforation
  - ◊ Nasal obstruction, laryngitis, hoarseness
  - ◊ Saddle nose
  - ◊ Keratitis, iridocyclitis
  - ◊ Painless inguinal and axillary lymphadenopathy
  - ◊ Testicular infiltrate and scarring - sterility
  - ◊ Gynecomastia
- Borderline leprosy
  - ◊ Increasing variability in the appearance of skin lesions
  - ◊ Papules and plaques may co-exist with macular lesions
  - ◊ Anesthesia is less prominent than in TT
  - ◊ Ear lobes slightly thickened, but eye brows and nasal region spared
  - ◊ Skin lesions become even more numerous in BL type but without the symmetry typical of polar LL
  - ◊ Skin lesions of BT generally resemble those of TT but are greater in number and have less well defined margins

CAUSES *Mycobacterium leprae*: an acid fast rod is the causal agent. Incubation period is frequently 3-5 yrs although a range of 6 months to several decades has been seen.

RISK FACTORS

- Close family contacts of untreated leprosy patients have 8-fold increased risk
- Compromised immunological status
- Poor socioeconomic status

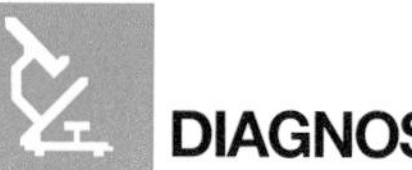

DIAGNOSIS

DIFFERENTIAL DIAGNOSIS

- Lupus erythematosus
- Lupus vulgaris
- Sarcoidosis
- Yaws
- Dermal leishmaniasis
- Other skin conditions
- Peripheral neuropathy
- Syringomyelia

LABORATORY

- Demonstration of acid-fast bacilli in skin smears made by scraped-incision method is strong evidence of leprosy
- Skin biopsy
- Histologic involvement of peripheral nerves pathognomonic
- Mild anemia, elevated ESR and hyperglobulinemia
- Lepromin test: Usually positive in TT and negative in LL poles. It has no diagnostic value since it gives false positives in nearly all normal adults.
- Serodiagnostic assay: Based on the detection of antibody to phenolic glycolipid 1, this assay has a sensitivity of over 95% in LL and about 30% in TT

Drugs that may alter lab results: N/A

Disorders that may alter lab results: N/A

PATHOLOGICAL FINDINGS

- TT: Noncaseating granulomas containing lymphocytes, epithelioid cells, and perhaps giant cells; bacilli are difficult to demonstrate
- LL: granulomas comprising macrophages, large foam (Virchow or lepra) cells, and many intracellular bacilli, frequently in spheroidal masses
- Borderline leprosy: granulomas change from an epithelioid cell predominance in BT to a macrophage predominance as the lepromatous pole is approached

SPECIAL TESTS

- Sero diagnostic assay
- Detection of *M. Leprae* in tissue by polymerase chain reaction

IMAGING N/A

DIAGNOSTIC PROCEDURES N/A

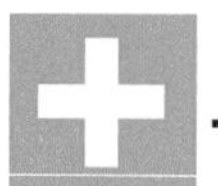

TREATMENT

APPROPRIATE HEALTH CARE

Outpatient usually, except in reactional states where inpatient care is called for

GENERAL MEASURES
- Manage with multidisciplinary approach, including orthopedic surgery, ophthalmology and physical therapy in addition to specific drugs
- Rigid soled foot wear or walking plaster casts may prevent plantar ulcers
- Physical therapy and casts prevent hand contractures
- Utilize vocational retraining and rehabilitation along with psychological support
- Immediate recognition and treatment of eye problems essential
- Manage mild reactional states such as reversal reaction and erythema nodosum leprosum (ENL) with bed rest, analgesics and sedatives. Severe reactions require corticosteroids, thalidomide or clofazimine. Specific therapy must be continued without interruption.

SURGICAL MEASURES
- Reconstructive surgery - nerve and tendon transplants, release of contractures and other cosmetic procedures can give more functional mobility and social acceptance
- Tarsorrhaphy or horizontal lid shortening for lagophthalmos with lid gap more than 5 mm or even lesser degree in patients with one eye. Cataract surgery with posterior chamber intraocular lens implantation to avoid glasses in patients with nasal bridge collapse.

ACTIVITY Dependent on severity of disease

DIET Nutritious balanced diet

PATIENT EDUCATION
- Educate about the indolent course of the disease; importance of therapeutic completion
- Information pamphlets and awareness to ease psychological trauma and stigma, emphasizing that a cure is possible with newer drug regimen
- Encourage case reporting since early treatment can prevent/reduce tissue damage and deformities

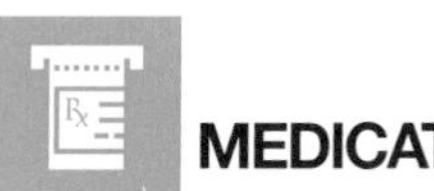

MEDICATIONS

DRUG(S) OF CHOICE
- Drugs and treatment duration are based on bacterial load (in skin smear) and clinical types. Multibacillary cases: bacterial load of 10 to the 11th power and clinical types BB, BL or LL. Paucibacillary cases: bacterial load of about 10 to the 6th power and clinical types TT, BT and indeterminate.
- Multibacillary standard regimen includes rifampin, clofazimine and dapsone:
  - ◊ Adult outside USA >35 kg
    - Rifampin 600 mg once a month
    - Clofazimine 300 mg once a mo+ 50 mg/d
    - Dapsone 100 mg/d
  - ◊ Adult outside USA < 35 kg
    - Rifampin 450 mg once a month
    - Clofazimine 300 mg once a mo+ 50 mg/d
    - Dapsone 50 mg/d
  - ◊ Children ages 10-14
    - Rifampin 450 mg once a month
    - Clofazimine 200 mg once a mo+ 50 mg qod
    - Dapsone 50 mg/d
  - ◊ Children underweight
    - Rifampin 12-15 mg/kg once a mo
    - Clofazimine 150 mg once a mo+ 50 mg qod
    - Dapsone 1-2 mg/kg/d
  - ◊ Adults in the USA (recommended regimen)
    - Rifampin 600 mg/d for 3 years
    - Dapsone 100 mg/d for life
    - Clofazimine is given in dapsone-resistant cases: 50-100 mg/d for life
- Paucibacillary standard regimen
  - ◊ Outside USA
    - Rifampin same doses as above
    - Dapsone 50-100 mg/d
  - ◊ In USA
    - Rifampin 600 mg a day for 6 mos
    - Dapsone 100 mg/d for 3-7 years
- The WHO recommends that the standard multidrug therapy (MDT) for multibacillary patients could be shortened to 12 months

Contraindications:
- Clofazimine and minocycline: pregnancy
- Ofloxacin: relative contraindication in children and adolescents
- Minocycline in pregnancy, during lactation and in children up to 5 years

Precautions:
- Hemolysis and methemoglobinemia are common untoward reactions to dapsone
- Screen for G6PD deficiency to prevent drug-induced hemolysis
- Reactionary states should be anticipated and treated aggressively
- Dapsone: GI upset, headaches, pruritus, agranulocytosis, fever, rash
- Clofazimine: GI upset and skin pigmentation
- Minocycline: reduce dose in renal damage

Significant possible interactions: Refer to manufacturer's literature for each drug

ALTERNATIVE DRUGS
- WHO recommended and widely used in countries where leprosy is endemic:
  - ◊ Rifampin 600 mg daily + ofloxacin 400 mg/d + minocycline 100 mg/d for up to 2 years (ROM)
  - ◊ Shorter duration of therapy in paucibacillary cases with the same combination has been successful

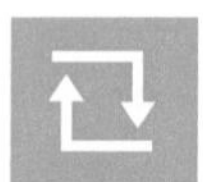

FOLLOWUP

PATIENT MONITORING
- Frequent follow-up visits until therapy course is stabilized, then monthly supervision
- Periodic CBC, renal and hepatic function

PREVENTION/AVOIDANCE
- Early case finding and chemotherapy to suppress infectiousness and control spread
- Examine family and other close contacts regularly for leprosy

POSSIBLE COMPLICATIONS
- Crippling of the hand and foot
- Trauma and secondary infection leading to loss of digits and extremities
- Corneal opacities and uveitis can lead to blindness
- Cataracts
- Lucio phenomenon - arteritis
- Secondary amyloidosis
- ENL: Rx with thalidomide 200 mg bid tapering to 50-100 mg/d in chronic patients
- Severe reversal reaction: prednisolone 40-60 mg/day, tapering slowly

EXPECTED COURSE/PROGNOSIS
Generally indolent, but may be interrupted by ENL and type 1 lepra reaction. Prognosis is good with early detection and therapy, especially with ROM.

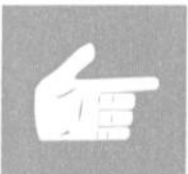

MISCELLANEOUS

ASSOCIATED CONDITIONS
HIV-positive patients with early or subclinical leprosy are more likely to develop overt disease. Concurrent leprosy may accelerate HIV-disease course.

AGE-RELATED FACTORS
Pediatric: Rare in infants under one year. Minocycline is contraindicated in children under age 5.
Geriatric: N/A
Others: N/A

PREGNANCY Clofazimine and minocycline contraindicated during pregnancy; dapsone may be used

SYNONYMS
- Hansen disease

ICD-9-CM
030.9 Leprosy, unspecified

SEE ALSO

OTHER NOTES Indeterminate, TT and perhaps BT classified as paucibacillary. BB, BL or LL are classified as multibacillary. The National Hansen's Disease Center, Carville, LA 70721 (504-642-4722) provides consultation for physicians.

ABBREVIATIONS
TT = Tuberculoid type leprosy
LL = Lepromatous leprosy
BT = Borderline tuberculoid
BL = Borderline lepromatous
BB = Mid-borderline type
ENL = Erythema nodosum leprosum

REFERENCES

- Jacobson RR, Krahenbuhl JL. Leprosy. Lancet 1999;353: 655-60
- Gelber RH. Leprosy (Hansen's disease). In: Fauci AS, et al, editors. Harrison's Principles of Internal Medicine. 15th ed. New York: McGraw-Hill; 2001. p.1035
- WHO Expert Committee on Leprosy: 7th Report. Geneva, World Health Organization,1998 (WHO Technical Report Series,No.874)
- Leprosy Rev 1998; 69 (1)
- World Health Organization. Leprosy - Global situition. Weekly Epidemiological Record. 2000; No 28, 14 July; 75:226-31
- Johnson GJ, Courtright P. Update on Ocular Leprosy. Workshop on Practical Eye Care Guidelines for Leprosy Patients. J Comm Eye Health 2001;14: 25-26
- Visschedijk J, van de Broek J, et al. Mycobacterium leprae--millennium resistant! Leprosy control on the threshold of a new era. Trop Med Int Health 2000;5(6):388-99

Web references: 3 available at www.5mcc.com
Illustrations N/A

Author(s):
V. Vasudeviah, BSc, MBBS

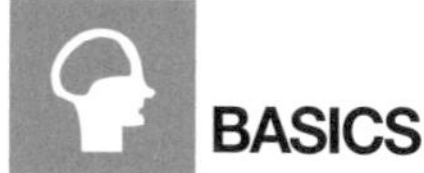

BASICS

DESCRIPTION Proliferation and accumulation of abnormal immature blood cell progenitors (blasts) in the bone marrow and other tissues. The outstanding characteristic is the development of marrow failure. Intracerebral leukostasis may develop if the blood blast count becomes greatly elevated.
Leukemia is classified according to the type of blast and according to the course, if untreated:
- Acute lymphoblastic leukemia (ALL)
- Acute nonlymphoblastic leukemia (ANLL)
- Chronic myelocytic leukemia (CML)
- Chronic lymphocytic leukemia (CLL)

System(s) affected: Hemic/Lymphatic/Immunologic
Genetics: Unknown, some are familial
Incidence/Prevalence in USA: The yearly incidence is 13.2:100,000 in males and 7.7:100,000 in females
Predominant age:
- 70% occurs in adults, mostly CLL and ANLL. 30% in children, mostly ALL.
- With the current cure rate especially good for childhood ALL, it is estimated that by the year 2010, one in 1,000 young adults (15-45 years of age) in the USA will be a childhood ALL survivor

Predominant sex: Males > Females

SIGNS & SYMPTOMS
- Mostly nonspecific and related to marrow failure or infiltration
- Fever
- Bleeding (e.g., petechiae, purpura, easy bruising, or oozing)
- Bone pain, pallor, fatigue
- Splenomegaly
- Hepatosplenomegaly
- Lymphadenopathy
- If CNS is involved, symptoms of increased intracranial pressure can be present
- Gingival swelling

CAUSES Precise causes unknown

RISK FACTORS
- Genetic and chromosomal abnormalities (e.g., trisomy 21, breakage and translocation, especially t9,22. Also AML, MLL, etc. genes)
- MLL gene for mixed lineage leukemia located on chromosome 11q23. Its abnormalities and rearrangements are easier detected with FISH (fluorescent in situ hybridization) or PCR (polymerase chain reaction). Most rearrangements in this gene result in aggressive AML, secondary AML (after chemotherapy), and infant leukemia. Example: t(11;19)(q23;p13) (MLL-ENL).
- t(12;21)(p13,q22) detected by FISH and by screening for TEL/AML1 rearrangement by PCR is now known to be the most common rearrangement in childhood ALL and carries a favorable prognosis.
- Radiation exposure
- Immunodeficiency states
- Chemical and drug exposure (nitrogen mustard and benzene)
- Preleukemia
- Cigarette smoking

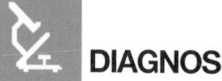

DIAGNOSIS

DIFFERENTIAL DIAGNOSIS
- Viral induced cytopenia, lymphadenopathy and organomegaly
- Immune cytopenias
- Drug induced cytopenias
- Other marrow failure and infiltrative diseases: aplastic, hypoblastic and refractory anemias; paroxysmal nocturnal hemoglobinuria; myelodysplastic syndromes, Gaucher disease, etc.

LABORATORY
- CBC, differential, platelets show subnormal RBC, neutrophils, and possibly subnormal platelets
- In some types, no circulating leukemic blasts are necessary to be present to establish the diagnosis. If 2 of the 3 above parameters are affected, or only one profoundly decreased, bone marrow failure should be ruled out.
- Reticulocyte count < 0.5
- Sedimentation rate usually elevated
- LDH and uric acid can be elevated
- Immunoglobulins IgG can be low or rarely elevated
- Coagulation profile can be normal or prolonged especially in promyelocytic leukemia (ANLL subtype)

Drugs that may alter lab results: Chemotherapy agents, especially corticosteroids. Don't prescribe these before finalizing the bone marrow studies. Some leukemic blasts are very sensitive and can have massive cell kill from as little as one dose of corticosteroids.

Disorders that may alter lab results: N/A

PATHOLOGICAL FINDINGS
- The marrow will be hypercellular and the normal architecture effaced
- The percentage of leukemic cells compared to the remainder of the cell population is usually more than 30%
- Liver, spleen, and kidneys can be enlarged and infiltrated with leukemic cells

SPECIAL TESTS Spinal tap may reveal fluid with leukemic cells

IMAGING
- Chest x-ray may reveal a large mediastinal mass
- Ultrasonography or CT scan of the abdomen may discover organomegaly

DIAGNOSTIC PROCEDURES
- Bone marrow studies are necessary to make the final diagnosis
- Aspirates are stained with a buffered Wright's stain and provide good resolution for cell morphology
- Biopsies are demineralized, sectioned and stained with hematoxylin-eosin (H&E) stain. They provide valuable information for cellularity, architecture, and megakaryocytic series.
- Marrow cell suspension used for:
  - ◊ Cytochemistries (e.g., myeloperoxidase and Sudan black are positive in myeloblasts)
  - ◊ Immunophenotyping especially useful for lymphoid leukemia and can indicate whether it is monoclonal or polyclonal, B lymphocytes or T lymphocytes, early or late, etc.
  - ◊ Chromosome studies will show the ploidy and/or the presence of a translocation which is of prognostic value
  - ◊ Immunofluorescent stain for terminal deoxyribonucleotidyl transferase (TdT), another marker that differentiates between myeloid and lymphoid blasts

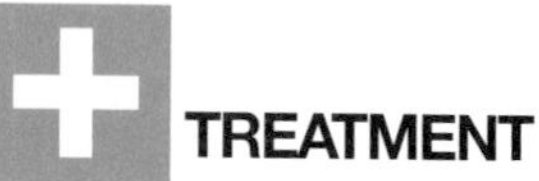

TREATMENT

APPROPRIATE HEALTH CARE
- Consult with a chemotherapist
- Induction for acute leukemia treatment requires inpatient care

GENERAL MEASURES
- Assessment of liver, heart, and kidney functions and performance status
- In acute leukemia induction, establish good hydration and urine flow (especially in ALL patients)
- Give platelet transfusion if platelet count is < 20,000 or if patient is having bleeding symptoms
- Avoid aspirin products
- Give packed red blood cells transfusion if patient is symptomatic from the anemia (e.g., orthostatic hypotension, dizziness, fatigue, hyperactive precordium) or if a cerebral or a cardiopulmonary problem is present
- If the absolute neutrophil count (ANC) < 1000, exert close temperature monitoring. (ANC = WBC x (Percentage of Polys + Bands) ÷ 100). If patient becomes febrile (even low grade fever), appropriate cultures should be taken and patient placed on broad spectrum IV antibiotics covering pseudomonas and gram positive bacteria.
- Isolation (when the ANC is low) has no value because majority of the infecting agents in this situation are the patient's own normal flora of the skin, mouth, or gut
- In promyelocytic leukemia (ANLL subtype), patients are especially at risk for DIC when treatment is started. Heparinization is indicated with close followup of coagulation parameters.

SURGICAL MEASURES
- Bone marrow transplant
  - ◊ Allogenic bone marrow transplantation in first remission for ANLL is advocated if a matched sibling is available. Autologous bone marrow transplant is also acceptable in first remission.
  - ◊ Allogenic or autologous bone marrow transplant is acceptable in first remission in high risk ALL, especially in adults. They are acceptable in second remission for childhood ALL.
  - ◊ Early studies using an allogenic non-related match donor seem to be promising and might replace the autologous route when a full sibling match is not available

ACTIVITY Ambulatory as tolerated. No intense or contact sports nor aspirin due to low platelets

DIET
- Ensure adequately balanced calorie/vitamin intake
- Follow weight closely

PATIENT EDUCATION
- Prognosis and treatment toxicity
- Leukemia Society of America: 33 Third Ave. New York, NY 10017, (212)573-8484
- NCI (Bethesda, Maryland) has pamphlets and telephone education
- "You and Leukemia, A Day At A Time" by Dr. Lynn S. Baker, W. B. Saunders Co.

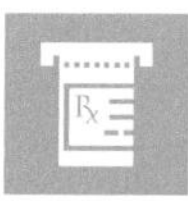

MEDICATIONS

DRUG(S) OF CHOICE
Change frequently as result of research
- ALL
  - ◊ Induction: vincristine plus prednisone plus asparaginase with or without doxorubicin or daunorubicin. CNS prophylaxis, intrathecal methotrexate with or without cranial irradiation. Add cyclophosphamide for adult ALL.
  - ◊ Maintenance: vincristine, prednisone, mercaptopurine (6-mercaptopurine) daily and methotrexate weekly for 2-3 years
  - ◊ Intensification with IV methotrexate without rescue for children or with IV cyclophosphamide, cytarabine, 6-mercaptopurine, 6-thioguanine with or without 3 weeks of induction like regimen is used for both adult and children ALL.
- ANLL
  - ◊ Induction: cytarabine plus daunorubicin, cytarabine plus idarubicin or cytarabine plus mitoxantrone. Idarubicin seems to be superior to daunorubicin in the treatment of ANLL. Yeast derived granulocyte-macrophage colony stimulating factor (GM-CSF) and granulocyte colony stimulating factor (G-CSF) do not stimulate leukemia cell growth; but help in the resolution of marrow hypoplasia associated with chemotherapy.
  - ◊ Maintenance: combined agents and high dose cytarabine (ARA-C) with timed sequence
- Promyelocytic leukemia:
  - ◊ All-trans-retinoic acid (ATRA) promotes maturation to normal granulocyte and provide remissions with lower toxicity
  - ◊ Arsenic is showing success in relapse
- CLL. An anti-CD33 monoclonal antibody has the potential for eradicating minimal residual disease.
  - ◊ Chlorambucil with or without prednisone used only if symptomatic or cytopenic. Fludarabine and cladribine (2-CDA), are showing great promise in refractory CLL. Fludarabine as a first line therapy was effective with 81% response rate and 2-CDA in a small study showed 85% response rate. New agents such as somatostatin analog, cyclosporine, theophylline have significant activity in CLL.
  - ◊ Added measurements for CLL management can include: splenectomy, leukophoresis, radiation therapy, pentostatin and 2'-deoxycoformycin
- Hairy cell leukemia. Interferon
- CML
  - ◊ Chronic phase, allogenic bone marrow transplantation. If not possible, busulfan, hydroxyurea, or interferon-alpha can prolong survival.
  - ◊ Acute phase - daunorubicin plus cytarabine plus vincristine plus prednisone with or without thioguanine, or
  - ◊ STI571 a specific inhibitor of the BCR-ABL (oncogene) tyrosine kinase has substantial activity in both chronic and blast crises in CML and in Philadelphia chromosome-positive ALL
  - ◊ High dose cytarabine with or without daunorubicin

Contraindications: No absolute contraindications

Precautions:
- Administration of chemotherapy agents should be by skilled and specifically trained individuals. IV vincristine, daunorubicin, and doxorubicin may lead to chemical burns in the event of extravasation.
- If liver injury, the toxicity of vincristine, anthracyclines and antimetabolites can be pronounced. If liver injury is advanced and hyperbilirubinemia is present, avoid those medications or reduce dosage.
- Avoid anthracyclines if patient has a pre-existing cardiac problem
- Close monitoring of the WBC's, polys, RBC and platelets is required especially in CML (chronic phase or ALL maintenance in order not to induce profound myelotoxicity
- Patients will be immunosuppressed during treatment. Avoid live vaccines. Administer varicella-zoster, or measles immunoglobulin as soon as exposure of a patient at risk becomes known.

Significant possible interactions: Allopurinol accentuates the toxicity of 6-mercaptopurine

ALTERNATIVE DRUGS N/A

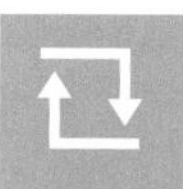

FOLLOWUP

PATIENT MONITORING
- Repeat bone marrow studies every week or every other week during induction of acute leukemia. Less frequently later. Also perform if a relapse is suspected.
- Follow uric acid level and urinary function
- Physical evaluation, including weight and blood pressure, should be done with every treatment and as frequently as once a week

PREVENTION/AVOIDANCE N/A

POSSIBLE COMPLICATIONS
- Side effects of chemotherapy
- Rarely in lymphoid leukemia, acute tumor lysis syndrome may develop leading to hyperuricemia, hyperkalemia, hyperphosphatemia, hypocalcemia, and/or uric acid nephropathy
- Late onset cardiomyopathy has been described in children treated with standard dose anthracyclines

EXPECTED COURSE/PROGNOSIS
- ALL remission rate is very good. In children, long term survival is the rule.
- AML remission rate is 60-80%, with only 20-40% long term survival
- CML invariably transforms into the acute phase within 2 years (median of 45 months). Afterward, survival rate is poor.
- CLL usually is asymptomatic for several years especially Rai, stages 0-II. In Rai's series the mean interval (in stages 0-II) is 5.3 years from diagnosis until therapy was needed. Median overall survival in CLL is thought to be 9 years.

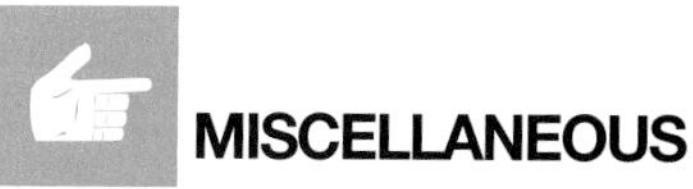

MISCELLANEOUS

ASSOCIATED CONDITIONS N/A

AGE-RELATED FACTORS
Pediatric: Tolerate intense treatments better

Geriatric:
- Do not tolerate allogenic bone marrow transplant. Age 50 is usual cut off for transplant.
- Autologous transplant may be tried in patients >50, if no organ failure is present and performance status is good
- Adding granulocyte-macrophage colony stimulating factor (GM-CSF) to induction for ANLL patients ≥ 60 years significantly reduced toxicity and made induction a feasible option in this patient profile

Others: N/A

PREGNANCY Chemotherapy is a viable option in the 2nd and 3rd trimesters.

SYNONYMS N/A

ICD-9-CM
202.40 Leukemic reticuloendotheliosis, unspecified site, extranodal and solid organ sites
204.00 Acute lymphoid leukemia without mention of remission
204.10 Chronic lymphoid leukemia
205.00 Acute myeloid leukemia without mention of remission
205.10 Chronic myeloid leukemia without mention of remission
206.00 Acute monocytic leukemia without mention of remission

SEE ALSO
Leukemia, acute lymphoblastic in adults (ALL)

OTHER NOTES N/A

ABBREVIATIONS
ALL = acute lymphoblastic leukemia
ANLL = acute nonlymphoblastic leukemia
CML = chronic myelocytic leukemia
CLL = chronic lymphocytic leukemia

REFERENCES

- Devita VT Jr, Helman S, Rosenberg SA, editors. Cancer: Principles & Practice of Oncology. 3rd ed. Philadelphia: J.B. Lippincott; 1989
- The Medical Letter on Drugs and Therapeutics: Drugs of Choice for Cancer Chemotherapy. Vol. (33) (issue 840), March 22, 1991
- Yearbook of Hematology, 1997. St. Louis, C.V. Mosby and Co, 1997

Web references: 0 available at www.5mcc.com
Illustrations 3 available

Author(s):
Mark R. Dambro, MD

Leukemia, acute lymphoblastic in adults (ALL)

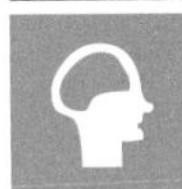

BASICS

DESCRIPTION A malignant proliferation and accumulation of immature lymphocytes
System(s) affected: Hemic/Lymphatic/Immunologic
Genetics: Increased incidence in children with Down syndrome or in rare familial diseases such as ataxia-telangiectasia, Bloom syndrome, Fanconi anemia, Klinefelter syndrome, and neurofibromatosis. Can rarely occur in adult identical twins.
Incidence/Prevalence in USA: 1000 adult cases/year
Predominant age: Median age is 35-40 years but incidence increases with age
Predominant sex: Male > Female (slightly)

SIGNS & SYMPTOMS
- Anemia - fatigue, shortness of breath, lightheadedness, angina, headache
- Thrombocytopenia - petechiae, ecchymoses, epistaxis, retinal hemorrhages
- Granulocytopenia - fever, infection
- Lymphocytosis - lymphadenopathy, hepato/splenomegaly, bone pain
- Immunosuppression
- Metabolic abnormalities - hyperuricemia, renal failure, increased lactate dehydrogenase (LDH)
- Central nervous system - cranial nerve palsies, confusion

CAUSES Unknown. Epstein-Barr virus is implicated in Burkitt leukemia/lymphoma.

RISK FACTORS
- Age over 60
- Incidence appears increased following exposure to chemical agents such as benzene or to radiation (but acute myeloid leukemia [AML] is more common)
- May follow aplastic anemia

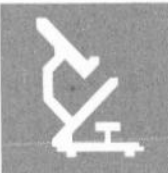

DIAGNOSIS

DIFFERENTIAL DIAGNOSIS
- Malignant disorders - other leukemias, especially AML; prolymphocytic leukemia; malignant lymphomas; multiple myeloma; bone marrow metastases from solid tumors (breast, prostate, lung, renal); myelodysplastic syndromes
- Nonmalignant disorders - aplastic anemia; myelofibrosis; autoimmune diseases (Felty syndrome, lupus); infectious mononucleosis; autoimmune thrombocytopenic purpura; leukemoid reaction to infection

LABORATORY
- Anemia - normochromic, normocytic
- Thrombocytopenia
- Peripheral blood lymphoblasts
- Elevated LDH
- Elevated uric acid

Drugs that may alter lab results: N/A

Disorders that may alter lab results: N/A

PATHOLOGICAL FINDINGS Diffuse replacement of marrow and lymph node architecture by sheets of malignant lymphoblasts

SPECIAL TESTS
- Immunophenotyping of marrow/blood lymphoblasts: B-lineage (CD19, CD20, CD24): T-lineage (CD2, CD5, CD7); CALLA ([common ALL antigen], CD10); human leukocyte antigen (HLA)-DR; terminal deoxynucleotidyl transferase (TdT); aberrant myeloid antigens (CD13); stem cell antigen (CD34)
- Cytochemical stains: Myeloperoxidase negative; Sudan black B usually negative; TdT positive; nonspecific esterase +/-; periodic acid Schiff (PAS) +/-
- Cytogenetics: Specific recurring chromosomal abnormalities have independent diagnostic and prognostic significance (hyperdiploidy > 50 chromosomes is favorable; the Philadelphia chromosome, t[9;22], the t[4;11], and the t[8;14] are unfavorable)
- Human leukocyte antigen (HLA) typing of patient and siblings for marrow transplantation

IMAGING
- Chest radiograph to evaluate for mediastinal mass or hilar adenopathy and for pulmonary infiltrates suggestive of infection
- Ultrasound exam to assess splenomegaly or renal enlargement suggestive of leukemic infiltration

DIAGNOSTIC PROCEDURES
- Bone marrow examination with aspiration, biopsy, immunophenotyping, cytochemistry, and cytogenetics
- Lymph node biopsy is rarely necessary but can be diagnostic
- Lumbar puncture should be done if neurological symptoms or signs are present. Repeat lumbar puncture after bone marrow remission is achieved to evaluate occult CNS involvement.

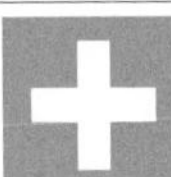

TREATMENT

APPROPRIATE HEALTH CARE
- Inpatient care during remission induction chemotherapy
- Post-remission therapy is usually outpatient
- Access to the resources and expertise of a major oncology center is important for appropriate support

GENERAL MEASURES Protective isolation from infection

SURGICAL MEASURES Surgical placement of a percutaneous silastic double-lumen central venous catheter

ACTIVITY Ambulatory as tolerated

DIET
- Nutritional support including intravenous hyperalimentation, if necessary
- Avoid alcohol

PATIENT EDUCATION
- Risks of infection, transfusion, chemotherapy
- Stop smoking

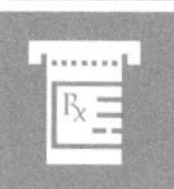

MEDICATIONS

DRUG(S) OF CHOICE

Optimal therapy is not yet known. All treatment regimens are still investigational, although clearly effective for some fraction of patients. CALGB protocol 9111 is an example of therapy (from Blood 1998; 92:1556-1564):

- Remission induction
  - ◊ Cyclophosphamide 1200 mg/square meter on day 1 (800 mg/m2 if > 60 years old)
  - ◊ Daunorubicin 45 mg/m2 on days 1, 2, and 3 (30 mg/m2 if > 60 years old)
  - ◊ Vincristine 2 mg on days 1, 8, 15, and 22
  - ◊ Asparaginase (L-asparaginase) 6000 units/m2 on days 5, 8, 11, 15, 18, and 22
  - ◊ Prednisone 60 mg/m2 on days 1-21 (days 1-7 if > 60 years old)
  - ◊ Filgrastim - G-CSF, 5 μg/kg/day SQ starting on day 4 has been shown to shorten the duration of neutropenia and improve the CR rate, especially in older patients
  - ◊ Imatinib mesylate 600-800 mg/day is effective alone and in combination with chemotherapy for Philadelphia chromosome positive ALL
- Consolidation (repeat twice in 8 weeks
  - ◊ Cyclophosphamide 1000 mg/m2 on day 1
  - ◊ Intrathecal (IT) methotrexate 15 mg with hydrocortisone 50 mg on day 1
  - ◊ Mercaptopurine (6-mercaptopurine) 60 mg/m2 on days 1-14
  - ◊ Cytarabine 75 mg/m2 SC on days 1-4 and 8-11
  - ◊ Vincristine 2 mg on days 15 and 22
  - ◊ Asparaginase 6000 units/m2 on days 15, 18, 22, and 25
- CNS prophylaxis and interim maintenance - 2400 cGy cranial irradiation
  - ◊ IT-methotrexate 15 mg with hydrocortisone 50 mg on days 1, 8, 15, 22, and 29
  - ◊ Mercaptopurine (6-mercaptopurine) 60 mg/m2 on days 1-70
  - ◊ Oral methotrexate 20 mg/m2 on days 36, 43, 50, 57, and 64
- Late intensification
  - ◊ Doxorubicin 30 mg/m2 on days 1, 8, and 15
  - ◊ Vincristine 2 mg on days 1, 8, and 15
  - ◊ Dexamethasone 10 mg/m2 on days 1-14
  - ◊ Cyclophosphamide 1000 mg/m2 on day 29
  - ◊ Thioguanine (6-thioguanine) 60 mg/m2 on days 29-42
  - ◊ Cytarabine 75 mg/m2 SC on days 29-32 and 36-39
- Prolonged maintenance
  - ◊ Vincristine 2 mg/month for 16 months
  - ◊ Prednisone 60 mg/m2 for 5 days with the vincristine
  - ◊ Mercaptopurine (6-mercaptopurine) 60 mg/m2/day for 16 months
  - ◊ Oral methotrexate 20 mg/m2/week for 16 months
- Philadelphia chromosome-positive ALL: imatinib mesylate (600-800 mg/day) is effective alone and in combination with chemotherapy

Contraindications: Doses and schedule may need to be altered for older patients and for concurrent infection and organ toxicity

Precautions:

- Tumor lysis syndrome (elevated uric acid, potassium, and phosphate with decreased calcium leading to renal failure, disseminated intravascular coagulation, and cardiac arrhythmias) may be prevented by administering allopurinol 300 mg/day. Begin 2 days before chemotherapy begins. Reduce doses if used with mercaptopurine or azathioprine. Give increased fluids. IV urate oxidase (Rasburicase); can be used to treat hyperuricemia rapidly
- Oral sulfamethoxazole-trimethoprim or aerosolized pentamidine is given for Pneumocystis carinii prophylaxis
- Profound immunosuppression. Take appropriate precautions when patient is neutropenic
- High dose cyclophosphamide causes severe nausea and vomiting. Use appropriate antiemetic regimen to prevent.
- Neurotoxicity, ileus with vincristine
- Asparaginase may cause severe allergic reactions as well as impaired pancreatic and liver function. Monitor serum glucose concentrations frequently and carefully. Pancreatitis or thrombosis may occur.

Significant possible interactions: N/A

ALTERNATIVE DRUGS
Other anthracyclines, investigational chemotherapy agents

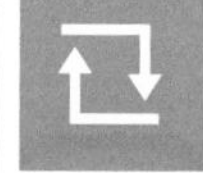

FOLLOWUP

PATIENT MONITORING
Daily during induction chemotherapy for metabolic and infectious complications. Weekly during remission consolidation chemotherapy. Monthly during maintenance therapy. Every 3 months thereafter.

PREVENTION/AVOIDANCE
N/A

POSSIBLE COMPLICATIONS

- Infections (pneumocystis carinii pneumonia, bacterial pneumonia or sepsis, fungal pneumonia)
- Bleeding
- Need for transfusions
- Sterility from treatment
- Arachnoiditis and CNS effects from intrathecal chemotherapy and irradiation
- Pancreatitis and liver dysfunction from chemotherapy
- Relapse of ALL in marrow or extramedullary sites (CNS, testis)

EXPECTED COURSE/PROGNOSIS

- 80-95% of patients < 60 years old will achieve a complete remission, and 35-60% will remain free of disease at 5 years
- Older patients (>60 years) do less well, but still 80% may achieve a complete remission
- Patients with unfavorable cytogenetic subtypes (especially t[9;22] and t[4:11]) should undergo allogeneic bone marrow transplantation in first remission if an HLA-identical donor were available

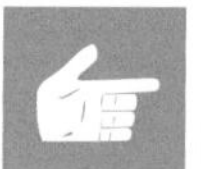

MISCELLANEOUS

ASSOCIATED CONDITIONS
N/A

AGE-RELATED FACTORS
Pediatric: Bone growth and IQ development may be affected by treatment

Geriatric: N/A

Others: N/A

PREGNANCY
Many chemotherapy drugs are teratogenic

SYNONYMS
Acute lymphocytic leukemia

ICD-9-CM
204.00 Acute lymphoid leukemia without mention of remission

204.01 Acute lymphoid leukemia in remission

SEE ALSO

OTHER NOTES
Burkitt leukemia/lymphoma (ALL-L3) - the outcome is clearly better if high dose methotrexate and alkylating agents are used for initial therapy. Only 18 weeks of treatment is required.

ABBREVIATIONS
HLA = human leukocyte antigen

REFERENCES

- Hoffman R, Benz EJ Jr, Shattil S, et al, eds. Hematology: Basic Principles and Practice. 3rd ed. New York: Churchill Livingstone; 2000
- Laport GF, Larson RA. Treatment of adult acute lymphoblastic leukemia. Semin in Oncology 1997;24:70-82
- Finiewicz KJ, Larson RA. Dose-intensive therapy for adult acute lymphoblastic leukemia. Semin in Oncology 1999;26:6-20
- Larson RA, Dodge RK, Linker CA, et al. A randomized controlled trial of filgrastim during remission induction and consolidation chemotherapy for adults with acute lymphoblastic leukemia. Blood 1998;92:1556-64
- Kantajian H, Hoelzer D, Larson RA, eds. Advances in the treatment of adult acute lymphocytic leukemia, Parts I and II. Hematol/Oncol Clin No Am 2000 and 2001
- Pui CH, Relling MV, Downing JR. Acute lymphoblastic leukemia. N Engl J Med 2004;350(15):1535-48

Web references: 7 available at www.5mcc.com

Illustrations N/A

Author(s):
Richard A. Larson, MD

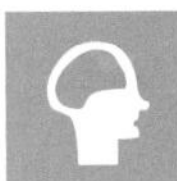

BASICS

DESCRIPTION A nonspecific clinical term used to describe a white patch in the oral mucosa which remains despite attempts to rub it off. It does not correlate with any specific microscopic findings and may be related to a variety of lesions, from benign hyperkeratosis to carcinoma.

System(s) affected: Gastrointestinal

Genetics: N/A

Incidence/Prevalence in USA:
- 3% of the adult population is affected, usually in men older than 40 years

Predominant age: 90% of lesions found in patients over 40 years of age

Predominant sex:
- Males > Female
- Some studies show no preference

SIGNS & SYMPTOMS
- Usually asymptomatic
- Location
  - ◊ 50% on tongue, mandibular alveolar ridge, and buccal mucosa
  - ◊ Also seen on maxillary alveolar ridge, palate and lower lip
  - ◊ Infrequently - floor of the mouth and retromolar areas
- Appearance
  - ◊ Varies from nonpalpable, faintly translucent white areas to thick, fissured, papillomatous, indurated lesions
  - ◊ May feel rough or leathery
  - ◊ Color may be white, gray, yellowish-white, or brownish-gray
  - ◊ Cannot be wiped off
  - ◊ Macular or plaque-like

CAUSES
- Tobacco use in any form
- Alcohol consumption
- Oral sepsis
- *Candida albicans*
- Human papilloma virus, types 11 and 15
- Actinic radiation
- Vitamin deficiency
- Syphilis
- Dental restorations
- Prosthetic dental appliances
- Alcoholism
- Estrogen therapy
- Chronic trauma or irritation

RISK FACTORS
- Age over 40
- Tobacco or alcohol use
- Repeated or chronic trauma or irritation to oral regions

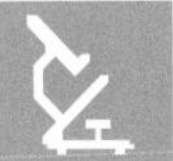

DIAGNOSIS

DIFFERENTIAL DIAGNOSIS
- White oral lesions that can be wiped away:
  - ◊ Candida
  - ◊ Aspirin burn
- White oral lesions that cannot be rubbed off:
  - ◊ Traumatic or frictional keratosis (e.g., linea alba)
  - ◊ Leukoedema
  - ◊ Galvanic keratosis
  - ◊ Lichen planus
  - ◊ Verrucous carcinoma
  - ◊ Lupus
  - ◊ Squamous cell carcinoma
  - ◊ Oral hairy leukoplakia, commonly on the lateral border of the tongue with a bilateral distribution
  - ◊ Leukokeratosis nicotina palati

LABORATORY N/A

Drugs that may alter lab results: N/A

Disorders that may alter lab results: N/A

PATHOLOGICAL FINDINGS
- Biopsy specimens range from hyperkeratosis to invasive carcinoma
- 6% at initial biopsy are invasive carcinoma
- 4% subsequently undergo malignant transformation
- Location is important: 60% on floor of mouth or lateral border of tongue are cancerous; rarely so on buccal mucosa

SPECIAL TESTS N/A

IMAGING N/A

DIAGNOSTIC PROCEDURES
Biopsy necessary to rule out carcinoma if lesion is persistent or unexplained

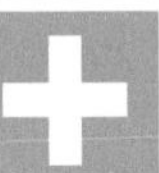

TREATMENT

APPROPRIATE HEALTH CARE
- Eliminate etiologic factors
- Reevaluate in 7-14 days
- Biopsy if lesion is persistent

GENERAL MEASURES
- Eliminate habitual lip biting
- Correct ill fitting dental appliances, bad restorations or sharp teeth
- Stop smoking and alcohol
- If dysplasia evident, remove lesion. Consider otolaryngologist referral.
- Some small lesions may respond to cryosurgery
- Beta-carotene may cause partial regression (experimental)
- For hairy tongue: Tongue brushing

SURGICAL MEASURES
- Excision is the treatment of choice for lesions exhibiting dysplasia or malignant transformation

ACTIVITY Full

DIET Regular

PATIENT EDUCATION
- If biopsy negative, stress importance of periodic and careful followup
- Dental referral to eliminate dental factors
- Stress importance of stopping tobacco and alcohol use
- Encourage participation in smoking cessation program

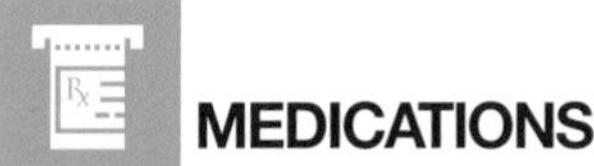

MEDICATIONS

DRUG(S) OF CHOICE
- Generally none needed
- Hairy leukoplakia
  - ◊ Acyclovir 2-4 gm/day systemically is effective, but the lesions recur when the treatment is stopped
  - ◊ Topical retinoids
  - ◊ Topical podophyllin 25% resin applied twice, one week apart, but the bad taste is poorly tolerated
- Leukoplakia
  - ◊ isotretinoin (Accutane) 1-2 mg/kg/day may lead to temporary remission, but side effects are poorly tolerated

Contraindications: N/A
Precautions: N/A
Significant possible interactions: N/A

ALTERNATIVE DRUGS N/A

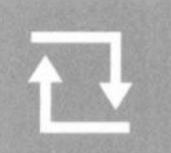

FOLLOWUP

PATIENT MONITORING Regular, close followup, even after successful treatment. Biopsy as needed.

PREVENTION/AVOIDANCE
- Avoid tobacco, alcohol, habitual biting
- Provide well-fitting dental prothesis
- Regular dental check-up to avoid bad restorations

POSSIBLE COMPLICATIONS
- Carcinoma
- New lesions may develop after treatment

EXPECTED COURSE/PROGNOSIS
- Curable if detected early
- 4-6% of initially benign lesions subsequently develop cancer
- More likely cancerous if on floor of mouth or lateral border of tongue

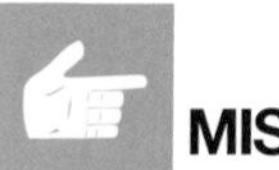

MISCELLANEOUS

ASSOCIATED CONDITIONS
- Leukokeratosis nicotina palati is rarely malignant
- HIV infection closely associated with hairy leukoplakia

AGE-RELATED FACTORS
Pediatric: N/A
Geriatric: More common in elderly
Others: Rare before age 40

PREGNANCY N/A

SYNONYMS N/A

ICD-9-CM
528.6 Leukoplakia of oral mucosa, including tongue

SEE ALSO
Epstein-Barr virus infections
HIV infection & AIDS

OTHER NOTES
- Uncommonly - other mucosal surfaces (vaginal, anal, etc.)
- Linea alba - a white line on the buccal mucosa, along the occlusal plane

ABBREVIATIONS N/A

REFERENCES

- Regezi JA, Sciubba JJ, Pogrel MA. Atlas of Oral and Maxillofacial Pathology. Philadelphia, WB Saunde5rs Co, 2000
- Yeats D, Burn J. Common Oral Mucosal Lesions in Adults. Amer Fam Phys 1991;44:2043-50
- Fitzpatrick T, et al. Color Atlas and Synopsis of Clinical Dermatology. 2nd Ed. New York, McGraw-Hill, 1992

Web references: 0 available at www.5mcc.com
Illustrations 1 available

Author(s):
Fady Faddoul, DDS, MSD

BASICS

DESCRIPTION A unique inflammatory disorder of the skin and mucous membranes. The disease is characterized by small flat, angular, violaceous, shiny, pruritic papules on the skin and white papules in the mouth. Onset abrupt or gradual. May be intermittent for years.
System(s) affected: Skin/Exocrine
Genetics: N/A
Incidence/Prevalence in USA: 450/100,000
Predominant age: 30-60 years, rare in children and the elderly
Predominant sex: Female > Male

SIGNS & SYMPTOMS
- Skin
  - ◊ Pruritus - often severe
  - ◊ Papules - 1-10 mm, shiny, flat
  - ◊ Color - violaceous, with white lace-like pattern (Wickham's striae) on papules. Wickham's striae best seen after topical application of mineral oil and if present, are almost pathognomonic for lichen planus.
  - ◊ Shape - polygonal or oval shaped
  - ◊ Arrangement - may be grouped, linear, annular, or scattered individual lesions.
  - ◊ Koebner's phenomenon is often seen
  - ◊ Distribution - ventral surface of wrists and forearms, glans penis, dorsa feet, groin, sacrum, shins and scalp. Hypertrophic (verrucous) lesions may occur on lower legs. An annular pattern may appear on trunk and mucous membranes. Linear arrangements of papules have been described.
- Mucous membranes
  - ◊ Mucous membrane involvement is seen in 40-60% of patients with skin lesions. 20% of patients have mucous membrane lesions only.
  - ◊ Milky-white papules with white lace-like pattern
  - ◊ Usually seen on buccal mucosa, but may appear on tongue, gingiva, palate, and lips
  - ◊ May be bullous or erosive
  - ◊ Painful, especially if ulcers present
  - ◊ Mucous membrane lesions may be precancerous (squamous cell carcinoma)
- Hair and nails
  - ◊ Scalp - atrophic scalp skin and destruction of hair follicles. May result in permanent patchy scarring alopecia.
  - ◊ Nails - (10%) may cause proximal to distal linear grooves and partial or complete destruction of nail bed with pterygium formation. Large toes most commonly affected.

CAUSES Etiology unknown. Possibly a disease of keratinization or an autoimmune disease. Emotional stress may antedate an attack.

RISK FACTORS Exposure to drugs or chemicals, graft versus host disease, or lupus erythematosus (LE-LP overlap syndrome)

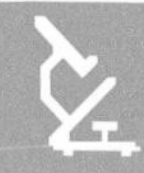

DIAGNOSIS

DIFFERENTIAL DIAGNOSIS
- Chemical exposure (chemicals used in color developing)
- Lichenoid drug eruption (chloroquine, quinacrine, gold salts, methyldopa, penicillamine, arsenic, bismuth, ACE inhibitors)
- Lichen nitidus
- Leukoplakia
- Psoriasis
- Candidiasis
- Squamous cell carcinoma; basal cell carcinoma
- Aphthous ulcers
- Herpetic stomatitis
- Secondary syphilis
- Scabies
- Pseudopelade

LABORATORY N/A

Drugs that may alter lab results: N/A

Disorders that may alter lab results: N/A

PATHOLOGICAL FINDINGS Inflammation with hyperkeratosis, increased granular layer, irregular acanthosis, basement-membrane thinning with "sawtoothing," hyaline bodies below the epidermis, band-like lymphocytic infiltrate of the upper dermis

SPECIAL TESTS N/A

IMAGING N/A

DIAGNOSTIC PROCEDURES Skin biopsy

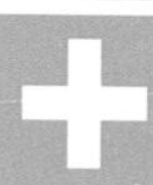

TREATMENT

APPROPRIATE HEALTH CARE Outpatient

GENERAL MEASURES
- Goal is to relieve itching with topical and systemic antipruritics
- Psoralens and ultraviolet A (PUVA) photochemotherapy may be helpful for generalized or resistant cases
- Behavior modification for stress reduction may prevent recurrence

SURGICAL MEASURES N/A

ACTIVITY Fully active

DIET No special diet

PATIENT EDUCATION Help with stress reduction if appropriate

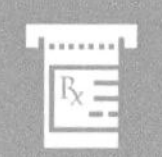

MEDICATIONS

DRUG(S) OF CHOICE
- Skin
  - ◊ Topical steroids (e.g., 0.1% triamcinolone acetonide) with occlusion
  - ◊ Intralesional corticosteroids, e.g., triamcinolone (Kenalog) 5-10 mg/mL) for hypertrophic lesions
  - ◊ Antihistamine (e.g., hydroxyzine, dosage - 25 mg q6h) if needed for itching
- Mucous membranes
  - ◊ Topical oral retinoids, e.g., 0.05% tretinoin (retinoic acid) in Orabase or topical oral corticosteroids (0.1% triamcinolone (Kenalog in Orabase) bid
  - ◊ Intralesional corticosteroids for erosive, painful lichen planus, e.g., 0.5-1.0 mL methylprednisolone (Depo-Medrol) 40 mg/mL
  - ◊ Oral retinoids - isotretinoin (Accutane) or etretinate (Tegison)

Contraindications: Patients with history of hypersensitivity to corticosteroids or retinoids

Precautions:
- Systemic absorption of steroids may result in hypothalamic-pituitary-adrenal axis suppression, Cushing syndrome, hyperglycemia, and glucosuria
- Increased risk with high potency - i.e., use over large surface area, prolonged use, occlusive dressings
- These medications are Category C teratogens. Avoid in pregnancy.
- Children may absorb a proportionally larger amount of topical steroid due to larger skin surface to weight ratio

Significant possible interactions: See manufacturer's profile of each drug

ALTERNATIVE DRUGS
- Oral prednisone - rarely used and only for a short course (e.g., prednisone 20 mg bid x 2-4 weeks)
- Cyclosporine may be used in severe cases, but cost and potential toxicity limits its use. Topical use for severe oral involvement refractory to other treatments.
- Thalidomide
- PUVA or narrow band UVB
- Griseofulvin
- Azathioprine
- Mycophenolate mofetil

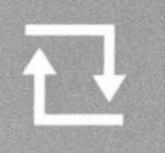

FOLLOWUP

PATIENT MONITORING Serial skin exams

PREVENTION/AVOIDANCE Reduce stress

POSSIBLE COMPLICATIONS
- Alopecia
- Nail destruction
- Squamous cell carcinoma of the mouth

EXPECTED COURSE/PROGNOSIS
- Spontaneous resolution in weeks is possible, but disease may persist for years - especially in the mouth and on shins
- There is a tendency toward relapse, especially with emotional stress
- Recurrence 12-20% especially in those with generalized involvement

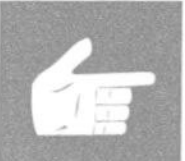

MISCELLANEOUS

ASSOCIATED CONDITIONS
- Hepatitis C
- Lichen nitidus
- Bullous pemphigoid
- Alopecia
- Myasthenia gravis
- Lupus erythematosus
- Biliary cirrhosis
- Vitiligo
- Ulcerative colitis
- Graft-versus-host reaction
- Morphea and lichen sclerosus et atrophicus

AGE-RELATED FACTORS
Pediatric: N/A
Geriatric: N/A
Others: N/A

PREGNANCY Avoid corticosteroids, retinoids

SYNONYMS
- Lichenoid eruptions

ICD-9-CM
697.0 Lichen planus

SEE ALSO

OTHER NOTES Remember the 5 p's of lichen planus - purple, planar, polygonal, pruritic papules

ABBREVIATIONS N/A

REFERENCES

- Habif T. Clinical Dermatology. 4th Ed. St. Louis, CV Mosby, 2004
- Fitzpatrick TB, et al. Color Atlas and Synopsis of Clinical Dermatology. 4th Ed. New York: McGraw-Hill; 2001
- Fitzpatrick TB, et al. Dermatology in General Medicine. 5th Ed. New York: McGraw-Hill; 1999
- Arnold HL Jr, Odom RB, James WD, editors. Andrews' Diseases of the Skin: Clinical pharmacology. 9th ed. Philadelphia: WB Saunders Co; 2000
- Rakel RE, editor. Conn's Current therapy. Philadelphia: WB Saunders Co; 2003
- Howard R. Adult skin disease in the pediatric patient. Dermatologic Clin 1998:16(3):593-608
- Miles DA. Diagnosis and management of oral lichen planus. Dermatologic Clin 1996;14(2):281-290

Web references: 1 available at www.5mcc.com
Illustrations 9 available

Author(s):
Marc Darr, MD

BASICS

DESCRIPTION Infection caused by the ubiquitous, weakly hemolytic, gram positive bacillus, Listeria monocytogenes, which is pathogenic to many animal species. Occurs most often in fetuses (disseminated infantile listeriosis), in neonates, and in immunosuppressed patients. Majority of adult patients have pre-existing disease (cirrhosis, lymphomas, solid tumors, AIDS, cancer therapy). Usual course - acute.
- In 2002, 46 culture-confirmed cases, 7 deaths and 3 miscarriages were linked to eating sliceable turkey deli meat

System(s) affected: Endocrine/Metabolic, Gastrointestinal, Hemic/Lymphatic/Immunologic, Nervous, Pulmonary, Renal/Urologic
Genetics: No known genetic pattern
Incidence/Prevalence in USA:
- 2500 serious illnesses; 500 deaths/year
- Pregnant women are about 20 times more likely than healthy adults to get listeriosis
- Persons with AIDS are almost 300 times more likely to develop infection

Predominant age: Neonates, elderly
Predominant sex: Male > Female

SIGNS & SYMPTOMS
- Asymptomatic
- Abdominal pain
- Adult respiratory distress syndrome
- Cervical lymphadenopathy
- Chills
- Conjunctivitis
- Decreased fetal movement
- Diarrhea
- Dysuria
- Fatigue
- Fever
- Hepatosplenomegaly
- Malaise
- Myalgia
- Nausea
- Pharyngitis
- Urinary frequency
- Vomiting
- Findings suggestive of meningitis - fever, headache, nausea and vomiting, stiff neck, delirium, coma
- Findings suggestive of sepsis - high fever and generalized severe illness without evidence of localized infection (in patients with alcoholism, malignancies, immunosuppression, AIDS)
- High risk patients with signs suggestive of listeriosis within one month of eating suspected or recalled foods should contact their physician

CAUSES Listeria monocytogenes, a small gram-positive bacillus; infection with other species of Listeria are rare. Illnesses can begin 2-8 weeks after eating contaminated food.

RISK FACTORS
- Age - fetus, neonates, elderly
- Metastatic malignant disease
- HIV infection
- Alcoholism
- Renal hemodialysis
- Pregnancy
- Immunosuppressed
- Exposure to infected animals (veterinarians, butchers, etc.). Animal-to-human transmission is rare.
- Ingesting contaminated food or drink (e.g., soft Mexican style cheese or feta cheese)

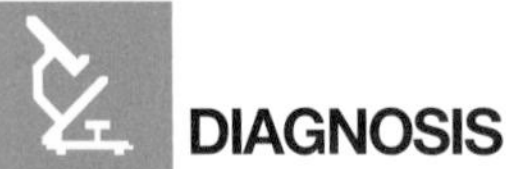

DIAGNOSIS

DIFFERENTIAL DIAGNOSIS
- Other infections - Staphylococcal, gram negative Klebsiella, Candida, cryptococcosis, viral
- Infantile listeriosis, E. coli, Group B streptococci
- Infectious mononucleosis

LABORATORY
- CSF
  - ◊ Gram stain - may reveal small, gram-positive rods or coccobacillary forms with "tumbling" motility. (Sometimes difficult to identify since organisms are not present in large numbers and may be confused with diphtheroids and other bacteria.)
  - ◊ Cell count - in most cases, the predominant cell type is the neutrophil; however, mononuclear cells may predominate. Counts range from 0-1200/mm3. RBC's frequently seen.
  - ◊ Protein concentration - within normal limits to 735 mg/dL
  - ◊ Glucose - within normal limits to undetectable
  - ◊ CSF cultures - demonstrates beta-hemolysis (L. monocytogenes grows well on 5% sheep's blood or chocolate agar)
  - ◊ Counterimmunoelectrophoresis (CIE) latex agglutination (LA) - possibly useful for differential diagnosis
- Other tests
  - ◊ Blood cultures should be done
  - ◊ CBC - peripheral WBC may show an elevated neutrophil count and/or left shift
  - ◊ Other cultures in newborn - cervical vaginal secretions and lochia from the mother; cord blood; grossly abnormal portions of the placenta, meconium, and exudate expressed from an incised skin papule of the neonate

Drugs that may alter lab results: Antibiotics

Disorders that may alter lab results: Cultures may be confusing in patients with mixed infections

PATHOLOGICAL FINDINGS
- Gross - multi-organ miliary granulomatosis
- Micro - nodular focal abscess
- Micro - necrotic amorphous basophilic debris
- Micro - increased tissue macrophages
- Micro - gram-positive bacilli
- Motile bacilli
- Chinese-letter aggregates

SPECIAL TESTS Specimens for serologic testing should be submitted to the local public health laboratory. In outbreaks, serotyping may be desirable.

IMAGING MRI with any patient having central nervous system symptoms

DIAGNOSTIC PROCEDURES Lumbar puncture

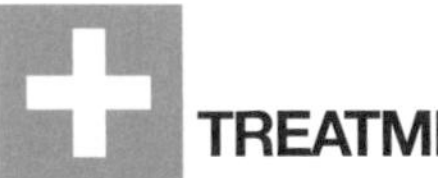

TREATMENT

APPROPRIATE HEALTH CARE Inpatient during acute phase

GENERAL MEASURES
- Bedrest
- Isolation if immunosuppressed
- Secretion precautions
- Respiratory assistance (if apneic, or CNS depressed)

SURGICAL MEASURES N/A

ACTIVITY Bedrest

DIET
- Acute case, total parenteral nutrition, nasogastric tube, or softer diet if tolerated
- As a preventive, avoid eating raw or partially cooked foods and soft cheeses. Warm leftovers thoroughly and wash raw vegetables before cooking.
- If high risk patient consumes recalled product, but does not develop symptoms within 1 month, no further treatment is needed. AN updated list of recalled food products can be found at the USDA website: www.fsis.usda.gov/OA/recalls/rec_intr.htm

PATIENT EDUCATION
- Dietary guidelines for avoidance in high risk patients
- CDC - National Center for Infectious Diseases; www.cdc.gov/ncidod/ncid.htm/

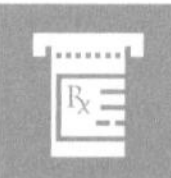

MEDICATIONS

DRUG(S) OF CHOICE

- Neonates - IV treatment 14-21 days:
  - ◊ Meningitis - for infants older than one month: ampicillin 300-400 mg/kg/day IV
  - ◊ Meningitis - neonate doses: < 2000 grams, less than 1 week old: ampicillin 50 mg/kg q12h. Older than 1 week: ampicillin 50 mg/kg every 8 hours. Plus gentamicin 7.5 mg/kg/day IV for 14 days. Discontinue gentamicin when cerebro-spinal fluid is sterile.
  - ◊ Alternate therapy for neonates - penicillin G 100,000-200,000 units/kg/d IV x 14-21 days plus gentamicin as above
  - ◊ Bacteremia or pneumonia - ampicillin 100-150 mg/kg/day (or penicillin G 200,000 units/kg/d IV) plus gentamicin 5.0 mg/kg/day. Discontinue gentamicin when blood cultures become negative.
- Pregnant women:
  - ◊ Ampicillin 2 gm IV q4h for 14-21 days plus gentamicin 120 mg IV q8h. Adjust for peak 5-6 mcg/mL.
- Immunocompromised/elderly patients:
  - ◊ Ampicillin 2 gm IV q4h plus ceftriaxone 2 gm IV q12h or cefotaxime 2 gm IV q6h plus vancomycin 500 mg IV q6h and dexamethasone .4 mg/kg IV q12h x 2 days; give first dose with first dose of antibiotic
- For endocarditis and typhoidal listeriosis:
  - ◊ Penicillin G 75,000-100,000 units/kg IV q4h and continue for 14 days after defervescence. plus tobramycin 2 mg/kg load, then adjust based on levels. Aim for peak at 5-6. Continue for 4 weeks after defervescence.
- For oculoglandular:
  - ◊ Erythromycin 30 mg/kg/day as 4 equal doses q6h and continue for 1 week after defervescence

Contraindications: Allergy to penicillins

Precautions: Cephalosporins are not adequate treatment. Refer to manufacturer's literature.

Significant possible interactions: Refer to manufacturer's literature

ALTERNATIVE DRUGS

- Trimethoprim-sulfamethoxazole may be the most effective treatment for adults because of its ability to penetrate cells. Total dose 10 mg/kg (based on trimethoprim component) in divided doses.
- Clarithromycin
- Ciprofloxacin

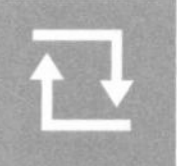

FOLLOWUP

PATIENT MONITORING

- Frequent arterial blood gases during acute phase
- Repeat lumbar puncture at 24-48 hours and at the end of treatment

PREVENTION/AVOIDANCE

- If pregnant, elderly or immune compromised: check USDA website for recalled foods
- Avoid handling livestock
- Avoid contaminated silage
- Avoid contaminated sewage
- Avoid raw or contaminated milk products
- Avoid soft cheeses (Mexican and feta)
- Wash carefully all raw vegetables
- Keep uncooked meats separate from vegetables
- Wash hands after handling uncooked foods
- Avoid foods from deli counter
- Cook leftovers, hot dogs, cold cuts, and deli meats until steaming hot before eating

POSSIBLE COMPLICATIONS

- Premature delivery
- Amnionitis
- Meningitis
- Septicemia
- Pulmonary abscess
- Hepatic abscess
- Placental abscess
- Splenic abscess
- Lymph node abscess
- Endocarditis
- Peritonitis
- Abortion
- Stillbirth
- Neonatal death

EXPECTED COURSE/PROGNOSIS

High mortality if symptomatic

MISCELLANEOUS

ASSOCIATED CONDITIONS

- Cirrhosis
- Lymphomas
- Solid tumors
- Immunodeficiencies
- Pregnancy

AGE-RELATED FACTORS

Pediatric:

- Infected fetuses are usually stillborn or premature. More than half are infected with lethal listeriosis.
- 50% mortality in treated neonates

Geriatric: Greater morbidity and mortality

Others: N/A

PREGNANCY

- Pregnant women are more susceptible to infection with Listeria monocytogenes; transmission to the fetus and neonates occurs with high mortality.
- Requires prompt and vigorous treatment to prevent transfer of disease to fetus (pregnant patient's symptoms may begin as a flu-like illness or be absent)

SYNONYMS

- Listeria monocytogenes
- Listerial disease

ICD-9-CM

027.0 Listeriosis

SEE ALSO

OTHER NOTES

- Notify laboratory at time of sending any specimen that listeriosis is a possibility
- Laboratory specimens must be sent to laboratory promptly (few organisms more difficult to culture)
- Need at least 10 cc of spinal fluid for culture
- Listeriosis is a reportable disease; report to CDC at 404-639-2215 or www.fsis.usda.gov/OA/recalls/reactv.htm
- Questions regarding safety of deli meat: USDA 800-535-4555
- More information online cdc.gov/foodnet

ABBREVIATIONS N/A

REFERENCES

- Linnan MJ, Mascola L, Lou X, May S, Salimen C, et al. Epidemic listeriosis associated with Mexican-style cheese. N Engl J Med 1988;319, 823:828
- Von Lichtenberg F. Pathology of Infectious Diseases. New York, Raven Press, 1988
- Southwick FS, Purich DL. Mechanisms of disease: Intracellular pathogenesis of listeriosis. NEJM 1996;334:770-76
- Update: Multi-state outbreak of listeriosis-United States, 1998-1999: MMWR 1999;47:1117-1118
- Mahoney, D. Listeriosis Outbreak linked to sliced deli turkey. Family Practice News. 2002;Nov 1, 2002.
- MMWR. 2002;51:950-951

Web references: 3 available at www.5mcc.com

Illustrations N/A

Author(s):

Susana May, MD, MPH

BASICS

DESCRIPTION Mechanical low back pain is a diagnosis of exclusion. It is generally a self-limiting condition of the aging spine, responsive to conservative measures including rest and pain management. Patients typically present with pain at the posterior belt line with occasional referred pain to the buttocks and/or posterior thighs. These symptoms often are the result of the mechanical stresses and functional demands placed on the low back area by everyday activities. The condition, for the vast majority of patients, is of short duration and complete recovery is the general rule. The primary goal of the clinician is to rule-out other more serious etiologies. It must be remembered that low back pain is a symptom, not a disease, and that the pathological basis of the pain frequently lies outside the spine.

System(s) affected: Musculoskeletal, Nervous
Genetics: N/A
Incidence/Prevalence in USA:
- 80% of Americans experience mechanical low back pain sometime in their lifetime
- One of the most common complaints for primary care visits
- Repetitive episodes are common

Predominant age: 25-99 years
Predominant sex: Male = Female

SIGNS & SYMPTOMS
- History
  - ◊ Onset of low back pain begins either suddenly after an injury or gradually over the next 24 hours
  - ◊ Variable pain at posterior belt-line, typically bilateral
  - ◊ Occasional radiation of pain to buttocks, and/or posterior thighs stopping at knees
  - ◊ Pain pattern referred rather than radicular
  - ◊ Back pain worse than leg pain
  - ◊ Pain aggravated by back motion, sitting, standing, lifting, bending and twisting
  - ◊ Pain relieved by rest (recumbency)
  - ◊ Bowel and bladder function preserved
- Physical findings
  - ◊ Normal motor, sensory, and reflex examinations
  - ◊ Decreased lumbar range of motion, tenderness to palpation, paraspinous musculature spasm common
  - ◊ Nerve root stretch tests are commonly negative
  - ◊ Straight leg raise and other tests causing spinal motion may increase low back pain, but not leg pain

CAUSES
- Normal aging process of musculoskeletal system aggravates an acute event
- Degenerative joint disease of LS spine

RISK FACTORS
- Age
- Activity
- Smoking
- Obesity
- Vibration, e.g., driving motor vehicles
- Sedentary lifestyle
- Psychosocial factors

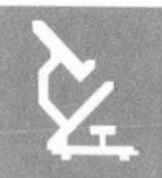

DIAGNOSIS

DIFFERENTIAL DIAGNOSIS
- Structural
  - ◊ Acute lumbar back pain
  - ◊ Chronic lumbar back pain
  - ◊ Low back strain/sprain
  - ◊ Herniated lumbar intervertebral disc
  - ◊ Degenerative disc disease
  - ◊ Degenerative segmental instability
  - ◊ Spinal stenosis
  - ◊ Spondylolisthesis
  - ◊ Fractures
- Inflammatory
  - ◊ Ankylosing spondylitis and related inflammatory spondylopathies
  - ◊ Infection: vertebral osteomyelitis, discitis
  - ◊ Rheumatoid arthritis
- Neoplastic
  - ◊ Primary tumors
  - ◊ Metastases
- Referred pain
  - ◊ Orthopaedic - osteoarthritis of hip
  - ◊ Sacroiliac joint disease
  - ◊ Gastrointestinal - duodenal ulcer, chronic pancreatitis, irritable bowel syndrome, diverticulitis
  - ◊ Genitourinary - pyelonephritis, nephrolithiasis, prostatism
  - ◊ Gynecological - pregnancy, endometriosis, ovarian cystic disease, pelvic inflammatory disease
  - ◊ Cardiovascular - abdominal aortic aneurysm, vascular claudication

LABORATORY
- Generally negative and not typically indicated with initial presentation
- Indications
  - ◊ Age > 50 years
  - ◊ Nonmechanical nature of pain
  - ◊ Atypical pain pattern or distribution
  - ◊ Persistent symptomatology remittent to conservative treatment measures
- Screening laboratory studies
  - ◊ CBC with differential
  - ◊ Sedimentation rate
  - ◊ Alkaline and acid phosphatase
  - ◊ Serum calcium
  - ◊ Serum protein electrophoresis

Drugs that may alter lab results: N/A

Disorders that may alter lab results: N/A

PATHOLOGICAL FINDINGS N/A

SPECIAL TESTS System directed investigation

IMAGING
- Plain radiographs
  - ◊ Not indicated to initiate conservative management program
  - ◊ Indicated for persistent symptoms > 1 week, patient age > 50 years, or suggestive history
  - ◊ Radiographs utilized to rule-out tumor or identify other disease process
  - ◊ Anteroposterior, lateral, spot lateral of L5-S1 and oblique x-rays are included in routine lumbo-sacral series
- Bone scan (scintigraphy)
  - ◊ Technetium-99m labeled phosphorus indicates active mineralization of bone
  - ◊ Rule-out tumor, trauma or infection

DIAGNOSTIC PROCEDURES MRI, CT/myelography only indicated with persistent symptoms, sciatica or the development of neurologic abnormalities

TREATMENT

APPROPRIATE HEALTH CARE Outpatient for majority

GENERAL MEASURES
- Initial short-term bedrest generally not recommended
- Short-term analgesics
- NSAIDs 10 day course initially, then prn
- Muscle relaxants 10 day course
- Physical therapy
- Manipulation

SURGICAL MEASURES N/A

ACTIVITY
- Restricted activities for 3-6 weeks
- Resume activities of daily living as soon as possible

DIET Weight reduction - if appropriate

PATIENT EDUCATION
- Home based exercise program
- Posture and body mechanics training
- "Back school" for chronic mechanical low back pain

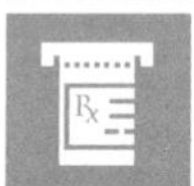

MEDICATIONS

DRUG(S) OF CHOICE Non-steroidal anti-inflammatory drugs: Ibuprofen, naproxen, salsalate, celecoxib, rofecoxib. Less expensive, equally efficacious.

Contraindications: Refer to manufacturer's product information

Precautions:
- History of ulcer disease
- Elderly patients
- Renal disease
- Cardiac disease

Significant possible interactions: Refer to manufacturer's product information

ALTERNATIVE DRUGS N/A

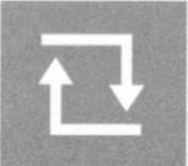

FOLLOWUP

PATIENT MONITORING Estimated duration of care 1-6 weeks

PREVENTION/AVOIDANCE
- Smoking cessation
- Weight reduction
- General physical condition
- Avoid aggravating tasks, e.g., heavy lifting, bending, twisting, sudden unexpected movements or combination of above

POSSIBLE COMPLICATIONS
- Incorrect diagnosis
- Chronic low back pain
- Narcotic addiction
- Persistent psychosocial impairment

EXPECTED COURSE/PROGNOSIS
- Resumption of normal activity without residual symptoms in most cases
- May be hindered by secondary gain issues

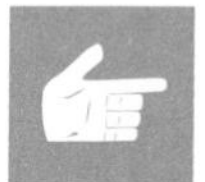

MISCELLANEOUS

ASSOCIATED CONDITIONS
- Deconditioning
- Obesity
- Psychosocial disease
- Compression fracture

AGE-RELATED FACTORS

Pediatric: Thorough work-up imperative

Geriatric: Tumors, degenerative conditions, fractures and stenosis more common

Others: N/A

PREGNANCY Commonly associated with low back pain and/or sciatica. Treatment is conservative.

SYNONYMS
- Low back syndrome
- Lumbar strain/sprain
- Lumbago

ICD-9-CM

722.2 Displacement of intervertebral disc, site unspecified, without myelopathy

722.6 Degeneration of intervertebral disc, site unspecified

724.2 Lumbago

724.5 Backache, unspecified

SEE ALSO

Lumbar (intervertebral) disk disorders

OTHER NOTES
- Adverse psychosocial factors to resolving back pain:
  - ◊ Pending litigation or compensation
  - ◊ Depressed or hostile patient
  - ◊ Prolonged use of narcotics or alcohol

ABBREVIATIONS N/A

REFERENCES

- American Academy of Orthopedic Surgeons: Clinical Policy; Low back musculoligamentous injury (sprain/strain). AAOS Bulletin 3638, April, 1991
- Macnab I, McCulloch J: Backache. 2nd Ed. Baltimore, Williams & Wilkins, 1986

Web references: 0 available at www.5mcc.com

Illustrations N/A

Author(s):

Michael J. Smith, MD

Robert A. Cheney, MD

BASICS

DESCRIPTION Many patients with low back pain have lumbar disk disease and involvement of surrounding spinal ligaments, muscles and skeleton. Over time may progress to disk degeneration, disk herniation, spinal narrowing and arthritic proliferation of the facet joint. Management is based on symptoms and disability, because the distinction between the normal aging of the spine and pathological findings are hard to distinguish.

- Non-radicular low back pain (acute and chronic) - low back pain remaining near belt-line caused by soft tissue or disk injury
- Radicular low back pain (acute and chronic) - neuropathic pain is to a greater degree in the buttocks, hips or legs rather than the back. There may or may not be signs of weakness, numbness, or loss of reflex. In younger patients, the source of the pain is likely to be mechanical compression or chemical irritation of a nerve root.
- Spinal stenosis is more likely to be the etiology of radicular pain in patients over 55 years

System(s) affected: Musculoskeletal, Nervous
Genetics: N/A
Incidence/Prevalence in USA:

- One of the most frequent complaints for which adults seek medical attention and second to the common cold for most time off work
- Lifetime prevalence of low back pain is 60-90%. The annual incidence is 5%. Among patients with acute back pain, 1% have nerve root symptoms.
- 95% of diseased disks are localized to L4-5 and L5-S1
- Less than 2% of patients with low back pain have infections, neoplasms, or inflammatory spondyloarthropathies

Predominant age: 25-45 years, first episode in 20's and 30's, infrequent before 20 years or after age 65
Predominant sex: Male = Female

SIGNS & SYMPTOMS

- Variable pain; usually dull, originating in back, extending below knee
- Pain may radiate (often unilaterally) in nerve root distribution
- Back pain decreases at night. Bedrest usually improves symptoms at least temporarily.
- Pain increases with sitting, standing
- Constitutional symptoms absent
- Sciatica can occur without back pain
- Often sensory aberrations in extremities, paresthesia and numbness
- Occasionally muscle group weakness
- Most disk ruptures are posterolateral and press upon lumbar nerve root with radiating pain
- Lumbar scoliosis possible, trunk tilted toward or away from affected side, depending on location of extrusion
- Paraspinal muscle spasm

CAUSES

- Trauma, major or minor
- Frequent lifting of objects weighing 25 pounds (11.3 kg) or more, especially if lifted with arms extended and knees straight, and body twisted
- Vibration; e.g., driving motor vehicles

RISK FACTORS

- Normal aging process after age 20 years
- Cigarette smoking
- Narrow lumbar vertebral canal (for prolapsed disk)
- Stress, muscle tension
- Obesity

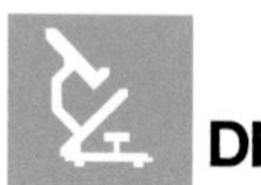

DIAGNOSIS

DIFFERENTIAL DIAGNOSIS

- Acute lumbosacral strain
- Chronic lumbosacral strain
- Spondylosis
- Spondylolisthesis
- Spinal arthritis
- Fibrositis
- Cauda equina syndrome
- Compression fracture
- Poor posture
- Bursitis
- Metastatic and primary tumors
- Vertebral infection
- Pain referred from hip, retroperitoneum, aneurysms, or pelvis (geriatrics), neurogenic claudication
- Signs and symptoms that suggest a more serious etiology are constitutional symptoms, night pain, recent infection, history of cancer, immunosuppression, IV drug use. Signs of cauda equina syndrome are peroneal anesthesia, bowel or bladder dysfunction, and severe lower extremity neurological losses

LABORATORY ESR or C-reactive protein - usually normal

Drugs that may alter lab results: N/A

Disorders that may alter lab results: N/A

PATHOLOGICAL FINDINGS Difficult to distinguish normal aging process of disk degeneration from specific lesions causing low back pain and sciatica

SPECIAL TESTS Electromyography - useful to exclude peripheral neuritis

IMAGING

- Lumbosacral plain films - rarely indicated just to initiate a conservative management program - indicated to rule out tumor or structural abnormality although presence of latter may not confirm source of pain
- Lumbosacral oblique views - controversial
- Magnetic resonance now preferred over CT scan and myelogram (for surgical candidate evaluation). Notes: disk herniation found in 20-35% and disk bulging in 56% of asymptomatic adults under 60 years.

DIAGNOSTIC PROCEDURES

- Sciatic stretch test - in supine position, elevation of affected leg (to 15-30% for severe, 30-60%, milder) elicits pain. Tip: can compare to sitting position to look for learned behavior.
- Laségue's sign - patient is supine, hip flexed, dorsiflexion of ankle accentuates sciatic pain or muscle spasm in posterior thigh
- Cross straight-leg-raising - elevating normal leg produces sciatica down other leg
- Doorbell sign - (insensitive) deep palpation of the spinous process over protruded disk reproduces sciatica
- Femoral stretch (for L2-3) in prone position, affected leg is extended from knee reproducing pain along femoral nerve
- Faber's test - (positive only for hip pain) in supine position, flexion, abduction and external rotation produces pain
- Neurologic defects of lower extremities and perineum will usually locate level of lesion. Test gait, reflexes, motor strength, muscle atrophy; pulses and abdominal bruits; rectal sphincter.

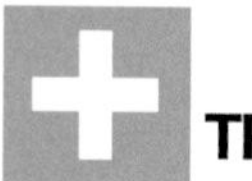

TREATMENT

APPROPRIATE HEALTH CARE Outpatient for majority. Inpatient for severe disability and/or surgery.

GENERAL MEASURES

- Conservative treatment is recommended for the first 6 weeks. Most herniated disks resorb over time, particularly large and extruded disks. For persistent pain and neurological deficits, consider evaluation for surgery. Surgery should not be delayed more than 6 months because of risk of chronic disability.
- Initial: minimize bedrest, ordinary activities as tolerated, local heat, pelvic traction, sedation, physical therapy (90% response)
- Manipulation therapy contraindicated with sciatica
- For chronic non-radicular pain: improve physical fitness with low impact aerobic exercise. Manipulation and physical therapy have shown benefit.
- Transcutaneous electrical nerve stimulation (TENS): very short-term benefit

SURGICAL MEASURES
- Gram positive antimicrobial prophylaxis recommended for all techniques
- Procedures available
  - ◊ Standard diskectomy
  - ◊ Microsurgical diskectomy. Open and micro techniques achieve highest relief of symptoms.
  - ◊ Percutaneous diskectomy. Other minimally invasive diskectomies are percutaneous suction, percutaneous laser, micro-endoscopic, and arthroscopic disk decompression. Success is critical to patient selection.
  - ◊ Chemonucleolysis - lower rate of benefit and occasional severe complications
  - ◊ Spinal fusion (arthrodesis) - indicated for spinal instability
- Absolute indications for diskectomy
  - ◊ Cauda equina syndrome
  - ◊ Progressive neurological deficit despite conservative treatment
- Relative indications for diskectomy
  - ◊ Intolerable pain
  - ◊ Multiple episodes of radiculopathy
  - ◊ Severe postural tilt
  - ◊ Persistent dysfunctional pain - these patients have been reported to improve more rapidly postoperatively but long term results show no difference from nonoperative treatment
  - ◊ Static neurological deficit - no reported difference between operative or nonoperative treatment for improvement in weakness or sensory disturbance
- Epidural steroid injection remains controversial

ACTIVITY
- After pain is controlled (2-4 days), begin progressive walking program. Short walks initially 4 times a day and lengthen as tolerated.
- Return to work as soon as possible with avoidance of high risk activities, e.g., heavy lifting, vibration, smoking

DIET Weight reduction if appropriate

PATIENT EDUCATION Good posture, proper body mechanics, physical fitness, physical therapy if appropriate

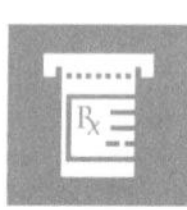

MEDICATIONS

DRUG(S) OF CHOICE
- Analgesics
- Non-steroidal anti-inflammatory drugs
- Mild sedatives
- Muscle relaxants not recommended

Contraindications: Refer to manufacturer's profile of each drug

Precautions: Elderly, hypertension, prior peptic ulcer disease or bleeding, renal disease, liver disease, cardiac dysfunction

Significant possible interactions: Refer to manufacturer's profile of each drug

ALTERNATIVE DRUGS N/A

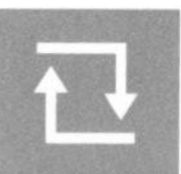

FOLLOWUP

PATIENT MONITORING Outpatient - return visit about 10 days following initial visit, should be improved. Follow pain history and neurological status. Thereafter monitor every 2 weeks until fully functional. Monitor exercise program.

PREVENTION/AVOIDANCE
- Modification of jobs to reduce exposure to known risk factors
- Selection of workers by such means as strength testing for certain jobs
- Avoid smoking
- Lessen obesity

POSSIBLE COMPLICATIONS
- Foot drop with weakness of anterior tibial, posterior tibial and peroneal muscles
- Loss of ankle jerk
- Bladder and rectal sphincter weakness with retention or incontinence
- Limitation of movement and restricted activity
- Narcotic addiction

EXPECTED COURSE/PROGNOSIS
- Acute low back pain (90%) and/or radiculopathy (60-80%) can be expected to recover spontaneously with conservative therapy
- Chronic nonradicular low back pain - most patients respond to conservative management such as manipulation, fitness, weight reduction, and education regarding back care
- Chronic radicular pain - good selection of surgical candidates have found satisfactory results (80% in long-term studies)

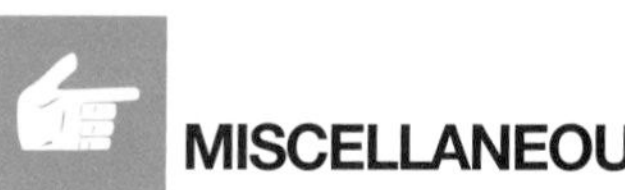

MISCELLANEOUS

ASSOCIATED CONDITIONS
- Poor physical conditioning/posture
- Obesity
- Osteoarthritis
- Osteoporosis
- Depression, other psychiatric disorders

AGE-RELATED FACTORS
Pediatric: Scoliosis, onset age 10 years, rarely symptomatic until adulthood. Detect difference in leg length.

Geriatric: Usually multifactorial lesions of spine. Degenerative spondylolisthesis (especially in women), spinal stenosis, and neurogenic claudication are more likely.

Others: N/A

PREGNANCY Commonly associated with low back pain and/or sciatica. Treatment is conservative.

SYNONYMS
- Degenerative disk disease
- Intervertebral disk dislocation

ICD-9-CM
722.10 Displacement of lumbar intervertebral disc without myelopathy
722.52 Degeneration of lumbar or lumbosacral intervertebral disc

SEE ALSO
Low back pain

OTHER NOTES
- Features which predict best surgical outcome (90-95% improvement when all three exist)
  - ◊ Definable neurological deficit
  - ◊ Pathology in imaging which correlates with deficit
  - ◊ Positive nerve root tension signs
- Adverse psychosocial factors to resolving back pain
  - ◊ Sciatica with predominant back symptoms
  - ◊ Pending litigation or compensation
  - ◊ Depressed or hostile patient
  - ◊ Low IQ or poorly educated may not be able to participate in assessment or decision
  - ◊ Prolonged use of narcotics or alcohol

ABBREVIATIONS N/A

REFERENCES

- Beaty JH, editor Orthopedic Knowledge Update, American Academy of Orthopedic Surgeons, 1997
- Kent OL, Haynor DR, Longstreth WT, Larson EB. The clinical efficacy of magnetic resonance imaging in neuroimaging. Ann Int Med 1994:120;856-871
- Frost H, Moffett JAK, Moser JS, Fairbank JCT. Randomized controlled trial for evaluation of fitness program for patients with chronic low back pain. Brit Med Jour 1995;310:151-159
- Malmivaara A, Hakkinen U, Aro T, Heinrichs MJ, et al. The treatment of acute low back pain - bed rest, exercises, or ordinary activity? NEJM 1995:332; 351-355

Web references: 0 available at www.5mcc.com

Illustrations N/A

Author(s):
Claudia A. Peters, MD

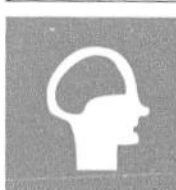

BASICS

DESCRIPTION A localized collection cavity of necrotic lung tissue and pus resulting from severe lung infection. Presentation can be acute or chronic (symptoms more than 4 weeks). Usual course is subacute progression of symptoms
System(s) affected: Pulmonary
Genetics: No known genetic pattern
Incidence/Prevalence in USA: Unknown, relatively rare, since advent of antibiotics
Predominant age: Mainly 4th-6th decades
Predominant sex: Male > Female (4:1)

SIGNS & SYMPTOMS
- Cough
- Sputum (purulent, foul-smelling, putrid, sour tasting)
- Fever
- Chest pain/pleurisy
- Dyspnea
- Malaise
- Diaphoresis
- Weight loss
- Anorexia
- Night sweats
- Hemoptysis
- Decreased breath sounds
- Crackles
- Wheezing
- Tachypnea
- Tachycardia
- Dullness to percussion
- Consolidation by auscultation
- Cavernous breath sounds
- Clubbing of digits

CAUSES
- Oral flora anaerobes (60-75% of cases)
  - ◊ Provetella
  - ◊ *Bacteroides sp.*
  - ◊ *Fusobacterium*
  - ◊ *Peptostreptococcus*
- Aerobes (10-20% of cases)
  - ◊ *Staphylococcus aureus*
  - ◊ *Streptococcus pyogenes*
  - ◊ *Klebsiella sp.*
  - ◊ *Pseudomonas aeruginosa*
  - ◊ *Streptococcus milleri*
- Atypical aerobes
  - ◊ Legionella
  - ◊ Nocardia
  - ◊ Actinomyces

RISK FACTORS
- Prone to aspiration of oral flora
  - ◊ Periodontal disease (gingivitis), dental abscess, dental surgery
  - ◊ Substance abuse, alcoholism
  - ◊ Epilepsy
  - ◊ CVA with oropharyngeal dysfunction
  - ◊ Sinusitis
  - ◊ General anesthetic with surgery
  - ◊ Dysphagia
  - ◊ Tracheal/nasogastric tube
  - ◊ Severe gastroesophageal reflux disease
  - ◊ Cerebral palsy
- Large bacterial burden
  - ◊ Necrotizing pneumonia
  - ◊ Bacteremia
  - ◊ Septic embolism (especially from endocarditis)
- Airway obstruction
  - ◊ Bronchial stenosis
  - ◊ Pulmonary embolism
  - ◊ Cavitary infarction
  - ◊ Lung neoplasia
  - ◊ Foreign body
- Immunosuppression conditions
  - ◊ Diabetes mellitus
  - ◊ HIV
  - ◊ Chronic steroid use

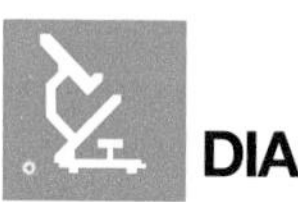

DIAGNOSIS

DIFFERENTIAL DIAGNOSIS
- Bronchogenic carcinoma
- Bronchiectasis
- Empyema with bronchopulmonary fistula
- Tuberculosis
- Mycotic lung infections
- Vasculitis
- Parasitic lung infections
- Infected pulmonary bulla
- Wegener granulomatosis
- Pulmonary sequestration
- Subphrenic or hepatic abscess with perforation into a bronchus
- Bronchogenic or parenchymal cyst
- Aspirated foreign body

LABORATORY
- Leukocytosis
- Anemia
- Hypoalbuminemia
- Sputum smear - mixed bacteria and neutrophils
- Sputum culture - mixed flora, anaerobes (not recommended)
- Pleural fluid - neutrophilia
- Blood culture - aerobes (often negative)

Drugs that may alter lab results: Prior antibiotics

Disorders that may alter lab results: N/A

PATHOLOGICAL FINDINGS
- Gross - solitary abscess
- Multiple abscesses
- Cavitation with necrosis

SPECIAL TESTS N/A

IMAGING
- Chest x-ray: consolidation with radiolucency, infiltrates, air fluid level, pleural effusion, mediastinal adenopathy
- CT: define location and extent (typical location is dependent segments such as posterior segments of upper lobes or superior segments of lower lobes

DIAGNOSTIC PROCEDURES
- Bronchoscopy if obstruction suspected
- Bronchoscopic protected brushing
- Bronchoalveolar lavage
- Transthoracic needle aspiration (rarely done)

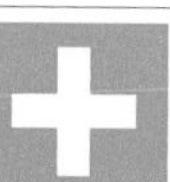

TREATMENT

APPROPRIATE HEALTH CARE Inpatient for monitoring and treatment

GENERAL MEASURES
- Postural drainage
- Nasotracheal suctioning if needed
- Prolonged course of antibiotics
- Pulmonary physiotherapy
- Bronchoscopy with selective therapeutic lavage (rarely done)

SURGICAL MEASURES
- Drainage with chest tube
- Pulmonary resection only if complications occur or patient fails therapy

ACTIVITY Reduced activity until x-ray evidence of clearing

DIET No restrictions

PATIENT EDUCATION Pulmonary physiotherapy techniques

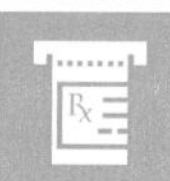

MEDICATIONS

DRUG(S) OF CHOICE Antibiotics according to culture and sensitivity results. For presumed anaerobes, clindamycin 600 mg every 6 hours IV, followed by 300 mg every 6 hours orally for 4 weeks.
Contraindications: Refer to manufacturer's literature.
Precautions: Refer to manufacturer's literature
Significant possible interactions: Refer to manufacturer's literature

ALTERNATIVE DRUGS
- Standard therapy has historically been penicillin G 1-2 million units IV every 4 hours until improved, followed by 1.2 million units (750 mg) orally every 6 hours for 3-4 weeks.
- Cefoxitin 2.0 gm IV q 8 hours
- Piperacillin-tazobactam 3.375 gm IV q 6 hours
- Ticarcillin-clavulanate 3.1 gm IV q 6 hours
- Metronidazole has not proven as effective as clindamycin, but is often recommended for use as an adjunctive therapy (500 mg IV q 6 hours
- Full course of therapy may be needed for 8 weeks

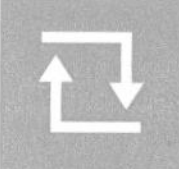

FOLLOWUP

PATIENT MONITORING Serial x-rays until resolution of cavity

PREVENTION/AVOIDANCE Treat predisposing diseases; aspiration precautions; treatment of periodontal diseases

POSSIBLE COMPLICATIONS
- Extension
- Empyema
- Massive hemoptysis
- Pneumothorax
- Brain abscess

EXPECTED COURSE/PROGNOSIS
- Clinical improvement with decrease in fever expected in 3-4 days after starting antibiotics
- Defervescence (resolution of fever) expected in 7-10 days
- Overall mortality 10-15%
- Prognosis depends on the underlying disease or immunosuppression
- Patients with primary abscess (otherwise healthy, typical aspiration) have cure rate of 90-95%
- Patients with secondary abscess (underlying neoplasm, obstruction, HIV) have 75% mortality
- Certain factors tend to have worse prognosis:
  - ◊ Large size of abscess (> 6 cm)
  - ◊ Anatomical obstruction
  - ◊ Right lower lobe location
  - ◊ Certain bacteriologic species - more violent (staph aureus, Klebsiella, pseudomonas)

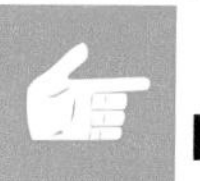

MISCELLANEOUS

ASSOCIATED CONDITIONS
- Pneumonia
- Alcoholism
- Empyema
- Tuberculosis

AGE-RELATED FACTORS
Pediatric: Occurs in children, Staphylococcus most common organism
Geriatric: Mortality higher in this age group
Others: N/A

PREGNANCY N/A

SYNONYMS Pulmonary abscess

ICD-9-CM
513.0 Abscess of lung

SEE ALSO
Pneumonia, bacterial

OTHER NOTES N/A

ABBREVIATIONS N/A

REFERENCES

- Bartlett JG: Anaerobic bacterial infections of the lung and pleural space. Clinical Infectious Diseases 1993;16;Suppl4:s248-255
- Murray JF, Nadel JA, eds: Textbook of Respiratory Medicine. 2nd Ed. Philadelphia, W.B. Saunders Co., 1994
- Guidiol F, Manresa F, Pallares R, et al: Clindamycin vs penicillin for anaerobic lung infections. Arch Int Med 1990;150:2525-2529
- Davis B, Systrom DM: Lung abscess: pathogenesis, diagnosis and treatment. Curr Clin Topics in Infect Dis 1998;18:252-273

Web references: 1 available at www.5mcc.com
Illustrations N/A

Author(s):
Sukanya Srinivasan, MD, MPH

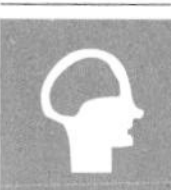

BASICS

DESCRIPTION Leading cause of cancer deaths in both men and women in the USA. The most common (bronchogenic carcinoma) may be divided into two broad categories:
- Non-small cell cancer (NSCLC)
  - ◊ Squamous cell cancer (epidermoid carcinoma) 20-30%
  - ◊ Adenocarcinoma
  - ◊ Large cell carcinoma
- Small cell cancer (oat cell carcinoma; SCLC) 20%
- Other less common primary malignancies of the lung include:
  - ◊ Mesothelioma
  - ◊ Carcinoid
  - ◊ Blastoma
  - ◊ Sarcoma
  - ◊ Melanoma
- NSCLC tumors are staged for treatment and prognostic purposes from stages 0 to IV. The definitions of each stage are dependent on the primary tumor (t), lymph node status (n), and presence of metastasis (m).
- SCLC tumors are staged on location of disease: limited to ipsilateral hemithorax (stages I-IIIB); or extensive if metastatic beyond hemithorax (stages IIIB and IV)

System(s) affected: Pulmonary
Genetics: 1.5-3 times increased risk in first degree relatives
Incidence/Prevalence in USA:
- 175,000 new cases per year
- 70/100,000 population
- 80% of new cases are NSCLC and 50% are metastatic at diagnosis
- Most common cancer world-wide (17.6% of cancers in men)

Predominant age: 50-70 years
Predominant sex: Male > Female

SIGNS & SYMPTOMS
- May be asymptomatic for majority of course
- Pulmonary
  - ◊ Cough (new or change in chronic cough)
  - ◊ Wheezing
  - ◊ Dyspnea
  - ◊ Hemoptysis
  - ◊ Pneumonia
- Constitutional
  - ◊ Bone pain
  - ◊ Excess fatigue
  - ◊ Weight loss
  - ◊ Fever
  - ◊ Anemia
  - ◊ Clubbing of digits
- Other presentations
  - ◊ Chest pain
  - ◊ Shoulder/arm pain
  - ◊ Dysphagia
  - ◊ Swelling of face or neck
  - ◊ Hoarseness

CAUSES Multifactorial; see risk factors

RISK FACTORS
- Smoking (attributable in 87% of cases)
- Passive - second hand smoke exposure
- Chronic obstructive pulmonary disease (COPD)
- Preexisting lung disease (pulmonary fibrosis)
- Environmental; occupational exposure
  - ◊ Asbestos exposure
  - ◊ Ionizing radiation
  - ◊ Atmospheric pollution
  - ◊ Gases: halogen ethers, radon, mustard gas, aromatic hydrocarbons
  - ◊ Metals: inorganic arsenic, chromium, nickel
- Possibly HIV (adenocarcinoma)

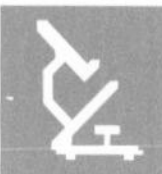

DIAGNOSIS

DIFFERENTIAL DIAGNOSIS
- Consider both pulmonary and extrapulmonary causes for symptoms
- Pulmonary
  - ◊ Chronic bronchitis
  - ◊ Granulomatous diseases (tuberculosis, sarcoidosis)
- Cardiac
  - ◊ Congestive heart failure
  - ◊ Cardiomyopathy

LABORATORY
- CBC with platelets (look for low H/H, high WBC)
- Basic metabolic panel (look for low Na, high K, high Ca)
- Liver enzymes
- Pro-time (PT), prothrombin (PTT)

Drugs that may alter lab results: None likely

Disorders that may alter lab results: None likely

PATHOLOGICAL FINDINGS
- Cancer cell type obtained from:
  - ◊ Cytology (sputum, pleural fluid, node aspirate, bronchial washing) particularly valuable in SCLC
  - ◊ Histology (tissue biopsies of nodes, nodules or masses)

SPECIAL TESTS
- Electrocardiogram
- Echocardiogram
- Stress testing (exercise or Persantine thallium scan if applicable)
- Pulmonary function studies
- Quality of life assessments
  - ◊ Karnofsky Performance Scale (KPS)
  - ◊ Eastern Cooperative Oncology Group (ECOG)

IMAGING
- Chest x-ray (important to compare with old films)
  - ◊ Nodule or mass, especially if calcified
  - ◊ Persistent infiltrate
  - ◊ Atelectasis
  - ◊ Mediastinal widening
  - ◊ Hilar enlargement
  - ◊ Pleural effusion
- CT scan of chest (with IV contrast)
  - ◊ Nodule or mass (central or peripheral)
  - ◊ Lymphadenopathy
- Other CT scans to look for metastatic disease
  - ◊ Brain - lesions may be necrotic, bleeding
  - ◊ Abdomen - hepatic or adrenal masses
- MRI or bone scan
  - ◊ Vertebral or bony metastases

DIAGNOSTIC PROCEDURES
- Needle biopsy under CT or fluoroscopic guidance
- Flexible fiberoptic bronchoscopy
- Cervical mediastinoscopy
- Video-assisted thoracoscopy
- Thoracotomy, when appropriate

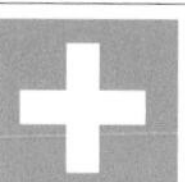

TREATMENT

APPROPRIATE HEALTH CARE
- Depends on tumor cell type and stage of disease at diagnosis
- Treatment options for NSCLC include:
  - ◊ Surgical resection
  - ◊ Chemotherapy
  - ◊ Radiation therapy
- Treatment options of SCLC include:
  - ◊ Chemotherapy
  - ◊ Radiation therapy

GENERAL MEASURES
- Relief of symptoms
- Pain relief as needed
- Discussions with patient and family about wishes for end-of-life care

SURGICAL MEASURES Resection for non-small cell cancer, when possible, stage I and II and some stage III. Resection of isolated, distant metastases has been achieved and may improve survival. Functional evaluation performed prior to surgery.

ACTIVITY No limitations; per patient tolerance

DIET No restrictions; good nutrition important during treatment

PATIENT EDUCATION
- American Lung Association
- American Cancer Society
- Web resources: www.lungcanceronline.org and www.cancer.about.com

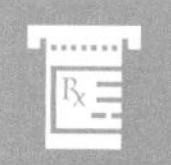

MEDICATIONS

DRUG(S) OF CHOICE
- NSCLC, chemotherapy. Indicated only in patients with a good functional status.
  - ◊ Cisplatin (Platinol) and cisplatin-based regimens are standard although response rates with cisplatin alone are <20% in stage IIIB/IV disease with a 3 year survival rate of 8%. Combination regimens can improve survival an average of 2 months with a 5-year survival rate improved by about 10% in stage III disease.
  - ◊ Etoposide (Toposar) beneficial in combination with cisplatin and radiation (becoming standard)
  - ◊ Newer agents include paclitaxel (Taxol), docetaxel (Taxotere), vinorelbine (Navelbine), gemcitabine (Gemzar), and irinotecan (Camptosar) either alone or as radiation sensitizers have led to response rates up to 40% in non-small cell tumors
- SCLC, chemotherapy. Excellent response, including complete remissions possible.
- Palliative measures
  - ◊ Analgesics: hydrocodone, morphine, fentanyl (Duragesic)
  - ◊ Dyspnea: oxygen, nebulized morphine, benzodiazepines [e.g., lorazepam (Ativan) 1-2 mg po, SL, SC, or pr q2-6 h]

Contraindications: Refer to manufacturer's instructions
Precautions: Refer to manufacturer's instructions
Significant possible interactions: Refer to manufacturer's instructions

ALTERNATIVE DRUGS N/A

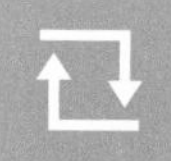

FOLLOWUP

PATIENT MONITORING
- Surgically resectable
  - ◊ First year each 3 months
  - ◊ Second year each 6 months
  - ◊ Third though fifth year once a year
- Surgically unresectable
  - ◊ As necessary for palliation
  - ◊ Consider early hospice referral
- Follow up CT scans as indicated

PREVENTION/AVOIDANCE
- Despite numerous studies, no cost effective screening measure has been found for lung cancer. Therefore, prevention via aggressive smoking cessation counseling and therapy is the cornerstone of patient management. 20-30% risk reduction within 5 years of cessation.
- Stop smoking; avoid second hand smoke exposure
- Avoid radon exposure
- Avoid occupational exposure to asbestos, metals
- Consider prophylaxis with retinoid, such as beta-carotene or antioxidants such as vitamin A or E

POSSIBLE COMPLICATIONS
- Development of metastatic disease to brain, bones and liver
- Local recurrence of disease
- Postsurgical complications
- Side effects of chemotherapy or radiation
  - ◊ Dysphagia (radiation-induced, fungal)
  - ◊ Infections
  - ◊ Bleeding
  - ◊ Radiation pneumonitis
- Superior vena cava syndrome
- Atelectasis
- Spinal cord compression
- Pulmonary abscess
- Horner syndrome
- Hypercalcemia (ectopic parathyroid hormone)
- Syndrome of inappropriate antidiuretic hormone (SIADH)
- Hypercoagulable state
- Terminal restlessness (anorexia, dyspnea

EXPECTED COURSE/PROGNOSIS
- Overall survival rate is 15%
- Stage I, 50% survival status postresection of squamous, adenocarcinoma or large cell
- Stage II, 33% survival status postresection for squamous and 20% for adenocarcinoma or large cell
- Stage IIIa, 15% survival status postresection for squamous
- Note: Presurgical staging is less accurate so survival figures are lower
- If nonresectable, prognosis is poor with mean survival of 8-14 months

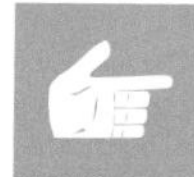

MISCELLANEOUS

ASSOCIATED CONDITIONS
- Hypertrophic pulmonary osteoarthropathy
- Eaton-Lambert syndrome
- Pulmonary emphysema
- Chronic bronchitis
- Pancoast syndrome (superior sulcus syndrome)

AGE-RELATED FACTORS
Pediatric: N/A
Geriatric: More common in elderly (> 75 years)
Others: N/A

PREGNANCY N/A

SYNONYMS
- Lung cancer

ICD-9-CM
162.9 Malignant neoplasm of bronchus and lung, unspecified

SEE ALSO
Restlessness

OTHER NOTES N/A

ABBREVIATIONS N/A

REFERENCES

- Hoffman PC, Mauer AM, Vokes EE. Lung cancer. Lancet 2000;355(9202):479-85
- Mountain CF. Revisions in the International System for Staging Lung Cancer. Chest 1997;111(6):1710-7
- Midthun DE, Jett JR. Clinical presentation of lung cancer. In: Pass, Hi, et al, eds. Lung Cancer: Principles and Practice. Philadelphia, Lippincott-Raven, 1996
- Bunn PA, Kelly K. Treatment of advanced non-small cell lung cancer: New combinations in the treatment of lung cancer. Chest 2000;117(4)
- Park BJ, Louie O, Altorki N. Staging and the surgical management of lung cancer. Radiologic Clinics of North America 2000;38(3)

Web references: 0 available at www.5mcc.com
Illustrations N/A

Author(s):
Sukanya Srinivasan, MD, MPH

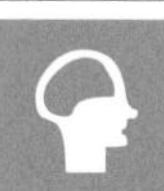

BASICS

DESCRIPTION Discoid lupus erythematosus (DLE) is the most common form of chronic cutaneous lupus. It is a chronic skin disease characterized by sharply marginated dull, red macules with adherent scales extending into areas of atrophy, telangiectasias, or follicular plugging.
- Localized DLE - more common form with lesions occurring on the face especially the malar areas, bridge of nose, lower lip, lower eyelids and ears
- Generalized DLE - lesions seen on upper extremities and thorax most often, along with usual sites for localized DLE

System(s) affected: Skin/Exocrine
Genetics: N/A
Incidence/Prevalence in USA:
- 3/100,000 Caucasian females; 8/100,000 black females
- 100/100,000

Predominant age: 25 to 45
Predominant sex:
- Localized DLE - Female > Male (3:1)
- Generalized DLE - Female > Male (9:1)

SIGNS & SYMPTOMS
- Red plaque-like lesions on face, thorax, or extensor aspect of upper extremities; rare below waist
- Older lesions atrophy and appear as smooth white or hyperpigmented scars with telangiectasias
- Scarring alopecia with scalp lesions
- "Carpet tack" appearance of skin when scale removed
- Lesions occasionally slightly pruritic or stinging
- Oral ulceration in 15 percent of patients
- Photosensitivity
- Koebner response (precipitation by cutaneous trauma)

CAUSES Unknown

RISK FACTORS Systemic lupus erythematosus (SLE)

DIAGNOSIS

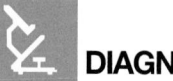

DIFFERENTIAL DIAGNOSIS
- Actinic keratoses
- Polymorphous light eruption
- Drug eruptions
- Sarcoid
- Cutaneous leishmaniasis
- Lupus vulgaris
- Seborrheic dermatitis
- Lichen planus
- Plaque psoriasis
- Rosacea
- Pemphigus erythematosus
- Tinea faciei
- Jessner-Kanof disease
- Granuloma faciale

LABORATORY
- Localized DLE: positive ANA in low titer (30%)
- Generalized DLE, may find, increased sedimentation rate, positive ANA (60-80%), positive SS-A (80%), positive SS-B (40%) autoantibodies, positive dsDNA (< 5%), leukopenia, hematuria and albuminuria if concomitant SLE

Drugs that may alter lab results: N/A

Disorders that may alter lab results: Concomitant SLE

PATHOLOGICAL FINDINGS
- Hyperkeratosis and parakeratosis
- Focal epidermal atrophy
- Hydropic degeneration of basal cell layer
- Edema, mucin, and inflammation of dermis
- Follicular plugging
- Basement zone thickened with strong periodic acid-Schiff reaction staining

SPECIAL TESTS Immunofluorescent staining of skin biopsies (lupus band test)

IMAGING N/A

DIAGNOSTIC PROCEDURES Skin biopsy

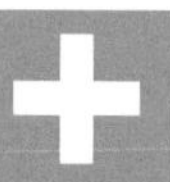

TREATMENT

APPROPRIATE HEALTH CARE Outpatient

GENERAL MEASURES Avoid sun exposure, avoid excessive heat, cold, or trauma

SURGICAL MEASURES N/A

ACTIVITY Full activity

DIET Regular

PATIENT EDUCATION
- Teach patients proper use of sunscreens and other measures to prevent sun exposure (e.g., wide-brimmed hats, long sleeves, etc.)
- Advise patient about symptoms of systemic lupus erythematosus (SLE) for which they should watch
- Griffith's Instructions for Patients, Philadelphia, Elsevier

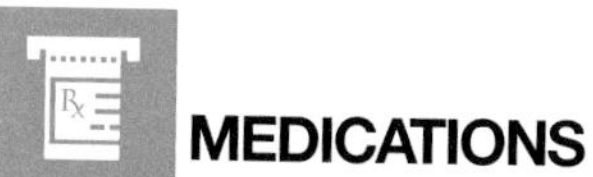

MEDICATIONS

DRUG(S) OF CHOICE

- Localized DLE:
  - ◊ Low to medium potency topical corticosteroid (eg, triamcinolone 0.1% bid) to all active lesions
  - ◊ If no response in 2-3 weeks, move to higher potency topical corticosteroid applied tid (eg, betamethasone) with or without occlusion
  - ◊ Intralesional corticosteroid (eg, triamcinolone 2.5-5 mg/mL for the face or 5-10 mg/mL elsewhere) for resistant lesions. Use 0.5 mL per 1 cm plaque.
- Generalized DLE:
  - ◊ Hydroxychloroquine 6.5 mg/kg per day. If no response after 3 months, switch to chloroquine 250 mg qd.
  - ◊ Short-term (1-2 weeks) of topical corticosteroids is helpful at the same time antimalarials are being started

Contraindications: Antimalarials such as hydroxychloroquine may have to be avoided in patients with preexisting retinal or hepatic disease. Do not give to individuals with G6PD deficiency. Quinacrine rarely causes hematologic cytopenia.

Precautions:

- Observe for skin atrophy with topical steroids especially with use on the face
- Patients on antimalarials should have an eye examination by an ophthalmologist at start of treatment and at 6 month intervals to monitor signs of retinal damage

Significant possible interactions: N/A

ALTERNATIVE DRUGS

- Localized DLE: Intralesional triamcinolone 2.5 mg/cc injected at monthly intervals. Prednisone 15 mg bid, then tapered after response.
- Generalized DLE: Quinacrine 100 mg qd, dapsone 100 mg qd, azathioprine 100 mg qd. Systemic retinoid (eg, etretinate 1 mg/kg); thalidomide is also effective.

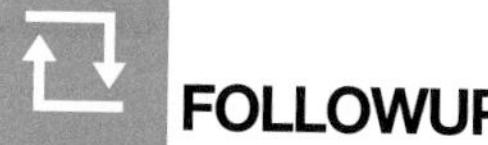

FOLLOWUP

PATIENT MONITORING

- Recheck patients once or twice per month
- Ophthalmology followup at 6 month intervals if patient on antimalarial
- If lesions subside, reduce dosage of antimalarials over 2-3 months, then discontinue

PREVENTION/AVOIDANCE Avoid sun exposure or excessive heat, cold, or skin trauma

POSSIBLE COMPLICATIONS Hypertrophic scarring, hypopigmentation (especially in blacks)

EXPECTED COURSE/PROGNOSIS

- 40% remit completely; 1-5% may develop systemic lupus (these patients usually have generalized DLE)
- Not life-threatening unless it turns into systemic type

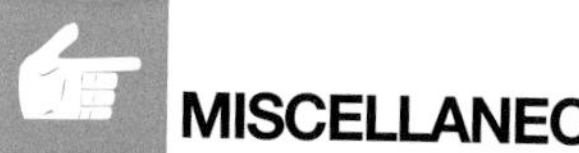

MISCELLANEOUS

ASSOCIATED CONDITIONS

- Systemic lupus erythematosus
- Mixed connective tissue disease (MCTD)
- Antiphospholipid syndrome

AGE-RELATED FACTORS

Pediatric: Neonatal lupus erythematosus is a syndrome of cutaneous lupus and/or congenital heart block. It is caused by transplacental passage of one of several maternal antibodies.
Geriatric: N/A
Others: N/A

PREGNANCY Be aware if systemic retinoids used, pregnancy category X

SYNONYMS

- Chronic cutaneous lupus erythematosus
- Subacute cutaneous lupus erythematosus (SCLE)

ICD-9-CM

695.4 Lupus erythematosus

SEE ALSO

Systemic lupus erythematosus (SLE)

OTHER NOTES N/A

ABBREVIATIONS N/A

REFERENCES

- Odom RB, James WD, Berger TG. Andrews' Diseases of the Skin. 9th ed. Philadelphia: WB Saunders; 2000
- Habif TP. Clinical Dermatology. 4th ed. New York: Mosby; 2004
- Lebwohl MG, et al, eds. Treatment of Skin Disease. 1st ed. New York: Mosby; 2002

Web references: 2 available at www.5mcc.com
Illustrations 8 available

Author(s):

Gary J. Silko, MD, MS

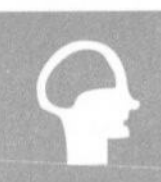

BASICS

DESCRIPTION A multisystem infection caused by the spirochete *Borrelia burgdorferi*, which is transmitted primarily by Ixodid ticks
- Stage 1, early localized Lyme disease, includes a characteristic expanding skin rash (erythema migrans) and constitutional flu-like symptoms
- Stage 2, early disseminated Lyme disease, may present with involvement of one or more organ systems. Neurologic (15%) and cardiac (8%) disease are most common.
- Stage 3, chronic Lyme disease, involves arthritis (50%) and chronic neurological syndromes

System(s) affected: Hemic/Lymphatic/Immunologic, Musculoskeletal, Skin/Exocrine
Genetics: HLA - haplotype DR4 or DR2 may be more susceptible to prolonged arthritis
Incidence/Prevalence in USA: Overall incidence 6.3/100,000. Highest prevalence in Connecticut, Rhode Island, New York, New Jersey, Pennsylvania, Wisconsin, Maryland and Minnesota.
Predominant age: Can occur in all ages, but most common in children ages 5-9 and in the 50-59 year age group
Predominant sex: Male > Female

SIGNS & SYMPTOMS
- Stage 1:
  - ◊ Erythema migrans (60-80%)
  - ◊ Fever
  - ◊ Headache
  - ◊ Myalgias
  - ◊ Arthralgias
  - ◊ Some patients may be asymptomatic
- Stage 2: (involvement of one or more organ systems)
  - ◊ Multiple erythema migrans
  - ◊ Facial palsies, or other cranial neuropathies
  - ◊ Aseptic meningitis
  - ◊ Heart block
  - ◊ Pericarditis
  - ◊ Orchitis, hepatitis, or iritis
  - ◊ Arthritis (usually large joint monarthritis)
- Stage 3:
  - ◊ Recurrent synovitis
  - ◊ Recurrent tendinitis and bursitis
  - ◊ Neuropsychiatric symptoms, may include: Psychotic behavior, memory loss, dementia, depression, sleep disorders
  - ◊ Encephalopathic symptoms: Headache, decreased memory, difficulty concentrating, confusion, fatigue
  - ◊ Symptoms mimicking other CNS diseases: Multiple sclerosis-like syndromes, stroke-like symptoms, vestibular neuronitis, transverse myelitis, parkinsonian symptoms
  - ◊ Peripheral neuropathic symptoms: Carpal tunnel syndrome, motor, sensory, or autonomic neuropathies
  - ◊ Ophthalmic manifestations: Iritis, keratitis, retinal vasculitis, optic neuritis
- In Europe, borrelia lymphocytoma and acrodermatitis chronica are manifestations of Lyme borreliosis, but rarely seen in the U.S.

CAUSES Infection with spirochete *Borrelia burgdorferi*, transmitted by the bite of Ixodid ticks

RISK FACTORS Exposure to tick infested area, most common from May to September

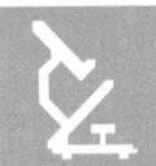

DIAGNOSIS

DIFFERENTIAL DIAGNOSIS
- Juvenile rheumatoid arthritis
- Viral syndromes
- Later stages may mimic many other diseases (see Signs and Symptoms)

LABORATORY
- ELISA for IgM and IgG B burgdorferi antibodies (frequently negative in stage 1 disease), followed by a Western blot test if positive
- Culture of CSF for B burgdorferi

Drugs that may alter lab results: Late stage disease with negative serology may be seen in patients who received early antibiotic treatment

Disorders that may alter lab results: False positive response has been seen with Rocky Mountain spotted fever, syphilis, systemic lupus erythematosus, and rheumatoid arthritis

PATHOLOGICAL FINDINGS Culture of *B. burgdorferi* from blood or skin biopsy specimens has a very low yield

SPECIAL TESTS N/A

IMAGING N/A

DIAGNOSTIC PROCEDURES
- Diagnosis is based on clinical features with exposure to a tick bite or endemic area
- Lumbar puncture when neurologic findings are present, with ELISA of CSF for *B. burgdorferi* antibodies

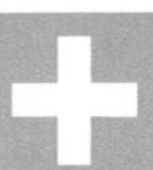

TREATMENT

APPROPRIATE HEALTH CARE
- Stage 1, clinical diagnosis, can be treated as an outpatient
- Stage 2 and 3 may require more intensive treatment, based on symptoms

GENERAL MEASURES Prevention of infection is possible by careful examination of skin for ticks after outdoor activities. Prompt removal of ticks may limit transmission. Clothing that covers the ankles should be worn in endemic areas, and the use of insect repellants is recommended.

SURGICAL MEASURES N/A

ACTIVITY No restriction

DIET No special diet

PATIENT EDUCATION
- In endemic areas, patients should be advised to protect themselves against tick exposure
- Information available from: American Lyme Disease Foundation, 293 Route 100, Suite 204, Somers NY 10589

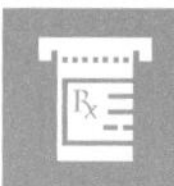

MEDICATIONS

DRUG(S) OF CHOICE

- Stage 1:
  - ◊ Doxycycline (Vibramycin) 100 mg po bid for 14-21 days (do not use in children under 12 or in pregnancy); or
  - ◊ Amoxicillin 500 mg po tid for 14-21 days, (pediatric dose 25-100 mg/kg/day)
  - ◊ Cefuroxime (Ceftin) axetil 500 mg bid for 14-21 days
- Stage 2:
  - ◊ Normal CSF, treat for 28 days - doxycycline 100 mg po bid; or
  - ◊ Amoxicillin 500 mg po tid
  - ◊ Short course of corticosteroids (5-7 days) may be helpful
  - ◊ With abnormal CSF, treat for 3-4 weeks - ceftriaxone (Rocephin) 2 g IV qd; or cefotaxime (Claforan) 2 g IV q 8 h; or penicillin G 20-24 million units/day IV
- Stage 3:
  - ◊ Oral treatment for 28 days with doxycycline 100 mg bid; or
  - ◊ Amoxicillin 500 mg tid
  - ◊ If oral treatment fails, IV treatment for 2-3 weeks with ceftriaxone 2 g qd; or cefotaxime 2 g q 8 hr; or penicillin G 20-24 million units/day IV

Contraindications:

- Allergy to agent
- Doxycycline contraindicated in children and in women who are pregnant or breast feeding

Precautions: Refer to manufacturer's profile of each drug

Significant possible interactions:

- Oral anticoagulants may need reduced dose
- Oral contraceptives may be less effective

ALTERNATIVE DRUGS

- Cefuroxime (Ceftin) 500 mg bid for stage 1 disease, or tid for stage 2 or 3 disease

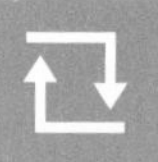

FOLLOWUP

PATIENT MONITORING Stage 2 and 3 disease requires careful monitoring over a period of months to years, based on severity of symptoms

PREVENTION/AVOIDANCE

- Awareness of the disease, protective clothing, and careful skin inspection with timely removal of ticks may reduce the incidence of disease. A 3 dose vaccine, LYMErix, is no longer available.
- Prophylactic treatment with one dose of 200 mg of doxycycline within 72 hours of a tick bite in endemic areas has been suggested

POSSIBLE COMPLICATIONS

- Recurrent synovitis, tendinitis, bursitis
- Chronic neurological symptoms
- Peripheral neuropathies
- See Signs and symptoms of Stage 3 disease

EXPECTED COURSE/PROGNOSIS

- Early treatment with antibiotics can shorten the duration of symptoms and prevent later disease
- Response of late stage disease is variable

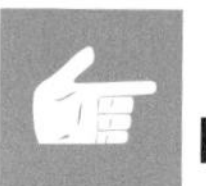

MISCELLANEOUS

ASSOCIATED CONDITIONS N/A

AGE-RELATED FACTORS

Pediatric: Drug of choice in pediatrics is amoxicillin. Tetracyclines are contraindicated.
Geriatric: N/A
Others: Ixodid ticks are commonly found on deer. Hunters may be at increased risk.

PREGNANCY Because *B. burgdorferi* can cross the placenta, pregnant patients with active disease should receive parenteral antibiotics. Doxycycline should not be used in pregnancy.

SYNONYMS Lyme arthritis

ICD-9-CM

088.81 Lyme disease

SEE ALSO

OTHER NOTES Ixodid ticks require white footed mice to complete their life cycle. Investigators have had some success in eradicating the ticks by providing permethrin laced cotton in areas where the mice forage for bedding material.

ABBREVIATIONS N/A

REFERENCES

- Lyme Disease-United States 2000. MMWR 2002;50:29-31, Mar 13
- Nadelman RB, Nowakowski J, Forseter G, et al: The clinical spectrum of early Lyme borreliosis in patients with culture-confirmed erythema migrans. Am J Med 1996;100;502-508
- Treatment of Lyme disease. Med Letter Drugs Ther 2000;42(1077):37-9
- Wormser GP. Practice guidelines for the treatment of Lyme disease. The Infectious Diseases Society of America. Clin Infect Dis 2000;31Suppl1:1-14
- Tick-Borne Diseases. Med Clin North Am 2002 Mar;86(2):205-349
- Stanek G, Strle F. Lyme borreliosis. Lancet 2003;362(9396):1639-47

Web references: 3 available at www.5mcc.com
Illustrations 3 available

Author(s):

Barbara A. Majeroni, MD

BASICS

DESCRIPTION Lymphogranuloma venereum (LGV) is a rare, systemic, sexually transmitted disease caused by the three most virulent strains or serovars of *Chlamydia trachomatis*, the same organism responsible for chlamydial urethritis

- Tender inguinal and/or femoral lymphadenopathy, usually unilateral, is the most common clinical manifestation in heterosexuals. Women and homosexual men might have proctocolitis or inflammatory involvement of perirectal lymphatic tissue. Painless vesicular or ulcerative lesions on the external genitalia may be seen in early disease and severe anogenital inflammation and scarring may result from untreated disease.
- Usually a disease of the tropics; especially Africa, but also seen in the Caribbean (Haiti and Jamaica), South America, East Asia and Indonesia. Chlamydial infections now require reporting in most states.

System(s) affected: Gastrointestinal, Hemic/Lymphatic/Immunologic, Reproductive
Genetics: N/A
Incidence/Prevalence in USA: Approximately 300 cases reported to CDC each year. The prevalence of anorectal LGV is increasing in the USA in male homosexuals.
Predominant age: Third decade; corresponds with average age of peak sexual activity
Predominant sex: Male > Female (5:1)

SIGNS & SYMPTOMS

Three stages:

- Primary:
  - ◊ Superficial lesions such as papules, vesicles, ulcers or erosions appear on the external genitalia 3-30 days after exposure. Lesions are painless and disappear in a few days leaving no scar. This stage often escapes notice.
- Secondary: the inguinal syndrome (bubonic stage) or hemorrhagic proctitis following rectal intercourse
  - ◊ Predominantly in men (Male : Female > 10:1)
  - ◊ Fever, chills, headache, myalgias
  - ◊ Inguinal syndrome: regional lymphadenopathy occurring a week to months after the primary stage
    - Buboes begin as a mass of firm, tender, enlarged, matted lymph nodes, often unilateral and eventually involving the overlying skin with erythema and adhesions. They may have a groove through them formed by the inguinal ligament. As the buboes enlarge:
    - The patient experiences severe groin pain and often walks with a limp
    - Within one to two weeks, the buboes may become fluctuant and rupture relieving the pain and leaving fistulas to drain, heal and scar. Sometimes buboes simply involute and form firm inguinal masses.
  - ◊ Proctitis:
    - Anal pruritus and a mucous rectal discharge
    - Multiple, discrete superficial ulcerations with irregular borders
    - Rectal pain and tenesmus
    - Rectal mucosa feels granular on digital exam
- Tertiary: the anogenital stage
  - ◊ Lymphatic obstruction or scarring
  - ◊ Genitalia or anorectal canal inflammation
  - ◊ Predominantly women and homosexual men. The rectal or vaginal mucosa can become involved after direct inoculation by receptive intercourse or may become involved through posterior lymphatic spread.
  - ◊ Lymphatic obstruction can produce either unusual perianal growths of lymphoid tissue resembling hemorrhoids or genital elephantiasis
  - ◊ Perirectal abscesses, ischiorectal and rectovaginal fistulas, anal fistulas, and rectal strictures or stenosis can occur

CAUSES Three of fifteen known strains of C. trachomatis described as serovars L1, L2, and L3 are responsible for LGV. While the strains of Chlamydia that cause urethritis appear to infect only squamocolumnar cells, LGV strains are more invasive and capable of replication in macrophages.

RISK FACTORS

- Unprotected intercourse, especially outside of a mutually monogamous and disease-free sexual relationship
- Anal intercourse
- Residing in or visiting tropical or developing countries
- With the increasing incidence of anorectal LGV in male homosexuals in the USA, LGV should be kept in mind when a patient presents with symptoms of proctocolitis
- Prostitutes

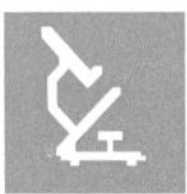

DIAGNOSIS

DIFFERENTIAL DIAGNOSIS

- Inguinal adenitis - chancroid, granuloma inguinale (Donovanosis), genital herpes or syphilis. In the USA, one or more of these is much more likely than LGV, especially if the diagnosed adenitis is associated with a prominent genital ulceration. Other causes of inguinal adenitis include cat-scratch disease, lymphoma, HIV, reactive adenopathy due to skin lesions on the lower extremities. Less common: lymphoproliferative buboes.
- Buboes or suppurative adenitis - chancroid, donovanosis, plague, tularemia, sporotrichosis, actinomycosis or tuberculosis
- Retroperitoneal adenitis - may present as lower abdominal pain with subsequent extensive differential diagnosis
- Proctitis - gonococcal and non-LGV chlamydial proctitis as well as antibiotic-induced and infectious proctitis. Also inflammatory bowel disease.
- Lymphatic obstruction - consider schistosomiasis or malignancy

LABORATORY

- Mild leukocytosis with relative lymphocytosis or monocytosis
- Elevated erythrocyte sedimentation rate
- VDRL/RPR and HIV testing should be considered

Drugs that may alter lab results: Antibiotics

Disorders that may alter lab results: Chlamydial urethritis

PATHOLOGICAL FINDINGS N/A

SPECIAL TESTS

- Bubo pus, saline injected into a bubo and re-aspirated, infected tissue or primary lesion scrapings, preserved in proper transport media (ask your lab), can be studied with Giemsa stain or by immunofluorescence for inclusion bodies. They can also be cultured on McCoy cells. Yield is about 30% for all of these methods.
- Immunoglobulin M microimmunofluorescence (MIF) is a test used frequently to diagnose chlamydial pneumonia among infants, but can also be used for LGV
- Antibody levels to L1, L2, and L3 serovars of C. trachomatis can also be measured with complement fixation although cross-reactivity with other Chlamydial organisms is possible.
- A fourfold rise in MIF titer to LGV antigen or a complement fixation titer above 1:64, with the proper clinical scenario, is probably LGV. Complement levels above 1:128 confirm the LGV diagnosis. These levels are reached early in the disease. Acute and convalescent titers usually do not vary much at six weeks.
- MIF titers are more sensitive and specific than the complement fixation test, however they are only used in specialized research labs and are not routinely available
- Frei's intradermal test is obsolete
- Polymerase chain reaction (PCR) testing - recently developed to diagnose LGV

IMAGING

- Computerized tomography for retroperitoneal adenitis. Lymphography does not outline buboes, but may demonstrate the extent of lymph node involvement
- Barium enema may reveal the characteristic elongated stricture of rectal LGV

DIAGNOSTIC PROCEDURES Aspiration or incision and drainage of bubo for culture

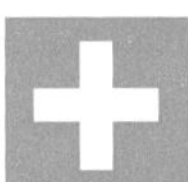

TREATMENT

APPROPRIATE HEALTH CARE Outpatient except for rare complications such as severe pain or for the surgical repair of complications. Surgery should only be attempted after antibiotic therapy.

GENERAL MEASURES Symptomatic treatment with non-steroidal anti-inflammatories should be offered in those not contraindicated. Local heat may provide some analgesia.

SURGICAL MEASURES In the acute bubonic stage, fluctuant nodes should be aspirated before they burst and the occasional abscess should be incised and drained. Otherwise surgery should be avoided until antibiotics have been administered. Fever abates rapidly and bubo pain usually responds within a few days after starting antibiotics.

ACTIVITY Sexual abstention pending treatment, otherwise limited only by symptoms

DIET No special diet unless tetracyclines utilized

PATIENT EDUCATION
- LGV is a sexually transmitted disease. The patient should be counseled about other sexually transmitted diseases and safe sex practices
- Sexual partner(s) should be treated, especially those with contact within 30 days before onset of symptoms
- Offer HIV and syphilis counseling and testing

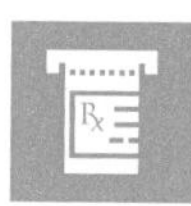

MEDICATIONS

DRUG(S) OF CHOICE
- For acute cases: Doxycycline 100 mg po bid for 21 days
- For chronic or relapsing cases: Consider longer course of therapy

Contraindications: Tetracycline allergy or sensitivity

Precautions:
- For patients taking tetracyclines longer than 21 days, leukocytosis, atypical lymphocytes, toxic granulation of granulocytes in the peripheral blood., and thrombopenic purpura (rare) may be observed
- Superinfections such as antibiotic-induced diarrhea may ensue
- Tetracyclines may cause photosensitization. Advise patients to use sunscreen.
- Avoid tetracyclines in pregnancy and children under 8
- Avoid any agents that chelate tetracycline. Allow 2 hours for gastric emptying prior to medication administration if any of these agents are taken.

Significant possible interactions:
- Avoid, when taking tetracyclines: milk and milk products, antacids, sodium bicarbonate, calcium and magnesium salts, silicate, iron preparations, and bismuth subsalicylate
- As opposed to the other tetracyclines, food does not otherwise interfere with absorption of doxycycline nor does doxycycline seem to have prolonged clearance in patients with impaired renal function
- Doxycycline's half-life is shortened from 20 to 7 hours in patients who are receiving chronic treatment with barbiturates or phenytoin and hence should be administered in the same dose three to four times a day in this group of patients

ALTERNATIVE DRUGS
- Erythromycin base 500 mg orally four times a day for 21 days, or
- Azithromycin 1.0 g orally once weekly for 3 weeks is likely effective, but data is lacking
- Tetracycline 500 mg po qid for 21 days or
- Sulfisoxazole 500 mg po qid for 21 days or equivalent sulfonamide course
- Chloramphenicol and rifampin have been used successfully

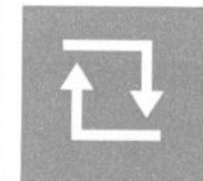

FOLLOWUP

PATIENT MONITORING
- Fever and bubo pain usually abate within 1 to 2 days after starting antibiotics. For persistent fever or malaise, monitor closely for complications such as abscesses or super-infections.
- Treatment has no effect on existing scar tissue, therefore monitor for surgical complications
- Dual infections with other sexually transmitted diseases are common - appropriate monitoring should be performed, especially for syphilis and HIV
- Patients should be followed until signs and symptoms resolve

PREVENTION/AVOIDANCE
- Treat sexual contact(s)
- Abstinence or mutual monogamy in a proven disease-free sexual relationship is the only prevention. Condoms should be worn with sexual activity outside of such relationships.
- Condoms may provide protection against genital-ano-genital transmission but have no impact on transmission between other sites

POSSIBLE COMPLICATIONS
- Scarring - including possible ureteral or bowel obstruction, persistent rectovaginal fistula or gross destruction of the anal canal, anal sphincter, or perineum. Repair of such complications as well as plastic repair of some of the complications of lymphatic obstruction such as genital elephantiasis are the more common surgical indications. Surgery should be performed only after antibiotic treatment.
- Mild rectal strictures can occasionally be dilated as an outpatient
- Squamous cell carcinoma has been associated with LGV

EXPECTED COURSE/PROGNOSIS
- Early treatment improves the prognosis
- Complete resolution of symptoms is usual if treatment is undertaken before scarring
- Reinfection and/or inadequate treatment may result in relapse

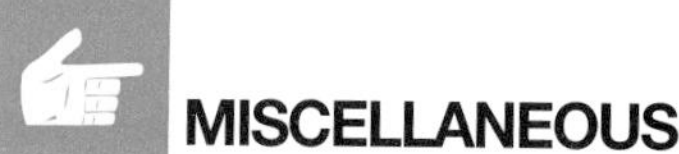

MISCELLANEOUS

ASSOCIATED CONDITIONS Any of the sexually transmitted diseases. Screening should be done for syphilis and HIV.

AGE-RELATED FACTORS
Pediatric: N/A
Geriatric: N/A
Others: N/A

PREGNANCY
- Congenital transmission does not occur, but infection may be acquired during passage through an infected birth canal
- Pregnant and lactating women should be treated with erythromycin regimen. Azithromycin may prove useful, but data is lacking. Doxycycline is contraindicated in pregnancy.

SYNONYMS
- Tropical bubo
- Climatic bubo
- Strumous bubo
- Poradenitis inguinalis
- Durand-Nicolas-Favre disease
- Lymphogranuloma inguinale
- Fourth or fifth or sixth venereal disease

ICD-9-CM
099.1 Lymphogranuloma venereum

SEE ALSO
Chancroid
Chlamydial sexually transmitted diseases
Herpes, genital
Syphilis

OTHER NOTES HIV infected patients with LGV should be treated with usual LGV regimen, but may require longer therapy

ABBREVIATIONS
HIV = human immunodeficiency virus
CDC = Centers for Disease Control
LGV = lymphogranuloma venereum
RPR = Rapid plasma reagin test for syphilis
VDRL = Venereal Disease Research Laboratory

REFERENCES
- Centers for Disease Control: 2002 Sexually transmitted diseases treatment guidelines. MMWR 51(RR-6), 2002
- Holmes KH, Mardh PA, Sparling PF, et al. Sexually Transmitted Diseases. 3rd ed. New York: McGraw Hill; 1999

Web references: 1 available at www.5mcc.com
Illustrations 2 available

Author(s):
Grant C. Fowler, MD

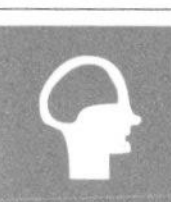

BASICS

DESCRIPTION Highly undifferentiated B cell lymphoma. It may involve sites other than lymph nodes or reticuloendothelial system, particularly bone marrow and central nervous system. Endemic areas - Central Africa; New Guinea. Rare in USA.
System(s) affected: Hemic/Lymphatic/Immunologic
Genetics: Translocation of chromosome 8 onto chromosome 14 (70%); c-myc activation
Incidence/Prevalence in USA: Rare
Predominant age: 3 months to 16 years
Predominant sex: Male > female

SIGNS & SYMPTOMS
- African:
  - ◊ Mouth pain
  - ◊ Loose teeth
  - ◊ Loose deciduous molars
  - ◊ Jaw mass
  - ◊ Anemia
- North American:
  - ◊ Abdominal mass
  - ◊ Abdominal pain

CAUSES Unknown; high association with Epstein-Barr virus

RISK FACTORS Living in endemic areas

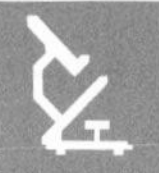

DIAGNOSIS

DIFFERENTIAL DIAGNOSIS N/A

LABORATORY
- Anemia
- Serum uric acid often elevated

Drugs that may alter lab results: N/A

Disorders that may alter lab results: N/A

PATHOLOGICAL FINDINGS
- Diffuse small round cell, non-cleaved lymphoma (Burkitt type)
- L3 morphology in B-cell leukemia
- High mitotic rate
- Starry sky pattern

SPECIAL TESTS
- Cytogenic studies - translocation between chromosomes 8 and 14
- Immunologic studies - presence of B cell markers (usually IgM) on cell surface

IMAGING CT scan

DIAGNOSTIC PROCEDURES
- Bone marrow aspiration
- Lumbar puncture
- Lymph node biopsy

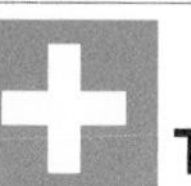

TREATMENT

APPROPRIATE HEALTH CARE
- Inpatient - for staging surgery and chemotherapy (may require ICU for advanced stages)
- Outpatient - after definitive treatment

GENERAL MEASURES
- Symptomatic treatment for respiratory, gastrointestinal, or psychosocial problems that may follow chemotherapy
- Be alert to increased risk for renal failure and life-threatening metabolic abnormalities due to tumor lysis

SURGICAL MEASURES
- Surgery for biopsy and staging

ACTIVITY As tolerated

DIET
- May have difficulty in swallowing or chewing (jaw involvement). Suggest small meals of a soft diet (protein milk shakes) to help prevent malnutrition.
- Adequate fluid intake

PATIENT EDUCATION
Leukemia Society of America
733 3rd Avenue
New York, NY 10017
(212)573-8424

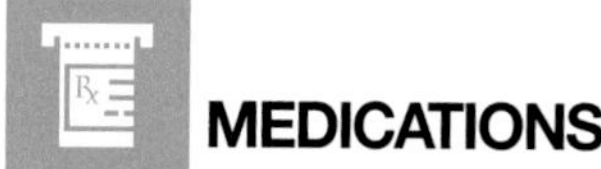

MEDICATIONS

DRUG(S) OF CHOICE Combination chemotherapy according to most recent protocols. Type and extent of therapy depends on stage of disease.
Contraindications: Refer to manufacturer's literature
Precautions: Myelosuppression, alopecia, mucositis, neurotoxicity with chemotherapy
Significant possible interactions: Refer to manufacturer's literature

ALTERNATIVE DRUGS Intensive chemotherapy with or without bone marrow transplantation for advanced case

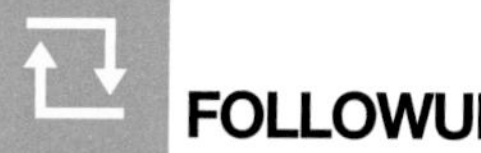

FOLLOWUP

PATIENT MONITORING
- For effects of chemotherapy
- Follow for detection of recurrence

PREVENTION/AVOIDANCE Avoid endemic areas

POSSIBLE COMPLICATIONS
- Tumor lysis syndrome with renal failure:
  - ◊ Hyperkalemia
  - ◊ Hyperphosphatemia
  - ◊ Hyperuricemia
  - ◊ Hypocalcemia
  - ◊ Tetany

EXPECTED COURSE/PROGNOSIS
- 95% of patients with localized disease experience long-term remission and possible cure
- With recent protocols, over 80% of patients with advanced stages have also been cured
- Without treatment, prognosis is grave

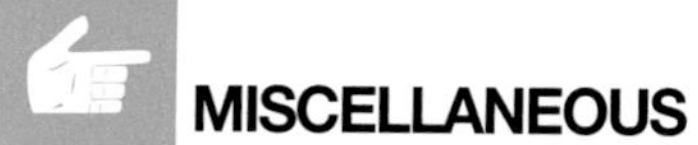

MISCELLANEOUS

ASSOCIATED CONDITIONS N/A

AGE-RELATED FACTORS
Pediatric: Common age group for this disorder
Geriatric: Unusual in this age group
Others: N/A

PREGNANCY N/A

SYNONYMS
- Monomorphic undifferentiated lymphoma
- African lymphoma
- Maxillary lymphosarcoma

ICD-9-CM
200.20 Burkitt tumor or lymphoma, unspecified site, extranodal and solid organ sites

SEE ALSO

OTHER NOTES N/A

ABBREVIATIONS N/A

REFERENCES

- Vietti T, Fernbach D, eds: Clinical Pediatric Oncology. 4th Ed. St. Louis, C.V. Mosby, 1992
- Williams WJ, et al: Hematology. 4th Ed. New York, McGraw-Hill, 1990
- Bennett JC, Plum F, eds: Cecil Textbook of Medicine. 20th Ed. Philadelphia, W.B. Saunders Co., 1996

Web references: 0 available at www.5mcc.com
Illustrations N/A

Author(s):
John J. Hutter, Jr., MD

BASICS

DESCRIPTION One definition of ARMD is pigmentary changes in the macula or typical drusen associated with visual loss to the 20/30 level or worse, not caused by cataract or other eye disease in individuals over 50 years of age. Other definitions do not include age or visual acuity criteria. ARMD is the leading cause of irreversible, severe visual loss in persons over 65 years of age.
- Stages:
  - ◊ Atrophic/nonexudative: drusen and/or pigmentary changes in the macula
  - ◊ Neovascular/exudative: growth of blood vessels underneath the retina

System(s) affected: Nervous

Genetics:
- The neovascular/exudative form is rare in blacks and more common in whites
- Genetic susceptibility may be a factor in senile macular degeneration, with approximately 1/4 of all senile cases being genetically determined

Incidence/Prevalence in USA:
- In the Framingham Eye Study (FES) drusen were noted in 25% of all participants who were ≥52 years of age. ARMD associated visual loss was noted in 5.7%.
- Prevalence increases with age. Over 75 years; one quarter of men and one third of women will have evidence of ARMD.
- The prevalence of severe visual loss from ARMD increases with age. 2.2% of patients over 65 years of age are blind in one or both eyes from ARMD.
- The atrophic/nonexudative stage accounts for 20% of cases of severe visual loss
- The neovascular/exudative stage accounts for 80% of cases of severe visual loss

Predominant age: FES prevalence rates:
- 1.6% of those individuals who were 52-64 years old
- 11% of those who were 65-74 years old
- 27.9% of those who were > 75 years

Predominant sex: Female > Male

SIGNS & SYMPTOMS
- Atrophic/nonexudative stage
  - ◊ Drusen
    - Small yellowish-white lesions
    - Can be subdivided into types such as hard drusen and soft drusen
  - ◊ Atrophy of the retinal pigment epithelium (RPE), a pigment layer underneath the retina
- Neovascular/exudative stage
  - ◊ Blood vessels growing underneath the retina from the choroid are called choroidal neovascular membranes (CNVMs) or subretinal neovascularization (SRN). The choroid is the vascular layer underneath the RPE.
    - Subretinal fluid
    - Exudates
    - Subretinal hemorrhage
    - Patients frequently notice distortion of central vision. On Amsler grid testing the horizontal or vertical lines may become broken, distorted or missing. Patients may notice straight lines appear crooked, e.g., telephone poles.
  - ◊ Disciform scar: An advanced stage resulting in a fibrovascular scar

CAUSES
- Visible light can result in the formation and accumulation of metabolic byproducts in the RPE which normally helps remove metabolic byproducts from the retina. The excess accumulation of these metabolic byproducts interferes with the normal metabolic activity of the RPE and can lead to the formation of drusen.
- The neovascular stage generally arises from the atrophic stage
- Most patients do not progress beyond the atrophic/nonexudative stage; however, those that do are at a greater risk to develop severe visual loss

RISK FACTORS
- Excess sunlight exposure
- Blue or light iris color
- Hyperopia
- History of cardiovascular disease (hypertension, circulatory problems)
- Short height
- History of lung infection
- Cigarette smoking
- Low dietary intake of antioxidant nutrients
- Family history

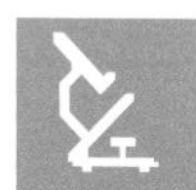

DIAGNOSIS

DIFFERENTIAL DIAGNOSIS
Idiopathic subretinal neovascularization, presumed ocular histoplasmosis syndrome, diabetic retinopathy, and hypertensive retinopathy

LABORATORY N/A

Drugs that may alter lab results: N/A

Disorders that may alter lab results: N/A

PATHOLOGICAL FINDINGS
- Drusen: deposits of hyaline material between the retinal pigment epithelium (RPE) and Bruch's membrane (the limiting membrane between the RPE and the choroid)
- Breaks in Bruch's membrane allows CNVMs to invade the RPE and grow into the subretinal space

SPECIAL TESTS
- Fluorescein angiography: Can detect CNVMs. This test helps to differentiate between atrophic and neovascular ARMD.
- Indocyanine green videoangiography: May be useful in identifying occult or hidden CNVM's

IMAGING N/A

DIAGNOSTIC PROCEDURES
- Daily Amsler grid testing
- Eye examination with detailed fundus examination
- Fluorescein angiography

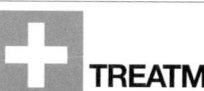

TREATMENT

APPROPRIATE HEALTH CARE Outpatient for laser treatment. Inpatient or outpatient for vitrectomy surgery.

GENERAL MEASURES
- Atrophic/nonexudative macular degeneration
  - ◊ No specific treatment alters the course
  - ◊ Free radical formation in the retina, induced by visible light may play a role in cellular damage that results in ARMD.
  - ◊ Vitamin A, E, C and beta-carotene may be useful in preventing cellular damage
  - ◊ Oral zinc may retard visual loss
  - ◊ Laser photocoagulation to treat drusen is being investigated
- Neovascular/exudative macular degeneration
  - ◊ The Macular Photocoagulation Study (MPS) demonstrated a treatment benefit for laser treatment of CNVMs which were 200 microns (200 microns = 0.2 mm) or greater from the center of the macula.
    - The MPS showed that the benefits of argon laser photocoagulation were greatest one year after treatment. At that time the proportion of eyes with severe visual loss was reduced 51% by treatment, from 43% in untreated eyes to 21% in treated eyes. The deterioration in treatment effect in the MPS is primarily due to recurrent CNVMs growing towards the center of the macula.
    - Fluorescein angiogram usually can determine whether a CNVM is present, if it is well defined, and if it is in a treatable position.
    - Recurrent CNVMs, after laser treatment, were seen in 59% of patients with ARMD. Recurrent CNVMs develop early after treatment; 73% of the recurrences occurred within the first year of treatment, usually within the first 6 months.
- Treatment of CNVMs from 1 to 199 microns from the center of the macula has been studied by the Age-Related Macular Degeneration Study-Krypton Laser (ARMDS-K). The benefit of laser treatment was greatest among patients without evidence of hypertension. No benefit was observed among patients who had highly elevated blood pressure and/or used antihypertensive medication.
  - ◊ Because patients in the ARMDS-K treatment group had CNVMs closer to the center of vision, the magnitude of treatment benefit after laser photocoagulation is smaller in the ARMDS-K treatment group than in the argon laser trial for CNVMs further away from the center of the macula.
  - ◊ Laser treatment can be applied to CNVMs directly underneath the center of vision; however, this can result in immediate worsening of vision. The long term benefits of laser treatment for these lesions makes this form of laser treatment an option.

- Vitrectomy has been used to remove CNVMs, but the benefits of this procedure are being studied
  - ◊ CNVMs can bleed spontaneously leaving blood underneath the retina. Vitrectomy to remove subretinal blood may be of benefit and should be performed within 7 days of the bleed. Tissue plasminogen activator (tPA) instilled into the eye, may help remove a subretinal hemorrhage. Intravitreal gas with or without tPA may be capable in some cases of displacing submacular blood.
- Macular translocation involves intentionally creating a retinal detachment and attempting to shift the macula away from the CNVM. Laser is then applied to the CNVM after the retina is translocated. This procedure is currently being refined and is associated with potential serious surgical risks.
- Patients need to be monitored (usually with fluorescein angiography) after laser treatment, for recurrent CNVMs. After treatment, patients should report changes in the Amsler grid or their vision
- Photodynamic therapy (PDT) with verteporfin reduces vision loss in patients with greater than 50% "classic" subfoveal CNVMs. Verteporfin is administered intravenously and diode laser at 689 nm is applied to the CNVM.
  - ◊ When PDT was used to treat predominately classic subfoveal CNVMs after 24 months of follow-up, 59% of the verteporfin-treated eyes versus 31% of the placebo-treated eyes lost fewer than 15 letters from baseline
  - ◊ In occult subfoveal CNVMs with no classic component, PDT significantly reduces the risk of moderate and severe vision loss
  - ◊ PDT treatment benefit may not only depend upon lesion type, but also upon lesion size and presenting visual acuity. The treatment benefit may be related to smaller lesion size and worse presenting visual acuity.
  - ◊ Patients should be informed that there is a small risk of acute, severe vision loss of approximately 4% after PDT
  - ◊ Intravitreal triamcinolone when combined with PDT may result in improved visual acuity for patients with CNVMs
- Low vision aids may be helpful
- Investigation/experimental treatments: transplanting of fetal RPE cells, laser treatment to drusen, low dose radiation therapy, transpupillary thermotherapy, via a diode laser at 810nm, for occult subfoveal CNVMs

SURGICAL MEASURES
See General Measures

ACTIVITY
Patients with the neovascular form of ARMD should avoid straining and anticoagulants if possible prior to laser treatment

DIET
- A diet high in vitamins A, E, C and beta-carotene along with zinc may be of benefit
- Eating dark green, leafy vegetables (spinach or collard greens) which are rich in carotinoids may decrease the risk of developing the neovascular/exudative stage
- May be a higher risk for ARMD with increasing intake of vegetable fat and monounsaturated and polyunsaturated fats, and linoleic acid. High concentrations of these substances tend to be found in highly processed, store-bought snack foods.
- Consumption of omega-3 fatty acids found in fish decreased the risk of ARMD when the intake of linoleic acid was low

PATIENT EDUCATION
- American Academy of Ophthalmology, 655 Beach Street, San Francisco, CA 94109-1336
- Visually impaired patients should check with their local low vision center for aids

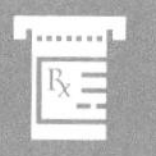

MEDICATIONS

DRUG(S) OF CHOICE
- Zinc and antioxidants may be of benefit. Zinc sulfate 100 mg bid with food has been recommended.
- Age-Related Eye Disease Study (AREDS) found that a high-dose regimen of vitamin and mineral supplements reduces progression of ARMD in some cases. Recommended daily doses: vitamin C 500 mg, vitamin E 400 1U, beta-carotene 15 mg, zinc oxide 80 mg, and cupric oxide 2 mg.

Contraindications: N/A

Precautions:
- Excess zinc ingestion can be associated with anemia and worsening of cardiovascular disease
- Exercise caution with beta-carotene use in smokers, may be a link to lung cancer

Significant possible interactions: N/A

ALTERNATIVE DRUGS
- Anecortave acetate is being tested in the treatment of exudative ARMD. This medicine is injected next to the eye, via a posterior juxtascleral injection.
- A VEGF (vascular endothelial growth factor) inhibitor which is injected into the eye is being tested in the treatment of exudative ARMD. Pegaptanib sodium (Macugen) is a compound that binds to and neutralizes VEGF.
- RhuFab is another promising anti-VEGF compound being tested in the treatment of exudative ARMD

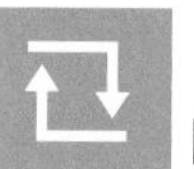

FOLLOWUP

PATIENT MONITORING
- Laser treated patients should be re-examined promptly if new visual symptoms occur
- The Amsler grid can aid in discovering visual disturbances
- Patients with soft drusen or pigmentary changes in the macula are at an increased risk of visual loss. They should be instructed that it is important to monitor their vision, such as by Amsler grid testing and subjective measures of visual acuity, such as reading vision and image clarity. If there are no new symptoms, follow-up examination in 6-12 months.
- Follow-up examination for patients at increased risk of visual loss may permit early detection of treatable lesions

PREVENTION/AVOIDANCE
- Ultraviolet protection for eyes
- Well balanced diet which includes zinc, vitamins A, E, C, and beta-carotene
- Routine ophthalmologic visits; q2-4 years for patients 40-64 and q1-2 years after age 65
- Daily Amsler grid testing
- Patients who take statin drugs, which modify lipid profiles, may have a reduced risk for ARMD

POSSIBLE COMPLICATIONS
Blindness

EXPECTED COURSE/PROGNOSIS
- Patients with bilateral soft drusen, and pigmentary changes in the macula, but no evidences of exudation, have an increased likelihood of developing CNVMs and subsequent visual loss
- Patients with bilateral drusen carry a cumulative risk of 14.7% over five years of suffering significant visual loss in one eye from the neovascular stage of ARMD.
- Patient's with neovascular stage in one eye and drusen in the opposite eye are at a risk of 5-14% annually of developing the neovascular stage in opposite eye with drusen
- High incidence of recurrence after laser treatment for CNVMs

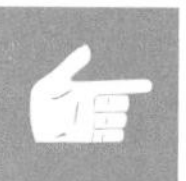

MISCELLANEOUS

ASSOCIATED CONDITIONS
- Presumed ocular histoplasmosis syndrome
- Exudative retinal detachment
- Vitreous hemorrhage
- Other causes of CNVMs

AGE-RELATED FACTORS
Pediatric: N/A

Geriatric: Prevalence will increase as population ages.

Others: N/A

PREGNANCY
N/A

SYNONYMS
- Senile macular degeneration
- Subretinal neovascularization

ICD-9-CM
362.51 Nonexudative senile macular degeneration
362.52 Exudative senile macular degeneration
362.57 Drusen (degenerative)

SEE ALSO

OTHER NOTES
N/A

ABBREVIATIONS
ARMD = age-related macular degeneration
SMD = senile macular degeneration
SRN = subretinal neovascularization
CNVM = choroidal neovascular membrane
RPE = retinal pigment epithelium
MPS = macular photocoagulation study
ARMDS-K = Age-related macular degeneration study-Krypton Laser
PDT = photodynamic therapy

REFERENCES

- Handwerger BA, Blodi BA, Chandra SR, et al. Treatment of submacular hemorrhage with low-dose intravitreal tissue plasminogen activator injection and pneumatic displacement. Arch Ophthalmol 2001;119;28-32
- Bressler NM. Photodynamic therapy of subfoveal choroidal neovascularization in age-related macular degeneration with verteporfin: two-year results of 2 randomized clinical trials-tap report 2. Arch Ophthalmol 2001;119(2):198-207
- Verteporfin therapy of subfoveal choroidal neovascularization in age-related macular degeneration: two-year results of a randomized clinical trial including lesions with occult with no classic choroidal neovascularization-verteporfin in photodynamic therapy report 2. Am J Ophthalmol 2001;131(5):541-60

Web references: 0 available at www.5mcc.com

Illustrations 4 available

Author(s):
Richard W. Allinson, MD

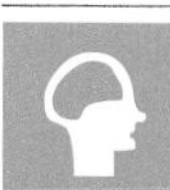

BASICS

DESCRIPTION Malaria is an acute and chronic protozoan infection transmitted by Anopheles mosquitoes to humans. There are four species of Plasmodium that cause human infection.

System(s) affected: Hemic/Lymphatic/Immunologic

Genetics: No known genetic pattern. Glucose-6-phosphate deficiency, sickle cell disease or trait, and hereditary ovalocytosis probably help protect against severe *P. falciparum* infection.

Incidence/Prevalence in USA:
- Most (> 99%) cases are imported. Very rare primary outbreaks in the U.S.
- Causes of all reported cases in the U.S. in 2002
  - ◊ *P. falciparum* 52%
  - ◊ *P. vivax* 25%
  - ◊ *P. malariae* 3%
  - ◊ *P. ovale* 3%

Predominant age: All ages

Predominant sex: Male = Female

SIGNS & SYMPTOMS
- Fever
- Malaise
- Chills
- Headache
- Nausea
- Splenomegaly (especially with chronic infection)
- Systolic hypotension
- *P. falciparum* (also known as malignant tertian malaria): Incubation period usually 12-14 days with subsequent high fevers every 48 hours within 2 months of infection. If large parasitemia, can lead to anemia, jaundice, thrombocytopenia, and vascular collapse. Other complications include gastroenteritis, central nervous system impairment, renal failure, and pulmonary edema. Associated with fatal outcome if severe infection.
- *P. vivax* (benign tertian malaria) and P. ovale: Incubation period up to 12 months with high fever every 48 hours. Dormant parasites may remain in the liver causing relapse months after the initial infection.
- *P. malariae* (benign quartan malaria): Incubation period approximately 35 days with high fevers every 72 hours. May become chronic and lead to nephrotic syndrome.

CAUSES
- *Plasmodium falciparum, P. malariae, P. vivax, P. ovale*

RISK FACTORS
- Usually traveling and/or living in endemic area (75% of *P. falciparum* cases from Sub-Sahara Africa)
- Rarely, blood transfusion or mother-to-fetus transmission

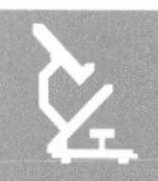

DIAGNOSIS

DIFFERENTIAL DIAGNOSIS
- Infections such as localized (abscess), viral (mononucleosis), rickettsial, and mycobacterial infections. Collagen vascular diseases including systemic lupus erythematosus, primary vasculitides, and mixed connective tissue diseases. Neoplasms such as lymphoma and leukemia. Other causes of tropical splenomegaly and blood dyscrasias.
- Severe *P. falciparum* infection may mimic acute hepatitis, acute hemolytic anemia, pneumonia and stroke

LABORATORY
- In uncomplicated infection:
  - ◊ Elevated liver function tests and lactate dehydrogenase (>50% of cases)
  - ◊ Thrombocytopenia (40%)
  - ◊ Anemia (25%)
  - ◊ Leukopenia (25%) vs leukocytosis (1-5%)

Drugs that may alter lab results: Antimalarial agents may reduce parasitemia

Disorders that may alter lab results: N/A

PATHOLOGICAL FINDINGS
- Malaria causes hemolysis
- If infection is severe, hemolysis of parasitized red blood cells activate pro-inflammatory cytokines causing sludging within the microcirculation and localized necrosis
- Edema, localized hemorrhage, and the presence of malarial pigments are frequent findings

SPECIAL TESTS
- Malarial smear thick and thin preparations obtained every 6-12 hours for 3 samplings. Microscopy to evaluate for parasite forms. (Best to obtain blood during or right after fever spike.)
- Other tests include species-specific PCR and the indirect fluorescent antibody (IFA) which is practical for the clinical laboratory

IMAGING N/A

DIAGNOSTIC PROCEDURES Malarial peripheral blood smear showing intracellular parasite forms

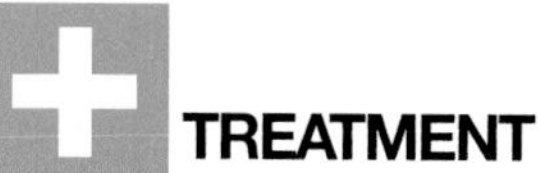

TREATMENT

APPROPRIATE HEALTH CARE Inpatient for most cases of falciparum malaria in nonimmune patients. Outpatient for others, except during acute phase if blood products or close observation is required.

GENERAL MEASURES In severe cases watch for complications, such as severe anemia and renal failure, otherwise supportive care

SURGICAL MEASURES N/A

ACTIVITY May resume activity as soon as the fever is under control. Avoid strenuous exercise if splenomegaly.

DIET No restrictions; as tolerated

PATIENT EDUCATION Prevention of future exposures. These measures include prevention of mosquito bites and malarial chemoprophylaxis.

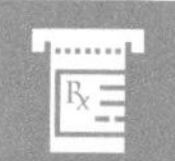

MEDICATIONS

DRUG(S) OF CHOICE

- Oral therapy for chloroquine-resistant *P. falciparum*
  - ◊ Quinine sulfate plus doxycycline or plus pyrimethamine-sulfadoxine (Fansidar) or plus tetracycline
    - Adults, quinine sulfate 650 mg salt tid for 3-7 days plus doxycycline 100 mg bid for 7 days or plus Fansidar 3 tablets on last day of quinine or plus tetracycline 250 mg qid for 7 days
    - Children, quinine sulfate 10 mg salt/kg (max 650 mg salt) tid for 3-7 days plus doxycycline (not for <8 years of age) 2 mg/kg bid for 7 days or plus Fansidar 1/2 tablet/10 kg on last day of quinine or plus tetracycline (not for < 8 years of age) 6.25 mg/kg qid for 7 days
  - ◊ Atovaquone-proguanil (Malarone) 250 mg/100 mg : adults, 2 tablets bid for 3 days. Children, 11-20 kg 1/2 adult tablet bid, 21-30 kg 1 adult tablet bid, 31-40 kg 1 1/2 adult tablets bid
- Oral therapy for *P. ovale*, *P. malariae*, chloroquine-sensitive *P. falciparum* and chloroquine-sensitive *P. vivax*
  - ◊ Chloroquine phosphate:
    - Adults, 600 mg base (1 gm salt) followed by 300 mg at 6, 24 and 48 hours
    - Children, 10 mg base/kg (max of 600 mg) then 5 mg/kg at 6, 24 and 48 hours
  - ◊ Primaquine phosphate (must be added to chloroquine therapy for cure of dormant forms of *P. vivax* and *P. ovale*)
    - Adults, 30 mg base (52.6 mg) daily for 2 weeks or 45 mg base (79 mg) weekly for 8 weeks
    - Children, 0.6 mg base/kg daily for 2 weeks
- Oral therapy for chloroquine-resistant *P. vivax*
  - ◊ Quinine sulfate plus doxycycline or plus tetracycline: see above for dosages
  - ◊ Mefloquine: adults 1250 mg once (usually divided as 750 mg, then 500 mg 8 hours later). Children 15 mg/kg, then 10 mg/kg 8 hours later.
- For severe infection requiring parenteral therapy
  - ◊ Quinidine gluconate: adults and children, 10 mg/kg in normal saline over 1-2 hours followed by 0.02 mg/kg/min continuous infusion or repeat initial dose every 8 hours until oral therapy can be started

Contraindications: Refer to manufacturer's literature

Precautions:

- Primaquine may cause hemolysis in patients with glucose-6-phosphate deficiency (G6PD); should be screened for if suspected
- Avoid Malarone in breast-feeding women and patients with severe renal impairment (cr cl. < 30 ml/min)
- Avoid mefloquine in patients with seizure, psychiatric illness or cardiac conduction abnormalities

Significant possible interactions: Refer to manufacturer's literature

ALTERNATIVE DRUGS
Oral therapy regardless of plasmodium species: mefloquine: adults, 1250 mg once (may divide as 750 mg and 500 mg over 12 hours); children, 15 mg/kg followed by 10 mg/kg at 12 hours

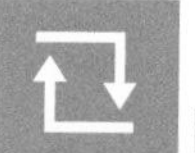

FOLLOWUP

PATIENT MONITORING
Watch for relapse of clinical symptoms

PREVENTION/AVOIDANCE

- Use malarial chemoprophylaxis when in an endemic area. In 2002, all deaths (8) in U.S. were of patients who did not take chemoprophylaxis appropriately.
- Oral chemoprophylaxis for areas with chloroquine-resistant Plasmodium species
  - ◊ Mefloquine (begin 1 week before arrival and continue for 4 weeks after leaving area):
    - Adults: 250 mg (1 tablet) weekly
    - Children: <15 kg 5 mg/kg; 15-19 kg 1/4 tablet weekly; 20-30 kg 1/2 tablet weekly; 31-45 kg 3/4 tablet weekly; >45 kg 1 tablet weekly
  - ◊ Malarone (begin 1-2 days before arrival and continue for 1 week after leaving area):
    - Adults: 250 mg / 100 mg (1 adult tablet) daily
    - Children: 11-20 kg 62.5 mg / 25 mg (1 pediatric tablet) daily; 21-30 kg 2 pediatric tablets daily; 31-40 kg 3 pediatric tablets daily; >40 kg 1 adult tablet daily
  - ◊ Doxycycline (begin 1-2 days before arrival and continue for 4 weeks after leaving area):
    - Adults: 100 mg daily
    - Children: 2 mg/kg daily, up to 100 mg daily (not for children < 8 years)
- Oral chemoprophylaxis for areas with chloroquine-sensitive Plasmodium species
  - ◊ Chloroquine phosphate (begin 1-2 weeks before arrival and continue for 4 weeks after leaving area):
    - Adults: 300 mg base (500 mg salt) weekly
    - Children: 5 mg base/kg weekly up to 300 mg base weekly
- Personal measures (variable efficacy)
  - ◊ DEET-containing insect repellent
  - ◊ Clothing that covers most of the body
  - ◊ Mosquito nets sprayed with permethrin
  - ◊ Air-conditioning

POSSIBLE COMPLICATIONS

- *P. falciparum*: if not treated early, may cause cerebral malaria, acute renal failure, acute gastroenteritis, pulmonary edema, massive hemolysis, and splenic rupture. Death from malaria is virtually limited to *P. falciparum* infection.
- *P. malariae*: nephrotic syndrome may develop in patients with chronic infection
- Other complications: seizures, anuria, delirium, coma, dysentery, algid malaria, blackwater fever, hyperpyrexia

EXPECTED COURSE/PROGNOSIS
Only *P. falciparum* infection carries a poor prognosis with high mortality if untreated. However, if diagnosed early and treated appropriately the prognosis is excellent.

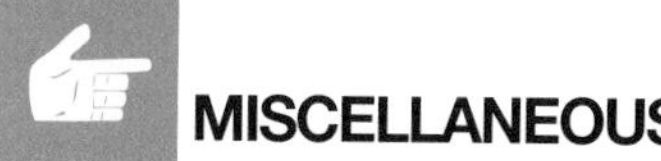

MISCELLANEOUS

ASSOCIATED CONDITIONS
N/A

AGE-RELATED FACTORS
Pediatric: N/A
Geriatric: More serious outcome in this age group
Others: N/A

PREGNANCY
Chloroquine is safe. Mefloquine is probably safe and is recommended if there is no effective alternative. Malarone, primaquine, tetracyclines, quinine and quinidine should not be used in pregnancy or in women breast-feeding.

SYNONYMS
N/A

ICD-9-CM
084.8 Blackwater fever
084.9 Other pernicious complications of malaria
084.5 Mixed malaria
084.1 Vivax malaria (benign tertian)
084.2 Quartan malaria
084.3 Ovale malaria
084.6 Malaria, unspecified
084.0 Falciparum malaria (malignant tertian)
771.2 Other congenital infections
573.2 Hepatitis in other infectious diseases classified elsewhere

SEE ALSO

OTHER NOTES

- Most areas of the world now have chloroquine-resistant *P. falciparum* (the form of malaria most prevalent world-wide). Some multi-drug resistant strains of *P. falciparum* and *P. vivax* are present in Southeast Asia.
- Current information regarding malaria treatment and prophylaxis is always available from Centers for Disease Control (CDC) in Atlanta, GA

ABBREVIATIONS
N/A

REFERENCES

- Freedman DO, editor. Travel Medicine. Inf Dis Clin NA 1998;12(2):267-284, 334-340, 364, 450-454
- Abramowicz A. Drugs for parasitic infections. Medical Letter 2002;44(1128):6-8. Online: www.medicalletter.com/freedocs/parasitic.pdf
- Centers for Disease Control and Prevention: Malaria Surveillance - United States, 2002. MMWR CDC Surveillance Summary 2004;53(SS01):21-34. Online: www.cdc.gov

Web references: 1 available at www.5mcc.com
Illustrations N/A

Author(s):
Beck Soderberg, MD

BASICS

DESCRIPTION
- Protein-calorie malnutrition (PCM) is present when sufficient energy and/or protein is not available to meet metabolic demands, leading to impairment in normal physiologic processes. PCM is classified according to degree of severity and by calculating the actual weight as a percentage of expected weight for height/length, using international standards (normal: 90-110%).
  - ◊ 1st degree: mild form characterized by growth failure in children and wasting in adults. Weight as a percentage of expected weight: 85-90%
  - ◊ 2nd degree: moderate form with additional biochemical changes, weight as a percentage of expected weight: 75-85%
  - ◊ 3rd degree: severe PCM with the development of additional clinical signs, weight as a percentage of expected weight: < 75%
- Kwashiorkor is a condition which develops when there is gross protein deficiency though nonprotein calorie intake may be adequate.
- Marasmus occurs with deficiency of both protein and calories.
- Disease-related malnutrition is common, often not detected, and worsens during a hospital stay. In burns, trauma and infection: release of cytokines such as interleukins, tumor necrosis factor (TNF) and interferons worsens the nutritional status.
- Malnutrition compromises posttransplant survival. Pretransplant nutritional assessment and support may improve transplant outcomes.

System(s) affected: Endocrine/Metabolic, Gastrointestinal, Hemic/Lymphatic/Immunologic, Musculoskeletal, Nervous
Genetics: N/A
Incidence/Prevalence in USA: Institutionalized elderly, hospital patients and children of the poor have a significant prevalence
Predominant age: Infants and younger children (age 1-2) are more susceptible to PCM. However, PCM may occur at all ages.
Predominant sex: Male = Female

SIGNS & SYMPTOMS
- Mild to moderate PCM
  - ◊ Weight loss and reduction in subcutaneous fat in adults
  - ◊ Stunted growth, wasted body habitus, delayed puberty and retarded cognitive and psychosocial development in children
  - ◊ Decreased hand grip strength
  - ◊ Impaired work capacity
  - ◊ Risk of intrauterine growth retardation when pregnant women have PCM
  - ◊ Reduced volume of breast milk with low fat content
- Severe PCM
  - ◊ Severe alterations in the body habitus
  - ◊ Muscle wasting in the extremities
  - ◊ Associated micronutrient deficiency features
  - ◊ Loss of subcutaneous fat
  - ◊ Atrophy of interosseus hand muscles and temporalis
  - ◊ Decreased skin elasticity
  - ◊ Impaired immunity and susceptibility to infections
  - ◊ Delayed wound healing and recovery
  - ◊ Decubitus ulcers
  - ◊ Dry, reddish-brown, sparse hair
  - ◊ Lethargy, early satiety, vomiting and constipation
  - ◊ Heart rate, BP and core body temperature may be subnormal
  - ◊ Marasmic infants show gross weight loss, growth retardation and wasting of subcutaneous fat and muscle
  - ◊ Kwashiorkor is characterized by generalized edema, flaky painful dermatoses, sparse hair with pigment changes, enlarged, fatty liver and petulant apathy

CAUSES
- Inadequate dietary intake
- Poor quality dietary protein
- Increased metabolic demands
- Increased nutrient losses

RISK FACTORS
- Nutritional
  - ◊ Prolonged and severe reduction of intake
  - ◊ Inadequate body reserves
  - ◊ Concurrent deficiencies of the other nutrients
  - ◊ Anorexia nervosa
- Underlying illnesses
  - ◊ Fever, infection, trauma, burns and other hypercatabolic states
  - ◊ Malabsorptive and maldigestive states
  - ◊ Protein-losing enteropathy, nephrotic syndrome, enteric fistulas
  - ◊ Metabolic disorders: Diabetes, hyperthyroidism
- Physiologic states in which requirements are increased
  - ◊ Pregnancy and lactation
  - ◊ Growth and development during infancy, childhood and adolescence

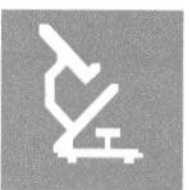

DIAGNOSIS

DIFFERENTIAL DIAGNOSIS
- Secondary growth failure due to malabsorption, congenital defects or deprivation
- Pellagra
- Nephritis or nephrosis
- Cardiac failure
- Disorders of glycogen metabolism
- Cystic fibrosis

LABORATORY
- Plasma albumin: Reduced
- Complete hemogram: Decreased lymphocyte count
- Serum chemistry
- Blood urea: Decreased
- Plasma transferrin: Decreased
- Plasma essential amino acids: Decreased
- Plasma betalipoprotein: Decreased
- Hypoglycemia with neuroglycopenia
- Plasma cortisol, GH: Increased, but insulin low

Drugs that may alter lab results: N/A

Disorders that may alter lab results: N/A

PATHOLOGICAL FINDINGS
- Marasmus

Muscle wasting and reduction in muscle mass due to gluconeogenesis. Mummified appearance. No edema. Fat depots reduced. Loss of subcutaneous fat.
- Kwashiorkor

Serum amino acid patterns distorted. Protein synthesis impaired. Hypoalbuminemia causes dependent edema. Impaired betalipoprotein synthesis causes fatty liver. Poor insulin response to glucose load. Growth, immune response, repair and production of enzymes and hormones are impaired in severe protein deficiency.

SPECIAL TESTS
- Triceps skin-fold thickness
- Mid-arm muscle area (MAMA)
- Protein index measurement
- Creatinine-height index
- Delayed-hypersensitivity index
- Prognostic-nutritional index (PNI)

IMAGING
Chest x-ray to rule out tuberculosis or other pulmonary infections

DIAGNOSTIC PROCEDURES
- History and physical examination
- MAMA = $[M - \pi(T)] \times [M - \pi(T)] \div 4\pi$

  where,
  M = mid-arm circumference (mm)
  T = triceps skin fold (mm)
  $\pi = 3.1415$

- Protein index = ratio of measured to predicted total body protein
- Creatinine-height index =

  Actual 24 hr urinary creatinine excretion ÷ normative value for height and sex

- Delayed hypersensitivity index: This index quantitates the amount of induration elicited by skin testing with a common antigen such as Candida, Trichophyton or mumps.

  Grading: 0 = < 0.5 cm; 1 = 0.5 cm; 2 = 1.0 cm

- Prognostic nutritional index is a weighted combination of 4 measures:

  PNI% = $158 - [1.66 \times A] - [0.78 \times T] - [2.0 \times F] - [5.8 \times D]$
  where,
  A = serum albumin (g/L)
  T = triceps skin fold (mm)
  F = serum transferrin (g/L)
  D = delayed hypersensitivity index

All the above indices should be compared with the normative values in standard charts

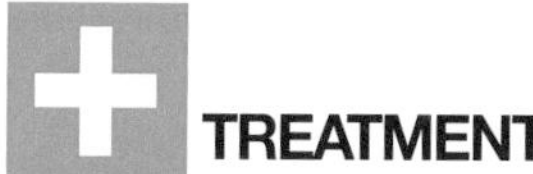

TREATMENT

APPROPRIATE HEALTH CARE
Inpatient care for severe anemia, dehydration, electrolyte imbalance and superimposed infections. Outpatient care for stabilized cases.

GENERAL MEASURES
- Fluid and electrolyte balance should be restored and maintained
- In severe kwashiorkor, IV or SC infusion of amino acids
- Low-lactose formulas have been helpful in some cases with diarrhea due to disaccharidases deficiency
- Diarrhea due to other causes should be identified and treated
- Supplementary vitamins and micronutrients as well as multiple antioxidants
- Mild anemia usually responds to oral protein, iron and folic acid supplements. Blood transfusion may be necessary in severe cases (Hb < 6 g/dL). Use oral iron with caution in kwashiorkor.

SURGICAL MEASURES N/A

ACTIVITY As tolerated

DIET
- Sufficient milk for infants and children to supply 2-5 g/kg/day protein. Lactic-acid fortified milk can be given.
- Adequate calories should be supplied by adding sugar and cereal to the milk diet (150-250 kcal/day)
- Gradual supplementation with high-energy foods such as candies, cake, puddings, meats, eggs and fruit juices
- Small, frequent feedings around the clock better tolerated in the early stages
- Prepared nutritional supplements available commercially are convenient

PATIENT EDUCATION
- Emphasis on nutrition education with the help of a dietitian
- Need for a balanced food intake
- Educate about the composition of nutritional products to ensure balanced intake
- Awareness about risk factors and need for timely nutritional supplements

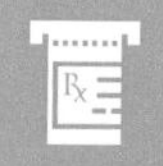

MEDICATIONS

DRUG(S) OF CHOICE
- Antibiotics may be indicated to treat infections
- Multivitamin-multimineral supplementation is required

Contraindications: N/A
Precautions: N/A
Significant possible interactions: N/A

ALTERNATIVE DRUGS N/A

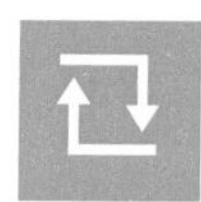

FOLLOWUP

PATIENT MONITORING
Initially periodic follow-up to ensure good nutritional status

PREVENTION/AVOIDANCE
- Emphasis on nutritional education and continuous nutritional care
- Routine record of height and weight
- Observe and record the patient's food intake
- Early recognition of increased nutritional needs during stress and infections
- Frequent interactions between physician, nurse and dietitian to assess nutritional needs
- Avoidance of risk factors when possible

POSSIBLE COMPLICATIONS
Death in the first few days of treatment is usually due to electrolyte imbalance, infection, hypothermia or circulatory failure. Stupor, jaundice, petechiae and low serum sodium are ominous signs.

EXPECTED COURSE/PROGNOSIS
- Mortality varies between 15-40%
- Recovery is more rapid in kwashiorkor than in marasmus. Disappearance of apathy, edema and anorexia are favorable signs.
- In adequately treated cases, liver recovers fully without subsequent cirrhosis, but GI malabsorption and pancreatic deficiency may remain
- Compromised cell-mediated immunity returns to normalcy with recovery
- Behavioral and mental retardation is marked in the severely malnourished child. It is related to the duration of malnutrition and to the age of onset. Relatively mild degree of mental retardation persists into school age.

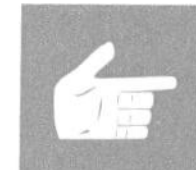

MISCELLANEOUS

ASSOCIATED CONDITIONS
- Malaria and other parasitic infections
- Multiple micronutrients deficiency
- Malabsorptive and maldigestive states

AGE-RELATED FACTORS
Pediatric:
Growth and development during infancy, childhood and adolescence increase nutritional requirements
Geriatric:
Institutionalized elderly are at special risk
Others: N/A

PREGNANCY
Pregnant women with mild to moderate PCM are at risk of delivering an infant with low weight/length for gestational age

SYNONYMS N/A

ICD-9-CM
260 Kwashiorkor
261 Nutritional marasmus
263.9 Unspecified protein-calorie malnutrition

SEE ALSO

OTHER NOTES N/A

ABBREVIATIONS
PCM = Protein - Calorie Malnutrition
PEM = Protein - Energy Malnutrition
MAMA = Mid - Arm Muscle Area
PNI = Protein Nutritional Index
TNF = tumor necrosis factor

REFERENCES

- Fauci AS, et al, editors. Harrison's Principles of Internal Medicine. 15th ed. New York: McGraw-Hill; 2001
- Garrow JS, James WPT, Ralph A, editors. Human Nutrition and Dietetics. 10th ed. New York: Churchill Livingstone; 2000
- Dempster WS, Sive AA, et al. Misplaced iron in kwashiorkor. Eur J Clin Nutr. 1995;49(3):208-10
- Hasse JM. Nutrition assessment and support of organ transplant recipients. J Parenter Enteral Nutr 2001;25(3):120-31

Web references: 1 available at www.5mcc.com
Illustrations N/A

Author(s):
V. Vasudeviah, BSc, MBBS

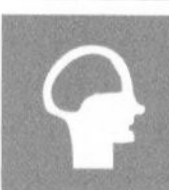

BASICS

DESCRIPTION A dominantly inherited disorder of connective tissue (elastic fibers) affecting primarily the musculoskeletal system, the cardiovascular system and the eye
System(s) affected: Endocrine/Metabolic, Musculoskeletal
Genetics: Autosomal dominant with high penetrance; 15% spontaneous mutation
Incidence/Prevalence in USA: 1 in 10,000 - 20,000 (estimated 1 in 15,000)
Predominant age: Congenital, so disorder is present from birth. However clinical manifestations do not usually become apparent until adolescence or young adulthood.
Predominant sex: No gender, ethnic or racial predilection

SIGNS & SYMPTOMS

- Musculoskeletal
  - ◊ Tall stature
  - ◊ Thin, gangly body habitus (limb length out of proportion to trunk)
  - ◊ Arachnodactyly i.e. long, thin fingers
  - ◊ Pectus deformity
  - ◊ High arched palate
  - ◊ Hyperextensible joints
  - ◊ Kyphoscoliosis
  - ◊ Joint laxity
- Cardiovascular
  - ◊ Aortic root dilatation
  - ◊ Aortic regurgitation
  - ◊ Aortic dissection
  - ◊ Mitral valve prolapse
  - ◊ Mitral regurgitation
- Ocular
  - ◊ Subluxation of lens, usually upward
  - ◊ Myopia
  - ◊ Retinal detachment (uncommon)
- Other
  - ◊ Easy bruising (uncommon)
  - ◊ Excessive bleeding (uncommon)
  - ◊ Sleep apnea
  - ◊ Uterine prolapse or urinary incontinence

CAUSES Genetic; at least 5% are obviously familial, the remainder arise from apparent spontaneous mutations

RISK FACTORS Advanced paternal age gives rise to a slightly increased risk only in those cases which are not clearly familial

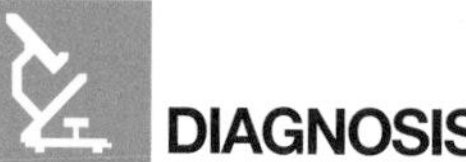

DIAGNOSIS

DIFFERENTIAL DIAGNOSIS Homocystinuria, contractural arachnodactyly, Ehlers-Danlos syndrome, Shprintzen-Goldberg syndrome, trisomy, all of which are rare conditions and all of which have clear cut distinguishing clinical features from the Marfan syndrome

LABORATORY

- There are no specific laboratory abnormalities in the Marfan syndrome
- It is recommended that suspected patients have urinary homocystine measured to rule out homocystinuria

Drugs that may alter lab results: N/A

Disorders that may alter lab results: N/A

PATHOLOGICAL FINDINGS

- Cystic medial necrosis of the aorta
- Myxomatous degeneration of the cardiac valves
- FBN1 gene on chromosome 15 codes for fibrillin, a large glycoprotein constituent of microfibrils. Mutations in this gene have been found in over 90% of patients with the Marfan syndrome, when tested.

SPECIAL TESTS Slit lamp examination is necessary to detect lens subluxation

IMAGING

- Plain x-rays of spine are necessary during growth years to detect and quantify scoliosis
- Annual screening echocardiograms are recommended beginning in adolescence in order to detect presymptomatic aortic root dilatation or valvular degeneration

DIAGNOSTIC PROCEDURES N/A

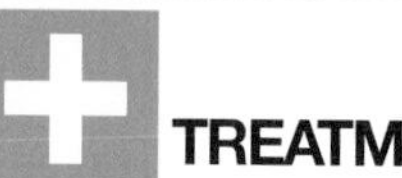

TREATMENT

APPROPRIATE HEALTH CARE Outpatient

GENERAL MEASURES Multidisciplinary approach including primary care physician, cardiologist, ophthalmologist and possibly orthopedic surgeon. A clinical geneticist if available, would be ideal as primary care physician.

SURGICAL MEASURES

- Many, if not most, of these patients will ultimately require reconstructive cardiovascular surgery
  - ◊ Aorta and aortic valve replacement
  - ◊ Mitral valve replacement

ACTIVITY

- Fully active unless limited by symptoms
- Several highly-trained athletes with the Marfan syndrome have suffered sudden death during competition leading to some concern that people with Marfan syndrome should be discouraged from participating in aerobically demanding sports

DIET No special diet

PATIENT EDUCATION Information available from the National Marfan Foundation, 382 Main St., Port Washington, NY 11959; 800-8MARFAN

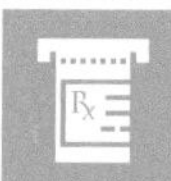

MEDICATIONS

DRUG(S) OF CHOICE
- No specific medical therapy is available, however drugs are used to try to prevent certain complications
- Propranolol or other beta-adrenergic blocking drugs are used to decrease the force of cardiac contraction, in the hope of delaying the development or progression of aortic root dilatation. The dosage of these drugs are adjusted to target heart rate, i.e., resting rate of 60 per minute, with a rise to no more than 80 per minute after moderate exertion.
- Calcium channel blockers have also been shown to retard aortic growth in children and adolescents
- Estrogen combined with progestogen has been used to induce puberty in pre-adolescent girls in an attempt to shorten the growth spurt thereby ameliorating scoliosis and preventing excessively tall stature. Do this only under the supervision of an endocrinologist.

Contraindications:
- Congestive heart failure, asthma, diabetes for the beta-adrenergic blocking drugs
- Thromboembolic disease for the estrogen/progestogen

Precautions: Refer to manufacturer's profile of each drug.

Significant possible interactions: Amphetamines, antihistamines, antidiabetics, oral contraceptives

ALTERNATIVE DRUGS N/A

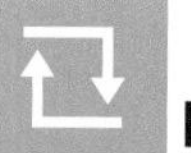

FOLLOWUP

PATIENT MONITORING
- Frequent examinations (at least twice a year) while growing, with particular attention to cardiovascular system and scoliosis
- When cardiac symptoms develop or aortic root diameter becomes > 50 mm, surgical intervention must be considered
- When lens subluxation is detected, surgical correction is possible. However a high incidence of glaucoma results, so surgery should be offered only to those who cannot be treated with corrective lenses.

PREVENTION/AVOIDANCE
- No prenatal diagnosis yet available, but presymptomatic diagnosis may be possible at research centers using linkage analysis techniques
- Each child has a 50% chance of inheriting the disorder from an affected parent. Clinical manifestations are variable, however, so children may be more or less severely affected.
- Antibiotic prophylaxis for endocarditis should be prescribed for all Marfan syndrome patients with either a heart murmur or echocardiographic evidence of valvular or aortic root abnormalities
- Especially tall athletes should be screened for aortic root dilation

POSSIBLE COMPLICATIONS
- Bacterial endocarditis
- Aortic dissection
- Aortic or mitral valve insufficiency
- Dilated cardiomyopathy
- Retinal detachment

EXPECTED COURSE/PROGNOSIS
- Life-threatening complications are cardiovascular. Before routine corrective surgery was available most Marfan syndrome patients died before reaching the age of 35.
- With appropriate surgical intervention most patients can live a normal life span

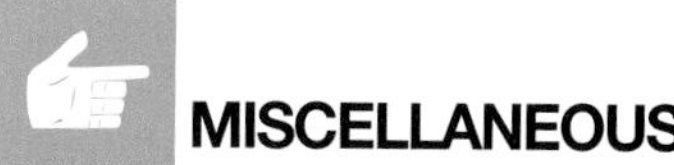

MISCELLANEOUS

ASSOCIATED CONDITIONS N/A

AGE-RELATED FACTORS
Pediatric: Early medical or surgical intervention may reduce the degree of scoliosis
Geriatric: N/A
Others: N/A

PREGNANCY
Pregnant women with the Marfan syndrome need to be managed as high-risk patients, preferably with involvement of a cardiologist. The outcome is usually excellent.

SYNONYMS N/A

ICD-9-CM
759.82 Marfan syndrome

SEE ALSO
Multiple endocrine neoplasia (MEN)

OTHER NOTES
Future trends - successful gene therapy in the mouse model may lead to human therapy

ABBREVIATIONS N/A

REFERENCES

- Cistulli PA, et al. Relationship between craniofacial abnormalities and sleep disturbed breathing in Marfan's syndrome. Chest 2001;120(5):1455-60
- Carley ME, et al. Urinary incontinence and pelvic organ prolapse in women with Marfan's syndrome. Am J Obstet Gynecol 2000;182(5):1021-3
- Gott VL, et al. Replacement of the aortic root in patients with Marfan's syndrome. New Engl J Med 1999;340(17):1307-13
- Kinoshita N, et al. Aortic root dilation among young competitive athletes. Am Heart J 2000;139(4):723-8
- Rossi-Foulkes R, et al. Phenotypic features and impact of beta-blocker or calcium channel antagonist therapy on aortic root lumen size in Marfan's syndrome. Am J Cardiol 1999;83(9):1364-8

Web references: 0 available at www.5mcc.com
Illustrations N/A

Author(s):
Timothy McCurry, MD
Michael Donahue, MD

BASICS

DESCRIPTION Chronic breast pain often occurring prior to menses. Breast pain could also be acute and caused by other problems such as breast abscess.
System(s) affected: Skin/Exocrine
Genetics: Familial tendency
Incidence/Prevalence in USA: Mild form is common; severe form is uncommon
Predominant age: > age 20; or until menopause
Predominant sex: Female

SIGNS & SYMPTOMS
- Breasts aching, heavy, or tender
- Enlarged breasts

CAUSES
- Associated with fibrocystic breast disease and premenstrual syndrome
- Hormonal influences; hormone replacement therapy
- Duct ectasia
- Trauma (including sexual)
- Macromastia

RISK FACTORS
- High saturated fat diet
- Tobacco use

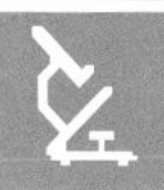

DIAGNOSIS

DIFFERENTIAL DIAGNOSIS
- The major alternate disease to consider is breast cancer, particularly if pain is localized
- Manipulation or trauma can also make symptoms worse
- Chest-wall pain or referred pain from splenomegaly must also be differentiated from mastalgia
- Sometimes concurrent with premenstrual syndrome
- Ductal ectasia of the breast

LABORATORY No relevant findings

Drugs that may alter lab results: N/A

Disorders that may alter lab results: N/A

PATHOLOGICAL FINDINGS Fibrocystic changes

SPECIAL TESTS
- Possibly TSH
- Prolactin if galactorrhea
- Pap test of discharge, if present

IMAGING Mammography to differentiate from breast cancer, not always required

DIAGNOSTIC PROCEDURES
- Cysts may need to be aspirated for symptom relief and diagnostic verification
- Biopsies may be indicated based on exam or mammography

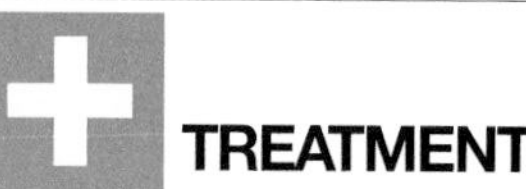

TREATMENT

APPROPRIATE HEALTH CARE Outpatient

GENERAL MEASURES
- Stop or modify current hormonal therapy
- Repeat examination may help establish any cyclic nodularity pattern
- Well-fitting support bra (maybe fitted by a professional).
- Reassurance (this is sufficient for most women)
- Weight reduction, if obese
- Stop smoking
- Relaxation training

SURGICAL MEASURES Reduction mammoplasty if cause is macromastia

ACTIVITY No restrictions

DIET
- Decreased fat intake to 20% of total calories

PATIENT EDUCATION
- Explain that breast pain does not mean the patient has cancer
- Explain relationship to menses

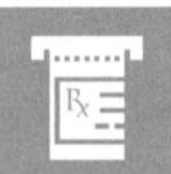

MEDICATIONS

DRUG(S) OF CHOICE
- No drugs are needed unless required by severity of symptoms
- Reassurance, acetaminophen, ibuprofen or topical NSAIDs may be all that is needed

Contraindications: Refer to manufacturer's profile of each drug
Precautions: Refer to manufacturer's profile of each drug
Significant possible interactions: Refer to manufacturer's profile of each drug

ALTERNATIVE DRUGS
- Agents often used, whose value has been questioned:
  - ◊ Diuretics (usually spironolactone) prior to menses
  - ◊ Vitamin E 600 IU/day
  - ◊ Evening primrose oil, includes high content of fatty acids, believed to decrease prostaglandin synthesis
  - ◊ Oral contraceptives may help some patients
  - ◊ Oral progesterones
- Other possibilities for refractory patients, used infrequently because of potential side effects:
  - ◊ Danazol 100 mg bid (possibly lower doses) - this may be the most effective. Major side effects - menstrual irregularities, weight gain, acne, hirsutism and voice change. May be used during luteal phase only. Approved by FDA for this indication.
  - ◊ Bromocriptine 2.5-5.0 mg/day. Major side effects - nausea, dizziness, orthostatic hypotension.
  - ◊ Tamoxifen 10 mg/day. Major side effects - cataracts, hepatocellular carcinoma, endometrial carcinoma. May be used during luteal phase only.
  - ◊ Gonadotropin-releasing hormone agonists - induces menopause

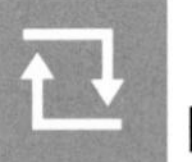

FOLLOWUP

PATIENT MONITORING
- As needed for patients not on prescription medications
- Time of followup will vary by type of prescription medication and patient problems

PREVENTION/AVOIDANCE See Risk Factors

POSSIBLE COMPLICATIONS N/A

EXPECTED COURSE/PROGNOSIS
- Premenstrual mastalgia increases with age, then generally stops at menopause unless on hormone replacement therapy
- Most patients will have control of symptoms without hormonal treatment
- Several months of hormonal treatment may lead to several more months of relief, but the mastalgia may recur

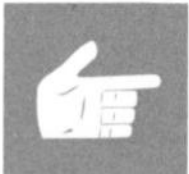

MISCELLANEOUS

ASSOCIATED CONDITIONS Premenstrual syndrome

AGE-RELATED FACTORS
Pediatric: N/A
Geriatric: N/A
Others: N/A

PREGNANCY N/A

SYNONYMS
- Mastodynia
- Breast pain

ICD-9-CM
611.71 Mastodynia

SEE ALSO
Premenstrual syndrome (PMS)

OTHER NOTES
- Cyclic mastalgia responds better than noncyclic mastalgia to treatment
- Effects of long-term hormonal treatment are unknown
- If other treatment fails, a final possibility is subcutaneous mastectomy (used rarely)
- Oophorectomy also provides relief and may be drastic treatment for some patients

ABBREVIATIONS N/A

REFERENCES

- Smith RL, Pruthi S, Fitzpatrick LA. Evaluation and management of breast pain. Mayo Clin Proc 2004;79(3):353-72
- Morrow M. The evaluation of common breast problems. Am Fam Phys 2000;61(8):2371-8, 2385
- Blommers J, de Lange-De Klerk ES, Kuik DJ, Bezemer PD, Meijer S. Evening primrose oil and fish oil for severe chronic mastalgia: a randomized, double-blind, controlled trial. Am J Obstet Gynecol 2002;187(5):1389-94

Web references: 0 available at www.5mcc.com
Illustrations N/A

Author(s):
Marjorie A. Bowman, MD, MPA

BASICS

DESCRIPTION Inflammatory process in the mastoid air cells

- Acute mastoiditis - acute suppurative inflammatory process, typically after acute otitis media. It is the most common complication of AOM.
- Chronic mastoiditis - usually associated with cholesteatoma and chronic ear disease

System(s) affected: Pulmonary
Genetics: No known genetic pattern
Incidence/Prevalence in USA: Unknown
Predominant age: Children, mainly less than 2 years old
Predominant sex: Male = Female

SIGNS & SYMPTOMS

- Otalgia
- Bulging erythematous tympanic membrane
- Post-auricular or supra auricular edema/mass
- Post-auricular or supra auricular erythema
- Post-auricular or supra auricular tenderness
- Protrusion of auricle
- Fever
- Increased WBC
- Possible otorrhea if perforated tympanic membrane
- Subperiosteal abscess
- Hearing loss
- Headache
- Displacement of pinna - outward and downward
- Tympanic membrane can be normal in 10% - suspect when symptoms of acute otitis media have lasted longer than 2 weeks

CAUSES

- Acute otitis media
- Inadequately treated suppurative otitis media
- Cholesteatoma
- Blockage of outflow tract of mastoid air cells (aditus ad antrum)
- Streptococcus pneumoniae

RISK FACTORS

- Cholesteatoma
- Recurrent acute otitis media
- Immunocompromised host

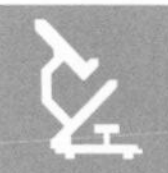

DIAGNOSIS

DIFFERENTIAL DIAGNOSIS

- Post-auricular inflammatory adenopathy
- Severe external otitis
- Post auricular cellulitis
- Benign neoplasm - aneurysmal bone cyst, fibrous dysplasia
- Malignant neoplasm - rhabdomyosarcoma
- HIV infection

LABORATORY CBC with differential - increased WBC

Drugs that may alter lab results: N/A

Disorders that may alter lab results: N/A

PATHOLOGICAL FINDINGS

- Inflammatory tissue in air cell system
- Granulation tissue
- Osteitis

SPECIAL TESTS Consider audiogram

IMAGING

- Plain mastoid films - clouding of mastoid air cells; can be negative
- CT scan if complication suspected. Cloud air cells - loss of bony septation of the air cell system.

DIAGNOSTIC PROCEDURES Myringotomy (also therapeutic)

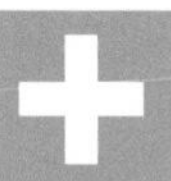

TREATMENT

APPROPRIATE HEALTH CARE Hospitalized during acute phase

GENERAL MEASURES

- Keep ear dry

SURGICAL MEASURES

- Myringotomy; placement of pressure equalization (PE) tube
- Culture material obtained at myringotomy
- Frequent cleaning of ear canal under microscope to assure PE tube patency and adequate drainage of middle ear
- IV antibiotics to cover the most common organisms
- Topical antibiotic drops are also usually used after insertion of PE tube
- If subperiosteal abscess present, it should be aspirated. If aspiration is not sufficient, incision and drainage should be performed.
- Mastoidectomy is reserved for those patients failing to respond to above measures within 18-72 hours or those with meningeal or intracranial complications

ACTIVITY Water precautions

DIET No special diet

PATIENT EDUCATION Griffith: Instructions for Patients; Philadelphia, W.B. Saunders Co.

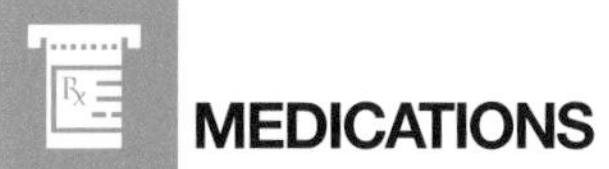

MEDICATIONS

DRUG(S) OF CHOICE
- IV antibiotics:
  - ◊ Directed against most common organisms - group A beta-hemolytic strep, *S. pneumonia*, *Haemophilus influenzae*, *M. catarrhatis*
  - ◊ In patients with cholesteatoma, consider *Proteus*, *Bacteroides* and occasional *S. aureus* and *Pseudomonas* organisms
  - ◊ IV antibiotics for adult - ampicillin, 1-2 gm q6h or ampicillin-sulbactam (Unasyn) or cefuroxime, 750 mg q8h, to ensure coverage of beta-lactamase producing organisms
  - ◊ IV antibiotics for children - ampicillin, 100-200 mg/kg/day divided q6h or cefuroxime, 750 mg q8h
- Topical/oral antibiotics:
  - ◊ Topical drops - neomycin-polymyxin B-hydrocortisone (Cortisporin) otic drops or gentamicin ophthalmic solution
  - ◊ Oral antibiotic - amoxicillin-clavulanate (Augmentin)

Contraindications: Refer to manufacturer's literature
Precautions: Refer to manufacturer's literature
Significant possible interactions: Refer to manufacturer's literature

ALTERNATIVE DRUGS
Other antibiotics depending on pathogen sensitivity

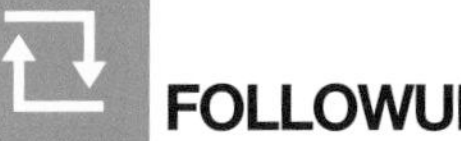

FOLLOWUP

PATIENT MONITORING
- Postoperative - audiogram after acute process subsided
- Frequent cleansing of ear canal to keep PE tube patent

PREVENTION/AVOIDANCE
- Adequate antibiotic treatment for acute otitis media
- Treatment of chronic eustachian tube dysfunction (PE tubes)
- Early identification of cholesteatoma

POSSIBLE COMPLICATIONS
- Subperiosteal abscess
- Gradenigo's syndrome (sixth nerve palsy, draining ear and retro-orbital pain)
- Bezold's abscess
- Sigmoid sinus thrombosis
- Meningitis
- Intracranial abscess epidural/subdural/intraparenchymal
- Periosteitis
- Osteitis
- Central venous sinus thrombosis

EXPECTED COURSE/PROGNOSIS
- Dependent on severity of disease
- Conductive hearing loss may require reconstructive surgery
- Expect to avoid complications with early treatment

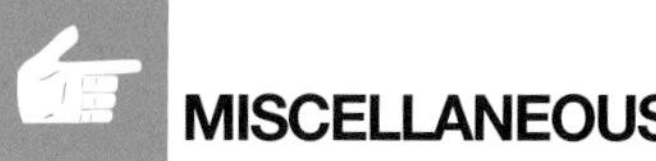

MISCELLANEOUS

ASSOCIATED CONDITIONS
N/A

AGE-RELATED FACTORS
Pediatric: N/A
Geriatric: N/A
Others: N/A

PREGNANCY
N/A

SYNONYMS
N/A

ICD-9-CM
383.00 Acute mastoiditis without complications
383.01 Subperiosteal abscess of mastoid
383.02 Acute mastoiditis with other complications
383.1 Chronic mastoiditis
383.9 Unspecified mastoiditis

SEE ALSO

OTHER NOTES
N/A

ABBREVIATIONS
PE = pressure equalization

REFERENCES

- Paparella MM, Shumrick DA, et al, eds. Otolaryngology. 4th ed. Philadelphia: W.B. Saunders Co; 1991
- Marx J, et al. Rosen's Emergency Medicine: Concepts and Clinical Practice. 5th ed. St. Louis: Mosby, Inc; 2002
- Mandell GL, editor. Principles and Practice of Infectious Diseases. 5th ed. New York: Churchill Livingstone; 2000
- Behrman RE, Kliegman M, eds: Nelson Textbook of Pediatrics. 16th ed. Philadelphia: W.B. Saunders Co; 2000

Web references: 0 available at www.5mcc.com
Illustrations N/A

Author(s):
Tadao Okada, MD, MPH

BASICS

DESCRIPTION An endemic and epidemic viral exanthematous infection of children and adults, worldwide in distribution. Many infections are subclinical, but this virus can potentially cause fetal infection with resultant birth defects.

System(s) affected: Hemic/Lymphatic/Immunologic, Nervous, Pulmonary, Skin/Exocrine

Genetics: Children with congenital rubella syndrome and children with insulin dependent diabetes mellitus share a high frequency of HLA-DR3 histocompatibility antigen and a high prevalence of islet cell antibodies

Incidence/Prevalence in USA:
- Before rubella vaccine was introduced in 1969, epidemics occurred at 6-9 year intervals. Sporadic outbreaks continue to occur in hospitals, colleges, prisons, prenatal clinics and isolated religious communities.
- In 2003 the incidence of postnatal rubella was 0.003 cases per 100,000 population. Presently, the source of the rubella outbreaks is from infected persons from countries where rubella is not included in routine immunization or just recently introduced schedules or administered in mass campaigns.

Predominant age: Children 5-9 years of age

Predominant sex: Male = Female

SIGNS & SYMPTOMS
- Postnatal rubella
  - ◊ Adenopathy - posterior auricular, posterior cervical, suboccipital
  - ◊ Low-grade fever
  - ◊ Exanthem - descending, maculopapular, may desquamate
  - ◊ Enanthem - soft palate petechiae (Forchheimer's sign)
  - ◊ Conjunctivitis
  - ◊ Splenomegaly, rarely
  - ◊ Coryza
  - ◊ Malaise
  - ◊ Headache
  - ◊ Polyarthralgia/polyarthritis, especially in young women
  - ◊ Asymptomatic (25%-50%)
- Congenital rubella: (T = Transient, P = Permanent, D = Developmental)
  - ◊ Cataracts (P)
  - ◊ Microphthalmia (P)
  - ◊ Chorioretinitis (P)
  - ◊ Patent ductus arteriosus (P)
  - ◊ Pulmonic stenosis (P,D)
  - ◊ Atrial and ventricular septal defects (P)
  - ◊ Sensorineural deafness (P,D)
  - ◊ Microcephaly (P)
  - ◊ Meningoencephalitis (T)
  - ◊ Mental retardation (P,D)
  - ◊ Low birth weight (T)
  - ◊ Purpuric ("blueberry muffin")

skin lesions (T)
  - ◊ Radiolucent bone disease (T)
  - ◊ Hepatosplenomegaly (T)
  - ◊ Large anterior fontanelle (T)
  - ◊ Language and behavior disorders (P,D)
  - ◊ Cryptorchidism (P)
  - ◊ Inguinal hernia (P)

CAUSES Rubella virus is a single-stranded RNA virus in the togavirus family. Traveling via airborne droplets of nasopharyngeal secretions, the virus replicates in the nasopharynx and regional lymph nodes during a 16-18 day incubation period. After invading the bloodstream, it may spread to skin and other distal organs or, transplacentally, to the developing fetus. Fetal viremia may then produce disseminated fetal infection. Organogenesis occurs 2 to 6 weeks postconception, so that infection is a maximum hazard (40-80% risk) to heart and eyes at that time. During the second trimester, the fetus develops increasing immunologic competence, making it less susceptible (10% risk) to the effects of intrauterine infection.

RISK FACTORS
- Inadequate immunization
- Immunodeficiency states
- Immunosuppressive therapy
- Pregnancy
- Crowded living conditions
- School, day care
- Late winter, spring seasons
- International travel aboard commercial airplanes, cruise ships

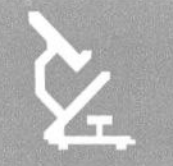

DIAGNOSIS

DIFFERENTIAL DIAGNOSIS
- Postnatal rubella
  - ◊ Measles virus (rubeola)
  - ◊ Scarlet fever
  - ◊ Infectious mononucleosis
  - ◊ Toxoplasmosis
  - ◊ Roseola infantum (exanthem subitum)
  - ◊ Erythema infectiosum (fifth disease)
  - ◊ Drug eruptions
  - ◊ Other exanthematous enteroviral infections
- Congenital rubella
  - ◊ Cytomegalovirus
  - ◊ Varicella-zoster virus
  - ◊ Picornaviruses (coxsackievirus, echovirus)
  - ◊ Poliovirus
  - ◊ Herpes simplex virus
  - ◊ Western equine virus
  - ◊ Measles virus (rubeola)
  - ◊ Hepatitis B virus
  - ◊ Mumps virus
  - ◊ Influenza virus
  - ◊ Toxoplasmosis
  - ◊ Congenital syphilis
  - ◊ Malaria

LABORATORY
- Postnatal rubella
  - ◊ Mild leukopenia with relative lymphocytosis
  - ◊ Fourfold rise in serum levels of antibody to rubella virus
  - ◊ Pharynx, nose and blood culture positivity to rubella virus
- Congenital rubella
  - ◊ Presence of rubella-specific IgM antibody in serum up to one year of age, at which time, IgG becomes the dominant antibody
  - ◊ Isolation of rubella virus from pharynx, blood, urine, cerebrospinal fluid

Drugs that may alter lab results: N/A

Disorders that may alter lab results: After re-exposure to rubella, a person with a low level of antibody from past infection or vaccination may experience an acute rise in antibody. This is not associated with a high incidence of contagion to others nor of fetal risk.

PATHOLOGICAL FINDINGS
- Inhibition of cellular growth after infection
- Fetal vasculitis
- Placental angiopathy
- Tissue necrosis

SPECIAL TESTS Cell-mediated immune responses (CMI) are impaired selectively in children with congenital rubella

IMAGING N/A

DIAGNOSTIC PROCEDURES Congenital rubella has been diagnosed by placental biopsy at 12 weeks

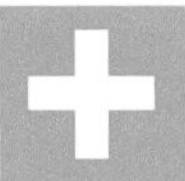

TREATMENT

APPROPRIATE HEALTH CARE Outpatient usually

GENERAL MEASURES
- Postnatal rubella - mild and self-limited. Treat for symptomatic relief.
- Congenital rubella - supportive, unless neurologic or hemorrhagic complications develop

SURGICAL MEASURES N/A

ACTIVITY
- For postnatal rubella - contact isolation for 7 days after onset of rash, bedrest is not necessary
- Contact isolation of congenitally infected infants for one year, unless nasopharyngeal and urine cultures after 3 months of age are negative for rubella virus

DIET No special diet

PATIENT EDUCATION
- Make every effort to avoid exposing infected patient to pregnant women
- JAMA Patient Page on Rubella located at www.jama.com go to Patient Page Index. Click on Previous Topics, Rubella (1/23-30/2002).

MEDICATIONS

DRUG(S) OF CHOICE Acetaminophen for fever every 4 hours if needed - 10-15 mg/kg/dose
Contraindications: N/A
Precautions: N/A
Significant possible interactions: N/A

ALTERNATIVE DRUGS None

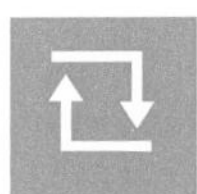

FOLLOWUP

PATIENT MONITORING
- Persons immune to rubella via natural infection or vaccine may be reinfected when re-exposed. This infection is usually asymptomatic and detectable only by serologic means.
- In congenital rubella, it is extremely important to detect auditory and visual impairment early, so that adequate education and counseling can begin
- Two-thirds of internationally adopted children entering the U.S. have no written records of overseas immunizations

PREVENTION/AVOIDANCE
- Rubella vaccine
  - ◊ A 2-dose schedule in combination with measles and mumps (MMR) is recommended for those born after 1956. The first dose is recommended at age 12-15 months; the second dose is recommended either at 4-6 years of age or at 11-12 years of age. Children with HIV should receive MMR vaccine at 12 months of age if no contraindications exist.
  - ◊ Recommended for susceptible individuals in the following groups: Prepubertal boys and girls, premarital or postpartum women, college students, day care personnel, health care workers, military personnel
  - ◊ It is contraindicated in: Pregnancy, immunodeficiency or immunocompromised state (except HIV), receipt within the last 3 months of immunoglobulin (Ig) or blood, severe febrile illness, or hypersensitivity to vaccine components
  - ◊ Persons who receive rubella vaccine do not transmit rubella to others, although the virus can be isolated from the pharynx
  - ◊ During outbreaks of rubella, serologic screening before vaccination is not recommended, because rapid vaccination is necessary to stop the spread of the disease
  - ◊ In 1997 Finland became the first country to be free of rubella; the result of an effective vaccination program
  - ◊ Strong evidence exists against the hypothesis that MMR vaccination causes autism
  - ◊ An investigational vaccine against measles, mumps, rubella and varicella (MMRV) shows similar efficacy to the currently licensed MMR vaccine. The two-dose response rate for rubella is 94.8% for MMRV vs. 92.8% for MMR.

POSSIBLE COMPLICATIONS
- Postnatal rubella
  - ◊ Postinfectious encephalitis (1/5,000 cases)
  - ◊ Thrombocytopenic purpura (1/3,000 cases)
  - ◊ Testicular pain
  - ◊ Mild hepatitis
- Congenital rubella
  - ◊ Spontaneous abortion
  - ◊ Stillbirth
  - ◊ Premature delivery
  - ◊ Progressive rubella panencephalitis
  - ◊ Endocrine disturbances (diabetes, thyrotoxicosis, hypothyroidism)
- Rubella vaccine
  - ◊ Lymphadenopathy
  - ◊ Fever
  - ◊ Rash
  - ◊ Arthritis/arthralgia (older girls, women)
  - ◊ Polyneuropathy
  - ◊ Idiopathic thrombocytopenic purpura (ITP)

EXPECTED COURSE/PROGNOSIS
- Postnatal rubella
  - ◊ Fever, 1-2 days
  - ◊ Rash, 3 days
  - ◊ Coryza, 5 days
  - ◊ Lymphadenopathy, 1 week
  - ◊ Arthralgia (when present), 2 weeks
  - ◊ Complete and full recovery without sequelae is the rule
- Congenital rubella
  - ◊ Varied and unpredictable spectrum of consequences, ranging from stillbirth to completely normal infancy and childhood
  - ◊ Disease characterized by chronic infection; infants may remain contagious for months after birth
  - ◊ Detectable levels of hemagglutination-inhibiting antibody (IgG) persist for years, then may decline. By age 5, 20% have no detectable antibody.
  - ◊ Overall mortality 10%; greatest during first 6 months
  - ◊ 70% of those with encephalitis develop residual neuromotor defects, including an autistic syndrome
  - ◊ Prognosis is excellent when only minor defects are present

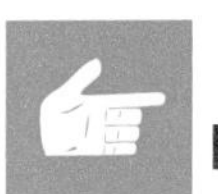

MISCELLANEOUS

ASSOCIATED CONDITIONS N/A

AGE-RELATED FACTORS
Pediatric:
- Postnatal rubella is a milder disease in children than it is in adults
- Adolescents and young adults currently account for about 60% of all new cases

Geriatric: N/A
Others: N/A

PREGNANCY
- Women vaccinated against rubella are advised not to become pregnant for at least 1 month. The vaccine-type virus can cross the placenta. However, no case of congenital rubella has occurred after inadvertent vaccination
- If a pregnant woman is exposed to rubella (native disease, not vaccine associated), obtain an antibody titer. Presence of antibody implies immunity and no risk. If antibody is not detectable, obtain a second titer in 3 weeks. If antibody is present in the second specimen, infection has occurred. If antibody is again negative, obtain a third titer in 3 more weeks (6 weeks after exposure). At this time, a negative test means that infection has not occurred; a positive test means that infection did occur, and the fetus is at risk for congenital rubella.
- Human immunoglobulin (gamma globulin) in prophylaxis of rubella during pregnancy does not prevent rubella or the congenital rubella syndrome in a predictable or reliable fashion
- A reliable PCR-based method of detecting viral RNA may allow much more rapid prenatal diagnosis of rubella virus infection. Routine use is not yet available.

SYNONYMS
- German measles
- Three-day measles

ICD-9-CM
056.9 Rubella without mention of complication
771.0 Congenital rubella

SEE ALSO
Measles, rubeola

OTHER NOTES Rubella vaccine is currently the only vaccine designed for the purpose of protecting someone other than the vaccine recipient

ABBREVIATIONS N/A

REFERENCES

- Committee on Infectious Diseases, Elk Grove, Illinois, AAP Red Book, ed. 26, 2003
- Revello MG, et al: Prenatal diagnosis of rubella virus infection by direct detection and semiquantitation of viral RNA in clinical samples by reverse transcription-PCR. J Clin Microbiol 1997;35:708-13
- Mandell GL, Bennett JE, Dolin R (eds). Mandell, Douglas, and Bennett's Principles and Practice of Infectious Diseases. 5th ed. Philadelphia: Churchill Livingstone; 2000
- Behrman RE, Kliegman RM, Jenson HB (eds). Nelson Textbook of Pediatrics. 17th ed. Philadelphia: W.B. Saunders Company; 2004
- Reef SE, Frey TK, Theall K, Abernathy E, et al. The changing epidemiology of rubella in the 1990s: on the verge of elimination and new challenges for control and prevention. JAMA 2002;287(4):464-72
- Schulte JM, Maloney S, Aronson J, San Gabriel P, et al. Evaluating acceptability and completeness of overseas immunization records of internationally adopted children. Pediatrics 2002;109(2):E22

Web references: 0 available at www.5mcc.com
Illustrations 1 available

Author(s):
Richard Viken, MD

BASICS

DESCRIPTION An acute epidemic viral exanthem which classically presents as a confluent erythematous maculopapular rash which begins over the head and spreads inferiorly to involve the trunk and extremities. The rash is preceded by the triad of cough, coryza, and conjunctivitis plus a pathognomonic enanthem (Koplik's spots).
System(s) affected: Hemic/Lymphatic/Immunologic, Pulmonary, Skin/Exocrine
Genetics: N/A
Incidence/Prevalence in USA: Number of cases peaked during 1990, 27,786; followed by marked decline, during 1997 the United States reported a provisional total of only 135 confirmed measles cases. Attack rate (# cases/100,000): 1991 - 3.82, 1992 - 0.87, 1993 - 0.12, 1994 - 0.37
Predominant age: Between 1985 and 1994, children ≤ 2 years constituted largest proportion of cases (≥ 90% of these unvaccinated). During a 7 week period in 1997, no indigenous cases were reported, suggesting an interruption of measles transmission.
Predominant sex: Male = Female

SIGNS & SYMPTOMS
- Incubation period:
  - ◊ 10+/-2 days from exposure to symptoms
  - ◊ 14 days average to onset of rash (range 7-18 days)
  - ◊ Patients contagious from 1-2 days before symptoms (3-5 days before rash) to 4 days after onset of rash, immunocompromised patients contagious for the duration of the illness
- Prodromal period:
  - ◊ Lasts 3+/-1 days
  - ◊ Classic triad (brassy cough, coryza, and conjunctivitis)
  - ◊ Fever
  - ◊ Malaise
  - ◊ Photophobia
  - ◊ Enanthem (Koplik's spots) - minute, whitish spots over buccal/labial mucosa; number rapidly increases and these coalesce. Underlying mucosa bright red and granular; spots appear 2 days before rash and resolve within 3 days after rash onset.
- Exanthem period:
  - ◊ Begins behind ears and at hairline
  - ◊ Spreads centrifugally from head to feet
  - ◊ Red, morbilliform, blanching rash
  - ◊ Discrete lesions become confluent
  - ◊ Confluence more prominent over upper body
  - ◊ Clearing begins after 3-4 days
  - ◊ Rash becomes coppery and nonblanching
  - ◊ Fever resolves 2-3 days after onset of rash
  - ◊ Pharyngitis
  - ◊ Lymphadenopathy
  - ◊ Croup, vomiting, and diarrhea (in young children)
  - ◊ Patients contagious from 2 days before symptoms to 4 days after onset of rash
- Modified illness:
  - ◊ Attenuated measles in partially immune patient
  - ◊ Secondary prior immune globulin, transplacental measles antibody, live vaccine failure
- Atypical measles:
  - ◊ Most cases secondary to natural infection following vaccination with killed vaccine (available in U.S. 1963-68; Canada until 1975)
  - ◊ Maculopapular rash begins distally and spreads centrally
  - ◊ Rash frequently is petechial, purpuric, or urticarial
  - ◊ Pulmonary involvement in all cases
  - ◊ Frequency decreasing

CAUSES Single antigenic type of a RNA Morbillivirus in the paramyxovirus family

RISK FACTORS Not being vaccinated

DIAGNOSIS

DIFFERENTIAL DIAGNOSIS
- Typical measles:
  - ◊ Any erythematous maculopapular rash
- Exanthems secondary to:
  - ◊ Drug eruptions
  - ◊ Infectious mononucleosis
  - ◊ Mycoplasma pneumoniae
  - ◊ Rubella
  - ◊ Erythema infectiosum
  - ◊ Roseola
  - ◊ Enteroviruses
- Atypical measles:
  - ◊ Rocky Mountain spotted fever
  - ◊ Drug eruptions
  - ◊ Anaphylactoid purpura
  - ◊ Mycoplasma pneumoniae infection

LABORATORY
- Viral isolation in tissue culture
- Detection of measles antigen in exfoliative cells by immunofluorescence
- Demonstration of measles specific IgM or substantial rise in IgG tilers between acute and convalescent sera

Drugs that may alter lab results: Immunosuppressive agents which may impair rise in specific antibody titers

Disorders that may alter lab results:
- Primary (severe combined immunodeficiency [SCID], etc.)
- Acquired immune deficiencies (HIV-1 infection, cancer chemotherapy)

PATHOLOGICAL FINDINGS
- Multinucleated giant cells
  - ◊ Reticuloendothelial types (Warthin-Finkeldey) in lymphoid tissues
  - ◊ Epithelial syncytial giant cells in skin, and respiratory mucosa
  - ◊ Damaged respiratory ciliated epithelium

SPECIAL TESTS N/A

IMAGING N/A

DIAGNOSTIC PROCEDURES N/A

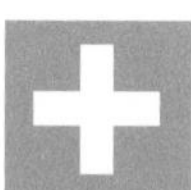

TREATMENT

APPROPRIATE HEALTH CARE Outpatient except when complications develop (encephalitis, pneumonitis)

GENERAL MEASURES
- Symptomatic therapy (i.e., antipyretics, antitussives, humidification, encourage oral fluids)
- Control
  - ◊ All cases should be placed in respiratory isolation until 4 days after the onset of the exanthem; immunocompromised patients should be isolated for the entire illness
  - ◊ Notify public health officials of suspected cases
  - ◊ Initiate preventive measures for all exposed susceptible persons or those at high risk for severe infection (i.e., symptomatic HIV infection, children less than 12 months)
  - ◊ Live measles vaccine can provide protection to susceptible persons if given within 72 hours postexposure
  - ◊ Immune globulin (Ig) given within 6 days postexposure can prevent or modify measles infection (0.25 mL/kg, maximum dose 15 mL; 0.5 mL/kg for immunocompromised patients)
  - ◊ Patients with symptomatic HIV infection should receive Ig regardless of prior immunization
  - ◊ Ig also indicated for susceptible household contacts of measles patient and pregnant women

SURGICAL MEASURES N/A

ACTIVITY Restricted during febrile phase

DIET As tolerated

PATIENT EDUCATION Avoid exposure to other children and potential secondary bacterial pathogens until respiratory symptoms resolve

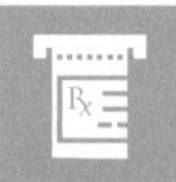

MEDICATIONS

DRUG(S) OF CHOICE
- No proven specific antiviral agent is available
- Following the onset of infection, immune globulin has no significant effect on symptoms and duration of illness
- Antibiotics reserved for bacterial superinfection

Contraindications: Steroids contraindicated
Precautions: N/A
Significant possible interactions: N/A

ALTERNATIVE DRUGS
- Vitamin A
  - ◊ 200,000 IU po per day for 2 days (100,000 IU between 6-12 months) has been shown to decrease the mortality and morbidity of severe measles in areas where vitamin A deficiency exists and mortality related to measles is ≥ 1%; efficacy in non-life-threatening infections not established
  - ◊ Vitamin A currently recommended for the following patients:
    - Children 6-24 months hospitalized with complications of measles
    - Children over 6 months with immunodeficiency, malabsorption, moderate to severe malnutrition, ophthalmologic evidence of vitamin A deficiency, or recent immigration from areas with vitamin A deficiency
- Ribavirin
  - ◊ Virus susceptible in vitro to ribavirin
  - ◊ Immunosuppressed children with severe measles have been treated with IV or aerosolized ribavirin, but no controlled data and not approved by FDA

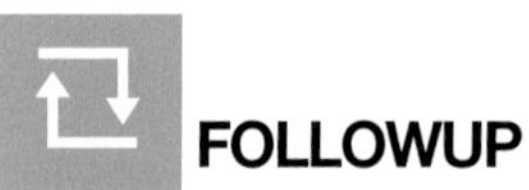

FOLLOWUP

PATIENT MONITORING
Not required unless complications develop

PREVENTION/AVOIDANCE
- Postexposure prophylaxis
  - ◊ Vaccine use - protective if given within 72 hours postexposure
  - ◊ Immune globulin (Ig) - prevents/modifies illness if given within 6 days postexposure. Dose - usually 0.25 mL/kg IM (for immunocompromised children 0.5 mL/kg IM) not to exceed 15 mL. Indicated for the following susceptible household contacts: Infants under 1 year, pregnant women, and immunocompromised persons, all HIV infected children and adolescents regardless of prior measles immunization status should if exposed receive IVIG (400 mg/kg) or IG prophylaxis (0.5 mL/kg) unless on monthly IVIG (last dose within the previous 3 weeks)
- Active immunization:
  - ◊ Live further-attenuated strain vaccine - only currently licensed vaccine available as monovalent vaccine or in combination with mumps and rubella i.e., measles and rubella (MR); measles, mumps and rubella (MMR)
- Indications:
  - ◊ Primary vaccination: Two doses of vaccine; 1st MMR at 12-15 months, 2nd dose of MMR SQ at school age (4-6 years). Two dose vaccination schedule mandated by need to compensate for primary vaccine failures and global efforts to eradicate measles. During outbreaks, monovalent measles vaccine may be given to infants > 6 months. These children must be vaccinated with MMR as above. For a comprehensive discussion of the complete use and control of measles outbreaks, the reader is referred to the first listing in References.
  - ◊ HIV infected children should be vaccinated while asymptomatic and before they develop profound immunosuppression. One case of a HIV infected young adult with advanced disease who developed measles vaccine virus associated pneumonitis post vaccination. The 2nd dose of vaccine may be given as early as 1 month after the 1st dose.
- Adverse events associated with vaccination (in 5-15% of susceptible vaccinees):
  - ◊ Fever (7-12 days after)
  - ◊ Transient rashes (in 5% of vaccinees)
  - ◊ Convulsions (most likely febrile)
  - ◊ Children with egg allergy are at low risk for anaphylactic reactions to MMR
  - ◊ Recent epidemiological evidence has not substantiated any linkage between MMR vaccine and autism

POSSIBLE COMPLICATIONS
- Otitis media (most common)
- Laryngotracheitis
- Bronchopneumonia - viral (Hecht's or giant cell pneumonitis) or bacterial in origin
- Encephalitis (incidence 1 per 1000)
- Hemorrhagic lesions ("black measles") of skin and bowel
- Thrombocytopenic purpura
- Myocarditis and pericarditis
- Subacute sclerosing panencephalitis - secondary to persistent infection following natural disease; disappearing as a result of mass vaccination

EXPECTED COURSE/PROGNOSIS
Self-limited; prognosis good

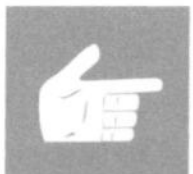

MISCELLANEOUS

ASSOCIATED CONDITIONS
- Primary measles in an immunosuppressed patient with leukemia or symptomatic HIV-1 infection may present with or without a rash and giant cell pneumonitis
- Giant cell pneumonitis
- Increased mortality with malnutrition
- Possible reactivation of latent tuberculosis secondary to measles

AGE-RELATED FACTORS
Pediatric: Infants have higher rate of complications than older children
Geriatric: N/A
Others: N/A

PREGNANCY
Increased fetal morbidity and mortality with infection during pregnancy

SYNONYMS
Rubeola

ICD-9-CM
055.9 Measles without mention of complication

SEE ALSO
Measles, rubella

OTHER NOTES
- Measles in developing countries
  - ◊ Major cause of childhood morbidity and mortality
  - ◊ Two types of severe disease:
    - Systemic fulminant illness
    - Prolonged illness with secondary infectious complications

ABBREVIATIONS
N/A

REFERENCES

- Measles. In Red Book 2000 Report of the Committee on Infectious Diseases, 385-396, American Academy on Pediatrics, 2000
- Measles Prevention: Recommendations of the Immunization Practices Advisory Committee (ACIP). Morbidity and Mortality Weekly Report, Recommendations and Reports. 38 (S-9):1-13, 1989
- Cherry J. Measles. In: Feigin R, Cherry J, editors. Textbook of Pediatric Infectious Diseases. 4th ed. Philadelphia: W.B. Saunders Co.; 1998

Web references: 0 available at www.5mcc.com
Illustrations N/A

Author(s):
Charles D. Mitchell, MD

BASICS

DESCRIPTION Malignant degeneration of cells from the melanocytic system. The overwhelming majority of melanoma arises in the skin, but it may also present as a primary lesion in any tissue pigmentation. Metastatic spread may be to any region in the body.
- Lentigo maligna - a cutaneous lesion that is the slowest growing malignant melanoma and has the least tendency to metastasize. Occurs most often on the face, beginning as a circumscribed macular patch of mottled pigmentation showing shades of dark brown, tan, or black, mostly in the elderly.
- Ocular - a malignant progressive lesion of the eye

System(s) affected: Skin/Exocrine

Genetics:
- Familial dysplastic nevus syndrome
- Lighter pigmented individuals
- Chromosomes 1, 6, 7, 9,10 most common affected
- Changes in oncogenes, suppressor genes growth factors and receptors have been noted

Incidence/Prevalence in USA:
- > 5/100,000
- 2% of all cancer deaths
- 1999 - 44,200 new cases, 7,300 deaths
- 2000 - 1 in 70 in US will be expected to have melanoma in their lifetime
- 2000 - 6th most common cancer in US

Predominant age:
- A median age is 53 with the highest annual incidence rate of any cancer in whites between the ages of 25-29 and in white males between 35-39
- Greater than 50% of all individuals with melanoma are between ages 20-40

Predominant sex: Male = Female

SIGNS & SYMPTOMS Any change in a pigmented lesion including hypo- or hyperpigmentation, bleeding, scaling, size change, texture change

CAUSES Under investigation. Probably radiation in the ultraviolet A+B range.

RISK FACTORS
- Heavy UVA and UVB exposure
- Previous pigmented lesions (especially dysplastic nevi)
- Fair complexioned, freckling, blue eyes and blonde hair
- Those with increased numbers of nevi
- Family history of melanoma
- Tanning bed use in ages < 30
- Changing nevus
- Large (> 5 cm) congenital nevi
- Other skin cancers
- Immunosuppression

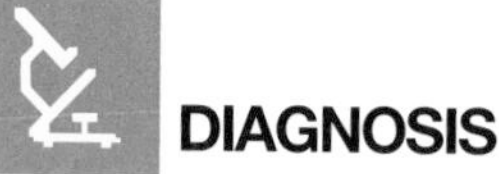

DIAGNOSIS

DIFFERENTIAL DIAGNOSIS
- Dysplastic nevi
- Vascular skin tumors
- Actinic keratosis
- Traumatic hematoma
- Lentigo
- Pigmented squamous cell and basal cell carcinomas, seborrheic keratoses, other changing nevi. It follows the ABCDE mnemonic which stands for (1) asymmetry, (2) border irregularity, (3) color variegation, and (4) diameter great than 6 millimeters with the location on whites being primarily back and lower leg, and on African Americans being hands, feet, and nails, (5) elevation above skin surface.

LABORATORY N/A

Drugs that may alter lab results: N/A

Disorders that may alter lab results: N/A

PATHOLOGICAL FINDINGS
- Gross pathologic features include four clinical types:
  - ◊ Superficial spreading melanoma - 70% of all cases
  - ◊ Nodular - 15% of all cases
  - ◊ Acral lentiginous - 2-8% of all cases
  - ◊ Lentigo-maligna - 4-10% of all cases; a small percentage are a melanotic
  - ◊ Note: Nodular melanoma is primarily vertical growth while the other three types are horizontal

SPECIAL TESTS The only special tests that exist for melanoma are those designed to follow metastatic disease

IMAGING Imaging studies are of benefit only in detecting metastatic disease which is usually to the brain, lymph nodes and lungs

DIAGNOSTIC PROCEDURES Surgical biopsy is the only form of appropriate diagnostic procedure

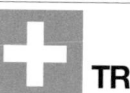

TREATMENT

APPROPRIATE HEALTH CARE Outpatient or inpatient surgery

GENERAL MEASURES The key to the cure of melanoma is prevention: Avoidance of blistering solar radiation and the use of a sunscreen when exposure is unavoidable

SURGICAL MEASURES
- The appropriate health care for melanoma is surgical excision. Much debate exists as to the extent of the margins of excision once diagnosis has been made. The tendency now is toward margins of 1 cm if the lesion is less than 1 mm thick. If thicker, then margins can be extended to 2 cm.
- Sentinel lymph node biopsy for lesions of 1-4 mm depth may benefit. However, increased survival has not been clearly demonstrated.
- Elective lymph node dissection (ELND) appears beneficial in patients age < 60 and thickness of lesion between 1.5-4 mm

ACTIVITY Avoid sun exposure

DIET No restrictions

PATIENT EDUCATION
- It is critical that a patient with a history of melanoma or dysplastic nevi syndrome has frequent total body examinations for any abnormal appearing or changing nevi
- National Cancer Institute, Department of Health And Human Services, Public Inquiries Section, Office of Cancer Communications, Building 31, Room 101-18, 9000 Rockville Pike, Bethesda, MD 20892, (301)496-5583

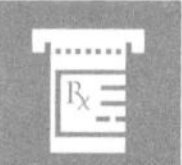

MEDICATIONS

DRUG(S) OF CHOICE
- No one chemotherapeutic agent has shown unequivocal benefit
- Adoptive immunotherapy with leukapheresis and IL-2 with LAK's (under investigation)
- Some benefit with vaccines containing melanoma associated antigens (MAAs) has occurred. No treatment has shown unequivocal benefit.
- Interferon alfa-2b is considered of possible benefit

Contraindications: Refer to manufacturer's literature
Precautions: Dacarbazine - myelosuppression, alopecia
Significant possible interactions: Refer to manufacturer's literature

ALTERNATIVE DRUGS
Many have been tried; recent trials show some promise

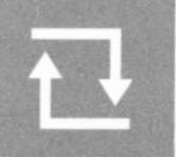

FOLLOWUP

PATIENT MONITORING
- Current recommendations after diagnosis of malignant melanoma are skin exams every 3-6 months
- Only chest x-rays on an annual basis have been shown to be of any benefit at all in that 6% of recurrences were detected. These findings did not appear to alter prognosis.
- The patient should conduct his/her own skin examinations on a weekly basis. They must be thorough.

PREVENTION/AVOIDANCE
Avoidance of prolonged and high altitude solar exposures and the use of sunscreens is critical. Those at high risk should do all they can to avoid sunburn especially during the adolescent years.

POSSIBLE COMPLICATIONS
- Metastatic spread
- Unsatisfactory cosmetic results following the primary surgery

EXPECTED COURSE/PROGNOSIS
- Prognosis is entirely based on staging of the initial lesion
- Staging (falls into two categories)
  - ◊ Breslow: This shows a 70% five-year survival of all patients who have no local or distant lymphatic spread.
  - ◊ Clark's staging depends on depth of invasion by skin layer. The best prognosis is for those lesions which are less than .85 mm (especially if restricted to the stratum granulosum or higher) which carry 95-100% five-year survival. Spread to lymphatics or regional lymph nodes carries less than a 5% five-year survival.
  - ◊ Women have a better prognosis than men
  - ◊ Truncal lesions have a poorer prognosis
  - ◊ With distant metastases, the disease is uniformly lethal

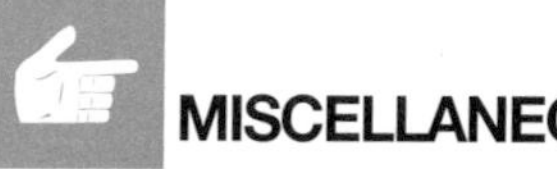

MISCELLANEOUS

ASSOCIATED CONDITIONS
As above

AGE-RELATED FACTORS
Pediatric: Rarely seen in pediatric age group
Geriatric: Lentigo maligna is most commonly seen in elderly patients who have had a slowly enlarging pigmented lesion, usually found on the face
Others: The most recent data on melanoma indicates that its highest incidence is between ages 30-50. However, it can occur at any age.

PREGNANCY
- Due to the facts that melanocyte-stimulating hormone (MSH) levels are markedly increased during pregnancy and that melanoma is one of the few carcinomas that can spread to the placenta, concern has been that pregnancy exacerbates melanoma. This has not been proven.
- If a person has had recent melanoma, many authors suggest waiting 1-2 years if further pregnancy is desired
- If invasion extends into the lymphatic structures, then further pregnancy is probably contraindicated

SYNONYMS
N/A

ICD-9-CM
172.9 Melanoma of skin, site unspecified

SEE ALSO

OTHER NOTES
- It is imperative for the physician to realize that any nevus or pigmented lesion that is in any way suspect should be excised. A full thickness total excisional biopsy must be sent for pathologic specimen and never to be curetted, electrodesiccated, or shaved.
- Any irregularly pigmented lesion in a preadolescent individual > 2 cm should be considered for excision

ABBREVIATIONS
N/A

REFERENCES

- Goldstein BG, Goldstein AO. Diagnosis and management of malignant melanoma. Am Fam Phys 2001;63(7):1359-68, 1374
- Symposium on Malignant Melanoma Parts II & IV. Mayo Clinic Prac 1997;72:356-371, 559-74
- Slominski A, Wortsman J, Carlson AJ, Matsuoka LY, Balch CM, Mihm MC. Malignant melanoma. Arch Pathol Lab Med 2001;125(10):1295-306

Web references: 0 available at www.5mcc.com
Illustrations 16 available

Author(s):
David P. Sealy, MD

BASICS

DESCRIPTION An inner ear (labyrinthine) disorder in which there is an increase in volume and pressure of the inner-most fluid of the inner ear (endolymph), resulting in recurrent attacks of hearing loss, tinnitus, vertigo, and fullness
- Usually unilateral, but in 10-50% may later involve the second ear
- Severity and frequency may diminish over the years, but with increasing loss of hearing. It is not a synonym for dizziness.

System(s) affected: Nervous
Genetics: N/A
Incidence/Prevalence in USA:
- No reliable figures are available to provide comprehensive numbers for incidence and prevalence by age and sex, but using incidence figures from a Swedish study conducted in 1973, it is estimated that the incidence of Ménière disease in the US is 46 (new cases/100,000/year). No figures for sex and age are available, but the disease is relatively equal in males and females, and is extremely rare in children.
- Using extrapolation, the estimated prevalence is 1,150 (cases/100,000 population)

Predominant age: Usual age of onset 20-60
Predominant sex: Male = Female

SIGNS & SYMPTOMS
- Hearing loss - low frequency, fluctuating
- Vertigo - spontaneous attacks, duration 20 minutes to several hours
- Ear fullness
- Occurs as attacks, with intervening remission
- During severe attacks
  - ◊ Pallor
  - ◊ Sweating
  - ◊ Nausea and vomiting
  - ◊ Falling
  - ◊ Prostration
  - ◊ All symptoms aggravated by motion
  - ◊ Between attacks may experience motion-related imbalance without vertigo

CAUSES
- Unknown. Best theory is inner ear response to variety of injuries (reduced middle ear pressure, allergy, endocrine disease, lipid disorders, vascular, viral, luetic).
- Recent theory is intracranial compression of balance nerve by blood vessel

RISK FACTORS
- Caucasian
- Stress
- Allergy
- Increased salt intake
- Noise

DIAGNOSIS

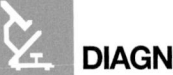

DIFFERENTIAL DIAGNOSIS
- Acoustic tumor
- Syphilis
- Perilymph fistula
- Multiple sclerosis
- Viral labyrinthitis
- Vertebrobasilar disease
- Other labyrinthine disorders producing same symptoms (Cogan's syndrome, benign positional vertigo, temporal bone trauma)

LABORATORY
- Lab studies done to rule out other conditions
- Serologic tests specific for Treponema pallidum - microhemagglutination (MHA), fluorescent treponemal antibody (FTA), Treponema immobilization test (TPI)
- Thyroid studies
- Lipid studies

Drugs that may alter lab results: Any medication that produces a significant degree of sedation is likely to affect vestibular testing and invalidate it

Disorders that may alter lab results: Many conditions may produce auditory and vestibular findings identical to those associated with Ménière disease, making it a diagnosis of exclusion. A low frequency sensorineural hearing loss (nerve loss as opposed to conductive loss) is seen on audiometry, and a reduced caloric response on caloric testing is usual.

PATHOLOGICAL FINDINGS Autopsy only. Shows dilation of inner ear fluid system (endolymph).

SPECIAL TESTS
- Otoscopy with air pressure applied to the tympanic membrane
- Auditory
  - ◊ Hearing test (audiometry using pure tone and speech) to show low frequency sensorineural [nerve] loss and impaired speech discrimination)
  - ◊ Tuning fork test (Weber and Rinne) to confirm validity of audiometry
  - ◊ Auditory Brainstem Response audiometry (ABR) to rule out acoustic neuroma
  - ◊ Electrocochleography (ECOG) may be useful to confirm etiology
- Vestibular
  - ◊ Spontaneous nystagmus (rapid rhythmic eye motion) seen visually. Must avoid eye fixation by having patient use 40 diopter glasses for test.
  - ◊ Caloric testing - electronystagmography (ENG) may show reduced caloric response. Can obtain reasonably comparable information with use of 0.8 cc ice water instilled in ear canal, then noting duration and frequency of resulting nystagmus with 40 diopter lenses in place. Reduced activity on either side is consistent with Ménière diagnosis, but is not diagnostic.

IMAGING MRI to rule out acoustic tumor, which can produce identical symptoms and findings

DIAGNOSTIC PROCEDURES N/A

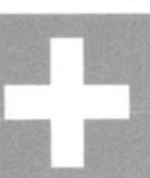

TREATMENT

APPROPRIATE HEALTH CARE Can usually be managed in outpatient setting. Inpatient for surgery.

GENERAL MEASURES
- Medications are given primarily for symptomatic relief of vertigo and nausea. There is no medication available that influences the disease process.
- For attacks, bedrest with eyes closed and protection from falling. Attacks rarely last longer than four hours.
- Streptomycin therapy for bilateral Ménière disease, when conventional management has failed. Streptomycin may be administered over a period of several days or weeks intentionally to damage the neuro-epithelium of the balance centers and reduce their function. Hearing must be carefully monitored during this time so that the treatment does not proceed to the point of damaging the hearing structures. This form of treatment should be administered only by an otolaryngologist and after careful patient education.

SURGICAL MEASURES
- Hearing good:
  - ◊ Endolymphatic sac surgery, either (1) decompression or (2) drainage of endolymph into mastoid or subarachnoid space
  - ◊ Alternative procedure is to cut the vestibular nerve (intracranial procedure)
  - ◊ A newer procedure involves placement of gentamicin through the tympanic membrane into the middle ear space
  - ◊ Another newer procedure is to place a ventilation tube through a myringotomy opening in the ear drum, and then use a pressure producing instrument called a Meniett device so as to apply pressure intermittently to the inner ear several times a day. This has been found helpful for the relief of dizziness, based on a large series of patients treated in Scandinavia.
- Hearing poor, but usable:
  - ◊ Can do sac procedure, nerve section, or gentamicin instillation depending on quality of hearing
  - ◊ Meniett device may also be used when hearing is poor
- Hearing not useful: Destruction of inner ear (labyrinthectomy)

ACTIVITY
- Limit activity during attacks
- Between attacks patient may be fully active, but this may be limited by (1) fear of impending attack, (2) unsteadiness following attacks, (3) ear fullness or tinnitus, or (4) hearing loss in involved ear that may severely limit the patient's ability to perform work duties or to participate in social life

DIET Limit total intake during attacks because of nausea. Otherwise diet is usually not a factor unless attacks are brought on by certain foods. A restricted salt diet may be useful in some cases.

PATIENT EDUCATION Many otolaryngologists keep booklets on Ménière disease as handouts. Ask your otolaryngology consultant for a supply.

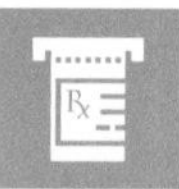

MEDICATIONS

DRUG(S) OF CHOICE

- Acute attack. For severe episode, one of the following may be used. Adult doses are indicated
  - ◊ Atropine 0.2-0.4 mg IV
  - ◊ Diazepam (Valium) 5-10 mg IV slowly
  - ◊ Transdermal scopolamine, 1 patch, or smaller segment of patch, applied to skin surface and not replaced sooner than 3 days
- Maintenance. Adult doses are indicated (frequently must be reduced to avoid sedating effects)
  - ◊ Meclizine (Antivert, Bonine) 25-100 mg orally, either at bedtime or in divided doses
  - ◊ Ergotamine-belladonna-phenobarbital (Bellergal Spacetabs), one q 12 hr
  - ◊ Diazepam (Valium), 2 mg (or less) tid

Contraindications:

- Atropine - cardiac disease, especially supraventricular tachycardia and other arrhythmias
- Scopolamine - children and elderly

Precautions:

- Sedating drugs should be used with caution, particularly in elderly people. The need to reduce the dosage is common. Patients should be cautioned not to operate motor vehicles when they are sedated.
- Atropine, scopolamine, and Bellergal should be used with particular caution. If not prescribed frequently, refer to manufacturer's literature.

Significant possible interactions:

- Bellergal - oral anticoagulants, tricyclic antidepressants, phenothiazines, narcotics, beta blockers, estrogens, and others
- Transdermal scopolamine - anticholinergics, belladonna products, antihistamines, tricyclic antidepressants, and others

ALTERNATIVE DRUGS

- Acute attack
  - ◊ Droperidol, 1.5-2.5 mg IV slowly (in hospital setting)
  - ◊ Promethazine (Phenergan) 12.5-25 mg IV slowly
  - ◊ Diphenhydramine (Benadryl) 50 mg IV slowly
  - ◊ Carbogen (5% carbon dioxide and 95% oxygen) by mask from tank
- Maintenance
  - ◊ Dimenhydrinate (Dramamine) 50 mg q4-6h po
  - ◊ Promethazine (Phenergan) 12.5-25 mg q4-6h po
  - ◊ Diphenidol (Vontrol) 25-50 mg tid po
  - ◊ Diphenhydramine (Benadryl), 25-50 mg q6-8h po. Maximum, 100 mg/24 hours
  - ◊ Chlorothiazide (Diuril) 500 mg daily po with potassium supplement

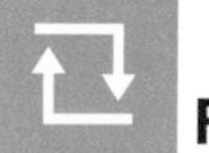

FOLLOWUP

PATIENT MONITORING The most common complaint by Ménière patients regarding prior treatment is that the primary care physician did not take the condition seriously and that he or she did not seem interested in providing ongoing care. Because of the emotional impact alone, these patients need close followup care. It is important to monitor the status of their hearing, since it is at risk, and to continue to consider the possibility of a more serious underlying problem such as an acoustic tumor.

PREVENTION/AVOIDANCE

- Reduce stress
- Reduce salt intake
- Don't smoke
- Avoid significant noise exposure, or use ear protectors
- Avoid use of ototoxic medications (aspirin, quinine, kanamycin, and many others)

POSSIBLE COMPLICATIONS

- Failure to diagnose acoustic neuroma
- Loss of hearing
- Injury during attack
- Inability to work

EXPECTED COURSE/PROGNOSIS

- Alternating attacks and remission
- Over time the balance problem tends to resolve, but the hearing worsens
- The great majority of patients can be managed successfully with medication. About 5-10% of patients require surgery for incapacitating vertigo.
- Very important not to overlook acoustic tumor, which produces an identical clinical picture

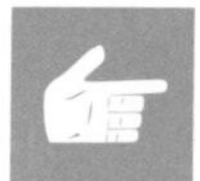

MISCELLANEOUS

ASSOCIATED CONDITIONS

- Cochlear hydrops (hearing problem only)
- Vestibular hydrops (balance problem only)
- Drop attacks

AGE-RELATED FACTORS

Pediatric: Unusual, but occasional. Dizziness in children likely to be on basis of significant central nervous system disease.
Geriatric: Less likely to occur in elderly. Patients exposed to loud noise levels over many years are more susceptible.
Others: Usual onset age 20-60

PREGNANCY Not a common problem, but difficult to treat because of risk of producing fetal abnormalities with medication

SYNONYMS

- Ménière syndrome
- Endolymphatic hydrops

ICD-9-CM

386.00 Meniere disease, unspecified

SEE ALSO

Labyrinthitis
Tinnitus

OTHER NOTES

- Hearing loss

ABBREVIATIONS N/A

REFERENCES

- Lucente FE, Gady HE. Essentials of Otolaryngology. 4th ed. Philadelphia, Lippincott Williams & Wilkins, 1999:116-125

Web references: 3 available at www.5mcc.com
Illustrations N/A

Author(s):
Gale Gardner, MD

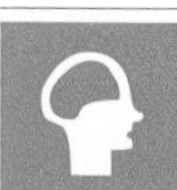

BASICS

DESCRIPTION Inflammation in response to bacterial infection of the pia-arachnoid and its fluid and the fluid of the ventricles. Meningitis is always cerebrospinal.
System(s) affected: Nervous
Genetics: Navajo Indian and American Eskimo may have genetic or acquired vulnerability to invasive disease
Incidence/Prevalence in USA: 3-10 cases per 100,000 population
Predominant age: Neonates, infants and geriatric aged
Predominant sex: Male = Female

SIGNS & SYMPTOMS
- Antecedent URI
- Fever
- Headache
- Meningismus
- Signs of cerebral dysfunction
- Vomiting
- Photophobia
- Seizures
- Nausea
- Rigors
- Profuse sweats
- Weakness
- Altered mental status
- Focal neurologic deficits
- Elderly have subtle findings commonly including confusion
- Meningococcemia has rash - macular and erythematous at first, then petechial or purpuric

CAUSES
Bacteria are divided into age groups to guide empiric therapy (parenthetical figures indicate relative incidence). Any organism can cause meningitis in any age group; therapy should be guided by culture whenever possible.
- Neonates (0-4 weeks)
  - ◊ *Group B or D Streptococcus* (70%)
  - ◊ *Listeria monocytogenes* (20%)
  - ◊ *Streptococcus pneumoniae* (10%)
  - ◊ *Escherichia coli*
  - ◊ *Non-group B Streptococcus*
- Infants (4-12 weeks)
  - ◊ *Neisseria meningitidis* (55%)
  - ◊ *Streptococcus pneumoniae* (40%)
  - ◊ *H. influenzae* (5%)
  - ◊ *Group B Streptococcus*
  - ◊ *Listeria monocytogenes*
  - ◊ *Escherichia coli*
- Children (3 months - 18 years)
  - ◊ *Neisseria meningitidis* (55%)
  - ◊ *Streptococcus pneumoniae* (30%)
  - ◊ *H. influenzae* (10%)
- Adults (>18 years)
  - ◊ *Streptococcus pneumoniae* (30-50%)
  - ◊ *Neisseria meningitidis* (10-35%)
  - ◊ *Staphylococci* (5-15%)
  - ◊ Gram-negative bacilli (e.g., *Escherichia coli*, *H. influenzae*; 1-10%)
  - ◊ *Streptococci* (5%)
  - ◊ *Listeria species* (5%)
  - ◊ *Haemophilus influenzae* (1-3%)

RISK FACTORS
- Immunocompromised host
- Alcoholism
- Neurosurgical procedure or head injury
- Abdominal surgery for gram-negative

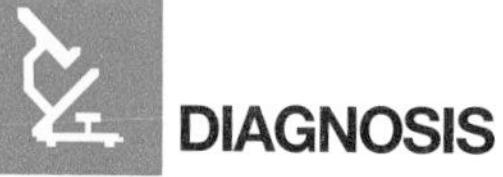

DIAGNOSIS

DIFFERENTIAL DIAGNOSIS
- Bacteremia
- Sepsis
- Brain abscess
- Seizures
- Other nonbacterial meningitides

LABORATORY
- Turbid CSF
- Neonates
  - ◊ > 10 WBC's in CSF
  - ◊ CSF: blood glucose ratio < 0.6
  - ◊ CSF protein >150 mg/dL (> 1500 mg/L)
- Infants/children
  - ◊ > 5 WBC's in CSF
  - ◊ CSF: blood glucose ratio < 0.6
  - ◊ CSF protein > 50 mg/dL (> 500 mg/L)
- Adults
  - ◊ 1000-100,000 WBC's in CSF
  - ◊ CSF: blood glucose ratio < 0.4
  - ◊ CSF protein > 45 mg/dL (usually 150-400 mg/dL)
  - ◊ Suspect ruptured brain abscess when WBC count is unusually high (> 100,000)
- In all age groups:
  - ◊ CSF opening pressure > 180 mm H2O (1.77 kPa)
  - ◊ CSF Gram stain + in 75% of untreated patients
  - ◊ CSF culture + 70-80% of the time
  - ◊ Blood culture + 40-60% of the time
  - ◊ CSF bacterial antigen test (sensitivity varies)

Drugs that may alter lab results: N/A

Disorders that may alter lab results: N/A

PATHOLOGICAL FINDINGS N/A

SPECIAL TESTS N/A

IMAGING
- CT scan of head if concern for increased intracranial pressure (ICP)
- Chest x-ray may reveal silent area of pneumonitis or abscess
- Sinus/skull x-rays may reveal cranial osteomyelitis, paranasal sinusitis or skull fracture
- Later in course, head CT scan, if hydrocephalus, brain abscess, subdural effusions or subdural empyema are considered

DIAGNOSTIC PROCEDURES
Lumbar puncture

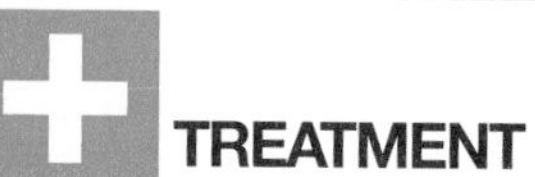

TREATMENT

APPROPRIATE HEALTH CARE
Inpatient often in ICU. If diagnosis is suspected, lumbar puncture should be done in office with antimicrobial therapy begun before transfer to hospital.

GENERAL MEASURES
- Appropriate antibiotic therapy
- Vigorous supportive care with constant nursing to ensure prompt recognition of seizures and prevention of aspiration
- Therapy for any coexisting conditions
- Measures to prevent hypothermia and dehydration

SURGICAL MEASURES N/A

ACTIVITY
As tolerated in hospital and on discharge

DIET
Regular as tolerated, except when SIADH complicates course

PATIENT EDUCATION
For patient education materials on this topic, contact: American Academy of Pediatrics, 141 Northwest Point Blvd., P.O. Box 927, Elk Grove Village, IL 60009-0927, (800)433-9016

MEDICATIONS

DRUG(S) OF CHOICE

- Empiric IV therapy until culture results available (consider local patterns of bacterial sensitivity). See Causes for age definitions and likely organisms.
- Treatment duration:
  - ◊ *N. meningitides*, *H. influenzae*: 7-10 days
  - ◊ *S. pneumoniae*: 10-14 days
  - ◊ *Group B Streptococcus*, *E. coli*, *L. monocytogenes*: 14-21 days
  - ◊ Neonates 12-21 days or at least 14 days after a repeat culture is sterile
- The following regimens are somewhat simplified but will adequately treat all patients while awaiting culture results. Additional subgroupings may simplify treatment in certain patients. Penicillin allergic patients present a special challenge not covered here.
- Corticosteroids. For all ages > 1 month and < 50 years corticosteroids decrease mortality and morbidity. Dexamethasone 0.15 mg/kg q6h, started 15-20 minutes before or with the antibiotic x 4 days. (N Engl J Med 324:1525, 1991)
- Antibiotics. Two IV regimens are presented; the first is usual therapy, the second is provided as an alternative is some settings
  - ◊ Ceftriaxone 100 mg/kg/d q12-24h (max 2 gm q12h) OR Cefotaxime 200 mg/kg/d q4-6h
  - ◊ Ampicillin 300-400 mg/kg/d q4h (max 2 gm q 3-4 h)
  - ◊ Vancomycin 10-15 mg/kg q12h (max 1500 mg q12h)

OR

- ◊ Neonates (give both)
  - Ampicillin 100-400 mg/kg/d divided q6-12h
  - Tobramycin 7.5 mg/kg/d q6-8h prematures or infants < 1 week, 2.5 mg/kg q12h
- ◊ Age > 4 weeks (give both)
  - Ampicillin 300-400 mg/kg/d divided q4-6h (max 2 gm q3-4h)
  - Chloramphenicol 75-100 mg/kg/d divided q6h

Contraindications: Allergies to specific antibiotic

Precautions:

- Ototoxicity from aminoglycoside

Significant possible interactions: Refer to manufacturer's literature

ALTERNATIVE DRUGS

- Antipseudomonal penicillins
- Aztreonam
- Quinolones (e.g., ciprofloxacin)
- Meropenem

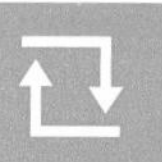

FOLLOWUP

PATIENT MONITORING Brainstem auditory evoked response (BAER) test should be done with infants prior to hospital discharge. Further followup will depend on its results and course of meningitis while in hospital.

PREVENTION/AVOIDANCE

- Prompt medical treatment for infections
- Strict aseptic techniques when treating patients with head wounds or skull fractures
- Look for evidence of CSF fistula in patients with recurrent meningitis

POSSIBLE COMPLICATIONS

- Seizures (20-30% during course of illness)
- Focal neurologic deficit
- Cranial nerve palsies (III, VI, VII, VIII) 10-20% of cases, usually disappear within a few weeks
- Sensorineural hearing loss (10% in children)
- Neurodevelopmental sequelae (subtle learning deficits 30%)
- Obstructive hydrocephalus
- Subdural effusions

EXPECTED COURSE/PROGNOSIS

- Overall case fatality 14%
  - ◊ *H. influenza* 5%
  - ◊ *Neisseria meningitidis* 10%
  - ◊ *Streptococcus pneumoniae* 25%

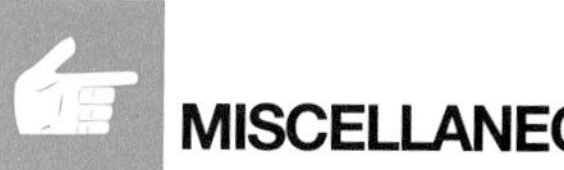

MISCELLANEOUS

ASSOCIATED CONDITIONS

Which worsen prognosis:

- Coma
- Seizures
- Alcoholism
- Old age
- Infancy
- Diabetes mellitus
- Multiple myeloma
- Head trauma

AGE-RELATED FACTORS

Pediatric: N/A

Geriatric: Several signs and symptoms may be less evident in elderly patients with other disorders (congestive heart failure, pneumonia)

Others: Different etiologic agents, antimicrobials and dosing, and CSF findings as listed above

PREGNANCY N/A

SYNONYMS N/A

ICD-9-CM

320.9 Meningitis due to unspecified bacterium

SEE ALSO

Meningitis, viral
Meningococcemia

OTHER NOTES N/A

ABBREVIATIONS N/A

REFERENCES

- Tunkel AR, Scheld WM. Issues in the management of bacterial meningitis. Am Fam Physician 1997;56(5):1355-62
- McIntyre PB, Berkey CS, King SM, et al. Dexamethasone as adjuvant therapy in bacterial meningitis. A meta-analysis of randomized clinical trials since 1988. JAMA 1997;278(11):925-31
- Anonymous: Therapy for children with invasive pneumococcal infections. American Academy of Pediatrics Committee on Infectious Diseases. Pediatrics 1997;99(2):289-99
- Odio CM, Faingezicht I, Paris M, et al. The beneficial effects of early dexamethasone administration in infants and children with bacterial meningitis. N Engl J Med 1991;324(22):1525-31
- van de Beek D, de Gans J, McIntyre P, Prasad K. Corticosteroids in acute bacterial meningitis. Cochrane Database Syst Rev. 2003;(3):CD004305. Comment in ACP J Club 2004;140(2):34
- de Gans J, van de Beek D; European Dexamethasone in Adulthood Bacterial Meningitis Study Investigators. Dexamethasone in adults with bacterial meningitis. N Engl J Med 2002;347(20):1549-56

Web references: 4 available at www.5mcc.com

Illustrations N/A

Author(s):
Paul R. Gordon, MD

BASICS

DESCRIPTION Viral infection of the meninges and spinal fluid. The usual cause is acute and may be relapsing. Peak incidence occurs in summertime.
System(s) affected: Nervous
Genetics: N/A
Incidence/Prevalence in USA: Average of 10,000 reported cases per year. Probably many more unreported.
Predominant age: May affect all ages, but most common in young adults
Predominant sex: Male = Female

SIGNS & SYMPTOMS
- Fever
- Headache, often severe
- Stiff neck
- Nausea and vomiting
- Photophobia
- Generalized aches and pains
- Occasional rash

CAUSES
- Coxsackie A, B
- ECHO virus (enteroviruses 70-75% of all cases)
- Poliovirus
- Lymphocytic choriomeningitis (LCM)
- Mumps
- Herpes (simplex and zoster)
- Epstein-Barr virus (EBV)
- Arthropod borne viruses
- Cytomegalovirus (CMV)
- Adenovirus

RISK FACTORS
- No specifics known
- Immunocompromised hosts may be more susceptible to CMV and adenovirus

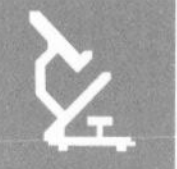

DIAGNOSIS

DIFFERENTIAL DIAGNOSIS
- Bacterial meningitis
- Encephalitis
- Acute encephalopathy
- Postinfectious encephalomyelitis
- Parameningeal infections (e.g., subdural empyema)
- Carcinomatous meningitis
- Meningeal leukemia
- Migraine headache
- Viral syndrome (e.g., influenza)
- Chemical meningitis
- Brain abscess
- Other infectious agents (TB, syphilis, ameba, leptospirosis)

LABORATORY
- CSF pleocytosis - usually predominantly mononuclear but may show more polys early on
- CSF cell count up to 3000-4000, but usually 50-200
- CSF - increased pressure
- CSF - serum antiviral antibody
- Elevated CSF protein, but usually < 150 mg/dL (< 1500 mg/L)
- CSF sugar usually normal (exceptions - herpes, mumps)
- Negative CSF Gram stain and culture for bacteria
- Negative CSF latex agglutination or CIEP for bacterial antigens
- Normal or mildly elevated WBC (blood)
- Viral cultures and/or antibody titers are seldom helpful

Drugs that may alter lab results: Pretreatment with antibiotics may result in a "partially treated" bacterial meningitis, mimicking viral meningitis

Disorders that may alter lab results:
- Diabetes (alteration in spinal fluid sugar)
- Pre-existing neurologic diseases (e.g., brain tumor, demyelinating disease) could affect CSF findings

PATHOLOGICAL FINDINGS Lymphocyte infiltration of meninges and ventricles

SPECIAL TESTS EEG in some cases, especially if encephalitis is a consideration

IMAGING
- CT scan or MRI scan of the brain
- Usually CT or MRI performed prior to lumbar puncture

DIAGNOSTIC PROCEDURES Lumbar puncture

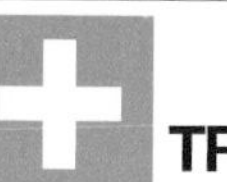

TREATMENT

APPROPRIATE HEALTH CARE
- Usually inpatient, depending on severity of symptoms
- Private room indicated with moderate sterile precautions. Stress hand washing.

GENERAL MEASURES
- Fever control
- IV fluids if oral intake is poor or vomiting is present

SURGICAL MEASURES N/A

ACTIVITY Bedrest initially, then activity as tolerated

DIET Determined by symptoms; may need to NPO due to nausea or vomiting, advance to clear fluids and regular diet as tolerated

PATIENT EDUCATION
- Discuss possibility, but low probability, of transmission to contacts
- Expected duration of illness (2-7 days)
- For patient education materials favorably reviewed on this topic, contact: American Academy of Pediatrics, 141 Northwest Point Blvd., P.O. Box 927, Elk Grove Village, IL 60009-0927, (800)433-9016

MEDICATIONS

DRUG(S) OF CHOICE
- Analgesics (adult doses)
  - ◊ Morphine 2-5 mg IV q3h
  - ◊ Nalbuphine (Nubain) 10 mg IM
  - ◊ acetaminophen-codeine or acetaminophen-oxycodone (Percocet), 1-2 q3h prn
- Antiemetics
  - ◊ Promethazine (Phenergan) 12.5-25 mg IV q4h
  - ◊ Prochlorperazine (Compazine) 10 mg IM q4h, in adults
- Antipyretics
  - ◊ Acetaminophen (Tylenol) 650 mg po or suppository q4h for adults. Approximately 60 mg per year of age in children or 10-15 mg/kg/dose.
- Antiviral agents are not indicated in the usual care of viral meningitis
- Antibiotics are not indicated for treatment of viral meningitis, but are often initiated until a diagnosis is firmly established. If all parameters suggest a viral etiology, it is usually prudent to treat symptomatically and follow the patient closely in the hospital setting. If in doubt, a broad spectrum antibiotic with good CSF penetration should be started intravenously. The choice may be dictated by local sensitivities, as well as a consideration of age related pathogens.

Contraindications: Refer to manufacturer's profile of each drug

Precautions:
- Aspirin should be avoided in children and adolescents due to a possible association with Reye syndrome
- Phenothiazines may produce a dystonic reaction, especially in adolescents

Significant possible interactions: Refer to manufacturer's profile of each drug

ALTERNATIVE DRUGS
Symptomatic relief may be provided by a variety of anti-emetics and analgesics (e.g., non-steroidal anti-inflammatory drugs)

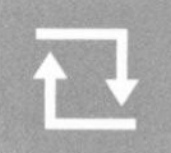

FOLLOWUP

PATIENT MONITORING
- Once the acute illness begins resolving, follow at least once within 7-10 days
- Repeat of lumbar puncture is not necessary unless the clinical course is atypical

PREVENTION/AVOIDANCE
N/A

POSSIBLE COMPLICATIONS
- Deafness
- Fatigue
- Irritability
- Muscle weakness
- Seizures (rare)

EXPECTED COURSE/PROGNOSIS
Complete recovery in 2-7 days; headaches and other uncomfortable symptoms may sometimes persist intermittently for 1-2 weeks

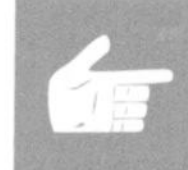

MISCELLANEOUS

ASSOCIATED CONDITIONS
Encephalitis

AGE-RELATED FACTORS
Pediatric: N/A
Geriatric: Viral meningitis is rarely seen in the elderly, and suspicions should be raised about an alternative diagnosis, e.g., carcinomatous meningitis
Others: N/A

PREGNANCY
N/A

SYNONYMS
- Abacterial meningitis
- Aseptic meningitis

ICD-9-CM
047.9 Unspecified viral meningitis

SEE ALSO
Encephalitis, viral
Meningitis, bacterial

OTHER NOTES
Enteroviruses and arthropod-borne viruses predominate in warm months; mumps usually occurs in the winter and spring, often in epidemics

ABBREVIATIONS
CIEP = counterimmunoelectrophoresis
CSF = cerebrospinal fluid

REFERENCES

- Mandell G, Douglas RG Jr, Bennett JE: Principles and Practice of Infectious Diseases. 4th Ed. New York, Churchill Livingstone, 1995
- Krugman S, Katz S, Gershon A, Wilfert C: Infectious Diseases of Children. 9th ed. New York, C.V. Mosby, 1990
- Rotbart HA: Enteroviral infections in the central nervous system. Clin Infect Dis 1995;20(4):971-81

Web references: 2 available at www.5mcc.com
Illustrations N/A

Author(s):
Gary M. Miller, MD

BASICS

DESCRIPTION The presence of *Neisseria meningitidis* in the blood. This encompasses a broad spectrum of clinical manifestations.
- Bacteremia without sepsis: the patient has upper respiratory symptoms only and recovers spontaneously without antibiotic
- Bacteremia without meningitis: the patient is acutely ill, may have skin manifestations (rashes, petechiae, ecchymosis) and hypotension
- Bacteremia with meningitis: this clinical picture of meningitis predominates (headache, decreased sensorium, neck rigidity). Patient may also have skin manifestations and hypotension.
- Bacteremia with acute arthritis dermatitis syndrome: the patient may have tenosynovitis typical of gonococcal etiology

System(s) affected: Cardiovascular, Endocrine/Metabolic, Hemic/Lymphatic/Immunologic, Musculoskeletal, Nervous, Renal/Urologic, Skin/Exocrine
Genetics: N/A
Incidence/Prevalence in USA: 1-3/100,000 population
Predominant age: Highest attack rate in infants ages 3 months to 1 year and then decreases with age; it may affect all ages
Predominant sex: Male = Female

SIGNS & SYMPTOMS
- Malaise
- Fever
- Chills, rigor
- Sore throat
- Cough
- Headache
- Changes in mental status - restlessness, agitation, confusion, delirium, lethargy, stupor, coma
- Myalgia
- Vomiting
- Convulsions
- Stiff neck
- Focal neurologic signs
- Tachycardia
- Tachypnea
- Hypotension
- Cyanosis
- Maculopapular rash
- Petechiae
- Ecchymosis, purpura
- Arthritis
- Tenosynovitis

CAUSES
- *Neisseria meningitidis*, a gram-negative diplococcus
  - ◊ At least 13 serotypes
  - ◊ Major serogroups: A, B, C, Y, W -135
  - ◊ Serogroup A may cause epidemics in many parts of developing
  - ◊ Serogroup C caused recent outbreaks in the U.S.
  - ◊ Serogroup B is predominant cause of meningococcemia in children <1 yr of age
  - ◊ Serogroup Y is becoming more common in the U.S.

RISK FACTORS
- Age 3 months to 1 year
- Late complement component deficiency (C5, C6, C7, C8 or C9)
- Household contacts
- Contacts in nurseries and day care centers
- Close quarters (e.g., dormitories, campus bars, and military barracks)

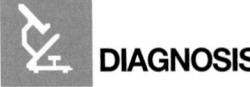

DIAGNOSIS

DIFFERENTIAL DIAGNOSIS
- Septicemia due to other microorganism
- Meningitis due to other pyogenic bacteria
- Gonococcemia
- Acute bacterial endocarditis
- Rocky Mountain spotted fever
- Hemolytic uremic syndrome
- Gonococcal arthritis dermatitis syndrome
- Influenza

LABORATORY
- Leukocytosis or leukopenia
- Left shift of leukocytes, toxic granulation
- Thrombocytopenia
- Lactic acidosis
- Prolonged prothrombin time
- Prolonged partial thromboplastin time
- Low fibrinogen
- Elevated fibrin degradation products
- Blood culture growing N. meningitidis
- Cerebrospinal fluid (CSF):
  - ◊ Cloudy
  - ◊ Increased WBC's with PMN's predominant
  - ◊ Gram stain showing gram-negative diplococci
  - ◊ Glucose to blood glucose ratio < 0.4
  - ◊ Protein > 45 mg/dL
  - ◊ Positive for N. meningitidis antigen
  - ◊ Culture grew N. meningitidis

Drugs that may alter lab results:
- Prior antibiotic administration may make blood and/or CSF culture negative
- Rifampin colors urine orange and may interfere with certain lab tests, e.g. urine dipstick

Disorders that may alter lab results: N/A

PATHOLOGICAL FINDINGS
- Disseminated intravascular coagulation
- Exudates on meninges
- PMN infiltration of meninges
- Hemorrhage of adrenal glands

SPECIAL TESTS N/A

IMAGING
CT scan of head if concern for space-occupying lesions

DIAGNOSTIC PROCEDURES
- Blood culture
- Lumbar puncture, done immediately after a brief history and physical examination, if meningitis suspected

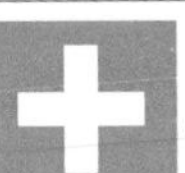

TREATMENT

APPROPRIATE HEALTH CARE
- If meningitis suspected, immediate lumbar puncture
- If lumbar puncture is delayed, administer antibiotic immediately
- Admit patient to ICU, if severe sepsis or meningitis suspected
- Droplet isolation, for 24 hours from the beginning of antibiotic therapy, is appropriate

GENERAL MEASURES
- Appropriate antibiotic
- Supportive care including IV fluids, oxygen when needed
- Close monitoring of patient for seizure activity
- Treat complications (e.g., DIC, ARDS, renal failure, adrenal failure)

SURGICAL MEASURES N/A

ACTIVITY
As tolerated depending on clinical condition

DIET
As tolerated depending on clinical condition

PATIENT EDUCATION
- Educate family and close contacts regarding risk of contracting meningococcal infections
- Educate healthcare personnel who are not at risk of contracting meningococcal infections

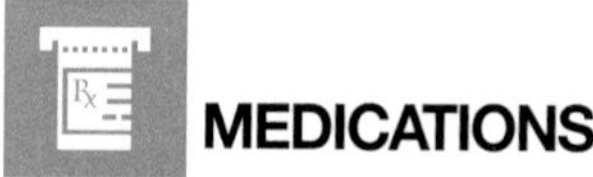

MEDICATIONS

DRUG(S) OF CHOICE
- In patients with severe mental changes, consider administering dexamethasone 0.15 mg/kg q 6h x 16 doses, starting 15 minutes before first dose of antibiotic
- When treating a patient with suspected meningitis, initiate early therapy with broad spectrum coverage such as a third generation cephalosporin plus vancomycin. Once *N. meningitidis* is identified, the drug of choice remains penicillin
- For meningitis - penicillin G 4 million units IV q 4h (children 0.25 mU/kg IV q 4-6h) or ampicillin 2 g IV q 4h (children 200-300 mg/kg IV q 6h)
- For other infections - use half the dose for meningitis
- Duration of treatment 7-10 days
- Chemoprophylaxis for close contacts (household members, personnel in nurseries, day care centers, nursing homes, dormitories and other closed institutions). Regimen: rifampin 600 mg (children 10 mg/kg) po q12h for 2 days or for adults only, one dose of ciprofloxacin 750 mg po. (No chemoprophylaxis is needed for casual contacts, health care personnel (except persons giving mouth-to-mouth resuscitation), schoolmates, office co-workers).

Contraindications: For patients with penicillin allergy, use alternate drugs

Precautions:
- Adjust dosage in patients with severe renal dysfunction
- Rifampin ingestion causes orange urine.

Significant possible interactions: Refer to manufacturer's literature

ALTERNATIVE DRUGS
- For meningitis - chloramphenicol 1 g IV q 6h (in children 75-100 mg/kg q 6h) or ceftriaxone 2 g IV q 12h (children 80-100 mg/kg q 12-24h)
  - ◊ Ceftriaxone should not be used in patients with history of anaphylactic reactions to penicillin (hypotension, laryngeal edema, wheezing, hives, etc.)
  - ◊ Chloramphenicol may cause aplastic anemia
- For other infections - ceftriaxone 1 g (children 40 mg/kg) IV q 24h

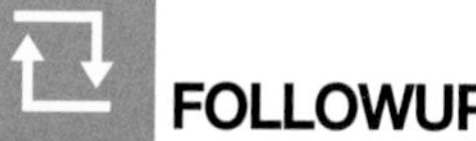

FOLLOWUP

PATIENT MONITORING In patients with neurologic deficits, follow-up with neurologist may be needed

PREVENTION/AVOIDANCE Before discharge, give patient rifampin 600 mg (children 10 mg/kg) po q 12h for 2 days to eradicate carriage or for adults only, one dose of ciprofloxacin 500-750 mg po

POSSIBLE COMPLICATIONS
- Disseminated intravascular coagulation
- Acute tubular necrosis
- Seizures
- Focal neurologic deficit
- Cranial nerve palsies
- Sensorineural hearing loss
- Obstructive hydrocephalus
- Subdural effusions
- Acute adrenal hemorrhage (Waterhouse-Friderichsen syndrome)

EXPECTED COURSE/PROGNOSIS
Overall mortality 10%

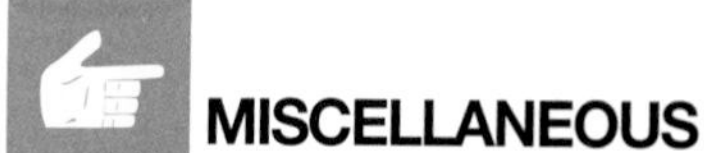

MISCELLANEOUS

ASSOCIATED CONDITIONS N/A

AGE-RELATED FACTORS
Pediatric: Age 3 months to 1 year - highest risk
Geriatric: Less common
Others: N/A

PREGNANCY N/A

SYNONYMS Spinal meningitis

ICD-9-CM
036.2 Meningococcemia
036.0 Meningococcal meningitis

SEE ALSO
Meningitis, bacterial
Sepsis

OTHER NOTES
- Vaccine containing polysaccharides of groups A, C, Y and W-135 is available for persons with late complement deficiency, anatomic or functional asplenia. Vaccination is also recommended for travelers to the Haj in Saudi Arabia and other areas with epidemic meningococcal disease (e.g., West Africa). It should also be considered for use in freshmen college students living in dormitories.

ABBREVIATIONS N/A

REFERENCES

- Apicella M. Neisseria meningitidis. In: Mandell GL, Bennett JR, Dolin R, eds. Principles and Practice of Infectious Diseases. 5th Ed. Philadelphia, Churchill Livingstone, 2000:2228-41
- Jackson LA, Schuchat A, Reeves MW, et al. Serogroup C meningococcal outbreaks in the United States. An emerging threat. JAMA 1995;273:383-389
- Imrey PB, Jackson LA, Ludwinski PH, et al. Outbreak of serogroup C meningococcal disease associated with campus bar patronage. Am J epidemiol 1996;143:624-630
- Meningococcal disease and college students. Recommendations of the Advisory Committee on Immunization Practices (ACIP). MMWR Morb Mortal Wkly Rep 2000;49(RR-7):1-20
- Rosenstein NE, Perkins BA, Stephens DS, Popovic T, Hughes JM. Meningococcal Disease. NEJM. 344(18), pp 1378-1388, 2001
- Diaz PS. The epidemiology and control of invasive meningococcal disease. Pediatric Infectious Disease Journal. 18(7):633-4, 1999

Web references: 0 available at www.5mcc.com
Illustrations N/A

Author(s):
Hans House, MD

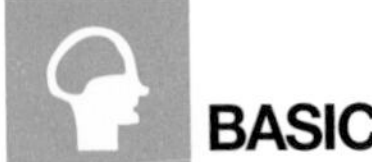

BASICS

DESCRIPTION
- Incomplete closure of the vertebral column during embryogenesis, resulting in exposure of meninges and spinal cord
- Always associated with the constellation of findings known as the Chiari II malformation which include: small posterior fossa, hindbrain herniation into the upper cervical spinal canal, dysgenesis or agenesis of the corpus callosum, neuronal migration disorders of varying degree, and hydrocephalus
- Chiari II abnormality associated with myelomeningocele, anencephaly, and encephalocele all belong to a group of disorders known as "neural tube defects." These serious congenital anomalies of the nervous system, which occur during the first 4 weeks of gestation, result from faulty formation of the neural tube.
- Post neurulation defects develop after 25 days of intrauterine life, ie, after neurulation is complete
  - ◊ Lesions include simple meningocele, lipomyelomeningocele, diastematomyelia, myelocystocele, neurenteric cyst, intraspinal and pelvic meningoceles
  - ◊ Characterized by intact skin over the underlying lesion

System(s) affected: Musculoskeletal, Nervous, Renal/Urologic, Skin/Exocrine

Genetics:
- Myelomeningocele and other neural tube defects (anencephaly and encephalocele) represent examples of multifactorial inheritance
- Parents of an affected infant have a 1:30 chance of producing a 2nd affected offspring. An affected patient, if able to have children, has a 3-4% chance of having an affected child. Parents with 2 affected children run the risk of 7-8% of having a third child so affected. 2nd degree relatives of an affected individual (nephews, nieces) have a 1:100 risk; the risk for 1st cousins is 1:200.
- Maternal folic acid deficiency is an environmental factor strongly associated with neural tube defects. (Serum from women with pregnancy complicated by a neural tube defect contains autoantibodies that bind folate receptors and block the cellular uptake of folate. Further study is warranted to assess whether the observed association between maternal antibodies against folate receptors and neural tube defects reflects a causal relation.)

Incidence/Prevalence in USA:
- Neural tube defects (also referred to as spina bifida) incidence in Caucasians is 1:700 live births
- Incidence among African-Americans is <1:3000

Predominant age: Congenital anomaly, apparent at birth

Predominant sex: Male = Female

SIGNS & SYMPTOMS
- The myelomeningocele is usually single and involves the lumbosacral spine
- Hydrocephalus requiring CSF diversion, occurs in > 80% of infants with the Chiari II abnormality and myelomeningocele
- The Chiari II malformation (hindbrain herniation into the upper cervical spinal canal) requires surgical decompression in some affected children
  - ◊ If symptomatic, can impair cranial nerve control of swallowing/respiration and, less frequently cause pyramidal signs
  - ◊ Syringomyelia, cystic expansion of the central spinal canal, is often present
  - ◊ Surgical hindbrain decompression, if done promptly after onset of symptoms of hindbrain compression, may reverse or arrest these symptoms (stridor, respiratory difficulties, laryngomalacia), but the latter syndromes are often confused with respiratory infections, thus delaying treatment

CAUSES
- Ultimate cause of spinal dysraphism is unclear
- Dysraphic malformations probably occur when environmental agents impact underlying hereditary risk factors

RISK FACTORS
- 1st trimester maternal valproic acid and derivatives (valproate sodium) use
- High risk pregnancy - previous children with spina bifida
- Insufficient maternal levels of folic acid
- >90% of spina bifida infants are the product of low-risk pregnancies

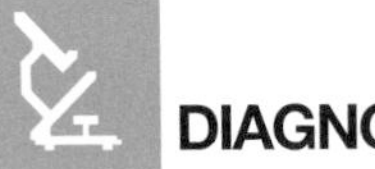

DIAGNOSIS

DIFFERENTIAL DIAGNOSIS N/A

LABORATORY
- Prenatal: maternal serum alpha-fetoprotein (AFP) levels - elevated AFP level at 16-18 weeks suggest fetal open neural tube defects, indicating further prenatal evaluation and genetic counseling
- Newborn: no specific lab studies indicated

Drugs that may alter lab results: N/A

Disorders that may alter lab results: N/A

PATHOLOGICAL FINDINGS N/A

SPECIAL TESTS
- Prenatal diagnosis
  - ◊ Amniocentesis: increased alpha-fetoprotein in amniotic fluid (by 14 weeks) suggests open neural tube defects
  - ◊ Ultrasound: hydrocephalus usually diagnosed readily. Other signs associated with Chiari II anomaly may be discernible (Banana sign, callosal anomalies, mega choroid plexus).
- Neonate
  - ◊ Neurological examination, including pinprick examination of trunk, legs, and perineum. Functional integrity present if stimulus causes purposeful limb movements, arousal, crying, anal wink, etc.

IMAGING
Neonate: cranial ultrasound most efficient way to assess ventricular size promptly; may demonstrate associated anomalies (callosal agenesis, etc)

DIAGNOSTIC PROCEDURES
- Neonate
  - ◊ Myelomeningocele is usually apparent on physical examination
  - ◊ Direct laryngoscopy is indicated for infants with stridor, an ominous sign suggesting the need for urgent CSF diversion and/or posterior fossa decompression
  - ◊ Cranial ultrasound at birth assesses the presence and severity of hydrocephalus and the need for prompt CSF diversion

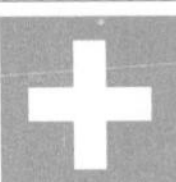

TREATMENT

APPROPRIATE HEALTH CARE Inpatient

GENERAL MEASURES
- Multidisciplinary approach: Pediatric neurosurgery, orthopedics, urology, nursing, social services, pediatrics and physical therapy
- Most patients with myelomeningocele have neurogenic bladder necessitating intermittent catheterization to prevent severe secondary urologic disorders

SURGICAL MEASURES
- Myelomeningocele repair - ideally within 24-48 hours of birth
- CSF diversion (usually ventriculoperitoneal shunt) usually required at birth or shortly thereafter
- Orthopedic correction of extremity and spinal deformities is more elective but requires evaluation early
- Infants with clinical evidence of hindbrain compression despite adequate CSF diversion require prompt posterior fossa decompression
- Prenatal (fetal) surgery to close myelomeningocele defects is being tested in several institutions, but remains an investigative procedure

ACTIVITY
- Determined by level of the lesion
- Optimized by physical therapists and multidisciplinary team

DIET
- Obesity a major cause of morbidity in myelomeningocele patients
- Modified as needed to facilitate bowel and bladder training

PATIENT EDUCATION
- Genetic counseling
- Signs and symptoms of shunt malfunction
- Bowel/bladder care
- Patient resources: Spina Bifida Association of America, 4590 MacArthur Blvd, Suite 250, Washington, DC 20007-4226; (800) 621-3141; e-mail sbaa@sbaa.org

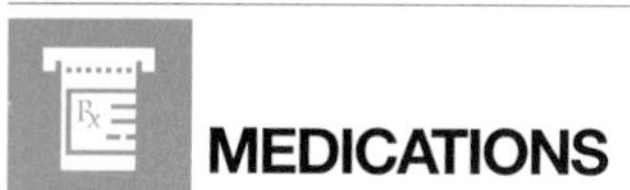

MEDICATIONS

DRUG(S) OF CHOICE N/A
Contraindications: N/A
Precautions: N/A
Significant possible interactions: N/A

ALTERNATIVE DRUGS N/A

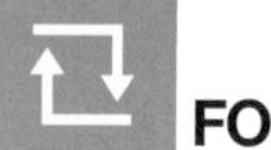

FOLLOWUP

PATIENT MONITORING Regular followup in spina bifida clinic, with multidisciplinary assessment including pediatrics, neurosurgery, orthopedics, and urology

PREVENTION/AVOIDANCE
- Adequate folate (0.4 mg/day) intake by sexually active women before pregnancy and through first trimester
- For women with prior NTD-affected pregnancy, give 4 mg/day of folate before conception and through first trimester

POSSIBLE COMPLICATIONS
- Late neurological deterioration due to tethering of spinal cord
- Shunt obstruction: headache, nausea and vomiting, visual disturbances, cognitive difficulty; the latter two problems may be chronic, unaccompanied by headache or vomiting
- Shunt obstruction may result in hydromyelia, which may manifest only with intrinsic muscle weakness of the hands
- Inadequate bladder hygiene can result in hydronephrosis progressing to renal failure
- Seizures may result from cortical migration disorders or herald shunt malfunction
- Myelomeningocele patients are at risk for latex allergy. Use latex precautions.

EXPECTED COURSE/PROGNOSIS
- >80% of treated patients with open neural tube defects have normal IQ
- Since 1970s, management techniques have improved, a result of the creation of multidisciplinary spina bifida clinics
- Shunt infection and malfunction less common, but still a major cause of morbidity
- Generally, early prediction of motor and intellectual outcome in neonates with Chiari II and myelomeningocele is hazardous
- Infants with head circumference > 50 cm at birth (eg, severe hydrocephalus) have dismal cognitive prognosis

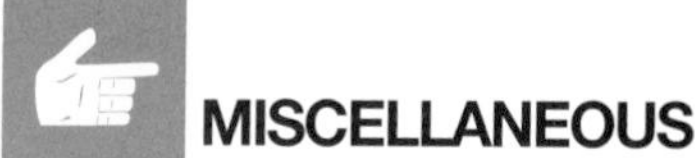

MISCELLANEOUS

ASSOCIATED CONDITIONS Infants with a "simple" meningocele may have associated intraspinal abnormalities requiring treatment

AGE-RELATED FACTORS
Pediatric: Congenital defect
Geriatric: N/A
Others: N/A

PREGNANCY Ultrasound key to the intrauterine diagnosis of this condition

SYNONYMS
- Myelomeningocele
- Spinal dysraphism
- Spina bifida
- Open neural tube defect

ICD-9-CM
741.00 Spina bifida with hydrocephalus, unspecified region
741.90 Spina bifida without mention of hydrocephalus, unspecified region

SEE ALSO

OTHER NOTES Decisions about performing operative procedures or letting the disorder "take its natural course" in severely affected infants presents serious ethical problems, usually the more aggressive course is best.

ABBREVIATIONS
ACM = Arnold Chiari malformation
NTD = Neural tube defect

REFERENCES

- Beuls E, Vanormelingen L, Van Aalst J, et al. The Arnold-Chiari type II malformation at midgestation. Pediatr Neurosurg 2003;39(3):149-58
- Czeizel AE, Dudas I. Prevention of the first occurrence of neural-tube defects by periconceptional vitamin supplementation. N Engl J Med 1992;327:1832-5
- American Academy of Pediatrics. Folic acid for the prevention of neural tube defects. Committee on Genetics. Pediatrics 1999;104(2 Pt 1):325-7
- McLone DG, Knepper PA. The cause of Chiari II malformation: a unified theory. Pediatr Neurosci 1989;15:1-12
- van Zalen-Sprock RM, van Vugt JM, van Geijn HP. First and early second trimester diagnosis of anomalies of the central nervous system. J Ultrasound Med 1995;14:603-10
- Rothenberg SP, da Costa MP, Sequeira JM, et al. Autoantibodies against folate receptors in women with a pregnancy complicated by a neural-tube defect. N Engl J Med 2004;350(2):134-42

Web references: 1 available at www.5mcc.com
Illustrations N/A

Author(s):
David Donahue, MD

BASICS

DESCRIPTION The cessation of spontaneous menstrual cycles
- Perimenopause: period of time where there is a decline in ovarian function. Although a woman may continue to have periodic uterine bleeding, such cycles may be anovulatory. During this time estrogen production diminishes and a woman may experience early signs of estrogen deficiency.
- Postmenopause: the period after menopause usually accounting for more than a third of a woman's total life
- Premature menopause: occurring before age 30 and may be associated with sex chromosome abnormalities

System(s) affected: Cardiovascular, Endocrine/Metabolic, Musculoskeletal, Reproductive
Genetics: N/A
Incidence/Prevalence in USA: Increasingly common as life span increases - currently affects over 30 million women
Predominant age:
- Average age is 51 in the U.S. (unrelated to the age of menarche) and virtually all women postmenopausal by age 58.

Predominant sex: Female only

SIGNS & SYMPTOMS
- Cessation of menses - either abruptly or preceded by a period of irregular cycles and/or diminished bleeding
- Vasomotor symptoms - hot flashes, sweating (85%)
- Psychologic symptoms - depression, nervousness, insomnia, decreases libido
- Vaginal atrophy - dyspareunia
- Urinary tract atrophy - stress or urge urinary incontinence
- Skin atrophy - wrinkles
- Osteoporosis - fractures (20% by age 85)
- Arteriosclerosis - coronary artery disease
- Breast tenderness
- Change in intensity and severity of migraines

CAUSES
- Physiologic - when due to depletion of oocytes
- Surgical - when due to removal of functioning ovaries because of disease or incidental to hysterectomy
- Medical - as a result of treatment of endometriosis (danazol [Danocrine] or GnRH analogues) or of breast cancer (antiestrogens). This etiology is reversible. May occur after cancer chemotherapy and be permanent or reversible.

RISK FACTORS
- Increasing age
- Pelvic surgery
- Sex chromosome abnormalities (eg, Turner syndrome)

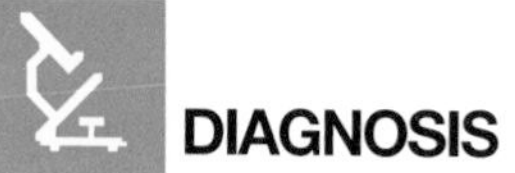

DIAGNOSIS

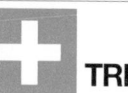

DIFFERENTIAL DIAGNOSIS
- Pregnancy
- Polycystic ovarian disease
- Microadenoma of pituitary
- Hypothalamic dysfunction
- Asherman's syndrome
- Obstruction of uterine outflow tract
- Sheehan syndrome

LABORATORY
- Usually none is required because patient's age and symptoms readily establish the diagnosis
- If the diagnosis is questionable in a young patient, an elevated serum FSH indicates ovarian failure (FSH greater than 40 mIU/mL [100 IU/L]). Measurement of LH is not necessary. Estradiol (E2) levels will be less than 30 pg/mL.
- Peripheral blood karyotype if age < 30

Drugs that may alter lab results:
- Estrogens
- Androgens
- Hormonal contraceptives

Disorders that may alter lab results: Temporary, reversible cessation of ovarian function, e.g., during chemotherapy

PATHOLOGICAL FINDINGS
- Atrophy of endometrium - virtually 100% if untreated. The uterus may seem smaller on bimanual examination.
- Atrophy of vagina - loss of rugae, appearance of petechiae - virtually 100% after several years if untreated
- Atrophy of urethra
- Osteoporosis - approximately 2% loss of bone mass/year. Most common in Caucasians and Orientals and least common in African-Americans.
- Arteriosclerosis
- Ovarian stroma only - or only a few inactive oocytes

SPECIAL TESTS
- Endometrial biopsy and/or D&C in patients who have intermenstrual or postmenopausal bleeding - may be accompanied by hysteroscopy. Investigation for endometrial cancer is necessary even in the presence of an atrophic vagina (usually the cause of the bleeding).
- Bleeding may also be evaluated by vaginal sonography; if double wall thickness of endometrial stripe is less than 5 mm, endometrial carcinoma is highly unlikely

IMAGING
- None for physiologic menopause
- MRI scan of head if pituitary tumor suspected

DIAGNOSTIC PROCEDURES
- Endometrial sampling if intermenstrual or post menopausal bleeding occurs
- Pap smear
- Bimanual pelvic examination
- Mammography annually
- Bone density determination of hip/spine

TREATMENT

APPROPRIATE HEALTH CARE Periodic office visits

GENERAL MEASURES
- To retard development of osteoporosis: adequate calcium intake; exercise; avoid smoking, avoid excessive alcohol or caffeine intake
- HRT for prophylaxis against osteoporosis, relief of vasomotor symptoms and urogenital atrophy. Exceptions are women with contraindications to therapy and obese women (who usually have sufficient endogenous estrogens produced by peripheral conversion of androgens by adipose tissue).
- HRT has a favorable effect on lipoproteins; elevates HDL and may retard progression of Alzheimer disease (no proof for prevention).

SURGICAL MEASURES N/A

ACTIVITY Active, weight-bearing exercise.

DIET Increased calcium intake, adequate Vitamin D, high fiber, low fat, decreased caffeine and alcohol intake

PATIENT EDUCATION
- American College of Obstetricians and Gynecologists (ACOG), 409 12th St. S.W., Washington, D.C. 20024, (800)673-8444; www.acog.com
- For a listing of sources for patient education materials favorably reviewed on this topic, physicians may contact: American Academy of Family Physicians Foundation, P.O. Box 8418, Kansas City, MO 64114, (800)274-2237, ext. 4400; www.familydoctor.org
- www. Menopause.com
- www.femalehealthlinks.com

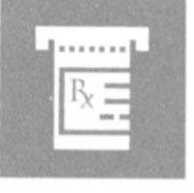

MEDICATIONS

DRUG(S) OF CHOICE
- Estrogens: commonly oral estrogen, conjugated (Premarin) or estradiol
  - ◊ For retarding osteoporosis 0.625 mg qd. Doses as low as 0.3 mg, used in conjunction with medroxyprogesterone and adequate calcium and vitamin D supplementation, is also effective.
  - ◊ If vasomotor symptoms persist at 0.625 mg, increase to 0.9 mg or 1.25 mg, however, optimal cardioprotective effect is 0.625 mg
- Progestogen: commonly medroxyprogesterone (Provera, Depo-Provera)
  - ◊ Because estrogens are carcinogenic to the endometrium, a progestogen should be added for its protective effect against endometrial cancer. (If the uterus has been removed, a progestogen is not needed.)
- Combination: conjugated estrogen-medroxyprogesterone (Prempro) or ethinyl estradiol-norethindrone (FemHRT) or estradiol-norethindrone (Activella)

- Bisphosphonates: only agents shown to reduce spine and nonspine fractures; commonly:
  - ◊ Alendronate (Fosamax) 10 mg qd or 70 mg every week
  - ◊ Risedronate (Actonel) 5 mg qd or 30 mg every week
- Calcium: 1500 mg elemental calcium per day
- Vitamin D: 600 to 800 IU per day
- Administration
  - ◊ Estrogens and progestogens may be administered continuously (no withdrawal bleeding expected) or cyclically
  - ◊ Common regimens: Premarin 0.625 mg + Provera 2.5 mg q day or Premarin 0.625 mg for 25 days per month + Provera 5 mg during the last 14 days of estrogen therapy OR Premarin 0.625 mg daily + Provera 5 mg during 14 days of month. Fixed combinations (Prempro, Premphase) may be convenient. Another option is Premarin and micronized progesterone.

Contraindications:
- Estrogen dependent malignancies
- Unexplained abnormal uterine bleeding
- History of thrombophlebitis
- Active liver disease
- Malignant melanoma

Precautions:
- Continuous combination therapy should not result in uterine bleeding
- Women on cyclic therapy may bleed normally only during those days when no therapy is given. Any other bleeding must be evaluated for the possibility of endometrial cancer.
- Higher doses of estrogen can cause hypercoagulability, breast tenderness, gall bladder disease and hypertension
- Combination estrogen/progestin therapy has been shown to increase risk of invasive breast cancer, coronary heart disease, stroke and pulmonary embolism after more than 5 years of use

Significant possible interactions: N/A

ALTERNATIVE DRUGS
- Other forms of estrogen used:
  - ◊ Oral: estropipate (Ogen) 0.625 mg, estradiol (Estrace) 1-2 mg
  - ◊ Transdermal: estradiol (Estraderm, Esclim, Vivelle, Alora, Climara) 0.05-0.1 mg/day applied twice weekly, or 0.05-0.1 mg/day applied weekly (Climara)
  - ◊ Vaginal: conjugated estrogens (Premarin cream) - best for local therapy of atrophic vaginitis only; blood levels are unpredictable.
  - ◊ Intramuscular: not recommended - may not be protective against coronary artery disease without first passing through the liver
- For women who cannot take estrogens - using progestogens (Depo-Provera) 150 mg IM every month is helpful in alleviating hot flashes. This may retard the development of osteoporosis, but is not helpful in preventing coronary artery disease or urogenital atrophy.
- Raloxifene (Evista) 60 mg/day has been shown to increase bone density, decrease vertebral and hip fractures and decrease risk of breast cancer
- Androgens/testosterone can increase libido and protect bone mass; can decrease triglyceride and HDL levels
- Clonidine (Catapres), oral or transdermal, may be used to treat vasomotor symptoms, but is not effective against other menopausal occurrences
- Calcitonin produces only a temporary increase in body calcium
- Phytoestrogens (soy isoflavone) act as selective estrogen receptor modulators; other alternative agents include black cohosh, garlic, catnip, belladonna, passion flower, chamomile
- Parathyroid hormone may increase bone density and decrease vertebral fractures

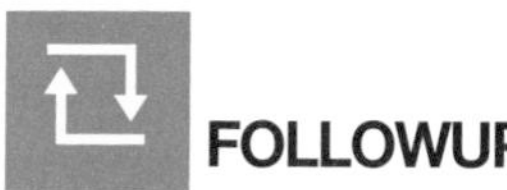

FOLLOWUP

PATIENT MONITORING
- Annual Pap smear, pelvic and breast exams
- Monthly breast self-examination
- Annual mammography
- Endometrial sampling in patients with abnormal bleeding

PREVENTION/AVOIDANCE
Menopause is a physiological process. It cannot be avoided, but the untoward effects can be moderated or eliminated by HRT.

POSSIBLE COMPLICATIONS
- Vasomotor symptoms
- Uncomfortable psychologic symptoms
- Vaginal atrophy
- Skin wrinkles
- Osteoporosis
- Arteriosclerosis
- Urinary tract symptoms

EXPECTED COURSE/PROGNOSIS
- If untreated
  - ◊ Ultimate disappearance of vasomotor symptoms - usually takes several years
  - ◊ Urogenital atrophy
  - ◊ Osteoporosis - possible fractures especially of the hip, vertebrae and wrists. Mortality associated with hip fractures is 15%.
  - ◊ Coronary artery disease - increased risk
- If treated
  - ◊ Minimal effects of estrogen deprivation
  - ◊ Slower bone loss and reduced incidence of coronary artery disease. Delayed appearance of Alzheimer disease

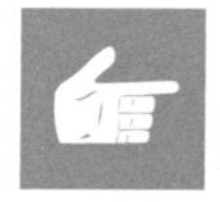

MISCELLANEOUS

ASSOCIATED CONDITIONS
Any medical problems that may occur with increasing age, especially osteoporosis

AGE-RELATED FACTORS
Pediatric: N/A
Geriatric: N/A
Others: N/A

PREGNANCY
Mutually exclusive

SYNONYMS
- Climacteric
- Ovarian failure

ICD-9-CM
627.0 Premenopausal menorrhagia
627.2 Symptomatic menopausal or female climacteric states
627.4 Symptomatic states associated with artificial menopause
716.30 Climacteric arthritis, site unspecified

SEE ALSO
Osteoporosis
Uterine bleeding postmenopausal

OTHER NOTES
- Estrogen replacement therapy is especially important in women having an early menopause, either spontaneous or surgical. Without such therapy, they may be at a significantly increased risk for osteoporosis.
- Following surgical menopause, vasomotor symptoms often appear very rapidly. Estrogen replacement therapy may be started in the early postoperative period.
- In perimenopausal women bothered by severe vasomotor symptoms, cyclic estrogen and progestogen therapy may be started even though the patient is still having periodic uterine bleeding

ABBREVIATIONS
ERT = estrogen replacement therapy
HRT = hormone replacement therapy
SERM = selective estrogen receptor modulator

REFERENCES

- Risks and benefits of estrogen plus progestin in healthy postmenopausal women: principal results From the Women's Health Initiative randomized controlled trial. JAMA 2002;288(3):321-33
- Cufson TM, Meuleman E. Managing menopause. Am Fam Phys 2000;61(5);1391-1400
- American Association of Clinical Endocrinologists. Guidelines for clinical procedures for management of menopause. Endoc Pract 1999;5(6):354-66
- Achilles C, Leppert PC. The menopausal woman. In: Leppert PC, Howard FM (editors). Primary Care for Women. Philadelphia, Lippincott-Raven, 1997:p97-102
- Grodstein F, et al. A prospective, observational study of postmenopausal hormone therapy and primary prevention of cardiovascular disease. Ann Intern Med 2000;133:933-41
- Recker R, et al. The effect of low-dose continuous estrogen and progesterone therapy with calcium and vitamin d on bone in elderly women. Ann Intern Med 1999;130:897-904

Web references: 1 available at www.5mcc.com
Illustrations N/A

Author(s):
Anna N. Maxey, MD
Michael A. Cooper, MD

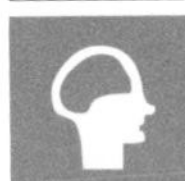

BASICS

DESCRIPTION Excessive amount or duration of menstrual flow, at more or less regular intervals
- Distinguish from, but may overlap with:
  - ◊ Metrorrhagia - irregular or frequent flow, noncyclic
  - ◊ Menometrorrhagia - frequent, excessive, irregular flow (menorrhagia plus metrorrhagia)
  - ◊ Polymenorrhea - frequent flow, cycles of 21 days or less
  - ◊ Intermenstrual bleeding - bleeding between regular menses
  - ◊ Dysfunctional uterine bleeding (DUB) - abnormal endometrial bleeding of hormonal cause and related to anovulation

System(s) affected: Reproductive
Genetics: N/A
Incidence/Prevalence in USA: Abnormal bleeding is common; prevalence varies with definition (endometrial carcinoma: about 40,000 new cases per year)
Predominant age:
- Menarche to menopause; about 50% of cases occur after 40 years of age
- Dysfunctional bleeding is fairly common in adolescence and near menopause

Predominant sex: Female only

SIGNS & SYMPTOMS
- "Excessive" menstrual flow defined subjectively varies greatly from woman to woman (average normal menstrual flow is about 30-40 mL per cycle)
- Useful historical features include:
  - ◊ Bleeding substantially heavier than the patient's usual flow
  - ◊ Bleeding lasting more than 7 days
  - ◊ Flow associated with passage of significant clots
  - ◊ Anemia
- The following symptoms tend to suggest that cycles are ovulatory:
  - ◊ Regular menstrual interval
  - ◊ Mid-cycle pain (mittelschmerz)
  - ◊ Dysmenorrhea
  - ◊ Premenstrual symptoms - breast soreness, mood changes, etc.
- Abdominal pain or cramps at other times of the cycle may be associated with structural causes:
  - ◊ Myomas
  - ◊ Polyps
  - ◊ Ovarian tumors
- Hirsutism or acne
  - ◊ May accompany polycystic ovarian syndrome

CAUSES
- Hypothyroidism
- Endometrial proliferation/excess/hyperplasia:
  - ◊ Anovulation, oligo-ovulation
  - ◊ Polycystic ovarian disease (PCOD)
  - ◊ Ovarian tumor
  - ◊ Obesity
  - ◊ Hormone (estrogen) therapy
- Endometrial atrophy:
  - ◊ Postmenopause
  - ◊ Prolonged progestin or oral contraceptive administration
- Local factors:
  - ◊ Endometrial polyps
  - ◊ Endometrial neoplasia
  - ◊ Adenomyosis/endometriosis
  - ◊ Uterine myomata (fibroids)
  - ◊ Intrauterine device (IUD)
  - ◊ Uterine sarcoma
- Coagulation disorders:
  - ◊ Thrombocytopenia, platelet disorders
  - ◊ von Willebrand disease
  - ◊ Leukemia
  - ◊ Ingestion of aspirin or anticoagulants
  - ◊ Renal failure/dialysis

RISK FACTORS
- Obesity
- Anovulation
- Estrogen administration (without progestin)
- Prior treatment with progestational agents or oral contraceptives increases the risk of endometrial atrophy, but decreases the risk of endometrial hyperplasia or neoplasia

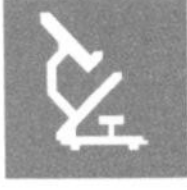

DIAGNOSIS

DIFFERENTIAL DIAGNOSIS
- Pregnancy complications:
  - ◊ Threatened abortion
  - ◊ Incomplete abortion
  - ◊ Ectopic pregnancy
- Nonuterine bleeding:
  - ◊ Cervical ectropion/erosion
  - ◊ Cervical neoplasia/polyp
  - ◊ Cervical or vaginal trauma
  - ◊ Condylomata
  - ◊ Atrophic vaginitis
  - ◊ Foreign bodies
- Pelvic inflammatory disease (PID):
  - ◊ Endometritis
  - ◊ Tuberculosis

LABORATORY
- Pregnancy test
- CBC to assess severity of blood loss, exclude thrombocytopenia and leukemia
- In selected cases:
  - ◊ TSH - elevated in hypothyroidism
  - ◊ Platelet count, bleeding time, prothrombin time (PT), partial thromboplastin time (PTT) for coagulation screen
  - ◊ Creatinine, BUN
  - ◊ Serum progesterone - 5-20 ng/mL (15.9-63.6 nmol/L) in luteal phase, < 1 ng/mL (< 3.18 nmol/L) in follicular phase or anovulatory cycle

Drugs that may alter lab results: Progestins used prior to endometrial biopsy may cause decidualization and obscure true diagnosis

Disorders that may alter lab results: N/A

PATHOLOGICAL FINDINGS Vary with cause: see Causes

SPECIAL TESTS Endometrial biopsy detects hyperplasia, dysplasia, or atrophy. If done prior to expected menses, may also help make the diagnosis of anovulation or luteal phase defect.

IMAGING
- Ultrasonography to evaluate adnexal masses or fibroids suspected from pelvic exam
- Transvaginal ultrasonography to measure thickness of endometrium may help distinguish bleeding due to atrophy from bleeding due to hyperplasia
- Computerized tomography used in investigation of potentially malignant pelvic masses

DIAGNOSTIC PROCEDURES
- Pelvic and rectal examination
- Pap smear
- Endometrial biopsy
- Diagnostic dilatation and curettage
- Hysteroscopy

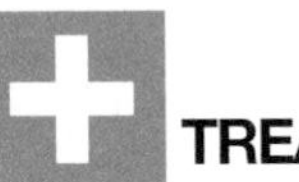

TREATMENT

APPROPRIATE HEALTH CARE
- Most cases can be managed as outpatients in office or emergency department
- Hospitalize for bleeding accompanied by orthostatic hypotension or hematocrit < 25%

GENERAL MEASURES
- Rule out pregnancy complications and non-uterine bleeding
- Treat severe or life-threatening bleeding acutely:
  - ◊ Intravenous estrogen
  - ◊ Curettage if necessary
  - ◊ Hysterectomy in extreme case
- Proceed to identify underlying cause of bleeding and treat to prevent recurrence
  - ◊ Hormonal therapy
  - ◊ Dilatation and curettage for hormone-unresponsive cases
  - ◊ Consider endometrial ablation or hysterectomy in persistent cases where fertility is not desired
  - ◊ Specific treatment for neoplasia, polyps, systemic disease, etc.
  - ◊ Patients who desire fertility may also need appropriate treatment for anovulation, endometriosis, myomata, etc.

SURGICAL MEASURES See general Measures

ACTIVITY As tolerated. Resting with feet elevated may be helpful.

DIET Iron supplementation may help correct for increased blood loss

PATIENT EDUCATION Information about side effects of medications

MEDICATIONS

DRUG(S) OF CHOICE
- For acute control of severe bleeding:
  - ◊ Estrogen, conjugated (Premarin) 25 mg IV every 4 hours up to 6 doses until bleeding abates
- For less severe bleeding or after control of acute bleeding:
  - ◊ Medroxyprogesterone acetate (Provera) 10-30 mg daily for 5-10 days
  - ◊ Any combination oral contraceptive, (usually one of the "high dose" oral contraceptives) one tablet 4 times a day for 5-7 days
- To prevent heavy bleeding in subsequent cycles:
  - ◊ Medroxyprogesterone acetate 10-20 mg daily for 10 days per month
  - ◊ Usual cyclic dose of a combination oral contraceptive
- For endometrial atrophy in postmenopausal woman:
  - ◊ Estrogen plus progesterone replacement therapy

Contraindications:
- To estrogen, oral contraceptives, or progestins:
  - ◊ Pregnancy
  - ◊ Breast or endometrial cancer
  - ◊ Thromboembolic disease, past or present
  - ◊ Impaired liver function

Precautions:
- Nausea and vomiting are common from IV estrogen; antiemetics are helpful
- Estrogen may precipitate acute intermittent porphyria or cholestatic jaundice in susceptible individuals

Significant possible interactions: Refer to manufacturer's profile of each drug

ALTERNATIVE DRUGS
- Non-steroidal prostaglandin-synthetase inhibitors (naproxen, mefenamic acid, ibuprofen, and others) can reduce blood loss with ovulatory cycles and reduce dysmenorrhea
- Norethindrone acetate (Aygestin) 2.5-10 mg daily for 10 days per month, during the assumed latter half of menstrual cycle
- Danazol and GnRH agonists are also effective therapies, but more likely to have adverse side effects
- Megestrol acetate (Megace) 40 mg daily for 10 days per month (caution required to prevent progression to endometrial carcinoma)
- Megestrol acetate (Megace) 40 mg daily continuously to treat atypical hyperplasia

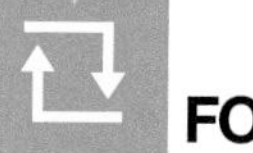

FOLLOWUP

PATIENT MONITORING
- Varies with cause of bleeding
- Medical treatment of hyperplastic/dysplastic endometrium should be followed by repeat biopsy to confirm that histologic structure has returned to normal

PREVENTION/AVOIDANCE
Pap smear and pelvic examination annually

POSSIBLE COMPLICATIONS
Anemia

EXPECTED COURSE/PROGNOSIS
- Varies with cause of bleeding
- Most patients with hormonal causes will respond to hormonal manipulation

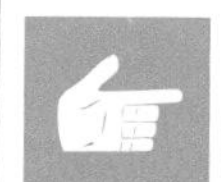

MISCELLANEOUS

ASSOCIATED CONDITIONS
Metrorrhagia; menometrorrhagia; androgenic disorders

AGE-RELATED FACTORS
Pediatric: Genital bleeding prior to puberty can result from trauma, foreign bodies, vaginal infection, or exogenous hormone administration

Geriatric: Genital atrophy may predispose to bleeding with minimal trauma. Neoplasm of ovary or endometrium must be ruled out.

Others:
- In adolescence, irregular bleeding due to anovulation and immaturity of the hypothalamic-pituitary-ovarian axis is common
- Beyond age 35-40, endometrial dysplasia and endometrial carcinoma are significant causes of bleeding. Obtain endometrial sampling before attempting hormonal treatment.

PREGNANCY
Bleeding in pregnancy is not menorrhagia. Complications of pregnancy or cervical/vaginal lesions should be considered.

SYNONYMS
N/A

ICD-9-CM
621.0 Polyp of corpus uteri
621.3 Endometrial cystic hyperplasia
621.8 Other specified disorders of uterus, NEC
626.2 Excessive or frequent menstruation
626.3 Puberty bleeding
626.4 Irregular menstrual cycle
626.6 Metrorrhagia
626.8 Disorders of menstruation and other abnormal bleeding from female genital tract, other
627.0 Premenopausal menorrhagia
627.1 Postmenopausal bleeding

SEE ALSO
Amenorrhea
Cervical dysplasia
Cervical malignancy
Cervical polyps
Cervicitis
Cervicitis, ectropion & true erosion
Dysmenorrhea
Menopause
Polycystic ovarian disease
Uterine myomas

OTHER NOTES
N/A

ABBREVIATIONS
N/A

REFERENCES

- Wentz AC. Abnormal Uterine Bleeding. In: Jones HW, ed. Novak's Textbook of Gynecology. 11th ed. Baltimore: Williams & Wilkins; 1988
- Cowan BD, Morrison JC. Management of abnormal genital bleeding in girls and women. N Engl J Med 1991;324(24):1710-15
- Dysfunctional uterine bleeding. In: Speroff L, Glass RH, Kase NG, eds. Clinical Gynecologic Endocrinology and Infertility. 6th ed. Baltimore: Williams & Wilkins; 1999: p575-93
- Carlson JM. Menorrhagia and Metrorrhagia. In: Friedman EA, ed. Gynecologic Decision Making. 2nd ed. Philadelphia: B.C. Decker; 1988
- Bonnar J, Sheppard B. Treatment of menorrhagia during menstruation. BMJ 1996;313:579-82

Web references: 1 available at www.5mcc.com

Illustrations N/A

Author(s):
Donald A. F. Nelson, MD

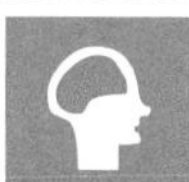

BASICS

DESCRIPTION Mental retardation (MR) is a symptom with multiple etiologies including chromosomal abnormalities, genetic defects, intrauterine, perinatal, neonatal, and postnatal causes. Mental retardation refers to substantial limitations in present functioning. It is characterized by significantly subaverage intellectual functioning, existing concurrently with related limitations in two or more of the following applicable adaptive skills areas: communication, self-care, home living, social skills, community use, self-direction, health and safety, functional academics, leisure and work. Cognitive and adaptive behavior deficits are manifested before age 18.

- Subgroups of mentally retarded:
  - ◊ Mild: IQ 55-69 (85%)
  - ◊ Moderate: IQ 40-54 (10%)
  - ◊ Severe: IQ 25-39 (5%)
  - ◊ Profound: IQ 0-24 (<1%)

System(s) affected: Nervous

Genetics:

- Autosomes: Trisomies and rearrangements - approximately 1500 variations are all associated with MR
- Sex chromosomes: 80 of 336 disorders cause MR
- Autosomal dominant: 180 of 3,000 disorders cause MR
- Autosomal recessive: 400 of 1,550 disorders cause MR

Incidence/Prevalence in USA: Incidence and prevalence are closely related to social, economic, and health conditions of the society. The general incidence of mental retardation in the United States has been estimated at 125,000 births per year by the American Association on Mental Retardation. This would correspond to approximately 3% of the population. The research on both incidence and prevalence of mental retardation in the US is exceedingly scant. A comprehensive Canadian study of the maritime Provinces found prevalences of 3.65 per 1000. Most professionals associated with the American Association on Mental Retardation accept a prevalence of 2.5% and they recognize that the prevalence varies with chronological age. Specifically, mildly retarded preschoolers are able to meet societies demands but are identified by the school system due to demands for cognitive processing. Conversely, once they leave the requirements of the educational system they may adapt to societies demands and the diagnosis need not apply.

Predominant age: By definition mental retardation occurs during the developmental period. Older adults who lose mental faculties are more accurately diagnosed as demented. Patients may present the MR after traumatic brain injury.

Predominant sex: Male > Female (1.5:1)

SIGNS & SYMPTOMS

- Profoundly and severely retarded children are frequently diagnosed at the time of birth or during the newborn period. Children with profound or severe retardation are more likely to have dysmorphic features.
- Moderately retarded children may go undiagnosed until they fail to meet normal developmental milestones
- Mildly retarded children may go undiagnosed until well into the school years

CAUSES

- Chromosomal abnormalities
  - ◊ Autosomal abnormalities
  - ◊ Trisomy, e.g., Down syndrome
  - ◊ Translocations
  - ◊ Inversions
  - ◊ Duplications
  - ◊ Deletions, e.g., Prader-Willi
- Sex chromosome abnormalities
  - ◊ Fragile X mutation
  - ◊ Turner syndrome
  - ◊ Klinefelter syndrome
  - ◊ Rett syndrome
  - ◊ Various multiple X and/or Y conditions
- Autosomal dominant conditions
  - ◊ Neurocutaneous syndromes, e.g., neurofibromatosis, tuberous sclerosis
- Autosomal recessive conditions
  - ◊ Amino acid metabolism, e.g., phenylketonuria, Maple syrup urine disease
  - ◊ Carbohydrate metabolism, e.g., galactosemia, fructosuria
  - ◊ Lipid metabolism
  - ◊ Tay-Sachs
  - ◊ Gaucher
  - ◊ Niemann-Pick, e.g., mucopolysaccharidosis
  - ◊ Purine metabolism, e.g., Lesch-Nyhan
  - ◊ Other, e.g., Wilson
- Multifactorial and sporadic conditions
  - ◊ Cornelia de Lange syndrome
  - ◊ Spinal cord disorders (spina bifida, Arnold-Chiari malformation)
  - ◊ Disorders of brain and skull
  - ◊ Prenatal factors
  - ◊ Rh incompatibility
  - ◊ Maternal infections - all the TORCH viruses - rubella, toxoplasmosis, cytomegalovirus, and herpes simplex)
  - ◊ Maternal diseases, e.g., diabetes mellitus, toxemia
  - ◊ Maternal substance abuse, e.g., alcohol use/abuse. Fetal alcohol syndrome is a leading environmental cause of mental retardation.
  - ◊ Prescription medications, such as Accutane or Dilantin
- Perinatal factors
  - ◊ Prematurity
  - ◊ Postmaturity
  - ◊ Birth injuries
  - ◊ High risk mothers
- Postnatal factors
  - ◊ Childhood diseases, e.g., meningitis, encephalitis, general inflammatory disease with high fever, hypothyroidism
  - ◊ Trauma, e.g., accidents, physical abuse, marked deprivation
  - ◊ Poisoning, e.g., lead, carbon monoxide, household products

RISK FACTORS

Risk factors for future offspring of the parent couple must be calculated based upon the specific etiology of related retarded individuals

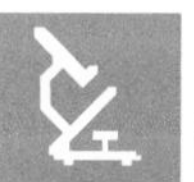

DIAGNOSIS

DIFFERENTIAL DIAGNOSIS

- Brain tumors
- Hearing and/or speech impairment
- Infantile autism
- Cerebral palsy
- Emotional disturbance
- Lack of environmental opportunities for appropriate development

LABORATORY

- Specific studies are available for those patients with identifiable genetic disease entities
- Chromosome studies
- Metabolic screens
- Amino acid
- Sugar substrates
- Molecular studies, e.g., DNA

Drugs that may alter lab results: N/A

Disorders that may alter lab results: N/A

PATHOLOGICAL FINDINGS

N/A

SPECIAL TESTS

- Individually administered measure of intellectual abilities
  - ◊ Measure utilized depends upon the age of the patient
  - ◊ Birth through 42 months: Bayley Scales of Infant Development-II
  - ◊ 2 years of age through adulthood: Stanford Binet (4th edition), Wechsler Scales
  - ◊ Preschool children: WPPSI-III
  - ◊ School age: WISC-III
  - ◊ Adults: WAIS-III, and an adaptive behavior scale. All patients need a measure of adaptive behavior. The Vineland Adaptive Behavior Scales are widely utilized.
  - ◊ Other measures are available; however, these are the most widely recognized and utilized measures of individual ability and adaptive behavior

IMAGING

N/A

DIAGNOSTIC PROCEDURES

See Special tests

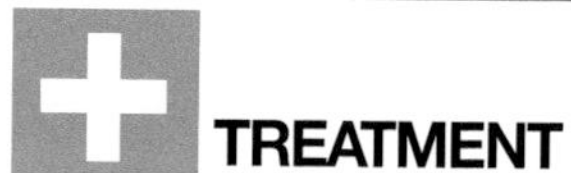

TREATMENT

APPROPRIATE HEALTH CARE
- Some specialized care may be necessary based upon the etiology of the retardation
- Care for the retarded is educational, not medical and should include early intervention

GENERAL MEASURES N/A

SURGICAL MEASURES N/A

ACTIVITY Full activity

DIET No research evidence supports the use of specific diets for mental retardation and/or Attention Deficit Hyperactivity Disorder (ADHD). Exception: Some metabolic and storage disorders, i.e., PKU.

PATIENT EDUCATION Parental education and consultation as to the development of appropriate behavioral and educational expectations are strongly advised. Families should be referred to the local Association for Retarded Citizens; web site www.thearc.org.

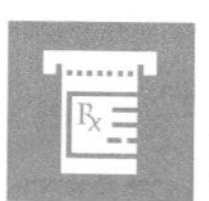

MEDICATIONS

DRUG(S) OF CHOICE None
Contraindications: N/A
Precautions: N/A
Significant possible interactions: N/A

ALTERNATIVE DRUGS N/A

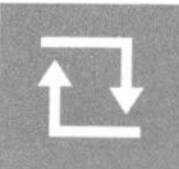

FOLLOWUP

PATIENT MONITORING Regular pediatric care

PREVENTION/AVOIDANCE N/A

POSSIBLE COMPLICATIONS Learning inappropriate behaviors

EXPECTED COURSE/PROGNOSIS
- Mild retardation: Social and communication skills appropriate for community functioning, basic job skills, and functional literacy
- Moderate mental retardation: Speech deficits, social awareness, personal care skills, i.e., dressing, feeding, washing, sheltered employment, group home living
- Severe mental retardation: Limited speech and language, poor motor development, in need of supervision
- Profound mental retardation: Neurological defect, poor cognitive social ability, absent speech, possible self harm, extended care
- Specific etiologies (e.g., Down syndrome and fragile X patients) show a decline in cognitive and adaptive behavior scores

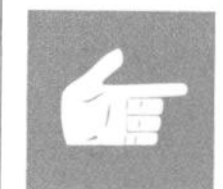

MISCELLANEOUS

ASSOCIATED CONDITIONS
- Speech problems
- Seizures
- Maladaptive behaviors
- Attention deficit hyperactivity disorder (ADHD):
  - ◊ Found with greater frequency among individuals with neuropsychological dysfunction
  - ◊ Treatment for ADHD among the mentally retarded is not unlike that for the "normal" population
  - ◊ Data indicates overuse of psychoactive substances to aid caretakers

AGE-RELATED FACTORS
Pediatric: N/A
Geriatric: N/A
Others: N/A

PREGNANCY Parents and first degree relatives could benefit from consultation with a genetic associate or counselor

SYNONYMS Mental deficiency

ICD-9-CM
317 Mild mental retardation
318.0 Moderate mental retardation
318.1 Severe mental retardation
318.2 Profound mental retardation
319 Unspecified mental retardation

SEE ALSO
Attention deficit/Hyperactivity disorder
Cerebral palsy
Down syndrome
Fragile X syndrome
Lead poisoning
Williams syndrome

OTHER NOTES
- Extensive family history to aid in diagnosis is mandatory
- Genetic referral in cases without known etiology is appropriate

ABBREVIATIONS
MR = mental retardation

REFERENCES

- Stevenson RE, Schwartz CE, Schroer RJ. X-Linked Mental Retardation. Oxford, Oxford University Press, 2000
- Gorlin RJ, Cohen MM, Hennekam RCM. Syndromes of the Head and Neck. 4th Ed. Oxford, Oxford University Press, 2001
- Baroff GS, Olley JG. Mental Retardation. 3rd Ed. Philadelphia, Brunner/Mazel, 1999
- Jones KL. Smith's Recognizable Patterns of Human Malformations. 5th Ed. Philadelphia, W. B. Saunders, 1997
- Weiderman HR, Kunze J. Clinical syndromes. 3rd Ed. English translation. London, Mosby-Wolfe, 1997
- Baraitser M, Winter RM. Color Atlas of Congenital Malformation Syndromes. London, Mosby-Wolfe, 1996

Web references: 5 available at www.5mcc.com
Illustrations N/A

Author(s):
Richard J. Simensen, PhD
Gene S. Fisch, PhD

BASICS

DESCRIPTION General term for pain of the plantar surface of the forefoot in the metatarsal head region
System(s) affected: Musculoskeletal
Genetics: N/A
Incidence/Prevalence in USA: Common
Predominant age: to 80's
Predominant sex: Female > Male

SIGNS & SYMPTOMS
- Acute, chronic or recurrent symptoms located in the region of the metatarsal heads usually on the plantar surface.
- Pain - often described like walking with a pebble in the shoe
- Swelling
- Tenderness of the metatarsal head(s) with pressure applied between the examiner and finger
- Calluses
- Erythema (occasionally)

CAUSES
- Abnormal pressure distribution plantar to the metatarsal heads
- General
  - ◊ Excessive or repetitive stress - high heels, ballet dancers, competitive athletes
  - ◊ Soft tissue dysfunction - intrinsic muscle weakness, laxity of the Lisfranc ligament
  - ◊ Abnormal foot posture - forefoot varus or valgus, cavus or equinus deformities, loss of the metatarsal arch, splay foot, pronated foot
  - ◊ Dermatologic - warts, callous
- Great toe
  - ◊ Hallux valgus (bunion), varus or rigidus
- Lesser metatarsals
  - ◊ Freiberg's infraction (aseptic necrosis of the metatarsal head usually in adolescents who jump or sprint)
  - ◊ Hammertoe or claw toe
  - ◊ Morton syndrome (long second metatarsal)

RISK FACTORS
- Obesity
- High heels or narrow shoes
- Competitive athletes for weight bearing sports (ballet, basketball, etc)
- Foot deformities (pes planus, pes cavus, tight Achilles, tarsal tunnel syndrome)

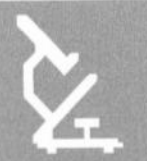

DIAGNOSIS

DIFFERENTIAL DIAGNOSIS
- Stress fracture (most commonly 2nd metatarsal)
- Morton neuroma (interdigital neuroma)
- Sesamoiditis or sesamoid fracture
- Arthritis (rheumatoid, inflammatory, osteoarthritis, septic)
- Infection (cellulitis, diabetic foot, Lyme disease, leprosy)
- Bone tumors (rare)
- Ganglion cyst
- Foreign body
- Vasculitis (diabetes)

LABORATORY Only if diagnosis is in question: ESR, RF, HLA Ag, VDRL, uric acid, glucose, CBC with differential.

Drugs that may alter lab results: N/A

Disorders that may alter lab results: Acute infections

PATHOLOGICAL FINDINGS Because of its two sesamoid bones the first metatarsal head usually carries 2/6 of the weight when walking. The normal metatarsal arch also assures this balance. The first metatarsal head has adequate padding to accommodate. A pronated splayfoot disturbs this balance, causing equal weight bearing on all metatarsal heads. Any foot deformity will also change the distribution of weight to areas of the foot that do not have sufficient padding.

SPECIAL TESTS N/A

IMAGING
- Weight-bearing films AP, lateral and oblique views. Occasionally metatarsal or sesamoid axial films (to r/o sesamoid fracture), or skyline view of the metatarsal heads - obtained with the metatarsophalangeal joints in dorsiflexion (to evaluate alignment).
- Bone scan if high index of suspicion of stress fracture

DIAGNOSTIC PROCEDURES N/A

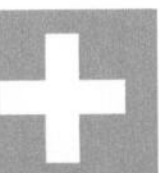

TREATMENT

APPROPRIATE HEALTH CARE
Outpatient

GENERAL MEASURES
- Relieve pain
  - ◊ Rest - temporary alteration of weight bearing activity, cane or crutch; for active patients, suggest an alternative exercise, cross train
  - ◊ Ice initially
  - ◊ Moist heat later
  - ◊ Taping or Gelcast
  - ◊ Stiff-soled shoes will act as a splint
- Relieve the pressure beneath the area of maximal pain:
  - ◊ Weight loss
  - ◊ Low heeled wide-toe-box shoes
  - ◊ Metatarsal pads and arch supports
  - ◊ Orthotics
  - ◊ Thick-soled shoes
- Improve flexibility and strength of the muscles of the foot:
  - ◊ Exercises (towel grasps and pencil curls)
  - ◊ Physical therapy - rarely

SURGICAL MEASURES If there is a correctable anatomical abnormality: bunionectomy, partial ostectomy, osteotomy, or surgical fusion

ACTIVITY
- Alteration of weight-bearing exercises may be temporarily necessary
- Use cross-training principles (bicycle or swimming instead of running for the acute phase)
- Gradual return to previous level of activities with arch support in running shoes

DIET N/A

PATIENT EDUCATION Instruct about proper shoes and gradual return to activity. See Web references for patient handout.

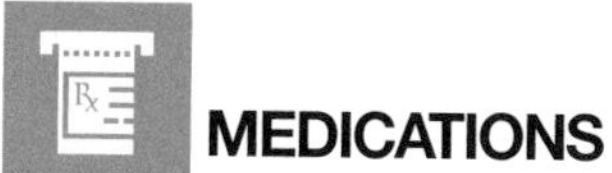

MEDICATIONS

DRUG(S) OF CHOICE

- NSAIDs (ibuprofen 800 mg tid 7-14 days or naproxen 500 bid 7-14 days)

Contraindications:

- GI bleed or ulcer

Precautions:

- Renal disease
- Hepatic disease
- Coagulation disorders

Significant possible interactions:

- Anticoagulants
- Digoxin
- Lithium
- Methotrexate
- Cyclosporin

ALTERNATIVE DRUGS COX 2 inhibitors

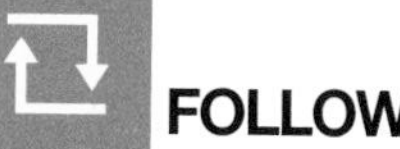

FOLLOWUP

PATIENT MONITORING Follow up visit at 2 weeks if not improved or worsened. If stress fracture has been ruled out and not improved after 6 months of conservative treatment consider surgical evaluation.

PREVENTION/AVOIDANCE Proper shoes.

POSSIBLE COMPLICATIONS Back, knee, and hip pain due to change in gait

EXPECTED COURSE/PROGNOSIS

The outcome is dependent on the severity of the problem and whether surgery is required to correct it

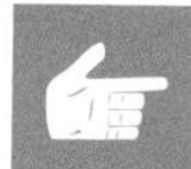

MISCELLANEOUS

ASSOCIATED CONDITIONS see Causes

AGE-RELATED FACTORS

Pediatric:

- Muscle imbalance disorders (Duchenne muscular dystrophy, etc) are a cause of foot deformities in children
- In adolescent females consider Freiberg's infraction (aseptic necrosis of the metatarsal head usually in adolescents who jump or sprint)

Geriatric:

- Arthritis should be ruled out early
- More frequent in older athletes and the aging.
- Symptoms are more pronounced.

Others: N/A

PREGNANCY

- Forefoot pain during pregnancy usually is secondary to the change in gait, increased weight, and joint laxity
- Well-fitting low-heeled shoes are especially important in this group of patients

SYNONYMS N/A

ICD-9-CM

726.70 Enthesopathy of ankle and tarsus, unspecified

SEE ALSO

Morton neuroma (interdigital neuroma)

OTHER NOTES N/A

ABBREVIATIONS N/A

REFERENCES

- Wu K. Morton neuroma and metatarsalgia. Curr Opin Rhuematol 2000;12:131-142
- Birrer R. Common foot problems in primary care. 2 Ed. Ch. 8: Metatarsals, Philadelphia, Hanley & Belfus, Inc., 1998:67-73
- vanWyngarden TM. The painful foot, Part I: Common forefoot deformities. Am Fam Phys 1997;55(5):1866-1876
- Merril D.P.M. Medical and Surgical Therapeutics of the Foot and Ankle. Part 4: Metatarsalgia. Baltimore, Williams & Wilkins, 1992: 384-390
- Cailliet R. Foot and Ankle Pain. 3 Ed. Philadelphia, F.A. Davis Co., 1997:141-147

Web references: 1 available at www.5mcc.com

Illustrations N/A

Author(s):

Frances Biagioli, MD

BASICS

DESCRIPTION

- Methanol is a solvent found in many commercial and industrial fluids like anti-freezes, windshield-washing fluids, paints, liquid fuels, and photocopying fluid. Methanol is commonly consumed by alcoholics who cannot find or purchase a source of ethyl alcohol. Rare intoxications occur after respiratory or environmental exposures.
- Fatal dose is 15-240 mL depending on concentration
- Peak blood levels occur 30-90 minutes after ingestion
- Methanol is mainly excreted by hepatic biotransformation into formaldehyde and formic acid that leads to retinal inflammation and blindness, acidosis, inebriation, and CNS depression.

System(s) affected: Gastrointestinal, Nervous
Genetics: N/A
Incidence/Prevalence in USA: 2418 methanol exposures reported in 2000, of which 209 were intentional. 12 deaths reported, one in a 3 month-old child
Predominant age: > 18 years primarily
Predominant sex: Male > Female (4:1)

SIGNS & SYMPTOMS

- Latent period after ingestion between 12 to 24 hours before onset of symptoms
- Initial CNS depression or inebriation depending on co-ingestion of ethyl alcohol. Co-ingestion of ethyl alcohol may delay onset of symptoms by 24 hours
- Common symptoms include visual disturbances, headache, lightheadedness, nausea, vomiting, abdominal pain, and dyspnea
- The presence of blurred vision and normal sensorium strongly suggests methanol intoxication
- Over 50% of patients complain of decreased visual acuity, photophobia, or feeling of "being in a snow field"
- Fundoscopic exam reveals retinal edema, hyperemia, or loss of physiological disk cupping. Other ocular findings include visual field defects and loss of pupillary reactions
- CNS symptoms include headache, vertigo, lethargy, confusion. Severe intoxications can present with coma and convulsions
- Gastrointestinal symptoms may include nausea, vomiting, and marked abdominal pain
- Pulmonary symptoms include Kussmaul respirations and pulmonary edema

CAUSES
Methanol ingestion

RISK FACTORS

- Alcoholism
- Epidemics may occur in institutionalized settings where ethyl alcohol is unavailable (i.e. prisons)

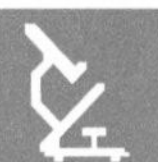

DIAGNOSIS

DIFFERENTIAL DIAGNOSIS

- Ingestion of other alcohols including ethyl alcohol, benzyl alcohol or isopropyl alcohol
- Other toxic ingestions including ethylene glycol, paraldehyde, salicylates, and formaldehyde
- Increased anion-gap metabolic acidosis caused by renal failure, diabetic ketoacidosis, and lactic acidosis

LABORATORY

- Serum methanol and ethanol concentrations, electrolytes, calcium, blood urea nitrogen & creatinine, osmolarity, hepatic aminotransferase enzymes, amylase, creatinine kinase, urinalysis, arterial blood gas
- Calculate anion gap and osmolar gap
- Calculated osmolarity is determined by (1.9[Na] + [BUN]/2.8 + [Glucose]/18). An osmolar gap exists if calculated osmolarity is greater than measured osmolarity by 10 mOsm/Kg H2O
- Increase anion-gap metabolic acidosis noted on arterial blood gas and serum electrolytes
- In acute intoxications serum methanol concentrations > 20mg/dL are associated with CNS effects; > 100 mg/dL are associated with visual defects; > 200 mg/dL are associated with death in untreated patients
- Methanol serum concentrations are not useful for treatment or prognosis decisions after the latency period since toxicity is determined by formic acid concentration in the blood
- MCV may increase due to generalized cellular swelling
- Elevated serum amylase may indicate the presence of pancreatitis

Drugs that may alter lab results: N/A

Disorders that may alter lab results: N/A

PATHOLOGICAL FINDINGS
Retinal edema, optic atrophy, bilateral putamen necrosis, pancreatitis

SPECIAL TESTS
Serum methanol concentration

IMAGING
CT or MRI scan of the brain if indicated by neurological exam. Brain imaging may reveal hypodensities in the putamen or caudate nucleus, cerebral edema, or cerebral hemorrhage

DIAGNOSTIC PROCEDURES
Visual evoked potentials and electroretinogram may give prognostic information about visual disturbances

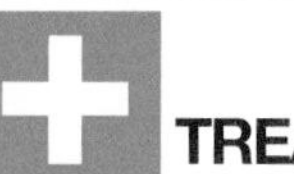

TREATMENT

APPROPRIATE HEALTH CARE

- Contact a regional poison control center for management recommendations
- All patients should be evaluated in a healthcare facility
- Evaluate and correct immediate life-threatening complications including airway, breathing, and circulation

GENERAL MEASURES

- Management priorities depend on the timing of presentation in relationship to ingestion or exposure
- Assess the magnitude of ingestion and inhibit methanol metabolism if ingestion is likely. Initial management is directed towards preventing metabolic acidosis and ophthalmologic complications
- Obtain laboratory studies
- Obtain intravenous access and administer isotonic fluids to maintain adequate urine output
- In general gastric decontamination with induced emesis, charcoal, or gastric lavage is **not** indicated unless a concomitant ingestion is known
- Ethanol or fomepizole should be administered as soon as possible in order to prevent hepatic biotransformation of methanol to formic acid. Ethanol is less expensive but more cumbersome to compound and administer. Fomepizole is easier to administer but is quite expensive.
- Sodium bicarbonate should be administered if serum pH < 7.2 to maintain pH > 7.3
- Folinic acid (Leucovorin) or folic acid may be administered
- Consider urgent hemodialysis when significant acidosis (pH < 7.2) unresponsive to therapy, deteriorating vital signs in spite of intensive support, renal failure, electrolyte imbalance, or serum methanol concentration > 50mg/dL

SURGICAL MEASURES
N/A

ACTIVITY
Restricted if patient is inebriated, has altered level of consciousness or visual impairments

DIET
No special diets. Thiamine supplementation in chronic alcoholics

PATIENT EDUCATION

- Anticipatory guidance for parents regarding storage of hazardous chemicals
- Patient education for chronic alcoholics concerning methanol toxicity
- Referral to alcoholic treatment program for patients with chronic alcohol abuse
- Other information can be obtained from the American Academy of Clinical Toxicology, 777 East Park Drive, P.O. Box 8820, Harrisburg, PA 17105-8820, or Agency for Toxic Substances and Diseases Registry, Division of Health Education, 1600 Clifton Road NE, Atlanta, GA 30333

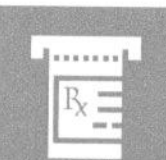

MEDICATIONS

DRUG(S) OF CHOICE

- Ethanol may be administered orally, if the gastrointestinal tract is functioning, or intravenously. A loading dose of 600-800 mg/kg followed by a maintenance dose of 66mg/kg/hr (non-drinker) or 154mg/kg/hr (ethanol abuser). Oral loading dose obtained by administering 2mL/kg body weight of 80 proof whiskey (31.6gm ethanol/100mL), may be administered as four 1 ounce oral doses in adults.
- Monitor serum ethanol concentrations q 1-2 hours to maintain at 100-150 mg/dL. Continue ethanol until serum methanol concentrations are <20 mg/dL and patient is asymptomatic with a normal serum pH.

3) Fomepizole . IV loading dose of 15mg/kg followed by IV boluses of 10mg/kg q 12 hours for 4 doses. If patient still symptomatic continue 15mg/kg q 12 hours until the methanol level is < 20mg/dL and patient is asymptomatic

4) Folinic acid (leucovorin). 1mg/kg (up to 50 mg) q 4 hrs until clinical endpoints reached. Alternatively folic acid, 50 mg IV q 4 hrs

Contraindications: Avoid ethanol if disulfiram used

Precautions:

- Avoid leucovorin with seizure disorders or vitamin B12 deficiency
- Avoid acetaminophen with ethanol use due to hepatotoxicity

Significant possible interactions:

- Do not use fomepizole and ethanol together
- Avoid metronidazole and procarbazine use within 72 hours of ethanol use - may cause disulfiram type reaction
- Avoid ethanol use with CNS depressants, anticonvulsants, SSRIs, antidepressants

ALTERNATIVE DRUGS N/A

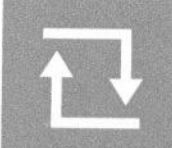

FOLLOWUP

PATIENT MONITORING

- Alcohol treatment program for chronic alcoholics
- Ophthalmology follow-up for patients with visual disturbances

PREVENTION/AVOIDANCE Avoid methanol containing fluids

POSSIBLE COMPLICATIONS

- Blindness and other visual disturbances
- Myoglobinuric renal failure
- Pancreatitis
- Parkinson-like syndrome

EXPECTED COURSE/PROGNOSIS

- Outcome varies depending on the time to presentation and quantity ingested
- Outcome is related to degree of acidosis, coma, or seizures at time of presentation
- In one study 19/51 patients died in an 11 year period.
- In a study from Ontario, Canada, 43 deaths in a 7 year period

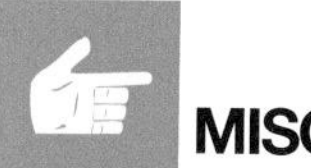

MISCELLANEOUS

ASSOCIATED CONDITIONS

- Alcoholism

AGE-RELATED FACTORS

Pediatric: Rare in this age group
Geriatric:
Others:

PREGNANCY Avoid ethanol during first trimester of pregnancy. May substitute fomepizole which is a Category C drug.

SYNONYMS N/A

ICD-9-CM

980.1 Methanol poisoning
E860.2 Accidental methanol poisoning
E950.9 Suicide attempt
E980.9 Undetermined methanol poisoning

SEE ALSO

Alcohol use disorders

OTHER NOTES Methanol also called: Methyl alcohol, wood alcohol, wood spirits, wood naphtha, carbinol, pyroligneous spirit

ABBREVIATIONS

MCV = mean corpuscular volume

REFERENCES

- Barceloux, DG. American Academy of Clinical Toxicology Practice Guidelines on the Treatment of Methanol Poisoning. Clinical Toxicology 2002;40(4):415-446
- Agency for Toxic Substances and Diseases Registry. Methanol Toxicity. Am Fam Phys. 1993;47(1):163-171
- Goldfrank LR, etal. Toxic Alcohols. In Toxicologic Emergencies, Seventh Edition, Lewis R. Goldfrank, editor; McGraw-Hill, New York, 2002

Web references: 1 available at www.5mcc.com
Illustrations N/A

Author(s):
Mark McConnell, MD

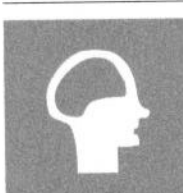

BASICS

DESCRIPTION Paroxysmal headache lasting 4-72 hours. Episodes vary in frequency from more than once a week to less than one per year with symptoms abating completely between attacks. Premonitory symptoms consisting of non-specific symptoms occur frequently hours to days before headache. Most frequent sub-types are:
- Without aura - (common migraine) defining over 80% of attacks
- With aura - (classic migraine) characterized by focal disruption of neurological function begins and ends prior to headache onset
- Variants of migraine include:
  - ◊ Transformed migraine - chronic headache pattern evolving from episodic migraine. Migraine-like attacks are superimposed on a daily or near-daily headache pattern, e.g., tension headache.
  - ◊ Basilar migraine - occipital headache, with aura symptoms of dysarthria, vertigo, tinnitus, ataxia, and bilateral paresis or bilateral paresthesias
  - ◊ Hemiplegic migraine - aura consisting of hemiplegia and/or hemiparesis
  - ◊ Ophthalmoplegic - palsy of the ipsilateral third cranial nerve during the headache phase
  - ◊ Retinal - symptoms of retinal vascular involvement during headache
  - ◊ Childhood periodic syndromes - (migraine equivalents) recurrent often cyclic episodes of symptoms
  - ◊ Status migrainous - persistent migraine which does not resolve spontaneously
  - ◊ Migrainous stroke - persistent or permanent neurologic deficits persisting beyond migraine attack usually with neuro-imaging changes
  - ◊ Chronic migraine - migraine-like headaches greater than 15 days a month for greater than 6 months

System(s) affected: Cardiovascular, Gastrointestinal, Musculoskeletal, Nervous

Genetics: > 80% of patients have positive family history. Identification of a chromosomal abnormality has been confirmed in familial hemiplegic migraine.

Incidence/Prevalence in USA:
- Adults: 18% of females, 6% of males
- Childhood unknown; may be significant

Predominant age: Childhood; increase in early adolescence, through 30s and 40s; decreases with age, attacks may persist into mature adulthood

Predominant sex:
- Male ≥ Female in childhood
- Female > Male (3:1) after menarche to mid-adult life
- Female > Male (2:1) in postmenopausal female populations

SIGNS & SYMPTOMS
- Five phases of a migraine; symptoms vary from patient to patient or from attack to attack within the same individual
- Premonitory symptoms (experienced by 50-80% of patients): A variety of "warnings" that precede migraine, frequently characterized by mood disruptions (e.g., euphoria, irritability, depression), fatigue, muscle tension, food craving, bloating, yawning, or subtle disruption of sensory processing. These symptoms are often not recognized by patients as associated with migraine.
- Aura: Visual disruptions are most common, including scotoma, hemianopsia, fortification spectra, geometric visual patterns, and occasionally hallucinations. Somatosensory disruption in face or upper extremities is also common. Headache typically begins within 1 hour of aura resolution.
- Headache: Headache usually begins with mild pain that escalates into a unilateral (30-40% bilateral), throbbing (40% non-throbbing) pain of 4-72 hours; intensified by movement; associated with systemic manifestations, e.g., nausea (87%), vomiting (56%), diarrhea (16%), photophobia (82%), phonophobia (78%), muscle tenderness (65%), lightheadedness (72%), vertigo (33%).
- Headache termination: Untreated, usually occurs with sleep; occasionally, vomiting or strong emotional experiences abort headache
- Postdrome: Headache pain resolved but another manifestation lingers on, such as, food intolerance, impaired concentration, fatigue, muscle soreness

CAUSES
- Etiology unknown; appears to be a genetically-linked, neuronal disease with vascular disruption as an epiphenomenon of underlying neurochemical disruption
- Serotonin, dopamine, glutamate and norepinephrine metabolism abnormalities may play a role
- Neurogenic inflammation and regional disruption of cerebral and/or extracranial blood flow may explain some clinical features

RISK FACTORS
- Specific foods, alcohol, missing meals, menstrual cycle, excessive sleep, fatigue, emotional stress, let down (relief of stress)
- Medications (estrogen replacement, BCPs, vasodilators)
- Family history of migraine
- Female gender
- Young age
- History of childhood cyclic vomiting, cyclic abdominal pain, motion sickness

DIAGNOSIS

DIFFERENTIAL DIAGNOSIS
- Other primary headache disorders
- Secondary headaches, such as tumor, infection, vascular pathology, or prescription or illicit drug, e.g., cocaine
- Drug seeking patients
- Psychiatric disease
- Rarely, migraine symptoms similar to certain forms of epilepsy

LABORATORY Only useful to rule out secondary causes of headache

Drugs that may alter lab results: N/A

Disorders that may alter lab results: N/A

PATHOLOGICAL FINDINGS
- Changes in blood serotonin levels and serotonin metabolites in the urine are reported
- Changes in regional blood flow
- Changes in sophisticated imaging studies

SPECIAL TESTS Only to rule out underlying pathology

IMAGING Occasionally required; indicated for new onset of headache for patient over age 50, and in patients with a change in established headache pattern

DIAGNOSTIC PROCEDURES Based on careful history and physical findings

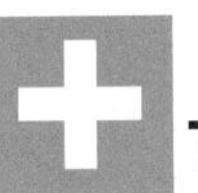

TREATMENT

APPROPRIATE HEALTH CARE Outpatient. For status migrainous or cases complicated by concurrent medical problems or significant medication-withdrawal issues, hospitalization may be required.

GENERAL MEASURES
- Compression to ipsilateral temporal artery or tender areas of scalp or neck
- Cold compresses to area of pain
- Rest with pillows comfortably supporting head or neck in area devoid of sensory stimulation, including light, sound, and odors
- Withdrawal from stressful surroundings
- Sleep is desirable
- Biofeedback and early psychologic intervention in appropriate cases or when pain behaviors are first identified
- Most patients manage attacks with self-care

SURGICAL MEASURES N/A

ACTIVITY In bed in a dark quiet environment

DIET Maintain fluid intake. Avoid dietary precipitants of migraine.

PATIENT EDUCATION
- Emphasize migraine can not be cured, but symptoms can be managed
- Encourage use of diary and patient education
- Emphasize proper use of all medications
- Encourage lifestyle modifications

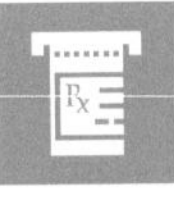

MEDICATIONS

DRUG(S) OF CHOICE
- 5-HT-1 agonists (triptans) intervention during the mild phase of headache offers greatest efficacy. For all triptans - oral tablets more effective in early mild headache phase; oral tablets slower in onset than injection or nasal spray; restore normal function for most; appropriate patient selection important.

◊ Sumatriptan (Imitrex), most effective during early mild headache phase of migraine. 6 mg self-administered injection with efficacy of 70-85%; nasal spray of 20 mg, or 25, 50 and 100 mg tablets with efficacy of 65%. 50 mg and 100 mg dose more effective than 25 mg. If initial injection fails to relieve migraine after 1 hour, don't repeat injection. If headache returns, repeat injection, nasal spray or oral tablets.
◊ Zolmitriptan (Zomig, Zomig-ZMT) 2.5 mg tablet at onset of migraine. 5 mg tablet available. Efficacy approximately 65%.
◊ Naratriptan (Amerge) 2.5 mg initially; 1 mg tablet available. Slower to act than other "triptans", but fewer adverse effects
◊ Rizatriptan (Maxalt) tablet and orally disintegrating tablet; initially 10 mg. 5 mg available and recommended for patients on propranolol. Efficacy similar to other "triptans". May have faster onset in moderate-severe headache.
◊ Almotriptan 6.25 or 12.5 mg tablet similar efficacy to other triptans
◊ Frovatriptan (Frova) 2.5 mg at onset; up to 3 doses (2.5 mg tablets) in 24 hr period
◊ Eletriptan (Relpax) 20 mg and 40 mg oral tablets; similar efficacy to other triptans

- Ergotamines
  ◊ Dihydroergotamine (DHE). Drug of choice in status migrainosus
    - Most effective ergotamine; available as IV, IM, or SC injection. Also available as nasal spray (Migranol)
    - 0.5-1 mg dose with up to 3 mg IM or 2 mg IV in 24 hours. Maximum weekly doses of 4-6 mg. Many protocols utilize antiemetic, such as, metoclopramide or prochlorperazine 5-10 mg IM or IV prior to DHE administration.
    - Dihydroergotamine (Migranal) nasal spray 2 mg intranasal (0.5 mg in each nostril repeated in 15 minutes). Low recurrence rate of migraine reported in trials.

  ◊ Ergotamine tartrate
    - Oral preparations contain 1 mg of ergotamine and 100 mg of caffeine. Two tablets at onset of symptoms. Repeat after 30 minutes up to maximum dose of 6 mg per day. Avoid chronic daily or near-daily use.
- Nonsteroidal anti-inflammatories: No clear superiority in efficacy established for any particular agent; early administration improves efficacy.
- Combination drugs
  ◊ Isometheptene - dichloralphenazone - acetaminophen (Midrin) 2 at onset then 1 q hr if needed up to 5 per 12 hour period

Contraindications:

- Avoid 5-HT-1 agonists (triptans) in coronary heart disease, peripheral vascular disease, uncontrolled hypertension, and complex migraine, such as basilar or hemiplegic migraine. Avoid within 2 wks of MAO usage (except Imitrex injection and Amerge tablets). Pregnancy category C.
- 5-HT-1 agonists (triptans) should not be used within 24 hours of an ergot derivative or a different 5-HT-1 agonists
- Selective 5-HT-1 agonists (triptans) pregnancy category C. Ergotamines pregnancy category X.
- Avoid NSAIDs if danger of gastric erosion, renal, or hepatic disease
- Avoid acetaminophen in hepatic disease or with alcohol consumption
- Avoid drugs containing narcotics or butalbital in addiction prone patients
- Avoid vasoconstrictors in uncontrolled hypertension, coronary heart disease, peripheral vascular disease
- Avoid sumatriptan, zolmitriptan, and rizatriptan within 2 weeks of MAO usage
- Avoid eletriptan within 72 hours of potent CYPA34 inhibitor such as ketoconazole, itraconazole, nefazodone, troleandomycin, or clarithromycin

Precautions:

- Administer ergotamines early
- Frequent use of acute treatment drugs may lead to changed migraine patterns
- Monitor use of aspirin and NSAIDs for dyspepsia
- Monitor use of drugs with addictive potential

Significant possible interactions:

- Other sedatives, analgesics, alcohol, vasoconstrictors including decongestants
- Ergotamine and macrolide antibiotics

ALTERNATIVE DRUGS

- Any analgesic, antiemetic, or sedative
- Narcotics including butorphanol (Stadol) are reserved for rescue therapy
- In emergency department: sumatriptan, DHE, adequate analgesics, antiemetic (chlorpromazine or prochlorperazine) and fluid replacement
- Other 5-HT-1 agonists
  ◊ A different route of delivery of 5-HT-1 agents or a different 5-HT-1 agent
  ◊ A wide variety of vasoconstrictors, analgesics, anti-inflammatories, antiemetics, and sedatives used alone or in combination are prescribed based on symptoms and other factors. Except for parenteral 5-HT-1 agonists and antiemetics, drugs are most effective when taken early in migraine attacks.

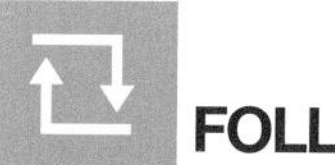

FOLLOWUP

PATIENT MONITORING

- Early intervention assist management
- Monitor frequency of attacks, pain behaviors. medication usage
- Encourage lifestyle modifications

PREVENTION/AVOIDANCE

- Avoid precipitants of attacks
- Prescribe biofeedback and psychologic intervention early if pain behavior evident
- Prophylactic therapy: If attacks significantly interfere with lifestyle or are not adequately controlled by appropriate acute interventions, daily prophylactic therapy may be appropriate. Regularly scheduled follow-up is mandatory.
  ◊ Propranolol (Inderal) 80-320 mg daily
  ◊ Atenolol (Tenormin) 50-100 mg daily
  ◊ Nadolol (Corgard) 40-80 mg daily
  ◊ Timolol (Blocadren) 10-20 mg daily
  ◊ Metoprolol (Lopressor) 100-450 mg daily
  ◊ Amitriptyline (Elavil) 10-150 mg daily
  ◊ Nortriptyline (Pamelor) 10-150 mg daily
  ◊ Verapamil (Calan, Isoptin) 80-120 mg daily
  ◊ Valproic acid (Depakene) or divalproex (Depakote) 250-1500 mg daily
  ◊ Cyproheptadine (Periactin) 4-16 mg daily
  ◊ Topiramate 100-200 mg
- Consultation/referral
  ◊ Obscure diagnosis, concomitant medical conditions, significant psychopathology
  ◊ Unresponsive to usual treatment
  ◊ Analgesic dependent headache patterns

POSSIBLE COMPLICATIONS

- Rare status migrainosus
- Rare cerebral ischemic events
- Iatrogenic effects of treatment

EXPECTED COURSE/PROGNOSIS

- With age - reduction in severity, frequency, and disability of attacks
- Most attacks subside within 72 hours

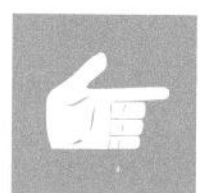

MISCELLANEOUS

ASSOCIATED CONDITIONS Depression, panic disorders, sleep disturbance, cerebral vascular disease, myocardial disease, peripheral vascular disease and seizure, irritable bowel syndrome

AGE-RELATED FACTORS

Pediatric: Recurrent abdominal pain and cyclic vomiting may predominate; attacks may be of shorter duration. Headache description by younger children may appear atypical.
Geriatric: Rare onset of non-cephalalgic migraine (aura without subsequent headache) after the age of 40. Possible relationship to transient global amnesia. Late onset of migraine requires diagnostic evaluation.
Others: Migraine affects all races, social classes, intelligence levels

PREGNANCY Attacks frequently diminish, especially in 2nd/3rd trimester. No treatment drug has FDA approval in pregnancy; ergotamines are contraindicated.

SYNONYMS

- Hemicrania
- Sick headache

ICD-9-CM

346.00 Classical migraine without mention of intractable migraine
346.21 Variants of migraine with intractable migraine, so stated
346.90 Migraine, unspecified without mention of intractable migraine
784.0 Headache

SEE ALSO

Headache, cluster
Headache, tension

OTHER NOTES N/A

ABBREVIATIONS N/A

REFERENCES

- Cady RK, Fox AW, editors. Treating the Headache Patient. New York: Marcel Dekker; 1995
- Sandler M, Collins GM, editors. Migraine: A Spectrum of Ideas. New York: Oxford University Press; 1990
- Raskin NH. Headache. 2nd ed. New York: Churchill Livingstone; 1986
- Dalessio DJ, editor. Wolff's Headache. 5th ed. New York: Oxford University Press; 1987

Web references: 2 available at www.5mcc.com
Illustrations N/A

Author(s):
Roger Cady, MD

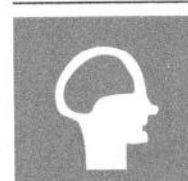

BASICS

DESCRIPTION Miliaria rubra or prickly heat is a papulovesicular eruption of eccrine sweat glands that often occurs in conditions of high heat and humidity
System(s) affected: Skin/Exocrine
Genetics: N/A
Incidence/Prevalence in USA: N/A
Predominant age: Common in infants, less common in adults
Predominant sex: Male = Female

SIGNS & SYMPTOMS
- Fine papules and vesicles on an erythematous base
- May become inflamed pustules (miliaria pustulosa)
- Prevalent in areas of friction caused by clothing and in areas of flexure
- In infants - trunk, diaper area, neck, groin, axilla, face
- Pilosebaceous follicles, palms, soles spared
- Lesions appear after individual has been in a hot humid environment, resulting in sweating
- Pruritus or prickly, mildly stinging sensation in affected areas

CAUSES
- Keratinous plugging of the sweat ducts as a result of toxins produced by resident bacteria
- This leads to rupture of sweat duct producing sweat retention vesicle

RISK FACTORS
- Hot humid environment
- Occlusive bandages
- Plastic undersheets
- High fever

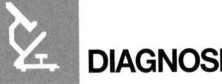

DIAGNOSIS

DIFFERENTIAL DIAGNOSIS
- Acne
- Folliculitis
- Viral exanthems
- Drug eruptions
- Erythema toxicum
- Yeast infections
- Pyogenic infections

LABORATORY N/A

Drugs that may alter lab results: N/A

Disorders that may alter lab results: N/A

PATHOLOGICAL FINDINGS
- Keratinous plugging of sweat ducts
- Sweat retention vesicle

SPECIAL TESTS N/A

IMAGING N/A

DIAGNOSTIC PROCEDURES Miliaria is a clinical diagnosis

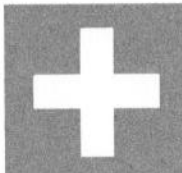

TREATMENT

APPROPRIATE HEALTH CARE Outpatient

GENERAL MEASURES
- Avoid wearing heavy, tight clothing or garments causing friction
- Avoid plastic or occlusive dressings/garments in hot environments
- Avoid excessive use of soap and contact with irritants
- Frequent cool baths with Aveeno colloidal, oatmeal or cornstarch
- Provide cool, dry environment for 8-10 hours a day
- Topical applications of lotions containing lanolin, calamine, boric acid and menthol

SURGICAL MEASURES N/A

ACTIVITY Avoid vigorous activity leading to sweating

DIET No special diet

PATIENT EDUCATION
- Cause of eruption/avoidance
- General measures for home care

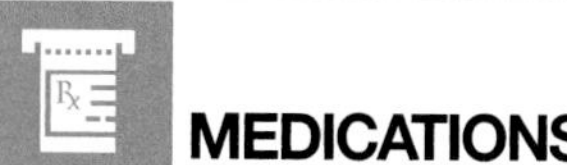

MEDICATIONS

DRUG(S) OF CHOICE

- Topical steroids to relieve pruritus - 0.1% betamethasone (Valisone) bid for 3 days
- Systemic antibiotics in cases of bacterial secondary infection - antibiotic effective against staphylococci, e.g., dicloxacillin 250 mg qid for 10 days (unless resistance)
- If sweating due to fever, antipyretic drugs may be useful

Contraindications: N/A
Precautions: Care with fluorinated steroid application in children. They may cause systemic effects.
Significant possible interactions: N/A

ALTERNATIVE DRUGS Over-the-counter preparations with menthol, camphor for pruritus, e.g., hydrocortisone (Sarna) or pramoxine (Prax)

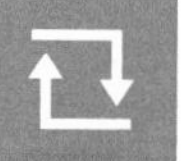

FOLLOWUP

PATIENT MONITORING As needed for persistence of symptoms

PREVENTION/AVOIDANCE

- See General measures
- Acclimatize slowly to hot weather

POSSIBLE COMPLICATIONS

- Secondary bacterial infections
- Miliaria profunda secondary to repeated miliaria rubra (can cause anhidrosis)

EXPECTED COURSE/PROGNOSIS

- Benign - responds to cooling
- Avoidance of causative agents is key

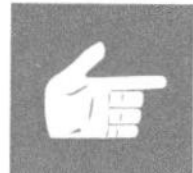

MISCELLANEOUS

ASSOCIATED CONDITIONS N/A

AGE-RELATED FACTORS

Pediatric: More common
Geriatric:

- Less common
- Backs of hospitalized patients

Others: N/A

PREGNANCY N/A

SYNONYMS Prickly heat

ICD-9-CM

705.1 Prickly heat

SEE ALSO

OTHER NOTES N/A

ABBREVIATIONS N/A

REFERENCES

- Bondi J, Jegasothy B, Lazarus G. Dermatology, Diagnosis and Therapy. Norwalk, CT: McGraw-Hill/Appleton & Lange; 1992

Web references: 2 available at www.5mcc.com
Illustrations 4 available

Author(s):

Aamir Siddiqi, MD

BASICS

DESCRIPTION A condition resulting from ingestion of excessive amounts of calcium and absorbable alkali (e.g., sodium bicarbonate and calcium carbonate) usually during self-treatment for peptic ulcer or gastroesophageal reflux
System(s) affected: Endocrine/Metabolic, Gastrointestinal, Renal/Urologic
Genetics: Unknown
Incidence/Prevalence in USA: Infrequent
Predominant age: 40-75 years
Predominant sex: Male = Female

SIGNS & SYMPTOMS
- Anorexia
- Band keratopathy
- Constipation
- Dehydration
- Depression
- Dizziness
- Food distaste
- Headache
- Irritability
- Mental status changes
- Myalgias
- Nausea
- Periarticular calcinosis
- Polydipsia
- Polyuria
- Vomiting
- Weakness

CAUSES Excess intake of milk and alkali as therapy for gastrointestinal problems accompanied with gastric hyperacidity (e.g., peptic ulcer, esophageal reflux)

RISK FACTORS
- Peptic ulcer
- Hiatal hernia
- Malignancies

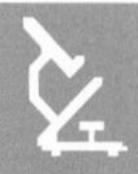

DIAGNOSIS

DIFFERENTIAL DIAGNOSIS Other causes of hypercalcemia, such as excessive osteolysis with malignant disease, vitamin intoxication, thyroid disease, sarcoidosis, thiazide diuretic treatment, hyperparathyroidism

LABORATORY
- Mild alkalosis
- Hypercalcemia
- Normocalciuria
- Decreased urine phosphate
- Increased BUN and serum creatinine
- Normal alkaline phosphatase

Drugs that may alter lab results: N/A

Disorders that may alter lab results: N/A

PATHOLOGICAL FINDINGS Nephrocalcinosis, ectopic calcification

SPECIAL TESTS N/A

IMAGING N/A

DIAGNOSTIC PROCEDURES N/A

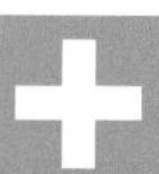

TREATMENT

APPROPRIATE HEALTH CARE Inpatient

GENERAL MEASURES
- Withdraw milk and alkali
- Treat the hypercalcemia
- Intravenous treatment to cause calcinosis (usually with sodium chloride solution)
- Goal of treatment: Maintain urine volume of 3 liters per day
- With significant renal insufficiency, employ renal dialysis

SURGICAL MEASURES N/A

ACTIVITY Bedrest during active treatment

DIET Increased fluid intake

PATIENT EDUCATION N/A

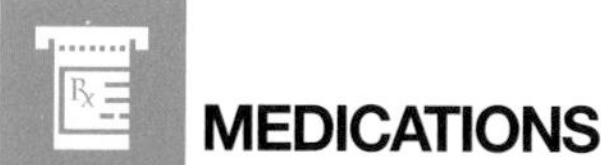

MEDICATIONS

DRUG(S) OF CHOICE
- To treat hypercalcemia: Isotonic sodium chloride 0.9% intravenously when serum calcium exceeds 15 mg/dL (3.75 mmol/L) (see Hypercalcemia), plus
- Furosemide 80-100 mgm IV q2 for 24 hours after volume depletion has been corrected

Contraindications: Refer to manufacturer's literature

Precautions: Replace sodium and potassium losses associated with furosemide use

Significant possible interactions: Refer to manufacturer's literature

ALTERNATIVE DRUGS
Disodium phosphate and monopotassium phosphate. HAZARDOUS - should be used only by experienced nephrologist and only if dialysis is unavailable.

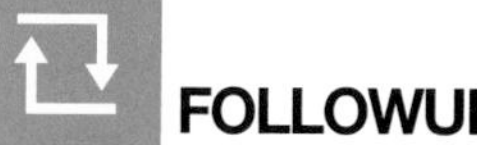

FOLLOWUP

PATIENT MONITORING
- Kidney function
- Fluid intake and output
- Urine electrolytes

PREVENTION/AVOIDANCE
Avoid excess milk and/or absorbable antacids

POSSIBLE COMPLICATIONS
- Renal failure
- Nephrocalcinosis

EXPECTED COURSE/PROGNOSIS
Favorable with appropriate therapy

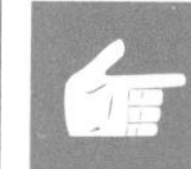

MISCELLANEOUS

ASSOCIATED CONDITIONS
- Peptic ulcer disease
- Hiatal hernia
- Gastroesophageal reflux
- Hyperparathyroidism
- Hypercalcemia of malignancy

AGE-RELATED FACTORS
Pediatric: N/A

Geriatric: Occurs predominantly in this age group

Others: N/A

PREGNANCY
N/A

SYNONYMS
- Burnett syndrome
- Milk poisoning
- Milk drinker's syndrome

ICD-9-CM
999.9 Other and unspecified complications of medical care, NEC

SEE ALSO

OTHER NOTES
N/A

ABBREVIATIONS
N/A

REFERENCES

- Wilson JD, Foster DW, eds: Williams' Textbook of Endocrinology. 8th ed. Philadelphia, Saunders, 1992
- Labhart A: Clinical Endocrinology: Theory & Practice. 2nd Ed. Springhouse, PA, Springer-Verlag, 1987

Web references: 0 available at www.5mcc.com

Illustrations N/A

Author(s):
Stanley G. Smith, MA, MB

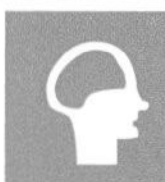

BASICS

DESCRIPTION Resistance to diastolic filling of the left ventricle due to valvular narrowing. In the adult, the most common etiology is rheumatic heart disease.
System(s) affected: Cardiovascular
Genetics: Congenital mitral stenosis is a rare congenital malformation, manifested in only 0.42% of children with congenital heart disease
Incidence/Prevalence in USA: The overall incidence of rheumatic heart disease is decreasing. The mitral valve is the valve most commonly affected with rheumatic heart disease.
Predominant age: Symptoms primarily occur in middle age (40-70 years)
Predominant sex: Female > Male

SIGNS & SYMPTOMS

- History:
  - ◊ History of murmur
  - ◊ History of rheumatic fever
  - ◊ History of pulmonary edema with pregnancy, exercise, infection or arrhythmia (commonly atrial fibrillation)
- Most common signs and symptoms:
  - ◊ Effort induced dyspnea
  - ◊ Palpitations
  - ◊ Effort fatigue
  - ◊ Hemoptysis (late)
  - ◊ Apical early diastolic low-pitched rumble often with presystolic accentuation (listen with bell of stethoscope in left lateral decubitus position)
  - ◊ Loud S1 (early in disease - as the valve becomes more stenotic and less mobile, this is less common)
  - ◊ Opening snap after S2 (may also diminish in intensity with increasing stenosis)
  - ◊ Right ventricle enlargement
- Other signs and symptoms:
  - ◊ Paroxysmal nocturnal dyspnea
  - ◊ Orthopnea
  - ◊ Recumbent cough
  - ◊ Hoarseness
  - ◊ Digital clubbing
  - ◊ Chest pain
  - ◊ Peripheral edema
  - ◊ Systemic embolization
  - ◊ Rales, atrial fibrillation, malar rash (rare)
  - ◊ Holosystolic murmur of mitral regurgitation may accompany the valvular deformity of mitral stenosis
  - ◊ If pulmonary hypertension is present: right ventricular lift, increased pulmonic second sound, a high pitched decrescendo diastolic murmur of pulmonic insufficiency (Graham Steell's murmur)
  - ◊ If right ventricular failure has developed: increased jugular venous distention, holosystolic murmur of tricuspid regurgitation at left sternal border, hepatomegaly and peripheral edema are often found
  - ◊ May also find associated aortic, or less commonly, tricuspid murmurs (due to aortic or tricuspid valve involvement with rheumatic heart disease)

CAUSES In the adult, mitral stenosis is almost always secondary to rheumatic heart disease. Rarely, congenital in etiology.

RISK FACTORS History of rheumatic fever

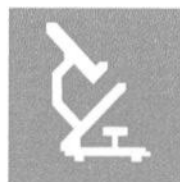

DIAGNOSIS

DIFFERENTIAL DIAGNOSIS The major differential diagnosis to be considered in a patient with the relatively characteristic findings of mitral stenosis is the uncommon atrial myxoma or vegetation due to endocarditis obstructing left ventricle (LV) inflow. Diastolic flow murmurs can be also heard in the absence of true stenosis due to increased flow across a normal valve. These murmurs are generally limited to early diastole and may be associated with anemia, thyrotoxicosis, shunts as well as with significant mitral regurgitation.

LABORATORY N/A

Drugs that may alter lab results: N/A

Disorders that may alter lab results: N/A

PATHOLOGICAL FINDINGS

- Scarring of the leaflets with fibrosis restricting valve mobility
- Retraction then leads to further valvular narrowing, often with a funnel shaped deformity
- Chordal involvement leads to fusion of the chords and obliteration of the interchordal spaces, further limiting LV inflow
- Left atrial dilatation
- Left atrial thrombi may be found
- Right ventricular hypertrophy
- Pulmonary arterial thickening

SPECIAL TESTS

- ECG:
  - ◊ Left atrial enlargement (manifested by broad, notched P waves in lead II with a negative terminal deflection of the P wave in lead V1)
  - ◊ Atrial fibrillation is commonly noted
  - ◊ With right ventricular hypertrophy, right axis deviation and a large R wave in V1 may be noted

IMAGING

- Chest x-ray:
  - ◊ Left atrial enlargement with straightening of the left heart border, a "double density", and elevation of the left main stem bronchus
  - ◊ Pulmonary venous patterns changes with redistribution of flow toward the apices
  - ◊ Prominent pulmonary arteries at the hilum with rapid tapering
  - ◊ Right ventricular enlargement
  - ◊ Kerley's B lines
  - ◊ Pulmonary edema pattern (late)

DIAGNOSTIC PROCEDURES

- Echocardiography: (2-D):
  - ◊ Mitral valve thickening with decreased diastolic excursion and "doming" of the anterior leaflet in diastole
  - ◊ Valvular calcification
  - ◊ Decreased mitral orifice as directly measured by planimetry
  - ◊ Enlarged left atrium
  - ◊ Right ventricular enlargement
  - ◊ Atrial thrombi
- Doppler:
  - ◊ Transvalvular pressure gradients
  - ◊ Calculated valve area
  - ◊ Concomitant mitral regurgitation (MR), pulmonary insufficiency (PI), tricuspid regurgitation (TR)
- Cardiac catheterization:
  - ◊ Increased left atrial or pulmonary capillary wedge pressure (PCWP)
  - ◊ Increased left atrial or PCWP to left ventricular pressure gradient
  - ◊ Calculated mitral valve orifice area
  - ◊ Calcified mitral valve
  - ◊ Concomitant mitral regurgitation
  - ◊ Presence of coronary artery disease

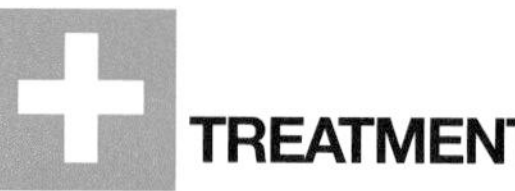

TREATMENT

APPROPRIATE HEALTH CARE Outpatient except for complications or surgery

GENERAL MEASURES

- Mitral stenosis is generally a progressive disease. The asymptomatic patient with non-critical mitral stenosis can be followed with appropriate evaluation.
- The patient should avoid unusual stresses (emotional and physical)
- All patients should receive endocarditis prophylaxis, prior to dental work or invasive procedures, regardless of age, etiology or severity of the stenosis (as recommended by the American Heart Association in Circulation, 1997; 96: 358-366)
- Patients who have mitral stenosis on the basis of rheumatic fever should also receive rheumatic fever prophylaxis (in addition to endocarditis prophylaxis) if under 35 years of age or continues to be in contact with young children
- If atrial fibrillation develops, it is important to slow the heart rate to allow more time for diastolic filling through the stenotic valve
- The development of pulmonary edema is often associated with atrial fibrillation and a rapid ventricular response. It is important to slow the heart rate. Cardioversion could be considered, particularly if the patient is chronically anticoagulated.
- Consider anticoagulation with warfarin (Coumadin) in all patients with mitral stenosis, particularly if a history of systemic embolism, or have atrial fibrillation or a large left atrium

SURGICAL MEASURES Surgical intervention: If the patient is eligible for a commissurotomy or balloon valvuloplasty, the onset of symptoms clearly referable to the mitral stenosis is generally considered an indication for early surgical intervention. If, however, the patient requires placement of a mitral valve prosthesis, often the timing of the surgical intervention is delayed until the symptoms are more severe.

ACTIVITY Adequate rest and reasonable physical activity

DIET Low salt

PATIENT EDUCATION Educate the patient about symptoms of mitral stenosis and report them should they occur

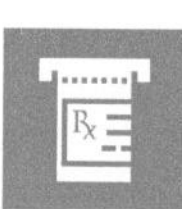

MEDICATIONS

DRUG(S) OF CHOICE

- Judicious addition of diuretics if symptoms indicate
- Atrial fibrillation - consider digoxin plus anticoagulation with warfarin (Coumadin). Beta or calcium channel blockers have been used in place of digoxin. Digoxin is used for rate control, not to convert to normal sinus rhythm.
- Rheumatic fever prophylaxis - preferably penicillin G benzathine, 1.2 million units IM every four weeks or penicillin V 250 mg twice daily
- Bacterial endocarditis prophylaxis - depends on procedure. For dental procedures - amoxicillin 2.0 g given orally 1 hour before procedure for adults without contraindications.

Contraindications: Penicillin allergy
Precautions: Refer to manufacturer's profile of each drug
Significant possible interactions: There are many when using the combination of warfarin and digoxin. Use caution when adding new medications. Refer to manufacturer's profile of each drug.

ALTERNATIVE DRUGS Erythromycin for rheumatic fever prophylaxis; Clindamycin for bacterial endocarditis prophylaxis

FOLLOWUP

PATIENT MONITORING Close regular visits for assessment of the gradually progressive symptoms

PREVENTION/AVOIDANCE

- Bacterial endocarditis prophylaxis for dental and invasive procedures continued for life
- Strep throat - treat appropriately when it occurs
- Rheumatic fever prophylaxis when indicated (See General Measures)

POSSIBLE COMPLICATIONS

- Thromboembolism from mitral stenosis is a major potential complication (anticoagulation therapy has lessened this risk substantially)
- Recurrent rheumatic fever
- Bacterial endocarditis
- Pulmonary hypertension
- Pulmonary edema

EXPECTED COURSE/PROGNOSIS

- Although a milder course is now seen in North America, the classic mitral stenosis history is 10 years from the episode of rheumatic fever to the development of a murmur, another 10 years until symptomatic and another 10 years for the patient to develop serious disability
- Operative mortality 1-2% for mitral commissurotomy; 2-5% for mitral valve replacement

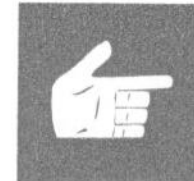

MISCELLANEOUS

ASSOCIATED CONDITIONS Congestive heart failure

AGE-RELATED FACTORS

Pediatric: N/A
Geriatric:

- Atrial fibrillation and complicating arterial embolism more common
- Though there is an increased risk for bleeding, anticoagulation therapy recommended (unless specifically contraindicated) due to high risk of embolism and valve thrombosis (especially if atrial fibrillation present)

Others: N/A

PREGNANCY

- Can cause marked deterioration in cardiac function due to hemodynamic changes associated with increased intravascular volume and heart rate, with decreased diastolic filling time
- The associated pulmonary hypertension also poorly tolerated in pregnancy

SYNONYMS N/A

ICD-9-CM

394.0 Mitral stenosis

SEE ALSO

OTHER NOTES N/A

ABBREVIATIONS N/A

REFERENCES

- Brandenburg RO, et al: Cardiology: Fundamentals and Practice, Chicago, Year Book Medical Publishers, 1987
- Dalen JE, Alpert JS: Valvular Heart Disease. 2nd Ed. New York, Little Brown, 1987
- Cotran RS, et al, eds: Robbins Pathological Basis of Disease. 4th Ed. Philadelphia, W.B. Saunders Co., 1989
- Hurst JW, et al: The Heart. 8th Ed. New York, McGraw-Hill, 1994

Web references: 1 available at www.5mcc.com
Illustrations N/A

Author(s):
Mark R. Dambro, MD

Mitral valve prolapse

BASICS

DESCRIPTION Mitral valve prolapse (MVP) = bulging of mitral valve leaflets into left atrium during systole. most often asymptomatic and nonprogressive. A subset of patients have MVP syndrome with signs and symptoms ranging from chest pain and fatigue to autonomic dysfunction (including syncope), cardiac dysrhythmias, strokes, and sudden death. Degeneration of prolapsing mitral valve with time sometimes occurs.

System(s) affected: Cardiovascular, Endocrine/ Metabolic, Nervous

Genetics: Autosomal dominant with variable expression. Part of inherited connective tissue disorders such as Marfan syndrome and Ehlers-Danlos syndrome.

Incidence/Prevalence in USA: Approximately 2.5-5% of the general population

Predominant age: Uncommon before adolescent growth spurt, usually detected in young adulthood

Predominant sex:
- Females > Males (under the age of 20)
- Females = Males (after age 20)
- Males more severely affected than females after age 50

SIGNS & SYMPTOMS
- Usually asymptomatic, nonprogressive, and benign; often an incidental finding on echocardiography - may be unrelated to presenting symptoms
- Subset of patients may have arrhythmias, emboli, endocarditis, severe mitral regurgitation, and sudden death.
- Characteristic systolic click (sound) and/or late systolic murmur, whose characteristics and timing change with body position and often fluctuate between exams.
- Chest pain: recurrent, located in left precordial and substernal areas, varies from instantaneous to hours in duration
- Fatigue
- Syncope/presyncope
- Dyspnea
- Body habitus: Thin, arm span greater than height, abnormal thoracic cage or spine including narrow AP chest and pectus excavatum, high arched palate, scoliosis
- "MVP" syndrome
  - ◊ Low body weight
  - ◊ Low blood pressure
  - ◊ Minor skeletal abnormalities
  - ◊ Orthostasis
  - ◊ Palpitations
  - ◊ Mitral regurgitation
  - ◊ Autonomic dysfunction: chest pain, panic attacks, anxiety
  - ◊ Neuroendocrine dysfunction
- Sudden death - autopsy studies show small vessel disease (including AV nodal coronary arteries) and cardiomyopathic changes of ventricle (especially septum), suggesting some cases of sudden death due to VT/VF from ischemia or scarring

CAUSES
- Primary disorder: inherited; mitral valve and supportive structures disproportionately large for left ventricle
- Secondary disorder:
  - ◊ Disorders of tissue structure: Marfan syndrome, Ehlers-Danlos, pseudoxanthoma elastica, osteogenesis imperfecta, myxomatous degeneration of connective tissue of the mitral valve
  - ◊ Connective tissue diseases: rheumatic endocarditis, SLE
  - ◊ Structural heart diseases: ruptured chordae tendineae, mitral stenosis, hypertrophic cardiomyopathy
  - ◊ Coronary artery disease
- Associated dysautonomia is cause of orthostasis and syncope, palpitations, anxiety, chest pain, fatigue, and dyspnea.
- Hypothesized that MVP = growth disorder: heart grows more than chest cavity causing mitral annulus distortion and leaflet prolapse

RISK FACTORS
- Positive family history
- Disorder of connective tissue/collagen
- Increased risk of complications
  - ◊ Male sex and age over 50
  - ◊ Posterior leaflet prolapse (associated with holosystolic murmur)
  - ◊ Mitral regurgitation (including exercise-induced MR)

DIAGNOSIS

DIFFERENTIAL DIAGNOSIS
- Click:
  - ◊ Ejection clicks
  - ◊ Opening snap (mitral/tricuspid stenosis)
  - ◊ Split S2
  - ◊ Ventricular aneurysm
  - ◊ Constrictive pericarditis causing pericardial knock
- Late systolic murmur:
  - ◊ Tricuspid valve prolapse
  - ◊ Papillary muscle dysfunction
  - ◊ Hypertrophic cardiomyopathy
  - ◊ VSD
- Auscultation - characteristic finding is a mid-systolic click; timing varies with LV load: standing, handgrip, Valsalva = earlier (click closer to S1); squatting, post-Valsalva = later (closer to S2)

LABORATORY N/A

Drugs that may alter lab results: N/A

Disorders that may alter lab results: N/A

PATHOLOGICAL FINDINGS
- Myxomatous degeneration of the mitral valve
- Thickened, redundant mitral valve leaflets

SPECIAL TESTS
- ECG
  - ◊ Usually normal
  - ◊ Inferior ST-T wave changes
  - ◊ Atrial arrhythmias, ventricular arrhythmias including complex arrhythmias, left atrial/ventricular enlargement secondary to mitral regurgitation
- Signal-averaged ECG helps predict ventricular and supraventricular arrhythmias

IMAGING Chest x-ray usually normal

DIAGNOSTIC PROCEDURES
- Echocardiogram (MVP may be an incidental discovery):
  - ◊ The most useful test for confirming and defining mitral valve prolapse. Diagnosis requires meeting criteria for displacement and thickness of valve leaflets.
  - ◊ Should not be used to screen for mitral valve prolapse. Clinically significant mitral valve prolapse usually obvious on physical exam. Silent mitral valve prolapse common and clinically insignificant.
  - ◊ Other valves may have myxomatous degeneration and prolapse. Echocardiogram evaluates the other valves as well.
  - ◊ Doppler echocardiogram detects and quantitates mitral regurgitation
  - ◊ Serial echocardiograms useful in following mitral regurgitation, LA/LV enlargement
- Tilt table studies useful to diagnose autonomic dysfunction causing light-headedness and syncope
- Signal-averaged ECG (SAECG) can detect patients at high risk of ventricular arrhythmias/sudden death
- Holter monitoring sometimes detects life-threatening arrhythmias. Atrial arrhythmias more common when mitral regurgitation present.
- EKG stress test:
  - ◊ Detects exercise-induced arrhythmias
  - ◊ Detects exercise-induced mitral regurgitation which is associated with higher risk
  - ◊ 50% false positive rate for ischemic changes
  - ◊ Repeating the stress test after beta blockers improves specificity

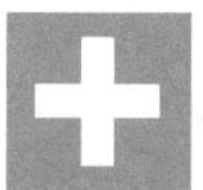

TREATMENT

APPROPRIATE HEALTH CARE Outpatient

GENERAL MEASURES 75% of cases have no increase in morbidity/mortality and no treatment required

SURGICAL MEASURES
- 25% of patients require valvular surgery after age 50, generally after long asymptomatic period
- Mitral valve and mitral annulus repair becoming preferred over mitral valve replacement

ACTIVITY
- Generally unrestricted
- Certain patients have arrhythmias precipitated by exercise which often respond to beta blockers
- Associated decreased intravascular volume may cause orthostasis and syncope with vigorous sports and/or dehydration
- Competitive sports should be avoided in patients with aortic root enlargement, unexplained syncope, uncontrolled tachyarrhythmias, etc.

DIET
- Adequate salt intake important: low baseline intravascular volume, abnormal renin-aldosterone response to volume depletion, and autonomic dysregulation limit compensatory response.
- Caffeine, alcohol, and cigarettes to be avoided with palpitations

PATIENT EDUCATION
- Assurance of usually benign course
- Patient information can be obtained from: American Heart Association, 7320 Greenville Avenue, Dallas, TX 75231, (214)373-6300
- On Health; http://onhealth.com

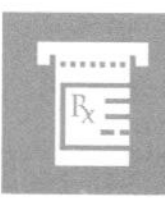

MEDICATIONS

DRUG(S) OF CHOICE
- Usually none needed.
- Beta-blockers (e.g. atenolol) helpful if palpitations severe.
- Aspirin indicated for TIA or atrial fibrillation (< 65 years old, no HTN or CHF)
- When indicated (see Prevention/Avoidance):
  - ◊ Antibiotics
  - ◊ Warfarin (Coumadin) for history of CVA or Afib plus >65 years old or history of HTN/CHF

Contraindications:
- Diuretics to be avoided (baseline low intravascular volume)
- Oral contraceptives to be avoided in patients with focal neurologic events

Precautions: Beta-blockers will increase fatigue and orthostasis/dizziness.

Significant possible interactions: Refer to manufacturer's literature

ALTERNATIVE DRUGS None

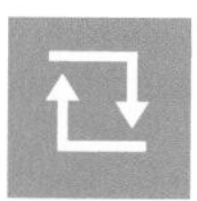

FOLLOWUP

PATIENT MONITORING
- Serial echocardiograms in patients with posterior leaflet prolapse, mitral regurgitation (including exercise-induced), thickened or redundant leaflets, increased left ventricular size.

PREVENTION/AVOIDANCE
- Endocarditis prophylaxis for auscultatory murmur or redundant, thickened leaflets by echocardiogram. Prophylaxis not needed in MVP without a murmur.
- Good dental hygiene
- Anticoagulation in patients with atrial fibrillation and atrial enlargement

POSSIBLE COMPLICATIONS
- Complication rate approximately 2% per year
- Sudden death - rare. Some cases of MVP associated with proteoglycan deposition (valves as well as extravalvular) and with small vessel disease, causing ventricular arrhythmias and sudden death.
- Uncommon and related to advancing age, male sex, atrial/ventricular size rather than to presence/absence of valvular prolapse:
  - ◊ Infective endocarditis
  - ◊ TIA
  - ◊ Stroke
  - ◊ Congestive heart failure
  - ◊ Heart block
  - ◊ Severe mitral regurgitation
  - ◊ Syncope

EXPECTED COURSE/PROGNOSIS
- 75% excellent with same morbidity/mortality as age-matched controls
- 25% progressive mitral regurgitation with a long (25 year) asymptomatic phase followed by rapid deterioration requiring valvular repair within a year once symptoms occur

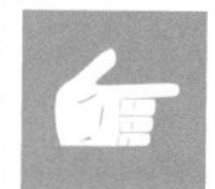

MISCELLANEOUS

ASSOCIATED CONDITIONS
< 5% of all mitral valve prolapse:
- Marfan syndrome
- Osteogenesis imperfecta
- Ehlers-Danlos syndrome
- Adult polycystic kidney disease
- Stickler syndrome
- Pseudoxanthoma elasticum
- Turner syndrome
- Rheumatologic diseases including SLE, PSS, MCTD
- Primary cardiac disorders including rheumatic endocarditis, mitral stenosis, hypertrophic cardiomyopathy, LV aneurysm, coronary artery disease, and congenital abnormalities
- Duchenne's muscular dystrophy
- Inherited disorders of metabolism (Hunter's, Hurler's, & Sanfilippo's syndromes)
- Autoimmune thyroid disease (including Grave's disease)

AGE-RELATED FACTORS
Pediatric: Rarely detected before adolescent growth spurt

Geriatric: Complications occur mostly in men over 50

Others: N/A

PREGNANCY
- Mitral valve prolapse itself not a contraindication to pregnancy.
- Connective tissue diseases (e.g., Marfan syndrome), especially with an enlarged aortic root, may be a contraindication to pregnancy
- Increased blood volume of pregnancy may improve symptoms of mitral valve prolapse

SYNONYMS
- Systolic murmur-click syndrome
- Mitral click murmur syndrome

ICD-9-CM
424.0 Mitral valve disorders
394.0 Mitral stenosis
394.1 Rheumatic mitral insufficiency
394.2 Mitral stenosis with insufficiency
394.9 Other and unspecified mitral valve diseases

SEE ALSO
Marfan syndrome
Mitral regurgitation due to papillary muscle dysfunction
Mitral regurgitation due to rheumatic fever
Mitral stenosis
Muscular dystrophy
Polycystic kidney disease
Systemic lupus erythematosus (SLE)
Turner syndrome

OTHER NOTES N/A

ABBREVIATIONS
MVP = mitral valve prolapse

REFERENCES

- Hurst JW, et al. The Heart. 8th Ed. New York, McGraw-Hill, 1994
- Bennett JC, Plum F, editors. Cecil Textbook of Medicine. 20th Ed. Philadelphia, W.B. Saunders Co., 1996
- Devereux RB. Recent developments in the diagnosis and treatment of MVP. Current Opinion Cardiol 1995; 10(2): 107-16
- Kim S, et al. Relationship between severity of MR and prognosis of MVP. Am Heart J 1996; 132(2(pt1)): 348-55
- Burke AF, Farb, et al. Fibromuscular dysplasia of small coronary arteries and fibrosis in the basilar ventricular septum in mitral valve prolapse. Am Heart J 1997;134(2):282-291
- Corrado D. Sudden death in young people. G Ital Cardiol 1997;27(11):1097-1105
- Bouknight DP, O'Rourke RA. Current management of mitral valve prolapse. Am Fam Physician 2000;61(11):3343-50,3353-4
- Freed LA, Levy D, et al. Prevalence and clinical outcome of mitral-valve prolapse. N Engl J Med 1999;341(1):1-7

Web references: 8 available at www.5mcc.com
Illustrations N/A

Author(s):
Jonathan Vinson, MD

BASICS

DESCRIPTION Common, benign viral skin disorder consisting of small umbilicated papules which tend to occur on the face, trunk and extremities in children and on the groin and genitalia in adults. Incubation period is 2 weeks to 2 months. In immunocompromised individuals (e.g., HIV infection), the lesions can be extensive and atypical. They are occasionally giant (up to 3 cm), involve face, neck and trunk, and are recalcitrant to treatment.
System(s) affected: Skin/Exocrine
Genetics: No known genetic pattern
Incidence/Prevalence in USA: Common
Predominant age: Children and young adults
Predominant sex: Male = Female

SIGNS & SYMPTOMS
- Discrete pearly to flesh colored firm papules
- Diameter 2 to 6 mm (rarely giant nodules up to 3 cm occur)
- Usually grouped in one or two areas
- Centrally umbilicated with erythematous base
- Lesions can be pruritic or tender
- Beneath umbilicated center is white curd-like core
- Distribution: Anywhere. Predilection for face, trunk and extremities in children and groin and genitalia in adults.

CAUSES DNA virus of the poxvirus group. The virus cannot be grown in cell cultures. Incubation period is 2 weeks to 2 months after contact.

RISK FACTORS
- Close personal contact with infected persons
- In children, transmission can occur from swimming pools
- In adults, sexual transmission is common
- Immunocompromised individuals

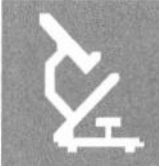

DIAGNOSIS

DIFFERENTIAL DIAGNOSIS
- Basal cell carcinoma
- Furunculosis
- Keratoacanthomas
- Warts
- Pyodermas (folliculitis, furunculosis)
- Pyogenic granuloma
- Vesicular skin disorders
- Disseminated mycosis in AIDS patients
- Lichen planus
- Lichen nitidus
- Bacillary angiomatosis

LABORATORY Virus particles cannot be cultured

Drugs that may alter lab results: N/A

Disorders that may alter lab results: N/A

PATHOLOGICAL FINDINGS
- Intracytoplasmic inclusion bodies in histological or cytological specimens
- Hypertrophied and hyperplastic epidermis

SPECIAL TESTS N/A

IMAGING N/A

DIAGNOSTIC PROCEDURES
- White, curd-like core easily expressed from beneath umbilication
- Biopsy

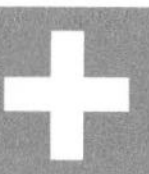

TREATMENT

APPROPRIATE HEALTH CARE Outpatient

GENERAL MEASURES Spontaneous resolution common in 6-24 months. Individual lesions often resolve in 2 months.

SURGICAL MEASURES
- The level of evidence for all surgical treatments is expert opinion or clinical experience. Options include:
  - ◊ Cryotherapy until halo of ice appears, and then thaw and repeat freeze
  - ◊ Curettage alone or followed by electrodesiccation under local or topical anesthesia
  - ◊ Expression of pearly core, either manually or using forceps
  - ◊ Piercing with an orange stick, with or without the application of tincture of iodine or phenol
- For recalcitrant lesions, especially in HIV infected patients, the use of lasers has been reported

ACTIVITY No restrictions

DIET No special diet

PATIENT EDUCATION Instructions for Patients, W.B. Saunders Co., Philadelphia

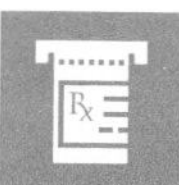

MEDICATIONS

DRUG(S) OF CHOICE
- Many medical regimens have been suggested for the treatment of Molluscum contagiosum, most of which have a level of evidence only of expert opinion or clinical experience. Options include:
  - ◊ Imiquimod cream - 1% or 5% applied topically 1 or 2 times daily 3 times a week for 4-16 weeks
  - ◊ Podofilox cream - 0.5% applied topically daily for up to 4 weeks
  - ◊ Potassium hydroxide - 5% or 10% applied topically twice daily for up to 6 weeks
  - ◊ Salicylic acid/lactic acid home treatments
  - ◊ Tretinoin cream or gel home treatments
  - ◊ Trichloroacetic acid treatment in the office
  - ◊ Podophyllin treatment in the office
- In addition, for recalcitrant lesions, especially in HIV infected patients, treatment with antiretrovirals such as cidofovir has been reported

Contraindications: Refer to manufacturer's literature
Precautions: Refer to manufacturer's literature
Significant possible interactions: Refer to manufacturer's literature

ALTERNATIVE DRUGS N/A

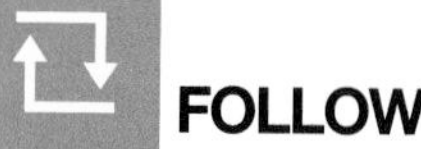

FOLLOWUP

PATIENT MONITORING Recheck in 4 to 6 weeks after treatment begun for development of new lesions. Two to 4 visits are often required for complete course of treatment (with office-based treatments).

PREVENTION/AVOIDANCE In adults, avoid sexual contact with infected individuals

POSSIBLE COMPLICATIONS
- Autoinoculation is common
- Contagious to others
- Immunocompromised individuals may have extensive infections

EXPECTED COURSE/PROGNOSIS
- Untreated, the condition is usually self limited. Individual lesions spontaneously involute in 2 months. Total resolution usually takes 6 to 24 months.
- Recurrences are uncommon in immunocompetent individuals, but may occur
- Lesions in HIV infected patients are more recalcitrant

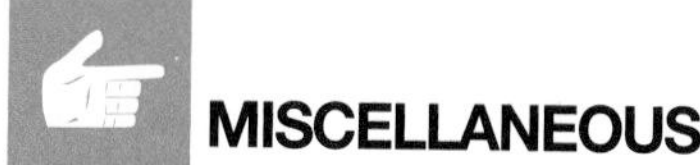

MISCELLANEOUS

ASSOCIATED CONDITIONS Occurs in 5-18% of patients with HIV infection

AGE-RELATED FACTORS
Pediatric: Commonly seen on face, trunk and extremities. May be spread through swimming pools.
Geriatric: N/A
Others: In adults, is often a sexually transmitted disease.

PREGNANCY N/A

SYNONYMS N/A

ICD-9-CM
078.0 Molluscum contagiosum

SEE ALSO

OTHER NOTES Spontaneous healing depends on triggering of a cell mediated immune response

ABBREVIATIONS N/A

REFERENCES

- Stulberg DL, Hutchinson AG. Molluscum contagiosum and warts. Am Fam Physician 2003;67(6):1233-40
- National guideline for the management of molluscum contagiosum. Clinical Effectiveness Group (Association of Genitourinary Medicine and the Medical Society for the Study of Venereal Diseases). Sex Transm Infect 1999;75 Suppl 1:S80-1
- Diven DG. An overview of poxviruses. J Am Acad Dermatol 2001;44(1);1-16
- Lewis EJ, Lam M, Crutchfield CE 3rd. An update on molluscum contagiosum. Cutis 1997;60(1):29-34

Web references: 1 available at www.5mcc.com
Illustrations 2 available

Author(s):
Nancy C. Elder, MD, MSPH

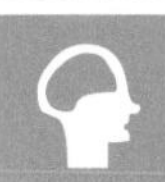

BASICS

DESCRIPTION Infectious mononucleosis, the classic triad of fever, lymphadenopathy, and pharyngitis is caused by the Epstein-Barr virus (EBV) in about 80% of cases. The majority of the remaining cases are due to cytomegalovirus (CMV) infection. Symptoms result from the effects on the lymphoreticular system. Transmission often attributed to kissing is via oropharyngeal/secretions/saliva. Incubation period is 30-50 days with the EBV replicating in the nasopharyngeal epithelial cells.

System(s) affected: Cardiovascular, Gastrointestinal, Hemic/Lymphatic/Immunologic, Nervous, Pulmonary

Genetics: Unknown; possibly related to severity of illness

Incidence/Prevalence in USA:
- Incidence is about 50/100,000/year in general population to 5,000/100,000/year in susceptible college students
- Lower socioeconomic status: 50-85% seropositive by age 4
- Middle-upper socioeconomic status: 14-50% seropositive by college age
- By young adult life, 90-95% of persons are antibody positive
- No clear seasonal incidence

Predominant age: 15-24; females 2 years earlier than males

Predominant sex: Male = Female

SIGNS & SYMPTOMS
- In most cases the clinical triad of sore throat (the most frequent complaint), fever, and lymphadenopathy (the most frequent finding) are present
- Lymphadenopathy (94%)
- Pharyngitis (84%)
- Sore throat (82%)
- Fever (76%)
- Malaise (57%)
- Splenomegaly (52%)
- Headache (51%)
- Anorexia (21%)
- Myalgias (20%)
- Chills (16%)
- Nausea, hepatomegaly, palatal exanthem, rash, jaundice, abdominal discomfort, cough, vomiting, arthralgias (all < 15%)

CAUSES
Epstein-Barr virus a double-stranded DNA herpes virus (≈80%); majority of remaining due to CMV

RISK FACTORS
- College and high school students
- Kissing
- 70-90% shed virus 2-6 months after initial infection
- 20-30% individuals shed virus after 6 months
- 10-20% culture rate from the oropharynx of normal adults and 50% from renal transplant and HIV positive patients
- Blood transfusion ("post pump perfusion syndrome"), due to CMV transmission

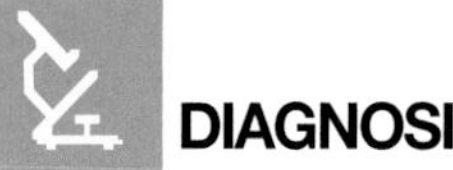

DIAGNOSIS

DIFFERENTIAL DIAGNOSIS
- Cytomegalovirus (CMV)
- Toxoplasmosis
- Rubella
- Adenovirus
- Herpes simplex
- Drug side effects
- Streptococcal pharyngitis
- Viral tonsillitis
- Vincent's angina
- Diphtheria
- Viral hepatitis A and B
- Lymphoma or leukemia
- Human herpesvirus -6
- Roseola
- Mumps
- Drug reactions
- Primary HIV infection

LABORATORY
- Positive EBV titers (IgG or IgM) (100%)
- Relative and absolute lymphocytosis (70%)
- Atypical monocytosis (90%)
- Elevated liver function tests (90%)
- Positive heterophil antibodies (90%)
- Thrombocytopenia (50%)
- Relative and absolute neutropenia (60-90%)
- Cryoproteins (90%)
- Monospot test useful as screen

Drugs that may alter lab results: N/A

Disorders that may alter lab results:
- CMV most frequently confused with EBV-induced mononucleosis. Majority of heterophile negative infectious mononucleosis due to CMV.
- Group A beta streptococcus often present (30%); does not rule out mononucleosis and deserves appropriate treatment

PATHOLOGICAL FINDINGS
- B-cell lymphocytes infected
- Polyclonal proliferation of B-cells
- Strong T-cell response

SPECIAL TESTS
- Heterophil antibody tests (Monospot or differential absorption). 40% of cases are positive in 1st week, 90% of cases are positive in 3rd week. Not helpful in children under age 5
- Specific EBV titers (use in heterophil negative or complications). Elevated in > 90% of cases at the onset of the disease.
  - ◊ Viral capsid antigen (VCA): IgG and IgM - peak at 3-4 weeks. IgG then declines, but persists for life. IgM declines rapidly and is undetectable by 3 months. High persisting IgG suggests remote infection, systemic lupus, chronic renal failure, Burkitt lymphoma, nasopharyngeal cancer, leukemia, sarcoidosis, cancer, AIDS, Hodgkin lymphoma, rheumatoid arthritis, and immunodeficiency state.
  - ◊ Early antigen (EA): Occur in 70-90%, persist 2-3 months. May persist in up to 20% of remote infections. High persisting titers might suggest: Pregnancy, immunodeficiency states, Hodgkin lymphoma, lymphoma, leukemia, AIDS, Burkitt, nasopharyngeal carcinoma.
  - ◊ Epstein-Barr nuclear antigen (EBNA): Develop after 2 months and persist indefinitely. E antigen in mononucleosis primarily. K antigen in nasopharyngeal carcinoma primarily. Absence suggests immunodeficiency.

IMAGING
- Ultrasound if clinically important. Useful for diagnosis and following splenomegaly.
- Commuted tomography (CT) best for imaging if splenic injury is suspected

DIAGNOSTIC PROCEDURES
- History and physical - fatigue, fever, splenomegaly, adenopathy, pharyngitis
- Heterophil antibodies - positive serology
- CBC/differential - abnormal white count
  - ◊ Absolute lymphocytosis (> 4,000 cells/cc)
  - ◊ Relative lymphocytosis (> 50%)
  - ◊ Atypical lymphocytosis (10-20% or more)

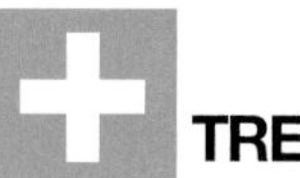

TREATMENT

APPROPRIATE HEALTH CARE Outpatient usually; 95% of patients recover uneventfully, without specific treatment

GENERAL MEASURES
- No specific treatment
- Quarantine not indicated
- General supportive measures
- Gargles
- Avoid vigorous splenic palpation

SURGICAL MEASURES
- Splenic rupture - inpatient observation with the ability to perform splenectomy if indicated
- Airway compromise - tonsillectomy or tracheostomy where clinically necessary

ACTIVITY
- Rest (bedrest possibly during acute phase)
- Avoid contact sports, heavy lifting, strenuous athletics (during first 2-3 weeks or as long as splenomegaly persists)
- Return to vigorous activity prior to 3 weeks from onset of symptoms should have documented resolution of splenomegaly by ultrasound (less than 14 cm)

DIET
- Healthy diet important
- To ease throat discomfort, patient may want to drink milk shakes, fruit juices and consume soft foods

PATIENT EDUCATION
- Convalescence may take several weeks
- Avoid stress
- Discuss feasibility of continuing with school or work
- Emphasize risk of splenic rupture from contact sports

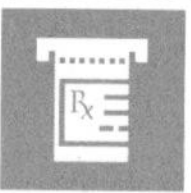

MEDICATIONS

DRUG(S) OF CHOICE
- Antibiotics for secondary infections only
- Analgesics
  - ◊ Acetaminophen (Tylenol)
  - ◊ Codeine
- Consider stool softeners to avoid constipation and its associated intra-abdominal pressure
- Steroids may be indicated in certain complications only - prednisone, 40-80 mg/d then less over 5-7 days. Consider in threatened airway obstruction, hemolytic anemia, and thrombocytopenia.
- Specific antiviral therapy is of no benefit to lessen symptoms; only decreases oral shedding of the virus during time of administration

Contraindications: Aspirin (associated with Reye syndrome)
Precautions: Refer to manufacturer's profile of each drug
Significant possible interactions: Refer to manufacturer's profile of each drug

ALTERNATIVE DRUGS N/A

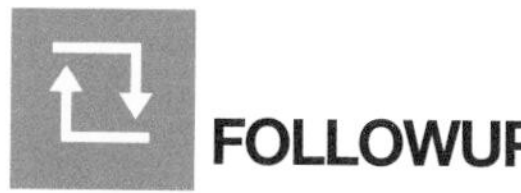

FOLLOWUP

PATIENT MONITORING
- Re-evaluate as needed based on clinical findings
  - ◊ Airway concerns
  - ◊ Splenomegaly
- Preferable documentation of resolution of splenomegaly before resuming contact sports

PREVENTION/AVOIDANCE
- Avoid saliva of infected persons
- DNA vaccine research in progress
- No blood donation for at least 6 months

POSSIBLE COMPLICATIONS
- Chronic EBV Infections (chronic fatigue syndrome- very controversial)
- Splenic rupture (rare, 0.1-0.5% of patients with proven mononucleosis)
- Hemolytic anemia (mild)
- Thrombocytopenic purpura
- Coagulopathy
- Aplastic anemia
- Hemolytic-uremic syndrome
- Seizures
- Cerebellar syndrome
- Nerve palsies
- Meningoencephalitis
- Optic neuritis
- Reye syndrome
- Coma
- Transverse myelitis
- Guillain-Barré syndrome
- Psychosis
- Pericarditis
- Myocarditis
- ECG changes
- Airway obstruction
- Pneumonitis
- Pleural effusion
- Pulmonary hemorrhage
- Hepatitis/liver necrosis
- Malabsorption
- Dermatitis
- Urticaria
- Erythema multiforme
- Glomerulonephritis
- Nephrotic syndrome
- Mild hematuria/proteinuria
- Conjunctivitis
- Episcleritis
- Uveitis
- ß-hemolytic streptococcal infections
- Staphylococcal infection
- Mycoplasma infection
- Bullous myringitis
- Orchitis
- Parotitis
- Monoarticular arthritis
- Jaundice

EXPECTED COURSE/PROGNOSIS
- Fever subsides in about 10 days
- Adenopathy and splenomegaly subside in about 4 weeks
- Children should be able to return to school when signs of infection have decreased, appetite returns, and alertness, strength, and sense of well-being allow.
- Death is uncommon (splenic rupture, blood dyscrasias, hypersplenism, or encephalitis)
- Potential role in some malignancies, especially in context of immune suppression

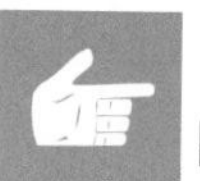

MISCELLANEOUS

ASSOCIATED CONDITIONS
Streptococcal pharyngitis

AGE-RELATED FACTORS
Pediatric:
- Children have subclinical or mild infections
- Most adolescents have clinically apparent infections

Geriatric: N/A
Others: N/A

PREGNANCY
No other specific recommendations

SYNONYMS
- Mono
- Infectious mononucleosis (IM)

ICD-9-CM
075 Infectious mononucleosis

SEE ALSO
Epstein-Barr virus infections

OTHER NOTES N/A

ABBREVIATIONS N/A

REFERENCES

- Braunwald E, et al, eds. Harrison's Principles of Internal Medicine. 15th Ed. New York: McGraw-Hill: 2001
- Safran D, Bloom GP. Spontaneous splenic rupture following mononucleosis. American Surgeon 1990;56(10):601-5 (VI:91093752)
- Schuler J, Horst F. Spontaneous splenic rupture - the role of nonoperative management. Arch Surg 1995;130:662-5
- Mandell GL, et al, eds. Principles and Practice of Infectious Disease, 5th ed. Churchill Livingstone, Inc. 2000
- Wick MJ, Woronzoff-Dashkoff KP, McGlennen RC. The molecular characterization of fatal infectious mononucleosis. Am J Clin Pathol 2002;117(4):582-8
- Burstin PP, Marshall CL. Infectious mononucleosis and bilateral peritonsillar abscesses resulting in airway obstruction. J Laryngol Otol 1998;112(12):1186-8
- Torre D, Tambini R. Acyclovir for treatment of infectious mononucleosis: a meta-analysis. Scand J Infect Dis 1999;31(6):543-7
- Berman MB, Nagel CE, Syed HJ, Morden RS. Spleen injury in sports, Part I: What diagnostic imaging can reveal. Phys Sports Med 1992;20(3):168-79
- Farley DR, Zietlow SP, Bannon MP, Farnell MB. Spontaneous rupture of the spleen due to infectious mononucleosis. Mayo Clin Proc 1992;67(9):846-53
- Maki DG, Reich RM. Infectious mononucleosis in the athlete. Diagnosis, complications, and management. Am J Sports Med 1982;10(3):162-73

Web references: 1 available at www.5mcc.com
Illustrations 2 available

Author(s):
W. Franklin Sease, Jr, MD

Morton neuroma (interdigital neuroma)

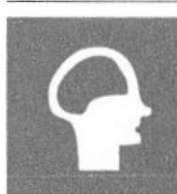

BASICS

DESCRIPTION Nerve swelling and inflammation of the digital nerve most commonly between the second and third metatarsal interspaces
System(s) affected: Musculoskeletal, Nervous
Genetics: N/A
Incidence/Prevalence in USA: Unknown
Predominant age: 20-50
Predominant sex: Female > Male (8:1)

SIGNS & SYMPTOMS

- Pain, cramping, or numbness of the forefoot with weight bearing or just after strenuous foot exertion
- Radiation to the toes
- Pain relieved with removing the shoe and massaging the foot
- Palpable nodule in the metatarsal interspace - occasional
- Positive Mulder's sign - a "click" and pain produced by squeezing the metatarsal heads together with one hand and simultaneously compressing the neuroma between the thumb and index finger of the other hand
- "Feels like I am walking on a marble"

CAUSES

- Excessive stress of the forefoot
- Repetitive trauma
- Congenitally enlarged plantar digital nerve

RISK FACTORS

- High heeled and narrow shoes
- Pronated foot (flat foot)
- Obesity
- Ballet dancing, basketball, aerobics, tennis, running, etc

DIAGNOSIS

DIFFERENTIAL DIAGNOSIS

- Stress fracture
- Arthritis
- Bursitis
- Foreign body

LABORATORY N/A

Drugs that may alter lab results: N/A

Disorders that may alter lab results: N/A

PATHOLOGICAL FINDINGS Chronic fibrosis and thickening of the digital nerve

SPECIAL TESTS Mulder's sign - a "click" and pain produced by squeezing the metatarsal heads together and simultaneously compressing the neuroma between the thumb and index finger of the other hand

IMAGING

- Radiographs may help rule out osseous pathology if diagnosis in question
- Ultrasound - hypoechoic nodule between the metatarsal interspace

DIAGNOSTIC PROCEDURES N/A

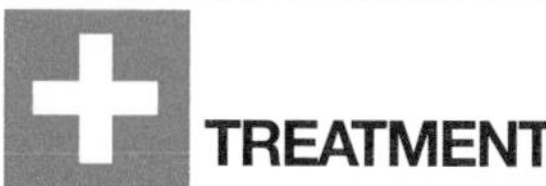

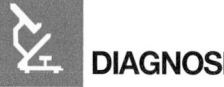

TREATMENT

APPROPRIATE HEALTH CARE Outpatient

GENERAL MEASURES

- Flat shoes with a roomy toe box
- Metatarsal pads - placed immediately proximal to the two involved metatarsal heads
- Corticosteroid injection into the dorsal part of the foot with medium- or long-acting steroid (betamethasone or methylprednisolone) mixed with local anesthetic (lidocaine)
- 80% respond to above measures

SURGICAL MEASURES Surgical removal of the neuroma (refractory cases)

ACTIVITY Modifying, shortening, or temporarily discontinuing standing, walking or running activities

DIET No restrictions

PATIENT EDUCATION Shoe wear. See Web references for patient handout.

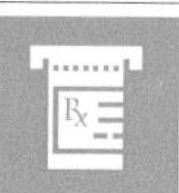

MEDICATIONS

DRUG(S) OF CHOICE Injectable steroids such as betamethasone phosphate/acetate or methylprednisolone - use if conservative measures fail
Contraindications: Refer to manufacture's literature
Precautions: Refer to manufacture's literature
Significant possible interactions: Refer to manufacture's literature

ALTERNATIVE DRUGS NSAIDs for temporary symptom relief

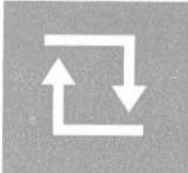

FOLLOWUP

PATIENT MONITORING If no improvement after 3 months of conservative treatment, consider corticosteroid injection. Repeat injection if no improvement after 2-4 weeks.

PREVENTION/AVOIDANCE Wide toe box and flat heeled shoes

POSSIBLE COMPLICATIONS Knee and hip pain related to a change in gait

EXPECTED COURSE/PROGNOSIS 40-50% improve after 3 months of conservative treatment, 45-50 % improve after steroid injection, 96% improve after surgery

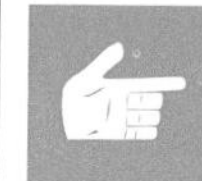

MISCELLANEOUS

ASSOCIATED CONDITIONS N/A

AGE-RELATED FACTORS
Pediatric: N/A
Geriatric: N/A
Others: N/A

PREGNANCY N/A

SYNONYMS
- Plantar digital neuritis

ICD-9-CM
355.6 Lesion of plantar nerve

SEE ALSO

OTHER NOTES N/A

ABBREVIATIONS N/A

REFERENCES

- Birrer R, DellaCorte M, Grisafi P. Common Foot Problems in Primary Care. 2nd Ed. Philadelphia, Hanley & Belfus, Inc., 1998:67-73
- vanWyngarden TM. The painful foot, Part I: Common forefoot deformities, Am Fam Phys 1997;55(5):1866-1876

Web references: 1 available at www.5mcc.com
Illustrations N/A

Author(s):
Frances Biagioli, MD

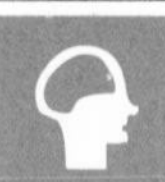

BASICS

DESCRIPTION Not a true sickness but a normal response to an abnormal situation in which there is a sensory conflict about body motion between the visual receptors, vestibular receptors and body proprioceptors. It can also be induced when patterns of motion differ from those previously experienced.
System(s) affected: Nervous
Genetics: N/A
Incidence/Prevalence in USA: N/A
Predominant age: N/A
Predominant sex: N/A

SIGNS & SYMPTOMS
- Nausea
- Vomiting
- Diaphoresis
- Pallor
- Hypersalivation
- Yawning
- Hyperventilation
- Anxiety
- Panic
- Malaise
- Fatigue
- Weakness
- Confusion

CAUSES Unknown

RISK FACTORS
- Motion (auto, plane, boat, amusement rides)
- Travel
- Visual stimuli (i.e. moving horizon)
- Poor ventilation (fumes, smoke, carbon monoxide)
- Emotions (fear, anxiety)
- Zero gravity
- Other illness or poor health

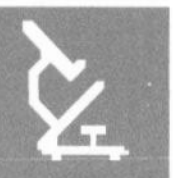

DIAGNOSIS

DIFFERENTIAL DIAGNOSIS
- Mountain sickness
- Vestibular disease
- Gastroenteritis
- Metabolic disorders
- Toxin exposure

LABORATORY N/A

Drugs that may alter lab results: N/A

Disorders that may alter lab results: N/A

PATHOLOGICAL FINDINGS N/A

SPECIAL TESTS N/A

IMAGING N/A

DIAGNOSTIC PROCEDURES N/A

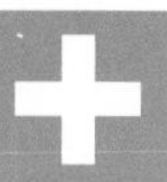

TREATMENT

APPROPRIATE HEALTH CARE Remove triggers or noxious stimuli

GENERAL MEASURES
- Minimize exposure (seat in middle of plane or boat)
- Improve ventilation
- Acupressure on the point PC6 is shown to reduce feelings of nausea, but not the incidence of vomtiing during pregnancy, after surgery, and in cancer chemotherapy. although no direct evidence is found for motion sickness. Point PC6 ('neiguan' in pericardium meridian): 2 cm proximal from the transverse crease of the palmar side of the wrist, between the tendons of m. palmaris longus and m. flexer radialis.

SURGICAL MEASURES N/A

ACTIVITY
- Semi-recumbent seating
- Fix vision at 45 degree angle above horizon
- Avoid fixation of vision on moving objects (i.e., waves)
- Avoid reading

DIET
- Decrease oral intake or take frequent small feedings
- Avoid alcohol

PATIENT EDUCATION N/A

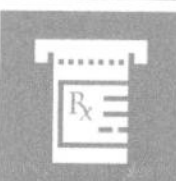

MEDICATIONS

DRUG(S) OF CHOICE
- Scopolamine transdermal where available; apply patch 6 hours before travel and replace every 3 days

or
- Dimenhydrinate (Dramamine); take 0.5-1 hour before travel; adults and adolescents 50-100 mg q4h, maximum 400 mg/day; children 6-12 years 25-50 mg q6-8h, maximum 150 mg/day; children 2-6 years 12.5-25 mg q6-8h, maximum 75 mg/day
- Meclizine (Antivert) 25-50 mg qd

Contraindications: Glaucoma

Precautions:
- Young children
- Elderly
- Pregnancy
- Urinary obstruction
- Pyloric obstruction

Significant possible interactions:
- Sedatives (antihistamines, alcohol, antidepressants)
- Anticholinergics (belladonna alkaloids)

ALTERNATIVE DRUGS
Ginger 940 mg or 1 gram; take 4 hours before travel; evidence controversial

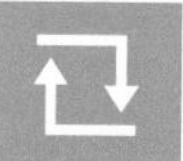

FOLLOWUP

PATIENT MONITORING
N/A

PREVENTION/AVOIDANCE
- Minimize exposure (seat in middle of plane or boat)
- Improve ventilation
- Semi-recumbent seating
- Fix vision at 45 degree angle above horizon
- Avoid fixation of vision on moving objects (i.e., waves)
- Avoid reading
- Minimize food intake prior to travel
- Increase airflow around the face
- Keep eyes fixed on still, distant objects

POSSIBLE COMPLICATIONS
- Hypotension
- Dehydration
- Depression
- Panic
- Syncope

EXPECTED COURSE/PROGNOSIS
- Symptoms should resolve when motion exposure ends
- Resistance to motion sickness seems to increase with age

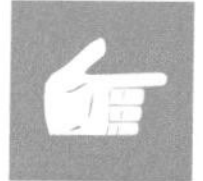

MISCELLANEOUS

ASSOCIATED CONDITIONS
N/A

AGE-RELATED FACTORS
Pediatric: Children more susceptible to motion sickness

Geriatric: Age confers some resistance to motion sickness

Others: N/A

PREGNANCY
N/A

SYNONYMS
- Car sickness
- Sea sickness
- Air sickness
- Space sickness
- Physiologic vertigo

ICD-9-CM
994.6 Motion sickness

SEE ALSO

OTHER NOTES
N/A

ABBREVIATIONS
N/A

REFERENCES

- Dundee JW, McMillan C. Positive evidence for P6 acupuncture antiemesis. Postgrad Med 1991;67:417-22
- Kohl RL, Calkins DS. Control of nausea & autonomic dysfunction with terfenadine, a peripherally acting antihistamine. Aviation, Space and Environmental Medicine 1991;62(5):392-6
- Rakel RE, ed: Conn's Current Therapy 2002. 54th Ed. Philadelphia, WB Saunders Co, 2002
- Goldman L, ed. Cecil's Textbook of Medicine. Philadelphia, WB Saunders; 1999
- Pizzorno JE. Textbook of Natural Medicine, 2nd Ed. New York, Churchill Livingstone; 1999
- Harris PE. Acupressure: a review of the literature. Complimentary Therapies in Medicine 1997;5(3):156-61

Web references: 1 available at www.5mcc.com

Illustrations N/A

Author(s):

Tadao Okada, MD, MPH

Multiple endocrine neoplasia (MEN)

BASICS

DESCRIPTION

Three subtypes of MEN are identified:

- MEN1 affects the parathyroid glands (hyperparathyroidism - 90% by age 40 years), the pancreatic islets (gastrinoma, insulinoma, glucagonoma, VIPoma, or pancreatic polypeptide-producing tumor), and the anterior pituitary (prolactinoma and GH-secreting tumors most commonly).
- MEN2A is a trio of medullary thyroid carcinoma (90%), pheochromocytoma (about 50%), and hyperparathyroidism (about 20-30%).
- MEN2B is defined by medullary thyroid carcinoma (90%) and pheochromocytoma (about 65%), marfanoid habitus, and mucosal and intestinal ganglioneuromatosis, but not hyperparathyroidism.

System(s) affected: Endocrine/Metabolic, Gastrointestinal

Genetics:

- Autosomal dominant.
- The gene responsible for MEN1 is a tumor suppressor gene located on chromosome 11q13 encoding the protein menin. Patients have germline mutations and develop tumors when there is a second hit to the other allele. 10% of mutations arise de novo. 10-20% of mutations are unable to be identified.
- The gene responsible for MEN2 is the proto-oncogene RET on chromosome 10q11.2. De novo mutations in 5% of MEN 2A and 50% of MEN 2B. No mutation identified in 2-5%.
- The degree of penetrance of MEN1 at age 20 years is about 43%.
- MEN2 is highly penetrant and should be diagnosed by mutation testing of RET by the age of 5 years. In children of patients with MEN2B, earlier diagnosis in the first year of life is recommended.

Incidence/Prevalence in USA: Prevalence in adults is about 1-250 per 100,000. Data for children are not available.

Predominant age: N/A

Predominant sex: Male > Female (2:1)

SIGNS & SYMPTOMS

- Hypercalcemia in hyperparathyroidism
- Hypoglycemia in insulinomas
- Abdominal pain in gastrinomas

CAUSES

- In MEN1, lack of functional menin interferes with its ability to act as a suppressor of JunD, a transcription factor important in cell growth
- In MEN2, mutations in RET cause it to function as an oncogene

RISK FACTORS

- Significant family history. In particular, consider screening for MEN2 in all patients who present with medullary thyroid carcinoma.
- Most hyperparathyroidism, pituitary tumors, and pancreatic islet cell tumors are sporadic, and only a few cases are related to MEN1

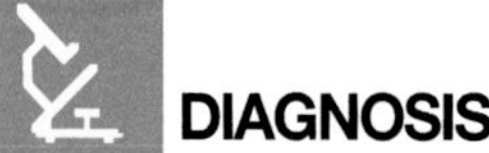

DIAGNOSIS

DIFFERENTIAL DIAGNOSIS

- Isolated tumors vs MEN syndromes

LABORATORY

Laboratory studies include investigations of the different tumor expression patterns.

- For MEN1:
  - ◊ Beginning at age 5 years: Annual fasting glucose, insulin, prolactin, and IGF-1
  - ◊ Beginning at age 8 years: Annual calcium, PTH
  - ◊ Beginning at age 20 years: Annual gastrin, chromogranin-A, glucagon, proinsulin
- For MEN2:
  - ◊ Calcitonin, plasma metanephrines or 24-hour urinary catecholamines or metanephrines, calcium and PTH

Drugs that may alter lab results: N/A

Disorders that may alter lab results: N/A

PATHOLOGICAL FINDINGS

- Hyperplasia of parathyroid glands
- Pancreatic microadenomas (mostly in the pancreatic tail)
- Duodenal tumors most often are gastrinomas staining positive for gastrin
- Diffuse hyperplasia of enterochromaffin-like (ECL) cells is found in the stomach
- Pituitary tumors are generally single in the anterior part of the gland
- Medullary thyroid carcinoma
- Unilateral or bilateral pheochromocytoma

SPECIAL TESTS N/A

IMAGING

In MEN1, abdominal CT scan (beginning at age 20 years) and brain MRI (beginning at age 5 years) every 3 years.

DIAGNOSTIC PROCEDURES

Biopsy as indicated

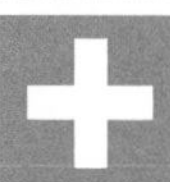

TREATMENT

APPROPRIATE HEALTH CARE

Outpatient with the exception of some inpatient stays for surgical therapy

GENERAL MEASURES

- Gastrinoma: The current treatment consists of proton pump inhibitors to reduce acid hypersecretion. Surgery is controversial.
- Insulinoma: Unresectable tumors are treated with diazoxide
- VIPoma: In unresectable tumors, octreotide may control diarrhea
- Prolactinoma: Dopamine agonists, such as bromocriptine or cabergoline
- Growth hormone-producing pituitary tumor: Transsphenoidal surgery or therapy with a growth hormone receptor antagonist

SURGICAL MEASURES

- Parathyroidectomy in hyperparathyroidism
- Thyroidectomy in medullary thyroid carcinoma. Prophylactic thyroidectomy in children with MEN2A by age 5 years, and with MEN2B by age 1 year.
- Partial pancreatectomy for tumors like insulinomas, glucagonomas, VIPomas
- Pheochromocytoma requires surgical excision under alpha-adrenergic blockade, starting 7-10 days prior to surgery
- Transsphenoidal pituitary surgery in some cases of pituitary tumors

ACTIVITY N/A

DIET N/A

PATIENT EDUCATION

- Counseling of inheritance pattern - 50% chance in siblings (unless de novo mutation) and children
- Importance of routine screening for tumor expression

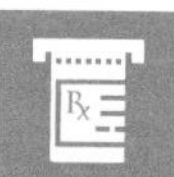

MEDICATIONS

DRUG(S) OF CHOICE

- Omeprazole (Prilosec) to reduce gastric acid secretion in gastrinomas
- Diazoxide (Hyperstat) to increase blood glucose in insulinomas
- Octreotide (Sandostatin) to decrease diarrhea in VIPomas
- Bromocriptine (Parlodel) or cabergoline (Dostinex) to treat prolactinomas

Contraindications: See manufacturer's literature
Precautions: See manufacturer's literature
Significant possible interactions: See manufacturer's literature

ALTERNATIVE DRUGS N/A

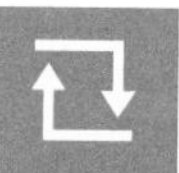

FOLLOWUP

PATIENT MONITORING Annual screening, lifelong.

PREVENTION/AVOIDANCE

- Monitor for tumor expression as under laboratory investigation. No prevention except for prophylactic thyroidectomy in children with MEN2A by age 5 years and with MEN2B by age 1 year.

POSSIBLE COMPLICATIONS Morbidity from development of tumors including nephrocalcinosis, osteoporosis, Zollinger-Ellison syndrome, complications from medullary thyroid carcinoma

EXPECTED COURSE/PROGNOSIS

Screening for tumors may reduce mortality, but there is no cure or prevention

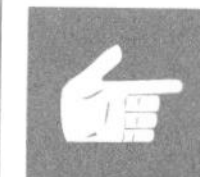

MISCELLANEOUS

ASSOCIATED CONDITIONS

- Tumors of the skin, adipose tissue, adrenal gland, and thymus may also occur in MEN1
- Cutaneous lichen amyloidosis and Hirschsprung's disease are associated with MEN2A

AGE-RELATED FACTORS

Pediatric:

- MEN1 onset typically before 40 years.
- In MEN2, medullary thyroid carcinoma presents in childhood. MEN 2A is highly penetrant and should be diagnosed by mutation testing of RET by the age of 5 years. If mutation test results are positive, subsequent prophylactic thyroidectomy with lymph node dissection is recommended. In children of patients with MEN2B, earlier diagnosis is recommended because the disease is even more aggressive, and thyroidectomy should be done in first year of life.

Geriatric: MEN syndromes typically present before age 40
Others: N/A

PREGNANCY May occur in patients after treatment of prolactinoma

SYNONYMS

- Multiple endocrine adenomatosis (MEA)
- Wermer syndrome
- Sipple syndrome
- Wagenmann-Froboese syndrome

ICD-9-CM

258.0 Polyglandular activity in multiple endocrine adenomatosis

SEE ALSO

Gastric malignancy
Hyperparathyroidism
Insulinoma
Marfan syndrome
Pheochromocytoma
Prolactinoma
Thyroid malignant neoplasia

OTHER NOTES N/A

ABBREVIATIONS N/A

REFERENCES

- Brandi ML, et al. Guidelines for diagnosis and therapy of MEN type 1 and type 2. J Clin Endocrinol Metab 2001 Dec;86(12):5658-71

Web references: 1 available at www.5mcc.com
Illustrations N/A

Author(s):

Caroline K. Buckway, MD

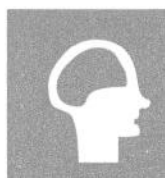

BASICS

DESCRIPTION Multiple myeloma (malignant tumor of plasma cells) is the most common primary malignancy of bone. It is the prototype of a monoclonal tumor cell proliferation that usually reveals monoclonal protein in the serum or urine of more than 90% of patients. The disease process encompasses a spectrum of localized and disseminated disease forms.
System(s) affected: Hemic/Lymphatic/Immunologic, Musculoskeletal, Nervous
Genetics: Occasional familial occurrence, indicating recessive heredity
Incidence/Prevalence in USA: Multiple myeloma accounts for approximately 1% of all types of malignant disease and slightly more than 10% of hematologic malignancies
Predominant age: Ages 40 to 80 (with a peak incidence in the 70's)
Predominant sex: Male = Female

SIGNS & SYMPTOMS

- The majority of patients (65%) present with bone pain
- Pathologic fracture occurs in approximately one-third of these patients
- Weakness and fatigue are common
- Bleeding (nose, gums), often evidenced by purpura or epistaxis, may occur in the presence of thrombocytopenia or secondary amyloidosis
- Recurrent infections may occur
- Patients may also present with renal insufficiency or renal failure
- Swelling on ribs, skull, sternum, vertebrae, clavicles, shoulder, pelvis
- Weight loss
- Hyperviscosity syndrome

CAUSES Unknown. There are tumor cells characteristic of plasma cells arising from bone marrow.

RISK FACTORS Family history of myeloma

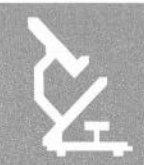

DIAGNOSIS

DIFFERENTIAL DIAGNOSIS

Metastatic carcinoma, primary malignancy of bone (sarcoma, lymphoma), metabolic bone disease, monoclonal gammopathy of undetermined significance (MGUS)

LABORATORY

- Anemia is present in 70% of the patients at the time of diagnosis. Nearly all patients will develop anemia as the disease progresses.
- Peripheral blood smear - rouleaux formation
- Serum protein electrophoresis - usually shows a spike or a localized band (M spike in approximately 80% of patients). Of these, 50% are IgG protein, 20% IgA, and 17% free monoclonal light chains (Bence Jones protein).
- Urine electrophoresis - positive about 70% of the time for light chains, but inconsistencies hinder diagnosis
- Hypercalcemia
- Decreased platelets
- Elevated sedimentation rate
- Elevated creatinine and BUN

Drugs that may alter lab results: N/A

Disorders that may alter lab results: N/A

PATHOLOGICAL FINDINGS

- Secondary amyloidosis
- Myeloma kidney

SPECIAL TESTS N/A

IMAGING

- Skeletal x-rays often show a radiolucent or a lytic lesion when the long bones are involved. The skull often shows punched-out lytic lesions with no sclerotic or reactive border. Periosteal reaction is uncommon. Vertebral compression fractures, with occasional extraosseous or extradural cord compression, are commonly seen.
- Although technetium-99 bone scans have often been described as cold, they will actually show some slight uptake increase in involved skeletal regions, particularly in the presence of fracture; however, the amount of uptake is far less than that demonstrated in other malignancies of bone
- MRI scans can be extremely valuable in determining the extent of marrow involvement as well as the difference between benign compression fractures and multiple myeloma lesions

DIAGNOSTIC PROCEDURES The laboratory test most likely to yield a definitive diagnosis is a bone marrow biopsy. The bone marrow will contain increased numbers of plasma cells at various stages of maturation.

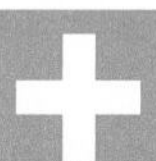

TREATMENT

APPROPRIATE HEALTH CARE Outpatient, except during intensive chemotherapy periods

GENERAL MEASURES

- Radiation therapy is limited to patients with intractable bone pain (failing chemotherapy)
- Patients with impending or pathologic fractures should have those fractures rigidly stabilized along with removal of the tumor, if possible. Patients with impending paraplegia secondary to spinal cord involvement should undergo immediate radiation therapy and bracing and/or surgical decompression and stabilization.

SURGICAL MEASURES N/A

ACTIVITY As tolerated

DIET No special diet

PATIENT EDUCATION American Cancer Society has literature available

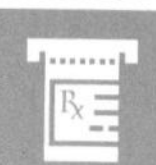

MEDICATIONS

DRUG(S) OF CHOICE Chemotherapy is the primary treatment for symptomatic multiple myeloma, but the ideal chemotherapy is unknown. The most common initial protocol management includes the oral administration of melphalan (Alkeran) and prednisone. This protocol produces an objective response in 50-60% of the patients. This is usually given in oral doses of 0.25 mg/kg/day for four days, along with 50 mg of prednisone bid for the same period of time. The dosage should be repeated every six weeks with leukocyte and platelet counts evaluated at three-week intervals.
Contraindications: Refer to manufacturer's profile of each drug
Precautions:
- Melphalan - myelosuppression is the major dose-limiting toxicity of this drug (mainly leukopenia, thrombocytopenia). Monitor CBC, platelets every 3 weeks.
- Prednisone - usual hazards of long-term corticosteroid administration. Refer to manufacturer's literature.

Significant possible interactions: Refer to manufacturer's profile of each drug

ALTERNATIVE DRUGS In the event of failure of the above-mentioned regimen, alternate protocols include
- ◊ Cyclophosphamide, carmustine (BCNU), vincristine, and prednisone
- ◊ VAD - combination of vincristine, doxorubicin (Adriamycin), and dexamethasone

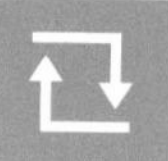

FOLLOWUP

PATIENT MONITORING CBC, platelets q 6 weeks

PREVENTION/AVOIDANCE N/A

POSSIBLE COMPLICATIONS
- Skeletal destruction
- Spontaneous fractures
- Secondary amyloidosis
- Renal insufficiency
- Recurrent infections (e.g., Streptococcus pneumoniae, Haemophilus influenzae)
- Hyperviscosity syndrome

EXPECTED COURSE/PROGNOSIS
- Average survival time varies considerably. The median survival of all patients is approximately 24 months. A significantly large number of patients survive for much longer periods of time with evidence of disease present.
- There are occasional temporary remissions with therapy
- Bone marrow transplantation should be considered in younger patients

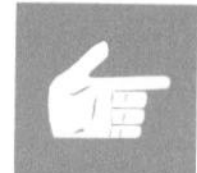

MISCELLANEOUS

ASSOCIATED CONDITIONS Multiple myeloma has an association with systemic amyloidosis in which the amyloid is derived from immunoglobulin light chains. In one autopsy series, 15% of the patients had generalized amyloidosis with deposits in the kidneys, spleen, adrenal bodies, and liver. Kidney involvement often leads to azotemia and secondary renal failure.

AGE-RELATED FACTORS
Pediatric: N/A
Geriatric: More common in older adults
Others: N/A

PREGNANCY N/A

SYNONYMS Myeloma, plasma cell

ICD-9-CM
203.00 Multiple myeloma without mention of remission

SEE ALSO

OTHER NOTES N/A

ABBREVIATIONS N/A

REFERENCES

- DeVita VT, Hellman S, Rosenberg SA: Cancer: Principles and Practices of Oncology. 6th Ed. Philadelphia, Lippincott Williams & Wilkins, 2001

Web references: 0 available at www.5mcc.com
Illustrations N/A

Author(s):
Mark C. Leeson, MD

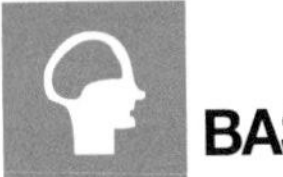

BASICS

DESCRIPTION Multiple sclerosis (MS) is a recurrent (occasionally progressive) inflammatory demyelinization of the white matter of the brain and spinal cord resulting in multiple and varied neurologic symptoms and signs. Usual course - intermittent, progressive and relapsing. It may pursue an acute or slowly progressive course. It is a major cause of disability in young adults.
System(s) affected: Nervous
Genetics: Appears to be a strong genetic component in determining susceptibility to the disease
Incidence/Prevalence in USA: 25,000 new cases each year
Predominant age: Young adult (16-40 years)
Predominant sex: Female > Male

SIGNS & SYMPTOMS
- Ataxia
- Babinski sign
- Blurred, double or loss of vision in a single eye; often triggered by retrobulbar neuritis and its visual sequelae
- Clonus
- Clumsiness
- Dysarthria
- Emotional lability
- Fatigue
- Genital anesthesia
- Hand paralysis
- Hemiparesis
- Hyperactive deep tendon reflexes
- Hyperesthesia
- Incoordination
- Loss of position sense
- Loss of vibration sense
- Monoparesis
- Ocular paralysis
- Paresthesias
- Sexual impotence in men
- Urinary frequency, hesitancy, incontinence
- Trigeminal neuralgia

CAUSES
- Unknown
- Autoimmune theory - supported by HLA linkage, hereditary pattern, immunocytes in plaques, changes in peripheral blood immunocytes
- Viral theory - supported by increasing incidence of disease at higher latitudes, clusters of cases with families, geographical clusters of cases, animal studies of infectious diseases of myelin
- Combined theory - autoimmune disorder triggered by environmental exposure to toxin or virus early in life

RISK FACTORS
- Living in temperate zone
- Northern European descent
- Family history of the disease

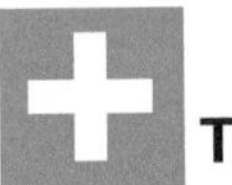

DIAGNOSIS

DIFFERENTIAL DIAGNOSIS
- Amyotrophic lateral sclerosis
- Behçet disease
- Brain stem tumors
- Central nervous system infections
- Cerebellar tumors
- Friedreich ataxia
- Hereditary ataxias
- Leukodystrophies
- Neurofibromatosis
- Pernicious anemia
- Progressive multifocal leukoencephalopathy
- Ruptured intervertebral disk
- Small cerebral infarcts
- Sarcoidosis
- Spinal cord tumors
- Syphilis
- Syringomyelia
- Systemic lupus erythematosus
- Vasculitides

LABORATORY
- Cerebrospinal fluid
  - ◊ Abnormal colloidal gold curve
  - ◊ Gamma globulin IgG elevated
  - ◊ Mild mononuclear pleocytosis (less than 40 cells/mL)
  - ◊ Myelin debris
  - ◊ Negative serology for syphilis
  - ◊ Protein normal or slightly elevated 50-100 mg/100 mL (50-100 mg/dL [500-1000 mg/L])
- Tests to exclude other disorders
  - ◊ Fluorescent treponemal antibody absorption (FTA-ABS)
  - ◊ Sedimentation rate
  - ◊ Screens for clinically suspected vasculitic disorders
  - ◊ Human T-lymphotropic virus-1 (HTLV-I) serology

Drugs that may alter lab results: N/A

Disorders that may alter lab results: N/A

PATHOLOGICAL FINDINGS
- Destruction of myelin sheaths of nerve fibers and axis cylinders, sparing axons, glia and other structures
- Atrophy of optic nerves and cerebral hemispheric white matter
- T-cell lymphocytes about venules

SPECIAL TESTS
- Visual evoked response (VER) - abnormal in 75-97% of definite MS cases
- Somatosensory evoked potentials - abnormal in 72-96% of cases
- Brain stem auditory evoked responses - abnormal in 57-65% of cases
- CSF
  - ◊ Oligoclonal bands
  - ◊ Increased IgG

IMAGING N/A
- MRI (more sensitive than CT) - may show many plaques
- CT scan (double-dose, delayed) - plaques

DIAGNOSTIC PROCEDURES
- No test specific to diagnose MS
- History, physical, CSF analysis, MRI, evoked potential studies, repeated observations over a period of time

TREATMENT

APPROPRIATE HEALTH CARE
- Outpatient as long as possible
- Long-term care facility for physical therapy or complications such as pyelonephritis

GENERAL MEASURES
- Remissions occur spontaneously and make treatment evaluations difficult
- Beta interferon 1a and 1b and glatiramer acetate represent breakthroughs in MS therapy
- Emotional support, encouragement
- Occupational therapy
- Urologic evaluation including any sexual dysfunction problems (impotence common in male patients)
- Self-catheterizations for inadequate bladder emptying (indwelling catheter may be necessary in a few patients)
- Custodial care, if patient cognitively impaired
- Physiotherapy to maintain range of movement and strength and to avoid contractures

SURGICAL MEASURES N/A

ACTIVITY
- Maintain activity, avoid overwork and fatigue
- Rest during periods of acute relapse

DIET If constipation a problem, high fluid intake, plus a high fiber diet

PATIENT EDUCATION For patient education materials favorably reviewed on this topic, contact: National Multiple Sclerosis Society, 205E 42nd Street, New York, NY 10017, (800)624-8236

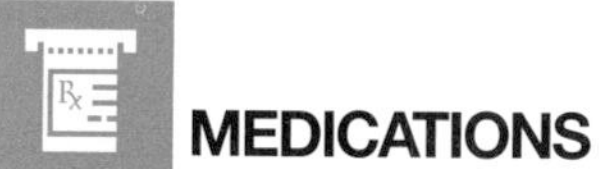

MEDICATIONS

DRUG(S) OF CHOICE

Drug therapy directed toward relieving symptoms

- Methylprednisolone: IV 1000 mg for 5 days followed by tapered oral prednisone for acute attacks, especially retrobulbar neuritis (recommended by some clinicians)
- Spasticity: baclofen, low dosage to start, 5 mg 1-3 times a day, increase as needed, or diazepam 2-5 mg qhs
- Constipation: stool softeners, bulk producing agents, laxative suppositories
- Urinary problems: propantheline 7.5 mg every 3-4 hours to start, increase to 15 mg 3-4 times a day plus 15-30 mg at bedtime; or oxybutynin chloride 5 mg 3-4 times a day
- Prophylactic antibiotics: for urinary infections
- Incoordination or tremors: no ideal therapy; may try beta-blockers (if not contraindicated), primidone, or clonazepam
- Depression and emotional lability: amitriptyline 10-25 mg at bedtime to start, increase as tolerated
- Paranoia or mania: haloperidol or lithium
- Musculoskeletal pain or discomfort: non-steroidal anti-inflammatories
- Hemifacial and dysesthesias: carbamazepine 100-200 once or twice a day to start, increase to total daily dosage of 600-1600 mg 3-4 times a day. Must monitor serum levels.
- Immunosuppressive agents (e.g., azathioprine, ACTH (adrenocorticotropic hormone), methylprednisolone, cyclophosphamide, interferons, cyclosporine) still investigational

Contraindications: Refer to manufacturer's literature

Precautions: Refer to manufacturer's literature

Significant possible interactions: Refer to manufacturer's literature

ALTERNATIVE DRUGS

- Oral steroids: Poor evidence for use alone
- Chronic fatigue: amantadine 200-300 mg/day (no specific evidence that this works)
- Baclofen 40-80 mg/day in divided doses for reduction of spasticity
- Interferon-beta approved for relapsing MS - 0.25 mg SC every other day
- Copolymer-1 approved for relapsing MS

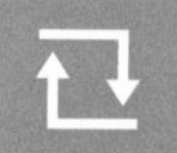

FOLLOWUP

PATIENT MONITORING Requires patient follow-up

PREVENTION/AVOIDANCE No known preventive measures. Avoid factors that may precipitate an attack, particularly stress from hot weather.

POSSIBLE COMPLICATIONS

- Coma
- Delirium
- Emotional lability
- Nystagmus
- Optic nerve atrophy
- Paraplegia
- Sexual impotence (men)
- Urinary tract infections

EXPECTED COURSE/PROGNOSIS

- Highly variable and unpredictable. Approximately 70% of patients lead active, productive lives with prolonged remissions.
- May disable the patient by early adulthood or cause death within months of onset
- Average duration exceeds 25 years
- 30% relapse in one year, 20% in 5-9 years, 10% in 10-30 years

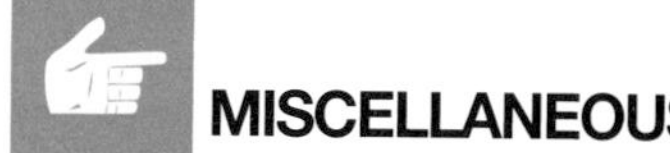

MISCELLANEOUS

ASSOCIATED CONDITIONS N/A

AGE-RELATED FACTORS

Pediatric: Unlikely before puberty
Geriatric: Remissions less frequent in this age group
Others: N/A

PREGNANCY A triggering factor for multiple sclerosis in some cases

SYNONYMS

- Disseminated sclerosis
- Insular sclerosis
- Neuromyelitis optica
- Devic disease

ICD-9-CM

340 Multiple sclerosis

SEE ALSO

OTHER NOTES

- Since the course is highly variable and unpredictable, avoid a hopeless outlook
- 30-40% of patients with optic neuritis alone eventually develop other signs

ABBREVIATIONS N/A

REFERENCES

- Sibley WA: Therapeutic claims in multiple sclerosis. 2nd Ed. New York, Demos, 1988
- Matthews WB, et al: McAlpine's Multiple Sclerosis. 2nd Ed. New York, Churchill Livingstone, 1991
- Adams RD, Victor M: Principles of Neurology. 5th Ed. New York, McGraw-Hill, 1993
- Rowlan LP, ed: Merritt's Textbook of Neurology. 9th Ed. Philadelphia, Williams & Wilkins, 1995
- Beck RW, et al: The effect of corticosteroids for acute optic neuritis on the subsequent development of multiple sclerosis. New Engl J Med 1994;329;24:1764-1769

Web references: 4 available at www.5mcc.com
Illustrations 1 available

Author(s):
Stanley G. Smith, MA, MB

BASICS

DESCRIPTION Acute generalized paramyxovirus infection usually presenting with unilateral or bilateral parotitis. Epidemics late winter and spring with transmission by respiratory secretions. Incubation is approximately 14 to 24 days.
System(s) affected: Hemic/Lymphatic/Immunologic, Reproductive, Skin/Exocrine
Genetics: N/A
Incidence/Prevalence in USA:
- 0.29/100,000 (725 per year)
- 0 .0064/100,000
- 90% of adults are seropositive even without history

Predominant age: 85% occur before age 15 years, but more severe in adults
Predominant sex: Male = Female

SIGNS & SYMPTOMS
- Parotid pain and swelling in one or both glands
- Rare prodrome of fever, neck muscle ache, malaise
- Initial parotid swelling just behind jaw
- Swelling peaks in 1-3 days, lasts 3-7 days
- Obscures angle of mandible
- Elevates earlobe
- Redness at opening of Stensen's duct
- Sour foods cause pain in the parotid gland region
- Moderate fever, usually not above 104°F (40.0°C). High fever is frequently associated with complications.
- Meningeal signs in 15%, encephalitis in 0.5%
- Rarely arthritis, orchitis, thyroiditis, mastitis, pancreatitis
- Rare maculopapular erythematous rash
- Up to 50% of cases may be asymptomatic
- Swelling in the sternal area, rare, but pathognomonic of mumps

CAUSES
- Mumps paramyxovirus
- Other viruses, such as Coxsackie (rare)

RISK FACTORS
- Highly contagious, 90% transmission rate for non-immune household contacts
- Urban epidemics, non-vaccinated population
- Usual communicable period is 24 hours before to 72 hours after onset of parotitis
- Incubation period usually 18 days
- Rubini strain mumps vaccine previously used in some areas of Europe and Asia is ineffective

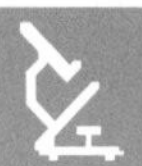

DIAGNOSIS

DIFFERENTIAL DIAGNOSIS
- Parainfluenza parotitis, other viruses
- Suppurative parotitis - often associated with Staphylococcus aureus (presence of Wharton's duct pus on massaging parotid gland nearly excludes diagnosis of mumps).
- Recurrent allergic parotitis
- Salivary calculus with intermittent swelling
- Lymphadenitis from any cause
- Cytomegalovirus parotitis in immunocompromised patients
- Mikulicz's syndrome (chronic, painless parotid and lacrimal gland swelling of unknown cause that occurs in tuberculosis, sarcoidosis, lupus, leukemia, and lymphosarcoma patients)
- Malignant or benign salivary gland tumors
- Drug-related parotid enlargement (iodides, guanethidine)
- Other causes of the complications of mumps (meningoencephalitis, orchitis, oophoritis, pancreatitis, polyarthritis, nephritis, myocarditis, prostatitis)
- Mumps orchitis must be differentiated from testicular torsion and from chlamydial or bacterial orchitis. (Testicular scan can be useful.)

LABORATORY
- Viral isolation from throat washings, urine, blood, or spinal fluid
- Serum amylase elevated
- Rise in paired antibodies: Anti-"S" antibodies peak early and may be seen at the time of presentation
- Cerebrospinal fluid (CSF) - leukocytosis
- Leukopenia

Drugs that may alter lab results: N/A

Disorders that may alter lab results: N/A

PATHOLOGICAL FINDINGS Periductal edema and lymphocytic infiltration

SPECIAL TESTS Rarely necessary, an easier salivary test for IgM is pending

IMAGING Useful to differentiate mumps orchitis from testicular torsion

DIAGNOSTIC PROCEDURES N/A

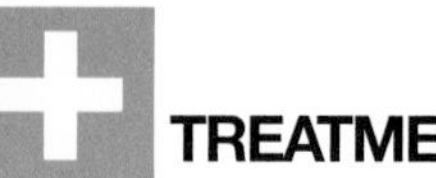

TREATMENT

APPROPRIATE HEALTH CARE
- Outpatient, if no complications
- High fever and testicular pain - may hospitalize for steroids or interferon

GENERAL MEASURES
- Supportive and symptomatic care
- For patients with orchitis, ice packs to scrotum can help relieve pain
- Scrotal support with adhesive bridge while recumbent and/or athletic supporter while ambulatory
- Use IV fluids if severe nausea or vomiting accompanies pancreatitis

SURGICAL MEASURES N/A

ACTIVITY Mumps orchitis - bedrest and local supportive clothing, such as wearing 2 pairs of briefs, or adhesive-tape bridge

DIET Liquids if cannot chew

PATIENT EDUCATION
- Must be out of school until no longer contagious - about 9 days after onset of pain
- Orchitis is common in older children but rarely results in sterility
- Immunization of family may protect against later exposures but not the present one

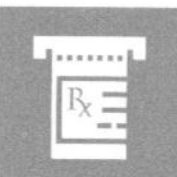

MEDICATIONS

DRUG(S) OF CHOICE Corticosteroids or a non-steroidal anti-inflammatory may diminish pain and swelling in acute orchitis and arthritis mumps, but usually not necessary. May use acetaminophen for fever and/or pain.

Contraindications: Refer to manufacturer's profile of each drug

Precautions: Avoid aspirin for pain in children. There may be an association of aspirin, virus infection, and Reye syndrome in children.

Significant possible interactions: Refer to manufacturer's profile of each drug

ALTERNATIVE DRUGS

- Mumps arthritis may improve with corticosteroids or a non-steroidal anti-inflammatory
- Interferon-alpha 2b for 7 days may be used in severe bilateral orchitis to prevent infertility

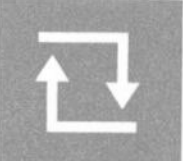

FOLLOWUP

PATIENT MONITORING Most cases will be mild. Monitor hydration status.

PREVENTION/AVOIDANCE

- 2 doses of live mumps vaccine or MMR recommended at 12-15 and 4-6 years of age. Vaccine is 95% effective. Adverse effects of vaccine: most common proven effect is ITP at an incidence of 3.3 per 100,000 doses.
- Immune globulin is not effective in preventing mumps
- Postexposure vaccination does not protect from recent exposure
- Isolate hospitalized patients until 9 days past onset

POSSIBLE COMPLICATIONS

- May precede, accompany, or follow salivary gland involvement and may occur (rarely) without primary involvement of the parotid gland
- Meningitis or encephalitis may present 10 days after first symptoms of illness. Aseptic meningitis is typically mild, but meningo-encephalitis may lead to seizures, paralysis, hydrocephalus or, in 2% of cases, death.
- Acute cerebellar ataxia has been reported after mumps infections; self-resolving in 2-3 weeks
- Cerebrospinal fluid (CSF) pleocytosis , usually lymphocytes found in 65% of cases with parotitis
- Orchitis common (30%) in postpubertal boys, starts within 8 days after parotitis, fever, swollen testis of 4 day duration, fertility impaired in 13% but absolute sterility is rare
- Oophoritis in 7% of postpubertal females, no decreased fertility
- Pancreatitis, usually mild
- Nephritis, thyroiditis, or arthralgias are rare
- Myocarditis - usually mild, but may depress ST segment, may be linked to endocardial fibroelastosis
- Deafness - 1/15,000 unilateral nerve deafness, may not be permanent
- Inflammation about the eye (rare)
- Dacryoadenitis, optic neuritis

EXPECTED COURSE/PROGNOSIS

- Complete recovery is usual, immunity is permanent
- Sensorineural hearing loss in 4% of adults - transient
- Rare recurrence after 2 weeks may be recurrent non-epidemic parotitis

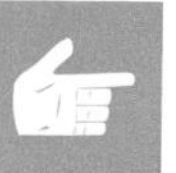

MISCELLANEOUS

ASSOCIATED CONDITIONS N/A

AGE-RELATED FACTORS

Pediatric:

- In adolescents - orchitis more common
- Most cases of acute epidemic mumps occur in children aged 5 to 15. Unusual in children less than 2 years. Most infants less than 1 year are immune.
- Less likely to develop complications

Geriatric: Most are immune

Others: Most complications occur in post-pubertal group

PREGNANCY

- No proven complications of vaccine, but theoretically should not vaccinate in pregnancy
- Disease may increase rate of spontaneous abortion in first trimester

SYNONYMS

- Epidemic parotitis
- Infectious parotitis

ICD-9-CM

072.9 Mumps without mention of complication

SEE ALSO

OTHER NOTES A portion of people infected with mumps virus have no parotid swelling and a clinically inapparent infection

ABBREVIATIONS N/A

REFERENCES

- Behrman RE, et al, eds. Nelson Textbook of Pediatrics. 17th Ed. Philadelphia, W.B. Saunders, 2003
- Report of the Committee on Infectious Diseases (Red Book). Elk Grove Village, Ill, American Academy of Pediatrics, 1997
- Casella R, Liebundgut B, Lehmann K, Gasser T. Mumps orchitis: report of a mini-epidemic. J Urol 1997;158:2158-2161
- CDC. Measles, Mumps, and Rubella - Vaccine Use and Strategies for Elimination of Measles, Rubella, and Congenital Rubella Syndrome and Control of Mumps. MMWR 1998;47:No. RR-8:6-15
- Peltola H, Davidkin I, Paunio M, et al. Mumps and rubella eliminated from Finland. JAMA 2000;284:2643-47
- Dale DC, Federman DD (eds). Scientific American Medicine. WebMD, New York, 2001
- Richard JL, Zwahlen M, Feuz M, Matter HC, et al. Comparison of the effectiveness of two mumps vaccines during an outbreak in Switzerland in 1999 and 2000: a case-cohort study. Eur J Epidemiol 2003;18(6):569-77
- Nussinovitch M, Prais D, Volovitz B, Shapiro R, Amir J. Post-infectious acute cerebellar ataxia in children. Clin Pediatr (Phila) 2003;42(7):581-4

Web references: 0 available at www.5mcc.com

Illustrations N/A

Author(s):

Frances Y. Wu, MD

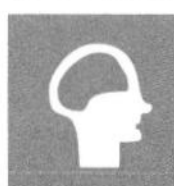

BASICS

DESCRIPTION Inherited progressive diseases of muscle with wide ranges of clinical expression.
Included:
- Congenital muscular dystrophy (CMD)
  - ◊ Merosin deficient
  - ◊ Merosin positive
  - ◊ With central nervous system abnormalities (CNS)
- Myotonic dystrophy
- Dystrophinopathies
  - ◊ Duchenne muscular dystrophy (DMD)
  - ◊ Becker muscular dystrophy (BMD)
- Limb girdle muscular dystrophy (LGMD)
- Emory-Dreifuss muscular dystrophy (EDMD)
- Fascioscapulohumeral muscular dystrophy (FSHD)

System(s) affected: Musculoskeletal, Nervous

Genetics:
- Xq28 recessive
  - ◊ EDMD 1 (encoding emerin)
- Autosomal dominant
  - ◊ LGMD 1 (A-E)
  - ◊ Myotonic dystrophy
  - ◊ EDMD 2 (1q21 encoding laminin A/C)
  - ◊ FSHD
- Autosomal recessive
  - ◊ LGMD 2 (A-J)
  - ◊ CMD
  - ◊ EDMD 1 (rare)
- Xp21 recessive
  - ◊ DMD
  - ◊ BMD

Incidence/Prevalence in USA:
- DMD: 1 in 3300 live male births
- BMD: 1 in 18000 live male births
- Congenital myotonic dystrophy: 1 per 10 000 births
- FSFHD: Prevalence of 1 in 20,000

Predominant age:
- Birth to infancy
  - ◊ CMD
- Infancy to early childhood
  - ◊ DMD, BMD, FSHD, EDMD
  - ◊ LGMD2
- Late childhood to adolescence
  - ◊ BMD, LGMD 1 and 2, FSHD
  - ◊ Myotonic dystrophy

Predominant sex: Male > Female

SIGNS & SYMPTOMS
- CMD and congenital myotonic dystrophy
  - ◊ Marked hypotonia and weakness, with feeding and respiratory difficulties. May present as neonatal arthrogryposis. Cardiac function is generally normal. Seizures are rare.
- DMD and BMD
  - ◊ Normal milestones until the child begins to walk
  - ◊ Progressive symmetric muscle weakness, proximal > distal, with inability to jump or climb stairs. Difficulty in rising to standing position - Gower's sign.
  - ◊ Pseudohypertrophy of calf muscles with heel cord contractures, toe walking, waddling gait and frequent falls
  - ◊ Inability to flex neck when lying supine helps to distinguish DMD from BMD
  - ◊ Initially a lumbar lordosis, later kyphosis and scoliosis with a progressive decline in vital capacity
- LGMD
  - ◊ LGMD 2: presents as DMD or BMD, particularly the sarcoglycanopathies (LGMD 2C-F)
  - ◊ LGMD 1: older onset, slower progression. Exception is LGMD 1C (caveolin mutations) and LGMD 1B (laminin A/C mutations) which may present in childhood.
- EDMD
  - ◊ Presents before 5 years of age with toe walking
  - ◊ Contractures develop before any significant weakness occurs, and typically involve the flexors of the arms and legs and cervical extensor muscles
  - ◊ Muscle weakness is mild and slowly progressive, initially involving humeral and peroneal muscles
  - ◊ Cardiac conduction abnormalities, usually in third decade
- FSHD
  - ◊ Facial weakness affecting eye closure and perioral muscles
  - ◊ Shoulder and proximal arm weakness with relative sparing of the biceps ("Popeye" arms). Inability to perform pushups, scapula winging, horizontal clavicles and forward sloping shoulders.
  - ◊ Muscle involvement is typically asymmetrical
  - ◊ Retinal vasculopathy and high tone sensorineural hearing loss present in some patients
- Myotonic dystrophy
  - ◊ Presents with weakness of the face, eyes, forearms and hands. (Proximal weakness may be seen in a later onset form: "Proximal myotonic myopathy.")
  - ◊ High forehead, receding hairline, open, triangular mouth and droopy eyelids
  - ◊ Sustained muscle contraction with percussion of the thenar eminence.
  - ◊ Difficulty in letting go (myotonia) after handshake. Myotonia worsened by cold.
  - ◊ Cataracts, cardiac conduction defects, gonadal dysfunction, personality changes

CAUSES
- CMD
  - ◊ Primary merosin deficiency: Chromosome 6q2. Laminin alpha2 gene mutation
- Myotonic dystrophy
  - ◊ Chromosome 19. CTG expansion affecting a protein kinase. Repeat size ranges from 50 to > 2000. The larger the repeat, the earlier the presentation.
  - ◊ Anticipation in successive generations may occur
- Dystrophinopathies
  - ◊ DMD: 96% with frame-shift mutation. 30% with new mutation
  - ◊ BMD: 70% with in-frame mutation
- LGMD
  - ◊ The most common LGMD in childhood are due to disruption of sarcolemmal proteins: part of a complex linking extracellular collagen with intracellular matrix proteins
- EDMD
  - ◊ EDMD 1: Chromosome Xq28. Most are nonsense mutations causing complete loss of emerin (nuclear membrane protein).
  - ◊ EDMD 2: Chromosome 1q21. Encodes laminin A/C (nuclear membrane protein). (Mutations within laminin A/C gene can also present as LGMD 1B, and cardiomyopathy with conduction block.)
- FSHD
  - ◊ Primary mechanism unknown. All patients have a reduction in the number of tandem repeats, of a tandem sequence termed D4Z4. Normal patients have more than 10 copies of this repeat. Patients with FSHD have 1-8 copies. Links to chromosome 4q35.

RISK FACTORS
- X-linked: affected male on maternal side of family (female carriers may rarely be symptomatic)
- Autosomal dominant - affected parent: Myotonic dystrophy more severe if mother is affected parent

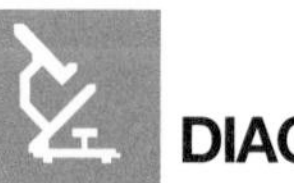

DIAGNOSIS

DIFFERENTIAL DIAGNOSIS
- Onset from birth to early infancy:
  - ◊ Encephalopathy, spinal muscular atrophy, infantile botulism, myasthenia gravis, congenital myopathies, metabolic myopathies, chromosomal disorders, paroxysmal disorders, neonatal spinal cord injury
- Onset from infancy to early childhood:
  - ◊ Mitochondrial myopathies, carnitine deficiency, acid maltase deficiency, spinal muscular atrophy, channelopathies
- Onset from childhood to adolescence:
  - ◊ Inflammatory myopathies, mitochondrial myopathies, spinal muscular atrophy, congenital and metabolic myopathies, channelopathies, myasthenia gravis

LABORATORY
- Creatine kinase
  - ◊ Marked elevation (more than 10 times the normal value) in DMD, BMD, LGMD
  - ◊ Mild to normal: CMD, myotonic dystrophy, FSHD, EDMD

Drugs that may alter lab results:
- Opiates (codeine, heroin, meperidine, morphine)
- Dexamethasone, ethanol, digoxin
- Furosemide, aminocaproic acid, halothane
- Imipramine, phenobarbital, lithium, clofibrate

Disorders that may alter lab results:
- Polymyositis/dermatomyositis
- Muscle trauma - exercise, seizures, IM injections, needle EMG
- Hypothyroidism, hyperthyroidism
- Myocardial infarction, stroke, sepsis, shock

PATHOLOGICAL FINDINGS
- Muscle biopsy
  - ◊ DMD/CMD: fiber splitting, centralized nuclei, necrosis and regeneration with increased fat and fibrous and connective tissues
  - ◊ LGMD: may show dystrophic changes as with DMD, or mild nonspecific myopathic changes
  - ◊ FSMD: highest yield in supraspinatus. Variability in fiber size, with cellular infiltrates and small, round, atrophic fibers.
  - ◊ EDMD: mild to moderate myopathic changes with type 1fiber atrophy

SPECIAL TESTS
- EMG:
  - ◊ Very helpful in workup to exclude neuropathies and disorders of the neuromuscular junction
  - ◊ In myotonic dystrophy high frequency repetitive, waxing and waning discharges ("Dive-bomber" effect).

IMAGING Brain MRI in merosin deficient CMD shows diffuse white matter changes resembling a leukodystrophy (represents a dysmyelinating process)

DIAGNOSTIC PROCEDURES

- Muscle biopsy
  - ◊ Biopsy moderately weak muscle (vastus lateralis, triceps, supraspinatus) not studied by needle EMG
  - ◊ Immunostaining: determines where the protein is present or absent. Useful in DMD, BMD, LGMD, CMD.
  - ◊ Western blot analysis allows the size and abundance of the protein to be determined. In DMD dystrophin content is <3% of normal; in BMD dystrophin content is <20% of normal.
  - ◊ Prenatal diagnosis:
    - DMD/BMD: Dystrophin studies in chorionic villous sampling and amniocytes; analysis of fetal RBC in maternal blood
    - CMD: direct mutation analysis of chorionic villous material or direct trophoblast staining for laminin alpha2 chain
  - ◊ Commercially available DNA testing: DMD/BMD, EDMD, FSHD, myotonic dystrophy

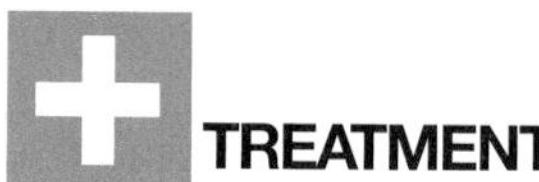

TREATMENT

APPROPRIATE HEALTH CARE Outpatient with team approach - neurologist, orthopedic surgeon, physical and occupational therapists, social worker, and orthotist

GENERAL MEASURES

- The broad goal of management is to lessen the impairments that result from disease and deter functional limitations and concomitant disability
  - ◊ Prevent contractures: active and passive stretching, physical therapy, positioning, splinting
  - ◊ Maintain muscle strength
  - ◊ Promote cardiopulmonary endurance
  - ◊ Maintain mobility and ambulation: bracing and walking aids
  - ◊ Monitor pulmonary and cardiac function
  - ◊ Vaccinations against influenza and pneumococcal infections when wheel chair bound and if on steroids

SURGICAL MEASURES Surgical release of contractures. Stabilization of the spine for scoliosis has no effect on the rate of decrease of respiratory function, but does decrease frequency of pneumonia and improves wheelchair comfort.

ACTIVITY Moderate exercise. Excessive demand can damage dystrophic muscle.

DIET Weight control is essential. Obesity adversely impacts on physical performance and respiratory function.

PATIENT EDUCATION

- Family and individual counseling
- Genetic counseling
- Printed material and clinical services available through the Muscular Dystrophy Association, 3561 E. Sunrise Dr., Tucson, AZ 85718; (800)221-1142; www.mdausa.org

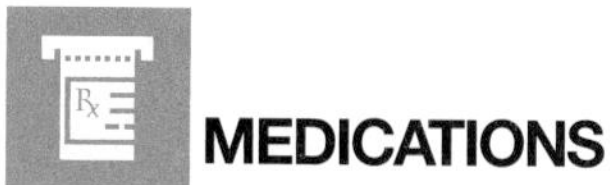

MEDICATIONS

DRUG(S) OF CHOICE Prednisone 0.75 mg/kg/day improves muscle strength in boys with DMD

Contraindications: N/A
Precautions: Monitor for side effects of long-term steroids. Includes osteopenia, weight gain, GI bleeding, hypertension, immunosuppression.
Significant possible interactions: N/A

ALTERNATIVE DRUGS N/A

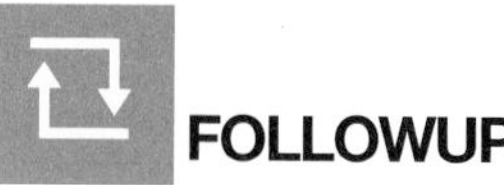

FOLLOWUP

PATIENT MONITORING

- Determined by interdisciplinary health team
- DMD: After age 11 years, yearly pulmonary function tests, EKG, CXR
- EDMD: Timely detection of cardiac conduction defects and early implantation of a pacemaker can be lifesaving.

PREVENTION/AVOIDANCE

- Maternal carrier status evaluation in DMD (80% sensitive) and BMD (60% sensitive) by creatine kinase levels
- DNA probes for carrier status determination and antenatal diagnosis in DMD and BMD
- PCR technology available for antenatal diagnosis of myotonic dystrophy due to myotonin mutation
- EDMD: Emerin determination in skin biopsies can be useful in identifying female carriers. Carriers are at substantial risk of having cardiac conduction defects.

POSSIBLE COMPLICATIONS

- Cardiac arrhythmias or myopathy
  - ◊ EDMD
  - ◊ BMD
  - ◊ DMD
  - ◊ Myotonic dystrophy
- Hypertension
  - ◊ FSHD
- Dysphagia or acute gastric dilation
  - ◊ DMD
  - ◊ Myotonic dystrophy
- Malignant hyperthermia
  - ◊ DMD
- Respiratory failure and early death
  - ◊ CMD (15%)
  - ◊ Congenital myotonic dystrophy (>50%)
- Endocrinopathies
  - ◊ Myotonic dystrophy
- Cataracts
  - ◊ Myotonic dystrophy
- Sensorineural hearing loss
  - ◊ FSHD
- Seizures and cerebral dysplasia
  - ◊ CMD with cerebral involvement
- Increase in fetal breech presentation in female carriers of DMD

EXPECTED COURSE/PROGNOSIS

- DMD and BMD
  - ◊ Progressive weakness, contractures, inability to walk
  - ◊ Kyphoscoliosis and progressive decline in vital capacity
  - ◊ Early death (Duchenne's 16 +/- 4 years; Becker's 42 +/- 16 years)
- CMD with brain involvement and congenital myotonic dystrophy
  - ◊ Progressive hypotonia and weakness
  - ◊ Respiratory failure and early death
- Other types
  - ◊ Slow progression and near normal life span

MISCELLANEOUS

ASSOCIATED CONDITIONS

- Mental retardation - DMD (25%), myotonic dystrophy with early onset
- Malignant hyperthermia may be seen in patients with DMD

AGE-RELATED FACTORS

Pediatric: N/A
Geriatric: N/A
Others: N/A

PREGNANCY Mother with myotonic dystrophy at increased risk for polyhydramnios, breech presentation and preterm labor

SYNONYMS

- Fukuyama muscular dystrophy
- Muscle-eye-brain disease
- Steinert disease

ICD-9-CM

359.0 Congenital hereditary muscular dystrophy
359.1 Hereditary progressive muscular dystrophy
359.2 Myotonic disorders

SEE ALSO

OTHER NOTES N/A

ABBREVIATIONS

CMD = Congenital muscular dystrophy
BMD = Becker's muscular dystrophy
FSHD = Fascioscapulohumeral muscular dystrophy
LGMD = Limb girdle muscular dystrophy
EDMD = Emory Dreifuss muscular dystrophy

REFERENCES

- Brooke MH. Clinician's View of Neuromuscular Disease. 2nd ed. Baltimore: Williams & Wilkins; 1986
- Crohn RD, Campbell KP. Molecular basis of muscular dystrophies. Muscle Nerve 2000;23:1456-71
- Darras BT, Jones HR. Diagnosis of pediatric neuromuscular disorders in the era of DNA analysis. Pediatr Neurol 2000;23:289-300
- Katirji B, et al. Neuromuscular Disorders in Clinical Practice. 1st ed. Boston: Butterworth-Heinemann; 2002
- Royden Jones H, De Vivo DC, Darras BT. Neuromuscular Disorders of Infancy, Childhood, and Adolescence: A Clinician's Approach. 1st ed. Boston: Butterworth-Heinemann, 2003

Web references: 4 available at www.5mcc.com
Illustrations N/A

Author(s):
Terence S. Edgar, MD
David A. Griesemer, MD

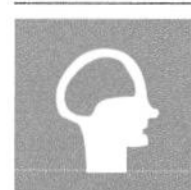

BASICS

DESCRIPTION
A disorder of the neuromuscular junction resulting in a pure motor syndrome characterized by weakness and fatigue particularly of the extraocular, pharyngeal, facial, cervical, proximal limb and respiratory musculature. Typical and neonatal forms are immunologically mediated. A number of congenital forms of obscure pathogenesis exist. Onset may be sudden and severe (myasthenic crisis) but, more typically, is mild and intermittent over many years.

System(s) affected: Hemic/Lymphatic/Immunologic, Musculoskeletal

Genetics:
- 15% of infants born to myasthenic mothers have neonatal myasthenia gravis, due to the transplacental passage of acetylcholine receptor antibodies. The condition completely resolves in weeks to months. Neonatal myasthenia gravis is not a genetic disorder.
- Infants with congenital myasthenia gravis syndromes are born to normal mothers. The onset is at birth or in early childhood. Inheritance is typically autosomal recessive. The condition is persistent.
- Typical adult and juvenile myasthenia gravis do have a familial predisposition (5% of cases) and an increased frequency of HLA-B8 and DR3.

Incidence/Prevalence in USA: 2-5/year/million; 3/100,000

Predominant age: Ages 20-40, but occurs at any age. Incidence in females peaks in the 3rd decade, in males in the 5th and 6th decades.

Predominant sex:
- Adults - Female > Male (3:2)
- Children - Female > Male (3:2)
- Children with myasthenia plus associated disease - Female > Male (5:1)

SIGNS & SYMPTOMS
- Ptosis
- Diplopia
- Facial weakness
- Fatigue on chewing
- Dysphagia
- Dysarthria
- Dysphonia
- Neck weakness
- Proximal limb weakness
- Respiratory weakness
- Generalized weakness

CAUSES Humoral immune-mediated injury of the post-synaptic neuromuscular junction acetylcholine receptors

RISK FACTORS
- Female
- Age 20-40
- Familial myasthenia gravis
- D-penicillamine ingestion
- Other autoimmune diseases

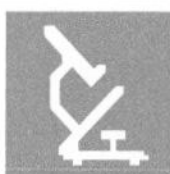

DIAGNOSIS

DIFFERENTIAL DIAGNOSIS
- Oculopharyngeal muscular dystrophy
- Thyrotoxic ophthalmopathy
- Other disorders of neuromuscular transmission (myasthenic syndrome, botulism)
- Polymyositis
- Other myopathies
- Guillain-Barre syndrome
- Intracranial focal lesions involving cranial nerves
- Multiple sclerosis
- Depression
- Chronic fatigue syndrome

LABORATORY
- Acetylcholine receptor antibody (AChR) - generalized myasthenia 80% positive; ocular myasthenia 50% positive; myasthenia + thymoma 100% positive; congenital myasthenia 0% positive; no clear correlation between antibody titer and disease severity
- Check thyroid function tests
- MuSK antibody - 40-70% of AChR negative patients have antibodies to MuSK

Drugs that may alter lab results: N/A

Disorders that may alter lab results: N/A

PATHOLOGICAL FINDINGS
- Muscle electron microscopy - receptor infolding and the tips of the folds are lost, synaptic clefts are widened
- Immunofluorescence - IgG antibodies and complement on receptor membranes

SPECIAL TESTS
- Motor nerve conduction velocity - normal
- Sensory nerve conduction velocity - normal
- Concentric needle (conventional) electromyography- normal in mild cases; low amplitude, short duration, polyphasic motor unit potentials with a varying morphology (may be called "myopathic")
- Repetitive nerve stimulation - shows a decremental response at 3Hz which is seen more frequently in the proximal, cervical or facial muscles. The decrement is less pronounced 30 seconds after a 30 second maximal voluntary contraction (post-tetanic facilitation) and most pronounced 120 seconds after the contraction (post-tetanic depression).
- Single fiber EMG (SFEMG) - highly sensitive but less specific, technically difficult to perform, limited availability. SFEMG assesses the temporal variability between two muscle fibers within the same motor unit (jitter). Myasthenia is one condition that increases jitter.
- Edrophonium (Enlon) test - initial dose is 2 mg IV, followed in 30 seconds by 3 mg, followed in 30 seconds by 5 mg to a maximum dose of 10 mg. A positive test is characterized by improvement of strength (of striated muscle) within 30 seconds of administration. False positives make a saline placebo control desirable. Atropine 0.4 mg IV may rarely be required as an antidote for severe bradycardia, but should always be available. Perform in a suitable setting with monitoring of EKG and vital signs and resuscitation capability.

IMAGING
- Chest CT scan - thymoma
- Chest MRI scan slightly less preferable because of movement

DIAGNOSTIC PROCEDURES
- History and physical
- Electrodiagnostic studies; repetitive nerve stimulation (RNS)
- Edrophonium (Enlon) test

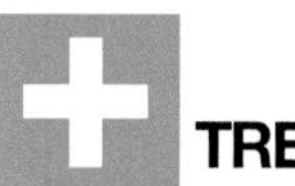

TREATMENT

APPROPRIATE HEALTH CARE
- Typically outpatient
- Inpatient care for plasmapheresis, intravenous gamma globulin, management of pulmonary infections, myasthenic or cholinergic crises

GENERAL MEASURES
- Management of myasthenia gravis is difficult and should be carried out by a neurologist with experience in the field.
- Three basic approaches to treatment, 1) being symptomatic, 2) being immunosuppressive and 3) being supportive. No or few patients should receive single therapeutic modality.
- Symptomatic therapy consists of reversal of weakness with an acetylcholinesterase inhibitor (eg pyridostigmine bromide; also available as slow release oral preparation), or neostigmine methylsulfate which can be administered parenterally. Symptomatic therapy does nothing to stop the ongoing immunologically mediated damage to the muscle receptor. An overdose of these agents may induce severe weakness known as a cholinergic crisis. Suspect cholinergic crisis if there are other signs of cholinergic overactivity (excessive secretions, diarrhea, bradycardia).
- Immunosuppressive or immunomodulatory therapy in some form is necessary. This includes thymectomy, corticosteroids, plasmapheresis, immunosuppressive drugs (mycophenolate, azathioprine, cyclophosphamide, cyclosporine) and/or intravenous human gamma globulin.
- Supportive therapy may be intermittently or occasionally eventually continually required; may include intubation, tracheostomy, artificial ventilation, respiratory therapy, administration of antibiotics, nasogastric tube and/or gastrostomy

SURGICAL MEASURES Thymectomy

ACTIVITY As tolerated. Heat and exercise both temporarily exacerbate symptoms.

DIET As tolerated

PATIENT EDUCATION Printed materials, reference lists and other forms of patient and family support available from:

1. Myasthenia Gravis Foundation, 2225 Riverside Plaza, #1540, Chicago, IL 60606, (800)541-5454; www.myasthenia.org
2. Muscular Dystrophy Association, 3300 E. Sunrise Drive, Tucson, AZ 85718-3208, (800)572-1717, (520)529-2000; www.mdausa.org

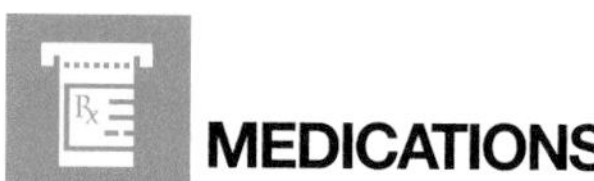

MEDICATIONS

DRUG(S) OF CHOICE

- Pyridostigmine bromide (Mestinon), 60 mg tablets and 180 mg sustained release tablets. Titrate dosage to clinical need. An average requirement would be 600 mg per day.
- Neostigmine methylsulfate (Prostigmin), 0.25, 0.5 and 1 mg/mL concentrations. Titrate dosage to clinical need. Starting dosages would be 0.5 mg SC or IM every 3 hours.
- Prednisone should be initiated usually on an inpatient basis, with a daily, followed by a switch to an alternate day, regimen. Start with a 60-80 mg/day, taper the dosage every 3 days. Switch to an alternate day regimen within 2 weeks, continue to taper very slowly attempting to establish the minimum dosage necessary to maintain remission. A typical maintenance dosage would be 35 mg every other day.
- Mycophenolate 2,000 mg/day
- Azathioprine or cyclophosphamide 150-200 mg per day.
- Immune globulin

Contraindications: Refer to manufacturer's literature

Precautions: Numerous. Avoid aminoglycosides and other drugs with potential for neuromuscular blockade which may precipitate weakness. Refer to manufacturer's literature.

Significant possible interactions: Numerous. Refer to manufacturer's literature.

ALTERNATIVE DRUGS Cyclosporine

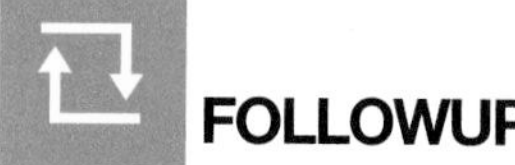

FOLLOWUP

PATIENT MONITORING

- Constant in an intensive care unit setting during myasthenic or cholinergic crises
- Inpatient in hospital during initiation of corticosteroids
- Outpatient follow-up every 3 months with stable patients

PREVENTION/AVOIDANCE Not possible

POSSIBLE COMPLICATIONS

- Acute respiratory arrest
- Chronic respiratory insufficiency
- Atelectasis, aspiration, pneumonia

EXPECTED COURSE/PROGNOSIS

Highly variable, ranging from remission to death. Mortality is probably less than 10%.

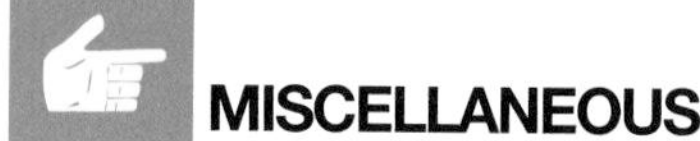

MISCELLANEOUS

ASSOCIATED CONDITIONS

- Thymoma
- Thymic hyperplasia
- Thyrotoxicosis
- Other autoimmune diseases

AGE-RELATED FACTORS

Pediatric: N/A
Geriatric: N/A
Others: Occurs in patients of all ages

PREGNANCY N/A

SYNONYMS N/A

ICD-9-CM

358.00 Myasthenia gravis without acute exacerbation
358.01 Myasthenia gravis with acute exacerbation

SEE ALSO

OTHER NOTES N/A

ABBREVIATIONS

MG = myasthenia gravis

REFERENCES

- Rowland LP, ed: Merritt's textbook of Neurology. 9th Ed. Philadelphia, Williams & Wilkins, 1995
- Kimura J: Electrodiagnosis in diseases of nerve and muscle: principles and practice. 2nd Ed. Philadelphia, F.A. Davis, 1989
- Snead OC, Benton JW, Dwyer D, et al: Juvenile myasthenia gravis. Neurology 1980;30:732-739
- Soliven BC, Lang DJ, Penn AS, et al: Seronegative myasthenia gravis. Neurology 1988;38:514-517

Web references: 1 available at www.5mcc.com
Illustrations N/A

Author(s):
Colin R. Bamford, MD

Myelodysplastic syndromes (MDS)

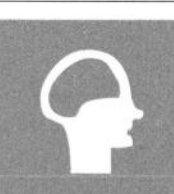

BASICS

DESCRIPTION A heterogeneous group of acquired hematopoietic stem cell disorders, characterized by cytologic dysplasia in the bone marrow and blood and by various combinations of anemia, neutropenia, and thrombocytopenia

- There is a natural progression of disease between categories as cellular maturation becomes more arrested and blast cells accumulate. There is a great deal of overlap between arbitrary diagnostic subgroups.
- Refractory anemia (RA) - < 5% blasts in marrow; < 1% blasts in blood
- Refractory anemia with ringed sideroblasts (RARS) - < 5% blasts in marrow; > 15% ringed sideroblasts; < 1% blasts in blood. Also known as acquired idiopathic sideroblastic anemia (AISA).
- Refractory anemia with excess of blasts (RAEB) - 5-20% blasts in marrow; < 5% blasts in blood.
- Refractory anemia with excess of blasts in transformation (RAEBT) - 20-30% blasts in marrow; or > 5% blasts in blood; or Auer rods present. This category is now generally considered to be acute myeloid leukemia (AML).
- Chronic myelomonocytic leukemia (CMMoL) - 1-20% blasts in marrow; < 5% blasts in blood with > 1000 monocytes/μl
- Refractory cytopenia - same as RA but with leukopenia or thrombocytopenia without anemia
- Refractory cytopenia with multi-lineage dysplasia (RCMD) - marked trilineage dysplasia but without excess of blasts
- Acute MDS with sclerosis - RAEB with marked myelosclerosis
- Refractory anemia with 5q minus syndrome - RA or RAEB with erythroid hyperplasia, mono- or biloculated megakaryocyte nuclei and normal or increased platelets. Incidence is 2:1 female > male. Characteristic interstitial deletion on the long arm of chromosome 5.
- Therapy-related (t-MDS) - seen 3-7 years after treatment with alkylating agents and/or radiation therapy. Evolves to acute myeloid leukemia (AML) over about 6 months.

System(s) affected: Hemic/Lymphatic/Immunologic
Genetics: Most are clearly clonal neoplasms by cytogenetics, G6PD isoenzyme analysis, or RFLP analysis. Mutations in RAS oncogene have been reported.
Incidence/Prevalence in USA: Apparent increased incidence (1-2/100,000/year) in recent years may be due to more accurate diagnosis
Predominant age: Median age is > 65 years; uncommon in children and young adults
Predominant sex: Male = Female

SIGNS & SYMPTOMS
- Anemia - fatigue, shortness of breath, lightheadedness, angina
- Leukopenia - fever, infection
- Thrombocytopenia - ecchymoses, petechiae, epistaxis, purpura
- Splenomegaly - uncommon; mild to moderate enlargement may be encountered, particularly in CMMOL
- Skin infiltrates

CAUSES Unknown

RISK FACTORS
- Primary MDS is associated with occupational exposure to petroleum solvents (benzene, gasoline)
- Secondary (therapy-related) MDS is associated with prior treatment with alkylating agents or radiation therapy

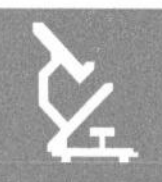

DIAGNOSIS

DIFFERENTIAL DIAGNOSIS
- Other malignant disorders - evolving acute myeloid leukemia (AML) or erythroleukemia; chronic myeloproliferative disorders (chronic myelogenous leukemia (CML), polycythemia vera, myeloid metaplasia with myelofibrosis); malignant lymphoma; metastatic carcinoma
- Nonmalignant disorders - aplastic anemia; autoimmune disorders (Felty syndrome, lupus); nutritional deficiencies (pyridoxine, vitamin B12, protein malnutrition); heavy metal intoxication; alcoholism; chronic liver disease; hypersplenism; chronic inflammation; recent cytotoxic therapy or irradiation; HIV infection; paroxysmal nocturnal hemoglobinuria (PNH).

LABORATORY
- Anemia - often macrocytic; occasional poikilocytosis, anisocytosis; variable reticulocytosis
- Granulocytopenia - hypogranular or agranular neutrophils with poorly condensed chromatin. Pelger-Huet anomaly with hyposegmented nuclei.
- Thrombocytopenia - occasionally giant platelets or hypogranular platelets
- Fetal hemoglobin - increased in 70%
- Sugar water (Ham's) test - increased RBC membrane sensitivity to complement lysis in some
- Flow cytometry to detect loss of CD59 on RBC, CD16 on granulocytes, and CD14 on monocytes; typical of paroxysmal nocturnal hemoglobinuria (PNH)
- Direct antiglobulin (Coombs) test - positive in some
- Paraprotein - present in some
- Erythropoietin - usually normal or physiologically compensated levels unless renal failure is present

Drugs that may alter lab results: N/A

Disorders that may alter lab results: N/A

PATHOLOGICAL FINDINGS
- Ineffective hematopoiesis with dysplasia in one or more cell lineages dominates the bone marrow picture in MDS. Marrow cellularity is usually normal or increased for the patient's age but may be hypoplastic in about 10%.
- Reticulin fibrosis is usually minimal except in therapy-related MDS
- Myeloblasts may be clustered in the inter-trabecular spaces, abnormal localization of immature precursors (ALIP)

SPECIAL TESTS
- Cytogenetics - at least half of patients with primary MDS and nearly all with therapy-related MDS have clonal chromosomal abnormalities (+8,-7,-5, del(5q), del(7q), del(20q), iso(17), and complex karyotypes). Detection of such a clonal abnormality establishes a diagnosis of neoplasm and rules out a nutritional, toxic, or autoimmune etiology.
- Granulocyte function tests - abnormal in half (decreased myeloperoxidase activity, phagocytosis, chemotaxis, and adhesion)
- Platelet function tests - impaired aggregation
- Marrow colony assays in vitro - results variable and correlate poorly with clinical course. Poor clonal growth may suggest more rapid evolution to AML.
- Immunophenotyping - nonspecific myeloid markers present. Occasionally evidence can be found for concomitant lymphoproliferative disorder. Loss of CD59 expression suggests PNH.

IMAGING Liver/spleen scan or CT although rarely necessary may disclose occult splenomegaly or lymphadenopathy

DIAGNOSTIC PROCEDURES
- Bone marrow aspiration, biopsy, and cytogenetics
- Review peripheral blood smear

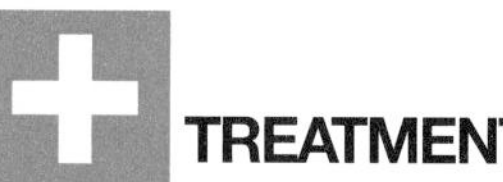

TREATMENT

APPROPRIATE HEALTH CARE Usually outpatient except when necessary to hospitalize for treatment of infection, blood transfusions, or intensive chemotherapy

GENERAL MEASURES
- Immunize for pneumococcal pneumonia and influenza and hepatitis B
- RBC transfusions to alleviate symptoms
- Platelet transfusions only for bleeding or prior to surgery, in order to avoid alloimmunization
- Early use of antibiotics for fever, even while culture results are pending, due to quantitative and qualitative granulocyte disorder
- Iron chelation therapy to avoid iron overload from chronic transfusions

SURGICAL MEASURES N/A

ACTIVITY As tolerated

DIET Reduce alcohol use. Reduce iron intake.

PATIENT EDUCATION
- Stop smoking
- Seek early medical attention for fever, bleeding, or symptoms of anemia
- Advise about the risks of chronic transfusion therapy

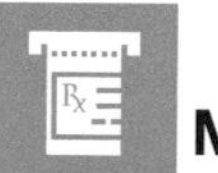

MEDICATIONS

DRUG(S) OF CHOICE

- Only 5-azacitidine has been proven more effective for these heterogeneous disorders than supportive care with antibiotics and transfusions as needed. Vitamins, iron, corticosteroids, androgens, or thyroid hormone are rarely helpful unless evidence of a specific deficiency exists.
- Clinical trials with 5-azacitidine, 75 mg/m2 SC for 7 days; repeated every 28 days, decreases RBC transfusion requirements and yields longer times to AML or death and improvements in quality of life.
- Intensive chemotherapy: younger patients with MDS may benefit from AML chemotherapy, especially if Auer rods are present, but toxicity may be severe for older patients. Remission durations are variable (median, about 1 year).
- Allogeneic bone marrow transplantation: recommended for younger patients with HLA-matched donors to eradicate the malignant clone and re-supply normal hematopoietic stem cells
- Aminocaproic acid (epsilon-aminocaproic acid, EACA) or tranexamic acid may benefit patients with chronic, severe thrombocytopenia and bleeding.

Contraindications: Cytotoxicity of chemotherapy may increase the risk of bleeding and infection and the need for transfusion support

Precautions: Aspirin, salicylates, and NSAIDs should be avoided

Significant possible interactions: N/A

ALTERNATIVE DRUGS

- Possible differentiating agents such as tretinoin (all-trans-retinoic acid); or homoharringtonine and other hematopoietic growth factors are under investigation
- Danazol or prednisone may benefit concomitant autoimmune thrombocytopenia
- Investigational agents: low doses of cytarabine or decitabine, 13-cis retinoic acid, interferon, cyclosporine, granulocyte-macrophage colony stimulating factor (GM-CSF) or granulocyte colony stimulating factor (G-CSF), interleukin-3 (IL-3)
- Agents, such as thalidomide, that inhibit production of tumor necrosis factor in the marrow are being investigated
- Amifostine may stimulate proliferation of normal hematopoiesis
- Topotecan has been reported to have cytotoxic benefit in CMMOL
- Revlimid has been reported to induce complete remissions in refractory anemia with del (5q) syndrome

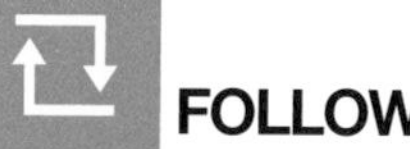

FOLLOWUP

PATIENT MONITORING At least monthly during supportive care. More frequently if receiving treatment.

PREVENTION/AVOIDANCE N/A

POSSIBLE COMPLICATIONS Infection, bleeding, complications of anemia and transfusions

EXPECTED COURSE/PROGNOSIS

- Median survival for RA and RARS is 5 years but may extend much longer. Refractory anemia with 5q minus syndrome is quite favorable.
- Median survival for RAEB, RAEBT, and CMMOL is about 1 year with half of patients evolving to AML and the other half dying of infection or bleeding

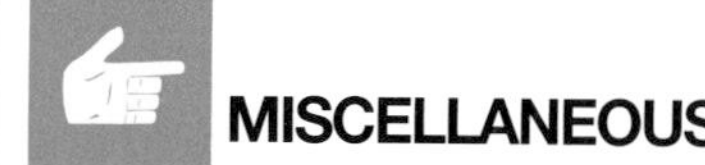

MISCELLANEOUS

ASSOCIATED CONDITIONS N/A

AGE-RELATED FACTORS

Pediatric: Monosomy 7 syndrome; juvenile chronic myelogenous leukemia

Geriatric: N/A

Others: N/A

PREGNANCY N/A

SYNONYMS

- Dysmyelopoietic syndrome
- Hemopoietic dysplasia
- Preleukemia
- Smoldering or subacute myeloid leukemia
- CMMoL; Chronic myelomonocytic leukemia
- CMML; Chronic myelomonocytic leukemia

ICD-9-CM

238.7 Neoplasm of uncertain behavior of other lymphatic and hematopoietic tissues

SEE ALSO

OTHER NOTES N/A

ABBREVIATIONS

PNH = paroxysmal nocturnal hemoglobinuria

REFERENCES

- Hoffman R, Benz EJ Jr, Shattil S, et al, eds: Hematology: Basic Principles and Practice. 3rd Ed. New York, Churchill Livingstone, 2000
- Greenberg P, Cox C, Le Beau MM, et al: International scoring system for evaluating prognosis in myelodysplastic syndromes. Blood 1997;89:2079-2088
- Thirman MJ, Larson RA: Therapy-related myeloid leukemia. Hematology/Oncology Clin of NA 1996;10:293-320
- Silverman LR, Demakos EP, Peterson BL, et al. Randomized controlled trial of azacitidine in patients with the myelodysplastic syndrome: a study of the cancer and leukemia group B. J Clin Oncol 2002;20(10):2429-40

Web references: 7 available at www.5mcc.com

Illustrations N/A

Author(s):
Richard A. Larson, MD

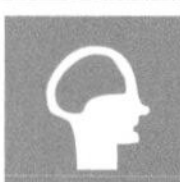

BASICS

DESCRIPTION The myeloproliferative disorders are neoplasms of the pluripotent hematopoietic stem cell. They include chronic myelogenous leukemia (CML), polycythemia vera (PV), chronic idiopathic myelofibrosis (CIMF), also known as agnogenic myeloid metaplasia or myelofibrosis with myeloid metaplasia, and essential thrombocytosis (ET). PV is discussed in another chapter.

- With each disorder, the proliferation of one particular cell line tends to dominate. There is a variable tendency for reactive proliferation of the bone marrow fibroblast, which is not a part of the malignant clone, resulting in myelofibrosis, and a variable tendency for termination in an acute leukemic phase. These disorders can mimic one another closely, CML is the only one that is readily distinguished from the others by the presence of the Philadelphia chromosome.
- CML
  - ◊ Characterized by splenomegaly and increased granulocytes, particularly neutrophils
  - ◊ Runs a generally mild course until it transforms to a frankly leukemic (blastic) phase
- CIMF
  - ◊ Characterized by extramedullary hematopoiesis in the spleen or multiple other organs, and myelofibrosis
  - ◊ Myelofibrosis appears to be a reaction to the presence of the abnormal, proliferating hematopoietic clone
- ET
  - ◊ Dominated clinically by a markedly elevated platelet count

System(s) affected: Hemic/Lymphatic/Immunologic

Genetics:
- CML - no genetic predisposition known
- CIMF - rare familial occurrence
- ET - may be familial

Incidence/Prevalence in USA:
- CML - annual incidence 1-2/100,000; incidence increases with age
- CIMF - annual incidence 0.5-1.5/100,000
- ET - annual incidence 1-2.5/100,000

Predominant age:
- CML - median age at diagnosis is 50-60
- CIMF; ET - median age at diagnosis is 60; distinct second peak incidence of ET occurs in younger patients, usually women, at about 30 years of age

Predominant sex:
- CML - Male > Female 1.4:1
- CIMF - Male = Female (No major sexual predilection)
- ET - Female > Male 1.3:1

SIGNS & SYMPTOMS
- General
  - ◊ Most are asymptomatic at the time of diagnosis
  - ◊ Vague constitutional symptoms
  - ◊ Hypermetabolic state (fever, sweating)
  - ◊ Acute gouty arthritis
  - ◊ Left-upper-quadrant abdominal pain or fullness from splenomegaly
- CML
  - ◊ Splenomegaly (palpable in 90% of patients)
- CIMF
  - ◊ Splenomegaly in virtually all patients, and can be massive
  - ◊ Hepatomegaly in 50%
  - ◊ Lymph node enlargement in 10%
  - ◊ Jaundice, edema, and ascites in 10-20%
  - ◊ Petechiae in up to 25%
- ET
  - ◊ May be asymptomatic in over 50%
  - ◊ Easy bruising, unusual bleeding after minor dental procedures, large-vessel bleeding in the absence of trauma
  - ◊ Transient ischemic attacks, or even frank strokes, may occur in patients with markedly elevated platelet counts

CAUSES Unknown. May be familial for some types.

RISK FACTORS
- Family history of myeloproliferative disorder (rare)
- CML - increased incidence in atomic bomb survivors and following radiation treatment of ankylosing spondylitis and cervical cancer

DIAGNOSIS

DIFFERENTIAL DIAGNOSIS
- CML
  - ◊ Leukemoid reaction
  - ◊ Chronic myelomonocytic leukemia which has features of both myeloproliferative and myelodysplastic syndromes
  - ◊ Low or absent leukocyte alkaline phosphatase (LAP) also seen in paroxysmal nocturnal hemoglobinuria
- CIMF
  - ◊ Spent PV (late stage of PV)
  - ◊ CML
  - ◊ Myelodysplastic syndrome (MDS) with fibrosis
  - ◊ Secondary myelofibrosis
- ET
  - ◊ Secondary thrombocytosis (including inflammation, iron deficiency, and neoplasia)
  - ◊ PV
  - ◊ CML

LABORATORY
- CML
  - ◊ Marked leukocytosis consisting of mature polymorphonuclear neutrophils and myelocytes or metamyelocytes
  - ◊ Chronic phase typically with less than 2% myeloblasts in peripheral blood and less than 5% blasts in the bone marrow
  - ◊ Blast crisis is defined when 20% or more blast cells are present in the bone marrow and/or peripheral blood
  - ◊ Basophilia
  - ◊ Elevated serum vitamin B12 level
  - ◊ Hyperuricemia
  - ◊ Markedly decreased leukocyte alkaline phosphatase (absent in 5-10% of patients)
- CIMF
  - ◊ Mild anemia - in more than 50% of patients at time of diagnosis, eventually in almost all patients, and is progressive
  - ◊ Leukocytosis in 30% of patients
  - ◊ Leukoerythroblastic blood picture in > 90% of cases
  - ◊ Leukopenia in 25%
  - ◊ Thrombocytopenia in 30%
  - ◊ Marked thrombocytosis (> 800,000/uL) in 12%
  - ◊ Occasional RBC autoantibodies
- ET - the WHO diagnostic criteria are:
  - ◊ Thrombocytosis persistently greater than 600,000 per mL /uL in the absence of an identifiable cause
  - ◊ Bone marrow biopsy showing increased numbers of enlarged, mature megakaryocytes
  - ◊ No evidence of PV (Normal total RBC mass
  - ◊ Presence of iron in the bone marrow, normal ferritin or normal MCV)
  - ◊ Absence of collagen fibrosis, minimal or absent reticulin fibrosis in bone marrow biopsy
  - ◊ Absence of the Philadelphia chromosome
  - ◊ No evidence of MDS
  - ◊ No evidence of reactive thrombocytosis

Drugs that may alter lab results: N/A

Disorders that may alter lab results: In CML, LAP rises during infection, glucocorticoid use, or successful therapy. False positive hyperkalemia can be seen in ET due to release of platelet potassium upon blood clotting

PATHOLOGICAL FINDINGS
- CIMF
  - ◊ Foci of extramedullary hematopoiesis may be seen in multiple organs including spleen, liver, kidneys, lymph nodes, adrenal glands, lungs, and spinal column
  - ◊ Bone marrow megakaryocytic hyperplasia and atypia, reticulin and/or collagen fibrosis, osteosclerosis (new bone formation). Bone marrow cellularity is variable depending on the degree of fibrosis.

SPECIAL TESTS CML > 95% of patients are Philadelphia chromosome positive (shortened chromosome 22 due to a reciprocal translocation between chromosomes 9 and 22). This translocation results in a fusion of the ABL gene on chromosome 9, to the BCR gene on chromosome 22.

IMAGING CIMF - radiographic osteosclerosis in 25-66% of patients, particularly in the axial skeleton and proximal long bones

DIAGNOSTIC PROCEDURES
- Peripheral blood smear
- Bone marrow aspiration and core biopsy
- Cytogenetic studies
- Molecular studies (RT-PCR to detect the BCR-ABL fusion gene)

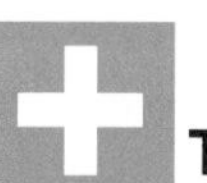

TREATMENT

APPROPRIATE HEALTH CARE N/A

GENERAL MEASURES
- Treatment to relieve symptoms and prevent infections
- Splenectomy has no impact on mortality, but is occasionally done for symptomatic relief. Extreme thrombocytosis, progressive and massive liver enlargement may ensue.
- CML
  - ◊ Molecularly targeted therapy (with imatinib mesylate)
  - ◊ Chemotherapy (for advanced phases of the disease)
  - ◊ Bone marrow transplantation is the only known curative option, with disease-free survival in 50-70%, and should be offered to young patients with HLA matched donors

- CIMF
  - ◊ No standard therapy
  - ◊ Rule out other treatable causes for anemia
  - ◊ Radiotherapy for symptomatic extramedullary hematopoietic tumors, or symptomatic splenomegaly
  - ◊ Successful bone marrow transplantation leads to the reversal of established fibrosis, and is the only known potential cure
- ET
  - ◊ Young, asymptomatic patients with platelet count < 1,500,000/uL generally not treated
  - ◊ Lower the platelet count in those > 60, history of thrombosis, or with other cardiovascular risk factors, or platelet count > 1,500,000/uL

SURGICAL MEASURES See General Measures

ACTIVITY Restrictions will be dependent on symptoms and progression of the disorder

DIET Maintain good nutrition

PATIENT EDUCATION
- Explanations about the disorder, treatment protocols, lab studies, and prognosis
- Symptoms of recurrence to watch for
- Importance of followup examinations

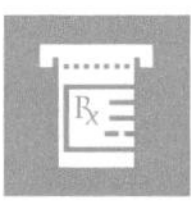

MEDICATIONS

DRUG(S) OF CHOICE
- CML
  - ◊ Imatinib mesylate (Gleevec), a potent inhibitor of the ABL tyrosine kinase, produces complete hematologic remissions in 95% and major cytogenetic remissions in 87% of newly diagnosed patients in chronic phase. Dosage - 400 mg/day in chronic phase CML, 600-800 mg/day in accelerated/blast phase disease
  - ◊ Interferon alpha produces 55% complete hematologic remissions, and 35% major cytogenetic remissions and has largely been replaced by imatinib as the treatment of choice for most patients
  - ◊ Allopurinol to control hyperuricemia - begin prior to hydroxyurea therapy
  - ◊ Hydroxyurea may be useful for controlling the excessive myelopoiesis at initial diagnosis in chronic phase disease, in conjunction with imatinib
  - ◊ Accelerated phase and blast crisis are usually treated with regimens designed for the treatment of acute leukemia. Imatinib mesylate induces hematologic remissions in 50% of patients with myeloid blast crises and major cytogenetic remissions in 16%. These responses tend to be transient in duration.
- ET
  - ◊ Hydroxyurea generally favored over alkylating agents for control of thrombocytosis, as it has little to no known leukemogenic potential
  - ◊ Anagrelide may also be used to control thrombocytosis, particularly in younger patients with ET

Interferon is also useful for cytoreduction and can be used safely in pregnancy
- CIMF
  - ◊ Anemia is treated with transfusions as required. Androgenic steroids - fluoxymesterone (Halotestin) 10 mg bid and prednisone 0.5 mg/kg/d may be useful for anemia. Erythropoietin (in patients with endogenous EPO levels of less than 100 IU/mL) and danocrine (Danazol) have also been used for treatment of anemia.
  - ◊ Hydroxyurea is useful for control of splenomegaly, thrombocytosis and leucocytosis
  - ◊ Investigational drug therapy should be considered since there is no standard therapy that significantly impacts mortality

Contraindications: N/A
Precautions: ET - prolonged administration of platelet-antiaggregating agents may increase the risk of gastrointestinal hemorrhage
Significant possible interactions: N/A

ALTERNATIVE DRUGS
- CIMF
  - ◊ Androgens and glucocorticoids may improve anemia
  - ◊ Corticosteroids if autoimmune hemolysis present
- ET
  - ◊ Aspirin, with or without dipyridamole, may prove useful in preventing thrombotic or ischemic symptoms in some patients
  - ◊ Erythromelalgia (described below) responds to rapid reduction of the platelet count or to administration of nonsteroidal anti-inflammatory agents

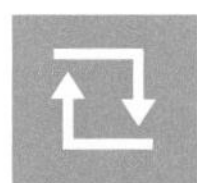

FOLLOWUP

PATIENT MONITORING Individualized and dependent on therapy, ongoing studies, and stage of the illness

PREVENTION/AVOIDANCE N/A

POSSIBLE COMPLICATIONS
- Transformation to acute leukemia
- Gout due to hyperuricemia
- Uric acid nephropathy
- CIMF
  - ◊ Portal hypertension
  - ◊ Splenic infarcts
  - ◊ Budd-Chiari syndrome
  - ◊ Pulmonary hypertension
  - ◊ Pleural or peritoneal effusions due to extramedullary hematopoiesis (EMH)
  - ◊ Paraspinal /epidural EMH
- ET
  - ◊ Thrombohemorrhagic complications in one third
  - ◊ Erythromelalgia (a vaso-occlusive syndrome with localized pain, burning, warmth of distal extremities - may progress to gangrene)

EXPECTED COURSE/PROGNOSIS
- CML
  - ◊ Median survival > 5 years from the time of diagnosis, approximately 12-18 months after development of the accelerated phase, and 3-6 months after developing blast crisis
  - ◊ Adverse prognostic factors include advanced age, degree of splenomegaly, elevated platelet count, degree of leukocytosis, presence of blasts or of large numbers of eosinophils or basophils, percent of immature cells in the marrow, and clonal evolution
  - ◊ 85% will die in blast crisis
- CIMF
  - ◊ Progressive splenomegaly, anemia and thrombocytopenia
  - ◊ Median survival is 5 years from the time of diagnosis
  - ◊ Usually die of hemorrhagic or thrombotic complications and infections, 10-20% terminate in a rapidly progressive form of acute leukemia
  - ◊ Adverse prognostic factors include hemoglobin of less than 10 gm/dL, leucocytosis (> 30,000/uL) or leukopenia (<10,000/uL), presence of peripheral circulating blasts, complex cytogenetic abnormalities, and hypercatabolic symptoms
- ET
  - ◊ Overall life expectancy only slightly shortened. Some studies indicate no significant difference in survival between patients and age/sex matched controls.

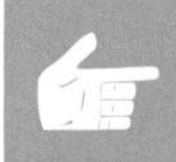

MISCELLANEOUS

ASSOCIATED CONDITIONS CIMF-Immunologic abnormalities have been reported including presence of antinuclear antibodies, elevated rheumatoid factor titers, presence of lupus anticoagulants, direct Coombs positivity and hypocomplementemia

AGE-RELATED FACTORS
Pediatric: Rare in the young
Geriatric: These disorders more often found in middle and later years
Others: N/A

PREGNANCY
- CML
  - ◊ Pregnancy does not affect the course of the disease
  - ◊ Greater than 95% of mothers survive to delivery, with greater than 80% fetal survival rate through gestation
  - ◊ Severe congenital defects have been reported with busulfan. Interferon alpha is safe during pregnancy for control of myeloproliferation.
- ET
  - ◊ Increased risk of 1st trimester abortion. No need to treat if asymptomatic.

SYNONYMS N/A

ICD-9-CM
205.10 Chronic myeloid leukemia without mention of remission
205.11 Chronic myeloid leukemia in remission
289.89 Other specified diseases of blood and blood-forming organs
238.7 Neoplasm of uncertain behavior of other lymphatic and hematopoietic tissues

SEE ALSO
Leukemia
Polycythemia vera

OTHER NOTES N/A

ABBREVIATIONS
CML = chronic myelogenous leukemia
PV = polycythemia vera
CIMF = chronic idiopathic myelofibrosis
ET = essential (hemorrhagic) thrombocythemia

REFERENCES

- Jaffe ES, Harris NL, Stein H, Vardiman JW (eds): World Health Organization Classification of Tumours. Pathology and Genetics of Tumours of Haematopoietic and Lymphoid Tissues. Lyon: IARC Press; 2001
- O'Brien SG, Guihot F, Larson RA et al. Imatinib compared with interferon and low dose cytarabine for newly diagnosed chronic-phase chronic myeloid leukemia. N Engl J Med.2003:348 (11):1048-50
- Tefferi A: Myelofibrosis with myeloid metaplasia. N Engl J Med 2000:342(17):1255-65
- Doll DC, et al, eds: Myeloproliferative disorders. Seminars in Oncology 1995;22(4):305-411

Web references: 3 available at www.5mcc.com
Illustrations N/A

Author(s):
Olatoyosi Odenike, MD

BASICS

DESCRIPTION Acute myocardial infarction (AMI) is the rapid development of myocardial necrosis resulting from a sustained and complete reduction of blood flow to a portion of the myocardium, produced by a superimposed thrombosis, generated by a ruptured atherosclerotic plaque

- Clinical consequences - dependent on the size and location of the infarction and the rapidity with which blood flow can be re-established by pharmacologic or mechanical modalities
- After total occlusion myocardial necrosis is complete in 4-6 hours. Flow to ischemic area must remain above 40% of pre-occlusion levels for that area to survive.
- Infarctions can be divided into Q-wave and non Q-wave, with the former being transmural and associated with totally obstructed infarct-related artery and the latter being non-transmural and associated with patent, but highly narrowed infarct-related artery
- Total occlusion of the left main coronary artery which usually supplies 70% of the LV mass is catastrophic and results in death in minutes

System(s) affected: Cardiovascular
Genetics: N/A
Incidence/Prevalence in USA: 600/100,000
Predominant age: Over 40
Predominant sex:
- Age 40-70: Male > Female
- Over age 70: Male = Female

SIGNS & SYMPTOMS
- Pain - arm, back, jaw, epigastrium, neck, chest
- Anxiety
- Lightheadedness, pallor, weakness, syncope
- Nausea, vomiting, diaphoresis
- Chest heaviness, tightness
- Cough, diaphoresis, dyspnea, rales, wheezing
- S4 heart sound
- Arrhythmias
- Hypertension, hypotension
- Jugular venous distention
- Cannon jugular venous A waves (in presence of heart block or right ventricular failure)

CAUSES
- Coronary thrombosis - most common cause due to ruptured plaque inducing platelet aggregation and then thrombosis has been identified as the initiating factor in most cases
- Coronary artery spasm
- Arteritis
- Embolic infarction
- Congenital coronary anomalies
- Oxygen supply - demand imbalance; carbon monoxide poisoning
- In situ thrombosis (e.g., polycythemia rubra vera, polyarteritis nodosa)
- Cocaine-induced vasospasm

RISK FACTORS
- Hypercholesterolemia (increased LDL; decreased HDL)
- Premature (<55) familial onset of coronary disease
- Smoking
- Diabetes mellitus
- Hypertension
- Sedentary life style
- Aging
- Hostile, frustrated personality
- Hypertriglyceridemia

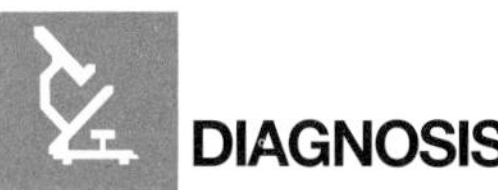

DIAGNOSIS

DIFFERENTIAL DIAGNOSIS
- Unstable angina pectoris - serial ECG and enzymes to differentiate
- Aortic dissection
- Pulmonary embolism
- Pleuro-pericarditis - differentially by history of postural improvement of pain and pleuritic component, plus presence of a pericardial or pleural friction rub and upward concave diffuse ST segment elevation on ECG
- Esophageal spasm - no ECG or enzyme elevations
- Pancreatitis and biliary tract disease
- Hyperventilation syndrome

LABORATORY
- Troponin I has been shown to be a specific indicator of myocardial infarction. It appears 3-6 hours after MI, peaks at 16 hours and decreases in 9-10 days.
- Creatine kinase (CK): rises following infarction; beginning in 4-8 hours; peaking in 18-24 hours and subsiding over 3-4 days. Is a specific indicator for myocardial necrosis, but has a 15% false positive rate.
- CK isoenzymes: MM, MB, and BB forms identified with skeletal muscle, BB in brain and kidney, and MB in cardiac. Elevation of CK-MB in serum is highly suggestive of myocardial infarction.
- LDH: rises above normal values within 24 hours of an acute MI and reaches a peak within 3-6 days and returns to baseline within 8-12 days. Can be used to date recent episode of acute MI well past the acute episode.
- ESR: rises above normal level within 3 days and may remain elevated for several weeks
- Leukocytes: rise within several hours after an MI, peak in 2-4 days, and are normal within 1 week

Drugs that may alter lab results: Refer to standard cardiology texts

Disorders that may alter lab results: Refer to standard cardiology texts

PATHOLOGICAL FINDINGS
- Myocardial necrosis
- Atherosclerosis, if etiologic
- Thrombosis; usually not seen because spontaneous thrombolysis occurs within 24 hours in most patients

SPECIAL TESTS
- Electrocardiography
  - ◊ ST segment elevation in a regional pattern - typical of acute transmural ischemia
  - ◊ ST segment depression with T-wave inversions - typical of subendocardial ischemia
  - ◊ New or presumably new bundle branch block
  - ◊ ST segment elevation and depression are early findings of myocardial ischemia. A significant percent of patients will have non-specific findings on presentation, such as peaked T-waves and ST-segment elevation less than 0.1 mv. A small percentage of patients, with transmural infarction, present with normal ECG.
  - ◊ Q-waves representing transmural myocardial necrosis appear with 24-48 hours
- Echocardiography
  - ◊ 2D and M-mode echocardiography useful in evaluating wall motion abnormalities in MI and overall left ventricular function
  - ◊ Useful in delineating and assessing mechanical complications, eg, mitral valve rupture or VSD, and later development of mural thrombus

IMAGING
- Chest x-ray
  - ◊ Findings dependent on severity of MI
- Radionuclide studies
  - ◊ Thallium scanning. Accumulates in viable myocardium.

DIAGNOSTIC PROCEDURES
- Angiography prior to procedures to re-establish coronary perfusion preferable to thrombolytics in first 12 hours. Early intervention rather than a "cooling off" observational period has been shown to be the safest approach by allowing early intervention.
- For suspected non-Q wave infarction (new ST segment depression or T-wave inversion and initial cardiac enzyme elevation) recommend procedural coronary intervention (PCI) with tirofiban or abciximab prior to cath.

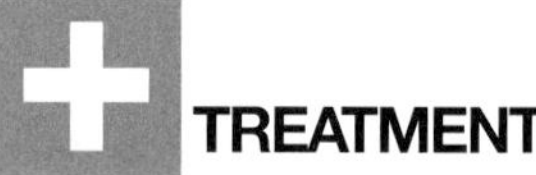

TREATMENT

APPROPRIATE HEALTH CARE Inpatient coronary care unit

GENERAL MEASURES
- General
  - ◊ Analgesia, prevention and treatment of electrical and mechanical complications, limitation of infarct size, and salvage of myocardium
- Arrhythmias
  - ◊ Ventricular tachycardia: DC countershock, lidocaine, or IV amiodarone (Cordarone)
  - ◊ Ventricular fibrillation: DC countershock and CPR/IV amiodarone (Cordarone)
  - ◊ Atrial flutter and fibrillation: digitalis or IV diltiazem (Cardizem) or verapamil. If hemodynamic compromise - DC countershock or rapid atrial pacing. May also use IV amiodarone (Cordarone)
  - ◊ Sinus bradycardia: no treatment unless accompanied by hypotension or hemodynamic compromise. Then treat with atropine and if ineffective, electrical pacing.

◊ Atrioventricular block: in inferior infarction requires transvenous pacing if patient hemodynamically compromised. In anterior infarction, pacing usually required as escape rhythm is unstable with ventricular asystole occurring quite suddenly.
◊ Cardiac cath followed by percutaneous transluminal coronary angioplasty (PTCA/stent) or coronary artery bypass grafting (CABG). Use clopidogrel as pretreatment. Abciximab plus unfractionated heparin when clinically indicated. Door-to-balloon time should be less than 90 minutes.

SURGICAL MEASURES
- Coronary reperfusion
  ◊ Emergency percutaneous transluminal angioplasty (PTCA) or stenting - mechanical form of coronary reperfusion. Recent studies suggest this technique is superior to intravenous thrombolysis if initiated within first 12 hours.
  ◊ Emergency surgical reperfusion - can be accomplished with low mortality.
- Pump failure
  ◊ Intra-aortic balloon counter pulsation

ACTIVITY
- Bedrest for first 24 hours; bedside commode
- Medically supervised rehabilitation plan

DIET Nothing by mouth until stable; later, low fat, low salt diet

PATIENT EDUCATION Printed patient information available from: American Heart Association, 7320 Greenville Avenue, Dallas, TX 75231, (214)373-6300

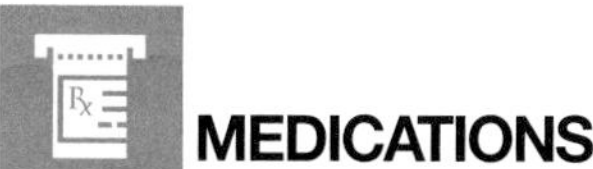

MEDICATIONS

DRUG(S) OF CHOICE
- Coronary reperfusion
  ◊ Aspirin 325 mg po acutely
  ◊ Alteplase (Activase); tissue plasminogen activator (tPA). 15 mg IV bolus, 50 mg over 30 minutes, then 35 mg over 60 minutes.
  ◊ Heparin by standard or weight-adjusted protocol or low molecular weight heparin - enoxaparin (Lovenox) 1 mg/kg q12hr SQ (preferred)
- Acute MI, general
  ◊ Nitrates 5 μg/min IV, increase slowly. Do not lower arterial blood pressure beyond 90 mm Hg. Change to oral or topical when patient stable.
  ◊ Oxygen, 2-4 L/minute
  ◊ Oxazepam 10 mg po or lorazepam 0.5 mg IV, if needed for sedation every 4-6 hours
  ◊ Morphine 2-6 mg IV q2-4h prn pain/sedation
  ◊ Metoprolol (Lopressor) 5 mg IV x 3, 5 minutes apart followed by 50 mg po q6h starting 15 minutes after last IV dose
  ◊ Stool softeners - milk of magnesia, docusate sodium (dioctyl sodium sulfosuccinate) 100 mg bid, etc. to avoid straining and constipation secondary to immobility and narcotic use
  ◊ Lidocaine 1-2 mg/kg once, then 1-4 mg/min. Use for ventricular arrhythmias only - not for arrhythmia prophylaxis.
- Post MI
  ◊ Beta-blockers reduce mortality
  ◊ Nitrates may be needed for angina
  ◊ ACE inhibitors prevent adverse remodeling, may improve longevity

Contraindications:
- Beta-blockers relatively contraindicated in CHF or incipient heart failure and bronchospasm. May use IV esmolol (Brevibloc), a short acting beta blocker, if uncertain.
- IV thrombolysis contraindicated in patients with active internal hemorrhage; recent head trauma, intracranial neoplasm, hemorrhagic CVA; pregnancy; persistent hypertension (>200/120); prolonged (>10 minutes) or traumatic CPR; diabetic hemorrhagic retinopathy; severe trauma or major surgery within 2 weeks; elderly (age > 80)

Precautions:
- Use IV thrombolysis cautiously in patients with active peptic ulcer or heme positive stools; known bleeding disorders or current use of anticoagulants; uncontrolled hypertension; prior exposure to Streptokinase or Streptococcal infection in last 6 months; Trauma or major surgery within 2 months.

Significant possible interactions: N/A

ALTERNATIVE DRUGS
- Thrombolytics
  ◊ Tenecteplase or reteplase
- Beta-blockers for acute arrhythmia
  ◊ Atenolol 5 mg IV over 5 minutes. Follow with a second dose 10 minutes later. Follow with 50 mg po in 10 minutes after the 2nd IV dose. Then q12h for at least 7 days.

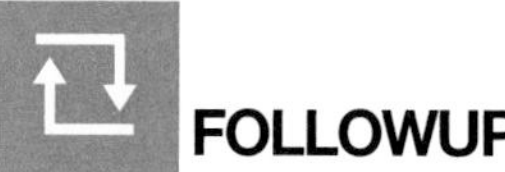

FOLLOWUP

PATIENT MONITORING
- Determined by needs of patient
- Early intervention if any one of the following: recurrent chest pain, CHF, hemodynamic instability, sustained V-tach, PCI within 6 months, prior CABG

PREVENTION/AVOIDANCE
- Avoid risk factors
- Aspirin 81 mg/day may be helpful
- Clopidogrel 75 mg day

POSSIBLE COMPLICATIONS
- Congestive heart failure
- Cardiogenic shock
- Myocardial rupture
- Left ventricular aneurysm
- Left ventricular thrombus and peripheral embolism
- Deep venous thrombosis and pulmonary embolism
- Pericarditis
- Dysrhythmias
- Mitral regurgitation
- Ventricular septal defect
- Dressler's syndrome
- Cardiac arrest
- Death

EXPECTED COURSE/PROGNOSIS
- Overall mortality rate is 10% during the hospital phase with an additional 10% mortality rate during the year after. More than 60% of the deaths occur within one hour of the onset of the event.

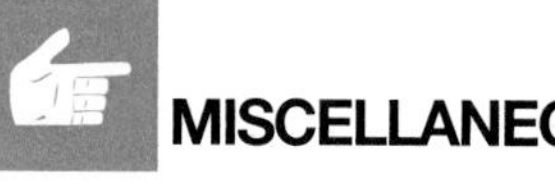

MISCELLANEOUS

ASSOCIATED CONDITIONS
- Abdominal aortic aneurysm
- Extracranial cerebrovascular disease
- Atherosclerotic peripheral vascular disease

AGE-RELATED FACTORS
Pediatric: N/A
Geriatric: All incidences of complications are higher
Others: N/A

PREGNANCY N/A

SYNONYMS
- Coronary thrombosis
- Coronary occlusion
- Heart attack

ICD-9-CM
410.00 Acute myocardial infarction of anterolateral wall, episode of care unspecified
410.90 Acute myocardial infarction of unspecified site, episode of care unspecified

SEE ALSO
Congestive heart failure
Ventricular standstill
Ventricular tachycardia (VT)

OTHER NOTES N/A

ABBREVIATIONS
CHF = congestive heart failure

REFERENCES

- Topol E, editor. Textbook of Cardiovascular Medicine. Philadelphia: Lippincott-Raven; 1997
- Braunwald E, Antman EM, Beasley JW, et al. American College of Cardiology/American Heart Association Task Force on Practice Guidelines (Committee on the Management of Patients With Unstable Angina). ACC/AHA guideline update for the management of patients with unstable angina and non-ST-segment elevation myocardial infarction--2002: summary article: a report of the American College of Cardiology/American Heart Association Task Force on Practice Guidelines (Committee on the Management of Patients With Unstable Angina). Circulation 2002;106(14):1893-900
- Cannon CP, Weintraub WS, Demopoulos LA. TACTICS (Treat Angina with Aggrastat and Determine Cost of Therapy with an Invasive or Conservative Strategy)-Thrombolysis in Myocardial Infarction 18 Investigators. Comparison of early invasive and conservative strategies in patients with unstable coronary syndromes treated with the glycoprotein IIb/IIIa inhibitor tirofiban. N Engl J Med 2001;344(25):1879-87

Web references: 0 available at www.5mcc.com
Illustrations N/A

Author(s):
Phil Lobstein, MD

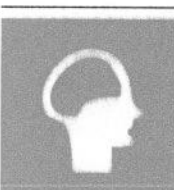

BASICS

DESCRIPTION A disorder of unknown etiology characterized by excessive sleepiness typically associated with cataplexy and other REM sleep phenomena, such as sleep paralysis and hypnagogic hallucinations. Commonly misconceived as representing low intelligence and/or poor motivation. The syndrome is frequently overlooked with an average of 15 years of symptoms prior to diagnosis. Onset is usually in teenage years.

System(s) affected: Nervous

Genetics:
- Autosomal recessive
- Increased incidence in families with positive history
- Incidence in first degree relative of index case is 1-2% (vs. 0.02% general population)
- Biologic marker HLA-DR2 allele on short arm of chromosome 6 in 100% of Caucasian patients; 1/3 normal subjects are also positive. 30% of black narcoleptic patients are non DR 2, but all with HLA-Dw1.

Incidence/Prevalence in USA: 1 in 3000 diagnosed

Predominant age: Mean age onset 18, 50% after age 40

Predominant sex: Male = Female

SIGNS & SYMPTOMS
- Tetrad: 10-20% with all symptoms
- All with excessive daytime sleepiness (EDS)
- Sleep attacks - primary symptom, most severe form of EDS
  - ◊ Instantaneous, irresistible REM sleep
  - ◊ First and most disabling symptom
  - ◊ Satisfied by naps lasting 5-10 minutes
  - ◊ Lasts minutes to hours
  - ◊ 1-8 naps per day, 24 hour duration of sleep normal
  - ◊ Increased in monotonous environment, warm environment, after a large meal, or with strong emotions
  - ◊ 20-25% of all patients with excessive somnolence
- Cataplexy (70%) auxiliary symptom
  - ◊ Sudden bilateral weakness of skeletal muscles
  - ◊ Provocation by sudden strong wave of emotion
  - ◊ Lack of impairment of consciousness and memory
  - ◊ Short duration (less than a few minutes)
  - ◊ Responsiveness to treatment with clomipramine and imipramine)
  - ◊ Can be limited to a particular muscle group, e.g., jaw droop with inability to speak; arm, neck or leg weakness
- Sleep paralysis - auxiliary symptom (50%)
  - ◊ When falling asleep or on awakening the patient wants to move but cannot
  - ◊ The brain wakes from sleep while the body remains in REM sleep
  - ◊ Lasts seconds to minutes
  - ◊ Patients are aware of events around them, but cannot open eyes or move
  - ◊ Can be preceded by hallucinatory phenomena
  - ◊ 50% of normal population have at least one episode (nonspecific)
- Hypnagogic hallucinations - auxiliary symptom (60%)
  - ◊ Vivid, frightening auditory or visual illusions or hallucinations at onset of sleep
  - ◊ Dream-like experiences that occur during wakefulness or suddenly at sleep onset
  - ◊ Characteristic hallucinations include seeing human or animal faces or feeling that someone else is in the room
- Disturbed nocturnal sleep (66%)
  - ◊ Normal total sleep with decreased sleep efficiency
  - ◊ More frequent transitions from wakefulness to sleep
  - ◊ Retrograde amnesic and automatic behavior lasting minutes to hours
  - ◊ Increased periodic leg movements (50%)

CAUSES
- Unknown; associated with loss of the neurotransmitter hypocretin-1 in CNS
- Possible involvement of the immune system
- 75% of narcoleptic patients - no detectable hypocretin in CSF

RISK FACTORS
- Head trauma
- CNS infectious disease
- Anesthesia
- Family history

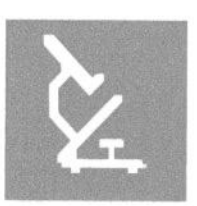

DIAGNOSIS

DIFFERENTIAL DIAGNOSIS
EDS present in 4% of population, most are not narcolepsy, causes include:
- Sleep apnea syndromes - 40-50% of those with excessive somnolence
- Epileptic seizures and syncope
- Idiopathic CNS hypersomnolence - 5-10% of those with excessive somnolence
- Nocturnal myoclonus
- Psychomotor seizures
- Abuse of sedative drugs
- Clinical diagnosis possible if cataplexy present

LABORATORY HLA-DR2

Drugs that may alter lab results: N/A

Disorders that may alter lab results: N/A

PATHOLOGICAL FINDINGS N/A

SPECIAL TESTS
- Nighttime polysomnography - monitoring of patients in a sleep laboratory will usually document fragmented sleep with a normal amount of REM sleep but a pattern of sleep onset REM. Polysomnography rules out other causes of excessive daytime sleepiness including sleep apnea syndromes and nocturnal myoclonus.
- Multiple sleep latency test (MSLT) - begins at least 90 minutes after nighttime test. Patient is monitored during 4-5 naps taken at two-hour intervals. The rapidity of sleep onset and type of sleep pattern are documented. A supportive test includes a mean sleep latency (time to fall asleep) of five minutes or less and at least two sleep-onset REM periods. Sensitivity 77%, specificity 97%, PPV 73%.
- HLA typing in ambiguous cases

IMAGING N/A

DIAGNOSTIC PROCEDURES
- REM periods during MSLT
- Diagnostic criteria - B and C, or A and D and E and G

A. Excessive sleepiness
B. Recurrent lapses into sleep daily for ≥ 3 months
C. Cataplexy
D. Associated features: sleep paralysis, hypnagogic hallucinations, disrupted sleep
E. Multiple sleep latency test abnormalities as described
F. Biologic markers (see Genetics)
G. Absence of medical or psychiatric disorder
H. CSF hypocretin-1 level low - 99% specificity, 87% sensitivity; useful in children unable to do MSLT

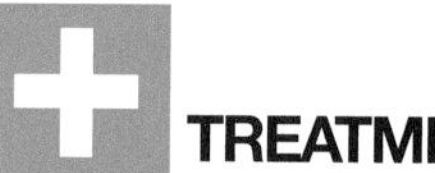

TREATMENT

APPROPRIATE HEALTH CARE
Inpatient for sleep laboratory analysis, outpatient for followup

GENERAL MEASURES
- Usually managed with medication
- Regularly scheduled time for naps may help in mild cases
- Regular sleep-wake schedule

SURGICAL MEASURES N/A

ACTIVITY
Exercise can sometimes decrease the number of sleep attacks. Seek to achieve optimal physical fitness.

DIET
No special diet, avoid alcohol

PATIENT EDUCATION
- Symptoms can spontaneously improve or worsen
- The American Narcolepsy Association, P.O. Box 1187, San Carlos, CA 94070, (800)327-6085
- Narcolepsy Sleep Disorder Association. Online newsletter at www.narcolepsy.com

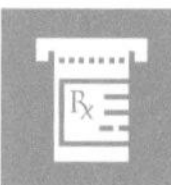

MEDICATIONS

DRUG(S) OF CHOICE

- Excessive daytime sleepiness
  - ◊ Non-amphetamines:
    - Modafinil (Provigil) 200 or 400 mg/day; structurally distinct from amphetamines. Start with 100 mg and increase over 3-4 days.
    - Selegiline - selective MAO-B inhibitor, 20-40 mg/day divided AM and noon; anticataplectic and effective for excessive daytime sleepiness
  - ◊ Amphetamines:
    - Methylphenidate (Ritalin) initial dose 30 mg/day divided 2-3/day; maximum dose 100 mg/day
    - Pemoline (Cylert) - longer half life 8-10 hours; initial dose 37.5 mg/day divided AM and noon; maximum dose 150 mg/day. Monitor liver function studies 4 weeks after start and then once a year.
    - Dextroamphetamine initial dose 15 mg/day divided 2-3/day; maximum dose 100 mg/day
    - Combination of long and short acting - pemoline plus single or multiple doses of methylphenidate
- Auxiliary symptoms (cataplexy, hypnagogic hallucination, sleep paralysis) - antidepressants suppress REM sleep
  - ◊ Imipramine 75-150 mg/day
  - ◊ Protriptyline 10-40 mg/day
  - ◊ Clomipramine 150-250 mg/day
  - ◊ Fluoxetine 20-60 mg/day
  - ◊ Sodium oxybate (Xyrem) - 6-9 gm/day po in 2 equal doses for cataplexy. Beginning dose is 4.5gm/day. Restricted access in U.S. (call 1-877-679-9736).

Contraindications: Stimulants in hypertensive patients

Precautions:

- Amphetamines
  - ◊ If patient develops tolerance to stimulants, switch drugs rather than increasing the dose - there is little cross-tolerance
  - ◊ Headaches, irritability, hypertension, psychosis, anorexia, habituation, rebound hypersomnia
  - ◊ Pemoline - less cardiovascular side effects, longer acting, liver toxicity, little abuse potential
- Other
  - ◊ Imipramine - dry mouth, sedation, urinary retention, impotence
  - ◊ Modafinil - less rebound hypersomnia; may become drug of choice; does not affect blood pressure; tolerance is limited; best if initial treatment; does not treat cataplexy; main side effect is headache
  - ◊ Selegiline - doses > 20 mg must be on low tyramine diet since it begins to lose selectivity
  - ◊ Patient may develop tolerance to the anticataplectic effect of tricyclic antidepressants and can get a rebound in cataplexy when withdrawn

Significant possible interactions: Combination of tricyclic antidepressants and stimulants can lead to significant hypertension

ALTERNATIVE DRUGS

- Excessive daytime sleepiness:
  - ◊ Propranolol 280-480 mg/day, good for patients during withdrawal from stimulants or patients with hypertension
  - ◊ Dextroamphetamines 5-60 mg/day
  - ◊ L-Tyrosine 64-120 mg/day
- Ancillary symptoms
  - ◊ Gamma-hydroxybutyrate 5.25-6.75 g during sleep, has little effect on sleep architecture of REM sleep but increases slow-wave sleep. Also has mild effect on excessive daytime sleepiness without tolerance development. Gamma-hydroxybutyrate can increase sleep walking by increasing slow-wave sleep.
  - ◊ Codeine 150 mg/day
  - ◊ Triazolam 0.25 mg improves nocturnal sleep quality

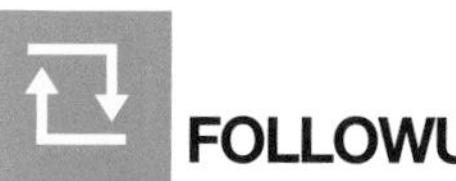

FOLLOWUP

PATIENT MONITORING

- Frequent blood pressure checks
- Followup every 6 months

PREVENTION/AVOIDANCE N/A

POSSIBLE COMPLICATIONS N/A

EXPECTED COURSE/PROGNOSIS

- Life-long disease
- Symptoms can worsen with aging
- In women, symptoms can improve after menopause

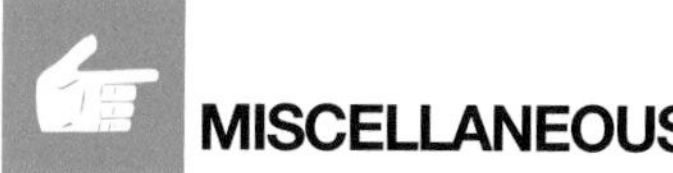

MISCELLANEOUS

ASSOCIATED CONDITIONS
Obstructive sleep apnea

AGE-RELATED FACTORS

Pediatric: Uncommon syndrome of childhood
Geriatric: Symptoms worsen with aging
Others: N/A

PREGNANCY N/A

SYNONYMS N/A

ICD-9-CM

347 Cataplexy and narcolepsy

SEE ALSO

Sleep apnea, obstructive

OTHER NOTES N/A

ABBREVIATIONS

- REM = rapid eye movement
- MSLT = multiple sleep latency test

REFERENCES

- Mitler M, Hajdukovic R, et al. Narcolepsy. Journal of Clinical Neurophysiology 1990;7(1):93-118
- Scharf M, Fletcher K, et al. Current pharmacologic management of narcolepsy. AFP 1988;38(1):143-8
- Nahmias J, Karetzky M. Current concepts in narcolepsy. New Jersey Medicine 1989;86:617-22
- Chaudhary B, Husain I. Narcolepsy. Jour Fam Prac 1993;36(2);207-13
- Standards of Practice Committee of the American Sleep Disorders Association. Practice parameters for the use of stimulants in the treatment of narcolepsy. Sleep 1994;17(4):348-51
- Parkes JD, Clift SJ, Dahlitz MJ. The narcoleptic syndrome. J of Psychiatry 1995;59(3):221-4
- Green P, Stillman M. Signs, symptoms, differential diagnosis, and management of narcolepsy. Arch Fam Med 1998;7:472-8
- Nishino S, Mignot E. Drug treatment of patients with insomnia and excessive daytime sleepiness. Clin Pharmacokinet 1999;37(4):305-30
- Feldman NT. Narcolepsy. South Med J 2003;96(3):277-82

Web references: 1 available at www.5mcc.com
Illustrations N/A

Author(s):

Jeffrey F. Minteer, MD

BASICS

DESCRIPTION Multisystem, potentially fatal disease, resulting from near suffocation secondary to submersion of a person's face or head. A form of ARDS with neurological complications. Approximately 10% of drowned patients die without actually aspirating. Most near drowning victims do not aspirate large volumes of fluid.

System(s) affected: Cardiovascular, Nervous, Pulmonary

Genetics: N/A

Incidence/Prevalence in USA:
- 8500 deaths yearly; 90,000 near-drowning victims
- Drowning is the 3rd leading cause of accidental death in the United States
- Leading cause of injury related death in children under 5

Predominant age: Teenagers and toddlers

Predominant sex: Male > Female

SIGNS & SYMPTOMS
- Altered level of consciousness or comatose
- Absent or thready pulse
- Tachypnea or agonal respirations
- Cyanosis
- Wheezing
- Hypothermia
- Poorly reactive, dilated and fixed pupils
- Poor peripheral perfusion
- Cough
- Abdominal distension

CAUSES
- Swimming accidents, scuba diving, water sports
- Hyperventilation before underwater swimming
- Boating mishaps
- Motor vehicle accidents (i.e., auto submerged in water)
- Suicide
- Drug overdose (including alcohol)
- Bathtub drowning in children less than 1 year
- Head trauma while swimming

RISK FACTORS
- Low socioeconomic class
- Alcohol
- Seizure disorder
- Inability to swim
- Improper pool fencing
- Inadequate adult supervision of children
- Cardiac arrhythmias
- Living in sunbelt states

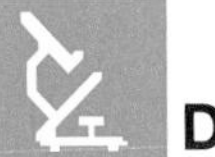

DIAGNOSIS

DIFFERENTIAL DIAGNOSIS The submersion may have resulted from loss of consciousness and accidentally falling into water because of another medical condition (i.e., head trauma, arrhythmia, seizure, etc.)

LABORATORY
- Salt water
  - ◊ Hypoxemia
  - ◊ Hypercarbia
  - ◊ Hypokalemia with significant aspiration
  - ◊ Mixed acidosis
  - ◊ Slight increase in serum sodium
  - ◊ Normal or minimally increased Hb
  - ◊ Rare albuminuria
  - ◊ Rare oliguria
  - ◊ Rare hemoglobinuria
  - ◊ Hypovolemia possibly, or hypervolemia
- Fresh water
  - ◊ Hypoxemia
  - ◊ Hypercarbia
  - ◊ Hypokalemia with significant aspiration
  - ◊ Mixed acidosis
  - ◊ Slight decrease in serum sodium
  - ◊ Normal or slightly decreased Hb
  - ◊ Albuminuria rarely
  - ◊ Oliguria rarely
  - ◊ Rare hemoglobinuria
  - ◊ Evidence of hemolysis

Drugs that may alter lab results: N/A

Disorders that may alter lab results: Any underlying condition that may alter normal fluid and electrolyte balance (i.e., congestive heart failure) or alter normal pulmonary function (i.e., emphysema)

PATHOLOGICAL FINDINGS
- "Dry lungs" 10% of time
- Loss of normal pulmonary architecture (fresh water). Alveolar consolidations, collapse, hyaline membrane formation, intrapulmonary shunting.
- Increased lung weight and intra-alveolar hemorrhages (salt water)
- Lung hyperexpansion
- Pneumonia, abscess and adult respiratory distress (ARDS) in those who survive only a few hours or days
- Renal - acute tubular necrosis
- Neurologic - cerebral edema

SPECIAL TESTS
- Lung compliance (reduced)
- Central venous pressure monitoring
- ECG
- EEG
- Calculation of V/Q mismatch, shunt, $AaDO_2$

IMAGING Chest x-ray may show pulmonary edema, consolidation from aspiration, atelectasis or pneumothorax

DIAGNOSTIC PROCEDURES N/A

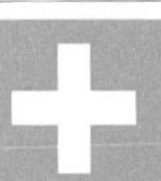

TREATMENT

APPROPRIATE HEALTH CARE Hospitalize all patients initially. Monitor patients in an Intensive Care setting except for those few who present to the emergency room in an alert condition without evidence of respiratory compromise. The incidence of delayed drowning is 5%. Therefore all patients who have had a significant submersion accident should be hospitalized for 24-48 hours.

GENERAL MEASURES
- Begin resuscitation at the scene. Remove from water quickly and place in normal CPR position.
- Support neck in case of spinal cord injury
- Supplemental oxygen
- Positive airway pressure - positive end-expiratory pressure (PEEP) or continuous positive airway pressure (CPAP) for persistent hypoxia
- Avoid abdominal thrust unless airway obstruction is present
- Monitor pH and adjust bicarbonate administration accordingly
- Monitor arterial oxygenation
- Avoid steroids
- Avoid prophylactic antibiotics
- Hyperventilate patient (keep $PaCO_2$ 25-30 mm HG)
- Warm hypothermic patients

SURGICAL MEASURES N/A

ACTIVITY Bedrest for at least the initial 24 hours

DIET N/A

PATIENT EDUCATION Proper water safety techniques may help to avoid this problem

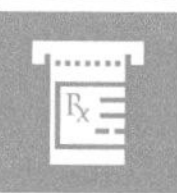

MEDICATIONS

DRUG(S) OF CHOICE
- All patients: Oxygen
- Unconscious patient without known pH: Sodium bicarbonate - 1.0 mEq/kg (1.0 mmol/kg)
- For bronchospasm: Aerosolized bronchodilator - albuterol (Proventil, Ventolin) 3cc of 0.083% solution OR 0.5mL of 0.5% solution diluted in 3cc saline
- Patients who develop pneumonia: Appropriate antibiotic based on sputum or endotracheal lavage culture
- Fresh water drowning patients with hemolysis: Transfusion may be necessary
- Prophylactic antibiotics and steroids are not helpful

Contraindications: Refer to manufacturer's profile of each drug

Precautions: Refer to manufacturer's profile of each drug

Significant possible interactions: Refer to manufacturer's profile of each drug

ALTERNATIVE DRUGS
- For bronchospasm
  - ◊ Aerosolized bronchodilator - metaproterenol (Alupent) 0.3 mL in 3 mL normal saline or levalbuterol (Xopenex) 0.63 mg or 1.25. mg
  - ◊ Aminophylline

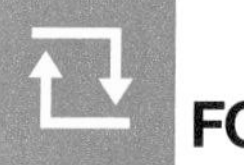

FOLLOWUP

PATIENT MONITORING
- Frequent check of vital signs
- Arterial blood gas monitoring
- Pulmonary artery catheter may be needed for hemodynamic monitoring
- Pulse oximeter for oxygen saturation trending
- Intracranial pressure monitoring in selected patients
- Serial chest x-rays
- Serum electrolyte determinations

PREVENTION/AVOIDANCE
- Proper adult supervision of children
- Knowledge of water safety guidelines
- Mandatory pool fencing
- Avoidance of alcohol or recreational drugs around water
- Swimming instruction at an early age
- Boating safety knowledge
- Personal flotation device (life preserver if necessary)

POSSIBLE COMPLICATIONS
- Early
  - ◊ Bronchospasm
  - ◊ Vomiting/aspiration
  - ◊ Hypoglycemia
  - ◊ Hypothermia
  - ◊ Seizure
  - ◊ Hypovolemia
  - ◊ Electrolyte abnormalities
  - ◊ Arrhythmia from hypoxia or hypothermia (rarely from electrolyte imbalance)
  - ◊ Hypotension
- Late
  - ◊ Adult respiratory distress syndrome
  - ◊ Anoxic encephalopathy
  - ◊ Pneumonia
  - ◊ Lung abscess/empyema
  - ◊ Renal failure
  - ◊ Coagulopathy
  - ◊ Sepsis
  - ◊ Barotrauma
  - ◊ Seizure

EXPECTED COURSE/PROGNOSIS
- Patients who are alert or mildly obtunded at the time they present to the hospital have an excellent chance for a full recovery
- Patients who are comatose or receiving CPR at the time of presentation or who have dilated and fixed pupils and no spontaneous respiratory activity have a more guarded and often poor prognosis
- Secondary drowning from neurogenic pulmonary edema may occur within 48 hours of initial presentation

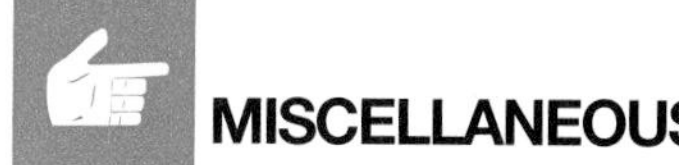

MISCELLANEOUS

ASSOCIATED CONDITIONS
- Cardiopulmonary arrest before the submersion
- Trauma, especially to the head causing altered mental status
- Seizure disorder
- Alcohol or drug overdose
- Hypothermia

AGE-RELATED FACTORS
Pediatric: Children frequently don't swim well
Geriatric: N/A
Others:
- Adolescents - may be intoxicated or using drugs
- Adults - most near-drownings are associated with boating accidents with or without alcohol

PREGNANCY N/A

SYNONYMS N/A

ICD-9-CM
994.1 Drowning and nonfatal submersion
518.5 Pulmonary insufficiency following trauma and surgery

SEE ALSO

OTHER NOTES
Accomplished swimmers may drown by hyperventilation before prolonged underwater swimming or by becoming fatigued following a particularly strenuous or long swim. Approximately 10% of victims drown without aspiration.

ABBREVIATIONS N/A

REFERENCES

- Wintemute G: Childhood Drowning and Near-Drowning in the United States. AJDC 1990;144:663
- Modell J, Graves S, Ketover A: Clinical Course of 91 Consecutive Near-Drowning Victims. Chest 1976;70:231
- Weinstein MD; Krieger BP. Near-drowning: epidemiology, pathophysiology, and initial treatment. J Emerg Med 1996;14(4):461-7
- Sachdeva RC. Near drowning. Crit Care Med 2002: 281-296

Web references: 0 available at www.5mcc.com
Illustrations N/A

Author(s):
Alan J. Cropp, MD

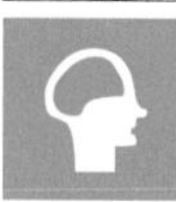

BASICS

DESCRIPTION Renal parenchymal damage and dysfunction associated with disordered uric acid metabolism. Several syndromes can present.

- Gout: Acute urate crystal-induced arthritis related to chronic hyperuricemia due to uric acid renal underexcretion in 80-90% and uric acid overproduction in 10-20%.
- Hyperuricemic acute renal failure: Precipitated by distal tubular obstruction resulting from acute massive overproduction of uric acid due to cell lysis. Serum uric acid usually greater than 15-20 mg/dL (0.88-1.18 mmol/L).
- Uric acid nephrolithiasis: Most commonly seen in gouty patients who are uric acid overproducers and have hyperuricosuria. Frequency of stone formation increases with increasing serum uric acid levels and urinary uric acid excretion rates. About 22% of gouty patients will form uric acid stones.
- Hyperuricemia of chronic renal failure: Occurs when creatinine clearance less than 15. Serum uric acid usually greater than 10 mg/dL. Secondary gout rare. Acute deterioration of renal function can be precipitated by an abrupt rise in serum uric acid.
- Chronic urate nephropathy: Renal insufficiency attributed to parenchymal damage secondary to medullary urate deposition. Bulk of evidence supports conclusion that typical gout or asymptomatic hyperuricemia are unlikely to lead to serious renal insufficiency. In patients with gout, renal insufficiency can usually be attributed to a complicating medical condition, most often hypertension, diabetes, renal vascular disease, obstructive uropathy, urinary tract infection or lead intoxication.

System(s) affected: Renal/Urologic
Genetics: N/A
Incidence/Prevalence in USA: Gout 0.3%, Hyperuricemia 5-10%
Predominant age: Adults
Predominant sex: Male > Female

SIGNS & SYMPTOMS

- Hyperuricemic acute renal failure
  - ◊ Precipitated by chemotherapy for leukemia or lymphoma
  - ◊ Precipitated by heat stress and exercise
  - ◊ Oliguria
  - ◊ Anuria
  - ◊ Anorexia, nausea, vomiting, encephalopathy and other manifestations of uremia
  - ◊ Hypertension
  - ◊ Anemia
  - ◊ Dehydration
- Uric acid nephrolithiasis
  - ◊ Flank pain
  - ◊ Groin pain
  - ◊ Micro or gross hematuria
  - ◊ Anorexia
  - ◊ Nausea
  - ◊ Vomiting
  - ◊ Dehydration
- Hyperuricemia of chronic renal failure
  - ◊ Established chronic renal failure with glomerular filtration rate (GFR) less than 15-20
  - ◊ Serum uric acid greater than 10 mg/dL chronically
  - ◊ Intercurrent cause of abrupt increase in serum uric acid
  - ◊ Acute decrease in GFR
  - ◊ Acute onset of uremic symptoms

CAUSES

- Primary
  - ◊ Congenital gout, hypertension and hyperuricemia (autosomal dominant)
  - ◊ Congenital HGPRT deficiency (X-linked recessive)
  - ◊ Congenital PRPP overactivity (X-linked recessive)
  - ◊ Congenital glycogen storage disease, type I
- Secondary
  - ◊ Lead intoxication
  - ◊ Diuretics
  - ◊ Cytotoxic chemotherapy in leukemia or lymphoma
  - ◊ Heat stress and exercise
  - ◊ Diabetic ketoacidosis
  - ◊ Starvation ketosis
  - ◊ Chronic myeloproliferative disease
  - ◊ Psoriasis

RISK FACTORS

- Sudden increase in uric acid load
- Dehydration
- Urine pH less than 5
- Hypertension
- Diabetes mellitus
- Renal insufficiency
- Renal vascular disease

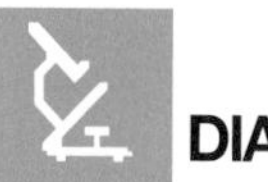

DIAGNOSIS

DIFFERENTIAL DIAGNOSIS Other causes of acute renal failure, other causes of nephrolithiasis, other causes of chronic renal failure

LABORATORY

- Gout and hyperuricemia
  - ◊ Hyperuricemia
  - ◊ Hyperuricosuria in 10-20%
  - ◊ Decreased urinary ammonia production
- Hyperuricemic acute renal failure
  - ◊ Serum uric acid greater than 15-20 mg/dL (0.88-1.18 mmol/L)
  - ◊ Rising BUN and creatinine
  - ◊ Urinary uric acid to creatinine ratio > 1
  - ◊ Uric acid crystals in urine
- Uric acid nephrolithiasis
  - ◊ Uric acid crystals in urine
  - ◊ Urinary uric acid greater than 600-700 mg (3.54-4.13 mmol) per 24 hours (hyperuricosuria) on purine-free diet
  - ◊ Hyperuricemia
  - ◊ Microhematuria
  - ◊ Pyuria
  - ◊ Positive urine culture
  - ◊ Stone composition uric acid or mixed uric acid and calcium oxalate or calcium phosphate
- Hyperuricemia of chronic renal failure
  - ◊ Acute exacerbation of hyperuricemia with serum uric acid greater than 10 mg/dL (0.59 mmol/L)
  - ◊ Acute on chronic BUN and creatinine elevations

Drugs that may alter lab results: N/A

Disorders that may alter lab results: N/A

PATHOLOGICAL FINDINGS

- Renal tophi-medullary monosodium urate deposits with inflammatory reaction and interstitial fibrosis
- Poor correlation between severity of renal pathology and severity of gout
- Tubulointerstitial nephritis with obstruction, recurrent infection or lead intoxication

SPECIAL TESTS Stone analysis

IMAGING

- IVP
- Renal ultrasound

DIAGNOSTIC PROCEDURES

- Cystoscopy and retrograde pyelography
- Renal biopsy

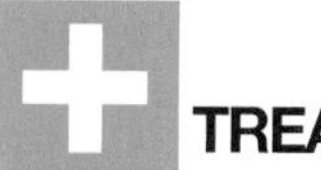

TREATMENT

APPROPRIATE HEALTH CARE

Outpatient except for complicated nephrolithiasis and hyperuricemic acute renal failure

GENERAL MEASURES

- Hydration to increase urine output
- Normalize serum uric acid
- Normalize renal uric acid excretion
- Decrease uric acid production
- Maintain urine pH greater than 6
- Antibiotic treatment of urinary tract infection
- Hyperuricemic acute renal failure:
  - ◊ IV hydration
  - ◊ Hemodialysis

SURGICAL MEASURES Uric acid nephrolithiasis: Cystoscopic or surgical stone removal for persistent ureteral obstruction

ACTIVITY Limited during attacks of acute gouty arthritis

DIET

- Purine restriction
- Protein restriction
- For nephrolithiasis, fluid intake adequate to produce urine output at least 2 L per day unless urine output is limited by acute or chronic renal failure
- In acute renal failure restrict sodium for hypertension and potassium for hyperkalemia

PATIENT EDUCATION Griffith, H.W.: Instructions for Patients. Philadelphia, W.B. Saunders Co., 1994

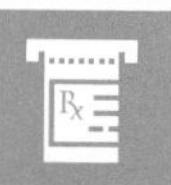

MEDICATIONS

DRUG(S) OF CHOICE

- Gout and hyperuricemia
  - ◊ Uricosuric agent - probenecid (Benemid) starting with 250 mg bid and doubling 7-10 day intervals up to 500-1000 mg bid (maximum 3 gm/day)
  - ◊ Xanthine oxidase inhibitor preferred for hyperuricosuria - allopurinol (Zyloprim) 200-300 mg/day.
  - ◊ Treatment of symptomatic or asymptomatic hyperuricemia with uric acid-lowering drugs has no apparent favorable or adverse effect with respect to development of renal insufficiency
- Hyperuricemic acute renal failure
  - ◊ Prevent by pretreating with allopurinol and hydrating patient prior to administration of chemotherapeutic agents for leukemia or lymphoma
  - ◊ Loop diuretic
  - ◊ IV alkalinizing solution
- Uric acid nephrolithiasis
  - ◊ Allopurinol 200-300 mg/day
  - ◊ Alkali to maintain urine pH 6.0-6.5 - sodium bicarbonate or potassium citrate-citric acid 0.5-1.5 mEq/kg in 5 or 6 divided doses
- Hyperuricemia of chronic renal failure
  - ◊ Allopurinol in patients with prior history of gout

Contraindications: Avoid uricosuric agents in patients with hyperuricosuria, uric acid nephrolithiasis or chronic renal failure

Precautions:

- Avoid abrupt decreases or increases in serum uric acid, which may precipitate acute gouty arthritis
- Administer colchicine 0.5-0.65 mg/day 1-4 times/week concomitantly with allopurinol first 2-3 months to prevent precipitation of acute gouty arthritis

Significant possible interactions: Phenylbutazone, diflunisal, aspirin (1-2 gm/day), contrast agents, glyceryl guaiacolate, pyrazinamide, ethambutol, ethanol, diuretics, ascorbic acid (high dose), nicotinic acid

ALTERNATIVE DRUGS Sulfinpyrazone (Anturane)

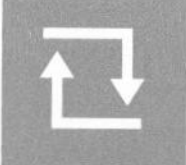

FOLLOWUP

PATIENT MONITORING

- Serum uric acid, urinary uric acid excretion, BUN and/or serum creatinine at least twice a year
- Blood pressure screening at least once a year

PREVENTION/AVOIDANCE

- Appropriate pretreatment prior to chemotherapy of leukemia or lymphoma
- Avoid factors that can cause abrupt or persistent increases of serum uric acid or urinary uric acid excretion
- Prompt treatment of urinary obstruction or infection
- Control blood pressure in hypertensives

POSSIBLE COMPLICATIONS

- Gout and hyperuricemia
  - ◊ No apparent renal complications
- Hyperuricemic acute renal failure
  - ◊ Irreversible renal failure (end-stage renal disease)
  - ◊ Residual renal insufficiency
  - ◊ Persistent renal tubular functional defects
- Uric acid nephrolithiasis
  - ◊ Urinary obstruction
  - ◊ Urinary infection
  - ◊ Renal insufficiency
- Hyperuricemia of chronic renal failure
  - ◊ Progression to end-stage renal failure

EXPECTED COURSE/PROGNOSIS

- With effective drug therapy and general management prognosis is excellent in patients with gout, hyperuricemia, or nephrolithiasis
- Development or progression of renal insufficiency should not occur unless due to underlying renal disease or associated medical conditions with adverse renal effects

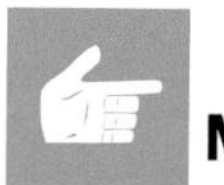

MISCELLANEOUS

ASSOCIATED CONDITIONS

- Hypertension
- Diabetes mellitus

AGE-RELATED FACTORS

Pediatric: Gout and uric acid nephrolithiasis may have onset in infancy or childhood with HGPRT deficiency or PRPP overactivity

Geriatric: Renal insufficiency more likely due to age and associated medical conditions

Others: N/A

PREGNANCY Women with nephrolithiasis have a slightly higher incidence of urinary tract infection, but no increase in stone formation rate

SYNONYMS N/A

ICD-9-CM

274.10 Gouty nephropathy, unspecified
274.11 Uric acid nephrolithiasis

SEE ALSO

OTHER NOTES N/A

ABBREVIATIONS N/A

REFERENCES

- Jacobson HR, Striker GE, Klahr S, editors. The Principles and Practice of Nephrology. Philadelphia: B.C. Decker, Inc.; 1995
- Brenner B, Rector F, editors. The Kidney. 6th Ed. Philadelphia: W.B. Saunders Co.; 2000
- Schrier RW, Gottschalk CW. Diseases of the Kidney. 6th ed. Boston: Little Brown & Co.;1997
- Rose BD, editor. Nephrology Up-To-Date [book on CD-ROM]. Up-To-Date, vol 8.1. Wellesley, 2000
- Puig JG, et al. Hereditary nephropathy associated with hyperuricemia and gout. Arch Int Med 1993;153:357

Web references: 0 available at www.5mcc.com

Illustrations N/A

Author(s):

Mark R. Dambro, MD

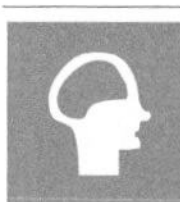

BASICS

DESCRIPTION A syndrome comprising glomerular proteinuria (3.5 g per 1.73m2 body-surface area/day), hypoalbuminemia, hypercholesterolemia and edema as a result of a primary renal disease or secondary to another disease process.

System(s) affected: Endocrine/Metabolic, Renal/Urologic

Genetics: N/A

Incidence/Prevalence in USA:
- Children - 2:100,000 new cases/year
- Adults - 3:100,000 new cases/year

Predominant age:
- Children - 1.5-6 years (MCD)
- Adults - all ages (FGS, MGN more common USA; IgG-IgA worldwide)

Predominant sex: Male = Female

SIGNS & SYMPTOMS
- Fluid retention: abdominal distention, ascites, edema, puffy eyelids, scrotal swelling, weight gain, shortness of breath
- Anorexia
- Hypertension
- Oliguria
- Orthostatic hypotension
- Retinal sheen
- Skin striae

CAUSES
- Primary renal disease
  - ◊ Fibrillary glomerulopathy (primary)
  - ◊ Focal glomerulonephritis
  - ◊ Focal glomerulosclerosis (FGS)
  - ◊ IgA nephropathy
  - ◊ Membranoproliferative glomerulonephritis (MPGN)
  - ◊ Membranous glomerulonephritis (MGN)
  - ◊ Mesangial proliferative glomerulonephritis
  - ◊ Minimal change disease (MCD)
  - ◊ Rapidly progressive glomerulonephritis (RPGN)
  - ◊ Congenital nephrotic syndrome
- Secondary renal disease. Associated primary renal disease shown in brackets:
  - ◊ Allergens (snake venoms, antitoxins, poison ivy, insect stings)
  - ◊ Amyloidosis
  - ◊ Carcinoma (bronchogenic, breast, colon, stomach, kidney) [MGN, etc]
  - ◊ Diabetes mellitus (most common)
  - ◊ Erythema multiforme
  - ◊ Fibrillary glomerulopathy (secondary: amyloid, cryoglobulins, multiple myeloma, chronic lymphocytic leukemia [CLL]
  - ◊ Henoch-Schönlein purpura
  - ◊ Heredofamilial (Alport's syndrome, Fabry disease)
  - ◊ Infections: ventriculoatrial shunt infection, bacterial endocarditis, HIV, HBV, HCV, schistosomiasis, TB, leprosy, post-strep GN (20% are nephrotic)
  - ◊ Leukemias
  - ◊ Lymphoma (Hodgkin [MCD], non-Hodgkin [MGN])
  - ◊ Focal glomerulosclerosis (reflux nephropathy, heroin abuse, nephron ablation, extensive glomerular scarring in acute glomerulonephritis, chronic renal allograft rejection, end stage kidney, morbid obesity, thromboembolism)
  - ◊ Malignant hypertension
  - ◊ Melanoma
  - ◊ Nephrotoxins and drugs (gold, penicillamine, mercury [MGN], NSAIDs [MCD] and interstitial nephritis
  - ◊ Polyarteritis nodosa
  - ◊ Preeclampsia
  - ◊ Sarcoid
  - ◊ Serum sickness
  - ◊ Sjögren syndrome
  - ◊ Systemic lupus erythematosus (SLE) [MGN, FGS, focal, mesangial, diffuse, proliferative]
  - ◊ Toxemia of pregnancy

RISK FACTORS
- Any of the disorders listed in causes
- Drug addiction (e.g. heroin [FGS])
- Hepatitis B and C, HIV, other infections
- Immunosuppression
- Nephrotoxic drugs
- Vesicoureteral reflux (FGS)
- Cancer (usually MGN, may be nil disease (MCD)
- Chronic analgesic use/abuse

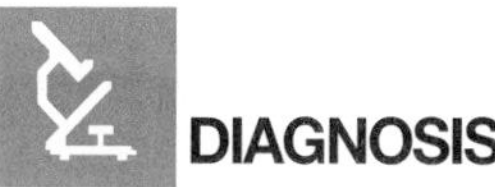

DIAGNOSIS

DIFFERENTIAL DIAGNOSIS See Causes. Is the disease predominantly nephrotic (protein without hematuria) such as MCD or MGN; or predominantly nephritic (protein plus blood) such as MPGN or FGS?

LABORATORY
- Hypoalbuminemia
- Hyperlipidemia
- Azotemia
- Hypercholesterolemia
- Urine
  - ◊ Proteinuria (> 3 gm/24 hr)
  - ◊ Glycosuria
  - ◊ Hematuria
  - ◊ Aminoaciduria
  - ◊ Granular casts
  - ◊ Hyaline casts
  - ◊ Fatty casts
  - ◊ Foamy appearance
  - ◊ Lipiduria

Drugs that may alter lab results: See causes

Disorders that may alter lab results: Many

PATHOLOGICAL FINDINGS
- Light microscopy
  - ◊ May see nothing (e.g., MCD)
  - ◊ Disease specific: sclerosis (e.g., FGS in diabetes)
- Immunofluorescence: Mesangial IgA (Henoch-Schönlein, IgG-IgA nephropathy). Other specific for disease.
- Electron microscopy (specific for disease as in subepithelial deposits of IgG in MGN)

SPECIAL TESTS
- Complement levels
- Antinuclear antibody, anti-dsDNA
- Serum protein electrophoresis (SPEP)
- Urine immune electrophoresis
- Blood cultures
- Diabetic testing
- HBV, HCV, HIV, RPR
- Fat pad biopsy
- Renal biopsy

IMAGING
- X-ray
- Ultrasound
- CT
- MRI or venography for renal vein thrombosis
- Fluorescein angiography (for retinopathy)

DIAGNOSTIC PROCEDURES N/A

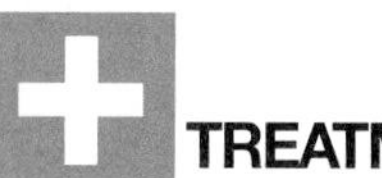

TREATMENT

APPROPRIATE HEALTH CARE Outpatient; inpatient , if complications

GENERAL MEASURES
- Treat infections vigorously (especially bacteriuria, endocarditis, peritonitis)
- Anticoagulant if thromboses
- Vaccines: Pneumococcal, influenza and H. influenzae
- Avoid excess sunlight
- Avoid nephrotoxic drugs
- Judicious use of diuretics
- Erythropoietin for anemia
- Consultation with nephrologist often required

SURGICAL MEASURES N/A

ACTIVITY As tolerated

DIET
- Normal protein (1 g/kg/day)
- Low fat (cholesterol)
- Reduced sodium
- Liberal potassium (unless hyperkalemic)
- Supplemental multivitamins and minerals, especially D and iron
- Fluid restriction if hyponatremic
- Caloric restriction if obese or diabetic

PATIENT EDUCATION
- Printed material for patients: National Kidney Foundation, 30 E. 33rd Street, Suite 1100, NY, NY 10016, (800)622-9010
  - ◊ "Childhood Nephrotic Syndrome" (Order #02-23NN)
  - ◊ "Diabetes and Kidney Disease" (Order #02-09CP) and "Focal Glomerulosclerosis" (Order #02-28NN)

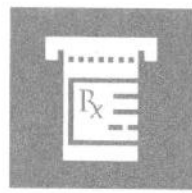

MEDICATIONS

DRUG(S) OF CHOICE
- ACE inhibitors to reduce proteinuria even in normotensive patients and to control hypertension if present. If intolerant of ACE I, use angiotensin II receptor blockers.
- For steroid-responsive disease (MCD and FGS), steroids dosed in consultation with nephrologist
- MGN patients with a poor prognosis: persistent, heavy proteinuria > 8 gm/day for > 6 months; elevated serum creatinine; hypertension; male sex; over age 50 or have a biopsy with sclerosis. Probably benefit from cytotoxic therapy (chlorambucil or cyclophosphamide). For hepatitis B glomerular disease - interferon. There are initial data for the use of cyclosporine.
- For edema
  - ◊ Most importantly salt restriction; then judicious thiazide, loop diuretics
  - ◊ If resistant, a combination of loop and distal diluting segment diuretics, e.g., metolazone, are synergistic
- Other nephrotic renal diseases: frequently relapsing MCD, RPGN, ?MGN, SLE
  - ◊ Bolus steroids and/or immune suppression (cyclophosphamide, mycophenolate mofetil, chlorambucil, cyclosporine)
  - ◊ Diet and cholesterol lowering drugs as needed
  - ◊ Anticoagulants for thrombotic events. There is data to suggest prophylactic oral anticoagulation in all cases of membranous GN (Kid Int. 1994;45:578-585).
  - ◊ Hypocalcemia from vitamin D loss should be treated with oral vitamin D (dihydrotachysterol) 0.2 mg q day

Contraindications: See manufacturer's literature
Precautions: See manufacturer's literature
Significant possible interactions: See manufacturer's literature

ALTERNATIVE DRUGS N/A

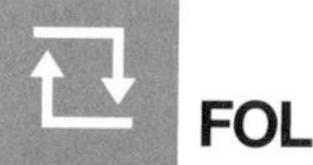

FOLLOWUP

PATIENT MONITORING Frequent monitoring for azotemia, hypertension, edema, nephrotoxicity, cholesterol, weight

PREVENTION/AVOIDANCE
- Avoid causative factors whenever possible
- Detect and treat infections vigorously. Infections may involve the common (Pneumococcus) to the unusual (Strongyloides), especially with immunosuppression.

POSSIBLE COMPLICATIONS
- Low levels of: 25-hydroxycholecalciferol, serum calcium, adrenocortical hormones, thyroid hormones
- Hypercoagulability, especially renal vein thrombosis
- Pulmonary emboli
- Hyperlipidemia
- Acute renal failure, progressive renal failure
- Protein malnutrition
- Infection
- Pleural effusion
- Ascites
- Iron deficiency (uncommon)

EXPECTED COURSE/PROGNOSIS
Varies with specific causes. Complete remission expected if basic disease is treatable (infection, malignancy, drug-induced). Otherwise may progress to dialysis dependence (e.g., diabetic glomerulosclerosis).

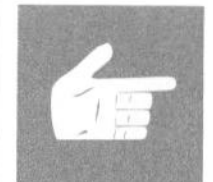

MISCELLANEOUS

ASSOCIATED CONDITIONS N/A

AGE-RELATED FACTORS
Pediatric: Relatively common in children aged 1.5-4 years (MCD)
Geriatric: Occurs in this age group. Prognosis is worse.
Others: N/A

PREGNANCY Toxemia of pregnancy may be nephrotic

SYNONYMS N/A

ICD-9-CM
581.9 Nephrotic syndrome with unspecified pathological lesion in kidney

SEE ALSO
Amyloidosis
Breast cancer
Colorectal malignancy
Diabetes mellitus, Type 1
Diabetes mellitus, Type 2
Endocarditis, infective
Glomerulonephritis, acute
HIV infection & AIDS
Multiple myeloma
Renal failure, acute (ARF)
Renal failure, chronic
Systemic lupus erythematosus (SLE)

OTHER NOTES N/A

ABBREVIATIONS
FGS = focal segmental glomerulosclerosis
MGN = membranous glomerulonephritis
MPGN = membranoproliferative glomerulonephritis
MCD = minimal change disease
RPGN = rapidly progressive glomerulonephritis

REFERENCES

- Klotman PE. HIV-associated nephropathy. Kid Int 1999;56:1161-76
- Madaio MP, Harrington JT. The diagnosis of glomerular diseases: acute glomerulonephritis and the nephrotic syndrome. Arch Intern Med 2001;161(1):25-34
- Muirhead N. Management of idiopathic membranous nephropathy: evidence-based recommendations. Kid Int (suppl) 1999;70:547-55
- Orth SR, Ritz E. The nephrotic syndrome. NEJM 1998;338:1202-11
- Remuzzi G, Schieppati A, Ruggenenti P. Clinical practice. Nephropathy in patients with type 2 diabetes. N Engl J Med 2002;346(15):1145-51
- Schwarz A. New aspects of the treatment of nephrotic syndrome. J Am Soc Nephrol 2001;12 Suppl 17:S44-7

Web references: 5 available at www.5mcc.com
Illustrations N/A

Author(s):
Neal S. Gold, MD

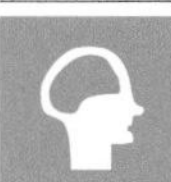

BASICS

DESCRIPTION A neoplasm of neural crest origin which may arise anywhere along the sympathetic ganglion chain or in the adrenal medulla. The most common tumor in children less than 1 year of age in the USA.

System(s) affected: Endocrine/Metabolic, Nervous

Genetics:
- Familial cases reported
- Genetic abnormalities in 80%
- Deletions in short arm of chromosome 1p36
- Amplification of n-myconcogene occurs on chromosome 2 (poor prognostic sign)

Incidence/Prevalence in USA:
- 27.8 cases/million children/year for 1st five years of life in USA; 8.7 cases/million in children/year for 1st 15 years of life in USA; Denmark: 1/12,000 - 14,000 live births; Japan: 1/15,000-18,749 infants
- Accounts for 6-10% of all childhood cancers
- 4th most common pediatric malignancy

Predominant age:
- 90% occur in 1st 8 years of life
- 60% occur in < 2 years of age
- Most common intra-abdominal malignancy in the newborn

Predominant sex: Slightly more common in boys than girls(1.2:1)

SIGNS & SYMPTOMS
- 50-60% present with metastatic disease
- Abdominal mass (50-75%)
- Weight loss
- Anemia
- Failure to thrive
- Abdominal pain and distension
- Bone pain
- Fever
- Diarrhea
- Hypertension (25%)
- Horner syndrome (ptosis, miosis, enophthalmos, heterochromia of iris)
- Orbital ecchymosis (panda eyes)
- Respiratory distress
- Dysphagia
- Paraplegia
- Cauda equina syndrome
- Flushing, sweating, irritability
- Cerebellar ataxia (chaotic nystagmus): dancing eye syndrome

CAUSES
- Genetic abnormalities in 80% of cases

RISK FACTORS
- Beckwith-Wiedemann syndrome
- Pancreatic islet cell dysplasia
- Maternal phenytoin treatment
- Fetal alcohol syndrome
- Hirschsprung's disease

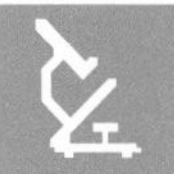

DIAGNOSIS

DIFFERENTIAL DIAGNOSIS
- Rhabdomyosarcoma
- Wilms' tumors
- Other tumors of neck, chest, abdomen and pelvis
- Hydronephrosis

LABORATORY
- CBC, platelet count
- Liver function studies
- Renal function studies
- Urinary catecholamines (85% secrete catecholamine metabolites)
- Uric acid
- Creatinine
- Magnesium, calcium
- LDH
- Electrolytes
- Bilirubin, SGOT, SGPT
- Gd2 monoclonal antibody levels
- Serum neuron-specific enolase
- Serum ferritin
- Bone marrow aspiration
- Assay for VIP

Drugs that may alter lab results: N/A

Disorders that may alter lab results: N/A

PATHOLOGICAL FINDINGS
- Small, dark, round cells
- Immature tumors tend to be large, red, lobular soft, friable
- Mature tumors are fibrous, contain calcification, hemorrhage, necrosis, cysts, rosettes, nerve filaments
- May be neuroblastoma, ganglioneuroblastoma, or benign neuroblastoma (depends on cell maturity)
- Favorable histology: Stroma-rich, well-differentiated and intermixed tumors
- Unfavorable histology: Stroma-rich nodular and stroma-poor, undifferentiated tumors
- Staging

Stage 1. Localized tumor with complete resection, with or without microscopic residual disease

Stage 2A. Localized tumor with incomplete gross excision, ipsilateral lymph node negative

Stage 2B. Localized tumor with or without complete excision, ipsilateral lymph nodes positive; contralateral lymph nodes negative

Stage 3. Unresectable tumor extending across midline or localized tumor with positive contralateral lymph nodes, or midline tumor with bilateral extension unresectable

Stage 4. Any primary tumor with distant metastases

Stage 4S. Localized primary tumor with dissemination limited to skin, liver, and/or bone marrow in infants < 1 year

- Amplification of n-myc oncogene (poor prognosis)
- Normal DNA ploidy - worse prognosis than hyperploidy

SPECIAL TESTS N/A

IMAGING
- Chest x-ray
- Skeletal survey (including orbital views)
- Bone scan
- CT or MRI of neck, chest, abdomen or pelvis (depending on location of tumor)
- Myelogram for neurologic symptoms

DIAGNOSTIC PROCEDURES
- Myelogram if needed
- Bone marrow aspiration

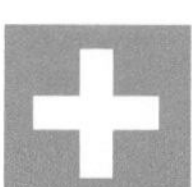

TREATMENT

APPROPRIATE HEALTH CARE Inpatient workup and treatment until stable and induction chemotherapy completed

GENERAL MEASURES
- Radiation therapy in Stage III over 1 year of age
- Chemotherapy for stage II and greater

SURGICAL MEASURES
- Surgical resection may be complete, incomplete or biopsy only (for Stage I, excision only)
- If resection incomplete or biopsy, chemotherapy followed by 2nd look operation
- Dumbbell extension through vertebral foramina, chemotherapy alone vs. laminectomy and decompression
- Stage IV-S: resection of primary tumor and chemotherapy
- Bone marrow transplantation considered in stages III & IV

ACTIVITY As tolerated

DIET No special diet

PATIENT EDUCATION
- Patient and family teaching regarding long term outlook
- Possibility of second malignancy
- Side effects of treatment

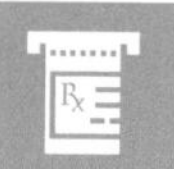

MEDICATIONS

DRUG(S) OF CHOICE
- Cyclophosphamide
- Melphalan
- Vincristine
- Dacarbazine
- Teniposide
- Etoposide
- Doxorubicin (Adriamycin)
- Cisplatin
- Peptichemio
- Carboplatin
- Ifosfamide [with mesna to protect against hemorrhagic cystitis]

Contraindications: See manufacturer's information
Precautions: See manufacturer's information
Significant possible interactions: See manufacturers information

ALTERNATIVE DRUGS
- By protocol
- Ondansetron (Zofran), dronabinol (Marinol), metoclopramide (Reglan), and others for nausea control

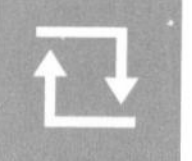

FOLLOWUP

PATIENT MONITORING
- Multi-agent chemotherapy every 3-4 weeks for 4 courses then re-evaluate with bone marrow or second look operation
- Follow every 3 months for 1st year, every 4 months for 2nd year, every 6 months for 3rd year, then at least yearly
- Follow with CT or MRI every 3-6 months initially, then yearly

PREVENTION/AVOIDANCE N/A

POSSIBLE COMPLICATIONS
- Nausea, vomiting
- Alopecia
- Bone marrow depression
- Immunosuppression
- Hemorrhagic cystitis
- Azotemia
- Diarrhea
- ADH secretion
- Local tissue necrosis
- Myocardiopathy
- Renal toxicity
- Hearing loss
- Hypocalcemia, hypomagnesemia

EXPECTED COURSE/PROGNOSIS
- Overall survival 58%
- Stage I - expected survival approximates 100%
- Stage II - Survival 75%
- Stage III - Survival 43%
- Stage IV - Survival 15%
- Stage IV-S - Survival 70-80%
- Normal DNA ploidy, n-myc amplifications, unfavorable histology indicates worse than usual prognosis for same tumor
- Infants under 1 year of age have better outcome
- Patients with cervical, pelvic, and mediastinal tumors have better prognosis than those with retroperitoneal, paraspinal or adrenal tumors
- Survival for those presenting with opsoclonus and nystagmus is nearly 90% (seen especially in mediastinal tumors in infants under 1 year of age)
- Neuron specific enolase level > 100 ng/mL correlates with advanced disease and reduced survival
- Serum LDH < 1500 IU/mL may indicate improved survival rate

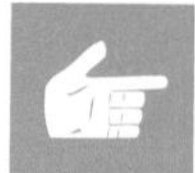

MISCELLANEOUS

ASSOCIATED CONDITIONS See Risk factors

AGE-RELATED FACTORS
Pediatric: Occurs only in children
Geriatric: N/A
Others: N/A

PREGNANCY N/A

SYNONYMS N/A

ICD-9-CM
194.0 Malignant neoplasm of adrenal gland
171.8 Malignant neoplasm of other specified sites of connective and other soft tissue
195.1 Malignant neoplasm of thorax

SEE ALSO

OTHER NOTES N/A

ABBREVIATIONS N/A

REFERENCES

- Ashcraft KW, Murphy JP, Sharp RJ, editors. Pediatric Surgery. 3rd ed. Philadelphia: W.B. Saunders Co; 2000
- Grosfeld JL, Rescorla F, West KW, Goldman J. Neuroblastoma in the First Year of Life: Clinical and Biologic Factors Influencing Outcome. Seminars in Pediatric Surgery 1993;2(1):37-46
- O'Neill JA, Rowe MI, Grosfeld JL, et al. Pediatric Surgery. 5th ed. St Louis: Mosby; 1998
- Matthay KK. Neuroblastoma: A clinical challenge and biological puzzle. CA Cancer Jour Clin 1995;45:179-182

Web references: 2 available at www.5mcc.com
Illustrations N/A

Author(s):
Timothy L. Black, MD

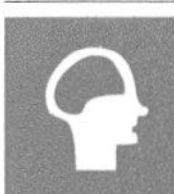

BASICS

DESCRIPTION A chronic dermatitis resulting from continued, repeated rubbing or scratching part of the skin
System(s) affected: Skin/Exocrine
Genetics: None known
Incidence/Prevalence in USA: Common
Predominant age: May occur at any age, but is uncommon in childhood. Peak incidence is between ages 30-50.
Predominant sex: Female > Male

SIGNS & SYMPTOMS
- Gradual onset
- Begins as a localized, pruritic patch of dermatitis
- Most commonly involves easily accessible areas, including nape of neck, lower legs, ankles, wrists, extensor surfaces of forearms, scalp, external ear, and anogenital region
- Nuchal and suboccipital regions more commonly affected in women
- Perineal region more commonly affected in men
- Pruritus that is out of proportion to the appearance of the lesion occurs paroxysmally, is usually worse at night, and may occur during sleep
- Lichenified, excoriated pruritic patches of skin
- Non-erythematous
- Accentuation of normal skin lines
- Vesicles or weeping are rare
- If cycle continues, verrucous thickening and changes in pigmentation may occur
- Moist scale, serum crusting or pustules suggest the presence of infection
- Scarring is rare except after serious secondary infections

CAUSES
- Idiopathic in many instances
- Some causes of apparent idiopathic disease may be secondary to a previously unrecognized dermatosis
- Secondary forms may begin as another pruritic skin disease which evolves into neurodermatitis after resolution of the primary dermatitis
- Primary dermatoses from which neurodermatitis may develop include lichen planus, stasis dermatitis, atopic dermatitis, contact dermatitis, psoriasis, tinea corporis, seborrheic dermatitis, xerosis and eczema
- Habitual scratching and resulting scratch-itch cycle lead to a chronic dermatosis. Scratching often occurs during sleep.
- Social stress or obsessive-compulsive personality trait may play a role in development of this disease

RISK FACTORS
- Any pre-existing pruritic dermatosis
- Obsessive-compulsive personality or anxiety
- Exposure to irritants

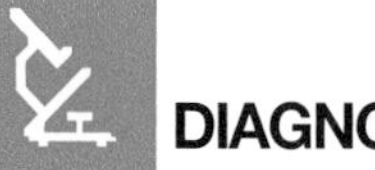

DIAGNOSIS

DIFFERENTIAL DIAGNOSIS
- Atopic dermatitis
- Contact dermatitis
- Cutaneous T-cell lymphoma
- Drug reaction
- Lichen planus
- Lichenified psoriasis
- Photodermatitis
- Stasis dermatitis
- Cutaneous amyloidosis
- Fungal infection
- Seborrheic dermatitis
- Lupus vulgaris (cutaneous tuberculosis)

LABORATORY None diagnostic. Appropriate tests to evaluate for other conditions.

Drugs that may alter lab results: N/A

Disorders that may alter lab results: N/A

PATHOLOGICAL FINDINGS
- Hyperkeratosis
- Acanthosis
- Lengthening of rete ridges
- Hyperplasia of all components of epidermis
- Chronic inflammatory infiltrate of dermis

SPECIAL TESTS None

IMAGING N/A

DIAGNOSTIC PROCEDURES Skin biopsy to evaluate for other conditions if no response to treatment

TREATMENT

APPROPRIATE HEALTH CARE Outpatient management

GENERAL MEASURES
- Patient education
- Treat pruritus to interrupt the scratch-itch cycle
- Occlusive dressings, especially at night, may be beneficial for preventing scratching and rubbing
- Nail trimming

SURGICAL MEASURES N/A

ACTIVITY As tolerated. Encourage exercise in those cases where stress may play a role.

DIET Regular

PATIENT EDUCATION
- Patients should understand the cause of this disease and their role in helping resolve the condition
- Various stress reduction techniques can also be used in those patients in whom stress plays a significant role
- Emphasize that scratching and rubbing must stop in order for lesions to heal

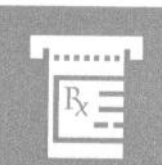

MEDICATIONS

DRUG(S) OF CHOICE
- Topical steroids
  - ◊ High potency steroids alone, such as 0.05% betamethasone dipropionate cream or 0.05% clobetasol propionate cream can be used initially, but these should not be used on the face, anogenital region, or intertriginous areas. They should be used on small areas only, and for no longer than two weeks.
  - ◊ An intermediate potency steroid such as 0.1% triamcinolone cream may be used initially under an occlusive dressing for one to two weeks instead
  - ◊ Switch to intermediate or low potency steroids alone as response allows
  - ◊ An intermediate potency steroid, such as 0.025% or 0.1% triamcinolone cream may be used for initial treatment of the face and intertriginous areas and for maintenance treatment of other areas. A low potency steroid, such as 1% hydrocortisone cream should be used for maintenance treatment of the face and intertriginous areas.
- Steroid tape (Cordran)
  - ◊ Optimized penetration
  - ◊ Provides some barrier to further trauma

Contraindications: High potency topical steroids are contraindicated for use on the face and intertriginous areas

Precautions: Topical and intralesional steroid therapy can cause epidermal and dermal atrophy as well as hypopigmentation

Significant possible interactions: N/A

ALTERNATIVE DRUGS
- Menthol 0.25% solution can help relieve pruritus
- Cold Burow's solution compresses: 1 packet of Domeboro powder in one quart ice cold water applied with a cloth for 15 minutes as needed
- Coal tar preparations are useful but cosmetically less appealing
- Topical doxepin cream 5%
- Topical capsaicin cream
- Oral antihistamines can be used for both their antipruritic and sedative effects.
- For resistant cases, consider a course of prednisone 40 mg/day for 2 weeks
- Intralesional corticosteroids: Inject 5-10 mg of Kenalog-10 (10 mg/ml) diluted with an equal amount of sterile saline intradermally or subcutaneously, directly under the lesion, using 26-30 gauge needle and Luer-Lok syringe. Spread solution around as needle is advanced. May repeat every 2-3 weeks as needed until resolution. Atrophy at injection site is a potential complication.
- Botulinum toxin A injected intradermally has been reported to produce a significant improvement in patients with recalcitrant pruritus
- Topical aspirin has been shown to be helpful
- Anxiolytics or tricyclic antidepressants (e.g., lorazepam or amitriptyline)
- Unna boot for barrier protection
- Oral antibiotics if secondary infection is present

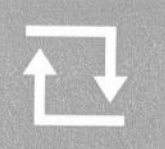

FOLLOWUP

PATIENT MONITORING Patients should be followed closely and regularly for response to therapy, complications from therapy, and secondary infections

PREVENTION/AVOIDANCE Avoid irritants and other known causative agents

POSSIBLE COMPLICATIONS
- Secondary infection
- Complications related to therapy, as mentioned in medication precautions

EXPECTED COURSE/PROGNOSIS
- Often chronic and recurrent
- The prognosis is good for those patients in whom the scratch-itch cycle can be broken
- After healing, the skin should have a normal appearance unless secondary infection has occurred

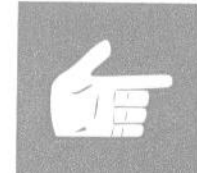

MISCELLANEOUS

ASSOCIATED CONDITIONS Prurigo nodularis is a nodular variety of the same disease process

AGE-RELATED FACTORS
Pediatric: Rare in pre-adolescents
Geriatric: Common > age 60
Others: N/A

PREGNANCY N/A

SYNONYMS
- Lichen simplex chronicus

ICD-9-CM
698.3 Lichenification and lichen simplex chronicus

SEE ALSO
Dermatitis, contact
Dermatitis, seborrheic
Dermatitis, stasis
Pruritus ani
Pruritus vulvae

OTHER NOTES N/A

ABBREVIATIONS N/A

REFERENCES

- Champion RH, et al. Rook/Wilkinson/Ebling Textbook of Dermatology. 6th ed. Oxford: Blackwell Science Inc; 1998
- Freedberg IM, et al. Fitzpatrick's Dermatology in General Medicine. 5th ed. New York: McGraw Hill; 1999
- Habif T. Clinical Dermatology. 4th Ed. St. Louis, CV Mosby, 2003
- Hall J. Sauer's Manual of Skin Diseases. 8th ed. Philadelphia: Lippincott Williams & Wilkins; 1999
- Heckmann M, Heyer G, Brunner B, Plewig G. Botulinum toxin type A injection in the treatment of lichen simplex: an open pilot study. J Am Acad Dermatol 2002;46(4):617-9
- Moschella SL, Hurley HJ. Dermatology. 3rd ed. Philadelphia: WB Sanders Co; 1992
- Odom RB, James W, Berger TG. Andrews' Diseases of the Skin. 9th ed. Philadelphia: W.B. Saunders Co.; 2000
- Orkin K, Maibach HI. Dermatology. San Mateo, CA: Appleton & Lange; 1991
- Pandhi D, Reddy BS. Lupus vulgaris mimicking lichen simplex chronicus. J Dermatol 2001;28(7):369-72
- Sams WM, Lynch PJ. Principles and Practice of Dermatology. 2nd ed. New York: Churchill Livingstone; 1996
- Yosipovitch G, Sugeng MW, Chan YH, Goon A, Ngim S, Goh CL. The effect of topically applied aspirin on localized circumscribed neurodermatitis. J Am Acad Dermatol 2001;45(6):910-3

Web references: 0 available at www.5mcc.com
Illustrations 6 available

Author(s):
Amy Y. Wang, MD

BASICS

DESCRIPTION The most common of the neurocutaneous syndromes (phakomatoses), consisting of Neurofibromatosis Type 1 (1 in 3,000) and Neurofibromatosis Type 2 (1 in 50,000). Although named similarly, and both autosomal dominant disorders, they are two distinctly different conditions with genes now identified on two separate chromosomes.
- Type 1 (NF 1) is also known as von Recklinghausen disease
- Type 2 (NF 2) is also known as bilateral acoustic neurofibromatosis

System(s) affected: Musculoskeletal, Nervous, Skin/Exocrine
Genetics:
- NF1: autosomal dominant inheritance. Nearly 50% of cases are attributed to new mutations. The NF 1 gene mapped to chromosome 17. Prenatal diagnosis possible.
- NF2: Autosomal dominant inheritance. The NF 2 gene mapped on chromosome 22.

Incidence/Prevalence in USA: NF 1 = 1/3,000; NF 2 = 1/50,000
Predominant age: N/A
Predominant sex: Male = Female

SIGNS & SYMPTOMS
- NF1: Two or more of the following:
  - ◊ Six or more café-au-lait macules measuring 5 mm or more in prepubertal individuals or 15 mm or more in adults (97%)
  - ◊ Two or more neurofibromata or plexiform neurofibroma (15%)
  - ◊ Axillary or inguinal freckling (91%)
  - ◊ Two or more Lisch nodules (30%)
  - ◊ Optic glioma (11-15% using MRI)
  - ◊ Characteristic osseous lesions such as sphenoid dysplasia, long bone cortical thinning, ribbon ribs, angular scoliosis (6%)
  - ◊ First degree relative with NF 1, according to above criteria
- NF2: When one or more present, diagnosis is likely:
  - ◊ Bilateral vestibular schwannomas
  - ◊ Family history of NF 2, plus unilateral 8th nerve mass or family history and any two of the following: neurofibroma, meningioma, glioma, schwannoma, and juvenile posterior subcapsular lenticular opacity.

CAUSES
- Congenital

RISK FACTORS
- Family history

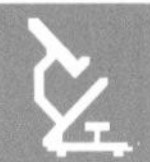

DIAGNOSIS

DIFFERENTIAL DIAGNOSIS
- NF1:
  - ◊ Familial café-au-lait spots (autosomal dominant) - no other NF1 features
- NF2:
  - ◊ Solitary acoustic neuroma (develops later in life and is not hereditary)

LABORATORY N/A

Drugs that may alter lab results: N/A

Disorders that may alter lab results: N/A

PATHOLOGICAL FINDINGS
- NF1: Generalized disorder of cells of neural crest origin

SPECIAL TESTS N/A

IMAGING See below

DIAGNOSTIC PROCEDURES
- NF1:
  - ◊ Dictated by findings and clinical evaluation
  - ◊ Slit lamp ocular exam
  - ◊ Radiology of skull and spine
  - ◊ Psychological testing
  - ◊ Characteristic x-ray findings such as sphenoid dysplasia, long bone cortical thinning, ribbon ribs, angular scoliosis (6%)
- NF2:
  - ◊ Clinical examination: skin, eye, and hearing
  - ◊ Audiologic evaluation: brain stem evoked response (BAER)
  - ◊ Radiologic examination: MRI of head
  - ◊ When one or more of the following are present, the diagnosis of NF 2 is likely:
    - Bilateral vestibular schwannomas
    - Family history of NF 2, plus unilateral 8th nerve mass or family history and any two of the following: neurofibroma, meningioma, glioma, schwannoma, and juvenile posterior subcapsular lenticular opacity

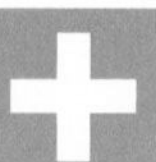

TREATMENT

APPROPRIATE HEALTH CARE Outpatient

GENERAL MEASURES
- Access to patient support groups
- Referral of patient to National NF Organization, local and state chapters
- NF1:
  - ◊ General outpatient follow-up of symptomatic patients for early identification of complications
  - ◊ Periodic exams with particular attention to CNS findings and close attention to any masses or focally arising "new" pain
  - ◊ Referral for psychosocial issues of family and affected individuals
  - ◊ Educational intervention for children with learning disabilities or ADHD (40%)
- NF2:
  - ◊ Annual neurologic examination
  - ◊ Annual ophthalmologic exam
  - ◊ Annual hearing examination or more frequently as necessitated
  - ◊ Hearing augmentation as needed
  - ◊ Speech therapy as needed
  - ◊ Counseling and education regarding insidious problems associated with hearing loss, balance, or sense of direction

SURGICAL MEASURES
- NF1: Surgical treatment if indicated for scoliosis, plexiform neurofibromata or malignancy
- NF2: excision of tumor as indicated

ACTIVITY
- NF2: Caution advised in swimming, diving, or climbing heights

DIET No restrictions

PATIENT EDUCATION
- Genetic counseling and patient education regarding future complications and decisions about family planning

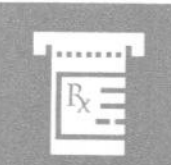

MEDICATIONS

DRUG(S) OF CHOICE

- NF1:
  - ◊ Anticonvulsants: for seizure control
  - ◊ Stimulant medications: for attention deficit hyperactivity disorder (ADHD)

Contraindications: N/A
Precautions: N/A
Significant possible interactions: caution necessary with these classes of drugs. Refer to manufacturer's profiles.

ALTERNATIVE DRUGS

Multiple clinical trials are recruiting patients with neurofibromatosis and progressive plexiform neurofibromas for experimental treatment with pharmaceutical agents (for more information see: http://www.clinicaltrials.gov/ct/search?term=Neurofibromatoses&submit=Search).

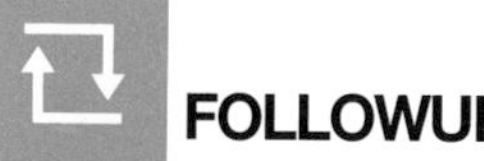

FOLLOWUP

PATIENT MONITORING

- Annual evaluation and periodic assessment for at risk individuals

PREVENTION/AVOIDANCE

- Genetic counseling

POSSIBLE COMPLICATIONS

- NF1:
  - ◊ Disfigurement: skin neurofibromata develop primarily on exposed areas
  - ◊ Scoliosis: common: most cases mild
  - ◊ CNS: A large head is common but rarely associated with hydrocephalus. Optic glioma or other CNS tumors arise usually during childhood (5-10%).
  - ◊ Learning disability: common; often diagnosed upon entering school. May be associated with attention deficit hyperactivity disorder (ADHD).
  - ◊ Rare Complications:
    - Mental retardation
    - Epilepsy
    - Hypertension
    - Variable onset of puberty
    - Slightly higher risk for malignancy (e.g. Wilms', leukemia, rhabdosarcoma)

EXPECTED COURSE/PROGNOSIS

- NF1: Variable; most patients have a mild expression and lead normal lives
- NF2: Variable

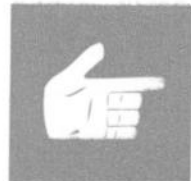

MISCELLANEOUS

ASSOCIATED CONDITIONS N/A

AGE-RELATED FACTORS

Pediatric: External stigmata subtle or absent in very young children
Geriatric: Cutaneous lesions and tumors increase in size and number with age
Others: N/A

PREGNANCY Genetic counseling

SYNONYMS

- Von Recklinghausen Disease (NF1)
- Bilateral acoustic neurofibromatosis (NF2)

ICD-9-CM

237.70 Neurofibromatosis, unspecified

SEE ALSO

Ataxia-telangiectasia
Tuberous sclerosis complex
von Hippel-Lindau disease

OTHER NOTES N/A

ABBREVIATIONS N/A

REFERENCES

- Listernick R, Charrow J: Neurofibromatosis type 1 in childhood. J Ped 1990;116;6:845-853
- Gutmann DH, et al: The diagnostic evaluation and multidisciplinary management of NF 1 and NF 2 JAMA 1997;278;1:51-57
- Martuza RL, Eldridge R: Neurofibromatosis 2. NEJM 1988;318(11):684-688
- North K. Neurofibromatosis type 1. Am J. Med Genet 2000;97;2:119-27
- Evans DG, Sainio M, Baser ME. Neurofibromatosis type 2. J Med Genet 2000;37(12):897-904

Web references: 4 available at www.5mcc.com
Illustrations N/A

Author(s):

Nuhad D. Dinno, MD

BASICS

DESCRIPTION Nocardiosis is an acute, subacute, or chronic infection occurring in cutaneous, pulmonary, and disseminated forms. Nocardiosis produces suppurative necrosis and abscess formation at sites of infection.

- Primary cutaneous nocardiosis presents as cutaneous infection (cellulitis or abscess), lymphocutaneous infection (similar to sporotrichosis), or subcutaneous infection (actinomycetoma)
- Pulmonary infection presents as an acute, subacute, or chronic pneumonitis
- Disseminated nocardiosis may involve any organ (lesions in the brain or meninges most frequent)

System(s) affected: Nervous, Pulmonary, Renal/ Urologic, Skin/Exocrine
Genetics: N/A
Incidence/Prevalence in USA: 0.4/100,000 (it is estimated that 500-1000 new cases occur per year)
Predominant age: All ages are susceptible, mean age at diagnosis is the fourth decade of life
Predominant sex: Males > Female (3:1)

SIGNS & SYMPTOMS

- Pulmonary nocardiosis:
  - ◊ Fever (70%)
  - ◊ Cough (52%)
  - ◊ Pleuritic chest pain (32%)
  - ◊ Dyspnea (16%)
  - ◊ Anorexia
  - ◊ Weight loss
  - ◊ Hemoptysis
  - ◊ Tachypnea
  - ◊ Rales
  - ◊ Central nervous system dysfunction in those with CNS involvement
  - ◊ Other focal infections in those with disseminated infection
- Cutaneous nocardiosis
  - ◊ Abscesses
  - ◊ Lymphadenopathy
- Disseminated nocardiosis
  - ◊ Confusion
  - ◊ Disorientation
  - ◊ Dizziness
  - ◊ Headache
  - ◊ Nausea and/or vomiting
  - ◊ Seizures
  - ◊ Shortness of breath

CAUSES Nocardiosis is caused by inhalation or traumatic inoculation of Nocardia species bacteria (predominantly *Nocardia asteroides*, but also *N. brasiliensis*, *N. caviae*, *N. farcinica*, *N. transvalensis*, *N. otitidiscavarium*, and *N. nova*) from soil

RISK FACTORS

- Most cases occur as opportunistic infection of immunocompromised hosts or hosts with predisposing pulmonary abnormalities
- Solid organ transplantation, chronic granulomatous disease of childhood, dysgammaglobulinemias, pemphigus, Cushing disease, hemochromatosis, cirrhosis, bronchiectasis, tuberculosis, sarcoidosis, anthrasilicosis, pulmonary alveolar proteinosis, lymphoma, leukemia, glucocorticoid and cytotoxic therapy, solid malignancies, and AIDS.
- Immunologically normal individuals can develop primary cutaneous disease days to weeks after receiving a wound contaminated with soil

DIAGNOSIS

DIFFERENTIAL DIAGNOSIS Includes other causes of acute, subacute, or chronic pneumonitis, particularly those occurring principally in immunocompromised hosts; tuberculosis, histoplasmosis, mixed bacterial lung abscess, and carcinoma

LABORATORY The diagnosis is established by observing the characteristic microscopical appearance of the organism in Gram stained and modified acid-fast stained preparations of sputum or pus or histopathologic samples. Confirmation is by culture of these same specimens.

Drugs that may alter lab results: N/A

Disorders that may alter lab results: N/A

PATHOLOGICAL FINDINGS Histopathology reveals a suppurative lesion with acute necrosis and abscess formation and the microorganism which may stain positive on acid fast stains

SPECIAL TESTS N/A

IMAGING

- X-ray - confluent bronchopneumonia with or without cavitation. Pleural effusion is common (up to 50%). Other chest x-ray presentations include masses, nodules, cavities, interstitial infiltrates.
- Imaging of the brain (CT or MRI) may reveal single or multiple intracranial abscesses, and is indicated in all patients with pulmonary nocardiosis. Other sites of focal infection may be identified by imaging in disseminated disease.

DIAGNOSTIC PROCEDURES If evaluation of sputum is nondiagnostic, bronchoscopy for bronchoalveolar lavage and transbronchial lung biopsy may prove valuable for diagnosis. Percutaneous aspiration of lung lesion is often useful.

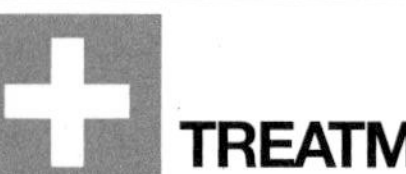

TREATMENT

APPROPRIATE HEALTH CARE Patients with moderate or severe illness generally require hospitalization

GENERAL MEASURES Respiratory support is often necessary in such hospitalized patients

SURGICAL MEASURES Surgical drainage of abscesses other than intrapulmonary abscesses is generally indicated if technically feasible

ACTIVITY Acute phase usually requires bedrest. Increase activity as condition improves.

DIET No special diet

PATIENT EDUCATION

- Not a contagious disease
- Advise patients of the need for long-term antimicrobial therapy to reduce the likelihood of relapse

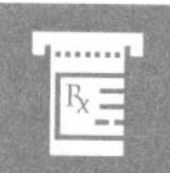

MEDICATIONS

DRUG(S) OF CHOICE

- Survival may be improved if a sulfa-containing regimen is used. Some prefer sulfadiazine because of possibly better CNS penetration. Sulfadiazine should be given as 4-8 gm po per day in 4 divided doses. Dosage should be adjusted to maintain sulfonamide serum levels in the range of 8-16 mg/dL.
- Some prefer to use trimethoprim-sulfamethoxazole. This agent must be used if parenteral sulfonamide therapy is required. Initial dose based on trimethoprim component: 640 mg trimethoprim daily. Base subsequent doses on sulfamethoxazole level. Dosage should provide equivalent sulfonamide dosing and levels as when a sulfonamide is used alone.
- Duration of therapy is usually 3 months for immunocompetent hosts and 6 months for those who are immunocompromised

Contraindications:

- Sulfonamides - in the last month of pregnancy (should only be used when the potential benefits outweigh the risks)
- All antimicrobial agents above are contraindicated in the presence of known hypersensitivity to the agent

Precautions: With the use of high dose sulfadiazine, high urine flow should be maintained to minimize risk of crystalluria. Generally, patient should be advised to drink 2-3 L/day.

Significant possible interactions:

- Sulfonamides can increase the therapeutic effects of oral anticoagulants, phenytoin, sulfonylurea hypoglycemic agents, methotrexate, and thiopental
- Decreased absorption of digoxin may be encountered

ALTERNATIVE DRUGS

- Alternatives for sulfonamide allergic patients include doxycycline or minocycline, ampicillin plus erythromycin, amikacin, imipenem, ß-lactam/ß-lactamase inhibitor combinations, and cefotaxime or ceftriaxone. Clinical experience with these alternative regimens is limited.
- Species specific trends in susceptibility have been identified
- For acutely ill, cefotaxime 1-2 gm IV every 8 hours plus imipenem 500 mg IV every 6 hours
- Selection of combination oral therapy should be based on microbiologic sensitivity testing

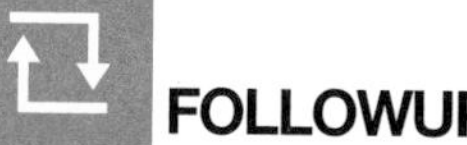

FOLLOWUP

PATIENT MONITORING

Patients on high dose sulfonamide therapy should have a complete blood count and assessment of hepatic and renal function performed at least every other week

PREVENTION/AVOIDANCE

N/A

POSSIBLE COMPLICATIONS

- Central nervous system infection (brain abscess or meningitis) (16%)
- Secondary cutaneous nocardiosis (13%)
- Septic arthritis (2%)
- Hematogenous osteomyelitis (1%)
- Other focal manifestations of disseminated infection (13%)

EXPECTED COURSE/PROGNOSIS

Overall modern mortality is 7-44%. In renal transplant recipients: overall mortality 25%, 0% mortality with isolated cutaneous involvement, 29% mortality with localized pleuropulmonary disease, 42% mortality with central nervous system involvement. In patients with the acquired immunodeficiency syndrome, mortality is 30%.

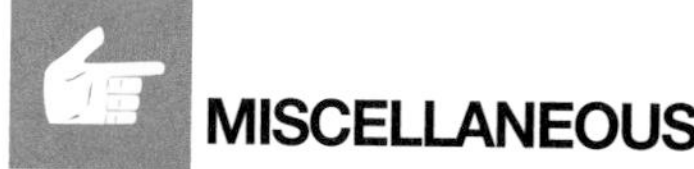

MISCELLANEOUS

ASSOCIATED CONDITIONS

See Risk factors

AGE-RELATED FACTORS

Pediatric: Reported association between chronic granulomatous disease of childhood and nocardiosis
Geriatric: N/A
Others: N/A

PREGNANCY

Sulfonamides - in the last month of pregnancy should only be used when the potential benefits outweigh the risks

SYNONYMS

N/A

ICD-9-CM

039.9 Actinomycotic infections of unspecified site

SEE ALSO

OTHER NOTES

Unusual nocardial infections: keratoconjunctivitis associated with contact lenses, peritonitis in patients on continuous ambulatory peritoneal dialysis, upper respiratory and digestive tract infections, pericarditis, hematogenous endophthalmitis, prosthetic joint infections, natural or prosthetic valve endocarditis

ABBREVIATIONS

N/A

REFERENCES

- Smego RA, Jr, Gallis HA. The clinical spectrum of Nocardia brasiliensis infetion in the United States. Rev Infect Dis 1984;6:164-80
- Kalb RE, Kaplan MH, Grossman ME. Cutaneous nocardiosis. J Am Acad Derm 198513:125-133
- Wilson JP, Turner HR, Kirchner KA, Chapman SW. Nocardial infection in renal transplant recipients. Medicine 1989;68:38-57
- Kim J, Minamoto GY, Grieco MH. Nocardial infection as a complication of AIDS: Report of six cases & review. Rev Infect Dis 1991;13:624-629
- Uttamchandani RB, Daikos GL, Reyes RR. Nocardiosis in 30 patients with advanced human immunodeficiency virus infection: clinical features and outcome. Clin Infec Dis 1994;181:348-53
- Mamelak AN, Obano WG, Flaherty JF, Rosenblum ML. Nocardial brain abscess: Treatment strategies and factors influencing outcome. Neurosurgery 1994;35:622-631
- Marrie TJ. Pneumonia caused by Nocardia Species. Sem Resp Infect 1994; 9:207
- Lerner Pl. Nocardiosis. Clin Infec Dis 1996;22:891-902

Web references: 0 available at www.5mcc.com
Illustrations 2 available

Author(s):

Brock D. Lutz, MD
Ronald A. Greenfield, MD

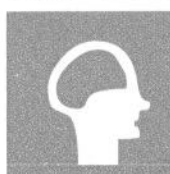

BASICS

DESCRIPTION A condition of increased body weight (consisting of both lean and fat tissue) that leads to increased morbidity and mortality. Also defined as weight 20% greater than an individual's desirable weight as defined by the Metropolitan Life Insurance Company or BMI ≥ 30. Overweight is defined as a BMI of 25 to 29.9. The table below reflects BMI values important in treatment decisions.
- Android obesity (male pattern or abdominal obesity) is higher risk and gynecoid obesity (female pattern or gluteal obesity) is lower risk for long-term health problems.

BMI Obesity threshold by height:

Height	BMI=27 Weight (lb/kg)	BMI=30 Weight (lb/kg)
5′ 0	138/63	153/70
5′ 2″	147/67	164/74
5′ 4″	157/71	174/79
5′ 6″	167/76	186/84
5′ 8″	177/81	197/89
5′ 10″	188/85	209/95
6′ 0″	199/90	221/100
6′ 2″	210/95	233/106
6′ 4″	221/101	246/112

System(s) affected: Endocrine/Metabolic, Gastrointestinal
Genetics: 25-30% of the variance in body fat is genetically transmitted
Incidence/Prevalence in USA:
- Ages 35-44: 1600/100,000 males; 1400/100,000 females
- Ages 65-74: 500/100,000 males; 400/100,000 females
- 25-35% of adult men and 30-40% of adult women (according to an NIH panel)

Predominant age: All ages
Predominant sex: Female > Male

SIGNS & SYMPTOMS Increased body weight and adipose tissue

CAUSES
- Multifactorial
- Rare genetic syndromes have been described
- Idiopathic obesity is assumed to be due to an imbalance between food intake and energy expenditure (physical activity and metabolic rate)
- Insulinoma
- Hypothalamic disorders
- Cushing syndrome
- Corticosteroid drugs

RISK FACTORS
- Parental obesity
- Pregnancy
- Sedentary lifestyle
- High fat diet
- Low socioeconomic status

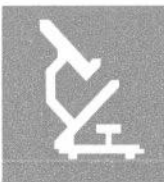

DIAGNOSIS

DIFFERENTIAL DIAGNOSIS N/A

LABORATORY
- Not needed for diagnosis
- Consider thyroid function tests
- Cardiac risk factors: serum cholesterol, triglycerides, glucose

Drugs that may alter lab results: N/A

Disorders that may alter lab results: Hypothyroidism

PATHOLOGICAL FINDINGS
- Hypertrophy and/or hyperplasia of adipocytes
- Cardiomegaly
- Hepatomegaly

SPECIAL TESTS
- Body mass index (BMI) = body weight (kg) divided by the square of body height (m). Obesity is BMI > 28 kg/m2.
- Determine fat distribution pattern by measuring waist circumference. Waist circumference greater than 40 in (102 cm) for men or 35 in (88 cm) for women is associated with increased risk for most obesity-related medical conditions.

IMAGING N/A

DIAGNOSTIC PROCEDURES N/A

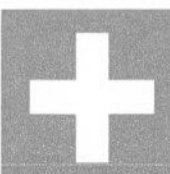

TREATMENT

APPROPRIATE HEALTH CARE Outpatient

GENERAL MEASURES
- Appropriate functions for the primary care physician include: assessment of degree of health risk from BMI and WHR (see Diagnosis); assessment of motivation to lose weight; helping patients to set goals of therapy; office counseling or referral to a registered dietitian or weight loss program for in depth counseling on diet, exercise, and behavior modification; and long term follow-up
- Many reputable commercial and community programs exist for obesity treatment. Desirable programs should include diets which meet the RDA for nutrients, exercise counseling, behavior modification, and provision for long term maintenance. Physicians can provide valuable additional monitoring and long term followup.

SURGICAL MEASURES Occasionally, treat patients with severe obesity (BMI > 40 kg/m2) with a gastric bypass or stapling procedure. This involves complex pre-surgical evaluation, surgery and followup and should be done in a center skilled in this treatment. Surgical treatment is the most effective long term weight loss treatment available for morbid obesity.

ACTIVITY
- Exercise alone rarely causes significant weight loss, but may improve long term results of weight loss treatment and should be an integral part of any weight loss program.
- Exercise regimens involve 30 minutes 5-7 times/week. Increasing calories expended in activities throughout the day is also important.
- Many patients may benefit from an "exercise prescription"

DIET
- Diet restriction is the cornerstone of obesity management
- Low-fat, high complex carbohydrate and high fiber diets have been most commonly recommended. Low carbohydrate diets have become popular recently, but long term data comparing the two diet approaches are not available.
- A 500 kcal (2.10 MJ) reduction in calorie per day intake will result in approximately 1 pound (.45 kg) weight loss per week
- Very low calorie diets (VLCD)
  - ◊ 400-800 kcal (1.68-3.35 MJ) per day are usually based on liquid formulas and cause more rapid weight loss
  - ◊ Complications of VLCD include: dehydration, orthostatic hypotension, fatigue, muscle cramps, constipation, headache, cold intolerance, and relapse after discontinuation
  - ◊ Contraindications of VLCD include: recent myocardial infarction or cerebrovascular accident, renal or hepatic disease, cancer, pregnancy, insulin-dependent diabetes mellitus, some psychiatric disturbances
  - ◊ Physician supervision is important for VLCD

PATIENT EDUCATION
- Educating the patient about the value of weight reduction is important
- Behavior modification can improve dietary adherence and long term results of weight loss and should be included in any weight loss program
- A self help brochure "On Your Way to Fitness" can be ordered for $1.00 per copy from Shape Up America, P.O. Box 9738, Bridgeport, CT 06699. It gives information for exercise self-assessment and increasing exercise for obese patients. Patients can also visit the web site www.shapeup.org.

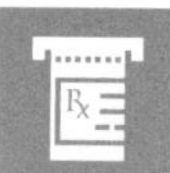

MEDICATIONS

DRUG(S) OF CHOICE
NIH guidelines suggest nonpharmacologic treatment for 6 months and then consideration of medication treatment for unsatisfactory weight loss in those with BMI > 30, or BMI > 27 with associated risk factors such as coronary heart disease, diabetes, sleep apnea, cigarette smoking, hypertension, hyperlipidemia (high LDL, or low HDL cholesterol), impaired fasting glucose, family history of premature CHD or age greater than 45 for men or 55 for women. Drug therapy is recommended as part of a program that includes diet, physical activity, and behavior therapy.
- Sibutramine 5-15 mg qd (starting dose 10 mg) is a serotonin and norepinephrine reuptake inhibitor classified as an appetite suppressant
- Orlistat 120 mg tid with meals is a lipase inhibitor which decreases absorption of dietary fat. Avoid fat soluble vitamin supplements within 2 hours of orlistat.

Contraindications:
- Sibutramine: uncontrolled hypertension, severe renal or hepatic dysfunction, narrow-angle glaucoma, history of substance abuse, symptomatic cardiovascular disease, congestive heart failure, arrhythmias, stroke, use of MAOI within 2 weeks.
- Orlistat: Chronic malabsorption syndromes, cholestasis

Precautions:
- Relapse after discontinuation of drug
- Sibutramine can cause elevations in pulse and blood pressure

Significant possible interactions:
- Concurrent use with general anesthetics may cause arrhythmias
- Serotonergic agents may cause "serotonin syndrome" in combination with sibutramine

ALTERNATIVE DRUGS
- Appetite suppressants recommended only for short term, "a few weeks only," treatment
  - ◊ Schedule IV drugs
    - Diethylpropion
    - Phentermine
    - Mazindol
  - ◊ Schedule II drugs
    - Phendimetrazine
    - Benzphetamine

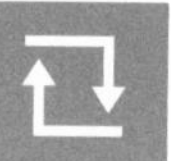

FOLLOWUP

PATIENT MONITORING Long term followup is crucial to prevent further weight gain or regain after weight loss

PREVENTION/AVOIDANCE Counseling in regular exercise and prudent diet with regular follow-up, especially in children and young adults and those with family history of obesity or diabetes mellitus

POSSIBLE COMPLICATIONS
- Increased mortality due largely to cardiovascular disease
- Diabetes mellitus
- Hypertension
- Hyperlipidemia
- Gall bladder disease with cholelithiasis
- Osteoarthritis
- Gout
- Thromboembolism
- Hypoventilation and sleep apnea syndromes
- Poor self-esteem
- Occupational discrimination

EXPECTED COURSE/PROGNOSIS
- Long term maintenance of weight loss is extremely difficult
- If patient is not motivated, successful weight loss is unlikely

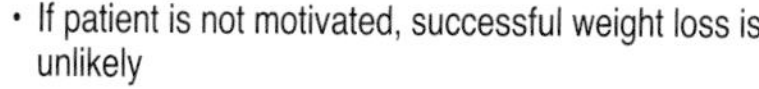

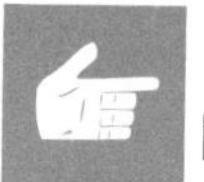

MISCELLANEOUS

ASSOCIATED CONDITIONS See Possible complications

AGE-RELATED FACTORS
Pediatric: Prevalence of obesity is increasing. Among other factors, decreased physical activity and increased television viewing have been implicated.
Geriatric: Desirable weights (those associated with the lowest risk of mortality) increase with age
Others: Pre-puberty and young adulthood appear to be sensitive periods for development of obesity

PREGNANCY Pregnancy is a common time for onset of, or increase in obesity

SYNONYMS
- Overweight
- Adiposis
- Adiposity

ICD-9-CM
278.00 Obesity, unspecified
278.01 Morbid obesity

SEE ALSO

OTHER NOTES N/A

ABBREVIATIONS
RDA = recommended daily allowance
BMI = body mass index

REFERENCES

- Gray DS. Obesity. In: Weiss BD, editor. 20 Common Problems in Primary Care. New York: McGraw-Hill; 1999. p.27-50
- The Practical Guide: Identification, Evaluation, and Treatment of Overweight and Obesity in Adults. Bethesda, MD: National Heart, Lung, and Blood Institute, North American Association for the Study of Obesity; 2000 (NIH publication no. 00-4048)
- Yanovski SZ, Yanovski JA. Obesity. N Engl J Med 2002;346(8):591-602
- Jones TF, Eaton CB. Exercise prescription. Am Fam Phys 1995;52(2):543-550

Web references: 3 available at www.5mcc.com
Illustrations N/A

Author(s):
David S. Gray, MD

BASICS

DESCRIPTION Psychiatric condition classified as an anxiety disorder in Diagnostic and Statistical Manual of Mental Disorders (DSM-IV-R) and characterized by recurrent, intrusive thoughts (obsessions) and ritualistic behaviors (compulsions)
- Obsessions and compulsions consume more than an hour per day and cause occupational/social impairment
- Patients know thoughts (obsessions) come from their own minds and are not imposed from outside (as in thought insertion). Thoughts are not associated with another disorder (for example, thought of food if an eating disorder is present).
- Compulsions are ritualistic behaviors designed to relieve the anxiety of obsessions
- Common obsessive themes:
  - ◊ Violence, such as harming a beloved child
  - ◊ Doubt, such as whether doors or windows locked or iron turned off
  - ◊ Blasphemous thoughts, such as in a devoutly religious person
  - ◊ Contamination, dirt or disease
  - ◊ Symmetry or orderliness
- Common rituals or compulsions:
  - ◊ Hand washing
  - ◊ Checking
  - ◊ Counting
  - ◊ Hoarding
  - ◊ Ordering, arranging
  - ◊ Repeaters - such as dressing rituals

System(s) affected: Nervous
Genetics: Positive family history in about 20% of cases, no mode of transmission identified
Incidence/Prevalence in USA: 2.5% lifetime prevalence, 1.5-2.1% one year prevalence
Predominant age: Mean age 20. 1/3 cases present by age 15, new cases after age 50 rare, 80% of cases before age 35
Predominant sex: Male = Female (males tend to present at a younger age)

SIGNS & SYMPTOMS
- Obsessions and/or compulsions that consume more than an hour a day and cause significant distress or impairment
- Obsessions (thoughts) are recurrent; patient attempts to ignore or neutralize thoughts with another thought or action
- Neither obsessions nor compulsions are related to another mental disorder
- Compulsions (actions) are repetitive, purposeful behaviors in response to thoughts in attempt to neutralize the thought - such as checking in response to doubt (locks, doors , windows or driving back over route to check for any possible damage inadvertently done while driving one's car)
- Repeated handwashing or ritualistic handwashing in response to fear of contamination
- 80-90% of patients have obsessions and compulsions
- 10-19% are pure obsessional
- 5% perform rituals until they "feel right" and may not have an identifiable obsession

CAUSES Dysregulation of neurotransmitter, serotonin

RISK FACTORS Greater concordance in monozygotic twins family history as above

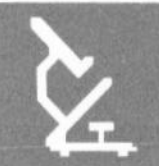

DIAGNOSIS

DIFFERENTIAL DIAGNOSIS
- Impulse control disorders: Compulsive gambling, sex or substance abuse - the "compulsive" behavior is not in response to obsessive thought and patient derives pleasure from the activity, unlike OCD where obsessions and compulsions are ego dystonic
- Depression: Can see brooding, but ideas not perceived as senseless as in OCD
- Schizophrenia: Patient perceives thought to be true and from an external source
- Obsessive compulsive personality disorder: Not to be confused with OCD. In personality disorder, traits are ego-syntonic. Traits include perfectionism, preoccupation with detail, trivia or procedure and regulation. Patient tends to be rigid, moralistic and stingy. Often traits are rewarded in patient's job as desirable traits.
- Generalized anxiety, phobic disorders, separation anxiety: Similar response of heightened anxiety, but presence of obsessions or rituals clarifies OCD diagnosis
- Anxiety disorder due to a general medical condition: may be obsessions or compulsions, are assessed to be a direct physiological consequence of a general medical condition

LABORATORY N/A

Drugs that may alter lab results: N/A

Disorders that may alter lab results: N/A

PATHOLOGICAL FINDINGS N/A

SPECIAL TESTS
- Yale Brown obsessive-compulsive scale (Y-BOCS)
- Maudsley obsessive-compulsive inventory (MOCI)
- Children's Yale Brown obsessive-compulsive scale (CY-BOCS)

IMAGING PET scan - abnormal metabolism in frontal cortex and caudate nuclei (not generally available other than in research centers)

DIAGNOSTIC PROCEDURES Psychiatric interview

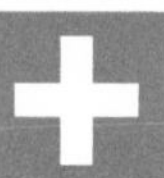

TREATMENT

APPROPRIATE HEALTH CARE Outpatient

GENERAL MEASURES
- Combine medications and cognitive behavior therapy
- Psychiatric referral for therapy (in vivo exposure and response prevention)
- Family psycho-education
- Parent behavior management training if OCD patient child/adolescent

SURGICAL MEASURES Psychosurgery (last resort)

ACTIVITY No restriction

DIET With use of phenelzine must have tyramine-free diet to prevent precipitation of hypertensive crisis

PATIENT EDUCATION
- Obsessive-Compulsive Foundation, P. O. Box 70, Milford, CT 06460-0070 (203) 878-5669 or (203) 874-3843 for recorded information
- Printed patient information available from: Obsessive-Compulsive Anonymous, P.O. Box 215, New Hyde Park, NY 11040, (516)741-4901

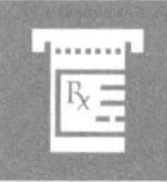

MEDICATIONS

DRUG(S) OF CHOICE

- Serotonin reuptake inhibitor, fluoxetine (Prozac)
  - ◊ Adults: begin with 20 mg/day q morning and increase every 4-6 weeks to obtain maximal clinical response. Dose range: 20-60 mg/day. Doses >20 mg/day should be divided.
  - ◊ Children: safety and efficacy has not been established for OCD
- Sertraline (Zoloft)
  - ◊ Adults: begin with 50 mg per day and increase every week until clinical response. Dose range: 50-200 mg per day. Doses > 100 mg/day should be divided.
  - ◊ Children: Begin with 25 mg per day, increase in 25 mg increments until clinical response
- Paroxetine (Paxil)
  - ◊ Adults: begin with 20 mg/day, increase weekly in 10 mg increments until maximal clinical response
  - ◊ Children: safety and efficacy has not been established for OCD
- Fluvoxamine (Luvox)
  - ◊ Adult - begin with 100 mg/day and increase every week until clinical response (dosage range 200-300 mg)
  - ◊ Children (8-17) - begin with 25 mg/day, increase in small increments (25-50 mg) until clinical response
- Clomipramine (Anafranil)
  - ◊ Adults - beginning at 25 mg/day and increased gradually to 100 mg over first 2 weeks. Then to 250 mg over next several weeks, as tolerated.
  - ◊ Children - beginning at 25 mg /day over first two weeks as in adults. Then titrated up to 3 mg/kg or 200 mg/day (which ever is smaller) over the next several weeks.

Contraindications:

- Absolute fluoxetine, paroxetine, and sertraline contraindications
  - ◊ Hypersensitivity to the selective serotonin re-uptake inhibitors
  - ◊ Within 14 days of MAO inhibitor
- Relative fluoxetine and sertraline contraindications
  - ◊ Severe liver impairment
  - ◊ Seizure disorders (lowers seizure threshold)
- Clomipramine is of the tricyclic antidepressant class, so carries same contraindications as drugs in that class
- Absolute clomipramine contraindications:
  - ◊ Within 6 months of myocardial infarction
  - ◊ Narrow angle glaucoma
  - ◊ 3rd degree AV block
  - ◊ Within 14 days of MAO inhibitor
- Relative clomipramine contraindications:
  - ◊ Prostatic hypertrophy (urinary retention)
  - ◊ Seizure disorder (lower seizure threshold)
  - ◊ 1st, 2nd degree AV block, bundle branch block and CHF (pro-arrhythmic effect)

Precautions:

- Drug should to be taken for a minimum of 10 weeks before considering it a treatment failure; could be several months before peak efficacy
- Because patients with OCD may have concomitant depression, suicide potential must be assessed
- Long half-life may be troublesome if patient has an adverse reaction
- May cause drowsiness and dizziness when therapy is initiated - warn patients about driving and heavy equipment hazards
- May alter glucose control by lowering blood glucose levels while on the medication and increase blood glucose after stopping the medication
- Tricyclic class of antidepressants dangerous in overdose

Significant possible interactions:

- Clomipramine
  - ◊ Not yet fully elucidated
  - ◊ May interfere with guanethidine, clonidine
  - ◊ Serum level increased if used concomitantly with haloperidol
  - ◊ Probable plasma increase if used with cimetidine, fluoxetine, methylphenidate
  - ◊ Increases serum level of phenobarbital
- Fluoxetine and sertraline
  - ◊ Causes increased concentrations of the following medications: warfarin, phenytoin, carbamazepine, diazepam, tricyclic antidepressants, and neuroleptics

ALTERNATIVE DRUGS N/A

FOLLOWUP

PATIENT MONITORING

- Y-BOCS
- MOCI

PREVENTION/AVOIDANCE N/A

POSSIBLE COMPLICATIONS

- Depression in 1/3 of OCD patients
- Avoidant behavior (phobic avoidance)
- Anxiety and panic-like episodes associated with obsessions

EXPECTED COURSE/PROGNOSIS

- Chronic waxing and waning course in majority
- 24-33% fluctuating course
- 11-14% phasic with periods of remission
- 54-61% chronic progressive course
- Early onset a poor outcome predictor

MISCELLANEOUS

ASSOCIATED CONDITIONS

- Depression
- Panic disorder
- Social phobia
- Phobia
- Tourette
- Alcoholism
- Substance abuse

AGE-RELATED FACTORS

Pediatric: Child/adolescent onset in 33%. At this age males outnumber females 3:1.
Geriatric: Diagnosis not generally made after age 50
Others: N/A

PREGNANCY

- Onset of OCD has been noted after delivery
- Safety of fluoxetine and clomipramine has not been established in pregnancy nor lactation

SYNONYMS

Obsessive compulsive neurosis

ICD-9-CM

300.3 Obsessive-compulsive disorders

SEE ALSO

Anxiety
Depression

OTHER NOTES

Not to be confused with obsessive compulsive personality disorder (see Differential Diagnosis)

ABBREVIATIONS

CY-BOCS = Children's Yale Brown obsessive compulsive scale
Y-BOCS = Yale Brown obsessive compulsive scale
OCD = obsessive compulsive disorder
MOCI = Maudsley obsessive-compulsive inventory

REFERENCES

- Diagnostic and Statistical Manual of Mental Disorders DSM-IV (Text Revision). 4th Ed . American Psychiatric Association, Washington, D.C., 2000
- Kaplan HI, Sadock BJ (eds). Comprehensive Textbook of Psychiatry. 7th Ed. Williams & Wilkins, Baltimore, MD, 2000
- Hohagen F. New perspectives in research and treatment of obsessive-compulsive disorder. Br J Psychiatry Suppl1998; (3 5):1-96
- Eddy MF, Walbroehl GS. Recognition and treatment of obsessive-compulsive disorder. Am Fam Phys 1998;57(7):1623-8, 1632-4
- AACAP. Practice parameters for the assessment and treatment of children and adolescents with obsessive-compulsive disorder. J Am Acad Child Adolesc Psychiatry 1998;37(10 Suppl):27S-45S

Web references: 4 available at www.5mcc.com
Illustrations N/A

Author(s):
Milisa Rizer, MD

BASICS

DESCRIPTION Chemical exposure to the eye can result in rapid, devastating, and permanent damage and is one of the true emergencies in ophthalmology
- Separate alkaline from acid chemical exposure:
  - ◊ Alkaline burns - more severe, alkali penetrates and saponifies tissues easily, may produce injury to lids, conjunctiva, cornea, sclera, iris, lens, and retina
  - ◊ Acid burns - usually acid does not damage internal structures since protein coagulation limits acid penetration. Injury often limited to lids, conjunctiva, and cornea.

System(s) affected: Nervous, Skin/Exocrine
Genetics: N/A
Incidence/Prevalence in USA: Estimated 300/100,000/year
Predominant age: 18-65
Predominant sex: Male > Female

SIGNS & SYMPTOMS
- Mild burns:
  - ◊ Pain and blurred vision
  - ◊ Eyelid skin erythema and edema
  - ◊ Corneal epithelial defects or superficial punctate keratitis
  - ◊ Conjunctival chemosis, hyperemia, and hemorrhages without perilimbal ischemia
  - ◊ Mild anterior chamber reaction
- Moderate to severe burns:
  - ◊ Severe pain and markedly reduced vision
  - ◊ Second and third degree burns of eyelid skin
  - ◊ Corneal edema and opacification
  - ◊ Corneal epithelial defects
  - ◊ Marked conjunctival chemosis and perilimbal blanching
  - ◊ Moderate anterior chamber reaction
  - ◊ Increased intraocular pressure
  - ◊ Local necrotic retinopathy
  - ◊ In alkaline burns, can have initial pain which later diminishes

CAUSES
- Alkali:
  - ◊ Ammonia (NH_3)
  - ◊ Lye (NaOH)
  - ◊ Magnesium hydroxide [$Mg(OH)_2$]
  - ◊ Potassium hydroxide (KOH)
  - ◊ Lime [$Ca(OH)_2$]
- Acids:
  - ◊ Hydrochloric (HCl)
  - ◊ Hydrofluoric (HF)
  - ◊ Acetic (CH_3COOH)
  - ◊ Nitrous (HNO_2)
  - ◊ Sulfuric (H_2SO_4)

RISK FACTORS
- Construction work (plaster, cement, whitewash)
- Use of cleaning agents (drain cleaners, ammonia)
- Automobile battery explosions (sulfuric acid)
- Industrial work (many possible agents)
- Alcoholism

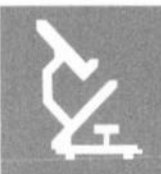

DIAGNOSIS

DIFFERENTIAL DIAGNOSIS
- Thermal burns
- Ocular cicatricial pemphigoid
- Other causes of corneal opacification
- Ultraviolet radiation keratitis

LABORATORY None

Drugs that may alter lab results: N/A

Disorders that may alter lab results: None

PATHOLOGICAL FINDINGS
- Precipitation of glycosaminoglycans causes corneal opacification
- Saponification of cell membranes causes cell death
- Cation binding to collagen results in hydration, thickening, and shortening of collagen fibrils. This can mechanically elevate intraocular pressure.

SPECIAL TESTS Measure pH of tear film with litmus paper or electronic probe (irrigating fluid with non-neutral pH [e.g., normal saline has pH of 4.5] may alter results)

IMAGING Not necessary unless suspicion of intraocular or orbital foreign body is present

DIAGNOSTIC PROCEDURES
- Careful slit lamp examination, fundus ophthalmoscopy, tonometry, and measurement of visual acuity
- Full extent of damage from alkaline burns may not be apparent until 48-72 hours after exposure

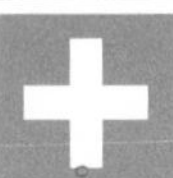

TREATMENT

APPROPRIATE HEALTH CARE Emergency room with inpatient admission and ophthalmology consultation, depending on severity

GENERAL MEASURES Copious irrigation and removal of corneal or conjunctival foreign bodies are always the initial treatment. Continue irrigation until the tear film is of neutral pH and pH is stable. Sweep the conjunctival fornices every 12-24 hours to prevent adhesions.

SURGICAL MEASURES
- Punctal occlusion for tear film preservation and corneal epitheliopathy
- Tarsorrhaphy for persistent epithelial defects
- Tissue adhesive (e.g., isobutyl cyanoacrylate) for impending or actual corneal perforation
- Conjunctival or limbal autograft transplantation for epithelial stem cell restoration
- Lamellar or penetrating keratoplasty for tectonic stabilization or visual rehabilitation
- Amniotic membrane transplantation, if no autogenous mucus membrane available

ACTIVITY Ambulatory

DIET Usual for patient

PATIENT EDUCATION
- Safety glasses
- Need for immediate ocular irrigation with any available water following chemical exposure to the eyes

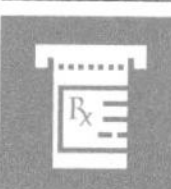

MEDICATIONS

DRUG(S) OF CHOICE

- Immediate treatment (any non-toxic irrigant):
  - ◊ In hospital setting, sterile water, normal saline, lactated Ringer's solution are effective
  - ◊ In the field, use what is available (tap water). Rapidity of irrigation is critical.
  - ◊ Irrigation is continued until pH of superior/inferior cul-de-sac is neutral
  - ◊ It is impossible to over-irrigate
- Further treatment: (depending on severity and associated conditions)
  - ◊ Topical prophylactic antibiotics: Any broad spectrum agent, e.g., bacitracin-polymyxin B (Polysporin) ointment q2-4h, ciprofloxacin (Ciloxan) drops q 2-4h, chloramphenicol (Chloroptic) ointment q2-4h
  - ◊ Tear substitutes: hydroxypropyl methylcellulose (Hypotears PF, Refresh Plus) drops q4h, carboxymethylcellulose (Refresh P.M.) ointment qhs
  - ◊ Cycloplegics for photophobia and/or uveitis: Cyclopentolate 1% tid, or scopolamine 1/4% bid
  - ◊ Anti-glaucoma for elevated intraocular pressure (IOP): latanoprost (Xalatan) 0.005% q24h or timolol (Timoptic) 0.5% bid or levobunolol (Betagan) 0.5% bid and/or acetazolamide (Diamox) 125-250 mg po q6h or methazolamide (Neptazane) 25-50 mg po bid and/or mannitol 20% 1-2 g/kg IV prn
  - ◊ Corticosteroids for intraocular inflammation: Prednisolone (Pred-Forte) 1% or equivalent q1-4h for 10-14 days; if severe, prednisone 20-60 mg po qd for 5-7 days. Taper rapidly if epithelium intact by this time.
  - ◊ Consider vitamin C (ascorbic acid) 500 mg po qid and/or acetylcysteine (Mucomyst) 10-20% top q4 h if corneal melting occurs

Contraindications: None

Precautions:

- For timolol and levobunolol - history of congestive heart failure or chronic obstructive pulmonary disease
- For acetazolamide and methazolamide - history of nephrolithiasis or metabolic acidosis
- For mannitol - history of congestive heart failure or renal failure
- For scopolamine - history of urinary retention
- Topical corticosteroids must be used with caution in the presence of damaged corneal epithelium as iatrogenic infection can occur. Daily follow-up or consultation with an ophthalmologist is recommended.

Significant possible interactions: Refer to manufacturer's literature

ALTERNATIVE DRUGS
Where available - topical fibronectin, epidermal growth factor, prokinase inhibitors

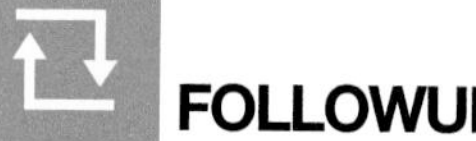

FOLLOWUP

PATIENT MONITORING

- Depending on severity of ocular injury, from daily to weekly visits initially
- May be inpatient
- If on mannitol or prednisone, consider frequent serum electrolytes

PREVENTION/AVOIDANCE
Safety glasses to safeguard uninvolved eye

POSSIBLE COMPLICATIONS

- Persistent epitheliopathy
- Fibrovascular pannus
- Corneal ulcer/perforation
- Progressive symblepharon and entropion
- Neurotrophic keratitis
- Glaucoma
- Cataract
- Hypotony
- Phthisis bulbi

EXPECTED COURSE/PROGNOSIS

- Depends on severity of initial injury
- Increasing amounts of limbal ischemia and corneal opacification correlate with poorer prognosis
- For severely injured eyes, permanent loss of vision is not uncommon
- Autologous cultivated corneal epithelium has been used for long term restoration of vision.
- Autologous nasal mucosal transplantation has also been successfully employed
- Use of amniotic membrane transplantation is being evaluated in clinical trials

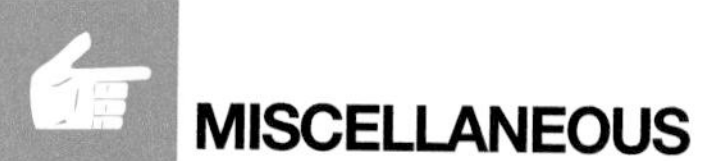

MISCELLANEOUS

ASSOCIATED CONDITIONS
Facial cutaneous chemical or thermal burns

AGE-RELATED FACTORS

Pediatric: N/A

Geriatric:

- Compromised ocular surface from keratitis sicca or other disease associated with poorer prognosis
- Compromised corneal endothelium or pre-existing glaucoma may also complicate clinical management

Others: N/A

PREGNANCY
N/A

SYNONYMS
Chemical ocular injuries

ICD-9-CM

940.2 Alkaline chemical burn of cornea and conjunctival sac

940.3 Acid chemical burn of cornea and conjunctival sac

SEE ALSO
Burns

OTHER NOTES
N/A

ABBREVIATIONS
N/A

REFERENCES

- Fraunfelder FT, Roy FH: Current Ocular Therapy. 5th Ed. Philadelphia, W.B. Saunders Co., 1999
- McCulley JP: Chemical Injuries. In: Smolin G, Thoft RA, eds. The Cornea: Scientific Foundations and Clinical Practice. New York, Little, Brown, 1987
- Shingleton BJ, Hersh PS, Kenyon KR: Eye Trauma. St. Louis, Mosby Year Book, 1991
- Ralph RA: Chemical Burns of the Eye. In: Tasman W, ed. Clinical Ophthalmology. Philadelphia, J.B. Lippincott, 1994

Web references: 2 available at www.5mcc.com

Illustrations N/A

Author(s):

Robert G. Fante, MD

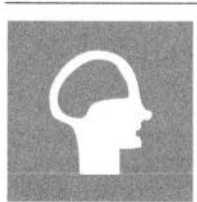

BASICS

DESCRIPTION Infection of nail by fungi (dermatophytes, Candida, molds).
System(s) affected: Skin/Exocrine
Genetics: N/A
Incidence/Prevalence in USA: 22-130 cases/1000 population
Predominant age:
- Dermatophytes common in adults; even molds in older adults

Predominant sex:
- Candidal: adult women

SIGNS & SYMPTOMS
- Dermatophytes: Commonly preceded by dermatophyte infection at another site; 80% involve toenails - especially hallux; simultaneous infection of finger and toe nails rare. Four clinical forms occur:
  - ◊ Distal subungual onychomycosis
    - Spreads from hyponychium to nailbed to nail-plate
    - Subungual hyperkeratosis
    - Subungual paronychia
    - Onycholysis
    - Nail dystrophy
    - Discoloration: yellow-brown
    - Bois vermoulu ("worm-eaten wood")
    - Onychomadesis
  - ◊ Lateral onychomycosis (common)
    - Yellowish discoloration lateral nail groove
    - Onycholysis, proximal or distal
  - ◊ Proximal onychomycosis (rare)
    - Hands or feet
    - Leukonychia: begins under posterior nail groove, spreading to nail plate and lunula
  - ◊ White superficial onychomycosis (rare)
    - Hallux preferentially affected
    - Infection of upper part of nail-plate
    - Opaque white spots on nail plate eventually merge to involve entire surface of the nail
- Candidal:
  - ◊ Hands 70% - especially dominant hand
  - ◊ Middle finger most common
  - ◊ Pain mild, unless secondarily infected
  - ◊ Pain increases on prolonged contact with water
  - ◊ Primarily affects tissue surrounding nail
  - ◊ Begins with cuticle detachment
  - ◊ Dark yellowish to blackish-brown zone along lateral border of nail
  - ◊ Secondary ungual changes - convex, irregular, striated nail-plate with dull rough surface
  - ◊ Onycholysis, especially on hands
  - ◊ Distal subungual onychomycosis may occur
  - ◊ Primary involvement of the nail-plate uncommon (thin, crumbly, opaque, brownish nail-plate deformed by transverse grooves)
  - ◊ Periungual edema/erythema may occur (club-shaped, bulbous fingertips)
  - ◊ Superficial white onychomycosis - young children
- Molds
  - ◊ More common over 60 years old
  - ◊ More common in nails of hallux
  - ◊ Resembles distal and lateral onychomycosis

CAUSES
- Dermatophytes (invade normal keratin)
  - ◊ *Trichophyton rubrum* - most common
  - ◊ *Trichophyton mentagrophytes* var. interdigitale - 25% as common as *T. rubrum* (most common pathogen for white superficial onychomycosis)
  - ◊ *Epidermophyton floccosum*, *T. violaceum*, *Microsporum* species less common
- Candida
  - ◊ 70% *Candida albicans*
  - ◊ *C. parapsilosis*, *C. tropicalis*, *C. krusei* (less common)
- Molds (invade altered keratin)
  - ◊ *Scopulariopsis brevicaulis*, *Hendersonula toruloidea*, *Aspergillus species*, *Alternaria tenuis*, *Cephalosporium*, *Scytalidium hyalinium*

RISK FACTORS
- Dermatophytes
  - ◊ Warmth, moisture, hyperhidrosis
  - ◊ Tight fitting shoes, rubber shoes
  - ◊ Peripheral vascular disease
  - ◊ Depressed cell-mediated immunity
  - ◊ Indirect contamination
- Candidal
  - ◊ Direct contamination - ano-vulvar, perirectal pruritus
  - ◊ Chemical or mechanical damage to cuticle
  - ◊ Maceration or occlusion
  - ◊ Contact with substances containing sugar
  - ◊ Hyperhidrosis
  - ◊ Chilblain
  - ◊ Cold hands (Raynaud phenomenon)
  - ◊ Psoriatic onycholysis
  - ◊ Diabetes mellitus
  - ◊ Hyperparathyroidism
  - ◊ Addison disease
  - ◊ Malnutrition
  - ◊ Malabsorption
  - ◊ Dyscrasias
  - ◊ Malignancies
  - ◊ Postoperative conditions
  - ◊ Altered immune function
- Molds
  - ◊ Soil contamination
  - ◊ Peripheral vascular disease
  - ◊ Overlapping toes
  - ◊ Onychogryphosis (deforming overgrowth of nails resulting in hooked or curved state)

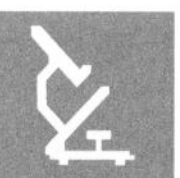

DIAGNOSIS

DIFFERENTIAL DIAGNOSIS
- Herpetic whitlow
- Eczema
- Pustular psoriasis
- Tumor
- Darier's disease
- Pityriasis rubra pilaris
- Trophic changes, peripheral vascular disease
- Endocrine disease
- Drugs; chemicals
- Trauma
- Alopecia areata
- Lichen planus
- Yellow-nail syndrome (icterus, carotenemia, lymphedema, amyloidosis)
- White acquired nail disease (trauma, acute infection, chronic disease, thallium or arsenic poisoning, hepatic cirrhosis, chronic hypo-albuminemia)
- Brown-black pigment (melanotic, hematoma)
- Green dyschromia (*Pseudomonas aeruginosa*, molds, eg, *penicillium*)
- Connective tissue disorders: dermatomyositis, scleroderma, Reiter

LABORATORY
- KOH preparation: clip or file away some of nail-plate as needed, collect scales from stratum corneum of most proximal area (beneath nail or crumbling nail itself with 1 mm curette), 5% KOH + gentle heat, 100% sensitive if > 2 preps examined
- Cultures - negative in 30% (secondary to loss of dermatophyte viability; improved by immediate culture on Sabouraud's and CC media)
- Histologic examination of keratin, punch or scalpel biopsy - proximal lesions with PAS stain
- All are influenced by quality of sampling
- CD4 < 450

Drugs that may alter lab results: Discontinue all topical medication several days before obtaining sample

Disorders that may alter lab results: N/A

PATHOLOGICAL FINDINGS Pathogens within the nail keratin

SPECIAL TESTS N/A

IMAGING N/A

DIAGNOSTIC PROCEDURES N/A

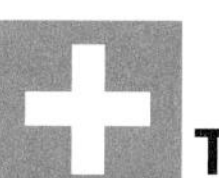

TREATMENT

APPROPRIATE HEALTH CARE
- Outpatient - unless secondary cellulitis/osteomyelitis

GENERAL MEASURES
- Avoid factors that promote fungal growth (heat, moisture)
- Treat underlying disease risk factors
- Treat other fungal infections
- Treat secondary infections

SURGICAL MEASURES
- Nail removal to remove infected keratin
  - ◊ Mechanical: soften with occlusive dressing with 40% urea gel, detach from nailbed with tweezers or file with abrasive paper/grinding stone
  - ◊ Chemical: protect peripheral tissue with adhesive strips, apply ointment of 30% salicylic acid, 40% urea or 50% potassium iodide under occlusive dressing
  - ◊ Surgical avulsion: for involvement of a few nails

ACTIVITY Restrictions based on promoting factors, underlying disease or secondary infection

DIET No special diet

PATIENT EDUCATION N/A

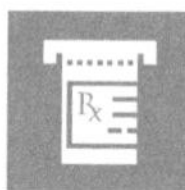

MEDICATIONS

DRUG(S) OF CHOICE
- Dermatophytes - local: Less effective than systemic, apply under occlusive dressing, may mix with keratinolytic chemicals
  - ◊ Imidazoles: Clotrimazole (Lotrimin, Mycelex), miconazole (Monistat), butoconazole, tioconazole, econazole (Spectazole), ketoconazole (Nizoral), sulconazole (Exelderm), oxiconazole (Oxistat), terbinafine (Lamisil)
  - ◊ Unsaturated fatty acid derivatives: Propionic acid, undecylenic acid; haloprogin (Halotex); tolnaftate (Tinactin)
  - ◊ Ciclopirox (Penlac) 8% topical lacquer for patients without lunula involvement
  - ◊ Amorolfine (Loceryl) 5% lacquer
- Dermatophytes - systemic:
  - ◊ Fluconazole (Diflucan) 300 mg po weekly for 6 months (pulse therapy), overall better tolerated than ketoconazole; expensive; reserve for extreme cases (disseminated disease, immunocompromised)
  - ◊ Itraconazole (Sporanox): 200 mg po bid for a week per month for 2 months for fingernails and 3-4 months for toenails (pulse therapy)
  - ◊ Terbinafine (Lamisil) 250 mg po qd for 3 months
- Candida:
  - ◊ Imidazole derivative
  - ◊ If bacterial infection present, use antibacterial plus anti-Candidal, e.g., nystatin (Mycostatin), topical amphotericin B (Fungizone), itraconazole (Sporanox) 200 mg po qd for 3 months, or fluconazole 300 mg po weekly for 6 months (pulse therapy)
- Mold:
  - ◊ 1% iodinated alcohol, benzoic acid, (Whitfield's ointment), silver nitrate, glutaraldehyde, imidazole derivatives, itraconazole

Contraindications:
- Griseofulvin: porphyria, hepatocellular failure, serious side effects (leukopenia, persistent anemia), pregnancy
- Ketoconazole: hepatocellular disease, pregnancy
- Fluconazole: hepatocellular failure, pregnancy

Precautions:
- Topical agents: use with caution on broken skin, vascular compromise, decreased sensation
- Griseofulvin: monitor for hepatic, renal, hematopoietic side effects; photo-sensitivity; lupus-like symptoms or exacerbation. Take with meals to enhance absorption.
- Ketoconazole: hepatotoxicity (may be severe or fatal), anaphylaxis may (rarely) occur with first dose, decreased testosterone levels
- Fluconazole: decrease dose in renal failure, hepatotoxicity

Significant possible interactions:
- Griseofulvin: warfarin, barbiturates, alcohol, oral contraceptives
- Ketoconazole: warfarin, rifampin, cyclosporine, phenytoin, terfenadine
- Fluconazole: phenytoin (Dilantin), cyclosporine, oral hypoglycemics, oral anticoagulants, rifampin, hydrochlorothiazide
- Itraconazole and ketoconazole require gastric acid for absorption - effectiveness reduced with antacids, H2 blockers, omeprazole, etc.

ALTERNATIVE DRUGS
- Dermatophytes - local: ciclopirox (Loprox, Penlac), naftifine (Naftin), cationic surfactants, e.g., benzalkonium chloride (Cetylcide), cetrimide, cetylpyridinium chloride (Ony-Clear, Fungoid)], halogenated / chlorinated / iodinated derivatives [chloramine, tincture of iodine], dyes [malachite green, crystal violet], mercury derivatives [thimerosal], phenols, glutaraldehyde
- Dermatophytes - systemic: griseofulvin (Fulvicin, Gris-PEG, Grisactin) ultramicrosize, usual adult dose 250-500 mg bid with meals for 6-12 months

FOLLOWUP

PATIENT MONITORING
- Topical agents: slow response expected; visits q 6-12 weeks
- Griseofulvin: CBC and liver function tests initially, then q 3 months
- Ketoconazole: liver function tests q 3 weeks for the first 3 months, then monthly
- Itraconazole and fluconazole - liver function tests at start and at 4 weeks
- Terbinafine - liver function and hematologic tests at start and at 4 weeks
- Treatment duration (months): fingernails 6-9, toenails 9-12, great toenail 12-24

PREVENTION/AVOIDANCE
- Keep affected area clean and dry
- Avoid rubber or other occlusive footwear
- Avoid tight or ill-fitting footwear
- Wear absorbent cotton socks - avoid wool or synthetic fibers
- Change clothing and towels frequently and launder in hot water

POSSIBLE COMPLICATIONS
- Secondary infections with progression to cellulitis/osteomyelitis

EXPECTED COURSE/PROGNOSIS
- Relapse common; prognosis especially poor if one hand, 2 feet or multiple nails involved
- 20-40% of nails fail to respond
- 40-70% of patients show long term relapse

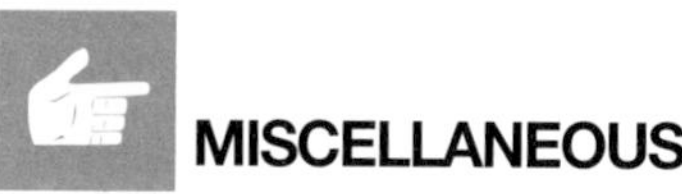

MISCELLANEOUS

ASSOCIATED CONDITIONS
- Immunodeficiency or chronic metabolic disease

AGE-RELATED FACTORS
Pediatric:
- Rare before puberty
- Candidal infection presents more commonly as superficial white onychomycosis

Geriatric:
- Mold onychomycosis more common
- Predisposing diseases more common
- Hepatic/renal reserve limited
- Decreased ability for topical self-treatment

Others: N/A

PREGNANCY Drug choices limited

SYNONYMS
- Tinea unguium
- Ringworm of the nail

ICD-9-CM
110.1 Dermatophytosis of nail
112.3 Candidiasis of skin and nails

SEE ALSO
HIV infection & AIDS

OTHER NOTES
- Onycholysis = detachment of nail-plate from nailbed
- Dystrophy = thickening, deformation, crumbling
- Onychomadesis = shedding of nail
- Leukonychia = yellowish-white spots

ABBREVIATIONS N/A

REFERENCES

- Mahoney JM, Bennet J, Olsen B.The diagnosis of onychomycosis. Dermatol Clin 2003;21:463-7
- Gupta AK, Ryder JE, Baran R. The use of topical therapies to treat onychomycosis. Dermatol Clin 2003;21:481-9
- Gupta AK, Ryder JE. The use of oral antifungal agents to treat onychomycosis. Dermatol Clin 2003;21:491-7
- Tosi A, Piraccini BM, Lorenzi S, Iorizzo M. Treatment of nondermatophyte mold and Candida onychomychosis. Dermatol Clin 2003;21:491-7

Web references: 0 available at www.5mcc.com
Illustrations 4 available

Author(s):
Samuel L. Moschella, MD

BASICS

DESCRIPTION End result of loss of ganglion cells or axons of the optic nerve
System(s) affected: Nervous
Genetics: Inherited forms may be autosomally recessive, autosomally dominant or X-linked recessive
Incidence/Prevalence in USA: Unknown
Predominant age:
- Inherited forms occur shortly after birth to the third decade
- Acquired forms tend to occur later

Predominant sex: Male > Female (inherited forms)

SIGNS & SYMPTOMS
- Loss of visual acuity
- Pallor of the optic disk
- Loss of pupillary reactions
- Visual field defects

CAUSES
- Glaucoma
- Post central retinal artery or vein occlusion
- Ischemic optic neuropathy
- Chronic optic neuritis
- Chronic papilledema
- Compression of the optic nerve or chiasm or tract by tumor or by aneurysm
- Trauma
- Syphilis
- Retinal degeneration (e.g., retinitis pigmentosa)
- Congenital optic atrophy
- Radiation neuropathy
- Drugs (amiodarone, chloroquine, ethambutol, oral contraceptives, streptomycin, vincristine)
- Thiamine deficiency
- HIV demyelinating disorders
- Graves disease
- Toxins (cyanide, lead, methanol)

RISK FACTORS
- Hereditary
  - ◊ Family history
- Acquired
  - ◊ Diabetes mellitus
  - ◊ Hypertension
  - ◊ Radiation exposure
  - ◊ Alcoholism
  - ◊ Renal failure
  - ◊ Arteriosclerosis

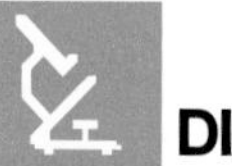

DIAGNOSIS

DIFFERENTIAL DIAGNOSIS
- Myopia
- S/p cataract extraction (no natural yellow color from the human lens)

LABORATORY
- CBC
- Antinuclear antibody (ANA)
- ESR
- Rapid plasma reagin (RPR)
- Fluorescent treponemal antibody absorption (FTA-ABS)
- Serological test for syphilis
- Heavy metal screen

Drugs that may alter lab results: N/A

Disorders that may alter lab results: N/A

PATHOLOGICAL FINDINGS N/A

SPECIAL TESTS
- Automated visual field test (i.e., Humphrey)
- Color vision testing
- Visual evoked potentials
- Fluoroscein angiography

IMAGING CT or MRI of head

DIAGNOSTIC PROCEDURES
- Carotid Doppler (adult acquired optic atrophy)
- Complete ophthalmologic exam including dilated evaluation of retina

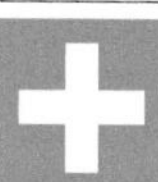

TREATMENT

APPROPRIATE HEALTH CARE Outpatient

GENERAL MEASURES
- Treat underlying cause (rarely possible)
- Discontinue causative drug if possible
- If pressure against optic nerve is cause, neurosurgery to relieve it may help if done early

SURGICAL MEASURES N/A

ACTIVITY Fully active

DIET No special diet

PATIENT EDUCATION
- Low vision counseling if bilateral
- Genetic counseling if inherited
- For patient education materials favorably reviewed on this topic, contact: National Eye Institute, Information Officer, Department of Health and Human Services, 9000 Rockville Pike, Bethesda, MD 20892, (301)496-5248

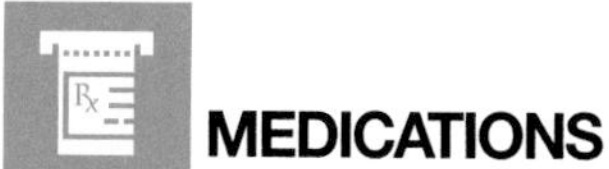

MEDICATIONS

DRUG(S) OF CHOICE None
Contraindications: N/A
Precautions: N/A
Significant possible interactions: N/A

ALTERNATIVE DRUGS Corticosteroids may briefly improve vision acuity when optic neuritis present. Long-term benefits unproven.

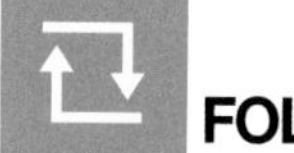

FOLLOWUP

PATIENT MONITORING Annual evaluations if stable

PREVENTION/AVOIDANCE
- Regular ophthalmologic exam in high risk groups
- Early aggressive management of treatable diseases such as Lyme disease or HIV with CMV infection

POSSIBLE COMPLICATIONS N/A

EXPECTED COURSE/PROGNOSIS
- Rarely possible to treat the underlying cause effectively
- Visual loss occurs over weeks to months
- Optic atrophy secondary to vascular, trauma, degenerative changes and some toxic causes has a very bad prognosis

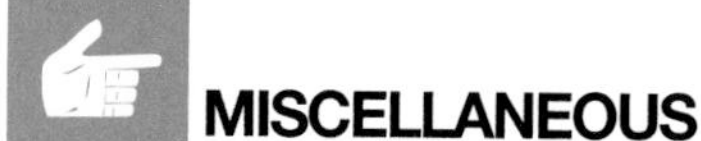

MISCELLANEOUS

ASSOCIATED CONDITIONS
- Inherited neurodegenerative conditions
  - ◊ Hereditary ataxia
  - ◊ Charcot-Marie-Tooth disease
  - ◊ Storage diseases
  - ◊ Leukodystrophies
- Multiple sclerosis
- Menke's syndrome

AGE-RELATED FACTORS
Pediatric: Optic atrophy in small children is difficult to recognize because disks normally have a pale appearance
Geriatric: None
Others: None

PREGNANCY None

SYNONYMS
- Leber's hereditary optic neuropathy

ICD-9-CM
377.10 Optic atrophy, unspecified

SEE ALSO

OTHER NOTES American Council of the Blind (800)424-8666

ABBREVIATIONS N/A

REFERENCES

- Miller NR. Walsh and Hoyt's Clinical Neuro-Ophthalmology. 4th ed. Baltimore: Lippincott Williams & Wilkins; 1988
- Fraunfelder FT, Roy FH. Current Ocular Therapy. 4th Ed. Philadelphia: WB Saunders Co; 1997e

Web references: 3 available at www.5mcc.com
Illustrations 1 available

Author(s):

William J. Moran, DO
Solomon Yigazu, MD

BASICS

DESCRIPTION Inflammation of the optic nerve
System(s) affected: Nervous
Genetics: N/A
Incidence/Prevalence in USA: 1:4 to 1:6 new cases annually per 100,000
Predominant age: Typically 18-50 years
Predominant sex: Female > Male

SIGNS & SYMPTOMS
- Decreased visual acuity, deteriorating from hours to days, usually reaching lowest level in one week
- Usually unilateral in adults, bilateral disease more common in children
- Tenderness of the globe, deep orbital pain or brow ache, especially with eye movement
- Central, cecocentral or arcuate visual field deficits
- Decreased color vision (dull or faded colors)
- Apparent dimness of light intensities
- Impairment of depth perception
- Increase in visual symptoms with increased body temperature and exercise (Uhthoff's symptom)
- May be either swollen optic disk (papillitis), most commonly seen in children, or normal optic disc
- Relative afferent pupillary defect (Marcus Gunn pupil)

CAUSES
- Idiopathic
- Multiple sclerosis
- Viral infections of childhood (measles, mumps, chickenpox)
- Other viral infections (mononucleosis, herpes zoster, encephalitis)
- Contiguous inflammation of the meninges, orbit, or sinuses
- Granulomatous inflammations (syphilis, tuberculosis, cryptococcus, sarcoidosis)
- Intraocular inflammations
- Lead toxicity
- Chronic high doses chloramphenicol
- Posterior uveitis
- Vascular lesions of optic nerve
- Tumors
- Fungal infections

RISK FACTORS N/A

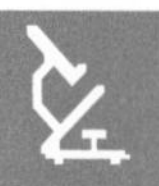

DIAGNOSIS

DIFFERENTIAL DIAGNOSIS
- Acute papilledema
- Anterior ischemic optic neuropathy
- Severe systemic hypertension
- Toxic/nutritional optic neuropathy
- Orbital tumor compressing the optic nerve
- Intracranial tumor pressing on the afferent visual pathway
- Leber's congenital optic neuropathy

LABORATORY
- CBC
- Antinuclear antibody (ANA)
- ESR
- Rapid plasma reagin (RPR)
- Fluorescent treponemal antibody absorption (FTA-ABS)
- Serological test for syphilis

Drugs that may alter lab results: N/A

Disorders that may alter lab results: N/A

PATHOLOGICAL FINDINGS N/A

SPECIAL TESTS
- Visual field test (preferably automated Humphrey or Octopus)
- Color vision testing

IMAGING
- Chest x-ray
- MRI head or CT head/orbits in atypical cases or when patient is not improving after 10-14 days and other tests are negative

DIAGNOSTIC PROCEDURES
- Check blood pressure
- Complete ophthalmologic exam including pupillary assessment, color vision evaluation with color plates, dilated retinal examination with optic nerve assessment
- Neurologic work-up

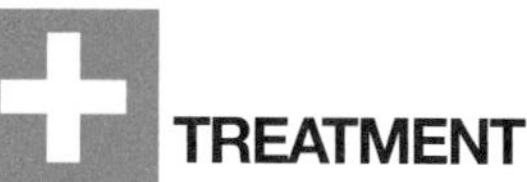

TREATMENT

APPROPRIATE HEALTH CARE Referral to an ophthalmologist

GENERAL MEASURES N/A

SURGICAL MEASURES N/A

ACTIVITY Fully active

DIET No special diet

PATIENT EDUCATION
- Reassurance about recovery of vision
- If felt to be secondary to demyelinating disease, patient should be informed of the risk of developing multiple sclerosis
- For patient education materials favorably reviewed on this topic, contact: National Eye Institute, Information Officer, Department of Health and Human Services, 9000 Rockville Pike, Bethesda, MD 20892, (301)496-5248

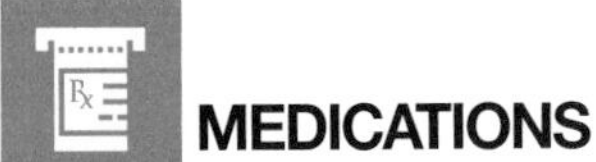

MEDICATIONS

DRUG(S) OF CHOICE For significant vision loss, corticosteroids may be indicated. These should be administered in conjunction with a neurology consult.
Contraindications: N/A
Precautions: N/A
Significant possible interactions: N/A

ALTERNATIVE DRUGS
- Pulse steroids: methylprednisolone 250 mg IV q6h x 12 doses in the hospital followed by prednisone 1 mg/kg/day po for 11 days, taper over 1-2 weeks
- Anti-ulcer medication is given with steroids

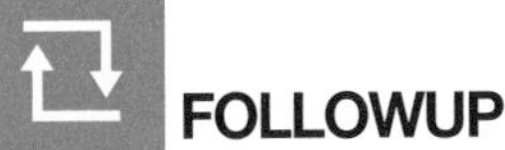

FOLLOWUP

PATIENT MONITORING Monthly followup to monitor visual changes

PREVENTION/AVOIDANCE N/A

POSSIBLE COMPLICATIONS Permanent loss of vision

EXPECTED COURSE/PROGNOSIS
- Visual acuity begins to improve 2-3 weeks after onset
- Improvement continues over several months and vision often returns to normal or near normal levels
- Those patients with poor vision and who receive IV steroids often recover faster
- When baseline vision is good, IV steroids have no beneficial effect

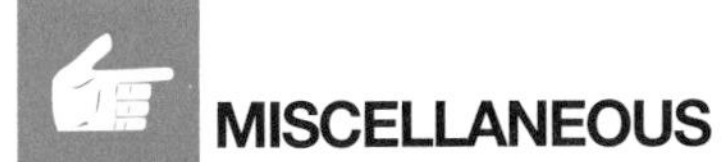

MISCELLANEOUS

ASSOCIATED CONDITIONS Over 50% of adult optic neuritis patients will develop multiple sclerosis

AGE-RELATED FACTORS
Pediatric: N/A
Geriatric: N/A
Others: N/A

PREGNANCY N/A

SYNONYMS
- Papillitis
- Retrobulbar neuritis

ICD-9-CM
377.30 Optic neuritis, unspecified

SEE ALSO
Multiple sclerosis

OTHER NOTES N/A

ABBREVIATIONS N/A

REFERENCES

- Optic neuritis treatment trial (ONTT) N Engl J Med 1992;326(9):581-8
- Sergott R, Brown M: Current concepts of the pathogenesis of optic neuritis associated with multiple sclerosis. Surv Ophthalmol 1988;33:108-116
- Miller N: Walsh and Hoyt's Clinical Neuro-Ophthalmology. 4th Ed. Baltimore, Williams & Wilkins, 1982
- Fraunfelder FT, Roy FH: Current Ocular Therapy. 3rd Ed. Philadelphia, W.B. Saunders Co., 1990

Web references: 0 available at www.5mcc.com
Illustrations 1 available

Author(s):
Laurel Powers, MD
David G. Pocock, MBBS

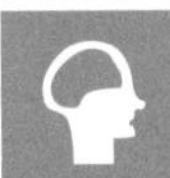

BASICS

DESCRIPTION Malignant tumors affecting the lip, tongue, floor of the mouth, salivary glands, inside of cheeks, gums, and palate. 90% of the neoplasms are squamous cell carcinomas and the remainder are lymphomas, melanomas, adenocarcinomas from minor salivary gland origin and sarcomas.
System(s) affected: Gastrointestinal
Genetics: N/A
Incidence/Prevalence in USA:
- 12/100,000 (30,300 new cases a year). 5000 persons die of this disease annually.
- Oral cavity neoplasms account for 4% of all cancers occurring in men and 2% in women
- High incidence in Asia, related to the habit of chewing betel nut, fresh betel leaf, and habitual reverse smoking in which the lighted end of the cigarette is held within the oral cavity

Predominant age: 50 and over. However, increasingly being seen in younger age group with the use of smokeless tobacco.
Predominant sex: Male > Female

SIGNS & SYMPTOMS
- Dysphagia
- Odynophagia
- Problems articulating
- Regurgitation of liquids secondary to nasopharyngeal incompetence from the tumor
- Ipsilateral otalgia from referred pain
- Friable granular exophytic and/or infiltrative mass or ulcer which frequently is tender and confused with infection. Usually has hard indurated margins by palpation which extend beyond the confines of the ulcer itself.
- Hard neck mass suggesting metastatic disease in the nodal chain along the internal jugular vein

CAUSES
- Tobacco use (smokeless or smoked)
- Use of snuff
- Excess alcohol consumption
- Exposure to ultraviolet light in the instances of lip carcinoma
- Riboflavin or iron deficiency anemia, and Plummer-Vinson syndrome associated with oral cancers
- Betel nut or leaf chewing

RISK FACTORS N/A

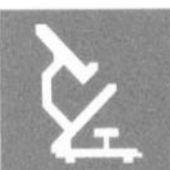

DIAGNOSIS

DIFFERENTIAL DIAGNOSIS
- Exudative tonsillitis (usually bilateral involvement)
- Stomatitis or glossitis secondary to infectious etiology, most commonly candidiasis
- Benign tumors of the oral cavity (slow growing and usually not erosive or ulcerative)
- Kaposi sarcoma
- Mycosis fungoides
- Premalignant lesions such as leukoplakia or erythroplasia
- Lichen planus

LABORATORY Liver function test to rule out metastasis to the liver

Drugs that may alter lab results: N/A

Disorders that may alter lab results:
- Alcoholism
- Hepatitis

PATHOLOGICAL FINDINGS Malignant changes characteristic of cell types

SPECIAL TESTS N/A

IMAGING
- Chest x-ray to rule out metastasis to the lungs
- Imaging bone scans if there is pain in the bones suggesting bone metastasis
- CT or MRI scan if clinical suggestion of intracranial or liver metastasis

DIAGNOSTIC PROCEDURES Transoral biopsy as an outpatient makes the definitive diagnosis

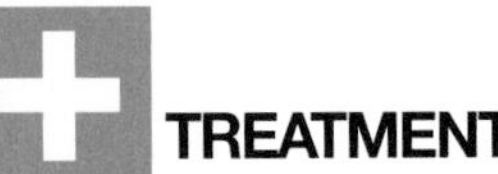

TREATMENT

APPROPRIATE HEALTH CARE
- Inpatient for surgery
- The treatment varies depending on location, i.e., tongue, buccal wall, pharynx, palate, lip

GENERAL MEASURES
- Unresectable lesions usually are treated with radiation therapy and/or chemotherapy for palliation
- Nutrition is of prime importance for normal wound healing should patient require surgery. Patients may need nasogastric and/or gastrostomy feedings if orally disabled.

SURGICAL MEASURES
- Wide resection with or without radiation therapy and/or chemotherapy is the treatment of choice
- Tracheotomy may be necessary if the patient has problems handling secretions or difficulty breathing

ACTIVITY As tolerated by patient's nutritional and physical status

DIET
- Depends on the extent of disease and whether the patient is able to chew or swallow
- Usually early lesions can be managed with a regular diet. As disease progresses, a soft diet is necessary.

PATIENT EDUCATION Literature is available from American Cancer Society

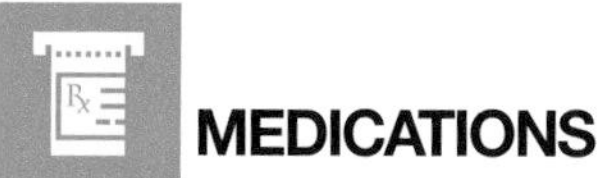

MEDICATIONS

DRUG(S) OF CHOICE Narcotics for pain relief
Contraindications: N/A
Precautions: N/A
Significant possible interactions: N/A

ALTERNATIVE DRUGS N/A

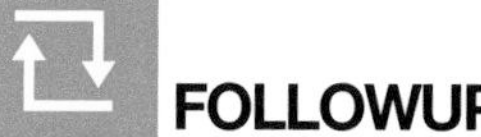

FOLLOWUP

PATIENT MONITORING Routine periodic head and neck exams to detect possible second primary or recurrence in the upper respiratory and digestive tract

PREVENTION/AVOIDANCE
- Avoidance of smoking or the use of smokeless tobacco
- Avoid alcohol use

POSSIBLE COMPLICATIONS
- Functional and/or cosmetic disabilities proportional to the degree of surgery and stage of tumor
- Stomatitis with or without candidiasis secondary to radiation therapy or chemotherapy
- Persistent dysphagia secondary to surgery or radiation therapy
- Persistent problems with articulation or deglutition depending on the amount of tongue resection

EXPECTED COURSE/PROGNOSIS
Early lesions with adequate treatment leads to a greater than 80% cure

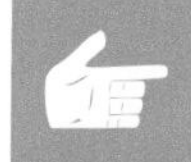

MISCELLANEOUS

ASSOCIATED CONDITIONS Leukoplakia or erythroplasia should be biopsied, since they are considered premalignant and associated with carcinoma at least 10% of the time

AGE-RELATED FACTORS None
Pediatric: N/A
Geriatric: Greater incidence after 50
Others: N/A

PREGNANCY N/A

SYNONYMS N/A

ICD-9-CM
145.9 Malignant neoplasm of mouth, unspecified
198.89 Secondary malignant neoplasm of other specified sites, other
230.0 Carcinoma in situ of lip, oral cavity and pharynx
210.4 Benign neoplasm of other and unspecified parts of mouth
235.1 Neoplasm of uncertain behavior of lip, oral cavity and pharynx

SEE ALSO

OTHER NOTES
- High incidence in Asia related to the habit of chewing the betel nut, fresh betel leaf, and habitual reverse smoking (lighted end is held within the oral cavity).

ABBREVIATIONS N/A

REFERENCES

- Cumming CW, Fredrickson JM, et al, eds. Otolaryngology Head and Neck Surgery, Vol 2. New York, C.V. Mosby Co, 1998

Web references: 2 available at www.5mcc.com
Illustrations 1 available

Author(s):
Roy R. Casiano, MD

BASICS

DESCRIPTION

- Dehydration and ongoing fluid losses from infectious gastroenteritis (GE) can be effectively treated with oral rehydration solutions (ORS), except in the most severe cases where initial parenteral fluid resuscitation is required. This therapy takes advantage of the coupled transport of sodium and glucose in the small intestine even during course of GE. Water follows osmotically after sodium entry. Potassium is passively absorbed via solvent drag. A glucose concentration of 2% allows maximal sodium absorption.
- ORS for rehydration should have a sodium content of about 75 mEq/L (75 mmol/L). Maintenance ORS, with sodium content of 40-50 mEq/L (40-50 mmol/L), are useful for mild dehydration and treatment of ongoing losses with a relatively low sodium content (e.g., rotavirus). Some investigators claim that high sodium diarrheal losses as from cholera require higher sodium content ORS (WHO solution = 90 mEq/L [90 mmol/L] Na). In 2002, the WHO reduced the sodium content of its ORS from 90 mEq/L to 75 mEq/L, and in 2003, the CDC endorsed this approach.

System(s) affected: Endocrine/Metabolic, Gastrointestinal
Genetics: N/A
Incidence/Prevalence in USA: N/A
Predominant age: Primarily infants and children; effective for all ages
Predominant sex: Male = Female

SIGNS & SYMPTOMS See Dehydration

CAUSES N/A

RISK FACTORS N/A

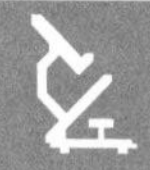

DIAGNOSIS

DIFFERENTIAL DIAGNOSIS N/A

LABORATORY N/A

Drugs that may alter lab results: N/A

Disorders that may alter lab results: N/A

PATHOLOGICAL FINDINGS N/A

SPECIAL TESTS N/A

IMAGING N/A

DIAGNOSTIC PROCEDURES N/A

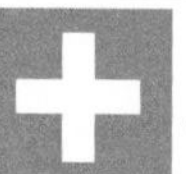

TREATMENT

APPROPRIATE HEALTH CARE Primarily outpatient. Designed to be administered by family members.

GENERAL MEASURES

- In developed countries, most diarrheal losses are low sodium. Consequently, maintenance ORS can be used for rehydration.
- Estimate replacement at 60 mL/kg for mild- and 80-100 mL/kg for moderate dehydration over the first 4-8 hours. Very important to replace any ongoing losses and add maintenance fluids.
- Replace ongoing stool losses with ORS. In infant, estimate 5-10 mL/kg per stool or weigh diapers.
- Add maintenance requirements to replacement:
  - ◊ Estimate:
    0-10 kg: 4 mL/kg/hr
    Plus 10-20 kg: 2 mL/kg/hr
    Plus > 20 kg: 1mL/kg/hr
  - ◊ Use maintenance ORS. Traditional clear fluids (e.g., fruit juice, soda) are inappropriate for oral rehydration therapy.
- If the patient has hypertonic dehydration, oral rehydration should be planned for 12-24 hours
- If vomiting occurs, small amounts of ORS given frequently is usually effective
- If patient is not vomiting and is alert, patient's thirst is excellent indicator of fluid needs
- ORS is not to be diluted
- Maintenance oral rehydration therapy begins when the deficit is replaced and provides for ongoing losses. Maintenance ORS or a combination of ORS and water or other clear liquids can be used.
- Effective at all ages. If child refuses because of taste, flavor with a commercial artificially sweetened flavoring, such as Nutrasweet flavored Kool-Aid; use approximately 1/4 teaspoon to 4 oz ORS.
- If necessary, rehydration by nasogastric tube is appropriate
- Effective at all ages: prepackaged ORS flavored freeze pops (often well accepted)
- Begin feeding as soon as rehydration achieved

SURGICAL MEASURES N/A

ACTIVITY As tolerated

DIET

- For breast feeding infants - mother should continue nursing
- For bottle fed babies - early institution of formulas. Lactose-free formulas rarely are required.
- Age appropriate - complex carbohydrate rich (eg, rice, bread, potato, cereal), low fat foods should be offered as soon as the dehydration deficit is replaced. Cow's milk can be added to diet after several days.

PATIENT EDUCATION

- Awareness and availability of ORS markedly diminishes morbidity from gastroenteritis
- Travelers concerned with severe diarrhea should carry ORS packets on trips

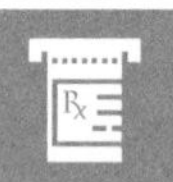

MEDICATIONS

DRUG(S) OF CHOICE

- The prototype ORS for dehydration due to cholera is the World Health Organization solution. When GE is unlikely to be caused by cholera, a lower sodium solution is advisable, especially in children.

WHO ORS:

- ◊ 1 liter of clean water
- ◊ 1/2 tsp sodium chloride (salt)
- ◊ 1/2 tsp trisodium citrate
- ◊ 1/4 tsp potassium chloride (salt substitute)
- ◊ 2 tbsp glucose

Notes:

- ◊ Glucose can be replaced by either sucrose (table sugar) or rice powder which are less expensive. Rice starch-based ORS decreases stool volume in cholera.
- ◊ Trisodium citrate can be replaced by sodium bicarbonate (baking soda)

Comparison of oral rehydration products:

Solution	Type†	Na+	K+	COH
WHO (1975)	R	90	20	20
WHO (2002)	R	75	20	13.5
Rehydralyte	R	75	20	25
Pedialyte	M	45	20	25
Enfalyte	M	50	25	30

† R = rehydration
M = maintenance
Na+ = Sodium (mEq/L or mmol/L)
K+ = Potassium (mmol/L)
COH = Carbohydrate (g/L)

Contraindications:

- Conditions predisposing to risk of aspiration: Altered consciousness, seizure activity, severe hypotension, shock
- Persistent vomiting (as in pyloric stenosis)
- Absent bowel sounds

Precautions:

- The ingredients should be provided in pre-mixed packets in order to avoid iatrogenic errors in mixing
- If water safety is questionable, it should be boiled or treated for purification
- Discard the solution after 12 hours if held at room temperature, or 24 hours if refrigerated
- After rehydration is complete, ORS's should not be used as the only fluid intake because the high sodium content may lead to hypernatremia

Significant possible interactions: N/A

ALTERNATIVE DRUGS N/A

FOLLOWUP

PATIENT MONITORING The patient needs to be frequently evaluated to ensure establishment of an improving clinical status and an adequate urine output

PREVENTION/AVOIDANCE N/A

POSSIBLE COMPLICATIONS Change to IV hydration if the patient has increasing weight loss (fluid deficit), clinical deterioration, or intractable vomiting.

EXPECTED COURSE/PROGNOSIS

- Rapid clinical improvement despite continuing diarrhea is the usual course
- The overall complication rate for oral rehydration is the same as that for parenteral rehydration in cases of mild and moderate dehydration.

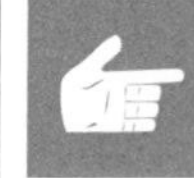

MISCELLANEOUS

ASSOCIATED CONDITIONS N/A

AGE-RELATED FACTORS N/A
Pediatric: See Diet
Geriatric: N/A
Others: N/A

PREGNANCY N/A

SYNONYMS N/A

ICD-9-CM

SEE ALSO

Cholera
Dehydration
Diarrhea, acute
Gastroenteritis, viral

OTHER NOTES Advantages of oral rehydration include a much lower cost, minimal storage requirements (for powder forms) and no need for sterile conditions

ABBREVIATIONS

GE = gastroenteritis
ORS = oral rehydration solutions

REFERENCES

- Nalin DR, Hirschhorn N, Greenough W 3rd, Fuchs GJ, Cash RA. Clinical concerns about reduced-osmolarity oral rehydration solution. JAMA 2004;291(21):2632-5
- Fonseca BK, Holdgate A, Craig JC. Enteral vs intravenous rehydration therapy for children with gastroenteritis: a meta-analysis of randomized controlled trials. Arch Pediatr Adolesc Med 2004;158(5):483-90
- Duggan C, Fontaine O, Pierce NF, Glass RI, Mahalanabis D, Alam NH, Bhan MK, Santosham M. Scientific rationale for a change in the composition of oral rehydration solution. JAMA 2004;291(21):2628-31
- Ramakrishna BS, Venkataraman S, et al. Amylase-resistant starch plus oral rehydration solution for cholera. N Engl J Med 2000;342(5):308-13
- Fontaine O, Gore S, Pierce N. Rice-based ORS for treating diarrhea. In: Cochrane Library, Issue I, 2002. Oxford: Update Software
- Hahn S, Kim S, Garner P. Reduced osmolarity oral rehydration solution for treating dehydration caused by acute diarrhoea in children. Cochrane Database Syst Rev 2002;(1):CD002847
- Finberg L. A commentary on the use of rational oral electrolyte therapy. Arch Pediatr Adolesc Med 1999;153(9):910-2
- Santosham M, et al. A double-blind clinical trial comparing WHO ORS with a reduced osmolarity solution containing amounts of sodium and glucose. J Pediatr 1996;128:45-51

Web references: 2 available at www.5mcc.com
Illustrations N/A

Author(s):
William A. Primack, MD
Charles N. Jacobs, MD

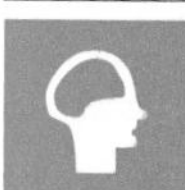

BASICS

DESCRIPTION The syndrome associated with traction apophysitis in adolescent boys and girls consisting of pain of the tibial tubercle with swelling
System(s) affected: Musculoskeletal
Genetics: Unknown
Incidence/Prevalence in USA: Not known, but common (13% of athletes in one Finnish study)
Predominant age:
- Females 10-16
- Males 11-18

Predominant sex: Male > Female

SIGNS & SYMPTOMS
- Unilateral or bilateral (30%) tibial tuberosity pain
- Pain exacerbated by exercise, especially jumping and landing after jumping
- Tibial tuberosity swelling
- Pain increased with knee extension against resistance or kneeling
- Knee pain with squatting or crouching
- Absence of effusion or condyle tenderness
- Erythema of tibial tuberosity

CAUSES Basic etiology unknown, but clearly exacerbated by exercise - jumping and pivoting sports are the worst; repetitive trauma the most likely source. Possible association with tight hip flexors, quadriceps and hamstring muscle groups.

RISK FACTORS
- Age between 11 and 18
- Male sex
- Rapid skeletal growth
- Involvement in repetitive jumping sports

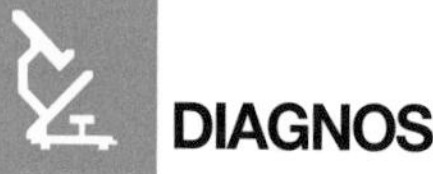

DIAGNOSIS

DIFFERENTIAL DIAGNOSIS
- Stress fracture of the proximal tibia
- Pes anserinus bursitis
- Quadriceps tendon avulsion
- Patellofemoral stress syndrome
- Chondromalacia patellae
- Proximal tibial neoplasm
- Osteomyelitis of the proximal tibia
- Tibial plateau fracture
- Sinding-Larson Johansson disease (patellar apophysitis)
- Patellar tendinitis

LABORATORY No blood tests indicated unless other diagnostic considerations are entertained

Drugs that may alter lab results: N/A

Disorders that may alter lab results: N/A

PATHOLOGICAL FINDINGS
- Osteochondritis of the tibial tubercle
- Heterotopic bone formation at insertion of the patellar tendon
- Bony fusion of the tibial metaphysis
- Inflammatory infiltrate of the epiphysis in severe cases
- Complete avulsion of the tibial tubercle with nonunion of the tubercle with the tibia - possible complication (extremely rare)

SPECIAL TESTS N/A

IMAGING
- X-ray imaging of the proximal tibia and knee may show heterotopic calcification in the patellar tendon. X-rays are rarely diagnostic.
- Calcified thickening of the tibial tuberosity with irregular ossification at insertion of tendon to tibial tubercle
- Bone scan may show increased uptake in the area of the tibial tuberosity; will have increased uptake in apophysis in any child, but may be more than opposite side
- Ultrasound is becoming an excellent alternative with characteristic findings and classifications

DIAGNOSTIC PROCEDURES N/A

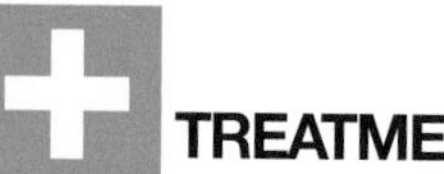

TREATMENT

APPROPRIATE HEALTH CARE Outpatient

GENERAL MEASURES
- Frequent ice applications post exercise with pain
- Rest
- Knee immobilization in extension (severe cases)
- In more severe cases, avoidance of activities that increase pain or swelling
- Quadriceps isometric strengthening, hip extensions, adductor strengthening, hamstring and quadriceps stretching exercises
- Patients with marked pronation may benefit from orthotics

SURGICAL MEASURES Débridement of a thickened cosmetically unsatisfactory tibial tubercle (rare) or removal of heterotopic bone

ACTIVITY Activity to be restricted to those activities not causing pain

DIET N/A

PATIENT EDUCATION
- Consider avoidance of jumping sports. Assure family that symptoms and findings will diminish with time and rest.
- OK to play sport with mild pain

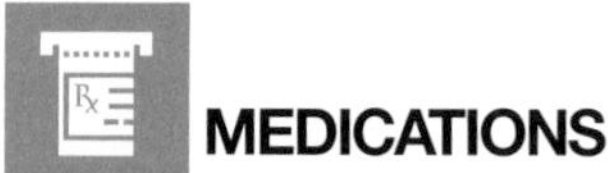

MEDICATIONS

DRUG(S) OF CHOICE None in particular, but all analgesics may be considered. NSAIDs are of minimal benefit; however narcotics are not recommended
Contraindications: N/A
Precautions: N/A
Significant possible interactions: N/A

ALTERNATIVE DRUGS
- More potent analgesics such as narcotics may be considered for short term use or in extreme situations
- No objective evidence to support the use of selenium in OSD

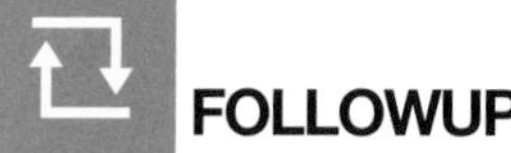

FOLLOWUP

PATIENT MONITORING Follow up on a prn basis for management of pain and disability

PREVENTION/AVOIDANCE
- Avoidance of those sports involving heavy quadriceps loading
- Patients may compete if the pain is minimal
- Increase hamstring and quadriceps flexibility

POSSIBLE COMPLICATIONS
- Nonunion of the tubercle to the tibia
- Upriding of the patella
- Patellar tendon avulsion
- Genu recurvatum
- Patellofemoral degenerative arthritis
- Patella alta
- Chondromalacia

EXPECTED COURSE/PROGNOSIS
Except in rare complicated cases, this is a self-limiting illness resolved within two years after full skeletal maturation. However, up to 60% of adults with prior Osgood-Schlatter disease will still report occasional symptoms and have pain with kneeling.

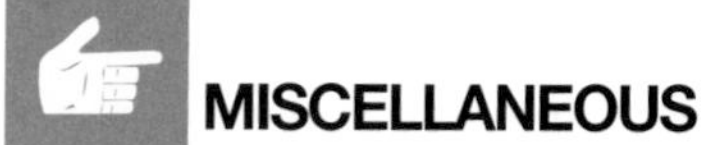

MISCELLANEOUS

ASSOCIATED CONDITIONS N/A

AGE-RELATED FACTORS
Pediatric: In skeletally mature boys and girls, with boys more frequent than girls
Geriatric: N/A
Others: Participants in sports involving heavy quadriceps activity

PREGNANCY N/A

SYNONYMS Osteochondritis of the tibial tubercle

ICD-9-CM
732.4 Juvenile osteochondrosis of lower extremity, excluding foot

SEE ALSO
Tendinitis

OTHER NOTES N/A

ABBREVIATIONS N/A

REFERENCES

- Outerbridge AR, Micheli LJ: Overuse injuries in the young athlete. Sports Med 1995;14(3):503-516
- Garrett WE Jr, et al. Principles and Practices of Primary Care Sports Medicine. Baltimore, Lippincott Williams & Wilkins, 2001:pp404-406

Web references: 2 available at www.5mcc.com
Illustrations N/A

Author(s):
David P. Sealy, MD

BASICS

DESCRIPTION Inflammatory focal or generalized condition of the skeleton characterized by rapid, chaotic bone resorption followed by equally chaotic and excessive bone formation. Leads to enlarged but weakened and highly vascularized bone which is painful, easily deformed and subject to fractures with minimal trauma. Cranial and vertebral involvement can also cause neurologic deficits.

System(s) affected: Musculoskeletal

Genetics: 15-50% of patients have one or more involved first order relatives with osteitis deformans. Recent data suggest an 18q locus is involved, but other chromosomal sites may also confer susceptibility.

Incidence/Prevalence in USA: 3% of Caucasian individuals above age 50 have at least one focus. Rare in African Americans and Asians.

Predominant age: Above age 50, occasional cases ages 20-50

Predominant sex: Male = Female

SIGNS & SYMPTOMS
- Frequently asymptomatic
- Bone pain
- Skeletal deformities
- Bowing of extremities
- Acetabular protrusion
- Headaches
- Head enlargement
- Fractures
- Secondary osteoarthritis
- Vertebral compression
- Neurologic deficits
- Osteoporosis circumscripta
- High output congestive heart failure (rare)
- Hypercalcemia (rare)
- Renal calculi (calcium, uric acid)
- Peyronie syndrome
- Angioid streaks (rare)
- Mottled retinal degeneration (rare)
- Increased skin temperature over affected areas
- Bone sarcomas (rare)
- Peripheral neuropathies
- Carpal/tarsal tunnel syndromes
- Valvular/endocardial calcification
- Accelerated atherosclerosis
- Gouty diathesis
- Hyperparathyroidism
- Sensorineural hearing loss
- Conductive hearing loss

CAUSES Unknown; best evidence to date is for slow virus infection in genetically susceptible individuals

RISK FACTORS None known

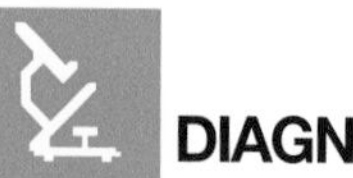

DIAGNOSIS

DIFFERENTIAL DIAGNOSIS
- Polyostotic fibrous dysplasia
- Osteitis fibrosis cystica (skeletal hyperparathyroidism)
- Primary bone neoplasms
- Osteolytic, osteoblastic metastases

LABORATORY
- Serum calcium - usually normal, rarely increased
- Serum alkaline phosphatase (total or bone specific) - usually increased
- Serum GGT - normal
- Serum osteocalcin (BGP) - usually increased
- Urinary pyridinoline collagen crosslinks - usually increased
- N- and C-telopeptide (collagen crosslinks) - usually increased in serum and urine

Drugs that may alter lab results:
- Vitamin D and its metabolites
- Hepatotoxic drugs

Disorders that may alter lab results:
- See Differential diagnosis
- Osteomalacia
- Liver disorders
- Traumatic fractures

PATHOLOGICAL FINDINGS
- Chaotic bone resorption at advancing edge of disease. Osteoclasts are large, contain 10-100 nuclei and have abnormal configuration.
- Electron photomicroscopically, the nuclei and cytoplasm contain myriads of inclusion bodies resembling viral nucleocapsids
- Later, excessive osteoblastic bone formation predominates with sclerotic bone containing cement lines forming mosaic pattern

SPECIAL TESTS
- Neurologic examination
- Audiogram, if skull involvement
- Visual field study, if skull involvement

IMAGING
- X-rays show irregular pattern of alternating bone formation and resorption in enlarged deformed bones. Resorptive fronts at advancing edge.
- Bone scans show intense uptake in focal pattern
- CT/MRI show extra-bony extension if sarcomatous degeneration occurs

DIAGNOSTIC PROCEDURES Bone biopsy needed only in confusing cases (rare)

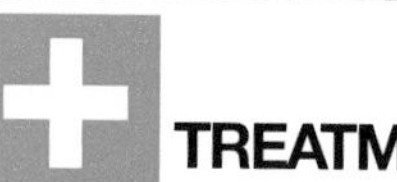

TREATMENT

APPROPRIATE HEALTH CARE Outpatient, except when intravenous treatment is used

GENERAL MEASURES
- Rarely, splints for severely resorbed areas with high risk of fracture
- Hearing aids for severe deafness; of some (but not great) value in sensorineural deafness

SURGICAL MEASURES
- Joint replacement (hip, knee) sometimes needed
- Osteotomy procedures for extreme deformity
- Decompression procedures (skull, spinal column) for acute neurologic deficits (rarely needed)
- Bone biopsy (rarely needed)
- Extirpative surgery for sarcomatous complications
- Open reduction of fractures

ACTIVITY
- Full activity to maintain function
- Avoid excessive mechanical stress on involved bones

DIET No special diet

PATIENT EDUCATION Paget Foundation, 120 Wall St., Suite 1602, New York, NY 10005 (212)509-5335; fax (212)509-8492; E-mail: pagetfdn@aol.com

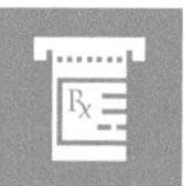

MEDICATIONS

DRUG(S) OF CHOICE
- Synthetic injectable salmon calcitonin (Miacalcin): 50 IU three times weekly to 100 IU qd, courses 1.5 to 3 years

or
- Etidronate (Didronel), 5 mg/kg/day (approximately 400 mg) x 6 mos (taken on an empty stomach). Rarely, 20 mg/kg/day x 1 month. Courses may be repeated after a 3-6 month rest period

or
- Alendronate (Fosamax) 40 mg/day (taken on an empty stomach) for 6 mos

or
- Risedronate (Actonel) 30 mg/day (taken on an empty stomach) for 2 months

or
- Pamidronate (Aredia) 60 mg/day by 4-6 hour infusions for 2-3 days. Alternately, 30 mg/day by 4-6 hour infusions once a week for 6 weeks. May be repeated several months later if effect wears off.
- Add non-steroidal anti-inflammatories (NSAIDs) to above drugs for secondary osteoarthritis. COX-2 inhibitors may be substituted.

Contraindications:
- Prior history of allergy or hypersensitivity
- For alendronate and risedronate, esophageal dysfunction, severe upper GI symptoms, GERD, etc.

Precautions:
- Adverse side effects may require ameliorative measures or temporary dose reduction
- Salmon calcitonin - nausea, vomiting, anorexia, flushing, rash, including urticaria (rare)
- Etidronate disodium - nausea, vomiting, diarrhea, increased bone pain
- Alendronate and risedronate - heartburn, epigastric pain, musculoskeletal pain. Take on an empty stomach with copious water. No food, beverages or other medications for 30-60 minutes. Remain upright for 1 hour.
- Pamidronate disodium - transient fever, leukopenia, hypocalcemia, headache, malaise, loss of appetite

Significant possible interactions: None

ALTERNATIVE DRUGS
NSAIDs or COX-2 inhibitors for mildly symptomatic disease in nonstrategic areas

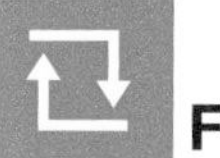

FOLLOWUP

PATIENT MONITORING
- Followup visits every 2-4 months during drug therapy; yearly if drugs not being used. Alkaline phosphatase (total or bone specific) before each visit.
- Repeat x-rays and bone scan every 3-5 years or as needed

PREVENTION/AVOIDANCE
Avoid excessive mechanical stress on afflicted bones to reduce chance of fractures and other complications

POSSIBLE COMPLICATIONS
Fractures, severe deformities, head enlargement, acetabular protrusion, carpal/tarsal tunnel syndromes, neurologic deficits, deafness, visual impairment, congestive heart failure (high output), renal calculi, Peyronie syndrome, sarcomatous degeneration

EXPECTED COURSE/PROGNOSIS
- Depends on severity, often asymptomatic
- Slow progression if untreated
- Significant amelioration with treatment (85% or greater)
- Poor prognosis if bone sarcoma develops

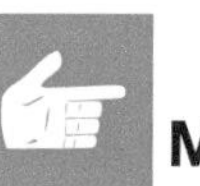

MISCELLANEOUS

ASSOCIATED CONDITIONS
- Hyperparathyroidism
- Gouty diathesis
- Secondary osteoarthritis
- Angioid streaks
- Mottled retinal degeneration
- Bone sarcoma (rare)
- Peyronie disease

AGE-RELATED FACTORS
Pediatric: N/A
Geriatric: Common
Others: More prevalent if ancestry Caucasian, especially United Kingdom, Northern Europe (excluding Scandinavia), Italy, Australia and New Zealand. Rare in African Americans and Asians.

PREGNANCY
N/A

SYNONYMS
Paget disease of bone

ICD-9-CM
731.0 Osteitis deformans without mention of bone tumor

SEE ALSO
Arthritis, osteo
Bone tumor, primary malignant
Hyperparathyroidism

OTHER NOTES
N/A

ABBREVIATIONS
N/A

REFERENCES

- Hadjipavlou A, Lander P, Srolovitz H, Enker IP. Malignant transformation in Paget's disease of bone. Cancer. 1992;70:2802-2808
- Morales-Piga AA, Rey-Rey JS, Corres-Gonzalez J, Garcia-Sagredo JM, Loopez-Abente G. Frequency and characteristics of familial aggregation of Paget's disease of bone. J Bone Miner Res. 1995;10:663-670
- Delmas PD, Meunier PJ: The management of Paget's disease of bone. NEJM 1997;336:558-566
- Wallach S. Identifying and controlling Paget's disease. J Musculoskel Med 1997;14(6):66-82
- Siris ES: Paget's disease of bone. Journal of Bone and Mineral Research 1998;13(7):1061-1065
- Ankrom MA, Shapiro JR: Paget's disease of bone (osteitis deformans). J Am Geriatr Soc 1998;46(8):1025-1033
- Noor M, Shoback D. Paget's disease of bone: diagnosis and treatment update. Curr Rheumatol Rep 2000;2(1):67-73
- Rothschild BM Paget's disease of the elderly. Compr Ther 2000;26(4):251-4

Web references: 1 available at www.5mcc.com
Illustrations N/A

Author(s):
Mark R. Dambro, MD

BASICS

DESCRIPTION Condition in which a segment of subchondral bone of any diarthrodial joint becomes separated from surrounding bone which can progress to include the cartilage and eventually to formation of a loose body in the affected joint.
System(s) affected: Musculoskeletal
Genetics: No distinct genetic pattern known, however bilateral lesions have been noted in up to 30% of patients
Incidence/Prevalence in USA: Unknown
Predominant age:
- 2 main age groups:
  - ◊ Young adults in their 2nd to 4th decades of life
  - ◊ Juvenile type which includes children and adolescents prior to physeal closure

Predominant sex: Male > Female (3:1)

SIGNS & SYMPTOMS
- Insidious or post-traumatic onset of pain, which improves with rest
- Pain may be associated with clicking, swelling, locking and stiffness
- May be associated with secondary muscle atrophy, effusion, and decreased range of motion
- Locking may be experienced if fragment detaches
- Pain usually defined as a deep ache

CAUSES
- Etiology unclear however it is most often associated with trauma or repetitive micro-trauma
- Most commonly effected joints are the knee, ankle, and elbow
  - ◊ Knee - overuse and with patellar dislocation, and with injury to the ACL
  - ◊ Elbow - overuse injury in overhead throwers and in female gymnasts
  - ◊ Ankle - frequently associated with history of previous ankle sprain
- Possible theories include vulnerability secondary to fragile blood supply of the physeal line

RISK FACTORS
- No clear genetic predisposition however up to 30% of lesions are bilateral
- Seen in active children and adults
- Multi-sport athletics, especially gymnastics and overhead sport participation

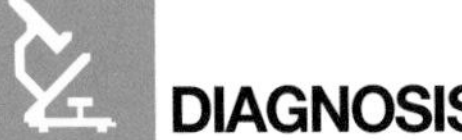

DIAGNOSIS

DIFFERENTIAL DIAGNOSIS
- In the knee: meniscal tear, patella-femoral pain syndrome
- Stress fracture
- Tendinopathy

LABORATORY No specific tests

Drugs that may alter lab results: N/A

Disorders that may alter lab results: N/A

PATHOLOGICAL FINDINGS
- Primary change in the bone
- Avascular necrosis occurs in a focal area
- Overlying cartilage changes are secondary to the bony changes
- Loss of subchondral bone support leads to degenerative cartilage changes - softening, and fibromatous fissuring
- Fragment may detach and become loose body within the effected joint
- Cartilage itself is without a vascular supply
- Healing occurs by vascular supply to bone which stimulates inflammation, repair and remodeling
- It is difficult to predict which lesions will go on to heal and remodel

SPECIAL TESTS N/A

IMAGING
- Plain radiographs are frequently normal
  - ◊ Knee - AP, lateral and "tunnel" view {most likely location for abnormality is in the lateral portion of the medial condyle}
  - ◊ Elbow - routine elbow series {common involvement of the humeral capitellum}
  - ◊ Ankle - AP, lateral, oblique and mortise view {lesions most commonly involve the posteromedial or anterolateral talus}
- MRI. Can delineate the bony lesion as well as involvement of cartilage and any fluid behind the fragment.
- CT scan - provides architectural description of bone lesion, providing less information than MRI
- Technetium 99 bone scan - may be useful in evaluation of healing potential, but this is controversial

DIAGNOSTIC PROCEDURES N/A

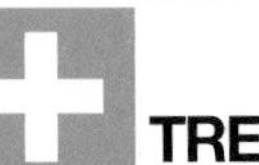

TREATMENT

APPROPRIATE HEALTH CARE Outpatient usually; inpatient for surgery

GENERAL MEASURES
- Goals of treatment - maintain smooth congruous joint surface. Alleviate pain. Prevent degenerative joint disease. Promote revascularization of necrotic fragment and regeneration of effected cartilage.
- There are no randomized controlled trials, however, in JOCD, non-surgical treatment initially is the norm
- Treatment options include a spectrum of alternatives from relative rest (removal from sport) to crutches (partial or non-weight bearing) to cylindrical casting and splinting

SURGICAL MEASURES Surgical treatment is utilized when conservative measures have failed or when physeal closure is approaching which carries a worse prognosis for healing (adult form). Surgical treatment includes drilling to increase blood supply and/or allograft insertion and requires an orthopedic consultation.

ACTIVITY
- Non-weight bearing, immobilization with intermittent maintenance of range of motion
- Follow closely for 12 weeks for healing
- Casting is utilized for 6 week intervals especially with JOCD due to issues of compliance

DIET No specific diet recommended

PATIENT EDUCATION
- Compliance with immobilization and possibility of further trauma should be emphasized especially with the younger athlete
- Many lesions heal without surgical intervention

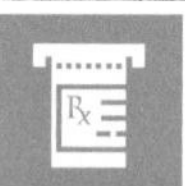

MEDICATIONS

DRUG(S) OF CHOICE NSAIDs or acetaminophen
Contraindications: N/A
Precautions: N/A
Significant possible interactions: N/A

ALTERNATIVE DRUGS N/A

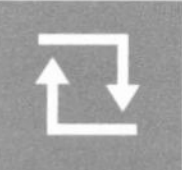

FOLLOWUP

PATIENT MONITORING Initially should be followed every 6 weeks with serial radiographs to check for healing and possible displacement. Expect healing in 4 to 6 months. In JOCD at one year radiographs may show no residual abnormality.

PREVENTION/AVOIDANCE No clear way to avoid its development.

POSSIBLE COMPLICATIONS
- Failure to revascularize and heal
- Displacement of fragment becoming loose body within a joint

EXPECTED COURSE/PROGNOSIS
- Patient age and degree of physeal closure has a significant effect on healing potential
- An incongruous joint surface may lead to degenerative changes in the future
- Clinical improvement may precede radiologic healing
- Fragment displacement may occur, in which case arthroscopy is indicated

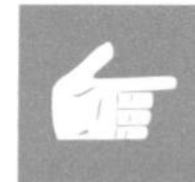

MISCELLANEOUS

ASSOCIATED CONDITIONS N/A

AGE-RELATED FACTORS
Pediatric: Multi-sport athletics especially gymnastics and overhead sport participation
Geriatric: N/A
Others: N/A

PREGNANCY N/A

SYNONYMS N/A

ICD-9-CM
732.7 Osteochondritis dissecans

SEE ALSO

OTHER NOTES N/A

ABBREVIATIONS N/A

REFERENCES

- Delee JD, Drez D, eds. Delee and Drez: Orthopedic Sports Medicine: Principles and Practice, 2nd ed. Philadelphia: WB Saunders; 2003:1273-79
- Birk GT, DeLee JC. Osteochondral injuries. Clinical findings. Clin Sports Med 2001;20(2):279-86
- Wall E, Von Stein D. Juvenile osteochondritis desicans. Orthopedic Clinics of North America 2003;34(3):341-53
- Bucholz R, ed. Rockwood and Green: Fractures in Adults and Fractures in Children. 4th ed. Philadelphia: Lippincott-Raven; 1996:289-93
- Rockwood CA, ed: Fractures in Children. 4th ed. Philadelphia: Lippincott-Raven; 1996:1290-94
- Cahill BR, Ahten SM. Osteochondral injuries of the knee. Clin Sports Med 2001;20(2):287-98

Web references: 0 available at www.5mcc.com
Illustrations N/A

Author(s):
Phyllis Montellese, MD

BASICS

DESCRIPTION Osteomalacia (referred to as rickets in children) is defined as an excess organic bone matrix secondary to defective or inadequate bone mineralization
System(s) affected: Musculoskeletal
Genetics: N/A
Incidence/Prevalence in USA: N/A
Predominant age: All ages. In adults, osteomalacia is usually a disease of the older population (50-80).
Predominant sex: Female > Male (slightly)

SIGNS & SYMPTOMS
- Bone pain, tenderness, muscle weakness
- Bone pain is dull and tends to be poorly localized, usually affecting the ribs and upper thighs
- Muscle weakness is usually proximal
- Other symptoms of malnutrition or an underlying problem such as chronic renal disease may also be clinically evident
- Weight loss
- Anorexia
- Tetany
- In young children - restlessness, poor sleep patterns, craniotabes, costochondral beading, bowlegs, kyphoscoliosis

CAUSES
- Can be caused by a wide variety of pathogenic processes, including, but not limited to, vitamin D deficiency (reduced exposure to sunlight, poor nutrition, malabsorption syndromes)
- Defective metabolism of parent vitamin D to active metabolites (drug-induced, i.e., anticonvulsants - phenytoin (Dilantin), chronic renal failure), hypophosphatemia (renal tubular acidosis, hypophosphatemic syndrome), miscellaneous (long-term hemodialysis, malnutrition, vitamin D-dependent rickets)

RISK FACTORS
- Poverty
- Inadequate nutrition and sunlight exposure

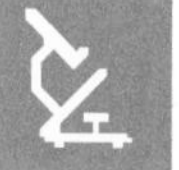

DIAGNOSIS

DIFFERENTIAL DIAGNOSIS
- Osteoporosis
- Metastatic bone disease
- Primary bone malignancies (lymphoma, myeloma)

LABORATORY
- Alkaline phosphatase - increased
- Serum calcium is low or normal (never high)
- Hypophosphatemia
- Aminoaciduria
- Acidosis
- Glucosuria
- Hypouricemia

Drugs that may alter lab results: N/A

Disorders that may alter lab results: N/A

PATHOLOGICAL FINDINGS
- Defective calcification of growing bone
- Hypertrophy of epiphyseal cartilages

SPECIAL TESTS N/A

IMAGING Radiographic changes are non-specific. Earliest manifestations are thinning of cortical bone. In long-term osteomalacia: bone softening (protrusio acetabuli), looser lines, stress fractures, and pathologic fractures.

DIAGNOSTIC PROCEDURES Bone biopsy and subsequent histopathologic evaluation deliver the most accurate diagnosis of osteomalacia. The biopsy is usually taken from the iliac crest, and both calcified, and non-calcified studies, as well as special stains (including von Kossa's stain) are helpful.

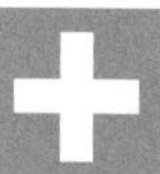

TREATMENT

APPROPRIATE HEALTH CARE Can be managed on an outpatient basis, except for complicating emergencies/fractures

GENERAL MEASURES
- Treatment of osteomalacia depends upon the cause, i.e., gastrointestinal, renal, or nutritional.
- For nutritional osteomalacia, calcium and vitamin D have been shown to correct the disease process
- Treatment can be monitored by observing simple bone biochemistry
- Treatment results depend on identifying and correcting the cause

SURGICAL MEASURES N/A

ACTIVITY Full activity is encouraged, including a neuroconditioning program

DIET
- Ensure adequate vitamin D intake
- Provide instructions for a high calcium diet and information on calcium supplements, if appropriate

PATIENT EDUCATION Educate family and patient on nutrition

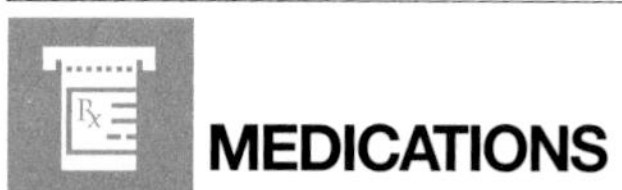

MEDICATIONS

DRUG(S) OF CHOICE For adults and uncomplicated rickets: vitamin D (ergocalciferol) 2000-4800 IU once a day for one month. Then reduce dose gradually.
Contraindications: N/A
Precautions: N/A
Significant possible interactions: N/A

ALTERNATIVE DRUGS
- IV calcium salts if tetany complicates. Single IM dose of 100,000 IU in adolescents each Fall.
- Alfacalcidol
- Calcitriol

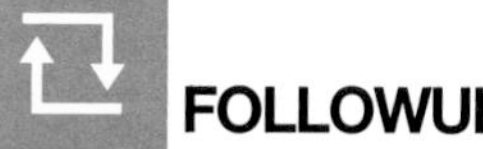

FOLLOWUP

PATIENT MONITORING Office visits every 6 months

PREVENTION/AVOIDANCE
- Adequate dietary intake of vitamin D
- Adequate sunlight exposure
- Fortified cow's milk

POSSIBLE COMPLICATIONS
- Fractures
- Osteomyelitis
- Renal failure
- Renal tubular acidosis
- Seizures
- Growth deformity; bowing long bones in children

EXPECTED COURSE/PROGNOSIS
Variable

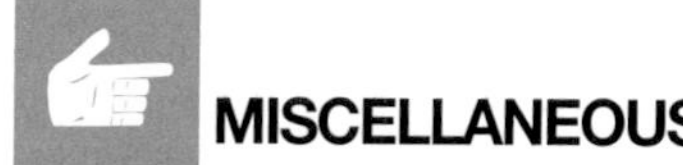

MISCELLANEOUS

ASSOCIATED CONDITIONS
- Chronic renal disease
- Epilepsy
- Malnutrition
- Previous gastric surgery
- Pregnancy-nutritional factors

AGE-RELATED FACTORS
Pediatric: N/A
Geriatric: Studies have suggested that vitamin D deficiency osteomalacia is a relatively common condition in the acutely ill elderly population, with an estimated prevalence of about 3-5%; however, it often goes undiagnosed
Others: N/A

PREGNANCY N/A

SYNONYMS Rickets

ICD-9-CM
268.2 Osteomalacia, unspecified

SEE ALSO

OTHER NOTES N/A

ABBREVIATIONS N/A

REFERENCES

- Mare GM, McKenna MJ, Frame B: Osteomalacia. Bone Mineral Res 1986;4:335

Web references: 0 available at www.5mcc.com
Illustrations N/A

Author(s):
Mark C. Leeson, MD

BASICS

DESCRIPTION Osteomyelitis is an acute or chronic infection of the bone and its structures caused most commonly by bacteria and rarely by other microorganisms. This infection may be acquired either by hematogenous, contiguous, or direct inoculation such as trauma or surgery.
System(s) affected: Musculoskeletal
Genetics: There is no genetic predisposition known in this disease
Incidence/Prevalence in USA: Uncommon
Predominant age: This infection is commonly seen in older adults; hematogenous is bimodal, also seen in infants and children
Predominant sex: Males > Females

SIGNS & SYMPTOMS
- Hematogenous long bone infection in children
  - ◊ Abrupt onset of high fever
  - ◊ Irritability
  - ◊ Malaise
  - ◊ Restriction of movement of the involved extremity
  - ◊ Signs of localized inflammation
- Hematogenous vertebral infection in adults
  - ◊ Illness is insidious and behaves more like a chronic infection
  - ◊ History of an acute bacteremic episode associated with infection of a specific organ may be found in some patients
- Contiguous and vascular insufficiency associated infection
  - ◊ Acute constitutional manifestations are seldom seen
  - ◊ Localized signs and symptoms of inflammation with or without drainage frequently found
- Chronic osteomyelitis
  - ◊ Non-healing ulcer or draining sinus
  - ◊ Constitutional symptoms, when present, indicate acute suppurative condition in the bone or surrounding tissues
- Prosthetic device associated infection
  - ◊ Infection may be acquired either by hematogenous route, or by contiguous foci such as local infection, operative contamination, or postoperative infection
  - ◊ Acute postoperative infection may present as fever, localized swelling, tenderness, and drainage
  - ◊ Chronic infection is characterized by joint discomfort, swelling, erythema, and joint dysfunction

CAUSES
- Acute hematogenous osteomyelitis
  - ◊ Staphylococcus aureus (most common)
  - ◊ Streptococcus, coagulase negative Staphylococcus, Haemophilus influenzae, and gram negative organisms (less common)
- Vertebral osteomyelitis
  - ◊ Staphylococcus aureus and gram negative enteric organisms (common)
  - ◊ Other microorganisms to consider include Mycobacterium tuberculosis, and fungi
- Contiguous focus osteomyelitis and vascular insufficiency osteomyelitis
  - ◊ Mixed aerobic/anaerobic microorganisms are frequently found
- Prosthetic device infection
  - ◊ Coagulase negative Staphylococcus, and S. aureus (most common)
  - ◊ Diphtheroids, and gram negative bacteria (less common)

RISK FACTORS
- Diabetes mellitus
- Sickle cell disease
- Other conditions which predispose to bone infarcts
- IV drug use
- Hemodialysis
- Local trauma
- Open fractures
- Presence of prosthetic orthopedic implant
- Vascular insufficiency
- Neuropathy

DIAGNOSIS

DIFFERENTIAL DIAGNOSIS
- Systemic infection from other source
- Aseptic bone infarction
- Localized inflammation or infection of overlying skin and soft tissues
- Neuropathic joint disease
- Fractures
- Gout

LABORATORY
- Definitive diagnosis is made by needle aspiration or bone biopsy and demonstration of the microorganism by culture or histology
- Blood culture may be positive in about 50% of younger patients with acute hematogenous disease
- Leukocyte count is usually elevated in the acute cases, but not in the chronic cases
- Sedimentation rate or c-reactive protein is usually elevated, but non-specific

Drugs that may alter lab results: Antimicrobial agents given before bone culture

Disorders that may alter lab results:
- Cultures from the sinus tract are unreliable because of frequent contamination
- Superficial cultures only helpful in identifying methicillin-resistant S. aureus

PATHOLOGICAL FINDINGS Inflammatory process of the bone with pyogenic bacteria

SPECIAL TESTS N/A

IMAGING
- No technique can absolutely confirm or exclude osteomyelitis
- Radiographic - routine x-ray (findings on plain x-ray often delayed for 10-14 days in acute infection)
- Radionuclide scanning (technetium, indium, or gallium) are also useful, but limited by low specificity
- CT with good resolution, artifact may decrease specificity
- MRI excellent, more expensive than other radiologic tests

DIAGNOSTIC PROCEDURES Needle biopsy or open bone biopsy for bacterial culture (which is the "gold standard"). However, antibiotic therapy within the past 2-4 weeks may prevent isolation of a specific pathogen.

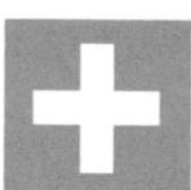

TREATMENT

APPROPRIATE HEALTH CARE Hospitalize the patient with suspected acute osteomyelitis for diagnostic work-up and initial treatment

GENERAL MEASURES Symptomatic treatment of pain

SURGICAL MEASURES
- Surgical drainage and removal of necrotic tissues are of utmost importance to effect cure
- In patients with vascular insufficiency or severe gangrenous infection, amputation may be the only effective treatment
- Revascularization may be an option for some patients

ACTIVITY Bedrest and immobilization of the involved bone and joint

DIET No restriction

PATIENT EDUCATION Stress need for long-term treatment and follow up

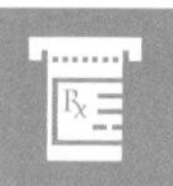

MEDICATIONS

DRUG(S) OF CHOICE

These are essentially empiric choices; recommendations based on data from a very small number of studies. Antimicrobial agent/agents based on susceptibility testing and known clinical efficacy. The duration of therapy for acute osteomyelitis should be at least 4-6 weeks. In chronic osteomyelitis, longer duration of therapy may be needed.

- Staphylococcus aureus and coagulase negative staphylococcus: nafcillin 2 g IV q4-6h. Vancomycin 1 g q12h for methicillin resistant Staph.
- Streptococcus spp.: penicillin G 2-4 million units q4h IV
- Enteric gram negative bacilli and Pseudomonas aeruginosa: piperacillin 4 g q4-6h IV, plus aminoglycoside
- Mixed aerobic/anaerobic infection (diabetic foot, bite wound): beta-lactamase inhibitor combination (ticarcillin-clavulanate 3.1 g q6h IV; ampicillin-sulbactam 3 g q6h IV); piperacillin-tazobactam 3.375 g q6h IV

Contraindications: Allergy
Precautions: In patients with renal or hepatic insufficiency, antimicrobial dose may need adjustment
Significant possible interactions: Refer to manufacturer's literature

ALTERNATIVE DRUGS

- Staphylococcus aureus and coagulase negative staphylococcus: clindamycin 600 mg IV q6h, nafcillin 2 g q4h, or cefazolin 1 g q8h IV, or vancomycin 1 g q12h
- Streptococcus spp.: penicillin G 2 million units q4h, cefazolin 1 g q8h IV, or clindamycin 600 mg q6h IV
- Enteric gram negative bacilli and Pseudomonas aeruginosa: ceftazidime 1 g q8h IV or ciprofloxacin [or other quinolone] 750 mg q12h orally.
- Mixed aerobic/anaerobic infection (diabetic foot, bite wound): clindamycin plus third generation cephalosporin or quinolone
- Home therapy often used - consider a simplified antibiotic regimen for outpatient use or oral therapy
- Some published studies recommend use of hyperbaric oxygen (HBO), but none are randomized, controlled trials

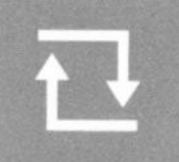

FOLLOWUP

PATIENT MONITORING Blood level of antimicrobial agents, serum antibacterial titers, sedimentation rate, repeat plain x-ray, CT or MRI to confirm healing

PREVENTION/AVOIDANCE Avoid further stress and weight bearing until healing

POSSIBLE COMPLICATIONS

- Abscess formation
- Bacteremia
- Fracture
- Loosening of the prosthetic implant
- Postoperative infection

EXPECTED COURSE/PROGNOSIS

- Cure of osteomyelitis with medical treatment is notoriously unpredictable especially when not accompanied by surgical debridement
- In patients with acute hematogenous osteomyelitis, the prognosis is usually good even without surgery. Cure takes about 6 weeks. X-ray improvement may take 3-6 months.
- The prognosis is improved if all infected bone has been removed

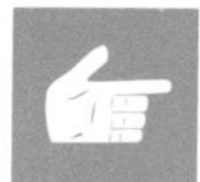

MISCELLANEOUS

ASSOCIATED CONDITIONS Listed with Causes

AGE-RELATED FACTORS

Pediatric: Occurs most often in 5-14 age group and more frequently in boys
Geriatric:

- Vertebral osteomyelitis more common
- Contiguous focus of infection more common
- Vascular insufficiency is most common cause of osteomyelitis in 50-70 age group (usually due to presence of associated conditions)

Others: N/A

PREGNANCY N/A

SYNONYMS N/A

ICD-9-CM

730.00 Acute osteomyelitis, site unspecified
730.10 Chronic osteomyelitis, site unspecified
526.4 Inflammatory conditions of jaws
376.03 Orbital osteomyelitis

SEE ALSO

OTHER NOTES N/A

ABBREVIATIONS N/A

REFERENCES

- Santiago Restrepo C, Gimenez CR, McCarthy K. Imaging of osteomyelitis and musculoskeletal soft tissue infections: current concepts. Rheum Dis Clin North Am 2003;29(1):89-109
- Stengel D, et al. Systematic review and meta-analysis of antibiotic therapy for bone and joint infections. Lancet 2001;1(3):175-88
- Carek PJ. Diagnosis and management of osteomyelitis. Amer Fam Phys 2001;63:2413-20
- Lew DP, Waldvogel FA. Osteomyelitis. N Engl J Med 1997;336(14):999-1007
- Tavakoli M. Diagnosis and management of osteomyelitis. Decision analytic and pharmacoeconomic considerations. Pharmacoeconomics 1999;16(6):627-47
- Lipsky BA. Current approach to diabetic foot infections. Curr Infect Dis Rep 1999;1(3):253-60
- Danville T, Jacobs RF. Management of acute hematogenous osteomyelitis in children. Pediatr Infect Dis J 2004 Mar;23:255-57

Web references: 0 available at www.5mcc.com
Illustrations 1 available

Author(s):
Jeffery T. Kirchner, DO

BASICS

DESCRIPTION Death of the cellular components of bony tissue
System(s) affected: Musculoskeletal
Genetics: The underlying condition of hemoglobinopathies, especially sickle cell disease, diabetes, and type II or IV hyperlipemia are inheritable and associated with a high incidence of osteonecrosis. Other forms have no proven genetic relationship.
Incidence/Prevalence in USA: Dependent upon the underlying condition
Predominant age: 3rd to 6th decade
Predominant sex: Male > Female

SIGNS & SYMPTOMS
- The symptoms may be acute as in osteonecrosis of sickle cell disease or renal transplant. Usually insidious in other forms. Diagnosis may not be made for two years after onset of symptoms.
- Pain, the prominent symptom, is made worse with activity
- Loss of motion of the affected joint
- Stiffness (especially early morning)
- Swelling if the involved joint is superficial
- Locking may occur if a loose body has developed
- Proximal femur is the most common site and more prevalent in males in the 3rd-6th decade
- The distal femur, especially the medial femoral condyle, is the second most frequent site. This area is unique in that night pain is a prominent early symptom. Most common in females in the 6th-7th decade.
- Other sites in decreasing frequency are the proximal humerus, talus, carpal lunate (Kienböck disease) and the humeral capitulum

CAUSES
- Idiopathic
- Fractures, especially the femoral neck
- Traumatic (fractures, dislocation)
- Dislocations
- Legg-Calvé-Perthes (seen in 6-12 year age group)
- Hemoglobinopathies (especially sickle cell disease)
- Metabolic (hemoglobinopathies, alcohol, steroids, renal failure/transplantation)

RISK FACTORS
- Gaucher disease - especially likely as a postoperative infection
- Diabetes mellitus
- Alcoholism - the most frequent cause
- Type II or IV hyperlipemia
- Cortisone therapy (may be seen with Cushing disease)
- Obesity
- Oral contraceptives
- Organ transplant, especially kidney
- Pregnancy
- Decompression sickness ("bends")
- Chronic pancreatitis
- Crohn disease
- Myeloproliferative disorders
- Radiation treatment
- Rheumatoid arthritis

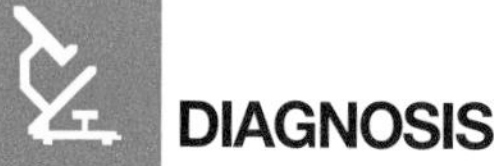

DIAGNOSIS

DIFFERENTIAL DIAGNOSIS
- Rheumatoid arthritis
- Osteoarthritis
- Femoral neck fracture
- Lumbar disk disease
- Muscle strain
- Groin injury
- Septic arthritis
- Secondary hyperparathyroidism

LABORATORY N/A

Drugs that may alter lab results: N/A

Disorders that may alter lab results: N/A

PATHOLOGICAL FINDINGS The subchondral fracture occurs during bone repair as necrotic bone is resorbed. Later, a collapse of the bone occurs with subsequent irregularities at the joint surface. This will eventually produce osteoarthritic changes.

SPECIAL TESTS Bone scan shows decreased bone uptake (sometimes increased uptake depending on the stage). Later, the uptake increases as reparative processes begin within the bone.

IMAGING
- Plain films of the epiphyseal region show arc-like subchondral radiolucent lesions, patchy lucent areas and sclerosis, osseous collapse, and preservation of the joint space. However, these abnormalities do not appear for several months after the onset of symptoms; therefore they are not a sensitive indicator of early disease. Furthermore, the initial features of osteonecrosis may simulate the aggressive pattern of bone destruction that accompanies malignancy or osteomyelitis.
- MRI will show a decreased signal intensity of the involved bone and is the most sensitive diagnostic exam

DIAGNOSTIC PROCEDURES The presence of a crescent sign is practically diagnostic (see Differential Diagnosis of osteonecrosis). It is caused by a subchondral fracture.

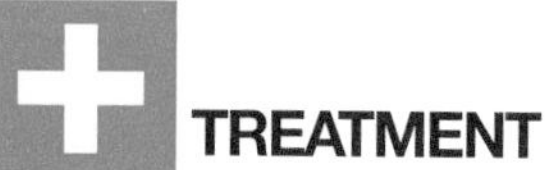

TREATMENT

APPROPRIATE HEALTH CARE Outpatient normally; inpatient if surgery indicated

GENERAL MEASURES
- The following conditions are ones that are amenable to treatment in order to decrease the accompanying incidence of osteonecrosis:
  - ◊ Alcoholism - abstinence is obvious, but quite difficult to attain
  - ◊ Dysbarism - new tables of decompression, if followed, will lower osteonecrosis incidence of divers
  - ◊ Transplant patients - decreased doses of cortisone and regulation of calcium and phosphorous metabolism
  - ◊ Sickle cell disease - treat a crisis vigorously with hydration, possible exchange transfusion and oxygenation, especially hyperbaric oxygen

SURGICAL MEASURES Bone grafts, arthroplasty, allografts and arthrodesis may be used, dependent upon the joint involved

ACTIVITY As tolerated

DIET No special diet

PATIENT EDUCATION The patient should be instructed in the use of crutches and/or canes when the lower extremity is involved. Proper use of a walking cane can decrease the pressure on the femoral head 20-30% when walking.

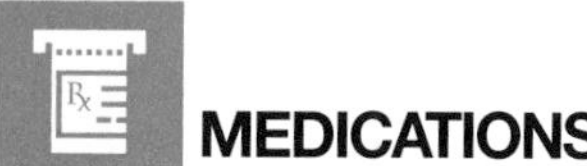

MEDICATIONS

DRUG(S) OF CHOICE

- NSAIDs - consistent with the underlying disease may be used for painful episodes
- Acetaminophen - 500 mg qid can be quite helpful in alleviating symptoms

Contraindications: See manufacturer's profile of each drug

Precautions: NSAIDs - if history of peptic ulcer is present, the use of ranitidine (Zantac) 150 mg bid or 300 mg hs can be given. Misoprostol (Cytotec) 100 μg bid will usually prevent gastritis (not needed with acetaminophen).

Significant possible interactions: See manufacturer's profile of each drug

ALTERNATIVE DRUGS

Other H2-receptor antagonists in patients with a history of peptic ulcer disease

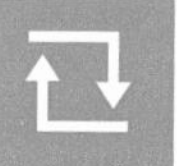

FOLLOWUP

PATIENT MONITORING

X-rays should be made every 12-18 months, more frequently if symptoms become more severe

PREVENTION/AVOIDANCE

Early diagnosis and treatment of underlying disease

POSSIBLE COMPLICATIONS

- Progression of disease
- The progression of osteonecrosis leads to osteoarthritis of the involved joint to a varying degree. Arthroplasty of the hip carries a much poorer prognosis than osteoarthritis alone. It should be postponed as long as possible.

EXPECTED COURSE/PROGNOSIS

Gaucher disease is associated with a high risk of infection following surgery

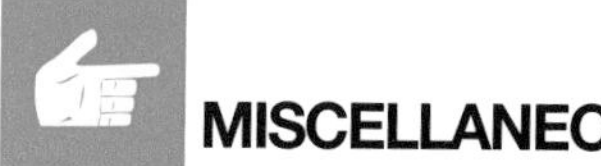

MISCELLANEOUS

ASSOCIATED CONDITIONS

N/A

AGE-RELATED FACTORS

Pediatric: Legg-Calvé-Perthes occurs in the 6-12 year age group. Prognosis is better in younger patients.

Geriatric: N/A

Others: N/A

PREGNANCY

Is a risk factor

SYNONYMS

- Idiopathic osteonecrosis
- Avascular necrosis
- Lunatomalacia, Kienböck disease
- Subchondral fracture

ICD-9-CM

730.10 Chronic osteomyelitis, site unspecified

SEE ALSO

Arthritis, osteo
Légg-Calvé-Pérthes disease

OTHER NOTES

N/A

ABBREVIATIONS

N/A

REFERENCES

- Greene WB, editor. Essentials of musculoskeletal care. 2nd ed. Rosemont, IL: American Academy of Orthopaedic Surgeons; 2001
- Ruddy S, Harris ED, Sledge CB, editors. Kelly's Textbook of Rheumatology. 6th ed. Philadelphia: WB Saunders Co; 2001
- Assuoline-Dayan Y, Chang C, Greenspan A, Shoenfeld Y, et al. Pathogenesis and natural history of osteonecrosis. Semin Arthritis Rheum 2002;32(2):94-124

Web references: 0 available at www.5mcc.com

Illustrations N/A

Author(s):
Richard Viken, MD

BASICS

DESCRIPTION A multifactorial skeletal disease characterized by severe bone loss, disruption of skeletal micro-architecture, and disturbed bone quality sufficient to predispose to atraumatic fractures of the vertebral column, upper femur, distal radius, proximal humerus, pubic rami and ribs. Five types recognized:
- Postmenopausal (Type I): The most common form in Caucasian and Asian women. Due to excessive and prolonged acceleration of bone resorption following menopausal loss of estrogen secretion.
- Involutional (Type II): Occurs in both sexes above age 75. Due to a subtle, prolonged imbalance between rates of bone resorption and formation. A mixture of Types I and II is common.
- Idiopathic: A rare form of primary osteoporosis occurring in premenopausal women and in men below age 75. Not related to secondary causes or risk factors predisposing to bone loss.
- Juvenile: A rare form of variable severity in prepubertal children. Self-limited with cessation of fractures at puberty.
- Secondary: Due to extrinsic factors

System(s) affected: Endocrine/Metabolic, Musculoskeletal

Genetics: Familial predisposition. More common in Caucasians and Orientals than in Black and Latino ethnic groups.

Incidence/Prevalence in USA:
- 30-40% cumulatively in women, 5-15% in men
- Prevalence of idiopathic and juvenile types unknown
- Secondary osteoporosis cumulatively 5-10%, both sexes

Predominant age: Elderly

Predominant sex: Female > Male

SIGNS & SYMPTOMS
- Back ache/pain; acute/chronic
- Loss of height
- Kyphosis/scoliosis
- Atraumatic fractures
- No peripheral bone deformities
- Sclerae not blue/green/grey
- Restrictive lung disease
- Gastrointestinal symptoms
- Depression, loss of self esteem
- Excess mortality, 15-20% during 1-5 years post acute fracture

CAUSES
- Postmenopausal (Type I): Hypoestrogenemia
- Involutional (Type II): Unknown
- Idiopathic: Unknown
- Juvenile: Unknown
- Secondary: Eating disorders, corticosteroid excess, rheumatoid arthritis, chronic liver/kidney disease, malabsorption syndromes, systemic mastocytosis, hyperparathyroidism, hyperthyroidism, elite athletes/ ballet dancers with hypoestrogenism, a variety of hypogonadal states, idiopathic hypercalciuria, chronic anticoagulant use, chronic anti-seizure medication and others
- Aging: Bone loss is a consequence of aging, however, osteoporosis occurs most severely in individuals who fail to achieve optimal skeletal mass at maturity or lose bone rapidly thereafter (e.g., excessive postmenopausal and/or involutional bone loss, or conditions/risk factors that increase bone loss).

RISK FACTORS
- Dietary - inadequate calcium or vitamin D; excessive phosphate/protein
- Physical - immobilization, sedentary lifestyle; elite athleticism in women leading to hypoestrogenism
- Social - alcohol, cigarettes, caffeine
- Medical - chronic diseases, malabsorption, endocrinopathies, (see also secondary osteoporosis in Description)
- Iatrogenic - corticosteroids, excess thyroid hormone replacement, chronic anticoagulant or anti-seizure medication use, chemotherapy, loop diuretics, radiation therapy
- Genetic/familial - suboptimal bone mass at maturity, "familial fast bone losers"

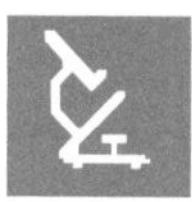

DIAGNOSIS

DIFFERENTIAL DIAGNOSIS
- Multiple myeloma
- Other neoplasms
- Osteomalacia
- Osteogenesis imperfecta tarda (Type I)
- Skeletal hyperparathyroidism (primary and secondary)
- Hyperthyroidism
- Mastocytosis (rare)

LABORATORY
- CBC, multi-panel tests usually normal
- Alkaline phosphatase (bone specific and total) may be transiently increased following fractures
- Serum and/or urine protein electrophoresis normal
- Thyroid function tests and urinary free cortisol normal in primary types
- Serum osteocalcin, if high, indicates high turnover type
- Urine calcium normal (except if idiopathic hypercalciuria)
- Serum and urinary pyridinoline and N- and C-telopeptide collagen crosslinks, if high, indicate high turnover type

Drugs that may alter lab results:
- Hepatotoxins: changes in total alkaline phosphatase
- Estrogens: changes in thyroid function tests

Disorders that may alter lab results:
- Multiple myeloma or other neoplasms
- Osteomalacia
- Hyperparathyroidism
- Hyperthyroidism

PATHOLOGICAL FINDINGS
- Reduced skeletal mass, trabecular bone more so than cortical bone. Thinned/loss of trabecular connections.
- Osteoclast and osteoblast number variable
- No evidence of other metabolic bone diseases and no increase in unmineralized osteoid
- Marrow normal or atrophic

SPECIAL TESTS N/A

IMAGING
- Plain film "early" changes: increased width of intervertebral spaces, relative accentuation of cortical plates, vertical striations of vertebral bodies
- Plain film "late" changes: cortical plate fractures, vertebral compression, wedge and crush fractures, peripheral fractures at ends of long bones, rib fractures
- Bone scan: increased uptake at previous fracture sites
- Bone mineral density (BMD). Data Analysis: Normative data for DXA, QUS, and QCT are incorporated into each instrument, allowing calculation of T and Z scores. T scores represent the number of standard deviations (SD) a measurement deviates from the mean for young normal (age 25-40) controls of same sex and in some cases, ethnic group. T scores indicate severity of bone loss as follows: T scores of ±1 SD are normal; a T score between -1 and -2 indicates an osteopenic state; T scores below -2 indicate established osteoporosis with high risk of fracture. Z scores indicate number of standard deviations compared to age matched controls; are not generally used to determine severity or need for treatment.
  - ◊ Whole body DXA: BMD of whole body
  - ◊ Central DXA: lumbar spine, upper femur
  - ◊ Peripheral (p) DXA: BMD of the calcaneus, distal tibia, and distal radius. Partial correlation with whole body and central DXA but does not accurately quantitate changes from baseline during treatment.
  - ◊ Quantitative CT (QCT): Quantitates either trabecular or cortical bone mass (or both) of lumbar spine. Use with other sites in development.
  - ◊ Quantitative ultrasound (QUS): Uses US attenuation at calcaneus. Correlates partially with whole body, central and peripheral DXA, but does not reflect changes during treatment. May be influenced by microarchitecture as well as BMD.

DIAGNOSTIC PROCEDURES Bone biopsy needed rarely, to rule out neoplasms and other metabolic bone diseases. Sometimes used to quantitate bone loss, utilizing quantitative histomorphometric techniques.

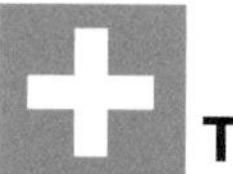

TREATMENT

APPROPRIATE HEALTH CARE
- Usually outpatient
- Inpatient care for acute back pain, especially for new vertebral fractures and for acute treatment of upper femoral and pelvic fractures
- Nursing home or home care may be needed following peripheral fractures

GENERAL MEASURES As required by pain and disability, e.g., heat, analgesics, physical therapy. Decrease falls. Avoid excessive psychotropic effects of drugs.

SURGICAL MEASURES N/A

ACTIVITY
- Maintain ambulation, walking 1 mile twice a day (if possible) swimming, tricycling
- Avoid exercises and maneuvers that increase compressive forces and mechanical stress on spine and peripheral bone sites
- Rehabilitation procedures for back muscle spasm, to increase agility (e.g., decrease falls), and encourage ambulation

DIET
- Reducing diet if overweight
- Calcium intake 1500 mg/day from all sources, if not hypercalciuric or with past medical history of calcium stones
- Avoid excess phosphate or protein intake, i.e., avoid phosphoric-acid-containing beverages and excess meat intake
- 600-1000 IU vitamin D daily from all sources

PATIENT EDUCATION Teaching resources and patient literature available from National Osteoporosis Foundation, 2100 M St., Suite 602, Washington, DC 20037

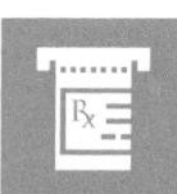

MEDICATIONS

DRUG(S) OF CHOICE
- Alendronate (Fosamax) 10 mg q AM on an empty stomach or 70 mg once a week
- Risedronate (Actonel) 5 mg q AM on an empty stomach
- Calcitonin (Miacalcin Nasal Spray) 200 IU intranasally; 1 puff per day, alternating nostrils or injectable calcitonin (Miacalcin) 100 IU SC qd or qod preferred, 50 IU qd or 3 times a week may be effective in high turnover types. Should be used in conjunction with adequate calcium and vitamin D.
- Raloxifene (Evista) 60 mg q day, a selective estrogen receptor modulator (SERM) with positive effects on BMD and fracture risk, but no stimulatory action on breast or uterus. Relative contraindications include hot flashes, history of thromboembolic conditions.

Contraindications:
- Calcitonins - none except allergy
- For alendronate and risedronate, esophageal dysfunction, severe upper GI symptoms, GERD
- HRT absolute - past medical history of endometrial or breast cancer (with estrogen receptors) or premalignant breast conditions
- HRT relative - medical history uncontrolled hypertension, thromboembolic conditions, edematous conditions, endometriosis, migraine, severe hepatic dysfunction; family history of breast or uterine cancer, breast cancer (without estrogen receptors)
- Raloxifene: past history thromboembolism disease (deep vein thrombosis)

Precautions:
- Calcitonins: none
- HRT: annual gynecology exam with Pap smear or endometrial biopsy, breast exam and mammography. Check BP twice a week during initiation of HRT.
- Alendronate and risedronate: take on empty stomach in the morning with 1-2 glasses of water. Nothing by mouth and remain seated or standing for 30 minutes to 1 hour.
- Raloxifene: may cause increased hot flashes, leg cramps

Significant possible interactions:
- Calcitonin - nasal decongestants
- Alendronate and risedronate - do not take other medications for 60 minutes after drug intake

ALTERNATIVE DRUGS
- Other bisphosphonates: etidronate (Didronel), pamidronate (Aredia) - inhibitors of bone resorption (not FDA approved)
- Sodium fluoride: stimulates bone formation, but effects on cortical bone uncertain. Sustained release preparations may be better tolerated.
- Tamoxifen: has some estrogen effects on bone without potential for breast stimulation. May stimulate uterus and cause other side effects.
- Hormone replacement therapy (HRT): reduce the rate of bone loss, but controversial
  - ◊ Estrogen-medroxyprogesterone (PremPro) q day
  - ◊ Estrogen, conjugated (Premarin) 0.625 mg q day, if post-hysterectomy. 0.3 mg q day is advocated as effective, but is not approved at this dose.
  - ◊ Estradiol (Estraderm) 0.05 mg q/day; patch applied biweekly; other estrogen patches may require only one weekly application
- Under study: androgens/anabolics, parathyroid hormone analogues, statins, other SERMs, other bisphosphonates, phytoestrogens

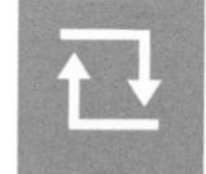

FOLLOWUP

PATIENT MONITORING
- Bimonthly initially, then q 6 months
- Periodic multiphasic screening, annual gynecological exam, breast exam, and mammography
- Annual or every other year BMD using same technique
- Repeat x-rays for acute pain, suspected fractures
- Serial serum or urinary pyridinoline or N- or C- telopeptide collagen cross-links, in selected patients

PREVENTION/AVOIDANCE
- General guidelines: Diet, exercise, calcium, vitamin D
- Prevention during the osteopenic phase (prolonged, usually asymptomatic phase prior to fracturing)
  - ◊ Identification of osteopenia
  - ◊ Correction of treatable medical conditions and other risk factors; will also help achieve optimal skeletal mass during development
  - ◊ HRT if postmenopausal and no absolute contraindications
  - ◊ Low dose alendronate (Fosamax) 5 mg qd, if no contraindications
  - ◊ Risedronate (Actonel), same dose (5 mg daily) as for treatment
  - ◊ Raloxifene (Evista) 60 mg qd

POSSIBLE COMPLICATIONS
- Severe disabling pain
- Dorsal/lumbar neurologic deficits secondary to vertebral fracture (rare)
- Respiratory and GI symptoms
- Invalidism/death secondary to complications

EXPECTED COURSE/PROGNOSIS
- With treatment, 80% of patients stabilize skeletal manifestations; increase bone mass, increase mobility, and have reduced pain
- 15% of vertebral and 20-40% upper femoral fractures may lead to chronic care and/or premature death

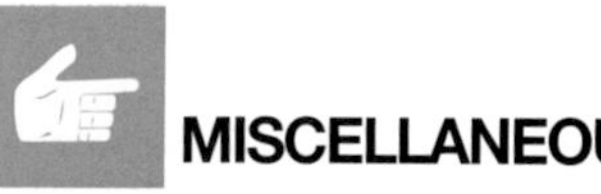

MISCELLANEOUS

ASSOCIATED CONDITIONS
- Corticosteroid excess
- Rheumatoid arthritis
- Chronic liver/kidney disease
- Malabsorption syndromes
- Systemic mastocytosis
- Hyperparathyroidism; Hyperthyroidism including iatrogenic
- Various hypogonadal states
- Seizure disorders under treatment
- Eating disorders

AGE-RELATED FACTORS
Pediatric: Juvenile osteoporosis not discussed herein
Geriatric: Postmenopausal/involutional/mixed types
Others: Primary types uncommon in African Americans. Patients with British, North European, Scandinavian, and Asian ancestry are most susceptible.

PREGNANCY Rare acute osteoporosis of pregnancy, not discussed herein

SYNONYMS N/A

ICD-9-CM
733.00 Osteoporosis, unspecified

SEE ALSO
Arthritis, rheumatoid (RA)
Cushing disease and syndrome
Hyperthyroidism
Malnutrition, protein-calorie

OTHER NOTES N/A

ABBREVIATIONS
BMD = bone mineral density
HRT = hormone replacement therapy

REFERENCES

- Lane JM, Russell L, Khan SN. Osteoporosis. Clinical Orthopaed & Related Research 2000;372:139-50
- Byers RJ, Hoyland JA, Braidman IP. Osteoporosis in men: a cellular endocrine perspective of an increasingly common clinical problem. J Endocrinol 2001;168(3):353-62

Web references: 1 available at www.5mcc.com
Illustrations N/A

Author(s):
Mark R. Dambro, MD

BASICS

DESCRIPTION Inflammation of the external auditory canal
- Acute diffuse otitis externa - the most common form, an infectious process usually bacterial, occasionally fungal (10%)
- Acute circumscribed otitis externa - synonymous with furuncle. Associated with infection of the hair follicle.
- Chronic otitis externa - same as acute diffuse, but of longer duration (greater than 6 weeks)
- Eczematous otitis externa - may accompany typical atopic eczema or other primary skin conditions
- Necrotizing "malignant" otitis externa - an infection which extends into the deeper tissues adjacent to the canal. May include osteomyelitis and cellulitis. Rare in children.

System(s) affected: Skin/Exocrine
Genetics: N/A
Incidence/Prevalence in USA:
- Unknown; incidence is higher in the summer months and warm, wet climates
- Acute, chronic and eczematous - common
- Necrotizing - uncommon

Predominant age: All ages
Predominant sex: Male = Female

SIGNS & SYMPTOMS
- Itching
- Plugging of the ear
- Otalgia
- Periauricular adenitis
- Erythematous canal
- Purulent discharge
- Eczema of pinna
- Cranial nerve involvement (VII, IX-XII) (rare)

CAUSES
- Acute diffuse otitis externa
  - ◊ Traumatized external canal (eg, from use of cotton tip swab)
  - ◊ Bacterial infection (90%) - pseudomonas (67% cases); staphylococcus; streptococcus; gram negative rods
  - ◊ Fungal infection (10%) - aspergillus (90% cases); Candida, Phycomycetes; Rhizopus; actinomyces; Penicillium
- Chronic otitis externa
  - ◊ Bacterial infection - pseudomonas
- Eczematous otitis externa (associated with primary skin disorder):
  - ◊ Eczema
  - ◊ Seborrhea
  - ◊ Psoriasis
  - ◊ Neurodermatitis
  - ◊ Contact dermatitis
  - ◊ Purulent otitis media
  - ◊ Sensitivity to topical medications
- Necrotizing otitis externa
  - ◊ Invasive bacterial infection - pseudomonas
  - ◊ Associated with Immunosuppression

RISK FACTORS
- Acute and chronic otitis externa
  - ◊ Traumatization of external canal
  - ◊ Swimming
  - ◊ Hot humid weather
  - ◊ Use of a hearing aid
- Eczematous
  - ◊ Primary skin disorder
- Necrotizing otitis externa in adults
  - ◊ Elderly
  - ◊ Diabetes mellitus
  - ◊ Debilitating disease
  - ◊ AIDS
- Necrotizing otitis externa in children (rare)
  - ◊ Leukopenia
  - ◊ Malnutrition
  - ◊ Diabetes mellitus
  - ◊ Diabetes insipidus

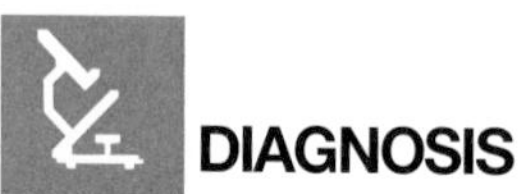

DIAGNOSIS

DIFFERENTIAL DIAGNOSIS
- Idiopathic ear pain
- Hearing loss
- Cranial nerve palsy (VII, IX-XII) with necrotizing otitis externa
- Wisdom teeth eruption
- Basal cell or squamous cell carcinoma

LABORATORY Gram stain and culture of canal discharge (occasionally helpful)

Drugs that may alter lab results: Antibiotic pretreatment

Disorders that may alter lab results: N/A

PATHOLOGICAL FINDINGS
- Acute and chronic otitis externa - desquamation of superficial epithelium of external canal with infection
- Eczematous otitis externa - pathologic findings consistent with primary skin disorder, secondary infection on occasion
- Necrotizing otitis externa - vasculitis, thrombosis and necrosis of involved tissues; osteomyelitis

SPECIAL TESTS N/A

IMAGING Radiologic evaluation of deep tissues in necrotizing otitis externa with high resolution CT, MRI, gallium scan and bone scan

DIAGNOSTIC PROCEDURES N/A

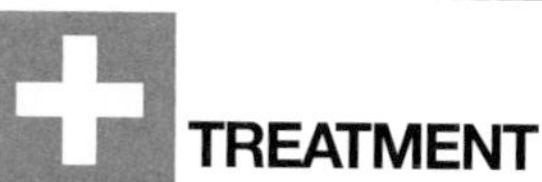

TREATMENT

APPROPRIATE HEALTH CARE Outpatient, except for resistant cases and necrotizing otitis externa

GENERAL MEASURES
- Thorough cleansing of external canal with suction
- Narcotic analgesics
- Antipruritic and antihistamines (eczematous form)
- Ear wick (Pope) for nearly occluded ear canal

SURGICAL MEASURES For necrotizing otitis externa or furuncle

ACTIVITY No restrictions

DIET No restrictions

PATIENT EDUCATION Discuss prevention

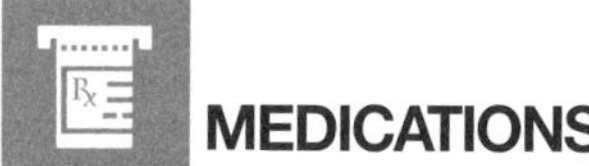

MEDICATIONS

DRUG(S) OF CHOICE
- Acute bacterial and chronic otitis externa
  - ◊ Topical therapy for approximately 5-7 days
    - 2% acetic acid (VoSol HC) fill ear canal qid OR
    - Neomycin-polymyxin B-hydrocortisone (Cortisporin); if the tympanic membrane is ruptured use the suspension, otherwise the solution can be used
  - ◊ Ciprofloxacin (Cipro) 0.3% and hydrocortisone suspension 3-4 drops BID
  - ◊ Ofloxacin (Floxin Otic) 0.3% solution 3-4 drops BID
  - ◊ Oral antibiotics are only indicated if there is associated otitis media or cellulitis of the outer ear
  - ◊ Analgesics: acetaminophen-hydrocodone (Vicodin)
- Fungal otitis externa
  - ◊ Topical therapy anti-yeast for Candida or yeast
    - 2% acetic acid 3-4 drops qid
    - Clotrimazole 1% solution
    - Itraconazole oral
  - ◊ Parenteral antifungal therapy - amphotericin B
  - ◊ Patients with Ramsay Hunt syndrome: acyclovir IV
- Eczematous otitis externa - topical therapy
  - ◊ Acetic acid 2% in aluminum acetate
  - ◊ 5% aluminum acetate (Burow's solution)
  - ◊ Steroid cream, lotion, ointment (e.g., triamcinolone 0.1% solution)
  - ◊ Antibacterial, if superinfected
- Necrotizing otitis externa
  - ◊ Parenteral antibiotics - antistaphylococcus and antipseudomonal
  - ◊ 4-6 weeks of therapy
  - ◊ Quinolones orally for 2-4 weeks

Contraindications:
- Hypersensitivity to topical or parenteral therapy
- Renal or hepatic failure when using amphotericin B

Precautions:
- Dosage adjustment for amphotericin B in patients with renal or hepatic dysfunction
- Sensitivity with neomycin

Significant possible interactions:
- Hypokalemia associated with amphotericin B may lead to digitalis toxicity
- Concurrent administration of nonabsorbable anions, such as carbenicillin, may exacerbate hypokalemia

ALTERNATIVE DRUGS
Azole antifungals for fungal otitis externa

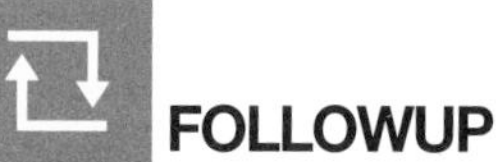

FOLLOWUP

PATIENT MONITORING
- Acute otitis externa
  - ◊ 48 hours after therapy instituted to assess improvement
  - ◊ At the end of treatment
- Chronic otitis externa
  - ◊ Every 2-3 weeks for repeated cleansing of canal
  - ◊ May require alterations in topical medication, including antibiotics and steroids
- Necrotizing otitis externa
  - ◊ Daily monitoring in hospital for extension of infection
  - ◊ Baseline auditory and vestibular testing at beginning and end of therapy

PREVENTION/AVOIDANCE
- Avoid prolonged exposure to moisture
- Utilize preventive antiseptics
  - ◊ Acidifying solutions with 2% acetic acid diluted 50/50 with water or isopropyl alcohol or 2% acetic acid with aluminum acetate (less irritating) after swimming
- Treat predisposing skin conditions
- Eliminate self-inflicted trauma to canal
- Diagnose and treat underlying systemic conditions
- Ear plugs
- Avoid trauma with swabs, etc.

POSSIBLE COMPLICATIONS
- Mainly a problem with necrotizing otitis externa. May spread to infect contiguous bone and CNS structures.
- Acute otitis externa may spread to pinna causing a chondritis

EXPECTED COURSE/PROGNOSIS
- Acute otitis externa - rapid response to therapy with total resolution
- Chronic otitis externa - with repeated cleansing and antibiotic therapy the majority of cases will resolve. Occasionally, surgical intervention is required for resistant cases.
- Eczematous otitis externa - resolution will occur with control of the primary skin condition
- Necrotizing otitis externa - can usually be managed with debridement and antipseudomonal antibiotics. Recurrence rate is 100% when treatment is inadequate. Surgical intervention may be necessary in resistant cases or if there is cranial nerve involvement. Mortality rate is significant, probably secondary to the underlying disease.

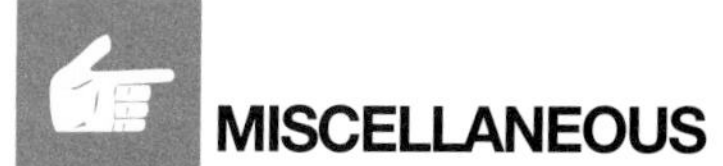

MISCELLANEOUS

ASSOCIATED CONDITIONS N/A

AGE-RELATED FACTORS N/A
Pediatric: N/A
Geriatric: N/A
Others: N/A

PREGNANCY N/A

SYNONYMS
- Swimmer's ear

ICD-9-CM
380.10 Infective otitis externa, unspecified

SEE ALSO
Ramsay Hunt syndrome, Type 1

OTHER NOTES N/A

ABBREVIATIONS N/A

REFERENCES

- Sander R. Otitis externa: a practical guide to treatment and prevention. Am Fam Physician 2001;63(5):927-36, 941-2
- Barker LR, Burton JR, Zieve PD, et al. editors. Principles of Ambulatory Medicine. 6th ed. Philadelphia: Lippincott Williams & Wilkins; 2003. p. 1689-90

Web references: 0 available at www.5mcc.com
Illustrations N/A

Author(s):
Douglas S. Parks, MD

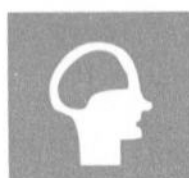

BASICS

DESCRIPTION Infection or inflammation of the middle ear
- Acute otitis media (AOM): Usually a bacterial infection accompanied by viral upper respiratory infection; rapid onset of signs and symptoms
- Recurrent AOM: 3 or more AOM in 6 months, or 4 or more AOM in 1 year
- Otitis media with effusion (OME): Persistent inflammation manifested as asymptomatic middle ear fluid that follows AOM or arises without prior AOM
- Chronic otitis media with or without cholesteatoma

System(s) affected: Nervous
Genetics: May be influenced by skull configuration or immunological defects
Incidence/Prevalence in USA: (Incidence) By age 7 years 93% of children have 1 or more AOM; 39% have 6 or more AOM; after AOM 10 to 20% still have OME 3 months later
Predominant age: Peak incidence age 6-18 months; declines after age 7 years; rare in adults. 75% of children have at least one episode by age 3.
Predominant sex: Male > Female (for AOM and recurrent AOM)

SIGNS & SYMPTOMS
- AOM:
  - ◊ Earache
  - ◊ Fever, although more often afebrile
  - ◊ Accompanying URI symptoms
  - ◊ Decreased hearing
  - ◊ Otorrhea if eardrum perforated
  - ◊ Unusual irritability
  - ◊ Difficulty in sleeping
  - ◊ Tugging at the ear
  - ◊ Loss of balance
  - ◊ Eardrum mobility decreased (as observed by pneumatic otoscopy)
  - ◊ Eardrum bulging, opaque, often yellowish or inflamed. Redness alone is not a reliable sign.
- AOM in infants:
  - ◊ May cause no symptoms in the first few months of life
  - ◊ Irritability is sometimes the only indication of earache
  - ◊ Eardrum bulging, opaque, often yellowish or inflamed. Redness alone not a reliable sign.
- OME:
  - ◊ Usually asymptomatic
  - ◊ Decreased hearing probably universal, but not always measurable, and rarely appreciated by parents
  - ◊ Eardrum often dull, but not bulging
  - ◊ Eardrum mobility decreased (as observed by pneumatic otoscopy)

CAUSES
- AOM, bacterial: A preceding viral upper respiratory infection produces eustachian tube dysfunction that is thought to promote bacterial infection via eustachian tube. Bacteriology:
  - ◊ Pneumococci: 30-35%
  - ◊ *Haemophilus influenzae*: 20-25%; 40% of these produce beta-lactamases that hydrolyze amoxicillin and some cephalosporins
  - ◊ *Moraxella (Branhamella) catarrhalis*: 10-15%; 90% of these produce beta-lactamases that hydrolyze amoxicillin and some cephalosporins
  - ◊ Group A streptococci: 3%
  - ◊ *Staphylococcus aureus*: 1-2%
  - ◊ Sterile/non-pathogens: 25-30%
- AOM, viral: Less than 10% of AOM infections are caused primarily by viruses (RSV, Parainfluenza, Influenza, enteroviruses, Adenovirus).
- OME:
  - ◊ 20-40% silent bacterial infection
  - ◊ Eustachian tube dysfunction thought important
  - ◊ Allergic causes rarely substantiated

RISK FACTORS
- Bottle feeds while supine
- Day care
- Formula feeding
- Smoking in household
- Male gender
- Family history of middle ear disease
- AOM in 1st year of life is a risk factor for recurrent AOM
- Sibling history of otitis media

DIAGNOSIS

DIFFERENTIAL DIAGNOSIS
- Tympanosclerosis
- Redness due to crying
- Earache with a normal ear exam may be caused by referred pain from the jaw or teeth

LABORATORY WBC higher in bacterial AOM than in sterile AOM

Drugs that may alter lab results: N/A

Disorders that may alter lab results: N/A

PATHOLOGICAL FINDINGS N/A

SPECIAL TESTS
- To document the presence of middle ear fluid - tympanometry, acoustic reflex measurement or acoustic reflectometry
- Hearing testing helpful to assess the need for early surgical intervention in OME
- Nasopharyngoscopy

IMAGING N/A

DIAGNOSTIC PROCEDURES Tympanocentesis for microbiologic diagnosis recommended for treatment failures, may be followed by myringotomy

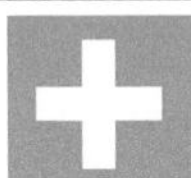

TREATMENT

APPROPRIATE HEALTH CARE Outpatient except when surgery is indicated

GENERAL MEASURES
- AOM: outpatient except for febrile infants < 2 months
- May use watchful waiting approach, treating symptoms without antibiotics for first 2-3 days. If symptoms persist, then amoxicillin is first line treatment.
- OME: presence of effusion without signs or symptoms of acute infection does not require antibiotics for initial treatment
- Antihistamine-decongestant preparations offer no added benefit to resolution of symptoms

SURGICAL MEASURES
- OME: Referral for surgery if: > 4-6 months bilateral OME, and/or > 6 months unilateral OME, and/or hearing loss > 25 decibels
- Recurrent AOM: Referral for surgery if > 2 or 3 AOM while on chemoprophylaxis. Tympanostomy tubes and adenoidectomy/adenotonsillectomy effective surgical procedures for OME and recurrent AOM, but not in all cases.

ACTIVITY No restrictions

DIET No special diet

PATIENT EDUCATION Avoidance of risk factors when possible

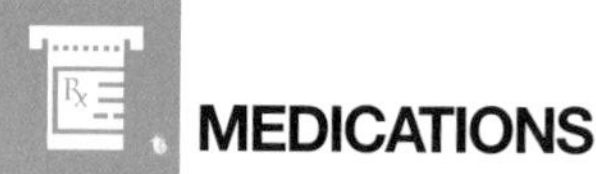

MEDICATIONS

DRUG(S) OF CHOICE

- AOM: Amoxicillin 40-45 mg/kg bid >age 2 years, 5-7 day course with no complications; probably the most effective of penicillins/cephalosporins against relatively resistant (but not highly resistant) pneumococci.
- Recurrent AOM: Only consider antibiotic prophylaxis for recurrent AOM (> 3 distinct, well documented episodes in 6 months). Amoxicillin 20 mg/kg daily for 3-6 months or until summer.
- OME: Antihistamines and decongestants ineffective, indications for steroids not defined, amoxicillin promotes resolution in 10-15% but effect is usually transitory - not recommended, no long term benefit.
- Note: if patient not toxic appearing, may choose to treat with antipyrine-benzocaine (Auralgan) drops and acetaminophen (Tylenol) as long as close follow up available. 81% of patients not treated with medication resolve.

Contraindications: Allergy to penicillins
Precautions: Refer to manufacturer's profile of each drug
Significant possible interactions: Refer to manufacturer's profile of each drug

ALTERNATIVE DRUGS

- Alternative drugs are indicated for the following AOM patients:
  - ◊ Patients with penicillin allergy
  - ◊ Persistent symptoms after 48-72 hrs of amoxicillin
  - ◊ AOM within 1 month of amoxicillin therapy
  - ◊ AOM with severe earache
  - ◊ Infants less than 6 months with high fever
  - ◊ Immunocompromised hosts
  - ◊ AOM due to *Chlamydia trachomatis* will respond to macrolides and sulfonamides
  - ◊ AOM due to *Mycoplasma pneumoniae* will respond to macrolides
- AOM: Alternative drugs (treat for 10 days):
  - ◊ Amoxicillin-clavulanate (Augmentin) 40 mg/kg/day of amoxicillin component tid - effective against resistant *H. influenzae* and *M. catarrhalis*, amoxicillin component effective against relatively resistant pneumococci
  - ◊ Cefaclor (Ceclor) 40 mg/kg/day bid or tid is less effective than other alternatives
  - ◊ Cefixime (Suprax) 8 mg/kg/day bid or single daily dose - effective against resistant *H. influenzae* and *M. catarrhalis* less effective than amoxicillin for pneumococci
  - ◊ Cefpodoxime (Vantin) 10 mg/kg/day bid - less effective in vivo against H. influenzae than other drugs
  - ◊ Ceftriaxone (Rocephin) 50 mg/kg IM single dose - effective against major pathogens, but expensive and painful so reserved for sick infants
  - ◊ Clarithromycin (Biaxin) 15 mg/kg/day divided bid - not effective in vivo against H. influenzae
  - ◊ Trimethoprim-sulfamethoxazole (Septra, Bactrim) 8 mg TMP/kg/day divided bid: up to 30% of pneumococci are resistant
  - ◊ Erythromycin-sulfisoxazole (Pediazole) 40 mg erythromycin component/kg/day divided qid - some strains of pneumococci are resistant
- Recurrent AOM:
  - ◊ Sulfisoxazole 75 mg/kg single daily dose for penicillin allergic patients
- Analgesics and antipyretics as needed

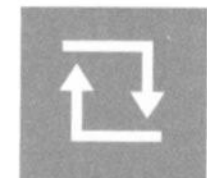

FOLLOWUP

PATIENT MONITORING

- AOM: Otoscopic examination 4 weeks after diagnosis
- OME: Monthly otoscopic or tympanometric exams as long as OME persists

PREVENTION/AVOIDANCE

- Breast-feeding decreases incidence of AOM
- Eliminate cigarette smoking in the household
- The heptavalent pneumococcal conjugate vaccine (PCV-78) [with nontoxic diphtheria-toxin analogue carrier protein, CRM197] is safe and efficacious in the prevention of acute otitis media caused by the serotypes included in the vaccine.

POSSIBLE COMPLICATIONS

- AOM: Perforation/otorrhea, acute mastoiditis, facial nerve paralysis, otitic hydrocephalus, meningitis, hearing impairment
- OME: Hearing loss, speech and language disabilities may occur with hearing impairment
- Recurrent AOM and OME: Atrophy and scarring of eardrum, chronic perforation and otorrhea, cholesteatoma, permanent hearing loss, chronic mastoiditis, brain abscess and other intracranial suppurative complications

EXPECTED COURSE/PROGNOSIS

- Children treated immediately with antibiotics had one less day of symptoms
- Symptoms of AOM (mostly otalgia) spontaneously resolve in 2/3 of children by 24 hours and in 80% at 2-7 days (NNT=17)
- AOM: Symptoms usually improve in 48-72 hrs; OME following AOM resolved in 90% by 3 months
- OME: Approximately 50% resolve after 8 weeks of observation
- Recurrent AOM and OME: Usually subsides in school age children; only a small percentage have complications

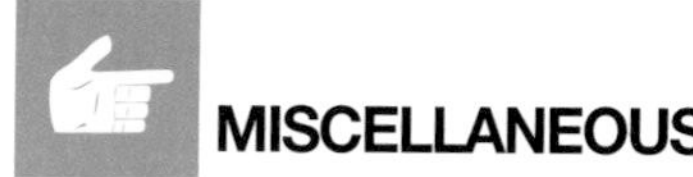

MISCELLANEOUS

ASSOCIATED CONDITIONS

- Upper respiratory infection
- Bacteremia
- Meningitis
- Allergies

AGE-RELATED FACTORS

Pediatric: Primarily a pediatric disease
Geriatric: N/A
Others: N/A

PREGNANCY N/A

SYNONYMS

- Secretory otitis media
- Serous otitis media

ICD-9-CM

381.00 Acute nonsuppurative otitis media, unspecified
382.00 Acute suppurative otitis media without spontaneous rupture of ear drum
382.9 Unspecified otitis media

SEE ALSO

OTHER NOTES In first few months of infancy, the eardrum is normally at an angle and less mobile in older adults

ABBREVIATIONS

AOM = acute otitis media
OM = otitis media
OME = otitis media with effusion
PCV-7 = heptavalent pneumococcal conjugate vaccine

REFERENCES

- Rosenfield RM, Vertrees JE, Carr J, et al. Clinical efficacy of antimicrobial drugs for acute otitis media: meta analysis of 5400 children from 33 randomized trials. J Pediatr 1994;124:355-67
- Stool SE, Berg AO, Bernan S, et al. Otitis media with effusion in young children. Clinical practice guideline. AHCPR Publication no 94-0622, 1994
- Kozyrsky AL, Hildes-Ripstein GE, et al. Treatment of acute otitis media with a shortened course of antibiotics. JAMA 1998;279(21):1736-41
- Eskola J, Kilpi T, Palmu A, et al. Efficacy of a pneumococcal conjugate vaccine against acute otitis media. N Engl J Med 2001;344(6):403-9
- McConaghy JR. The evaluation and treatment of children with acute otitis media. J Fam Pract 2001;50(5):457-9, 463-5

Web references: 3 available at www.5mcc.com
Illustrations N/A

Author(s):
J. C. Chava-Zimmerman, MD

Otosclerosis (otospongiosis)

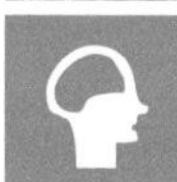

BASICS

DESCRIPTION A primary bone dyscrasia involving the otic capsule. It is the leading cause of conductive hearing loss in adults.

- Histologic otosclerosis: Asymptomatic form in which abnormal bone spares vital structures of the ear
- Clinical otosclerosis: Abnormal spongy bone involves ossicular chain or other structures leading to altered physiology

System(s) affected: Nervous

Genetics:

- 60% of those affected give positive family history
- Appears to be transmitted by autosomal dominant gene with variable penetrance

Incidence/Prevalence in USA:

- 4-8% among Caucasians; 1% among African-Americans (histologic form)
- Caucasians 5000/100,000; Blacks 1000/100,000 (histologic form)

Predominant age: Clinical onset usually in early 20's. Peak incidence fourth and fifth decades.

Predominant sex: Female > Male (2:1)

SIGNS & SYMPTOMS

- Progressive conductive hearing loss, usually with well preserved speech discrimination. May have sensorineural hearing loss with cochlear involvement.
- Carhart's notch: A dip in bone conductive threshold at 2000 Hz. on audiometric testing
- Schwartze's sign: Reddish hue on promontory upon otoscopic examination
- Patients often soft spoken and aware they seem to hear better in noisy environments

CAUSES Unknown; fluoride metabolism felt by some authorities to play a role in etiology

RISK FACTORS Unknown

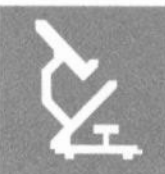

DIAGNOSIS

DIFFERENTIAL DIAGNOSIS

- Chronic suppurative otitis media
- Serous otitis media
- External auditory canal occlusion
- Ossicular chain disruption
- Congenital fixation of stapes
- Presbycusis
- Advanced otosclerosis mimics sensorineural deafness

LABORATORY N/A

Drugs that may alter lab results: N/A

Disorders that may alter lab results: N/A

PATHOLOGICAL FINDINGS

- Gross: Off-white to reddish bone formation, most often located anterior to the oval window and extending to involve the stapedial footplate. Sometimes covers entire oval window (obliterative). May be found anywhere in otic capsule. Bilateral in 75% of cases.
- Micro: "Spongy" appearing bone with increased vascular spaces. Osteoblasts and osteoclasts are plentiful.

SPECIAL TESTS Tuning fork and audiometric testing for conductive and/or sensorineural hearing loss. Will lateralize to more impaired ear with Weber's test.

IMAGING Coaxial or computerized tomography sometimes helpful

DIAGNOSTIC PROCEDURES N/A

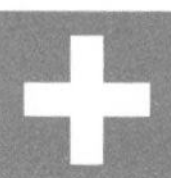

TREATMENT

APPROPRIATE HEALTH CARE Inpatient for surgery. Outpatient if surgery not feasible.

GENERAL MEASURES Hearing aids

SURGICAL MEASURES

- Surgical correction (stapedectomy): Usually involves mobilization or removal of the stapedial foot plate with placement of a stapes prosthesis. Recent procedural innovations have involved use of lasers.
- Relative indications for surgery include: Negative Rinne's test (air-bone audiometric gap at least 20 dB); bilateral involvement

ACTIVITY No restrictions

DIET No special diet

PATIENT EDUCATION

- Because speech discrimination is usually preserved, patients should be advised of the possible benefit from hearing aids (as an alternative or adjunct to surgery)
- Mayo Foundation for Medical Education and Research, Section of Patient and Health Education, Sieber Subway, Rochester, MN 55905, (507)284-8140

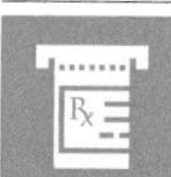

MEDICATIONS

DRUG(S) OF CHOICE No specific drug therapy but sodium fluoride, vitamin D and calcium gluconate have been tried, especially in cases of predominantly sensorineural hearing loss
Contraindications: Refer to manufacturer's literature
Precautions: Refer to manufacturer's literature
Significant possible interactions: Refer to manufacturer's literature

ALTERNATIVE DRUGS N/A

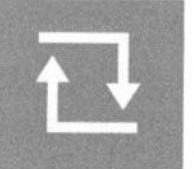

FOLLOWUP

PATIENT MONITORING Interval audiometric testing

PREVENTION/AVOIDANCE N/A

POSSIBLE COMPLICATIONS Surgical risks include chorda tympani nerve injury, tympanic membrane laceration, ossicular chain disruption, otitis media and externa, labyrinthitis, granuloma formation, perilymph fistulae, and total deafness ("dead ear")

EXPECTED COURSE/PROGNOSIS
Progressive hearing loss if not treated. Surgery improves hearing by at least 15 dB in 90% of cases.

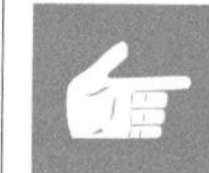

MISCELLANEOUS

ASSOCIATED CONDITIONS
- Van der Hoeve's syndrome (rare triad of osteogenesis imperfecta, blue sclera, and otospongiosis)
- Tinnitus
- Vertigo

AGE-RELATED FACTORS
Pediatric: N/A
Geriatric: Important differential diagnosis for presbycusis
Others: N/A

PREGNANCY Progression may accelerate during pregnancy. Some women first notice hearing loss at this time.

SYNONYMS N/A

ICD-9-CM
387.9 Otosclerosis, unspecified

SEE ALSO
Hearing loss

OTHER NOTES N/A

ABBREVIATIONS N/A

REFERENCES

- English GM: Otolaryngology: A Textbook. New York, Harper & Rowe, 1976
- Lee KJ: Essential Otolaryngology: Head & Neck Surgery. 4th Ed. New Hyde Park, NY, Medical Examination Pub. Co., 1987
- Weber PC, Klein AJ. Hearing loss. Med Clin North Am 1999;83(1):125-37

Web references: 0 available at www.5mcc.com
Illustrations N/A

Author(s):
Jeffrey D. Wolfrey, MD

BASICS

DESCRIPTION A variety of malignancies that arise from the epithelium (85-90%), stromal cells, or germ cells, or are metastatic to the ovary. These include:
- Epithelial:
  - ◊ Serous (Fallopian tube-like epithelium)
  - ◊ Mucinous (Cervical and GI mucinous epithelium)
  - ◊ Endometrioid (Endometrial epithelium)
  - ◊ Clear cell (Mesonephroid)
  - ◊ Brenner (Transitional cell epithelium)
  - ◊ Carcinosarcoma and mixed mesodermal
- Stromal:
  - ◊ Granulosa cell tumor
  - ◊ Theca cell tumor
  - ◊ Sertoli-Leydig cell tumors
  - ◊ Gynandroblastoma
  - ◊ Lipid cell tumor
- Germ cell:
  - ◊ Teratoma (mature [e.g., dermoid cyst] and immature)
  - ◊ Dysgerminoma
  - ◊ Embryonal carcinoma
  - ◊ Gonadoblastoma
  - ◊ Endodermal sinus tumor
  - ◊ Embryonal carcinoma
  - ◊ Choriocarcinoma
- Metastatic disease from:
  - ◊ Breast
  - ◊ Endometrium
  - ◊ Lymphoma
  - ◊ Gastrointestinal tract (Krukenberg tumor)

System(s) affected: endocrine/metabolic, gastrointestinal, Reproductive

Genetics:
- For a woman who has a first-degree relative with a history of ovarian cancer, her risk for disease increases from 1.4% to 5%. With 2 or more such relatives lifetime risk is 7%. In families with hereditary ovarian cancer syndrome (site-specific familial ovarian cancer syndrome, breast-ovarian cancer syndrome, and Lynch syndrome II) risk rises to 40-50%. Transmission is autosomal dominant. These syndromes are associated with a variety of mutations in BRCA-1 and BRCA-2, and commercial screens for these genes are available. The clinical utility of such screening is under study. Patients with germ-line mutations of BRCA-1 appear to have better survival rates compared to patients who do not. The over-expression of certain oncogenes (her-2/neu, K-ras, c-myc) and of a mutant form of the tumor suppression factor p53 are associated with poor outcome.
- A history of breast cancer impacts risk for ovarian cancer significantly. In women diagnosed with breast cancer prior to the age of 40, the risk for ovarian cancer increases 60%. If this same woman has a family history of either breast or ovarian cancer in a first-degree relative, then her risk for ovarian cancer increases 17-fold more than a woman without breast cancer. Consequently, women with onset of breast cancer prior to the age of 40 should be monitored closely for the possibility of ovarian cancer.

Incidence/Prevalence in USA:
- 1/56 women develop disease
- 26,500 new cases/yr, 14,500 deaths/year
- Leading cause of gynecologic cancer death in women. Mortality of ovarian cancer has not decreased significantly during the last six decades.

Predominant age:
- Epithelial: 40-75 years
- Germ cell malignancies: usually observed in patients < 20 yrs.

Predominant sex: Females only

SIGNS & SYMPTOMS Often vague and nonspecific and often relate to pressure on surrounding abdominopelvic organs.
- Vague gastrointestinal symptoms
- Bloating and dyspepsia
- Sense of abdominal fullness
- Increased abdominal girth
- Abdominopelvic cramping
- Occasional vaginal discharge
- Irregular vaginal bleeding
- Urinary frequency in absence of infection
- Fatigue
- Ascites
- Cul-de-sac and/or pelvic nodularity
- Pelvic mass
- Dyspareunia
- Weight loss/loss of appetite
- Severe pain secondary to ovarian rupture (with hemoperitoneum) or torsion. Most commonly seen with germ cell tumors.
- Precocious puberty (choriocarcinoma, embryonal carcinoma)
- Hirsutism in androgen secreting germ cell tumors

CAUSES Unknown

RISK FACTORS Family history; multiple genetic factors. Environmental factors as yet undefined. Professional occupations and jobs requiring administrative roles are associated with an increased incidence of ovarian cancer; possibly because of delayed childbearing, but race and socioeconomic factors also likely play parts.

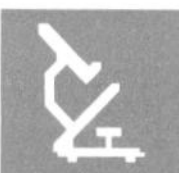

DIAGNOSIS

DIFFERENTIAL DIAGNOSIS
- Gastrointestinal or other gynecologic malignancies
- Irritable bowel syndrome
- Colitis
- Hepatic failure with ascites
- Diverticulitis
- Tubo-ovarian abscess
- Uterine fibroids
- Pelvic kidney

LABORATORY
- CA-125 (normal < 35 u/mL); not a good screening test
- Liver function tests (LFTs) to rule out hepatic involvement
- CBC
- Urinalysis
- Carcinoembryonic antigen (CEA) if gastrointestinal primary suspected
- Chorionic gonadotropin (beta-hCG [dysgerminoma, choriocarcinoma, embryonal carcinoma]), alpha-fetoprotein (endodermal sinus tumor, embryonal carcinoma), or LDH (dysgerminoma), or inhibin (granulosa cell tumor)

Drugs that may alter lab results: N/A

Disorders that may alter lab results: CA-125 may be elevated with benign gynecologic disease (endometriosis, peritonitis, myomas, PID, Meigs' syndrome) and with CHF, pancreatitis, SLE, liver disease

PATHOLOGICAL FINDINGS At surgery, most common type will be epithelial ovarian cancer and most common subtype will be serous cystadenocarcinoma

SPECIAL TESTS N/A

IMAGING Pelvic ultrasound, CXR, mammogram. Abdominopelvic CT scan with contrast, IVP, and barium enema only as warranted.

DIAGNOSTIC PROCEDURES
- Surgery is definitive
- Paracentesis for cytology is no longer advised
- Endometrial biopsy if mass associated with menstrual abnormalities

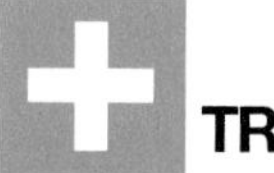

TREATMENT

APPROPRIATE HEALTH CARE Inpatient

GENERAL MEASURES N/A

SURGICAL MEASURES
- Surgical staging and optimal debulking are critical. New emphasis has been placed on maximal cytoreduction of tumor burden (enhances effectiveness of adjuvant therapy and associated with longer survival). Chemotherapy and/or radiotherapy as recommended.
- For epithelial malignancies staging, tumor excision/debulking includes:
  - ◊ Peritoneal fluid (or washings from peritoneal lavage) is aspirated and cytology evaluated
  - ◊ Omentum is biopsied or completely excised in the presence of tumor implants
  - ◊ Peritoneal surfaces, the inferior aspect of the diaphragm, liver surface, and the small intestine and bowel are inspected and palpated for tumor.
  - ◊ Cytologic smear of right hemidiaphragmatic undersurface
  - ◊ Biopsy of adhesions
  - ◊ Biopsy of paracolic recesses, pelvic side-walls, and bladder cul-de-sac
  - ◊ Pelvic and para-aortic lymph node biopsy
  - ◊ TAH-BSO and extirpation of all associated masses as feasible
- For germ cell cancers (which are less likely to be bilateral)
  - ◊ Salpingo-oophorectomy (unilateral if only one ovary involved) in young patient
  - ◊ Careful staging, including lymph node dissection, may be adequate. Adjuvant therapy for higher stage or grade or with recurrence, depending on tumor type.
  - ◊ In patients with early stage 1 ovarian cancer, the use of carboplatin- and cisplatin-based adjuvant chemotherapy improves recurrence-free survival by 37% over 5.5 years of follow-up. Most of this benefit is restricted to patients who are adequately staged and thus at increased risk for residual disease.

ACTIVITY As tolerated

DIET
- High protein diet
- Follow serum protein closely with significant ascites

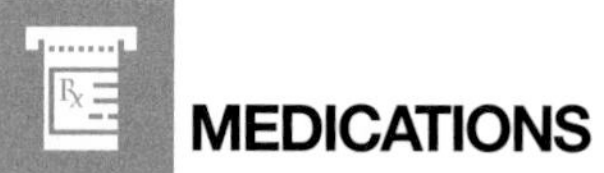

MEDICATIONS

DRUG(S) OF CHOICE Oral contraceptives decrease risk for forming new ovarian cysts
Contraindications: Those established for OCPs (e.g., hypercoagulable state or history of DVT, ischemic heart disease, history of CVA, hypertension, hepatic adenoma)
Precautions: N/A
Significant possible interactions: N/A

ALTERNATIVE DRUGS N/A

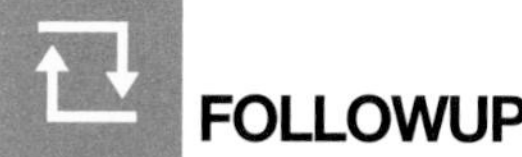

FOLLOWUP

PATIENT MONITORING
- Most require only yearly exams
- Varies by diagnosis

PREVENTION/AVOIDANCE
- Although oral contraceptives do not appear to increase rates of cyst resorption, they do decrease risk for forming new ovarian cysts
- A large British cohort of 5,479 women demonstrated that the resection of benign cysts has no impact on future risk for ovarian cancer

POSSIBLE COMPLICATIONS Complications of untreated dermoid and mucinous cysts may include rupture and pseudomyxoma peritonei

EXPECTED COURSE/PROGNOSIS
Complete cure

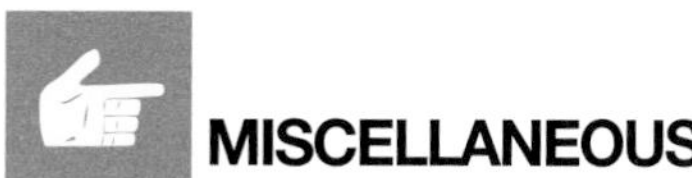

MISCELLANEOUS

ASSOCIATED CONDITIONS N/A

AGE-RELATED FACTORS
Pediatric: Malignancy must be ruled out in premenarchal patients
Geriatric: Because incidence of malignancy increases with age, postmenopausal patients warrant comprehensive evaluation and follow-up.
Others: N/A

PREGNANCY The majority of cysts discovered during pregnancy are corpus luteum or follicular cysts. The two most commonly encountered tumors during pregnancy are cystadenomas (serous or mucinous) and dermoid cysts.

SYNONYMS N/A

ICD-9-CM
220 Benign neoplasm of ovary

SEE ALSO

OTHER NOTES N/A

ABBREVIATIONS N/A

REFERENCES

- Hillard PA. Benign diseases of the female reproductive tract: symptoms and signs. In: Berek, J.S., Adashi EY, Hillard PA, eds. Novak's Gynecology. 12th Ed. Baltimore, Williams & Wilkins, 1996
- Steinkampt MP, Hammond KR, Blackwell RE. Hormonal treatment of functional ovarian cysts: a randomized, prospective study. Fertil Steril 1990;54:775-77
- Turan C, Zorlu CG, et al. Expectant management of functional ovarian cysts: an alternative to hormonal therapy. Int J Gynaecol Obstet 1994;47:257-60
- Benacerrif BR, Finkler NJ, et al. Sonographic accuracy in the diagnosis of ovarian masses. J Reprod Med 1990;35:491-495.
- Bird C, et al. Benign neoplasms of the ovary. In Sciarra J, Droegemueller W, eds. Clinical Gynecology. Philadelphia, JB Lippincott, 1990
- DiSaia PJ, Creasman, WT. Clinical Gynecologic Oncology. 5Th ed. Mosby, St Louis, 1997
- Drake J. Diagnosis and management of the adnexal mass. Amer Fam Phys 1998;57: 2471-2476
- Jones, HW. Ovarian cysts and tumors. In: Jones HW, Wentz, AC, Burnett, LS, eds: Novak's Textbook of Gynecology. 11th ed. Baltimore, Williams and Wilkins, 1988
- Mishell DR. Noncontraceptive benefits of oral contraceptives. J Reprod Med 1993;38: 1021-29
- Crayford TJB, Rawson H, et al. Benign ovarian cysts and ovarian cancer: a cohort study with implications for screening. Lancet 2000;355:1060-63

Web references: 0 available at www.5mcc.com
Illustrations N/A

Author(s):
Peter P. Toth, MD, PhD

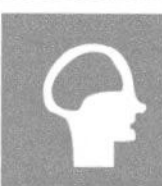

BASICS

DESCRIPTION Rare type of carcinoma that appears unilaterally as dermatitis of the nipple, representing an extension to the epidermis of an underlying carcinoma of a mammary duct.
System(s) affected: Skin/Exocrine
Genetics: No known genetic pattern
Incidence/Prevalence in USA:
- 1000-4000 new cases each year
- Approximately 1-2% of all cases of breast cancer

Predominant age: 40-75
Predominant sex: Female

SIGNS & SYMPTOMS
- Nipple skin changes that do not respond to conservative treatment
- Nipple itching
- Nipple burning
- Nipple oozing
- Nipple bleeding
- Eczematoid nipple changes
- Breast mass
- Nipple fissures
- Nipple ulceration
- Local hyperemia
- Local edema

CAUSES Unknown

RISK FACTORS
- Same as for non-heritable breast carcinoma
  - ◊ Early menarche
  - ◊ Late menopause
  - ◊ Nulliparity
  - ◊ First birth after age 30
  - ◊ Family history of breast cancer
  - ◊ History of radiation exposure
  - ◊ History of alcohol use
  - ◊ Proliferative benign breast disease

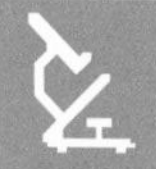

DIAGNOSIS

DIFFERENTIAL DIAGNOSIS
- Eczema
- Psoriasis
- Skin tumors (e.g., Bowen disease)
- Squamous cell carcinoma
- Basal cell carcinoma

LABORATORY N/A

Drugs that may alter lab results: N/A

Disorders that may alter lab results: N/A

PATHOLOGICAL FINDINGS
- Micro - malignant cell invasion of the epidermis with large pale staining cells
- Underlying ductal adenocarcinoma

SPECIAL TESTS N/A

IMAGING Mammography - useful, but cannot exclude malignancy without clinicopathological correlation

DIAGNOSTIC PROCEDURES Any chronic or non-healing nipple lesion should be biopsied

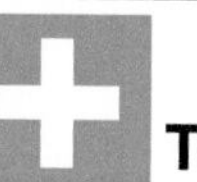

TREATMENT

APPROPRIATE HEALTH CARE Treatment of the underlying breast cancer with surgery. Additional adjuvant chemotherapy and/or radiation therapy dependent on cancer histology, size and stage.

GENERAL MEASURES
- Radiotherapy
- Chemotherapy
- Hormonal manipulation

SURGICAL MEASURES To be determined by surgeon

ACTIVITY Full activity

DIET No special diet

PATIENT EDUCATION National Cancer Institute, Department of Health And Human Services, Public Inquiries Section, Office of Cancer Communications, Building 31, Room 101-18, 9000 Rockville Pike, Bethesda, MD 20892, (301)496-5583

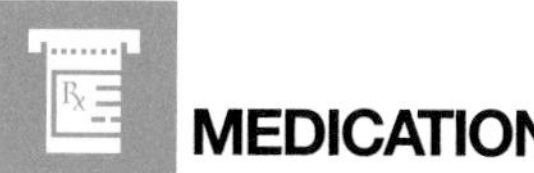

MEDICATIONS

DRUG(S) OF CHOICE
- Chemotherapy per oncology study protocols
  - ◊ Doxorubicin (Adriamycin) based regimen
  - ◊ CMF - cyclophosphamide, methotrexate, 5-fluorouracil
  - ◊ Tamoxifen
  - ◊ Paclitaxel (Taxol)

Contraindications: Refer to manufacturer's literature
Precautions: Refer to manufacturer's literature
Significant possible interactions: Refer to manufacturer's literature

ALTERNATIVE DRUGS N/A

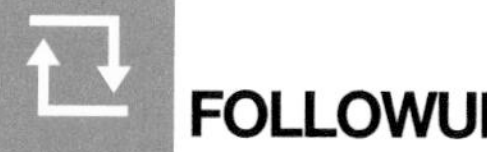

FOLLOWUP

PATIENT MONITORING
- Routine screening for women over age 40
  - ◊ Annual mammogram
  - ◊ Monthly self-exams
  - ◊ Annual physician exams

PREVENTION/AVOIDANCE None known

POSSIBLE COMPLICATIONS Metastases

EXPECTED COURSE/PROGNOSIS
- Dependent on stage of underlying breast carcinoma

Ten year survival for Paget disease:

Stage		10yr†
1	< 2 cm tumor; - nodes	70-95%
2	> 2 cm tumor or + nodes	40-45%
3	> 5 cm tumor; + nodes or fixed nodes	10-15%
4	Metastatic disease	<5%

†10 year disease-free survival

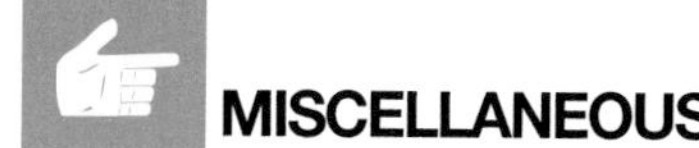

MISCELLANEOUS

ASSOCIATED CONDITIONS Underlying carcinoma

AGE-RELATED FACTORS
Pediatric: N/A
Geriatric: N/A
Others: N/A

PREGNANCY N/A

SYNONYMS N/A

ICD-9-CM
174.0 Malignant neoplasm of female breast, nipple and areola
174.9 Malignant neoplasm of female breast, unspecified

SEE ALSO
Breast cancer

OTHER NOTES Extramammary Paget disease can also occur

ABBREVIATIONS N/A

REFERENCES

- Bland KI, Copeland EM, eds: The Breast. Philadelphia, W.B. Saunders Co., 1998
- Fitzpatrick TB, et al, eds: Dermatology In General Medicine. 5th Ed. New York, McGraw-Hill, 1999
- DeVita VT Jr, Hellman S, Rosenberg A, eds: Cancer: Principles and Practices of Oncology. 5th Ed. Philadelphia, J.B. Lippincott, 1997

Web references: 2 available at www.5mcc.com
Illustrations N/A

Author(s):
Mark Horattas, MD

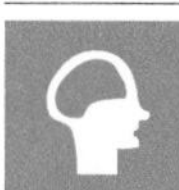

BASICS

DESCRIPTION Pancreatic malignancies represent only 3% of all cancers but are the 5th leading cause of cancer deaths in the United States. 90% of all pancreatic tumors are adenocarcinomas.
- Pancreatic cancers include exocrine tumors (adenocarcinoma, cystadenocarcinoma and acinar cell carcinoma) and endocrine/islet cell tumors (insulinoma, gastrinoma and other secretory tumors).
- Exocrine tumors are divided into two broad categories:
  - ◊ Periampullary lesions - most commonly adenocarcinoma of head of the pancreas. Of lesser frequency are malignant lesions of ampulla, duodenum and common bile duct. Lesions in these areas characterized by jaundice, weight loss and abdominal pain.
  - ◊ Lesions of body and tail - account for twenty-five percent of adenocarcinomas of pancreas. Due to retroperitoneal location and distance from common bile duct, lesions are usually large at diagnosis. Common symptoms are weight loss and pain.
  - ◊ Endocrine tumors are rare. 85% of these tumors secrete biologically active substances resulting in specific clinical syndromes.

System(s) affected: Gastrointestinal
Genetics: More common in blacks, diabetic patients
Incidence/Prevalence in USA:
- Approximately 28,000 new cases diagnosed per year
- Varies among ethnic groups, highest in Blacks and Hawaiians

Predominant age: Mean age in males = 63 years, females = 67 years
Predominant sex: Male > Female (1.5-2:1)

SIGNS & SYMPTOMS
- Weight loss (90%)
- Pain (80%)
- Jaundice (70%)
- Anorexia (60%)
- Pruritus (40%)
- Diabetes mellitus (20%)
- Malnutrition (75%)
- Hepatomegaly (65%)
- Palpable gallbladder (25%)
- Abdominal tenderness (20%)
- Mass (10%)
- Ascites (5%)

CAUSES
- No known etiology, though many associations
- Association with chronic pancreatitis is controversial

RISK FACTORS
- Probable: Race, diabetes mellitus, tobacco
- Possible: Environmental/occupational exposures, dietary lipids, also is possible genetic predisposition in individuals with chronic familial pancreatitis, Peutz-Jeghers syndrome and familial polyposis

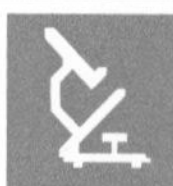

DIAGNOSIS

DIFFERENTIAL DIAGNOSIS
- Choledocholithiasis
- Pancreatitis
- Pancreatic pseudocyst
- Cholangiocarcinoma
- Carcinoma of the ampulla of Vater
- Duodenal neoplasms
- Endocrine tumors of pancreas
- Miscellaneous malignancies with extrinsic bile duct compression
- Biliary tract stricture
- Choledochal cyst

LABORATORY
- Bilirubin level mean of 15 mg/dL (256.5 μmol/L) in patients with jaundice due to pancreatic cancer; considerably higher than that in patients with benign diseases (choledocholithiasis, strictures)
- Patients with recent onset of jaundice with bilirubin greater than 10 mg/dL (171.0 μmol/L) should be considered to have neoplastic obstruction of common bile duct until proven otherwise
- Alkaline phosphatase elevated in most patients. Mean of 550 U/L not significantly different from level in patients with bile duct obstruction from benign disease
- Anemia present in approximately 60% of patients
- Stool occult blood present in approximately 90% of patients with periampullary tumors
- Elevated amylase found in less than 5% of patients
- Specific enzymes (gastrin, insulin) may be elevated when endocrine/islet cell tumor present
- Tumor markers:
- No tumor markers can be considered definitive in screening and detecting patients with pancreatic cancer. Is no single marker with excellent sensitivity and specificity.
- CA 19-9 is primary marker used at present. Approximately 80% of patients with pancreatic cancer have serum CA 19-9 levels above 37 mcg/ml. Serum CA 19-9 is also elevated in patients with acute pancreatitis (30%), chronic pancreatitis (10%), biliary tract disease (20%) and chronic liver disease (20%).
- Carcinoembryonic antigen (CEA) is elevated in about 50% of patients, the majority of whom are nonresectable for cure.

Drugs that may alter lab results: N/A

Disorders that may alter lab results: N/A

PATHOLOGICAL FINDINGS
- Adenocarcinoma (90%)
- Acinar cell carcinoma (1.2%)
- Other (0.8%)
- Uncertain (9.2%)

SPECIAL TESTS Pancreatic juice - for cytology and CEA, CA 19-9 assays

IMAGING
- Some controversy as to best imaging option as accuracy varies with site and size of tumor
- Helical CT scan: considered most useful imaging technique with sensitivity of 90% and specificity of 95%.
- Abdominal ultrasound: useful initial screen in patients presenting with jaundice. Falling out of favor because not useful for staging and accuracy is operator dependent and limited by overlying bowel.
- Endoscopic retrograde cholangiopancreatography (ERCP): Most useful in patients with suspected cancer in whom CT or US does not reveal a mass lesion within the pancreas and in those in whom the differential diagnosis includes chronic pancreatitis. Allows for biopsy, sampling of pancreatic juice and pancreatic duct cytology.
- MRI/MRCP: Sensitivity/specificity similar to ERCP
- Endoscopic ultrasonography: Is being increasingly studied as diagnostic tool. Appears useful in diagnosis of small tumors (<2-3 cm in diameter) and allows for fine needle aspiration of tissue during exam. Accuracy is operator dependent.

DIAGNOSTIC PROCEDURES
- Biopsy:
  - ◊ CT-guided percutaneous needle aspiration has sensitivity of 85% with specificity of approximately 100% in pancreatic adenocarcinoma. Few complications and extremely low risk of tract seeding.
  - ◊ Endoscopic ultrasound (EUS) guided fine needle biopsy gaining popularity for diagnosis/staging
  - ◊ Pseudocyst aspiration can differentiate benign pseudocysts from cystadenocarcinoma. Fluid in cystadenocarcinoma has low amylase, high CEA and lactate dehydrogenase (LDH) levels, and malignant cells are usually present.
  - ◊ Liver biopsy may be useful in patients with hepatic metastases
  - ◊ Laparoscopy/laparoscopy with ultrasonography with biopsy is becoming a popular technique and is likely to be more frequently used in the future for staging

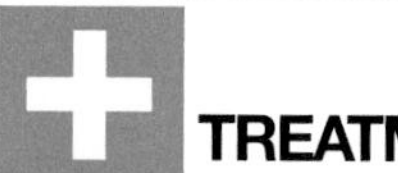

TREATMENT

APPROPRIATE HEALTH CARE Inpatient for testing, preliminary therapy, surgery or other protocols

GENERAL MEASURES
- Management highly variable and influenced by the overall health of the patient, presence of metastases, and location and size of tumor
- Analgesia
- Management of pruritus
- Control of diabetes (usually "brittle") if total pancreatectomy performed
- Non-operative procedures
  - ◊ Biliary decompression by use of endoprostheses, transhepatic drainage catheters
  - ◊ Celiac blockade and epidural catheter placement for analgesia
  - ◊ Chemotherapy - multiple protocols
  - ◊ Radiation therapy - external beam (intraoperative - largely investigational)
  - ◊ Duodenal endoprosthesis for malignant duodenal obstruction

SURGICAL MEASURES
- Pancreaticoduodenectomy (Whipple procedure)
- Total pancreatectomy
- Regional pancreatectomy - resection pancreas, portal vein, regional nodes, subtotal gastrectomy
- Biliary decompression for unresectable disease - T-tube, bilio-enteric anastomoses
- Gastrojejunostomy for gastric outlet obstruction in unresectable disease

ACTIVITY Ad lib

DIET As tolerated. Serve small frequent meals.

PATIENT EDUCATION Printed patient information available from: National Cancer Institute, Department of Health And Human Services, Public Inquiries Section, Office of Cancer Communications, Building 31, Room 101-18, 9000 Rockville Pike, Bethesda, MD 20892, (301)496-5583

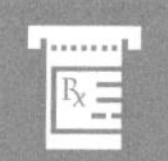

MEDICATIONS

DRUG(S) OF CHOICE
- Analgesics
- Management of pruritus, e.g., phenothiazines or cholestyramine
- Chemotherapy - multiple protocols
- Antacids
- Pancreatic enzymes
- Diabetes control

Contraindications: N/A
Precautions: N/A
Significant possible interactions: N/A

ALTERNATIVE DRUGS N/A

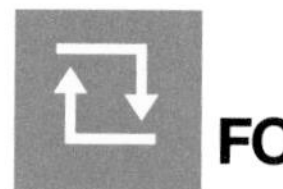

FOLLOWUP

PATIENT MONITORING Variable

PREVENTION/AVOIDANCE Avoid tobacco

POSSIBLE COMPLICATIONS
- Pain
- Jaundice
- Malnutrition
- Diabetes - especially in patients undergoing total pancreatectomy
- Operative mortality - varies from 10-40%

EXPECTED COURSE/PROGNOSIS
- Overall 5 year survival rate is <5% given high likelihood of metastasis at time of diagnosis and is <1% if tumor is non-resectable at the time of diagnosis
- Only treatment modality with potential for cure is surgical resection. Only 15-20% of patients are found to have potentially resectable disease at time of diagnosis.

Annual survival for patients with "resectable" pancreatic cancer:

Resection Performed?	1yr	2yr	3yr
Yes	48%	24%	17%
No	23%	9%	6%

Notes:
(1) 5yr survival rate if tumor is resectable & node negative, 25-30%
(2) 5 yr survival rate if tumor is resectable and node positive, 10%
(3) Median survival after resection, 18-20 months

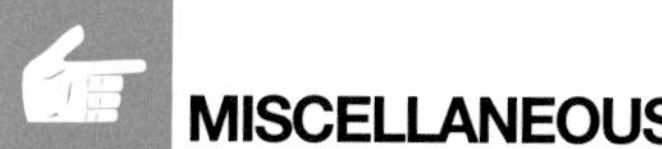

MISCELLANEOUS

ASSOCIATED CONDITIONS
- Diabetes
- Other findings associated with metastases, e.g., superior vena cava syndrome, Horner syndrome

AGE-RELATED FACTORS
Pediatric: N/A
Geriatric: More common in this age group, particularly males
Others: N/A

PREGNANCY N/A

SYNONYMS N/A

ICD-9-CM
157.0 Malignant neoplasm of head of pancreas
157.9 Malignant neoplasm of pancreas, part unspecified

SEE ALSO
Pancreatitis

OTHER NOTES N/A

ABBREVIATIONS
CEA = carcinoembryonic antigen
CA = cancer antigen

REFERENCES

- American Gastroenterological Association Technical Review on the Epidemiology, Diagnosis, and Treatment of Pancreatic Ductal Adenocarcinoma. May, 1999
- Niederhurer, JE, Brennan, MF, Menck, HR. The National Cancer Data Base report on pancreatic cancer. Cancer 1995;76:1671.
- Schwartz SI, Shires GT, Spencer FC, Storer EH, eds. Principles of Surgery. New York, McGraw-Hill Book Company, 1999
- Howard JM, Jordan GL, Reber HA, eds. Surgical Diseases of the Pancreas. Philadelphia, Lea and Febiger, 1987

Web references: 0 available at www.5mcc.com
Illustrations N/A

Author(s):
Mark Hickman, MD

BASICS

DESCRIPTION

- Acute pancreatitis - an acute inflammatory process of the pancreas with variable involvement of regional or remote tissues
  - ◊ Inflammatory episode with symptoms related to intrapancreatic activation of enzymes with pain, nausea and vomiting, and associated intestinal ileus
  - ◊ It varies widely in severity, complications and prognosis
- Chronic pancreatitis - irreversible
  - ◊ Progressive destruction of the pancreas
  - ◊ Results in both exocrine and endocrine deficiencies
  - ◊ Pain, maldigestion and diabetes mellitus are the major features

System(s) affected: Gastrointestinal

Genetics: Hereditary pancreatitis is a very rare condition with an autosomally dominant inheritance pattern

Incidence/Prevalence in USA: Acute - 19/10,000; chronic 8.3/10,000

Predominant age:

- Acute pancreatitis - none
- Chronic pancreatitis - 35-45 years (usually related to alcohol)

Predominant sex: Male = Female

SIGNS & SYMPTOMS

- Similar to an acute abdomen of any cause
- Abdominal pain - epigastric, may radiate into back
- Nausea and/or vomiting
- Other
  - ◊ Fever
  - ◊ Hypotension/shock
  - ◊ Jaundice
  - ◊ Ileus
  - ◊ Pleural effusion
- Special (rare)
  - ◊ Flank discoloration (Grey Turner sign)
  - ◊ Umbilical discoloration (Cullen's sign)

CAUSES

- Gallstones/microlithiasis
- Alcohol
- Trauma/surgery
- Post ERCP
- Medications
  - ◊ AIDs therapy
  - ◊ Antimicrobials
  - ◊ Diuretics
  - ◊ Therapy for inflammatory bowel disease
  - ◊ Immunosuppressants
  - ◊ Neuropsychiatric therapies
  - ◊ Others
- Metabolic
  - ◊ Hypertriglyceridemia
  - ◊ Hypercalcemia
  - ◊ Renal failure
- Hereditary
- Systemic lupus erythematosus
- Infections
  - ◊ Mumps
  - ◊ Coxsackie B
  - ◊ Hepatitis A and B
  - ◊ Ascariasis
  - ◊ Salmonella
- Penetrating peptic ulcer (rare)
- Cystic fibrosis and CFTR gene mutations
- Tumors (eg, ampullary)
- Idiopathic
- Pancreas divisum
- Scorpion venom
- Sphincter of Oddi dysfunction
- Vascular disease

RISK FACTORS See Causes

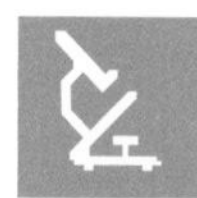

DIAGNOSIS

DIFFERENTIAL DIAGNOSIS

- Acute pancreatitis
  - ◊ Penetrating or perforated peptic ulcer
  - ◊ Acute cholecystitis
  - ◊ Choledocholithiasis
  - ◊ Macroamylasemia, macrolipasemia
  - ◊ Mesenteric vascular obstruction and/or infarction
  - ◊ Perforation of a viscus
  - ◊ Intestinal obstruction
  - ◊ Aortic aneurysm
- Chronic pancreatitis
  - ◊ Pancreatic cancer
  - ◊ Other malabsorptive processes
  - ◊ Other cause of biliary obstruction

LABORATORY

- None 100% sensitive or specific
- Acute pancreatitis
  - ◊ Elevated serum amylase (amylase P)
  - ◊ Elevated serum lipase
  - ◊ Elevated (mild) alanine aminotransferase (ALT) and/or aspartate aminotransferase (AST) - when associated with alcoholic hepatitis or choledocholithiasis
  - ◊ Elevated alkaline phosphatase (mild) - when associated with alcoholic hepatitis or choledocholithiasis
  - ◊ Hyperbilirubinemia - when associated with alcoholic hepatitis or choledocholithiasis
  - ◊ Glucose increased - in severe disease
  - ◊ Calcium decreased - in severe disease
  - ◊ WBC 10,000 - 25,000
- Chronic pancreatitis
  - ◊ Sometimes normal
  - ◊ Hyperglycemia
  - ◊ Steatorrhea
  - ◊ Flare-ups may mimic acute pancreatitis
  - ◊ Elevated alkaline phosphatase, bilirubin

Drugs that may alter lab results: Insulin and corticosteroids

Disorders that may alter lab results:

- Biliary tract disease
- Penetrating peptic ulcer
- Intestinal obstruction
- Intestinal ischemia/infarction
- Ruptured ectopic pregnancy
- Renal insufficiency
- Burns
- Macroamylasemia, macrolipasemia

PATHOLOGICAL FINDINGS

- Acute pancreatitis: autodigestion of the pancreas, interstitial edema, hemorrhage, cell and fat necrosis
- Chronic pancreatitis: calcification, fibrosis

SPECIAL TESTS N/A

IMAGING

- Acute pancreatitis
  - ◊ Plain film of abdomen - signs of ileus
  - ◊ Chest x-ray - pleural effusion
  - ◊ Ultrasound/CT scan of abdomen/MRI
  - ◊ Endoscopic retrograde cholangiopancreatography (ERCP)
- Chronic pancreatitis
  - ◊ X-ray of abdomen - pancreatic calcification
  - ◊ Ultrasound and/or CT scan of abdomen - pseudocyst formation/calcification
  - ◊ ERCP/MRCP - ductal deformity, retained common bile duct (CBD) stone, pancreatic duct stones and strictures
  - ◊ Endoscopic ultrasound

DIAGNOSTIC PROCEDURES

- Acute pancreatitis
  - ◊ CT guided aspiration of necrotic areas
  - ◊ ERCP for common duct stone removal
- Chronic pancreatitis (tests of endocrine function)
  - ◊ Secretin stimulation test
  - ◊ Secretin/chymotrypsin
  - ◊ Serum trypsinogen
  - ◊ Stool chymotrypsin
  - ◊ Stool elastase
  - ◊ Stool fat

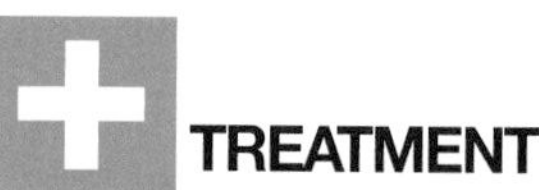

TREATMENT

APPROPRIATE HEALTH CARE

- Acute pancreatitis - hospitalization, unless very mild and able to maintain oral intake
- Chronic pancreatitis - outpatient except for complications

GENERAL MEASURES

- Acute pancreatitis
  - ◊ P - pain control: meperidine
  - ◊ A - arrest shock: IV fluids
  - ◊ N - nasogastric tube for vomiting
  - ◊ C - calcium monitoring
  - ◊ R - renal evaluation
  - ◊ E - ensure pulmonary function
  - ◊ A - antibiotics
  - ◊ S - surgery or special procedures in selected cases
- Chronic pancreatitis
  - ◊ Pain - alcohol abstinence, analgesia (avoid narcotics if possible), celiac ganglion block, surgery, pancreatic enzyme preparations
  - ◊ Maldigestion - pancreatic enzyme supplements, H2-blockers
  - ◊ Diabetes mellitus - insulin

SURGICAL MEASURES

- Acute pancreatitis
  - ◊ Infected necrosis
  - ◊ Peritoneal lavage
- Chronic pancreatitis
  - ◊ Pain
  - ◊ Pseudocyst drainage

ACTIVITY

- Acute pancreatitis - usually bedrest although sitting in a chair may be more comfortable. Advance as able.
- Chronic pancreatitis - not restricted

DIET
- Acute pancreatitis: begin diet after pain, tenderness and ileus have resolved; small amounts of high carbohydrate, low fat and low protein foods. Advance as tolerated. NPO or nasogastric tube, if vomiting.
- TPN if oral not tolerated (no lipids if triglycerides increased)
- Chronic pancreatitis: small meals high in protein. Adjust if diabetes mellitus is present.

PATIENT EDUCATION For patient education materials favorably reviewed on this topic, contact: National Digestive Diseases Information Clearinghouse, Box NDDIC, Bethesda, MD 20892, (301)468-6344

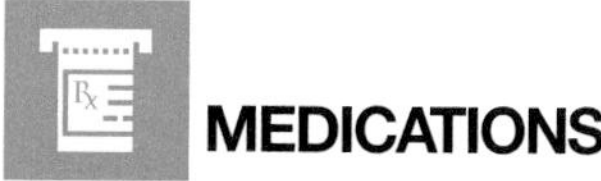

MEDICATIONS

DRUG(S) OF CHOICE
- Acute pancreatitis
  - ◊ Meperidine (Demerol) 50-100 mg IM/IV every 3-4 hours
- Antibiotics
- Somatostatin
- Chronic pancreatitis
  - ◊ Analgesics: acetaminophen (Tylenol), acetaminophen-oxycodone (Tylox), acetaminophen-hydrocodone (Vicodin), propoxyphene napsylate
  - ◊ Pancreatic enzyme (Pancrease MT, Creon) supplements
  - ◊ H2-blockers (reducing gastric acid increases availability of pancreatic enzymes)

Contraindications:
- Nor-meperidine, a metabolite of meperidine, may accumulate following several days of round-the-clock dosing. May cause mental status changes or seizures.
- Antibiotic allergy

Precautions: Narcotic addiction
Significant possible interactions: Refer to manufacturer's profile of each drug

ALTERNATIVE DRUGS N/A

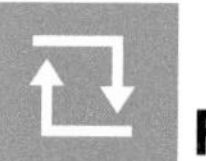

FOLLOWUP

PATIENT MONITORING
- Assure alcohol abstinence
- Follow and correct any etiologic cause - hypertriglycerides, choledocholithiasis
- Persistent elevation of amylase weeks after acute pancreatitis suggests possibility of pseudocyst - should perform imaging study

PREVENTION/AVOIDANCE
- Avoid alcohol
- Correct underlying causes, i.e., lipids, drug use, ARDS

POSSIBLE COMPLICATIONS
- Acute pancreatitis
  - ◊ Infection
  - ◊ Pseudocyst
  - ◊ Abscess
  - ◊ Systemic
    - Encephalopathy
    - Fat necrosis
    - Splenic hematuria
- Chronic pancreatitis
  - ◊ Pseudocyst/abscess
  - ◊ Duodenal/biliary stenosis
  - ◊ Fistulae
  - ◊ Cancer (4% lifetime risk)
  - ◊ Diabetes
  - ◊ Splenic vein thrombosis

EXPECTED COURSE/PROGNOSIS
- Acute pancreatitis: 85-90% resolve spontaneously, 3-5% mortality
  - ◊ Poor prognosis indicated by:
    - On admission: age > 55 years, WBC > 16,000/mm, blood glucose > 200 mg/dL (11.1 mmol/L), serum LDH > 2 x normal, serum SGOT > 6 x normal
    - Within 48 hours: hematocrit decrease > 10%, serum calcium < 8 mg/dL, BUN increase > 5 mg/dL, arterial pO2 < 60 mm Hg, base deficit > 4 mEq/L, fluid retention > 6L
- Chronic pancreatitis: may have recurrent episodes of "acute pancreatitis", slow progression, may "burn out" with resolution of symptoms. Narcotic addiction frequent.

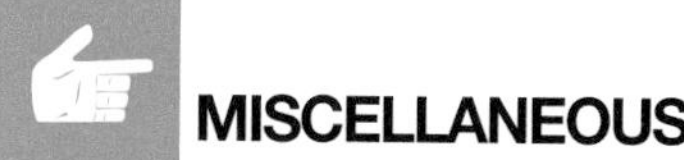

MISCELLANEOUS

ASSOCIATED CONDITIONS N/A

AGE-RELATED FACTORS
Pediatric: Mumps, sometimes complicated by pancreatitis
Geriatric: Vascular disease
Others: N/A

PREGNANCY Acute fatty liver of pregnancy

SYNONYMS N/A

ICD-9-CM
577.0 Acute pancreatitis
577.1 Chronic pancreatitis

SEE ALSO
Alcohol use disorders
Choledocholithiasis
Peptic ulcer disease
Pseudocyst pancreas
Systemic lupus erythematosus (SLE)

OTHER NOTES N/A

ABBREVIATIONS N/A

REFERENCES

- Feldman M, Friedman L, Sleisenger M, editors. Gastrointestinal Disease: Pathophysiology, Diagnosis, Management. 7th Ed. Philadelphia: WB Saunders Co; 2002
- Frank B, Gottlieb K. Amylase normal, lipase elevated: is it pancreatitis? Am J Gastrol 1999;94(2):463-9
- Pitchumoni CS. Chronic pancreatitis: pathogenesis and management of pain. J Clin Gastrol 1998;279(2):101-7
- Powell JJ, Miles R, Siriwardena AK. Antibiotic prophylaxis in the initial management of severe acute pancreatitis. Br J Surg 1998;85(5)582-7
- Lillemoe KD, Yeo CJ. Management of complications of pancreatitis. Curr Prob in Surg 1998;35(1):1-98
- Naruse S, Kitagawa M, et al. Chronic pancreatitis: overview of medical aspects. Pancreas 1998;16(3):323-8
- Watanabe S. Acute pancreatitis. overview of medical aspects. Pancreas 1998;16(3):307-11
- Greenfeld JI, Harmon, CM. Acute pancreatitis. Curr Opin In Pediatr 1997;9(3):260-4

Web references: 1 available at www.5mcc.com
Illustrations N/A

Author(s):
Duane C. Roe, MD

BASICS

DESCRIPTION An adult-onset neurodegenerative disorder of the extrapyramidal system characterized by a combination of tremor at rest, rigidity and bradykinesia. The diagnosis requires therapeutic response to levodopa which implies normal striatal neurons. This is the only neurodegenerative disease which is treatable long-term.
System(s) affected: Musculoskeletal, Nervous
Genetics: May be a genetic role with risk 2.95-fold in patients with positive family history in late onset disease; 7.76-fold increase in early onset disease (<50)
Incidence/Prevalence in USA: 50,000 per year; 0.3% 55-64, 1% 65-74, 3.1% 75-84; 4.3% 85-94
Predominant age: Age 60 with 5% between the ages of 21 and 39
Predominant sex: Male > Female (1.4:1)

SIGNS & SYMPTOMS
- Cardinal signs
  - ◊ Tremor (4-8 Hz) in repose: Diagnostic, but not required; relieved with activity, concentration, and sleep; increases with stress; 10% of patients present with only tremor, 30% present without; most begin with unilateral tremor.
  - ◊ Bradykinesia: required for diagnosis; most disabling symptom; movement initiation difficult, can be overcome with will; causes the gait and postural abnormalities
  - ◊ Rigidity: lead pipe type; cog-wheeling with tremor
- Other associated signs and symptoms
  - ◊ Speech is poorly enunciated, low volume, clipped
  - ◊ Ocular abnormalities: Decreased blinking, blepharospasm, impaired upward gaze
  - ◊ Seborrhea
  - ◊ Dysautonomia with constipation, incontinence, sexual dysfunction
  - ◊ Depression in 2/3 of patients
  - ◊ Dementia in 20% of patients; more common in patients whose disease onset was bilateral - mild to moderate, 90% with Folstein MMSE >15
  - ◊ Gait disturbances including no arm swing, en mass turning, problems getting up from chair, festination, freezing
  - ◊ Leaning posture
  - ◊ Propulsion or retropulsion
  - ◊ Micrographia
  - ◊ Mask faces
  - ◊ Neglect of swallowing with drooling
  - ◊ Excessive daytime sleepiness increases with severity of disease and medication use
- Hoehn and Yahr scale of disability in Parkinson disease
  - ◊ Stage 1 unilateral, minimal functional impairment
  - ◊ Stage 2 bilateral without impairment of balance
  - ◊ Stage 3 bilateral, positive instability, physically independent
  - ◊ Stage 4 severe disability, can walk or stand without assist, but markedly incapacitated
  - ◊ Stage 5 wheelchair bound or bedridden unless aided

CAUSES
- Unknown
- Loss of dopaminergic neurons in the substantia nigra with rate of loss 1% per year in patients with Parkinson versus 0.5% in normal aging.
- Probably not genetic rather toxic or infectious
- Known toxins: MPTP, pesticides. Other non-dopaminergic neurons can be affected.

RISK FACTORS
- Unknown in the idiopathic disease
- Association between smoking and increased caffeine intake and reduced risk for Parkinson disease has been reported

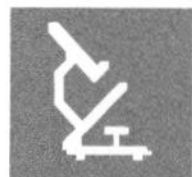

DIAGNOSIS

DIFFERENTIAL DIAGNOSIS
- Parkinsonism: bradykinesia and occasionally tremor with little or no response to levodopa indicating that the striatal neurons are also degenerated
  - ◊ Progressive supranuclear palsy
  - ◊ Multisystem atrophy
  - ◊ Alzheimer with extrapyramidal features
  - ◊ Side effects of neuroleptic medications
  - ◊ Infectious - postencephalitic
  - ◊ Vascular - lacunar state
  - ◊ Toxins
  - ◊ Metabolic - Wilson disease: onset <40
- Benign essential tremor: positive family history and relief with alcohol

LABORATORY N/A

Drugs that may alter lab results: N/A

Disorders that may alter lab results: N/A

PATHOLOGICAL FINDINGS
Typical changes that allow precise pathological diagnosis. Lewy bodies.

SPECIAL TESTS N/A

IMAGING
- CT or MRI help rule out other disorders
- PET scanning

DIAGNOSTIC PROCEDURES
Diagnostic criteria:
- Clinically possible - any one of:
  - ◊ Rest tremor
  - ◊ Rigidity
  - ◊ Bradykinesia
- Clinically probable - any 2 of:
  - ◊ Rest tremor
  - ◊ Rigidity
  - ◊ Bradykinesia
  - ◊ Impaired postural reflexes, or

One of first three displaying asymmetry
- Clinically definite - any 3 of:
  - ◊ Rest tremor
  - ◊ Rigidity
  - ◊ Bradykinesia
  - ◊ Impaired postural reflexes, or
  - ◊ Any 2 of above with one of first 3 displaying asymmetry

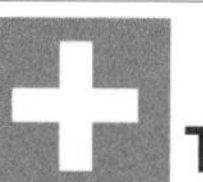

TREATMENT

APPROPRIATE HEALTH CARE
Outpatient

GENERAL MEASURES
- Drugs have therapeutic and toxic effects
- Acute worsening may indicate depression, non-compliance or supervening illness
- Course is progressive with or without drugs. Life-long therapy directed toward symptom control - treat disability
- Investigate for drug-induced cause; if found, discontinue drug. Symptom resolution may take weeks to months.
- Physical, occupational and speech therapy
- Physical limitations require adjustments in the home, e.g., special chairs, elevated toilet seat, eating utensils, dressing oneself

SURGICAL MEASURES
- Adrenal medullary transplants, fetal midbrain with substantia nigra neurons - unproven
- Thalamotomy - akinesia
- Stereotactic pallidotomy - akinesia
- Deep brain stimulation subthalamic nucleus - dyskinesia, tremor response 88%; may worsen pre-existing psychiatric disorders; less "off" problems, less "on" dyskinesias, and 50% reduction of medications

ACTIVITY
Maintain activity to whatever degree possible; use cane for walking

DIET
- Small frequent meals if difficulty in eating
- High liquid intake important; high bulk foods
- Reduced protein diet is unnecessary

PATIENT EDUCATION
- Local support groups
- United Parkinson Foundation, 360 W. Superior St., Chicago, IL 60610, 312-664-2344
- American Parkinson Disease Foundation, 1250 Hyland Blvd., Staten Island, NY 10305, 800-223-2732

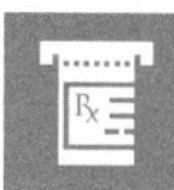

MEDICATIONS

DRUG(S) OF CHOICE
- Levodopa-carbidopa (Sinemet): may be initial drug of choice in older patients with more severe symptoms; although neuro-vegetative symptoms such as speech disorders and falls are resistant to levodopa
  - ◊ Sinemet SR 50-200 (start with 1/2 tab) qid after food. Increase by 100 mg levodopa per day until desired effect or side effects occur. If early morning symptoms, add Sinemet 25-100 immediate release one half hour before arising.
  - ◊ If switching to the SR, increase daily dose by 25%
  - ◊ Add agonist if "wear off" or dyskinesia appears or when 800-1000 mg levodopa SR per day being taken

- Dopamine agonists. Low potency; long half-life; reduces wearing-off effects of levodopa. Add when levodopa > 500 mg/day. early monotherapy may reduce levodopa use and long-term effects. May be initial drug of choice in younger patients with milder symptoms. May slow progression of the disease vs. L-Dopa.
  - ◊ Bromocriptine - start with 1.25 mg qd or bid
  - ◊ Pergolide - 0.05 mg/d for 2 days and increase by 0.1 mg/d q 3 days x 12 days. If higher doses needed, then increase by 0.25 mg q 3 days. Mean dose is 3 mg.
  - ◊ Pramipexole non-ergoline 0.125 mg tid, max 4.5 mg/day; useful for drug-resistant tremor
  - ◊ Ropinirole non-ergoline. 0.25 mg tid, max 24 mg/day
  - ◊ Titrate the levodopa-carbidopa combination downward as these agents are added such that 1 mg of bromocriptine equals 10 mg of levodopa and 1 mg of pergolide equals 10 mg of bromocriptine
- MAO inhibitors. Blocks metabolism of dopamine. May be neuro-protective. Added to levodopa to diminish motor fluctuations.
  - ◊ Selegiline 5 mg - start with 1/2 tab qAM and 1/2 q noon; increase to 5 mg bid. If add to levodopa-carbidopa, lower dosage 20%.
- Anticholinergics. For tremor and rigidity in early stages or as an adjunct (30% improvement in 50% of patients). Not recommended for patients > age 65.
  - ◊ Trihexyphenidyl (Artane): 1 mg/day, increase by 2 mg every 3 days until 6-10 mg/day
  - ◊ Benztropine (Cogentin): 1-2 mg/day. Start with 0.5 mg/day and increase slowly by 0.5 mg every 6 days. Maximum 6 mg/day.
- Amantadine, mode of action unknown
  - ◊ Similar to anticholinergics; improves bradykinesia and rigidity; rapid onset 48-72h
  - ◊ Synergistic with L-dopa; reduces dyskinesia
  - ◊ 100-200 mg/day
- COMT inhibitor
  - ◊ Reduces peripheral metabolism of levodopa permitting increase brain concentration
  - ◊ Use as adjunct to L-dopa as in dopamine agonists
  - ◊ May decrease motor fluctuation in late stage disease and reduce early wearing off of levodopa, requires fewer daily doses of levodopa
  - ◊ Tolcapone - 100 mg tid, max 1200 mg/day
  - ◊ Entacapone - 100 mg tid, max 1200 mg/day

Contraindications: Refer to manufacturer's literature

Precautions:

- L-dopa/carbidopa - late effects
  - ◊ Time related dosage problems occur in 50% of patients in 4-5 years
  - ◊ Dyskinesias probably secondary to receptor hypersensitivity.
    - Inter dose dyskinesia: occurs at peak level of drug 2 hours after immediate release form, limb choreoathetosis and grimacing; change to sustained release, reduce levodopa dose plus add agonist or clozapine 100-200 mg.
    - Diphasic dyskinesia: mobile dystonia of limbs occurs as the dose is rising and falling; increase individual dose or subcutaneous apomorphine pulses.
    - "Off" period dyskinesia: may begin as early morning dystonia (foot); reduce inter-dose interval or switch to sustained release or agonist
  - ◊ Wear-off phenomena: usually occurs 3-4 hours after last dose. Usually first sign of drug-response problems caused by increased severity of nigral degeneration. Use sustained release form with an agonist or selegiline.
  - ◊ On/off phenomena: 15-20% of patients develop severe fluctuation of response. Long-term high dose levodopa may be cause. Try low protein diet, slow release preparations, continuous subcutaneous infusions, or enteral infusion into duodenum. Also can decrease dose until on-off phenomena disappears and then restart drug. COMT inhibitors increase "on" time and reduce "off" time
  - ◊ Hourly liquid preparation - 10 tablets 25-100 plus 2g ascorbic acid crystals in 1L of tap water; 75 mL in AM, then 35-50 mL/hr
  - ◊ Freezing: find a visual clue to "step over" or counting numbers in head
  - ◊ Psychiatric side effects: confusion, hallucinations (well-formed visual or auditory) paranoia, nightmares. If mainly at night, reduce last evening dose or try clozapine.
- Agonists
  - ◊ Somnolence (27%), nausea, nightmares, agitation, orthostatic hypertension, hallucinations (17%), edema (14%)
  - ◊ Raynaud phenomena in doses > 30 mg/day, edema, hypertension, worsening CHF
  - ◊ If stopped abruptly, can result in a syndrome resembling neuroleptic malignant syndrome
- MAO inhibitor: Anxiety/sleep disturbance
- Anticholinergics: Confusion, constipation, urinary retention, dry mouth and glaucoma
- Dopamine release stimulator: Confusion, hallucinations, edema, livedo reticularis, and worsening CHF

Significant possible interactions: Most have additive therapeutic and side effects

ALTERNATIVE DRUGS

- Tricyclic antidepressants for night time sedation and associated depression (50% of patients with Parkinson)
- Antioxidants or vitamin E have shown no definite benefit
- Selective COMT inhibitors
- Apomorphine as agonist or for "freezing" (use limited by adverse effects [vomiting] and need for parenteral administration)
- Clozapine: 70-200 mg/day can suppress frequency of dyskinesia and increase "on" time; also useful for hallucinations. Side effects include sedation and sialorrhea, and most serious, agranulocytosis. Use 50 mg or less per day for drug-induced psychosis.
- Donepezil 5-10 mg/day well tolerated, improved cognitive impairment
- Modafinil 100-200 mg q AM may improve excessive daytime sleepiness

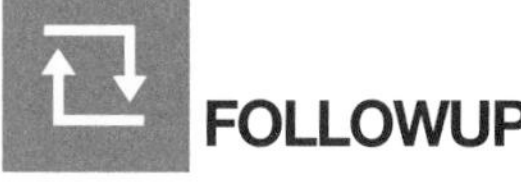

FOLLOWUP

PATIENT MONITORING Life-long for medication adjustment and physical therapy

PREVENTION/AVOIDANCE Avoid drugs known to cause tardive dyskinesia, such as: Fluphenazine, perphenazine, prochlorperazine, thiopropazate, trifluoperazine, promazine, thioridazine, haloperidol, droperidol, benperidol, fluspirilene, pimozide, trifluperidol, chlorprothixene, clopenthixol, thiothixene

POSSIBLE COMPLICATIONS Dementia, depression, aspiration pneumonia, falls, freezing, dyskinesias; also associated with a twofold increase risk of death

EXPECTED COURSE/PROGNOSIS

- More rapid progression: Older at disease onset; dementia
- Milder disease, the predominant feature is tremor

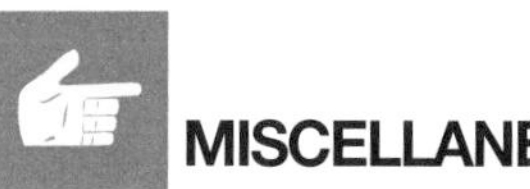

MISCELLANEOUS

ASSOCIATED CONDITIONS Psychosis; depression

AGE-RELATED FACTORS

Pediatric: May occur as secondary parkinsonism in this age group
Geriatric: Common among elderly
Others: N/A

PREGNANCY N/A

SYNONYMS

- Paralysis agitans
- Shaking palsy

ICD-9-CM

332.0 Paralysis agitans

SEE ALSO

Benign essential tremor syndrome
Dementia
Depression

OTHER NOTES New approaches in treatment undergoing study

ABBREVIATIONS

COMT = catechol-O-methyltransferase

REFERENCES

- Poewe WH, Wenning GK. The natural history of Parkinson's disease. Neurology 1996;47(3):s146-s51
- Krauss JK, Jankovic J. Surgical treatment of Parkinson's disease. Am Fam Phys 1996;54(5):1621-8
- Stacy M. Pharmacotherapy for advanced Parkinson's. Pharmacotherapy 2000;20(1):85-165
- Stern M. Parkinson's Disease: Early Diagnosis and Management. J Fam Pract 1993;36:439-46
- Koller WC, Calne DB, editors. Strategies for treating complications of levodopa therapy. Neurology 1994;44(Suppl 16)
- Siderowf A, Stern M. Update on Parkinson disease. Ann Intern Med 2003;138(8):651-8

Web references: 2 available at www.5mcc.com
Illustrations N/A

Author(s):

Jeffrey F. Minteer, MD

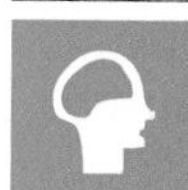

BASICS

DESCRIPTION Infectious inflammation of the folds of skin surrounding the fingernail or toenail. May be acute or chronic.
System(s) affected: Skin/Exocrine
Genetics: No known genetic pattern
Incidence/Prevalence in USA: Common
Predominant age: All ages
Predominant sex: Female > Male (3:1)

SIGNS & SYMPTOMS
- Separation of nail fold from nail plate
- Red, painful swelling of skin around nail plate
- Purulent
- Secondary changes of nail plate
- Green changes in nail (pseudomonas)

CAUSES
- Acute - Staphylococcus aureus. Less frequently by Streptococci and Pseudomonas
- Chronic - Candida albicans. Less frequently by fungi - dermatophytes and occasionally, by molds (Scytalidium Fusarium)

RISK FACTORS
- Acute - trauma to skin surrounding nail, ingrown nails
- Chronic - frequent immersion of hands in water (cooks, chefs, bartenders), diabetes mellitus

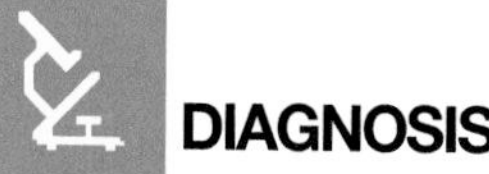

DIAGNOSIS

DIFFERENTIAL DIAGNOSIS
- Herpetic whitlow
- Felon
- Reiter disease
- Psoriasis

LABORATORY
- Gram stain
- Culture and sensitivity
- KOH preparation plus fungal culture

Drugs that may alter lab results: Use of over-the-counter antimicrobials or antifungals

Disorders that may alter lab results: N/A

PATHOLOGICAL FINDINGS N/A

SPECIAL TESTS None

IMAGING N/A

DIAGNOSTIC PROCEDURES N/A

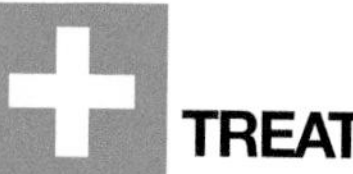

TREATMENT

APPROPRIATE HEALTH CARE Outpatient

GENERAL MEASURES
- Acute - warm compresses or vinegar soaks, elevation
- Chronic - keep fingers dry

SURGICAL MEASURES Incision and drainage (I&D) of abscess, if present. If there is a subungual abscess or ingrown nail present, will need partial or complete removal of nail.

ACTIVITY Full activity

DIET No special diet

PATIENT EDUCATION Chronic - keep fingers dry

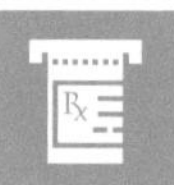

MEDICATIONS

DRUG(S) OF CHOICE
- Acute (if diabetic, suppurative or more severe cases):
  - ◊ Dicloxacillin 125-500 mg q6h
  - ◊ Cloxacillin 250-500 mg q6h
  - ◊ Erythromycin 500 mg q6h
  - ◊ Cephalexin (Keflex) 250 mg q6h
- Chronic:
  - ◊ Bacterial - mupirocin (Bactroban)
  - ◊ Yeast or dermatophyte - topical imidazoles (econazole, ketoconazole, terbinafine
- Systemic:
  - ◊ Itraconazole (Sporanox) 200 mg/day for 90 days (may have longer action because incorporated in nail plate). Pulse therapy may be useful: 200 mg BID for 7 days, repeated monthly for 2 months
  - ◊ Terbinafine (Lamisil) 250 mg q/d x 6 weeks (fingernails) or 12 weeks (toenails)
  - ◊ Fluconazole (Diflucan) 150 mg/week for 4-6 months

Contraindications: Allergy to antibiotic
Precautions: Erythromycin may cause significant gastrointestinal upset
Significant possible interactions:
- Erythromycin affects levels of theophylline and effects of carbamazepine, digoxin and corticosteroids. Cardiac toxicity with terfenadine or astemizole.
- Ketoconazole, astemizole, itraconazole, fluconazole - terfenadine, statin drugs

ALTERNATIVE DRUGS
Antipseudomonal drugs, e.g., third generation cephalosporin, aminoglycosides

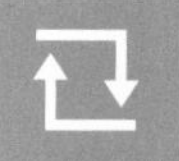

FOLLOWUP

PATIENT MONITORING
Routine followup until healed

PREVENTION/AVOIDANCE
- Chronic - avoid frequent wetting of hands, wear rubber gloves with cloth liner
- Good diabetic control

POSSIBLE COMPLICATIONS
- Acute - subungual abscess
- Chronic - secondary ridging, thickening and discoloration of nail, nail loss

EXPECTED COURSE/PROGNOSIS
With adequate treatment and prevention, healing can be expected

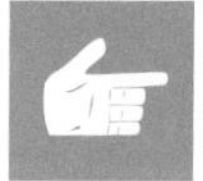

MISCELLANEOUS

ASSOCIATED CONDITIONS
Diabetes mellitus

AGE-RELATED FACTORS
Pediatric: Anaerobes may be involved in cases with thumb/finger sucking
Geriatric: N/A
Others: N/A

PREGNANCY
N/A

SYNONYMS
- Eponychia
- Perionychia

ICD-9-CM
681.02 Onychia and paronychia of finger
112.3 Candidiasis of skin and nails

SEE ALSO
Onychomycosis

OTHER NOTES
May be considered work-related in bartenders, waitresses, nurses and others who often wet their hands

ABBREVIATIONS
N/A

REFERENCES

- Fitzpatrick TB, et al, eds. Dermatology in General Medicine. 5th Ed. New York, McGraw-Hill, 1999
- Moschella SC, Hurley HJ, eds. Dermatology. 3rd Ed. Philadelphia, W.B. Saunders Co., 1992
- Baran R, Dawber RPR, eds. Diseases of the Nail and Their Management. 2nd Ed. Boston, Blackwell Scientific, 1994

Web references: 0 available at www.5mcc.com
Illustrations 2 available

Author(s):
Larry Millikan, MD

BASICS

DESCRIPTION Human parvovirus B19 is the primary cause of erythema infectiosum (EI, or fifth disease). It also causes aplastic anemia in patients with increased RBC turnover (e.g., sickle cell anemia), chronic anemia in immunodeficient individuals, and arthritis and arthralgias in normal hosts. There is also the potential for intrauterine infection after maternal parvovirus B19 infection.

System(s) affected: Hemic/Lymphatic/Immunologic, Musculoskeletal, Renal/Urologic, Skin/Exocrine

Genetics: Erythrocyte P antigen-negative individuals are resistant to infection

Incidence/Prevalence in USA: Extremely common; 50% of adults have evidence of prior infection. Most common as community epidemics in winter and spring in non-tropical regions.

Predominant age:
- Infection is common in childhood; approximately 2-11% of children under 11 years of age are parvovirus B19 seropositive
- Peak age for EI is 4-12 years

Predominant sex: Male = Female

SIGNS & SYMPTOMS
- In adults, asymptomatic infection or unrecognized illness is the most common manifestation
- Erythema infectiosum (EI)
  - ◊ Incubation period 4-14 days
  - ◊ Epidemics often occur in late spring every 2-4 years
  - ◊ No preclinical symptoms most commonly. Fever is absent or low grade.
  - ◊ Onset of rash noted first on the face ("slapped cheek appearance") with diffuse erythema of the face followed 1-4 days later by a second stage of a lacy reticular rash on the trunk and limbs
  - ◊ A third stage of the rash is characterized by marked evanescence and recrudescence, sometimes associated with bathing, exercise, or sun exposure
  - ◊ Pruritus and mild arthralgia may occur
  - ◊ Headache, pharyngitis, coryza, myalgia, arthralgias, arthritis, and GI disturbances are more frequent and severe in adults
- Joint disease
  - ◊ In adults, 80% of patients may manifest arthritis and/or arthralgia
  - ◊ In children, joint symptoms are less common
  - ◊ Knees, hands, and ankles (frequently symmetrical) are most commonly involved
  - ◊ Joint symptoms usually subside within 3 weeks but may persist for months and may be associated with the onset of juvenile rheumatoid arthritis. Joint destruction generally not seen.
- Transient aplastic crisis
  - ◊ Seen in patients with chronic hemolysis, such as sickle cell anemia, spherocytosis, thalassemia, and pyruvate kinase deficiency
  - ◊ Aplastic event is self-limited with reticulocytes reappearing in 7-10 days and full recovery in 2-3 weeks
  - ◊ In those children with sickle-cell hemoglobinopathies and heredity spherocytosis, fever is the most common symptom (73%), and rash is highly unlikely
- Chronic anemia
  - ◊ Seen in immunodeficient individuals
  - ◊ No manifestations of fever, rash, or joint symptoms usually
- Fetal/neonatal infection
  - ◊ Risk of transplacental spread of virus approximately 33% in infected mothers
  - ◊ Clinical manifestations range from asymptomatic seroconversion (most commonly), no seroconversion, second trimester fetal death, or stillbirth secondary to severe anemia and the development of fetal hydrops
  - ◊ B19 infection should always be suspected in cases of nonimmune hydrops
  - ◊ The principal organ involved in the fetus is the bone marrow: RBC survival is shortened and profound anemia can result from B19 induced erythroid bone marrow aplasia
  - ◊ A pregnant woman with a new rash or arthralgia should be tested for parvovirus B19
  - ◊ Risk of fetal loss in pregnancy is highest in first trimester B19 infection (9%)
  - ◊ Anemia is the most common manifestation of later infection
  - ◊ In one study, 84% of B19 infected pregnant women who carried to term delivered normal infants
  - ◊ No known long-term developmental problems in infant survivors
- Glove-sock syndrome: severe petechial and ecchymotic rash in hand-foot distribution with associated febrile tonsillopharyngitis

CAUSES
- Small (20-25 mm), nonenveloped, single stranded DNA virus. It is the only known parvovirus to infect humans and belongs to the family Parvoviridae.
- In EI, the period of viral shedding precedes the development of the rash, suggesting the pathogenesis of the rash is immune related
- In fetal infection, maternal viremia with transplacental passage is the source of infection. Respiratory secretions and rarely blood products are sources of human spread of virus.

RISK FACTORS
- Aplastic crisis - increased RBC turnover (e.g., sickle cell anemia)
- Chronic anemia - immunodeficient individuals
- Intrauterine infection - pregnant, nonimmune woman

DIAGNOSIS

DIFFERENTIAL DIAGNOSIS
- Rubella
- Enteroviral disease
- Systemic lupus erythematosus
- Drug reaction
- Lyme disease
- Rheumatoid arthritis

LABORATORY
- Anemia with reticulocytopenia
- Serum IgM antibody to B19 is usual method of confirming diagnosis. During acute infection B19 IgM persists for 1-2 months (less in neonates).
- To exclude congenital B19 in infants with negative B19 IgM, one must follow an infant's B19 IgG serology in the first year of life
- Maternal serum alpha-fetoprotein may be increased in fetuses with hydrops fetalis

Drugs that may alter lab results: N/A

Disorders that may alter lab results: N/A

PATHOLOGICAL FINDINGS
- Skin biopsy usually normal or mild inflammation, usually consisting of perivascular infiltrations of mononuclear cells
- In hydrops fetalis, may see intranuclear inclusions in nucleated red blood cells
- In stillbirths, virus can be detected in all tissues

SPECIAL TESTS
- Antigen detection in tissue or fluids by nucleic acid hybridization or polymerase chain reaction is available on an investigational basis in many academic centers
- B19 cannot be grown in traditional tissue culture systems, but can be detected by enzyme immunoassays, immune fluorescence and Western blot assays

IMAGING Maternal infection - fetal ultrasound

DIAGNOSTIC PROCEDURES Amniotic fluid and chorionic villus sampling may be useful diagnostically in investigation of some maternal infections

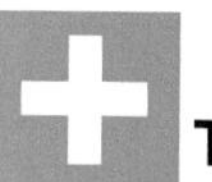

TREATMENT

APPROPRIATE HEALTH CARE
- Outpatient management for EI
- Inpatient for aplastic crisis, other severe manifestations

GENERAL MEASURES None

SURGICAL MEASURES N/A

ACTIVITY
- Unrestricted for EI
- Arthritis patients may require physical therapy/exercise program

DIET No special diet

PATIENT EDUCATION
- Patients with chronic hemolytic diseases should be aware of risks for aplastic crisis if exposed to EI
- Pregnant women should avoid exposure to patients with active or chronic infections. However, most adults have already had inapparent infection are therefore not at risk. Exclusion of pregnant women from the workplace where EI is occurring is not recommended.
- Children with symptoms are not infectious and may attend child care or school (e.g., transmission of virus occurs in the asymptomatic interval between infection and symptom expression)
- Immunocompromised patients (eg, receiving chemotherapy) are at increased risk of infection

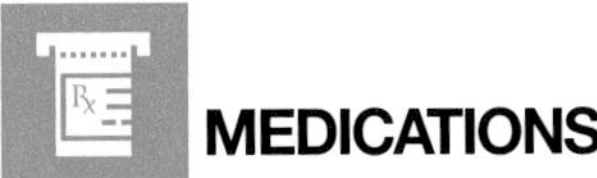

MEDICATIONS

DRUG(S) OF CHOICE
- No therapy needed usually
- Immune globulinl (IVIG) IV has been used successfully for refractory anemias, especially with AIDS
- Cessation of immunosuppressive therapy has allowed some patients to clear chronic infections
- Red blood cell transfusions may be required for aplastic crisis
- Anti-inflammatory agents may alleviate arthritic symptoms

Contraindications: None

Precautions:
- Contact and respiratory isolation for patients hospitalized with aplastic crisis
- EI not contagious once rash has appeared

Significant possible interactions: None

ALTERNATIVE DRUGS
None

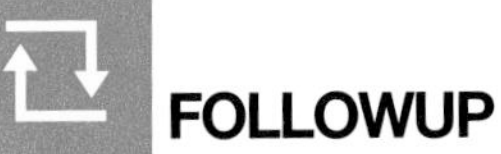

FOLLOWUP

PATIENT MONITORING
Periodic blood counts for anemic patients

PREVENTION/AVOIDANCE
- Standard hygienic practices can minimize spread
- Because EI is so common, it is not possible to avoid exposure completely. Also, period of contagion is before clinical illness (rash) appears.
- Pregnant health care workers should avoid caring for patients with aplastic crises
- Pregnant child care workers are at some increased risk; however, exclusion from the work place will not eliminate this risk, and therefore is not recommended

POSSIBLE COMPLICATIONS
Rare, but more commonly seen in adults than children
- Arthritis
- Persistent anemia
- Hemophagocytic syndrome
- Pneumonitis
- Encephalopathy
- Stroke
- Reports of congenital anomalies and chronic fatigue syndrome, but no clear-cut association
- Glomerulonephritis and other renal diseases have been reported in both immunocompromised and immunocompetent patients
- Nephrotic syndrome
- Hepatitis
- Neuropathies
- Rarely associated temporally in Henoch-Schonlein purpura (HSP) or vasculitis diseases in children
- Myocarditis/pericarditis

EXPECTED COURSE/PROGNOSIS
- Usually self-limited
- Joint symptoms subside in weeks (often by 2 weeks)
- About 20% of infections result in delayed virus elimination and viremia persisting for several months to years
- Full recovery from aplastic crisis in 2-3 weeks

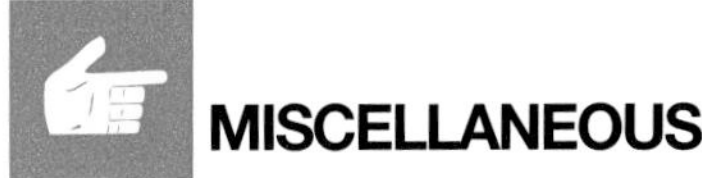

MISCELLANEOUS

ASSOCIATED CONDITIONS
None

AGE-RELATED FACTORS
Pediatric: N/A

Geriatric: None known

Others:
- School-related epidemic and non-immune household contacts have a secondary attack rate of 50%
- Health care workers have a secondary attack rate of 35% with the highest rate being among nurses exposed to children with aplastic crises
- Antibody prevalence: age and percent

1-5 = 2-15%
6-9 = 20-40%
11-19 = 35-60%
> 50 = > 75%

PREGNANCY
See Prevention/Avoidance

SYNONYMS
- Fifth disease
- Erythema infectiosum

ICD-9-CM
057.0 Erythema infectiosum (fifth disease)

SEE ALSO
Abortion, spontaneous
Anemia, sickle cell
Arthritis, rheumatoid (RA)
Henoch-Schönlein purpura
Systemic lupus erythematosus (SLE)

OTHER NOTES
N/A

ABBREVIATIONS
EI = erythema Infectiosum

REFERENCES

- Al-Khan A, Caligiuri A, Apuzzio J. Parvovirus B-19 infection during pregnancy. Infect Dis Obstet Gynecol. 2003;11(3):175-9
- Kellermayer R, Faden H, Grossi M. Clinical presentation of parvovirus B19 infection in children with aplastic crisis. Pediatr Infect Dis J. 2003 Dec;22(12):1100-1
- Harris JW. Parvovirus B19 for the hematologist. Am J Hematol 1992;39:119
- van Elsacker-Niele AM, Kroes AC. Human parvovirus B19: relevance in internal medicine. Neth J Med 1999;54(6):221-30
- Taylor G, Drachenberg C, Faris-Young S. Renal involvement of human parvovirus B19 in an immunocompetent host. Clin Infect Dis 2001;32(1):167-9
- Manaresi E, Gallinella G, Gentilomi G, et al. Humoral immune response to parvovirus B19 and serological diagnosis of B19 infection. Clin Lab 2002;48(3-4):201-5
- Katta R. Parvovirus B19: a review. Dermatol Clin 2002;20(2):333-42
- Seishima M, Oyama Z, Yamamura M. Two-year follow-up study after human parvovirus b19 infection. Dermatology 2003;206(3):192-6

Web references: 0 available at www.5mcc.com

Illustrations 4 available

Author(s):
Benjamin Barankin, MD

BASICS

DESCRIPTION Patent ductus arteriosus (PDA) is the failure of the ductus arteriosus to close after birth. 75% of time occurs as isolated defect.
System(s) affected: Cardiovascular
Genetics: No Mendelian inheritance. 1% chance of PDA in infant if one parent affected.
Incidence/Prevalence in USA: 8/1000 live births
Predominant age: Infancy
Predominant sex: Female > Male (2-3:1)

SIGNS & SYMPTOMS

- Children
    - ◊ Failure to grow
    - ◊ Recurrent respiratory infections
    - ◊ Easy fatigability
    - ◊ Dyspnea on exertion
- Adult
    - ◊ Leg fatigue
    - ◊ Fatigue
    - ◊ Shortness of breath
    - ◊ Angina
    - ◊ Syncope
- Signs (left-to-right shunt)
    - ◊ Rough systolic murmur
    - ◊ Continuous "machinery" murmur
    - ◊ Thrill at left upper sternal border
    - ◊ Bounding pulse with wide pulse pressure
    - ◊ Prominent, displaced apical impulse
    - ◊ Systolic ejection click
    - ◊ Diastolic flow murmur (across mitral valve)
    - ◊ Excessive sweating
    - ◊ Tachypnea, tachycardia, rales if failure ensues
- Signs (right-to-left shunt)
    - ◊ Cyanosis, especially lower extremities
    - ◊ Clubbing
    - ◊ Diastolic Graham-Steele murmur (pulmonic insufficiency)
    - ◊ Right ventricular heave
    - ◊ Polycythemia

CAUSES

- Prematurity
- Congenital
- Hypoxia
- Prostaglandins

RISK FACTORS

- Premature birth
- High altitudes
- Maternal rubella
- Coexisting cardiac anomalies
- Any condition resulting in hypoxia (pulmonary, hematologic, etc.)

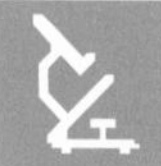

DIAGNOSIS

DIFFERENTIAL DIAGNOSIS

- Venous hum
- Total anomalous pulmonary venous return
- Ruptured sinus of Valsalva
- Arteriovenous communications
- Anomalous origin of left coronary artery from pulmonary artery
- Absence or atresia of pulmonary valve
- Aortic insufficiency with ventricular septal defect
- Peripheral pulmonary stenosis (maternal rubella)
- Truncus arteriosus
- Aortopulmonary fenestration
- Coronary artery fistula

LABORATORY Arterial blood gas

Drugs that may alter lab results: None

Disorders that may alter lab results: None

PATHOLOGICAL FINDINGS

- Left ventricular and atrial enlargement
- Patent ductus may have abnormal intima (maternal rubella)

SPECIAL TESTS

- ECG in children and adults may show left ventricle and left atrial hypertrophy
- ECG in infants usually normal

IMAGING

- Echocardiography/Doppler
- Contrast echocardiography
- Radionuclide angiography
- Magnetic resonance imaging (MRI)
- Chest x-ray usually normal in infants
- Chest x-ray in children and adults (shunt vascularity, calcifications, left ventricle and left atrial enlargement, dilated ascending aorta, dilated pulmonary arteries)

DIAGNOSTIC PROCEDURES

- Cardiac catheterization and angiography - will demonstrate the shunt and determine the amount of shunt, pulmonary pressures, and other coexisting cardiac abnormalities
- Echocardiography - left atrial enlargement
- Doppler - displays direction of shunt and size of the patent ductus

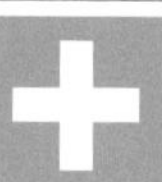

TREATMENT

APPROPRIATE HEALTH CARE Inpatient surgery

GENERAL MEASURES

- Small, asymptomatic shunts may not need closure
- Pulmonary support
- Oxygen to correct hypoxia
- Sodium and fluid restriction
- Correction of anemia (hematocrit > 45)

SURGICAL MEASURES

- Surgical transection and ligation for moderate/large shunts
- Transfemoral catheter technique to occlude PDA with foam plastic plug or double umbrella

ACTIVITY As tolerated

DIET No special diet

PATIENT EDUCATION Discuss prematurity and explain different treatments of premature infants and full-term infants

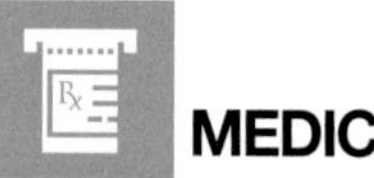

MEDICATIONS

DRUG(S) OF CHOICE
- Ibuprofen 10mg/kg on day 3 of life, 5mg/kg/day for 2 days.
- Oxygen
- Diuretics
- Antibiotic prophylaxis if not surgically repaired

Contraindications:
- To treatment with indomethacin
  - ◊ Renal dysfunction
  - ◊ Overt bleeding
  - ◊ Shock
  - ◊ Necrotizing enterocolitis
  - ◊ Myocardial ischemia

Precautions: With indomethacin treatment - oliguria, hyponatremia

Significant possible interactions: Refer to manufacturer's profile of each drug

ALTERNATIVE DRUGS
- Indomethacin 0.2-0.25 mg/kg/dose IV preferred. Repeat every 12-24 hours x 3 doses. (Decreased efficacy in term infants; not effective in children or adults.)
- Alprostadil

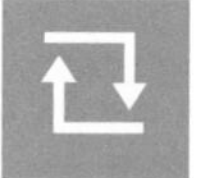

FOLLOWUP

PATIENT MONITORING
- Annual, routine followup after closure
- Shunts that have not been closed should be followed more closely

PREVENTION/AVOIDANCE N/A

POSSIBLE COMPLICATIONS
- Left heart failure
- Pulmonary hypertension
- Right heart hypertrophy and failure
- Eisenmenger's physiology
- Bacterial endocarditis
- Myocardial ischemia
- Necrotizing enterocolitis

EXPECTED COURSE/PROGNOSIS
- Spontaneous closure after 3 months is rare
- Before 3 months, closure in premature infants is 75%
- Before 3 months, closure in term infants is 40%
- Best postoperative results if closed before age 3 years
- Increased pulmonary vascular resistance and pulmonary hypertension more common if closed after age 3 years
- No firm statistics but decreased survival for large shunts

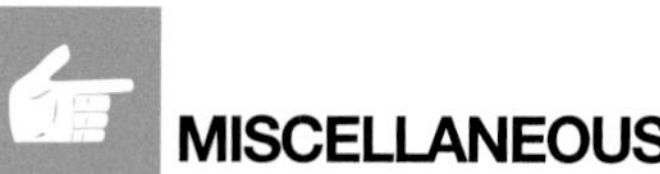

MISCELLANEOUS

ASSOCIATED CONDITIONS
- Coarctation of the aorta
- Pulmonary valve stenosis or atresia
- Peripheral pulmonary stenosis (maternal rubella)
- Aortic stenosis
- Ventricular septal defect
- Necrotizing enterocolitis
- Club feet, cataracts, blindness, systemic arterial stenosis (associated with maternal rubella)

AGE-RELATED FACTORS
Moderate to large shunts usually diagnosed in infancy or childhood. Small shunts occasionally diagnosed in adults.

Pediatric:
- Symptoms and signs depend largely on size of shunt
- Some infants with coexisting cardiac anomalies benefit temporarily from a patent ductus to provide shunting to the lungs (right heart obstructions) or periphery (coarctation of the aorta). This benefit is short lived, so definitive treatment should proceed as soon as feasible

Geriatric: Good results expected with repair age 50-70 years

Others: N/A

PREGNANCY
- Women with small to moderate sized ductus and left-to-right shunt can expect an uncomplicated pregnancy
- High risk in those with high pulmonary resistance and right-to-left shunt

SYNONYMS
- Aorticopulmonary shunt
- Aorticopulmonary communication

ICD-9-CM
747.0 Patent ductus arteriosus

SEE ALSO

OTHER NOTES
No need for antibiotic prophylaxis after surgical repair

ABBREVIATIONS N/A

REFERENCES

- Adams FH, Emmanouilides GC, Riemenschneider TA: Moss' Heart Disease in Infants, Children and Adolescents. 5th Ed. Baltimore, Williams & Wilkins, 1995
- Braunwald E, ed. Heart Disease: A Textbook of Cardiovascular Medicine. 5th Ed. Philadelphia, W.B. Saunders Co., 1996
- Makowitz JS, et al: Transcatheter versus surgical closure of patent ductus arteriosus. New Engl J Med 1994;330(14);1014
- Overneire BV, Smets K, Lecoutere D, et al. A Comparison of Ibuprofen and Indomethacin for Closure of Patent Ductus Arteriosus. N Engl J Med 2000 Sep 7 (to be published)

Web references: 0 available at www.5mcc.com

Illustrations N/A

Author(s):
Ricardo Samson, MD

BASICS

DESCRIPTION Pediculosis is an infestation by lice

- Characteristics of lice:
  - ◊ Feed solely on human blood by piercing the skin, injecting saliva, and then sucking blood
  - ◊ Move quickly
  - ◊ A mature adult female lays 3-6 eggs (nits) a day. Nits are 0.8 mm long, white, and appear cemented to the base of the hair.
  - ◊ Nits may survive three weeks when removed from host
- Two species of lice infest humans:
  - ◊ *Pediculus humanus* has two subspecies, the head louse (capitis), and the body louse (corporis). Both species are smaller than 2 mm, are flat, wingless, and have three pairs of legs that attach closely behind the head.
  - ◊ *Phthirus pubis* (pubic or crab louse): resembles a sea crab and has widespread claws on the 2nd and 3rd legs.

System(s) affected: Skin/Exocrine
Genetics: No genetic pattern
Incidence/Prevalence in USA: 6-12 million a year
Predominant age:
- Pubic lice - most common in adults
- Head lice - most common in children, 3-10 years

Predominant sex: Female > Male

SIGNS & SYMPTOMS
- *Pediculosis capitis* (head lice)
  - ◊ Found most often on the back of the head and neck and behind the ears (warmer areas of the hair)
  - ◊ Nits are white spheres found on the hair shaft. They cannot be moved.
  - ◊ Itching common, mostly at night
  - ◊ Scratching can cause inflammation and secondary bacterial infection
  - ◊ Eyelashes may be involved
- Pediculosis corporis (body louse)
  - ◊ Poor hygiene
  - ◊ Adult lice and nits in the seams of clothing
  - ◊ Pruritus
  - ◊ Secondary infection
  - ◊ Uninfected bites present as red papules, 2-4 mm in diameter, with an erythematous base
- *Phthirus pubis* (pubic louse)
  - ◊ Anogenital pruritus
  - ◊ May have no symptoms during 30-day incubation period
  - ◊ Nits are present at the base of hair shafts
  - ◊ Delay in treatment may lead to development of groin infection, and regional adenopathy
  - ◊ Pubic hair most common site
  - ◊ Lice may spread to hair around anus, abdomen, axillae, chest, beard, eyebrows, and eyelashes
  - ◊ Infested adult patients may spread lice to eyelashes of children. This may induce blepharitis.

CAUSES Infestation by lice

RISK FACTORS
- *Pediculosis corporis* - overcrowded sleeping quarters
- *Phthirus pubis* - sexual contact
- Immunosuppression
- Sharing combs, hats, clothing, and bed linen, etc.
- Close personal contact
- Poor personal hygiene

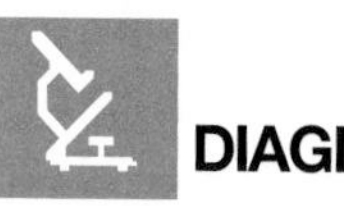

DIAGNOSIS

DIFFERENTIAL DIAGNOSIS
- Scabies and other mite species that can cause cutaneous reactions in humans
- Dandruff for head lice

LABORATORY N/A

Drugs that may alter lab results: N/A

Disorders that may alter lab results: N/A

PATHOLOGICAL FINDINGS N/A

SPECIAL TESTS
- Careful examination of hair shafts under the microscope
- Lice and nits can easily be seen under a microscope. Nits cannot be moved from hair shaft.
- On Wood's lamp exam, live nits fluoresce white, empty nits fluoresce gray
- Examination of the seams of clothing reveals body lice and their eggs

IMAGING N/A

DIAGNOSTIC PROCEDURES
- History and physical exam
- Microscopic exam

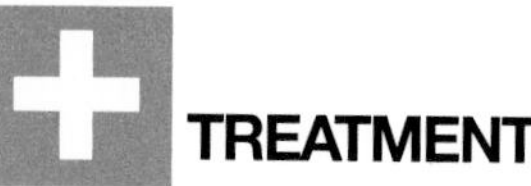

TREATMENT

APPROPRIATE HEALTH CARE Outpatient

GENERAL MEASURES
- Nit removal:
  - ◊ After treatment with shampoo or lotion, nits remain in scalp or pubic hair
  - ◊ Nits are best removed with a very fine comb (nit comb). Removal may be made easier by soaking the hair in a solution of equal parts water and white vinegar and wrapping wet scalp in a towel for at least 15 minutes.
  - ◊ Repeat treatment periodically as needed for stubborn nits
  - ◊ All family contacts possibly infested with head lice should be treated concomitantly
  - ◊ Discarding the clothes or washing them in hot water
  - ◊ Evaluate for other sexually transmitted diseases (for pubic lice)

SURGICAL MEASURES N/A

ACTIVITY No restrictions

DIET No special diet

PATIENT EDUCATION
- Poor hygiene is not a risk factor in acquiring pediculosis capitis
- Printed patient information available from: Mayo Foundation for Medical Education and Research, Section of Patient and Health Education, Sieber Subway, Rochester, MN 55905, (507)284-8140

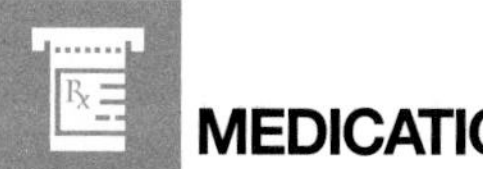

MEDICATIONS

DRUG(S) OF CHOICE

- Head lice - many topical preparations are effective. 1% lindane may be used but may have to be repeated in one week. 1% permethrin or pyrethrin are effective. They should be applied and washed off after 10 minutes.
- Pubic lice - treatments available include synergized pyrethrins, or permethrin. These can be used either as the shampoo left on for 10 minutes or the lotion which can be left on for several hours for best results.
- Body lice - best treated with synergized pyrethrins lotion applied once and left on for several hours
- Eyelash infestation - treated by careful manual removal of lice and nits, or by application of petroleum jelly three or four times a day for 5 days
- In rare cases, oral TMP/SMX can be used

Contraindications: Avoid lindane in premature infants, infants and pregnant women

Precautions:

- Pediculicides should never be used to treat eyelash infections
- Accidental ingestion and gross overuse of lindane may be associated with CNS toxicity. Use carefully in immunocompromised patients.
- Lindane - use properly to avoid neurotoxicity

Significant possible interactions: N/A

ALTERNATIVE DRUGS

For resistant head lice, shaving the head or oral antibiotics may be indicated

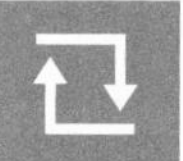

FOLLOWUP

PATIENT MONITORING

As needed

PREVENTION/AVOIDANCE

- Proper hygiene
- Careful followup in schools by public health nurses may help prevent recurrence and spread of head lice
- Washing combs, brushes, hats, coats, collars, sheets, pillow cases, etc., will help to prevent reinfestation by head lice
- Safe sex (pubic lice)

POSSIBLE COMPLICATIONS

- Persistent itching may be caused by too-frequent use of the pediculicide
- Secondary bacterial infections

EXPECTED COURSE/PROGNOSIS

- With appropriate treatment over 90% cure rate
- Recurrence common, mainly from reinfection, failure to comply with treatment

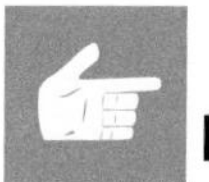

MISCELLANEOUS

ASSOCIATED CONDITIONS

- Pubic lice are readily transmitted by sexual contact, with a 90% transmission rate. Up to 1/3 of patients have at least one concomitant sexually transmitted disease.
- Eyelash infestation on a child may be a sign of sexual abuse

AGE-RELATED FACTORS

N/A

Pediatric: N/A

Geriatric: N/A

Others: Typhus, relapsing fever, and trench fever are spread by body lice during wartime and in underdeveloped countries

PREGNANCY

N/A

SYNONYMS

- Lice
- Crabs

ICD-9-CM

132.9 Pediculosis, unspecified

SEE ALSO

HIV infection & AIDS
Typhus fevers

OTHER NOTES

N/A

ABBREVIATIONS

N/A

REFERENCES

- Habif T. Clinical Dermatology. 4th Ed. St. Louis, CV Mosby, 2004

Web references: 2 available at www.5mcc.com

Illustrations N/A

Author(s):
George E. Kikano, MD

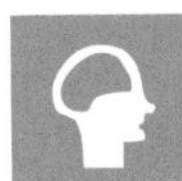

BASICS

DESCRIPTION PID is a clinical syndrome caused by the ascent of microorganisms from the vagina and endocervix to the endometrium, fallopian tubes, ovaries, and contiguous structures. PID is a broad term that includes a variety of upper genital tract infections, unrelated to pregnancy or surgical procedures, such as salpingitis, salpingo-oophoritis, endometritis, tubo-ovarian inflammatory masses, and pelvic or diffuse peritonitis.

- Pathogenesis: The precise mechanism by which microorganisms ascend from the lower genital tract is not known. One possibility is that chlamydial or gonococcal endocervicitis alters the defense mechanisms of the cervix allowing ascent of the vaginal flora with or without the original pathogen. Other possibilities suggest that polymicrobial infection can occur without *N. gonorrhoeae* or *C. trachomatis*. Factors that predispose to the ascent of bacteria include the use of an intrauterine device (IUD) and the hormonal and physical changes associated with menstruation.

System(s) affected: Reproductive
Genetics: N/A
Incidence/Prevalence in USA: Estimated 1 million women are treated each year; 100-200/100,000
Predominant age: One-third younger than 20 years, two-thirds younger than 25 years
Predominant sex: Female only

SIGNS & SYMPTOMS
- May be asymptomatic
- Lower abdominal pain
- Fever and malaise
- Vaginal discharge
- Irregular bleeding
- Urinary discomfort, proctitis
- Nausea and vomiting
- Abdominal tenderness
- Tenderness with cervical motion
- Adnexal tenderness
- Unilateral or bilateral tender adnexal mass

CAUSES
Bacteriology - multiple organisms act as etiologic agents in PID and most cases are polymicrobial. *Chlamydia trachomatis*, *Neisseria gonorrhoeae*, and a wide variety of aerobic and anaerobic bacteria are recognized as etiologic agents. *Mycoplasmas* have also been implicated but their role is less clear. The proportion of cases infected with chlamydia or gonorrhea varies widely depending on the population studied. The most common anaerobes include *Bacteroides*, *Peptostreptococcus*, and Peptococcus species. The organisms involved in bacterial vaginosis are similar to the nongonococcal, nonchlamydial bacteria often found in the upper genital tract of women with PID, but the relationship between these conditions is unclear.

RISK FACTORS
- Sexually active, reproductive age
- Most common in adolescents
- Multiple sexual partners
- Use of an IUD, greatest risk in first few months after insertion
- Previous history of PID; 20-25% will have a recurrence
- Chlamydial or gonococcal cervicitis; 8-10% will develop PID
- Gonococcal salpingitis occurs commonly within 7 days of onset of menses
- Condoms and vaginal spermicides lessen the risks of PID
- Oral contraceptives may reduce the risk of PID

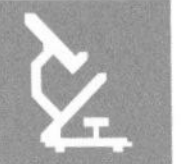

DIAGNOSIS

DIFFERENTIAL DIAGNOSIS
- Appendicitis
- Ectopic pregnancy
- Ovarian torsion
- Hemorrhagic or ruptured ovarian cyst
- Endometriosis
- Irritable bowel syndrome
- Somatization disorder

LABORATORY
- Pregnancy test
- Leukocyte count greater than 10,000 cells per mm3
- Endocervical gram stain for gram-negative intracellular diplococci
- ESR of 15 mm/hour or higher
- Endocervical culture for gonorrhea
- Endocervical culture or antigen test for chlamydia
- Plasma cell endometritis on endometrial biopsy

Drugs that may alter lab results: N/A

Disorders that may alter lab results: N/A

PATHOLOGICAL FINDINGS N/A

SPECIAL TESTS
- Culdocentesis with culture of aspirated material
- Diagnostic laparoscopy with culture of fallopian tubes

IMAGING Pelvic ultrasound

DIAGNOSTIC PROCEDURES
- PID diagnosis is elusive and even asymptomatic patients are at risk for sequelae. Diagnosis incorrect in up to a third of women diagnosed. Laparoscopic diagnosis best but impractical as routine and generally reserved for problem situations. In general, wiser to over-treat lower tract genital infection than to miss an upper tract infection.
- Suggested criteria for diagnosis (sufficient for empiric treatment):
  - ◊ Uterine/adnexal tenderness, or
  - ◊ Cervical motion tenderness
- Additional criteria:
  - ◊ Temperature greater than or equal to 38°C
  - ◊ WBC greater than or equal to 10,500/mm3
  - ◊ Purulent material by culdocentesis
  - ◊ Adnexal mass
  - ◊ ESR > 15 mm/hour
  - ◊ Laboratory evidence of gonorrhea or chlamydia
  - ◊ Elevated C-reactive protein
- Definitive criteria:
  - ◊ Histopathologic endometritis on biopsy
  - ◊ Adnexal abscess on sonography
  - ◊ Laparoscopic evidence of PID

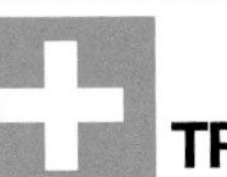

TREATMENT

APPROPRIATE HEALTH CARE
- Outpatient, normally
- Hospitalization recommended in the following situations:
  - ◊ Uncertain diagnosis
  - ◊ Surgical emergencies cannot be excluded, e.g., appendicitis
  - ◊ Suspected pelvic abscess
  - ◊ Pregnancy
  - ◊ Adolescent patient with uncertain compliance with therapy
  - ◊ Severe illness
  - ◊ Cannot tolerate outpatient regimen
  - ◊ Failed to respond to outpatient therapy
  - ◊ Clinical follow-up within 72 hours of starting antibiotics cannot be arranged
  - ◊ HIV-infected

GENERAL MEASURES
- Avoidance of sex until treatment is completed
- Insure that sex partners are referred for appropriate evaluation and treatment. Partners should be treated, irrespective of evaluation, with regimens effective against chlamydia and gonorrhea.

SURGICAL MEASURES
- Reserved for failures of medical treatment and for suspected ruptured adnexal abscess with resulting acute surgical abdomen
- Conservative surgery preferred. This allows a 10-15% postoperative fertility rate.
- Hysterectomy and adnexectomy for older patients with completed childbirth
- Failure of medical therapy generally associated with adnexal abscess which may be amenable to transabdominal or transvaginal drainage under guidance by ultrasonography, computerized tomography, or laparoscopy

ACTIVITY According to severity of illness

DIET According to severity of illness

PATIENT EDUCATION Information on written materials for patient distribution can be obtained from local and state health departments or from Information Services, CDC, E06, Atlanta, GA 30333, (404)639-1819

MEDICATIONS

DRUG(S) OF CHOICE
Several antibiotic regimens are highly effective with no single regimen of choice, but coverage should include chlamydia, gonorrhea, anaerobes, gram-negative rods, and streptococci. The CDC regimens that follow are recommendations and the specific antibiotics named are examples.
- Parenteral; regimen A
  - ◊ Cefoxitin 2 g IV every 6 hours or cefotetan IV 2 g every 12 hours (or other cephalosporins such as ceftizoxime, cefotaxime, and ceftriaxone) plus doxycycline 100 mg orally or IV every 12 hours
  - ◊ Therapy for 24 hours after clinical improvement and doxycycline continued after discharge for a total of 10-14 days
- Parenteral; regimen B
  - ◊ Clindamycin 900 mg IV every 8 hours plus gentamicin loading dose IV or IM (2 mg/kg of body weight) followed by a maintenance dose (1.5 mg/kg) every 8 hours
  - ◊ Therapy for 24 hours after clinical improvement with doxycycline after discharge as above, or clindamycin 450 mg orally qid for a total of 14 days
- Outpatient treatment; regimen A
  - ◊ Ofloxacin 400 mg orally bid for 14 days or levofloxacin 500 mg orally once daily for 14 days with or without metronidazole 500 mg orally bid for 14 days
- Outpatient treatment; regimen B
  - ◊ Cefoxitin 2 g IM plus probenecid, 1 g orally, concurrently or ceftriaxone 250 mg IM or equivalent cephalosporin plus doxycycline 100 mg orally bid for 10-14 days with or without metronidazole 500 mg orally bid for 14 days

Contraindications: Refer to manufacturer's profile of each drug
Precautions: Refer to manufacturer's profile of each drug
Significant possible interactions: Refer to manufacturer's profile of each drug

ALTERNATIVE DRUGS
Many other antibiotic regimens have been proposed and used with success. For example, tobramycin in place of gentamicin, tetracycline in place of doxycycline.

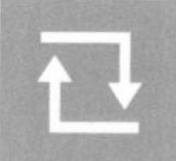

FOLLOWUP

PATIENT MONITORING
- Close observation of clinical status, in particular for fever, symptoms, level of peritonitis, white cell count
- Follow adnexal abscess size and position with ultrasonography

PREVENTION/AVOIDANCE
- Educational programs about safe sex practices
- Education, particularly for those who have had an episode of PID
- IUD contraindicated in women with history of PID or lifestyle associated with STD
- Oral contraceptive appears to decrease risk of PID in cases with cervicitis and the PID cases which do occur are generally less severe
- Barrier contraceptives, especially condoms, and spermicidal creams or sponges provide protection, the extent of which is not well documented
- Insure evaluation and treatment of sex partners
- Comply with management instructions
- Seek medical care early when genital lesions or discharge appear
- Seek routine check-ups for STD if in non-mutually monogamous relationship(s)

POSSIBLE COMPLICATIONS
- A tubo-ovarian abscess will develop in approximately 7-16% of patients
- Recurrent infection occurs in 20-25% of patients
- Risk of ectopic pregnancy increased by 7-10-fold to about 8% of women who have had PID
- Tubal infertility in 15, 35, and 55% of women after one, two, and three episodes of PID, respectively
- Chronic pelvic pain in 20% related to adhesion formation, chronic salpingitis, or recurrent infections

EXPECTED COURSE/PROGNOSIS
- Wide variation with good prognosis if early, effective therapy instituted and further infection avoided
- Poor prognosis related to late therapy and continued unsafe lifestyle

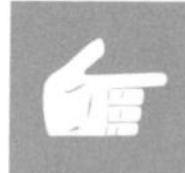

MISCELLANEOUS

ASSOCIATED CONDITIONS
- In PID patients with an IUD in situ, especially if an adnexal abscess is present, the possibility of actinomyces infection requiring penicillin treatment must be kept in mind
- The IUD is contraindicated in women with a previous episode of PID
- Rupture of an adnexal abscess is rare but life-threatening. Early surgical exploration is mandatory.
- Chlamydia or gonococcal perihepatitis may occur with PID. This combination is termed the Curtis-Fitz-Hugh Syndrome.

AGE-RELATED FACTORS
Pediatric:
- PID is rare before puberty
- Adolescents are highly vulnerable to sexually transmitted diseases (STD) including PID. Early vigorous therapy to prevent infertility is especially important in this age group.

Geriatric: PID is rare after menopause, although postmenopausal adnexal abscess is a well-documented entity
Others: N/A

PREGNANCY
PID is rare during pregnancy but occurs occasionally and the possibility must be kept in mind

SYNONYMS
- Salpingitis
- Salpingo-oophoritis
- Adnexitis
- Pyosalpinx
- Tubo-ovarian abscess
- Pelvic peritonitis

ICD-9-CM
614.9 Unspecified inflammatory disease of female pelvic organs and tissue

SEE ALSO
Chlamydial sexually transmitted diseases
Gonococcal infections
Syphilis

OTHER NOTES N/A

ABBREVIATIONS N/A

REFERENCES

- Pelvic inflammatory disease: Guidelines for prevention and management. MMWR. 40:1-25, 1991
- 2002 Guidelines for treatment of sexually transmitted diseases MMWR. 51-RR-6
- Beigi RH, Wiesenfeld HC. Pelvic inflammatory disease: new diagnostic criteria and treatment. Obstet Gynecol Clin North Am. 2003;30(4):777-93

Web references: 0 available at www.5mcc.com
Illustrations N/A

Author(s):
Michel E. Rivlin, MD

BASICS

DESCRIPTION Chronic benign bullous eruption considered to be an autoimmune disease. Most frequently affects people over 60.
System(s) affected: Hemic/Lymphatic/Immunologic, Skin/Exocrine
Genetics: HLA typing does not reveal any typical pattern
Incidence/Prevalence in USA: Uncommon
Predominant age: Greater than 60 years
Predominant sex: Female > Male

SIGNS & SYMPTOMS
- Large bullae 2 to 5 cm in diameter. Occasional tiny, herpetiform peripheral vesicles.
- Bullae that arise from normal-appearing skin (sometimes) or erythematous skin (usually)
- Bullae stay intact for many days
- Located on extremities at first, trunk later
- Occasionally located on the scalp, palms, and soles; mucous membranes (infrequently)
- Intact blisters outnumber erosions (reverse is true with pemphigus)
- Clear fluid fills bullae (usually)
- Blood tinged fluid in bullae (sometimes)
- Itching (sometimes severe)
- Some patients are asymptomatic
- 10-20% of skin surface is continuously involved
- Pruritus may antedate onset of blisters (weeks to months)

CAUSES Autoimmune disorder

RISK FACTORS
- Female, age over 60
- Drug associated: furosemide, phenacetin, various penicillins

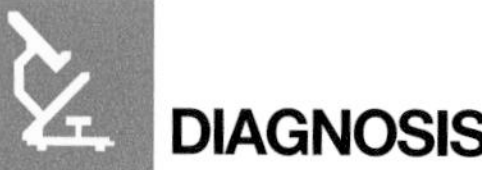

DIAGNOSIS

DIFFERENTIAL DIAGNOSIS
- Pemphigus
- Bullous erythema multiforme
- Dermatitis herpetiformis
- Drug eruptions
- Epidermolysis bullosa acquisita
- Porphyria cutanea tarda
- Bullosis diabeticorum
- Paraneoplastic pemphigus (almost all patients have a malignant tumor; most commonly lymphoma)

LABORATORY
- Circulating autoantibodies in 70% directed at the basement membrane (by immunofluorescence). These can be demonstrated in serum or skin.
- Demonstration of antibodies directed toward bullous pemphigoid antigens BP230 (BPAG1) and BP180 (BPAG2)

Drugs that may alter lab results: N/A

Disorders that may alter lab results: N/A

PATHOLOGICAL FINDINGS
- Bullae located in a subepidermal location
- Light microscopy reveals subepidermal blister with perilesional inflammation containing many eosinophils and mononuclear cells; eosinophilic spongiosis; and a variant described as cell poor
- Immunofluorescent studies - deposition of C3 (100%) and IgG (65-90%) in lamina lucida

SPECIAL TESTS N/A

IMAGING N/A

DIAGNOSTIC PROCEDURES
- History and physical
- Biopsy and immunofluorescence studies - essential for precise diagnosis

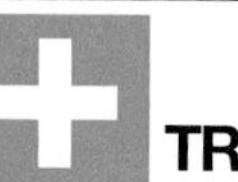

TREATMENT

APPROPRIATE HEALTH CARE Outpatient, unless significant complications

GENERAL MEASURES
- Soak active lesions to debride and remove crusts
- Analgesic mouth washes (see Medications)
- Plasmapheresis can be considered

SURGICAL MEASURES N/A

ACTIVITY Depends on severity of disease and/or complications

DIET Liquid. Regular diet when tolerated.

PATIENT EDUCATION
- Use of oral analgesics
- Teach side effects and adverse reactions of steroids

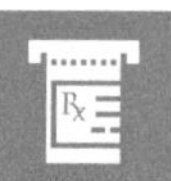

MEDICATIONS

DRUG(S) OF CHOICE

- Initially, a 3 week intensive trial of topical class I topical steroid (eg, clobetasol propionate cream) is warranted. However, if there is no significant and promising response, then institute adjunctively one of the following systemic therapies.
  - ◊ Prednisone 60-80 mg qAM. Gradually taper in several weeks to maintenance level of 20-40 mg per day. Attempt switch to alternate day treatment.
  - ◊ Tetracycline 2 gm/day plus niacinamide 1.5 gm/day
  - ◊ Dapsone 100-200 mg/day (check G6PD before therapy)
- Consider adjunctive drugs and infrequently as monotherapy:
  - ◊ Azathioprine (Imuran) 100-150 mg to reduce prednisone maintenance therapy dosage or even as only drug to maintain control of the disease (rarely monotherapy)
  - ◊ Methotrexate 10-25 mg per week as another adjunctive drug (can be monotherapy)
  - ◊ Mycophenolate mofetil (CellCept) 500-1000 mg bid po (can be monotherapy)
- Topical and intralesional corticosteroids may be sufficient for patients with localized disease
- Oral analgesics prn:
  - ◊ Elixir of diphenhydramine (Benadryl) for oral ulcers
  - ◊ Lidocaine (Xylocaine) viscous
  - ◊ Dyclonine solution

Contraindications: Refer to manufacturer's literature

Precautions: Some patients (who have only occasional lesions) can be managed without the need for internal medication

Significant possible interactions: Refer to manufacturer's literature

ALTERNATIVE DRUGS

- Cyclophosphamide (Cytoxan)
- Cyclosporine (Sandimmune, Neoral) for resistant cases
- Immune globulin IV
- Erythromycin
- Steroids IV, pulsed

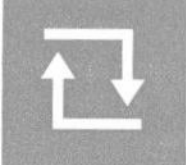

FOLLOWUP

PATIENT MONITORING

- Dapsone (GGPD, methemoglobinemia, methemoglobinuria, CBC, platelets, SGOT and alkaline phosphatase
- Methotrexate (liver and renal function and CBC)
- Mofetil (CBC and GI intolerance)
- Cyclosporine (blood pressure, BUN, creatinine, uric acid and magnesium)

PREVENTION/AVOIDANCE N/A

POSSIBLE COMPLICATIONS

- Superimposed infection (may result in death in elderly debilitated patient)
- Complications of steroid therapy
- Rare associated malignancy
- Untreated severe disease can be fatal

EXPECTED COURSE/PROGNOSIS

- A chronic disease of unpredictable duration and frequency of relapse
- Old lesions heal rapidly as new lesions appear
- Accompanying debilitation not as great as with pemphigus

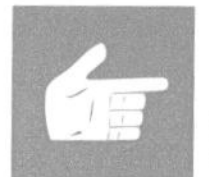

MISCELLANEOUS

ASSOCIATED CONDITIONS May have an associated malignancy

AGE-RELATED FACTORS

Pediatric: Not a problem in pediatric age group
Geriatric: Older people with pemphigoid may have higher than expected rate of malignancy
Others: N/A

PREGNANCY N/A

SYNONYMS Pemphigoid

ICD-9-CM

694.5 Pemphigoid

SEE ALSO

OTHER NOTES N/A

ABBREVIATIONS N/A

REFERENCES

- Habif T. Clinical Dermatology. 4th Ed. St. Louis, CV Mosby, 2004
- Stearns RS. Bullous pemphigoid therapy - think globally act locally. N Engl J Med 2002;346:364-7
- Borradori L, Bernard P. Pemphigoid Group in Dermatology, editors: Bolgna J, Jorizzo J, Rapini RP, et al. Mosby, New York, 2003;463-77
- Musasin DF, Anhalt GJ. Bullous disease in elderly. Clin Geriatr Med 2002;18:43-58
- fantaine J, Joly P, Roujeau. Treatment of bullous pemphigoid. J Dermatol 2003;30:83-90

Web references: 0 available at www.5mcc.com
Illustrations 6 available

Author(s):
Samuel L. Moschella, MD

BASICS

DESCRIPTION Uncommon, debilitating, potentially fatal skin disorder characterized by painful intraepidermal bullae that appear on normal appearing skin without surrounding inflammation, often starting in the mouth
System(s) affected: Gastrointestinal, Skin/Exocrine
Genetics: HLA-A10 and HLA-DR4 and HLA-DRW6 antigens; higher incidence among persons of Jewish or Mediterranean descent
Incidence/Prevalence in USA: Rare
Predominant age: 30-60 years of age
Predominant sex: Male = Female

SIGNS & SYMPTOMS
- Oral mucous membrane lesions (particularly in the posterior mouth) often precede the cutaneous lesions (sometimes by several weeks or months)
- Lesion distribution - upper trunk or back initially. Gradual extension to face, groin, and axillae.
- Bullae arise from normal appearing skin
- Multiple shallow erosions which heal slowly
- Blisters are fragile
- Intact bullae are found only on the first day or two of their existence
- After blister roof breaks, a bright red or crusted shallow erosion follows which requires weeks or months to heal
- Outer layer of skin can easily be rubbed off (Nikolsky's sign)

CAUSES An autoimmune disorder with specific IgG antibodies and sometimes complement arising from bone marrow plasma cells which are deposited at sites of epidermal cell damage; a few cases from captopril, penicillamine, piroxicam, penicillin, phenobarbital, pyritinol, heroin

RISK FACTORS
- Genetic factors (more common in persons of Jewish or Mediterranean descent)
- Medications (particularly penicillamine)

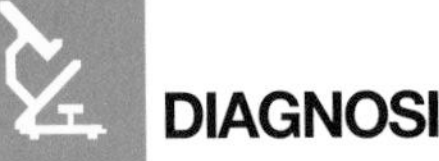

DIAGNOSIS

DIFFERENTIAL DIAGNOSIS
- Eczematous disorders
- Herpes
- Tinea
- Varicella-zoster
- Erythema multiforme
- Bullous impetigo
- Pemphigoid
- Dermatitis herpetiformis
- Drug eruptions
- Transient acantholytic dermatosis
- Haley and Haley disease
- Paraneoplastic pemphigus

LABORATORY
- Autoantibody titers (by immunofluorescent studies) 80-90%
- Titer corresponds to severity of the disease. Increasing titer found prior to relapse.

Drugs that may alter lab results: N/A

Disorders that may alter lab results: N/A

PATHOLOGICAL FINDINGS
- Causative antigens are located on the exterior surface of the cytoplasmic membrane of epithelial cells
- Biopsy shows acantholytic intraepidermal bullae
- IgG deposition in the epidermal intercellular space is found 100% of time in perilesional skin

SPECIAL TESTS N/A

IMAGING N/A

DIAGNOSTIC PROCEDURES
- Biopsy of lesions
- Light microscopy - suprabasal cleft formation and acantholysis

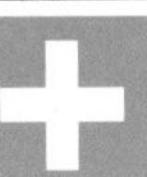

TREATMENT

APPROPRIATE HEALTH CARE Depends on severity of the disease and medical status of patient

GENERAL MEASURES
- May require reverse isolation procedures
- Topical treatment to prevent oozing skin from adhering to bed sheets
- Soak active lesions to debride and remove crusts
- Analgesic mouth washes (see Medications)
- Plasmapheresis, or cyclosporine, if patient fails to respond to an adequate trial of recommended regimens

SURGICAL MEASURES N/A

ACTIVITY As severity of disease and medical status of patient dictates

DIET Liquid or soft for patient with mouth lesions. Regular diet when tolerated.

PATIENT EDUCATION
- Use of oral analgesics
- Teach side effects and adverse reactions of steroids

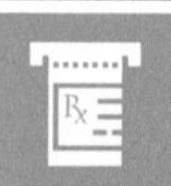

MEDICATIONS

DRUG(S) OF CHOICE
- Prednisone: high doses 60-100 mg, higher if necessary. Start at 80 mg, increase by 50% every 7 days until no new blisters. Reduce to every other day dosage when possible. Taper over 6-8 months to every other day maintenance therapy, usually continued for years.
- Consider concomitant immunosuppressants, such as azathioprine 2-3 mg/kg/day, less effective than cyclophosphamide, but less toxic. Use with steroid, or cyclophosphamide 1-3 mg/kg/day - second best therapy, more toxic.
- Severe cases may require combination plasmapheresis, cyclophosphamide and prednisone or immune globulin
- Oral analgesics prn, choose one:
  - ◊ Diphenhydramine (Benadryl) elixir
  - ◊ Lidocaine (Xylocaine) viscous
  - ◊ Dyclonine solution or lozenges

Contraindications: Refer to manufacturer's literature
Precautions: Refer to manufacturer's literature
Significant possible interactions: Refer to manufacturer's literature

ALTERNATIVE DRUGS
- Gold therapy (with or without concomitant corticosteroids)
- Dapsone controls some cases
- Methotrexate often helpful, but too toxic due to need for high doses
- Chlorambucil
- Cyclosporine
- Gold
- Tetracycline with niacinamide (worth a trial in mild cases)
- Mofetil (CellCept) as concomitant therapy and rarely as a monotherapy
- Immune globulin (IVIG) IV in cases where adjunctive therapy not effective with prednisone, or significant side effects from systemic corticosteroids (such as prednisone). It has been effective as monotherapy; however, it is very costly.
- Rituximab (Rituxan), a chimeric anti-CD 20 monoclonal antibody (MAb); a valuable treatment for refractory pemphigus

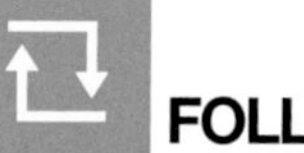

FOLLOWUP

PATIENT MONITORING
- Frequent visits during acute phases
- If immunosuppressants prescribed, monitor blood levels frequently
- In elderly patients, chest x-ray to rule out reactivation of old tuberculosis, test urine daily for glycosuria

PREVENTION/AVOIDANCE N/A

POSSIBLE COMPLICATIONS
- Steroid complications that can lead to morbidity and mortality
- Inadequate nutrition and debilitation due to pain of oral lesions
- Sepsis/death for untreated or poorly controlled cases

EXPECTED COURSE/PROGNOSIS
- Chronic. Inevitably fatal if not treated.
- 10% fatality with vigorous treatment
- Ruptured bullae require weeks to heal

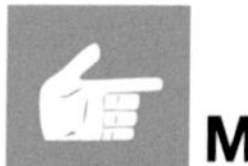

MISCELLANEOUS

ASSOCIATED CONDITIONS
- Thymomas
- Other internal malignancies
- Other autoimmune diseases

AGE-RELATED FACTORS
Pediatric: Unusual in this age group
Geriatric:
- This is the age group in which pemphigus is most likely to occur
- Close followup is needed for elderly patients on high doses of steroids

Others: N/A

PREGNANCY N/A

SYNONYMS Pemphigus

ICD-9-CM
694.4 Pemphigus

SEE ALSO

OTHER NOTES
- Atypical presentation - pemphigus foliaceus has infrequent oral lesions and is not as debilitating
- In mild disease, gold salts alone can sometimes produce remission. This has the obvious advantage of avoiding immunosuppression, However, not uniformly beneficial and no controlled trials.

ABBREVIATIONS N/A

REFERENCES

- Fitzpatrick TB, et al, eds: Dermatology In General Medicine. 3rd Ed. New York, McGraw-Hill, 1987
- Habif T. Clinical Dermatology. 4th Ed. St. Louis, CV Mosby, 2004
- Olson GL: Blistering disorders: which ones can be deadly? Postgrad Med 1994;46(1):53-64
- Thevolet J: Pemphigus: past, present and future. Dermatology 1994;189(sup2):26-29
- Huilgol SC, Black MM: Management of the immunobullous disorders. II pemphigus. Clinical & Experimental Dermatology 1995;20:283-293
- Dupuy A, Viguier M, Bedang C, et al. Treatment of refractory pemphigus vulgaris with rituximab (anti-CD20 monoclonal antibody). Arch Dermatol 2004;140:91-96

Web references: 0 available at www.5mcc.com
Illustrations 8 available

Author(s):
Samuel L. Moschella, MD

BASICS

DESCRIPTION A chronic ulcer in the lining of the gastrointestinal tract.
- Duodenal ulcer (DU): Most located in the duodenal bulb. Multiple ulcers, and if distal to the bulb raise the possibility of Zollinger-Ellison syndrome.
- Gastric ulcer (GU): Much less common than DU (in NSAID absence). Commonly located along lesser curvature of the antrum near the incisura and in the pre-pyloric area.
- Esophageal ulcers: A peptic ulcer in the distal esophagus may be part of Barrett's epithelial change due to chronic reflux of gastroduodenal contents
- Ectopic gastric mucosal ulceration: May develop in patients with Meckel diverticula or other sites of ectopic gastric mucosa

System(s) affected: Gastrointestinal

Genetics: Higher incidence with HLA-B12, B5, Bw35 phenotypes, identical twins

Incidence/Prevalence in USA:
- DU: 4 times more common than GU. Lifetime prevalence = 10% for men; 5% for women (gender gap is closing). 200,000-400,000 new DU cases/annually.
- GU: 87,500 new cases annually. Incidence of new GU in adults; 50/100,000

Predominant age:
- DU 25-75 years (rare before age 15)
- GU peak incidence age 55-65; rare < age 40

Predominant sex:
- DU: Male > Female (slightly)
- GU: Male = Female (female predominance among NSAID users)

SIGNS & SYMPTOMS
- In adults (DU)
  - ◊ Gnawing or burning epigastric pain 1-3 hours after meals, relieved by food, antacids, or antisecretory agents
  - ◊ Nocturnal pain causing early morning awakening
  - ◊ Epigastric pain in 60-90% (often vague discomfort, cramping, hunger pangs). Non-specific dyspeptic complaints (belching, bloating, abdominal distention, food intolerance) in 40-70%.
  - ◊ Up to 1/3 of adults >60 years old do not report abdominal pain
  - ◊ Symptomatic periods occur in clusters lasting a few weeks followed by symptom-free periods for weeks to months. Some seasonal occurrence (spring and fall).
  - ◊ Early satiety, anorexia, weight loss, abnormal saline load test, succussion splash, gastric retention of barium, nausea, vomiting suggest pyloric obstruction
  - ◊ Heartburn (suggesting reflux disease)
  - ◊ Sudden, severe mid-epigastric pain radiating to right shoulder, peritoneal signs and free peritoneal air may indicate perforation
  - ◊ Dizziness, syncope, hematemesis or melena suggest hemorrhage
- In adults (GU)
  - ◊ Symptom complex similar to DU
  - ◊ NSAID-induced ulcers often silent; perforation or bleeding may be initial presentation
  - ◊ Epigastric pain following a meal an uncommon finding; early satiety, nausea, vomiting suggest gastric outlet obstruction
  - ◊ Weight loss can occur with either benign or malignant gastric ulcers
- In children (DU)
  - ◊ Positive family history in 50% of early onset DU patients (under age 20)
  - ◊ May account for chronic abdominal pain syndrome in young children
  - ◊ Gastric outlet obstruction from ulcer must be distinguished from congenital infantile hypertrophic pyloric stenosis (seen within the first month after birth along with visible peristalses and a palpable pyloric mass)

CAUSES
Etiology of DU and GU is multifactorial. H. pylori gastritis is present in >80% of DU and >60% of GU.
- Imbalance between aggressive factors (e.g., gastric acid, pepsin, bile salts, pancreatic enzymes) and defensive factors maintaining mucosal integrity (e.g., mucus, bicarbonate, blood flow, prostaglandins, growth factors, cell turnover) which may relate to H. pylori infection
- Ulcerogenic drugs (e.g., NSAIDs)
- Zollinger-Ellison syndrome
- Other hypersecretory syndromes
- Retained gastric antrum

RISK FACTORS
- Strongly associated: Drugs (e.g., NSAID use), family history of ulcer, Zollinger-Ellison syndrome (gastrinoma), cigarettes (>1/2 pack/day)
- Possibly associated: Corticosteroids (high dose and/or prolonged therapy); blood group O; HLA-B12, B5, Bw35 phenotypes; stress; lower socioeconomic status; manual labor
- Poorly or not associated: Dietary spices, alcohol, caffeine, acetaminophen
- Lifetime risk for PUD in H. pylori infected individuals is 15%
- Annual risk of DU developing in H. pylori - positive individual ≤1%

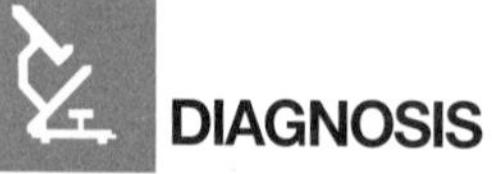

DIAGNOSIS

DIFFERENTIAL DIAGNOSIS
- Non-ulcer dyspepsia
- Gastric carcinoma
- H. pylori-associated gastritis (without ulcer)
- Gastroesophageal reflux (with or without esophagitis)
- Crohn disease (gastroduodenal)
- Pancreatitis
- Variant angina pectoris
- Cholelithiasis syndrome
- Atrophic gastritis

LABORATORY
- Anemia uncommon in absence of hemorrhage. Fecal occult blood requires colonic evaluation before attributing positive test to ulcer alone (especially in patients > 40 years).
- Elevated serum gastrin (to rule out Zollinger-Ellison syndrome)
- Gastric analysis (to rule out achlorhydria, acid hypersecretion)
- Secretin stimulation test (paradoxical rise seen in ZE)
- Serum pepsinogen

Drugs that may alter lab results: Antisecretory medications may give falsely low gastric analysis or elevated gastrin

Disorders that may alter lab results: N/A

PATHOLOGICAL FINDINGS
- Helicobacter pylori gastritis, atrophic gastritis, mucosa-associated lymphoid tissue (MALT)
- Ulcer crater usually > 5 mm diameter; extends through the mucosa (in contrast to stress-related ulceration)

SPECIAL TESTS Serology, stool antigen, rapid urease test or urea breath test for H. pylori

IMAGING
- Endoscopy more accurate than radiography
- Radiographic features of benign GU include ulcer projecting beyond the lumen, radiolucent band (Hampton line) paralleling ulcer base, radiating folds

DIAGNOSTIC PROCEDURES
- Endoscopy (accuracy > 95%)
- Barium meal (accuracy 70-90%)
- Mucosal biopsy, cytology (excludes malignancy in > 99%)
- Exploratory laparotomy
- Histology, blood antibody, stool antigen or urea breath test for H. pylori
- Current recommendations for diagnosing H. pylori in PUD
  - ◊ New onset PUD by endoscopy or radiography: rapid urease test (RUT) or specimen obtained by biopsy of the antrum or serum antibody; if negative, perform histology, stool antigen or urea breath test (UBT)
  - ◊ History of uncomplicated PUD or those receiving maintenance antisecretory therapy for suspected PUD: nonendoscopic detection method; if negative, maintenance therapy can be discontinued; confirm negative H. pylori status by UBT or stool antigen 2-4 weeks later
  - ◊ New onset ulcer-like dyspepsia under age 50 without alarm symptoms: blood antibody testing, UBT or stool antigen. Over age 50 or any patient with alarm symptoms should have endoscopy and RUT or histology.

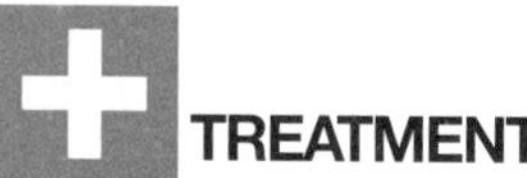

TREATMENT

APPROPRIATE HEALTH CARE
- H. pylori should be sought in all patients with new onset PUD, those with a history of PUD, those with MALT-lymphoma or in otherwise healthy patients with ulcer-like dyspepsia
- Empiric treatment for young healthy patients with dyspepsia, otherwise endoscopy or barium meal for suspected complications, weight loss, persistent vomiting, etc., or symptom onset after age 50 years
- A noninvasive "test and threat" strategy for H. pylori in patients with ulcer-like dyspepsia results in an equivalent outcome compared to prompt endoscopy
- Patients with nonulcer dyspepsia are unlikely to benefit from H. pylori therapy
- Emergency endoscopy and hospitalization for suspected ulcer bleeding
- ICU care for severe hemorrhage

GENERAL MEASURES
- Reduce use of NSAIDs and psychic stress
- Avoid or eliminate cigarette smoking

SURGICAL MEASURES For bleeding complication, obstruction or perforation

ACTIVITY Fully active in uncomplicated

DIET Regular meals; avoid dietary irritants

PATIENT EDUCATION National Digestive Diseases Information, Box NDDIC, Bethesda, MD 20892, (301)468-6344

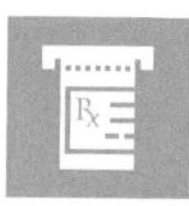

MEDICATIONS

DRUG(S) OF CHOICE
- Acid suppression
  - ◊ H2 blocker: ranitidine or nizatidine 150 bid or 300 mg hs; cimetidine 400 mg bid or 800 mg hs; famotidine 150 mg bid or 300 mg hs for 8-12 weeks
  - ◊ Proton pump inhibitor, e.g., omeprazole 20 mg, lansoprazole 15 mg qd, rabeprazole 20 mg, esomeprazole 40 mg, or pantoprazole 40 mg daily for 4 weeks
- Eradication of Helicobacter pylori (HP), single antibiotic regimens discouraged. Currently optimal HP eradication regimens:
  - ◊ Proton pump inhibitor bid plus 2 antibiotics (e.g., clarithromycin 500 mg bid and amoxicillin 1 gm bid for 14 days)
  - ◊ Ranitidine-bismuth-citrate 400 mg bid plus clarithromycin 500 mg bid and amoxicillin 1 gm bid for 14 days
  - ◊ Alternative antibiotics: Tetracycline, metronidazole, rifampin
  - ◊ 2nd line regimen for treatment failures using rabeprazole, levofloxacin and rifabutin with or without bismuth subcitrate for 7 days had an eradication rate of 91%
- Other:
  - ◊ Treatment of H. pylori-negative ulcers: Most are due to NSAIDs; treat acutely with proton pump inhibitor for 4-12 weeks. Optimally, the NSAID should be discontinued, or switch to selective cox-2 inhibitor
  - ◊ Unhealed refractory ulcers: higher doses of H2 blockers or proton pump inhibitors or surgery and exclude surreptitious NSAID or salicylate use
- Reduced risk of recurrent ulcer bleeding after endoscopic therapy followed by 72 hour IV infusion of omeprazole
- Successful management of ZES with IV pantoprazole when po not possible

Contraindications: Known hypersensitivity to the drug or another member of the class

Precautions:
- Renal insufficiency (GFR < 30 mL/min): reduce H2 blocker dose by 50%. Avoid magnesium-containing antacids
- Give sucralfate distant from meals
- Bacterial resistance: clarithromycin 10%, amoxicillin 1-2%, metronidazole 3%
- Antibiotic-related side effects:
  - ◊ Diarrhea (10%): change amoxicillin to tetracycline
  - ◊ Nausea/vomiting (20%)
  - ◊ Unpleasant taste with clarithromycin
  - ◊ Rash (5%): stop antimicrobial
  - ◊ Pseudomembranous colitis (< 1%): treat with vancomycin
  - ◊ Anaphylaxis, Stevens-Johnson syndrome (rare)

Significant possible interactions:
- Cimetidine interacts with many drugs (e.g., theophylline, warfarin, phenytoin, lidocaine) via inhibition of cytochrome P-450 isozymes, leading to reduced drug clearance; avoid cimetidine with interacting drugs.
- Ranitidine and famotidine rarely associated with increased theophylline levels; nizatidine not associated with drug interactions
- Omeprazole may prolong the elimination of diazepam, warfarin and phenytoin
- Sucralfate reduces absorption of tetracycline, norfloxacin, ciprofloxacin, and theophylline leading to subtherapeutic levels

ALTERNATIVE DRUGS
- Alternative ulcer healing drugs
  - ◊ Sucralfate 1 gm qid or 2 gm bid for 4-8 wks
  - ◊ Antacids, e.g., magnesium hydroxide, aluminum hydroxide 1 and 3 hours after meals (4-7 doses daily)

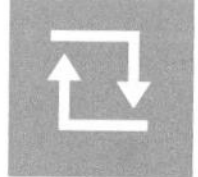

FOLLOWUP

PATIENT MONITORING
- Eradication of H. pylori: Expected in >90% (with 2 antibiotic regimen)
  - ◊ Confirm eradication by CLOtest biopsy, histology, urea breath test, or stool antigen (has high predictive value on day 7 after treatment) in patients who remain symptomatic or relapse
  - ◊ Blood antibody less useful in the immediate post-treatment period
  - ◊ Treatment failure: use different antimicrobial regimen or test for sensitivity
- Acute DU: monitor clinical response. No need to repeat endoscopy or x-ray exam to document healing unless recurrence or complication suspected.
- Acute GU: confirm healing (endoscopy after 6-12 weeks for cytology and biopsy of poorly or unhealed ulcer to rule out malignancy)
- Symptomatic response to therapy does not preclude malignancy

PREVENTION/AVOIDANCE
- Eradication of HP: recurrence < 10% in the first year, off of all therapies
- Maintenance therapy (using proton pump inhibitor or H2 blocker) suppresses ulcer relapse indefinitely while treatment is continued - however, relapses occur in most patients who remain HP positive off therapy
- Bleeding ulcers require continued maintenance therapy (e.g., H2 blocker or PPI if H. pylori not eradicated
- NSAID-related ulcers: avoid salicylates and NSAIDs. If NSAIDs needed, add misoprostol (Cytotec) or proton pump inhibitor.
- To reduce ulcer risk, eradicate H. pylori prior to start of NSAIDs
- Selective COX-2 NSAIDs (eg celecoxib, rofecoxib) produce significantly fewer GI ulcers; consider for use in patients at risk for ulceration
- Eradication of H. pylori proven to reduce risk of gastric cancer

POSSIBLE COMPLICATIONS
- Hemorrhage in up to 25% of cases (initial presentation in 10%)
- Perforation occurs in < 5%, usually related to NSAID use
- Gastric outlet obstruction occurs in up to 5% of patients with duodenal or pyloric channel ulcers. Men predominate.
- Risk of gastric adenocarcinoma increased up to 9 fold in H. pylori infected patients

EXPECTED COURSE/PROGNOSIS
- Ulcer relapse rates after H. pylori eradication low; suspect surreptitious NSAID use
- Reinfection rates < 1% per year
- Risk of rebleeding after successful H. pylori therapy is extremely low
- NSAID-related ulcers occur less commonly after H. pylori eradication
- Intractability now rare
- Regression or resolution of atrophic gastritis or low-grade MALT-lymphoma with successful H. pylori eradication

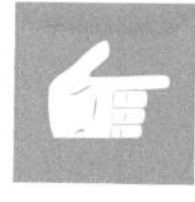

MISCELLANEOUS

ASSOCIATED CONDITIONS
- Zollinger-Ellison syndrome (gastrinoma)
- Systemic mastocytosis
- MEN Type 1
- COPD, chronic renal failure, cirrhosis, hyperparathyroidism, carcinoid syndrome, polycythemia rubra vera, basophilic leukemia, porphyria cutanea tarda

AGE-RELATED FACTORS
Pediatric: Uncommon before puberty; hemorrhage and perforation more common

Geriatric: N/A

Others: N/A

PREGNANCY PUD unusual in gestation; safety of H2 blockers and PPIs not established; studies with cimetidine, ranitidine and omeprazole suggest safe use if needed. Sucralfate and antacids appear safe.

SYNONYMS
- Duodenal ulcer
- Gastric ulcer
- Helicobacter pylori gastritis

ICD-9-CM
532.90 Duodenal ulcer, unspecified as acute or chronic, without mention of hemorrhage, perforation, or obstruction

531.90 Gastric ulcer, unspecified as acute or chronic, without mention of hemorrhage, perforation, or obstruction

SEE ALSO
Pyloric stenosis

Zollinger-Ellison syndrome

OTHER NOTES N/A

ABBREVIATIONS N/A

REFERENCES

- Suerbaum S, Michetti P. Helicobacter pylori infection. N Engl J Med 2002;347(15):1175-86

Web references: 2 available at www.5mcc.com

Illustrations N/A

Author(s):

James H. Lewis, MD

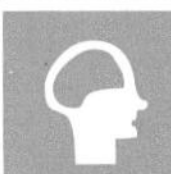

BASICS

DESCRIPTION The clinical manifestations of disease processes involving the pericardium
- Acute pericarditis: an inflammatory process from a wide spectrum of etiologies of the pericardium with or without associated effusion. The most common etiology is idiopathic or nonspecific pericarditis.
- Pericardial tamponade: cardiac compression from pericardial effusion causing hemodynamic compromise and disruption of compensatory mechanisms
- Constrictive pericarditis: thickening and adherence of the pericardium to the heart after chronic inflammation

System(s) affected: Cardiovascular
Genetics: Unknown
Incidence/Prevalence in USA: 2% penetration trauma develop tamponade
Predominant age: Adolescents and young adults
Predominant sex: Male > Female

SIGNS & SYMPTOMS
- Acute pericarditis
  - ◊ Chest pain, typically sharp, retrosternal with radiation to the trapezial ridge
  - ◊ Pain frequently sudden in onset, with inspiration or movement
  - ◊ Pain reduced by leaning forward and sitting up
  - ◊ Splinted breathing
  - ◊ Odynophagia
  - ◊ Fever
  - ◊ Myalgia
  - ◊ Anorexia
  - ◊ Anxiety
  - ◊ Pericardial friction rub
  - ◊ Cardiac arrhythmias often intermittent, supraventricular tachycardia (SVT)
  - ◊ Tachypnea
  - ◊ Localized rales
- Pericardial tamponade
  - ◊ Dyspnea
  - ◊ Tachycardia
  - ◊ Distended jugular neck veins
  - ◊ Cyanosis
  - ◊ Relative or absolute hypotension
  - ◊ Quiet precordium with little palpable cardiac activity
  - ◊ Pericardial friction rub
  - ◊ Lungs clear
  - ◊ Ewart's sign - dullness and bronchial breathing between the tip of the left scapula and vertebral column
  - ◊ Rapid thready pulse
  - ◊ Varying degrees of consciousness
  - ◊ Pulsus paradoxus: > 10 mm Hg (1.33 kPa) decrease in systolic pressure with inspiration
  - ◊ Beck's triad - distended neck veins, hypotension and muffled heart sounds
- Constrictive pericarditis
  - ◊ Asymptomatic, early
  - ◊ Dyspnea, pulmonary congestion
  - ◊ Fatigue very common
  - ◊ Peripheral edema
  - ◊ Hepatomegaly
  - ◊ Ascites
  - ◊ Jugular venous distention - elevated, deep Y trough (not seen in tamponade)
  - ◊ Kussmaul's sign - inspiratory increase in jugular venous pressure
  - ◊ Pericardial "knock" - follows S2 by 0.06-0.12 sec, increases with squatting
  - ◊ Hypovolemia may mask the signs of constriction

CAUSES
- Idiopathic
- Viral: Coxsackie, echo, adenovirus, Epstein-Barr, mumps
- Bacterial: Haemophilus (especially children), Staphylococcus, Pneumococcus, Salmonella, Meningococcus, Lyme disease, Legionella, Mycoplasma
- Fungal: Candida, Histoplasmosis, Aspergillus, Nocardia
- Mycobacterial: Mycobacterium tuberculosis
- Parasites, protozoa
- Neoplastic: Breast, lung, lymphoma, mesothelioma
- Drug-induced: Procainamide, hydralazine, bleomycin, phenytoin, minoxidil, mesalamine, azathioprine and perhaps others
- Connective tissue disease: Systemic lupus erythematosus, rheumatoid arthritis, scleroderma, acute rheumatic fever
- Radiation
- Myocardial infarction, Dressler's
- Postpericardiotomy
- Uremia
- Myxedema
- Cholesterol pericarditis
- Aortic dissection
- Sarcoidosis
- Pancreatitis
- Inflammatory bowel disease
- AIDS
- Chylopericardium
- Familial - autosomal recessive (Mulibrey nanism)

RISK FACTORS
- Chest trauma

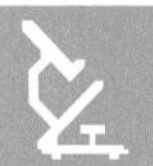

DIAGNOSIS

DIFFERENTIAL DIAGNOSIS
- Acute myocardial infarction
- Pneumonia with pleurisy
- Pulmonary emboli
- Aortic dissection
- Pneumothorax
- Mediastinal emphysema
- Cholecystitis
- Pancreatitis
- Esophageal perforation, rupture, inflammation or tear

LABORATORY
- Leukocytosis and increased ESR
- May see elevated creatine kinase (CK), lactate dehydrogenase (LDH), serum glutamic-oxaloacetic (SGOT)

Drugs that may alter lab results: N/A

Disorders that may alter lab results: N/A

PATHOLOGICAL FINDINGS
Micro: acute inflammation

SPECIAL TESTS
4 stages in pericarditis
- Electrocardiogram - electrical alternans in tamponade
- Echocardiogram - determines fluid, RA or RV collapse
- Right heart catheterization - equalization of mean and diastolic pressure in all wave forms

IMAGING
- Chest x-ray - small pleural effusion, transient infiltrates; "water bottle" silhouette in large associated pericardial effusion
- Chest CT or MRI in suspected constrictive pericarditis may reveal calcified or thickened pericardium; delineate effusions

DIAGNOSTIC PROCEDURES
- Pericardiocentesis
- Pericardial biopsy

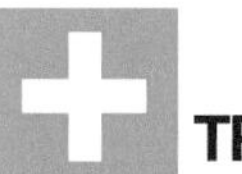

TREATMENT

APPROPRIATE HEALTH CARE
- Outpatient unless signs of complications
- Inpatient with complications (hemodynamic compromise or effusion present)

GENERAL MEASURES N/A

SURGICAL MEASURES Pericardiectomy may be required if drugs are not effective

ACTIVITY No restrictions; limited by patients symptoms only

DIET No restriction. If patient overweight, suggest a weight loss program.

PATIENT EDUCATION Since 15% of patients have a recurrence, must educate for return of symptoms and followup

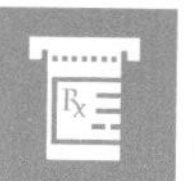

MEDICATIONS

DRUG(S) OF CHOICE

Uncomplicated: aspirin 650 mg q4h. If effective, continue for 2 weeks.

Contraindications: Hypersensitivity to aspirin, known coagulopathy

Precautions: Use with caution in patients with asthma, nasal polyps, severe carditis, pregnancy in the third trimester, history of GI disturbances or bleeding, bleeding disorders or diathesis, telangiectasis, anticoagulation, renal or hepatic dysfunction

Significant possible interactions: Acetaminophen, acetazolamide, ammonium chloride, antacids, aurothioglucose, chlorpropamide, cimetidine, corticosteroids, diclofenac, dicumarol, diltiazem, dipyridamole, etodolac, flurbiprofen, ibuprofen, indomethacin, insulin, ketorolac, meclofenamate, mefenamic acid, methotrexate, metoclopramide, naproxen, nitroglycerin, nizatidine, penicillin G, phenprocoumon, phenylbutazone, phenytoin piroxicam, probenecid, protirelin, quinidine, spironolactone, sulfinpyrazone, sulfonylureas, sulindac, suprofen, tolmetin, valproic acid, warfarin

ALTERNATIVE DRUGS

- Ibuprofen 400-600 mg q6h for 2 weeks
- Indomethacin 25-75 mg q6-8h for 2 weeks
- Colchicine 1 mg q day
- Prednisone 60 mg q day x 2-3 days and quickly taper (last resort) over 2-4 weeks. Risk of recurrence with withdrawal.

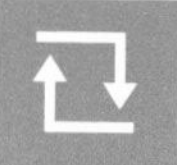

FOLLOWUP

PATIENT MONITORING

- Followup patients in office in 2 weeks and re-evaluate cardiac status and symptomatology
- Repeat chest x-ray and electrocardiogram should be considered at 4 weeks

PREVENTION/AVOIDANCE N/A

POSSIBLE COMPLICATIONS

- Pericardial tamponade
- Recurrence of pericarditis
- Non-compressive effusion
- Chronic, constrictive pericarditis

EXPECTED COURSE/PROGNOSIS

- The majority of patients have complete resolution of pain and symptoms during the 2 weeks of therapy
- Fifteen per cent will have at least one recurrence in the first few months
- A rare patient may become refractory and require corticosteroids or pericardiectomy
- The hemodynamic effects of effusions depends on the volume and rapidity of development
- A very small percentage of patients can develop signs of right sided heart failure secondary to constriction. These patients are best treated with pericardiectomy.

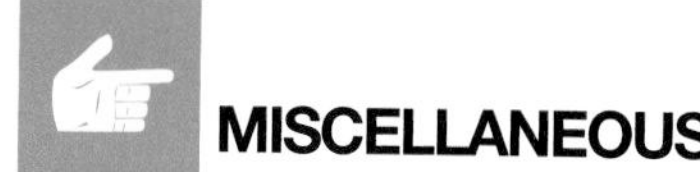

MISCELLANEOUS

ASSOCIATED CONDITIONS Dependent on etiology

AGE-RELATED FACTORS

Pediatric: N/A
Geriatric: N/A
Others: N/A

PREGNANCY N/A

SYNONYMS Acute nonsuppurative pericarditis

ICD-9-CM

420.91 Acute idiopathic pericarditis
420.99 Other acute pericarditis

SEE ALSO

OTHER NOTES N/A

ABBREVIATIONS N/A

REFERENCES

- Bennett JC, Plum F, eds: Cecil Textbook of Medicine. 20th Ed. Philadelphia, W.B. Saunders Co., 1996
- Shabetai R: Diseases of the Pericardium. Cardio Clinics Nov;1990
- Estok DE, et al: Cardiac tamponade in patients with AIDS: a review of pericardial disease in patients with HIV infection. Mt Sinai J Med 1998;65:33-39
- Pawsat DE, et al: Inflammatory disorders of the heart. pericarditis, myocarditis, and endocarditis. Emerg Med Clin of NA 1998;16:665-681

Web references: 3 available at www.5mcc.com
Illustrations N/A

Author(s):

Darell E. Heiselman, DO

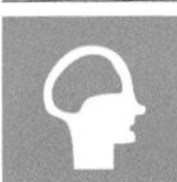

BASICS

DESCRIPTION Acute inflammation of the visceral and parietal peritoneum
System(s) affected: Cardiovascular, Endocrine/ Metabolic, Gastrointestinal
Genetics: No known genetic pattern
Incidence/Prevalence in USA: Common
Predominant age: None
Predominant sex: Male > Female

SIGNS & SYMPTOMS
- Acute abdominal pain
- Fever
- Nausea
- Vomiting
- Constipation
- Abdominal pain exacerbated by motion
- Abdominal distention
- Dyspnea
- Diffuse abdominal rebound
- Generalized abdominal rigidity
- Decreased bowel sounds
- Abdominal hyper-resonance to percussion
- Hypotension
- Tachycardia
- Tachypnea
- Dehydration
- Ascites

CAUSES
- Primary - spontaneous bacterial peritonitis
  - ◊ Ascites associated with cirrhosis, nephrotic syndrome
- Secondary
  - ◊ Following abdominal trauma
  - ◊ Penetrating wounds
  - ◊ Continuous ambulatory peritoneal dialysis
  - ◊ Perforation of bowel
  - ◊ Appendicitis
  - ◊ Colitis - infectious, inflammatory
  - ◊ Peptic ulcer perforation
  - ◊ Gangrene of the bowel
  - ◊ Diverticulitis
  - ◊ Pancreatitis
  - ◊ Postoperative (intra-abdominal surgery)
  - ◊ Acute cholecystitis

RISK FACTORS
- Recent surgery
- Cirrhosis, frequently secondary to alcoholism
- Corticosteroid medication
- Nephrotic syndrome
- Continuous ambulatory peritoneal dialysis

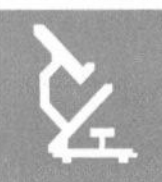

DIAGNOSIS

DIFFERENTIAL DIAGNOSIS
- Abscess formation (subdiaphragmatic, subhepatic, peritoneal, pelvic)
- Other causes of ileus (volvulus, intussusception)
- Mesenteric adenitis
- Appendicitis
- Pancreatitis

LABORATORY
- Positive culture of peritoneal aspirate
- Leukocytosis
- Increased BUN
- Hemoconcentration
- Positive blood culture
- Metabolic acidosis
- Respiratory acidosis
- elevated amylase
- Ascitic fluid analysis

Drugs that may alter lab results: Antibiotics prior to blood studies

Disorders that may alter lab results: N/A

PATHOLOGICAL FINDINGS
- Peritoneum - generalized fibrinopurulent exudate
- Peritoneum - polymorphonuclear infiltration

SPECIAL TESTS N/A

IMAGING
- Abdominal film: free air in peritoneal cavity, large bowel dilatation, small bowel dilatation, intestinal wall edema
- Chest x-ray: elevated diaphragm
- CT: intra-abdominal mass, ascites
- Sonograph: intra-abdominal mass, ascites

DIAGNOSTIC PROCEDURES N/A

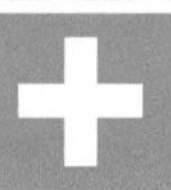

TREATMENT

APPROPRIATE HEALTH CARE Inpatient with intensive care as indicated

GENERAL MEASURES
- Treat paralytic ileus (nasogastric decompression)
- Treat dehydration
- Antibiotics are started empirically to cover a broad spectrum of organisms. The choice of antibiotic may be altered after culture results are obtained.
- Respiratory support if needed
- IV fluids
- Blood transfusions (sometimes)

SURGICAL MEASURES Treat underlying condition(s) and infection (by surgery if necessary)

ACTIVITY Bedrest until infection is under control

DIET
- IV fluids and electrolytes
- Oral feedings only after return of bowel sounds, and passage of flatus and/or feces
- Total parenteral nutrition may be necessary

PATIENT EDUCATION N/A

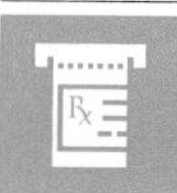

MEDICATIONS

DRUG(S) OF CHOICE
- Spontaneous peritonitis
  - ◊ Ampicillin IV plus gentamicin
  - ◊ Third generation cephalosporin (ceftriaxone)
  - ◊ Ticarcillin-clavulanate, piperacillin-tazobactam, ampicillin-sulbactam
- Secondary peritonitis
  - ◊ Must cover against anaerobic organisms and gram-negative aerobic/facilitative organisms
  - ◊ Agents active against anaerobic organisms include cefoxitin, cefotetan, ticarcillin-clavulanate, piperacillin-tazobactam, ampicillin-sulbactam, imipenem
- Associated with chronic ambulatory peritoneal dialysis
  - ◊ Vancomycin plus gentamicin instilled in peritoneal cavity

Contraindications: Refer to manufacturer's literature
Precautions: Refer to manufacturer's literature
Significant possible interactions: Refer to manufacturer's literature

ALTERNATIVE DRUGS
- Antibiotics, other than those mentioned, if indicated by culture of blood or peritoneal fluid
- Meperidine 50-100 mg IM

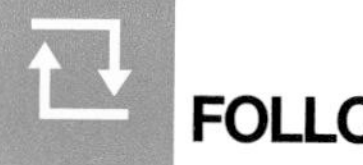

FOLLOWUP

PATIENT MONITORING Frequent monitoring acutely

PREVENTION/AVOIDANCE Prophylactic antibiotics during abdominal surgery

POSSIBLE COMPLICATIONS
- Hypovolemic consequences
- Septicemia
- Septic shock
- Acute renal failure
- Acute respiratory insufficiency
- Liver failure
- Abscess formation

EXPECTED COURSE/PROGNOSIS
- Fully developed paralytic ileus requires 48 hours for recovery
- Mortality dependent on - age, duration, cause, and on pre-existing conditions

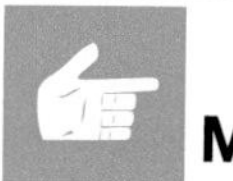

MISCELLANEOUS

ASSOCIATED CONDITIONS
- Abscesses: Subdiaphragmatic, subhepatic, peritoneal, pelvic
- Ileus

AGE-RELATED FACTORS
Pediatric: Get pediatric and surgical consultation, if available
Geriatric: Mortality greater in this age group. Symptoms may be muted.
Others: N/A

PREGNANCY Ruptured ectopic pregnancy may lead to peritonitis

SYNONYMS N/A

ICD-9-CM
567.2 Other suppurative peritonitis
567.9 Unspecified peritonitis

SEE ALSO
Appendicitis, acute
Crohn disease
Diverticular disease
Ectopic pregnancy
Pancreatitis

OTHER NOTES N/A

ABBREVIATIONS N/A

REFERENCES

- Gilbert DN, Moellering RC Jr, Sande MA. The Sanford Guide to Antimicrobial Therapy-2000. 13th ed. Hyde Park, VT: Antimicrobial Therapy, Inc.; 2000
- Fauci AS, et al, editors. Harrison's Principles of Internal Medicine. 14th ed. New York: McGraw Hill;1998
- Mandell GL, Bennett JE, Dolin R, editors. Principles and Practices of Infectious Disease. 5th ed. Philadelphia: Churchill Livingstone; 2000

Web references: 0 available at www.5mcc.com
Illustrations N/A

Author(s):
Alan Adelman, MD, MS

BASICS

DESCRIPTION Infection with abscess formation and collection of pus in the space between the anterior and posterior tonsillar pillars and the superior pharyngeal constrictor muscle. Usually follows an episode of acute pharyngitis or tonsillitis.
System(s) affected: Gastrointestinal, Pulmonary
Genetics: N/A
Incidence/Prevalence in USA: Estimated 45,000 cases yearly (30 cases per 100,000 person-years)
Predominant age: Can occur in all age groups, with greatest incidence in adolescents and young adults 15-30 years of age
Predominant sex: Male = Female

SIGNS & SYMPTOMS
- Extreme sore throat or neck pain
- Odynophagia
- Dysphagia
- Fever greater than 38° C
- Trismus
- "Hot potato voice" (thickened, muffled voice)
- Drooling and pooling of saliva in the mouth
- Tonsillar exudates are uncommonly seen
- Erythematous, edematous tonsil
- Asymmetry of the oropharynx with inferior and medial displacement of the infected tonsil often with contralateral deviation of the uvula
- Cervical adenopathy

CAUSES
Polymicrobial infection is the rule in peritonsillar abscess and multiple bacteria will likely be grown from cultures of drained pus. *Streptococcus* species are the most common pathogens.
- Aerobic bacteria
  - ◊ *Streptococcus pyogenes*
  - ◊ *Streptococcus milleri* group
  - ◊ *Haemophilus influenzae*
  - ◊ Viridans streptococci
  - ◊ Neisseria species
  - ◊ *Staphylococcus aureus*
- Anaerobic bacteria
  - ◊ Fusobacterium
  - ◊ Peptostreptococcus
  - ◊ Prevotella
  - ◊ Bacteroides

RISK FACTORS
- Prior episodes of tonsillitis
- Age (young are more susceptible)

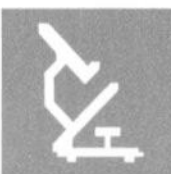

DIAGNOSIS

DIFFERENTIAL DIAGNOSIS
- Peritonsillar cellulitis
- Tonsillar abscess
- Infectious mononucleosis (EBV infection)
- Aspiration of foreign body
- Dental infection
- Salivary gland infection
- Cervical adenitis
- Mastoiditis
- Internal carotid artery aneurysm

LABORATORY
- Leukocytosis
- Culture of pathogens from aspirated or drained pus to identify organism(s)

Drugs that may alter lab results: N/A

Disorders that may alter lab results: N/A

PATHOLOGICAL FINDINGS N/A

SPECIAL TESTS N/A

IMAGING
- Ultrasonography will show a discrete abscess cavity if present. Computed tomography (CT scanning), best performed with contrast, will also show a discrete abscess cavity. Edema of the surrounding tissues can also be seen on CT scan.

DIAGNOSTIC PROCEDURES Incision and drainage of pus, via needle aspiration or an operative procedure under general anesthesia or conscious sedation.

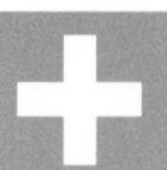

TREATMENT

APPROPRIATE HEALTH CARE Inpatient. Same day surgery is possible in some cases with outpatient management

GENERAL MEASURES
- Intravenous rehydration
- Pain control

SURGICAL MEASURES
Small studies indicate that rates of success are equivalent between needle aspiration and operative incision and drainage.
- Needle aspiration with ultrasound or CT guidance
- Operative incision and drainage when needle aspiration is too difficult due to trismus or lack of patient cooperation
- Immediate tonsillectomy at the time of incision and drainage (known as quinsy tonsillectomy) has decreased in favor, due to increased risk of hemorrhage and overall low rates of abscess recurrence without tonsillectomy
- Delayed tonsillectomy (known as interval tonsillectomy) has also fallen from favor, due to the low rates of recurrent abscess

ACTIVITY As tolerated

DIET No restrictions, liquid diet may be tolerated best until pain improves

PATIENT EDUCATION Important to complete course of antibiotics

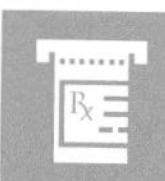

MEDICATIONS

DRUG(S) OF CHOICE

Penicillin remains the standard antimicrobial therapy with initial therapy delivered parenterally. Tailor therapy to cultured pathogens as possible. If organisms other than oral *Streptococci* are suspected, expanded therapy may be indicated. With growing concern for beta-lactamase producing organisms, antibiotics with beta-lactamase inhibitors or cephalosporins may be preferred. If Fusobacterium or Bacteroides are implicated, additional anaerobic therapy with metronidazole may be indicated with increasing resistance to penicillin among these pathogens.

- Penicillin G 1-4 million units IV q 4 hours, OR
- Benzathine Penicillin G 1.2 million units IM x 1, OR
- Benzathine Penicillin G 900,000 units and Procaine Penicillin G 300,000 units IM x 1

Followed by

- Penicillin V 500 mg (25-50 mg/kg for children) tid to complete 10-14 days of total therapy
- For penicillin allergic patients, erythromycin ethyl succinate 300 to 400 mg tid, or
- Cephalexin 250-500 mg tid

If resistant organisms (including oral anaerobes) are suspected, add to the above oral therapy:

- Metronidazole 500 mg tid-qid or
- Clindamycin 150-450 mg tid-qid

Alternatively:

- Amoxicillin-Clavulanate (Augmentin) 500 mg tid or 875 mg bid or
- Cefuroxime 500 mg bid (or other second or third generation cephalosporin) and metronidazole 500 mg tid-qid

Contraindications: Allergy to specific antibiotic
Precautions: Refer to manufacturer's profile of each drug
Significant possible interactions: Refer to manufacturer's profile of each drug

ALTERNATIVE DRUGS N/A

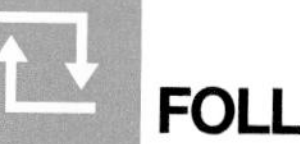

FOLLOWUP

PATIENT MONITORING

- Follow-up to ensure resolution of symptoms and tonsillar inflammation
- Lack of improvement may indicate antibiotic-resistant pathogens or residual abscess necessitating repeat drainage

PREVENTION/AVOIDANCE N/A

POSSIBLE COMPLICATIONS

- Airway obstruction
- Spread to parapharyngeal or retropharyngeal spaces
- Septic jugular vein thrombosis
- Brain abscess
- Sepsis

Possible complications of incision and drainage:

- Pulmonary aspiration of blood and pus with bronchopneumonia
- Tonsillar hemorrhage
- Perforation of the carotid artery

EXPECTED COURSE/PROGNOSIS

- Symptoms will improve rapidly after incision and drainage and appropriate antibiotics
- Pain and inflammation may persist for up to a week after treatment
- Recurrent peritonsillar abscess does occur, but is rare

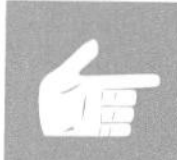

MISCELLANEOUS

ASSOCIATED CONDITIONS

- Pharyngitis
- Tonsillitis
- Peritonsillar cellulitis
- Septic jugular vein thrombophlebitis (Lemierre syndrome)

AGE-RELATED FACTORS

Pediatric: N/A
Geriatric: N/A
Others: N/A

PREGNANCY N/A

SYNONYMS

- Quinsy

ICD-9-CM

475 Peritonsillar abscess

SEE ALSO

Epiglottitis
Pharyngitis

OTHER NOTES N/A

ABBREVIATIONS

N/A

REFERENCES

- Dunne, AA, et al: Peritonsillar abscess - critical analysis of abscess tonsillectomy. Clin Otolaryngol. 2003 Oct;28(5):420-4
- Herzon, FS: Peritonsillar abscess: incidence, current management practices, and a proposal for treatment guidelines. Laryngoscope. 1995 Aug;105(8 Pt 3 Suppl 74):1-17
- Johnson, RJ, et al: An evidence-based review of the treatment of peritonsillar abscess. Otolaryngol Head Neck Surg 2003;128:332-43
- Schraff, S, et al: Peritonsillar abscess in children: a 10-year review of diagnosis and management. Int J Pediatr Otorhinolaryngol. 2001 Mar;57(3):213-8
- Steyer TE: Peritonsillar abscess: diagnosis and treatment: Am Fam Physician. 2002 Jan 1;65(1):93-6

Web references: 0 available at www.5mcc.com
Illustrations N/A

Author(s):

Matthew R Leibowitz, MD

BASICS

DESCRIPTION A group of conditions, with onset at or before adolescence, characterized by enduring patterns of maladaptive and dysfunctional behavior that deviate markedly from one's culture and social environment leading to functional impairment and distress to the individual, coworkers and the family. These behaviors are perceived by the patient to be "normal" and "right" and they have little insight as to their responsibility for these behaviors. These conditions are classified based on the predominant symptoms and their severity.

System(s) affected: Nervous

Genetics: Major character traits inherited; others result from a combination of genetics and environment

Incidence/Prevalence in USA:
- Prevalence 12%
- In male prisoners the prevalence of antisocial personality disorder is about 60%

Predominant age: Starts in adolescence and early twenties and persists throughout one's life

Predominant sex: No difference as a whole; some personality disorders are more common in females and others are more common in males

SIGNS & SYMPTOMS
- Criteria for a personality disorder include an enduring pattern of:
  - ◊ Inner experience and behavior manifesting in two or more of the following areas: cognition, affectivity, interpersonal functioning, or impulse control
  - ◊ Inflexibility and pervasiveness across a broad range of personal and social situations
  - ◊ Significant distress or impairment in social, occupational, or other important areas of functioning
  - ◊ Onset can be traced to adolescence or early adulthood
  - ◊ Not better accounted for as a manifestation or consequence of another mental disorder
  - ◊ Not due to the direct physiological effects of a substance, such as a drug of abuse, or a medication, or a general medical condition, such as a head trauma
- Personality disorders (PD) are classified into three major clusters
  - ◊ Cluster A : eccentricism and oddness
    - Paranoid PD: unwarranted suspiciousness and distrust of others, defensive, guarded, and overly sensitive
    - Schizoid PD: emotional, cold, or detached, apathetic to criticism or praise, socially isolated
    - Schizotypal PD: eccentric behavior, odd belief system, perceptions and speech, social isolation, and general suspiciousness
  - ◊ Cluster B: dramatic, emotional, or erratic behavioral patterns
    - Antisocial PD: aggressive, impulsive, irritable, irresponsible, dishonest, deceitful, and at times reckless disregard for safety of self or others
    - Borderline PD: pervasive pattern of unstable interpersonal relationships, self image, with high impulsivity from early adulthood. Intense fear of abandonment, mood swings, poor self-esteem, chronic boredom, and feelings of inner emptiness.
    - Histrionic PD: excessive emotionality and attention seeking in a variety of contexts. Needs to be the center of attention with self-dramatizing behaviors; suggestive with flowing and impressionistic speech.
    - Narcissistic PD: grandiosity, a need for affirmation and for admiration from others. Lack of empathy for other people's pain or discomfort. Grandiose sense of self-importance and preoccupation with fantasies of success, power, brilliance, beauty or ideal love. Belief that the individual is special, unique and deserves special treatment. At times they may show arrogance, haughty behaviors, or attitudes.
  - ◊ Cluster C: anxiety, excessive worry, fear and different patterns to cope with these emotions
    - Avoidant PD: social inhibition, feelings of inadequacy, and hyper-sensitivity to negative evaluation. Avoidance of occupational and interpersonal activities that involve the risk of criticism by others. They avoid taking chances and risks involving significant interpersonal contact, preoccupied with fears of being criticized and rejected, and view themselves as socially inept, and personally unappealing or inferior to others.
    - Dependent PD: excessive need to be taken care of that leads to submissive, clinging behavior, and fears of separation. Needs constant and repeated reassurance and guidance by others. Difficulties making decisions with the activities of daily living. Avoids expressing disagreements with others due to fear of losing support and approval. Usually seeks out strong and confident people as friends or spouses and feels more secure in such relationships.
    - Obsessive-Compulsive PD (OCPD): pre-occupation with cleanliness, orderliness, perfectionism, and control of events and people at the expense of flexibility, openness, and efficiency. Preoccupation with excessive details, rules, lists, order, organization, and schedules to the extent that the major point of the activity is lost. Exhibits perfectionism that interferes with task completion. Indecisive, over conscientious, scrupulous, and rigid about matters of morality, ethics, or values. Reluctant to delegate tasks at work or home and some are unable to discard worn out or worthless objects even if they have no sentimental value.
    - PD, not otherwise specified: a mixture of characteristics from other PDs without a predominant pattern compatible with above categories. It can also be used for specific personality disorders not mentioned in the APA classification (DSM-IV-TR) such as depressive PD, masochistic PD, passive-aggressive PD and others.

CAUSES
Environmental and genetic factors

RISK FACTORS
- Positive family history
- Pregnancy risk factors
  - ◊ Nutritional deprivation
  - ◊ Use of alcohol or drugs
  - ◊ Viral and bacterial Infections
- Dysfunctional family with child abuse and neglect

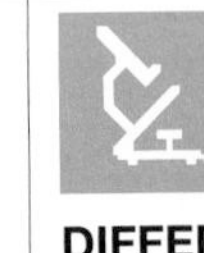

DIAGNOSIS

DIFFERENTIAL DIAGNOSIS
- Medical disorders (e.g., brain diseases) with behavioral changes
- Other psychiatric disorders, with similar symptoms, have a specific time of onset signifying a change from a previously different pattern of behavior or have a difference in self-perception
  - ◊ In obsessive compulsive disorder (OCD), symptoms are ego-dystonic, i.e., are perceived as foreign and unwanted. In addition, OCD has a pattern of relapse and perhaps remission.
  - ◊ In obsessive compulsive personality disorder (OCPD), symptoms are perceived as desirable behaviors (ego-syntonic) that the patient feels proud of and wants others to emulate. In addition, OCPD has a life-long pattern (i.e., without significant relapse or remission).

LABORATORY TSH, VDRL, CBC, CMP, HIV

Drugs that may alter lab results: N/A

Disorders that may alter lab results: N/A

PATHOLOGICAL FINDINGS N/A

SPECIAL TESTS Psychological testing, e.g., MMPI-II

IMAGING CT scan, and MRI of the brain may be necessary in newly developed symptoms to rule out organic brain disease (e.g., frontal lobe tumor)

DIAGNOSTIC PROCEDURES
- Comprehensive interview and mental status examination
- Interview of relatives and friends helpful in establishing the enduring pattern of behavior

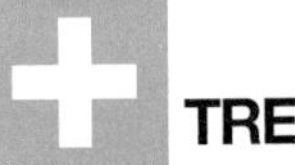

TREATMENT

APPROPRIATE HEALTH CARE Outpatient individual psychotherapy and group therapy

GENERAL MEASURES
- Long term psychotherapy and cognitive behavior therapy
- Group therapy is helpful in the utilization of therapeutic confrontation and increasing one's awareness and insight regarding the damaging effects of dysfunctional behavior patterns

SURGICAL MEASURES N/A

ACTIVITY Regular physical exercise helps in coping with stress and the activities of daily living

DIET Emphasize variety of healthy foods, avoid obesity

PATIENT EDUCATION Bibliotherapy and writing therapy, specific assignments and watching certain movies to better understand the nature and origin of one's specific condition are helpful
- The movie "As Good As It Gets" illustrates someone with obsessive compulsive behaviors and their impact on activities of daily living and relationships with family and friends
- The movie series "The Godfather" is an example of several characters with anti-social personality disorder and how this affects their interpersonal relationships and their own physical and mental health

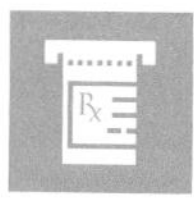

MEDICATIONS

DRUG(S) OF CHOICE
- No specific drugs treat personality disorders, however, specific medications can reduce the intensity, frequency, and dysfunctionality of certain behaviors, thoughts, and feelings
- Symptom management:
  - ◊ Mini-psychosis (associated with paranoid, schizoid, and schizotypal personality disorders). Atypical antipsychotics: clozapine (Clozaril), risperidone (Risperdal), quetiapine (Seroquel), olanzapine (Zyprexa), ziprasidone (Geodon), and aripiprazole (Abilify). Start with a low dose gradually adjusting to the patient's needs.
  - ◊ Anxiety. Anxiolytics: benzodiazepines, buspirone, and the SSRIs
  - ◊ Depressed mood. Anti-depressants: SSRIs

Contraindications: Refer to manufacturer's profile of each drug

Precautions:
- Risperidone and ziprasidone may be associated with hyperglycemia and ketoacidosis

Significant possible interactions: Refer to manufacturer's profile of each drug

ALTERNATIVE DRUGS Mood stabilizers (e.g., lithium carbonate, divalproex [Depakote] and anti-epileptic drugs may be helpful

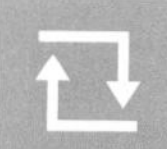

FOLLOWUP

PATIENT MONITORING
- If substance abuse is suspected, check drug screens
- Infrequent sessions, with relative or friends, helpful in monitoring progress and behavior changes

PREVENTION/AVOIDANCE N/A

POSSIBLE COMPLICATIONS
- Disruptive family life with frequent divorces and separations, alcoholism, substance abuse and drug addiction
- Disruptive behaviors in the work place may cause absenteeism, loss of productivity, and loss of self support
- Violation of the law and disregard for the concerns and rights of others

EXPECTED COURSE/PROGNOSIS
Personality disorders are enduring patterns of behavior throughout one's lifetime and are not easily responsive to treatment

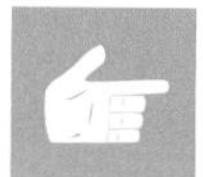

MISCELLANEOUS

ASSOCIATED CONDITIONS Depression, other psychiatric disorders in patient and family members

AGE-RELATED FACTORS
Pediatric: History of childhood neglect, abuse, and trauma are not uncommon

Geriatric: Coping with stresses of elderly life difficult

Others: N/A

PREGNANCY Adds pressure in coping with the activities of daily living

SYNONYMS
- Character disorders
- Character pathology

ICD-9-CM
301.9 Unspecified personality disorder
301.50 Histrionic personality disorder, unspecified
300.3 Obsessive-compulsive disorders
301.0 Paranoid personality disorder
301.20 Schizoid personality disorder, unspecified
301.22 Schizotypal personality
301.6 Dependent personality disorder
301.7 Antisocial personality disorder
301.81 Narcissistic personality
301.82 Avoidant personality
301.83 Borderline personality

SEE ALSO
Obsessive compulsive disorder

OTHER NOTES N/A

ABBREVIATIONS
OCPD = obsessive compulsive personality disorder
OCD = obsessive compulsive disorder

REFERENCES

- American Psychiatric Association. Diagnostic and Statistical Manual of Mental Disorders: Text Revision. 4th ed. Washington DC: American Psychiatric Press; 2000
- Bienvenu OJ, Stein MB. Personality and anxiety disorders: a review. J Personal Discord 2003;17(2):139-51
- Cloninger CR. Personality and Psychopathology. Washington DC: American Psychiatric Press; 1999
- Coid J. Epidemiology, public health and the problem of personality disorder. Br J Psychiatry Suppl 2003;44: S3-10
- Ekselius L, Tillfors M, et al. Personality disorders in the general population: DSM-IV and ICD-10 defined prevalence as related to sociodemograhpic profile. Pers Individ Dif 2001;30(2): 320-331
- Endler NS, Kocovski NL. Personality disorders at the crossroads. J Personal Discord 2002;16(6):487-502
- Jablensky A. The classification of personality disorders: critical review and need for rethinking. Psychopathology 2002;35(2-3):112-6
- Kendell RE. The distinction between personality disorder and mental illness. Br J Psychiatry 2002;180:110-5
- Links PS, Boggild A, Sarin N. Psychopharmacology of personality disorders: review and emerging issues. Curr Psychiatry Rep 2001;3(1):70-6
- Moran P. The epidemiology of antisocial personality disorder. Soc Psychiatry Psychiatr Epidemiol 1999; 34(5):231-42
- Newton-Howes G, Tyrer P. Pharmacotherapy for personality disorders. Expert Opin Pharmacother 2003;4(10):1643-49
- Ogrodniczuk JS, Piper WE. Day treatment for personality disorders: a review of research findings. Harv Rev Psychiatry 2001;9(3):105-17
- Parker G, Both L, et al. Defining disordered personality functioning. J Personal Disord 2002;16(6):503-22
- Piper WE, Ogrodniczuk JS. Psychotherapy of personality disorders. Curr Psychiatry Rep 2001;3(1):59-63
- Rizvi SL, Linehan MM. Dialectical behavior therapy for personality disorders. Curr Psychiatry Rep 2001;3(1):64-9
- Sater N, Samuels JF et al. Epidemiology of personality
- disorders. Curr Psychiatry Rep 2001;3(1):41-5
- Torgersen S, Kringlen E, Cramer V. The prevalence of personality disorders in a community sample. Arch Gen Psychiatry 2001;58(6):590-6
- Widiger TA, Chaynes K. Current issues in the assessment of personality disorders. Curr Psychiatry Rep 2003;5(1):28-35

Web references: 0 available at www.5mcc.com
Illustrations N/A

Author(s):
Moshe S. Torem, MD

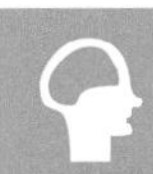

BASICS

DESCRIPTION Pertussis or whooping cough is a highly communicable, respiratory bacterial infection. Characteristically, it produces a paroxysmal spasmodic cough, ending in prolonged high-pitched inspiratory whoop or crow. Transmission is by direct contact and patients are contagious for 3 weeks. Incubation period averages 7 to 14 days (maximum 3 weeks). Usual course - acute, but protracted (lasts 4-12 weeks after catarrhal period).

System(s) affected: Pulmonary

Genetics: N/A

Incidence/Prevalence in USA:
- 1.74 cases/100,000 people
- Annual average cases - 3,500, with 10 deaths
- Occurs in 3-5 year cycles
- 80% of nonimmune household contacts contract disease
- Increasing as immunization rates decline.

Predominant age: 3 months-6 years (infants comprise about half of the cases)

Predominant sex: Female > Male

SIGNS & SYMPTOMS
- Cough paroxysms
- Staccato cough
- Mild fever
- Rhinorrhea
- Anorexia
- "Whoop" cough
- Apnea, episodic
- Posttussive inspiratory gasp
- Posttussive emesis

CAUSES
- *Bordetella pertussis*
- *Bordetella parapertussis* and *Bordetella bronchiseptica* produce a similar, but milder, clinical illness.

RISK FACTORS
- Unimmunized children
- Contact with an infected person
- Epidemic exposure
- Pregnancy

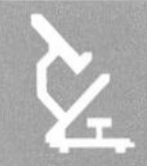

DIAGNOSIS

DIFFERENTIAL DIAGNOSIS
- Common cold
- Adenoviral syndromes
- Mycoplasma
- Chlamydia
- Bronchiolitis
- Influenza
- Bacterial pneumonias
- Cystic fibrosis
- Tuberculosis
- Interstitial pneumonitis
- Foreign body

LABORATORY
- WBC: elevated (15,000-60,000) with marked lymphocytosis
- Bordetella pertussis culture on Bordet-Gengou culture medium (takes 10-14 days)
- DFA has variable sensitivity and low specificity
- PCR assay rapid, sensitive, specific
- Culture and PCR negative after 4 weeks of illness

Drugs that may alter lab results: N/A

Disorders that may alter lab results: N/A

PATHOLOGICAL FINDINGS
- Focal emphysema
- Mucopurulent exudate
- Patchy ulceration of respiratory epithelium

SPECIAL TESTS N/A

IMAGING Chest x-ray - focal atelectasis, peribronchial cuffing, emphysema

DIAGNOSTIC PROCEDURES Nasal swab

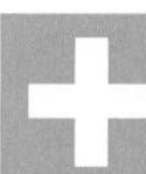

TREATMENT

APPROPRIATE HEALTH CARE Hospitalization for seriously ill infants. Outpatient for milder cases.

GENERAL MEASURES
- General supportive, skilled nursing care
- Isolation and quarantine for 4 weeks; 5 days after erythromycin started
- Parenteral fluid therapy if needed
- Oxygen
- Careful observation for apnea in young infants, and, to avoid stimuli that trigger paroxysms
- Mechanical ventilation
- Nutritional support - may require tube feedings in infants

SURGICAL MEASURES N/A

ACTIVITY Rest during active phase in quiet environment

DIET Encourage extra fluids. May need to provide small frequent meals to assure adequate nutrition.

PATIENT EDUCATION For patient education materials favorably reviewed on this topic, contact: American Academy of Pediatrics, 141 Northwest Point Blvd., P.O. Box 927, Elk Grove Village, IL 60009-0927, (800)433-9016

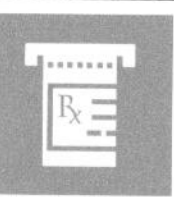

MEDICATIONS

DRUG(S) OF CHOICE
- Erythromycin, 40-50 mg/kg/day divided doses q 6 h for 14 days; drug of choice, maximum 2 g/day
- Azithromycin, 10 mg/kg/day in 1 dose for five days, maximum 60 mg/day, for 5 days
- Clarithromycin, 15-20 mg/kg/day in 2 divided doses, maximum 1 g/day, for 7 days
- Penicillins and cephalosporins not effective
- Other antibiotics for bacterial complications such as bronchopneumonia or otitis media
- Antibiotics do not alter course of illness unless given very early, however they prevent transmission.

Contraindications: Do not use cough suppressants

Precautions: Erythromycin may be associated with hypertrophic pyloric stenosis in infants under 2 weeks of age, but still should be used

Significant possible interactions: N/A

ALTERNATIVE DRUGS
- Steroids and/or theophylline have been suggested for treatment of severely ill patients (their effectiveness and potential hazards require further controlled studies)
- Beta-2 agonists (e.g., albuterol) may help with cough paroxysms
- Trimethoprim-sulfamethoxazole

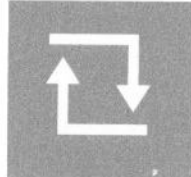

FOLLOWUP

PATIENT MONITORING
- Intensive care unit may be necessary for severely ill infants
- Older children and adults with mild cases do not need to be confined to bed or admitted to hospital

PREVENTION/AVOIDANCE
- Respiration isolation of infected persons until treated with erythromycin 5 days
- Immunization for all infants, usually combined with diphtheria and tetanus toxoids (DTaP). Immunization or booster not recommended after age 7 years.
- Erythromycin - (40 mg/kg/day in 4 divided doses, maximum 2 g/day for 14 days, for all household and close contacts (e.g., day-care)
- Immediately immunize all unimmunized contacts under age 7
- Observe contacts for symptoms for 21 days after exposure
- Classroom prophylaxis not recommended

POSSIBLE COMPLICATIONS
- Can infect up to 80% of household members who are not immune
- Death, especially in infants
- Pneumonia
- Encephalopathy
- Coma
- Otitis media
- Tuberculosis activation
- Epistaxis
- Hernia
- Re-induction of paroxysmal coughing (for several months) especially with upper respiratory infections
- Seizures
- Cerebral hemorrhage
- Weight loss
- Hemoptysis
- Atelectasis

EXPECTED COURSE/PROGNOSIS
Complete recovery

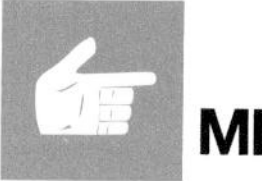

MISCELLANEOUS

ASSOCIATED CONDITIONS
- Otitis media
- Bronchopneumonia
- Failure to thrive
- Swallow dysfunction

AGE-RELATED FACTORS
Pediatric: Most serious and highest mortality in infants less than 6 months of age (death usually due to complications)

Geriatric: May be more serious in this age group

Others: N/A

PREGNANCY N/A

SYNONYMS
Whooping cough

ICD-9-CM
033.9 Whooping cough, unspecified organism

SEE ALSO
Adenovirus infections
Bronchiolitis
Common cold
Cystic fibrosis
Failure to thrive (FTT)
Immunizations
Influenza
Otitis media
Pneumonia, bacterial
Tuberculosis

OTHER NOTES
- Do not use cough suppressants
- Reporting of selected adverse reactions with certain vaccines is now required by the National Childhood Vaccine Injury Act of 1986. Toll-free information number - (800)822-7967.

ABBREVIATIONS
DFA = direct fluorescent antibody
PCR = polymerase chain reaction

REFERENCES

- Mandell GL, ed. Principles and Practice of Infectious Diseases. 4th Ed. New York: Churchill Livingstone; 1995
- Centers for Disease Control. National Childhood Vaccine Injury Act: Requirements for permanent vaccination records and for reporting of selected events after vaccination. MMWR 1988;37:197-200
- Red Book: 2003 Report of the Committee on Infectious Diseases. 26th ed. Elk Grove, IL: American Academy of Pediatrics; 2003.p.472-86

Web references: 2 available at www.5mcc.com

Illustrations N/A

Author(s):
Nancy N. Dambro, MD

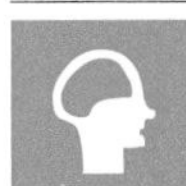

BASICS

DESCRIPTION Inflammation of the pharynx most commonly caused by acute infection. Group A streptococcus is a focus of diagnosis due to its potential for preventable rheumatic sequelae. Chronic low grade symptoms usually related to reflux disease or vocal abuse.
System(s) affected: Gastrointestinal
Genetics: Individuals with a positive family history of rheumatic fever have a higher risk of rheumatic sequelae following an untreated group A beta hemolytic streptococcal infection
Incidence/Prevalence in USA:
- Estimated 30 million cases diagnosed yearly
- 11% of all school age children visit a physician annually with pharyngitis
- 12-25% of sore throats seen by physicians
- Incidence of rheumatic fever is decreasing with estimate of 64 cases per 100,000

Predominant age:
- Pharyngitis occurs in all age groups
- Streptococcal infection has greatest incidence 5 to 18 years of age

Predominant sex: Male = Female

SIGNS & SYMPTOMS
- Sore throat
- Enlarged tonsils
- Pharyngeal erythema
- Tonsillar exudates
- Soft palate petechiae
- Cervical adenopathy
- Absence of cough, hoarseness, or lower respiratory symptoms
- Fever (> 102.5°F [39.1°C] suggests Streptococcus)
- Scarlet fever rash: punctate erythematous macules with reddened flexor creases and circumoral pallor (Streptococcal pharyngitis)
- Gray pseudomembrane found in diphtheria and occasionally, mononucleosis
- Characteristic erythematous based clear vesicles in herpes stomatitis
- Anorexia
- Chills
- Malaise
- Headache
- Conjunctivitis, more commonly with adenovirus infections

CAUSES
- Acute - bacterial:
  - ◊ Group A beta-hemolytic streptococci
  - ◊ Neisseria gonorrhoeae
  - ◊ Corynebacterium diphtheriae (diphtheria)
  - ◊ Haemophilus influenzae
  - ◊ Moraxella (Branhamella) catarrhalis
  - ◊ Group C and G streptococcus, rarely
- Acute - virus:
  - ◊ Rhinovirus
  - ◊ Adenovirus
  - ◊ Parainfluenza virus
  - ◊ Coxsackievirus
  - ◊ Coronavirus
  - ◊ Echovirus
  - ◊ Herpes simplex virus
  - ◊ Epstein-Barr virus (mononucleosis)
  - ◊ Cytomegalovirus
- Chronic
  - ◊ More likely non-infectious
  - ◊ Irritation from post-nasal discharge of chronic allergic rhinitis or reflux
  - ◊ Chemical irritation or smoking
  - ◊ Neoplasms and vasculitides

RISK FACTORS
- Group A beta hemolytic streptococcal epidemics occur
- Age (young are more susceptible)
- Family history
- Close quarters, such as in new military recruits
- Immunosuppression
- Fatigue
- Smoking
- Excess alcohol consumption
- Oral sex
- Diabetes mellitus
- Recent illness

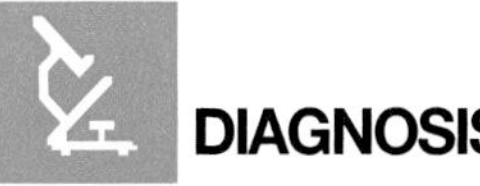

DIAGNOSIS

DIFFERENTIAL DIAGNOSIS
- See causative factors
- Sore throat can be seen with leukopenia

LABORATORY
- Blood agar throat culture from swab. Bacitracin disc sensitivity of hemolytic colonies suggest group A streptococci. Specific antibody identification available.
- Rapid screening for streptococci can be done from throat swab with antigen agglutination kits. 5-10% false negatives lead some to suggest routine backup of all negatives with blood agar culture. Newer optical immunoassay tests are more sensitive.
- Leukocytosis (if bacterial)

Drugs that may alter lab results: N/A

Disorders that may alter lab results: N/A

PATHOLOGICAL FINDINGS Culture of pathogens to identify causes

SPECIAL TESTS
- Special tests usually done only if history is suggestive
- Screening for gonococcal infection requires warm Thayer-Martin plate
- Viruses can be cultured in special media
- Mono spot test for Epstein-Barr virus
- Gram stain can be suggestive
- Streptococcal isolates can be immunologically typed

IMAGING N/A

DIAGNOSTIC PROCEDURES History and physical probably only 50% accurate. Laboratory required unless in epidemic setting.

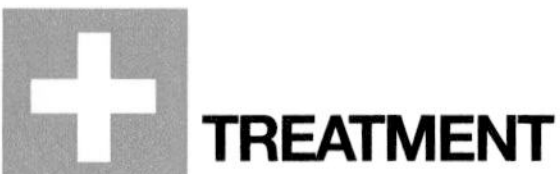

TREATMENT

APPROPRIATE HEALTH CARE Outpatient

GENERAL MEASURES
- Salt water gargles
- Acetaminophen
- Dyclonine lozenges
- Cool-mist humidifier

SURGICAL MEASURES N/A

ACTIVITY As tolerated

DIET No restrictions. Encourage extra fluids.

PATIENT EDUCATION
- Important to complete 10 day course of antibiotics regardless of symptom response
- Patients presumed to be non-infectious after 24 hours of antibiotic coverage

MEDICATIONS

DRUG(S) OF CHOICE
For streptococcal pharyngitis, penicillin is the standard. All choices should have complete 10 day course.
- Penicillin V 250 mg tid (25-50 mg/kg/day), or
- For penicillin allergic patients, erythromycin ethylsuccinate 300 to 400 mg tid (30 mg/kg/day), or
- Cephalexin 250 mg tid (30 mg/kg/day)

Contraindications: Allergy to specific antibiotic
Precautions: Refer to manufacturer's profile of each drug
Significant possible interactions: Refer to manufacturer's profile of each drug

ALTERNATIVE DRUGS
- Treatment of carrier state is difficult, usually requiring addition of rifampin to penicillin regimen
- Penicillin is the treatment most documented to prevent rheumatic sequelae but cephalosporins have lower rate of bacteriologic failure
- Bacterial eradication rates ≥ 10 days therapy with penicillin have been achieved with 6 days of amoxicillin and 5 days with various cephalosporins
- The newer macrolides, azithromycin and clarithromycin, are also effective against streptococcal pharyngitis, but more expensive. The chief advantage of azithromycin is its 5 day course with 10 day effective duration.
- Other cephalosporins are generally effective for streptococcal pharyngitis, but more expensive than cephalexin

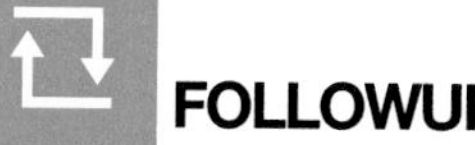

FOLLOWUP

PATIENT MONITORING
- Routine followup cultures not necessary
- Telephone consult for duration of symptoms

PREVENTION/AVOIDANCE
Avoid contact with infected people

POSSIBLE COMPLICATIONS
- Rheumatic fever
- Post-streptococcal glomerulonephritis
- Peritonsillar abscess
- Systemic infection
- Otitis media
- Mastoiditis
- Septicemia
- Rhinitis
- Sinusitis
- Pneumonia

EXPECTED COURSE/PROGNOSIS
- Streptococcal pharyngeal infection runs a 5-7 day course with peak of fever at 2-3 days
- Symptoms will resolve spontaneously without treatment, but rheumatic complications are still possible
- Suppurative complications such as peritonsillar abscess require surgical intervention

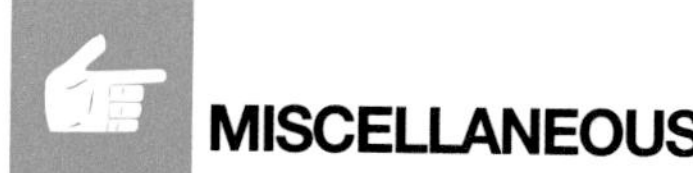

MISCELLANEOUS

ASSOCIATED CONDITIONS
N/A

AGE-RELATED FACTORS
Pediatric: N/A
Geriatric: N/A
Others: N/A

PREGNANCY
N/A

SYNONYMS
- Sore throat
- Tonsillitis
- Streptococcal throat

ICD-9-CM
462 Acute pharyngitis
463 Acute tonsillitis
472.1 Chronic pharyngitis
474.00 Chronic tonsillitis
034.0 Streptococcal sore throat
034.1 Scarlet fever

SEE ALSO
Herpes simplex
Mononucleosis
Rheumatic fever

OTHER NOTES
Unless clinical presentation is unusual, treatment is based on presence or absence of group A streptococci

ABBREVIATIONS
N/A

REFERENCES

- Pichichero ME: Controversies in the treatment of streptococcal pharyngitis. Amer Fam Phys 1990;42(6):1558-1560
- Goldman L, Ausiello D, eds: Cecil Textbook of Medicine. 22nd ed. Philadelphia, WB Saunders Co, 2004
- Bisno AL, et al: Diagnosis and management of group A streptococcal pharyngitis: a practice guideline. Clin Infect Dis 1997;25(3):574-583
- Pichichero ME, Cohen R: Shortened course of antibiotic therapy for acute otitis media, sinusitis and tonsillopharyngitis. Pediatr infect Dis 1997;16(7):680-695

Web references: 1 available at www.5mcc.com
Illustrations N/A

Author(s):
David E. Burtner, MD

BASICS

DESCRIPTION Catecholamine-producing tumor. In 90% of cases, the tumors are found in the adrenal medulla, but may also be found in other tissues derived from neural crest cells.

System(s) affected: Endocrine/Metabolic

Genetics: N/A

Incidence/Prevalence in USA:
- 0.01% to 0.1% of the hypertensive population

Predominant age: Any age, peak incidence ages 30 to 60 years

Predominant sex: Male = Female

SIGNS & SYMPTOMS
- Paroxysmal spells (the "5 P's")
  - ◊ Pressure - sudden increase in blood pressure
  - ◊ Pain - headache, chest and abdominal pain
  - ◊ Perspiration
  - ◊ Palpitation
  - ◊ Pallor
- Additional symptoms
  - ◊ Constipation
  - ◊ Tremor
  - ◊ Weight loss
  - ◊ Anxiety
- Signs
  - ◊ Hypertension - paroxysmal in half of the patients
  - ◊ Orthostatic hypotension
  - ◊ Grade II to IV retinopathy
  - ◊ Fever
  - ◊ Hyperglycemia
  - ◊ Hypercalcemia
  - ◊ Erythrocytosis
  - ◊ 10% of patients are asymptomatic

CAUSES
- Catecholamine-producing tumor - "Rule of 10:"
  - ◊ 10% are extra-adrenal
  - ◊ 10% are multiple or bilateral
  - ◊ 10% are malignant
  - ◊ 10% recur after surgical removal
  - ◊ 10% occur in children
  - ◊ ≥10% are familial
  - ◊ 10% present as adrenal incidentalomas

RISK FACTORS
- Familial pheochromocytoma
- Multiple endocrine neoplasia types II A and B
- Neurofibromatosis, type 1
- Von Hippel-Lindau syndrome
- Familial paraganglioma

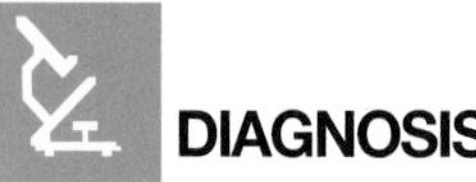

DIAGNOSIS

DIFFERENTIAL DIAGNOSIS
- Labile essential hypertension
- Anxiety and panic attacks
- Paroxysmal cardiac arrhythmia
- Thyrotoxicosis
- Menopausal syndrome
- Hypoglycemia
- Mastocytosis
- Withdrawal of adrenergic-inhibiting medications
- Angina
- Hyperventilation
- Migraine headache
- Amphetamine or cocaine use
- Sympathomimetic ingestion

LABORATORY
- Elevated 24-h urine metanephrine
- Elevated 24-h urine or plasma catecholamines measured by high performance liquid chromatography (HPLC)
- Elevated fractionated plasma metanephrines
- If results equivocal or normal, repeat 24-hr urine collection with a spell

Drugs that may alter lab results:
- Increased by:
  - ◊ Amphetamines
  - ◊ Tricyclic antidepressants
  - ◊ Clonidine or other drug withdrawal
  - ◊ Labetalol
  - ◊ Ethanol
  - ◊ Methyldopa
  - ◊ Sotalol
  - ◊ Levodopa
- Decreased by:
  - ◊ Central alpha-2 agonists
  - ◊ Reserpine

Disorders that may alter lab results: Major physical stress (e.g., surgery, stroke)

PATHOLOGICAL FINDINGS Catecholamine-producing tumor in the adrenal medulla, para-aortic sympathetic chain, wall of the urinary bladder, sympathetic chain in the neck or mediastinum

SPECIAL TESTS Clonidine suppression test, suppression/provocative tests

IMAGING
- Computerized abdominal imaging (MRI preferred over CT)
- I-123: I-metaiodobenzylguanidine scan
- In-111: pentetreotide scan

DIAGNOSTIC PROCEDURES N/A

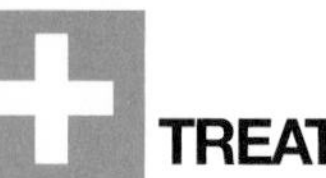

TREATMENT

APPROPRIATE HEALTH CARE Inpatient surgery

GENERAL MEASURES
- Combined alpha- and beta-adrenergic blockade
- Cardiovascular and hemodynamic variables must be monitored closely

SURGICAL MEASURES
- High risk surgical procedure
- Experienced surgeon/anesthesiologist team required

ACTIVITY No limitations

DIET High in salt content preoperatively

PATIENT EDUCATION National Adrenal Disease Foundation (NADF), 505 Northern Blvd, Great Neck, NY 11021; 516-407-4992; e-mail: nadf@aol.com

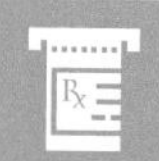

MEDICATIONS

DRUG(S) OF CHOICE
- Combined alpha- and beta-adrenergic blockade required preoperatively
- Initiate alpha-blockade first - phenoxybenzamine (Dibenzyline) 10 mg daily and increase by 10-20 mg every 2 days as needed to control blood pressure and paroxysmal spells (average dose is 0.5-1.0 mg/kg daily)
- Beta-blockade after alpha-blockade is established - propranolol (Inderal) 10 mg q 6 hrs initially and increase as necessary to control tachycardia
- Acute hypertensive crises should be treated with phentolamine (Regitine) or nitroprusside administered intravenously

Contraindications: Beta-adrenergic blockade in patients with asthma, sinus bradycardia and greater than first degree block, or congestive heart failure. Avoid beta-blockers with intrinsic sympathomimetic activity

Precautions:
- Beta-adrenergic blockade alone may result in more severe hypertension due to the unopposed alpha-adrenergic stimulation; patients should be cautioned about postural hypotension
- Beta-adrenergic blockade is initiated at low doses of a short acting agent due to the possible side effect of pulmonary edema in the patient with catecholamine myocardiopathy

Significant possible interactions: For beta-adrenergic blockade - verapamil, phenytoin, phenobarbitone, rifampin, chlorpromazine, cimetidine

ALTERNATIVE DRUGS
- Alpha-adrenergic blocking agents - prazosin (Minipress), terazosin (Hytrin), doxazosin (Cardura)
- Beta-adrenergic blocking agents - nadolol (Corgard), atenolol (Tenormin), metoprolol (Lopressor)
- Combined beta- and alpha-adrenergic blocker - labetalol (Normodyne, TranDate)
- Catecholamine synthesis inhibitor - metyrosine (Demser)

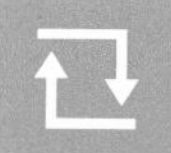

FOLLOWUP

PATIENT MONITORING
- Daily blood pressure monitoring prior to surgery
- Intra-operative hemodynamic monitoring
- Two weeks postoperatively - 24-h urine for measurement of catecholamines and metanephrines; if normal, re-check annually, indefinitely

PREVENTION/AVOIDANCE N/A

POSSIBLE COMPLICATIONS
- Postural hypotension with alpha-adrenergic blockade
- Pulmonary edema with beta-adrenergic blockade
- Intra-operative hypertensive crisis

EXPECTED COURSE/PROGNOSIS
- The survival rate after removal of a benign pheochromocytoma is nearly that of age- and sex-matched controls
- For malignant pheochromocytoma, the 5-year survival rate is less than 50%

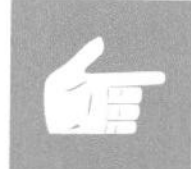

MISCELLANEOUS

ASSOCIATED CONDITIONS
- Multiple endocrine neoplasia type IIA (medullary thyroid carcinoma and primary hyperparathyroidism)
- Multiple endocrine neoplasia type IIB (medullary thyroid carcinoma and mucosal neuromas)
- Neurofibromatosis, type 1
- Von Hippel-Lindau syndrome (retinal angiomatosis and cerebellar hemangioblastoma)
- Familial paraganglioma
- Ataxia-telangiectasia
- Tuberous sclerosis
- Sturge-Weber syndrome
- Cholelithiasis
- Renal artery stenosis

AGE-RELATED FACTORS
Pediatric: N/A
Geriatric: N/A
Others: N/A

PREGNANCY
- First and second trimester - surgical resection
- Third trimester - cesarean section and removal of the pheochromocytoma in the same operation

SYNONYMS Paraganglioma

ICD-9-CM
194.0 Malignant neoplasm of adrenal gland
227.0 Benign neoplasm of adrenal gland

SEE ALSO
Hypertension, essential
Multiple endocrine neoplasia (MEN)

OTHER NOTES
All patients with paroxysmal spells and hypertension or with difficult to control hypertension should be screened

ABBREVIATIONS
HPLC = high performance liquid chromatography

REFERENCES
- Young WF Jr: Pheochromocytoma: 1926-1993: Trends in Endocrinology and Metabolism 1993;4:122
- Bravo EL, Gifford RW: Pheochromocytoma: Diagnosis, localization, and management. N Engl J Med 1984;311:1298
- Young WF Jr: Spells: In search of a cause. Mayo Clin Proc 1995;70:757-765

Web references: 1 available at www.5mcc.com
Illustrations 2 available

Author(s):
William F. Young, Jr, MD

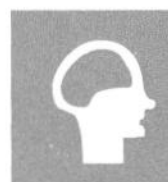

BASICS

DESCRIPTION
- Phimosis: tightness of the penile foreskin which prevents it from being drawn back from over the glans
- Paraphimosis: constriction of glans penis by proximally placed phimotic foreskin

System(s) affected: Renal/Urologic, Reproductive, Skin/Exocrine
Genetics: N/A
Incidence/Prevalence in USA: 1% of males over 16 years of age
Predominant age: Infancy and adolescence
Predominant sex: Male only

SIGNS & SYMPTOMS
- Phimosis
  - ◊ Unretractable foreskin
  - ◊ Pain on erection
  - ◊ Superimposed balanitis
- Paraphimosis
  - ◊ Penile pain
  - ◊ Drainage
  - ◊ Ulceration
  - ◊ Swelling

CAUSES
- Phimosis
  - ◊ "Physiologic" - present at birth and resolves spontaneously during the first 2-3 years of life by nocturnal erections which slowly dilate the phimotic ring
  - ◊ Congenital - unresolved physiologic phimosis
  - ◊ Acquired - recurrent infection or irritation
- Paraphimosis
  - ◊ Foreskin not pulled back over the glans after cleaning, cystoscopy or catheter insertion

RISK FACTORS
- Phimosis
  - ◊ Poor hygiene
  - ◊ Diabetes
  - ◊ Frequent diaper rash in infant
- Paraphimosis
  - ◊ Presence of foreskin
  - ◊ "Inexperienced" health care provider, i.e., leaving foreskin retracted after catheter placement

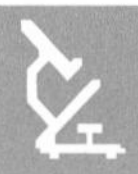

DIAGNOSIS

DIFFERENTIAL DIAGNOSIS Penile lymphedema which can be related to insect bites, trauma or allergic reactions

LABORATORY N/A

Drugs that may alter lab results: N/A

Disorders that may alter lab results: N/A

PATHOLOGICAL FINDINGS N/A

SPECIAL TESTS N/A

IMAGING N/A

DIAGNOSTIC PROCEDURES N/A

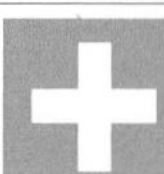

TREATMENT

APPROPRIATE HEALTH CARE Outpatient except for complications

GENERAL MEASURES
Paraphimosis: Reduction if possible (should be done with the patient sedated). Place the middle and index fingers of both hands on the engorged skin proximal to the glans. Place both thumbs on glans and with gentle pressure pushing on the glans and pulling on foreskin, attempt reduction. If unsuccessful, a dorsal slit will be necessary with eventual circumcision after the edema resolves.

SURGICAL MEASURES
- Phimosis: Circumcision
- Paraphimosis: Dorsal slit with subsequent circumcision

ACTIVITY No sexual activity following circumcision until healing is complete

DIET No limitations

PATIENT EDUCATION If the patient is uncircumcised, appropriate hygiene and care of the foreskin is necessary to prevent phimosis and paraphimosis

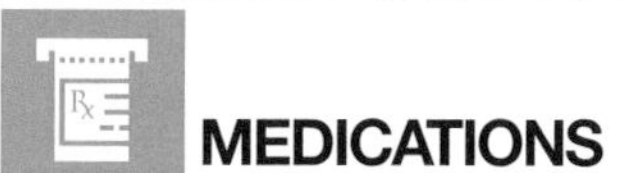

MEDICATIONS

DRUG(S) OF CHOICE N/A
Contraindications: N/A
Precautions: N/A
Significant possible interactions: N/A

ALTERNATIVE DRUGS N/A

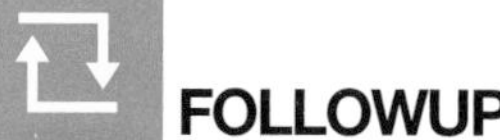

FOLLOWUP

PATIENT MONITORING 1 week after reduction of paraphimosis and 1 to 2 weeks after a circumcision

PREVENTION/AVOIDANCE Good patient and parental education

POSSIBLE COMPLICATIONS
- Unreduced paraphimosis can lead to gangrene of the glans
- Posthitis (inflammation of the prepuce)

EXPECTED COURSE/PROGNOSIS
Complete resolution if treatment is carried out effectively

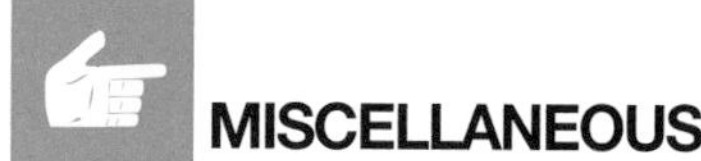

MISCELLANEOUS

ASSOCIATED CONDITIONS N/A

AGE-RELATED FACTORS
Pediatric:
- Recurrent balanitis, either chemical or infectious, can lead to an acquired phimosis
- Forced reduction of a physiologic foreskin can lead to chronic scarring and acquired phimosis

Geriatric: Recurrent infection and irritations (condom catheters) can lead to phimosis
Others: N/A

PREGNANCY N/A

SYNONYMS N/A

ICD-9-CM
605 Redundant prepuce and phimosis

SEE ALSO

OTHER NOTES N/A

ABBREVIATIONS N/A

REFERENCES

- Kelalis PP, King LR, Belman AB: Clinical Pediatric Urology. 3rd Ed. Philadelphia, W.B. Saunders Co., 1991
- Stringer MD, Oldham KT, Mouriquand PD, Howard ER: Pediatric Surgery and Urology: Long Term Outcomes. Philadelphia, WB Saunders Co., 1998

Web references: 0 available at www.5mcc.com
Illustrations N/A

Author(s):
James P. Miller, MD
Timothy L. Black, MD

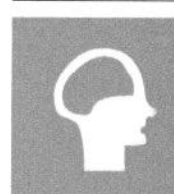

BASICS

DESCRIPTION A persistent irrational fear of a specific object, activity or situation that results in a compelling desire to avoid the perceived fear. Psychiatric conditions classified in Diagnostic and Statistical Manual of Mental Disorders (DSM-IV-R) as anxiety disorders. When confronted with the phobic stimulus, patient reacts with intense anxiety, usually realizes the fear is excessive or exaggerated. When a fear causes significant distress and interferes with normal functions of life, then it is considered a psychiatric disorder.
- Agoraphobia: Fear of being trapped in a situation where escape is impossible or difficult. Fear centers on (1) fear of being alone, (2) fear of being away from home and (3) fear of being in a place from where escape is difficult - seen most often in association with panic disorder.
- Simple phobia: Fear of a discrete stimulus such as animals, insects, heights, flying, closed spaces (claustrophobia), blood-injury phobia
- Social phobia: Fear of humiliation or embarrassment in social situations where person may be under scrutiny by others, e.g., performance anxiety, speaking in public, or fear of using public toilets

System(s) affected: Nervous
Genetics: No consistent genetic pattern
Incidence/Prevalence in USA: 1 month prevalence of all phobic conditions: 6.2%; lifetime prevalence: 12.5%
Predominant age:
- Agoraphobia - onset 18-35 (mean 24)
- Simple phobia fear of animals - onset usually in childhood (mean 4.4 years)
- Simple phobia fear of heights, claustrophobia - 4th decade
- Other simple phobias - mean 22.7 years
- Social phobia - late childhood, adolescence (mean 19 years)

Predominant sex:
- Female > Male, overall phobias
- Male = Female, social phobia

SIGNS & SYMPTOMS
- Extreme anxiety when exposed to phobic stimulus
- Tremors
- Palpitations
- Sweating
- Blushing
- Dyspnea
- Dizziness
- Associated nausea

CAUSES
- Persistence or exaggeration of learned response, learned initially as a protective mechanism (such as avoidance of large dogs by small children)
- Social - learned maladaptive anxiety response to social situation

RISK FACTORS
- For all phobias - presence of another psychiatric disorder
- Separation anxiety in childhood
- Introverted or dependent personality

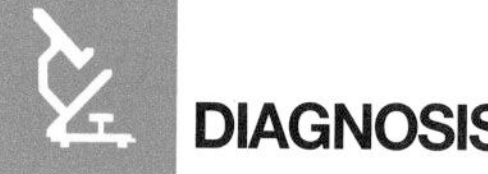

DIAGNOSIS

DIFFERENTIAL DIAGNOSIS
- For agoraphobia:
  - ◊ Paranoid and psychotic states
  - ◊ PTSD (post-traumatic stress disorder)
  - ◊ Depression - but do not see the other aspects of depression (anhedonia, loss of appetite and libido, sleep disturbance-early morning awakening, frequent night awakening, difficulty falling asleep)
- For simple phobia:
  - ◊ Schizophrenia - avoidance can be seen but usually in response to a delusion and patient does not realize that fear is excessive. Schizophrenia is intimately intertwined with delusion.
  - ◊ PTSD - phobic avoidance seen and is associated with the original trauma
  - ◊ Obsessive compulsive disorder (OCD) - avoidance associated with obsessions (such as dirt avoidance)
- For social phobia:
  - ◊ Avoidant personality disorder - central fear in avoidant personality disorder is that of rejection, not of humiliation or embarrassment as in social phobia
  - ◊ Paranoid personality disorder
  - ◊ Schizophrenia

LABORATORY None

Drugs that may alter lab results: N/A

Disorders that may alter lab results: N/A

PATHOLOGICAL FINDINGS N/A

SPECIAL TESTS None

IMAGING N/A

DIAGNOSTIC PROCEDURES
- Careful history and observation of the patient
- Description of the behavior by patient, family or friends
- Psychiatric examination

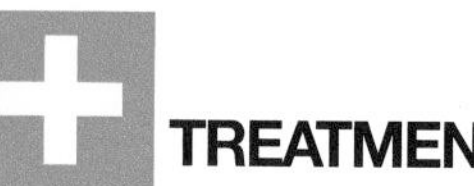

TREATMENT

APPROPRIATE HEALTH CARE Outpatient

GENERAL MEASURES
- Agoraphobia:
  - ◊ Behavioral treatment
  - ◊ Graduated exposure
  - ◊ Different treatment required when agoraphobia is associated with panic disorder
- Simple phobia:
  - ◊ In vivo or graduated exposure
  - ◊ Fear of flying specifically - benzodiazepine
- Social phobia:
  - ◊ Social skills training
  - ◊ Graduated exposure
  - ◊ Performance anxiety or situations where patient in a circumscribed setting - beta blocker

SURGICAL MEASURES N/A

ACTIVITY No restriction

DIET Consider restriction of stimulants - such as caffeine, nicotine, xanthines, sympathomimetics, which can overdrive anxiety. Phenelzine - requires tyramine free diet.

PATIENT EDUCATION
- Cognitive therapy
- Phobia clinic or group therapy, if available
- Anxiety Disorders of America; website www.adaa.org

MEDICATIONS

DRUG(S) OF CHOICE
- Agoraphobia - none recommended
- Simple phobia - none recommended, except for fear of flying. A benzodiazepine, such as alprazolam, may help. Initial dose as low as 0.25 mg titrated upward as needed.
- Social phobia (acute) - beta-blocker, e.g., propranolol (Inderal) 20-40 mg, 45-60 minutes before anticipated performance, atenolol 50-100 mg/day for more generalized social phobia
- Social phobia (chronic) - sertraline 50-150 mg/day, phenelzine, a MAO inhibitor, up to 60 mg/day, if social phobia more generalized and requires more constant medication (as opposed to the sporadic treatment for performance anxiety)

Contraindications:
- Beta-blocker - asthma or bronchospasm, congestive heart failure, bradycardia
- Phenelzine - not with other antidepressants, tyramine in diet, decongestants, diet pills, meperidine (Demerol), dextromethorphan, levodopa, and sympathomimetics

Precautions:
- Do not abruptly discontinue alprazolam due to potential for withdrawal seizures
- Monitor blood pressure in patients taking beta-blockers
- Consult drug information before using phenelzine

Significant possible interactions:
- Phenelzine - significant dietary restrictions due to potential for hypertensive crisis; avoid sympathomimetics, TCAs, fluoxetine and other SSRIs, CNS depressants
- Consult drug information sources before adding new medications in patients

ALTERNATIVE DRUGS N/A

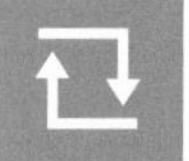

FOLLOWUP

PATIENT MONITORING Outpatient as needed

PREVENTION/AVOIDANCE N/A

POSSIBLE COMPLICATIONS
- Avoidance behavior
- Episodic alcohol, barbiturate and anxiolytic abuse/overuse and dependence as patients try to self-medicate to ameliorate symptoms
- Development of mild depression

EXPECTED COURSE/PROGNOSIS
- Agoraphobia - usually associated with panic disorder, chronic. Often patient becomes more and more homebound as condition continues.
- Simple phobia - some spontaneously remit as person ages (as in some simple phobias of childhood), alternatively some become chronic. Impairment can be minimal if object can be avoided (such as snakes). Although improvement occurs with in vivo exposure, phobia can recur after successful treatment.
- Social phobia - chronic course

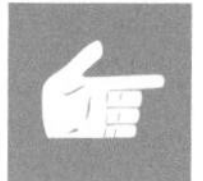

MISCELLANEOUS

ASSOCIATED CONDITIONS
- For all phobias - depression, substance abuse
- Social and agoraphobia - panic attacks or panic disorder

AGE-RELATED FACTORS
Pediatric: Animal phobia mean age of onset 4.4 years
Geriatric: N/A
Others: N/A

PREGNANCY No data

SYNONYMS N/A

ICD-9-CM
300.20 Phobia, unspecified
300.21 Agoraphobia with panic attacks
300.22 Agoraphobia without mention of panic attacks
300.23 Social phobia
300.29 Other isolated or simple phobias

SEE ALSO
Anxiety
Depression
Dissociative disorders
Obsessive compulsive disorder
Post-traumatic stress disorder (PTSD)
Schizophrenia

OTHER NOTES N/A

ABBREVIATIONS
PTSD = post-traumatic stress disorder

REFERENCES

- Diagnostic and Statistical Manual of Mental Disorders (DSM-IV-R). 4th Ed. American Psychiatric Association, Washington, DC, 2000
- Cutis GC, et al. Specific fears and phobias. Epidemiology and classification. Brit J Psych 1998;173:212-7

Web references: 1 available at www.5mcc.com
Illustrations N/A

Author(s):
Brian J. Murray, MD

BASICS

DESCRIPTION Light-induced eruptions seen in a pattern of photo-distribution
- Phototoxic reactions - result of the acute toxic effect on skin of ultraviolet light alone (sunburn) or together with a photosensitizing substance (non-allergic)
- Photoallergic eruptions - a form of allergic dermatitis resulting from combined effects of a photosensitizing substance (drugs or chemical) plus ultraviolet light (immunologic/delayed hypersensitivity)
- Polymorphous light eruption (PLE) - chronic, intermittent light-induced eruption with erythematous papules, urticaria, or vesicles on areas exposed to sunlight

System(s) affected: Skin/Exocrine
Genetics: Predisposition occurs in inbred populations (e.g., Pima Indians)
Incidence/Prevalence in USA: > 115 chemical agents used topically in the U.S. are known to cause photodermatitis
Predominant age: All ages
Predominant sex: Male = Female

SIGNS & SYMPTOMS
- Phototoxic
  - ◊ Erythema
  - ◊ With increasing severity - vesicles and bullae
  - ◊ Classic example - sunburn
  - ◊ Nails may exhibit onycholysis
  - ◊ Chronic - epidermal thickening, elastosis, telangiectasia and pigmentary changes
  - ◊ Sharp lines of demarcation between involved and uninvolved skin (sunlight exposure)
  - ◊ Phototoxic eruption due to topicals - area of application
  - ◊ Usually develops shortly after sun exposure
  - ◊ Hyperpigmentation may follow resolution
  - ◊ Pain
- Photoallergic
  - ◊ Papules with erythema and occasionally vesicles
  - ◊ Area exposed to light with less distinct borders
  - ◊ Usually delayed - 24 hours or more after exposure
  - ◊ May spread to unexposed areas
  - ◊ Pruritus
- Polymorphous light eruption (PLE)
  - ◊ Erythematous papules
  - ◊ Occasionally urticaria or vesicles
  - ◊ Scattered over sun exposed areas with normal skin in between
  - ◊ Can spread to non-exposed areas
  - ◊ Often flares in spring or early summer
  - ◊ Desensitization affect (less over the course of the summer)
  - ◊ Burning or pruritus may precede lesions

CAUSES
- Sunlight
- Phenothiazines
- Diuretics
- Tetracyclines
- Sulfonamides
- Oral contraceptives
- Topicals - psoralens, coal tars, photo-active dyes (eosin, acridine orange)
- 5-fluorouracil
- Quinine
- Sunscreens containing paraaminobenzoic acid (PABA)

RISK FACTORS
- Job related exposure to sunlight
- Light and fair colored skin

DIAGNOSIS

DIFFERENTIAL DIAGNOSIS Systemic lupus erythematosus

LABORATORY Antinuclear antibody (ANA) to rule out systemic lupus erythematosus

Drugs that may alter lab results: N/A

Disorders that may alter lab results: N/A

PATHOLOGICAL FINDINGS Nonspecific

SPECIAL TESTS
- Photo-testing - exposing patient to UV light
- Photopatch testing - applying suspected agents and chemicals to patient's skin
- Skin biopsy - to rule out other disorders

IMAGING N/A

DIAGNOSTIC PROCEDURES Physical examination and medical history

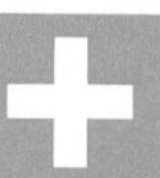

TREATMENT

APPROPRIATE HEALTH CARE Outpatient

GENERAL MEASURES
- Avoid sunlight/limit exposure
- Protective clothing/sunscreens
- Ice packs/cold water compresses

SURGICAL MEASURES N/A

ACTIVITY Avoid sunlight

DIET No special diet

PATIENT EDUCATION
- Avoidance of sunlight
- Avoidance of photosensitizing drugs
- Protective clothing (eg, Hats, long sleeves)
- Sunscreens > 15 SPF

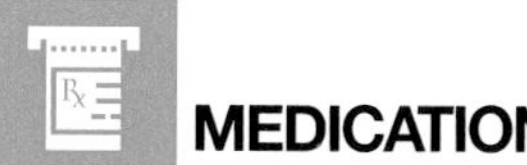

MEDICATIONS

DRUG(S) OF CHOICE
- Topical corticosteroids (betamethasone valerate 0.1% cream)
- NSAIDs (indomethacin 25 mg tid; aspirin; others)
- Prednisone for severe reactions

(0.5-1 mg/kg/d) for 3-10 days
- Antihistamines for pruritus (hydroxyzine 25-50 mg qid)
- Sunscreens (> 15 SPF) for prevention. Use broad-spectrum sunscreen to block both UVA and UVB. PABA may aggravate photodermatitis in sensitized patients (due to the sulfa moiety).

Contraindications: Refer to manufacturer's profile of each drug
Precautions: Refer to manufacturer's profile of each drug
Significant possible interactions: Refer to manufacturer's profile of each drug

ALTERNATIVE DRUGS N/A

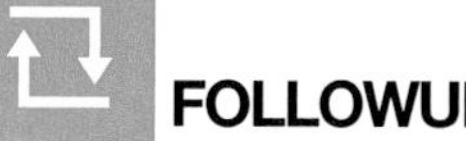

FOLLOWUP

PATIENT MONITORING
As necessary for persistence or recurrence

PREVENTION/AVOIDANCE
- Sunlight avoidance/protective clothing
- Identification and avoidance of causative drugs (see under Causes)
- Sunscreens - apply before exposure
  - ◊ Zinc oxide - opaque, cosmetically less acceptable
  - ◊ Chemical - use sun-protective factor > 15 for maximum protection; substantively resistant to sweat and swimming; cosmetically more acceptable

POSSIBLE COMPLICATIONS N/A

EXPECTED COURSE/PROGNOSIS
Good with avoidance/protection measures

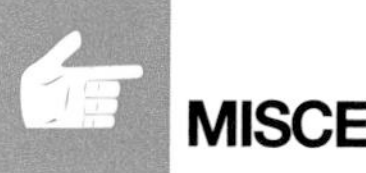

MISCELLANEOUS

ASSOCIATED CONDITIONS
- Sunlight aggravation of systemic lupus
- Persistent light reactivity
- Actinic reticuloid

AGE-RELATED FACTORS N/A
Pediatric: N/A
Geriatric: More likely to experience adverse reactions to causative drugs
Others: N/A

PREGNANCY N/A

SYNONYMS
- Sun poisoning
- Sun allergy

ICD-9-CM
692.79 Other dermatitis due to solar radiation
692.9 Contact dermatitis and other eczema due to unspecified cause

SEE ALSO

OTHER NOTES N/A

ABBREVIATIONS
NSAID = nonsteroidal anti-inflammatory drug

REFERENCES

- Bondi J, Jegasothy B, Lazarus G. Dermatology, Diagnosis and Therapy. Norwalk, CT: McGraw-Hill/Appleton & Lange; 1992

Web references: 2 available at www.5mcc.com
Illustrations 2 available

Author(s):
Aamir Siddiqi, MD

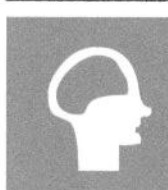

BASICS

DESCRIPTION Intestinal infection with *Enterobius vermicularis*. Characterized by perianal itching, usually worse at night.
System(s) affected: Gastrointestinal, Skin/Exocrine
Genetics: N/A
Incidence/Prevalence in USA: Approximately 20% of young children (ages 5-10)
Predominant age: 5 to 14
Predominant sex: Female > Male

SIGNS & SYMPTOMS
- Perianal itching
- Perineal itching
- Vulvovaginitis
- Enuresis
- Abdominal pain
- Insomnia

CAUSES The intestinal nematode *Enterobius (Oxyuris) vermicularis*

RISK FACTORS
- Institutionalization (50-90% of institutionalized children have pinworms)
- Crowded living conditions
- Poor hygiene
- Warm climate

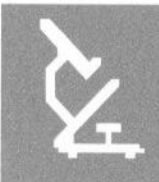

DIAGNOSIS

DIFFERENTIAL DIAGNOSIS
- Idiopathic pruritus ani
- Atopic dermatitis
- Contact dermatitis
- Psoriasis
- Lichen planus
- Infection with human papilloma virus
- Herpes simplex
- Fungal infections
- Erythrasma
- Scabies
- Vaginitis

LABORATORY N/A

Drugs that may alter lab results: N/A

Disorders that may alter lab results: N/A

PATHOLOGICAL FINDINGS Identification of ova on low power microscopy or direct visualization of the female worm (10 mm in length). Ova are asymmetric, flattened on one side, and measure 30 by 60 μm.

SPECIAL TESTS
- Transparent tape test - a piece of transparent cellophane tape is adhered to the perianal skin in the early morning and then affixed to a microscope slide. This procedure must be performed at least 3 times to achieve 90% sensitivity. Alternatively, anal swabs or Swube Tubes (a pinworm paddle coated with adhesive material) can also be useful.
- Flashlight to perianal region at night for direct observation
- Digital rectal examination with saline slide preparation of stool on gloved finger

IMAGING N/A

DIAGNOSTIC PROCEDURES N/A

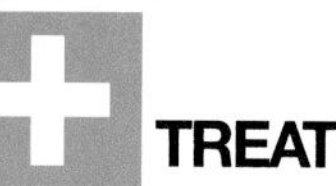

TREATMENT

APPROPRIATE HEALTH CARE Outpatient

GENERAL MEASURES
- All symptomatic family members should be treated simultaneously
- Bedclothes and underwear of infected individuals should be washed in hot water at the time of treatment (ova can remain viable for 2-3 weeks in a moist environment)
- Strict hand washing can help prevent fecal-oral transmission
- Practice good hygiene (showers, nail cleaning)
- Topical use of antipruritic creams or ointments may help relive itching in the perianal region

SURGICAL MEASURES N/A

ACTIVITY No restrictions

DIET No restrictions

PATIENT EDUCATION For patient education materials on this topic: Centers for Disease Control, Department of Health and Human Services, Office of Public Affairs, Atlanta, GA 30333, (404)329-3534

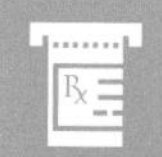

MEDICATIONS

DRUG(S) OF CHOICE
- Some clinicians recommend repeat treatment after 2 weeks. Occasionally, recalcitrant cases may require retreatment every 2 weeks for 4-6 cycles.
- Mebendazole (Vermox) chewable tablet 100 mg as a single dose. Use with caution in children < age 2

or
- Albendazole 400 mg orally as a single dose

or
- Pyrantel pamoate (Antiminth) oral suspension 11 mg/kg as a single dose. Maximum dose 1 gram. Use with caution in children < age 2

Contraindications: Refer to manufacturer's profile of each drug

Precautions:
- All family members should be treated
- Take medicine on empty stomach
- May cause diarrhea and/or nausea

Significant possible interactions: Refer to manufacturer's profile of each drug

ALTERNATIVE DRUGS N/A

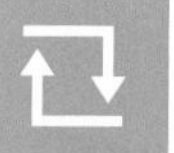

FOLLOWUP

PATIENT MONITORING Unnecessary unless symptoms do not abate following drug therapy

PREVENTION/AVOIDANCE
- Careful hand washing, keep nails short and clean
- Wash anus and genitals at least once a day, preferably in a shower
- Don't scratch anus or put fingers near nose or mouth

POSSIBLE COMPLICATIONS
- Perianal scratching may cause impetigo or excoriation
- Young girls - vulvovaginitis, urethritis, endometritis, salpingitis
- Urinary tract infections

EXPECTED COURSE/PROGNOSIS
- Asymptomatic carriers are common
- Symptomatic infections are cured > 90% of the time with drug therapy
- Reinfection is common

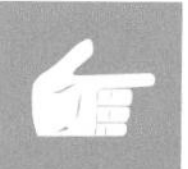

MISCELLANEOUS

ASSOCIATED CONDITIONS Pruritus ani

AGE-RELATED FACTORS
Pediatric: More common in children and more likely to get reinfected

Geriatric: N/A

Others: N/A

PREGNANCY Drug therapy is contraindicated in pregnancy

SYNONYMS Enterobiasis

ICD-9-CM
127.4 Enterobiasis

SEE ALSO
Pruritus ani

OTHER NOTES N/A

ABBREVIATIONS N/A

REFERENCES

- Bennett JC, Plum F, editors Cecil Textbook of Medicine. 20th Ed. Philadelphia: WB Saunders Co; 1996
- Berman RE, et al, editors. Nelson Textbook of Pediatrics. 15th Ed. Philadelphia: WB Saunders Co; 1996
- Sanford JP, et al. Guide to Antimicrobial Therapy. New York: Pfizer; 2003
- Feigin RD, Cherry JD, editors. Textbook of Pediatric Infectious Diseases. 4th Ed. Philadelphia: WB Saunders Co; 1998

Web references: 3 available at www.5mcc.com

Illustrations N/A

Author(s):
Steven Eisenstein, MD

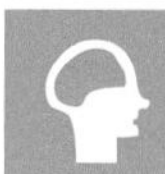

BASICS

DESCRIPTION A chronic skin disorder characterized by one or more groups of poorly marginated, pale pink or tan/white patches and plaques that appear on the cheeks, neck and lateral arms of children and young adults
System(s) affected: Skin/Exocrine
Genetics: Unknown, but is primarily seen in children with a genetic predisposition to atopic disease
Incidence/Prevalence in USA: Common, exact incidence unknown. Common, especially in dark-skin individuals in sunnier climates
Predominant age: 90% are between ages 6-12. Rare after 25.
Predominant sex: Male = Female

SIGNS & SYMPTOMS
- Description - small, ill-defined pale pink or tan/white patches 1/2 to 3 cm size
- Rash evolves from pink patch to white macule with fine scale to smooth hypopigmented macule
- Location - cheeks and lateral arms
- Number - 1-12 or more patches
- Palpation - smooth or slightly rough, and dry
- Appearance - pinpoint white papules (representing accentuation and keratinization of follicular orifices)
- Scale is either invisible or fine and light
- More common in dark skinned individuals
- Usually asymptomatic
- Pruritic (rare)
- More apparent in summertime in light skinned individuals
- Lesions do not tan in summer
- Even a small amount of sunlight exposure causes lesions to redden

CAUSES
- Unknown. Maybe part of an atopic diathesis.
- Possibly defects in melanin production or transfer

RISK FACTORS Children with a genetic predisposition to atopic disease

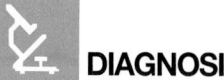

DIAGNOSIS

DIFFERENTIAL DIAGNOSIS
- Pityriasis versicolor
- Vitiligo
- Milia
- Keratosis pilaris
- Indeterminate or uncharacteristic leprosy

LABORATORY N/A

Drugs that may alter lab results: N/A

Disorders that may alter lab results: N/A

PATHOLOGICAL FINDINGS Irregular melanin pigmentation of basal layer, follicular plugging, follicular spongiosis, and atrophic sebaceous glands

SPECIAL TESTS Negative KOH skin scraping

IMAGING N/A

DIAGNOSTIC PROCEDURES History and physical exam. Atopic diathesis is of diagnostic significance.

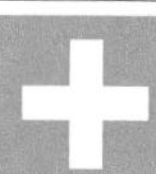

TREATMENT

APPROPRIATE HEALTH CARE Outpatient

GENERAL MEASURES No truly effective therapy available. Lubricating cream application may improve roughness and/or dryness.

SURGICAL MEASURES N/A

ACTIVITY No restrictions

DIET No special diet

PATIENT EDUCATION Stress long-term chronicity and permanent resolution in second or third decade of life

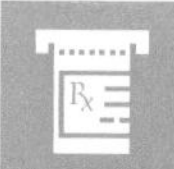

MEDICATIONS

DRUG(S) OF CHOICE

- Coal tar preparations - Alphosyl, Estar, Balnetar, applied topically once or twice a day. Treatment is not mandatory.
- Topical steroids if needed to reduce redness due to sunburn or spontaneous inflammation
- Note: Neither will change the pigmentation, but may improve pruritus, roughness and/or dryness, if the lubricating cream is not sufficient
- Phototherapy (eg, UVB) for extensive involvements in adults only
- Anecdotal evidence supports use of Lacticare HC 1% (Lac-Hydrin + 1% hydrocortisone lotion)

Contraindications: N/A
Precautions: Refer to manufacturer's literature
Significant possible interactions: N/A

ALTERNATIVE DRUGS Tacrolimus or picrolimus have been used off label for pityriasis alba

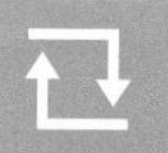

FOLLOWUP

PATIENT MONITORING As needed only if lesions become symptomatic

PREVENTION/AVOIDANCE No known preventive measures

POSSIBLE COMPLICATIONS None expected

EXPECTED COURSE/PROGNOSIS Permanent resolution during second or third decade of life

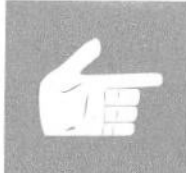

MISCELLANEOUS

ASSOCIATED CONDITIONS Atopic dermatitis

AGE-RELATED FACTORS

Pediatric: More common in children 3 to 10 years
Geriatric: Rare in this age group
Others: N/A

PREGNANCY N/A

SYNONYMS

- Pityriasis streptogenes
- Pityriasis simplex
- Pityriasis sicca faciei
- Erythema streptogenes
- Furfuraceous impetigo

ICD-9-CM

696.5 Other and unspecified pityriasis

SEE ALSO

Keratosis, actinic
Tinea versicolor
Vitiligo

OTHER NOTES N/A

ABBREVIATIONS N/A

REFERENCES

- Habif T. Clinical Dermatology. 4th ed. St. Louis: CV Mosby; 2004
- Sams WM, Lynch PJ, eds. Principles and Practices of Dermatology. 2nd ed. New York: Churchill Livingstone; 1996
- Fitzpatrick TB, et al, eds. Dermatology in General Medicine. 5th ed. New York: McGraw-Hill, 1999
- Arnold KL, Odom RB, James WD. Andrews' Diseases of the Skin. 9th Ed. Philadelphia, W.B. S;unders Co., 2000
- Halder RM, Nandedkar MA, Neal KW. Pigmentary disorders in ethnic skin. Dermatol Clin 2003;21(4):617-28
- Galen EB. Pityriasis alba. Cutis 1998;61(1):11-13

Web references: 0 available at www.5mcc.com
Illustrations 2 available

Author(s):

Mitchell S. King, MD
Jasmine Chao, DO

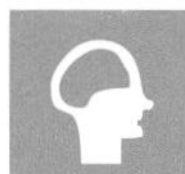

BASICS

DESCRIPTION An idiopathic self-limited skin eruption characterized by widespread papulosquamous lesions
System(s) affected: Skin/Exocrine
Genetics: Less than 5 percent of those affected give a positive family history
Incidence/Prevalence in USA: Relatively common but exact frequency unknown
Predominant age: 10-35, but occurs in all age groups
Predominant sex: Male = Female

SIGNS & SYMPTOMS
- Salmon to light brown oval plaques with fine scales centrally and "collarette" of loose scales along borders
- Lesions average 1-2 cm in diameter and usually spare face, hands and feet in adults
- Lesions frequently oriented along skin cleavage lines in "Christmas tree" pattern
- Eruption often preceded by 2-6 cm "herald patch" of similar appearance days to weeks before generalized rash
- Mild pruritus, rarely severe
- Fever and malaise rare
- Variant forms include purpuric, urticarial, and vesicular lesions

CAUSES Unknown, may be a viral agent or an autoimmune disorder. Several studies have implicated herpesviruses, but other research has not confirmed this association.

RISK FACTORS Unknown

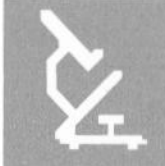

DIAGNOSIS

DIFFERENTIAL DIAGNOSIS
- Secondary syphilis
- Viral exanthems
- Drug rashes
- Psoriasis
- Parapsoriasis
- Eczema
- Lichen planus
- Tinea corporis

LABORATORY WBC normal. No specific lab markers. Serology to rule out syphilis.

Drugs that may alter lab results: N/A

Disorders that may alter lab results: N/A

PATHOLOGICAL FINDINGS Chronic inflammation with cytolytic degeneration of keratinocytes adjacent to Langerhans cells

SPECIAL TESTS KOH preparation to distinguish from tinea corporis

IMAGING N/A

DIAGNOSTIC PROCEDURES N/A

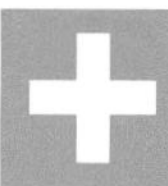

TREATMENT

APPROPRIATE HEALTH CARE Outpatient

GENERAL MEASURES
- Symptomatic treatment
- Topical antipruritics as needed
- Ultraviolet therapy has been used but a controlled study showed minimal benefit
- Lukewarm oatmeal baths (not hot as it can intensify itching)

SURGICAL MEASURES N/A

ACTIVITY Full activity with good skin hygiene to prevent secondary infection

DIET N/A

PATIENT EDUCATION
- Reassurance as to self-limited nature of condition
- Printed patient information available from: American Academy of Dermatology (708) 330-0230

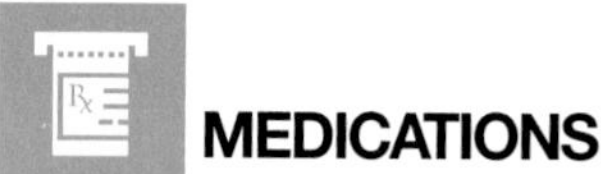

MEDICATIONS

DRUG(S) OF CHOICE
- Topical steroids to reduce itching, if needed
  - ◊ Triamcinolone 0.1% cream
- Oral antihistamines
  - ◊ Diphenhydramine (Benadryl) 25 mg tid
  - ◊ Chlorpheniramine 8 mg tid

Contraindications: N/A
Precautions: N/A
Significant possible interactions: N/A

ALTERNATIVE DRUGS Erythromycin showed apparent benefit in one trial

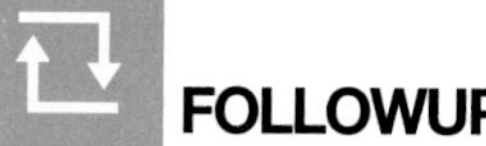

FOLLOWUP

PATIENT MONITORING
- Check syphilis serology
- Return visit for reevaluation, if lesions persist longer than 8-10 weeks

PREVENTION/AVOIDANCE N/A

POSSIBLE COMPLICATIONS Secondary infection (e.g., impetigo)

EXPECTED COURSE/PROGNOSIS
Gradual resolution in 1-14 weeks (usually 2-6)

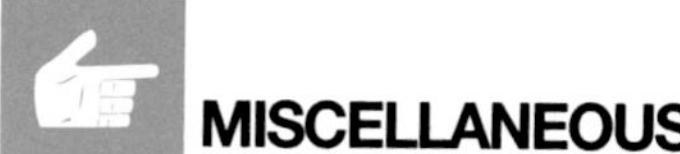

MISCELLANEOUS

ASSOCIATED CONDITIONS N/A

AGE-RELATED FACTORS
Pediatric: Face, distal extremities more often involved in children and lesions may be more papular
Geriatric: N/A
Others: N/A

PREGNANCY N/A

SYNONYMS N/A

ICD-9-CM
696.3 Pityriasis rosea

SEE ALSO
Dermatitis, exfoliative
Pityriasis alba
Tinea versicolor

OTHER NOTES N/A

ABBREVIATIONS N/A

REFERENCES

- Fitzpatrick TB, et al, editors. Dermatology in General Medicine. 5th Ed. New York: McGraw-Hill;
- Habif T. Clinical Dermatology. 4th Ed. St. Louis, CV Mosby, 2004
- Cheong WK, Wong KS: Pityriasis Rosea. Singapore Medical Jour 1989
- Leenutaphong V, Jiamton S. UVB phototherapy for pityriasis rosea: a bilateral comparison study. J Am Acad Dermatol 1995;33(6):996-9
- Sharma PK, Yadav TP, Gautam RK, et al. Erythromycin in pityriasis rosea: A double-blind, placebo-controlled clinical trial. J Am Acad Dermatol 2000;42(2 Pt 1):241-4
- Drago F, Ranieri E, Malaguti F, et al. Human herpesvirus 7 in patients with pityriasis rosea. Electron microscopy investigations and polymerase chain reaction in mononuclear cells, plasma and skin. Dermatology 1997;195(4):374-8
- Kempf W, Adams V, Kleinhans M, et al. Pityriasis rosea is not associated with human herpesvirus 7. Arch Dermatol 1999;135(9):1070-2

Web references: 0 available at www.5mcc.com
Illustrations 10 available

Author(s):
Jeffrey D. Wolfrey, MD

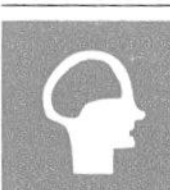

BASICS

DESCRIPTION Placental implantation in the lower uterine segment in advance of the presenting fetal part.
- Total previa: placenta covers entire cervical os
- Partial previa: placenta covers part of the cervical os
- Marginal previa: placental edge just reaches cervical os
- Low lying placenta: placental edge is in the lower uterine segment but does not encroach on the cervical os

System(s) affected: Cardiovascular, Reproductive
Genetics: N/A
Incidence/Prevalence in USA: 0.5% to 0.8% of all pregnancies, approximately 4/1,000 births; low lying placenta 4-8% in early pregnancy with < 10% persisting to term
Predominant age: Childbearing ages
Predominant sex: Female only

SIGNS & SYMPTOMS
- Typically painless bright red bleeding 2nd or 3rd trimester
- Average time of first bleed, 27-32 weeks
- Contractions variably present
- First bleed usually self limited
- Maternal hemodynamic status consistent with clinical blood loss estimate
- Complete previas may bleed earlier and not "migrate"

CAUSES Prior uterine insult or injury or other uterine factors

RISK FACTORS
- Prior previa (4%-8%)
- First subsequent pregnancy following a cesarean section delivery
- Multiparity (5% in grand multiparous patient)
- Advanced maternal age
- Multiple gestation
- Smoking
- Cocaine use
- Male fetus
- C-section odds ratio (OR)
  - ◊ Primipara with one C-section OR=1.28 (95% confidence interval [CI] 0.82-1.99)
  - ◊ Multipara with 4 or more deliveries and one C-section OR=1.72 (95% CI 1.12-2.64)
  - ◊ Multipara with >4 deliveries and >4 C-sections OR=8.76 (95% CI 1.58-48.53)
- Induced abortion
  - ◊ Sharp curettage - three or more procedures OR=2.9 (95% CI 1.0-8.5)
  - ◊ Vacuum aspiration - not associated with increased risk of placenta previa

DIAGNOSIS

DIFFERENTIAL DIAGNOSIS Abruptio placentae, vasa previa, vaginal and cervical causes including marked "bloody show" and infections

LABORATORY
- Maternal blood type and Rh
- Hemoglobin and hematocrit
- Platelet count
- PT, PTT, fibrinogen
- Type and cross match packed RBC (at least three units)
- Apt test: To determine fetal origin of blood (as in vasa previa). Mix vaginal blood with small amount tap water to cause hemolysis, centrifuge for several minutes, mix 1 cc of 1% NaOH with each 5 cc of the pink-hemoglobin-containing supernatant, observing pink fluid if fetal hemoglobin, and yellow-brown if adult origin.
- Wright's stain applied to a slide smear of vaginal blood looking for nucleated RBC's which are usually from cord blood and not adult blood
- L/S ratio for fetal maturity if needed

Drugs that may alter lab results: Drugs altering cell counts or clotting studies

Disorders that may alter lab results:
- Coagulopathies from other causes
- Red cell and hemoglobin disorders from other causes

PATHOLOGICAL FINDINGS
- Normocytic, normochromic anemia with acute bleed
- Coagulopathy rare, but may occur
- Positive Kleihauer-Betke if fetal/maternal transfusion

SPECIAL TESTS
- Kleihauer-Betke if concerned about fetal-maternal transfusion
- Bedside clot test: Draw red top tube from mother and observe for clot quality at 7-10 minutes. If there is no clot or if clot is friable may indicate disseminated intravascular coagulation (DIC).

IMAGING
- External sector sonography with moderately full and empty bladder
- Vaginal probe sonography may be done if not actively bleeding. Place the probe just inside vaginal os and use 5 or 6.5-MHz transducers.
- Magnetic resonance imaging (MRI) accurate, but more expensive, less available, and time consuming

DIAGNOSTIC PROCEDURES
- If placental location unknown and sonography not available, a double setup bimanual vaginal exam may be done in operating room with complete cesarean section readiness
- Careful vaginal speculum exam is not contraindicated and allows checking for cervical or vaginal source of bleeding, fern and nitrazine testing, cultures, and fluid for determining bleeding source
- Since fibrin degradation products rise in pregnancy, these levels are less helpful

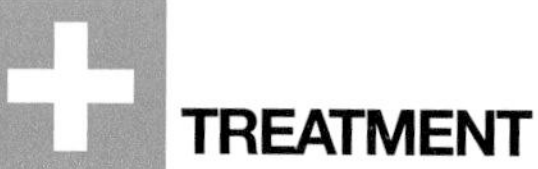

TREATMENT

APPROPRIATE HEALTH CARE
- Inpatient observation at bedrest initially; once stable, and preterm, may be followed as outpatient
- May consider transfer to high risk center based on condition and local services

GENERAL MEASURES
- Optimizing maternal stability while delaying delivery, if possible, or if preterm to improve perinatal outcome
- Cesarean section indicated for partial or complete previa if fetus is mature or if the situation is urgent and the fetus is immature
- A trial of labor may be considered with anterior marginal previa, including oxytocin (Pitocin) augmentation IV
- Amniocentesis for L/S ratio for maturity as needed
- IV fluid support, oxygen, transfusions of packed RBC's, platelets and fresh frozen plasma if needed
- External fetal and labor monitoring
- Other intervention or observation based on maternal condition
- DIC risk low unless massive bleed. Follow coagulation studies and give fresh frozen plasma (FFP), platelets as needed, or cryoprecipitate if fibrinogen < 100-150 mg/dL (< 1.0-1.5 g/L).
- Transfuse platelets at < 20,000 or < 50,000 if surgery needed
- Low lying posterior marginal previa associated with dystocia and greater need for cesarean section
- Blood volume increased in pregnancy; can lose > 30% maternal blood volume before shock findings
- Central line placement only after checking coagulation studies
- May use sector probe with condom at introitus if vaginal probe unavailable
- With significant hemorrhage, Rh negative women should receive Rho(D) immune globulin (Rhogam) with each bleed

SURGICAL MEASURES Cervical cerclage may reduce risk of delivery before 34 weeks (RR=0.45 [95% CI 0.23-0.87]) or birth weight less than 2kg RR=0.34 (0.14-0.83) or low 5-minute Apgar score RR=0.19 (0.04-1.00)

ACTIVITY
- Bedrest
- Pelvic rest; intercourse abstinence, avoid douching

DIET NPO initially, then based on delivery decisions

PATIENT EDUCATION
- First bleed rarely fatal
- Rebleed risk with activity or cervical stimulation
- Greatest cause of perinatal mortality is prematurity
- Risks and conditions associated with previa

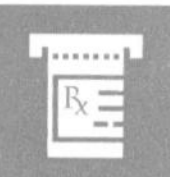

MEDICATIONS

DRUG(S) OF CHOICE
- For IV fluids: Lactated Ringer's or saline
- Oxygen for all, since O2 consumption up 20% in pregnancy and fetus is more prone to hypoxia
- Fresh frozen plasma and platelets as needed
- Cryoprecipitate and fibrinogen if above unsuccessful
- Tocolytics may have role in certain preterm patients, but tachycardia of ß-agonists (terbutaline) and risk of placental hypoperfusion with calcium channel blockers may make MgSO4 the drug of choice. For MgSO4, use 4 grams IV load and 1-4 grams/hour as indicated.

Contraindications:
Avoid tocolytics with term infant or unstable mother

Precautions:
- Beta-agonists and calcium channel blockers may complicate clinical picture
- Cryoprecipitate and fibrinogen may increase infection transmission risk

Significant possible interactions: Refer to manufacturer's profile of each drug

ALTERNATIVE DRUGS
- Ritodrine (Yutopar) IV may be an alternate beta-agonist, but carries same concerns as terbutaline

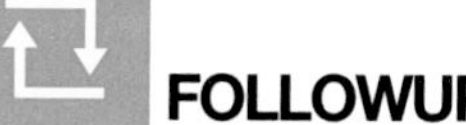

FOLLOWUP

PATIENT MONITORING
- Inpatient followup
- Outpatient care with frequent visits

PREVENTION/AVOIDANCE
- Decrease activity to avoid rebleeding
- All vaginal exams, sexual intercourse, douching, or other vaginal manipulation may cause rebleeding

POSSIBLE COMPLICATIONS
- Maternal mortality is rare with cesarean section available. Greatest fetal risk is preterm delivery.
- History of prior C-section and/or general anesthesia increases risk for need of transfusion
- Attempted tocolysis may compromise maternal status
- Rebleeding risk may be more risky than delivery and management
- If previa present after 30 weeks, there is greater risk of persisting previa
- Placental accreta strongly associated with placenta previa (up to 15% of patients). Higher incidence in women with placenta previa and multiple prior cesarean sections.
- Vasa previa
- IUGR - 16% incidence
- Congenital anomalies: Most common major anomalies of the central nervous system, cardiovascular system, respiratory and gastrointestinal tracts.
- Fetal anemia and Rh isoimmunization

EXPECTED COURSE/PROGNOSIS
- If term and complete or partial: Cesarean delivery
- If term and anterior marginal: Trial of labor may be okay
- If preterm and maternal and fetal status stable: May observe and delay delivery

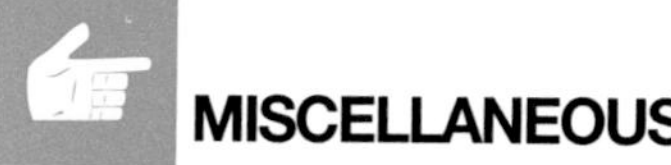

MISCELLANEOUS

ASSOCIATED CONDITIONS
- Abnormal presentations such as oblique and/or transverse lie
- Persistent high fetal station
- Postpartum hemorrhage
- Increased incidence of small for gestational age (SGA) babies with previas

AGE-RELATED FACTORS
Pediatric: N/A
Geriatric: N/A
Others: Advanced maternal age increases risk

PREGNANCY As above

SYNONYMS N/A

ICD-9-CM
641.00 Placenta previa without hemorrhage, unspecified
641.10 Hemorrhage from placenta previa, unspecified
641.20 Premature separation of placenta, unspecified
762.1 Premature separation of placenta (when causing newborn complications)

SEE ALSO
Abruptio placentae

OTHER NOTES N/A

ABBREVIATIONS
DIC = disseminated intravascular coagulation
L/S ratio = lecithin/sphingomyelin ratio
PT = prothrombin time
PTT = partial thromboplastin time

REFERENCES

- Neilson JP. Interventions for suspected placenta praevia (Cochrane Review). In: The Cochrane Library, Issue 2, 2002. Oxford: Update Software
- Royal College of Obstetricians and Gynecologists. Placenta Praevia: diagnosis and management. London: RCOG, 2000. (Green-top guideline No 27.)
- Cunningham FG, et al: Williams Obstetrics. 21st ed. McGraw-Hill Professional; 2001
- Creasy RD, Resnik R: Maternal - Fetal Medicine. 5th ed. WB Saunders Company; 2003
- Baron F, et al: Placenta previa, placenta abruptio. Clin Ob Gyn, Vol 41, No3, 1998;527-532
- Frederiksen MC, Glassenberg R, Stika CS. Placenta previa: a 22-year analysis. Am J Obstet Gynecol 1999;180(6 Pt 1):1432-7
- Faiz AS, Ananth CV. Etiology and risk factors for placenta previa: an overview and meta-analysis of observational studies. J Matern Fetal Neonatal Med. 2003;13(3):175-90
- Johnson L, Mueller B, Daling J.The relationship of placenta previa and history of induced abortion. Int J Gynaecol Obstet. 2003;81(2):191-8
- Gilliam M, Rosenberg D, Davis F. The likelihood of placenta previa with greater number of cesarean deliveries and higher parity. Obstet Gynecol. 2002;99(6):976-80

Web references: 1 available at www.5mcc.com
Illustrations N/A

Author(s):
Sandra M. Sulik, MD

BASICS

DESCRIPTION
- Acute infection
- Sporadic limited geographic distribution, especially Third World nations and Southwestern USA
- Epidemics associated with war, famine, and disaster
- Disease of rats and other small vertebrates
- Transmitted to humans by rat flea or human flea
- Occasional transmission to humans handling infected tissues
- Occasional human to human transmission by pulmonary secretions
- Recently shown that infected cats may transmit disease to humans by bite, licking or scratch
- Yersinia pestis as a bio-weapon has been described

System(s) affected: Hemic/Lymphatic/Immunologic, Pulmonary, Skin/Exocrine
Genetics: N/A
Incidence/Prevalence in USA: Few cases annually in Southwestern states, usually Spring, Summer, Fall
Predominant age: N/A
Predominant sex: Male = Female

SIGNS & SYMPTOMS
- Bubonic plague
  - ◊ Acute onset after 2-8 days incubation
  - ◊ Fever
  - ◊ Chills
  - ◊ Weakness
  - ◊ Headache
  - ◊ Bubo - painful, very tender enlargement of regional lymph node(s) draining inoculation site. Overlying edema. Typically, absence of overlying skin lesion, ascending lymphangitis.
  - ◊ Skin lesions - pustules, vesicles, eschars in area of flea bite(s), purpura
- Septicemic plague
  - ◊ Features of bubonic plague
  - ◊ Occasional occurrence without bubo
  - ◊ Hypotension
  - ◊ Hepatosplenomegaly
  - ◊ Delirium
  - ◊ Seizures in children
  - ◊ Shock
- Secondary pneumonic plague
  - ◊ Features of bubonic and septicemic plague
  - ◊ Cough
  - ◊ Chest pain
  - ◊ Hemoptysis
- Primary pneumonic plague
  - ◊ Acute onset within hours to one day after inhalation of bacteria
  - ◊ Fever
  - ◊ Chills
  - ◊ Cough
  - ◊ Chest pain
  - ◊ Dyspnea
  - ◊ Hemoptysis
  - ◊ Lethargy
  - ◊ Hypotension
  - ◊ Shock

CAUSES
- Yersinia pestis, transmitted by bite of a flea from an infected rodent; secondary - other infected animal or human contact
- Untreated bubonic plague may progress to secondary pneumonic type which can be transmitted by contaminated respiratory droplets

RISK FACTORS
- Exposure to rats and fleas
- Close contact with infected cat
- Close contact with pneumonic plague patient
- Plague bacillus in laboratory
- Hunters who skin wild animals
- Potential agent of bioterrorism
- Occupational risk: field workers, animal researchers and others exposed in endemic regions

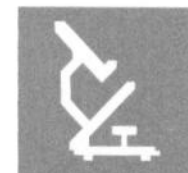

DIAGNOSIS

DIFFERENTIAL DIAGNOSIS Other causes of fulminant bacteremia, pneumococcal sepsis, meningococcemia; other causes of acute suppurative lymphadenitis (bubo), or rapidly progressive pneumonitis

LABORATORY
- Elevated white cell count, predominantly mature and immature neutrophils. Leukemoid reaction sometimes.
- Stained smears of aspirate of bubo, sputum, peripheral blood reveal gram-negative coccobacilli with bipolar staining, "safety pin" appearance
- Aspirate, blood, sputum cultures (infusion broth, blood and MacConkey agar) grow typical bacteria. Public health authorities arrange definitive identification and serological followup.

Drugs that may alter lab results: Antibiotics - prior use of antibiotics

Disorders that may alter lab results: N/A

PATHOLOGICAL FINDINGS Acute lymphadenitis with inflammation dominated by neutrophils, necrosis, masses of plague bacilli, seropurulent pericarditis

SPECIAL TESTS Low platelet number; evidence of disseminated intravascular coagulation may be seen

IMAGING Chest x-ray - patchy or confluent pulmonary consolidation in pneumonic plague

DIAGNOSTIC PROCEDURES N/A

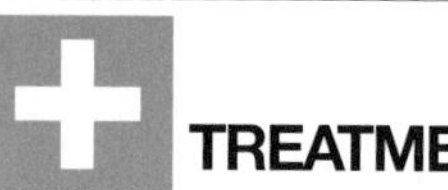

TREATMENT

APPROPRIATE HEALTH CARE
- Hospitalization. For suspected pneumonic plague, respiratory isolation until 48 hours after initial effective therapy or after sputum negative.
- Notify public health authorities

GENERAL MEASURES
- Do not create aerosol
- Handle blood and bubo aspirate with gloves
- Notify laboratory to take precautions
- Intravenous fluids as required
- Hot, moist compresses for buboes

SURGICAL MEASURES N/A

ACTIVITY Bedrest until convalescent

DIET As tolerated during recovery

PATIENT EDUCATION
- Avoid contact with wild animals
- Reduce rat and flea population in environment

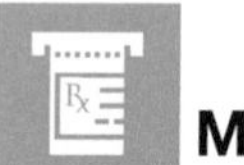

MEDICATIONS

DRUG(S) OF CHOICE

- Aminoglycoside (gentamicin 5.1 mg/kg/day or streptomycin 15 mg/kg)
- If condition allows oral medication: tetracycline 25-50 mg/kg/day, equally divided, every 6 hours for 10 days
- For meningitis: chloramphenicol 25 mg/kg followed by 60 mg/kg in 4 equally divided doses, daily for 10 days
- Fluoroquinolones (levofloxacin, ofloxacin) and third generation cephalosporins (cefotaxime) may also be effective

Contraindications: Tetracyclines - contraindicated in pregnancy and ages under 8

Precautions:

- Reduce dose of aminoglycoside for renal impairment
- Pregnant women and those with hearing disorders (aminoglycosides)
- Chloramphenicol associated with hematologic toxicity

Significant possible interactions: N/A

ALTERNATIVE DRUGS

None demonstrated to be as effective or less toxic

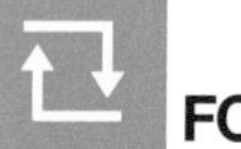

FOLLOWUP

PATIENT MONITORING

- CBC for hematologic toxicity of chloramphenicol
- Aminoglycoside blood levels if indicated
- Clinical testing for antibiotic toxicity if indicated

PREVENTION/AVOIDANCE

- Avoid contact with vectors, infected tissue or aerosol, e.g., pneumonic plague case
- Killed vaccine for people at high risk to reduce risk and/or severity; tetracycline prophylaxis. Vaccine available from C.D.C., Atlanta.

POSSIBLE COMPLICATIONS

- Progression of bubonic form to septicemic and pneumonic forms
- Necrosis of bubo may require aspiration or incision and drainage
- Pericarditis
- Adult respiratory distress syndrome
- Meningitis
- Death

EXPECTED COURSE/PROGNOSIS

- Untreated plague mortality > 50%; 100% in primary pneumonic plague
- Plague may be fulminant, e.g., exposure, first symptoms and death in one day in primary pneumonic plague. Must not delay treatment of suspected cases until laboratory-confirmed diagnosis. Delay of initial therapy beyond 24 hours after onset of primary pneumonic plague regularly followed by death.

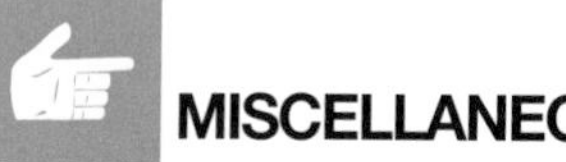

MISCELLANEOUS

ASSOCIATED CONDITIONS

N/A

AGE-RELATED FACTORS

N/A

Pediatric: N/A

Geriatric: N/A

Others: N/A

PREGNANCY

N/A

SYNONYMS

Black death

ICD-9-CM

020.0 Bubonic plague
020.2 Septicemic plague
020.5 Unspecified pneumonic plague
020.3 Primary pneumonic plague
020.4 Secondary pneumonic plague

SEE ALSO

OTHER NOTES

N/A

ABBREVIATIONS

N/A

REFERENCES

- Butler T. Yersinia Species (including Plague). In: Mandell GL, Bennett JF, Dolin R, editors. Principles and Practice of Infectious Diseases. 5th edition. New York: Churchill Livingstone; 2000
- Leggiadro RJ. The threat of biological terrorism: a public health and infection control reality. Infect Control Hosp Epidemiol 2000;21:53-6
- Kilonzo BS. Plague epidemiology and control in eastern and southern Africa during the period 1978 to 1997. Central African J Med 1999;45:70-76
- Gratz NG. Emerging and re-surging vector-borne diseases. Ann Rev Entomol 1999;44:51-75
- Titball RW, Leary SE. Plague. Br Med Bull 1998;54:625-33
- Perry RD, Fetherston JD. Yersinia pestis--etiologic agent of plague. Clin Microbiol Rev 1997;10:35-6
- Frean JA, Arntzen L, Capper T, et al. In vitro activities of 14 antibiotics against 100 human isolates of Yersinia pestis from a southern African plague focus. Antimicrob Agents Chemother 1996;40(11):2646-7
- Anonymous. Human plague in 1995. Weekly Epidemiological Record 1997;S72:344-347
- Inglesby TV, Dennis DT, Henderson DA, et al. Plague as a biological weapon: medical and public health management. Working Group on Civilian Biodefense. JAMA 2000;283(17):2281-90
- Dennis DT, Chow CC. Pediatr Infect Dis J. 2004 Jan;23(1):69-71
- Kohler W, Kohler M. Plague and rats, the "plague of the Philistines", and: what did our ancestors know about the role of rats in plague. Int J Med Microbiol. 2003 Nov;293(5):333-340

Web references: 4 available at www.5mcc.com

Illustrations N/A

Author(s):

D. W. MacPherson, MD

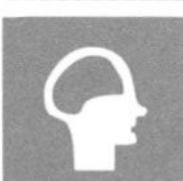

BASICS

DESCRIPTION A pleural effusion occurs when there is excessive fluid released into the pleural space or if there is lymphatic obstruction precluding normal drainage. Under normal conditions there is a small volume of pleural fluid in the pleural space which functions as a lubricant. Under pathological conditions, effusions develop and are classified as either transudates or exudates. Transudates are due to an imbalance between hydrostatic and oncotic pressures (as in hepatic cirrhosis, congestive heart failure, nephrotic syndrome, and obstruction of the superior vena cava). Exudates are secondary to a disturbance of the systems regulating pleural fluid formation and absorption/drainage (as in bacterial, viral, or fungal infection, rheumatologic disease, or malignancy). Distinguishing between these types of effusions, when etiology is uncertain or if there is inadequate response to therapy, can be helpful.
System(s) affected: Cardiovascular, Pulmonary
Genetics: N/A
Incidence/Prevalence in USA: Not known
Predominant age: Can occur at any age
Predominant sex: Male = Female

SIGNS & SYMPTOMS
- None in small volume effusion
- Pleuritic chest pain and referred abdominal or shoulder pain
- Cough, may be productive or nonproductive, depending on etiology
- Chest wall splinting
- Dyspnea
- Tachypnea, particularly with lung compression or more severe infections
- Diminished chest wall excursion
- Decreased tactile fremitus
- Dullness to percussion over effusion
- Diminished or absent breath sounds
- Friction rub
- Chills
- Mediastinal shift (on chest radiograph)
- Weight loss
- Night sweats
- Hemoptysis
- Anorexia
- General malaise

CAUSES
- Congestive heart failure, effusion usually bilateral, but if unilateral R > L.
- Hypoalbuminemic states (cirrhosis, nephrotic syndrome)
- Constrictive pericarditis
- Dressler's syndrome with pericardial effusion
- Infection: parapneumonic effusion or empyema. Etiologic agents include bacteria, viruses, fungi, Mycoplasma, parasites, and tuberculosis. Empyema usually caused by polymicrobial anaerobic infection, Pseudomonas, Staphylococcus aureus, Escherichia coli, and occasionally Streptococcus pneumoniae.
- Pulmonary embolism/infarction
- Neoplastic processes: mesothelioma from asbestos exposure, bronchogenic carcinoma, breast carcinoma, lymphoma, leukemia, metastatic disease
- Rheumatologic disease (systemic lupus erythematosus, rheumatoid arthritis)
- Pancreatitis (left-sided exudate with high amylase concentration)
- Esophageal rupture
- Drug reaction, possibly accompanied by eosinophilia
- Uremia
- Atelectasis
- Meig syndrome
- Subdiaphragmatic abscess
- Cirrhosis with ascites
- Chylous or pseudochylous effusion (thoracic duct injury)
- Trauma leading to intrapleural hemorrhage
- Idiopathic

RISK FACTORS N/A

DIAGNOSIS

DIFFERENTIAL DIAGNOSIS See causes

LABORATORY
- Leukocytosis with bandemia
- Anemia
- Hypoalbuminemia
- ANA titer
- Rheumatoid factor
- Pancreatic enzymes
- CA-125
- CA-19-9
- Creatinine/BUN
- Aerobic/anaerobic blood cultures
- Microbial cultures of pleural effusion fluid

Drugs that may alter lab results: N/A

Disorders that may alter lab results: N/A

PATHOLOGICAL FINDINGS See causes

SPECIAL TESTS
- Evaluation of pleural fluid withdrawn by thoracentesis. Transudates and exudates must be distinguished. A transudate has none of the following characteristics; however, an exudate must meet one:
  - ◊ Pleural fluid protein/serum protein
  - ◊ Pleural fluid LDH/serum LDH > 0.6
  - ◊ Pleural fluid LDH > 2/3 upper limit of that in serum
- All exudates must be evaluated for:
  - ◊ Differential cell count
  - ◊ Amylase level
  - ◊ Glucose level
  - ◊ Comprehensive microbiologic culturing and Gram staining. If infection is suspected, the effusion should be evaluated for aerobic and anaerobic bacteria, mycobacteria, protozoa, fungi, and parasites, as appropriate. Tuberculosis effusions may be associated with elevations in lysozyme and adenosine deaminase.
  - ◊ Cytology for tumor cells
  - ◊ Triglyceride levels > 110 mg/dL are consistent with chylothorax
- Additional studies: pH, RBC count (hemorrhagic effusion if > 100,000/cc, consider trauma as etiology for effusion)
- In the absence of a known primary tumor and/or there is a high index of suspicion for malignancy, the cells harvested from an effusion can be evaluated for a variety of tumor markers (VIM, CD-15, CA19-9, CA-125, CEA, HBME-I, etc)

IMAGING
- Chest radiography: AP and lateral decubitus views
- Thoracic ultrasound
- CT scan

DIAGNOSTIC PROCEDURES
- Pleural biopsy if suspicion of tuberculosis or neoplasm
- Thoracentesis
- Thoracoscopy (provides direct view of both parietal and visceral aspects of pleura)

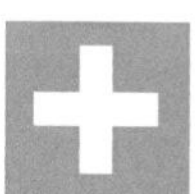

TREATMENT

APPROPRIATE HEALTH CARE Inpatient

GENERAL MEASURES
- Supportive care
  - ◊ Supplemental oxygen
  - ◊ IV fluid hydration
  - ◊ Chest physiotherapy
  - ◊ Therapeutic/diagnostic thoracentesis
- Antibiotics
  - ◊ Empirically by age/social circumstances and modified by blood and pleural effusion fluid culture results
- Empyema
  - ◊ Consider antibiotics alone with close monitoring in children
  - ◊ Antibiotics with chest tube drainage in adults
  - ◊ Pleurectomy in cases of trapped lung
- Pleural fluid loculation
  - ◊ May inject 250,000 units of streptokinase or 100,000 units of urokinase intrapleurally to dissolve fibrin meshes creating loculation. If unsuccessful, then either thoracoscopic adhesiolysis or decortication via thoracotomy are indicated.
- Malignancy
  - ◊ Consider treatment of primary source. However, most malignancies accompanied by malignant pleural effusions are advanced and cure is unlikely with chemotherapeutic intervention.
  - ◊ If effusion is causing dyspnea, perform therapeutic thoracentesis and, if fluid reaccumulates rapidly, then place chest tube for continuous drainage.
  - ◊ Other therapeutic interventions include placement of a pleuroperitoneal shunt and chemical pleurodesis
- Chylothorax - radiation therapy if from malignant cause or surgical repair of thoracic duct trauma.
- Hemothorax - diagnosed if hematocrit of pleural fluid > 50% that seen in blood. Usually caused by trauma or rupture of a tumor. Drainage via tube thoracostomy indicated. If bleeding persists or is of high volume then emergent thoracotomy is indicated

SURGICAL MEASURES See General Measures

ACTIVITY As tolerated

DIET Depends on clinical circumstances

PATIENT EDUCATION American Lung Association, 1740 Broadway, New York, New York 10038

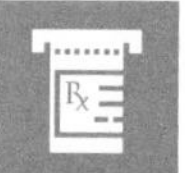

MEDICATIONS

DRUG(S) OF CHOICE
- Antimicrobial therapy according to pathogens and associated sensitivities
- Chemical pleurodesis with doxycycline 500 mg, bleomycin 60 units, or talc in a slurry, as indicated. The patient should be provided intravenous narcotic analgesia, as this procedure can cause considerable pain. Pleurodesis can be extremely effective therapy for preventing nonmalignant recurrent effusions. If pleurodesis fails, the patient may be offered pleural abrasion, though this is not commonly performed.
- Chemotherapy according to current oncologic protocols
- Steroids and non-steroidal anti-inflammatory drugs for rheumatologic and inflammatory etiologies
- Diuresis as appropriate for effusions secondary to congestive heart failure and ascites

Contraindications: Refer to manufacturer's drug profiles
Precautions: Refer to manufacturer's drug profiles
Significant possible interactions: Refer to manufacturer's drug profiles

ALTERNATIVE DRUGS N/A

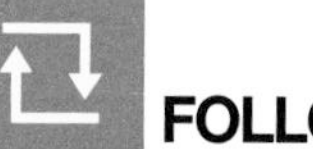

FOLLOWUP

PATIENT MONITORING
- Serial chest radiographs, with frequency/interval determined by patient status/diagnosis
- Pulmonary function testing as indicated
- Serum studies, echocardiography, renal/hepatic function tests as indicated to monitor for stability/progression of nonmalignant/noninfectious factors precipitating effusions

PREVENTION/AVOIDANCE N/A

POSSIBLE COMPLICATIONS
- Chronic empyema
- Drainage through chest wall - pleurocutaneous fistula
- Bronchopleural fistula
- Toxic shock syndrome

EXPECTED COURSE/PROGNOSIS
Mortality rate around 20% for exudative effusions; worse for elderly patients or those with serious underlying conditions

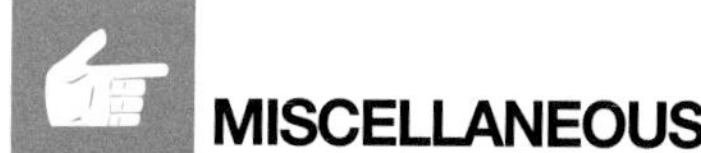

MISCELLANEOUS

ASSOCIATED CONDITIONS N/A

AGE-RELATED FACTORS N/A
Pediatric: N/A
Geriatric: N/A
Others: N/A

PREGNANCY N/A

SYNONYMS N/A

ICD-9-CM
511.9 Unspecified pleural effusion
511.1 Pleurisy with effusion, with mention of a bacterial cause other than tuberculosis
197.2 Secondary malignant neoplasm of pleura

SEE ALSO

OTHER NOTES N/A

ABBREVIATIONS N/A

REFERENCES

- Dowdeswell I. Pleural Diseases. In Internal Medicine (Stein J et al., eds). 5th Ed. St. Louis, Mosby, 1998
- Kendig R, Chernick V. Disorders of the Respiratory Tract in Children 5th Ed. Philadelphia, WB Saunders Co., 1990
- Light RW: Disorders of the pleura, mediastinum and diaphragm. In: Fauci AS, et al, eds: Harrison's Textbook of Internal Medicine. New York, McGraw Hill, 1998

Web references: 0 available at www.5mcc.com
Illustrations N/A

Author(s):
Peter P. Toth, MD, PhD

BASICS

DESCRIPTION An acute, bacterial infection of the lung parenchyma. Infection may be community-acquired or nosocomial (hospital acquired by an inpatient for at least 48 hours or inpatient in the previous 3 weeks). Most commonly, community-acquired disease is caused by *Streptococcus pneumoniae* or *Mycoplasma pneumoniae*. Hospital-acquired pneumonia is usually due to gram negative rods (60%, such as Pseudomonas) or Staphylococcus (14.5%).
System(s) affected: Pulmonary
Genetics: No known genetic pattern
Incidence/Prevalence in USA:
- Incidence - community-acquired: 1200 cases/100,000 population per year
- Incidence - nosocomial: 800 cases/100,000 admissions per year

Predominant age: Age extremes
Predominant sex: Male > Female

SIGNS & SYMPTOMS
- Cardinal signs and symptoms
  - ◊ Cough and fever
  - ◊ Chest pain (pleuritic)
  - ◊ Chill, with sudden onset
  - ◊ Dark, thick or bloody (rusty) sputum
- Respiratory
  - ◊ Signs of consolidation
    - Rales
    - Egophony
  - ◊ Signs of pleural involvement
    - Decreased breath sounds
    - Dullness to percussion
    - Friction rub
- Signs of respiratory distress
  - ◊ Tachypnea/tachycardia (or bradycardia)
  - ◊ Cyanosis
- Central nervous system
  - ◊ Mentation changes to include anxiety, confusion and restlessness
- Gastrointestinal
  - ◊ Abdominal pain
  - ◊ Anorexia

CAUSES
- Sources
  - ◊ Aspiration from the oropharynx
  - ◊ Inhalation
  - ◊ Hematogenous spread
- Bacterial pathogens
  - ◊ *Streptococcus pneumoniae* (pneumococcus)
  - ◊ *Haemophilus influenzae*
  - ◊ *Mycoplasma pneumoniae*
  - ◊ *Staphylococcus aureus*
  - ◊ *Legionella pneumophila*
  - ◊ *Chlamydia pneumoniae, C. psittaci*
  - ◊ *Moraxella catarrhalis* (Branhamella catarrhalis)
  - ◊ *Pseudomonas aeruginosa*
  - ◊ *Klebsiella pneumoniae* (and other gram-negative rods)
  - ◊ Anaerobes

RISK FACTORS
- Tobacco smoking
- Recent/concurrent viral infections
- Hospitalization to include mechanical ventilation, antecedent antibiotics, NG tubes
- Age extremes
- Alcoholism
- AIDS or other immunosuppression
- Renal failure
- Cardiovascular disease
- Functional asplenia
- Chronic obstructive pulmonary disease
- Diabetes mellitus
- Malnutrition
- Malignancy
- Altered level of consciousness or gag (e.g., seizures, stroke, neuromuscular disease, etc.)
- Occupational exposure
- Poorly implemented infection control practices (poor handwashing)
- Postoperative atelectasis

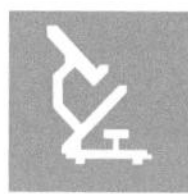

DIAGNOSIS

DIFFERENTIAL DIAGNOSIS Other causes of infectious pneumonitis: Viruses (human metapneumovirus, SARS coronavirus, respiratory syncytial, adenovirus, CMV, parainfluenza, influenzae A and B, varicella, measles, rubella, hantavirus); Nocardia; Fungi (Blastomyces, Cryptococcus, Aspergillus, Histoplasma, Coccidioides, Pneumocystis carinii); Protozoans (Toxoplasma); Rickettsia (Coxiella burnetii - Q fever). Also tuberculosis, pulmonary embolism with infarction, bronchiolitis obliterans with organizing pneumonia (BOOP), pulmonary contusion, pulmonary vasculitis, acute sarcoid, hypersensitivity pneumonitis, ARDS, pneumothorax, and other causes.

LABORATORY
- CBC - leukocytosis with an immature shift on differential; ESR, CRP
- Chem - hyponatremia (SIADH)
- ABG - hypoxemia
- ABG - hypocapnia initially, then hypercapnia
- Blood culture - positive in 10-20% of adult patients and 7% of pediatric patients with community-acquired pneumonia (partially because many have been pre-treated with antibiotics), 8-20% nosocomial pneumonia

Drugs that may alter lab results: Antecedent antibiotics

Disorders that may alter lab results: Refer to lab test reference

PATHOLOGICAL FINDINGS
- Lung:
  - ◊ Segmental, lobar, or multifocal peribronchial consolidation
  - ◊ Positive gram stain for bacteria

SPECIAL TESTS
- Decubitus CXR to investigate for empyema or parapneumonic effusion
- Gram stain and culture of pleural fluid
- pH of pleural fluid (iced, airless sample sent to blood gas laboratory)
- Urine legionella antigen (in ICU/severe cases)
- Tuberculin skin test (PPD) - for hilar adenopathy or upper respiratory infection

IMAGING
- CXR (with lateral decubitus views if pleural effusion present)
  - ◊ Lobar or segmental consolidation (air bronchogram)
  - ◊ Bronchopneumonia
  - ◊ Interstitial infiltrate
  - ◊ Pleural effusion (free-flowing or loculated)
- Ultrasound recommended to check for location and presence of loculations before thoracentesis

DIAGNOSTIC PROCEDURES
- Gram stain and culture of sputum (induced, if necessary)
- Nasotracheal suctioning for culture
- Transtracheal aspirate for culture
- Bronchoscopy with bronchoalveolar lavage or protected telescoping catheter brushing for culture
- Thoracentesis for pleural fluid studies
- Blood culture, especially if hospitalized - prior to antibiotics

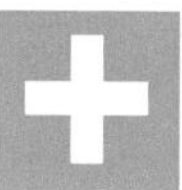

TREATMENT

APPROPRIATE HEALTH CARE
- Community-acquired - outpatient for mild case, inpatient for moderate to severe case such as hypoxemia, altered mental status, hypotension, significant co-morbid illness, and age extremes.
- Nosocomial - patients already hospitalized

GENERAL MEASURES
- Empiric antimicrobial therapy for most likely pathogen(s)
- Consider oxygen for patients with cyanosis, hypoxia, dyspnea, circulatory disturbances or delirium
- Mechanical ventilation for respiratory failure
- Hydration
- Analgesia for pain
- Electrolyte correction
- Respiratory isolation if TB is a possibility

SURGICAL MEASURES N/A

ACTIVITY Bedrest and/or reduced activity during acute phase

DIET
- Nothing by mouth if there is incipient respiratory failure
- Consider soft, easy-to-eat foods

PATIENT EDUCATION National Jewish, 1400 Jackson, Denver, CO 80206; 800222-lung (5864); www.nationaljewish.org/medfacts/pneumonia.html or www.medlineplus.gov

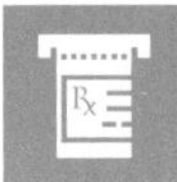

MEDICATIONS

DRUG(S) OF CHOICE

- Initial therapy
  - ◊ Usually empiric for most likely pathogens given clinical scenario (if specific etiology is identified, adjust antimicrobial therapy)
  - ◊ Otherwise healthy young adult with mild community-acquired pneumonia: erythromycin 500 po q6h; in those intolerant of erythromycin and in smokers [to treat H. influenzae], consider the new macrolides or doxycycline 100 mg bid
  - ◊ Older patients or patients with preexistent illnesses, with mild community-acquired pneumonia: pneumococcal-active fluoroquinolone or amoxicillin-clavulanate with erythromycin or other macrolide
  - ◊ Patients with community-acquired pneumonia requiring hospitalization: a specific cephalosporin (cefotaxime, ceftriaxone or cefuroxime) or ampicillin-sulbactam plus macrolide; or a pneumococcal-active fluoroquinolone alone
  - ◊ For nosocomial pneumonia: either ceftazidime or an antipseudomonal penicillin (piperacillin, mezlocillin, or ticarcillin) plus an aminoglycoside. Vancomycin should be considered if strong suspicion of *Staphylococcus aureus*.
- Therapy for specific organisms
  - ◊ *S. pneumoniae*: penicillin G or oral amoxicillin. If high incidence of penicillin resistant *S. pneumoniae* in the area, consider pneumococcal-active fluoroquinolone
  - ◊ *H. influenzae*: trimethoprim-sulfamethoxazole. For severe infections - cefotaxime, ceftriaxone, or carbapenems
  - ◊ *S. aureus*: nafcillin or vancomycin (if high incidence of methicillin resistant *S. aureus*)
  - ◊ Klebsiella species: carbapenems or 3rd generation cephalosporin
  - ◊ Pseudomonas: aminoglycoside plus antipseudomonal penicillin or ceftazidime
  - ◊ *Moraxella catarrhalis*: 2nd generation cephalosporin (cefuroxime axetil) or ß-lactam/ß-lactamase inhibitors
  - ◊ *Chlamydia pneumoniae*: doxycycline, fluoroquinolone
  - ◊ *Mycoplasma pneumoniae*: doxycycline
  - ◊ *Legionella pneumophila*: fluoroquinolone or azithromycin
  - ◊ Anaerobes: clindamycin or ß-lactam/ß-lactamase inhibitors

Contraindications: Allergy or likely cross-allergy to the prescribed antibiotic
Precautions: Possible significant sodium overload with antipseudomonal penicillins
Significant possible interactions: Refer to manufacturer's literature

ALTERNATIVE DRUGS

- *S. pneumoniae*: macrolide, doxycycline; cefotaxime, ceftriaxone or cefuroxime, linezolid
- *H. influenzae*: cefuroxime; fluoroquinolones; extended macrolides; beta-lactam/beta-lactamase inhibitor
- *S. aureus*: a first generation cephalosporin; clindamycin; linezolid
- Klebsiella: fluoroquinolone
- Pseudomonas: carbapenems, aztreonam, cefepime
- *Moraxella catarrhalis*: trimethoprim- sulfamethoxazole; fluoroquinolone; cefixime, extended macrolide
- *Chlamydia pneumoniae*: clarithromycin; azithromycin; erythromycin
- *Mycoplasma pneumoniae*: clarithromycin; erythromycin; azithromycin or fluoroquinolone
- *Legionella pneumophila*: clarithromycin; erythromycin; doxycycline

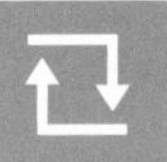

FOLLOWUP

PATIENT MONITORING

- If outpatient therapy, daily assessment of the patient's progress, and reassessment of therapy if clinical worsening or no improvement in 48-72 hours
- CXR take time to clear and may not show clearing, even though patient is improving. Repeat study about 6 weeks after recovery to verify the pneumonia was not caused by an obstructing endobronchial lesion in selected patients (smokers and older patients).
- Repeating the cultures after treatment has been started is unnecessary unless there has been treatment failure or if treating TB

PREVENTION/AVOIDANCE

- Reduce risk factors where possible (quit smoking)
- Bedridden and postoperative patients - deep breathing and coughing exercises; prevent aspiration during nasogastric tube feedings
- Avoid indiscriminate use of antibiotics during minor viral infections
- Annual influenza vaccine for high risk individuals
- Polyvalent pneumococcal vaccine

POSSIBLE COMPLICATIONS

- Empyema
- Pulmonary abscess
- Superinfections
- Multiple organ dysfunction syndrome (MODS)
- Adult respiratory distress syndrome (ARDS)
- Post-pneumonic atelectasis may occur in 5-10% of children

EXPECTED COURSE/PROGNOSIS

- Usual course - acute. In otherwise healthy individual, improvement seen and fever resolved in 1-3 days; sometimes up to 1 week
- Overall mortality is about 5% in community acquired; (≈15% if hospitalized and < 1% if not hospitalized) 25-40% in nosocomial
- Poorest prognosis - age extremes, positive blood cultures, low WBC, presence of associated disease, immunosuppression respiratory failure, inappropriate antecedent antibiotics, delayed treatment >8 hours

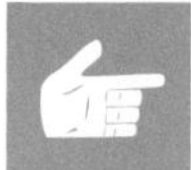

MISCELLANEOUS

ASSOCIATED CONDITIONS

- Tobacco smoking
- Alcoholism
- Upper respiratory infection

AGE-RELATED FACTORS

Pediatric: Morbidity and mortality high in children under age 1
Geriatric: Morbidity and mortality high if > 70, especially with associated disease or risk factor
Others: N/A

PREGNANCY N/A

SYNONYMS

- Lobar pneumonia
- Classic pneumococcal pneumonia

ICD-9-CM

481 Pneumococcal pneumonia [Streptococcus pneumoniae pneumonia]
486 Pneumonia, organism unspecified

SEE ALSO

Pneumonia, mycoplasma
Pneumonia, viral
Rhodococcus infections

OTHER NOTES Pneumococcal vaccine for all adults over age 65 and children over 2 years (and adults) with risk (cardio, pulmonary or metabolic disorders); strongly consider in all adults age 50 and older.

ABBREVIATIONS N/A

REFERENCES

- Bartlett JG, Dowell SF, et al. Practice guidelines for the management of community-acquired pneumonia in adults. Infectious Diseases Society of America. Clin Infect Dis 2000;31(2):347-82
- American Thoracic Society. Hospital acquired pneumonia in adults: diagnosis, assessment of severity, initial antimicrobial therapy, and preventive strategies. Am J Res Crit Care 1996;153:1711-25
- Bartlett JG, Mundy LM. Community-acquired pneumonia. N Engl J Med 1995;333:1618-24
- American Thoracic Society. Guidelines for the management of adults with community acquired pneumonia. Am J Respir Crit Care 2001;163:1730-54
- British Thoracic Society. Guidelines for the Management of Community Acquired Pneumonia in Adults. Thorax 2001;56(Suppl4):IVI-64

Web references: 0 available at www.5mcc.com
Illustrations N/A

Author(s):

James K. Radike, MD
Ronald A. Greenfield, MD

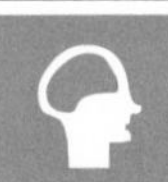

BASICS

DESCRIPTION Interstitial pneumonia caused by extensive infection of the lungs and bronchi, particularly the lower lobes of the lungs, by Mycoplasma pneumoniae. Usual course - acute. Incubation period is about 18-21 days and includes prodromal symptoms.
- Little seasonal variation of incidence, therefore a greater percentage of pneumonia in summer and fall are from Mycoplasma. Epidemics in communities tend to be prolonged (over many months) and occur every 4-5 years.

System(s) affected: Pulmonary
Genetics: None
Incidence/Prevalence in USA:
- 130 cases/100,000 people
- Estimated to be most common cause of pneumonia in school children and young adults (without chronic underlying condition). The incidence varies considerably each year. Major outbreaks are repeated every 3-5 years.

Predominant age: Ages 5-15, but occurs at any age
Predominant sex: Male > Female

SIGNS & SYMPTOMS
- Gradual onset with upper respiratory infection symptoms that progress
- Most will develop fever, cough, headache, sore throat, rales, and wheeze
- Many will develop myalgias, nasal congestion, chest pain
- Some will develop pleural effusion, pleural friction rub, cervical adenopathy, bullous myringitis, skin rash

CAUSES Mycoplasma pneumoniae infection

RISK FACTORS
- Close community living (e.g., hospitals, prisons, military bases, fraternity houses). Some of largest outbreaks have been in army recruits.
- Family exposure
- Immunocompromised patients

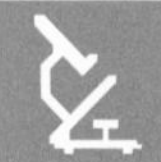

DIAGNOSIS

DIFFERENTIAL DIAGNOSIS
- Viral pneumonia
- Bacterial pneumonia (including plague and tularemia in severe cases)
- Fungal pneumonias
- *Pneumocystis carinii* pneumonia
- Chlamydia pneumonia, TWAR or psittaci
- Legionella pneumonia
- Tuberculosis

LABORATORY
- Positive cold agglutinins (titer of 1:1024 or greater; or rising fourfold) in 50% of infections
- *M. pneumoniae* culture (requires 7-10 days)
- Complement fixation serologic assay shows fourfold rise in titer at 2-4 weeks after symptom onset
- IgM antibody to M. pneumoniae in 80% of patients after 1-2 weeks of illness (enzyme immunoassay)
- Detection of M. pneumoniae DNA by PCR testing of nasopharyngeal aspirate

Drugs that may alter lab results: N/A

Disorders that may alter lab results: N/A

PATHOLOGICAL FINDINGS Absence of bacterial pathogens on Gram stain and culture of sputum or transtracheal aspirate. Mycoplasma is a fastidious and slow-growing organism.

SPECIAL TESTS N/A

IMAGING Chest x-ray - diffuse interstitial infiltrates; small bilateral pleural effusion present in 25% of cases

DIAGNOSTIC PROCEDURES N/A

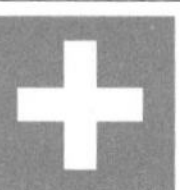

TREATMENT

APPROPRIATE HEALTH CARE Outpatient usually; inpatient if symptoms severe

GENERAL MEASURES N/A

SURGICAL MEASURES N/A

ACTIVITY Rest during acute phase

DIET Drink plenty of fluids

PATIENT EDUCATION Printed patient information available from American Lung Association, 1740 Broadway, New York, NY 10019, (212)315-8700; www.lungusa.org

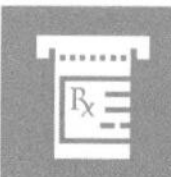

MEDICATIONS

DRUG(S) OF CHOICE
- Erythromycin - children 30-50 mg/kg/day for 10-14 days; adults 500 mg every 6 hours for 10-14 days
- Clarithromycin - children 15 mg/kg/d for 10-14 days; adults 500 mg bid for 10-14 days or azithromycin - children 10 mg/kg po first day, 5 mg/kg po for days 2-5; adults 500 mg first day, then 250 mg every day for 5 days.
- Consider 3 weeks of therapy if patient has persistent cough or airway reactivity
- Penicillins are ineffective against M. pneumoniae

Contraindications: Refer to manufacturer's literature
Precautions: Refer to manufacturer's literature
Significant possible interactions: Erythromycin and other macrolides inhibit the cytochrome P-450 microsomal enzyme system and can reduce elimination of other drugs such as carbamazepine, phenytoin, lovastatin, and theophylline. Prolongation of the QT interval and ventricular tachycardia have occurred in some patients receiving astemizole or terfenadine concomitantly with erythromycin.

ALTERNATIVE DRUGS
- Doxycycline 100 mg PO bid if older than 9 years
- Levofloxacin shows good activity against Mycoplasma
- Adjunctive drugs - albuterol inhaler, 2 puffs qid for wheezing
- Children 9 yr and older - doxycycline 100 mg po bid

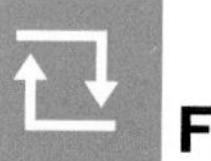

FOLLOWUP

PATIENT MONITORING
- Phone or in person followup
- Clearing of chest x-ray should be documented if the patient is older than 50. In smokers, document a clear x-ray in 6-8 weeks.

PREVENTION/AVOIDANCE
Highly contagious, M pneumoniae is carried in respiratory droplets. Consider isolation of active cases in closed communities (schools, camps, military bases). Azithromycin prophylaxis (standard 5 day course) may lower attack rate.

POSSIBLE COMPLICATIONS
Note: All complications are rare except reactive airway disease, hemolytic anemia, and erythema multiforme.
- Reactive airway disease
- Hemolytic anemia
- Erythema multiforme
- Meningoencephalitis
- Polyneuritis
- Polyarthritis
- Stevens-Johnson syndrome
- Pericarditis
- Myocarditis
- Respiratory distress syndrome
- Cerebral ataxia
- Thromboembolic phenomena
- Pleural effusion
- Nephritis

EXPECTED COURSE/PROGNOSIS
- Mycoplasma infection symptoms usually resolve in about 2 weeks
- Some constitutional symptoms may persist for several weeks
- With correct therapy, even most severe cases can expect complete recovery

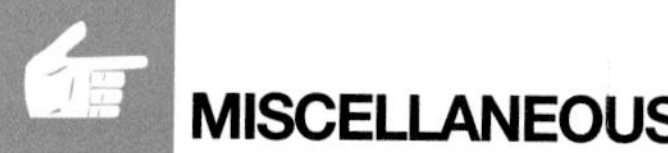

MISCELLANEOUS

ASSOCIATED CONDITIONS
N/A

AGE-RELATED FACTORS
Pediatric:
- Unusual in infants
- M. pneumoniae is associated with an increased incidence of asthma attacks in older children

Geriatric: Unusual in this age group
Others: N/A

PREGNANCY
Tetracycline contraindicated in pregnancy

SYNONYMS
- Primary atypical pneumonia (PAP)
- Eaton agent pneumonia
- Cold agglutinin-positive pneumonia

ICD-9-CM
483.0 Mycoplasma pneumoniae

SEE ALSO
Pneumonia, bacterial
Pneumonia, Pneumocystis (PCP)
Pneumonia, viral

OTHER NOTES
N/A

ABBREVIATIONS
N/A

REFERENCES

- Luthan-Sadler BA, Morell VW. Viral and atypical pneumonias. Primary Care 1996;23:837-848
- Block S, Hedrick J, et al. Mycoplasma pneumonia and chlamydia pneumonia in pediatric community acquired pneumonia. Ped Infect Dis 1995;14:471-477
- O'Handley JG, Gray LD. The incidence of Mycoplasma pneumoniae. J Am Board Fam Pract 1997;10:425-9
- Hyde TB, Gilbert M, Schwartz SB, et al. Azithromycin prophylaxis during a hospital outbreak of Mycoplasma pneumoniae pneumonia. J Infect Dis 2001;183(6):907-12

Web references: 0 available at www.5mcc.com
Illustrations N/A

Author(s):
George R. Bergus, MD

BASICS

DESCRIPTION A pneumonia arising in immunosuppressed persons caused by *Pneumocystis jiroveci*. This is one of the most common opportunistic infections occurring in patients with human immunodeficiency virus (HIV) infections. Pneumocystis infection can cause organ involvement and disseminated disease as well as pneumonia.
System(s) affected: Pulmonary
Genetics: N/A
Incidence/Prevalence in USA: PCP is the AIDS indicator disease in 43% of patients; with effective prophylaxis and antiretroviral therapy - incidence is decreasing
Predominant age:
- In HIV infected children, not taking prophylaxis, median age of onset is 5 months of age
- In HIV infected adults, PCP may occur at any age

Predominant sex: Male > Female (reflecting prevalence of HIV infection)

SIGNS & SYMPTOMS
- Usually insidious but occasionally abrupt in onset
- Dyspnea on exertion progressing to continuous dyspnea
- Weakness, fatigue, malaise
- Fever, chills
- Cough - non-productive or productive of scant white or clear sputum
- Tachypnea
- Extrapulmonary Pneumocystis may occur (visceral, cutaneous, eyes) particularly in patients on aerosolized pentamidine for prophylaxis

CAUSES The ubiquitous *Pneumocystis jiroveci* may cause infection in normal hosts (65-100% of young children have positive serology) but will rarely cause symptoms in immunocompetent individuals. Studies suggest person to person transmission possible.

RISK FACTORS
- Immunodeficiency (premature infants, neoplasia, congenital, acquired or drug-induced immunodeficiency states, CD4 counts < 200 in adults)
- Patients with a history of previous PCP

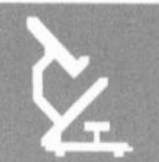

DIAGNOSIS

DIFFERENTIAL DIAGNOSIS
- Tuberculosis
- *Mycobacterium avium intracellulare*
- Viral pneumonias
- Fungal pneumonias
- Lymphoid interstitial pneumonitis (in children)
- Bacterial pneumonia
- CMV pneumonia (cytomegalovirus)

LABORATORY
- Serum LDH frequently elevated (mean elevation of 362 IU)
- Arterial blood gases reveal hypoxemia and increased alveolar-arterial gradient (varies with severity of disease)
- Sputum induced with inhaled 3-5% hypertonic saline may reveal pneumocystis on cytologic evaluation using various stains. An IF (immunofluorescence) technique is also available. (Sensitivity may be as high as 78% in labs with experienced personnel.)
- CD4 cell count generally below 200 in HIV infected patients with PCP.

Drugs that may alter lab results: Inhaled pentamidine used to prevent PCP may change radiographic picture to infiltrates in predominantly upper-lobe distribution

Disorders that may alter lab results: N/A

PATHOLOGICAL FINDINGS Pneumonitis caused by presence of organism and inflammatory response

SPECIAL TESTS Gallium scanning of the lungs is highly sensitive for PCP but is not very specific. May be useful when sputum studies are inconclusive and bronchoscopy is not available.

IMAGING
- Chest x-ray
  - ◊ Shows bilateral diffuse interstitial or perihilar infiltrate in 75% of cases
  - ◊ May also show a normal chest x-ray, unilateral disease, pleural effusions, abscesses or cavitations, pneumothorax, and lobar consolidations
  - ◊ Upper lobe infiltrates may be present in patients on pentamidine prophylaxis

DIAGNOSTIC PROCEDURES
- Fiberoptic bronchoscopy with broncho-alveolar lavage or transbronchial biopsy is the preferred method of diagnosis when sputums are negative
- Open lung biopsy is rarely required
- A PCR test for pneumocystis may be useful in the future (on sputum, bronchoalveolar fluid)

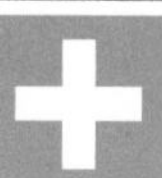

TREATMENT

APPROPRIATE HEALTH CARE Outpatient in mild cases, otherwise inpatient

GENERAL MEASURES Oxygen therapy often necessary

SURGICAL MEASURES N/A

ACTIVITY As tolerated

DIET No special diet

PATIENT EDUCATION For patient education materials on this topic, contact: American Lung Association, 1740 Broadway, New York, NY 10019, (212)315-8700 or Project Inform - http://www.projinf.org

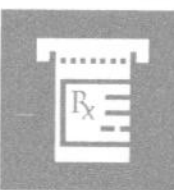

MEDICATIONS

DRUG(S) OF CHOICE
- Trimethoprim-sulfamethoxazole (Bactrim, Septra) 15 mg/kg/day of trimethoprim component po in 3 divided doses or IV for 21 days. Reduce dose of trimethoprim-sulfamethoxazole in patients with renal failure.
- Adjunctive corticosteroid (prednisone or methyl prednisolone) therapy begun within 72 hours of diagnosis decreases mortality in AIDS patients (adults and children) with moderate to severe PCP (those with pO2<70 mmHg)

Contraindications: Use with care in pregnant patient and infants less than 2 months

Precautions:
- History of sulfa allergy
- A high percentage of patients with AIDS will develop intolerance to trimethoprim/ sulfamethoxazole. Especially common are dermatologic reactions, hematologic toxicity, or fever.
- Avoid sunlight

Significant possible interactions: Phenytoin, oral anti-coagulants, oral sulfonylureas, digitalis

ALTERNATIVE DRUGS
- Pentamidine 4 mg/kg/day IV for 21 days
- Dapsone 100 mg po daily plus trimethoprim 15 mg/kg/day po in 3-4 divided doses. Check G6PD level before beginning dapsone as hemolysis may result.
- Clindamycin 300-400 mg po qid for 21 days plus primaquine 30 mg po daily for 21 days
- Trimetrexate glucuronate 45 mg/m2 IV qd over 60-90 minutes with leucovorin 20 mg/m2 IV or po q6h - continue for 72 hours after last dose of trimetrexate. Recommended course of therapy is 21 days of trimetrexate and 24 days of leucovorin. Doses may need to be adjusted for hematologic toxicity - monitor CBC/differential and platelets.
- Atovaquone suspension 750 mg bid for 21 days

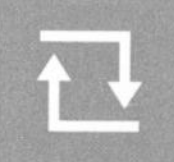

FOLLOWUP

PATIENT MONITORING Serum LDH, pulmonary function tests and arterial blood gases generally normalize with treatment

PREVENTION/AVOIDANCE
- All AIDS patients with a history of PCP (or CD4 cells < 200 or evidence of immunodeficiency) require prophylaxis with daily trimethoprim-sulfamethoxazole (double-strength), daily dapsone (100 mg) or monthly aerosolized pentamidine (300 mg). In patients intolerant of TMP-SMX, consider a rechallenge or desensitization with TMP-SMX; various protocols exist.
- Prophylaxis may be discontinued in patients on antiretroviral therapy when CD4 cells > 200 for over 3 months
- All babies born to HIV infected mothers need to be on prophylaxis after the first month of life. Drug of choice is TMP-SMX; 150 mg/m2/day (TMP component) 3 times weekly (on consecutive days). This should be continued until the baby is proven HIV negative or for the first year of life, after which CD4 cell count may be used to guide prophylaxis.

POSSIBLE COMPLICATIONS
- Respiratory failure
- Pneumothorax (even after successful treatment)
- Extrapulmonary pneumocystis (especially in patients on inhaled pentamidine prophylaxis)

EXPECTED COURSE/PROGNOSIS
- Mortality from first episode PCP is 10-15%. With prophylactic therapy, mean survival has increased.
- 40% of patients with PCP will have a recurrence without prophylaxis

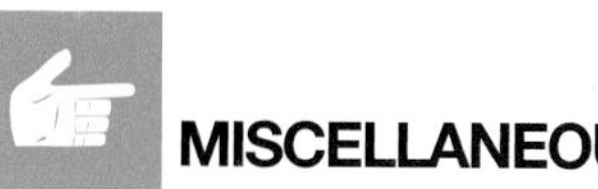

MISCELLANEOUS

ASSOCIATED CONDITIONS
- AIDS
- HIV infection

AGE-RELATED FACTORS
Pediatric:
- Early onset (5 months of age) and high mortality (median survival 1 month)
- Important to distinguish from lymphoid interstitial pneumonitis (LIP) as treatment and prognosis differ
- PCP prophylaxis with TMP-SMX, dapsone or pentamidine for all HIV positive children less than 1 year old is recommended. For older HIV positive children, prophylaxis individualized based on CD4 counts (see Prevention/Avoidance section).

Geriatric: N/A

Others: N/A

PREGNANCY Trimethoprim-sulfamethoxazole has been used for treatment and prophylaxis. Avoid pentamidine.

SYNONYMS
- Pneumocystosis
- Pulmonary pneumocystosis
- Interstitial plasma cell pneumonia
- Pneumocystis carinii pneumonia

ICD-9-CM
136.3 Pneumocystosis

SEE ALSO
HIV infection & AIDS

OTHER NOTES DNA analysis has revealed multiple species of Pneumocystis and the organism causing disease in humans was renamed *P. jiroveci* from *P. carinii* in 1999.

ABBREVIATIONS
LDH = lactate dehydrogenase
G6PD = glucose 6-phosphate dehydrogenase
TMP-SMX = trimethoprim-sulfamethoxazole

REFERENCES

- Miller RF, Mitchell DM. <I>Pneumocystis carinii</I> pneumonia. Thorax 1995;50:191-200
- Sistek CJ, et al. Adjuvant corticosteroid therapy for <I>Pneumocystis carinii</I> pneumonia in AIDS patients. Ann Pharmacother 1992;9:1127-1133
- Simonds RJ, Hughes WT, Feinberg J, et al. Preventing <I>Pneumocystis carinii</I> pneumonia in persons infected with human immunodeficiency virus. Clin Infect Dis 1995;21(suppl 1):544-548
- Gluckstein D, Ruskin J. Rapid oral desensitization to trimethoprim-sulfamethoxazole: use in prophylaxis for <I>Pneumocystis carinii</I> pneumonia in patients with AIDS who were previously intolerant of TMP-SMX. Clin Infect Dis 1995;20:849-53
- Dohn MN, White ML, Vigdorth EM, et al. Geographic clustering of <I>Pneumocystis carinii</I> pneumonia in patients with HIV infection. Am J Respir Crit Care Med 2000;162(5):1617-21
- 2001 USPHS/IDSA Guidelines for the Prevention of Opportunistic Infections in Persons Infected with Human Immunodeficiency Virus;July, 2001 (Draft Revisions to MMWR 1999;48:NoRR10
- Stringer JR, Beard CB, Miller RF, Wakefield AE. A new name (<I>Pneumocystis jiroveci</I>) for Pneumocystis from humans.
- Emerg Infect Dis. 2002;8(9):891-6

Web references: 2 available at www.5mcc.com

Illustrations N/A

Author(s):
Cynthia Gail Carmichael, MD

BASICS

DESCRIPTION Inflammatory disease of the lungs. Most viral pneumonia results from exposure of a nonimmune individual to infected aerosolized secretions.

System(s) affected: Pulmonary

Genetics: No known genetic pattern

Incidence/Prevalence in USA:
- Approximately 90% of childhood pneumonia is viral
- 4-39% of pneumonia in adults has been attributed to viral etiologies in different series
- Prevalence is unknown and variable due to seasonal variation, though more common in winter months
- Mixed infections with bacterial pathogens common

Predominant age:
- More common in children than in adults

Predominant sex: Male = Female

SIGNS & SYMPTOMS
- Fever
- Chills
- Cough (with or without purulent sputum production)
- Dyspnea
- Pulmonary rales and rhonchi
- Altered breath sounds
- Pleurisy
- Friction rub
- Headache
- Myalgias
- Malaise
- Gastrointestinal symptoms

CAUSES
- Influenza A, B and C
- Parainfluenza 1, 2, 3, and 4
- Respiratory syncytial virus (RSV, especially in young children)
- Adenovirus
- Cytomegalovirus (CMV), particularly in immunocompromised patients)
- Varicella (chickenpox)
- *Herpes simplex*
- Enterovirus
- Coronavirus
- Rubeola (measles)
- Epstein-Barr virus
- Hanta virus

RISK FACTORS
- Immunocompromised
- Living in close quarters
- Seasonal - epidemic upper respiratory illness
- Elderly
- Cardiac disease
- Chronic pulmonary disease
- Recent upper respiratory infection
- Travel to endemic area (Hantavirus and SARS)

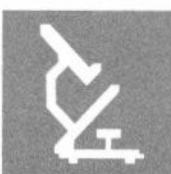

DIAGNOSIS

DIFFERENTIAL DIAGNOSIS
- Bacterial pneumonia (especially atypical etiologies: *Chlamydia pneumoniae* and *Psittaci*, *Mycoplasma pneumoniae*, *Legionella pneumophila*)
- Pulmonary edema
- *Pneumocystis carinii* pneumonia (PCP)
- Aspiration pneumonia
- Hypersensitivity pneumonitis
- Bronchial carcinoma with lymphangitic spread
- Bronchiolitis obliterans with organizing pneumonia (BOOP)
- Pulmonary embolus/infarction
- Cystic fibrosis (in infants)
- Severe acute respiratory syndrome (SARS-CoV)

LABORATORY
- Sputum gram stain and culture to identify bacterial co-pathogens if present
- Appropriate direct fluorescent antibody from throat nasopharyngeal washings (children) or swab (adults), tracheal aspirate, or bronchoalveolar lavage specimens (HSV, VZV, influenza A and B, RSV, adenovirus)
- Viral culture
- Cytopathology (CMV, HSV, Rubeola)
- Normal or near normal granulocyte count, occasionally leukopenic with increased lymphocyte percentage
- Hypoxemia with severe disease
- Hemoconcentration (Hanta virus)
- Serology (4-fold rise in acute vs convalescent titers)
- Polymerase chain reaction (PCR) detection if available

Drugs that may alter lab results: N/A

Disorders that may alter lab results: Coronavirus antibody or RT-PCR if SARS possible

PATHOLOGICAL FINDINGS
- Heavy lungs
- Enlarged regional lymph nodes
- Cytoplasmic inclusion bodies (CMV)
- Intranuclear inclusion bodies (adenovirus, CMV, herpes virus, varicella)
- Intense inflammatory reaction with mononuclear cells
- Multinucleated giant cells (parainfluenza virus, Rubeola, HSV, varicella)

SPECIAL TESTS N/A

IMAGING
- CXR - interstitial or alveolar infiltrates, peribronchial thickening, pleural effusion

DIAGNOSTIC PROCEDURES
- Nasopharyngeal throat swab
- Tracheal aspiration (seldom needed)
- Bronchoscopy with bronchoalveolar lavage (BAL)
- Serologic testing for hantavirus. Enzyme immunoassay (EIA) available from health departments.
- Information on SARS for clinicians: cdc.gov/ncidod/sars/clinicians.htm

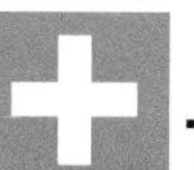

TREATMENT

APPROPRIATE HEALTH CARE
Outpatient for most cases. Inpatient for infants under 4 months of age or elderly, or for any patient with diffuse, severe infection (hypoxemia, hypercarbia, hypotension or shock, adult respiratory distress syndrome) or significant comorbidity (CHF, CAD, COPD, etc.)

GENERAL MEASURES
- Encourage coughing and deep breathing exercises to clear secretions
- Careful disposal of secretions/universal precautions
- Hydration
- Respiratory isolation for varicella which is highly contagious (i.e., negative pressure)

SURGICAL MEASURES N/A

ACTIVITY
- Rest

DIET
- Increase fluids, high calorie, high protein, soft diet

PATIENT EDUCATION
For patient education materials on this topic, contact: American Lung Association, 1740 Broadway, New York, NY 100919, 800-LUNG-USA

MEDICATIONS

DRUG(S) OF CHOICE
- Amantadine (Symmetrel): influenza A (not effective for influenza B) - effective only in first 24-48 hours
  - ◊ Age < 10: 4-8 mg/kg/day in 2 divided doses. Not to exceed 150 mg/day.
  - ◊ Age 10-65: 100 mg orally q12 h (adults may be given a loading dose of 200 mg initially)
  - ◊ Age > 65: 100 mg orally once a day
- Acyclovir (Zovirax): pulmonary infections involving herpes simplex, herpes zoster or varicella
  - ◊ Adults 5 mg/kg IV q8h for HSV pneumonia and 10 mg/kg IV q8h for varicella pneumonia
  - ◊ Children 250 mg/square meter body surface area IV q8h
- Ganciclovir (Cytovene): CMV infection, HSV infection
  - ◊ 5 mg/kg IV 12h
- Ribavirin (Virazole): RSV, possibly Hanta and influenza B virus (20 mg/mL via continuous aerosol administration for 12-18 hours/day for 3-7 days). Indicated only in severe RSV infections, given via small particle aerosol generator (SPAG).
- Zanamivir (Relenza) - influenza A and B
  - ◊ Age > 12: 10 mg (2 inhalations) inhaled by mouth q 12 h for 5 days
- Oseltamivir (Tamiflu) - influenza A and B
  - ◊ Age > 18: 75 mg by mouth q 12 h for 5 days. Dose adjusted to 75 mg q 24 h for creatinine clearance < 30 mL/min.

Contraindications: Refer to manufacturer's literature

Precautions:
- Amantadine should be used cautiously in patients with liver disease, epilepsy, renal disease, eczematoid rash, and those with a history of psychotic illness
- Ribavirin is teratogenic and should not be administered by pregnant health-care personnel; its cost is high and benefit marginal

Significant possible interactions: Refer to manufacturer's literature

ALTERNATIVE DRUGS
- Rimantadine (Flumadine), an amantadine analog, is equally effective as amantadine and has fewer CNS adverse effects. Useful for Influenza A. Effective only in first 24-48 hours.
- Antibiotics for superimposed bacterial infections.
- Foscarnet (Foscavir) for CMV, HSV, varicella infections, 60 mg/kg IV q8h
- Immune globulin (IVIG) IV may increase response in non-AIDS, immunosuppressed patients with CMV pneumonia. Dose and dosage regimen not well established, but 500 mg/kg IV qod x 10 doses may be beneficial.

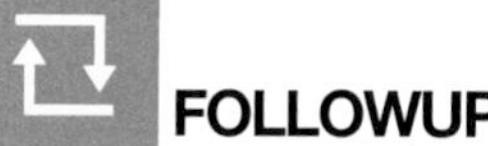

FOLLOWUP

PATIENT MONITORING
- Physical examinations, CXR
- Oxygenation if illness severe enough for hospitalization

PREVENTION/AVOIDANCE
- Influenza A and B vaccine: Use for patients with chronic cardiovascular lung disease, residents of chronic care facilities, medical personnel with extensive contact with high risk patients, people over 50 years of age or those with chronic diseases, immunosuppressed patients including all those with HIV, healthcare workers, and people in frequent contact with high risk person
- For those patients unable to receive influenza vaccine (egg allergy or other) and are at high risk because of age, co-morbid illness, or other risk factor, amantadine or rimantadine can be given throughout the infectious season if tolerated
- For those who did not receive the vaccine and have been exposed to influenza, or there is an influenza A outbreak, amantadine or rimantadine may also be taken for 2 weeks until vaccination has produced immunity
- Health care workers who are pregnant need to take proper precautions to avoid infectious patients
- Measles vaccine
- Varicella vaccine

POSSIBLE COMPLICATIONS
- Superimposed bacterial infections such as S. pneumoniae, S. aureus, H. influenzae and others
- Respiratory failure requiring mechanical ventilation
- Adult respiratory distress syndrome (ARDS)
- Reye syndrome after influenza in children

EXPECTED COURSE/PROGNOSIS
Usually favorable prognosis with illness lasting several days to a week. Post-viral fatigue is common. However, death can occur, especially in pediatric or bone-marrow transplant adenovirus infections or in elderly influenza infections.

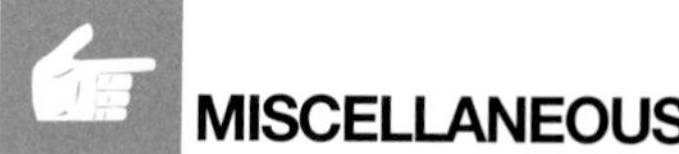

MISCELLANEOUS

ASSOCIATED CONDITIONS
- Bacterial pneumonias
- Fungi, Pneumocystis carinii in immunosuppressed patients

AGE-RELATED FACTORS
Pediatric: Adenovirus infections in children are serious. More serious RSV infections are almost always seen in infants and immunocompromised patients.
Geriatric: Greatest morbidity and mortality
Others: N/A

PREGNANCY Should avoid contact with persons who may have viral infections. Consider vaccination if woman will be > 3 months pregnant during influenza season.

SYNONYMS N/A

ICD-9-CM
480.9 Viral pneumonia, unspecified

SEE ALSO
Bronchiolitis obliterans & organizing pneumonia
Severe acute respiratory syndrome (SARS)

OTHER NOTES N/A

ABBREVIATIONS
RSV = respiratory syncytial virus
PCP = Pneumocystis carinii pneumonia
ARDS = adult respiratory distress syndrome
BOOP = bronchiolitis obliterans with organizing pneumonia
CMV = cytomegalovirus
PCR = polymerase chain reaction
SARS = severe acute respiratory syndrome
SARS-CoV = SARS-associated coronavirus

REFERENCES
- Mandell GL, ed: Principles and Practice of Infectious Diseases. 4th Ed. New York, Churchill Livingstone, 1995
- Fields BN, ed: Virology. 2nd Ed. New York, Raven Press, 1990
- Greenburg SB: Viral Pneumonia. Infectious Disease Clinics of North America. vol. 5 (3), September 1991
- Gorbach SL, ed: Infectious Diseases. Philadelphia, W.B. Saunders Company, 1992

Web references: 1 available at www.5mcc.com
Illustrations N/A

Author(s):
Gene W. Voskuhl, MD

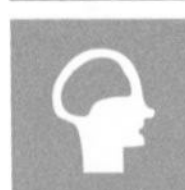

BASICS

DESCRIPTION Accumulation of air or gas between the parietal and visceral pleurae.
- Spontaneous pneumothorax - may be primary or secondary
  - ◊ Primary in young (early 20s) and otherwise healthy patients; rare after age 40
  - ◊ Secondary - as a complication of an underlying lung disease (COPD, cystic fibrosis, AIDS, TB)
- Traumatic pneumothorax (closed and open) - may coexist with hemothorax
- Tension pneumothorax - inspired air accumulates into pleural space with no means of escape. Like "check valve" mechanism. More air increases lung compression and causes hypoxia/hemodynamic compromise.

System(s) affected: Cardiovascular, Pulmonary
Genetics: No known genetic pattern, possible congenital predisposition in thin, tall young men; especially in Marfan
Incidence/Prevalence in USA: 9/100,000
Predominant age: Adults 20-40 years
Predominant sex: Male > Female

SIGNS & SYMPTOMS
- Pleuritic chest pain
- Cough
- Dyspnea
- Cyanosis
- Moderate to severe - profound respiratory distress, shock, circulatory collapse
- Asymmetry of respirations
- Diminished breath sounds on affected side
- Referred pain to shoulder
- Tachycardia
- Rapid, shallow breathing
- Hyperresonance to percussion
- Subcutaneous emphysema/crepitus over chest wall and neck
- Tension pneumothorax - weak, rapid pulse, pallor, neck vein distention, anxiety, tracheal deviation

CAUSES
- Perforation of the visceral pleura and entry of gas from the lung
- Gas generated by microorganisms in an empyema
- Penetration of the chest wall, diaphragm, mediastinum, or esophagus
- Blunt trauma to thorax

RISK FACTORS
- Trauma (broken rib, ruptured bronchus, perforated esophagus)
- Rupture of superficial lung bulla following cough or blowing a musical instrument
- Strenuous activity
- Flying (high altitude) after loss of pressurization
- Diving (at ascension or rapid decompression)
- Pneumoconioses
- Tuberculosis
- Pneumonia due to TB, Klebsiella, Staph aureus
- Subpleural Pneumocystis carinii pneumonia (PCP) (in AIDS patients on PCP prophylaxis via pentamidine aerosol)
- Bronchial obstruction
- COPD (particularly emphysema)
- Asthma
- Neoplasms
- Endometriosis (during menstruation)
- Rare diseases (Marfan, Ehlers-Danlos)
- Rupture of an infected abscess
- Lymphangioleiomyomatosis
- Cystic fibrosis
- Cigarette smoking
- Procedures including intubation central line placement, liver biopsy, mechanical ventilation, thoracentesis and acupuncture

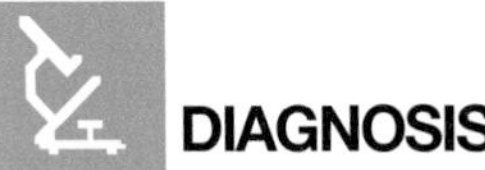

DIAGNOSIS

DIFFERENTIAL DIAGNOSIS
- Pleurisy
- Pericarditis
- Myocardial infarction
- Pulmonary embolism
- Diaphragmatic hernia
- Stomach herniation through diaphragm
- Dissecting aneurysm
- Flail chest
- Hemothorax
- Angina pectoris
- Asthma
- COPD exacerbation

LABORATORY
- Arterial blood gases in significant pneumothorax
  - ◊ pH < 7.35
  - ◊ pO2 < 80 mm Hg (10.6 kPa)
  - ◊ pCO2 > 45 mm Hg (6.0 kPa)

Drugs that may alter lab results: N/A

Disorders that may alter lab results: N/A

PATHOLOGICAL FINDINGS N/A

SPECIAL TESTS N/A

IMAGING
- Chest x-ray (obtain inspiration and expiratory views):
  - ◊ Air without lung markings peripherally, mediastinal shift to contralateral side
  - ◊ Small pneumothorax may be evident only with expiratory or lateral decubitus film
  - ◊ Upright CXR - as little as 50 mL of pleural gas can be visible
  - ◊ Lateral decubitus view - as little as 5 mL of pleural gas is visible
  - ◊ Supine CXR - ≈500 mL of pleural gas is needed for definitive diagnosis
  - ◊ Tension pneumothorax - can see mediastinum shift to opposite side
- Ultrasound - helpful in major trauma patients where CXR may be limited (in early stages of use)

DIAGNOSTIC PROCEDURES Careful history and physical. The physical findings depend on size of pneumothorax.

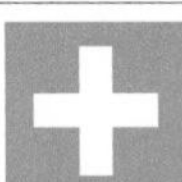

TREATMENT

APPROPRIATE HEALTH CARE
- Outpatient - lung collapse less than 30%, no dyspnea, no signs of tension pneumothorax, no underlying lung disease
- Inpatient - if more than 30% collapse, tension pneumothorax or underlying lung disease
- Tension pneumothorax is a medical emergency. Decompress as soon as possible.

GENERAL MEASURES
- Outpatient
  - ◊ Bed rest
- Inpatient
  - ◊ Monitoring blood pressure, pulse rate, respirations
  - ◊ Oxygen at high concentration will accelerate rate of absorption by 4 times
  - ◊ Treatment of any underlying condition
- Serial radiographs to document improvement
- Open pneumothorax - place dressing over wound. Secure only on three sides to avoid tension pneumothorax.

SURGICAL MEASURES
- Simple aspiration - first step for primary spontaneous pneumothorax unless unstable. Insert 16 gauge cannula into 2nd anterior intercostal space at midclavicular line and attach a 3-way stopcock and 60 mL syringe. Withdraw air manually until no more can be aspirated. Close stopcock and CXR after 4 hours. Remove if re-expanded. Observe 2 more hours.
- Thoracotomy tube (16F to 22F) - Usually first step for secondary spontaneous pneumothorax. Insert in 4th, 5th or 6th intercostal space at midaxillary line and connect underwater seal. Clamp after 12 hours of no bubbles.
- Tension pneumothorax - immediate decompression. Insert 19 gauge or larger needle into the second intercostal space at midclavicular line over superior aspect of rib to avoid vessels. and attach a 3-way stopcock. Use a large syringe to withdraw air. Follow with chest tube.
- Recurrent pneumothorax (more often occurs with larger pneumothoraces)
  - ◊ Consider thoracoscopy or thoracotomy following 2 or more spontaneous pneumothoraces, if lungs not expanded after 7 days therapy or persistent bronchopleural fistula. Also consider surgical correction for occupation or avocation that would put person at risk if pneumothorax recurs (eg, pilot, diver).
  - ◊ Consider pleurodesis with talc or other agents

ACTIVITY
- Bed rest until re-expanded
- No air travel until x-ray normal
- Athletes with pneumothorax may return to their sport after 2-3 weeks of rest as symptoms allow; athletes requiring inpatient care should have a follow up chest radiograph before returning to sport

DIET No special diet

PATIENT EDUCATION Stop smoking

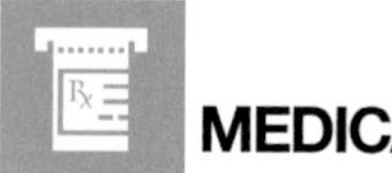

MEDICATIONS

DRUG(S) OF CHOICE
- Pleurodesis for recurrent pneumothorax:
  - ◊ Intrapleural doxycycline, 5 mg/kg in a total volume of 50 mL. Intrapleural doxycycline is painful so premedicate with short-acting benzodiazepine and give 4 mg/kg lidocaine in a total volume of 50 mL intrapleurally before doxycycline is injected.
  - ◊ Intrapleural talc, 5g in 250 mL isotonic saline; more effective than tetracycline derivatives, but safety concerns exist

Contraindications: If patient a possible candidate for future lung transplant, do not do sclerosing pleurodesis (sclerosing agents increase risk of bleeding at surgery so patients are not eligible for transplant)

Precautions:
- Talc procedure precipitated respiratory distress syndrome in 2 reports
- Pain at time of intrapleural instillation and post-procedure is the most common side effect. Premedicate with benzodiazepine and/or narcotic.

Significant possible interactions: Refer to manufacturer's literature

ALTERNATIVE DRUGS
None

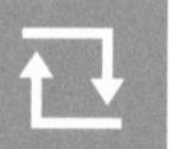

FOLLOWUP

PATIENT MONITORING
- Outpatient management should include follow up chest x-ray to document resolution of pneumothorax. Typically in several days.
- Blood pressure, respiratory rate, arterial blood gases, for hospitalized patients
- After simple aspiration - clamp chest tube for 24 hours, then remove if no recurrence on x-ray. If lung not fully re-expanded after 7 days, consider persistent air leak/bronchopleural fistula.

PREVENTION/AVOIDANCE
No preventive measures known, but patients may avoid some risk factors, e.g., exposure to high altitudes, flying in unpressurized aircraft, scuba diving, smoking

POSSIBLE COMPLICATIONS
- Re-expansion pulmonary edema following suction
- Bronchopleural fistulae requiring surgical repair
- Surgery indicated following 2 spontaneous pneumothoraces on the same side
- Myocardial infarction (MI)
- Respiratory arrest

EXPECTED COURSE/PROGNOSIS
- Air reabsorbed from small spontaneous pneumothorax in a few days
- Air reabsorbed from larger air space in 2-4 weeks
- Risk of recurrence is 30-50%

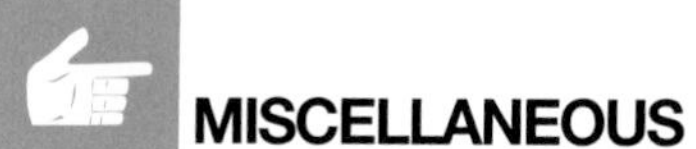

MISCELLANEOUS

ASSOCIATED CONDITIONS
Listed with Causes

AGE-RELATED FACTORS
Pediatric: Unusual in this age group except following trauma. Can see in neonates with respiratory distress syndrome and meconium aspiration.
Geriatric: Higher morbidity and mortality
Others: N/A

PREGNANCY
A known, but unusual complication of labor and delivery. It should be suspected in the pregnant patient with dyspnea and chest pain.

SYNONYMS
N/A

ICD-9-CM
512.0 Spontaneous tension pneumothorax
512.1 Iatrogenic pneumothorax
512.8 Other spontaneous pneumothorax

SEE ALSO

OTHER NOTES
Chest pain may simulate an acute MI or acute abdomen

ABBREVIATIONS
MI = myocardial infarction

REFERENCES

- Chan SS. Emergency bedside ultrasound to detect pneumothorax. Acad Emerg Med.2003;10(1):91-4
- Baumann MH, Strange C, Heffner JE, et al. Management of spontaneous pneumothorax: an American College of Chest Physicians Delphi consensus statement. Chest 2001;119(2):590-602
- Massad G, Thomas P, Wihlm JM. Minimally invasive management for first and recurrent pneumothorax. Ann Thorac Surg 1998;66:592-9
- Tschopp JM, Brutsche M, Frey JG. Treatment of complicated spontaneous pneumothorax by simple talc pleurodesis. Thorax 1997;52:329-32
- Sadikot RT, Greene T, Meadows K, Arnold AG. Recurrence of primary spontaneous pneumothorax. Thorax 1997;52:805-9
- Light RW. Management of spontaneous pneumothorax. Ann rev Respir Dis 1993;148:245
- Miller AC, Harvey JE. Guidelines for the management of spontaneous pneumothorax. Br Med J 1993;307:114
- Baumann MH. The clinician's perspective on pneumothorax management. Chest 1997;112:822-28
- Safran MR, McKeag DB, Van Camp SP, eds. Manual of Sports Medicine. Philadelphia: Lippincott-Raven; 1998

Web references: 3 available at www.5mcc.com
Illustrations N/A

Author(s):
Carrie A. Jaworski, MD
Shagun Saggar, MD

BASICS

DESCRIPTION Acute illness, symptomatic cases present as aseptic meningitis. Only a small number of cases with residual neurologic disease. Most symptomatic cases have nonspecific manifestations of infection. Illness is biphasic, paralysis occurs in second phase. Paralytic disease occurs with rapid onset. Spread by direst contact - fecal/oral. More common in warm months. Virus secreted for weeks in stool.

- Three types
  - ◊ Encephalitic - coma
  - ◊ Bulbar - cranial nerve paralysis
  - ◊ Spinal - arm(s) and leg(s) weakness

System(s) affected: Musculoskeletal, Nervous
Genetics: N/A
Incidence/Prevalence in USA: Now rare
Predominant age: 3 months-16 years; rarely adults
Predominant sex: Male = Female

SIGNS & SYMPTOMS

- Nonspecific
- Meningitis
- Neurologic symptoms

CAUSES

- Poliovirus 3 serotypes
- Poliomyelitis can occur in other infections, such as West Nile virus

RISK FACTORS

- Living in areas where sanitation and hygiene are poor
- Low socioeconomic status
- Increasing age, if not immunized
- Pregnancy
- Recent tonsillectomy
- Inoculation (e.g., DPT injection)

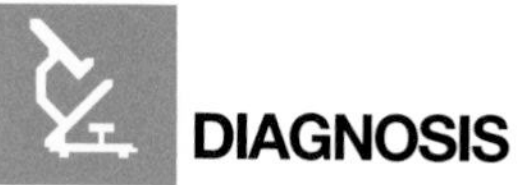

DIAGNOSIS

DIFFERENTIAL DIAGNOSIS

- Guillain-Barré syndrome
- Mumps, herpes, coxsackievirus infection
- Aseptic meningitis/encephalitis
- Tick paralysis

LABORATORY

- Pleocytosis
- Increased protein
- Normal glucose
- Serology
- Virus culture - should be done when suspected

Drugs that may alter lab results: N/A

Disorders that may alter lab results: N/A

PATHOLOGICAL FINDINGS

- Spinal cord - perivascular cuffing, abnormal motor nuclei, chromatolysis of motor neurons, intermediate column inflammation, posterior column inflammation
- Diffuse mononuclear infiltrate
- Abnormal anterior horn cells
- Hypothalamic lesion
- Thalamic lesion
- Brainstem lesion
- Vestibular nuclei lesions
- Cerebellar deep nuclei lesions
- Reticular formation lesions
- Cortical motor area lesions
- Cerebral edema
- Edematous cord

SPECIAL TESTS Spinal fluid virus isolation from throat (early in disease) and/or feces (early and late in the disease)

IMAGING N/A

DIAGNOSTIC PROCEDURES Viral culture of CSF, stool and throat

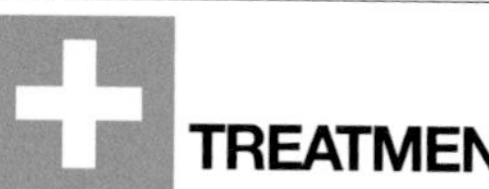

TREATMENT

APPROPRIATE HEALTH CARE Inpatient for acute phase. Outpatient or rehabilitation facility for therapy.

GENERAL MEASURES

- Provide bed that has firm mattress, footboard, foam rubber pads or sandbags. Change positions frequently. Give good skin care.
- Mechanical ventilation, if required
- Management of fecal impaction and urinary retention. Catheterization may be necessary.
- Nonnarcotic analgesics
- Hot, moist packs
- Physical therapy
- Public health - all suspected cases, report immediately to public health department

SURGICAL MEASURES Tracheostomy is frequently required in respiratory paralysis

ACTIVITY

- Bedrest during active phase. With paralysis, may require an extended period.
- Long-term rehabilitation plan - using physical therapy, braces, special shoes, possibly orthopedic surgery. Team effort with doctors, physical and occupational therapists, and social worker or psychiatrist, if necessary.

DIET Be sure patient has adequate well-balanced diet. May require tube feedings.

PATIENT EDUCATION For patient education materials favorably reviewed on this topic, contact: International Polio Network, 4502 Maryland Avenue, St. Louis, MO 63108, (314)361-0475

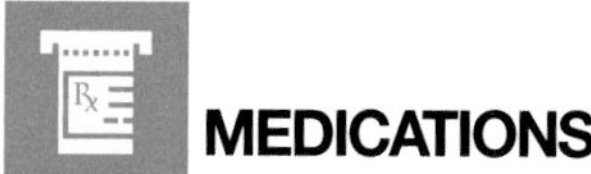

MEDICATIONS

DRUG(S) OF CHOICE
- Aspirin or other nonnarcotic analgesics
- Antibiotics, if other infection develops
- Parasympathomimetic (bethanechol) may help patient with urinary retention, 10-50 mg po bid-qid. Up to 100 mg qid may be required.
- New anti enteroviral agents may be useful

Contraindications: Refer to manufacturer's literature
Precautions: Bethanechol - adverse affects are rare, but may occur if dose increased. Includes colicky feeling, urinary urgency, skin flushing.
Significant possible interactions: Refer to manufacturer's literature

ALTERNATIVE DRUGS N/A

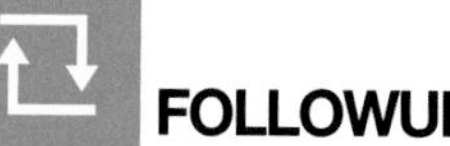

FOLLOWUP

PATIENT MONITORING
Individualized depending on severity and long-term physical therapy requirements

PREVENTION/AVOIDANCE
- Poliovirus vaccines; any inactivated vaccine recommended in USA. Disease may soon be eradicated. Travelers may still need IPV. Recommendations are country/region specific.

POSSIBLE COMPLICATIONS
- Urinary tract infection
- Atelectasis
- Pneumonia
- Myocarditis
- Postpoliomyelitis progressive muscular atrophy (PPMA) - characterized by progressive weakness beginning 30 years or more after an attack of poliomyelitis. Many adult survivors of childhood polio now with late complications.
- Postpoliomyelitis motor neuron disease - occurs many years after acute poliomyelitis, less common than PPMA
- Vaccine-associated paralytic poliomyelitis (VAPP) is a rare complication of OPV use

EXPECTED COURSE/PROGNOSIS
- Often irreversible paralysis; less than 5% mortality during acute disease
- Increased mortality over age 40
- Poor recovery for totally paralyzed muscle groups
- Good recovery for partially paralyzed muscle groups

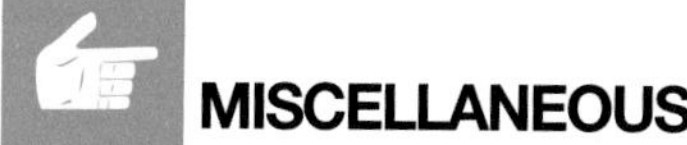

MISCELLANEOUS

ASSOCIATED CONDITIONS N/A

AGE-RELATED FACTORS
Pediatric: Most common in this age group. Polio is an extremely rare infection in U.S. since introduction of effective vaccines. (See Immunizations topic).
Geriatric: Extremely rare. Primary vaccination not recommended (except when traveling to endemic areas).
Others: N/A

PREGNANCY
A risk factor for developing polio

SYNONYMS
- Infantile paralysis
- Acute anterior poliomyelitis
- Acute lateral poliomyelitis

ICD-9-CM
045.1 Acute poliomyelitis with other paralysis

SEE ALSO
Immunizations
Tick paralysis

OTHER NOTES
Wild type polio non-existing in America. Polio left in 6 countries in Asia and Africa. WHO has a goal to eradicate the disease by the end of 2004.

ABBREVIATIONS
WHO = World Health Organization

REFERENCES

- Bennett JC, Plum F, eds. Cecil Textbook of Medicine. 20th Ed. Philadelphia, W.B. Saunders Co., 1996
- Mandell GL, ed. Principles and Practice of Infectious Diseases. 4th Ed. New York, Churchill Livingstone, 1995

Web references: 0 available at www.5mcc.com
Illustrations N/A

Author(s):
Mark M. Shelton, MD

BASICS

DESCRIPTION Polyarteritis nodosa (PAN) presents pathologically as an ongoing segmental inflammatory, necrotizing vasculitis response within the media of small and medium sized muscular arteries
- Organ involvement - kidney, GI tract, skin, muscles, joints, genitourinary tract, peripheral and central nervous system, heart, testes, epididymis and ovaries
- One of the vasculitic syndromes which vary in involvement from mild, self-limited skin lesions to severe systemic isolated and combined, multi-organ dysfunction and death
- Although heterogeneity and "overlap" manifestations abound, PAN is classified as a systemic necrotizing vasculitis

System(s) affected: Cardiovascular, Gastrointestinal, Musculoskeletal, Nervous, Renal/Urologic, Skin/Exocrine
Genetics: Unknown
Incidence/Prevalence in USA: 9-17/1,000,000
Predominant age: Childhood to geriatric age groups. Mean is 50 years.
Predominant sex: Male > Female (2.5:1)

SIGNS & SYMPTOMS
- General (often nonspecific) - multisystem involvement
  - ◊ Fever
  - ◊ Weakness
  - ◊ Weight loss
  - ◊ Malaise
  - ◊ Myalgia
  - ◊ Livido reticularis
  - ◊ Headache
  - ◊ Abdominal pain and vague discomfort
- Related to organ system involved (may dominate clinical picture and course)
  - ◊ Renal - hypertension, hematuria (usually microscopic), proteinuria, progressive renal failure
  - ◊ Musculoskeletal - myalgia, migratory arthralgia and arthritis
  - ◊ Skin - purpura, urticaria, subcutaneous hemorrhages, polymorphic rashes, subcutaneous nodules (uncommon but characteristic), persistent livedo reticularis and Raynaud phenomenon (rare)
  - ◊ Gastrointestinal - recurrent and severe pain, hepatomegaly, nausea, vomiting and bleeding. Cholecystitis, acute abdomen.
  - ◊ Lung - Hilar adenopathy, patchy infiltrates, reticular or nodular lesions, often fleeting
  - ◊ CNS - seizures, CVA's, headache, papillitis, altered mental states
  - ◊ Peripheral nervous system - mononeuritis multiplex
  - ◊ Cardiac - pericarditis, CHF associated with hypertension and/or myocardial infarction
  - ◊ Genitourinary - usually asymptomatic but may have testicular, epididymal, ovarian pain. Neurogenic bladder reported, glomerulonephritis.

CAUSES
- Unclear. Suggestive evidence for immunological involvement.
  - ◊ Endothelial COH antibodies
  - ◊ Antineutrophilic cytoplasmic antibody (ANCA)
  - ◊ Tissue deposition of immune complexes
  - ◊ Hepatitis B antigenemia in 30% of cases
  - ◊ Hepatitis B antigen in circulating immune complexes
  - ◊ Hepatitis B antigen, complement and IgM demonstrated in vascular walls
  - ◊ Hepatitis C association

RISK FACTORS N/A

DIAGNOSIS

DIFFERENTIAL DIAGNOSIS
- Systemic lupus erythematosus
- Multiple sclerosis
- Atrial myxoma
- Dissecting aneurysm
- Cryoglobulinemia
- Subacute endocarditis
- Trichinosis
- Some rickettsial diseases
- Microscopic polyangiitis
- Other vasculitis
- The key differences from other necrotizing vasculitides are lack of granuloma formation, sparing of veins and pulmonary arteries

LABORATORY
- Non specific:
  - ◊ Abnormal urine sediment
  - ◊ Rheumatoid factor
  - ◊ Endothelial cell antibodies
  - ◊ High neutrophil count
  - ◊ Eosinophilia rare. Suggests granulomatous involvement when present
  - ◊ Anemia of chronic disease
  - ◊ Elevated sedimentation rate and C-reactive protein
  - ◊ Hypergammaglobulinemia
  - ◊ Hepatitis B surface antigen positive in 10-50% of cases (strong circumstantial evidence)
  - ◊ Hepatitis C antibody or HCV RNA
- Specific
  - ◊ Mainly based on pathological findings of biopsy material from involved organs
  - ◊ Necrotizing arteritis
  - ◊ Careful examinations of biopsies from "acute abdomens", especially in males between the second and fourth decade
  - ◊ Anti-neutrophil cytoplasm antibodies (ANCA); rare

Drugs that may alter lab results:
- Corticosteroids, cytotoxic agents

Disorders that may alter lab results: Allergic reactions and other immunologic disorders

PATHOLOGICAL FINDINGS
- Necrotizing inflammation with fibrinoid necrosis, in various stages, of small and medium muscular arteries. Segmental in distribution, often seen at bifurcations and branchings. Involvement of venules not seen in classic PAN.
- Acute lesions show infiltration of polymorphonuclear cells through vessel wall and perivascular area
- Subsequent proliferation, degeneration, appearance of monocytes, necrosis with thrombosis and infarction of the involved tissue. Aneurysmal dilatations characteristic.
- Aortic dissection reported attributed to necrotizing vasculitis of the vasa vasorum
- Peripheral nerves positive 50-70%
- GI vessels 50% (at autopsy)
- Gall bladder and appendix 10%
- Muscle vessels 50%
- Testicle often positive when males are symptomatic

SPECIAL TESTS Angiographic demonstration of aneurysmal changes of small and medium sized arteries involving renal hepatic and mesenteric arteries represents strong evidence supporting the diagnosis

IMAGING Angiography: Mesenteric artery aneurysm, renal aneurysm, hepatic aneurysm, intestinal aneurysm

DIAGNOSTIC PROCEDURES Arterial or organ biopsy

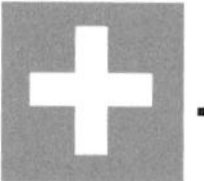

TREATMENT

APPROPRIATE HEALTH CARE Depends on extent and involvement of specific organs

GENERAL MEASURES The same as those needed for patients under treatment with steroids (high risk of infections), cytotoxic agents and plasmapheresis. Biologic agents under study.

SURGICAL MEASURES Biopsy; surgery for organ complication such as ischemic bowel

ACTIVITY As tolerated

DIET Low salt if hypertensive

PATIENT EDUCATION Arthritis Foundation, 1314 Spring Street N.W., Atlanta, GA 30309, (800)283-7800

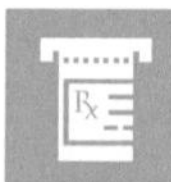

MEDICATIONS

DRUG(S) OF CHOICE

- Favorable results reported with prednisone and cyclophosphamide. Reports differ as to the benefits of adding plasmapheresis.
- Other immunosuppressive agents: (azothioprine (Imuran)
- Plazma exchange (efficacy not established)
- High dose IV pulse steroids
- Hepatitis B vaccine may be considered for the amelioration of any subsequent development of life-threatening complications of hepatitis B virus-associated polyarteritis nodosa

Contraindications: Refer to manufacturer's profile of each drug

Precautions: Refer to manufacturer's profile of each drug

Significant possible interactions: Refer to manufacturer's profile of each drug

ALTERNATIVE DRUGS N/A

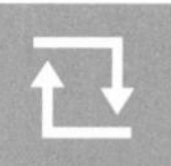

FOLLOWUP

PATIENT MONITORING

- CBC, urinalysis, renal and liver profiles
- Careful monitoring for infection
- Delayed appearance of neoplasms
- Angiographic changes may improve rapidly with combination steroid/cyclophosphamide therapy
- Acute phase reactants such as Interleukin-6 and C-reactive protein may be useful in diagnosis and monitoring activity level during treatment and followup

PREVENTION/AVOIDANCE N/A

POSSIBLE COMPLICATIONS

- Glomerulonephritis
- Renal failure
- Thrombosis
- Infarction
- Tissue/organ necrosis
- Stroke
- Myocardial infarct
- Mononeuritis multiplex

EXPECTED COURSE/PROGNOSIS

- Expected course of untreated polyarteritis nodosa is poor
- 5 year survival rate 13%
- Steroid and cytotoxic therapy treatment may increase percentage survival rate significantly.
- Renal and GI signs most serious prognostic factors
- Patients with microscopic polyangiitis

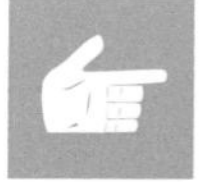

MISCELLANEOUS

ASSOCIATED CONDITIONS

- Churg-Strauss syndrome
- Benign cutaneous periarteritis nodosa (bears watching and investigating because not necessarily benign)
- Hepatitis B
- Hepatitis C

AGE-RELATED FACTORS

Pediatric: N/A

Geriatric: N/A

Others: N/A

PREGNANCY One case report suggests that if a patient attains remission before becoming pregnant, the chance of a successful delivery is reasonable

SYNONYMS

- Periarteritis
- Panarteritis
- Necrotizing arteritis

ICD-9-CM

446.0 Polyarteritis nodosa

SEE ALSO

Hepatitis B
Hepatitis C

OTHER NOTES

- Recommended reading: Jennette JC, Falk RJ. Small vessel vasculitis in N Engl J Med 1997: 337(21) 1512-1523

ABBREVIATIONS N/A

REFERENCES

- Soto O, Conn DL. Polyarteritis nodosa and microscopic polyangiitis. In: Hochberg MC, Silman AJ, et al, eds. Rheumatology. 3rd ed. St. Louis: Mosby; 2003. p.1611-21
- Lightfoot RW Jr, Michel BA, Bloch DA, Hunder GG, Zvaifler NJ, McShane DJ, Arend WP, Calabrese LH, Leavitt RY, Lie JT, et al. The American College of Rheumatology 1990 criteria for the classification of polyarteritis nodosa. Arthritis Rheum 1990;33(8):1088-93
- Guillevin L, Lhote F, Gayraud M, Cohen P, Jarrousse B, Lortholary O, Thibult N, Casassus P. Prognostic factors in polyarteritis nodosa and Churg-Strauss syndrome. A prospective study in 342 patients. Medicine (Baltimore) 1996;75(1):17-28
- Gayraud M, Guillevin L, le Toumelin P, Cohen P, Lhote F, Casassus P, Jarrousse B; French Vasculitis Study Group. Long-term followup of polyarteritis nodosa, microscopic polyangiitis, and Churg-Strauss syndrome: analysis of four prospective trials including 278 patients. Arthritis Rheum 2001;44(3):666-75
- Braunwald E, et al, eds. Harrison's Principles of Internal Medicine. 15th Ed. New York: McGraw-Hill; 2001
- Bennett JC, eds. Cecil Textbook of Medicine. 21st ed. Philadelphia: WB Saunders Co; 2001
- Iino T, et al: Polyarteritis nodosa. J Rheumatol 1992;19(10):1632-36
- Nakayama H. Distinct response interleukin-6 and other laboratory parameters to treatment in a patient with polyarteritis nodosa. Angiology 1992;43(6):512-6
- Garanger TA, et al. Anti-neutrophil cytoplasmic antibodies in patient's with the American College of Rheumatology criteria for pain. Autoimmunity 1995;20(1):33-7

Web references: 0 available at www.5mcc.com

Illustrations N/A

Author(s):

Eric P. Gall, MD

BASICS

DESCRIPTION Inherited disorders characterized by the development and growth of cysts in the kidneys; lined by epithelium, filled with fluid or semi-solid debris; accounts for 5-10% of patients with end stage renal disease
System(s) affected: Renal/Urologic
Genetics: See Causes
Incidence/Prevalence in USA: 1/200-1/1000
Predominant age: Usually diagnosed by age 45
Predominant sex: Male = Female

SIGNS & SYMPTOMS
- Hypertension
- Hematuria; microscopic or macroscopic
- Palpable kidneys
- Hepatomegaly
- Abdominal pain
- Flank pain (60%)
- Headache
- Nocturia
- Dysuria
- Urinary frequency
- Polyuria

CAUSES
- Inherited autosomal dominant abnormality linked to chromosome 16. 90% penetrance by age 90 in gene carriers. A second gene on chromosome 4 recently identified. Rare autosomal recessive form exists in neonates. Offspring of affected individuals with 50% chance of acquiring disease. Can be detected in amniocentesis.
- Acquired polycystic kidney disease - found in 50% of patients on dialysis > 3 years

RISK FACTORS Dialysis

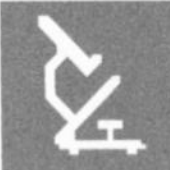

DIAGNOSIS

DIFFERENTIAL DIAGNOSIS
- Simple cysts
- Nephronophthisis-medullary cystic disease
- Medullary sponge kidney

LABORATORY
- Hematocrit - elevated in 5% of cases
- Urinalysis - may have hematuria and mild proteinuria
- Serum creatinine - may be elevated
- Kidney stones - usually calcium oxalate

Drugs that may alter lab results: N/A

Disorders that may alter lab results: N/A

PATHOLOGICAL FINDINGS N/A

SPECIAL TESTS
- Gene linkage analysis
  - ◊ Helpful for suspected cases with nondiagnostic imaging
  - ◊ Expensive
  - ◊ Requires other family members

IMAGING
- Ultrasonography: > 5 cysts in the renal cortex or medulla of each kidney, in children, 2 or more cysts in either kidney
- CT scan more sensitive
- 85% of patients can be detected by age 25

DIAGNOSTIC PROCEDURES N/A

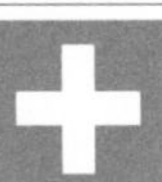

TREATMENT

APPROPRIATE HEALTH CARE Outpatient except for complicating emergencies (infected cysts require 2 weeks IV antibiotics then long-term oral antibiotics)

GENERAL MEASURES
- Pain - bed rest and analgesics
- Hematuria (due to ruptured cyst) - bed rest, sedation, IV hydration

SURGICAL MEASURES
Renal transplant, by age 6-8 years, for autosomal recessive form

ACTIVITY Avoid contact activities that may damage enlarged organs.

DIET Low protein diet may retard progression of renal disease.

PATIENT EDUCATION
- Genetic counseling is critical
- Avoidance of nephrotoxic drugs

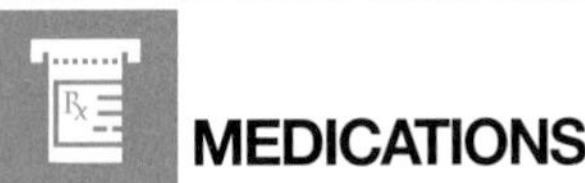

MEDICATIONS

DRUG(S) OF CHOICE
- No drug therapy available for polycystic kidney disease
- Hypertension - ACE inhibitors; avoid diuretics (possible adverse effects with cyst formation)

Contraindications: N/A
Precautions: N/A
Significant possible interactions: N/A

ALTERNATIVE DRUGS N/A

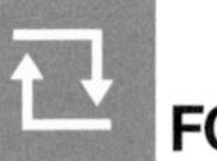

FOLLOWUP

PATIENT MONITORING Serum creatinine and blood pressure monitoring twice a year; more frequently as disease progresses

PREVENTION/AVOIDANCE Genetic counseling

POSSIBLE COMPLICATIONS
- Progression to renal failure
- Renal calculi in up to 30%
- Cyst infection
- Cyst rupture

EXPECTED COURSE/PROGNOSIS
- The disease is slowly progressive and has a variable outcome
- End stage renal disease occurs in 70% of patients by age 65
- Acquired disease with 5% adenocarcinoma, cysts regress after renal transplant, once nonazotemic

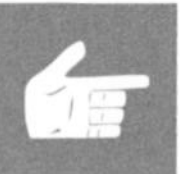

MISCELLANEOUS

ASSOCIATED CONDITIONS
- Cerebral aneurysms present in 10-40% of patients
- Colonic diverticula in 80%
- Liver cysts in approximately 50%
- Pancreatic and ovarian cysts
- Mitral valve prolapse in 26%

AGE-RELATED FACTORS
Pediatric: N/A
Geriatric: Renal insufficiency in 50% of patients by age 70, accounts for 5-10% of dialysis patients.
Others: Hypertension is secondary to high renin. Responds to angiotensin converting enzyme (ACE) inhibitors.

PREGNANCY Higher frequency of new onset hypertension than in women without polycystic kidney disease. No adverse effect on the course of the polycystic kidney disease in asymptomatic patients. Patients with hypertension, proteinuria or renal insufficiency are at increased risk of complications. Also an increase in hepatic cysts with pregnancy (rarely a problem).

SYNONYMS N/A

ICD-9-CM
753.12 Polycystic kidney, unspecified type
753.13 Polycystic kidney, autosomal dominant
753.14 Polycystic kidney, autosomal recessive

SEE ALSO
Renal calculi
Renal failure, chronic

OTHER NOTES N/A

ABBREVIATIONS N/A

REFERENCES

- Welling LW, Granthem JJ: Cystic and developmental diseases of the kidney. In: Brenner BM, Rector FC, eds. The Kidney. Philadelphia, W.B. Saunders, 1991
- Chapman AB, Johnson A, Gabow PA, Schrier RW: The renin-angiotensin-aldosterone system and autosomal dominant polycystic kidney disease. N Engl J Med 1990;323:1091-1096
- Beebe DK: Autosomal dominant polycystic kidney disease. Amer Fam Phys 1996;53(3):925-931

Web references: 1 available at www.5mcc.com
Illustrations N/A

Author(s):
Douglas M. Hoy, MD

BASICS

DESCRIPTION Polycystic ovarian disease (PCOD) is characterized by a state of chronic oligo-ovulation and/or anovulation culminating in oligomenorrhea and/or amenorrhea
System(s) affected: Endocrine/Metabolic, Reproductive, Skin/Exocrine
Genetics: Probably transmitted genetically, especially if associated with 21-hydroxylase deficiency or other enzyme deficiencies
Incidence/Prevalence in USA: 6% of premenopausal women
Predominant age: Women of reproductive age
Predominant sex: Female only

SIGNS & SYMPTOMS
- Amenorrhea
- Oligomenorrhea
- Obesity
- Hirsutism
- Acne
- Dysfunctional uterine bleeding
- Infertility
- Acanthosis nigricans
- Hypertension
- Virilism
- Enlarged ovaries
- Enlarged clitoris
- Deep voice
- Seborrhea

CAUSES Disruption of hypothalamic-pituitary-ovarian axis (high normal luteinizing hormone and low normal follicle stimulating hormone leading to ovarian hyperandrogenism and follicular atresia and anovulation) or secondary to increased levels of insulin or increased sensitivity to normal levels of insulin

RISK FACTORS
- Endometrial hyperplasia
- Endometrial carcinoma
- Obesity
- Hypertension
- Diabetes mellitus
- Breast cancer
- Infertility

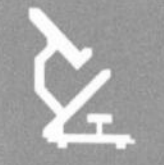

DIAGNOSIS

DIFFERENTIAL DIAGNOSIS
- Cushing syndrome
- HAIR-An syndrome (hyperandrogenism, insulin resistance, acanthosis nigricans)
- Testosterone-producing ovarian or adrenal tumor
- Prolactin-producing pituitary adenoma
- Hyperthecosis
- Adult-onset adrenal hyperplasia
- Partial congenital adrenal hyperplasia (21-hydroxylase deficiency)
- Endometrial hyperplasia
- Endometrial carcinoma
- 11 beta-hydroxylase deficiency
- 17beta-hydroxysteroid dehydrogenase deficiency
- Acromegaly
- Drug-induced hirsutism, oligoovulation (danazol, steroids)

LABORATORY
- Luteinizing hormone/follicle stimulating hormone (LH/FSH) ≥ 2.5-3.0/1
- Testosterone increased, but less than 200 ng/dL (6.94 nmol/L)
- Dehydroepiandrosterone sulfate (DHEA-S) increased, but less than 800 μg/dL (20.8 μmol/L)
- Dehydroepiandrosterone (DHEA) increased
- 17-OH progesterone increased
- Estrone increased
- Androstenedione increased
- Sex hormone binding globulin decreased
- Prolactin increased slightly
- Increased fasting insulin levels and possibly elevation in fasting glucose; plasminogen activator inhibitor-1

Drugs that may alter lab results:
- Oral contraceptives
- Steroids
- Antidepressants

Disorders that may alter lab results: N/A

PATHOLOGICAL FINDINGS
- Ovary usually enlarged with a smooth white glistening capsule
- Ovarian cortex lined with follicles in all stages of development but most are atretic
- Theca cell proliferation with an increase in the stromal compartment

SPECIAL TESTS
- Fasting serum glucose and insulin level to rule out insulin resistance and glucose intolerance
- Overnight dexamethasone suppression test (Decadron 1 mg po at 11:00PM and fasting serum cortisol at 8:00AM the next morning) to rule out Cushing syndrome

IMAGING Pelvis ultrasound revealing enlarged ovaries with multiple small follicular cysts

DIAGNOSTIC PROCEDURES
- History and physical examination
- Endometrial biopsy to rule out hyperplasia and or carcinoma

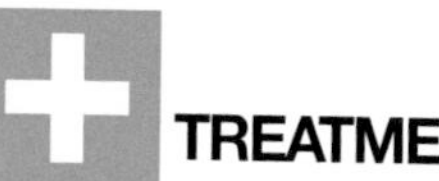

TREATMENT

APPROPRIATE HEALTH CARE
- Outpatient
- Inpatient, if surgery for wedge resection recommended (rare)
- Laser drilling (controversial as may cause adhesions)

GENERAL MEASURES No ideal treatment exists. Treatment must be individualized according to the needs and desires of the patient.

SURGICAL MEASURES Ovarian wedge resection and laparoscopic laser drilling controversial and rarely used today

ACTIVITY Full activity

DIET Regular (weight loss recommended, if overweight)

PATIENT EDUCATION Counsel the patient regarding the risk of endometrial and breast carcinoma, insulin resistance and diabetes mellitus, obesity and infertility

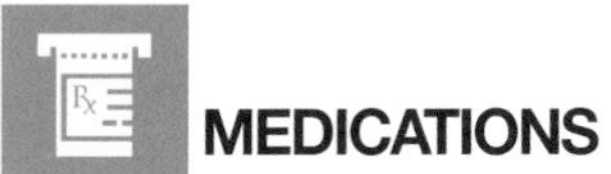

MEDICATIONS

DRUG(S) OF CHOICE
- If pregnancy not desired:
  - ◊ Cyclic withdrawal bleeding with medroxyprogesterone (Provera) 10 mg po x 12-14 days/month

or
  - ◊ Low dose oral contraceptives
- If pregnancy desired:
  - ◊ Ovulation induction with clomiphene (Clomid, Serophene)

or
  - ◊ Human menopausal gonadotropins - menotropins (Pergonal, Humegon, Repronex)

or
  - ◊ Pure follicle-stimulating hormone (Follistim, Gonal-F) with or without the addition of gonadotropin releasing hormone (GnRH) agonist - leuprolide (Lupron) or nafarelin (Synarel), or in a combination with GnRH antagonist - cetrorelix (Cetrotide) or ganirelix (Antagon)
  - ◊ Metformin (Glucophage) 500 mg po daily, bid, tid have been shown to improve hyperandrogenism and restore ovulation. Use from cycle day 1 and stop with ovulation. Many times the drug is continued throughout the 1st trimester or the entire pregnancy if there is a history of spontaneous abortion or glucose intolerance. Refer to a perinatologist for high-risk opinion.

Contraindications: None, but if using oral contraceptive agents to prevent sequelae of anovulation, be aware of contraindications

Precautions:
- Risks of multiple fetuses with clomiphene citrate is 8%
- Risks of multiple fetuses with HMG, FSH is 25%
- Risk of severe ovarian hyperstimulation syndrome (OHS) is less than 1%
- Diarrhea and GI symptoms with metformin
- Check liver function monthly with troglitazone

Significant possible interactions: Refer to manufacturer's profile of each drug

ALTERNATIVE DRUGS
- Bromocriptine if prolactin is elevated
- Prednisone or dexamethasone (Decadron) if DHEA-S is elevated

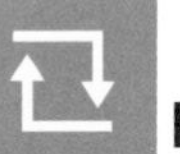

FOLLOWUP

PATIENT MONITORING Monitor patient frequently throughout the menstrual cycle depending upon which drug combination is utilized for ovulation induction

PREVENTION/AVOIDANCE Prevent endometrial and breast carcinoma

POSSIBLE COMPLICATIONS
- Multiple pregnancies
- Ovarian hyperstimulation syndrome (OHS)
- Oral contraceptives are not without risk

EXPECTED COURSE/PROGNOSIS
- Prognosis for fertility is excellent depending upon other fertility factors
- Proper treatment and followup of chronic anovulation can prevent endometrial hyperplasia and/or carcinoma

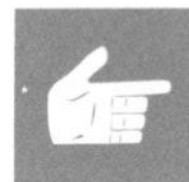

MISCELLANEOUS

ASSOCIATED CONDITIONS
- Obesity
- Hypertension
- Endometrial hyperplasia and/or carcinoma
- Breast carcinoma
- Diabetes mellitus
- HAIR-An syndrome
- Infertility
- Hyperthecosis

AGE-RELATED FACTORS
Pediatric: May begin at puberty
Geriatric: N/A
Others: N/A

PREGNANCY Does not cure the syndrome

SYNONYMS
- Stein-Leventhal syndrome
- Polycystic ovary syndrome

ICD-9-CM
256.4 Polycystic ovaries
628.0 Female infertility associated with anovulation

SEE ALSO
Amenorrhea
Fertility problems
Forbes-Albright syndrome

OTHER NOTES
- Drug costs high
- Monitoring (ultrasounds, estradiols) costs high

ABBREVIATIONS
OHS = ovarian hyperstimulation syndrome
HMG = human menopausal gonadotropins
FSH = follicle stimulating hormone

REFERENCES
- Danforth DM, Scott JR, et al, editors: Obstetric and Gynecology. 9th ed. Philadelphia: Lippincott Williams & Wilkins; 2003

Web references: 0 available at www.5mcc.com
Illustrations N/A

Author(s):
Nicholas J. Spirtos, DO

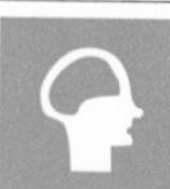

BASICS

DESCRIPTION A clonal cell hematologic malignant disorder with excessive erythroid, myeloid and megakaryocytic elements in the bone marrow. It is one of a group of myeloproliferative disorders.
System(s) affected: Hemic/Lymphatic/Immunologic
Genetics: Unknown genetic pattern (some suggestion that a chromosomal abnormality may be involved)
Incidence/Prevalence in USA: 0.5 per 100,000
Predominant age: Middle to late years, mean is 60 years (range 15-90)
Predominant sex: Male > Female (slightly)

SIGNS & SYMPTOMS
- Early stages may produce no symptoms
- Headaches
- Tinnitus
- Vertigo
- Blurred vision
- Epistaxis
- Increased blood viscosity
- Spontaneous bruising
- Upper GI bleeding
- Peptic ulcer disease
- Arterial and venous occlusive events
- Pruritus
- Sweating
- Weight loss
- Plethora (face, hands, feet)
- Splenomegaly
- Hepatomegaly
- Hyperhistaminemia
- Bone pain (ribs and sternum)
- Bone tenderness (ribs and sternum)

CAUSES Unknown, all three hematopoietic cell lines originate in a single clone

RISK FACTORS
- Jewish ancestry (may have increased frequency)
- Familial history (rare)

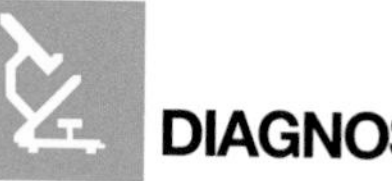

DIAGNOSIS

DIFFERENTIAL DIAGNOSIS
- Secondary polycythemias
- Hemoglobinopathy
- Spurious polycythemia

LABORATORY
- Tests used for diagnosis of polycythemia vera
  - ◊ A1: Increased RBC mass - female ≥ 32 mL/kg, male ≥ 36 mL/kg
  - ◊ A2: Normal arterial oxygen saturation (≥ 92%)
  - ◊ A3: Splenomegaly
  - ◊ B1: Thrombocytosis platelet count > 400,000/μL
  - ◊ B2: Leukocytosis > 12,000/μL
  - ◊ B3: Leukocyte alkaline phosphatase increased
  - ◊ B4: Increased serum B12 or increased unsaturated vitamin B12 binding capacity (UB12CB)
- Diagnosis acceptable with following combinations:
  - ◊ A1 + A2 + A3
  - ◊ A1 + A2 + any 2 from B category (splenomegaly absent in about 25% of patients)
- Other lab findings
  - ◊ Hyperuricemia
  - ◊ Hypercholesterolemia
  - ◊ Elevated blood histamine level

Drugs that may alter lab results: Diuretics may cause a spurious polycythemia

Disorders that may alter lab results: Excessive use of alcohol or tobacco

PATHOLOGICAL FINDINGS
- Plethoric congestion in all organs and tissues
- Major vessels contain thick, viscous blood
- Sinuses of spleen packed with red blood cells

SPECIAL TESTS Bone marrow aspiration (red cell hyperplasia, absent iron stores) and biopsy (fibrosis during spent phase of the disease)

IMAGING CT - splenomegaly

DIAGNOSTIC PROCEDURES Bone marrow aspiration - hyperplastic and panmyelosis

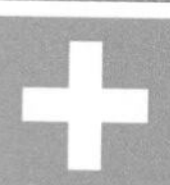

TREATMENT

APPROPRIATE HEALTH CARE Outpatient

GENERAL MEASURES
Individualized management necessary. Dependent on many factors - age, disease duration, disease phenotype, complications, disease activity.
Currently, phlebotomy is mainstay of therapy. Beyond that, differences exist among authorities about use and effectiveness of myelosuppressives.
- Phlebotomy
  - ◊ To reduce hematocrit to approximately 45%
  - ◊ Performed as often as every 2 or 3 days until normal hematocrit reached. Phlebotomies of 250-500 m/L. Reduce to 250-350 m/L in elderly patients or patients with cardiovascular disease.
  - ◊ Concomitant therapy possibilities, e.g., some form of myelosuppression, radioactive phosphorus (in elderly patients), hydroxyurea
  - ◊ Phlebotomy repeated as necessary for maintenance
  - ◊ If patient cannot tolerate phlebotomy - chemotherapy (hydroxyurea is the least mutagenic agent) or radiation therapy
- Other therapy
  - ◊ Maintain hydration
  - ◊ Pruritus therapy
  - ◊ Manage thrombotic or hemorrhagic complications the same as with nonpolycythemic patient
  - ◊ Uric acid reduction therapy

SURGICAL MEASURES N/A

ACTIVITY No restrictions

DIET
- No special diet (iron replacement not necessary)
- Phlebotomy regimen will produce pica, resulting in craving for crisp green vegetables (lettuce, celery) and ice

PATIENT EDUCATION
- Lifelong maintenance
- Complications to watch for

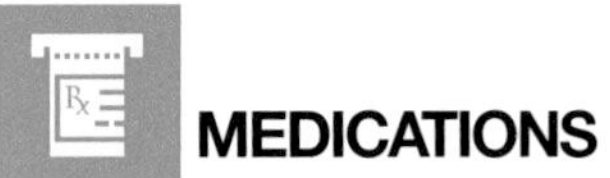

MEDICATIONS

DRUG(S) OF CHOICE
- Adjunctive
  - ◊ Allopurinol 300 mg/day for uric acid reduction
  - ◊ Cyproheptadine for pruritus, 4-16 mg as needed
  - ◊ H2-receptor blockers or antacids for GI hyperacidity
- Myelosuppression
  - ◊ Radioactive phosphorous in selected cases
  - ◊ Busulfan or alkylating agents (e.g., hydroxyurea)
  - ◊ Low-dose aspirin or anagrelide; aspirin is controversial in view of bleeding risk, but small doses may be given if required
  - ◊ Note: Refer to hematologist/oncologist for dosages and instructions

Contraindications: Refer to manufacturer's literature
Precautions: Refer to manufacturer's literature
Significant possible interactions: Refer to manufacturer's literature

ALTERNATIVE DRUGS
- Myelosuppression: chlorambucil, some authors believe contraindicated
- Interferon-alpha (IFN-a) may be an effective alternative to present forms of treatment and is under investigation

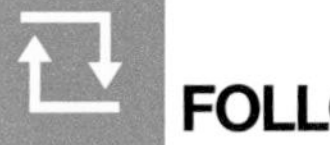

FOLLOWUP

PATIENT MONITORING
- Frequent during early treatment until satisfactory hematocrit is reached
- Monitor hematocrit often and phlebotomize when needed

PREVENTION/AVOIDANCE No known preventive measures

POSSIBLE COMPLICATIONS
- Uric acid stones
- Secondary gout
- Vascular thromboses (major cause of death)
- Transformation to leukemia
- Hemorrhage
- Peptic ulcer
- Increased risk for complications and mortality from surgery procedures. Assess risk-benefits and assure optimal control of disorder before any elective surgery.

EXPECTED COURSE/PROGNOSIS
- Median survival without treatment - 6 to 18 months following diagnosis
- Survival up to 10 years with treatment
- Some patients live, symptom-free, for 20 or more years

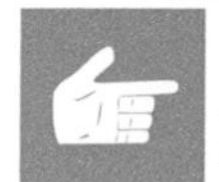

MISCELLANEOUS

ASSOCIATED CONDITIONS
- Budd-Chiari syndrome
- Mesenteric artery thrombosis

AGE-RELATED FACTORS
Pediatric: Rare in this age group
Geriatric: Phlebotomies and other therapies need to be adjusted for patients over 70
Others: N/A

PREGNANCY Treat with phlebotomy alone

SYNONYMS
- Primary polycythemia
- Vaquez disease
- Polycythemia, splenomegalic
- Vaquez-Osler disease

ICD-9-CM
238.4 Polycythemia vera

SEE ALSO
Myeloproliferative disorders

OTHER NOTES N/A

ABBREVIATIONS N/A

REFERENCES

- Beutler E, Lichtman MA, et al. eds. Williams Hematology. 6th Ed. New York, McGraw-Hill, 2000
- Conley CL. Polycythemia vera, diagnosis and treatment. Hosp Practice 1987;22:107

Web references: 1 available at www.5mcc.com
Illustrations N/A

Author(s):
Stanley G. Smith, MA, MB

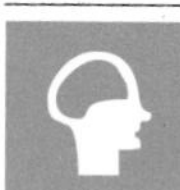

BASICS

DESCRIPTION A clinical syndrome characterized by aching and stiffness of the shoulder and hip girdle muscles affecting older patients, associated with an elevated ESR, lasting over 1 month and responsive to low dose steroids
System(s) affected: Hemic/Lymphatic/Immunologic, Musculoskeletal
Genetics: Associated with HLA determinants
Incidence/Prevalence in USA: Approximate prevalence 50/100,000 patients over age 50/year
Predominant age: 60 or older. Incidence increases with age (rare under 50 years old).
Predominant sex: Females > Male (2:1)

SIGNS & SYMPTOMS
- Onset - abrupt or insidious
- Pain and stiffness shoulder and hip girdle
- Usually symmetrical
- Symptoms more common in the morning
- Gel phenomena (stiffness after prolonged inactivity)
- Constitutional symptoms - fatigue, malaise, depression, weight loss, low grade fever
- Arthralgias/arthritis (non inflammatory)
- No weakness (pain may limit strength)
- Muscle tenderness mild to moderate
- No muscle atrophy
- Decreased range-of-motion of joints on active motion usually due to pain
- May have signs and symptoms of giant cell arteritis (seen in approximately 15% of patients)
- Mild synovitis hands and wrists

CAUSES Unknown

RISK FACTORS
- Age greater than 50
- Presence of giant cell arteritis

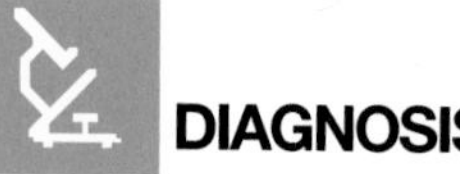

DIAGNOSIS

DIFFERENTIAL DIAGNOSIS
- Rheumatoid arthritis
- Other connective tissue disease
- Fibromyalgia
- Giant cell arteritis
- Depression
- Polymyositis/dermatomyositis (check CPK, aldolase)
- Thyroid disease
- Viral myalgia
- Osteoarthritis
- Occult infection
- Occult malignancy (extensive search usually not necessary)
- Myopathy (steroid, alcohol, electrolyte depletion)

LABORATORY
- ESR (Westergren) elevation greater than 50
- Anemia - normochromic/normocytic
- Creatine phosphokinase (CPK)- normal
- Rheumatoid factor (RF) - negative (5-10% patients over 60 will have positive RF without RA)
- Mild elevations in liver function tests

Drugs that may alter lab results: Prednisone

Disorders that may alter lab results: Disorders causing acute phase reactants can elevate ESR (e.g., infection, neoplasm, renal failure)

PATHOLOGICAL FINDINGS
- None in muscle biopsy or type II fiber atrophy without inflammation
- Mild non-specific synovitis

SPECIAL TESTS Temporal artery biopsy if symptoms of giant cell arteritis

IMAGING N/A

DIAGNOSTIC PROCEDURES
- In patients with symptoms suggesting giant cell arteritis a temporal artery biopsy may be indicated
- Negative muscle enzymes
- Elevated Westergren sedimentation rate

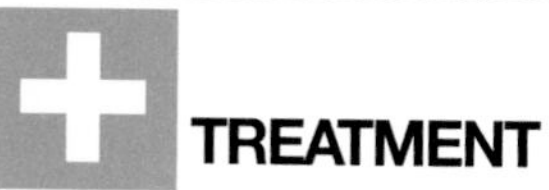

TREATMENT

APPROPRIATE HEALTH CARE Outpatient

GENERAL MEASURES Physical therapy for range-of-motion exercises if necessary

SURGICAL MEASURES N/A

ACTIVITY Do not exercise excessively to cause exertion

DIET
- Adequate calcium and electrolyte intake (1500 mg/day)
- Regular diet

PATIENT EDUCATION
- Precautions regarding steroid use
- Instruct the patient about symptoms of giant cell arteritis and to report them immediately
- For a listing of sources for patient education materials favorably reviewed on this topic, physicians may contact: American Academy of Family Physicians Foundation, P.O. Box 8418, Kansas City, MO 64114, (800)274-2237, ext. 4400
- Excellent materials also available from Arthritis Foundation, http://www.arthritis.org/

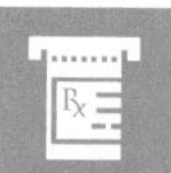

MEDICATIONS

DRUG(S) OF CHOICE

- Prednisone
  - ◊ 10 mg/day initially (average initial effective dose 10-15 mg/d)
  - ◊ Usually dramatic (diagnostic) response.
  - ◊ May increase to 20 mg if no immediate response
  - ◊ Begin slow taper at 4-6 weeks by only 1 mg every 1-4 weeks to a dose of 5-7.5 mg. Continue at this dose for approximately 18 months to 2 years, if no recurrence of symptoms.
  - ◊ After 18-24 months of treatment, attempt to taper by 1 mg every 2-4 weeks until drug discontinued. Patient may, however, require steroids for 3 or more years.
  - ◊ Increase prednisone for recurrence of symptoms (relapse common).
- Nonsteroidal anti-inflammatory drugs (NSAIDs) often not helpful

Contraindications: Use steroids with caution in patients with chronic heart failure, diabetes mellitus, systemic fungal or bacterial infection. Must treat infections concurrently if steroids are absolutely necessary.
Precautions: Long term steroid use associated with several significant adverse effects including sodium and water retention, exacerbation of chronic heart failure, hypokalemia, increased susceptibility to infection, osteoporosis, cataracts, avascular necrosis. Patients may develop temporal arteritis while on low dose corticosteroid treatment for polymyalgia. This requires immediate increase in dose to 60 mg (see topic on Temporal arteritis). Alternate day steroids not effective.
Significant possible interactions: Refer to manufacturer's literature

ALTERNATIVE DRUGS
NSAIDs have been used, rarely successful

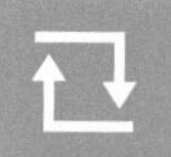

FOLLOWUP

PATIENT MONITORING

- Follow monthly initially and during taper of medication, every 3 months otherwise
- Follow ESR as steroids tapered
- Followup with patient for symptoms of giant cell arteritis. Educate patient to report such symptoms immediately (headache, visual and neurologic symptoms).

PREVENTION/AVOIDANCE
N/A

POSSIBLE COMPLICATIONS

- Medication - complications related to steroid use
- Disease - exacerbation of disease with taper of steroids; development of giant cell arteritis (may occur when PMR is being adequately treated)

EXPECTED COURSE/PROGNOSIS

- Average length disease is 3 years (range 1-10 years)
- Exacerbation if steroids tapered too fast
- Prognosis very good if treated (may gradually remit even if no treatment)
- Relapse common

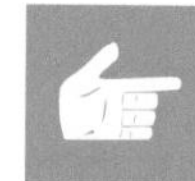

MISCELLANEOUS

ASSOCIATED CONDITIONS

- Giant cell arteritis
- Temporal arteritis

AGE-RELATED FACTORS
Pediatric: Does not occur in this age group
Geriatric: Incidence increases with age
Others: N/A

PREGNANCY
N/A

SYNONYMS

- Senile rheumatic disease
- Forestier-Certonciny syndrome
- Polymyalgia rheumatica syndrome
- Rhizomelic pseudoarthrosis

ICD-9-CM
725 Polymyalgia rheumatica

SEE ALSO
Arthritis, osteo
Arthritis, rheumatoid (RA)
Depression
Fibromyalgia
Giant cell arteritis
Polymyositis/dermatomyositis

OTHER NOTES
Westergren ESR is the preferred laboratory technique. If other types of ESR studies are used (e.g., Wintrobe) the guidelines listed in this chapter cannot be used for abnormal levels.

ABBREVIATIONS
PMR = polymyalgia rheumatica
NSAIDs = non-steroidal anti-inflammatory drugs

REFERENCES

- Hunder GG. Giant Cell Arteritis and Polymyalgia Rheumatica. Chapt 78. In: Ruddy S, Harris ED, Sledge CB, eds. Textbook of Rheumatology. 6th Ed. Philadelphia, W.B. Saunders Co., 2001:1155-64
- Weyland CM, Goronzy JJ. Polymyalgia rheumatica and giant cell arteritis. Chapt 88. In: Koopman WJ, ed: Arthritis and Allied Disorders. 14th ed. Philadelphia, Lippincott Williams & Wilkins, 2001
- Hazelman BL. Polymyalgia rheumatica and giant cell arteritis. In: Hochberg MC, Silman AJ, Smolen JS, Weinblatt ME, Weisman MH. Rheumatology, 3rd ed. Edinburgh: Mosby; 2003. p. 1623-1633

Web references: 2 available at www.5mcc.com
Illustrations N/A

Author(s):
Eric P. Gall, MD

BASICS

DESCRIPTION Systemic connective tissue disease characterized by inflammatory and degenerative changes in proximal muscles sometimes accompanied by characteristic skin rash.
- If skin manifestations are associated, it is designated as dermatomyositis
- Different types of myositis include:
  - ◊ Idiopathic PM
  - ◊ Idiopathic DM
  - ◊ Childhood PM/DM
  - ◊ PM/DM with malignancy
  - ◊ PM/DM as an overlap
  - ◊ Inclusion body myositis
  - ◊ HIV associated myopathy

System(s) affected: Cardiovascular, Musculoskeletal, Pulmonary, Skin/Exocrine
Genetics: Mild association with HLA-DR3, HLA-DRw52
Incidence/Prevalence in USA: Estimated at 0.5-0.8 new cases/100,000; 1-2 patients/100,000
Predominant age: 5-15 years, 40-60 years
Predominant sex: Female > Male (2:1)

SIGNS & SYMPTOMS
- Symmetrical proximal muscle weakness causing:
  - ◊ Difficulty when arising from sitting or lying positions
  - ◊ Difficulty kneeling
  - ◊ Difficulty climbing stairs
  - ◊ Difficulty descending stairs
  - ◊ Difficulty raising arms
- Joint pain/swelling
- Dysphagia
- Respiratory impairment
- Decreased deep tendon reflexes of proximal muscle groups
- Muscle swelling, stiffness, induration
- Rash over face (eyelids, nasolabial folds), upper chest, dorsal hands, (especially knuckle pads), fingers ("mechanic's hands")
- Periorbital edema
- Calcinosis cutis (childhood cases)
- Mesenteric arterial insufficiency/infarction (childhood cases)
- Cardiac impairment; arrhythmia, failure

CAUSES
- Unknown; potential factors:
  - ◊ Inciting viral infection
  - ◊ T cell activation
  - ◊ Cytokine release
  - ◊ Immune-mediate muscle destruction
  - ◊ Genetic predisposition
  - ◊ HTLV I

RISK FACTORS Family history of autoimmune disease or vasculitis

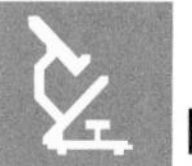

DIAGNOSIS

DIFFERENTIAL DIAGNOSIS
- Vasculitis
- Progressive systemic sclerosis
- Systemic lupus erythematosus
- Rheumatoid arthritis
- Muscular dystrophy
- Eaton-Lambert syndrome
- Sarcoidosis
- Amyotrophic lateral sclerosis
- Endocrine disorders
  - ◊ Thyroid disease
  - ◊ Cushing syndrome
- Infectious myositis (viral, bacterial, parasitic)
- Drug-induced myopathies
  - ◊ Cholesterol lowering agents
  - ◊ Colchicine
  - ◊ Corticosteroids
  - ◊ Ethanol
  - ◊ Chloroquine
  - ◊ Zidovudine (AZT)
- Electrolyte disorders (magnesium, calcium, potassium)
- Heritable metabolic myopathies

LABORATORY
- Increased creatine kinase (CK)
- Increased aldolase
- Increased SGOT/AST
- Increased LDH
- Myoglobinuria
- Increased ESR
- Positive rheumatoid factor (less than 50% of patients)
- Positive ANA (more than 50% of patients)
- Leukocytosis (less than 50% of patients)
- Anemia (less than 50% of patients)
- Hyperglobulinemia (less than 50% of patients)
- Increased creatinine (less than 50% of patients)
- Myositis specific antibodies have been described in a minority of patients - most are anti-synthetase antibodies, anti-Jo-1 is the most common and has been found in about 20% of patients; associated with an increased incidence of interstitial lung disease

Drugs that may alter lab results: N/A

Disorders that may alter lab results: Liver disease and hemolysis may cause increased AST/SGOT, LDH

PATHOLOGICAL FINDINGS
- Micro - muscle fiber degeneration
- Micro - phagocytosis of muscle debris
- Micro - perifascicular muscle fiber atrophy
- Micro - inflammatory cell infiltrates in adult form
- Micro (electron microscopy) - inclusion bodies (inclusion body myositis only)
- Sarcoplasmic basophilia
- Muscle fiber increased in size
- Vasculopathy (childhood PM/DM)

SPECIAL TESTS
- ECG - arrhythmias, conduction disturbances
- Electromyography (EMG) - muscle irritability, low amplitude potentials, polyphasic action potentials, fibrillations
- Muscle biopsy (deltoid or quadriceps femoris)

IMAGING
- Chest x-ray: pulmonary interstitial disease
- MRI being used more often to assess muscle edema and inflammation, possibly to guide biopsy, and follow activity of disease

DIAGNOSTIC PROCEDURES Diagnosis usually relies on 4 findings - weakness, CPK elevation, abnormal EMG, findings on muscle biopsy. Presence of skin rash of dermatomyositis also helpful.

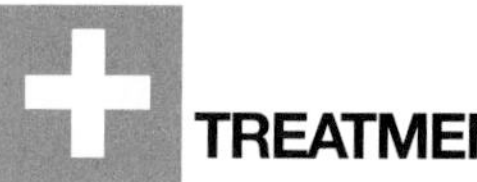

TREATMENT

APPROPRIATE HEALTH CARE Outpatient

GENERAL MEASURES
- Search for malignancy in all adults
- Follow serum muscle enzymes carefully

SURGICAL MEASURES N/A

ACTIVITY
- Curtailed until after inflammation subsides
- Range-of-motion exercises to prevent contractures

DIET No special diet

PATIENT EDUCATION Muscular Dystrophy Association, 3561 E. Sunrise Dr., Tucson, AZ 85718. Telephone (800)221-1142.

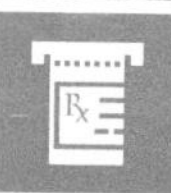

MEDICATIONS

DRUG(S) OF CHOICE
- Prednisone 40-60 mg/day initially in divided doses. Consolidate doses and reduce prednisone slowly when enzyme levels are normal. Probably need to continue 5-10 mg/day for maintenance.
- For steroid refractory cases:
  - ◊ Azathioprine 1.0 mg/kg (arthritis dose) once or twice a day. Maintain at lowest possible dose.
  - ◊ Methotrexate 10-25 mg weekly useful in some steroid-resistant cases
- Rash of dermatomyositis may require topical steroids, oral hydroxychloroquine

Contraindications: Refer to manufacturer's literature. Methotrexate contraindicated in patients with previous liver disease, current alcohol use, pregnancy.

Precautions:
- Prednisone - adverse effects associated with long-term steroid use include adrenal suppression, sodium, water retention, hypokalemia, osteoporosis, cataracts, increased susceptibility to infection
- Azathioprine - adverse effects include bone marrow suppression, increased LFT's, increased susceptibility to infection
- Methotrexate - adverse effects include stomatitis. bone marrow suppression, pneumonitis, and risk of liver fibrosis and cirrhosis with prolonged use

Significant possible interactions: Refer to manufacturer's literature

ALTERNATIVE DRUGS
Other immunosuppressant drugs such as cyclophosphamide, chlorambucil, cyclosporine can be added to steroids. Immune globulin IV added to steroids being evaluated in resistant cases, also tacrolimus. Combination methotrexate and azathioprine may also be useful in refractory cases.

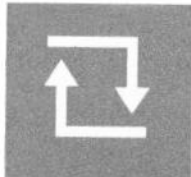

FOLLOWUP

PATIENT MONITORING
- Serial serum muscle enzyme testing
- Any adult should be studied for malignancy
- Monitor for steroid-induced metabolic complications (hypokalemia, hypertension, hyperglycemia, etc.)
- Bone densitometry and consideration of calcium, vitamin D, and Alendronate (Fosamax) therapy
- If azathioprine, methotrexate or other immunosuppressant used, then appropriate laboratory monitoring should be done periodically.

PREVENTION/AVOIDANCE
N/A

POSSIBLE COMPLICATIONS
- Pneumonia
- Infection
- Myocardial infarction
- Carcinoma (especially breast, lung)
- Severe dysphagia
- Respiratory impairment due to muscle weakness, interstitial lung disease
- Aspiration pneumonitis
- Steroid myopathy
- Steroid induced diabetes, hypertension, hypokalemia, osteoporosis

EXPECTED COURSE/PROGNOSIS
- 30% residual weakness
- 20% persistent active disease
- 75% 5-year survival
- Survival worse for women and African-Americans, and patients with associated cancer
- Most patients improve with therapy
- 50% have full recovery
- Possibly relapsing
- Inclusion body myositis tends to be more steroid-refractory and includes more distal weakness

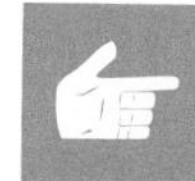

MISCELLANEOUS

ASSOCIATED CONDITIONS
- Malignancy
- Progressive systemic sclerosis
- Vasculitis
- Systemic lupus erythematosus
- Other connective tissue disorders

AGE-RELATED FACTORS
Pediatric:
- Childhood dermatomyositis occurs
- May be possible to discontinue prednisone gradually after a year or so

Geriatric:
- Rare after age 60
- Elderly male patient with polymyositis more likely to have underlying neoplasm

Others: N/A

PREGNANCY
N/A

SYNONYMS
- Myositis

ICD-9-CM
710.3 Dermatomyositis
710.4 Polymyositis

SEE ALSO
Osteoporosis

OTHER NOTES
Classification of types of myositis: Childhood dermatomyositis, primary idiopathic dermatomyositis, dermatomyositis or polymyositis associated with malignancy, primary polymyositis, myositis associated with overlap syndrome. Inclusion-body myositis represents a variant with atypical presentation and variable response to therapy.

ABBREVIATIONS
N/A

REFERENCES

- Kelley W, et al. Textbook of Rheumatology. 5th Ed. Philadelphia, W.B. Saunders Co., 1997
- Villalba L, et al. Treatment of refractory myositis. A randomized crossover trial of two new cytotoxic regimens. Arthritis Rheum 1998;41:392-9
- Kagen LJ, ed. Inflammatory disorders of muscle. Rheum Dis Clin of No Amer 1994;20:811-1057
- Plotz PH, et al. Myositis: Immunologic contributions to understanding cause, pathogenesis, and therapy. Ann Int Med 1995;122:715-724
- Wortman RL. Diseases of Skeletal Muscle, Philadelphia, Lippincott Williams & Wilkins, 2000

Web references: 2 available at www.5mcc.com
Illustrations 4 available

Author(s):
Christopher M. Wise, MD

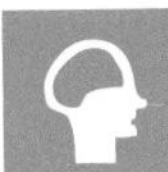

BASICS

DESCRIPTION Several heme synthesis pathway enzyme deficiencies with overproduction and accumulation of intermediate metabolic products and resultant neuropsychiatric-abdominal or dermatologic symptoms and syndromes. All more common in Caucasians than Blacks or Asians.
- Porphyria cutanea tarda (PCT) - dermatologic
- Acute intermittent porphyria (AIP) - pyrroloporphyria; neuropsychiatric-abdominal
- Protoporphyria (PP) - erythropoietic or hepatoerythropoietic; mild dermatologic
- Variegate porphyria (VP) - South African porphyria, prevalence in S. Africa is 1/400
- Hereditary coproporphyria (HCP) - neuropsychic, occasionally dermatologic
- Porphobilinogen synthetase deficiency (PBD) - delta-aminolevulinic aciduria; neuropsychiatric-abdominal
- Congenital erythropoietic porphyria (CEP) - Günther's disease; severe dermatologic
- Other rare genetic variants reported

System(s) affected: Gastrointestinal, Hemic/Lymphatic/Immunologic, Skin/Exocrine

Genetics:
- Autosomal dominant - PCT (< 20% of cases), AIP, PP, VP, HCP
- Autosomal recessive - PBD, CEP
- Latency common with variable expression, many asymptomatic or minimally symptomatic carriers
- PCT also sporadic and acquired (> 80% of cases)
- The pathogenesis of any inherited porphyria has now been defined at the molecular level. It is clear there is a great deal of genetic heterogeneity in each porphyria.

Incidence/Prevalence in USA:
- PCT - 1/10,000
- AIP, PP, VP - 1/10,000 to 1/100,000
- HCP - less than 1/100,000
- PBD, CEP - very rare

Predominant age:
- CEP - early childhood
- PP - older childhood
- AIP, VP, HCP, PBD - young adult
- PCT - middle age

Predominant sex:
- PP, CEP - male = female
- PCT - seen more commonly in male
- AIP, VP, HCP, PBD - seen more commonly in female

SIGNS & SYMPTOMS
- All usually reversible, lasting days to weeks
- May be permanent
- Urine may turn dark red or brown on standing (word porphyria from Greek porphyra = purple)
- Abdominal:
  - ◊ Rather severe abdominal pain, occasionally in back and extremities
  - ◊ Generalized more often than localized
  - ◊ Often colicky
  - ◊ Can mimic acute abdomen
  - ◊ No fever should be present
  - ◊ Chronic constipation common
  - ◊ Severity of symptoms often out of proportion to physical findings
- Neurologic:
  - ◊ Essentially anything
  - ◊ Includes sensory and motor systems
  - ◊ Includes autonomic nervous system
  - ◊ May include seizures
  - ◊ May lead to quadriplegia and/or respiratory paralysis with death
- Psychiatric:
  - ◊ Essentially anything
  - ◊ Psychosis most common
  - ◊ Visual hallucinations common
  - ◊ Disorientation frequent
  - ◊ Chronic depression frequent
- Dermatologic:
  - ◊ Photosensitivity
  - ◊ Scrapes, ulcerations, blisters with minimal trauma
  - ◊ Hyperpigmentation, especially hands and face
  - ◊ Scarring frequent
  - ◊ Facial hypertrichosis
  - ◊ CEP - mutilating, with hemolysis, erythrodontia, splenomegaly
  - ◊ PP - occasional hepatic disease, including hepatic failure

CAUSES
- Genetic enzyme deficiencies
- PCT - uroporphyrinogen decarboxylase
- AIP - porphobilinogen deaminase
- PP - ferrochelatase
- VP - protoporphyrinogen oxidase
- HCP - coproporphyrinogen oxidase
- PBD - porphobilinogen synthetase
- CEP - uroporphyrinogen III synthetase (cosynthetase)
- Acquired PCT causes:
  - ◊ Hepatitis C virus - strong association
  - ◊ Heavy alcohol use
  - ◊ Decreased enzyme associated with steroids and hormones
  - ◊ Specific exposure to poly-halogenated hydrocarbons (e.g., hexachlorobenzene)
  - ◊ Lead poisoning may alter pathways
  - ◊ HIV
  - ◊ Ascorbic acid deficiency?

RISK FACTORS
- Multiple precipitating factors, especially AIP, VP, HCP
- Drugs (e.g., barbiturates and sulfas in AIP)
- Estrogens, especially oral contraceptives
- Steroids
- Liver disease
- Menstrual cycles
- Infection
- Fasting
- Heavy alcohol use
- Hexachlorobenzene exposure

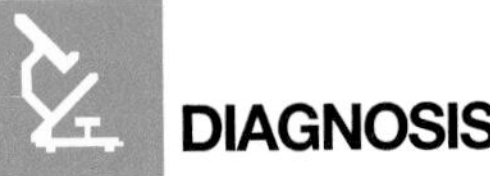

DIAGNOSIS

DIFFERENTIAL DIAGNOSIS
- Vast and protean
- Pseudoporphyria - rare syndrome, indistinguishable from PCT, due to some NSAIDs (eg, nabumetone and naproxen) and flutamide

LABORATORY
- Urine for porphyrins during acute attack. Urine may be normal at other times.
- Individual enzyme activity in erythrocytes or other body cells/tissues
- Stool for porphyrins in PP, VP, HCP, CEP
- Bile for porphyrin in VP
- Plasma for fluorescence emission spectroscopy in VP
- Saliva for porphyria in PCT
- Erythrocyte uroporphyrin in CEP
- PP exception - urine unremarkable. Test erythrocyte protoporphyrin.
- Ferritin typically elevated in PCT due to increased iron stores

Drugs that may alter lab results: Unknown

Disorders that may alter lab results:
- Numerous conditions may cause slight increase in porphyrinuria, but patients asymptomatic
- Acute liver disease
- Hepatoma
- Hodgkin lymphoma
- Multiple neurologic diseases

PATHOLOGICAL FINDINGS N/A

SPECIAL TESTS Genetic studies when applicable

IMAGING N/A

DIAGNOSTIC PROCEDURES N/A

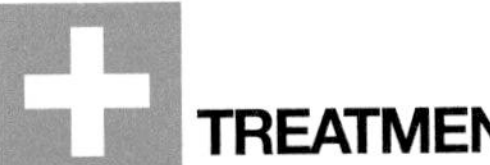

TREATMENT

APPROPRIATE HEALTH CARE Outpatient, except for crises

GENERAL MEASURES
- Neuropsychiatric-abdominal - avoid drugs, alcohol, known toxins
- Dermatologic - shade, protective clothing; avoid skin trauma; PCT - phlebotomy weekly to monthly may help prevent
- CEP - consider bone marrow transplantation

SURGICAL MEASURES N/A

ACTIVITY Normal, except dermatologic avoid sun

DIET Neuropsychiatric - large quantities of carbohydrates have been reported to help

PATIENT EDUCATION Porphyria Foundation, P.O. Box 22712, Houston, TX 77227, (713)266-9617

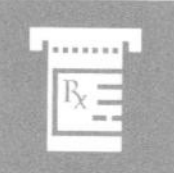

MEDICATIONS

DRUG(S) OF CHOICE
- Neuropsychiatric-abdominal
  - ◊ Intravenous glucose 400 grams daily for one to two days
  - ◊ Hematin (ferriprotoporphyrin IX, hemin [Panhematin]) IV 1-4 mg/kg/d over 10-15 minutes x 3-14 days
  - ◊ Epilepsy - consider clonazepam or gabapentin
  - ◊ Depression - consider selective serotonin re-uptake inhibitors
- Dermatologic:
  - ◊ Oral carotenoids, e.g., beta-carotene (Solatene), 30 mg, 1-10 capsules per day

Contraindications: Known sensitivity to drug
Precautions: Hematin - phlebitis at IV site, reduced clotting ability
Significant possible interactions: None

ALTERNATIVE DRUGS
- PCT - chloroquine 125 mg twice weekly, or hydroxychloroquine 250 mg tid, in conjunction with phlebotomy
- PCT with hepatitis C virus - interferon beneficial for both
- In vitro gene therapy has been successful for CEP and PP
- PCT - thalidomide being studied
- AIP - LHRH analogues being studied
- Menstruating women - hematin premenstrual; cycle suppressors, e.g., luteinizing hormone releasing hormone (LHRH) analogues
- Autonomic manifestations - beta blockers
- Other symptoms - treat symptomatically

Note: AIP - antioxidants ineffective

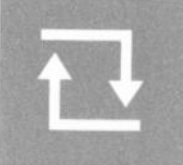

FOLLOWUP

PATIENT MONITORING Individualized

PREVENTION/AVOIDANCE
- Avoid precipitating drugs
  - ◊ Alcohol
  - ◊ Barbiturates
  - ◊ Carbamazepine
  - ◊ Chlorpropamide
  - ◊ Danazol
  - ◊ Ergots
  - ◊ Estrogens and progestins
  - ◊ Ethchlorvynol
  - ◊ Glutethimide
  - ◊ Griseofulvin
  - ◊ Mephenytoin
  - ◊ Meprobamate
  - ◊ Methotrexate
  - ◊ Methyprylon
  - ◊ Metoclopramide
  - ◊ Phenytoin
  - ◊ Pyrazolones
  - ◊ Succinimides
  - ◊ Sulfonamide antibiotics
  - ◊ Valproic acid
- Eat an adequate diet with high carbohydrate intake

POSSIBLE COMPLICATIONS See list in Signs and Symptoms

EXPECTED COURSE/PROGNOSIS
- In all porphyrias:
  - ◊ Patients who are asymptomatic or minimally symptomatic - unaffected longevity
  - ◊ Patients who are more symptomatic - treatable and do well
  - ◊ Neurologic complications (e.g., peripheral neuropathy, neurosis or hemiplegia), at times permanent
- In AIP
  - ◊ Acute attacks have 25% mortality
  - ◊ Increased risk of hepatocellular carcinoma
- Acquired PCT
  - ◊ HIV
  - ◊ Hepatitis C virus
  - ◊ Hepatic malignancies

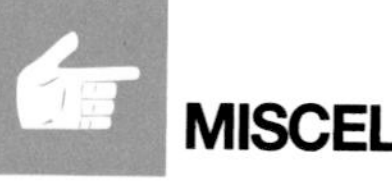

MISCELLANEOUS

ASSOCIATED CONDITIONS N/A

AGE-RELATED FACTORS
Pediatric: N/A
Geriatric: N/A
Others: N/A

PREGNANCY Unpredictable disease activity

SYNONYMS
- Delta-aminolevulinic aciduria
- Erythropoietic porphyria
- Günther disease
- Hepatoerythropoietic porphyria
- Pyrroloporphyria
- South African porphyria

ICD-9-CM
277.1 Disorders of porphyrin metabolism

SEE ALSO

OTHER NOTES Some drugs considered safe - acetaminophen, amiodarone, aspirin, atropine, bromides, chlorpromazine, diazepam (in small doses), dicumarol, digoxin, diphenhydramine, ether, glucocorticoids, guanethidine, heparin, insulin, lithium, magnesium, neostigmine, nitrous oxide, penicillin and derivatives, phenothiazines, promethazine, narcotic analgesics, propranolol, streptomycin, succinylcholine, thiazides

ABBREVIATIONS
PCT = Porphyria cutanea tarda
AIP = Acute intermittent porphyria
PP = Protoporphyria
VP = Variegate porphyria
HCP = Hereditary coproporphyria
PBD = Porphobilinogen synthetase deficiency
CEP = Congenital erythropoietic porphyria

REFERENCES

- Braunwald E, et al, editors. Harrison's Principles of Internal Medicine. 15th Ed. New York: McGraw-Hill; 2001. p.2261-2267
- Bennett JC, Plum F, editors. Cecil Textbook of Medicine. 20th ed. Philadelphia: WB Saunders Co; 1996
- Kelly WN, et al, editors. Textbook of Internal Medicine. 3rd ed. New York: Lippincott-Raven; 1997. p.880-882

Web references: 0 available at www.5mcc.com
Illustrations 5 available

Author(s):
Emil S. Dickstein, MD

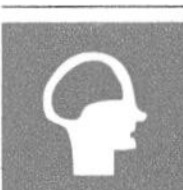

BASICS

DESCRIPTION Increased portal venous pressure (> 10 mm Hg.) that occurs in association with splanchnic vasodilatation, portosystemic collateral formation and a hyperdynamic circulation. Course is generally progressive and may produce one or more devastating clinical disorders.
System(s) affected: Cardiovascular, Gastrointestinal, Nervous
Genetics: No known genetic patterns except those associated with specific hepatic diseases that cause portal hypertension
Incidence/Prevalence in USA: Unknown. (Incidence of bleeding from gastroesophageal varices is approximately 120 episodes per 100,000 population per year.)
Predominant age: Adult
Predominant sex: Male > Female

SIGNS & SYMPTOMS
May be general or related to specific complications
- General
  - ◊ Splenomegaly
  - ◊ Caput medusa
  - ◊ Umbilical bruit
  - ◊ Hemorrhoids
  - ◊ Spider angiomata
  - ◊ Gynecomastia
  - ◊ Testicular atrophy
  - ◊ Digital clubbing
  - ◊ Palmar erythema
- Gastroesophageal varices
  - ◊ Hematemesis
  - ◊ Melena
  - ◊ Anemia
  - ◊ Hypotension
  - ◊ Tachycardia
- Ascites
  - ◊ Distended abdomen
  - ◊ Fluid wave
  - ◊ Shifting percussion dullness
- Hepatic encephalopathy
  - ◊ Confusion
  - ◊ Asterixis
  - ◊ Hyperreflexia
- Hepatorenal syndrome
  - ◊ Oliguria

CAUSES
May be intrahepatic or extrahepatic
- Cirrhosis present. Accounts for > 90% of cases.
  - ◊ Alcoholic
  - ◊ Viral (HBV, HCV, HGV)
  - ◊ Wilson disease
  - ◊ Hemochromatosis
  - ◊ Primary biliary cirrhosis
  - ◊ Schistosomiasis
- Cirrhosis not present.
  - ◊ Portal vein thrombosis
  - ◊ Hepatic vein obstruction (Budd-Chiari syndrome)
  - ◊ Right ventricular failure
  - ◊ Myeloproliferative disorders

RISK FACTORS Many different chronic liver diseases and hepatotoxins

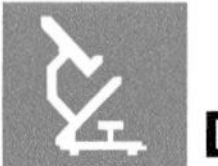

DIAGNOSIS

DIFFERENTIAL DIAGNOSIS
Usually related to specific complications/presentations.
- Gastroesophageal varices with hemorrhage vs:
  - ◊ Portal hypertensive gastropathy
  - ◊ Hemorrhagic gastritis
  - ◊ Peptic ulcer disease
  - ◊ Mallory-Weiss tear
- Ascites vs:
  - ◊ Spontaneous bacterial peritonitis
  - ◊ Pancreatic ascites
  - ◊ Peritoneal carcinomatosis
  - ◊ Tuberculous peritonitis
  - ◊ Nephrotic syndrome
  - ◊ Cardiac ascites
- Hepatic encephalopathy vs:
  - ◊ Delirium tremens
  - ◊ Intracranial hemorrhage
  - ◊ Sedative abuse
  - ◊ Uremia
- Hepatorenal syndrome vs
  - ◊ Drug nephrotoxicity
  - ◊ Renal tubular necrosis

LABORATORY
Non-specific changes associated with underlying disease.
- Hypersplenism
  - ◊ Anemia
  - ◊ Leukopenia
  - ◊ Thrombocytopenia
- Hepatic dysfunction
  - ◊ Hypoalbuminemia
  - ◊ Hyperbilirubinemia
  - ◊ Elevated alkaline phosphatase
  - ◊ Elevated liver enzymes
  - ◊ Abnormal clotting factors (PT, PTT.)
- Gastrointestinal bleeding
  - ◊ Iron deficiency anemia
  - ◊ Elevated serum ammonia
- Hepatorenal syndrome
  - ◊ Elevated serum creatinine, BUN
  - ◊ Urine Na < 20 mEq/L (< 20 mmol/L)

Drugs that may alter lab results: N/A

Disorders that may alter lab results: N/A

PATHOLOGICAL FINDINGS Specific for underlying disease

SPECIAL TESTS Specific for underlying disease

IMAGING
- UGI series. May outline varices in esophagus and stomach.
- CT scan and ultrasound. May detect cirrhosis, splenomegaly, ascites and varices.
- Duplex-Doppler (ultrasound.) Can determine presence and direction of flow in portal and hepatic veins. Useful in diagnosing portal vein and/or shunt thrombosis.
- Angiography. Demonstrates cork-screwing of intrahepatic vessels (cirrhosis); can identify varices and vascular anomalies.
- Contrast-enhanced MR angiography may be imaging modality of choice. Can provide three dimensional information about the patency of the portal vein and the presence of collateral pathways.

DIAGNOSTIC PROCEDURES
- Endoscopy. Can diagnose esophageal and gastric varices and portal hypertensive gastropathy or can directly visualize other bleeding sites (peptic ulcers, gastritis, Mallory-Weiss tears.)
- Hepatic venous wedge pressure. Correlates with portal pressure; risk of variceal bleeding is increased if HVWP > 12 mm./Hg.

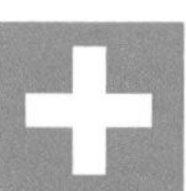

TREATMENT

APPROPRIATE HEALTH CARE Inpatient

GENERAL MEASURES
- Treat underlying disease and support metabolic/nutritional needs.
- Avoid sedatives; may precipitate encephalopathy
- Transfuse packed RBCs as needed. Use caution; circulation is already hyperdynamic.
- Correct coagulopathy. Administer vitamin K and/or fresh-frozen plasma.
- Limit sodium administration; cirrhotic patients avidly retain sodium

SURGICAL MEASURES
- Liver transplantation may be recommended for selected patients with far-advanced hepatic disease. Other less aggressive approaches are available for specific complications of portal hypertension.
- Gastroesophageal varices with hemorrhage
  - ◊ Endoscopic variceal sclerosis
  - ◊ Endoscopic variceal banding
  - ◊ Portacaval shunting
  - ◊ Transjugular intrahepatic portosystemic shunt (TIPS)
- Ascites refractory to medical management
  - ◊ Large volume paracentesis
  - ◊ Peritoneovenous shunt
  - ◊ Transjugular intrahepatic portosystemic shunt (TIPS)

ACTIVITY Bed rest for acute complications (bleeding, encephalopathy or hepatorenal syndrome)

DIET Restrict sodium and protein

PATIENT EDUCATION N/A

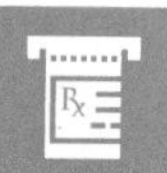

MEDICATIONS

DRUG(S) OF CHOICE
- Therapy for variceal hemorrhage:
  - ◊ For acute control: intravenous somatostatin or octreotide - synthetic analogue
  - ◊ Alternative: vasopressin; but, has more complications (decreased by addition of nitroglycerin)
  - ◊ For prevention of recurrence: propranolol
- Therapy for encephalopathy:
  - ◊ Lactulose. Induces diarrhea and traps intracolonic ammonia.
  - ◊ Neomycin. Reduces bacterial production of nitrogenous substances in colon.
- Therapy for ascites:
  - ◊ Furosemide (Lasix)
  - ◊ Spironolactone.

Contraindications: Vasopressin is a systemic vasodilator and may cause hypotension, bradycardia and cardiac and peripheral ischemia. Cardiac monitoring is advisable.
Precautions: Vasopressin may cause hypertension, bradycardia, arrhythmias. Patient must be on a cardiac monitor while receiving this drug. Co-administration of nitroprusside may reduce cardiotoxicity.
Significant possible interactions: Refer to manufacturer's literature

ALTERNATIVE DRUGS
Terlipressin (Glypressin) - more selective splanchnic vasoconstrictor and may be associated with fewer complications. Studies are continuing.

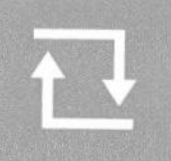

FOLLOWUP

PATIENT MONITORING
Acute complications of portal hypertension require intensive monitoring of vital signs and organ function. Long-term management includes regular follow-up of all affected organ systems.

PREVENTION/AVOIDANCE
Abstinence from alcohol. Adequate and appropriate nutrition.

POSSIBLE COMPLICATIONS
As described above

EXPECTED COURSE/PROGNOSIS
- Variceal bleeding: 50% re-bleed, usually within 2 years unless portal pressure is reduced by shunt or TIPS procedure
- Ascites: Generally recurs. Frequency and severity can be reduced if salt restriction is observed.
- Hepatic encephalopathy. Often recurs especially if re-bleeding develops. Low protein diet advised.

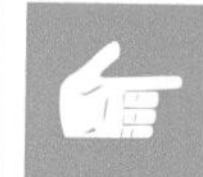

MISCELLANEOUS

ASSOCIATED CONDITIONS
As described above

AGE-RELATED FACTORS
Pediatric: Uncommon. Generally different etiology than in adults.
- Intrahepatic
  - ◊ Biliary atresia
  - ◊ Viral hepatitis
  - ◊ Metabolic liver disease.
- Extrahepatic
  - ◊ Congenital anomalies of portal vein
  - ◊ Neonatal omphalitis (umbilical vein catheterization, sepsis, abdominal trauma)

Geriatric: Mortality and complication rate are increased
Others: N/A

PREGNANCY
N/A

SYNONYMS
N/A

ICD-9-CM
572.3 Portal hypertension

SEE ALSO
Cirrhosis of the liver
Hepatitis A
Hepatitis B
Hepatitis C

OTHER NOTES
- Other treatment approaches (inadequately studied with non-control protocols)
  - ◊ Transhepatic obliteration of varices
  - ◊ Concomitant treatment with non-selective beta-adrenergic blockers

ABBREVIATIONS
N/A

REFERENCES

- Sleisenger MH, Fortran JS, eds. Gastrointestinal Disease: Pathophysiology, Diagnosis, Management. 5th ed. Philadelphia: WB Saunders Co; 1994
- Jaffe DL, Chung RT, Friedman LS. Management of portal hypertension and its complications. Med Clin N Am 1996;80:1021-34
- D'Amico G, Pietrosi G, Tarantino I, Pagliaro L. Emergency sclerotherapy versus vasoactive drugs for variceal bleeding in cirrhosis: a Cochrane meta-analysis. Gastroenterology. 2003;124(5):1277-91
- Teran JC, Imperiale TF, Mullen KD, et al. Primary prophylaxis of variceal bleeding in cirrhosis: a cost-effectiveness analysis. Gastroent 1997;112:473-82
- Lake JR. The role of transjugular shunting in patients with ascites. N Engl J Med 2000;342(23):1745-7

Web references: 1 available at www.5mcc.com
Illustrations N/A

Author(s):
Wayne H. Schwesinger, MD

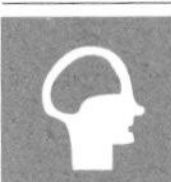

BASICS

DESCRIPTION

- CNS dysfunction occurring after minor head injury with or without initial loss of consciousness. The primary cause is diffuse axonal injury and small vessel injury. Diffuse axonal injury is a result of shearing forces caused by rapid deceleration, flexion-extension injury, and rotatory injury. Neuronal injury continues for 6-12 hours secondary to free radical formation and other factors.
- Occurs in up to 50% of patients with mild traumatic brain injury (TBI)
- Most patients recover within 12 weeks but 15% with minor TBI will be symptomatic at 1 year and some never become asymptomatic
- By definition, these patients have an initial GCS of 13-15
- Concussion Grades:
  - ◊ 1: transient confusion, no LOC, duration of mental status changes < 15 minutes
  - ◊ 2: transient confusion, no LOC, duration of mental status change > 15 minutes
  - ◊ 3: any LOC (including seizures), either brief or prolonged

System(s) affected: Nervous
Genetics: N/A
Incidence/Prevalence in USA: 180/100,000 with 27/100,000 being persistent
Predominant age: 15-24 years. Patients over 55 are more likely to have persistent deficits
Predominant sex: Female > Male

SIGNS & SYMPTOMS

- Chronic headache; some may be severe. May be bandlike, migraine-like, on the vertex of the head, or ill-defined with patchy pain involvement secondary to post-traumatic nerve injury.
- Chronic neck pain
- Dizziness or vertigo
- Poor concentration
- Memory deficits
- Personality changes
- Irritability, depression, anxiety
- Decrease in ability to smell or taste (5%)
- Sleep-wake disturbances
- Other cognitive disturbances
- Positive Dix-Hallpike test (nystagmus and/or vertigo induction with certain head motions) in traumatic vestibulopathy

CAUSES Falls, motor vehicle accidents (MVA), assault, etc

RISK FACTORS Those that predispose to falls, MVA, etc. including drugs and alcohol. Additionally, there is some association with litigation, female gender, preexisting headaches, and low socioeconomic status. However, these factors account for only a minority of the cases (eg, men are almost as likely as women to have symptoms, patients without pending litigation are almost as likely as those with pending litigation to have symptoms, etc.)

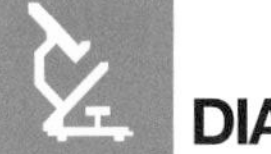

DIAGNOSIS

DIFFERENTIAL DIAGNOSIS N/A

LABORATORY N/A

Drugs that may alter lab results: N/A

Disorders that may alter lab results: N/A

PATHOLOGICAL FINDINGS Diffuse axonal injury has been demonstrated on post mortem specimens

SPECIAL TESTS

- Neuropsychometric testing will demonstrate subtle abnormalities not demonstrable on instruments such as mini mental status exam

Glasgow Coma Score (GCS):

```
Best Eye Response (E)
  1 No eye opening
  2 Eye opening to pain
  3 Eye opening to verbal command
  4 Eyes open spontaeously
Best Verbal Response (V)
  1 No verbal response
  2 Incomprehensible words
  3 Inappropriate words
  4 Confused
  5 Oriented
Best Motor Response (M)
  1 No motor response
  2 Extension to pain
  3 Flexion to pain
  4 Withdrawal from pain
  5 Localizing pain
  6 Obeys commands
-------------------------------------
(1) Score GCS with componenets (e.g.
E2V3M4 = GCS 9).
(2) Interpretation: >12 mild brain in-
jury; 9-12 moderate injury; <9 severe
injury.
```

IMAGING

- CT scan is usually normal
- MRI may show small petechial hemorrhages or focal cortical contusions. SPECT scanning may show small areas of focal edema. MRI and SPECT scanning should be considered research tools at this time since the diagnosis is primarily clinical.

DIAGNOSTIC PROCEDURES N/A

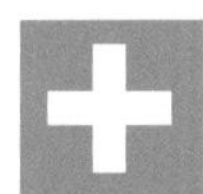

TREATMENT

APPROPRIATE HEALTH CARE An outpatient setting with involvement of a primary care physician, neurologist, and psychologist as appropriate. Many cases can be handled solely by the patient's primary care physician.

GENERAL MEASURES

- Address the patient's symptoms such as neck pain, headaches, depression, etc. using the usual medications
- Involvement of vocational rehabilitation may be necessary
- Behavioral therapy, etc. can be tried, but there is no good evidence that this is effective

SURGICAL MEASURES N/A

ACTIVITY Sports activity, etc., should be limited based on degree of injury. Parents and coaches will often try to return an athlete to sports competition prematurely. The American Academy of Neurology has published these guidelines (226 MMWR March 14, 1997). A second impact syndrome phenomenon occurs. The second injury, while in and of itself may be mild, is cumulative with the first and may be fatal. Recommendations are verbatim from MMWR.

- Grade 1 concussion:
  - ◊ Management: the athlete should be removed from sports activity, examined immediately and at 5-minute intervals, and allowed to return that day to the sports activity only if post-concussive symptoms (headache, vomiting, etc.) resolve within 15 minutes. Any athlete who incurs a second Grade 1 concussion on the same day should be removed from sports activity until asymptomatic for 1 week.
- Grade 2 concussion:
  - ◊ Management: The athlete should be removed from sports activity and examined frequently to assess the evolution of symptoms, with more extensive diagnostic evaluation if the symptoms worsen or persist for > 1 week. The athlete should return to sports activity only after asymptomatic for 1 full week. Any athlete who incurs a Grade 2 concussion subsequent to a Grade 1 concussion on the same day should be removed from sports activity until asymptomatic for 2 weeks.
- Grade 3 concussion:
  - ◊ Management: the athlete should be removed from sports activity for 1 full week without symptoms if the loss of consciousness is brief or 2 full weeks without symptoms if the loss of consciousness is prolonged. If still unconscious or if abnormal neurologic signs are present at the time of initial evaluation, the athlete should be transported by ambulance to the nearest hospital emergency department. An athlete who suffers a second Grade 3 concussion should be removed from sports activity until asymptomatic for 1 month. Any athlete with an abnormality on computerized tomography (CT) or magnetic resonance imaging (MRI) of brain consistent with brain swelling, contusion, or other intracranial pathology should be removed from sports activities for the season and discouraged from future return to participation in contact sports.

DIET N/A

PATIENT EDUCATION Discussion with patient and family about long term prospects, etc.

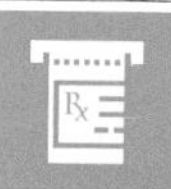

MEDICATIONS

DRUG(S) OF CHOICE
- Sleep disorders/depression/headache:
  - ◊ Amitriptyline in age appropriate doses or other tricyclic drug
  - ◊ SSRIs are less well studied in PCS, but can be used for depression
  - ◊ Benzodiazepines should be avoided if possible
- Neck pain/headache:
  - ◊ NSAIDs
  - ◊ Avoid narcotics if possible

Contraindications: Allergy to medication

Precautions:
- NSAIDs may cause ulcer disease, elevated blood pressure, renal dysfunction and bleeding among other side effects
- Tricyclics can cause arrhythmias and should not be used in the suicidal patient; tricyclics can also cause urinary retention, constipation and other anticholinergic side effects

Significant possible interactions:
- NSAIDs: warfarin, ACE inhibitors, and lithium.
- Ibuprofen-oral hypoglycemics: hypoglycemia
- Tricyclics: multiple drug interactions including cimetidine and MAOIs. Check a drug reference.
- SSRI-MAOI: should never be given together; risk of serotonin syndrome. These may also cause tricyclic toxicity when used together.

ALTERNATIVE DRUGS N/A

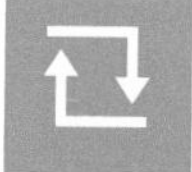

FOLLOWUP

PATIENT MONITORING As needed. Each case is individualized.

PREVENTION/AVOIDANCE Discussing the avoidance of drugs and alcohol with teens at the time of a sports physical. Discussion of seat-belt use.

POSSIBLE COMPLICATIONS Loss of source of income and resulting problems such as loss of house, strain on the family, etc.

EXPECTED COURSE/PROGNOSIS
Those not better by 1 year will probably not get better. It is of note that the resolution of litigation does not generally result in improvement of this disorder. Outcome correlates better with length of post traumatic amnesia than GCS.

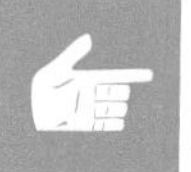

MISCELLANEOUS

ASSOCIATED CONDITIONS See Risk factors

AGE-RELATED FACTORS
Pediatric: Tend to improve more quickly
Geriatric: Tend not to improve
Others: Those over age 55 are more likely to have permanent deficits

PREGNANCY N/A

SYNONYMS N/A

ICD-9-CM
310.2 Postconcussion syndrome

SEE ALSO
Brain injury, traumatic
Cervical spine injury
Depression
Migraine

OTHER NOTES Consider a repeat head CT within the first couple of weeks if symptoms persist. The symptoms of PCS can also be due to subdural hemorrhages.

ABBREVIATIONS
TBI = traumatic brain injury
LOC = loss of consciousness
MVA = motor vehicle accident
PCS = post concussive syndrome
GCS = Glasgow Coma Score
SPECT = single photon emission computed tomography

REFERENCES

- Alexander MP: Mild traumatic brain injury: pathophysiology, natural history, and clinical management. Neurology 1995;45:1253-1260
- Borczuk P. Neurologic emergencies: Mild head trauma. Emergency Clinics of NA 1997;15(3):653-679
- Rees PM. Contemporary Issues in Mild Traumatic Brain Injury. Arch Phys Med Rehabil 2003;84:1885-94

Web references: 0 available at www.5mcc.com
Illustrations N/A

Author(s):
Dana Collaguazo, MD
Hans House, MD

Post-traumatic stress disorder (PTSD)

BASICS

DESCRIPTION A condition seen in people who experienced an event that would be extremely distressing to most human beings, e.g., serious threat to one's life, physical or psychological integrity; serious threat or harm to one's children, spouse, siblings, parents or other close relatives or friends; sudden destruction of one's home or community; seeing another person who has recently been (or is being) injured or killed as a result of a man-made violent act or natural disaster.
- Response involved intense fear, helplessness, or horror. Note: In children, this may be expressed by disorganized or agitated behavior.
- Symptoms did not exist prior to the trauma, and symptoms persist for at least one month
- Acute PTSD is < 3 months
- Chronic form is > 3 months
- Subtype PTSD: delayed onset of the symptoms > 6 months after the event

System(s) affected: Nervous
Genetics: N/A
Incidence/Prevalence in USA: Up to 30% of disaster victims develop PTSD. Lifelong prevalence in general population ranges from 1-14%.
Predominant age: The elderly and the very young are more vulnerable
Predominant sex: Adult women are more inclined to ask for help. Young boys may be more vulnerable to trauma than girls. Most men with PTSD have experienced combat or exposure to trauma on the job. Most women with PTSD have a history of rape or being physically assaulted.

SIGNS & SYMPTOMS
- The event is persistently re-experienced in one or more of the following ways:
  - ◊ Recurrent and intrusive distressing recollections (flashbacks) of the event, including images, thoughts or perceptions. Note: In young children repetitive play may occur in which themes or aspects of the trauma are expressed.
  - ◊ Recurrent distressing dreams of the event. Note: In children, there may be frightening dreams without recognizable content.
  - ◊ Acting or feeling as if the traumatic event were recurring (includes a sense of reliving the experience, illusions, hallucinations, and dissociative flashback episodes, including those that occur on awakening or when intoxicated). Note: In young children, trauma-specific reenactment may occur.
  - ◊ Intense psychological distress at exposure to internal or external cues that symbolize or resemble an aspect of the traumatic event
  - ◊ Physiological reactivity on exposure to internal or external cues that symbolize or resemble an aspect of the traumatic event, such as increased heart rate, changes in blood pressure, discoloration of the skin, blurred vision, hyperperistalsis in smooth muscle, nausea, vomiting, diarrhea, urinary urgency, etc.
- Persistent avoidance of the stimuli associated with the trauma, or numbing of general responsiveness (not present before the trauma) as indicated by three (or more) of the following:
  - ◊ Efforts to avoid thoughts, feelings or conversations associated with the trauma
  - ◊ Efforts to avoid activities, places or people that arouse recollections of the trauma
  - ◊ Inability to recall an important aspect of the trauma (psychogenic amnesia)
  - ◊ Markedly diminished interest or participation in significant activities (in young children, loss of recently acquired developmental skills such as toilet training or language skills)
  - ◊ Feelings of detachment or estrangement from others
  - ◊ Restricted range of affect (e.g., unable to have loving feelings)
  - ◊ Sense of a foreshortened future (e.g., does not expect to have a career, marriage, or a normal life span)
- Persistent symptoms of increased arousal (not present before the trauma), as indicated by two or more of the following:
  - ◊ Difficulty falling or staying asleep (insomnia)
  - ◊ Irritability or outbursts of anger
  - ◊ Difficulty in concentrating
  - ◊ Hypervigilance
  - ◊ Exaggerated startle response
- Others:
  - ◊ Duration of the disturbance > 1 month
  - ◊ Disturbance causes clinically significant distress or impairment in social, occupational, or other important areas of functioning

CAUSES Events which are insults to one's personal integrity, self-esteem and security are psychologically traumatic and may lead to PTSD

RISK FACTORS
- History of childhood abuse, neglect or dysfunctional families, and children of alcoholic parents
- Individuals born with a smaller hippocampus

DIAGNOSIS

DIFFERENTIAL DIAGNOSIS
- Organic mental disorders
- Generalized anxiety disorder
- Phobic disorders
- Depressive disorder
- Panic disorder
- Conversion disorder
- Somatization disorder
- Personality disorders
- Substance and chemical dependency

LABORATORY N/A

Drugs that may alter lab results: N/A

Disorders that may alter lab results: N/A

PATHOLOGICAL FINDINGS Character pathology as shown on the Minnesota multiple personality inventory (MMPI)

SPECIAL TESTS
- Neuropsychological testing is helpful in cases of dementia and more subtle cognitive dysfunction
- EEG (results may be altered by any drug affecting EEG patterns such as - sleeping pills, antidepressants, neuroleptics and other psychotropic medications)
- Psychological testing and a thorough mental status examination
- Sleep studies
- Through an examination and interview, assisted by hypnosis or IV amobarbital (Amytal) or similar substances, traumatic material may be uncovered in patients with amnesia.
- Tests may be affected by withdrawal or intoxication from drugs and alcohol; any organic brain syndromes (e.g., multiple infarct dementia, forms of epilepsy)

IMAGING MRI of the head focusing on the size of the hippocampus

DIAGNOSTIC PROCEDURES
- Psychiatric examination
- Psychological testing
- Note: Acute Stress Disorder is similar to PTSD but lasts between 2 and 30 days and occurs within 4 weeks of the event.

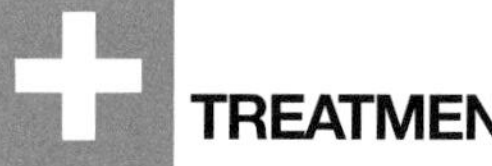

TREATMENT

APPROPRIATE HEALTH CARE
- Most treatment is done on an outpatient basis
- Suicidal or dysfunctional with activities of daily living patients should be hospitalized

GENERAL MEASURES
- As indicated by the patient's general condition, treatment includes individual psychotherapy, group therapy, hypnotherapy, narcoanalysis and narcosynthesis, and behavior therapy
- Crisis intervention shortly after the traumatic event is very valuable for the immediate distress and may prevent the development of a chronic or delayed form of PTSD
- Relaxation exercises
- Eye movement desensitization and reprocessing (EMDR) may help in some cases

SURGICAL MEASURES N/A

ACTIVITY
- As indicated by patient's physical condition
- Restoration of regular sleep is essential in cases of insomnia

DIET A healthy diet of complex carbohydrates, proteins, and multivitamins and minerals. Avoid fatty foods.

PATIENT EDUCATION Lenore Terr: Too Scared to Cry. Harper & Row, NY, 1990

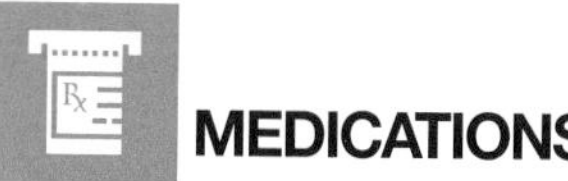

MEDICATIONS

DRUG(S) OF CHOICE
- Selective serotonin reuptake inhibitors (SSRI):
  - ◊ Fluoxetine 20-80 mg/day
  - ◊ Sertraline 50-200 mg/day
  - ◊ Paroxetine 20-60 mg/day
  - ◊ Citalopram 20-60 mg/day
  - ◊ Venlafaxine 75-325 mg/day
  - ◊ Escitalopram 10-20 mg/day
- TCAs:
  - ◊ Doxepin 50-150 mg/day
  - ◊ Nortriptyline 30-100 mg/day
  - ◊ Imipramine 50-300 mg/day
  - ◊ Desipramine 50-300 mg/day
  - ◊ Amitriptyline 50-300 mg/day
  - ◊ Trimipramine 50-300 mg/day
  - ◊ Protriptyline 15-60 mg/ day
  - ◊ Amoxapine 50-300 mg/day
  - ◊ Maprotiline 50-225 mg/day (increased risk of seizures with higher doses)
- MOAIs:
  - ◊ Phenelzine 45-75 mg/day is useful in PTSD patients with panic attacks
- Others:
  - ◊ Trazodone 100-400 mg/day, given mostly at bedtime in patients with insomnia
  - ◊ Bupropion 100-450 mg/day
  - ◊ Neuroleptics - small doses are helpful in selective patients
  - ◊ Benzodiazepines should be used selectively and with caution

Contraindications:
- Allergic reactions to specific drugs
- Use with caution in alcoholic patients with poor liver functions

Precautions:
- Do not mix TCAs with MOAIs
- Long-term use of benzodiazepines may lead to increased tolerance and drug dependency

Significant possible interactions: MOAIs may interact with other antidepressants, sympathomimetics such as pseudoephedrine and any foods with tyramine or its precursors

ALTERNATIVE DRUGS
- Clomipramine 75-250 mg/day or fluvoxamine 100-300 mg/day or fluoxetine 20-80 mg/day in patients with obsessive compulsive symptoms has been helpful in some cases
- Buspirone 30-80 mg/day has been found helpful in cases with severe anxiety
- Propranolol and clonidine have been used with limited results to control the psychophysiological hyperactivity during intense flashbacks
- Mirtazapine (Remeron) 15-45 mg given at bed time has been helpful in patients with insomnia, poor appetite and weight loss
- Prazosin (Minipress) for nightmares

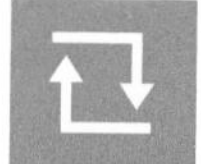

FOLLOWUP

PATIENT MONITORING Psychotherapy for at least one hour per week is necessary in the first phase of treatment

PREVENTION/AVOIDANCE Crisis intervention immediately after the traumatic event may prevent the development of chronic PTSD

POSSIBLE COMPLICATIONS Alcohol and substance abuse, depression, suicide, self-inflicted violence and reenactment of trauma

EXPECTED COURSE/PROGNOSIS
- The lack of crisis intervention immediately following the trauma may lead to the persistence of symptoms. If symptoms last less than 3 months, the patient is still in the acute form of PTSD. If symptoms persist over 3 months, patients may develop chronic PTSD which may lead to loss of job, marital conflicts, total disability and repeated and/or lengthy hospitalizations with severe morbidity.
- If the onset of symptoms is at least 6 months or more after the original traumatic event, the patient suffers from a delayed onset type
- The more chronic and delayed the onset, the worse the prognosis. Early treatment in acute phase associated with better prognosis.

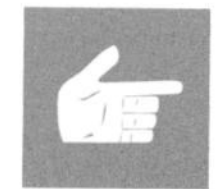

MISCELLANEOUS

ASSOCIATED CONDITIONS Personality disorders such as borderline personality disorder, depression, panic disorder, anxiety disorder, and dissociative disorders

AGE-RELATED FACTORS
Pediatric: Young children are susceptible to abuse and neglect; can develop chronic PTSD with failure to progress and grow in healthy way
Geriatric: Have fewer social support resources; adjustment to trauma less flexible; more sensitive to medication and need dose adjustment.
Others: N/A

PREGNANCY Avoid psychotropics in the first trimester. Focus on non-pharmacologic treatment techniques such as psychotherapy, hypnotherapy, relaxation therapy, etc.

SYNONYMS
- Trauma syndrome
- Battle fatigue
- Shell shock
- Post-disaster syndrome
- Trauma survivor's syndrome
- Traumatic neurosis

ICD-9-CM
293.9 Unspecified transient organic mental disorder
308.3 Other acute reactions to stress

SEE ALSO

OTHER NOTES N/A

ABBREVIATIONS
MOAIs = monoamine oxidase inhibitors
TCA = tricyclic antidepressant
EMDR = eye movement desensitization and reprocessing

REFERENCES

- Yehuda R. Risk and resilience in posttraumatic stress disorder. J Clin Psychiatry. 2004;65 Suppl 1:29-36
- Davidson JR. Long-term treatment and prevention of posttraumatic stress disorder. J Clin Psychiatry. 2004;65 Suppl 1:44-8
- Lecrubier Y. Posttraumatic stress disorder in primary care: a hidden diagnosis. J Clin Psychiatry. 2004;65 Suppl 1:49-54
- Ballenger JC, Davidson JR, Lecrubier Y, Nutt DJ, Marshall RD, Nemeroff CB, Shalev AY, Yehuda R. Consensus statement update on posttraumatic stress disorder from the international consensus group on depression and anxiety. J Clin Psychiatry. 2004;65 Suppl 1:55-62
- Rasmusson AM, Vythilingam M, Morgan CA 3rd. The neuroendocrinology of posttraumatic stress disorder: new directions. CNS Spectr. 2003;(9):651-6, 665-7
- Liberzon I, Phan KL. Brain-imaging studies of posttraumatic stress disorder. CNS Spectr. 2003;8(9):641-50
- Loveland Cook CA, Flick LH, Homan SM, Campbell C, McSweeney M, Gallagher ME. Posttraumatic stress disorder in pregnancy: prevalence, risk factors, and treatment. Obstet Gynecol. 2004;103(4):710-7
- Shapiro F, Maxfield L. Eye Movement Desensitization and Reprocessing (EMDR): information processing in the treatment of trauma. J Clin Psychol. 2002;58(8):933-46
- Yehuda R, Marshall R, Penkower A, Wong C. Pharmacological Treatment for Post traumatic Stress Disorder. In: Natham P, Gorman JM, eds. A Guide to Treatments That Work. 2nd Ed. London, England, Oxford University; 2002; p411-445
- Foa EB, Davidson JRT, Frances A, Ross R. Expert consensus treatment guidelines for post-traumatic stress disorder. A guide for patients and families. J Clin Psychiatry 1999:60;Suppl 1-8
- van der Kolk BA, McFarlane AC, Van der Hart O. Psychotherapy for Post-raumatic Stress Disorder and Other Trauma-related Disorders. In: Stein DJ. Hollander E, eds. Textbook of Anxiety Disorders. Washington DC, American Psychiatric Publishing Co; 2002. p403-411
- Van derKolk, et al. Traumatic stress: the effects of overwhelming experiences on mind, body, and society. New York, Guilford Press 1996
- Field LH. Post-traumatic stress disorder; a reappraisal. J of the Royal Soc of Med. 1999;92:35-37
- Rauch SL, et al. A symptom provocation study of PTSD using PET and script driven imagery. Arch Gen Psychiatry. 1996;53:380-387
- Burton JK, Marshall RD. Categorizing fear and the role of trauma in a clinical formulation. Am J of Psychiatry 1999;156:761-766
- Yul W. Post-traumatic stress disorder. Archives of Disease in Childhood. 1999;80:107-109
- Yehuda R. Biological factors associated with susceptibility to post traumatic stress disorder. Canadian J of Psychiat 1999;44:34-39
- Hampton MR, Frombach I. Women's experience of traumatic stress in cancer treatment. Health Care for Women Internat 2000;21(1):67-76
- Weintraub D, Ruskin PE. Posttraumatic stress disorder in the elderly: A review. Harvard Rev Psychiatry 1999;7:144-52
- Hembree EA, Foa EB. Posttraumatic stress disorder: psychological factors and psychosocial interventions. J Clin Psychiatr 2000;61 Suppl 7:33-9
- Focus on past-traumatic stress disorder. J Clin Psychiatr 2000;61 Suppl 5:33-9
- Briere J. Child Abuse Trauma: Theory and Treatment of the Lasting Effects. Newbury Park, CA, Sage, 1992

Web references: 1 available at www.5mcc.com
Illustrations N/A

Author(s):
Moshe S. Torem, MD

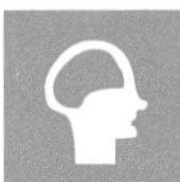

BASICS

DESCRIPTION Postpartum depression, postpartum blues and postpartum psychosis are the three main behavioral conditions that may take place in women following the delivery.
System(s) affected: Nervous
Genetics: N/A
Incidence/Prevalence in USA: 10-15% of new mothers develop postpartum depression.
Predominant age: Women of reproductive age. It has been described in mothers adopting a baby.
Predominant sex: Female

SIGNS & SYMPTOMS
Most women will have some of these symptoms, not all
- Depressed mood
- Sadness
- Crying spells
- Fatigue
- Sleep disturbances (insomnia or hypersomnia)
- Appetite disturbances (poor appetite or excessive eating)
- Poor concentration
- Feelings of helplessness
- Feelings of hopelessness
- Fears of harming the baby
- Lack of interest in the baby
- Feelings of guilt and inadequacy
- Feelings of worthlessness and low self-esteem
- Fears of harming oneself
- Sudden mood swings
- Lability of affect
- Excessive concern with the baby's health
- Poor libido, no interest in sex
- Anxiety symptoms
- Feelings of gloom and doom
- Dizziness and rapid breathing
- Heart palpitations
- Obsessive and intrusive thoughts

CAUSES
Unknown. Perhaps multifactorial, including: biological-genetic predisposition in terms of brain chemistry, sudden drop in estrogen and progesterone levels at delivery, socioeconomic stress

RISK FACTORS
- Previous episodes of postpartum depression
- Previous episodes of depression
- History of depression during pregnancy
- Family history of depression
- Early childhood losses
- Growing up with alcoholic dysfunctional parents
- Unwanted pregnancy
- Presence of socioeconomic stress
- Lack of social and family support system

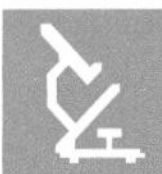

DIAGNOSIS

DIFFERENTIAL DIAGNOSIS
- Baby blues
- Postpartum psychosis
- Postpartum anxiety/panic disorder
- Postpartum obsessive compulsive disorder
- Hypothyroidism
- Sleep apnea

LABORATORY
- TSH
- Estrogen and progesterone levels may be helpful (often low)

Drugs that may alter lab results: N/A

Disorders that may alter lab results: N/A

PATHOLOGICAL FINDINGS N/A

SPECIAL TESTS
- Polysomnograms for sleep apnea and/or daytime sleepiness. Sleep EEG to confirm short REM latency prognosticating a better response to antidepressants.
- Psychological testing for personality/character disorders and provide clues for the best choice of nonpharmacological therapies

IMAGING Head CT/MRI rarely needed

DIAGNOSTIC PROCEDURES
- Neuropsychological testing
- Projective psychological testing
- Beck, Hamilton and Zung depression inventories may provide information on the severity of the depression and suicidal risks

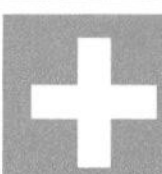

TREATMENT

APPROPRIATE HEALTH CARE
- Most patients respond to outpatient individual psychotherapy in combination with pharmacotherapy
- Support/therapy groups helpful
- Assess for homicidal and suicidal ideations
- Visiting nurse services can provide direct observations of the mother regarding safety issues and bonding
- Assess (consider psychiatrist consultation) patients for psychotic symptoms - if psychotic delusions or hallucinations present, immediate hospitalization needed. The psychotic mother should not be left alone with the baby.

GENERAL MEASURES
- Proper sleep and rest for the new mother are very important for stable mood.
- Patient education and bibliotherapy for the patient and her family are helpful and valuable
- ECT: Some patients who cannot tolerate the antidepressant medication, or who are actively engaged in suicidal self-destructive behaviors or who have a previous history of responding favorably to ECT should be seriously considered for treatment with ECT

SURGICAL MEASURES N/A

ACTIVITY Based on patients physical condition

DIET
- Good nutrition and hydration
- The addition of a multivitamin with minerals may be helpful

PATIENT EDUCATION
- Patient and family education helpful
- Encourage the patient to read, for example:
  - ◊ "That Isn't What I Expected: Overcoming Postpartum Depression" by Karen R. Kleinman and Valerie Davis Radkin, 1994
  - ◊ "Sleepless Days: One Woman's Journey Through Postpartum Depression" by Susan Kushner Resnick, 2000
  - ◊ "A Mother's Tears: Understanding the Mood Swings that Follow Childbirth", by Arlene M. Huysman, 1998
  - ◊ "Overcoming Postpartum Depression and Anxiety", by Linda Sebastian, 1998.

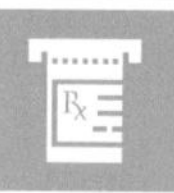

MEDICATIONS

DRUG(S) OF CHOICE
- SSRIs are effective and safe and are also effective for patients with depression and OCD symptoms.
  - ◊ Fluoxetine (Prozac) 20-80 mg/day (most activating of all SSRIs)
  - ◊ Sertraline (Zoloft) 50-200mg/day (sedating)
  - ◊ Paroxetine (Paxil) 20-60mg/day (sedating)
  - ◊ Citalopram (Celexa) 20-60mg/day
  - ◊ Fluvoxamine (Luvox) 25-200mg/day (effective for postpartum depression associated with OCD)
- Tricyclic antidepressants are effective and less expensive. Lethal in overdoses and have unfavorable side effects with less tolerance compared to the SSRIs.
- Bupropion (Wellbutrin) 150-450mg/day in patients with depression plus psychomotor retardation, hypersomnia, low energy, general slowing and hyperphagia with weight gain. Bupropion does not cause weight gain nor sexual dysfunction. It is highly activating and safe in the SR (slow release) form.
- Nefazodone (Serzone) 150-600mg/day with sedating effects but without causing sexual dysfunction nor weight gain nor REM sleep interruption.
- Mirtazapine (Remeron) 15-45mg/day given at bedtime. Non-SSRI antidepressant helps with sleep restoration and in patients with weight loss. No sexual dysfunction side effects.
- Venlafaxine (Effexor) is a dual action antidepressant that blocks the reuptake of serotonin in doses of up to 150mg/day and then blocks the reuptake of norepinephrine in doses of 150-450mg/day. The new XR (extended release) is given once daily and is also effective for the control of anxiety.

Contraindications:
- Known drug allergy
- Some antidepressants are excreted in breast milk

Precautions: Avoid tricyclic antidepressants in mothers with a known history of suicide attempts by overdose.
- Use non-SSRIs very cautiously in nursing mothers, carefully assessing the risk benefit

Significant possible interactions:
- Avoid the use of the above antidepressants with an MAO inhibitors
- For a patient who may have a coexisting medical illness and who may need a quick change from one antidepressant to another due to drug interactions, sertraline or citalopram may be a better choice

ALTERNATIVE DRUGS
- Lithium carbonate or valproic acid, may be added as a mood stabilizer and to augment antidepressant effect. However, both may be teratogenic in case of a new pregnancy. Buspirone (Buspar) may be added for the control of anxiety and for antidepressant augmentation.

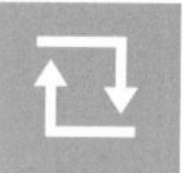

FOLLOWUP

PATIENT MONITORING
If psychotic symptoms present observe quality and safety of mother's interaction with baby. Home observation and monitoring helpful.

PREVENTION/AVOIDANCE
- Routinely assess women in the third trimester for depression, to identify depression and begin treatment before or immediately after delivery.
- Self-rating depression scales (e.g., Zung depression scale or the Beck depression scale) helpful

POSSIBLE COMPLICATIONS
- Self inflicted violence and suicide attempts
- Psychotic delusions
- Neglect of baby
- Harm to the baby

EXPECTED COURSE/PROGNOSIS
Generally good. Improvement expected within a few months to a year. Some patients, particularly those with personality disorders, develop chronic depression requiring long term treatment.

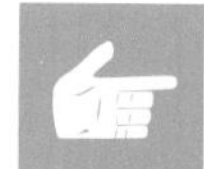

MISCELLANEOUS

ASSOCIATED CONDITIONS
- Bipolar mood disorder
- Depressive disorder not otherwise specified
- Dysthymic disorder
- Cyclothymic disorder

AGE-RELATED FACTORS
Pediatric: N/A
Geriatric: N/A
Others:
- Teenage mothers are more susceptible.

PREGNANCY N/A

SYNONYMS
- Postnatal depression
- Post gestational depression

ICD-9-CM
648.44 Mental postpartum condition or complication

SEE ALSO
Baby blues
Depression
Postpartum anxiety/panic disorder
Postpartum obsessive compulsive disorder
Postpartum psychosis

OTHER NOTES N/A

ABBREVIATIONS N/A

REFERENCES

- Austin MP, Lumley J. Antenatal screening for postnatal depression: a systematic review. Acta Psychiatr Scand 2003;107(1):10-7
- Bloch M, Daly RC, Rubinow DR. Endocrine factors in the etiology of postpartum depression. Compr Psychiatry 2003;44(3):234-46
- McCoy SJ, Beal JM, Watson GH. Endocrine factors and postpartum depression. A selected review. J Reprod Med 2003;48(6):402-8
- Henshaw C. Mood disturbance in the early puerperium: a review. Arch Women Ment Health 2003;6 Suppl 2: S33-42
- Seyfried LS, Marcus SM. Postpartum mood disorders. Int Rev Psychiatry 2003;15(3):231-42
- Ogrodniczuk JS, Piper WE. Preventing postnatal depression: a review of research findings. Harv Rev Psychiatry 2003;11(6):291-307
- Tammentie T, Tarkka MT, Astedt-Kurki P, Paavilainen E, Laippala P. Family dynamics and postnatal depression. J Psychiatr Ment Health Nurs 2004;11(2):141-9
- Winsner KL, Parry, BL, Piontek CM. Postpartum depression. New Engl J Med 2002;347(3):194-9
- Torem MS. Psychopharmacology for office gynecology. In: Curtis MG, Hopkins MP, editors. Glass's Office Gynecology. Baltimore: Williams & Wilkins; 1999. p. 519-548
- Pajer K. New strategies in the treatment of depression in women. J Clin Psychiatry 1995;56: 30-7
- Corral MK, Dernetra AK. Bright light therapy's effect on postpartum depression. Am J Psych 2000;157: 303-4
- Hagen EH. The Functions of postpartum depression. Evolution and Human Behavior 1999;20:325-59
- Crouch M. The evolutionary context of postnatal depression. Human Nature 1999;10:163-82
- Steinberg SI, Bellavance F. Characteristics and treatment of women with postpartum depression. Int J of Psychiatry in Medicine 1999;20:209-33
- Milgram J, et al. Treating postnatal depression: A psychological approach for health care practitioners. New York: John Wiley & Sons; 1999
- O'Hara MV. Post-partum 'blues', depression and psychosis; a review. J Psychosom Obstetrical Gynecology 1987;7:205-27
- Holden JM. Postnatal depression: its nature, effects and identification using the Edinburgh Postnatal Depression Scale. Birth 1991;18:211-21
- Suri R, Burt VK. The assessment and treatment of postpartum psychiatric disorders. J Pract Psychiatry Behavior Health 1997;3:67-77
- Wisner KL, Perel JM, Peindl KS, Hanusa BH, Findling RL, Rapport D. Prevention of recurrent postpartum depression: a randomized clinical trial. J Clin Psychiatry 2001 Feb;62(2):82-6
- Georgiopoulos AM, Bryan TL, Wollan P, Yawn BP. Routine screening for postpartum depression. J Fam Pract 2001 Feb;50(2):117-22
- Marcus SM, Barry KL, Flynn HA, Tandon R, Greden JF. Treatment guidelines for depression in pregnancy. Int J Gynaecol Obstet 2001 Jan;72(1):61-70

Web references: 1 available at www.5mcc.com
Illustrations N/A

Author(s):
Moshe S. Torem, MD

BASICS

DESCRIPTION Hypertension associated with proteinuria, edema, and acute excessive weight gain developing during pregnancy after 20 weeks gestation
System(s) affected: Cardiovascular, Nervous, Reproductive
Genetics: N/A
Incidence/Prevalence in USA: About 7% of first-time mothers and 1-2% of subsequent pregnancies
Predominant age:
- Young, primigravida women
- Women over 35 years of age

Predominant sex: Female only

SIGNS & SYMPTOMS
- Elevated BP (> 140/90 [18.6/12 kPa] or increased 30 [4 kPa] systolic or increased 15 [2 kPa] diastolic) recorded on 2 BP readings 6 hours apart
- Proteinuria (> 300 mg/24 hours or > 1 gram/L)
- Edema
- Rapid excessive weight gain (> 5 lb/week) (2.3 kg/week)
- Epigastric pain
- Headache
- Hyperreflexia
- Visual disturbances
- Apprehension
- Retinal arteriolar spasm
- Papilledema
- Retinal cotton-wool exudate
- Amnesia
- Oliguria
- Anuria

CAUSES
- Altered cardiovascular reactivity
- Increased capillary permeability
- Widespread endothelial dysfunction
- Microthrombi
- Hypertension

RISK FACTORS
- Familial incidence
- Lower socioeconomic
- Multiple fetuses
- Teenage
- Collagen disorders
- Females > 35 years old
- Primigravida
- First subsequent pregnancy with a different father
- Diabetes mellitus of pregnancy
- Chronic hypertension
- Hydatid mole
- Fetal hydrops
- History of renal disease

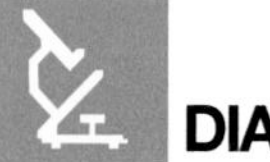

DIAGNOSIS

DIFFERENTIAL DIAGNOSIS
- Chronic hypertension
- Pregnancy worsened hypertension
- Pregnancy induced hypertension

LABORATORY
- Proteinuria (> 300 mg/24 hrs or > 1 gram/L)
- Uric acid increased (mild increase > 5.5 mg/dL [0.32 mmol/L]);

(severe increase > 9.5 mg/dL [0.56 mmol/L])
- Thrombocytopenia
- Creatinine clearance < 90 mL/min/1.73m2 (0.87 mL/s/m2)
- Increased BUN (> 16 mg/dL [5.7 mmol/L])
- Increased creatinine (> 1.0 mg/dL [88 μmol/L])
- Abnormal increased liver function tests
- Increased fibrin degradation products
- Increased PT
- Decreased fibrinogen
- Granular casts in urine
- Red blood cell casts in urine
- Renal tubular cell casts in urine
- White blood cell casts in urine
- Increased urine specific gravity
- Increased T4
- Decreased fibrinogen
- Disseminated intravascular coagulation
- Hyperbilirubinemia

Drugs that may alter lab results: N/A

Disorders that may alter lab results: Chronic renal disease

PATHOLOGICAL FINDINGS
- Fibrin deposits in kidneys
- Fibrin deposits in liver with necrosis and periportal hemorrhages
- Placental vascular abnormalities

SPECIAL TESTS N/A

IMAGING N/A

DIAGNOSTIC PROCEDURES 24 hour urine for protein

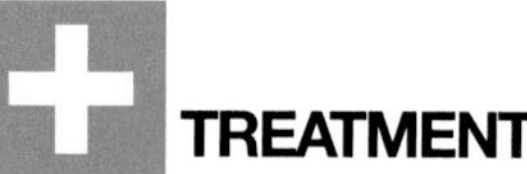

TREATMENT

APPROPRIATE HEALTH CARE
- Outpatient care if mild
- Inpatient care if deterioration
- Delivery of fetus as soon as possible if severe
- Admit to hospital if blood pressure > 160/110 (21.3/14.6 kPa), proteinuria > 5 gm/24 hr, oliguria, cerebral or visual disturbances (scotoma, blurred vision), severe headache, altered consciousness, pulmonary edema, thrombocytopenia, impaired liver function tests, epigastric pain

GENERAL MEASURES
- If outpatient, keep a daily weight record; use a home test to check for proteinuria
- If outpatient, twice a week blood pressure tests

SURGICAL MEASURES N/A

ACTIVITY
- Bedrest on left side
- Ambulatory only to void

DIET
- Salt restriction is not good because the patient is in an intravascular contracted state
- Protein 80-100 gm/day

PATIENT EDUCATION
- Excessive weight gain (>25-30 lb [11.4-13.6 kg]) should be avoided during pregnancy

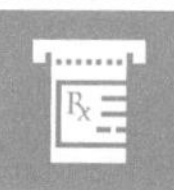

MEDICATIONS

DRUG(S) OF CHOICE For seizure prophylaxis - magnesium sulfate (MgSO4) loading dose 4 grams IV in 200 mL normal saline over 20-30 min. Maintenance dose - 1-2 grams/hr IV.

Contraindications: Refer to manufacturer's profile of each drug

Precautions:

- Therapeutic magnesium levels are 4-7 mEq/L (2-3.5 mmol/L)
- Toxicity (flushing, sweating, hyporeflexia, flaccid paralysis, CNS depression, oliguria, decreased cardiac function)
- Continue 24 hour postpartum
- Toxicity therapy with 10% calcium gluconate, 1 gram over 2-3 minutes plus oxygen
- Give oxytocin (Pitocin) postpartum to prevent bleeding (60 unit/L at 50 cc/hr)
- Keep urine flow > 25 cc/hr
- Recheck reflexes often. They may be hypoactive, but should be present.

Significant possible interactions: Refer to manufacturer's profile of each drug

ALTERNATIVE DRUGS

- Hypertension:
  - ◊ Hydralazine (Apresoline) 5-10 mg IV q 20-30 minutes, or
  - ◊ Diazoxide 30 mg minidose if refractory to hydralazine
  - ◊ Avoid nitroprusside (decreased uterine blood flow plus possible lethal fetal cyanide levels)
- Seizures:
  - ◊ MgSO4 - not as effective for treatment of seizures as it is for prophylaxis
  - ◊ Diazepam (Valium) 10 mg IV followed by 10 mg IM q4h if MgSO4 unavailable or ineffective

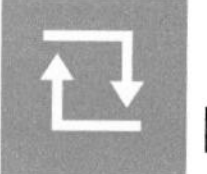

FOLLOWUP

PATIENT MONITORING

- Keep urine output > 25 cc/hr
- Continue MgSO4 for 24 hr postpartum
- Give oxytocin (Pitocin) postpartum to prevent bleeding (60 unit/L at 50 cc/hr)

PREVENTION/AVOIDANCE

- Weight control
- Large scale studies do not support low dose aspirin for prevention
- High dose calcium (1gm/day) has not been shown to prevent preeclampsia in low risk women

POSSIBLE COMPLICATIONS

- Eclampsia (seizures) - 0-2%
- Hypertensive crisis
- Acute pyelonephritis
- Acute fatty liver
- Acute pulmonary edema
- HELLP syndrome (5-10%)

EXPECTED COURSE/PROGNOSIS

- Prevention of seizures
- Delivery of viable fetus
- Estimated 30-300 deaths/1000 births depending on neonatal support capabilities

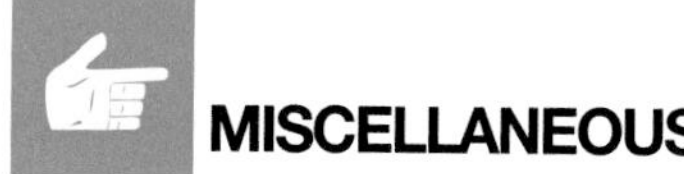

MISCELLANEOUS

ASSOCIATED CONDITIONS Abruptio placenta

AGE-RELATED FACTORS

Pediatric: Increased incidence in teenagers
Geriatric: N/A
Others: Older pregnant females (> 35 years old) have increased incidence

PREGNANCY N/A

SYNONYMS

- Pregnancy-induced hypertension
- Toxemia of pregnancy

ICD-9-CM

642.40 Mild or unspecified pre-eclampsia, unspecified
642.50 Severe pre-eclampsia, unspecified

SEE ALSO

Eclampsia (toxemia of pregnancy)

OTHER NOTES N/A

ABBREVIATIONS

MgSO4 = magnesium sulfate

REFERENCES

- Burrow GN, Ferris TF, eds: Medical complications during pregnancy. 4th ed. Philadelphia: WB Saunders; 1995:p1-28
- Cunningham FG, MacDonald PC, Gant NF, eds: Williams' Obstetrics. 20th ed. Norwalk, CT: Appleton and Lange; 1997
- Fisher S: J of Clin Investigation 1997;5
- Caritis S, et al: Low-dose aspirin to prevent preeclampsia in women at high risk. National Institute of Child Health and Human Development Network of Maternal-Fetal Medicine Units. N Engl J Med 1998;338(11):701-5

Web references: 0 available at www.5mcc.com
Illustrations N/A

Author(s):

Stoney A. Abercrombie, MD

BASICS

DESCRIPTION Labor occurring prior to the completion of 36 weeks' gestation
System(s) affected: Reproductive
Genetics: N/A
Incidence/Prevalence in USA: 8-12% of all births in the USA
Predominant age: Childbearing
Predominant sex: Female only

SIGNS & SYMPTOMS
- Regular uterine contractions, with or without pain, continuing for 1 hour
- Dull, low backache, pressure, or pain
- Intermittent lower abdominal or thigh pain
- Intestinal cramping, with or without diarrhea or indigestion
- Change in vaginal discharge
- Contractions every 5-10 minutes
- Dilatation of the cervix greater than 1 cm
- Effacement of the cervix more than 50%
- Signs of ruptured membranes (pH paper turns blue; fern positive)

CAUSES
- Infections (UTI, pyelonephritis, pneumonia)
- Subclinical chorioamnionitis (intra-amniotic infections from aerobes, anaerobes, mycoplasma, and ureaplasma)
- Uterine abnormalities (incompetent cervix, leiomyomata; septa, diethylstilbestrol DES exposure)
- Over-distention (by multiple gestation or hydramnios)
- Premature rupture of membranes
- Trauma
- Iatrogenic
- Abruption of placenta
- Immunopathology (eg, antiphospholipid antibodies)

RISK FACTORS
- Prior preterm delivery
- Multiple gestation
- Bacterial vaginosis
- Three or more first-trimester abortions
- Previous second-trimester abortion
- Cervical incompetence
- Abdominal surgery during pregnancy
- Uterine or cervical anomalies
- Placenta previa
- Premature placental separation (trauma or drug abuse - especially cocaine)
- Fetal abnormalities
- Hydramnios
- Serious maternal infection
- Vaginal bleeding in pregnancy
- Prepregnancy weight less than 45 kg (100 lb), BMI < 20
- Single parent
- No prenatal care
- Lower socioeconomic status
- Substance abuse (e.g., cocaine, tobacco)
- IUGR

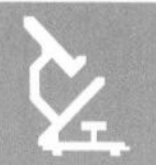

DIAGNOSIS

DIFFERENTIAL DIAGNOSIS Dehydration, urinary tract infections, round ligament pain, viral gastroenteritis, lumbosacral muscular back pain, vaginal infections, Braxton-Hicks contractions, adnexal torsion, severe constipation, appendicitis

LABORATORY
- Urinalysis and urine culture for evaluation of urinary tract infection
- Bacterial vaginosis evaluation
- Vaginal-rectal-perineal culture for group B strep
- Drug screen when appropriate
- CBC with differential
- Electrolytes, creatinine and BUN for dehydration

Drugs that may alter lab results: N/A

Disorders that may alter lab results: N/A

PATHOLOGICAL FINDINGS Placental inflammation. Acute inflammation usually caused by infection. Chronic inflammation caused by immunopathology. Abruption.

SPECIAL TESTS Consider amniocentesis if ≥32 weeks' gestation for evaluation of lecithin/sphingomyelin (L/S) ratio and phosphatidalglyceral (PG). If L/S ratio is greater than 2:1, and PG is present, hyaline membrane disease is unlikely. Also consider amniocentesis to evaluate for intra-amniotic infection (cell count with differential; glucose; gram stain; aerobic, anaerobic, mycoplasma and ureaplasma cultures.

IMAGING
- Consider uterine ultrasound to quantitate gestational age, estimated fetal weight, multiple gestations, amount of amniotic fluid, and fetal growth
- Transvaginal ultrasound to evaluate cervical length and dilatation

DIAGNOSTIC PROCEDURES
- Uterine monitoring for at least two hours or until contractions stop
- Speculum vaginal examination for signs of infection (purulent discharge, opaque membranes) and cultures
- pH and fern testing for ruptured membranes
- Digital cervical examination for effacement and dilatation (if membranes intact)
- Fetal fibronectin swabs, obtained from the posterior vaginal fornix after 22 weeks' gestation. If results are positive (≥ 50 ng/mL), patient is at an increased risk of preterm birth (sensitivity 23%, specificity 97%). If negative, consider avoiding complicated or high-risk interventions.

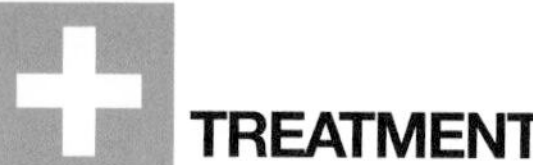

TREATMENT

APPROPRIATE HEALTH CARE Outpatient or inpatient depending on circumstances

GENERAL MEASURES
- Treat underlying risk factors with appropriate measures (antibiotics for infections, hydration for dehydration)
- If delivery is inevitable, but not immediate, consider transport to a tertiary care center or hospital equipped with a neonatal intensive care unit
- If mother is at 24-34 weeks' gestation and has no evidence of infection, administer glucocorticoids to reduce incidence of neonatal respiratory distress, intraventricular hemorrhage and necrotizing enterocolitis

SURGICAL MEASURES For malpresentation or fetal compromise, consider cesarean delivery if labor is progressing

ACTIVITY
- Pelvic rest (no douching or sexual intercourse)
- Bedrest. Discontinue work or other physical activities.
- Hospitalization may be necessary if on intravenous tocolysis or if bedrest is impossible at home

DIET Liquids only or npo, if delivery becomes imminent

PATIENT EDUCATION Call physician or proceed to hospital whenever contractions last over an hour, low back pain that comes and goes, change in vaginal discharge, "menstrual cramping." or intestinal cramping. In the presence of risk factors, patient should be counseled early in pregnancy.

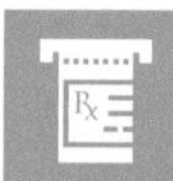

MEDICATIONS

DRUG(S) OF CHOICE

- Hydrate with 500 mL D5NS or D5LR for first half hour
- For tocolysis, protocols include:
  - ◊ Terbutaline 0.25 mg subcutaneously every 30 minutes up to 3 doses until contractions stop. Then 0.25 SQ every 6 hours for 4 doses (optional). Consider oral terbutaline 2.5-5 mg every 4-6 hours. If contractions persist or pulse is greater than 120, change to another tocolytic.
  - ◊ Magnesium sulfate solution of 40 g per 1000 mL of D5NS. Bolus 4-6 g over 20 min, then begin infusion at 2 g/hr, increasing by 0.5 g/hr every 15-30 min to a maximum of 4 g/hr; check reflexes and serum magnesium levels (therapeutic is 6-8 mg/dL [2.47-3.29 mmol/L]). Stop for significant side effects. When tocolysis occurs, decrease dose by 0.5 g/hr each hour to a minimum of 2 g/hr and then consider switch to oral therapy after 12 -24 hours.
- Antibiotics for group B strep prophylaxis pending cultures
- Glucocorticoids to reduce incidence of neonatal respiratory distress, protocols include:
  - ◊ Betamethasone 12 mg IM two doses 24h apart

  or

  - ◊ Dexamethasone 6 mg IM bid x 4 doses

  or

  - ◊ Betamethasone 12 mg IM single dose can be repeated after 7 days as long as preterm delivery is likely; discontinue at 34 weeks gestation

Contraindications:

- Severe preeclampsia, hemorrhage, chorioamnionitis, advanced labor, intrauterine growth retardation, fetal heart decelerations or lethal fetal abnormalities
- Relative contraindications to terbutaline include maternal cardiac rhythm disturbance or poorly controlled diabetes or thyrotoxicosis
- Relative contraindications to magnesium sulfate are myasthenia gravis, hypocalcemia, renal failure, or concurrent use of calcium channel blockers

Precautions:

- Palpitations, nausea, intractable vomiting, pulse greater than 140, decreased urine output
- Long-term terbutaline may adversely affect glucose tolerance. Consider repeating glucose screen if using terbutaline for more than 1 week.

Significant possible interactions: Pulmonary edema from rehydration fluids and tocolytic agents, nifedipine and magnesium sulfate

ALTERNATIVE DRUGS

- Nifedipine 10 mg po q 20 minutes x 3 doses, then 10 mg every hour. Check blood pressure often and avoid hypotension. Concurrent use with magnesium sulfate is contraindicated.
- Indomethacin: 100 mg suppository per rectum q 12 hours x 2 doses, then 25 mg every 8 hours. Use no more than 72 hours due to risk of premature closure of ductus arteriosus, oligohydramnios, and necrotizing enterocolitis.

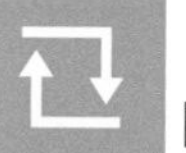

FOLLOWUP

PATIENT MONITORING

- Weekly office visits and cervical checks or cervical ultrasound for those at high risk for preterm labor
- Ambulatory external tocodynamometry has not yet been proven efficacious for prevention of preterm labor
- Treating bacterial vaginosis in second trimester with metronidazole 250 mg tid for 7 days, erythromycin base 333 mg tid for 14 days; alternatively, using clindamycin 300 mg bid for 7 days may reduce risk of premature delivery
- Controversy exists on whether maintenance tocolysis is useful, especially with negative fetal fibronectin testing
- The role of cervico-vaginal fetal fibronectin testing to assist risk assessment is controversial
- Fetal fibronectin vaginal swabs if symptoms recur - to reassess risk of preterm birth

PREVENTION/AVOIDANCE

- Patient education at each visit in 2nd and 3rd trimester for those at risk; for general population, periodically during the 2nd and 3rd trimester
- Consider cerclage placement before 22 week's gestation for those at high risk because of an incompetent cervix or progressive cervical shortening

POSSIBLE COMPLICATIONS

Labor resistant to tocolysis; pulmonary edema

EXPECTED COURSE/PROGNOSIS

If membranes are ruptured and no infection, manage expectantly, but delivery often occurs within 3-7 days. If membranes are intact, treat until 36-37 weeks, gestational age.

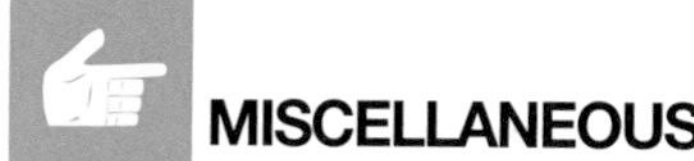

MISCELLANEOUS

ASSOCIATED CONDITIONS

See Risk Factors

AGE-RELATED FACTORS

N/A

Pediatric: N/A
Geriatric: N/A
Others: N/A

PREGNANCY

By definition, a problem of pregnancy

SYNONYMS

Preterm labor

ICD-9-CM

644.20 Early onset of delivery, unspecified as to episode of care or not applicable
644.21 Early onset of delivery, delivered with or without mention of antepartum condition

SEE ALSO

OTHER NOTES

N/A

ABBREVIATIONS

IUGR = intrauterine growth retardation

REFERENCES

- Goepfert AR, Goldenberg RL, Mercer B, et al. The preterm prediction study: quantitative fetal fibronectin values and the prediction of spontaneous preterm birth. The National Institute of Child Health and Human Development Maternal-Fetal Medicine Units Network. Am J Obstet Gynecol 2000;183(6):1480-3
- Iams JD. Preterm Birth. In: Gabbe SG, editor. Obstetrics - Normal and Preterm Pregnancies. 4th ed. New York: Churchill Livingston; 2002

Web references: 2 available at www.5mcc.com
Illustrations N/A

Author(s):
Cathryn Heath, MD
John C. Smulian, MD, MPH

Premenstrual syndrome (PMS)

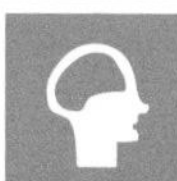

BASICS

DESCRIPTION Premenstrual syndrome is a constellation of symptoms that occurs prior to menstruation and is severe enough to interfere significantly with the patient's life. DSM-IV-R diagnosis is premenstrual dysmorphic disorder when the dominant symptoms are emotional.
System(s) affected: Endocrine/Metabolic, Nervous, Reproductive
Genetics: Unknown, probably familial incidence
Incidence/Prevalence in USA: Almost all women have some symptoms prior to menses (this is not PMS). About 5% have actual PMS.
Predominant age: Childbearing years, increasing with years
Predominant sex: Females only

SIGNS & SYMPTOMS
Symptoms can involve any organ system but the following are more common:
- Depressed mood
- Mood swings
- Irritability
- Difficulty concentrating
- Fatigue
- Edema
- Breast tenderness
- Headaches
- Sleep disturbances

CAUSES Unknown, presumed hormonal; perhaps interacting with neurotransmitters

RISK FACTORS
- Premenstrual exacerbations can occur with other diseases (i.e., depression)
- Caffeine and high fluid intake exacerbate PMS symptoms
- Stress may precipitate
- PMS increases with age
- History of depression
- Tobacco use

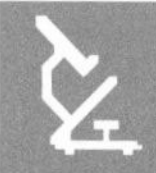

DIAGNOSIS

DIFFERENTIAL DIAGNOSIS The major differentials are psychiatric syndromes, particularly depressive disorders and/or dysthymia. Other entities may be suggested by history or physical.

LABORATORY There are no laboratory tests which confirm or refute PMS. History and physical may disclose a need for specific laboratory tests.

Drugs that may alter lab results: N/A

Disorders that may alter lab results: N/A

PATHOLOGICAL FINDINGS N/A

SPECIAL TESTS N/A

IMAGING N/A

DIAGNOSTIC PROCEDURES Patients complete questionnaires over a minimum of two months to confirm premenstrual exacerbation of symptoms and lack of substantial symptoms in the follicular phase

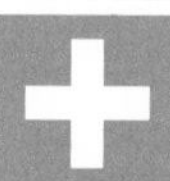

TREATMENT

APPROPRIATE HEALTH CARE Outpatient

GENERAL MEASURES
- Increase daily exercise
- Eat regular, balanced meals
- Stop smoking
- Get regular sleep
- Stress reduction techniques
- Cognitive behavioral therapy (may provide better long-term effect than SSRIs)
- Support groups
- Light therapy

SURGICAL MEASURES N/A

ACTIVITY
- No restrictions
- Exercise is recommended

DIET Low-salt; low-caffeine; low-fat; frequent, small meals; high complex carbohydrates

PATIENT EDUCATION Explain PMS and treatment

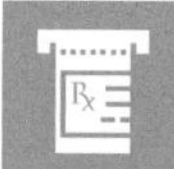

MEDICATIONS

DRUG(S) OF CHOICE

No single drug works for all women. Drugs that are used with varying degrees of success are listed.

- Antidepressants [fluoxetine (Prozac, Sarafem), sertraline, clomipramine, citalopram or nortriptyline], particularly for patients with depressive symptoms. Antidepressants can work when used only during the luteal phase of the menstrual cycle.
- Elemental calcium 1000 mg/day
- Diuretics (usually spironolactone) during luteal phase
- Symptomatic treatment of pain (ibuprofen or acetaminophen)
- Vitamin B6 in modest doses (50 mg bid, may be toxic in higher doses)
- Vitamin E: up to 600 IU/day
- Evening primrose oil, high content of fatty acids, 500 mg qd to 1000 mg tid for breast tenderness, believed to decrease prostaglandin synthesis
- Oral contraceptives may help
- Bromocriptine 2.5 mg tid at time of symptoms and danazol 100 mg bid may also work for breast tenderness, but have more side effects
- Danazol for the total PMS symptom complex
- Gonadotropin-releasing hormone agonists with or without concurrent estrogens/progestins
- L-tryptophan 2 g three times a day

Contraindications: Refer to manufacturer's profile of each drug

Precautions: Refer to manufacturer's profile of each drug

Significant possible interactions: Refer to manufacturer's profile of each drug

ALTERNATIVE DRUGS N/A

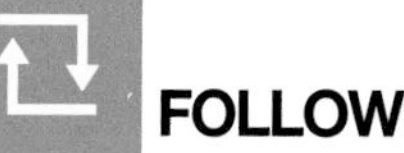

FOLLOWUP

PATIENT MONITORING See patient to provide general support and further patient education

PREVENTION/AVOIDANCE N/A

POSSIBLE COMPLICATIONS N/A

EXPECTED COURSE/PROGNOSIS

Many patients can have their symptoms adequately controlled. Disappears at menopause.

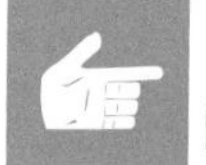

MISCELLANEOUS

ASSOCIATED CONDITIONS N/A

AGE-RELATED FACTORS

Pediatric: N/A
Geriatric: N/A
Others: N/A

PREGNANCY N/A

SYNONYMS

- Premenstrual dysphoric disorder
- PMDD

ICD-9-CM

625.4 Premenstrual tension syndromes

SEE ALSO

Mastalgia

OTHER NOTES Treatment may need to be continued for a long time. PMS sometimes continues after hysterectomy. Effects of long-term hormonal treatment unknown.

ABBREVIATIONS N/A

REFERENCES

- Practice Bulletin. The American College of Obstetricians and Gynecologists. Management of Premenstrual Syndrome. Clinical Management Guidelines No. 15, April 2000
- Grady-Weliky TA. Clinical practice. Premenstrual dysphoric disorder. N Engl J Med 2003;348(5):433-8
- Wyatt KM, Dimmock PW, O'Brien PM. Selective serotonin reuptake inhibitors for premenstrual syndrome. Cochrane Database Syst Rev 2002;(4):CD001396
- Hunter MS, Ussher JM, Browne SJ, et al. A randomized comparison of psychological (cognitive behavior therapy), medical (fluoxetine) and combined treatment for women with premenstrual dysphoric disorder. J Psychosom Obstet Gynaecol 2002;23(3):193-9

Web references: 1 available at www.5mcc.com
Illustrations N/A

Author(s):

Marjorie A. Bowman, MD, MPA

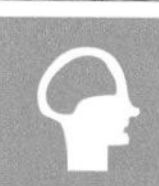

BASICS

DESCRIPTION A localized site of skin breakdown and continuum of tissue damage more likely to develop when soft tissue is compressed between bone and an external surface for prolonged time. A common and serious complication affecting usually frail, disabled, acutely ill or immobile elderly patients, especially within long-term care settings. Most common sites are over bony prominences, such as elbows, hips, heels, outer ankles, and base of spine (coccyx and sacrum with highest incidence). Over 95% of ulcers develop on lower part of body. Median length of hospital stay to treat pressure sore is 46 days. Risk of death in elderly patient increases fourfold when sores heal and sixfold when sores do not heal. Need to categorize pressure ulcers by location, stage, and size; and, presence of exudate, granulation tissue, eschar, or infection.

System(s) affected: Skin/Exocrine

Genetics: N/A

Incidence/Prevalence in USA:
- 10-17% of all hospitalized, 20-40% of all nursing home patients, 20% occur in the home
- 2 million new patients each year
- Incidence is 43/100,000 population every year; 65% of elderly with femoral fractures; 33% of critical care patients, and over 60% prevalence among quadriplegic patients and orthopedic patients
- Estimated prevalence in nursing home residents ranges from 2.6-24%

Predominant age: 60-70% are over age 70; age >85 at greatest risk

Predominant sex: Female > Male (due to survival differential); cost to heal pressure ulcer ranges from $5,000-$40,000

SIGNS & SYMPTOMS
- Stage I - non-blanching erythema, warmth, tenderness
- Stage II - skin breakdown limited to dermis, excoriation, blistering, drainage, more sharply defined erythema, variable skin temperature, local swelling or edema
- Stage III - ulcer formation into subcutaneous tissues, crater formation, slough, eschar, and/or drainage
- Stage IV - ulcers extend beyond deep fascia into muscle or bone, decayed area may be larger than visibly apparent wound, osteomyelitis or sepsis may be present, granulation tissue and epithelialization may be present at wound margins

CAUSES
- Uneven application of pressure over a bony hard site; high pressure (over 60-70 mm Hg) applied for two hours produces irreversible tissue ischemia and necrosis
- Shearing forces which develop when a seated person slides toward floor or toward foot of bed if supine
- Frictional forces which develop when pulling a patient across a bed sheet
- Moisture from incontinence or perspiration can increase the friction between two surfaces

RISK FACTORS
- Immobility (e.g., quadriplegia)
- Spinal cord injuries
- Malnutrition and low body weight
- Hypoalbuminemia (< 3.5 g/dL)
- Previous pressure ulcer
- Extended time in hospital or nursing home
- Fecal incontinence
- Urinary incontinence (moisture)
- Bone fracture (especially femoral)
- Vitamin C deficiency
- Low diastolic blood pressure
- Elder abuse
- Friction during transfers
- Age-related skin changes, such as diminished pain perception, thinning of epidermis, loss of dermal vessels, altered barrier properties, reduced immunity, and slowed wound healing
- Anemia
- Infections
- Peripheral vascular disease
- Decreased oxygen perfusion
- Dementia
- Malignancies
- Diabetes mellitus
- Cerebral vascular accidents
- Dry skin (low humidity, < 40%, and cold)
- Fractures
- Edema
- Assessment scales for evaluating risk factors include: Norton, Braden (Braden Q version for children), Waterlow and Walsall

DIAGNOSIS

DIFFERENTIAL DIAGNOSIS
- Stasis or ischemic ulcers
- Vasculitides
- Cancers
- Radiation injury
- Pyoderma gangrenosum and other dermatologic conditions

LABORATORY
- Culture of wound if there is evidence of infection (surrounding erythema, purulent drainage, foul odor)
- White blood cell count and differential if fever is present (greater than 37°C)
- Erythrocyte sedimentation rate
- If above tests positive, blood and urine cultures to identify causative agents

Drugs that may alter lab results: N/A

Disorders that may alter lab results: N/A

PATHOLOGICAL FINDINGS Extensive necrosis of affected part

SPECIAL TESTS N/A

IMAGING Plain radiographs if bone involvement suspected

DIAGNOSTIC PROCEDURES N/A

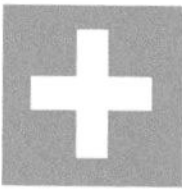

TREATMENT

APPROPRIATE HEALTH CARE
- An interdisciplinary approach usually indicated in nursing home, inpatient or home care settings if trained supervision available
- Wound healing from inflammation to remodeling is dependent on energy and protein synthesis
- Complications will require inpatient setting to treat systemic infection, extensive debridement or skin grafting

GENERAL MEASURES
- Improve overall nutritional status (adequate protein intake)
- Clean wound each time dressing is changed to remove dead tissue, excess fluid and other debris
- Avoid rolling the patient, and prop heels off bed
- Insufficient evidence whether sterile technique is better than clean dressing change in reducing infection risk or improving healing time.
- Healing enhanced with body temperature maintained at 37°C (97.7°F) and an acidic pH
- Never use antiseptics and skin cleansers (eg, Betadine) which harm the tissue
- Surgery for wounds not responding to treatment within 2-4 weeks
- Débridement of necrotic pressure ulcers using occlusive dressings, hydrotherapy, proteolytic enzymes, or surgical or laser débridement
- Pressure reduction products such as specialized beds and repositioning every two hours to relieve pressure at site of ulceration (air-fluidized or low-air-loss beds); static-pressure and foam mattresses, water mattresses, sheepskins, and egg-crate mattresses are less expensive devices.
- Avoid agents that delay wound healing, such as topical corticosteroids, hydrogen peroxide, povidone iodine solution, and hypochlorite solutions
- Avoid saline dressings that interrupt fragile wound healing
- Control of fecal and/or urine incontinence
- Inadequate data to support use of electromagnetic therapy

Specific measures by stage as follows:
- Stage I: Nonblanchable erythema of intact skin
  - ◊ Relieve pressure (floatation or airflow mattress/bed)
  - ◊ Use moisture barrier lubricant, transparent bio-occlusive dressings (Opsite) or Granulex Spray on reddened areas
  - ◊ Keep all skin areas clean and dry
  - ◊ Assess skin every 8-12 hours
- Stage II: Partial thickness skin loss of epidermis, dermis, or both; presents as abrasion, blister or crater
  - ◊ Use dry 4 x 4's to cleanse pressure sore followed by topical antibiotic
  - ◊ Apply protective barrier film to unbroken skin surrounding pressure sore
  - ◊ Apply occlusive hydrocolloid dressing (Duoderm)
  - ◊ Repeat every three days
  - ◊ Loosely pack wound
  - ◊ Whirlpools useful for debriding necrotic wounds
- Stage III: Full thickness skin loss through subcutaneous tissue down to but not through underlying fascia; presents as deep crater with or without undermining adjacent tissue
  - ◊ Scrub and debride with dry gauze and gels for autolytic débridement
  - ◊ Re-rinse wound
  - ◊ Blot excess moisture with dry 4 x 4 gauze
  - ◊ Apply protective barrier film
  - ◊ Apply skin care product (occlusive hydrocolloid dressing, granules, or paste)
  - ◊ If wound highly exudative, use absorption dressing (exudate absorbers) and change daily; consider wound culture
  - ◊ For necrotic wounds, consider high-pressure injection using 35-mL syringe and 19-gauge angiocatheter
- Stage IV: Full thickness skin loss with exposure or destruction extended to muscle, bone and/or other supportive structure
  - ◊ If eschar present, needs debridement or wait for sloughing

◊ Blot excess moisture with 4 x 4 dry gauze
◊ Apply protective barrier film to unbroken skin surrounding sore
◊ Moisten packing gauze (Kerlix) in saline and pack wound
◊ Apply outer dressing
◊ Negative pressure therapy (vacuum-assisted closure device)
◊ Surgical intervention for definitive treatment of deep and complicated pressure ulcers, such as myocutaneous flaps, split-thickness skin grafts and primary closure

SURGICAL MEASURES See under various stages in General Measures

ACTIVITY
- Any activity consistent with patient's ambulatory status and relief of pressure on wound
- Perform passive range-of-motion exercises for patient or encourage patient to do active exercises if possible

DIET
- Oral high-calorie and high-protein supplements, including daily multivitamin with 100% RDA
- Vitamin A to aid epithelialization and fibroblast stimulation, vitamin C (500 mg/day) to aid collagen synthesis and tensile strength, zinc (15 mg/day) for protein synthesis, copper for collagen production and cross-linking, manganese for collagen and ground substance

PATIENT EDUCATION
- Patient Care 1993; 27(7):65-66
- National Action Group for the Prevention and Treatment of Decubitus Ulcers, P.O. Box 1098, Union City, CT 06770
- AHCPR publications - No. 92-0048, Preventing Pressure Ulcers: A Patient's Guide and No. 95-0654, Treating Pressure Sores: Consumer's Guide; 800-358-9295
- Patient information handout from: Findley D: Practical management of pressure ulcers. Amer Fam Phys 1996;54(3):1519-1536

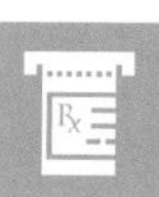

MEDICATIONS

DRUG(S) OF CHOICE
- Clindamycin or gentamicin for complications such as cellulitis, osteomyelitis, or sepsis
- Supplements - vitamin C 500 mg twice a day, zinc sulfate
- Antibiotic prophylaxis for bacterial endocarditis if valvular lesions present
- Two week trial of topical antimicrobials (e.g., silver sulfadiazine or triple antibiotics) should be used only for a clean superficial ulcer not healing or producing moderate amount of exudate; cultures are necessary to determine whether antifungal (miconazole, clotrimazole, or haloprogin) or specific antibacterial agents (silver sulfadiazine, neomycin-polymyxin B-bacitracin, gentamicin, mupirocin 2%) are indicated
- Enzymatic debridement agents such as collagenase (Santyl), trypsin (Granulex), fibrinolysin-deoxyribonuclease (Elase), papain (Panafil) or sutilains (Travase) used with a moisture barrier to protect surrounding normal tissue
- Profore pressure bandages for venous stasis, changed every 4-7 days
- Recommended dressings include Saran Wrap, polyurethane films (Op-site, Tegaderm), absorbent hydrocolloid dressings (Duoderm, Comfeel Ulcus)
- Recombinant human platelet-derived growth factor [e.g., becaplermin (Regranex) gel] for diabetic neuropathic ulcers extending through the dermis

Contraindications: Refer to manufacturer's literature
Precautions: Refer to manufacturer's literature
Significant possible interactions: Refer to manufacturer's literature

ALTERNATIVE DRUGS
Miscellaneous treatments
- Calendula ointment or a 5% flower extract with allantoin stimulates new epithelial growth in surgical wounds
- Two drops of tea tree oil in 8 ounces of water - used as a rinse to decrease risk of infection
- Marshmallow root ointment over wound daily
- Nerve growth factor
- Electrical stimulation
- Anabolic hormones (injectable and oral) may promote weight gain, esp. LBM, limited evidence effective in nonhealing wounds, consider testosterone, testosterone analogs (eg, oxandrolone), or growth hormone (IGF-1).
- Unproven alternate therapies include - sterile maggots, hyperbaric oxygen, low-energy laser irradiation, ultrasound therapy

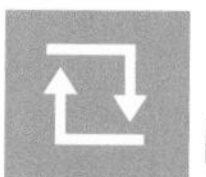

FOLLOWUP

PATIENT MONITORING
- Frequent evaluation of all patients with history of pressure sores, especially if limited mobility. Include nutritional status and dietary intervention.
- Early identification of areas of skin redness to prevent subsequent breakdown
- Skin cleansing as soon as soiled and at routine intervals
- Home telemedicine to assess treatment

PREVENTION/AVOIDANCE
- Up to 95% of all pressure ulcers are preventable
- Assess nutrient status and provide required macro- and micronutrients, by oral route, enteral, or parenteral if necessary
- Resistance exercise to speed up LBM growth
- Pressure reducing support surfaces (eg, high-density, 4 inch foam overlays)
- Keep the skin clean and dry by using mild soap, warm water and moisturizer
- Early identification of at risk individuals and elimination of risk factors (risk assessment tools: Brader Scale for Predicting Pressure Sore Risk for nursing home patients and The Norton Scale for hospitalized patients)
- Underpads (non-cloth) to absorb moisture
- Quality nursing care
- Early interdisciplinary supportive care - include staff, patient, family/caregiver
- Nutritional assessment of patient, 24-hour dietary recall and serum pre-albumin, especially if cannot take food by mouth or has experienced involuntary change in weight
- Frequent patient repositioning if immobile - every hour if wheelchair bound and every 2 hours if bedridden
- Positioning devices
- Functional assessment of patient and treatment of incontinence
- Frequent physical examination of skin areas affected by pressure, moisture, shearing or friction sources
- Use mattress overlays, thick air seat cushions and high specification mattresses and beds to reduce pressure on pressure points, especially for hospitalized patients

POSSIBLE COMPLICATIONS
- Growth of resistant organisms if antibiotics used inappropriately
- Sepsis, cellulitis, septic arthritis, sinus tract or abscess, squamous cell carcinoma in ulcer
- Osteomyelitis in up to 25% of nonhealing ulcers
- Gangrene
- Increased incidence of death annually

EXPECTED COURSE/PROGNOSIS
- Though pressure ulcers are associated with an increased rate of mortality, with good medical care, most can be expected to heal
- In a recent study among long-term care hospital patients, 79% of pressure sores improved and 40% completely healed during a six-week followup period using ordinary therapies

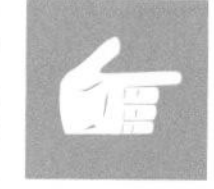

MISCELLANEOUS

ASSOCIATED CONDITIONS
- Malnutrition
- Fecal and/or urinary incontinence
- Immobility
- Impaired mental status
- Skin atrophy
- Low body weight
- Compromised immune states

AGE-RELATED FACTORS
Pediatric: N/A
Geriatric: Over 60% occur in elderly
Others: N/A

PREGNANCY N/A

SYNONYMS
- Decubitus ulcer
- Bedsore
- Trophic ulcer
- Pressure sore

ICD-9-CM
707.0 Decubitus ulcer

SEE ALSO

OTHER NOTES N/A

ABBREVIATIONS N/A

REFERENCES

- Dharmarajan TS, Ahmed S. The growing problem of pressure ulcers. Evaluation and management for an aging population. Postgrad Med 2003;113(5):77-8, 81-4, 88-90

Web references: 3 available at www.5mcc.com
Illustrations N/A

Author(s):
Evan W. Kligman, MD

BASICS

DESCRIPTION Painful and/or abnormally prolonged penile erection
System(s) affected: Reproductive
Genetics: N/A
Incidence/Prevalence in USA: Unknown
Predominant age: Young adult
Predominant sex: Male only

SIGNS & SYMPTOMS
- Penile erection that is persistent, prolonged, painful, and tender
- Urination difficult during erection
- Loss of sexual function if treatment is not prompt and effective
- Low flow or ischemic priapism - glans penis flaccid
- High flow or arterial priapism - glans penis rigid

CAUSES
- Intracavernosal injections of vasoactive drugs for erectile dysfunction; most common cause
- Pelvic vascular thrombosis
- Prolonged sexual activity
- Sickle cell anemia
- Leukemia
- Other blood dyscrasias
- Pelvic hematoma or neoplasia
- Cerebrospinal tumors
- Tertiary syphilis
- Bladder calculus
- Injury to penis
- Urinary tract infections, especially prostatitis, urethritis, cystitis
- Several drugs suspected as causing priapism, such as chlorpromazine, prazosin, trazodone, and certain corticosteroids, anticoagulants, antihypertensives
- Intracavernous fat emulsion

RISK FACTORS
- Dehydration

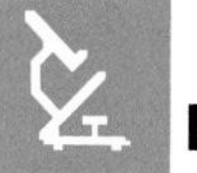

DIAGNOSIS

DIFFERENTIAL DIAGNOSIS List with Causes

LABORATORY
- CBC
- Sickle prep and hgb electrophoresis
- Coagulation profile
- Platelet count
- Urinalysis

Drugs that may alter lab results: N/A

Disorders that may alter lab results: N/A

PATHOLOGICAL FINDINGS
- Pelvic vascular thrombosis
- Partial thrombosis of corpora cavernosa
- Corpus spongiosum, glans penis: No involvement
- Arterial priapism will show arteriocavernous fistula

SPECIAL TESTS N/A

IMAGING
- Penile doppler testing may be necessary to differentiate high-flow from low-flow priapism

DIAGNOSTIC PROCEDURES Physical examination

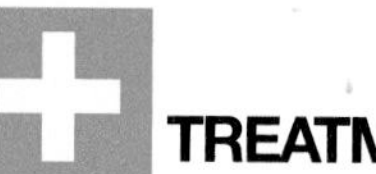

TREATMENT

APPROPRIATE HEALTH CARE Inpatient

GENERAL MEASURES
- Reassurance about outcome if warranted
- Continuous caudal or spinal anesthesia if etiology is neurogenic
- Treat any underlying cause
- In sickle cell anemia: Intravenous hydration; partial exchange or repeated transfusions to reduce percent of sickle cells below 50%
- Pain relief

SURGICAL MEASURES
- Introduction of 12 or 16 gauge needles into corpora cavernosa (best done by urologist if available)
  - ◊ First: aspiration of 20-30 cc of blood from corpora cavernosum with 12-16 gauge needle
  - ◊ Then: if caused by injected vasodilator, use intracavernous injection of 10-25 mg ephedrine sulfate or 5-10 μg epinephrine or 125-250 μg phenylephrine
  - ◊ May repeat one time in 20-30 minutes if no response
- Create fistula between glans and corpus cavernosum (with biopsy needle by urologist)
- Semipermanent diversion by saphenous shunt from one or both corpora
- Cavernosa-spongiosum shunt to permit reestablishment of pelvic circulation

ACTIVITY Bedrest until relieved

DIET N/A

PATIENT EDUCATION
- Information about long-term outlook, referral for counseling
- Reduction of vasoactive drug therapy, if responsible for priapism and elimination of offending drugs if causal

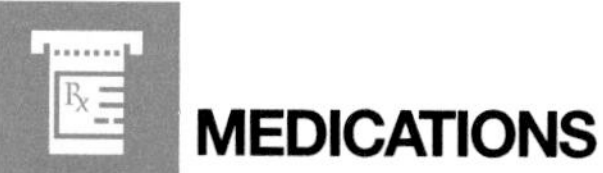

MEDICATIONS

DRUG(S) OF CHOICE
- Narcotics for pain if needed
- Vasoconstrictors may be injected after dilution, e.g., metaraminol 1 mg into the penis

Contraindications: Refer to manufacturer's literature
Precautions: Refer to manufacturer's literature
Significant possible interactions: Refer to manufacturer's literature

ALTERNATIVE DRUGS N/A

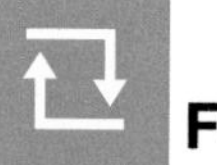

FOLLOWUP

PATIENT MONITORING
Close followup after surgery

PREVENTION/AVOIDANCE
- Avoid dehydration
- Avoid excessive sexual stimulation
- Avoid causative drugs (see Causes) when possible

POSSIBLE COMPLICATIONS
- Erectile dysfunction (impotence)

EXPECTED COURSE/PROGNOSIS
- Even with excellent treatment, detumescence may require several weeks
- Impotence is likely

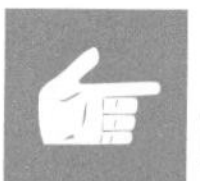

MISCELLANEOUS

ASSOCIATED CONDITIONS
Sickle cell anemia

AGE-RELATED FACTORS
Pediatric: > 85% likelihood of sickle cell in African American children
Geriatric: Treatment more difficult and less likely successful
Others: N/A

PREGNANCY N/A

SYNONYMS N/A

ICD-9-CM
607.3 Priapism

SEE ALSO
Anemia, sickle cell
Erectile dysfunction

OTHER NOTES N/A

ABBREVIATIONS N/A

REFERENCES

- Smith DR: General Urology. 15th Ed. Los Altos, CA, Lange Medical Publications, 2000
- Tanagho EA, McAninch JW, eds: Smith's General Urology. 12th Ed. Norwalk, CT, Appleton & Lange, 1988
- Harmon WJ and Nehra A: Priapism: Diagnosis and Management. Mayo Clinic Proceedings 12 (4) April 1997: 350-355.
- Burnett AL. Pathophysiology of priapism: dysregulatory erection physiology thesis. Journal of Urology 170(1), July 2003, pp. 26-34

Web references: 0 available at www.5mcc.com
Illustrations N/A

Author(s):
Bruce Block, MD

BASICS

DESCRIPTION Pulmonary arterial hypertension of unknown cause, where secondary causes have been ruled out. Three pathologic subtypes have been identified: (1) thrombotic (56%), (2) plexogenic (28%), (3) veno-occlusive (16%).
System(s) affected: Cardiovascular, Pulmonary
Genetics: 7% familial; autosomal dominant with variable expression and "genetic anticipation"
Incidence/Prevalence in USA: 1-2 cases/million. 1% of all causes of cor pulmonale at autopsy. 0.5-2% of patients with portal hypertension or HIV
Predominant age: Mean age 34-36 years; second incidence peak in males 50-59 years
Predominant sex: Female > Male (3:1)

SIGNS & SYMPTOMS
- Loud P2 (> 80%)
- Right ventricular lift (> 80%)
- Dyspnea (> 75%)
- Murmur of tricuspid insufficiency (50-80%)
- Increased jugular venous pressure (50-80%)
- Right ventricular S4 (50-80%)
- Chest pain (> 50%)
- Fatigue (> 50%)
- Palpitations (< 50%)
- Syncope; dizziness (< 50%)
- Cough (< 50%)
- Raynaud phenomenon (< 10%)
- Hepatomegaly (< 50%)
- Pulmonic ejection click (< 50%)
- Right ventricular S3 (< 50%)
- Murmur of pulmonic insufficiency (< 50%)
- Lower extremity edema (< 50%)
- Superficial thrombophlebitis (5%)

CAUSES
- Unknown; possible pulmonary arteriolar hyperactivity and vasoconstriction; occult thromboembolism; possible autoimmune (high frequency antinuclear antibodies)
- In Europe, reports of PPH associated with anorectic agent aminorex fumarate in late 1960's; tainted rapeseed oil
- HIV positive patients may have an increased incidence of primary pulmonary hypertension
- Anorectic agents (fenfluramine and dexfenfluramine)
- Amphetamines

RISK FACTORS Female sex

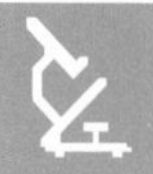

DIAGNOSIS

DIFFERENTIAL DIAGNOSIS
- Pulmonary parenchymal disease (COPD, asthma, pulmonary fibrosis, granulomatous disease, malignancy)
- Pulmonary vascular disease (pulmonary thromboembolism, collagen vascular disease, pulmonary arteritis, schistosomiasis, sickle cell disease)
- Cardiac disease (cardiomyopathy, valvular heart disease, congenital heart disease, persistent fetal circulation, pulmonary venous hypertension)
- Other disorders of respiratory function (sleep apnea syndromes, neuromuscular diseases, pleural diseases, thoracic cage abnormalities)
- IV drug abuse

LABORATORY
- ANA positive (1/3 of patients)

Drugs that may alter lab results: Hydralazine, procainamide, isoniazid, etc.

Disorders that may alter lab results: Many other diseases, e.g., lupus, scleroderma

PATHOLOGICAL FINDINGS
- Medial hypertrophy and arterial thrombosis are common in all subtypes
- Plexogenic pulmonary arteriopathy (30-70%): laminar "onion skin" intimal proliferation, focal medial disruption, aneurysmal dilatation
- Microthromboemboli (20-50%)
- Veno-occlusive disease (10-15%)

SPECIAL TESTS
- ECG: right ventricular hypertrophy and right axis deviation
- Pulmonary function testing: arterial hypoxemia, reduced diffusion capacity, hypocapnia
- V/Q scan: must rule out proximal pulmonary artery emboli
- Exercise test: reduced maximal O2 consumption, high minute ventilation, low anaerobic threshold, reduced maximal oxygen pulse, increased DO2A-a. Correlation to severity of disease with 6 minute walk test.

IMAGING
- Chest x-ray: enlarged central pulmonary arteries with pulmonary arterial branches attenuated. Right ventricular enlargement a late finding. If increased interstitial markings, consider lung parenchymal disease or veno-occlusive disease.
- Echo-Doppler: right ventricular enlargement and overload; important to rule out underlying cardiac disease such as atrial septal defect with secondary pulmonary hypertension or mitral stenosis
- Ultra fast CT: sensitivity probably equal to pulmonary angiogram with lower contrast dose

DIAGNOSTIC PROCEDURES
- Chest x-ray, pulmonary function tests, arterial blood gases, and V/Q scan should be done
- Cardiac catheterization: right heart catheterization is necessary to measure pulmonary artery pressures and hemodynamics; rule out underlying cardiac disease and response to vasodilator therapy
- Pulmonary angiography: should be done if segmental or larger defect on V/Q scan. Caution in pulmonary hypertension as can lead to hemodynamic collapse; use low osmolar agents, subselective angiograms.
- Lung biopsy: not recommended

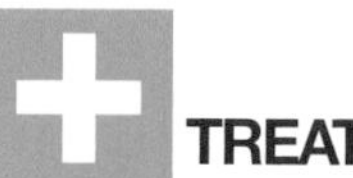

TREATMENT

APPROPRIATE HEALTH CARE
- Medical therapy is first line and primarily palliative; health care is guided by clinical status
- Hospitalization with invasive monitoring is needed to screen vasodilator responsiveness and initiate vasodilator therapy
- There is a national registry established by the National Heart, Lung, and Blood Institute

GENERAL MEASURES
- Primary modalities are oxygen supplementation, vasodilators, anticoagulants, and treatment of heart failure (e.g., diuretics)
- Oxygen supplementation is indicated for rest, exercise, or nocturnal hypoxemia
- The acute response to vasodilators may improve survival; hydralazine, calcium channel blockers and prostacyclin

SURGICAL MEASURES
- Surgical procedures - patients with documented large vessel thromboembolic disease should be considered for pulmonary thrombectomy
- Heart-lung or lung transplantation is an option for appropriate patients when medical therapy has failed
- Blade-balloon atrial septostomy

ACTIVITY Restricted; exercise worsens pulmonary vascular resistance

DIET Low salt with heart failure

PATIENT EDUCATION
- Need to discuss prognosis; options such as transplantation
- Avoidance of pregnancy

MEDICATIONS

DRUG(S) OF CHOICE

- Medical therapy may be guided by suspected subtype:
  - ◊ Plexogenic (clear lung fields, normal perfusion scan) - vasodilators potentially useful. Vasodilators - calcium channel blockers, first line, may be more effective in high doses. Other agents: ACE-inhibitors, alpha-antagonists, hydralazine - none shown to improve survival.
  - ◊ Thrombotic (clear lung fields, patchy perfusion scan) - anticoagulants potentially useful. Anticoagulants - warfarin, heparin, antiplatelet agents.
  - ◊ Veno-occlusive (pulmonary venous congestion, patchy perfusion scan) - vasodilators probably useless

All types: Heart failure may be treated with diuretics. Digoxin use controversial - not shown to be beneficial or detrimental. Digoxin may adversely affect exercise capacity due to increase in pulmonary vascular resistance.

- Chronic vasodilator therapy
  - ◊ Nifedipine, diltiazem
  - ◊ Prostacyclin
  - ◊ Hydralazine
  - ◊ Isoproterenol
  - ◊ Terbutaline
  - ◊ Prazosin
  - ◊ Phentolamine
  - ◊ Phenoxybenzamine
- Screening for responsiveness
  - ◊ Prostacyclin
  - ◊ Iloprost; stable analog of prostacyclin
  - ◊ Acetylcholine
  - ◊ Adenosine
  - ◊ Nitric oxide
  - ◊ Nitroprusside
  - ◊ Isoproterenol
  - ◊ Hydralazine
  - ◊ Phentolamine
- Anticoagulation: 2 small studies suggest prolonged survival. Warfarin with INR ≈2.0.

Contraindications: Avoid warfarin in patients with syncope or hemoptysis

Precautions: Vasodilator therapy and response should be evaluated with invasive monitoring. Short acting agents such as prostacyclin, adenosine, or acetylcholine are useful for screening.

Significant possible interactions: Refer to manufacturer's literature

ALTERNATIVE DRUGS N/A

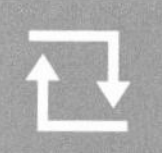

FOLLOWUP

PATIENT MONITORING Frequent

PREVENTION/AVOIDANCE None

POSSIBLE COMPLICATIONS Thromboembolism, heart failure, sudden death

EXPECTED COURSE/PROGNOSIS

- Mean survival 2-3 years from time of diagnosis, 75% mortality at 5 years, although survival is quite variable as learned from the NIH registry.
- Mean age at diagnosis 34 years
- Mode of death:
  - ◊ Right heart failure 63%
  - ◊ Indeterminate 15%
  - ◊ Pneumonia 7%
  - ◊ Sudden death 7%
  - ◊ Cardiac death 5%
- Poor prognostic factors:
  - ◊ PaO2 < 63%
  - ◊ RA pressure > 20 mm Hg
  - ◊ Cardiac index < 2 L/min/m2
  - ◊ Mean pulmonary arterial pressure > 85 mm Hg
  - ◊ New York Heart Assn. (NYHA) class 3 or 4
  - ◊ Raynaud phenomenon

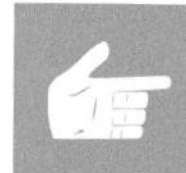

MISCELLANEOUS

ASSOCIATED CONDITIONS

- Portal hypertension
- Systemic lupus erythematosus
- HIV
- Raynaud

AGE-RELATED FACTORS

Pediatric: N/A
Geriatric: N/A
Others: N/A

PREGNANCY Must be avoided; high mother and fetal wastage

SYNONYMS Primary pulmonary vascular disease

ICD-9-CM

416.0 Primary pulmonary hypertension

SEE ALSO

Cor pulmonale
Pulmonary embolism

OTHER NOTES N/A

ABBREVIATIONS

V/Q = ventilation-perfusion ratio

REFERENCES

- Palevsky HE, Fishman AP: The management of primary pulmonary hypertension. JAMA 1991;265:1014-1020
- Hawkins JW, Dunn MI: Primary pulmonary hypertension in adults. Clinical Cardiology 1990;13:382-387
- Rich S: Primary pulmonary hypertension. In: Isselbacher KJ, et al, eds. Harrison's Principles of Internal Medicine. 13th Ed. McGraw-Hill, New York, 1994
- Cremona G, Higenbottom T: Role of prostacyclin in the treatment of pulmonary hypertension. AF Cardio 1995;75(3):67A-71A
- Olschewski H, Walmrath D, Schermuly R, Ghofrani A, Grimminger F, Seeger W. Aerosolized prostacyclin and iloprost in severe pulmonary hypertension. Ann Intern Med 1996 May 1;124(9):820-4

Web references: 0 available at www.5mcc.com
Illustrations N/A

Author(s):

Darell E. Heiselman, DO

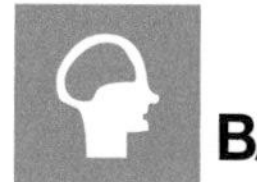

BASICS

DESCRIPTION An acute or chronic inflammation of the rectal mucosa
System(s) affected: Gastrointestinal
Genetics: Higher incidence in Jews
Incidence/Prevalence in USA: 0.5-3/100,000 (ulcerative proctitis)/10-30/100,000 (ulcerative proctitis)
Predominant age: Adult
Predominant sex: Male > Female

SIGNS & SYMPTOMS
- Rectal and/or perianal discomfort
- Rectal bleeding and/or mucous discharge
- Diarrhea
- Tenesmus
- Urgency
- Constipation
- Fever
- Weight loss

CAUSES
- Idiopathic
- Rectal gonorrhea
- Crohn disease
- Syphilis (usually secondary)
- Nonspecific sexually transmitted infection
- *Herpes simplex*
- Chlamydia
- Papillomavirus
- Amebiasis
- *Lymphogranuloma venereum*
- Ischemia
- Radiation therapy
- Toxins (e.g., hydrogen peroxide enemas)
- Vasculitis

RISK FACTORS
- Rectal intercourse
- Radiation
- Rectal injury
- Rectal medications
- Jewish heritage

DIAGNOSIS

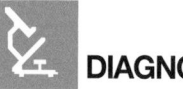

DIFFERENTIAL DIAGNOSIS
- Traumatic proctitis
- Radiation proctitis
- Ulcerative colitis
- Crohn disease
- Infections such as shigellosis or amebiasis

LABORATORY
- Serological tests for syphilis, ameba
- Smear, culture from rectal wall
- Stool cultures

Drugs that may alter lab results: N/A

Disorders that may alter lab results: N/A

PATHOLOGICAL FINDINGS
- Inflammation of rectal mucosa
- Ulceration
- Disruption of crypts

SPECIAL TESTS N/A

IMAGING N/A

DIAGNOSTIC PROCEDURES
- Flexible sigmoidoscopy
- Biopsy for histology, culture, viral studies, chlamydia culture
- Colonoscopy to exclude more proximal involvement

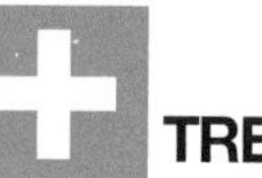

TREATMENT

APPROPRIATE HEALTH CARE Outpatient, unless severe and refractory to usual measures

GENERAL MEASURES
- Treatment depends upon the cause
- Rectal gram stains have significant false-negative rate and if clinician has strong suspicion of gonorrheal proctitis, empiric treatment warranted while culture results pending
- Avoidance of causative factors
- Sitz baths may provide some relief

SURGICAL MEASURES N/A

ACTIVITY No restrictions

DIET No special diet

PATIENT EDUCATION Counseling regarding HIV infection risk

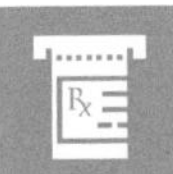

MEDICATIONS

DRUG(S) OF CHOICE
- Ulcerative proctitis - topical steroids (enemas or foam), mesalamine (Rowasa, 5-ASA, 5-aminosalicylic acid) enemas or suppositories; oral mesalamine (Asacol, Pentasa), olsalazine (Dipentum), sulfasalazine; systemic steroids when refractory to above drugs
- Gonorrheal - IM ceftriaxone 250 mg in a single dose plus doxycycline 100 mg orally bid for 7 days
- Herpetic - oral acyclovir 200-400 mg 5 times a day for 10 days
- Chlamydial - oral tetracycline 500 mg tid or doxycycline 100 mg bid

Contraindications: Refer to manufacturer's literature
Precautions: Refer to manufacturer's literature
Significant possible interactions: Refer to manufacturer's literature

ALTERNATIVE DRUGS For gonorrheal - in patients unable to take ceftriaxone - IM spectinomycin 2 g in a single dose or ciprofloxacin 500 mg orally in a single dose. Perform culture 4-7 days after treatment to verify efficacy of treatment.

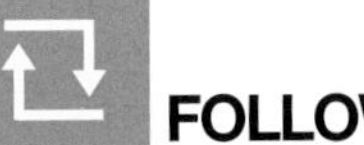

FOLLOWUP

PATIENT MONITORING Follow until completely healed and monthly thereafter for 6 months

PREVENTION/AVOIDANCE Safe sex, if sexually transmitted

POSSIBLE COMPLICATIONS
- Chronic ulcerative colitis
- Fistulae/abscess formation
- Treatment failure (may be as much as 35% in gonorrhea proctitis)
- Perforation

EXPECTED COURSE/PROGNOSIS
Satisfactory cure or control with appropriate treatment

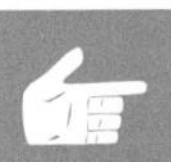

MISCELLANEOUS

ASSOCIATED CONDITIONS
- Syphilis
- Gonorrhea
- Other sexually transmitted disease
- Prostate cancer (radiation therapy)

AGE-RELATED FACTORS
Pediatric:
- Not common, but if found, is more apt to spread to full-blown disease in more proximal areas of the colon
- Consider sexual abuse, if gonorrheal infection

Geriatric: Slower to heal, consider ischemia
Others: N/A

PREGNANCY N/A

SYNONYMS N/A

ICD-9-CM
569.49 Other specified disorders of rectum and anus, other

SEE ALSO
Crohn disease
Gonococcal infections
Herpes simplex
Lymphogranuloma venereum
Syphilis
Ulcerative colitis

OTHER NOTES N/A

ABBREVIATIONS N/A

REFERENCES

- Wexner SD: Sexually transmitted diseases of the colon, rectum, and anus. The challenge of the nineties. Dis Colon Rectum 1990;33:1048-62
- Kirsner JB, Shorter G, eds: Diseases of the Colon, Rectum and Anal Canal. Baltimore, Williams & Wilkins, 1989
- Rompalo A. Diagnosis and treatment of sexually acquired proctitis and proctocolitis: an update. Clin Infec Dis 1999;28(suppl1):s84-90
- Swaroop VS, Gostout CJ. Endoscopic treatment of radiation proctopathy. J Clin Gastroenterol 1998;27:36-40
- Strong S, Fazio V. Crohn's disease of the colon, rectum and anus. Surg Clin NA 1993;73:933-63

Web references: 6 available at www.5mcc.com
Illustrations N/A

Author(s):
Philip E. Jaffe, MD

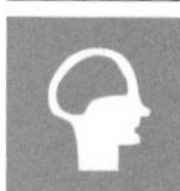

BASICS

DESCRIPTION The prostate is composed of acinar glands and their ducts arranged in a radial fashion with the stroma containing blood vessels, lymphatics and nerves. 95% of prostate cancers are acinar adenocarcinomas.
- TNM staging
  - ◊ T1 Clinically inapparent tumor not palpable or visible by imaging
  - ◊ T1a Tumor incidental histological finding in 5% or less of tissue resected
  - ◊ T1b Tumor incidental histological finding in more than 5% of tissue resected
  - ◊ T1c Tumor identified by needle biopsy (eg, because of elevated PSA)
  - ◊ T2 Tumor confined within the prostate†
  - ◊ T2a Tumor involves one lobe
  - ◊ T2b tumor involves both lobes
  - ◊ T3 Tumor extends through the prostatic capsule††
  - ◊ T3a Extracapsular extension (unilateral or bilateral)
  - ◊ T3b Tumor invades seminal vesicle(s)
  - ◊ T4 Tumor is fixed or invades adjacent structures other than seminal vesicles; bladder neck, external sphincter, rectum, levator muscles, and/or pelvic wall

† Tumor found in one or both lobes by needle biopsy, but not palpable or visible by imaging, is classified as T1c

†† Invasion into the prostatic apex or into (but not beyond) the prostatic capsule is not classified as T3, but as T2

System(s) affected: Reproductive
Genetics: Unknown
Incidence/Prevalence in USA:
- Incidence: 200/100,000 men per year
- Approximately 30% of 30 year old men and 70% of 80 year old men have pathologically discernible intraepithelial neoplasia of the prostate giving this condition a very high prevalence

Predominant age: Sixth or seventh decade; mean age at diagnosis is 71 years
Predominant sex: Male only

SIGNS & SYMPTOMS
- May be asymptomatic early or late in the course of disease
- Induration of the prostate on digital rectal exam
- Hard prostate, localized or diffuse
- Bladder outlet symptoms
- Acute urinary retention
- Hematuria (rare)
- Urinary tract infection (usually unrelated)
- Bone pain
- Weight loss
- Anemia
- Shortness of breath
- Lymphedema
- Neurologic symptoms
- Lymphadenopathy

CAUSES Unknown

RISK FACTORS
- Genetic predisposition (risk of prostatic cancer increases if a malignancy has occurred in a first degree relative)
- Endogenous hormonal influences
- Exposure to chemical carcinogens
- Sexually transmitted diseases
- Male over 60 years of age
- Increased risk with vasectomy has been newly proposed but is unsupported

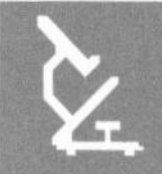

DIAGNOSIS

DIFFERENTIAL DIAGNOSIS
- Benign nodule prostate growth
- Prostate stones
- Nodular whorls of adenoma
- Seminal vesicle enlargement

LABORATORY
- Prostate specific antigen (PSA), elevated
- Free PSA - low in cancer (Catalana, et al: JAMA 1995;274:1213-1220)
- Alkaline phosphatase, elevated with metastasis
- Urine cytology, rarely helpful

Drugs that may alter lab results: None

Disorders that may alter lab results:
- Rectal manipulation will not significantly increase PSA
- Prior liver or bone disease

PATHOLOGICAL FINDINGS
- Size and shape of prostatic acini almost always altered
- Small closely packed interposed stroma
- Eosinophilic crystalloids present
- Architecture disrupted
- Cells invade perineural space

SPECIAL TESTS
- Prostate specific antigen (PSA)
- Free PSA

IMAGING
- Bone scan, positive with metastasis
- Skeletal survey, positive with metastasis
- Lymph node aspiration, positive with metastasis
- Computerized tomography of pelvic lymph nodes, positive with metastasis
- Prostatic ultrasound
- Magnetic resonance imaging of little value

DIAGNOSTIC PROCEDURES
- Biopsy, fine needle aspiration or core
- Ultrasound
- Lymph node aspiration
- Lymph node biopsy (dissection)
- Laparoscopic lymph node dissection

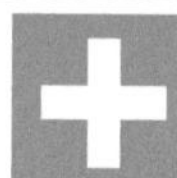

TREATMENT

APPROPRIATE HEALTH CARE
- Inpatient for surgery, outpatient for other treatment
- Main options for clinically localized prostate cancer treatment are:
  - ◊ Radical prostatectomy
    - Retropubic
    - Perineal
    - Laparoscopic
    - Robotic (robotic assisted laparoscopic)
  - ◊ External beam radiation therapy
  - ◊ Brachytherapy (seed implementation)

GENERAL MEASURES
- Treatment - consider age factor
- T1a - observation may be appropriate
- T1b, T1c - candidate for prostatectomy, external beam radiation, brachytherapy
- T2a, T2b - prostatectomy, external beam radiation, brachytherapy
- T3 - possible prostatectomy, possible radiation
- T4 - hormonal (androgen) ablation, palliative therapy if needed

SURGICAL MEASURES
- Under age 70, aggressive therapy for cure
- Orchiectomy (reduces serum testosterone by 90%)

ACTIVITY Full activity

DIET No special diet

PATIENT EDUCATION Printed material available from:
- American Cancer Society
- National Kidney & Urologic Diseases Information Clearinghouse, Box NKUDIC, Bethesda, MD 20893, (301)468-6345

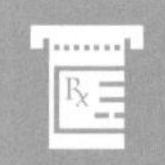

MEDICATIONS

DRUG(S) OF CHOICE

- In androgen-dependent tumors a reduction in serum testosterone is helpful in reducing tumor size, bone pain, and for improving survival. Orchiectomy is the simplest androgen ablation method, however, medical castration can alternatively be utilized.
- CAB or MAB (combined or maximum androgen blockade). Often recommended although some studies have shown no survival advantage over orchiectomy alone. Reduction in pain (54% versus 37% in patients with orchiectomy alone) is significant, although the side effects of the anti-androgens (hot flashes, night blindness, diarrhea, etc.) may be troublesome.
- For androgen ablation (medical castration), **in patients without orchiectomy**:
  - ◊ Leuprolide (Lupron) 1 mg subcutaneously daily or 7.5 mg IM depot monthly or 30 mg IM depot-4 months sustained q 4 months
  - ◊ Goserelin (Zoladex) 3.6 mg q month
- Nonsteroidal anti-androgens (to block testosterone produced outside the testes, i.e., used with androgen ablation or orchiectomy)

Contraindications: None

Precautions:

- Flare phenomenon with metastatic disease
- Fluid retention
- Nausea
- Vomiting
- Hot flashes
- Liver enzyme changes

Significant possible interactions: Refer to manufacturer's profile of each drug.

ALTERNATIVE DRUGS

- Chemotherapy considered experimental. Many combinations of chemotherapeutic agents have been tried - none have been effective to date.
  - ◊ Mitoxantrone (Novantrone)12mg/m2 IV q 3 weeks + prednisone 5mg bid po appears to reduce pain and reduces PSA levels in some patients
- Other nonsteroidal anti-androgens
  - ◊ Bicalutamide (Casodex) 50 mg qd
  - ◊ Flutamide (Eulexin) 250 mg tid (no survival advantage over bicalutamide and has increased diarrhea, Antabuse effects, and occasional elevations of liver enzymes)
  - ◊ Nilutamide (Nilandron) give 50 mg on day of castration and for 30 days, then continue at 150 mg qd (compared to bicalutamide has more side effects including diarrhea, occasional interstitial pneumonitis, and light-dark adaptation problems)

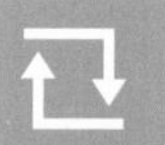

FOLLOWUP

PATIENT MONITORING

- Routine clinical examination every 3 months for 1 year, then every 6 months for a year
- Annual examinations indefinitely
- PSA every 3 months for 1 year, every 6 months 1 year, then yearly
- Other studies dependent on rising PSA

PREVENTION/AVOIDANCE None

POSSIBLE COMPLICATIONS

- Cardiac failure
- Phlebitis
- Pathologic fracture

EXPECTED COURSE/PROGNOSIS

- Early diagnosis and treatment of lesions should be curable
- Advanced disease favorable prognosis if endocrine sensitive
- Advanced unresponsive disease progresses in 18 months average

Ten year survival for prostate cancer by stage:

Stage	TNM	10-year Survival
A	T1	NC
B	T2	75%
C	T3	55%
D	N1-2	(70% at 7yr)
D	M1	15%

NC = no change from general population

Five year survival after treatment† (Lancet 1995) for prostate cancer:

Time	--- Treatment --- Castration	CAB
40 months	58%	56%
5 years††	23%	26%

† Includes patients with advanced disease
†† Projected survival, no statistical difference

Survival in prostate cancer without treatment (Denmark 1979-1983: Natural history of Prostate Cancer):

Time	% of patients surviving††
1 year	80%
5 years	38%
10 years	17%

† Includes all patients; both early and advanced disease
†† 62% of patients died primarily of prostate cancer; 38% died from other causes

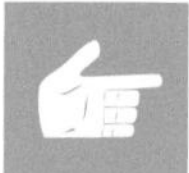

MISCELLANEOUS

ASSOCIATED CONDITIONS N/A

AGE-RELATED FACTORS

Pediatric: N/A
Geriatric: N/A
Others: N/A

PREGNANCY N/A

SYNONYMS

Carcinoma of the prostate

ICD-9-CM

185 Malignant neoplasm of prostate

SEE ALSO

OTHER NOTES N/A

ABBREVIATIONS

PSA = Prostate specific antigen

REFERENCES

- Walsh PC, Gittes RF, Perlmutter AD. Campbell's Urology. 7th Ed. Philadelphia, W.B. Saunders Co., 1997
- Miglari R, Muscas G, Murru M, Verdacchi T, De Benedetto G, De Angelis M. Antiandrogens: a summary review of pharmacodynamic properties and tolerability in prostate cancer therapy. Arch Ital Urol Androl 1999;71(5):293-302
- Tyrrell CJ. Controversies in the management of advanced prostate cancer. Br J Cancer 1999;79(1):146-55
- Tannock IR, et al. Chemotherapy with mitoxantrone plus prednisone or prednisone alone for symptomatic hormone-resistant prostate cancer: A Canadian randomized trial with palliative end points. J Clin Oncol 1996;14(6):1756-64
- Sarosdy MF. Which is the optimal antiandrogen for use in combined androgen blockade of advanced prostate cancer? The transition from a first- to second-generation antiandrogen. Anticancer Drugs 1999;10(9):791-6
- Borre M, Nerstrom B, Overgaard J. The natural history of prostate carcinoma based on a Danish population treated with no intent to cure. Cancer 1997;80:917-28

Web references: 2 available at www.5mcc.com
Illustrations N/A

Author(s):

Kevin Spear, MD

BASICS

DESCRIPTION Benign adenomatous growth of prostate which may result in bladder outlet obstruction
System(s) affected: Renal/Urologic, Reproductive
Genetics: Genetic factors may be involved. Risk higher if father had clinical BPH in his 50's.
Incidence/Prevalence in USA:
- Universal pathologic phenomenon seen in older men
- No hard evidence suggesting racial predisposition

Predominant age:
- Rarely seen in men < 40
- Seen in 50% of men > 50; 80% of men > 70

Predominant sex: Male only

SIGNS & SYMPTOMS
Prostate size correlates poorly with symptoms
- Obstructive symptoms: Due to mechanical obstruction and/or detrusor muscle decompensation
  - ◊ Decrease force or caliber of stream
  - ◊ Hesitancy
  - ◊ Post-void dribbling
  - ◊ Sensation of incomplete bladder emptying
  - ◊ Overflow incontinence
  - ◊ Inability to voluntarily stop stream
  - ◊ Urinary retention
- Irritative symptoms: Due to incomplete bladder emptying and/or detrusor muscle instability
  - ◊ Frequency
  - ◊ Nocturia
  - ◊ Urgency
  - ◊ Urge incontinence
- Other symptoms and signs:
  - ◊ Gross hematuria
  - ◊ Observation of weak stream
  - ◊ Distended bladder (> 150 cc in order to detect by percussion)
  - ◊ Increased post-void residual (> 100 cc)
  - ◊ Prostate enlarged (normal 20 gram prostate - size of horse chestnut)
  - ◊ Clinical clues suggesting renal failure due to obstructive uropathy (edema, pallor, pruritus, ecchymoses, nutritional deficiencies, etc.)
  - ◊ American Urological Association (AUA) symptom index score > 7

CAUSES Exact etiology unknown, but evidence suggests BPH arises from a systemic hormonal alteration which may or may not act in combination with growth factors stimulating stromal or glandular hyperplasia. Environmental and hereditary factors influence development of clinical BPH. Lower incidence of BPH in Japanese and Chinese.

RISK FACTORS
- Intact testes (BPH rare in eunuchs)
- Aging (thus, rare in men < 40 years old)
- Dietary and environmental may be implicated

DIAGNOSIS

DIFFERENTIAL DIAGNOSIS
- Obstructive conditions:
  - ◊ Prostate cancer
  - ◊ Urethral stricture or valves
  - ◊ Bladder neck contracture (acquired or congenital)
  - ◊ Anterior or posterior urethral valves
  - ◊ Mullerian duct cysts
  - ◊ Inability of bladder neck or external sphincter to relax appropriately during voiding
- Non-obstructive conditions:
  - ◊ Neurogenic bladder (detrusor denervation)
  - ◊ Myogenic cause (detrusor muscle failure)
  - ◊ Medications (parasympatholytics, sympathomimetics, etc.)
  - ◊ Psychogenic
- Irritative conditions:
  - ◊ Neurogenic bladder
  - ◊ Inflammatory disorders (prostatitis, urethritis, radiation cystitis, interstitial cystitis, etc.)
  - ◊ Neoplasm (bladder carcinoma, especially carcinoma in situ)
  - ◊ Detrusor overactivity (OAB)

LABORATORY
- BPH is a pathologic diagnosis - lab data is only suggestive
- Urinalysis: pyuria if stones or infection present, pH changes due to chronic residual urine
- Elevated serum creatinine (if obstructive uropathy present)
- Urine culture positive (sometimes due to chronic residual urine)
- Prostate specific antigen (PSA) may be elevated but usually < 10 ng/mL (10 μg/L)
- Increased post-void residual (> 100 mL)
- Acute urinary retention, transurethral instrumentation may elevate the PSA

Drugs that may alter lab results:
- Finasteride (Proscar) may lower the PSA

Disorders that may alter lab results:
- Acute urinary retention, prostatitis, urinary tract instrumentation or prostatic infarction may elevate the PSA

PATHOLOGICAL FINDINGS Confirmation obtained by biopsy, resection or extirpation surgery. 5 types: Stromal (fibrous), fibromuscular, muscular ("leiomyoma"), fibroadenoma, fibroadenoma.

SPECIAL TESTS
- Transrectal prostate ultrasound gives volumetric estimate of gland
- Needle biopsy (to rule out cancer)
- Have patient complete IPSS (International Prostate Symptom Score)
  - ◊ Mild symptoms (score 0-7): Offer watchful waiting only
  - ◊ Moderate symptoms (score 8-19) to severe symptoms (score 20-35): Offer treatment options

IMAGING
- Ultrasound - increase postvoid residual, prostate or hydronephrosis
- CT scan or MRI of pelvis - enlarged prostate
- IVP - increased post-void residual, large prostatic impression on bladder, trabeculated bladder, bladder diverticula, upper tract dilation, bladder stones

DIAGNOSTIC PROCEDURES
- Uroflow - volume voided per unit time. Peak flow < 10 mL/sec suggests obstruction (accurate when voided volume is > 150 mL). May be low if bladder contractility is impaired.
- Pressure-flow curve (urine flow versus voiding pressures) - decreased urine flow and increased pressure indicates obstruction
- Cystoscopy demonstrates presence, configuration and site of obstructive tissue - helps to show stricture, stones. May help determine best therapy option.
- Post-void residual (PVR) by catheterization or bladder ultrasound; PVR >150 associated with increased risk of retention

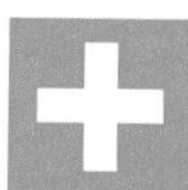

TREATMENT

APPROPRIATE HEALTH CARE Inpatient or outpatient treatment required, either for surgery or medical treatment. Inpatient emergent treatment required to manage fluid and electrolyte abnormalities of obstructive uropathy.

GENERAL MEASURES
- Avoid large boluses of oral or IV fluids or alcohol intake
- Avoid prolonged periods of not voiding
- Avoid sympathomimetic or anticholinergic medications (e.g., cold/flu preparations)
- Urethral catheterization or clean intermittent catheterization if in retention

SURGICAL MEASURES
- Surgery (indicators to determine necessity)

One of the following:
  - ◊ Urinary retention due to prostatic obstruction, recurrent
  - ◊ Intractable symptoms due to prostatic obstruction (gauged by AUA symptom index; score at least > 8)
  - ◊ Obstructive uropathy (renal insufficiency)
  - ◊ Recurrent or persistent urinary tract infections due to prostatic obstruction
  - ◊ Recurrent gross hematuria due to enlarged prostate
  - ◊ Bladder calculi
  - ◊ Medical therapy indicated when surgery indicators not met
- Surgical procedures - minimally invasive
  - ◊ Interstitial laser coagulation (ILC)
  - ◊ High frequency focused ultrasound (HIFU)
  - ◊ Transurethral needle ablation (TUNA)
  - ◊ Transurethral microwave thermotherapy (TUMT)
  - ◊ Water-induced thermotherapy (WIT)
  - ◊ Prostate stenting
  - ◊ Transurethral balloon dilation (TUDP)
  - ◊ Transurethral ethanol ablation of prostate
- Surgical procedures - more invasive
  - ◊ TURP
  - ◊ Open prostatectomy
  - ◊ Transurethral laser ablation, laser-induced prostatectomy or laser enucleation of prostate
  - ◊ Transurethral vaporization of prostate

ACTIVITY No restriction

DIET Avoid caffeinated or alcoholic beverages, excessively spiced foods

PATIENT EDUCATION
- The Prostate Book, published by Krames Communications, 312 90th St, Daly City, CA 94015-1898
- National Kidney & Urologic Diseases Information Clearinghouse, Box NKUDIC, Bethesda, MD 20893, (301)468-6345

MEDICATIONS

DRUG(S) OF CHOICE

- Indicated when no strong indication for surgery exists or patient declines surgery
- Alpha adrenergic antagonist: terazosin (Hytrin) 1-10 mg/day, doxazosin (Cardura) 1-8 mg/day, tamsulosin (Flomax) 0.4-0.8 mg/day, alfuzosin (Uroxatral) 10 mg qd
- Hormonal (anti-androgens) agents: finasteride (Proscar) a 5-alpha reductase inhibitor, 5 mg/day works best for larger prostates; dutasteride (Avodart) 0.5 mg/day, turosteride, flutamide (Eulexin) and leuprolide (Lupron) are rarely used; phytotherapy (e.g., serenoa repens [saw palmetto], similar to finasteride in efficacy)
- Combination therapy of alpha blocker plus 5-alpha reductase inhibitor is superior to monotherapy

Contraindications:

- Use alpha adrenergic antagonists with caution in patients with cardiac or cerebrovascular disease or those who operate machinery. Give the first dose at bedtime to avoid orthostatic hypotension
- Hormones may cause impotence (less with flutamide) and lower the PSA
- The semen of men taking finasteride may cause effects on the fetus of pregnant sex partners
- Alpha blockers contraindicated with PDE V inhibitor vardenafil (Levitra) used for erectile dysfunction

Precautions: Refer to manufacturer's profile of each drug

Significant possible interactions:

- Tamsulosin-cimetidine: do not administer together
- Alpha blockers should not be taken within 4 hours of taking sildenafil

ALTERNATIVE DRUGS

- Saw palmetto (serenoa repens) - has been demonstrated to improve symptoms. Mechanism of action not fully identified.
- South African stargrass, a beta-sitosterol, improves IPSS score, decreases nocturia and frequency and increases flow rate

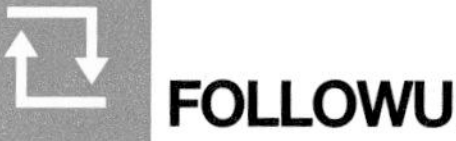

FOLLOWUP

PATIENT MONITORING

- Symptom index (IPSS) monitored every 3-12 months
- Digital rectal exam yearly
- PSA yearly
- Bladder scan post-void residual every 3-12 months

PREVENTION/AVOIDANCE

Appears to be part of the aging process

POSSIBLE COMPLICATIONS

- Urinary retention (acute or chronic)
- Bladder stones
- Prostatitis
- Renal failure
- Hematuria
- Erectile dysfunction in men with lower urinary tract symptoms (LUTS)

EXPECTED COURSE/PROGNOSIS

- Symptoms improve or stabilize in 70-80% of patients; 20-30% require treatment because of worsening symptoms
- 11-33% men with BPH have occult prostate cancer

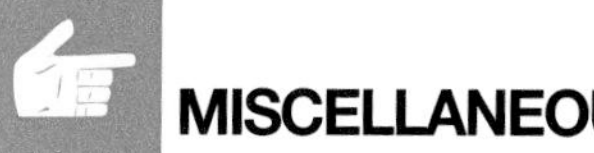

MISCELLANEOUS

ASSOCIATED CONDITIONS

N/A

AGE-RELATED FACTORS

Pediatric: N/A
Geriatric: Much more prevalent in elderly men
Others: N/A

PREGNANCY

N/A

SYNONYMS

- Prostatic hyperplasia
- Prostatic hypertrophy

ICD-9-CM

600.90 Hyperplasia of prostate, unspecified, without urinary obstruction
600.91 Hyperplasia of prostate, unspecified, with urinary obstruction

SEE ALSO

OTHER NOTES

N/A

ABBREVIATIONS

IPSS = International Prostate Symptom Score
IVP = intravenous pyelogram
AUA = American Urological Association

REFERENCES

- Proceedings of 94th annual American Urological Association Meeting, Dallas, 1999
- McConnel JD: Benign prostatic hypertrophy. In: Walsh PC, et al, eds. Campbell's Urology. Philadelphia, W.B. Saunders Co., 1998
- Kirby RS, McConnel JD: Benign prostatitis hypertrophy, Fast Facts. Oxford, Health Press, 1997
- Kapoor DA, Reddy PK: Surgical alternatives to TURP in the management of BPH. AUA Update Series 1993;3(12)
- McConnell JD, Roehrborn CG, Bautista OM, et al. Medical Therapy of Prostatic Symptoms (MTOPS) Research Group. The long-term effect of doxazosin, finasteride, and combination therapy on the clinical progression of benign prostatic hyperplasia. N Engl J Med 2003;349(25):2387-98
- Braeckman J. The extract of Serenoa repens in the treatment of benign prostatic hyperplasia: a multicenter open study. Curr Ther Res 1994;55:776-85
- Wilt T, Ishani A, MacDonald R. Serenoa repens for benign prostatic hyperplasia (Cochrane Review). In: The Cochrane Library, 2004(1)

Web references: 0 available at www.5mcc.com
Illustrations N/A

Author(s):

Pamela I. Ellsworth, MD
William Merriam, MD

BASICS

DESCRIPTION One of several inflammatory and/or painful conditions affecting the prostate gland
- Acute bacterial prostatitis; NIH Class I. Generally associated with urinary tract infection, has characteristically abrupt onset
- Chronic bacterial prostatitis; NIH Class II. Major cause of recurrent bacteriuria, less fulminant
- Chronic prostatitis/pelvic pain syndrome (CPPS); NIH Class III
  - ◊ Inflammatory; NIH Class IIIa. Inflammatory cells in prostatic secretions, post-prostate massage urine or seminal fluid
  - ◊ Noninflammatory; NIH Class IIIb. Similar to chronic bacterial, but bacterial culture negative
- Asymptomatic inflammatory prostatitis; NIH class IV. Incidental finding during prostate biopsy for infertility, cancer workup

NIH classification of prostatitis:

Trad. Class	VB2 Cult	VB2 WBC	EPS Cult	EPS WBC	NIH Class
ABP	+	+	+	+	I
CBP	+	+	+	+	II
NBP	0	0	0	+	IIIa
Pdyn*	0	0	0	0	IIIb
Asymt	+-	+	+-	+	IV

* Pdyn = prostatodynia

System(s) affected: Renal/Urologic, Reproductive
Genetics: No known genetic pattern
Incidence/Prevalence in USA: Common
Predominant age:
- Mostly ages 30-50, sexually active
- Chronic more common in ages over 50

Predominant sex: Male only

SIGNS & SYMPTOMS
- Acute bacterial
  - ◊ Fever; chills
  - ◊ Tense, boggy, very tender and warm prostate
  - ◊ Low back pain, myalgias
  - ◊ Prostatodynia, perineal pain
  - ◊ Frequency
  - ◊ Urgency
  - ◊ Dysuria
  - ◊ Nocturia
  - ◊ Bladder outlet obstruction
- Chronic bacterial
  - ◊ Symptoms often absent
  - ◊ Prostatodynia, perineal pain
  - ◊ Dysuria, irritative voiding
  - ◊ Lower abdominal pain
  - ◊ Low back pain
  - ◊ Scrotal pain
  - ◊ Penile pain
  - ◊ Pain on ejaculation
  - ◊ Hematospermia
- Chronic prostatitis/pelvic pain syndrome (inflammatory/noninflammatory)
  - ◊ Prostatodynia, perineal pain
  - ◊ Dysuria, irritative voiding
  - ◊ Lower abdominal pain
  - ◊ Low back pain
  - ◊ Scrotal pain
  - ◊ Penile pain
  - ◊ Pain on ejaculation
  - ◊ Hematospermia

CAUSES
- Bacterial
  - ◊ Ascending infection through urethra
  - ◊ Refluxing urine into prostate ducts
  - ◊ Direct extension or lymphatic spread from rectum
  - ◊ Hematogenous spread
  - ◊ Calculi serving as nidus for infection
  - ◊ Aerobic gram negative bacteria (*Escherichia coli, Pseudomonas, Klebsiella, Proteus*), *N. gonorrhea, Enterobacteriaceae, Burkholderia pseudomallei*)
  - ◊ Miscellaneous - *Chlamydia trachomatis*
  - ◊ Gram positive bacteria (*Streptococcus faecalis, Staphylococcus. aureus*)
  - ◊ Organisms suspected, but unproven (*Staphylococcus epidermidis*, Micrococci, non-group D streptococcus, Diphtheroids)
  - ◊ Uncommon: *Mycobacterium tuberculosis*, parasitic, Mycoses (blastomycosis, coccidioidomycosis, cryptococcus, histoplasmosis, paracoccidiomycosis, candidiasis)
- Nonbacterial
  - ◊ Non-relaxation (spasm) of the internal urinary sphincter and pelvic floor striated muscles leading to increased prostatic urethral pressure and intraprostatic urinary reflux, leading theory
  - ◊ Ureaplasma, *Trichomonas vaginalis*, and Chlamydia postulated, but not proven

RISK FACTORS
- Male sex
- Age over 50
- Prostatic calculi
- Urinary tract infection
- Trauma
- Dehydration
- Sexual abstinence
- Chronic indwelling catheter
- HIV positive
- Urethral stricture

DIAGNOSIS

DIFFERENTIAL DIAGNOSIS
- Cystitis (bacterial, interstitial)
- Urethritis
- Pyelonephritis
- Malignancy
- Obstructive calculus
- Foreign body
- Acute urinary retention

LABORATORY
- Fractional urine examination (4 glass test). (Note: Avoid vigorous massage of the prostate in acute bacterial prostatitis secondary to induced iatrogenic bacteremia.)
  - ◊ Specimen collection
    - VB1: Initial 10 mL urine from urethra
    - VB2: Next 200 mL discarded, then midstream from bladder
    - EPS: Then, expressed prostate secretion
    - VB3: Urine after prostate massage.
  - ◊ Specimen handling
    - Urinalysis, culture, sensitivities, gram stain on all samples
    - pH of EPS
    - Bacterial antigen-specific IgA and IgG levels in EPS
    - Wet mount of EPS
  - ◊ Interpretation
    - Over 10-15 white cells per high powered field suggests bacterial prostatitis
    - Macrophages containing fat (oval bodies) suggests bacterial prostatitis
    - Positive culture in EPS or VB3 but not VB1 or VB2 diagnostic of bacterial prostatitis
    - In acute bacterial prostatitis, serum and EPS fluid bacterial antigen-specific IgA and IgG can be detected immediately after the onset of infection. Level decline over 6-12 months after successful antibiotic therapy.
    - Bacteria count generally less in chronic prostatitis
    - In chronic bacterial prostatitis, no serum IgG elevation is seen, whereas EPS fluid IgA and IgG levels are increased. With antibiotic therapy, IgG levels return to normal in several months, but IgA levels remain elevated for 2 years.
    - Prostatic fluid alkaline in chronic bacterial prostatitis
    - White blood cells with a negative culture (although false negative cultures are not uncommon) suggests non-bacterial prostatitis
    - No abnormal findings with chronic prostatitis without inflammation (this misnomer refers to patients with symptoms such as perineal pain, ejaculatory pain, and lower abdominal pain but who do not have inflammatory changes on lab studies)
- PSA level increased with acute prostatitis. (Do not order for prostate cancer screening until at least one month after prostatitis treated.)

Drugs that may alter lab results: Antibiotics

Disorders that may alter lab results: N/A

PATHOLOGICAL FINDINGS Inflammatory changes (except prostatodynia)

SPECIAL TESTS N/A

IMAGING
- CT or ultrasound, if malignancy or abscess suspected
- Transrectal ultrasound (if prostatic calculi or abscess suspected)

DIAGNOSTIC PROCEDURES
- Needle biopsy or aspiration for culture
- Urodynamic testing (prostatodynia)
- Cystoscopy (in persistent nonbacterial prostatitis to rule out bladder cancer, interstitial cystitis)

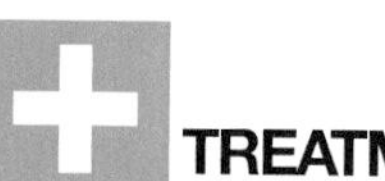

TREATMENT

APPROPRIATE HEALTH CARE
- Inpatient (proven or suspected abscess, urosepsis, immunocompromised)
- Outpatient, if nontoxic

GENERAL MEASURES
- Analgesics
- Antipyretics
- Stool softeners
- Hydration
- Sitz baths to relieve pain and spasm
- Suprapubic catheter for severe urinary retention
- Psychotherapy if sexual dysfunction
- Neuromodulation, acupuncture, heat therapy, antidepressants, antianxiolytics, analgesics

SURGICAL MEASURES Surgical resection for intractable chronic disease, or to drain an abscess; transurethral microwave thermotherapy for chronic nonbacterial prostatitis

ACTIVITY Bedrest in severe cases

DIET N/A

PATIENT EDUCATION
- Printed patient information available from:
National Kidney & Urologic Diseases Information Clearinghouse, Box NKUDIC, Bethesda, MD 20893, (301)468-6345

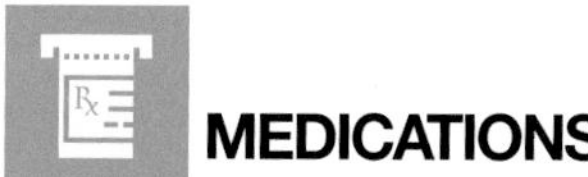

MEDICATIONS

DRUG(S) OF CHOICE
- Acute bacterial (outpatient):
  - ◊ If urine shows gram positive cocci, amoxicillin 500 mg po tid x 30 days, otherwise, use
  - ◊ Trimethoprim-sulfamethoxazole (Septra-DS) BID for 30 days
- Acute bacterial (inpatient): Ampicillin 1-3 gram IV divided q6h plus aminoglycoside - gentamicin 2.0 mg/kg loading dose; 1.7 mg/kg q8h maintenance
- Chronic bacterial: A fluoroquinolone (e.g., ofloxacin 300 mg bid, ciprofloxacin 500 mg bid) for 4-12 weeks
- Chronic prostatitis/pelvic pain syndrome without inflammation
  - ◊ Alpha-adrenergic blocking agents (e.g., terazosin (Hytrin) 1 mg po qHS increased slowly to a maximum of 10 mg qD) may be useful
  - ◊ Diazepam 2-10 mg po BID with pelvic floor dysfunction
- Analgesics, NSAIDs
- Antipyretics
- Stool softeners

Contraindications: Drug allergies
Precautions:
- Renal disease
- Hepatic disease
- Elderly may not tolerate higher dose benzodiazepines
- G6PD deficiency may manifest with sulfonamides or NSAIDs

Significant possible interactions: Fluoroquinolones with magnesium/aluminum antacids, theophylline, probenecid, NSAIDs, warfarin

ALTERNATIVE DRUGS
- Carbenicillin with aminoglycoside, erythromycin, tetracycline, cephalexin, fluoroquinolones, dicloxacillin, nafcillin IV, vancomycin IV
- Finasteride (in patients older than 45 years old, category IIIa inflammatory CP/CPPS, or enlarged prostate glands)
- Pentosan polysulfate (Elmiron) 100mg TID, in patients with suprapubic discomfort associated with frequency and urgency
- Nonbacterial: May benefit from erythromycin, doxycycline, trimethoprim-sulfamethoxazole

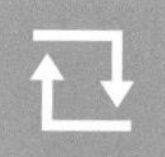

FOLLOWUP

PATIENT MONITORING
- Acute bacterial - urinalysis and culture 30 days after initiating treatment
- Chronic bacterial - urinalysis and culture every 30 days (may take several months)
- The symptom index from the National Institutes of Health-Chronic Prostatitis Symptom Index (NIH-CPSI) encompasses 13 items that are tabulated into three domain scores: (1) pain, (2) urinary symptoms, and (3) quality of life. Reference: http://www.niddk.nih.gov/fund/divisions/kuh/useful-tools/english-nih-cpsi.pdf

PREVENTION/AVOIDANCE Suppression therapy may benefit patient with chronic bacterial prostatitis

POSSIBLE COMPLICATIONS
- Abscess (more common if HIV infected)
- Sepsis, bacteremia
- Urinary retention
- Epididymitis
- Chronic bacterial prostatitis (with acute prostatitis)

EXPECTED COURSE/PROGNOSIS
Often prolonged and difficult to cure. Studies with 55-97% cure rate depending on population and drug used.

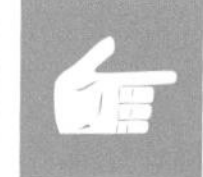

MISCELLANEOUS

ASSOCIATED CONDITIONS
- Prostatic hypertrophy
- Cystitis
- Urethritis

AGE-RELATED FACTORS
Pediatric: None
Geriatric: Consider prostatic hypertrophy and urinary retention more seriously
Others: N/A

PREGNANCY N/A

SYNONYMS N/A

ICD-9-CM
601.0 Acute prostatitis
601.1 Chronic prostatitis

SEE ALSO
Interstitial cystitis
Prostatic cancer
Prostatic hyperplasia, benign (BPH)
Urinary tract infection in males

OTHER NOTES
- Prostatodynia: pain in the area of prostate. Sometimes inaccurately designated as a diagnosis.

ABBREVIATIONS
VB = voided bladder
EPS = expressed prostate secretion
CPPS = chronic prostatitis/pelvic pain syndrome

REFERENCES

- Nickel JC, Downey J, Ardern D, Clark J, Nickel K. Failure of Monotherapy Strategy for Difficult Chronic Prostatitis/Chronic Pelvic Pain Syndrome. J Urology 2004; 172(2): 551-554
- Shoskes DA, Hakim I, Gboniem G and Jackson CL. Long-term results of multimodal therapy for chronic prostatitis/chronic pelvic pain syndrome. J Urol 2003; 169: 1406
- McNaughton Collins M, MacDonald R, Wilt TJ. Diagnosis and treatment of chronic abacterial prostatitis: a systematic review. Ann Intern Med 2000;133(5):367-81
- Walsh PC, Retnick AB, Vaughan ED, Wein AJ, eds. Campbell's Urology. 7th ed. Philadelphia: W.B. Saunders; 1997
- Mandell GL, Douglas RG, Bennett JE, eds. Principles and Practice of Infectious Diseases. 5th ed. New York: Churchill; 1999
- Nickel JC. Research guidelines for chronic prostatitis: consensus report from the first National Institutes of Health International Prostatitis Collaborative Network. Urology 1999;54(2):229-33.
- Nickel JC. Prostatitis: evolving management strategies. Urol Clin North Am 1999;26(4):737-51.
- Nickel JC. Effective office management of chronic prostatitis. Urol Clin North Am 1998;25(4):677-84
- Krieger JN, Nyberg L Jr, Nickel JC. NIH consensus definition and classification of prostatitis. JAMA 1999;282(3):236-7
- Game X, Vincendeau S, Palascak R, et al. Total and free serum prostate specific antigen levels during the first month of acute prostatitis. Eur Urol 2003;43(6):702-5

Web references: 3 available at www.5mcc.com
Illustrations N/A

Author(s):
Gary A. Goforth, MD

BASICS

DESCRIPTION Intense chronic itching in the anal and perianal skin. Usual course - acute. Chronic pruritus ani is a symptom, not a diagnosis or disease.
System(s) affected: Skin/Exocrine
Genetics: No known genetic pattern
Incidence/Prevalence in USA: Common
Predominant age: All ages
Predominant sex: Male > Female (4:1)

SIGNS & SYMPTOMS
- Primary
  - ◊ Rectal itching
  - ◊ Anal erythema
- Secondary

Secondary infections with yeast, fungus, and/or bacteria are possible after prolonged scratching
  - ◊ Anal itching
  - ◊ Anal fissures
  - ◊ Maceration
  - ◊ Lichenification
  - ◊ Excoriations

CAUSES
- Dermatologic disorders
  - ◊ Allergies (soap, topical anesthetics, oral antibiotics)
  - ◊ Fistulas
  - ◊ Fissures
  - ◊ Neoplasms
  - ◊ Psoriasis
  - ◊ Eczema
  - ◊ Seborrheic dermatitis
  - ◊ Contact dermatitis
- Infections
  - ◊ Pinworms and other worms
  - ◊ Scabies
  - ◊ Pediculosis
  - ◊ Candidiasis
  - ◊ Tinea
- Other
  - ◊ Poor hygiene (fecal material allowed to dry on the skin)
  - ◊ Diabetes mellitus
  - ◊ Chronic liver disease
  - ◊ Diarrheic alkalotic irritation
  - ◊ Trauma from scented toilet paper

RISK FACTORS
- Overweight
- Hairy, tendency to perspire a great deal
- Anxiety-itch-anxiety cycle

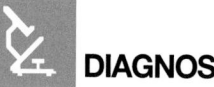

DIAGNOSIS

DIFFERENTIAL DIAGNOSIS
- Allergies
- Psoriasis
- Atopic dermatitis
- Fungus infection
- Bacterial infection
- Parasites
- Hyperhidrosis
- Diabetes mellitus
- Liver disease
- Neoplasia
- Anxiety

LABORATORY
- Glycosuria
- Hyperglycemia
- Skin scraping, yeast
- Fungi
- Parasites
- Stool - ova plus parasites

Drugs that may alter lab results: N/A

Disorders that may alter lab results: N/A

PATHOLOGICAL FINDINGS Excoriation of epithelial layer of skin

SPECIAL TESTS Blood sugar levels

IMAGING N/A

DIAGNOSTIC PROCEDURES
- Inspection
- Anoscopy biopsy (to exclude neoplasia)

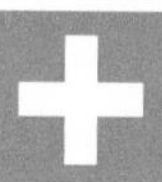

TREATMENT

APPROPRIATE HEALTH CARE Outpatient

GENERAL MEASURES
- Treat predisposing factors, such as parasites, diabetes, liver disease, cryptitis, scabies, pediculosis
- Resist overly meticulous use of soap and rubbing
- Avoid tight clothing and under clothing
- Cleanse anal area after bowel movements with moistened absorbent cotton and plain water; baby wipes may be a convenient alternative
- Dust anal area with non-medicated talcum powder
- If unable to completely empty rectum with defecation, use small plain water enema (infant bulb syringe) after each bowel movement. This may prevent postevacuation soilage and irritation.

SURGICAL MEASURES N/A

ACTIVITY Avoid getting overheated

DIET If suspicious of food allergy, eliminate as a trial: Coffee, beer, cola, vitamin C tablets in excessive doses, spices, citrus fruits

PATIENT EDUCATION See information in General Measures

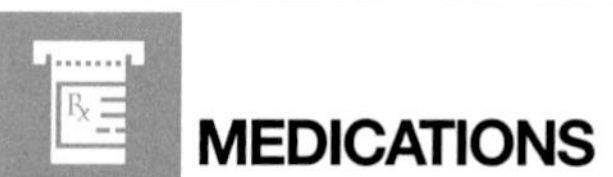

MEDICATIONS

DRUG(S) OF CHOICE
- Specific treatment for allergies, micro-organisms, bacteria and worm infestation
- For symptomatic treatment - hydrocortisone cream 1% applied sparingly, usually at night. If severe, may need to apply several times a day. Discontinue when itching subsides.

Contraindications: Refer to manufacturer's literature
Precautions: Refer to manufacturer's literature
Significant possible interactions: Refer to manufacturer's literature

ALTERNATIVE DRUGS N/A

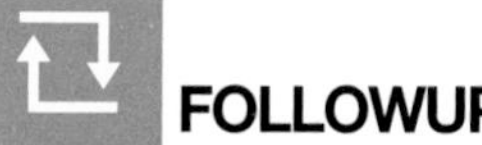

FOLLOWUP

PATIENT MONITORING As needed

PREVENTION/AVOIDANCE
- Avoid topical agents
- Avoid laxatives
- Avoid tight underclothing made from synthetic material
- Practice good hygiene
- Use talcum powder
- Possibly lactobacillus acidophilus (tablets or in milk); possibly malt soup extract
- Eat yogurt when taking broad-spectrum antibiotics

POSSIBLE COMPLICATIONS
- Secondary bacterial infection
- Chronicity
- Excoriation
- Lichenification

EXPECTED COURSE/PROGNOSIS
- Depends upon etiology; usually good
- May be persistent and recurrent

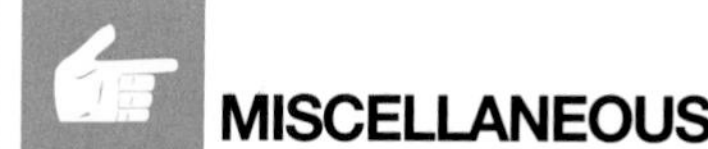

MISCELLANEOUS

ASSOCIATED CONDITIONS
- Diabetes mellitus
- Psoriasis
- Hyperhidrosis
- Parasite infestations
- Hemorrhoids

AGE-RELATED FACTORS
Pediatric:
- Usually secondary to enterobiasis, anal fissures, other local inflammatory lesions, or coarse or moist undergarments. Nocturnal itching may be due to pinworms.
- Exposure to sunlight or dry heat may be helpful for infants with inflamed anal area

Geriatric: Common in this age group
Others: N/A

PREGNANCY N/A

SYNONYMS N/A

ICD-9-CM
698.0 Pruritus ani

SEE ALSO
Pinworms
Pruritus vulvae

OTHER NOTES N/A

ABBREVIATIONS N/A

REFERENCES

- Feldman M, Scharschmidt, BF, eds. Sleisenger and Fordtran's Gastrointestinal and Liver Disease: Pathophysiology/Diagnosis/ Management. 6th ed. Philadelphia, WB Saunders, 1998
- Kirsner JB, Shortet G, eds: Diseases of the Colon, Rectum and Canal. Baltimore, Williams & Wilkins, 1988

Web references: 0 available at www.5mcc.com
Illustrations N/A

Author(s):
Stanley G. Smith, MA, MB

BASICS

DESCRIPTION Pruritus vulvae is both a symptom and a pathologic process affecting the vulva. It is a symptom of underlying disease in the vast majority of the patients. As a primary diagnosis, it consists of irritation and vulvar itching without an underlying pathologic etiology.

System(s) affected: Skin/Exocrine
Genetics: Unknown
Incidence/Prevalence in USA: The exact incidence is unknown, although most women will complain of vulvar pruritus at some time during their life
Predominant age:
- Any age can be affected
- In young girls, it is usually caused by an infection
- Frequent in postmenopausal women

Predominant sex: Female only

SIGNS & SYMPTOMS
- Constant itching of the vulva
- Constant burning of the vulva

CAUSES
- Infectious causes - vaginal yeast infections, Gardnerella, other vaginal infections, and yeast dermatitis of the vulva itself
- Urinary tract infections will produce vulvar burning on occasion
- Vulvar vestibulitis (inflammation of the vestibular glands) produces a constant burning with pruritus and dyspareunia
- Human papilloma virus (HPV) has been associated with burning and itching of the vulva
- Vulvar tissues are estrogen sensitive. Estrogen deprivation can produce burning and itching.
- A search for underlying malignancy should be paramount. Carcinoma in situ (Bowen disease) and invasive malignancy will often be associated with pruritus.
- Changes in the epidermis, such as lichen sclerosis et atrophicus (LSA) (thinning of the vulvar tissues and homogenization at the basement membrane) or hyperkeratosis of the vulva produce pruritus
- Anal incontinence with fecal soilage produces pruritus
- Excessive heat produces symptoms from sweat and irritation
- Environmental and dietary irritants such as nylon, soaps, perfumes, and over-zealous cleansing can produce symptoms
- Dietary irritants include methylxanthines (coffee, cola), tomatoes, peanuts

RISK FACTORS N/A

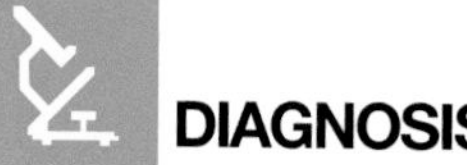

DIAGNOSIS

DIFFERENTIAL DIAGNOSIS
- The diagnosis of primary idiopathic vulvar pruritus must be made by exclusion
- A search for infectious causes should be undertaken with treatment of yeast and other vaginitis
- Biopsy of any abnormal-appearing epithelium on the vulva to insure that malignant changes are not present
- Only when all other factors have been ruled out can the diagnosis primary idiopathic vulvar pruritus be established

LABORATORY
- Vaginal secretions can be evaluated by wet mount (NaCl for trichomonas or Gardnerella, and KOH for yeast). Cultures seldom required.
- Gram stain of the vagina is non-diagnostic as multiple organisms are present in the normal flora

Drugs that may alter lab results: N/A

Disorders that may alter lab results: N/A

PATHOLOGICAL FINDINGS These are related to the underlying etiology. In primary vulvar pruritus, no changes will be noted. If HPV is present, these changes will be seen in the cornified layer of the squamous epithelium.

SPECIAL TESTS Whenever necessary, biopsy of the vulva should be used to establish the primary diagnosis

IMAGING N/A

DIAGNOSTIC PROCEDURES Biopsy when needed

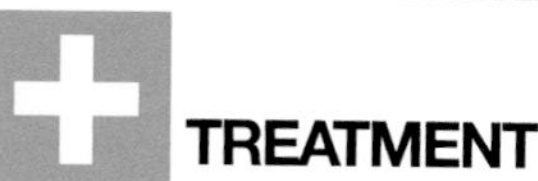

TREATMENT

APPROPRIATE HEALTH CARE Outpatient

GENERAL MEASURES
- Treatment of any underlying cause must be undertaken
- In cases of idiopathic primary vulvar pruritus, conservative measures include sitz baths, topical steroid creams, avoidance of chemical irritants and dietary changes
- When conservative measures fail, advanced cases can be treated with alcohol block or laser

SURGICAL MEASURES Bowen disease and premalignant changes are treated with excision or laser vaporization

ACTIVITY Unlimited

DIET A trial of dietary alteration should be attempted for idiopathic pruritus. Coffee and caffeine-containing beverages should be avoided. Other foods to avoid include tomatoes, peanuts.

PATIENT EDUCATION See Prevention/Avoidance

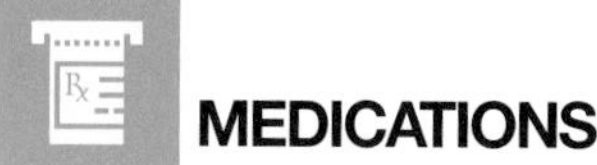

MEDICATIONS

DRUG(S) OF CHOICE
- Infectious sources should be treated with appropriate antimicrobials or antifungals
- Lichen sclerosis is treated with 2% testosterone in petrolatum
- Hyperkeratotic lesions are treated with topical steroid
- Idiopathic primary vulvar pruritus can be treated with topical steroids such as triamcinolone (Kenalog) or desoximetasone (Topicort) cream

Contraindications: N/A
Precautions: N/A
Significant possible interactions: N/A

ALTERNATIVE DRUGS N/A

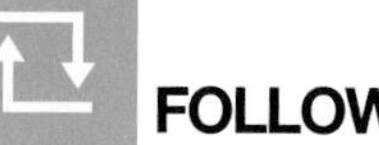

FOLLOWUP

PATIENT MONITORING These women should be followed closely for the development of premalignant or malignant changes within the area of pruritus

PREVENTION/AVOIDANCE
- Irritants to the vulva such as perfumes, soaps (use non-allergenic) or perfume douches must be avoided
- Only cotton underwear should be worn
- No tight fitting clothes or nylon pantyhose

POSSIBLE COMPLICATIONS Chronic course

EXPECTED COURSE/PROGNOSIS
- Vulvar pruritus can be kept under control with conservative measures and topical steroids
- When it advances to uncontrollable symptoms, alcohol block or laser may be necessary

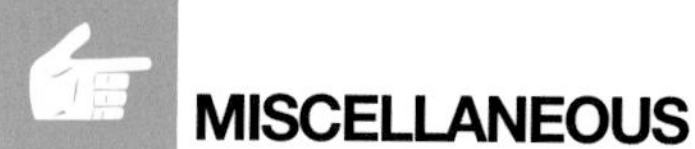

MISCELLANEOUS

ASSOCIATED CONDITIONS N/A

AGE-RELATED FACTORS
Pediatric: N/A
Geriatric: More frequent
Others: N/A

PREGNANCY N/A

SYNONYMS
- Vulvar pruritus
- Vulvodynia
- Burning vulva syndrome

ICD-9-CM
698.1 Pruritus of genital organs

SEE ALSO

OTHER NOTES N/A

ABBREVIATIONS N/A

REFERENCES

- McKay M. Vulvodynia vs. pruritus vulvae. Clin Obstet Gynecol 1985;28:123-33
- Smith L, Henricks D, McCullah R. Prospective studies on the etiology and treatment of pruritus ani. Dis Colon Rectum 1982;25:258-363
- Hopkins MP. Anatomy and pathology of the vulva and vagina. In: Rebar R, Baker V, eds. Gynecology & Obstetrics, An Integrated Approach. New York: Churchill Livingstone; 1993
- Hopkins MP. Benign and preinvasive lesions of the vulva and vagina. In: Copeland LJ, ed. Textbook of Gynecology. 2nd ed. Philadelphia: W B Saunders Co; 2000

Web references: 0 available at www.5mcc.com
Illustrations N/A

Author(s):
Michael P. Hopkins, MD, MEd

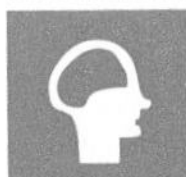

BASICS

DESCRIPTION Foreign body inflammatory reaction surrounding an ingrown hair (usually in beard area, especially submandibular region, but can occur on scalp, axilla, or pubic area if these sites are shaved or plucked). Characterized by red papule/pustule at point of entry. A mechanical problem.
System(s) affected: Skin/Exocrine
Genetics: Curly haired people, especially Blacks
Incidence/Prevalence in USA: Widespread. Incidence of 45% in black soldiers who shave. Adult male blacks - 50,000/100,000; adult male Caucasians - 3000-5000/100,000.
Predominant age: Postpubertal, middle age (40-75)
Predominant sex: Male > Female

SIGNS & SYMPTOMS
- Tender exudative, erythematous follicular papules or pustules in beard area (less commonly in scalp, axilla, pubic areas)
- Range from 2-4 mm in size
- Painful upon shaving
- Alopecia
- Lusterless brittle hair

CAUSES
- Reentry penetration of skin by external pointed tip of growing curved whisker, or sharp tipped whisker can grow into follicular wall if shaved too close
- Plucking of hair can cause abnormal hair growth in injured follicles

RISK FACTORS
- Curly hair
- Shaving too close with multiple razor strokes
- Plucking hairs
- Black race

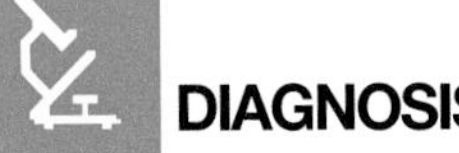

DIAGNOSIS

DIFFERENTIAL DIAGNOSIS
- Bacterial folliculitis
- Impetigo

LABORATORY N/A

Drugs that may alter lab results: N/A

Disorders that may alter lab results: N/A

PATHOLOGICAL FINDINGS
- Clinical pathology - follicular papules and pustules
- Histopathology - because of its curvature, the advancing hair's sharp-tipped free end causes an epidermal invagination as it approaches the skin. This is accompanied by inflammation and often an intra-epidermal abscess. As hair enters dermis, more severe inflammation occurs with downgrowth of epidermis in an attempt to ensheath hair. An abscess forms within the pseudofollicle and a foreign body reaction forms at the tip of invading hair.

SPECIAL TESTS Culture of pustules - usually sterile. May show coagulase-negative micrococcus (normal skin flora).

IMAGING N/A

DIAGNOSTIC PROCEDURES Clinical diagnosis

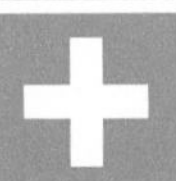

TREATMENT

APPROPRIATE HEALTH CARE Outpatient

GENERAL MEASURES
- Acute treatment
  - ◊ Dislodge embedded hair with sterile needle
  - ◊ Discontinue shaving until red papules have resolved (minimum 3-4 weeks)
  - ◊ Massage beard area with washcloths, coarse sponge or brush several times daily
  - ◊ Systemic antibiotics if secondary infections present

SURGICAL MEASURES N/A

ACTIVITY Unlimited

DIET No restrictions

PATIENT EDUCATION
- Dunn 88, Pseudofolliculitis Barbae, pages 170-172
- American Family Physician (see References)
- Cutis, Vol 61, June 1998, pages 355-356

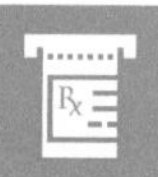

MEDICATIONS

DRUG(S) OF CHOICE
- Topical or systemic antibiotic for secondary infection
  - ◊ Application of clindamycin (Cleocin-T) solution bid
  - ◊ Low doses erythromycin or tetracycline 250 mg bid
  - ◊ Administer until papule/pustule resolution
- Mild cases
  - ◊ 5% benzoyl peroxide - apply after shaving
  - ◊ 1% hydrocortisone cream - apply at bedtime
- Moderate disease - chemical depilatories
  - ◊ Disrupt cross-linking of disulfide bonds of hair causing blunt hair tip
  - ◊ Apply no more frequently than every 3rd day - 2% barium sulfide (Magic Shave) or calcium thioglycolate (Surgex)
- Moderate disease - adjunct treatment
  - ◊ Tretinoin (Retin-A) liquid/cream, applied daily or every other day

Contraindications:
- Clindamycin - history of regional enteritis or ulcerative colitis; history of antibiotic associated colitis
- Erythromycin, tetracycline, tretinoin hypersensitivity only

Precautions:
- Clindamycin - colitis, eye burning and irritation, skin dryness, pregnancy category B
- Erythromycin - cautious use in patients with impaired hepatic function, GI side effects especially abdominal cramping, pregnancy category B
- Tetracycline - permanent discoloration of teeth if given during last half of pregnancy
- Tretinoin - severe skin irritation, pregnancy category C
- Benzoyl peroxide - skin irritation and dryness, allergic contact dermatitis
- Hydrocortisone cream - local skin irritation, skin atrophy with prolonged use

Significant possible interactions:
- Erythromycin - increases theophylline and carbamazepine levels, decreases clearance of warfarin; cardiac toxicity with terfenadine and astemizole
- Tetracycline - depresses plasma prothrombin activity (therefore need to decrease warfarin dosages)

ALTERNATIVE DRUGS Topical application of glycolic acid lotion (8% buffered glycolic acid in a suitable carrier, either oil-in-water lotion or a non-lipid soap) twice daily. This treatment may allow shaving comfortably every day.

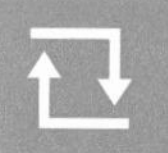

FOLLOWUP

PATIENT MONITORING As needed. Educate patient on curative and preventive treatment.

PREVENTION/AVOIDANCE
- Mild cases
  - ◊ Use tiny plastic hook for removing ingrown hairs before shaving
  - ◊ Shave either with a manual adjustable razor at coarsest settings (avoids close shaves), a single edge blade razor (The Bump-Fighter), a foil guarded razor (PFB razor), electric triple "O" head razor, or electric hair clipper with polyester skin cleansing pad (Buf-Puf by Riker Labs)
  - ◊ Purchase "Bump Fighter" razor through ASR Consumer products (www.asrco.com)
  - ◊ Shave beard in direction of hair growth
  - ◊ Do not stretch skin when shaving
  - ◊ Use correct shaving cream/gel (Ef-Kay Shaving Gel, Edge Shaving Gel, Aveeno Therapeutic Shave Gel, Easy Shave Medicated Shaving Cream)
  - ◊ Consider 5% benzoyl peroxide after shaving and application of 1% hydrocortisone cream at bedtime (or Lacticare HC lotion after shaving)
- Moderate cases
  - ◊ Chemical depilatories (barium sulfide), (Magic Shave Powder)
  - ◊ Consider 0.05% tretinoin (Retin-A) liquid or cream
  - ◊ Consider eflornithine HCl (Vaniqa) cream
- Severe cases
  - ◊ Laser therapy - experimental
  - ◊ Avoidance of shaving completely
  - ◊ Electrolysis to destroy remaining hair follicles - controversial
- Use "collar extender" (JC Penney)

POSSIBLE COMPLICATIONS
- Scarring (occasionally keloidal)
- Foreign body granuloma formation
- Disfiguring postinflammatory hyperpigmentation
- Impetiginization of inflamed skin

EXPECTED COURSE/PROGNOSIS
- Course is recurrent if preventative measures not followed
- Prognosis is poor in presence of progressive scarring and foreign body granuloma formation

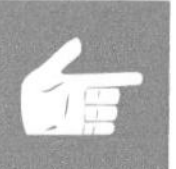

MISCELLANEOUS

ASSOCIATED CONDITIONS Keloidal folliculitis

AGE-RELATED FACTORS
Pediatric: N/A
Geriatric: N/A
Others: N/A

PREGNANCY Do not use tretinoin (Retin-A), tetracycline, benzoyl peroxide

SYNONYMS
- Chronic sycosis barbae
- Pili incarnati
- Folliculitis barbae traumatica
- Razor bumps

ICD-9-CM
704.8 Other specified diseases of hair and hair follicles

SEE ALSO
Folliculitis
Impetigo
Tinea barbae

OTHER NOTES N/A

ABBREVIATIONS N/A

REFERENCES

- Perry PK, Cook-Bolden FE, Rahman Z, et al. Defining pseudofolliculitis barbae in 2001: a review of the literature and current trends. J Am Acad Dermatol 2002;46(2 Suppl Understanding):S113-9
- Lever WF, Schaumburg-Lever G: Histopathology of the Skin. Philadelphia, J.B. Lippincott, 1990
- Dunn JF Jr: Pseudofolliculitis Barbae. Amer Fam Phys 1988;9
- Habif T. Clinical Dermatology. 4th Ed. St. Louis, CV Mosby, 2004
- Sams W Jr, Lynch P: Principles and Practice of Dermatology. New York, Churchill Livingstone, 1990
- Perricone NV: Treatment of pseudofolliculitis barbae with topical glycolic acid: A report of two studies. Cutis 1993;52(4):232-235
- Lewis CW, Coquilla BH: Management of pseudofolliculitis barbae. Military Medicine, Vol 160, May 1995
- Crutchfield CE III. The causes and treatment of pseudofolliculitis barbae. Cutis 1998;61(6):351-6
- Ross EV. Lasers in the military for cutaneous disease and wound healing. Dermatol Clin 1999;17(1):135-50

Web references: 1 available at www.5mcc.com
Illustrations N/A

Author(s):
W. Paul Slomiany, MD

BASICS

DESCRIPTION An acute inflammatory arthritic disease usually involving large joints which primarily affects the elderly and is caused by calcium pyrophosphate dihydrate (CPPD) crystal deposition in joints. Associated with chondrocalcinosis.
- CPPD crystal deposition may cause a progressive degenerative arthritis in numerous joints
- CPPD crystal deposition may cause a more insidious, smoldering, symmetrical, polyarthritis which is similar to rheumatoid arthritis

System(s) affected: Endocrine/Metabolic, Musculoskeletal

Genetics:
- Uncommonly seen in familial pattern with autosomal dominant inheritance (< 1% of cases)
- Most cases sporadic

Incidence/Prevalence in USA: Unknown, primarily a disease of the elderly; chondrocalcinosis is present 1 in 10 in ages 60-75, over age 80 in 1 in 3. Only a small percentage develop pseudogout.

Predominant age: 80% of patients > than 60

Predominant sex: Male = Female

SIGNS & SYMPTOMS
- Acute pain and swelling of one or more joints. Knee is involved in one-half of all attacks, ankle, wrist and shoulder also common.
  - ◊ Inflammation, joint effusion, limitation of motion
  - ◊ 50% associated with fever
  - ◊ Any other synovial joint may be involved including first metatarsophalangeal
- Can present with a chronic progressive arthritis upon which acute inflammation attacks are superimposed
- Progressive degenerative arthritis in numerous joints including: wrists, metacarpophalangeal, hips, shoulders, elbows, and ankles without inflammatory attacks also seen
- Low grade inflammatory arthritis with multiple symmetrical joint involvement (mimics rheumatoid arthritis) < 5% of cases

CAUSES
- Acute inflammatory reaction to CPPD crystals shed into synovial cavity
- Physical and chemical changes in aging cartilage that favor crystal growth

RISK FACTORS
- Aging
- Trauma
- Pseudogout will often occur as a complication in patients hospitalized for other medical and surgical illnesses
- Metabolic diseases (10% or less of the cases)
  - ◊ Hyperparathyroidism
  - ◊ Hemochromatosis
  - ◊ Gout
  - ◊ Hypophosphatasia
  - ◊ Hypothyroidism
  - ◊ Ochronosis
  - ◊ Wilson disease
  - ◊ Amyloidosis
  - ◊ Hypomagnesemia

DIAGNOSIS

DIFFERENTIAL DIAGNOSIS
- Illness that may cause an acute inflammatory arthritis in a single or multiple joint(s): Gout, septic arthritis or trauma
- Other illnesses that may present with an acute inflammatory arthritis: Reiter syndrome, Lyme disease, acute rheumatoid arthritis

LABORATORY
- Elevated sedimentation rate
- Leukocytosis with mild left shift

Drugs that may alter lab results: N/A

Disorders that may alter lab results: N/A

PATHOLOGICAL FINDINGS CPPD crystal deposition in articular cartilage, synovium, ligaments and tendons

SPECIAL TESTS
- Synovial fluid analysis consistent with an inflammatory effusion:
  - ◊ Cell count from 2000 to 100,000 WBC/mL
  - ◊ Differential predominantly neutrophils (80-90%)
  - ◊ Wet prep with polarized microscopy may demonstrate small numbers of weakly positively birefringent crystals in the fluid and within neutrophils, false negative rate is high
- Metabolic studies
  - ◊ To exclude an underlying cause should always be obtained in patients under age 50 and considered in the elderly
  - ◊ Serum calcium
  - ◊ Serum phosphorus
  - ◊ Serum alkaline phosphatase
  - ◊ Serum parathormone
  - ◊ Serum iron, total iron binding capacity, and serum ferritin
  - ◊ Serum magnesium
  - ◊ Serum thyroxine and thyroid stimulating hormone (TSH) level

IMAGING
- X-rays of joints
  - ◊ May demonstrate punctate and linear calcification in articular hyaline or fibrocartilage: Knees, hips, symphysis pubis, and wrists most often affected, may also be found in asymptomatic individuals
  - ◊ In the chronic destructive indolent form of the disease: Subchondral cyst formation, fragmentation with formation of intra-articular radiodense bodies in joints not typically affected by degenerative joint disease.

DIAGNOSTIC PROCEDURES
- Aspiration of joint fluid with synovial fluid analysis required for proper confirmation of pseudogout; aspiration may relieve symptoms and speed resolution of inflammatory process

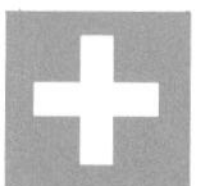

TREATMENT

APPROPRIATE HEALTH CARE
- If septic arthritis is considered possible, inpatient care may be required for empiric antibiotic therapy pending culture results
- If patient does not have adequate support system inpatient care may be required until patient is able to walk

GENERAL MEASURES
- Rest and elevate affected joint(s)
- Apply moist warm compresses to affected joints

SURGICAL MEASURES N/A

ACTIVITY
- Non-weight bearing on affected joint while painful. Use crutches or walker.
- Perform isometric exercises to maintain muscle strength during the acute stage, i.e., quadriceps isometric contractions and leg lifts, if knee affected
- Begin range of motion of joint as inflammation and pain subside
- Resume weight bearing when pain subsides

DIET No special diet

PATIENT EDUCATION Specific instructions on exercise and activity

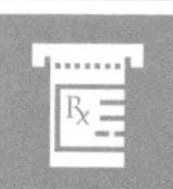

MEDICATIONS

DRUG(S) OF CHOICE

- Non-steroidal anti-inflammatory drugs (choose one of the following):
  ◊ Indomethacin (Indocin) 50 mg tid with food
  ◊ Naproxen (Naprosyn) 500 mg bid with food
  ◊ Sulindac (Clinoril) 150-200 mg bid with food
  ◊ Ibuprofen (Motrin) 600-800 mg tid-qid with food. Maximum of 3.2 gm daily.
  ◊ Other NSAIDs at anti-inflammatory doses are effective. The COX-2 inhibitors celecoxib and rofecoxib are not FDA approved for treatment of crystal-induced arthritis but should be effective especially for patients with gastrointestinal ulcers or traditional NSAID intolerance. Use celecoxib (Celebrex) 200 mg bid or rofecoxib (Vioxx) 50 mg q day.

Contraindications:

- History of hypersensitivity to NSAIDs or aspirin
- Active peptic ulcer disease or history of recurrent upper gastrointestinal lesions
- Use with extreme caution when impaired renal function exists. Monitor serum creatinine.

Precautions:

- May interfere with platelet aggregation and prolong bleeding time. This effect is much shorter lived than with aspirin.
- May cause fluid retention and worsen congestive heart failure
- Abnormal liver function tests may develop in approximately 15% of patients. Discontinue if findings worsen or systemic manifestations occur.
- Serious gastrointestinal bleeding can occur without warning. Follow patient carefully for internal bleeding. Administer misoprostol 200 μg qid in patients with a history of peptic ulcer disease.

Significant possible interactions:

- May blunt the antihypertensive effects of angiotensin converting enzyme inhibitors
- May prolong the prothrombin time in patients taking oral anticoagulants
- Avoid concomitant usage of aspirin
- May blunt the diuretic effect of furosemide and hydrochlorothiazide
- May increase plasma lithium level in patients taking lithium carbonate
- May increase methotrexate levels

ALTERNATIVE DRUGS

- Intra-articular instillation of methylprednisolone acetate, 20-80 mg for large joints; 10-40 mg for medium joints. Available in 20, 40 and 80 mg/mL ampules.
- Oral prednisone. Begin at 40-60 mg/day and taper over 10 days
- Intravenous colchicine 2 mg IV; may repeat 0.5 mg IV q6h; not to exceed 4 mg in 24 hours (oral colchicine ineffective). Contraindication: significant bone marrow dysfunction, renal insufficiency (creatinine clearance < 10 mL/min), biliary obstruction, sepsis.

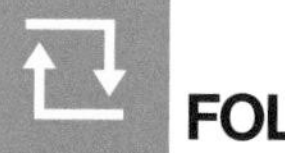

FOLLOWUP

PATIENT MONITORING Reevaluate patient for response to therapy 48-72 hours after treatment instituted. Reexamine 1 week later, then as needed.

PREVENTION/AVOIDANCE None known

POSSIBLE COMPLICATIONS

- Erosive destructive arthritis in pattern of joints not usually affected by degenerative joint disease
- Recurrences may occur and a destructive arthritis may complicate CPPD

EXPECTED COURSE/PROGNOSIS

- Acute attack usually resolves in 10 days. Prognosis for resolution of acute attack is excellent.
- Some patients experience progressive joint damage with functional limitation

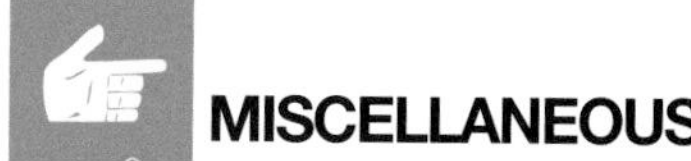

MISCELLANEOUS

ASSOCIATED CONDITIONS Consider in patients with pseudogout - hyperparathyroidism, hemochromatosis, gout, hypophosphatasia, hypothyroidism, ochronosis, Wilson disease, amyloidosis, hypomagnesemia

AGE-RELATED FACTORS

Pediatric: Not seen in children
Geriatric: Most cases are in patients over 60
Others: N/A

PREGNANCY N/A

SYNONYMS

- Calcium pyrophosphate deposition disease

ICD-9-CM

712.10 Chondrocalcinosis due to dicalcium phosphate crystals, site unspecified
712.20 Chondrocalcinosis due to pyrophosphate crystals, site unspecified
712.30 Chondrocalcinosis, unspecified, site unspecified

SEE ALSO

Arthritis, osteo
Arthritis, psoriatic
Arthritis, rheumatoid (RA)
Gout

OTHER NOTES N/A

ABBREVIATIONS

CPPD = calcium pyrophosphate deposition disease

REFERENCES

- Agudelo C, Wise C. Crystal-Associated Arthritis in the Elderly. Rheu Clin NA 2000;26:527-46
- Segal JB, Albert D. Diagnosis of crystal induced arthritis by synovial fluid examination for crystals: Lessons from an imperfect test. Arthritis Care Res 1999;12:376-80
- Sack K. Monoarthritis: Differential Diagnosis. Am j of Med 1997;102(Suppl 1A):305-395
- Schumacher H. Crystal induced arthritis: an overview. Am J of Med 1996;100(2A):465-525

Web references: 2 available at www.5mcc.com
Illustrations N/A

Author(s):

Paul T. Cullen, MD

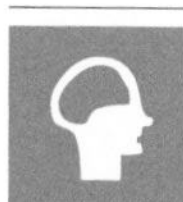

BASICS

DESCRIPTION Inflammatory bowel disorder associated with antibiotic use. May be mild diarrhea, or move through several stages to a severe colitis. Usual course - acute, relapsing.

System(s) affected: Gastrointestinal

Genetics: No known genetic factors

Incidence/Prevalence in USA:
- Epidemic or endemic in hospitals and nursing homes
  - ◊ Nursing homes: 2-8%
  - ◊ Hospitals: 7-15%
- Community: 6.7/100,000 patients treated with antibiotics
- Healthy adults: 5% colonized with C. difficile
- Hospitalized patients: 10-20% are colonized
- Neonates: 40% are colonized

Predominant age: 40-75 years

Predominant sex: Male = Female

SIGNS & SYMPTOMS
- Diarrhea (classically watery, green, foul-smelling, bloody)
- Abdominal tenderness, pain, cramps
- Fever (up to 8% report fever only)
- Nausea and vomiting
- Hypovolemia/dehydration
- Hypoalbuminemia

CAUSES Pathogenic *Clostridium difficile* toxins (A & B). *Clostridium difficile* is the most common nosocomial pathogen of the GI tract.

RISK FACTORS
- Antibiotic exposure (prior 6 weeks) particularly: clindamycin, lincomycin, ampicillin, cephalosporins. However, may also rarely occur with penicillins, erythromycin, sulfa-trimethoprim, chloramphenicol, tetracycline. In fact, nearly all antibiotics have been implicated.
- Cancer chemotherapy: fluorouracil, methotrexate, combination regimens.
- Recent surgery, especially bowel surgery
- Uremia or hemolytic-uremic syndrome
- Intestinal ischemia
- Shock
- Tube feedings
- Enemas
- GI stimulants
- Stool softener
- H2 blockers and antacids
- Immunocompromise (e.g., low CD4)
- Prolonged hospitalization
- Advancing age
- Hirschsprung
- Inflammatory bowel disease

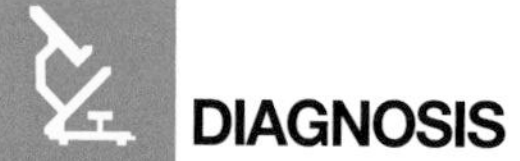

DIAGNOSIS

DIFFERENTIAL DIAGNOSIS
- Other enteric pathogens
- Nonspecific inflammatory bowel diseases

LABORATORY
- Fecal leukocytosis
- Leukocytosis
- ELISA for *C. difficile* toxin, positive
- Culture

Drugs that may alter lab results: N/A

Disorders that may alter lab results: A high percentage of infants are normal carriers of *C. difficile* and are positive for toxin B

PATHOLOGICAL FINDINGS
- Mild, nonspecific colitis without plaques
- Gross - yellow-white plaques on colonic and small intestinal mucosa
- Micro - pseudomembrane arising from point of superficial ulceration
- Micro - fibrin
- Micro - thick confluent pseudomembrane
- Polymorphonuclear cells

SPECIAL TESTS
- Sigmoidoscopy - may be normal in 10-33%
- Colonoscopy may show involvement of the rectum and sigmoid colon and occasionally only right colon and/or distal ileum. Some patients do not have pseudomembrane.

IMAGING
- Abdominal film - distorted haustral markings, colonic distention
- CT - thickened or edematous colonic wall with pericolonic inflammation
- Note: Avoid barium enemas

DIAGNOSTIC PROCEDURES Endoscopic visualization and sample collection

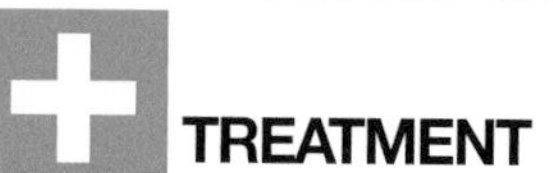

TREATMENT

APPROPRIATE HEALTH CARE
- Outpatient for most patients
- Inpatient for severe or patients with co-morbidities

GENERAL MEASURES
- Fluid replacement
- Fluid plus electrolyte therapy
- Discontinue antimicrobial agent
- Avoid anti-diarrheal agents
- Successful in 25%
- Do not treat asymptomatic carriers

SURGICAL MEASURES
- Colectomy, not diversion, may be required
- 1-3% of patients with severe colitis require emergency colectomy because of impending perforation, severe ileus with megacolon, or refractory septicemia

ACTIVITY Bedrest during acute phase

DIET Nothing by mouth during fulminant phase

PATIENT EDUCATION N/A

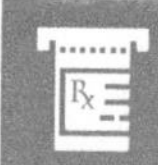

MEDICATIONS

DRUG(S) OF CHOICE

If drugs are not able to be taken orally, give via NG, enema, or direct instillation by colostomy/ileostomy or IV

- Metronidazole (Flagyl) 500 mg po tid for 10-14 days
- Vancomycin
  - ◊ 125 mg po qid (only for severe or resistant cases) for 10-14 days
  - ◊ May increase dose to 500 mg qid if diarrhea, fever, and leukocytosis fail to abate after 48 hours
  - ◊ Severely ill patients who do not respond to oral vancomycin may benefit from addition of IV metronidazole 500 mg q8 hours
- Teicoplanin 50 mg po qid for 3 days then 100 mg bid for 4 days

Contraindications: Refer to manufacturer's literature

Precautions: Avoid antiperistaltic drugs such as diphenoxylate, atropine, loperamide to reduce risk of toxic megacolon

Significant possible interactions: Alcohol and metronidazole. Refer to manufacturer's literature.

ALTERNATIVE DRUGS

- Bacitracin 250,000 units qid
- For flora repletion: Lactobacilli capsules or Saccharomyces boulardii enema of mixed colonies
- For chronic recurrences, adjunct therapy with full colon irrigation with Golytely

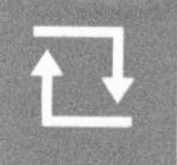

FOLLOWUP

PATIENT MONITORING

Careful monitoring through fulminant phase

PREVENTION/AVOIDANCE

- Judicious use of antimicrobial agents
- Keep courses of antibiotics as brief as possible
- Avoidance of recurrences
  - ◊ Prolonged therapy
  - ◊ Lactobacillus
  - ◊ Repletion of other organisms which compete with *C. Difficile*
  - ◊ In children, some success with IV gamma globulin

POSSIBLE COMPLICATIONS

- Reactive arthritis; Reiter syndrome
- Hypoalbuminemia
- Ascites
- Dehydration, hypovolemia, shock
- Bowel perforation
- Toxic megacolon
- Ileus relapses - 20% due to vegetative spores
- Death

EXPECTED COURSE/PROGNOSIS

- If treated, usual improvement in 3 days and virtually all patients recover
- Resistance to antibiotic therapy (metronidazole or vancomycin) is rare. Failure to respond to treatment may reflect noncompliance with therapy, misdiagnosis, underlying IBD or irritable bowel syndrome or malabsorption.
- Relapses occur in 10-25% of cases of *C. difficile* colitis
  - ◊ Symptoms usually appear a few days after completing therapy, but may appear up to 30 days later
  - ◊ For treatment, repeat a 10-14 day course of metronidazole 500 mg tid
- Untreated, 10-30% mortality
- In severely ill, colectomy sometimes required
- Significant morbidity and mortality in critical ill patients
- Poor prognostic factors: hypoalbuminemia, rapid fall in albumin, over 3 antibiotics, persistent *C. difficile* toxin after 7 days of treatment

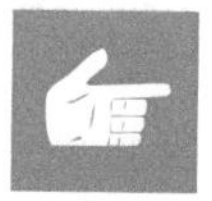

MISCELLANEOUS

ASSOCIATED CONDITIONS

- Surgery
- Spinal fracture
- Intestinal obstruction
- Colon cancer

AGE-RELATED FACTORS

Pediatric:

- Unusual in children, but does occur
- Most infants are carriers; may become invasive in children with malignancy or Hirschsprung disease

Geriatric: The elderly have a higher mortality rate from pseudomembranous colitis

Others: N/A

PREGNANCY

Serious complication if it occurs during pregnancy

SYNONYMS

- Antibiotic associated colitis
- Pseudomembranous enterocolitis

ICD-9-CM

008.45 Intestinal infections due to Clostridium difficile

SEE ALSO

OTHER NOTES

N/A

ABBREVIATIONS

N/A

REFERENCES

- Fekety R, Akshay S: Diagnosis and treatment of Clostridium difficile. JAMA 1993;269:71-75
- Leung D, et al: Treatment with intravenously administered gamma globulin of chronic relapsing colitis induced by Clostridium difficile toxin. Jour of Pediatr 1991;118:633-7
- Bartlett JG: Antibiotic-associated diarrhea. Clinical Infect Dis 1992;15:573-81
- Fualman S, et al: Clostridial difficile invasion & toxin circulation in fatal pediatric pseudomembranous colitis. Amer J Clin Pathol 1990;94:410-6
- McFarland L, Surawicz C, Stamm W: Risk factors for C. difficile carriage and C. difficile associated diarrhea in a cohort of hospitalized patients. J of Infect Dis 1990;162:678-84
- Ramaswamy R, et al: Prognostic criteria in Clostridium difficile colitis. Amer J Gastro 1996;91(3):460-4
- Hirschorn LR, et al: Epidemiology of community-acquired Clostridium difficile-associated diarrhea. J Infec Dis 1994;169:127-33
- Chatila W, Constantine M: Clostridium difficile causing sepsis and an acute abdomen in critically ill patients. Crit Care Med 1995;23(6):1146-1150
- Walker KJ, et al: Clostridium difficile colonization in residents in long-term care facilities: prevalence and risk factors. J Amer Geriatric Soc 41(9):940-6
- Simor AE, et al: Infection due to Clostridium difficile among elderly residents of a long term care facility. Clin Infec Dis 1993;17(4):672-8
- Reinke C, Messik CR: Update on Clostridium-difficile-induced colitis, Part 2. Amer J Hosp Pharm 1994;51(15):1892-901
- Tumbarello M, et al: Clostridium difficile-associated diarrhoea in patients with human immunodeficiency virus infection: a case control study. European J Gastro & Hepatol 1995;7(3):259-63
- Wenisch C, et al: Comparison of vancomycin, teicoplanin, metronidazole and fusidic acid for the treatment of Clostridium difficile associated diarrhea. Clin Infec Dis 1996;5:813-818
- Grundfest, et al: Clostridium difficile colitis in the critically ill. Dis of Colon Rectum 1996;6:619-623
- Liacouras CA, Piecol DA: Whole bowel irrigation as an adjunct to the treatment of chronic relapsing Clostridium difficile colitis. J Clin Gastroenterology 1996;22(3):186-189

Web references: 0 available at www.5mcc.com

Illustrations N/A

Author(s):

J. C. Chava-Zimmerman, MD

BASICS

DESCRIPTION Psittacosis is the clinical manifestation of a respiratory infection with the bacteria *Chlamydia psittaci*. The infection is virtually always contracted from an infected bird. Human to human transmission is rare.
- Pneumonia, bronchitis and fever of unknown origin (FUO) are most common diagnoses
- Can range from sub-clinical respiratory infection to severe systemic infection. Severity of illness may vary with strain of *C. psittaci*.

System(s) affected: Pulmonary
Genetics: No known genetic predisposition
Incidence/Prevalence in USA:
- .04-.08/100,000. 100-200 cases/year reported to Centers for Disease Control. True incidence probably greater.
- Outbreaks may occur, usually associated with occupational exposure to infected turkeys or ducks

Predominant age: Adults
Predominant sex: Male = Female

SIGNS & SYMPTOMS
- Onset usually acute but may be insidious
- Fever (often > 39°C)
- Chills
- Cough (may develop later, usually non-productive)
- Headache (may be severe)
- Malaise
- Anorexia
- Myalgias
- Confusion
- Vomiting and/or diarrhea
- Abdominal pain
- Pleuritic chest pain
- Hemoptysis
- Dyspnea without wheezing
- Arthralgias
- Sore throat
- Hoarseness
- Epistaxis
- Photophobia
- Tachycardia
- Retractions
- Flaring
- Cyanosis
- Crepitations more common than signs of consolidation
- Auscultation may be normal even with pneumonia
- Relative bradycardia
- Tender hepatomegaly and splenomegaly
- Horder's spots (faint, reddish brown, blanching rash)
- Petechiae

CAUSES Infection with *Chlamydia psittaci*

RISK FACTORS Exposure to infected bird(s), usually a pet pigeon or parakeet, or occupational exposure at a turkey or duck processing plant. Infected birds may appear healthy. Incubation period is 5-15 days. Human-to-human transmission possible, but rare.

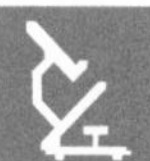

DIAGNOSIS

DIFFERENTIAL DIAGNOSIS
- Consider other common bacterial respiratory pathogens including
  - ◊ *Streptococcus pneumoniae*
  - ◊ *Haemophilus influenzae*
  - ◊ *Klebsiella pneumoniae*
  - ◊ *Chlamydia pneumoniae*
  - ◊ *Mycoplasma pneumoniae*
  - ◊ *Legionella* species
- Typhoid fever, Q fever, brucellosis

LABORATORY
- Leukocyte count often normal or low
- Erythrocyte sedimentation rate (ESR) usually elevated
- Sputum usually negative by gram stain and routine culture
- Proteinuria possible during febrile period
- Liver enzymes may be elevated
- Increased IgG, IgM, IgA
- Leukocytes with left shift
- Hypoxemia
- Hypocapnia
- Eosinophilia

Drugs that may alter lab results: Serologic response may be blunted by early treatment with tetracycline

Disorders that may alter lab results: N/A

PATHOLOGICAL FINDINGS
- Alveolar phagocyte and lymphocyte infiltrate
- Granuloma formation
- Bronchial wall thickening
- Type III and IV immune complex deposition
- Diffuse miliary nodules

SPECIAL TESTS
- Culture requires special facilities and is rarely done
- Sera for serology should be collected 2 to 3 weeks apart (3-4 weeks for micro-immunofluorescence, and a second convalescent sera at 6-8 weeks if the pattern is uninterpretable)
- Complement fixation (CF) test most common serologic test for psittacosis, but is also positive with *C. pneumoniae* (a much more common respiratory pathogen) and *C. trachomatis* infections
- A fourfold rise in CF titer is diagnostic of an acute infection with Chlamydia
- A single or stable CF titer of > 1:64 suggests a recent infection
- The species specific micro-immunofluorescence test for *C. psittaci* is preferred, but not as widely available as the CF test

IMAGING
- Chest radiograph often shows patchy alveolar infiltrates of interstitial pneumonitis and small nodular densities
- Lobar consolidation also common
- Hilar adenopathy
- Pleural effusion possible but usually scanty
- Radiographic abnormalities may persist for several months after successful treatment

DIAGNOSTIC PROCEDURES N/A

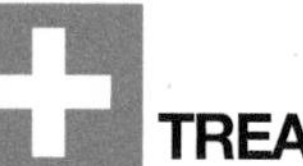

TREATMENT

APPROPRIATE HEALTH CARE
- Outpatient
- Patients with dyspnea, hypoxia, confusion or other signs or severe disease should be hospitalized

GENERAL MEASURES
- History of avian exposure (particularly to a sick bird) is key to making early diagnosis
- Treatment depends primarily on severity of respiratory symptoms. Severely ill patients may require oxygen, intravenous fluids and antibiotics.
- While human to human transmission is rare, sputum and respiratory secretion precautions should be observed

SURGICAL MEASURES N/A

ACTIVITY Based on disease severity. No disease-specific restrictions.

DIET No special diet

PATIENT EDUCATION American Lung Association, 1740 Broadway, New York, NY 10019, (800)586-4872

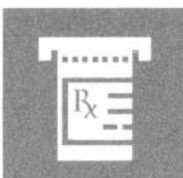

MEDICATIONS

DRUG(S) OF CHOICE

- Doxycycline (Vibramycin) 100 mg po bid for 14-21 days or 100 mg IV q12h
- Tetracycline 500 mg po qid for 14-21 days. If severely ill, tetracycline 5-7.5 mg/kg q12h IV.
- Clarithromycin (Biaxin) 500 mg q12h (length of treatment not established for psittacosis)

Contraindications: History of allergic reaction to the medication

Precautions: Tetracycline and doxycycline - avoid dairy products and sun exposure. Reduce dosage in renal failure. Avoid using in pregnancy or in children less than 8 years old (causes permanent discoloration of teeth).

Significant possible interactions: Refer to manufacturer's profile of each drug

ALTERNATIVE DRUGS

- Erythromycin also has in vitro activity and can be used at doses of 500 mg po qid for 14 to 21 days
- Azithromycin (Zithromax) 500 mg on first day; then 250 mg qd (length of treatment not established for psittacosis)
- Rifampin (Rifadin, Rimactane) has in vitro activity and has been used in doses of 600 to 1200 mg po per day with erythromycin to treat endocarditis due to *C. psittaci*
- Beta-lactam (penicillin based) antibiotics not effective

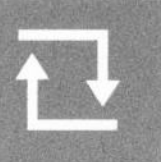

FOLLOWUP

PATIENT MONITORING Determined by severity of illness in the acute period. No disease-specific monitoring.

PREVENTION/AVOIDANCE

- Report to local health department
- Identify source of the infection if possible
- Public health surveillance of poultry flocks and pet shops
- Prophylactic antibiotic treatment with doxycycline (100 mg po qd for 10 days) has been advocated for people with known exposure

POSSIBLE COMPLICATIONS

- Meningitis and encephalitis
- Endocarditis, pericarditis and myocarditis
- Renal failure
- Erythema nodosum
- Sinusitis
- Respiratory failure
- Hepatitis
- Reactive arthritis (rare)
- Disseminated intravascular coagulation (rare)
- Valvular heart disease (rare)
- Spontaneous abortion (rare)
- Thyroiditis (rare)
- Pancreatitis (rare)
- Transverse myelitis (rare)

EXPECTED COURSE/PROGNOSIS

- Mortality rate less than 1% with appropriate treatment
- Patients usually respond within 24 to 48 hours following initiation of appropriate antibiotic therapy
- Full recovery may take weeks to months
- Relapse may occur necessitating second course of antibiotics
- Chest radiograph may not return to normal for up to 4 months

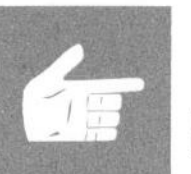

MISCELLANEOUS

ASSOCIATED CONDITIONS None known

AGE-RELATED FACTORS

Pediatric: Uncommon in pediatric age group
Geriatric: Mortality rate may be higher in elderly or debilitated patients
Others: None

PREGNANCY Spontaneous abortion has been reported with infection with some *C. psittaci* strains, primarily acquired from contact with sheep

SYNONYMS

- Ornithosis
- Bird breeder's disease
- Bird fancier's lung

ICD-9-CM

073.9 Ornithosis, unspecified
495.8 Other specified allergic alveolitis and pneumonitis

SEE ALSO

Chlamydia pneumoniae
Q fever

OTHER NOTES

- Incubation period ranges from 5 to 40 days; usually 7 to 15 days
- No persistent immunity to reinfection

ABBREVIATIONS N/A

REFERENCES

- Gregory DW, Schaffner W. Psittacosis. Sem Resp Infect 1997;12:7-11
- Schlossberg D. Chlamydia psittaci (psittacosis). In: Mandell Gl, Bennett JE, Dolin R, editors. Principles and Practices of Infectious Disease. 5th ed. New York: Churchill Livingstone; 2000. p.2004-6

Web references: 0 available at www.5mcc.com
Illustrations N/A

Author(s):

David H. Thom, MD, PhD

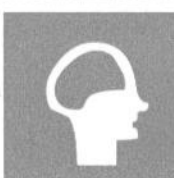

BASICS

DESCRIPTION Genetically determined (sporadic) common, chronic, epidermal proliferative disease. Clinically characterized by erythematous, dry scaling patches, recurring remissions and exacerbations. Flares may be related to systemic and environmental factors. Usual course - acute, chronic; unpredictable.
- Clinical forms:
  - ◊ Discoid or plaque psoriasis - most common, patches appear on scalp, trunk and limbs, nails may be pitted and/or thickened
  - ◊ Guttate psoriasis - occurs most frequently in children, numerous small papules over wide area of skin, but greatest on the trunk
  - ◊ Pustular psoriasis - small pustules over the body or confined to one area (i.e., palms and soles) or arranged in annular patterns (especially children)
  - ◊ Inverse, flexural psoriasis - affects the flexural areas, lesions are moist and without scales (common in older people)
  - ◊ Erythroderma (exfoliative psoriasis or red man syndrome) - patients skin turns red, may result from a flare of pre-existing dermatosis
  - ◊ Ostraceous - grossly hyperkeratotic

System(s) affected: Skin/Exocrine
Genetics:
- Genetic predisposition (probably polygenic)
- Type I psoriasis - young, strong family history = more aggressive disease
- Type 2 psoriasis - older, no family history = more stable disease
- Higher incidence in Caucasians and atopic families
- Increased incidence of human leukocyte antigens (HLA antigens)

Incidence/Prevalence in USA: 1000-2000 cases/100,000 people in the U.S.
Predominant age: Two peaks of onset, age 16-22 and age 57-60; can develop in infants
Predominant sex: Male = Female

SIGNS & SYMPTOMS
- Arthritis
- Pruritus
- Silvery scales on red plaques
- Knee-elbow-scalp distribution
- Stippled nails and pitting
- Positive Auspitz sign (underlying pinpoints of bleeding following scraping)
- Koebner phenomenon (psoriatic response in previously unaffected area 1-2 weeks after skin injury)

CAUSES Possible genetic error in mitotic control. Activation of lymphocytes (antigen? autoimmune?). Epidermal cell cycle 10 times shorter than normal, leading to epidermal hyperproliferation.

RISK FACTORS
- Local trauma; local irritation
- Infection (streptococcal pharyngitis can stimulate acute guttate psoriasis, HIV)
- Endocrine changes
- Stress (physical and emotional)
- Sudden withdrawal of systemic and/or potent topical steroids
- Alcohol use
- Obesity

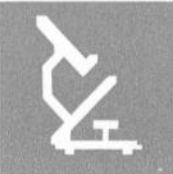

DIAGNOSIS

DIFFERENTIAL DIAGNOSIS
- Scalp - seborrheic dermatitis
- Body folds - intertrigo or candidiasis
- Diaper dermatitis
- Nails - onychomycosis
- Trunk - pityriasis rosea, pityriasis rubra pilaris, tinea corporis
- Squamous cell carcinoma
- Secondary and tertiary syphilis
- Cutaneous lupus erythematosus
- Eczema (nummular)
- Lichen planus
- Localized scratch dermatitis (lichen simplex chronicus)
- Mycosis fungoides
- Reiter disease
- Subcorneal pustulosis
- Pustular eruptions (aseptic and septic)
- Majocchi granuloma

LABORATORY
- Negative rheumatoid factor
- Latex fixation test
- Leukocytosis and increased sedimentation rate, especially in pustular psoriasis
- Fungal studies - may show a superimposed infection
- Uric acid increases in 10-20%
- In severe cases, anemia, B12, folate and iron deficiency can be present

Drugs that may alter lab results: N/A

Disorders that may alter lab results: N/A

PATHOLOGICAL FINDINGS
- Parakeratosis (focal), especially with neutrophils
- Hyperkeratosis
- Hypogranulosis
- Epidermal hyperplasia
- Elongation and thickening of rete ridges
- Thin epidermis above dermal papillae
- Spongiform pustule of Kogoj
- Munro's microabscess
- Abnormal mitoses
- Dilated tortuous capillary loops
- "Squirting" papillae

SPECIAL TESTS Biopsy

IMAGING N/A

DIAGNOSTIC PROCEDURES Usually diagnosis accomplished by inspection, occasionally biopsy required

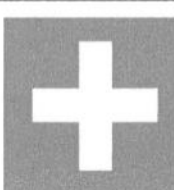

TREATMENT

APPROPRIATE HEALTH CARE
- Outpatient usually
- May require inpatient for severe or resistant cases. Emergency: Severe and unstable forms like acute pustular psoriasis (Von Zumbusch) or acute erythroderma.

GENERAL MEASURES
- Solar radiation
- Mild disease: ultraviolet radiation (UVA/UVB)
- Medication to soften scale, followed by soft brush while bathing
- Oatmeal baths for itching
- Tar shampoos
- Avoid excessive sun exposure
- Desert climates may provide a favorable effect
- Wet dressings may help relieve pruritus
- For extensive, recalcitrant psoriasis, a referral to a specialist in psoriatic therapy is suggested

SURGICAL MEASURES N/A

ACTIVITY No restrictions

DIET No special diet

PATIENT EDUCATION
- Provide patient reassurance and anxiety relief to the extent possible
- Assurance to patient and family the condition is non-contagious
- For patient education materials, physicians may contact: American Academy of Family Physicians, (800)274-2237, ext. 4406
- National Psoriasis Foundation, (800)723-9166; fax (503)245-0626; E-mail 76135.2746@comserve.com

MEDICATIONS

DRUG(S) OF CHOICE
- Mild to moderate disease:
  - ◊ Emollients bid: soft yellow paraffin or aqueous cream; petrolatum or Aquaphor cream greasier and more effective
  - ◊ Topical, **low potency** corticosteroids on delicate skin (eg, face, genitals or flexures). Alclometasone dipropionate, triamcinolone acetonide 0.025%, hydrocortisone 2.5%
  - ◊ Topical, **medium potency** corticosteroids (fluticasone propionate, triamcinolone acetonide 0.1%, hydrocortisone valerate, mometasone furoate usually for lesions on the torso) tid-qid (overnight occlusion with plastic wrap will hasten resolution). Switching products prevents tachyphylaxis. Non-fluorinated is less atrophogenic.
  - ◊ Topical, **strong potency** corticosteroids - betamethasone dipropionate, halcinonide, fluocinonide, desoximetasone
  - ◊ Topical, **super potency** corticosteroids - augmented betamethasone dipropionate, diflorasone diacetate, clobetasol propionate, halobetasol propionate. Limit use to 2 weeks if possible, avoid occlusive dressings. Taper to prevent rebound. Usually reserved for recalcitrant plaques or lesions on palms or soles of feet.
  - ◊ Intralesional corticosteroid: 2-5 mg/mL triamcinolone acetonide
  - ◊ Coal tar (Estar, PsoriGel) may be beneficial when alternated with topical steroids. Apply and air dry for 15 minutes before going to bed or apply in AM for 15 minutes, then shower. Tar bath preparations for widespread involvement.

◊ Keratolytic agents to decrease scale: salicylic acid 6% gel (or 2-10% salicylate acid ointment) bid several weeks. Even 20% for 2 weeks, except in children. alpha hydroxy acid, glycolic acid or lactic acid. Alternate keratolytics with other topicals.
◊ Corticosteroid solutions, betamethasone valerate mousse and tar shampoos - scalp lesions
◊ Ultraviolet lamps and sun light effective. May be best treatment option during pregnancy or in young children.
◊ UVB + emollients in erythemogenic dose in fair-skinned patients - less toxic than PUVA
◊ Anthralin ointment 1% or higher applied for 5-30 minutes, then washed off, useful adjunctive treatment. Use prior to ultraviolet light (UVA, UVB). Indicated for quiescent or chronic psoriasis, contraindicated in acute or actively inflamed psoriatic eruptions. Start with 0.1%, gradually increase to 3.5%. Irritates unaffected skin, protect areas with zinc oxide or petrolatum. Avoid face, eyes, mucous membranes. New preparation - Micanol delivers drug at body temperature so staining household items minimized.

- Severe disease:
  ◊ Triamcinolone, intralesional - mix with procaine or normal saline for concentrate of 4 mg/mL. Administer with syringe or dermajet. Effective in treating solitary resistant plaques and psoriasis involving the nails.
  ◊ Vitamin D analogs (calcipotriene ointment 0.005% for moderate plaque psoriasis). Results may not be maximal for 2 months. Too irritating for facial lesions. Watch for hypercalcemia if large quantity used. Weekly cumulative dose < 100-120 gram. Associated with little or no tachyphylaxis. Calcipotriene is inactivated by salicylic acid, ammonium lactate lotion and hydrocortisone valerate 0.2% ointment. Halobetasol proprionate 0.05% and 5% tar gel are compatible.
  ◊ Acitretin (Soriatane) - oral retinoid (active metabolite of etretinate) replaces etretinate (Tegison) which had 120 day half life. Safe for use on face. Also treats pustular and erythrodermic psoriasis not responding to standard treatment. Fetotoxic. Contraception needed one month before, during and for at least 3 years after treatment. Ethanol may convert acitretin to etretinate so no ethanol while using acitretin. Women should refrain from drinking alcohol for 2 months after treatment stopped.
  ◊ Tazarotene (Tazorac) - for psoriasis involving up to 20% body surface area. Avoid face and groin due to irritation. Daily or every other day treatment. Retinoid induced dermatitis major side effect.
  ◊ Oral corticosteroids only for severe or life-threatening disease (risk of rebound)
  ◊ Isotretinoin: may work on some patients
  ◊ PUVA oral (psoralen plus ultraviolet light) - very effective, but causes skin-aging, cataracts and increases risk of skin cancers
  ◊ Bath PUVA - topical psoralen applied 5 min to 2 hours before UVA. Better for soles, palms, ie, localized disease, because less nausea of systemic psoralens. May cause severe local phototoxic reaction and patchy pigmentation.
  ◊ Goeckerman regimen - black tar/UVB all day treatment. Psoriasis Day Treatment Programs.
  ◊ Methotrexate - single weekly dose (up to 25 mg) or 2.5-5 mg q12h for 3-4 days per week, but precautions necessary. Hydroxyurea for methotrexate failure. Azathioprine and intralesional cyclosporine, not common.
  ◊ Cyclosporine or tacrolimus [S/E of paresthesias, diarrhea]: only for recalcitrant psoriasis (possible nephrotoxicity)
    - Cyclosporine: regimens for short-term use only, perhaps alternating with other agents. Gradual taper over 12 weeks when stopping minimizes relapse.

Contraindications: Refer to manufacturer's literature
Precautions: Refer to manufacturer's literature
Significant possible interactions: Refer to manufacturer's literature

ALTERNATIVE DRUGS
- RePUVA (acitretin plus PUVA)
- Mycophenolate mofetil (CellCept) 250-500 mg qid for recalcitrant disease (hematologic and hepatic toxicity, teratogenic; check CBC weekly during first month, twice monthly second and third month, then monthly; contraception needed)
- Thioguanine - anti-metabolite. Risk of myelosuppression. Check CBC and platelets q 2 wks, and q wk with dose increase
- Narrow band UV-B therapy (311-nm)
- Combined systemic treatments - MTX or hydroxyurea + PUVA, acitretin or MTX, or calcipotriene + UVB
- Sequential therapy
  ◊ Clearance phase - 1 month class 1 topical steroid every AM, calcipotriene qhs + cyclosporine 4-5 mg/kg/day
  ◊ Transition phase - 1 month calcipotriene bid weekdays, class 1 topical steroids bid weekend and gradually acitretin
  ◊ Maintenance phase - until remission; calcipotriene bid then taper; continue acitretin; taper and stop cyclosporine

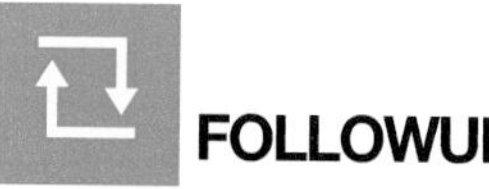

FOLLOWUP

PATIENT MONITORING
- Continuous supportive care
- Medications used require close followup. Certain lab studies necessary. Long-term use of topicals not recommended.
- With methotrexate therapy check CBC, SGOT, albumin every month. Some recommend liver biopsy before treating or 3 months after treatment started and then regularly (usually every 2 years) based on a cumulative methotrexate dose of 1.5 grams.

PREVENTION/AVOIDANCE
- Avoid alcoholic beverages
- Avoid irritating drugs
- Avoid stimulating drugs (lithium, ACE inhibitors, beta-adrenergic blockers, tetracycline, NSAIDs, amiodarone, morphine, procaine, potassium iodide, salicylates, sulfapyridine, sulfonamides and penicillin. Pustular flares may occur with steroids).
- Avoid antimalarial medications (aminoquinolone compounds)

POSSIBLE COMPLICATIONS
- Pustular psoriasis
- Exfoliative erythrodermatitis
- Rebound when corticosteroids discontinued
- Topical corticosteroid thinning of skin, striae, masking local infection, hypopigmentation and tachyphylaxis
- Hypercalcemia with excessive calcipotriene
- Salicylism possible in children with high dose topical salicylic acid.

EXPECTED COURSE/PROGNOSIS
- Usually benign
- Life-threatening forms do occur
- May be refractory to treatment

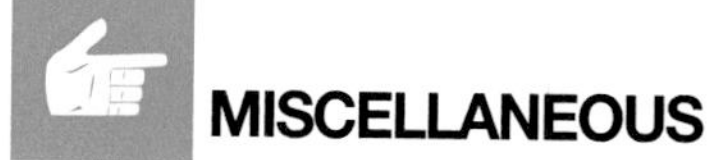

MISCELLANEOUS

ASSOCIATED CONDITIONS
- Extensive erythrodermic psoriasis may accompany AIDS
- Arthritis
- Psoriatic arthritis
- Myopathy
- Enteropathy
- Spondylitic heart disease
- Acute anterior uveitis

AGE-RELATED FACTORS
Pediatric: Onset common <10, rarely <3; disease may be atypical in its course
Geriatric:
- 3% of patients acquire psoriasis > 65
- Many drugs (eg, beta-blockers) can exacerbate psoriasis
- If using cytotoxic medications for treatment of psoriasis, closely follow hepatic and renal functions, and creatinine clearance
- Elderly may have difficulty applying topicals on all affected body parts

Others: N/A

PREGNANCY
Unpredictable effect on disease. Avoid tars, topical corticosteroids, calcipotriene, and systemic therapies. Etretinate is fetotoxic.

SYNONYMS
N/A

ICD-9-CM
696.1 Other psoriasis
696.2 Parapsoriasis

SEE ALSO

OTHER NOTES
N/A

ABBREVIATIONS
N/A

REFERENCES

- Burrall B, Dijkstra J, Lowe N, Maibach H: Psoriasis therapies: Old, new and borrowed. Patient Care 1995;10:38-65
- Greaves MW, Weinstein GD: Treatment of psoriasis. NEJM 1995;332(9):581-588
- Habif T. Clinical Dermatology. 4th Ed. St. Louis, CV Mosby, 2004
- Abel E: Diagnosis of drug induced psoriasis. Seminars in Dermatology 1992;11(4)
- Jegasothy B, et al: Tacrolimus (FK 506): A new therapeutic agent for severe recalcitrant psoriasis. Arc Dermatol 1992;128
- Moschella S, et al, eds: Dermatology. 3rd Ed. Philadelphia, W.B. Saunders Co., 1992

Web references: 1 available at www.5mcc.com
Illustrations 15 available

Author(s):
Sean Herrington, MD

BASICS

DESCRIPTION Bacterial infection of the genital tract following delivery. Endometritis (infection of the endometrium), is the most common infection. Less common are infections of the myometrium and parametrial tissues, vaginal and cervical infections, perineal cellulitis, pelvic cellulitis, septic pelvic vein thrombophlebitis and parametrial phlegmon.

System(s) affected: Reproductive

Genetics: N/A

Incidence/Prevalence in USA:
- Vaginal deliveries - <3%
- Cesarean sections - <10%
- Accounts for 7% of maternal deaths
- Fourth leading cause of maternal mortality

Predominant age: N/A

Predominant sex: Female only

SIGNS & SYMPTOMS
- Oral temperature >38.7°C (101.6°F) in first 24 hours post-partum or
- Oral temperature >38°C (100.4°F) in two of first 10 days post-partum (excluding first 24 hours)
- Uterine tenderness on exam
- Other localized tenderness on exam
- Ileus
- Tachycardia
- Chills, malaise, headache, anorexia
- Abdominal or localized pain
- Purulent or malodorous lochia
- Note: Group A or Group B strep bacteremia may have no localizing signs

CAUSES
- The risk of endometritis increases 5-30 fold following Cesarean delivery
- Endometritis commonly follows chorioamnionitis
- Other infections follow trauma to the perineum, vagina, cervix and uterus
- Infection is nearly always polymicrobial and involves organisms that have ascended from the lower genital tract:
  - ◊ Aerobic isolates in 70% - *S. faecalis*, *S. agalactiae*, *S. viridans*, *Staphylococcus aureus*, *E. coli*, *Klebsiella sp.*, *Proteus sp.*, *Gardnerella vaginalis*
  - ◊ Anaerobic isolates in 80% - *Peptococcus sp.*, *Peptostreptococcus sp.*, *Clostridium sp.*, *Bacteroides bivius*, *B. fragilis*, *Fusobacterium sp.*
  - ◊ Other - genital mycoplasmas - role in endometritis is unclear
  - ◊ *Chlamydia trachomatis* - responsible for some late (2-10 days) post-partum endometritis (see alternative drugs)
  - ◊ Range of number of isolates is 1-8

RISK FACTORS
- Cesarean section
- Pre-existing chorioamnionitis
- Multiple vaginal examinations
- Indigent status
- Bacterial vaginosis or group B strep colonization of genital tract
- Prolonged rupture of membranes, prolonged labor and the use of internal fetal monitoring have been shown to be significant factors in univariate but not multivariate analysis

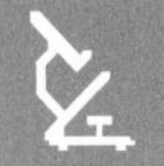

DIAGNOSIS

DIFFERENTIAL DIAGNOSIS
- Fever from other sources
  - ◊ Urinary tract infection
  - ◊ Viral syndrome
  - ◊ Dehydration
  - ◊ Pneumonia
  - ◊ Wound infection
  - ◊ Thrombophlebitis
  - ◊ Thyroid storm
  - ◊ Mastitis

LABORATORY
- CBC - interpret with care as physiologic leukocytosis may be as high as 20,000
- Blood cultures - if sepsis is suspected
- Amniotic fluid gram stain - usually polymicrobial
- Uterine tissue cultures - difficult to obtain without contamination
- Genital tract cultures and rapid test for group B strep - may be done when patient is in labor
- Note: Diagnosis is usually made clinically

Drugs that may alter lab results: N/A

Disorders that may alter lab results: N/A

PATHOLOGICAL FINDINGS
- Microscopic sections of uterine lining show superficial layer of infected necrotic tissue
- Thrombosis of any of the pelvic veins including the vena cava
- Phlegmon on leaves of the broad ligament
- Abscess

SPECIAL TESTS N/A

IMAGING
- If patient is not responsive to antibiotics
  - ◊ CT or MRI for pelvic vein thrombophlebitis
  - ◊ U/S, CT or MRI for abscess, pelvic masses or deep-seated wound infection

DIAGNOSTIC PROCEDURES Paracentesis or culdocentesis with culture - rarely necessary

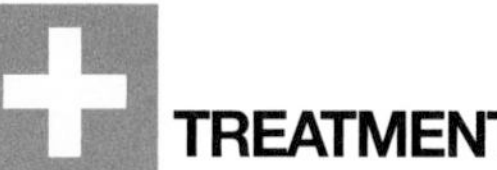

TREATMENT

APPROPRIATE HEALTH CARE
- Inpatient for severe infection
- Low grade endometritis may respond to outpatient treatment with oral antibiotics (see alternative drugs)
- Most infections (94%) occur after hospital discharge

GENERAL MEASURES
- IV antibiotics and close observation for severe infections
- Open and drain infected wounds
- Normalize fluid status
- Note: Amnioinfusion during labor may decrease infections when membranes have been ruptured for more than 6 hours.

SURGICAL MEASURES
- Curettage of retained products of conception
- Surgery to establish drainage of abscess
- Surgery to decompress the bowel
- Surgical drainage of a phlegmon is not advised unless suppurative

ACTIVITY As tolerated

DIET As tolerated although may be limited by ileus.

PATIENT EDUCATION
Call doctor if fever >38°C (100.4°F) post-partum or other symptoms of infection (see Signs and Symptoms)

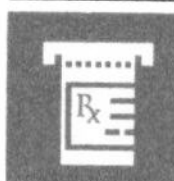

MEDICATIONS

DRUG(S) OF CHOICE

- Cefoxitin 2 gm IV q6hrs. Add ampicillin 2 gm IV q6hrs if clinical failure after 48 hours.
- Cefotetan 2 gm IV q12hrs. Add ampicillin 2 gm IV q6hrs if clinical failure after 48 hours.
- Piperacillin 4 gm IV q6hrs
- Ampicillin-sulbactam (Unasyn) 2/1 gm IV q6hr
- Clindamycin 600-900 mg IV q8hr plus gentamicin 5 mg/kg IV q24hrs (traditional 'gold standard' but may cause nephrotoxicity, ototoxicity, pseudomembranous colitis, diarrhea [in up to 6%] and may require gentamicin peak and trough levels)
- Note: Base therapy on cultures, sensitivities, and clinical response

Contraindications:

- Drug allergy
- Renal failure (aminoglycosides)
- Avoid chloramphenicol, sulfa, tetracyclines, and fluoroquinolones before delivery and if breast-feeding

Precautions:

- Chloramphenicol rarely causes bone marrow suppression
- Clindamycin and other antibiotics occasionally cause pseudomembranous colitis

Significant possible interactions: Refer to manufacturer's literature

ALTERNATIVE DRUGS

- Metronidazole 7.5 mg/kg IV q6hr plus gentamicin 2 mg/kg IV qd (see above)
- Amoxicillin-clavulanate (Augmentin) 500/125 mg po tid for mild infections as outpatient
- Clindamycin 300-450 mg po qid for penicillin allergic outpatients with mild infections
- Note: Consider adding a macrolide antibiotic (for chlamydia coverage) for infections occurring after 48 hours
- Note: Heparin may be indicated for septic pelvic vein thrombophlebitis - requires 10 days at full anticoagulation

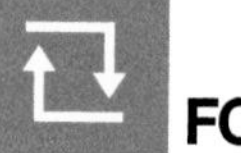

FOLLOWUP

PATIENT MONITORING

- Individualize according to severity
- IV antibiotics can be stopped when afebrile for 24 - 48 hours
- Oral antibiotics on discharge are not necessary except in cases of bacteremia

PREVENTION/AVOIDANCE

- Treat chorioamnionitis during labor
- Treat prophylactically with cefazolin for C/S deliveries after the cord is clamped
- Avoid unnecessary vaginal exams
- Avoid retained placental fragments or membranes

POSSIBLE COMPLICATIONS

- Resistant organisms
- Pelvic abscess
- Septic pelvic vein thrombosis
- Septic shock
- Death

EXPECTED COURSE/PROGNOSIS

- With supportive therapy and appropriate antibiotics most patients improve within a few days
- If no improvement on antibiotics, consider retained placental fragments or membranes, abscess, wound infection, hematoma, cellulitis, phlegmon or septic pelvic vein thrombosis

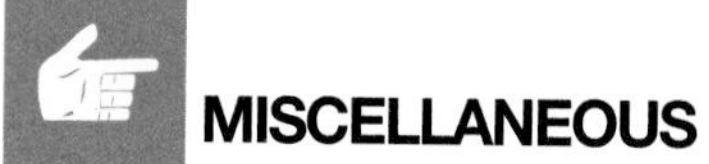

MISCELLANEOUS

ASSOCIATED CONDITIONS

- Chorioamnionitis

AGE-RELATED FACTORS

Pediatric: N/A
Geriatric: N/A
Others: N/A

PREGNANCY

A complication of pregnancy

SYNONYMS

- Post-partum infection
- Endometritis
- Endoparametritis
- Endomyometritis
- Myometritis
- Endomyoparametritis
- Metritis
- Metritis with pelvic cellulitis

ICD-9-CM

670.04 Major puerperal infection, postpartum condition or complication

SEE ALSO

OTHER NOTES N/A

ABBREVIATIONS N/A

REFERENCES

- Deborah S. Yokoe, et. al. Epidemiology of and Surveillance for Postpartum Infections. Emerg Infec Dis 7(5), 2001
- Hamadeh G, et al. Postpartum fever. Amer Fam Phys 1995;52(2):531-538
- Casey BM, Cox SM. Chorioamnionitis and endometritis. Infect Dis Clin of NA 1997;11(1):203-222
- Creasy RK, Resnick R. Maternal-Fetal Medicine. 4th Ed. Philadelphia, WB Saunders Co., 1999
- Yokoe DS, Christiansen CL, Johnson R, et al. Epidemiology of and surveillance for postpartum infections. Emerg Infect Dis 2001;7(5):837-41
- French LM, Smaill FM. Antibiotic regimens for endometritis after delivery (Cochrane Review). In: The Cochrane Library, Issue1, 2004, Chichester, UK: John Wiley & Sons. Ltd.

Web references: 1 available at www.5mcc.com
Illustrations N/A

Author(s):
Carol Cordy, MD

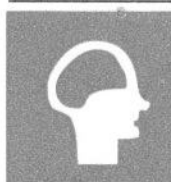

BASICS

DESCRIPTION Pulmonary interstitial and/or alveolar fluid accumulation that results when the forces moving fluid out of the pulmonary capillary exceed the forces restraining that fluid
System(s) affected: Cardiovascular, Pulmonary
Genetics: Multifactorial
Incidence/Prevalence in USA: Approximately 150,000 persons per year in U.S. affected with non-cardiogenic pulmonary edema
Predominant age: Middle age and elderly
Predominant sex: Male = Female

SIGNS & SYMPTOMS
- Respiratory
  - ◊ Shortness of breath
  - ◊ Dyspnea with exertion
  - ◊ Orthopnea, paroxysmal nocturnal dyspnea
  - ◊ Cough, often accompanied by pink or blood-tinged and frothy sputum
  - ◊ Wheezing, rhonchi, gurgles
  - ◊ Moist, crepitant rales noted initially at bases and progressing to apices
  - ◊ Breathlessness, air hunger
  - ◊ Noisy respirations
  - ◊ Tachypnea
  - ◊ Dilated alae nasi
  - ◊ Inspiratory retraction of the intercostal spaces and/or supraventricular fossae
  - ◊ Cheyne-Stokes respirations
- Cardiovascular
  - ◊ Tachycardia
  - ◊ Elevated jugular venous pulse
  - ◊ Increased P2
  - ◊ S3
  - ◊ S4
  - ◊ Nocturnal angina
  - ◊ Pulsus alternans or presence of valvular heart disease
- General
  - ◊ Weakness, fatigue
  - ◊ Other symptoms depending on etiology
  - ◊ Anxiety
  - ◊ Diaphoretic, cold, ashen, or cyanotic skin
  - ◊ Lower extremity edema

CAUSES
- Cardiogenic
  - ◊ Left heart failure
  - ◊ Ischemic heart disease
  - ◊ Acute myocardial infarction
  - ◊ Aortic and mitral valvular disease
  - ◊ Hypertensive heart disease
  - ◊ Cardiomyopathy
  - ◊ Volume overload
  - ◊ Arrhythmias
  - ◊ Endocarditis
  - ◊ Myocarditis
  - ◊ Congenital heart disease
  - ◊ Acute rheumatic fever and rheumatic heart disease
  - ◊ Septal defects
  - ◊ Cardiac tamponade
  - ◊ High cardiac output states (e.g., thyrotoxicosis, beriberi)
- Non-cardiogenic
  - ◊ Shock
  - ◊ Multiple trauma
  - ◊ Infection/sepsis (especially pneumonia)
  - ◊ Liquid aspiration (e.g., drowning, gastric contents)
  - ◊ Inhaled toxic gases
  - ◊ Pulmonary lymphatic obstruction
  - ◊ Drug overdose (especially narcotics)
  - ◊ High-altitude illness
  - ◊ Pancreatitis
  - ◊ Embolism (thrombus, fat, air, amniotic fluid)
  - ◊ Neurogenic
  - ◊ Hematologic and immunologic disorders
  - ◊ Disorders associated with high negative pleural pressure
  - ◊ Radiation pneumonitis
  - ◊ Disseminated intravascular coagulation
  - ◊ Eclampsia
  - ◊ Decreased plasma oncotic pressure (e.g., hypoalbuminemia)
  - ◊ After cardioversion, anesthesia, or cardiopulmonary bypass
  - ◊ Oxygen toxicity
  - ◊ ARDS
  - ◊ Renal failure

RISK FACTORS Dependent on etiology

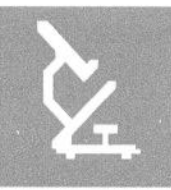

DIAGNOSIS

DIFFERENTIAL DIAGNOSIS
Important to distinguish between cardiogenic and non-cardiogenic pulmonary edema
- Pneumonia
- Asthma
- COPD exacerbation
- Pulmonary embolism
- Hyperventilation syndrome

LABORATORY
- None specific for pulmonary edema; laboratory abnormalities (e.g., troponin, natriuretic peptide, amylase, etc.) may point to underlying etiology
- Hypoxemia
- Hypocarbia
- Respiratory alkalosis
- Increased A-a gradient
- Leukocytosis

Drugs that may alter lab results: Administered oxygen may complicate arterial blood gas interpretation

Disorders that may alter lab results: Underlying pulmonary disease from an unrelated etiology may complicate arterial blood gas interpretation

PATHOLOGICAL FINDINGS
- Cardiogenic
  - ◊ Heavy, wet, subcrepitant lungs
  - ◊ Intra-alveolar granular pink precipitate
  - ◊ Alveolar microhemorrhages and hemosiderin-laden macrophages
  - ◊ "Brown induration," chronic passive congestion
  - ◊ Hypostatic bronchopneumonia
- Non-cardiogenic
  - ◊ Heavy, firm, red, and boggy lungs
  - ◊ Interstitial and intra-alveolar edema, inflammation, fibrin deposition, hemorrhage, and patchy atelectasis
  - ◊ Hyaline membrane formation
  - ◊ Interstitial and intra-alveolar fibrosis

SPECIAL TESTS
- Arterial blood gas
- Electrocardiogram
- Pulmonary function tests
- Mixed venous oxygen saturation

IMAGING
- Two-dimensional echocardiography with Doppler may be useful in some cases of cardiogenic pulmonary edema (e.g., valvular heart disease, systolic vs. diastolic dysfunction)
- Chest x-ray (may be difficult or impossible to differentiate cardiogenic from non-cardiogenic pulmonary edema)
  - ◊ Cardiogenic chest x-ray; Interstitial edema, cardiomegaly, pulmonary venous redistribution, Kerley's B lines, alveolar edema (initially perihilar), pleural effusions (more common)
  - ◊ Non-cardiogenic chest x-ray; alveolar edema, cardiomegaly absent, pulmonary venous redistribution absent, pleural effusions less common

DIAGNOSTIC PROCEDURES
- Swan-Ganz catheter may help differentiate cardiogenic from non-cardiogenic pulmonary edema
- Cardiac catheterization - occasionally beneficial

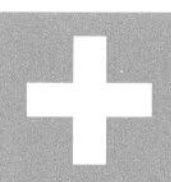

TREATMENT

APPROPRIATE HEALTH CARE Generally inpatient or intensive care; outpatient for mildest forms

GENERAL MEASURES
- Treat underlying condition
- Patient sitting, with legs dangling
- Oxygen
- Rotating tourniquets or phlebotomy selectively
- Mechanical ventilation, often requiring positive end-expiratory pressure support
- Rapid reduction in altitude in cases of high altitude pulmonary edema

SURGICAL MEASURES N/A

ACTIVITY Bedrest in most cases

DIET Low sodium diet

PATIENT EDUCATION
- Low sodium, fluid restriction
- Symptoms and signs of pulmonary edema
- Importance of medical compliance

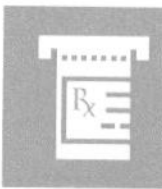

MEDICATIONS

DRUG(S) OF CHOICE

- Acute cardiogenic pulmonary edema
  - ◊ Morphine sulfate 2-5 mg IV
  - ◊ Furosemide 20-80 mg IV
  - ◊ Nitroglycerin paste 1-2 inches
  - ◊ In selected cases: Nitroglycerin drip beginning at 5 μg/min and increasing by 5-10 μg/min every few minutes, titrating to blood pressure, etc. Nitroprusside IV drip beginning at 10 μg/min and increasing by 5-10 μg/min every few minutes, titrating to blood pressure, etc. Dobutamine 2 μg/kg/min IV titrating to blood pressure, cardiac output, pulmonary capillary wedge pressure, etc.
- Chronic management of cardiogenic pulmonary edema
  - ◊ Furosemide 20-400 mg daily
  - ◊ Angiotensin converting enzyme inhibitors (e.g., captopril 6.25-25 mg po tid, lisinopril 2.5-20 mg po qd, enalapril 2.5-15 mg po qd-bid)
  - ◊ Digoxin 0.125-0.25 mg po qd
  - ◊ Carvedilol 3.125-25 mg po bid
  - ◊ Isosorbide dinitrate 10-60 mg po tid-qid
  - ◊ Thiazide diuretics (e.g., hydrochlorothiazide [HCTZ] 25-50 mg po qd)
  - ◊ Spironolactone 25-200 mg daily
- Non-cardiogenic pulmonary edema
  - ◊ Oxygen
  - ◊ Selected cardiovascular drugs to optimize tissue oxygen delivery

Contraindications: Refer to manufacturer's profile of each drug

Precautions:

- Avoid liberal intravenous fluids, especially normal saline or lactated Ringer's
- Avoid use of carvedilol and other beta blockers in decompensated cardiac failure, bronchospastic disease, second or third degree AV block, sick sinus syndrome and severe bradycardia
- Avoid calcium channel blockers and other negative inotropic agents in the setting of cardiogenic pulmonary edema
- Avoid high forced inspiratory O2 (FiO2) > 50% for prolonged periods of time if possible
- Avoid prolonged administration of nitroprusside due to risk of cyanide toxicity. If nitroprusside administered for > 72 hrs, obtain a thiocyanate level.

Significant possible interactions: Additive hypotensive effects of nitrates, afterload reducers, diuretics, etc.

ALTERNATIVE DRUGS

- Chlorothiazide
- Metolazone
- Acetazolamide
- Bumetanide
- Potassium-sparing diuretics
- Other ACE inhibitors

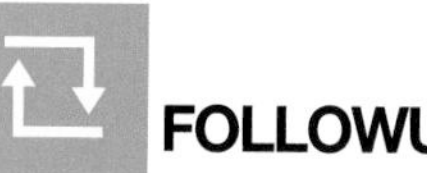

FOLLOWUP

PATIENT MONITORING

- Inpatient
  - ◊ Serial arterial blood gases or pulse oximetry, often in the intensive care unit with one-on-one nursing
  - ◊ Strict measurement of intake and output
  - ◊ Attention to optimal fluid management
  - ◊ Attention to optimal ventilator settings
  - ◊ Serial chest x-rays
- Outpatient
  - ◊ Attention to clinical status
  - ◊ Serial weights to assess fluid accumulation

PREVENTION/AVOIDANCE Compliance with medications and diet

POSSIBLE COMPLICATIONS

- Death
- Reversible or irreversible organ ischemia
- Pulmonary fibrosis, particularly with non-cardiogenic pulmonary edema

EXPECTED COURSE/PROGNOSIS

- Dependent on underlying etiology
- Mortality approximately 50-60% for non-cardiogenic pulmonary edema and up to 80% for cardiogenic shock

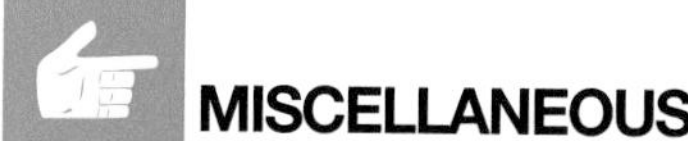

MISCELLANEOUS

ASSOCIATED CONDITIONS (see Causes)

AGE-RELATED FACTORS

Pediatric: Usually secondary to lung immaturity, congenital heart disease, or associated with trauma
Geriatric: Higher mortality
Others: N/A

PREGNANCY Pulmonary edema may occur as a complication of tocolytic therapy with magnesium sulfate, terbutaline or ritodrine

SYNONYMS N/A

ICD-9-CM

428.1 Left heart failure
518.4 Acute edema of lung, unspecified

SEE ALSO

Altitude illness
Congestive heart failure
Respiratory distress syndrome, adult

OTHER NOTES N/A

ABBREVIATIONS

ARDS = adult respiratory distress syndrome

REFERENCES

- Ingram RH, Braunwald E. Pulmonary edema. In: Braunwald E, editor. Heart disease - A Textbook of Cardiovascular Medicine. 6th ed. Philadelphia: WB Saunders Co; 2001
- Braunwald E, et al. Harrison's Textbook of Internal Medicine. 15th ed. New York: McGraw-Hill Inc; 2001

Web references: 0 available at www.5mcc.com
Illustrations N/A

Author(s):
Peter Kozisek, MD

Pulmonary embolism

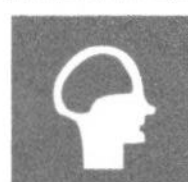

BASICS

DESCRIPTION Pulmonary embolism occurs when venous thrombi in the deep venous system of the legs dislodge and enter the pulmonary arterial circulation
- Pulmonary embolism presents as three different syndromes
  - ◊ Acute cor pulmonale - due to massive pulmonary embolism, obstructing > 60-75% of the pulmonary circulation
  - ◊ Pulmonary Infarction - occurs in patients with submassive pulmonary embolism with complete obstruction of a distal branch of the pulmonary circulation
  - ◊ Acute unexplained dyspnea - occurs in patients who do not develop acute cor pulmonale or pulmonary infarction

System(s) affected: Cardiovascular, Pulmonary
Genetics: Hypercoagulability
Incidence/Prevalence in USA:
- 600,000-700,000 cases/year
- 100,000-200,000 deaths/year

Predominant age: Very rare in children, incidence increases with advancing age
Predominant sex: Male = Female

SIGNS & SYMPTOMS
- Acute cor pulmonale
  - ◊ Syncope
  - ◊ Hypotension or cardiac arrest
  - ◊ Dyspnea
  - ◊ Anxiety
  - ◊ Tachypnea
  - ◊ Tachycardia
  - ◊ Distended neck veins
  - ◊ S3 gallop
  - ◊ Clear lungs on auscultation
  - ◊ ± Signs of deep venous thrombosis
  - ◊ ECG - S1Q3T3 pattern or incomplete right bundle branch block
  - ◊ Chest x-ray - usually normal
  - ◊ Arterial blood gases (room air) decreased PO2, decreased PCO2
- Pulmonary infarction
  - ◊ Pleuritic chest pain
  - ◊ Dyspnea
  - ◊ ± Hemoptysis
  - ◊ Tachypnea
  - ◊ Lungs - rales, wheezes and/or signs of pleural effusion
  - ◊ ± Signs of deep venous thrombosis
  - ◊ ECG - normal
  - ◊ Chest x-ray - elevated hemidiaphragm, infiltrate or small pleural effusion
  - ◊ Arterial blood gases (room air) - normal or decreased PO2, decreased PCO2, alkalosis
- Acute unexplained dyspnea
  - ◊ Dyspnea
  - ◊ ± Anxiety
  - ◊ ± Tachycardia
  - ◊ Tachypnea
  - ◊ Clear lungs
  - ◊ ± Signs of deep venous thrombosis
  - ◊ ECG - usually normal
  - ◊ Chest x-ray - normal

CAUSES
- Hypercoagulability
- Deep vein thrombosis responsible for 95% of pulmonary embolism

RISK FACTORS
- Prolonged immobility
- Advanced age
- Congestive heart failure
- Malignancy
- Stroke
- Pregnancy
- Oral contraceptives
- Postoperative
- Trauma to legs
- Obesity

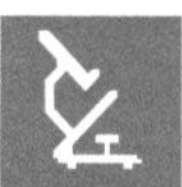

DIAGNOSIS

DIFFERENTIAL DIAGNOSIS
- Pneumonia
- Myocardial infarction
- Congestive heart failure
- Viral pleuritis

LABORATORY N/A

Drugs that may alter lab results: N/A

Disorders that may alter lab results: N/A

PATHOLOGICAL FINDINGS Pulmonary infarction

SPECIAL TESTS N/A

IMAGING
- The diagnosis is confirmed by V/Q lung scan (multiple segmental or lobar perfusion defects with normal ventilation), or pulmonary angiogram (intraluminal filling defects and/or arterial cutoffs)
- Chest x-ray may reveal parenchymal infiltrate, pleural effusion

Weight-based heparin dosing:

aPTT	Bolus† (U/kg)	Hold††	Rate (/hr)	Repeat aPTT
Initial	80	NO	18	6 hrs
<35	80	NO	+4	6 hrs
35-45	40	NO	+2	6 hrs
46-70	none	NO	no change	in AM
71-90	none	NO	-2	6 hrs
91-120	none	60 min	-3	6 hrs
>120	HOLD INFUSION & CALL PHYSICIAN			

†Maximum heparin dose 7,500 units
††If bleeding, regardless of PTT results, hold heparin and call physician

DIAGNOSTIC PROCEDURES
- Lung scan
- Pulmonary angiogram
- Echocardiogram
- Spiral CT scan
- D-Dimer
- Ultrasound of legs
- Diagnosis suspected on basis of signs and symptoms consistent with one of the three syndromes in a patient with deep venous thrombosis (DVT) or with risk factors for DVT

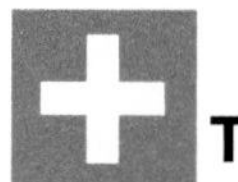

TREATMENT

APPROPRIATE HEALTH CARE Hospitalization, ICU if hemodynamically unstable; selected stable patients may be treated as outpatient

GENERAL MEASURES
- Designed to maintain adequate cardiovascular and pulmonary function and to prevent recurrence of emboli
- Oxygen therapy as needed

SURGICAL MEASURES
- Interruption of inferior vena cava may be indicated in patients who can not take anticoagulants or those who have recurrent emboli despite anticoagulant therapy
- In patients with massive embolism who have persistent hypotension, pulmonary embolectomy may be life saving despite a mortality of approximately 30%. An alternative to embolectomy is thrombolytic therapy in patients without a contraindication.

ACTIVITY
- Bed rest, move legs frequently
- Ambulation when patient stable

DIET No special diet, need to maintain adequate nutrition and fluids

PATIENT EDUCATION N/A

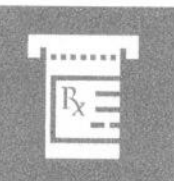

MEDICATIONS

DRUG(S) OF CHOICE
- Low molecular weight heparin by subcutaneous injection qd or bid for at least 5 days or
- Intravenous heparin by continuous infusion, at dose to prolong partial thromboplastin time to 1.5-2.0 times control for five days. Usual regimen requires beginning with 80 units/kg load followed by 18 unit/kg/hr. Check PTT 6 hours after beginning infusion, then daily.
- Warfarin beginning day one or day two of hospitalization for at least three months. Warfarin dose adjusted to prolong prothrombin time to an INR of 2.5 (range 2.0 to 3.0).
- In event of hypotension requiring vasopressors in a patient with angiographically documented pulmonary embolism, pulmonary embolectomy or intravenous thrombolytic agents may be required

Contraindications: Refer to manufacturer's profile of each drug

Precautions:
- Refer to manufacturer's profile of each drug
- The major complication of heparin is the possibility of hemorrhage. If PTT is appropriately adjusted, the major hemorrhage rate should be low.

Significant possible interactions: Refer to manufacturer's profile of each drug

ALTERNATIVE DRUGS
- Thrombolytics (streptokinase, urokinase, tissue plasminogen activator [tPA])

FOLLOWUP

PATIENT MONITORING After hospital discharge, prothrombin time should be prolonged to an INR of 2.5 (range 2.0 to 3.0). Warfarin should be continued 3-6 months. In patients with continuous predisposition to DVT, it should be continued indefinitely.

PREVENTION/AVOIDANCE Recognition of patients with multiple risk factors for deep venous thrombosis and implementation of prophylactic therapy including low dose heparin, warfarin or leg compression devices

POSSIBLE COMPLICATIONS
- Pulmonary infarction
- Acute cor pulmonale
- Recurrent deep venous thrombosis or pulmonary embolism, post phlebitic syndrome
- Treatment failure requiring surgical venous interruption

EXPECTED COURSE/PROGNOSIS
With appropriate therapy hospital mortality is less than 5%. Long-term prognosis determined by coexisting disease(s).

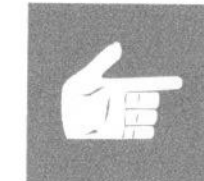

MISCELLANEOUS

ASSOCIATED CONDITIONS
- Deep vein thrombosis
- Occult cancer (lung, GI tract, breast, uterus, prostate)

AGE-RELATED FACTORS
Pediatric: Quite rare
Geriatric: More common, more often fatal.
Others: N/A

PREGNANCY Risk of occurrence during pregnancy and puerperium

SYNONYMS N/A

ICD-9-CM
415.19 Pulmonary embolism and infarction, other

SEE ALSO
Thrombosis, deep vein (DVT)

OTHER NOTES N/A

ABBREVIATIONS N/A

REFERENCES

- Hyers TM, Agnelli G, Hull RD, et al. Antithrombotic therapy for venous thromboembolic disease. Chest 2001;119(1 Suppl):176S-193S
- Rippe JM, et al, eds. Intensive Care Medicine. 2nd Ed. New York, Little, Brown, 1991:308-316
- Raschke, et al. The Weight Based Heparin Dosing Nomogram Compared with a 'Standard Care' Nomogram. Ann Int Med, 1993;119:874-81

Web references: 1 available at www.5mcc.com
Illustrations N/A

Author(s):
James E. Dalen, MD, MPH

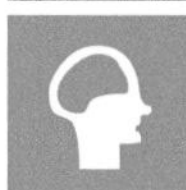

BASICS

DESCRIPTION A congenital deformity consisting of obstruction to right ventricular outflow at the pulmonic valve level
System(s) affected: Cardiovascular
Genetics: N/A
Incidence/Prevalence in USA: 10% of congenital heart disease
Predominant age: Newborn, but often asymptomatic for years
Predominant sex: Male = Female

SIGNS & SYMPTOMS
- History of heart murmur since birth
- Acyanotic
- Dyspnea and fatigue are the most frequent symptoms
- Occasionally dizziness or syncope occurs, particularly exertional, due to the low fixed cardiac output
- Chest pain can occur
- Myocardial infarction of the hypertrophied right ventricle has been noted
- Prominent A wave of the jugular venous pulse
- Right ventricular impulse
- Midsystolic murmur (increased duration and later peaking with increased severity)
- Pulmonic ejection sound
- Soft, delay in P2
- Occasional tricuspid regurgitation

CAUSES
- Congenital
- Rubella embryopathy

RISK FACTORS Family history

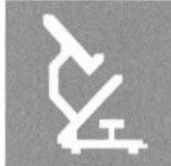

DIAGNOSIS

DIFFERENTIAL DIAGNOSIS
- Dysplastic pulmonic valve stenosis
- Discrete infundibular stenosis
- Subinfundibular obstruction
- Isolated pulmonary artery stenosis
- Supravalvar pulmonary stenosis
- Tetralogy of Fallot (Pink)

LABORATORY N/A

Drugs that may alter lab results: N/A

Disorders that may alter lab results: N/A

PATHOLOGICAL FINDINGS N/A

SPECIAL TESTS ECG - generally sinus rhythm, occasional supraventricular arrhythmias, tall peaked P waves, rightward axis, severity correlates with R/S ratio in leads V1 and V6, right ventricular hypertrophy

IMAGING
- X-ray - post stenotic dilatation of the pulmonary trunk, prominence of right atrium and ventricle
- Echocardiogram - mobile dome, thickened pulmonic valve, post stenotic dilatation of the pulmonary trunk, small valve annulus; continuous wave Doppler provides an estimate of the transvalvular gradient
- Color-flow Doppler - delineates area of obstruction, defects pulmonary regurgitation

DIAGNOSTIC PROCEDURES
- Cardiac catheterization
  - ◊ Not indicated in mild pulmonic stenosis
  - ◊ Essential in severe pulmonic stenosis
  - ◊ Used to assess morphology of the right ventricle, pulmonary outflow tract and the pulmonary arteries
  - ◊ Also used to rule out associated lesions e.g., atrial septal defect (ASD), though echocardiography may suffice.

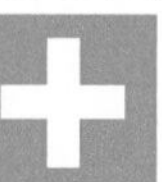

TREATMENT

APPROPRIATE HEALTH CARE Usually outpatient. Inpatient, if surgery indicated.

GENERAL MEASURES
- Though infective endocarditis is rare, SBE prophylaxis is advisable
- Diagnostic treatment for critical pulmonary stenosis in newborns
- Intervention
  - ◊ None required for mild pulmonic stenosis
  - ◊ Intervention of asymptomatic patients with moderate PS is controversial. At minimum, regular assessment is advisable.

SURGICAL MEASURES Percutaneous balloon valvotomy (preferred) or surgical pulmonic valvotomy required for patient with severe obstruction

ACTIVITY No specific prescription. The lesion, if significant, will limit activity.

DIET No specific regimen

PATIENT EDUCATION American Heart Association, 7320 Greenville Avenue, Dallas, TX 75231, (214)373-6300

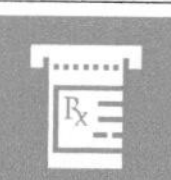

MEDICATIONS

DRUG(S) OF CHOICE
- No specific regimen in the absence of congestive heart failure
- Endocarditis prophylaxis

Contraindications: Refer to manufacturer's literature
Precautions: Refer to manufacturer's literature
Significant possible interactions: Refer to manufacturer's literature

ALTERNATIVE DRUGS N/A

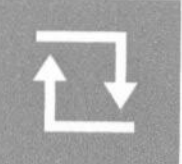

FOLLOWUP

PATIENT MONITORING
- Postoperative (or post-balloon valvotomy) Doppler ultrasound suggested at approximately 1 year after procedure
- Post valvotomy SBE prophylaxis still required
- Regular followup assessment for patients not undergoing surgical correction

PREVENTION/AVOIDANCE N/A

POSSIBLE COMPLICATIONS
- Up to 10% late mortality following valvotomy in critical pulmonary stenosis in neonates
- Slower recovery in those with chronic severe right ventricular hypertrophy
- Post valvotomy pulmonic regurgitation reported in up to 50% (variable severity)
- Residual ASD or patent foramen ovale
- Persistent repolarization abnormalities on ECG associated with severe postoperative pulmonic regurgitation
- Late atrial arrhythmias

EXPECTED COURSE/PROGNOSIS
Outcome following either balloon or surgical valvotomy is excellent in general

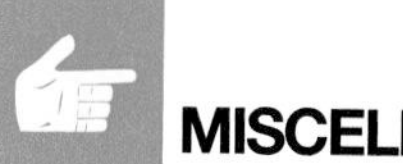

MISCELLANEOUS

ASSOCIATED CONDITIONS Other cardiac abnormalities, e.g., ventricular and atrial septal defects

AGE-RELATED FACTORS
Pediatric: Congenital disorder
Geriatric: N/A
Others: N/A

PREGNANCY In asymptomatic young women with mild to moderate PS, pregnancy is generally well tolerated

SYNONYMS Pulmonic stenosis

ICD-9-CM
424.3 Pulmonary valve disorders
746.02 Stenosis, congenital

SEE ALSO
Tetralogy of Fallot

OTHER NOTES N/A

ABBREVIATIONS
- SBE = subacute bacterial endocarditis
- PS = pulmonic stenosis

REFERENCES

- Braunwald E, ed. Heart Disease: A Textbook of Cardiovascular Medicine. 5th Ed. Philadelphia, W.B. Saunders Co., 1996
- Liberthson R: Congenital Heart Disease: Diagnosis & Management in Children and Adults. Boston, Little Brown & Co., 1989
- Perloff J: Clinical Recognition of Congenital Heart Disease. 4th Ed. Philadelphia, WB Saunders Co, 1994

Web references: 0 available at www.5mcc.com
Illustrations N/A

Author(s):
Ricardo Samson, MD

BASICS

DESCRIPTION

- Acute pyelonephritis is a syndrome caused by an infection of the pyelocaliceal system, producing localized flank or back pain combined with systemic symptoms such as fever, chills and prostration. It is accompanied by bacteriuria, and often by bacteremia, which can progress to "septic shock" and death.
- Chronic pyelonephritis is the pathological result of progressive inflammation on the renal interstitium and tubules, and the radiologic diagnosis of the renal scarring and destructive changes in the caliceal system that are presumed to be caused by bacterial infection, vesicoureteral reflux, or both.

System(s) affected: Renal/Urologic
Genetics: N/A
Incidence/Prevalence in USA:

- Community acquired acute pyelonephritis - 15.7 per 100,000/per year
- Hospital acquired acute pyelonephritis - 7.3 per 10,000 hospital persons

Predominant age: All ages, especially > 50
Predominant sex: Female > Male

SIGNS & SYMPTOMS

- In adults
  - ◊ Fever; above 38.5°C
  - ◊ Chills
  - ◊ Unilateral vs. bilateral pain in the lumbar flank area
  - ◊ Malaise
  - ◊ Myalgia
  - ◊ Anorexia
  - ◊ Nausea
  - ◊ Vomiting
  - ◊ Diarrhea
  - ◊ Headache
  - ◊ Dysuria
  - ◊ Frequency
  - ◊ Urgency
  - ◊ Suprapubic discomfort
  - ◊ Flank pain on palpation
  - ◊ From no physical findings to septic shock
- In infants and children
  - ◊ Sepsis
  - ◊ Fever
  - ◊ Irritability
  - ◊ Poor skin perfusion
  - ◊ Inadequate weight gain or weight loss
  - ◊ Gastrointestinal symptoms
  - ◊ Jaundice to gray skin color
  - ◊ Flank mass
  - ◊ Enuresis
  - ◊ Vaginal discharge, vulval soreness or pruritus in girls

CAUSES

- *E. coli* (≈75%)
- Other gram-negative rods, *Proteus mirabilis*, *Klebsiella* and *Enterobacter* account for 10-15%
- Enterococcus
- Staphylococcus - epidermis, saprophyticus (number two cause in young women) and aureus
- *Leptospira*
- *Salmonella typhi*
- Mycoplasma
- Anaerobes

RISK FACTORS

- Underlying urinary tract abnormalities
- Indwelling catheter
- Nephrolithiasis
- Diabetes mellitus
- Immunocompromised conditions
- Elderly, institutionalized women
- Acute pyelonephritis within the prior year
- Prostatic enlargement
- Recent urinary tract instrumentation
- Childhood UTI
- Symptoms longer than 7 days at presentation

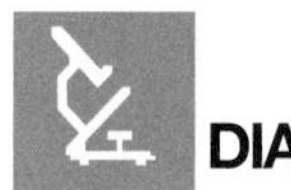

DIAGNOSIS

DIFFERENTIAL DIAGNOSIS

- Renal infarction
- Acute renal vein thrombosis
- Acute renal artery dissection
- Obstructive uropathy
- Acute glomerulonephritis
- Acute bacterial pneumonia
- Myocardial infarction
- Acute hepatitis
- Cholecystitis
- Acute pancreatitis
- Appendicitis
- A perforated viscus
- Splenic infarct
- Aortic dissection
- Acute pelvic inflammatory disease
- Kidney stone
- Ectopic pregnancy

LABORATORY

- Urine culture (> 100,000 colony-forming units [CFU/mL]) and sensitivities
- Urine gram stain
- Pyuria
- The leukocyte esterase test in the urine
- Leukocyte casts
- Hematuria and mild proteinuria
- Leukocytosis
- Blood culture(s)

Drugs that may alter lab results: Antibiotics

Disorders that may alter lab results: N/A

PATHOLOGICAL FINDINGS

- Acute:
  - ◊ Abscess formation with neutrophils
  - ◊ Glomeruli spared
  - ◊ The area of the infection is wedge-shaped toward the medulla
- Chronic:
  - ◊ Fibrosis
  - ◊ Reduction in renal tissue
  - ◊ Scarring
  - ◊ Calyceal clubbing, dilatation and distortion

SPECIAL TESTS

- Bladder washout
- Antibody coated bacteria or ACB test

IMAGING 67gallium or 131I-Hippuran scanning

DIAGNOSTIC PROCEDURES

- If febrile for longer than 72 hours or if obstruction/anatomic abnormality suspected
  - ◊ Cystoscopy with ureteral catheterization
  - ◊ Contrast-enhanced computerized tomography (CT) - spiral more sensitive than conventional
  - ◊ Ultrasound
  - ◊ Intravenous pyelogram (IVP)

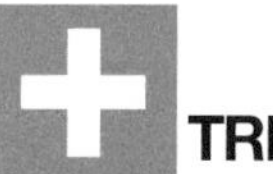

TREATMENT

APPROPRIATE HEALTH CARE

- Outpatient therapy if mild to moderate illness (not pregnant, no nausea or vomiting; fever and pain not severe), no risk factors, and tolerating oral hydration and medications.
- Inpatient therapy for severe illness (pregnant, high fevers, severe pain, marked debility, intractable vomiting, possible urosepsis) or risk factors

GENERAL MEASURES

- Intravenous fluids when needed
- Broad-spectrum antibiotics initially, tailoring therapy to culture and sensitivity results
- Analgesics and antipyretics
- Urinary analgesics (e.g., phenazopyridine 200 mg tid) for severe dysuria

SURGICAL MEASURES Percutaneous drainage of abscess if necessary

ACTIVITY As tolerated

DIET Encourage fluid

PATIENT EDUCATION Griffith's Instructions for Patients; Philadelphia, Elsevier

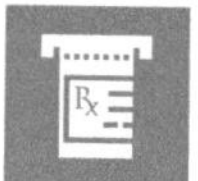

MEDICATIONS

DRUG(S) OF CHOICE

Severe Illness: IV therapy until afebrile 48 hours and tolerating oral hydration and medications, then oral agents to complete 2 weeks

- IV agents (assuming normal creatinine clearance):
  - ◊ Cefotaxime I g q 12 hours up to 2 g q 4 hours
  - ◊ Ceftriaxone 1-2 g q day
  - ◊ Cefoxitin 2 g q 8 hours
  - ◊ Ciprofloxacin 400 mg q 12 hours
  - ◊ Levofloxacin 500 mg q day
  - ◊ Moxifloxacin 400 mg qd
  - ◊ Gatifloxacin 400 mg qd
  - ◊ Piperacillin-tazobactam 3.375 g q 6 hours
  - ◊ Ticarcillin-clavulanate 3.1 g q 6 hours
  - ◊ Gentamicin 3-5 mg/kg of body weight q day (with or without ampicillin I g q 6 hours). Consider once daily dosing for synergy with ampicillin.
  - ◊ Trimethoprim-sulfamethoxazole 160-800 mg q 12 hours (Note: Up to 30% *E. coli* resistant to ampicillin and trimethoprim/sulfamethoxazole in community acquired infections). If enterococcus suspected based on gram stain, ampicillin plus low-dose once daily gentamicin is a reasonable empiric choice, unless penicillin allergic, then use vancomycin. Do not use a third generation cephalosporin for suspect or proven enterococcal infection.
- Oral agents:
  - ◊ Moxifloxacin 400 mg q day
  - ◊ Ciprofloxacin 500 mg q 12 hours
  - ◊ Ciprofloxacin ER 1000 mg q day
  - ◊ Levofloxacin 500 mg q day
  - ◊ Norfloxacin 400 mg q 12 hours
  - ◊ Gatifloxacin 400 mg q day
  - ◊ Cephalexin 500 mg qid
  - ◊ Amoxicillin-clavulanate 875/125 mg q 12 hours or 500/125 mg tid

Contraindications:

- Allergies to penicillin, sulfa, or other agents listed
- Fluoroquinolones contraindicated in adolescents, children and pregnant women
- Nitrofurantoin does not achieve reliable tissue levels for pyelonephritis treatment

Precautions:

- Most antibiotics require adjustments in dosage with renal insufficiency
- Follow aminoglycoside levels and renal function

Significant possible interactions: The absorption of most quinolone antibiotics is decreased in the presence of iron, aluminum, zinc, magnesium and calcium containing products (eg, multivitamins, antacids, sucralfate, etc)

ALTERNATIVE DRUGS N/A

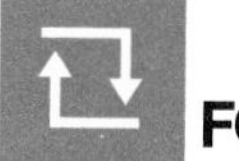

FOLLOWUP

PATIENT MONITORING

- Response within 48 hours (95% of patients): discharge on oral agent (see above) after patient is afebrile for 48 hours to complete 2 weeks
- No response within 48 hours (5% of patients): reevaluate, review cultures; CT (spiral CT most sensitive), IVP or ultrasound; adjust therapy as needed; may need urological consult
- Mild/moderate Illness - oral therapy for 2 weeks as outpatient: ciprofloxacin, gatifloxacin, levofloxacin, norfloxacin, cephalexin, amoxicillin/clavulanate. (Up to 30% *E. coli* resistance to ampicillin and trimethoprim/sulfamethoxazole in community acquired UTIs.) If enterococcus suspected based on urine gram stain, add amoxicillin to fluoroquinolone pending culture and sensitivity.
- All patients: follow-up urine analysis 1 to 2 weeks after completing therapy; if persistent hematuria despite eradication of infection, refer for urologic evaluation
- Women: routine follow-up cultures not recommended unless symptoms resolve but recur within 2 weeks; obtain urine culture, sensitivity, gram stain and CT or renal ultrasound. If symptoms resolve but recur after 2 weeks, treat as sporadic episode of pyelonephritis, unless 2 or more recurrences, then urologic evaluation necessary.
- Men, children, adolescents, patients with recurrent infections, patients with risk factors: repeat cultures 1 to 2 weeks after completing therapy; urologic evaluation after first episode of pyelonephritis and with recurrences.

PREVENTION/AVOIDANCE N/A

POSSIBLE COMPLICATIONS

- Kidney abscess
- Metastatic infection: skeletal system, endocardium, eye, meningitis with subsequent seizures
- Septic shock and death
- Chronic renal insufficiency
- Complications of antibiotics

EXPECTED COURSE/PROGNOSIS

95% respond in 48 hours

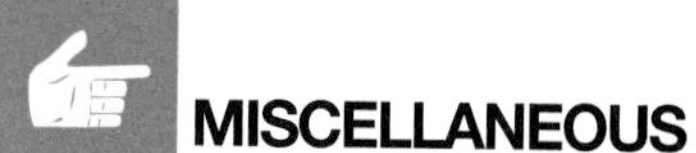

MISCELLANEOUS

ASSOCIATED CONDITIONS N/A

AGE-RELATED FACTORS

Pediatric: Nonspecific systems, jaundice, enuresis, sepsis

Geriatric:

- May present as confusion
- Characteristics may change

Others: N/A

PREGNANCY

- The most common medical complications requiring hospitalization
- May complicate the pregnancy course and produce low weight babies

SYNONYMS

- Acute upper urinary tract infection

ICD-9-CM

590.00 Chronic pyelonephritis without lesion of renal medullary necrosis
590.01 Chronic pyelonephritis with lesion of renal medullary necrosis
590.10 Acute pyelonephritis without lesion of renal medullary necrosis
590.11 Acute pyelonephritis with lesion of renal medullary necrosis
590.80 Pyelonephritis, unspecified

SEE ALSO

Urinary tract infection in females
Urinary tract infection in males

OTHER NOTES N/A

ABBREVIATIONS N/A

REFERENCES

- Hooton TM, Stamm WE. Diagnosis and treatment of uncomplicated urinary tract infections. Infect Dis Clin North Am 1997;11(3):551-81
- Bacheller CD, Bernstein JM. Urinary tract infections. Med Clin North Am 1997;81(3):719-30
- Orenstein R, Wong ES. Urinary tract infections in adults. Am Fam Phys 1999;59:1225-34
- Roberts JA. Management of pyelonephritis and upper urinary tract infections. Urol Clin North Am 1999;26(4):753-63
- Warren JW, Abrutyn E, Hebel JR, et al. Guidelines for antimicrobial treatment of uncomplicated acute bacterial cystitis and acute pyelonephritis in women. Infectious Diseases Society of America (IDSA). Clin Infect Dis 1999;29(4):745-58
- Gaspari R, Bosker G. Urinary tract infection: Risk stratification, clinical evaluation and evidence-based antibiotic therapy - year 2003 update. In: Bosker G, editor. Infectious Disease Update Year 2003. Atlanta, GA: American Health Consultants; 2003. p.1-21

Web references: 2 available at www.5mcc.com
Illustrations N/A

Author(s):
John Spangler, MD, MPH
Julienne K. Kirk, PharmD

BASICS

DESCRIPTION A progressive stenosis of the pyloric canal occurring in infancy
System(s) affected: Gastrointestinal
Genetics: Multifactorial inheritance risk; recurrence risk 3-9% if first degree relative affected
Incidence/Prevalence in USA: 1/300-1/1000 live births (male 1/150 live births; female 1/750 live births)
Predominant age: Infancy; onset usually at 3-4 weeks of age, rarely in the newborn period or as late as 5 months of age
Predominant sex: Male > Female (5:1)

SIGNS & SYMPTOMS
- Intermittent, non-bilious, projectile vomiting of increasing frequency and severity
- Initially hunger, later weakness
- Epigastric distention
- Visible gastric peristalsis, sometimes retrograde
- Palpable tumor (olive) in right upper quadrant
- Jaundice, occasional
- Late signs: dehydration, weight loss
- Diminished stools

CAUSES
- Obscure, sometimes familial; 6% risk of recurrence if either parent had pyloric stenosis, much higher if the mother was affected

RISK FACTORS 2.5 times more common in Caucasians than in blacks

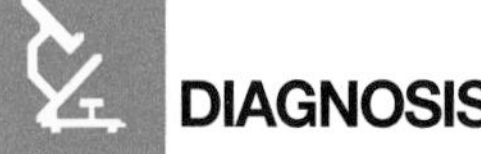

DIAGNOSIS

DIFFERENTIAL DIAGNOSIS
- Inexperienced or inappropriate feeding
- Gastroesophageal reflux
- Gastritis
- Congenital adrenal hyperplasia, salt-losing
- Pyloric diaphragm
- Pylorospasm

LABORATORY
- Early - evidence hypochloremic alkalosis, with low serum chloride and high bicarbonate
- Later - may have acidosis with low bicarbonate and low potassium
- Elevated unconjugated bilirubin level

Drugs that may alter lab results: N/A

Disorders that may alter lab results: N/A

PATHOLOGICAL FINDINGS Concentric hypertrophy of pyloric muscle

SPECIAL TESTS Abdominal ultrasound by experienced radiologist will usually outline the pyloric tumor

IMAGING
- Upright plain film of abdomen may reveal dilated stomach (filled with fluid and/or air) and relative lack of air in intestines
- Ultrasound (first choice if available) shows thickened and elongated pyloric muscle
- Barium swallow (performed only when diagnosis is not clinically clear) reveals strong gastric contractions and elongated, narrow pyloric canal (string sign); now rarely performed if ultrasound available

DIAGNOSTIC PROCEDURES None

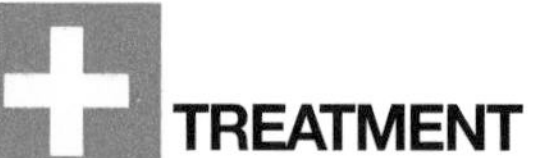

TREATMENT

APPROPRIATE HEALTH CARE
- Inpatient
- Surgery: Fredet-Ramstedt pyloromyotomy

GENERAL MEASURES N/A

SURGICAL MEASURES Surgery must be preceded by preoperative preparation, including: Empty stomach with nasogastric tube, fluid replacement, correction of electrolyte imbalance

ACTIVITY N/A

DIET
- No preoperative feeding
- No feeding for 8-16 hours postoperative
- Gradual increase in feedings thereafter
- Should reach full feedings 48-72 hours after surgery

PATIENT EDUCATION Instructions about preoperative and postoperative care

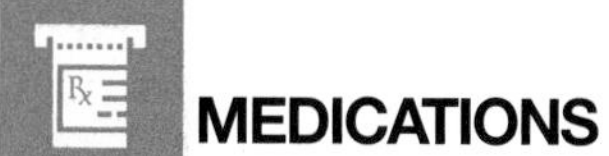

MEDICATIONS

DRUG(S) OF CHOICE N/A
Contraindications: N/A
Precautions: N/A
Significant possible interactions: N/A

ALTERNATIVE DRUGS N/A

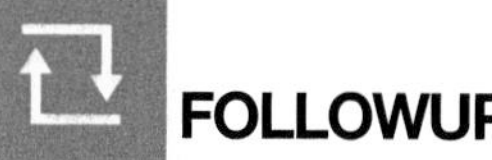

FOLLOWUP

PATIENT MONITORING Routine pediatric health maintenance

PREVENTION/AVOIDANCE N/A

POSSIBLE COMPLICATIONS
- No long term morbidity
- Occasional postoperative wound infection with staph aureus

EXPECTED COURSE/PROGNOSIS
Complete recovery with catch-up growth and weight gain

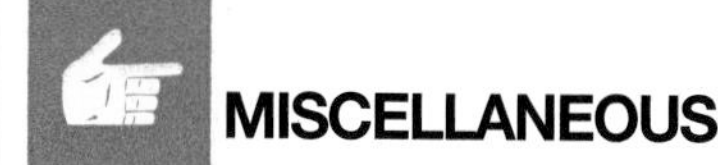

MISCELLANEOUS

ASSOCIATED CONDITIONS
- Usually none
- Rarely
  - ◊ Hiatal hernia
  - ◊ Esophageal atresia
  - ◊ Malrotation
  - ◊ Gastroesophageal reflux

AGE-RELATED FACTORS
Pediatric: N/A
Geriatric: N/A
Others: N/A

PREGNANCY N/A

SYNONYMS
- Infantile hypertrophic pyloric stenosis

ICD-9-CM
537.0 Acquired hypertrophic pyloric stenosis
750.5 Congenital hypertrophic pyloric stenosis

SEE ALSO

OTHER NOTES N/A

ABBREVIATIONS N/A

REFERENCES

- Walker, Durie, Hamilton, Walker-Smith, Watkins. Pediatric Gastrointestinal Disease, 2nd ed. CV Mosby, 1996.
- Garcia VF, Randolph TG: Pyloric Stenosis: Diagnosis and Management. Pediatrics in Review 1990;11:292-296
- Dolgin SE: Pyloric stenosis. In: FD Burg (ed): Gellis and Kagan's Current Pediatric Therapy. Philadelphia, WB Saunders, 1999

Web references: 0 available at www.5mcc.com
Illustrations N/A

Author(s):
Kurt J. Wegner, MD

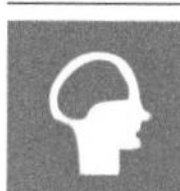

BASICS

DESCRIPTION A rapidly progressive infection of the central nervous system caused by an RNA virus and affecting mammals, including humans
- The disease is essentially 100% fatal once symptoms develop in prodrome stage
- Infection can be prevented by prompt, postexposure treatment of persons bitten by, or otherwise exposed to, animals known, or suspected to be, carrying the disease

System(s) affected: Nervous
Genetics: N/A
Incidence/Prevalence in USA: 0-5 cases per year in humans (most associated with bites of insectivorous bats although patients rarely recall exposure); about 7000 cases per year in animals (about 45% in raccoons); about 30,000 postexposure treatments. In US citizens - rate of rabies < 0.001/100,000/year.
Predominant age: Any
Predominant sex: Male = Female

SIGNS & SYMPTOMS
Usually proceed through four stages, although they may overlap
- Incubation
  - ◊ The incubation period is the time between bite and first symptoms of disease. This time is between one and three months in 2/3 of the cases. Sometimes can be as short as 6 days or longer than 6 years. It is shortest in patients with extensive bites about the head and trunk.
  - ◊ No symptoms except bite trauma
- Prodrome
  - ◊ Lasts 2 to 10 days
  - ◊ Pain or paresthesia at the bite site is the most specific symptom at this stage
  - ◊ Symptoms are often extremely variable and nonspecific, including fever, headache
  - ◊ May be referable to any of a number of organ systems
  - ◊ May suggest any of a number of common infections
- Acute neurologic period
  - ◊ Lasts 2 to 10 days
  - ◊ Symptoms referable to central nervous system dominate clinical picture
  - ◊ Generally takes one of two forms
  - ◊ Furious rabies: Episodes of hyperactivity last about 5 minutes and include hydrophobia, aerophobia, hyperventilation, hypersalivation and autonomic instability interspersed with periods of normalcy
  - ◊ Paralytic rabies: Paralysis dominates clinical picture, may be ascending (like Guillain-Barré syndrome) or affect one or more limbs differentially
- Coma
  - ◊ Last hours to days; with intensive care, may rarely last months
  - ◊ May evolve over a few days following acute neurologic period
  - ◊ May be sudden, with respiratory arrest
- Death
  - ◊ Usually occurs within three weeks of onset as result of complications
  - ◊ Only 4 survivors reported in the world's literature

CAUSES Rabies virus, a neurotropic virus present in saliva of infected animals

RISK FACTORS
For exposure to rabies:
- Professions or activities that may expose a person to wild or domestic animals, e.g., animal handlers, some lab workers, veterinarians, spelunkers (cave explorers)
- International travel to countries where canine rabies is endemic (most common risk factor)
- In the United States, most cases appear due to exposure to bats

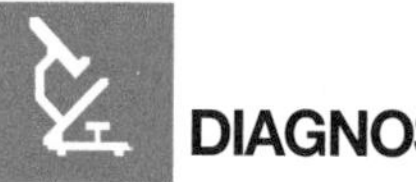

DIAGNOSIS

DIFFERENTIAL DIAGNOSIS
- Any rapidly progressive encephalitis; important to exclude treatable causes of encephalitis, especially herpes
- Diagnosis should be considered if there is a bite by an animal capable of transmitting the disease or travel to rabies endemic country; however, most patients in the U.S. do not recall exposure

LABORATORY
- WBC count in cerebrospinal fluid (CSF) exam may be normal or show moderate pleocytosis
- CSF protein may be normal or moderately elevated
- Viral isolation from saliva or CSF
- Serum CSF for rabies antibody
- Corneal smear stains positive by immunofluorescence in 50% of patients

Drugs that may alter lab results: Immunosuppressive agents

Disorders that may alter lab results: None

PATHOLOGICAL FINDINGS Encephalitis may be found in brain biopsy, but abnormal findings may be confined to parts (brainstem, midbrain, cerebellum) only examined postmortem

SPECIAL TESTS
- Only available in state and federal reference laboratories
- Rabies antibody titer should be obtained on serum and CSF
- Skin biopsy from nape of neck should be obtained for direct fluorescent antibody examination
- Saliva culture for rabies virus

IMAGING Normal, or nonspecific findings consistent with encephalitis

DIAGNOSTIC PROCEDURES
- Spinal tap
- Skin biopsy to detect rabies antigen in hair follicles

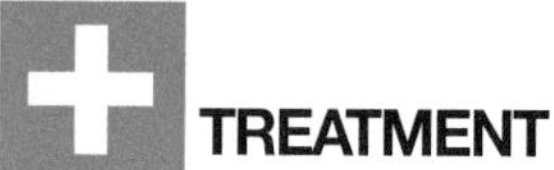

TREATMENT

APPROPRIATE HEALTH CARE
- Suspect rabies encephalitis - inpatient with isolation
- Exposure to rabies - inpatient if wounds serious; outpatient for prophylactic treatment

GENERAL MEASURES
- Since there is no treatment for clinical rabies, this section is directed at prevention of disease following exposure to potentially rabid animals
- Persons who observe abnormal behavior in any wildlife species should contact animal control or animal rescue agencies and should avoid approaching or handling these animals
- Physicians should evaluate each possible exposure to rabies and consult with local or state public health officials about the need for rabies prophylaxis
  - ◊ In the United States, raccoons, skunks, bats, foxes, coyotes are the animals most likely to be infected, but any carnivore can carry the disease
  - ◊ Postexposure prophylaxis should be considered for any person who reports direct contact with bats, unless it is known that an exposure did not occur.
- Outside the United States, dogs are a main reservoir especially in developing countries
- Before specific antirabies treatment is initiated, consider: Types of exposure (bite or non-bite), epidemiology of rabies in involved species, circumstances of biting incident and vaccination status of exposing animal

SURGICAL MEASURES N/A

ACTIVITY As tolerated

DIET No restrictions

PATIENT EDUCATION
- Avoid wild and unknown domestic animals
- Seek treatment promptly if bitten
- Thorough wound cleansing with soap is first line of treatment
- Pre-exposure vaccination if at risk of inapparent or unrecognized exposure to rabies inside or outside the United States

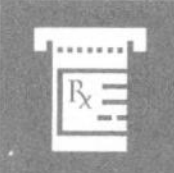

MEDICATIONS

DRUG(S) OF CHOICE

- Postexposure prophylaxis regimen (do all 3)
  - ◊ Local wound treatment: Immediate and thorough washing of all bite wounds and scratches with soap and water
  - ◊ Passive vaccination: rabies immune globulin (RIG, Hyperab) administered once - 20 IU/kg body weight (formula is applicable for all ages). If anatomically feasible, all of the RIG should be thoroughly infiltrated in the area around the wound. Any remaining RIG should be administered IM. RIG should never be administered in the same syringe or into the same anatomical site as vaccine.
  - ◊ Active vaccination: rabies vaccine, human diploid cell (HDCV) or Rabies vaccine adsorbed (RVA) or purified chick embryo cell vaccine (PCEC) IM in the deltoid. For children, the anterolateral aspect of the thigh is acceptable. Gluteal area should never be used for vaccine injections. Give the first dose, 1 mL, as soon as possible after exposure; one additional dose should be given on days 3, 7, 14, and 28.

For previously vaccinated patients, two IM doses (1 mL each) of vaccine should be administered, one immediately and one 3 days later. RIG not necessary in these patients.

- Preexposure vaccination: For persons in high risk groups, such as veterinarians, animal handlers, certain laboratory workers, and persons spending time in foreign countries where rabies is enzootic
  - ◊ Primary preexposure: IM vaccination regimen consists of three 1.0 mL injections of HDCV or RVA given in deltoid area, one each on days 0, 7, and 28. HDCV may also be given in intradermal (ID) doses, administered with a special syringe developed for that purpose (Imovax Rabies I.D. Vaccine); the 0.1 mL ID dose is administered in the deltoid area, follow the same schedule as for IM doses. Recently, the manufacturer discontinued production of Imovax rabies I.D.
  - ◊ Preexposure boosters: For persons at frequent risk of exposure to rabies, serum should be tested every 2 years. A preexposure booster (1.0 mL IM) should be administered if this is less than acceptable level. If titer cannot be obtained, a booster can be administered instead.

Contraindications: None for postexposure treatment
Precautions: About 6% of persons develop mild serum sickness reaction following HDCV boosters. Mild local and systemic reactions are very common following vaccination. Mild reactions should not be a cause for interruption of immunization.
Significant possible interactions: Antibody response may be suppressed by diseases that suppress immune system

ALTERNATIVE DRUGS None

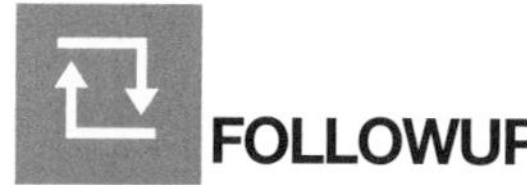

FOLLOWUP

PATIENT MONITORING After primary vaccination, serologic testing only necessary if patient has disease or takes medications that may suppress immune system

PREVENTION/AVOIDANCE See Treatment

POSSIBLE COMPLICATIONS None

EXPECTED COURSE/PROGNOSIS No postexposure failures reported in the United States since the 1970's

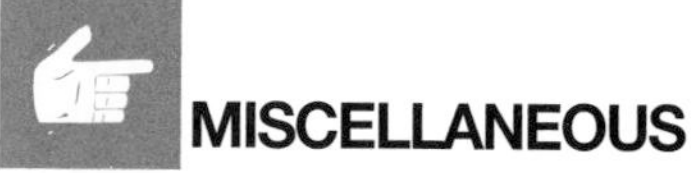

MISCELLANEOUS

ASSOCIATED CONDITIONS N/A

AGE-RELATED FACTORS

Pediatric: N/A
Geriatric: N/A
Others: N/A

PREGNANCY N/A

SYNONYMS Hydrophobia

ICD-9-CM

071 Rabies
V01.5 Rabies exposure
V04.5 Need for prophylactic vaccination and inoculation against rabies

SEE ALSO

Animal bites

OTHER NOTES N/A

ABBREVIATIONS

- RIG = rabies immune globulin
- HDCV = human diploid cell rabies vaccine
- RVA = rabies vaccine adsorbed
- PCEC = purified chick embryo cell vaccine

REFERENCES

- Fishbein DB. Rabies in humans. In: Baer G, ed. Natural History of Rabies. 2nd Ed. Boca Raton, CRC Press, 1991:519-549
- Bleck TP, Rupprecht CE. Rabies virus. In: Mandell GI, et al. Principles and Practice of Infectious Disease. 5th Ed. New York, Churchill Livingstone, 2000
- Rabies Prevention - United States, 1999. Morbidity and Mortality Weekly Reports 1999;48(RR-1):1-20
- Noah DL, Drenzek CL, Smith JS, et al. Epidemiology of human rabies in the United States, 1980-1996. Ann Intern Med 1998;128:922-30

Web references: 2 available at www.5mcc.com
Illustrations N/A

Author(s):

Daniel B. Fishbein, MD

BASICS

DESCRIPTION Any somatic or genetic disruption of function or form caused by electromagnetic waves or accelerated atomic particles
- Acute radiation sickness: Symptoms occurring within 24 hours of exposure
- Chronic radiation syndrome: Symptoms occurring greater than 24 hours after exposure, and generally over an extended time
- Radiation measures
  - ◊ 1 rad is the absorption of 100 ergs of energy by 1 gram of tissue
  - ◊ 100 rads = 1 gray (Gy)
  - ◊ The REM (Radiation Equivalent Man) unit was developed because different tissues have different sensitivities to radiation. 1 REM (Radiation Equivalent Man) is radiation dose in rads multiplied by a relative biologic effectiveness factor for the tissue involved. 100 REM = 1 sievert (Sv).
- Radiation includes:
  - ◊ Electromagnetic emissions. Energy (and hence penetration) is inversely proportional to wave length, eg x-rays, gamma rays
  - ◊ Particles. Alpha particles are the nuclei of helium atoms and beta particles are electrons. Both have low penetrance externally but are dangerous if ingested. Neutrons are damaging and penetrate well. Includes electrons, protons, alpha particles, neutron, negative pi-mesons, and heavy charged ions.

System(s) affected: Cardiovascular, Gastrointestinal, Hemic/Lymphatic/Immunologic, Musculoskeletal, Nervous, Pulmonary, Renal/Urologic, Reproductive, Skin/Exocrine

Genetics: Females tolerate better than males. The exception is pregnant females with risk of fetal injury at low dose.

Incidence/Prevalence in USA:
- Most acute radiation injury is related to accidents or radiation therapy
- 400,000 patients receive radiation therapy yearly for malignancies
- Accidents are sporadic and usually involve small numbers of individuals
- Historically:
  - ◊ 120,000 individuals developed acute radiation syndrome in Japan as a result of nuclear explosions
  - ◊ 7,266 natives of the Marshall Islands were exposed to radiation due to errors in judging winds after a nuclear test in the South Pacific
  - ◊ Chernobyl accident in Russia in 1986 where an estimated 50,000 individuals received at least 0.5 Sv of exposure.

Predominant age: N/A

Predominant sex: N/A

SIGNS & SYMPTOMS
- Acute radiation exposure is divided into several syndromes:
  - ◊ Less than 200 rads = no disease. There may be some nausea more than 3 hours after the event. Nausea is not a reliable sign of exposure since most people involved in an accident of this type will complain of some nausea when questioned.
  - ◊ 200-1000 rads = hematopoietic syndrome. Acute nausea and vomiting within 3 hours. Acute granulocyte elevation, then lymphopenia, then thrombocytopenia and neutropenia, then anemia. Peak lowering of platelets and granulocytes at 3 weeks (resolving in 12 weeks). Lymphopenia may last years. Survivors may get lung or kidney changes months after. Death rate 0-80% depending on dose received and treatment. Ld 50 for humans is 650 rads.
  - ◊ 1000-5000 rads = gastrointestinal syndrome. Nausea and vomiting 30-60 minutes postexposure. Loss of the villus structure of small bowel. Severe GI bleeding, diarrhea and abdominal pain develop in 3 days and precede the hematopoietic syndrome. Death due to blood loss or gram negative sepsis. Survivors usually die late of bone marrow suppression. Death rate 80-100%.
  - ◊ Over 5000 rads = neurovascular syndrome or "Spock syndrome". After a 15-30 minute asymptomatic period; tremors, ataxia, vomiting, hypotension, seizures and death. Death rate 100%.

CAUSES
- Nuclear weapons
- Industrial accidents
- Nuclear power accidents
- Radiation therapy

RISK FACTORS
- Young patients more susceptible than old
- Men more sensitive than women
- Debilitated more susceptible than healthy

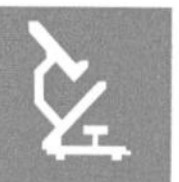

DIAGNOSIS

DIFFERENTIAL DIAGNOSIS
Was the patient exposed to radiation?
- Acute viral illness or anxiety cause nausea and vomiting
- Blast or heat cause skin redness
- Chemical exposure causes blistering, pain

LABORATORY
- Lymphocyte count at 48 hours post event
  - ◊ Over 1500 = trivial or no exposure
  - ◊ Over 1000 = survival without treatment
  - ◊ 500-1000 = survival with treatment
  - ◊ 100-400 = death without bone marrow transplant
  - ◊ Under 100 = certain death

Drugs that may alter lab results: Chemotherapeutic agents cause bone marrow suppression identical to radiation exposure

Disorders that may alter lab results: N/A

PATHOLOGICAL FINDINGS
- Hypocellular marrow with the hematopoietic syndrome
- The GI syndrome with loss of villus margin and sloughing of villus structure
- Late cases with fibrosis of lung, liver and kidney tissues
- Loss of hair indicates exposure of 350 rads and is complete at 700 rads

SPECIAL TESTS Total body dosimetry may suggest dose of compound ingested. Most radioisotopes are not excreted well.

IMAGING N/A

DIAGNOSTIC PROCEDURES N/A

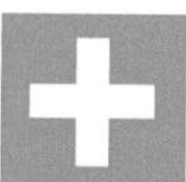

TREATMENT

APPROPRIATE HEALTH CARE Inpatient

GENERAL MEASURES
- Step 1 is decontamination to reduce external radiation and collateral exposure
- IV fluids, antinauseants and bedrest
- Platelet, RBC and WBC transfusion if needed
- Antibiotics for sepsis and neutropenia
- Treatment of collateral injuries such as burns and lacerations only after decontamination

SURGICAL MEASURES
- Debridement of all wounds to decontaminate
- All surgery within two days before loss of white cell and platelet function
- Bone marrow transplant for severe exposure

ACTIVITY Isolation techniques for immune system injury

DIET As tolerated. Hyperalimentation for severe GI syndromes.

PATIENT EDUCATION Recommend genetic counseling and screening to persons who have been exposed to significant amounts of radiation

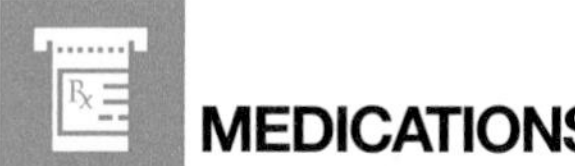

MEDICATIONS

DRUG(S) OF CHOICE
- Supportive therapy
  - ◊ Antibiotics for enteric organisms for GI syndrome, e.g., trimethoprim-sulfamethoxazole, ciprofloxacin
  - ◊ Broad spectrum antibiotics for infections common with bone marrow suppression, e.g., neutropenia
  - ◊ If radioactive iodine - potassium iodide (SSKI) in doses proportional to the exposure
  - ◊ If radioactive phosphorus - use parenteral magnesium sulfate
  - ◊ Nonspecific ingestions - use laxatives to increase GI transit rate

Contraindications: Refer to manufacturer's literature
Precautions: Refer to manufacturer's literature
Significant possible interactions: Refer to manufacturer's literature

ALTERNATIVE DRUGS N/A

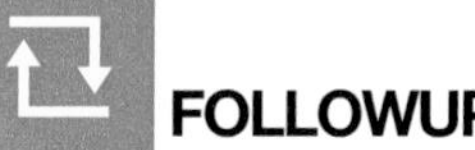

FOLLOWUP

PATIENT MONITORING
- Daily CBC, platelet, granulocyte, lymphocyte counts
- Stools for blood
- Vital signs q4h looking for sepsis

PREVENTION/AVOIDANCE
Follow safety procedures

POSSIBLE COMPLICATIONS
- Long-term fibrosis of kidneys, liver and lung. Occur within 6 months of acute exposure and with as little as 300 rads of exposure.
- Radiation exposure can induce malignancies
- Increased long-term risk of leukemia (acute lymphocytic or chronic myelogenous)
- Multiple myeloma and cancers of the breast, esophagus, stomach, colon, lung, ovary, bladder, thyroid
- Sterility

EXPECTED COURSE/PROGNOSIS
- Patients surviving 12 weeks have excellent prognosis but should be monitored for long-term complications
- Hair lost usually returns within 2 months

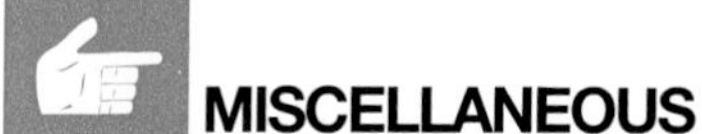

MISCELLANEOUS

ASSOCIATED CONDITIONS N/A

AGE-RELATED FACTORS
Pediatric: More sensitive to injury
Geriatric: Less sensitive to injury
Others: N/A

PREGNANCY
Injury to fetus likely

SYNONYMS N/A

ICD-9-CM
990 Radiation effects, unspecified

SEE ALSO

OTHER NOTES N/A

ABBREVIATIONS N/A

REFERENCES

- Bennett JC, Plum F, eds: Cecil Textbook of Medicine. 20th Ed. Philadelphia, W.B. Saunders Co., 1996
- Kissane JM, ed: Anderson's pathology. 9th Ed. St. Louis, Mosby, 1990
- Cotran RS, Ramzi S, et al, eds: Robbins Pathological Basis of Disease. 5th Ed. Philadelphia, Saunders 1994
- Fauci AS, ed: Harrison's Principles of Internal medicine. 15th ed. New York, McGraw-Hill, 2001

Web references: 2 available at www.5mcc.com
Illustrations 2 available

Author(s):
Mark R. Dambro, MD

BASICS

DESCRIPTION

- Definitions (legal definitions may vary from state to state)
  - ◊ Sexual contact - intentional touching of a person's intimate parts (including thighs) or the clothing covering such areas, if it is construed as being for the purpose of sexual gratification
  - ◊ Sexual conduct - vaginal intercourse between a male and female, or anal intercourse, fellatio, or cunnilingus between persons regardless of sex
  - ◊ Rape - any sexual penetration, however slight, using force or coercion against the person's will
  - ◊ Sexual imposition - similar to rape but without penetration or the use of force (i.e., non-consenting sexual contact)
  - ◊ Gross sexual imposition - non-consenting sexual contact with the use of force
  - ◊ Corruption of a minor - sexual conduct by an individual 18 years old or greater with an individual less than 16 years of age
  - ◊ Most states have expanded rape statutes to include: marital rape, date rape, shield laws

System(s) affected: Nervous, Reproductive

Genetics: N/A

Incidence/Prevalence in USA:

- Over 100,000 cases of alleged rape reported in US every year
- Estimated that only 1 in 5 to 1 in 10 adult cases reported
- Estimated only 1 in 15 to 1 in 20 pediatric cases reported
- Estimated incidence of reported rape is 80/100,000 females (7% of violent crime)
- One in three women will be a victim of sexual assault in her lifetime
- One in four women will experience rape or attempted rape during her college years
- The majority of rape victims either know or have some acquaintance with their attackers

Predominant age:

- Majority of adult victims are female in teens and 20's, (reported as high as 97 years)
- Pediatric victims may be either gender with predominance of females. Reported as young as 2 months.
- Increasing numbers of adult male victims presenting for treatment

Predominant sex: Female > Male

SIGNS & SYMPTOMS

- In adults
  - ◊ History of sexual penetration
  - ◊ Sexual contact, or sexual conduct without consent and/or with the use of force
- In pediatrics
  - ◊ Actual observation of, or suspicion of, sexual penetration, sexual contact, or sexual conduct
  - ◊ Signs include evidence of the use of force and/or evidence of sexual contact (e.g., presence of semen and/or sperm)

CAUSES Listed with Description

RISK FACTORS

- Numerous
- About 50% of rapes occur in the home, with 1/3 of these involving a male intruder

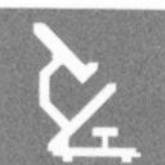

DIAGNOSIS

DIFFERENTIAL DIAGNOSIS Consenting sex among adults

LABORATORY

- Record results of wet mount noting the presence or absence of sperm and, if present, whether or not it is motile or immotile
- If indicated, a serum or urine pregnancy test should be obtained and the results recorded
- Drug/alcohol testing as indicated by history and/or physical findings
- Testing and/or specimen collection as indicated and in compliance with state requirements

Drugs that may alter lab results: N/A

Disorders that may alter lab results: N/A

PATHOLOGICAL FINDINGS N/A

SPECIAL TESTS N/A

IMAGING N/A

DIAGNOSTIC PROCEDURES

- History:
  - ◊ Avoid questioning which implies the patient is at fault
  - ◊ Record in patient's own words in so far as possible. Include date, approximate time, and general location as best possible. Document physical abuse other than sexual. Describe all types of sexual contact whether actual or attempted. History of alcohol and/or drugs before or after alleged incident.
  - ◊ Document time of last activity which could possibly alter specimens (e.g., bath, shower, or douche). Thorough gynecologic history is mandatory including last menstrual period (LMP), last consenting sexual contact, contraceptive practice, and prior gynecologic surgery.
- Physical examination:
  - ◊ Use of drawings and/or photographs is encouraged. Use of UV light (Wood's lamp) to detect seminal stains on clothing or skin. Document all signs of trauma or unusual marks. Documentation of mental status/emotional state.
  - ◊ Complete genital-rectal examination including evidence of trauma, secretions, or discharge. Use of a non-lubricated, water moistened speculum is mandatory since commonly used lubricants may destroy evidence.

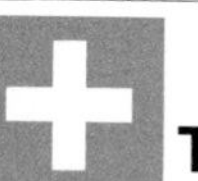

TREATMENT

APPROPRIATE HEALTH CARE

- Contact appropriate social services agency
- Majority of adult victims can be treated as outpatients unless associated trauma (physical or mental) requires admission
- Majority of pediatric sexual assault/abuse victims will require admission or outside placement until appropriate social agency can evaluate home environment

GENERAL MEASURES

- Providing health care to victims of sexual assault/abuse requires special sensitivity and privacy
- All such cases MUST be reported immediately to the appropriate law enforcement agency
- With the victim's permission, utilize personnel from local support agencies (e.g., Rape Crisis Center). When available, use of in-house Social Services is extremely helpful to victim/family.
- Sedation and tetanus prophylaxis should be utilized when indicated
- Venereal disease prevention for gonorrhea/Chlamydia should be administered
- A discussion of possible pregnancy and pregnancy termination should be held with the victim. If hospital policy precludes such a discussion, then information about this option should be offered the victim via the followup mechanisms.
- Suspected HIV and hepatitis B exposure and testing should be discussed with the victim and be in keeping with hospital, regional and state policies/protocols. The initial HIV test should be completed within seven days of the suspected exposure.
- Sexual assault nurse examiner (SANE) programs have been shown to be beneficial especially in large cities and metropolitan areas with multiple emergency departments of varying capability and staff training/experience

SURGICAL MEASURES N/A

ACTIVITY No restrictions

DIET No restrictions

PATIENT EDUCATION

- Information and help available from local rape crisis support organizations
- National Institute of Mental Health, Public Inquiries Branch, Office of Scientific Information, Department of Health and Human Services, Parklawn Bldg., Room 15C-05, 5600 Fishers Lane, Rockville, MD 20857, (301)443-4513

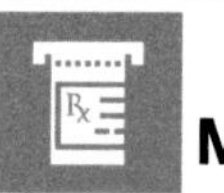

MEDICATIONS

DRUG(S) OF CHOICE
- Gonorrhea: ceftriaxone 250 mg IM once or cefpodoxime 200 mg po or ciprofloxacin 500 mg po or ofloxacin 400 mg po or spectinomycin 2 g IM
- Chlamydia: azithromycin (Zithromax) 1.0 g po single dose; or doxycycline 100 mg po bid or tetracycline 250 mg qid for 10 days. If the patient is pregnant, erythromycin should be used, 500 mg every 6 hours.
- Specific treatment for bacterial vaginosis if present - metronidazole 500 mg po bid for 7 days; or metronidazole 2 g po single dose (considered less efficacious than 7 day therapy)
- If pregnancy prophylaxis is given, consider progestin + estrogen - Ovral 4 pills total or Lo/Ovral 8 pills total. Half total pills taken within 72 hours of alleged event; half total pills 12 hours after first dose.
- HIV - currently there is lack of evidence supporting postexposure prophylaxis (PEP) after sexual assault except for specific high-risk circumstances. Regimen is lamivudine-zidovudine (Combivir) bid for 28 days; or zidovudine 300 mg plus lamivudine 150 mg bid for 28 days.
- Hepatitis B - if prevalent in area or assailant known high-risk, then hepatitis B immune globulin (HBIG) 0.06 mL/kg IM single dose and initiate 3 dose HBV immunization series
- Note - gonorrhea and chlamydia medications may be given concomitantly

Contraindications: Refer to manufacturer's literature
Precautions: Refer to manufacturer's literature
Significant possible interactions: Refer to manufacturer's literature

ALTERNATIVE DRUGS
- Gonorrhea: norfloxacin, ampicillin/probenecid, or amoxicillin/probenecid. Note: Be aware of drug resistance in your region. In NE Ohio, for example, a 20% resistance of gonorrhea to ciprofloxacin has been reported.

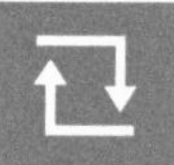

FOLLOWUP

PATIENT MONITORING
- The patient should be seen in seven to ten days for followup care, including pregnancy testing, and counseling by a gynecologist or appropriate gynecologic clinic
- Close examination for vaginitis and treatment if necessary
- Followup test for syphilis and gonorrhea should occur in five to six weeks
- Followup testing for HIV and hepatitis B should occur in six months
- Telephone numbers of counseling agency(ies) which can provide counseling/legal services to the patient should be provided
- Consider Sexual Assault Nurse Examiner (SANE) if available in area

PREVENTION/AVOIDANCE
- Scope of rape prevention is too complex and too broad to be discussed in these pages. True prevention will require many changes.
- Women may benefit from assertiveness training and self-defense training

POSSIBLE COMPLICATIONS
- Sexually transmitted disease and subsequent treatment
- Pregnancy (with the possibility of abortion)
- Trauma (physical and mental)
- Post-traumatic stress disorder (PTSD)

EXPECTED COURSE/PROGNOSIS
- Acute phase (usually 1-3 weeks following rape) - shaking, pain, wound healing, mood swings, appetite loss, crying. Also feelings of grief, shame, anger, fear, revenge or guilt.
- Late or chronic phase female victim may develop fear of intercourse, fear of men, nightmares , sleep disorders, daytime flashbacks, fear of being alone, loss of self-esteem, anxiety, depression, post-traumatic stress syndrome
- Recovery may be prolonged. Patients who are able to talk about their feelings seem to have a faster recovery.

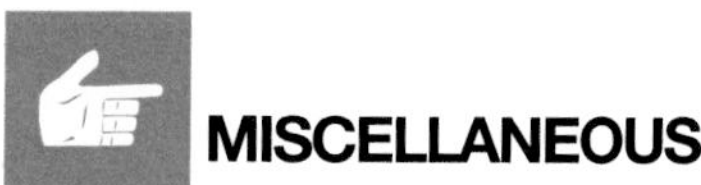

MISCELLANEOUS

ASSOCIATED CONDITIONS N/A

AGE-RELATED FACTORS
Pediatric: Assurance to the child that he or she is a good person and was not the cause of the incident
Geriatric: N/A
Others: N/A

PREGNANCY
Baseline pregnancy test conducted. Pregnancy prevention discussed with patient.

SYNONYMS
- Sexual assault
- Rape trauma

ICD-9-CM
V71.5 Observation following alleged rape or seduction
959.19 Other injury of other sites of trunk
959.9 Injury, unspecified site

SEE ALSO
Chlamydial sexually transmitted diseases
Gonococcal infections
Hepatitis B
Hepatitis C
HIV infection & AIDS
Post-traumatic stress disorder (PTSD)
Syphilis

OTHER NOTES
- Rape is a legal term and the examining physician is encouraged to use terminology such as "alleged rape" or "alleged sexual conduct".
- In majority of states, wife may now accuse husband of rape if they are estranged and living apart
- Since "consent defense" is common, documentation of evidence supporting the use of force or the administration of drugs/alcohol is imperative
- The use of a protocol is encouraged to assure every victim a uniform, comprehensive evaluation regardless of the expertise of the examining physician. The protocol must ensure that all evidence is properly collected and labeled, chain-of-custody is maintained, and the evidence is sent to the most appropriate forensic laboratory.
- All medical records must be well documented and legible
- All medical personnel must be willing and able to testify on behalf of the patient

ABBREVIATIONS N/A

REFERENCES
- American College of Emergency Physicians. Evaluation and management of the sexually assaulted or sexually abused patient. Dallas: ACEP; 1999
- Tintinalli JE, ed. Emergency Medicine: A Comprehensive Study Guide. 5th ed. New York: McGraw-Hill; 2000
- Rosen P, ed. Emergency Medicine Concepts and Clinical Practice. 4th ed. St. Louis: Mosby; 1998
- Hogan TM, Uyenishi AA. Sexual assault: medical and legal implications of the emergency care of adult victims. Emer Med Prac 2003;5(3)

Web references: 0 available at www.5mcc.com
Illustrations N/A

Author(s):
Daniel T. Schelble, MD

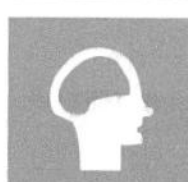

BASICS

DESCRIPTION Bilaterally occurring vasospastic disorder manifested by intermittent attacks of extreme pallor, then cyanosis of the fingers (rarely, of the toes) brought on by cold exposure. With warming, vasodilatation and intense redness develops, followed by swelling, throbbing, paresthesias. Resolves with warming. May accompany emotional upset. Thumbs rarely involved. 13% may progress to atrophy of digital fat pads, ischemic ulcers of fingertips. 50% idiopathic or primary Raynaud disease, 50% secondary (Raynaud phenomenon).

- Disease: progressive, symmetrical. Involves fingers; rarely toes. Ages 15 to 45. Spasm is more frequent, more severe with time. No gangrene; rarely ulcerates. Diagnose only after 2 years if no underlying associated disease. May be associated with coronary vasospasm or primary pulmonary hypertension. No histologic abnormality found in digital arteries.
- Phenomenon: may be unilateral, asymmetric; may affect only one or two fingers. Underlying condition usually identifiable with time. Usually has a worse morbidity and prognosis than primary disease.

System(s) affected: Hemic/Lymphatic/Immunologic, Musculoskeletal, Skin/Exocrine
Genetics: Little information available, but some suggest a dominant inheritance pattern. One study suggests there is a 5-fold increase in Raynaud in family members of a Raynaud patient. (Arthritis Rheum 1996; 39:1189-91)
Incidence/Prevalence in USA: 4 to 10% of population (based on reporting of characteristic color changes, cold intolerance)
Predominant age: After 40
Predominant sex:

- Female > Male (4:1 in primary form)
- Male = Female (secondary form)

SIGNS & SYMPTOMS

- Pallor/whiteness of fingertips with cold exposure, followed by cyanosis, then redness and pain with warming
- Ulceration of finger pads, progressing to autoamputation in severe, prolonged cases (10-13% of cases)
- Normal physical exam in primary; may show signs of underlying vasospastic or autoimmune disease in secondary form

CAUSES Unknown. May involve increased sensitivity of alpha-2-adrenergic receptors in digital vessels in primary type. Serotonin receptors (5-HT2 type) may be involved in secondary Raynaud. Platelet and blood viscosity abnormalities also implicated.

RISK FACTORS

- Smoking (men only)
- Existing autoimmune or connective tissue disorder
- Alcohol use (women only)
- Unopposed estrogen therapy was associated with higher incidence of Raynaud phenomenon in postmenopausal women. Not seen in women receiving combined hormone therapy.
- Helicobacter pylori may play a role in vascular diseases including Raynaud phenomenon. Some patients showed significant improvement following eradication of H. pylori.

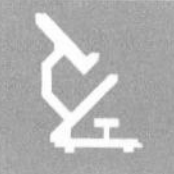

DIAGNOSIS

DIFFERENTIAL DIAGNOSIS

- Thromboangiitis obliterans (Buerger disease) - primarily affects men; involves legs and feet; less than 5% have hand involvement, 90% have Raynaud; smoking related
- Rheumatoid arthritis
- Progressive systemic sclerosis (scleroderma) - 90% have Raynaud; Raynaud may precede other symptoms by years
- Systemic lupus
- Carpal tunnel syndrome
- Thoracic outlet syndrome
- CREST syndrome (calcinosis cutis, Raynaud phenomenon, esophageal dysmotility, sclerodactyly and telangiectasia)
- Cryoglobulinemias
- Waldenström macroglobulinemia
- Acrocyanosis
- Polycythemia
- Occupational injury (especially from vibrating tools, masonry work, etc.)
- Drugs (beta-blockers, clonidine, ergotamine, methysergide, amphetamines, bromocriptine, bleomycin, vinblastine, cisplatin, cyclosporine).

LABORATORY Tests for underlying secondary causes (CBC, ESR, RA, ANA, immunoelectrophoresis, esophageal motility studies)

Drugs that may alter lab results: N/A

Disorders that may alter lab results: N/A

PATHOLOGICAL FINDINGS Histology of skin biopsy correlates poorly with clinical presentation. May show edema, necrotizing or non-necrotizing vasculitis, and/or perivasculitis.

SPECIAL TESTS

- Cold challenge test to elicit characteristic color changes in hands
- Nailfold capillaroscopy to detect enlarged, irregular capillary loops of other connective tissue diseases (primary Raynaud should show normal vasculature)

IMAGING Rarely, cases may demonstrate osteolysis of distal metaphyseal portions of phalanges, tapering and calcification of soft tissues

DIAGNOSTIC PROCEDURES Diagnosis largely determined by history, provocative exposure to cold

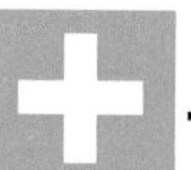

TREATMENT

APPROPRIATE HEALTH CARE Outpatient management usually sufficient

GENERAL MEASURES

- Dress warmly, wear gloves, avoid cold
- No smoking
- Avoid beta-blockers, amphetamines, ergot alkaloids, sumatriptan
- Biofeedback techniques to teach patients to increase hand temperature
- Finger guards over ulcerated fingertips

SURGICAL MEASURES Cervical sympathectomy effect is transient - symptoms return in 1 to 2 years

ACTIVITY Avoidance of situations in which exposure to cold is likely; avoid vibrating tools

DIET No special diet

PATIENT EDUCATION Emphasis on smoking cessation. Avoidance of aggravating factors (trauma, vibration, cold, etc.).

MEDICATIONS

DRUG(S) OF CHOICE
- Nifedipine 30-90 mg daily (sustained release form). (May only be needed during winter). Up to 75% experience improvement.
- Symptomatic responses do not correlate with objective evidence of improvement

Contraindications: Allergy to drug, pregnancy, congestive heart failure
Precautions: May cause headache, dizziness, lightheadedness, hypotension
Significant possible interactions:
- Increases serum level of digoxin - monitor digoxin levels closely after nifedipine added
- Cimetidine increases nifedipine level - may require dosage adjustment
- May increase prothrombin time in patients taking warfarin

ALTERNATIVE DRUGS
- Amlodipine, isradipine, nicardipine, and felodipine also appear to be effective and may be associated with fewer adverse effects
- Use of diltiazem, verapamil, reserpine, methyldopa, prazosin have equivocal support in literature
- Captopril studies suggest benefit, but need further evaluation (not FDA approved)
- Parenteral and oral prostacyclin have offered subjective improvement, but the effect is short-lived and not statistically significant
- Nitroglycerin patches may also be helpful, but limited by the incidence of severe headache

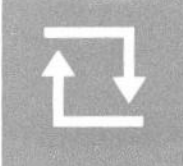

FOLLOWUP

PATIENT MONITORING
- Management of fingertip ulcers, including rapid treatment of infection
- Continue to observe for signs of associated illnesses, since Raynaud may precede overt development of these conditions by an average of 11 years

PREVENTION/AVOIDANCE
- Avoid trauma to fingertips
- Avoid exposure to cold
- Smoking cessation

POSSIBLE COMPLICATIONS
Gangrene, autoamputation of fingertips

EXPECTED COURSE/PROGNOSIS
- Prolonged course with recurrent ischemia, ulceration
- In case of secondary phenomenon, many eventually develop hallmarks of underlying disease
- Between 12-50% of Raynaud patients developed a secondary disorder, many of which were connective-tissue diseases

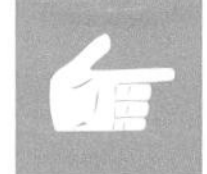

MISCELLANEOUS

ASSOCIATED CONDITIONS
- Lupus
- Rheumatoid arthritis
- Scleroderma
- Polymyositis
- Sjögren
- Occlusive vascular disease
- Cryoglobulinemia
- Use of vibrating tools

AGE-RELATED FACTORS
Pediatric: Associated with systemic lupus erythematosus and scleroderma in children
Geriatric: Appearance of Raynaud after 40 almost always indicates an underlying disease
Others: N/A

PREGNANCY
N/A

SYNONYMS
N/A

ICD-9-CM
443.0 Raynaud syndrome

SEE ALSO
Sjögren syndrome

OTHER NOTES
N/A

ABBREVIATIONS
N/A

REFERENCES

- Isselbacher KJ, et al, eds: Harrison's Principles of Internal Medicine. 13th Ed. New York, McGraw-Hill, 1994
- Maricq HR, et al: Prevalence of Raynaud phenomenon in the general population. A preliminary study by questionnaire. J Chronic Dis 1986;39:423
- Coffman JD: Raynaud's phenomenon: an update. Hypertension 1991;17:593
- Gasbarrini A, et al: Helicobacter pylori eradication ameliorates primary Raynaud's phenomenon. Dig Dis Sci 1998;43(8):1641-5
- Palesch YY, et al: Association between cigarette and alcohol consumption and Raynaud's phenomenon. J Clin Epidemiol 1999;52(4):321-8
- Williams HJ, et al: Early undifferentiated connective tissue disease (C7D). VI. An inception cohort after 10 years: disease remissions and changes in diagnoses in well established and undifferentiated CTD. J Rheumatol 1999;26(4)-816-25
- Fraenkel L, et al: Different factors influencing the expression of Raynaud's phenomenon in men and women. Arthritis Rheum 1999;42(2):306-10
- Sturgill MG, Seibold JR: Rational use of calcium-channel antagonists in Raynaud's phenomenon. Curr Opin Rheumatol 1998;10(6):584-8
- Lekakis J, et al: Short-term estrogen administration improves abnormal endothelial function in women with systemic sclerosis and Raynaud's phenomenon. Am Heart J 1998; 136(5):905-12
- Fraenkel L, et al: The association of estrogen replacement therapy and the Raynaud phenomenon in postmenopausal women. Ann Intern Med 1998;129(3):208-11
- Spencer-Green G: Outcomes in primary Raynaud phenomenon: a meta-analysis of the frequency, rates, and predictors of transition to secondary diseases. Arch Intern Med 1998;158(6):595-600

Web references: 0 available at www.5mcc.com
Illustrations 2 available

Author(s):
Mark R. Dambro, MD

BASICS

DESCRIPTION Protrusion of the rectum through the anus
- Partial prolapse - involves only mucosa. This frequently follows anal operative procedures. (Radial rectal folds prolapsed through anus).
- Complete prolapse - involves the entire rectal wall (procidentia). This type occurs most commonly as a spontaneous event in children and complication of other disorders in the elderly. (Concentric rectal folds prolapsed through anus).

System(s) affected: Gastrointestinal
Genetics: Unknown
Incidence/Prevalence in USA: 4.2:1000 overall; 10:1000 after age 65 years
Predominant age: 2 years in children, 60-70 years in adults
Predominant sex: Male > Female (5:1 in adults, and a slight predominance in children)

SIGNS & SYMPTOMS
- Children
  - ◊ Sensation of anal mass
  - ◊ Pain
  - ◊ Rectal bleeding
  - ◊ Protruding mass
- Adults
  - ◊ Anorectal pain or discomfort during defecation
  - ◊ Feeling of incomplete evacuation
  - ◊ Rectal and urinary incontinence
  - ◊ Rectal bleeding or discharge

CAUSES
- Children
  - ◊ Idiopathic (most common)
  - ◊ Abnormal innervation of levator ani muscle complex, puborectalis or anal sphincters or abnormal anatomic relationships of these muscle groups
- Adults
  - ◊ Diastasis of levator ani
  - ◊ Loose endopelvic fascia
  - ◊ Loss of normal horizontal position of rectum
  - ◊ Weak anal sphincter

RISK FACTORS
- Myelomeningocele
- Exstrophy of the bladder
- Cystic fibrosis
- Chronic constipation or diarrhea
- Imperforate anus
- Multiple sclerosis
- Stroke/paralysis
- Dementia

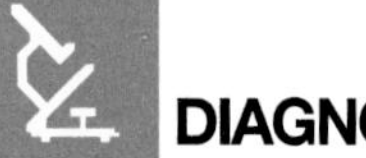

DIAGNOSIS

DIFFERENTIAL DIAGNOSIS
- Intussusception
- Rectal polyps
- Hemorrhoids

LABORATORY N/A

Drugs that may alter lab results: N/A

Disorders that may alter lab results: N/A

PATHOLOGICAL FINDINGS N/A

SPECIAL TESTS Evaluate for cystic fibrosis

IMAGING Barium enema is useful in selected cases of recurrent rectal prolapse

DIAGNOSTIC PROCEDURES Sigmoidoscopy is useful in recurrent prolapse to rule out rectal lesions

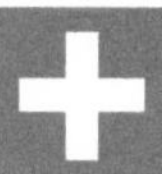

TREATMENT

APPROPRIATE HEALTH CARE Outpatient, unless complications occur or surgical intervention required

GENERAL MEASURES
- Acute
  - ◊ Prompt manual reduction of prolapse
  - ◊ Treatment of diarrhea or constipation

SURGICAL MEASURES
- Recurrent
  - ◊ Sub-mucosal injection of 5% phenol in glycerine in four quadrants under general anesthesia (outpatient)
  - ◊ Linear electrocauterization (inpatient)
  - ◊ Transabdominal Ripstein's procedure (suspension of rectum from sacrum by means of artificial material)
  - ◊ Posterior sagittal rectal suspension and levator repair
  - ◊ Ivalon sponge wrap procedure
  - ◊ Anterior resection of rectum
  - ◊ Transabdominal proctopexy (no artificial material used)
  - ◊ Perineal rectosigmoidectomy
  - ◊ Thiersch's wire (outpatient procedure; may be modified by using Marlex or Silastic strip instead of wire); used more commonly in children and elderly, poor-risk adults
  - ◊ Gracilis Sling procedure

ACTIVITY Full activity, when able

DIET High fiber

PATIENT EDUCATION
- Particular reassurance to parents of infants with prolapse regarding benign nature of problem and high rate of spontaneous resolution
- Diet instructions
- Teach measures to avoid constipation
- Teach family/patient to reduce prolapse

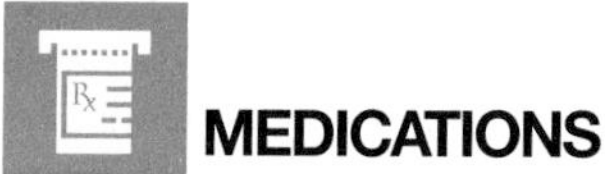

MEDICATIONS

DRUG(S) OF CHOICE
- Mineral oil
- Stool softeners
- Lactulose

Contraindications: N/A
Precautions: N/A
Significant possible interactions: N/A

ALTERNATIVE DRUGS N/A

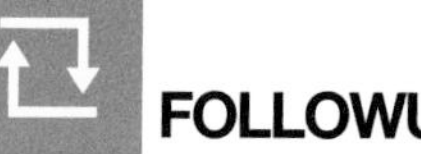

FOLLOWUP

PATIENT MONITORING Monthly visits until possible need for surgery has been determined or until prolapse has resolved

PREVENTION/AVOIDANCE Avoid constipation and diarrhea

POSSIBLE COMPLICATIONS
- Mucosal ulcerations
- Necrosis of rectal wall

EXPECTED COURSE/PROGNOSIS
- Spontaneous resolution expected in most children
- 5-10% recurrence rate for most procedures
- Good prognosis with treatment

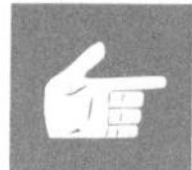

MISCELLANEOUS

ASSOCIATED CONDITIONS
- Cystic fibrosis
- Myelomeningocele
- Exstrophy of the bladder
- Chronic constipation or diarrhea
- Imperforate anus
- Paraplegia
- Stroke
- Incontinence

AGE-RELATED FACTORS
Pediatric: Idiopathic most common type of rectal prolapse in children
Geriatric: Common problem in the elderly
Others: N/A

PREGNANCY N/A

SYNONYMS N/A

ICD-9-CM
569.1 Rectal prolapse

SEE ALSO
Hemorrhoids
Intussusception

OTHER NOTES N/A

ABBREVIATIONS N/A

REFERENCES

- Ashcraft KW, Garred JL, Holder TM, et al. Rectal prolapse: 17 year experience with the posterior repair and suspension. J Ped Surg 1990;25(9):992-995
- Ashcraft KW, Murphy JP, Sharp RJ, editors. Pediatric Surgery. 3rd ed. Philadelphia: W.B. Saunders Co; 2000
- Schwartz SI, Shires GT, Spencer FC, et al, editors. Principles of Surgery. 7th ed. New York: McGraw-Hill Book Co; 1999
- O'Neill JA, Rowe MI, Grosfeld JL, et al. Pediatric Surgery. 5th ed. St Louis: Mosby; 1998

Web references: 1 available at www.5mcc.com
Illustrations N/A

Author(s):
Timothy L. Black, MD
James P. Miller, MD

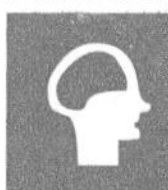

BASICS

DESCRIPTION An inability of the eye to produce a focused image on the fovea or central part of the retina

- Emmetropia: When light rays are in perfect focus, the image being viewed is seen clearly
- Ametropia: Any refractive error of the eye which prevents normal focusing of the image
- Hyperopia: When the cornea of the eye is too flat or the eye is too short, light rays fall in focus behind the retina, and an individual is "farsighted"
- Myopia: When the cornea is too steep or the length of the eyeball is too long, light rays fall short of the retina, and the eye is "nearsighted"
- Presbyopia: The natural tendency of the crystalline lens to harden or become sclerotic, limiting the focusing of the eye on near objects (accommodation). The human crystalline lens thickens with age. By the age of 40, most people do not have enough room within the eye to allow normal excursion of the lens and accommodation: viewing of near objects are blurred and reading glasses are required.
- Astigmatism: When the cornea is steeper in one meridian more than the other or the globe is not round (oval or almond-shaped), visual blurriness occurs

System(s) affected: Nervous
Genetics: Refractive errors are inherited
Incidence/Prevalence in USA: 70% of the general population have some form of ametropia
Predominant age: Refractive errors are present at birth, but not usually detected until puberty
Predominant sex: Male = Female

SIGNS & SYMPTOMS

- Difficulty seeing objects at a distance
- Difficulty focusing on near objects
- Difficulty reading
- Squinting
- Headaches (from squinting)
- In children:
  - ◊ Rubbing the eyes
  - ◊ Sitting close to TV or computer screen
  - ◊ Problems in sports; particularly declining performance
  - ◊ Declining grades
  - ◊ Preference for front row seating
  - ◊ Covering an eye while reading

CAUSES

- Developmental (most common)
- Ocular trauma
- Iatrogenic (e.g. post cataract removal)

RISK FACTORS N/A

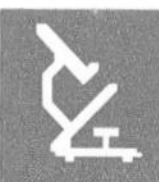

DIAGNOSIS

DIFFERENTIAL DIAGNOSIS

- Corneal disease
- Cataract
- Retinal abnormalities
- Diseases of the optic nerve

LABORATORY N/A

Drugs that may alter lab results: N/A

Disorders that may alter lab results: N/A

PATHOLOGICAL FINDINGS N/A

SPECIAL TESTS

- Pinhole vision test: To distinguish a refractive error from an organic cause of visual blurring, have the patient look through a pinhole in a card without a corrective lens. Patient's with a pure refractive error improve their vision since the pinhole blocks nonparallel and unfocusable rays of light.

IMAGING N/A

DIAGNOSTIC PROCEDURES

- Methods:
  - ◊ Objective streak retinoscopy can be used to measure the degree of refractive error in spherocylinder correction for the proper spectacle or contact lens
  - ◊ Antimuscarinic agents, e.g., cyclopentolate (Cyclogyl), tropicamide (Mydriacyl) applied topically paralyze the ciliary body, preventing accommodation. Cycloplegic refraction can then be performed.
- Age-related testing:
  - ◊ Newborns should be examined for general eye health; ophthalmologic evaluation indicated for any discovered problems
  - ◊ Vision screening should occur at each well child visit
  - ◊ Visual acuity testing should be performed at approximately 3 1/2 years
  - ◊ Visual acuity and motility testing should be performed at age 5
  - ◊ Visual acuity should be retested prior to obtaining a driver's license, at age 40, and every 2-4 years until age 65, when evaluations are recommended every 1-2 years

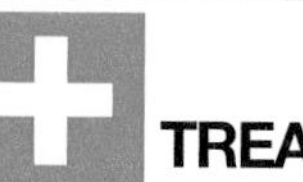

TREATMENT

APPROPRIATE HEALTH CARE Outpatient

GENERAL MEASURES

- Spectacle lenses (glasses)
- Soft and hard contact lenses

SURGICAL MEASURES

- Laser-assisted in-situ keratomileusis (LASIK), FDA approved 1997. A superficial corneal flap is created with the keratome and the excimer laser removes a small amount of tissue thus reshaping the cornea. Corrects all refractive errors. Healing is rapid since re-epithelialization is not needed. Considered an adjunctive procedure for use with the excimer laser.
- Older methods now superseded by LASIK
  - ◊ Radial keratotomy (RK),. With topical anesthesia, using a surgical keratome, multiple (4-8) radial incisions are placed onto the surface of the peripheral cornea to flatten the central, optical zone. The length, depth and proximity of the incision to the central optical zone determines its effect, and degree of correction obtained. Radial keratotomy is safe and effective and corrects nearsightedness, astigmatism or a combination of both, after the age of 18 when the prescription has stabilized.
  - ◊ Photorefractive keratectomy (PRK). Surface corneal tissue is removed, with the excimer laser, to re-shape the cornea thus correcting nearsightedness, farsightedness, or astigmatism. Risks and disadvantages include pain, keratitis, and potential scarring. Healing requires 3 months with topical antibiotics and steroids with associated risks of glaucoma, cataract, and chronic inflammation.
  - ◊ Automated lamellar keratoplasty (ALK). A microsurgical dermatome removes a layer of the superficial cornea to induce flattening. Investigational.
- Excimer laser. The laser photoablates corneal tissue from the central visual axis, thus flattening it. Following the procedure, the cornea must re-epithelialize. Healing takes several months, during which there is a mild haze and blurring of vision. FDA approved Oct, 1995.
- Implantable contact lens (ICL). A thin, plastic lens is permanently implanted in the posterior chamber between the iris and the human crystalline lens. All refractive errors can be corrected. Risks include damage to the natural lens during surgery, cataract formation, and intraocular inflammation or infection; investigational
- Several scleral expansion procedures - presently under investigation - are methods to increase the space within the ciliary body by surgical means to restore lens movement and accommodation
- Bifocal intraocular lenses (IOLS)
- Accommodative intraocular lenses are presently under investigation for the treatment of presbyopia

ACTIVITY N/A

DIET N/A

PATIENT EDUCATION
- All patients should have their eyes examined when starting school, and periodically thereafter
- The options of eyeglasses, contact lenses and permanent surgical correction of refractive errors should be considered
- Aggressive control of diabetes mellitus should be encouraged

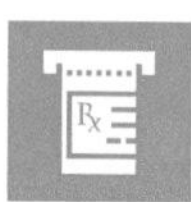

MEDICATIONS

DRUG(S) OF CHOICE N/A
Contraindications: N/A
Precautions: Antimuscarinic agents may induce acute glaucoma, via acute angle closure
Significant possible interactions: N/A

ALTERNATIVE DRUGS N/A

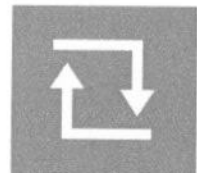

FOLLOWUP

PATIENT MONITORING
- Routine annual adult eye exams in individuals < age 40 are not indicated
- Individuals with risks will need ocular exams as indicated by their conditions

PREVENTION/AVOIDANCE N/A

POSSIBLE COMPLICATIONS
- Amblyopia
- Poor school performance

EXPECTED COURSE/PROGNOSIS
Good if discovered early and corrected appropriately.

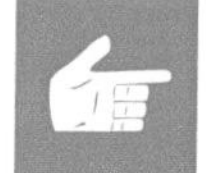

MISCELLANEOUS

ASSOCIATED CONDITIONS
Patients with diabetes mellitus have fluctuating myopia as a result of poorly controlled blood glucose and concomitant swelling of the crystalline lens

AGE-RELATED FACTORS
Pediatric: Refractive errors can be detected early in life
Geriatric: Presbyopia occurs in later life
Others: Individuals over the age of 40 are more likely to experience presbyopia or normal loss of accommodation which occurs with age, necessitating the use of reading glasses for close work

PREGNANCY
It is not unusual for refractive errors to be temporarily worsened during pregnancy due to hormonal changes in tear function and corneal swelling

SYNONYMS N/A

ICD-9-CM
367.0 Hypermetropia
367.1 Myopia
367.4 Presbyopia
367.21 Regular astigmatism

SEE ALSO

OTHER NOTES
Fax-On-Demand service of American Academy of Ophthalmology for policy statement and patient education materials (908)935-2761

ABBREVIATIONS N/A

REFERENCES

- Kershner RM: Lessons from the Practice: The Gift of Sight - A Guide to Understanding Your Eyes. Thorofare, NJ, Slack, Inc., 1994
- Infant and Children's Vision Screening. American Academy of Ophthalmology - Policy Statement (#812), June, 1991
- Frequency of Ocular exams. American Academy of Ophthalmology - Policy Statement (#808), Sept, 1990

Web references: 0 available at www.5mcc.com
Illustrations N/A

Author(s):
Robert M. Kershner, MD

BASICS

DESCRIPTION A classic triad of features including arthritis, conjunctivitis, and urethritis or cervicitis. Epidemiologically similar to other reactive arthritis syndromes characterized by sterile inflammation of joints from infections originating at non-articular sites. A fourth feature may be buccal ulceration or balanitis. (It is possible for only two features to be present.)
- Two forms:
  - ◊ Sexually transmitted; symptoms usually begin 7-14 days after exposure
  - ◊ Post-dysentery

System(s) affected: Musculoskeletal, Renal/Urologic, Skin/Exocrine
Genetics: HLA-B27 tissue antigen present in 60-80% of patients
Incidence/Prevalence in USA: 0.24-1.5% incidence after epidemics of bacterial dysentery; complicates 1-2% cases of non-gonococcal urethritis
Predominant age: 20-40 years
Predominant sex: Male > Female

SIGNS & SYMPTOMS
- Musculoskeletal:
  - ◊ Asymmetric arthritis (especially knees, ankles, MTP joints)
  - ◊ Enthesopathy (inflammation at tendinous insertion into bone) such as plantar fasciitis, digital periostitis, Achilles tendinitis
  - ◊ Spondyloarthropathy (spine and sacroiliac joint involvement)
- Urogenital tract:
  - ◊ Urethritis
  - ◊ Prostatitis
  - ◊ Occasionally cystitis
  - ◊ Balanitis
  - ◊ Cervicitis - usually asymptomatic
- Eye:
  - ◊ Conjunctivitis of one or both eyes
  - ◊ Occasionally scleritis, keratitis, corneal ulceration
  - ◊ Rarely uveitis and iritis
- Skin:
  - ◊ Mucocutaneous lesions (small, painless, superficial ulcers on oral mucosa, tongue, glans penis)
  - ◊ Keratoderma blennorrhagica (hyperkeratotic skin lesions of palms and soles and around nails)
- Cardiovascular:
  - ◊ Occasionally pericarditis, murmur, conduction defects, aortic incompetence
- Nervous system:
  - ◊ Rarely peripheral neuropathy, cranial neuropathy, meningoencephalitis, neuropsychiatric changes
- Constitutional:
  - ◊ Fever, malaise, anorexia, weight loss
  - ◊ Can appear seriously ill (fever, rigors, tachycardia, exquisitely tender joints)

CAUSES
- *Chlamydia trachomatis* the usual causative organism of postvenereal variety
- Dysenteric form following enteric bacterial infection due to Shigella, Salmonella, Yersinia, and Campylobacter organisms. This form more likely in women, children and the elderly.

RISK FACTORS
- Sexual intercourse 7-14 days prior to illness
- Food poisoning or bacterial dysenteric outbreak

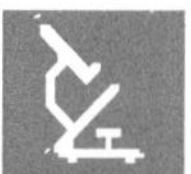

DIAGNOSIS

DIFFERENTIAL DIAGNOSIS
- For specific diagnosis, arthritis associated with urethritis for longer than one month
- Rheumatoid arthritis
- Ankylosing spondylitis
- Arthritis associated with inflammatory bowel disease
- Psoriatic arthritis
- Juvenile rheumatoid arthritis
- Bacterial arthritis including gonococcal

LABORATORY
- Blood
  - ◊ WBC 10,000-20,000
  - ◊ Neutrophilic leukocytosis
  - ◊ Elevated erythrocyte sedimentation rate
  - ◊ Moderate normochromic anemia
  - ◊ Hypergammaglobulinemia
- Synovial fluid
  - ◊ WBC 1000-8000 cells/mm3
  - ◊ Bacterial culture negative
- Collaborative tests
  - ◊ Cultures or serology positive for Chlamydia trachomatis, or stools positive for Salmonella, Shigella, Yersinia or Campylobacter support the diagnosis

Drugs that may alter lab results: Antibiotics may affect isolation of the bacterial pathogens

Disorders that may alter lab results: N/A

PATHOLOGICAL FINDINGS
- A seronegative spondyloarthropathy (similar to ankylosing spondylitis, enteric arthritis and psoriatic arthritis)
- Villous formation in joints
- Joint hyperemia
- Joint inflammation
- Prostatitis
- Seminal vesiculitis
- Skin biopsy similar to psoriasis
- Non-specific conjunctivitis

SPECIAL TESTS Histocompatibility antigen HLA-B27 positive in 60-80% of cases in non-HIV related Reiter syndrome

IMAGING
- X-ray
  - ◊ Periosteal proliferation, thickening
  - ◊ Spurs
  - ◊ Erosions at articular margins
  - ◊ Residual joint destruction
  - ◊ Syndesmophytes (spine)
  - ◊ Sacroiliitis

DIAGNOSTIC PROCEDURES N/A

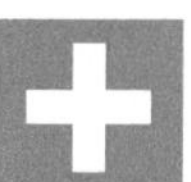

TREATMENT

APPROPRIATE HEALTH CARE Inpatient possibly, during acute phase

GENERAL MEASURES
- Treatment is symptomatic
- No treatment necessary for conjunctivitis. Iritis may require treatment.
- Treatment unnecessary for mucocutaneous lesions
- Physical therapy during recovery phase
- Arthritis may be prominent and disabling during the acute phase

SURGICAL MEASURES N/A

ACTIVITY Bedrest until joint inflammation subsides

DIET No special diet

PATIENT EDUCATION
- Teach home physical therapy techniques
- For a listing of sources for patient education materials favorably reviewed on this topic, physicians may contact: American Academy of Family Physicians Foundation, P.O. Box 8418, Kansas City, MO 64114, (800)274-2237, ext. 4400
- Arthritis Foundation, 1314 Spring Street N.W., Atlanta, GA 30309, (404)872-7100

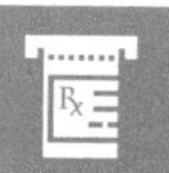

MEDICATIONS

DRUG(S) OF CHOICE
- Symptomatic management - NSAIDs including indomethacin, naproxen; intraarticular or systemic corticosteroids for refractory arthritis and enthesitis
- Specific treatment of pathogenic microorganism should be attempted:
  - ◊ C. trachomatis - doxycycline 100 mg po bid for 7-14 days
  - ◊ Salmonella, Shigella, Yersinia Campylobacter infections - ciprofloxacin 500 mg po bid for 5 days (course may be extended to 14-28 days to eradicate chronic carrier state). Note: emerging antimicrobial resistance may limit effectiveness in treatment and bacterial clearance.
- For gastrointestinal upset - antacids
- For iritis - intraocular steroids
- For keratitis - topical steroids

Contraindications:
- Gastrointestinal bleeding
- Patients with peptic ulcer, gastritis, ulcerative colitis
- Renal insufficiency

Precautions: Refer to manufacturer's literature
Significant possible interactions: Refer to manufacturer's literature

ALTERNATIVE DRUGS
- Aspirin or other NSAIDs
- Sulfasalazine is promising, but not yet approved
- Methotrexate or azathioprine in severe cases (still experimental and not approved or agreed to be effective. Contraindicated, if HIV related Reiter).
- Consultation with specialist recommended when considering immunomodulatory agents such as sulfasalazine, methotrexate or azathioprine
- Role of antibiotics under investigation, maybe helpful in some cases

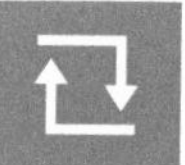

FOLLOWUP

PATIENT MONITORING Monitor clinical response to medications. Surveillance for complications of therapy, sulfasalazine, immunosuppressives.

PREVENTION/AVOIDANCE N/A

POSSIBLE COMPLICATIONS
- Chronic or recurrent disease in 5-50%
- Ankylosing spondylitis develops in 30-50% of HLA-B27 positive patients
- Urethral strictures
- Cataracts and blindness
- Aortic root necrosis

EXPECTED COURSE/PROGNOSIS
- Urethritis within 1-15 days after sexual exposure
- Onset of Reiter syndrome within 10-30 days of infection
- Mean duration 19 weeks
- Poor prognosis associated with local disease involving heel, eye or heart

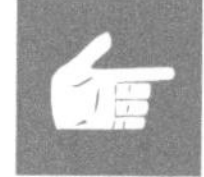

MISCELLANEOUS

ASSOCIATED CONDITIONS
- Prior shigellosis
- Salmonellosis
- Yersinia infection
- Mycoplasma or ureaplasma infection
- Chlamydia urethritis
- HIV infection

AGE-RELATED FACTORS
Pediatric: Enteric etiology more likely than chlamydia
Geriatric: Enteric etiology more likely than sexually transmitted
Others: N/A

PREGNANCY No special considerations other than usual precautions regarding drugs

SYNONYMS
- Idiopathic blennorrheal arthritis
- Arthritis urethritica
- Urethro-oculo-synovial syndrome
- Fiessinger-Leroy-Reiter disease

ICD-9-CM
099.3 Reiter disease

SEE ALSO
Ankylosing spondylitis
Arthritis, psoriatic
Behçet syndrome

OTHER NOTES No evidence to support on effect of antibiotics on the development and long-term outcome of Reiter syndrome

ABBREVIATIONS N/A

REFERENCES

- Mandell GL, Bennett JF, Dolin R, eds. Principles and Practice of Infectious Diseases. 5th Ed. New York: Churchill Livingstone; 2000
- Barth WF. Segal K. Reactive arthritis (Reiter's syndrome). Am Fam Phys 1999;60:499-503, 507
- Bryant GA. Reiter's syndrome. Orthopaedic Nursing 1998;17:57-62
- Amor B. Reiter's syndrome. Diagnosis and clinical features. Rheum Dis Clin North Am 1998;24:677-695
- Banares A, Hernandez-Garcia C, Fernandez-Gutierrez B, Jover JA. Eye involvement in the spondyloarthropathies. Rheum Dis Clin North Am 1998;24:771-84.
- Wollenhaupt J. Zeidler H. Undifferentiated arthritis and reactive arthritis. Curr Opin in Rheumatol 1998;10:306-13
- Olivieri I. Barozzi L. Padula A. De Matteis M. Pavlica P. Clinical manifestations of seronegative spondyloarthropathies. Euro J Radiol 1998;27(Suppl 1):S3-6
- Kean WF, MacPherson DW. Reiter's syndrome. In: Bellamy N, editor. Prognosis in the Rheumatic Diseases. London: Kluwer Academic Publishers; 1991
- McCormack WM, Rein MF. Urethritis. In: Mandell GL, Douglas RG, Bennett JE, editors. Principles and Practice of Infectious Diseases. 5th Ed. New York: Churchill Livingstone; 2000
- Hughes RA, Keat AC. Reiter's syndrome and reactive arthritis: A current view. Sem in Arthritis and Rheumatism 1994;24(3):190-210
- Smieja M, MacPherson DW, Kean et al. Randomised, blinded, placebo controlled trial of doxycycline for chronic seronegative arthritis. Ann Rheum Dis 2001;60(12):1088-94
- Neumann S, Kreth F, Schubert S, Mossner J, Caca K. Reiter's syndrome as a manifestation of an immune reconstitution syndrome in an HIV-infected patient: successful treatment with doxycycline. Clin Infect Dis. 2003 Jun 15;36(12):1628-1629
- Schneider JM, Matthews JH, Graham BS. Reiter's Syndrome. Cutis. 2003 Mar;71(3):198-200
- Parker CT, Thomas D. Reiter's syndrome and reactive arthritis. J Am Osteopath Assoc. 2000 Feb;100(2):101-104
- Toivanen P, Toivanen A. Two forms of reactive arthritis? Ann Rheum Dis. 1999 Dec;58(12):737-741
- Barth WF, Segal K. Reactive arthritis (Reiter's syndrome). Am Fam Physician. 1999 Aug;60(2):499-503, 507
- Kiss S, Letko E, Qamruddin S, Baltatzis S, Foster CS. Long-term progression, prognosis, and treatment of patients with recurrent ocular manifestations of Reiter's syndrome. Ophthalmology. 2003 Sep;110(9):1764-1769

Web references: 1 available at www.5mcc.com
Illustrations 3 available

Author(s):
D. W. MacPherson, MD

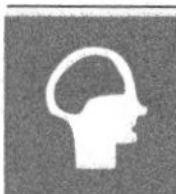

BASICS

DESCRIPTION Condition related to the presence of stones in the urinary tract. Stones form in the proximal tract and migrate distally, commonly lodging at three points along the ureter:
- Ureteropelvic junction
- Pelvic brim, as ureter crosses the iliac vessels
- Ureterovesical junction

System(s) affected: Renal/Urologic
Genetics:
- Familial tendency
- Some cases of hypercalciuria-autosomal dominant metabolic defect
- Cystinuria-autosomal recessive metabolic defect of amino acid transport

Incidence/Prevalence in USA:
- 1-4/1000 annual incidence
- 5-12% lifetime incidence
- Higher incidence in the "stone belt" (southeastern USA)
- Recurrence rate - 50% in five years

Predominant age: 20-40
Predominant sex: Male > Female (≈3:1), except for struvite (infection) stones which are more common in females

SIGNS & SYMPTOMS
- Renal colic
  - ◊ Sudden onset
  - ◊ Agonizing flank pain, waxing and waning
  - ◊ Radiation to lower abdomen, groin, testicles, or labia
  - ◊ Causes patient to be restless
- Tachycardia
- Diaphoresis
- Nausea, with or without vomiting
- Abdominal tenderness, on deep palpation
- Ileus
- Costovertebral angle tenderness
- Hematuria
- Urinary frequency
- Chills, fever, pyuria (if infection present)
- Asymptomatic stones may be found on abdominal radiograph done for other reasons

CAUSES
- Metabolic abnormalities (a patient may show more than one)
  - ◊ Supersaturation of urine with stone-forming salts
    - Hypercalciuria (>300 mg/24hr): 40-60% of cases
    - Hyperuricosuria (>750 mg/24hr): 20-35% of cases
    - Hyperoxaluria (>40 mg/24hr): 10-20% of cases
    - Cystinuria (>250 mg/L): 1-2% of cases
  - ◊ Reduced inhibitors of stone formation
    - Hypocitraturia (<320 mg/day): 10-40% of cases
    - Hypomagnesuria
    - Abnormal nephrocalcin, or other glycoprotein defects (Tamm-Horsfall protein, glycosaminoglycan, uropontin, crystal matrix protein)
- Infection with urease-producing organisms (mostly Proteus): 10-20% of cases
- Alterations in urinary pH
  - ◊ pH<5.5 leads to uric acid stones
  - ◊ pH>7.5 seen with struvite stones

RISK FACTORS
- Low urine output (<1100 ml/24hr)
- Strenuous work
- Dehydration
- Diet high in protein, oxalate, salt
- Medications
  - ◊ Antacids
  - ◊ Vitamins A, C, D
  - ◊ Triamterene
  - ◊ Ritonavir, indinavir
  - ◊ Some sulfa drugs
  - ◊ Carbonic anhydrase inhibitors
  - ◊ Some antiepileptic drugs
  - ◊ Corticosteroids
  - ◊ Acetazolamide
- Immobility
- Weightlessness (as in space travel)

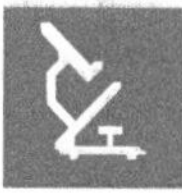

DIAGNOSIS

DIFFERENTIAL DIAGNOSIS
- Acute abdomen
- Acute lumbosacral strain, ruptured lumbar disc
- Aortic aneurysm
- Ectopic pregnancy
- Endometriosis
- Gastroenteritis
- Malingering or drug seeking behavior
- Pancreatitis
- Peptic ulcer disease
- Pyelonephritis or perinephric abscess
- Salpingitis
- Ureteral clot or sloughed papilla (secondary to diabetes, infection, analgesic abuse)

LABORATORY
- CBC
- Urinalysis
  - ◊ Hematuria
  - ◊ Crystals
  - ◊ pH
  - ◊ Pyuria, bacteruria
- Urine culture, if indicated
- Chemistry profile
- Parathyroid hormone, if calcium elevated
- For patients with recurrent episode (4 to 8 weeks after acute episode):
  - ◊ 24 hour urine collection for volume, calcium, creatinine, uric acid, oxalate, citrate, sodium, magnesium
  - ◊ If abnormal, consider repeating same tests on 24 hour urine after one week of dietary restrictions

Drugs that may alter lab results: Allopurinol, diuretics, Pyridium

Disorders that may alter lab results: Other underlying infections, renal abnormalities

PATHOLOGICAL FINDINGS
- Stone analysis:
  - ◊ Calcium oxalate: 36-70%
  - ◊ Calcium phosphate: 6-20%
  - ◊ Mixed calcium stones: 11-31%
  - ◊ Uric acid: 6-17%
  - ◊ Struvite ("triple phosphate" or "infection") stone: 6-20%
  - ◊ Cystine: 0.5-3%

SPECIAL TESTS Nitroprusside test on urine if cystinuria suspected

IMAGING
- Plain film of abdomen (KUB): 80-90% of stones are at least partially radiopaque
- IVP
- Ultrasound, especially if allergic to contrast dye
- Helical CT scan - becoming procedure of choice where available

DIAGNOSTIC PROCEDURES Antegrade or retrograde pyelogram - rarely needed except in possible case of allergy to contrast dye

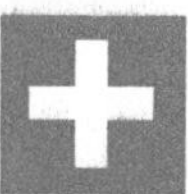

TREATMENT

APPROPRIATE HEALTH CARE
- Outpatient management possible for 80-90%
- Inpatient management and urology consult if:
  - ◊ Intractable pain, nausea, or vomiting
  - ◊ Signs of infection
  - ◊ Imaging studies show non-functioning kidney, solitary or horseshoe kidney, or urine extravasation
  - ◊ Stone larger than 6 mm

GENERAL MEASURES
- Pain control
- Hydration (2-3 L/day)
- Strain urine to recover the stone

SURGICAL MEASURES
- Cystoscopy with basket extraction or laser lithotripsy
- Extracorporeal shock wave lithotripsy
- Percutaneous lithotripsy or nephrolithotomy
- Open removal-required in less than 5% of patients

ACTIVITY As tolerated

DIET
- During acute episode-push fluids
- To reduce likelihood of recurrence:
  - ◊ Fluid intake of 2 L/day (eight 8 ounce glasses/day besides meals)
  - ◊ Moderate protein intake (60 gm/day)
  - ◊ Moderate salt intake (3-4 gm/day)
  - ◊ Avoid foods high in oxalate (spinach, rhubarb, beans, peanuts, tea, chocolate, cola)
  - ◊ Avoid excess vitamin C (intake should be <1000 mg/day total)
  - ◊ Significant restriction of calcium intake is not recommended (1000-1500 mg/day probably reasonable)
  - ◊ For cystine stones, reduce methionine in diet

PATIENT EDUCATION
- Instruction in straining urine
- Fluid and dietary instruction

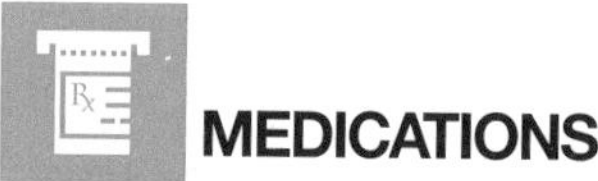

MEDICATIONS

DRUG(S) OF CHOICE
- Acute therapy:
  - ◊ Oral NSAIDs (ibuprofen 600-800 mg tid)
  - ◊ Oral narcotics (acetaminophen-codeine, acetaminophen-hydrocodone, acetaminophen-oxycodone)
  - ◊ Oral indomethacin 50 mg qid (also available as a suppository)
  - ◊ Injectable meperidine 50-100 mg or morphine 10-15 mg q3-4h
- Maintenance therapy:
  - ◊ Calcium stones: hydrochlorothiazide (HCTZ) or chlorthalidone 25-50 mg/day or bid (consider potassium citrate 20 mEq bid or amiloride 5-10 mg/day to avoid low potassium); indapamide 2.5 mg/day; neutral phosphate 500 mg tid or qid with meals
  - ◊ Uric acid stones: potassium citrate 20 mEq bid to maintain urine pH 6-7; allopurinol 300 mg/day
  - ◊ Cystine stones: potassium citrate titrated to achieve urine pH>7.5; tiopronin 200-500 mg bid; penicillamine (d-penicillamine) 1-2 gm/day
  - ◊ Struvite stones: antibiotics for 3 to 4 months after removal of stone; acetohydroxamic acid 250 mg tid or qid

Contraindications: Renal failure - neutral phosphate, d-penicillamine; pregnancy, lactation- tiopronin, d-penicillamine, acetohydroxamic acid; medication allergy

Precautions: Monitor CBC, liver and renal function with tiopronin, d-penicillamine; monitor CBC, renal function with acetohydroxamic acid

Significant possible interactions: See manufacturer's profile of each drug

ALTERNATIVE DRUGS
Ketorolac po, IM or IV for pain (short term use only)

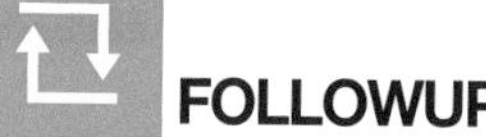

FOLLOWUP

PATIENT MONITORING
- Acute episode:
  - ◊ Signs of infection
  - ◊ Repeat KUB radiograph or ultrasound every 1-2 weeks
  - ◊ Consider urologic referral if not resolved in 2-4 weeks
  - ◊ Strain urine until stone passed

PREVENTION/AVOIDANCE
- Recurrent stones:
  - ◊ Fluid intake to maintain urine output >2L/day
  - ◊ Dietary compliance
  - ◊ Struvite stones: periodic culture to confirm sterile urine

POSSIBLE COMPLICATIONS
- Hydronephrosis
- Infection/sepsis
- Renal impairment, especially in struvite stones (most "malignant" of the stones)
- Related to ESWL:
  - ◊ Skin bruising
  - ◊ Perinephric hematoma
  - ◊ Hematuria
  - ◊ Hypertension (possibly)

EXPECTED COURSE/PROGNOSIS
- Overall, 80-90% of stones pass spontaneously
  - ◊ 50% of 5-6 mm stones pass
  - ◊ Most stones >10 mm require surgical removal
- Recurrence - 50% in 5 years

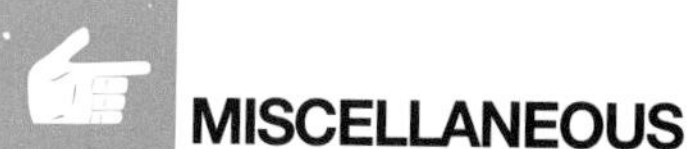

MISCELLANEOUS

ASSOCIATED CONDITIONS
- Crohn disease
- Gout
- Jejunoileal bypass, ileostomy, ileal conduit
- Laxative abuse
- Medullary sponge kidney
- Milk-alkali syndrome
- Myeloproliferative disorder
- Paraplegia/neurogenic bladder
- Primary hyperparathyroidism
- Renal tubular acidosis (type I)
- Sarcoidosis

AGE-RELATED FACTORS
Pediatric: Rare; consider inborn error of metabolism
Geriatric: N/A
Others: N/A

PREGNANCY
Consider urologic referral

SYNONYMS
- Nephrolithiasis
- Kidney stone

ICD-9-CM
592.0 Calculus of kidney

SEE ALSO
Urolithiasis

OTHER NOTES
Black males have fewer stones than white males (approximately 1:3)

ABBREVIATIONS
CBC = complete blood count
KUB = kidney, ureter, bladder
IVP = intravenous pyelogram
CT = computerized tomography
NSAID = non-steroidal anti-inflammatory drug
HCTZ = hydrochlorothiazide
ESWL = extra-corporeal shock wave lithotripsy

REFERENCES

- Portis AJ, Sundaram CP. Diagnosis and initial management of kidney stones. Am Fam Physician 2001;63(7):1329-38
- Goldfarb DS, Coe FL. Prevention of recurrent nephrolithiasis. Am Fam Phys 1999;60(8):2269-76
- Pak CYC. Kidney stones. Lancet 1998;351:1797-1800
- Saklayen MG. Medical management of nephrolithiasis. Med Clin N Am 1997;81(3):785-99
- Wasserstein AG. Nephrolithiasis: acute management and prevention. Dis Mon 1998;44(5):196- 213

Web references: 0 available at www.5mcc.com
Illustrations N/A

Author(s):
Rich Londo, MD

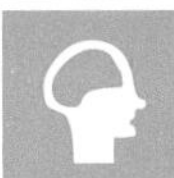

BASICS

DESCRIPTION Renal cell carcinoma represents 2-3% of all cancers and 2% of all cancer deaths; 9th most common male malignant tumor; 13th most common female malignant tumor. Characterized by obscure and varied presentations including paraneoplastic syndromes, vascular findings, and uncommon metastatic sites. Paraneoplastic and vascular syndromes do not indicate incurability or unresectability. Early, aggressive surgical management provides the best opportunity for cure.

System(s) affected: Renal/Urologic

Genetics:
- Oncogenes localized to the short arm of chromosome 3 may have etiologic implications. Chromosome 3p12-p26 are specific for clear cell RCC; 4% of RCC is familial.
- People with HLA antigen types Bw44 and DR8 are prone to develop renal cancer. These are rare familial renal carcinomas.

Incidence/Prevalence in USA:
- 30,000 new cases/year (1998); 11,600 deaths /year
- Men: 9.6/100,000
- Women: 4.2/100,000

Predominant age: 5th and 6th decades

Predominant sex: Male > Female (2:1)

SIGNS & SYMPTOMS
- Diverse and obscure presentations, "the internist's tumor"
- Solid renal masses, most 6-7 cm (incidentally discovered in asymptomatic patient due to increased use of CT and MRI)
- Hematuria 50-60%
- Elevated erythrocyte sedimentation rate 50-60%
- Abdominal mass 24-45%
- Anemia 21-41%
- Flank pain 35-40%
- Hypertension 22-38%
- Weight loss 28-36%
- Pyrexia 7-17%
- Hepatic dysfunction 10-15%
- Classic triad: (hematuria, abdominal mass, flank pain) only 9% of cases
- Hypercalcemia 3-6%
- Erythrocytosis 3-4%
- Scrotal varicoceles 2-11% (most are left sided)
- Patients with vena caval thrombus present with lower extremity edema, new varicocele, dilated superficial abdominal veins, albuminuria, pulmonary emboli, right atrial mass or non-function of the involved kidney

CAUSES Unknown

RISK FACTORS
- Smoking (doubles likelihood of RCC)
- Obesity (linear relationship in women)
- Urban environment
- Cadmium
- Asbestos
- Petroleum byproducts
- Herpes simplex virus exposure
- Phenacetin or analgesic abuse for transitional cell of the renal pelvis

DIAGNOSIS

DIFFERENTIAL DIAGNOSIS
- Benign renal masses (i.e. renal hamartomas)
- Hydronephrosis
- Polycystic kidneys
- Renal tuberculosis
- Renal calculi
- Renal infarction
- Benign renal cyst
- Transitional cell carcinoma (rare)

LABORATORY
- Increased plasma fibrinogen
- Anemia (21-41% of patients)
- Polycythemia
- Hematuria
- Alkaline phosphate may be elevated
- Increased erythrocyte sedimentation rate
- Urine - neoplastic cells
- Hypercalcemia
- Increased renin
- Transitional cell cancer (rare)

Drugs that may alter lab results: N/A

Disorders that may alter lab results: N/A

PATHOLOGICAL FINDINGS
- Renal cell tends to bulge out from the cortex producing a mass effect
- 48% of renal cell carcinomas measure < 5 cm and is grossly yellow to yellow/orange due to its high lipid content in the clear cell variety. Average renal cell size has been decreasing due to incidental discovery.
- Small tumors are homogenous
- Large tumors may have areas of necrosis and hemorrhage
- A pseudocapsule covers some tumors
- Tumor thrombi into the vena cava generally do not invade the vena caval wall
- 5 distinct subtypes:
  - ◊ Clear cell (75-85%; proximal tubule)
  - ◊ Chromophilic (12-14%; proximal tubule)
  - ◊ Chromophobic (4-6%; intercalated cells)
  - ◊ Oncocytic (2-4%; intercalated cells)
  - ◊ Collecting duct tumors (1%; medullary collecting duct)

SPECIAL TESTS
- Arteriography (rarely needed) - for tumors larger than 10 cm, it may identify parasitic capsular vessels for early control
- Cystoscopy - to rule out bladder cancer
- ECG as needed

IMAGING
- IVP remains part of primary evaluation for hematuria. CT and ultrasound are the mainstays for evaluation of suspected renal mass.
- Ultrasonography - if there appears to be a mass on IVP, confirms the presence of a lesion and determines whether it is solid or cystic. Cystic lesions may either be observed or subjected to percutaneous cyst puncture.
- CT scan and, occasionally, arteriography - if solid or complex masses upon ultrasonography require further evaluation. 3% of RCC are bilateral by CT scan.
  The most common alteration with RCC is deletion of chromosome 3p. Recent evidence implicates gene p53 on chromosome 17p13.1 to be critical in renal cell carcinogenesis.
- Rapid sequence CT can demonstrate tumor enhancement
- MRI has not been shown to be superior to CT for tumors smaller than 8 cm, for larger tumors it may have advantage in delineating the vena cava
- Bone scans are indicated if the alkaline phosphatase is elevated or the patient has bone pain
- Brain CT is indicated if the patient has neurologic symptoms

DIAGNOSTIC PROCEDURES
- Simple cyst need not be aspirated unless painful
- Calcified cysts may contain renal cell cancer and therefore require open renal biopsy of the wall of the cyst or partial nephrectomy
- Hemorrhagic cyst - aspiration cytology may be helpful but needle biopsy of solid masses is to be discouraged, particularly if the patient has a normal contralateral kidney
- In solitary kidneys, open renal biopsy with wedge resection (not enucleation) can be performed if mass is ≤ 4 cm
- Doppler flow ultrasound of the renal veins or CT (thin cuts) that shows the renal vein entering the vena cava can be used to rule out tumor thrombus
- Venogram - when tumor thrombus is identified. The venogram can demonstrate when the thrombus goes above the hepatic veins or diaphragm (i.e., rarely cardiopulmonary bypass needed to remove the thrombus above the diaphragm at the time of nephrectomy).

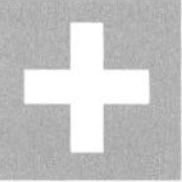

TREATMENT

APPROPRIATE HEALTH CARE Inpatient

GENERAL MEASURES N/A

SURGICAL MEASURES
- Surgery is indicated. Cytotoxic drug therapy has been only erratically effective. Lesions are fairly radiation resistant.
- Maintain hydration during iodine injection diagnostic studies to prevent acute tubular necrosis
- Consider a mechanical bowel preparation to ease the nephrectomy
- Consider antibiotic bowel preparation for larger tumors (> 10 cm) where possible bowel injury or resection may be more likely
- Exploration wedge resection for solitary kidney or tumors less than 4 cm, otherwise radical nephrectomy in the face of a normal contralateral kidney is preferred
- Usual preoperative pulmonary toilet, pulmonary function tests if indicated
- Renal cell carcinoma (85% of renal parenchymal malignant tumors) - CT solid mass larger than 3 cm, radical nephrectomy if there is a normal contralateral kidney; smaller than 3 cm, wedge resection. Intraoperative Doppler ultrasound is undergoing study to determine the optimum partial nephrectomy approach to small tumors. Laparoscopy nephrectomy is still investigational.

- Angiomyolipoma (80% of tuberous sclerosis patients have these benign tumors) - classic CT findings, may be followed with CT
- Hemorrhage into a cyst - aspiration cytology
- Complex cyst (calcified cyst wall or irregular wall) - open cyst wall biopsy if cytology is inconclusive
- Transitional cell carcinoma of the renal pelvis or calyces - nephroureterectomy
- Oncocytoma - larger than 3 cm, radical nephrectomy
- Sarcoma - wide excision
- Adult Wilms' tumor - radical nephrectomy for unilateral disease
- Metastasis (lymphoma > lung > breast > stomach) - depends on prognosis of primary tumor; nephrectomy for uncontrolled bleeding
- Cortical adenoma smaller than 3 cm (7-22% at autopsy) - wedge resection

ACTIVITY
- No special preoperative activity
- Postoperatively - as tolerated; full activity in 8 weeks

DIET
Low protein diet for patients with proteinuria

PATIENT EDUCATION
- Preoperative nursing education is indicated for pulmonary toilet
- Pre-anesthesia education is needed if the patient is to have a patient controlled analgesia pump or epidural catheter for postoperative pain relief
- Printed patient information available from: National Kidney & Urologic Diseases Information Clearinghouse, Box NKUDIC, Bethesda, MD 20893, (301)468-6345
- CancerNet (cancernet.nci.nih.gov)

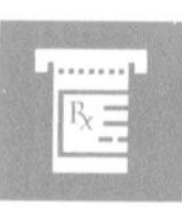

MEDICATIONS

DRUG(S) OF CHOICE
- For advanced renal cell carcinoma - interleukin-2 (IL-2) plus lymphokine-activated killer (LAK), or IL-2 alone, includes 4% complete responders and 11% partial responders. Dose schedules are under study.

Contraindications: N/A
Precautions: IUL monitoring for IL-2
Significant possible interactions: IL-2 associated with capillary leak syndrome (CLS)

ALTERNATIVE DRUGS
- Hormones - progesterone agents yield a 5-10% response rate
- Chemotherapy - vinblastine alone or with lomustine (CCNU) yields a 10-15% response rate

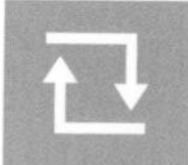

FOLLOWUP

PATIENT MONITORING
- One CT scan of the abdomen and renal fossa can be done 3-6 months later, particularly if the capsule or lymph nodes are positive, to monitor recurrences and repeat resection if needed for flank pain or mass
- For partial nephrectomy - renal ultrasound every 6 months for 3 years, then annually
- Chest x-rays to rule out pulmonary metastasis are performed quarterly for 2 years, then less often
- Skeletal x-rays and bone scan can be useful in detecting skeletal metastasis but should only be obtained if patient complains of bone pain or an alkaline phosphatase elevation
- Postoperative followup may be possible with plasma transcobalamin II or serum haptoglobin level to detect or monitor recurrences

PREVENTION/AVOIDANCE
- Do not smoke; smoking may contribute to 1/3 of all cases
- Eat a sensible diet
- Avoid stress, asbestos, cadmium, and petroleum distillates

POSSIBLE COMPLICATIONS
- Paraplegia can result with little warning from spinal vertebral metastasis
- CNS metastasis are not uncommon
- Approximately 30% of patients with RCC have metastatic disease when the diagnosis is established. The most common sites of metastasis are the lung (50-60%), bone (30-40%), regional nodes (15-30%), brain (10%) and adjacent organs (10%).

EXPECTED COURSE/PROGNOSIS

Five year survival for renal cell cancer (Robson's staging):

	Stage	5 yr†
Small tumor	I	60-70%
Large tumor	I	60-70%
Perinephric fat	II	50-65%
Renal vein	IIIa	50-60%
IVC involvement††	IIIa	5-35%
Adjacent structure	IVa	0-5%
Single node	IIIb	35%
Multiple nodes	III	5-35%
Fixed nodes	IIIb	5%
Distant metastases	IVb	0-5%

Five year survival for renal cell cancer (TNM staging):

	Stage	5 yr†
Small tumor	T1	60-70%
Large tumor	T2	60-70%
Perinephric fat	T3	50-65%
Renal vein	T3b	50-60%
IVC involvement††	T3c	5-35%
Adjacent structure	T4a	0-5%
Single node	N1	35%
Multiple node	N2	5-35%
Fixed nodes	N3	5%
Distant metastases	M1	0-5%

† 5 year survival
††Infradiaphragmatic vena caval

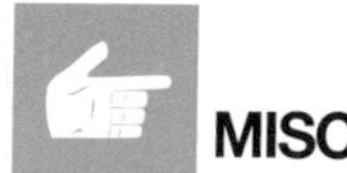

MISCELLANEOUS

ASSOCIATED CONDITIONS
- Von Hippel-Lindau disease (30-45% of these patients develop renal cell)
- Adult polycystic kidney disease
- Horseshoe kidney
- Acquired renal cystic disease from chronic renal failure

AGE-RELATED FACTORS
Pediatric: Extremely rare in children
Geriatric: Most commonly presents in the 5th and 6th decade
Others: N/A

PREGNANCY
N/A

SYNONYMS
- Kidney cancer
- Hypernephroma
- Grawitz tumor
- Hypernephroid cancer

ICD-9-CM
189.0 Malignant neoplasm of kidney, except pelvis

SEE ALSO

OTHER NOTES
N/A

ABBREVIATIONS
RCC = renal cell carcinoma
IVC = inferior vena cava

REFERENCES

- Resnick MY. Current Therapy in Genitourinary Surgery. 2nd Ed. St. Louis, Mosby-Year Book Publishers, 1992
- Novick AC, Streem SB, et al. Conservative surgery for renal cell carcinoma; A single center experience with 100 patients. J Urol 1989;141:835
- Novick AC. Partial nephrectomy gaining wider acceptance as alternative treatment in surgery for RCC. The Kidney Cancer Jour 1994;1(2)
- Franklin JR, Figlin R, Belldegrun A. Renal cell carcinoma: basic biology and clinical behavior. Seminars in Urologic Oncology 1996;14(4):208-215/230-243
- Riglin RA. Renal cell carcinoma: management of advanced disease. J Urol 1999 Feb;161(2):381-6; discussion 386-7
- Brenner B, Rector F, editors. The Kidney. 6th Ed. Philadelphia: W.B. Saunders Co.; 2000
- Spencer W, Novick AC, et al: Conservative surgery for transitional cell carcinoma of the renal pelvis. J Urol 1988;139:507

Web references: 1 available at www.5mcc.com
Illustrations N/A

Author(s):
Marc Rucquoi, MD

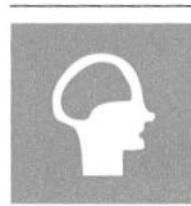

BASICS

DESCRIPTION A syndrome of rapidly deteriorating kidney function with the accumulation of nitrogenous wastes
System(s) affected: Cardiovascular, Renal/Urologic
Genetics: No known genetic pattern
Incidence/Prevalence in USA: 5% of patients admitted to the hospital develop ARF; 10-15% of ICU patients develop ARF; 2-7% post open heart patients develop ARF; 50% of hospital ARF is iatrogenic.
Predominant age: All ages (average age increasing)
Predominant sex: Male = Female

SIGNS & SYMPTOMS
- Anorexia
- Asterixis
- Back pain
- Coma
- Delirium
- Diarrhea
- Dyspnea
- Ecchymosis
- Edema
- Encephalopathy
- Epistaxis
- Fasciculation
- Fatigue
- GI hemorrhage
- Headache
- Hiccups
- Hyperpnea
- Hypertension
- Left ventricular failure
- Lethargy
- Muscle cramps
- Myoclonus
- Nausea
- Oliguria
- Pericarditis
- Petechiae
- Purpura (vasculitis)
- Rales
- Rash (acute interstitial nephritis)
- Retinopathy
- Seizure
- Somnolence
- Tachycardia
- Tachypnea
- Uriniferous odor
- Vomiting
- Weakness
- Xerostomia

CAUSES
- Pre-renal (30-60% of all cases)
  - ◊ Hypovolemia
  - ◊ Ineffective circulating volume: Congestive heart failure, cirrhosis, nephrotic syndrome and early sepsis
- Renal
  - ◊ Tubular, interstitial: Acute interstitial nephritis (AIN) (drugs, infection); nephrotoxins; acute tubular necrosis; reflex anuria; contrast media (40-70% of all cases)
  - ◊ Glomerular: Rapidly progressive (crescentic) glomerulonephritis (RPGN) (Immunofluorescence biopsy staining: linear, immune complex or pauci-immune); pregnancy (2%); systemic lupus erythematosus
- Vascular
  - ◊ Ischemic nephropathy (renal artery stenosis)
  - ◊ Dissecting aortic aneurysm
  - ◊ Ruptured abdominal aortic aneurysm
- Post-renal
  - ◊ Obstruction (See topic for Hydronephrosis) (1-10% of all cases)

RISK FACTORS
- Surgery (especially with increased age, elevated creatinine, simultaneous cardiac valve and bypass surgery)
- Volume depletion (especially in diabetes)
- Aminoglycoside therapy, congestive heart failure, contrast exposure, septic shock
- Nephrotoxic drugs (e.g., ACE inhibitors in renal artery stenosis)
- Rhabdomyolysis
- Administration of contrast (parenteral) in susceptible individuals
- Dopamine and mannitol appear to increase the risk of acute renal failure in some groups; particularly patients with diabetes mellitus.

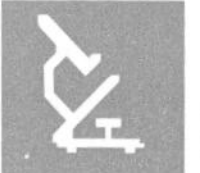

DIAGNOSIS

DIFFERENTIAL DIAGNOSIS See causes

LABORATORY
- Urinalysis
  - ◊ Proteinuria
  - ◊ Hematuria
  - ◊ Brown granular urinary casts
  - ◊ Urinary renal tubular epithelial cells
- Urine sediment
  - ◊ Coarse granular casts
  - ◊ Renal tubular epithelial cells
  - ◊ Eosinophils (AIN?)
  - ◊ Red cell or hemoglobin casts (RPGN)
  - ◊ Crystals (lithiasis, obstruction)
- Urine electrolytes/osmolality
  - ◊ Increased urine sodium (> 20 mEq/L [>20 mmol/L]), increased fractional excretion of sodium (> 3%) (e.g., renal).

Calculation: Fractional excretion of sodium = [(urine Na+/serum Na+) / (urine creatinine/serum creatinine)] X 100
  - ◊ Urine isotonic to plasma
  - ◊ Low urine sodium < 10 mEq/L (< 10 mmol/L), low fractional excretion of sodium (≤ 1%), concentrate urine osmolality (≥ 500 mOsm/liter) (e.g., pre-renal)
- Other
  - ◊ Azotemia
  - ◊ Decreased creatinine clearance
  - ◊ Hyperosmolarity
  - ◊ Hyperphosphatemia
  - ◊ Hyperkalemia
  - ◊ Decreased serum bicarbonate
  - ◊ Increased plasma volume
  - ◊ Decreased hemoglobin
  - ◊ Decreased hematocrit
  - ◊ Hypocapnia
  - ◊ Increased serum magnesium
  - ◊ Acidemia (increased anion gap)
  - ◊ Increased serum amylase/lipase
  - ◊ Hyponatremia
  - ◊ Hypocalcemia
  - ◊ Increased serum uric acid
  - ◊ Increased bleeding time
  - ◊ Impaired phagocytic function

Drugs that may alter lab results: Too many to list

Disorders that may alter lab results: Too many to list

PATHOLOGICAL FINDINGS
- Kidney biopsy:
  - ◊ Not particularly helpful in acute tubular necrosis (ATN)
  - ◊ Diagnostic in AIN and RPGN
  - ◊ In acute ischemic or toxic injury, necrosis or apoptosis of renal tubular cells

SPECIAL TESTS
- Angiogram (renal vascular disease)
- Cystoscopy - retrograde
- Bleeding time

IMAGING
- Obstruction - renal scan, CT scan
- Kidney ultrasound
  - ◊ Renal cause: "Medical" renal disease (renal echogenicity = liver), normal size kidneys, kidney size disparity: ischemia
  - ◊ Post renal cause - hydronephrosis

DIAGNOSTIC PROCEDURES Renal biopsy (ARF, unknown cause), diagnostic for AIN, RPGN

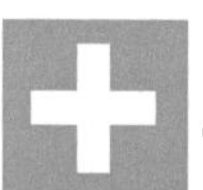

TREATMENT

APPROPRIATE HEALTH CARE Inpatient and intensive care

GENERAL MEASURES
- Correction of underlying hemodynamic abnormalities, especially volume
- Hemodialysis as soon as diagnosis of uremia is established (or continuous renal replacement therapy). The use of biocompatible membranes (e.g., polymethyl methylacrylate) as opposed to cuprophane results in a higher rate of recovery of renal function, more rapid recovery and better patient survival.
- Decrease catabolism
- Convert oliguria to nonoliguria
- Daily weight
- Correct reversible causes (volume and mannitol)
- Modify dosages of renal excreted drugs (see under Medications - Precautions)
- If drug induced, discontinue offending agent
- Meticulous aseptic technique
- Continuous arteriovenous hemofiltration
- Intravenous human immunoglobulin G
- Correct easy bleeding with DDAVP, estrogen and cryoprecipitate
- Question prednisone in AIN
- Hyperkalemia - severe (1 amp Ca gluconate IV); other IV insulin + glucose, if acidosis also present (1 amp NaHCO3) Kayexalate po 15-60 gm/day if gastrointestinal tract functions
- Mannitol - alkaline diuresis in rhabdomyolysis

SURGICAL MEASURES N/A

ACTIVITY As tolerated

DIET
- Restrict fluids to volume of urine output plus 500 mL/day
- Eliminate potassium if serum level increased
- Oral and IV amino acids
- Increase carbohydrates to decrease catabolism
- Alimentation to decrease catabolism

PATIENT EDUCATION
National Kidney & Urologic Diseases Information Clearinghouse, Box NKUDIC, Bethesda, MD 20893, (301)468-6345 and The National Kidney Foundation, Inc., 30 East 33rd Street, NY, NY 10016. "What Everyone Should Know About Kidneys and Kidney Disease" (Order #01-01BP - English), (Order #01-02BP -Spanish).

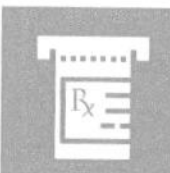

MEDICATIONS

DRUG(S) OF CHOICE Prior to fixed renal failure: IV volume expansion with normal saline followed by mannitol, furosemide (Lasix), and calcium channel blockers. Low dose dopamine has not been shown to have a beneficial effect on survival. Volume expansion alone is beneficial in contrast injury. Dopamine-1 selective agonists may have promise for future treatment.
Contraindications: N/A
Precautions:
- Pharmacokinetics of all drugs used during renal failure should be reviewed for appropriate adjustment. For example, antiarrhythmic drugs:
  - ◊ Quinidine: decrease dose, closely monitor drug level
  - ◊ Procainamide: avoid in renal failure
  - ◊ Disopyramide: reduction in maintenance dose
  - ◊ Mexiletine: no dose adjustment-liver metabolized, etc.

Significant possible interactions: Nonsteroidals plus other nephrotoxic drugs, male gender, increasing age, cardiovascular comorbidity and recent hospitalization are synergistic in causing ARF

ALTERNATIVE DRUGS N/A

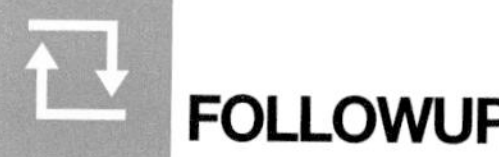

FOLLOWUP

PATIENT MONITORING As needed

PREVENTION/AVOIDANCE
- See risk factors
- Allopurinol prior to chemotherapy for hematologic malignancy
- Hydration most important, especially prior to contrast and chemotherapy
- Non biocompatible membranes
- Hypotension

POSSIBLE COMPLICATIONS
- Sepsis - infection (leading cause of mortality)
- Convulsions
- Edema
- Pulmonary edema
- Congestive heart failure
- Hyperkalemia
- Paralysis
- Arrhythmias
- Death (50%)
- Pericarditis/tamponade
- Uremia
- Bleeding
- Hypotension

EXPECTED COURSE/PROGNOSIS
Recover usually in days to 6 weeks. High mortality rate (5-80%) depending on cause/multi-organ involvement, and age.

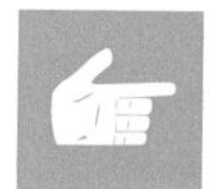

MISCELLANEOUS

ASSOCIATED CONDITIONS
- Hyperphosphatemia
- Hydronephrosis
- Muscle injury
- Congestive heart failure
- Cirrhosis
- Malignant hypertension
- Vasculitis
- Bacterial infections
- Drug reactions
- Hypercalcemia
- Hyperuricemia
- Sepsis
- Severe trauma
- Burns
- Transfusion reactions
- Internal bleeding

AGE-RELATED FACTORS
Pediatric: Congenital
Geriatric: Greater occurrence in this age group especially after surgery
Others: N/A

PREGNANCY
- Infected uterus (e.g., C. welchii [C. perfringens])
- Toxemia and a related obstetric complication
- Cortical necrosis
- Postpartum renal failure

SYNONYMS N/A

ICD-9-CM
584.9 Acute renal failure, unspecified

SEE ALSO
Hepatorenal syndrome
Hydronephrosis
Multiple myeloma
Renal failure, chronic
Reye syndrome
Rhabdomyolysis
Rocky Mountain spotted fever

OTHER NOTES N/A

ABBREVIATIONS
ATN = acute tubular necrosis
AIN = acute interstitial nephritis
RPGN = rapidly progressive glomerulonephritis
ACE = angiotensin converting enzyme

REFERENCES

- Humes HD: Acute renal failure - the promise of new therapies. N Engl J Med 1997;336:870871
- Klahr S, Miller SB: Acute oliguria. NEJM 1998;338:671-675
- Alkhunaizi AM, Schrier RW: Management of acute renal failure: new perspectives. Am J Kid Dis 1996;28:315-328
- Thadoni R, Pascual M, Bonventre JV: Acute renal failure. N Engl J Med 1996;334:1448-1460
- Gutthann SP, Rodriguez LAG, Raiford DS, et al: Nonsteroidal drugs and the risk of hospitalization. Arch Int Med 1996;156:2433-2439
- Nolon CR, Anderson RJ: Hospital-acquired acute renal failure. J Am Soc Nephrol 1998;9:710-718
- Rao TK: Acute renal failure syndromes in human immunodeficiency virus infection. Semin in Nephrol 1998;18(4):378-395
- Nissenson AR: Acute renal failure: definition and pathogenesis. Kid Intl 1998;53(suppl66):s7-s10
- Andreussi VE, Fuiano G, Stanziale P, et al: Role of renal biopsy in the diagnosis and prognosis of acute renal failure. Kid Intl 1998;53(suppl66):s91-s95

Web references: 6 available at www.5mcc.com
Illustrations N/A

Author(s):
Mark R. Dambro, MD

BASICS

DESCRIPTION The result of any renal injury that decreases renal excretory and regulatory function chronically. Characteristic findings: nitrogen retention, acidosis, and anemia.

System(s) affected: Endocrine/Metabolic, Hemic/Lymphatic/Immunologic, Renal/Urologic

Genetics:

- Compared to general population, African Americans 3.9 x more likely to have end stage renal disease (ESRD) (irreversible, dialysis dependent) and 6.7 x more likely to have hypertensive ESRD
- Hereditary renal diseases can lead to chronic renal failure in children and some adults (Alport syndrome, autosomal recessive polycystic kidney disease)
- Autosomal dominant polycystic kidney disease is a relatively common cause of chronic renal failure in adults affecting approximately 10% of dialysis population (mutation on short arm chromosome 16)

Incidence/Prevalence in USA:

- Common (estimated 160,000 persons per year are treated for ESRD). Prevalence in USA: 2.8/100,000 people in USA (estimate) with a chronic elevation of creatinine greater than 2.0 mg/dL (176.8 μmol/L).
- Most common causes: diabetes, hypertension, HIV-associated

Predominant age: All ages - much more common in adults. In children, chronic renal failure affects between 2 and 6 per 1 million population. The elderly represent approximately 1/3 of new patients with ESRD from 1988-1991.

Predominant sex: Male = Female

SIGNS & SYMPTOMS

- Anemia (normochromic, normocytic)
- Anorexia
- Confusion (late sign)
- Depression
- Emotional lability
- Encephalopathy
- Endocrine dysfunction (thyroid, pituitary)
- Fatigue on slight exertion
- Hypertension
- Insomnia
- Intractable hiccups
- Metallic taste in mouth
- Muscle cramps, muscle twitching
- Nausea, vomiting
- Neuropathy
- Nocturia, polyuria
- Pruritus
- Seizures (late sign)
- Serositis
- Skin dry
- Stomatitis

CAUSES

- Renal parenchymal: Glomerular: membranous nephropathy, membranoproliferative glomerulonephritis, systemic lupus erythematosus, focal glomerulosclerosis, diabetes mellitus, proliferative glomerulonephritis, amyloidosis, Alport syndrome, connective tissue disease.
- Interstitial-tubular: Heavy metals, drugs, nephrotoxins, multiple myeloma, hypertension, gout(?), thrombotic microangiopathies, oxalate deposition, infection, renal artery stenosis or ischemic stenosis, connective tissue disease, autosomal dominant polycystic kidney disease, congenital.
- Post-renal: See hydronephrosis causes
- Pre-renal: Cirrhosis, cardiac, volume, nephrotic, drugs (e.g., NSAIDs)

RISK FACTORS

- Volume depletion
- Contrast (diabetes, myeloma)
- Circulatory failure
- Urinary tract obstruction
- Analgesic abuse
- Untreated hypertension
- Diabetes mellitus
- The greater the proteinuria, the quicker the progression of CRF
- Cigarette smoking

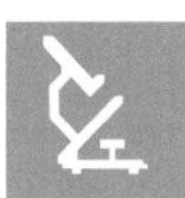

DIAGNOSIS

DIFFERENTIAL DIAGNOSIS See causes

LABORATORY

- Urine
  - ◊ Proteinuria
  - ◊ Casts
  - ◊ Microalbuminuria
  - ◊ Spot urine for protein/creatinine ratio
  - ◊ Electrolytes
  - ◊ 24 hour for protein, creatinine clearance
- Blood:
  - ◊ Normochromic, normocytic anemia
  - ◊ Thrombocytopenia
  - ◊ Increased bleeding time
- Chemistry:
  - ◊ Azotemia
  - ◊ Elevated ammonia
  - ◊ Type IV hyperlipidemia
  - ◊ Decreased active Vitamin D
  - ◊ Increased parathyroid hormone
  - ◊ Elevated glucose, insulin resistance
  - ◊ Elevated phosphate
  - ◊ Elevated potassium
  - ◊ Elevated sulfate
  - ◊ Elevated uric acid
  - ◊ Reduced calcium
  - ◊ Serum CO_2 content - 15-20 mEq/L (15-20 mmol/L)

Drugs that may alter lab results:

- Cimetidine
- Trimethoprim
- Cefazolin: increase creatinine

Disorders that may alter lab results: Ketosis may artificially raise creatinine

PATHOLOGICAL FINDINGS N/A

SPECIAL TESTS

- Complement studies
- Antinuclear antibody
- Serum protein electrophoresis
- Urine immune electrophoresis
- Hepatitis B surface antigen
- Hepatic C antigen
- HIV testing

IMAGING

- Ultrasound - decreased kidney size, may show obstructed ureter and bladder outlet (diabetic kidneys and ADPKD kidneys are not small)
- CT scan

DIAGNOSTIC PROCEDURES Kidney biopsy

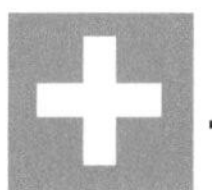

TREATMENT

APPROPRIATE HEALTH CARE Inpatient or outpatient depending on severity

GENERAL MEASURES

- Main goal is to slow progression
- Treat any aggravating cause aggressively (salt and water depletion, nephrotoxins, congestive heart failure, infection, hypercalcemia, urinary obstruction)
- Careful prescription of drugs (renal dosing; avoid use of nephrotoxin agents)
- Treat anemia with erythropoietin (HCT ≤ 30%)
- Use ACE inhibitors or receptor blockers to decrease proteinemia aggressively
- Dialysis: hemodialysis, peritoneal dialysis, transplant
- Strong emphasis on optimization of pre-ESRD care
- Vitamin D (active) and calcium supplements (dihydrotachysterol 0.2-0.4 mg q day); calcium acetate tablets with meals tid
- Strict control of blood pressure. For patients with proteinuria > 1 gm/d ≤ 125/75; < 1 gm/d 130/80. ACE inhibitors in diabetes mellitus.
- Earlier referral to a nephrologist decreases mortality on dialysis
- Control glucose in diabetics
- Reduce contrast-induced damage in diabetics with hydration, acetylcysteine
- Vaccines: Pneumococcal, influenza and H. influenzae
- Smoking cessation
- Treat dyslipidemia (goal LDL < 100)

SURGICAL MEASURES Transplantation

ACTIVITY Restricted only by patient's condition

DIET
- Adequate caloric intake
- Restricted protein (insufficient evidence for restriction below 0.8 g/kg/day)
- Restricted intake of phosphate
- Water intake limited to maintain serum sodium concentration of 135 to 145 mEq/L
- Sodium restriction if volume expanded
- Potassium restriction if hyperkalemic
- Vitamin supplementation (avoid extra-dietary intake of magnesium)
- Strict dietary restrictions in the elderly may not be necessary, since they often have a low protein and salt intake
- Referral to dietician

PATIENT EDUCATION
- For patient education materials favorably reviewed on this topic, contact: National Kidney and Urologic Diseases Information Clearinghouse, Box NKUDIC, Bethesda MD 20893. (301)468-6345
- The National Kidney Foundation, Inc. 30 East 33rd Street, New York, New York 10016. "Bone Disease in Chronic Renal Failure" (Order #02-27CP), "Diabetes and Kidney Disease" (Order #02-09CP). "Drug Abuse Can Hurt Your Kidneys" (Order #02-22N) or "Nutrition and Changing Kidney Function" (Order #0401).

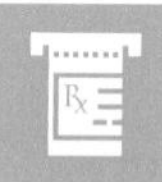

MEDICATIONS

DRUG(S) OF CHOICE
- Calcium-based phosphate binders and vitamin D to maintain PO4 and calcium levels
- Erythropoietin for anemia, approximately 100-150 units/kg thrice weekly IV or subcutaneous
- Salt restriction and diuretics for edema. Thiazides do not work at glomerular filtration rate (GFR) < 30 cc/min (creatinine > 2.5 mg/dL).
- Antihypertensives. For diabetic CRF, angiotensin converting enzyme inhibitors slow progression to dialysis dependence. Avoid dihydropyridine calcium channel blockers as sole agents.
- Muscle cramps: Vitamin E
- Pruritus: Skin moisturizers, diphenhydramine, activated charcoal
- Bleeding: DDAVP, cryoprecipitate, dialysis in uremia

Contraindications: Refer to manufacturer's literature

Precautions:
- Monitor serum electrolytes carefully
- Monitor loop diuretic use to avoid volume depletion
- Adjust all renally-excreted medications

Significant possible interactions: Refer to manufacturer's literature

ALTERNATIVE DRUGS
- Multivitamin preparation excluding fat-soluble vitamins and magnesium-containing products
- Angiotensin II receptor blockers may also be utilized in lieu of ACE I

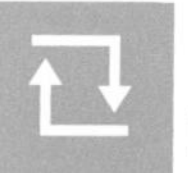

FOLLOWUP

PATIENT MONITORING
- Blood, urine, chemistries and clinical status
- Blood pressure, volume monitored frequently
- Diagnose uremia and then dialyze

PREVENTION/AVOIDANCE
- Avoid nephrotoxic drugs when possible (especially iodinated contrast, NSAIDs)
- Treat all disorders known to lead to chronic renal failure
- Many drugs require dosage reduction to prevent toxicity
- Avoid volume depletion

POSSIBLE COMPLICATIONS
- Anemia
- Changes in calcium and phosphorous metabolism
- Lipid disorders, accelerated hypertension
- Pericarditis-tamponade
- Serositis
- Increased magnesium
- Platelet dysfunction, bleeding
- Pseudogout, gout
- Hypothyroidism
- Infections
- Hyperkalemia
- Acidosis
- Hyponatremia
- Metabolic calcification
- Spontaneous abortion
- Infertility
- Impotence
- GI mucosal ulcerations
- GI A-V malformations
- Seizures
- Fractures
- Fluid overload

EXPECTED COURSE/PROGNOSIS
Serious, chronic, mortality > 20% despite careful attention to fluid and electrolyte balance or other treatment

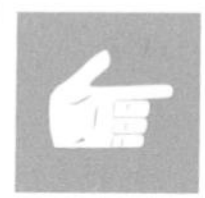

MISCELLANEOUS

ASSOCIATED CONDITIONS
See conditions listed under Risk factors

AGE-RELATED FACTORS
Pediatric:
- Main causes in children include congenital renal and urinary tract malformations (signs appear before age 5), glomerular and hereditary renal diseases (signs appear between ages 5-15)
- Medical management much more difficult in children
- When develops in infancy, growth impairment more profound than when develops in otherwise healthy teenager

Geriatric:
- Highest incidence, highest morbidity, highest mortality. Renal disease is secondary to many age-dependent illnesses.
- Rule out such potentially reversible causes as urinary tract obstruction (particularly in men), renal arterial occlusion, hypercalcemia, use of nephrotoxic agents
- Older patients may tolerate dialysis quite well

Others: N/A

PREGNANCY
Pregnancy to term less common in CRF. Fertility and libido disturbed in CRF.

SYNONYMS
- Uremia
- CRF
- End stage renal disease
- CRI

ICD-9-CM
585 Chronic renal failure

SEE ALSO
Hydronephrosis
Nephrotic syndrome
Polycystic kidney disease
Renal failure, acute (ARF)

OTHER NOTES
N/A

ABBREVIATIONS
CRF = chronic renal failure
ESRD = end-stage renal disease

REFERENCES
- Eschbach JW. Current concepts of anemia management in chronic renal failure: impact of NKF-DOQI. Semin Nephrol 2000;20(4):320-9
- Klotman PE. HIV-associated nephropathy. Kid Int 1999;56:1161-76
- Levey AS. Clinical practice. Nondiabetic kidney disease. N Engl J Med 2002;347(19):1505-11
- McCarthy JT. A practical approach to the management of patients with CRF. Mayo Clin Prac 1999;74:269-73
- Palmer BF. Renal dysfunction complicating the treatment of hypertension. N Engl J Med 2002;347(16):1256-61
- Pereria BJ. Optimization of pre-ESRD care: the key to improved dialysis outcomes. Kid Int 2000;57:351-65
- Remuzzi G, Schieppati A, Ruggenenti P. Clinical practice. Nephropathy in patients with type 2 diabetes. N Engl J Med 2002;346(15):1145-51
- Safian RD, Textor SC. Renal-artery stenosis. N Engl J Med 2001;344(6):431-42
- Tepel M, van der Giet M, Schwarzfeld C, Laufer U, Liermann D, Zidek W. Prevention of radiographic-contrast-agent-induced reductions in renal function by acetylcysteine. N Engl J Med 2000;343(3):180-4

Web references: 3 available at www.5mcc.com

Illustrations 3 available

Author(s):
Neal S. Gold, MD

BASICS

DESCRIPTION A group of disorders characterized by an abnormality of renal tubular acidification, which results in hyperchloremic acidosis and a normal anion gap. Several types have been identified:
- Classic distal RTA (type I): usually secondary to impaired ability to secrete hydrogen ions into the distal tubule or collecting duct. Urine pH > 5.5.
- Proximal RTA (type II): due to impaired bicarbonate reabsorption in the proximal tubule. Bicarbonate spills into the urine at lower than normal plasma bicarbonate concentrations. If the plasma bicarbonate level is low enough (typically between 15-18), the urine may be acidified (pH < 5.5), in contrast to type I.
- Type III: no longer considered a distinct entity
- Distal hyperkalemic RTA (type IV): several subtypes are recognized but all are characterized by aldosterone resistance or deficiency. This leads to hyperkalemia (not seen in types 1 or 2) along with acidosis. The urine pH may be < 5.5.

System(s) affected: Endocrine/Metabolic, Renal/Urologic

Genetics:
- Type I RTA: Autosomal dominant or recessive. May occur in association with other genetic diseases such as Ehlers-Danlos syndrome, hereditary elliptocytosis, or sickle-cell nephropathy. Autosomal recessive form associated with sensorineural deafness.
- Type II RTA: Autosomal dominant form is rare. Autosomal recessive form is associated with ophthalmologic abnormalities and mental retardation. Occurs in Fanconi syndrome, which is associated with several genetic diseases (cystinosis, Wilson disease, tyrosinemia, hereditary fructose intolerance, Lowe syndrome, galactosemia, glycogen storage disease, metachromatic leukodystrophy).
- Type IV RTA: Some cases familial such as pseudohypoaldosteronism type I (autosomal dominant)

Incidence/Prevalence in USA: N/A
Predominant age: occurs at all ages
Predominant sex: Male > Female in type II RTA with isolated defect in bicarbonate reabsorption

SIGNS & SYMPTOMS
- Failure to thrive in children
- Anorexia, nausea
- Vomiting
- Weakness due to potassium loss
- Polyuria due to potassium loss
- Rickets in children
- Osteomalacia in adults
- Constipation
- Polydipsia

CAUSES
- Type I
  - ◊ Genetic - autosomal dominant
  - ◊ Genetic - autosomal recessive associated with sensorineural deafness
  - ◊ Sporadic
  - ◊ Ehlers-Danlos syndrome
  - ◊ Hematologic diseases: sickle cell disease, hereditary elliptocytosis
  - ◊ Hypercalciuria
  - ◊ Vitamin D intoxication
  - ◊ Medullary cystic disease
  - ◊ Glycogenosis type III
  - ◊ Autoimmune disease
  - ◊ Diseases causing nephrocalcinosis
  - ◊ Fabry disease
  - ◊ Wilson disease
  - ◊ Drug induced (amphotericin B, lithium, analgesics)
  - ◊ Toxin induced (toluene, glue)
  - ◊ Hypergammaglobulinemic syndrome
  - ◊ Obstructive uropathy
  - ◊ Chronic pyelonephritis
  - ◊ Renal transplantation
  - ◊ Leprosy
  - ◊ Hepatic cirrhosis
  - ◊ Malnutrition
- Type II
  - ◊ Diseases associated with Fanconi syndrome (see Genetics)
  - ◊ Sporadic
  - ◊ Multiple myeloma and other dysproteinemic states
  - ◊ Heavy metal poisoning (cadmium, lead, mercury)
  - ◊ Medications: acetazolamide, sulfanilamide, ifosfamide, outdated tetracycline)
  - ◊ Autoimmune disease
  - ◊ Amyloidosis
  - ◊ Interstitial renal disease
  - ◊ Nephrotic syndrome
  - ◊ Congenital heart disease
  - ◊ Defects in calcium metabolism (hyperparathyroidism)
- Type IV
  - ◊ Lupus nephropathy
  - ◊ Diabetic nephropathy
  - ◊ Obstructive nephropathy
  - ◊ Nephrosclerosis due to hypertension
  - ◊ Tubulointerstitial nephropathies
  - ◊ Addison disease
  - ◊ Acute adrenal insufficiency
  - ◊ Pseudohypoaldosteronism (end organ resistance to aldosterone)
  - ◊ Gordon syndrome
  - ◊ Sickle cell nephropathy

RISK FACTORS N/A

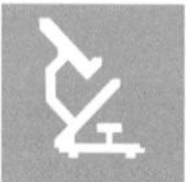

DIAGNOSIS

DIFFERENTIAL DIAGNOSIS
- Anion gap must be normal. If not, look for causes of metabolic acidosis other than RTA. (As in mnemonic MUDPILES: Metabolic disease or methanol ingestion, uremia, diabetic ketoacidosis, paraldehyde ingestion, iron or isoniazid ingestion, lactic acidosis, ethylene glycol ingestion, salicylate ingestion.)
- Diarrhea with bicarbonate loss in stools
- Acidosis of chronic renal failure
- Urinary diversion (ureterosigmoidostomy, ileal conduit)
- Ingestion of hydrochloric acid, ammonium chloride, lysine HCL, excess calcium or magnesium chloride
- Small bowel, pancreatic or biliary fistulas

LABORATORY
- Electrolytes reveal hyperchloremic metabolic acidosis
- Plasma anion gap normal (anion gap=plasma Na-(Cl+CO2)). Normal values: neonates <18; infants and children <16; adolescents and adults <14).
- Hypokalemia or normokalemia
  - ◊ Type I
  - ◊ Type II
- Hyperkalemia - type IV
- BUN and creatinine usually normal (rules out renal failure as cause of acidosis)
- Urine pH - not acidified (pH >5.5) despite metabolic acidosis in type I
- Urine culture - rule out UTI with urea splitting organism (may elevate pH) and chronic infection
- Urine anion gap, an estimate of urine ammonium excretion (urine Na+K-Cl on random urine). Measure before treatment. Most useful if measured when patient is acidotic. Results tend to be:
  - ◊ Negative in bicarbonate losses secondary to diarrhea
  - ◊ Negative in UTI due to urea splitting organism
  - ◊ Positive in type I
  - ◊ Positive in type IV
- Urine calcium
  - ◊ Typically normal in type II
  - ◊ High in type I

Drugs that may alter lab results:
- Diuretics
- Sodium bicarbonate
- Cholestyramine

Disorders that may alter lab results: N/A

PATHOLOGICAL FINDINGS
- Nephrocalcinosis, nephrolithiasis
- Rickets, osteomalacia
- Findings of underlying disease causing RTA

SPECIAL TESTS
- May be helpful to measure urine pH on fresh specimens with pH meter for increased accuracy instead of dipstick. Place oil over urine to avoid loss of carbon dioxide if pH cannot be measured quickly.
- Urine ammonium excretion (anion gap is indirect measurement of this, but is not as accurate)
- Ammonium chloride (NH4+) loading to evaluate acid excretion
- Bicarbonate titration curves

IMAGING Not needed except to rule out underlying conditions such as nephrocalcinosis or complications

DIAGNOSTIC PROCEDURES N/A

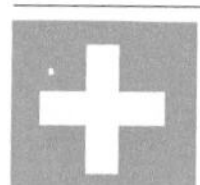

TREATMENT

APPROPRIATE HEALTH CARE
- Outpatient
- Inpatient if acidosis severe, patient unreliable, persistent emesis, infant with severe failure to thrive

GENERAL MEASURES Treatment with appropriate medications to correct acidosis

SURGICAL MEASURES If distal RTA IV is due to obstructive uropathy, may require surgical intervention

ACTIVITY As tolerated

DIET Varies with type of acidosis

PATIENT EDUCATION
- National Kidney & Urologic Diseases Information Clearinghouse, Box NKUDIC, Bethesda, MD 20893, (301)468-6345; http://www.niddk.nih.gov/health/kidney/.
- National Kidney Foundation; http://www.kidney.org

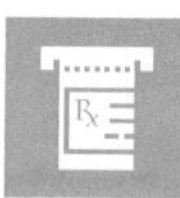

MEDICATIONS

DRUG(S) OF CHOICE
Provide oral alkali to raise serum bicarbonate to normal. Start at a low dose and increase until serum bicarbonate is normal. Give as sodium bicarbonate or citrate mixtures (1 mEq citrate = 1 mEq HCO3) such as Bicitra (1 mEq Na, 1 mEq Citrate/mL, no K) or Polycitra (1 mEq Na, 1 mEq K, 2 mEq citrate/mL) depending on need for potassium. Sodium bicarbonate tablets available (7.7 mEq HCO3/tab)
- Type I: typical doses 1-4 mEq/kg/day oral alkali divided tid-qid, unless bicarbonate wasting present, in which case much larger doses required. May require potassium supplementation if serum potassium low.
- Type II: typical doses 5-10 mEq/kg/day alkali. May be difficult to control and require doses divided 4-6 doses/day. May require potassium supplementation if serum potassium low.
- Type IV: 1-5 mEq/kg/day alkali divided bid-tid. Avoid potassium. In some cases furosemide used to lower potassium levels, but avoid if patient wastes salt. Fludrocortisone - 0.1-0.3 mg/day, if mineralocorticoid deficient.

Contraindications: Refer to manufacturer's literature
Precautions: Sodium bicarbonate may cause flatulence as carbon dioxide is formed, whereas citrate mixtures are metabolized to bicarbonate in the liver, thereby avoiding gas production.
Significant possible interactions: N/A

ALTERNATIVE DRUGS
- Hydrochlorothiazide an adjunct in type II after maximal alkali replacement, but may exacerbate already existing kaliuresis

FOLLOWUP

PATIENT MONITORING
- Varies with patient response. Suggested: electrolytes every 2-4 weeks at onset of therapy, every 2 weeks for one or two months once bicarbonate concentration normal, then monthly for several months
- Monitor underlying disease as indicated
- Poor compliance common due to tid-qid alkali dosing schedule

PREVENTION/AVOIDANCE
- Careful use or avoidance of causative agents listed above

POSSIBLE COMPLICATIONS
- Nephrocalcinosis
- Hyper- or hypokalemia
- Nephrolithiasis
- Rickets
- Osteomalacia
- Hypercalciuria

EXPECTED COURSE/PROGNOSIS
- Prognosis dependent on the associated disease, otherwise good with therapy
- Transient forms of all types of RTA may occur

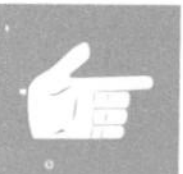

MISCELLANEOUS

ASSOCIATED CONDITIONS
- Type I in children - hypercalciuria leading to rickets, nephrocalcinosis
- Type I in adults - autoimmune diseases such as Sjögren disease
- Type II - Fanconi syndrome: A generalized tubular defect with bicarbonaturia, aminoaciduria, glycosuria, phosphaturia
- Type IV: obstructive uropathy, renal insufficiency, diabetic nephropathy

AGE-RELATED FACTORS
Pediatric: N/A
Geriatric: N/A
Others: N/A

PREGNANCY N/A

SYNONYMS N/A

ICD-9-CM
588.8 Other specified disorder resulting from impaired renal function
270.0 Disturbances of amino-acid transport

SEE ALSO
Fanconi syndrome
Hyperkalemia
Sjögren syndrome
Wilson disease

OTHER NOTES N/A

ABBREVIATIONS N/A

REFERENCES

- Morris RC, Ives HE. In: Brenner BM, ed: Brenner & Rector's: The Kidney. 5th Ed. Philadelphia, WB Saunders Co., 1996:1779-84
- Chesney RW. In: Bennett, ed: Cecil Textbook of Medicine. 20th Ed. Philadelphia, WB Saunders Co., 1996:594-9
- Rodriguez-Soriano J. New insights into the pathogenesis of renal tubular acidosis--from functional to molecular studies. Pediatr Nephrol 2000;14(12):1121-36
- Chiang M, Hill LL. Renal tubular acidosis. In: Oski FA, ed: Principles and Practices of Pediatrics. 2nd Ed. Philadelphia, JB Lippincott, 1994:1810-8
- Carey CF, Hans L, eds. Washington Manual of Medical Therapeutics. 29th ed. Philadelphia, Lippincott Williams & Wilkins, 1998:55-9

Web references: 2 available at www.5mcc.com
Illustrations N/A

Author(s):
David E. Hall, MD
Richard F. Salmon, DO

BASICS

DESCRIPTION ARDS is defined as the abrupt onset of respiratory distress accompanied by 3 components: severe hypoxemia, bilateral pulmonary infiltrates on chest radiograph and absence of clear evidence of heart failure or volume overload. Disease severity ranges from acute lung injury (ALI) to full blown adult respiratory distress syndrome (ARDS). In addition, it is often progressive.
System(s) affected: Cardiovascular, Pulmonary
Genetics: Flores and Pavlovic suggest that pulmonary surfactant and its components may provide markers to identify ARDS subgroups and provide a basis for identifying at risk groups and study potential treatments
Incidence/Prevalence in USA: 1.5-8.3 cases/100,000/year
Predominant age: All ages
Predominant sex: Male = Female

SIGNS & SYMPTOMS
- Most patients demonstrate similar clinical and pathologic features regardless of the cause of the acute lung injury. There are 3 phases:
  - ◊ Acute exudative phase characterized by profound hypoxia and associated with inflammation with infiltration of inflammatory and proinflammatory mediators and diffuse alveolar damage.
  - ◊ Fibrosing alveolitis phase coincides with recovery or after about 1 -2 weeks. Patients continue to be hypoxic, have increased dead space and decreased compliance.
  - ◊ Resolution may require 6 - 12 months. Residual respiratory concerns are outlined in the section on prognosis.
- Signs and symptoms:
  - ◊ Tachypnea and tachycardia during the first 12 to 24 hours
  - ◊ Moist and cyanotic skin
  - ◊ Breathing difficulty with intercostal and accessory respiratory muscles
  - ◊ Dramatic increase in work of breathing
  - ◊ High-pitched end-expiratory crackles are heard throughout all lung fields
  - ◊ Increased agitation
  - ◊ Lethargy, then obtundation
  - ◊ Hypoxemia may be present long before clinical signs

CAUSES
- Recent studies have revealed a number of mediators are involved in the initiation and perpetuation of ARDS
  - ◊ Cytokines (tumor necrosis factor, interleukin 1, interleukin 6)
  - ◊ Complement activation
  - ◊ Coagulation activation
  - ◊ Platelet - activating factor
  - ◊ Oxygen radicals
  - ◊ Lipoxygenase pathways (Leukotrienes C4, D4 and E4)
  - ◊ Neutrophil proteases
  - ◊ Nitric oxide - may be deleterious or advantageous
  - ◊ Endotoxin
  - ◊ Cyclooxygenase pathway products (thromboxane A2, prostacyclin)
- Systemic inflammatory response with activation of the previous mediators can occur with direct or indirect injury to the lung
  - ◊ Direct
    - Aspiration
    - Pulmonary infections (bacterial, fungal, viral and protozoan)
    - Air, fat or amniotic fluid emboli (e.g., long bone fractures)
    - Near-drowning
    - Pulmonary contusion
    - Inhalation of toxic gases (oxygen, smoke, NH_3, chlorine, plastics, phosgene, cadmium)
  - ◊ Indirect
    - Sepsis (gram negative, gram positive, fungi, tuberculous, Pneumocystis pneumonia)
    - Shock (hemorrhage, cardiogenic, septic, anaphylactic)
    - Transfusions
    - Trauma (e.g., head injury, burns
    - Overdose
    - Pancreatitis, severe
    - Eclampsia
    - Carcinomatosis
    - Leukoagglutinin reaction

RISK FACTORS
- Systemic sepsis (40% risk of progression to ALI or ARDS)
- Multiple predisposing disorders increases risk
- Chronic alcohol abuse
- Chronic lung disease
- Low serum pH

DIAGNOSIS

DIFFERENTIAL DIAGNOSIS Cardiogenic pulmonary edema

LABORATORY
- ALI: $PaO_2/FiO_2 \leq 300$
- ARDS: $PaO_2/Fio_2 \leq 200$
- Bronchoalveolar lavage shows evidence of substantial inflammation

Drugs that may alter lab results: N/A

Disorders that may alter lab results:
- Multiple pulmonary emboli
- Cardiogenic pulmonary edema
- Severe chronic obstructive pulmonary disease
- Severe pneumonia

PATHOLOGICAL FINDINGS
- Lungs show exudative phase, early proliferative phase or late proliferative phase
- Interstitial and alveolar edema
- Inflammatory cells and erythrocytes spill into interstitium and the alveolus
- Type I cells are destroyed, leaving a denuded basement membrane
- Protein-rich fluid fills the alveoli
- Type II alveolar cells appear unaltered initially
- Type II cells begin to proliferate within 72 hours of initial insult
- The type II cells cover the denuded basement membrane
- Aggregates of plasma proteins, cellular debris, fibrin and surfactant remnants form hyaline membranes
- Over next 3-10 days, alveolar septum thickens by proliferating fibroblasts, leukocytes and plasma cells
- Capillary injury begins to occur
- Hyaline membranes begin to reorganize
- Fibrosis becomes apparent in respiratory ducts and bronchioles

SPECIAL TESTS
- Invasive vital sign, cardiac output and PAWP monitoring
- ABGs

IMAGING
- CXR: linear opacities, consistent with evolving fibrosis
- Chest CT: diffuse interstitial opacities and bullae

DIAGNOSTIC PROCEDURES
- Pulmonary artery catheterization to demonstrate:
  - ◊ Normal pulmonary arterial occlusion pressure (PAOP)
  - ◊ Note: The main point of this study is to determine if the PAOP is inconsistent with cardiogenic pulmonary edema. A low PAOP with low serum albumin may lead to cardiogenic etiology. The patient with chronic congestive heart failure may have high wedge, but still develop ARDS.

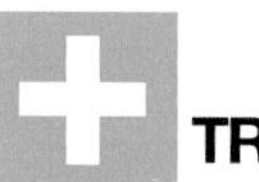

TREATMENT

APPROPRIATE HEALTH CARE Intensive care unit

GENERAL MEASURES
- Treat underlying etiology (sepsis, pneumonia, shock) as appropriate
- Prevent complications (e.g., gastrointestinal bleeding, nosocomial infections, thromboembolus)
- Corticosteroids have not been shown to add benefit during the acute phase, but may have value in patients with established ARDS
- Support ventilation utilizing lung protection strategies (i.e., low tidal volume and PEEP)
- Consider paralyzing agents (to improve compliance and decrease barotrauma) if patient is fighting ventilator. Initiate anxiolytics when instituting treatment with paralytic agents.
- Maintain oxygen delivery and avoid supranormal oxygen delivery
- Recruitment maneuvers may be helpful
  - ◊ High level continuous PEEP
  - ◊ Intermittent sighs
  - ◊ Intermittent and stepwise high PEEP and fixed pressure control maneuver
  - ◊ Prone positioning

- Measure CO with each PEEP change. If CO decreases, give fluids to regain adequate CO and allow additional PEEP adjustments if necessary. A pulmonary artery catheter may be helpful in assessing left ventricular function, CO, oxygen delivery and consumption. It is necessary if high levels of PEEP are used.
- Fluid and hemodynamic management
  - ◊ Maintain intravascular volume at lowest level consistent with adequate perfusion (assessed by metabolic acid-base balance and renal function)
  - ◊ If perfusion is inadequate after restoration of intravascular volume (e.g., septic shock), vasopressor is indicated
  - ◊ Increase oxygen content with packed red blood cells transfusions as necessary
- Provide appropriate nutritional support
- Extraordinary management
  - ◊ Extracorporeal membrane oxygenation (ECMO)
  - ◊ High-frequency ventilation
  - ◊ Pressure controlled inverse ratio ventilation (PCIRV)
  - ◊ Extracorporeal CO2 removal with low frequency ventilation

SURGICAL MEASURES N/A

ACTIVITY Bedrest

DIET Nutritional support

PATIENT EDUCATION N/A

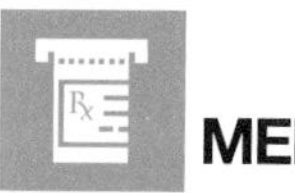

MEDICATIONS

DRUG(S) OF CHOICE

No single or combination of drugs prevents or treats ARDS. Treatment is supportive while addressing the underlying cause.

- Inotropic agents - dobutamine to maintain adequate cardiac output after appropriate fluid resuscitation fails to restore perfusion
- Vasodilators - nitroprusside, ACE inhibitors, hydralazine. (Only if BP is adequate.)
- Anxiolytics (e.g., lorazepam)
- Deep-vein thrombosis prophylaxis
- Ulcer prophylaxis
- Inhaled or systemic beta-agonists may be helpful during the resolution phase

Contraindications: See manufacturer's profile of each drug
Precautions: See manufacturer's profile of each drug
Significant possible interactions: See manufacturer's profile of each drug

ALTERNATIVE DRUGS

- Corticosteroids: short term use during the acute phase has not been shown to be effective. However, some data suggest that sustained therapy in patients with established ARDS may be beneficial, therefore a short course of high dose glucocorticoids could be considered in a patient with severe, unresolving disease.
- Atrial natriuretic polypeptide (ANP): control trials have been done and results are pending
- Antioxidants, such as procysteine have had conflicting results in patients with ARDS
- Pulmonary surfactant: has been successful in infants with neonatal respiratory distress syndrome. However there is insufficient data to recommend its use in adults. Clinical trials are ongoing.
- Vasodilators: nitric oxide, sodium nitroprusside, hydralizine, alprostadil and prostacyclin have not been shown to be beneficial
- Recombinant human activated protein C [drotrecogin alfa (Xigris)]. Published trials suggest benefit for patients with severe sepsis. Further trials are ongoing to determine appropriate patient selection.

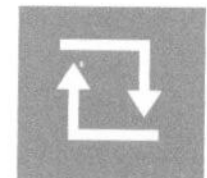

FOLLOWUP

PATIENT MONITORING

- Vital capacity and static lung compliance are important measures of mechanics
- Daily labs until no longer critical
- CXR to assess - endotracheal tube placement; the possible development of barotrauma; the presence of infiltrates; PA catheter migration
- Swan-Ganz catheter - to help assess 02 delivery and consumption; monitor cardiac output

PREVENTION/AVOIDANCE N/A

POSSIBLE COMPLICATIONS

- Multiple organ dysfunction syndrome (MODS)
- Death
- Permanent lung disease
- Oxygen toxicity
- Barotrauma
- Superinfection

EXPECTED COURSE/PROGNOSIS 36% mortality rate. Failure of lung function to improve in the first week of treatment portends a poor prognosis. Most survivors will regain normal or near normal pulmonary function within 6-12 months. However, general health and respiratory-related quality of life and pulmonary function decrements may occur. Residual impairment of respiratory mechanics include mild restriction, mild obstruction, impaired DLCO or gas exchange abnormalities with exercise. Survivors who required prolonged ventilatory support as well as those with severe disease are more likely to have persistent respiratory abnormalities.

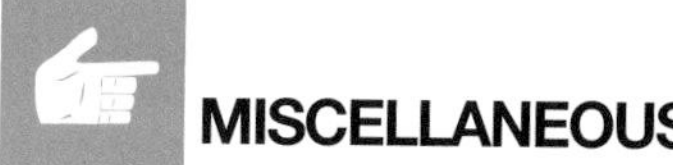

MISCELLANEOUS

ASSOCIATED CONDITIONS N/A

AGE-RELATED FACTORS N/A
Pediatric: N/A
Geriatric: Increasing mortality with increasing age
Others: N/A

PREGNANCY N/A

SYNONYMS

- Shock lung
- Wet lung
- Noncardiac pulmonary edema

ICD-9-CM

786.09 Dyspnea and respiratory abnormalities, other
518.5 Pulmonary insufficiency following trauma and surgery
518.82 Other pulmonary insufficiency, NEC

SEE ALSO

Congestive heart failure
Pneumonia, bacterial
Shock, circulatory

OTHER NOTES N/A

ABBREVIATIONS

PEEP = positive end-expiratory pressure

REFERENCES

- Ware, LB, Matthay, MA, Medical Progress: The Acute Respiratory Distress Syndrome, NEJM, 342(18);2000:1334-49
- Petrucci, N, Iacovelli, W, Ventilation with lower tidal volumes versus traditional tidal volumes in adults for acute lung injury and acute respiratory distress syndrome, Cochrane Database of Systemic Reviews, Cochrane Library, Vol 3, 2003
- ICD-9-CM Professional: for Physicians, Vol 1 & 2, 6th edition 2004, Hast, AAC, Hopkins, CA, Ingenex Inc 2003
- Kallet,, RH, Hass, CF, Adult respiratory Distress Syndrome, Part 1, Respiratory Clinics of North America, 9(3) 2003 WB Saunders, Phil
- Kallet, RH, Hass, CF, Adult Respiratory Distress Syndrome Part 2, Respiratory Clinics of North America 9(4) 2003
- Flores, J, Palovic, J, Genetics of Acute Respiratory Distress Syndrome: Challenges, Approaches, Surfactant Proteins as Candidate Genes, Sem in Resp & CCM, 24(2) 2003: 161-68
- Bernard GR, Margolis BD, Shanies HM, Ely EW, Wheeler AP, Levy H, Wong K, Wright TJ; Extended Evaluation of Recombinant Human Activated Protein C United States Investigators. Extended evaluation of recombinant human activated protein C United States Trial (ENHANCE US): a single-arm, phase 3B, multicenter study of drotrecogin alfa (activated) in severe sepsis. Chest 2004;125(6):2206-16

Web references: 0 available at www.5mcc.com
Illustrations N/A

Author(s):
Mary Cataletto, MD

BASICS

DESCRIPTION Serious disorder of prematurity, with clinical manifestation of respiratory distress. Pulmonary surfactants that are deficient at birth cause diffuse lung atelectasis. Must differentiate from pneumonia, sepsis, meconium aspiration.
System(s) affected: Pulmonary
Genetics: No known genetic pattern
Incidence/Prevalence in USA: Common
Predominant age: Neonatal
Predominant sex: Male = Female, although usually more severe in males

SIGNS & SYMPTOMS
- Onset within few hours after birth
- Delayed, weak cry
- Expiratory grunt
- Frothing at lips
- Intercostal, sternal retractions
- Nasal flaring
- Rapid respiratory rate
- Respiratory excursions decreased
- Rales
- Cyanosis
- Peripheral edema
- Oliguria

CAUSES
- Prematurity
- Deficient pulmonary surfactants in the neonatal period
- Possible pulmonary ischemia

RISK FACTORS
- Premature infants born prior to 37 weeks gestation
- Infants born of diabetic mothers
- More common and more severe with greater prematurity
- Fetal asphyxia
- Multiple births

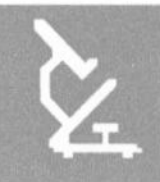

DIAGNOSIS

DIFFERENTIAL DIAGNOSIS
- Early group B streptococcal pneumonia
- Transient tachypnea of newborn
- Meconium aspiration pneumonia
- Sepsis with group B streptococcus pneumonia

LABORATORY
- Amniotic fluid:
  - ◊ Lecithin:sphingomyelin ratio (L:S ratio < 2)
  - ◊ Absence of phosphatidyl glycerol
  - ◊ Surfactant production deficient
- Features of respiratory, metabolic acidosis
- Arterial blood gases - hypoxemia and hypercarbia

Drugs that may alter lab results: Artificial or human surfactant; betamethasone

Disorders that may alter lab results: N/A

PATHOLOGICAL FINDINGS
- Voluminous, noncrepitant, purplish red lungs
- Dilatation right heart and vena cava
- Possible patent ductus
- Extensive resorptive atelectasis
- Hyaline membranes

SPECIAL TESTS
- Monitor arterial blood gases

IMAGING
- X-ray - reticulogranular appearance of lung fields demonstrating:
  - ◊ Diffuse atelectasis
  - ◊ Air bronchograms

DIAGNOSTIC PROCEDURES N/A

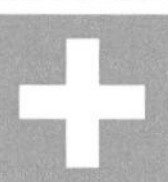

TREATMENT

APPROPRIATE HEALTH CARE Inpatient - intensive care

GENERAL MEASURES
- Warm, humidified, oxygen enriched gases by hood
- CPAP
- Positive pressure ventilation per ET tube
- Monitor respiratory and circulatory status carefully
- Umbilical artery catheter placed for monitoring blood pressure and sampling arterial blood gases
- Transcutaneous monitors to measure O2 and CO2 tension
- Pulse oximetry
- Radiant infant warmer
- Tube feedings or hyperalimentation
- High-frequency ventilation. Choices include conventional ventilation at faster-than-normal rates; high-frequency jet ventilation; high-frequency oscillation.
- Relationship between using surfactant and high-frequency ventilation still being studied
- Extracorporeal membrane oxygenation (ECMO) measure of last resort. Its use is still uncommon and there are risks associated. Not available for infants under 2 kg.

SURGICAL MEASURES N/A

ACTIVITY None; may require sedation or paralysis while on ventilator

DIET Special premature formula or parenteral alimentation

PATIENT EDUCATION For patient education materials favorably reviewed on this topic, contact: American Lung Association, 1740 Broadway, New York, NY 10019, (212)315-8700

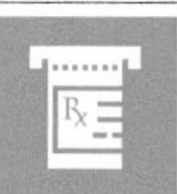

MEDICATIONS

DRUG(S) OF CHOICE Beractant (Survanta): bovine surfactant. Dose: 2.6-8.0 mL depending on patient's weight (see Manufacturer's Dosing Table). Other surfactant preparations available. Prophylaxis: as soon as possible after birth. Therapeutic: when signs and symptoms of RDS appear.
Contraindications: Refer to manufacturer's literature
Precautions: Do not administer beractant into a mainstem bronchus. Check endotracheal tube placement before administration. Be prepared for rapidly changing lung compliance; peak ventilator pressures may need to be reduced immediately.
Significant possible interactions: Refer to manufacturer's literature

ALTERNATIVE DRUGS N/A

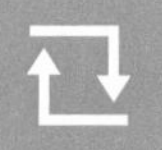

FOLLOWUP

PATIENT MONITORING
- Continuous monitoring in an intensive care nursery
- Should have stable vital signs and pulse oximetry before discharge

PREVENTION/AVOIDANCE
- Prevention of premature birth
- Systemic betamethasone given to mother when fetal lung profile is immature; at least 24 hours before delivery

POSSIBLE COMPLICATIONS
- Intraventricular hemorrhage
- Intracranial pathology
- Tension pneumothorax
- Retinopathy of prematurity
- Apnea
- Chronic lung disease - bronchopulmonary dysplasia (BPD) - 5-20%

EXPECTED COURSE/PROGNOSIS
- Course
  - ◊ Acute, possibly fatal within 48 hours in 20-30%, increasing with lower birth weights, especially < 1,000 grams.
  - ◊ In larger prematures, course may be brief and uncomplicated, with recovery in 1 week
- Prognosis
  - ◊ Successful outcome expected in tertiary care centers in children older than 28 weeks gestation
  - ◊ Chronic lung disease, bronchopulmonary dysplasia (BPD), frequent in severe cases, especially after prolonged artificial ventilation
  - ◊ Careful postdischarge follow-up needed, including monitoring of oxygen saturation, growth and development

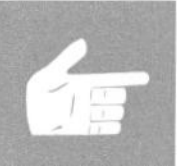

MISCELLANEOUS

ASSOCIATED CONDITIONS N/A

AGE-RELATED FACTORS
Pediatric: A disorder of the neonatal period
Geriatric: N/A
Others: N/A

PREGNANCY N/A

SYNONYMS
- Hyaline membrane disease
- RDS
- Surfactant deficiency

ICD-9-CM
770.89 Other respiratory problems after birth

SEE ALSO

OTHER NOTES N/A

ABBREVIATIONS
CPAP = continuous positive airway pressure

REFERENCES

- Avery GB, Fletcher MA, MacDonald MG, eds. Neonatology: Pathophysiology and Management of the Newborn. 5th ed. Philadelphia: Lippincott Williams & Wilkins; 1999
- Hageman JR. Neonatology update. The Pediat Clinics of North America, Philadelphia: WB Saunders Co; 1998

Web references: 0 available at www.5mcc.com
Illustrations N/A

Author(s):
Kurt J. Wegner, MD

BASICS

DESCRIPTION
- RSV causes respiratory illness
  - ◊ Adults: URI's
  - ◊ Infants and children: bronchitis, bronchiolitis, pneumonia
  - ◊ Leading cause of pediatric admissions for respiratory illness

System(s) affected: Pulmonary
Genetics: None known
Incidence/Prevalence in USA: Common in winter. Almost all persons infected one or more times during lifetime.
Predominant age: Birth to age 2
Predominant sex:
- Males = females as outpatients
- 2:1 males/females in hospital

SIGNS & SYMPTOMS
- Cold signs and symptoms (mild disease)
  - ◊ Fever
  - ◊ Cough
  - ◊ Coryza
  - ◊ Congestion
  - ◊ Otitis media
  - ◊ Malaise
- Bronchitis/bronchiolitis/pneumonia
  - ◊ Cough
  - ◊ Chest congestion, rales/rhonchi
  - ◊ Wheezing
  - ◊ Dyspnea
  - ◊ Hypoxia
  - ◊ Cyanosis
- Vomiting

CAUSES
Infection with RSV

RISK FACTORS
- Impaired immunity
  - ◊ AIDS
  - ◊ Chemotherapy
  - ◊ Other types of impaired immunity
- Occupational exposure
  - ◊ Day care workers
  - ◊ Pediatric hospital staff
  - ◊ School teachers
- Neonatal/congenital conditions
  - ◊ Congenital cardiac anomalies
  - ◊ Respiratory distress syndrome
  - ◊ Premature birth
- Low socioeconomic status
- More common in urban vs. rural areas

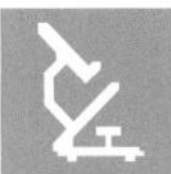

DIAGNOSIS

DIFFERENTIAL DIAGNOSIS
- Mild illness/upper respiratory tract
  - ◊ Colds (non RSV)
  - ◊ Allergic rhinitis
  - ◊ Sinusitis
  - ◊ Croup
- Severe illness/lower respiratory tract
  - ◊ Asthma
  - ◊ Bronchitis
  - ◊ Bronchiolitis
  - ◊ Pneumonia

LABORATORY
- WBC may be normal to elevated
- Positive RSV antigen test on nasal washings

Drugs that may alter lab results: None

Disorders that may alter lab results: None

PATHOLOGICAL FINDINGS
Lymphocytic peribronchiolar infiltrates (autopsy)

SPECIAL TESTS
N/A

IMAGING
- Chest x-ray
  - ◊ Hyperinflation - most common, characteristic finding
  - ◊ Interstitial infiltrates - fairly common
  - ◊ Segmental or lobar consolidation in pneumonia
  - ◊ Pleural fluid

DIAGNOSTIC PROCEDURES
None

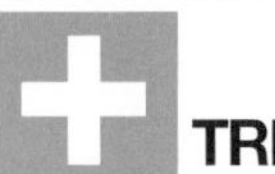

TREATMENT

APPROPRIATE HEALTH CARE
Outpatient for mild cases; inpatient for severe disease or for those with underlying disorders. Illness can last from days to several weeks.

GENERAL MEASURES
- Outpatient
  - ◊ Rest/supportive care
  - ◊ Bronchodilators - albuterol nebulizer/inhaler
  - ◊ Monitor oxygenation-pulse oximeter
- Inpatient
  - ◊ Oxygen
  - ◊ Bronchodilators - albuterol nebulizer q4h
  - ◊ Respiratory isolation
  - ◊ Ribavirin
  - ◊ Antibiotics for secondary bacterial pneumonia
  - ◊ Monitor arterial blood gases/pulse oximeter
  - ◊ Use of steroids is controversial; may help in some cases
- Avoid exposing others
  - ◊ Remove from day care/school until well
  - ◊ Good hand washing practices
  - ◊ Respiratory isolation in hospital

SURGICAL MEASURES
N/A

ACTIVITY
Decreased household activity/rest

DIET
- Maintain nutrition
- Avoid over-hydration (may increase lung congestion)

PATIENT EDUCATION
- Printed patient information available from: ICN Pharmaceuticals, Inc., ICN Plaza, 3300 Hyland Ave., Costa Mesa, CA 92626 "All about RSV: a guide for parents."
- RSV Info Center - http://www.rsvinfo.com

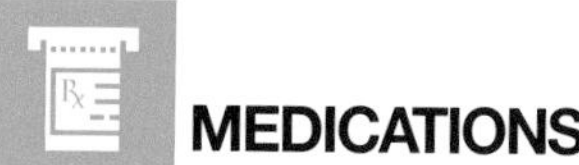

MEDICATIONS

DRUG(S) OF CHOICE
- Ribavirin 20 mg/mL mist 12-18 hours/day for 3-7 days. (Can shorten duration and severity of illness.)
- Bronchodilators - albuterol nebulizer q4h (dose appropriate for age)
- Antibiotics for secondary bacterial infections/pneumonia
  - ◊ Appropriate to particular pathogen
  - ◊ Prophylactic use of antibiotics controversial
- Potential use of RSV immune globulin in high risk infants

Contraindications: See specific drug related information
Precautions: Avoid exposure of pregnant/potentially pregnant women to ribavirin
Significant possible interactions: See specific drug information

ALTERNATIVE DRUGS
- Antibiotic appropriate to identified or suspected bacterial pathogen
- Theophylline use all right, but not recommended

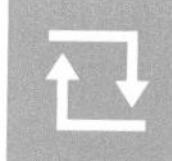

FOLLOWUP

PATIENT MONITORING
- Uneventful resolution is the norm
- No special monitoring is needed as illness resolves
- May want to educate parents about SIDS - avoid prone sleeping in infants

PREVENTION/AVOIDANCE
- Avoid exposure to those ill with RSV
- Good hand washing practices (since hand-nose and hand-eye transmission is common)
- Avoid rubbing the eyes (common RSV inoculation route)
- Use of palivizumab (Synagis) recommended for preemies < 35 weeks and infants with bronchopulmonary dysplasia prior to and during RSV season (Fall, Winter, Spring). Dose 15 mg/kg of body weight IM monthly.

POSSIBLE COMPLICATIONS
- Pneumonia
- Sudden infant death
- Death from severe lower respiratory tract infections
- Possible residual lung damage

EXPECTED COURSE/PROGNOSIS
- Usually resolves within two weeks without sequelae
- Hospitalization rate of children ill with RSV varies from 1:50 to 1:200 (children < 2 years old)

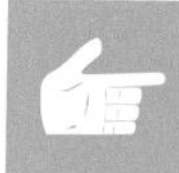

MISCELLANEOUS

ASSOCIATED CONDITIONS
- Asthma is worse with RSV and vice versa
- SIDS may be a sequelae of RSV

AGE-RELATED FACTORS
Pediatric: Most common under age 2
Geriatric: N/A
Others: Increasing immunity with subsequent infections by RSV usually results in less serious illness

PREGNANCY
- Avoid ribavirin therapy in pregnancy
- Healthcare workers who may be pregnant should avoid exposure to ribavirin

SYNONYMS N/A

ICD-9-CM
480.1 Pneumonia due to respiratory syncytial virus

SEE ALSO
Bronchiolitis
Bronchitis, acute
Pneumonia, bacterial
Pneumonia, viral

OTHER NOTES N/A

ABBREVIATIONS
- RSV = respiratory syncytial virus
- SIDS = sudden infant death syndrome
- URI = upper respiratory infection

REFERENCES

- Mandell GL, ed: Principles and Practice of Infectious Diseases. 4th Ed. New York, Churchill Livingstone, 1995
- Rudolph AM, ed: Rudolph's Pediatrics 19th Ed. Norwalk, CT, Appleton & Lange, 1991
- Gilchrist S, et al: National surveillance for RSV, U.S., 1985-1990. J Inf Dis 1994;170:986-990
- Levin MJ: Treatment & prevention options for RSV infections. J Pediatr 1994;124:322-325
- Groothuis J, et al: Prophylactic administration of RSV immune globulin to high risk infants and young children. New Engl J Med 1993;329:1524-1530

Web references: 0 available at www.5mcc.com
Illustrations N/A

Author(s):
Joseph G. Ewing, MD

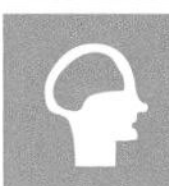

BASICS

DESCRIPTION Restless leg syndrome (RLS) and periodic limb movement disorder (PLMD) are two separate but related intrinsic disorders of sleep
- RLS is a neurological movement disorder diagnosed strictly by the following four criteria:
  - ◊ There is a conscious urge to move the legs (focal akathisia) usually accompanied or caused by uncomfortable or unpleasant sensations in the legs that persist without movement or a counter stimulus. The sensation is described as creepy, crawly, creeping or any other unpleasant adjectives and cannot be ignored.
  - ◊ The urge to move or unpleasant sensations begin or worsen when the patient is at rest or inactive (sitting or lying down)
  - ◊ The urge or sensation is relieved or reduced by movement but returns quickly when movement stops
  - ◊ The sensation or urge is worse in the evening or night than during the day or occur only at night or in the evening
- PLMD is diagnosed on the basis of the above clinical history plus the recorded evidence of periodic limb movements in sleep (PLMS). There are brief (0.5 to 9 seconds in duration) dystonic leg movements (dorsiflexion of the foot and extension of the great toe). There must be four consecutive movements separated by at least four but not more than 90 seconds to define an episode. Most episodes will have a regular rhythm (15-20 seconds) and last for several minutes. Evidence of sleep disturbance may be in the form of delayed sleep onset, fragmented sleep stages, absence of expected delta sleep stages or K-complexes associated with EMG or other EEG signs of arousal. A diagnosis of RLS excludes PLMD whereas a diagnosis of RLS includes PLMD.

System(s) affected: Musculoskeletal, Nervous

Genetics:
- RLS: 3-5 times greater prevalence among first degree relatives of RLS patients than in people without RLS

Incidence/Prevalence in USA:
- Common sleep disorder

Predominant age:
- PLMS
  - ◊ Occurs commonly in the elderly (less commonly in children), in patients with other sleep disorders (narcolepsy, obstructive sleep apnea), and end-stage renal disease
  - ◊ Present in 85% of patients with RLS
- RLS
  - ◊ Elderly; rare in children; there is a bimodal distribution
  - ◊ Onset before age 50 results in a more insidious onset with more affected first degree relatives
  - ◊ Onset after age 50 is associated with more abrupt and more severe symptoms

Predominant sex: N/A

SIGNS & SYMPTOMS
- RLS - inability to tolerate immobility or leg confinement on trips in cars, airplanes, etc.
- PLMS - may present as insomnia of either inability to initiate or sustain sleep

CAUSES
- RLS - primarily idiopathic, secondary iron deficiency
- PLMS - primarily idiopathic, secondary causes (RLS, REM behavior disorder, narcolepsy, uremia, synucleinopathies [Parkinson disease, multiple system atrophy, diffuse Lewy body disease])

RISK FACTORS
- Chemical agents
  - ◊ Caffeine may aggravate
  - ◊ Antidepressants may induce or aggravate PLMS and RLS (trazodone, bupropion [Wellbutrin] and nefazodone are exceptions)
  - ◊ Dopamine antagonists that cross the blood-brain barrier (most antipsychotics), metoclopramide, calcium channel blockers, theophylline, and adrenergics are among those agents reported to aggravate symptoms
  - ◊ Withdrawal from sedatives/narcotics can augment symptoms
- Diseases
  - ◊ Primary neurological disorders should be considered. Among most common are peripheral neuropathies, radiculopathies, neurodegenerative disease, or, another movement disorder such as Parkinson disease. A higher incidence occurs in association with narcolepsy and sleep apnea.
  - ◊ Metabolic disorders
    - A much higher incidence of PLMS/RLS has been reported in diabetes
    - Electrolyte deficiencies which may involve K, Ca, or Mg. (low normal values may indicate a low tissue level)
    - Anemia (low tissue iron or low serum ferritin)
    - Uremic/renal failure patients will have a high percentage of PLMS/RLS symptoms

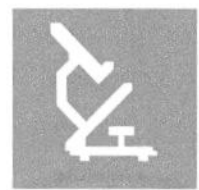

DIAGNOSIS

DIFFERENTIAL DIAGNOSIS
- RLS
  - ◊ Akathisia produced by dopamine receptor blockers
  - ◊ Painful legs and moving toes, usually caused by direct trauma
  - ◊ Fasciculations from upper motor neuron disease
  - ◊ Leg cramps
- PLMS
  - ◊ Sleep jerks or hypnic jerks are normal and occur more frequently in sleep deprived individuals
  - ◊ Myoclonic epilepsy disappears in sleep

LABORATORY
- Fasting glucose
- Electrolytes Na, K, Ca, Mg
- Ferritin
- B12, folate levels
- BUN, creatinine

Drugs that may alter lab results: N/A

Disorders that may alter lab results: N/A

PATHOLOGICAL FINDINGS N/A

SPECIAL TESTS
- RLS - none; actigraphy can be helpful in measuring severity
- PLMS - nocturnal polysomnography (NPSG)

IMAGING N/A

DIAGNOSTIC PROCEDURES
- RLS is diagnosed by history alone, though excessive leg movements will be seen with nocturnal polysomnography
- PLMS: affected individuals are often unaware and diagnosis by NPSG is appropriate

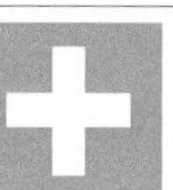

TREATMENT

APPROPRIATE HEALTH CARE Outpatient

GENERAL MEASURES
- RLS and PLMD - essentially the same measures are effective. All the dopaminergic drugs work to some degree.
- Eliminate aggravating factors
  - ◊ Good sleep hygiene (adequate and regular time in bed)
  - ◊ Avoid CNS stimulants (caffeine, chocolate, tea, etc.)
  - ◊ Avoid dopamine antagonists
  - ◊ Avoid antidepressants (nefazodone [Serzone], trazodone and bupropion [Wellbutrin]) are best used)
  - ◊ Exercise before 7 pm
  - ◊ Ferrous sulfate if ferritin is < 50 mcg/mL

SURGICAL MEASURES N/A

ACTIVITY
- Regular mild to moderate exercise

DIET N/A

PATIENT EDUCATION
- The Restless Legs Syndrome Foundation Inc. publishes the "Nightwalkers Newsletter" and provides useful information and identifies support groups. Address is 819 2nd St, SW, Rochester MN 55902-9872; 800-757-7563; http://www.rls.org; fax 507-287-6312; e-mail rlsfoundation@rls.org
- National Sleep Foundation, 1522 K St NW, Suite 500, Washington, DC 20005-1253
- Sleep Thief by Virginia Wilson is recommended reading. Contact Galaxy Books Inc., P.O. Box 1421 Orange Park FL 32067

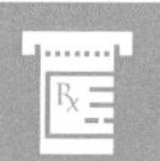

MEDICATIONS

DRUG(S) OF CHOICE
Three major classes of drugs are used:
- Dopaminergic agonists are the treatment of choice.
- Moderate to severe cases
  - ◊ Pramipexole (Mirapex) - start at 0.125 mg and increase by 0.125 mg steps every 2-3 days until symptoms are controlled. Reassess at 0.5 mg. Take 1-2 hours before symptoms occur.
  - ◊ Ropinirole (Requip) - same treatment protocol but start at 0.25 mg and reassess at 1.0 mg
  - ◊ Carbidopa-levodopa (Sinemet) - mild or intermittent symptoms. Use PRN. Stop if symptoms worsen (augmentation)
- Severe cases
  - ◊ Increase dose of pramipexole or ropinirole
  - ◊ Consider opioids
- Benzodiazepines do not suppress movements in most patients but allow greater sleep continuity.
  - ◊ Clonazepam 0.5-2.0 mg, but temazepam, diazepam and shorter acting benzodiazepines may be effective
- Opiates and synthetic narcotics actually reduce the number of movements and are the drugs of choice after failure or intolerance to dopaminergic agents
  - ◊ Hydrocodone 5 mg before hs can be quite effective. Propoxyphene, codeine, oxycodone, pentazocine, methadone are effective in equivalent doses.

Contraindications: Refer to manufacturer's literature
Precautions: Refer to manufacturer's literature
Significant possible interactions: Refer to manufacturer's literature

ALTERNATIVE DRUGS
- Agents reported to be effective in selected individuals or subgroups include:
  - ◊ Mineral supplements (when indicated)
  - ◊ Quinine - circulatory
  - ◊ Carbamazepine, valproic acid (Depakote), gabapentin, propranolol, clonidine - uremia
  - ◊ Baclofen - motor neuron disease
  - ◊ Gamma-hydroxybutyrate, 5-hydroxytryptophan, vitamin B12 and folate - anemia
  - ◊ Paradoxically, tricyclics - painful neuropathy

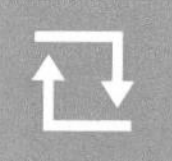

FOLLOWUP

PATIENT MONITORING
- Visits at 2 week intervals until stable; then at 6-12 months
- Iron levels should be checked after several weeks if supplemental iron is recommended to be certain that hemochromatosis is not induced

PREVENTION/AVOIDANCE N/A

POSSIBLE COMPLICATIONS
- Tolerance may develop to medications after months to years and necessitate change to another agent
- Augmentation of RLS into daytime symptoms may develop particularly with use of carbidopa/levodopa in which case it should be reduced while adding another agent in increments
- Side effects may occur with any medication and are usually dose related
- Electrolyte and iron supplementation in excess can have serious consequences

EXPECTED COURSE/PROGNOSIS
- Periods of spontaneous remission may occur
- RLS and PLMS tend to worsen with age

MISCELLANEOUS

ASSOCIATED CONDITIONS
- Sleep deprivation

AGE-RELATED FACTORS
Pediatric: RLS may be misdiagnosed as growing pains or ADHD in younger patients
Geriatric: Increased incidence in geriatric patients
Others: RLS/PLMS may occur at any age but usually after age 30.

PREGNANCY
PLMS often occur during pregnancy and resolve afterward.

SYNONYMS N/A

ICD-9-CM
333.99 Other and unspecified extrapyramidal diseases and abnormal movement disorders, other

SEE ALSO

OTHER NOTES
Extremely rare, RLS symptoms in the torso or arms have been reported

ABBREVIATIONS
RLS = restless leg syndrome
PLMS = periodic limb movement disorder
NPSG = nocturnal polysomnography

REFERENCES

- Allen RP, Earley CJ. Defining the phenotype of the restless legs syndrome using age-of-symptom-onset. Sleep Med 2000; 1(1):11-19
- Allen RP. Advances in diagnosis and treatment of the restless legs syndrome and periodic limb movements in sleep. 1997, 11th Annual Associated Professional Sleep Societies Meeting
- Chesson Al Jr, Wise M, Davila D, et al. Practice parameters for the treatment of restless legs syndrome and periodic limb movement disorder. Sleep 1999;22(7):961-6
- Kryger MH, Roth T, Dement W. Principles and Practice of Sleep Medicine, 2nd ed. Philadelphia: W. B. Saunders Co; 1994
- Lin SC, Kaplan J. Burger CD, Fredrickson PA. Effect of pramipexole in treatment of resistant restless legs syndrome. Mayo Clinic Proceedings 1998;73:497-500
- Hening W, Allen R, et al. The treatment of restless legs syndrome and periodic limb movement disorder. Sleep 1999;22(7):970-82
- Wilson VN. Sleep Thief; Restless Legs Syndrome. Orange Park, FL: Galaxy Books, Inc, 1996
- AAmerican Sleep Disorders Association. The international classification of sleep disorders, revised: diagnostic and coding manual. Rochester, MN: American Sleep Disorders Association; 1997
- Restless Legs Syndrome: Detection and management in primary care. National Heart, Lung, and Blood Institute Working Group on Restless Legs Syndrome. Am Fam Physician 2000;62:108-14

Web references: 2 available at www.5mcc.com
Illustrations N/A

Author(s):
Edgar A. Lucas, PhD
John R. Burk, MD
Kristyna Hartse, PhD
Sandra Knaur, MSN

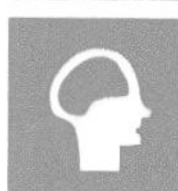

BASICS

DESCRIPTION Excess physical or psychologic agitation often associated with specific physical abnormalities or existential conflict. When associated with pre-terminal events, sometimes called terminal restlessness.
System(s) affected: Nervous
Genetics: N/A
Incidence/Prevalence in USA: N/A
Predominant age: N/A
Predominant sex: Male=Female

SIGNS & SYMPTOMS
- Sleep disturbances
- Inability to concentrate
- Non-purposeful motor activity
- Inability to relax
- Some clinicians include: delirium (a change in level of consciousness)

CAUSES
- Delirium
  - ◊ Medications (especially polypharmacy, and also steroids, narcotics, anticholinergics)
  - ◊ Sensory deprivation (e.g., ICU psychosis)
  - ◊ Alzheimer disease
  - ◊ AIDS (57% have delirium at the time of death)
  - ◊ Brain tumor; primary or metastatic
  - ◊ Endocrinopathies (thyroid, adrenal dysfunction)
  - ◊ Electrolyte imbalance
  - ◊ Hepatic encephalopathy
  - ◊ Korsakoff syndrome
  - ◊ Neurosyphilis and other CNS infections
  - ◊ Nutritional deficiency
- Myoclonus
  - ◊ High dose morphine
  - ◊ Prolonged meperidine use
  - ◊ Lowered seizure threshold (metoclopramide, phenothiazines, haloperidol, antihistamines, TCAs, anticholinergics, hypoxia, dehydration, electrolyte abnormalities)
- Extrapyramidal symptoms (EPS)
  - ◊ Phenothiazines
  - ◊ Haloperidol
  - ◊ Metoclopramide
- Hypoxia
- Inadequately treated pain, especially in the non-verbal patient
- Anxiety
- Pruritus
- Urinary or fecal retention
- Medication/drugs effects
  - ◊ Benzodiazepine withdrawal
  - ◊ Corticosteroids
  - ◊ Cocaine
  - ◊ Alcohol
  - ◊ Narcotics
- Existential issues
  - ◊ Unresolved existential issues
  - ◊ Death anxiety
    - Past-related regret (unfulfilled aspirations; low self-esteem)
    - Future-related regret (anticipation of failure to achieve important goals)
    - Meaningfulness of death (fear of unknown; concept of death)

RISK FACTORS N/A

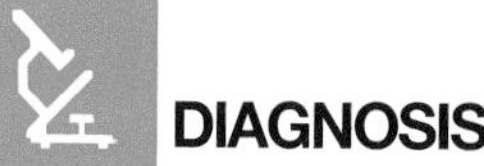

DIAGNOSIS

DIFFERENTIAL DIAGNOSIS
N/A

LABORATORY
- Electrolytes, calcium, glucose, oxygen (hyponatremia, hypercalcemia, hypoglycemia, oximetry)
- VDRL, TSH, HIV, LFTs, drug screen if cause of restlessness not obvious

Drugs that may alter lab results: N/A

Disorders that may alter lab results: N/A

PATHOLOGICAL FINDINGS N/A

SPECIAL TESTS
- Restlessness Scale (to be completed by patient, family, and/or staff)
  - ◊ 0 - no restlessness
  - ◊ 1 - mild agitation
  - ◊ 2 - moderate agitation
  - ◊ 3 - severe agitation without delirium
  - ◊ 4 - moderate agitation with delirium
  - ◊ 5 - severe agitation with delirium
- Mini Mental Status Exam (MMSE)
- Delirium Rating Scale
- Review unfinished spiritual and/or interpersonal conflicts
- Pain assessment

IMAGING
- MRI/CT of brain

DIAGNOSTIC PROCEDURES
- Physical exam
  - ◊ Rectal exam for fecal impaction
  - ◊ Abdominal exam and/or bladder catheterization for urinary retention

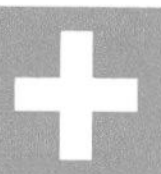

TREATMENT

APPROPRIATE HEALTH CARE
Terminal restlessness is best cared for in a quite, supportive environment, often in the patient's home. Hospice team care is often helpful.

GENERAL MEASURES
- Treatment goals
  - ◊ Identify and address physical and/or existential issues to reduce restlessness
  - ◊ Support family members and caregivers in dealing with restlessness, especially terminal restlessness
- Eliminate unnecessary medications
  - ◊ CNS stimulants (e.g., albuterol, theophylline)
  - ◊ Anticholinergics (scopolamine, tricyclic antidepressants)
- Physical modalities
  - ◊ Limit extraneous stimuli including loud noises and bright lights
  - ◊ Teach rhythmic breathing and relaxation techniques
  - ◊ Provide a quiet, well-lit room with familiar objects (pictures of family or friends, keepsakes, etc.)
- Psychosocial modalities
  - ◊ Frequent re-orientation to person, place, and time
  - ◊ Supportive listening
  - ◊ Guided imagery
  - ◊ Music therapy
  - ◊ Massage; gentle touch
  - ◊ Recognize caregiver fatigue and provide appropriate respite care
- Spiritual modalities
  - ◊ Provide for clergy visits for prayer or exploration of spiritual and other existential issues
    - Spiritual assessment
    - Patient and family counsel
    - Offer prayer for existential resolution (e.g., Sinner's Prayer for Christians, confession, etc.)
    - Preparation for death (Last Rites for Catholics, etc.)

SURGICAL MEASURES N/A

ACTIVITY
- Rarely, physical restraint or 24 hour bedside assistance is needed
- Indwelling urinary bladder catheter, for persistent urinary retention

DIET
- Avoid caffeine and other CNS stimulants

PATIENT EDUCATION
- Education of family and patient regarding the events surrounding the terminal patient, prior to terminal events, may reduce the severity of restlessness

MEDICATIONS

DRUG(S) OF CHOICE
- Antipsychotics
  ◊ Haloperidol (Haldol) 0.5-5mg q6-12h po, pr, IM, or SC
  ◊ Risperidone (Risperdal) 1 mg BID po
- Narcotics for pain control as needed
  ◊ Hydrocodone
  ◊ Morphine
- Oxygen, when hypoxia is present

Contraindications: N/A

Precautions:
- Use caution when combining CNS-acting drugs
- Barbiturates increase benzodiazepine levels
- Antipsychotics may induce EPS which may be mistaken for primary restlessness. Treat EPS with benztropine (Cogentin) 1-4mg BID, if the antipsychotics are relieving disturbing hallucinations or other symptoms causing restlessness.
- Risperidone may be associated with hyperglycemia and ketoacidosis

Significant possible interactions: N/A

ALTERNATIVE DRUGS
- Benzodiazepines: induce quiet sedation, but do not improve cognition or sensorium
  ◊ Lorazepam (Ativan) 1-2mg q4h po, pr, or IV
  ◊ Midazolam (Versed) .25-3mg/hour via SC infusion
- Beta blockers reduce physical manifestations of autonomic hyperactivity
  ◊ Atenolol (Tenormin) 25-50 mg/day
- Methotrimeprazine (Levoprome) 12.5-50mg q4-8h is more sedating than haloperidol (oral not available in the U.S.)
- Barbiturates in sedative or hypnotic doses may be helpful, but have a low safety margin, especially when used with narcotics.
  ◊ Pentobarbital (Nembutal) 100mg IM or pr

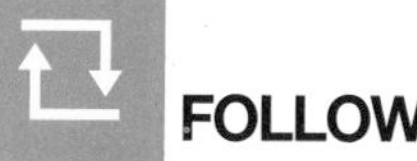

FOLLOWUP

PATIENT MONITORING
- Regular assessment and re-evaluation of the causes of restlessness

PREVENTION/AVOIDANCE
See General Measures and Patient Education sections

POSSIBLE COMPLICATIONS N/A

EXPECTED COURSE/PROGNOSIS
- Terminal restlessness, by definition, is a pre-terminal event
- Causes other than the pre-terminal condition will determine the response to therapy and course

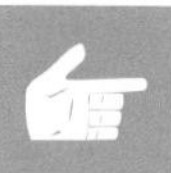

MISCELLANEOUS

ASSOCIATED CONDITIONS
- Depression
- Dementia
- Terminal anguish (suspect this as a cause of restlessness in patients without cognitive failure, hallucinations, or delusions)

AGE-RELATED FACTORS
Pediatric:
- Pain, psychologic, and existential issues may be more difficult to assess in this age group

Geriatric:
- EPS more frequent in this group
- Anticholinergic effects (dry mouth, urinary retention, delirium, etc.) may be troublesome

Others: N/A

PREGNANCY N/A

SYNONYMS N/A

ICD-9-CM
799.2 Nervousness

SEE ALSO
Anxiety
Delirium

OTHER NOTES N/A

ABBREVIATIONS
EPS = extrapyramidal symptoms
TCA = tricyclic antidepressant

REFERENCES

- Kuebler KK. The Hospice and Palliative Care Clinical Practice Protocols: Terminal Restless, Hospice and Palliative Nurses Association (APNA), 1997
- Doyle D, Hanks GWC, MacDonald N editors. Oxford Textbook of Palliative Medicine, 2nd edition, Oxford University Press, 1998
- Trzepacz PT, Baker RW, Greenhouse J. A symptom rating scale for delirium. Psychological Research, 1988; 23:89-97
- Tomer A, Eliason G. Toward a Comprehensive Model of Death Anxiety, Death Studies (20), 343-365, 1996
- Johanson GA. Physician's Handbook of Symptom Relief in Terminal Care, 4th ed, 1994

Web references: 0 available at www.5mcc.com
Illustrations N/A

Author(s):
Mark R. Dambro, MD

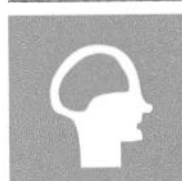

BASICS

DESCRIPTION Separation of the sensory retina from the underlying retinal pigment epithelium.
- Rhegmatogenous retinal detachment (RRD): Is the most common type. It occurs when the fluid vitreous gains access to the subretinal space through a break in the retina (Greek rhegma, rent).
- Exudative or serous detachment: Occurs in the absence of a retinal break, usually in association with inflammation or a tumor.
- Traction detachment: Vitreoretinal adhesions mechanically pull the retina from the retinal pigment epithelium. The most common cause is proliferative diabetic retinopathy.

System(s) affected: Nervous
Genetics: Most cases are sporadic
Incidence/Prevalence in USA:
- 1/10,000 per year in patients who have not had cataract surgery
- 1-3% of patients after cataract surgery will develop a retinal detachment

Predominant age: The incidence increases with age.
Predominant sex: Male > Female (3:2)

SIGNS & SYMPTOMS
- Flashes (photopsia)
- Floaters
- Visual field loss
- Pigmented cells within the vitreous "tobacco dust"
- Central vision will be preserved if the macula is not detached
- Poor visual acuity (20/200 or worse) with loss of central vision when macula is detached.
- Elevation of retina associated with one or more retinal tears in RRD or elevation of the retina without tears in exudative detachment
- In 3-10% of patients with presumed RRD, no definite retinal break is found
- Tenting of the retina without retinal tears in traction detachment

CAUSES
- Traction from a posterior vitreous detachment (PVD) causes most retinal tears. With aging, vitreous gel liquefies leading to the separation of the vitreous from the retina. The vitreous gel remains attached at the vitreous base, in the retinal periphery, resulting in vitreous traction producing tears in the retinal periphery.
- PVD associated with vitreous hemorrhage has a high incidence of retinal tears
- Exudative detachment:
  - ◊ Tumors
  - ◊ Inflammatory diseases (Harada's, posterior scleritis)
  - ◊ Miscellaneous (central serous retinopathy, uveal effusion, malignant hypertension)
- Traction detachment:
  - ◊ Proliferative diabetic retinopathy
  - ◊ Cicatricial retinopathy of prematurity
  - ◊ Proliferative sickle cell retinopathy
  - ◊ Penetrating trauma

RISK FACTORS
- Myopia (greater than 5 diopters)
- Aphakia or pseudophakia
- PVD and associated conditions (aphakia, inflammatory disease and trauma)
- Trauma
- Retinal detachment in fellow eye
- Lattice degeneration. Lattice degeneration is a vitreoretinal abnormality found in 6-10% of the general population
- Glaucoma. 4-7% of patients with retinal detachment have chronic open angle glaucoma
- Vitreoretinal tufts. Peripheral retinal tufts are caused by focal areas of vitreous traction.
- Meridional folds. Redundant retina usually found in the supranasal quadrant

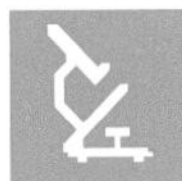

DIAGNOSIS

DIFFERENTIAL DIAGNOSIS Retinoschisis (splitting of the retina). Vitreous cell or vitreous hemorrhage are rarely found in the vitreous with retinoschisis, whereas they are commonly seen in RRD. Retinoschisis usually has a smooth surface and is dome shaped; whereas, RRD often has a corrugated, irregular surface.

LABORATORY N/A

Drugs that may alter lab results: N/A

Disorders that may alter lab results: N/A

PATHOLOGICAL FINDINGS Elevation of the neurosensory retina from the underlying retinal pigment epithelium.

SPECIAL TESTS
- Visual field testing. Differentiate between a RRD and retinoschisis. An absolute scotoma is seen in retinoschisis whereas a RRD causes a relative scotoma.
- Ultrasonography can demonstrate a detached retina and may be helpful when the retina can not be visualized directly (cataracts, etc).

IMAGING Fluorescein dye leakage can be seen in exudative retinal detachment caused by central serous retinopathy and other inflammatory conditions

DIAGNOSTIC PROCEDURES
- Slit lamp examination
- Dilated fundus examination with binocular indirect ophthalmoscopy

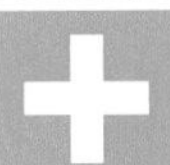

TREATMENT

APPROPRIATE HEALTH CARE Referral to an ophthalmologist for examination and treatment, if indicated

GENERAL MEASURES
- Not all retinal tears or breaks need to be treated. Flap tears or horseshoe tears in symptomatic patients (that is patients with flashes or floaters) frequently are treated. Operculated holes in symptomatic patients are sometimes treated. Atrophic holes in symptomatic patients are rarely treated.
- Lattice degeneration with or without holes within the lattice in an asymptomatic patient with prior retinal detachment in the fellow eye may be prophylactically treated.
- Flap retinal tears in asymptomatic patients are frequently treated prophylactically
- Exudative detachments are usually managed by treatment of the underlying disorder
- Traction detachments usually managed by observation. If the fovea is involved, then a vitrectomy is needed

SURGICAL MEASURES
- Timing of repairs
  - ◊ Macula attached: within 24 hours. If the detachment is peripheral and does not have features suggestive for rapid progression (such as large and/or superior tears) then repair can be performed within a few days.
  - ◊ Macula recently detached: within 10 days of development of a macula-off retinal detachment
  - ◊ Old macular detachment: elective repair within 2 weeks
- If a retinal break has lead to the development of a retinal detachment, then surgery will be needed. Surgical options (and combinations) include:
  - ◊ Demarcation laser treatment.
  - ◊ Pneumatic retinopexy. Head positioning is required postoperatively.
  - ◊ Scleral buckle.
  - ◊ Vitrectomy.
  - ◊ Perfluorocarbon liquids for giant tears (circumferential tears 90° or larger)
  - ◊ Silicone oil for complex repairs
- Anesthesia. Usually with local anesthesia.
- RRD may have more than one break. If any retinal break is not closed at the time of surgery, the surgery will fail.
- Additional surgery may be required if the retina redetaches secondary to a new retinal break or due to proliferative vitreoretinopathy (PVR).

ACTIVITY Bedrest prior to surgery. Postoperatively, if an intraocular gas has been used, the patient may need specific head positioning and should not travel to high altitudes.

DIET NPO if surgery is imminent

PATIENT EDUCATION American Academy of Ophthalmology, 655 E. Beach Street, San Francisco, California 94109-1336

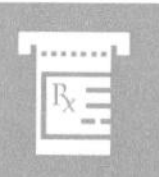

MEDICATIONS

DRUG(S) OF CHOICE
- Intraocular gases
  - ◊ Air
  - ◊ Perfluoropropane (C3F8)
  - ◊ Sulfur hexafluoride (SF6)
- Perfluorocarbon liquids
- Silicone oil

Contraindications: Patients with poorly controlled glaucoma.

Precautions: Expanding intraocular gas bubble increases intraocular pressure, therefore, avoid higher altitudes

Significant possible interactions: Nitrous oxide used in general anesthesia can expand an intraocular gas bubble

ALTERNATIVE DRUGS Steroids can cause worsening of central serous retinopathy

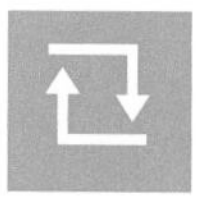

FOLLOWUP

PATIENT MONITORING
- Alert ophthalmologist immediately:
  - ◊ Symptoms of PVD and detachment (new onset of floaters or flashes, increase in floaters or flashes, sudden shower of floaters, curtain or shadow in the peripheral visual field, or reduced vision)
- Patients with an acute symptomatic PVD associated with mild vitreous hemorrhage should be reexamined in 3-4 weeks by the ophthalmologist. The development of a retinal detachment is unlikely if no retinal tears are present on reexamination in 3-4 weeks.
- A patient with an acute symptomatic PVD, even in the absence of vitreous hemorrhage, vitreous pigment or detectable retinal break, may need to be reexamined in 3-4 weeks by the ophthalmologist, depending on clinical circumstances such as aphakia or myopia, because retinal breaks may develop over time.
- If an acute symptomatic PVD is associated with gross vitreous hemorrhage which interferes with complete visualization of the retinal periphery by indirect ophthalmoscopy, then a patient should be reexamined at short intervals with indirect ophthalmoscopy until the entire retinal periphery can be observed.
- If the examiner is not certain that the retina is detached in the presence of opaque media, ultrasonography should be performed

PREVENTION/AVOIDANCE
- Patients at risk for a retinal detachment should have regular ophthalmologic examination

POSSIBLE COMPLICATIONS
- PVR is the most common cause of failed retinal detachment repair. 10-15% of patients, whose retinas reattach initially after retinal surgery, will subsequently re-detach; usually within 6 weeks due to cellular proliferation and contraction on the retinal surface.
- Partial or total loss of vision due to macular detachment and/or PVR
- Moderate to severe forms of PVR are usually treated with pars plana vitrectomy and fluid-gas exchange. If a segmental scleral buckle was placed at the initial procedure, then this will need to be revised.
- Scleral buckles may erode the overlying conjunctiva and lead to an infection

EXPECTED COURSE/PROGNOSIS
- RRD:
  - ◊ 90% of retinal detachments can be reattached successfully after one or more surgical procedures. Postoperative visual acuity depends primarily on the status of the macula preoperatively. Also important is the length of time between the detachment and the repair (75% of macular detachments of less than one week will obtain a final visual acuity of 20/70 or better).
  - ◊ 87% of eyes with a retinal detachment not involving the macula attain a visual acuity of 20/50 or better postoperatively. 37% of eyes with a detached macula preoperatively attain 20/50 or better vision postoperatively.
  - ◊ In 10-15% of successfully repaired retinal detachments not involving the macula preoperatively, visual acuity does not return to the preoperative level. This decrease is secondary to complications such as macular edema or macular pucker.
- Tractional retinal detachment:
  - ◊ When not involving the fovea, the patient can usually be observed since it is uncommon for these to extend into the fovea.
- Exudative retinal detachment:
  - ◊ Management is usually nonsurgical
  - ◊ The presence of shifting fluid is highly suggestive of an exudative retinal detachment. Fixed retinal folds which are indicative of PVR are rarely seen in exudative retinal detachment. If the underlying condition is treated the prognosis is generally good.

MISCELLANEOUS

ASSOCIATED CONDITIONS
- Lattice degeneration
- High myopia
- Cataract surgery
- Glaucoma
- History of retinal detachment in the fellow eye
- Trauma

AGE-RELATED FACTORS
Pediatric: Usually associated with underlying vitreoretinal disorders and/or retinopathy of prematurity

Geriatric:
- Posterior vitreous detachment
- Cataract surgery

Others: N/A

PREGNANCY Pre-eclampsia/eclampsia may be associated with exudative retinal detachment. No intervention is indicated, provided hypertension is controlled, prognosis is usually good.

SYNONYMS N/A

ICD-9-CM
361.00 Retinal detachment with retinal defect, unspecified
379.21 Vitreous degeneration
361.2 Serous retinal detachment
361.81 Traction detachment of retina
362.63 Lattice degeneration of retina
361.30 Retinal defect, unspecified

SEE ALSO
Retinopathy, diabetic

OTHER NOTES N/A

ABBREVIATIONS
RRD = rhegmatogenous retinal detachment
PVD = posterior vitreous detachment
PVR = proliferative vitreoretinopathy

REFERENCES

- Tani P, Robertson, DM, Langworthy A: Prognosis for Central Vision and Anatomic Reattachment in Rhegmatogenous Retinal Detachment with Macula Detached. Am J Ophthalmol 1981;92:611-620
- The American Academy of Ophthalmol. Ophthalmic Procedure Assessment: The Repair of Rhegmatogenous Retinal Detachments. Ophthalmology 1996;103:1313-1324
- The American Academy of Ophthalmol. Preferred Practice Pattern: Retinal Detachment 1990: 1-17
- The American Academy of Ophthalmol: Preferred Practice Pattern: Management of Posterior Vitreous Detachment, Retinal Breaks, and Lattice Degeneration 1998:1-24
- Regillo CD, Benson WE: Retinal Detachment Diagnosis and Management. 3rd ed. Philadelphia, J.B. Lippincott Co., 1998
- Vitrectomy with Silicone Oil or Perfluoropropane Gas in Eyes with Severe Proliferative Vitreoretinopathy: Results of a Randomized Clinical Trial. Silicone Study Report 2. Arch Ophthalmol 1992;110:780-792
- Hassan TS, Sarrafizadeh R, Ruby AJ, et al. The effect of duration of macular detachment on results after the scleral buckle repair of primary, macula-off retinal detachments. Ophthalmology 2002;109: 146-152
- Vrabec TR, Baumal CR. Demarcation laser photocoagulation of selected macula-sparing rhegmatogenous retinal detachments. Ophthalmol 2000;107(6):1063-7

Web references: 0 available at www.5mcc.com
Illustrations 7 available

Author(s):
Richard W. Allinson, MD

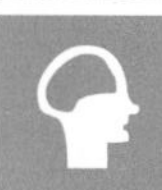

BASICS

DESCRIPTION Retinitis pigmentosa is characterized by poor night vision, constricted visual fields, bone spicule-like pigmentation of the fundus, and electroretinographic evidence of photoreceptor cell dysfunction.

System(s) affected: Nervous

Genetics:
- Autosomal dominant - 20%
- Autosomal recessive - 37%
- X-linked recessive - 4.5%
- Sporadic - 38.5%

Incidence/Prevalence in USA: RP affects approximately 1 in 4,000 people in the US

Predominant age:
- X-linked RP has the earliest onset of the major hereditary types and many X-linked patients are legally blind by age 30
- Autosomal dominant RP has a later onset than autosomal recessive or X-linked recessive RP
- Leber congenital amaurosis which is a variant of RP presents at birth
- Late onset RP typically is asymptomatic and unrecognized until age 40 or 50

Predominant sex: Male > female

SIGNS & SYMPTOMS
- Headache and light flashes are the most common initial complaints
- Night blindness (nyctalopia)
- Bone spicule pigmentation in the retina
- Retinal arteriolar narrowing
- Optic nerve head pallor, "waxy pallor"
- Progressive visual field loss
- Central visual acuity is usually preserved until the end stages of retinitis pigmentosa
- Most patients are myopic
- Posterior subcapsular cataracts are common in all forms of retinitis pigmentosa
- Cystoid macular edema
- Optic nerve head drusen
- Electroretinogram (ERG) changes
- Retinal neovascularization
- RP associated with an exudative retinal vasculopathy. Fundus findings would include serous retinal detachment, lipid deposition in the retina and telangiectatic vascular anomalies.
- Variants of RP exists with unusual or regional distribution including:
- Sectorial RP
- Pigmented paravenous atrophy
- Unilateral RP

CAUSES
- The genetic mutations responsible for RP have been identified in some families with RP, primarily those with the autosomal dominant form
- Mutations in the rhodopsin gene account for about 30% of cases with autosomal dominant RP
- Another 4-6% of autosomal dominant RP is due to a mutation in the gene for a photoreceptor protein, peripherin/RDS

RISK FACTORS Family history

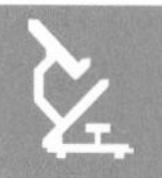

DIAGNOSIS

DIFFERENTIAL DIAGNOSIS
Bone spicule-like retinal pigmentation and retinal atrophy are nonspecific findings and can result from conditions other than retinitis pigmentosa
- Infections
- Syphilis
- Rubella
- Inflammation (severe uveitis)
- Choroidal vascular occlusion
- Toxicity (chloroquine or thioridazine)
- Choroideremia
- Gyrate atrophy of choroid and retina (10 to 20 fold elevation of plasma ornithine levels)
- Systemic metabolic disorders such as Refsum disease and abetalipoproteinemia
- Kearns-Sayre syndrome. Usually presents in adolescents. It is characterized by progressive external ophthalmoplegia, the first sign usually being ptosis, pigmentary degeneration of the retina and a cardiac conduction defect which may cause complete heart block.
- Cone-rod dystrophy. Characterized by bilateral and symmetric loss of cone function in the presence of reduced rod function.
- Cone dystrophy characterized by marked abnormality in cone function with some or no rod involvement.
- Congenital stationary night blindness
- Oguchi disease
- Fundus albipunctatus
- Trauma

LABORATORY
- Elevated plasma levels of phytanic acid in Refsum disease
- Acanthocytosis of red blood cells in peripheral blood smear in abetalipoproteinemia. This is an autosomal recessive disorder in which abetalipoprotein B is not synthesized, leading to fat malabsorption and deficiencies of fat soluble vitamins. Therapy with vitamin A and E can improve retinal function.
- Syphilitic neuroretinitis can be diagnosed by performing a FTA-ABS or MHA-Tp
- Elevated plasma ornithine levels in gyrate atrophy of the choroid and retina. Usually a 10-20 fold elevation of plasma ornithine levels.

Drugs that may alter lab results: N/A

Disorders that may alter lab results: N/A

PATHOLOGICAL FINDINGS
- Disappearance of the rods, cones and outer nuclear layers in the retina.
- Bone spicule formation in the retina is secondary to the migration of retinal pigment epithelial cells into the overlying retina

SPECIAL TESTS
- Electroretinography (ERG). Photoreceptors generate reduced amplitude a- and b-waves in RP. Rod and cone responses may be undetectable in advanced RP.
- Visual field testing. A ring scotoma in the mid periphery may be identified. The ring scotoma generally starts as a group of isolated scotomas in the area 20-25° from fixation. Long after the entire peripheral field is gone, there remains a small island of intact central visual field.
- Fluorescein angiography can demonstrate cystoid macular edema.
- Fundus photography to document the status of the retina.
- Hearing tests in patients complaining of hearing loss such as patients with Usher syndrome (RP with hearing loss).

IMAGING N/A

DIAGNOSTIC PROCEDURES N/A

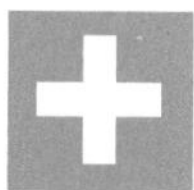

TREATMENT

APPROPRIATE HEALTH CARE Outpatient

GENERAL MEASURES
- Supportive
- Genetic counseling
- Low vision aids
- Educating the patient

SURGICAL MEASURES
- The efficacy of the "Cuban" therapy, which is electric stimulation, autotransfused ozonized blood, and ocular surgery has not been proven to be of benefit
- Macular grid laser photocoagulation may be of benefit for patients with cystoid macular edema secondary to RP
- Research is being done on photoreceptor transplantation, gene therapy, and implantation of a visual prosthesis. The inner retinal neurons may be preserved after death of photoreceptors in RP, which could make some of these experimental procedures feasible one day.

ACTIVITY Full activity. Caution should be exercised because of the reduced peripheral vision and poor night vision.

DIET No special diet

PATIENT EDUCATION
- Counsel patients to help them understand RP and its genetics
- RP is a slowly progressive, chronic disease; patients do not go blind rapidly and total blindness is not a frequent end-point of this disease
- RP Foundation Fighting Blindness, Executive Plaza One, Suite 800, 11350 McCormick Road, Hunt Valley, MD 21031-1014, (800)683-5555
- The American Academy of Ophthalmology, 655 E. Beach Street, San Francisco, CA 94109-1336, (415)561-8540

MEDICATIONS

DRUG(S) OF CHOICE
- Vitamin A 15,000 IU q day (retinal degeneration slowed as measured by ERG/visual fields). [Note: beta-carotene not a suitable substitute; not studied in patients under age 18]
- Vitamin E 400 IU q day results in faster retinal degeneration and is not recommended
- Acetazolamide may be of benefit in the treatment of cystoid macular edema which may occur in RP. 500 mg/day in a sustained release capsule was found to be more effective than 250 mg/day.

Contraindications: Women who are pregnant or considering pregnancy should not take more than 8,000 IU of vitamin A per day. There is an increased incidence of birth defects in babies born to women who ingest higher dosages of vitamin A during pregnancy. Women should consult their obstetrician.
Precautions: Avoid vitamin A supplement dosages >15,000 IU per day as higher dosages can cause liver damage
Significant possible interactions: N/A

ALTERNATIVE DRUGS N/A

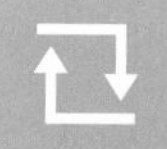

FOLLOWUP

PATIENT MONITORING
- Ophthalmic examinations every 1-2 years
- Check for complications (cataracts, etc.)

PREVENTION/AVOIDANCE
- Genetic counseling
- There is no conclusive evidence that demonstrates that the amount of light modifies the course of RP. A study in which one eye was covered with an opaque lens did not show any difference in disease progression compared to the fellow eye.
- Ultraviolet-absorbing sunglasses and brimmed hats are recommended when patients are at the beach or in the snow.

POSSIBLE COMPLICATIONS
- Cataract
- Cystoid macular edema
- Loss of visual field
- Poor night vision
- Blindness

EXPECTED COURSE/PROGNOSIS
- Reassurance about the slow course of RP
- Most of the deafness in Usher syndrome is congenital. It is unlikely that an RP patient who is not born deaf will go deaf later in his life.
- RP severity varies with inheritance pattern
- Autosomal recessive form has an early age of onset and may have severely constricted visual fields by age 20. Tends toward more rapid progression as compared to autosomal dominant RP; also increased incidence of cataracts.
- X-linked RP is similar in clinical presentation to autosomal recessive RP
- Autosomal dominant RP generally has less severe findings initially than autosomal recessive RP; symptoms may not occur until 30 years of age
- Good central vision usually preserved. If the central visual field radius is >30°, >90% of patients will have visual acuities of 20/40 or better. If the central visual field radius is smaller than 10°, 30% of patients will have a visual acuity of 20/40 or better.

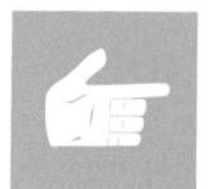

MISCELLANEOUS

ASSOCIATED CONDITIONS
- With systemic disorders:
  - ◊ Usher syndrome. RP and congenital sensorineural hearing impairment.
  - ◊ Laurence-Moon-Biedl syndrome (also called the Bardet-Biedl syndrome) is an autosomal recessive disorder associated with retinal dystrophy, mental retardation, obesity, hypogonadism, and postaxial polydactyly.
  - ◊ Cockayne syndrome. This is an autosomal recessive disorder in which children at the age of one or two years present with retinal dystrophy, sensorineural deafness, cerebellar dysfunction, dementia, and ultraviolet light photosensitivity.

AGE-RELATED FACTORS
Pediatric: Leber congenital amaurosis is characterized by severely reduced vision from birth and impaired ERG responses from both cones and rods. Most cases are autosomal recessive.
Geriatric: Late onset RP is asymptomatic; generally unrecognized until age >40
Others: N/A

PREGNANCY
Remember risk of teratogenicity of high intake vitamin A during pregnancy

SYNONYMS
- Rod-cone dystrophy
- Retinal dystrophy

ICD-9-CM
362.74 Pigmentary retinal dystrophy

SEE ALSO
Cataract
Laurence-Moon-Biedl syndrome

OTHER NOTES N/A

ABBREVIATIONS
RP = eetinitis pigmentosa
ERG = electroretinogram

REFERENCES

- Berson EL, Remulla JFC, Rosner B, et al. Evaluation of patients with retinitis pigmentosa receiving electric stimulation, ozonated blood, and ocular surgery in Cuba. Arch Ophthalmol 1996;114:560-3
- Pagon RA. Retinitis pigmentosa. Surv Ophthalmol 1988;33:137-77
- Madreperla SA, et al: Visual acuity loss and retinitis pigmentosa: relationship to visual field loss. Arch Ophthalmol 1990;108:358-64
- Rothman KJ, Moore LL, Singer MR, et al. Teratogenicity of high vitamin A intake. NEJM 1995;333:1369-73
- Berson EL, Rosner B, Sandberg MA, et al. A randomized trial of vitamin A and vitamin E supplements for retinitis pigmentosa. Arch Ophthalmol 1993;111:751-72
- Fishman GA, Gilbert LD, Fisella RG, et al. Acetazolamide for treatment of chronic cystoid macular edema in retinitis pigmentosa. Arch Ophthalmol 1989;107:1445-52
- Santos A, Humayun M, de Juan E, et al. Preservation of the inner retina in retinitis pigmentosa: a morphometric analysis. Arch Ophthalmol 1997;115:511-5
- Newsome DA, Blacharski P. Grid Photocoagulation for macular edema in patients with retinitis pigmentosa. Am J Ophthalmol. 1987;103:161-6
- Fishman GA, Gilbert LD, Fisella RG, et al. Acetazolamide for treatment of chronic cystoid macular edema in retinitis pigmentosa. Arch Ophthalmol 1989;107:1445-52
- Rothman KJ, et al: Teratogenicity of high vitamin A intake. N Engl J Med 1995;333:1369-73
- Berson EL, Rosner B, Sandberg, MA, et al. A randomized trial of vitamin A and vitamin E supplementation for retinitis pigmentosa. Arch Ophthalmol 1993;111:761-72

Web references: 0 available at www.5mcc.com
Illustrations 1 available

Author(s):
Richard W. Allinson, MD

BASICS

DESCRIPTION Noninflammatory retinal disorder characterized by retinal capillary closure and microaneurysms. Retinal ischemia leads to release of a vasoproliferative factor stimulating neovascularization on the retina, optic nerve, or iris.
- Most patients with diabetes mellitus will develop diabetic retinopathy. It is the leading cause of new cases of legal blindness among Americans between the ages of 20-64.
- Diabetic retinopathy can be divided into three stages:
  - ◊ Background diabetic retinopathy
  - ◊ Preproliferative diabetic retinopathy
  - ◊ Proliferative diabetic retinopathy

System(s) affected: Nervous
Genetics: N/A
Incidence/Prevalence in USA:
- Approximately 6.6% of the population between ages 20-74 has diabetes
- Approximately 25% of the diabetic population has some form of diabetic retinopathy
- Diabetic retinopathy accounts for approximately 10% of new cases of blindness each year

Predominant age:
- Peak incidence of Type I, juvenile onset diabetes mellitus, is between the ages of 12-15
- Peak incidence of Type II, adult onset, between the ages of 50-70
- The incidence of diabetic retinopathy is directly related to the duration of diabetes
- In children less than 10 years of age, it is unusual to see diabetic retinopathy, regardless of the duration of diabetes
- The risk of developing diabetic retinopathy increases after puberty
- Almost all diabetics will develop background retinopathy if they have had diabetes for at least 20 years
- Two-thirds of juvenile-onset diabetics who have had diabetes for at least 35 years will develop proliferative diabetic retinopathy, and one-third will develop macular edema. The proportions are reversed for adult-onset diabetes.

Predominant sex:
- Male = Female - juvenile onset diabetes mellitus
- Female > Male: non-insulin-dependent diabetes mellitus

SIGNS & SYMPTOMS
- Background diabetic retinopathy
  - ◊ Microaneurysms
  - ◊ Intraretinal hemorrhage
  - ◊ Macular edema
  - ◊ Lipid deposits
- Preproliferative diabetic retinopathy
  - ◊ Nerve fiber layer infarctions (cotton wool spots)
  - ◊ Venous beading
  - ◊ Venous dilation
  - ◊ Intraretinal microvascular abnormalities (IRMA)
  - ◊ Extensive retinal hemorrhage
- Proliferative diabetic retinopathy
  - ◊ New blood vessel proliferation (neovascularization) on the retinal surface, optic nerve, and iris

CAUSES Related to the development of diabetic microaneurysms and microvascular abnormalities.

RISK FACTORS
- Duration of diabetes mellitus (usually over 10 years)
- Poor glycemic control
- Pregnancy
- Renal disease
- Systemic hypertension
- Smoking
- Elevated serum lipid levels are associated with an increased risk of retinal lipid deposits (hard exudates)
- Proteinuria

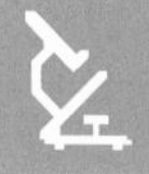

DIAGNOSIS

DIFFERENTIAL DIAGNOSIS Other causes of retinopathy, e.g., radiation retinopathy, retinal venous obstruction, and hypertensive retinopathy.

LABORATORY N/A

Drugs that may alter lab results: N/A

Disorders that may alter lab results: N/A

PATHOLOGICAL FINDINGS
- Increased capillary permeability
- Microaneurysms
- Hemorrhages in retina
- Exudates in retina
- Capillary nonperfusion

SPECIAL TESTS Fluorescein angiography: Demonstrates retinal nonperfusion, retinal leakage, and proliferative diabetic retinopathy

IMAGING N/A

DIAGNOSTIC PROCEDURES
Eye examination: Measurement of visual acuity and documentation of the status of the iris, lens, vitreous and fundus

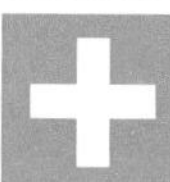

TREATMENT

APPROPRIATE HEALTH CARE Inpatient or outpatient surgery for vitrectomy; outpatient for laser treatment

GENERAL MEASURES
- The Early Treatment Diabetic Retinopathy Study demonstrated that systemic aspirin did not prevent the development of proliferative diabetic retinopathy, or reduce the risk of visual loss associated with diabetic retinopathy
- Microvascular complications, including proliferative diabetic retinopathy are significantly increased when blood-sugar levels are equal to or greater than 200 mg/dL
- Poor glycemic control is associated with an increased risk, both for developing diabetic retinopathy and with its progression, regardless of the type of diabetes, insulin-dependent or non-insulin dependent
- Cataracts are more common among diabetics. Try to delay cataract surgery in diabetics with retinopathy until the symptoms are more severe than in non-diabetics; cataract surgery can cause retinopathy to worsen

SURGICAL MEASURES
- Laser treatment: Recommended for patients with proliferative diabetic retinopathy and for patients with clinically significant macular edema
- The Diabetic Retinopathy Study demonstrated panretinal photocoagulation overall reduced the rate of severe visual loss from 15.9% in untreated eyes to 6.4% in treated eyes. In certain subgroups of eyes with proliferative diabetic retinopathy, the incidence of severe visual loss in untreated eyes was as high as 36.9% with a follow-up of 2 years.
- The Early Treatment Diabetic Retinopathy Study (ETDRS) demonstrated that eyes with clinically significant diabetic macular edema benefitted from focal laser treatment. Clinical significant diabetic macular edema is defined as the following:
  - ◊ 1. Thickening of the retina within 500 microns of the center of the macula
  - ◊ 2. Hard exudates within 500 microns of the center of the macula associated with thickening of the adjacent retina
  - ◊ 3. A zone of retinal thickening 1 disc area or larger within 1 disc diameter of the center of the macula
- Patients with clinically significant diabetic macular edema (CSDME) and high risk proliferative disease can have simultaneous focal and panretinal photocoagulation without adversely affecting the visual outcome
- Vitrectomy may benefit some cases of diffuse macular edema
- Intravitreal triamcinolone may be helpful for diabetic macular edema that fails to respond to focal laser treatment
- Cryoretinopexy can be used instead of laser treatment in certain cases to decrease the neovascular stimulus and treat proliferative diabetic retinopathy
- Vitrectomy: Recommended for patients with severe proliferative diabetic retinopathy, traction retinal detachment involving the macula, and nonclearing vitreous hemorrhage. In eyes undergoing vitrectomy for severe proliferative diabetic retinopathy, the percentage of eyes with a visual acuity of 10/20 or better was greater in the group that underwent early vitrectomy versus conventional management.
- Vitrectomy can be considered after 1 month for a vitreous hemorrhage decreasing the vision to the 5/200 level or worse

ACTIVITY As tolerated

DIET Follow prescribed diabetic diet

PATIENT EDUCATION
- Patient information available from the American Diabetes Association - (800)232-3472 or local office
- American Academy of Ophthalmology, 655 Beach St., San Francisco, CA 94109-1336
- Stress importance of strict blood glucose control through diet, exercise, drugs/insulin and monitoring of blood glucose

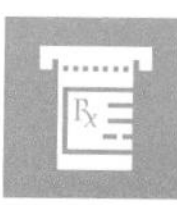

MEDICATIONS

DRUG(S) OF CHOICE
- None are specific for retinopathy. See Other Notes. Lisinopril, an angiotensin-converting enzyme (ACE) inhibitor, was found to slow the progression of retinopathy in insulin dependent diabetes.
- An oral therapy for diabetic retinopathy is being tested. Protein kinase C-beta (PKC-beta) is an enzyme activated by hyperglycemia and is associated with the development of vascular dysfunction. Inhibition of PKC-beta could help reduce the retinal vascular complications from diabetes.
- Nutritional antioxidant intake of vitamins C, E and beta-carotene has no protective effect on diabetic retinopathy
- The lipid lowering drug atorvastatin may reduce the severity lipid deposits in patients with CSDME with type II diabetes and dyslipidemia

Contraindications: N/A
Precautions: N/A
Significant possible interactions: N/A

ALTERNATIVE DRUGS N/A

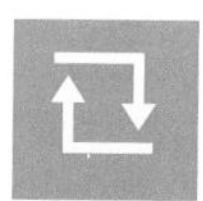

FOLLOWUP

PATIENT MONITORING
- Scheduled eye examinations by an ophthalmologist:
  - ◊ The diabetic patient with no diabetic retinopathy should be followed yearly
  - ◊ Patients with background diabetic retinopathy should be followed at least every six months
  - ◊ Patients with preproliferative diabetic retinopathy should be followed at least every three to four months
  - ◊ Patients with active proliferative diabetic retinopathy should be followed at least every two to three months

PREVENTION/AVOIDANCE
- Careful monitoring and control of blood glucose
- Routine visits to an ophthalmologist

POSSIBLE COMPLICATIONS Blindness

EXPECTED COURSE/PROGNOSIS If treated early, outlook good. If treatment delayed, blindness may result.

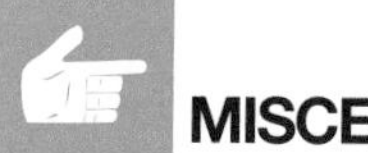

MISCELLANEOUS

ASSOCIATED CONDITIONS
- Glaucoma
- Cataracts
- Retinal detachment
- Vitreous hemorrhage
- Disc edema (diabetic papillopathy); can occur in type I or type II diabetes

AGE-RELATED FACTORS
Pediatric: N/A
Geriatric: Prevalence will increase as population ages and diabetic patients live longer
Others: N/A

PREGNANCY
- Pregnancy can exacerbate diabetic retinopathy
- Any woman with diabetes who becomes pregnant should be examined in the first trimester. She should be examined at least every three months until parturition.

SYNONYMS N/A

ICD-9-CM
362.01 Background diabetic retinopathy
362.02 Proliferative diabetic retinopathy

SEE ALSO
Diabetes mellitus, Type 1
Diabetes mellitus, Type 2

OTHER NOTES
- The Diabetes Control and Complications Trial (DCCT) recommends that for most patients with insulin-dependent diabetes mellitus, blood glucose levels should be as close to the nondiabetic range as is safe to do so, to reduce the risk and rate of progression of the diabetic retinopathy
- In the DCCT, insulin-dependent diabetics were randomly assigned into either conventional or intensive insulin treatment. Conventional treatment consisted of one or two daily insulin injections, with daily self-monitoring of urine or blood glucose. Intensive treatment consisted of insulin administered three or more times daily by injection or an external pump, with self-monitored blood glucose levels measured at least four times per day.
- The DCCT demonstrated intensive insulin therapy reduced the risk of macular edema and retinal neovascularization
- In the DCCT, intensive insulin therapy was more effective in reducing the risk of progression of diabetic retinopathy in the less advanced stages. However, advanced diabetic retinopathy also benefited from the intensive insulin.
- The DCCT demonstrated improvement in diabetic retinopathy was more likely to occur with intensive insulin therapy in insulin-dependent diabetes

ABBREVIATIONS
- BDR = background diabetic retinopathy
- PPDR = preproliferative diabetic retinopathy
- PDR = proliferative diabetic retinopathy
- CSDME = clinically significant diabetic macular edema

REFERENCES

- Diabetic Retinopathy Study Research Group: Indications for photocoagulation treatment of diabetic retinopathy. DRS Report No. 14. Int Ophthal Clin, 1987, 27:239-253
- Early Treatment Diabetic Retinopathy Study Research Group: Photocoagulation for Diabetic Macular Edema. ETDRS Report No. 1. Arch Ophthalmol, 1985; 103:1796-1806
- Early vitrectomy for severe proliferative diabetic retinopathy in eyes with useful vision: Results of a randomized trial diabetic retinopathy vitrectomy study. Report No. 3. The Diabetic Retinopathy Vitrectomy Study Research Group. Ophthalmol 1988;95:1307-1320
- The Diabetes Control and Complications Trial Research Group: The effect of intensive diabetes treatment on the progression of diabetic retinopathy in insulin-dependent diabetes mellitus. Arch Ophthalmol 1995;113:36-51
- Diabetic Retinopathy Vitrectomy Study Research Group: Early vitrectomy for severe vitreous hemorrhage in diabetic retinopathy: Two year results of a randomized trial. Diabetic retinopathy Vitrectomy Study Report 2. Arch Ophthalmol 1985;103:1644-1651
- Regillo CD, Brown GC, Savino PJ, et al. Diabetic papillopathy: Patient characteristics and fundus findings. Arch Ophthalmol 1995;113:889-895
- Browning DJ, Zhang Z, Benfield M, et al. The effect of patient characteristics on response to focal laser treatment for diabetic macular edema. Ophthalmol 1997;104:466-472
- Klein R, Klein BEK, Moss SE, et al. The Wisconsin epidemiologic study of diabetic retinopathy XVII. The 14-year incidence and progression of diabetic retinopathy and associated risk factors in type 1 diabetes. Ophthalmol 1998;1801-1815
- Mayer-Davis EJ, Bell RA, Reboussin BA, et al. Antioxidant nutrient intake and diabetic retinopathy: The San Luis Valley Diabetic Study. Ophthalmol 1998:2264-2270
- Pendergast SD, Hassan TS, Williams GA, et al. Vitrectomy for diffuse diabetic macular edema associated with a taut premacular posterior hyaloid. Am J Ophthalmol 2000;130(2):178-86
- Martidis A, Duker JD, Greenberg PB, et al. Intravitreal triamcinolone for refractory diabetic macular edema. Ophthalmol 2002:109;920-927
- Gupta A, Gupta V, Thapar S, Bhansali A. Lipid-lowering drug atorvastatin as an adjunct in the management of diabetic macular edema. Am J Ophthalmol 2004;137(4):675-82

Web references: 0 available at www.5mcc.com
Illustrations 5 available

Author(s):
Richard W. Allinson, MD

BASICS

DESCRIPTION Retinopathy of prematurity (ROP) is a proliferative disorder of the retinal blood vessels in premature infants. The normal retinal vascularization occurs nasally at approximately 36 weeks of gestation and temporally at approximately 40 weeks of gestation.

System(s) affected: Nervous

Genetics: Black infants appear less susceptible

Incidence/Prevalence in USA:
- One third of infants weighing < 1500 grams at birth may show evidence of retinopathy of prematurity
- 65.8% of infants weighing less than 1251 grams at birth, and 81.6% of those weighing less than 1000 grams
- Babies with a birth weight of 1001-1500 grams, 2.2% will develop cicatricial changes as a complication of ROP and 0.5% of them will be blind
- 5.1 % of premature infants with birth weights < 1251 grams will have vision of 20/200 or worse after 5 1/2 years of follow-up

Predominant age: Premature infants

Predominant sex: Male = Female

SIGNS & SYMPTOMS
Acute ROP is classified as follows:
- Location:
  - ◊ Zone I: posterior retina within a 60 degree circle centered on the optic nerve
  - ◊ Zone II: extends from the edge of Zone I to the nasal ora anteriorly
  - ◊ Zone III: is the residual temporal crescent of retina anterior to Zone II
- Extent: number of clock hours involved
- Degree of abnormal vascular response observed:
  - ◊ Stage 1: the development of a demarcation line between the vascularized and nonvascularized retina
  - ◊ Stage 2: the presence of a demarcation line that extends out of the plane of the retina (ridge)
  - ◊ Stage 3: a ridge with extraretinal fibrovascular proliferation
  - ◊ Stage 4: subtotal retinal detachment
  - ◊ Stage 5: total retinal detachment
- "Plus" disease is characterized by the tortuosity of the retinal vasculature in the posterior fundus

CAUSES Oxidative processes, influenced by high levels of arterial oxygen, in immature retina, may be an important causative factor

RISK FACTORS
- Low birth weight
- Prematurity
- Supplemental oxygen. Once the retina becomes fully vascularized, oxygen will not affect the retina.
- Supplemental oxygen given to premature infants with moderate retinopathy of prematurity will not make the retinopathy worse

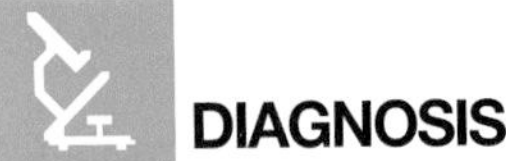

DIAGNOSIS

DIFFERENTIAL DIAGNOSIS
- Retinoblastoma
- Congenital cataracts
- Norrie disease
- Incontinentia pigmenti
- Familial exudative vitreoretinopathy
- Ocular toxocariasis
- Coat disease
- Persistent hyperplastic primary vitreous
- X-linked retinoschisis

LABORATORY N/A

Drugs that may alter lab results: N/A

Disorders that may alter lab results: N/A

PATHOLOGICAL FINDINGS
- Peripheral retinal nonperfusion
- Retinal neovascularization
- Retinal hemorrhages
- Retinal detachment

SPECIAL TESTS N/A

IMAGING N/A

DIAGNOSTIC PROCEDURES
- An ophthalmologist skilled in the detection of this disorder should examine all infants with a birth weight ≤ 1500 grams or with a gestational age of 28 weeks or less
- Infants with a birth weight over 1500 grams and who are clinically unstable and are felt to be at high risk by their pediatrician or neonatologist should have an ophthalmologic exam to detect ROP
- The American Academy of Pediatrics, the American Association for Pediatric Ophthalmology and Strabismus and the American Academy of Ophthalmology recommend the initial eye exam should be performed between 4-6 weeks of chronological age or between 31-33 weeks postconceptional age (gestational age at birth plus chronological age)
- Analysis of the natural history data from the Multicenter Trial Of Cryotherapy for Retinopathy of Prematurity (CRYO-ROP) study and the Light Reduction in Retinopathy (LIGHT-ROP) study have provided the following recommendations:
  - ◊ Eye exams for infants at risk for ROP should commence by 31 weeks postmenstrual age or 4 weeks chronological age, whichever is later
  - ◊ Acute-phase ROP screening can be terminated when 1 of the following 3 end points has been achieved: 1) Infant's attainment of 45 weeks postmenstrual age without the development of prethreshold ROP or worse, 2) Progression of retinal vascularization into zone III without previous zone II ROP, and 3) Full retinal vascularization.
- Follow-up exams are performed until the retina is fully vascularized

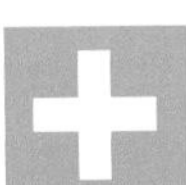

TREATMENT

APPROPRIATE HEALTH CARE Treatment usually is performed in the neonatal intensive care unit or as an outpatient or inpatient as the child grows older

GENERAL MEASURES
- The multicenter trial of cryotherapy demonstrated a favorable outcome for eyes treated at threshold (Stage 3+ retinopathy of prematurity) versus control eyes
- Stage 3 retinopathy defined as a ridge of extraretinal fibrovascular proliferation
- A plus sign is added to the ROP stage number when retinal vascular tortuosity is noted in the posterior fundus
- Threshold disease was defined as at least 5 contiguous or 8 cumulative clock hours of Stage 3 associated with retinal vascular tortuosity in the posterior segment of the eye ("plus" disease)
- When threshold disease is detected in infants, ablative therapy should be considered in at least one eye within 72 hours of diagnosis
- Using Teller Acuity Card assessment an unfavorable outcome was noted in 35.0% of the treated eyes compared with 56.3% of the control eyes, at one year in the multicenter trial of cryotherapy
- The development of ROP is not influenced by reducing ambient light exposure for a short period of time in premature babies
- There is a 50% reduction in unfavorable outcomes (retinal detachment, partial retinal detachment, or fold through the macula) in infants treated at threshold. Fewer than 20% infants with a favorable outcome after treatment of threshold disease will have a visual acuity of 20/40 or better. The Multicenter Study of Early Treatment for Retinopathy of Prematurity (ETROP) will study if earlier treatment by retinal ablation to the avascular retina in high risk eyes with prethreshold disease will result in better vision than in eyes treated at the conventional threshold point.
- The Early Treatment of Retinopathy of Prematurity (ETROP) study demonstrated that premature infants at high risk of vision loss from retinopathy of prematurity retain better vision when therapy is administered early than when treatment is held until the traditional threshold. The eyes assigned early treatment had a significantly reduced likelihood of poor vision, from 19.5% to 14.5%, at about 1 year of age.
  - ◊ In the ETROP study patients received treatment with laser therapy, but cryotherapy was also allowed
  - ◊ Eyes with high-risk prethreshold ROP or type 1 ROP were treated. Type 1 ROP was defined as zone I with any stage of ROP with plus disease (dilation and tortuosity of posterior pole retinal vessels in at least 2 quadrants, usually 6 or more clock-hours); zone I, stage 3 ROP with or without plus disease; zone II, stage 2 or 3 ROP with plus disease.
  - ◊ Serial exams should be performed on eyes with type 2 ROP, which is defined as zone I, stage 1 or 2 ROP without plus disease; zone II, stage 3 ROP without plus disease. Treatment should be considered for an eye with type 2 ROP when progression to type 1 ROP or threshold ROP occurs. Eyes with low-risk prethreshold type 2 ROP received follow-up every 2 to 4 days for at least 2 weeks until the ROP regressed or progressed to high-risk prethreshold disease.

SURGICAL MEASURES
- Transscleral cryotherapy to the avascular retina when applied to high risk eyes can reduce the incidence of sight threatening complications. The multicenter trial of cryotherapy has shown that treatment of high risk eyes reduces the incidence of unfavorable outcomes by 46%.
- The multicenter trial of cryotherapy demonstrated an unfavorable outcome, defined as posterior retinal detachment, retinal fold involving the macula, or retrolental tissue, was significantly less frequent in eyes undergoing cryotherapy

- The results at one year from the multicenter trial of cryotherapy demonstrated an unfavorable outcome in 25.7% of eyes that received cryotherapy compared with 47.4% of control eyes
- The results at 10 years from the multicenter trial of cryotherapy for retinopathy of prematurity demonstrated the following: 20/200 or worse vision occurred in 44.4% of treated eyes versus 62.1% of control eyes and an unfavorable outcome for the fundus status was found in 27.2% of treated eyes versus 47.9% of control eyes. The incidence of total retinal detachment remained stable in the treated eyes from the 5 1/2 year report to the 10 year report at 22.0%, while the incidence to total retinal detachment in the control eyes increased from 38.6% at 5 1/2 years to 41.4% at 10 years.
- In eyes treated with cryotherapy for severe ROP, the cryotherapy did not change the refractive error status of the treated eyes compared to control eyes
- Laser treatment applied to the avascular retina in high risk eyes can reduce the incidence of sight-threatening complications; cataract formation and serous retinal detachment are possible complications
- Diode laser treatment is becoming the primary treatment modality as it may be better tolerated and probably results in better vision, less myopia, and less retinal dragging compared to eyes treated with cryotherapy
- Threshold ROP had a reduced rate of progression in eyes with zone 2 disease when a dense, near confluent, pattern of diode laser treatment was applied versus a less dense pattern of diode laser treatment
- Intravenous fentanyl is a good analgesic agent to use when performing laser treatment with scleral depression on preterm infants
- After 10 years of follow-up eyes treated with laser were 5.2 times more likely to have 20/50 or better vision that eyes treated with cryotherapy
- After 10 years of follow-up eyes treated with laser had a mean vision of 20/66, compared to eyes treated with cryotherapy which had a mean vision of 20/182.
- Scleral buckling can reduce progression from stage 4 to 5 ROP. The encircling 240 band can be divided at 3 months after surgery if it is felt the retina will remain attached.
- Vitrectomy and/or scleral buckling can be used to treat retinal detachment associated with ROP. Emphasis should be placed on prevention of retinal detachment in premature infants, because of the poor visual outcome after a lensectomy-vitrectomy procedure for retinal detachment due to ROP.

ACTIVITY N/A

DIET N/A

PATIENT EDUCATION
- Expectant mothers should avoid behavioral and environmental risk factors associated with low birth weight. These include smoking, alcohol and other substance abuse, and poor nutrition.
- American Academy of Ophthalmology, 655 Beach St., San Francisco, CA 94109-1336

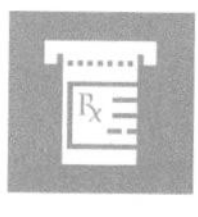

MEDICATIONS

DRUG(S) OF CHOICE
- Vitamin E prophylaxis is controversial; it may reduce the severity, but not the incidence of ROP
- Extremely low birth weight infants receiving prophylactic treatment with calf lung surfactant extract have a lower incidence of any stage when compared with control infants

Contraindications: N/A
Precautions: N/A
Significant possible interactions: N/A

ALTERNATIVE DRUGS N/A

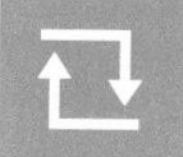

FOLLOWUP

PATIENT MONITORING
- Close follow-up of patients with ROP is required
- Follow-up exams after the initial examination are performed every 2-4 weeks until the retina is fully vascularized or until the ROP regresses
- Follow-up exams are performed every 1-2 weeks if "prethreshold" disease is present. Prethreshold disease is characterized by the following:
  - ◊ Zone I, any stage
  - ◊ Zone II, Stage 2 (ridge) with "plus" disease
  - ◊ Zone II, Stage 3 (ridge) with extraretinal fibrovascular proliferation
- Exam infants with zone I ROP at least weekly until involution of ROP occurs and normal vascularization proceeds to zone II.
- In some cases of regressed ROP, cicatrization can develop and is associated with variable degrees of fibrosis. This can lead to vitreoretinal traction and subsequent retinal detachment from formation of a retinal hole.
- Retinal detachment secondary to cicatricial ROP can occur during the midteens; long term follow-up of ROP cicatricial cases is indicated

PREVENTION/AVOIDANCE See Patient Education

POSSIBLE COMPLICATIONS
- Retinal detachment
- Retinal fold involving the macula
- Vitreous hemorrhage
- Angle closure glaucoma
- Amblyopia
- Strabismus
- Myopia

EXPECTED COURSE/PROGNOSIS
- Spontaneous regression occurs over a period of weeks or months in most cases. Spontaneous regression occurs in approximately 85% of eyes.
- The earliest sign of regression is the growth of blood vessels beyond the demarcation line into previously avascular retina
- Some cases of ROP do not regress spontaneously without sequela, but progress. A gradual transition then occurs from active ROP to cicatricial ROP which is associated with varying degrees of fibrosis and vitreoretinal traction which can lead to retinal detachment.

MISCELLANEOUS

ASSOCIATED CONDITIONS Neonatal respiratory distress syndrome

AGE-RELATED FACTORS
Pediatric: N/A
Geriatric: N/A
Others: N/A

PREGNANCY N/A

SYNONYMS
- ROP
- Retrolental fibroplasia

ICD-9-CM
362.21 Retrolental fibroplasia

SEE ALSO

OTHER NOTES N/A

ABBREVIATIONS
- ROP = retinopathy of prematurity
- RLF = retrolental fibroplasia

REFERENCES

- Ben-Sir I, Nissenkorn I, Kremer I. Retinopathy of Prematurity. Surv Ophthalmol 1988;33:1-16
- Cryotherapy for retinopathy of prematurity cooperative group. Multicenter trial of cryotherapy for retinopathy of prematurity. Preliminary results. Arch Ophthalmology 1988;106:471-9
- The committee for the classification of retinopathy of prematurity. An international classification of retinopathy of prematurity. Arch Ophthalmology 1984;102:1130-4
- Screening examination of premature infants for retinopathy of prematurity: a joint statement of the American Academy of Pediatrics, the American Association for Pediatric Ophthalmology and Strabismus, and the American Academy of Ophthalmology 1997;104:888-9
- Quinn GE, Dobson V, Barr CC, et al. Visual acuity of eyes after vitrectomy for retinopathy of prematurity: follow-up at 5 1/2 years. Ophthalmology 1996;103:595-600
- Trese M. Scleral buckling for retinopathy of prematurity. Ophthalmology 1994;101:23-6
- Reynolds JD, Hardy RJ, Kennedy KA, et al. Lack of efficacy of light reduction in preventing retinopathy of prematurity. NEJM 1998;338:1572-6
- The STOP ROP multicenter Study Group. Supplemental oxygen for retinopathy of prematurity. Pediatrics 2000;105:295-310
- Quinn GE, Dobson V, Siatkowski R, et al. Does cryotherapy affect refractive error? Results from treated versus control eyes in the cryotherapy for retinopathy of prematurity trial. Ophthalmology 2001;108(2):343-7
- Banach MJ, Ferrone PJ, Trese MD. A comparison of dense versus less dense diode laser photocoagulation patterns for threshold retinopathy of prematurity. Ophthalmology 2000;107:324-7
- Good WV, Hardy RJ. The multicenter study of early treatment for retinopathy of prematurity (ETROP). Ophthalmol 2001;108:1013-14
- Ng EY, Connolly BP, McNamara JA, et al. A comparison of laser photocoagulation with cryotherapy for threshold retinopathy of prematurity at 10 years. Part 1. Visual function and structural outcome. Ophthalmol 2002:109:928-35
- Connolly BP, Ng EY, McNamara JA, et al. A comparison of laser photocoagulation with cryotherapy for threshold retinopathy of prematurity at 10 years. Part 2. Refractive Outcome. Ophthalmol 2002:109;936-41
- Multicenter trial of cryotherapy for retinopathy of prematurity. Natural History ROP: Ocular outcome at 5 V2 years in premature infants with birth weights less than 1251 grams. Arch Ophthalmol 2002:120;595-99
- Multicenter trial of cryotherapy for retinopathy of prematurity. Ophthalmological outcomes at 10 years. Arch Ophthalmol 2001:119;1110-18
- Cryotherapy for retinopathy of prematurity cooperative group. Multicenter trial of cryotherapy for retinopathy of prematurity: one year outcome - structure and function. Arch Ophthalmol 1990;108:1408-16
- Reynolds JD, Dobson V, Quinn GE, et al. Evidence-based screening criteria for retinopathy of prematurity: natural history data from the CRYO-ROP and LIGHT-ROP studies. Arch Ophthalmol 2002;120(11):1470-6

Web references: 0 available at www.5mcc.com
Illustrations N/A

Author(s):
Richard W. Allinson, MD

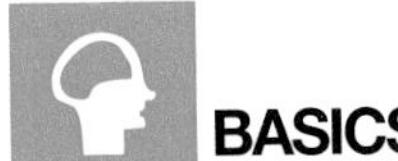

BASICS

DESCRIPTION Acute encephalopathy with cerebral edema and fatty infiltration of the liver. Occurs in previously healthy children, often associated with an antecedent viral infection such as varicella or influenza. Markedly decreased in incidence since late 1970's when association with aspirin use and Reye syndrome made. Most cases currently seen are "Reye-like syndrome" (RLS) caused by inborn error of metabolism or toxin (see Differential Diagnosis).
System(s) affected: Gastrointestinal, Nervous
Genetics: No known genetic pattern
Incidence/Prevalence in USA: Currently very rare
Predominant age: Infants, children, adolescents. Peak incidence at 6 years of age. Most cases between 4-12 years of age.
Predominant sex: Male = Female

SIGNS & SYMPTOMS
- Symptoms reflected in clinical staging system
  - ◊ I: Vomiting, sleepy, lethargic
  - ◊ II: Confusion, delirium, hyperpnea, irritability, combative, hyperreflexia, altered muscle tone
  - ◊ III: Obtunded, light coma and seizures, decorticate rigidity, loss of oculocephalic reflexes, intact pupillary reflex
  - ◊ IV: Coma, decerebrate posturing spontaneously or in response to painful stimuli, seizures, fixed pupils
  - ◊ V: Coma, flaccid paralysis, loss of deep tendon reflexes, seizures, respiratory arrest, isoelectric EEG

CAUSES Unknown - mitochondrion is major site of injury

RISK FACTORS
- Pediatric age group
- Viral illness, especially varicella, influenza A
- Use of preparations containing aspirin, salicylates, and/or salicylamides
- More common in rural and suburban areas

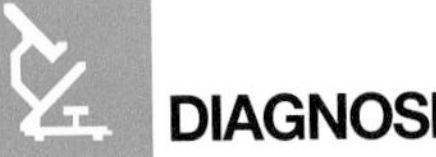

DIAGNOSIS

DIFFERENTIAL DIAGNOSIS
- Acute encephalopathy without hepatic abnormalities
  - ◊ Encephalitis, meningitis, diabetes mellitus, drug overdose, poisoning, psychiatric illness
- Acute toxic encephalopathy with hepatic abnormalities (Reye-like syndrome)
  - ◊ Inherited metabolic disorders
    - Organic acidurias with defects in hepatic fatty acid oxidation
    - Fatty acid metabolism defects: Acyl-CoA dehydrogenase, carnitine deficiency
    - Urea cycle defects: carbamyl phosphate synthetase, ornithine transcarbamylase
    - Fructosemia
  - ◊ Drug ingestions
    - Valproate, aspirin
  - ◊ Toxin ingestion (produce Reye-like syndrome)
    - Margosa oil, hopantenate, aflatoxin, hypoglycin (akee fruit), Jamaican vomiting sickness

LABORATORY
- Usually severe elevations of AST (SGOT) and ALT (SGPT)
- Hypoglycemia
- Normal or slightly elevated bilirubin or alkaline phosphatase
- Elevated ammonia
- Prolonged prothrombin time - often not responsive to Vitamin K
- Increased CSF pressure without pleocytosis (< 8 leukocytes per cubic millimeter)
- Mixed respiratory alkalosis and metabolic acidosis
- Hyperaminoacidemia (glutamine, alanine, lysine)

Drugs that may alter lab results: N/A

Disorders that may alter lab results: N/A

PATHOLOGICAL FINDINGS
- Slightly enlarged, firm, yellow liver with fat droplets throughout
- Characteristic liver biopsy with foamy cytoplasm with microvesicular fat - may need special preparation
- Uniformly severe mitochondrial injury

SPECIAL TESTS EEG

IMAGING N/A

DIAGNOSTIC PROCEDURES
- Liver biopsy
- CSF pressure measurement

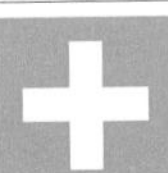

TREATMENT

APPROPRIATE HEALTH CARE Medical emergency requiring immediate hospitalization

GENERAL MEASURES
- Supportive depending on severity of illness
- IV glucose and close monitoring of blood or serum glucose (to prevent severe hypoglycemia)
- Hyperventilation, mannitol, barbiturates to reduce intracranial pressure
- Minimize noise and other CNS stimulation (to prevent increases in intracranial pressure)
- Vitamin K, fresh frozen plasma, platelets as needed
- Mechanical ventilation
- Dialysis to reduce high ammonia levels and/or residual salicylate

SURGICAL MEASURES
- Decompression craniotomy may be necessary

ACTIVITY Complete bedrest

DIET Nothing by mouth

PATIENT EDUCATION Printed material from the National Reye Syndrome Foundation, P.O. Box 829, Byron, OH 43506-0829, (800)233-7393

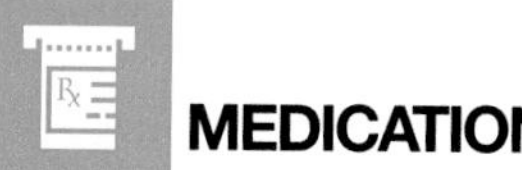

MEDICATIONS

DRUG(S) OF CHOICE
All treatment is supportive.
- 10-15% glucose IV
- Vitamin K
- For increased intracranial pressure, for example:
  - ◊ Mannitol 0.5-1.0 gm/kg IV, as long as there is urine output
  - ◊ Dexamethasone 0.5 mg/kg/day
  - ◊ Barbiturates

Contraindications: Mannitol - do not use if patient has no renal output
Precautions: Mannitol and poor renal output may result in vascular overload and pulmonary edema
Significant possible interactions: Refer to manufacturer's literature

ALTERNATIVE DRUGS N/A

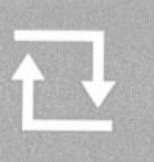

FOLLOWUP

PATIENT MONITORING Will depend on specific residual effects; may require care of physicians, nurses, psychologists, physical, occupational and/or speech therapists

PREVENTION/AVOIDANCE
- Avoidance of salicylates in children with viral illness
- Recognition of early symptoms of the disease

POSSIBLE COMPLICATIONS
See Signs and Symptoms also.
- Aspiration pneumonia
- Respiratory failure
- Cardiac dysrhythmia/arrest
- Inappropriate vasopressin excretion
- Diabetes insipidus
- Cerebral edema
- Seizures

EXPECTED COURSE/PROGNOSIS
- Majority will have mild illness without progression. Prognosis related to degree of cerebral edema and ammonia level on admission.
- Possible neurologic sequelae include problems with attention, concentration, speech, language, fine and gross motor skills - more common with higher stages

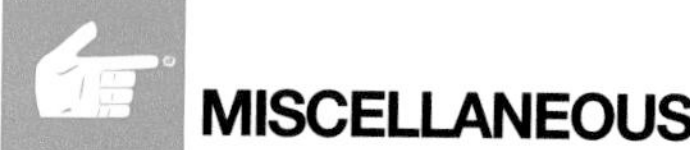

MISCELLANEOUS

ASSOCIATED CONDITIONS N/A

AGE-RELATED FACTORS
Pediatric: Especially in infants under age 2, essential to make correct diagnosis; rule out other causes of Reye-like syndrome (see Differential Diagnosis section)
Geriatric: N/A
Others: N/A

PREGNANCY N/A

SYNONYMS White liver disease

ICD-9-CM
331.81 Reye syndrome

SEE ALSO
Encephalitis, viral
Hepatic encephalopathy

OTHER NOTES N/A

ABBREVIATIONS N/A

REFERENCES

- Monto J. The disappearance of Reye's syndrome - a public health triumph. NEJM 1999;340:1423-4
- Belay E, Bresee J, Holman R, et al. Reye's syndrome in the United States from 1981 through 1997. NEJM 1999;340:1377-82
- Balistreri W. Reye syndrome and 'Reye-like' diseases. In: Behrman RE, Kliegman RM, Arvin A, eds. Nelson Textbook of Pediatrics. Philadelphia: WB Saunders Co; 1996. p .1144-5
- Visentin M, Salmona M, Tacconi MT. Reyes and Reye-like syndrome, Drug related diseases? Drug Met Rev 1995;27:517-39
- Green A, Hall S. Investigation of metabolic disorders resembling Reye's syndrome. Arch Dis Child 1992;67:1313-7
- Glasgow JF, Middleton B. Reye syndrome-insights on causation and prognosis.Arch Dis Child 2001;85(5):351-3

Web references: 1 available at www.5mcc.com
Illustrations N/A

Author(s):
William A. Primack, MD

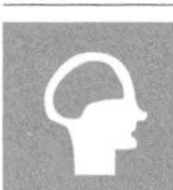

BASICS

DESCRIPTION Antibody-mediated destruction of red blood cells that bear Rh surface antigens by individuals who lack the antigens and have become isoimmunized ("sensitized") to them. Can occur with transfusion of incompatible blood. More commonly seen in the Rh-positive fetus or infant of an Rh-negative mother.
System(s) affected: Hemic/Lymphatic/Immunologic
Genetics: Complex autosomal inheritance of polypeptide Rh antigens. Two closely related genes RHD and RHCE carry an assortment of alleles: Dd, Cc, Ee. Individuals who express the D antigen (also called Rho or Rho[D]) are considered Rh positive, as are those expressing the weak D (Du) variant.
Individuals lacking the D antigen are Rh negative. Antibodies may be produced to C, c, D, E, or e in individuals lacking the specific antigen; only D is strongly immunogenic. Isoimmunization to Rh antigens is not inherited.
Incidence/Prevalence in USA:
- 15% of Caucasian population and smaller fractions of other races are Rh negative
- Risk of isoimmunization during or after an Rh-positive pregnancy has been up to 15%, but seems to be decreasing to less than 5% in recent studies
- Only 1-2% of isoimmunizations occur antepartum
- With Rho(D) immune globulin prophylaxis, risk of sensitization is reduced to less than 1% of susceptible pregnancies

Predominant age: Childbearing
Predominant sex: Female only

SIGNS & SYMPTOMS
- Hemolytic transfusion reaction in recipient of Rh-incompatible blood
- Jaundice of newborn
- Kernicterus
- Congenital or fetal anemia
- Fetal hydrops
- Fetal death in utero

CAUSES
- Transfusion of Rh-positive blood to Rh-negative recipient
- Maternal exposure to fetal Rh antigens, either antepartum or intrapartum

RISK FACTORS
- Any Rh-positive pregnancy in Rh-negative woman
- Induced abortion
- Spontaneous abortion
- Ectopic pregnancy
- Amniocentesis, chorionic villus sampling
- Fetomaternal hemorrhage (fetal death in utero)
- Fetal manipulation, external version
- Cesarean delivery
- Maternal trauma
- Placental abruption
- Placenta previa
- Manual placental removal

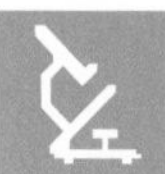

DIAGNOSIS

DIFFERENTIAL DIAGNOSIS
- ABO incompatibility
- Other blood group (non-Rh) isoimmunization
- Nonimmune fetal hydrops
- Hereditary spherocytosis
- Red cell enzyme defects

LABORATORY Positive indirect Coombs' test (antibody screen) during pregnancy

Drugs that may alter lab results: Prior administration of D immune globulin may lead to weakly (false) positive indirect Coombs' test in mother and direct Coombs' test in infant

Disorders that may alter lab results: N/A

PATHOLOGICAL FINDINGS N/A

SPECIAL TESTS
- Paternal blood typing
- Kleihauer-Betke test to quantify an acute fetal-maternal bleed

IMAGING N/A

DIAGNOSTIC PROCEDURES N/A

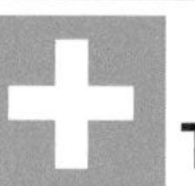

TREATMENT

APPROPRIATE HEALTH CARE Outpatient, ambulatory management in most cases. Because of the specialized, somewhat hazardous treatment measures involved, pregnancies usually managed at tertiary care level.

GENERAL MEASURES
- See Patient Monitoring also
- Depending on severity of involvement, treatment of newborn or fetus may include:
  - ◊ Phototherapy
  - ◊ Transfusion after delivery
  - ◊ Exchange transfusion
  - ◊ Diuretics and digoxin for hydrops
  - ◊ Early delivery
  - ◊ Intrauterine transfusion

SURGICAL MEASURES N/A

ACTIVITY N/A

DIET N/A

PATIENT EDUCATION Griffith: Instructions for Patients; Philadelphia, 1994 W.B. Saunders Co.

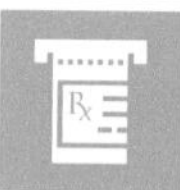

MEDICATIONS

DRUG(S) OF CHOICE

- For prophylaxis:

Rho(D) immune globulin (RhIG, RhoGAM, Gamulin Rh) given to unsensitized, Rh-negative women following:
  - ◊ Spontaneous abortion
  - ◊ Induced abortion
  - ◊ Ectopic pregnancy
  - ◊ Antepartum hemorrhage
  - ◊ Amniocentesis
  - ◊ Chorionic villus sampling
  - ◊ Routinely at 28 weeks
  - ◊ Within 72 hours after delivery of Rh-positive infant
- Dose:
  - ◊ 50 mcg dose for events up to 12 weeks gestation
  - ◊ 300 mcg dose for events after 12 weeks
  - ◊ Higher doses may be required in the event of a large fetal - maternal hemorrhage (> 30 mL whole blood)

Contraindications: Patient with known severe reaction to human globulin. Refer to manufacturer's profile.

Precautions: Refer to manufacturer's profile

Significant possible interactions: N/A

ALTERNATIVE DRUGS N/A

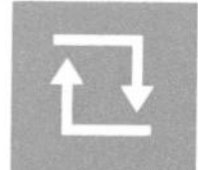

FOLLOWUP

PATIENT MONITORING

- Antibody titer measured every few weeks during pregnancy. A titer of 1:16 or greater indicates need for further testing.
- Amniocentesis for amniotic fluid bilirubin levels
- Umbilical blood sampling (cordocentesis) for fetal blood type, hematocrit, reticulocyte count, presence of erythroblasts
- Fetal heart rate testing/ultrasonography to assess fetal status
- Amniocentesis for fetal lung maturity

PREVENTION/AVOIDANCE

- Blood typing (ABO and Rh) on all pregnant women
- Antibody screening early in pregnancy
- Rh immune globulin prevents only sensitization to the D antigen
- Follow prophylaxis routine listed in Medications for unsensitized, Rh-negative women

POSSIBLE COMPLICATIONS

- Pregnancy loss from umbilical blood sampling
- Pregnancy loss from intrauterine transfusion
- Fetal distress requiring emergent delivery

EXPECTED COURSE/PROGNOSIS

- With appropriate monitoring and treatment, infants born of severely affected pregnancies have a survival rate of greater than 80%
- Fetuses with hydrops have a higher mortality rate
- Disease is likely to be more severe in affected subsequent pregnancies
- Even with severe disease, the neurologic outcome of survivors is generally good

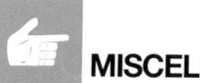

MISCELLANEOUS

ASSOCIATED CONDITIONS

- Hemolytic disease of newborn
- Hydrops fetalis
- Neonatal jaundice
- Kernicterus

AGE-RELATED FACTORS

Pediatric: N/A
Geriatric: N/A
Others: N/A

PREGNANCY N/A

SYNONYMS

- Rh isoimmunization
- Rh alloimmunization
- Rh sensitization

ICD-9-CM

656.10 Rh isoimmunization in pregnancy, unspecified
656.20 Isoimmunization in pregnancy from other and unspecified blood-group incompatibility, unspecified
773.0 Rh hemolytic disease in fetus or newborn
773.1 ABO hemolytic disease in fetus or newborn
773.2 Other hemolytic disease in fetus or newborn
773.3 Isoimmune hydrops fetalis
773.4 Kernicterus due to isoimmunization
773.5 Isoimmune late anemia

SEE ALSO

Anemia, hemolytic
Erythroblastosis fetalis
Jaundice

OTHER NOTES N/A

ABBREVIATIONS N/A

REFERENCES

- Crosby WM, Block MF, Morgan MA. Rh (and other) isoimmunization. In: Dilts PV, Sciarra JJ, eds. Gynecology and Obstetrics. Philadelphia, JB Lippincott Co, 1994: vol2,chap52
- Perkins JT. Hemolytic Disease of the Newborn. In: Gleicher N, ed. Principles and Practice of Medical Therapy in Pregnancy. 2nd Ed. Norwalk, CT, Appleton & Lange, 1992
- Socol ML. Management of blood group isoimmunization. In: Gleicher N, ed. Principles and Practice of Medical Therapy in Pregnancy. 2nd Ed. Norwalk, CT, Appleton & Lange, 1992
- Management of Isoimmunization in Pregnancy. ACOG Technical Bulletin, 148, Oct 1990
- Prevention of D Isoimmunization. ACOG Technical Bulletin, 147, Oct 1990
- Giblett ER. Blood groups and blood transfusion. In: Braunwald E, et al, eds. Harrison's Principles of Internal Medicine. 12th Ed. New York, McGraw-Hill Inc., 1991
- Agre P, Cartron J. Molecular biology of the Rh antigens. Blood 1991;78(3):551-63

Web references: 4 available at www.5mcc.com
Illustrations N/A

Author(s):

Donald A. F. Nelson, MD

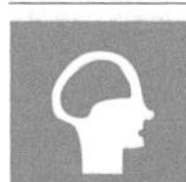

BASICS

DESCRIPTION A syndrome resulting from damage to skeletal muscle with the resultant appearance of free myoglobin in the circulation. Myoglobin is then filtered by the glomerulus and appears in the urine. Elevated urinary levels of myoglobin can lead to acute renal failure.

System(s) affected: Cardiovascular, Gastrointestinal, Musculoskeletal, Nervous, Renal/Urologic

Genetics: Certain inherited disorders of fatty acid metabolism (Carnitine Palmityltransferase deficiency - autosomal recessive) and glycogen storage diseases (phosphofructokinase deficiency autosomal recessive; phosphoglycerate kinase deficiency is the only of these categories which is X-linked recessive) are inherited and lead to muscle injury with exercise which may eventuate rhabdomyolysis and acute renal failure.

Incidence/Prevalence in USA: Unknown (estimate: at Harborview Medical Center, a Seattle municipal hospital, rhabdomyolysis accounts for approximately 10-15% of ARF cases, per Zager RA)

Predominant age: Depends on the etiology for rhabdomyolysis, i.e., inherited disorders lead to rhabdomyolysis at a younger age but other etiologies may occur at any time - trauma or rhabdomyolysis secondary to infection.

Predominant sex: M > F; because of greater incidence of trauma in males

SIGNS & SYMPTOMS Rhabdomyolysis may present with obvious muscle injury and swelling on examination, e.g., crush injury, compartment syndrome; or muscle exam may be completely negative despite severe rhabdomyolysis/myoglobinuria. The signs and symptoms with renal failure are the same as those for acute tubular necrosis (ATN) from other etiologies.

CAUSES
- Metabolic, electrolytes - hypokalemia, hypophosphatemia, myopathies, inherited disorders of fatty acid metabolism (i.e., acyl-CoA dehydrogenase deficiency), glycogen storage diseases (e.g., phosphorylase b-kinase deficiency) and others (lactate dehydrogenase A deficiency)
- Polymyositis
- Dermatomyositis
- Malignant hyperthermia
- Neuroleptic malignant syndrome (anesthesia, phenothiazines, MAO inhibitors)
- Muscle exertion (physical, secondary to convulsions or to heat injury)
- Trauma-crush syndromes and pseudo-crush syndrome
- Muscle ischemia secondary to arterial occlusion or insufficiency
- Burns
- Repetitive muscle injury (bongo drumming, torture)
- Status epilepticus
- Hyperosmolality
- Head injury
- Infections
  - ◊ Viral (influenza A, Epstein-Barr virus, measles, varicella, etc.)
  - ◊ Bacterial - Legionnaires
  - ◊ Septicemia
  - ◊ Parasites (malaria)
- Toxic muscle injury
  - ◊ Alcohol induced
  - ◊ Tetanus
  - ◊ Snake venom (viper bite) and rattlesnake
  - ◊ Carbon monoxide exposure
- Drug abuse
  - ◊ Crack-cocaine, heroin, amphetamine abuse, "ecstasy", ketamine
- Drug overdoses
  - ◊ Theophylline, INH, acetaminophen
  - ◊ Lipid lowering agents (clofibrate, gemfibrozil in combination with HMG-CoA reductase inhibitors, HMG-CoA reductase inhibitors and cyclosporine or itraconazole, possibly cyclosporine alone)
  - ◊ Any drug that leads to neuroleptic malignant syndrome
- Carcinoma - acute necrotizing myopathy of carcinoma
- Diabetes mellitus; ketoacidosis
- Extreme lithotomy position for extended periods
- Extended periods of muscle pressure
  - ◊ After allogenic bone marrow transplant
  - ◊ Hyponatremia or correction thereof
  - ◊ Hypothyroidism
  - ◊ Water intoxication
  - ◊ Hypokalemia

RISK FACTORS See Causes

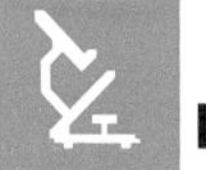

DIAGNOSIS

DIFFERENTIAL DIAGNOSIS
- For acute renal failure with rhabdomyolysis - any disease that causes acute tubular necrosis can be confused with rhabdomyolysis
- Renal pigment injury from hemoglobin resembles pigment injury from myoglobin

LABORATORY
- Muscle enzyme elevations (creatinine kinase, aldolase, and lactic dehydrogenase)
- Marked elevations of potassium and phosphorus from muscle injury
- Hypocalcemia during oliguria with hypercalcemia occasionally during the recovery phase from acute tubular necrosis (in fact, hypercalcemia during recovery from ATN is almost diagnostic of rhabdomyolysis and myoglobulin tubular injury)
- Urinalysis - dipstick positive for blood without red cells in sediment is very suggestive of pigment injury from either hemoglobin or myoglobin; coarsely granular, pigmented casts
- Urine or serum myoglobin levels may be helpful, but normal levels do not rule out pigment injury
- Extreme hyperuricemia may be present and actually can cause acute uric acid nephropathy in the setting of rhabdomyolysis
- When measured, vitamin D levels are decreased in the oliguric phase of rhabdomyolysis
- Reversible hepatic dysfunction occurs

Drugs that may alter lab results: None

Disorders that may alter lab results: Hemoglobin may be confused with myoglobin on dipstick

PATHOLOGICAL FINDINGS Muscle necrosis; kidney-myoglobin renal injury looks like ATN from other causes

SPECIAL TESTS
- Hypocalcemia during the oliguric phase helps but is not diagnostic of rhabdomyolysis
- Extreme hyperkalemia, hyperphosphatemia and hyperuricemia is very suggestive of rhabdomyolysis

IMAGING Any renal imaging is similar as for other etiologies of ATN

DIAGNOSTIC PROCEDURES A good index of clinical suspicion with evidence of muscle damage on exam or by lab tests make the diagnosis likely

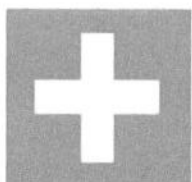

TREATMENT

APPROPRIATE HEALTH CARE Inpatient

GENERAL MEASURES
(See also topic on acute renal failure)
- Dialysis will be necessary for severe renal failure
- Caution: Diagnose muscle entrapment or compartment syndromes (anterior compartment rhabdomyolysis may require surgical intervention and relief of pressure to stop rhabdomyolysis - anterior tibial, soleus, lateral thigh or gluteus maximus)
- Severe hypocalcemia with symptoms (Chvostek's and Trousseau's) during the oliguric phase would benefit from intravenous calcium gluconate and intravenous vitamin D (Calcijex). Symptomatic hypocalcemia is rare.

SURGICAL MEASURES Relief of compartment syndrome by fasciotomy to preserve muscle viability and nerve function

ACTIVITY Physical exertion can lead to rhabdomyolysis and less exertion is tolerated in people with metabolic myopathies mentioned above. (See Genetics and Causes.)

DIET When acute renal failure occurs from rhabdomyolysis, protein restriction to lower BUN, potassium restriction to lower potassium and volume restriction with anuria are essential

PATIENT EDUCATION Specific for possible causes

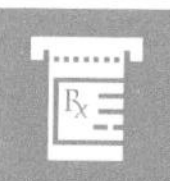

MEDICATIONS

DRUG(S) OF CHOICE

- When rhabdomyolysis is identified, appropriate intervention may prevent renal failure
  - ◊ Volume expansion attempt to increase urine output to approximately 150 cc/hr (3 mL/kg/hr), strong support for aggressive and early fluid replacement
  - ◊ IV mannitol as a bolus - 12.5 to 25 grams (0.25-0.5 g/kg); not to exceed approximately 50 grams in 24 hours; or as a constant infusion of 20% mannitol to a total of 25-50 g in 24 hours
  - ◊ Alkalinization of the urine decreases myoglobin tubular injury (sodium bicarbonate to increase urine pH above 6.5)
- When renal failure supervenes from rhabdomyolysis, severe hyperkalemia may be life threatening. Treatment is based on EKG changes (tall, thin T waves; P-R prolongation; QRS widening; P wave flattening).
  - ◊ Calcium gluconate IV 1-2 amps (0.5 mL of 10% calcium gluconate = 4 mg elemental calcium; give 4 mg/kg/hr x 4 hrs). Remember that bicarbonate administration may lead to alkalosis and worsening hypocalcemia.
  - ◊ If acidosis is present 1-2 amps (2-3 mL/kg) sodium bicarbonate IV
  - ◊ If tolerated oral sodium polystyrene sulfonate (Kayexalate) as much as 20 grams (1 gm/kg)
  - ◊ insulin and glucose; tall peaked T waves-treatment resembles wide QRS.
  - ◊ Dialysis may then become necessary to remove potassium.
- Vitamin D and calcium were mentioned above

Contraindications: See manufacturer's literature
Precautions: See Causes, especially drug combinations
Significant possible interactions: N/A

ALTERNATIVE DRUGS N/A

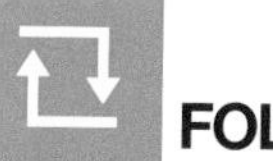

FOLLOWUP

PATIENT MONITORING

- Contingent on primary disease. Some cases (crush injury) are accidental and will not occur again.
- Contingent on disease - essential for metabolic myopathies
- There have been reports of interstitial nephritis many years after rhabdomyolysis from heat stroke and exertion

PREVENTION/AVOIDANCE

- Avoidance of situations leading to rhabdomyolysis (see Causes) prevent the injury
- Avoidance of metabolic states (hypokalemia) and drug combinations that lead to rhabdomyolysis (gemfibrozil and HMG-CoA reductase inhibitors) are necessary

POSSIBLE COMPLICATIONS Death especially from hyperkalemia or renal failure. With dialysis and supportive care, prognosis much better.

EXPECTED COURSE/PROGNOSIS

Contingent on primary cause of rhabdomyolysis and contingent on recovery from acute renal failure without complications (infection, GI bleeding, cardiac standstill from hyperkalemia)

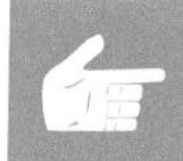

MISCELLANEOUS

ASSOCIATED CONDITIONS See Causes

AGE-RELATED FACTORS

Pediatric: Inherited myopathies and trauma more common
Geriatric: N/A
Others: N/A

PREGNANCY N/A

SYNONYMS Myoglobinuria with renal failure

ICD-9-CM

728.88 Rhabdomyolysis

SEE ALSO

Renal failure, acute (ARF)

OTHER NOTES N/A

ABBREVIATIONS

ATN = acute tubular necrosis
MAO = monoamine oxidase

REFERENCES

- Homis E. Prophylaxis of acute renal failure in patients with rhabdomyolysis. Ren Fail 1997;19:283-85
- Singh U, Schels WM. Infectious etiologies of rhabdomyolysis: three case reports and review. CID 1996;22:642-49
- Knochel JP. in Current Therapy in Nephrology and Hypertension. Glassock RJ, ed. St Louis, Mosby, 1998
- Rutecki GW, Ognibene AJ, Geib JD. Rhabdomyolysis in antiquity: from ancient descriptions to scientific explications. The Pharos of AOA 1998;61:18-22
- Slater MS, Mullins RJ. Rhabdomyolysis and myoglobinuric failure in trauma and surgical patients: a review. J Amer Coll Surg
- 1998;186(6)693-716
- Szewczyk D, Ovadia P, Abdullah F, et al. Pressure-induced rhabdomyolysis and acute renal failure. J of trauma
- Trimarchi H, Gonzalez J, Olivero J. Hyponatremia-associated rhabdomyolysis, Nephron 1999;82:274-7

Web references: 4 available at www.5mcc.com
Illustrations N/A

Author(s):

Mark R. Dambro, MD

BASICS

DESCRIPTION Rheumatic fever is an inflammatory disease, possibly autoimmune in nature. Rheumatic fever involves many tissues, including the heart, joints, skin, and central nervous system. Preceding infection of the upper respiratory tract with group A Streptococcus is a prerequisite to the development of acute rheumatic fever.
- Rheumatic fever can cause permanent cardiac valvular disease as well as acute cardiac decompensation.
- Recurrences are common if not prevented with "prophylactic" antibiotic treatment. In recent years there have been multiple reports of recurrences in adults as well as children.

System(s) affected: Cardiovascular, Hemic/Lymphatic/Immunologic, Musculoskeletal, Nervous, Skin/Exocrine
Genetics: A specific genetic marker that correlates with susceptibility to rheumatic fever has not been found, but the disease is known to occur in families
Incidence/Prevalence in USA:
- The incidence of rheumatic fever in the United States has been showing an overall decline for decades. In the 1970's it was a rare disease with an incidence of 0.5-1.88 cases per 100,000. However, since the mid-1980's there has been a resurgence of cases with multiple "outbreaks" having been reported in the U. S.
- The incidence calculated based on recent outbreaks has been as high as 18.1 per 100,000 in children aged 5-17 years

Predominant age: Most common in children ages 5-15. Recurrences can be seen in adulthood.
Predominant sex: Male = Female

SIGNS & SYMPTOMS
- Joint symptoms ranging from arthralgias to frank arthritis (75%)
- Joints involved are medium to large, e.g., ankles, knees, wrists
- Joint involvement is classically migratory
- Joint symptoms usually disappear in 3-4 weeks without permanent deformities
- Carditis (65%), mild or severe with murmurs
- Cardiac involvement may include pericarditis, myocarditis, and/or valvular insufficiency. Appears within 2 weeks and lasts 6 weeks to 6 months.
- Valvular damage may be permanent
- P-R prolongation on ECG
- Erythema marginatum (classic rash) < 5%
- Subcutaneous nodules (painless, hard swellings overlying bony prominences) 5-10%
- Chorea is often a late finding but may be a presenting complaint. It occurs in 10-15% of patients, and its duration is not altered by treatment.
- Fever 101-104°F (38.3-40.0°C)
- Abdominal pain is common. It may be severe.
- Epistaxis (historically important, but rarely seen in acute rheumatic fever)
- Facial tics
- Facial grimace

CAUSES
- Autoimmune mechanisms
- A preceding upper respiratory infection with group A Streptococcus is a prerequisite

RISK FACTORS
- Crowded living, school or working conditions
- Tendency to upper respiratory infections

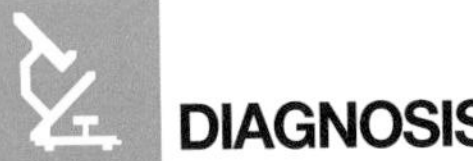

DIAGNOSIS

DIFFERENTIAL DIAGNOSIS Lupus, juvenile rheumatoid arthritis, infectious arthritis, viral myocarditis, innocent murmurs, Tourette syndrome, Kawasaki syndrome

LABORATORY
- Increased acute phase reactants, including sedimentation rate (ESR) and C-reactive protein (CRP)
- Bacteriological or serological evidence of group A streptococcal infection, antistreptolysin O (ASO), Streptozyme, or anti-deoxyribonuclease B (DNase)
- Anemia

Drugs that may alter lab results: Prior treatment with aspirin or steroids

Disorders that may alter lab results: N/A

PATHOLOGICAL FINDINGS
- Subcutaneous nodules have a characteristic histological appearance
- Pericardial effusion
- Fibrinous pericardium

SPECIAL TESTS N/A

IMAGING
- Chest x-ray
- Echocardiogram (reveals pericardial effusion and documents valvular disease)

DIAGNOSTIC PROCEDURES
- Throat cultures for Group A beta-hemolytic streptococci
- Diagnosis is dependent on fulfilling the modified Jones criteria of two major manifestations or one major and two minor manifestations. In either case, there must be evidence of preceding group A streptococcal infection. The five major criteria are carditis, arthritis, chorea, erythema marginatum, subcutaneous nodules. The minor criteria include fever, arthralgia (cannot use if arthritis was used as a major criteria), previous rheumatic fever, acute phase labs, prolonged P-R interval on EKG.

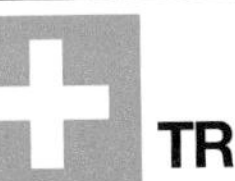

TREATMENT

APPROPRIATE HEALTH CARE
- Outpatient
- Initial hospitalization may be helpful to diagnose and establish stability of the patient

GENERAL MEASURES
- Mainstay of therapy is anti-inflammatory
- Patients with arthritis - therapy for relief of pain
- Patients with carditis - suppress inflammation
- Patients with arrhythmias - treat with appropriate agents

SURGICAL MEASURES N/A

ACTIVITY
- Initial bedrest with activity increasing gradually as tolerated
- Advance activity cautiously if there is evidence of carditis

DIET Regular; low sodium initially if the patient has carditis

PATIENT EDUCATION Information available from the American Heart Association

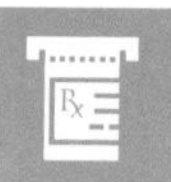

MEDICATIONS

DRUG(S) OF CHOICE
- If patient has carditis with cardiomegaly, start prednisone, 2 mg/kg/day (maximum 60 mg) for two weeks then taper over two weeks. Start aspirin at beginning of steroid taper. Continue aspirin for 6 weeks.
- If no cardiomegaly, start aspirin 60 mg/kg/day (to maintain salicylate level of 20-25μg/mL), 75-100 mg/kg/day for children, for 4-6 weeks
- Treat initially with penicillin as if active streptococcal infection is present, then begin prophylaxis. See Followup.
- Chorea may require treatment with haloperidol

Contraindications: Specific drug allergies

Precautions:
- Usual steroid side effects
- Extrapyramidal effects can occur with haloperidol

Significant possible interactions: Refer to manufacturer's profile of each drug

ALTERNATIVE DRUGS
- Sulfadiazine may be used for prophylaxis in penicillin allergic patients. Patients who take sulfadiazine should take at least 2 liters of fluid daily to guard against sulfadiazine crystalluria.
- Naproxen at a dose of 15-20 mg/kg/day, divided twice daily, for children, has been found to be safe and effective in rheumatic fever and has less adverse reactions than aspirin

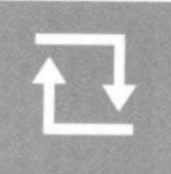

FOLLOWUP

PATIENT MONITORING Each week initially, then every 6 months

PREVENTION/AVOIDANCE
- Patients will need to be on prophylactic penicillin throughout childhood and possibly indefinitely during adulthood. Monthly injections of 1.2 million units of benzathine penicillin intramuscularly is the preferred treatment.
- Adults should be treated for a minimum of five years after an attack. Some treat adults indefinitely if there has been valvular disease. Oral penicillin V-K, 125 mg twice daily is an alternative to monthly injections. In the event of penicillin allergy, sulfadiazine, 500 mg daily for children weighing less than 30 kg or 1 gm daily for all others may be used.
- If patients have valvular damage from acute rheumatic fever, they will require bacterial endocarditis prophylaxis for dental and other high risk procedures

POSSIBLE COMPLICATIONS
- Subsequent attacks of acute rheumatic fever secondary to streptococcal reinfection
- Carditis
- Mitral stenosis
- Congestive heart failure

EXPECTED COURSE/PROGNOSIS
Sequelae limited to the heart and dependent of severity of carditis during an acute attack

MISCELLANEOUS

ASSOCIATED CONDITIONS N/A

AGE-RELATED FACTORS
Pediatric: More common in children
Geriatric: N/A
Others: N/A

PREGNANCY Residual valvular disease may be exacerbated by pregnancy. Refer pregnant patient to cardiologist for assistance in management.

SYNONYMS N/A

ICD-9-CM
390 Rheumatic fever without mention of heart involvement

SEE ALSO

OTHER NOTES N/A

ABBREVIATIONS N/A

REFERENCES

- Behrman RE, Kliegman RM, Jenson HB, editors. Nelson Textbook of Pediatrics. 17th ed. Philadelphia: W.B. Saunders Company; 2003
- Ferrieri P. Acute rheumatic fever. The come-back of a disappearing disease. Am J Dis Child 1987;141(7):725-7
- Quinn RW. Comprehensive review of morbidity and mortality trends for rheumatic fever, streptococcal disease, and scarlet fever: the decline of rheumatic fever. Rev Infect Dis. 1989;11(6):928-53
- daSilva NA. Acute rheumatic fever. Still a challenge. Rheumatol Dis Clin NA 1997;23(3)545-68
- Hashkes PJ, Tauber T, et al; Pediatric Rheumatlogy Study Group of Israel. Naproxen as an alternative to aspirin for the treatment of arthritis of rheumatic fever: a randomized trial. J Pediatr 2003;143(3):399-401
- Milojevic DS, Ilowite NT. Treatment of rheumatic diseases in children: special considerations. Rheum Dis Clin North Am 2002;28(3):461-82

Web references: 1 available at www.5mcc.com
Illustrations N/A

Author(s):
H. Gratin Smith, MD

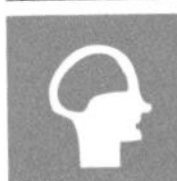

BASICS

DESCRIPTION Immediate and delayed reactions to airborne allergens, beginning with the generation and presence of specific antigen-responsive IgE antibody receptors on mast cells of the nasal mucosa
- An antigen-antibody chemical union initiates a cascade of events in the mast cell culminating in its degranulation and production of a melange of inflammatory mediators including histamine, heparin, leukotrienes, prostaglandins, proteases and platelet activating factor
- An immediate symptomatic response occurs followed by a more prolonged, persistent late phase reaction. This involves the infiltration into the reactive region of eosinophils, neutrophils, basophils and mononuclear cells
- May be seasonal or perennial depending on climate and individual response and the offending antigens
- Seasonal responses usually to grasses, trees and weeds
- Perennial responses usually house dust mites, mold antigens and animal body products

System(s) affected: Hemic/Lymphatic/Immunologic, Pulmonary, Skin/Exocrine

Genetics: Complex, but strong genetic determination present

Incidence/Prevalence in USA: 10-25% of the population affected

Predominant age:
- Onset usually in first 4 decades with declining tendency with advancing age
- Mean age onset approximately 10 years

Predominant sex: Male = Female

SIGNS & SYMPTOMS
- Nasal stuffiness and congestion
- Rhinorrhea usually clear
- Pruritus of nose, eyes and palate
- Sneezing, often paroxysmal
- Injection and watering of eyes
- Postnasal drainage
- Mouth breathing
- Fatigue or malaise
- Dark circles under eyes, "allergic shiners"
- Transverse nasal crease from rubbing nose upwards

CAUSES
- Inhalant allergens:
  - ◊ Perennial: house dust mites, molds, animal dander, cockroach

Seasonal: tree, grass and weed pollens
  - ◊ Occupational: latex, plant products (such as baking flour), sensitizing chemicals

RISK FACTORS
- Family history
- Repeated exposure to offending antigen
- Exposure to multiple offending allergens
- Presence of other allergies, e.g., atopic dermatitis, asthma, urticaria
- Non-compliance to appropriate therapeutic measures

DIAGNOSIS

DIFFERENTIAL DIAGNOSIS
- Nonallergic rhinitis with eosinophilia syndrome (NARES)
- Vasomotor rhinitis
- Chronic sinusitis
- IgA deficiency with recurrent sinusitis
- Nasal polyps and tumor
- Reactive rhinitis of recumbency
- Cribriform plate defect with cerebrospinal fluid leakage (rule out by testing watery discharge for sugar)
- Foreign body
- Hormonal: pregnancy, thyroid disorder, oral contraceptives
- Medications
  - ◊ Rebound effect associated with continued use of topical decongestant drops and sprays
  - ◊ Aldosterone converting enzyme inhibitors
  - ◊ Chronic aspirin use
- Septal/anatomical obstruction
- Chronic rhinitis digitorum

LABORATORY
- CBC with differential. May have slight increase in eosinophils but often normal with uncomplicated rhinitis.
- Nasal probe smear with cytologic exam for eosinophils
- Increase IgE level. Determine specific allergen sensitivity with allergen skin testing or RAST.

Drugs that may alter lab results:
- Corticosteroids will ablate eosinophilia

Disorders that may alter lab results:
- Secondary infections may alter differential and decrease nasal eosinophils
- Parasitic infestations with more marked eosinophilia

PATHOLOGICAL FINDINGS
- Nasal washing/scraping
  - ◊ Eosinophils predominate
  - ◊ Basophils
  - ◊ May see mast cells
- Nasal mucosa
  - ◊ Submucosal edema but intact without evidence of destruction
  - ◊ Eosinophilic infiltration
  - ◊ Granulocytes to lesser extent
  - ◊ Increased amount of tissue water with poor staining of ground substance
  - ◊ Congested mucous glands and goblet cells

SPECIAL TESTS
- Skin tests using suspected antigens

Either technique manifests a positive reaction by inducing an expanding wheal and flare reaction. Special training recommended and available treatment for anaphylaxis mandatory
  - ◊ Prick or puncture: a superficial injury to the epidermis with application of diluted test antigen
  - ◊ Intradermal: Introduction of diluted material between layers of skin raising a 4 mm wheal using a 25 or 27 gauge needle
- Radioallergosorbent test (RAST)
  - ◊ More expensive and used especially in cases where skin testing not practical, e.g., in atopic dermatitis and dermatographia
- Audiometry
  - ◊ For deficits and base line evaluation
  - ◊ Rhinoscopy - particularly useful to visualize intranasal anatomy, posterior pharyngeal structures including adenoids and larynx

IMAGING Sinus film when indicated. Check for complete opacity, fluid level and mucosal thickening. Sinus imaging using CT may be preferable.

DIAGNOSTIC PROCEDURES Appropriate diagnostic prick test kits available.

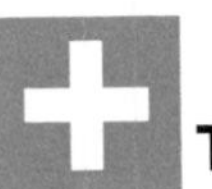

TREATMENT

APPROPRIATE HEALTH CARE Outpatient

GENERAL MEASURES
- Patient education, assurance and understanding important
- Limit exposure to offending allergen
- Try to establish specific cause(s) - history and appropriate skin testing
- Intensity of treatment determined by severity of disease
- Allergen immunotherapy (allergy shots/desensitization):
  - ◊ Usually reserved for seasonal allergies uncontrollable with drugs and not responding to environmental adjustment.
  - ◊ Specific allergen extract is injected subcutaneously in increasing doses to patient tolerance as determined by local reaction
  - ◊ Patient response should be evaluated each season or year

SURGICAL MEASURES Septoplasty when deviation significant enough to interfere with benefits of medication.

ACTIVITY No specific restrictions. Emphasize avoiding activity in areas of allergen exposure.

DIET No special diet unless concomitant food reactions suspected and evaluated

PATIENT EDUCATION Printed material available from many sources including: Asthma & Allergy Foundation of America. 1717 Massachusetts Ave., Suite 305, Washington, DC 20036, (800)7-ASTHMA; website www.aafa.org.

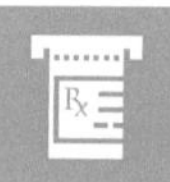

MEDICATIONS

DRUG(S) OF CHOICE

Most patients present because of inability to control symptoms with avoidance of allergens or with over the counter medications. Antihistamines (second generation have a favorable side effects profile) are considered first line therapy for most patients. Topical nasal corticosteroids are usually considered second line therapy, but should be used in patients with more severe nasal symptoms. Consider allergen immunotherapy when usual pharmaceutical therapy fails or in patients with comorbidities or complications. Cromolyn is sometimes surprisingly helpful but a patient may have already tried this OTC agent.

- Antihistamines (H1 antagonists):
  - ◊ First generation: side effects include sedation, performance impairment, anticholinergic effects. Includes 5 major classes:
    - Ethanolamines - diphenhydramine (Benadryl), clemastine (Tavist)
    - Alkylamine - chlorpheniramine, brompheniramine
    - Ethylenediamines - tripelennamine (PBZ)
    - Piperazines - hydroxyzine (Atarax)
    - Phenothiazines - promethazine (Phenergan), methdilazine (Tacaryl)
  - ◊ Second generation (considered non-sedating)
    - Loratadine (Claritin)
    - Desloratadine (Clarinex)
    - Fexofenadine (Allegra)
    - Cetirizine (Zyrtec)
    - Intranasal: azelastine (Astelin)
- Decongestants
  - ◊ Oral, e.g., pseudoephedrine
  - ◊ Topical drops or sprays, e.g., phenylephrine
  - ◊ Topical ophthalmic for annoying conjunctival itching
- Mast cell stabilizers
  - ◊ Cromolyn (Nasalcrom)
  - ◊ Olopatadine (Patanol), cromolyn (Opticrom); topical ophthalmics for conjunctival itching
- Leukotriene antagonist
  - ◊ Montelukast (Singulair)
- Steroids
  - ◊ Intranasal
    - Beclomethasone (Beconase AQ, Vancenase AQ)
    - Flunisolide (Nasalide, Nasarel)
    - Triamcinolone (Nasacort)
    - Budesonide (Rhinocort)
    - Mometasone (Nasonex)
    - Fluticasone (Flonase)
  - ◊ Systemic. Only in urgent, selected cases and only for short-term use.
- Physiologic saline solution may be comforting

Contraindications:

- Antihistamines may precipitate urinary retention in males with prostatism and/or hypertrophy
- Decongestants if congestion is a "rebound" phenomenon
- Discourage decongestants if hypertension a problem

Precautions:

- The elderly often require less aggressive treatment and will more frequently present with non-allergic rhinitis
- Warn patients that first generation antihistamines are associated with somnolence and may impair performance

Significant possible interactions: Refer carefully to manufacturer's literature for interactions

ALTERNATIVE DRUGS

Combinations with decongestants

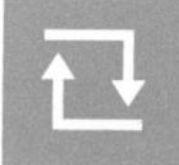

FOLLOWUP

PATIENT MONITORING

- Initiate patient education, supplementing with available videotapes and/or literature

PREVENTION/AVOIDANCE

- Avoidance - most patients with inhalant allergy have problems controlling their symptoms totally with allergen avoidance
- Air conditioning and limited outside exposure during season helpful
- Instructions as to the best housekeeping tactics and control for dust mites in patients sensitive to this allergen helpful
- Exposure to all animal contacts minimized. Discourage house pets.
- Avoid environmental irritants, e.g., smoke and fumes
- Air cleaners
- Use of allergy control covers especially on mattresses and pillows

POSSIBLE COMPLICATIONS

- Secondary infection
- Otitis media
- Sinusitis
- Epistaxis
- Nasopharyngeal lymphoid hyperplasia
- Decreased pulmonary function
- Asthma
- Continue to suspect effects of medications
- Facial changes (see Signs and Symptoms)

EXPECTED COURSE/PROGNOSIS

- Maximal, beneficially acceptable control of symptoms should be the goal
- Treatment tailored to each individual case.
- Immune system changes over time often associated with lessening of symptoms of allergic rhinitis. Therefore early, adequate control important.

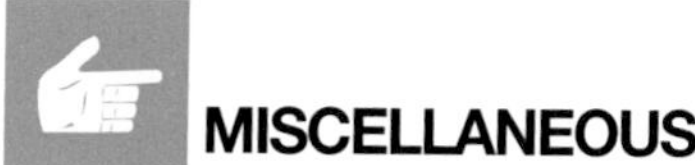

MISCELLANEOUS

ASSOCIATED CONDITIONS

- Other IgE mediated conditions, e.g., asthma and atopic dermatitis

AGE-RELATED FACTORS

Pediatric:

- Consider allergy as principle cause of persistent rhinitis
- Family understanding and involvement important
- Environmental control requires a cooperative effort and may include carpet and drape removal, removal of house plants, pet control, etc.

Geriatric:

- Increased medication side effects
- Number and specific types of allergens causing symptoms may change
- Symptoms may decrease by 4th-5th decade (not a hard rule)

Others: N/A

PREGNANCY

Physiological changes of pregnancy may aggravate all types of rhinitis including allergic, vasomotor, nonallergic rhinitis with eosinophilia and chronic irritable airways

SYNONYMS

- Hay fever
- Pollinosis
- IgE mediated rhinitis

ICD-9-CM

477.9 Allergic rhinitis, cause unspecified

SEE ALSO

Conjunctivitis, acute

OTHER NOTES

N/A

ABBREVIATIONS

N/A

REFERENCES

- Dykewicz MS. Rhinitis and sinusitis. J Allergy Clin Immunol 2003;111(2 Suppl):S520-9
- Dykewicz MS, Fineman S, Skoner DP, et al. Diagnosis and management of rhinitis: complete guidelines of the Joint Task Force on Practice Parameters in Allergy, Asthma and Immunology. American Academy of Allergy, Asthma, and Immunology. Ann Allergy Asthma Immunol 1998;81(5 Pt 2):478-51
- Wilson AM, O'Byrne PM, Parameswaran K. Leukotriene receptor antagonists for allergic rhinitis: a systematic review and meta-analysis. Am J Med 2004;116(5):338-44

Web references: 3 available at www.5mcc.com

Illustrations N/A

Author(s):

Stanley Fineman, MD

BASICS

DESCRIPTION Rocky Mountain spotted fever (RMSF) is an acute, potentially fatal febrile illness caused by *Rickettsia rickettsii* and transmitted by tick bite. The primary pathology is a vasculitis due to direct endothelial cell invasion by rickettsiae. The cardinal clinical features are headache, fever, and a centripetal rash which is often petechial.
System(s) affected: Cardiovascular, Musculoskeletal, Nervous, Skin/Exocrine
Genetics: N/A
Incidence/Prevalence in USA: About 600 new cases are reported each year in the USA. There is considerable geographic variability; most cases are reported from south Atlantic and south central states. Peak incidence is in late spring and summer.
Predominant age: Highest incidences occur among children and young adults, primarily due to environmental exposure patterns. All ages are susceptible.
Predominant sex: Male > Female (due to more frequent outdoor activity by males)

SIGNS & SYMPTOMS
- Fever (100%)
- Rash (macular, maculopapular, petechial) (90-100%)
- Headache (65%)
- Rash (petechial) (50%)
- Headache, fever, rash (50-60%)
- Other neuropsychiatric symptoms (40-50%)
- Nausea, vomiting (30-50%)
- Headache, fever, petechial rash (33%)
- Abdominal pain (30%)
- Myalgias (30%)
- Hepatosplenomegaly (30%)
- Lymphadenopathy (25%)
- Arthralgias (10%)
- Cough (15%)
- Central nervous system dysfunction (stupor, confusion, coma, focal abnormalities) (10-30%)

CAUSES RMSF is caused by *Rickettsia rickettsii* which is transmitted by the bite of ticks (*Amblyomma americanum*, *Dermacentor andersoni*, *Dermacentor variabilis*). Rarely by direct inoculation of tick blood into open wounds or conjunctivae.

RISK FACTORS
- Outdoor activity during warm months
- Contact with outdoor pets or wild animals

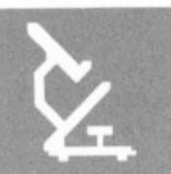

DIAGNOSIS

DIFFERENTIAL DIAGNOSIS
- Viral exanthems (measles, rubella, etc.)
- Meningoencephalitis (viral meningitis or encephalitis, bacterial meningitis)
- Typhus, rickettsialpox
- Ehrlichiosis
- Lyme disease
- Meningococcemia
- Leptospirosis

LABORATORY
- Nonspecific laboratory changes
  - ◊ Thrombocytopenia
  - ◊ WBC normal, increased, or decreased
  - ◊ Anemia (mild)
  - ◊ Hyponatremia (usually mild)
  - ◊ CSF protein and WBC modestly elevated (lymphocytic predominance), glucose usually normal
  - ◊ Prolonged PT, PTT; decreased fibrinogen; elevated fibrin degradation products (FDP) (uncommon)

Drugs that may alter lab results: Early treatment may blunt antibody response

Disorders that may alter lab results: N/A

PATHOLOGICAL FINDINGS
- The principal pathological abnormality is a systemic vasculitis
- Rickettsiae may be demonstrated within endothelial cells by DFA or electron microscopy
- Petechiae due to the vasculitis may be seen on various organ surfaces (e.g., liver, brain, epicardium)
- Secondary thromboses and tissue necrosis may be seen

SPECIAL TESTS
- Specific laboratory diagnosis
  - ◊ Serum Proteus Ox-19 antibody; fourfold increase (acute and convalescent) or solitary titer > 1:320 (relatively specific)
  - ◊ Serum complement fixation (CF) antibody: fourfold increase or solitary titer > 1:16
  - ◊ Serum indirect fluorescent antibody (IFA): fourfold increase or solitary titer > 1:64
  - ◊ Direct fluorescent antibody (DFA) test on skin biopsy (not widely available)

IMAGING Other than nonspecific pneumonic infiltrates which may be seen on routine chest x-ray, imaging procedures are rarely helpful

DIAGNOSTIC PROCEDURES
- Tissue (primarily skin) biopsy can be helpful if rapid DFA or electron microscopy are available
- Diagnosis is usually presumptive, based upon a compatible syndrome in a patient with exposure history in an endemic area; confirmation is obtained by subsequent serology
- Polymerase chain reaction diagnosis currently not reliable

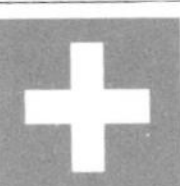

TREATMENT

APPROPRIATE HEALTH CARE
- Patients with the full clinical presentation or who are moderately ill should usually be hospitalized
- Patients with mild disease are treated presumptively as outpatients. Close followup is important in identifying complications.

GENERAL MEASURES
- Oxygen therapy and assisted ventilation for pulmonary complications, if necessary
- Good mouth care
- Blood transfusions for anemia
- Turning bed-confined patient frequently
- Watch patient closely for signs of renal failure

SURGICAL MEASURES N/A

ACTIVITY Bed rest until symptoms subside

DIET Critically ill patients may require IV nutrition. In others, small frequent meals may be necessary to maintain nutritional levels.

PATIENT EDUCATION See information in Prevention/Avoidance

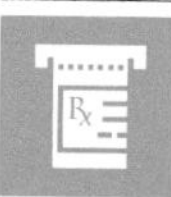

MEDICATIONS

DRUG(S) OF CHOICE

- For adults (choose one of the following)
  - ◊ Doxycycline 200 mg po initially, followed by 100 mg po bid for 7-10 days; same dosage IV; 100 mg q24h in renal failure (see Contraindications)
  - ◊ Tetracycline 500 mg po q6h for 7-10 days; should not be used in renal failure (see Contraindications)
  - ◊ Chloramphenicol 20 mg/kg IV q6h (4 gm per day maximum); same dose in renal failure (oral chloramphenicol is not available in the U.S.)
- For children (choose one of the following)
  - ◊ Chloramphenicol 20 mg/kg IV q6h
  - ◊ Doxycycline 2.0-2.5 mg/kg po q12h for 7-10 days; 4.4 mg/kg IV initially, followed by 2.2 mg per kg IV q12h (see Precautions)
  - ◊ Tetracycline 10 mg per kg po q6h for 7-10 days (see Contraindications)
- The duration of therapy is 7-10 days, or for 2 days after fever subsides

Contraindications:
- Pregnant women - doxycycline and tetracyclines are contraindicated because they may cause severe hepatic disease in the mother and retarded bone growth in the fetus

Precautions:
- Patients taking doxycycline or tetracyclines should minimize sun exposure to avoid photosensitization
- Infants or children with liver disease taking chloramphenicol should have serum drug levels monitored
- Chloramphenicol may rarely cause idiosyncratic, nonreversible, aplastic anemia
- Doxycycline and tetracycline may cause staining of permanent teeth when given to children less than 9 years old. This risk appears to be minimal if no more than 5 courses of therapy are administered prior to age 9.

Significant possible interactions: Absorption of tetracyclines may be inhibited if they are ingested with milk products, iron preparations, or antacids containing aluminum or magnesium

ALTERNATIVE DRUGS
There are no currently available or adequately studied alternative drugs

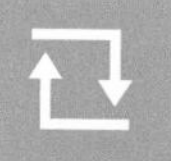

FOLLOWUP

PATIENT MONITORING

- If patients are not hospitalized, they should be seen every 2-3 days until symptoms have fully resolved
- CBC, creatinine, electrolytes should be monitored

PREVENTION/AVOIDANCE

- People who go into tick-infested areas can take measures to prevent infection
  - ◊ Occlusive clothing should be worn and insect repellants applied
  - ◊ After possible exposure, all body areas should be carefully inspected for ticks, especially legs, groin, external genitalia, belt lines. Likelihood of infection increases with the duration of tick attachment.
  - ◊ Ticks should be removed from humans or animals with caution; gloves should be worn or instruments used to minimize direct contact. Place a drop of oil, alcohol, gasoline or kerosene on the tick first. Hands should be washed thoroughly afterwards.

POSSIBLE COMPLICATIONS

- Encephalopathy, usually transient (30-40%)
- Seizures, focal neurologic signs (10%)
- Renal insufficiency (10%)
- Hepatitis (10%)
- Congestive heart failure (5%)
- Respiratory failure (5%)

EXPECTED COURSE/PROGNOSIS

- When treated promptly, the usual prognosis is excellent with resolution of symptoms over several days and no sequelae
- Mortality is rare with prompt institution of appropriate therapy
- If complications develop (see above), the course may be more severe and long-term sequelae may be present, particularly neurologic sequelae

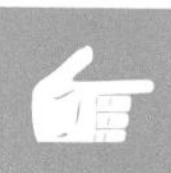

MISCELLANEOUS

ASSOCIATED CONDITIONS N/A

AGE-RELATED FACTORS
Pediatric: N/A
Geriatric: Mortality risk higher
Others: N/A

PREGNANCY
- Chloramphenicol is the preferred therapy in pregnancy
- Transplacental transmission has not been demonstrated

SYNONYMS N/A

ICD-9-CM
082.0 Spotted fevers

SEE ALSO
Ehrlichiosis

OTHER NOTES
Treatment should be initiated on the basis of clinical diagnosis or skin biopsy. Treatment should not be delayed for serologic confirmation.

ABBREVIATIONS N/A

REFERENCES

- Kirk JL, Fine DP, Sexton, DJ, Muchmore HG. Rocky Mountain spotted fever. A clinical review based on 48 confirmed cases, 1943-1986. Medicine 1990;69:35-45
- Melnick CG, Bernard KW, D'Angelo L. Rocky Mountain spotted fever: Clinical, laboratory, and epidemiological features of 262 cases. J Infect Dis 1984;150:480-8
- Archibald LK, Sexton DJ. Long-term sequelae of Rocky Mountain spotted fever. Clin Infect Dis 1995;20:1122-5
- Abramson JS, Givner LB. Should tetracycline be contraindicated for therapy of presumed Rocky Mountain spotted fever in children less than 9 years of age? Pediatr 1990;86:123-4
- Cale DF, McCarthy MW. Treatment of Rocky Mountain spotted fever in children. Ann Pharmacother 1997;31:492-4
- Stallings SP. Rocky Mountain spotted fever and pregnancy: a case report and review of the literature. Obstet Gynecol Surv 2001;56(1):37-42

Web references: 2 available at www.5mcc.com
Illustrations N/A

Author(s):
Brock D. Lutz, MD
Ronald A. Greenfield, MD

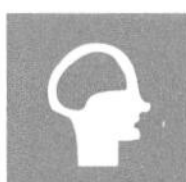

BASICS

DESCRIPTION An acute disease of infants or very young children with an incubation period of about 5-15 days. Characteristically, it causes first a high fever, followed by the appearance of an eruption (whose appearance is similar to that of measles) simultaneously with, or following defervescence. Transmission now believed to be via contact of salivary secretions from adults shedding HHV-6.
System(s) affected: Endocrine/Metabolic, Skin/Exocrine
Genetics: No known genetic pattern
Incidence/Prevalence in USA:
- Unknown
- More likely to occur in spring and fall

Predominant age: Infants and very young children (6 months to 3 years); 90% before age 2
Predominant sex: Male = Female

SIGNS & SYMPTOMS
- Abrupt fever without apparent cause (103-105°F [39.4-40.5°C]) for 3-5 days
- Sudden drop of fever. As fever disappears, skin rash begins (lasts hours to days).
- Anorexia
- Irritability
- Inflammation of the tympanic membranes
- Listlessness
- Does not appear seriously ill
- Maculopapular, nonpruritic rash, first appearing on the trunk, that blanches on pressure
- Rash appears as very slightly elevated, rose-pink papules that appear profusely on trunk, arms and neck; mild on face and legs
- Rash fades within a few hours to 2 days
- Febrile convulsions during height of fever (10-15%)
- Lymphadenopathy in cervical and posterior auricular regions
- Spleen enlarged (uncommon)

CAUSES A communicable DNA virus, human herpesvirus-6B (HHV-6B)

RISK FACTORS
- Day care center
- Exposure to infected infant

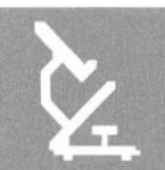

DIAGNOSIS

DIFFERENTIAL DIAGNOSIS
- Enterovirus infection
- Fifth disease
- Rubella
- Measles
- Sepsis
- Otitis media
- UTI
- Meningitis
- Drug eruption

LABORATORY
- CBC - leukopenia with relative lymphocytosis; thrombocytopenia
- Urinalysis
- IgM, IgG (fourfold increase IgG for diagnosis) for human herpesvirus-6 (HHV-6)
- PCR (serum) for HHV-6 qualitative and quantitative can be performed
- Blood culture for HHV-6

Drugs that may alter lab results: N/A

Disorders that may alter lab results: N/A

PATHOLOGICAL FINDINGS None

SPECIAL TESTS N/A

IMAGING Chest x-ray negative

DIAGNOSTIC PROCEDURES Careful physical examination. Roseola should be suspected if it is known to be in the community and the child presents with a high temperature. HHV-6-IgM - diagnostic for acute infection. HHV-6 by PCR found in CSF and in saliva.

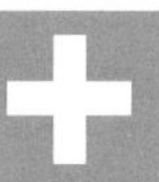

TREATMENT

APPROPRIATE HEALTH CARE Outpatient

GENERAL MEASURES
- Symptomatic
- Tap water baths to cool excess temperature elevation
- Lightweight clothing
- Maintain normal room temperature

SURGICAL MEASURES N/A

ACTIVITY Rest until rash appears and fever breaks

DIET Encourage fluids

PATIENT EDUCATION
- Infection is self-limiting
- If seizures occur, they will not cause brain damage and will cease after fever subsides

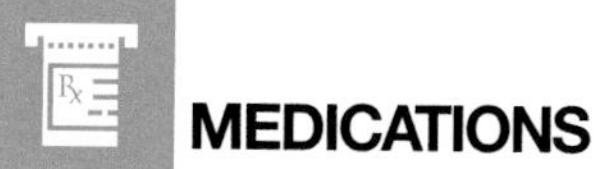

MEDICATIONS

DRUG(S) OF CHOICE
- Antipyretics for excessively high fever. Avoid aspirin. Instead use acetaminophen, 10-15 mg/kg/q4h to a maximum of 2.6 g/24h. (Aspirin may enhance the risk of Reye syndrome.)
- Phenobarbital may be considered for seizure

Contraindications: N/A
Precautions: N/A
Significant possible interactions: N/A

ALTERNATIVE DRUGS No clinical trials to date evaluating antiviral agents, but in-vitro data does exist

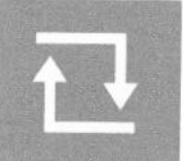

FOLLOWUP

PATIENT MONITORING None after typical rash appears

PREVENTION/AVOIDANCE None

POSSIBLE COMPLICATIONS
- Febrile seizures
- Encephalitis (rare)
- Meningitis
- Hepatitis

EXPECTED COURSE/PROGNOSIS
- Course - acute, benign, complete recovery without sequelae
- One attack usually confers permanent immunity
- Reactivation in immunocompromised patients is possible

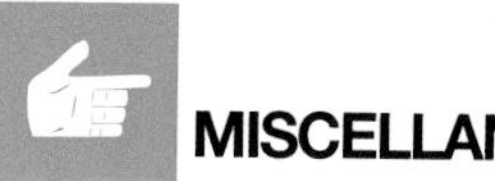

MISCELLANEOUS

ASSOCIATED CONDITIONS N/A

AGE-RELATED FACTORS
Pediatric: A disease of infants and very young children
Geriatric: N/A
Others: N/A

PREGNANCY N/A

SYNONYMS
- Exanthem subitum
- Pseudorubella
- Sixth disease

ICD-9-CM
057.8 Other specified viral exanthemata

SEE ALSO

OTHER NOTES N/A

ABBREVIATIONS N/A

REFERENCES

- Caserta MT, et al. Human herpesvirus 6. Clin Infect Dis 2001;33:829-33
- Asano Y, Yoshikawa T, Suga S, Kobayashi I, et al. Clinical features of infants with primary human herpesvirus 6 (roseola infantum). Pediatrics 1994;93:104-8
- Kimberlin DW. Human herpesvirus 6 and 7: identification of newly recognized viral pathogens and their association with human disease. Pediatr Infect Dis 1998;17:59-68
- Leach CT. Human herpesvirus-6 and -7 infections in children: agents of roseola and other syndromes. Curr Opin Pediatr 2000;12(3):269-74
- Dockrell DH, et al. Human herpesvirus 6. Mayo Clin Proc 1999;74:163-70

Web references: 0 available at www.5mcc.com
Illustrations N/A

Author(s):
Jeffery T. Kirchner, DO

Roundworms, intestinal

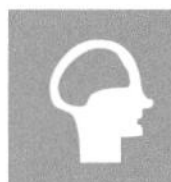

BASICS

DESCRIPTION Intestinal roundworms (nematodes) have adult stages infecting the intestinal tract of man. Larval stages may exist elsewhere in the body. Except for Trichinella spiralis, which is encysted in muscle; egg and/or larval stages can be isolated from the intestinal canal.
- Nematodes parasitizing the intestinal tract of man:
  - ◊ Enterobius vermicularis (pinworm)
  - ◊ Trichuris trichiura (whipworm)
  - ◊ Ascaris lumbricoides (large roundworm of man)
  - ◊ Necator americanus (hookworm)
  - ◊ Ancylostoma duodenale (hookworm)
  - ◊ Strongyloides stercoralis
  - ◊ Trichostrongylus
  - ◊ Trichinella spiralis (trichinosis)

System(s) affected: Cardiovascular, Gastrointestinal, Musculoskeletal, Nervous, Pulmonary, Renal/Urologic

Genetics: N/A

Incidence/Prevalence in USA:
- Up to 40% of children may have pinworms
- Trichinella 4-20%
- Others mostly in Southern regions
- Incidence of intestinal obstruction with ascaris is 2/1000
- Incidence of ascaris reportedly decreasing in the US, presumably due to improved sanitation

Predominant age: All ages; pinworm infestations more common in children

Predominant sex: Male = Female

SIGNS & SYMPTOMS
- Lung Invasion:
  - ◊ Fever
  - ◊ Cough
  - ◊ Blood-tinged sputum
  - ◊ Wheezing
  - ◊ Rales
  - ◊ Dyspnea
  - ◊ Substernal pain
  - ◊ Pulmonary consolidations
  - ◊ Eosinophilia
  - ◊ Urticaria
  - ◊ Asthma
  - ◊ Angioneurotic edema
  - ◊ Brain, kidney, eye, spinal cord, etc. (rare)
- Intestinal invasion:
  - ◊ May be asymptomatic (small number)
  - ◊ Abdominal pain (usually vague)
  - ◊ Abdominal cramps/colic
  - ◊ Diarrhea
  - ◊ Rarely vomiting
  - ◊ Occasionally constipation
- Muscle and other tissue invasion: (Trichinosis)
  - ◊ Myalgias
  - ◊ Fever
  - ◊ Edema and spasm
  - ◊ Periorbital and facial edema
  - ◊ Photophobia
  - ◊ Sweating
  - ◊ Conjunctivitis
  - ◊ Weakness or prostration
  - ◊ Pain on swallowing
  - ◊ Subconjunctival, retinal and nail hemorrhages
  - ◊ Rashes and formication
  - ◊ Encephalitis, myocarditis, nephritis
  - ◊ Pneumonia, meningitis, neuropathy

CAUSES
- Ingestion of mature eggs in fecally contaminated food or drink
- Larval penetration of skin (hookworm)

RISK FACTORS
- Low standard of hygiene
- Poor sanitation
- Human feces fertilizer

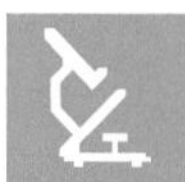

DIAGNOSIS

DIFFERENTIAL DIAGNOSIS
- Pulmonary ascariasis with eosinophilia - consider asthma, Löffler's syndrome, eosinophilic pneumonia, systemic lupus erythematosus, Hodgkin disease, and other parasitic causes (tropical pulmonary eosinophilia, toxocariasis, strongyloidiasis, hookworm, paragonimiasis)
- Worm-induced GI diseases - consider other causes of pancreatitis, appendicitis, diverticulitis, duodenitis, esophagitis, cholecystitis
- Anemia/hypoproteinemia (hookworm) - consider other etiology
- Neurohelminthiasis - consider other causes of CNS infection or mass lesion

LABORATORY
- Based on characteristics of eggs or larvae in stool or adult worm, if passed
- Cellophane-tape impression for pinworms
- Eosinophilia
- Larvae in sputum or adult worms seen on radiologic studies (uncommon)

Drugs that may alter lab results: N/A

Disorders that may alter lab results: N/A

PATHOLOGICAL FINDINGS
Characteristic eggs/worms

SPECIAL TESTS Serologic tests not useful

IMAGING Ultrasound is useful in the diagnosis of ascariasis as cause of biliary tract disease

DIAGNOSTIC PROCEDURES
- Stool exams
- Cellophane-tape impression

TREATMENT

APPROPRIATE HEALTH CARE Outpatient

GENERAL MEASURES None other than medications to eradicate the worms

SURGICAL MEASURES N/A

ACTIVITY No restrictions

DIET No special diet

PATIENT EDUCATION Avoid fecally contaminated food, water, and soil

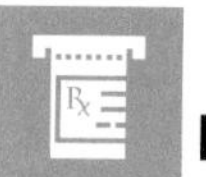

MEDICATIONS

DRUG(S) OF CHOICE

- Enterobius vermicularis (pinworm) - mebendazole (Vermox) 100 mg single dose, or albendazole 400 mg once, or pyrantel pamoate 11 mg/kg once (maximum of 1 g), repeat after 2 weeks (all dosages for adult and pediatrics)
- Trichuris trichiura (whipworm) - mebendazole 100 mg bid x 3 days or 500 mg once (all dosages for adults and children)
- Ascaris lumbricoides (large roundworm of man), mebendazole 100 mg bid x 3 days or 500 mg once or pyrantel pamoate 11 mg/kg once (maximum of 1 g) (all dosages for adult and pediatrics), or albendazole 400 mg once
- Necator americanus (hookworm), Ancylostoma duodenale (hookworm) - mebendazole 100 mg bid x 3 days or pyrantel pamoate 11 mg/kg (maximum of 1 g) x 3 days (all dosages for adult and pediatrics), or albendazole 400 mg once
- Trichostrongylus - pyrantel pamoate 11 mg/kg once (maximum of 1 g) or mebendazole 100 mg bid x 3 day (all dosages for adult and pediatrics)
- Trichinella spiralis - mebendazole 200-400 mg tid x 3 days, then 400-500 mg tid x 10 days (adult dosage) plus steroids if severe symptoms
- Strongyloides stercoralis - thiabendazole 50 mg/kg/d in 2 doses (maximum of 3 g a day) for 2 days (adult and pediatric), or ivermectin (Mectizan) 200 mcg/kg/day x 1-2 days (also effective against co-existing ascaris, trichuris, enterobius). Superior to benzimidazoles for this indication.
- Note: FDA may consider certain uses of above drugs investigational, consult Medical Letter or appropriate drug reference

Contraindications: Refer to manufacturer's profile of each drug
Precautions: Refer to manufacturer's profile of each drug
Significant possible interactions: Refer to manufacturer's profile of each drug

ALTERNATIVE DRUGS

- Trichuris trichiura (whipworm) - albendazole 400 mg once (adults and children). Note - albendazole investigational for this purpose
- Strongyloides stercoralis - albendazole 400 mg daily x 3 days

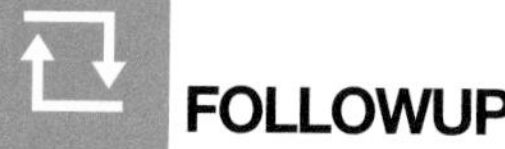

FOLLOWUP

PATIENT MONITORING Followup stool studies at 2 weeks and retreat if necessary

PREVENTION/AVOIDANCE Good hygiene and sanitation

POSSIBLE COMPLICATIONS

- Vomiting worms
- Cholangitis - migration to common bile duct
- Pancreatitis - migration to pancreatic duct
- Appendicitis - migration to appendix
- Diverticulitis - migration to diverticula
- Liver abscess
- Intestinal obstruction
- Volvulus
- Intussusception
- Bowel penetration
- Anemia (hookworm)
- Hypoproteinemia (hookworm)
- CNS infection (Strongyloides)

EXPECTED COURSE/PROGNOSIS

Good for light to moderate infections. Ascariasis should always be treated due to the risk of migrating adult worms.

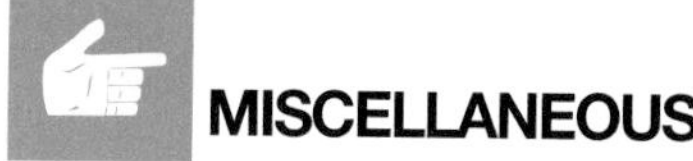

MISCELLANEOUS

ASSOCIATED CONDITIONS N/A

AGE-RELATED FACTORS Affects all ages
Pediatric: Children commonly infected
Geriatric: N/A
Others: N/A

PREGNANCY Benzimidazoles (mebendazole, albendazole, thiabendazole) should not be used; ivermectin has shown little teratogenic potential, and has provided an effective therapy though benefits should clearly outweigh risks

SYNONYMS N/A

ICD-9-CM

127.0 Ascariasis

SEE ALSO

Intestinal parasites
Roundworms, tissue

OTHER NOTES HIV infected patients have a higher risk of dissemination (e.g., strongyloides) and "standard" treatment failure therefore they may require prolonged, repeated, or alternative therapies

ABBREVIATIONS N/A

REFERENCES

- Strickland GT. Hunter's Tropical Medicine. 8th ed. Philadelphia: WB Saunders Co; 2000
- Jong EC. Travel & Tropical Medicine Manual. 3rd ed. Philadelphia: WB Saunders Co; 2003
- Steffen R. Manual of Travel Medicine & Health. 2nd ed. Ontario, Canada: BC Decker; 2003
- Drugs for Parasitic Infections. The Medical Letter. Vol 40 (issue 1071) Jan 2, 1998
- Jensenius M. Hookworm disease: A differential diagnosis in iron deficiency anemia. Tidsskrift for den Norske Laegeforening 1995;115(3):367-9
- Hardman JG, et al, eds. Goodman & Gilman's: The Pharmacological Basis of Therapeutics. 10th ed. New York: McGraw-Hill; 2001

Web references: 1 available at www.5mcc.com
Illustrations N/A

Author(s):

James F. Broomfield, MD

BASICS

DESCRIPTION Tissue roundworms (nematodes) affect man when the adults or larval stages infect certain tissues. Infective larval stages are transmitted to man by arthropod vectors or from the soil. Once in human tissue, worms mature over 6-12 months and survive as long as 15 years. Symptoms depend on tissue infected.
- Filarial infections
  - ◊ *Wuchereria bancrofti* (bancroftian filariasis)
  - ◊ *Brugia malayi* (Malayan filariasis)
  - ◊ *Brugia timori* (Timorian filariasis)
  - ◊ Loa loa (eye worm)
  - ◊ *Onchocerca volvulus* (river blindness, onchocerciasis)
  - ◊ *Mansonella perstans*
  - ◊ *Mansonella ozzardi* (Ozzard filariasis)
  - ◊ *Mansonella streptocerca*
- Other tissue nematode infections
  - ◊ *Dracunculus medinensis* (guinea worm, dracunculosis)
  - ◊ *Ancylostoma braziliense* (cutaneous larva migrans, creeping eruption)
  - ◊ *Toxocara canis* or *cati* (visceral larva migrans, toxocariasis)
- Distribution
  - ◊ Over 300 million people are exposed to lymphatic filariasis in India and SE Asia; 30 million to onchocerciasis
  - ◊ *W. bancrofti*: Tropics worldwide
  - ◊ *B. malayi*: Southeast Asia
  - ◊ *B. timori*: Indonesia
  - ◊ L. loa: Africa
  - ◊ *O. volvulus*: Africa, Central and South America
  - ◊ *M. perstans*: Africa, South America
  - ◊ *M. ozzardi*: Africa
  - ◊ *M. streptocerca*: Central and South America
  - ◊ *D. medinensis*: Africa, Asia
  - ◊ *A. braziliense*: Tropics and Subtropics worldwide
  - ◊ *T. canis/cati*: Over 50 countries worldwide, especially warmer tropical and subtropical regions

System(s) affected: Cardiovascular, Gastrointestinal, Hemic/Lymphatic/Immunologic, Musculoskeletal, Nervous, Renal/Urologic, Skin/Exocrine

Genetics: N/A

Incidence/Prevalence in USA:
- Visceral larva migrans - 4-30% seroprevalence has been reported, highest in southeastern United States
- Others - unknown

Predominant age: All ages, but children more commonly infected

Predominant sex: Male = Female

SIGNS & SYMPTOMS
- Lymphatic filariasis (*W. bancrofti*, *B. malayi*, *B. timori*)
  - ◊ Inflammatory signs - pain, tenderness, swelling, erythema
  - ◊ Filarial adenolymphangitis
  - ◊ Filarial orchitis
  - ◊ Funiculitis and epididymitis
  - ◊ "Filarial" and "Elephantoid" fever
  - ◊ Filarial abscess
  - ◊ Obstructive signs - lymph varices, lymph scrotum, hydrocele
  - ◊ Lymphedema and elephantiasis
  - ◊ Chyluria
  - ◊ Filarial hypereosinophilia (tropical pulmonary eosinophilia)
- Loiasis (L. loa)
  - ◊ Calabar swellings - recurrent subcutaneous inflammation/swelling
  - ◊ Eye worm - adult or larvae migrate under conjunctiva
  - ◊ Eosinophilia (may exceed 70%)
  - ◊ Fever, irritability, urticaria and pruritus
- Onchocerciasis (O. volvulus)
  - ◊ Dermatitis
  - ◊ Nodules
  - ◊ Lymphadenitis
  - ◊ Ocular changes - intraocular microfilariae, punctate keratitis, sclerosing keratitis, anterior uveitis chorioretinitis, optic neuritis, optic atrophy, glaucoma, blindness (river blindness)
- Other filarial syndromes (M. ozzardi, M. perstans, M. streptocerca)
  - ◊ Headaches, coldness, pruritus, and articular swelling/arthritis
  - ◊ Eosinophilia and vague allergic signs
  - ◊ Chronic dermatitis and macules can be confused with leprosy
  - ◊ Lymphadenopathy
- Dracunculiasis (D. medinensis, guinea worm disease)
  - ◊ Allergic manifestations - erythema, urticaria, pruritus, nausea, vomiting, giddiness, syncope, and occasional fever)
  - ◊ Local lesions - papule, sterile blister, ulceration, abscesses
  - ◊ Worm protrusion
- Toxocariasis (T. canis/cati, visceral or ocular larva migrans)
  - ◊ Eosinophilia
  - ◊ Visceral larva migrans
  - ◊ Ocular larva migrans
- Cutaneous larva migrans (A. braziliense, creeping eruption)
  - ◊ Itching and red papules
  - ◊ Serpiginous track
  - ◊ Edema and acute inflammation
  - ◊ Scars
  - ◊ Secondary infection

CAUSES Larvae introduced into human host by arthropod vector or infected soil

RISK FACTORS
- Geographic exposure to arthropod vectors
- Fishermen or women washing clothes have increased risk of 'river blindness'
- Contact with infected soil in cutaneous larva migrans (hence plumber's itch, sandworm, duck hunter's itch)

DIAGNOSIS

DIFFERENTIAL DIAGNOSIS
- Other causes of tissue inflammation (i.e., lymphangitis, epididymitis, dermatitis, conjunctivitis, blisters, pleuritis, peritonitis, pericarditis, encephalitis, nephropathy, cardiomyopathy, etc.)
- Nonfilarial causes of lymphangitis:
  - ◊ Acute bacterial lymphangitis
  - ◊ Phlebitis
  - ◊ Unusual - plague, anthrax, TB, lymphogranuloma inguinale
- Nonfilarial causes of lymphedema, chyluria, and elephantiasis:
  - ◊ Infiltrative or granulomatous process: Tumor, fungus, TB, leprosy
  - ◊ Chronic venostasis or phlebitis
  - ◊ Cardiac insufficiency
  - ◊ Nutritional deficiencies
  - ◊ Hereditary (Milroy disease)
  - ◊ Lateritious soil obstructing lymphatics

LABORATORY Examination of larvae or adult worms taken from the tissue; characteristic microfilariae on blood smear; eosinophilia. Distinction of species by larval exam is challenging and may require expert examination. Onchocerciasis is identified by skin snip/biopsy showing larval.

Drugs that may alter lab results: N/A

Disorders that may alter lab results: N/A

PATHOLOGICAL FINDINGS Characteristic eggs/worms/larvae in tissue

SPECIAL TESTS Skin snip, nodulectomy, slit-lamp exam, and Mazzotti, test may be helpful in onchocerciasis

IMAGING Occasional worms seen on x-ray

DIAGNOSTIC PROCEDURES Microfilariae on blood smear or other body fluids; clinical observations; serologies (e.g., ELISA)

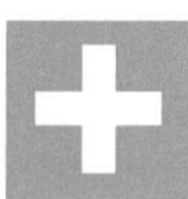

TREATMENT

APPROPRIATE HEALTH CARE Outpatient

GENERAL MEASURES
- Identify cause and treat accordingly
- Best treatment - direct removal of worm from tissue with caution not to break the worm
- Treat secondary infections

SURGICAL MEASURES Long-standing lymphatic filariasis due to W. bancrofti and B. malayi may require surgical intervention to increase lymphatic drainage. This is unusual, and likely seen in long-term residents of endemic areas, subjected to extensive exposure to parasite.

ACTIVITY No restrictions. If edema a problem, may want to elevate legs while sitting.

DIET No special diet

PATIENT EDUCATION
- Avoid bites by arthropod vectors, insect repellants and other protective measures, e.g., proper clothing
- Avoid rivers and streams and soils known to be infected

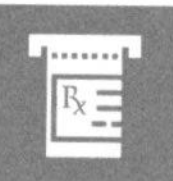

MEDICATIONS

DRUG(S) OF CHOICE

- Visceral larva migrans (Toxocara): diethylcarbamazine (DEC) 6 mg/kg/d in 3 doses x7-10 days for adult and pediatric
- Cutaneous larva migrans (Ancylostoma braziliense): thiabendazole topical and/or albendazole 400 mg qday x3 days for adults and children. Topical 15% thiabendazole in a water soluble cream base is the treatment of choice given low toxicity and high cure rate (98%). Ivermectin 150-200 mcg/kg once is effective.
- Filariasis (W. bancrofti, B. malayi):
  - ◊ Diethylcarbamazine: Adult: day 1) 50 mg po after meals; day 2) 50 mg tid; day 3) 100 mg tid; days 4-14) 6 mg/kg/d in 3 doses. Children: day 1) 1 mg/kg po after meals; day 2) 1 mg/kg tid; day 3) 1-2 mg/kg tid; days 4-14) 6 mg/kg/d in 3 doses.
- Loa, loa
  - ◊ Diethylcarbamazine: as above except days 4-21: 9 mg/kg/day in 3 doses (adults and children)
  - ◊ Antihistamines and steroids: may be useful to reduce allergic response to disintegration of microfilaria
- Onchocerciasis: ivermectin (Mectizan) 150 μg/kg po once, repeated every 6-12 months for adults and children can prevent blindness. Treatment with ivermectin only kills the larval worms, responsible for pathology, not the adult worms producing the larvae. Thus, treatment must be continued over a period of years until the adult worms die.
- Mansonella ozzardi: ivermectin 6 mg in single dose has been effective. Diethylcarbamazine is not effective.
- Mansonella perstans: mebendazole 100 mg bid x 30 days (approved drug, but considered investigational for this condition)
- Guinea worm (Dracunculus): metronidazole 250 mg tid x 10 days for adult; 25 mg/kg/d (max 750 mg/d) in 3 doses x 10 days for children. Metronidazole does not cure the infection, but rather decreases the reaction to worm products. Cure is achieved only through physical removal of the adult worm.
- Note: FDA may consider certain uses of above drugs investigational and some may not be available in USA. Contact Parasitic Disease Drug Service, Parasitic Diseases Branch, Center for Disease Control, Atlanta 30333, (404)488-4240.

Contraindications: Refer to manufacturer's information
Precautions: Children, pregnancy, lactation
Significant possible interactions: Refer to manufacturer's profile of each drug

ALTERNATIVE DRUGS

- Visceral larva migrans (Toxocara): albendazole 400 mg bid x3-5 days for adults and children or mebendazole 100-200 mg bid x5 days for adults and children
- Filariasis (W. bancrofti, B. malayi): Ivermectin (available from the CDC Drug Services 404-639-3670) 150 mcg/kg as a single dose is highly effective against microfilaria but does not kill adult worms. More effective when combined with albendazole 400 mg.
- Onchocerciasis: DEC has been used, but causes bad reactions, likely due to rapid killing of the larval worms with sudden release of large amounts of worm antigens. DEC is obsolete for this indication. Suramin, a drug used in the treatment of trypanosomiasis, is effective at killing the adult worms, but severe side effects prevent its use for onchocerciasis.

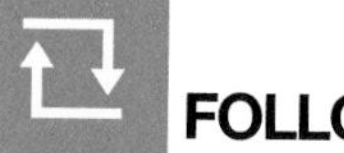

FOLLOWUP

PATIENT MONITORING N/A

PREVENTION/AVOIDANCE

- Avoid sources of infection (arthropod bites, rivers/streams, or contaminated soils)
- Diethylcarbamazine (DEC) 300 mg once weekly has been used successfully in Peace Corps' workers for prophylaxis against L. loa
- Prophylaxis with ivermectin is under investigation
- Public health activities such as vector control

POSSIBLE COMPLICATIONS

- Depends upon type of worm
- Onchocerciasis - blindness
- Visceral worms - hepatitis, splenomegaly, pleuritis, peritonitis, eosinophilic granuloma or other organ damage as larvae migrate for up to 6 months
- Filariasis - lymphatic destruction leading to severe edema (elephantiasis)
- Neurohelminthiasis: CNS migrations and infection

EXPECTED COURSE/PROGNOSIS

- Good for light to moderate infections; depends on organ infected and extent of infection
- Long-term DEC treatment and immunomonitoring of filaria patients are essential in endemic areas to arrest and prevent pathology

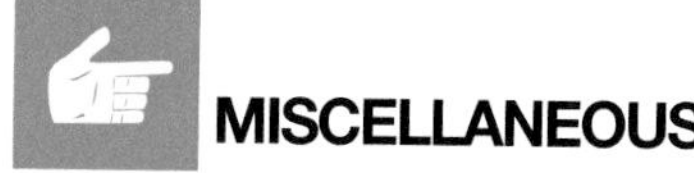

MISCELLANEOUS

ASSOCIATED CONDITIONS N/A

AGE-RELATED FACTORS

Pediatric: Children commonly infected
Geriatric: N/A
Others: Presence of onchocerciasis increases with age

PREGNANCY N/A

SYNONYMS

- Nematodes

ICD-9-CM

127.0 Ascariasis

SEE ALSO

Roundworms, intestinal

OTHER NOTES N/A

ABBREVIATIONS N/A

REFERENCES

- Strickland GT. Hunter's Tropical Medicine. 8th ed. Philadelphia: WB Saunders Co; 2000
- Jong EC. Travel & Tropical Medicine Manual. 3rd ed. Philadelphia: WB Saunders Co; 2003
- Warren KS, Mahmoud AAF: Tropical and Geographic Medicine. New York: McGraw-Hill; 1990
- Drugs for Parasitic Infections. Medical Letter. New Rochelle, NY, Medical Letter, Inc Jan 2, 1998;Vol 40 (1017)
- Steffen R. Manual of Travel Medicine & Health. 2nd ed. Ontario, Canada: BC Decker; 2003
- Padrigel UM, et al: Immunomonitoring of filarial patients during DEC therapy in an endemic area: A seven year followup. Jour Tropical Med & Hygiene 1995;98(1):52-6
- Cook GC. Manson's Tropical Diseases. 21st ed. PHiladelphia: WB Saunders; 2002

Web references: 1 available at www.5mcc.com
Illustrations 1 available

Author(s):

James F. Broomfield, MD

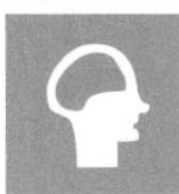

BASICS

DESCRIPTION A systemic disorder caused by acute and/or chronic intoxication from salicylate containing medications.
- Following accidental or intentional exposure, toxic actions of salicylates include:
  - ◊ Stimulation of the CNS respiratory center
  - ◊ Uncoupling of oxidative phosphorylation
  - ◊ Inhibition of Krebs cycle dehydrogenases
  - ◊ Stimulation of gluconeogenesis
  - ◊ Increased lipolysis and lipid metabolism
  - ◊ Inhibition of aminotransferases
  - ◊ Cyclooxygenase inhibition and decreased production of clotting factors
  - ◊ Irritation of the gastric mucosa and stimulation of the CNS chemoreceptor trigger zone.
- These actions cause sequential and progressively severe physiologic abnormalities with increasing doses of salicylates, time following exposure, duration of chronic exposure, extremes of age, and presence of concurrent medical conditions; abnormalities include:
  - ◊ Respiratory alkalosis accompanied by progressive metabolic acidosis
  - ◊ Hyperpyrexia
  - ◊ Gastrointestinal, renal, pulmonary, and skin losses of body fluids and electrolytes
  - ◊ Initial hyperglycemia followed by hypoglycemia, particularly CNS hypoglycemia
  - ◊ Abnormal hemostasis and coagulation.
- The clinical presentation of patients with salicylate toxicity can range from minor symptoms to a syndrome initially indistinguishable from septic shock with multiple organ failure, including encephalopathy and adult respiratory distress syndrome (ARDS). The very young and elderly are particularly prone to develop severe toxicity, as are those with chronic intoxication. Also, conditions causing concurrent acidosis may increase tissue concentrations of salicylate and result in greater morbidity and mortality.

System(s) affected: Cardiovascular, Endocrine/Metabolic, Gastrointestinal, Hemic/Lymphatic/Immunologic, Musculoskeletal, Nervous, Pulmonary, Renal/Urologic, Skin/Exocrine

Genetics: N/A

Incidence/Prevalence in USA:
- > 20,800 ingestions of salicylate containing medications reported to poison control centers in 2002
- 67 deaths in 2002, none in children < 6

Predominant age: Occurs in children and adults at any age; over 73% of cases are in children > 5 and adults

Predominant sex: Male = Female

SIGNS & SYMPTOMS
- Acute intoxication
  - ◊ Symptoms vary with the amount ingested, usually begin within 3-8 hours of ingestion, and progress more rapidly in children:
    - < 150 mg/kg, minimal symptoms
    - 150-300 mg/kg, moderate symptoms
    - 300-500 mg/kg, severe symptoms
    - > 500 mg/kg, potentially fatal
  - ◊ Nausea and vomiting
  - ◊ Hyperpnea
  - ◊ Tachypnea
  - ◊ Hyperpyrexia
  - ◊ Tinnitus
  - ◊ Disorientation
  - ◊ Coma
  - ◊ Convulsions
  - ◊ Cardiac arrhythmias
  - ◊ Hypotension
  - ◊ Pulmonary edema
- Chronic intoxication
  - ◊ Signs and symptoms similar to acute intoxication may occur
  - ◊ Onset of symptoms is usually gradual
  - ◊ Signs and symptoms may be advanced at diagnosis and include severe hypotension and ARDS
  - ◊ Neurologic symptoms often predominate, particularly in the elderly, and include agitation, confusion, stupor, hyperactivity, paranoia, bizarre behavior, dysarthria, restlessness

CAUSES
- Accidental or intentional ingestion of salicylates or salicylate containing medications
- Percutaneous absorption of dermatologic medications containing salicylate
- Breast feeding by mothers ingesting salicylate containing medications
- Teething gels containing salicylates

RISK FACTORS
- Dehydration
- Conditions causing metabolic or respiratory acidosis
- Extremes of age - the very young and elderly
- Psychiatric illness
- History of previous toxic ingestions or suicide attempts
- Concurrent oral poisoning with other substances
- Concurrent use of acetazolamide (Diamox)

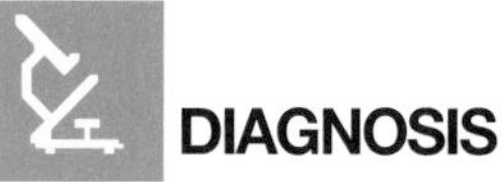

DIAGNOSIS

DIFFERENTIAL DIAGNOSIS
- All ages: infection, sepsis, DKA, other causes of metabolic acidosis
- In the elderly: delirium, CVA, myocardial infarction, ethyl alcohol (EtOH) intoxication, congestive heart failure

LABORATORY
- Serum salicylate levels initially on all patients to confirm the diagnosis. Following acute ingestions, check levels 6 or more hours after ingestion and repeat q2h until levels are declining and the patient's condition has stabilized.
- Acid-base abnormalities common; usually respiratory alkalosis or mixed respiratory alkalosis and metabolic acidosis. Metabolic acidosis often predominates in chronic or severe acute poisonings and in poisonings in young children.
- Increased anion gap, especially in acute poisonings and salicylate-only poisonings
- Initial hyperglycemia may be followed by hypoglycemia
- Electrolyte abnormalities such as hyper- or hyponatremia, and hypokalemia common
- Findings consistent with dehydration are common including an increased BUN/Cr ratio
- PT may be increased
- Liver function abnormalities may be present
- Proteinuria, renal function abnormalities may be present
- Stool guaiac testing may be positive
- Occasional hypouricemia

Drugs that may alter lab results:
- Diflunisal (Dolobid) may cross react with assay of salicylate concentration
- Medications affecting similar organ systems including oral anticoagulants and hypoglycemic agents

Disorders that may alter lab results: Concurrent medical conditions involving similar organ systems

PATHOLOGICAL FINDINGS None specific for salicylate intoxication; associated findings include:
- Gastrointestinal = antral and prepyloric ulcers; small bowel ulcerations with enteric coated salicylates
- Renal = interstitial nephritis, acute tubular necrosis, minimal change nephrotic syndrome
- Pulmonary = non-cardiogenic pulmonary edema

SPECIAL TESTS N/A

IMAGING
- Chest X-ray: non-cardiogenic pulmonary edema; variable severity, from mild to ARDS
- Abdominal plain film: nonspecific bowel gas pattern with retained contrast in chronic bismuth subsalicylate ingestion

DIAGNOSTIC PROCEDURES None, other than correlating serum salicylate concentration with the clinical presentation.
- Following acute ingestions, the significance of the serum salicylate level can be estimated by using the Done nomogram (Temple AR. Acute and chronic effects of aspirin toxicity and their treatment. Arch Intern Med 1981;141:364-9). However, the nomogram's usefulness in managing patients is limited and it may underestimate the severity of poisonings in patients with:
  - ◊ Illnesses accompanied by dehydration and/or acidosis
  - ◊ Chronic exposure to salicylates
  - ◊ Ingestion of enteric coated or sustained release medications
  - ◊ Unknown time of ingestion

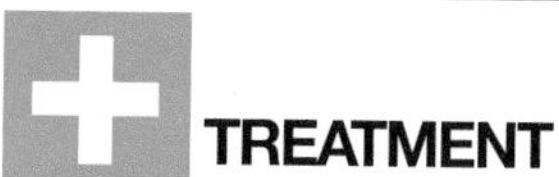

TREATMENT

APPROPRIATE HEALTH CARE
Evaluate all patients at a healthcare facility; outpatient for non-toxic accidental ingestions; inpatient for toxic and intentional ingestions

GENERAL MEASURES
- Prevent further absorption:
  - ◊ Gastric lavage, within 1 hour of ingestion
  - ◊ Activated charcoal after gastric emptying
  - ◊ Ipecac is no longer recommended for routine use at home or in health care facilities
- Fluid/electrolyte balance: IV fluids to restore intravascular volume and prevent hypoglycemia. With hypotension give isotonic fluid until orthostatic changes no longer present; the fluids should contain at least 5% dextrose unless hyperglycemia is a problem. Normal saline or a mixture of .45% NaCl with 1 ampule of sodium bicarbonate (50 mEq $NaHCO_3$) may be administered at 10-15 mL/kg/hr for 1-2 hours, depending on the degree of acidosis. When blood pressure stable, fluid management is directed toward alkalinizing the urine to enhance salicylate excretion, preventing CNS hypoglycemia, and treating fluid and electrolyte abnormalities.
- Enhance elimination:
  - ◊ Alkaline diuresis (urine pH >7.5) and prevention of hypoglycemia can usually be maintained by an initial bolus of $NaHC0_3$, 2 mEq/kg intravenously, followed by an infusion of 1000 cc D5W plus three ampules of $NaHC0_3$ (50 mEq $NaHC0_3$/ampule) at 1.5 to 2 times maintenance rate. Potassium should be added for potassium levels below 4.0 mEq/L. Serum electrolytes and glucose should be monitored frequently and the urine pH checked hourly until stable at > 7.5. Arterial blood gases should be monitored after 2-4 hours to ensure the blood pH is no more than 7.5. Patients with cardiovascular compromise should be monitored closely for fluid overload. Alkalinization can be discontinued when the salicylate level decreases into the therapeutic range.
  - ◊ Hemodialysis should be considered in poisonings with markedly elevated salicylate levels (> 100 mg/dL in acute poisonings, > 40-60 mg/dL in chronic poisonings), acidosis unresponsive to alkalinization and diuresis, renal and/or hepatic dysfunction with impaired salicylate clearance, noncardiac pulmonary edema, and persistent, severe CNS symptoms.

SURGICAL MEASURES
N/A

ACTIVITY
Bedrest initially

DIET
No special diet

PATIENT EDUCATION
- Education of parents/caregivers during well child visits
- Education of patients on chronic salicylate therapy
- Anticipatory guidance for caregivers, family, and cohabitants of potentially suicidal patients
- Patient brochure (item 1515): Child Safety: Keeping your home safe for your baby. American Academy of Family Physicians, 11400 Tomahawk Creek Parkway, Leawood, KS 66211-2672

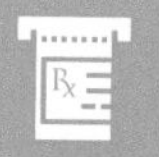

MEDICATIONS

DRUG(S) OF CHOICE
- Emergency facility/hospital:
  - ◊ Patients evaluated within 1 hour of ingestion may have their stomachs evacuated by gastric lavage
  - ◊ Repeat activated charcoal every 4 hours (1 g/kg each dose) until passage of a charcoal stool
  - ◊ Bicarbonate is used to alkalinize the urine (pH >7.5) and, when appropriate, to correct severe systemic acidosis (for pH < 7.1)
  - ◊ Give dextrose-containing IV solution to prevent hypoglycemia; CNS hypoglycemia may be present despite a normal serum glucose

Contraindications: Medication allergies

Precautions:
- Intravascular overload may result from injudicious use of sodium bicarbonate, particularly in patients with cardiovascular compromise
- Dextrose should not be given to patients with severe hyperglycemia

Significant possible interactions: N/A

ALTERNATIVE DRUGS
N/A

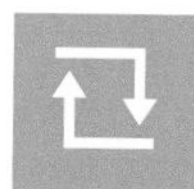

FOLLOWUP

PATIENT MONITORING
- Fluid, acid base, blood glucose, and electrolyte status until stable; urine pH (to enhance elimination of salicylate)
- Psychiatric followup after intentional ingestions

PREVENTION/AVOIDANCE
- Patient and parent/caregiver education essential. See Patient Education.
- Emergency telephone numbers

POSSIBLE COMPLICATIONS
- Non-cardiogenic pulmonary edema, including development of ARDS
- Rare following recovery from poisoning

EXPECTED COURSE/PROGNOSIS
- Complete recovery with early therapy
- Clinical course and prognosis are worse in the very young and elderly, chronic intoxications, and in patients with concurrent conditions which cause dehydration and/or acidosis

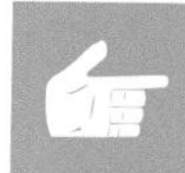

MISCELLANEOUS

ASSOCIATED CONDITIONS
Reye syndrome with salicylate use and varicella or influenza viral infection

AGE-RELATED FACTORS
Pediatric: Acidosis is often more severe in the very young, particularly in chronic or repeated therapeutic dose poisonings

Geriatric:
- Increased risk for chronic toxicity because of decreased renal function
- Increased risk for bleeding or perforated gastric ulcers in patients over 70 years

Others: N/A

PREGNANCY
- No teratogenic effect in humans
- Salicylates may cause premature closure of ductus arteriosus in fetus
- Increased risk of ante and intrapartum hemorrhage

SYNONYMS
N/A

ICD-9-CM
965.1 Poisoning by salicylates (aspirin)

SEE ALSO

OTHER NOTES
N/A

ABBREVIATIONS
ARDS = adult respiratory distress syndrome
DKA = diabetic ketoacidosis

REFERENCES

- American Academy of Pediatrics Committee on Injury, Violence, and Poison Prevention. Poison treatment in the home. American Academy of Pediatrics Committee on Injury, Violence, and Poison Prevention. Pediatrics 2003;112(5):1182-5
- Shannon M. Ingestion of toxic substances by children. N Engl J Med 2000;342(3):186-91
- Watson WA, Litovitz TL, Rodgers GC Jr, et al. 2002 annual report of the American Association of Poison Control Centers Toxic Exposure Surveillance System. Am J Emerg Med 2003;21(5):353-421

Web references: 0 available at www.5mcc.com

Illustrations N/A

Author(s):
Lars C. Larsen, MD

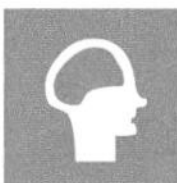

BASICS

DESCRIPTION The formation of stones in intraglandular or extraglandular ducts of submandibular, parotid, sublingual, or minor salivary glands.
System(s) affected: Gastrointestinal
Genetics: No known genetic pattern
Incidence/Prevalence in USA: Not uncommon, but reliable incidence figures not available; 1% in autopsy series, most of these asymptomatic
Predominant age: Middle to old age; uncommon in children
Predominant sex: Male > Female (slight predominance)

SIGNS & SYMPTOMS
- Initial symptoms, consistent with partial duct obstruction:
  - ◊ Episodic or variable unilateral swelling and tenderness of the affected gland,
  - ◊ Worse just before meals, then tapering off till the next meal
- Symptoms of complete duct obstruction:
  - ◊ Persistent swelling and pain
- Symptoms of commonly associated sialadenitis:
  - ◊ Fever, sweats, chills
  - ◊ Acute and severe worsening of localized pain and swelling
  - ◊ Acute general malaise
- Signs when not associated with sialadenitis:
  - ◊ Unilateral localized swelling
  - ◊ Boggy tender mass associated with affected gland in acute obstruction
  - ◊ Firm to hard mass associated with gland fibrosis in chronic obstruction
  - ◊ Palpable and/or visible stone in distal duct (in 1/2 to 1/3 of cases, and more often with submandibular stones than parotid stones)
  - ◊ No saliva expressed, or scant, cloudy, thick, mucinous saliva expressed on milking duct
- Signs in association with sialadenitis:
  - ◊ Fever, tachycardia
  - ◊ Generalized toxicity
  - ◊ Diffuse, tender, hot swelling associated with affected gland
  - ◊ Otherwise palpable stone now obscured by swelling and acute pain

CAUSES
- Submandibular gland/ducts are involved in more than 80% of cases, thought to be due to:
  - ◊ Tortuous course of these ducts
  - ◊ Flow of saliva in these ducts is "up hill"
  - ◊ Submandibular saliva has higher concentration of calcium and is more viscous
- General causes of salivary gland stones:
  - ◊ Any mechanical hindrances to normal flow of saliva
    - Acute or chronic inflammation in or around duct
    - Scarring or stenosis of duct (trauma, surgery, past stone damage)
    - Altered or tortuous duct path (from extrinsic masses, surgery or previous obstruction)
    - Presence of food particles or organic debris in duct as an obstruction and/or nidus of stone formation
  - ◊ Alteration of saliva quality
    - Dehydration
    - Anticholinergic medications (including those with anticholinergic side effects such as tricyclic antidepressants and phenothiazines)
    - Chronic parotitis, Sjögren syndrome, cystic fibrosis

RISK FACTORS
- Sources for alterations in gland function and duct anatomy, as mentioned above
- Previous stone formation
- Local irradiation
- Chronic, debilitating illness
- Poor oral hygiene

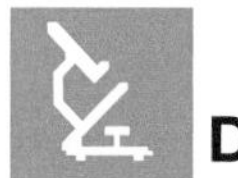

DIAGNOSIS

DIFFERENTIAL DIAGNOSIS
- Sialadenitis
- Lymphadenitis
- Salivary neoplasms (80% benign in parotid, 50% benign in submandibular gland)
- Foreign body in duct or soft tissue
- Neoplasms of adjacent oral or neck tissues
- Other facial/dental soft tissue infections (eg dissecting dental abscess)

LABORATORY
- WBC, acute phase reactants, and serum amylase may be elevated if associated with sialadenitis

Drugs that may alter lab results: N/A

Disorders that may alter lab results: N/A

PATHOLOGICAL FINDINGS
- Submandibular glands/ducts involved in 80% of cases, parotid in 15%, and remainder in sublingual and minor salivary glands
- In acute cases without sialadenitis:
  - ◊ Acute ductal and glandular inflammation
- In chronic cases:
  - ◊ Ductal ectasia, stenosis, scarring, thickening
  - ◊ Metaplasia of duct lining
  - ◊ Periductal chronic inflammation
  - ◊ Glandular fibrosis and atrophy
  - ◊ Multiple stones in intra- and extra- glandular ducts
- Stones vary in size from <1 mm to >10 mm and show alternating layers of mineralization (predominantly calcium salts) and organic material (mucinous material, lipids, cellular debris)

SPECIAL TESTS N/A

IMAGING
- Due to differences in mineralization, 80% of SMG stones are radiopaque, but 80% of parotid stones are radiolucent
- Plain head and neck radiographs
- Dental occlusive films
- Ultrasound (particularly useful in acute parotid sialadenitis with swelling and pain)
- MR imaging is investigational and promising. Does not visualize stones, but shows ducts as with sialography.
- CT - "CT reconstruction" most sensitive technique, showing presence of stones or differentiating multiple stones when other imaging methods fail
- Xerography

DIAGNOSTIC PROCEDURES
- Fine needle aspiration if glandular neoplasm is high in the differential diagnosis
- Surgical excision may be needed to differentiate chronic ductal squamous metaplasia from low-grade mucoepidermoid carcinoma
- Sialoendoscopy under development

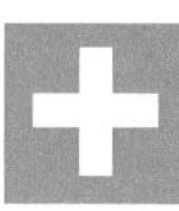

TREATMENT

APPROPRIATE HEALTH CARE
- Outpatient for conservative treatment or minor surgical procedures
- Inpatient for salivary gland excision or for treating associated severe sialadenitis

GENERAL MEASURES
- Small stones close to the ductal orifice are often removed with a conservative approach:
  - ◊ Sialagogues (eg hard sour candy) to stimulate salivary flow
  - ◊ Gentle ductal massage, from gland to ductal orifice
  - ◊ Ductal dilatation (lacrimal probe and/or lacrimal punctum dilator)
  - ◊ Incision of ductal papilla if stone is hung up just inside the orifice
  - ◊ For more proximal SMG stones still within 1.25 cm from orifice (Wharton's duct) the duct may be incised longitudinally from the orifice and the stone expressed by massage
  - ◊ Penicillinase-resistant staphylococcal antibiotic coverage, particularly if duct instrumented or incised
- In setting of acute sialadenitis:
  - ◊ Hydration
  - ◊ Sialagogues
  - ◊ Local heat
  - ◊ Release of a distal obstructing stone as above, if palpable
  - ◊ Attempted proximal-to-distal expression of pus after release of obstruction
  - ◊ Full course of penicillinase-resistant staph coverage (IV therapy in hospital for severely ill or elderly)
  - ◊ Extracorporeal shock-wave lithotripsy (ECSWL) has been effective in treating >50% of the parotid stones not cleared with conservative measures

SURGICAL MEASURES
- A more extensive procedure by a surgical specialist, such as proximal duct dissection or gland excision, is appropriate for:
  - ◊ Any but most distal parotid stones, particularly if ECSWL not available or ineffective
  - ◊ Proximal stone with high grade obstruction
  - ◊ Chronic or recurrent sialadenitis with glandular fibrosis and/or ductal scarring and stenosis
  - ◊ Multiple stones
  - ◊ Neoplasm is a consideration

ACTIVITY No restrictions

DIET Until specific therapy initiated
- Liberal oral water intake for hydration
- Reduce other oral intake to reduce pain
- Particularly avoid Sialagogues to reduce pain
- No specific dietary measures required after therapy

PATIENT EDUCATION
- General management principles and diet as above
- Avoid OTC anticholinergic medications as discussed below
- Bring early signs of recurrence to medical attention

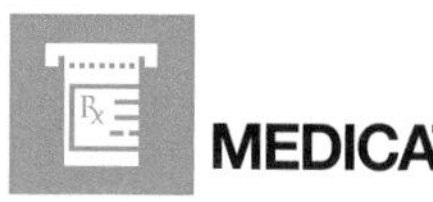

MEDICATIONS

DRUG(S) OF CHOICE
- Antibiotics, if infection present
  - ◊ Amoxicillin-clavulanate (Augmentin) 500 mg tid
  - ◊ Cefuroxime (Ceftin)
- Analgesic: codeine, NSAID, etc

Contraindications: Hypersensitivity to drugs chosen

Precautions:
- Refer to manufacturer's literature for drugs chosen
- Prescribed or OTC anticholinergics may predispose to, or accelerate stone formation

Significant possible interactions: Refer to manufacturer's literature

ALTERNATIVE DRUGS
Erythromycin 250 mg qid

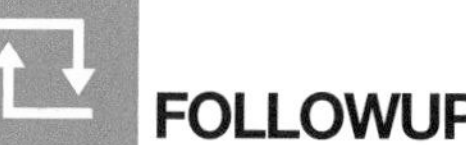

FOLLOWUP

PATIENT MONITORING
- Close post-procedure or post-surgical surveillance for infection
- Close follow-up during treatment of sialadenitis to ensure resolution of infection
- Patient education to seek early medical attention for symptoms of recurrence

PREVENTION/AVOIDANCE
- Treat any associated conditions
- Avoid anticholinergics
- Good hydration
- Good oral hygiene

POSSIBLE COMPLICATIONS
- Ductal scarring after stone passage, after instrumentation or surgery
- Infection associated with stone itself or with surgical procedures
- Salivary gland fibrosis and atrophy from duct obstruction or infection
- Salivary fistula after surgical procedure

EXPECTED COURSE/PROGNOSIS
- The majority of patients with uncomplicated stones who are successfully treated early in the process do not have recurrences
- A previous stone may damage the duct, setting up conditions for more stones
- Recurrence, particularly with multiple proximal stones, may warrant gland excision

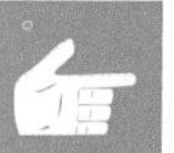

MISCELLANEOUS

ASSOCIATED CONDITIONS
- Sialadenitis
- Chronic anticholinergics
- Poor oral hygiene
- Sjögren syndrome
- Cystic fibrosis
- Oral trauma

AGE-RELATED FACTORS
Pediatric: N/A
Geriatric: Multiple chronic illnesses, multiple anticholinergics, dehydration
Others: N/A

PREGNANCY N/A

SYNONYMS Sialolithiasis

ICD-9-CM
527.5 Sialolithiasis

SEE ALSO
Sialadenitis
Sjögren syndrome

OTHER NOTES Multiple stones in 20% of cases. In past, stones were felt to be secondary to altered calcium metabolism, but this has not been demonstrated.

ABBREVIATIONS N/A

REFERENCES

- Pollack CV, Severance HW. Sialolithiasis: case studies and review. J Emerg Med 1990;8:561-5
- McKenna JP, Bostock DJ, McMenamin PG. Sialolithiasis. Am Fam Physician 1987;36:119-25
- McGurk M, Escudier M. Removing salivary gland stones. Br J Hosp Med 1995;54:184-5
- Raymond AK, Batsakis JG. Angiolithiasis and sialolithiasis in the head and neck. Ann Otol Rhinol Laryngol 1992;101:455-7
- Iro H, Zenk J, Waldfahrer F, et al. Extracorporeal shock wave lithotripsy of parotid stones. Ann Otol Rhinol Laryngol 1998;107:860-4
- Stanley MW, Bardales RH, Beneke J, et al. Sialolithiasis: differential diagnostic problems in fine-needle aspiration cytology. Am J Clin Pathol 1996;106:229-33
- Williams MF. Sialolithiasis. Otolaryngolog Clin NA 1999;32:819-34
- Yousem DM, Kraut MA, Chalian AA. Major salivary gland imaging. Radiology 2000;216(1):19-29

Web references: 0 available at www.5mcc.com
Illustrations 1 available

Author(s):
Douglas C. Woolley, MD

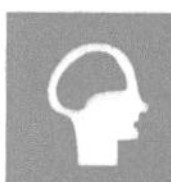

BASICS

DESCRIPTION Neoplasms benign or malignant of the major (parotid, submaxillary, sublingual) salivary glands or the minor (intra-oral, pharyngeal, nasal) salivary glands. Most tumors are discrete masses although some may manifest as diffuse enlargement of the gland or submucosal intraoral swelling. Malignant tumors are characterized by local recurrence and perineural spread (adenoid cystic), or local recurrence and lymph node metastases (mucoepidermoid, adenocarcinoma, squamous cell carcinoma).
- Types
  - ◊ Pleomorphic adenoma (most common tumor) - 45% overall
  - ◊ Monomorphic adenoma - 12% overall
  - ◊ Mucoepidermoid carcinoma - 12% overall
  - ◊ Adenoid cystic - 6% overall
  - ◊ Less frequent lesions are - adenocarcinoma, squamous cell carcinoma, acinic cell carcinoma, oxyphilic adenomas, Warthin's tumor
- Distribution of neoplasms
  - ◊ Generally, the smaller the salivary gland is, the higher the probability of malignancy if a tumor is found in it.
  - ◊ Parotid (80% benign, 20% malignant) - 70% are pleomorphic adenoma; 10% are monomorphic adenoma; 12% are mucoepidermoid carcinoma; 5% are adenoid cystic
  - ◊ Submandibular (60% benign, 40% malignant) - 40% are pleomorphic adenoma; 10% are mucoepidermoid carcinoma; 20% are adenoid cystic carcinoma
  - ◊ Minor salivary glands (40% benign, 60% malignant) - 40% are pleomorphic adenoma; 25% are mucoepidermoid carcinoma; 25% are adenoid cystic carcinoma

System(s) affected: Gastrointestinal, Nervous
Genetics: Increased incidence of adenocarcinoma of parotid in Eskimos, otherwise no known genetic pattern
Incidence/Prevalence in USA: The incidence is 1-3 per 100,000 per year. 3% of new tumors, 5% of all head and neck neoplasms.
Predominant age: Malignant - age 55; benign - age 45
Predominant sex:
- Pleomorphic adenoma: Female > Male
- Other adenomas: Male = Female

SIGNS & SYMPTOMS
- Discrete mass in anatomic area - 96% (malignant)
- Elevation of earlobe
- Pain 12-25% (malignant); 2.5% (benign)
- Trigeminal paresthesias
- Facial nerve palsy or dysfunction 8-26% (malignant)
- Fixation to masseter and pterygoids 17% (malignant)
- Skin ulceration 9% (malignant)
- Cervical lymph node metastases 20% (malignant)
- Pharyngeal mass (representing deep lobe tumors of the parotid gland)

CAUSES
- Unknown
- Possible ionizing radiation
- Epstein-Barr virus

RISK FACTORS Tobacco smoke and excess alcohol intake associated with Warthin tumor

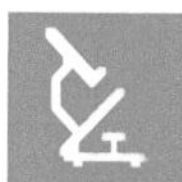

DIAGNOSIS

DIFFERENTIAL DIAGNOSIS
- Metabolic causes (diabetes, vitamin deficiencies, EtOH, gout)
- Drugs (thioureas, iodine)
- Inflammatory masses
- Parotid and submandibular lymph nodes
- Mikulicz's syndrome
- Salivary gland stones
- Torus palatinus (minor)
- Necrotizing sialometaplasia (minor)
- Cervical lymph nodes
- Sjögren syndrome
- Sarcoidosis
- Lymphadenopathy with AIDS

LABORATORY
- Autoimmune studies
- Fractionated amylase (inflammation)

Drugs that may alter lab results: None known

Disorders that may alter lab results: None known

PATHOLOGICAL FINDINGS Of 100 parotid masses, 70 will be non-neoplastic, 21 will be benign neoplasms, and 9 will be malignant neoplasms

SPECIAL TESTS
- Technetium-99 (Warthin's tumor)
- Ultrasound (inflammatory or malignant)
- Sialography (for calculi or chronic parotitis)

IMAGING
- Chest x-ray - Sjögren, metastases
- CT: provides detail of tumor invasion, temporal bone or mandibular destruction
- MRI: provides definition of soft tissue, and any evidence of perineural invasion or intracranial extension. Also discriminates tumor from mucus and bone marrow invasion.
- PET: uses radionuclide-labeled radiotracers for detection of malignancy in the early stages. Also useful in detecting tumor recurrences and differentiating soft tissue damage secondary to radiation from inflammatory changes.

DIAGNOSTIC PROCEDURES
- Fine needle aspiration. There has been concern regarding this procedure, as there may be tumor seeding via the needle track. However, local tumor growth or metastatic tumor spread from tumor seeding is rare.
- Superficial lobectomy
- Staging is based on tumor size (T0-T4), nodal status (N0-N3) and metastasis (M0-M1). Staging ranges from stage 1 (T0, N0, M0) to stage IVc (any T, any N, M1)

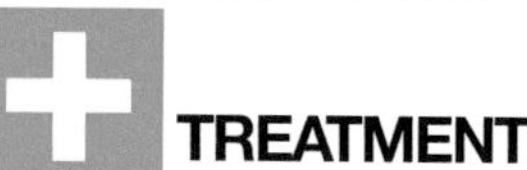

TREATMENT

APPROPRIATE HEALTH CARE Inpatient

GENERAL MEASURES
- Inpatient procedures with usual nursing care
- Drain parotid bed
- Usually 1-2 day hospitalization

SURGICAL MEASURES
- Benign tumors - superficial or total conservative (nerve-sparing) parotidectomy depending on site of tumor
- Malignant tumors - total parotidectomy, or sialadenectomy with adjuvant radiotherapy to parotid base of skull with/without neck depending on histology. Preservation of facial nerve unless involved by tumor.
- Cervical lymphadenectomy if palpable nodes or elective neck dissection in squamous cell carcinoma, high grade mucoepidermoid carcinoma or high grade adenocarcinoma
- Elevate head of bed postoperative
- Suction drainage x 1-2 days
- Suture line care with antibiotic ointment
- Radiation and oncological measures:
  - ◊ Post-operative irradiation (via fast neutron beam) is utilized for larger and high-grade carcinoma
  - ◊ Chemotherapy is reserved for metastatic disease or locally advanced and unresectable tumors

ACTIVITY Moderate restriction for 1 day

DIET Non-stimulating liquid

PATIENT EDUCATION
- Basic cancer followup
- Recurrent masses
- Trigeminal nerve symptoms
- Frey syndrome (gustatory sweating)
- Facial nerve symptoms (paresis)

MEDICATIONS

DRUG(S) OF CHOICE N/A
Contraindications: N/A
Precautions: N/A
Significant possible interactions: N/A

ALTERNATIVE DRUGS N/A

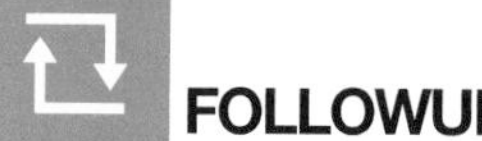

FOLLOWUP

PATIENT MONITORING
- For malignancy - once every 4 months the first year, once every six months subsequent 3 years, once per year subsequently
- For benign tumors - once per year for five years

PREVENTION/AVOIDANCE No known etiologic agents

POSSIBLE COMPLICATIONS
- Frey syndrome (gustatory sweating) occurs symptomatically in about 20% of patients undergoing parotidectomy
- Hematoma with possible posterior displacement of tongue and airway obstruction if the major branch of the lingual artery (supplying the submandibular gland) is injured
- Facial neurapraxia from surgery should resolve within six months, even with use of adjuvant radiotherapy
- Cosmetic deformity of moderate facial flattening on side of parotidectomy
- Injury to hypoglossal or lingual nerve during submandibular resection
- Pleomorphic adenoma may recur, if inadequately excised, since it has pseudopods throughout the lobe

EXPECTED COURSE/PROGNOSIS
- By tumor type:
  - ◊ Parotid pleomorphic adenoma - untreated will demonstrate malignant degeneration in 2-10% over 20 years. Treated adequately, parotid pleomorphic adenoma has 1.5% recurrence rate. Extension of pseudopods of tumor beyond the tumor mass increases the risk of recurrent disease. Malignancy prognosis depends on stage.
  - ◊ Adenoid cystic - parotid 5 year survival 73%, 15 year 21%; submandibular 5 year 50%, 15 year 0%; palate 5 year 80%, 15 year 38%
  - ◊ Adenocarcinoma - are aggressive tumors with a tendency for local recurrence (38%), regional lymph node metastasis (33%) and dissemination to lungs, bone and liver; 5 year survival 78%, 20 year 41%
  - ◊ Mucoepidermoid - low-grade 5 year survival 81%, 15 year 48%, high-grade 5 year survival 46%, 15 year 25%
  - ◊ Squamous cell carcinoma - rare tumor with 50% incidence of cervical lymph node metastasis and local recurrence, 5 year 18%, 15 years 0%
- 5 year survival rate for stages I-IV and cause specific survival (CSS)
  - ◊ Stage I - 75% (CSS, 86%)
  - ◊ Stage II - 59% (CSS, 66%)
  - ◊ Stage III - 57% (CSS, 53%)
  - ◊ Stage IV - 28% (CSS, 32%)

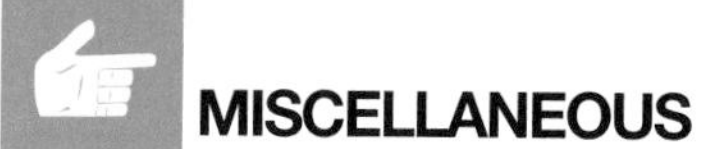

MISCELLANEOUS

ASSOCIATED CONDITIONS None known

AGE-RELATED FACTORS
Pediatric: Colon hemangioma is the most common benign tumor in pediatric population accounting for 25-60%, followed by pleomorphic adenoma. Mucoepidermoid most common malignant.
Geriatric: N/A
Others: N/A

PREGNANCY Not affected

SYNONYMS N/A

ICD-9-CM
142.0 Malignant neoplasm of parotid gland
142.1 Malignant neoplasm of submandibular gland
142.2 Malignant neoplasm of sublingual gland
142.9 Malignant neoplasm of salivary gland, unspecified

SEE ALSO
Sjögren syndrome

OTHER NOTES N/A

ABBREVIATIONS N/A

REFERENCES

- Coleman JJ: Salivary gland disorders. In: Jurkiewicz MJ, Krizek TJ, et al, eds. Plastic Surgery: Principles and Practices. St. Louis, C.V. Mosby Co.; 199:1
- Edgerton MT, Angel MF, Morgan RF. The mouth, tongue, jaw and salivary glands. In: Sabiston Jr D, ed. Textbook of Surgery: the Biological Basis of Modern Surgical Practice. 14th ed. Phildelphia: WB Saunders; 1991
- Ward MJ, Levine PA. Salivary gland tumors. In: Close LG, Larson DL, Shah JP, eds. Essentials of Head and Neck Oncology. 1st ed. New York: Thieme; 1998
- Rankow RM, Polayes IM. Diseases of the Salivary Glands. Philadelphia: W.B. Saunders; 1976
- Batsakis JG: Tumors of the Head and Neck. Clinical and Pathological Considerations. 3rd ed. Baltimore: Lippincott Williams and Wilkins; 2000

Web references: 0 available at www.5mcc.com
Illustrations 1 available

Author(s):
Bruce T. Vanderhoff, MD
Jacob Varghese, MD

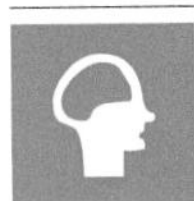

BASICS

DESCRIPTION Disease caused by any serotype of the genus Salmonella. Clinical syndromes include enterocolitis (75%), bacteremia (10%), enteric fever (10%) (see Typhoid fever), localized infection outside gastrointestinal tract (5%) and an asymptomatic carrier state (< 1%). Organisms invade gut mucosa, producing inflammatory, cytotoxic response. Organisms can then disseminate into systemic circulation via lymphatics. Infective dose and host defenses dictate extent of disease.

System(s) affected: Gastrointestinal

Genetics: Molecular studies have determined the total genome DNA sequence for a particular multi-drug resistant human Salmonella serotype

Incidence/Prevalence in USA:
- 800 cases/100,000 population/year. Peak frequency July-November. Salmonella isolations represent only 1-10% of actual yearly incidence. Second only to Campylobacter as cause of bacterial diarrheal illness. Each year, an average of 55 outbreaks of Salmonella infections are reported to CDC.
- Infants: 130/100,000
- Adults: 6/100,000
- Use of e-mail in outbreak investigations has proved to be speedy and cost effective in amassing a critical amount of data needed for public health action

Predominant age:
- High prevalence in persons > 70 or < 20
- Highest in infants < 1 year

Predominant sex: Male = Female

SIGNS & SYMPTOMS
- Acute uncomplicated illness
  - ◊ Nausea, vomiting, diarrhea
  - ◊ Abdominal cramps
  - ◊ Headache, myalgias
  - ◊ Fever to 102°F (39°C)
- Protracted disease
  - ◊ Persistent fever
  - ◊ Arthritis, reactive or septic
  - ◊ Osteomyelitis
  - ◊ Sacroiliitis
  - ◊ Wound infection, soft tissue abscesses
  - ◊ Meningitis
  - ◊ Arteritis
  - ◊ Endocarditis, pericarditis
  - ◊ Pneumonia, lung abscess, empyema
  - ◊ Hypovolemia
  - ◊ Splenic (abscess)
  - ◊ Hepatic (abscess)
  - ◊ Urogenital tract infection

CAUSES
- Ingestion of contaminated food - (poultry, beef, eggs, dairy products) or water
- Person-to-person and/or fecal-oral spread
- Contact with animal reservoirs - poultry, cows, pigs, birds, sheep, seals, donkeys, lizards, snakes, pets (e.g., turtles, cats, dogs, mice, guinea pigs, hamsters)
- Iatrogenic contamination - blood transfusion, endoscopy
- Contact with asymptomatic chronic carrier (e.g., day care center)
- Achlorhydria - gastroduodenal surgery, idiopathic
- Ulcerative colitis
- Systemic lupus erythematosus
- Schistosomiasis
- Cholelithiasis
- Nephrolithiasis
- Drugs - antibiotics, purgatives, opiates
- Intentional contamination of restaurant food through criminal mischief has been reported

RISK FACTORS
- Impaired gastric acidity-H2 blockers, antacids, gastrectomy, achlorhydria
- Hemolytic anemias - sickle-cell, malaria, bartonellosis
- Malignancy - lymphoma, leukemia, disseminated carcinoma
- Immunosuppression - AIDS, steroids, other immunosuppressants, chemotherapy, radiation
- Pets with high fecal carriage rates for salmonella, especially reptiles (e.g., snakes, iguanas)
  - ◊ Antibiotic treatment of the animal is not recommended, due to temporary effect only

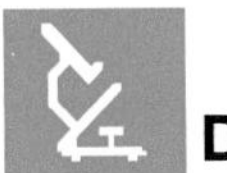

DIAGNOSIS

DIFFERENTIAL DIAGNOSIS
- Viral gastroenteritis
- Other bacterial enteritis (e.g., shigellosis, cholera)
- Other bacterial sources or systemic and localized sepsis (e.g., meningococci, staphylococci)
- Pseudomembranous colitis
- Inflammatory or granulomatous bowel disease
- Appendicitis
- Cholecystitis
- Perforated viscus

LABORATORY
- Enterocolitis
  - ◊ Fecal leukocytes positive
  - ◊ Stool culture positive for Salmonella species
  - ◊ WBC normal or decreased
  - ◊ Blood cultures negative
- Bacteremia
  - ◊ Blood cultures positive
  - ◊ Stool cultures negative
- Local infections
  - ◊ Polymorphonuclear leukocytosis
  - ◊ Tissue site culture positive
- Asymptomatic carrier state
  - ◊ Stool culture positive for more than 1 year
  - ◊ Urine culture may be positive with certain serotypes

Drugs that may alter lab results: Antibiotics used early may lead to false-negative cultures and blunted immunologic response

Disorders that may alter lab results: N/A

PATHOLOGICAL FINDINGS
- Mucosal ulceration, hemorrhage and necrosis
- Reticuloendothelial hyperplasia and hypertrophy
- Focal organ and soft tissues abscesses

SPECIAL TESTS
- Serologic tests identify particular clinical syndromes and serve as epidemiologic markers
- A rapid test (TUBEX) used in children to detect anti-Salmonella IgM antibodies was found to be 92.6% sensitive and 94.8% specific

IMAGING Angiography in patients over 50 with bacteremia. To rule out presence of infected aneurysm, particularly of aorto-iliac vessels.

DIAGNOSTIC PROCEDURES N/A

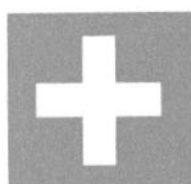

TREATMENT

APPROPRIATE HEALTH CARE
- Outpatient for uncomplicated enterocolitis and carrier state
- Inpatient for bacteremia and extra-intestinal infection (11% hospitalization rate)
- Do not wait for stool culture results before initiating important therapeutic decisions

GENERAL MEASURES
- Correct fluid and electrolyte deficits
- Control symptoms (pain, nausea, vomiting)

SURGICAL MEASURES
- Surgical drainage and vascular bypass procedures for infected tissue sites
- When biliary tract disease is present, the best results are obtained with the combination of cholecystectomy and a 10-14 day course of parenteral antibiotics (see Drug(s) of Choice - bacteremia) initiated before surgery

ACTIVITY As tolerated

DIET Oral rehydration solution during diarrhea phase; advance to normal diet as tolerated

PATIENT EDUCATION Food Safety and Inspection Service, Office of Public Awareness, Department of Agriculture, Rm. 1165-S, Washington, DC 20205, (202)447-9351

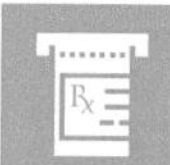

MEDICATIONS

DRUG(S) OF CHOICE

- Enterocolitis uncomplicated:
  - None recommended
- Enterocolitis complicated: (by age extremes, immunosuppression, underlying cardiovascular abnormalities, prosthetic orthopedic devices, hemolytic anemia)
  - Adults
    - Ciprofloxacin (Cipro) 500 mg PO bid for 5-7 days; or
    - Norfloxacin (Noroxin) 400 mg PO q12 hours for 3-7 days; or
    - Azithromycin (Zithromax) 1.0 gm PO once, then 500 mg PO qd for 6 days
  - Children
    - Ampicillin 50-100 mg/kg/24h in 4 divided doses for 10-14 days; or
    - Trimethoprim-sulfamethoxazole (Bactrim, Septra) 10 mg-50 mg/kg/24h in 2 divided doses for 10-14 days
- Bacteremia:
  - Adults
    - Ciprofloxacin (Cipro) 400 mg IV bid or 500 mg PO bid for 7 days; or
    - Ceftriaxone (Rocephin) 2 gm IV/IM qd for 7 days
  - Children
    - Ampicillin 200 mg/kg/24h in 4 divided doses for 10-14 days; or
    - Trimethoprim-sulfamethoxazole (Bactrim, Septra) 10 mg-50 mg/kg/24h in 2 divided doses for 10-14 days; or
    - Chloramphenicol 75 mg/kg/24h in 4 divided doses for 10-14 days
- Localized infection:
  - Same as for bacteremia
  - In sustained bacteremia or prolonged local infection, antibiotics can be given PO for 4-6 weeks (substitute trimethoprim-sulfamethoxazole for cefotaxime, using 2-4 double strength (DS) tablets given tid)
- Chronic carrier state:
  - Ampicillin 2-4 gm/day plus probenecid 1-2 gm/day, both divided into 4 PO doses, for 6 weeks; or
  - 40-160 mg/day trimethoprim and 200-800 mg/day sulfamethoxazole divided into 2 doses for 6 weeks
  - Consider ciprofloxacin 500 mg PO bid for 4 weeks, or norfloxacin (Noroxin) 400 mg PO bid for 4 weeks, if gallstones are present

Contraindications: Known drug allergy

Precautions:

- Use bowel motility inhibitors (Lomotil, Imodium) with caution, if at all
- Monitor blood levels of chloramphenicol in neonates and infants
- Ampicillin-resistant strains increasing; now at 15-30% in US. Some strains are rapidly becoming multidrug resistant.

Significant possible interactions:

- Ampicillin failure rate is 75% in chronic carriers with gallbladder disease
- Fluoroquinolone resistance has been observed in some Salmonella serotypes common to swine and humans. Use of fluoroquinolones in food animals is implicated.
- Ceftriaxone resistance has been reported in Taiwan and fluoroquinolone resistance in Japan

ALTERNATIVE DRUGS Fluoroquinolones - ciprofloxacin (Cipro), ofloxacin (Floxin) gaining favor in management of gastroenteritis, osteomyelitis and carrier state. Use is restricted to nonpregnant adults only. For gastroenteritis in children > 1 year, consider furazolidone (Furoxone) 2.5 mg/kg PO qid for 5 days.

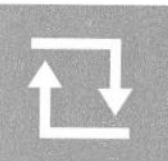

FOLLOWUP

PATIENT MONITORING Repeat stool culture at 5 months (40% of children negative, 90% of adults negative) and at 1 year (> 99% of all patients negative)

PREVENTION/AVOIDANCE

- Proper hygiene in production, transport and storage of food
- Control of animal reservoir, especially by avoiding contact with animal feces
- Hand washing emphasized
- No vaccine available to oppose salmonellosis
- The US Dept of Agriculture endorses a program to spray newly hatched chicks with benign bacterial species in order to prevent gut colonization with Salmonella

POSSIBLE COMPLICATIONS

- Toxic megacolon
- Hypovolemic shock
- Metastatic abscess formation
- Acute or chronic hydrocephalus

EXPECTED COURSE/PROGNOSIS

- Prognosis for enterocolitis is excellent. Exceptions - in the very young (7.0% fatal), the very old (8.7% fatal) and the debilitated and/or institutionalized (2.3% fatal).
- Prognosis for meningitis or endocarditis is poor, unless effective treatment given early
- Mortality is increased with multidrug resistant strain

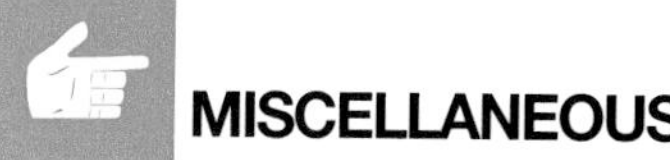

MISCELLANEOUS

ASSOCIATED CONDITIONS The frequency of reactive arthritis after various Salmonella outbreaks is approximately 10%

AGE-RELATED FACTORS

Pediatric: Children, especially neonates, more likely to become chronic carriers
Geriatric: Patients over 60 also have high carrier rate presumably due to biliary sequestration of organisms
Others: Contaminated marijuana is important source of infection, particularly in young adults

PREGNANCY Consult obstetrician regarding antibiotics. Keep a low threshold for hospital admission.

SYNONYMS N/A

ICD-9-CM

003.0 Salmonella gastroenteritis

SEE ALSO

Gastroenteritis, viral
Typhoid fever

OTHER NOTES If one member of a household becomes infected with salmonellosis, the chance of at least one other member becoming infected is 60%. The CDC has identified Salmonella as a Category B biological terrorism agent: moderately easy to disseminate, causing moderate morbidity/low mortality, requiring specific enhancements of the CDC's diagnostic capacity and disease surveillance capabilities.

ABBREVIATIONS

CDC = Centers for Disease Control

REFERENCES

- Gilbert DN, Moellering RC, Eliopoulos GM, Sande MA. The Sanford Guide to Antimicrobial Therapy. 34th ed. Dallas: Antimicrobial Therapy, inc.; 2004
- Behrman RE, Kliegman RM, Jenson HB, eds. Nelson Textbook of Pediatrics. 17th ed. Philadelphia: W.B. Saunders Company; 2004
- Mandell GL, Bennett JE, Dolin R (eds). Mandell, Douglas, and Bennett's Principles and Practice of Infectious Diseases. 5th ed. Philadelphia: Churchill Livingstone; 2000
- Case records of the Massachusetts General Hospital. Weekly clinicopathological exercise. Case 16-2001. A 17-year-old girl with worsening abdominal pain, fever, and diarrhea after a recent cesarean section. NEJM 2001 May 24;344:1622-1627
- Helms M, Vastrup P, Gerner-Smidt P, Molbak K. Excess mortality associated with antimicrobial drug-resistant Salmonella typhimurium. Emerg Infect Dis 2002;8(5):490-5
- Feldman M, Friedman LS, Sleisenger MH, editors. Sleisenger & Fordtran's Gastrointestinal and Liver Disease. 7th ed. Philadelphia: WB Saunders Co; 2002
- Oracz G, Feleszko W, Golicka D, Maksymiuk J, et al. Rapid diagnosis of acute Salmonella gastrointestinal infection. Clinical Infectious Diseases 2003;36:112-5

Web references: 1 available at www.5mcc.com
Illustrations N/A

Author(s):
Richard Viken, MD

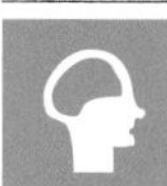

BASICS

DESCRIPTION Non-infectious multisystem disease of unknown cause, commonly affecting young and middle-age adults. Frequently presents with bilateral hilar adenopathy, pulmonary infiltrates, ocular and skin lesions. Other organs may be involved, including liver, spleen, lymph nodes, heart, and central nervous system.
System(s) affected: Cardiovascular, Gastrointestinal, Hemic/Lymphatic/Immunologic, Pulmonary
Genetics: Although world-wide in distribution, increased prevalence found in Scandinavians, Japanese, Irish females, and African American women
Incidence/Prevalence in USA: 30-80 per 100,000
Predominant age: 20-60 years
Predominant sex: Female > Male

SIGNS & SYMPTOMS
- Patients may be asymptomatic
- Cough
- Shortness of breath
- Skin (new lesions)
- Pain or irritation of eyes
- General fatigue, malaise
- Fever
- Night sweats
- Bell palsy

CAUSES Unknown

RISK FACTORS None known

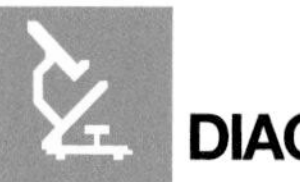

DIAGNOSIS

DIFFERENTIAL DIAGNOSIS
- Infectious granulomatous disease such as tuberculosis and fungal infections
- Foreign body reactions
- Lymphoma
- Other malignancies associated with lymphadenopathy
- Berylliosis

LABORATORY
- Lymphopenia, anemia, or leukopenia can be seen in over half of the patients
- Abnormal liver function, especially increased alkaline phosphatase is frequently encountered
- Hypercalciuria occurs in up to 10% of patients, with hypercalcemia less frequent

Drugs that may alter lab results: Prednisone will lower serum-angiotensin converting enzyme and normalize Gallium scan. ACE inhibitors will lower serum ACE level.

Disorders that may alter lab results: Hyperthyroidism and diabetes will increase serum angiotensin converting enzyme level

PATHOLOGICAL FINDINGS Noncaseating epithelioid granulomas without evidence of fungal or mycobacterial infection

SPECIAL TESTS
- Serum angiotensin converting enzyme (ACE) is elevated in over 60% of patients
- Gallium scan uptake in chest, lymph nodes, and parotids may be seen in active disease
- Characteristically in active disease, bronchoalveolar lavage (BAL) fluid has an increased percentage of lymphocytes, specifically CD4 positive (T-helper/inducer lymphocytes)
- Ophthalmologic exam

IMAGING
- Routine CXR are staged using Scadding's classification:
  - ◊ Stage 0 = normal
  - ◊ Stage 1 = hilar adenopathy alone
  - ◊ Stage 2 = hilar adenopathy plus parenchymal infiltrates
  - ◊ Stage 3 = parenchymal infiltrates alone
  - ◊ Stage 4 = pulmonary fibrosis
- Gallium scan will be positive in areas of acute disease
- Computerized tomography may enhance appreciation of lymph nodes and high resolution CT scan shows peribronchial disease
- Positive emission transmission (PET) scan can indicate areas of disease activity in lungs, lymph nodes, and other areas of the body

DIAGNOSTIC PROCEDURES
- Bronchoscopy with transbronchial biopsy and bronchoalveolar lavage is often performed to diagnose lung disease
- Mediastinoscopy, skin or lymph node biopsy (if needed to establish diagnosis)
- When available, Kveim-Siltzbach skin test can be performed. This test is fairly sensitive (approximately 80%) and highly specific (> 95%). Unfortunately, the antigen is not generally available.

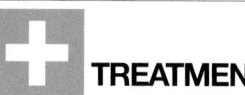

TREATMENT

APPROPRIATE HEALTH CARE Outpatient

GENERAL MEASURES
- The disease may require no specific therapy in the asymptomatic individual or may treat for specific indications, such as cardiac, central nervous system, ocular, or hypercalcemia
- Treatment of pulmonary and skin manifestations usually done on the basis of impairment

SURGICAL MEASURES N/A

ACTIVITY Generally no limitations

DIET
- Avoid high calcium diets
- In patients on corticosteroids, avoid high salt foods

PATIENT EDUCATION Generally stress the benign nature of the disease and the fact that it is not contagious to others and is not malignant

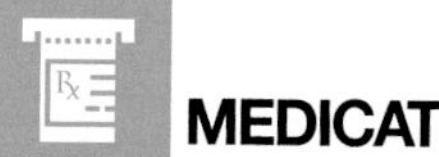

MEDICATIONS

DRUG(S) OF CHOICE
- Systemic corticosteroids in the symptomatic individual, usually prednisone initially 40 mg every day or every other day. Treatment with tapering doses of prednisone for at least one year.
- In patients with skin or ocular disease, topical steroids may be effective

Contraindications: Patients with known problems with corticosteroids
Precautions: Careful monitoring in patients with diabetes mellitus and/or hypertension
Significant possible interactions: Refer to manufacturer's profile of each drug

ALTERNATIVE DRUGS
- Methotrexate 10 mg per week, hydroxychloroquine (Plaquenil) 100-400 mg per day, azathioprine 50-100 mg per day. Use of immunosuppressants such as methotrexate or azathioprine will require careful, regular monitoring of complete blood count.
- Thalidomide has been used for chronic skin lesions. The anti-TNF agent infliximab has also been used in some refractory cases.

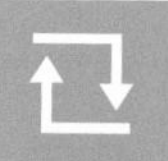

FOLLOWUP

PATIENT MONITORING
- Patients on prednisone for symptoms should be seen every month or two while on therapy
- Patients not requiring therapy should be seen regularly (every three months) for at least the first two years after diagnosis
- CXR and pulmonary function tests are useful for monitoring for pulmonary changes
- Serum angiotensin converting enzyme level is used by some to follow disease activity. In patients with an initially elevated ACE level, it should fall towards normal while on therapy or when the disease resolves.

PREVENTION/AVOIDANCE None known

POSSIBLE COMPLICATIONS
- Patients may develop significant respiratory involvement including cor pulmonale
- Other organs, especially the heart (congestive heart failure, arrhythmias), eyes (rarely blindness) and central nervous system can be involved with serious consequences. Fortunately, cardiac, ocular, and CNS involvement usually manifests itself early on in patients with these manifestations of the disease.

EXPECTED COURSE/PROGNOSIS
- 50% of patients will have spontaneous resolution within two years
- 25% will have significant fibrosis but no further worsening of disease after two years
- 25% (higher in some populations, including African Americans) will have chronic disease
- Patients on corticosteroids for more than 6 months have a greater chance of having chronic disease

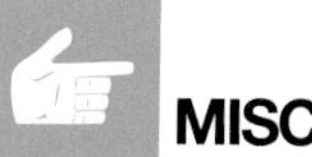

MISCELLANEOUS

ASSOCIATED CONDITIONS None known

AGE-RELATED FACTORS
Pediatric: Rare
Geriatric: Less than 5% of patients with active disease are 60 years or older
Others: Sarcoidosis is a disease of youth to middle age

PREGNANCY No increased incidence

SYNONYMS
- Lofgren syndrome (erythema nodosum, hilar adenopathy plus uveitis)
- Besnier-Boeck disease
- Boeck sarcoid
- Schaumann disease

ICD-9-CM
135 Sarcoidosis

SEE ALSO

OTHER NOTES N/A

ABBREVIATIONS N/A

REFERENCES

- Statement on sarcoidosis. Joint Statement of the American Thoracic Society (ATS), the European Respiratory Society (ERS) and the World Association of Sarcoidosis and Other Granulomatous Disorders (WASOG) adopted by the ATS Board of Directors and by the ERS Executive Committee, February 1999. Am J Respir Crit Care Med 1999;160(2):736-55
- Sharma OP: Sarcoidosis. Dis Month 1990;36:469-535.3
- Lower LL, Baughman RP. Prolonged use of methotrexate for sarcoidosis. Arch Int Med 1995;155:846-51
- Baughman RP, Lower EE. Steroid-sparing alternatives for sarcoidosis. Clin Chest Med 1997;18:853-64
- Baughman RP, Lower EE, du Bois RM. Lancet 2003;361(9363):1111-8

Web references: 0 available at www.5mcc.com
Illustrations 4 available

Author(s):
Robert P. Baughman, MD

BASICS

DESCRIPTION A contagious disease caused by infestation of the skin by the mite *Sarcoptes scabiei*, var. hominis
System(s) affected: Skin/Exocrine
Genetics: N/A
Incidence/Prevalence in USA: Common, although number of cases per year is declining as the epidemic, which began in 1971, passed its peak (1986). Worldwide incidence is 300 million cases per year.
Predominant age: Children and young adults
Predominant sex: Male = Female

SIGNS & SYMPTOMS
- Generalized itching (often severe)
- Nocturnal pruritus
- Burrows in finger webs and sides of fingers
- Excoriated and non-excoriated papules on hands, flexor surfaces of wrist, elbow, anterior axillary folds, waistline, penis, scrotum and buttocks
- Vesicles and papules (discrete)
- Secondary erosions or excoriations
- Pustules (if secondarily infected)
- Scaling
- Erythema
- Nodules in covered areas (buttocks, groin, axillae)
- Atypical infestations in immunosuppressed patients

CAUSES *Sarcoptes scabiei*, var. hominis

RISK FACTORS
- Personal skin-to-skin contact, e.g., sexual promiscuity, crowding, poverty, nosocomial infection
- Immunocompromised patients including HIV/AIDS
- Atopic eczema

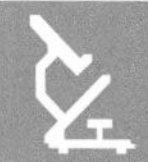

DIAGNOSIS

DIFFERENTIAL DIAGNOSIS
- Atopic dermatitis
- Dermatitis herpetiformis
- Eczema
- Insect bites
- Papular urticaria
- Pediculosis corporis
- Pityriasis rosea
- Prurigo
- Pyoderma
- Seborrheic dermatitis
- Syphilis

LABORATORY CBC (although rarely needed) will frequently demonstrate eosinophilia

Drugs that may alter lab results: N/A

Disorders that may alter lab results: N/A

PATHOLOGICAL FINDINGS Skin biopsy of a nodule (although rarely performed) will reveal portions of the mite in the corneal layer

SPECIAL TESTS N/A

IMAGING N/A

DIAGNOSTIC PROCEDURES
- Examination of skin with magnifying lens - look for typical burrows in finger webs, on flexor aspects of the wrists, and penis. Look for a dark point at the end of the burrow (the mite). The mite can be extracted with a 25 gauge needle and examined microscopically.
- Mineral oil mounts - place a drop of mineral oil over a suspected lesion. Non-excoriated papules or vesicles may also be sampled. Scrape the lesion with a #15 surgical blade. Examine under a microscope for mites, eggs, egg casings or feces. Scraping from under fingernails may often be positive.
- Potassium hydroxide (KOH) wet mount - transfer skin scrapings directly to a glass slide, add a drop of KOH, and apply a cover slip. Examine the slide for diagnostic material. If none is evident, heat slide gently to separate squamous cells and reexamine.
- Burrow ink test - if burrows are not obvious, apply blue black ink to an area of rash. Wash off the ink with alcohol. A burrow should remain stained and become more evident. Then apply mineral oil, scrape and observe microscopically as previously noted.

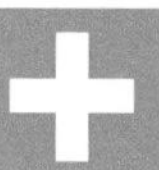

TREATMENT

APPROPRIATE HEALTH CARE Outpatient

GENERAL MEASURES
- Treat all intimate contacts and close household and family members
- Wash all clothing, bed linen, and towels in a normal wash cycle

SURGICAL MEASURES N/A

ACTIVITY Full activity

DIET No special diet

PATIENT EDUCATION
- Patient instruction sheet "Scabies" in Epstein: Common Skin Disorders, page P-95 (see References)
- Griffith's Instructions for Patients, Philadelphia, Elsevier
- Schmitt: Instructions for Pediatric Patients, Philadelphia, W.B. Saunders Co.

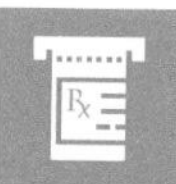

MEDICATIONS

DRUG(S) OF CHOICE

- Permethrin (Elimite) 5% cream: considered by many to be the drug of choice for scabies. Cream is applied into the skin from the neck to the soles of the feet with particular attention given to skin creases. It is left on for 8 to 14 hours, then thoroughly washed off. Thirty grams is usually adequate for an adult. A second application 1 week later is sometimes recommended.
- Lindane (Kwell, Scabene) 1%: available in lotion, cream and shampoo. The cream or lotion should be applied to all skin surfaces from the neck down and washed off 8 to 12 hours later. Two applications 1 week apart are recommended.
- Crotamiton (Eurax) 10%: cream is applied into the skin from the head to the soles of the feet and left on for 8 to 14 hours, then thoroughly washed off. It is felt to be less toxic than lindane, but perhaps slightly less effective, therefore, application 2 nights in a row is advised.

Contraindications: Lindane should be avoided in children who are premature, malnourished or emaciated and those with severe underlying skin disease or a history of seizure disorders.

Precautions:

- Patients should be cautioned not to overuse the medication when applying it to the skin
- For medications other than permethrin, patients should use a second application only when specifically advised to do so by their physician
- Lindane should be used cautiously in immunocompromised patients

Significant possible interactions: Avoid lindane for patients on medications that lower the seizure threshold, such as tricyclic antidepressants

ALTERNATIVE DRUGS

- Precipitated sulfur 6% in petroleum: applied to the entire body from the neck down for 3 nights. It is malodorous and messy, but is thought to be safer than lindane, especially in infants under age 6 months and safer than permethrin in infants under age 2 months.
- Ivermectin (Mectizan) 100-200 μg/kg in combination with topical scabicide for HIV-positive patients

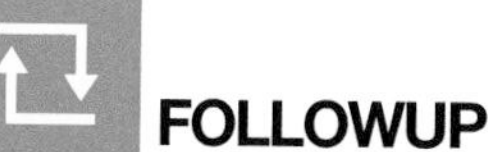

FOLLOWUP

PATIENT MONITORING Recheck patient at weekly intervals only if rash or itching persists. Scrape new lesions and retreat if mite or products found.

PREVENTION/AVOIDANCE N/A

POSSIBLE COMPLICATIONS

- Eczema
- Pyoderma
- Postscabetic pruritus
- Nodular scabies

EXPECTED COURSE/PROGNOSIS

- Lesions begin to regress in 1 to 2 days along with the worst itching
- Some itching and dermatitis commonly persists for 10 to 14 days and can be treated with antihistamines and/or topical or oral corticosteroids
- Nodular lesions may persist for several weeks, perhaps necessitating intralesional or systemic steroids
- Some instances of lindane resistant scabies have now been reported. These do respond to permethrin.

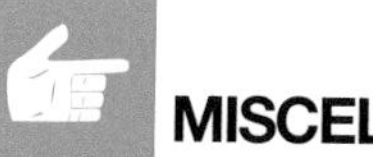

MISCELLANEOUS

ASSOCIATED CONDITIONS N/A

AGE-RELATED FACTORS

Pediatric:

- Infants often have more widespread involvement. They are occasionally infested on the face and scalp (rare for adults). Vesicular lesions on the palms and soles are also more commonly seen. When treating infants with permethrin, the entire body should be treated.
- The FDA recommends caution when using lindane in patients who weigh less than 50 kg. It is not recommended for infants and is contraindicated in premature infants.

Geriatric: The elderly often itch more severely, despite fewer cutaneous lesions. Elderly at risk for extensive infestations, perhaps related to a decline in cell-mediated immunity. May see back involvement in those who are bedridden.

Others: N/A

PREGNANCY Permethrin and lindane are category B drugs. Until more information is available precipitated sulfur appears to be the safest treatment in pregnant or lactating women.

SYNONYMS N/A

ICD-9-CM

133.0 Scabies

SEE ALSO

Insect bites & stings

OTHER NOTES N/A

ABBREVIATIONS N/A

REFERENCES

- Epstein E. Common Skin Disorders. 5th ed. Philadelphia: WB Saunders; 2001
- Odom RB, James WD, Berger TG. Andrews' Diseases of the Skin. 9th ed. Philadelphia: WB Saunders; 2000
- Lebwohl MG, et al, eds. Treatment of Skin Disease. 1st ed. New York: Mosby; 2002
- Weston WL, Lane AT, Morelli JG. Color Textbook of Pediatric Dermatology. 3rd ed. St. Louis: Mosby; 2002

Web references: 2 available at www.5mcc.com

Illustrations 5 available

Author(s):

Gary J. Silko, MD, MS

BASICS

DESCRIPTION "Streptococcal sore throat with a rash." A childhood disease characterized by high fever, pharyngitis, and rash caused by Group A beta-hemolytic streptococci (GAS) pyogenes that produce erythrogenic toxin. Incubation period 1-7 days, duration of illness 4-10 days.
System(s) affected: Gastrointestinal, Skin/Exocrine
Genetics: N/A
Incidence/Prevalence in USA: Up to 10% of GAS pharyngitis
Predominant age: 6-12 years
Predominant sex: Male = Female

SIGNS & SYMPTOMS
- Prodrome 1-2 days
  - ◊ Sore throat
  - ◊ Headache
  - ◊ Vomiting
  - ◊ Abdominal pain (may mimic acute abdomen)
  - ◊ Fever (up to 40°C or 103.6°F)
- Oral exam
  - ◊ "Beefy red" tonsils and pharynx with or without exudate
  - ◊ Petechiae on palate
  - ◊ White coating on tongue "White strawberry tongue" appears on days 1-2. This sheds by day 4-5 leaving a "Red strawberry tongue" - shiny, red with prominent papillae.
- Exanthem (appears within 1-5 days)
  - ◊ Orange-red punctate skin eruption with sandpaper-like texture - "sunburn with goose pimples"
  - ◊ Initially, chest and axillae, then spreads to abdomen and extremities; prominent in skin folds (axillae, groin, buttocks)
  - ◊ Flushed face with circumoral pallor
  - ◊ Transverse red streaks in skin folds of abdomen, antecubital space, and axillae: "Pastia's lines"
  - ◊ Desquamation begins on face after 7-10 days and proceeds over trunk to hands and feet; may persist for 6 weeks
  - ◊ In severe cases, small vesicular lesions (miliary sudamina) may appear on abdomen, hands, feet

CAUSES
- Hypersensitivity to erythrogenic toxins produced by GAS
- Site of GAS infection: Usually tonsils, may occur with skin infection
- Staphylococcus aureus may also produce erythrogenic toxin - "staphylococcal scarlet fever." May be mild form of toxic shock syndrome or scalded skin syndrome.

RISK FACTORS
- Winter/spring seasons
- Age - school age children - by age 10, 80% have antibodies to erythrogenic toxin
- Contact with infected individual
- Crowded living conditions, eg, lower socioeconomic status, military, child care

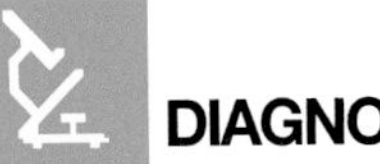

DIAGNOSIS

DIFFERENTIAL DIAGNOSIS
- Measles
- Rubella
- Infectious mononucleosis
- Roseola
- Severe sunburn
- Secondary syphilis
- Arcanobacterium haemolyticum
- Toxic shock syndrome
- Staphylococcal scalded skin syndrome
- Kawasaki disease
- Drug hypersensitivity
- Mycoplasma pneumonia
- Viral exanthem

LABORATORY
- Throat culture definitive diagnosis
- Rapid Strep antigen tests - diagnostic if positive, but sensitivity only 50-90%, so must do throat culture if negative result
- Serologic tests (includes antistreptolysin O titer and streptozyme tests) - confirm recent GAS infection; not helpful for diagnosis of acute disease

Drugs that may alter lab results:
- Prior antibiotic therapy may result in negative throat culture
- Penicillin within 5 days of symptoms can delay/abolish anti-streptolysin O response

Disorders that may alter lab results: N/A

PATHOLOGICAL FINDINGS N/A

SPECIAL TESTS N/A

IMAGING N/A

DIAGNOSTIC PROCEDURES N/A

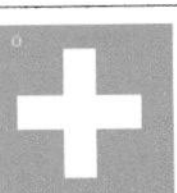

TREATMENT

APPROPRIATE HEALTH CARE Outpatient except for severe suppurative complications

GENERAL MEASURES Supportive care

SURGICAL MEASURES tonsillectomy may be recommended with recurrent bouts of pharyngitis

ACTIVITY Fully active

DIET No special diet

PATIENT EDUCATION Must take antibiotics for full course; brief delay in initiating treatment awaiting throat culture results does not increase the risk of rheumatic fever.

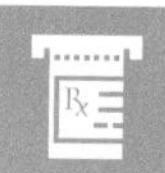

MEDICATIONS

DRUG(S) OF CHOICE
- Penicillin (oral; penicillin V and others) for 10 days
  - ◊ 125 mg po tid for under 60 lb/27 kg; 250 mg tid for others; bid dosing may also be effective.
  - ◊ If compliance questionable, use penicillin, benzathine (Bicillin LA): single IM dose 600,000 units for under 60 lb/27 kg; 1,200,000 million units for others
- Acetaminophen for fever and comfort

Contraindications: Penicillin allergy
Precautions: Refer to manufacturer's profile of each drug
Significant possible interactions: Refer to manufacturer's profile of each drug

ALTERNATIVE DRUGS
- Erythromycin estolate (20-40 mg/kg/day divided tid or qid or erythromycin ethyl succinate (40-50 mg/kg/day divided tid or qid) for 10 days. Maximum dose: 1 gm/day.
- Newer macrolides
  - ◊ Azithromycin (Zithromax, Z pak): Adults - 500 mg the first day, then 250 mg qd for 4 days; Children over 2 years - 12 mg/kg/day (maximum of 500 mg) for 5 days
  - ◊ Clarithromycin (Biaxin): Adults - 250 mg bid for 10 days; Children over 6 months - 7.5 mg/kg bid for 10 days
- Oral cephalosporins; many are effective, but first generation are less expensive.
  - ◊ Cephalexin 40 mg/kg/day divided tid. Maximum: 250 mg tid for 10 days.
  - ◊ Cefadroxil 30 mg/kg/day divided bid. Maximum: 500 mg bid for 10 days.
- Clindamycin 20 mg/kg/day divided tid for 10 days
- Tetracyclines and sulfonamides should not be used

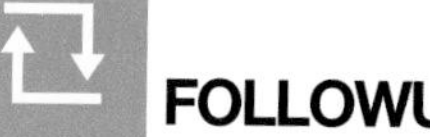

FOLLOWUP

PATIENT MONITORING
- Routine follow-up throat cultures not needed unless patient is symptomatic.
- Since GAS uniformly susceptible to penicillin; bacteriologic treatment failures possibly due to:
  - ◊ Poor compliance
  - ◊ Beta-lactamase oral flora hydrolyzing penicillin
  - ◊ GAS carrier state and concurrent viral rash (require no treatment)

PREVENTION/AVOIDANCE
- GAS spread by contact with respiratory secretions. Avoid if possible.
- Children should not return to school or day care until after 24 hours of antibiotic therapy
- Prophylactic penicillin not recommended after exposure to scarlet fever

POSSIBLE COMPLICATIONS
- Suppurative
  - ◊ Sinusitis
  - ◊ Otitis media/mastoiditis
  - ◊ Cervical adenitis
  - ◊ Peritonsillar abscess/retropharyngeal abscess
  - ◊ Pneumonia
  - ◊ Septicemia/meningitis/osteomyelitis/septic arthritis
- Non-suppurative
  - ◊ Rheumatic fever (penicillin prevents RF when started as long as 10 days after onset of acute GAS infection)
  - ◊ Glomerulonephritis (prevention even after adequate treatment of GAS is less certain)
  - ◊ "Streptococcal toxic shock syndrome": Fever, hypotension, disseminated intravascular coagulation (DIC); cardiac, liver, kidney dysfunction.

EXPECTED COURSE/PROGNOSIS
- With penicillin, course may be shortened by 12-24 hours
- Can have recurrent attacks

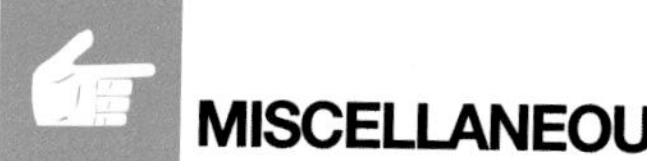

MISCELLANEOUS

ASSOCIATED CONDITIONS
- Pharyngitis
- Impetigo
- Puerperal sepsis

AGE-RELATED FACTORS
Pediatric: Rare in infancy
Geriatric: N/A
Others: N/A

PREGNANCY N/A

SYNONYMS Scarlatina

ICD-9-CM
034.1 Scarlet fever

SEE ALSO
Pharyngitis

OTHER NOTES N/A

ABBREVIATIONS
GAS = Group A beta-hemolytic streptococci

REFERENCES

- Committee on Infectious Diseases of Amer Acad Ped. (Red Book). 573-589, 2003
- Behrman R, Kliegman R, Arvin A: Nelson's Textbook of Pediatrics. 17th Ed. Philadelphia, WB Saunders Co., 2003
- Bisno AL, Gerber MA, Gwaltney JM, Kaplan EL, Schwartz RN: Diagnosis and management of group A streptococcal pharyngitis: a practice guideline. Clin Inf Dis 1997;25:574-583

Web references: 0 available at www.5mcc.com
Illustrations 1 available

Author(s):
Mitchell S. King, MD

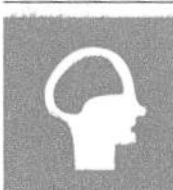

BASICS

DESCRIPTION Major psychiatric disorder with prodrome, active and residual symptoms involving disturbances (lasting at least 6 months) in:
- Appearance (deteriorated)
- Speech (loosened association)
- Behavior (grossly disorganized)
- Perception (hallucinations)
- Thinking (delusions)

System(s) affected: Nervous
Genetics: Genetic predisposition
Incidence/Prevalence in USA:
- Lifetime (1%). Highest prevalence in lower socioeconomic classes.
- 1.1% of the population > 18 years of age; similar rates in all countries

Predominant age: Onset typically before age 45
Predominant sex: Male = Female; onset earlier in males (early-mid 20's) than females (late 20's)

SIGNS & SYMPTOMS
- Withdrawal from reality
- Delusions (false personal beliefs)
- Reference (people or things have unusual significance)
- Others can hear your thoughts, put thoughts into you or control you; grandiose or religious delusions
- Hallucinations - usually auditory
- Illusions - incorrectly interpreted sensory stimuli
- Affect - flat or blunted
- Thought processes - loose associations (thoughts don't follow)
- Much speech but convey little information
- Extremes of gross overactivity to stupor with mutism

CAUSES Unknown - not initiated or maintained by an organic factor. Probably a complex interaction between inherited and environmental factors.

RISK FACTORS Biologic relative with schizophrenia (if first degree relative, risk is 8%)

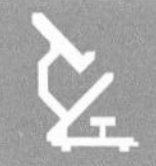

DIAGNOSIS

DIFFERENTIAL DIAGNOSIS
- Organic mental disorder - characterized by JOMAC (a mnemonic that stands for impaired Judgment, Orientation, Memory, Affect and Concentration). Disorientation, in particular indicates organicity. Organic mental disorders may be due to trauma, infection, tumor, metabolic, endocrine, intoxication (psychoactive substance use), epilepsy, neurological disorders, etc.
- Organic delusional syndrome - secondary to substance use/abuse (e.g., amphetamines, LSD, or phencyclidine) may have identical symptoms
- Mood disorders - especially bipolar disorder (manic depressive disorder); schizoaffective disorder; mood disorders with psychotic features
- Psychotic disorder due to general medical condition: delusions and/or hallucinations are the direct physiological consequence of a general medical condition
- Cultural belief system

LABORATORY
- No test available to indicate schizophrenia
- Laboratory tests needed to rule out organicity - may include CBC, blood chemistries, thyroid screen, urinalysis, vitamins (B12, folate, thiamine), blood and urine for drugs and alcohol
- Others for: heavy metals - ceruloplasmin, urine porphobilinogen

Drugs that may alter lab results: N/A

Disorders that may alter lab results: N/A

PATHOLOGICAL FINDINGS N/A

SPECIAL TESTS
- Psychological - Bender Gestalt, intelligence testing (WAIS-R), MMPI-2; neuropsychological testing
- EEG - to rule out seizure disorder, brain damage, etc.

IMAGING CT and MRI to rule out organicity

DIAGNOSTIC PROCEDURES Lumbar puncture

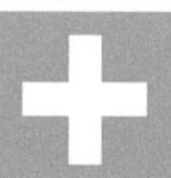

TREATMENT

APPROPRIATE HEALTH CARE
- Usually hospitalize initially for organic workup and for treatment of psychotic symptoms
- Outpatient if not dangerous to self or others, able to cooperate with treatment, and supportive family: community treatment and case management
- Family intervention: psycho-education

GENERAL MEASURES Ensure safety of patient and others - may act on delusional thinking

SURGICAL MEASURES N/A

ACTIVITY Establish safe hospital environment

DIET No special diet

PATIENT EDUCATION
- Education and support groups for patient and family available from National Alliance for the Mentally Ill (NAMI), 2101 Wilson Blvd., Suite 302, Arlington, VA 22201, (703)524-7600
- National Mental Health Association, National mental Health Information Center, 1021 Prince St, Alexandria, VA 22314-2971; 800-969-6642
- Smoking cessation: American Cancer Society; American Lung Association

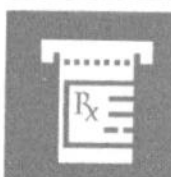

MEDICATIONS

DRUG(S) OF CHOICE
- Two main groups
  - ◊ Conventional: chlorpromazine, fluphenazine, trifluoperazine, perphenazine, thioridazine, haloperidol, thiothixene
  - ◊ Atypical: risperidone, clozapine, olanzapine, quetiapine, ziprasidone
- Medication choice based on clinical and subjective response: if
  - ◊ Sensitivity to extrapyramidal adverse effects: atypical
  - ◊ Tardive dyskinesia: clozapine
  - ◊ Poor compliance/high risk of relapse: injectable form of long-acting antagonist (haloperidol or fluphenazine)
- Usual oral daily dose (mg); initial dose may be lower
  - ◊ Chlorpromazine 200 mg bid
  - ◊ Fluphenazine 10 mg qd
  - ◊ Trifluoperazine 10 mg bid
  - ◊ Perphenazine 25 mg/day divided bid or tid
  - ◊ Thioridazine 150 mg bid
  - ◊ Haloperidol 5 mg bid
  - ◊ Thiothixene 10 mg bid
  - ◊ Risperidone 4 mg qd
  - ◊ Clozapine 100-200 mg tid
  - ◊ Olanzapine 15-25 mg qd
  - ◊ Quetiapine 200-300 mg bid
  - ◊ Ziprasidone 40-80 mg bid
  - ◊ Aripiprazole 10-30 mg qd

Contraindications: Refer to manufacturer's profile of each drug

Precautions:
- For acute side effects of neuroleptic - dystonic reaction (especially of head and neck) - diphenhydramine (Benadryl) 25-50 mg IM
- For pseudoparkinsonism reaction - trihexyphenidyl (Artane) 2 mg bid (may be increased to 15 mg/day if needed) or benztropine (Cogentin) 0.5 bid (range: 1-4 mg/day)
- Neuroleptic malignant syndrome-hyperthermia, severe extrapyramidal effect and autonomic dysfunction (hypertension, tachycardia, diaphoresis and incontinence)
- Risperidone and ziprasidone may be associated with hyperglycemia and ketoacidosis

Significant possible interactions: Refer to manufacturer's profile of each drug

ALTERNATIVE DRUGS
- Clozapine (Clozaril) 25 mg qd or bid
  - ◊ Increase slowly to dose of 300-400 mg given tid; do not exceed 900 mg/day
  - ◊ Serious toxicity of agranulocytosis mandates weekly CBC; obtain WBC before initiating therapy; withhold clozapine if < 3,500; if < 2,000, discontinue immediately; reserve for therapy resistant patients.
  - ◊ Effective in treatment of refractory patients
- Benzodiazepines:
  - ◊ May be effective adjuncts to antipsychotics during acute phase of illness
  - ◊ Withdrawal reactions can include psychosis, seizures
  - ◊ Schizophrenic patients vulnerable to abuse/addiction
- Anticonvulsants:
  - ◊ May be effective adjuncts to patients with EEG abnormalities suggestive of seizure activity and those with agitated/violent behavior

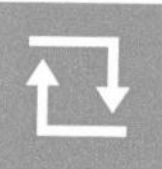

FOLLOWUP

PATIENT MONITORING Continue medication as well as psychiatric therapies (individual, group, family), vocational rehabilitation, social skills training, day treatment

PREVENTION/AVOIDANCE N/A

POSSIBLE COMPLICATIONS
- Side effects of neuroleptics especially risk of tardive dyskinesia with chronic use
- Self-inflicted trauma
- Combative behavior toward others
- High risk of suicide

EXPECTED COURSE/PROGNOSIS
- Chronic course - remission and exacerbations
- Guarded prognosis, complete remission not common
- The negative symptoms (consisting of decreased ambition, energy, emotional responsiveness and social withdrawal) are often most difficult to treat

MISCELLANEOUS

ASSOCIATED CONDITIONS N/A

AGE-RELATED FACTORS
Pediatric: Unusual before puberty
Geriatric: Those who survive enter into a chronic phase
Others: Onset in 30's - more paranoid type

PREGNANCY Use of haloperidol (most studies support its safety); complications of being on neuroleptics

SYNONYMS N/A

ICD-9-CM
295.90 Unspecified schizophrenia, unspecified

SEE ALSO

OTHER NOTES N/A

ABBREVIATIONS
WAIS-R = Wechsler Adult Intelligence Scale, Revisited
MMPI-2 = Minnesota Multiphasic Personality Inventory, Revised

REFERENCES

- Kaplan HI, Sadock BJ (eds). Comprehensive Textbook of Psychiatry. 7th Ed. Baltimore, Williams & Wilkins, 2000
- American Psychiatric Association: Diagnostic and Statistical Manual of Mental Disorders DSM-IV-TR (Text Revised). 4th Ed. Washington, DC, 2000
- American Psychiatric Association. Practice guidelines for the treatment of patients with schizophrenia. Am J Psychiatry 1997;154(suppl):1-63
- Mojtabai R, Nicholson RA, Carpenter BN. Role of psychosocial treatments in management of schizophrenia: a meta-analytic review of controlled outcome studies. Schizophr Bull 1998; 24(4):569-87
- AACAP Practice parameters for the assessment and treatment of children and adolescents with schizophrenia. American Academy of Child and Adolescent Psychiatry. J Am Acad Child Adolesc Psychiatry 1997;36(10 suppl):1775-1935
- The Medical Letter on Drugs and Therapeutics. Aripiprazole (Abilify) for Schizophrenia. The Medical Letter 2003 Feb 17;45(1150):15-16

Web references: 7 available at www.5mcc.com
Illustrations N/A

Author(s):
Milisa Rizer, MD

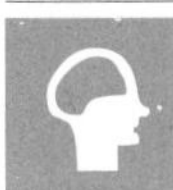

BASICS

DESCRIPTION Scleritis is an inflammation of the scleral outer coat of the eye
System(s) affected: Nervous
Genetics: None
Incidence/Prevalence in USA: Scleritis is uncommon
Predominant age: None
Predominant sex: Male = Female

SIGNS & SYMPTOMS
- Redness and inflammation of the sclera
- Pain ranging from mild discomfort to extreme localized tenderness

CAUSES The most common cause of scleritis is in association with collagen vascular diseases such as rheumatoid arthritis

RISK FACTORS Individuals with autoimmune disorders, and chronic rheumatoid arthritis are most at risk

DIAGNOSIS

DIFFERENTIAL DIAGNOSIS
- Conjunctivitis
- Episcleritis
- "Pink eye"
- Iritis
- Trauma

LABORATORY
- Rheumatoid factor
- ANA, and HLA serotyping may help aid in the diagnosis
- Elevated sedimentation rate

Drugs that may alter lab results: None

Disorders that may alter lab results: None

PATHOLOGICAL FINDINGS
- Nodules can form on the sclera which demonstrate fibrinoid necrosis of the sclera
- There may or may not be adjacent inflammation
- The scleritis may be diffuse, nodular, or necrotizing
- If the posterior region of the globe is involved, adjacent swelling of orbital tissues may occur

SPECIAL TESTS N/A

IMAGING CT scan of the orbit may help differentiate the extensiveness and location of scleritis

DIAGNOSTIC PROCEDURES History and physical examination

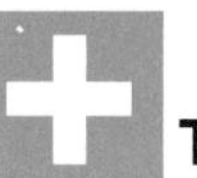

TREATMENT

APPROPRIATE HEALTH CARE Outpatient

GENERAL MEASURES
- Treatment of the inflammation usually with systemic steroids is required
- All of the immunosuppressants and antimetabolites used for autoimmune and collagen vascular disorders may be of help in active scleritis

SURGICAL MEASURES N/A

ACTIVITY No restrictions

DIET No special diet

PATIENT EDUCATION N/A

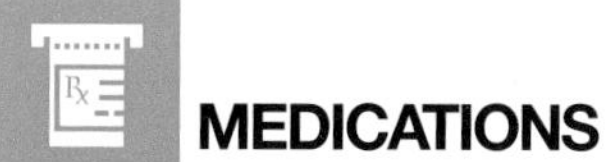

MEDICATIONS

DRUG(S) OF CHOICE Prednisone is the mainstay of treatment including both topical, periocular, and systemic administration
Contraindications: None
Precautions: Scleritis can progress to ocular perforation which may be hastened with periocular steroid injection
Significant possible interactions: Refer to manufacturer's literature

ALTERNATIVE DRUGS Non-steroidal anti-inflammatory medications

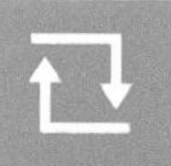

FOLLOWUP

PATIENT MONITORING The patient should be followed very closely in the active stage of inflammation to assess the effectiveness of therapy

PREVENTION/AVOIDANCE None

POSSIBLE COMPLICATIONS
- Increased intraocular pressure
- Cataract and glaucoma can result as a result of treatment
- Ocular perforation can occur in severe stages

EXPECTED COURSE/PROGNOSIS
- Scleritis is indolent, chronic, and often times progressive
- Recurrent bouts of inflammation occur

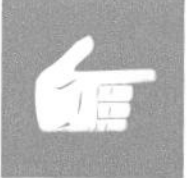

MISCELLANEOUS

ASSOCIATED CONDITIONS
- Sjögren syndrome
- Pseudo tumor

AGE-RELATED FACTORS
Pediatric: N/A
Geriatric: N/A
Others: N/A

PREGNANCY N/A

SYNONYMS N/A

ICD-9-CM
379.00 Scleritis, unspecified

SEE ALSO
Sjögren syndrome

OTHER NOTES N/A

ABBREVIATIONS N/A

REFERENCES

- Merrill GM: Diseases of The Cornea. Boston, Little, Brown, 1990

Web references: 0 available at www.5mcc.com
Illustrations N/A

Author(s):
Robert M. Kershner, MD

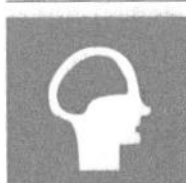

BASICS

DESCRIPTION Scleroderma (systemic sclerosis [SSc]) is a chronic disease of unknown etiology, characterized by diffuse fibrosis, degenerative changes, and vascular abnormalities in the skin, articular structures and other organs (kidneys, lung, heart, gastrointestinal and skeletal muscles). The majority of manifestations have vascular features (e.g., Raynaud phenomenon), but frank vasculitis is rarely seen. It can range from a mild disease, affecting the skin, to a systemic disease that can cause death in a few months.
- Divided into two major clinical variants:
  - ◊ Diffuse - distal and maximal extremity and truncal skin thickening
  - ◊ Limited - restricted to the fingers, hands and face. CREST syndrome (calcinosis, Raynaud phenomenon, poor esophageal mobility, sclerodactyly, telangiectasia) closely analogous with limited scleroderma.

System(s) affected: Cardiovascular, Gastrointestinal, Musculoskeletal, Pulmonary, Renal/Urologic, Skin/Exocrine
Genetics: Familial clustering is rare, but has been seen
Incidence/Prevalence in USA: 1/100,000
Predominant age:
- Young adult (16-40 years); middle age (40-75 years)
- Symptoms usually appear in the 3rd to 5th decade

Predominant sex: Female > Male (4:1)

SIGNS & SYMPTOMS
- Skin
  - ◊ Digital ulcerations
  - ◊ Tightness, swelling, thickening of digits
  - ◊ Hyperpigmentation, hypopigmentation
  - ◊ Narrowed oral aperture
  - ◊ Pruritus
  - ◊ Scaling of skin
  - ◊ Subcutaneous calcinosis
- Peripheral vascular system
  - ◊ Raynaud phenomenon
  - ◊ Telangiectasia
- Joints, tendons and bones
  - ◊ Flexion contractures
  - ◊ Friction rub on tendon movement
  - ◊ Hand swelling
  - ◊ Joint stiffness
  - ◊ Polyarthralgia
  - ◊ Sclerodactyly
- Muscle
  - ◊ Proximal muscle weakness
  - ◊ Weakness
- Gastrointestinal tract
  - ◊ Dysphagia
  - ◊ Esophageal reflux
  - ◊ Malabsorptive diarrhea
  - ◊ Nausea and vomiting
  - ◊ Weight loss
  - ◊ Xerostomia
- Kidney
  - ◊ Hypertension
- Pulmonary
  - ◊ Dry crackles at lung bases
  - ◊ Dyspnea
- Nervous system
  - ◊ Peripheral neuropathy
  - ◊ Trigeminal neuropathy

CAUSES
- Unknown
- Possible alterations in immune response
- Possibly some association with quartz mining, quarrying, vinyl chloride, hydrocarbons, toxin exposure, rape seed oil
- Treatment with bleomycin has caused a scleroderma-like syndrome

RISK FACTORS Unknown

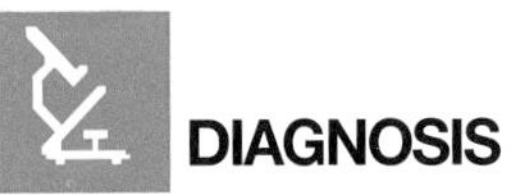

DIAGNOSIS

DIFFERENTIAL DIAGNOSIS
- Sclerodermatomyositis
- Mixed connective tissue disease
- Toxic oil syndrome (Madrid, 1981, affecting 20,000 people)
- Eosinophilia-myalgia syndrome
- Diffuse fasciitis with eosinophilia
- Scleredema of Buschke's

LABORATORY
- Increased ESR
- Normocytic anemia
- Normochromic anemia
- Positive ANA, often with a nucleolar pattern
- Anti-centromere antibody
- Anti-Scl-70 (topoisomerase antibody)
- Albuminuria
- Microscopic hematuria
- Eosinophilia
- Hemolysis
- Hypergammaglobulinemia
- Decreased maximum breathing capacity
- Increased residual volume
- Diffusion defect
- Positive rheumatoid factor test (33%)

Drugs that may alter lab results: N/A

Disorders that may alter lab results: N/A

PATHOLOGICAL FINDINGS
- Skin: edema, fibrosis or atrophy (late stage)
- Lymphocytic infiltrate around sweat glands
- Loss of capillaries
- Endothelial proliferation
- Hair follicle atrophy
- Synovium - pannus formation, fibrin deposits in tendons
- Kidney - small kidneys, intimal proliferation in interlobular arteries
- Heart - endocardial thickening, myocardial interstitial fibrosis, ischemic band necrosis
- Enlarged heart
- Cardiac hypertrophy
- Lung - interstitial pneumonitis, cyst formation
- Interstitial fibrosis
- Bronchiectasis
- Esophagus - esophageal atrophy, fibrosis

SPECIAL TESTS
- Skin biopsy - compact collagen fibers in the reticular dermis and hyalinization and fibrosis of arterioles. Thinning of epidermis with loss of rete pegs and atrophy of dermal appendages. Accumulation of mononuclear cells is also seen.
- ECG - low voltage; possibly nonspecific abnormalities
- Lung function tests - decreased diffusion and vital capacity
- Nail fold capillary loop abnormalities

IMAGING
- Hand x-ray - acto-osteolysis, soft tissue atrophy, subcutaneous calcinosis
- Upper GI - distal esophageal dilatation, atonic esophagus, esophageal dysmobility, duodenal diverticula
- Barium enema - colonic diverticula, megacolon
- Chest x-ray - diffuse reticular pattern, bilateral basilar pulmonary fibrosis
- Gallium-67 lung scan - can be positive in early interstitial disease
- High resolution CT scan for detecting alveolitis - giving a "ground glass" appearance or "honeycomb" pattern in fibrosis

DIAGNOSTIC PROCEDURES N/A

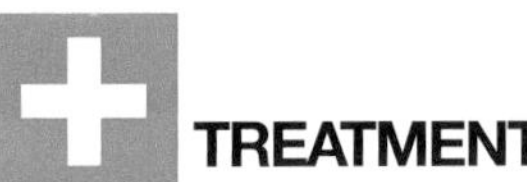

TREATMENT

APPROPRIATE HEALTH CARE Outpatient. Inpatient possibly for some surgical procedures.

GENERAL MEASURES
- Treatment is symptomatic and supportive
- Esophageal dilatation for strictures
- Avoid cold, dress appropriately for the weather
- Avoid smoking (crucial)
- For chronic digital ulcerations - débridement after soaking in half-strength hydrogen peroxide solution, digital plaster to immobilize
- Physical therapy to maintain function and promote strength
- Avoid finger sticks (e.g., blood tests)
- Be wary of air conditioning
- Heat therapy to relieve joint stiffness
- Elevation of the head of the bed during sleep may help relieve gastrointestinal symptoms
- Skin - use softening lotions, ointments, bath oils to help prevent dryness and cracking
- Dialysis may be necessary in renal crisis

SURGICAL MEASURES Some success with gastroplasty for correction of gastroesophageal reflux

ACTIVITY Stay as active as possible, but avoid fatigue

DIET
- Soft, bland diet with frequent small meals
- Drink plenty of fluids with meals

PATIENT EDUCATION
- Printed patient information available from: Scleroderma Federation, 1725 York Avenue, No. 29F, New York, NY 10128, (212)427-7040
- Advise patient to report any abnormal bruising or non-healing abrasions
- Assist patient in smoking cessation, if needed

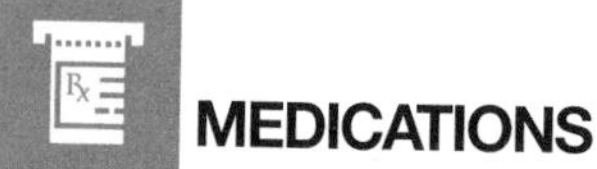

MEDICATIONS

DRUG(S) OF CHOICE

- There are no drug therapies of proven value, except for ACE inhibitors for hypertensive renal crisis
- Corticosteroids - for disabling myositis, pulmonary alveolitis or mixed connective tissue disease
- NSAIDs - for joint or tendon symptoms
- Antibiotics - for secondary infections in bowel
- Antacids or cimetidine - for gastric reflux
- Dipyridamole (Persantine) or aspirin - antiplatelet therapy
- Hydrophilic skin ointments - skin therapy
- Topical clindamycin or erythromycin or silver sulfadiazine (Silvadene) cream - may prevent recurrent infectious cutaneous ulcers; use systemic antibiotic therapy for active infections
- Consider immunosuppressives - used alone or with plasmapheresis for treatment of life-threatening or potentially crippling scleroderma or interstitial pneumonitis
- Vasoactive agents and antihypertensives - for Raynaud phenomenon
- Penicillamine (d-penicillamine) - reduce skin thickening and delay the rate of new visceral involvement (anecdotally)
- Angiotensin-converting enzyme (captopril) - for kidney disease

Contraindications: Refer to manufacturer's literature
Precautions: Refer to manufacturer's literature
Significant possible interactions: Refer to manufacturer's literature

ALTERNATIVE DRUGS Many other drugs are currently under investigation, but no evidence of real benefits as yet

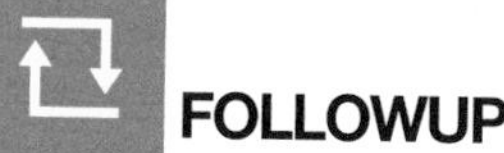

FOLLOWUP

PATIENT MONITORING Frequent to monitor end organ involvement and medications and offer encouragement

PREVENTION/AVOIDANCE None

POSSIBLE COMPLICATIONS

- Renal failure
- Respiratory failure
- Flexion contractures
- Disability
- Esophageal dysmotility
- Reflux esophagitis
- Arrhythmia
- Megacolon
- Pneumatosis intestinalis
- Obstructive bowel
- Cardiomyopathy
- Death

EXPECTED COURSE/PROGNOSIS

- Variable
- Possible improvement, but incurable
- Prognosis is poor if cardiac, pulmonary or renal manifestations present early

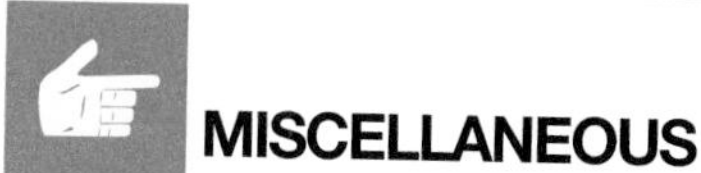

MISCELLANEOUS

ASSOCIATED CONDITIONS

- Rheumatoid arthritis
- Systemic lupus erythematosus
- Polymyositis
- Overlap connective tissue disease

AGE-RELATED FACTORS

Pediatric: Rare in this age group
Geriatric: Not rare until after age 75
Others: N/A

PREGNANCY N/A

SYNONYMS

- Progressive systemic sclerosis
- Morphea
- PSS

ICD-9-CM

710.1 Systemic sclerosis

SEE ALSO

OTHER NOTES N/A

ABBREVIATIONS N/A

REFERENCES

- Kelley WN, Harris ED, Ruddy S, Sledge CB, eds: Textbook of Rheumatology. 5th Ed. Philadelphia, W.B. Saunders, 1997
- Koopman WJ, eds: Arthritis and Allied Disorders. 13th Ed. Philadelphia, Lea & Febiger, 1997
- Kippel JH, Dippe PR, eds: Rheumatology, St. Louis, Mosby, 1994

Web references: 1 available at www.5mcc.com
Illustrations 9 available

Author(s):

Michael Tutt, MD

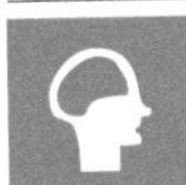

BASICS

DESCRIPTION A seizure is a sudden change in cortical electrical activity, manifested through motor, sensory, or behavioral changes, with or without an alteration in consciousness

System(s) affected: Nervous

Genetics: Genetically predisposed with variable penetrance. Family history increases risk three fold. A great deal will be understood concerning genetics and seizure disorder in the near future.

Incidence/Prevalence in USA:
- 2.5 million with seizure disorder/4 million people have had one or more seizures
- 181,000 people with first seizure/yr
- 45,000 new cases under the age of 15/yr
- 600,000 people over the age of 65 have a seizure disorder
- 33% over 75 years of age have had at least one lifetime seizure

Predominant age: Pediatric and geriatric populations most commonly present with new onset seizure disorder. Drug and or drug withdrawal seizures should be strongly considered in the adult population.

Predominant sex: Male = Female

SIGNS & SYMPTOMS
- General
  - ◊ Fever - indicative of infectious etiology
  - ◊ Focal neurologic finding - may indicate tumor or localized injury to the brain
  - ◊ Papilledema - suggestive of increased intracranial pressure
  - ◊ Hemorrhagic eye grounds - suggests underlying hypertension
  - ◊ Meningismus - may be present with meningitis
  - ◊ Headache - sometimes associated with infectious or hemorrhagic causes of seizures
- Generalized seizures
  - ◊ Absence - loss of consciousness or posture
  - ◊ Myoclonic - repetitive muscle contractions
  - ◊ Tonic-clonic - sustained contraction followed by rhythmic contractions of all four extremities
- Partial seizures
  - ◊ Simple - focal seizures without alteration of awareness/consciousness
  - ◊ Complex - focal seizures with alteration of awareness/consciousness
- Febrile seizures (see separate chapter on febrile seizures)
  - ◊ Occurs between three months and five years of age.
  - ◊ Fever without evidence of any other defined cause for seizures
  - ◊ If febrile seizures occur in the first year, the recurrence rate is 51%
  - ◊ If febrile seizures occur in the second year, they recurrence rate is 25%
  - ◊ 88% of all recurrences of febrile seizures occur in the first two years
  - ◊ The earlier the age of onset, the more likely repetitive febrile seizures will occur
  - ◊ Recurrent febrile seizures probably do not increase the risk of epilepsy
- Status epilepticus (see separate chapter)
  - ◊ Repetitive generalized seizures without return to consciousness between seizures
  - ◊ Considered a neurological emergency

CAUSES
- Brain tumor
- Cerebral hypoxia (breath holding, carbon monoxide poisoning, anesthesia)
- Cerebrovascular accident (infarct or hemorrhage)
- Convulsive or toxic agents (lead, alcohol, picrotoxin, strychnine)
- Eclampsia
- Exogenous factors (sound, light, cutaneous stimulation)
- Fever (see chapter on febrile seizures)
- Head injury
- Heat stroke
- Infection
- Metabolic disturbances
- Withdrawal from, or hereditary intolerance of, alcohol

RISK FACTORS
- Susceptibility to seizures determined by a complex interplay between genetic factors and acquired brain disorders
- Children delivered breech have a prevalence rate of 3.8% compared with 2.2% in children delivered vertex

DIAGNOSIS

DIFFERENTIAL DIAGNOSIS
- Infancy (0-2)
  - ◊ Perinatal hypoxia
  - ◊ Birth injury
  - ◊ Metabolic - hypoglycemia, hypocalcemia, hypomagnesemia, vitamin B6 deficiency, phenylketonuria
  - ◊ Acute infection
- Childhood (2-10)
  - ◊ Febrile seizure
  - ◊ Idiopathic
  - ◊ Acute infection
  - ◊ Trauma
- Adolescent (10-18)
  - ◊ Idiopathic
  - ◊ Trauma
  - ◊ Drug and alcohol withdrawal
  - ◊ Arteriovenous malformations
- Early adulthood (18-25)
  - ◊ Idiopathic
  - ◊ Drug and alcohol withdrawal
  - ◊ Trauma
- Middle age (25-60)
  - ◊ Drug and alcohol withdrawal
  - ◊ Trauma
  - ◊ Tumor
  - ◊ Vascular disease
- Late adulthood (over 60)
  - ◊ Vascular disease
  - ◊ Tumor
  - ◊ Degenerative disease
  - ◊ Metabolic - hypoglycemia, uremia, hepatic failure, electrolyte abnormality

LABORATORY
- Serum tests - glucose, sodium, potassium, calcium, phosphorus, magnesium, BUN, ammonia
- Anticonvulsant levels - inadequate level of anticonvulsant medication is the most common cause of recurrent seizures in children, and many adults
- Drug and toxic screens - include alcohol
- Complete blood count - helpful in evaluating infection

Drugs that may alter lab results:
- Anticonvulsant therapy may dramatically affect the EEG results
- Levels of anticonvulsants may be altered by a variety of common medications such as erythromycin, sulfonamides, warfarin, and cimetidine, as well as alcohol

Disorders that may alter lab results: Pregnancy decreases serum concentration. Frequent monitoring and dosage adjustments are necessary.

PATHOLOGICAL FINDINGS MRI may identify a lesion responsible-that is, a nidus for seizure activity

SPECIAL TESTS
- Electroencephalogram (EEG) A negative EEG does not rule out a seizure disorder. Sleep deprivation is helpful prior to EEG to identify positive spike wave formations.
- Video EEG monitoring is helpful in differentiating psychomotor nonepileptiform seizures (PNES)

IMAGING
- MRI of brain - superior in evaluation of the temporal lobes
- CT scan of brain - indicated routinely in work-up of tonic-clonic seizures

DIAGNOSTIC PROCEDURES Stereotactic investigation may prove beneficial for the 10% of seizures recalcitrant to pharmaceutical therapy

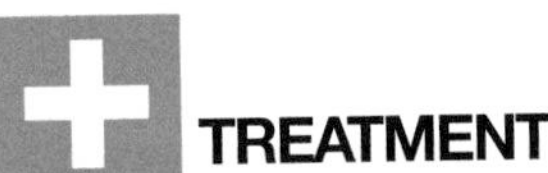

TREATMENT

APPROPRIATE HEALTH CARE Outpatient therapy is usually sufficient except for status epilepticus

GENERAL MEASURES Protect the patient's airway, and if possible protect the patient from physical harm

SURGICAL MEASURES Many academic centers are finding success with stereo tactic surgery for seizures that fail traditional therapy

ACTIVITY Uncontrolled seizures should encourage the avoidance of heights and swimming. State driving laws can be located at www.epilepsyfoundation.org.

DIET Regular

PATIENT EDUCATION
- Stress the importance of medication compliance, avoidance of alcohol and recreational drugs
- Printed patient information available from: Epilepsy Foundation of America, 4351 Garden City Drive, Landover, MD 20785-2267, (800)EFA-1000; www.epilepsyfoundation.org

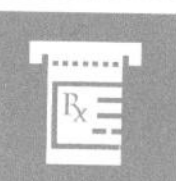

MEDICATIONS

DRUG(S) OF CHOICE
- Selection of medications from seizure groups below, with attention toward potential side effects is preferred as is monotherapy whenever possible.
  - ◊ Generalized seizures - tonic-clonic
    - Phenytoin (Dilantin): 200-400 mg/day in 1-3 doses; therapeutic range 10-20 mcg/ml
    - Carbamazepine (Tegretol) 100-200 mg/day in 1-2 doses; therapeutic range: 4-12 mcg/ml
    - Valproic acid (Depakene): 750-3000 mg/day in 1-3 doses begin at 15 mg/kg/day; therapeutic range 50-150 mcg/ml
  - ◊ Generalized seizures - absence
    - Ethosuximide (Zarontin): 250-1500 mg/day in 1-2 doses; therapeutic range 40-100 mcg/ml
    - Valproic acid - see above
  - ◊ Partial seizures
    - Phenytoin (Dilantin)
    - Carbamazepine (Tegretol)
    - Phenobarbital

Contraindications: Refer to manufacturer's profile of each drug
Precautions: Doses should be based on individual's response and drug levels where available
Significant possible interactions: Refer to manufacturer's profile of each drug

ALTERNATIVE DRUGS
- Felbamate (Felbatol) 1200 mg/day in 3-4 divided doses, max 3600 mg/day
- Gabapentin (Neurontin) 300 mg hs, then 2-3 divided doses, max 2400-3600 mg/day
- Lamotrigine (Lamictal) 25-50 mg/day. Adjust in 100 mg increments q1-2 weeks to 300-500 mg/day in 2 divided doses
- Methsuximide (Celontin) 300 mg/day for first week, increase 300 mg/3weeks,Max. 1200 mg daily
- Oxcarbazepine (Trileptal) 300 mg bid, increase 300 mg/3 days; maintenance 1200 mg/day
- Primidone (Mysoline) 100-125 mg hs, adjust to max 2000 mg/day in two doses
- Tiagabine (Gabitril) 4 mg/day adjust weekly to max 56 mg/day
- Topiramate (Topamax) 50 mg/day adjust weekly to effect. 400 mg/day in two doses max 1600 mg/day

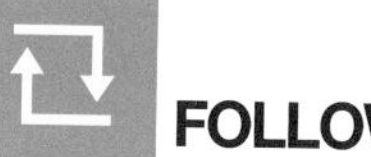

FOLLOWUP

PATIENT MONITORING
- Regular monitoring of anticonvulsant levels
- CBC as indicated
- Monitor medication side effects and adverse reactions

PREVENTION/AVOIDANCE Maintain adequate epileptic drug therapy, continue efforts at insuring compliance and/or access to medication

POSSIBLE COMPLICATIONS Drug toxicity

EXPECTED COURSE/PROGNOSIS
- Dependant on type of seizure disorder
- Seizure activity may become quiescent. After a seizure free two-year period, withdrawal of therapy may be considered. 33% relapse rate should be expected in following three years.

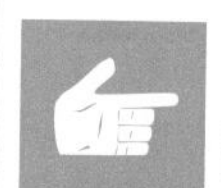

MISCELLANEOUS

ASSOCIATED CONDITIONS
- Infections
- Tumors
- Drug abuse
- Metabolic disorders
- Trauma

AGE-RELATED FACTORS
Pediatric: Breast-feeding is not contraindicated in mothers taking anticonvulsant medication, however drug levels can be measured if sedation occurs in the infant
Geriatric: Fractures from falls are more common in the osteopenic age range
Others: N/A

PREGNANCY Serum levels of anticonvulsants may decline, frequent monitoring recommended. There is a two-fold increased risk of congenital malformation in mothers taking anticonvulsant medications.

SYNONYMS
- Convulsions
- Epilepsy
- Fits
- Spells
- Attacks

ICD-9-CM
780.39 Other convulsions
345.10 Generalized convulsive epilepsy without mention of intractable epilepsy
779.0 Convulsions in newborn

SEE ALSO
Seizures, febrile
Status epilepticus

OTHER NOTES The International League Against Epilepsy (ILAE) is currently making progress in a new 5-axis classification system for seizure disorder, which will include genetics, characterization, and disability for seizure disorder syndromes

ABBREVIATIONS N/A

REFERENCES
- Chang BS, Lowenstein DH. Epilepsy. N Engl J Med 2003;349:1257-66
- Annegers JF. The epidemiology of epilepsy. In: Wyllie E, ed. The treatment of epilepsy: principles and practice. 3rd ed. Philadelphia: Lippencot Williams & Wilkins; 2001.p.131-8
- Mengel MB, Schwiebert LB, eds. Ambulatory Medicine: Primary care Famlies. 4th ed. New York: McGraw-Hill; 2004
- Goldstein LH. Assessment of patients with psychogenic non-epileptiform seizures. J Neurol Neurosurg Psychiatry 2004;75(5):667-8
- Commission on Classification and Terminology of the International League Against Epilepsy. Proposal for revised classification of epilepsies and epileptic syndromes. Epilepsia 1989;30(4):389-99

Web references: 3 available at www.5mcc.com
Illustrations N/A

Author(s):
Shawn H. Blanchard, MD
William L. Toffler, MD

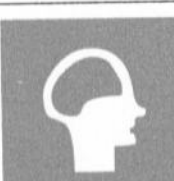

BASICS

DESCRIPTION Seizure occurring with fever in infancy or childhood without evidence of other underlying cause. Seizures secondary to other CNS events like meningitis, tumor, or afebrile convulsive history excluded from this topic.
- Simple febrile seizure - single episode in 24 hours, lasting less than 15 minutes and generalized tonic-clonic activity. Accounts for 85% of febrile seizures.
- Complex febrile seizure - multiple episodes in 24 hours with focalizing findings and lasting more than 15 minutes. Accounts for 15% of febrile seizures.

System(s) affected: Nervous
Genetics: Uncertain but may be autosomal dominant with variable expression and incomplete penetrance
Incidence/Prevalence in USA: Approximately 2500/100,000. 2-5% of all children, comprising 30% of all childhood seizures.
Predominant age: Age of onset is 6 months to 6 years; 95% occur by 5 years; peak at 2 years
Predominant sex: Male > Female (slightly)

SIGNS & SYMPTOMS
- Fever usually 39°C (102.2°F) or greater
- Tonic-clonic convulsive activity
  - ◊ Generalized with simple seizure or focal with complex event
  - ◊ Usually occurs within hours of fever onset
  - ◊ The seizure is the initial sign of illness in 25% of patients
  - ◊ Duration is less than 15 minutes with simple seizures; longer with complex episodes
  - ◊ Average frequency is once in 24 hours with simple; more with complex

CAUSES
- Fever may lower seizure threshold in susceptible children
- Temperature usually greater than 39°C (102.2°F), but rate of change may be more important than temperature
- Viral illnesses: Upper respiratory infections, roseola infantum, influenza A, gastroenteritis
- Bacterial infections: Shigella, salmonella, otitis media
- Mumps, measles, rubella immunization (MMR) within prior 7-10 days or diphtheria, pertussis, tetanus immunization (DPT) within prior 48 hours

RISK FACTORS Febrile seizure in sibling raises risk 2-3 times

DIAGNOSIS

DIFFERENTIAL DIAGNOSIS
- Febrile delirium
- Febrile shivering with pallor and perioral cyanosis
- Breath holding spell during fever event
- Afebrile seizure occurring during fever event
- Acute meningitis presenting with seizure
- Head injury and fever
- Drug induced seizures
- Sudden discontinuance of anticonvulsants

LABORATORY
- First episode: CBC, calcium, glucose, magnesium, electrolytes (especially sodium), urinalysis, blood culture, BUN, creatinine
- A toxicologic screen may be indicated in unclear cases
- First episode or under 1 year old, consider a lumbar puncture to rule out meningitis

Drugs that may alter lab results: N/A

Disorders that may alter lab results: Infections

PATHOLOGICAL FINDINGS N/A

SPECIAL TESTS EEG may be indicated: If recurrent frequent febrile seizures, those with focal findings, complex type, underlying neurological disorder, family history of afebrile seizures, delayed awakening after event, or if this is first event after age 3. Perform EEG 2-4 weeks after event. EEG not indicated for simple febrile seizure when there is a ready explanation for fever and recovery is quick.

IMAGING CT scan of brain for complex types, focal findings, underlying neurological disorder, or prolonged recovery phase

DIAGNOSTIC PROCEDURES
- Lumbar puncture - should be considered in children:
  - ◊ Younger than 18 months of age, no other cause of fever
  - ◊ With duration of illness > 48 hours
  - ◊ With complex seizures
  - ◊ With suspicious symptoms like lethargy, irritability or vomiting
  - ◊ With suspicious physical findings including nuchal rigidity, bulging fontanelles, Kernig's or Brudzinski's signs, and/or altered sensorium
- Simple seizures - lasting < 15 minutes, generalized, no postictal period, single episode in 24 hours
- Complex seizures - lasting > 15 minutes, focalizing signs, prolonged postictal period, multiple episodes in 24 hours

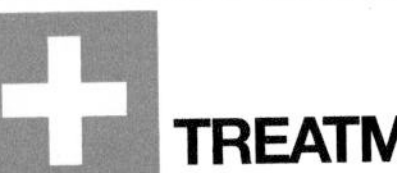

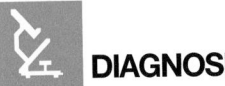

TREATMENT

APPROPRIATE HEALTH CARE Emergency room or extended observation based on clinical situation, seizure type and whether first or subsequent event

GENERAL MEASURES
- Supportive care
- If seizure ended and simple type with recovery progressing, determine fever source so underlying cause can be treated
- Tepid sponge bath to lower temperature
- If seizure less than 10 minutes, supportive measures with laying on side, protecting from injury, maintaining airway, low flow oxygen

SURGICAL MEASURES N/A

ACTIVITY Bedrest during observation interval

DIET Nothing by mouth until status clarified

PATIENT EDUCATION
- Parents need much support
- Febrile seizures do not cause developmental delay
- Febrile seizures do not cause retardation
- Febrile seizures do not cause behavioral abnormalities
- Febrile seizures do not cause death
- Recurrence risk 30%, if first seizure at less than 12 months of age and 50% if greater than 12 months of age. Risk of epilepsy only slightly increased from the normal pediatric population.
- Educate parents about methods to reduce possible harm during a seizure

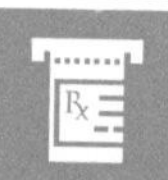

MEDICATIONS

DRUG(S) OF CHOICE

- Rectal or oral acetaminophen for fever 10-15 mg/kg/dose or ibuprofen 10 mg/kg/dose
- Anticonvulsants rarely indicated. See topic Status epilepticus for treatment of prolonged seizures.
- Oxygen

Contraindications: Allergy to drug
Precautions: Respiratory compromise needing support or intubation
Significant possible interactions: N/A

ALTERNATIVE DRUGS

- Phenobarbital 10-15 mg/kg IV, slower onset of action and may cause respiratory depression and hypotension
- Phenytoin 10-15 mg/kg IV, slower onset of action and may cause cardiac arrhythmias and hypotension
- Valproic acid 40-60 mg/kg in equal parts water - 5 cm rectally is longer acting but may cause hepatotoxicity in under 2 year age group, slower onset of action

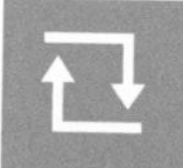

FOLLOWUP

PATIENT MONITORING Based on the site, severity, and origin of the fever.

PREVENTION/AVOIDANCE

- Acetaminophen 10 mg/kg orally or rectally or ibuprofen 10 mg/kg - temperature greater than 38°C (100.5°F) rectal
- May use intermittent prophylactic rectal diazepam for fever greater than 38.5°C (101.3°F); 5 mg if under 3 years or 7.5 mg 3 to 6 years or 0.5 mg/kg (up to 15 mg), repeated every 12 hours for 4 doses total
- Continuous prophylaxis is controversial; may consider for high risk child with strong family history, multiple recurrences, complex events, or underlying neurological abnormalities until 1 year after last seizure. Phenobarbital 3-5 mg/kg/day may be used but often causes behavioral problems; valproic acid 30-40 mg/kg/day may be tried but may cause severe hepatotoxicity.

POSSIBLE COMPLICATIONS

- Febrile seizures do not cause death, retardation, behavioral problems nor developmental delays
- Risk of epilepsy is approximately 2-4% in simple febrile seizures (highest risk exists in children with abnormal neurodevelopmental status, family history of febrile seizures and complex feature)
- If an anticonvulsant drug is used (eg multiple recurrences), the typical duration of therapy is one year (period with highest recurrence risk)
- Significant predictors of increased risk for recurrence
    - ◊ Shorter duration of fever prior to initial seizure
    - ◊ Lower temperature
    - ◊ Younger age at onset < 12 months
    - ◊ Family history of febrile seizures
    - ◊ Multiple initial seizures
    - ◊ Several seizures within first 24 hours

EXPECTED COURSE/PROGNOSIS

- 33% develop recurrent febrile seizures, 50% if first episode before 12 months, 45% if two involved siblings
- 95% of recurrences occur within 1 year

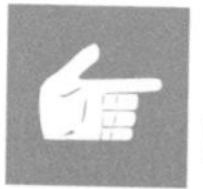

MISCELLANEOUS

ASSOCIATED CONDITIONS

- Examine child for port wine stain over trigeminal nerve with Sturge-Weber syndrome, adenoma sebaceum and hypopigmented skin of tuberous sclerosis, and café-au-lait spots and subcutaneous nodules of neurofibromatosis
- Bacterial meningitis that manifests as an apparent febrile seizure is extremely low (0-0.6%)

AGE-RELATED FACTORS

Pediatric: Range 3 months to 5 years with 95% by age 5 and peak incidence at age 2 years
Geriatric: N/A
Others: N/A

PREGNANCY N/A

SYNONYMS

- Febrile convulsions
- Febrile fits

ICD-9-CM

780.31 Febrile convulsions

SEE ALSO

Seizure disorders
Status epilepticus

OTHER NOTES

- Intermittent phenobarbital prophylaxis not recommended
- Phenytoin and carbamazepine are ineffective for prophylaxis
- No evidence that preventing recurrent febrile seizures prevents epilepsy
- Critical to distinguish between simple and complex events
- Postictal sleepiness is common; if marked may indicate underlying pathology

ABBREVIATIONS N/A

REFERENCES

- McAbee GN, Wark JE. A practical approach to uncomplicated seizures in children. Am Fam Phys 2000;62(5):1109-16
- Berg AT, Shinnar S, Hauser WA, et al.A prospective study of recurrent febrile seizures. N Engl J Med 1992;327(16):1122-7
- Al-Eissa YA. Lumbar puncture in the clinical evaluation of children with seizures associated with fever. Pediatr Emerg Care 1995;11(6):347-50
- Leung AKC: Febrile Convulsions: How dangerous are they? Postgraduate Medicine 1991;89(5):217-224
- Applegate MS, Lo W: Febrile Seizures: Current Concepts Concerning Prognosis and Clinical Management. Journal of Family Practice 1989;29(4):422-428
- Sexton ME: Childhood Seizures. AAFP Home Study Audio Series, Sept. 1991

Web references: 0 available at www.5mcc.com
Illustrations N/A

Author(s):
J. C. Chava-Zimmerman, MD
Pushpa Krishnasami, MD

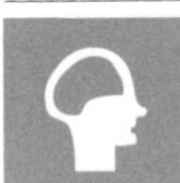

BASICS

DESCRIPTION The systemic response to infection; it encompasses a broad array of clinical manifestations and overlaps with inflammatory reactions to other clinical insults (e.g., severe trauma or burn)
- Bacteremia: Bacteria in the blood; may have no accompanying symptoms
- Systemic inflammatory response syndrome (SIRS): inflammatory reaction to different clinical insults manifest by two of the following: (1) temperature >38°C or < 36°C, (2) heart rate > 90/min; (3) respiratory rate >20/min or PaCO2 < 32 mm Hg, and (4) WBC count > 12,000/mm3, < 4,000/mm3 or > 10% immature forms (bends)
- Sepsis: SIRS with documented infection (typically bacterial)
- Septic shock: Sepsis induced hypotension (systolic BP < 90 mmHg or ≥ 40 mmHg drop from baseline) despite adequate fluid resuscitation plus hypoperfusion abnormalities (oliguria, lactic acidosis, acute change in mental status)
- Multiple organ dysfunction syndrome (MODS): altered organ function in an acutely ill patient - requires intervention to maintain homeostasis

System(s) affected: Cardiovascular, Endocrine/Metabolic, Gastrointestinal, Hemic/Lymphatic/Immunologic, Nervous, Pulmonary, Renal/Urologic
Genetics: Single nucleotide polymorphisms i.e., cytokine and cytokine receptor genes influence risk for development of sepsis and risk of mortality from sepsis
Incidence/Prevalence in USA: 300/100,000 persons/year
Predominant age: All ages
Predominant sex: Male > Female (1.28:1)

SIGNS & SYMPTOMS
- Fever
- Chills, rigors
- Myalgias
- Changes in mental status - restlessness, agitation, confusion, delirium, lethargy, stupor, coma
- Tachycardia
- Tachypnea
- Hypotension
- Skin lesions - erythema, petechiae, ecthyma gangrenosum, embolic lesions
- Signs and symptoms related to site of primary infection:
  - ◊ Respiratory tract - cough, sputum production, dyspnea, chest pain
  - ◊ Urinary tract - dysuria, flank pain, frequency, urgency
  - ◊ Intra-abdominal source - nausea, vomiting, diarrhea, constipation, abdominal pain
  - ◊ Central nervous system - stiff neck, headache, photophobia, focal neurologic signs
- Signs and symptoms related to end organ failure:
  - ◊ Pulmonary - cyanosis
  - ◊ Renal - oliguria, anuria
  - ◊ Hepatic - jaundice
  - ◊ Cardiac - congestive heart failure

CAUSES
- Specific etiologic agents include:
  - ◊ Gram positive organisms - most commonly *Staphylococcus spp*, *Streptococcus spp*, *Enterococcus spp*
  - ◊ Gram negative organisms - most commonly *Escherichia coli*, *Klebsiella spp*, *Proteus spp*, *Pseudomonas spp*
  - ◊ Fungi - most commonly *Candida spp*
  - ◊ Other agents - anaerobes. Also, see Differential diagnosis.
- Common sources of septicemia include:
  - ◊ Lungs
  - ◊ Urinary tract
  - ◊ Intra-abdominal focus - biliary tree, abscess, peritonitis
  - ◊ Intravascular catheters
  - ◊ Skin - cellulitis, decubitus ulcer, gangrene
  - ◊ Heart valves

RISK FACTORS
- Age extremes (very old and very young)
- Impaired host (see associated conditions)
- Indwelling catheters - intravascular, urinary, biliary, etc.
- Complicated labor and delivery - premature and/or prolonged rupture of membranes, etc.
- Certain surgical procedures

DIAGNOSIS

DIFFERENTIAL DIAGNOSIS
- Viral diseases (influenza, dengue and other hemorrhagic viruses, Coxsackie B virus)
- Rickettsial diseases (Rocky Mountain spotted fever, endemic typhus)
- Spirochetal diseases (leptospirosis, relapsing fever [Borrelia sp], Jarisch-Herxheimer reaction in syphilis)
- Protozoal diseases (Toxoplasma gondii, Trypanosoma cruzi, Pneumocystis carinii, Plasmodium falciparum)
- Collagen vascular diseases, vasculitides, myocardial infarction, pulmonary embolus, thrombotic thrombocytopenic purpura/hemolytic-uremic syndrome, thyrotoxicosis, adrenal insufficiency (Addison disease), dissecting aortic aneurysm, multiple trauma, third-degree burn

LABORATORY
- Positive blood cultures
- Positive cultures from other sites (sputum, urine, cerebrospinal fluid [CSF], etc.)
- Gram stain of clinical specimens (sputum, urine, CSF, etc.)
- Common:
  - ◊ Leukocytosis
  - ◊ Proteinuria
  - ◊ Hypoxemia
  - ◊ Eosinopenia
  - ◊ Hypoferremia
  - ◊ Hyperglycemia
  - ◊ Hypocalcemia
  - ◊ Mild hyperbilirubinemia
- Less common:
  - ◊ Lactic acidosis
  - ◊ Leukopenia
  - ◊ Azotemia
  - ◊ Thrombocytopenia
  - ◊ Prolonged prothrombin time
  - ◊ Anemia
  - ◊ Hypoglycemia

Drugs that may alter lab results: Prior antibiotic use

Disorders that may alter lab results: N/A

PATHOLOGICAL FINDINGS
- Inflammation at primary site of infection
- Disseminated intravascular coagulation
- Non-cardiogenic pulmonary edema

SPECIAL TESTS
- Antigen detection systems - counterimmunoelectrophoresis (CIE) and latex agglutination tests (pneumococcus, H. influenzae type B, group B streptococcus, meningococcus)
- Gram stain of buffy coat smears occasionally useful

IMAGING
- X-rays (e.g., chest)
- Ultrasound, CT scan, or MRI may be useful in delineating sites of infection

DIAGNOSTIC PROCEDURES
- Aspiration of potentially infected body fluids (pleural, peritoneal, CSF) when appropriate
- Biopsy, drainage of potentially infected tissues (abscess, biliary tree, etc.) when appropriate

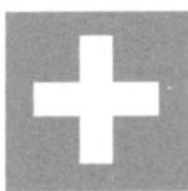

TREATMENT

APPROPRIATE HEALTH CARE
- Hospitalization
- Intensive care treatment of patients with shock, respiratory failure

GENERAL MEASURES
- Removal or drainage of septic foci
- Correction of metabolic abnormalities (hypoxemia, hyperglycemia, hypoglycemia, severe acidemia [pH < 7.10])
- Mechanical ventilation for respiratory failure
- Transfusion of RBC, platelets, and/or fresh frozen plasma for bleeding
- Volume replacement followed by pressors for hypotension
- Stress ulcer and deep venous thrombosis prophylactic measures
- Insulin therapy to keep serum glucose < 150 mg/dl

SURGICAL MEASURES Drainage of infected sites, débridement of necrotic tissues

ACTIVITY Bedrest

DIET NPO initially; intravenous hyperalimentation appropriate in some severely malnourished patients and in patients who will be unable to receive enteral alimentation within the week

PATIENT EDUCATION N/A

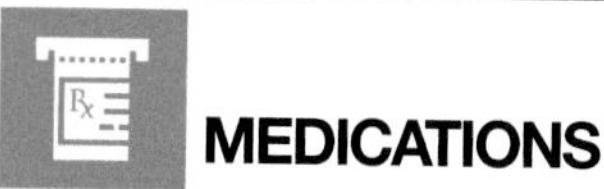

MEDICATIONS

DRUG(S) OF CHOICE
- Antibiotic coverage should be broad initially and directed against organisms associated with identified septic foci. After culture results are available, treatment should be more organism-specific. Knowledge of the antibiotic susceptibility patterns of local pathogens extremely important.
- Neonatal (< 7 days old) sepsis - ampicillin 300 mg/kg/d in 3 divided doses and gentamicin (Garamycin) 5 mg/kg/d in 2 divided doses
- Non-immunocompromised child - cefotaxime (Claforan) 200 mg/kg/d in 4 divided doses
- Non-immunocompromised adult - cefotaxime (Claforan) 1-2 gm q8-12 or ticarcillin-clavulanate (Timentin) 3.1 g q6h plus gentamicin 5 mg/kg/day in 1-3 divided doses
- Neutropenic host - cefepime (Maxipime) 1-2 gm q12h, and gentamicin (Garamycin) or tobramycin 3-5 mg/kg/d in 2-3 divided doses; vancomycin (Vancocin) is added when there is an obvious catheter-related infection or a known gram positive bacteremia or if there is an increased likelihood of infection with resistant gram positive organisms.

Contraindications: History of anaphylaxis or other allergic reaction to the antibiotic

Precautions: Dose adjustments required in renal failure

Significant possible interactions:
- Aminoglycosides - increased nephrotoxicity with enflurane, cisplatin and possibly vancomycin; increased ototoxicity with loop diuretics; increased paralysis with neuromuscular blocking agents
- Ampicillin - increased frequency of rash with allopurinol

ALTERNATIVE DRUGS
- Intravenous hydrocortisone (200-300 mg/day in 3-4 divided doses) may benefit patients who require vasopressor therapy to maintain an adequate blood pressure. Higher doses of corticosteroids should not be used.
- Many other drug combinations are possible to get adequate coverage
- Antifungals
- Antimicrobials for anaerobic infections
- Antipseudomonals
- Drotrecogin alfa (Xigris) - 24 mcg/kg/hr for 96 hrs in patients with severe sepsis (APACHE score >24). Do not use in patients with increased risk of bleeding, thrombocytopenia with platelets < 30,000, sepsis-induced organ dysfunction for >24 hours, hypercoagulable states, chronic renal or hepatic failure, children or pregnancy. Very expensive.

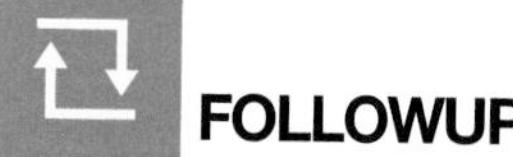

FOLLOWUP

PATIENT MONITORING
- Depends upon source of infection, underlying disease(s)
- Peak and trough drug levels for aminoglycosides
- BUN, creatinine, electrolytes and complete blood counts at least twice weekly; more frequently if unstable

PREVENTION/AVOIDANCE
- Vaccination - pneumococcal (geriatric patients, patients with certain chronic diseases), *Haemophilus influenzae* type B (infants, young children)
- Gamma globulin (for hypo- or agammaglobulinemic patients)
- Hand washing by hospital personnel, appropriate catheter care, etc., for hospitalized patients

POSSIBLE COMPLICATIONS
- Death
- Adult respiratory distress syndrome (ARDS)
- Multi-organ failure (cardiac, pulmonary, renal, hepatic)
- Disseminated intravascular coagulation (DIC)
- Gastrointestinal hemorrhage

EXPECTED COURSE/PROGNOSIS
Even with optimal care, mortality will be 10-50% overall; this is increased in patients with neutropenia, diabetes, alcoholism, renal failure, respiratory failure, hypogammaglobulinemia, certain etiologic agents (e.g., Pseudomonas aeruginosa), a delay in appropriate antimicrobial therapy, and those patients at the age extremes

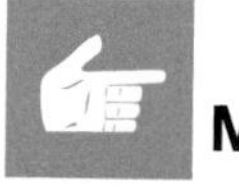

MISCELLANEOUS

ASSOCIATED CONDITIONS
- Neutropenia
- Diabetes mellitus
- Alcoholism
- Leukemia, lymphoma, and solid tumors
- Cirrhosis
- Burns
- Multiple trauma
- Intravenous drug abuse
- Malnutrition
- Complement deficiencies
- Hypo- or agammaglobulinemia
- Splenectomy
- HIV infection

AGE-RELATED FACTORS
Pediatric: Screen newborns for infection due to prolonged rupture of membranes (> 24 h), maternal fever, prematurity

Geriatric:
- Often more difficult to diagnose clinically in the elderly
- Change in mental status/behavior may be only early manifestation

Others: N/A

PREGNANCY Beta lactam antibiotics, aminoglycosides, erythromycin are considered safe

SYNONYMS
- Septicemia
- Sepsis neonatorum

ICD-9-CM
038.9 Unspecified septicemia

SEE ALSO
Candidiasis
Endocarditis, infective
Listeriosis
Meningitis, bacterial
Pneumonia, bacterial
Pyelonephritis
Rocky Mountain spotted fever
Toxic shock syndrome
Tularemia

OTHER NOTES High dose steroids of no benefit

ABBREVIATIONS N/A

REFERENCES
- Bone RC, Balk RA, Cerra FB, Dellinger RP, Knaus WA, et al. Definitions for sepsis and organ failure and guidelines for the use of innovative therapies in sepsis. The ACCP/SCCM Consensus Conference Committee. American College of Chest Physicians/Society of Critical Care Medicine. Chest 1992;101:1644-55
- Wheeler AP, Bernard GR. Treating patients with severe sepsis. N Engl J Med 1999;340:207-14
- Hotchkiss RS, Karl IE. The pathophysiology and treatment of sepsis. N Engl J Med 2003;348(2):138-50
- Dellinger RP, Carlet JM, Masur H, Gerlach H, Calandra T, Cohen J, et al. Surviving Sepsis Campaign Management Guidelines Committee. Surviving sepsis campaign guidelines for management of severe sepsis and septic shock. Crit Care Med 2004;32(3):858-73

Web references: 2 available at www.5mcc.com

Illustrations 5 available

Author(s):
Robert L. Atmar, MD

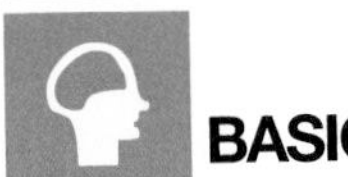

BASICS

DESCRIPTION Allergic reaction to foreign serum or drugs, usually appearing 5-14 days after administration of the allergen. Characterized by fever, arthralgias, skin rash and lymphadenopathy.
System(s) affected: Cardiovascular, Gastrointestinal, Hemic/Lymphatic/Immunologic, Musculoskeletal, Skin/Exocrine
Genetics: N/A
Incidence/Prevalence in USA: Common
Predominant age: All ages
Predominant sex: Male = Female

SIGNS & SYMPTOMS
- History of antibiotic therapy (especially penicillin and related drugs)
- History of injection of horse serum or other species serum
- Fever
- Arthralgias (particularly TM joint)
- Malaise
- Pruritus
- Nausea
- Vomiting
- Abdominal pain
- Splenomegaly
- Myalgias
- Extremity weakness
- Sneezing
- Coughing
- Dyspnea
- Melena
- Cutaneous eruptions
- Facial swelling
- Lymphadenopathy
- Urticaria
- Joint effusion
- Myocarditis (rare)
- Palpable purpura

CAUSES
- IgG antibodies that form soluble complexes with the antigen to cause an immune complex (type III) reaction
- Drugs (penicillin, cephalosporins, sulfonamides, thiouracils, iodinated dyes, streptomycin)
- Tetanus toxoid
- Rabies antiserum
- Release of vasoactive substance
- Rabbit antiserum
- Crotalidae antivenin

RISK FACTORS Previous exposure to injection of foreign protein (reaction usually occurs sooner than the expected 5-14 days)

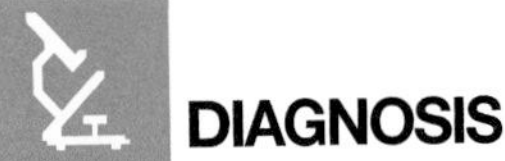

DIAGNOSIS

DIFFERENTIAL DIAGNOSIS
- Periarteritis nodosa
- Anaphylaxis
- Drug hypersensitivity

LABORATORY
- Eosinophilia
- Proteinuria
- Decreased C3
- Decreased C4
- Increased ESR
- Mixed IgG-IgM cryoprecipitates

Drugs that may alter lab results: N/A

Disorders that may alter lab results: N/A

PATHOLOGICAL FINDINGS Nodular lesions in segments of arteries resembling periarteritis nodosa

SPECIAL TESTS Test all persons prior to administering a foreign serum (see Prevention/avoidance)

IMAGING N/A

DIAGNOSTIC PROCEDURES N/A

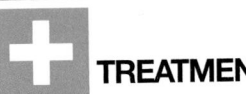

TREATMENT

APPROPRIATE HEALTH CARE Inpatient, if severe; outpatient for mild cases

GENERAL MEASURES Treat symptomatically. Usually self-limited.

SURGICAL MEASURES N/A

ACTIVITY Bed rest during acute illness

DIET No special diet

PATIENT EDUCATION N/A

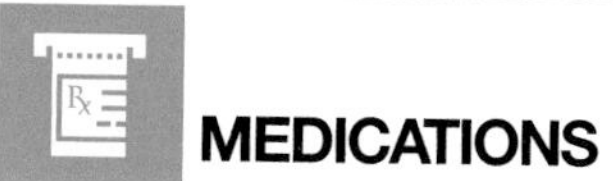

MEDICATIONS

DRUG(S) OF CHOICE
- Antihistamine of choice for urticaria and generalized pruritus
- Aspirin 0.6-1.5 grams orally q 4h

Contraindications: Refer to manufacturer's literature
Precautions: Refer to manufacturer's literature
Significant possible interactions: Refer to manufacturer's literature

ALTERNATIVE DRUGS Prednisone - 40 mg/day orally if simpler medicines do not bring symptomatic relief. Prednisone also used if peripheral neuritis or myocarditis (rare) develops.

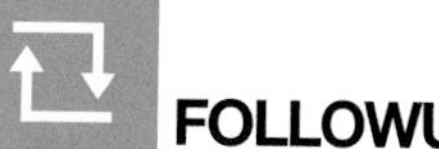

FOLLOWUP

PATIENT MONITORING During acute illness, monitor closely for signs of myocarditis or peripheral neuritis

PREVENTION/AVOIDANCE
- Special caution in patients who need foreign serum if they have history of asthma, hay fever, urticaria or other allergic symptoms
- Testing in patients with no previous exposure or allergic history: Before administering a foreign protein - prick test with 1:10 dilution. If this is negative, 0.02 mL of 1:10 dilution given intracutaneously.
- Testing in patients with previous exposure or allergic history: Test first with 1:1000 dilution
- If skin test is positive and serum treatment is essential, then desensitization is necessary

POSSIBLE COMPLICATIONS
- Vasculitis
- Neuropathy
- Glomerulonephritis (rare)
- Anaphylaxis
- Shock
- Death

EXPECTED COURSE/PROGNOSIS
Favorable; self-limiting with 2-3 weeks for recovery

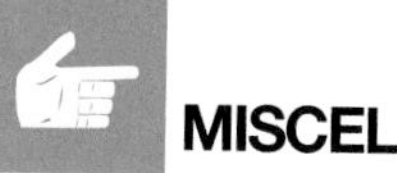

MISCELLANEOUS

ASSOCIATED CONDITIONS Drug hypersensitivity

AGE-RELATED FACTORS
Pediatric: N/A
Geriatric: N/A
Others: N/A

PREGNANCY N/A

SYNONYMS
- Inoculation reaction
- Protein sickness

ICD-9-CM
999.5 Other serum reaction

SEE ALSO

OTHER NOTES Horse antiserum still used in treatment of botulism, diphtheria, venomous snake bites, spider bites. Antilymphocyte or antilymphocyte serum is used to suppress immune reactions to transplanted organs.

ABBREVIATIONS N/A

REFERENCES

- Isselbacher KJ, et al, eds: Harrison's Principles of Internal Medicine. 14th Ed. New York, McGraw-Hill Inc., 1998
- Virella G: Hypersensitivity reactions. Immunology Series 1993;58:329

Web references: 0 available at www.5mcc.com
Illustrations N/A

Author(s):
Brian J. Murray, MD

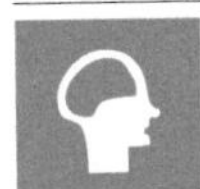

BASICS

DESCRIPTION Difficulty getting or staying sexually aroused, reaching orgasm too quickly, difficulty or inability to reach orgasm, inability to relax, lack of interest in sex, distaste or revulsion with sex, too little foreplay, too little tenderness after intercourse.

- Most women who have orgasms do not do so invariably during intercourse, and some mistakenly think this is dysfunction
- Four major types:
  - ◊ Disorder of desire - both hypo- and hyper- (initiation and response), global desire disorder, couple desire discrepancy, situational desire disorder - these must be evaluated in the context of the relationship overall
  - ◊ Disorder of arousal
  - ◊ Dyspareunia, vaginismus
  - ◊ Orgasmic disorders - primary and secondary, during masturbation or coitus, situational or partner specific

System(s) affected: Nervous, Reproductive
Genetics: N/A
Incidence/Prevalence in USA:

- 1 in 5 women is sexually dissatisfied, and two thirds of women report some degree of sexual dysfunction. Only one third of anorgasmic women in general think it is a problem.
- Overall prevalence for dysfunction is 15-30% of all women. Desire disorders are complaint of 30-55% of individual patients presenting to clinics, and 31% of couples; arousal disorders present in about 14-48% in community studies. Orgasmic disorders probably the most common; about 10% primary, and up to 65-80% secondary in community studies.
- There are many barriers to seeking help, so data for prevalence incomplete; barriers include stigma of exposing sexual inadequacy, fear of unknown therapy, e.g., of having to perform before a therapist.

Predominant age: Can occur in post-pubertal age group; women's ability to experience orgasm increases gradually from puberty; in later teens nearly half have not had orgasm; by mid-thirties, about 10% have not
Predominant sex: Female (heterosexual, homosexual, and bisexual women)

SIGNS & SYMPTOMS

- Complaint to health care provider (if the clinician inquires, over twice as many are revealed than if clinician waits for patient to mention)
- Infertility
- Marital conflict
- Family dysfunction

CAUSES

- Inter-relational difficulties and conflict regarding intimacy
- Anxiety
- Survivor of sexual abuse, including incest
- Alcohol
- Drug use, including prescription medications (e.g., MAO inhibitors, tricyclic antidepressants, beta-blockers, especially SSRI antidepressants [Prozac, Paxil, Zoloft, etc.])
- Proximity of other people in household (mother-in-law)
- Anorgasmia can be due to diabetes
- Spinal cord damage
- Hormonal imbalance?
- Thyroid disease
- Sexual frequency myths
- Control issues in the relationships
- Dyspareunia, including vaginal dryness causing interference with lubrication, secondary to infection or endocrine
- There is little endocrine data on women with sexual dysfunction

RISK FACTORS Couple discrepancies in - expectations, cultural backgrounds, attitudes toward sexuality in family of origin, previous sexual trauma, low self-esteem

DIAGNOSIS

DIFFERENTIAL DIAGNOSIS

- Medication side effects. Psychotropics, monoamine oxidase inhibitors, tricyclic and other antidepressants.
- Marital dysfunction including domestic violence
- Decreased sensation secondary to back or nerve disease
- Multiple sclerosis
- Abdominal surgery (can interfere with pelvic innervation)
- Depression
- Vaginitis
- Decreased vaginal lubrication secondary to hormonal imbalance
- Pregnancy
- Anatomic or congenital abnormalities
- Pseudodyspareunia (use of complaint of pain to distance from partner)

LABORATORY As needed to identify infections and other medical causes

Drugs that may alter lab results: N/A

Disorders that may alter lab results: N/A

PATHOLOGICAL FINDINGS Varied if any

SPECIAL TESTS May need life experiences or some other psychological inventory to evaluate couple. (Alcohol, marijuana or other illicit drug use may make these evaluations unreliable.)

IMAGING N/A

DIAGNOSTIC PROCEDURES N/A

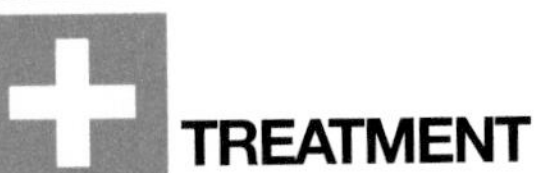

TREATMENT

APPROPRIATE HEALTH CARE Outpatient

GENERAL MEASURES

- For childhood trauma - scripting, psychotherapy, cognitive restructuring
- For anorgasmia - directed masturbation and "homework" with partners
- For prescription drug causes - reduced dosages, or change to different medication
- Other - family therapy, sensate conditioning; referral to specialized sex therapy

SURGICAL MEASURES N/A

ACTIVITY Varies with couple

DIET Weight reduction if needed for either partner

PATIENT EDUCATION Information about normal sexual function and human reproductive anatomy and function and changes expected with aging

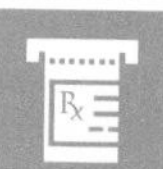

MEDICATIONS

DRUG(S) OF CHOICE These are usually multifactorial psychosocial conditions. Using medications doesn't address the cause of the problem and can make it worse.
Contraindications: N/A
Precautions: N/A
Significant possible interactions: N/A

ALTERNATIVE DRUGS
- Postmenopausal women
  - ◊ Adding testosterone to hormone replacement therapy may increase sexual desire
- Premenopausal women
  - ◊ Some data suggests testosterone may be low with decreased libido. No clear studies inidicate testosterone replacement as beneficial.

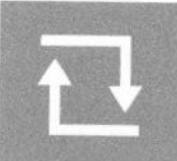

FOLLOWUP

PATIENT MONITORING Varies with patient

PREVENTION/AVOIDANCE Sex education starting in elementary years, early intervention in dysfunctional family or incest

POSSIBLE COMPLICATIONS Marital or family stress, breakup and divorce

EXPECTED COURSE/PROGNOSIS Lack of desire is the most difficult to treat (less than 50% successful by patient report), and success is sometimes less optimal than patient's initial wish. Best predictors are desire to change and overall healthy relationship.

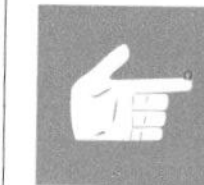

MISCELLANEOUS

ASSOCIATED CONDITIONS Marital stress

AGE-RELATED FACTORS
Pediatric: N/A
Geriatric:
- Societal expectations about geriatric sexuality, (especially the myth older women aren't sexually active) can cause distress if patient has sexual desires or sexual experience
- Normal physiologic changes in aging are misinterpreted as dysfunction

Others: Sex role stereotypes

PREGNANCY Often affects but the effect varies depending on the patient and couple's beliefs about pregnancy and the problem

SYNONYMS
- Hypoactive sexual desire disorder
- Sexual aversion disorder
- Female sexual arousal disorder
- Inhibited female orgasm

ICD-9-CM
302.70 Psychosexual dysfunction, unspecified
302.72 Psychosexual dysfunction with inhibited sexual excitement
302.73 Psychosexual dysfunction with inhibited female orgasm
302.76 Psychosexual dysfunction with functional dyspareunia

SEE ALSO
Vaginismus

OTHER NOTES
- Women must feel safe in order to let go and lose some control to experience orgasm
- Performance anxiety makes males ejaculate prematurely, while it inhibits orgasm in women
- Simple lack of knowledge about anatomy and physiology of sex can lead to problems

ABBREVIATIONS N/A

REFERENCES

- Leiblum SR, Rosen RC: Principles and Practice of Sex Therapy: Update for the 1990's. New York, The Guilford Press, 1989
- Wincze JP, Carey MP: Sexual Dysfunction: A Guide for Assessment and Treatment. New York, The Guilford Press, 1991
- Bancroft J: Human Sexuality and Its Problems. 2nd Ed. New York, Churchill Livingstone, 1989

Web references: 0 available at www.5mcc.com
Illustrations N/A

Author(s):
S. Shevaun Duiker, MD

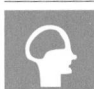

BASICS

DESCRIPTION Inadequate tissue perfusion (oxygen supply) resulting in organ dysfunction, cellular and organ damage and, if not corrected quickly, death.
Classification of shock:
- Hypovolemic shock - cardiac output is severely reduced due to loss of intravascular volume. Most often caused by blood loss.
- Cardiogenic shock - cardiac output is severely reduced due to a loss of myocardial muscle function, valvular dysfunction or arrhythmia. Most often caused by large myocardial infarctions.
- Obstructive shock - cardiac output is severely reduced by vascular obstruction of venous return to the heart (vena cava syndrome), compression of the heart, (pericardial tamponade, tension pneumothorax) or outflow from the heart (aortic dissection, pulmonary embolism)
- Distributive shock - maldistribution of blood flow
- Venous pooling (most often due to spinal shock or drug overdose) behaves much like hypovolemic shock, cardiac output severely reduced because blood is pooled in peripheral veins rather than being returned to the heart
- High output or vasodilating shock (most often due to sepsis or septic like states such as toxic shock) is unique in that cardiac output is normal or elevated, but not distributed appropriately, resulting in over perfusion of some tissues and underperfusion (to the point of critical ischemia) of other tissues.

System(s) affected: Cardiovascular
Genetics: Unknown
Incidence/Prevalence in USA: N/A
Predominant age: All ages. Determined by underlying diseases causing shock. More frequent and less well tolerated in the elderly.
Predominant sex: Male = Female

SIGNS & SYMPTOMS
- Underlying disease
  - ◊ Upper gastrointestinal (UGI) bleeding (ulcer pain, hematemesis, melena)
  - ◊ Sepsis (fever, chills, myalgia)
  - ◊ Pyelonephritis (urosepsis): dysuria, CVA tenderness, fever, chills, myalgia
  - ◊ Myocardial infarction (chest pain, diaphoresis, nausea, vomiting, S4 or S3 gallop, new heart murmur, rales due to pulmonary edema)
- Underperfusion of organ systems:
  - ◊ Brain: confusion, anxiety, agitation, coma only if severe
  - ◊ Kidney: oliguria
  - ◊ Skin: peripheral cyanosis, sluggish capillary refill, mottling, coolness, may be overly perfused (flushed) in high output (septic) shock
  - ◊ GI: absence of bowel sounds
  - ◊ Circulation: thready pulses, tachycardia, hypotension (mean arterial pressure < 60 torr or systolic pressure < 90 torr or blood pressure > 40 torr less than usual blood pressure in chronic hypertension), secondary cardiac ischemia (ST depression) or heart failure may occur due to underperfusion of the heart during shock. Jugular-venous distention (JVD), pulsus paradoxus in pericardial tamponade.

CAUSES
- Hypovolemic shock
  - ◊ Blood loss due to trauma or gastrointestinal bleeding
  - ◊ Third space loss of plasma volume (pancreatitis, bowel obstruction, infarction, anaphylaxis)
  - ◊ Diarrhea (e.g., in cholera-like states)
  - ◊ Burns
- Cardiogenic shock
  - ◊ Acute myocardial infarction (> 40% of LV mass)
  - ◊ Arrhythmia (heart block, ventricular tachycardia, atrial fibrillation with rapid ventricular response, etc.)
  - ◊ Acute valvular dysfunction (mitral valve due to papillary muscle rupture following inferior MI's or chordal rupture) aortic or mitral valve due to bacterial endocarditis
  - ◊ Ventricular septal rupture following anterior/septal MI's
- Obstructive shock
  - ◊ Pericardial tamponade
  - ◊ Inferior/superior vena caval obstruction usually due to neoplasms
  - ◊ Aortic dissection
  - ◊ Massive pulmonary embolism
- Distributive shock
  - ◊ Venous pooling due to a loss of venous tone caused by loss of sympathetic nervous system activity (e.g., acute spinal injury, general or spinal anesthesia or overdose of sedative drugs)
  - ◊ High output shock is due to sepsis, toxic shock or anaphylaxis (once plasma volume normalized)

RISK FACTORS N/A

DIAGNOSIS

DIFFERENTIAL DIAGNOSIS N/A

LABORATORY
- Specific to shock
  - ◊ Elevated lactate (> 2 mmol/L) indicates anaerobic metabolism due to tissue underperfusion
  - ◊ Reduced mixed venous P02 (< 28 mm Hg) (< 3.7 kPa) obtained from the pulmonary artery indicates vigorous extraction of oxygen from tissues due to underperfusion
- Underlying diseases responsible for shock
  - ◊ ECG, CPK (serial), troponin
  - ◊ CXR
  - ◊ Arterial blood gases
  - ◊ Gram stain and culture of infected sites
  - ◊ Blood cultures
  - ◊ CBC (serial determination of Hgb/Hct in bleeding patients)

Drugs that may alter lab results: N/A

Disorders that may alter lab results: N/A

PATHOLOGICAL FINDINGS N/A

SPECIAL TESTS
- Endoscopy/Radioisotope bleeding scan: localize ongoing bleeding which may direct surgical intervention. The endoscopist may intervene directly via the endoscope. (e.g., injection of sclerosants into varices or ulcers).
- Echocardiogram: valvular failure, pericardial effusions, echo-guided pericardiocentesis
- Pulmonary artery (Swan-Ganz) catheterization: serial measurement of cardiac output, central venous, pulmonary arterial and pulmonary arterial occlusion pressures (left atrial pressure) and vascular resistance. Mixed venous blood gases can be drawn from the catheter. Indicated when the etiology of shock is uncertain, in cardiogenic and septic shock, or when initial therapy of shock fails to provide for rapid correction of perfusion failure.

IMAGING
- Chest CT, VQ scan, and/or pulmonary angiogram: pulmonary embolism

DIAGNOSTIC PROCEDURES N/A

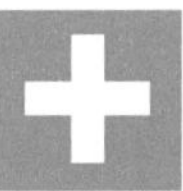

TREATMENT

APPROPRIATE HEALTH CARE
- Emergency room or intensive care unit
- Continuous electrocardiographic monitoring with frequent assessment of blood pressure, respiratory status, and urine output

GENERAL MEASURES
- Therapy must proceed quickly before extensive damage to vital organs occur. Therapy is directed simultaneously to correct both the deficit in tissue perfusion and the underlying disease causing shock (see Associated conditions).
- Maintain SaO2 > 95% with supplemental oxygen. Intubate and mechanically ventilate if patient cannot oxygenate adequately or has markedly increased breathing effort (excessive oxygen cost of breathing).
- Maintain pH between 7.3 and 7.5 to preserve vascular responsiveness to endogenous or exogenous catecholamines
- Correct plasma volume deficits rapidly by volume expanders consisting of isotonic saline (NS or Ringer's lactate) with or without colloid (albumin 5% or hydroxyethyl starch 6%)
- Packed red blood cell transfusion to correct or prevent anemia. HgB maintained at or above 10 grams/dl.
- Administer coagulation factors (fresh frozen plasma, cryoprecipitate) and platelets if coagulopathy (prolonged PT, PTT or platelet count < 50,000) is present in a patient who is bleeding
- Tachyarrhythmias (other than sinus tachycardia) should be promptly corrected by electro-cardioversion. Insert transvenous pacemaker to correct bradyrhythmias.
- Vasopressors to correct hypotension or low cardiac output due to myocardial failure or hypotension due to low vascular resistance
- End points of resuscitation: adequate blood pressure (> 60 mm Hg [8.0 kPa] mean or > 90 mm Hg [12.0 kPa] systolic or within 40 mm Hg [5.32 kPa] of patient's normal blood pressure). Patient is awake/alert, urine output adequate, heart rate < 100, warm skin with brisk capillary refill, bowel sounds present. Lactate < 2 mmol/L, mixed venous PO2 > 30 mm Hg.

SURGICAL MEASURES N/A

ACTIVITY Bedrest

DIET N/A until stable

PATIENT EDUCATION N/A

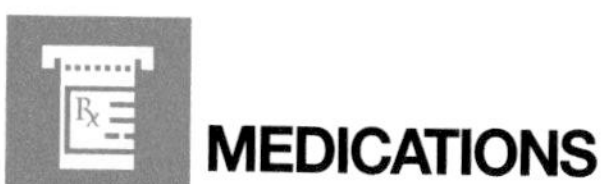

MEDICATIONS

DRUG(S) OF CHOICE

- Dopamine > 4 μg/kg/min: augments contractility, and cardiac output (beta-1) and increased heart rate. Increases blood pressure by a combination of increased cardiac output and vasoconstriction (alpha).
- Norepinephrine up to 2 μg/kg/min: augments blood pressure by increasing vascular resistance (alpha). Cardiac output in septic shock maintained or increased (beta-1).
- Phenylephrine 20-200 μg/min: see norepinephrine
- Dobutamine 5-10 μg/kg/min augments contractility and cardiac output (beta-1). Does not raise blood pressure because of vasodilation (beta-2).
- Corticosteroids/vasopressin

Contraindications: Refer to manufacturer's profile of each drug

Precautions:

- Myocardial oxygen consumption is increased by increased heart rate, afterload, and contractility
- Pressors can increase myocardial ischemia if present and may precipitate or worsen tachyarrhythmias. Use in lowest possible dose for as limited period of time as possible

Significant possible interactions: Refer to manufacturer's profile of each drug

ALTERNATIVE DRUGS N/A

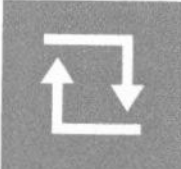

FOLLOWUP

PATIENT MONITORING Careful monitoring in intensive care

PREVENTION/AVOIDANCE Shock is best avoided by prompt recognition and treatment of underlying diseases which cause shock (e.g., early antibiotic therapy for infections)

POSSIBLE COMPLICATIONS

- Multiple organs may be damaged by underperfusion during shock
- Acute tubular necrosis
- Ischemic hepatitis
- Ischemic bowel
- Disseminated intravascular coagulopathy
- Adult respiratory distress syndrome (ARDS)
- Encephalopathy and/or cerebrovascular accident

EXPECTED COURSE/PROGNOSIS

- Mortality is determined by a complex interaction of primary disease causing shock, age, coexisting chronic disease and shock severity as marked by the number of acute organ system failures that follow shock
- Best outcome (> 90% survival) in young patient with transient shock due to trauma or gastrointestinal blood loss without chronic irreversible illnesses
- Poor outcome (> 90% mortality) in elderly patient with septic shock, underlying chronic liver disease, who develops acute renal failure, ARDS, and coagulopathy

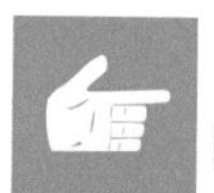

MISCELLANEOUS

ASSOCIATED CONDITIONS

- Gastrointestinal blood loss: may require endoscopic or surgical intervention if bleeding doesn't spontaneously cease, e.g., electrocoagulation or injecting sclerosant for bleeding peptic ulcers, sclerotherapy in esophageal varices
- Sepsis: empiric antibiotic therapy; activated protein C may reduce mortality by 25% in severe septic shock with end organ failure. Hydrocortisone (50 mg q 6 hours or equivalent for 5-7 days and vasopressin (0.01-0.04 units per minute) improves blood pressure and reduces vasopressin dependence and (perhaps) mortality in septic shock. Consider when patients do not improve in response to fluids, antibiotics, and low doses of vasopressors.
- Cardiogenic shock: therapy should help reduce cardiac ischemia (oxygen, nitrates) and accomplish rapid reperfusion of injured, but potentially viable, myocardium (thrombolysis with fibrinolytic agents, balloon angioplasty of stenotic vessels or surgical bypass grafting). A balloon pump may temporize by providing improved coronary blood flow during and following diagnostic testing and revascularization therapy. If shock is due to acute failure of the mitral or aortic valve, surgical valve replacement may be lifesaving.
- Pulmonary embolism
- Cardiac tamponade

AGE-RELATED FACTORS

Pediatric: N/A
Geriatric: Prognosis more guarded
Others: N/A

PREGNANCY N/A

SYNONYMS N/A

ICD-9-CM

785.50 Shock, unspecified
785.51 Cardiogenic shock
785.59 Shock without mention of trauma, other

SEE ALSO

Anaphylaxis
Cardiac tamponade
Myocardial infarction
Peptic ulcer disease
Pulmonary embolism
Sepsis

OTHER NOTES N/A

ABBREVIATIONS N/A

REFERENCES

- Parillo JE: Shock. In: Braunwald E, et al, editors. Harrison's Principles of Internal Medicine. 12th Ed. New York: McGraw-Hill, Inc; 1991
- Schuster DP, Lefrah SS. Shock. In: Civetta JF, et al, editors. Critical Care. Philadelphia: J.B. Lippincott Corp; 1988. p.891-908
- Bernard GR, Vincent JL, Laterre PF, et al. Efficacy and safety of recombinant human activated protein C for severe sepsis. N Engl J Med 2001;344(10):699-709
- Cooper MS, Stewart PM. Corticosteroid insufficiency in acutely ill patients. N Engl J Med 2003;348(8):727-34
- Holmes CL, Patel BM, Russell JA, Walley KR. Physiology of vasopressin relevant to management of septic shock. Chest 2001;120(3):989-1002

Web references: 0 available at www.5mcc.com
Illustrations N/A

Author(s):

Mark R. Dambro, MD

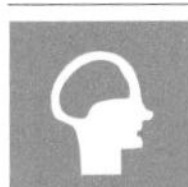

BASICS

DESCRIPTION Inflammation of the salivary glands from nonspecific bacterial infection or inflammation most often arises in the excretory duct. The parotid is the most commonly affected gland with invasion of bacteria from the oral cavity. Inflammation may also follow trauma, spread of infection from adjoining tissues, and via hematogenous routes during bacteremia. Inflammation may lead to stone formation (sialolithiasis) or an obstructed duct may lead to inflammation of the gland. Stones are more commonly associated with the submaxillary glands. Recurrent infections or other chronic inflammatory processes can lead to decreased gland function with resulting xerostomia.
System(s) affected: Gastrointestinal, Skin/Exocrine
Genetics: Unknown
Incidence/Prevalence in USA: Most commonly seen in debilitated patients
Predominant age: N/A
Predominant sex: N/A

SIGNS & SYMPTOMS
- Enlarged, painful salivary gland
- Purulent discharge from duct orifice
- Red, painful duct orifice
- Fever
- Xerostomia
- Decreased salivary secretion (aptyalism)

CAUSES
- Bacteria from the oral cavity are the most common infectious cause of sialadenitis.
- The causative agents of the following diseases may also infect a salivary gland to cause sialadenitis:
  - ◊ Mumps
  - ◊ Actinomycosis
  - ◊ Tuberculosis
  - ◊ Syphilis
  - ◊ CMV
  - ◊ Cat-scratch disease

RISK FACTORS
- Dehydration
- Fever
- Hypercalcemia
- Severely debilitated patient
- Treatment with radiation or chemotherapy for underlying malignant disease

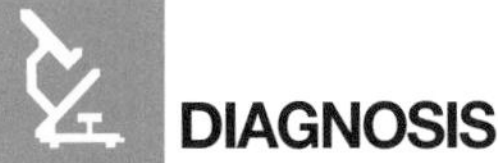

DIAGNOSIS

DIFFERENTIAL DIAGNOSIS
Decreased salivary secretion is associated with:
- Drugs:
  - ◊ Tricyclic antidepressants (amitriptyline, etc.)
  - ◊ Phenothiazines (chlorpromazine, fluphenazine, thioridazine, prochlorperazine, etc.)
  - ◊ Anticholinergics
- Myxedema
- Plummer-Vinson disease
- Pernicious anemia
- Febrile diseases
- Neuropsychiatric disorders
- Mikulicz disease (benign lymphoepithelial lesion)

Enlarged glands may be the result of a variety of neoplasms including:
- Pleomorphic adenoma
- Mucoepidermoid carcinoma
- Other tumor types can also occur very rarely (lipoma, neurofibroma, fibrosarcoma, melanoma, lymphocytoma, Hodgkin, etc.)

Also, obesity results in what appears to be enlarged parotids, but the bilateral nature and non-progressive course should help differentiate this from malignant neoplasms.

LABORATORY N/A

Drugs that may alter lab results: N/A

Disorders that may alter lab results: N/A

PATHOLOGICAL FINDINGS
With chronic infection of the gland:
- Enlarged gland
- Ductal dilatation with retention of saliva
- Acinar atrophy or dilated and filled with mucus
- Purulent/seropurulent exudate within the duct
- Glandular replacement by fibrotic tissue
- Infiltration with leukocytes

SPECIAL TESTS N/A

IMAGING Radiographs may reveal a stone in sialolithiasis

DIAGNOSTIC PROCEDURES
- Digital manipulation of the duct may express pus from the ductal orifice

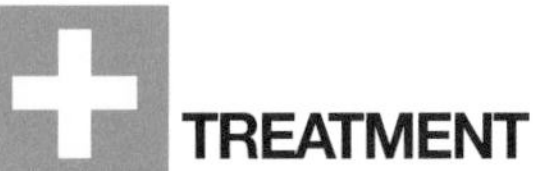

TREATMENT

APPROPRIATE HEALTH CARE Outpatient

GENERAL MEASURES Heating pad and/or cool compresses may be comforting

SURGICAL MEASURES
- Superficial parotidectomy in patients with chronic nonspecific sialadenitis. Complications include temporary (or permanent) facial nerve weakness, neuromas, but a reduction in symptoms can be expected.

ACTIVITY Unrestricted

DIET Avoid pain-producing sialagogues (lemon, etc.) during an acute episode

PATIENT EDUCATION N/A

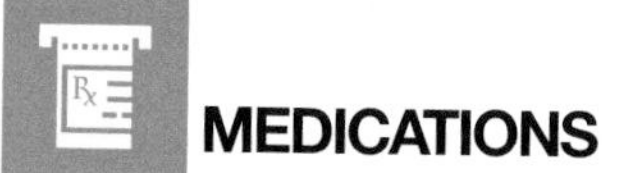

MEDICATIONS

DRUG(S) OF CHOICE
- Antibiotics
  - ◊ Penicillin V (Pen VK) 250-500 mg QID
  - ◊ Erythromycin 250 mg QID
  - ◊ Amoxicillin-clavulanate (Augmentin) 500 mg TID
  - ◊ Cefuroxime (Ceftin)
- Analgesic: codeine, hydrocodone, NSAIDs, etc

Contraindications: N/A
Precautions: N/A
Significant possible interactions: N/A

ALTERNATIVE DRUGS N/A

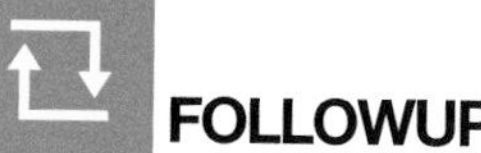

FOLLOWUP

PATIENT MONITORING N/A

PREVENTION/AVOIDANCE N/A

POSSIBLE COMPLICATIONS
Occasional loss of salivary function

EXPECTED COURSE/PROGNOSIS
Complete recovery and good prognosis

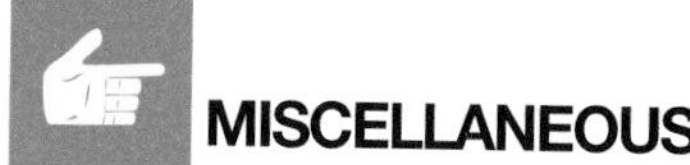

MISCELLANEOUS

ASSOCIATED CONDITIONS
- Rheumatoid arthritis (Sjögren syndrome)
- Sarcoidosis (Herrfordt syndrome)

AGE-RELATED FACTORS
Pediatric: Rare in children
Geriatric: N/A
Others: N/A

PREGNANCY N/A

SYNONYMS
- Sialadenosis

ICD-9-CM
527.2 Sialadenitis

SEE ALSO
Sjögren syndrome

OTHER NOTES N/A

ABBREVIATIONS
CMV = cytomegalovirus

REFERENCES

- Bhatty MA, Piggot RA, Soames JV, McLean NR. Chronic non-specific parotid sialadenitis. Br J Plast Surg 1998 Oct;51(7):517-21

Web references: 0 available at www.5mcc.com
Illustrations N/A

Author(s):
James F. Broomfield, MD

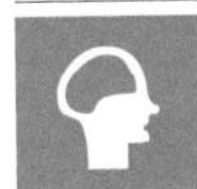

BASICS

DESCRIPTION Pneumoconiosis (fibrogenic) caused by inhaling silica dust (in the form of quartz, cristobalite, or tridymite)
- Chronic (classical) silicosis can be simple or complicated
- Chronic simple silicosis (sim sil) is asymptomatic, nonprogressive once exposure ends, and consists solely of small round radiographic pulmonary opacities
- Chronic complicated silicosis (comp sil) has progressively worsening symptoms and enlarging pulmonary opacities, even after exposure ends.
- Subacute silicosis (sub sil) develops after 3-6 years of high exposure, and resembles chronic complicated silicosis
- Acute silicosis (ac sil) develops within a couple years of massive exposure and is clinically distinct from the other forms

System(s) affected: Pulmonary
Genetics: No known genetic pattern
Incidence/Prevalence in USA: Unknown
Predominant age: 40-75
Predominant sex: Male > Female

SIGNS & SYMPTOMS
- Sim sil
  - ◊ Asymptomatic
  - ◊ Cough and mild dyspnea typically accompany, and are due to smoking or occupational bronchitis
- Comp sil; sub sil
  - ◊ Chest tightness
  - ◊ Cough
  - ◊ Dyspnea
  - ◊ Expectoration
  - ◊ Signs and symptoms of right heart failure as cor pulmonale develops
- Ac sil
  - ◊ Dry cough
  - ◊ Fever
  - ◊ Severe dyspnea

CAUSES
- Sim sil: 10-12 years of exposure to silica dust
- Comp sil: > 20 years of exposure
- Sub sil: 3-6 years of heavy exposure
- Ac sil: < 2 years of massive exposure

RISK FACTORS
- Industrial activities that involve cutting, polishing, or shearing rock, or involve the use of sand, including:
  - ◊ Metal mining (copper, silver, gold, lead, hard coal)
  - ◊ Foundries
  - ◊ Pottery making
  - ◊ Sandstone cutting
  - ◊ Granite cutting

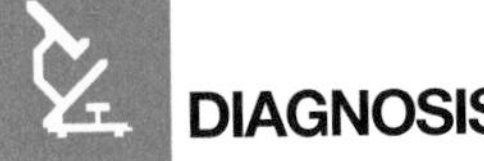

DIAGNOSIS

DIFFERENTIAL DIAGNOSIS
- Sim sil
  - ◊ Sarcoidosis
  - ◊ Radiographic egg shell calcifications also seen in sarcoidosis and Hodgkin disease
- Comp sil, sub sil
  - ◊ Coal worker pneumoconiosis
  - ◊ Consider especially when consolidations are rapidly progressive, unilateral, or cavitating - tuberculosis, neoplasia, fungal pneumonia
- Ac sil
  - ◊ Alveolar proteinosis

LABORATORY
- Hypoxemia
- Hypercarbia

Drugs that may alter lab results: N/A

Disorders that may alter lab results: N/A

PATHOLOGICAL FINDINGS
- Lung
  - ◊ Pleural adhesions
  - ◊ Pleural thickening
  - ◊ Gray-black subpleural nodules
  - ◊ Blackened lung
  - ◊ Leathery lung
  - ◊ Concentric layers of dense connective tissue
  - ◊ Cellular infiltrate
  - ◊ Ischemic degeneration of central nodule
  - ◊ Metachromatic silica particles

SPECIAL TESTS
- Pulmonary function testing is normal in simple silicosis. Other forms show decreased pulmonary compliance, decreased lung volumes, decreased diffusing capacity.
- International Labor Office (ILO) classification system for quantification of chest radiograph abnormalities.
- Yearly PPD

IMAGING
Chest x-ray:
- Sim sil
  - ◊ Egg shell calcification in hilar and mediastinal lymph nodes
  - ◊ Small round opacities, initially in upper lobes
- Comp sil, sub sil
  - ◊ Pulmonary opacities > 1 cm
  - ◊ Opacities form bilateral conglomerate shadows (progressive massive fibrosis)
  - ◊ Opacities initially peripheral, later migrate towards hilum.
  - ◊ Opacities may cavitate (rule out tuberculosis!)

CT:
- May be helpful in identifying nodules

DIAGNOSTIC PROCEDURES
- Bronchoscopy
- Detailed occupational history
- Open lung biopsy

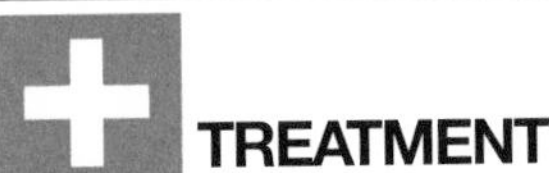

TREATMENT

APPROPRIATE HEALTH CARE Prevention - respiratory protective devices for unavoidable short-term exposure

GENERAL MEASURES
- No known effective treatment
- Postural drainage
- Mist inhalation
- Chest physical therapy
- Breathing exercises

SURGICAL MEASURES
- Lung transplantation
- Whole lung lavage remains investigational

ACTIVITY Maintain regular exercise program

DIET
- No special diet
- Increase fluid intake

PATIENT EDUCATION Printed patient information available from: American Lung Association, 1740 Broadway, New York, NY 10019, (212)315-8700

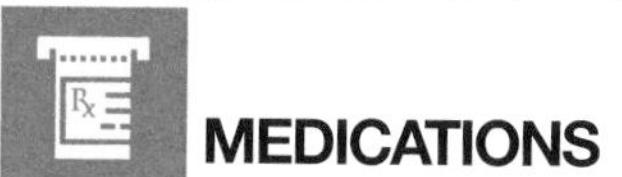

MEDICATIONS

DRUG(S) OF CHOICE
- None specific for silicosis
- Isoniazid, 300 mg/d for one year, if tuberculin skin test is positive
- Silicotuberculosis requires at least 3 anti-tuberculous drugs initially, including rifampin

Contraindications: Avoid sedatives and hypnotics
Precautions: Refer to manufacturer's literature
Significant possible interactions: Refer to manufacturer's literature

ALTERNATIVE DRUGS
Antifibrinogenic agents remain investigational

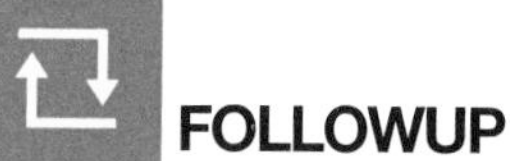

FOLLOWUP

PATIENT MONITORING
- Monitor for heart failure and hypoxemia
- Treat intercurrent infections aggressively

PREVENTION/AVOIDANCE
Avoid dust exposure; substitute other materials for silica

POSSIBLE COMPLICATIONS
- Progressive massive fibrosis
- Respiratory infection
- Pneumothorax
- Emphysema
- Cor pulmonale
- Right heart failure
- Mycobacterial infections
- Fungal infections

EXPECTED COURSE/PROGNOSIS
- Sim sil - remains asymptomatic and does not progress if exposure ends
- Comp sil; sub sil - progressive pulmonary fibrosis with cor pulmonale and right heart failure, even after exposure ends.

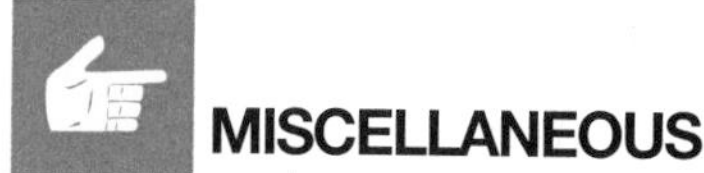

MISCELLANEOUS

ASSOCIATED CONDITIONS
- Tuberculosis
- Caplan syndrome

AGE-RELATED FACTORS
Pediatric: Unusual
Geriatric: Symptoms and complications more severe
Others: N/A

PREGNANCY
N/A

SYNONYMS
N/A

ICD-9-CM
502 Pneumoconiosis due to other silica or silicates

SEE ALSO
Chronic obstructive pulmonary disease & emphysema
Cor pulmonale
Pneumothorax
Tuberculosis

OTHER NOTES
Silica - formula for calculating the threshold limit value (TLV) for respirable dust: TLV (threshold limit value) = (10 mg per cu meter/% SiO2) + 2

ABBREVIATIONS
Ac sil = Acute silicosis
Comp sil = Chronic complicated silicosis
Sim sil = Chronic simple silicosis
Sub sil = Subacute silicosis

REFERENCES

- Silicosis and Silicate Disease Committee. Diseases associated with exposure to silica and non-fibrous silicate materials. Arch Pathol Lab Med 1988;112:673
- Banks DE, et al: Strategies for the treatment of pneumoconiosis. Occup Med 1993;8(1):205-232

Web references: 3 available at www.5mcc.com
Illustrations N/A

Author(s):
Robert P. Baughman, MD

BASICS

DESCRIPTION Acute sinusitis is a symptomatic inflammation of the paranasal sinuses of less than 4 weeks duration occurring as a result of impaired drainage and retained secretions. Subacute when symptomatic from 4-12 weeks. Chronic when symptomatic for greater than 12 weeks. Acute exacerbation of chronic disease when worsening of already symptomatic patient.

System(s) affected: Pulmonary
Genetics: No known genetic pattern
Incidence/Prevalence in USA:
- 16% of population annual diagnosis of sinusitis
- Fifth leading reason for antibiotic prescriptions
- Approximately 5% of office visits for young adults
- Incidence of both acute and chronic sinusitis increases in the latter part of childhood
- Incidence increases up to age 75 and then decreases

Predominant age: All ages
Predominant sex: Both sexes equally

SIGNS & SYMPTOMS
- Symptoms predictive of bacterial sinusitis:
  - ◊ Persistent duration of symptoms for at least one week
  - ◊ Purulent nasal discharge
  - ◊ Maxillary tooth or facial pain (especially if unilateral)
  - ◊ Unilateral maxillary sinus tenderness
  - ◊ Worsening of symptoms after initial improvement
- Other associated symptoms:
  - ◊ Headache
  - ◊ Retro-orbital pain
  - ◊ Otalgia
  - ◊ Hyposomia
  - ◊ Halitosis
  - ◊ Chronic cough
- Symptoms indicating urgency:
  - ◊ Orbital pain
  - ◊ Visual disturbances, especially diplopia
  - ◊ Periorbital swelling or erythema
  - ◊ Facial swelling or erythema
  - ◊ Mentation change
- Predictive physical examination findings:
  - ◊ Purulent rhinorrhea
- Other associated signs
  - ◊ Edematous nasal mucosa
  - ◊ Nasal obstruction/polyps
- Signs indicating urgency or complications:
  - ◊ Visual changes
  - ◊ Abnormal extraocular movements
  - ◊ Periorbital edema or erythema
  - ◊ Change in mental status

CAUSES
- Viral - vast majority (rhinovirus, coronavirus, influenzae A & B, parainfluenzae virus, RSV, adenovirus and enterovirus)
- Bacterial - complicates 0.2% to 2% of viral cases
  - ◊ Risk is over diagnosis of bacterial and encouragement of resistance to antibiotics
  - ◊ *Streptococcus pneumoniae*, *Haemophilus influenzae* most common bacterial etiologies
- Fungal

RISK FACTORS
- Viral upper respiratory infection
- Anatomical abnormalities
  - ◊ Tonsillar and adenoid hypertrophy
  - ◊ Turbinate hypertrophy
  - ◊ Deviated septum
  - ◊ Nasal polyps
  - ◊ Cleft palate
- Barotrauma
- Dental infections and procedures
- Immunodeficiency & HIV disease
- Cystic fibrosis
- Asthma and allergies
- For fungal infection:
  - ◊ Diabetics
  - ◊ Leukemia
  - ◊ Neutropenia
  - ◊ High-dose steroids
  - ◊ Transplant recipients
  - ◊ Congenital T-cell Immunodeficiencies

DIAGNOSIS

DIFFERENTIAL DIAGNOSIS
- Viral URI
- Dental disease
- Cystic fibrosis
- Wegener granulomatosis
- HIV infection
- Kartagener syndrome
- Immotile cilia syndrome
- Neoplasm

LABORATORY
- Sedimentation rate > 19 mm/hr
- C-reactive protein > 10 mg/L

Drugs that may alter lab results: N/A

Disorders that may alter lab results: N/A

PATHOLOGICAL FINDINGS
- Inflammation
- Edema
- Thickened mucosa
- Impaired ciliary function
- Inflammatory metaplasia to ciliated columnar cells
- Relative acidosis and hypoxia within sinuses
- Polyps

SPECIAL TESTS Nasal endoscopy

IMAGING
- Routine use of sinus radiography discouraged because (1) the presence of 3 or more clinical findings may have similar diagnostic accuracy of imaging and (2) imaging ability to distinguish bacterial from viral sinusitis is limited.
- Complete opacification with air-fluid levels most specific.
- Mucosal thickening has low specificity.
- The presence of sinus fluid or sinus opacity on standard radiography yields moderate sensitivity (76%) and specificity (79%) when compared to sinus puncture
- Limited coronal CT of sinuses - most useful in evaluation of repeated or recurrent sinusitis, i.e., 3-4 annual episodes or failure to respond to medical therapy

DIAGNOSTIC PROCEDURES
- History and physical exam sufficient for majority of cases of sinusitis
- Transnasal endoscopic or sublabial maxillary antrum aspiration culture are gold standards, but generally performed only in selected cases

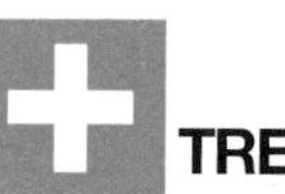

TREATMENT

APPROPRIATE HEALTH CARE
- Outpatient
- Hospitalization for complications (meningitis, orbital cellulitis or abscess, brain abscess)

GENERAL MEASURES
- Adequate hydration (8-10 glasses water daily)
- Steam inhalation 20-30 minutes tid or use of facial steamer
- Saline irrigation or saline nose drops
- Sleep with head of bed elevated
- Avoid exposure to cigarette/cigar/pipe smoke, fumes
- Avoid dehydrants (caffeine and alcohol)
- Antibiotics indicated when purulent rhinorrhea or worsening symptoms last more than 5-10 days

SURGICAL MEASURES
- If medical therapy fails, consider sinus irrigation to wash out inspissated material
- Functional endoscopic sinus surgery is the preferred treatment for medically recalcitrant cases
- Absolute surgical indications:
  - ◊ Massive nasal polyposis
  - ◊ Acute complications: subperiosteal or orbital abscess, frontal soft tissue spread of infection)
  - ◊ Mucocele or mucopyocele
  - ◊ Invasive or allergic fungal sinusitis
  - ◊ Suspected obstructing tumor
  - ◊ CSF rhinorrhea

ACTIVITY
- Adequate rest, otherwise no restrictions

DIET
- No special diet

PATIENT EDUCATION
- Call back if no significant improvement within one week, symptoms worsen, or symptoms such as headache, neck stiffness, visual changes, nausea or vomiting occur
- Educate patient on potential major side effects of selected medications
- For patient education materials favorably reviewed on this topic, contact:
  - ◊ American College of Allergy, Asthma & Immunology, 85 West Algonquin Road, Suite 550, Arlington Heights, IL 60005, 1-847-427-1200
  - ◊ Smoots E. American Family Physician 1998; 58(5):1805-6 (see www.aafp.org)

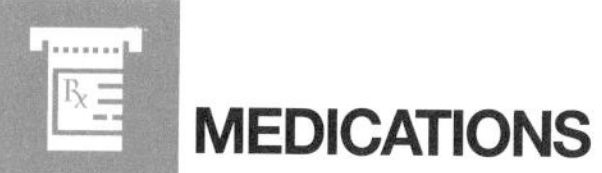

MEDICATIONS

DRUG(S) OF CHOICE

- Antibiotics. Several recent randomized controlled trials and meta-analyses suggest antibiotics have slight advantage over placebo, with most patients improving without such therapy. Newer agents not shown superior, yet studies may have underestimated antibiotic resistance. Major issue is accurate diagnosis of bacterial from viral infection. Recommendation is to reserve antibiotics use for those patients with moderate to severe disease.
- Initial therapy with no allergies or intolerance to beta-lactam:
  - ◊ Amoxicillin-clavulanate (Augmentin) 875 mg/125 mg po q12 hr and 80-90 mg/kg amoxicillin plus 6.4 mg/kg clavulanate per day daily for 10-14 days (in areas of higher beta-lactam resistance)
  - ◊ Amoxicillin 500 mg-1gm tid for 10-14 days in adults and 80-90 mg/kg per day divided q 8 hr for 10-14 days in children
  - ◊ Cefpodoxime (Vantin) 200 mg po 12 hrs for 10 days and 10 mg/kg/day divided bid in children
  - ◊ Cefuroxime (Ceftin) axetil 250 mg q 12 hr or 30 mg/kg/day divided q 12 hr in children up to 1 gm daily for suspension.
- Initial therapy if allergic to beta-lactam:
  - ◊ Trimethoprim-sulfamethoxazole (TMP-SMX) 160 mg/800 mg po q 12 hr in adults or 8-12 mg/kg/day of TMP component in children divided q 12 hr
  - ◊ Azithromycin (Zithromax) for children 10 mg/kg on day-1; 5 mg/kg on days 2-5
  - ◊ Clarithromycin 15 mg/kg day for children divided bid; in adults, extended-release 1,000 mg once qd for 14 days
  - ◊ Levofloxacin (Levaquin) 500 mg qd for 10-14 days; safety not established for children under age 18
  - ◊ Moxifloxacin (Avelox) 400 mg once daily for 10-days; safety not established for children under age 18
- Switch therapy if no resolution after minimum of 72-hr antibiotic use or previous antibiotics within 4-6 weeks:
  - ◊ Amoxicillin/clavulanate (Augmentin) as above
  - ◊ Use of TMP-SMX as above
  - ◊ Use of one of the cephalosporins above
  - ◊ Use of one of the fluoroquinolones above
  - ◊ Combination therapy with amoxicillin plus one of the cephalosporins above
- Lack of response to three weeks of antibiotics, consider: Waters view film, limited coronal CT scan or ENT referral
- Decongestants. Useful for first 3-5 days
  - ◊ Pseudoephedrine HCL 60 mg q 4-6 hours, not to exceed 4 doses in 24 hours (avoid or monitor closely in patients with hypertension)
  - ◊ Phenylephrine 2-3 sprays in each nostril q 4-6 hours; for 2-3 days
  - ◊ Oxymetazoline (Afrin) < 4 days use
- Analgesics: acetaminophen, aspirin, NSAIDS, acetaminophen-codeine

Contraindications:

- Refer to manufacturer's literature for drug contraindications

Precautions:

- Decongestants can exacerbate hypertension
- Prolonged use of topical decongestants (> 4-days) may precipitate rhinitis medicamentosa
- Major side effect of sulfonamides is Steven-Johnson syndrome: inform patients to report any mucous membrane ulcerations

Significant possible interactions:

- Warfarin (Coumadin): Increased effect of warfarin with TMP-SMX resulting in marked increase in INR and PT. Similar effect can also be seen with use of macrolides.

ALTERNATIVE DRUGS

- Allergies may be a predisposing factor; some patients report benefits from the use of antihistamine agents or nasal steroids [fluticasone (Flonase), beclomethasone (Beconase AQ, Vancenase AQ)] with underlying asthma or allergies; use established if underlying history of asthma
- Antihistamines
  - ◊ Loratadine (Claritin) 10 mg/day for all patients over age 6
  - ◊ Fexofenadine (Allegra) 60 mg bid in adults
  - ◊ Chlorpheniramine (Chlor-Trimeton) 0.35 mg/kg/day divided q6h or 8 mg tid in adults
- Leukotriene inhibitors (Singular, Accolate) may be indicated in patients with concomitant asthma

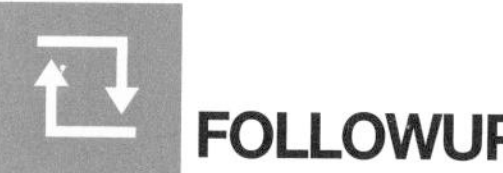

FOLLOWUP

PATIENT MONITORING

- Return if no improvement after completion of first course of antibiotics
- Report skin rash during use of antibiotics
- Instruct for proper use of adjunctive medications (nasal steroids, antihistamines)

PREVENTION/AVOIDANCE

- No documented evidence for prevention measures

POSSIBLE COMPLICATIONS

- Brain abscess
- Cavernous sinus thrombosis
- Meningitis
- Osteomyelitis
- Orbital cellulitis
- Subdural empyema

EXPECTED COURSE/PROGNOSIS

- Alleviation of symptoms within 72 hours with complete resolution within 10 days

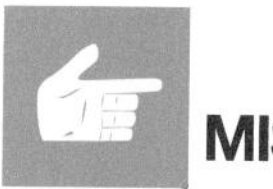

MISCELLANEOUS

ASSOCIATED CONDITIONS

- Allergic Rhinitis
- Asthma
- Bronchitis
- Otitis Media
- Pharyngitis

AGE-RELATED FACTORS

Pediatric:

- Average 6-8 colds per year; more frequent may indicate or place at risk for bacterial sinusitis
- Adenoid hypertrophy may complicate chronic sinusitis
- Chronic sinusitis indicates a need to search for underlying cause, eg., nasal deformities, or infected and hypertrophied adenoids

Geriatric:

- More difficult to heal in this age group

Others: N/A

PREGNANCY

- TMP-SMX = Category B; during term = Category D; can be used during lactation except for premature infants, those with hyperbilirubinemia and those with G-6-PD deficiency; avoid in children < 2, those with severe asthma or allergies; hemolytic anemia may occur in patients with G-6-PD deficiency
- Azithromycin = Category B; clarithromycin = Category C
- Penicillins listed as Category B; they are excreted in low concentrations into breast milk and can cause symptoms

SYNONYMS

Rhinosinusitis

ICD-9-CM

473.9 Unspecified sinusitis (chronic)
473.0 Chronic maxillary sinusitis
461.9 Acute sinusitis, unspecified
461.2 Acute ethmoidal sinusitis
461.1 Acute frontal sinusitus
461.0 Acute maxillary sinusitis
461.3 Acute sphenoidal sinusitus
461.8 Other acute sinusitis
117.9 Other and unspecifed mycoses

SEE ALSO

Asthma
Common cold
Rhinitis, allergic
Temporomandibular joint (TMJ) syndrome
Wegener granulomatosis

OTHER NOTES

- Resistance of S. pneumoniae and H. influenzae is increasing with prevalence rates estimated to be 25% and 40% in some localities
- Generally self-limited infections

ABBREVIATIONS

CSF = cerebrospinal fluid
TMP-SMX = trimethoprim-sulfamethoxazole
URI = upper respiratory infection

REFERENCES

- Antimicrobial treatment guidelines for acute bacterial rhinosinusitis. Sinus and Allergy Health Partnership. Otolaryngol Head Neck Surg 2000;123(1 Pt 2):5-31
- Engels EA, Terrin N, Barza M, Lau J. Meta-analysis of diagnostic tests for acute sinusitis. J Clin Epidemiol 2000;53(8):852-62
- Varonen H, Makela M, Savolainen S , et al. Comparison of ultrasound, radiography, and clinical examination in the diagnosis of acute maxillary sinusitis: a systematic review. J Clin Epidemiol 2000;53(9):940-8
- Williams JW, Aguilar C, Makela M, et al. Antibiotics for acute maxillary sinusitis. Cochrane Database Syst Rev 2000;(2):CD000243
- Snow V, Mottur-Pilson C, Hickner JM. Principles of appropriate antibiotic use for acute sinusitis in adults. Ann Intern Med 2001;134(6):495-7
- Hickner JM, Bartlett JG, Besser RE, et al. Principles of appropriate antibiotic use for acute rhinosinusitis in adults: background. Ann Intern Med 2001;134(6):498-505
- AHCPR. Diagnosis and treatment of acute bacterial rhinosinusitis. Rockville (MD): Agency for Health Care Policy and Research; 1999

Web references: 3 available at www.5mcc.com
Illustrations N/A

Author(s):

A. Peter Catinella, MD

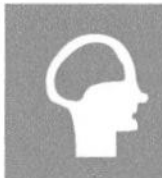

BASICS

DESCRIPTION Repetitive episodes of upper airway occlusion during sleep, often with oxygen desaturation. Nearly always associated with snoring. Apneas often terminate with a snort or gasp. Repetitive apneas produce sleep disruption, leading to excessive daytime sleepiness (EDS). Usual course is chronic.
System(s) affected: Cardiovascular, Nervous, Pulmonary
Genetics: Hereditary factors unknown. Familial patterns sometimes seen.
Incidence/Prevalence in USA: 4% of middle-age and older males; 2% middle-age and older females
Predominant age: Middle-age
Predominant sex: Males > Females (60-40%)

SIGNS & SYMPTOMS
- Cardinal symptom is excessive daytime sleepiness (EDS)
- Loud snoring
- Complaints of disrupted sleep
- Repetitive awakenings with transient sensation of shortness of breath or for unclear reasons
- Tired and unrefreshed upon A.M. awakening
- Witnessed apneas at night
- Complaints of poor concentration, memory problems, irritability
- Morning headaches
- Short-tempered
- Decreased libido is also common
- Depression
- Systemic and pulmonary hypertension

CAUSES Upper airway narrowing may be due to obesity, enlarged tonsils or uvula, low soft palate, redundant tissue in soft palate or tonsillar pillars, large or posteriorly located tongue or craniofacial abnormalities. Anatomical narrowing superimposed upon a coexistent abnormality of neurological control of upper airway muscle tone or ventilatory control during sleep.

RISK FACTORS
- Obesity
- Nasal obstruction (due to polyps, rhinitis or deviated septum)
- Hypothyroidism
- Macroglossia
- Micrognathia (retrognathia)
- Acromegaly
- Persons with hypertension, cardiovascular or arteriovascular disease or alveolar hypoventilation have a much higher risk of obstructive sleep apnea (OSA)
- Alcohol intake before bedtime

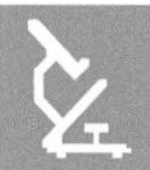

DIAGNOSIS

DIFFERENTIAL DIAGNOSIS
- Other causes of EDS such as narcolepsy, idiopathic daytime hypersomnolence, inadequate sleep time, depressive episodes with EDS, periodic limb movements of sleep
- Respiratory disorders with nocturnal awakenings such as asthma, COPD, CHF
- Central sleep apnea may mimic OSA
- Sudden nocturnal awakenings due to panic attacks
- Sleep-related choking or laryngospasm
- Gastroesophageal reflux may also present with similar symptoms
- Sleep associated seizures (temporal lobe epilepsy)

LABORATORY
- Polycythemia (occasional) reflects the degree of nocturnal hypoxemia due to OSA
- Thyroid function should be evaluated to rule out concomitant hypothyroidism
- Daytime hypercapnia occasionally seen

Drugs that may alter lab results: Benzodiazepines or other sedatives can accentuate the severity of apnea seen on sleep study

Disorders that may alter lab results: N/A

PATHOLOGICAL FINDINGS
- Anatomically small upper airway common
- CNS abnormalities rare

SPECIAL TESTS
- Echocardiography may demonstrate right and/or left ventricular enlargement or pulmonary hypertension
- Polysomnogram (nighttime sleep study) including O2 saturation, CO2
- Multiple sleep latency testing (MSLT) provides an objective measurement of daytime sleepiness

IMAGING
- Cephalometric measurements from lateral head and neck x-rays are occasionally useful if surgery is contemplated
- MRI, CT scans or fiberoptic evaluation of upper airway occasionally helpful

DIAGNOSTIC PROCEDURES
- Nighttime sleep study (polysomnogram)
  - ◊ Shows repetitive episodes of cessation or marked reduction in airflow despite continued respiratory efforts
  - ◊ These apneic episodes must last at least 10 seconds and occur 10-15 times per hour to be considered clinically significant
  - ◊ Polysomnogram demonstrates severity of hypoxemia, sleep disruption and cardiac arrhythmias associated with OSA and elevated end tidal CO2

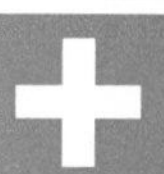

TREATMENT

APPROPRIATE HEALTH CARE Outpatient for treatment or sleep study; inpatient for surgery

GENERAL MEASURES
- For patients with significant EDS and 15-20 apneas per hour or more, CPAP is probably the best treatment
- If OSA present only when supine - keep patient off the back (e.g., tennis ball sewn on nightshirt or fanny-pack with tennis balls worn at back)
- Mild to moderate OSA - surgery (tonsillectomy or uvulopalatopharyngoplasty [UPPP]), dental appliances or nasal continuous positive airway pressure (CPAP)
- Moderate to severe OSA - CPAP or BiPAP (biphasic positive airway pressure) is the standard therapy
- Avoid driving if EDS significant
- No alcohol within 6 hours of bedtime
- Avoid sedatives and sleeping pills

SURGICAL MEASURES Severe OSA that is not controllable with nasal CPAP or UPPP - tracheostomy or craniofacial surgery (mandibular advancement)

ACTIVITY Significantly sleepy patients should not drive motor vehicle or operate equipment with risk for injury until treated

DIET Obese patients must lose weight. All patients must avoid weight gain and alcohol.

PATIENT EDUCATION
- Stress the fact that obesity can be the cause of OSA and weight loss may "cure" the condition
- Necessity to avoid alcohol and sedatives
- Stress the dangers of driving while suffering EDS

MEDICATIONS

DRUG(S) OF CHOICE Medications are generally not effective in treating OSA. However, protriptyline 10-30 mg/d or fluoxetine 20-60 mg can occasionally be useful adjunct in the management of OSA (especially OSA in REM sleep) and to improve EDS.
Contraindications: None
Precautions: May cause or exacerbate narrow angle glaucoma or urinary retention. Use with caution in patients with supraventricular tachycardia.
Significant possible interactions: See manufacturer's profile of each drug

ALTERNATIVE DRUGS Medroxyprogesterone is helpful in Pickwickian patients with both daytime alveolar hypoventilation and OSA

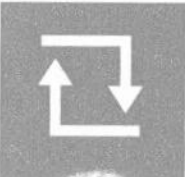

FOLLOWUP

PATIENT MONITORING Physician followup improves compliance with CPAP therapy. Observe for return of snoring, EDS, or sleep disruption which may indicate inadequate control of apneas.

PREVENTION/AVOIDANCE See Patient Education

POSSIBLE COMPLICATIONS
- Untreated OSA can be associated with development of pulmonary hypertension, ventricular arrhythmias, cor pulmonale, CHF
- Significant morbidity and mortality due to accidents caused by EDS and inattentiveness
- Acute blood pressure elevations

EXPECTED COURSE/PROGNOSIS
- With appropriate control of apneas, EDS dramatically improves quickly
- All therapeutic measures other than surgery and aggressive weight loss in obese patients are methods of apnea control, rather than cure. Lifelong compliance with weight loss or nasal CPAP are necessary for therapy of OSA.
- Untreated, OSA appears to progress in severity
- Death due to OSA usually secondary to arrhythmias, cardiac ischemia or hypertensive complications, or motor vehicle accidents

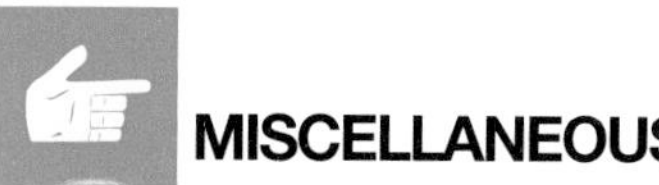

MISCELLANEOUS

ASSOCIATED CONDITIONS
- Hypertension
- Arteriosclerotic vascular disease
- Coronary arterial disease
- Diabetes
- Obesity
- Nasal obstructive problems
- Acromegaly
- Hypothyroidism

AGE-RELATED FACTORS
Pediatric:
- OSA not as common in pediatric age group. If present, often due to tonsillar enlargement, craniofacial abnormalities. Response to tonsillectomy often good. Abnormal apnea/hypopnea index is different in children; >1-2 per hour is abnormal. Children may have obstructive hypoventilation with elevated pCO2 so that EtCO2 should be monitored during study.
- Pediatric OSAS: sweating, FTT, hyperactivity, poor school performance in early/later school years neuro and cranio-facial=high risk. Adenotonsillectomy relieves S&S in ≈70% of children. Whereas ≈10% of children snore regularly, only 1-2% are estimated to have OSAS.
- Seen commonly in children with neuromuscular diseases, such as cerebral palsy, spinal muscular atrophy

Geriatric: OSA appears to increase in frequency after middle age and after the menopause in women. Often coexists with other health problems in the elderly.
Others: N/A

PREGNANCY Rare

SYNONYMS
- Pickwickian syndrome
- Sleep apnea syndrome
- Nocturnal upper airway occlusion

ICD-9-CM
780.57 Other and unspecified sleep apnea

SEE ALSO

OTHER NOTES OSA rare in premenopausal women unless there is coexistent morbid obesity or neurologic/craniofacial abnormalities

ABBREVIATIONS
- CPAP = continuous positive airway pressure
- BiPAP = bilevel positive airway pressure
- UPPP = uvulopalatopharyngoplasty
- EDS = excessive daytime sleepiness
- OSA = obstructive sleep apnea

REFERENCES

- Kryger MH. Principles and Practice of Sleep Medicine. 3rd ed. Philadelphia: WB Saunders Co; 2000
- Thorpy MJ. Handbook of Sleep Disorders. New York: Marcel Dekker Inc; 1990

Web references: 0 available at www.5mcc.com
Illustrations N/A

Author(s):
Mary E. Klink, MD

BASICS

DESCRIPTION The senses of smell and taste allow full appreciation of the flavor and palatability of foods and also serve as an early warning system against toxins, polluted air, smoke and spoiled food products. Physiologically, the chemical senses aid in normal digestion by triggering gastrointestinal secretions. Smell or taste dysfunction can have a significant impact on quality of life. Loss of smell occurs more frequently than loss of taste, and patients frequently confuse the concepts of "flavor loss" (as a result of smell impairment) with "taste loss" (impaired ability to sense *sweet*, *sour*, *salty* or *bitter*).
- Smell - depends on the functioning of cranial nerve I (olfactory nerve) and cranial nerve V (trigeminal nerve).
- Taste - depends on the functioning of cranial nerves 7, 9, 10. Because of these multiple pathways, total loss of taste (ageusia) is rare.

System(s) affected: Nervous
Genetics: Smell and taste disturbances may be related to genetically-associated underlying diseases (eg, Kallmann's syndrome, Alzheimer disease, migraine, and rheumatologic and endocrine disorders)
Incidence/Prevalence in USA: Estimated > 2 million; 200,000 visit a physician each year
Predominant age:
- Chemosensory loss is age-dependent
  - ◊ Age > 80 - 80% have major olfactory impairment; nearly 50% are anosmic
  - ◊ Ages 65-80 - 60% have major olfactory impairment; nearly 25% are anosmic
  - ◊ Age < 65 - 1-2% have smell impairment

Predominant sex: Male > Female (men also begin to lose ability to smell earlier in life than women)

SIGNS & SYMPTOMS
- Problems with smell and taste
- Weight loss
- Malnutrition
- Impaired immunity
- Worsening of medical illness
- Increased use of sugar and salt to compensate for diminished senses of smell and taste

CAUSES
- Smell and/or taste disturbances
  - ◊ Nutritional factors (malnutrition, vitamin deficiencies, liver disease, anemia)
  - ◊ Endocrine disorders (thyroid disease, diabetes mellitus, renal disease)
  - ◊ Head trauma
  - ◊ Migraine headache (gustatory aura, olfactory aura)
  - ◊ Sjögren syndrome
  - ◊ Toxic chemical exposure
  - ◊ Industrial agent exposure
  - ◊ Aging
  - ◊ Medications (see below)
  - ◊ Neurodegenerative diseases (multiple sclerosis, Alzheimer disease, cerebrovascular accident, Parkinson disease)
  - ◊ Infections (upper respiratory infection, oral and perioral infections, candidiasis, *Coxsackievirus*, acquired immunodeficiency syndrome, viral hepatitis, herpes simplex virus)
- Possible causes of smell disturbance:
  - ◊ Nasal and sinus disease (allergies, rhinitis, rhinorrhea)
  - ◊ Cigarette smoking
  - ◊ Cocaine abuse (intranasal)
  - ◊ Radiation treatment of head and neck
  - ◊ Congenital conditions
  - ◊ Neoplasm (brain tumor, nasal polyps, intranasal tumor)
  - ◊ Systemic lupus erythematosus
  - ◊ Bell palsy
  - ◊ Oral or perioral skin lesion
  - ◊ Damage to cranial nerves 1 or 5
- Possible causes of taste loss:
  - ◊ Oral appliances
  - ◊ Dental procedures
  - ◊ Intraoral abscess
  - ◊ Gingivitis
  - ◊ Damage to cranial nerves 7, 9 or 10
- Selected medications that reportedly alter smell and taste:
  - ◊ Antibiotics: ampicillin, azithromycin (Zithromax), ciprofloxacin (Cipro), clarithromycin (Biaxin), griseofulvin (Grisactin), metronidazole (Flagyl), ofloxacin (Floxin), tetracycline, terbinafine (Lamisil)
  - ◊ Anticonvulsants: carbamazepine (Tegretol), phenytoin (Dilantin)
  - ◊ Antidepressants: amitriptyline (Elavil), clomipramine (Anafranil), desipramine (Norpramin), doxepin (Sinequan), imipramine (Tofranil), nortriptyline (Pamelor)
  - ◊ Antihistamines and decongestants: chlorpheniramine, loratadine (Claritin), pseudoephedrine
  - ◊ Antihypertensives and cardiac medications: acetazolamide (Diamox), amiloride (Midamor), betaxolol (Betoptic), captopril (Capoten), diltiazem (Cardizem), enalapril (Vasotec), hydrochlorothiazide (Esidrix) and combinations, nifedipine (Procardia), nitroglycerin, propranolol (Inderal,) spironolactone (Aldactone)
  - ◊ Anti-inflammatory agents: auranofin (Ridaura), colchicine, dexamethasone (Decadron), gold (Myochrysine), hydrocortisone, penicillamine (Cuprimine)
  - ◊ Antimanic drug: lithium
  - ◊ Antineoplastics: cisplatin (Platinol), doxorubicin (Adriamycin), methotrexate (Rheumatrex), vincristine (Oncovin)
  - ◊ Antiparkinsonian agents: levodopa (Larodopa; with carbidopa: Sinemet)
  - ◊ Antipsychotics: clozapine (Clozaril), trifluoperazine (Stelazine)
  - ◊ Antithyroid agents: methimazole (Tapazole), propylthiouracil
  - ◊ Lipid-lowering agents: fluvastatin (Lescol), lovastatin (Mevacor), pravastatin (Pravachol)
  - ◊ Muscle relaxants: baclofen (Lioresal), dantrolene (Dantrium)

RISK FACTORS N/A

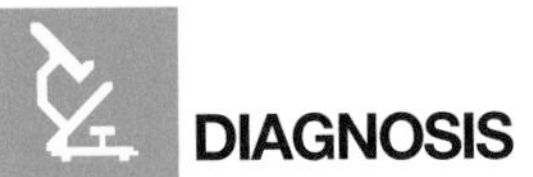

DIAGNOSIS

DIFFERENTIAL DIAGNOSIS
- Epilepsy (gustatory aura)
- Epilepsy (olfactory aura)
- Memory impairment
- Psychiatric conditions

LABORATORY
- Hematocrit
- Hemoglobin
- White blood cell count
- Blood urea nitrogen
- Blood glucose
- Creatinine
- Blood glucose
- Bilirubin
- Alkaline phosphatase
- Prothrombin time
- Erythrocyte sedimentation rate
- Altered thyroid function tests
- Eosinophil count
- Immunoglobulin E

Drugs that may alter lab results: N/A

Disorders that may alter lab results: N/A

PATHOLOGICAL FINDINGS N/A

SPECIAL TESTS
- Olfactory tests:
  - ◊ Smell identification test - evaluates the ability to identify 40 microencapsulated "scratch and sniff" odorants
  - ◊ Three-item forced-choice microencapsulated Pocket Smell Test
  - ◊ Brief smell identification test
  - ◊ Squeeze-bottle odor threshold test kit
- Taste tests (more difficult because no convenient standardized tests are presently available).
  - ◊ Solutions containing sucrose (sweet), sodium chloride (salty), quinine (bitter) and citric acid (sour) are helpful.
  - ◊ Electrogustometry. A portable, battery-powered device delivers small currents to different parts of the tongue to obtain threshold and suprathreshold measures.

IMAGING
- Plain radiographs have substantial limitations; rarely useful
- CT scanning is the most useful and cost-effective technique for assessing sinonasal disorders and is superior to MRI in evaluation of bony structures. Coronal CT scans are particularly valuable in assessing paranasal anatomy.
- MRI is useful in defining soft tissue disease; therefore, it is technique of choice to image the olfactory bulbs, tracts, and cortical parenchyma

DIAGNOSTIC PROCEDURES
- Medical history
- Physical examination

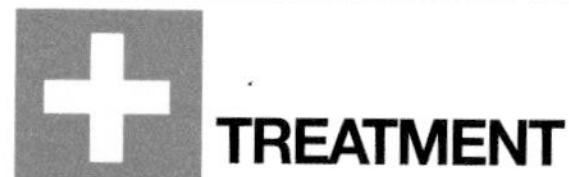

TREATMENT

APPROPRIATE HEALTH CARE Outpatient usually

GENERAL MEASURES
- Appropriate treatment for underlying cause
- Quit smoking
- Some drug-related dysgeusias can be reversed with cessation of the offending agent
- Eliminate exposures (eg, volatile gases, toxins, repeated use of oxygen-liberating mouthwashes)
- Stop repeated oral trauma (eg, appliances, tongue biting behaviors)
- Proper nutritional and dietary assessment
- Formal dental evaluation

SURGICAL MEASURES If needed for treatment of underlying cause

ACTIVITY N/A

DIET
- Patients should be cautioned not to overindulge as compensation for the bland taste of food. For example, patients with diabetes may need help in avoiding excessive sugar intake as an inappropriate way of improving food taste.
- Patients with chemosensory impairment should use measuring devices when cooking, not "cook by taste"
- Optimizing food texture, aroma, temperature and color may improve the overall food experience when taste is limited

PATIENT EDUCATION
- Patients with permanent smell dysfunction need to develop adaptive strategies for dealing with hygiene, appetite, safety and health
  - ◊ Check smoke detectors frequently
  - ◊ Use electric instead of gas appliances (if anosmic)
  - ◊ Check food expiration dates frequently; discard old food

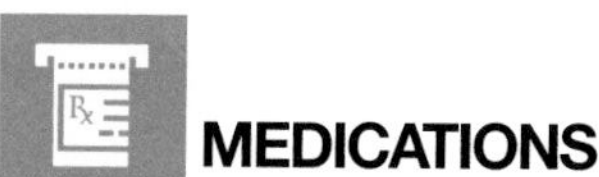

MEDICATIONS

DRUG(S) OF CHOICE
- Corticosteroids topically (e.g., aqueous nasal spray) or systemically (eg, oral prednisone) may be helpful. Prednisone - 60 mg per day for four days, with the dosage tapered by 10 mg each day thereafter.
- Artificial saliva (eg, Xero-Lube) may be helpful in patients with xerostomia
- Pilocarpine (Salagen) 5-10 mg po tid may help with dry mouth/xerostomia. Response may take 6-12 weeks.
- Chlorhexidine (Peridex) 0.12% oral rinse may help with gingivitis or dysgeusias
- Zinc and vitamin (A, B-complex) when deficiency suspected

Contraindications: N/A
Precautions: N/A
Significant possible interactions: N/A

ALTERNATIVE DRUGS N/A

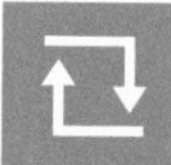

FOLLOWUP

PATIENT MONITORING Patients with persistent smell and taste complaints may need to be referred to an otolaryngologist, a neurologist or a subspecialist at a smell and taste center

PREVENTION/AVOIDANCE
- Avoid exposures to chemicals, smoke, and radiation
- Maintain good oral and nasal health with routine visits to the dentist
- Eat a well-balanced diet for optimal nutrition

POSSIBLE COMPLICATIONS Permanent loss of ability to smell or taste

EXPECTED COURSE/PROGNOSIS
- In general, the olfactory system regenerates poorly after a head injury. Most patients who recover smell function subsequent to head trauma do so within 12 weeks of injury.
- Patients who quit smoking typically have improved olfactory function and flavor sensation over time
- Many taste disorders (dysgeusias) resolve spontaneously within a few years of onset
- Conditions such as radiation-induced xerostomia and Bell palsy generally improve over time

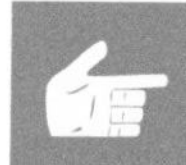

MISCELLANEOUS

ASSOCIATED CONDITIONS Smell and taste disturbances are primarily symptoms; it is essential to look for possible underlying cause

AGE-RELATED FACTORS
Pediatric: Delayed puberty in association with anosmia (with or without midline craniofacial abnormalities, deafness, and renal abnormalities) suggests the possibility of Kallmann's syndrome
Geriatric: Aging is a cause of smell/ taste deficits, should consider as diagnosis of exclusion
Others: N/A

PREGNANCY Uncommon cause for smell and taste disturbances. Many women report increased sensitivity to odors during pregnancy, as well as an increased dislike for bitter and a preference for salt substances.

SYNONYMS
- Burning mouth syndrome

ICD-9-CM

SEE ALSO

OTHER NOTES N/A

ABBREVIATIONS
fMRI = functional MRI
SPECT = single photon emission computed tomography

REFERENCES

- Bromley SM. Smell and taste disorders: a primary care approach. Amer Fam Phys 2000;61(2):427-36
- Deems DA, Doty RL, Settle RG, Moore-Gillon V, Shaman P, Mester AF, et al. Smell and taste disorders, a study of 750 patients from the University of Pennsylvania Smell and Taste Center. Arch Otolaryngol Head Neck Surg 1991;117:519-28

Web references: 0 available at www.5mcc.com
Illustrations N/A

Author(s):
Steven M. Bromley, MD

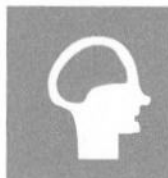

BASICS

DESCRIPTION Symptom complex occurring following human envenomation by a snake of the family Crotalidae (pit vipers)
- These include those of the genus Crotalus (rattlesnakes), Agkistrodon (moccasins) and Sistrurus (pygmy rattlesnakes). Occurs most commonly in southeastern and southwestern US.
- These snakes characteristically have triangular-shaped heads, eyes with elliptical pupils, and small heat-sensing facial pits located between the nostril and the eye

System(s) affected: Cardiovascular, Hemic/Lymphatic/Immunologic, Nervous, Skin/Exocrine
Genetics: N/A
Incidence/Prevalence in USA: 3.2/100,000. 8,000 bites/year (20-25% of bites do not result in envenomation)
Predominant age: 19-30 years
Predominant sex: Male > Female

SIGNS & SYMPTOMS
- These vary by species; prevalence as stated refers to family as whole
- Fang marks (may be two or only one) (>90%)
- Pain out of proportion to puncture wound (>50%)
- Edema of site, progressing proximally up extremity (>50%)
- Weakness, dizziness (>50%)
- Numbness/tingling in extremity, in mouth, tongue (>50%)
- Ecchymosis of skin, vesiculations around bite (>50%)
- Tachycardia (>50%)
- Nausea/vomiting (<50%)
- Hypo/Hypertension (<50%)
- Muscle fasciculations (<50%)
- Mental status changes including coma (<25%)
- Elevated creatine kinase (CK)

CAUSES Pit viper venom is a complex mixture which contains cytotoxins, hemotoxins, neurotoxins, and cardiotoxins

RISK FACTORS
- Risk taking behaviors
- Acute ethanol intoxication or intoxication with other drugs which impair judgment

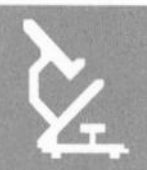

DIAGNOSIS

DIFFERENTIAL DIAGNOSIS Bite of non-venomous snake, bite of venomous species other than from Crotalidae family

LABORATORY
- CBC (Hgb/Hct decreased in < 50%)
- PT/INR (prolonged in > 50%)
- Fibrinogen (decreased in < 50%), fibrin degradation products (increased in < 50%)
- Urinalysis - glycosuria (< 50%), proteinuria (< 25%), hematuria (< 25%)
- Decrease in blood platelets (< 50%)
- Type and crossmatch "to hold" in severe envenomations
- Electrolytes, blood urea nitrogen, creatinine
- Creatine kinase in severe envenomations
- Serum ethanol level if suspicious

Drugs that may alter lab results: Anticoagulants

Disorders that may alter lab results: N/A

PATHOLOGICAL FINDINGS N/A

SPECIAL TESTS N/A

IMAGING N/A

DIAGNOSTIC PROCEDURES If suspicious of developing compartment syndrome, measure compartment pressures (rarely needed)

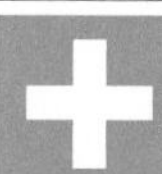

TREATMENT

APPROPRIATE HEALTH CARE Patients with true envenomations and resulting signs/symptoms need emergency department evaluation with admission if necessary

GENERAL MEASURES
- Support vital signs
- Reassurance
- Remove rings and constrictive items proximal to site of envenomation
- Place affected injured part at level of heart
- Evaluate all pre-hospital care. If tourniquet has been placed in pre-hospital setting, sudden removal could "bolus" patient with venom.
- Obtain toxicology consultation by contacting American Association of Poison Centers (AAPCC) Regional Poison Information Center for your area
- Level 1:
  - ◊ If local signs of edema are confined to area of bite without any other symptom of envenomation, place intravenous line of crystalloid at maintenance rates (if no history of renal or heart disease requiring fluid restriction) and draw laboratory studies
  - ◊ Place reference marks for measuring circumference of extremity at 10 cm and 20 cm proximal to site of envenomation
  - ◊ Measure every 15 minutes and trace leading edge of swelling
  - ◊ Give tetanus toxoid, if needed
  - ◊ Pain relief
  - ◊ Repeat laboratory studies in six hours. If all remain normal and swelling does not progress, observe 8-12 hours then follow as outpatient.
  - ◊ If swelling progresses or systemic signs and symptoms appear will need admission and further therapy (progresses to Level 2)
- Level 2:
  - ◊ If edema, vesiculations, erythema progress beyond the immediate bite area or there are associated systemic signs/symptoms or laboratory abnormalities (as above), all therapy as in Level 1 above plus intravenous antivenin
  - ◊ Intensive care monitoring may be necessary in most institutions
  - ◊ Repeat laboratory evaluations every 6 hours initially until stable, then less frequently
  - ◊ Continue to monitor vital signs and circumference of affected part

SURGICAL MEASURES N/A

ACTIVITY Bedrest with extremity elevated

DIET Nothing by mouth initially

PATIENT EDUCATION
- Snake bite prevention and first aid
- Avoid elective surgery, dental work, contact sports or anticoagulant medications (including aspirin) after discharge

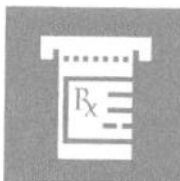

MEDICATIONS

DRUG(S) OF CHOICE
- Crotalidae polyvalent immune Fab (Ovine)
  - ◊ No skin test necessary
  - ◊ 10 mL sterile water added to each vial. Swirl only (do not shake) so as to not denature proteins.
  - ◊ Add 4 to 6 reconstituted vials to normal saline to make total volume of 250 mL
  - ◊ Infuse intravenously slowly for the first 10 minutes then increase rate to 250 mL/hr to run remainder over 60 minutes
  - ◊ After first infusion complete, if all signs / symptoms of envenomation have not ceased, then up to two more doses of 4 to 6 vials should be given until initial control is achieved
  - ◊ After initial control of symptoms, three maintenance doses of 2 vials should be administered at 6, 12, and 18 hours following time of initial control
- Pain relief with opiate (e.g., morphine sulfate .1 - .2 mg/kg/dose q 2 - 6 hrs prn pain) or acetaminophen (10 - 15 mg/kg/dose q 4 - 6 hrs prn pain; max 4 g/day in adults). Avoid aspirin.
- Appropriate tetanus toxoid
- Intravenous fluids and standard therapies for the treatment of hypotension

Contraindications: N/A

Precautions:
- Papain is used in the manufacturing process, patients with papaya allergies may be at risk for allergic reaction
- Have equipment and medications readily at hand to treat anaphylaxis. Although 15 - 20 % of patients have had reactions during infusion no anaphylaxis has been noted.
- Avoid aspirin or other anticoagulants

Significant possible interactions: N/A

ALTERNATIVE DRUGS Blood products only necessary for coagulopathies with clinical bleeding, not for treatment of laboratory abnormalities

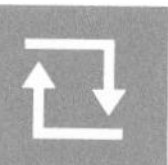

FOLLOWUP

PATIENT MONITORING
- First return visit within 48 hours, then as clinically indicated
- Physical therapy referral should be made early for optimal outpatient intervention

PREVENTION/AVOIDANCE
- Use of preventive measures if handling snakes
- In snake-infested areas
  - ◊ Wear protective shoes and clothing when walking
  - ◊ Do not insert hands or feet into cracks or crevices or hollow logs
  - ◊ Carry a flashlight if walking at night

POSSIBLE COMPLICATIONS
- Serum sickness from antivenin therapy
- Local wound infection
- Bleeding after discharge from hospital. Patients should be told to report nosebleeds, excessive bleeding after brushing teeth, blood in stools or vomitus, excessive menstrual bleeding.

EXPECTED COURSE/PROGNOSIS If properly treated, mortality is very rare. Morbidity rare.

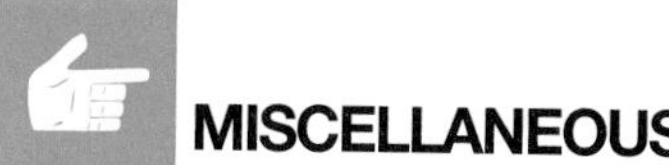

MISCELLANEOUS

ASSOCIATED CONDITIONS Underlying health of patient

AGE-RELATED FACTORS
Pediatric: Course may be more severe
Geriatric: Course may be more severe
Others: N/A

PREGNANCY N/A

SYNONYMS
- Snakebite
- Venomous snakebite
- Pit viper snake bite

ICD-9-CM
989.5 Toxic effect of venom

SEE ALSO
Snake envenomations: Elapidae

OTHER NOTES N/A

ABBREVIATIONS N/A

REFERENCES

- Ellenhorn MJ, Barceloux DG. Medical Toxicology: Diagnosis and Treatment of Human Poisoning. New York, Elsevier 1988;1113-1126
- Russell FE. Snake Venom Poisoning. Philadelphia, J.B. Lippincott, 1980
- Kurecki BA, Brownlee HJ. Venomous snakebites in the United States. J Fam Prac 1987;25(4):386-392

Web references: 0 available at www.5mcc.com
Illustrations N/A

Author(s):
Gregory G. Gaar, MD

BASICS

DESCRIPTION Symptom complex occurring following human envenomation by a snake of the family Elapidae

- In the US these include the genera Micrurus and Micruroides, commonly called "Coral Snakes." The Sonoran or Arizona coral snake is found mainly in Arizona (Micruroides euryxanthus), the Texas coral snake (Micrurus fulvius tenere) in Texas, Arkansas, and Louisiana, and the eastern coral snake (Micrurus fulvius fulvius) throughout the Southeastern US.
- The snakes have a characteristic rounded head with round pupils. Coloration is important in that in the U.S. broad rings of red and black are separated by narrow rings of yellow. ("Red on yellow, kill a fellow; red on black, venom lack.")
- Unlike Crotalidae envenomations, local signs and symptoms are mild in envenomation of Elapidae, even those which prove to be severe envenomations. Neurologic symptoms may be delayed; they have been reported to develop up to 12 or more hours after the envenomation.

System(s) affected: Nervous, Skin/Exocrine
Genetics: N/A
Incidence/Prevalence in USA: Unknown
Predominant age: 19-30 years
Predominant sex: Male > Female

SIGNS & SYMPTOMS

- Fang marks; may be shallow or appear as scratch (> 75%)
- Local swelling (<50%)
- Numbness/change in sensation (< 50%)
- Nausea/vomiting (< 50%)
- Weakness (< 25%)
- Dizziness (< 15%)
- Diplopia (< 15%)
- Muscle fasciculations (< 15%)

CAUSES Venom is primarily a neurotoxin. Little or no cytotoxin to cause local tissue reaction.

RISK FACTORS Coral snakes are nocturnal and timid. Therefore they rarely bite humans. They must be deliberately provoked to bite.

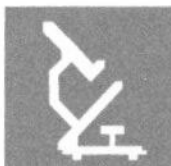

DIAGNOSIS

DIFFERENTIAL DIAGNOSIS

- Bite of other venomous snake (Crotalidae) without envenomation ("dry bite")
- Bite of a non-venomous snake

LABORATORY

- Creatine kinase (CPK) often elevated
- Blood ethanol level often elevated
- Laboratory not diagnostic

Drugs that may alter lab results: N/A

Disorders that may alter lab results: N/A

PATHOLOGICAL FINDINGS N/A

SPECIAL TESTS Measurement of tidal volume serially might help in early recognition of decreasing ventilatory function

IMAGING N/A

DIAGNOSTIC PROCEDURES N/A

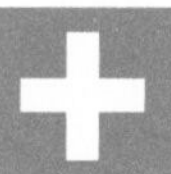

TREATMENT

APPROPRIATE HEALTH CARE All patients with suspected coral snake envenomation need Emergency Department evaluation

GENERAL MEASURES

- All patients who have (1) confirmed bite by a snake identified as a coral snake, (2) history of the snake's having chewed on the person, and, (3) visible fang marks which pierce the epidermis, should be admitted to hospital for intensive care monitoring
- In this group of patients, perform a skin test for horse serum sensitivity. If negative, antivenin to Micrurus fulvius fulvius should be given early, even if there are no neurologic signs or symptoms present.
- If skin test is positive, and neurological symptoms are rapidly progressing, admission to ICU is indicated
- Give tetanus toxoid, if needed
- Support vital signs, intubation may be necessary if respiratory compromise ensues
- Good supportive care with cardiac, respiratory, neurological monitoring
- Reassurance
- Immobilize extremity and keep at level of atria
- Contact AAPCC Regional Center for your area

SURGICAL MEASURES N/A

ACTIVITY Bedrest initially. May need physical therapy in severe cases of envenomation.

DIET Nothing by mouth initially

PATIENT EDUCATION N/A

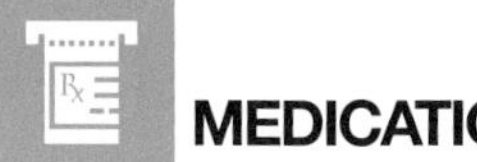

MEDICATIONS

DRUG(S) OF CHOICE
- No antivenin is available for Micruroides euryxanthus
- Antivenin to the North American coral snake (Micrurus fulvius fulvius antivenin)
  - ◊ Is available commercially. It is a horse serum product and is effective only for the envenomation of the Texas and eastern coral snakes (Micrurus fulvius tenere and Micrurus fulvius fulvius).
  - ◊ If patients meet the criteria above (see General Measures), skin test should be performed according to directions taken from package insert. If negative, 4-6 vials of the antivenin should be reconstituted and diluted into 250 mL of normal saline. Begin infusion at 3-5 mL/hr and, if no systemic reaction occurs, increase until a rate of 1 diluted vial is being given every thirty minutes.
  - ◊ If skin test is positive the literature is not clear about specific recommendations, however pretreatment with diphenhydramine (Benadryl) [1mg/kg/dose q6h IV; adults 25-50 mg IV], steroids [e.g., methylprednisolone (Solu-Medrol) 1-2 mg/kg/dose q8h IV], and other antihistamines (e.g., cimetidine 10 mg/kg/dose IV; adults 300 mg IV) may allow for infusion of antivenin. In this instance, obtain toxicology consultation from the American Association of Poison Control Centers (AAPCC) certified Poison Information Center for your area.
  - ◊ Envenomations with more severe sequelae or prolonged sequelae may require larger doses of antivenin. Unfortunately it is impossible to specify dosage more specifically.

Contraindications: History of allergy to horse serum
Precautions: Have equipment and medications readily at hand to treat anaphylaxis
Significant possible interactions: N/A

ALTERNATIVE DRUGS
- Steroid use is controversial. [If used, methylprednisolone (Solu-Medrol) 1-2 mg/kg/dose IV q8h]

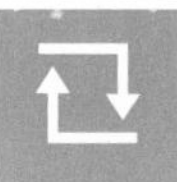

FOLLOWUP

PATIENT MONITORING First return visit within 48 hours, then as clinically indicated

PREVENTION/AVOIDANCE
- Use of preventive measures if handling snakes
- In snake-infested areas:
  - ◊ Wear protective shoes and clothing when walking
  - ◊ Do not insert hands or feet into cracks or crevices or hollow logs
  - ◊ Carry a flashlight if walking at night

POSSIBLE COMPLICATIONS
- Serum sickness from antivenin therapy (perhaps in 10% or more)
- Local wound infection
- Aspiration pneumonia

EXPECTED COURSE/PROGNOSIS
- Neurologic deterioration may progress despite antivenin administration. Complete paralysis can occur.
- Early, elective intubation during progression of paralysis may help to prevent aspiration pneumonia
- Discharge should not occur until the patient has made neurologic recovery to the point that there is no concern of respiratory failure
- Muscle strength may not return to normal for 4-6 weeks
- Long-term morbidity rare
- Mortality does occur even with antivenin therapy

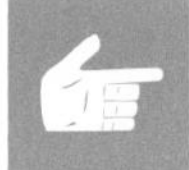

MISCELLANEOUS

ASSOCIATED CONDITIONS N/A

AGE-RELATED FACTORS
Pediatric: Not well described
Geriatric: Morbidity and danger of mortality is greater
Others: N/A

PREGNANCY N/A

SYNONYMS
- Neurotoxic snake bite
- Snakebite

ICD-9-CM
989.5 Toxic effect of venom

SEE ALSO
Snake envenomations: Crotalidae

OTHER NOTES N/A

ABBREVIATIONS N/A

REFERENCES

- Kitchens CS, Van Mierop LHS. Envenomation by the eastern coral snake (Micrurus fulvius fulvius). JAMA 1987;258(12):1615-1618
- Russell FE. Snake Venom Poisoning. Philadelphia, J.B. Lippincott, 1980
- Ellenhorn MJ, Barceloux DG. Medical Toxicology: Diagnosis and Treatment of Human Poisoning. New York, Elsevier, 1988:1127-1128

Web references: 0 available at www.5mcc.com
Illustrations N/A

Author(s):
Gregory G. Gaar, MD

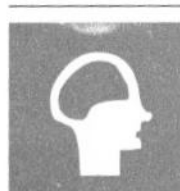

BASICS

DESCRIPTION Subacute or chronic fungal infection occurring in 4 forms: cutaneous or lymphocutaneous, pulmonary, osteo-articular, or disseminated; and rarely musculoskeletal (joint and tendon by puncture wounds). Most likely to occur in farmers, horticulturists, gardeners. Cutaneous lesions occur 20-90 days after cutaneous inoculation.
System(s) affected: Hemic/Lymphatic/Immunologic, Musculoskeletal, Skin/Exocrine
Genetics: No known genetic pattern
Incidence/Prevalence in USA: N/A
Predominant age: Adults
Predominant sex: Male > Female (mostly due to occupational exposure)

SIGNS & SYMPTOMS
- Cutaneous or lymphocutaneous:
  - ◊ Characteristic skin lesions, beginning as an inoculation chancre, or erythematous plaque with satellite, small papule, painless, movable, subcutaneous nodules in a linear distribution. Lesions progress to larger nodules which may ulcerate and drain. Affects primarily upper extremities.
  - ◊ Additional lesions spread proximally along lymphatics
- Pulmonary
  - ◊ Cough, occasionally productive
  - ◊ Cavitary lung disease
  - ◊ Hilar adenopathy
  - ◊ Signs and symptoms indistinguishable from other chronic pneumonias
- Osteo-articular
  - ◊ Subacute or chronic inflammatory arthritis, often monoarticular, may persist for many years
  - ◊ Signs and symptoms of osteomyelitis
  - ◊ Generally afebrile
- Disseminated
  - ◊ Multifocal skin lesions
  - ◊ Polyarticular arthritis
  - ◊ Weight loss
  - ◊ Chronic lymphocytic meningitis

CAUSES Infection with *Sporothrix schenckii*, a fungus found in soil, sphagnum peat moss, and decaying vegetation. Infection acquired by direct inoculation (usual) or inhalation (rare).

RISK FACTORS
- Gardening - contact with mulch, sphagnum moss, hay, timber, thorny bushes
- Occupations handling gardening materials, such as nursery workers, landscapers, florists, carpenters
- Animal handlers (transmission from animals, especially cats, to humans has been documented)
- Immunocompromised (drugs or HIV infection)
- Alcoholism (pulmonary and disseminated)
- HIV/AIDS patients are at increased risk for disseminated disease including the central nervous system

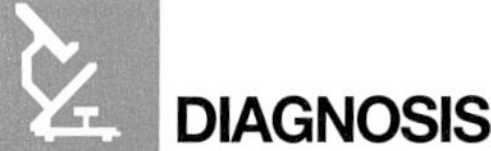

DIAGNOSIS

DIFFERENTIAL DIAGNOSIS
- Cutaneous or lymphocutaneous
  - ◊ Sporotrichoid nocardiosis
  - ◊ Leishmaniasis
  - ◊ Chromomycosis
  - ◊ Atypical mycobacterial infection (*M. marinum, M. chelonei, M. kansasii*)
  - ◊ Tularemia
  - ◊ Plague
- Pulmonary
  - ◊ Tuberculosis
  - ◊ Sarcoidosis
  - ◊ Chronic fungal pneumonia
  - ◊ Neoplasm
  - ◊ Atypical mycobacterial infection (*M. avium* complex, *M. kansasii*)
  - ◊ Rhodococcus equi
  - ◊ Nocardia spp
- Osteoarticular
  - ◊ Rheumatoid arthritis
  - ◊ Bacterial arthritis/osteomyelitis

LABORATORY
- Culture of *S. schenckii* in sputum, pus, synovial fluid or bone drainage
- Organism found with difficulty with PAS and Gomori stains of skin or other biopsied lesions
- Serum antibody tests may be useful for extracutaneous disease

Drugs that may alter lab results: Antifungal drugs

Disorders that may alter lab results: N/A

PATHOLOGICAL FINDINGS Granulomas with central necrosis

SPECIAL TESTS Immunohistochemical staining of biopsy specimens

IMAGING Chest and skeletal x-rays

DIAGNOSTIC PROCEDURES
- Careful history and physical
- Culture of draining lesions
- Culture of inflammatory joint effusions or sputum
- Biopsy if diagnosis not confirmed

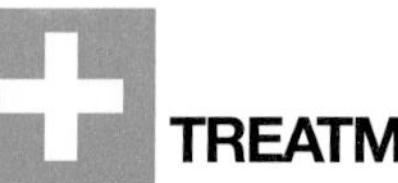

TREATMENT

APPROPRIATE HEALTH CARE
- Many patients can be managed on outpatient basis
- Hospitalization for adjunctive surgical procedures or initiation of amphotericin B therapy

GENERAL MEASURES
- Local heat application useful for cutaneous and lymphocutaneous disease
- Keep cutaneous lesions clean
- Repeated drainage of infected joints may be indicated

SURGICAL MEASURES
- Synovectomy of infected joints may be indicated
- Surgical débridement of osteomyelitis usually indicated

ACTIVITY No restrictions

DIET No special diet

PATIENT EDUCATION Patients should be advised of the nature of the infection, the toxicities associated with therapy, and the need for sustained therapy

MEDICATIONS

DRUG(S) OF CHOICE
- Cutaneous or lymphocutaneous disease:
  - ◊ Itraconazole 100-200 mg qd for 3-6 mo
  - ◊ Potassium iodide saturated solution (SSKI) is an alternative treatment. Initially 5 drops orally tid increased by 1 drop each dose to 40-50 drops tid as tolerated for 3-6 mos. Dilute in a beverage to disguise taste.
- Pulmonary:
  - ◊ Amphotericin B for extensive or life-threatening disease
  - ◊ Itraconazole 200 mg bid for non-life-threatening disease
  - ◊ Surgical resection combined with antifungals when feasible
- Osteoarticular:
  - ◊ Itraconazole 200 mg bid for 12 mo
- Meningeal and disseminated:
  - ◊ Amphotericin B
- AIDS
  - ◊ Amphotericin B until clinical improvement, then itraconazole 200 mg bid for life

Contraindications: SSKI contraindicated in tuberculosis

Precautions:
- Amphotericin B can cause fever, chills, nausea and vomiting. Refer to manufacturer's literature for precautions, adverse effects and interactions.
- SSKI requires extra care if patient also has tuberculosis, kidney disease, renal dysfunction or hyperthyroidism. Can cause folliculitis and tender, swollen salivary glands.
- Itraconazole capsule absorption may be decreased with concomitant administration of antacids or gastric acid secretion suppressors

Significant possible interactions:
- SSKI taken concurrently with amiloride, spironolactone or triamterene may result in hyperkalemia
- Itraconazole taken with terfenadine or astemizole may result in life-threatening cardiac dysrhythmias

ALTERNATIVE DRUGS
- Ketoconazole 400 mg orally daily may be effective alternative therapy in immunocompetent hosts
- Fluconazole 800 mg per day orally is an alternative therapy in patients unable to receive itraconazole therapy

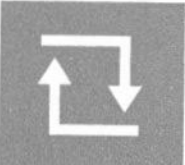

FOLLOWUP

PATIENT MONITORING
- Check for compliance with long-term drugs (SSKI should be continued for 1-2 months after lesions heal)
- Hepatic enzyme tests should be monitored periodically in patients receiving itraconazole treatment for > 1 month

PREVENTION/AVOIDANCE
- Avoid endemic areas
- Wear gloves when working in soil

POSSIBLE COMPLICATIONS
- Secondary bacterial infection
- Bone and joint deformities from osteoarticular disease

EXPECTED COURSE/PROGNOSIS
- Prognosis is excellent for complete recovery from cutaneous or lymphocutaneous infections
- Other disease forms demonstrate a chronic indolent course and are variably responsive to therapy
- AIDS patients often have a poor outcome

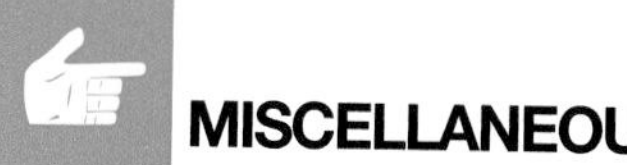

MISCELLANEOUS

ASSOCIATED CONDITIONS See Risk Factors

AGE-RELATED FACTORS
Pediatric: Rare
Geriatric: N/A
Others: N/A

PREGNANCY N/A

SYNONYMS
- Schenck's disease
- Rose gardener's disease

ICD-9-CM
117.1 Sporotrichosis

SEE ALSO

OTHER NOTES Rare ocular disease due to direct inoculation

ABBREVIATIONS N/A

REFERENCES

- Winn RE. Sporotrichosis. Infect Dis Clinic North Am 1988;2:899
- Mandell GL, ed. Principles and Practice of Infectious Diseases. 5th ed. New York: Churchill Livingstone; 2000
- Sharkey-Mathis PK, Kauffman CA, Graybill JR, Stevens DA, Hostetler JS, Cloud G, Dismukes WE & other members of the NIAID Mycoses Study Group. Treatment of sporotrichosis with itraconazole. Am J Med 1993;95:279
- Kauffman CA, Papps PG, McKinsey DS, Greenfield RA, Perfect JR, Cloud GA, et al. Treatment of Lymphocutaneous and Visceral Sporotrichosis with Fluconazole. Clin Infect Dis 1996;22:46
- Kauffman CA, Haijeh R. Chapman SW. For the Mycoses Study Group. Practice Guidelines for the Management of Patients with Sporotrichosis. Clin Infect Dis 2000;30:684-7

Web references: 3 available at www.5mcc.com
Illustrations N/A

Author(s):
Linda J. Machado, MD
Ronald A. Greenfield, MD

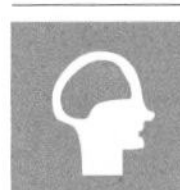

BASICS

DESCRIPTION
- Sprain: complete or partial ligamentous injury, either within the body of the ligament or at the site of attachment to bone. It may be classified as Grade I, II, or III. Grades I and II are incomplete tears and differ in severity; Grade III is complete dissolution of the ligamentous connection. Physical exam is key to the diagnosis. Usually secondary to trauma (falls, twisting injuries or motor vehicle accidents).
- Strain: partial or complete disruption of the muscle or tendon, usually associated with overuse injuries.

System(s) affected: Musculoskeletal
Genetics: N/A
Incidence/Prevalence in USA:
- Total incidence including spine, upper and lower extremities probably occurs in close to 80% of all athletes sometime in their career
- Prevalence - approximately 30,000

Predominant age:
- Sprains- any age where patient is physically active
- Strains - usually 15-40

Predominant sex: Male > Female

SIGNS & SYMPTOMS
- Swelling
- Pain
- Erythema and/or ecchymosis
- Tenderness
- Gait disturbances if severe
- Decreased range of motion of joint and joint instability

CAUSES
- Falls
- Motor vehicle accident
- Trauma
- Excessive exercise or inadequate warm-up and stretching prior to activity
- Poor conditioning

RISK FACTORS
- Change in or improper shoe gear, protective gear, or environment (e.g., surface)
- Inappropriate sudden increase in training schedule

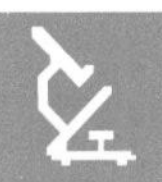

DIAGNOSIS

DIFFERENTIAL DIAGNOSIS
- Sprains (ligament tears) must be differentiated from strains (muscle-tendon unit tears), although this is difficult and often the diagnosis is strain/sprain
- Tendonitis
- Bursitis
- Bony injuries
- Rarely, muscle hematomas account for some of the signs and symptoms of strains

LABORATORY N/A

Drugs that may alter lab results: N/A

Disorders that may alter lab results: N/A

PATHOLOGICAL FINDINGS N/A

SPECIAL TESTS
- Exam under anesthesia
- Arthroscopy in some cases
- For ankle, anterior drawer test, which tests the integrity of the anterior talofibular ligament

IMAGING
- Ankle films - only required if there is pain in malleolar zone and

1. Bone tenderness posterior edge or tip of lateral malleolus

or

2. Bone tenderness posterior edge or tip of medial malleolus

or

3. Unable to bear weight, both immediately and in emergency department

- Foot films - only required if there is midfoot zone pain and

1. Bone tenderness at base of 5th metatarsal

or

2. Bone tenderness at navicular

or

3. unable to bear weight, both immediately and in emergency department

- X-rays to rule out bony injury. Stress views may be helpful.
- CT scan of the affected area
- MRI
- Exam under anesthesia in difficult cases

DIAGNOSTIC PROCEDURES
- Sprains/strains
  - ◊ Grade I - pain/tenderness without loss of motion
  - ◊ Grade II - pain/tenderness; ecchymosis with some loss of range of motion
  - ◊ Grade III - pain/tenderness; swelling and ecchymosis and complete loss of range of motion

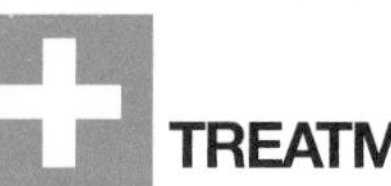

TREATMENT

APPROPRIATE HEALTH CARE Outpatient

GENERAL MEASURES
History and physical exam along with treatment of the worst possible suspected injury
- Acutely
  - ◊ RICE therapy - Rest, Ice, Compression, Elevation
    - Elastic bandage wrap (Ace) is comfortable
    - Jones dressing for more severe injuries
  - ◊ Orthosis (splint) for pain relief and stability; air cast type devices provide effective stability and pain relief
  - ◊ Crutches and crutch gait training

SURGICAL MEASURES
- Casting and surgery reserved for select Grade III injuries

ACTIVITY
- Bed rest for acute injuries
- Physical therapy for more severe injuries
- Elevate joint while sleeping

DIET Weight loss if obesity etiologic

PATIENT EDUCATION
- Instructions on how to wrap with elastic bandage
- Prevention of injury

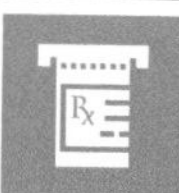

MEDICATIONS

DRUG(S) OF CHOICE
- NSAIDs: ibuprofen 200-800 mg TID, naproxen 375-500 mg BID, indomethacin 25-50 mg TID
- Narcotics for severe pain, e.g., acetaminophen-hydrocodone (Vicodin)

Contraindications: Refer to manufacturer's profile of each drug
Precautions: Refer to manufacturer's profile of each drug
Significant possible interactions: Refer to manufacturer's profile of each drug

ALTERNATIVE DRUGS
- Analgesic balms
- Capsaicin (Dolorac, Zostrix) cream 0.025% or capsaicin (Zostrix-HP) cream 0.075%: apply qid

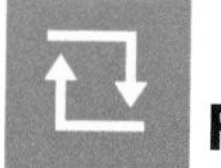

FOLLOWUP

PATIENT MONITORING After initial treatment, consider rehabilitation. Direct emphasis towards limiting swelling and providing a pain-free full range of motion.

PREVENTION/AVOIDANCE
- Maintaining a reasonable level of physical fitness
- Avoidance of excessive physical stresses and wearing of proper exercise gear (particularly shoes). Using proper equipment for the activity.
- Knowledge of the risks associated with the intended activity
- Appropriate conditioning, warm-up and cool-down exercises

POSSIBLE COMPLICATIONS
- Chronic joint instability
- Arthritis

EXPECTED COURSE/PROGNOSIS
With appropriate treatment and rest, 6-8 weeks or longer for recovery, depending on severity of injury

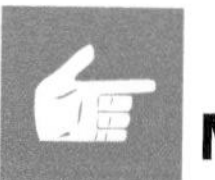

MISCELLANEOUS

ASSOCIATED CONDITIONS Hemarthrosis, stress, avulsion, or other fractures, syndesmotic injuries, contusions, wounds, dislocations

AGE-RELATED FACTORS
Pediatric: Sprains and strains accounted for 24% of injuries in an analysis of 1,124 sports injuries of children in a study done in West Germany, 1980-82
Geriatric: More likely to see associated bony injuries due to decreased joint flexibility and prevalence of osteoporosis and osteopenia
Others: N/A

PREGNANCY N/A

SYNONYMS N/A

ICD-9-CM
848.9 Sprain and strain, site unspecified

SEE ALSO
Tendinitis

OTHER NOTES N/A

ABBREVIATIONS
NSAID = non-steroidal anti-inflammatory drug

REFERENCES

- Kvist M, Kujala VM, Heinonen OJ, Vuori IV, Aho AJ, Pajulo O, Hintsa A, Parvinen T: Sports related injuries in children. IJSM 1989;10(2):81-86
- Strong WB, Stanitski EL, Smith RE, Wilmore JH: Diagnosis and treatment of ankle sprains. AJDC 1990;144:809-814
- Ruda S: Sports Nursing. In Nursing Clinics of North America. Philadelphia, W.B. Saunders Co., Mar, 1991
- Stiell I.G, McKnight D, Greenberg GH, et al: Implementation of the Ottawa ankle rules. JAMA 1994;271(11):827-832

Web references: 0 available at www.5mcc.com
Illustrations N/A

Author(s):
Timothy Robinson, DO
Brenda Oshea-Robinson, RPAC

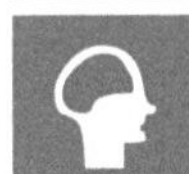

BASICS

DESCRIPTION Epileptic seizure longer than 30 minutes or absence of full recovery of consciousness between seizures. Tonic/clonic (grand mal or generalized convulsive) status epilepticus (SEp) is the most common and most serious form. SEp is a life-threatening emergency; begin treatment if seizure lasts >5-10 min. Rapid control of SEp is critical to success.
System(s) affected: Nervous
Genetics: Unknown
Incidence/Prevalence in USA: 18-50 cases per 100,000 per year; 1/3 as unprovoked first seizure, 1/6 in patients with known epilepsy, 1/2 secondary to acute CNS insult
Predominant age: > 50% of new cases of SEp occur in young children. Incidence is 2 times higher in elderly.
Predominant sex: Male = Female

SIGNS & SYMPTOMS
- Depend on the duration and type of seizure
- Recurrent generalized (tonic-clonic) convulsions: May be preceded by aura. Tonic phase (stiffening) for 30 to 45 seconds. Clonic phase (rhythmic jerking) for 2-5 minutes. No intervening consciousness before seizure recurs. See OTHER NOTES for additional types of SEp: focal, non-convulsive, and neonatal.
- Associated autonomic phenomena: Excess catecholamine secretion resulting in glandular hypersecretion, piloerection, hyperthermia, cyclic pupillary dilation, and prolonged apnea (may lead to cyanosis)
- Metabolic changes: Lactic acidosis, carbon dioxide narcosis, hyperkalemia, hyperglycemia - followed by hypoglycemia
- Cardiac changes: Hypertension (may be followed by hypotension), arrhythmias, high output failure
- Respiratory changes: Increased secretions, lax tongue, possible-airway obstruction, pulmonary edema, aspiration
- Renal complications: Acute tubular necrosis from myoglobinuria after rhabdomyolysis
- Cerebrovascular changes: Loss of autoregulation, focal ischemia, cerebral edema, Todd's paralysis may occur
- Postictal findings: Fever, tachycardia, mydriasis, conjugate deviation of eyes, decreased corneal reflex, positive Babinski's sign, fecal and urinary incontinence and tongue, cheek, or lip lacerations or injury

CAUSES
- Febrile convulsions (especially in children)
- Acute CNS injury - trauma, infection, mass/vascular lesion, metabolic disorder or anticonvulsant withdrawal/noncompliance
- Idiopathic
- Intoxication - cocaine, TCAs, isoniazid, chloroquine
- Chronic CNS injury - previous trauma, stroke, infection, encephalopathy (hypoxic or other chronic or degenerative type)

RISK FACTORS
- Known seizure disorder plus any precipitating insult. Prior history of SEp (recurrence rate is 17% in children; 50% in those with neurologic abnormality).
- Porphyria

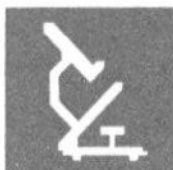

DIAGNOSIS

DIFFERENTIAL DIAGNOSIS
- Pseudostatus may occur with pseudoseizures; avoid dangerous therapy
- While tonic/clonic status is usually apparent, comatose or paralyzed patients and other forms of status require neurologic exam and EEG

LABORATORY Glucose, electrolytes, CBC, CPK, calcium, magnesium, phosphate, and osmolarity; ABGs; toxicology screen; carboxyhemoglobin; anticonvulsant levels; liver/renal function.

Drugs that may alter lab results: N/A

Disorders that may alter lab results: N/A

PATHOLOGICAL FINDINGS Variable

SPECIAL TESTS EEG will differentiate pseudoseizures, will reveal non-convulsive status, and will confirm successful treatment. Check EEG on any patient not awake 30 minutes after seizure.

IMAGING Non-contrast CT scan in new onset seizure, MRI if more detail needed

DIAGNOSTIC PROCEDURES Lumbar puncture (particularly if meningitis is suspected). CAUTION - intracranial pressure may be increased.

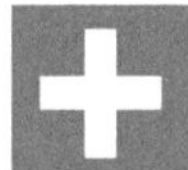

TREATMENT

APPROPRIATE HEALTH CARE Tonic/clonic SEp is an emergency; treat if seizure lasts >5-10 min. Simultaneous goals are: stop seizure, find etiology, and treat secondary complications.

GENERAL MEASURES
- Manage airway, breathing and circulation (ABCs). Monitor pulse oximetry, end-tidal CO2, blood pressure, ECG and temperature. Give oxygen. Intubate and hyperventilate if hypoventilation, hypoxia and/or hypercarbia occur or if aspiration is a concern.
- Observe and confirm the fit is SEp
- Pursue available drug history
- Establish IV (or intraosseous line for a child)
- Obtain initial lab studies
- Stop the seizure

SURGICAL MEASURES Experimental

ACTIVITY Protect the patient from injury. Place on side. Clear airway secretions. Prevent tongue laceration.

DIET NPO

PATIENT EDUCATION Epilepsy Foundation (800)EFA-1000; www.efa.org

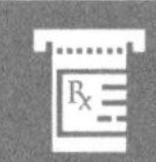

MEDICATIONS

DRUG(S) OF CHOICE Depend on the type of seizure. Approach tonic-clonic SEp as follows: (For other types, see Other Notes.)
Stabilization: Continue "ABC" assessment and monitoring. Intubate if needed. Prevent hypotension with vasopressors (e.g., dopamine). Treat fever.
- Thiamine: 100mg IV or IM (adults only)
- 50% dextrose - if blood sugar is low or cannot be measured; give 50mL IV (for child - use D25W; give 2 mL/kg slowly)
- Naloxone (Narcan): if pupils are myotic or drug overdose suspected; give 2mg IV (for child - 0.1 mg/kg IV, up to 2 mg slowly)
- Pyridoxine: If isoniazid poisoning is suspected
- Antibiotics: If meningitis is strongly suspected
- Intubation: if needed, use rocuronium bromide 0.6mg/kg (a short-acting non-depolarizer)

To stop seizures IV available:
- Start with:
  - ◊ Lorazepam (Ativan): 0.05-0.15 mg/kg IV at 1-2mg/min to maximum of 8mg (for child 0.05-0.1 mg/kg IV at <2mg/min to maximum of 4mg). May repeat q 10 min X 2.

(Some prefer diazepam [see Alternative Drugs below]).
- If SEp persists, after 5 minutes add:
  - ◊ Fosphenytoin (Cerebyx), prodrug of phenytoin: 15-20mg phenytoin equivalents (PE)/kg IV at < 150mgPE/min. May add 5-10 mgPE/kg IV. Maintenance 4-6mgPE/kg/day IV or IM (for child same as adult doses - see Precautions.)
- If these fail, add:
  - ◊ Phenobarbital (Luminal): 10-20 mg/kg IV (in saline) at 50-100mg/min (use lower rate for old age or cardiac history); may repeat dose of 4-6 mg/kg IV until no seizures or total dose of 1-2 grams. (For child - 20mg/kg IV at 1 mg/kg/min, maximum 30mg/kg.)

To stop seizures if IV not available:
- Intraosseous infusion in small children for benzodiazepines, fosphenytoin and phenobarbital - doses are the same as IV
- Rectal diazepam: 0.5-1.0mg/kg (child - 20 mg maximum) use the gel (Diastat) or IV solution (this benzodiazepine has less respiratory depression)
- Sublingual lorazepam: use IV dose
- IM fosphenytoin: dose same as IV (slow)
- Midazolam (Versed): 0.2mg/kg IM or 0.5mg/kg intranasal or buccal (onset 5-10 min, brief duration)

If seizures persist (refractory status):
- Admit to ICU and induce drug coma (anesthesia). Use infusion of short acting agent (benzodiazepine, propofol, or barbiturate) to obtain a burst suppression pattern EEG and stop seizures. Requires intubation, continuous respiratory support, cardiovascular and EEG monitoring, and (often) blood pressure support. Adjust to keep EEG at BSup. Maintain infusion for 12 to 24 h, then withdraw gradually.
- Use midazolam (Versed): 0.2-0.5mg/kg slow IV bolus injection, followed by 0.5-10mcg/kg/min IV drip titrated to BSup. Tachyphylaxis may develop.
- OR, propofol (Diprivan): 3-5mg/kg IV, followed by 1-15mg/kg/hr IV titrated to BSup (in elderly, reduce initial dose by half)
- OR, thiopental (Pentothal): Induction with 3-6mg/kg in divided doses, then add 50 mg IV q 2-5 min to produce BSup. Maintain with IV drip of 0.2% solution; start at 2-5mg/kg/hr and adjust based on EEG

Contraindications:
- Review current package inserts
- Benzodiazepines (diazepam, lorazepam, midazolam) - in acute narrow-angle glaucoma
- Barbiturates - in acute intermittent porphyria
- Propofol - in allergy to soybean oil, egg, lecithin, or glycerol.
- Valproic acid in hepatic disease and pregnancy

Precautions:
- Reduce dosage of depressants in patients with shock, coma or alcohol intoxication
- Most drugs listed may exacerbate porphyria; exceptions are lorazepam, midazolam and propofol
- Benzodiazepines - apnea may occur with rapid IV injection, especially with barbiturates. Reduce dose in the chronic pulmonary patient, renal failure, the elderly and hepatic insufficiency.
- Diazepam - venous thrombosis/phlebitis
- Phenobarbital - caution in pulmonary insufficiency, hepatic disease and pregnancy. Withdrawal seizures may occur following abrupt termination of high doses. Increase the dosing interval in renal failure. Reduce dose in severe liver disease.
- Propofol - strict aseptic technique required. May cause stinging discomfort on injection. Prolonged use in children may cause lactic acidosis and systemic collapse. Safety not established for child <3 y/o.
- Fosphenytoin (Cerebyx). Though recommended by authors, safety not established for children. Monitor ECG for arrhythmias, prolonged QT interval, and hypotension. If these occur, decrease rate of administration. Use with caution in pregnancy (increased risk of malformations and may lead to vitamin K deficiency bleeding problems in both mother and newborn), liver disease, hyperglycemia, and elderly patients. Abrupt withdrawal may precipitate status. Overdose may cause paradoxical inefficacy.
- Phenytoin - similar to fosphenytoin but greater toxicity and cardiovascular suppression
- Valproic acid - may affect platelet function and increase the effect of anti-platelet agents

Significant possible interactions:
- CNS depressants: depression enhanced
- Phenobarbital: reduced efficacy of quinidine and warfarin; induces metabolism of phenytoin
- Fosphenytoin/phenytoin: increased serum levels and toxicity of warfarin, disulfiram, phenylbutazone, and isoniazid. Decrease dose with renal insufficiency; monitor free levels if possible.
- Valproic acid - increased toxicity of phenytoin/fosphenytoin

ALTERNATIVE DRUGS
- Medium acting benzodiazepine - diazepam (Valium): 0.2-0.5mg/kg IV at 5mg/min up to a dose of 30mg (for child 0.3 mg/kg at <2mg/min IV or up to 10 mg). Repeat q 5 min X 3. May wear off quickly.
- Phenytoin: doses are same as fosphenytoin (mg for mgPE) but must be given more slowly (<1 mg/kg/min) to lessen toxicity and cardiovascular suppression
- Second line drugs:
  - ◊ Pentobarbital: 10-15mg/kg IV loading dose over 1 hr, followed by continuous infusion of 0.5-10mg/kg/hr; adjust based on EEG.
  - ◊ Lidocaine (Xylocaine): 1-3mg/kg IV bolus; if effective, drip 3-10mg/kg/hr IV
  - ◊ Valproic acid: clinical pilot studies have used 15-40mg/kg IV loading dose over 5-10 min, followed by 1-5mg/kg/hr
- Investigational drugs:

Isoflurane, desflurane by inhalation; etomidate by continuous IV infusion; chlormethiazole by IV infusion; nimodipine; ketamine, NMDA antagonist-IV as neuroprotectants; topiramate PO; levetiracetam; lamotrigine

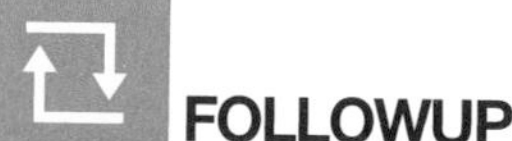

FOLLOWUP

PATIENT MONITORING Therapeutic blood levels of anticonvulsants

PREVENTION/AVOIDANCE
- Establish maintenance regimen of anticonvulsants
- Encourage compliance

POSSIBLE COMPLICATIONS
- Morbidity/mortality related to the acute CNS insult, stress, injury from repeated seizures
- Causes of death - cardiopulmonary arrest, renal failure, hyperthermia, aspiration pneumonia, the underlying pathology or the treatment instituted
- Anticonvulsants cause respiratory and cardiovascular depression

EXPECTED COURSE/PROGNOSIS
Mortality is 6-18% (3-6% in children; increases to 50% in those over 80 years) and is improving. Usually related to the underlying cause. Prolonged seizures (> 30 min) may cause neurologic injury or death. Seizure >4 hr, mortality = 50%; >12 hr = 80%.

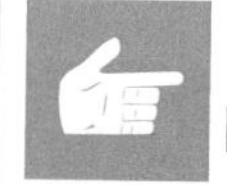

MISCELLANEOUS

ASSOCIATED CONDITIONS Etiology varies by age group. In adults, usually related to a known condition, e.g., established epilepsy, alcohol withdrawal or acquired CNS lesion (especially frontal).

AGE-RELATED FACTORS
Pediatric: Lower mortality rate. More likely present in SEp as their first seizure due to febrile seizure; new onset epilepsy (idiopathic); CNS infection; metabolic derangement.
Geriatric: More likely to have SEp secondary to a change in drug therapy (noncompliance, drug interaction or toxicity); tend to have localized (often frontal lobe) CNS lesions.
Others: Neonatal status is most often related to meningitis or metabolic disorders (deficiencies of calcium, magnesium, or pyridoxine); needs careful workup for cause

PREGNANCY
- Fosphenytoin/phenytoin - use with caution (increased risk of malformations in first trimester)
- Phenobarbital - use with caution
- Valproate - increased risk of neural tube defects

SYNONYMS Status convulsivus

ICD-9-CM
345.3 Epilepsy, grand mal status
345.71 Epilepsia partialis continua, with intractable epilepsy, so stated
345.2 Epilepsy, petit mal status

SEE ALSO
Seizure disorders
Seizures, febrile

OTHER NOTES
Additional categories of status:
- Focal convulsive status:
  - ◊ Focal motor status - starts distally with clonic jerking in ascending pattern; eyes and head deviate to side opposite the focus; may progress to generalized status; underlying CNS pathology is common. Treat like tonic-clonic SEp. May respond to carbamazepine.
  - ◊ Epilepsia partialis continua - rapid focal jerking; no loss of consciousness; worsened by voluntary movements; may persist for hours to days; poor response to therapy; often associated with underlying pathology. Pentobarbital and lorazepam recommended.
  - ◊ Myoclonic status - sudden spasmodic contraction of limbs; usually secondary to widespread neurologic or metabolic dysfunction; consciousness usually maintained. Treat with lorazepam.
- Non-convulsive status:
  - ◊ Complex partial status (psychomotor status) short seizures with automatisms (eg, lip smacking, random eye movements, chewing, staring); followed by post-ictal confusion. May respond to carbamazepine. With status, treat like tonic-clonic SEp.
  - ◊ Absence status - varies from mild lethargy to severe confusion, 10 second duration, no aura, eyes flutter and turn upward, with irregular myoclonic jerks, automatisms, no post-ictal confusion; may progress to generalized status. If so, treat as tonic-clonic status.
  - ◊ In coma - may occur as late stage of a prolonged seizure or in ICU patient with altered consciousness. Use EEG for diagnosis. Consider treating as tonic/clonic SEp.
- Neonatal status epilepticus - subtle multifocal, clonic, tonic, and myoclonic features; risk of intracerebral hemorrhage; common causes meningitis, CNS injury, malformation, and metabolic disorders (deficiencies of calcium, magnesium, pyridoxine).

ABBREVIATIONS
SEp = status epilepticus
BSup = burst suppression
PE = phenytoin equivalents
TCA = tricyclic antidepressant

REFERENCES

- ACEP Clinical Policies Committee; Clinical Policies Subcommittee on Seizures. Clinical Policy: Critical Issues in the Evaluation and Management of Adult Patients Presenting to the Emergency Department With Seizures. Annals of Emergency Medicine 2004; 43(5):605-625
- Manno EM. New management strategies in the treatment of status epilepticus. Mayo Clin Proc 2003;78(4):508-18
- Rosenow F, Arzimanoglou A, Baulac M. Recent developments in treatment of status epilepticus: a review. Epileptic Disord 2002;4 Suppl 2:S41-51
- Chapman MG, Smith M, Hirsch NP. Status epilepticus. Anaesthesia 2001;56(7):648-59
- Bleck TP. Refractory status epilepticus in 2001. Arch Neurol 2002;59(2):188-9
- Shepherd SM. Management of status epilepticus. Emerg Med Clin North Am 1994;12(4):941-61
- Canadian Pediatric Society Statement: Management of the pediatric patient with generalized convulsive status epilepticus in the emergency department. Paediatrics & Child Health 1996;1(2):151-155

Web references: 5 available at www.5mcc.com
Illustrations N/A

Author(s):
Jeff Ray Gibson, Jr., MD

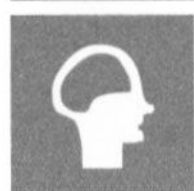

BASICS

DESCRIPTION Until recently Stevens-Johnson syndrome (SJS) was considered to be the same as erythema multiforme major, a severe form of erythema multiforme in which more than one mucosal surface was involved. Now it is thought that erythema multiforme spectrum is a single entity. The milder form, also known as erythema multiforme-Hebra, either has no mucous membrane involvement, or may involve one mucous membrane. The more severe form is erythema multiforme major, involving more than one mucus membrane. In both these variants, it is a self limited hypersensitivity reaction, usually to a preceding viral infection, and has an excellent prognosis. SJS is a generalized hypersensitivity reaction, usually to a drug, in which the skin and mucus membrane lesions are early manifestation. It may progress to its more severe form, toxic epidermal necrolysis which has a high morbidity and up to 40% mortality.
System(s) affected: Cardiovascular, Hemic/Lymphatic/Immunologic, Nervous, Renal/Urologic, Skin/exocrine
Genetics: Possibly associated with HLA-B15
Incidence/Prevalence in USA: Difficult to estimate because of confusion with erythema multiforme major, perhaps 0.1/100,000, or less
Predominant age: More common in children and young adults
Predominant sex: Males > Females (2:1)

SIGNS & SYMPTOMS
- There is usually a preceding illness for which medication was given
- Sudden onset with rapid progressive pleomorphic rash which includes petechiae, vesicles, bullae
- The condition is classified as SJS if epidermal detachment affects less than 10% of the skin, as toxic epidermal necrolysis (TEN) if epidermal detachment exceeds 30%, or if it exceeds 10% in the absence of discrete skin lesions. Cases with discrete skin lesions and between 10% and 30% epidermal detachment are in the overlap between SJS and TEN.
- Vesicles and ulcers on the mucous membranes, especially of the mouth and throat

Burning sensation of the skin and sometimes of the mucous membranes
- Usually no pruritus
- Fever 39-40°C (102-104°F)
- Headache
- Malaise
- Arthralgias
- Epistaxis
- Crusted nares
- Conjunctivitis
- Corneal ulcerations
- Erosive vulvovaginitis or balanitis
- Cough productive of thick purulent sputum
- Tachypnea/respiratory distress
- Albuminuria/hematuria
- Arrhythmias
- Pericarditis
- Congestive heart failure
- Mental status changes
- Electrolyte disturbance
- Seizures
- Coma
- Sepsis

CAUSES
- Often unknown
- Medications - especially sulfonamides, penicillins, anticonvulsants, salicylates, non-steroidal anti-inflammatory drugs (especially the "oxicams", e.g., piroxicam, tenoxicam, meloxicam, isoxicam), methazolamide, carvedilol and anti-neoplastic chemotherapy
- Vaccines - diphtheria/typhoid, bacillus Calmette Guerin (BCG), oral polio vaccine (OPV)
- Mycoplasma pneumonia infection

RISK FACTORS
- Patients with HIV infection appear to be predisposed to developing SJS in response to their medications
- Craniotomy or cranial radiation therapy when prophylactic phenytoin or carbamazepine are prescribed
- Previous history of SJS
- Male sex

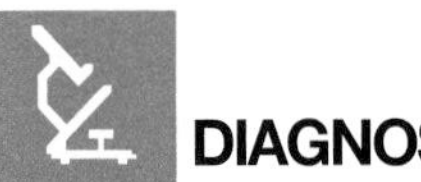

DIAGNOSIS

DIFFERENTIAL DIAGNOSIS
- Exfoliative dermatitis
- Linear IgA bullous dermatosis
- Staphylococcal scalded skin syndrome
- Acute generalized exanthematic pustulosis
- Pemphigus (paraneoplastic)
- Generalized fixed drug eruption
- Erythema multiforme major
- Burns
- Pressure blisters (coma, barbiturates)

LABORATORY Culture or serological tests for suspected sources of infection

Drugs that may alter lab results: N/A

Disorders that may alter lab results: N/A

PATHOLOGICAL FINDINGS Compared with the mainly inflammatory changes in erythema multiforme, necrotic changes predominate in SJS and TEN. There is a cell poor infiltrate in which macrophages and dendrocytes predominate with a strong immunoreactivity for TNF-alpha.

SPECIAL TESTS None

IMAGING N/A

DIAGNOSTIC PROCEDURES Skin biopsy

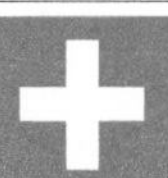

TREATMENT

APPROPRIATE HEALTH CARE Since this disease can progress quickly, all patients should be admitted. If the sloughed skin exceeds 10% of the body surface, consideration should be given to transferring the patient to a burns unit. Bronchiolitis, adult respiratory distress syndrome or multi-organ damage may require care in an intensive care unit.

GENERAL MEASURES
- Withdrawal of any suspected medication, and treatment of any underlying disease
- Meticulous care of damaged skin
- Reverse isolation when epidermal loss is extensive
- Maintenance of fluid, electrolyte and protein balance
- Plasmapheresis
- Adequate calorie intake, parenteral nutrition if necessary
- Oral hygiene with mouthwashes of warm saline, or solution of diphenhydramine, lidocaine, and kaolin suspension
- Ophthalmological consultation and monitoring for corneal damage

SURGICAL MEASURES Sterile débridement of areas of extensive epidermal loss. Application of biosynthetic dressings such as Biobrane to denuded areas. Long-term damage to the vulva, vagina or cornea may need surgical repair.

ACTIVITY Bed rest until clinically stabilized

DIET As tolerated. Increased fluid intake is recommended. IV nutritional support may be needed.

PATIENT EDUCATION
- The patient should be kept informed of the progress of the disease, and the treatment options available
- Recurrences are possible. Etiologic agents should be identified if possible, and avoided indefinitely.

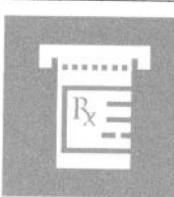

MEDICATIONS

DRUG(S) OF CHOICE

- Administration of steroids is controversial. If there is no clear benefit within a few days, they should be withdrawn.
- Experimental treatments that appear to have been useful include:
  - ◊ Recombinant granulocyte colony stimulating factor
  - ◊ Cyclophosphamide
  - ◊ Cyclosporine
  - ◊ immune globulin IV, in HIV positive patients
- Although not FDA approved, immune globulin IV has been reported as beneficial both for treatment and prophylaxis

Contraindications: Particularly avoid steroids in diabetic or immunosuppressed patients or those with chronic infections.

Precautions: Refer to the manufacturer's profile for each drug

Significant possible interactions: Refer to manufacturer's profile of each drug

ALTERNATIVE DRUGS

- Acyclovir for herpetic infections
- Erythromycin or related antibiotic for Mycoplasma infections (empiric use of antibiotics is not recommended)

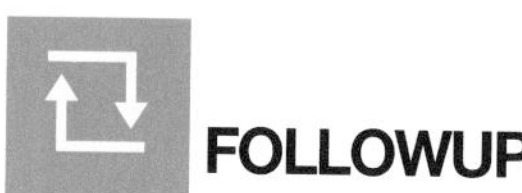

FOLLOWUP

PATIENT MONITORING

- Secondary or intercurrent infections
- Dehydration
- Electrolyte imbalance
- Malnutrition
- End-organ damage

PREVENTION/AVOIDANCE

- It is rarely possible to anticipate a first attack
- Avoid re-exposure to the presumed cause
- Although not FDA approved, immune globulin IV has been reported as beneficial both for treatment and prophylaxis

POSSIBLE COMPLICATIONS

- Secondary infections
- Sepsis
- Pneumonia
- Adult respiratory distress syndrome
- Bronchiolitis obliterans in children
- Dehydration/electrolyte disturbance
- Acute tubular necrosis
- Corneal ulceration or iritis
- Arrhythmias
- Death in about 15% of untreated cases of SJS, and up to 40% of TEN

EXPECTED COURSE/PROGNOSIS

- Disease may have a rapid onset, or may evolve slowly over 1-2 weeks, with resolution over 4-6 weeks
- There may be scarring of the skin or mucous membranes, especially of the vulva
- There may be blindness or corneal opacities in 7-20% of patients
- Risk of recurrence may be a s high as 37%
- Death occurs in 5-15% of patients with SJS, and up to 40% of patients with TEN

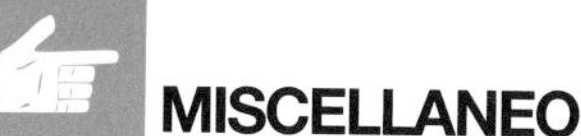

MISCELLANEOUS

ASSOCIATED CONDITIONS

- Stevens-Johnson syndrome and toxic epidermal necrolysis are associated conditions
- Mycoplasma pneumonia has been described as an infectious precursor

AGE-RELATED FACTORS

Pediatric: Rare under 3 years; more common in children and young adults

Geriatric: TEN has a greater mortality in older patients

Others: N/A

PREGNANCY

Reported as a possible predisposing condition

SYNONYMS

- Ectodermosis erosiva pluriorificialis
- Febrile mucocutaneous syndrome
- Herpes iris
- Erythema polymorphe

ICD-9-CM

695.1 Erythema multiforme

SEE ALSO

Burns
Erythema multiforme
Pemphigoid, bullous
Pemphigus vulgaris
Respiratory distress syndrome, adult

OTHER NOTES

N/A

ABBREVIATIONS

SJS = Stevens-Johnson syndrome
TEN = toxic epidermal necrolysis

REFERENCES

- Mockenhaupt M, et al. The risk of Stevens-Johnson syndrome and toxic epidermal necrolysis associated with nonsteroidal antiinflammatory drugs: a multinational perspective. Journal of Rheumatology 2000;30(10):2234-40
- Hockett KC. Stevens-Johnson syndrome and toxic epidermal necrolysis: oncological considerations. [Review] Clinical Journal of Oncology Nursing 2004;81(1):27-30, 55
- Baba M, et al. The anticonvulsant hypersensitivity syndrome. Journal of the European Academy of Dermatology and Venereology 2003;17(4):399-401
- Jones DH, et al. Journal of the American Osteopathic Association 2004;104(4):157-63
- Herbert AA, Bogle MA. Intravenous immunogloblin prophylaxix for recurrent Stevens-Johnson syndrome. Journal of the American Academy of Dermatology 2004;50(2):286-8
- Metry DW, et al. Use of intravenous immunoglobulin in children with Stevens-Johnson syndrome and toxic epidermal necrolysis: seven cases and review of the literature. Pediatrics 2003;112(6 Pt 1):1430-6
- Saunders Electronic Atlas of Dermatology. Philadelphia, WB Saunders Co, 1996
- Mockenhaupt M, Schopf E: Epidemiology of drug-induced severe skin reactions. Seminars in Cutaneous Medicine and Surgery 1996;15(4):236-243
- Shirato S, et al: Stevens-Johnson syndrome induced by methazolamide treatment. Archives of Ophthalmology 1997;115(4):550-553
- Kowalski BJ, Cody RJ: Stevens-Johnson syndrome associated with carvedilol therapy. American Journal of Cardiology 1997;80(5):669-670
- Tay YK, et al: Mycoplasma pneumonia infection is associated with Stevens-Johnson Syndrome, not erythema multiforme (von Hebra). Journal of the American Academy of Dermatology 1996;35(5pt1):757-760
- Revuz JE, Roujeau JC: Advances in toxic epidermal necrolysis. Seminars in Cutaneous Medicine & Surgery 1966;15(4):258-266
- Paquet P, Pierard GE: Erythema multiforme and toxic epidermal necrolysis: a comparative study. American Journal of Dermatopathology 1997;19(2):127-132
- Criton S, et al: Toxic epidermal necrolysis - a retrospective study. International Journal of Dermatology 1997;36(12):923-925
- Engelhardt SL, et al: Toxic epidermal necrolysis: an analysis of referral patients and steroid usage. Journal of Burn Care and Rehabilitation 1997;18(6):520-524
- Yarbrough DR 3rd: Treatment of toxic epidermal necrolysis in a burn center. Journal South Carolina Medical Association 1997;93(9):347-350
- Khoo AK, Foo CL: Toxic epidermal necrolysis in a burns center. Burns 1996;22(4):275-278
- Wallis C, McClymont W: Toxic epidermal necrolysis with adult respiratory distress syndrome. Anaesthesia 1995;50(9):801-803
- Bradley T, et al: Toxic epidermal necrolysis: a review and report of the successful use of Biobrane for early wound coverage. Annals of Plastic Surgery 1995;35(2)124-132
- Kakourou T, et al: Corticosteroid treatment of erythema multiforme major (Stevens-Johnson syndrome in children. European Journal of Pediatrics 1997;156(2):90-93

Web references: 0 available at www.5mcc.com
Illustrations 2 available

Author(s):
Lewis C. Rose, MD

BASICS

DESCRIPTION Syncope due to transient complete heart block and resulting severe bradycardia or asystole with hypotension
System(s) affected: Cardiovascular, Nervous
Genetics: No known genetic pattern
Incidence/Prevalence in USA: Undocumented
Predominant age: Most commonly, greater than 40 years of age
Predominant sex: Male = Female

SIGNS & SYMPTOMS
- Acute bradycardia
- Hypotension
- Paleness
- Altered sensorium or loss of consciousness, unrelated to position or exertion
- Acute onset of syncopal or near syncopal symptoms (with or without palpitations)

CAUSES
- Medications:
  - ◊ Calcium channel blockers
  - ◊ Beta blockers
  - ◊ Sotalol
  - ◊ Digoxin
  - ◊ Clonidine
  - ◊ Propafenone (Rythmol); a class IC antiarrhythmic
- Other causes:
  - ◊ Myocardial ischemia involving the AV node
  - ◊ Infiltrative or fibrosing diseases involving the heart and its conduction system
  - ◊ Degeneration of the AV node secondary to aging
  - ◊ Neuromuscular diseases (e.g., myotonic muscular dystrophy or Kearns-Sayre syndrome)

RISK FACTORS
- Use of the above mentioned medications
- Coronary artery disease
- History of previous AV nodal dysfunction
- Acute myocardial infarction (especially acute right coronary artery occlusion)
- Amyloidosis
- Chagas disease
- Connective tissue diseases involving the heart (e.g., systemic lupus erythematosus, rheumatoid arthritis)

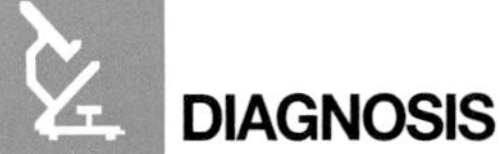

DIAGNOSIS

DIFFERENTIAL DIAGNOSIS
- Seizures
- Transient ischemia attacks
- Orthostatic hypotension
- Vasovagal attacks
- Neurocardiogenic syncope
- Cardiac arrhythmias
  - ◊ Ventricular tachycardia
  - ◊ Supraventricular tachycardia
  - ◊ Re-entrant tachycardia
  - ◊ Wolff-Parkinson-White syndrome
  - ◊ Sinus arrest
  - ◊ Sinus exit block
  - ◊ "Sick-sinus syndrome"
  - ◊ Transition from normal sinus rhythm to atrial fibrillation or from atrial fibrillation to normal sinus rhythm

LABORATORY
- Serum digoxin level
- Cardiac enzymes

Drugs that may alter lab results: None

Disorders that may alter lab results: Transient or long-standing renal failure may falsely elevate cardiac enzymes (creatine kinase)

PATHOLOGICAL FINDINGS N/A

SPECIAL TESTS N/A

IMAGING Transthoracic cardiac 2d-echo if infiltrative disease is suspected

DIAGNOSTIC PROCEDURES
- Cardiac coronary catheterization to rule out coronary ischemia
- Electrophysiologic testing to assess status of AV nodal conduction
- Myocardial biopsy if infiltrative disease is suspected
- ECG, event monitor or Holter monitor demonstrating (transient) complete heart block with slow or no ventricular escape
- Tilt table testing to rule out a neurogenic etiology for bradycardia and syncope

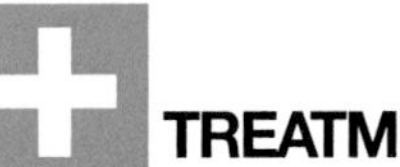

TREATMENT

APPROPRIATE HEALTH CARE
- Inpatient assessment in a monitored setting
- Continuing treatment - ambulatory

GENERAL MEASURES
- Cardiac monitoring
- Trans-thoracic pacer availability
- Atropine by the bedside

SURGICAL MEASURES
- Consider temporary pacemaker placement
- Permanent pacemaker placement, if etiology of transient complete heart block not reversible

ACTIVITY As tolerated after assessment

DIET Regular

PATIENT EDUCATION Once the diagnosis has been made and pacemaker has been implanted (if indicated) patient should be instructed in pacemaker guidelines

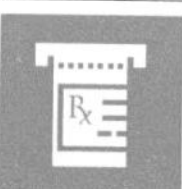

MEDICATIONS

DRUG(S) OF CHOICE
- For symptomatic bradyarrhythmias:
  - ◊ For acute bradyarrhythmias - atropine, 1 mg IV push to be given during the complete heart block with hypotension; may be repeated once for a total dosage of 2 mg
  - ◊ Epinephrine, 1 mg 1:10,000 IV push to be given during the complete heart block if associated with asystole; may be repeated every 5 minutes
  - ◊ Isoproterenol drip, 1 mg in 250 cc D5W or normal saline to be started at 5 micrograms per minute if patient maintains bradycardia and hypotensive after atropine given; may titrate drip as necessary

Contraindications: Use of epinephrine in bradycardia patient with a normal blood pressure may precipitate hypertensive crisis
Precautions: Possible tachycardiac response to the above mentioned medications
Significant possible interactions: None

ALTERNATIVE DRUGS N/A

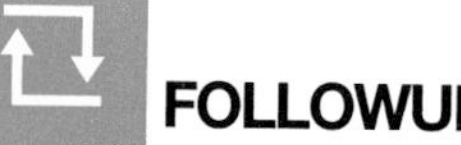

FOLLOWUP

PATIENT MONITORING
- Routine pacemaker checks, if permanent pacemaker implanted
- Followup Holter and/or event, monitor within two weeks after causal medications have been discontinued
- Discontinuation of driving, heavy machinery operation and being at unprotected heights pending normal followup

PREVENTION/AVOIDANCE
Avoidance of taking any drug similar to those causing the complete heart block

POSSIBLE COMPLICATIONS
- Protracted bradycardia with hypotension leading to end-organ damage or death
- Loss of consciousness while operating machinery or at unprotected heights

EXPECTED COURSE/PROGNOSIS
Once diagnosis is made and appropriate treatment is implemented (e.g., pacemaker insertion), prognosis is excellent and further difficulty not expected

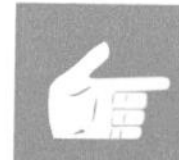

MISCELLANEOUS

ASSOCIATED CONDITIONS
- Myocardial ischemia
- Acute myocardial infarction
- Systemic manifestations of connective tissue disease
- Unreliable self-administration of medications
- Neuromuscular disease

AGE-RELATED FACTORS
Pediatric: N/A
Geriatric: More common problem in this age group
Others: N/A

PREGNANCY
Rare during pregnancy

SYNONYMS
Drop attacks

ICD-9-CM
426.9 Conduction disorder, unspecified

SEE ALSO
Amyloidosis
Complete heart block
Myocardial infarction
Seizure disorders
Sinus bradycardia

OTHER NOTES N/A

ABBREVIATIONS N/A

REFERENCES

- Brandenburg RO, Fuster V, Giuliani ER, McGoon DC: Cardiology: Fundamentals and Practice. Chicago, Year Book Medical Publishers, 1987
- Braunwald E, ed. Heart Disease: A Textbook of Cardiovascular Medicine. 5th Ed. Philadelphia, W.B. Saunders Co., 1996

Web references: 0 available at www.5mcc.com
Illustrations N/A

Author(s):
David J. Framm, MD

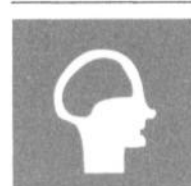

BASICS

DESCRIPTION Generalized inflammation of the oral mucosa of many possible etiologies
System(s) affected: Skin/Exocrine
Genetics: N/A
Incidence/Prevalence in USA:
- Herpetic stomatitis, hand-foot-and-mouth disease, and recurrent aphthous stomatitis are very common
- Herpangina is fairly common as are nicotinic and denture related stomatitis. The remaining causes are uncommon or rare.

Predominant age:
- Herpetic-primary infections - children
- Hand-foot-and-mouth disease - children
- Vincent's stomatitis - teenagers and young adults
- Behçet disease - young adults
- Herpangina - children
- Others - N/A

Predominant sex: Male = Female

SIGNS & SYMPTOMS
- General:
  - ◊ Depends on etiology
  - ◊ Varies from minimal to severe pain
  - ◊ Many have multiple intraoral ulcers from 1 mm to several centimeters in diameter
  - ◊ Some with constitutional symptoms - fever, malaise, headache
- Allergic stomatitis:
  - ◊ Intense shiny erythema
  - ◊ Slight swelling
  - ◊ Itching
  - ◊ Dryness
  - ◊ Burning
- Vincent's infection:
  - ◊ Necrotic ulceration of interdental papillae and mucous membrane
- Thrush (candidiasis):
  - ◊ White patches, slightly raised (resembling milk curds)
  - ◊ Distribution - tongue, buccal mucosa, palate, gums, tonsils, larynx, pharynx, GI tract, skin; commonly seen in infants, immunocompromised patients; patients on long-term antibiotics, corticosteroids, and anti-neoplastic treatment
- Pseudomembranous stomatitis:
  - ◊ Membrane-like exudate
- Mucous lesions accompanying systemic disease:
  - ◊ Mucous patches (syphilis)
  - ◊ Strawberry (measles)
  - ◊ Koplik's spots (measles)
  - ◊ Ulcers (erythema multiforme)
  - ◊ Smooth, fire-red, painful (pellagra)

CAUSES
- Allergy - foods, drugs, contact (some erythema multiforme)
- Vitamin deficiency - riboflavin (angular stomatitis)
- Viral - herpes simplex I and II (herpetic stomatitis), Coxsackie A (herpangina and hand-foot-and-mouth disease)
- Smoking (nicotinic stomatitis)
- Hormonal (possibly recurrent ulcerative stomatitis)
- Uncertain (recurrent aphthous stomatitis, Vincent's stomatitis, recurrent scarifying stomatitis, Behçet disease, angular stomatitis, gangrenous stomatitis, erythema multiforme)
- Bacterial (scarlatina)
- Uremic (uremic/nephritic)
- Dentures

RISK FACTORS Listed with Causes

DIAGNOSIS

DIFFERENTIAL DIAGNOSIS
- Squamous cell cancer
- Herpetic stomatitis
- Hand-foot-and-mouth disease
- Recurrent aphthous stomatitis
- Vincent's stomatitis
- Nicotinic stomatitis
- Denture related stomatitis
- Erythema multiforme/Stevens-Johnson syndrome
- Recurrent ulcerative stomatitis
- Recurrent scarifying stomatitis
- Behçet disease
- Angular stomatitis
- Noma (gangrenous stomatitis)
- Scarlatina (scarlet fever)
- Herpangina
- Uremic
- Pemphigus/pemphigoid

LABORATORY
- Hematologic profile
- Tzanck test of historic interest only
- Serologic test for syphilis

Drugs that may alter lab results: N/A

Disorders that may alter lab results: N/A

PATHOLOGICAL FINDINGS Biopsy suspicious lesions or lesions that fail to heal or chronically recur to rule out cancer or vasculitis

SPECIAL TESTS N/A

IMAGING N/A

DIAGNOSTIC PROCEDURES Biopsy if persistent/recurrent/suspicious

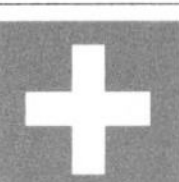

TREATMENT

APPROPRIATE HEALTH CARE Outpatient, unless severe

GENERAL MEASURES
- In most cases treatment is symptomatic only
- Severe cases may require parenteral fluids, particularly in children
- Topical anesthesia
- Analgesics
- Oral rinses such as 1/2 strength hydrogen peroxide
- Mycostatin, if superinfected with candida
- Stop smoking

SURGICAL MEASURES N/A

ACTIVITY As tolerated by patient

DIET May need to avoid spicy, sharp, hard, and dry foods

PATIENT EDUCATION Griffith: Instructions for Patients; Philadelphia, W.B. Saunders Co.

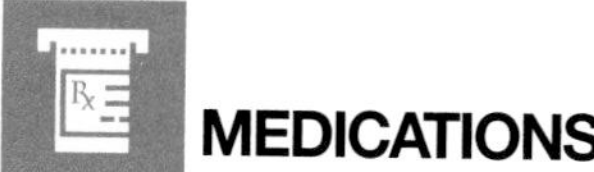

MEDICATIONS

DRUG(S) OF CHOICE

- Steroids and cytotoxic drugs for Behçet disease
- 2% viscous lidocaine (Xylocaine) for local discomfort
- Liquid diphenhydramine (Benadryl) po, or swish and spit
- Antibiotics for gangrenous stomatitis
- Antifungal ointment, e.g., nystatin (Mycostatin) for candida complicating angular stomatitis
- For candidiasis - nystatin oral suspension 400,000 units (4 mL) qid for 10 days. Use as oral rinse, then swallow.
- Acyclovir - 200-800 mg 5 times a day for 7-14 days for herpetic stomatitis
- Sucralfate (Carafate) - suspension 1 tsp swish in mouth or place on ulcers 4 times a day (is helpful)

Contraindications: Allergy to specific medication

Precautions: Toxic dose of topical lidocaine uncertain, but likely only 25-33% of infiltration dose - may have significant absorption from open ulcers or mucous membrane

Significant possible interactions: Refer to manufacturer's literature

ALTERNATIVE DRUGS Steroid oral rinses or topical preparations for aphthous ulcers

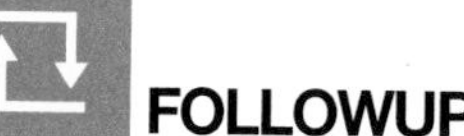

FOLLOWUP

PATIENT MONITORING Lesions need to be followed until resolved. If they fail to resolve, continuously recur, or appear suspicious, biopsy may be needed to establish a diagnosis.

PREVENTION/AVOIDANCE Avoid causative factors

POSSIBLE COMPLICATIONS

- Recurrent scarifying stomatitis may result in intraoral scarring with restriction of oral mobility
- Behçet disease may result in visual loss, pneumonia, colitis, vasculitis, large artery aneurysms, thrombophlebitis, or encephalitis
- Gangrenous stomatitis may lead to death
- Scarlet fever may result in cardiac disease
- Herpetic stomatitis may be complicated by ocular or CNS involvement

EXPECTED COURSE/PROGNOSIS

- Herpetic - self-limited with resolution in 7-14 days
- Hand-foot-and-mouth disease - same as herpetic
- Recurrent aphthous - 7-14 day course per episode
- Vincent's - may progress to fascial space infection with airway compromise or sepsis
- Nicotinic - will resolve with cessation of smoking
- Denture - will resolve with careful oral hygiene and daytime denture wear only
- Erythema multiforme - resolution in 2-3 weeks
- Stevens-Johnson: resolution in about 6 weeks with adequate supportive care
- Recurrent ulcerative - as the name implies, these recur over time, but the overall prognosis is good
- Recurrent scarifying - occasional patients suffer continuous ulcers, others recur with eventual scarring. The prognosis is otherwise good.
- Behçet disease - may recur for several years. Prognosis for vision is poor. Overall prognosis is related to other aspects of the disease.
- Angular - after correction of mechanical problems, allergic disorders, and nutritional deficiencies the prognosis is good
- Gangrenous - this is the most serious stomatitis, requiring aggressive treatment with IV antibiotics and débridement to avoid death
- Scarlatina - the prognosis is related to other manifestations of the disease
- Herpangina - 7-14 day course with total resolution
- Uremic - depends on the underlying renal disease

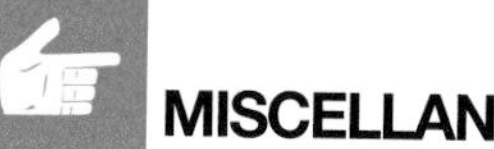

MISCELLANEOUS

ASSOCIATED CONDITIONS AIDS - associated with severe lesions

AGE-RELATED FACTORS

Pediatric: Certain etiologies more likely in the pediatric population: Herpetic-primary, hand-foot-and-mouth disease, herpangina

Geriatric: Certain etiologies more likely in the geriatric population, e.g., dentures

Others: N/A

PREGNANCY May bring on recurrent ulcerative stomatitis

SYNONYMS N/A

ICD-9-CM

528.0 Stomatitis
054.2 Herpetic gingivostomatitis
528.2 Oral aphthae
101 Vincent angina

SEE ALSO

OTHER NOTES N/A

ABBREVIATIONS N/A

REFERENCES

- Moran WJ: Diseases of the mouth. In: Rakel E, ed. Conn's Current Therapy, Philadelphia, W.B. Saunders Co., 1990
- Teele DW: Inflammatory diseases of the mouth and pharynx. In: Paparella MM, Shumrick DA, eds. Otolaryngology. Philadelphia, W.B. Saunders Co., 1980:974-1017

Web references: 0 available at www.5mcc.com

Illustrations 11 available

Author(s):
Mark R. Dambro, MD

BASICS

DESCRIPTION The sudden onset of a focal neurological deficit resulting from either infarction or hemorrhage within the brain
System(s) affected: Cardiovascular, Nervous
Genetics: Inheritance is polygenic with a tendency to clustering of risk factors within families
Incidence/Prevalence in USA: Incidence 150/100,000 ; prevalence 550/100,000
Predominant age: Risk increases over age 45 and is highest in the seventh and eighth decades
Predominant sex: Male > Female (3:1), but equalizes after menopause

SIGNS & SYMPTOMS
- Carotid circulation (hemispheric): Hemiplegia, hemianesthesia, neglect, aphasia, visual field defects; less often headaches, seizures, amnesia, confusion
- Vertebrobasilar (brainstem or cerebellar): Diplopia, vertigo, ataxia, facial paresis, Horner syndrome, dysphagia, dysarthria
- Impaired level of consciousness
- Cerebellar lesion in patients with headache, nausea, vomiting and ataxia

CAUSES
- Ischemic: Carotid atherosclerotic disease with artery-to-artery thromboembolism
- Cardiac: Cardioembolism secondary to valvular (mitral valve) pathology; mural hypokinesias or akinesias with thrombosis (acute anterior myocardial infarctions or congestive cardiomyopathies); cardiac arrhythmia (atrial fibrillation)
- Hypercoagulable states: Antiphospholipid antibodies, factor V leiden deficiency, deficiency of protein S, protein C; presence of antithrombin 3, oral contraceptives
- Other causes: Spontaneous and post-traumatic (i.e., chiropractic manipulation) artery dissection, fibromuscular dysplasia, vasculitis, drugs (cocaine, amphetamines)
- Hemorrhagic
- Hypertension: may cause damage to putamen, internal capsule, cerebellum, brainstem, corona radiata
- Amyloid (congophilic) angiopathy: Lobar (cortical) hemorrhages in the elderly
- Vascular malformations: Arteriovenous malformation, cavernous angioma, venous angioma and capillary angioma

RISK FACTORS
- Age
- Hypertension
- Cardiac disease
- Smoking
- Diabetes
- Antiphospholipid antibodies
- Family history
- Atrial fibrillation
- Hyperlipidemia
- Homocystinemia

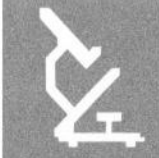

DIAGNOSIS

DIFFERENTIAL DIAGNOSIS
- Migraine
- Focal seizure
- Tumor
- Subdural hematoma
- Hypoglycemia; hyperglycemia; hypercalcemia

LABORATORY N/A

Drugs that may alter lab results: N/A

Disorders that may alter lab results: N/A

PATHOLOGICAL FINDINGS N/A

SPECIAL TESTS
- Duplex carotid ultrasonography
- Cerebral angiography
- ECG
- Transthoracic echocardiogram (TTE); if normal and a cardiac source is suspected, followup with transesophageal echocardiogram
- Holter monitoring
- EEG for suspected seizure
- International normalized ratio (INR) and partial thromboplastin time (PTT). Coumadin prolongs PT.
- Antiphospholipid antibodies
- Cardiac enzymes

IMAGING Acute phase:
- CT of head
- MRI scan of brain with diffusion weighted imaging, MRA of brain and neck vessels

DIAGNOSTIC PROCEDURES N/A

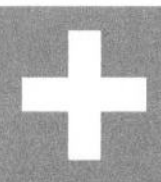

TREATMENT

APPROPRIATE HEALTH CARE
- Acute phase: Inpatient care, preferably in a stroke unit
- Surgical therapy: In medically fit patients with non-disabling stroke, carotid endarterectomy is indicated for stenosis of > 70% on side ipsilateral to stroke; medical therapy for < 50% stenosis, 50-69% depends on risk factors

GENERAL MEASURES
- Maintain oxygenation
- Monitor cardiac rhythm for 48 hours
- Control hyperglycemia (keep glucose < 220 mg/dL [12.1 mmol/L])
- Treat blood pressure > 185/110 if patient will be or has been treated with IV tPA
- Do not treat elevated blood pressure unless acute end-organ dysfunction (encephalopathy, myocardial ischemia, aortic dissection, ARF)
- Prevent hyperthermia
- Early introduction of physiotherapy and ambulation
- Subcutaneous heparin 5,000 units subcutaneously every 12 hours

SURGICAL MEASURES N/A

ACTIVITY Ambulate as soon as possible

DIET
- Alert with no dysphagia: Diet as tolerated (no added salt if hypertensive)
- Alert with dysphagia: Pureed dysphagia diet or nasogastric feeding tube if indicated

PATIENT EDUCATION National Stroke Association, 9707 E. Easter Ln, Englewood, CO 80112 (800-STROKES)

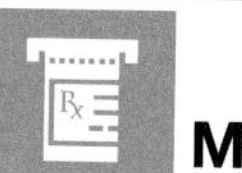

MEDICATIONS

DRUG(S) OF CHOICE
- IV tissue plasminogen activator (tPA) 0.9 mg/kg in highly selected cases within 3 hours of ischemic stroke
- Enteric coated aspirin (EC ASA) 50-325 mg/day

or
- Dipyridamole-aspirin (Aggrenox) - extended release, 200 mg/25 mg capsule po bid; more efficacious than aspirin alone
- Clopidogrel (Plavix)75 mg/day is ticlopidine's descendent, has fewer side effects, but shows an only slight advantage over ASA
- Warfarin - INR adjusted dose. For patients with atrial fibrillation and cardioembolic stroke.

Contraindications:
- EC ASA - active peptic ulcer disease, hypersensitivity to aspirin, patients who had bronchospastic reaction to ASA or other non-steroidal anti-inflammatory drugs
- Ticlopidine - known hypersensitivity to the drug, presence of hematopoietic disorders, presence of a hemostatic disorder, conditions associated with active bleeding, severe liver dysfunction
- Warfarin - intolerance or allergy, dementia, liver disease, active bleeding, pregnancy, recent head injury

Precautions:
- EC ASA - may aggravate pre-existing peptic ulcer disease, may worsen symptoms in some patients with asthma
- Ticlopidine - 2.4% of patients develop neutropenia (0.8% severe neutropenia) which is reversible with cessation of drug; monitor blood counts every 2 weeks for the first 3 months
- Clopidogrel and ticlopidine - TTP can occur
- Warfarin - poor balance, alcohol/drug abuse, age > 80

Significant possible interactions:
- EC ASA - may potentiate effects of anticoagulants and sulfonylurea, hypoglycemic agents
- Ticlopidine - digoxin plasma levels decreased 15%, theophylline half-life increased from 8.6 to 12.2 hours
- Warfarin - ASA, NSAIDs, antibiotics, tranquilizers

ALTERNATIVE DRUGS
- Ticlopidine (Ticlid) 250 mg po bid - has fallen out of favor due to unfavorable side effect profile, risk of neutropenia and need for CBC monitoring

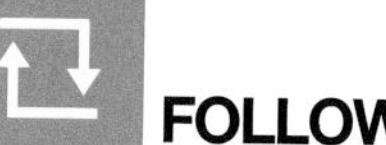

FOLLOWUP

PATIENT MONITORING
Follow every 3 months for first year then yearly

PREVENTION/AVOIDANCE
- Stop smoking
- Control blood pressure, diabetes, hyperlipidemia
- Use alcohol in moderation, if at all
- Regular exercise
- Maintain positive psychological outlook
- Maintain weight control
- Antiplatelet drugs
- Angiotensin converting enzyme (ACE) inhibitors
- Statins
- Treat homocystinemia with vitamin B6, vitamin B12, and folic acid
- Anticoagulation when cardioembolism is the suspected cause

POSSIBLE COMPLICATIONS
- Shoulder subluxation
- Hyperextension knee injury
- Depression
- Sympathetic dystrophy

EXPECTED COURSE/PROGNOSIS
- Variable depending on severity of stroke
- Posterior circulation strokes have a higher acute mortality rate but generally make a better functional recovery than hemispheric strokes

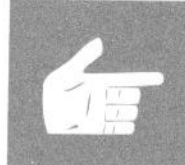

MISCELLANEOUS

ASSOCIATED CONDITIONS
Major cause of death in first five years after a stroke is cardiac disease

AGE-RELATED FACTORS
Pediatric:
- Cardiac (especially developmental abnormalities)
- Metabolic: Homocystinuria, Fabry disease

Geriatric: Amyloid (congophilic) angiopathy is most prevalent in elderly, especially if patient also has dementia

Others: Adults < 45 years old most likely to have a cardiac source of embolism

PREGNANCY
- Parturition may increase risk of rupture for aneurysm; amniotic fluid embolism may cause stroke at time of delivery
- Postpartum period associated with increased risk for cerebral venous thrombosis

SYNONYMS
- Cerebrovascular accident
- CVA
- Reversible ischemic neurological accident
- RIND

ICD-9-CM
431 Intracerebral hemorrhage
434.11 Cerebral embolism with cerebral infarction
436 Acute, but ill-defined, cerebrovascular disease

SEE ALSO
Stroke rehabilitation
Transient ischemic attack (TIA)

OTHER NOTES
N/A

ABBREVIATIONS
N/A

REFERENCES
- Hachinski V (ed): Stroke. Lancet 1998;352:(suppl III):1-30
- Hachinski V: Brain Attack: The Clinical Handbook. Meducom International,1999

Web references: 2 available at www.5mcc.com
Illustrations N/A

Author(s):
Vladimir Hachinski, MD, DSc
Bart Demaerschalk, MD

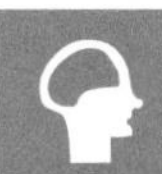

BASICS

DESCRIPTION Stroke rehabilitation involves restoration of function after medical and neurologic stability have been achieved
- Cerebrovascular diseases and/or disorders that affect central nervous system function by compromising delivery of blood or by hemorrhage resulting in ischemia, necrosis and gliosis
- Anterior lesions in the cerebrovascular system affect the arteries that supply the cerebral hemispheres and cause thrombotic strokes
- Posterior lesions affect arteries that supply the brain stem and yield crossed motor and/or sensory signs and symptoms of hemorrhagic strokes
- Both anterior and posterior lesions can cause sudden death, but the lower in the central nervous system the lesion, or the more incomplete the lesion, or the more hemorrhagic the lesion, the higher the chance for neurologic return and also for second, etc., strokes

System(s) affected: Cardiovascular, Nervous
Genetics: Similar to the probability of developing hypertension or coronary artery disease
Incidence/Prevalence in USA: 459/100,000
Predominant age: Over 45
Predominant sex: Male > Female

SIGNS & SYMPTOMS
- Variable - depends upon the arterial system affected
- Hemiparesis
- Hemianesthesia
- Unilateral central facial palsy
- Homonymous hemianopsia
- Aphasia, apraxia (if the dominant cerebral hemisphere is involved)

CAUSES
- Coronary artery disease
- Hypertension
- Cerebral arteriosclerosis
- Cardiac thrombus embolus
- Foreign body embolus
- Frequently, the combination of gout, diabetes, hypertension has been untreated for some 5-10 years before the onset of the stroke disorder
- aneurysms and arteriovenous malformations

RISK FACTORS
- Many are lifestyle oriented and preventable. Factors include coffee ingestion, cigarette smoking, obesity, inactivity, hyperactivity to the point of exhaustion, emotional lability, sexual hyperactivity, starvation, antidepressant or diet reduction medication, alcohol or recreational drug habituation, unusual stress states.
- Ethnicity may be a risk factor but relationships to factors above first must be clarified
- Overly aggressive treatment of diabetes with insulin, hypoglycemia
- Vasculitis; immune, infections, associated with malignancy

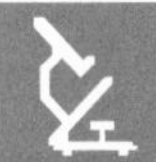

DIAGNOSIS

DIFFERENTIAL DIAGNOSIS
- Infection, tumor, bleeding disorders, endocrinologic, metabolic, gastrointestinal, toxic, etc.
- Different types of stroke disorders can occur in one patient
- Liver failure with/without transplantation can be associated with cognitive deficits that persist even after transplantation
- Brain tumors often present as stroke syndromes with significant personality and/or aphasic disorders and relatively less obvious weakness or spasticity upon examination

LABORATORY
- CBC
- Blood alcohol level
- Spinal fluid for routine studies (only if indicated)
- Urinalysis
- RPR
- ANA for collagen vascular disorders
- Consider quantitative immunoelectrophoresis with the combination of stroke disorders, anemia, hypertension
- Carotid flow studies

Drugs that may alter lab results: N/A

Disorders that may alter lab results: N/A

PATHOLOGICAL FINDINGS Thrombotic, hemorrhagic, mixed, combinations can be present

SPECIAL TESTS
- Somatosensory, auditory, and visual evoked potential technology can monitor neurologic recovery.
- EEG sometimes useful in evaluating seizure disorders
- Cardiovascular stress testing to evaluate the extent of coronary artery disease
- Serum glucose level

IMAGING
- Scanning - CT, MRI and PET scanning give good data about anatomy, blood flow, and metabolic activity
- Serial exams can delineate the course of this disease and reveal hydrocephalus or brain tumors
- Total body bone scans can help diagnose reflex sympathetic dystrophy (hand shoulder syndrome)

DIAGNOSTIC PROCEDURES
- Spinal taps, myelography, pneumoencephalography, angiography all have special indications and contraindications at this time. None are routinely used.
- Electrodiagnosis for neuritis, radiculitis in specialized centers if available
- Endovascular procedures have great diagnostic implications.

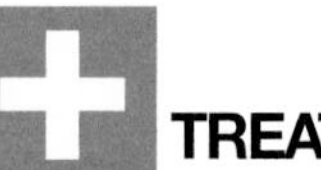

TREATMENT

APPROPRIATE HEALTH CARE
Referral to a full service rehabilitation center - a rehabilitation medicine team can make the difference between independence and dependency. Refer when medically and neurologically stable.

GENERAL MEASURES
- Full service rehabilitation center characteristics: Comparison with national standards for admission, process, discharge, and followup care; closed units; regular team meetings to discuss long and short term objectives; quality assurance system in place; accreditation by Commission on Accreditation of Rehabilitation Facilities.
- Use deep heat (e.g., ultrasound, prolonged hydrotherapy) with caution in patients with reduced sensation and/or taking anticoagulants
- Use hydrotherapy and/or isometric exercise cautiously in patients with limited cardiopulmonary reserve
- In patients able to respond to the protocols after surgery, restorative, tendon transplant, or nerve transplants may be of value
- Cardiac precautions and a CPR team may be required during exercise programs since obese, hypertensive, or patients with coronary artery disease are at increased risk. Real-time monitoring might be required.
- Open units, especially in investor owned, private rehabilitation centers, need to be closely monitored for outcome and cost/benefit ratio type productivity quality
- Inpatient rehab in acute rehab units is probably not necessary for stable, uncomplicated strokes (can be done as outpatient)
- Check and adjust serum glucose level if necessary

SURGICAL MEASURES
- Microcatheter and microsurgical technology have been used to clip, embolize or reset aneurysms and other lesions.
- Applied cardioangiographic technology has generated new endovascular treatment procedures.

ACTIVITY
- Physical therapy, occupational therapy, speech pathology, psychology, nursing therapy should be delivered to the patient for at least three hours/day throughout the inpatient stay.
- The patient must be able to tolerate this vigorous activity level. If the patient becomes medically or neurologically unstable during the inpatient stay, a 48 hour leeway is usually built into the system. After that period, therapy must resume or the patient must be returned to an acute hospital bed. Most stroke acute rehabilitation units are usually able to deliver this type of functional return within one month of inpatient stay, although length of stay is individually determined.
- While most rehabilitative efforts take place within a very short time after ictus, successful rehabilitative efforts have taken place as long as five years later

DIET Depends upon other medical conditions, but control of hypertension and diabetes is important

PATIENT EDUCATION

- Stroke is usually an unnecessary illness. Major risk factors are nearly all preventable. The difficulty that arises is that the patient's life style must be changed. Aerobic daily exercise, diet and a balanced conditioning program will significantly lower stroke risk. Patients mount a great deal of active and passive resistance.
- The progressive physical and mental deterioration noted with hypertension and/or coronary artery disease is not inevitable
- Family pressure and support is helpful to interest the patient in his/her health in a consistent and sustained manner
- Disuse will add subsequent complications and sequelae
- Second complex strokes - patients with second ictus and/or renal failure, heart failure or cor pulmonale might require 20-30 days inpatient rehab in a skilled nursing facility before disposition

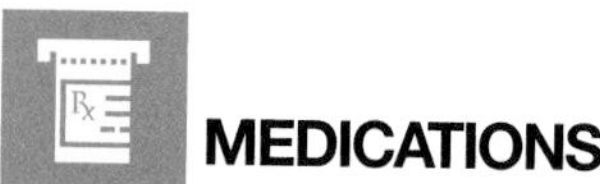

MEDICATIONS

DRUG(S) OF CHOICE

- Use only what is absolutely necessary. Sleeping medications, such as flurazepam, can accumulate over time in stroke patients.
- As needed for underlying disorders (e.g., hypertension, heart disease) or for complications (e.g., seizures, deep vein thrombosis, pneumonitis).
- Once neurological and medical stability have been achieved, depression can be treated with a serotonin inhibitor antidepressant, e.g., sertraline HCL 50 mg every morning.
- For thrombotic strokes or for patients with a high risk of this type of stroke, anticoagulant medications are important

Contraindications: Refer to manufacturer's profile of each drug

Precautions:

- Four or more medications will often have interactions; polypharmacy is frequent
- Antihypertensive medication can generate orthostatic hypotension
- Antidepressant medication can lower the seizure threshold and interact with antihypertensive medications
- Muscle relaxants, tranquilizers, major neuroleptic medication can confuse, delay return of memory and cognition, sedate, occasionally agitate, and obliterate spontaneous thought
- Unnecessary medications, such as antihistamines, should be withdrawn due to risk of hypertension
- Elderly patients regularly require lower dosages of the above medications
- Most common cause of resistance to hypertensive medication is patient's failure to take medicine

Significant possible interactions:

- NSAIDs can adversely interact with psychotropic medication, can generate hypertension/GI bleeding
- Some NSAIDs contain sulfa drugs which will cause allergic reactions
- Too aggressive treatment of hypertension can yield hypotension and extend the stroke

ALTERNATIVE DRUGS

- Reflex sympathetic dystrophy (shoulder-hand syndrome) - can be treated with tizanidine (Zanaflex) 4-8 mg every hs and botulinum (Myobloc) injections
- Flexor spasms in spasticity - to help control, tizanidine 4-8 mg every hs, diazepam 5 mg bid and/or baclofen 10 mg tid
- For spasticity in those not tolerating systemic medication: either intrathecal baclofen by pump or botulinum toxin IM administration

FOLLOWUP

PATIENT MONITORING

- Within the month following discharge, the patient and family should be seen in an outpatient group "alumni" day coordinated with an interdisciplinary outpatient clinic appointment
- If outpatient therapy is rendered, the team therapist(s) should meet with the physician regularly to rate progress and discuss long- and short-term objectives
- For first uncomplicated stroke patients - once the acute rehab is completed, the rest of the rehab can be accomplished as an outpatient or in a day care program

PREVENTION/AVOIDANCE

See Risk factors and Patient education

POSSIBLE COMPLICATIONS

- Reflex sympathetic dystrophy syndromes - such as hand/shoulder syndrome - are nonspecific complications and last for 12 weeks before subsiding to adhesive capsulitis
- Tendonitis-bursitis-capsulitis may coexist with prolonged paralysis. Prolonged range-of-motion and neuromuscular re-education exercises help retard functional deterioration of the limb. Electrical stimulation and biofeedback for control and relaxation have also been used, but the treatment of choice is restoration of function.
- Diabetes, alcohol intake will add peripheral neuritis. Diabetes could also be associated (especially in males) with gout and hypertension
- Many patients develop osteoporosis - especially on side of paresis. The normal side can develop osteoarthritis.
- Repeat strokes from lack of hypertension and/or artery disease control

EXPECTED COURSE/PROGNOSIS

- Generally good, although pneumonia, respiratory failure, heart failure, and myocardial infarction occur more frequently after stroke
- Outcome studies have shown that acute rehab center programs generate 33% more functional improvement than comparable skilled nursing facilities, but tend to also cost more
- Too early discharges can often be associated with suboptimal functional recovery

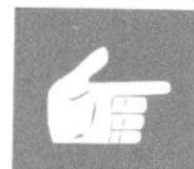

MISCELLANEOUS

ASSOCIATED CONDITIONS

- Hypertension
- Coronary artery disease
- Diabetes mellitus
- Gout
- Atherosclerosis
- Smoking
- Alcoholism

AGE-RELATED FACTORS

Pediatric: Aneurysms, hypertension, tumors, trauma

Geriatric: Heart disease, vascular disease, hypertension

Others: See Risk factors

PREGNANCY

Hypertension in pregnancy can lead to stroke

SYNONYMS

N/A

ICD-9-CM

438.9 Unspecified late effects of cerebrovascular disease

SEE ALSO

Brain injury - post acute care issues
Stroke (Brain attack)

OTHER NOTES

N/A

ABBREVIATIONS

N/A

REFERENCES

- Kaplan PE, Cailliet R, Kaplan C. Stroke Rehabilitation. Boston: Butterworth; 2002
- Clinchot DM, Kaplan PE, et al. Cerebral aneurysms and arteriovenous malformations. Arch Phys Med Rehabil 1994;75:1342-51
- Kaplan PE, Clinchot DM, Firnett JA. Cognitive deficits after hepatic transplantation. Brain Injury 1996;10:599-607
- Clinchot DM, Bogner JA, Kaplan PE. Cerebral aneurysms. Arch Phys Med Rehabil 1997;78:346-349

Web references: 3 available at www.5mcc.com

Illustrations N/A

Author(s):
Paul E. Kaplan, MD

BASICS

DESCRIPTION Subarachnoid hemorrhage is the extravasation of blood into the subarachnoid space particularly of the basal cisterns and into the cerebral spinal fluid pathways.
- Traumatic: More common and it is related to head trauma
- Spontaneous: Rare. 50-60% of spontaneous subarachnoid hemorrhages are due to intracranial saccular aneurysms.

System(s) affected: Nervous
Genetics: N/A
Incidence/Prevalence in USA:
Spontaneous: Incidence is 10.9/100,000 per year
Predominant age:
- The majority of subarachnoid hemorrhages due to aneurysms occur in the fourth to seventh decades
- Subarachnoid hemorrhage due to arteriovenous (AV) malformation appears more commonly in the second, third, and fourth decades

Predominant sex: Subarachnoid hemorrhage due to aneurysm occurs slightly more commonly in females (55%).

SIGNS & SYMPTOMS
- Abrupt onset of headache associated with stiff neck and photophobia
- May or may not lose consciousness
- May develop focal neurological deficits such as hemiparesis or a dilated pupil
- Subhyaloid hemorrhages are more common in anterior communicating artery aneurysms

CAUSES
- Trauma
- Intracranial saccular aneurysm
- Intracranial A-V malformation
- Hypertension
- Rarely tumors and blood dyscrasias.

RISK FACTORS
- Intracranial aneurysms associated with coarctation of the aorta
- AV malformations
- Polycystic disease of the kidneys
- Fibromuscular dysplasia of the renal arteries
- Hypertension is not necessarily associated with saccular aneurysms, but is associated with rupture of an existing aneurysm

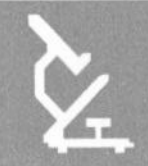

DIAGNOSIS

DIFFERENTIAL DIAGNOSIS
- Intracerebral hematomas
- Meningitis
- Acute (usually first) migrainous attacks and thunderclap headaches

LABORATORY N/A

Drugs that may alter lab results: N/A

Disorders that may alter lab results: N/A

PATHOLOGICAL FINDINGS N/A

SPECIAL TESTS N/A

IMAGING
- CT scan:
  - ◊ The diagnosis is established in more than 95% of the cases with a CT scan. This demonstrates blood in the basal cisterns and may help in localizing the source of hemorrhage.
  - ◊ It also can rule out mass effect so that if this study is negative a spinal puncture can be safely performed
  - ◊ A small percentage of subarachnoid hemorrhages will be missed on the CT scan. If CT negative and clinical suspicion high, a lumbar puncture should be performed to evaluate for blood.
- Cerebral angiography
  - ◊ Following the establishment of the diagnosis of subarachnoid hemorrhage, it is imperative to find out the source of bleeding, therefore, cerebral angiography is used to identify the source of hemorrhage such as a saccular aneurysm or AV malformation
  - ◊ High definition MRA (magnetic resonance angiography) occasionally will establish the diagnosis, but angiography is still the gold standard for planning surgery
- Other
  - ◊ It must be remembered that occasional hemorrhage may occur from an AV malformation of the spinal cord or a vascular tumor in the spinal arachnoid space. Therefore, if no source of subarachnoid hemorrhage is found intracranially, consideration might be made for studies involving the subarachnoid space which would include MRI spinal scanning or myelography.

DIAGNOSTIC PROCEDURES See above

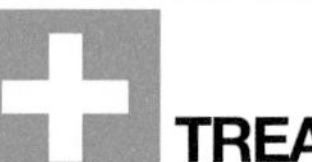

TREATMENT

APPROPRIATE HEALTH CARE Initial therapy is carried out in the Intensive Care Unit

GENERAL MEASURES
- The treatment is directed to prevent complications of subarachnoid hemorrhage which include rebleeding, hydrocephalus, and cerebral vasospasm
- Vasospasm is treated with generous volume expansion and hypertension to promote cerebral perfusion after the aneurysm has been obliterated. This is not wise if an aneurysm is untreated.
- Once the patient has stabilized and recovered from the initial hemorrhage, then a vigorous rehabilitation program is indicated

SURGICAL MEASURES
- If the source of hemorrhage such as an aneurysm can be readily obliterated, this reduces the risk of rebleeding and allows more vigorous treatment with fluid and hypertensive therapy of cerebral vasospasm
- Hydrocephalus should be treated with cerebral spinal fluid drainage and may require permanent shunting procedures
- AV malformations may be obliterated with embolization and surgery
- Radiosurgery shows promise in the treatment of small deep AV malformations
- Endovascular obliteration of aneurysms is being performed in selected centers

ACTIVITY Strict bedrest until source of hemorrhage is eliminated

DIET N/A

PATIENT EDUCATION N/A

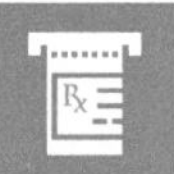

MEDICATIONS

DRUG(S) OF CHOICE
- Nimodipine
  - ◊ Has been used at 60 mg q4h for the prevention of cerebral vasospasm
  - ◊ Therapy should begin as soon as possible
  - ◊ The capsule contents may be given via NG tube if patient can't swallow

Contraindications: Hypotension is contraindication in patients with vasospasm

Precautions:
- Quiet room
- Reduce stress
- Control blood pressure until source of hemorrhage eliminated
- Stool softeners to prevent straining

Significant possible interactions: Refer to manufacturer's profile

ALTERNATIVE DRUGS Nicardipine

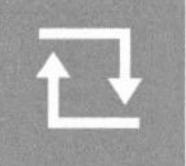

FOLLOWUP

PATIENT MONITORING As needed

PREVENTION/AVOIDANCE Incidental aneurysms have a risk of hemorrhage of 1-2% per year so prophylactic surgery or endovascular treatment may be indicated

POSSIBLE COMPLICATIONS
- Death
- Paralysis

EXPECTED COURSE/PROGNOSIS
- Approximately 25-30% of the patients will die from a spontaneous subarachnoid hemorrhage due to an aneurysm. The highest morbidity is secondary to cerebral vasospasm.
- If the aneurysm can be successfully obliterated and the vasospasm treated effectively, satisfactory outcome occurs in approximately 50-65% of patients
- Approximately 25-30% of aneurysms will be multiple. It is advisable to treat multiple aneurysms during the same procedure, but if this is not possible, treatment is directed at the aneurysm most likely to have hemorrhaged.
- Further surgical procedures may be necessary to obliterate additional aneurysms
- AV malformations do not have as high morbidity and mortality associated with the hemorrhage. Both untreated aneurysms and AV malformations are likely to bleed at about 2% per year. Therefore in the younger age groups, incidentally found A-V malformations and aneurysms may require aggressive treatment.

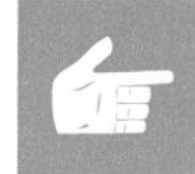

MISCELLANEOUS

ASSOCIATED CONDITIONS N/A

AGE-RELATED FACTORS
Pediatric: N/A

Geriatric: In the elderly patient, incidental aneurysms and AV malformations may best be followed since the chance of hemorrhage is only 2% per year

Others: In younger and middle-aged people, surgery is recommended

PREGNANCY
In the pregnant female, increased blood pressure and blood volume may predispose to hemorrhages. Under life-threatening situations, surgical or endovascular procedures can be performed on a pregnant patient. However, with AV malformations, a less lethal lesion compared to aneurysms it may be worthwhile to allow the pregnancy go to term.

SYNONYMS N/A

ICD-9-CM
430 Subarachnoid hemorrhage

852.00 Subarchnoid hemorrhage following injury without mention of open intracranial wound, unspecified state of consciousness

SEE ALSO

OTHER NOTES N/A

ABBREVIATIONS
AV = arteriovenous

REFERENCES

- Weir B, ed. Aneurysm Affecting the Nervous System. Baltimore, Williams & Wilkins, 1987
- Sahs AL, Perret G, Nishioka H, eds. Intracranial and Subarachnoid Hemorrhage: A Cooperative Study. Philadelphia, J.B. Lippincott Co, 1969
- Youmans JR, ed. A Comprehensive Reference Guide to the Diagnosis and Management of Neurosurgical Problems. 3rd Ed. Philadelphia, W.B. Saunders Co., 1990
- Carter LP, Spetzler RF, eds. Neurovascular Surgery. New York, McGraw-Hill, 1995

Web references: 0 available at www.5mcc.com

Illustrations N/A

Author(s):
L. Philip Carter, MD

Subclavian steal syndrome

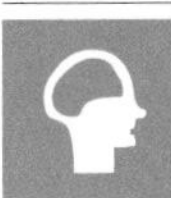

BASICS

DESCRIPTION Origin of the subclavian artery becomes compromised causing a reversal of flow in the branches of the first portion of the subclavian artery as a means of supplying blood to the upper extremity, especially during exercise. This may result in symptoms of vertebral-basilar insufficiency.

System(s) affected: Cardiovascular, Musculoskeletal, Nervous

Genetics: N/A

Incidence/Prevalence in USA:
- 17% incidence (only 2.5% with angiographic steal documented)
- 70% are left subclavian

Predominant age:
- > 55 years - atherosclerotic etiology
- <30 years - 90% of Takayasu arteritis

Predominant sex: Male > Female (2:1)

SIGNS & SYMPTOMS
- Most common - vertigo or presyncope following upper extremity exercise. The reversal of flow down the ipsilateral vertebral artery results in a relative vertebral-basilar insufficiency
- Less common - weakness and clumsiness of an extremity, loss of vision, homonymous hemianopsia, ataxia and drop attacks
- Arm claudication following minimal exercise.
- Reduced blood pressure of > 20 mm Hg in involved arm
- Symptoms should be reproducible by exercising the arm

CAUSES
- Arteriosclerosis obliterans of the proximal subclavian artery in 95% of cases
- Less common causes of obstruction: dissecting aneurysm of aortic arch, trauma, embolus and Takayasu arteritis

RISK FACTORS
- Smoking
- Hypertension
- Diabetes
- Hyperlipidemia

DIAGNOSIS

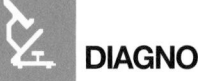

DIFFERENTIAL DIAGNOSIS
- Intracranial vascular disease
- Carotid artery disease
- Vertebral artery disease
- Brain tumor
- Subdural hematoma

LABORATORY
- Noninvasive measurement of blood pressure in upper extremities
- Arteriogram of arch vessels with delayed films of vertebral arteries
- ESR elevated, CBC (thrombocytosis), ECG (ischemic pattern), and chest X-ray (widening of thoracic aorta) if Takayasu arteritis is suspected

Drugs that may alter lab results:
- Prednisone

Disorders that may alter lab results: N/A

PATHOLOGICAL FINDINGS
- Absent or diminished pulses in ipsilateral arm
- Reduced blood pressure (> 20 mm Hg) (> 2.7 kPa) when compared to contralateral arm

SPECIAL TESTS Pulse volume recording of upper extremities

IMAGING
- Duplex scanning of extracranial vessels
- Arteriography

DIAGNOSTIC PROCEDURES Arteriography

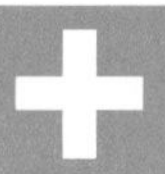

TREATMENT

APPROPRIATE HEALTH CARE Outpatient unless vascular surgery anticipated

GENERAL MEASURES Reduce cholesterol levels, if appropriate, with diet or medication

SURGICAL MEASURES
- Carotid-subclavian bypass
- Balloon angioplasty
- Stent insertion

ACTIVITY Reduced exercise of arms

DIET Low cholesterol diet, if appropriate

PATIENT EDUCATION
- Prevent injury to arm
- Reduce exercise to arm

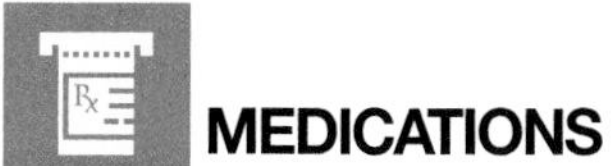

MEDICATIONS

DRUG(S) OF CHOICE None
Contraindications: N/A
Precautions: N/A
Significant possible interactions: N/A

ALTERNATIVE DRUGS N/A

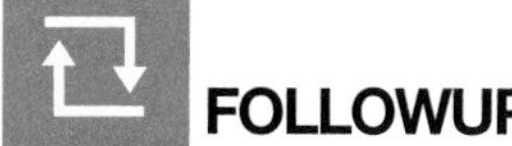

FOLLOWUP

PATIENT MONITORING Annual physical to include blood pressure in both arms

PREVENTION/AVOIDANCE N/A

POSSIBLE COMPLICATIONS Completed stroke

EXPECTED COURSE/PROGNOSIS
Good

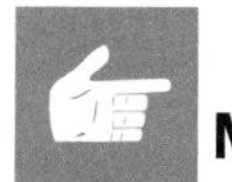

MISCELLANEOUS

ASSOCIATED CONDITIONS
- Carotid artery disease
- Heart disease
- Arteriosclerosis

AGE-RELATED FACTORS
Pediatric: N/A
Geriatric: Older patient more likely to have arteriosclerosis
Others: Younger patients affected if condition secondary to Takayasu arteritis

PREGNANCY N/A

SYNONYMS N/A

ICD-9-CM
435.2 Subclavian steal syndrome

SEE ALSO
Arteriosclerosis obliterans
Takayasu syndrome

OTHER NOTES N/A

ABBREVIATIONS
ESR = erythrocyte sedimentation rate
CBC = complete blood count
ECG = electrocardiogram

REFERENCES

- Rutherford RB: Vascular Surgery. 5th ed. Philadelphia, W.B. Saunders Co., 1999
- Sabiston DC Jr: Essentials of Surgery. Philadelphia, W.B. Saunders Co., 1987

Web references: 1 available at www.5mcc.com
Illustrations N/A

Author(s):
Aaron T. Yu, MD

BASICS

DESCRIPTION The accumulation of blood in the subdural space

- Acute subdural hematoma: The most severe form, usually the result of trauma involving acceleration or deceleration head injury and commonly associated with parenchymal brain injury. Hematoma age is three days or less.
- Chronic subdural hematoma: Often the result of trivial head injury in older patients, one-fourth to one-half have no history of head trauma. Hematoma is classically older than three weeks and is associated with an encapsulating membrane.
- Subacute subdural hematoma: Appearing 4-21 days from maturation of acute subdural hematoma

System(s) affected: Cardiovascular, Nervous

Genetics: N/A

Incidence/Prevalence in USA:

- Acute subdural hematoma: 1-2/100,000
- Chronic subdural hematoma: 1-2/100,000
- Acute subdural hematoma in newborn infants and children are relatively infrequent, occurring approximately 25% as often as in adults. Chronic subdural hematomas occur in children of all ages. However, chronic subdural hematomas present a peak incidence at about 6 months and rarely, after 1 year of age.

Predominant age:

- Acute subdural hematoma - < age 60 years
- Chronic subdural hematoma - > age 50 years

Predominant sex: Male > Female

SIGNS & SYMPTOMS

- Acute subdural hematoma:
  - ◊ Altered level of consciousness 99%
  - ◊ Pupillary irregularity (usually it is unilateral to hematoma) 47-53%
  - ◊ Hemiparesis (usually contralateral to hematoma) 34-47%
  - ◊ Decerebrate posturing or flaccid motor exam 47%
  - ◊ Papilledema 16%
  - ◊ Cranial nerve VI palsy 5%
- Chronic subdural hematoma:
  - ◊ Impaired consciousness 53%
  - ◊ Hemiparesis 45%
  - ◊ Papilledema 24%
  - ◊ Cranial nerve III abnormality 11%
  - ◊ Hemianopsia 7%
  - ◊ Infants often present with an accelerated increase in head size with or

without irritability, poor feeding, occasional vomiting or tension of the anterior fontanelle (60% of cases).

  - ◊ Infants may present with seizures

CAUSES

- Acute subdural hematoma
  - ◊ High velocity acceleration or deceleration head injury resulting in tearing of the bridging veins between cerebral cortex and the dural venous sinuses
  - ◊ Injury to surface of brain with bleeding from injured cortical vessels
- Chronic subdural hematoma
  - ◊ Often from a trivial head injury in adults. In children, may be caused by

unrecognized/unreported trauma, abuse, or rarely birth trauma.

  - ◊ A balance between recurrent bleeding from the hematoma membrane and

resorption determines the ultimate size of the hematoma

RISK FACTORS

- Acute subdural hematoma
  - ◊ 5-22% of severe head trauma
  - ◊ High velocity acceleration or deceleration head injury (motor vehicle accidents, falls, blunt head trauma)
  - ◊ Suspected non-accidental trauma (SNAT) in infants
- Chronic subdural hematoma
  - ◊ Chronic alcoholism
  - ◊ Epilepsy
  - ◊ Coagulopathy/anticoagulation therapy
  - ◊ Cerebral spinal fluid shunt for hydrocephalus
  - ◊ Rarely metastatic carcinoma to subdural space

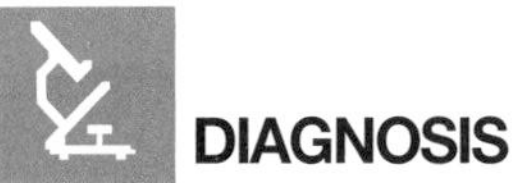

DIAGNOSIS

DIFFERENTIAL DIAGNOSIS

- Acute subdural hematoma and other forms of intracranial hematoma (epidural hematoma, cerebral contusion/hematoma)
- Chronic subdural hematoma
- Dementia
- Stroke
- Transient ischemic attack
- Brain tumor
- Subdural empyema
- Meningitis

LABORATORY

- Acute subdural hematoma - consumptive coagulopathy due to underlying parenchymal injury diagnosed with elevated PT and PTT, elevated fibrin degradation products, decreased fibrinogen, decreased platelet level, and extended bleeding time
- Chronic subdural hematoma - predisposing factors such as coagulopathy or anticoagulation therapy producing appropriate abnormalities in bleeding time or coagulation parameters. Subtherapeutic anticonvulsant levels in patients with epilepsy. Serum ethanol level in alcoholics.

Drugs that may alter lab results: Anticoagulants (e.g., warfarin)

Disorders that may alter lab results: DIC and other coagulopathies (e.g., hemophilia)

PATHOLOGICAL FINDINGS

- Acute subdural hematoma - this is a fresh hemorrhage
- Chronic subdural hematoma - there is a liquefied hematoma, an outer membrane beneath the dura after one week, and an inner membrane between the hematoma and arachnoid after three weeks. Cytology examination may reveal metastatic carcinoma cells on rare occasions to be associated with the hemorrhage.

SPECIAL TESTS EEG for seizures and intensive care consisting of continuous cardiac monitoring often in conjunction with continuous monitoring of intra-arterial pressure and intracranial pressure (ventriculostomy or intraparenchymal or subdural pressure monitoring probe)

IMAGING

- Acute subdural hematoma - the imaging study of choice is the CT head scan (with intravascular contrast if hemoglobin is less than or equal to 9 gm/dQ. Axial view demonstrates a hyperdense, cresenteric, extra-axial collection usually adjacent to inner table.
- Chronic subdural hematoma - a CT head scan is also preferred. Usually

hematomas evolve from isodense to hypodense by three weeks. A MRI head scan is often necessary for hematomas isodense with brain due to the mixture of chronic hematoma with recurrent hemorrhage.

DIAGNOSTIC PROCEDURES N/A

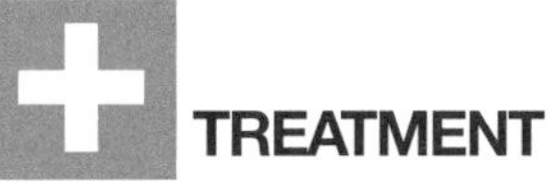

TREATMENT

APPROPRIATE HEALTH CARE Inpatient

GENERAL MEASURES

- Acute subdural hematoma
  - ◊ Medically, the management consists of controlling elevated intracranial pressure with osmotic and loop diuretics and hyperventilation to induce hypocapnia (PaCO2 of 22-28 mm Hg [2.9-3.7 kPa])
- Subacute subdural hematoma
  - ◊ Maintenance of adequate airway and ventilation and support of cardiovascular system to promote normal cerebral perfusion
  - ◊ Treatment of multi-system trauma and precautions for cervical and other spine injury

SURGICAL MEASURES

- Acute subdural hematoma
  - ◊ Emergent craniotomy is indicated for evacuation of hematomas causing significant mass effect
- Subacute subdural hematoma
  - ◊ If patient is neurologically stable, surgery may be delayed until hematoma matures and becomes chronic at which time a burr hole drainage can be performed
  - ◊ Subacute hematomas causing significant mass effect and neurological deficit may require craniotomy for evacuation
- Chronic subdural hematoma - burr hole drainage of hematoma. Some

neurosurgeons leave a catheter in the subdural space for 24 hours after the operation.

ACTIVITY
- Acute subdural hematoma - the patient will need the head of the bed elevated to reduce intracranial pressure and flexion of lower body avoided until thoracic, lumbar, or sacral spine injuries are ruled out. The patient should be maintained in a rigid cervical collar until the cervical spine is cleared radiographically.
- Chronic subdural hematoma - the head of the bed is flat and appropriate precautions are taken if a spinal injury is present

DIET
- Most patients with acute subdural hematoma require enteral or total parenteral nutrition initially
- Depending on level of consciousness, patients with chronic subdural hematoma can usually have the diet advanced to regular food as tolerated

PATIENT EDUCATION The National Institute of Neurological and Communicative Disorders and Stroke (NINDS), The National Institutes of Health, Bethesda, MD 20892

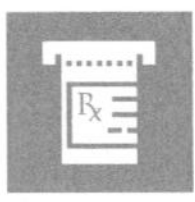

MEDICATIONS

DRUG(S) OF CHOICE
- Acute subdural hematoma:
  - ◊ Prior to surgical therapy, management of cerebral edema and elevated intracranial pressure may require mannitol 20% solution 0.5-1.0 gm/kg followed by 0.25-0.75 gm/kg every 4-6 hours. If a loop diuretic is used in conjunction with mannitol, furosemide (Lasix) 0.5 mg/kg IV is administered. Check serum osmolality every 8 hours and serum electrolytes at least daily. A 5% or 25% albumin preparation (Plasmanate) may be used either as a continuous or an intermittent infusion to augment osmotherapy as needed.
  - ◊ Seizure prophylaxis includes phenytoin (Dilantin) 1000 mg load (50 mg/min IV) with ECG monitoring followed by 100 mg IV every 8 hours or as needed to maintain therapeutic blood levels (10-20 μg/mL [40-79 μmol/L]). Dilantin therapy should be converted to the oral route as soon as possible to avoid cardiovascular complications of IV Dilantin administration.
  - ◊ In the chronic subdural hematoma, medical management alone is frequently unsuccessful and entails risks of neurological deterioration. When small and asymptomatic, however, it may be appropriate to treat such patients conservatively with observation as some chronic subdural hematomas have been known to resolve spontaneously. Steroids may be helpful in some patients, if not otherwise contraindicated.

Contraindications: Refer to manufacturer's literature

Precautions: Refer to manufacturer's literature

Significant possible interactions: Refer to manufacturer's literature

ALTERNATIVE DRUGS N/A

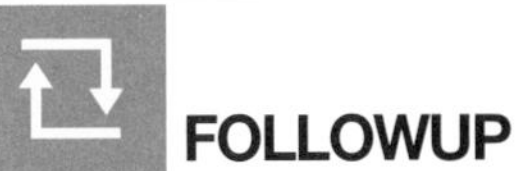

FOLLOWUP

PATIENT MONITORING
- Anticonvulsant levels should be checked approximately every 3-6 months after initiation
- Consider discontinuing anticonvulsant if patient has no seizures for at least one year
- EEG may be complimentary in the decision making process for discontinuation of anticonvulsants

PREVENTION/AVOIDANCE
- Acute subdural hematoma
  - ◊ Trauma prevention programs
- Chronic subdural hematoma
  - ◊ Alcoholism prevention
  - ◊ Medical and surgical management of epilepsy
  - ◊ Conservative use of anticoagulation therapy
  - ◊ Medium or high pressure ventriculoperitoneal shunt valves in at risk patients with hydrocephalus

POSSIBLE COMPLICATIONS
- Acute subdural hematoma - immediate postoperative complications include elevated intracranial pressure and brain edema, new or recurrent hematoma, infection, and seizures (in approximately one-third of cases)
- Chronic subdural hematoma - recurrent hematoma in up to 50% of cases (can be alleviated by the use of subdural drainage catheters), infection (subdural empyema, wound), and seizures in up to 10% of cases

EXPECTED COURSE/PROGNOSIS
- Acute subdural hematoma - mortality is greater then 50%. Significant neurological disability and impairment of function is seen in most surviving patients. Outcome highly dependent on presurgical neurological status. Seizure prophylaxis is usually required for at least one year.
- Chronic subdural hematoma - mortality is less than 10%. Most patients resume preoperative functional status. Outcome highly dependent on pre-surgical neurological status.

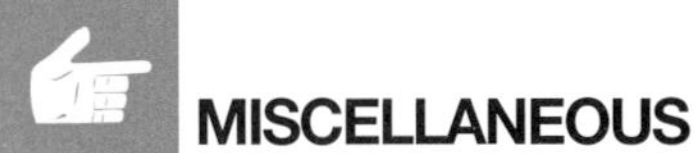

MISCELLANEOUS

ASSOCIATED CONDITIONS
- Acute subdural hematoma
  - ◊ Multi-system trauma
  - ◊ Cervical spinal cord injury
  - ◊ Injury to the thoracic, lumbar, or sacral spine
  - ◊ Disseminated intravascular coagulation
  - ◊ Epilepsy
- Chronic subdural hematoma
  - ◊ Alcoholism
  - ◊ Epilepsy
  - ◊ Coagulopathy
  - ◊ Cerebral spinal fluid shunt
  - ◊ Birth trauma
  - ◊ Child abuse
  - ◊ Rarely metastatic carcinoma

AGE-RELATED FACTORS
Pediatric: N/A

Geriatric:
- Cerebral atrophy is common and predisposes to subdural hematomas
- Insidious onset of symptoms may lead to misdiagnosis of dementia, tumor or depression

Others:
- Acute subdural hematoma - lower mortality in patients less than 40 years of age compared to those older then 40 years of age
- Chronic subdural hematoma - majority of patients are older than 50 years of age

PREGNANCY N/A

SYNONYMS Subdural hemorrhage

ICD-9-CM
852.30 Subdural hemorrhage following injury with open intracranial wound, unspecified state of consciousness

SEE ALSO

OTHER NOTES N/A

ABBREVIATIONS N/A

REFERENCES

- Francel PC, Park TS, Shaffrey ME, Jane JA. Diagnosis and treatment of moderate and severe head injuries in infants and children. In: Youmans JR, ed. Neurological surgery. 4th Ed. Philadelphia, W.B. Saunders, 1996 p1730-66
- Greenberg MS. Handbook of neurosurgery. 4th Ed. Florida, Greenberg Graphics, 1997
- Samudrala S, Cooper PR. Traumatic intracranial hematomas. In: Wilkins RH, Rengachary SS, eds. Neurosurgery. 2nd ed. New York, McGraw-Hill, 1996 p2797-807

Web references: 11 available at www.5mcc.com

Illustrations N/A

Author(s):

Oren N. Gottfried, MD

Martin E. Weinand, MD

BASICS

DESCRIPTION Any localized collection of pus below the diaphragm and in contact with the diaphragm
System(s) affected: Gastrointestinal, Pulmonary
Genetics: N/A
Incidence/Prevalence in USA: N/A
Predominant age: N/A
Predominant sex: N/A

SIGNS & SYMPTOMS
- High spiking fever with chills and sweating
- Abdominal tenderness
- Ileus
- Anterior abdominal wall erythema
- Abdominal pain
- Tachycardia
- Chest pain
- Nausea
- Dyspnea
- Localized tenderness on palpation
- Pleural effusion
- Elevation of diaphragm
- Shoulder pain
- Hiccups
- Tenderness when compressing lower ribs
- Rales at lung base

CAUSES
- Complications of abdominal surgery cause 50%
- Penetrating trauma
- Gastrointestinal perforations - appendicitis, diverticulitis
- Organisms: Escherichia, Streptococcus, Proteus, Klebsiella, Bacteroides fragilis, cocci, Clostridium

RISK FACTORS
- Operative procedure with significant contamination
- Patients with chronic disease - cirrhosis, renal failure, malnutrition
- Patients on corticosteroids, chemotherapy, radiotherapy
- Myelosuppression

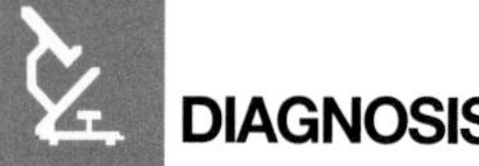

DIAGNOSIS

DIFFERENTIAL DIAGNOSIS
- Other intra-abdominal abscesses
- Empyema

LABORATORY
- White blood count
- Blood cultures
- Automated chemical profile

Drugs that may alter lab results: N/A

Disorders that may alter lab results: N/A

PATHOLOGICAL FINDINGS N/A

SPECIAL TESTS N/A

IMAGING
- CT scan
- Ultrasound
- Plain films of chest and abdomen display elevation and immobility of right diaphragm, fluid in right costophrenic sulcus; air-fluid level in subphrenic space
- Gallium scan

DIAGNOSTIC PROCEDURES CT or ultrasound directed aspiration

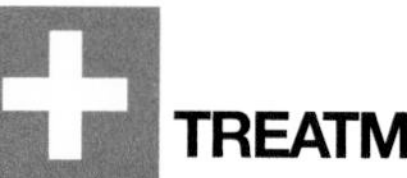

TREATMENT

APPROPRIATE HEALTH CARE Inpatient

GENERAL MEASURES
- Antibiotics
- Supportive care - nutrition, monitoring, oxygenation, hydration
- Swan-Ganz catheter if unstable
- Mechanical ventilation if necessary
- Vasopressors if indicated

SURGICAL MEASURES
- Adequate drainage of abscess - percutaneous and/or surgical
- Percutaneous drainage not advised if (1) abscess is multiloculated, (2) drainage route would traverse bowel, uncontaminated peritoneal or pleural space, (3) source of continued contamination still present, (4) fungal infection, (5) pus too viscous
- Surgical drainage mandated if patient fails to respond to percutaneous drainage in 24 to 48 hours

ACTIVITY As tolerated

DIET NPO until intestinal function returns

PATIENT EDUCATION N/A

MEDICATIONS

DRUG(S) OF CHOICE
Broad spectrum antibiotics based on culture and sensitivity
- Aminoglycosides (tobramycin or gentamicin) 1.5-2.0 mg/kg loading dose
- Amikacin 5-7.5 mg/kg loading dose (very expensive)
- Plus clindamycin 600 mg IV q6h,

or
- Metronidazole (Flagyl) loading dose 15 mg/kg and maintenance dose 7.5 mg/kg q6h

Contraindications: Known allergy to antibiotics
Precautions:
- Aminoglycosides are ototoxic and nephrotoxic - follow BUN, creatinine and serum blood levels (peak and trough)
- Prolong dosing interval to achieve appropriate trough level; especially in renal failure
- Adjust dose for desired peak level
- Dosage adjustments in renal failure not needed for metronidazole since it is metabolized by the liver

Significant possible interactions: N/A

ALTERNATIVE DRUGS
- Cefoxitin 2 gm IV q4-6h
- Cefoperazone 1-2 gm IV q12h
- Cefotaxime 1 gm IV q6-8h
- Mezlocillin 3 gm IV q4h

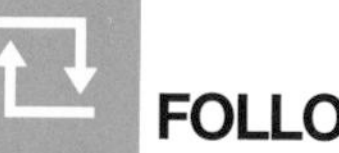

FOLLOWUP

PATIENT MONITORING
- Frequent evaluation after discharge up to six weeks
- White blood counts regularly
- Chest x-rays until normal

PREVENTION/AVOIDANCE N/A

POSSIBLE COMPLICATIONS
- Mortality - 10 to 90% if not adequately drained
- Multi-system organ failure
- Recurrent abscess
- Hemorrhage
- Bowel obstruction
- Wound dehiscence
- Continuing sepsis
- Pneumonia
- Pleural effusion
- Suppurative pylephlebitis

EXPECTED COURSE/PROGNOSIS
- Death if abscess is not adequately drained or patient vigorously supported

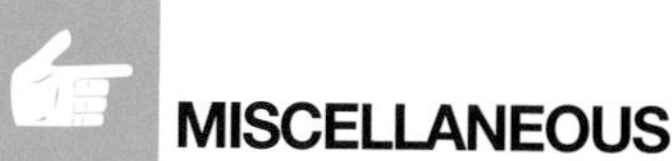

MISCELLANEOUS

ASSOCIATED CONDITIONS
- Multi-system organ failure
- Systemic sepsis
- Fistula

AGE-RELATED FACTORS
Pediatric: N/A
Geriatric: Worse prognosis
Others: N/A

PREGNANCY N/A

SYNONYMS Subdiaphragmatic abscess

ICD-9-CM
998.59 Other postoperative infection

SEE ALSO

OTHER NOTES N/A

ABBREVIATIONS N/A

REFERENCES

- Hau T, et al: Diagnosis and Treatment of Abdominal Abscesses, Current Problems in Surgery, Vol. XXI No. 7, Chicago, Year Book Medical Publishers, 1984

Web references: 0 available at www.5mcc.com
Illustrations N/A

Author(s):
Gary B. Williams, MD

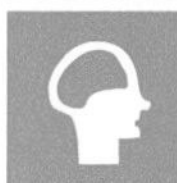

BASICS

DESCRIPTION
- Any pattern of substance use causing significant physical, mental, or social dysfunction
- Substances of abuse include:
  - ◊ Alcohol
  - ◊ Amphetamines (black beauties, truck drivers, hearts, uppers, speed)
  - ◊ Anabolic steroids (nandrolone [Durabolin], oxandrolone); testosterone (Depo-testosterone)
  - ◊ Barbiturates (barbs, red birds, yellow jackets)
  - ◊ Benzodiazepines (downers, candy, tranks, Xanax)
  - ◊ Cannabinoids: hashish, marijuana (dope, grass, joint, pot, reefer, sinsemilla, weed)
  - ◊ Cocaine (coke, crack, blow, rocks, snow)
  - ◊ Codeine (Cody, school boy)
  - ◊ Fentanyl (Apache, China girl, dance fever, jackpot, TNT)
  - ◊ Flunitrazepam (Rohypnol, Mexican Valium, roofies)
  - ◊ Gamma-hydroxybutyrate (GHB, liquid ecstasy, woman's Viagra)
  - ◊ Heroin (diacetylmorphine; horse, junk, smack, white horse, brown sugar)
  - ◊ Inhalants (gasoline, glue, paint thinners, nitrous oxide)
  - ◊ Ketamine (cat Valium, Special K, Vitamin K, Kit-Kat)
  - ◊ Lysergic acid diethylamide (LSD; acid, microdot, cubes, yellow sunshine)
  - ◊ Mescaline, psilocybin (cactus, mushrooms, peyote)
  - ◊ Methadone (Methadose)
  - ◊ Methamphetamines (crank, crystal, ice, fire, speed; and "designer drugs": Adam, clarity, ecstasy, Eve, MDMA, XTC, lover's speed)
  - ◊ Methaqualone (Quaalude, mandrex)
  - ◊ Methylphenidate (Ritalin, JIF, Skippy, MPH)
  - ◊ Morphine (M, Miss Emma, monkey, white stuff)
  - ◊ Nicotine (tobacco)
  - ◊ Opium (Paregoric, big O, block)
  - ◊ Oxycodone, hydrocodone, hydromorphone, meperidine, propoxyphene
  - ◊ Phencyclidine (PCP; angel dust, hog, love boat, peace pill, supergrass, ozone, wack)
- Substance abuse (DSM-IV criteria): A maladaptive pattern of substance use manifested by one (or more) of the following:
  - ◊ Failure to fulfill major obligations at work, at school, or home
  - ◊ Recurrent use in hazardous situations
  - ◊ Recurrent substance-related legal problems
  - ◊ Continued substance use despite substance-related social or interpersonal problems
- Substance dependence (DSM-IV criteria): A maladaptive pattern of substance use manifested by 3 (or more) of the following:
  - ◊ Tolerance
  - ◊ Withdrawal
  - ◊ Using the substance more than intended
  - ◊ Persistent desire or attempts to cut down or to stop
  - ◊ Much time is spent obtaining, using, or recovering from the substance
  - ◊ Social, occupational or recreational activities are sacrificed for substance use
  - ◊ Continued use despite substance-related physical or psychological problems

System(s) affected: Cardiovascular, Endocrine/Metabolic, Nervous

Genetics: The dopamine system in the ventral tegmental area of the brain is activated during the use of virtually all drugs of abuse. Substances of abuse affect dopamine, acetylcholine, GABA, norepinephrine, opioid, and serotonin receptors. Variant alleles of these receptors probably account for interpersonal differences in susceptibility to substance use disorders.

Incidence/Prevalence in USA:
- 36% have used illicit drug at least once
- 14.0 million or 6.3% (10.4-25.4% for ages 12-17) have used in past month
- 1 in 6 males ages 18-25 currently use marijuana

Predominant age: 16-25

Predominant sex: Male > Female

SIGNS & SYMPTOMS
- History of infections, e.g., endocarditis, hepatitis B or C, tuberculosis, sexually transmitted diseases, or recurrent pneumonia
- Social or behavioral problems, including chaotic relationships and/or employment
- Frequent visits to emergency department
- Criminal incarceration
- History of blackouts or morning tremor, insomnia, mood swings, chronic pain, repetitive trauma
- Dilated or constricted pupils, reduced pupillary response to light
- Needle marks on skin
- Perforation of the nasal septum (with cocaine use)
- Cardiac dysrhythmias, pathologic murmurs,
- Anxiety, fatigue, depression, psychosis
- Sexual assault with GHB, Rohypnol

CAUSES
Multifactorial including genetic, environmental

RISK FACTORS
- Male gender, young adult
- Depression, anxiety
- Other substance use disorders
- Family history
- Peer or family use or approval
- Low socioeconomic status
- Unemployment
- Accessibility of substances of abuse
- Family dysfunction or trauma
- Antisocial personality disorder
- Academic problems, school dropout
- Criminal involvement

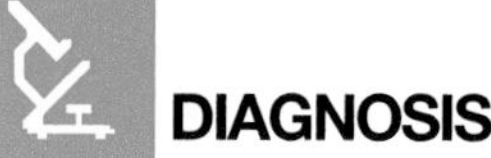

DIAGNOSIS

DIFFERENTIAL DIAGNOSIS
- Delirium, agitation
- Depression, anxiety, or other mental states
- Metabolic causes of altered mental status (hypoxia, hypoglycemia, infection, thiamine deficiency, hypothyroidism, thyrotoxicosis)
- Medication interactions or side effects

LABORATORY
- Blood alcohol concentration
- Urine drug screen, confirmatory tests
- Approximate detection limits:
  - ◊ Alcohol: 6-10 hours
  - ◊ Amphetamines and variants: 2-3 days
  - ◊ Barbiturates: 2-10 days
  - ◊ Benzodiazepines: 1-6 weeks
  - ◊ Cocaine: 2-3 days
  - ◊ Heroin: 1-1.5 days
  - ◊ LSD, psilocybin: 8 hours
  - ◊ Marijuana: 1 day - 4 weeks
  - ◊ Methadone: 1 day - 1 week
  - ◊ Opioids: 1-3 days
  - ◊ PCP: 7-14 days
  - ◊ Anabolic steroids: oral = 3 weeks, injectable = 3 months, nandrolone = 9 months
- For altered mental status consider CBC, glucose, chemistry panel, TSH, T4, RPR, UA, Head CT scan, CXR, EKG, lumbar puncture, pulse oximetry/ABG, blood cultures
- HIV, Hepatitis B and C screens

Drugs that may alter lab results: N/A

Disorders that may alter lab results: N/A

PATHOLOGICAL FINDINGS
N/A

SPECIAL TESTS
- History (often unreliable) and physical; substance abuse screening tests
- CAGE questionnaire (used for alcoholism)
  - ◊ Have you ever felt you should cut down on your drinking?
  - ◊ Have people annoyed you by criticizing your drinking?
  - ◊ Have you ever felt bad or guilty about your drinking?
  - ◊ Have you ever had a drink first thing in the morning to steady your nerves or to get rid of a hangover (eye-opener)?

More than 2 "yes" answers is 74-89% sensitive, 79-95% specific for alcohol use disorder; less sensitive for early problem drinking or heavy drinking

- Rost, et al screening:
  - ◊ Have you misused one of these substances (see DESCRIPTION) more than 5 times in your life?
  - ◊ Have you ever found that you needed to increase your use of a substance in order to get the same effect?
  - ◊ Have you ever had emotional or psychological problems from using drugs - like feeling crazy or paranoid or uninterested in things?

IMAGING
Echocardiography for endocarditis

DIAGNOSTIC PROCEDURES
N/A

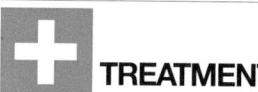

TREATMENT

APPROPRIATE HEALTH CARE
- Outpatient usually by individual physicians or substance abuse clinics
- Inpatient for medical comorbidities, history of severe withdrawal such as seizures, disorientation, threat of harm to self or others

GENERAL MEASURES
- Behavioral and cognitive therapy
- Community reinforcement
- Interventional counseling
- Nonjudgmental, medically-oriented attitude
- Self-help groups to aid recovery (Alcoholic Anonymous, other 12 step programs)
- Support groups for family members (Al-Anon and Alateen)
- Monitoring for infectious diseases and other complications

SURGICAL MEASURES N/A

ACTIVITY
Unrestricted - unless suicidal, homicidal, psychotic, disoriented, or otherwise incompetent

DIET
Patients often malnourished; emphasize good nutrition

PATIENT EDUCATION
- National Clearinghouse for Alcohol and Drug Information: (800) 729-6686 or http://www.health.org
- Center for Substance Abuse Treatment: 800-662-HELP
- National families in Action (404)248-9676 or http://www.nationalfamilies.org
- Alcoholics Anonymous: literature, crisis hot line, from local chapter or http://www.alcoholics-anonymous.org
- Cocaine Anonymous
- Narcotics Anonymous
- Rational Recovery
- Secular Organizations for Sobriety

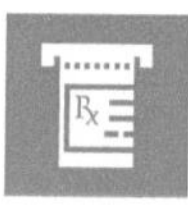

MEDICATIONS

DRUG(S) OF CHOICE
- Methadone - 15-20 mg PO qd (max 120 mg) only in specially licensed clinics (or when hospitalized) for detoxification and maintenance therapy for opioid (e.g., heroin) dependence
- L-alpha-acetylmethadol (LAAM) - also for opioid therapy, longer acting than methadone, given 3 times weekly
- Naltrexone (ReVia) - 50 mg PO qd; or 100 mg Mon, Wed + 150 mg Fri; blocks opioid euphoria and reduces craving for alcohol
- Clonidine 0.1-0.2 mg PO q4-6 hrs or transdermal patch for opioid withdrawal
- Valproic acid, carbamazepine - useful for benzodiazepine taper, withdrawal
- Bupropion 150 mg PO bid, nicotine replacement systems (patches, gum) to aid in smoking cessation
- Buprenorphine 300 mcg IM q 4 hr prn to alleviate opiate withdrawal symptoms
- Buspirone 5-15 mg PO bid or imipramine 25-75 mg PO bid to help discontinuation of long-term benzodiazepine use
- Adjuncts to therapy:
  - ◊ Thiamine 100 mg IV for presenting alcohol use disorder or depressed mental status of unknown cause
  - ◊ Fluoxetine, nefazodone - for comorbid depressive states, may decrease metabolism rate of benzodiazepines and valproic acid
  - ◊ Lithium - for comorbid bipolar affective states
  - ◊ Non-benzodiazepine anxiolytics, sedatives (hydroxyzine, diphenhydramine, trazodone, imipramine, amitriptyline, buspirone)
  - ◊ Use all medications in conjunction with psychosocial, behavioral interventions

Contraindications: Naltrexone - pregnancy, hepatic failure, acute hepatitis
Precautions: Clonidine may cause hypotension
Significant possible interactions: Naltrexone - opioid medications (naltrexone will precipitate or exacerbate withdrawal symptoms)

ALTERNATIVE DRUGS
None approved for cocaine or other stimulants

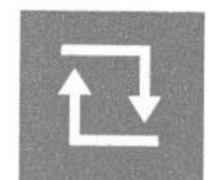

FOLLOWUP

PATIENT MONITORING
- Verify patient's compliance with the substance abuse treatment program
- Following treatment, follow-up on medical issues and provide support for continued abstinence

PREVENTION/AVOIDANCE
- Reduce risks through education
- Early identification and aggressive early intervention (mild substance use disorders respond better to treatment intervention)

POSSIBLE COMPLICATIONS
- Hepatitis, HIV, tuberculosis
- Subacute bacterial endocarditis
- Many other infectious diseases
- Malnutrition
- Social problems including arrest
- Poor marital adjustment and violence
- Depression, schizophrenia
- Serious harm to self and others
- Sexual assault with GHB, Rohypnol
- Overdoses resulting in seizures, arrhythmias, cardiac and respiratory arrest, coma, death

EXPECTED COURSE/PROGNOSIS
- Success rates vary widely
- Patients who stay in treatment for longer periods of time (at least a year) have a higher success rate
- Counseling combined with drug therapy appears to be more successful than either one alone

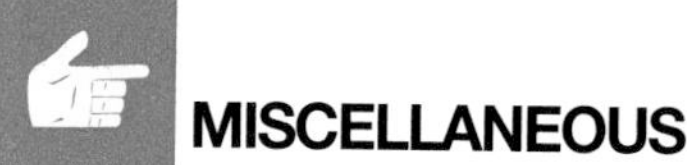

MISCELLANEOUS

ASSOCIATED CONDITIONS
- Depression
- Personality disorders
- Bipolar affective disorder

AGE-RELATED FACTORS
Pediatric: 10.4-25.4% ages 12-17 reported use in the past month
Geriatric: Alcohol, prescription drug interactions
Others: N/A

PREGNANCY
Substance abuse may cause major problems that can lead to fetal abnormality, morbidity, and death of infant and mother

SYNONYMS
- Drug abuse
- Drug dependence
- Substance abuse

ICD-9-CM
304.00 Opioid type dependence, unspecified
304.10 Barbiturate and similarly acting sedative or hypnotic dependence, unspecified
304.20 Cocaine dependence, unspecified
305.20 Cannabis abuse, unspecified
305.40 Barbiturate and similarly acting sedative or hypnotic abuse, unspecified
305.50 Opioid abuse, unspecified
305.60 Cocaine abuse, unspecified

SEE ALSO
Alcohol use disorders

OTHER NOTES N/A

ABBREVIATIONS
DSM-IV = Diagnostic and Statistical Manual of Mental Disorders, 4th edition

REFERENCES

- National Institute on Drug Abuse: The Sixth Triennial Report to Congress: Drug Abuse and Addiction Research. DHHS, 1999
- National Institute on Drug Abuse: Principles of Drug Addiction Treatment: A Research-Based Guide. DHHS, 1999
- The National Household Survey on Drug Abuse. Substance Abuse and Mental Health Services Administration, DHHS, 2000
- Kosten TR, O'Connor PG. Management of drug and alcohol withdrawal. N Engl J Med 2003;348(18):1786-95

Web references: 3 available at www.5mcc.com
Illustrations 1 available

Author(s):
S. Lindsey Clarke, MD

BASICS

DESCRIPTION The sudden death of an infant under one year of age which remains unexplained after a thorough case investigation, including performance of a complete autopsy, examination of the death scene, and review of the clinical history. SIDS was first formally defined in 1969 and the definition was revised in 1989.

System(s) affected: Cardiovascular, Endocrine/Metabolic, Nervous, Pulmonary

Genetics: Emerging evidence for genetic risk factors, especially related to impaired brainstem regulation of breathing or other autonomic control

Incidence/Prevalence in USA: (for 2001)
- All races: 0.56/1000 live births (2,236 cases/yr)
- White non-Hispanic: 0.53/1000 live births (1,221 cases/yr)
- Black non-Hispanic: 1.14/1000 live births (688 cases/yr)
- Hispanic: 0.27/1000 live births (232 cases/yr)
- Native American: 1.46/1000 live births (61 cases/yr)

Predominant age: Uncommon in first month of life, peak occurs in infants between 2 and 4 months, 80% of deaths occur by 6 months

Predominant sex: Males > Females (52-60% of SIDS cases are males)

SIGNS & SYMPTOMS These babies generally appear healthy, or may have had a minor upper respiratory or gastrointestinal infection in the last 2 weeks of life

CAUSES
- There are many theories about the cause of SIDS. There may be subtle developmental abnormalities resulting from pre- and/or perinatal brain injury.
- Possible causes:
  - ◊ Abnormalities in respiratory control and arousal responsiveness
  - ◊ Central and peripheral nervous system abnormalities
  - ◊ Cardiac arrhythmias
  - ◊ Rebreathing in face down position on soft surface leading to hypoxia and hypercarbia
  - ◊ SIDS may occur when one or more environmental risk factors interact with one or more genetic risk factors

RISK FACTORS
- Most SIDS deaths occur in children who are "low-risk." However, there are several risk factors associated with SIDS:
  - ◊ Race: Native Americans and African Americans have highest incidence
  - ◊ Season - late fall and winter months
  - ◊ Time of day - between midnight and 6 AM
  - ◊ Activity - during sleep
  - ◊ Low birth weight; intrauterine growth retardation (IUGR)
  - ◊ Poverty
- Maternal factors: decreased age, decreased education, maternal use of cigarettes or drugs (cocaine, opiates) during pregnancy, higher parity, inadequate prenatal care
- Respiratory or gastrointestinal infection in recent past
- Sleep practices - prone and side sleep position, heavier clothing and bedding, soft bedding
- Passive cigarette smoke exposure after birth
- No pacifier use

DIAGNOSIS

DIFFERENTIAL DIAGNOSIS
- Suffocation
- Abnormalities of fatty acid metabolism (e.g., deficiency of medium-chain acyl-CoA dehydrogenase, or of carnitine)
- Homicide
- Dehydration/electrolyte disturbance

LABORATORY
- Pneumocardiograms have been abandoned in the workup
- Postmortem laboratory tests are done to rule out other cause of death (e.g., electrolytes to rule out dehydration and electrolyte imbalance). In SIDS, there are no consistently abnormal laboratory tests.

Drugs that may alter lab results: N/A

Disorders that may alter lab results: N/A

PATHOLOGICAL FINDINGS
- Characteristic findings on postmortem examination:
  - ◊ Frothy discharge, sometimes blood-tinged, from nostrils and mouth in majority
  - ◊ Petechiae on surface of lungs, heart and thymus gland in 50-85% (but not unique to SIDS)
  - ◊ Pulmonary congestion and edema often present
  - ◊ Morphologic markers of hypoxia: Increased gliosis in brain stem, retention of periadrenal brown fat, and hematopoiesis in the liver - present to varying degrees, not confirmed by all studies

SPECIAL TESTS N/A

IMAGING X-rays are taken to rule out possible child abuse

DIAGNOSTIC PROCEDURES
- Because the diagnosis of SIDS is often one of "exclusion," it is crucial to do a thorough death scene investigation and case review, in addition to the autopsy and lab tests

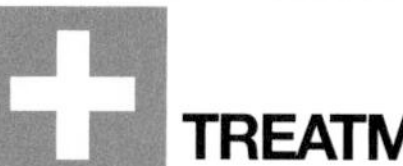

TREATMENT

APPROPRIATE HEALTH CARE
- Because a SIDS death is sudden and the cause is unknown, SIDS cannot be "treated." However, there are some measures that may be effective in reducing the risk of SIDS:
  - ◊ Maternal avoidance of cigarette and illicit drug use during pregnancy
  - ◊ Avoidance of the prone and side sleep position, excessive bed clothing and soft bedding, such as pillows, comforters, or soft mattress
  - ◊ Avoidance of passive cigarette smoke exposure
  - ◊ A crib conforming to federal safety standards is the most desirable sleeping location
  - ◊ Avoidance of bed-sharing with the infant, particularly adults other than the parent(s) or other children. Bed-sharing should be avoided if mother has used cigarettes, drugs or alcohol. Bed-sharing on couches is very dangerous and should never be done.
  - ◊ Infants who sleep in the same room as their parents (without bed-sharing) have a lower risk of SIDS
- Studies from U.S., Europe, Australia and New Zealand indicate significant SIDS rate reductions with reductions in prone sleep position. Because infants placed on their side may turn during sleep to the prone position, it is now believed that back position is best.
- It is critical that all people caring for infants, including day care providers, be instructed in these risk reduction measures

GENERAL MEASURES N/A

SURGICAL MEASURES N/A

ACTIVITY N/A

DIET N/A

PATIENT EDUCATION
- Family counseling (see Expected Course/Prognosis))
- SIDS Alliance, Baltimore, MD, (800)221-SIDS
- Back to Sleep Information Line, (800)505-CRIB (sponsored by the U.S. Public Health Service to provide information to parents and health providers about their recommendations to place infants on back, and general information about SIDS)
- National SIDS Resource Center, Vienna, VA, (703)902-1249
- SIDS Network, Ledyard, CT, (800)560-1454
- Association of SIDS and Infant Mortality Programs, Baltimore, MD, (410)706-5062

MEDICATIONS

DRUG(S) OF CHOICE N/A
Contraindications: N/A
Precautions: N/A
Significant possible interactions: N/A

ALTERNATIVE DRUGS N/A

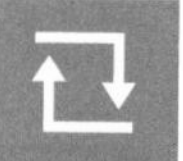

FOLLOWUP

PATIENT MONITORING Some authorities recommend cardiopulmonary monitoring in siblings of prior SIDS victims. There is no evidence that use of monitors prevents SIDS, and recent research calls this practice into question even more so.

PREVENTION/AVOIDANCE N/A

POSSIBLE COMPLICATIONS N/A

EXPECTED COURSE/PROGNOSIS
- SIDS deaths have a powerful impact on families and their functioning. Physicians play an important role in providing immediate information about SIDS and sensitive counseling to limit parents' misinformation and feelings of guilt.
- Counseling needs of families vary from short-term to long-term; support groups are helpful to many couples. Physicians need to be familiar with resources available in their communities to help families mourning a SIDS death. Parents need to be counseled about subsequent pregnancies. They need to be advised of the most current recommendations regarding sleep position and other infant care practices during subsequent pregnancies.
- Follow-up counseling, including review of the autopsy report with the family after some time has passed, will be important to help with understanding this condition and to alleviate the tremendous guilt these families experience.

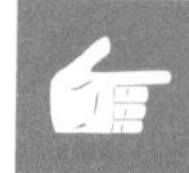

MISCELLANEOUS

ASSOCIATED CONDITIONS N/A

AGE-RELATED FACTORS N/A
Pediatric: Occurs in infants only
Geriatric: N/A
Others: N/A

PREGNANCY N/A

SYNONYMS
- Crib death
- Cot death

ICD-9-CM
798.0 Sudden infant death syndrome

SEE ALSO

OTHER NOTES N/A

ABBREVIATIONS N/A

REFERENCES

- Hauck FR, Hunt CE. Sudden infant death syndrome in 2000. Curr Probl Pediatr 2000;30:241-61
- Horchler JN, Morris RR. The SIDS and Infant Death Survival Guide. Information and Comfort for Grieving Family and Friends and Professionals Who Seek to Help Them. Hyattsville, MD: SIDS Educational Services; 2003
- Willinger M, James LS, Catz C. Defining the sudden infant death syndrome (SIDS): Deliberations of an expert panel convened by the National Institute of Child Health and Human Development. Pediatr Pathol 1991;11:677-84
- Byard RW, Krous HF, editors. Sudden Infant Death Syndrome - Problems, Progress and Possibilities, London: Arnold; 2001
- Changing concepts of sudden infant death syndrome: implications for infant sleeping environment and sleep position. American Academy of Pediatrics. Task Force on Infant Sleep Position and Sudden Infant Death Syndrome. Pediatrics 2000;105(3 Pt 1):650-6
- American Academy of Pediatrics, Committee on Fetus and Newborn. Apnea, sudden infant death syndrome, and home monitoring. Pediatrics 2003;111:914-17

Web references: 7 available at www.5mcc.com
Illustrations N/A

Author(s):
Fern R. Hauck, MD, MS

BASICS

DESCRIPTION Completed suicide refers to self-inflicted death. Attempted suicide refers to potentially lethal acts which do not result in death and non-lethal, attention-seeking gestures (e.g., superficial cuts on wrists).

System(s) affected: Nervous
Genetics: No known genetic pattern
Incidence/Prevalence in USA:
- 10-12 in 100,000. Ninth leading cause of death in US adults. Second leading cause of death among children and adolescents.
- Approximately 28,000 completed suicides yearly in US accounting for 2% of all deaths
- Attempted suicide is ten times more frequent than completed suicides
- Subpopulation incidence
  - ◊ Ages 5-14 - 8/100,000
  - ◊ Ages 15-24 - 13.1/100,000

Predominant age: Highest in elderly (> 65 years) and adolescent age period (15-24 years)
Predominant sex:
- Male > Female - complete suicide (3:1)
- Female > Male - attempted suicide (3:1)

SIGNS & SYMPTOMS
- Hopelessness about future
- Suicidal thoughts with organized plan and intent
  - ◊ Suicide note
  - ◊ Giving away personal possessions
  - ◊ Quitting a job
- Major depression (screen for symptoms)
  - ◊ Change in sleep
  - ◊ Loss of interest
  - ◊ Loss of energy
  - ◊ Loss of concentration
  - ◊ Loss of appetite
  - ◊ Diminished psychomotor activity
  - ◊ Guilt
  - ◊ Suicidal ideations
- Psychosis
  - ◊ Ask about command auditory hallucinations to kill oneself

CAUSES
- Combination of psychiatric illness and social circumstances. Most patients have active psychiatric illness.
- Major depression and bipolar disorder account for 50% of completed suicides
- Alcoholism and drug abuse disorders account for 25% of completed suicides
- Schizophrenia and other psychotic disorders account for 10% of completed suicides

RISK FACTORS
- Psychiatric
  - ◊ Mood disorders (major depression, bipolar), alcoholism, drug abuse, psychotic disorders, personality disorders
  - ◊ Family history of suicide
  - ◊ History of previous suicide attempt
  - ◊ Medical diagnosis of terminal illness (cancer, AIDS), chronic intractable pain, chronic and disabling illness (renal dialysis patient)
  - ◊ Hopelessness about future
- Epidemiologic
  - ◊ Sex - males three times females
  - ◊ Age - adolescent and geriatric population (males peaking at 75 years, females peaking at 55 years)
  - ◊ Race - American Indian, Caucasian
  - ◊ Marital status - single > divorced, widowed > married
- Psychologic
  - ◊ History of recent loss (loved one, job, etc.)
  - ◊ Loss of social supports
  - ◊ Important dates (holidays, birthdays, anniversaries, etc.)
- Review mnemonic for risk factors = SAD PERSONS
  - ◊ S = sex
  - ◊ A = age
  - ◊ D = depression
  - ◊ P = previous attempt
  - ◊ E = ethanol abuse
  - ◊ R = rational thinking loss
  - ◊ S = social support loss
  - ◊ O = organized plan
  - ◊ N = no spouse
  - ◊ S = sickness
  - ◊ If five risk factors present, consider very high suicidal risk

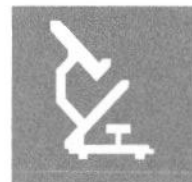

DIAGNOSIS

DIFFERENTIAL DIAGNOSIS
- Psychiatric
  - ◊ Mood disorders (major depression, bipolar)
  - ◊ Alcohol intoxication and other drug abuse
  - ◊ Psychotic disorders (e.g., schizophrenia)
  - ◊ Personality disorder (e.g., borderline)
  - ◊ Organic mental disorders (e.g., dementia, delirium)
  - ◊ Adjustment disorders
  - ◊ Panic disorders
  - ◊ Post-traumatic stress disorder
- Medical
  - ◊ Hypothyroidism
  - ◊ Cushing disease/syndrome
  - ◊ Addison disease
  - ◊ Hypopituitarism
- Other (medications associated with depression)
  - ◊ Antihypertensives (methyldopa, reserpine, clonidine)
  - ◊ Corticosteroids
  - ◊ Opiates
  - ◊ Anti-tuberculous agents (isoniazid, ethionamide, cycloserine)
  - ◊ Anabolic steroid withdrawal
  - ◊ Barbiturates
  - ◊ Benzodiazepines
  - ◊ Cocaine withdrawal
  - ◊ Amphetamine withdrawal

LABORATORY There are no laboratory tests to determine who will commit suicide. Patients who have completed violent suicides were found to have low CSF levels of 5-Hydroxyindoleacetic acid (5-HIAA), a serotonin metabolite. Other findings have included: increased CSF methoxyhydroxyphenylglycol (MHPG), nonsuppression of dexamethasone suppression test (DST), low platelet MAO (mono amine oxidase), low platelet serotonin, high platelet serotonin-2 receptor responsiveness.

Drugs that may alter lab results: N/A

Disorders that may alter lab results: N/A

PATHOLOGICAL FINDINGS Patients who have completed violent suicides were found to have low CSF levels of 5-Hydroxyindoleacetic acid (5-HIAA), a serotonin metabolite

SPECIAL TESTS N/A

IMAGING N/A

DIAGNOSTIC PROCEDURES N/A

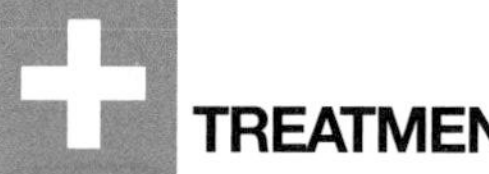

TREATMENT

APPROPRIATE HEALTH CARE
- Admit to psychiatric ward (voluntarily/involuntarily) if patient is severely depressed, intoxicated, psychotic or status post serious suicide attempt
- Admit to general hospital for acute medical care with psychiatric consultation
- Consider outpatient treatment with scheduled followup appointment if patient has social support system and no evidence of severe depression, psychosis or intoxication
- If unsure or patient is high risk (i.e., five positive risk factors - SAD PERSONS), admit to hospital for further observation and evaluation

GENERAL MEASURES
- All patients with suicide threats, gestures or attempts should be screened for suicide risk factors and have a full mental status exam and psychiatric consultation
- Ensure patient safety by least restrictive method (i.e., remove potentially dangerous objects, provide one-to-one constant observation, medication, 2-4 point restraints)
- Diagnose and treat underlying psychiatric and medical disorder
- Electroconvulsive therapy provides rapid, safe, and effective treatment option for severely depressed, acutely suicidal patients

SURGICAL MEASURES N/A

ACTIVITY Suicide precautions; q 15 minute checks; one-to-one observation; 2-4 point restraints

DIET N/A

PATIENT EDUCATION
- For a listing of sources for patient education materials favorably reviewed on this topic, physicians may contact: American Academy of Family Physicians Foundation, P.O. Box 8418, Kansas City, MO 64114, (800)274-2237, ext. 4400

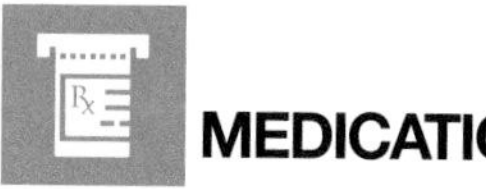

MEDICATIONS

DRUG(S) OF CHOICE
- Treat underlying psychiatric and medical illness
- Antidepressants, psychostimulants, carbamazepine, valproic acid, or lithium for mood disorders
- New generation antidepressants including selective serotonin reuptake inhibitors ([SSRIs], e.g., fluoxetine [Prozac], paroxetine [Paxil], sertraline [Zoloft]) and bupropion (Wellbutrin) and venlafaxine (Effexor) are less likely to be lethal with overdose attempts
- A minimum of two weeks required to obtain response from antidepressants
- Neuroleptic medications (e.g., haloperidol, risperidone, olanzapine) for psychotic symptoms
- Benzodiazepines (e.g., lorazepam) for anxiety symptoms
- Agitated, combative and intoxicated patients in the emergency room:
  - ◊ May require sedation with benzodiazepines (e.g., lorazepam 2 mg IM/IV) and/or neuroleptics (e.g., haloperidol 2-5 mg IM/IV)
  - ◊ Clinical response typically seen within 20-30 minutes
  - ◊ If no response, increase previous dose (e.g., 4-10 mg haloperidol)

Contraindications: Avoid tricyclic antidepressants in patient with evidence of 2°, 3° AV block or left bundle branch block ECG
Precautions:
- Use smaller doses in elderly patients
- Risperidone may be associated with hyperglycemia and ketoacidosis

Significant possible interactions:
- Hypertensive crisis if MAO inhibitor antidepressants given in combination with medications containing sympathomimetic amines; tyramine-rich food; meperidine (Demerol); tricyclic antidepressants
- Overdose of SSRIs may produce serotonergic syndrome (hyperthermia, confusion) which may be managed with cyproheptadine

ALTERNATIVE DRUGS N/A

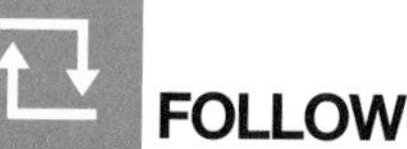

FOLLOWUP

PATIENT MONITORING
- Weekly (or more often if needed) outpatient followup appointments
- Prescribe only a weekly supply of antidepressants or other psychotropic medications at each appointment

PREVENTION/AVOIDANCE
- Provide crisis hot-line phone number and nearest crisis emergency room location
- Mobilize social support system and inform family and friends of options if patient becomes more suicidal
- Instruct patient to avoid any alcohol consumption

POSSIBLE COMPLICATIONS Brief period of increased suicide risk as depression resolves and patient's energy and initiative returns

EXPECTED COURSE/PROGNOSIS
- 15% of suicidal, depressed patients will ultimately complete suicide
- 82% of suicide victims have seen a doctor within the previous six months
- Approximately one-half of suicide victims have seen a doctor within one month of their death
- The key to a favorable course and prognosis is early recognition of risk factors, early diagnosis and treatment of a psychiatric disorder, and appropriate intervention and followup

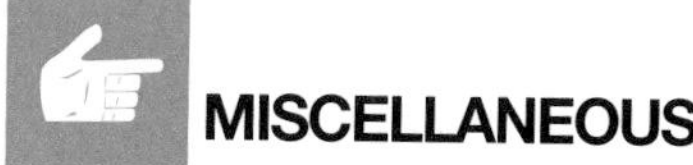

MISCELLANEOUS

ASSOCIATED CONDITIONS Depression

AGE-RELATED FACTORS
Pediatric: Increasing suicide rate in adolescents. Suicide is second leading cause of death in adolescents.
Geriatric: Increasing rate with increasing age (women peak at 55 years, men peak at 75 years)
Others: N/A

PREGNANCY N/A

SYNONYMS N/A

ICD-9-CM
E950.5 Suicide and self-inflicted poisoning by unspecified drug or medicinal substance

SEE ALSO
Alcohol use disorders
Depression
Schizophrenia

OTHER NOTES
- Overdose is the most common method for suicide attempts
- Shooting is the most common method for completed suicides
- Men prone to more violent suicides (i.e., shooting, jumping, hanging)
- Jumping most common method of suicide among patients in a general medical/surgical hospital

ABBREVIATIONS N/A

REFERENCES

- Hackett TP, Cassem NH. MGH Handbook of General Hospital Psychiatry. 2nd Ed. New York, PSG Publishing Company, Inc., 1987
- Talbott JA, Hales RE, Yudofsky SC. Textbook of Psychiatry. Washington, DC, American Psychiatric Press, Inc., 1988
- Patterson WM, Dohn HH, et al. Evaluation of suicidal patients, THE SAD PERSONS Scale, Psychosomatics, 1983
- Mann J, Oquendo M, Underwood M, et al. The neurobiology of suicide risk: a review for the clinician. J of Clin Psychiatry 1999;60(suppl2):7-11
- Shaffer D, Craft L. Methods of adolescent suicide prevention. J of Clin Psychiatry 1999;60(suppl2):70-76
- Miller-Oerlinghausen B, Bergöfer A. Antidepressants and suicide risk. J of Clin Psychiatry 1999;60(supl2):94-99

Web references: 3 available at www.5mcc.com
Illustrations N/A

Author(s):
M. Beatriz Currier, MD
Edwin J. Olsen, MD, MBA

BASICS

DESCRIPTION Partial or complete obstruction of the superior vena cava, 90% extrinsic, 70% from neoplasm (most frequently bronchogenic carcinoma), also thrombosis, fibrosis, invasion and aneurysm causing suffusion, varying degrees of airway obstruction and/or cyanosis of the face, neck, arms and occasionally chest and upper abdomen. Usual course - acute; usually 28 days from onset of symptoms to diagnosis.
System(s) affected: Cardiovascular, Pulmonary
Genetics: N/A
Incidence/Prevalence in USA: N/A
Predominant age: Young adult (16-40 years); middle age (40-60 years)
Predominant sex: Male > Female

SIGNS & SYMPTOMS
- Feeling of fullness in the head (ears and eyes) (81%)
- Facial edema/arm edema (78%)
- Jugular venous distension (75%)
- Prominent veins over chest (73%)
- Dyspnea (59%)
- Cough (37%)
- Dilated retinal vessels, conjunctival edema, proptosis
- Horner syndrome
- Facial plethora, cyanosis
- Stridor, paralyzed vocal cord
- Non-pitting edema in neck (Stoke's collar)
- Truncal swelling
- Tachypnea, wheezing
- Altered consciousness
- Visual symptoms
- Dysphagia, hoarseness
- Easy fatigability
- Chest pain
- Orthopnea

CAUSES
- Obstruction of venous drainage of upper part of chest and neck. Sudden occlusion can cause rapid development of cerebral edema, intracranial thrombosis and death.
- Lung cancer, bronchogenic carcinoma/small cell
- Lymphoma
- Thymoma
- Fungus infections
- Breast cancer
- Other malignancies
- Iatrogenic (including catheter-induced)
- Thyroid goiter
- Syphilitic aneurysm
- Tuberculous mediastinitis
- Primary superior vena caval thrombosis
- Pericardial constriction
- Idiopathic sclerosing mediastinitis

RISK FACTORS HIV infection

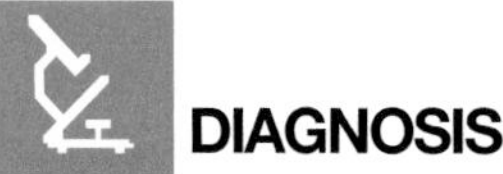

DIAGNOSIS

DIFFERENTIAL DIAGNOSIS
- Aortic aneurysm
- Tuberculosis, Histoplasmosis
- Fungal infections

LABORATORY Sputum cytology-malignant cells

Drugs that may alter lab results: N/A

Disorders that may alter lab results: N/A

PATHOLOGICAL FINDINGS Sputum cytology, occasionally thoracentesis, bone marrow, lymph node biopsy, bronchoscopy or thoracotomy confirm - malignant cells.

SPECIAL TESTS Increased central venous pressure (CVP), usually 20-50 mm Hg.

IMAGING
- Chest x-ray abnormal in 96% with mediastinal widening in 51% and right hilar mass in 48%
- MRI, CT scan, and/or tomography - mediastinal mass, superior mediastinal mass, pulmonary lesion, superior vena cava obstruction, hilar adenopathy, pleural effusion.
- Tc 99m scan - block to flow of contrast material into right heart, large collateral veins
- Venography - superior vena cava obstruction

DIAGNOSTIC PROCEDURES
- Bronchoscopy (diagnostic in 54%)
- Thoracentesis, thoracotomy, lymph node biopsy, as indicated

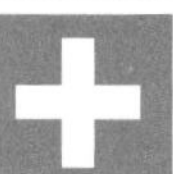

TREATMENT

APPROPRIATE HEALTH CARE Inpatient, intensive care

GENERAL MEASURES
- Chemotherapy (treatment of choice for high grade lymphomas, general tumors and small cell lung cancer)
- Intravascular stenting
- Radiotherapy
- Neoadjuvant chemoradiotherapy and then resection
- Thrombolytic therapy if catheter-induced

SURGICAL MEASURES Superior vena cava reconstruction for benign processes may be considered. Case report stage IIIB non-small cell lung cancer treatment response with chemoradiation, then resection.

ACTIVITY Bedrest (head of bed elevated)

DIET As tolerated, possibly salt restriction

PATIENT EDUCATION As appropriate

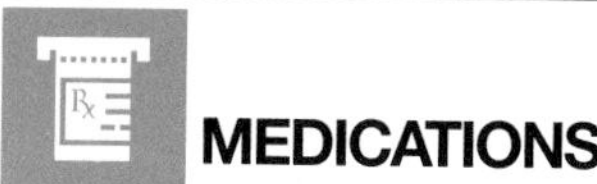

MEDICATIONS

DRUG(S) OF CHOICE
- Chemotherapy for cancer
- Steroids for some malignancies, especially if cerebral or laryngeal edema
- Antifungal or antitubercular medications according to underlying cause
- Consider diuretics
- Anticoagulation role unclear
- Fibrinolytics (e.g., urokinase) for thrombosis

Contraindications: Refer to manufacturer's literature
Precautions: Refer to manufacturer's literature
Significant possible interactions: Refer to manufacturer's literature

ALTERNATIVE DRUGS Streptokinase, tPA

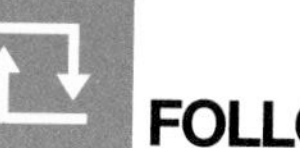

FOLLOWUP

PATIENT MONITORING Linked to cause. If infection, monitor for evaluation of antimicrobial treatment. If malignant, monitor response to radiotherapy or chemotherapy.

PREVENTION/AVOIDANCE No preventive measures known

POSSIBLE COMPLICATIONS Complications of underlying disease

EXPECTED COURSE/PROGNOSIS
High probability of response; prognosis linked to cause; 20% 1-year survival for lung cancer; 50% 2-year survival for lymphoma. 85% neoplastic cases better in 3 weeks with radiation therapy, but symptoms usually recur.

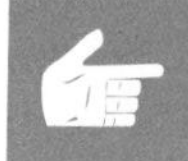

MISCELLANEOUS

ASSOCIATED CONDITIONS
- Breast cancer
- Lung cancer
- HIV infection
- Hyperthyroidism
- Tuberculosis, histoplasmosis
- Lymphoma

AGE-RELATED FACTORS
Pediatric: N/A
Geriatric: N/A
Others: N/A

PREGNANCY Must treat underlying condition despite pregnancy

SYNONYMS
- Superior mediastinal syndrome
- Superior vena cava obstruction

ICD-9-CM
459.2 Compression of vein

SEE ALSO

OTHER NOTES N/A

ABBREVIATIONS N/A

REFERENCES

- Roberts JR, Bueno R, Sugarbaker DJ. Multimodality treatment of malignant superior vena cava syndrome. Chest 1999;116;(3):835-7
- Laguna DE, Gazapo NT: Superior vena cava syndrome: a study based on 81 cases. Am Med Interna 1998;15(9):470-475
- Sculier JP, Feld R: Superior Vena Cava Obstruction Syndrome: Recommendations for Management. In Cancer Treat Rev 1985;12:209
- DeVita VT Jr, Hellman S, Rosenberg SA, eds: Cancer: Principles and Practices of Oncology. 3rd Ed. Philadelphia, J.B. Lippincott, 1989
- Bennett JC, Plum F, eds: Cecil Textbook of Medicine. 20th Ed. Philadelphia, W.B. Saunders Co., 1996
- Schwartz SI, ed: Principles of Surgery. 4th Ed. New York, McGraw-Hill, 1984
- Wilkinson P, MacMahon J, Johnston L: Stenting and superior vena caval syndrome. Irish J Med Sci 1995;164(2):128-131
- Yim CD, Sane SS, Bjarnason H. Superior vena cava stenting. Radiol Clin North Am 2000;38(2):409-24

Web references: 0 available at www.5mcc.com
Illustrations N/A

Author(s):
Sean Herrington, MD

BASICS

DESCRIPTION Approximately 5-20% of adults will have one or more episodes of syncope by age 75. The disorder accounts for about 1% of hospital admissions and about 3% of emergency room visits. Its annual incidence in the institutionalized elderly is about 6%.

System(s) affected: Cardiovascular, Nervous
Genetics: N/A
Incidence/Prevalence in USA: 6% in persons over age 75 (incidence)
Predominant age: Elderly
Predominant sex: N/A

SIGNS & SYMPTOMS

Transient loss of consciousness characterized by unresponsiveness, loss of postural tone, and spontaneous recovery

CAUSES

- Cardiac - obstruction to outflow:
  - ◊ Aortic stenosis
  - ◊ Hypertrophic cardiomyopathy
  - ◊ Pulmonary embolus
- Cardiac - arrhythmias:
  - ◊ Ventricular tachycardia
  - ◊ Sick sinus syndrome
  - ◊ 2nd and 3rd degree AV block
- Non-cardiac:
  - ◊ Reflex mediated vasovagal, situational (micturition, defecation, cough)
  - ◊ Orthostatic hypotension
  - ◊ Drug induced
  - ◊ Neurologic: Seizures, transient ischemic attack
  - ◊ Carotid sinus
  - ◊ Psychogenic

RISK FACTORS

- Patients with heart disease
- Patients taking following drugs:
  - ◊ Antihypertensives
  - ◊ Vasodilators (including calcium channel blockers, ACE inhibitors, and nitrates)
  - ◊ Phenothiazines
  - ◊ Antidepressants
  - ◊ Antiarrhythmics
  - ◊ Diuretics

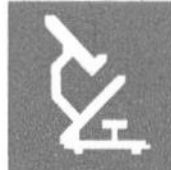

DIAGNOSIS

DIFFERENTIAL DIAGNOSIS

- Drop attacks
- Coma
- A careful history, physical examination and an ECG are more important than other investigations in determining a diagnosis. Make sure that the patient or witness (if present) is not talking about vertigo, coma, or drop attacks. Prodromal manifestations of sudden weakness, nausea, and sweating, especially in circumstances provoking strong emotion, are diagnostic of vasovagal syncope. Syncope of sudden onset with no prodrome or brief premonitory symptoms suggest a cardiac cause. Vasovagal syncope does not occur when the patient is horizontal; cardiac syncope can occur in any position. Syncope with exertion suggests a cardiac cause.

Physical exam should be directed to blood pressure and pulse, both lying and standing. Check for a cardiac murmur or a focal neurologic abnormality.

After a careful evaluation, including diagnostic procedures and special tests, the cause of syncope will be found in only 50-60% of patients.

LABORATORY Rarely helpful. Less than 2% have hyponatremia, hypocalcemia, hypoglycemia or renal failure causing seizures.

Drugs that may alter lab results: N/A

Disorders that may alter lab results: N/A

PATHOLOGICAL FINDINGS N/A

SPECIAL TESTS

- If history and physical suggestive of ischemic, valvular or congenital heart disease - echocardiogram, cardiac catheterization
- If CNS disease suspected - EEG, head CT, head MRI. These tests should not be ordered unless there are hints of CNS disease on history or physical examination.

IMAGING Lung scan or helical CT of the thorax if history and physical examination suggestive of pulmonary embolism

DIAGNOSTIC PROCEDURES

- ECG monitoring, either in the hospital or ambulatory (Holter), is useful in 4-15% of patients. Arrhythmias are frequently documented, but rarely associated with syncope. Monitoring should be done in patients with heart disease, and in patients with recurrent syncope. Patient activated intermittent loop recorders, which the patient activates after regaining consciousness, can record 4-5 minutes of retrograde ECG rhythm. These have been helpful in patients with recurrent syncope with a diagnostic yield between 24-47%.
- Electrophysiologic studies (EPS) have been positive in 18-75% of patients. Induction of ventricular tachycardia and dysfunction of the His-Purkinje system are the two most common abnormalities. Although there is the problem of knowing whether the arrhythmia noted or induced during the study is the cause of syncope, EPS should be done in patients with heart disease or recurrent syncope.
- The following findings are probable causes of syncope:
  - ◊ Sustained ventricular tachycardia
  - ◊ Sinus node recovery time 3 seconds or more
  - ◊ Pacing-induced infranodal block
  - ◊ H-V interval greater than 100 msec
- Carotid hypersensitivity should be considered in patients with syncope on head turning, especially with head turning while wearing tight collar, and in patients with neck tumors and neck tissue scars. The technique is not standardized. One side should be massaged at a time for 20 seconds with constant monitoring of pulse and blood pressure. Atropine should be readily available.
- Tilt testing, with and without isoproterenol infusion, is a provocative test for vasovagal syncope which is not standardized, but has been reported positive (symptomatic hypotension and bradycardia) in 26-87% of patients. However, the test has been reported positive in 0-45% of control subjects. The role of this test in the workup of patients with syncope of unknown origin is not known, and should be done only in patients in which cardiac causes of syncope have been excluded. Patients with a positive tilt test often respond to beta-blocker treatment.
- Psychiatric evaluation should be considered in patients with multiple episodes of syncope (greater 5/year) who do not have heart disease. Anxiety, depression, alcohol and drug abuse can be associated with syncope.

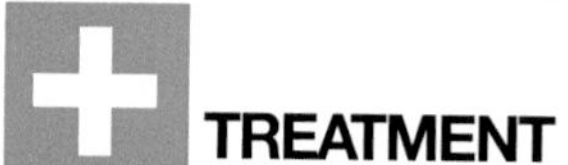

TREATMENT

APPROPRIATE HEALTH CARE
- Patients with heart disease should be admitted to the hospital for evaluation
- Elderly patients without previously recognized heart disease should be admitted if the physician thinks that a cardiac cause of syncope is likely
- Patients without heart disease, especially young patients (less 60 years old), can be safely worked up as outpatients

GENERAL MEASURES
No specific measures

SURGICAL MEASURES
N/A

ACTIVITY
Fully active unless severe cardiac disease

DIET
No specific diet unless heart disease

PATIENT EDUCATION
- Reassure the patient that most cardiac causes of syncope can be treated, and that patients with non-cardiac causes do well, even if the cause of syncope is never discovered
- The physician and patient should carefully consider whether the patient should continue to drive while syncope is being evaluated. Physicians should be aware of the pertinent laws in their own state.

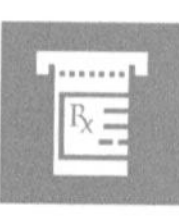

MEDICATIONS

DRUG(S) OF CHOICE
- Antiarrhythmic drugs for documented arrhythmias occurring simultaneously with syncope or symptoms of presyncope. Asymptomatic arrhythmias do not require treatment.
- The decision to treat patients on the basis of arrhythmias or conduction abnormalities provoked or detected during EPS is even more problematic. Does the arrhythmia or conduction abnormality have anything to do with the patient's symptoms? Most would treat a patient with provoked sustained ventricular tachycardiac with an antiarrhythmic drug that suppressed the arrhythmia during the study. Many recommend pacemaker implantation in patients with H-V intervals greater than 100 msec, pacing induced infranodal block, or sinus node recovery time of 3 sec or more. The rationale basis for such treatment is that recurrent syncope is less frequent in those patients with positive EPS who are treated than it is in those who have negative EPS.

Contraindications: N/A
Precautions: N/A
Significant possible interactions: N/A

ALTERNATIVE DRUGS
N/A

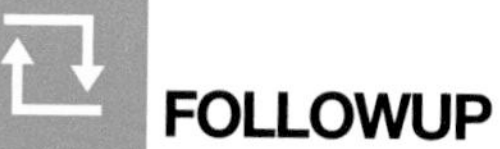

FOLLOWUP

PATIENT MONITORING
- Frequent followup visits for patients with cardiac causes of syncope, especially patients on antiarrhythmic drugs
- Patients with an unknown cause of syncope rarely (5%) have a diagnosis made during followup

PREVENTION/AVOIDANCE
Avoid Risk factors

POSSIBLE COMPLICATIONS
- Trauma from falling
- Death - see prognosis

EXPECTED COURSE/PROGNOSIS
- Cumulative mortality at 2 years:
  - ◊ Low (2-5%) - young patients (< 60) with a non-cardiac cause or unknown cause of syncope.
  - ◊ Intermediate (20%) - older patients (> 60) with a non-cardiac or unknown cause of syncope.
  - ◊ High (32-38%) - patients with cardiac cause of syncope.

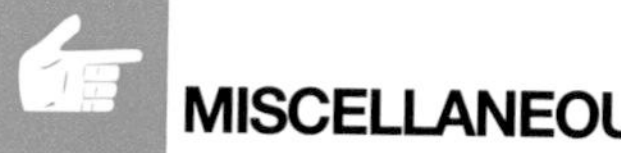

MISCELLANEOUS

ASSOCIATED CONDITIONS
See Causes

AGE-RELATED FACTORS
Pediatric: Rare in this age group
Geriatric: More common in this age group, prognosis worse in older patients
Others: N/A

PREGNANCY
N/A

SYNONYMS
N/A

ICD-9-CM
780.2 Syncope and collapse

SEE ALSO
Aortic valvular stenosis
Atrial septal defect (ASD)
Carotid sinus syndrome
Complete heart block
Idiopathic hypertrophic subaortic stenosis (IHSS)
Patent ductus arteriosus
Primary pulmonary hypertension
Pulmonary embolism
Seizure disorders
Stokes-Adams attacks
Ventricular tachycardia (VT)

OTHER NOTES
N/A

ABBREVIATIONS
N/A

REFERENCES

- Schnipper JL, Kapoor WN. Diagnostic evaluation and management of patients with syncope. Med Clin North Am 2001;85(2):423-56
- Linzer M, Gang EH, Estes NA, Wang P, Vonpenan V, Kapoor WN: Diagnosing syncope part 1: Value of history, physical examination and electrocardiography. The Clinical Efficacy of Assessment Project of the American College of Physicians. Ann Int Med 1997;126:989-996
- Linzer M, Gang EH, Estes NA, Wang P, Vonpenan V, Kapoor WN: Diagnosing syncope part 2: Unexplained syncope. The Clinical Efficacy of Assessment Project of the American College of Physicians. Ann Int Med 1997;127:76-86

Web references: 0 available at www.5mcc.com
Illustrations N/A

Author(s):
Ricardo Samson, MD

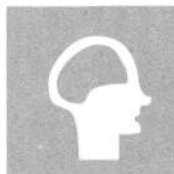

BASICS

DESCRIPTION A proliferative disorder of unknown etiology affecting synovial lined joints, tendon sheaths or bursa. Occurs in diffuse or focal forms which have a quite different prognosis.
System(s) affected: Musculoskeletal
Genetics: N/A
Incidence/Prevalence in USA: Two occurrences per 1 million population
Predominant age:
- Diffuse form appears more commonly in the 3rd and 4th decades
- Focal is more common in the 5th and 6th decades

Predominant sex:
- Diffuse form: Male = Female
- Focal form: Female > Male

SIGNS & SYMPTOMS
- Diffuse form:
  - ◊ Unilateral and monoarticular with 80% occurring in the knee and affecting the hip, ankle and shoulder in decreasing order
  - ◊ Mild and progressive pain in involved joint
  - ◊ History of trauma (30% of cases)
  - ◊ Recurrent swelling and tenderness to palpation of involved joint
  - ◊ Increased skin temperatures over involved joint
- Focal form:
  - ◊ More common in tendon than joints
  - ◊ Involves the tendons of the hand and feet, usually, rarely the wrist and ankle or a major joint
  - ◊ Presents as slow growing, painless mass
  - ◊ Most common cause of tumor in hand, second to ganglion
- Chronic, inflammatory:
  - ◊ Unusual monoarticular presentation

CAUSES Unknown, possibly repeated local hemorrhages

RISK FACTORS N/A

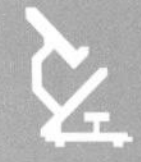

DIAGNOSIS

DIFFERENTIAL DIAGNOSIS
- Diffuse form (if soft tissue swelling is the main finding):
  - ◊ Synovioma - frequently calcifies
  - ◊ Synovial hemangioma - usually occurs in childhood and often associated with cutaneous hemangioma
  - ◊ Lipoma - boggy fullness to palpation and absence of serosanguinous fluid on aspiration
  - ◊ Unusual mono-articular presentation for other forms of chronic, inflammatory arthritis
- Diffuse form (if multiple subchondral cysts on x-ray are the main finding):
  - ◊ Degenerative joint disease - cysts occur on weight bearing surfaces only, while cysts of PVNS may occur anywhere in joints. Osteophytes common in degenerative arthritis, absent in PVNS.
  - ◊ Tuberculous arthritis is characterized by severe juxta-articular osteoporosis
  - ◊ Amyloid arthropathy is usually symmetrical and more common in the upper extremities. The joint space is preserved.
  - ◊ Synovial chondromatosis - presence of punctate calcifications along the margin. (Occurs 60-70% of time.)
- Focal form:
  - ◊ Ganglion - contains jelly-like fluid on aspiration
  - ◊ Dupuytren nodules - not attached to tendon sheath and therefore does not move with tendon

LABORATORY Aspiration of a serosanguineous fluid from a joint in the absence of trauma is highly suggestive of diffuse pigmented villonodular synovitis (fluid can be clear, however). Aspirated joint fluid may contain high cholesterol.

Drugs that may alter lab results: N/A

Disorders that may alter lab results: N/A

PATHOLOGICAL FINDINGS The synovium shows proliferation into villi or nodules with subsynovial cellular infiltrate that includes fibroblasts, lymphocytes and lipid-laden macrophages (foam cells)

SPECIAL TESTS N/A

IMAGING
- The CT scan may be helpful, but MRI has the best potential for being diagnostic due to the presence of hemosiderin and fat within the abnormal tissue present in the joint
- X-ray shows soft tissue swelling of involved joints. Subchondral cysts and pressure erosions are limited mostly to the hip. The absence of osteophytes and juxta-articular osteoporosis is significant.

DIAGNOSTIC PROCEDURES
- Arthroscopy usually reveals characteristic synovial changes and allows definitive biopsy
- An arthrogram is not usually diagnostic
- Radioisotopes and ultrasound studies are also usually not definitive

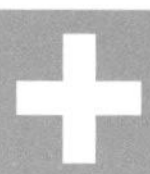

TREATMENT

APPROPRIATE HEALTH CARE Inpatient or outpatient surgery

GENERAL MEASURES N/A

SURGICAL MEASURES
- Diffuse form - total synovectomy is the usual recommended treatment, but has a recurrence rate of 25-40%. X-ray therapy alone or combined with synovectomy has been tried, again with high recurrence rate. Recently, intra-articular injections of radioisotopes, in particular yttrium-90, has been tried and shows some early promise, but evaluation of this is incomplete.
- Focal form - local excision results in cure

ACTIVITY No restrictions

DIET No special diet

PATIENT EDUCATION N/A

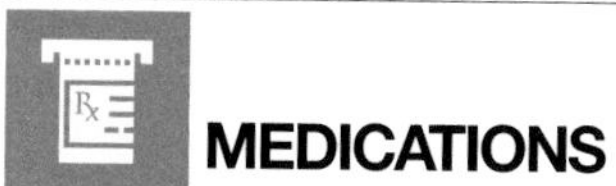

MEDICATIONS

DRUG(S) OF CHOICE None
Contraindications: N/A
Precautions: N/A
Significant possible interactions: N/A

ALTERNATIVE DRUGS N/A

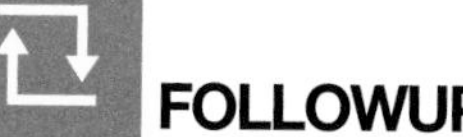

FOLLOWUP

PATIENT MONITORING Patients should be followed twice annually after treatment of the diffuse form by history and physical examination. X-rays yearly, especially if the hip is involved.

PREVENTION/AVOIDANCE N/A

POSSIBLE COMPLICATIONS Osteoarthritis, especially in the hip joint

EXPECTED COURSE/PROGNOSIS
- Good in focal type
- Guarded in the diffuse form with recurrences of disease common as well as joint dysfunction

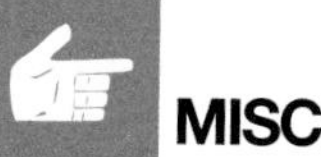

MISCELLANEOUS

ASSOCIATED CONDITIONS N/A

AGE-RELATED FACTORS
Pediatric: N/A
Geriatric: N/A
Others: N/A

PREGNANCY N/A

SYNONYMS
- Xanthoma
- Benign synovioma
- Giant cell tumor of tendon sheath
- Fibroxanthoma
- PVNS

ICD-9-CM
719.20 Villonodular synovitis, site unspecified

SEE ALSO
Arthritis, rheumatoid (RA)

OTHER NOTES N/A

ABBREVIATIONS PVNS = pigmented villonodular synovitis

REFERENCES

- Flandry JB, Hughston JS: Pigmented Villonodular Synovitis. Current Concepts and Review, 1987

Web references: 0 available at www.5mcc.com
Illustrations N/A

Author(s):
R. Bruce Hall, MD

BASICS

DESCRIPTION A sexually transmitted infection, characterized by sequential stages (acute, subacute or chronic), with the spirochete, *Treponema pallidum*

- Infectious syphilis consists of a primary stage and a secondary stage. It may also include neurosyphilis (central nervous system involvement). If untreated, the infectious stage may be followed by a latent stage.
- Latent syphilis is an asymptomatic phase in an untreated patient, characterized by positive specific treponema Ab test with normal CSF. Early latent is less than 1 year and late latent is more than 1 year after onset of infection.
- Neurosyphilis may occur at any stage in syphilis. Primary, secondary stages usually asymptomatic; tertiary stage is symptomatic.
- Tertiary (or late syphilis) stage is late generalized syphilis
- Congenital is syphilis acquired in utero

System(s) affected: Cardiovascular, Nervous, Reproductive, Skin/Exocrine

Genetics: N/A

Incidence/Prevalence in USA:

- 1989 - 18.4/100,000 new cases
- 2000 - 2.1/100,000 (lowest rates since reporting started in 1941). Still greater than Healthy People 2010 objective of 0.2/100,000.
- 2001 - 2.2/100,000. First documented rise since 1990. Rise only in men. CDC attributes to high risk subpopulation of men who have sex with men. Rates for women and non-Hispanic blacks have declined.
- 2002 - 2.4/100,000.

Predominant age: Sexually active years

Predominant sex: Male > Female (2.1:1)

SIGNS & SYMPTOMS

- Infectious syphilis - primary
  - ◊ Chancre begins as a painless papule which erodes to a 0.3 to 2 cm non-tender ulcer with a hard edge and clean, yellow base (unless untreated, secondarily infected) 9 to 90 days after exposure (median 3 weeks)
  - ◊ Usually found on genitalia or area exposed to partner's ulcer. Frequently solitary, may be multiple, may have regional lymphadenopathy.
  - ◊ Heals with scarring in 3 to 6 weeks with or without treatment; 75% of patients having no further symptoms
  - ◊ 1/3 will progress to chronic stages
- Infectious syphilis - secondary
  - ◊ 25% of patients enter this stage 2-6 weeks after exposure, may overlap with chancre
  - ◊ Often characterized by a rash that is generalized polymorphic, palpable lesions with "fresh cut ham" color, non-pruritic, usually not bullous or vesicular, classically involves palms and soles. Active bacteria present in the rash; contact with broken skin can spread the infection.
  - ◊ Resolves spontaneously in 2-6 weeks in most patients
  - ◊ May wax and wane between secondary and latent stages for years
  - ◊ Patchy alopecia of scalp, eyebrows and beard common
  - ◊ Condyloma lata - large gray-to-white lesions involving warm, moist area of body, such as mucus membranes in mouth, perineum
  - ◊ Generalized lymphadenopathy and flu-like symptoms occur early with rash
  - ◊ Rarely may be accompanied by nephritis, meningitis, uveitis, hepatitis
  - ◊ Mild hepatosplenomegaly often noticeable
- Latent syphilis
  - ◊ Characterized by positive serology but no signs or symptoms
  - ◊ Patient is not infectious after one year, but may relapse to infectious secondary stage if untreated (25% in first year, small percent second year, none after that)
- Tertiary syphilis - 1/3 of patients with secondary syphilis go on to tertiary syphilis. Bacteria can damage the heart, eyes, brain, CNS, bones and joints.
  - ◊ Cardiovascular - can have asymptomatic murmur, left heart failure, aneurysms of ascending thoracic aorta or aortic valve regurgitation
  - ◊ Deep cutaneous - gummas are destructive granulomatous pockets that can occur anywhere
  - ◊ Orthopedic (Charcot's joints, osteomyelitis) complications (rare with antibiotics)
  - ◊ Serologies often negative
- Neurosyphilis
  - ◊ Can be any stage with CNS involvement, eye, ear symptoms
  - ◊ General paresis
- Congenital syphilis
  - ◊ Young infants
    - Snuffles (mucopurulent rhinitis)
    - Failure to thrive
    - Rhinitis
    - Lymphadenopathy
    - Jaundice
    - Anemia
    - Hepatosplenomegaly
    - Nephrosis
    - Meningitis
    - Rash (the hallmark) similar to secondary syphilis in adults, but may be bullous or vesicular
  - ◊ Children
    - Hutchinson teeth
    - Saber shins
    - Charcot joints
    - Deafness
    - Interstitial keratitis

CAUSES *Treponema pallidum*

RISK FACTORS

- Multiple sexual partners
- Exposure to infected body fluids
- IV drug use
- Infants may be exposed transplacentally

DIAGNOSIS

DIFFERENTIAL DIAGNOSIS

- Primary syphilis - chancroid, lymphogranuloma venereum, granuloma inguinale, herpes, Behçet syndrome, trauma
- Secondary syphilis - pityriasis rosea, guttate psoriasis, drug eruption
- Positive serology, asymptomatic - previously treated syphilis, biological false positive, other spirochetal disease (yaws, pinta)

LABORATORY

- Requires either demonstration of organisms on microscopy or positive serology on blood or cerebrospinal fluid (CSF)
- Organism may not be cultured, but diagnosis is never made on clinical signs and symptoms alone
- Nontreponemal tests: Venereal Disease Research Laboratory (VDRL) or rapid plasma reagin (RPR) are characterized as follows:
  - ◊ Relatively inexpensive, primary screening test
  - ◊ Positive within 7 days of exposure
  - ◊ Titer decreases with time or treatment
  - ◊ Used to monitor therapy: fourfold rise in titer indicates new infection while failure to decrease fourfold within one year is treatment failure; always use the same test (VDRL or RPR). Since some patients stay serofast followup can be difficult.
  - ◊ False-positive common, especially in autoimmune disorders and certain viral infections, but positives are highly suggestive even without clinical signs and symptoms (confirm with fluorescent treponemal antibody absorption [FTA-ABS])
  - ◊ Titer ≥ 1:64 even without confirming test is probably diagnostic of acute syphilis or other treponematoses
  - ◊ Labs need to titer tests to final end point (not report as ">1:512" for example) to make best use of results in monitoring therapy response
  - ◊ Beware of prozone phenomenon - negative results due to very high titers of antibody. Test diluted serum sample, as well, to declare a given specimen as negative.
- Treponemal tests: Fluorescent treponemal antibody absorption (FTA-ABS), microhemagglutination *Treponema pallidum* (MHA-TP)
  - ◊ More expensive, used to confirm diagnosis
  - ◊ Usually positive for life after treatment
  - ◊ Due to unusual nontreponemal test results in HIV infected patients, these tests may be needed to absolutely rule out syphilis
- Lumbar puncture for CSF serologies (plus WBC, protein, glucose) should be done:
  - ◊ In cases of latent syphilis where duration is unknown or non-penicillin therapy is planned
  - ◊ Whenever neurological symptoms are present
  - ◊ In treatment failures
  - ◊ In patients with positive HIV tests
  - ◊ If other evidence of active syphilis is present (aortitis, gumma, iritis)
  - ◊ If serum nontreponemal antibody titer is >1:32
  - ◊ Children with syphilis, after the newborn period, should be tested to rule out neurosyphilis
  - ◊ VDRL, not RPR is used on CSF. May be negative in neurosyphilis. Highly specific/not sensitive.
  - ◊ Negative FTA-ABS or MHA-TP on CSF excludes neurosyphilis
  - ◊ Positive FTA-ABS or MHA-TP on CSF not diagnostic because high false positive rate

Drugs that may alter lab results: Many drugs reported to cause false-positive, but this is relatively uncommon with a good history

Disorders that may alter lab results:

- Rheumatic (SLE: false-positive)
- Acute febrile illness
- HIV infection
- Pregnancy
- Mycoplasma
- Malaria

PATHOLOGICAL FINDINGS Aneurysm, osteomyelitis, gummas in late cases

SPECIAL TESTS

- Dark field microscopy
- Immunofluorescence
- Skin biopsy to demonstrate *T. pallidum* in tissue

IMAGING Only in late cases as indicated

DIAGNOSTIC PROCEDURES Specialized test available from Center for Disease Control (CDC) to confirm false-positive if necessary

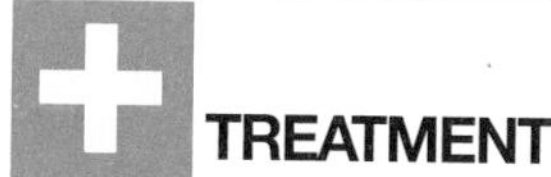

TREATMENT

APPROPRIATE HEALTH CARE Outpatient, except for initiating IV penicillin or desensitization

GENERAL MEASURES
- Baseline serologies prior to treatment to monitor its success
- Prompt institution of antibiotics
- Symptomatic treatment of the chancres and rash of secondary syphilis (for patient's comfort only) includes baths, antihistamines, etc. Chancres require only routine cleansing with water and mild soap.
- Neurosyphilis
  - ◊ Harder to treat in HIV patients
  - ◊ Can occur up to 20 years after infection

SURGICAL MEASURES N/A

ACTIVITY
- Full activity, but no sexual contacts until declared cured

DIET No special diet

PATIENT EDUCATION
- Need to trace and treat all sexual contacts of the patient
- Keep followup appointments to monitor success of therapy
- Advise patient to avoid intercourse until treatment is complete
- Local health department can provide literature and contact tracing

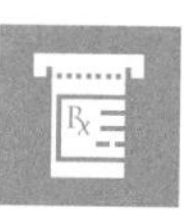

MEDICATIONS

DRUG(S) OF CHOICE
- Parenteral penicillin G is drug of choice for all stages (for patients allergic to penicillin see Other Notes)
- Primary, secondary and early latent less than one year:
  - ◊ Benzathine penicillin G, 2.4 million units IM for 1 dose
  - ◊ In penicillin allergic patients: doxycycline 100 mg po bid x 2 weeks or tetracycline 500 mg po qid x 2 weeks. Ceftriaxone (Rocephin) 1 gm IM qd x 10 days is a newer alternative used by some clinicians.
- Late latent ≥ 1 year and tertiary syphilis (not neurosyphilis)
  - ◊ Benzathine penicillin G, 2.4 million units IM weekly for 3 doses
  - ◊ In penicillin allergic patients: should attempt desensitization and treatment with penicillin. Doxycycline 100 mg po bid x 4 weeks or tetracycline 500 mg po qid x 4 weeks.
- Neurosyphilis: penicillin G 3-4 million units IV q4 hours x 10-14 days or aqueous procaine penicillin G (APPG) 2.4 million units IM qd x 10-14 days with probenecid 500 mg PO qid.
- Congenital syphilis: aqueous crystalline penicillin G 50,000 units/kg/dose IV q 8-12 hours x 10-14 days or APPG 50,000 units/kg IM x 10-14 days. If negative CSF serologies, 50,000 units/kg benzathine penicillin G in one IM injection.
- Children (after newborn period): 50,000 units/kg IM up to adult dose of 2.4 million units as a single dose. Late latent = 50,000 units/kg IM as 3 doses at 1 week intervals.
- Pregnancy and syphilis: treatment same as nonpregnant patients. Some recommend a second dose of 2.4 million units benzathine penicillin G 1 week after initial dose especially in third trimester or with secondary syphilis.
- Epidemiologic treatment for contacts without symptoms, treat as primary after baseline serologies are obtained

Contraindications: Allergy to penicillin
Precautions:
- HIV infected and pregnant patients may show poor response to recommended IM doses. Use IV therapy for all treatment failures in these patients.
- Do NOT give benzathine or procaine penicillins IV

Significant possible interactions: See manufacturers literature

ALTERNATIVE DRUGS N/A

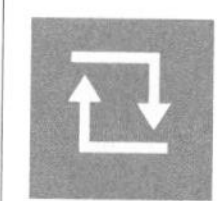

FOLLOWUP

PATIENT MONITORING
- Repeat serologies at 3, 6, and 12 months after treatment. If more than one year's duration, check at 24 months. Do serological studies more frequently in HIV infected patients.
- Clinical response = decrease in VDRL titers: primary and secondary VDRL decrease of 2 tubes at 6 months, 3 at 12 months, 4 at 24 months. In neurosyphilis, response = fourfold or greater decrease in VDRL over 6-12 months.
- Retreat for persistent clinical signs or recurrence, a fourfold rise in titers, or a failure of initially high (> 1:32) to decrease to < 1:8 at 12-24 months

PREVENTION/AVOIDANCE
- Discuss safe sex; use of condoms

POSSIBLE COMPLICATIONS
- Cardiovascular disease
- Central nervous system disease
- Membranous glomerulonephritis
- Paroxysmal cold hemoglobinemia
- Meningitis, tabes dorsalis
- Organ damage that cannot be reversed
- Jarisch-Herxheimer reaction, marked by fever, chills, headache, myalgias, new rash is common on starting treatment (of primary or secondary disease; less common with tertiary) due to the lysis of treponemes and should not be confused with a reaction to antibiotics. It is managed with antihistamines and antipyretics.

EXPECTED COURSE/PROGNOSIS
- Excellent in all cases except late syphilis complications and a few HIV infected patients
- Syphilis in HIV patient: HIV considered in any patient with syphilis. More often false-negative treponema and non-treponema tests and the serologic response to therapy is less predictable. Patient with early syphilis more treatment failures, higher incidence of neurosyphilis. Follow-up is important.

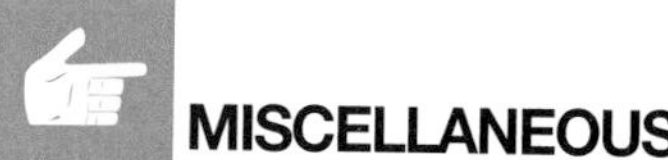

MISCELLANEOUS

ASSOCIATED CONDITIONS
- Other sexually transmitted diseases
- HIV infection and hepatitis B (strongly urge patients treated for syphilis to obtain screenings for both)

AGE-RELATED FACTORS
Pediatric: In non-congenital cases, must consider possible child abuse
Geriatric: N/A
Others: N/A

PREGNANCY
- Early detection is imperative, all expectant mothers should have serologies as part of routine prenatal care in the first trimester. If high exposure risk, repeat in second trimester and at delivery.
- Jarisch-Herxheimer reaction may induce preterm labor or fetal distress, but still need to treat

SYNONYMS
- Lues
- The Great Imitator

ICD-9-CM
097.9 Syphilis, unspecified

SEE ALSO
Chlamydial sexually transmitted diseases
Gonococcal infections
Pelvic inflammatory disease (PID)

OTHER NOTES
- Many experts urge more aggressive treatment than standard regimens in all patients and strongly advocate the use of penicillin rather than any alternative antibiotic.
- Penicillin allergic patients should undergo desensitization, particularly in neurosyphilis, HIV infected, and pregnant patients.

ABBREVIATIONS
CSF = cerebrospinal fluid
FTA-ABS = fluorescent treponemal antibody absorption
MHA-TP = microhemagglutination *Treponema pallidum*
VDRL = Venereal Disease Research Laboratory
RPR = rapid plasma reagin

REFERENCES
- Centers for Disease Control and Prevention. Primary and secondary syphilis - United States, 2002. MMWR Morb Wkly Rep 2003;21(46):117-20
- Centers for Disease Control and Prevention. Sexually transmitted diseases: Treatment guidelines 2002. MMWR Morb Mortal Wkly Rep 2002:51(RR-6):18-30
- Guarino CD. Syphilis in pregnancy and infancy: ongoing but treatable. Family Prac Recertification 2003;25(2):67-73
- Drugs for Sexually Transmitted Diseases. Medical Letter, 37:964, Dec 1995

Web references: 4 available at www.5mcc.com
Illustrations 3 available

Author(s):
Carrie A. Jaworski, MD
Aarthi Anand, MD

Systemic lupus erythematosus (SLE)

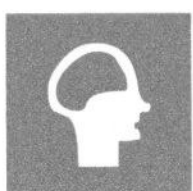

BASICS

DESCRIPTION A multi-system, autoimmune inflammatory condition characterized by a fluctuating, chronic course. Varies from mild to severe and may be lethal (CNS and renal forms).

System(s) affected: Endocrine/Metabolic, Gastrointestinal, Hemic/Lymphatic/Immunologic, Musculoskeletal, Nervous, Renal/Urologic, Skin/Exocrine

Genetics: Markers: HLA-B8; HLA-DR2; HLA-DR3

Incidence/Prevalence in USA: 20/100,000

Predominant age: All ages, but 30-50 are most common

Predominant sex: Female > Male (10:1)

SIGNS & SYMPTOMS

- Arthritis
- Fever
- Anorexia
- Malaise
- Weight loss
- Skin lesions
- Oral ulcers
- Eye pain and/or redness
- Chest pain and/or shortness of breath
- Pallor
- Nausea, vomiting, diarrhea
- Muscles - tenderness, aching and stiffness
- Headaches and visual problems
- Psychosis/delirium

CAUSES

- Most cases are idiopathic
- Drugs - drug induced lupus is clinically different from idiopathic SLE

RISK FACTORS

- Race - blacks, Hispanics, Asians, and Native Americans have higher prevalence than whites.
- Genetic markers - HLA-B8, HLA-DR2, HLA-DR3.
- Hereditary complement deficiency especially C1q. C1r. C1s, C4 and C2
- Polymorphisms in the Fc gammaRIIa and Fc gammaRIIIa gene may be important risk factor in SLE

DIAGNOSIS

DIFFERENTIAL DIAGNOSIS

- SLE mimics numerous systemic conditions, especially those involving inflammation
- Many other disorders mimic SLE - rheumatoid arthritis, mixed connective tissue disease (MCTD), scleroderma, metastatic malignancy, fever of unknown origin, psychogenic rheumatism and many cutaneous rashes. No one test or biopsy is pathognomonic.

LABORATORY

- Positive antinuclear antibody (ANA)
- Anti-double standard DNA (dsDNA), anti-Sm, false-positive VDRL, or positive LE preparation. These tests have either high sensitivity (ANA, false-positive VDRL) or specificity (anti-dsDNA, anti-Sm and LE preparation) and are included as American Rheumatology Association (ARA) criteria for the diagnosis of SLE along with the clinical features.
- Sedimentation rate is nonspecific, but valuable in assessing activity of SLE
- Anemia
- Anticardiolipin antibody
- Leukopenia
- Lymphopenia
- Abnormal urinary sediment
- Proteinuria
- Increased prothrombin time
- Hypoalbuminuria
- Thrombocytopenia
- Increased serum creatinine
- Positive Coombs test

Drugs that may alter lab results: N/A

Disorders that may alter lab results: N/A

PATHOLOGICAL FINDINGS Connective tissue disorders affecting skin, blood vessels, serous and synovial membranes

- Collagenous swelling
- Fibrinoid change
- Cellular necrosis
- Periarterial sclerosis
- Granulomatous reaction
- Infiltration of polymorphonuclear leukocytes, plasma cells, lymphocytes in walls of small vessels, arterioles of skin, spleen, glomeruli, endocardium pericardium, brain
- Hematoxylin bodies resembling those in LE cells
- Vegetation on heart valves

SPECIAL TESTS

- Complement levels, immune complex assays (cryoglobulins, Raji cell test, C1q precipitins)
- Coagulation studies (lupus anticoagulant)
- Biopsy of skin, kidney and peripheral nerves may reveal typical histopathology

IMAGING

- Cerebral angiography in CNS lupus
- Chest x-ray for pulmonary infiltration, pleural effusion
- MRI to detect CNS lupus
- Echocardiogram for pericardial effusion

DIAGNOSTIC PROCEDURES

- American Rheumatology Association (ARA) criteria are a combination of any 4 manifestations of the 11 listed
  - ◊ Malar (butterfly) rash
  - ◊ Discoid rash
  - ◊ Photosensitivity
  - ◊ Oral/nasopharyngeal ulcers
  - ◊ Nonerosive arthritis
  - ◊ Pleuritis or pericarditis
  - ◊ Renal disorder - proteinuria or cylindruria
  - ◊ Neurologic disorder - psychosis or seizures
  - ◊ Hematologic disorder - hemolytic anemia, leukopenia (less than 4,000), lymphopenia (less than 1,500), thrombocytopenia (less than 100,000)
  - ◊ Immunologic disorder
  - ◊ Positive antinuclear antibody (ANA) in absence of drugs known to cause positive ANA

Note: While the above criteria are required for proper epidemiologic classification of SLE, in practical situations, the combination of a multi-system inflammatory illness, positive antinuclear antibody (ANA) and absence of a better diagnosis often represents the most practical way to make a clinical diagnosis

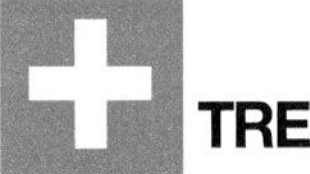

TREATMENT

APPROPRIATE HEALTH CARE Outpatient with regular monitoring

GENERAL MEASURES

- Avoidance of or protection from ultraviolet light by using sunscreens, hats, etc.
- Early intervention when infections occur
- Energy conservation
- Stress avoidance/management

SURGICAL MEASURES N/A

ACTIVITY

- As active as possible
- Those with arthritis may be limited by their pain, but active exercises are to be encouraged

DIET No special diet unless for complications such as renal failure

PATIENT EDUCATION Printed materials available on lupus from the Arthritis Foundation, 1314 Spring Street N.W., Atlanta, GA 30309, (404)872-7100; and from the Lupus Foundation of America, 1717 Massachusetts Avenue, NW, Suite 203, Washington, DC 20036, (800)558-0121

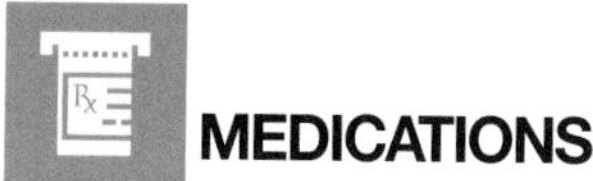

MEDICATIONS

DRUG(S) OF CHOICE
No one drug of choice available. Treatment is symptomatic with certain exceptions. Use of local steroids for cutaneous manifestations, NSAIDs for minor arthritis symptoms, low dose steroids for minor discomfort and high dose steroids for major inflammatory disease.
- Immunosuppressants are indicated for renal disease and severe disease in other organs
- NSAIDs: minor arthritis
- Sunscreen and topical steroids for cutaneous lupus
- Hydroxychloroquine 310 mg (400 mg of the sulfate salt) qd for more significant arthritis or dermal lupus
- Prednisone 30-60 mg qd for major symptoms in one or more organ systems
- Cyclophosphamide 0.5 gm/m2 IV monthly together with prednisone 60 mg po qd tapering to 10 mg every other day after 4 months for glomerulonephritis
- Methotrexate 5-25 mg oral or subcutaneous, weekly in 1 single dose has been effective as a "steroid sparer" for arthritis, rash, serositis or fever
- Immune globulin IV pulse has been effective in the temporary treatment of SLE thrombocytopenia
- Heparin or warfarin (Coumadin) in obvious thrombotic disease and/or CNS symptoms, when associated with a positive "lupus anticoagulant" test or anticardiolipin antibody

Contraindications: Refer to manufacturer's profile of each drug
Precautions: Ensure good hydration when administering cyclophosphamide due to possibility of hemorrhagic cystitis
Significant possible interactions: Refer to manufacturer's profile of each drug

ALTERNATIVE DRUGS N/A

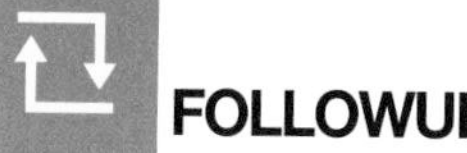

FOLLOWUP

PATIENT MONITORING
- Follow acute flares frequently, (weekly to monthly) for adjustment of medication based on clinical impression. Laboratory parameters are of limited value. CBC useful in hematologic lupus. Serum creatinine or renal clearance tests of value in renal lupus. Sedimentation rate often helps determine adequate suppression of symptoms or development of a remission.
- The confirming tests for lupus (ANA titers, anti-DNA titers, complement levels, etc.) are usually not helpful in follow-up assessment
- Use of continuing medication depends upon symptoms. Exception is in the case of renal lupus for which it has been shown that a defined course of monthly IV cyclophosphamide has been of value.
- Baseline ophthalmological exam and yearly exam while on hydroxychloroquine

PREVENTION/AVOIDANCE
- Avoiding sun exposure is only necessary for approximately one sixth of SLE patients (those who self report such sensitivity)
- Routine vaccinations are safe and appropriate for SLE patients
- Drugs known to induce SLE in normal individuals are not necessarily contraindicated in patients who have idiopathic SLE

POSSIBLE COMPLICATIONS
Fever, vasculitis, panniculitis, myositis, avascular necrosis of bone, endocarditis, pulmonary fibrosis, renal failure, organic brain syndromes, peripheral neuropathy, stroke syndromes, pancreatitis and elevated liver enzymes, infertility, ascites, venous thrombosis, seizures

EXPECTED COURSE/PROGNOSIS
- Most patients with lupus follow a course of remissions and exacerbations. Many experience spontaneous permanent remission.
- Treatment of renal lupus (the most serious form) with immunosuppressors, renal dialysis, and renal transplantation, has increased the five year life expectancy to over 90%. For those patients surviving the first two years of disease, life expectancy is essentially normal.
- In patients with drug-induced lupus, symptoms should gradually decrease upon discontinuation of the suspected agent.

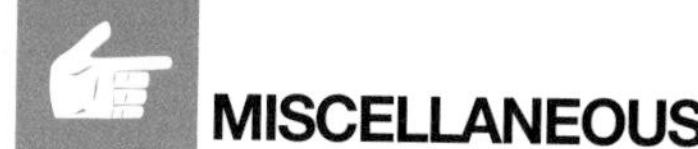

MISCELLANEOUS

ASSOCIATED CONDITIONS
Other autoimmune diseases - rheumatoid arthritis, hypothyroidism, diabetes

AGE-RELATED FACTORS
Pediatric: Stroke syndromes frequently seen in children
Geriatric:
- Higher percentage of males involved among the elderly
- Since "false-positive ANA" reaches 15% in the elderly, caution in interpretation is required in this age group

Others: N/A

PREGNANCY
- Onset of lupus and lupus flares are more common during pregnancy
- Fetal loss is increased for mothers with lupus
- Newborns of mothers who have lupus are more likely to have cardiac arrhythmias
- Specialists' collaboration during pregnancy is indicated

SYNONYMS
- SLE
- Disseminated lupus erythematosus

ICD-9-CM
710.0 Systemic lupus erythematosus

SEE ALSO
Anemia, autoimmune hemolytic
Glomerulonephritis, membranous

OTHER NOTES N/A

ABBREVIATIONS N/A

REFERENCES

- Kelley WN, Harris ED, Ruddy S, Sledge CB: Textbook of Rheumatology. 4th Ed. Philadelphia, W.B. Saunders Co., 1993
- Kippel JH, Dippe PA, eds: Rheumatology, St. Louis, Mosby, 1994
- Tan FK, Arnett FC: The genetics of lupus. Curr Opin in Rheumatol 1998;10(4):399-408
- Godfrey T, et al: Therapeutic advances in SLE. Curr Opin in Rheumatol 1998;10(4):435-41

Web references: 1 available at www.5mcc.com
Illustrations 5 available

Author(s):
Michael Tutt, MD

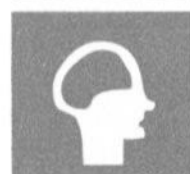

BASICS

DESCRIPTION Tapeworms (cestodes, flatworms) can be parasitic in humans. Adult worms consist of a head (scolex), which attaches to the host's GI tract; the neck (germinal region); and a segmented body (strobila), with individual segments (proglottid) containing sets of male and female reproductive organs that produce eggs. The life cycle of all but one tapeworm (*Hymenolepis nana*) requires an intermediate host, where they grow as larval forms in tissue that is then ingested by the final host, where it subsequently develops into an adult. *Hymenolepis nana* can complete all stages of development in humans, helping to make it the most common tapeworm in humans.
Most tapeworm infections are confined to the GI tract, however somatic disease can occur with *Taenia solium* eggs being ingested (cysticercosis), or with echinococcus infections, making infections with these more serious. Neurocysticercosis is the most common inpatient disorder due to parasite infection. Tapeworms/their usual intermediate host/and type of infection in humans/description include:

Tapeworm intermediate hosts:

Name	Host
D. latum	fresh water fish
D. caninum	dog, cat, fleas
E. granulosis	human, sheep, cow, dog
E. multilocularis	fox, coyotes, cats, rodents
H. diminuta	rodent, insects
H. nana	human, rodent, insects
T. saginata	cow
T. solium	pig

- *Taenia saginata*/beef/intestinal worm. 2-4 months after ingestion to become adult tapeworm. 3-10 meters long. Usually single tapeworm. Proglottids are motile and can crawl out of anus. May live 30 years.
- *Taenia solium*/pork/a.) intestinal worm, b.) Cysticercosis, a somatic infection/2-4 months to become adult worm. 3 meters long, occasionally multiple. Proglottids not motile. May live up to 25 years. Ingestion of encysted larvae (cysticerci) cause intestinal tapeworm. Ingestion of *T. solium* eggs causes cysticercosis. Eggs look identical to *T. saginata* eggs.
- *Diphyllobothrium latum* and other species/fresh water fish/intestinal worm/longest adult tapeworm - up to 25 meters. Matures to adult in 3-5 weeks.
- *Hymenolepis nana*/rodent, insects, or human /intestinal worm/ Mature to adult worms in 10-12 days. Seldom exceeds 40 mm long. Proglottids rarely seen in stool. Eggs can autoinfect individual, or occasionally insects (especially meal worms). Fecal oral transmission possible. Lifespan 4-10 weeks, but autoinfection can perpetuate infection. Usually self cleared by adolescence.
- *Echinococcus granulosis* and *Echinococcus multilocularis*/humans, sheep, cattle are intermediate hosts with dogs the definitive hosts for granulosis. Foxes, coyotes or cats are definitive hosts for multilocularis with rodents the intermediate hosts. Somatic infections: a.) hydatid disease of liver, spleen, etc., b.) alveolar hydatid disease/Adult worm lives in dogs (or rodents), human ingests eggs, larvae hatch and are carried through circulation to various organs such as liver and lungs where develop into hydatid cysts which enlarge causing symptoms perhaps 5-20 years later.
- *Hymenolepis diminuta*/rodents and insects/intestinal worm/90 cm long. Humans rare accidental host by swallowing contaminated mealworms or grain beetles in grain.
- *Dipylidium caninum*/dogs and cats and fleas/intestinal worm/10-70 cm long. Motile proglottids, shape of cucumber seeds, can crawl out anus. Rare accidental infection of humans from ingesting infected flea that came from dogs or cats.

System(s) affected: Gastrointestinal, Nervous
Genetics: N/A
Incidence/Prevalence in USA: Occurs infrequently. More often associated with immigrant population and ethnic groups with certain cultural eating habits. Can be endemic when fecal contamination enters water or food supplies.
Predominant age: All ages affected. *Hymenolepis nana* and *H. diminuta* more common in children.
Predominant sex: Male = Female

SIGNS & SYMPTOMS

- *Taenia saginata* (beef tapeworm): Generally asymptomatic. Often noted by passing eggs or proglottids, which can occasionally be felt crawling out of anus. Mild gastrointestinal symptoms may occur (one third) - nausea, abdominal pain, change in appetite, weakness, weight loss, allergic symptoms urticaria, pruritus.
- *Taenia solium* (pork tapeworm):
  - ◊ Intestinal worm - generally asymptomatic, noted passing eggs or proglottids (which are not motile). Occasional minor abdominal complaints similar to *T. saginata*.
  - ◊ Larval migration - Cysticercosis - most common to brain and skeletal muscle. Neurologic manifestations such as new onset of seizures, focal neurologic deficits, hydrocephalus, headache, vomiting, visual changes, dizziness.
- *Diphyllobothrium latum* (fish tapeworm): Generally asymptomatic, noted passing eggs, vomiting segment of worm, or occasionally passing proglottid segments. Occasionally mild abdominal discomfort, weight loss. Worm has marked affinity for vitamin B12, 40% decreased B12 levels, 2% megaloblastic anemia with glossitis, rare B12 associated neurologic symptoms.
- *Hymenolepis* nana (dwarf tapeworm): Usually asymptomatic. If heavy infection: anorexia, abdominal pain, and diarrhea.
- *Echinococcosis* (hydatid disease): Symptoms related to growth of cyst. Liver cysts - abdominal pain, RUQ mass, obstructive jaundice. Cyst rupture - fever, urticaria, pruritus, anaphylaxis. Pulmonary cyst, cough, chest pain, hemoptysis. Other organs possible - bone with pathologic fractures, CNS - space-occupying lesions, heart - conduction defects, pericarditis.
- *Hymenolepis diminuta* (rodent tapeworm): Most asymptomatic. Pass eggs in stool, proglottids disintegrate. Headache, mild GI symptoms - anorexia, nausea, cramps diarrhea.
- *Dipylidium caninum* (dog tapeworm): Most asymptomatic. Occasionally abdominal pain, diarrhea, anal pruritus, urticaria. May observe proglottid in diaper or stool.

CAUSES Eating the infective form of the parasite either by eating contaminated food such as undercooked beef, pork, fish, or infected insects that may be in cereals or grains, or through fecal-oral contamination.

RISK FACTORS

- Taenia's: Eating raw or undercooked beef or pork, particularly in Africa, Latin America, Middle East, Central Asia, India
- Cysticercosis: Presence of a tapeworm carrier in close environment. Water contaminated with sewage.
- *Diphyllobothrium*: Eating raw or undercooked fish, particularly in northern Europe
- *Hymenolepis nana*: More frequent in children, institutionalized, malnourished, immunodeficient
- *Echinococcus granulosis*: Keeping dogs around sheep and goats highest risk for hydatid cyst disease
- *Echinococcus multilocularis*: Contact with foxes, coyotes - such as hunters, trappers, veterinarians; mostly found in northern latitudes

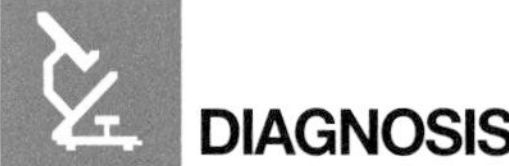

DIAGNOSIS

DIFFERENTIAL DIAGNOSIS

- Non-tapeworm gastroenteritis
- Irritable bowel syndrome
- Intestinal obstruction
- Cholecystitis or biliary obstruction
- B12 deficiency from non-tapeworm etiologies
- Tumors (abscesses, malignant, benign, etc.)
- Idiopathic epilepsy

LABORATORY

- Mild to moderate eosinophilia, increased IgE
- Microscopic analysis of eggs or proglottids
- Macrocytic, megaloblastic anemia rarely with diphyllobothriasis

Drugs that may alter lab results: N/A

Disorders that may alter lab results: N/A

PATHOLOGICAL FINDINGS

- Intestinal tapeworms - no pathological findings
- Cysticercosis: Cysts, 5-10 mm in soft tissue. Calcified cysts in CNS, muscle.
- Echinococcus: Hydatid cyst in liver, lung, other tissues

SPECIAL TESTS

- Stool evaluation of O&P
- Microscopic evaluation of proglottid collected in water or saline
- Antibody testing by ELISA to differentiate *T. saginata* eggs from *T. solium*
- Enzyme-linked immunoelectrotransfer blot (EITB) - test of choice for cysticercosis, echinococcus
- DNA probes for *T. saginata* or *T. solium*
- Consider serologic testing if identify *T. solium* eggs or proglottids (as autoinfection possible, which can cause cysticercosis)
- Serologic testing for echinococcus

IMAGING

- Intestinal tapeworms occasionally seen by small bowel enteroclysis
- Cysticercosis: start with CT; MRI may be used as adjunct if CT unclear
- Echinococcus cysts: start with ultrasound; CT scan may also be used.

DIAGNOSTIC PROCEDURES

- Occasional excisional biopsy of cysticercosis cyst
- Perianal inspection for eggs or proglottids

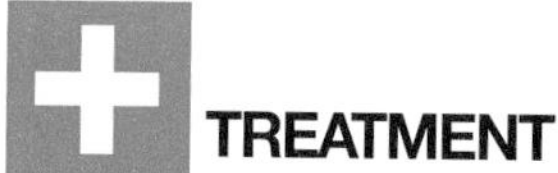

TREATMENT

APPROPRIATE HEALTH CARE Outpatient unless complications from cysts

GENERAL MEASURES
- Treatment of large percentage of population in endemic area can help
- Treatment of all immigrants from endemic countries with albendazole is being explored
- General supportive care during treatment
- Good hygienic measures should be employed
- Asymptomatic cysticercosis may resolve spontaneously without treatment, however, antiparasitic therapy of parenchymal cysts may reduce the number of seizures with generalization. Treatment may induce an inflammatory response and symptoms.

SURGICAL MEASURES
- Cysticercosis and hydatid cysts have been removed surgically, with care not to leak fluid.
- Hydatid cysts: Surgery may be necessary based on location of cyst. Surgical risks may make medical therapy preferred particularly if the cyst is not in a troublesome location. Surgery generally involves total pericystectomy or partial resection of affected organ, with albendazole pretreatment for one month. Follow surgery with albendazole.

ACTIVITY As tolerated

DIET As tolerated

PATIENT EDUCATION
- Proper cooking of beef, pork, fish
- Proper freezing of meat or fish
- Good hand washing
- Treatment of infected animals and flea prevention

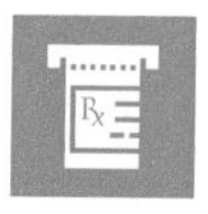

MEDICATIONS

DRUG(S) OF CHOICE
- Praziquantel (Droncit):
  - ◊ Single dose of 5-10 mg/kg (generally 10 mg/kg) for taeniasis, diphyllobothriasis, dipylidium infection and most other intestinal cestodes (cure rate > 95%)
  - ◊ Single dose of 25 mg/kg for *H. nana* adults or children (cure rate >95%)
  - ◊ 50-100 mg/kg/day tid x 14-30 days for children and adults for cysticercosis
- Niclosamide: Single dose of 2 gm for adult or 50 mg/kg for children for diphyllobothriasis, taeniasis and dipylidium infection (cure rate 90% for taeniasis and slightly less for diphyllobothriasis)
- Albendazole (Zentel):
  - ◊ Dose: > 60 kg, 400 mg bid with meals; < 60 kg, 15 mg/kg/day bid (maximum 800 mg/day)
  - ◊ For echinococcus hydatid cysts, give for 28 days, 14 days off, repeat for 3 cycles. Can be 1-6 months.
  - ◊ For neurocysticercosis, drug of choice, give 8-30 days, but examine for retinal lesions first; may repeat
- Steroids and anticonvulsants for neurocysticercosis
- PAIR therapy (puncture, aspiration, injection of a scolicidal, re-aspiration) compares favorably with surgery for echinococcosis

Contraindications: Prior sensitivity
Precautions:
- Niclosamide: Occasional nausea and abdominal pain, diarrhea, drowsiness, dizziness
- Praziquantel: Mild but frequent dizziness, myalgias, nausea, diarrhea, abdominal pain
- Albendazole: Occasional diarrhea and abdominal pain. Rare leukopenia, increased serum transaminase levels.

Significant possible interactions: Phenytoin and carbamazepine can induce metabolism of praziquantel by cytochrome P-450 causing treatment failures. Cimetidine, dexamethasone and praziquantel can increase concentration of albendazole. Corticosteroids may decrease concentration of praziquantel.

ALTERNATIVE DRUGS Niclosamide: 2 gm, then 1 gm qd X 5 more days for *H. nana*

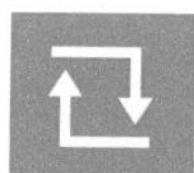

FOLLOWUP

PATIENT MONITORING Examine several stool specimens for O&P at sufficient interval to allow regrowth of worms: 3 months for *Taenia* species and 1 month for others. Follow neurocysticercosis to resolution with CT.

PREVENTION/AVOIDANCE
- Treatment of infected animals, populations and screening household contacts, immigrants
- Improved sewage treatment
- See Patient Education

POSSIBLE COMPLICATIONS
- Larval form of *T. solium* can cause system-wide cysticercosis, including neurocysticercosis (etiologic in up to 25% of cases of new-onset seizures in indigenous areas)
- Echinococcus hydatid cysts may occur causing abnormalities in the organ involved. Cyst rupture can cause spread of disease and anaphylaxis.
- B12 deficiency with *D. latum*
- Proglottid of *T. saginata* can rarely obstruct appendix, pancreatic and bile ducts
- *D. latum* can occasionally cause intestinal obstruction, cholangitis, cholecystitis

EXPECTED COURSE/PROGNOSIS
- Cure of > 95% of intestinal tapeworms with medications, occasionally requiring a second treatment
- *H. nana* often self-cured by adolescence
- *E. multilocularis* often severe or fatal
- Prognosis of systemic cysts influenced by their location

MISCELLANEOUS

ASSOCIATED CONDITIONS N/A

AGE-RELATED FACTORS
Pediatric: *H. nana*, highest among children with fecal-oral spread. *H. diminuta*, and *Dipylidium caninum* more common in children, as more likely to accidentally ingest insects.
Geriatric: N/A
Others: N/A

PREGNANCY N/A

SYNONYMS N/A

ICD-9-CM
122.9 Echinococcosis, other and unspecified
123.8 Other specified cestode infection
123.9 Cestode infection, unspecified

SEE ALSO

OTHER NOTES Vaccination of pigs to *T. Solium* is being explored

ABBREVIATIONS
O&P = ova and parasites

REFERENCES

- Isselbacher KJ, et al, editors. Harrison's Principles of Internal Medicine 13th Edition, New York: McGraw-Hill; 1994
- Liu LX, Weller PF. Antiparasitic Drugs. New Eng J of Med 1996;334(18): 1178-1184
- Miranda A. Neurocysticercosis. Amer Fam Phys 1993;47(5):1193-1197
- Schantz PM. Tapeworms (cestodiasis). Gastroenterol Clin of No Amer 1996;25(3):637-653
- Wyngaarden JB, Smith LH, Bennett JC, editors. Cecil Textbook of Medicine. 19th Ed. Philadelphia: W.B. Saunders Co; 1992
- The Medical Letter On Drugs and Therapeutics. Drugs For Parasitic Infections. Mark Abramowicz, editor. New Rochelle (NY): The Medical Letter, Inc.; April 2003
- Garcia HH, et al. A Trial of Antiparasitic Treatment to Reduce the Rate of Seizures Due to Cerebral Cysticercosis. New Eng J of Med 2004;350(3):249-258

Web references: 2 available at www.5mcc.com
Illustrations N/A

Author(s):
Kenton Voorhees, MD

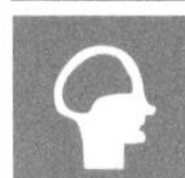

BASICS

DESCRIPTION Teething is the eruption of the deciduous teeth which most children experience without difficulty. It is a natural, gradual and predictable process but the timetable varies from baby to baby.

- Deciduous teeth
  - ◊ Most deciduous teeth begin to erupt at 5-7 months of age and teething is completed by 2-3 years
  - ◊ The mandibular central incisors erupt first, then the two or four maxillary incisors followed by the lower lateral incisors
  - ◊ After a few months, the four molars appear (lower ones at 12 months, the upper ones at 14 months)
  - ◊ After the cuspid teeth appear at 16-18 months of age the second molars erupt at 25-33 months
  - ◊ About 25% normal babies may have delayed eruption of teeth until 4 or 6 teeth simultaneously appear after their first birthday
  - ◊ Premature babies erupt teeth according to their gestational age rather than chronological age. If teething seems particularly delayed, refer patient to a pediatric dentist.
- Teeth in neonates
  - ◊ One in 2000 neonates are born with a tooth (appears to be familial)
  - ◊ These neonatal teeth may be loose but most are the normal deciduous lower central incisors and can persist
  - ◊ Mild ulceration in the sublingual area has been reported in 18% of these babies
  - ◊ Because of the potential for aspiration there is some controversy about elective removal of the loose teeth (most pediatric dentists would remove these teeth if they are loose)

System(s) affected: Gastrointestinal
Genetics: N/A
Incidence/Prevalence in USA: N/A
Predominant age: Birth to 2 1/2 years
Predominant sex: N/A

SIGNS & SYMPTOMS

- A large percent of babies have no signs or symptoms of teething
- Excessive drooling and chewing on fingers begins at 3-4 months of age. This is also the time that normal hand-mouth stimulation increases salivation.
- A small red or white spot may appear over the swollen gum just prior to tooth eruption
- Local inflammation, swelling and occasional hemorrhage can be found on the involved gums
- Discomfort may be noted more with the eruption of the first tooth, the molars and/or with the simultaneous eruption of multiple teeth
- Restlessness, irritability, disturbed sleep, changes in feeding patterns, nasal discharge, mild cough, chin rash, fever, diarrhea, pulling of ear and rubbing of the cheeks have been reported by parents. It is impossible to document that these are caused by teething, so parents and health providers should consider other possible etiologies so as not to miss or delay diagnosing an illness.

CAUSES N/A

RISK FACTORS N/A

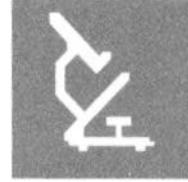

DIAGNOSIS

DIFFERENTIAL DIAGNOSIS

Herpetic gingivostomatitis - infants with fever, irritability, sleeplessness and difficulty feeding may have underlying infection caused by herpes simplex virus. Some of these infants with positive culture may not have evidence of inflammation or ulceration expected in gingivitis.

LABORATORY N/A

Drugs that may alter lab results: N/A

Disorders that may alter lab results: N/A

PATHOLOGICAL FINDINGS N/A

SPECIAL TESTS N/A

IMAGING N/A

DIAGNOSTIC PROCEDURES N/A

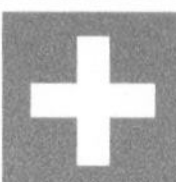

TREATMENT

APPROPRIATE HEALTH CARE

Outpatient

GENERAL MEASURES

- Treatment for teething include reassurance for the parents and symptomatic relief, if needed
- Provide the infant with a safe, one piece teething ring, clean cloth or pacifier for gumming
- Rub the involved swollen gums if the baby appears to be comforted
- Cool fluids may be offered but avoid frozen foods or objects. These could cause thermal damage to the tissues.
- Toast, cookies, bagels and crackers are offered by some parents for teething, but parents must observe carefully to prevent choking
- Avoid over-the-counter preparations for teething such as lidocaine (Xylocaine 2%, Baby Ora-Gel, Num-zit Gel, Num-zit Liquid, Anbesol). Misuse, overuse and sensitivity have been reported.
- Avoid the use of alcohol
- For the infant with low grade fever, irritability and/or inflamed gums (where other comforting measures have not been of help) - acetaminophen, in proper doses (10-15 mg/kg/dose every 4 hours prn), can be used intermittently
- Gum hematomas that erupt appear as a blue cyst. Most do not require medical intervention. Be sure there are no other signs of a bleeding disorder.
- Breast feeding babies may attempt to chew on the nipple at the end of sucking while teething but can be taught not to bite. Breast feeding can continue after teeth are present.
- Advise parents to avoid: Sugared pacifiers, painted furniture which may contain lead, tying teething ring with cord around the infant's neck, and imported fluid-filled teething rings

SURGICAL MEASURES N/A

ACTIVITY

No restrictions

DIET

No special diet

PATIENT EDUCATION

- Parents should be cautioned not to misinterpret teething as the cause of any systemic manifestation. The health provider should be consulted for any systemic complaints.
- The ABC's of Teething, Am Academy of Pediatric Dentistry, Public Relations Manual

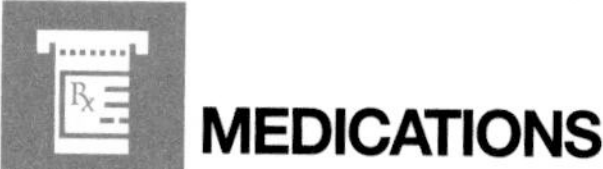

MEDICATIONS

DRUG(S) OF CHOICE N/A
Contraindications: N/A
Precautions: N/A
Significant possible interactions: N/A

ALTERNATIVE DRUGS N/A

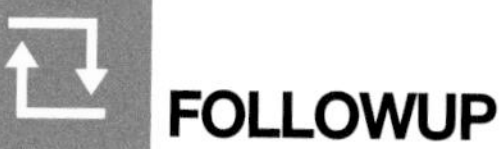

FOLLOWUP

PATIENT MONITORING N/A

PREVENTION/AVOIDANCE N/A

POSSIBLE COMPLICATIONS N/A

EXPECTED COURSE/PROGNOSIS
Normal progression through the teething process without illness

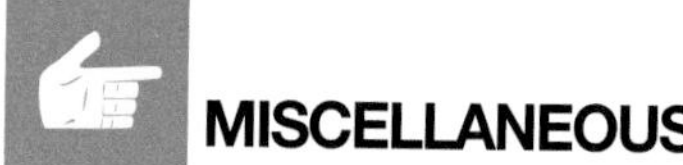

MISCELLANEOUS

ASSOCIATED CONDITIONS N/A

AGE-RELATED FACTORS
Pediatric: N/A
Geriatric: N/A
Others: N/A

PREGNANCY N/A

SYNONYMS N/A

ICD-9-CM
520.7 Teething syndrome

SEE ALSO

OTHER NOTES N/A

ABBREVIATIONS N/A

REFERENCES

- King NM, Lee A: Prematurely erupted teeth in the newborn infant. J Ped, 1989;114:807
- Gardiner J: Erupted teeth in the newborn. Proc Roy Soc Med, 1961;4:504
- Falkner F: Deciduous tooth eruption. Archives Disease of Childhood, 1957;32:386-391
- Seward M: General disturbances attributed to the eruption of human primary dentition. J of Dent for Children, 1972;39(3):178-183
- Golden N, Takieddine F, Hirsch V: Teething age - prematurely born infants. Am J of Dis of Child, 1981;135:903-904
- McDonald RE: Eruption of the teeth, local, systematic and congenital factors that influence the process. In: Dentistry for the Child and Adolescent. 5th Ed. St. Louis, C.V. Mosby Co., 1987:189-196
- King DL, Steinhauer W, Garcia-Godoy F, Elkins CO: Herpetic gingivostomatitis and teething difficulty in infants. Pediatric Dentistry 1992;14:82-85

Web references: 1 available at www.5mcc.com
Illustrations N/A

Author(s):
Dan Doss, DDS

BASICS

DESCRIPTION Syndrome characterized by pain and tenderness in the jaw muscles, sound and/or pain over the temporomandibular joint (TMJ), with limitation of mandibular movement
System(s) affected: Musculoskeletal
Genetics: N/A
Incidence/Prevalence in USA: Symptoms or signs of TMJ dysfunction are present in up to one half of the population but only 5-25% seek treatment
Predominant age: Symptoms more common age 30-50
Predominant sex: Female > Male (3:1)

SIGNS & SYMPTOMS
- Facial and/or TMJ pain
- Locking or catching of the jaw
- TMJ noises - clicking, grinding, popping
- Headache
- Earache
- Neck pain

CAUSES
- TMJ synovitis
- TMJ disc derangement
- Hyper- or hypomobile TMJ
- Occluso-muscular dysfunction (bruxism)
- Masticatory muscle spasm
- Trauma
- Poorly fitting dentures

RISK FACTORS
- Chronic oral habits such as clenching or grinding of the teeth
- Osteoarthritis, rheumatoid arthritis
- Dental malocclusion
- Fibrositis
- Psychosocial stress

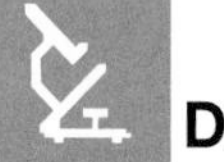

DIAGNOSIS

DIFFERENTIAL DIAGNOSIS
- Condylar fracture/dislocation
- Trigeminal neuralgia
- Dental or periodontal conditions
- TMJ neoplasm

LABORATORY N/A

Drugs that may alter lab results: N/A

Disorders that may alter lab results: N/A

PATHOLOGICAL FINDINGS
- Condylar head displacement
- Anterior disc displacement
- Posterior capsulitis
- Loosening of disc and capsular attachments
- Chondroid metaplasia of disc leading to disc perforation and degeneration

SPECIAL TESTS Jaw range of motion (opening, closing, lateral, protrusive) and masticatory muscle strength

IMAGING
- Single-contrast videoarthrography demonstrates joint dynamics and disc movement
- Panoramic dental radiographs
- MRI - noninvasive study for disc position. Information gained helps in deciding conservative versus surgical management.

DIAGNOSTIC PROCEDURES Arthroscopy

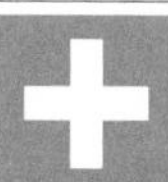

TREATMENT

APPROPRIATE HEALTH CARE Outpatient treatment

GENERAL MEASURES
- Jaw rest
- Local heat therapy
- Anti-inflammatory medications
- Muscle relaxants
- Analgesics
- Correction of malocclusion with orthodontic appliance
- Stress reduction
- Behavior modification to eliminate tension-relieving oral habits
- Buccal separator orthodontic appliance
- Linearly polarized, near-infrared irradiation

SURGICAL MEASURES N/A

ACTIVITY Jaw rest

DIET Soft diet to reduce chewing

PATIENT EDUCATION
- Be aware of any teeth-clenching or grinding habits, and relax the jaw by disengaging the teeth
- Avoid wide uncontrolled opening such as yawning
- Management of stress. Behavioral modification counseling may be helpful.

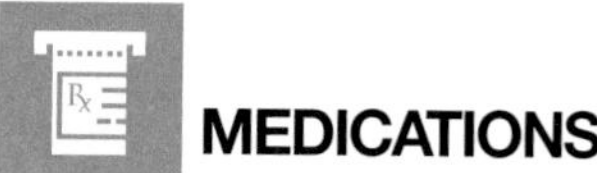

MEDICATIONS

DRUG(S) OF CHOICE
- Non-steroidal anti-inflammatory drugs (NSAIDs) - no single drug more efficacious than another
- Botulinum toxin

Contraindications:
- History of anaphylaxis to aspirin
- Peptic ulcer disease
- Renal insufficiency

Precautions:
- Peptic ulcers, gastritis or GI bleeding may occur with chronic use
- May cause acute interstitial nephritis
- Drug accumulation with renal insufficiency
- Liver function abnormalities in up to 15% of patients

Significant possible interactions:
- Albumin-bound drugs - displacement of either drug
- Warfarin - increased prothrombin time
- Lithium - increased lithium plasma level
- Furosemide - decreased natriuretic effect
- Propranolol - decreased antihypertensive effect

ALTERNATIVE DRUGS Analgesic agents; muscle relaxants

FOLLOWUP

PATIENT MONITORING
- Ongoing assessment of clinical response to conservative therapies (NSAIDs, behavior modification, occlusal splints) is necessary
- A surgical procedure to correct disc displacement or replace a damaged disc may be indicated only if the patient has not responded to conservative treatment

PREVENTION/AVOIDANCE Elimination of tension-relieving oral habits and reducing overall muscle tension

POSSIBLE COMPLICATIONS
- Secondary degenerative joint disease
- Chronic TMJ dislocation
- Loss of joint range of motion
- Depression and chronic pain syndromes

EXPECTED COURSE/PROGNOSIS
- With conservative therapy, symptoms resolve in 3/4 of the cases within three months
- Patients benefit the most from a comprehensive treatment approach including correction of occlusal discrepancies, restoration of normal muscle function, pain control, stress management and behavior modification

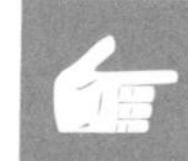

MISCELLANEOUS

ASSOCIATED CONDITIONS Cranio-mandibular disorders

AGE-RELATED FACTORS
Pediatric: N/A
Geriatric: N/A
Others: N/A

PREGNANCY No association

SYNONYMS
- Myofascial pain-dysfunction (MPD) syndrome

ICD-9-CM
524.60 Temporomandibular joint disorders, unspecified

SEE ALSO
Bruxism

OTHER NOTES N/A

ABBREVIATIONS N/A

REFERENCES

- Wright EF, Schiffman EL. Treatment alternatives for patients with masticatory myofacial pain. J ADA 1995;126(7):1030-1039
- dosSantos J. Supportive conservative therapies for temporomandibular disorders. Dental Clin NA 1995;39(2):459-477
- Laskin DM. Putting order into temporomandibular disorders. J Oral Maxillofacial Surg 1998;56(2):121
- Mock D. The differential diagnosis of temporomandibular joint disorders. J Orofac Pain 1999;13(4):246-250
- Kuttila S, Kuttila M, Le Bell Y, Alanen P, Jouko S. Aural symptoms and signs of temporomandibular disorder in association with treatment need and visits to a physician. Laryngoscope 1999;109(10):1669-73
- Pankhurst CL. Controversies in the aetiology of temporomandibular disorders. Part 1. Temporomandibular disorders: all in the mind? Prim Dent Care 1997;4(1):25-30
- Bush FM, Harkins SW, Harrington WG. Otalgia and aversive symptoms in temporomandibular disorders. Ann Otol Rhinol Laryngol 1999;108(9):884-92
- Schwartz MB, Freund BB. Treatment of temporomandibulr disorders with botulinum toxin. Clin J Pain Nov/Dec 2002;18(6)suppl:S198-S203
- Yokoyama K, Sugiyama K. Temporomandibular joint pain analgesia by linearly polarized near-infrared irradiation. Clin J Pain Mar 2001; 17(1):47-51

Web references: 0 available at www.5mcc.com
Illustrations N/A

Author(s):
Scott A. Fields, MD

BASICS

DESCRIPTION Inflammation of tendon occurring usually at its point of insertion into bone or at the point of muscular origin. The inflammation can extend to adjacent bursal tissue.
System(s) affected: Musculoskeletal
Genetics: N/A
Incidence/Prevalence in USA: Common
Predominant age: None
Predominant sex: Male > Female (slightly)

SIGNS & SYMPTOMS
- Pain overlying the point of inflammation. This is usually worsened by active motion, but can be present at rest.
- Tenderness over the affected tendon
- Mild erythema and increased heat of overlying skin, especially if the tendon is superficial as in the case of the tendo Achilles

CAUSES Usually related to repetitive activity or trauma, but can be without obvious cause

RISK FACTORS Professional athletes and manual laborers are especially prone to tendinitis due to repetitive use

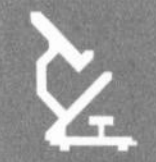

DIAGNOSIS

DIFFERENTIAL DIAGNOSIS
- Avulsion of the tendon - may occur with loss of function of the affected muscle. X-rays may show a portion of bone avulsed with the tendon, though this is not constant.
- Bursitis - can be impossible to differentiate, especially since the two conditions may coexist
- Infectious tenosynovitis - this occurs largely in the hand. The tenderness and swelling are located along the synovial lines proximally, instead of the insertion. Pain is more marked as is swelling and erythema. The sedimentation rate and white count will usually be elevated.
- Arthritis - the joint may be swollen. Tenderness and pain are in the joint proper in contrast to tendinitis which will be localized to the side of the joint where tendon insertion occurs.

LABORATORY Normal

Drugs that may alter lab results: N/A

Disorders that may alter lab results: N/A

PATHOLOGICAL FINDINGS Tendinitis is usually associated with some degenerative changes in the tendon under microscopic examinations with presence of fibrinoid, mucoid or hyaline degeneration of the connective tissue

SPECIAL TESTS Sonogram - this can be an accurate examination when done with real-time machines. Dynamics of the tendon during contraction may be obtained. Exert care that the ultrasound beam does not cross the tendon obliquely.

IMAGING The CT scan and MRI have replaced even arthrography of the shoulder in most instances. In case where diagnosis is in doubt, especially as regards tendon integrity, an MRI can be obtained and this will usually identify tears, partial tears, inflammation, or tumors. MRI cannot show irregularities of the tendon sheath itself however, and will not diagnose stenosing tenosynovitis or minimal tenosynovitis, unless fluid is present.

DIAGNOSTIC PROCEDURES N/A

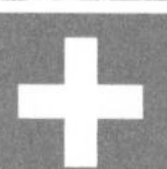

TREATMENT

APPROPRIATE HEALTH CARE Outpatient

GENERAL MEASURES Treatment goals are to relieve pain, reduce inflammation, rest the joint

SURGICAL MEASURES N/A

ACTIVITY
- In acute phases the involved muscle and tendon should be put at rest. Use slings and splints for the upper extremity. Use braces, canes and/or crutches for the lower limbs.
- Physical therapy, once patient is free of pain

DIET No special diet

PATIENT EDUCATION
- Explanation of the problem
- Instructions for use of supportive devices (e.g., crutches, slings)

MEDICATIONS

DRUG(S) OF CHOICE
- Anti-inflammatory drugs:
  - ◊ NSAIDs - all have about the same efficacy and the one which is most familiar to the prescriber can be used e.g., piroxicam (Feldene) 10 mg daily or indomethacin (Indocin) 25 or 50 mg tid after meals. Ibuprofen is a low-cost NSAID available over-the-counter.
  - ◊ Corticosteroids - injectable, 40 mg of methylprednisolone (Depo-Medrol) accompanied by 4-6 cc of 1% or 2% lidocaine (Xylocaine) often results in dramatic relief. Never inject tendon, only into tendon sheath or surrounding bursa. (Careful preparation of the skin using Betadine or similar surgical prep is mandatory to prevent infection.)

Contraindications: A tendon should never be injected with a local anesthetic and/or cortisone to allow participation in an athletic event. This can result in complete rupture of the tendon.
Precautions: See manufacturer's profile of each drug
Significant possible interactions: See manufacturer's profile of each drug

ALTERNATIVE DRUGS N/A

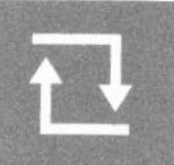

FOLLOWUP

PATIENT MONITORING Symptoms will usually subside within a few days after treatment

PREVENTION/AVOIDANCE After adequate rest and treatment, prevention of recurrences is important. Splints such as circular bands for forearm extension tendinitis or patella tendinitis may be useful.

POSSIBLE COMPLICATIONS
- Tendon rupture or avulsion fractures may occur
- Repeated exacerbations of pain. This is probably the most common indication for MRI to confirm the diagnosis and determine the extent of attenuation of the tendon.

EXPECTED COURSE/PROGNOSIS
The great majority subside without complications

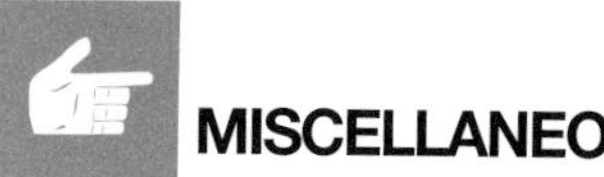

MISCELLANEOUS

ASSOCIATED CONDITIONS Bursitis, arthritis - osteophytes may be a factor in traumatizing tendons if located adjacent to a tendon

AGE-RELATED FACTORS
Pediatric: A prevalent form of tendinitis is patellar tendinitis associated with inflammation of the tibial apophysis. Known as Osgood-Schlatter disease, it is seen in adolescents especially during a growth spurt. Splinting with a patella band and restricted activity usually alleviate symptoms. However, some are recalcitrant and may require steroid injections and even surgery with splitting of the patella tendon.
Geriatric: N/A
Others: N/A

PREGNANCY N/A

SYNONYMS N/A

ICD-9-CM
726.90 Enthesopathy of unspecified site

SEE ALSO
Osgood-Schlatter disease

OTHER NOTES N/A

ABBREVIATIONS N/A

REFERENCES

- Fornage BD, Rifkin MD: Ultrasonic examinations of tendons. Radiologic Clinics of North America 1988;26(1):87-107
- Baker KS, Gilula LA: Current Role of tenography and bursography. American Journal of Roentgenography 1990;154(7):129-137
- Lawrence BD, et al: Recent advances in magnetic resonance imaging of the knee. Radiologic Clinics of North America 1990;28(1)

Web references: 0 available at www.5mcc.com
Illustrations N/A

Author(s):
R. Bruce Hall, MD

BASICS

DESCRIPTION Primary testicular neoplasms may arise from any testicular or adnexal cell component. They are divided into germinal (90-95%) and non-germinal tumors. The germinal tumors, discussed here, are further divided into seminomatous and non-seminomatous types (embryonal, teratoma, choriocarcinomas, yolk sac).
- Clinical staging - Skinner/Walter Reed
  - ◊ A: tumor limited to testis and cord
  - ◊ B: tumor of testis and retroperitoneal nodes
  - ◊ B1: <6 nodes all less than 2 cm
  - ◊ B2: > 6 nodes > 2 cm in diameter
  - ◊ B3: positive retroperitoneal nodes > 5 cm in diameter (bulky)
  - ◊ C: metastases above diaphragm or involving abdominal solid organs

System(s) affected: Reproductive
Genetics: Weak influence
Incidence/Prevalence in USA:
- 1-2% of all neoplasms in male
- 2.3-6.3 cases/year per 100,000 men (less common in African-Americans - 0.9 cases/year per 100,000)
- In adults, germ cell types comprise 90-95% of testicular cancers; in children, they represent only 60-75%

Predominant age: Peak incidence - age 20-40; smaller peaks between age 0-10 years and > 60
Predominant sex: Male only

SIGNS & SYMPTOMS
- In adults
  - ◊ Testicular nodule or swelling most common
  - ◊ Sensation of fullness or heaviness of scrotum, may be interpreted as "pain"
  - ◊ Previously "small" testicle enlarging to size of "normal" contralateral one
  - ◊ Firm, non-tender mass within confines of tunica albuginea usually palpably distinct from cord structures
  - ◊ Acute or chronic epididymitis/epididymo-orchitis resulting in delay of diagnosis (10%)
  - ◊ Manifestations due to metastasis e.g., neck mass (supraclavicular node), respiratory symptoms (lung metastasis), low back pain (nerve root or psoas irritation), uni- or bilateral lower extremity swelling (iliac or caval thrombosis or obstruction) palpable abdominal mass.
  - ◊ Hydrocele (10-20%)
  - ◊ Gynecomastia (may or may not be due to elevated hormones) (5%)
  - ◊ Rapid tumor growth resulting in hemorrhage and necrosis
- In children
  - ◊ Non-tender, non-painful scrotal mass
  - ◊ Non-transilluminable, large, non-tender testicle
  - ◊ Hydrocele (15-20%)
  - ◊ With hormonally active tumors, the scrotal exam may be unrevealing

CAUSES No real clear cause and effect relations identified

RISK FACTORS
- Caucasian race; especially Scandinavian background
- Higher social status
- Unmarried
- Rural resident
- History of cryptorchism (even if previously repaired) - only undisputed risk factor
- Positive HIV
- Weak associations
  - ◊ Maternal ingestion of hormones during 1st trimester
  - ◊ Intersex disorders in genotypic male with dysgenetic gonad, trauma (no hard evidence of significant risk factor)
  - ◊ Atrophy of any cause

DIAGNOSIS

DIFFERENTIAL DIAGNOSIS
- Hernia
- Hydrocele
- Hematoma
- Spermatocele
- Syphilitic gumma
- Varicocele
- In children - epidermoid/dermoid cyst, para-testicular rhabdomyosarcoma, macroorchidism, torsion
- Epididymitis

LABORATORY
Serum markers should be performed pre and post-operatively
- Alpha-fetoprotein (AFP) - serum half life is 5-7 days; levels elevated by pure embryonal carcinoma, teratocarcinoma, yolk sac tumor or combinations of these three, but not by pure choriocarcinoma or seminoma
- Beta human chorionic gonadotropin (beta-HCG) - serum half life is 24-36 hours; elevated by all choriocarcinoma, 40-60% embryonal carcinoma; 5-10% pure seminomas have detectable levels of beta-HCG (usually < 500 ng/mL)
- Placental alkaline phosphatase (PLAP) - may be marker of choice for seminoma. 70-90% patients with recurrent or disseminated seminomas have elevated PLAP.
- Lactate dehydrogenase (LDH) - too ubiquitous to be specific. May be direct relationship between elevated LDH levels and tumor burden. Elevated LDH may be sole biochemical abnormality in 10% of patients with persistent or recurrent non-seminomatous tumors.

Drugs that may alter lab results: N/A

Disorders that may alter lab results:
- AFP alterations may be caused by - benign liver disease; telangiectasia and tyrosinemia; malignancies of the liver, pancreas, stomach and lung; heavy marijuana smoking
- PLAP may be elevated by heavy tobacco smoking
- Beta-HCG - pancreatic, stomach, kidney, breast and bladder cancers

PATHOLOGICAL FINDINGS Basically, two different groups based on germinal vs. non-germinal and seminomatous vs. non-seminomatous types

SPECIAL TESTS N/A

IMAGING
- Scrotal ultrasound - see mass clearly originating within testis with echo-texture pattern (hypoechoic) distinct from surrounding normal testicular tissue. Echo-texture may be mixed.
- For staging:
  - ◊ Chest x-ray - good PA and lateral
  - ◊ CT scan - very accurate; able to define pelvic retroperitoneal and mediastinal lymphadenopathy as well as to detect abdominal visceral and lung metastases
  - ◊ Pedal lymphangiography (LAG) - is sensitive in picking up lymph node involvement intra-abdominally but not as accurate as CT scan in picking up upper para aortic nodes or visceral involvement
  - ◊ MRI - still largely experimental

DIAGNOSTIC PROCEDURES
- Transinguinal scrotal exploration with biopsy and/or radical orchiectomy (testicle and spermatic cord excised) makes definite diagnosis, helps stage, and decrease tumor size
- Transscrotal open or percutaneous biopsy or trans-scrotal orchiectomy contraindicated secondary to anatomical trespassing into different lymph drainage system

TREATMENT

APPROPRIATE HEALTH CARE Inpatient and outpatient

GENERAL MEASURES

Radical orchiectomy and adjuvant measures:

- Both seminomatous and non-seminomatous tumors are chemosensitive and have good chemotherapeutic response. Seminomas are extremely radiosensitive.
- Treatment for seminomas by stage:
  - ◊ A: irradiation, 2500 R to ipsilateral inguinal, iliac chains and bilateral periaortic/pericaval nodes to level of diaphragm versus observation (experimental)
  - ◊ B2: same as A, with irradiation using 600-1000 R to positive nodes
  - ◊ B3: chemotherapy - if post-chemotherapy lymph nodes persists more than 3 cm in diameter, then a retroperitoneal lymph node biopsy is added (43% of cases have viable tumor present) and further chemotherapy given if viable tumor found. If < 3 cm, observe.
  - ◊ C: primary chemotherapy
- Treatment for non-seminomatous germ cell tumor by stage:
  - ◊ A: nerve sparing staging and therapeutic retroperitoneal lymph node dissection (RPLND) alone versus observation (careful followup protocol)
  - ◊ B1 (microscopic metastasis in 1-6 nodes, < 2 cm): observation if serum markers negative
  - ◊ B2 (microscopic metastases in > 6 nodes or grossly positive nodes, 2-6 cm): observation or two courses of chemotherapy
  - ◊ B3 (nodes > 6 cm or tumor extension outside nodes): initially 4 courses of chemotherapy. If complete response based on CT scan, serum markers, and no teratoma seen in original specimen, then observe. If partial response, do retroperitoneal lymph node dissection and tumor excision plus 2 more courses of chemotherapy. If tumor cannot all be excised, salvage chemotherapy.
- Children: radical orchiectomy plus initial AFP level
  - ◊ If age ≤ 1 year and AFP rapidly normalizes, no metastases: observe for 2 years with AFP and CXR
  - ◊ If AFP doesn't normalize or CT shows suspicious lymph nodes and CXR negative: do RPLND
  - ◊ If lymph nodes are positive and chest x-ray negative: chemotherapy; if CXR positive for solitary lesion, add surgery
  - ◊ If CXR shows several lesions - give radiation
  - ◊ If age > 1 year: chemotherapy

SURGICAL MEASURES

- All patients receive radical orchiectomy for diagnosis and excellent local control

ACTIVITY As tolerated

DIET No special diet

PATIENT EDUCATION

- Discuss patient's concerns about sterility, impotence, testicular prostheses, hormone supplements
- Patient education material available from American Cancer Society

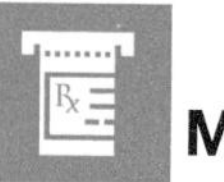

MEDICATIONS

DRUG(S) OF CHOICE

- Commonly used chemotherapeutic agents include cisplatin + etoposide ± bleomycin, paclitaxel (Taxol)
- Salvage chemotherapy includes cyclophosphamide (Cytoxan), ifosfamide [with mesna to protect against hemorrhagic cystitis], carboplatin, chemotherapy intensification with granulocyte colony stimulating factor (G-CSF) or autologous bone marrow transplant (BMT)
- In children - vincristine, dactinomycin (actinomycin-D), cyclophosphamide, doxorubicin (Adriamycin)

Contraindications: N/A

Precautions:

- Cisplatin - nephrotoxicity, ototoxicity, neurotoxicity
- Etoposide - marrow suppression, leukemia
- Cyclophosphamide/ifosfamide - hemorrhagic cystitis
- Bleomycin - pulmonary fibrosis
- Adriamycin - marrow suppression
- Vincristine - marrow suppression, neuromuscular toxicity
- Carboplatin - ototoxicity
- Taxol - neuropathy

Significant possible interactions: Refer to manufacturer's literature

ALTERNATIVE DRUGS

- Ondansetron (Zofran), dronabinol (Marinol), metoclopramide (Reglan), and others for nausea control

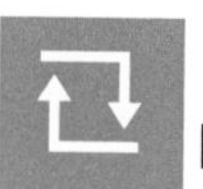

FOLLOWUP

PATIENT MONITORING

- First year - markers and chest x-ray every month, physical exam (emphasizing nodes) every 2 months
- After 1 year - markers and chest x-ray every 2 months and physical exam every 4 months
- After 2 years - markers and chest x-ray and physical exam every 6-12 months
- If patient had teratoma at diagnosis, need to followup for at least 5 years and get CT scan every year for 3 years
- Annual ultrasound of remaining testicle

PREVENTION/AVOIDANCE N/A

POSSIBLE COMPLICATIONS

- RPLND treatment - loss of seminal emission (prevented by using nerve-sparing RPLND), atelectasis, hypoalbuminemia
- Radiation treatment - radiation nephritis, enteritis
- Non-seminomatous tumors are more likely to have metastatic disease than seminomas (50-70% vs. 25%, respectively)

EXPECTED COURSE/PROGNOSIS

Usually complete cure in patients with limited disease, 70-80% cure in patients with advanced disease

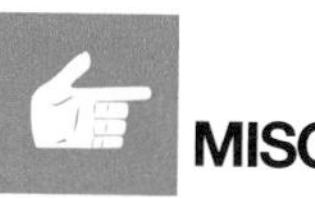

MISCELLANEOUS

ASSOCIATED CONDITIONS N/A

AGE-RELATED FACTORS

Pediatric: Rare in childhood (only 2% of all solid tumors in childhood)
Geriatric: N/A
Others: N/A

PREGNANCY N/A

SYNONYMS N/A

ICD-9-CM

186.0 Malignant neoplasm of undescended testis
186.9 Malignant neoplasm of testis, other and unspecified

SEE ALSO

OTHER NOTES N/A

ABBREVIATIONS

AFP = alpha-fetoprotein
Beta-HCG = beta human chorionic gonadotropin
LDH = lactate dehydrogenase
PLAP = placental alkaline phosphatase
RPLND = retroperitoneal lymph node dissection
G-CSF = granulocyte cell stimulating factor
BMT = bone marrow transplant

REFERENCES

- Leibovitch I: Annual ultrasound screening of remaining testicle following radical orchiectomy for testicular cancer. Multi-center trial proceedings of 94th annual American Urological Association Meeting, Dallas, 1999
- Skinner EC: In: Walsh PC, et al, eds. Campbell's Urology. Philadelphia, W.B. Saunders Co., 1998
- Klein EA: Tumor Markers in Testis Cancer. The Urologic Clinics of North America 1993;20(1):67
- Motzer RJ, Bosl GJ: Role of adjuvant chemotherapy in patients with Stage II, nonseminomatous germ cell tumors. The Urologic Clinics of North America 1993;20(1):111

Web references: 1 available at www.5mcc.com
Illustrations N/A

Author(s):
Mark R. Dambro, MD

BASICS

DESCRIPTION Twisting of testis and spermatic cord resulting in acute ischemia.
- Intravaginal torsion: occurs within tunica vaginalis
- Extravaginal torsion: involves twisting of testis, cord and processus vaginalis (especially in newborns) and in undescended testes

System(s) affected: Reproductive
Genetics: Unknown
Incidence/Prevalence in USA: 1:160 males
Predominant age: Occurs from newborn period to 7th decade; 2/3 of cases occur in 2nd decade, with peak at age 14 years; 2nd peak in neonates
Predominant sex: Males only

SIGNS & SYMPTOMS
- Scrotum is enlarged, red, and edematous
- First symptom is pain (sudden or gradual onset, increasing in severity)
- Nausea and vomiting are common
- Fever may occur
- Testicle exquisitely tender
- Testis may be high in scrotum with a transverse lie
- Absence of cremasteric reflex

CAUSES
- Torsion is usually spontaneous and idiopathic
- History of trauma in 20% of patients
- 1/3 have had prior episodic testicular pain
- Contraction of cremasteric muscle or dartos may play a role and is stimulated by trauma, exercise, cold, sexual stimulation
- Possible alterations in testosterone levels during nocturnal sex response cycle; possible elevated testosterone levels in neonates
- Testis must have inadequate, incomplete or absent fixation within scrotum

RISK FACTORS
- May be more common in winter
- Paraplegia

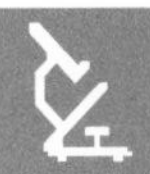

DIAGNOSIS

DIFFERENTIAL DIAGNOSIS
- Epididymo-orchitis
- Incarcerated/strangulated inguinal hernia
- Acute hydrocele
- Traumatic hematoma
- Idiopathic scrotal edema
- Torsion appendix testis
- Acute varicocele
- Testicular tumor
- Henoch-Schönlein purpura
- Scrotal abscess
- Leukemic infiltrate

LABORATORY Urinalysis may be helpful (usually not)

Drugs that may alter lab results: N/A

Disorders that may alter lab results: N/A

PATHOLOGICAL FINDINGS
- Venous thrombosis
- Tissue edema and necrosis
- Arterial thrombosis

SPECIAL TESTS N/A

IMAGING Ultrasound may confirm testicular swelling, and with Doppler, is diagnostic

DIAGNOSTIC PROCEDURES
- Doppler ultrasonic flow detection demonstrates absent or reduced blood flow with torsion, increased flow with inflammatory process (only reliable in 1st 12 hrs.)
- Radionuclide testicular scintigraphy with technetium 99m. pertechnetate demonstrates absent/decreased vascularity in torsion, increased vascularity with inflammatory processes (including torsion of appendix testes)

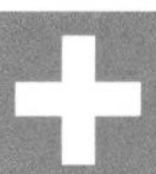

TREATMENT

APPROPRIATE HEALTH CARE
- Manual reduction - may be successful, facilitated by Lidocaine 1% (plain) injection at level of external ring. Must always be followed by orchidopexy.
- Surgical exploration via scrotal approach with detorsion, evaluation of testicular viability, orchidopexy of viable testicle, orchiectomy of non-viable testicle.

GENERAL MEASURES N/A

SURGICAL MEASURES
- Bilateral testicular fixation is recommended
- At least 3-4 point fixation with nonabsorbable sutures
- Excision of window of tunica albuginea with suture to dartos fascia
- Any testis that is not clearly viable (and obvious) should be removed.

ACTIVITY As tolerated

DIET Regular

PATIENT EDUCATION Possibility of testicular atrophy in salvaged testis with depressed sperm counts

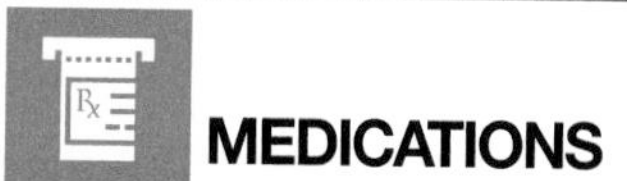

MEDICATIONS

DRUG(S) OF CHOICE N/A
Contraindications: N/A
Precautions: N/A
Significant possible interactions: N/A

ALTERNATIVE DRUGS N/A

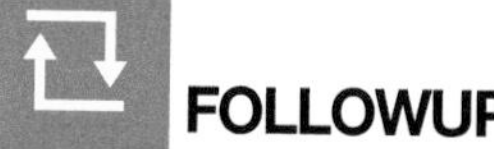

FOLLOWUP

PATIENT MONITORING
- Postoperative visit at 1-2 weeks
- Yearly visits until puberty to evaluate for atrophy

PREVENTION/AVOIDANCE N/A

POSSIBLE COMPLICATIONS
- Possible testicular atrophy
- Abnormal spermatogenesis
- Infertility

EXPECTED COURSE/PROGNOSIS
- Testicular salvage directly related to duration of torsion (85-97% if less than 6 hours, less than 10% if greater than 24 hrs)
- 80-94% may have depressed spermatogenesis related to duration of ischemic injury (possibly related to autoimmune - mediated injury)
- As many as 2/3 of salvaged testicles may atrophy in first 2-3 years post torsion

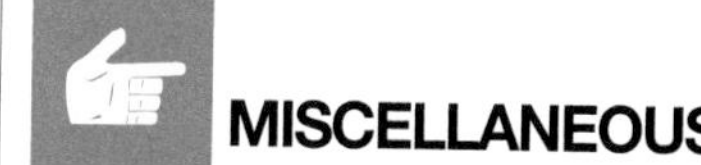

MISCELLANEOUS

ASSOCIATED CONDITIONS N/A

AGE-RELATED FACTORS N/A
Pediatric: Most common at age 14
Geriatric: Rare in this age group
Others: N/A

PREGNANCY N/A

SYNONYMS N/A

ICD-9-CM
608.2 Torsion of testis

SEE ALSO

OTHER NOTES N/A

ABBREVIATIONS N/A

REFERENCES

- Ashcraft KW. Pediatric Urology. Philadelphia, W.B. Saunders Co, 1990.
- Ashcraft KW, Murphy JP, Sharp RJ, eds. Pediatric Surgery. 3rd Ed. Philadelphia, W.B. Saunders Co., 2000
- Kelalis PP, King LR, Belman AB. Clinical Pediatric Urology. 3rd Ed. Philadelphia, W.B. Saunders Co, 1992.

Web references: 1 available at www.5mcc.com
Illustrations N/A

Author(s):
Timothy L. Black, MD

BASICS

DESCRIPTION Severe illness characterized by intermittent tonic spasms of voluntary muscles. Toxin enters the central nervous system along the peripheral nerves or is blood borne. Tetanospasmin binds at synapses and blocks inhibitors. Usual course is acute.
System(s) affected: Nervous
Genetics: N/A
Incidence/Prevalence in USA: Rare
Predominant age: Over 70% of cases in persons > 50 years of age
Predominant sex: Male = Female

SIGNS & SYMPTOMS
- Arrhythmias
- Asphyxia
- Convulsions
- Cyanosis
- Drooling
- Dysphagia
- Fluctuating hypertension
- Hydrophobia
- Hyperhidrosis
- Hyperpyrexia
- Hyperreflexia
- Hypotension
- Irritability
- Low-grade fever
- Muscular rigidity
- Muscular spasticity
- Nuchal rigidity
- Opisthotonos
- Pain at wound site
- Painful tonic convulsions
- Risus sardonicus (fixed smile)
- Stiffness of the jaw
- Sudden bradycardia
- Sudden cardiac arrest
- Tachycardia
- Tingling at wound site
- Trismus
- Wound history (may be absent)

CAUSES
- Infection with Clostridium tetani
- Neurotoxin produced by Clostridium tetani
- Tetanospasmin (an exotoxin)

RISK FACTORS
- Burns
- Drug addiction (parenteral)
- Ear infection (with tympanic membrane perforation)
- Early postpartum with an infected uterus
- Exposure of open wounds to soil and animal feces
- Frostbite
- Newborn (umbilicus stump entry)
- Skin ulcers
- Surgical wounds
- Age > 50 years
- Traumatic wound

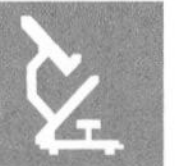

DIAGNOSIS

DIFFERENTIAL DIAGNOSIS
- Dental abscess
- Subarachnoid hemorrhage
- Seizure disorder
- Meningoencephalitis
- Peritonsillar abscess
- Dystonic reaction to phenothiazines
- Hypocalcemic tetany
- Strychnine poisoning
- Alcohol withdrawal

LABORATORY
- Polymorphonuclear leukocytosis
- Culture of Clostridium tetani from wound (may not be positive even if tetanus is the problem)

Drugs that may alter lab results: N/A

Disorders that may alter lab results: N/A

PATHOLOGICAL FINDINGS N/A

SPECIAL TESTS
- ECG - supraventricular tachycardia
- Multifocal ventricular ectopia
- Bradycardia
- EEG sleeping pattern
- Culture of wound infrequently recover C. tetani

IMAGING N/A

DIAGNOSTIC PROCEDURES N/A

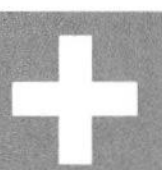

TREATMENT

APPROPRIATE HEALTH CARE Intensive care

GENERAL MEASURES
- Wound excision
- Quiet observation
- Intubation
- IV hydration
- Catheterize the bladder
- Prevent jarring of bed or drafts

SURGICAL MEASURES Tracheostomy if needed

ACTIVITY Absolute bedrest with sedation

DIET Nothing by mouth until well

PATIENT EDUCATION Griffith: Instructions for Patients. Philadelphia, W.B. Saunders Co.,1994

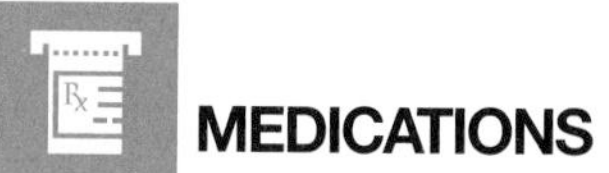

MEDICATIONS

DRUG(S) OF CHOICE

- Anticonvulsants
- Diazepam for muscle rigidity
- Pancuronium bromide (administered by anesthesiologist) plus ventilation
- Tetanus toxoid in a previously immunized patient
- Tetanus immune globulin (TIG) 3000 units to 6000 units IM. May infiltrate the area around the wound with a portion of the dose.
- Penicillin G - 2 million units IV q6h. In a penicillin allergic patient, use doxycycline 100 mg q12h, or clindamycin 150-300 mg IV q6h.

Contraindications: Refer to manufacturer's literature

Precautions: Refer to manufacturer's literature. Do not use tetanus immune globulin intravenously.

Significant possible interactions: Refer to manufacturer's literature

ALTERNATIVE DRUGS Equine tetanus antitoxin 50,000 units IM - only if tetanus immune globulin (human) is not available

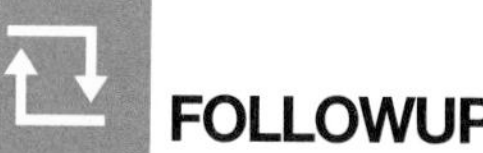

FOLLOWUP

PATIENT MONITORING Careful observation in intensive care

PREVENTION/AVOIDANCE Active immunization with tetanus toxoid; wound débridement; passive immunization with tetanus immune globulin; acellular vaccine; benzathine penicillin; penicillin G; erythromycin

POSSIBLE COMPLICATIONS

- Respiratory arrest
- Cardiac failure
- Pulmonary emboli
- Bacterial infection
- Dehydration
- Vertebral fractures
- Airway obstruction
- Anoxia
- Urinary retention
- Constipation
- Pneumonia
- Rhabdomyolysis

EXPECTED COURSE/PROGNOSIS

- 25-50% mortality
- Poor prognostic factors:
  - ◊ Form of tetanus
  - ◊ Incubation period
  - ◊ Onset period
  - ◊ Patient's age
  - ◊ Severity of symptoms
  - ◊ Heart wound
- Recovery is complete if patient survives

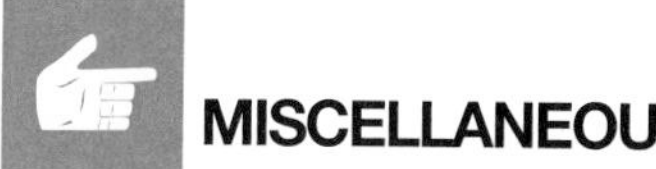

MISCELLANEOUS

ASSOCIATED CONDITIONS N/A

AGE-RELATED FACTORS

Pediatric:

- Mortality high in young
- Infection may enter through umbilical cord

Geriatric: Mortality high in elderly and may not have adequate immunizations.

Others: N/A

PREGNANCY

- Must treat vigorously despite pregnancy
- Infection may enter uterus postpartum
- Tetanus toxoid probably safe, but few data available

SYNONYMS Lockjaw

ICD-9-CM

037 Tetanus

SEE ALSO

Anaerobic & necrotizing infections
Immunizations
Meningitis, bacterial

OTHER NOTES N/A

ABBREVIATIONS N/A

REFERENCES

- von Behring E, Kitasato S. Uber das Zustandelkommen der Diphtherie-Immunität und der Tetanus-Immunität bei Thieren. Dtsch Med Wochenschr 1890;16:1113
- Centers for Disease Control, Tetanus: United States 1981-1984. MMWR, 1985;34:602
- Mandell GL, ed. Principles and Practice of Infectious Diseases. 4th Ed. New York, Churchill Livingstone, 1995
- Lugauer S, Heininger U, Cherry JD, Stehr K. Long-term clinical effectiveness of an acellular pertussis component vaccine and a whole cell pertussis component vaccine. Eur J Pediatr 2002;161(3):142-6

Web references: 0 available at www.5mcc.com

Illustrations N/A

Author(s):

Abdulrazak Abyad, MD, MPH

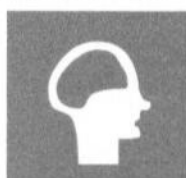

BASICS

DESCRIPTION Large ventricular septal defect (VSD) associated with right ventricular outflow obstruction (infundibular and/or valvular pulmonic stenosis), right ventricular (RV) hypertrophy and an overriding aorta
- Pathophysiology dependent primarily on severity of right ventricular outflow tract obstruction
- Right and left ventricular pressures are generally equal (VSD is proximal to level of RV obstruction, therefore, RV pressures are elevated)
- Right to left shunting is typical

System(s) affected: Cardiovascular, Pulmonary
Genetics: Familial occurrence, components indicating dominant hereditary
Incidence/Prevalence in USA:
- 5-10% of all congenital heart disease. Most common cardiac cyanotic anomaly after age 1.
- 40 per 100,000 live births

Predominant age: Newborn
Predominant sex: Male > Female (slightly)

SIGNS & SYMPTOMS
- With mild RV outflow tract obstruction a left to right shunt predominates, and the patient is acyanotic = ("Pink" tetralogy of Fallot)
- Cyanosis with severe RV outflow tract obstruction (generally recognized early)
- Exertional dyspnea, poor exercise tolerance
- Lower birth weight, retarded growth
- Clubbing and polycythemia commonly in children
- Squatting position, typical following exertion (allows increased systemic vascular resistance, lessening right to left shunting)
- No typical facies
- Scoliosis is common
- Normal arterial and jugular venous pulses
- Systolic thrill along the left sternal border
- Early systolic ejection sound (aortic)
- Single S2 (decreased P2)
- Systolic ejection murmur due to flow across narrowed RV outflow tract
- May auscultate the continuous diminished murmur of bronchial collateral vessels
- Right aortic arch in 30%
- Atrial septal defect (ASD) in 15%
- Anomalous coronary arteries in 2-10%
- Retinal engorgement
- Hemoptysis
- Aortic ejection click

CAUSES Unknown

RISK FACTORS
- Documented increased incidence with increased maternal age
- Occasional familial occurrence

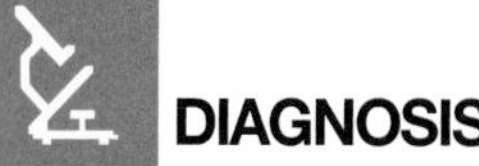

DIAGNOSIS

DIFFERENTIAL DIAGNOSIS
- Fallot's tetralogy with absent pulmonic valve
- Fallot's tetralogy with absent pulmonary artery
- Pseudotruncus arteriosus

LABORATORY N/A

Drugs that may alter lab results: N/A

Disorders that may alter lab results: N/A

PATHOLOGICAL FINDINGS
- Anterior deviation of the infundibular septum, resulting in malalignment with the muscular septum, creating a ventricular septal defect
- Malposition of the infundibular septum, which encroaches on the right ventricular outflow tract, resulting in an increased aortic root size
- Aortic root rotated into overriding position

SPECIAL TESTS
- ECG
  - ◊ Right axis deviation, right ventricular hypertrophy, subsequent right ventricular conduction abnormality
  - ◊ Sinus rhythm in general, however, some may develop atrial fibrillation or flutter

IMAGING
- Chest x-ray
  - ◊ In children, typically a small boot-shaped heart (coeur en sabot) with diminished pulmonary blood flow
  - ◊ Prominent right ventricle
  - ◊ Possibly a right sided aortic arch and knob
  - ◊ Normal (or perhaps decreased) pulmonary vascularity in approximately 50% adults
- 2D echocardiogram/Doppler echocardiogram
  - ◊ 2D images demonstrate the VSD, overriding aorta, extent and location of the infundibular obstruction, assessment of pulmonic valve, right ventricular hypertrophy, and coronary anatomy, additional ventricular septal defects, and peripheral branch pulmonic arteries
  - ◊ Doppler echocardiogram allows quantification of the outflow gradient
  - ◊ Color-flow Doppler provides assessment of the VSD
  - ◊ Coronary anatomy

DIAGNOSTIC PROCEDURES
- Cardiac catheterization
  - ◊ Assesses pulmonary annulus size and pulmonary arteries
  - ◊ Assesses severity of right ventricular outflow obstruction
  - ◊ Locates position of VSD and its size
  - ◊ Rules out possible coronary artery anomalies

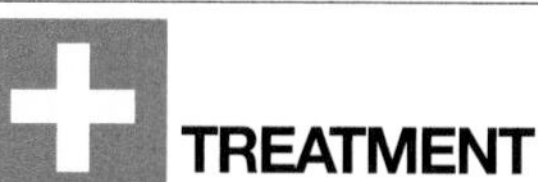

TREATMENT

APPROPRIATE HEALTH CARE Inpatient for diagnosis and surgery

GENERAL MEASURES
- Good dental hygiene
- Endocarditis prophylaxis

SURGICAL MEASURES
- Palliative surgical therapy
  - ◊ It is important to emphasize that complete repair is the preferable modality of treatment
  - ◊ Blalock-Taussig shunt or modified shunt (subclavian to pulmonary artery)
  - ◊ Pott's procedure (descending aorta to pulmonary artery)
  - ◊ Waterston's shunt (ascending aorta to pulmonary artery)
- Total correction surgical therapy
  - ◊ Includes patch closure of VSD and relief of right ventricular outflow obstruction

ACTIVITY As tolerated

DIET Salt restriction

PATIENT EDUCATION American Heart Association, 7320 Greenville Avenue, Dallas, TX 75231, (214)373-6300

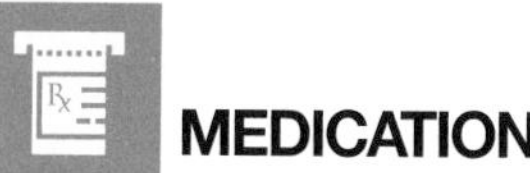

MEDICATIONS

DRUG(S) OF CHOICE No specific drug therapy in the absence of heart failure
Contraindications: N/A
Precautions: N/A
Significant possible interactions: N/A

ALTERNATIVE DRUGS N/A

FOLLOWUP

PATIENT MONITORING
- Postoperative (or post-balloon valvotomy) Doppler ultrasound suggested at approximately 1 year from procedure
- Post-valvotomy SBE prophylaxis still required
- Regular followup assessment for patients not undergoing surgical correction

PREVENTION/AVOIDANCE N/A

POSSIBLE COMPLICATIONS
- Erythrocytosis may develop secondary to chronic hypoxemia (risk for thrombosis, thrombotic CVA and paradoxical emboli)
- Increased risk for brain abscess, acute gouty arthritis
- Infective endocarditis
- Cerebrovascular thrombosis
- Delayed puberty
- Postoperatively
  - ◊ Residual right ventricular outflow obstruction
  - ◊ Residual VSD
  - ◊ Pulmonic regurgitation
  - ◊ Ventricular arrhythmias
  - ◊ Right bundle branch block quite common
  - ◊ Left anterior hemiblock
  - ◊ Infective bacterial endocarditis

EXPECTED COURSE/PROGNOSIS
Fatal if not surgically corrected

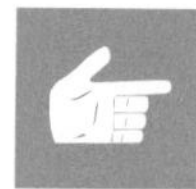

MISCELLANEOUS

ASSOCIATED CONDITIONS
- Stenotic pulmonary artery
- Patent ductus arteriosus
- Atrial septal defect
- Iron deficiency anemia

AGE-RELATED FACTORS
Pediatric: Congenital disorder
Geriatric: N/A
Others: N/A

PREGNANCY Well tolerated after total surgical correction

SYNONYMS N/A

ICD-9-CM
745.2 Tetralogy of Fallot

SEE ALSO

OTHER NOTES N/A

ABBREVIATIONS
- VSD = ventricular septal defect
- RV = right ventricle

REFERENCES

- Braunwald E, ed. Heart Disease: A Textbook of Cardiovascular Medicine. 5th Ed. Philadelphia, W.B. Saunders Co., 1996
- Liberthson R: Congenital Heart Disease: Diagnosis & Management in Children and Adults. Boston, Little Brown, 1989
- Perloff J: Clinical Recognition of Congenital Heart Disease. 4th Ed. Philadelphia, W.B. Saunders Co., 1994

Web references: 0 available at www.5mcc.com
Illustrations N/A

Author(s):
Mark R. Dambro, MD

BASICS

DESCRIPTION A group of inherited disorders that affect the synthesis of hemoglobin. In beta-thalassemia, there is deficient synthesis of beta globin, while in alpha-thalassemia, there is deficient synthesis of alpha globin. This leads to deficient hemoglobin accumulation, resulting in hypochromic and microcytic red cells. Abnormality of the red cells is the most characteristic feature of the thalassemias.
Thalassemia is prevalent in the Mediterranean region, Middle East and Southeast Asia, and among ethnic groups originating from these areas
- Types
  - ◊ Beta-thalassemia major (Cooley's anemia) - severe anemia, growth retardation, hepatosplenomegaly, bone marrow expansion and bone deformities. Transfusion therapy necessary to sustain life.
  - ◊ Thalassemia intermedia - milder form. Transfusion therapy may not be needed.
  - ◊ Thalassemia trait (alpha or beta) - mild anemia with microcytosis and hypochromia. No transfusion therapy needed.
- Varieties unique to Southeast Asians include hemoglobin H disease (a more severe form of alpha thalassemia) and hemoglobin E/beta thalassemia which often mimics Beta thalassemia major in its severity. Both alpha and beta thalassemia trait (minor) are frequent in African-Americans but symptomatic thalassemia is very rare.

System(s) affected: Hemic/Lymphatic/Immunologic

Genetics:
- Inherited in an autosomal recessive pattern
- Inheritance of one defective gene = milder type of thalassemia, two defective genes = severe type of thalassemia

Incidence/Prevalence in USA:
- Approximately 1000 patients with severe thalassemia
- The incidence of thalassemia trait within the ethnic groups involved ranges from 3-5%

Predominant age: Symptoms start to appear 3-6 months after birth

Predominant sex: Male = Female

SIGNS & SYMPTOMS
(Thalassemia trait has no signs or symptoms)
- Pallor
- Poor growth
- Inadequate food intake
- Fatigue
- Shortness of breath
- Splenomegaly
- Jaundice
- Maxillary hyperplasia
- Dental malocclusion
- Cholelithiasis
- Pathologic fractures

CAUSES Genetic

RISK FACTORS Family history

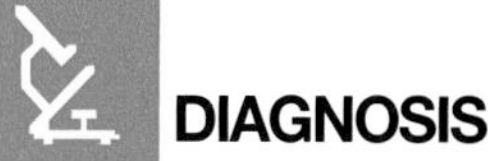

DIAGNOSIS

DIFFERENTIAL DIAGNOSIS
- Iron deficiency
- Other hemoglobinopathies
- Other hemolytic anemias

LABORATORY
- Hemoglobin
  - ◊ Elevated Hb A2 levels in beta-thalassemia trait
  - ◊ Elevated Hb A2, elevated Hb F, reduced or absent Hb A1 in beta-thalassemia major or intermedia
- Peripheral blood
  - ◊ Pronounced microcytosis
  - ◊ Anisocytosis
  - ◊ Hypochromia
  - ◊ Punctate basophilic stippling
  - ◊ High percentage of target cells
  - ◊ Reticulocyte count elevated
- Hematocrit
  - ◊ 28-40% in alpha-thalassemia trait and beta-thalassemia trait
  - ◊ May fall to less than 10% in beta-thalassemia major

Drugs that may alter lab results: N/A

Disorders that may alter lab results:
Parvovirus B19 infection may produce "aplastic crisis" and severe reticulocytopenia

PATHOLOGICAL FINDINGS
- Bone marrow hyperactivity
- Iron deposits in heart muscle
- Hepatic siderosis

SPECIAL TESTS
Bone marrow aspiration

IMAGING
Skull x-ray: thickened diploë of skull, osteoporosis

DIAGNOSTIC PROCEDURES
Family history

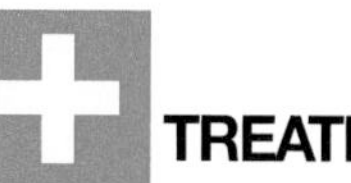

TREATMENT

APPROPRIATE HEALTH CARE Outpatient for mild cases. Inpatient for transfusion therapy.

GENERAL MEASURES
- Mild cases require no therapy
- Thalassemia intermedia - normally no therapy necessary unless hemoglobin levels fall to a dangerous level, then may need transfusion therapy
- Patients with severe thalassemia
  - ◊ Maintain the mean hemoglobin level of at least 9.3 g/dL (1.4 mmol/L) with a regular transfusion schedule (transfusions of about 15 mL per kg at 3-5 week intervals)
  - ◊ Folate supplementation
  - ◊ Treat infections promptly
- Iron overload
  - ◊ Patients receiving transfusion therapy increase total body iron 4 times over the normal amount
  - ◊ Therapy is iron chelation

SURGICAL MEASURES
- Splenectomy
  - ◊ May be needed if hypersplenism causes a marked increase in the transfusion requirement
  - ◊ Recommendation is to defer surgery until patient is 4-6 years of age (due to increased infection risk)
  - ◊ Administer polyvalent pneumococcal vaccine one month prior to splenectomy
  - ◊ Prophylaxis with a daily regimen of penicillin
- Bone marrow transplantation
  - ◊ Available for selected patients with a matched sibling or unrelated donor
  - ◊ Cures the disease, but may be associated with significant mortality and morbidity

ACTIVITY
- Avoid strenuous activities (e.g., football, soccer)
- Acceptable activity levels will need to be determined on an individual basis depending on severity of disorder

DIET
- Avoid iron-rich foods (meats such as liver, and some cereals)
- Drinking tea may possibly help reduce iron

PATIENT EDUCATION
- Genetic counseling
- Teach parents signs of hepatitis, iron overload
- Printed patient information available from: Cooley Anemia Foundation, 105 E. 22nd St., Suite 911, New York, NY 10010, (212)598-0911

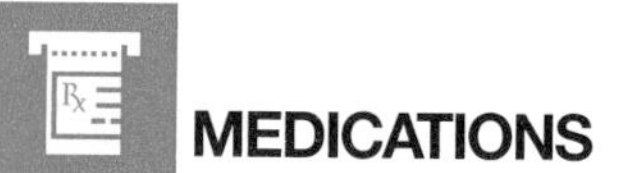

MEDICATIONS

DRUG(S) OF CHOICE
- Antibiotics for infection
- Folic acid supplements
- Iron chelation with deferoxamine (Desferal). Continuous subcutaneous or intravenous infusion with a small infusion pump 40 mg per kg per day (about a 10 hour period). Usually started before 5-8 years of age.

Contraindications: Refer to manufacturer's literature
Precautions: Refer to manufacturer's literature
Significant possible interactions: Refer to manufacturer's literature

ALTERNATIVE DRUGS N/A

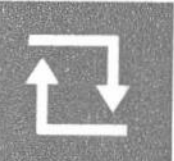

FOLLOWUP

PATIENT MONITORING Life-long monitoring necessary because both the therapy and disease progression have numerous possible complications

PREVENTION/AVOIDANCE
- Prenatal information
  - ◊ Genetic counseling
  - ◊ Prenatal diagnosis - study of beta globin genes performed on fetal cell DNA obtained by amniocentesis after 14 weeks
- Complication prevention
  - ◊ Evaluation for thalassemia by 1 year of age for offspring of adult thalassemia patients
  - ◊ Avoidance of infections
  - ◊ Prompt treatment of infections (after splenectomy, patients should maintain a supply of ampicillin to take if symptoms of infection appear)
  - ◊ Periodic dental checkups
  - ◊ Avoidance of activities that could result in bone fractures

POSSIBLE COMPLICATIONS
- Chronic hemolysis
- Susceptibility to infections after splenectomy
- Infections from blood transfusion
- Intercurrent infections
- Worsening of anemia during infections
- Jaundice
- Leg ulcers
- Cholelithiasis
- Pathologic fractures
- Impaired growth rate
- Delayed or absent puberty
- Hepatic siderosis
- Hemolytic anemia
- Splenomegaly
- Cardiac disease from iron overload
- Aplastic and megaloblastic crises

EXPECTED COURSE/PROGNOSIS
- Outlook varies depending on type
- Thalassemia major patients live an average of 17 years, some into their mid-twenties. Effective iron chelation is improving longevity.
- Thalassemia minor patients live a normal life span

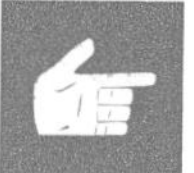

MISCELLANEOUS

ASSOCIATED CONDITIONS See Possible complications

AGE-RELATED FACTORS
Pediatric: A disorder of childhood
Geriatric: N/A
Others: N/A

PREGNANCY Genetic counseling - advised for parents or other relatives of a child with thalassemia and for any individual with beta-thalassemia minor

SYNONYMS
- Mediterranean anemia
- Hereditary leptocytosis
- Thalassemia major and minor
- Cooley anemia

ICD-9-CM
282.49 Other thalassemia

SEE ALSO

OTHER NOTES N/A

ABBREVIATIONS N/A

REFERENCES

- Nathan DG, Oski F, eds: Hematology of Infancy and Childhood. Philadelphia, W.B. Saunders Co., 1997
- Fosburg MT, Nathan DG: Treatment of Cooley's anemia. Blood 1990;76:435

Web references: 0 available at www.5mcc.com
Illustrations N/A

Author(s):
Mark R. Dambro, MD

Thoracic outlet syndrome

BASICS

DESCRIPTION A constellation of symptoms that affect the head, neck, shoulders and upper extremities caused by compression of the neurovascular structures (ie, cords of brachial plexus and subclavian artery and vein) at the thoracic outlet
- May be due to congenital bony, muscular, or tendon anomalies; post traumatic, following clavicular or cervical spine injures; or idiopathic, without discernible cause

System(s) affected: Cardiovascular, Musculoskeletal, Nervous

Genetics: N/A

Incidence/Prevalence in USA: Unknown

Predominant age:
- Neurologic type (95%) - 20-60 years
- Venous type (4%) - 20-35 years
- Arterial type (1%) (atherosclerosis) - young adult or older than 50

Predominant sex:
- Neurologic type - Female > Male (3.5:1)
- Venous type - Male > Female
- Arterial type - Male = Female

SIGNS & SYMPTOMS
- General symptoms
  - ◊ Positive costoclavicular maneuver
  - ◊ Positive hyperabduction maneuver
  - ◊ Positive Adson's maneuver (head rotation to the affected side with slight cervical extension)
  - ◊ Positive elevated arm stress test
  - ◊ Tenderness to percussion or palpation of supraclavicular area
  - ◊ Worsening of symptoms with elevation of arm, overhead extension of arms, or with arms extended forward (e.g., driving a car, typing, carrying objects). Prompt disappearance of symptoms with arm returning to neutral position.
  - ◊ Supraventricular bruit
- Neurologic type, upper plexus (C4-C7)
  - ◊ Pain and paresthesias in head, neck, mandible, face, temporal area, upper back/chest, outer arm and hand in a radial nerve distribution
  - ◊ Occipital and orbital headache
- Neurologic type, lower plexus (C8-T1)
  - ◊ Pain and paresthesias in axilla, inner arm and hand in an ulnar nerve distribution, often nocturnal
  - ◊ Hypothenar and interosseous muscle atrophy
- Venous type
  - ◊ Arm claudication
  - ◊ Cyanosis
  - ◊ Swelling
  - ◊ Distended arm veins
- Arterial type
  - ◊ Digital vasospasm
  - ◊ Thrombosis/embolism
  - ◊ Aneurysm
  - ◊ Gangrene
- Morley test: Brachial plexus compression test in the supraclavicular area from the scalene triangle. A "positive" response is the reproduction of an aching sensation and typical localized paresthesia.
- One-minute Roos test: A thoracic outlet shoulder girdle "stress test." Shoulders and arms are braced in a 90° abducted and externally rotated position; patient is required to clench and relax fists repetitively for on minute. A positive test is one that reproduces the symptom.

CAUSES
- Upper thoracic neurovascular bundle compression
- Cervical rib
- Taut anomalous scalene muscles
- Elongated C7 transverse process
- Poor posture
- Pancoast's tumor
- Atherosclerotic plaques within vessels
- Subclavian muscle
- Fibrous and ligamentous bands
- Costocoracoid tendon
- Callous bone formation from fractured clavicle or first rib
- Aberrant tissue
- Neck trauma

RISK FACTORS
- Exuberant callus after fracture of clavicle or first rib
- Exostosis of clavicle or first rib
- Postural abnormalities (e.g., drooping of shoulders, scoliosis)
- Body building, with increased muscular bulk in thoracic outlet area
- Rapid weight loss combined with vigorous physical exertion and/or exercise
- Occupational exposure
  - ◊ Computer users
  - ◊ Musicians
  - ◊ Repetitive work involving shoulders, arms, hands

DIAGNOSIS

DIFFERENTIAL DIAGNOSIS
- Cervical disk syndrome
- Carpal tunnel syndrome
- Orthopedic shoulder problems (shoulder strain, rotator cuff injury, tendinitis)
- Cervical spondylitis
- Ulnar nerve compression at the elbow and hand
- Multiple sclerosis
- Spinal cord tumor or disease
- Angina pectoris
- Migraine
- Reflex sympathetic dystrophy
- C8 radiculopathies

LABORATORY N/A

Drugs that may alter lab results: N/A

Disorders that may alter lab results: N/A

PATHOLOGICAL FINDINGS
- Bony abnormalities (cervical rib, anomalous first thoracic rib)
- Abnormal muscles
- Congenital fibromuscular bands

SPECIAL TESTS
- Plethysmography with previously mentioned maneuvers
- Doppler and duplex ultrasound if venous obstruction suspected
- Ulnar and median nerve conduction velocity studies (< 70 m/sec is abnormal)
- Venogram and arteriogram if presents with edematous changes in upper extremity

IMAGING
- X-ray (chest x-ray, oblique C-spine)
- Arteriogram or venogram - if arterial or venous obstruction, aneurysm or emboli are suspected
- CT scan - if cord compression lesions (disc and/or tumor) are suspected
- Helical CT
- 3-D MR angiography

DIAGNOSTIC PROCEDURES
- Thoracic outlet syndrome (TOS) is a clinical diagnosis
- Anterior scalene muscle injections are useful in confirming the diagnosis and in determining which patients may respond favorably to surgery

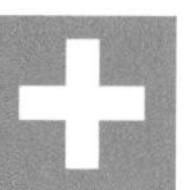

TREATMENT

APPROPRIATE HEALTH CARE
- Outpatient for conservative treatment
- Inpatient if surgery required

GENERAL MEASURES
- Conservative
  - ◊ If no vascular involvement is present and/or if no loss of function or lifestyle is present due to severity of symptoms, conservative therapy may be undertaken for 2-3 months
  - ◊ Improvement can be expected in 60% of patients
  - ◊ Exercise program to promote shoulder muscle function
  - ◊ Physical therapy for postural faults
  - ◊ Cervical collar, traction
  - ◊ Weight loss if axillary folds are causing compression

SURGICAL MEASURES
- Operative - if vascular involvement is present and/or if there is loss of function or lifestyle secondary to severity of symptoms and if conservative therapy fails after 2-3 months
- Resection of first rib or cervical ribs (transaxillary, supraclavicular, posterior approaches)
- Excision of adhesive bands via transaxillary approach
- Anterior scalenectomy

ACTIVITY
- Light activity with arm and hand encouraged
- No straining or heavy activity for 3 months

DIET N/A

PATIENT EDUCATION
- Physical therapy following surgery
- Postural exercises
- NSAIDs may improve pain
- Ergonomic work station
- Surgery if conservative treatment not successful

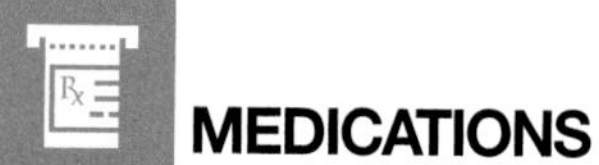

MEDICATIONS

DRUG(S) OF CHOICE
- Analgesics
- Muscle relaxants
- Antispasmodics

Contraindications: Refer to manufacturer's profile of each drug
Precautions: Refer to manufacturer's profile of each drug
Significant possible interactions: Refer to manufacturer's profile of each drug

ALTERNATIVE DRUGS N/A

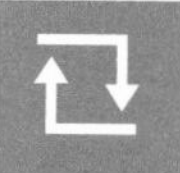

FOLLOWUP

PATIENT MONITORING Office follow-up visits e.g., q3 weeks x 2

PREVENTION/AVOIDANCE N/A

POSSIBLE COMPLICATIONS
- Postoperative shoulder, arm, hand pain and paresthesias in 10%, usually responds to physiotherapy
- 1.5-2% of patients will have symptomatic recurrences 1 month to 7 years postoperatively (usually within 3 months)
- 0.5-1% of patients have brachial plexus injury, probably due to intraoperative traction
- Re-operation indicated for symptomatic recurrence with long posterior remnant of first rib (posterior approach) or with disrupted fibrous adhesions (transaxillary approach)
- Venous obstruction or arterial emboli; usually responds to thrombolytics

EXPECTED COURSE/PROGNOSIS
- 60% improve with appropriate physiotherapy program
- 90% have excellent or good early results with surgery
- 70-80% have no recurrence at 5 years and 10 years

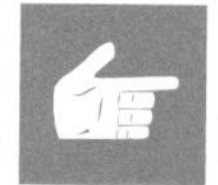

MISCELLANEOUS

ASSOCIATED CONDITIONS N/A

AGE-RELATED FACTORS N/A
Pediatric: N/A
Geriatric: N/A
Others: N/A

PREGNANCY Generalized tissue fluid accumulations and postural changes could aggravate symptoms

SYNONYMS
- Scalenus anticus syndrome
- Cervical rib syndrome
- Costoclavicular syndrome
- TOS

ICD-9-CM
353.0 Brachial plexus lesions

SEE ALSO

OTHER NOTES 2-3 months trial of physiotherapy always indicated except in presence of obvious bony abnormality

ABBREVIATIONS N/A

REFERENCES

- Axelrod DA, Proctor MC, Geisser ME, et al. Outcomes after surgery for thoracic outlet syndrome. J Vasc Surg 2001;33(6):1220-5
- Gillard J, Perez-Cousin M, Hachulla E, et al. Diagnosing thoracic outlet syndrome: contribution of provocative tests, ultrasonography, electrophysiology, and helical computed tomography in 48 patients. Joint Bone Spine 2001;68(5):416-24
- Ursche HC, Rassuk MA. Thoracic Outlet Syndromes. In: Sabiston DC, Spencer FC, eds. Surgery of the Chest. 5th Ed. Philadelphia, W.B. Saunders Co.,1990
- Roos DB. Thoracic Outlet Nerve Compression. In: Ruthford RB, ed. Vascular Surgery. 3rd Ed. Philadelphia, W.B. Saunders Co.,1989
- Dale WQ. Thoracic outlet compression syndrome. Arch Surg 1982;117:1437
- Stallworth JM. Thoracic Outlet Compression Syndromes. In: Haimoviei H, ed. Vascular Surgery. 3rd Ed. Norwalk, Appleton & Lange,1989
- Novak CB, Mackinnon SE. Thoracic outlet syndrome. Orthopedic Clinics of NA 1996;27:747-762
- Oates SD, Daley RA. Thoracic outlet syndrome. Hand Clinics 1996;12:705-728
- Jordan SE. Diagnosis of thoracic outlet syndrome using electrophysiologically guided scalene blocker. Am Vasc Surg 1998;12:260-264
- Functional anatomy of the thoracic outlet: evaluation with spinal CT. Thoracic Radiology 1997;295:843-851
- Wilbourn AJ. Thoracic outlet syndrome. Neurol Clin 1999;17(3):477-97
- Dymarkowski R, Bosmans H, Marchal G, Bogaert J. Three dimensional MR angiography in the evaluation of thoracic outlet syndrome. Amer J of Roentgenol 1999;173:1005-08
- Sanders RJ, Hammond SL. Management of cervical ribs and anomalous first ribs causing neurogenic thoracic outlet syndrome. J Vas Surg 2002;36(1): 51-6
- Kai Y, Oyama M, Kurose S, Inadome T, Oketani Y, Masuda Y. Neurogenic thoracic outlet syndrome in whiplash injury. J Spinal Disord 2001;14(6):487-93
- Pascarelli EF, Hsu YP. Understanding work-related upper extremity disorders: clinical findings in 485 computer users, musicians, and others. J Occup Rehabil 2001;11(1):1-21

Web references: 0 available at www.5mcc.com
Illustrations N/A

Author(s):
Violet Siwik, MD

Thromboangiitis obliterans (Buerger disease)

BASICS

DESCRIPTION Nonatherosclerotic segmental occlusion of small and medium sized arteries and veins caused by inflammatory changes in these vessels. It primarily occurs in men who smoke.
System(s) affected: Cardiovascular
Genetics: Greater prevalence of HLA-A54, HLA-A9 and HLA-B5. Familial cases reported rarely.
Incidence/Prevalence in USA: 13/100,000
Predominant age: 20 to 40 years
Predominant sex: Male > Female (3:1). Increasing numbers of women are being diagnosed, presumably due to increased smoking.

SIGNS & SYMPTOMS

Symptoms tend to wax and wane in early disease and are often asymmetric. Symptoms may be gradual or have a sudden onset related to impaired vasculature. Usually more than one limb involved.

- Ulceration of digits; pain may be disabling
- Coldness in feet and/or fingers
- Cold sensitivity
- Paresthesias (numbness, tingling, burning, hypoesthesia) of feet and/or fingers
- Intermittent claudication in arch of foot or leg (rarely hand, forearm)
- Persistent extremity pain (may be worse at rest)
- Paroxysmal "electric shock" pain of ischemic neuropathy
- Raynaud phenomenon
- Postural color changes (pallor on elevation; rubor on dependency)
- "Buerger color" - cyanosis of hands and feet
- Migratory superficial phlebitis
- Tender skin nodules on extremities
- Impaired distal pulses; proximal pulses normal
- Foot edema
- Gangrene

CAUSES

(Postulated)

- Smoking
- Genetic factors
- Autoimmune disorder with cell mediated sensitivity to types I and III human collagens (both are normal constituents of blood vessels)
- Impaired peripheral endothelium-dependent vasodilation. Nonendothelium mechanisms of vasodilation are intact.
- Arsenic content of tobacco

RISK FACTORS

- Smoking tobacco
- Occasional cases is users of smokeless tobacco and snuff
- Incidence higher in Israel, Middle East, Eastern Europe, Japan, India, Far East than in North America and Western Europe
- More common in countries with heavy use of tobacco

DIAGNOSIS

DIFFERENTIAL DIAGNOSIS

- Peripheral neuropathy
- Peripheral atherosclerotic disease
- Arterial embolus and thrombosis
- Idiopathic peripheral thrombosis
- Hypercoagulable states
- Other causes of vasculitis
- SLE
- Scleroderma
- Occupational trauma
- Repetitive trauma
- Cervical rib
- Livedo reticularis
- Raynaud disease
- Acrocyanosis
- Ergotism
- Frostbite
- Neurotrophic ulcers
- Reflex sympathetic dystrophy
- Metatarsalgia
- Gout
- Periarteritis nodosa
- Juvenile temporal arteritis with eosinophilia
- Polyarteritis
- Carpal tunnel syndrome
- Takayasu arteritis (Japanese young women)
- CREST syndrome

LABORATORY Routine laboratory studies show no changes characteristic of this disorder. Auto-antibodies to collagen and circulating immune complexes may be present, but are considered a research tool only. Homocysteine may be elevated but is not diagnostic.

Drugs that may alter lab results: N/A

Disorders that may alter lab results: N/A

PATHOLOGICAL FINDINGS

- Segmental inflammatory thrombosis of both arteries and veins
- Histologic findings may vary between acute, intermediate, and chronic stages of the disease
- Histologic sine qua non - granulomas with collections of neutrophils in the organizing thrombus. The vessel wall is relatively spared. Wall sparing distinguishes thromboangiitis obliterans from arteriosclerosis and other systemic vasculitis which show striking wall disruption.
- Acute lesions show occlusive, highly cellular inflammatory thrombi with less inflammation in vessel wall. PMNs, microabscesses and multinucleated giant cells may be present.
- Intermediate lesions show organizing thrombus
- Chronic lesions show recanalized thrombus and perivascular fibrosis

SPECIAL TESTS

- Doppler ultrasound (not specific)
- Point scoring systems may help clarify clinical diagnosis

IMAGING

- Arteriogram or digital-subtraction angiography (DSA)
  - ◊ Multiple areas of segmental occlusion of small to medium arteries of arms and legs
  - ◊ "Skip" areas may be demonstrated
  - ◊ Numerous collateral vessels around occluded segments may give a characteristic "cork screw" appearance
  - ◊ Larger arteries are spared. More serious disease distally.
  - ◊ No apparent source of emboli

DIAGNOSTIC PROCEDURES

- History and physical examination
- Allen test may be abnormal
- Studies of nerve conduction velocity (to exclude neuropathy)
- Echocardiography (to exclude emboli)

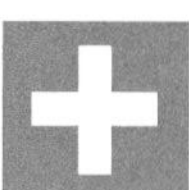

TREATMENT

APPROPRIATE HEALTH CARE

- Outpatient
- Inpatient if surgery needed for gangrene
- Inpatient for dorsal or lumbar sympathectomy if indicated

GENERAL MEASURES

- Stop smoking (mandatory)
- Protect against trauma (poor fitting shoes)
- Protect against infections
- Protect against vasoconstriction from cold or drugs
- Eliminate exposure to thermal damage
- Eliminate exposure to chemical damage (iodine, carbolic acid, salicylic acid)
- Thrombolytic therapy of occlusive thrombus and angioplasty are experimental

SURGICAL MEASURES

- Amputation for non-healing ulcers, gangrene or intractable pain. Should preserve as much limb as possible. Rarely required.
- Omental autotransplantation has been successful in treating ulcers
- Infrainguinal bypass
- In severe disease, a lumbar sympathectomy to increase blood supply to the skin
- Spinal cord stimulator
- Direct revascularization of distal arteries is not practical. Distal target vessel is usually not available.

ACTIVITY Restricted by symptoms. Use a bed cradle (non-heated) to prevent pressure from bed linens.

DIET No restrictions

PATIENT EDUCATION

- Must stop smoking
- Remove possibilities of exposure to others in the environment who smoke
- Nicotine replacement may keep the disease active
- Use heel pads or foam rubber boots
- See General Measures

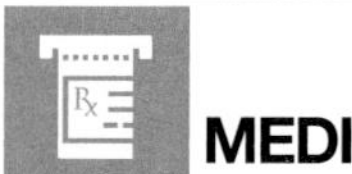

MEDICATIONS

DRUG(S) OF CHOICE
- Medications are not a substitute for discontinuance of smoking
- Antibiotics for infected digital ulcers and osteomyelitis
- Iloprost, a prostacyclin analogue, promotes ulcer healing (available in Europe)
- Urokinase or streptokinase selectively infused into occluded artery
- Intramuscular endothelial growth factor gene therapy
- No form of medical treatment has been shown to be effective (including steroids, calcium channel blockers, reserpine, pentoxifylline, vasodilators, antiplatelet drugs, anticoagulants)

Contraindications: Refer to manufacturer's literature
Precautions: Refer to manufacturer's literature
Significant possible interactions: Refer to manufacturer's literature

ALTERNATIVE DRUGS Calcium channel blocking agents such as nifedipine may allow vasodilatation, but have not been proven effective.

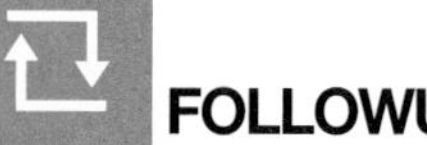

FOLLOWUP

PATIENT MONITORING Frequent history and physical examinations

PREVENTION/AVOIDANCE Never smoke

POSSIBLE COMPLICATIONS
- Ulcerations
- Gangrene
- Need for amputation
- Rare occlusion of cerebral, coronary, renal, splenic, mesenteric, pulmonary, iliac arteries and aorta

EXPECTED COURSE/PROGNOSIS
- Occasional remissions
- Unremitting progression if patient continues to smoke
- Death rare; normal survival curve

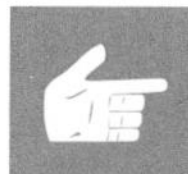

MISCELLANEOUS

ASSOCIATED CONDITIONS N/A

AGE-RELATED FACTORS
Pediatric: Not a problem in this age group
Geriatric: Not common in this age group, but diagnosis in the elderly is increasing
Others: N/A

PREGNANCY N/A

SYNONYMS
- Buerger disease
- TAO

ICD-9-CM
443.1 Thromboangiitis obliterans (Buerger disease)

SEE ALSO

OTHER NOTES May be difficult to differentiate from some types of atherosclerosis, systemic emboli or idiopathic peripheral thromboses

ABBREVIATIONS N/A

REFERENCES

- Case records of the Mass. General Hospital. Weekly clinicopathological exercises. case 16-1989. A 36 year-old man with peripheral vascular disease. New Eng J Med 1989;20;320(16):1068-76
- Olin JW, et al. The changing clinical spectrum of thromboangiitis obliterans (Buerger's disease). Circulation Supplement IV 1990;82(5)
- Dale DC, Federman DD, eds. Scientific American Medicine. New York, Scientific American, Inc 1998
- Olin JW. Thromboangiitis obliterans (Buerger's disease). N Engl J Med 2000;343(12):864-9

Web references: 1 available at www.5mcc.com
Illustrations N/A

Author(s):
Rick Kellerman, MD

BASICS

DESCRIPTION Superficial thrombophlebitis is an inflammatory condition of the veins with secondary thrombosis.

- Septic (suppurative) thrombophlebitis types:
  - ◊ Iatrogenic
  - ◊ Infectious, mainly syphilis and psittacosis
- Aseptic thrombophlebitis types:
  - ◊ Primary hypercoagulable states - disorders with measurable defects in the proteins of the coagulation and/or fibrinolytic systems
  - ◊ Secondary hypercoagulable states - clinical conditions with a risk of thrombosis

System(s) affected: Cardiovascular

Genetics:
- Septic - no known genetic pattern
- Antithrombin III deficiencies - autosomal dominant
- Proteins C and S deficiency - autosomal dominant with variable penetrance
- Disorders of fibrinolytic system - congenital defects inheritance variable
- Dysfibrinogenemia - autosomal dominant
- Factor XII deficiency - autosomal recessive

Incidence/Prevalence in USA:
- Septic
  - ◊ Up to 10% of all nosocomial infections
  - ◊ Incidence of catheter-related thrombophlebitis is 88/100,000
  - ◊ Develops in 4-8% if cut down is performed
- Aseptic primary hypercoagulable state
  - ◊ Antithrombin III and heparin cofactor II deficiency incidence is 50/100,000
- Aseptic secondary hypercoagulable state
  - ◊ Trousseau incidence in malignancy 5-15%
  - ◊ Trousseau in pancreatic carcinoma 50%
  - ◊ In pregnancy 49-fold increased incidence of phlebitis
  - ◊ Superficial migratory thrombophlebitis in 27% of patients with thromboangiitis obliterans

Predominant age:
- Septic
  - ◊ More common in childhood
- Aseptic primary hypercoagulable state
  - ◊ Antithrombin III and heparin cofactor II deficiency - neonatal period, but first episode usually at age 20-30 years
  - ◊ Proteins C and S - before age 30
- Aseptic secondary hypercoagulable state
  - ◊ Mondor disease: women, ages 21-55 years
  - ◊ Thromboangiitis obliterans onset: 20-50 years

Predominant sex:
- Suppurative:
  - ◊ Male = Female
- Aseptic
  - ◊ Mondor - Female > Male (2:1)
  - ◊ Thromboangiitis obliterans - Female > Male (1-19% of clinical cases)

SIGNS & SYMPTOMS
- Swelling, tenderness, redness along the course of the veins
- May look like cellulitis or erythema nodosa
- Fever in 70% of patients
- Warmth, erythema, tenderness, or lymphangitis in 32%
- Sign of systemic sepsis in 84% in suppurative
- Red, tender cord
- Pain

CAUSES
- Septic
  - ◊ Staphylococcus aureus in 65-78%
  - ◊ Enterobacteriaceae, especially Klebsiella
  - ◊ Multiple organisms in 14%
  - ◊ Anaerobic isolate rare
  - ◊ Candida spp.
  - ◊ Cytomegalovirus in AIDS patients
- Aseptic primary hypercoagulable state
  - ◊ Antithrombin III and heparin II deficiency
  - ◊ Protein C and protein S deficiency
  - ◊ Disorder of tissue plasminogen activator
  - ◊ Abnormal plasminogen and co-plasminogen
  - ◊ Dysfibrinogenemia
  - ◊ Factor XII deficiency
  - ◊ Lupus anticoagulant and anticardiolipin antibody syndrome
- Aseptic secondary hypercoagulable states
  - ◊ Malignancy (Trousseau syndrome: Recurrent migratory thrombophlebitis). Most commonly seen in - metastatic mucin or adenocarcinomas of the GI tract (pancreas, stomach, colon and gall bladder); lung, prostate, ovary.
  - ◊ Pregnancy
  - ◊ Oral contraceptive
  - ◊ Infusion of prothrombin complex concentrates
  - ◊ Behçet disease
  - ◊ Buerger disease
  - ◊ Mondor disease

RISK FACTORS
- Nonspecific
  - ◊ Immobilization
  - ◊ Obesity
  - ◊ Advanced age
  - ◊ Postoperative states
- Septic
  - ◊ Intravenous catheter
  - ◊ Duration of intravenous catheterization (68% of cannulae have been left in place for 2 days)
  - ◊ Cutdowns
  - ◊ Cancer, debilitating diseases
  - ◊ Steroid
  - ◊ Incidence is 40 times higher with plastic cannula (8%) than with steel or scalp cannulas (0.2%)
  - ◊ Thrombosis
  - ◊ Dermal infection
  - ◊ Burned patients
  - ◊ Lower extremities intravenous catheter
  - ◊ Intravenous antibiotics
  - ◊ AIDS
  - ◊ Varicose veins
- Antithrombin II and heparin cofactor II deficiency
  - ◊ Pregnancy
  - ◊ Oral contraceptives
  - ◊ Surgery; trauma; infection
- In pregnancy
  - ◊ Increased age
  - ◊ Hypertension
  - ◊ Eclampsia
  - ◊ Increased parity
- Thromboangiitis obliterans
  - ◊ Persistent smoking
- Mondor disease
  - ◊ Breast abscess
  - ◊ Antecedent breast surgery
  - ◊ Breast augmentation
  - ◊ Reduction mammoplasty

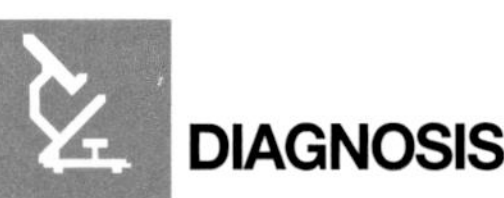

DIAGNOSIS

DIFFERENTIAL DIAGNOSIS
- Cellulitis
- Erythema nodosa
- Cutaneous polyarteritis nodosa
- Sarcoid
- Kaposi sarcoma
- Hyperalgesic pseudothrombophlebitis

LABORATORY
- Septic
  - ◊ Bacteremia in 80-90%
  - ◊ Culture of IV fluid bag
  - ◊ Leukocytosis
- Aseptic
  - ◊ Acute phase reactant
  - ◊ Factor levels
  - ◊ Thrombin activity
  - ◊ Platelet function test

Drugs that may alter lab results: In septic, broad spectrum antibiotics

Disorders that may alter lab results: N/A

PATHOLOGICAL FINDINGS
- The affected vein is enlarged, tortuous, and thickened
- Associated perivascular suppuration and/or hemorrhage
- Vein lumen may contain pus and thrombus
- Endothelial damage, fibrinoid necrosis and thickening of the vein wall

SPECIAL TESTS Leukocyte imaging

IMAGING
- Septic and aseptic
  - ◊ Ultrasound of veins reveal an increase in the diameter of the lumen
  - ◊ Chest x-ray - multiple peripheral densities or a pleural effusion consistent with pulmonary embolism, abscess, or empyema
  - ◊ Bone and gallium scan - for associated subperiosteal abscess in septic thrombophlebitis
  - ◊ Evaluation of complications (deep vein thrombosis and others)

DIAGNOSTIC PROCEDURES Skin biopsy

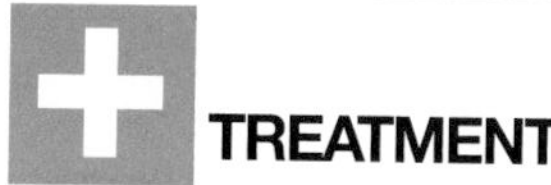

TREATMENT

APPROPRIATE HEALTH CARE
- Septic - inpatient
- Aseptic - outpatient

GENERAL MEASURES
- Heat application
- Extremity elevation

SURGICAL MEASURES
- Septic
  - ◊ Excision of the involved vein segment and all involved tributaries
  - ◊ Excision from ankle to groin may be required in some burn patients
  - ◊ If systemic symptoms persist after vein excision, re-exploration is necessary with removal of all involved veins
  - ◊ Drainage of contiguous abscesses
  - ◊ Remove all cannulae
- Aseptic
  - ◊ Mondor disease, consider surgical transection of the phlebitic cord
  - ◊ Management of underlying conditions

ACTIVITY Bedrest

DIET No restrictions

PATIENT EDUCATION
- Avoid trauma
- Be alert to change in skin color
- Be alert to tenderness over extremities

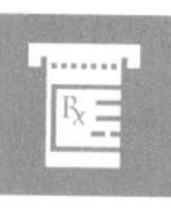

MEDICATIONS

DRUG(S) OF CHOICE
- Septic
  - ◊ Initially: semisynthetic penicillin (e.g., nafcillin 2 g IV q6h) plus an aminoglycoside (e.g., gentamicin, 1.0-1.7 mg/kg IV)
  - ◊ Duration of therapy is empiric
  - ◊ If due to Candida albicans, consider a short course of amphotericin B, approximately 200 mg cumulative dose
  - ◊ If osteomyelitis documented, antibiotic therapy for at least 6 weeks
- Aseptic general
  - ◊ Non-steroidal anti-inflammatories
  - ◊ Oral anticoagulant warfarin
  - ◊ Systemic anticoagulant heparin
  - ◊ Low molecular weight heparin
- Antithrombin III and heparin cofactor II deficiency
  - ◊ IV heparin
  - ◊ Antithrombin III concentrate
  - ◊ Prophylaxis: warfarin, oxymetholone
- Proteins C and S
  - ◊ Long-term warfarin, lower dose, no loading
- Disorder of tissue plasminogen activator
  - ◊ Phenformin and ethylestrenol
  - ◊ Stanozolol and phenformin
  - ◊ Stanozolol alone
  - ◊ Ethylestrenol alone
- Dysfibrinogenemia
  - ◊ Acute attack - anticoagulation
  - ◊ Prophylaxis - stanozolol
- Abnormal plasminogen and plasminogenemia
  - ◊ Acute attack - anticoagulation
  - ◊ Prophylaxis - warfarin
- Factor XII deficiency
  - ◊ Standard therapy
- Lupus anticardiolipin
  - ◊ Prophylaxis - warfarin
- Trousseau syndrome
  - ◊ Heparin
- For pregnancy
  - ◊ Heparin
- Behçet disease
  - ◊ Phenformin
  - ◊ Ethylestrenol
  - ◊ Stanozolol
- Thromboangiitis obliterans
  - ◊ Stop smoking
  - ◊ Pentoxifylline

Contraindications: Refer to manufacturer's literature

Precautions: Refer to manufacturer's literature

Significant possible interactions: Refer to manufacturer's literature

ALTERNATIVE DRUGS
- Factor XII deficiency - streptokinase or alteplase [tissue plasminogen activator (tPA)]
- Behçet - oral anticoagulants plus cyclosporine
- Thromboangiitis obliterans - corticosteroid, antiplatelets and vasodilating drugs

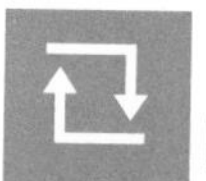

FOLLOWUP

PATIENT MONITORING
- Septic
  - ◊ Routine WBC and differential and culture
  - ◊ Repeat culture from the phlebitic vein
- Aseptic
  - ◊ Clinical followup to rule out secondary complications
  - ◊ Repeat of blood studies for fibrinolytic system, platelets and factors

PREVENTION/AVOIDANCE
- Use of scalp vein cannulae
- Avoidance of lower extremity cannulations
- Insertion under aseptic conditions
- Secure anchoring of the cannulae
- Replacement of cannulae, connecting tubing, and IV fluid every 48-72 hrs
- Neomycin-polymyxin B-bacitracin ointment in cutdown

POSSIBLE COMPLICATIONS
- Septic: Systemic sepsis, bacteremia (84%); septic pulmonary emboli (44%); metastatic abscess formation; pneumonia (44%); subperiosteal abscess of adjacent long bones in children
- Aseptic: Deep vein thrombosis; thromboembolic phenomena

EXPECTED COURSE/PROGNOSIS
- Septic high mortality (50%), if untreated
- Aseptic
  - ◊ Usually benign course; recovery 7-10 days
  - ◊ Antithrombin III and heparin cofactor deficiency; recurrence rate is 60%
  - ◊ Proteins C and S, recurrence rate 70%
  - ◊ Prognosis depends on development of DVT and early detections of complications
  - ◊ Aseptic thrombophlebitis can be isolated, recurrent or migratory

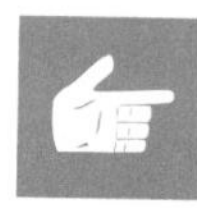

MISCELLANEOUS

ASSOCIATED CONDITIONS Varicose veins, manifestation of systemic disease, hyper-coagulable states, surgery, trauma, burns, obesity, pregnancy

AGE-RELATED FACTORS
Pediatric: Subperiosteal abscesses of adjacent long bone may complicate

Geriatric: Septic thrombophlebitis is more common, prognosis poorer

Others: N/A

PREGNANCY
- Associated with increased risk of aseptic superficial thrombophlebitis
- Warfarin and NSAIDs are contraindicated

SYNONYMS
- Phlebitis
- Phlebothrombosis

ICD-9-CM
451.0 Phlebitis and thrombophlebitis of superficial vessels of lower extremities

451.2 Phlebitis and thrombophlebitis of deep vessels of lower extremities, unspecified

SEE ALSO
Thrombosis, deep vein (DVT)

OTHER NOTES N/A

ABBREVIATIONS DVT = deep vein thrombosis

REFERENCES

- Samlaskie CP, James WD: Superficial thrombophlebitis II. Secondary hypercoagulable states. J Am Acad Dermato 1990;23(1)1-18
- Samlaskie CP, James WD: Superficial thrombophlebitis I. Primary hypercoagulable states. J Am Acad Dermatol 1990;22:975-89
- Mandell GL, ed: Principles and Practice of Infectious Diseases. 4th Ed. New York, Churchill Livingstone, 1995

Web references: 0 available at www.5mcc.com

Illustrations N/A

Author(s):
Abdulrazak Abyad, MD, MPH

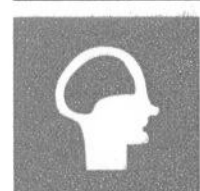

BASICS

DESCRIPTION Development of single or multiple blood clots within the deep veins of the extremities or pelvis, usually accompanied by inflammation of the vessel wall. The major clinical consequence is embolization, usually to the lung, that is frequently life-threatening.
System(s) affected: Cardiovascular
Genetics: Inherited thrombophilic states increase risk for venous thromboembolic disease
Incidence/Prevalence in USA: Common (approximately 250,000 hospitalizations and 50,000 deaths from complications of venous thromboembolic disease)
Predominant age: Mean age of 60 (increasing age is an independent risk factor)
Predominant sex: Male > Female (1.2 : 1)

SIGNS & SYMPTOMS
- Many cases are completely asymptomatic, diagnosed after embolization
- Physical exam is only 30% accurate for DVT
- Limb pain (common)
- Limb swelling (common)
- Leg pain on dorsiflexion of the foot (Homan sign; unreliable test for DVT)
- Palpable tender cord in affected limb (uncommon)
- Warmth of skin over area of thrombosis (uncommon)
- Redness of skin over area or thrombosis (uncommon)
- Fever (uncommon, except in septic thrombophlebitis)
- Non-tender swelling of collateral superficial veins (uncommon)
- Massive edema with cyanosis and ischemia; a medical emergency (Phlegmasia cerulea dolens, rare)
- Pain on percussion of the medial tibia (Lisker sign)
- Pain on compression of the calf against the tibia in the anteroposterior plane (Bancroft or Moses sign)

CAUSES
- Venous stasis
- Injury to vessel wall
- Abnormalities of coagulation

RISK FACTORS
- Clinical risk factors:
  - ◊ Increasing age
  - ◊ Trauma, especially long bone fractures or crush injuries
  - ◊ Surgery (most commonly orthopedic, gastrointestinal, and genitourinary)
  - ◊ Prolonged immobility
  - ◊ Pregnancy, especially the puerperium
  - ◊ Indwelling central venous catheters
  - ◊ Travel (> 4 hours)
  - ◊ Hormone replacement therapy
  - ◊ Tamoxifen therapy
  - ◊ Selective estrogen receptor modulator therapy (SERMs; raloxifene [Evista])
  - ◊ High altitude (> 14,000 feet)
- Pathological risk factors:
  - ◊ Prior DVT or pulmonary embolism
  - ◊ Inherited hypercoagulable states (thrombophilic states)
    - Factor V Leiden mutation resulting in resistance to activated protein C
    - Prothrombin mutation (G20210A)
    - Hyperhomocysteinemia
    - Protein C deficiency
    - Protein S deficiency
    - Antithrombin III deficiency
    - Homocysteinuria (rare)
  - ◊ Other hypercoagulable states
    - Antiphospholipid syndrome (lupus anticoagulant, anticardiolipin antibodies)
    - Elevated factor VIII, IX, XI
    - Elevated fibrinogen
    - Elevated vonWillebrand factor
  - ◊ Malignancy
  - ◊ Obesity
  - ◊ Nephrotic syndrome
  - ◊ Polycythemia vera
  - ◊ Homocystinuria (rare)
  - ◊ *Campylobacter jejuni* bacteremia (very rare)
  - ◊ Myeloproliferative disorders
  - ◊ Vitamin deficiencies (B6, B12, folate)
  - ◊ Heparin-induced thrombocytopenia
  - ◊ Acute myocardial infarction
  - ◊ Neurologic disease with paralysis (acute spinal cord injury, CVA)

DIAGNOSIS

DIFFERENTIAL DIAGNOSIS
- Cellulitis
- Ruptured synovial cyst (Baker cyst)
- Lymphedema
- Extrinsic compression of vein by tumor or enlarged lymph nodes
- Pulled, strained, or torn muscle
- Compartment syndrome
- Localized allergic reaction
- Filariasis (in developing countries)

LABORATORY
- D-dimer (sensitive but not specific; has a high negative predictive value)
- Baseline labs: CBC, platelet count, aPTT, PT/INR
- Labs for idiopathic (no known inciting event) DVT
  - ◊ First tier of testing: Factor V Leiden, G20210A prothrombin, serum homocysteine, factor VIII level, and lupus anticoagulant
  - ◊ Second tier of testing: Protein C and S antigen levels, antithrombin activity, and anticardiolipin antibodies

Drugs that may alter lab results:
- Heparin, estrogens may lower antithrombin III levels
- Coumadin affects protein C and protein S function so may interfere with functional assays of these proteins

Disorders that may alter lab results:
- Thrombosis itself lowers antithrombin III levels so any workup for antithrombin III deficiency must be performed after patient has completed therapy
- Syphilis and systemic lupus erythematosus are associated with increased antiphospholipid antibodies

PATHOLOGICAL FINDINGS
- Clot consisting predominantly of red blood cells, with some platelets and fibrin attached to vessel wall at one end with proximal end floating free in the lumen. Varying degrees of inflammation of the vessel wall are present.
- DVT may be the "sentinel" event for an underlying malignancy or thrombophilia

SPECIAL TESTS N/A

IMAGING
- Imaging studies are necessary to diagnose or rule out suspected DVT
- Compression ultrasonography; noninvasive, highly sensitive and specific for popliteal and femoral thrombi. Disadvantages include poor ability to detect calf vein thrombi, does not identify clots in pelvic veins or vena cava, is operator-dependent, does not distinguish acute from chronic thrombi, and is difficult to distinguish extrinsic vein compression from intravenous clot.
- Contrast venography is the gold standard test (i.e., most sensitive and specific) but should not be the initial screening tool. Disadvantages include discomfort, technical difficulty and small risk of morbidity.
- Impedance plethysmography (IPG); probably as accurate as duplex ultrasound, less operator dependency, but poor at detecting calf vein thrombi. Not widely available.
- Magnetic resonance venography: as accurate as contrast venography; may be useful for patients with contraindications to IV contrast material
- 125 I-fibrinogen scan; detects only active clot formation; very good at detecting ongoing calf thrombi. Major disadvantage is that it takes 4 hours for results. This test has generally been supplanted by contrast ultrasonography and IPG.

DIAGNOSTIC PROCEDURES N/A

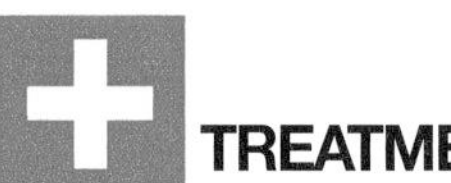

TREATMENT

APPROPRIATE HEALTH CARE Patients with complicated DVT (see Medications Section) should usually be admitted, others can be managed as outpatients

GENERAL MEASURES For hospitalized patient - intravenous anticoagulation, a brief period of bedrest, and close observation for embolic events

SURGICAL MEASURES When anticoagulants and thrombolytics are contraindicated, filtering devices ("umbrellas") can be inserted into the vena cava to "trap" emboli before reaching the lungs. Very large clots can be surgically removed in certain circumstances.

ACTIVITY Bedrest for 1-2 days, then gradual resumption of normal activity, with avoidance of prolonged immobility

DIET No special diet, however patients taking warfarin need to be aware that foods high in vitamin K can affect their PT

PATIENT EDUCATION
- Advise women taking estrogen of the risks, and the common symptoms of thromboembolic disease
- Advise women with an inherited or acquired thrombophilia or a history of thrombosis to avoid oral contraceptives and hormone replacement therapy
- Women with personal or family history of thrombosis should be offered screening for inherited or acquired thrombophilias (clotting disorders)
- Discourage prolonged immobility

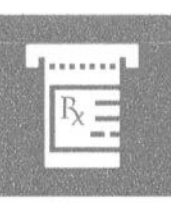

MEDICATIONS

DRUG(S) OF CHOICE
DVT is "complicated" if any of these are present: evidence of pulmonary embolism, recent surgery, peptic ulcer disease, malignant hypertension, increased risk of falling, extensive proximal DVT, heparin allergy or history of heparin-induced thrombocytopenia, known bleeding disorder, active bleeding, comorbid illness with high risk of bleeding, renal insufficiency, pregnancy, known protein C or S deficiency, noncompliance, poor followup, inadequate home support, inaccessibility to outpatient monitoring, morbid obesity, age < 18 years, age > 75 years, and severe leg pain and swelling.

- Uncomplicated DVT : LMWH (can be administered in an outpatient setting) [enoxaparin (Lovenox) 1 mg/kg/dose bid SC; dalteparin (Fragmin)]. No laboratory monitoring required.
- Complicated DVT
  - ◊ Heparin 80 units/kg IV bolus followed by continuous infusion starting at 18 units/kg/hr. Adjust dosage to aPTT of 2-3x control OR
  - ◊ Enoxaparin (Lovenox) either 1mg/kg/dose bid SC or 1.5mg/kg/qd SC. No laboratory monitoring required.
- Maintenance therapy: Warfarin (Coumadin) may be started on the first day, once therapeutic anticoagulation is reached, 5mg qDay and adjusting based on prothrombin time (PT) with a target PT of 1.5-2x control. Continue heparin until target PT level is achieved (INR 2-3). For patients with contraindications to warfarin, LMWH or heparin can be continued SC for the duration of treatment.
- Dalteparin (Fragmin) is approved for DVT prophylaxis

Contraindications:
- Severe active bleeding, neurosurgical procedure within 30 days, pregnancy (warfarin only), previous adverse reaction to the drug (other than bleeding, which is a known side effect)
- Relative contraindications: Recent hemorrhage, recent surgical procedure other than neurosurgery, history of significant peptic ulcer disease, recent nonembolic stroke

Precautions:
- Observe patient for signs of embolization, further thrombosis or bleeding
- Avoid IM injections. Periodically check stool and urine for occult blood, monitor complete blood counts including platelets.
- Heparin - thrombocytopenia and/or paradoxical thrombosis with thrombocytopenia
- Warfarin - necrotic skin lesions (typically breasts, thighs, buttocks)
- LMWH - adjust dosage in renal insufficiency

Significant possible interactions:
- Agents that intensify the response to oral anticoagulants: Alcohol, allopurinol, amiodarone, anabolic steroids, androgens, many antimicrobials, cimetidine, chloral hydrate, disulfiram, all NSAIDs, sulfinpyrazone, tamoxifen, thyroid hormone, vitamin E, ranitidine, salicylates, acetaminophen
- Agents that diminish the response to anticoagulants: Aminoglutethimide, antacids, barbiturates, carbamazepine, cholestyramine, diuretics, griseofulvin, rifampin, oral contraceptives

ALTERNATIVE DRUGS
- Thrombolytic agents (urokinase, streptokinase, alteplase [tissue plasminogen activator]) are effective in dissolving clots and are currently investigational for treatment of DVT. In current clinical practice should be reserved for massive thromboembolic disease. The same contraindications apply as to anticoagulants.
- If warfarin is contraindicated, heparin can be given in the ambulatory setting by intermittent SC self-injection (see Pregnancy)

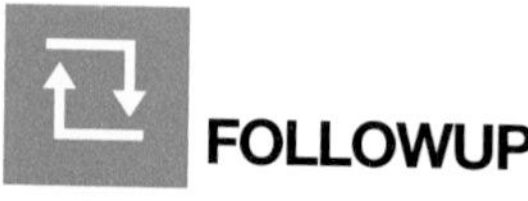

FOLLOWUP

PATIENT MONITORING
- Heparin: aPTT monitored several times a day until dose stabilizes. Discontinue heparin if platelets < 75,000
- Warfarin: PT/INR daily until target achieved, then weekly for several weeks, then (if stable) monthly
- Duration of treatment with warfarin after venous thrombotic event
  - ◊ 3 months of warfarin
    - Event provoked by surgery, trauma or immobilization
  - ◊ 6 months of warfarin
    - First unprovoked event
    - Event provoked by pregnancy, peripartum, or OCPs/HRT
    - Proximal vein thrombosis
    - Pulmonary embolism provoked by surgery, trauma or immobilization
    - Age > 45 with DVT
    - Heterozygous for Factor V Leiden with event
    - Heterozygous for G20210A prothrombin mutation with event
  - ◊ 6-18 months of warfarin. Active cancer, continued immobilization, venous insufficiency, Protein C/S deficiency, or elevated factor VIII
  - ◊ Indefinite treatment with warfarin
    - Recurrent DVT, PE or other thrombotic event
    - Life threatening event (large PE, limb threatening DVT)
    - Cerebral or visceral vein thrombosis
    - Antithrombin deficiency with event
    - Homozygous for Factor V Leiden with event
    - Combined clotting disorders (eg, Factor V Leiden plus elevated homocysteine) with event
    - Antiphospholipid antibodies with event
- Monitoring with LMWH: No monitoring required, however in select patients (eg, those with severe renal insufficiency, morbid obesity) an antifactor Xa activity level may help guide titration of therapy. This assay is limited by controversy over its correlation to therapeutic efficacy and ability to predict hemorrhage in high risk patients.
- Investigate significant bleeding (eg, hematuria or GI hemorrhage) since anticoagulant therapy may unmask a pre-existing lesion (e.g., cancer, peptic ulcer disease, or arteriovenous malformation)

PREVENTION/AVOIDANCE
- Avoid prolonged immobility
- Low-estrogen birth control pills when possible
- Surgical patients need active prophylaxis: Low dose SC heparin with dosage adjusted to slightly prolong the aPTT, low dose warfarin, LMWH and intermittent mechanical compression of the legs reduce the risks of DVT.
- Dalteparin (Fragmin) is approved for DVT prophylaxis

POSSIBLE COMPLICATIONS
- Pulmonary embolism (fatal in 10-20%)
- Arterial embolism ("paradoxical embolization") with AV shunting
- Chronic venous insufficiency
- Post-phlebitic syndrome (pain and swelling in affected limb without new clot formation)
- Treatment-induced hemorrhage
- Soft tissue ischemia associated with massive clot and very high venous pressures - phlegmasia cerulea dolens (very rare but is a surgical emergency)

EXPECTED COURSE/PROGNOSIS
- About 20% of untreated proximal (ie, above the calf) DVTs progress to pulmonary emboli and 10-20% of those are fatal. With aggressive anticoagulant therapy the mortality is decreased five to tenfold.
- DVT confined to the infrapopliteal veins has a small risk of embolization. However these can propagate into the proximal system - follow with serial IPG or duplex ultrasound. Some recommend full anticoagulation therapy for all patients with calf vein DVT because of a 25% one-year risk of developing chronic venous insufficiency.
- Skin necrosis is a possibility in patients with protein C deficiency who also take warfarin

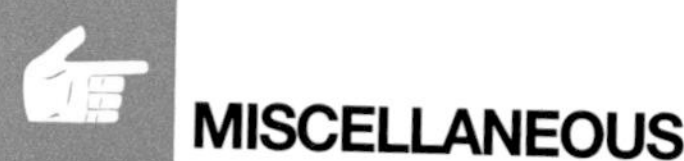

MISCELLANEOUS

ASSOCIATED CONDITIONS
- Malignant neoplasm (1/5 of all venous thromboembolic disease)
- Mild to moderate hyperhomocysteinemia
- Inherited thrombophilias
- Antiphospholipid antibody syndrome
- Budd-Chiari syndrome (hepatic vein thrombosis)
- Renal vein thrombosis

AGE-RELATED FACTORS
Pediatric: In this age group, patients with DVT in absence of preceding trauma should be worked up for inherited coagulopathy
Geriatric: More common because predisposing conditions are more common
Others: N/A

PREGNANCY
- Warfarin (Coumadin) is a teratogen and is therefore contraindicated in pregnancy. Treat pregnant women with DVT with full dose heparin initially followed by subcutaneous heparin starting at 15,000 units twice daily with target aPTT of 1.5-2x control.
- Warfarin is considered safe with breast-feeding
- Septic thrombophlebitis, usually associated with childbirth, requires antibiotic therapy as well as anticoagulation

SYNONYMS
Deep venous thrombophlebitis

ICD-9-CM
451.19 Phlebitis and thrombophlebitis of deep vessels of lower extremities, other
415.19 Pulmonary embolism and infarction, other
453.8 Embolism and thrombosis of other specified veins
289.81 Primary hypercoagulable state
289.82 Secondary hypercoagulable state

SEE ALSO
Antithrombin deficiency
Factor V Leiden
Protein C deficiency
Protein S deficiency
Prothrombin 20210 (Mutation)
Pulmonary embolism

OTHER NOTES
N/A

ABBREVIATIONS
DVT = deep vein thrombosis
IPG = impedance plethysmography
INR = international normalized ratio
LMWH = low molecular weight heparin
aPTT = activated partial thromboplastin time
AV = arteriovenous

REFERENCES

- Brown DF. Treatment options for deep venous thrombosis. Emerg Med Clin North Am 2001;19(4):913-23
- Collet JP, Montalescot G, Fine E, et al. Enoxaparin in unstable angina patients who would have been excluded from randomized pivotal trials. J Am Coll Cardiol 2003;41:8-14
- Heit JA: Risk factors for venous thromboembolism. Clin Chest Med 2003;24(1):1-12

Web references: 0 available at www.5mcc.com
Illustrations N/A

Author(s):
Rob Tiller, MD

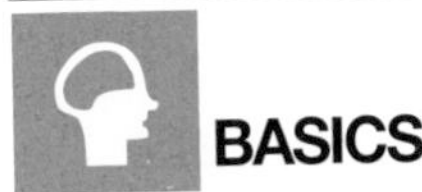

BASICS

DESCRIPTION Cystic remnant of thyroid descent in the neck
System(s) affected: Endocrine/Metabolic, Skin/Exocrine
Genetics: N/A
Incidence/Prevalence in USA: N/A
Predominant age: 50% less than 10 years, 65% less than 20 years of age
Predominant sex: Male = Female

SIGNS & SYMPTOMS
- Midline neck mass
- Non-tender, unless infected
- Rises in the neck with tongue protrusion
- 80% juxtaposed to the hyoid bone

CAUSES Failure of obliteration of the thyroglossal duct following descent of the thyroid in the 6th week of fetal life

RISK FACTORS None

DIAGNOSIS

DIFFERENTIAL DIAGNOSIS
- Ectopic midline thyroid
- Dermoid cyst
- Thyroid adenoma of isthmus or pyramidal lobe
- Lymphadenitis

LABORATORY None

Drugs that may alter lab results: N/A

Disorders that may alter lab results: N/A

PATHOLOGICAL FINDINGS Cyst lined with stratified squamous or pseudostratified ciliated columnar epithelium. Thyroid tissue seen in 10-45% of cysts.

SPECIAL TESTS N/A

IMAGING
- Ultrasound
- Thyroid scan if midline ectopic thyroid or thyroid nodule is suspected

DIAGNOSTIC PROCEDURES N/A

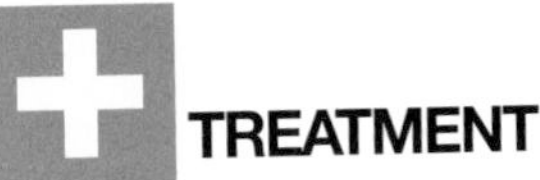

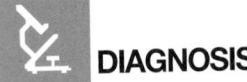

TREATMENT

APPROPRIATE HEALTH CARE Outpatient surgery

GENERAL MEASURES N/A

SURGICAL MEASURES
- Once diagnosed, the excision can be done with Sistrunk procedure. This requires removal of the center portion of the hyoid bone to minimize recurrence.
- If the cyst is infected, it should be initially treated (antibiotics and local heat) or drained. After resolution of the inflammation, excision should be performed.

ACTIVITY Unrestricted

DIET Unrestricted

PATIENT EDUCATION
- Reassurance to family about absence of malignancy
- Patient may require thyroid medication for life, if ectopic, midline thyroid mistakenly removed

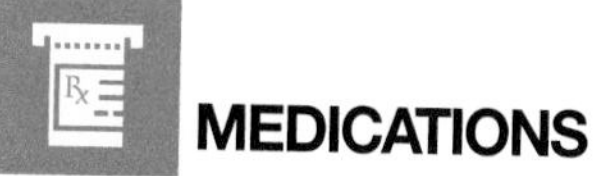

MEDICATIONS

DRUG(S) OF CHOICE None. All thyroglossal duct cysts should be surgically removed.
Contraindications: N/A
Precautions: N/A
Significant possible interactions: N/A

ALTERNATIVE DRUGS N/A

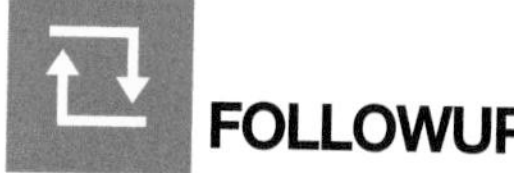

FOLLOWUP

PATIENT MONITORING 1-2 weeks after drainage or resection

PREVENTION/AVOIDANCE N/A

POSSIBLE COMPLICATIONS Infection and malignant degeneration if not excised

EXPECTED COURSE/PROGNOSIS
Resolution with resection (less than 5% recurrence using the Sistrunk procedure)

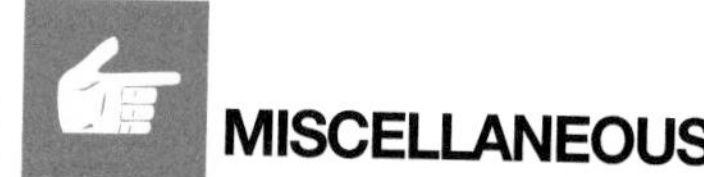

MISCELLANEOUS

ASSOCIATED CONDITIONS None

AGE-RELATED FACTORS
Pediatric: N/A
Geriatric: N/A
Others: N/A

PREGNANCY N/A

SYNONYMS N/A

ICD-9-CM
759.2 Congenital anomalies of other endocrine glands

SEE ALSO

OTHER NOTES N/A

ABBREVIATIONS N/A

REFERENCES

- Welch KJ, Randolph JG, Ravitch MM, et al, eds: Pediatric Surgery. 4th Ed. New York, Year Book Medical Publishers, 1986

Web references: 1 available at www.5mcc.com
Illustrations N/A

Author(s):
James P. Miller, MD
Timothy L. Black, MD

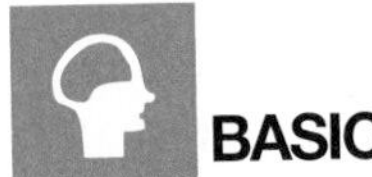

BASICS

DESCRIPTION Autologous growth of thyroid nodules with potential for metastases
- Papillary carcinoma - most common variety, 60-70% of thyroid tumors. May be associated with radiation exposure. Tumor contains psammoma bodies. Metastasizes by lymphatic route (30% at time of diagnosis).
- Follicular carcinoma - 10-20% of thyroid tumors. The incidence has been decreasing since the addition of dietary iodine. It occurs usually in females over 40 years of age. Metastasizes by the hematogenous route.
- Hürthle cell carcinoma - usually in patients over 60 years of age. Radioresistant. Composed of distinct large eosinophilic cells with abundant cytoplasmic mitochondria.
- Medullary carcinoma - arises from parafollicular cells, C-cells. 2-5% of all thyroid tumors. 25-35% are associated with multiple endocrine neoplasia (MEN) syndromes which can be familial or sporadic. Calcitonin is a chemical marker.
- Anaplastic carcinoma - 3% of thyroid tumors, usually in patients over 60 years of age
- Other - lymphoma, sarcoma, or metastatic (renal, breast or lung)

System(s) affected: Endocrine/Metabolic
Genetics:
- Medullary - autosomal dominant with MEN syndrome
- Others - none known

Incidence/Prevalence in USA: 0.0051/100,000 (16,100 new cases per year); < 1,200 deaths per year from thyroid cancer
Predominant age: Usually over 40 years of age
Predominant sex: Female > Male (2.6:1)

SIGNS & SYMPTOMS
- Painless hard, fixed neck mass (in advanced cases; otherwise soft to hard masses)
- Hoarseness
- Dysphagia
- Cervical lymphadenopathy
- Dyspnea

CAUSES Unknown

RISK FACTORS
- Family history
- Neck irradiation (6-2000 rads) - papillary carcinoma
- Iodine deficiency - follicular carcinoma
- MEN syndrome - medullary carcinoma
- Previous history of less than a total thyroidectomy for malignancy - anaplastic carcinoma

DIAGNOSIS

DIFFERENTIAL DIAGNOSIS
- Multinodular goiter
- Thyroid adenoma
- Thyroglossal duct cyst
- Thyroiditis
- Thyroid cyst
- Ectopic thyroid

LABORATORY Thyroid function tests usually normal

Drugs that may alter lab results: N/A

Disorders that may alter lab results: N/A

PATHOLOGICAL FINDINGS
- Papillary - psammoma bodies, anaplastic epithelial papillae
- Follicular - anaplastic epithelial cords with follicles
- Hürthle cell - large eosinophilic cells with granular cytoplasm
- Medullary - large amounts of amyloid stroma
- Anaplastic - small cell and giant cell undifferentiated tumors

SPECIAL TESTS
- Medullary carcinoma - calcitonin level (normal is less than 300 pg/mL [300 ng/L])
- Thyroglobulin level - post operative tumor marker
- DNA content of tumors from biopsy specimen. Diploid content has a better prognosis.

IMAGING
- Thyroid scan - cold nodules are more suspicious of malignancy
- Ultrasound - solid mass is more suspicious of malignancy
- CT and MRI can be useful to evaluate large substernal masses and recurrent soft tissue masses

DIAGNOSTIC PROCEDURES
- Fine needle aspiration
- Surgical biopsy/excision
- Laryngoscopy, if vocal cord paralysis is suspected

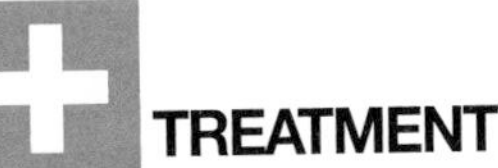

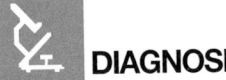

TREATMENT

APPROPRIATE HEALTH CARE Inpatient

GENERAL MEASURES N/A

SURGICAL MEASURES
- Papillary carcinoma - lobectomy with isthmectomy (if lesion < 1.5 cm) or total thyroidectomy, and removal of suspicious lymph nodes
- Follicular carcinoma and Hurthle cell - total thyroidectomy and removal of suspicious lymph nodes
- Medullary carcinoma - total thyroidectomy with central node dissection. Unilateral or bilateral modified radical neck dissection if lateral nodes are histologically positive.
- Anaplastic carcinoma - aggressive en bloc thyroidectomy. Often times tracheostomy required.

ACTIVITY As tolerated

DIET Avoid iodine deficiency

PATIENT EDUCATION
National Cancer Institute
Building 31, Room 101-18
9000 Rockville Pike
Bethesda, MD 20892
(301)496-5583

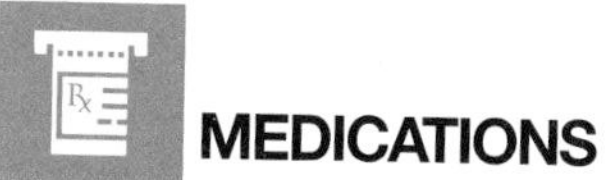

MEDICATIONS

DRUG(S) OF CHOICE
- Post operatively will require thyroid replacement to suppress serum TSH level:
  - ◊ Levothyroxine (T4, Synthroid) 100-200 μg/day or
  - ◊ Liothyronine (T3, Cytomel) 50-100 μg/day

Contraindications: N/A
Precautions: N/A
Significant possible interactions:
- Amphetamines
- Anticoagulants
- Tricyclic antidepressants
- Antidiabetic medications
- Aspirin
- Barbiturates
- Beta adrenergic blockers
- Cholestyramine
- Colestipol
- Oral contraceptives
- Digitalis preparation
- Ephedrine
- Estrogens
- Methylphenidate
- Phenytoin

ALTERNATIVE DRUGS N/A

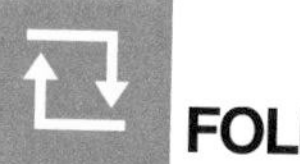

FOLLOWUP

PATIENT MONITORING
- Thyroid scan at 6 weeks and administration of I131 for any visible uptake evidence of residual thyroid tissue (after total thyroidectomy) or lymph node disease is treated with radioactive iodine
- At 6 months and then yearly the patient should have a thyroid scan and chest x-ray
- Papillary and follicular - a thyroglobulin level should be done yearly
- Medullary - calcitonin level should be done yearly with pentagastrin stimulation
- The thyroid scan and thyroglobulin level should be done with the patient in the hypothyroid state induced by 6 week withdrawal of levothyroxine or 2-3 week withdrawal of liothyronine

PREVENTION/AVOIDANCE
- Physical exam in high risk group
- Calcium infusion or pentagastrin stimulation test in high risk MEN patients

POSSIBLE COMPLICATIONS Recurrence of tumor

EXPECTED COURSE/PROGNOSIS
- Papillary carcinoma - overall mortality 3-8%
- Follicular carcinoma - overall 80% 5 year survival rate, 77% 10 year survival rate. Histologically microinvasive tumors parallel papillary tumor results while grossly invasive tumors do far worse.
- Hürthle cell carcinoma - 93% 5 year survival rate, and 83% survival rate overall. Grossly invasive tumors - survival is less than 25%.
- Medullary carcinoma - negative nodes 90% 5 year survival rate and 85% 10 year survival rate; with positive nodes 65% 5 year survival rate and 40% 10 year survival rate
- Anaplastic carcinoma - survival unexpected

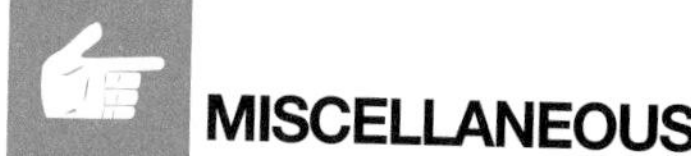

MISCELLANEOUS

ASSOCIATED CONDITIONS Medullary carcinoma - pheochromocytoma, hyperparathyroidism, ganglioneuroma of the GI tract, neuromata of mucosal membranes

AGE-RELATED FACTORS
Pediatric: Over 60% of thyroid nodules are malignant
Geriatric: Risk of malignancy increases over age 60
Others: N/A

PREGNANCY N/A

SYNONYMS
- Follicular carcinoma of the thyroid
- Papillary carcinoma of the thyroid
- Hürthle cell carcinoma of the thyroid
- Anaplastic cell carcinoma of the thyroid

ICD-9-CM
193 Malignant neoplasm of thyroid gland
198.89 Secondary malignant neoplasm of other specified sites, other

SEE ALSO
Multiple endocrine neoplasia (MEN)

OTHER NOTES N/A

ABBREVIATIONS MEN = multiple endocrine neoplasia

REFERENCES

- Bell RM: Thyroid carcinoma. Surg Clin North Am 1986;66:13
- Lennquist S: The Thyroid Nodule, Surg Clin North Am 1987;66:213-232
- Gagel RF, Goepfert H, Callender RL: Changing Concepts in the Pathogenesis and Management of Thyroid carcinoma, CA Cancer J Clin 1996;46:261-283

Web references: 2 available at www.5mcc.com
Illustrations N/A

Author(s):

James P. Miller, MD
Timothy L. Black, MD

BASICS

DESCRIPTION A variety of inflammatory thyroid disorders that can cause thyroid enlargement and thyroid atrophy. May lead to hypothyroidism or hyperthyroidism. Complete resolution can occur.

- Hashimoto disease - the most common form, an autoimmune disease, often presenting as an asymptomatic diffuse goiter. Often first detected after thyroid atrophy and hypothyroidism have occurred and occasionally as hyperthyroidism ("Hashitoxicosis").
- Granulomatous thyroiditis ("subacute") - probably related to viral infection and usually presenting with thyroid pain (which may be severe), involving one or both thyroid lobes, accompanied by hyperthyroidism, followed by a phase of mild hypothyroidism and then to permanent resolution to normal
- "Silent" thyroiditis - characterized by lack of pain, one form of which is characterized by spontaneously resolving hypothyroidism and/or hyperthyroidism often associated with pregnancy. Another form has the characteristics of granulomatous thyroiditis without the pain.
- Rare forms of thyroiditis
  - ◊ Suppurative, due to bacterial infection of the thyroid
  - ◊ Radiation due to ingested radionuclides or external irradiation
  - ◊ Riedel thyroiditis: dense infiltration of fibrous tissue into thyroid gland and surrounding structures of unknown cause
- One form is postpartum onset of goiter and/or hypothyroidism that may resolve spontaneously. Another is painless granulomatous thyroiditis.

System(s) affected: Endocrine/Metabolic
Genetics: N/A
Incidence/Prevalence in USA:

- Not known definitively
- Lymphocytic thyroiditis increases with age, probably up to 10% over age 65
- Granulomatous thyroiditis much less common, has an epidemic pattern

Predominant age: All ages, postpuberty
Predominant sex: Female > Male

SIGNS & SYMPTOMS

- Lymphocytic thyroiditis
  - ◊ Insidious onset of goiter, often detected incidentally
  - ◊ Slow onset of hypothyroidism
  - ◊ Association with other autoimmune diseases
- Granulomatous thyroiditis
  - ◊ Pain, tenderness and enlargement of one or both thyroid lobes
  - ◊ Malaise, fever
  - ◊ Mild to moderate symptoms of hyperthyroidism
  - ◊ History of recent respiratory infection

CAUSES

- Hashimoto disease
  - ◊ Autoimmune response of thyroid tissue
  - ◊ Genetic susceptibility
- Granulomatous thyroiditis
  - ◊ Chronic inflammatory response of thyroid tissue
  - ◊ Preceding infection with any of a variety of viruses

RISK FACTORS

- Hashimoto disease
  - ◊ Positive family history of thyroid disease or other autoimmune disease
  - ◊ Preceding autoimmune diseases including type I diabetes, primary adrenal insufficiency, rheumatoid arthritis, pregnancy/delivery
- Granulomatous thyroiditis
  - ◊ Recent viral respiratory infection
  - ◊ Other known cases in the community

DIAGNOSIS

DIFFERENTIAL DIAGNOSIS

- Hashimoto disease
  - ◊ Simple goiter
  - ◊ Iodine-deficient goiter (especially in endemic areas)
  - ◊ Early Graves disease
  - ◊ Lithium induced goiter
- Granulomatous thyroiditis
  - ◊ Infections of oropharynx and trachea
  - ◊ Hemorrhage into a thyroid cyst
  - ◊ Subacute systemic illness
  - ◊ Suppurative thyroiditis

LABORATORY

- Hashimoto disease
  - ◊ Elevated anti-thyroid antibodies (especially high titers of anti-TPO antibodies)
  - ◊ Free thyroxine index (FTI, normal 4.5-12) less than 5 with TSH greater than 5 mcg/dl (normal 0.5-5 mcg/dl)
  - ◊ Thyroid radioactive iodine uptake (RAIU) variable with scintiscan showing patchy distribution of radioiodine
  - ◊ Positive cytopathology of fine needle aspirate or positive formal biopsy
- Granulomatous thyroiditis
  - ◊ Elevated erythrocyte sedimentation rate
  - ◊ Normal or moderately elevated WBC without a granulocyte shift to band forms
  - ◊ FTI greater than 12, TSH undetectable, RAIU less than 5% in 24 hours (often nil) early in course. FTI less than 4.5 with RAIU above normal (greater than 35% in 24 hours in USA) late in course

Drugs that may alter lab results:

- Thyroid
- Corticosteroids
- Iodine containing drugs and contrast media
- Lithium
- Amiodarone

Disorders that may alter lab results:

- Iodine-deficiency
- Non-thyroidal illness

PATHOLOGICAL FINDINGS

- Hashimoto disease
  - ◊ Lymphocytic infiltration
  - ◊ Oxyphilic changes in follicular cells
  - ◊ Fibrosis
  - ◊ Atrophy
- Granulomatous thyroiditis
  - ◊ Giant cells
  - ◊ Mononuclear cell infiltrate

SPECIAL TESTS

- Immunometric assays
- Anti-thyroid antibody titers
- Complete blood count with differential count
- Erythrocyte sedimentation rate

IMAGING

- Thyroid radioiodine uptake and scan in granulomatous thyroiditis
- Ultrasonography if hemorrhage into thyroid cyst suspected

DIAGNOSTIC PROCEDURES Needle biopsy in confusing cases

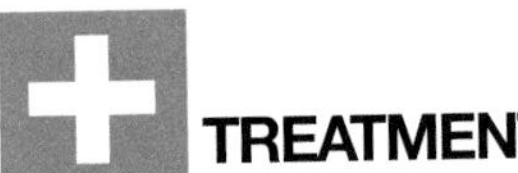

TREATMENT

APPROPRIATE HEALTH CARE Outpatient

GENERAL MEASURES

- Analgesics for pain
- Corticosteroids for severe granulomatous thyroiditis

SURGICAL MEASURES N/A

ACTIVITY Fully active

DIET No special diet

PATIENT EDUCATION N/A

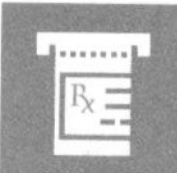

MEDICATIONS

DRUG(S) OF CHOICE
- Hashimoto disease
  - ◊ Levothyroxine if hypothyroid or goitrous. Generic levothyroxine may not be bioavailable. Carafate, iron preparations may decrease levothyroxine availability. Begin with 25 or 50 μg/day and titrate to TSH suppression to lower limit of assay normal range.
  - ◊ Propylthiouracil and propranolol if thyrotoxic and symptomatic
- Granulomatous thyroiditis:
  - ◊ Analgesics, e.g., codeine for pain
  - ◊ Propranolol 40 mg q6h for symptomatic hyperthyroidism
  - ◊ Levothyroxine 80 μg per 100 lbs (45.5 kg) body wt/day if hypothyroid phase is symptomatic
  - ◊ Prednisone once daily in lowest effective dose, for severe symptoms
- Maintenance:
  - ◊ Optimal levothyroxine dose can be established by measuring TSH at 6-8 week intervals until dosage level causes TSH to be at the lower level of normal for the assay used

Contraindications:
- Propylthiouracil - allergy or hypersensitivity to analgesics/narcotics
- Propranolol - insulin therapy, asthma
- Prednisone - adverse reactions
- Levothyroxine - none

Precautions: Reduce doses of corticosteroids, propranolol and narcotics as soon as feasible

Significant possible interactions: Sucralfate (Carafate) and iron preparations may decrease levothyroxine availability

ALTERNATIVE DRUGS
Methimazole for propylthiouracil

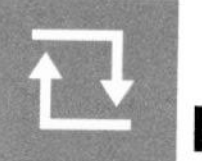

FOLLOWUP

PATIENT MONITORING
- Repeat thyroid function tests every 3-12 months in Hashimoto disease
- Repeat thyroid function tests every 3-6 weeks in granulomatous thyroiditis until permanently euthyroid

PREVENTION/AVOIDANCE
N/A

POSSIBLE COMPLICATIONS
Treatment induced hypothyroidism or hyperthyroidism

EXPECTED COURSE/PROGNOSIS
- Hashimoto disease - persistent goiter, eventual thyroid failure
- Granulomatous thyroiditis - eventual return to normal over weeks or months

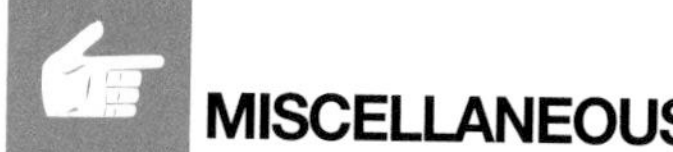

MISCELLANEOUS

ASSOCIATED CONDITIONS
Other autoimmune diseases with Hashimoto disease including type I diabetes, primary adrenal insufficiency, premature ovarian failure

AGE-RELATED FACTORS
Pediatric: N/A
Geriatric: Remission of granulomatous thyroiditis may be slower in the elderly
Others: N/A

PREGNANCY
- Avoid radioisotope scanning
- Avoid hypothyroidism
- Minimize use of antithyroid drugs

SYNONYMS
- Lymphocytic thyroiditis
- Granulomatous thyroiditis
- Silent thyroiditis

ICD-9-CM
245.0 Acute thyroiditis

SEE ALSO
Hyperthyroidism
Hypothyroidism, adult

OTHER NOTES
N/A

ABBREVIATIONS
- RAIU = radioactive iodine uptake
- FTI = free thyroxine index
- TSH = thyroid stimulating hormone

REFERENCES

- Burman KD. Thyroiditis. Wellesley, MA: UpToDate: 2004
- DeGroot LW, Larsen PR, Hennemann G. The Thyroid and its Diseases. 6th ed. New York: Churchill Livingston; 1996
- Jacobson DL, et al. Epidemiology and estimated population burden of selected autoimmune diseases in the United States. Clin Immunol Immunopathol 1997;84(3):223-43
- Stagnaro-Green A. Recognizing, understanding, and treating postpartum thyroiditis. Endocrinol Metab Clin North Am 2000;29(2):417-30
- Muller AF, Drexhage HA, Berghout A. Postpartum thyroiditis and autoimmune thyroiditis in women of childbearing age: recent insights and consequences for antenatal and postnatal care. Endocr Rev 2001;22(5):605-30
- Lo JC, Loh KC, Rubin AL, Cha I, Greenspan FS. Riedel's thyroiditis presenting with hypothyroidism and hypoparathyroidism: dramatic response to glucocorticoid and thyroxine therapy. Clin Endocrinol (Oxf) 1998;48(6):815-8

Web references: 0 available at www.5mcc.com
Illustrations N/A

Author(s):
Richard P. Levy, MD

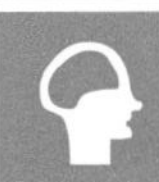

BASICS

DESCRIPTION A fungal infection of the scalp often called "ringworm." The infection results from contact with infected persons or animals. It is contagious and may become epidemic. Affected areas of the scalp can show characteristic black dots resulting from broken hairs.

System(s) affected: Skin/Exocrine

Genetics: N/A

Incidence/Prevalence in USA: Although still common, the incidence and prevalence have markedly dropped over the past 30 years

Predominant age: Children particularly ages 3 to 9. Adult infection is rare.

Predominant sex: Male = Female

SIGNS & SYMPTOMS

- Infection commonly begins with round patches of scale (alopecia less common)
- Frequently, infection will take on the patterns of chronic scaling with little inflammation or marked inflammation and alopecia. Less frequently, patients will present with multiple patches of alopecia and characteristic black dot pattern of broken hairs. Extreme inflammation results in kerion (exudative pustular nodulation).

CAUSES

- 90% *Trichophyton tonsurans*
- 10% *Microsporum species* (*canis*, *audouinii*, *gypseum*)

RISK FACTORS

- Day-care centers or schools
- Living in confined quarters
- Poor hygiene
- Immunosuppression

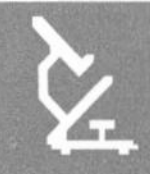

DIAGNOSIS

DIFFERENTIAL DIAGNOSIS

- Psoriasis and seborrhea dermatitis are most often confused with tinea capitis
- Pyoderma
- Alopecia areata and trichotillomania
- Aphasia cutis congenita

LABORATORY

- Microscopy of a KOH preparation of hairs from affected area can show arthrospores that appear within hair shafts
- Fungal culture of hairs from affected areas allows the infection to be confirmed and the causative organism to be identified

Drugs that may alter lab results: N/A

Disorders that may alter lab results: N/A

PATHOLOGICAL FINDINGS

- Chronic inflammation
- Superficial infection producing lesions with follicular pustules, abscess
- Hyphae in follicles, keratin of skin

SPECIAL TESTS Viewed under a Wood's lamp, the 10% of infections caused by *Microsporum species* will fluoresce a light green. 90% of tinea capitis infections, those caused by *Trichophyton*, will NOT fluoresce.

IMAGING N/A

DIAGNOSTIC PROCEDURES N/A

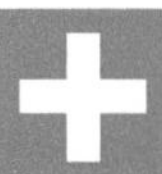

TREATMENT

APPROPRIATE HEALTH CARE Outpatient

GENERAL MEASURES

- Careful hand washing
- Launder towels, clothing, head wear of infected individual
- Check other family members

SURGICAL MEASURES N/A

ACTIVITY No restrictions

DIET No special diet except persons treated with griseofulvin should not be on a restricted fat diet

PATIENT EDUCATION

- KidsHealth at the AMA: www.ama-assn.org/insight/h_focus/nemours/infectio/childhd/fungi.htm
- Information from your family doctor: http://familydoctor.org/handouts/316.html

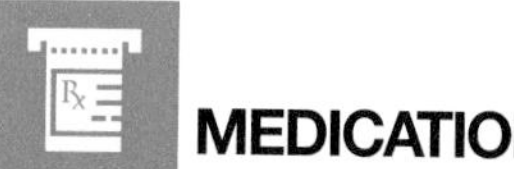

MEDICATIONS

DRUG(S) OF CHOICE

- Griseofulvin (Fulvicin P/G, Fulvicin U/F, Gris-PEG) - preferred treatment
  - ◊ Micro-sized preparation
  - ◊ Available in 125 mg, 250 mg and 500 mg tablets and 125 mg/5 mL suspension
  - ◊ Dose at 10 mg/kg/day taken bid or as single daily dose up to 500 mg/day for 6-12 weeks
- Itraconazole (Sporanox)
  - ◊ Matches griseofulvin in treatment and is better tolerated
  - ◊ 3-5 mg/kg/day, but most studies have used 100 mg daily for 6 weeks in children over 2 years of age
- Oral terbinafine (Lamisil) - for 2-4 weeks
  - ◊ 62.5 mg po qd for children < 20 kg
  - ◊ 125 mg po qd for children 20-40 kg
  - ◊ 250 po qd for adults and children > 40 kg

Contraindications:

- Griseofulvin contraindicated in patients with porphyria because of increased risk of hepatotoxicity

Precautions:

- Griseofulvin
  - ◊ Headache in up to 10% of patients initially but generally resolves after first week of treatment
  - ◊ Abdominal bloating, dyspepsia, and diarrhea also common
  - ◊ Hypersensitivity and liver toxicity rare. The manufacturer recommends monitoring liver functions while on griseofulvin but due to rarity of hepatotoxicity many physicians choose to forgo any testing.
- Itraconazole
  - ◊ Side effects - nausea, vomiting, diarrhea, headache, dizziness, abnormal hepatic function tests, rare significant liver toxicity (appears safer than ketoconazole)

Significant possible interactions: Griseofulvin accentuates the effect of alcohol and increases the metabolism of warfarin and oral contraceptives.

ALTERNATIVE DRUGS

- Oral terbinafine (Lamisil) - 250 mg for 2 weeks for *T. tonsurans*. Faster cure rate and lower recurrence than griseofulvin.
- If kerion is present, prednisone 1 mg/kg/d can be added to antifungal therapy for 5-10 days

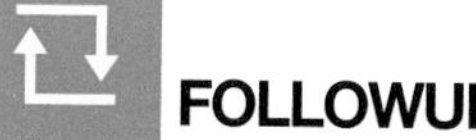

FOLLOWUP

PATIENT MONITORING Recheck after two weeks of therapy to document improvement and after the 6 week course of therapy. Patients might need liver function monitoring - see medication precautions.

PREVENTION/AVOIDANCE

- Good personal hygiene
- Don't share head wear
- Identification and treatment of infected individuals and household pets

POSSIBLE COMPLICATIONS Permanent scarring and hair loss from kerion

EXPECTED COURSE/PROGNOSIS

Without treatment lesions will usually spontaneously heal in 6 months. Lesions with marked inflammation will spontaneously resolve much more rapidly but are more likely to leave scarring.

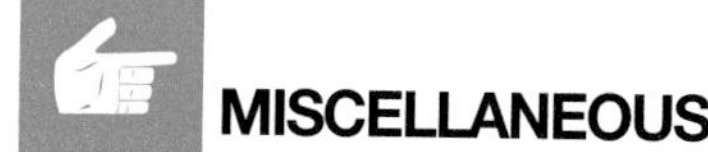

MISCELLANEOUS

ASSOCIATED CONDITIONS N/A

AGE-RELATED FACTORS

Pediatric: Highest incidence in this age group
Geriatric: N/A
Others: N/A

PREGNANCY Oral antifungals are contraindicated in pregnancy

SYNONYMS Scalp ringworm

ICD-9-CM

110.0 Dermatophytosis of scalp and beard

SEE ALSO

Alopecia
Tinea corporis

OTHER NOTES N/A

ABBREVIATIONS N/A

REFERENCES

- Temple ME. Pharmacotherapy of tinea capitis. J Am Board Fam Pract 1999;12(3):236-42
- Frieden IJ, Howard R. Tinea capitis: epidemiology, diagnosis, treatment and control. J Am Acad Dermatol 1994;31:542-6
- Friedlander SF. The evolving role of itraconazole, fluconazole and terbinafine in the treatment of tinea capitis. Pediatr Infect Dis J 1999;18(2):205-10
- Stein DH. Tineas - superficial dermatophyte infections. Pediatr Rev 1998;19:368-72
- Friedlander SF, et al. Terbinafine in the treatment of Trichophyton tinea capitis. Pediatrics 2002;109:602-7
- Gupta AK, Adam P, Dlova N, et al. Therapeutic options for the treatment of tinea capitis caused by Trichophyton species: griseofulvin versus the new oral antifungal agents, terbinafine, itraconazole, and fluconazole.
- Pediatr Dermatol 2001;18(5):433-8

Web references: 2 available at www.5mcc.com
Illustrations 4 available

Author(s):

George R. Bergus, MD

BASICS

DESCRIPTION Scaling plaque characterized by a sharply defined annular pattern with peripheral activity and central clearing. Papules and occasionally pustules/vesicles present at border, and less commonly in center. Affects face, trunk, and extremities.
- Zoophilic infections are acquired from animals
- Anthropophilic infections acquired from personal contact or fomites

System(s) affected: Skin/Exocrine
Genetics: There is evidence for genetic susceptibility in some people
Incidence/Prevalence in USA: Fairly common
Predominant age: All ages
Predominant sex: Male = Female

SIGNS & SYMPTOMS
- Characteristic rash and mild pruritus
- Scaling plaques that are circular, bright red, sharply marginated, occur singly or in groups of 3-4
- Each plaque is less than 5 cm in diameter
- Plaques are solid, but annular forms occur
- Patient may experience intense itching
- Hyperpigmentation (occasionally)

CAUSES Fungal infection due to dermatophyte, e.g., Trichophyton rubrum (most common). Microsporum canis often results in multiple lesions.

RISK FACTORS
- Warm climates
- Direct contact with an active lesion on a human, an animal, or rarely from soil
- Working with animals
- Immunosuppression including prolonged use of topical steroids

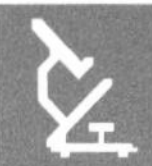

DIAGNOSIS

DIFFERENTIAL DIAGNOSIS
- Pityriasis rosea
- Eczema
- Contact dermatitis
- Syphilis
- Psoriasis
- Subacute lupus erythematosus
- Elastosis perforans serpiginosa
- Erythema annulare
- Gyrate erythemas, especially centrifugum
- Erythema multiforme
- Erythema migrans

LABORATORY Potassium hydroxide preparation of skin scrapings. Fungal culture may be obtained, but is not generally necessary.

Drugs that may alter lab results: N/A

Disorders that may alter lab results: N/A

PATHOLOGICAL FINDINGS Branching hyphae with septa on potassium hydroxide preparation

SPECIAL TESTS
- Tinea corpora does not fluoresce with Wood's light
- Culture on Sabouraud's medium - sample by scraping or vigorous rubbing of a cotton swab on the lesion, then rolled/rubbed on the medium

IMAGING N/A

DIAGNOSTIC PROCEDURES
- Skin scraping:
  - ◊ Use No.15 blade and place several small scrapings of the active border on glass slide with coverslip
  - ◊ Apply 10-20% potassium hydroxide and heat gently without boiling
  - ◊ Let stand for 5 minutes and examine for septate, branching hyphae. Use lowered condenser and dim light to enhance contrast. Hyphae may be accentuated with a commercial fungal stain or a drop of blue ink.

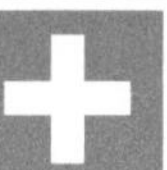

TREATMENT

APPROPRIATE HEALTH CARE Outpatient

GENERAL MEASURES Proper hygiene

SURGICAL MEASURES N/A

ACTIVITY Avoid contact sports, e.g., wrestling for 2 days while starting treatment

DIET Unrestricted diet

PATIENT EDUCATION Avoid contact with suspected lesions. Be careful with animal contacts.

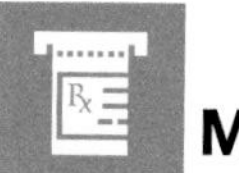

MEDICATIONS

DRUG(S) OF CHOICE

- Topical antifungal creams - miconazole (Monistat-Derm) or clotrimazole (Lotrimin, Mycelex) applied bid for 2 weeks. Also ketoconazole (Nizoral) applied qd for 2 weeks. To prevent relapse should use for one week after resolution. Also econazole (Spectazole) and allylamines, e.g., naftifine (Naftin, Lamisil). For added benefit, wash with antifungal shampoo ketoconazole (Nizoral Shampoo) prior to use of cream.
- For resistant, extensive and/or invasive infections, oral agents are recommended for 4 weeks. Oral ultramicrosize griseofulvin (e.g., Gris-PEG) 7 mg/kg/day in children over 2 years; 375 mg/day in adults. Oral itraconazole, in lieu of ketoconazole - less toxic and less drug side effects. Although not indicated, itraconazole (Sporanox) is effective at 200 mg/day for 7 days.
- Terbinafine (Lamisil) 250 mg/d for 2-4 weeks
- Fluconazole (Diflucan) 150-300mg (one dose weekly for 2 weeks)

Contraindications: Known hypersensitivity to agent

Precautions:

- Ketoconazole contains a sulfite and should be avoided in sulfite sensitive people. There is a 1:10,000 reported incidence of hepatotoxicity with oral ketoconazole. Baseline liver function tests should be obtained prior to initiating oral ketoconazole and patients should be followed closely.
- Terbinafine - gastrointestinal side effects; rare hepatotoxicity and hematologic changes

Significant possible interactions: Griseofulvin induces hepatic enzymes that metabolize warfarin and other drugs. H2 blockers and antacids reduce ketoconazole absorption. Ketoconazole is an enzyme inhibitor and may cause drug toxicity (case report of apparent terfenadine toxicity causing ventricular arrhythmia). Ketoconazole also significantly increases cyclosporine levels.

ALTERNATIVE DRUGS N/A

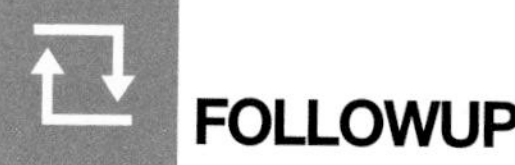

FOLLOWUP

PATIENT MONITORING Necessary for invasive disease or prolonged treatment with oral ketoconazole

PREVENTION/AVOIDANCE Avoid contact with suspicious lesions

POSSIBLE COMPLICATIONS

- Bacterial super-infection
- Generalized, invasive dermatophyte infection

EXPECTED COURSE/PROGNOSIS

Resolution without sequelae in 1-2 weeks of therapy

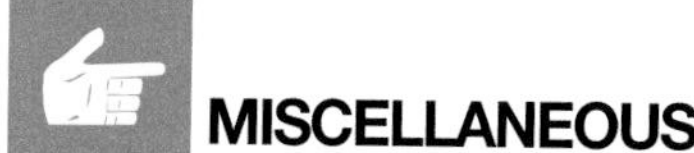

MISCELLANEOUS

ASSOCIATED CONDITIONS Other tineas - pedis, cruris, capitis, barbae, and manus

AGE-RELATED FACTORS

Pediatric: N/A
Geriatric: N/A
Others: N/A

PREGNANCY N/A

SYNONYMS

- Ringworm
- Tinea circinata

ICD-9-CM

110.5 Dermatophytosis of the body

SEE ALSO

Tinea capitis
Tinea cruris
Tinea pedis

OTHER NOTES N/A

ABBREVIATIONS N/A

REFERENCES

- Habif T. Clinical Dermatology. 4th ed. St. Louis: CV Mosby; 2004
- Fitzpatrick TB et al: Color Atlas and Synopsis of Clinical Dermatology. 4th ed. New York: McGraw-Hill; 2000

Web references: 2 available at www.5mcc.com
Illustrations 6 available

Author(s):
Samuel L. Moschella, MD

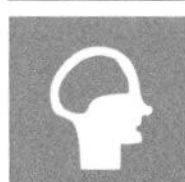

BASICS

DESCRIPTION A superficial fungal infection of the groin area caused by a group of fungi known as dermatophyte infections may result from three genera of fungi: *Microsporum*, *Trichophyton* and, *Epidermophyton*.

- Tinea cruris is characterized by development of well marginated erythematous half-moon shaped plaques in the crural folds which spread to the upper thighs. The advancing border is well-defined often with fine scaling and sometimes includes vesicular eruptions. The lesions are usually bilateral and do not include the scrotum or penis, but may migrate to the buttock and gluteal cleft area.

System(s) affected: Skin/Exocrine
Genetics: N/A
Incidence/Prevalence in USA: Common
Predominant age: Any age (rare prior to puberty)
Predominant sex: Male > Female

SIGNS & SYMPTOMS

- Lesions may be asymptomatic but more frequently are quite pruritic
- Acute inflammation may result from wearing occlusive clothing
- Chronic scratching may result in an eczematous appearance
- Previous application of topical steroids may alter the appearance causing a more extensive eruption with irregular borders and erythematous papules. This modified form is called tinea incognito.

CAUSES

- *Trichophyton rubrum*, *Trichophyton mentagrophytes*, and *Epidermophyton floccosum* are most common causative dermatophytes

RISK FACTORS

- Summer months and/or increased sweating
- Wearing wet clothing
- Wearing multiple layers of clothing
- Depression of cell mediated immune response (atopic individuals, AIDS, etc.)
- Obesity

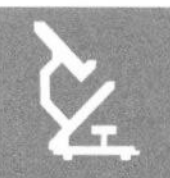

DIAGNOSIS

DIFFERENTIAL DIAGNOSIS

- Intertrigo-inflammatory process of moist opposed skin folds, often including infection with bacteria yeast, and fungi. Painful longitudinal fissures occur in the creases of skin folds.
- Erythematous-diffuse brown scaly

noninflammatory plaque with irregular borders often involving the groin. Caused by bacterial infection with *Corynebacterium minutissimum*. Fluoresces coral-red with Wood's lamp.

- Seborrheic dermatitis of the groin
- Psoriasis of the groin
- Candidiasis of the groin
- Acanthosis nigricans

LABORATORY

- Fungal culture using Sabouraud's dextrose agar or dermatophyte test medium (DTM)
- Potassium hydroxide preparation of skin scrapings from the dermatophyte leading border shows translucent branching, rod-shaped hyphae

Drugs that may alter lab results:

- Partial treatment with antifungal preparations
- Topical steroid treatment may confuse diagnosis by causing tinea incognito

Disorders that may alter lab results:
Pruritus with extensive itching

PATHOLOGICAL FINDINGS

Skin biopsy showing fungal hyphae in the epidermis

SPECIAL TESTS

Wood's lamp exam reveals no fluorescence

IMAGING N/A

DIAGNOSTIC PROCEDURES

Potassium hydroxide, (KOH) preparation of skin scrapings form leading border

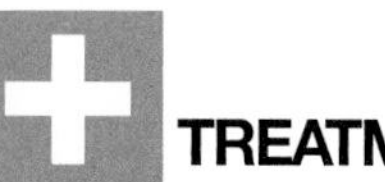

TREATMENT

APPROPRIATE HEALTH CARE

Outpatient

GENERAL MEASURES

- Avoid predisposing conditions, keep area as dry as possible
- Topical steroid preparations should not be used

SURGICAL MEASURES N/A

ACTIVITY Full activity

DIET No restrictions

PATIENT EDUCATION

Explanation of the causative agents, predisposing factors, and prevention measures

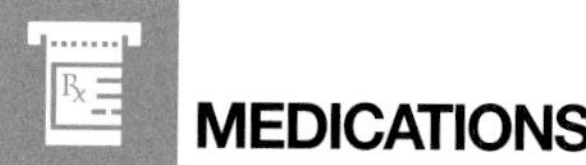

MEDICATIONS

DRUG(S) OF CHOICE

- Topical azole antifungal compounds:
  - ◊ econazole (Spectazole), ketoconazole (Nizoral) are usually applied bid for 2-3 weeks
  - ◊ Terbinafine (Lamisil), now an OTC compound can be applied once or twice daily for 1-2 weeks
  - ◊ Butenafine (Mentax) applied once daily for 2 weeks is also very effective

Contraindications: Oral itraconazole (Sporanox) is contraindicated with the following drugs: astemizole (Hismanal), triazolam (Halcion), lovastatin (Mevacor), simvastatin (Zocor). But pravastatin (Pravachol) can be given with itraconazole. These compounds should not be given during pregnancy.
Precautions: N/A
Significant possible interactions: N/A

ALTERNATIVE DRUGS

- Oral antifungal agents are effective, but not indicated in uncomplicated tinea cruris. If topical therapy fails one may consult a dermatologist for possible oral therapy. Griseofulvin can be given 500 mg po once per day for 1-2 weeks.
- The following oral regimens have been reported in the medical literature as being effective, but currently are not specifically approved by the FDA for tinea cruris:
  - ◊ Oral terbinafine (Lamisil) 250 mg per day for one week
  - ◊ Oral itraconazole (Sporanox) 100 mg bid once and repeated one week later
  - ◊ Oral fluconazole (Diflucan) 150 mg once per week for four weeks
- Topical terbinafine 1% solution has recently been studied and appears effective as a once daily application for 1 week

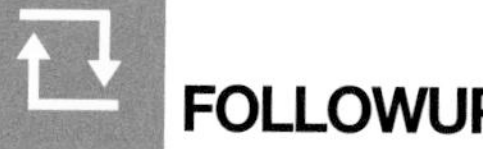

FOLLOWUP

PATIENT MONITORING

- Liver function testing prior to therapy and at regular intervals during the course of therapy for those patients requiring oral terbinafine, fluconazole itraconazole, and griseofulvin

PREVENTION/AVOIDANCE

Avoidance of risk factors

POSSIBLE COMPLICATIONS

Secondary bacterial function

EXPECTED COURSE/PROGNOSIS

Excellent prognosis for cure with therapy

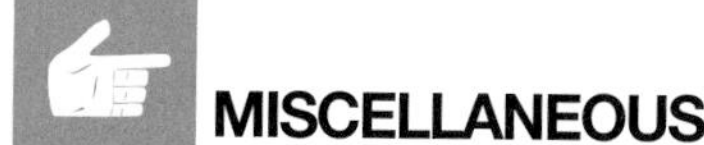

MISCELLANEOUS

ASSOCIATED CONDITIONS

None

AGE-RELATED FACTORS

Pediatric: Rare in pediatric population prior to puberty
Geriatric: More common due to increase in risk factors
Others: N/A

PREGNANCY Rare

SYNONYMS

- Jock itch
- Ring worm

ICD-9-CM

110.3 Dermatophytosis of groin and perianal area

SEE ALSO

Acanthosis nigricans

OTHER NOTES N/A

ABBREVIATIONS N/A

REFERENCES

- Elewski B. Cutaneous Fungal Infections 2nd ed. Boston: Blackwell Science; 1998
- Nozickova M, et al. A comparison of the efficiency of oral fluconazole 150 mg /week vs. 50 mg/day in the treatment of tinea corporis, cruris, pedis, and cutaneous candidiasis. Int J. Dermatol 1998;37(9):703-5
- Farag A, et al. One week therapy with oral terbinafine in cases of tinea cruris/corporis. Br J Dermatol 1994;131(5):684-6
- Lesher JL Jr, et al. Butenafine 1% cream in the treatment of tinea cruris. J Am Acad Dermatol 1997;36(2pt1):520-4
- Fitzpatrick TB, et al. Color Atlas and Synopsis of Clinical Dermatology. 3rd ed. New York: McGraw-Hill, Inc; 1997
- Physician's Desk Reference. 53rd ed. New York, Medical Economics, 1999:2174-5
- Lebwohl M, Elewski B, Eisen D, Savin RC. Efficacy and safety of terbinafine 1% solution in the treatment of interdigital tinea pedis and tinea corporis or tinea cruris. Cutis 2001;67(3):261-6
- Sanmano B, et al. Abbreviated oral itraconazole therapy for tinea corporis and tinea cruris. Mycoses 2003;46(8):316-21

Web references: 3 available at www.5mcc.com
Illustrations 2 available

Author(s):
Glenn Russo, MD

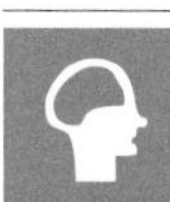

BASICS

DESCRIPTION Tinea pedis is a superficial infection of the feet caused by dermatophytes. It is the most common dermatophyte infection encountered in clinical practice.
System(s) affected: Skin/Exocrine
Genetics: No known genetic pattern
Incidence/Prevalence in USA: Approximately 4% of the population
Predominant age: All ages, but most common in ages 20-50
Predominant sex: Male > Female

SIGNS & SYMPTOMS
- Strong odor
- Hyperkeratosis
- Itching
- Scaling (chronic)
- Maceration/ulceration
- Vesicles/bullae (acute)
- Primarily in interdigital spaces, especially 4th and 5th
- May involve soles, arch and sides of feet (moccasin distribution)
- May be associated with nail plate cellulitis, destruction, discoloration, thickening and crumbling

CAUSES
- *Trichophyton mentagrophytes* (acute)
- *Trichophyton rubrum* (chronic)
- *Trichophyton tonsurans*
- Epidermophyton floccosum

RISK FACTORS
- Hot, humid weather
- Occlusive footwear
- Immunosuppressed patients
- Prolonged application of topical steroids

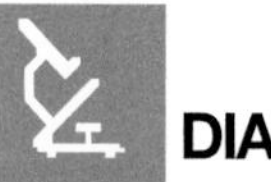

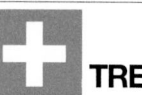

DIAGNOSIS

DIFFERENTIAL DIAGNOSIS
- Interdigital type - erythrasma, impetigo, pitted keratolysis, candida intertrigo
- Moccasin type - psoriasis vulgaris, eczematous dermatitis, pitted keratolysis
- Inflammatory/bullous type - impetigo, allergic contact dermatitis, dyshidrotic eczema, bullous disease

LABORATORY
- Direct microscopic examination (KOH)
- Culture (Sabouraud's medium)
- Wood's lamp exam

Drugs that may alter lab results: N/A

Disorders that may alter lab results: N/A

PATHOLOGICAL FINDINGS
- Septate and branched mycelia on KOH
- Culture - dermatophyte

SPECIAL TESTS N/A

IMAGING N/A

DIAGNOSTIC PROCEDURES Culture

TREATMENT

APPROPRIATE HEALTH CARE Outpatient

GENERAL MEASURES
- Treatment is generally with topical antifungal medications
- Soaking with aluminum chloride 30% or aluminum subacetate for 20 minutes bid
- After soaking or bathing, patient should carefully remove or debride dead or thickened tissues
- Chronic or extensive disease or nail involvement requires oral antifungal medication - systemic therapy

SURGICAL MEASURES N/A

ACTIVITY Avoid sweating feet

DIET No restrictions

PATIENT EDUCATION See Prevention/Avoidance

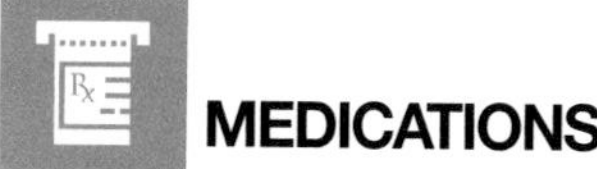

MEDICATIONS

DRUG(S) OF CHOICE
- Acute treatment
  - ◊ Aluminum acetate (Burow's solution, Domeboro) soak (1 pack Domeboro to 1 quart warm water)
  - ◊ Antifungal cream of choice bid after soaks. Note: antifungal cream plus cortisone cream [eg, clotrimazole-betamethasone (Lotrisone)] may be helpful initially.
- Chronic treatment
  - ◊ Antifungal cream bid
  - ◊ May try systemic antifungal therapy (consider if concomitant onychomycosis or after failed topical treatment)
- Systemic antifungal
  - ◊ Itraconazole (Sporanox) 200 mg PO bid for 14 days (cure rate > 90%)
  - ◊ Terbinafine (Lamisil) 250 mg PO qd for 14 days
- If concomitant onychomycosis
  - ◊ Itraconazole 200 mg PO bid for first week of month for 4 months. Monitoring LFT recommended.
  - ◊ Terbinafine (Lamisil) 250 mg PO qd for 12 weeks or pulse dosing - 500 mg PO qd for first week of month for 4 months. Not recommended if creatinine clearance < 50 mL/min.

Contraindications:
- Griseofulvin - patients with porphyria, hepatocellular failure, and in patients with a history of hypersensitivity to griseofulvin
- Itraconazole pregnancy category C

Precautions:
- Griseofulvin - should be used only in severe cases. Periodic monitoring of organ system functioning, including renal, hepatic, and hematopoietic. Possible photosensitivity reactions. Lupus erythematosus, lupus-like syndromes, or exacerbation of existing lupus erythematosus have been reported.
- Note: All systemic antifungal drugs have potential hepatotoxicity - ranging from low to high

Significant possible interactions:
- Griseofulvin - decreases the activity of warfarin-type anticoagulants. Barbiturates usually depress griseofulvin activity. The effect of alcohol may be potentiated, producing such effects as tachycardia and flush.
- Itraconazole and ketoconazole require gastric acid for absorption - effectiveness reduced with antacids, H2 blockers, omeprazole, etc. Take with acidic beverage such as Coca Cola if on antacids.

ALTERNATIVE DRUGS
- Systemic antifungal
  - ◊ Fluconazole 150 mg, 1 tablet every week for 1-4 weeks (noted in 1997 Sanford Guide - 70% cure, however not an FDA approved indication)
  - ◊ Griseofulvin 660-750 mg/day for 21 days

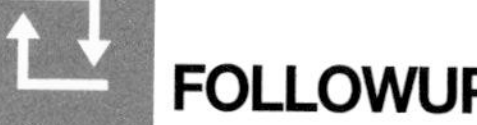

FOLLOWUP

PATIENT MONITORING
As needed

PREVENTION/AVOIDANCE
- Good personal hygiene
- Wearing rubber or wooden sandals in community showers or bathing places
- Careful drying between the toes after showering or bathing. Blow dry the feet with a hair dryer (removes excess water from the outer layer of skin and is more effective than drying with a towel).
- Changing socks and shoes frequently
- Applying drying or dusting powder
- Topical antiperspirants
- Put socks on before underwear to avoid spreading to groin

POSSIBLE COMPLICATIONS
- Secondary bacterial infections
- Eczematoid changes

EXPECTED COURSE/PROGNOSIS
Control, but not completely cured. Symptoms continue indefinitely with periods of relative quiescence.

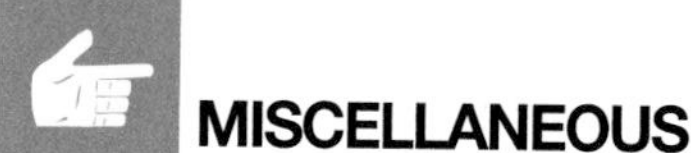

MISCELLANEOUS

ASSOCIATED CONDITIONS
- Hyperhidrosis
- Onychomycosis

AGE-RELATED FACTORS
Pediatric: Rare in younger children (common in teens)
Geriatric: Elderly are more susceptible to outbreaks because of changes in the distal tissues resulting from peripheral vascular disease and immunocompromised
Others: N/A

PREGNANCY
N/A

SYNONYMS
Athlete's foot

ICD-9-CM
110.4 Dermatophytosis of foot

SEE ALSO
Dermatitis, contact
Dyshidrosis

OTHER NOTES
N/A

ABBREVIATIONS
N/A

REFERENCES

- Residents' Prescribing Reference. New York, Prescribing Reference, 2001
- Fitzpatrick TB, et al. Color Atlas and Synopsis of Clinical Dermatology. 3rd Ed. New York, McGraw-Hill, 1997
- Sober AJ, Fitzpatrick TB, eds. Year Book of Dermatology. St. Louis, C.V. Mosby, 1994
- Helm KF, et al. Atlas of Differential Diagnosis in Dermatology. New York, Churchill Livingstone, 1998
- Hall JC, ed. Sauer's Manual of Skin Diseases. 8th ed. Philadelphia, Lippincott Williams & Wilkins, 2000
- Gilbert DN, Moellering RC, Sande MA, eds. Sanford Guide to Antimicrobial Therapy. Vienna, Antimicrobial Therapy, Inc., 2001
- Crissey JT. Common dermatophyte infections. A simple diagnostic test and current management. Postgrad Med 1998;103(2):191-2, 197-200, 205

Web references: 3 available at www.5mcc.com
Illustrations 6 available

Author(s):
J. C. Chava-Zimmerman, MD

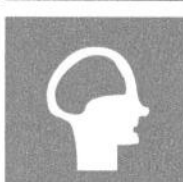

BASICS

DESCRIPTION Multiple patches on skin, generally asymptomatic. Ranges in color, usually white to brown. In blacks, lesions may be hyperpigmented. Probably the most common superficial mycosis.
System(s) affected: Skin/Exocrine
Genetics: No known genetic pattern
Incidence/Prevalence in USA: Common
Predominant age: Teenagers and young adults
Predominant sex: Male = Female

SIGNS & SYMPTOMS
- Versicolor = various colors. Sun exposed areas - lesions usually white; on covered areas - they are often brown or red-brown.
- Distribution - (sebum-rich areas) chest, shoulders, back
- Appearance - sharply marginated 3 or 4 mm in diameter with centrifugal growth and coalescence
- Scale - fine, visible only with scraping
- Itching (rare)
- More prominent in summer
- Periodic recurrence

CAUSES
- Pityrosporum ovale (formerly Malassezia furfur), also known as Malassezia globosa
- Variations in skin lipid formation

RISK FACTORS
- High heat
- High humidity
- Excessive sweating
- HIV infection

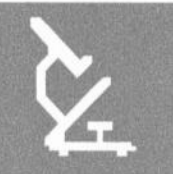

DIAGNOSIS

DIFFERENTIAL DIAGNOSIS Other skin diseases with white patches and plaques including:
- Pityriasis alba
- Vitiligo
- Seborrheic dermatitis
- Nummular eczema

LABORATORY Routine lab not usually necessary

Drugs that may alter lab results: N/A

Disorders that may alter lab results: N/A

PATHOLOGICAL FINDINGS
- Short stubby fungal hyphae
- Y-shaped hyphae
- Small round spores in clusters on hyphae

SPECIAL TESTS KOH preparation to visualize budding yeast forms and club-shaped hyphae

IMAGING N/A

DIAGNOSTIC PROCEDURES Wood's lamp - golden fluorescence or pigment changes

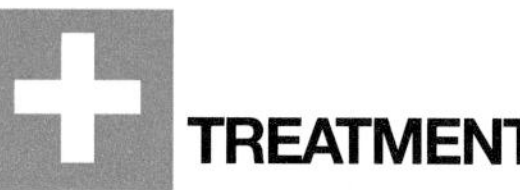

TREATMENT

APPROPRIATE HEALTH CARE Outpatient

GENERAL MEASURES
- Apply prescribed topical medications to affected parts with cotton balls
- Repeat treatment each spring prior to sun exposure

SURGICAL MEASURES N/A

ACTIVITY No restrictions

DIET No special diet

PATIENT EDUCATION For patient education materials favorably reviewed on this topic, contact: American Academy of Dermatology, 930 N. Meacham Rd., P.O. Box 4014, Schaumberg, IL 60168-4014, (708)330-0230

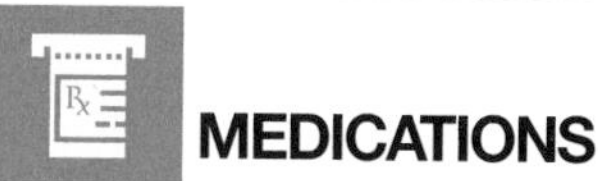

MEDICATIONS

DRUG(S) OF CHOICE
- Selenium sulfide shampoo (Excel and Selsun), allowed to dry for 10 minutes prior to showering daily for 1 week or allowed to remain on body for 12-24 hours before showering once a week for 4 weeks

or
- Clotrimazole topical (Lotrimin) bid for several weeks,

or
- Miconazole (Micatin, Monistat) bid for several weeks,

or
- Ketoconazole (Nizoral) cream bid for several weeks or terbinafine (Lamisil) solution of 1% bid for 1 week
- Ketoconazole 2% shampoo applied to damp skin and left on for 5 minutes for 1 or 3 days

or
- Terbinafine 1% solution bid 1 week

or
- Terbinafine (Lamisil DermGel) once daily for 1 week

Contraindications: Ketoconazole contraindicated in pregnancy
Precautions: N/A
Significant possible interactions: N/A

ALTERNATIVE DRUGS
- Ketoconazole (rarely needed and has significant adverse reactions): 400 mg in a single dose or 200 mg/day for one week
- Ketoconazole shampoo can be used weekly for maintenance
- Itraconazole 200 mg/day for one week
- Sulfur-salicylic acid (Sebulex) soap or shampoo can be used chronically for prophylaxis

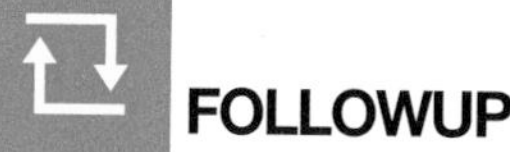

FOLLOWUP

PATIENT MONITORING Recheck each spring

PREVENTION/AVOIDANCE N/A

POSSIBLE COMPLICATIONS None expected

EXPECTED COURSE/PROGNOSIS
Recurs almost routinely

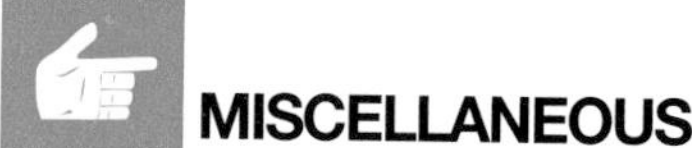

MISCELLANEOUS

ASSOCIATED CONDITIONS N/A

AGE-RELATED FACTORS
Pediatric: Usually occurs after puberty (except in tropical areas)
Geriatric: Not common in this age group
Others: N/A

PREGNANCY N/A

SYNONYMS Pityriasis versicolor

ICD-9-CM
111.0 Pityriasis versicolor

SEE ALSO

OTHER NOTES
- Warn patients that whiteness will remain for several months after treatment
- Treat again each spring prior to tanning season

ABBREVIATIONS N/A

REFERENCES

- Lynch PJ: Dermatology for the House Officer. 3rd Ed. Baltimore, Williams & Wilkins, 1994
- Savin R: Diagnosis and treatment of tinea versicolor. J Fam Prac 1996;43(2):127
- Drake LA. Guidelines of care for superficial mycotic infections of the skin: Pityriasis (tinea) versicolor. Guidelines/Outcomes Committee.
- American Academy of Dermatology. J Am Acad Dermatol 1996;34(2 Pt 1):287-9

Web references: 3 available at www.5mcc.com
Illustrations 4 available

Author(s):
Kathryn Reilly, MD, MPH

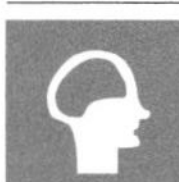

BASICS

DESCRIPTION Rotation and tilting of head caused by primary pathology of the neck muscles or secondary to head and neck disorders. The condition may be congenital or acquired.

System(s) affected: Musculoskeletal, Nervous

Genetics: No known genetic pattern

Incidence/Prevalence in USA: Uncommon

Predominant age:

- Congenital - newborn
- Acquired - under age 10, and adults 30-60

Predominant sex: Male = Female

SIGNS & SYMPTOMS

- Rotation and tilting of the head to the affected side (right side 80%), chin rotates to the opposite side
- Intermittent painful spasms of sterno-cleidomastoid, trapezius and other neck muscles
- With congenital form, the first sign may be a firm, nontender, palpable enlargement of the sternocleidomastoid muscle that is visible at birth
- An early sign in acquired form is stiffness of neck muscles

CAUSES

- Congenital
  - ◊ Injury to sternocleidomastoid muscle on one side at birth
  - ◊ Possible malposition of head in utero
  - ◊ Prenatal injury
- Acquired
  - ◊ Muscular damage from inflammatory disease (myositis, lymphadenitis)
  - ◊ Cervical spine injuries
  - ◊ Ocular disorder
  - ◊ Organic CNS disorder
  - ◊ Psychogenic
  - ◊ Tumor
  - ◊ Cervical spondylosis
  - ◊ Vestibular dysfunction

RISK FACTORS

- Traumatic delivery, including breech
- Acquired
  - ◊ Inflammation
  - ◊ Neurologic disorder
  - ◊ Optical disorder
  - ◊ Trauma

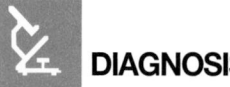

DIAGNOSIS

DIFFERENTIAL DIAGNOSIS

- Bony
  - ◊ Rotatory subluxation
  - ◊ Trauma
  - ◊ Cervical disk disorder
  - ◊ Congenital scoliosis
  - ◊ Tumor
- Infection
  - ◊ Central nervous system infections
  - ◊ Abscess of cervical lymph node(s)
  - ◊ Pharyngeal infection
- Neurogenic
  - ◊ Cervical dystonia
  - ◊ Basal ganglia disease
- Non-osseous
  - ◊ Ophthalmologic disorders
  - ◊ Vestibular disorders
  - ◊ Myositis involving cervical muscles
  - ◊ Soft tissue trauma
  - ◊ Soft tissue tumor

LABORATORY N/A

Drugs that may alter lab results: N/A

Disorders that may alter lab results: N/A

PATHOLOGICAL FINDINGS N/A

SPECIAL TESTS N/A

IMAGING

- Radiographs to rule out skeletal abnormality (appearance may be subtle)
- CT or MRI of cervical spine to aid in differential diagnosis, especially for acquired cases

DIAGNOSTIC PROCEDURES

- History and physical examination

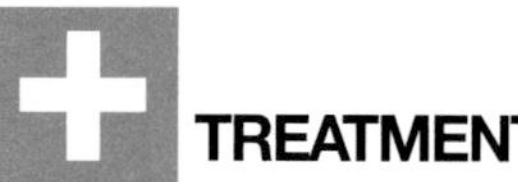

TREATMENT

APPROPRIATE HEALTH CARE

- Outpatient
- Specialty consultation as appropriate (eg, orthopedic, ENT)

GENERAL MEASURES

- Congenital - physical therapy
- Acquired
  - ◊ If less than 1 week in duration - soft collar and rest
  - ◊ If less than 1 month duration - traction
- Psychiatric treatment if there is an emotional disorder

SURGICAL MEASURES Congenital: operative division of involved muscle if physical therapy (eg, passive stretching) is unsuccessful by one year of age

ACTIVITY No restrictions

DIET No special diet

PATIENT EDUCATION For congenital, training of parents to perform massage and range of motion exercises

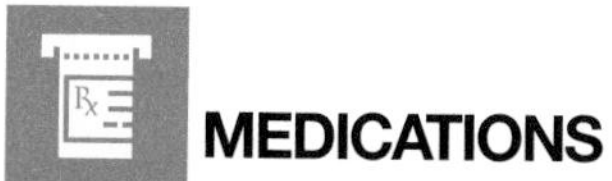

MEDICATIONS

DRUG(S) OF CHOICE None indicated, other than analgesics for pain. If the torticollis has been drug induced, treatment can include diphenhydramine or diazepam.
Contraindications: N/A
Precautions: N/A
Significant possible interactions: N/A

ALTERNATIVE DRUGS Botulinum toxin (Ortholinum) injections are being studied for spastic form

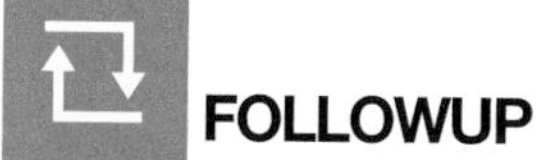

FOLLOWUP

PATIENT MONITORING
- Periodic followup to assess progress
- In acquired form (e.g., infection or traumatic), weekly assessments

PREVENTION/AVOIDANCE No preventive measures known

POSSIBLE COMPLICATIONS
- Movement disorders
- Postural disorders
- Dental malocclusion
- Facial asymmetry in congenital cases

EXPECTED COURSE/PROGNOSIS
Good prognosis for correctable pathology

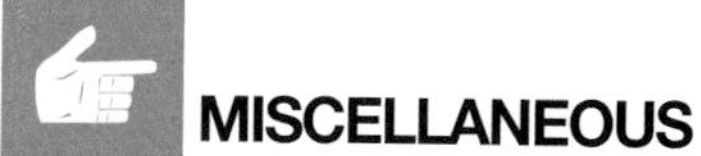

MISCELLANEOUS

ASSOCIATED CONDITIONS
- Difficult delivery in congenital cases

AGE-RELATED FACTORS
Pediatric: Congenital variety, associated with injury at time of birth that without treatment, becomes a fibrous cord
Geriatric: N/A
Others: N/A

PREGNANCY Associated with breech birth

SYNONYMS
- Spasmodic torticollis
- Wryneck

ICD-9-CM
333.83 Spasmodic torticollis
754.1 Certain congenital musculoskeletal deformities of sternocleidomastoid muscle
300.11 Conversion disorder

SEE ALSO

OTHER NOTES Torticollis means "rotation", anterocollis means "tilting"

ABBREVIATIONS N/A

REFERENCES

- Herring JA, ed. Tachdjian's Pediatric Orthopaedics. 3rd ed. Philadelphia: WB Saunders, 2001
- Lovell WW, Morrissy BT, et al (eds). Lovell and Winter's Pediatric Orthopaedics. 5th ed. Philadelphia: Lippincott Williams & Wilkins Publishers; 2001
- Epps HR, Salter RB. Orthopedic conditions of the cervical spine and shoulder. Pediatr Clin North Am 1996;43(4):919-31

Web references: 1 available at www.5mcc.com
Illustrations N/A

Author(s):
Francisco G. Valencia, MD
Patrick C. Henderson, MD

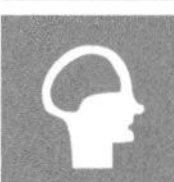

BASICS

DESCRIPTION Gilles de la Tourette syndrome is a hereditary, chronic neurological disorder consisting of various motor and vocal tics. Tics are sudden, involuntary, brief, repetitive, stereotypic motor movements. Symptoms begin in childhood and the location, number, frequency and complexity of tics change over time.
System(s) affected: Nervous
Genetics: Genetic predisposition, frequent familial history of tic disorders. Thought to be autosomal dominant with incomplete and sex-specific penetrances. Tourette is concordant in identical twins and discordant in fraternal twins.
Incidence/Prevalence in USA: 0.1 to 0.5 cases per 1,000. It is estimated that there are one million sufferers of Tourette in the U.S.
Predominant age: 2-15 years in 95% of cases, average age is 6 years
Predominant sex: Males 3 times more frequent than females

SIGNS & SYMPTOMS
- Tics occur many times throughout the day and they change over time. May have only one tic at a time.
- Multiple motor tics such as: facial grimacing, blinking, head or neck twitching, tongue protruding, sniffing, touching
- Vocal tics such as grunts, snorts, throat clearing or barking and more complex vocal tics with echolalia (repeating the last words of someone else), palilalia (repeating one's own words), coprolalia (use of obscenities) or copropraxia (use of obscene gestures)
- Tics usually worsen with stress and are most severe in the day and infrequent with sleep. When absorbed in a physical activity the tics are less severe or abate.
- Tics may persist for a few months and remiss then reoccur with a new motor tic

CAUSES Possibly a gene defect that results in variable phenotypic expressions including Tourette and chronic tic disorder, obsessive-compulsive disorders, attention deficit hyperactivity disorder. Pathology in the basal ganglia is suspected. Dopamine hypothesis suggests abnormal regulation of dopamine release and uptake may be the cause.

RISK FACTORS Increased prevalence in family members. Studies reveal 15 to 80% of patients have a family history of Tourette, often undiagnosed.

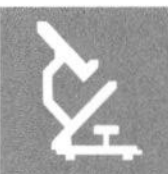

DIAGNOSIS

DIFFERENTIAL DIAGNOSIS
- Chronic-tic disorder (present for greater than 12 months and involves either motor or phonic tics)
- Huntington disease
- Post-infectious encephalitis
- Drug intoxication
- Wilson disease
- Cerebral palsy
- Sydenham chorea
- Head trauma
- Hyperthyroidism

LABORATORY N/A

Drugs that may alter lab results: N/A

Disorders that may alter lab results: N/A

PATHOLOGICAL FINDINGS N/A

SPECIAL TESTS
- EEG studies may reveal nonspecific abnormalities in 50%
- EMG studies reveal short bursts of muscle activity

IMAGING N/A

DIAGNOSTIC PROCEDURES A good history makes the diagnosis; physical exam is typically normal. Most are diagnosed by parents, relatives or friends who are knowledgeable.

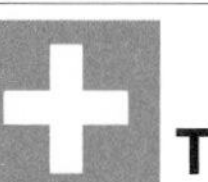

TREATMENT

APPROPRIATE HEALTH CARE Neurologic evaluation for therapy

GENERAL MEASURES Patients are clinically heterogeneous and may have mild, moderate or very disturbing tics. Encourage a supportive environment, educate family and friends. The majority of patients require no medication. Adjustments may be required in work and school schedule to accommodate behaviors. Ignore outbursts and motor and vocal tics. Punishing the child rarely suppresses the present tic and classically provokes new tics which may be more problematic.

SURGICAL MEASURES N/A

ACTIVITY No restrictions, encourage exercise

DIET N/A

PATIENT EDUCATION Printed patient information available from:
Tourette Syndrome Association (TSA)
42-40 Bell Blvd., Bayside, NY 11361-2861
National Hotline (800) 237-0717

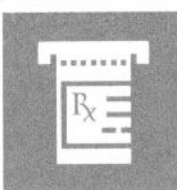

MEDICATIONS

DRUG(S) OF CHOICE

- Haloperidol: The most frequently used; start at 0.25 mg at bedtime and slowly increase by 0.25 mg every few weeks up to minimum dosage calculated by weight. Side effects common, including lethargy and cognitive impairment.
- Clonidine: May help attention deficit disorders as well. Start at 0.05 mg/day and slowly increase by 0.05 mg every few weeks to 0.20 mg/day, given in divided doses. It may take many months to see an effect. Side effects common, such as sedation, will decrease with time.

Contraindications:

- Haloperidol
  - ◊ CNS depression
  - ◊ CNS disease
  - ◊ Allergy
  - ◊ Pregnancy
- Clonidine
  - ◊ Allergy
  - ◊ Pregnancy
  - ◊ Hypotension

Precautions:

- Haloperidol
  - ◊ Not recommended under age 3
  - ◊ Not recommended during pregnancy
  - ◊ Glaucoma
  - ◊ Seizure disorders
  - ◊ Thyrotoxicosis
- Clonidine
  - ◊ Myocardial diseases
  - ◊ Renal failure
- Risperidone may be associated with hyperglycemia and ketoacidosis

Significant possible interactions:

- Haloperidol
  - ◊ Possible increase toxicity with lithium
  - ◊ Antagonized by anticholinergics
  - ◊ May decrease anticoagulant effects
  - ◊ May decrease guanethidine effects
  - ◊ Potentiates CNS depression, especially if used with other CNS agents
- Clonidine
  - ◊ Potentiates CNS depressants
  - ◊ Antagonized by tricyclic antidepressants

ALTERNATIVE DRUGS

- Fluoxetine may alleviate the obsessive-compulsive symptoms. Naltrexone has been shown to be effective, but not recommended for long-term use due to its toxicity. A specific dopamine d2 antagonist, pimozide, has been shown to be effective in reducing tics, but its potential cardiotoxicity and need for periodic EKGs renders it a less likely choice for use.
- Other dopamine receptor antagonists that have been used include - thiothixene, risperidone, tiapride, trifluoperazine, fluphenazine
- Other agents used include - calcium channel blockers, benzodiazepines, alpha adrenergic receptor agonists (clonidine) and dopamine depletors

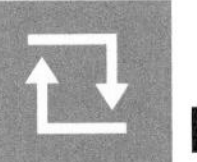

FOLLOWUP

PATIENT MONITORING Observe for associated attention deficit disorder or obsessive-compulsive disorders

PREVENTION/AVOIDANCE N/A

POSSIBLE COMPLICATIONS N/A

EXPECTED COURSE/PROGNOSIS

Clinically, symptoms wax and wane and new tics commonly develop. Up to 50% of patients show marked improvement during the teenage years. If tics abate, they do not usually reoccur in adulthood. If tics persist past age 15 then they tend to remain chronically.

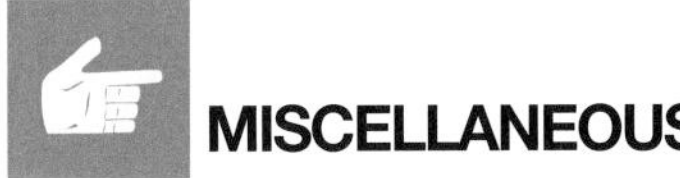

MISCELLANEOUS

ASSOCIATED CONDITIONS

- Up to 50% develop attention deficit disorders and/or obsessive-compulsive disorders
- Phobias

AGE-RELATED FACTORS

Pediatric: Childhood onset, 90% by age 10
Geriatric: N/A
Others: None after age 21, by definition

PREGNANCY N/A

SYNONYMS N/A

ICD-9-CM

307.23 Gilles de la Tourette disorder

SEE ALSO

OTHER NOTES N/A

ABBREVIATIONS N/A

REFERENCES

- American Psychiatric Association. Diagnostic and Statistical Manual of Mental Disorders (DSM-IV-R). 4th Ed. Washington, DC, 2000
- Arzimanoglou AA. Gilles de la Tourette syndrome. J Neurology 1998;245:761-5
- Bagheri MM, Kerbeshian J, Burd J. Recognition and management of Tourette's syndrome and tic disorders. Am Fam Phys 1999;59(8):2263-71
- Jankovic J. Tourette's syndrome. NEJM 2001;345(16):1184-92

Web references: 1 available at www.5mcc.com
Illustrations N/A

Author(s):

Brian J. Murray, MD

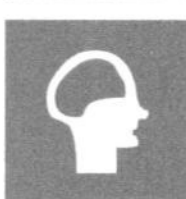

BASICS

DESCRIPTION An acute multisystem illness associated with *Staphylococcus aureus* infections and characterized by the sudden onset of high fever, peculiar skin rash with desquamation, and shock

- Menstrual toxic shock: associated with menstruation and tampon use
- Nonmenstrual toxic shock: more common than the menstrual form; associated with postoperative wounds, barrier contraception, etc. Can occur in children, men, and women.

System(s) affected: Cardiovascular, Endocrine/ Metabolic, Skin/Exocrine
Genetics: No specific mode of inheritance is recognized
Incidence/Prevalence in USA: 0.22 to 1.23 cases per 100,000
Predominant age: All ages, but especially 30-60 years
Predominant sex: Female > Male (3:2)

SIGNS & SYMPTOMS

- Almost always present (> 80%)
  - ◊ Temperature > 38.9°C (102°F)
  - ◊ Erythroderma
  - ◊ Diffuse macular rash
  - ◊ Skin desquamation a few days after rash appears
  - ◊ Shock, orthostatic hypotension or syncope
  - ◊ Nausea or vomiting
- Commonly present (20-80%)
  - ◊ Headache
  - ◊ Confusion or agitation
  - ◊ Acute respiratory distress syndrome
  - ◊ Meningismus
  - ◊ Pharyngeal erythema
  - ◊ Vaginitis or vaginal discharge
  - ◊ Conjunctivitis
  - ◊ Periorbital edema
  - ◊ Strawberry tongue
  - ◊ Non-pitting edema
  - ◊ Myalgia
  - ◊ Oliguria
  - ◊ Arthralgia
  - ◊ Diarrhea
- Rarely present (< 20%)
  - ◊ Arthritis
  - ◊ Lymphadenopathy
  - ◊ Hepatosplenomegaly
  - ◊ Cardiomyopathy
  - ◊ Pericarditis
  - ◊ Photophobia
  - ◊ Seizure

CAUSES *Staphylococcus aureus* exotoxins, especially toxic shock syndrome toxin-1 (TSST-1), and staphylococcal enterotoxins A, B and C (SEA, SEB, SEC)

RISK FACTORS

- High
  - ◊ Absence of antibody to TSS toxin-1
  - ◊ Infection with *Staphylococcus aureus* which produces TSST-1
  - ◊ Continuous use of super absorbency tampons during menstruation
  - ◊ Nasal surgery with packing
- Moderate
  - ◊ Use of regular absorbency tampons during menstruation
  - ◊ Use of contraceptive sponge
- Low
  - ◊ Alternating use of tampons and pads during menstruation
  - ◊ Intrauterine contraceptive device
  - ◊ Surgical wound infections
  - ◊ Early postpartum state

DIAGNOSIS

DIFFERENTIAL DIAGNOSIS

- Streptococcal scarlet fever
- Toxic strep syndrome
- Drug reactions
- Rocky Mountain spotted fever
- Leptospirosis
- Kawasaki disease
- Staphylococcal scalded skin syndrome
- Meningococcal or possibly gram negative sepsis
- Measles, rubeola

LABORATORY

- Microbiologic:
  - ◊ Positive culture for Staphylococcus aureus from vagina or surgical wound (> 90%)
  - ◊ Nasal or perineal carriage of Staphylococcus aureus
  - ◊ Positive blood culture for Staphylococcus aureus (uncommon)
- Hematologic: (50-90%)
  - ◊ Granulocytosis with increased band forms
  - ◊ Lymphopenia
  - ◊ Normocytic, normochromic anemia
  - ◊ Thrombocytopenia
  - ◊ Coagulopathy
- Biochemical: (50-90%)
  - ◊ Hypoalbuminemia
  - ◊ Abnormal electrolytes
  - ◊ Hypocalcemia
  - ◊ Hypomagnesemia
  - ◊ Hypophosphatemia
  - ◊ Increased SGOT
  - ◊ Increased SGPT
  - ◊ Increased CPK
  - ◊ Increased BUN
  - ◊ Increased serum creatinine
  - ◊ Increased calcitonin
  - ◊ Increased serum bilirubin
  - ◊ Abnormal urine sediment

Drugs that may alter lab results: N/A

Disorders that may alter lab results: N/A

PATHOLOGICAL FINDINGS

- Subepidermic cleavage plane in the skin
- Minimal inflammatory reaction in tissues
- Lymphocyte depletion in lymph nodes
- Cervico-vaginal ulcerations

SPECIAL TESTS

- Absent serum antibodies to TSST-1, SEA, SEB or SEC
- Detection of TSST-1 or SEA-SEC in *Staphylococcus aureus* isolate

IMAGING No unusual or characteristic findings

DIAGNOSTIC PROCEDURES No specific diagnostic test is currently available

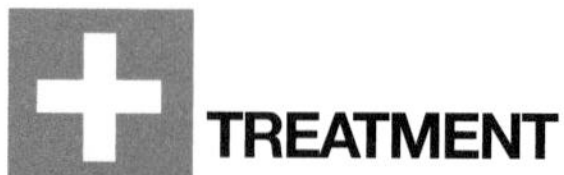

TREATMENT

APPROPRIATE HEALTH CARE Inpatient, admission to intensive care for monitoring

GENERAL MEASURES

- Removal of tampon or other vaginal foreign bodies
- Fluid resuscitation
- Management of renal or cardiac insufficiency
- Mechanical ventilation if necessary

SURGICAL MEASURES Surgical drainage of loculated infections

ACTIVITY Bed rest throughout acute illness

DIET As tolerated

PATIENT EDUCATION Advise patient regarding possible sequelae or recurrence

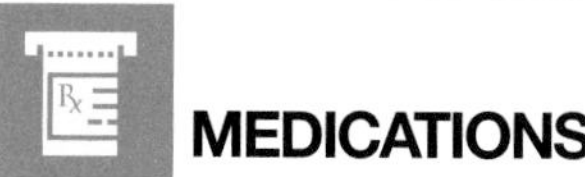

MEDICATIONS

DRUG(S) OF CHOICE
- Treatment of shock or hypotension
  - ◊ Fluid replacement
  - ◊ Dopamine
  - ◊ Steroids or naloxone have not been proven to be of value
- Eradication of *Staphylococcus aureus*
  - ◊ Oxacillin or nafcillin 100 mg/kg/day every 6 hours

Contraindications: Penicillin allergy
Precautions:
- Rash, diarrhea, seizures
- Reduce oxacillin dosage in patients with severe renal failure. Not necessary to reduce nafcillin dose for renal dysfunction.

Significant possible interactions: See manufacturer's profile of each drug

ALTERNATIVE DRUGS
- Clindamycin 25 mg/kg/day q 8 hours for patients allergic to penicillin
- Vancomycin 30 mg/kg/day q 6 hours
- Toxin neutralization. Benefit in humans is unproven, but animal and in vitro studies support this approach.
  - ◊ Immune globulin IV 0.4 g/kg over 6 hours

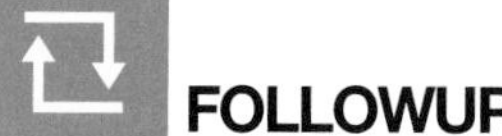

FOLLOWUP

PATIENT MONITORING
- Admit to intensive care if in shock
- Daily vital signs until patient is afebrile and normotensive

PREVENTION/AVOIDANCE
- Avoidance of continuous tampon use during menstruation
- Avoidance of super absorbency tampons
- Encourage frequent tampon changes during the day
- Use sanitary napkins at night
- Early medical attention to infected wounds

POSSIBLE COMPLICATIONS
- Common (> 20%)
  - ◊ Acute renal failure
  - ◊ Adult respiratory distress syndrome
  - ◊ Menorrhagia
  - ◊ Alopecia
  - ◊ Nail loss
- Rare (< 20%)
  - ◊ Disseminated intravascular coagulation
  - ◊ Ataxia, toxic encephalopathy
  - ◊ Memory impairment
  - ◊ Cardiomyopathy
  - ◊ Protracted malaise

EXPECTED COURSE/PROGNOSIS
- Mortality 3-9%
- Recurrence 10-15%

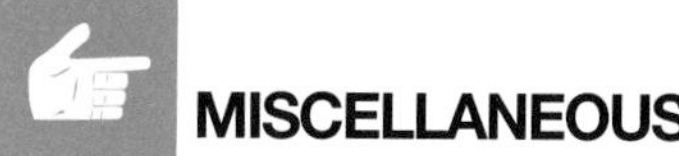

MISCELLANEOUS

ASSOCIATED CONDITIONS Staphylococcal infections

AGE-RELATED FACTORS
Pediatric: May occur as a complication of chickenpox
Geriatric: Cellulitis or surgical wound infections
Others: None

PREGNANCY Postpartum infections, especially postcesarean section wound infection, or episiotomy infections

SYNONYMS Staphylococcal scarlet fever

ICD-9-CM
040.82 Toxic shock syndrome

SEE ALSO
Measles, rubeola
Pancreatitis
Rocky Mountain spotted fever
Scarlet fever

OTHER NOTES Streptococcal toxic shock syndrome or toxic strep syndrome may be clinically indistinguishable from staphylococcal toxic shock

ABBREVIATIONS N/A

REFERENCES

- Whiting JL, Chow AW: Toxic shock syndrome. In: Rakel RE, ed. Conn's Current Therapy. Philadelphia, W.B. Saunders Co., 1990:972-975
- See RH, Chow AW: Microbiology of TSS: overview. Rev Infect Dis 1989;11(suppl 1):S55-S60
- Reingold AL: Toxic shock syndrome: An update. Am J Obstet Gynecol 1991;165(suppl):1236-1239
- Barry W, et al: Intravenous immunoglobulin therapy for Toxic Shock Syndrome. JAMA 1992;267:3315-3316
- Kain KC, Schulzer M, Chow AW: Clinical spectrum of nonmenstrual toxic shock syndrome (TSS): Comparison with menstrual TSS by multivariate discriminant analyses. Clin Infect Dis 1993;16:100-106

Web references: 1 available at www.5mcc.com
Illustrations 1 available

Author(s):
Anthony W. Chow, MD

BASICS

DESCRIPTION Infection with the protozoan Toxoplasma gondii. Four types:
- Congenital toxoplasmosis: Acute infection of mother during gestation that is passed to fetus. Often asymptomatic, effects on fetus are more severe in first trimester infection.
- Ocular toxoplasmosis: Important cause of chorioretinitis, usually resulting from congenital infection but remaining asymptomatic until second or third decade of life. Uncommon in acquired disease in immunocompetent patients.
- Acute toxoplasmosis in immunocompetent host: Acute self-limiting asymptomatic or mildly symptomatic infection in normal host
- Acute toxoplasmosis in immunocompromised host: Primary or reactivation infection that can be a life-threatening disseminated infection involving many organ systems such as heart, lung, liver, but especially the central nervous system

System(s) affected: Cardiovascular, Gastrointestinal, Nervous, Pulmonary, Skin/Exocrine
Genetics: No known genetic pattern
Incidence/Prevalence in USA:
- Up to 70% of healthy adults are seropositive
- Seroconversion rate for women of childbearing age is 0.8% per year
- Affects more than 3500 newborns in U.S. each year

Predominant age: All ages
Predominant sex: Male = Female

SIGNS & SYMPTOMS
- Congenital toxoplasmosis
  - ◊ Most severe when maternal infection occurs early in pregnancy
  - ◊ No signs or symptoms of infection (67%)
  - ◊ Chorioretinitis (15%)
  - ◊ Intracranial calcifications (10%)
  - ◊ Cerebrospinal fluid pleocytosis and elevated protein (20%)
  - ◊ Anemia, thrombocytopenia, jaundice at birth
  - ◊ Microcephaly
  - ◊ Affected survivors may have mental retardation, seizures, visual defects, spasticity, other severe neurologic sequelae
- Ocular toxoplasmosis
  - ◊ Chorioretinitis - focal necrotizing retinitis
  - ◊ Yellowish white elevated cotton patch with indistinct margins
  - ◊ May be small clusters of lesions
  - ◊ Congenital disease is usually bilateral
  - ◊ Acquired disease is usually unilateral
  - ◊ Symptoms include blurred vision, scotoma, pain, photophobia
- Acute toxoplasmosis in immunocompetent host
  - ◊ 80-90% are asymptomatic
  - ◊ Cervical lymphadenopathy with discrete, usually non-tender nodes, less than 3 cm in diameter
  - ◊ Fever, malaise, night sweats, myalgias
  - ◊ Sore throat
  - ◊ Maculopapular rash
  - ◊ Retroperitoneal and mesenteric lymphadenopathy with abdominal pain may occur
  - ◊ Chorioretinitis
- Acute toxoplasmosis in immunocompromised host
  - ◊ May be newly acquired or reactivation disease
  - ◊ Central nervous system disease (50%)
  - ◊ Encephalitis, meningoencephalitis or mass lesions
  - ◊ Hemiparesis, seizures, mental status changes
  - ◊ Visual changes
  - ◊ May have signs and symptoms as seen in immunocompetent host
  - ◊ Myocarditis, pneumonitis

CAUSES
- Etiologic agent for each of the clinical syndromes is Toxoplasma gondii
- Congenital disease is passed transplacentally from newly infected mother to fetus during pregnancy
- Other syndromes may result from newly acquired infection or reactivation of latent infection
- Ingestion of meats or foods containing cysts or oocysts present in cat feces
- Infection can be transmitted by blood transfusion or organ transplantation

RISK FACTORS
- Immunocompromised hosts especially those with defects in cellular immunity such as AIDS, lymphoma, high dose corticosteroids
- Risk of transplacental transmission is greatest during third trimester but disease is more severe if acquired during first trimester

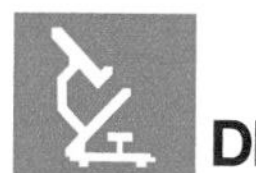

DIAGNOSIS

DIFFERENTIAL DIAGNOSIS
- Congenital toxoplasmosis: Other members of TORCH syndrome (rubella, cytomegalovirus, herpes simple), syphilis, Listeria, other infectious encephalopathies, erythroblastosis fetalis, sepsis
- Ocular toxoplasmosis: Tuberculosis, syphilis, leprosy, ocular histoplasmosis
- Acute toxoplasmosis (normal and immunocompromised): Must consider lymphoma, infectious mononucleosis, cytomegalovirus, cat scratch disease, sarcoidosis, tuberculosis, tularemia, metastatic carcinoma, leukemia
- Toxoplasma encephalitis: Tuberculosis, fungal diseases, vasculitis, progressive multifocal leukoencephalopathy (PML), brain abscess, tumor, herpes encephalitis, CNS lymphoma, *Nocardia* spp

LABORATORY
- Demonstration of Toxoplasma organism in blood, body fluids or tissue is evidence of infection
- Isolation of Toxoplasma from placenta is diagnostic of congenital infection
- Lymphocyte transformation to Toxoplasma antigens is indicator of previous Toxoplasma infection in adults
- Detection of Toxoplasma antigen in blood or body fluids by ELISA technique indicates acute infection
- PCR for detection of Toxoplasma DNA in body fluids and tissues is useful in the diagnosis of ocular, cerebral, disseminated, and especially intrauterine infection
- Several serologic tests used in diagnosis, some measuring IgM and others IgG antibody
- Sabin-Feldman dye test is a sensitive and specific neutralization test, measures IgG antibody, is the standard reference test for toxoplasmosis, but requires live Toxoplasma organisms, so is not available in most labs. High titers suggest acute disease.
- Indirect fluorescent antibody test (IFA) measures same antibodies as dye test. Titers parallel dye test titers.
- IgM fluorescent antibody test detects IgM antibodies with first week of infection but titers fall within a few months
- Indirect hemagglutination test measures a different antibody than dye test. Titers tend to be higher and remain elevated longer.
- Double-sandwich IgM ELISA is more sensitive and specific than other IgM tests
- Negative tests for IgM antibodies during the first two trimesters excludes recently acquired infection

Drugs that may alter lab results: None

Disorders that may alter lab results:
- Antinuclear antibodies and rheumatoid factor may cause false positive serologic test
- Pregnancy may cause false negative hemagglutination test

PATHOLOGICAL FINDINGS
- Lymph node histology shows triad of:
  - ◊ Reactive follicular hyperplasia
  - ◊ Irregular clusters of epithelioid histiocytes encroaching on and blurring the margins of the germinal centers
  - ◊ Focal distention of sinuses with monocytoid cells

SPECIAL TESTS
- Antibody levels in aqueous humor or cerebrospinal fluid may reflect local antibody production and infection at these sites
- Amniocentesis at 20-24 weeks in suspected congenital disease

IMAGING
- CT scan of head in cerebral toxoplasmosis
- Ultrasound of fetus at 20-24 weeks
- MRI scan of head in cerebral toxoplasmosis

DIAGNOSTIC PROCEDURES
- Lymph node biopsy showing characteristic pathologic triad
- Brain biopsy in CNS disease and demonstration of organisms by peroxidase-antiperoxidase technique
- Empiric therapy for CNS mass lesions in HIV patients with response on 2 week followup imaging study is presumptive evidence for diagnosis

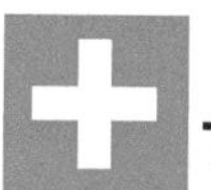

TREATMENT

APPROPRIATE HEALTH CARE
- Outpatient for acquired disease in immunocompetent host and ocular toxoplasmosis
- Inpatient initially for CNS toxoplasmosis and acute disease in immunocompromised host

GENERAL MEASURES
- Usually no treatment in asymptomatic hosts except in child under 5
- Symptomatic patients should be treated until immunity is assured

SURGICAL MEASURES N/A

ACTIVITY Level of activity dependent on severity of disease and organ systems involved

DIET No special diet

PATIENT EDUCATION
- Infected mother must be completely informed of potential consequences to fetus
- Explain prevention methods, e.g., protecting children's play area from cat litter
- Additional materials available from:
- National Institute of Allergy and Infectious Disease, Department of Health and Human Services, Bldg. 31, Rm 7A-32, 9000 Rockville Pike, Bethesda, MD 20892, (301)496-5717

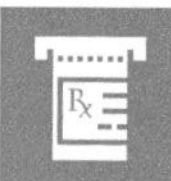

MEDICATIONS

DRUG(S) OF CHOICE

- Acute toxoplasmosis in immunodeficient host:
  ◊ Sulfadiazine (Microsulfon) 100 mg/kg/day up to 8 grams/day plus pyrimethamine (Daraprim) 200 mg the first day, then 25-50 mg/day plus leucovorin (folinic acid) 10 mg/day for several weeks followed by maintenance therapy with the same drugs at lower dosage for several months
- Ocular toxoplasmosis: Above regimen for 1-2 months
- Acute toxoplasmosis in pregnant women: Above regimen may be used after the 16th week of pregnancy
- Congenital toxoplasmosis: Sulfadiazine 100 mg/kg/day plus pyrimethamine 1 mg/kg every 2 days plus leucovorin (folinic acid) 5 mg every 2 days

Contraindications:

- Pyrimethamine should not be used in first trimester of pregnancy
- Known hypersensitivity to pyrimethamine or sulfadiazine (Note: many HIV positive patients have a sulfa sensitivity)

Precautions:

- Bone marrow toxicity an important problem while treating toxoplasmosis
- Use with caution in patients with possible folate deficiency
- Use with caution in patients with renal or hepatic dysfunction
- Sulfonamides may increase anticoagulant effect of warfarin (Coumadin)
- Sulfonamides may increase phenytoin (Dilantin) levels
- Sulfonamides may increase hypoglycemic effect of oral hypoglycemic agents
- Adequate hydration is essential since sulfadiazine is poorly soluble and may crystallize in the urine

Significant possible interactions: Sulfonamides may interact with phenytoin, warfarin (Coumadin) and oral hypoglycemic agents

ALTERNATIVE DRUGS

- In pregnancy - Spiramycin 3 g/day for 3 weeks, then 2 weeks off, then repeat 5 week cycles throughout pregnancy. Drug not yet FDA approved in U.S. Contact manufacturer - Rhone-Poulenc, Inc., CN5266, Princeton, NJ 08543-5266.
- Clindamycin 900-1200 mg tid IV has been used for ocular and CNS toxoplasmosis alone and in combination with pyrimethamine. May be as effective as the sulfa/pyrimethamine combination, but with fewer adverse effects.
- Corticosteroids (prednisone 1-2 mg/kg/day) may be added for macular chorioretinitis or CNS infection
- Atovaquone (Mepron), azithromycin (Zithromax) and clarithromycin (Biaxin) - promising new agents for CNS toxoplasmosis

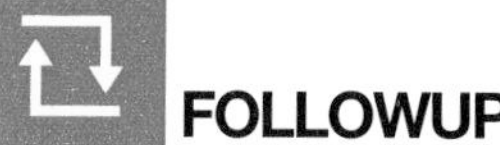

FOLLOWUP

PATIENT MONITORING

- Followup visits every 2 weeks until stable, then monthly during therapy
- CBC weekly for first month, then every 2 weeks
- Renal and liver function tests monthly

PREVENTION/AVOIDANCE

Prevention is important in seronegative pregnant women and immunodeficient patients. Avoid eating raw meat, unpasteurized milk, uncooked eggs and avoid contact with cat feces.

POSSIBLE COMPLICATIONS

- Seizure disorder or focal neurologic deficits in CNS toxoplasmosis
- Partial or complete blindness with ocular toxoplasmosis
- Multiple complications may occur with congenital toxoplasmosis including mental retardation, seizures, deafness and blindness

EXPECTED COURSE/PROGNOSIS

- Immunodeficient patients often relapse if treatment is stopped
- Treatment may prevent the development of untoward sequelae in both symptomatic and asymptomatic infants with congenital toxoplasmosis

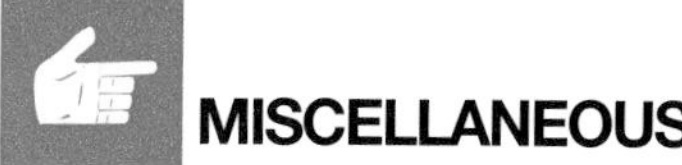

MISCELLANEOUS

ASSOCIATED CONDITIONS

Cellular immune compromised patients, especially those with AIDS, have a higher incidence of toxoplasmosis

AGE-RELATED FACTORS

Pediatric: With acute congenital toxoplasmosis, children often die in the first month of life. Subacute congenital disease may not be observed until some time after birth, when symptoms start to appear.
Geriatric: Acquired infection. Often reactivation disease more likely.
Others: None

PREGNANCY

- Have serum examined for Toxoplasma antibodies. Those with negative titers should take extra precautions to avoid contact with cats, not to eat raw meat and wash all fruits and vegetables carefully.
- For toxoplasmosis infection during pregnancy, refer patient to specialist

SYNONYMS N/A

ICD-9-CM

130.9 Toxoplasmosis, unspecified
771.2 Other congenital infections

SEE ALSO

OTHER NOTES N/A

ABBREVIATIONS N/A

REFERENCES

- Mandell G, ed. Principles and Practice of Infectious Diseases. 5th Ed. New York, Churchill Livingstone, 2000
- Katkama C, et al. Pyrimethamine-clindamycin vs. pyrimethamine-sulfadiazine in acute and long term therapy for toxoplasmic encephalitis in patients with AIDS. Clin Infect Dis 1996;22(2):268-75
- Montoya JG, Liesenfeld O. Toxoplasmosis. Lancet. 2004;363(9425):1965-76

Web references: 1 available at www.5mcc.com
Illustrations 2 available

Author(s):
William G. Gardner, MD

BASICS

DESCRIPTION
- Acute, potentially life-threatening infraglottic bacterial infection following a primary viral infection, usually parainfluenzae or influenza viruses
- Also called membranous tracheitis or pseudomembranous croup
- Direct laryngoscopy reveals subglottic edema compounded by thick, purulent exudate in the larynx, trachea, and bronchi sometimes causing pseudomembranes

System(s) affected: Pulmonary
Genetics: No known genetic predisposition
Incidence/Prevalence in USA: True incidence is unknown; first cases described prior to 1950, a resurgence of cases has been noted since 1979; fall/winter predominance
Predominant age: Mean age 54 months; range 3 weeks to 168 months; infections in adolescents and adults have been reported
Predominant sex: Some studies have shown a male to female ratio as high as 5:1. Others have shown a 1:1 ratio.

SIGNS & SYMPTOMS
- Barking, "brassy" cough
- Inspiratory stridor
- Variable degree of respiratory distress
- Child is usually lying flat
- Fever > 38°C (100.4°F)
- Toxic-appearing
- There is a gradual progression of mild upper airway symptoms over 1 hour to six days to an acute, febrile phase of rapid respiratory decompensation
- Voice and cry are usually normal
- Absence of drooling and dysphagia help distinguish it from epiglottitis
- Does not respond to aerosolized epinephrine (unlike patients with croup)
- Subglottic edema
- If intubated for viral croup, pre-membranous tracheitis "web" can obstruct the distal airway beyond the E-T tube

CAUSES
- Staph aureus (most common pediatric cause)
- *H. influenzae* type b
- Strep pyrogenes/group A strep
- *M. catarrhalis*
- Peptostreptococcus
- Strep pneumoniae
- Klebsiella
- Neisseria

RISK FACTORS
- Periods of increased seasonal activity of respiratory viruses
- Case reports following adenoidectomy

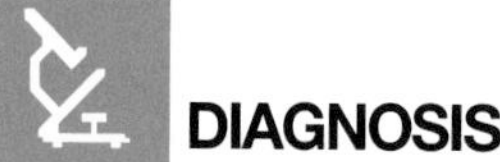

DIAGNOSIS

DIFFERENTIAL DIAGNOSIS
- Laryngotracheobronchitis (viral)
- Epiglottitis
- Foreign body
- Retropharyngeal abscess
- Pneumonia
- Asthma
- Spasmodic croup
- Diphtheritic laryngitis

LABORATORY
- Elevated WBC count with predominance of PMNs
- Band cells often present
- Blood cultures are usually negative

Drugs that may alter lab results: N/A

Disorders that may alter lab results: N/A

PATHOLOGICAL FINDINGS
- Mucosal destruction and/or local immunodeficiency caused by viral infection may predispose to bacterial infection
- Intense inflammation, sloughing of subglottic epithelium, and profuse mucopurulent secretions which compromise the airway and which make airway management very difficult

SPECIAL TESTS Rapid antigen tests are available for bacteria and viruses in some centers

IMAGING
- AP and lateral neck radiographs show subglottic and tracheal narrowing with haziness and radiopaque linear or particulate densities (crusts)
- In patients with risk of acute respiratory obstruction, either do not obtain radiographs or monitor carefully
- Often see pneumonic infiltrates

DIAGNOSTIC PROCEDURES
- Endoscopy is diagnostic and demonstrates severe inflammation of the subglottic region and trachea with copious mucopurulent secretions and sloughed epithelium that separates from the tracheal wall in sheets
- Obtain Gram stain, aerobic and anaerobic cultures of tracheal secretions

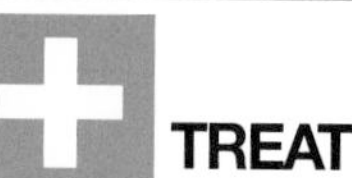

TREATMENT

APPROPRIATE HEALTH CARE ICU

GENERAL MEASURES
- Constitutes a true pediatric emergency
- Maintain airway - this is often very difficult due to copious secretions
- Hydration, humidification, antibiotics
- Endotracheal or nasotracheal intubation will usually be needed, especially in infants and children under the age of 4. Much less likely to need intubation if child older than 8. Another advantage of intubation is ability to clear trachea and bronchi of secretions and pseudomembranes.
- Vigorous pulmonary toilet to clear airway of secretion
- Does not respond to epinephrine

SURGICAL MEASURES
- Tracheotomy may be necessary
- Membrane may require surgical removal

ACTIVITY Complete bed rest

DIET Parenteral nutrition or nasogastric tube feeding if intubated. Oral nutrition otherwise.

PATIENT EDUCATION Usually requires 3-7 days of hospitalization with complete recovery expected

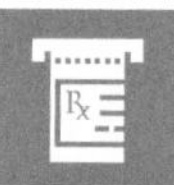

MEDICATIONS

DRUG(S) OF CHOICE
- Nafcillin 150 mg/kg/day divided QID plus cefotaxime 150 mg/kg/day in 4-6 divided doses; maximum of 2 grams q6h
- Vancomycin for MRSA
- Ceftriaxone 75 mg/kg/day divided BID plus ampicillin-sulbactam 300 mg/kg/day divided QID
- Best single drug choice: ticarcillin-clavulanate 3.1g IV q 4-6 hours for adults, 150 mg/kg/d IV q 12 hours for children (max 18-24 g/d)
- Does not respond to epinephrine
- Narrow the regimen when pathogens and sensitivities available

Contraindications: Refer to manufacturer's literature
Precautions: Refer to manufacturer's literature
Significant possible interactions: See manufacturer's literature

ALTERNATIVE DRUGS
For patients with penicillin allergy: Clindamycin 40 mg/kg/day divided QID plus chloramphenicol 75 mg/kg/day divided QID

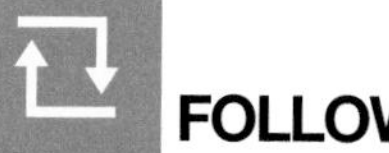

FOLLOWUP

PATIENT MONITORING
ICU care with cardiopulmonary monitoring

PREVENTION/AVOIDANCE
N/A

POSSIBLE COMPLICATIONS
- Postintubation subglottic stenosis
- Cardiopulmonary arrest
- Pneumonia
- Toxic shock syndrome secondary to enterotoxin-producing staphylococci

EXPECTED COURSE/PROGNOSIS
- With vigorous airway management with or without intubation for up to 7 days, complete recovery is expected
- Cardiopulmonary arrest and death have occurred

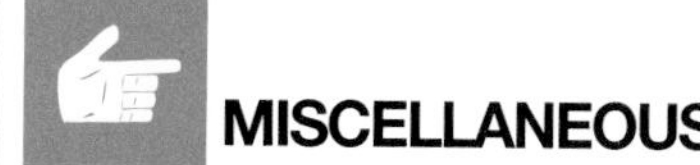

MISCELLANEOUS

ASSOCIATED CONDITIONS
Consider anatomic abnormalities or foreign body as well as recent pharyngeal or laryngeal surgery

AGE-RELATED FACTORS
Pediatric: Typically affects children ages 3-5
Geriatric: N/A
Others: N/A

PREGNANCY
Scrupulous handwashing is recommended

SYNONYMS
- Pseudomembranous croup
- Membranous tracheitis

ICD-9-CM
464.10 Acute tracheitis without mention of obstruction
464.20 Acute laryngotracheitis without mention of obstruction
464.11 Acute tracheitis with obstruction
464.21 Acute laryngotracheitis with obstruction

SEE ALSO
Bronchiolitis
Common cold
Epiglottitis

OTHER NOTES
N/A

ABBREVIATIONS
ED = Emergency department
LTS = Laryngotracheobronchitis

REFERENCES

- Bernstein T, Brilli R, Jacobs B. Is bacterial tracheitis changing? A 14-month experience in a pediatric intensive care unit. Clin Infect Dis 1998;27(3):458-62
- Cunningham MJ: The old and new of acute laryngotracheal infections. Clinical Pediatrics 1992;31(1):56-64
- Berhman RE, Kliegman RM, Jenson HB, eds. Nelson Textbook of Pediatrics. 16th ed. Philadelphia: Saunders; 2000
- Burns JA, Brown J, Ogle JW. Group A streptococcal tracheitis associated with toxic shock syndrome. Pediatr Infect Dis J 1998;17(10):933-5
- Brook I. Aerobic and anaerobic microbiology of bacterial tracheitis in children. Clin Infect Dis 1995;20 Suppl 2:S222-3
- Eid NS, Jones VF. Bacterial tracheitis as a complication of tonsillectomy and adenoidectomy. J Pediatr 1994;125(3):401-2

Web references: 0 available at www.5mcc.com
Illustrations N/A

Author(s):
Bruce T. Vanderhoff, MD
Gabriel Neal, MD

BASICS

DESCRIPTION A cytotoxic, hemolytic reaction that occurs after administration of blood or blood components, resulting in hemolysis of donor's or recipient's RBC's (usually the latter). Reactions may be immune or nonimmune, and can vary from a mild to a fatal consequence. (Infection risks outweigh immune risks.)
System(s) affected: Cardiovascular, Hemic/Lymphatic/Immunologic
Genetics: No known genetic pattern
Incidence/Prevalence in USA: Uncommon
Predominant age: All ages
Predominant sex: Female > Male

SIGNS & SYMPTOMS
- Immediate (intravascular) hemolytic transfusion reaction:
  - ◊ Anxiety
  - ◊ Flushing
  - ◊ Tachycardia
  - ◊ Hypotension
  - ◊ Chest or back pain
  - ◊ Dyspnea
  - ◊ Fever
  - ◊ Chills
  - ◊ Note: symptoms are masked in anesthetized patient
- Delayed (extravascular) hemolytic transfusion reaction:
  - ◊ Fever
  - ◊ Anemia (2-14 days after transfusion)
  - ◊ Jaundice

CAUSES
- Immune reactions - incompatibility within ABO system
- A nonhemolytic febrile reaction due to immune sensitivity to leukocytes, platelets, plasma constituents
- Hemolytic reactions:
  - ◊ Transfusion of mismatched blood
  - ◊ Destruction of donor erythrocytes by recipient incompatible isoantibodies
  - ◊ Isosensitization by repeated transfusions
  - ◊ Isosensitization by prior pregnancies
  - ◊ Universal blood donor type considered dangerous unless thoroughly checked for agglutination titer
  - ◊ Acquisition of B antigen by Group A individuals with colon cancer

RISK FACTORS
- Multiple blood transfusions
- Rh negative mother
- Multiple pregnancies

DIAGNOSIS

DIFFERENTIAL DIAGNOSIS
- Other causes of acute hemolysis
  - ◊ Autoimmune diseases
  - ◊ Hemoglobinopathies
  - ◊ Red blood cell enzyme defects
  - ◊ Bacterial contamination of stored blood

LABORATORY
- Positive direct antiglobulin test (Coombs)
- Plasma obtained 2-4 hours after lysis is red or pink, indicating free hemoglobin
- Increased BUN, creatinine
- Elevated serum bilirubin (mild)
- Wine-colored urine indicating hemoglobinuria
- Reduced serum haptoglobin

Drugs that may alter lab results: N/A

Disorders that may alter lab results: N/A

PATHOLOGICAL FINDINGS N/A

SPECIAL TESTS
Blood bank evaluation for immune reactions

IMAGING N/A

DIAGNOSTIC PROCEDURES N/A

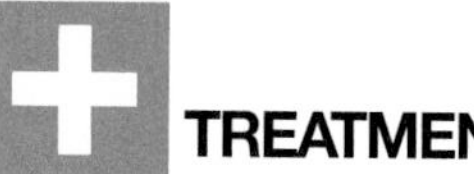

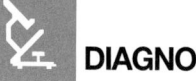

TREATMENT

APPROPRIATE HEALTH CARE
Inpatient

GENERAL MEASURES
- Stop transfusion immediately upon first sign of reaction
- Substitute infusion with normal saline at 150-300 mL per hour
- Check paperwork for any clerical error (usual cause of an ABO-incompatible transfusion)
- Monitor vital signs
- Maintain urine flow at 100 mL/hr for 6-8 hours or until hemoglobinuria clears
- Recognize and treat disseminated intravascular coagulation if it occurs
- Posttransfusion blood sample and discontinued blood to blood bank for investigation
- Maintain systolic blood pressure above 100 mm Hg

SURGICAL MEASURES N/A

ACTIVITY
Bedrest

DIET
As tolerated

PATIENT EDUCATION N/A

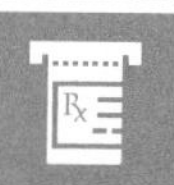

MEDICATIONS

DRUG(S) OF CHOICE
- Oxygen as needed
- Epinephrine for wheezing and/or dyspnea
- Corticosteroids to reduce inflammation
- Adequate colloid or crystalloid (may need 1000 mL/hr normal saline for 2-3 hours) to maintain systolic blood pressure above 100 mm Hg
- Mannitol not of proven value
- Dopamine effective against hypotension and impaired renal perfusion
- Heparinization, at moderate doses, is indicated if DIC present
- Diuretic: furosemide 80-120 mg IV or ethacrynic acid 50 mg IV

Contraindications: Refer to manufacturer's literature
Precautions: Refer to manufacturer's literature
Significant possible interactions: Refer to manufacturer's literature

ALTERNATIVE DRUGS
Diphenhydramine to combat cellular histamine release from mast cells

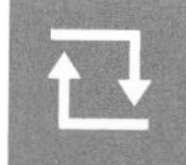

FOLLOWUP

PATIENT MONITORING
Until hemolytic signs are gone

PREVENTION/AVOIDANCE
- History of patient's responses to previous transfusions
- Risk/benefit of any transfusion needs to favor benefit
- Autologous transfusion
- Careful typing and crossmatch, double-check all data available
- Identity of unit of blood is carefully checked before administered
- Close observation of the patient during the transfusion
- Consider leukocyte depleted blood in people with history of recurrent febrile reactions
- Avoid prophylactic antipyretics
- Use of genotype specific RBCs in sickle cell anemia

POSSIBLE COMPLICATIONS
- Uremia, oliguria, anuria
- Right heart failure

EXPECTED COURSE/PROGNOSIS
- Usual course - acute
- Usually no harm if transfusion is stopped at onset of manifestations
- Severe - mortality 50%

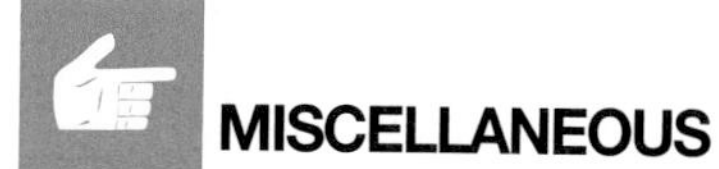

MISCELLANEOUS

ASSOCIATED CONDITIONS
- Disseminated intravascular coagulation
- Acute renal failure

AGE-RELATED FACTORS
Pediatric: Reaction greater and outlook poorer in the very young
Geriatric: Outlook more grave in the elderly
Others: N/A

PREGNANCY
N/A

SYNONYMS
N/A

ICD-9-CM
999.8 Other transfusion reaction

SEE ALSO
Anemia, autoimmune hemolytic
Anemia, hemolytic
Anemia, sickle cell
Disseminated intravascular coagulation (DIC)
Renal failure, acute (ARF)

OTHER NOTES
N/A

ABBREVIATIONS
N/A

REFERENCES
- Lee RG, Bithell TC, et al: Wintrobe's Clinical Hematology. 9th Ed. Philadelphia, Lea & Febiger, 1993
- Huestis DW, Bove JR, Case S: Practical Blood Transfusion. 4th Ed. Boston, Little, Brown and Co., 1988

Web references: 0 available at www.5mcc.com
Illustrations N/A

Author(s):
Bruce G. Bellamy, MD

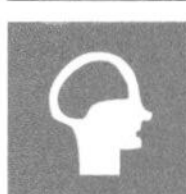

BASICS

DESCRIPTION The sudden onset of a focal and transient (< 24 hours) neurological deficit due to brain ischemia
System(s) affected: Nervous
Genetics: Inheritance is polygenic with a tendency to clustering of risk factors within families
Incidence/Prevalence in USA: Incidence 30/100,000
Predominant age: Risk increases over age 45 and is highest in the seventh and eighth decades
Predominant sex: Male > Female (3:1)

SIGNS & SYMPTOMS
- Carotid circulation (hemispheric) - monocular visual loss, hemiplegia, hemianesthesia, neglect, aphasia, visual field defects; less often headaches, seizures, amnesia, confusion
- Vertebrobasilar (brainstem or cerebellar) - bilateral visual obscuration, diplopia, vertigo, ataxia, facial paresis, Horner syndrome, dysphagia, dysarthria
- Cerebellar or brainstem lesion in patients with headache, nausea, vomiting and ataxia

CAUSES
- Carotid atherosclerotic disease with artery to artery thromboembolism
- Small, deep, vessel disease associated with hypertension
- Cardiac - cardioembolism secondary to valvular (mitral valve) pathology; mural hypo- or akinesias with thrombosis (acute anterior myocardial infarctions or congestive cardiomyopathies); cardiac arrhythmia (atrial fibrillation)
- Hypercoagulable states - antiphospholipid antibodies, deficiency of protein S, protein C. Presence of antithrombin 3, oral contraceptives.
- Other causes - spontaneous and post-traumatic (i.e., chiropractic manipulation) arterial dissection, fibromuscular dysplasia

RISK FACTORS
- Age
- Hypertension
- Cardiac disease
- Smoking
- Diabetes
- Antiphospholipid antibodies
- Family History
- Hypercholesterolemia
- Atrial fibrillation
- Homocystinemia

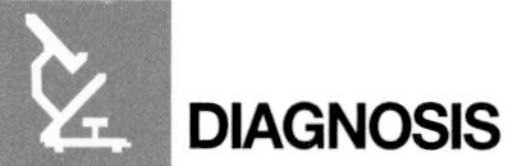

DIAGNOSIS

DIFFERENTIAL DIAGNOSIS
- Migraine (hemiplegic)
- Focal seizure (Todd's paralysis)
- Hypoglycemia
- Todd's paralysis

LABORATORY N/A

Drugs that may alter lab results: N/A

Disorders that may alter lab results: N/A

PATHOLOGICAL FINDINGS N/A

SPECIAL TESTS
- Duplex carotid ultrasonography
- Cerebral angiography
- ECG
- Transthoracic echocardiogram (TTE); if normal and a cardiac source is suspected, follow with transesophageal echocardiogram
- Holter monitoring
- EEG for suspected seizure
- INR and partial thromboplastin time (PTT) (Coumadin prolongs INR)
- Antiphospholipid antibodies

IMAGING
- Acute phase - CT of head
- Angiography - carotid arterial stenosis
- Digital substraction - stenosis
- MRI brain
- MRA brain and blood vessels

DIAGNOSTIC PROCEDURES MRI brain and diffusion weighted imaging

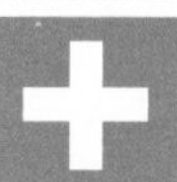

TREATMENT

APPROPRIATE HEALTH CARE Acute phase: Outpatient for investigations; inpatient for surgery and high risk groups

GENERAL MEASURES
- Strict control of medical risk factors, e.g., diabetes, hypertension, hyperlipidemia, cardiac disease
- Antithrombotic therapy
- Counseling towards cessation of smoking

SURGICAL MEASURES In medically fit patients with non-disabling stroke, carotid endarterectomy (CEA) is indicated for stenosis of 70-99% on side ipsilateral to stroke; CEA is of modest benefit for carotid stenosis of 50-69% and depends on risk factors. The North American Symptomatic Carotid Endarterectomy Trial (NASCET) showed no benefit of CEA above medical therapy alone in stenosis of <50%.

ACTIVITY No restrictions

DIET As appropriate to underlying medical problems (diabetic diet, low fat diet, low salt diet etc.)

PATIENT EDUCATION National Stroke Association, 9707 E. Easter Ln, Englewood, CO 80112 (800-STROKES)

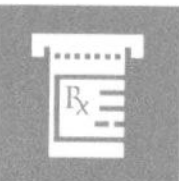

MEDICATIONS

DRUG(S) OF CHOICE
- Enteric coated aspirin (EC ASA) 50-325 mg/day,

or
- Clopidogrel (Plavix) 75 mg daily; ticlopidine's descendent has fewer side effects, and shows a slight advantage over ASA
- Dipyridamole-aspirin (Aggrenox) - extended release, 200 mg/25 mg capsule po bid; more efficacious than aspirin alone, but more costly
- Warfarin - INR adjusted dose. For patients with atrial fibrillation and cardioembolic stroke.

Contraindications:
- EC ASA - active peptic ulcer disease, hypersensitivity to aspirin, patients who had bronchospastic reaction to ASA or other non-steroidal anti-inflammatory drugs
- Ticlopidine - known hypersensitivity to the drug, presence of hematopoietic disorders, presence of a hemostatic disorder, conditions associated with active bleeding, severe liver dysfunction
- Warfarin - intolerance or allergy, dementia, liver disease, active bleeding, pregnancy, recent head injury

Precautions:
- EC ASA - may aggravate pre-existing peptic ulcer disease, may worsen symptoms in some patients with asthma
- Ticlopidine - 2.4% of patients develop neutropenia (0.8% severe neutropenia) which is reversible with cessation of drug. Monitor blood counts every 2 weeks for the first 3 months.
- Clopidogrel and ticlopidine - TTP can occur
- Warfarin - poor balance, alcohol/drug abuse, age > 80

Significant possible interactions:
- EC ASA - may potentiate effects of anticoagulants and sulfonylurea, hypoglycemic agents
- Ticlopidine - digoxin plasma levels decreased 15%, theophylline half-life increased from 8.6 to 12.2 hours
- Warfarin - ASA, NSAIDs, antibiotics, tranquilizers

ALTERNATIVE DRUGS Ticlopidine (Ticlid) 250 mg po bid; fallen out of favor due to unfavorable side effect profile

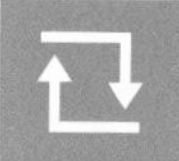

FOLLOWUP

PATIENT MONITORING Followup every 3 months for first year then yearly

PREVENTION/AVOIDANCE
- Stop smoking
- Control blood pressure, diabetes, hyperlipidemia
- Antiplatelet therapy
- Angiotensin converting enzyme (ACE) inhibitors
- Statins
- Treat homocystinemia with vitamin B6, vitamin B12, and folic acid
- Anticoagulation when cardioembolism is the suspected cause

POSSIBLE COMPLICATIONS
- Stroke
- Seizure
- Trauma if patient experiences sudden fall due to weakness

EXPECTED COURSE/PROGNOSIS
5-20% risk of stroke on ipsilateral side within one year and cumulative thereafter. Frequency increases with addition of multiple risk factors and severity of carotid stenosis.

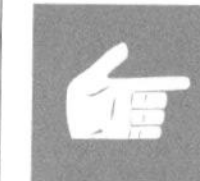

MISCELLANEOUS

ASSOCIATED CONDITIONS
- Atrial fibrillation
- Major cause of death in first five years after a TIA is cardiac disease

AGE-RELATED FACTORS
Pediatric:
- Cardiac (especially developmental abnormalities)
- Metabolic - homocystinuria, Fabry disease

Geriatric: Atrial fibrillation is a frequent cause of TIA among the elderly

Others: Adults < 45 years old most likely to have a cardiac source of embolism

PREGNANCY A hypercoagulable state is associated with pregnancy and parturition

SYNONYMS
- Mini-stroke

ICD-9-CM
435.9 Unspecified transient cerebral ischemia

SEE ALSO
Stroke (Brain attack)

OTHER NOTES N/A

ABBREVIATIONS N/A

REFERENCES

- Hachinski V, ed. Stroke. Lancet 1998;352(suppl3):1-30
- Hachinski V. Brain attack: The Clinical Handbook. Meducom International, 1999

Web references: 0 available at www.5mcc.com
Illustrations N/A

Author(s):

Vladimir Hachinski, MD, DSc
Vivek Jain, MD

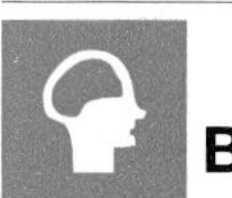

BASICS

DESCRIPTION
- Trichinosis is a parasitic disease that develops after ingesting infected pork or other meat containing viable cysts of *Trichinella spiralis*, a nematode, with rarer cases attributable to several different species of *Trichinella*. The cysts remain viable and can cause disease when the infected meat is undercooked. Most common outbreaks are attributable to undercooked pork, wild boar meat, homemade and commercial sausage, bear, walrus and other wild animal meats. Horsemeat has become another important source in the European Union.
- Enteric phase, phase 1: Cysts are broken down by digestive acid and pepsin in the stomach freeing larvae which develop into mature adult worms in the upper to middle small intestine, taking about one week after ingestion and may last 3 to 5 weeks
- Systemic phase, phase II: Female worms then release newborn larvae that migrate through blood vessels and lymphatics to multiple organ systems, occurring 2 to 3 weeks after ingestion and may last for 2 months
- Muscular encystment phase, phase III: Larvae become encysted in striated skeletal and sometimes cardiac muscle, where they form a nurse cell which functions to nourish it and protect it from host immunity. This complex can survive in humans up to 30 years. The intramuscular cysts usually eventually calcify.

System(s) affected: Gastrointestinal, Musculoskeletal

Genetics: N/A

Incidence/Prevalence in USA: From 1991-1996, an average of 38 cases were reported annually in the United States. Only 15 cases were reported in 2000. Most mild cases probably are undiagnosed, based on autopsy studies.

Predominant age: Cases have been reported from all age groups. It occurs most frequently in ages 20-49.

Predominant sex: Male = Female

SIGNS & SYMPTOMS
Signs and symptoms begin within one week of ingesting infected meat.
- Common symptoms (and can occur concurrently):
  - ◊ Diarrhea (mostly phase I)
  - ◊ Abdominal Cramping (mostly phase I)
  - ◊ Fever (mostly phase II and III)
  - ◊ Myalgias (mostly phase II and III)
  - ◊ Eosinophilia (mostly phase II and III)
  - ◊ Periorbital edema (mostly phase II and III)
  - ◊ Weakness (mostly phase II and III
- Symptoms depend on the number of ingested infective larvae, and the phase of the parasitic invasion. Light infections,<10 larvae per gram of muscle, usually asymptomatic. Heavy infections, >50 larvae per gram of muscle can be life threatening. Skeletal muscle (gastrocnemius, masseter, diaphragm, biceps, lower back, extraocular muscles, jaw and neck) is the most frequent site of symptoms due to larval migration, however in severe cases there can be myocardial damage, pulmonary infiltration and focal neurologic damage.
- Less common symptoms (mostly phase II and III):
  - ◊ Conjunctivitis
  - ◊ Subconjunctival hemorrhage
  - ◊ Retinal hemorrhages
  - ◊ Maculopapular rash
  - ◊ Splinter hemorrhages
  - ◊ Headache
  - ◊ Photophobia
  - ◊ Pneumonitis
  - ◊ Tachycardia
  - ◊ Heart failure
  - ◊ Pericardial effusion
  - ◊ CNS involvement

CAUSES Eating undercooked meat that is infected with viable *Trichenella* cysts.

RISK FACTORS
- Access to wild game, homemade pork products, noncommercial sources of meat
- Eating pigs that were fed uncooked garbage
- Under cooking pork
- Eating wild game inadequately cooked or frozen
- Ethnic groups from Southeast Asia raising their own pork or favoring partially cooked pork products.
- Higher incidence in Alaska and northeastern United States.

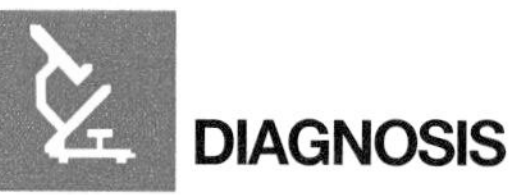

DIAGNOSIS

DIFFERENTIAL DIAGNOSIS
- Acute rheumatic fever
- Arthritis, angioedema
- Botulism
- Collagen vascular disease
- Dermatomyositis
- Encephalitis
- Eosinophilia-myalgia syndrome
- Gastroenteritis
- Idiopathic hypereosinophilic syndrome
- Idiopathic polymyositis
- Influenza
- Meningitis
- Pneumonitis
- Polyarteritis nodosa
- Polymyositis
- Typhoid fever
- Tuberculosis

LABORATORY
- Eosinophilia (>600/cubic millimeter), with leukocytosis
- Increased creatine phosphate kinase (CPK)
- Increased lactate dehydrogenase (LDH)
- Hypergammaglobulinemia
- Elevated erythrocyte sedimentation rate (several weeks)
- Urinalysis may show myoglobinuria

Drugs that may alter lab results: Rare increases in SGOT with thiabendazole

Disorders that may alter lab results: N/A

PATHOLOGICAL FINDINGS Larvae on muscle biopsy (often gastrocnemius), however absence of larvae does not exclude diagnosis. Rarely find worm in stool.

SPECIAL TESTS
- Serologic tests for *T. spiralis*, IgM and IgG
- ELISA (enzyme linked immunosorbent assay) IgM and IgG
- Bentonite flocculation after 3rd week for parasite specific antibody
- Indirect immunofluorescence
- Complement fixation
- DNA testing [RAPD (random amplified polymorphic DNA), PCR (polymerase chain reaction)]
- Antibody levels are often not detectable until 3-5 weeks post infection
- Antibody peaks 3rd month
- Antibody testing 15-22% false negative in phase 1
- Paired specimens helpful, 1-2 months apart. Look for fourfold increase in titer.
- Antibody remains detectable 2-3 years

IMAGING
- CT may help see calcified muscle cysts
- MRI may help in evaluation of neurologic complications
- Chest x-ray may detect patchy infiltrates
- Extremity x-ray may show calcified densities

DIAGNOSTIC PROCEDURES Muscle biopsy of gastrocnemius or deltoid with at least 1 gram of muscle, including examination between compressed slides (higher detection rate)

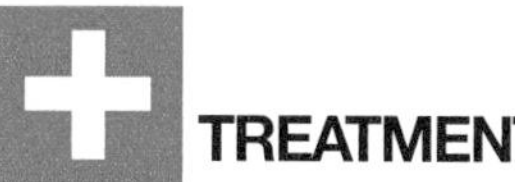

TREATMENT

APPROPRIATE HEALTH CARE
- Outpatient unless complications such as cardiac, pulmonary, or neurological
- May call CDC for appropriate diagnostic tests (404-639-3311).

GENERAL MEASURES Bedrest, antipyretics and analgesics.

SURGICAL MEASURES Pacemaker has been required on occasion for severe myocarditis

ACTIVITY As tolerated. Bedrest may help muscular pain.

DIET As tolerated

PATIENT EDUCATION
- Manage complications as appropriate
- Measures at prevention
- Cook potentially contaminated meat such as pork to 170°F (77°C), no longer pink
- Freeze at -15°C for 21 days (longer if meat is >15 cm thick), however *Trichinella* larvae in wild game may be resistant to freezing
- Do not feed hogs uncooked garbage

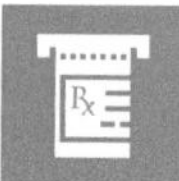

MEDICATIONS

DRUG(S) OF CHOICE

- For early intestinal phase (presenting in first 1-2 weeks), to treat adult worms:
  - ◊ Mebendazole may be used 200-400 mg tid x 3 days, then 400-500 mg tid for 10 days, adults and children
  - ◊ Albendazole 400 mg bid x 8-14 days, adults and children
- No drugs are very effective against larvae once encysted in muscle, however they may halt further dissemination
- Call CDC for current dosage and recommendation (404)639-3311
- Corticosteroids such as prednisone 40 to 60 mg/day for 3-5 days and then tapered as symptoms subside may be helpful in severe cases, particularly to help decrease inflammation when signs of myocarditis, neurologic disease, pulmonary insufficiency, or severe myositis

Contraindications: Corticosteroids have been reported to be contraindicated in the intestinal phase, as they could prolong this phase

Precautions: Minimal experience exists with the use of medications in small children and in pregnancy. Mebendazole should not be given in the first trimester, and any medications should only be used if felt absolutely necessary.

Significant possible interactions: Carbamazepine or alcohol may decrease the effect of mebendazole. Cimetidine may increase the level of mebendazole.

ALTERNATIVE DRUGS

Thiabendazole, which used to be the drug of choice at 25 mg/kg bid x 1 week, maximum dose 1.5 gm, has been replaced by the above drugs because they have fewer side effects, and are equally effective.

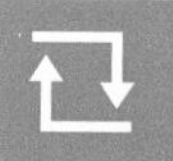

FOLLOWUP

PATIENT MONITORING

Monitor for signs and symptoms of complications such as cardiac, neurological and pulmonary

PREVENTION/AVOIDANCE

Avoid eating undercooked pork and game meat. Prolonged freezing may also be effective, but less so for wild game meat.

POSSIBLE COMPLICATIONS

- Meningitis
- Subcortical infarcts
- Encephalitis
- Myocarditis with congestive heart failure
- Nephritis
- Glomerulonephritis
- Sinusitis
- Pneumonitis

EXPECTED COURSE/PROGNOSIS

- Most infections are asymptomatic, short-lived and generally have uneventful recovery without medication
- Encysted larvae remain viable for several years
- Prognosis is good in most cases, although 5-10% of cases can be severe
- There is no clear evidence that chronic trichinosis exists
- Less than 1% of cases can be fatal, generally around the 4th-8th week, as a result of cardiac failure or pneumonia

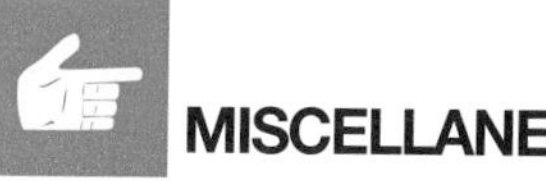

MISCELLANEOUS

ASSOCIATED CONDITIONS

N/A

AGE-RELATED FACTORS

Pediatric: N/A
Geriatric: N/A
Others: N/A

PREGNANCY

Although not much information, there is one case of a woman 16 weeks pregnant who delivered a normal child without complications or evidence of problems

SYNONYMS

Trichinellosis
Trichinelliasis

ICD-9-CM

124 Trichinosis

SEE ALSO

OTHER NOTES

N/A

ABBREVIATIONS

N/A

REFERENCES

- Bailey TM, Schantz PM. Trends in the incidence and transmission patterns of trichinosis in humans in the United States: comparisons of the periods 1975-1981 and 1982-1986. Rev Infect Dis 1990;12(1):5-11
- Clausen MR, et al. Trichinella infection and clinical disease. QJ Med 1996;89(8):631-6
- McAuley JB, et al. Trichinosis surveillance, United States, 1987-1990. Morbidity and Mortality Weekly Report CDC Surveillance Summary 1992:40:35-42
- Stack PS. Trichinosis, Still a public health threat. Postgraduate Medicine 1995;97(6):137-9/143-4

Web references: 2 available at www.5mcc.com
Illustrations N/A

Author(s):
Kenton Voorhees, MD

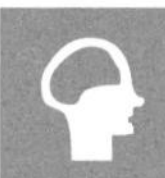

BASICS

DESCRIPTION Trichomonas is a protozoan parasite found in men and women at genitourinary sites

System(s) affected: Renal/Urologic, Reproductive

Genetics: N/A

Incidence/Prevalence in USA:
- Makes up 10-25% of vaginal infections
- 300/100,000 women/year for first time diagnosis of trichomoniasis; 600/100,000 women/year for any diagnosis for trichomoniasis
- In sexually active adult women: 2,000/100,000 in a family planning clinic; 35,000/100,000 in a STD clinic

Predominant age:
- Young and middle aged adults
- Rare until onset of sexual activity
- Not uncommon in postmenopausal women

Predominant sex: Both affected, but women more commonly symptomatic

SIGNS & SYMPTOMS
- Female
  - ◊ 40% can be asymptomatic at time of diagnosis
  - ◊ Symptoms typically begin or worsen at time of menstrual period
  - ◊ Vaginal discharge (75%, usually copious, watery and pooling, can be frothy)
  - ◊ Vulvovaginal irritation (50%)
  - ◊ Dysuria (50%)
  - ◊ Vaginal odor (10%)
  - ◊ A "strawberry cervix" from punctate hemorrhages (5% of cases)
  - ◊ Vaginal hyperemia
  - ◊ Dyspareunia
  - ◊ Suprapubic discomfort
  - ◊ Cervical erosion
- Male
  - ◊ Most are asymptomatic
  - ◊ Symptomatic (20%)
    - Urethral discharge
    - Dysuria
    - Epididymitis (rare)

CAUSES
- Trichomonas vaginalis is a pear shaped protozoan which is a facultative anaerobe. It is usually sexually transmitted although a non-venereal route is possible as the organism survives for several hours in a moist environment.
- Transmission is rarely seen in female children of infected women
- Incubation period is 3-28 days

RISK FACTORS Multiple sexual partners

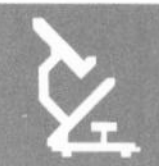

DIAGNOSIS

DIFFERENTIAL DIAGNOSIS
- Female - vaginal candidiasis, bacterial vaginosis. Cervical inflammation can lead to the mistaken diagnosis of cervicitis.
- Male - chlamydia urethritis

LABORATORY
- Female
  - ◊ Wet prep is 60-70% sensitive and highly specific. Sensitivity is reduced with loss of motility due to cooling, low inoculum size and rapid scanning of the slide. Specificity is about 100%.
  - ◊ Vaginal pH is > 4.5 in 90% of women
  - ◊ Wet prep usually shows many more PMN's than epithelial cells
- Male
  - ◊ A wet prep and culture of urethral discharge after prostatic exam is 50-80% sensitive

Drugs that may alter lab results: N/A

Disorders that may alter lab results: N/A

PATHOLOGICAL FINDINGS N/A

SPECIAL TESTS
- Culture has a sensitivity of greater than 95% but takes 4-7 days
- ELISA and direct fluorescent antibody tests are available and are 80-90% sensitive
- Pap smear has a 60% sensitivity and 99% specificity
- Rapid diagnostic kits using PCR DNA probes have sensitivity of 97% and specificity of 98%

IMAGING N/A

DIAGNOSTIC PROCEDURES N/A

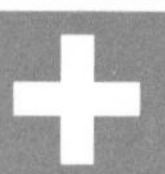

TREATMENT

APPROPRIATE HEALTH CARE Outpatient

GENERAL MEASURES Education about the venereal aspect of the infection

SURGICAL MEASURES N/A

ACTIVITY Sexual activity should not be resumed until patient and partner are both treated

DIET Should abstain from alcohol if metronidazole used for therapy

PATIENT EDUCATION
- Discussion about safe sex during health maintenance visits
- National Institutes of Health: www. niaid.nih.gov//factsheets/stdvag.htm
- Planned Parenthood: www.plannedparenthood.org/womenshealth/vaginitis.htm
- Family Doctor web site: http://familydoctor.org/handouts/275.html
- American Social Health Association: www.ashastd.org/std/vaginit.html

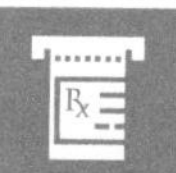

MEDICATIONS

DRUG(S) OF CHOICE

- Metronidazole: adult dose 2 grams at one time or 500 mg bid for 7 days. The routines are effective in women but the one time dose has a higher failure rate in men. All sexual partners need treatment.

Contraindications: First trimester pregnancy or allergy to the antibiotic

Precautions: Avoid metronidazole or reduce the dosage in patients with liver failure

Significant possible interactions: Ethanol, warfarin, disulfiram, phenobarbital

ALTERNATIVE DRUGS

- For treatment failure after metronidazole, CDC recommends 2 grams m qd for 3-5 daysetronidazole
- Clotrimazole: 100 mg vaginal tablets hs for 14 days. Cure rate is 20-25% but symptoms will be reduced in most women.
- Alternatively, saline or vinegar douching can be tried

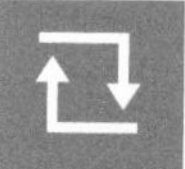

FOLLOWUP

PATIENT MONITORING Monitor target symptoms. No followup is needed if symptoms resolve with treatment.

PREVENTION/AVOIDANCE Practice safe sex by using condoms. Trichomonas can be identified in 30-40% of the male sexual partners of infected women.

POSSIBLE COMPLICATIONS Recurrent infections

EXPECTED COURSE/PROGNOSIS

Prognosis is good but recurrent infection raises possibility of non-compliance with therapy, reinfection, or infection with a resistant organism. If resistance is suspected, try metronidazole 2 g every day for 3-5 days

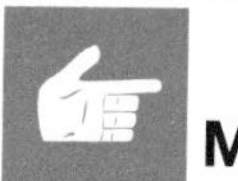

MISCELLANEOUS

ASSOCIATED CONDITIONS Other sexually transmitted diseases

AGE-RELATED FACTORS

Pediatric: Very uncommon in prepubertal (confirmed diagnosis should raise concern of sexual abuse)
Geriatric: Older people remain at risk for Trichomonas
Others: N/A

PREGNANCY Do not use metronidazole in the first trimester. Treatment of infection in pregnancy does not prevent preterm labor.

SYNONYMS

- Trick
- Trichomonal urethritis

ICD-9-CM

131.9 Trichomoniasis, unspecified
131.01 Trichomonal vulvovaginitis
131.00 Urogenital trichomoniasis, unspecified

SEE ALSO

Abnormal Pap smear
Vulvovaginitis, bacterial

OTHER NOTES N/A

ABBREVIATIONS N/A

REFERENCES

- CDC. 2002 Sexually transmitted disease treatment guidelines. MMWR 2002;51(RR-6):1-84
- Forna F, Gulmezogly AM. Interventions for treating trichomoniasis in women. Cochrane Data Base Syst Rev 2003(2):cd000218
- Schweke JR. Metronidazole utilization in the obstetric gynecologic patient. Sex Trans Dis 1995;22:370-76
- Sobel JK. Vaginitis. N Engl J Med 1997;337:1896-903
- Klebanoft MA, et al. Failure of metronidazole to prevent preterm labor. N Engl J Med 2001;345:487-93

Web references: 1 available at www.5mcc.com
Illustrations N/A

Author(s):

George R. Bergus, MD

BASICS

DESCRIPTION A disorder of the sensory nucleus of the 5th cranial nerve (trigeminal nerve), producing episodic, paroxysmal, severe lancinating pain lasting seconds to minutes followed by a pain free period in the distribution of one or more of its divisions. Often precipitated by stimulation of well-defined, ipsilateral trigger zones, usually perioral, perinasal, occasionally intraoral (eg washing, shaving).
System(s) affected: Nervous
Genetics: N/A
Incidence/Prevalence in USA: 16/100,000
Predominant age: Over age 50, peak age 60, rare before age 35
Predominant sex: Female > Male (2:1)

SIGNS & SYMPTOMS
- Unilateral (< 4% bilateral, rarely at the same time; bilateral mostly in MS), symptoms rarely present at night
- Excruciating lip pain
- Excruciating gum pain
- Excruciating cheek pain
- Paroxysmal facial pain
- Wincing
- Pain elicited by tickle or touch
- Flushing
- Lacrimation
- Salivation
- Pain "bursts" several seconds to minutes with refractory period after
- Right > left side preference
- 2nd > 3rd >> 1st (less than 5%) division trigeminal nerve most commonly affected

CAUSES
- When present, most commonly compression of the trigeminal nerve by anomalous arteries or veins of the posterior fossa, usually the superior cerebral artery compressing the trigeminal root.
- Etiology classification
  - ◊ Idiopathic
  - ◊ Secondary - disseminated sclerosis; cerebellopontine angle tumors, e.g., meningioma; tumors of the 5th nerve, e.g., neuroma, vascular malformations

RISK FACTORS Unknown

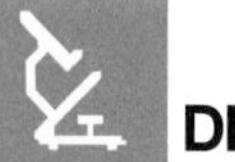

DIAGNOSIS

DIFFERENTIAL DIAGNOSIS
- Other forms of neuralgia usually have sensory loss. The presence of sensory loss nearly excludes the diagnosis of trigeminal neuralgia (if younger patient frequently is MS).
- Neoplasia in the cerebellopontine angle
- Vascular malformation of the brain stem
- Demyelinating lesion (of all patients with MS, 10% have facial pain first, other MS symptoms may not appear for 6 years)
- Vascular insult
- Migraine
- Chronic meningitis
- Acute polyneuropathy
- Atypical odontalgia
- SUNCT syndrome (short lasting, unilateral, neuralgiform pain with conjunctival injection)

LABORATORY N/A

Drugs that may alter lab results: N/A

Disorders that may alter lab results: N/A

PATHOLOGICAL FINDINGS
- Semilunar ganglion - inflammatory changes
- Degenerative changes

SPECIAL TESTS N/A

IMAGING N/A

DIAGNOSTIC PROCEDURES MRI or CT scan - neoplasm in cerebellopontine angle must be ruled out. Special MRA technique of collapsed MRA superimposed on routine spin echo T-1 weighted images.

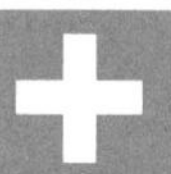

TREATMENT

APPROPRIATE HEALTH CARE Outpatient

GENERAL MEASURES
- Drug treatment is first approach. Invasive procedures for patients who cannot tolerate, or fail to respond to, drug treatment.
- Avoidance of stimulation (air, heat, cold) of trigger zones (lips, cheeks, gums)
- 4% tetracaine dissolved in 0.5% bupivacaine nerve block (only a few case reports to date)
- 25-50% of TN patients eventually fail medical treatment
- Alcohol block or glycerol injection into the trigeminal cistern - unpredictable side effects (dysesthesia and anesthesia dolorosa); temporary

SURGICAL MEASURES
- Microvascular decompression of the 5th cranial nerve at its entrance to (or exit from) the brainstem (70-90% effective)
- Partial sensory rhizotomy
- Peripheral block or section of 5th nerve proximal to the Gasserian ganglion
- Gamma knife radiosurgery (minimally invasive, 77% significant relief)
- Balloon compression of the Gasserian ganglion (especially effective for 1st division TN pain)
- Peripheral nerve ablation
  - ◊ Radiofrequency thermocoagulation (possibly 90-97% partial or complete relief; recurrence rate is unknown)
  - ◊ Neurectomy
  - ◊ Cryotherapy - good initial results; considerable relapse rate

ACTIVITY Full activity

DIET No special diet

PATIENT EDUCATION Instruct regarding medication dosage and side effects

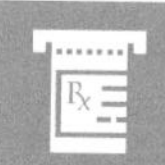

MEDICATIONS

DRUG(S) OF CHOICE Carbamazepine (Tegretol) starting dose 100-200 mg bid; effective dose usually 200 mg qid; 1200 mg/day maximum. By 3 years, 30% no longer helped. Most common side effect is sedation.

Contraindications: MAO inhibitors taken concurrently

Precautions: Use with caution in presence of liver disease

Significant possible interactions: Macrolide antibiotics with Carbamazepine. Oral anticoagulants, anticonvulsants, tricyclics, oral contraceptives, steroids, digitalis, INH, MAO inhibitors, methyprylon nabilone, nizatidine, other H2 blockers, phenytoin, propoxyphene, benzodiazepines, calcium, channel blockers.

ALTERNATIVE DRUGS

- Phenytoin (Dilantin) 300-400 mg/day (synergistic with carbamazepine)
- Baclofen (Lioresal) 10-80 mg/day; start at 5-10 mg tid with food (as adjunct with phenytoin or carbamazepine): drowsiness, weakness,`nausea, vomiting
- Gabapentin (Neurontin) 100 mg tid or 300 mg qhs, increased up to 300-600 mg tid-qid
- Lamotrigine - (10% rash)
- Chlorphenesin carbamate (Maolate) 800-2400 mg/day: drowsiness, (as adjunct with phenytoin and/or carbamazepine)
- Oxcarbazepine (Trileptal) - derivative of carbamazepine also similar to gabapentin. Faster with less drowsiness. Decreases serum sodium.
- Clonidine - stimulates inhibitory bulbospinal pain pathways that are norepinephrine dependent. Second line after anticonvulsants and/or antidepressants.
- Antidepressants, especially used with anticonvulsants. Particularly effective for atypical forms of TN - amitriptyline, fluoxetine, trazodone.
- Clonazepam (Klonopin): frequently causes drowsiness and ataxia
- Mexiletine (Mexitil). Experimental for this condition.
- Narcotics - controversial
- Capsaicin cream (not standard therapy; anecdotal evidence)
- Pimozide (Orap) superior to carbamazepine in one study of 48 patients, but it is an antipsychotic drug with extrapyramidal affects, dystonia and tardive dyskinesia. High side effect profile.
- Valproic acid (Depakene, Depakote)

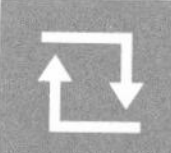

FOLLOWUP

PATIENT MONITORING

- Carbamazepine and/or phenytoin serum levels
- If carbamazepine is prescribed: CBC and platelets at baseline then weekly for a month, then monthly for 4 months, then every 6-12 months if dose stable (regimens for monitoring vary)
- CBC as needed

PREVENTION/AVOIDANCE Reduce drugs after 4-6 weeks to determine if condition is in remission, resume at previous dose if pain recurs. Withdraw drugs slowly after several months again to check for remission or if lower dose of drugs can be tolerated.

POSSIBLE COMPLICATIONS Mental and physical sluggishness, dizziness with carbamazepine

EXPECTED COURSE/PROGNOSIS

Exacerbations in fall and spring; otherwise good

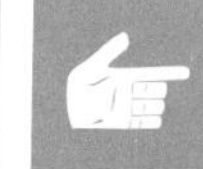

MISCELLANEOUS

ASSOCIATED CONDITIONS

- Sjögren syndrome
- Rheumatoid arthritis
- Chronic meningitis
- Facial migraine
- Acute polyneuropathy
- Multiple sclerosis
- Hemifacial spasm
- Pretrigeminal neuralgia

AGE-RELATED FACTORS

Pediatric: Unusual in childhood
Geriatric: N/A
Others: N/A

PREGNANCY N/A

SYNONYMS

- Tic douloureux
- Fothergill neuralgia
- Trifacial neuralgia

ICD-9-CM

350.1 Trigeminal neuralgia

SEE ALSO

Headache, cluster
Migraine
Sjögren syndrome

OTHER NOTES N/A

ABBREVIATIONS N/A

REFERENCES

- Vaillancourt PD, Largevin HM. Painful peripheral neuropathies. Med Clin NA 1999;83(3):627-42
- Bell WE: Orofacial Pain. 4th Ed. Chicago, Year Book Medical Publishers, 1989
- Adams RD, Victor M: Principles of Neurology. 5th Ed. New York, McGraw-Hill, 1993
- Sweet WH: The treatment of trigeminal neuralgia (tic douloureux). New Engl J Med 1986;174-177
- Moller AR: The cranial nerve vascular compression syndrome: A review of treatment. Acta Neurochirurgica 1991;113:18-23
- Merrill R, Graff-Radford SB: Trigeminal neuralgia: How to rule out the wrong treatment. JADA 1992;123:63-68
- Smith LH Jr, Bennett C: Trigeminal neuralgia. In: Wyngaarden JB, ed. Cecil Textbook of Medicine. Philadelphia, W.B. Saunders Co., 1992
- Fields HL: Treatment of trigeminal neuralgia (editorial). NEJM 1996;334(17):1125-1126

Web references: 2 available at www.5mcc.com
Illustrations N/A

Author(s):
Sean Herrington, MD

BASICS

DESCRIPTION Malabsorption syndrome of unknown etiology that occurs primarily in the tropics and subtropics. Characteristics include protein malnutrition and folic acid anemia. Usual course - relapsing without treatment. Symptoms may appear years after leaving an endemic area.
- Endemic areas - tropical regions only, Far East, India, Caribbean and the Middle East. Distribution is sporadic.
- The presence of normal jejunal biopsy nearly excludes this diagnosis

System(s) affected: Gastrointestinal, Hemic/Lymphatic/Immunologic
Genetics: N/A
Incidence/Prevalence in USA: Unknown
Predominant age: None
Predominant sex: Male = Female

SIGNS & SYMPTOMS
- Fatigue
- Asthenia
- Weight loss, pallor
- Diarrhea
- Abdominal cramps
- Borborygmus
- Night blindness
- Stomatitis
- Glossitis
- Cheilosis
- Anorexia
- Steatorrhea
- Hyperkeratosis
- Edema
- Abdominal distension
- Hyperpigmentation
- Koilonychia

CAUSES
- Unknown
- Possible dietary deficiency
- Possible infectious agent
- Vitamin deficiency (folate), B12
- Food toxins (rancid fats)
- Toxigenic strains of coliform bacteria

RISK FACTORS Parasitic infestation

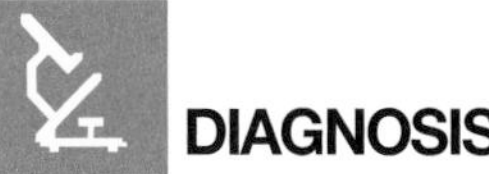

DIAGNOSIS

DIFFERENTIAL DIAGNOSIS
- Other causes of megaloblastic anemia
- Other malabsorption syndromes
- Celiac disease
- Inflammatory bowel disease
- Giardiasis
- Strongylosis
- Other infectious causes:
  - ◊ Coccidial isospora
  - ◊ Capillaria philippinensis
  - ◊ Cryptosporidium

LABORATORY
- Megaloblastic anemia in 60% of cases
- Steatorrhea
- Decreased D-Xylose
- Decreased serum iron
- Decreased calcium
- Decreased folic acid
- Decreased serum vitamin B12
- Decreased serum carotene
- Decreased cholesterol, albumin
- Deficiency of magnesium
- Deficiency of alpha-tocopherol

Drugs that may alter lab results: N/A

Disorders that may alter lab results: N/A

PATHOLOGICAL FINDINGS
- Jejunal biopsy - mild villous atrophy, increased villous crypts, mononuclear cell infiltration
- Patients may have chronic atrophic gastritis and nonspecific colopathy
- Serum motilin and enteroglucagon levels are increased in fasting and postprandially

SPECIAL TESTS N/A

IMAGING
- Mild jejunal dilatation
- Jejunal fold coarsening
- Flocculation and segmentation of Barium meal

DIAGNOSTIC PROCEDURES
- Duodenal/jejunal biopsy - not specific
- Malabsorption of at least two nutrients is considered essential for diagnosis
- D- Xylose, fat and radiolabeled vitamin B12 are used to test for absorptive capacity
- Stool microscopy
- Imaging - not specific

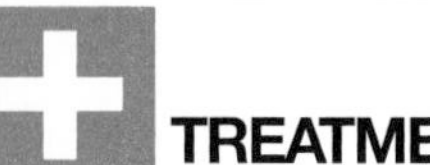

TREATMENT

APPROPRIATE HEALTH CARE Outpatient

GENERAL MEASURES
- Replace deficiencies, such as vitamin B12 and folic acid
- Control of diarrhea
- Fluid and blood replacement

SURGICAL MEASURES N/A

ACTIVITY No restrictions

DIET No special diet (gluten-free diets do not improve this disease)

PATIENT EDUCATION Written patient information available from:
National Digestive Diseases Information Clearinghouse
Box NDDIC
Bethesda, MD 20892
(301)654-3810

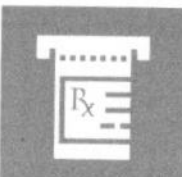

MEDICATIONS

DRUG(S) OF CHOICE
- Vitamin B12 1000 mcg SC for several days, then monthly thereafter for 6 months
- Folic acid 5 mg po daily
- Tetracycline 250 mg qid for 1-2 months, then half doses for up to 6 months. Occasionally, longer course is required.
- Combination folic acid and B12 plus tetracycline or sulfonamide

Contraindications: Allergy to tetracycline or oxytetracycline

Precautions:
- Use with caution in patients with lupus, myasthenia gravis, kidney or liver disease
- Don't take with milk, antacids or iron preparations
- Don't use during pregnancy
- Don't use in children under age 8

Significant possible interactions:
- Antacids, anticoagulants, bismuth subsalicylate
- Oral contraceptives
- Lithium

ALTERNATIVE DRUGS
- Oxytetracycline
- Nonabsorbable sulfonamides

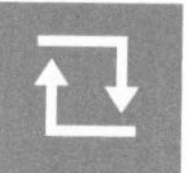

FOLLOWUP

PATIENT MONITORING As needed for symptoms

PREVENTION/AVOIDANCE N/A

POSSIBLE COMPLICATIONS
- Malabsorption
- Relapse if medication regimen is stopped too soon

EXPECTED COURSE/PROGNOSIS
- Good with appropriate treatment
- Recurrences can happen in native residents treated in the tropics

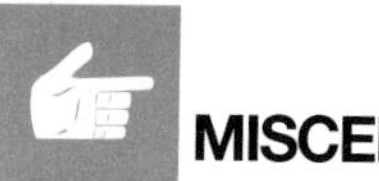

MISCELLANEOUS

ASSOCIATED CONDITIONS N/A

AGE-RELATED FACTORS
Pediatric: Don't treat with tetracycline
Geriatric: N/A
Others: N/A

PREGNANCY Don't treat with tetracycline during pregnancy

SYNONYMS N/A

ICD-9-CM
579.1 Tropical sprue

SEE ALSO
Celiac disease
Diarrhea, chronic
Whipple disease

OTHER NOTES N/A

ABBREVIATIONS N/A

REFERENCES

- Sleisenger MH, Fordtran JS, eds. Gastrointestinal and Liver Disease: Pathophysiology, Diagnosis, Management. 7th ed. Philadelphia: WB Saunders Co.; 2002
- Mandell GL, ed. Principles and Practice of Infectious Diseases. 5th ed. New York: Churchill Livingstone; 2000

Web references: 1 available at www.5mcc.com
Illustrations N/A

Author(s):
Abdulrazak Abyad, MD, MPH

BASICS

DESCRIPTION A common disease transmitted by inhaling airborne bacilli from a person with active tuberculosis (TB). The bacilli multiply in the alveolus and are carried by macrophages, lymphatics and blood to distant sites (eg. lung pleura, brain, kidney and bone). Tissue hypersensitivity usually halts infection within 10 weeks.

- Latent tuberculosis infection (LTBI) is asymptomatic, noninfectious and usually detected by a positive skin test
- TB: active disease - occurs in 10% of infected individuals without preventive therapy. Chance of disease increases with immunosuppression and is highest for all individuals within 2 years after infection - 85% of cases are pulmonary which is infectious.
- Primary TB: disease resulting from the initial pulmonary infection which the immune system is unable to control
- Recrudescent TB: active disease occurring after a period of latent asymptomatic infection
- Miliary TB: disseminated disease

System(s) affected: Endocrine/Metabolic, Gastrointestinal, Hemic/Lymphatic/Immunologic, Musculoskeletal, Nervous, Pulmonary, Renal/Urologic
Genetics: N/A
Incidence/Prevalence in USA: Decreasing overall incidence of TB: 5.1/100,0000, but greater among high risk
Predominant age:

- Primary infection - any age, especially pediatric
- Recrudescent disease - adults and elderly

Predominant sex: Male > Female

SIGNS & SYMPTOMS

- Cough
- Hemoptysis
- Fever and night sweats
- Weight loss
- Malaise
- Adenopathy
- Pleuritic chest pain
- Hepatosplenomegaly
- Renal, bone or CNS disease are late findings

CAUSES *Mycobacterium tuberculosis*, *Mycobacterium bovis*, and *Mycobacterium africanum*

RISK FACTORS

- For infection: Urban, homeless, minority, migrant workers; institutional (eg, prison, nursing home); close contact with infected individual; immigrant within 5 years (Asia, Africa, Latin America); healthcare workers
- For disease: HIV; recent infection; IV drug abuse; lymphoma; diabetes mellitus; chronic renal failure; malnutrition; steroids, immunosuppressive drugs; silicosis; gastrectomy; cancer of head, neck or lung

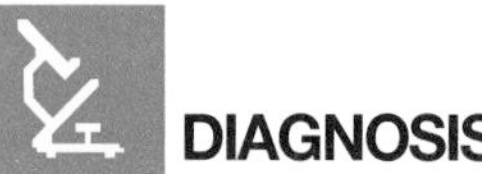

DIAGNOSIS

DIFFERENTIAL DIAGNOSIS

- Other pneumonias
- Lymphomas
- Fungal infections, especially other atypical Mycobacteria or Nocardia

LABORATORY

- Nonspecific laboratory findings include anemia, monocytosis, thrombocytosis, hypergammaglobulinemia, SIADH and sterile pyuria

Drugs that may alter lab results:

- BCG: false-positive skin test but unreliable and should not influence decision to treat LTBI
- Steroids: false-negative skin test

Disorders that may alter lab results: False-negative skin test: Recent viral infections, new (<10 weeks) infection, severe malnutrition, HIV, anergy, age < 6 months, overwhelming TB

PATHOLOGICAL FINDINGS

- Granulomas with foci of caseating necrosis surrounded by epithelioid histiocytes and giant cells, in turn surrounded by lymphocytes
- AFB stains positive

SPECIAL TESTS

- Persons with TB should be tested for HIV; if positive, get CD4 count
- Baseline liver enzymes, bilirubin, creatinine, CBC with platelet count. If using ethambutol, baseline visual acuity and color discrimination. Test for hepatitis B and C if high risk.
- If extrapulmonary suspected, urine, CSF, bone marrow and liver biopsy for culture

IMAGING

- CXR with primary disease: may show infiltrate with or without effusion atelectasis or adenopathy
- With recrudescent TB: cavitary lesions and upper lobe disease with hilar adenopathy common. Diffuse miliary pattern possible with appearance of "millet seeds".
- HIV: atypical findings with primary infection - right upper lobe atelectasis
- CXR useful to rule out TB in asymptomatic infected persons
- CT chest - good sensitivity

DIAGNOSTIC PROCEDURES

- PPD: 5 units (0.1cc) intermediate strength intradermal volar forearm. Measure induration at 48-72 hrs.
  - ◊ PPD positive if induration:
    - > 5 mm and HIV infection (or suspected), immunosuppressed, recent close TB contact, clinical evidence of active or old disease on chest x-ray
    - > 10 mm and age < 4 yrs or other risk factors
    - > 15 mm and age > 4 yrs and no risk factors
  - ◊ PPD negative if induration:
    - < 5 mm on initial test and, if indicated, on second test. Utilize 2-step test if patient has had no recent PPD, age > 55 years, nursing home resident, prison inmate, or healthcare worker (administer a second intradermal test 1-3 weeks after initial test; measure and interpret as usual)
- For suspected pulmonary TB, obtain at least 3 morning sputum samples for AFB stain and culture - use aerosol induction, gastric aspirate (children) or bronchoalveolar lavage if needed
- AFB stain can give a presumptive diagnosis
- Culture confirms diagnosis; 4-6 weeks on solid media or 2 weeks on BACTEC broth system
- Direct nucleic acid amplification approved if AFB stain positive and < 7 days of antiTB treatment, provides rapid accurate detection, but expensive
- Culture and sensitivity guide treatment

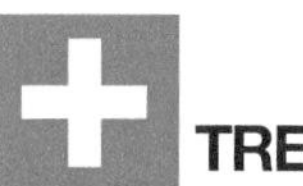

TREATMENT

APPROPRIATE HEALTH CARE

- For active disease, treatment in the initial 2 month phase usually includes INH, RIF, PZA, EMB (for alternatives, see treatment algorithms). Two drugs are used in the continuation phase for 4-7 months, usually INH/RIF with choices based on clinical criteria.
- Treatment adherence plans using directly observed treatment or DOT (5 days/week) have the highest completion rates. DOT must be used for non-daily regimens, children, HIV, drug abuse, relapse or adherence not assured.
- For active TB and HIV+, note special precautions
- For inactive pulmonary TB on chest x-ray, use INH for 9 months

GENERAL MEASURES Prescribing physician is responsible for treatment completion determined by total number doses taken, not just duration

SURGICAL MEASURES For extra pulmonary complications (spinal cord compression, constrictive pericarditis)

ACTIVITY

- As tolerated. Respiratory isolation for infectious pulmonary TB until clinical response and 3 ABF smears are negative.
- Children without cough and negative sputum smears: no isolation required after treatment started

DIET Regular. Consider pyridoxine supplement.

PATIENT EDUCATION

- Teach pathogenesis, emphasize importance of drug therapy, warn of effects and/or interactions, and find contacts
- Inform local health department

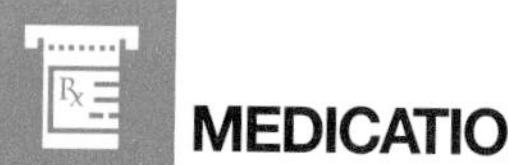

MEDICATIONS

DRUG(S) OF CHOICE

- Isoniazid (INH) - scored tabs 50/100/300 mg, syrup 10 mg/mL, or aqueous solution 100 mg/mL
  - ◊ Daily dose: adult 300 mg; pediatric 10-15 mg/kg (maximum 300 mg)
  - ◊ Twice weekly: adult 15 mg/kg; pediatric 20-30 mg/kg (maximum 900 mg)
  - ◊ Weekly: adult 15 mg/kg (maximum 900 mg)
  - ◊ Consider adding pyridoxine 10-50 mg/day
- Rifampin (RIF) capsules (150/300 mg, powder for oral suspension, or IV aqueous
  - ◊ Daily dose: adult 600 mg; pediatric dose 10-20 mg/kg (maximum 600 mg)
  - ◊ Twice weekly: adult 600 mg; pediatric 10-20 mg/kg (maximum 600 mg)
- Pyrazinamide (PZA), scored 500 mg
  - ◊ Daily dose: adult 15-25 mg/kg (maximum 2 gm); pediatric 15-30 mg/kg (maximum 2 gm)
  - ◊ Twice weekly: adult 50 mg/kg; pediatric 50 mg/kg (maximum 4 gm)
- Rifabutin (Mycobutin) capsules 150 mg (pediatric not approved)
  - ◊ Daily dose: adult 300 mg
  - ◊ Twice weekly: adult 300 mg
- Rifapentine (Priftine) tablet 150 mg (pediatric not approved); must be given with other medications
  - ◊ Twice weekly dose: adult 600 mg (may be sufficient for HIV negative, noncavitary TB, and negative sputum at second month)
- Ethambutol (EMB) - tablets 100/400 mg bacteriostatic
  - ◊ Daily dose: 15-20 mg/kg, with maximum of 1.6 gm
  - ◊ Twice weekly: 50 mg/kg, with maximum of 4 gm

Contraindications:

- RIF: avoid if patient taking antiretrovirals
- Ethambutol: because of optic neuritis, avoid ethambutol unless patient old enough to cooperate for visual acuity and color testing.

Precautions:

- INH, RIF or PZA may cause hepatitis
- Follow liver function if the patient has history of liver dysfunction or new signs develop
- RIF - colors urine, tears and secretions orange. Can permanently stain contact lenses.
- INH - peripheral neuritis and hypersensitivity possible. Consider pyridoxine.
- PZA - may increase uric acid
- EMB - may cause optic neuritis; follow monthly vision and color tests

Significant possible interactions: Rifamycins alter the level of phenytoin, antivirals and other drugs metabolized by the liver and may inactivate birth control pills (recommend a barrier method). Monitor and adjust doses as needed.

ALTERNATIVE DRUGS

- Steroids - use only with concurrent anti-TB therapy. Recommended for meningitis or pericarditis.
- Other antituberculous drugs, especially quinolones, may be useful for multidrug resistant TB (MDRTB)
- Combination tablets enhance adherence
- Streptomycin (caution: ototoxicity and nephrotoxic; don't use in pregnancy)

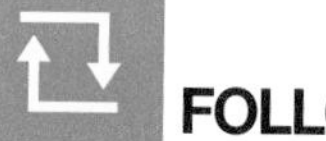

FOLLOWUP

PATIENT MONITORING

- Assess monthly for treatment adherence and adverse effects
- Check liver enzymes if symptomatic, HIV positive, chronic liver disease, alcohol use, pregnant or postpartum, and modify drugs if needed
- During TB therapy - obtain sputum culture monthly until two consecutive specimens are negative
- If culture positive after 2 months of therapy, reassess drug sensitivity and initiate DOT
- CXR at 3 months

PREVENTION/AVOIDANCE

- Identify and treat contagious persons. Notify public health department and hospital infection control if admitted
- Inpatient - use personal sealed respirators, negative pressure ventilation, ultraviolet
- Ambulatory patients use mask and tissues
- Not infectious if: favorable clinical response after 2-3 weeks of therapy and 3 AFB smears are negative.

POSSIBLE COMPLICATIONS

- Cavitary lesions can be secondarily infected
- Spread to susceptible persons of all ages
- Drug resistance - suspect if immigrant, drug resistant source or noncompliant

EXPECTED COURSE/PROGNOSIS

Generally few complications and full resolution if drugs taken for full course as prescribed

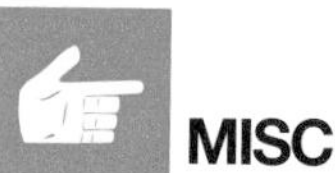

MISCELLANEOUS

ASSOCIATED CONDITIONS HIV infection (emphasize DOT; most recommendations remain the same)

AGE-RELATED FACTORS

Pediatric:

- Emphasize DOT
- Caution with ethambutol
- Children on medication may attend school
- Disseminated TB more common in infants; prompt treatment with 4 drugs if TB suspected
- Congenital infection may occur with miliary TB of maternal bacillemia, endometritis or amniotic aspiration. If suspected, get PPD, CXR, LP, culture placenta and infant, then start treatment promptly
- Protocol for newborn with mother/household contact with infection or disease
  - ◊ If mother or household contact has LTBI: skin test all household members and treat any with positive PPD
  - ◊ Contact has abnormal CXR: separate infant until infectious status known; if not contagious, monitor infant PPD
  - ◊ Mother with disease and possibly contagious: evaluate infant for congenital TB and test for HIV; separate newborn until member is noninfectious
  - ◊ If congenital TB suspected, treat as above
  - ◊ If no congenital disease, start INH and repeat PPD after 8-12 weeks.: If positive, reassess infant and finish 6 months INH. If PPD is negative, and source is noninfectious, stop INH and monitor infant.
- Consider BCG

Geriatric:

- Symptoms may be more subtle and may be attributed to associated conditions or to aging
- Side effects of INH more pronounced

Others: N/A

PREGNANCY

- Treat active TB in pregnant woman with INH, rifampin and ethambutol; add pyridoxine
- Avoid streptomycin
- Use PZA with caution
- Breast-feeding okay while taking TB drugs

SYNONYMS

- Consumption

ICD-9-CM

011.90 Pulmonary tuberculosis, unspecified

SEE ALSO

Tuberculosis, CNS
Tuberculosis, latent

OTHER NOTES

- BCG vaccine, live attenuated *Mycobacterium bovis*
  - ◊ 50% efficacy for pediatric and adult pulmonary TB
  - ◊ In USA, consider BCG for children with negative PPD and HIV tests with unavoidable high risk and for health care workers at high risk for drug resistant infection
  - ◊ Abscess, ulceration and regional lymphadenitis occur in 1-2%, osteitis and fatal infection can occur in immunosuppressed
  - ◊ Used more commonly in developing countries to prevent complications of TB

ABBREVIATIONS

PPD = purified protein derivative
BCG = Bacillus Calmette-Guérin
DOT = directly observed treatment
LTBI = latent tuberculosis infection

REFERENCES

- Centers for Disease Control: Screening for tuberculosis and tuberculosis infection in high-risk populations. MMWR 2000;49(No.RR-6):1-51
- ATS. Diagnostic Standards and Classification of Tuberculosis in Adults and Children. Am J Respir Crit Care Med 2000;161(4 Pt 1):1376-95
- Report of the Committee on Infectious Diseases (Red Book). Elk Grove Village, Ill, American Academy of Pediatrics, 2003
- CDC Prevention and treatment of tuberculosis among patients infected with human immunodeficiency virus: principles and revised recommendations. MMWR 1998;47(No. RR-20)
- American Thoracic Society/Centers for Disease Control and Prevention/Infectious Diseases Society of America: Treatment of Tuberculosis. MMWR 2003;52(No. RR-11)

Web references: 4 available at www.5mcc.com
Illustrations N/A

Author(s):

Gregory Snyder, MD

BASICS

DESCRIPTION

- Tuberculosis (TB) of the CNS is a granulomatous infection of brain, meninges or spinal cord caused by *Mycobacterium tuberculosis*. Clinical forms include intracranial tuberculoma, tuberculous meningitis (TBM), spinal tuberculoma and spinal tuberculous arachnoiditis.
- Pathophysiology: Tuberculous infection spreads hematogenously to the CNS generally from a primary pulmonary focus. Infection starts as a subpial or subependymal cortical focus (Rich focus) resulting in a intraparenchymal granuloma eventually giving rise to intracerebral mass lesions (intracerebral tuberculomas) or will rupture, discharging organisms into the subarachnoid space and giving rise to basal lepto and pachymeningitis. Meningitis causes hydrocephalus and cranial neuropathies. Hydrocephalus is either communicating or obstructive (at foramina of Luschka and Magendie). Tuberculous vasculitis involves the lenticulostriate and thalamo-perforatoring arteries and can cause small infarcts in the deep gray nuclei and deep white matter.
- Uncommon manifestations of CNS tuberculosis: en-plaque granulomas, tuberculous abscesses, pituitary tuberculosis and tuberculous ventriculitis. Spinal cord infection is less common, but results in arachnoiditis, focal intramedullary tuberculomas, intramedullary abscesses and syringomyelia.

System(s) affected: Endocrine/Metabolic, Nervous

Genetics: Host immune response related to incompletely understood genetic factors

Incidence/Prevalence in USA:

- In the US: The incidence of TB is 5.3/100,000. CNS involvement: 2-5% in immunocompetent patients with TB and 10-15% in AIDS-related TB. CNS tuberculomas account for about 1% of all intracranial mass lesions.
- Internationally: Rates of TB and tuberculous meningitis (TBM) increasing, especially in countries of Africa and Asia affected by the HIV pandemic. Incidence is 544 and 757 new patients per 100,000 in Africa and India, respectively. CNS tuberculomas account for about 20% of all intracranial mass lesions.

Predominant age:

- Intracranial tuberculomas: 70% patients < 30 years; uncommon < 4 years
- Tuberculous meningitis (TBM): Highest incidence in first 3 years of life; uncommon < 6 months

Predominant sex: Male = Female

SIGNS & SYMPTOMS

- Seizures (85% of patients)
- Signs and symptoms of raised ICP (70%)
  - ◊ Headaches
  - ◊ Vomiting
  - ◊ Lethargy
  - ◊ Papilledema
  - ◊ Slowly progressive in 50% of all patients
- Symptoms of focal mass lesion (70%)
  - ◊ Weakness
  - ◊ Hemiparesis
  - ◊ Ataxia
  - ◊ Cranial nerve palsy
- Pyrexia (20 to 25%)
- Signs of extra-cranial TB (33%)
- Rare signs: Scalp swelling, homonymous hemianopia, unilateral proptosis, CSF rhinorrhea, amenorrhea, behavioral problems, Brown-Sequard syndrome

CAUSES

- *Mycobacterium tuberculosis*
- *Mycobacterium avium* complex, in immunosuppressed patients (e.g., AIDS)

RISK FACTORS

- CNS TB more common in immunosuppressed (e.g., older, younger, HIV, diabetes, steroids or cytotoxic drugs).
- Emigrants from TB-endemic areas
- History of pulmonary TB
- Exposure to population with high rates of TB (e.g., health care professionals, prison workers)

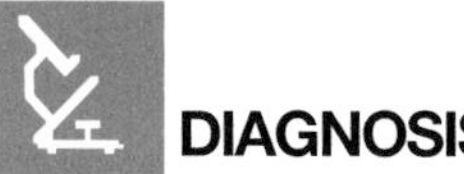

DIAGNOSIS

DIFFERENTIAL DIAGNOSIS

- TBM
  - ◊ Meningitis (chronic, fungal, bacterial, carcinomatous)
  - ◊ Sarcoidosis
- Intracranial tuberculoma
  - ◊ Granulomas (cysticercus, sarcoid, fungal)
  - ◊ Pyogenic abscess
  - ◊ Metastasis
  - ◊ Glioma
- Spinal tuberculoma
  - ◊ Intramedullary tumors
  - ◊ Syringomyelia
  - ◊ Spinal abscess
  - ◊ Myelitis

LABORATORY

- General labs
  - ◊ PPD positive in 85% of immunocompetent patients
  - ◊ ESR raised in 15% patients
- CSF study in TBM
  - ◊ Mild non-specific increase in protein content
  - ◊ Lymphocytic pleocytosis
  - ◊ Normal or slightly low glucose
  - ◊ Tubercle bacilli found on direct smear in 10 -15%
  - ◊ Difficult to isolate in cultures and time consuming
- CSF study in tuberculoma
  - ◊ Isolated from subarachnoid space due to thick capsule, so no CSF changes seen, except in 3 to 10% where TBM can co-exist with tuberculomas

Drugs that may alter lab results:

- Steroids may alter CSF findings and give false-negative skin tests
- ATT may alter CSF findings

Disorders that may alter lab results:

- Immunodeficient states (e.g., HIV) may give false-negative skin tests

PATHOLOGICAL FINDINGS

- In TBM
  - ◊ Thick tubercular exudates seen in the basal cisterns and Sylvian fissures
  - ◊ Hydrocephalus common, can be obstructive in acute phase due to exudates
  - ◊ In chronic phase hydrocephalus is due to vascular adhesive arachnoiditis
  - ◊ Watershed infarcts are seen due to obliteration of perforators
- In tuberculoma
  - ◊ Well-defined avascular lesions composed of a necrotic caseous centre surrounded by a tuberculous granulation tissue made of fibroblasts, epithelioid cells, Langhans giant cells and lymphocytes. TB bacilli can be present in this granulation tissue.
  - ◊ Surrounding brain shows edema, thrombosed vessels, swollen astrocytes and degenerated nerve cells. Smaller satellite tuberculomas may surround the main mass.
  - ◊ Calcifications can occur in a concentric ring at the margins
  - ◊ Occurs at any site in brain; may adhere to dura
  - ◊ Unusual forms of tuberculomas are:
    - Grapelike clusters of tuberculomas
    - Meningeal tuberculomatosis
    - Cystic tuberculoma
    - Tuberculous abscess
    - Extensive edematous encephalopathy with a small tuberculoma
    - Transdural spread to calvarium
- Special comments
  - ◊ Tuberculous bacilli difficult to culture from tuberculomas
  - ◊ Immunohistochemical demonstration of mycobacterial antigen is possible from tuberculoma tissue

SPECIAL TESTS

- Dot Enzyme Linked Immunosorbent assay (Dot ELISA) may detect MTB antigens (MTB antigen 5) and anti-mycobacterial antibodies in the CSF (60% sensitive and 100% specific).
- Latex particle agglutination test of CSF
- PCR of CSF has high sensitivity (75%)
- Direct nucleic acid amplification techniques like amplified *Mycobacterium tuberculosis* direct test (MTD) when used with Ziehl-Neelsen (ZN) staining of CSF has high accuracy

IMAGING

- Skull radiography not helpful
- Ultrasound. In infants with patent fontanel, follow-up examination of hydrocephalus rather than CT, thereby reducing radiation dose.
- CT scan
  - ◊ Lesions 1.5 cm in diameter identifiable
  - ◊ Tuberculomas are isodense or slightly hyperdense and enhance strongly with contrast in the shape of a concentric ring (sometimes as a disc)
  - ◊ Calcification can be peripheral or central. Central calcification in peripheral ring enhancing lesion gives the 'target sign'. 50-60% tuberculomas are multiple. Surrounding low-attenuation white matter edema common. Edema more marked in TB abscesses.
  - ◊ Exudates in basal cisterns, hydrocephalus, infarcts and white matter edema are commonly seen in TBM
  - ◊ Contrast enhancement of meninges, especially thick and irregular in basal meninges, is seen in 71% of cases of TBM
  - ◊ Pan-ventricular hydrocephalus is seen in 72% of cases
  - ◊ Periventricular lucencies in TBM may be due to inflammatory process and may not necessarily indicate raised ICP.
- MRI scan
  - ◊ In TBM, more sensitive in demonstrating early infarcts than CT
  - ◊ Solid tuberculomas isointense with grey matter on T1-weighted images and hyperintense on T2. Central necrosis better seen as central hyperintensity on T2-weighted images. Surrounding edema seen hyperintense on T2.

DIAGNOSTIC PROCEDURES

- Lumber and ventricular punctures
  - ◊ Avoid lumbar sampling of CSF in acute phase of TBM or in intracranial tuberculomas with raised ICP
- CT guided stereotactic brain biopsy: helpful in differentiating tuberculomas from other space occupying lesions (SOLs); diagnostic yield ≈ 85%

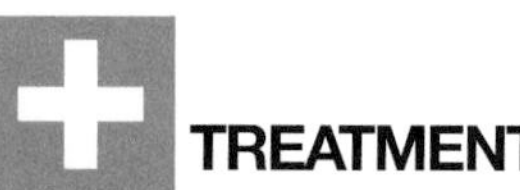

TREATMENT

APPROPRIATE HEALTH CARE

Often inpatient

GENERAL MEASURES

- To look for other foci of infection (pulmonary and other extra-pulmonary sites) and start appropriate treatment
- Care needs to be taken so that patient may not harm himself during an episode of seizure

- In TBM neuropsychological surveillance is essential
- If associated with AIDS, proper treatment of AIDS required

SURGICAL MEASURES

- TBM
  - ◊ Surgical diversion of CSF when TBM associated with symptomatic raised ICP (VP shunt preferred. VA shunt not preferred due to auto-immune reactions to tuberculous proteins, higher chance of lower end obstruction and chronic pulmonary hypertension from the shunt.)
  - ◊ Occasionally double shunts (one in each lateral ventricles or one in lateral and one in fourth ventricle) are needed
  - ◊ Rarely optic-chiasmal arachnoiditis may need optic nerve decompressions
  - ◊ Endoscopic release of intra-ventricular septae useful in loculated hydrocephalus
  - ◊ External ventricular drainage is used in patients with very poor neurological status who are toxic
- TUBERCULOMA
  - ◊ Surgical intervention when
    - No response to ATT
    - Diagnosis is in doubt
    - Obstructive hydrocephalus present
    - Elevated ICP threatening life or vision
  - ◊ Surgical procedures
    - Craniotomy and complete removal
    - Craniectomy and partial removal
    - Decompressive craniectomy
    - Chiasmal decompression for intrasellar tuberculomas
    - Stereotactic guidance for decompression of brain stem tuberculomas
- OTHER FORMS
  - ◊ Tuberculous abscesses can be aspirated under stereotactic guidance
  - ◊ Thick walled, single and located in non-eloquent areas can be excised during craniotomy
  - ◊ Intramedullary spinal tuberculomas with impending paraplegia: excision or decompression
  - ◊ Pituitary TB due to the diagnostic problems need a trans-sphenoidal decompression

ACTIVITY

- Appropriate restriction if seizures is a major symptom
- No isolation required

DIET Nutritious balanced diet with pyridoxine supplementation (10 to 40 mg/day)

PATIENT EDUCATION To explain the nature of problem, importance of drug therapy, importance of seizure prophylaxis, course of disease, side effects of drugs and interactions

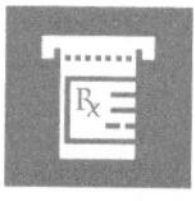

MEDICATIONS

DRUG(S) OF CHOICE

ANTITUBERCULOUS MEDICATIONS

- First line agents used in CNS TB are:
  - ◊ Isoniazid (INH) 300 mg/day (3-10 mg/kg) po or IM
  - ◊ Rifampicin (RIF) 450-600 mg/day (10 mg/kg) po
  - ◊ Ethambutol (ETB) 15 mg/kg po
  - ◊ Pyrazinamide (PZA). 20 30 mg/kg po
- Second line drugs include:
  - ◊ Streptomycin (SM) 1 gm/day (20-25 mg/kg) IM
  - ◊ Ethionamide 15 mg/kg po
- Other drugs: kanamycin, capreomycin, cycloserine, ciprofloxacin, and ofloxacin
- Usual regimen: INH + RIF + PZA for 3 to 4 months followed by INH + RIF for 15-18 months.
- Other drugs added when resistance suspected
- Continue ATT (anti-tuberculous therapy) 1.5-3 years for optimal response
- Intrathecal SM is controversial

CORTICOSTEROIDS

- Steroids are used in patients with raised ICP or severe cerebral edema as noted on the CT scan (dexamethasone 4 mg q6h IV)
- Usually a short course is needed, occasionally long term steroids are essential
- Useful in children < 1 year or in severely ill children with TBM
- Intrathecal steroids useful in patients with spinal block due to spinal arachnoiditis

ANTICONVULSANTS

- High incidence of seizures in tuberculomas mandates the routine use of anticonvulsants
- Phenytoin or carbamazepine commonly used. Dosage adjusted according to serum levels.

Contraindications:

- INH - liver disease
- RIF - patient taking retrovirals, jaundice, pregnancy
- PZA - liver disease
- SM - pregnancy
- ETB - optic neuritis

Precautions:

- INH - peripheral neuritis, psychosis, lupus syndrome, hepatitis, convulsions, optic neuritis
- RIF - hepatitis, colors urine, gastric symptoms
- PZA - hepatitis, may increase uric acid
- SM - ototoxicity and nephrotoxicity
- ETB - optic neuritis, color blindness, peripheral neuritis
- Ultra-short chemotherapy (2 months of triple therapy and 4 month of double therapy) not recommended

Significant possible interactions: INH can interact with phenytoin metabolism and produce toxicity

ALTERNATIVE DRUGS

- Rifabutin instead of RIF in patients taking retroviral drugs
- Add quinolone (e.g., ciprofloxacin) if response is partial in tuberculoma

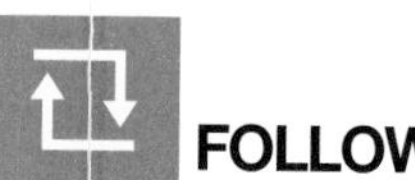

FOLLOWUP

PATIENT MONITORING

- Liver enzymes
- Monthly vision and color tests if on ETB
- Anticonvulsant medication serum levels
- Head circumference in children with TBM
- Contrast enhanced CT scan in patients with tuberculoma on medical treatment every 3 to 6 months until complete resolution
- Hormonal evaluation (e.g., TSH, cortisol, prolactin, etc.) in patients with pituitary TB

PREVENTION/AVOIDANCE

- Prevention of pulmonary TB
- Aggressive and complete ATT to prevent recurrence

POSSIBLE COMPLICATIONS

- Visual deterioration
- Focal deficits
- Cognitive deterioration
- Paraplegia
- Hormonal deficiencies
- Shunt block
- Shunt infection
- Systemic side effects of ATT

EXPECTED COURSE/PROGNOSIS

- Initial reports of 10 to 27% mortality have improved in recent times in intracranial tuberculomas
- In TBM prognosis depends on level of consciousness on initial presentation, presence and degree of exudates and presence of hydrocephalus

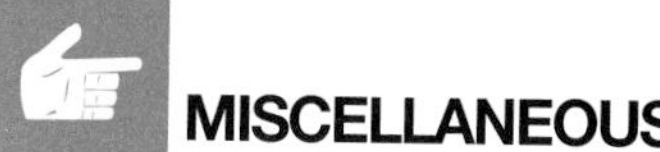

MISCELLANEOUS

ASSOCIATED CONDITIONS

- HIV
- Deep cerebral infarcts
- TB osteomyelitis of spine

AGE-RELATED FACTORS

Pediatric: Emergent surgical intervention if has signs of raised ICP in TBM
Geriatric: Cerebral metastases can mimic tuberculomas on imaging studies. Mortality higher in elderly with TBM.
Others: N/A

PREGNANCY

- Avoid streptomycin
- Anticonvulsants to be properly chosen
- Breast feeding is okay

SYNONYMS N/A

ICD-9-CM

013.0 Tuberculous meningitis
013.2 Tuberculoma of brain
013.4 Tuberculoma of spinal cord

SEE ALSO

Tuberculosis

OTHER NOTES

Clinical Grading for TBM:

Grade	Symptoms	Mortality
I	Headaches, vomiting, fever with normal sensorium and no neurodeficits	20%
II	Normal sensorium with neurodeficits	35%
III	Altered sensorium but easily arousable	50%
IV	Deeply comatose, decerebrate or decorticate posturing	100%

ABBREVIATIONS

TBM = tuberculous meningitis
ICP = intracranial pressure
CT = computerized tomography
ATT = anti-tuberculous therapy
CSF= cerebrospinal fluid
SOL = space occupying lesion
PPD = purified protein derivative
ESR = erythrocyte sedimentation rate
VA = ventriculo-atrial
VP = ventriculo-peritoneal
PCR = polymerase chain reaction

REFERENCES

- Palur R, Rajshekhar V, Chandy MJ, Joseph T, Abraham J. Shunt surgery for hydrocephalus in tuberculous meningitis: a long-term follow-up study. J Neurosurg 1991;74(1):64-9

Web references: 0 available at www.5mcc.com
Illustrations N/A

Author(s):
Milind Deogaonkar, MD

BASICS

DESCRIPTION A common infection transmitted by inhaling airborne bacilli from a person with active tuberculosis (TB). The bacilli multiply in the alveolus and are carried by macrophages, lymphatics and blood to distant sites (eg. lung pleura, brain, kidney and bone). Tissue hypersensitivity usually halts infection within 10 weeks.

- Latent tuberculosis infection (LTBI) is asymptomatic, noninfectious and usually detected by a positive skin test (evidence of prior tuberculosis infection by PPD or CXR, but acid-fast bacilli (AFB) smear and culture are negative and CXR does not suggest active TB).
- TB: active disease - occurs in 10% of infected individuals without preventive therapy. Chance of disease increases with immunosuppression and is highest for all individuals within 2 years after infection - 85% of cases are pulmonary which is infectious.
- Recrudescent TB: active disease occurring after a period of latent asymptomatic infection

System(s) affected: Hemic/Lymphatic/Immunologic, Pulmonary

Genetics: N/A

Incidence/Prevalence in USA:
- 15 million have latent infection

Predominant age:
- Primary infection - any age, especially pediatric
- Recrudescent disease - adults and elderly

Predominant sex: Male > Female

SIGNS & SYMPTOMS None

CAUSES *Mycobacterium tuberculosis*, *Mycobacterium bovis*, and *Mycobacterium africanum*

RISK FACTORS
- Urban, homeless
- Minority
- Migrant workers
- Institutional (eg, prison, nursing home)
- Close contact with infected individual
- Immigrant within 5 years (Asia, Africa, Latin America)
- Healthcare workers
- HIV infection immunosuppression

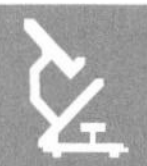

DIAGNOSIS

DIFFERENTIAL DIAGNOSIS Fungal infections, especially other atypical Mycobacteria or Nocardia

LABORATORY
- None routinely recommended

Drugs that may alter lab results:
- BCG: false-positive skin test but unreliable and should not influence decision to treat LTBI
- Steroids: false-negative skin test
- Measles vaccine may suppress tuberculin activity; recommend simultaneous PPD and measles vaccine; if not simultaneous defer PPD 4-6 weeks after measles vaccine

Disorders that may alter lab results: False-negative skin test: Recent viral infections, new (<10 weeks) infection, severe malnutrition, HIV, anergy, age < 6 months, overwhelming TB

PATHOLOGICAL FINDINGS N/A

SPECIAL TESTS HIV test recommended to assess risk for active TB

IMAGING
- CXR required to rule out TB in asymptomatic infected persons
- CT chest - good sensitivity

DIAGNOSTIC PROCEDURES
- PPD: 5 units (0.1cc) intermediate strength intradermal volar forearm. Measure induration at 48-72 hrs.
  - ◊ PPD positive if induration:
    - > 5 mm and HIV infection (or suspected), immunosuppressed, recent close TB contact, clinical evidence of active or old disease on chest x-ray
    - > 10 mm and age < 4 yrs or other risk factors
    - > 15 mm and age > 4 yrs and no risk factors
  - ◊ PPD negative if induration:
    - < 5 mm on initial test and, if indicated, on second test. Utilize 2-step test if patient has had no recent PPD, age > 55 years, nursing home resident, prison inmate, or healthcare worker (administer a second intradermal test 1-3 weeks after initial test; measure and interpret as usual)
- Multiple puncture test (TINE) not recommended

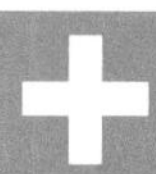

TREATMENT

APPROPRIATE HEALTH CARE
- Treat LTBI at any age if: HIV, close contact, recent converter (< 2 years), IV drug use, abnormal CXR, high risk medical condition or other high risk group. Use INH daily for 9 months (preferred) or accepted alternative:
  - ◊ INH twice weekly for 9 months with DOT (directly observed treatment)
  - ◊ INH daily or twice weekly for 6 months with DOT
  - ◊ Rifampin plus pyrazinamide daily for 2 months or twice weekly for 2-3 months; special monitoring for hepatic toxicity required (preferred if INH resistance)
  - ◊ Rifampin daily for 4 months
- For inactive pulmonary TB on chest x-ray, use INH for 9 months
- Consider INH resistance
- Recommend DOT if adherence not assured

GENERAL MEASURES Careful reevaluation required. Only change to twice weekly dosing if using DOT.

SURGICAL MEASURES N/A

ACTIVITY
- As tolerated
- No isolation required

DIET Regular. Consider pyridoxine (10-50 mg/day) supplement.

PATIENT EDUCATION
- Teach pathogenesis, emphasize importance of drug therapy, warn of effects and/or interactions, and find contacts
- Inform local health department

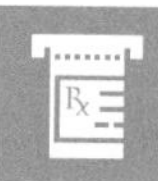

MEDICATIONS

DRUG(S) OF CHOICE

- Isoniazid (INH) - scored tabs 100 mg, 300 mg or syrup 10 mg/mL
  - ◊ Daily dose: adult 300 mg; pediatric 10-20 mg/kg (maximum 300 mg)
  - ◊ Twice weekly: adult 15 mg/kg; pediatric 20-40 mg/kg (maximum 900 mg)
  - ◊ Consider pyridoxine 10-50 mg/day
- Rifampin (RIF) capsules (150/300 or syrup 10 mg/mL)
  - ◊ Daily dose: adult 600 mg; pediatric dose 10-20 mg/kg (maximum 600 mg)
  - ◊ Twice weekly: adult 600 mg; pediatric 10-20 mg/kg (maximum 600 mg)
- Pyrazinamide (PZA), scored 500 mg
  - ◊ Daily dose: adult 15-25 mg/kg (maximum 2 gm); pediatric 15-30 mg/kg (maximum 2 gm)
  - ◊ Twice weekly: adult 50 mg/kg; pediatric 50 mg/kg (maximum 4 gm)
- Rifabutin capsules 150 mg
  - ◊ Daily dose: adult 300 mg
  - ◊ Twice weekly: adult 300 mg

Contraindications: N/A

Precautions:

- INH, RIF or PZA may cause hepatitis
- Follow liver function if the patient has history of liver dysfunction or new signs develop
- RIF - colors urine, tears and secretions orange. Can permanently stain contact lenses.
- INH - peripheral neuritis and hypersensitivity possible. Consider pyridoxine.
- PZA - may increase uric acid

Significant possible interactions: RIF alters the level of phenytoin (Dilantin), antivirals and other drugs metabolized by the liver and may inactivate birth control pills (recommend a barrier method)

ALTERNATIVE DRUGS N/A

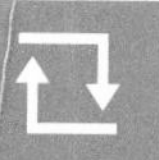

FOLLOWUP

PATIENT MONITORING

- During preventive therapy (for LTBI) - monthly visits to assess adherence to regimen and monitor for hepatitis and neuropathy
- If patient remains asymptomatic, a repeat CXR is not needed
- Check liver enzymes if symptomatic, HIV positive, chronic liver disease, alcohol use, pregnant or postpartum, and modify drugs if needed
- RIF plus PZA treatment of LTBI requires special monitoring - dispense only 2 week supply of RIF-PZA. Reevaluate in person at 2, 4, 6, and 8 weeks; test liver enzymes and bilirubin at baseline 2, 4, 6 weeks. Stop treatment if bilirubin above normal or symptoms of hepatitis with enzymes above normal or enzymes 5 times normal.

PREVENTION/AVOIDANCE

- Targeted tuberculin testing for high risk groups only
- Identify and treat contagious persons

POSSIBLE COMPLICATIONS

- Recrudescent TB

EXPECTED COURSE/PROGNOSIS

Generally few complications and full resolution if drugs taken for full course as prescribed

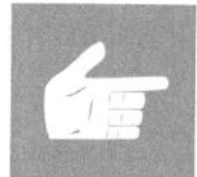

MISCELLANEOUS

ASSOCIATED CONDITIONS HIV infection (see special protocols)

AGE-RELATED FACTORS

Pediatric:

- Protocol for newborn with mother/household contact with infection or disease
  - ◊ If mother or household contact has LTBI: skin test all household contacts and treat any with positive PPD
  - ◊ If contact has abnormal CXR: separate infant until infectious status known; if not contagious, monitor infant PPD
  - ◊ If mother with disease and possibly contagious: evaluate infant for congenital TB and test for HIV; separate newborn until mother is noninfectious
  - ◊ If congenital TB suspected, treat
  - ◊ If no congenital disease, start INH and repeat PPD after 3-4 months. If positive, reassess infant and finish 9 months INH. If PPD is negative, and source is noninfectious, stop INH and monitor infant.
- Consider BCG

Geriatric:

- Should have a PPD prior to entering a chronic-care facility using two step protocols
- Side effects of INH more pronounced

Others: N/A

PREGNANCY

- Avoid pyrazinamide
- Treat LTBI in pregnancy if recent infection or HIV positive (use INH with pyridoxine and monitor liver enzymes) otherwise may postpone until postpartum
- Breast-feeding okay while taking TB drugs

SYNONYMS N/A

ICD-9-CM

795.5 Non-specific reaction to tuberculin skin test without active tuberculosis (PPD positive)

SEE ALSO

Tuberculosis

OTHER NOTES

- BCG vaccine, live attenuated *Mycobacterium bovis*. Used more commonly in developing countries to prevent complications of TB

ABBREVIATIONS

PPD = purified protein derivative
BCG = Bacillus Calmette-Guérin
DOT = directly observed treatment
LTBI = latent tuberculosis infection

REFERENCES

- American Thoracic Society. Targeted tuberculin testing and treatment of latent tuberculosis infection. Am J Respir Crit Care Med 2000;161:S221-S247
- Centers for Disease Control: Screening for tuberculosis and tuberculosis infection in high-risk populations. MMWR 2000;49(No.RR-6):1-51
- American Thoracic Society. Treatment of tuberculosis and tuberculosis infections in adults and children. Am J Respir Crit Care Med 1994;149:1359-1374
- Report of the Committee on Infectious Diseases (Red Book). Elk Grove Village, Ill, American Academy of Pediatrics, 1997
- Centers for Disease Control. Core curriculum on tuberculosis - what the clinician should know, 1994
- Dutt AK. Tuberculosis. Part 1 and 2. Disease-A-Month 1997;43(3 & 4)
- CDC Prevention and treatment of tuberculosis among patients infected with human immunodeficiency virus: principles and revised recommendations. MMWR 1998;47(No. RR-20)

Web references: 0 available at www.5mcc.com

Illustrations N/A

Author(s):

Gregory Snyder, MD

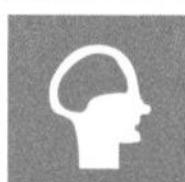

BASICS

DESCRIPTION One of the neurocutaneous syndromes (phakomatoses). A genetic developmental disorder with variable presentations, a broad clinical spectrum and multi-organ involvement. Organ systems may be few and subtle, but can encompass multiple types of cutaneous lesions and tumor formation in the central nervous system, skin, retina, heart, lung, viscera, liver, kidney, bone, teeth and nails. Other phakomatoses include neurofibromatosis, Sturge-Weber disease, von Hippel-Lindau syndrome, and ataxia-telangiectasia.

System(s) affected: Cardiovascular, Musculoskeletal, Nervous, Pulmonary, Renal/Urologic, Skin/Exocrine

Genetics:
- Autosomal dominant with variable penetrance
- Two thirds are the result of a new gene mutation
- Two chromosomal loci are mapped; TSC1 (locus 9q34) and TSC2 (locus 16p13.3)

Incidence/Prevalence in USA: Reported to affect 1 in 6,000 in the general population

Predominant age: Clinical expression is variable, and diagnosis may be delayed. Usually diagnosed during the first decade.

Predominant sex: Male = Female (but autism more common in males)

SIGNS & SYMPTOMS
- Most cases have more than one of the following: Angiofibromata (labeled as adenoma sebaceum and ranging from 0.1-1.0 cm) and often present as facial lesions in a "butterfly" distribution (80%)
  - ◊ Hypopigmented areas mainly on trunk and extremities often the first sign (ash-leaf spots). Present at birth or shortly after (50%).
  - ◊ Seizure disorders including myoclonic (90%)
  - ◊ Renal cysts (50-80%)
  - ◊ Pulmonary lymphangiomatosis (<10%)
  - ◊ CNS periventricular calcifications (50-80%)
  - ◊ Retinal astrocytomas and hamartomas (50-80%)
  - ◊ Cardiac rhabdomyomas (50%)
  - ◊ Mental retardation (60-70%)
  - ◊ Autism (10-20%)
  - ◊ Ungual fibromas, multiple (20%)
  - ◊ Dental pits
  - ◊ Liver hamartomas (10%)

CAUSES Congenital

RISK FACTORS Family history

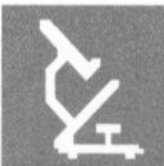

DIAGNOSIS

DIFFERENTIAL DIAGNOSIS
- Polycystic kidney disease, renal hamartomas
- Other causes of seizure disorders, mental retardation, autistic behavior, traumatic ungual fibromata
- Other neurocutaneous syndromes (phakomatoses)

LABORATORY
- Present day diagnostic criteria mainly confined to clinical evaluations
- Abnormal electroencephalogram
- Search for reliable molecular marker and gene is promising

Drugs that may alter lab results: N/A

Disorders that may alter lab results: N/A

PATHOLOGICAL FINDINGS
- Nodular lesions made up largely of irregular groups of glial fibrils, ganglion cells and atypical cells seeming to result from faults in developing tissue combinations as in hamartomas
- Lesions may be sparse at birth
- Calcification of subependymal lesions may not occur until several months after birth
- Facial angiofibromas, ungual fibromas, renal angiomyolipomas are quite specific lesions which may develop months after birth
- 1% present with tuberous sclerosis lymphangioleiomyomatosis and are usually women of reproductive age
- Not practical to have age specific criteria

SPECIAL TESTS Must rely on clinical diagnostic criteria pending development of reliable molecular marker

IMAGING
- Magnetic resonance imaging (MRI)and CT scanning have become major diagnostic techniques
- With gadolinium enhancement, MRI provides more detailed imaging of characteristic subependymal nodules and cortical white matter tubers
- Fetal cardiac rhabdomyomas can be seen in late gestation sonography.

DIAGNOSTIC PROCEDURES
- Woods lamp evaluation for ash-leaf spots.
- EEG
- Biopsy of indeterminate lesions
- MRI with gadolinium contrast
- Renal CT, ultrasound
- Echocardiography
- Molecular testing generally available on research basis only, although it is available on a clinical basis to families with known TSC1 or TSC2 mutation.

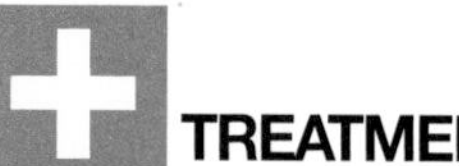

TREATMENT

APPROPRIATE HEALTH CARE
Outpatient care, except for complications for severely involved manifestations or uncontrolled seizures

GENERAL MEASURES
- Team approach with neurological, orthopedic, surgical and radiological involvement
- Physical, occupational and speech therapy
- Social work for home care, and vocational training support
- Periodic reassessment in at-risk families
- Genetic counseling for patient and family
- Neurosurgical consideration for uncontrollable seizures

SURGICAL MEASURES Surgical excision of tumors where and when appropriate

ACTIVITY Determined by degree and complexity of involvement

DIET No restrictions. A ketogenic diet has been used for seizure control.

PATIENT EDUCATION
- Precautions related to seizures
- Updated information available from: National Tuberous Sclerosis Association, Inc., 8181 Professional Place, Suite 110, Landover, MD 20785 (800) 225-6872, E-mail ntsa@ntsa.org, Web site www.ntsa.org

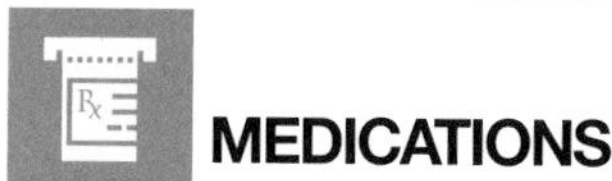

MEDICATIONS

DRUG(S) OF CHOICE
- Anticonvulsants for seizure control
- Antibiotic prophylaxis for surgery if indicated

Contraindications: N/A

Precautions: Refer to manufacturer's profile of each drug

Significant possible interactions:
- Knowledge of anticonvulsant used is necessary to avoid drug interactions especially with antibiotics
- Refer to manufacturer's profile of each drug

ALTERNATIVE DRUGS N/A

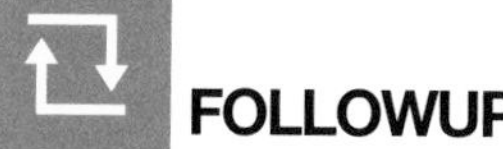

FOLLOWUP

PATIENT MONITORING
- Clinical features of proband periodically reviewed and updated
- Periodic reassessment of at-risk individuals

PREVENTION/AVOIDANCE Genetic counseling

POSSIBLE COMPLICATIONS See Signs and Symptoms

EXPECTED COURSE/PROGNOSIS
Variable; decreased longevity compared to general population

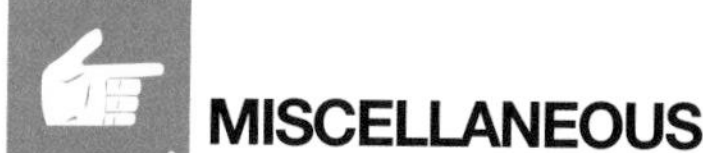

MISCELLANEOUS

ASSOCIATED CONDITIONS N/A

AGE-RELATED FACTORS
Pediatric: N/A
Geriatric: N/A
Others: Stigmata may be present at, or shortly after birth or may become apparent in late childhood or adulthood

PREGNANCY
- Genetic counseling
- Prenatal testing by ultrasonography for tumors is available, but sensitivity is unknown. Prenatal DNA analysis is available to families previously enrolled in a research protocol.

SYNONYMS Bourneville disease

ICD-9-CM
759.5 Tuberous sclerosis

SEE ALSO
Ataxia-telangiectasia
Neurofibromatosis (Types 1 & 2)
Sturge-Weber disease
von Hippel-Lindau disease

OTHER NOTES N/A

ABBREVIATIONS
- TS = tuberous sclerosis
- TSC = tuberous sclerosis complex

REFERENCES

- Aicardi J. Tuberous Sclerosis. International Pediatrics 1993;8:2:171-175
- Perspective Newsletter, National Tuberous Sclerosis Association, Inc., Spring/Summer/Fall/ Winter Publications
- Roach ES, DiMario FJ, Kandt RS, Northup H. Tuberous sclerosis consensus conference: recommendations for diagnostic evaluation. J Child Neurol 1999;14(6):401-7
- Caldemeyer KS, Mirowski GW. Tuberous Sclerosis. Part 1 Clinical and central nervous system findings. J Am Acad Dermatol 2001;45(3):448-9
- Baker P, Piven J, Sato Y. Autism and tuberous sclerosis complex: prevalence and clinical features J Autism Dev Disord 1998;28:279-85

Web references: 2 available at www.5mcc.com
Illustrations N/A

Author(s):
Nuhad D. Dinno, MD

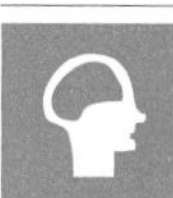

BASICS

DESCRIPTION Acute infection with Francisella tularensis. Incubation averages 3-4 days; ranges from 1-21 days. May be ulceroglandular, glandular, typhoidal, oculoglandular, or oropharyngeal.
System(s) affected: Cardiovascular, Hemic/Lymphatic/Immunologic, Pulmonary, Skin/Exocrine
Genetics: N/A
Incidence/Prevalence in USA: (Incidence) 0.1 per 100,000
Predominant age: All ages
Predominant sex: Male > Female

SIGNS & SYMPTOMS
- Nearly all cases have fever, chills, fatigue, malaise
- Ulceroglandular (3/4 of cases)
  - ◊ Non-healing ulcer
  - ◊ Regional adenopathy
  - ◊ Failure of cephalosporin treatment
- Glandular
  - ◊ Localized adenopathy
  - ◊ No ulcer
- Typhoidal
  - ◊ Systemic febrile illness
  - ◊ Fulminating sepsis
  - ◊ Pleuropulmonary disease
  - ◊ No ulcer
- Oropharyngeal
  - ◊ Exudative pharyngitis
  - ◊ Membranous pharyngitis
  - ◊ Cervical adenopathy
- Oculoglandular
  - ◊ Purulent conjunctivitis
  - ◊ Preauricular adenopathy
  - ◊ Cervical adenopathy

CAUSES
- Inoculation of F. tularensis via:
  - ◊ Tick bite
  - ◊ Deer fly bite
  - ◊ Cat bite
  - ◊ Aerosol inhalation
  - ◊ Contact with infected carcass (can penetrate unbroken skin)
  - ◊ Ingestion

RISK FACTORS
- Location in endemic area; > 50% USA cases in AR, MO, OK, TN, TX; also in SD, MT, TN, KS, CO, IL
- Outdoor work
- Rural residence
- Game handling
- Laboratory work
- Considered a potential bioweapon

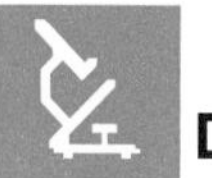

DIAGNOSIS

DIFFERENTIAL DIAGNOSIS
- Ulceroglandular/glandular
  - ◊ Staphylococcal infections
  - ◊ Streptococcal infections
  - ◊ Cat-scratch disease
  - ◊ Pasteurella infections
  - ◊ Lymphogranuloma venereum
  - ◊ Sporotrichosis
  - ◊ Plague
  - ◊ Toxoplasmosis
- Typhoidal
  - ◊ Legionellosis
  - ◊ Rocky Mountain spotted fever
  - ◊ Ehrlichiosis
  - ◊ Borreliosis (including Lyme disease)
  - ◊ Infectious mononucleosis
  - ◊ Non-typhoid salmonellosis
  - ◊ Typhoid fever
  - ◊ Brucellosis
  - ◊ Q fever
  - ◊ Psittacosis
  - ◊ Tick-borne typhus
  - ◊ Viral pneumonia
- Oropharyngeal
  - ◊ Streptococcal pharyngitis
  - ◊ Viral pharyngitis
  - ◊ Diphtheric pharyngitis
  - ◊ Infectious mononucleosis

LABORATORY
- Fourfold rise in antibody titer (peak in 4-8 weeks)
- Convalescent titer of 160 or greater
- Delayed growth on specific media or blood culture
- Elevated ESR
- Normal WBC, left shift
- PCR, investigational

Drugs that may alter lab results: N/A

Disorders that may alter lab results: Brucella antibodies may cross-react

PATHOLOGICAL FINDINGS
- Necrotic areas in liver, spleen, other organs
- Caseating granulomata
- Microscopic foci with PMNs, macrophages, giant cells

SPECIAL TESTS
- Referral to specialized lab
- Pleomorphic Gram-negative coccobacilli
- Metabolic profile of isolate
- Specific immunofluorescent stain
- Culture ulcer

IMAGING Chest x-ray may show ill-defined infiltrates, lobar consolidation, or pleural effusion

DIAGNOSTIC PROCEDURES
- Lymph node aspiration
- Thoracentesis
- Thorough history of patient's contact with wild rodents or exposure to arthropod vectors

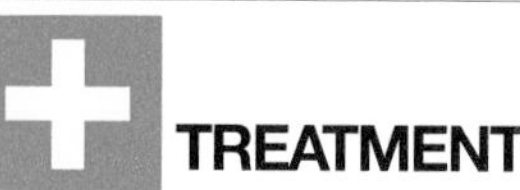

TREATMENT

APPROPRIATE HEALTH CARE Inpatient or outpatient depending on severity.

GENERAL MEASURES
- Isolation not needed for patient, but handle secretions carefully
- Hydration, fever control, antibiotics
- Wet saline dressings for skin lesions
- Recovery requires intact cell-mediated immunity

SURGICAL MEASURES Incision and drainage of abscesses

ACTIVITY As tolerated

DIET As tolerated, high caloric, easily digestible

PATIENT EDUCATION
- Person-to-person transmission not documented
- See Prevention/Avoidance
- Vaccine for high-risk persons; contact CDC

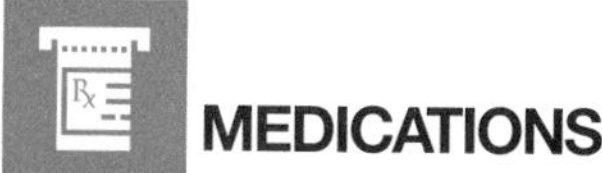

MEDICATIONS

DRUG(S) OF CHOICE
- Streptomycin 15-20 mg/kg IM per day, divided bid for 7-14 days (may be difficult to obtain)
- Gentamicin - 3-5 mg/kg/day divided bid dosing may be possible

Contraindications:
- Known hypersensitivity, pregnancy
- Doxycycline or ciprofloxacin are considered drugs of choice in mass casualty situation (such as biowarfare). Prophylactic use in postexposure period is suggested, even in children.

Precautions:
- Long-term therapy may produce eighth nerve damage
- Reduce dose for known renal dysfunction
- Long-term therapy may produce renal dysfunction
- Use with care post-anesthesia (respiratory paralysis), and in patients with myasthenia gravis

Significant possible interactions: Other aminoglycosides, cephaloridine, polymyxin B, amphotericin B, colistin, muscle relaxants, paralyzing anesthetic agents

ALTERNATIVE DRUGS
- Fluoroquinolones - successful treatment reports increasing. More success reported in USA. Maybe serovar specific.
- Chloramphenicol - may be difficult to obtain
- Tetracyclines - associated with higher relapse rate
- 3rd generation cephalosporins - high relapse rate or failure rate

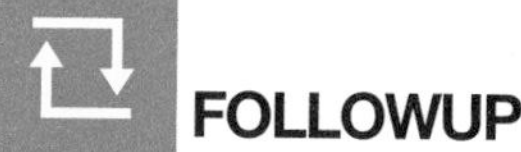

FOLLOWUP

PATIENT MONITORING
- Monitor eighth nerve function in long-term therapy
- Monitor renal function in long-term therapy

PREVENTION/AVOIDANCE
- Tick repellents
- Remove tick by grasping near mouthparts
- Avoid squeezing body of embedded tick
- Wear gloves while dressing game
- Avoid contact if game appeared ill
- Lab workers - vaccine possibly protective. Wear protective hoods.
- Cook wild game thoroughly

POSSIBLE COMPLICATIONS
- Lung abscess
- Adult respiratory distress syndrome
- Hepatic dysfunction
- Rhabdomyolysis
- Renal failure
- Osteomyelitis, meningitis, endocarditis, pericarditis, peritonitis
- Mediastinitis

EXPECTED COURSE/PROGNOSIS
- Cure complete if treated early and vigorously
- Immunity is lifelong
- Mortality is 1-3%, higher in typhoidal-type disease

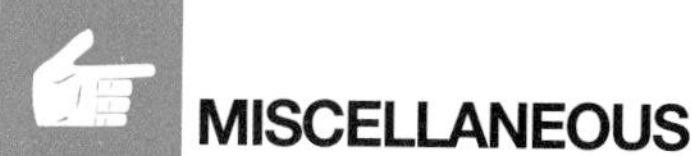

MISCELLANEOUS

ASSOCIATED CONDITIONS
- Other arthropod-borne diseases
- Tularemic conjunctivitis
- Bacteremia
- Atypical pneumonia

AGE-RELATED FACTORS
Pediatric: Often affected
Geriatric: Complications more likely, mortality rate higher
Others: More likely to occur in outdoor-type, young adult males

PREGNANCY
Streptomycin may cause fetal 8th nerve damage

SYNONYMS
- Rabbit fever
- Deer-fly fever
- Pasteurella tularensis
- Bacterium tularense
- Tick fever
- Ohara disease
- Francis disease

ICD-9-CM
021.9 Unspecified tularemia

SEE ALSO
Bartonella infections
Diphtheria
Ehrlichiosis
Lymphogranuloma venereum
Plague
Psittacosis
Q fever
Rocky Mountain spotted fever
Toxoplasmosis
Typhus fevers

OTHER NOTES
Incidence higher in summer and fall. Has received mention as a biological weapon.

ABBREVIATIONS
N/A

REFERENCES

- Mandell GL, Bennett JE, Dolin R, eds. Principles and Practice of Infectious Diseases. 5th Ed. New York, Churchill Livingstone, 2000
- Feigin RD, Cherry JD. Textbook of Pediatric Infectious Disease. 4th Ed. Philadelphia, W.B. Saunders Co., 1998
- Dennis DT, Inglesby TV, Henderson DA, et al. Tularemia as a biological weapon: medical and public health management. JAMA 2001;285(21):2763-73

Web references: 1 available at www.5mcc.com
Illustrations N/A

Author(s):
J. Gregory Elders, MD

BASICS

DESCRIPTION Edema of hands and feet and excess skin of the neck (webbing) are presenting features during infancy. As children, girls are short and may have left sided heart or aortic abnormalities. Primary amenorrhea or delayed onset of puberty with short stature are important clues during adolescence.
System(s) affected: Cardiovascular, Endocrine/Metabolic, Musculoskeletal, Nervous, Renal/Urologic, Reproductive
Genetics: usually sporadic
Incidence/Prevalence in USA: 40 per 100,000 female births
Predominant age: All ages
Predominant sex: Female only

SIGNS & SYMPTOMS
Frequencies are for classic 45,X and vary with other chromosomal abnormalities associated with Turner syndrome
- Short stature (98%)
- Gonadal dysgenesis (95%)
- Lymphedema (70%)
- Broad chest (75%)
- Hypoplastic, wide-spaced nipples (78%)
- Prominent, anomalous ears (70%)
- High palate (82%)
- Short neck (80%)
- Webbing of neck (65%)
- Low hairline (80%)
- Cubitus valgus (75%)
- Short fourth metacarpal (65%)
- Nail hypoplasia (75%)
- Excess nevi (70%)
- Renal anomalies (60%)
- Heart malformations (30%)
- Hearing impairment (70%)

CAUSES Monosomy for all or part of the X chromosome can result in symptoms consistent with Turner syndrome

RISK FACTORS Familial chromosome translocations involving the X chromosome increase the risk of conceiving a child with Turner syndrome

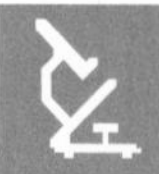

DIAGNOSIS

DIFFERENTIAL DIAGNOSIS
- Short stature
  - ◊ Noonan syndrome
  - ◊ Hypothyroidism
  - ◊ Familial short stature
  - ◊ Léri-Weill syndrome
  - ◊ Brachydactyly E
  - ◊ Growth hormone deficiency
  - ◊ Glucocorticoid excess
  - ◊ Klippel-Feil anomaly
  - ◊ Short stature due to chronic disease
- Amenorrhea or delayed puberty
  - ◊ Pure gonadal dysgenesis
  - ◊ Stein-Leventhal syndrome
  - ◊ Primary/secondary amenorrhea
- Lymphedema
  - ◊ Hereditary congenital lymphedema
  - ◊ Milroy disease
  - ◊ Lymphedema with recurrent cholestasis
  - ◊ Lymphedema with intestinal lymphangiectasia
- Other
  - ◊ Multiple pterygium syndrome
  - ◊ Pseudo-hypoparathyroid

LABORATORY
- Chromosome analysis (a buccal smear is not adequate to rule out Turner)
- At puberty FSH and LH levels may approach castration levels. FSH may be transiently high in infancy

Drugs that may alter lab results: N/A

Disorders that may alter lab results: N/A

PATHOLOGICAL FINDINGS
- Ovarian dysgenesis (> 90%)
- Renal: horseshoe kidney, double collecting system (60%)
- Cardiac: bicuspid aortic valve, coarctation of aorta, valvular aortic stenosis (70% with heart defects also have coarctation)
- Bone dysplasia (> 50%)
- Gonadoblastomas in X/XY mosaics

SPECIAL TESTS
- Upper/lower extremity blood pressures
- ECG

IMAGING
- Renal ultrasound
- Cardiac ultrasound

DIAGNOSTIC PROCEDURES N/A

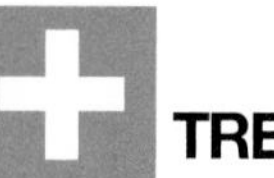

TREATMENT

APPROPRIATE HEALTH CARE Outpatient

GENERAL MEASURES
Once diagnosis is confirmed by karyotype, the following measures are appropriate:
- Cardiology evaluation to include upper and lower extremity blood pressures, and echocardiography. If an abnormality exists, prophylactic antibiotics may be indicated (e.g., dental procedures).
- Renal ultrasound or intravenous pyelography
- Thyroid function test and antithyroid antibodies
- Routine hearing examination
- Treat gonadal failure in girls who do not enter puberty spontaneously
  - ◊ Replacement therapy: begin with one to two years of low dose estrogen followed by larger dose estrogens cycled with progesterone
  - ◊ Maintenance therapy: Birth control pills, after menses and secondary sexual characteristics are established. Continue into the late forties.
  - ◊ Routine gynecologic evaluation indicated
  - ◊ Infertility is the general rule, but alternatives such as in vitro fertilization and embryo transfer may be options
- Growth retardation has been managed with sex hormone replacement, anabolic agents, and human recombinant growth hormone (hrGH). Some patients increase final height attainment with hrGH treatment. Start hrGH therapy (0.05 mg/kg SC qDay) before significant growth deceleration occurs (between 3-10 years of age).
- Intelligence is usually normal. Problems may exist in non-verbal areas such as imagining objects in relationship to one another. If concerns about school performance arise, they should be evaluated and treated.
- Regular physician visits are recommended. Be aware of the social and emotional problems associated with issues such as short stature and infertility.

SURGICAL MEASURES
- Removal of gonads in X/XY individuals
- Physical appearance may be enhanced by plastic surgery for inner canthal folds, protruding auricles and webbed neck.

ACTIVITY Normal other than limitations that may be placed on individuals with similar cardiac or renal abnormalities.

DIET Normal, but there is a tendency toward obesity

PATIENT EDUCATION
- Families and patients need a thorough explanation of the condition and its management, especially in regards to sexual development and growth. Jones/Smith suggest advising patient between age 8 and adolescence that she will probably not bear children.
- Excellent patient educational materials include:
  - ◊ Plumridge D: Good things come in small packages: the whys and hows of Turner Syndrome. Crippled Children's Division, University of Oregon Health Sciences Center, Portland, OR 97203.
  - ◊ Rieser PA, Underwood LE: Turner syndrome: a guide for families. Turner Syndrome Society, York University, ASB 006, 4700 Keele St., Downsview, Ontario, Canada, M3J 1P3, (416)667-3773 or Turner Syndrome Society, 3539 Tonkawood Rd., Minnetonka, MN 55345, (612)938-3118

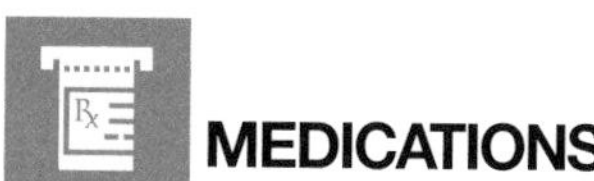

MEDICATIONS

DRUG(S) OF CHOICE N/A
Contraindications: N/A
Precautions: N/A
Significant possible interactions: N/A

ALTERNATIVE DRUGS N/A

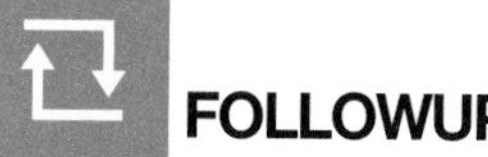

FOLLOWUP

PATIENT MONITORING
- Regular measurement of growth parameters
- Regular blood pressure checks
- Annual urinalysis if renal abnormality is present
- Monitor for signs of hypothyroidism
- Regular hearing testing
- Regular eye exams
- Consider screening for occult blood loss
- Regular cardiac exams with sonography of the aortic root in adult women

PREVENTION/AVOIDANCE Prenatal detection is available for high risk couples (who carry chromosomal translocations or who have had an affected child). There is no in utero treatment, but pregnancy termination is an option if a fetus with Turner syndrome is identified

POSSIBLE COMPLICATIONS Complications are related to associated abnormalities

EXPECTED COURSE/PROGNOSIS
Most girls with Turner syndrome can be expected to lead reasonably normal lives with appropriate medical management

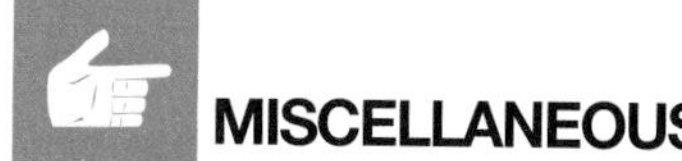

MISCELLANEOUS

ASSOCIATED CONDITIONS
- Hashimoto thyroiditis
- Hypothyroidism
- Alopecia
- Vitiligo
- Gastrointestinal vascular malformations
- Gastrointestinal disorders
- Carbohydrate intolerance
- Aortic dissection in adults
- Deafness

AGE-RELATED FACTORS
Pediatric: N/A
Geriatric: N/A
Others: N/A

PREGNANCY N/A

SYNONYMS
- Ullrich-Turner syndrome
- Bonnevie-Ullrich
- XO syndrome
- Monosomy X
- Short stature-sexual infantilism
- Gonadal dysgenesis

ICD-9-CM
758.6 Gonadal dysgenesis

SEE ALSO
Amenorrhea
Coarctation of the aorta
Hypothyroidism, adult
Thyroiditis

OTHER NOTES N/A

ABBREVIATIONS N/A

REFERENCES

- Frias JL, Davenport ML. The Committee on Genetics and the Section on Endocrinology. Health Supervision for Children With Turner Syndrome. Pediatrics 2003; 111: 692-702.
- Ranke MB, Saenger P. Turner's syndrome. Lancet 2001;358(9278):309-14
- Hall JG, Gilchrist DM. Turner's syndrome and its variants. Pediatr Clin NA 1990;37(6):1421-40
- Jones KL. Smith's Recognizable Patterns of Human Malformation. Philadelphia: WB Saunders Co; 1997
- Sanger P. Turner syndrome. N Engl J Med 1996;335(23):1749-54

Web references: 2 available at www.5mcc.com
Illustrations N/A

Author(s):
John R Waterson, MD, PhD

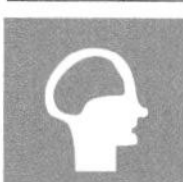

BASICS

DESCRIPTION Typhoid fever is an acute systemic illness unique to humans caused by Salmonella typhi. It is a classic example of enteric fever caused by the Salmonella family of bacteria.
- It is endemic in some developing nations where sanitation is suboptimal. Majority of cases in North America are acquired after travel to endemic areas.
- Mode of transmission is fecal-oral through ingestion of contaminated food (commonly poultry), water and milk. Incubation period varies from 7 to 21 days.

System(s) affected: Gastrointestinal, Pulmonary, Skin/Exocrine
Genetics: N/A
Incidence/Prevalence in USA: 300-500 cases per year
Predominant age: All ages
Predominant sex: Male = Female

SIGNS & SYMPTOMS
- Fever
- Headache
- Malaise
- Abdominal discomfort/bloating/constipation
- Diarrhea (less common)
- Dry cough
- Confusion/lethargy
- Rose spot (transient erythematous maculopapular rash in anterior thorax or upper abdomen)
- Splenomegaly
- Hepatomegaly
- Cervical adenopathy
- Relative bradycardia
- Conjunctivitis

CAUSES *Salmonella typhi*

RISK FACTORS Must be considered in any patient presenting with fever after tropical travel or exposed to chronic carrier

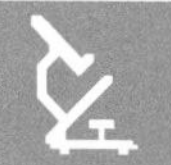

DIAGNOSIS

DIFFERENTIAL DIAGNOSIS
- Malaria
- "Enteric fever-like" syndrome caused by Yersinia enterocolitica, Yersinia pseudotuberculosis, and Campylobacter sp.
- Enteric fever caused by non-typhi Salmonella
- Infectious hepatitis
- Atypical pneumonia
- Infectious mononucleosis
- Subacute bacterial endocarditis
- Tuberculosis
- Brucellosis
- Q fever

LABORATORY
- Definitive diagnosis by isolation of S. typhi from blood. Isolation of S. typhi in sputum, urine or stool is presumptive diagnosis in typical clinical presentation.
- Serology is nonspecific and usually not useful
- If multiple blood cultures are negative or in patients with prior antibiotic therapy, diagnostic yield is better with bone marrow culture
- Anemia, leukopenia (neutropenia), thrombocytopenia or evidence of DIC (disseminated intravascular coagulopathy) are supportive evidence. Elevated liver enzymes are commonly seen.

Drugs that may alter lab results:
- Prior antibiotic therapy
- Vaccination

Disorders that may alter lab results: N/A

PATHOLOGICAL FINDINGS Classically, mononuclear proliferation involving lymphoid tissue of intestinal tract especially Peyer's patch in terminal ileum

SPECIAL TESTS N/A

IMAGING Consider serial plain abdominal films for evidence of intestinal perforation

DIAGNOSTIC PROCEDURES Bone marrow aspirate for culture is rarely indicated

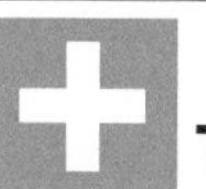

TREATMENT

APPROPRIATE HEALTH CARE
- Inpatient if acutely ill
- Outpatient for less ill patient or for carrier

GENERAL MEASURES
- Fluid and electrolyte support
- Strict isolation of patient's linen, stool and urine
- Monitor clinically and consider serial plain abdominal films for evidence of perforation, usually in the third to fourth week of illness
- Indication for treatment must be determined on an individual basis. Factors to be considered are age, public health (food handler, chronic care facilities, medical personnel), intolerance to antibiotics, and evidence of biliary tract disease.
- For hemorrhage - need blood transfusion and shock management

SURGICAL MEASURES Cholecystectomy may be warranted in carriers with cholelithiasis, relapse after therapy, or intolerance to antimicrobial therapy

ACTIVITY Bedrest initially, then as tolerated

DIET If abdominal symptoms severe, nothing by mouth. With improvement, normal low-residue diet, possibly enriched in calories.

PATIENT EDUCATION
- Discussion of chronic carrier state and its complications
- For family members, travelers or workers at risk, provide hygiene education, possibly vaccination

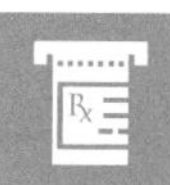

MEDICATIONS

DRUG(S) OF CHOICE
- Chloramphenicol: Children - 50 mg/kg/d po qid x 2 weeks; adult dose - 50 mg/kg per day, divided q6h x 2 weeks,

or
- Ampicillin: Children - 100 mg/kg/d qid po x 2 weeks; adults - 500 mg q6h x 2 weeks,

or
- Ciprofloxacin 500 mg po bid x 2 weeks, indicated in MDR-T, has been successfully and safely used in children

or
- Ceftriaxone 1-2 gm IV qd x 2 weeks,

or
- Furazolidone 7.5 mg/kg/d po x 10 days; in uncomplicated MDR-T; safe in children; efficacy > 85% cure
- Chronic carrier state
  - ◊ Is treated with ampicillin 4-5 gram/day plus probenecid 2 grams/day qid x 6 weeks (for patients with normal functioning gallbladder without evidence of cholelithiasis)
  - ◊ Ciprofloxacin 500 mg po bid x 4-6 weeks is also efficacious

Note: Chloramphenicol resistance - reported in Mexico, South America, Central America, Southeast Asia, India, Pakistan, Middle East and Africa

Contraindications: Refer to manufacturer's profile of each drug

Precautions: Rarely, Jarisch-Herxheimer reaction post antimicrobial therapy

Significant possible interactions: Refer to manufacturer's profile of each drug

ALTERNATIVE DRUGS
- Trimethoprim-sulfamethoxazole

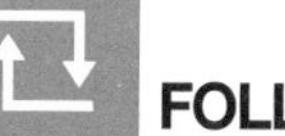

FOLLOWUP

PATIENT MONITORING
See General Measures

PREVENTION/AVOIDANCE
- For high risk travel to an endemic area, consider vaccination for typhoid:
  - ◊ Parenteral ViCPS or capsular polysaccharide typhoid vaccine (Typhim Vi)

OR
  - ◊ Ty21a or live oral typhoid vaccine (Vivotif Berna), particularly if traveler will have prolonged risk (>4 weeks)
- Avoid tap water, salad/raw vegetables, unpeeled fruits, dairy products in tropical travel
- Avoid poultry or poultry products left unrefrigerated for prolonged period of time
- Consider vaccination for workers exposed to *S. typhi*, household or intimate exposure to a carrier of *S. typhi*

Typhoid fever vaccines:

Name (type)	Dosing	Protection (1,2)
†Ty21a (3)	One capsule qOD for 4 doses	40-65% up to 7 yrs
†† ViCPS (4)	Single IM dose	50-75% up to 3 yrs

† Do not give to children < 6 yrs of age
†† Do not give to children < 1 yr of age
(1) little data for travelers from developed countries
(2) any protection can be overwhelmed by a large inoculum
(3) oral, live attenuated vaccine
(4) capsular polysaccharide vaccine

POSSIBLE COMPLICATIONS
- Intestinal hemorrhage and perforation in distal ileum
- Patient may become chronic carrier state (up to 3%) defined as persistent stool excretor for longer than 1 year
- Predilection for seeding in the biliary tract exists and may become a focus for relapse of typhoid fever. Most common in female and the elderly (> 50 years old).
- Osteomyelitis especially in sickle cell anemia, systemic lupus erythematosus, hematologic neoplasms and immunosuppressed hosts
- Endovascular infection in the elderly and in patients with history of bypass operation or aneurysm
- Rarely, endocarditis or meningitis

EXPECTED COURSE/PROGNOSIS
Overall prognosis good with therapy. < 2% mortality rate; 15% relapse rate with some antibiotic treatments; 3% bowel perforation

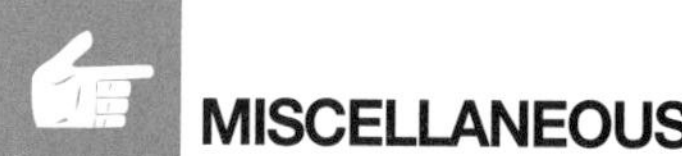

MISCELLANEOUS

ASSOCIATED CONDITIONS
N/A

AGE-RELATED FACTORS
Pediatric: Disease more critical in infants, but may be milder in children
Geriatric: Disease more serious in elderly
Others: N/A

PREGNANCY
Ciprofloxacin relative contraindicated in pregnancy

SYNONYMS
- Typhoid
- Typhus abdominalis
- Enteric fever

ICD-9-CM
002.0 Typhoid fever
002.9 Paratyphoid fever, unspecified

SEE ALSO

OTHER NOTES
N/A

ABBREVIATIONS
N/A

REFERENCES

- Mandell GL, ed: Principles and Practice of Infectious Diseases. 5th Ed. New York, Churchill Livingstone, 2000
- Miller SI, Pegues DA. Salmonella Species (including Salmonella typhi). In: Mandell GL, Bennett JF, Dolin R, eds. Principles and Practice of Infectious Diseases. 5th Ed. New York. Churchill Livingstone, 2000
- Akalin HE. Quinolones in the treatment of typhoid fever. Drugs 1999;58(Suppl 2):52-4.
- Peter G, des Vignes-Kendrick M, Eickhoff TC, Fine A, Galvin V, Levine MM, et al. Lessons learned from a review of the development of selected vaccines. Pediatrics 1999;104:942-50
- Thompson RF, Bass DM, Hoffman SL. Travel vaccines. Infect Dis Clin North Am 1999;13:49-67
- Dick L. Travel medicine: helping patients prepare for trips abroad. Am Fam Physician 1998;58:383-98,401-2
- Rowe B, Ward LR, Threlfall EJ. Multidrug-resistant Salmonella typhi: a worldwide epidemic. Clin Infect Dis 1997;24(Suppl(1):S106-9
- Yoon J, Segal-Maurer S, Rahal JJ. An outbreak of domestically acquired typhoid fever in Queens, NY. Arch Intern Med. 2004 Mar 8;164(5):565-567

Web references: 5 available at www.5mcc.com
Illustrations N/A

Author(s):
D. W. MacPherson, MD

BASICS

DESCRIPTION Acute infectious diseases caused by three species of rickettsiae
- Epidemic typhus - human to human transmission by body louse. Primarily in circumstances such as refugee camps, war, famine and disaster. Recrudescent disease, occurring years after initial infection can be source of human outbreak. Flying squirrels also reservoir.
- Endemic (murine) typhus - infection of rodents. To humans by rat flea.
- Scrub typhus - infection of chiggers and of rodents. To humans by the chigger. Primarily in Asia and the Western Pacific.

System(s) affected: Endocrine/Metabolic, Hemic/Lymphatic/Immunologic, Pulmonary, Skin/Exocrine
Genetics: N/A
Incidence/Prevalence in USA:
- Epidemic typhus - rare
- Endemic typhus - fewer than 100 cases annually, primarily in gulf states, especially South Texas, underreporting suspected
- Scrub typhus - travelers returning from endemic areas, only (rare)

Predominant age: N/A
Predominant sex: N/A

SIGNS & SYMPTOMS
- General
  - ◊ Acute onset
  - ◊ Fever
  - ◊ Chills
  - ◊ Headache
  - ◊ Myalgia
  - ◊ Malaise
  - ◊ Diffuse organ involvement, e.g., intestine, liver, heart, kidneys, brain
- Epidemic typhus
  - ◊ Incubation period about 1 week
  - ◊ Macular or maculopapular rash beginning on trunk about fifth day of illness
  - ◊ Nonproductive cough
  - ◊ Pulmonary infiltrates
- Endemic typhus
  - ◊ Incubation period 1-2 weeks
  - ◊ Macular or maculopapular rash beginning on trunk third to fifth day of illness
- Scrub typhus
  - ◊ Incubation period 1-3 weeks
  - ◊ Eschar at bite site
  - ◊ Regional lymphadenopathy
  - ◊ Generalized lymphadenopathy
  - ◊ Splenomegaly
  - ◊ Macular or maculopapular rash beginning on trunk about the fifth day of illness
  - ◊ Relative bradycardia early in disease
  - ◊ Ocular pain
  - ◊ Conjunctival injection

CAUSES
- Epidemic typhus by Rickettsia prowazekii
- Endemic typhus by R. typhi
- Scrub typhus by R. tsutsugamushi

RISK FACTORS
- Exposure to vectors, e.g., travel to certain countries
- Elderly may have more severe disease
- Laboratory worker

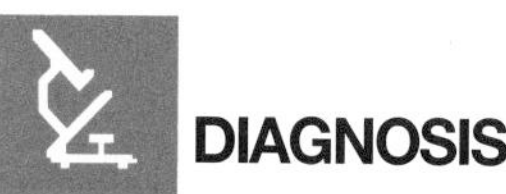

DIAGNOSIS

DIFFERENTIAL DIAGNOSIS
- Any acute febrile disease
- Rocky Mountain spotted fever
- Meningococcemia
- Bacterial meningitis
- Boutonneuse fever (R. conorii)
- Measles
- Rubella
- Toxoplasmosis
- Leptospirosis
- Typhoid fever
- Dengue
- Relapsing fever
- Secondary syphilis
- Viral syndromes - mononucleosis, acute retro-viral syndrome, etc.

LABORATORY
- WBC usually normal
- Abnormalities reflecting the particular organs affected
- Weil-Felix serological reaction may be positive; test limited to mid-illness or after, and by low sensitivity and non-specificity. Epidemic and endemic typhus, fourfold titer rise or titer > 1/320 to OX-19. Scrub typhus, fourfold rise in titer to OX-K.
- Hyponatremia in severe cases
- Hypoalbuminemia in severe cases

Drugs that may alter lab results: Prior antibiotic use

Disorders that may alter lab results: N/A

PATHOLOGICAL FINDINGS Diffuse vasculitis

SPECIAL TESTS Specific serological test showing a rising antibody titer. Isolation of rickettsia should be undertaken only in special laboratories to minimize risk of laboratory acquired infection.

IMAGING N/A

DIAGNOSTIC PROCEDURES N/A

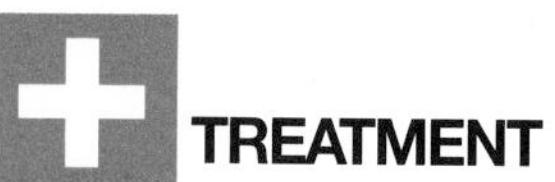

TREATMENT

APPROPRIATE HEALTH CARE Outpatient unless severely ill

GENERAL MEASURES
- Protect agitated patient from injury
- Skin and mouth care
- Supportive care for the severely ill, directed to the complications

SURGICAL MEASURES N/A

ACTIVITY Bedrest during acute stages, otherwise as tolerated

DIET As tolerated

PATIENT EDUCATION Prevention information to travelers

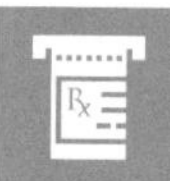

MEDICATIONS

DRUG(S) OF CHOICE

- Treatment should begin when diagnosis is reasonably likely and continue until improved and afebrile for a minimum of 48 hours
- Children over 8 years and adults:
  - ◊ Tetracycline , or a congener, orally 25 mg per kg initially, and then 25 mg per kg daily in equally divided doses every 6 hours
  - ◊ If severely ill, may use doxycycline IV, adults 100 mg every 12 hours, children >8 years 5 mg per kg in 24 hours (maximum of 200 mg/24 hrs)
- Children under 8 years, pregnant women or if typhoid fever is possible cause of illness:
  - ◊ Chloramphenicol orally 50 mg per kg initially, and then 50 mg per kg daily in equally divided doses every 6 hours
  - ◊ If severely ill, chloramphenicol sodium succinate intravenously 20 mg per kg initially infused in 30-45 minutes, and then 50 mg per kg daily infused in equally divided doses every 6 hours until orally tolerable.

Contraindications: N/A
Precautions: Refer to manufacturer's profile of each drug
Significant possible interactions: Refer to manufacturer's profile of each drug

ALTERNATIVE DRUGS

- Doxycycline single oral dose of 100 or 200 mg in refugee camps, disasters or limited medical services
- Isolated reports indicate that erythromycin and ciprofloxacin are effective

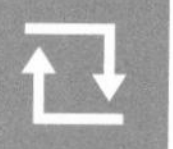

FOLLOWUP

PATIENT MONITORING Severely ill patients should be observed regularly in hospital. Outpatients checked periodically as improvement is evident.

PREVENTION/AVOIDANCE

- Avoid vectors for each disease, e.g., scrub typhus; wear protective clothing and use insect repellents, endemic typhus; practice ectoparasite and rodent control, and epidemic typhus; delousing and cleaning of clothing
- Epidemic typhus vaccine considered for persons at high risk of exposure

POSSIBLE COMPLICATIONS

- Consequences of specific organ system involvement in the second week, e.g., azotemia, meningoencephalitis, seizures, delirium, coma, myocardial failure, hyponatremia, hypoalbuminemia, hypovolemia, and shock
- Death

EXPECTED COURSE/PROGNOSIS

- Recovery expected if treatment is instituted before complications
- Relapses may follow treatment, especially if initiated within 48 hours of onset (this is not an indication to delay treatment). Relapses treated same as primary disease.
- Without treatment the mortality is 40-60% in epidemic, 1-2% in endemic, and up to 30% in scrub typhus. Mortality higher among the elderly.

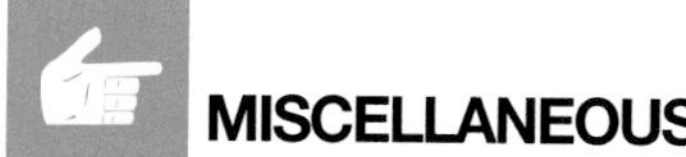

MISCELLANEOUS

ASSOCIATED CONDITIONS N/A

AGE-RELATED FACTORS

Pediatric: N/A
Geriatric: N/A
Others: N/A

PREGNANCY N/A

SYNONYMS

- Louse-borne typhus
- Brill-Zinsser disease
- Murine typhus

ICD-9-CM

080 Louse-borne [epidemic] typhus
081.0 Murine [endemic] typhus
081.1 Brill disease

SEE ALSO

OTHER NOTES

- Severe headache often intractable and not eased by the usual drugs
- Report case to Health Department

ABBREVIATIONS N/A

REFERENCES

- Mandell GL, Bennett JF, Dolin R, eds. Principles and Practice of Infectious Diseases. 5th Ed. New York, Churchill Livingstone, 2000
- Raoult D, Roux V. The body louse as a vector of re-emerging human diseases. Clin Infect Dis 1999;29:888-11
- Azad AF, Beard CB. Rickettsial pathogens and their arthropod vectors. Emerg Infect Dis 1998;4:179-86
- Azad AF, Radulovic S, Higgins JA, Noden BH, Troyer JM. Flea-borne rickettsioses: ecologic considerations. Emerg Infect Dis 1997;3:319-27
- Dumlev JS, Taylor JP, Walker DH. Clinical and laboratory features of murine typhus in south Texas, 1980 through 1987. JAMA 1991;266:1365-70
- Walker DH, et al. Emerging bacterial zoonotic and vector-borne diseases: ecological and epidemiological factors. JAMA 1996;275:463-9
- Watt G, Parola P. Scrub typhus and tropical rickettsioses. Curr Opin Infect Dis. 2003 Oct;16(5):429-436

Web references: 2 available at www.5mcc.com
Illustrations N/A

Author(s):

D. W. MacPherson, MD

BASICS

DESCRIPTION An inflammatory disease of the colon mucosa, always more intense in the rectum and usually involving the entire colon in a contiguous manner. At least 95% have rectal involvement, 50% have disease limited to rectum and sigmoid, 30-40% have disease beyond the sigmoid but not of the entire colon and 20% have pancolitis.
System(s) affected: Gastrointestinal
Genetics: Family aggregates common, positive family history in 8-11%. More likely vertical than horizontal. More common in Jews.
Incidence/Prevalence in USA: 70-150 per 100,000. Incidence 6-8 new cases per 100,000 population.
Predominant age: Between ages of 15 and 35 years. There is a second and smaller peak in the 7th decade.
Predominant sex: Male = Female

SIGNS & SYMPTOMS
- Bloody diarrhea
- Abdominal pain
- Fever
- Weight loss
- Arthralgias and arthritis (15-20%)
- Spondylitis (3-6%)
- Ocular complications (4-10%) includes episcleritis, uveitis, cataracts, keratopathy, marginal corneal ulceration, and central serous retinopathy
- Erythema nodosum
- Pyoderma gangrenosum
- Aphthous ulcers of mouth (5-10%)
- Asymptomatic fatty liver common - occasional hepatomegaly
- Pericholangitis (uncommon)
- Primary sclerosing cholangitis (1-4%)
- Cirrhosis of liver (1-5%)
- Bile duct carcinoma
- Thromboembolic disease (1-6%)
- Pericarditis (rare)
- Amyloidosis (rare)

CAUSES Unknown. Major hypotheses include allergy to dietary components, or abnormal immune responses to bacterial or self-antigens.

RISK FACTORS
- None known
- Higher incidence in Jews and those with positive family history
- Negative association with smoking

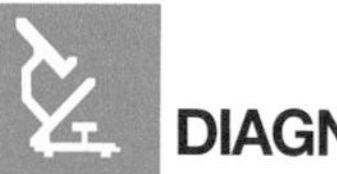

DIAGNOSIS

DIFFERENTIAL DIAGNOSIS
- Other sources of rectal bleeding including hemorrhoids, neoplasms, colonic diverticula, A-V malformation, Crohn disease
- Infectious causes of diarrhea including bacteria (Enterotoxigenic E. coli, E. coli 0157:H7, Salmonella, Shigella, Aeromonas, Plesiomonas), parasitic (Entamoeba histolytica)
- "Gay bowel" syndrome causes (*Herpes simplex*, *Chlamydia trachomatis*, *Cryptosporidium*, *Isospora belli*, cytomegalovirus, and other infectious causes as listed above)
- Antibiotic associated diarrhea
- Radiation proctitis
- Ischemic proctitis and colitis

LABORATORY
- Nonspecific. Usually reflects the degree of severity of the bleeding and inflammation.
- Anemia may reflect chronic disease as well as iron deficiency from blood loss
- Leukocytosis during exacerbation
- Elevated sedimentation rate and C-reactive protein
- Electrolyte abnormalities, especially hypokalemia
- Hypoalbuminemia
- Elevated liver function tests
- pANCA (perinuclear antineutrophil cytoplasmic antibody) is elevated in 85% of cases of ulcerative colitis and 15% of Crohn disease. Antiglycan antibody is elevated in 75% of Crohn disease, 5% ulcerative colitis. This pair of markers in the blood help distinguish which disease is present in obscure cases.

Drugs that may alter lab results: N/A

Disorders that may alter lab results: N/A

PATHOLOGICAL FINDINGS Inflammation of the colonic mucosa with ulcerations. These appear hyperemic and hemorrhagic. Rectum involved 95% of time. The inflammation extends proximally in a continuous fashion, but for a variable distance. May affect terminal ileum - referred to as "backwash ileitis."

SPECIAL TESTS None

IMAGING
- Air contrast barium enema
- Plain abdominal films are invaluable in management of acute complications of ulcerative colitis and should be immediately available in all patients who show tenderness of the colon, fever, and leukocytosis. Permits the early diagnosis of toxic megacolon and perforation and planning of appropriate treatment. Toxic megacolon is most severe near the cecum and is present when diameter exceeds 12 cm.

DIAGNOSTIC PROCEDURES
- Sigmoidoscopy, may include biopsy
- Colonoscopy, may include biopsy for evaluation for premalignant features; also used to differentiate from Crohn disease, and to investigate abnormalities that appear on radiography, such as stricture or mass lesions. Colonoscopy useful to define the extent of involvement and specific segments involved as this has bearing on therapy and prognosis.

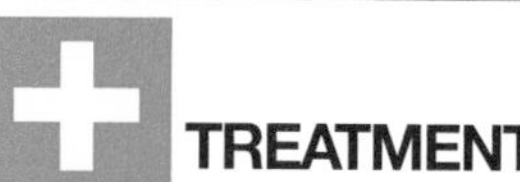

TREATMENT

APPROPRIATE HEALTH CARE Outpatient, except for severe exacerbations which may require hospitalization

GENERAL MEASURES Goal is to control inflammation, prevent complications, replace nutritional losses and blood volume

SURGICAL MEASURES
- Emergency surgery for massive hemorrhage, perforation, and toxic dilatation of the colon that does not respond to treatment in 72 hours
- Elective surgery is required for cancer, for persistent multisite mucosal dysplasia, and for patients refractory to all other forms of therapy
- Total colectomy with ileostomy pouch cures the disease
  - ◊ Patients prefer a continent ileostomy (J-pouch) emptying through the rectum, or rarely subtotal colectomy with their ileum connected to their rectal stump.
  - ◊ With the continent ileostomy operations "Pouchitis" occurs in about 10% with erratic partial response to antibiotics. If any colonic mucosa is retained there is a risk of future cancer of the colon.

ACTIVITY Full activity as tolerated

DIET No specific diet; milk products not withheld unless an associated lactase deficiency exists

PATIENT EDUCATION
- Close doctor/patient relationship encouraged
- Self-help organizations such as:

National Foundation for Ileitis and Colitis
444 Park Avenue S., 11th Floor, New York, NY 10016-7374, (800)343-3637

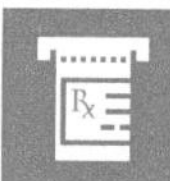

MEDICATIONS

DRUG(S) OF CHOICE
- Sulfasalazine is treatment of choice both for mild flare-ups and for the chronic treatment used to decrease the frequency of relapses (dosage range 1-4 grams daily)
- Disease limited to the rectum (proctitis) or to the left side of the colon and rectum (proctosigmoiditis) may be treated topically with steroid enemas or mesalamine (5-aminosalicylic acid, 5-ASA) enemas and suppositories
- Oral or parenteral corticosteroids are used for more severe flare-ups (e.g., prednisone 40-60 mg qd, gradually tapered off over two months) - never chronic
- Approximately 10% of patients have chronic disease activity and require continuous low - moderate steroid doses
- Newer agents include oral 5-ASA derivatives
- Immunomodulators such as azathioprine, mercaptopurine (6-mercaptopurine), methotrexate, and cyclosporine are of use in patients failing to respond to steroids and 5-ASA drugs or who cannot be weaned from high toxic doses of steroids. Most experience is with azathioprine and mercaptopurine. See discussion under Crohn disease for safe use of these agents. Toxic megacolon is treated with high dose prednisone intravenously and antibiotics covering colon bacteria. If patient already on prednisone >30 mg/day, cyclosporine is used. Daily plain films of the abdomen are obtained until there is improvement. If dilatation of colon increases or treatment has failed to attain reversal in 72 hours, emergency colectomy is indicated.
- Antimicrobial agents (anti-mycobacteriums and metronidazole) sometimes useful in Crohn disease but not in ulcerative colitis
- Antidiarrheal agents, diphenoxylate-atropine and loperamide may be used to help control diarrhea, but require careful monitoring since they may precipitate toxic megacolon

Contraindications:
- Allergy to any of above agents
- Refer to manufacturer's profile of each drug

Precautions: Use of antidiarrheal agents in severe disease could precipitate toxic megacolon

Significant possible interactions: Refer to manufacturer's profile of each drug

ALTERNATIVE DRUGS
- Budesonide is a less toxic steroid almost totally cleared by the liver. It is used in children, and patients who attain a good response to prednisone but cannot be weaned in order to avoid toxicity.
- Several preparations of 5-ASA exist, but results seem best with sulfasalazine in full dose
- Infliximab is not effective in glucocorticoid resistant disease

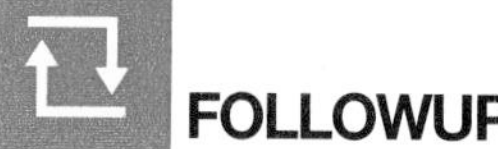

FOLLOWUP

PATIENT MONITORING Regularly scheduled appointments are important to evaluate for disease activity, appearance of complications, and the psychological and social well being of the patient

PREVENTION/AVOIDANCE
- Patients retaining colon are at risk for colon cancer. Daily 300 mg aspirin and in those with sclerosing cholangitis daily ursodeoxycholic acid 10 mg/kg have been shown to be preventive.
- Colonoscopic evaluation for cancer surveillance with biopsy evaluation of the mucosa for evidence of dysplasia must be performed every 1-2 years after the disease has been present for 7-8 years. This is particularly important in pancolitis. Low grade dysplasia warrants more frequent evaluation (e.g., every 3-6 months) and high grade dysplasia (or low grade dysplasia within a mass) warrant consideration of colectomy.
- Annual liver tests
- Cholangiography for cholestasis

POSSIBLE COMPLICATIONS
- Perforation
- Toxic megacolon
- Liver disease
- Stricture formation (less than Crohn disease)
- Colon cancer (may occur in as many as 30% of those with pancolitis for 25 years). Incidence of cancer is cumulative and begins after 7-8 years of disease; risk may be considerably less in left sided disease.

EXPECTED COURSE/PROGNOSIS
- Course extremely variable; mortality for initial attack approximately 5%. Approximately 75-85% of patients experience relapse, and up to 20% in some studies eventually require colectomy.
- Colon cancer risk is the single most important risk factor affecting long-term prognosis
- Left-sided colitis and ulcerative proctitis have very favorable prognosis with probable normal life span

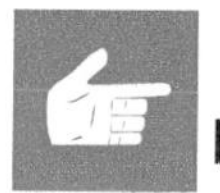

MISCELLANEOUS

ASSOCIATED CONDITIONS
- Extracolonic manifestations occur in 10 to 15% of patients
- Arthritic include large joint arthritis, sacroiliitis and ankylosing spondylitis. Infliximab has had a favorable response in treating these conditions.
- Pyoderma gangrenosum and some other skin conditions. Infliximab has helped.
- Episcleritis and uveal tract disease occurs
- Sclerosing cholangitis occurs. Helped with ursodeoxycholic acid.

AGE-RELATED FACTORS
Pediatric:
- Approximately 20% of patients are 21 years or younger
- Cancer surveillance is important since occurrence of cancer relates to the duration and extent of disease, whether frequently symptomatic or not

Geriatric: Increased mortality with initial attack in patients over 60

Others: N/A

PREGNANCY
- Outcome of pregnancy similar to general population. One study showed 30% of those with inactive disease at onset of pregnancy relapsed and 14% did so in first trimester.
- Treatment with sulfasalazine does not seem to affect outcome of pregnancy
- Recommend patient delay pregnancy until time when disease is inactive

SYNONYMS Idiopathic proctocolitis

ICD-9-CM
556.9 Ulcerative colitis, unspecified

SEE ALSO
Crohn disease
Diarrhea, acute
Diarrhea, chronic
Intestinal parasites

OTHER NOTES N/A

ABBREVIATIONS N/A

REFERENCES

- Almogy G, Bodian CA, Greenstein AJ. Surgery for late-onset ulcerative colitis: predictors of short-term outcome. Scandinavian J Gastroenterology 2002;37:11025-8
- Su C, Salzberg BA, Lewis JD, Deren JJ,et al. Efficacy of anti-tumor necrosis factor therapy in patients with ulcerative colitis. Amer J of Gastoenterol 2002;97:2577-84
- Sood A, Midha V, Sood N, Awasthi G. A prospective, open-label trial assessing dexamethasone pulse therapy in moderate to severe ulcerative colitis. J of Clin Gastroenterol 2002;35:328-31
- Su C, Lichtenstein GR. Recent developments in inflammatory bowel disease. Med Clin of No Amer 2002;86:1497-1523
- Rubin G, Hungin AP, Chinn D, et al. Long-term aminosalicylate therapy is under-used in patients with ulcerative colitis: a cross-sectional survey. Alimentary Pharmacol & Therapeu 2002;16:1889-93
- Lindgren S, Lofberg R, Bergholm L, et al. Effect of budesonide enema on remission and relapse rate in distal ulcerative colitis and proctitis. Scand J of Gastroenterol 2002;37:705-10
- Gionchetti P, Amadini C, Rizzello F, et al. Review article: treatment of mild to moderate ulcerative colitis and pouchitis. Alimentary Pharmacol and Therapeu 2002;16:Suppi 4:13-9
- Judge TA, Lewis JD, Lichtenstein GR. Colonic dysplasia and cancer in inflammatory bowel disease. Gastrointes Endoscopy Clinics of No Amer 2002;12:495-523
- Sutherland L, Roth D, Beck P, May G, Makiyama K. Oral 5-aminosallicylic acid for maintenance of remission in ulcerative colitis. Cochrane Database of Systematic Reviews 2002;4:CDO00544

Web references: 1 available at www.5mcc.com
Illustrations 3 available

Author(s):
Frank L. Iber, MD

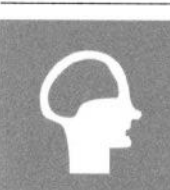

BASICS

DESCRIPTION Syndrome of urethral inflammation marked by painful urination and discharge. Usually a sexually transmitted disease (STD); other causes not uncommon. Untreated cases may gradually resolve, but complications, such as urethral stricture in males or pelvic inflammatory disease (PID) in women, may then ensue.
System(s) affected: Renal/Urologic
Genetics: N/A
Incidence/Prevalence in USA: Very common - over 830,000 cases of chlamydia and 350,000 cases of gonorrhea reported in 2002
Predominant age: Sexually active, 15-24 years old
Predominant sex: Classic symptoms more commonly reported by males; incidence in females probably equal

SIGNS & SYMPTOMS
- Both sexes may be asymptomatic carriers of the causative organisms
- In males - abrupt onset of symptoms 3 to 5 days after exposure to an infected sexual partner.
- In females - classic urethral syndrome often not present. Infections which cause simple urethritis in males will often have symptoms besides dysuria, including vaginal discharge and cervicitis.
- Dysuria - pain throughout urination
- Urethral discharge - may be profuse and purulent in acute GC, or scanty, evident only with milking of the urethra with other causes
- Urethral itching or tenderness
- Tenderness, edema and inflammation of the urethral meatus, especially in women
- Dyspareunia
- Vaginitis, cystitis, cervicitis in women
- Proctitis, pharyngitis, conjunctivitis may also be present (sexual history is important)
- Lymphadenopathy or fever are not part of the syndrome and suggest another diagnosis
- Bloody discharge - rarely seen and suggests another diagnosis
- Suprapubic or abdominal pain suggest another diagnosis or presence of complications, e.g. PID, prostatitis, or cystitis

CAUSES
- Predominantly *Neisseria gonorrhea* and *Chlamydia trachomatis* infection, often together.
- Less common infectious agents include:
  - ◊ *Ureaplasma urealyticum*
  - ◊ *Trichomonas vaginalis*
  - ◊ Herpes virus
  - ◊ *Mycoplasma genitalium*
- Non-infectious causes - generally rare:
  - ◊ Foreign bodies
  - ◊ Soaps
  - ◊ Shampoos
  - ◊ Douches
  - ◊ Spermicides
  - ◊ Catheters
  - ◊ Urethral instrumentation
  - ◊ Manual stimulation

RISK FACTORS
- Multiple sexual partners
- History of other STD
- Unprotected intercourse

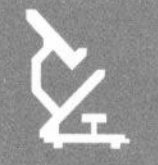

DIAGNOSIS

DIFFERENTIAL DIAGNOSIS
- Other urinary tract infections - cystitis, epididymitis, prostatitis, PID, pyelonephritis
- Atrophy, especially in postmenopausal women
- Stevens-Johnson syndrome
- Reiter syndrome - arthritis, uveitis and urethritis.
- Wegener granulomatosis can have urethritis as one of its manifestations

LABORATORY
- Gram stain of discharge: intracellular gram-negative diplococci strongly indicates GC; five or more WBC's/HPF indicates urethritis
- Cultures or reagin detection: DNA probe is probably the best screening test. Cultures can be difficult to obtain correctly but allow for antimicrobial sensitivity testing. PCR on urine more sensitive and specific but costly. Can get PCR on sample from Thin Prep test. Negatives may be false results or indicate another infecting organism.
- Urinalysis: If indicated, sample discharge before patient voids, usually normal in cases of simple urethritis. First void urine often positive for leukocyte esterase and should have ten or more WBC/HPF in urethritis.
- Urine culture: Performed only if Gram stain of discharge is unremarkable or unobtainable
- Wet prep of discharge: may reveal Trichomonas, usually reserved in males for those who fail adequate treatment for GC and Chlamydia.
- Syphilis, HIV and hepatitis B serology as indicated to rule out concomitant STDs

Drugs that may alter lab results: Recent treatment with antibiotics may lead to false negative results

Disorders that may alter lab results: N/A

PATHOLOGICAL FINDINGS Urethral strictures (untreated GC), intraurethral lesions (venereal warts, congenital anomalies)

SPECIAL TESTS N/A

IMAGING None needed

DIAGNOSTIC PROCEDURES Urethrocystoscopy for cases with suspected foreign body, intraurethral warts

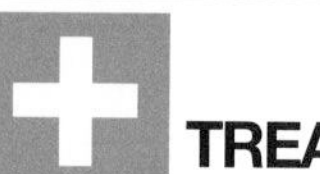

TREATMENT

APPROPRIATE HEALTH CARE
- Most cases can be treated in the outpatient setting
- Single dose regimens can be directly observed in the office for noncompliant or high-risk patients
- Antibiotics should not be withheld until culture (test) results are known, rather they should be initiated as soon as cultures (samples) have been collected
- Treatment should cover both gonorrhea and chlamydia since they cause the majority of cases and often coexist
- Patients with persistent symptoms and signs after adequate treatment should be
  - ◊ Evaluated and/or treated for Trichomonas
  - ◊ Retreated with the original regimen if not compliant
  - ◊ Treated with an alternative regimen for 14 days if *U. urealyticum* is suspected (tetracycline resistance in ≤ 10% of isolates)

GENERAL MEASURES Identification and treatment of sexual partners. All sexual partners within the previous 60 days should be investigated and treated.

SURGICAL MEASURES N/A

ACTIVITY Full activity, no sexual intercourse until seven days after single dose therapy or completion of seven-day therapy

DIET Avoid alcohol with metronidazole

PATIENT EDUCATION
- Handouts available online at www.familydoctor.org.
- Most important to emphasize need for compliance with therapy and treatment of sexual partners. Patients should be urged to undergo screening for other STDs.

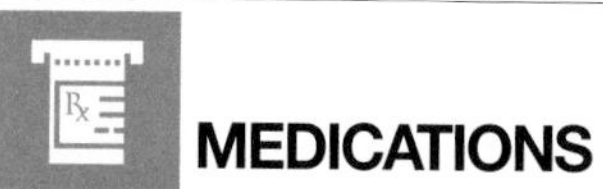

MEDICATIONS

DRUG(S) OF CHOICE
- Gonorrhea
  - ◊ Cefixime 400 mg PO x 1
  - ◊ Ceftriaxone 125 IM x 1
- Chlamydia
  - ◊ Azithromycin 1 g PO x 1
  - ◊ Doxycycline 100 mg PO bid x 7 days
- Trichomonas
  - ◊ Metronidazole 2 grams PO x 1 or 250 mg tid for 7 days
- Recurrent and resistant urethritis
  - ◊ Metronidazole 2mg PO x1 plus erythromycin base 500mg PO qid x 7 days or erythromycin ethylsuccinate 800mg PO qid x 7 days

Contraindications: Sensitivity to any of the indicated medications. Pregnant patients should not receive tetracyclines.

Precautions: Patients taking tetracyclines need to be told of the possibility of increased sensitivity to sunlight

Significant possible interactions: Tetracyclines should not be taken with milk products or antacids. Oral contraceptives may be rendered ineffective by oral antibiotics. Patients and partners should use a back-up method of birth control for remainder of the cycle.

ALTERNATIVE DRUGS
- Gonorrhea - due to the spread of quinolone resistant *N. gonorrhea* from the Pacific and Asia, quinolones are no longer recommended treatment in individuals who have acquired GC from that area. Fluoroquinolones are also not recommended as first line therapy for people in Hawaii and California and men who have sex with men due to endemic spread of quinolone resistant GC. Resistance to penicillin and tetracycline has been reported in up to one third of isolates of *N. gonorrhea*.
- Ciprofloxacin 500 mg PO x 1
- Ofloxacin 400 mg PO x 1
- Levofloxacin 250 mg PO x 1
- Others available, but offer no particular advantage to drugs of choice
- Chlamydia
  - ◊ Erythromycin base 500 mg PO qid x 7 days
  - ◊ Erythromycin ethylsuccinate 800 mg PO qid x 7 days
    - If intolerant of high dose erythromycin - erythromycin base 250 mg PO qid x 14 days or erythromycin ethylsuccinate 400 mg PO qid x 14 days
  - ◊ Ofloxacin 300 mg PO bid x 7 days
  - ◊ Levofloxacin 500 mg PO qd x 7 days

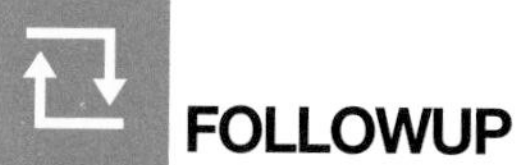

FOLLOWUP

PATIENT MONITORING Patients should be instructed to return if symptoms persist or recur after completing treatment. Test of cure cultures not usually required unless pregnant.

PREVENTION/AVOIDANCE Safer sex protection techniques, treatment of all sexual partners

POSSIBLE COMPLICATIONS
- Stricture formation
- Epididymitis
- PID in women
- Disseminated gonococcal infection
- Gonococcal meningitis
- Gonococcal endocarditis
- Perinatal transmission (Chlamydia conjunctivitis, Chlamydia pneumonia, ophthalmia neonatorum)
- Reiter syndrome

EXPECTED COURSE/PROGNOSIS If diagnosis is firmly established, appropriate medications prescribed and patient is compliant with treatment, there will be relief of symptoms within days and the problem will resolve without sequelae

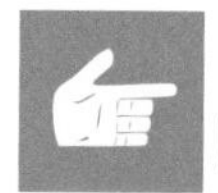

MISCELLANEOUS

ASSOCIATED CONDITIONS Other STDs - patients should be strongly urged to undergo testing for syphilis, hepatitis B, and HIV

AGE-RELATED FACTORS
Pediatric: Proven cases of GC, Chlamydia or Trichomonas should raise the question of sexual abuse
Geriatric: N/A
Others: None

PREGNANCY Tetracyclines and quinolones are contraindicated. Avoid erythromycin estolate because of an increased risk of cholestatic jaundice. Otherwise use the standard treatment recommendations. Seven day therapy for Chlamydia favored in pregnancy but single dose still recommended.

SYNONYMS N/A

ICD-9-CM
597.80 Urethritis, unspecified
597.81 Urethral syndrome NOS
098.0 Acute gonoccal infection of lower genitourinary tract
098.2 Chronic gonococcal infection of lower genitourinary tract
099.41 Chlamydia trachomatis
099.40 Other nongonococcal urethritis (NGU), unspecified
099.49 Other nongonococcal urethritis (NGU), other specified organism
131.02 Trichomonal urethritis
099.3 Reiter disease

SEE ALSO
Chlamydial sexually transmitted diseases
Epididymitis
Gonococcal infections
Pelvic inflammatory disease (PID)
Prostatitis
Urinary tract infection in females
Urinary tract infection in males
Vulvovaginitis, bacterial
Vulvovaginitis, candidal

OTHER NOTES For patients who present without symptoms stating that a sexual partner was treated for this problem: Obtain specimens for lab tests, but treat this patient before the results are available (due to the high prevalence of the illness and the possibility of false-negative test results). Use any of the regimens discussed in Medications section.

ABBREVIATIONS
STD = sexually transmitted disease
GC = gonococcal
PID = pelvic inflammatory disease
HPF = high power field

REFERENCES

- Sexually transmitted diseases treatment guidelines for 2002. Centers for Disease Control and Prevention. MMWR May 10, 2002;51(RR06):1-80
- Summary of notifiable diseases-United States, 2002. Centers for Disease Control and Prevention. MMWR 2004 Apr 30;51(No 53):1-88
- Kodner C. Sexually transmitted infections in men. Prim Care 2003 Mar;30(1):173-91
- Increases in fluoroquinolone-resistant Neisseria gonorrhoeae - Hawaii and California, 2001. Centers for Disease Control and Prevention. 2002 Nov 22;51(No 46):1041-1044
- Increases in fluoroquinolone-resistant Neisseria gonorrhoeae among men who have sex with men-United States, 2003, and revised recommendations for gonorrhea treatment, 2004. Centers for Disease Control and Prevention. 2004 Apr 30;53(No 16):335-338

Web references: 3 available at www.5mcc.com
Illustrations N/A

Author(s):
J. Christopher Graves, MD

Urinary incontinence

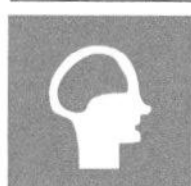

BASICS

DESCRIPTION Urinary incontinence is the involuntary loss of urine from the bladder. It can occur while asleep or awake. The amount of urine lost can vary greatly. The condition comes to medical attention when it is perceived to be a social and/or hygiene problem by the patient or caregiver.
System(s) affected: Renal/Urologic, Skin/Exocrine
Genetics: Unknown
Incidence/Prevalence in USA:
- Women (community-dwelling)
  - ◊ 10% < age 65
  - ◊ 35% > age 65
- Men (community-dwelling)
  - ◊ 1.5% < age 65
  - ◊ 22% > age 65
- Institutionalized > 65 years of age: 30-50%
- Prevalence in U.S.: 1:20 people

Predominant age: Elderly
Predominant sex: Female > Male

SIGNS & SYMPTOMS
- Involuntary loss of urine
- May be associated with urinary urgency, frequency, and nocturia

CAUSES
- Overactive bladder
  - ◊ Idiopathic
  - ◊ Neurogenic (stroke, dementia, Parkinson disease, multiple sclerosis)
  - ◊ Inflammatory (infection, tumors, stones, diverticula)
- Stress urinary incontinence
  - ◊ Genuine (Types 0, 1, 2): pelvic floor muscle weakness, urethral hypermobility
  - ◊ Intrinsic sphincteric deficiency (Type 3): post-TURP, post-radical prostatectomy, prior urethral/pelvic surgery
- Mixed: stress plus urge incontinence
- Overflow incontinence
  - ◊ Bladder outlet obstruction (BPH, urethral stricture, pelvic prolapse)
  - ◊ Neurogenic bladder (diabetes, spinal cord injury, multiple sclerosis)
- Transient/Reversible
  - ◊ Delirium, infection, atrophic urethritis/vaginitis, excessive urine output, restricted mobility, stool impaction (DIAPPERS)

RISK FACTORS
- Increasing age
- Female sex/estrogen deficiency
- Prostatic hypertrophy (males)
- Multiparity (females)
- Dementia
- Stroke
- Diabetes
- Spinal cord injury
- Multiple sclerosis
- Obesity
- Hysterectomy
- Vaginal childbirth
- Functional impairment

DIAGNOSIS

DIFFERENTIAL DIAGNOSIS
- Urinary tract infection
- Vaginal discharge (women)
- Urethral discharge (men)
- Medication effect (diuretics, alcohol, caffeine, anticholinergics, beta-agonists, calcium channel blockers, alpha-adrenergic blockers, anti-parkinson drugs, ACE inhibitors)
- Polyuria (diabetes, excessive water intake)

LABORATORY
- Urinalysis - generally normal. May show glycosuria (diabetes), proteinuria (glomerular disease), white blood cells (infection), red blood cells (tumor), or bacteria (infection).
- Urine culture - will be positive in urinary tract infection

Drugs that may alter lab results:
- Diuretics (low urine specific gravity)
- Antibiotics (negative urine culture)

Disorders that may alter lab results:
Disorders producing abnormal lab results generally contribute to the problem of incontinence

PATHOLOGICAL FINDINGS
- Relate to the primary cause of incontinence
- Intrinsic urinary sphincter disorder
- Prostatic hypertrophy
- Neurogenic bladder
- Bladder tumors

SPECIAL TESTS
- Urodynamic evaluation
  - ◊ Uroflowmetry - poor flow rate may be indicative of obstruction or poor detrusor contractility
  - ◊ Cystometrogram: may show abnormal sphincter pressure or bladder function
  - ◊ Pressure flow: high pressure with low flow may indicate obstruction
  - ◊ Video: visualization to rule out diverticulum, reflux
  - ◊ EMG: assesses sphincteric activity

IMAGING
- Renal ultrasound: rule out hydronephrosis
- Bladder scan or ultrasound post-void residual: may show increased residual urine (normally < 50 cc); ultrasound can assess bladder wall thickness and rule out bladder stones
- IVP - may show renal pathology, rarely needed
- Voiding cystourethrogram - may show bladder and/or urethral pathology

DIAGNOSTIC PROCEDURES
- The diagnosis is generally made by history
- Physical examination of men should include palpation of abdomen (for distended bladder), digital rectal exam (for prostatic hypertrophy/cancer/fecal impaction) and neurological exam
- Physical exam of women should include palpation of abdomen (for distended bladder), vaginal speculum and bimanual pelvic exam (for genitourinary pathology), rectal exam (for fecal impaction) and neurologic exam
- Assess lower extremities for edema
- It is sometimes helpful to ask the patient to reproduce the activities (e.g., coughing, sneezing, laughing) which result in loss of urine
- Urinary diaries over 2-3 days

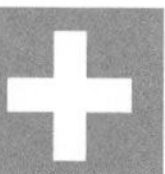

TREATMENT

APPROPRIATE HEALTH CARE Outpatient

GENERAL MEASURES
The least invasive and least dangerous procedure that is appropriate for the patient should be the first choice when treating urinary incontinence.
- All primary conditions relating to urinary incontinence should be identified and treated specifically (e.g., urinary tract infection, bladder tumors, prostatic hypertrophy, diabetes)
- Good perineal hygiene
- Pelvic floor (Kegel) exercises
- Biofeedback/behavioral training
- Intermittent catheterization (selected patients)
- Incontinence pads
- Indwelling catheterization (selected patients); rarely
- Condom catheters (male patients)
- Treatment for fecal impaction
- Electrical stimulation (selected patients)
- Vaginal cones

SURGICAL MEASURES
- Male patients with overflow incontinence secondary to prostatic hypertrophy benefit from prostatic reduction (e.g., transurethral resection of the prostate). Men with post-radical prostatectomy incontinence and post-TURP incontinence may benefit from bulking agents, artificial sphincters or other surgical procedures
- Female patients with stress incontinence may benefit from bladder suspension/sling procedures
- Female patients with poor urethral tone may benefit from periurethral bulking agents or sphincter implants
- Evolving surgical therapies include neurostimulators, detrusor myectomy

ACTIVITY Full activities should be encouraged

DIET
- No special diet
- In situations where access to bathroom facilities is limited, may want to avoid high volume fluid intake
- Caffeine may aggravate overactive bladder symptoms by increasing urine volume and by an irritant effect on the bladder

PATIENT EDUCATION
- Should be directed at the general problem, as well as underlying diseases
- Should include instructions regarding good general nutrition and exercise practices
- Rational toileting schedule, based on the pattern of incontinence
- Easy access to toilet facilities
- Pelvic floor (Kegel) exercises
- Bladder training - timed voiding and double voiding to ensure regular and complete bladder emptying

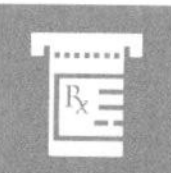

MEDICATIONS

DRUG(S) OF CHOICE

- Overactive bladder
  - ◊ Oxybutynin (Ditropan XL) 5-30 mg qd
  - ◊ Oxybutynin (Ditropan) 2.5-5 mg qid
  - ◊ Flavoxate (Urispas) 100-200 mg tid
  - ◊ Imipramine (Tofranil) 25-50 mg tid
  - ◊ Tolterodine (Detrol IR) 1-2 mg bid
  - ◊ Tolterodine (Detrol LA) 2-4 mg qd
  - ◊ Trospium chloride (Sanctura) 20 mg bid
- Sphincter incompetence
  - ◊ Pseudoephedrine (Sudafed) 30-60 mg tid
  - ◊ Imipramine (Tofranil) 25-50 mg tid
- Prostatic enlargement
  - ◊ Doxazosin (Cardura) 1-8 mg qd
  - ◊ Terazosin (Hytrin) 1-10 mg qd
  - ◊ Tamsulosin (Flomax) 0.4-0.8 mg qd
  - ◊ Finasteride (Proscar) 5 mg qd
  - ◊ Dutasteride (Avodart) 0.5 mg qd

Contraindications:

- Should be reviewed for each specific medication prior to initiating
- Anticholinergic agents are contraindicated in patients with glaucoma, decreased GI motility or bladder outlet obstruction (e.g., prostatic hypertrophy)

Precautions:

- Use smallest dose possible in elderly patients
- Common side effects include: Dry mouth, blurred vision, constipation, postural hypotension (alpha-blockers), cognitive dysfunction

Significant possible interactions: Will vary for each of the drugs listed

ALTERNATIVE DRUGS

- Oral or topical estrogens for stress incontinence associated with atrophic vaginitis
- Prostaglandin inhibitors
- Calcium antagonists
- Desmopressin (DDAVP) nasal spray (nocturnal enuresis)

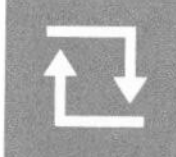

FOLLOWUP

PATIENT MONITORING

- Biweekly at first (while exercises are being learned and medication dosage is being adjusted), then quarterly once incontinence is under control
- Ask about side effects of medication
- Check for orthostatic hypotension (in patients using alpha-blockers)
- Consider measuring intraocular pressure in high risk patients

PREVENTION/AVOIDANCE

- Instruct women in routine use of Kegel exercises after childbirth
- Regular pelvic examination of female patients to detect pelvic pathology
- Regular rectal examination in male patients to detect prostatic pathology

POSSIBLE COMPLICATIONS

- Urinary tract infections
- Hydronephrosis (with atonic bladder or outlet obstruction)
- Renal failure (with obstructive hydronephrosis)
- Bladder calculi
- Skin irritation or infection
- Increased incidence of falls and fractures in elderly with overactive bladder
- Adverse drug events

EXPECTED COURSE/PROGNOSIS

- Prognosis is generally good. Most patients can achieve an increase in bladder control with appropriate medical/behavioral management.
- Some feel sphincter incompetence is best treated surgically

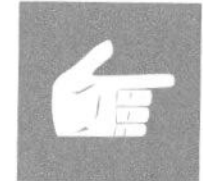

MISCELLANEOUS

ASSOCIATED CONDITIONS N/A

AGE-RELATED FACTORS

Pediatric: Neurogenic, congenital, and idiopathic overactive bladder also occurs in children
Geriatric: This problem most commonly seen in older patients
Others: N/A

PREGNANCY

Stress incontinence can occur during pregnancy

SYNONYMS

- Transient incontinence
- Urge incontinence
- Overflow incontinence
- Stress incontinence

ICD-9-CM

788.30 Urinary incontinence, unspecified

SEE ALSO

Prostatic hyperplasia, benign (BPH)
Urethritis
Urinary tract infection in females
Urinary tract infection in males

OTHER NOTES N/A

ABBREVIATIONS N/A

REFERENCES

- Wilson L, Brown JS, Shin GP, Luc KO, Subak LL. Annual direct cost of urinary incontinence. obstetrics and gynecology 2001;98:398-406
- Abrams P, Cardozo L, Khoury S, Wein. A, eds. Incontinence. 2nd ed. Plymouth UK: Health Publication Ltd; 2002
- Borello-France D, Burgio KL. Nonsurgical treatment of urinary incontienence. Clinical Obstet and Gynecol 2004;47(1):70-82
- Fine P, Antonini TG, Appell R. Clinical evaluation of women with lower urinary tract dysfunction. Clinical Obtet & Gynecol 2004;47(1):44-52

Web references: 0 available at www.5mcc.com
Illustrations N/A

Author(s):
Pamela I. Ellsworth, MD
Alexander Berry, MD

BASICS

DESCRIPTION Inflammation of the bladder mucosa. This topic refers primarily to infectious cystitis. Other urinary tract infections are discussed elsewhere.
System(s) affected: Renal/Urologic
Genetics: N/A
Incidence/Prevalence in USA: 3-8% of women have bacteriuria at any given time. 30% of females have at least one UTI; 7 million doctor visits a year
Predominant age: Young adults and older
Predominant sex: Female

SIGNS & SYMPTOMS

Note: Any or all may be present
- Burning during urination
- Pain during urination
- Urgency (sensation of need to urinate frequently)
- Frequency
- Sensation of incomplete bladder emptying
- Blood in urine
- Lower abdominal pain or cramping
- Offensive odor of urine
- Nocturia

CAUSES Acute infection, usually with gram negative bacteria (E. coli in >90% of uncomplicated cystitis).

RISK FACTORS

- Previous urinary tract infection
- Diabetes mellitus
- Pregnancy
- More frequent or vigorous sexual activity than usual
- Use of spermicides or diaphragm
- Underlying abnormalities of the urinary tract such as tumors, calculi, strictures, incomplete bladder emptying, etc.

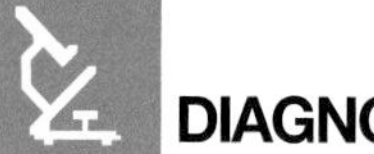

DIAGNOSIS

DIFFERENTIAL DIAGNOSIS

- Vaginitis
- Sexually transmitted diseases causing urethritis or pyuria
- Hematuria from causes other than infection (e.g., neoplasia, calculi)
- Interstitial cystitis
- Psychological dysfunction

LABORATORY

- Urinalysis demonstrating pyuria (more than 10 neutrophils per high power field on microscopic exam). Leukocyte esterase dipsticks also useful for detecting pyuria but fail to detect pyuria in up to 20% of patients, and false positives occur from vaginal leukocytes.
- Urinalysis demonstrating bacteriuria (any amount on unspun urine, or 10 rod-shaped bacteria per high power field on centrifuged urine). Nitrite dipsticks also useful (and 94% specific), but fail to detect bacteriuria in 30-50% of patients. Nitrite dipsticks may be negative in patients who do not eat meat.
- Urine culture demonstrating growth of single species of bacteria. Suspect contaminated specimen when culture shows multiple types of bacteria.

Drugs that may alter lab results: N/A

Disorders that may alter lab results: N/A

PATHOLOGICAL FINDINGS N/A

SPECIAL TESTS N/A

IMAGING

- For all infants and may be indicated for older patients with recurrent infections:
  - ◊ Ultrasound imaging is first choice test
  - ◊ For infants and children, obtain ultrasound and if ureteral dilation detected, obtain either voiding cystourethrogram or isotope cystogram to detect reflux

DIAGNOSTIC PROCEDURES

- Suprapubic bladder aspiration or urethral catheterization to obtain urine specimen from infants
- Urethral catheterization to obtain urine specimen from children and adults if voided urine suspected of being contaminated
- Classic symptoms in non-pregnant young adult female with first episode of UTI require no urine culture for diagnosis. Obtain urinalysis and culture in other age groups, if repeat episode, if pregnant, or if symptoms not classic.
- Some recent research suggests the most cost-effective approach is empiric treatment without lab tests in non-pregnant premenopausal women with symptoms of UTI and no risks for complicated infection

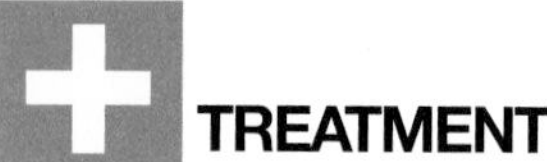

TREATMENT

APPROPRIATE HEALTH CARE Outpatient, except for complicated or upper tract infections

GENERAL MEASURES

- Maintain good hydration
- One-fourth of women with simple UTI experience a second UTI within six months, and half at some time during lifetime. Patients with multiple recurrent UTI and no underlying urinary tract abnormality may receive long-term prophylactic antibiotic treatment. Trimethoprim-sulfamethoxazole and nitrofurantoin commonly used.
- Patients with chronic indwelling urinary catheters always have colonization of urine, usually with multiple bacterial species. This should not be treated unless symptomatic with fever, sepsis, or other systemic symptoms.
- Preliminary studies indicate that Vaccinium macrocarpon (Cranberry Juice) may help prevent and treat UTIs by inhibiting bacterial adherence to bladder epithelium

SURGICAL MEASURES N/A

ACTIVITY Avoid sexual intercourse when symptoms present

DIET No special diet

PATIENT EDUCATION

- Take antibiotic as directed
- Return if symptoms not resolved or markedly improved within 48 hours
- Return if fever, chills, or flank pain develop
- If taking prophylactic antibiotics, take at bedtime

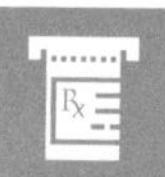

MEDICATIONS

DRUG(S) OF CHOICE

- First, rare, or infrequent UTI in older children, adolescents, and adults who are nonpregnant, nondiabetic, afebrile, nonimmunocompromised and have no abnormality of the urinary tract (i.e., uncomplicated). New studies show 3 day therapy is OK for children.
  - ◊ 3 day treatment with fluoroquinolone or trimethoprim-sulfamethoxazole (TMP-SMX) Increasing resistance being reported to TMP-SMX. It is the preferred treatment if local sensitivity patterns indicate low resistance rates.
- Postcoital
  - ◊ Single-dose TMP-SMX or cephalexin may reduce frequency of UTI in sexually active women
- Pregnant patients
  - ◊ 10-14 day or longer treatment with pregnancy-safe antibiotic chosen based on culture/sensitivity results. May begin with cephalosporin, amoxicillin, or other antibiotic while awaiting culture/sensitivity results.
- All other patients
  - ◊ 10-14 day treatment with antibiotic chosen based on culture/sensitivity results. May begin with fluoroquinolone, TMP-SMX, cephalosporin or other antibiotic while awaiting culture/sensitivity results.

Contraindications: Refer to manufacturer's literature. Fluoroquinolones not safe during pregnancy or for treatment of children. TMP/SMX use in pregnancy not desirable (especially in 3rd trimester), but appropriate in some circumstances.
Precautions: Refer to manufacturer's literature
Significant possible interactions: Refer to manufacturer's literature

ALTERNATIVE DRUGS Change antibiotic if indicated by culture/sensitivity results

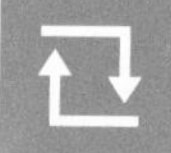

FOLLOWUP

PATIENT MONITORING

- First or rare UTI: In young or middle-age, nonpregnant adult female requires no followup if patient cured after 3 day therapy. If not resolved within two to three days, obtain culture/sensitivity and change antibiotic accordingly.
- All other patients should have post-treatment urine culture to document eradication of infection

PREVENTION/AVOIDANCE

- Maintain good hydration
- Women with frequent or intercourse-related UTI should empty bladder immediately before and following intercourse and consider postcoital antibiotic treatment
- Avoid feminine hygiene sprays and scented douches
- Wipe urethra from front to back

POSSIBLE COMPLICATIONS

- Pyelonephritis or sepsis
- Renal abscess
- Acute urinary outlet obstruction

EXPECTED COURSE/PROGNOSIS

Symptoms resolve within 2-3 days after starting treatment in almost all patients

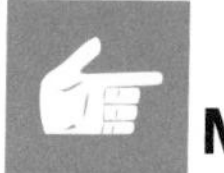

MISCELLANEOUS

ASSOCIATED CONDITIONS Described under Risk Factors

AGE-RELATED FACTORS

Pediatric: Infants and young children with cystitis are at higher risk of pyelonephritis
Geriatric:

- Elderly may have bacteriuria without symptoms; generally does not require treatment if urinary tract otherwise normal
- Elderly more apt to have underlying urinary tract abnormality
- Acute UTI sometimes associated with incontinence or mental status changes in the elderly

Others: N/A

PREGNANCY UTI during pregnancy always requires culture/sensitivity and usually requires 10-14 day treatment. Following treatment of acute infection, pregnant women often receive prophylactic antibiotics for the remainder of pregnancy.

SYNONYMS Cystitis

ICD-9-CM

595.0 Acute cystitis

SEE ALSO

Pyelonephritis

OTHER NOTES N/A

ABBREVIATIONS N/A

REFERENCES

- Bent S, Nallamouthu BK, Simel DL, Fihn SD, Saint S. Does this woman have an acute uncomplicated urinary tract infection. JAMA 2002;287(20):2701-10
- Barry HG, Ebell MH, Hickner J. Evaluation of suspected urinary tract infection in ambulatory women: a cost-utility analysis of office-based strategies. J of Fam Prac 1997;44:49-60
- Ebell MH, Barry NC. Urinary tract infection. In: Weiss BD, ed. 20 Common Problems in Primary Care. New York, McGraw-Hill, 1999
- Gupta K, Scholes D, Stamm WE. Increasing prevalence of antimicrobial resistance among uropathogens causing acute uncomplicated cystitis in women. JAMA 1999;281:736-38
- Stamm WE, Hooton T. Management of urinary tract infections in adults. New Eng J Med 1993;329:1328-34
- Huang ES, Stafford RS. National patterns in the treatment of urinary tract infections in women by ambulatory care physicians. Arch Intern Med. 2002 Jan 14;162(1):41-7

Web references: 2 available at www.5mcc.com
Illustrations N/A

Author(s):

Barry D. Weiss, MD

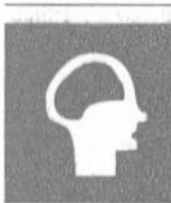

BASICS

DESCRIPTION Cystitis is an infection of the lower urinary tract, usually resulting from a single gram-negative enteric bacteria. (See separate chapters for information on prostatitis, pyelonephritis, and non-gonococcal urethritis.)
System(s) affected: Renal/Urologic
Genetics: No specific genetic pattern
Incidence/Prevalence in USA: Not common
Predominant age: Increases with age. Uncommon in men under 50. 8 infections/10,000 men, ages 21-50.
Predominant sex: Male only (for this discussion)

SIGNS & SYMPTOMS
- Urinary frequency
- Urinary urgency
- Dysuria
- Hesitancy
- Slow urinary stream
- Dribbling of urine
- Nocturia
- Suprapubic discomfort
- Low back pain
- Hematuria
- Systemic symptoms (chills, fever) present with concomitant pyelonephritis or prostatitis

CAUSES
- Escherichia coli (80% of infections)
- Klebsiella
- Enterobacter
- Proteus
- Pseudomonas
- Serratia
- Streptococcus faecalis and Staphylococcus

RISK FACTORS
- Benign prostatic hypertrophy
- Cognitive impairment
- Fecal incontinence
- Urinary incontinence
- Anal intercourse
- Recent urologic surgery, catheterization
- Infection of the prostate or kidney
- Urinary tract instrumentation
- Immunocompromised host
- Outlet obstruction

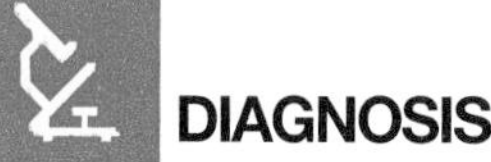

DIAGNOSIS

DIFFERENTIAL DIAGNOSIS
- Anatomic or functional pathology
- Urethritis
- Infections in other sites of the genitourinary tract (e.g., epididymis)

LABORATORY
- Pyuria
- Bacteriuria
- Urine dipstick leukocyte esterase (75-90%, sensitivity, 95% specificity), and nitrate (35-85% sensitivity, 70% specificity)
- Urine culture - 10/high power colonies of pathogens (or counts > 100,000 bacteria/mL of urine) confirms diagnosis (Escherichia coli, Klebsiella, Pseudomonas, other agents). Lower counts can also be indicative of infection, especially in presence of pyuria.
- Segmented bacteriologic localization cultures
  - ◊ VB1 - collect 5-10 mL of urine of patient's initial voiding
  - ◊ VB2 - then a sample of sterile midstream urine is obtained
  - ◊ EPS - prostatic massage performed, and expressed prostatic secretion is collected from the meatus
  - ◊ VB3 - patient completes voiding and 4th sample is collected
  - ◊ Cultures and sensitivity collected from each specimen

Drugs that may alter lab results: Antibiotics prior to culture

Disorders that may alter lab results: N/A

PATHOLOGICAL FINDINGS Depends on site of infection

SPECIAL TESTS Urologic investigations necessary to rule out other disorders

IMAGING Intravenous pyelography, cystoscopy, ultrasound

DIAGNOSTIC PROCEDURES Careful history and physical

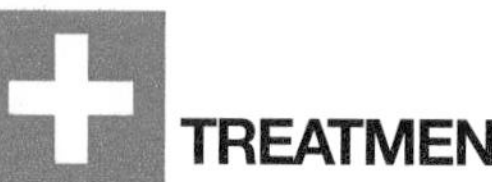

TREATMENT

APPROPRIATE HEALTH CARE Outpatient, except for acute illness with toxicity or kidney failure

GENERAL MEASURES
- Hydration and analgesia if required
- Discontinue sexual activity until cured
- Patient with indwelling catheters
  - ◊ If asymptomatic bacterial colonization - no need to treat (sterilization of urine not possible and resistant organisms can take up residence)
  - ◊ If symptomatic of acute infection - institute treatment

SURGICAL MEASURES N/A

ACTIVITY Activity as tolerated.

DIET No special diet

PATIENT EDUCATION For patient education materials favorably reviewed on this topic, contact: National Kidney Foundation, 30 E. 33rd Street, Suite 1100, New York, NY 10016, (212)889-2210

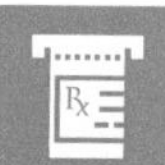

MEDICATIONS

DRUG(S) OF CHOICE
- Acute UTI , first infection, no risk factors for treatment: 7-10 days of oral antibiotics either empirically or based on cultures and sensitivity results. For empiric therapy, trimethoprim-sulfamethoxazole (SMX-TMP) bid will usually treat the most likely pathogens.
- Complicated or recurrent UTI: 14-21 days of antibiotics based on antimicrobial sensitivities with repeat urine check after treatment

Contraindications: Refer to manufacturer's information
Precautions: Refer to manufacturer's information
Significant possible interactions: Refer to manufacturer's information

ALTERNATIVE DRUGS
According to culture and sensitivity results and patient's history

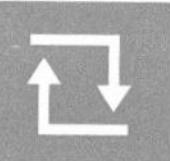

FOLLOWUP

PATIENT MONITORING
Close followup until clinically well and repeat urinalysis after treatment

PREVENTION/AVOIDANCE
- Prompt treatment of predisposing factors
- Catheter use only when necessary. If needed, use aseptic technique and closed system, with removal as soon as possible.

POSSIBLE COMPLICATIONS
- Pyelonephritis
- Ascending infection
- Recurrent infection

EXPECTED COURSE/PROGNOSIS
Clearing of infections with appropriate antibiotic treatment

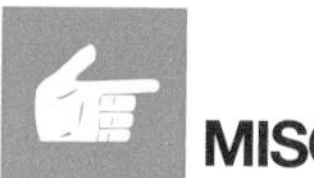

MISCELLANEOUS

ASSOCIATED CONDITIONS
- Acute bacterial pyelonephritis
- Chronic bacterial pyelonephritis
- Urethritis
- Prostatitis
- Prostatic hypertrophy
- Prostate cancer

AGE-RELATED FACTORS
Pediatric: Usually associated with obstruction to normal flow of urine, such as vesicoureteral reflux
Geriatric: Bacteriuria is common in the elderly, appears related to functional status and is usually transient. If asymptomatic bacteriuria is noted, no treatment is needed.
Others: N/A

PREGNANCY
N/A

SYNONYMS
- UTI
- Cystitis

ICD-9-CM
595.0 Acute cystitis
595.1 Chronic interstitial cystitis
595.2 Other chronic cystitis

SEE ALSO
Prostatic cancer
Prostatic hyperplasia, benign (BPH)
Prostatitis
Pyelonephritis

OTHER NOTES
N/A

ABBREVIATIONS
N/A

REFERENCES

- Lipsky BA. Urinary tract infections in men. Epidemiology, pathophysiology, diagnosis, and treatment. Ann Intern Med 1989;110:138-150
- Finn SD. Urinary tract infections - diagnosis and treatment in women and men. Consultant 1992;10:43-58
- Hooton TM, Stamm WE. Management of acute uncomplicated urinary tract infection in adults. Med Clin of North Am 1991;75(2);339-57
- Khan AJ, Schaffer HA, Evans H. Urinary tract infections in adolescent boys. J Nat Med A 1996;88(1):25-26
- Hutton J, Hughes M, Raymond CH. Management of bacterial urinary tract infections in adults. Ann Pharm 1994;28(11):1264-1272
- Harrington RD, Hooton TM. Urinary tract infection risk factors and gender. J Gend Specif Med 2000 Nov-Dec;3(8):27-34
- Lipsky BA. Managing urinary tract infections in men. Hosp Pract (Off Ed) 2000;35(1):53-9; discussion 59-60
- Naber KG, Bergman B, Bishop MC, et al. Urinary Tract Infection (UTI) Working Group of the Health Care Office (HCO) of the European Association of Urology (EAU). EAU guidelines for the management of urinary and male genital tract infections. Urinary Tract Infection (UTI) Working Group of the Health Care Office (HCO) of the European Association of Urology (EAU). Eur Urol 2001;40(5):576-88

Web references: 2 available at www.5mcc.com
Illustrations N/A

Author(s):
Scott A. Fields, MD

BASICS

DESCRIPTION The state describing the presence of calculi within the urinary system. Commonly known as kidney stones.
System(s) affected: Renal/Urologic
Genetics: Familial tendency
Incidence/Prevalence in USA: 70-210 in 100,000 population. 2%-5% of population in lifetime.
Predominant age: Peak 20-30. Range 20-60.
Predominant sex: Male > Female (4:1)

SIGNS & SYMPTOMS
- Usually sudden onset
- Severe agonizing pain, costovertebral angle to groin depending on stone location
- Patient in constant motion, no comfort
- Nausea with or without vomiting
- Diaphoresis
- Tachycardia
- Intestinal ileus
- Abdominal guarding and rebound (rare)
- Tenderness to deep abdominal palpation, usually at CVA
- Lower tract stone with frequency, urgency, dysuria
- Fever, with infection
- Hematuria
- Pyuria, with infection
- May be asymptomatic if stone stays within kidney

CAUSES
- Calcium oxalate/calcium phosphate 65%-85%
  - ◊ Supersaturation from any cause
  - ◊ Dehydration
  - ◊ Increased absorption
  - ◊ Increased calcium excretion - familial
  - ◊ Renal tubular acidosis
  - ◊ Hyperparathyroidism
  - ◊ Chronic bowel disease with absorptive disorders
  - ◊ Poor GI citrate absorption
  - ◊ Excessive oral vitamin D or C
  - ◊ Alkaline urinary pH
  - ◊ Chronic use of calcium antacids
  - ◊ Diet high in calcium or oxalate
  - ◊ Malignancy
  - ◊ Hyperthyroidism
  - ◊ Chronic steroid therapy
  - ◊ Thiazide diuretics
- Struvite (staghorn calculus) 15%-20%
  - ◊ Infection
  - ◊ Alkaline urine
- Uric acid 5%
  - ◊ Hereditary
  - ◊ Gout
  - ◊ Chronic bowel disease
  - ◊ High purine diet
  - ◊ Acidic urine, very low pH
  - ◊ Malignancy with chemotherapy
- Cystine 1%-3%
  - ◊ Hereditary homocystinuria

RISK FACTORS
- Family history
- Climate, hot
- Work in hot environment
- Poor fluid consumption
- Diet high in oxalate, purine, calcium
- Excessive vitamins
- Malignancy
- Sarcoidosis
- Gout
- Thiazide diuretics
- Bowel or kidney disease

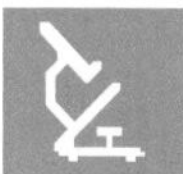

DIAGNOSIS

DIFFERENTIAL DIAGNOSIS
- Pyelonephritis
- Clot or sloughed papillae (secondary to diabetes, infection, analgesic abuse)
- Drug-seeking addiction
- Acute abdomen
- Gynecological problems
- Diverticulitis
- Abdominal aortic aneurysm

LABORATORY
- Urinalysis: Hematuria nearly 100%; if pH < 5.5 means uric acid, if pH > 7.5 means struvite
- Chemistries: Calcium, phosphorus, electrolytes, uric acid, creatinine, magnesium
- Parathyroid hormone: If serum calcium high
- Urine cystine: If stone not visible on plain x-ray
- Urine culture: If pyuria or fever

Drugs that may alter lab results: Pyridium may alter urinalysis

Disorders that may alter lab results: See Causes and Risk Factors

PATHOLOGICAL FINDINGS Stone analysis: 60-80% calcium base, 15-20% struvite, 5% uric acid, 1-3% cystine

SPECIAL TESTS Stone analysis

IMAGING
- Plain kidney, ureter and bladder (KUB) x-ray: 60-80% visible with some calcium
- Intravenous pyelogram (IVP): Standard for urolithiasis; also shows kidney function
- Ultrasound: Technique varies, if good has equal sensitivity and specificity to IVP
- Spiral CT scan (becoming primary); can still miss a small stone. Good for other causes of the pain.
- New MRI study being explored. Good results, but usually not timely. Shows renal function and stones.

DIAGNOSTIC PROCEDURES Retrograde pyelogram, if necessary for high grade obstruction or poor visualization on IVP

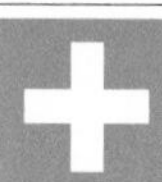

TREATMENT

APPROPRIATE HEALTH CARE
- 80% outpatient only, most pass in 48 hrs
- 20% hospitalization and urology referral
- Stone size and likelihood of passing spontaneously
  - ◊ < 4 mm - 80%
  - ◊ 4-6 mm - 59%
  - ◊ > 6 mm - 21%

GENERAL MEASURES
- Reassurance
- Strain urine
- Hydration
- Pain control
- Refer to urologist for: Intractable pain, obstruction, size > 6 mm, infection, dehydration, failure to progress, stone growth, single kidney, persistent gross hematuria, pregnancy, severe renal disease
- Hospitalize for:
  - ◊ Pain - intractable - parenteral medications
  - ◊ Persistent vomiting
  - ◊ High grade fever
  - ◊ Obstruction with infection
  - ◊ Solitary kidney with obstruction

SURGICAL MEASURES
- Extracorporeal shock wave lithotripsy: Stone in renal pelvis or upper 2/3 ureter, size < 2 cm, noninfected, no coagulopathy
- Urethroscopy: Lower 1/3 ureter, normal anatomy present. Newer graspers available for upper ureter.
- Percutaneous nephrolithotomy: Renal collecting system or upper 2/3 ureter, size > 2 cm, ureter stricture, cystine or uric acid stones, struvite, infection, obesity - may be used with intracorporeal lithotripsy
- Open surgery: Less than 5% of patients, complex anatomy, obstruction, large infected struvite stone
- Urethroscopy with lithotripsy available for lower 1/3 ureter
- Stenting for upper 1/3 or lower 1/3 ureter

ACTIVITY Bedrest, if necessary during acute phase. No restrictions after stone passes.

DIET
- Normal diet, 8 oz. water every 1 hour while awake, and if possible every 2 hours during sleep hours
- If uric acid stones, less protein in diet and take sodium bicarbonate to alkalinize urine

PATIENT EDUCATION
- Instructions on urine straining, dietary advice
- See Patient Care, August 15, 1990, p.42

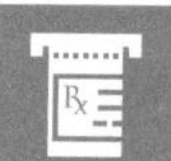

MEDICATIONS

DRUG(S) OF CHOICE

- Acute therapy:
  - ◊ Pain control (in office) - IM meperidine (Demerol) or morphine or buprenorphine (Buprenex), etc.
  - ◊ 3 day supply pain control - acetaminophen-oxycodone (Percocet), pentazocine (Talwin), acetaminophen-hydrocodone (Vicodin), etc.
  - ◊ Uric acid stone - potassium citrate (Urocit-K), 60-80 mEq/d (30-40 mmol/d) to keep urine pH 6.5-7.0. Check urine pH qid.
  - ◊ Cystine stone - penicillamine (Cuprimine, Depen) 1-4 g/d, K-citrate (Urocit-K) 60 mEq/d (30 mmol/d)
  - ◊ Infected stones - antibiotics for complicated pyelonephritis
- Maintenance therapy:
  - ◊ Hypercalciuria - sodium cellulose phosphate 10-15 g/d (2.5-5.0 grams with each meal), hydrochlorothiazide (HCTZ) 50 mg bid, K-citrate 15-20 mEq (7.5-10 mmol) bid
  - ◊ Uric acid - allopurinol (Zyloprim) 300 mg/d, K-citrate 20-30 mEq bid
  - ◊ Cystine - K-citrate 30 mEq (15 mmol) bid, penicillamine 1-4 g/d

Contraindications:

- Penicillamine with pregnancy, renal failure, aplastic anemia, hypersensitivity reaction
- Avoid potassium citrate with renal insufficiency

Precautions: Penicillamine requires regular CBC with differential counts, urinalysis, liver function tests

Significant possible interactions: Refer to manufacturer's profile of each drug

ALTERNATIVE DRUGS

Individualize to any underlying metabolic etiology found

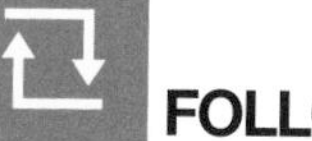

FOLLOWUP

PATIENT MONITORING

- Acute urolithiasis:
  - ◊ Strain urine until stone or 72 hours after symptoms cease
  - ◊ Repeat urinalysis 2-3 days
  - ◊ Repeat KUB x-ray and or IVP/CT scan/ultrasound if no stone passed
  - ◊ Stone analysis
  - ◊ KUB x-ray at 3-6 months and at 1 year, if no new stone, then no further followup needed
- Recurrent urolithiasis:
  - ◊ 24 hour urine: volume, pH, calcium, phosphorus, sodium, uric acid, oxalate, citrate, creatinine clearance
  - ◊ Measure parathyroid hormone (PTH)
  - ◊ Calcium restricted diet test for urine calcium level with 24 hour urine

PREVENTION/AVOIDANCE

- Hydration with urine > 2 liters a day (including nocturia once nightly)
- Dietary calcium < 1 g/d (being questioned if correct)
- Also should correct any zinc deficiency to help solubility

POSSIBLE COMPLICATIONS

- Hydronephrosis or kidney damage
- Infection and sepsis

EXPECTED COURSE/PROGNOSIS

- 80% will pass in 48-72 hours with outpatient therapy
- Recurrence - 10% 1 year, 35% 5 years, 50% 10 years

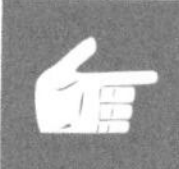

MISCELLANEOUS

ASSOCIATED CONDITIONS

See Causes section

AGE-RELATED FACTORS

Pediatric: Homocystinuria or other hereditary disorder

Geriatric: N/A

Others: N/A

PREGNANCY

Urology referral

SYNONYMS

- Nephrolithiasis
- Kidney stone
- Renal colic

ICD-9-CM

592.9 Urinary calculus, unspecified

SEE ALSO

Renal calculi

OTHER NOTES

N/A

ABBREVIATIONS

KUB = kidney, ureter, bladder

IVP = intravenous pyelogram

HCTZ = hydrochlorothiazide

REFERENCES

- Coe FL, Parks JH, Asplin JR: The pathogenesis and treatment of kidney stones. New Eng J Med 1992;327(46):1141-1152
- Resnick MI, ed: The Urologic Clinics of North America: urolithiasis. Philadelphia, WB Saunders Co, 1997;2:1-185
- Rakel RE, ed: Conn's Current Therapy. Philadelphia, WB Saunders Co., 1997:727-732
- Goldfarb DS, Coe FL. Prevention of recurrent nephrolithiasis. Am Fam Physician 1999;60(8):2269-76
- Manthey DE. Nephrolithiasis. Emerg Med Clin North Am 2001;19(3):633-54

Web references: 0 available at www.5mcc.com

Illustrations N/A

Author(s):

William H. Billica, MD

BASICS

DESCRIPTION Itchy rash. Single or multiple superficial pale papules and plaques with red halo. Subside within 24 hours; no scars or change in pigmentation. May be recurrent.
- Acute urticaria
  - ◊ Response to many stimuli
  - ◊ IgE-mediated histamine release from mast cells
  - ◊ Sometimes idiosyncratic response to drug exposure
  - ◊ Subsides over several hours
- Chronic urticaria: Persists > 6 weeks (30% of cases). Not mediated by IgE. Multiple types:
  - ◊ Cold urticaria - from cooling and then rewarming. Can be fatal (cold immersion with massive histamine release). Also a familial form with fever, chills, arthralgia, myalgia, headache, lymphocytosis.
  - ◊ Cholinergic urticaria - heat urticaria. Small (5-10 mm) wheals on upper trunk from overheating, hot shower; often adolescents ans young adults
  - ◊ Exercise-induced urticaria - from extreme exercise; presents as cholinergic urticaria, angioedema, wheezing, hypotension. Often associated with eating food to which patient is allergic.
  - ◊ Dermatographism - linear, itchy, red wheal and flare resulting from scratching or rubbing the skin
  - ◊ Solar urticaria - result of exposure to sunlight. Several types, by wavelength of light which induces reaction. Majority react to ultraviolet. Onset in minutes; subsides in 1-2 hours.
  - ◊ Delayed pressure urticaria - deeper and more painful urticaria, occurs 2-6 hours after pressure to skin (elastic, shoes, etc.)
  - ◊ Aquagenic urticaria - rare. Small wheals after contact with water at any temperature.
- It is common for one form of physical urticaria to overlap with another
- Idiopathic urticaria
  - ◊ Acute or chronic

System(s) affected: Skin/Exocrine
Genetics: No consistent genetic pattern known
Incidence/Prevalence in USA: 1 in 1000. Affects 15-20% of population at some time during life.
Predominant age: All ages. Acute form mainly in children, young adults.
Predominant sex: Male = Female (chronic forms more often in older women)

SIGNS & SYMPTOMS
- Seen alone or with angioedema
- May occur with generalized anaphylactic reaction, potentially fatal
- Single or multiple raised, blanched, central wheals surrounded by red flare
- Intensely pruritic
- May occur anywhere on body
- Variably sized, 1-2 mm to 15-20 cm or larger; sometimes confluent
- Rapid onset, resolves spontaneously in less than 48 hours

CAUSES
- Allergic or non-allergic; massive histamine release from mast cells in superficial dermis
- Drug reaction (any drug) either from allergy or idiosyncrasy
- Aspirin, NSAID's seem to trigger by inhibiting cyclo-oxygenase, without IgE
- Food or food additive allergy
- Allergy to peanuts and/or tree nuts a leading cause of severe (sometimes fatal) food-induced allergic reactions. Affects 1% of the general population. Other foods that cause hives are chocolate, fish, tomatoes, eggs, fresh berries, milk. Also food additives and preservatives.
- Inhalant, contact, or ingestant allergy
- Transfusion reaction
- Insect bite, sting
- Infection - viral upper respiratory infections (especially in children) and infectious mononucleosis, viral hepatitis; bacterial (strep throat, sinusitis, dental abscess, otitis); vaginitis; fungal (tineas); helminthic; protozoan. Helicobacter pylori has been increasingly associated with, and its eradication may stop, chronic urticaria.
- Collagen vascular disease (cutaneous vasculitis, serum sickness, lupus)
- Thyroid autoimmunity often associated. Administering thyroid hormone may alleviate chronic urticaria in hypothyroid patients with autoantibodies.
- Physical trauma (heat, cold, sunlight, etc.)
- Emotional stress (reported; little supporting evidence)
- Histamine-releasing autoantibodies have been identified in some cases of chronic idiopathic urticaria
- In childhood acute urticaria, infection (especially urinary tract) is the most frequently documented cause (49%), followed by drugs (5%), and food allergies (3%).
- In chronic urticaria, physical factors are the leading cause (53%). Urticaria management should include a survey of certain infectious agents (E. coli, C. pneumonia, H. pylori) in addition to a detailed history.

RISK FACTORS Listed with Causes

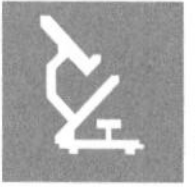

DIAGNOSIS

DIFFERENTIAL DIAGNOSIS
- Insect bites
- Morbilliform drug eruptions
- Erythema multiforme
- Vasculitis and polyarteritis
- Systemic lupus erythematosus
- Urticaria pigmentosa (mastocytosis). Pink lesions urticate when scratched (Darier's sign).
- Bullous pemphigoid (urticarial stage)

LABORATORY
- More likely to discover the cause of acute than of chronic urticaria. Routine lab screening not helpful in diagnosing chronic urticaria.
- Cause found in only 10-25% of chronic cases
- Food and drug reactions - elimination diets, challenges with suspected agents
- Inhalant allergens - skin tests, radioallergosorbent (RAST)
- Idiopathic for > 6 weeks - CBC, skin biopsy, ESR, urinalysis, ANA
- 40-50% of patients with chronic urticaria have a cutaneous autoimmune disorder mediated by autoantibodies to the IgE receptor on mast cells
- Blood eosinophilia should prompt stool examination for O & P

Drugs that may alter lab results: Antihistamines, H2-blockers, tricyclic antidepressants

Disorders that may alter lab results: N/A

PATHOLOGICAL FINDINGS Edema, vasculitis and/or perivasculitis involving only superficial dermis

SPECIAL TESTS
- Cold urticaria - ice cube test (place ice cube on skin 5 minutes, observe 10-15 minutes)
- Cholinergic or exercise-induced: exercise challenge; methacholine skin test (local reaction to 0.01 mg in 0.05 ml saline intradermally. 50% false negatives).
- Dermatographism - scratch skin with piece of tongue blade, observe
- Solar - expose to defined wavelengths of light. Must rule out erythropoietic protoporphyria.
- Delayed pressure: apply 5-10 pound sandbag for 3 hours, observe
- Aquagenic - apply tap water at different temperatures
- Vibratory: apply vibration 4-5 minutes with a lab mixing device, observe
- Infection - pharyngeal culture, antistreptolysin (ASO) titer, rapid plasma reagin (RPR), parasitology, liver function tests, mononucleosis test
- Autoimmune - antinuclear antibody (ANA), rheumatoid arthritis (RA), complement, cryoglobulins, serum protein electrophoresis

IMAGING N/A

DIAGNOSTIC PROCEDURES Skin biopsy beneficial only in ruling out urticarial vasculitis

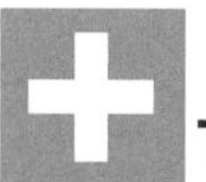

TREATMENT

APPROPRIATE HEALTH CARE Don't work up acute cases (results usually inconclusive)

GENERAL MEASURES Cool moist compresses help to control itching

SURGICAL MEASURES N/A

ACTIVITY As desired. Avoid overheating.

DIET As desired. Avoid foods implicated as possible etiologic agents.

PATIENT EDUCATION Avoidance if etiology is apparent. Antihistamines if accidentally re-exposed.

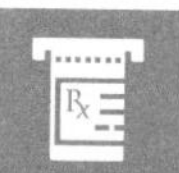

MEDICATIONS

DRUG(S) OF CHOICE

- First generation antihistamines
  - ◊ Older children and adults: hydroxyzine or diphenhydramine, 25-50 mg q6h
  - ◊ Children under six: diphenhydramine 12.5 mg (elixir) q6-8h (5 mg/kg/day)
- Second generation H1 blockers are more expensive, about as effective as older antihistamines, but are less sedating (14% of patients, still less than 1st generation drugs), because they do not cross the blood-brain barrier.
  - ◊ Fexofenadine (Allegra) 60 mg bid
  - ◊ Loratadine (Claritin) 10 mg daily
  - ◊ Acrivastine (Semprex) 8 mg tid
  - ◊ Cetirizine (Zyrtec)10 mg daily. More sedating than others in this class.

Contraindications: Danazol not for use in childhood, pregnancy.

Precautions:

- Drowsiness with first generation drugs
- Second generation H1 blockers of little benefit in delayed pressure urticaria or urticarial vasculitis; should be used with caution in pregnancy and the elderly

Significant possible interactions: Refer to manufacturer's profile of each drug

ALTERNATIVE DRUGS

- Doxepin (Sinequan), tricyclic antidepressant with strong H1 and H2 blocking properties; very effective for urticaria (10 to 25 mg at bedtime). Sedation limits usefulness during the day.
- H2-blockers (cimetidine, ranitidine, etc.) may be mildly helpful in chronic urticaria
- Corticosteroids for unresponsive cases (not acutely), e.g., prednisone 40 mg daily for 5-7 days, followed by taper as antihistamines are introduced. Often used in delayed pressure urticaria.
- Cyproheptadine is an antihistamine and antiserotonergic agent, which may be particularly beneficial in cold urticaria
- Cyclosporine is the best studied immunosuppressive therapy; effective (2.5-5 mg/kg/day) and steroid sparing
- Leukotriene antagonists are safe and worth trying in chronic, unresponsive cases
- IVIG, plasmapheresis, sulfasalazine, dapsone, and hydroxychloroquine require further study

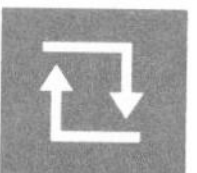

FOLLOWUP

PATIENT MONITORING No followup for initial episode. Evaluate if symptoms persist or recur.

PREVENTION/AVOIDANCE If etiology identified, avoidance is best solution

POSSIBLE COMPLICATIONS Severe systemic allergic reaction (bronchospasm, anaphylaxis)

EXPECTED COURSE/PROGNOSIS
70% better in < 72 hours. 30% chronic. 20% have attacks for > 20 years. Becomes chronic in 75% of patients with both urticaria and angioedema.

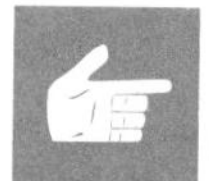

MISCELLANEOUS

ASSOCIATED CONDITIONS Angioedema, anaphylaxis

AGE-RELATED FACTORS
Pediatric: Acute isolated incidents are more frequent, chronic urticaria is rare.
Geriatric: Less likely to occur in this age group
Others: N/A

PREGNANCY Chronic urticaria

SYNONYMS Hives

ICD-9-CM
708.8 Other specified urticaria

SEE ALSO
Anaphylaxis
Angioedema

OTHER NOTES Same pathophysiology for urticaria and angioedema - localized anaphylaxis causes vasodilatation, vascular permeability of skin (urticaria) or subcutaneous tissue (angioedema)

ABBREVIATIONS N/A

REFERENCES

- Sackesen C, Sekerel BE, Orhan F, Kocabas CN, Tuncer A, Adalioglu G. The etiology of different forms of urticaria in childhood. Pediatr Dermatol. 2004 Mar-Apr;21(2):102-8
- Grattan CE, et al. Chronic urticaria. J Am Acad Dermatol 2002;46(5):645-57
- Heymann WR: Chronic urticaria and angioedema associated with thyroid autoimmunity; review and therapeutic implications. J Am Acad Dermatol 1999;40(2pt1):229-232
- Kozel MM, et al: The effectiveness of a history-based diagnostic approach in chronic urticaria and angioedema. Arch Dermatol 1998;134(12):1575-80
- Kumar SA, Martin BL: Urticaria and angioedema: diagnostic and treatment considerations. J Am Osteopath Assoc 1999;99(3suppl):s1-4
- Mortureux P, et al: Acute urticaria in infancy and early childhood: a prospective study. Arch Dermatol 1998;134(3):319-23
- Sabroe RA, et al: Chronic idiopathic urticaria: comparison of the clinical features of patients with and without anti-Fc epsilon RI or anti-IgE autoantibodies. J Am Acad Dermatol 1999;40(3):443-50
- Sicherer SH, et al: Clinical features of acute allergic reactions to peanut and tree nuts in children. Pediatrics 1998;102(1):e6
- Wedi B, et al: Prevalence of helicobacter pylori-associated gastritis in chronic urticaria. Int Arch Allergy Immunol 1998;116(4):288-94
- Zuberbier T. Urticaria. Allergy 2003;58(12):1224-34

Web references: 1 available at www.5mcc.com
Illustrations 8 available

Author(s):

Benjamin Barankin, MD

Uterine corpus malignancy

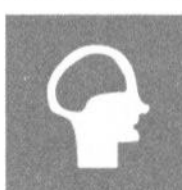

BASICS

DESCRIPTION
- Endometrial cancer: Malignancy of the endometrial lining of the uterus. Tumor grade - low, moderate, high. Cell types - adenocarcinoma, adenosquamous (benign or malignant squamous elements), clear cell, papillary serous.
- Sarcomas:
  - ◊ Mixed müllerian sarcoma - heterologous elements not native to the müllerian systems, such as cartilage or bone; homologous elements native to the mullerian system
  - ◊ Endometrial stromal sarcoma develops from the stromal component of the endometrium
  - ◊ Leiomyosarcoma develops in the myometrium or in a myoma (fibroid)

System(s) affected: Reproductive
Genetics: Unknown
Incidence/Prevalence in USA: Most common gynecologic malignancy, 35,000 new cases per year
Predominant age:
- Endometrial cancer - postmenopausal (mid fifties to mid sixties). Also can occur in young women in their twenties and thirties with polycystic ovarian disease or chronic anovulation.
- Sarcomas - forties to sixties

Predominant sex: Female only

SIGNS & SYMPTOMS
- Endometrial cancer:
  - ◊ Postmenopausal bleeding is the most frequent sign. Any spotting should lead to evaluation.
  - ◊ Pap smear is rarely positive
  - ◊ Occasionally a patient will pass tissue that will render a diagnosis
- Sarcoma:
  - ◊ Mixed müllerian sarcoma - bleeding and prolapsing tissue
  - ◊ Leiomyosarcoma - increasing size of presumed uterine myomas
  - ◊ D&C rarely diagnostic

CAUSES
- Unopposed estrogen due to:
  - ◊ Polycystic ovarian disease
  - ◊ Obesity
  - ◊ Chronic anovulation
  - ◊ Estrogen replacement therapy. (Estrogen replacement without concomitant progesterone increases the risk 70 times. When progesterone is added the risk does not decrease to zero but decreases to that of the population in general).
- Tamoxifen. Increases risk similar to that for unopposed estrogen.
- Sarcomas:
  - ◊ Etiology unknown

RISK FACTORS
- Early menarche
- Late menopause
- Nulliparity
- Hypertension and diabetes are probably associated with underlying obesity

DIAGNOSIS

DIFFERENTIAL DIAGNOSIS
- Atypical complex hyperplasia (a premalignant lesion of the endometrium)
- Bleeding from cervical cancer
- Ovarian cancer invading the uterus
- Adenocarcinoma of the cervix
- Endometriosis

LABORATORY
- Liver function tests
- CA-125 can be elevated when intra-abdominal disease is present

Drugs that may alter lab results: N/A

Disorders that may alter lab results: A biopsy of a pregnant uterus can produce tissue which has a hyperplastic or premalignant appearance

PATHOLOGICAL FINDINGS
- Stage I - confined to corpus
  - ◊ A. Confined to endometrium
  - ◊ B. Less than 50% myometrial invasion
  - ◊ C. More than 50% myometrial invasion
- Stage II
  - ◊ A. Endocervical involvement (microscopic)
  - ◊ B. Cervical stromal invasion (macroscopic)
- Stage III
  - ◊ A. Uterine serosal/adnexal involvement/positive peritoneal cytology
  - ◊ B. Vaginal metastases
  - ◊ C. Involved pelvic/para aortic lymph nodes
- Stage IV
  - ◊ A. Extension to involve the mucosa of the bladder or rectum
  - ◊ B. Distant metastatic disease or inguinal node involvement
- Stages are also subgrouped according to histologic grade:
  - ◊ GI - Well differentiated
  - ◊ G2 - Moderately differentiated
  - ◊ G3 - Poorly differentiated

SPECIAL TESTS Any that may be indicated preoperatively

IMAGING
- Chest x-ray - the most common site of metastases is the lungs. Rarely does this malignancy go to the bone or the liver except in advanced disease.
- CT scan, bone scan, liver spleen scan - not part of the routine evaluation, but may be needed occasionally
- Mammogram (endometrial cancer is associated with breast cancer)
- Barium enema (endometrial cancer is associated with colon cancer)
- MRI has been reported to accurately show the depth of myometrial penetration, but this is not always cost-effective
- Vaginal ultrasound can show increased endometrial echoes prior to D & C, which will lead to the diagnosis

DIAGNOSTIC PROCEDURES
- Office endometrial biopsy (90% accurate). If this is negative, a D & C is necessary. Endometrial stromal sarcoma and leiomyosarcoma are rarely diagnosed preoperatively.
- D & C (99% accurate)

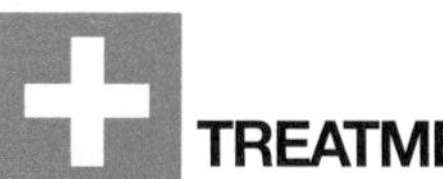

TREATMENT

APPROPRIATE HEALTH CARE Inpatient surgery

GENERAL MEASURES
- Radiation is used to prevent the recurrence of tumor at the vaginal cuff
- When distant metastatic disease occurs, progesterone produces a 30% response rate. Active chemotherapeutic agents are cisplatin and Adriamycin.

SURGICAL MEASURES
- Surgical procedure is abdominal exploration with extrafascial total abdominal hysterectomy, bilateral salpingo-oophorectomy, cytology, pelvic and para-aortic node sampling
- Surgery is followed by radiation therapy in high-risk patients who have Stage 1B disease or greater, or for patients with poorly differentiated tumors regardless of stage. There is no adjuvant therapy that has been shown to be effective after surgery and radiation.

ACTIVITY Patients are usually ambulatory and able to resume full activity by six weeks after surgery

DIET Unrestricted unless they are undergoing radiation

PATIENT EDUCATION
- The American Cancer Society in the local community
- American College of Obstetricians & Gynecologists (ACOG), 409 12th St., SW, Washington, DC 20024-2188, (800)762-ACOG

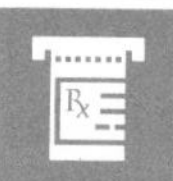

MEDICATIONS

DRUG(S) OF CHOICE
- There are no drugs as adjuvant therapy
- Premalignant lesions in young women or in patients unsuitable for hysterectomy can be treated with megestrol (Megace), 160 mg qd x 3 months. This is followed by repeat D & C to ascertain whether the hyperplasia has resolved.
- Metastatic disease is treated with high dose progesterone, or doxorubicin (Adriamycin) or cisplatin

Contraindications:
- Progestational agents can cause significant fluid retention in 5-10% of patients
- Patients with congestive heart failure must be observed closely

Precautions: Usual precautions with chemotherapeutic agents. Refer to manufacturer's profile of each drug.

Significant possible interactions: Refer to manufacturer's profile of each drug

ALTERNATIVE DRUGS
- Ondansetron (Zofran), dronabinol (Marinol), metoclopramide (Reglan), and others for nausea control

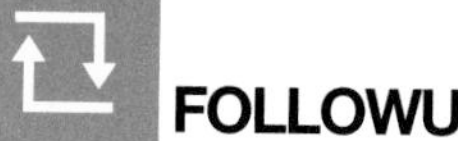

FOLLOWUP

PATIENT MONITORING
- Pap smear every 3 months for two years, then every 6 months for 3 years
- Chest x-ray once a year

PREVENTION/AVOIDANCE
- In young women who are obese or anovulatory, endometrial cancer can be reduced by cyclic progesterone to prevent unopposed estrogen or by taking birth control pills
- Estrogen replacement therapy should always include progestational agents unless the woman has undergone hysterectomy

POSSIBLE COMPLICATIONS Those attendant upon major abdominal surgery

EXPECTED COURSE/PROGNOSIS

Five year survival for uterine malignancy:

Grade	Survival
Ia G1	98%
Ib G2	85%
Ic G3	60%
IIa/b	60%
III	40%
IV	15%

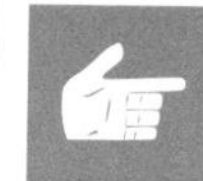

MISCELLANEOUS

ASSOCIATED CONDITIONS
- Obese patients with endometrial cancer should be screened annually because of increased risk of breast and colon cancer
- Patients who have breast or colon cancer are at increased risk for endometrial cancer. Granulosa cell tumors of the ovary produce estrogen and these patients will have an increased risk of endometrial cancer.

AGE-RELATED FACTORS
Pediatric: N/A

Geriatric: Older (especially obese) patients may be at high risk for surgery. Alternative radiation therapy can be considered.

Others: If preserving fertility is desired - young anovulatory women, polycystic ovarian patients with atypical complex hyperplasia, or patients with well differentiated endometrial cancer can be treated with progestational agents x 3 months followed by D&C

PREGNANCY This malignancy is not associated with pregnancy

SYNONYMS
- Uterine cancer
- Endometrial cancer
- Corpus cancer

ICD-9-CM
182.0 Malignant neoplasm of corpus uteri, except isthmus
182.8 Malignant neoplasm of other specified sites of body of uterus
182.1 Malignant neoplasm of body of uterus, isthmus
180.0 Malignant neoplasm of body of cervix uteri, endocervix

SEE ALSO
Cervical malignancy

OTHER NOTES N/A

ABBREVIATIONS N/A

REFERENCES

- Hopkins MP: Benign and Malignant Diseases of the Uterus. In: Willson JR, ed. Obstetrics and Gynecology. St. Louis, Mosby Year Book, 1991
- Hopkins MP. Endometrial hyperplasia and adenocarcinoma of the endometrium. In: Copeland LJ, ed. Textbook of gynecology. 2nd ed. Philadelphia, PA: W B Saunders Co; 2000. chapters 57 & 58.

Web references: 1 available at www.5mcc.com
Illustrations N/A

Author(s):
Michael P. Hopkins, MD, MEd
Eric L. Jenison, MD

BASICS

DESCRIPTION Uterine leiomyomas are well circumscribed, pseudo-encapsulated benign tumors composed mainly of smooth muscle but with varying amounts of fibrous connective tissue

- Three major types:
  - ◊ Submucous: 5% of total, susceptible to abnormal uterine bleeding, infection and occasionally protrude from cervix
  - ◊ Subserous: Common, may become pedunculated and rarely parasitic
  - ◊ Intramural: Common, may cause marked uterine enlargement

System(s) affected: Reproductive
Genetics: N/A
Incidence/Prevalence in USA: 4-11% of all women, 20% of all women over 35 years of age and 40% of women over 50 years of age
Predominant age: Fourth and fifth decades
Predominant sex: Female only

SIGNS & SYMPTOMS
- Majority are asymptomatic and are only suspected from pelvic examination
- Most common symptom is abnormal uterine bleeding. Hypermenorrhea most common. Secondary anemia with associated symptomatology may result.
- Pressure on bladder may result in suprapubic discomfort, urinary frequency
- Pressure on rectosigmoid may result in low back pain
- Edema and varicosities of the lower extremities may result from large tumors
- Pain may result from twisted, pedunculated myomas or degenerating, hemorrhagic or infected myomas
- Infertility may result from submucous myomas or with distortion of uterine cavity
- Rapid growth particularly in perimenopausal or post-menopausal may indicate sarcoma

CAUSES
- May arise from totipotential cells normally giving rise to muscle and connective tissue cells
- May arise from small immature smooth muscle cell nests
- Positive correlation with estrogen stimulation, i.e., not seen before menarche, may grow rapidly during pregnancy, with use of oral estrogen, and with estrogen producing tumors. Myomas regress following pregnancy and after menopause.

RISK FACTORS
- Later reproductive and perimenopausal age groups
- 3-9 times higher among African-Americans

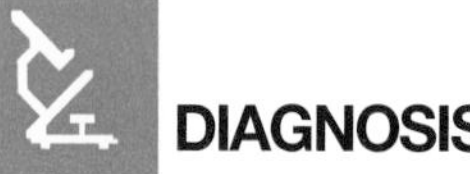

DIAGNOSIS

DIFFERENTIAL DIAGNOSIS
- Intrauterine pregnancy
- Ovarian tumor
- Cecal or sigmoid tumor
- Appendiceal abscess
- Diverticulitis
- Pelvic kidney
- Urachal cyst

LABORATORY
- Pregnancy test
- CBC, differential count
- CA-125 - may be slightly elevated in some cases of uterine myomas, but generally is more useful in differentiating myomas from various gynecologic adenocarcinomas

Drugs that may alter lab results: N/A

Disorders that may alter lab results: N/A

PATHOLOGICAL FINDINGS
- Myomas are usually multiple and vary in size and location. Have been reported up to 100 pounds (45 kg).
- Gross pathology reveals firm tumors with characteristic whorl-like trabeculated appearance. A thin pseudo-capsular layer is present.
- Microscopic appearance reveals bundles of smooth muscle mixed with varying amounts of connective tissue elements running in different directions
- Cellular variant has a preponderance of muscle cells. Mitoses are rare.
- May undergo various types of degeneration:
  - ◊ I - Hyaline degeneration. Very common, eventually results in liquefaction and cyst formation.
  - ◊ II - Calcification. Late result of circulatory impairment to myomas.
  - ◊ III - Infection and suppuration. Submucous myomas most prone to infection and may lead to sepsis.
  - ◊ IV - Necrosis. Pedunculated subserous fibroids most prone to necrosis secondary to torsion.
  - ◊ V - Sarcomatous change. Incidence ranges from 1.0 to 0.1% of clinically apparent myomas.

SPECIAL TESTS N/A

IMAGING
- Ultrasonography shows characteristic hypoechoic appearance
- Saline infusion hysterosonography may help to distinguish submucous myomas
- CT scan, MRI may help to differentiate complex cases
- Intravenous pyelogram (IVP)
- Barium enema

DIAGNOSTIC PROCEDURES
- Presumptive diagnosis by abdominal and pelvic examination: Firm, smooth nodules or masses arising from uterus. Masses are mobile without pain.
- Fractional D & C aids in ruling out cervical, uterine carcinomas
- Hysteroscopy may help diagnose submucous myomas
- Laparoscopy may be useful in complex cases and in ruling out other pelvic pathology

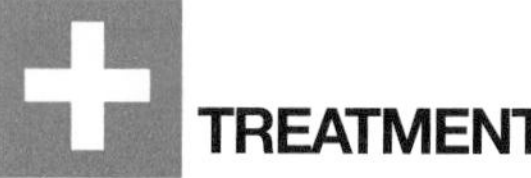

TREATMENT

APPROPRIATE HEALTH CARE Outpatient usually; inpatient for some surgical procedures

GENERAL MEASURES
- Treatment must be individualized
- Patients with minimal symptoms may be managed with iron preparations and analgesics
- Conservative management: Asymptomatic myomas of less than 14 weeks' size gestation should be closely observed with pelvic examinations and ultrasonography at 3-6 month intervals, as long as size stable. Usually regress after menopause.
- Nonsurgical therapies
  - ◊ Luteinizing hormone releasing hormone (LHRH) agonists induce an abrupt artificial menopause with cessation of bleeding and shrinkage of myomas. Not recommended for more than six months. May be useful in perimenopausal patients or as an adjunct in preparation for surgery.
  - ◊ Myolysis by needle cautery or cryotherapy. Long term outcome is unknown
  - ◊ Uterine artery embolization average 50% shrinkage; painful
  - ◊ Endometrial ablation for hypermenorrhea

SURGICAL MEASURES
- Surgical management is indicated in the following situations:
  - ◊ Excessive uterine size (> 14 weeks gestation) or excessive rate of growth (except during pregnancy)
  - ◊ Submucous location if associated with hypermenorrhea
  - ◊ Pedunculated myomas may undergo torsion, pain, necrosis and hemorrhage
  - ◊ Symptomatic from pressure on bladder or rectum
  - ◊ If differentiation from ovarian mass is not possible
  - ◊ If there is associated pelvic disease, i.e., endometriosis, pelvic inflammatory disease, etc.
  - ◊ If infertility or habitual abortion is likely due to the anatomic location of the myoma
- Surgical procedures:
  - ◊ Hysteroscopic or laparoscopic cautery or laser myoma resection can be performed in selected cases
  - ◊ Myomectomies may be performed in younger women desiring to maintain fertility
  - ◊ Hysterectomy, either vaginal or abdominal, is procedure of choice for symptomatic women no longer desiring fertility
  - ◊ Preliminary Pap smear and endometrial sampling or D & C must be performed to rule out malignant or premalignant conditions

ACTIVITY

- Following hysteroscopic or laparoscopic myoma resection, bedrest 24 hours, no sexual intercourse for two weeks
- Following laparotomy for myomectomy or hysterectomy, 3-5 days hospital, followed by limited activity and no sexual intercourse for one month

DIET No restrictions

PATIENT EDUCATION ACOG (American College of Obstetricians and Gynecologists) pamphlet entitled "Uterine Fibroids," ACOG p-074

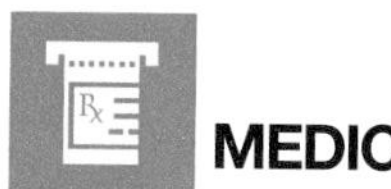

MEDICATIONS

DRUG(S) OF CHOICE

- Luteinizing hormone releasing hormone (LHRH) agonists such as nafarelin (Synarel Nasal Spray), goserelin (Zoladex Depot), leuprolide (Lupron Depot)
  - ◊ Induce abrupt, artificial menopause and render patients asymptomatic
  - ◊ Induce atrophy of myomas by up to 40% within 2-3 months
  - ◊ May be valuable as a preoperative adjunct to myomectomy or hysterectomy by allowing recovery of anemia, donation of autologous blood and possibly converting abdominal to vaginal hysterectomy, thereby decreasing postoperative pain, hospitalization, and morbidity. Generally used two to three months prior to surgery.
  - ◊ Not recommended for use longer than six months because of osteoporosis
  - ◊ Following discontinuation, myomas return within 60 days to pretherapy size
- Patients with minimal symptoms
  - ◊ May be managed conservatively with iron preparations and analgesics
  - ◊ Progestins such as norethindrone, 10 mg daily, or medroxyprogesterone (Depo-Provera) 200 mg IM, once monthly, may reduce the amount of blood flow. They do not reduce myoma size.

Contraindications:

- Progestins - history of thromboembolic phenomenon
- LHRH agonists - history of osteoporosis

Precautions: LHRH agonists induce acute menopausal symptoms: hot flashes, night sweats, insomnia, emotional lability, and osteoporosis

Significant possible interactions: Refer to manufacturer's profile of each drug

ALTERNATIVE DRUGS N/A

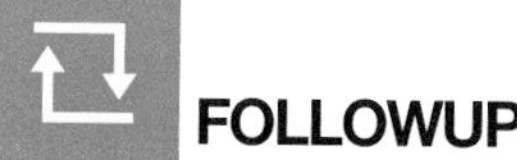

FOLLOWUP

PATIENT MONITORING

- Newly diagnosed uterine myoma, if symptomatic or excessive size, 2-3 months with pelvic exam and ultrasonography
- Consider CA-125 antigen
- Monitor hemoglobin and hematocrit, if uterine bleeding excessive
- If uterine size and symptoms stable, monitor every 6 months

PREVENTION/AVOIDANCE Excessive growth during estrogen stimulation, i.e., birth control pills, postmenopausal estrogen replacement therapy and pregnancy

POSSIBLE COMPLICATIONS

- Complications during pregnancy include abortion; premature labor; second trimester rapid myoma growth leading to degeneration and pain; third-trimester fetal dystocia during labor and delivery
- Previous myomectomy patients in labor may develop uterine rupture. C-section is recommended if entered endometrial cavity during myomectomy.
- May mask other gynecologic malignancies, i.e., uterine sarcoma, ovarian cancer

EXPECTED COURSE/PROGNOSIS

- Following myomectomy, 40% pregnancy rate in patients previously infertile
- At least 10% myomas recur following myomectomy

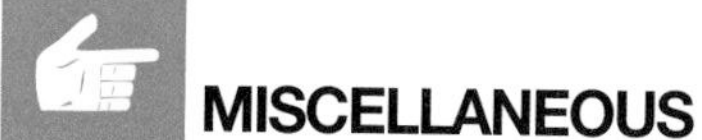

MISCELLANEOUS

ASSOCIATED CONDITIONS Endometrial carcinoma also associated with high unopposed estrogen stimulation

AGE-RELATED FACTORS

Pediatric: N/A

Geriatric: In postmenopausal patients with newly diagnosed uterine myoma or enlarging uterine myomas, highly suspect uterine sarcoma or other gynecologic malignancy

Others:

- Not seen in premenarchal females
- Incidence increases with each decade during reproductive years and is highest in perimenopausal age group

PREGNANCY See associations above

SYNONYMS

- Fibroids
- Myoma
- Fibromyoma
- Myofibroma
- Fibroleiomyoma

ICD-9-CM

218.0 Submucous leiomyoma of uterus

SEE ALSO

OTHER NOTES N/A

ABBREVIATIONS N/A

REFERENCES

- Zacur HA, Murray AA, Tulandi T, Verkauf BS. Myomas: advances in diagnosis and treatment. Contem OB/Gyn 1999;44(2):84-108
- Cunningham FG, MacDonald PC, Gant NF, eds. Williams' Obstetrics. 20th Ed. Norwalk, CT, Appleton and Lange, 1997
- Ryan KJ, Berkowitz R, Barbieri RL. Kistners' Gynecology: Principles & Practice. 6th Ed. Chicago, Year Book Publishers, 1995
- Jones HW III, Wentz AC, Burnett LS. Novak's Textbook of Gynecology. 12th Ed. Baltimore, Williams and Wilkins, 1996
- ACOG (American College of Obstetricians and Gynecologists) pamphlet entitled 'Uterine Fibroids,' ACOG p-074
- Rock JA, Thompson JD. Leiomyomata uteri and myomectomy. In: Thompson JD, Rock JA (eds): Telinde's Operative Gynecology. 8th ed. Philadelphia, Lippincott-Raven, 1997
- Verkauf BS. Myomectomy as a fertility-promoting procedure. Infertil & Reprod Med Clin NA 1996;1:69-89
- Goodwin SC, Vedantham S, McLucas B, et al. Preliminary experience with uterine artery embolization for uterine fibroids. J Vasc Interv Radiol 1997;8:517-526

Web references: 0 available at www.5mcc.com

Illustrations N/A

Author(s):

Eric L. Jenison, MD

Michael P. Hopkins, MD, MEd

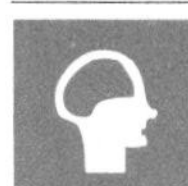

BASICS

DESCRIPTION Uterine prolapse occurs when the integrity of supporting structures is lost. This allows the uterus to descend into the vagina. In advanced cases, complete protrusion with inversion of the vagina occurs.
- Prior to menopause, the degree and severity of prolapse is usually related to the number of children and the difficulty of childbirth. After menopause, atrophy and loss of tissue integrity further leads to prolapse.

System(s) affected: Gastrointestinal, Renal/Urologic, Reproductive

Genetics:
- Common among Caucasian races
- Less common among Asians and African Americans and particularly uncommon in South African Bantus and West Africans

Incidence/Prevalence in USA: Approximately 1 in 10 women will experience some degree of prolapse

Predominant age: Peri- and post-menopausal female

Predominant sex: Female only

SIGNS & SYMPTOMS
- Pelvic pressure and low back pain
- As prolapse progresses, eventually a bulging is noticed as a result of protrusion
- Dyspareunia
- Difficulty with urination or defecation

CAUSES
- Advancing age and vaginal childbirth are the most important factors
- The incidence of prolapse increases with the frequency and difficulty of vaginal deliveries. Less than 2% of prolapse occurs in nulliparous women.
- Other causes of prolapse include connective tissue disorders with lax tissue, i.e., Marfan syndrome and neurogenic disorders, i.e., multiple sclerosis, cloacal agenesis, chronic constipation, pelvic tumors or ascites and chronic coughing from chronic lung disease
- Patients who have undergone radical vulvectomy with loss of the external supporting structures have a higher rate of prolapse

RISK FACTORS
- Childbirth, particularly multiple parity
- Advancing age
- Caucasian race
- Various connective tissue and neurogenic disorders
- Conditions resulting in increased intra-abdominal pressure, such as obesity, abdominal or pelvic tumors, pulmonary disease with chronic coughing, chronic constipation
- Occupations requiring heavy lifting

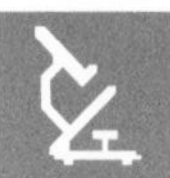

DIAGNOSIS

DIFFERENTIAL DIAGNOSIS N/A

LABORATORY
- Evaluation of renal function to rule out ureteral obstruction
- Urinalysis to rule out urinary tract infection

Drugs that may alter lab results: N/A

Disorders that may alter lab results: N/A

PATHOLOGICAL FINDINGS
- Hyperkeratosis of the cervical and vaginal tissues occur with prolapse beyond the introitus due to chronic irritation and drying. As the irritation becomes more pronounced, bleeding and ulceration occur.
- Degrees of prolapse:
  - ◊ First degree prolapse - to the ischial spine
  - ◊ Second degree prolapse - to the introitus
  - ◊ Third degree prolapse - just beyond the introitus
  - ◊ Fourth degree prolapse - complete uterine and vaginal inversion involving bladder and bowel

SPECIAL TESTS N/A

IMAGING
- Intravenous pyelogram to rule out ureteral obstruction in complete uterine prolapse (optional)
- Pelvic ultrasound or CT scan to rule out other pelvic pathology, if suspected (optional)

DIAGNOSTIC PROCEDURES
- If ulceration or bleeding is present, Pap smears and appropriate cervical and endometrial biopsies should be done to rule out concomitant malignancies
- IDiagnosis is by physical and pelvic examination. With coughing and straining, the cervix will prolapse toward introitus or beyond. The patient may need to be examined in the standing as well as lying position for diagnosis.

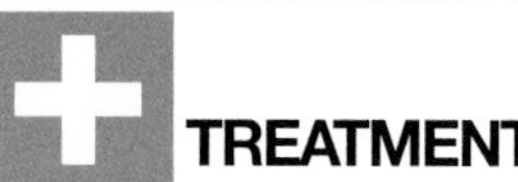

TREATMENT

APPROPRIATE HEALTH CARE
- Outpatient
- Inpatient when surgery is necessary

GENERAL MEASURES
- Treatment depends on multiple variables including the severity of prolapse, age, sexual activity, associated pelvic pathology and desire for future fertility
- Treatment of first and second degree prolapse is expectant unless patient is symptomatic
- Mildly symptomatic patients and poor surgical candidates - can be treated nonoperatively with perineal (Kegel) exercises, estrogen replacement and vaginal pessaries. Estrogen replacement restores healthy vaginal mucosa and promotes healing.

SURGICAL MEASURES
- Surgically able patients without additional pelvic pathology - vaginal hysterectomy with or without enterocele, cystocele, rectocele repair and vaginal vault suspension
- For patients who desire to maintain reproductive function - uterine suspension (rarely performed) with vaginal repair or Manchester procedure are options
- Elderly, non-sexually active women - can be treated with a colpocleisis or vaginal obliteration procedure

ACTIVITY Heavy lifting or significant increases in intra-abdominal pressure will lead to worsening of prolapse or recurrence after surgical correction. Lifting should therefore be restricted.

DIET Unlimited. Avoid constipation.

PATIENT EDUCATION
- Kegel exercises when applicable
- American College of Obstetricians & Gynecologists (ACOG), 409 12th St., SW, Washington, DC 20024-2188, (800)762-ACOG

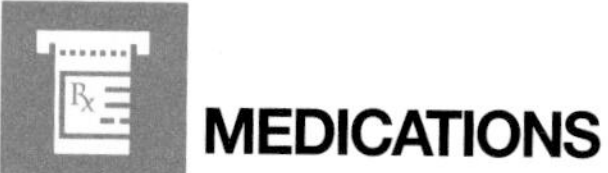

MEDICATIONS

DRUG(S) OF CHOICE Estrogen replacement therapy (oral or vaginal cream) can increase the blood supply to the vaginal tissues and in mild cases increase supporting tissue strength to a point where surgery or pessary use may be avoided

Contraindications: Those associated with the use of estrogen. Refer to manufacturer's literature.

Precautions: If estrogen therapy is utilized and the uterus is present, progesterone should be utilized to offset the potential of endometrial carcinoma

Significant possible interactions: Refer to manufacturer's literature

ALTERNATIVE DRUGS None

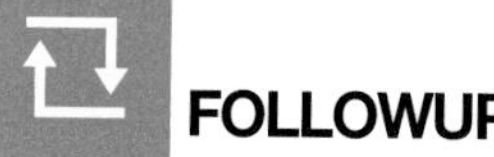

FOLLOWUP

PATIENT MONITORING
- Expectant management is appropriate with periodic follow-up examinations
- If a pessary is placed, it should be removed, cleaned and replaced each month or more often

PREVENTION/AVOIDANCE
- Kegel exercises will increase the strength of the pelvic diaphragm muscles and may provide some pelvic support
- Weight loss and proper management of conditions that would increase abdominal pressure help to prevent prolapse

POSSIBLE COMPLICATIONS
- Ureteral obstruction and renal failure
- Incarceration of bowel herniations
- Pessary use - may not always be effective, and may cause discomfort, ulcers, infection

EXPECTED COURSE/PROGNOSIS
- It is expected that as patients age, the incidence and severity of prolapse will increase
- Surgical correction usually successful

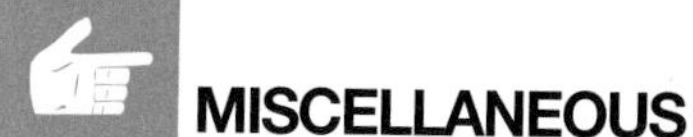

MISCELLANEOUS

ASSOCIATED CONDITIONS Cystocele, rectocele, enterocele and vaginal vault prolapse are often associated with uterine prolapse

AGE-RELATED FACTORS
Pediatric: Prolapse in newborn has been reported, but is rare and usually associated with congenital disorders and neuropathies

Geriatric: This is largely a disease of aging and will be much higher as the population ages

Others: N/A

PREGNANCY This disorder in large part results from vaginal childbirth and the distention and distortion of supporting tissues with childbirth

SYNONYMS
- Uterine prolapse
- Genital prolapse
- Genital relaxation
- Uterine descensus
- Total or partial procidentia
- Dropped uterus

ICD-9-CM
618.1 Uterine prolapse without mention of vaginal wall prolapse
618.4 Uterovaginal prolapse, unspecified
618.9 Unspecified genital prolapse

SEE ALSO

OTHER NOTES N/A

ABBREVIATIONS N/A

REFERENCES

- Nichols DH, Randall CL: Vaginal Surgery. 4th Ed. Baltimore, Williams & Wilkins, 1996
- Ryan KJ, Berkowitz R, Barbieri RL: Kistner's Gynecology: Principles and Practice. 6th Ed. Chicago, Year Book Medical Publishers, Inc., 1995
- American College of Obstetricians & Gynecologists (ACOG), 409 12th St., SW, Washington, DC 20024-2188, (800)762-ACOG
- Nichols DH: Gynecologic and Obstetric Surgery. 1st ed. St Louis, MO, CV Mosby, 1993
- Thompson JD, Rock JA: Telinde's Operative Gynecology. 8th ed. Philadelphia, Lippincott-raven, 1997
- Mishell DR, Stenchever MA, et al: Comprehensive Gynecology. 3rd ed. St Louis, CV Mosby, 1997
- Mann WJ, Stovall TG: Gynecologic Surgery. 1st ed. New York, Churchill Livingstone, 1996

Web references: 0 available at www.5mcc.com

Illustrations N/A

Author(s):
Eric L. Jenison, MD
Michael P. Hopkins, MD, MEd

BASICS

DESCRIPTION Uveitis is a nonspecific term used to describe any intraocular inflammatory disorder. Symptoms vary depending on depth of involvement and associated conditions.
- Anterior uveitis - refers to ocular inflammation limited to the iris (iritis) alone or iris and ciliary body (iridocyclitis)
- Intermediate uveitis - refers to inflammation of the structures just posterior to the lens (pars planitis or peripheral uveitis)
- Posterior uveitis - refers to inflammation of the choroid (choroiditis), retina (retinitis), or vitreous near the optic nerve and macula

System(s) affected: Nervous
Genetics: No specific pattern for uveitis in general; iritis: 50-70% of patients are HLA-B27 positive
Incidence/Prevalence in USA:
- Anterior uveitis most common (8.2 cases/100,000 annual incidence)
- Iritis is 4 times more prevalent than posterior uveitis

Predominant age: All ages
Predominant sex: Male = Female (except for HLA-B27 anterior uveitis male > female (2.5:1)

SIGNS & SYMPTOMS
- Anterior uveitis (approximately 80% of patients with uveitis)
  - ◊ Decreased visual acuity
  - ◊ Generally acute in onset
  - ◊ Deep eye pain
  - ◊ Photophobia (consensual)
  - ◊ Conjunctival vessel dilation
  - ◊ Perilimbal (circumcorneal) dilation of episcleral and scleral vessels (ciliary flush)
  - ◊ Small pupillary size of affected eye
  - ◊ Frequently unilateral (95% of HLA-B27 associated cases)
  - ◊ Bilateral involvement and systemic symptoms (fever, fatigue, abdominal pain) may be associated with interstitial nephritis
  - ◊ Systemic disease is most likely to be associated with anterior uveitis (53% of patients found to have systemic disease in one study)
- Intermediate and posterior uveitis
  - ◊ Decreased visual acuity
  - ◊ Generally insidious in onset
  - ◊ More commonly bilateral
  - ◊ Posterior inflammation will generally cause minimal pain or redness unless associated with an iritis

CAUSES
- Infectious - may result from viral, bacterial, parasitic, or fungal etiologies
- Suspected immune-mediated - possible autoimmune or immune-complex mediated mechanism postulated in association with systemic (especially rheumatologic) disorders
- Isolated eye disease
- Idiopathic (approximately 25%)
- Masquerade syndromes - diseases such as malignancies that may be mistaken for inflammation of the eye

RISK FACTORS No specific risk factors. Higher incidence seen with specific associated conditions.

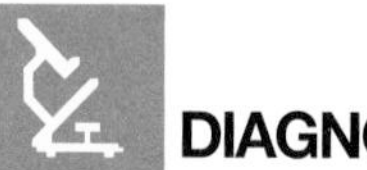

DIAGNOSIS

DIFFERENTIAL DIAGNOSIS
- Conjunctivitis
- Episcleritis
- Scleritis
- Keratitis
- Acute angle-closure glaucoma

LABORATORY
- No specific test for the diagnosis of uveitis. Tests for etiologic factors or associated conditions should be based on history and physical examination.
- CBC, BUN, creatinine (interstitial nephritis)
- HLA-B27 typing (ankylosing spondylitis, Reiter syndrome)
- ANA, ESR (SLE, Sjögren syndrome)
- VDRL, FTA (syphilis)
- PPD (tuberculosis)
- Lyme serology (Lyme disease)

Drugs that may alter lab results: N/A

Disorders that may alter lab results: Immune deficiency

PATHOLOGICAL FINDINGS Keratic precipitates, inflammatory cells in anterior chamber or vitreous, synechiae (fibrous tissue scarring between iris and lens), macular edema, perivasculitis of retinal vessels

SPECIAL TESTS Slit lamp examination and indirect ophthalmoscopy are necessary for precise diagnosis

IMAGING
- Chest x-ray (sarcoidosis, histoplasmosis, tuberculosis, lymphoma)
- Sacroiliac x-ray (ankylosing spondylitis)

DIAGNOSTIC PROCEDURES Slit lamp examination

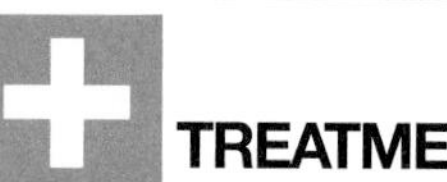

TREATMENT

APPROPRIATE HEALTH CARE Outpatient with urgent ophthalmologic consultation

GENERAL MEASURES
- Medical therapy best initiated following full ophthalmologic evaluation
- Treatment of underlying cause, if identified
- Cycloplegia
- Anti-inflammatory therapy

SURGICAL MEASURES N/A

ACTIVITY Full activity

DIET No special diet

PATIENT EDUCATION
- Instructions on proper method for instilling eye drops
- Wear dark glasses, if photophobia a problem
- Medication side effects to watch for and report

MEDICATIONS

DRUG(S) OF CHOICE

- Homatropine hydrobromide (Isopto) 2% ophthalmic solution - 2 gtts to the affected eye bid, or as often as every 3 hours if necessary, plus
- Prednisolone acetate 1% ophthalmic suspension - 2 gtts to the affected eye every 1 hour initially, tapering to qid with improvement

Contraindications:

- Hypersensitivity to the medication or component of the preparation
- Cycloplegia is contraindicated in patients known to have, or predisposed to, glaucoma
- Topical corticosteroid therapy is contraindicated in uveitis secondary to infectious etiologies

Precautions:

- Homatropine hydrobromide may produce adverse systemic antimuscarinic effects. Use extreme caution in infants and young children because of increased susceptibility to systemic effects.
- Topical corticosteroids may increase intraocular pressure. Prolonged use may cause cataract formation and exacerbate existing herpetic keratitis which may masquerade as iritis.

Significant possible interactions: Refer to manufacturer's profile of each drug

ALTERNATIVE DRUGS

- Cycloplegia - scopolamine hydrobromide 0.25% (Isopto Hyoscine) up to 3 times daily, or cyclopentolate hydrochloride 1% (Cyclogyl)
- Anti-inflammatory - prednisolone sodium phosphate 1% (Ocu-Pred Forte), dexamethasone sodium phosphate 0.1% (Ocu-Dex), and dexamethasone suspension
- Systemic non-steroidal anti-inflammatory agents may provide some benefit

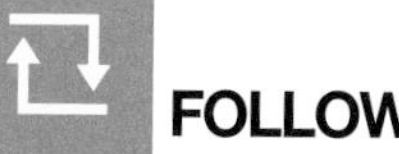

FOLLOWUP

PATIENT MONITORING

- Ophthalmologic followup as recommended by consultant
- Schedule for complete history and physical to evaluate for associated systemic disease

PREVENTION/AVOIDANCE N/A

POSSIBLE COMPLICATIONS

- Loss of vision as a result of the following:
  - ◊ Keratic precipitate deposition on the corneal or lens surfaces
  - ◊ Increased intraocular pressure, acute angle-closure glaucoma
  - ◊ Formation of synechiae
  - ◊ Cataract formation
  - ◊ Vasculitis with vascular occlusion, retinal infarction
  - ◊ Macular edema
  - ◊ Optic nerve damage

EXPECTED COURSE/PROGNOSIS

- Dependent upon the presence of causal diseases, or associated conditions
- Uveitis resulting from infections (systemic or local) tend to resolve with eradication of the underlying infection
- Uveitis associated with seronegative arthropathies tend to be acute (lasting less than 3 months) and frequently recurrent

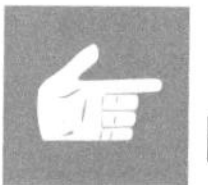

MISCELLANEOUS

ASSOCIATED CONDITIONS

- Viral infections: HIV, herpes simplex, herpes zoster, cytomegalovirus
- Bacterial infections: Tuberculosis, leprosy, Propionibacterium, syphilis, leptospirosis, brucellosis, Lyme disease, Whipple disease
- Parasitic infections: Toxoplasmosis, acanthamebiasis, toxocariasis, cysticercosis, onchocerciasis
- Fungal infections: Histoplasmosis, coccidioidomycosis, candidiasis, aspergillosis, sporotrichosis, blastomycosis, cryptococcosis
- Suspected immune-mediated: Ankylosing spondylitis, Behçet disease, Crohn disease, drug or hypersensitivity reaction, interstitial nephritis, juvenile rheumatoid arthritis, Kawasaki disease, multiple sclerosis, psoriatic arthritis, Reiter syndrome, relapsing polychondritis, sarcoidosis, Sjögren syndrome, systemic lupus erythematosus, ulcerative colitis, vasculitis, vitiligo, Vogt-Koyanagi (Harada) syndrome
- Isolated eye disease: Acute multifocal placoid pigmentary epitheliopathy, acute retinal necrosis, bird-shot choroidopathy, Fuch heterochromatic cyclitis, glaucomatocyclitic crisis, lens-induced uveitis, multifocal choroiditis, pars planitis, serpiginous choroiditis, sympathetic ophthalmia, trauma
- Masquerade syndromes: Leukemia, lymphoma, retinitis pigmentosa, retinoblastoma

AGE-RELATED FACTORS

Pediatric: Infection should be the primary consideration. Allergies and psychological factors (depression, stress) may serve as a trigger factor.
Geriatric: The inflammatory response to systemic disease may be suppressed
Others: N/A

PREGNANCY

May be of importance in the selection of medications

SYNONYMS

- Iritis
- Iridocyclitis
- Choroiditis
- Retinochoroiditis
- Chorioretinitis
- Anterior uveitis
- Posterior uveitis
- Pars planitis
- Panuveitis

ICD-9-CM

364.3 Unspecified iridocyclitis

SEE ALSO

Conjunctivitis, acute
Glaucoma, primary angle-closure
Keratitis, superficial punctate
Scleritis
Sjögren syndrome

OTHER NOTES

- Synonyms are anatomic descriptions of the focus of the uveal inflammation
- Severe or unresponsive uveitis may require therapy including periocular injection of corticosteroids, systemic corticosteroids, cytotoxic agents (azathioprine, cyclophosphamide, chlorambucil and methotrexate), immunosuppressive agents (cyclosporine), immunomodulatory agents (sulfasalazine), or tumor necrosis factor inhibitors (infliximab, etanercept)

ABBREVIATIONS

gtt = drop

REFERENCES

- Smith JR, Rosenbaum JT. Management of uveitis: a rheumatologic perspective. Arthritis Rheum 2002;46(2):309-18
- McCluskey PJ, Towler HM, Lightman S. Management of chronic uveitis. BMJ. 2000;320(7234):555-8
- Schiffman RM, Jacobsen G, Whitcup SM. Visual functioning and general health status in patients with uveitis. Arch Ophthalmol. 2001;119(6):841-9
- Rosenbaum JT: An algorithm for the systemic evaluation of patients with uveitis: guidelines for the consultant. Semin Arthritis Rheum 1990;19(4):248-57

Web references: 0 available at www.5mcc.com
Illustrations N/A

Author(s):

William L. Toffler, MD

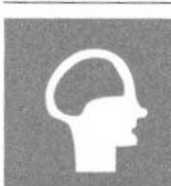

BASICS

DESCRIPTION Adenosis is a term used to describe non-epithelialized columnar glandular epithelium in the vagina. At approximately the 15th week of embryological development, the müllerian system, which forms the upper two-thirds of the vagina, fuses with the invaginating cloaca, which forms the lower vagina. Squamous metaplasia from the cloacal region then produces a squamous epithelium through the vagina. Adenosis occurs when this squamous epithelium fails to completely epithelialize the vagina.

System(s) affected: Reproductive

Genetics: Unknown

Incidence/Prevalence in USA: Adenosis is relatively common, affecting 10-20% of young females studied. As maturation progresses with puberty, epithelialization occurs.

Predominant age:
- Teenage years. From puberty to approximately age twenty, epithelialization occurs.
- By age thirty, it is extremely rare to have adenosis present

Predominant sex: Female only

SIGNS & SYMPTOMS A clear, watery vaginal discharge which is the glandular epithelium producing a small amount of mucus

CAUSES
- In the vast majority of young females, the etiology is incomplete squamous metaplasia. This occurs as a natural phenomenon and resolves with age.
- In diethylstilbestrol (DES) exposed females, the incidence of adenosis is higher and the etiology presumably is from the effect of the DES on the developing embryological system

RISK FACTORS Diethylstilbestrol (DES) exposed females

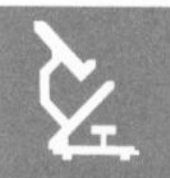

DIAGNOSIS

DIFFERENTIAL DIAGNOSIS A thorough evaluation for adenocarcinoma of the vagina arising in adenosis should be done. A biopsy may be necessary to ensure that the process represents only benign adenosis. Colposcopy of the upper vagina aids in choosing the areas for biopsy. On visual inspection, adenosis appears as a fine, raised, reddened, granular type tissue.

LABORATORY
- When extensive adenosis is present
  - ◊ Four-quadrant Pap smear of the vagina should be obtained
  - ◊ Initial colposcopy performed
  - ◊ Once squamous metaplasia is complete, four quadrant pap smear need not be performed

Drugs that may alter lab results: N/A

Disorders that may alter lab results: N/A

PATHOLOGICAL FINDINGS Biopsy will show benign glandular epithelium, which has not yet undergone squamous metaplasia. Biopsies in the areas of ongoing squamous metaplasia will be typical for this process.

SPECIAL TESTS N/A

IMAGING N/A

DIAGNOSTIC PROCEDURES
- Four quadrant Pap smear should be liberally utilized to isolate quadrants of the vagina which may contain abnormalities. This can be followed by colposcopy and biopsy.
- Colposcopy should be used to outline areas of adenosis and insure that no malignancy is present

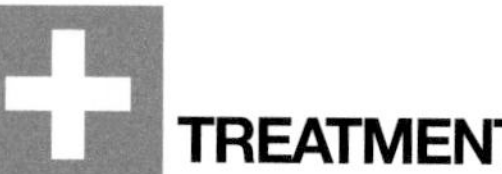

TREATMENT

APPROPRIATE HEALTH CARE Outpatient

GENERAL MEASURES
- Unless malignancy is present, conservative treatment is indicated
- In the vast majority of young females with this condition, it will resolve with expectant management

SURGICAL MEASURES Aggressive therapy such as laser or surgical excision is only necessary if premalignant or malignant changes arise

ACTIVITY
- No limitations
- It is not necessary to avoid intercourse or placing objects in the vagina

DIET No special diet

PATIENT EDUCATION The patient should be educated that in the vast majority of situations this is benign and expectant management is all that is necessary
- American College of Obstetricians & Gynecologists (ACOG), 409 12th St., SW, Washington, DC 20024-2188, (800)762-ACOG

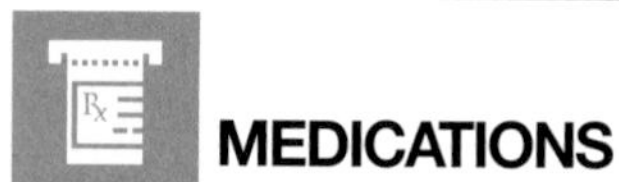

MEDICATIONS

DRUG(S) OF CHOICE N/A
Contraindications: N/A
Precautions: N/A
Significant possible interactions: N/A

ALTERNATIVE DRUGS N/A

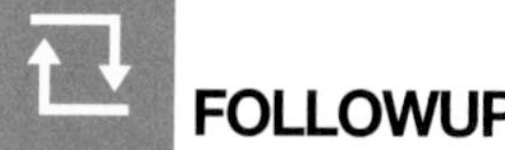

FOLLOWUP

PATIENT MONITORING
- Initial evaluation consists of four-quadrant vaginal Pap smear, cervical Pap smear and colposcopy of the upper vagina and cervix
- If the initial colposcopy is normal, a yearly four-quadrant Pap smear of the vagina and Pap smear of the cervix is all that is necessary

PREVENTION/AVOIDANCE N/A

POSSIBLE COMPLICATIONS N/A

EXPECTED COURSE/PROGNOSIS
- It is expected that the vast majority of patients will have squamous metaplasia with complete resolution of the adenosis
- The rare patient, 1:1,000 to 1:10,000, may develop adenocarcinoma in the adenosis and will require definitive therapy as for vaginal cancer

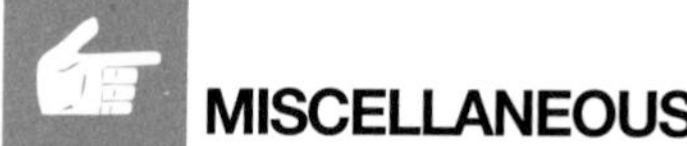

MISCELLANEOUS

ASSOCIATED CONDITIONS
- DES exposure
  - ◊ Adenosis from DES exposure should lead to an evaluation of other DES related abnormalities
  - ◊ The greatest risk to the patient is from müllerian tract anomalies. These include cervical abnormalities with cervical hood, ridges, shortened cervix and incompetent cervix.
  - ◊ Patients with a known DES exposure should have the reproductive tract evaluated prior to conception
  - ◊ The vast majority of patients with adenosis have not been DES exposed and do not require evaluation of the reproductive system
  - ◊ DES was last used to prevent spontaneous abortion in approximately 1970. This is a problem of decreasing importance.

AGE-RELATED FACTORS
Pediatric: N/A
Geriatric:
- Adenosis is a disorder of the young female. By the time of menopause the vagina and cervix should be completely epithelialized.
- The presence of glandular epithelium in the postmenopausal patient is an indication for excision and close evaluation for the possibility of a well-differentiated adenocarcinoma

Others: N/A

PREGNANCY
Pregnancy produces a wide eversion of the transformation zone of the cervix. This will occasionally become so widely everted that it will extend onto the vaginal fornices leading to the impression of adenosis. This will resolve after the pregnancy is completed.

SYNONYMS N/A

ICD-9-CM
752.49 Other congenital anomalies of cervix, vagina, and external female genitalia

SEE ALSO

OTHER NOTES N/A

ABBREVIATIONS N/A

REFERENCES

- Sandberg EC: The incidence and distribution of occult vaginal adenosis. Am J Obstet Gynecol 1968;101:322-34
- Hopkins MP: Vaginal Neoplasms. In: Copeland LJ, ed. Textbook of Gynecology. Philadelphia, W.B. Saunders Co., 1993

Web references: 0 available at www.5mcc.com
Illustrations N/A

Author(s):

Michael P. Hopkins, MD, MEd
Eric L. Jenison, MD

BASICS

DESCRIPTION Vaginal bleeding during pregnancy has many causes and ranges in severity from mild (with normal pregnancy outcome) to life-threatening for both infant and mother. The bleeding can vary from scant to excessive, from brown to bright red, and can be painless or painful. The different causes can be divided into vaginal, cervical and uterine factors. The differential diagnosis is guided by the gestational age of the pregnancy.

System(s) affected: Cardiovascular, Reproductive

Genetics: No known genetic pattern

Incidence/Prevalence in USA: Common

Predominant age: Childbearing

Predominant sex: Female only

SIGNS & SYMPTOMS
- Bleeding can vary from scant to excessive
- Color of blood varies from brown to bright red
- May be painless or painful
- Patient reports bleeding from vagina

CAUSES
- Vaginal or cervical causes can occur throughout the pregnancy, and usually are no threat to the pregnancy. They include:
  - ◊ Vaginal infection or trauma
  - ◊ Cervicitis-infections or non-infections
  - ◊ Cervical polyp
  - ◊ Cervical neoplasia
  - ◊ Hyperemia of cervix (increased blood flow from pregnancy)
  - ◊ Post coital bleeding - usually cervical source
- Bleeding from above the cervix is a concern because it can be life threatening to mother and/or fetus. In determining the cause it is helpful to separate first trimester bleeding from later pregnancy bleeding.
  - ◊ First trimester bleeding causes include:
    - Implantation bleeding-benign
    - Ectopic pregnancy
    - Threatened or spontaneous abortion
    - Molar pregnancy
    - Subchorionic bleed
  - ◊ Second of third trimester bleeding causes include:
    - Placenta previa (non-painful)
    - Placenta abruption (painful, contraction usually present)
    - Subchorionic bleed
- Many times the cause is unknown. Up to 50% of first trimester bleeding, no cause is ever found.

RISK FACTORS
- Cervical or vaginal infections
  - ◊ Multiple sexual partners
  - ◊ Previous history of STD or PID
- Cervical dysplasia
  - ◊ Previous history of abnormal pap
- Placenta previa
  - ◊ Previous history of previa
  - ◊ Previous cesarean section
  - ◊ History of uterine surgery including D&C
- Placental abruption
  - ◊ Previous history of abruption (increases risk by 10%)
  - ◊ Hypertension
  - ◊ Preeclampsia
  - ◊ Multiple gestation
  - ◊ Smoking
  - ◊ Cocaine use

DIAGNOSIS

DIFFERENTIAL DIAGNOSIS
- Hematuria from UTI, kidney stones
- Bleeding hemorrhoids
- Rectal bleeding from lower GI bleed - extremely rare in pregnancy

LABORATORY
- Blood work based on dating of pregnancy, previous tests, and need for further diagnosis
- Blood type and screen. If not known already, needs to be done on all women.
- Rh negative patients that bleed during pregnancy will need Rho(d) immune globulin (RhoGAM), to prevent mother from becoming sensitized if exposed to infant's Rh positive blood. In third trimester bleeding, the mother may lose significant amounts of blood and require transfusion.
- Quantitative beta-human chorionic gonadotropin (Q HCG). This can be used in early pregnancy when ultrasound is not able to diagnose cause. Ultrasound should be able to see an intrauterine pregnancy (IUP) when Q HCG >2000. Levels can be followed serially every couple of days. Levels fall in spontaneous abortion, are extremely high in molar pregnancy, and rise gradually in ectopic or intrauterine pregnancy. This level usually doubles in 48 hours in normal pregnancy, and failure to double is concerning for ectopic. Once Q HCG level is greater than 2000 an ultrasound should be performed to confirm diagnosis. When spontaneous abortion is suspected but no definitive diagnosis by either ultrasound or pathology confirmation of products of conception, then following Q HCG weekly until level is <25 is advised to exclude possible undiagnosed ectopic. If dropping levels start to rise reconsider ectopic pregnancy. In molar pregnancy, after surgical evacuation of productions of conception, monthly Q HCG are followed for one year to rule out the possibility of choriocarcinoma. During this time the patient should be instructed to not get pregnant.
- Other labs are based on severity of bleeding:
  - ◊ CBC - may be done to assess severity, when bleeding profuse
  - ◊ Bleeding time, fibrinogen, fibrin split products - rarely necessary. DIC reported rarely in missed abortion.

Drugs that may alter lab results: N/A

Disorders that may alter lab results: N/A

PATHOLOGICAL FINDINGS Depends on cause

SPECIAL TESTS N/A

IMAGING
- Ultrasound (USN) is the diagnostic test of choice. A gestational sac can be seen at 5-6 weeks, fetal heart tone can be observed by 8-9 weeks. USN is diagnostic of molar pregnancy with 98% accuracy. In later pregnancy USN locates the placenta and may show degree of placental separation in abruption.
- Serial ultrasound may be required in early pregnancy

DIAGNOSTIC PROCEDURES
- It is important to evaluate whether bleeding is coming from genital tract or from other near by structures
- Association of bleeding with other activities or symptoms may aid in the diagnosis, eg, following bowel movement, after intercourse, associated with abdominal cramping
- In first trimester bleeding: pelvic exam is performed to confirm bleeding from cervical os, and if any adnexal masses. If pregnancy is greater than 8 weeks USN should be done to confirm IUP. If no IUP and USN not confirmatory for ectopic, then serial Q HCG are followed. If pelvic pain and concern for ectopic high but not confirmed by USN a laparoscopy or laparotomy may be performed to make a diagnosis.
- In second or third trimester bleeding - locate placenta by ultrasound prior to pelvic exam. If placenta previa, do not perform bimanual or speculum exam unless set up for immediate cesarean delivery.

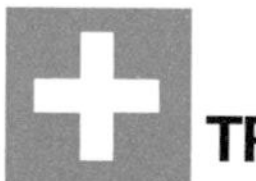

TREATMENT

APPROPRIATE HEALTH CARE
- In first trimester bleeding most patients can be managed as outpatient
- In late pregnancy bleeding, most patients need inpatient monitoring

GENERAL MEASURES
- In late pregnancy bleeding, the amount of bleeding and presence of maternal or fetal compromise indicates whether emergent cesarean section is performed or whether conservative measures are appropriate until greater fetal lung maturity can be obtained
- Threatened abortion: Bedrest and nothing in the vagina. If bleeding is severe, hospitalization and close observation. Type and screen for possible transfusion

SURGICAL MEASURES
- If ectopic or molar pregnancy is diagnosed immediate surgical treatment is appropriate
- Some early ectopic pregnancies can be treated medically if certain criteria are met
- Inevitable or incomplete abortion: D&C (usually suction)
- If completeness of abortion is in doubt, then D&C and removal of retained products
- Cesarean section for placenta previa or placental abruption

ACTIVITY Bedrest; no coitus, no douching

DIET No restrictions

PATIENT EDUCATION
- Patient should be instructed to report any increase in the amount and frequency of bleeding and should seek immediate care if experiencing abdominal pain or sudden increased bleeding. She should bring for examination any tissue passed vaginally.
- Grief counseling is appropriate if pregnancy loss is inevitable
- American College of Obstetricians & Gynecologists (ACOG), 409 12th St., SW, Washington, DC 20024-2188, (800)762-ACOG

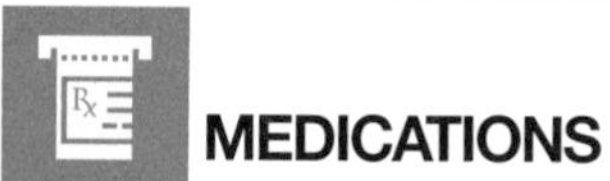

MEDICATIONS

DRUG(S) OF CHOICE Rho(d) immune globulin if mother Rh negative and significant bleeding from uterus
Contraindications: N/A
Precautions: N/A
Significant possible interactions: N/A

ALTERNATIVE DRUGS Tocolytics in suspected premature labor

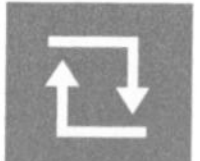

FOLLOWUP

PATIENT MONITORING Daily to weekly depending on diagnosis and severity of bleeding

PREVENTION/AVOIDANCE N/A

POSSIBLE COMPLICATIONS
- Anemia
- Shock
- Fetal or maternal death
- Infection
- Choriocarcinoma or invasive mole in the case of hydatidiform mole
- Premature delivery of infant with associated complications
- Coagulopathy (extremely rare)

EXPECTED COURSE/PROGNOSIS
Depends on the cause of vaginal bleeding, the severity of bleeding and the rapidity of diagnosis. Maternal mortality is 1 in 826 of ectopic pregnancies.

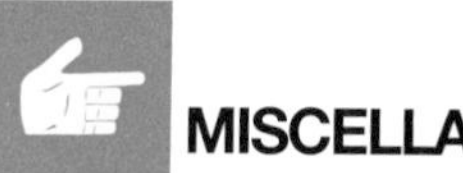

MISCELLANEOUS

ASSOCIATED CONDITIONS Depends on cause of vaginal bleeding

AGE-RELATED FACTORS
Pediatric: N/A
Geriatric: N/A
Others: N/A

PREGNANCY A complication of pregnancy

SYNONYMS N/A

ICD-9-CM
630 Hydatidiform mole
633.90 Unspecified ectopic pregnancy without intrauterine pregnancy
634.90 Spontaneous abortion without mention of complication, unspecified
641.10 Hemorrhage from placenta previa, unspecified
641.20 Premature separation of placenta, unspecified

SEE ALSO
Abnormal Pap smear
Abortion, spontaneous
Abruptio placentae
Cervical dysplasia
Cervical malignancy
Cervical polyps
Cervicitis
Cervicitis, ectropion & true erosion
Chlamydial sexually transmitted diseases
Ectopic pregnancy
Placenta previa
Premature labor
Trichomoniasis
Vaginal malignancy
Vulvovaginitis, bacterial
Vulvovaginitis, candidal

OTHER NOTES N/A

ABBREVIATIONS N/A

REFERENCES

- American College of Emergency Physicians: Clinical policy for the initial approach to patients presenting with a chief complaint of vaginal bleeding. Ann Emerg Med 1997;29(3):435-458
- Signore CC: Second trimester vaginal bleeding: correlation of ultrasonographic findings with perinatal outcome. Am J Ob Gyn 1998:179(2):336-40
- Cunningham FG, MacDonald PC, Gant NF, eds: Williams' Obstetrics. 19th Ed. Norwalk, CT, Appleton and Lange, 1993
- Danforth DM, Scott JR., et al, eds: Obstetrics and Gynecology. 6th Ed. Philadelphia, J.B. Lippincott, 1990

Web references: 0 available at www.5mcc.com
Illustrations N/A

Author(s):
Kimberle Vore, MD

BASICS

DESCRIPTION
- Vaginal intraepithelial neoplasia (carcinoma in situ): A premalignant phase with full thickness neoplastic changes in the superficial epithelium. However there is no invasion through the basement membrane.
- Invasive malignancies: Vaginal malignancies are squamous cell in 90% of the patients and the remaining 10% are adenocarcinomas, sarcomas and melanomas. The clear cell carcinoma is a subtype of adenocarcinoma.
- To be classified as a vaginal malignancy, only the vagina can be involved. If the cervix or the vulva is involved, then the tumor is classified as a primary cancer arising from the cervix or the vulva.

System(s) affected: Reproductive
Genetics: No known genetic pattern
Incidence/Prevalence in USA: This is one of the rarest of all gynecological malignancies
Predominant age:
- Carcinoma in situ - mid-forties to sixties
- Invasive squamous cell malignancy - mid-sixties to seventies
- Adenocarcinoma - any age range, fifties is mean age
- Mixed müllerian sarcomas and leiomyosarcomas in the adult population - mean age sixty
- Sarcoma botryoides and embryonal sarcomas - occur in the pediatric population

Predominant sex: Female only

SIGNS & SYMPTOMS
- Abnormal bleeding is the most common symptom. This results from a fungating tumor present in the vagina.
- Dyspareunia
- Postcoital bleeding can result from direct trauma to the tumor
- Pain along with symptoms and signs of hydroureter are late findings when tumor has spread into the paravaginal tissues and extends to the pelvic side wall
- In the pediatric population, sarcomas can present either as a mass protruding from the vagina or as abnormal genital bleeding

CAUSES
- Women with a history of cervical malignancy have a higher probability of developing squamous cell malignancy in the vagina after hysterectomy
- The human papilloma virus (HPV) has been associated with vulvovaginal, cervical, adenocarcinoma and squamous cell carcinoma
- Smokers have a higher incidence
- Clear cell adenocarcinoma of the vagina in young women has been associated with diethylstilbestrol (DES) exposure. The incidence, however, is exceedingly rare estimated at 1:1,000 to 1:10,000 DES exposed females.
- Metastatic lesions can involve the vagina from the other gynecologic organs
- Renal cell carcinoma and breast cancer can metastasize to the vagina (rarely)

RISK FACTORS
- History of squamous cell cancer of the cervix or vulva
- Smoking
- Multiple sex partners

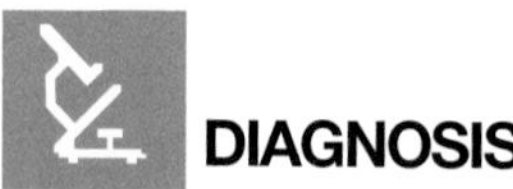

DIAGNOSIS

DIFFERENTIAL DIAGNOSIS
- Vaginal intraepithelial neoplasia (VAIN) involves premalignant changes that do not infiltrate beyond the basement membrane
- Adequate biopsies ensure that invasive lesions are not overlooked. Invasive lesions penetrate the basement membrane and cannot be treated conservatively. Other malignancies such as endometrial, cervix, bladder or colon cancer can invade directly into the vagina or metastasize to the vagina.
- In the childbearing age, trophoblastic disease should be considered. The vagina is a common site of metastases. Biopsy will usually provide a clue to the primary site.

LABORATORY Cytology will usually be positive when an obvious lesion is present

Drugs that may alter lab results: N/A

Disorders that may alter lab results: N/A

PATHOLOGICAL FINDINGS
- Stage 0 - carcinoma in situ
- Stage I - infiltrative tumor not involving the paravaginal tissues
- Stage II - paravaginal extension but not to the side wall
- Stage III - paravaginal extension to the side wall
- Stage IVA - tumor involving the bladder or the rectum
- Stage IVB - distant metastatic disease

SPECIAL TESTS N/A

IMAGING
- Chest x-ray - lung metastases are a late finding.
- IVP - to evaluate for ureteral obstruction
- CAT scan to evaluate the retroperitoneum and especially the lymph nodes in the pelvic and periaortic area
- Lymphangiography is also useful for evaluation of the lymph node status
- Barium enema to rule out rectal invasion

DIAGNOSTIC PROCEDURES
- Colposcopy with directed biopsies for small lesions
- Wide excision under anesthesia of superficial disease may be necessary to insure that invasive cancer is not present
- Cystoscopy to rule out bladder invasion
- Sigmoidoscopy to rule out rectal invasion

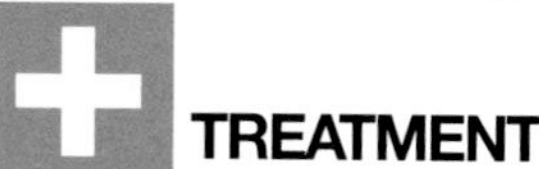

TREATMENT

APPROPRIATE HEALTH CARE Outpatient or inpatient depending on treatment

GENERAL MEASURES
- Carcinoma in situ can be treated by a variety of methods: Laser vaporization under microscopic guidance; fluorouracil (Efudex) intravaginal cream; partial vaginectomy
- There is no effective chemotherapy for squamous cell malignancy of the vagina
- In all tumor types, metastatic disease from the vagina to other sites is only minimally responsive to chemotherapy

SURGICAL MEASURES
- Whenever there is a doubt as to the presence or absence of invasive disease, vaginectomy must be performed
- Invasive lesions are usually treated by radiation therapy, but stage I lesions can be treated with radical hysterectomy, radical vaginectomy with pelvic lymph node dissection
- If the lesion involves the lower vagina, inguinal node dissection must also be done as cancer involving the lower vagina can metastasize to the groin region
- Sarcomas are treated by radiation therapy followed by pelvic exenteration if persistent disease is present
- Childhood sarcomas are treated with chemotherapy followed by local resection. Childhood sarcomas are responsive to multi-agent combination chemotherapies.

ACTIVITY
- The patients are usually ambulatory and able to resume full activity by six weeks after surgery
- Most patients are fully active while receiving radiation therapy

DIET Unrestricted unless they are undergoing radiation

PATIENT EDUCATION
- This is an uncommon malignancy and these patients should be treated by a physician familiar and experienced with this malignancy
- Printed patient information available from: American College of Obstetricians & Gynecologists, 409 12th St., SW, Washington, DC 20024-2188, (800)762-ACOG

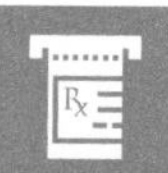

MEDICATIONS

DRUG(S) OF CHOICE

- With one exception, there are no chemotherapeutic agents to which this tumor is responsive. The exception is the childhood sarcomas, which have been treated with combinations of:
  - ◊ Vincristine
  - ◊ Dactinomycin (actinomycin-D)
  - ◊ Cyclophosphamide (Cytoxan)
  - ◊ Cisplatin
  - ◊ Etoposide (VP-16)
- Adjuvant chemotherapy has no proven benefit in squamous cell or adenocarcinoma of the vagina
- Carcinoma in situ can be eradicated in 90% of patients with fluorouracil (Efudex) cream 5% applied bid x 2 hours x 7 days, then qd x 7 days, repeated in six weeks

Contraindications:

- Prior to treatment the diagnosis must be established with certainty
- If there is any doubt that a process beyond in situ disease exists, vaginectomy must be performed. Because these patients are often elderly, aggressive therapy is limited by the patient's performance status and ability to tolerate radical surgery, chemotherapy or radiation.

Precautions: Refer to manufacturer's literature

Significant possible interactions: Refer to manufacturer's literature

ALTERNATIVE DRUGS

- Ondansetron (Zofran), dronabinol (Marinol), metoclopramide (Reglan), and others for nausea control

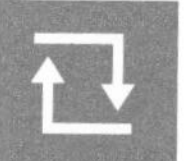

FOLLOWUP

PATIENT MONITORING

- Pelvic examination and Pap smear every 3 months for 2 years and then every 6 months for subsequent 3 years
- Chest x-ray once a year

PREVENTION/AVOIDANCE

- A Pap smear should be performed for all women on a yearly basis, even after hysterectomy
- Premalignant changes discovered on Pap smear screening should be followed up with colposcopy, biopsy and treatment. This needs to be undertaken by a physician well trained in the diagnosis and treatment of vaginal disease.
- Patients with a history of in situ or invasive disease of the cervix and/or the vulva should be followed at close intervals for development of disease in the vagina

POSSIBLE COMPLICATIONS

Those associated with major abdominal surgery or radiation therapy

EXPECTED COURSE/PROGNOSIS

- Stage and 5 year survival
  - ◊ I - 60%
  - ◊ II - 40%
  - ◊ III - 20%
  - ◊ IVA - 5%
  - ◊ IVB - 0%

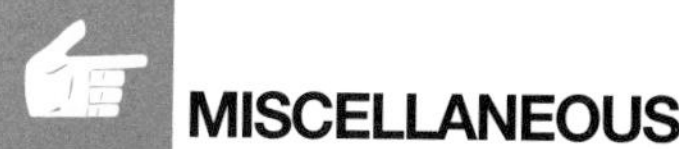

MISCELLANEOUS

ASSOCIATED CONDITIONS

Due to the field effect, patients with vaginal cancer are more likely to develop malignancy in the cervix or vulva and should be followed closely

AGE-RELATED FACTORS

Pediatric: Childhood sarcomas can be treated in a conservative fashion with multi-modality therapy. This avoids the loss of the young child's bladder and/or rectum.

Geriatric: Older patients, many with a long smoking history, are at a higher risk for surgery

Others:

- Younger patients, who have not completed their family, can occasionally be treated with limited resection and localized radiation to the area
- Premenopausal women, who desire to retain ovarian function, are better candidates for radical surgery for early stage disease

PREGNANCY

This malignancy is not associated with pregnancy

SYNONYMS

- Bowen disease
- Vaginal intraepithelial neoplasia (VAIN)

ICD-9-CM

184.0 Malignant neoplasm of vagina

SEE ALSO

OTHER NOTES

N/A

ABBREVIATIONS

N/A

REFERENCES

- Hopkins MP: Vaginal Neoplasms. In: Copeland LJ, ed. Textbook of Gynecology. Philadelphia: W.B. Saunders Co; 1993.
- Peters WA, Kumar NB, Morley GW: Carcinoma of the vagina: Factors influencing treatment outcome. Cancer 1985;55(4):892-97
- Hopkins MP. Vaginal neoplasms. In: Copeland LJ, ed. Textbook of gynecology. Philadelphia: W B Saunders Co; 2000. chapter 54.

Web references: 1 available at www.5mcc.com

Illustrations N/A

Author(s):

Michael P. Hopkins, MD, MEd

Eric L. Jenison, MD

BASICS

DESCRIPTION Involuntary painful contraction of perineal muscles prior to or during vaginal intercourse. The experience of or even the anticipation of pain on vaginal entry causes theses muscles to contract, occluding the vaginal opening and causing further pain when penetration is attempted.
System(s) affected: Reproductive
Genetics: N/A
Incidence/Prevalence in USA: 6-8% of women in some studies report complete vaginismus and up to 30% some degree of vaginismus
Predominant age: Postpubertal
Predominant sex: Female

SIGNS & SYMPTOMS
- Inability to allow entry for vaginal sexual intercourse secondary to involuntary muscle spasms
- Reluctance or avoidance of pelvic examination
- Relationship discord or difficulty
- Infertility
- Sexual satisfaction may be independent of sexual function!

CAUSES
- Primary: Often multifactorial
  - ◊ Negative messages about sex and sexual relations in upbringing may cause phobic reaction
  - ◊ Poor body image of genital area
  - ◊ History of sexual trauma, although rates of vaginismus appear to be similar in sexually abused and un-abused populations of women (studies show incidence of sexual abuse of women to be from 12-40%)
- Secondary
  - ◊ New onset of infection
  - ◊ Surgical or post delivery scarring
  - ◊ Endometriosis
  - ◊ Inadequate vaginal lubrication

RISK FACTORS
- Previous sexual trauma, but rates appear to be similar in abused and non-abused women
- Often associated with other sexual dysfunctions

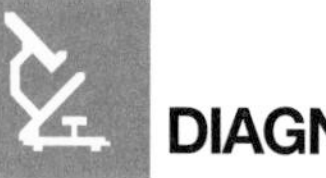

DIAGNOSIS

DIFFERENTIAL DIAGNOSIS
- Dyspareunia

LABORATORY N/A

Drugs that may alter lab results: N/A

Disorders that may alter lab results: N/A

PATHOLOGICAL FINDINGS Rarely found in primary vaginismus, but may be varied such as endometriosis or scarring in secondary vaginismus

SPECIAL TESTS Psychiatric consultation if not responsive to primary physician's therapy or if primary provider not comfortable with caring for sexual problems

IMAGING N/A

DIAGNOSTIC PROCEDURES
- General and sexual history
- At some point, a careful pelvic examination to rule out medical cause

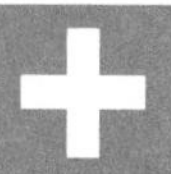

TREATMENT

APPROPRIATE HEALTH CARE Outpatient care

GENERAL MEASURES
- Can often treat vaginismus successfully without defining/treating its etiologies
- No published controlled studies on success of psychotherapy for vaginismus
- Patient education as noted below on pelvic anatomy and sexual function
- Kegel's exercises to control perineal muscles
- Stepwise vaginal desensitization exercises:
  - ◊ A) with vaginal dilators (patient inserts/controls), or
  - ◊ B) with woman's own finger(s) (promotes sexual self-awareness)
- Valsalva can help with vaginal entry
- Advance to husband's fingers with patient's control
- Coitus after achieving largest vaginal dilator or 3 fingers; important to begin with sensate focused exercises/sensual caressing without necessarily a demand for coitus
  - ◊ A) Female superior at first; passive (non-thrusting); female directed
  - ◊ B) Later, thrusting may be okay

SURGICAL MEASURES Contraindicated

ACTIVITY Simple techniques of gentle, progressive, patient-controlled vaginal dilation

DIET No special diet

PATIENT EDUCATION
- Education about pelvic anatomy, nature of the vaginal spasms, normal adult sexual function
- Hand held mirror can help the woman visually learn to tighten and loosen perineal muscles
- Important to teach the partners that the spasms are not under conscious control and are not a reflection on the relationship or a woman's feelings about her partner
- Instruction in techniques for vaginal dilation
- Resources
  - ◊ American College of Obstetricians & Gynecologists (ACOG), 409 12th St., SW, Washington, DC 20024-2188, (800)762-ACOG
  - ◊ Valins L. When a Woman's Body Says No to Sex: Understanding and Overcoming Vaginismus. New York: Penguin, 1992.

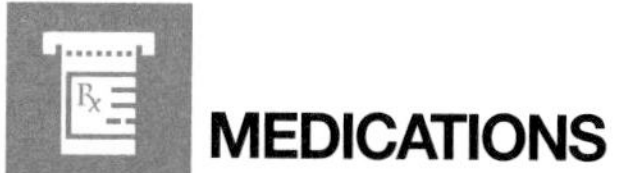

MEDICATIONS

DRUG(S) OF CHOICE N/A
Contraindications: Anxiolytics, especially benzodiazepines
Precautions: N/A
Significant possible interactions: N/A

ALTERNATIVE DRUGS N/A

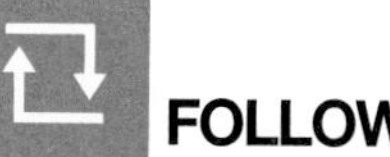

FOLLOWUP

PATIENT MONITORING General preventive health care

PREVENTION/AVOIDANCE N/A

POSSIBLE COMPLICATIONS Precipitation of memory of incest prior to patient's readiness to deal with it

EXPECTED COURSE/PROGNOSIS
- Some studies show high degrees of success (58-70%) with behavioral interventions
- History of sexual abuse does not predict outcome negatively or positively

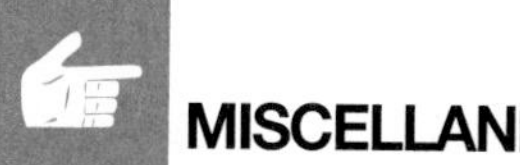

MISCELLANEOUS

ASSOCIATED CONDITIONS
- Marital stress, family dysfunction
- Dyspareunia

AGE-RELATED FACTORS Vaginismus is generally primary, e.g. happens with first attempt at intercourse
Pediatric: N/A
Geriatric: N/A
Others: N/A

PREGNANCY Pregnancy can occur in patients with vaginismus via perineal ejaculation

SYNONYMS N/A

ICD-9-CM
306.51 Psychogenic vaginismus

SEE ALSO
Dyspareunia
Sexual dysfunction in women

OTHER NOTES N/A

ABBREVIATIONS N/A

REFERENCES

- Biswas A: Vaginismus and outcome of treatment: Human Sexuality and Sexual Dysfunction 1995;24:755-758
- Heiman JR: Evaluating sexual dysfunctions: Primary Care of Women. Norwalk, CT, Appleson and Lange, 1995
- Read S, King M, Watson J: Sexual dysfunction in primary medical care. Journal of Public Health Medicine, Oxford University Press 1997;19(4):387-391
- Sarwer D, Durlak J: A field trial of the effectiveness of behavioral treatment for sexual dysfunctions. Journal of Sex and Marital Therapy 1997;23(2):87-97

Web references: 0 available at www.5mcc.com
Illustrations N/A

Author(s):
Kay A. Bauman, MD, MPH

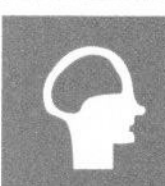

BASICS

DESCRIPTION Elongated, dilated, tortuous superficial veins with congenitally absent valves, or valves that have become incompetent. Affects legs where reverse flow occurs when dependent.
System(s) affected: Cardiovascular, Skin/Exocrine
Genetics: Familial, dominant, x-linked
Incidence/Prevalence in USA: About 20% of adults
Predominant age: Middle age
Predominant sex: Female > Male (5:1)

SIGNS & SYMPTOMS
- Sometimes asymptomatic
- Leg muscular cramp
- Dilatation, tortuosity of superficial veins chiefly in the lower extremities
- Edema of affected limb
- Leg aching
- Fatigue
- Symptoms worse during menses
- Pain if varicose ulcer develops

CAUSES
- Faulty valves in one or more perforator veins in the lower leg causing secondary incompetence at the saphenofemoral junction
- Deep thrombophlebitis
- Increased venous pressure from any cause
- Congenital valvular incompetence
- Trauma (should consider AV fistula - listen for bruit)
- In many individuals, no cause or precipitating factor found

RISK FACTORS
- Pregnancy
- Occupations requiring prolonged standing, restrictive clothing (e.g., very tight girdles)
- Obesity

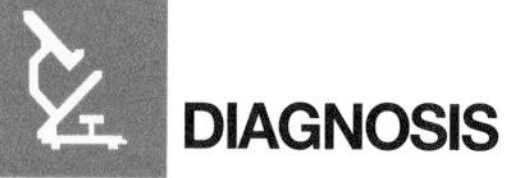

DIAGNOSIS

DIFFERENTIAL DIAGNOSIS
- Nerve root compression
- Arthritis
- Peripheral neuritis
- Telangiectasia - smaller, visible blood vessels that are permanently dilated
- Deep vein thrombosis

LABORATORY None helpful

Drugs that may alter lab results: N/A

Disorders that may alter lab results: N/A

PATHOLOGICAL FINDINGS
- Elongation and tortuosity of veins
- Medial fibrosis of veins
- Disappearance or atrophy of valves

SPECIAL TESTS Trendelenburg's test, Perthes test

IMAGING N/A

DIAGNOSTIC PROCEDURES
- Clinical inspection
- Duplex scanning, venous Doppler study, photoplethysmography, light reflection rheography, air plethysmography, and other vascular testing should be reserved for those patients who have venous symptoms and/or large (>4 mm in diameter) vessels or large numbers of spider telangiectasia indicating venous hypertension

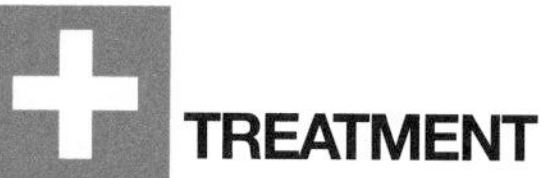

TREATMENT

APPROPRIATE HEALTH CARE Outpatient

GENERAL MEASURES
- Conservative methods
  - ◊ Frequent rest periods with legs elevated
  - ◊ Lightweight, elastic compression hosiery. Best put on before getting out of bed.
  - ◊ Avoid girdles and other restrictive clothing
  - ◊ If stasis ulcers present, use warm, wet dressings
- Spider veins (idiopathic telangiectases)
  - ◊ Fine intracutaneous angiectasis
  - ◊ May be extensive/unsightly
  - ◊ Eliminate with intracapillary injections of 1% solution of sodium tetradecyl sulfate (or hypertonic saline 23.4%) using a fine-bore needle
  - ◊ Subsequent treatments may be required until optimal results attained

SURGICAL MEASURES
- Surgical and other methods
  - ◊ If there is pain, recurrent phlebitis, skin changes, or for cosmetic improvement for severe cases
  - ◊ Ligation and stripping of the saphenous vein
  - ◊ Injection of sclerosing solution
  - ◊ Stab evulsion phlebectomy (procedure with shorter recovery time)
  - ◊ For extensive fibrosis - excision of the entire area, followed by skin graft may be necessary
  - ◊ Laser or radiofrequency therapy

ACTIVITY
- Avoid long periods of standing
- Appropriate exercise routine as part of conservative treatment
- Walking regimen after sclerotherapy is important to help promote healing
- Apply elastic stockings before lowering legs from the bed
- Never sit with legs hanging down

DIET
- No special diet
- Weight loss diet recommended, if obesity a problem

PATIENT EDUCATION
- Inform patients that the surgery or sclerotherapy may not prevent development of varicosities and that the procedure may need to be repeated in later years
- For patient education materials favorably reviewed on this topic, contact: National Heart, Lung & Blood Institute, Communications & Public Information Branch, National Institutes of Health, Building 31, Room 41-21, 9000 Rockville Pike, Bethesda, MD 20892, (301)496-4236

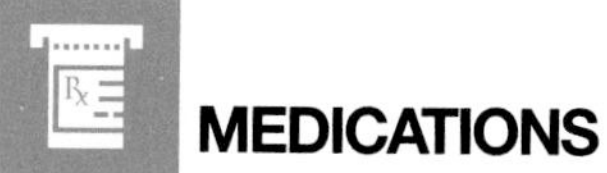

MEDICATIONS

DRUG(S) OF CHOICE Injection sclerotherapy with compression to totally obliterate the vein by fibrosis. Sclerosant is sodium tetradecyl sulfate 1-3% solution. Bandages remain 3 weeks or longer.
Contraindications: Refer to manufacturer's literature
Precautions: No oral contraceptives for at least 6 weeks prior to sclerotherapy because of their thrombogenic effect
Significant possible interactions: Refer to manufacturer's literature

ALTERNATIVE DRUGS Antibiotics for infected varicose ulcers

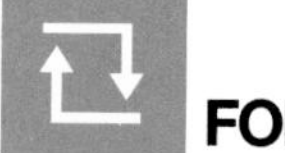

FOLLOWUP

PATIENT MONITORING Until surgery or conservative therapy brings maximal benefit

PREVENTION/AVOIDANCE N/A

POSSIBLE COMPLICATIONS
- Petechial hemorrhages
- Chronic edema
- Superimposed infection
- Varicose ulcers
- Pigmentation
- Eczema
- Recurrence after surgical treatment
- Scarring or nerve damage from stripping technique

EXPECTED COURSE/PROGNOSIS
- Usual course - chronic
- Prognosis - favorable with appropriate treatment

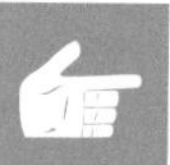

MISCELLANEOUS

ASSOCIATED CONDITIONS
- Stasis dermatitis
- Stasis ulcer

AGE-RELATED FACTORS
Pediatric: Unlikely in this age group
Geriatric:
- More common, usually valvular degeneration, but may be secondary to chronic venous deficiency
- Recommended therapy - elastic support hose and frequent rests with legs elevated rather than ligation and stripping

Others: N/A

PREGNANCY Frequent problem. Use of elastic stockings recommended for individuals who have a history of varicosities or when activities involve a great deal of standing.

SYNONYMS N/A

ICD-9-CM
454.1 Varicose veins of lower extremities with inflammation

SEE ALSO
Dermatitis, stasis

OTHER NOTES N/A

ABBREVIATIONS N/A

REFERENCES

- Berkow R, et al, eds. Merck Manual. 17th Ed. Rahway, NJ, Merck Sharp & Dohme, 1997
- Guidelines of care for sclerotherapy treatment of varicose and telangiectatic leg veins. American Academy of Dermatology. J Am Acad Dermatol 1996 Mar;34(3):523-8
- Ellis H, Taylor P. Varicose Veins. 3rd Ed. London, Greenwich Medical Media, 1999

Web references: 1 available at www.5mcc.com
Illustrations N/A

Author(s):
Joseph A. Florence, MD

BASICS

DESCRIPTION Congenital or acquired defect of the interventricular septum that allows communication of blood between the left and right ventricles. Other than bicuspid aortic valve, this is the most common congenital heart malformation reported in infants and children. It also occurs as a complication of acute myocardial infarctions (MI). Blood flow across the defect is typically left to right and depends on the size of the defect and the pulmonary vascular resistance (PVR). Prolonged shunting of blood can lead to pulmonary hypertension and eventually reversal of flow across the defect, and to cyanosis (Eisenmenger's complex).
System(s) affected: Cardiovascular
Genetics: Multifactorial etiology; autosomal dominant and recessive transmission have been reported
Incidence/Prevalence in USA:
- Congenital - 100-500 of 100,000 live births
- Acute myocardial infarctions - estimated to complicate 1-3%

Predominant age: Infants and children
Predominant sex: Male = Female (male > female if secondary to myocardial infarction)

SIGNS & SYMPTOMS
- Depend on the degree of shunting across the defect
- Respiratory distress, tachypnea, tachycardia
- Diaphoresis with feeds, poor weight gain in infants
- Forceful apical impulse
- Thrill along the left lower or midsternal borders
- High-frequency holosystolic murmur
- S3
- Increased intensity of P2
- Elevated jugular venous pressure
- Diastolic rumble due to increased flow across the mitral valve
- If pulmonary hypertension exists: cyanosis with exertion
- If Eisenmenger's complex is present: cyanosis and clubbing

CAUSES
- Congenital
- In adults, secondary to myocardial infarction

RISK FACTORS
- Congenital
  - ◊ 4.2% risk of sibling being affected
  - ◊ 4.0% of offspring being affected
- Post-acute myocardial infarctions
  - ◊ First MI
  - ◊ Limited coronary artery disease
  - ◊ Hypertension
  - ◊ Most frequent within first week after myocardial infarction (MI)
  - ◊ Occur in 1-2% of MI, most commonly after anterior MI

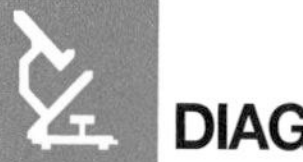

DIAGNOSIS

DIFFERENTIAL DIAGNOSIS
- Any disease with left-to-right shunt, such as large patent ductus arteriosus or atrial septal defect
- Children - Tetralogy of Fallot
- Adults - acute mitral regurgitation

LABORATORY None specific

Drugs that may alter lab results: N/A

Disorders that may alter lab results: N/A

PATHOLOGICAL FINDINGS
- Congenital VSD's (4 major anatomical types):
  - ◊ Membranous (70%)
  - ◊ Muscular (20%)
  - ◊ Atrioventricular canal type (5%)
  - ◊ Supracristal (5%; higher percent in Oriental population)
- Postmyocardial infarction VSD's
  - ◊ Involve predominantly the muscular septum

SPECIAL TESTS
- ECG may suggest severity of VSD. Initially, left ventricular hypertrophy and left atrial enlargement may be evident. With pulmonary hypertension, right ventricular hypertrophy and right atrial enlargement may be seen.
- After surgical repair, right bundle branch block and left anterior hemi-block are common

IMAGING
- Chest x-ray may demonstrate increased pulmonary vascularity and/or cardiomegaly
- Two-dimensional echocardiogram for visualization
- Color-flow Doppler, for detection of ventricular septal defect jet

DIAGNOSTIC PROCEDURES
- Cardiac catheterization (left and right heart) can establish the diagnosis, quantitate degree of shunting
- Demonstration of an oxygen saturation step-up (>8 mm Hg [1.1 kPa]) from the right atrium to the distal pulmonary artery with Swan-Ganz catheter

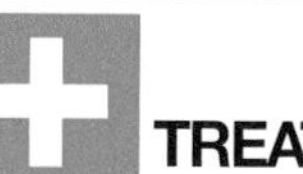

TREATMENT

APPROPRIATE HEALTH CARE
- Outpatient, until surgical repair is indicated
- Inpatient in setting of acute MI
- Inpatient for treatment of severe congestive heart failure

GENERAL MEASURES N/A

SURGICAL MEASURES
- Surgical closure is indicated if the pulmonic to systemic flow is > 1.5:1
- Congenital VSD surgery is usually performed before the child enters school or earlier, if hemodynamically indicated
- In the post-MI setting, afterload reduction, inotropic support and intra-aortic balloon pump may be used to stabilize the patient prior to surgery

ACTIVITY As tolerated

DIET Low sodium

PATIENT EDUCATION
- Endocarditis prophylaxis
- Parents need support and instructions for prevention of complications until the child is ready for surgery

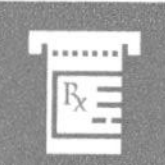

MEDICATIONS

DRUG(S) OF CHOICE

- Antibiotic prophylaxis
- Pediatric
  - ◊ Furosemide 1-2 mg/kg dose PO/IV qd-bid
  - ◊ Digoxin:
    - Infants < 2 years old 10 mcg/kg/day PO divided bid
    - Children 2-10 years old 5-10 mcg/kg/day PO divided bid
    - Children > 10 years old 2-5 mcg/kg/day PO divided bid
  - ◊ Spironolactone 1-2 mg/kg/day divided qd-bid
  - ◊ Captopril 0.1-0.4 mg/kg/dose po given q6-24h. (max 6 mg/kg/24h)
- Adult
  - ◊ Nitroglycerin drip beginning at 5 μg/kg/min and increasing by 5 μg/kg/min every few minutes, then by up to 20 μg/kg/min and titrate effect blood pressure, cardiac output, etc.
  - ◊ Nitroprusside beginning at 10 μg/min and increasing by 5-10 μg/min every few minutes, titrating to blood pressure, cardiac output, etc.
  - ◊ Angiotensin converting enzyme (ACE) inhibitors (e.g., captopril 6.25-25 mg po tid or lisinopril 2.5-20 mg po qd or enalapril 2.5-15 mg po qd or bid)
  - ◊ Hydralazine 10-100 mg po qid
  - ◊ Dobutamine 2.5-10 μg/kg/min titrating to cardiac output and systemic resistance (SVR)
  - ◊ Dopamine 5-10 μg/kg/min titrating to cardiac output and SVR

Contraindications: Drugs that increase peripheral vascular resistance may increase right-to-left shunting
Precautions: Hypotension
Significant possible interactions: Refer to manufacturer's profile of each drug

ALTERNATIVE DRUGS
Diuretics and digoxin may also be beneficial in certain circumstances

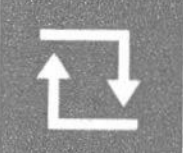

FOLLOWUP

PATIENT MONITORING
Close followup (at least every 6 months) of a congenital VSD is necessary until primary intracardiac repair is performed to ensure that significant pulmonary hypertension does not develop

PREVENTION/AVOIDANCE

- For adults, avoid risk factors for myocardial infarction and obtain evaluation before pregnancy

POSSIBLE COMPLICATIONS

- Congestive heart failure
- Infective endocarditis
- Aortic insufficiency
- Sudden death
- Hemoptysis
- Chest pain
- Cerebral abscess
- Paradoxical emboli
- Cardiogenic shock
- Heart block may rarely accompany surgical closure
- Pulmonary hypertension

EXPECTED COURSE/PROGNOSIS

- Congenital
  - ◊ Course is variable depending on the size of the VSD
  - ◊ 25-45% of small VSD will close spontaneously by age 3
  - ◊ With large VSD - CHF, failure to thrive in infancy, necessitating surgical repair
  - ◊ 4% of patients with VSD develop infective endocarditis by the third or fourth decade of life
  - ◊ Progressive pulmonary vascular disease and pulmonary hypertension are the most feared complications of VSD caused by left-to-right shunting, and may eventually lead to reversal of the shunt (Eisenmenger's complex). Death usually occurs in the fourth decade of life if untreated.
- Postmyocardial infarction
  - ◊ 80-90% mortality in the first two weeks with medical management alone
  - ◊ Prognosis worse with inferior MI compared to anterior MI

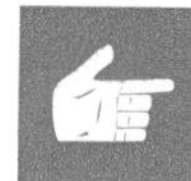

MISCELLANEOUS

ASSOCIATED CONDITIONS

- Congenital
  - ◊ Tetralogy of Fallot
  - ◊ Aortic valvular deformities, especially aortic insufficiency
  - ◊ Down syndrome (Trisomy 21), endocardial cushion defect
  - ◊ Transposition of the great arteries
  - ◊ Coarctation of the aorta
  - ◊ Tricuspid atresia
  - ◊ Truncus arteriosus
  - ◊ Patent ductus arteriosus
  - ◊ Atrial septal defect
  - ◊ Pulmonic stenosis
  - ◊ Subaortic stenosis
- Adult
  - ◊ Coronary artery disease

AGE-RELATED FACTORS
Pediatric: Congenital
Geriatric: Almost entirely associated with myocardial infarction
Others: N/A

PREGNANCY

- May exacerbate symptoms and signs with a congenital VSD
- Tolerated during pregnancy if the septal defect is small

SYNONYMS
N/A

ICD-9-CM
745.4 Ventricular septal defect

SEE ALSO
Down syndrome
Myocardial infarction
Tetralogy of Fallot

OTHER NOTES
N/A

ABBREVIATIONS
N/A

REFERENCES

- Friedman WF, Perloff JK. Congenital heart disease in infancy and childhood. In: Braunwald E, ed. Heart Disease. 4th Ed. Philadelphia, W.B. Saunders Co., 1992
- Hillis DL, Lange RA, Winniford MD, Page RL: Manual of Clinical Problems in Cardiology. New York, Little, Brown and Co., 1995
- Radford MJ, et al: Ventricular septal rupture: a review of clinical and physiologic features and an analysis of survival. Circulation 1981;64(3)
- McDaniel NL. Ventricular and atrial septal defects. Pediatr Rev 2001;22(8):265-70

Web references: 0 available at www.5mcc.com
Illustrations N/A

Author(s):
Ricardo Samson, MD

BASICS

DESCRIPTION Vitamin deficiency syndromes develop slowly and are difficult to diagnose. Vitamins can not be synthesized by humans and therefore must be supplied by diet. Vitamins are required for maintenance of optimal health and prevention of chronic diseases. Multiple deficiencies of vitamins occur more frequently than a deficiency in a single vitamin. Vitamin classification follows:
- Fat-soluble
  - ◊ Vitamin A (retinol)
  - ◊ Vitamin D (vitamin D2 = ergocalciferol; vitamin D3 = cholecalciferol)
  - ◊ Vitamin E
  - ◊ Vitamin K (K1 = phytomenadione; K2 = menaquinone; K3 = menadione)
- Water-soluble
  - ◊ Vitamin B1 (thiamine)
  - ◊ Vitamin B2 (riboflavin)
  - ◊ Vitamin B3 (niacin, nicotinic acid, niacinamide)
  - ◊ Vitamin B6 (pyridoxine)
  - ◊ Vitamin B12 (cobalamin)
  - ◊ Vitamin C (ascorbic acid)

System(s) affected: Endocrine/Metabolic
Genetics:
- Hereditary vitamin D-dependent rickets - autosomal recessive syndrome
- Thiamine-dependent beriberi - rare hereditary metabolic disorder
- Pernicious anemia

Incidence/Prevalence in USA: Unknown
Predominant age: Elderly
Predominant sex: Male = Female

SIGNS & SYMPTOMS
- Vitamin (A) (retinol)
  - ◊ Early - dryness of conjunctiva (xerosis)
  - ◊ Bitot's spots (small whites spots on conjunctiva)
  - ◊ Loss of appetite, growth retardation and anemia commonly found in children
  - ◊ Late - keratomalacia (ulceration & necrosis of cornea), endophthalmitis, blindness
- Vitamin B 1 (thiamine)
  - ◊ Infantile beriberi - occur in infants breast-fed by thiamine deficient mothers
  - ◊ "Wet beriberi" - cardiovascular symptoms - peripheral vasodilation, high output failure and dyspnea tachycardia
  - ◊ "Dry beriberi" - neurological symptoms symmetrical motor and sensory peripheral neuropathy with, paresthesias, loss of reflexes
  - ◊ Wernicke encephalopathy - nystagmus, ophthalmoplegia, truncal ataxia, confusion
  - ◊ Korsakoff syndrome - amnesia, impaired learning, confabulation
- Vitamin B3 (niacin [nicotinic acid] niacinamide)
  - ◊ Anorexia, weakness, irritability, mouth soreness, glossitis, stomatitis, weight loss
  - ◊ Dermatitis seen symmetrically in sun exposed areas, skin is dry dark and scaly
  - ◊ Dementia, insomnia, irritability, apathy, confusion, memory loss, psychosis, hallucination
  - ◊ Diarrhea
  - ◊ Death
- Vitamin B12 (cobalamin)
  - ◊ Anorexia, diarrhea, glossitis
  - ◊ Peripheral nerves - paresthesias
  - ◊ Posterior column - difficulty with balance
  - ◊ Confusion, memory loss, disorientation
  - ◊ Dementia
- Vitamin C (ascorbic acid)
  - ◊ Scurvy - develops in children between 6- 24 months
  - ◊ Early - weakness, malaise
  - ◊ Late - perifollicular hemorrhage and hyperkeratotic papules, petechia, purpura, splinter hemorrhages, bleeding gums, hematomas, subperiosteal hemorrhages
  - ◊ Terminal - edema, oliguria, neuropathy, intracranial, hemorrhage, death
- Vitamin E (alpha-tocopherol)
  - ◊ RBC hemolysis, creatinurias ceroid deposition in muscle
  - ◊ Areflexia, gait disturbances ophthalmoplegia
- Vitamin K (K1 - phytomenadione; K2 - menaquinone; K3 - menadione)
  - ◊ Early - hemolytic disease of newborn (HDN) seen within first 24 hours of birth
  - ◊ Classic - seen within 7-14 days of birth - bleeding from skin gut, circumcision site
  - ◊ Late - seen 2-12 weeks after birth, intracranial hemorrhage

CAUSES
- Inadequate dietary intake
- Impaired absorption or storage

RISK FACTORS
- Social and psychological - social isolation, depression, alcohol abuse, elder abuse and neglect, institutionalization, poverty, inadequate assistance with eating, eating disorders (anorexia/bulimia), loss of spouse or caretaker
- Physical - chronic disease (eg cancer), poorly fitting/missing dentures, reduced calorie intake with advanced age, impaired mobility, memory and attention disorders, neurological impairment of chewing or swallowing
- Others
  - ◊ Parenteral nutrition, malabsorption, bile deficiency, dialysis, chronic protein-calorie undernutrition, drug interactions, infants, elderly, laxative abuse, genetic disorder (abetalipoproteinemia) (vitamin E), intestinal parasites, food faddism, gastrointestinal surgery
  - ◊ Increased physiologic demands of pregnancy, hemolytic anemia, and exfoliative skin diseases

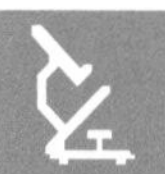

DIAGNOSIS

DIFFERENTIAL DIAGNOSIS
- Vitamin A deficiency - retinitis pigmentosa
- Vitamin B1 deficiency - polyneuropathy
- Vitamin B2 deficiency - other causes of seborrheic dermatitis and ocular lesions
- Vitamin D - infantile scurvy; congenital syphilis; chondrodystrophy; readily distinguishable disorders (cretinism, hydrocephalus, poliomyelitis, etc.); convulsions due to other causes
- Vitamin K - liver damage, anticoagulant or salicylate therapy, other disorders that produce hemorrhagic symptoms (scurvy, allergic purpura, leukemia, thrombocytopenia)
- Niacin - other causes of stomatitis, glossitis, diarrhea, dementia
- Vitamin B12 - other causes of myelodysplasia

LABORATORY
- Vitamin A - serum levels below normal
- Vitamin BI - elevated blood pyruvate
  - ◊ Decreased urinary thiamin excretion
  - ◊ Erythrocyte transketolase activity > 15-20%
- Vitamin B2
  - ◊ Erythrocyte glutathione reductase coefficient >1.2 - 1.3
  - ◊ Lower serum levels of plasma and red cell plasma
  - ◊ Lower urinary excretion of riboflavin
- Vitamin B3 (niacin)
  - ◊ Lower levels of N-methylnicotinamide
  - ◊ Lower levels of serum and Red cell NAD and NADP
- Vitamin B6 - lower levels of pyridoxal in blood (normal - 50 ng/ml)
- Vitamin B 12
  - ◊ Serum levels <150 pg/ml
  - ◊ MCV 110-140 fl, ovalocytes, hypersegmented neutrophils, decreased reticulocyte count, pancytopenia
  - ◊ Bone marrow - erythroid hyperplasia
  - ◊ Increased LDH - increased indirect bilirubin
  - ◊ Schilling test
- Vitamin C - levels <0.1 mg/dl
- Vitamin D - plasma calcium level < 7.5 mg/dL (1.88 mmol/L); low plasma vitamin D sterols; inorganic phosphate serum levels < 3 mg/dL (0.97 mmol/L); serum citrate levels, 2.5 mg/dL; alkaline phosphate < 4 Bodansky units/100 mL
- Vitamin E - serum levels < 0.8 mg/dL (18.5 μmol/L) (adults)
- Vitamin K - prothrombin time 25% longer than normal range (diagnostic for vitamin deficiency after ruling out other disorders), PIUKA II test

Drugs that may alter lab results: Refer to laboratory test reference

Disorders that may alter lab results: Refer to laboratory test reference

PATHOLOGICAL FINDINGS N/A

SPECIAL TESTS N/A

IMAGING N/A

DIAGNOSTIC PROCEDURES History and physical

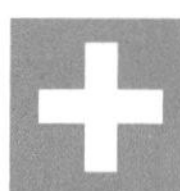

TREATMENT

APPROPRIATE HEALTH CARE Outpatient usually. Inpatient in severe cases.

GENERAL MEASURES
- Treatment of any underlying causes
- Oral or parenteral vitamin therapeutic replacement
- Maintenance vitamin supplement as required
- For vitamin D deficiency - adequate exposure to sunlight

SURGICAL MEASURES N/A

ACTIVITY As tolerated

DIET
- For dietary deficiencies - provide nutritional counseling with emphasis on appropriate foods and the proper methods for their preparation
- Abstain from alcohol

PATIENT EDUCATION
- Refer patients to appropriate social service agencies if socioeconomic factors contribute to deficient diet
- Emphasis on compliance with vitamin supplementation regimens
- Help with alcohol or smoking cessation

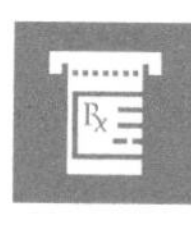

MEDICATIONS

DRUG(S) OF CHOICE
- Vitamin A: retinol, carotene, or beta-carotene. Acute deficiencies require aqueous vitamin A solution IM.
- Vitamin B1: oral thiamine 5-30 mg tid depending on deficiency. Acute symptoms: 100 mg IV q day. Maintenance: supplemental B complex vitamin.
- Vitamin B2: oral riboflavin 10-30 mg/day in divided doses until patient response is evident, then decrease to 2-4 mg/day until recovered. May be given IM 5-20 mg/day.
- Vitamin B3: confirmed deficiencies require niacinamide 300-500 mg/day in divided doses by mouth or IV. Supplemental B complex vitamins and dietary increase in foods high in niacin.
- Vitamin B6: oral or parenteral replacement for confirmed deficiency. Prophylactic doses for epileptic children. Women on oral contraceptives may need supplement, pyridoxine 2.5-10 mg po.
- Vitamin B12
  - ◊ 100 mg IM - qd x one week
  - ◊ 100 mg IM - qd x one month
  - ◊ 100 mg IM - qd x lifetime
- Vitamin C (ascorbic acid): daily doses of 100-200 mg in synthetic form or in orange juice for mild scurvy, doses up to 500 mg/day in severe disease
- Vitamin D (cholecalciferol, ergocalciferol): oral doses. For rickets refractory to vitamin D, include 25-hydroxy-cholecalciferol, active form of vitamin D.
- Vitamin E: oral or parenteral replacement with a water soluble vitamin E supplement, 60-70 units/day for adult, 1 unit/kg/day for children
- Vitamin K1: 10 mg (adult dose) phytonadione (Mephyton) for hypoprothrombinemia given subcutaneously or IM. For non-emergency, give oral dose 5-20 mg. A single dose of 0.5-1 mg IM or SC for newborns.

Contraindications: Refer to manufacturer's literature
Precautions: Refer to manufacturer's literature
Significant possible interactions: Refer to manufacturer's literature

ALTERNATIVE DRUGS
- In Vitamin D deficiency: Calcitriol (Rocaltrol) 0.25 mcg q day, increasing weekly to maintenance of 1 mcg q day (1 mg - 40,000 units)

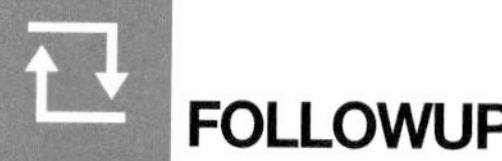

FOLLOWUP

PATIENT MONITORING As needed depending on severity of problem

PREVENTION/AVOIDANCE
- Proper nutrition
- Supplemental vitamins if needed
- Reduce risk factors that lead to deficiency where possible
- Vitamin D deficiency - adequate exposure to sunlight (30 minutes several times a week)
- Postoperative vitamin K for patients are NPO
- Neonates - should receive vitamin K1 IM, subcutaneously or orally to prevent hemolytic disease of the newborn

POSSIBLE COMPLICATIONS
- Vitamin A deficiency - mortality high in advanced cases; eye lesions are a threat to vision
- Vitamin B1 (thiamine) deficiency - cardiac beriberi and Wernicke-Korsakoff syndrome may be fatal if left untreated
- Vitamin B6 chronic deficiency - may increase risk of kidney stone formation
- Vitamin D deficiency - skeletal deformities, greenstick fractures, bone pain
- Excessive synthetic vitamin K may lead to hemolytic anemia and kernicterus in infants

EXPECTED COURSE/PROGNOSIS
With proper diagnosis and adequate therapy, expect full recovery without complications

MISCELLANEOUS

ASSOCIATED CONDITIONS N/A

AGE-RELATED FACTORS
Pediatric:
- Vitamin D deficiency rickets is now rare in the U.S., but may occur in breast-fed infants who do not receive a vitamin D supplement, or in infants fed a formula with a nonfortified milk base
- Vitamin E deficiency in infants usually results from formulas high in polyunsaturated fatty acids that are fortified with iron but not vitamin E
- Vitamin E - seen with severe malabsorption, genetic disorder of abetalipoproteinemias, children with cholestatic liver disease, biliary atresia or cystic fibrosis
- Vitamin K deficiency - common among newborns

Geriatric: More likely to have multiple risk factors that can lead to vitamin deficiencies
Others: N/A

PREGNANCY Women should take a supplemental multivitamin tablet that contains at least 60 mg of elemental iron and 1.0 mg of folic acid

SYNONYMS N/A

ICD-9-CM
269.2 Unspecified vitamin deficiency
264.9 Unspecified vitamin A deficiency
266.9 Unspecified vitamin B deficiency
265.1 Other and unspecified manifestations of thiamine deficiency
266.0 Ariboflavinosis
266.1 Vitamin B6 deficiency
266.2 Other B-complex deficiencies
267 Absorbic acid deficiency
268.9 Unspecified vitamin D deficiency
269.1 Deficiency of other vitamins
269.0 Deficiency of vitamin K
776.0 Hemorrhagic disease of newborn

SEE ALSO

OTHER NOTES Alcohol withdrawal - initial therapy of alcohol withdrawal should include B vitamins, especially thiamine to avoid causing neurological complications

ABBREVIATIONS N/A

REFERENCES

- Machlin LJ, ed: Handbook of Vitamins. 2nd Ed. New York, Marcel Dekker, 1990
- Shils ME, Young VR, eds: Modern Nutrition in Health and Disease. 7th Ed. Philadelphia, Lea & Febiger, 1988
- Konis AB: Vitamin deficiency in the elderly. NY State Dent J;1991
- Tierney LM, et al: Current Medical Diagnosis & Treatment. 38th Ed. New York, Appleton & Lange, 1999
- Rakel RE: Conn's Current Therapy. Philadelphia, WB Saunders Co, 1997
- Champe PC: Lippincott's Illustrated Review: Biochemistry. 2nd Ed. 1994, Philadelphia, Lippincott Williams & Wilkins

Web references: 0 available at www.5mcc.com
Illustrations N/A

Author(s):
Chandramohan Batra, MD

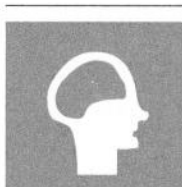

BASICS

DESCRIPTION

- An acquired, slowly progressive depigmenting condition in small or large areas of the skin due to the disappearance of previously active melanocytes
  - ◊ Focal (including segmental) vitiligo - one to a few scattered macules, occasionally in a dermatomal distribution
  - ◊ Generalized vitiligo - many widespread macules (most common form)
  - ◊ Universal vitiligo - little remaining normal pigment
  - ◊ Acrofacial - affects distal fingers and facial orifices

System(s) affected: Skin/Exocrine
Genetics: Autosomal dominant with variable expression and incomplete penetrance. Positive family history in 30% of cases.
Incidence/Prevalence in USA: 500-1000/100,000
Predominant age: All ages: 50% begin before age 20
Predominant sex: Male = Female

SIGNS & SYMPTOMS

- Loss of pigment
- Locally increased sunburning
- Predilection for acral areas and around orifices such as eyes, mouth, anus
- Pruritus (10%)
- Premature graying (35%)
- Koebner phenomenon (aggravation by trauma)

CAUSES Etiology is unclear, but is thought to be an autoimmune reaction to preexisting melanocytes

RISK FACTORS

- Positive family history
- Autoimmune disorders including hemolytic anemia and adrenal insufficiency
- Major life crisis or illness

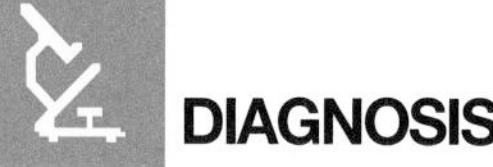

DIAGNOSIS

DIFFERENTIAL DIAGNOSIS

- Any condition that causes acquired hypomelanosis:
  - ◊ Tinea versicolor
  - ◊ Leprosy
  - ◊ Lupus erythematosus
  - ◊ Pityriasis alba
  - ◊ Atopic dermatitis
  - ◊ Albinism
  - ◊ Alopecia areata
  - ◊ Chemical exposure (phenols, arsenic, chloroquine, hydroquinone)
  - ◊ Steroid exposure
  - ◊ Retinoic acid use
  - ◊ Tuberous sclerosis
  - ◊ Neurofibromatosis
  - ◊ Melanocytic nevi (halo nevi)
  - ◊ Tumor regression of malignant melanoma
  - ◊ Piebaldism
  - ◊ Hypopituitarism
  - ◊ Hyperthyroidism
  - ◊ Morphea
  - ◊ Lichen sclerosis

LABORATORY

- Routine blood and urine studies are usually normal in the absence of associated diseases in adults
- In children screen for autoimmune diseases with TSH, CBC, and fasting glucose

Drugs that may alter lab results: N/A

Disorders that may alter lab results: N/A

PATHOLOGICAL FINDINGS Complete absence of melanocytes in skin biopsy. At the margins one may see a few lymphocytes and large melanocytes with abnormal melanosomes.

SPECIAL TESTS N/A

IMAGING N/A

DIAGNOSTIC PROCEDURES

- Examination under Wood's light accentuates the hypopigmented areas, especially in light-skinned individuals
- Skin scraping and a potassium hydroxide (KOH) preparation can be examined microscopically to rule out tinea versicolor

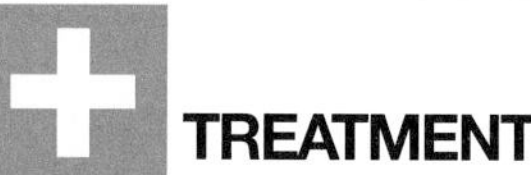

TREATMENT

APPROPRIATE HEALTH CARE Outpatient except in rare cases of surgical skin-grafting or transplantation

GENERAL MEASURES

- Sun exposure can accentuate the difference between normal and abnormal skin, so for cosmetic reasons patients may wish to avoid this
- Skin dyes and cosmetics may be used as cover-ups

SURGICAL MEASURES N/A

ACTIVITY Full activity

DIET No special diet

PATIENT EDUCATION

- Reassure patient that in absence of associated autoimmune illness the problem is purely cosmetic. Successful cosmetic cover-up is usually quite simple. Some areas offer vitiligo support groups.
- Information available through National Vitiligo Foundation, P.O. Box 6337, Tyler TX 75711; (903)531-0074

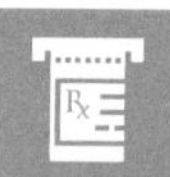

MEDICATIONS

DRUG(S) OF CHOICE
- Focal or segmental vitiligo: Begin with a mid-potency steroid cream applied daily for 3-4 months. If no response, advance to high potency steroids. Clobetasol (Temovate) cream applied qd for 2 months (every other day on the face). Treatment may be resumed following a 1 to 4 month respite. Alternatively topical psoralens applied in a 1% solution followed in 90 minutes by ultraviolet exposure (UVA). Caution for subsequent exposure to light (sunburn).
- Generalized vitiligo: Oral systemic steroids, e.g., betamethasone 5 mg given 2 days in a row, then held the remainder of the week. This pattern continued for 2-4 months minimizes side effects and is effective in arresting the disease in many patients. Oral trimethylpsoralen or methoxsalen (Oxsoralen-Ultra, 8-MOP) and UVA over a 12-24 month period. Alternatively depigmenting the remaining normal skin with monobenzone, a hydroquinone derivative, 20% cream may be elected. It should be applied twice daily for 3-6 months.

Contraindications:
- Absolute contraindications to use of psoralen compounds: Idiosyncratic reaction to psoralens, photosensitive disease (e.g., systemic lupus erythematosus, albinism, porphyria), invasive squamous cell carcinoma, melanoma, aphakia
- Relative contraindications to use of psoralen compounds: Cardiac disease, hepatic dysfunction, multiple basal cell carcinomas, prior radiation therapy, prior arsenic therapy

Precautions:
- Watch for skin atrophy and telangiectasias when using topical steroids, especially on the face
- Watch for photosensitizers with UVA treatment
- Severe burns possible with topical psoralens. Partially avoided with - 1:10 or 1:50 dilution of psoralens.
- Psoralen plus UVA (PUVA) cannot be used for children less than 12 years of age due to immaturity of the ocular lens
- Patients undergoing PUVA therapy should have a screening ophthalmologic examination to rule out subclinical retinal pigmentary disease that is frequently associated with vitiligo

Significant possible interactions: Other photosensitizers, e.g., tetracyclines and retinoic acid

ALTERNATIVE DRUGS
- Patients with unresponsive focal vitiligo may be candidates for mini-grafting with or without PUVA therapy
- Narrow band UVB phototherapy is also being tried
- Levamisole 150 mg 2 days/week for several months has been effective in patients with limited or slowly-spreading disease

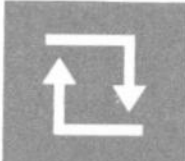

FOLLOWUP

PATIENT MONITORING
- With PUVA therapy, CBC, liver, renal function tests, and an ANA should be done every 6 months.
- With topical steroids, follow at monthly intervals to avoid steroid-atrophy of the skin.

PREVENTION/AVOIDANCE
While undergoing all therapies, avoid excessive sun exposure

POSSIBLE COMPLICATIONS
- Phototoxic reactions ranging from mild to severe with PUVA
- Skin atrophy and telangiectasias with topical steroids
- Contact dermatitis can occur with use of depigmenting agents and cosmetic covers

EXPECTED COURSE/PROGNOSIS
- Only 5% spontaneously repigment
- Best results are with PUVA therapy where 70% have repigmentation of head and neck area, less in other body areas. Lower percentages respond to topical therapy.
- There is no response in at least 20% of cases, especially long-standing cases
- Once repigmentation occurs it usually persists

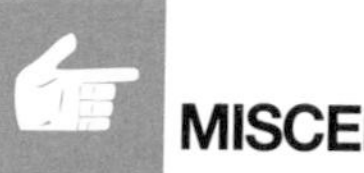

MISCELLANEOUS

ASSOCIATED CONDITIONS
- Addison disease
- Alopecia areata
- Chronic mucocutaneous candidiasis
- Diabetes mellitus (insulin dependent)
- Hypoparathyroidism
- Melanoma
- Pernicious anemia
- Polyglandular autoimmune syndrome
- Thyroid disorders (hyper- and hypothyroidism) - 30% of patients with vitiligo
- Uveitis
- Halo nevi

AGE-RELATED FACTORS
Pediatric: Childhood vitiligo is a distinct subset of vitiligo. Higher incidence of focal vitiligo. Also higher incidence of autoimmune and endocrine disease. Response is poor to topical PUVA therapy, but can be tried. Topical steroids may be prescribed, e.g., desonide 0.05% cream every day for 4 months.
Geriatric: NA
Others: N/A

PREGNANCY
Treatment with topical or oral psoralens is contraindicated

SYNONYMS
- Hypomelanosis
- Depigmentation

ICD-9-CM
709.00 Dyschromia, unspecified

SEE ALSO
Arsenic poisoning
Hyperthyroidism
Hypothyroidism, adult
Pityriasis alba
Tinea versicolor

OTHER NOTES
If PUVA therapy considered, dermatologic consultation should be considered

ABBREVIATIONS
CBC = complete blood count

REFERENCES

- Odom RB, James WD, Berger TG. Andrews' Diseases of the Skin. 9th ed. Philadelphia: WB Saunders; 2000
- Habif TP. Clinical Dermatology. 4th ed. New York: Mosby; 2004
- Lebwohl MG, et al, eds. Treatment of Skin Disease. 1st ed. New York: Mosby; 2002

Web references: 2 available at www.5mcc.com
Illustrations 5 available

Author(s):
Gary J. Silko, MD, MS

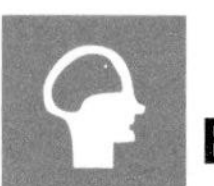

BASICS

DESCRIPTION
- Carcinoma in situ (Bowen disease). Premalignant changes involving the squamous epithelium of the vulva.
- Squamous cell carcinoma - invasive squamous cell carcinoma is the most common malignancy involving the vulva (85% of the patients). The malignancy can be well, moderately or poorly differentiated.
- Other invasive cell types include melanoma, Paget disease, adenocarcinoma, adenocystic carcinoma, small cell carcinoma and sarcomas. Sarcomas are usually leiomyosarcoma and probably arise at the insertion of the round ligament in the labium majus.

System(s) affected: Reproductive
Genetics: No known genetic pattern
Incidence/Prevalence in USA: Invasive vulvar malignancy is a rare gynecologic malignancy accounting for approximately 2,000 new cases per year in the USA
Predominant age:
- In situ disease - mean age, forties
- Invasive malignancy - mean age, sixties with a range of twenties to nineties

Predominant sex: Female only

SIGNS & SYMPTOMS
- In situ disease - a small raised area associated with pruritus
- Invasive malignancy - an ulcerated, non-healing area; as lesions become large, bleeding occurs with associated pain and foul smelling discharge
- In far advanced diseases - the patients can develop rectal bleeding or urethral obstruction
- Large involved inguinal lymph nodes are also associated with advanced disease

CAUSES
- Patients with cervical cancer are more likely to develop vulvar cancer at a later date. This is due to the so-called field effect with a carcinogen involving the lower genital tract.
- Human papilloma virus (HPV) has been associated with squamous cell abnormalities of the cervix, vagina and the vulva but has not been proven to be the causative agent
- Smoking is associated with squamous cell disease of the vulva possibly from direct irritation of the vulva by the transfer of tars and nicotine on the patient's hands or from systemic absorption of carcinogen

RISK FACTORS
- Old age. Invasive disease is rarely seen before age forty and the majority of the patients are elderly.
- In situ disease can occur at any age but is rarely seen before the age of twenty-five

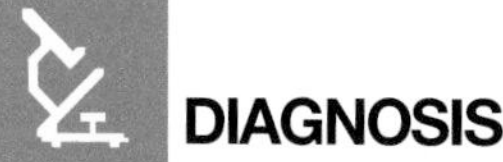

DIAGNOSIS

DIFFERENTIAL DIAGNOSIS
- The definitive diagnosis for vulvar lesions is made by biopsy. Infectious processes can present as ulcerative lesions and include syphilis, lymphogranuloma venereum and granuloma inguinale.
- Crohn disease can present as an ulcerative area on the vulva
- Rarely, lesions can metastasize to the vulva

LABORATORY
- Squamous cell antigen can be elevated with invasive disease
- Hypercalcemia can occur when metastatic disease is present

Drugs that may alter lab results: N/A

Disorders that may alter lab results: N/A

PATHOLOGICAL FINDINGS
- A surgical staging system is used for vulvar cancer
  - TNM Classification = tumor, node, and metastases:
    - ◊ T1 - tumor less than or equal to 2.0 cm
    - ◊ T2 - tumor greater than 2.0 cm
    - ◊ T3 - lower urethra or vagina involved
    - ◊ T4 - upper urethra, bladder, or rectum involved
    - ◊ N0 - nodes negative
    - ◊ N1 - unilateral positive lymph nodes
    - ◊ N2 - bilateral positive lymph nodes
    - ◊ M0 - no metastatic disease
    - ◊ M1 - distant metastatic disease, positive pelvic lymphs node
- International Federation of Obstetrics and Gynecology Classification using TNM:
  - ◊ Stage I - T1, N0, M0
  - ◊ Stage II - T2, N0, M0
  - ◊ Stage III - T1-3, N1, M0; T3, N0-I, M0
  - ◊ Stage IVA - T1-3, N2, M0
  - ◊ Stage IVB - any T, any N, any M

SPECIAL TESTS N/A

IMAGING
- Chest x-ray to evaluate for metastatic disease to lungs
- CAT scan to evaluate pelvic lymph node status and periaortic lymph node status

DIAGNOSTIC PROCEDURES
- Office vulvar biopsy; vulvar punch biopsy should be done to establish the diagnosis
- Wide excision can be performed for carcinoma in situ and any lesion where there is doubt should be further excised for definitive diagnosis to insure that invasive disease is not coexistent with the carcinoma in situ
- Cystoscopy and sigmoidoscopy should be performed if there is a question of invasion into the urethra, bladder or rectum

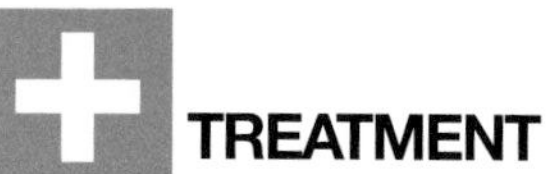

TREATMENT

APPROPRIATE HEALTH CARE Inpatient for treatment

GENERAL MEASURES
- Radiation therapy is used as adjuvant therapy for patients with positive inguinal lymph nodes
- In advanced malignancy involving the urethra and rectum, concomitant cisplatin/5-FU chemotherapy with radiation produces significant decrease in size of the primary tumor, usually obviating the need for pelvic exenteration

SURGICAL MEASURES
- In situ disease can be treated with wide excision or laser vaporization of the affected area. Laser vaporization is preferable in the younger patient while wide excision is preferable in the elderly patient where the risk of invasive disease is also higher.
- Invasive disease is treated primarily by radical vulvectomy and bilateral groin node dissection
- In selected patients, pelvic lymphadenectomy can be performed. If the pelvic lymph nodes are negative, radiation therapy can be avoided.
- Pelvic exenteration provides effective therapy for advanced or recurrent malignancies involving the bladder or rectum after radiation
- Radical vulvectomy and bilateral groin node dissection can be performed through three separate incisions
- Unilateral lesions can be treated with radical hemivulvectomy and unilateral groin node dissection. These modified techniques provide fewer complications and better cosmetic results.

ACTIVITY The patients are usually ambulatory and able to resume full activities by six weeks after surgery unless wound breakdown occurs

DIET Unrestricted, unless undergoing radiation

PATIENT EDUCATION Two complications are common with radical vulvectomy and bilateral groin node dissection, which is the usual treatment of this disease. In the immediate postoperative period, approximately 50% of patients will experience breakdown of the wound. This requires aggressive wound care by visiting nurses approximately twice a day. The wounds usually will granulate and heal over a period of six to ten weeks. Approximately 15-20% of the patients experience some form of mild to moderate lymphedema after the groin node dissection. The patients should be instructed in use of leg elevation and support hose. Less than 1% of the patients will experience severe debilitating lymphedema.
- American College of Obstetricians & Gynecologists (ACOG), 409 12th St., SW, Washington, DC 20024-2188, (800)762-ACOG

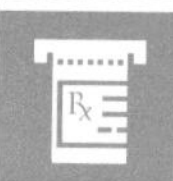

MEDICATIONS

DRUG(S) OF CHOICE
- There are no curative drugs
- As an adjuvant therapy, fluorouracil (Efudex) cream for in situ disease can produce occasional results, but the regimen is not well tolerated because of the excoriation and irritation of the vulva. Adjuvant chemotherapy has not proven to be effective in this disease.
- Metastatic disease, especially in the subcutaneous tissues of the leg or abdomen will produce hypercalcemia, which is treated in the usual medical fashion for hypercalcemia

Contraindications: Elderly patients - if chemotherapeutic agents are used, pay close attention to the patient's performance status and ability to tolerate aggressive chemotherapy
Precautions: The usual precautions for chemotherapy agents. Refer to manufacturer's literature.
Significant possible interactions: Refer to manufacturer's literature

ALTERNATIVE DRUGS N/A

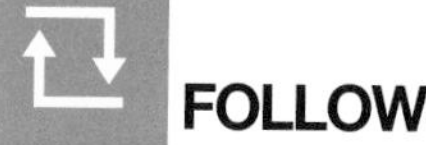

FOLLOWUP

PATIENT MONITORING
- Clinical examination of the groin nodes and vulvar area every 3 months for 2 years, then every 6 months for 3 years
- Chest x-ray should be obtained once a year

PREVENTION/AVOIDANCE
- Any woman complaining of symptoms related to the vulva should have a close examination and biopsies made of appropriate areas
- The vulva can be washed with 3% acetic acid to highlight areas. Areas of white raised epithelium should be biopsied.
- Patients with new onset of pruritus should be biopsied in the area of pruritus
- Liberal biopsy must be used to diagnose in situ disease prior to invasion and to diagnose early invasive disease
- The patient should not be treated for presumed benign conditions of the vulva without full examination and biopsy
- When symptoms persist, reexamination and rebiopsy should be undertaken
- The treatment of benign condyloma of the vulva has not been shown to decrease the eventual incidence of in situ or invasive disease of the vulva

POSSIBLE COMPLICATIONS
The major complications from radical vulvectomy and groin node dissection are wound breakdown, lymphedema and urinary stress incontinence

EXPECTED COURSE/PROGNOSIS
- The five year survival is based on stage:
  - ◊ Stage I 90%
  - ◊ Stage II 85%
  - ◊ Stage III 70%
  - ◊ Stage IVA 25%
  - ◊ Stage IVB 5%

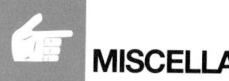

MISCELLANEOUS

ASSOCIATED CONDITIONS
- The patients with invasive vulvar cancer are often elderly and have associated medical conditions
- High rate of other gynecologic malignancies. Patients should be evaluated for these.

AGE-RELATED FACTORS
Pediatric: N/A
Geriatric:
- Older patients with associated medical problems are at high risk for radical surgery. The surgery, however, is external, usually well-tolerated and is the treatment of choice.
- In the very elderly, palliative vulvectomy provides relief of symptoms for ulcerating symptomatic advanced disease

Others:
- More limited surgery
  - ◊ Has been undertaken for invasive lesions especially in young patients to preserve the clitoris and sexual function
  - ◊ Radical vulvectomy with groin node dissection through separate incisions provides better cosmetic results than the en bloc technique
  - ◊ Radical hemivulvectomy can also be utilized for smaller lesions

PREGNANCY
This malignancy is not associated with pregnancy

SYNONYMS
- Bowen disease
- Vulvar cancer

ICD-9-CM
184.4 Malignant neoplasm of vulva, unspecified

SEE ALSO

OTHER NOTES N/A

ABBREVIATIONS N/A

REFERENCES

- Hopkins MP: Disease of the vulva. In: Willson JR, ed. Obstetrics & Gynecology. St. Louis, C.V. Mosby Co., 1991
- Hopkins MP, Reid GC, Vettrano I, Morley GW: Squamous cell carcinoma of the vulva: Prognostic factors influencing survival. Gynecol Oncol 1991;43:113-7
- Hopkins MP. Vulvar neoplasms. In: Copeland LJ, ed. Textbook of gynecology. 2nd ed. Philadelphia: W B Saunders Co; 2000. chapter 53.

Web references: 1 available at www.5mcc.com
Illustrations N/A

Author(s):
Michael P. Hopkins, MD, MEd
Eric L. Jenison, MD

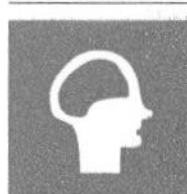

BASICS

DESCRIPTION A syndrome where H2O2 producing lactobacilli are replaced by anaerobic bacteria
System(s) affected: Reproductive
Genetics: N/A
Incidence/Prevalence in USA: As low as 4% in unselected populations; up to 33% in STD clinics; up to 44% in patients with vaginitis
Predominant age: N/A
Predominant sex: Female

SIGNS & SYMPTOMS
- Unpleasant vaginal odor, musty or fishy, exacerbated immediately after intercourse
- Thin gray-white vaginal discharge, mildly adherent to vaginal walls
- 10-30% with vaginal/vulvar irritation
- 10% with frothy discharge.

CAUSES
- Polymicrobial; *Gardnerella vaginalis*, Mobiluncus species, Mycoplasma hominis, Peptostreptococcus, other various anaerobes, including Prevotella, Bacteroides, and Fusobacterium
- There is a shift from a healthy lactobacilli based endogenous flora to an anaerobically based endogenous flora
- Rectal reservoir of organisms leading to autoinfection

RISK FACTORS
- Controversial regarding multiple sexual partners
- IUD

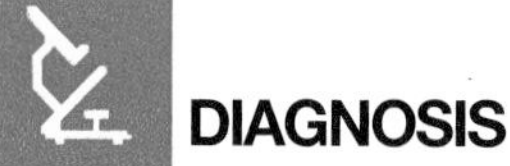

DIAGNOSIS

DIFFERENTIAL DIAGNOSIS
- Gonorrhea
- Chlamydial infection
- Trichomoniasis
- *E. coli* vaginitis
- Staphylococci vaginitis
- Fungal vaginitis
- Trophic vaginitis

LABORATORY
- Affirm VP microprobe
- PH paper (pH > 4.5)
- Wet prep - clue cells in > 10-20% of epithelial cells, fewer WBC's than epithelial cells
- 10% KOH - "whiff test" transient amine or fishy odor
- Gram stain indicating absence of lactobacilli
- May be seen on cytology
- Culture difficult for mycoplasma, not useful

Drugs that may alter lab results: Recent douching

Disorders that may alter lab results: N/A

PATHOLOGICAL FINDINGS Biopsies demonstrate no histologic evidence of inflammation

SPECIAL TESTS N/A

IMAGING N/A

DIAGNOSTIC PROCEDURES N/A

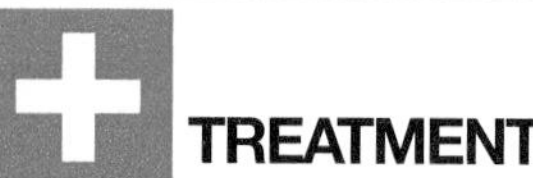

TREATMENT

APPROPRIATE HEALTH CARE Outpatient

GENERAL MEASURES Consider repletion of lactobacilli

SURGICAL MEASURES N/A

ACTIVITY No restrictions

DIET No restrictions

PATIENT EDUCATION N/A

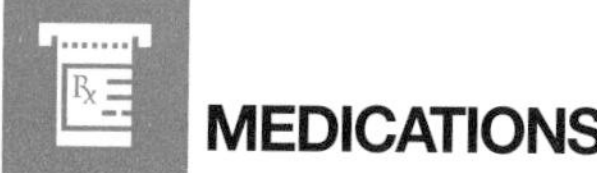

MEDICATIONS

DRUG(S) OF CHOICE

- Metronidazole (Flagyl) 500 mg PO bid for 7 days

or

- Metronidazole vaginal gel 0.75% - 5 gm intravaginally daily for 7 days

or

- Clindamycin 2% vaginal cream 5 gm intravaginally daily for 7 days

Contraindications: Refer to manufacturer's literature

Precautions: Refer to manufacturer's literature

Significant possible interactions: Metronidazole and alcohol

ALTERNATIVE DRUGS

- Metronidazole 2 g PO single dose
- Clindamycin 300 mg PO daily for 7 days
- Clindamycin ovules 100 g intravaginally at bedtime for 3 days (clindamycin creams less effective than metronidazole)

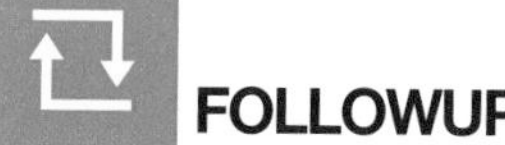

FOLLOWUP

PATIENT MONITORING None indicated

PREVENTION/AVOIDANCE

- Good hygiene
- Use of condoms for sexual intercourse

POSSIBLE COMPLICATIONS

- Uncommon but include
  - ◊ Adnexal tenderness
  - ◊ PID
  - ◊ Intrauterine infections
  - ◊ Chorioamnionitis
  - ◊ Post abortion PID
  - ◊ Postpartum endometritis
  - ◊ Pelvic abscesses
  - ◊ Vaginitis emphysematous
  - ◊ Rare extravaginal disease
  - ◊ Pre-term labor
  - ◊ Premature rupture of membranes
  - ◊ Chorioamnionitis
  - ◊ Newborn infections, including scalp electrode sites, abscesses, and 1 reported case of meningitis
  - ◊ Fetal loss
- Post-hysterectomy infection, septicemia, gaseous crepitation in wound

EXPECTED COURSE/PROGNOSIS Relapses fairly common, can be decreased by increased colonization of lactobacilli

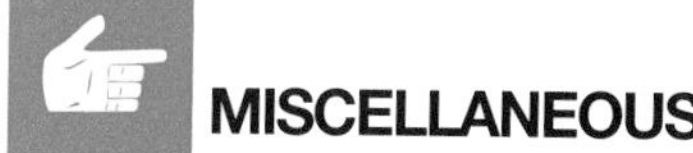

MISCELLANEOUS

ASSOCIATED CONDITIONS N/A

AGE-RELATED FACTORS

Pediatric: N/A
Geriatric: N/A
Others: N/A

PREGNANCY All symptomatic women and those who have had preterm delivery should be treated. Avoid creams. Metronidazole 250 mg PO tid for 7 days or clindamycin 300 mg orally twice a day for 7 days.

SYNONYMS

- Gardnerella vaginosis
- Bacterial vaginosis
- Nonspecific vaginitis
- Haemophilus vaginitis
- Corynebacterium vaginitis

ICD-9-CM

616.10 Vaginitis and vulvovaginitis, unspecified

SEE ALSO

OTHER NOTES N/A

ABBREVIATIONS N/A

REFERENCES

- Centers for Disease Control and Prevention. 1998 guidelines for treatment of sexually transmitted diseases. MMWR Morb Mortal Wkly Rep 2002;MMWR 51(RR06):1-80
- Ray A, et al: Non-specific vaginitis vis-a-vis Gardnerella vaginalis. J of Communicable Dis 1990;22(4)
- Herbst A, Mishell D Jr, Stenchever A, Droegemueller W: Comprehensive Gynecology. 2nd Ed. C.V. Mosby Yearbook, 1992
- Caitlin BW: Gardnerella vaginalis: Characteristics, clinical considerations and controversies. Clinical Microbiology Review 1992;5(3):213-217
- Kharsany AB, Hosen AA, Vanden Ende J: Antimicrobial susceptibility of Gardnerella vaginalis. Antimicrobial Agents and Chemotherapeutics 1993;37(12):2733-2735
- Reed B, Eyler A: Vaginal infections: Diagnosis and management. Amer Fam Phys 1993;47(8)
- Briselden AM, Hillier SL: Evaluation of affirm VP microbial identification test for Gardnerella vaginalis and trichomonas vaginalis. J Clin Microbiology 1994;32(1):148-152
- Curry SL, Barclay: Benign disorders of the vulva-vagina. In: DeCherry & Perroll, eds. Current Obstetric & Gynecologic Diagnosis & Treatment. 8th Ed. Norwalk, Appleton & Lang, 1994
- Majeroni BA: Bacterial vaginosis: An update. American Family Physician 1998;57(6)

Web references: 2 available at www.5mcc.com

Illustrations N/A

Author(s):

J. C. Chava-Zimmerman, MD

BASICS

DESCRIPTION Vulvar pruritus and/or burning, often with abnormal vaginal discharge

System(s) affected: Reproductive, Skin/Exocrine

Genetics: N/A

Incidence/Prevalence in USA:
- 40% of vulvovaginitis is caused by Candida
- 16% of non-pregnant premenopausal women are asymptomatic carriers

Predominant age: Menarche to menopause

Predominant sex: Female only

SIGNS & SYMPTOMS
- Intense vulvar itching
- Thick curd-like vaginal discharge
- Dyspareunia at times
- Erythema of vulva
- Erythema, pain and pruritus of crural and perineal area
- Thick white patches appear attached to vaginal mucosa
- Inflamed vulvar skin

CAUSES
Overgrowth of Candida species (*C. albicans, C. glabrata, C. tropicalis*) in vagina

RISK FACTORS
- Pregnancy
- Diabetes mellitus
- Antibiotic therapy
- Corticosteroid therapy
- Immunosuppressed states
- HIV infection
- Occlusive synthetic underpants and undergarments
- Hypothyroidism
- Oral contraceptive medications (low dose usually not a cause of increased infection risk)
- Anemia
- Zinc deficiency

DIAGNOSIS

DIFFERENTIAL DIAGNOSIS
- Trichomonas vaginitis
- Gonorrheal vaginitis - in prepubertal girls
- Pinworm vaginitis
- Contact dermatitis/vaginitis

LABORATORY
- Yeast, spores, and/or pseudohyphae on smear with 10% KOH solution
- Culture findings on Nickerson's or Sabouraud's media; usually only indicated for recurrent infections
- Vaginal pH < 4.5

Drugs that may alter lab results: N/A

Disorders that may alter lab results: N/A

PATHOLOGICAL FINDINGS N/A

SPECIAL TESTS N/A

IMAGING N/A

DIAGNOSTIC PROCEDURES
- Smear of discharge with 10% KOH solution
- Pap smear

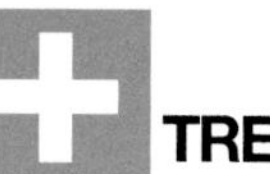

TREATMENT

APPROPRIATE HEALTH CARE
Outpatient

GENERAL MEASURES
- Remove foreign body if one present
- Consider povidone-iodine (Betadine, Operand) douche 15 to 30 mL/L (2 tbsp/qt) of water for symptomatic relief until specific therapy is effective
- If urination causes burning, have the patient
  - ◊ Urinate through a tubular device such as a toilet-paper roll or plastic cup with the end cut out
  - ◊ Pour warm water over vaginal area while urinating
- Insist on strict diabetic control if patient is diabetic

SURGICAL MEASURES N/A

ACTIVITY
- Avoid overexertion, heat, and excessive sweating
- Delay sexual relations until symptoms clear

DIET
Limit sweets (sucrose) and dairy products (lactose) in recurrent infections

PATIENT EDUCATION
- Keep the genital area clean. Use plain unscented soap.
- Take showers rather than tub baths
- Wear cotton underpants with a cotton crotch. Avoid clothing made from non-ventilating materials, including most synthetic underclothing. Avoid tight-fitting jeans or slacks
- Sleep in loose gown without underpants
- Don't sit around in wet clothing - especially a wet bathing suit
- Avoid frequent douches
- Avoid broad-spectrum antibiotics when possible
- After urinating or bowel movements, cleanse by wiping or washing from front to back (vagina toward anus)
- Lose weight, if obese
- American College of Obstetricians & Gynecologists (ACOG), 409 12th St., SW, Washington, DC 20024-2188, (800)762-ACOG

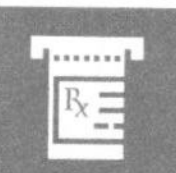

MEDICATIONS

DRUG(S) OF CHOICE
- Fluconazole (Diflucan): 150 mg po once
- Miconazole nitrate (Monistat): one suppository q night x 3, or miconazole vaginal cream q night x 7, or
- Butoconazole nitrate (Femstat): vaginal cream q night x 3, or
- Terconazole (Terazol): one suppository or vaginal cream q night x 3, or
- Clotrimazole (Gyne-Lotrimin): two 100 mg tablets intravaginally x 3 days or cream each night x 7 days

Contraindications: N/A

Precautions:
- Use fluconazole with caution in patients with liver disease

Significant possible interactions: Refer to manufacturer's profile of each drug

ALTERNATIVE DRUGS
- Retreat with different agent, if recurrence
- Course of oral nystatin; 100,000 units tid for 2 weeks
- Topical gentian violet 1% aqueous solution painted onto vagina weekly until infection resolves (usually 2-3 weeks)
- Boric acid 600 mg in gelatin capsule inserted vaginally daily for 2 weeks.

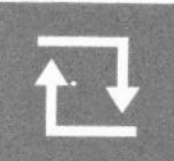

FOLLOWUP

PATIENT MONITORING Generally no specific followup needed. If symptoms persist, then repeat pelvic exam and culture.

PREVENTION/AVOIDANCE
- Follow instructions under patient education
- For recurrences consider reinfection from sexual partner(s). Examine and treat sex partner for Candida balanitis and oral Candida if vaginitis recurs.
- Review Risk Factors

POSSIBLE COMPLICATIONS Secondary bacterial infections of the vagina or vulva

EXPECTED COURSE/PROGNOSIS
- Complete cure with vigorous treatment
- Recurrences are common

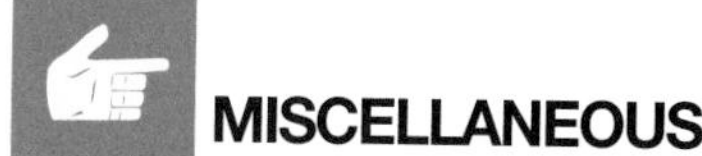

MISCELLANEOUS

ASSOCIATED CONDITIONS Sexually transmitted diseases

AGE-RELATED FACTORS
Pediatric: Less common before puberty
Geriatric: N/A
Others: N/A

PREGNANCY Common

SYNONYMS
- Monilial vulvovaginitis

ICD-9-CM
112.1 Candidiasis of vulva and vagina

SEE ALSO

OTHER NOTES N/A

ABBREVIATIONS N/A

REFERENCES

- Jones HW, Wentz-Colston A, eds: Novak's Textbook of Gynecology. 11th Ed. Baltimore, Williams & Wilkins Co., 1988
- Kaufman RH, Faro S, (eds: Benign Diseases of the Vulva and Vagina. 4th Ed. St. Louis, Mosby-Year Book, 1994
- Sobel J. Vulvovaginitis, when candida becomes a problem. Dermatologic Clinics 1998;16(4):763-69

Web references: 0 available at www.5mcc.com
Illustrations N/A

Author(s):
Albert T. Shiu, MD

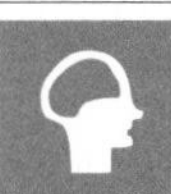

BASICS

DESCRIPTION Decreased blood flow with a thinning and atrophy of the female genital tissue. Changes from estrogen deficiency occur throughout the body. The genital tissues are hormone responsive. Estrogen deficient vulvovaginitis is frequently associated with urinary incontinence.
System(s) affected: Reproductive
Genetics: No known genetic pattern
Incidence/Prevalence in USA: This disorder will affect all women, to some degree, unless estrogen replacement therapy is provided
Predominant age: This is predominantly a problem of the postmenopausal female. The average age of menopause in the United States is 52.5 years.
Predominant sex: Female only

SIGNS & SYMPTOMS
- Vaginal dryness
- Decreased vaginal secretions
- Dyspareunia
- Vulva undergoes a thinning of the epidermis along with decreased integrity of the supporting structures. The thinning and atrophy often produces pruritus.

CAUSES
- Estrogen deficiency
  - ◊ Menopause (surgical or natural)
  - ◊ Ovariectomy
  - ◊ Radiation of the pelvis

RISK FACTORS
- Estrogen deficient states accompanying metabolic disorders
- Vaginal infections with bacteria and fungi

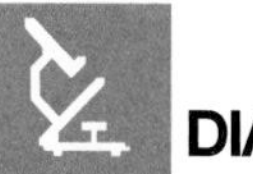

DIAGNOSIS

DIFFERENTIAL DIAGNOSIS
- Malignancy
- Vulvar dystrophies

LABORATORY
- Cytology for maturation index will show a low maturation index, signifying a decreased turnover of the cells from the decreased estrogen effect
- In the perimenopausal or menopausal female, follicle stimulating hormone (FSH) will be elevated and estradiol will be decreased

Drugs that may alter lab results:
- Estrogen therapy will alter the maturation index
- Digoxin has estrogen-like properties
- Tamoxifen (Nolvadex) can produce menopausal type symptoms but also can act on genital tissues as a weak estrogen agonist. Symptoms can vary.
- Drugs used to treat endometriosis or uterine bleeding such as progestins, Danazol or gonadotropin releasing hormone (GnRH) agonists can produce a pseudomenopause which is reversible

Disorders that may alter lab results: N/A

PATHOLOGICAL FINDINGS Thinning of the cornified squamous layer of both the vulva and the vagina

SPECIAL TESTS N/A

IMAGING N/A

DIAGNOSTIC PROCEDURES
- Examination of the vagina and the vulva for maturation index
- FSH level to confirm menopause
- Estradiol level to evaluate circulating estrogen level

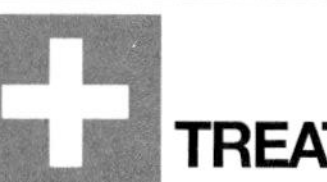

TREATMENT

APPROPRIATE HEALTH CARE Outpatient

GENERAL MEASURES
- Estrogen replacement therapy (ERT) will alleviate and reverse the symptoms and the thinning of the squamous epithelial layer. Replacement therapy leads to an increased blood supply to the genital tissues.
- Symptomatic relief, if needed, e.g., cool baths or compresses

SURGICAL MEASURES N/A

ACTIVITY No restriction

DIET No special diet

PATIENT EDUCATION
- American College of Obstetricians & Gynecologists (ACOG), 409 12th St., SW, Washington, DC 20024-2188, (800)762-ACOG

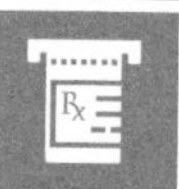

MEDICATIONS

DRUG(S) OF CHOICE
- A wide variety of preparations are available:
  - ◊ Estrogen, conjugated (Premarin) 0.625 mg daily
  - ◊ Estradiol (Estrace) 1 mg daily
  - ◊ Estradiol (Estraderm) patch 0.05 mg, changed twice weekly
  - ◊ If the uterus is not removed, progesterone should be considered. This can be added as medroxyprogesterone (Provera) 2.5 mg daily or 10 mg for 10 days of each month.
  - ◊ Conjugated estrogen vaginal cream (2-4 g/day intravaginally)

Contraindications:
- Estrogen therapy is contraindicated in patients with a history of breast cancer or estrogen positive tumor receptors
- A history of uterine malignancy is a relative contraindication

Precautions: Refer to manufacturer's literature
Significant possible interactions: Refer to manufacturer's literature

ALTERNATIVE DRUGS
N/A

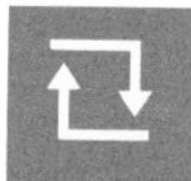

FOLLOWUP

PATIENT MONITORING The patient should be instructed that symptoms should resolve within 30-60 days. If they do not, reevaluation and reexamination for other causes should be undertaken.

PREVENTION/AVOIDANCE N/A

POSSIBLE COMPLICATIONS Those associated with estrogen replacement - postmenopausal bleeding, nausea, headache, libido changes, thrombophlebitis

EXPECTED COURSE/PROGNOSIS Excellent. The vast majority of symptoms will be relieved with estrogen replacement therapy.

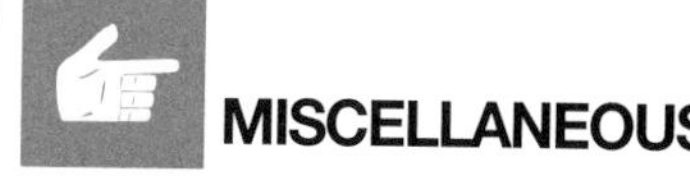

MISCELLANEOUS

ASSOCIATED CONDITIONS None

AGE-RELATED FACTORS
Pediatric: N/A
Geriatric: N/A
Others: N/A

PREGNANCY The lactating postpartum woman with high levels of prolactin are in a hypo-estrogenic state. These women should be instructed to use lubrication for symptoms of dyspareunia. The symptoms will resolve when breast-feeding is stopped.

SYNONYMS N/A

ICD-9-CM
616.10 Vaginitis and vulvovaginitis, unspecified

SEE ALSO

OTHER NOTES The obese patient, especially those weighing more than 100 pounds (45 kg) over the ideal body weight, have higher levels of circulating estrogen and thus may have fewer symptoms. (Androstenedione is converted to estrone in peripheral adipose tissue and when there is an abundance of adipose, higher estrone levels are present.)

ABBREVIATIONS N/A

REFERENCES

- Cunningham FG, MacDonald PC, Gant NF, eds: Williams Obstetrics. 19th Ed. Norwalk CT, Appleton & Lange, 1993
- Novak ER, et al, eds: Novak's Textbook of Gynecology. 11th Ed. Baltimore, Williams & Wilkins, 1988

Web references: 0 available at www.5mcc.com
Illustrations N/A

Author(s):
Michael P. Hopkins, MD, MEd
Eric L. Jenison, MD

BASICS

DESCRIPTION Irritation and/or inflammation of the vulva and/or vagina frequently associated with vaginal discharge
System(s) affected: Reproductive, Skin/Exocrine
Genetics: Not well studied
Incidence/Prevalence in USA: Common
Predominant age: Toddlers to menarche
Predominant sex: Female only

SIGNS & SYMPTOMS
- Irritation and erythema of vulva
- Vaginal discharge
- Offensive odor
- Itching
- Excoriation
- Bleeding

CAUSES
- Most often due to:
  - ◊ Poor hygiene, may lead to labial agglutination
  - ◊ Primary infection elsewhere, e.g., otitis media, pharyngitis
- Most common specific organisms:
  - ◊ Group A beta-hemolytic streptococci; *Streptococcus pyogenes*, Streptococcus pneumoniae
  - ◊ *E. coli*
  - ◊ *Staphylococcus aureus*
  - ◊ *Haemophilus influenzae*
- Less common specific organisms:
  - ◊ Pinworms
  - ◊ *Sarcoptes scabiei* (scabies)
  - ◊ *Candida sp* - most common with immunocompromised, antibiotic therapy, or diapers
- Systemic illnesses:
  - ◊ Measles
  - ◊ Chickenpox
  - ◊ Stevens-Johnson syndrome
  - ◊ Inflammatory conditions, e.g., Reiter syndrome
- Localized vulvar disease:
  - ◊ Seborrheic dermatitis
  - ◊ Psoriasis
  - ◊ Atopic dermatitis
  - ◊ Contact dermatitis
  - ◊ Lichen sclerosus et atrophicus
- Other:
  - ◊ Urethral prolapse
  - ◊ Ectopic ureter
  - ◊ Sexual abuse (gonorrhea, chlamydia, trichomoniasis, herpes). In one study, 4% of girls not suspected to have sexual abuse had positive cultures for gonorrhea.
  - ◊ Other trauma
  - ◊ Foreign body
  - ◊ Tumors or polyps
  - ◊ Masturbation
  - ◊ Genital tract malformations
  - ◊ Polyps or tumors

RISK FACTORS
- Co-existing pharyngitis or other systemic conditions
- Faulty hygiene
- Trauma

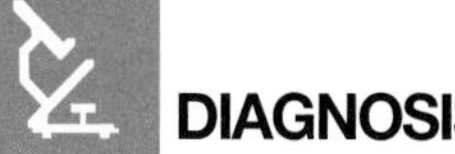

DIAGNOSIS

DIFFERENTIAL DIAGNOSIS
- Contact dermatitis
- Eczema
- Psoriasis

LABORATORY
- Culture for bacteria, fungi or viruses
- Gram stain
- Tape examination for pinworms
- Potassium hydroxide and saline smears

Drugs that may alter lab results: N/A

Disorders that may alter lab results: N/A

PATHOLOGICAL FINDINGS N/A

SPECIAL TESTS Exploration of vagina for foreign body may be necessary in long-standing vaginal discharge

IMAGING N/A

DIAGNOSTIC PROCEDURES Visualization of the vagina may be necessary using a nasal speculum or infant laryngoscope. If blood or foul-smelling discharge is present, visualization is mandatory. Place child in knee-chest position for best result. Hold buttocks apart and slightly upward.

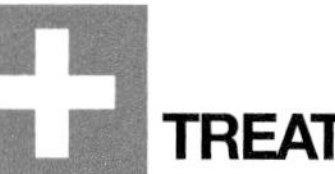

TREATMENT

APPROPRIATE HEALTH CARE Outpatient (except where systemic illness requires hospital care)

GENERAL MEASURES
- Hygiene:
  - ◊ Wipe front-to-back after elimination
  - ◊ Avoid bubble baths and other irritating products
  - ◊ Clean daily with mild soap and water, drying gently with soft towel or cool hair dryer
  - ◊ Apply bland ointments for protection of the skin, if necessary

SURGICAL MEASURES N/A

ACTIVITY Normal

DIET N/A

PATIENT EDUCATION As noted above under General measures

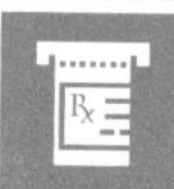

MEDICATIONS

DRUG(S) OF CHOICE
- For empiric treatment, amoxicillin 20 mg/kg/day for 7 days; in areas of high prevalence of resistant H. flu, amoxicillin-clavulanate (Augmentin) 20 mg/kg/day
- Estrogen deficiency with labial adhesion/agglutination - estrogen, conjugated cream to fused area nightly for two weeks
- Specific organisms on culture:
  - ◊ Group A beta-Streptococcus, Streptococcus pneumoniae - penicillin V (Pen Vee K) 25-50 mg/kg/day, maximum of 3 gm/day, divided qid x 10 days
  - ◊ *H. influenzae* - amoxicillin 20-40 mg/kg/day x 7 days; amoxicillin-clavulanate 20 mg/kg/day
  - ◊ *Staphylococcus aureus* - cephalexin 25-50 mg/kg/day, divided qid x 7-10 days or dicloxacillin 12.5-25 mg/kg/day x 7-10 days
  - ◊ *Candida spp* - topical nystatin (Mycostatin), miconazole, clotrimazole or terconazole

Contraindications: Allergy to proposed treatment
Precautions: Avoid potential allergens/topical sensitizers if possible
Significant possible interactions: See manufacturer's profile of each drug

ALTERNATIVE DRUGS
- Topical corticosteroids for pruritus, avoid long-term use

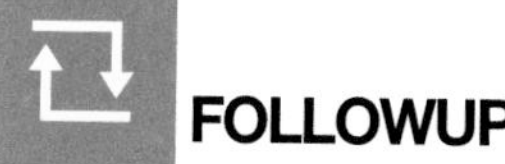

FOLLOWUP

PATIENT MONITORING Only if symptoms do not respond to treatment

PREVENTION/AVOIDANCE
- Perineal hygiene
- Avoidance of irritants and tight or occlusive, non-breathable clothing
- White, unscented toilet paper

POSSIBLE COMPLICATIONS Labial agglutination or adhesions

EXPECTED COURSE/PROGNOSIS
Usually clears with appropriate treatment with no permanent sequelae (if not due to underlying disease such as psoriasis, etc.)

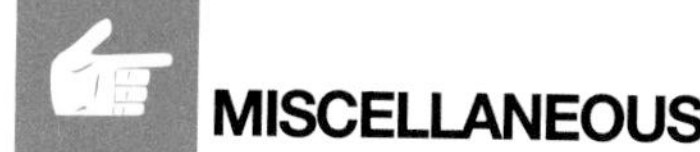

MISCELLANEOUS

ASSOCIATED CONDITIONS N/A

AGE-RELATED FACTORS
Pediatric:
- Usual adult vulvitis/vaginitis organisms are rare in the prepubertal child
- Lack of estrogen causing thin vaginal mucosa which is more susceptible to trauma and infection

Geriatric: N/A
Others: N/A

PREGNANCY N/A

SYNONYMS
- Vaginitis
- Vulvitis

ICD-9-CM
616.10 Vaginitis and vulvovaginitis, unspecified

SEE ALSO

OTHER NOTES N/A

ABBREVIATIONS N/A

REFERENCES

- Vandeven AM, Emans SJ. Vulvovaginitis in the child and adolescent. Pediatric Rev 1993;14:141-7
- Pierce AM, Hart CA. Vulvovaginitis: causes and management. Arch Dis Child 1992;67:509-512
- Jones R. Childhood vulvovaginitis and vaginal discharge in general practice. Family Practice 1996;13(4):369-72
- Shapiro RA, Schubert CJ, Siegel RM. Neisseria gonorrhea infections in girls younger than 12 years of age evaluated for vaginitis. Pediatrics 1999:104(6) e72
- Paek SC, Merritt D, Mallory SB. Pruritus vulvae in prepubertal children. J Am Acad Dermatol 2001;44:795-802

Web references: 0 available at www.5mcc.com
Illustrations N/A

Author(s):
Janice E. Daugherty, MD

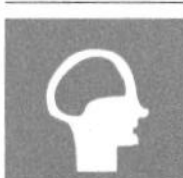

BASICS

DESCRIPTION Warts are painless, benign skin tumors characterized by an area of well circumscribed epithelial thickening. Most people develop warts on their hands or feet at sometime in their lives. They are most common in childhood, with 4-20% of school children having warts at any one time. The DNA papillomavirus is causative and is passed by direct contact with an infected person or from recently shed virus kept intact in a moist, warm environment. Five types of warts are caused by specific genotypes of HPV:
- Common wart (verruca vulgaris)
- Plantar wart (verruca plantaris)
- Flat wart (verruca plana)
- Venereal wart (condyloma acuminatum); see separate topic in book
- Epidermodysplasia verruciformis

System(s) affected: Skin/Exocrine
Genetics: N/A
Incidence/Prevalence in USA: 7-10% of the population
Predominant age: Young adults and children
Predominant sex: Female > Male

SIGNS & SYMPTOMS
- Verruca vulgaris: Rough surfaced, raised, skin-colored papules 5-10 mm in diameter. They may coalesce into a mosaic 1-3 cm in diameter. Most frequently seen on hands.
- Verruca plantaris: Rough surfaced (although smoother than the common wart), flat, skin-colored papules not infrequently attaining 2-3 cm in diameter
- Verruca plana: Slightly elevated, flat-topped, skin-colored papules 1-3 mm in diameter sometimes in a linear arrangement often on hands and face
- Condyloma acuminatum: thin, flexible, tall, papules sometimes demonstrating a confluent growth resembling cauliflower. They do not have the visible or palpable keratin of the previous warts. In infants, laryngeal papillomatosis may occur if condyloma is transmitted during vaginal delivery.
- Epidermodysplasia verruciformis: Flat, reddish lesions on the hands and shoulders presenting in childhood with lifelong persistence

CAUSES Human papilloma virus (HPV)

RISK FACTORS
- AIDS and other immunosuppressive diseases (e.g., lymphomas)
- Immunosuppressive drug use
- Atopic dermatitis
- Locker room use
- Skin trauma

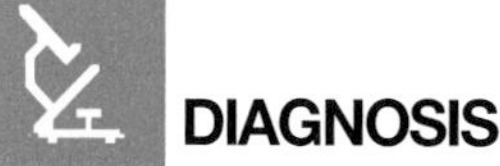

DIAGNOSIS

DIFFERENTIAL DIAGNOSIS
- Corns (on paring, a single "eye" of keratin is observed, whereas a wart shows hemorrhagic spots or "roots")
- Scar tissue
- Molluscum contagiosum (central umbilication and, after curettage, the characteristic pearl)
- Condyloma lata (flat warts of syphilis)
- Seborrheic keratoses

LABORATORY HPV cannot be cultured

Drugs that may alter lab results: N/A

Disorders that may alter lab results: N/A

PATHOLOGICAL FINDINGS
- Papillomavirus found in the nuclei and nucleoli of the stratum granulosum and keratin layers of the epidermis.
- Plantar warts have rete pegs (a downward proliferation of epidermal ridges).
- Thrombosed dermal capillaries

SPECIAL TESTS
Definitive diagnosis can be achieved with the following, but are not clinically relevant for most presentations:
- Electron microscopy
- Immunohistochemical study
- Nucleic acid hybridization

IMAGING N/A

DIAGNOSTIC PROCEDURES
- Paring or débridement and simple visualization will be diagnostic in most cases.
- The use of intuitive clinical diagnosis generally results in excellent specificity, sensitivity, and positive predictive and negative predictive values for recognizing the presence of common viral warts (verrucae vulgaris) according to a published study

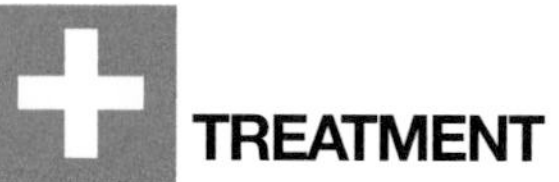

TREATMENT

APPROPRIATE HEALTH CARE Outpatient

GENERAL MEASURES
- The clinical management of verrucae vulgaris is often challenging and no ideal treatment currently exists
- If warts are increasing or painful, they should be treated
- Spontaneous remissions are common (more likely in children than adults), probably related to a host immune response
- Conservative, nonscarring treatments are preferred. Each treatment is associated with a 60-70% cure rate. Cure is achieved when skin lines are restored to a normal pattern.

SURGICAL MEASURES
- Pretreat with anesthetic cream such as EMLA
- Cryotherapy - often preferred because scar formation is minimized. Freezing periungual warts may result in nail deformation.
- Excision with electrocautery, laser ablation, curettage (the virus may be found in smoke so masks should be worn)
- Disfiguring scars and wart recurrence are problems

ACTIVITY If plantar warts are on weight-bearing surface, they may cause significant discomfort and subsequent decrease in activity

DIET N/A

PATIENT EDUCATION Infectious nature should be discussed; keep warts covered while under treatment to avoid auto-inoculation and transmission to others.

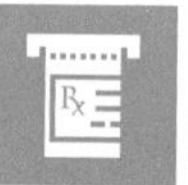

MEDICATIONS

DRUG(S) OF CHOICE

- Benign neglect - safe cost effective treatment option except when warts are extensive, spreading, symptomatic
- Hyperthermia - safe and inexpensive approach; immerse affected area into 45°C water bath for 30 minutes three times per week
- Chemotherapy - all treatments begin by paring the wart, then soaking the area in warm water to moisten the wart
  - ◊ Topical retinoids: tretinoin (retinoic acid, Retin-A) for flat warts, less scarring than cryotherapy or surgical approaches; may be best for warts on the face. Apply bid for 4-6 weeks.
  - ◊ Lactic-salicylic acid (Duofilm): daily treatment for about 3 months
  - ◊ Salicylic acid (Trans-Ver-Sal) in a transdermal delivery system : daily treatment for about 6 weeks
  - ◊ Salicylic acid in propylene glycol; rub into warts each night
  - ◊ Combination cantharidin; 30% salicylic acid, 2% podophyllin, and 19% cantharidin in flexible collodion: apply thin coat, occlude 4-6 hours (or less if painful), then wash off; blisters when form require roof to be removed, debridement of base, and antibiotic cream applied: multiple applications at 2-4 week intervals
  - ◊ Imiquimod; for external genital and perianal warts; apply 5% cream (250 mg single use packets) three times/week at bedtime. Wash off after 6-10 hours. May be used for up to 16 weeks. May weaken condoms and diaphragms.
  - ◊ Induction of delayed type hypersensitivity with dinitrochlorobenzene, or squaric acid dibutylester: apply 2% solution to light shielded area every 2-3 weeks until sensitivity reaction occurs; then apply lower concentration to affected areas. Effective in management of multiple and resistant warts in children.
  - ◊ Occlusion - the easiest and least expensive; cover the wart with a waterproof tape and leave on for a week. Remove and leave open for 12 hours then re-tape if wart is still present. The environment under the tape does not foster viral growth. May be the best for periungual warts.

Contraindications: See specific treatments. Vascular insufficiency is a relative contraindication to some treatments.

Precautions: Avoid normal skin when using the topical chemicals

Significant possible interactions: N/A

ALTERNATIVE DRUGS

- Chemotherapy
  - ◊ Benzoyl peroxide: apply bid for 4-6 weeks
  - ◊ Bleomycin - intradermal injection, is expensive and causes severe pain, but has a 75% cure rate
  - ◊ Cimetidine - 30-40 mg/kg divided tid for 3 months. 86% of patients will have partial or complete regression.
  - ◊ 24% podophyllin applied weekly to anogenital warts, or 5% podofilox (Condylox) self-applied twice daily for 3 days each week for 1 month
  - ◊ Others - dichloroacetic acid, trichloroacetic acid, podophyllin, 5-fluorouracil, silver nitrate, idoxuridine (Herplex Liquifilm), formaldehyde, glutaraldehyde
- Immunotherapy
  - ◊ Dinitrochlorobenzene (DNCB) - should be considered a last resort because of side effects and possible mutagenicity
  - ◊ Interferon - intralesional for urogenital warts
  - ◊ Interferon-alpha - systemic for genital warts
  - ◊ Interferon-beta or gamma - systemic for disseminated verruca vulgaris
- Imiquimod (Aldara) applied daily
- Photodynamic therapy with topical 5-aminolevulinic acid followed by irradiation with incoherent light for recalcitrant warts has shown beneficial results
- Consider pulsed-dye laser therapy. It is performed at 585 nm for up to 4 treatments at 1 month intervals. Complete response averages 66% compared to 70% for conventional type therapies.

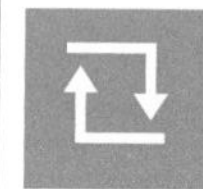

FOLLOWUP

PATIENT MONITORING

One third of the warts of epidermodysplasia may become malignant

PREVENTION/AVOIDANCE

- Cover warts under treatment. Avoid the wound fluid after cryotherapy.
- Use personal footwear in locker room settings

POSSIBLE COMPLICATIONS

- Auto-inoculation
- Scar formation
- Chronic pain after plantar wart removal and scar formation
- Nail deformity after injury to nail matrix

EXPECTED COURSE/PROGNOSIS

Good; complete resolution with or without treatment

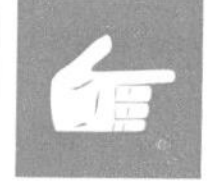

MISCELLANEOUS

ASSOCIATED CONDITIONS

- Acquired immunodeficiency syndrome
- Renal transplantation
- Other conditions with immunosuppression
- Lewandowsky-Lutz disease (associated with epidermodysplasia)

AGE-RELATED FACTORS

Pediatric: Generally more prevalent in children

Geriatric: Less common in non-immunocompromised adults

Others: N/A

PREGNANCY

Podophyllin is contraindicated

SYNONYMS

N/A

ICD-9-CM

078.10 Viral warts, unspecified

SEE ALSO

Condyloma acuminata
Warts, plantar

OTHER NOTES

N/A

ABBREVIATIONS

HPV = Human papilloma virus

REFERENCES

- Bolton RA: Warts. Am Fam Phys 1991;43(6):2049-2056
- Lynch PJ: Dermatology for the House Officer. 3rd Ed. Baltimore, Williams & Wilkins, 1994
- Sams W, et al: Principles and Practices of Dermatology. 2nd Ed. New York, Churchill Livingston, 1996
- Ordoukhanian E: Warts and molluscum contagiosum; beware of treatments worse than the disease. Postgrad Med 1997;2:223-235
- Siegfried EC: Warts on children: an approach to therapy. Ped Annuals 1996;2:79-90
- Gaspari AA, et al: Successful treatment of a generalized human papillomavirus infection with granulocyte-macrophage colony-stimulating factor and interferon gamma immunotherapy in a patient with a primary immunodeficiency and cyclic neutropenia. Arch of Dermatol 1997;133(4):491-96
- Anonymous. Tackling warts on the hands and feet. Drug Ther Bull 1998;36(3):22-4
- Stender IM, Na R, Fogh H, Gluud C, Wulf HC. Photodynamic therapy with 5-aminolaevulinic acid or placebo for recalcitrant foot and hand warts: randomised double-blind trial. Lancet 2000;355(9208):963-6
- Young R, Jolley D, Marks R. Comparison of the use of standardized diagnostic criteria and intuitive clinical diagnosis in the diagnosis of common viral warts (verrucae vulgaris). Arch Dermatol 1998;134(12):1586-9
- Micali G, Nasca MR, et al. Use of squaric acid dibutylester (SADBE) for cutaneous warts in children. Pediatr Dermatol 2000;17(4):315-8
- Robson KJ, Robson KJ, et al. Pulsed-dye laser versus conventional therapy in the treatment of warts: a prospective randomized trial. J Am Acad Dermatol 2000;43(2 Pt 1):275-80
- Silverberg NB, Lim JK, Paller AS, Mancini AJ. Squaric acid immunotherapy for warts in children. J Am Acad Dermatol 2000;42(5 Pt 1):803-8

Web references: 2 available at www.5mcc.com

Illustrations 10 available

Author(s):

David G. Pocock, MBBS

BASICS

DESCRIPTION Discrete or grouped firm keratotic masses on the sole of the foot initiated by a viral infection of keratinocytes
System(s) affected: Skin/Exocrine
Genetics: Unknown
Incidence/Prevalence in USA: Widespread; 2000/100,000
Predominant age: Any age, although more common in children and young adults
Predominant sex: Female > Male (slightly)

SIGNS & SYMPTOMS
- Foot pain
- Discrete or grouped masses on sole of foot with disruption of normal skin markings
- Generally occur at pressure points
- Rough, hyperkeratotic surface with brown-black dots (thrombosed capillaries)
- Callus formation
- Leg or back pain (distortion of posture)

CAUSES Human papillomavirus type 1; less commonly types 2 and 4

RISK FACTORS
- AIDS
- Atopic dermatitis
- Lymphomas
- Patient taking immunosuppressive drugs

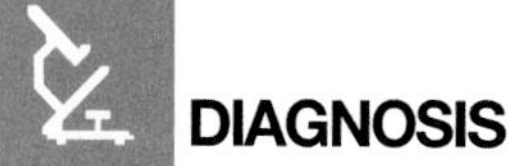

DIAGNOSIS

DIFFERENTIAL DIAGNOSIS
- Corns (clavi)
- Calluses
- Black heel (ruptured capillaries)

LABORATORY N/A

Drugs that may alter lab results: N/A

Disorders that may alter lab results: N/A

PATHOLOGICAL FINDINGS Acanthotic epidermis with hyperkeratosis, papillomatosis, and parakeratosis

SPECIAL TESTS N/A

IMAGING N/A

DIAGNOSTIC PROCEDURES
- Inspection usually confirms the diagnosis
- If cannot distinguish between callus and wart, can examine with a magnifying lens. The wart should demonstrate a highly organized mosaic pattern.
- When pared down have a soft central core and bleeding points (unlike calluses)

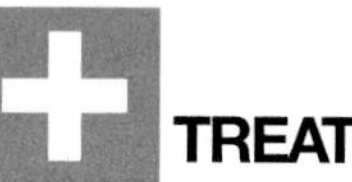

TREATMENT

APPROPRIATE HEALTH CARE
- Outpatient cryotherapy at weekly intervals
- Repeated parings at weekly intervals with or without use of a keratolytic is also an option. Most successful appears to be curettage and chemical cautery (with phenol or trichloroacetic acid) or light electrocautery. (Note: extreme care must be exercised with this procedure because excessive cautery or curettage can cause a painful scar.)

GENERAL MEASURES
- If warts are asymptomatic, no treatment is necessary. However patient may be at risk for spread of warts.
- Warm soaks followed by patient's paring of the top layer of skin on repeated occasions may speed disappearance
- Patient may use pumice stone, emery board or a blade
- Over-the-counter keratolytics containing salicylic acid may help. The advised procedure is paring of skin followed by warm soaks, and finally application of a few drops of keratolytic daily.
- Hyperthermia - hot water immersion (113°F) 1/2-3/4 hour 2-3 times per week for 16 treatments is effective for some patients
- Other measures include use of a heel bar or appropriate padding to relieve pressure points where warts tend to aggregate

SURGICAL MEASURES
- Cryotherapy - application of liquid nitrogen is often effective. It usually requires at least 4 applications at weekly or biweekly intervals. Aggressive cryotherapy may cause blistering or even scarring, so light applications with two freeze-thaw cycles are preferred.
- Blunt dissection - a simple surgical procedure is effective and usually nonscarring. It requires inserting a blunt dissector between the wart and normal skin and separating the wart using short, firm stroke.
- CO2 laser surgery - used for recalcitrant warts

ACTIVITY Ambulatory unless warts or treatment is painful

DIET No special diet

PATIENT EDUCATION
- In Epstein: Common Skin Disorders, patient instructions, pages P-129 (see References)
- Griffith's Instructions for Patients, Philadelphia, Elsevier
- American Academy of Dermatology (708)330-0230

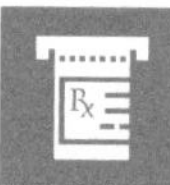

MEDICATIONS

DRUG(S) OF CHOICE
- No effective antiviral wart medications currently exist. Keratolytics (over-the-counter or prescription) and a variety of chemotherapeutic acids may be used.
- Salicylic acid - see General Measures for instructions
- 40% salicylic acid plasters - available as Mediplast. It is supplied in 3 by 4 inch sheets which are cut to the size of the wart and the sticky surface applied to the wart. They are removed every 1 to 2 days, the white keratin peeled and a fresh plaster applied.
- Chemotherapy, dichloroacetic acid and trichloroacetic acid kits are available. Callus is pared and the surrounding skin is protected by a ring of petrolatum. The wart(s) are coated with acid which is then worked into the wart with a sharp toothpick. Procedure should be repeated at weekly intervals.
- Transdermal salicylates (Trans-Plantar)
- Vesicants containing cantharidin (Cantharone, Verrusol) applied in the office, allowed to dry and then covered with occlusive tape for 24 hours

Contraindications: Infection, vascular insufficiency

Precautions:
- If the dermis is damaged with any of the above procedures, a scar may result which can be permanently painful
- Care should be taken to avoid excessive contact with normal skin when using keratolytics or chemotherapy
- Avoid bleomycin treatment during pregnancy
- Imiquimod has not been studied in patients under age 18

Significant possible interactions: N/A

ALTERNATIVE DRUGS
- Bleomycin injected intralesionally q 2 weeks
- Imiquimod (Aldara) 5% cream applied daily after soaking. It appears to be more effective when occluded and when in combination with other treatments such as cryotherapy or keratolytics.
- Alternative procedures include laser therapy (various)

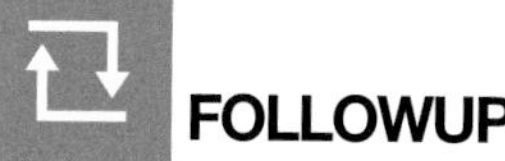

FOLLOWUP

PATIENT MONITORING With any treatment modality, followup weekly

PREVENTION/AVOIDANCE Use rubber footwear in communal shower areas

POSSIBLE COMPLICATIONS
- Scarring with overly aggressive treatment
- A rare type of verrucous carcinoma, epithelioma cuniculatum, is thought to arise from these warts

EXPECTED COURSE/PROGNOSIS
The course of plantar warts is like that of other varieties of warts, i.e., highly variable. Most resolve spontaneously in weeks to months.

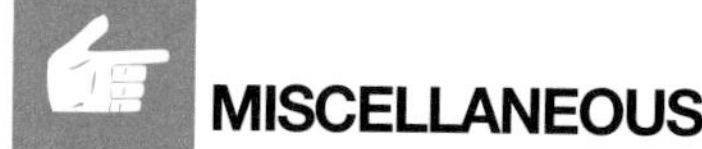

MISCELLANEOUS

ASSOCIATED CONDITIONS N/A

AGE-RELATED FACTORS
Pediatric: Duration of warts is generally shorter in children than in adults

Geriatric: N/A

Others: N/A

PREGNANCY
- Avoid bleomycin treatments

SYNONYMS Verruca plantaris

ICD-9-CM
078.19 Other specified viral warts

SEE ALSO
Condyloma acuminata
Warts

OTHER NOTES N/A

ABBREVIATIONS N/A

REFERENCES

- Epstein E. Common Skin Disorders. 5th ed. Philadelphia: WB Saunders Co; 2001
- Odom RB, James WD, Berger TG. Andrews' Diseases of the Skin. 9th ed. Philadelphia: WB Saunders; 2000
- Habif TP. Clinical Dermatology. 4th ed. New York: Mosby; 2004

Web references: 3 available at www.5mcc.com

Illustrations 2 available

Author(s):
Gary J. Silko, MD, MS

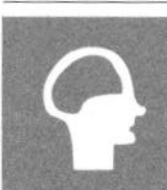

BASICS

DESCRIPTION A multisystem disease characterized by granulomatous vasculitis involving multiple organs. The characteristic "triad" of involvement includes the upper airway (otitis, sinusitis, nasal mucosa), lung, and kidney. Other organ systems involved include skin, joints, nervous system (peripheral or central).
- As the condition progresses untreated, upper airway erosions, necrotic pulmonary nodules, and renal failure are common, and, without treatment, mortality rate is high

System(s) affected: Cardiovascular, Gastrointestinal, Nervous, Pulmonary, Renal/Urologic, Skin/Exocrine

Genetics:
- Increased presence in HLA-B8
- Increased presence in HLA-DR2

Incidence/Prevalence in USA: Incidence estimated at approximately 0.4/100,000; prevalence 3/100,000

Predominant age: Mean age of onset in mid-40's, but has been described in all age groups

Predominant sex: Male > Female (3:2)

SIGNS & SYMPTOMS
- Pulmonary infiltrates (71%)
- Sinusitis (67%)
- Arthralgia/arthritis (44%)
- Fever (34%)
- Cough (34%)
- Otitis (25%)
- Rhinitis (22%)
- Hemoptysis (18%)
- Ocular inflammation (16%)
- Weight loss (16%)
- Skin rash (13%)
- Epistaxis (11%)
- Renal failure (11%)
- Chest pain, anorexia, proptosis, dyspnea, oral ulcers, hearing loss, headache (all < 10%)

CAUSES No known etiology. Autoimmune phenomena and immune complex deposition in arterial walls are implicated as pathogenetic factors. Triggering infectious agents, yet unidentified, may be involved.

RISK FACTORS None identified

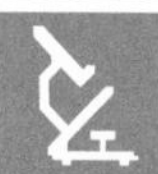

DIAGNOSIS

DIFFERENTIAL DIAGNOSIS
- Infectious otitis and sinusitis (bacterial or fungal)
- Midline granuloma or other upper airway malignancy
- Relapsing polychondritis
- Fungal or tuberculous pulmonary infections, (Goodpasture syndrome)
- Other vasculitic syndromes (including polyarteritis nodosa, lymphomatoid granulomatosis, Churg-Strauss vasculitis, and overlap vasculitis syndromes)
- Any disease associated with necrotizing and crescentic glomerulonephritis, sarcoidosis

LABORATORY
- Anemia, leukocytosis, and thrombocytosis common during active phases of disease
- Erythrocyte sedimentation rate (ESR) usually markedly elevated (75%)
- Rheumatoid factor present in low to moderate titer in up to 50%
- Hematuria and/or cellular casts with moderate range proteinuria
- Renal insufficiency, mild to moderate at first, but frequently progresses to end-stage renal disease

Drugs that may alter lab results: Corticosteroids and cytotoxic drugs, used to treat the disease, may cause normalization of most abnormal laboratory findings

Disorders that may alter lab results: See disorders listed under Differential Diagnosis

PATHOLOGICAL FINDINGS
- Upper airways: Granulomatous inflammation frequently seen, although not specific unless showing actual vasculitis
- Lung: Granulomatous arteritis involving vessels of all sizes, classically medium-sized arteries
- Kidney: Necrotizing and crescentic glomerulonephritis without immunofluorescent staining (pauci-immune) is common, granulomatous vasculitis rarely seen
- Skin: Vasculitic lesions, from leukocytoclastic vasculitis of small vessels; granulomatous arteritis seen occasionally

SPECIAL TESTS Antibodies to neutrophilic cytoplasmic antigens with a cytoplasmic pattern of staining (c-ANCA) are detected in a majority (60-90%) of patients. Such pattern of staining is highly specific (90+%) for this diagnosis. A similar finding, with perinuclear staining (p-ANCA), is nonspecific, but frequently seen in patients with other vasculitic syndromes or isolated necrotizing glomerulonephritis.

IMAGING
- Upper airways: Chronic otitis and sinusitis, often with evidence of erosion into bony structures - seen on plain x-rays
- CT scans of sinuses useful in demonstrating mucosal and bony involvement
- Lungs: X-rays show nodular pulmonary densities, often with central necrosis and cavitation. Local infiltrates, or more diffuse interstitial involvement also described, as are radiographic findings of pulmonary hemorrhage.

DIAGNOSTIC PROCEDURES
- Renal biopsy may give findings consistent with diagnosis, although not always definitive
- Sinus or upper airway mucosal biopsy often helpful, although findings are often nonspecific
- Open lung biopsy most likely to confirm granulomatous arteritis
- Diagnosis best made by demonstration of granulomatous arteritis of involved organ, although compatible renal lesion in setting of chronic destructive sinusitis and/or pulmonary nodules can be used to make a presumptive diagnosis
- A positive serologic test for c-ANCA in proper clinical setting felt to be diagnostic by many

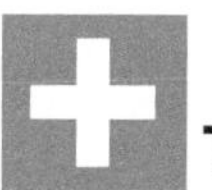

TREATMENT

APPROPRIATE HEALTH CARE
- Patients are usually ill enough with fever, sinus or pulmonary involvement, or renal disease to require hospitalization for diagnostic tests (to rule out infectious causes) and appropriate biopsies
- An occasional patient can be managed as an outpatient

GENERAL MEASURES Careful attention to upper airway drainage, and supportive measures for pulmonary, renal, or neurologic involvement

SURGICAL MEASURES N/A

ACTIVITY No specific restrictions. Fatigue, fever, and weight loss usually limit activity.

DIET Vigorous nutritional support may be needed early in illness

PATIENT EDUCATION
- Nutritional and drug counseling when patient is able to return home
- Wegener Granulomatosis Support Group, P.O. Box 28660, Kansas City, MO 64188

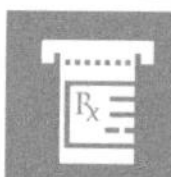

MEDICATIONS

DRUG(S) OF CHOICE
- Prednisone - given initially in high doses (60-100 mg/day). After initial 2-4 weeks may be tapered to alternate-day regimen. Then gradually discontinued over 2-6 months in most patients, depending on clinical course.
- Cyclophosphamide - in critically ill patient, may be given initially at a dose of 4 mg/kg/day IV for 2-3 days, then continued at 2 mg/kg/day orally. In stable patient, may be started at 2 mg/kg/day orally. Dosage may need to be adjusted, based on patient response and toxicity (usually bone marrow suppression). Usually continued for 1-2 years after patient felt to be in remission, and tapered slowly, with careful monitoring for reactivation of disease.
- Methotrexate 15-25 g/week orally - has been shown in a recent trial to be successful in maintaining remission in patients treated with cyclophosphamide

Contraindications: No absolute contraindications, although diabetes, hypertension, metabolic bone disease are relative contraindications to prednisone

Precautions:
- Careful monitoring if taking corticosteroids
- Consider reducing dose of cyclophosphamide in patient with baseline leukopenia, renal insufficiency

Significant possible interactions:
- Prednisone may interfere with hypoglycemics, antihypertensives
- Cyclophosphamide may increase risk of other drugs with potential for bone marrow toxicity

ALTERNATIVE DRUGS
- Azathioprine: in patients with history of severe bone marrow toxicity or hemorrhagic cystitis from cyclophosphamide
- Trimethoprim-sulfamethoxazole (TMP-SMX) has been used alone with success in some patients with limited (usually upper airway) disease, and has some potential as adjunctive therapy with prednisone and cyclophosphamide
- Methotrexate: in some patients without renal involvement and may be useful in maintaining remission in patients with stable disease, as an alternative to chronic cyclophosphamide therapy
- Etanercept currently being evaluated in clinical trials

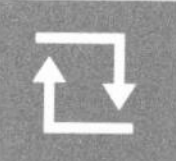

FOLLOWUP

PATIENT MONITORING
- Early, careful monitoring of upper airway, pulmonary, and renal manifestations for response to therapy
- Monitor blood pressure, glucose, potassium for steroid effects
- Frequent (every 2-4 weeks) CBC with differential to monitor for bone marrow toxicity from cyclophosphamide. Leukopenia most common. Dose needs to be reduced if peripheral WBC < 3000/ mm3.
- Monitor urinalysis for potential of hemorrhagic cystitis from cyclophosphamide. Consider cystoscopy for persistent or recurrent hematuria, especially later in course of treatment.

PREVENTION/AVOIDANCE
- Calorie and salt reduction in patients on prednisone
- High fluid intake to prevent hemorrhagic cystitis from cyclophosphamide
- Give cyclophosphamide dose in morning to decrease amount of drug present overnight in bladder.

POSSIBLE COMPLICATIONS
- Disease related
  - ◊ Destructive nasal lesions with "saddle nose" deformity
  - ◊ Deafness from refractory otitis
  - ◊ Necrotic pulmonary nodules with hemoptysis
  - ◊ Interstitial lung disease
  - ◊ Renal failure
  - ◊ Foot drop from peripheral nerve disease
  - ◊ Skin ulcers, digital and limb gangrene from peripheral vascular involvement
- Drug related
  - ◊ Prednisone - weight gain, hyperglycemia, hypertension, hypokalemia, skin thinning and bruising, infection, osteoporosis
  - ◊ Cyclophosphamide - bone marrow suppression (especially leukopenia, neutropenia), alopecia, hemorrhagic cystitis, mucosal membrane irritation, sterility and premature gonadal failure, secondary malignancies (especially leukemias) with long term therapy. Risk of bladder cancer is 5% (10 years) and 16% (15 years) after first treatment, and is related to previous cystitis.

EXPECTED COURSE/PROGNOSIS
- Without treatment, almost uniformly fatal with 10% 2 year survival and mean survival of 5 months
- With aggressive treatment, survival improved to 75-90% at 5 years
- Treatment-related toxicity is significant, especially from long-term cyclophosphamide. After 1-2 years of disease-free interval, cyclophosphamide is usually tapered, although some patients demonstrate disease re-activation during this phase.

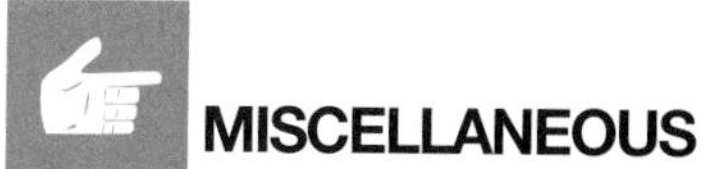

MISCELLANEOUS

ASSOCIATED CONDITIONS None

AGE-RELATED FACTORS
Pediatric: N/A
Geriatric: N/A
Others: N/A

PREGNANCY
- Rarely reported. Pregnancy should be considered only when patient is disease-free and off therapy.
- Cyclophosphamide often causes sterility and is potentially teratogenic

SYNONYMS N/A

ICD-9-CM
446.4 Wegener granulomatosis

SEE ALSO
Goodpasture syndrome, pulmonary component
Goodpasture syndrome, renal component
Polyarteritis nodosa

OTHER NOTES N/A

ABBREVIATIONS
c-ANCA = antibodies to neutrophilic cytoplasmic antigens with cytoplasmic staining pattern
p-ANCA = antibodies to neutrophilic cytoplasmic antigens with perinuclear staining pattern

REFERENCES

- Hoffman GS, et al: Wegener's granulomatosis: an analysis of 158 patients. Ann of Intern Med 1992;115:488-498
- Hoffman GS: Editorial-Treatment of Wegener's granulomatosis: time to change the standard of care? Arthritis Rheum 1997;40:2099-2104
- Langford CA, et al. A staged approach to the treatment of Wegener's granulomatosis. Induction of remission with glucocorticoids and daily cyclophosphamide switching to methotrexate for remission maintenance. Arthritis Rheum 1999;42:2666-73
- Nolle B, et al: Anticytoplasmic autoantibodies: Their immunodiagnostic value in Wegener's granulomatosis. Ann Intern Med 1989;111:28
- Lieberman KV, Churg A: Wegner's granulomatosis. In: Churg A, Churg J, eds. Systemic Vasculitides. New York, Igaku-Shoin, 1991
- Hoffman GS, Specks V: Review: Antineutrophilic cytoplasmic antibodies. Arthritis Rheum 1998; 41:1521-1537

Web references: 1 available at www.5mcc.com
Illustrations 1 available

Author(s):
Christopher M. Wise, MD

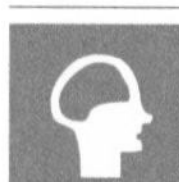

BASICS

DESCRIPTION Williams syndrome is an unusual multisystem neurodevelopmental disorder typified by characteristic craniofacial features, mild microcephaly, mild to moderate mental retardation with a distinctive cognitive-behavioral profile, connective tissue abnormalities, growth retardation, supravalvular aortic stenosis, peripheral pulmonary stenosis, renal artery stenosis, limited joint movement and transient hypercalcemia. Its occurrence is sporadic, although familial autosomal dominant cases have been infrequently reported.
System(s) affected: Cardiovascular, Endocrine/Metabolic, Musculoskeletal, Nervous, Renal/Urologic
Genetics: The pattern of occurrence is nearly always sporadic and observed in both sexes, although there are several reported cases of familial transmission as an autosomal dominant mutation. The phenotypic expression is somewhat varied and associated with a hemizygous microdeletion of ≈1.6 Mb in the 7q11.23 region which includes the elastin (ELN) and LIM-kinase (LIMK) gene.
Incidence/Prevalence in USA: Affected individuals have been estimated at 1:20,000 live births
Predominant age: Life-long condition
Predominant sex: Male=Females

SIGNS & SYMPTOMS

- The signs and symptoms observed in the classic case of WS may be diagnostic but the clinical presentation is somewhat varied
- Early childhood: Global developmental delay albeit with seemingly normal speech and expressive language
  - ◊ Hyperacusis
  - ◊ Characteristic craniofacial features
    - Elfin-like facial appearance
    - Medial eyebrow flare and stellate irises
    - Wide mouth
    - Long flat philtrum
    - Upturned nose with a flat nasal bridge
    - Dental anomalies
    - Mild microcephaly
  - ◊ Characteristic clinical features
    - Supravalvar aortic stenosis
    - Peripheral pulmonary stenosis
    - Renal artery stenosis
    - Infantile hypercalcemia
    - Growth retardation and short stature
    - Slender limbs and trunk
  - ◊ Characteristic cognitive/behavioral features
    - Weakness in abstract/visual reasoning
    - Highly developed expressive language skills
    - Low levels of daily living skills
    - Age-related decreases in IQ scores
- Postpubertal males and females
  - ◊ Characteristic clinical features
    - Hypertension
    - Lordosis and/or limited joint movement
  - ◊ Characteristic behavioral features
    - Anxiety
    - Depression and suicidal ideation

CAUSES Microdeletion in the 7q11.23 region produced by unequal crossing over

RISK FACTORS Possible familial transmission as an autosomal dominant mutation

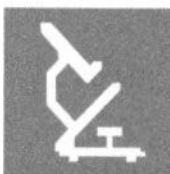

DIAGNOSIS

DIFFERENTIAL DIAGNOSIS Rule out uncomplicated hypercalcemia or supravalvular aortic stenosis

LABORATORY Molecular-genetic (DNA) evaluation is the diagnostic test of choice and can determine the size of the deletion

Drugs that may alter lab results: N/A

Disorders that may alter lab results: N/A

PATHOLOGICAL FINDINGS N/A

SPECIAL TESTS Affected individuals require cognitive, behavioral, psychological and educational evaluations to develop individual education programs

IMAGING N/A

DIAGNOSTIC PROCEDURES N/A

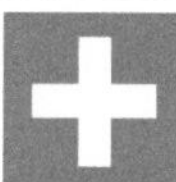

TREATMENT

APPROPRIATE HEALTH CARE Affected individuals will generally need life-long adult supervision. Early intensive educational intervention and behavior modification should be implemented.

GENERAL MEASURES

- Early detection will permit early intervention and intensive behavioral training
- Treatment for hypercalcemia by controlling dietary intake of calcium and vitamin D
- Ophthalmological evaluations are recommended for problems associated with visual acuity
- Preventive dentistry to reduce risk of malocclusion
- Continual monitoring of cardiovascular anomalies and for hypertension
- Filtered ear protection for hyperacusis

SURGICAL MEASURES Treatment for aortic, pulmonary or renal artery stenoses if needed

ACTIVITY Full activity unless cardiovascular stenoses are problematic

DIET For hypercalcemia, control intake of calcium and vitamin D

PATIENT EDUCATION

- The patient and family should receive genetic evaluation and counseling
- Patient and family should contact the Williams Syndrome Association, Box 297, Clawson, MI 48017, (800) 806-1871; website: www.williams-syndrome.org

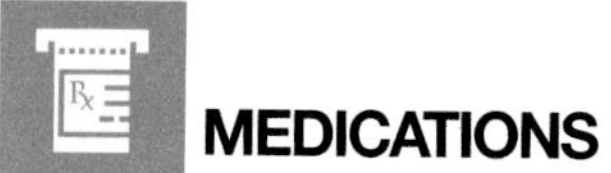

MEDICATIONS

DRUG(S) OF CHOICE Medication for hypertension and for hyperparathyroidism
Contraindications: N/A
Precautions: N/A
Significant possible interactions: N/A

ALTERNATIVE DRUGS N/A

FOLLOWUP

PATIENT MONITORING Regular pediatric care and general health maintenance with particular attention to endocrine, renal and cardiovascular function

PREVENTION/AVOIDANCE Genetic counseling and evaluation, especially among high-functioning patients, about pregnancies. Prenatal diagnosis is available.

POSSIBLE COMPLICATIONS
- Learning problems, especially in abstract/visual reasoning
- Behavioral problems concerning indifference to personal safety
- Post-pubescent anxiety and depression
- Risk of cardiovascular disease and/or renal dysfunction

EXPECTED COURSE/PROGNOSIS
- Individuals may need life-long supervision
- Life span may be affected by renal dysfunction; or, hypertension resulting from supravalvar stenosis and/or peripheral pulmonary stenosis

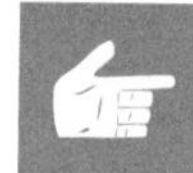

MISCELLANEOUS

ASSOCIATED CONDITIONS
- Developmental delay
- Growth retardation
- Cardiovascular dysfunction
- Renal dysfunction
- Attention deficit disorder (ADD)
  - ◊ Frequently associated with neuropsychological dysfunction
  - ◊ Treatment for ADD is similar to methods used in the general population

AGE-RELATED FACTORS
Pediatric: Infantile hypercalcemia
Geriatric: N/A
Others: N/A

PREGNANCY Patient and family should receive genetic evaluation and counseling as prenatal diagnosis is available

SYNONYMS
- Williams-Beuren syndrome
- Fanconi type idiopathic infantile hypercalcemia
- Elfin facies syndrome

ICD-9-CM
758.9 Conditions due to anomaly of unspecified chromosome

SEE ALSO
Attention deficit/Hyperactivity disorder
Down syndrome
Fragile X syndrome
Hyperparathyroidism
Hypertension, essential
Mental retardation

OTHER NOTES N/A

ABBREVIATIONS
ADD = attention deficit disorder

REFERENCES
- Anderson PE, Rourke BP. Williams Syndrome. In: White BP, editor. Syndrome of Nonverbal Learning Disabilities. New York: Guilford Press; 1995
- Bayes M, Perez-Juardo LA. Williams-Beuren Syndrome. In: Fisch GS, editor. Genetics and Genomics of Neurobehavioral Disorders. Totowa, NJ: Humana Press; 2003

Web references: 1 available at www.5mcc.com
Illustrations N/A

Author(s):
Gene S. Fisch, PhD

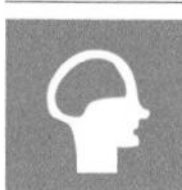

BASICS

DESCRIPTION An embryonal renal neoplasm containing blastema, stromal or epithelial cell types usually affecting children before the 5th year.x
System(s) affected: Renal/urologic
Genetics: Several congenital anomalies are known to be associated with Wilms tumor. A two stage mutational model has been proposed: occurrence in either hereditary form or sporadic form. Patients with aniridia have a deletion of the short arm of chromosome 11 (11p13).
Incidence/Prevalence in USA:
- 0.69/100,000 people in the U.S. 8 cases/million children under 15 year of age.
- Most common renal malignancy in childhood

Predominant age: Median age of 36.5 months
Predominant sex: Female > Male (1.1 : 1)

SIGNS & SYMPTOMS
- Usually asymptomatic
- Palpable upper abdominal mass
- Abdominal pain
- Fever
- Anemia
- Rarely, signs of acute abdomen with free intraperitoneal rupture
- Cardiac murmur
- Hepatosplenomegaly
- Ascites
- Prominent abdominal wall veins
- Varicocele
- Gonadal metastases

CAUSES
- Hereditary or sporadic forms of genetic mutation
- Familial form: autosomal dominant trait with incomplete penetrance (1%)
- Potential of paternal occupational exposure (machinists, welders, motor vehicle mechanics, auto body repairmen)

RISK FACTORS
- Aniridia (600 times greater than normal risk)
- Hemihypertrophy (100 times greater than normal risk)
- Cryptorchidism
- Hypospadias
- Duplicated renal collecting systems
- Wiedemann-Beckwith syndrome
- Drash syndrome
- Klippel-Trenaunay syndrome
- Familial occurrence
- Paternal occupation (see Causes)

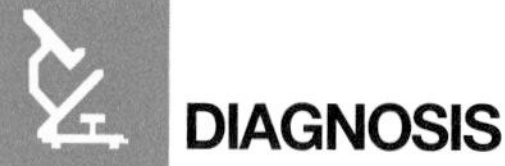

DIAGNOSIS

DIFFERENTIAL DIAGNOSIS
- Neuroblastoma
- Hepatic tumors
- Sarcoma
- Rhabdoid tumors

LABORATORY
- Urinalysis (occasional hematuria)
- CBC (anemia)
- LDH
- Plasma renin (rarely helpful)
- Urine catecholamines

Drugs that may alter lab results: N/A

Disorders that may alter lab results: N/A

PATHOLOGICAL FINDINGS
- Favorable findings (mortality of 7%)
  - ◊ Bulky lesion, well-encapsulated
  - ◊ Focal areas of hemorrhage and necrosis
  - ◊ Absence of anaplasia and sarcomatous cell types
  - ◊ Presence of blastema, stomal and epithelial elements
- Unfavorable histology (mortality rate of 57%)
  - ◊ Anaplasia - markedly enlarged and multipolar mitotic figures 3-fold enlargement of nuclei in comparison with adjacent similar nuclei, hyperchromasia of enlarge nuclei. Anaplasia may be diffuse or focal.
  - ◊ Sarcomatous changes - are now considered to be separate from Wilms, not subtypes. (Mortality of 64%)
- Nephroblastomatosis
  - ◊ Considered premalignant

SPECIAL TESTS N/A

IMAGING
- Chest x-ray
- KUB (presence of linear calcifications)
- Abdominal ultrasound - gives best information about tumor extension into IVC
- CT (with IV and oral contrast) of chest and abdomen
- IVP rarely helpful

DIAGNOSTIC PROCEDURES Occasionally bone marrow aspiration necessary to distinguish from neuroblastoma

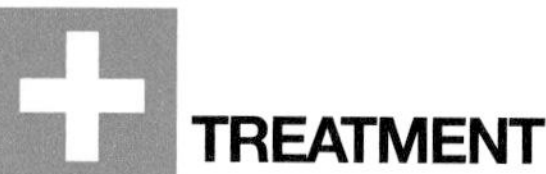

TREATMENT

APPROPRIATE HEALTH CARE
- In-patient work-up and treatment until stable postoperative and induction chemotherapy completed

GENERAL MEASURES
- Chemotherapy
- Radiation therapy in Stage II, unfavorable histology, Stage II and Stage IV

SURGICAL MEASURES
- Examination (visual and manual) of contralateral kidney
- Radical nephroureterectomy and biopsies as needed to provide precise staging information
- Sampling of any enlarged lymph nodes
- Identification of any retained tumor with titanium clips.
- Tumor should be given to pathologist fresh, not in formalin
- Vertical midline incision if tumor extension to right atrium present (possible use of cardiopulmonary bypass)
- With bilateral Wilms tumors, biopsy, then chemotherapy and 2nd look operation 6 weeks to 6 month later for partial bilateral nephrectomy if possible

ACTIVITY As tolerated

DIET No special diet

PATIENT EDUCATION
- Patient and family teaching regarding long-term outlook
- Possibility of second malignancy
- Side effects of chemotherapy, radiation therapy

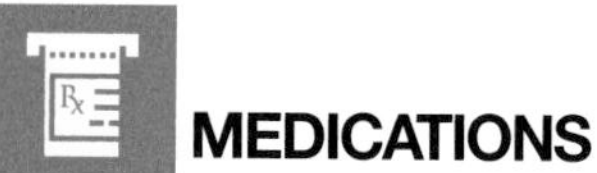

MEDICATIONS

DRUG(S) OF CHOICE
- Dactinomycin (actinomycin-D)
- Vincristine
- Doxorubicin
- Cyclophosphamide (Cytoxan)

Contraindications: Refer to manufacturer's literature
Precautions: Refer to manufacturer's literature
Significant possible interactions: Refer to manufacturer's literature

ALTERNATIVE DRUGS
- Doxorubicin (Adriamycin)
- Cyclophosphamide

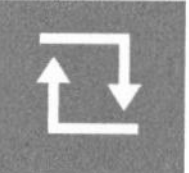

FOLLOWUP

PATIENT MONITORING
- Multidrug chemotherapy every 3-4 weeks for 16 weeks - 15 months depending on stage
- Every 4 months for 1 year, every 6 months for 2nd - 3rd year, yearly after that
- CBC, CT chest and abdomen with each visit

PREVENTION/AVOIDANCE N/A

POSSIBLE COMPLICATIONS
- 1-2% will develop second malignant neoplasms (leukemia, lymphoma, hepatocellular carcinoma, soft tissue sarcoma)
- High risk of low birth weight infants, perinatal mortality in offspring of female survivors of Wilms tumor
- Chest is usual site of recurrence
- Occurrence of second malignant neoplasms in 2% of patients 7-34 years after treatment

EXPECTED COURSE/PROGNOSIS
- With favorable histology, 91% survival
- With diffuse anaplasia, 20% survival
- With focal anaplasia, 64% survival
- With rhabdoid features, 19% 3 year survival
- Staging
  - ◊ I - tumor limited to kidney, completely excised
  - ◊ II - Tumor extends beyond kidney, completely excised
  - ◊ III - Residual non-hematogenous tumor confined to abdomen (lymph nodes positive, spillage of tumor, peritoneal implants, extension beyond resection region)
  - ◊ IV - Hematogenous metastases
  - ◊ V - Bilateral renal involvement

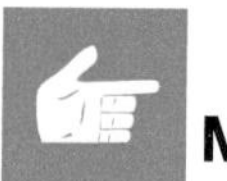

MISCELLANEOUS

ASSOCIATED CONDITIONS See risk factors

AGE-RELATED FACTORS Occurs only in children
Pediatric: N/A
Geriatric: N/A
Others: N/A

PREGNANCY N/A

SYNONYMS
- Nephroblastoma

ICD-9-CM
189.0 Malignant neoplasm of kidney, except pelvis

SEE ALSO

OTHER NOTES
- Mesoblastic nephroma - distinguished only by histology. Age usually under 6 months. Essentially benign although metastases have been reported; tends to be locally invasive. Operative spillage may lead to recurrence. No chemotherapy or radiotherapy needed with complete excision.
- Nephroblastomatosis - considered premalignant; may present as nodularity of one or both kidneys; treated with biopsy and local excision (renal tissue sparing)

ABBREVIATIONS N/A

REFERENCES

- Ashcraft KW, Murphy JP, Sharp RJ, eds. Pediatric Surgery. 3rd Ed. Philadelphia, W.B. Saunders Co., 2000
- Shochat SJ: Wilms' Tumor: Diagnosis and Treatment in the 1990's. Seminars in Pediatric Surgery 1993;2(1):59-68
- O'Neill JA, Rowe MI, Grosfeld JL, et al: Pediatric Surgery. 5th ed., St Louis, Mosby, 1998

Web references: 2 available at www.5mcc.com
Illustrations N/A

Author(s):
Timothy L. Black, MD

BASICS

DESCRIPTION Males affected by this rare x-linked genetic disorder display combined immunodeficiency, microcytic thrombocytosis and eczema leading to life threatening infections and bleeding complications. Average life span is 11 years. The syndrome has variable expression. XLT is a related but milder form with mostly platelet defects.

System(s) affected: Hemic/Lymphatic/Immunologic, Skin/Exocrine

Genetics:
- Family history in >60%
- X-Linked recessive trait
- WASP and XLT genes located at X/11.22
  - ◊ Codes for cytoplasmic protein that signals cell membrane structure changes required for activation of blood cells

Incidence/Prevalence in USA: 1 in 4 million live male births

Predominant age: Onset at birth, most diagnosed by 24 months

Predominant sex: Male > Female
- Rarely females develop WAS
  - ◊ Some carriers express disease
  - ◊ Other have different but related gene defect

SIGNS & SYMPTOMS
- Neonatal:
  - ◊ Excessive bleeding from circumcision
  - ◊ Bloody diarrhea
  - ◊ Petechiae and purpura
- Childhood:
  - ◊ Eczema with secondary skin infections
  - ◊ Recurrent bacterial infections
  - ◊ Viral infections
  - ◊ Hepatosplenomegaly
  - ◊ Autoimmune vasculitis and hemolytic anemia

CAUSES
- Hematopoietic cells express WASP
  - ◊ Defective WASP fails to organize membrane activation
  - ◊ Membranes don't form normal actin cytoskeletons
  - ◊ Altered motility and inability to change cell shapes inhibits normal functions
- Platelets are intrinsically abnormal
  - ◊ Accelerated destruction, sequestered in spleen
- T cells show decreased responsiveness to antigens
- B cells show abnormal antibody production

RISK FACTORS
- Family history of WAS
- History of congenital defects

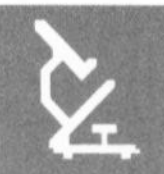

DIAGNOSIS

DIFFERENTIAL DIAGNOSIS May be difficult in infancy before immune changes present
- ITP other causes of TCP
- Severe Atopic Disease
- Acute lymphoblastic anemia
- Other causes of immunodeficiency
  - ◊ SCID, HIV
- Leukemias or marrow aplasias

LABORATORY
- Platelets abnormal at birth
  - ◊ <30,000, MPV 2/3 normal
- B cell and T cell changes over time
  - ◊ WBC count fall by age 6
  - ◊ Low IgM, Normal IgG, High IgA and IgE
  - ◊ Decreased response to capsular antigens
  - ◊ Low CD 8 counts in 61%
  - ◊ Decreased delayed hypersensitivity responses
  - ◊ Decreased mitogenic responses

Drugs that may alter lab results: Antibiotics

Disorders that may alter lab results: Infections

PATHOLOGICAL FINDINGS
- Hyperplasia of lymphoreticular system
- Vasculitic changes with multiple thromboses of small arterioles of kidney, lung, pancreas, brain

SPECIAL TESTS
- Genetic testing for WASP
- Carrier identification

IMAGING Not helpful

DIAGNOSTIC PROCEDURES
- Bone marrow aspiration to exclude leukemia and aplastic conditions and to HLA type for bone marrow transplantation
- Gene mapping of mutation in affected or female carriers
- Chorionic villus sampling for in utero diagnosis

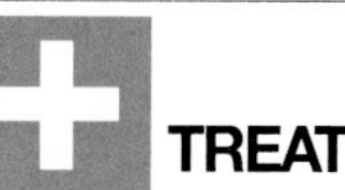

TREATMENT

APPROPRIATE HEALTH CARE
- Inpatient for acute infections
- No live virus vaccination

GENERAL MEASURES
- HLA typed bone marrow or umbilical cord blood stem cell transplant restores all abnormalities with an 85% cure rate
- Crossmatched platelets
- Irradiated, CMV negative blood products
- Aggressive antibiotic therapy for infections
- Prophylactic antibiotics

SURGICAL MEASURES Splenectomy can transiently improve TCP but increases the risk of infection

ACTIVITY
- Plan activities to help normal development
- Avoid contact sports and prevent head injuries
- Avoid crowds

DIET No special diet

PATIENT EDUCATION
- Patient/parent counseling to cope with disease and outcome
- Genetic testing and counseling for family

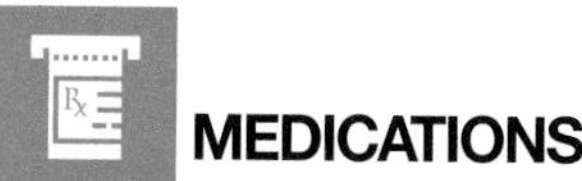

MEDICATIONS

DRUG(S) OF CHOICE
- Immunoglobulin infusions
- Prophylactic penicillin after splenectomy
- Antibiotics as indicated by culture
- Topical steroids for eczema
- Parenteral steroids, vincristine or plasmapheresis for autoimmune complications
- Interleukin-2 can increase platelet counts while waiting stem cell transplantation

Contraindications: Refer to manufacturer's literature

Precautions: Corticosteroids in immunosuppressed patients. Refer to manufacturer's literature

Significant possible interactions: Refer to manufacturer's literature

ALTERNATIVE DRUGS N/A

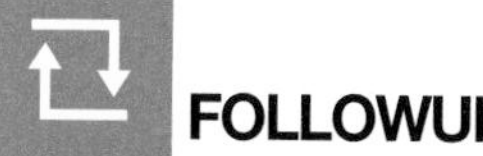

FOLLOWUP

PATIENT MONITORING
As needed for therapy, monitor for infections, for progression of disease, complications

PREVENTION/AVOIDANCE
- Genetics counseling
  - ◊ Identify carriers
  - ◊ Prenatal diagnosis

POSSIBLE COMPLICATIONS
- Severe infections especially after splenectomy
- Hemorrhage, cerebral common
- Malignancies (lymphoreticular, leukemia, Kaposi)
- Nephropathy
- Autoimmune disease in 40% can be aggressive
- Malabsorption syndrome

EXPECTED COURSE/PROGNOSIS
- Usual course is acute and chronic infections with progressive decrease in immune status.
- Average life expectancy is 11 years with more living past twenty with bone marrow transplant. Transplant therapy can restore all abnormalities. Causes of death have been infection (50%), bleeding (27%), malignancies (12%).

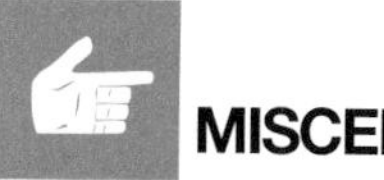

MISCELLANEOUS

ASSOCIATED CONDITIONS
- Lymphomas, brain is primary site in 50%, nephropathy, other lymphoreticular tumors

AGE-RELATED FACTORS
Pediatric:
- Onset at birth
- First year infections with encapsulated bacteria: respiratory, meningitis, sepsis
- Later infections occur with opportunistic organisms and virus

Geriatric: None have survived this long

Others: N/A

PREGNANCY N/A

SYNONYMS
- Aldrich syndrome
- Immunodeficiency-2

ICD-9-CM
279.12 Wiskott-Aldrich syndrome

SEE ALSO
Idiopathic thrombocytopenic purpura (ITP)
Immunodeficiency diseases
Leukemia

OTHER NOTES N/A

ABBREVIATIONS
WAS = Wiskott-Aldrich syndrome
XLT = x-linked thrombocytopenia
WASP = Wiskott-Aldrich syndrome protein
TCP = thrombocytopenia
SCID = severe combined Immunodeficiency

REFERENCES

- Klein C, Nguyen D, Liu CH, et al. Gene therapy for Wiskott-Aldrich syndrome: rescue of T-cell signaling and amelioration of colitis upon transplantation of retrovirally transduced hematopoietic stem cells in mice. Blood 2003;101(6):2159-66
- Ming JE. Syndromic immunodeficiencies with humoral defects. Immunol Allergy Clin North Am 2001;21(1):91-111
- Elder ME. T-cell immunodeficiencies. Pediatr Clin North Am 2000;47(6):1253-74
- Ochs HD. The Wiskott-Aldrich syndrome. Isr Med Assoc J 2002;4(5):379-84
- Braithwaite K, Abu-Ghosh A, Anderson L, Cairo MS. Treatment of severe thrombocytopenia with IL-11 in children with Wiskott-Aldrich syndrome. J Pediatr Hematol Oncol 2002;24(4):323-6
- Nonoyama S, Ochs HD. Wiskott-Aldrich syndrome. Curr Allergy Asthma Rep 2001;1(5):430-7

Web references: 1 available at www.5mcc.com

Illustrations N/A

Author(s):
Patricia Borman, MD

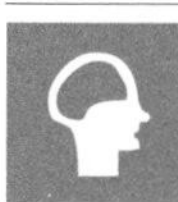

BASICS

DESCRIPTION Constellation of growth retardation, hypogonadism, cell mediated immune dysfunction, and skin changes related to decreased zinc
System(s) affected: Endocrine/Metabolic, Nervous, Skin/Exocrine
Genetics: Usually acquired, but rarely acrodermatitis enteropathica (autosomal recessive) and associated with sickle cell anemia (autosomal recessive)
Incidence/Prevalence in USA: Unknown
Predominant age: All ages, most often adolescent
Predominant sex: Male = Female

SIGNS & SYMPTOMS
- Mild deficiency
  - ◊ Hypogeusia
  - ◊ Decreased dark adaptation
  - ◊ Decreased lean body mass
- Moderate deficiency
  - ◊ All of the above
  - ◊ Diarrhea
  - ◊ Growth retardation
  - ◊ Hypogonadism (especially male)
  - ◊ Mental lethargy
  - ◊ Anergy
  - ◊ Rough skin
  - ◊ Delayed wound healing
  - ◊ Glucose intolerance
  - ◊ Impaired cell mediated immunity
- Severe deficiency
  - ◊ All of the above
  - ◊ Bullous pustular dermatitis
  - ◊ Weight loss
  - ◊ Dwarfism
  - ◊ Emotional instability
  - ◊ Tremors
  - ◊ Ataxia
  - ◊ Alopecia
  - ◊ Death

CAUSES
- Increased requirements
  - ◊ Pregnancy
  - ◊ Lactation
  - ◊ Rapid growth phase of childhood
  - ◊ Burns
  - ◊ Major trauma
- Increased losses
  - ◊ Diabetes
  - ◊ Cirrhosis
  - ◊ Renal disease
  - ◊ Malabsorption states, e.g., inflammatory bowel diseases
  - ◊ Sickle cell anemia
- Decreased absorption
  - ◊ Acrodermatitis enteropathica, an autosomal recessive deficiency in the enzyme required for intestinal absorption
  - ◊ Geophagia
  - ◊ Chelating agents
  - ◊ Parasitism
  - ◊ Diet high in phytates
- Insufficient dietary intake
  - ◊ Vegetarianism
  - ◊ Parenteral hyperalimentation without supplementation
  - ◊ Breast feeding
  - ◊ Suboptimal zinc conditions in diet (rare)
  - ◊ Alcoholism

RISK FACTORS
- High milk consumption
- Low socioeconomic status

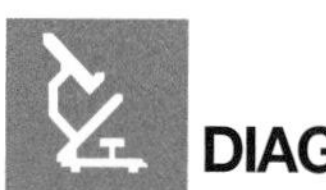

DIAGNOSIS

DIFFERENTIAL DIAGNOSIS
- Congenital dwarfism
- Failure to thrive in infants
- Primary hypogonadism
- Mental retardation

LABORATORY
- Plasma zinc levels decreased (in moderate to severe zinc deficiency)
- Erythrocyte or leukocyte zinc levels more adequately assess tissue stores, but these are more costly and not widely available
- Hair or fingernail zinc levels not useful

Drugs that may alter lab results: N/A

Disorders that may alter lab results: N/A

PATHOLOGICAL FINDINGS N/A

SPECIAL TESTS N/A

IMAGING N/A

DIAGNOSTIC PROCEDURES N/A

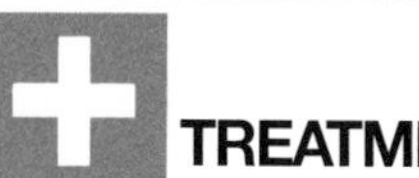

TREATMENT

APPROPRIATE HEALTH CARE Outpatient

GENERAL MEASURES N/A

SURGICAL MEASURES N/A

ACTIVITY Full activity

DIET
- Balanced omnivorous diet
- Avoid excessive intake of foods with high phytate content, (e.g., cereals)

PATIENT EDUCATION Dietary consultation

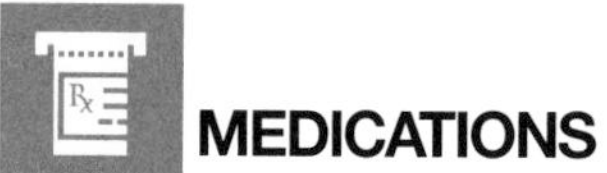

MEDICATIONS

DRUG(S) OF CHOICE
- Zinc gluconate or zinc sulfate 25-50 mg po qd for 6-9 months
- 4-6 mg of elemental zinc qd added to hyperalimentation in adult patient, may increase to 12 mg qd if suspect ongoing heavy zinc losses, e.g., burns or major trauma
- In pediatric patients, 0.02-0.04 mg zinc/kg/day in hyperalimentation
- Prenatal vitamins with minerals during pregnancy and lactation to prevent deficiency

Contraindications: None
Precautions: Avoid large (> 20 mg elemental zinc) parenteral doses
Significant possible interactions: N/A

ALTERNATIVE DRUGS N/A

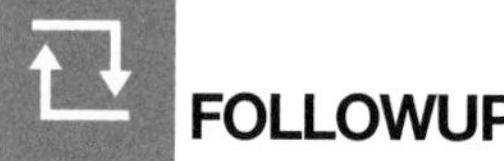

FOLLOWUP

PATIENT MONITORING Clinical status such as improved outlook, weight gain, resolution of symptoms

PREVENTION/AVOIDANCE
- Adequate diet
- Supplementation when indicated (see Medications)

POSSIBLE COMPLICATIONS N/A

EXPECTED COURSE/PROGNOSIS Immediate improvement in clinical status. Full resolution of signs and symptoms.

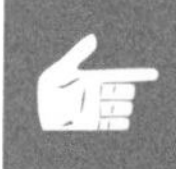

MISCELLANEOUS

ASSOCIATED CONDITIONS
- Sickle cell anemia
- Pregnancy and lactation
- Alcoholism
- Malabsorption
- Parenteral hyperalimentation
- In the older patient, diabetes, cirrhosis, those taking diuretics

AGE-RELATED FACTORS
Pediatric: Zinc deficiency may cause failure to thrive, impair growth and development of secondary sexual characteristics
Geriatric:
- Zinc deficiency may cause poor night vision leading to falls; poor wound healing or chronic skin ulcer; loss of taste which may cause worsening nutrition
- Elderly persons living in institutions may have low zinc intake

Others: N/A

PREGNANCY Requirements increase; deficiency may cause spontaneous abortion, inadequate weight gain

SYNONYMS N/A

ICD-9-CM
269.3 Mineral deficiency, NEC
686.8 Other specific local infections of skin & subcutaneous tissue

SEE ALSO
Acrodermatitis enteropathica
Alcohol use disorders
Anemia, sickle cell
Failure to thrive (FTT)

OTHER NOTES N/A

ABBREVIATIONS N/A

REFERENCES

- Tasman-Jones C: Disturbances of trace mineral metabolism. In: Wyngaarden JB, et al, eds. Cecil Textbook of Medicine. 19th Ed. Philadelphia, W.B. Saunders Co., 1992
- Ronaghy H: World Review Nutr. Diet 1987:54

Web references: 1 available at www.5mcc.com
Illustrations 3 available

Author(s):
Clyde L. Harris, MD

Zollinger-Ellison syndrome

BASICS

DESCRIPTION
- A triad of
  - ◊ Markedly elevated gastric acid secretion
  - ◊ Peptic ulcer disease
  - ◊ A gastrinoma or non-beta islet cell tumor of the pancreas or duodenal wall which produces gastrin
- Gastrinomas (at time of diagnosis) may be single or multiple (1/2-2/3), large or small, benign or malignant (2/3), sporadic (70-75%) or associated with multiple endocrine neoplasia (MEN 1)(25-30%)

System(s) affected: Endocrine/Metabolic, Gastrointestinal

Genetics: 25-30% occur in association with the MEN 1 syndrome

Incidence/Prevalence in USA: 1 per million per year

Predominant age: Middle age (30-65)

Predominant sex: Male > Female (3:2)

SIGNS & SYMPTOMS
- Abdominal pain >80%
- Epigastric pain
- Reflux esophagitis
- Vomiting unresponsive to standard therapy
- Diarrhea including while fasting 40-70%
- Peptic ulcer disease
- Weight loss
- Hepatomegaly with metastasis
- Steatorrhea
- Endoscopic findings including esophagitis, duodenal ulceration with multiple ulcers and prominent gastric and duodenal folds
- Complications of severe peptic ulcer disease including hemorrhage, perforation and obstruction
- Signs of MEN 1 including those of hypercalcemia hyperparathyroidism and Cushing syndrome.

CAUSES Gastrinoma equally distributed between the head of the pancreas and the first or second portion of the duodenum. May also be found rarely in the mesentery, peritoneum, spleen, skin or mediastinum (possibly metastasis with primary not identified).

RISK FACTORS
- MEN 1
- Family history of ulcer disease

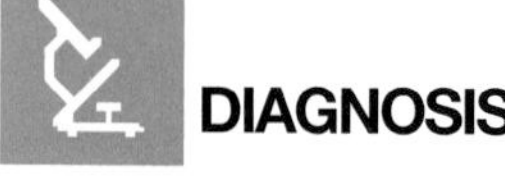

DIAGNOSIS

DIFFERENTIAL DIAGNOSIS
- Elevated serum gastrin with hypochlorhydria/achlorhydria
  - ◊ Atrophic gastritis
  - ◊ Drug induced
  - ◊ Gastric cancer
  - ◊ Pernicious anemia
  - ◊ Postvagotomy
- Elevated serum gastrin with normal or increased gastric acid
  - ◊ Antral G-cell hyperfunction
  - ◊ Chronic renal failure
  - ◊ H. pylori infection
  - ◊ Gastric outlet obstruction
  - ◊ Retained gastric antrum
- Consider gastrinoma in all patients with:
  - ◊ Recurrent or refractory ulcer disease
  - ◊ Gastric hypertrophy and ulcers
  - ◊ Duodenal and jejunal ulcers
  - ◊ Ulcers and diarrhea
  - ◊ Ulcers and kidney stones
  - ◊ Hypercalcemia and ulcers
  - ◊ Pituitary disease
  - ◊ Family history of ulcer disease or endocrine tumors suggestive of MEN 1

LABORATORY
- Elevated serum gastrin-fasting (>1000 pg/mL with ulcers diagnostic, >200 pg/mL with ulcers suggestive)
- Elevated basal gastric acid output >15 mEq/hr (>15 mmol/hr)
- Elevated serum pepsinogen-I levels
- Gastric pH <2.0 with elevated gastrin
- Check serum calcium, phosphorous, cortisol and prolactin (to R/O MEN 1)

Drugs that may alter lab results: H2 blockers and proton pump inhibitors may increase gastric pH

Disorders that may alter lab results: N/A

PATHOLOGICAL FINDINGS
- 90% of gastrinomas found in gastric triangle (borders are bile duct, junction of 2nd and 3rd portion of duodenum, junction of head and body of pancreas)
- Almost 50% in head of pancreas
- Almost 50% in wall of 1st or 2nd portion of duodenum (more likely to be small, solitary)
- 2/3 malignant in both sites (defined by behavior not histology)
- 50% of gastrinomas stain positive for ACTH, VIP, insulin or neurotensin (in decreasing order of incidence)
- 1/3 of patients have metastasis on presentation with regional nodes > liver > bone. More rarely seen metastasis to peritoneum, spleen, skin and mediastinum.
- Duodenal, jejunal and gastric ulcers which are often multiple
- Gastric and duodenal mucosal fold thickening
- Hyperplasia of antral gastrin producing cells
- Histology similar in appearance to carcinoid

SPECIAL TESTS
- Preferred test is secretion stimulation test- gastrin level increases > 200 pg/mL (>200 ng/L)
- Gastric secretory studies - basal acid output
- Alternative test is calcium infusion test-gastrin level increases > 400 pg/mL (test less specific and is more dangerous because of IV calcium infusion)

IMAGING
- Used to localize tumor for possible resection
- Abdominal CT scan (finds 30-38% of primary tumors and 42-70% of liver metastases)
- Abdominal ultrasound (finds 20% of primary tumors and 46% of liver metastases)
- Abdominal angiography (finds 40-50% of primaries)
- Endoscopic ultrasound (finds 41-58% of primary tumors). When combined with somatostatin receptor scintigraphy finds 69-86% of primary tumors.
- Abdominal MRI (finds 30-45% of primaries and 70-90% of liver metastases)
- Somatostatin receptor scintigraphy (finds 70% of primaries and 92% of liver metastases)
- Somatostatin receptor scintigraphy is most sensitive, combining with CT or MRI and angiography will find around 75% of primaries
- Sella turcica imaging can help if MEN 1 suspected to look for pituitary tumors

DIAGNOSTIC PROCEDURES
Endoscopy may see tumors in duodenal wall, multiple ulcers including jejunal ulcers and prominent gastric and duodenal folds.

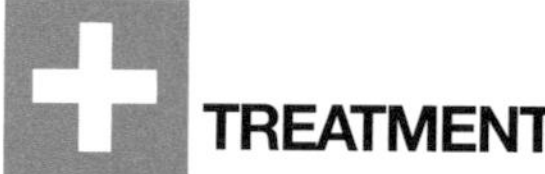

TREATMENT

APPROPRIATE HEALTH CARE
- Advise daily care based on symptoms
- Appropriate surveillance of basal gastric acid output to monitor anti-acid secretory therapy
- Appropriate surveillance postoperatively to look for metastasis

GENERAL MEASURES
- Advanced imaging initially to assess for possible resection
- Surgical removal when primary can be identified and as an adjunct for symptom control
- Medical treatment for symptom control when primary not found or metastasis present on diagnosis

SURGICAL MEASURES
- Laparotomy to search for resectable tumors (especially in the pancreas and duodenal wall) unless have liver metastasis on presentation or MEN 1
- Definitive therapy-removal of gastrinomas when found (surgery finds 95% of tumors, 5 year cure 40% when all can be removed)
- Total gastrectomy was formerly used to stop acid production before pharmacologic therapy available, now seldom done
- Vagotomy in some patients will reduce acid secretion and improve therapeutic effect of medication. May allow decrease dose of medication.
- In MEN 1 parathyroidectomy by lowering calcium may decrease acid production and decrease antisecretory drug use. Gastrinomas generally benign but multiple and not usually cured by surgery.

ACTIVITY As tolerated

DIET Restrict foods which aggravate symptoms

PATIENT EDUCATION Inform as to nature of disease and prognosis

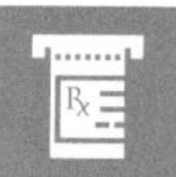

MEDICATIONS

DRUG(S) OF CHOICE
- General guidelines
  - ◊ Heal 80-85% of ulcers
  - ◊ While medications heal ulcers, they nearly always recur. While doses may be adjusted, need to plan on life long medication use.
  - ◊ Dosages frequently exceed usual doses for treatment of ulcers by 4-8 fold. Start at lower recommended dose below and titrate up to resolution of symptoms or maximum listed below.
  - ◊ If hyperparathyroidism present because of MEN 1, must correct hypercalcemia.
  - ◊ Proton pump inhibitors (PPI) first line treatment. May need to add H2 blockers.
- Proton pump inhibitors (PPI)
  - ◊ Omeprazole 60-120 mg/d
  - ◊ Lansoprazole 60-180 mg/d (doses>120 mg need to be divided bid)
  - ◊ Rabeprazole 60-100 mg/qd up to 60 mg bid
  - ◊ Pantoprazole po 40-240 mg/d; IV 80-120 mg/q12h
- H2 blockers
  - ◊ Cimetidine 300 mg q6h, up to 1.25-5.0 gm/day
  - ◊ Ranitidine 150 mg q 12 hrs, up to 6 gm/day
  - ◊ Famotidine 20 mg at bedtime up to 800 mg/day

Contraindications:
- Known hypersensitivity to the drug
- H2-blockers-androgen effects, drug interactions due to Cytochrome P-450 stimulation
- Omeprazole-none
- Lansoprazole-none

Precautions:
- Adjust doses for renal and geriatric patients depending on drug
- Gynecomastia reported with high dose cimetidine (>2.4 gm/d)
- Proton pump inhibitors may induce a profound and long lasting effect on gastric acid secretion, thereby affecting the bioavailability of drugs dependent on low gastric pH (eg, ketoconazole, ampicillin, iron)

Significant possible interactions: Refer to the drug manufacturer's literature.

ALTERNATIVE DRUGS
- Octreotide appears helpful in slowing growth of liver metastasis. May produce regression in some cases. Octreotide-LAR can be given every 28 days.
- Chemotherapy regimens of streptozocin, 5-fluorouracil and doxorubicin show only limited response
- Interferon shows more limited response; may be useful in combination with octreotide

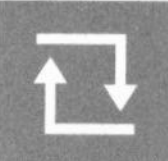

FOLLOWUP

PATIENT MONITORING
- Usual close follow-up necessary after any surgery, in addition need to monitor over time for evidence of metastasis
- Careful dose titration needed of medical therapy to control symptoms
- Gastric acid analysis to maintain basal gastric acid output to <10 mEq/hr (<2 mEq/hr if have complications such as perforation or esophagitis)

PREVENTION/AVOIDANCE Screen first degree relatives of patients with MEN 1

POSSIBLE COMPLICATIONS
- Complications of peptic ulcer disease (bleeding, perforation, obstruction)
- 2/3 of gastrinomas are malignant with metastasis
- Other substances may be produced by the tumor such as ACTH (5-8% of patients) with resulting Cushing syndrome
- Possible decrease in B-12 levels with long-term PPI use

EXPECTED COURSE/PROGNOSIS
- Overall survival rate- 5 year=62-75%, 10 year=47-53%
- Prognosis improves if complete surgical removal of tumor possible
- If liver metastasis present on initial surgery, 5 year survival 30-40%, 10 year 25%

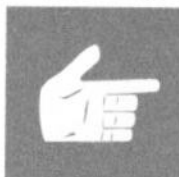

MISCELLANEOUS

ASSOCIATED CONDITIONS
- MEN 1: hyperparathyroidism, prolactinomas, other pituitary tumors
- Insulinoma
- Carcinoid tumors

AGE-RELATED FACTORS
Pediatric: There are cases reported in teenagers which are very aggressive.
Geriatric: Consider diagnosis in patient with persistent or recurring peptic ulcer disease. Is less aggressive disease if appears after 65 years.
Others: N/A

PREGNANCY Cases reported. Influences medication choices and surgical timing.

SYNONYMS
- Z-E syndrome
- Pancreatic ulcerogenic tumor syndrome
- Multiple endocrine neoplasia, partial
- Ulcerogenic islet cell tumor

ICD-9-CM
251.5 Abnormality of secretion of gastrin

SEE ALSO

OTHER NOTES N/A

ABBREVIATIONS
- MEN = multiple endocrine neoplasia
- ACTH = adrenocorticotropic hormone
- VIP = vasoactive intestinal polypeptide
- PPI = proton pump inhibitors

REFERENCES

- Pisegna JR. Zollinger Ellison Syndrome and Other Hypersecretory States. In: Feldman M, Friedman L, Sleisenger MH, editors. Sleisenger and Fortran's Gastrointestinal and Liver Disease. 7th ed. Philadelphia: WB. Saunders Co; 2002. p.782-92
- Alexander H, Fraker, et al. Prospective study of somatostatin receptor scintigraphy and its effect on operative outcome in patients with Zollinger-Ellison syndrome. Annals of Surgery 1998;228:2 228-38
- Yu F, Venzon DJ, Serrano J, Goebel SU, et al. Prospective study of the clinical course, prognostic factors, causes of death, and survival in patients with long-standing Zollinger-Ellison syndrome. J Clin Oncol 1999;17(2):615-30
- Feldman M. Peptic ulcer disease. In: Dale DC, Federman DD, editors. Scientific American Medicine. New York: Scientific American, Inc; 1999;4:II:3-4,8,11
- Jensen RT. Zollinger-Ellison syndrome. In: Goldman L, Bennett JC, editors. Cecil Textbook of Medicine. 21st ed. Philadelphia: WB Saunders Co; 2000. p.684-6

Web references: 1 available at www.5mcc.com
Illustrations N/A

Author(s):
Douglas S. Parks, MD

Section 2

Short Topics

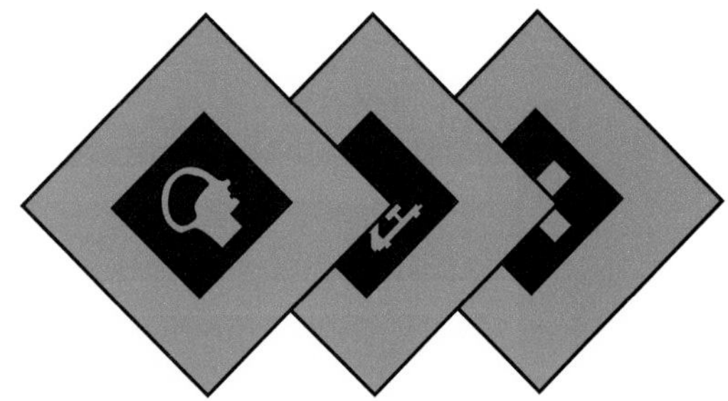

Acanthosis nigricans

DESCRIPTION A circumscribed melanosis consisting of a brown pigmented velvety verrucosity or fine papillomatosis appearing in the axillae and other body folds. Occurs in association with endocrine disorders, underlying malignancy, administration of certain drugs, or as in inherited disorder. Usual course - chronic.

CAUSES
- congenital
- associated with malignant disease
- obesity
- idiopathic

TREATMENT
- treat underlying cause
- malignancy workup

ICD-9-CM
701.2 Acquired acanthosis nigricans

Acoustic neuroma

DESCRIPTION A tumor arising from Schwann cells of the 8th cranial nerve (most often the vestibular division, rather than the acoustic division). Neurofibromatosis type II strongly predisposes patients to acoustic neuromas. Symptoms include unilateral hearing loss and other neurologic findings when the tumor compresses the cerebellum, pons, or facial nerve.

SYNONYMS
- Acoustic schwannoma

CAUSES
- Unknown

TREATMENT
- Surgical excision

ICD-9-CM
225.1 (M9560/0) Benign neoplasm of cranial nerves

Acquired adrenogenital syndrome

DESCRIPTION A condition of adults that is acquired or congenital in which excessive output of adrenal androgenic hormones causes virilization. The effects depend on age. Usual course - chronic; progressive.

CAUSES
- androgen producing tumors
- adrenal adenoma
- adrenal adenocarcinoma

TREATMENT
- surgery

ICD-9-CM
255.2 Adrenogenital disorders

Acrodermatitis enteropathica

DESCRIPTION Previously fatal disorder resulting from malabsorption of zinc. Characteristics: psoriasiform dermatitis, hair loss, paronychia, diarrhea, and growth retardation. Symptoms begin in infants just after weaning.

SYNONYMS
- Danbolt-Closs syndrome
- Brandt syndrome

CAUSES
- zinc deficiency
- defective zinc absorption

TREATMENT
- oral elemental zinc

ICD-9-CM
686.8 Other specific local infections of skin & subcutaneous tissue

Acromegaly

DESCRIPTION A disorder due to excessive secretion of pituitary growth hormone, characterized by progressive enlargement of the head and face, hands and feet, and thorax. Usual course - progressive.

SYNONYMS
- Acromegalia
- Eosinophilic adenoma syndrome

CAUSES
- growth hormone excess from pituitary adenoma

TREATMENT
- transsphenoidal resection
- heavy particle irradiation
- radiotherapy
- bromocriptine

ICD-9-CM
253.0 Acromegaly and gigantism

Actinomycosis of the kidney

DESCRIPTION Infectious bacterial disease that appears in 4 clinical forms - abdominal, cervicofacial, thoracic, and generalized. The generalized form can involve the kidneys as well as other organs. Characteristics - back pain, lethargy, weight loss, fever, hematuria. Usual course - acute.

CAUSES
- retrograde infection by actinomyces israelii

TREATMENT
- antibiotics
- drainage

ICD-9-CM
039.2 Actinomycotic infections, abdominal

Actinomycosis of the thorax

DESCRIPTION Infectious bacterial disease affecting the thorax and lungs. It also occurs in three other forms that include abdominal, cervicofacial and generalized. Usual course - progressive.

CAUSES
- actinomyces infection
- oral commensal
- aspiration of infected material
- impaired consciousness
- alcoholism

TREATMENT
- prolonged antibiotic therapy
- surgical drainage of suppurative lesions

ICD-9-CM
039.1 Actinomycotic infections, pulmonary

Adenocarcinoma of the bladder

DESCRIPTION Malignant growth in the bladder with characteristic hematuria, dysuria, urinary frequency, weight loss and suprapubic mass. Usual course - progressive.

CAUSES
- cystitis glandularis
- exstrophy of the bladder

TREATMENT
- segmental bladder resection
- total cystectomy

ICD-9-CM
188.9 Malignant neoplasm of bladder, part unspecified

Adenocarcinoma of the colon

DESCRIPTION The colon and rectum account for more new cases of cancer each year than any other site, exclusive of the lung. The incidence increases with age and peaks at 60-75. Characteristics - melena, diarrhea, rectal mass, iron deficiency anemia. Usual course - progressive.

CAUSES
- familial polyposis
- chronic ulcerative colitis
- possibly low fiber, high fat diet
- granulomatous colitis

TREATMENT
- surgery
- radiotherapy
- palliative chemotherapy

ICD-9-CM
153.9 Malignant neoplasm of colon, unspecified

Adenocarcinoma of the endometrium

DESCRIPTION Third rank in frequency of malignancies affecting women after breast and colon. Usually postmenopausal. Peak incidence between 50 and 60 years. Characteristics - positive Pap smear, menometrorrhagia, postmenopausal bleeding, perimenopausal bleeding. Usual course - progressive.

SYNONYMS
- Fundal carcinoma
- Corpus carcinoma
- Endometrial cancer

CAUSES
- irregular menses
- late menopause
- obesity
- diabetes mellitus
- hypertension
- infertility
- prolonged unopposed exogenous estrogen
- polycystic ovary disease

TREATMENT
- hysterectomy
- radiotherapy
- hormonal therapy with progesterone

ICD-9-CM
182.0 Malignant neoplasm of corpus uteri, except isthmus

Adenocarcinoma of the gallbladder

DESCRIPTION The most frequent cause of extrabiliary obstruction. Characteristics - nausea, vomiting, abdominal pain, anorexia, jaundice, hepatomegaly, enlarged gallbladder.

CAUSES
- cholelithiasis
- calcified gallbladder

TREATMENT
- surgical resection
- palliative radiotherapy
- palliative chemotherapy

ICD-9-CM
156.0 Malignant neoplasm of gallbladder

Adenocarcinoma of the rectum

DESCRIPTION A slow-growth rate malignancy that depends on routine examination to discover before symptom-producing size. Most common symptom is blood passage at the time of bowel movement. All rectal bleeding should raise suspicion of cancer until proven otherwise. Usual course - progressive; surgical cure.

CAUSES
• ulcerative colitis
• previous rectal cancer
• familial polyposis

TREATMENT
• surgery
• radiotherapy

ICD-9-CM
154.1 Malignant neoplasm of the rectum

Adenoid hyperplasia

DESCRIPTION An enlargement of the adenoidal tissue of the nasopharynx. Normally small at birth (2-3 cm), adenoidal tissue grows until child reaches adolescence, and then begins to atrophy slowly. With adenoid hyperplasia, however, this tissue continues to grow. Symptoms can include cough, earache, restlessness, headache, impaired taste or smell, mouth breathing, sleep apnea, snoring, chronic sinusitis, hyponasal voice, purulent rhinorrhea.

SYNONYMS
• adenoid hypertrophy

CAUSES
• unknown; factors that contribute: heredity, chronic infection, chronic nasal congestion, persistent allergy, insufficient aeration, inefficient nasal breathing, and repeated infections

TREATMENT
• antibiotics
• adenoidectomy

ICD-9-CM
474.12 Hypertrophy of adenoids alone

Adrenoleukodystrophy

DESCRIPTION A sphingolipidosis which combines the features of leukodystrophy and Addison disease. A rare, sex-linked recessive metabolic disorder that occurs in boys. Characteristics include - adrenal atrophy and widespread cerebral demyelinization. Usual course - progressive.

SYNONYMS
• sudanophilic leukodystrophy with adrenal atrophy
• Addison-Schilder disease
• Siemerling-Creutzfeldt disease
• diffuse cerebral sclerosis with adrenocortical atrophy
• Addison disease with cerebral sclerosis
• Sex-linked metachromatic leukodystrophy

CAUSES
• unknown biochemical enzyme defect

TREATMENT
• hormone replacement therapy
• dietary therapy

ICD-9-CM
330.0 Leukodystrophy

Afibrinogenemia, congenital

DESCRIPTION Hereditary recessive disorder characterized by failure of synthesis of adequate amounts of fibrinogen causing blood to be incoagulable. Symptoms include bruising, epistaxis, easy post-traumatic bleeding.

CAUSES
• no fibrinogen
• no factor I

TREATMENT
• transfusion
• cryoprecipitate
• plasma
• whole blood

ICD-9-CM
286.3 Congenital deficiency of other clotting factors

Agammaglobulinemia, acquired

DESCRIPTION Heterogenous disorder characterized by onset of recurrent bacterial infections in 2nd and 3rd decade, resulting from drastic decrease in Ig and antibody levels. It affects males and females equally and does not interfere with normal lifespan. Usual course - chronic.

SYNONYMS
• late-onset agammaglobulinemia
• common variable immunodeficiency

CAUSES
• Unknown, but most patients have defective synthesis or release of immunoglobulins.

TREATMENT
• maintenance gamma globulin
• fresh frozen plasma acutely

ICD-9-CM
279.06 Common variable immunodeficiency

Agranulocytosis

DESCRIPTION Reduction of blood neutrophil (granulocyte) count, leading to increased susceptibility to bacterial and fungal infection. Acute, severe neutropenia due to impaired production is often life-threatening. Characteristics - fever, fatigue, sore throat, buccal ulcers, dyspnea, tachycardia. Usual course - acute.

SYNONYMS
• malignant neutropenia
• primary granulocytopenia
• agranulocytic angina

CAUSES
• ionizing radiation, benzene, antimetabolites, nitrogen mustards, aminopyrine, phenothiazines, sulfonamides, chloramphenicol
• typhoid, paratyphoid, influenza, measles, rickettsia, cachexia, septicemia

TREATMENT
• eliminate etiological agent
• antibiotics
• supportive measures

ICD-9-CM
288.0 Agranulocytosis

Agranulocytosis, infantile genetic

DESCRIPTION Rare, hereditary and congenital disease, including familial neutropenia, cyclic neutropenia, pancreatic insufficiency with neutropenia, and several other disorders combining impaired neutrophil production and severe immune deficiency. Characteristics include fever, recurrent skin and respiratory infections, cough. Usual course - progressive; chronic; spontaneous remission.

SYNONYMS
• Kostmann syndrome

CAUSES
• defective bone marrow microenvironment
• progenitor defect

TREATMENT
• antibiotics
• bone marrow transplantation

ICD-9-CM
288.0 Agranulocytosis

Ainhum

DESCRIPTION A condition occurring chiefly in Black people in tropical countries. Characteristics - linear constriction of a toe, especially the little toe, which by its contraction gradually amputates the toe. Usual course - progressive; leading to amputation. Endemic areas - tropics; Africa.

SYNONYMS
• dactylolysis spontanea
• fibrous bands

CAUSES
• unknown

TREATMENT
• surgery
• Z-plasty
• relaxing incision
• amputation
• control infection

ICD-9-CM
136.0 Ainhum

Albright syndrome with precocious puberty

DESCRIPTION Fibrous dysplasia (cystic bone lesion) involving several bones plus cutaneous pigmentation and endocrine abnormalities. Characteristics - limb deformity, femoral fracture. Usual course - chronic; progressive.

SYNONYMS
• polyostotic fibrous dysplasia
• McCune-Albright syndrome
• osteitis fibrosa cystica

CAUSES
• Unknown

TREATMENT
• hyperthyroidism therapy
• adrenalectomy
• surgery

ICD-9-CM
756.54 Polyostotic fibrous dysplasia of bone

Alcaptonuria

DESCRIPTION Inborn aminoacidopathy due to defective homogentisate 1,2-dioxygenase. The accumulation of homogentisic acid leads to homogentisic aciduria causing the urine to turn dark brown on standing or alkalinization. Other characteristics include ochronosis and arthritis Usual course - asymptomatic until adulthood; progressive.

SYNONYMS
• homogentisic aciduria

CAUSES
• homogentisic acid oxidase activity
• increased homogentisic acid

TREATMENT
• supportive rehabilitation

ICD-9-CM
270.2 Other disturbances of aromatic amino acid metabolism

Alveolar proteinosis of the lung

DESCRIPTION Rare disease of unknown etiology characterized by filling of alveolar spaces with granular, periodic acid-Schiff (PAS)- positive material consisting of phospholipids and proteins. Age predilection is 20 to 60 years. It predominantly occurs in previously healthy males or females. Usual course - progressive.

SYNONYMS
• pulmonary alveolar proteinosis

CAUSES
- Unknown

TREATMENT
- total lung lavage under general anesthesia
- steroids not indicated

ICD-9-CM
516.0 Pulmonary alveolar proteinosis

SEE ALSO
- Cor pulmonale

Amaurosis, congenital

DESCRIPTION A cone-rod abiotrophy causing blindness or amblyopia at birth; frequently found in Holland and Sweden. Usual course - stable; gradual deterioration.

SYNONYMS
- congenital retinal blindness
- amaurosis congenita of Leber
- heredoretinopathia congenita

CAUSES
- unknown

TREATMENT
- none

ICD-9-CM
362.76 Dystrophies primarily involving the retinal pigment epithelium

Amaurosis fugax

DESCRIPTION Acute, transient episode of blindness or partial blindness, lasting ten minutes or less.

CAUSES
- retinal arteriolar emboli

TREATMENT
- medical:
  - ◊ control hypertension
  - ◊ antithrombotic medications
  - ◊ aspirin
  - ◊ dipyridamole
- surgical:
  - ◊ carotid endarterectomy

ICD-9-CM
362.34 Transient arterial occlusion

SEE ALSO
- Glaucoma, primary angle-closure
- Glaucoma, primary open-angle
- Retinal detachment
- Transient ischemic attack (TIA)

Amebic meningoencephalitis

DESCRIPTION A rare and often fatal, acute, febrile, purulent meningoencephalitis caused by usually free-living soil and water amebas of the genera Naegleria, Acanthamoeba, or Hartmannella. Generally seen in young persons who swim in contaminated fresh water. Also seen in a less fulminant form in older persons and in immunocompromised persons. Usual course: acute.

CAUSES
- naegleria
- acanthamoeba
- Hartmanella

TREATMENT
- amphotericin B
- miconazole
- rifampin

ICD-9-CM
006.5 Amebic brain abscess

Aminoaciduria

DESCRIPTION Impairment of renal tubular transport of amino acids.

SYNONYMS
- cystinuria
- dibasic aminoaciduria
- Hartnup disease
- iminoglycinuria
- dicarboxylate aminoaciduria

CAUSES
- Unknown

TREATMENT
- diet management
- high fluid intake
- lithotomy
- penicillamine
- nicotinamide

ICD-9-CM
270.9 Unspecified disorder of amino-acid metabolism

Anemia, acquired sideroblastic

DESCRIPTION A microcytic (or normocytic), hypochromic anemia due to inadequate or abnormal utilization of intracellular iron for hemoglobin synthesis, despite adequate or increased amounts of iron within the mitochondria of the developing red blood cell precursors. Peripheral blood shows polychromatic, stippled, targeted red blood cells. Usual course - slowly progressive.

CAUSES
- idiopathic
- antituberculous drugs
- alcohol
- chloramphenicol

TREATMENT
- avoid precipitating drug
- avoid alcohol
- treat consequences

ICD-9-CM
285.0 Sideroblastic anemia

Anemia due to chronic disease

DESCRIPTION The second most common anemia in the world. The major characteristic is that the marrow erythroid mass fails to expand appropriately in response to microcytic anemia from whatever cause. The defect, then, is one of decreased red blood cell production. The symptoms are primarily those of the underlying disease, such as rheumatoid arthritis, infections, or cancer. Usual course - chronic.

CAUSES
- chronic inflammation: iron metabolism abnormality
- defective RBC production
- inability to compensate for decreased red blood cell life span

TREATMENT
- treat underlying condition

ICD-9-CM
285.9 Anemia, unspecified

Anemia due to folate deficiency

DESCRIPTION Decreased red blood cells and hemoglobin content due to impaired production. This is one form of megaloblastic anemia characterized by decreased red blood cells and decreased serum folate.

SYNONYMS
- nutritional macrocytic anemia
- tropical macrocytic anemia

CAUSES
- malnutrition
- inadequate folate intake
- malabsorption of folate
- increased demand for folate
- drugs

TREATMENT
- folic acid supplements
- avoid precipitating drug

ICD-9-CM
281.2 Folate-deficiency anemia

Anemia, hemolytic

DESCRIPTION A general term covering a large group of anemias in which there is a shortened life span of the red blood cells (normal = 120 days). Most hemolysis occurs extravascularly in the spleen, liver, and bone marrow.

- Characteristics - signs and symptoms include chills, fever, pain in the back and abdomen, prostration, shock, jaundice, splenomegaly, hemoglobinuria, hemosiderinuria, reticulocytosis

CAUSES
- G6PD deficiency
- Intrinsic abnormalities of red blood cell contents (hemoglobin or enzymes) or membrane
- Serum antibodies, trauma in circulation, infectious agents
- Temporary failure of red blood cell production
- Autoantibodies against red cell antigens, idiopathic or secondary to autoimmune diseases
- Drug-induced (penicillin type or methyldopa type)

TREATMENT
- individualized to specific hemolytic disorders. Modalities may include splenectomy and iron replacement.

ICD-9-CM
282.9 Hereditary hemolytic anemia, unspecified
283.9 Acquired hemolytic anemia, unspecified

Anemia, myelophthisic

DESCRIPTION Anemia characterized by appearance of immature myeloid and nucleated erythrocytes in the peripheral blood, resulting from infiltration of the bone marrow by foreign or abnormal tissue. Usual course - progressive.

SYNONYMS
- myelopathic anemia
- leukoerythroblastosis
- secondary myelofibrosis

CAUSES
- hematologic consequences of marrow infiltration
- lymphoma
- leukemias
- myelomas
- metastatic carcinoma
- tuberculosis
- lipid storage diseases
- fungus infection
- granulomatous disorders

TREATMENT
- treat underlying condition
- supportive measures
- splenectomy if hypersplenism

ICD-9-CM
285.8 Other specified anemias

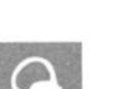

Anhidrosis

DESCRIPTION Abnormal deficiency of sweat. Other characteristics - malaise, easy fatigability, headache, nausea, warmth, dry skin, tachycardia.

CAUSES
- senile skin

- radiodermatitis
- acrodermatitis chronica atrophica
- scleroderma
- lichen sclerosis et atrophica
- spinal cord lesions
- quinacrine toxicity
- miliaria
- sympathectomy
- peripheral neuropathy
- sympathetic ganglion antagonists
- hereditary anhidrotic ectodermal dysplasia
- acetylcholine antagonists
- hysteria
- brainstem, pontine or medulla tumors
- Franceschetti-Jadassohn syndrome
- Fabry disease

TREATMENT
- symptomatic

ICD-9-CM
705.0 Anhidrosis

Anorectal fissure

DESCRIPTION An acute tear or chronic ulcer in the stratified squamous epithelium of the anal canal. Symptoms include rectal pain and bleeding with defecation.

SYNONYMS
- Anal fissure
- Fissure in ano
- Anal ulcer

CAUSES
- Unknown. Probably traumatic laceration from a hard or large stool with secondary infection.

TREATMENT
- Stool softeners; psyllium seed laxatives
- glycerin suppositories
- warm sitz baths
- surgery if conservative measures fail

ICD-9-CM
565.0 Anal fissure

Anthracosis

DESCRIPTION Usually asymptomatic form of pneumoconiosis caused by deposition of coal dust in the lungs. Usual course - progressive; chronic. Endemic areas - urban areas.

CAUSES
- inhalation of atmospheric particles
- inhalation of soot

TREATMENT
- none

ICD-9-CM
500 Coal workers pneumoconiosis

Anthrax of the intestine

DESCRIPTION Highly infectious disease of animals, (especially ruminants) that is rarely transmitted to man by contact with the animals or their products. Anthrax infection also occurs in a cutaneous form. Characteristics - fever, malaise, hematemesis, anorexia, abdominal pain, bloody diarrhea. Usual course - acute.

CAUSES
- Bacillus anthracis
- ingestion of bacillus
- contaminated meat

TREATMENT
- penicillin
- tetracycline

ICD-9-CM
022.2 Gastrointestinal anthrax

Anthrax of the lung

DESCRIPTION Highly infectious disease of animals (especially ruminants) that is rarely transmitted to man by contact with the animals or their products. Characteristics - fever, malaise, cough, myalgia, dyspnea, headache. This infection can be severe enough to be fatal. Usual course - acute; 3-4 day incubation. (Rare in U.S.)

SYNONYMS
- woolsorter disease
- anthrax pneumonia

CAUSES
- bacillus anthracis
- inhalation

TREATMENT
- penicillin
- streptomycin
- hydration

ICD-9-CM
022.1 Pulmonary anthrax

Anthrax of the skin

DESCRIPTION Highly infectious disease of animals, especially ruminants. Transmitted to man by contact with the animals or their products. Cutaneous form begins as a red-brown papule that enlarges with peripheral erythema, vesiculation, and induration, followed by ulceration and local lymphadenopathy. Usual course - acute.
Endemic areas - Haiti; South Africa; Asia.

SYNONYMS
- cutaneous anthrax
- charbon
- malignant pustule
- Siberian ulcer
- malignant edema
- splenic fever
- milzbrand
- ragpicker's disease

CAUSES
- bacillus anthracis
- skin contact

TREATMENT
- penicillin
- tetracycline
- erythromycin
- hydrocortisone

ICD-9-CM
022.0 Cutaneous anthrax

SEE ALSO
- Anthrax of the lung

Aortic regurgitation

DESCRIPTION Retrograde flow from the aorta into the left ventricle through incompetent aortic cusps. Symptoms include dyspnea, shortness of breath, palpitations, orthopnea. Usual course - acute; chronic.

SYNONYMS
- aortic valve insufficiency

CAUSES
- bacterial endocarditis, aortic dissection, ankylosing spondylitis, aortic stenosis, rheumatic fever, giant cell arteritis, syphilis, Marfan syndrome, osteogenesis imperfection, Reiter syndrome, rheumatoid arthritis, cystic medial necrosis, sinus of Valsalva aneurysm, hypertension, arteriosclerosis, myxomatous degeneration of valve, dissection of aorta, bicuspid aortic valve

TREATMENT
- aortic valve replacement

ICD-9-CM
424.1 Aortic valve disorders

Apert syndrome

DESCRIPTION Autosomal dominant mutation characterized by acrocephalosyndactyly and mental retardation. Usual course - chronic; progressive.

SYNONYMS
- acrocephalosyndactyly

CAUSES
- unknown
- probable early bridging of mesenchymal blastema
- probable early bridging of bone hypoplasia

TREATMENT
- supportive
- orthopedic surgery
- maxillofacial surgery
- neurosurgery

ICD-9-CM
755.55 Acrocephalosyndactyly

Argininosuccinicaciduria

DESCRIPTION Presence in urine of argininosuccinic acid, characteristic of a condition resulting from an inborn error of metabolism (autosomal recessive) and accompanied by mental retardation, failure to thrive, ataxia, seizures. Usual course - progressive.

SYNONYMS
- argininosuccinicacidemia
- argininosuccinase deficiency

CAUSES
- argininosuccinase deficiency

TREATMENT
- decrease urea precursors
- decrease ureapoiesis
- decrease nitrogen waste production

ICD-9-CM
270.6 Disorders of urea cycle metabolism

Arsenic poisoning

DESCRIPTION Toxic condition caused by exposure to arsenic. Characteristics - throat constriction, dysphagia, burning gastrointestinal pain, vomiting, diarrhea, dehydration, pulmonary edema, renal failure, liver failure. Usual course - acute; chronic.

CAUSES
- pentavalent arsenic salt
- trivalent arsenic salt
- arsine gas

TREATMENT
- dimercaprol
- induce vomiting
- gastric lavage
- milk
- penicillamine
- hemodialysis

ICD-9-CM
985.1 Toxic effect of arsenic and its compounds

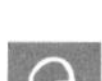

Arteriosclerosis obliterans

DESCRIPTION Arteriosclerosis in which proliferation of the intima leads to occlusion of the lumen of the arteries.
Usual course - progressive

CAUSES
- atherosclerosis

TREATMENT
- exercise
- weight loss
- avoid tobacco smoking
- angioplasty
- surgery

• lumbar sympathectomy

ICD-9-CM
440.9 Generalized and unspecified atherosclerosis

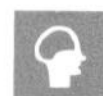

Ascites, chylous

DESCRIPTION The presence of chyle in the peritoneal cavity as a result of anomalies, injuries, or obstruction of the thoracic duct. Characteristics - abdominal pain, fullness, discomfort, distention, shortness of breath, nausea, weight gain.

SYNONYMS
• chylous peritonitis

CAUSES
• abdominal neoplasm
• lymphoma
• abdominal lymphatic obstruction
• trauma
• intestinal obstruction
• chylous cyst rupture
• Hodgkin disease

TREATMENT
• paracentesis

ICD-9-CM
789.5 Ascites

Astrocytoma

DESCRIPTION A tumor composed of astrocytes characterized by hemiparesis, cranial nerve palsy, personality changes, headache, seizures, and mentation change. Usual course - progressive.

SYNONYMS
• Astrocytic glioma
• Astroglioma

CAUSES
• tuberous sclerosis

TREATMENT
• grade I: surgery
• combined surgery plus radiotherapy
• grade II: combined surgery plus radiotherapy
• grade III: combined surgery plus radiotherapy

ICD-9-CM
191.9 Malignant neoplasm of brain, unspecified

Ataxia-telangiectasia

DESCRIPTION One of the neurocutaneous syndromes and progressive multisystem disorder characterized by cerebellar ataxia, skin and conjunctival telangiectasia, recurrent infections of sinuses and lungs, and variable immunologic disease. Affected are predisposed to malignancy. Death usually occurs during childhood. Ataxia can be confused with cerebral palsy.

SYNONYMS
• Louis-Bar syndrome
• Cerebello-oculocutaneous telangiectasia

CAUSES Autosomal recessive disorder; gene locus at chromosome region 11q22.3

TREATMENT
• Management of complications
• Genetic counseling of family
• Supportive measures

ICD-9-CM
334.8 Other spinocerebellar diseases
334.9 Spinocerebellar disease, unspecified

Author(s)
Nuhad D. Dinno, MD

Atrial flutter

DESCRIPTION Atrial rate 240-400 beats per minute. QRS complexes uniform in shape, irregular in rate. P waves may have saw-toothed configuration.

CAUSES
• postoperative revascularization
• digitalis toxicity
• pulmonary embolism
• valvular heart disease
• congestive heart failure

TREATMENT
• Digoxin (except when due to digitalis toxicity), quinidine, propranolol
• Cardioversion
• Atrial pacemaker

ICD-9-CM
427.32 Atrial flutter

Atrial myxoma

DESCRIPTION A benign tumor composed of primitive connective tissue cells forming a gelatinous growth, usually pedunculated. Symptoms include dyspnea of effort, weight loss, fatigue, low-grade fever, polyneuritis, nausea, syncopal attacks. Usual course: progressive.

CAUSES
• unknown

TREATMENT
• surgical excision of mass

ICD-9-CM
212.7 Benign neoplasm of heart

Atypical mycobacterial infection

DESCRIPTION Disease caused by mycobacteria other than the tubercle and lepra bacillus. The illnesses are similar both pathologically and clinically to tuberculosis. Usual course - acute; progressive.
Endemic areas: Central USA; Texas; England; Wales; Southeastern USA

CAUSES
• Mycobacterium ulcerans
• Mycobacterium kansasii
• Mycobacterium avium intracellulare
• Mycobacterium xenopi
• Mycobacterium szulgai

TREATMENT
• rifampin
• ethambutol
• isoniazid
• surgery
• minocycline
• trimethoprim-sulfamethoxazole
• ethionamide
• pyrazinamide
• cycloserine

ICD-9-CM
031.9 Unspecified diseases due to mycobacteria

Baby blues

DESCRIPTION Baby blues is a transient self-limiting condition that affects about 50-80% of new mothers. It begins within the first week following delivery and is usually resolved within 4 weeks. It is characterized by lability of affect, tearfulness, irritability, restlessness, sleep disturbance, general fatigue and feelings of being overwhelmed. Some cases of postpartum depression may present initially as "baby blues" but if the symptoms do not respond to reassurance and support and last for more than four weeks, the diagnosis of postpartum depression should be considered. Moreover, mothers who experience "baby blues": typically do not present symptoms of suicidal thoughts or feelings of guilt, which are not uncommon in mothers with postpartum depression.

SYNONYMS
• Maternity blues

CAUSES N/A

TREATMENT
• Reassurance and support

ICD-9-CM
648.44 Mental postpartum condition or complication

Author(s)
Moshe S. Torem, MD

Balantidiasis

DESCRIPTION Infection by protozoan parasites of the genus Balantidium. B. coli may cause diarrhea and dysentery in man, with ulceration of the colon mucosa. Usual course - acute. Endemic areas - tropical areas.

CAUSES
• balantidium coli

TREATMENT
• tetracycline
• iodoquinol

ICD-9-CM
007.0 Balantidiasis

Balkan nephritis syndrome

DESCRIPTION A chronic progressive nephritis seen in a large percentage of the population living in the endemic areas of Yugoslavia, Romania, Bulgaria.

CAUSES
• unknown
• possible environmental toxin

TREATMENT
• treat renal failure
• avoid endemic areas

ICD-9-CM
582.89 Nephritis, interstitial, chronic

Bartter syndrome

DESCRIPTION Hypertrophy and hyperplasia of the juxtaglomerular cells producing hypokalemic alkalosis and hyperaldosteronism. Characteristics - absence of hypertension in the presence of markedly increased plasma renin concentrations and insensitivity to the pressor effects of angiotensin. Usually affects children, is perhaps hereditary, and may be associated with other congenital anomalies, such as short stature and mental retardation.

CAUSES
• unknown
• primary renal potassium wasting
• defective renal tubular potassium transport
• defective renal tubular chloride transport

TREATMENT
• liberal dietary potassium and sodium chloride
• potassium supplementation
• spironolactone, indomethacin, ibuprofen, aspirin, captopril, propranolol

ICD-9-CM
255.13 Bartter syndrome

Beckwith-Wiedemann syndrome

DESCRIPTION A syndrome of multiple defects characterized primarily by umbilical hernia, macroglossia, and gigantism and secondarily by visceromegaly, hypoglycemia, ear abnormalities, etc. Usual course - acute.

SYNONYMS
• Beckwith syndrome

- Wiedemann II syndrome
- Exomphalos-macroglossia-gigantism syndrome

CAUSES
- unknown

TREATMENT
- steroids; feeding manipulations; non-ketogenic diet high in calories
- surgery

ICD-9-CM
759.89 Other specified congenital anomalies

Benign essential tremor syndrome

DESCRIPTION A fine-to-coarse slow, rhythmic tremor, primarily affecting the hands, head and voice, with a frequency of 4-12 times per second. Affected body part may be in movement or held in one position. The tremor may begin at any age, most often affects upper extremities and can be aggravated by anxiety, stress, fatigue and cold. Tends to increase with age; generally no disability; treatment often unnecessary.

SYNONYMS
- presenile tremor syndrome
- familial tremor

CAUSES
- exact cause is unknown
- inherited as an autosomal dominant trait in about 50% of cases

TREATMENT
- extra rest may help
- propranolol or primidone
- benzodiazepines
- ingestion of a small amount of alcohol provides short-term relief

ICD-9-CM
333.1 Essential and other specified forms of tremo
r

Beriberi heart disease

DESCRIPTION A form of beriberi caused by a deficiency of thiamine characterized by cardiac failure and edema, but without extensive nervous system involvement.

SYNONYMS
- vitamin B1 deficiency heart disease
- wet beriberi

CAUSES
- chronic alcoholism
- thiamine deficiency
- malnutrition

TREATMENT
- thiamine
- diuretics
- digoxin

ICD-9-CM
265.0 Beriberi

Beriberi nervous system syndrome

DESCRIPTION Usual course - chronic; progressive; generally associated with beriberi heart disease; often progresses to cerebral beriberi

CAUSES
- thiamine deficiency
- malnutrition
- chronic alcoholism
- fever
- high carbohydrate intake
- thyrotoxicosis
- dialysis
- diuresis

TREATMENT
- intramuscular thiamine
- water-soluble vitamin repletion

ICD-9-CM
265.0 Beriberi

SEE ALSO
- Beriberi heart disease
- Korsakoff psychosis
- Neuritis/neuralgia

Bezoar

DESCRIPTION Concretions of swallowed hair, fruit or vegetable fibers, or similar substances found in the alimentary canal. Usual course - acute.

CAUSES
- partial gastrectomy
- autonomic neuropathy
- accumulation of vegetable fibers
- accumulation of hairs

TREATMENT
- phytobezoars: cellulose digestion, papain digestion, lavage, surgery
- trichobezoars: lavage, surgery

ICD-9-CM
938 Foreign body in digestive system, unspecified

Bezold abscess

DESCRIPTION Sore throat and nuchal rigidity caused by insufficiently treated otitis media. Named after Friedrich Bezold, an otologist from Munich. Usual course - chronic.

SYNONYMS
- subperiosteal abscess of the temporal bone
- bezold mastoiditis

CAUSES
- insufficiently treated otitis media

TREATMENT
- antibiotics
- surgical drainage

ICD-9-CM
383.01 Subperiosteal abscess of mastoid

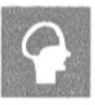

Bladder tumors

DESCRIPTION
- The second most common site for tumors of the urinary tract. Most bladder tumors occur in men aged 50 and over. Common types include transitional cell carcinoma (the most common) type), epidermoid tumors, adenocarcinoma, and sarcoma with systemic disease.
- Characteristics - symptoms include hematuria, urinary frequency, urgency, dysuria, reduced force and size of the urinary stream, suprapubic pain, and sometimes a palpable suprapubic mass. Should rule out renal calculi, cystitis, nephritis. Measures to confirm diagnosis include cystoscopy, biopsy, CT scan, ultrasound.

CAUSES
- Unknown. Risk factors include alcoholism, tobacco smoking, radiation exposure.

TREATMENT
- tumor staging
- surgery
- radiation therapy
- hormone therapy
- immunotherapy
- chemotherapy

ICD-9-CM
188.9 Malignant neoplasm of bladder, part unspecified

Bloom syndrome

DESCRIPTION Autosomal recessive syndrome developing during infancy. Characteristics include erythema and telangiectasia (in a butterfly distribution on the face), photosensitivity, and dwarfism. Usual course - chronic; onset in infancy; decreased infection rate with age. Information available - Bloom Syndrome Registry 212-570-3075.

SYNONYMS
- congenital telangiectatic erythema

CAUSES
- chromosomal breakage
- chromosomal instability
- sister chromatid exchanges
- chromosomal aberrations

TREATMENT
- sunscreens
- symptomatic
- cancer therapy as necessary

ICD-9-CM
757.39 Other specified congenital anomalies of skin, other

Blue diaper syndrome

DESCRIPTION Defect in tryptophan absorption in which the urine contains abnormal indoles, giving it a blue color. This is similar to Hartnup disease. Usual course - chronic.

SYNONYMS
- familial hypercalcemia; with nephrocalcinosis and indicanuria
- tryptophan malabsorption

CAUSES
- defective tryptophan absorption

TREATMENT
- low tryptophan diet
- definitive treatment unknown

ICD-9-CM
270.0 Disturbances of amino-acid transport

Boutonneuse fever

DESCRIPTION A febrile disease of the Mediterranean area, the Crimea, Africa and India, due to infection with Rickettsia conorii.
Usual course - acute; 5-7 day incubation period
Endemic areas: Mediterranean littoral; Africa; Indian subcontinent

SYNONYMS
- African tick typhus
- African tick-borne fever

CAUSES
- Rickettsia conorii
- tick bite
- rodent reservoir
- dog reservoir

TREATMENT
- chloramphenicol
- tetracycline

ICD-9-CM
082.1 Boutonneuse fever
087.1 Tick-borne relapsing fever

Bowen disease

DESCRIPTION An epidermal hyperplasia (often occurring in multiple primary sites), which may progress to squamous cell carcinoma

SYNONYMS
- precancerous dermatosis
- intradermal epidermoid carcinoma
- carcinoma in-situ

• intraepidermal squamous cell carcinoma

CAUSES
• sun damage
• arsenic

TREATMENT
• surgical excision
• topical 5-fluorouracil

ICD-9-CM
239.2 Neoplasms of unspecified nature of bone, soft tissue, and skin

Brill disease

DESCRIPTION Recrudescence of epidemic typhus occurring years after the initial infection in which the etiologic agent Rickettsia prowazekii persists in body tissues in an inactive state (up to 70 years). Usual course - relapsing. Endemic areas - worldwide.

SYNONYMS
• Brill-Zinsser disease
• recrudescent typhus

CAUSES
• persistent rickettsia prowazekii in human reservoirs
• prior epidemic typhus fever

TREATMENT
• tetracycline
• chloramphenicol
• pediculicides

ICD-9-CM
081.1 Brill disease

Broncholithiasis

DESCRIPTION Condition in which calculi (broncholiths) are present within the lumen of the tracheobronchial tree.

SYNONYMS
• calculi of bronchus
• bronchopulmonary lithiasis

CAUSES
• usually a late complication of a granulomatous disease

TREATMENT
• antibiotics
• endoscopic removal
• surgery

ICD-9-CM
518.89 Other diseases of lung, NEC

Brown-Sequard syndrome

DESCRIPTION Syndrome due to damage of one half of the spinal cord, resulting in ipsilateral paralysis and loss of discriminatory and joint sensation, and contralateral loss of pain and temperature sensation.

SYNONYMS
• hemiparaplegic syndrome
• spastic spinal monoplegia syndrome

CAUSES
• spinal trauma
• unilateral spinal cord lesion
• spinal cord tumors
• spinal cord radiation
• spinal cord compression

TREATMENT
• surgery
• decompression

ICD-9-CM
344.89 Other specified paralytic syndrome

Bruxism

DESCRIPTION The grinding and clenching of teeth (usually performed during sleep) which may lead to occlusal trauma. It is common in persons of all ages (approximately 15% of children and as many as 96% of adults). Clinically, bruxism commonly accompanies the stress of marital strife, school examinations or work difficulties; it may resolve when these stresses lessen. A genetic predisposition may exist.

SYNONYMS
• tooth grinding

CAUSES
• unknown
• associated with stress, occlusal disorders, allergies and sleep position

TREATMENT
• biofeedback exercises
• changes in sleep position
• drug therapy, e.g., diazepam, methocarbamol, injections of botulinum toxin
• psychotherapy
• hypnotherapy
• physical therapy
• occlusal orthotics
• stress reduction
• coping techniques

ICD-9-CM
306.8 Other specified psychophysiological malfunction

Budd-Chiari syndrome

DESCRIPTION Symptomatic occlusion or obstruction of the hepatic veins, causing hepatomegaly, abdominal pain and tenderness, intractable ascites, mild jaundice, portal hypertension and liver failure. The onset may be acute. In cases of complete occlusion, death may occur within days of onset. More often, there is a chronic course with survival for months or years.

SYNONYMS
• hepatic vein thrombosis

CAUSES
• trauma
• oral contraceptives
• polycythemia rubra vera
• paroxysmal nocturnal hemoglobinuria
• hypercoagulable state
• pyrrolizine alkaloids

TREATMENT
• portacaval shunt

ICD-9-CM
453.0 Budd-Chiari syndrome

Byssinosis

DESCRIPTION An occupational airway disorder (in which bronchial constriction occurs); common to those who come in contact with crude cotton, hemp or flax. Characterized by chest tightness, wheezing, dyspnea that develop on the first day after a weekend or vacation away from the work environment; symptoms decrease during the week and by the end of the week, the individual is symptom-free.

CAUSES
• inhalation of substance; dust component not positively identified

TREATMENT
• discontinue exposure

ICD-9-CM
504 Pneumonopathy due to inhalation of other dust

Campylobacter infections

DESCRIPTION Campylobacter species are small, gram-negative, curved or spiral bacilli associated with enteritis and systemic disease in humans. Outbreaks have been associated with day care centers, contaminated water supplies and raw milk. C. jejuni frequently causes acute enteritis (can be mild or severe), C. coli causes diarrhea and C. fetus causes bacteremia and meningitis in immunocompromised patients and may cause maternal fever, abortion, stillbirth, and severe neonatal infection. Helicobacter pylori (previously called Campylobacter pylori) has been associated with gastritis and peptic ulcer disease.

CAUSES
• contact with infected animals
• contaminated food and water
• improperly cooked poultry
• person-to-person spread via fecal-oral route

TREATMENT
• fluid and electrolyte replacement
• erythromycin (in children)
• tetracycline (in adults)
• note: trimethoprim-sulfamethoxazole and ampicillin are ineffective against Campylobacter

ICD-9-CM
008.43 Intestinal infections due to Campylobacter

Carcinoid syndrome

DESCRIPTION A symptom complex associated with carcinoid tumors (argentaffinoma). Characteristics - attacks of severe cyanotic flushing of the skin that lasts from minutes to days; watery stools; bronchoconstrictive attacks; sudden drop in blood pressure; edema; ascites. Symptoms are caused by the tumor secreting serotonin prostaglandins, and other biologically active substances.

SYNONYMS
• Thorson-Bioerck syndrome
• argentaffinoma syndrome
• flush syndrome
• Cassidy-Scholte syndrome

CAUSES
• tumor
• overproduction of serotonin

TREATMENT
• medical management of symptoms
• appropriate treatment of tumor

ICD-9-CM
259.2 Carcinoid syndrome

Carcinoid tumor

DESCRIPTION Yellow, circumscribed tumor occurring in the small intestine, appendix, stomach or colon. Usually asymptomatic. Usual course - progressive.

SYNONYMS
• argentaffinoma
• carcinoid
• argentaffin carcinoid tumor

CAUSES
• multiple endocrine neoplasia, type 1
• regional enteritis
• Gardner syndrome

TREATMENT
• surgical excision
• antihormonal therapy as needed
• radiation therapy

ICD-9-CM
238.9 Neoplasm of uncertain behavior, site unspecified

Cardiospasm

DESCRIPTION Failure to relax the smooth muscle fibers of the esophagus. Usual course - chronic; progressive.

SYNONYMS
- achalasia
- megaesophagus
- esophageal dyssynergia

CAUSES
- unknown
- impairment of postganglionic innervation of esophagus

TREATMENT
- soft foods
- sedatives
- nitrates
- anticholinergics
- calcium channel blockers
- balloon dilatation
- myotomy

ICD-9-CM
530.0 Achalasia and cardiospasm

Caroli disease

DESCRIPTION Congenital dilatation of the intrahepatic bile ducts. Characteristics - abdominal pain, fever, intermittent jaundice, hepatomegaly. Usual course - chronic; progressive; relapsing.

CAUSES
- congenital dilatation of intrahepatic bile ducts
- intrahepatic stones
- biliary obstruction

TREATMENT
- antibiotics
- surgery not indicated

ICD-9-CM
751.69 Other congenital anomalies of gallbladder, bile ducts, and liver

Cauda equina syndrome

DESCRIPTION Dull aching pain of the perineum, bladder, and sacrum, generally radiating in a sciatic fashion, with associated paresthesias and paralysis, due to compression of the spinal nerve roots. Usual course - chronic.

SYNONYMS
- cauda equina pseudo-claudication

CAUSES
- lumbar spondylosis with cauda equina compression
- congenital narrowing of lumbar canal

TREATMENT
- decompressive laminectomy
- rest

ICD-9-CM
344.60 Cauda equina syndrome without mention of neurogenic bladder
344.61 Cauda equina syndrome with neurogenic bladder

Cavernous sinus thrombosis

DESCRIPTION Infection of the venous channels that drain the orbit and face. Characteristics - symptoms include exophthalmos, papilledema, headache, convulsions, septic temperature curve. Prognosis is grave.

CAUSES Direct extension of infection from the orbit and face. Risk factors include diabetes mellitus and immunosuppression.

TREATMENT
- hospitalization, intensive care, IV fluids, and intense intravenous antibiotic treatment

ICD-9-CM
325 Phlebitis and thrombophlebitis of intracranial venous sinuses

Chagas disease

DESCRIPTION An acute, subacute or chronic form of trypanosomiasis occurring widely in Central and South America, transmitted by bites of reduviid bugs. Usual course - acute; chronic; progressive.
Endemic areas: western hemisphere; Mexico to Central America; South America; identified mammalian reservoirs in USA

SYNONYMS
- Brazilian trypanosomiasis

CAUSES
- inoculation of trypanosoma cruzi
- congenital breast milk
- transfusion-related infection

TREATMENT
- no definitive treatment
- nifurtimox in acute phase
- metronidazole
- pacemaker
- esophageal dilatation
- gastrointestinal surgery

ICD-9-CM
086.2 Chagas disease without mention of organ involvement

Charcot joint

DESCRIPTION Neuropathic arthropathy associated with certain chronic disorders. Usual course - chronic; progressive.

SYNONYMS
- neuropathic arthropathy
- tabetic osteoarthropathy
- neuropathic joint disease

CAUSES
- peripheral neuropathy
- diabetes
- tertiary syphilis
- tabes dorsalis
- syringomyelia
- myelomeningocele

TREATMENT
- immobilization
- reduction of weight-bearing
- surgical arthrodesis

ICD-9-CM
094.0 Tabes dorsalis
713.5 Arthropathy associated with neurological disorders

Charcot-Marie-Tooth disease

DESCRIPTION Progressive neuropathic (peroneal) muscular atrophy, usually autosomal dominant. Characteristics - cramps, paresthesias, leg and hand weakness, difficulty in walking. Usual course - chronic; progressive.

CAUSES
- hereditary

TREATMENT
- leg braces

ICD-9-CM
356.1 Peroneal muscular atrophy

Cheese-worker lung

DESCRIPTION A pathologic condition caused by inhalation of mold that grows on cheese. Usual course - acute; subacute; chronic.

SYNONYMS
- cheese-washer's lung

CAUSES
- antigens of aspergillus clavatus
- antigens of penicillium casei
- breathing cheese mold

TREATMENT
- avoid causative agents
- tapered steroids suppress alveolitis
- chronic disease: long-term steroids

ICD-9-CM
495.8 Other specified allergic alveolitis and pneumonitis

SEE ALSO
- Eosinophilic pneumonias

Chiari-Frommel syndrome

DESCRIPTION Persistent lactation and amenorrhea following pregnancy.
Usual course - chronic

SYNONYMS
- Frommel Disease
- Amenorrhea-galactorrhea syndrome

CAUSES
- microadenoma of the pituitary

TREATMENT
- treat underlying disorder

ICD-9-CM
676.60 Galactorrhea associated with childbirth, unspecified

Chikungunya

DESCRIPTION A self-limited dengue-like illness caused by an alphavirus transmitted by mosquitoes of the genus Aedes, principally occurring in Southeast Asia and Africa. Usual course - acute.

CAUSES
- group A arbovirus
- alphavirus
- arthropod-borne
- mosquito vector
- Aedes aegypti

TREATMENT
- supportive
- bed rest
- non-salicylate antipyretics
- analgesics
- anti-inflammatory agents
- physiotherapy
- anticonvulsants
- rehydration

ICD-9-CM
066.3 Other mosquito-borne fever

Chloasma

DESCRIPTION Sharply demarcated, blotchy, brown, macules found in a symmetric distribution over the cheeks and forehead and sometimes on the neck or upper lip. Frequently occurs during pregnancy, at menopause, and in patients taking oral contraceptives. Same type may be seen in patients with chronic liver disease. Usual course - variable; chronic; relapsing.

SYNONYMS
- melasma
- mask of pregnancy

CAUSES
- oral contraceptives plus ultraviolet light
- pregnancy plus ultraviolet light
- endocrine dysfunction
- cosmetics
- Mesantoin
- diphenylhydantoin

TREATMENT
• avoid sun exposure
• avoid oral contraceptives
• delivery
• discontinue implicated drug
• discontinue implicated cosmetic
• topical bleaching agents

ICD-9-CM
709.00 Dyschromia, unspecified

Chondroma

DESCRIPTION Benign tumor of cartilage cells. Usual course - progressive; curable

SYNONYMS
• true chondroma
• enchondroma
• chondromyxoma

CAUSES
• cartilaginous exostoses

TREATMENT
• block excision of tumor
• combined surgery plus radiotherapy
• palliative radiotherapy for advanced disease

ICD-9-CM
213.9 Benign neoplasm of bone and articular cartilage, site unspecified

Chromomycosis

DESCRIPTION Systemic infectious fungus disease caused by Hormodendrum pedrosoi, H. compactum, or Phialophora verrucosa. Characteristics - slowly develop into large papillomatous vegetations that frequently ulcerate. Usual course - chronic. Endemic areas - worldwide; most common in tropical and subtropical areas; Brazil; Costa Rica.

SYNONYMS
• dermatomycosis
• verrucous dermatitis
• phaeohyphomycosis
• cystic chromomycosis
• cerebral chromomycosis

CAUSES
• traumatic inoculation of saprophytic soil fungi
• phialophora fungi
• Fonsecaea fungi
• cladosporium fungi

TREATMENT
• successful in inverse relation to duration and extent of infection
• antifungals: amphotericin B, flucytosine, ketoconazole
• anthelmintic: thiabendazole

ICD-9-CM
117.2 Chromoblastomycosis

Chromophobe adenoma of the pituitary

DESCRIPTION Tumor of anterior lobe of the pituitary gland whose cells do not stain with either acid or base dyes. The tumor may be non- functioning or may be associated with hyperpituitarism including acromegaly or Cushing syndrome. Usual course - progressive.

CAUSES
• increased incidence after bilateral adrenalectomy

TREATMENT
• radiotherapy for small tumors
• surgery with postoperative radiotherapy for large tumors

ICD-9-CM
227.3 Benign neoplasms of pituitary gland and craniopharyngeal duct (pouch)

Chronic pain disorder

DESCRIPTION Perceived pain that continues longer than 6 months without an accompanying injury or illness; or there is a medical problem, but it does not have a major role in causing the pain. Patients have often tried numerous medications and a variety of doctors in seeking a solution. Standard pain treatment brings only minimal relief. Characteristics include pain that is described as stinging, burning, aching. The pain may come and go, vary in intensity, duration, location and radiating pattern (moving from one body part to another); the pain may begin suddenly and increase in severity over days to weeks. Anxiety and depression are often present.

SYNONYMS
Somatoform pain disorder

CAUSES Unknown

TREATMENT
• Counseling, biofeedback, hypnosis
• Medications in some cases
• Group therapy

ICD-9-CM
306.9 Unspecified psychophysiological malfunction

Cirrhosis, cardiac

DESCRIPTION Fibrosis of the liver following central hemorrhagic necrosis associated with congestive heart failure. Usual course - chronic.

SYNONYMS
• posthepatic cirrhosis

CAUSES
• right ventricular failure
• tricuspid stenosis
• rheumatic heart disease
• cardiomyopathy
• constrictive pericarditis

TREATMENT
• fluid restriction
• diuretics
• sodium restriction
• digitalis
• rest

ICD-9-CM
571.5 Cirrhosis of liver without mention of alcohol

Cirrhosis, macronodal

DESCRIPTION Disorganization of liver structure by widespread fibrosis characterized by connective tissue bands of varying thickness and by nodules that vary in size and contain portal spaces and terminal hepatic veins. Characteristics - anorexia, fatigue, jaundice, right upper quadrant pain, ascites. Usual course - chronic; progressive.

SYNONYMS
• postnecrotic liver cirrhosis
• toxic cirrhosis
• posthepatic cirrhosis
• necrotic liver cirrhosis

CAUSES
• unknown
• possible sequela of viral hepatitis
• phosphorus intoxication
• poisons
• infection
• metabolic disorders

TREATMENT
• treat complications
• avoid drugs
• protein restriction

ICD-9-CM
571.5 Cirrhosis of liver without mention of alcohol

Cirrhosis, primary biliary

DESCRIPTION Fibrosis of the liver due to obstruction or infection of the major extra- or intrahepatic bile ducts. Characteristics include jaundice, abdominal pain, steatorrhea, and enlargement of the liver and spleen.

SYNONYMS
• Hypertrophic cirrhosis of Hanot
• Hanot syndrome
• Cholangiolitic biliary cirrhosis

CAUSES
• autoimmune

TREATMENT
• corticosteroids
• azathioprine
• penicillamine
• colchicine

ICD-9-CM
571.6 Biliary cirrhosis

SEE ALSO
• Sjögren syndrome

Colorado tick fever

DESCRIPTION A febrile illness characterized by chills, aches, vomiting, leucopenia, and sometimes encephalitis; caused by a retrovirus transmitted by the tick Dermacentor andersoni. Usual course - 3 to 7 day incubation period after tick bite; acute onset; brief symptom-free interval; second febrile illness. Endemic areas - Rocky Mountain area; western Canada.

SYNONYMS
• American mountain tick fever
• mountain tick fever

CAUSES
• arbovirus transmitted by bite of hard-shelled wood tick (dermacentor andersoni)

TREATMENT
• supportive therapy

ICD-9-CM
066.1 Tick-borne fever

Complete heart block

DESCRIPTION Characteristics - QRS interval normal (nodal pacemaker); wide and bizarre (ventricular pacemaker). No relationship between P waves and QRS complexes. No constant P-R interval.

CAUSES
• Myocardial infarction or ischemic heart disease, post-surgical valve replacement, hypoxia with syncope as with Stokes-Adams syndrome, digitalis toxicity

TREATMENT
• pacemaker

ICD-9-CM
426.0 Atrioventricular block, complete

Cor triloculare biatriatum

DESCRIPTION Three chambered heart

SYNONYMS
• single ventricle
• univentricular heart
• double inlet ventricle

CAUSES
• unknown

TREATMENT
• palliative surgery
• corrective surgery
• medical treatment of cardiac failure

ICD-9-CM
745.3 Common ventricle septal defect

Cornelia de Lange syndrome

DESCRIPTION A congenital syndrome in which severe mental retardation is associated with many abnormalities such as short stature, brachycephaly, low-set ears, webbed neck, bushy eyebrows and flat hands. Possible autosomal dominant; autosomal recessive; chromosomal mutation.

SYNONYMS
- typus degenerativus amstelodamensis
- Amsterdam dwarf syndrome of de Lange
- Brachman de Lange syndrome

CAUSES
- genetic

TREATMENT
- dependent on congenital heart disease or respiratory failure

ICD-9-CM
759.89 Other specified congenital anomalies

Cowden syndrome

DESCRIPTION Autosomal dominant hereditary disease. Characteristics - ectodermal neoplasia, microstomia, trichilemmomas of the face, acral verrucous papules. Usual course - chronic; progressive.

SYNONYMS
- multiple hamartoma syndrome

CAUSES
- ectodermal neoplasia
- mesodermal neoplasia
- malignant transformation

TREATMENT
- surgical
- chemotherapy when applicable

ICD-9-CM
759.6 Other hamartoses, NEC

Craniopharyngioma

DESCRIPTION A tumor arising from cell rests derived from the hypophyseal stalk, frequently associated with increased intracerebral pressure, and showing calcium deposits in the capsule or the tumor proper. Usual course - progressive.

SYNONYMS
- Rathke pouch tumor
- suprasellar cyst
- pituitary epidermoid tumor
- ameloblastoma
- pituitary adamantinoma

CAUSES
congenital in origin

TREATMENT
- surgery
- radiotherapy
- hormone replacement therapy

ICD-9-CM
237.0 Neoplasm of uncertain behavior of pituitary gland and craniopharyngeal duct

Creutzfeldt-Jakob disease

DESCRIPTION Rare, usually fatal, transmissible spongiform encephalopathy, occurring in middle life in which there is partial degeneration of the pyramidal and extrapyramidal systems accompanied by progressive dementia, tremor, muscle wasting, athetosis and spastic dysarthria. Usual course - progressive; 15-20 months incubation; 6 months average duration. Four subtypes described: classic, iatrogenic, familial, and new variant (nvCJD). The latter was first described in the United Kingdom in 1996 and has been linked to bovine spongiform encephalopathy (BSE), also known as "mad cow disease."

SYNONYMS
- spastic pseudosclerosis
- corticostriatal-spinal degeneration
- transmissible virus dementia

CAUSES
- Scrapie PrP (prion protein)

TREATMENT
- effective treatment unknown
- experimentally amantadine
- experimentally vidarabine

ICD-9-CM
046.1 Jakob-Creutzfeldt disease

SEE ALSO
- Kuru

REFERENCES

- Fagih B. Reuse of angioplasty catheters and risk of Creutzfeldt-Jakob disease. Am Heart J 1999 Jun;137(6):1173-8

Crigler-Najjar syndrome

DESCRIPTION Two distinct, inherited, syndromes marked by deficiencies of hepatic glucuronyl transferase. Both produce non-hemolytic unconjugated hyperbilirubinemia with jaundice.
- Type I is an autosomal recessive form. Kernicterus may develop at any age (homozygotes develop severe hyperbilirubinemia in the first few days of life). Survival into childhood is possible with intensive therapy. Patients have no response to phenobarbital.
- Type II, Arias syndrome, is an autosomal dominant form; one parent will have elevated bilirubin. Kernicterus has been reported in infants, but hyperbilirubinemia may be consistent with physiologic jaundice. Patients are responsive to phenobarbital.

SYNONYMS
- congenital hyperbilirubinemia
- glucuronyl transferase deficiency type I
- familial unconjugated hyperbilirubinemia

CAUSES
- no uridine diphosphoglucuronic transferase

TREATMENT
- exchange transfusion
- phototherapy
- cholestyramine
- phenobarbital (in Type II)

ICD-9-CM
277.4 Disorders of bilirubin excretion

Cryptosporidiosis

DESCRIPTION A gastrointestinal infection characterized by watery diarrhea and cramps, sometimes severe, produced by protozoa of the genus Cryptosporidium. Other characteristics include weight loss, nausea, vomiting and fever. Disease is self-limiting except in the immunocompromised, where it is typically chronic and may be fatal. The number of cases continues to rise.

CAUSES
- Cryptosporidium spp

TREATMENT
- no known effective therapy
- rehydration
- discontinuance of immunosuppressive drugs
- good hygiene

ICD-9-CM
136.9 Unspecified infectious and parasitic diseases

Cyanide poisoning

DESCRIPTION Cyanide inhibits mitochondrial cytochrome oxidase, resulting in decreased oxidative metabolism and oxygen utilization. Exposure to cyanide gas produces symptoms within seconds, oral absorption delays symptoms to perhaps 30 minutes. Cyanide is rapidly absorbed from mucosal surfaces and intact skin. A lethal dose of potassium cyanide is approximately 200 mg and of hydrocyanic acid (produced by exposing cyanide to stomach hydrochloric acid), approximately 50 mg. Decontaminate affected surfaces after donning appropriate protective gear (latex gloves not sufficient). Do not give mouth to mouth resuscitation.

CAUSES
- Cyanide gas, soluble cyanide salts, insoluble cyanide salts

TREATMENT
- General supportive care, high-dose oxygen
- Antidotal therapy (Lilly cyanide antidote kit) with amyl nitrite, 30 seconds of each minute with a new ampule each 3 minutes; sodium nitrite, 3% solution IV; sodium thiosulfate, 25% solution IV
- Consider hyperbaric oxygen
- Intubation may be needed

ICD-9-CM
987.7 Toxic effect of hydrocyanic acid gas
989.0 Toxic effect of hydrocyanic acid and cyanides

REFERENCES

- Fauci, Braunwald, et al. Editors, Harrison's Principles of Internal Medicine, 14th edition, 1998

Cyclosporiasis

DESCRIPTION A parasitic disease caused by Cyclospora cayetanensis transmitted by contaminated food and water (person-to-person transmission is unlikely). Low prevalence in U.S. Cases reported in Central and South America, Australia, Southeast Asia, Africa, and Europe. Infection occurs in warmer months. Incubation period 1-11 days. Onset often abrupt with symptoms of watery diarrhea, fatigue, anorexia, myalgia, abdominal cramps, flatus, nausea, fever; duration 9-43 days with periods of remission /relapse. Prolonged course typical in immunocompromised patients. Current diagnosis and detection methods have poor sensitivity and specificity.

CAUSES Cyclospora cayetanensis (a coccidian)

TREATMENT
- Trimethoprim-sulfamethoxazole

ICD-9-CM
007.5 Cyclosporiasis

Dehydration

DESCRIPTION Extracellular fluid volume depletion. Routes of loss are from the gastrointestinal tract, urinary tract, and skin.
- Characteristics - signs and symptoms include diminished skin turgor, diminished intraocular tension, dry shrunken tongue, low central venous pressure (measured from neck veins), postural hypotension, tachycardia, disorientation, shock, increased hematocrit.

CAUSES Excessive loss of fluid from the gastrointestinal tract, urinary tract and skin. Conditions favoring excess loss include vomiting, diarrhea, gastric suction, excessive sweating, dialysis, chronic renal failure, salt-wasting renal disease, interstitial nephritis, myeloma, acute real failure, diuretic therapy, diabetes mellitus with ketoacidosis or extreme glycosuria, Bartter syndrome, adrenal disease (glucocorticoid deficiency), hypoaldosteronism.

TREATMENT
- fluid and electrolyte replacement
- discontinue diuretics

ICD-9-CM
276.5 Volume depletion

Delirium tremens

DESCRIPTION Severe alcohol withdrawal syndrome characterized by agitation, violence, anxiety, insomnia, muscle cramps, tremor, delusion, hallucinations, ataxia, fever, with clearing beginning in 12-24 hours up to 2-10 days. Usual course - acute; relapsing.

SYNONYMS
- alcohol withdrawal delirium

CAUSES
- cessation in alcohol consumption after heavy alcohol ingestion

TREATMENT
- benzodiazepines
- barbiturates
- beta-adrenergic blockers

ICD-9-CM
291.0 Alcohol withdrawal delirium

Dengue fever

DESCRIPTION Acute, self-limited disease. Characteristics include fever, prostration, headache, myalgia, rash, lymphadenopathy, leukopenia, Caused by four antigenically related but distinct types of the dengue virus. Endemic areas are tropics and subtropics.

SYNONYMS
- breakbone fever

CAUSES
- Aedes aegypti mosquito vector
- group B arbovirus
- flavivirus

TREATMENT
- symptomatic
- supportive if hemorrhagic

ICD-9-CM
061 Dengue

Diffuse esophageal spasm

DESCRIPTION Retching, chest pain, dysphagia, and regurgitation associated to esophageal motor dysfunction. Usual course - progressive; intermittent.

CAUSES
- esophageal motor dysfunction

TREATMENT
- anticholinergics
- nitrates
- esophageal dilatation

ICD-9-CM
530.5 Dyskinesia of esophagus

DiGeorge syndrome

DESCRIPTION An embryonic fault in the derivation of the thymus and parathyroid glands. Also with defects in the aortic arch and heart, hypoplastic mandible, defective ears, and short philtrum. Marked variability occurs, but patient with this syndrome must have both parathyroid dysfunction (lack of PTH) and T-cell dysfunction.

SYNONYMS
N/A

CAUSES
- congenital

TREATMENT
- thymic transplantation

ICD-9-CM
279.11 DiGeorge syndrome

Diphtheria of the skin

DESCRIPTION Occurs when any disruption of the skin becomes colonized by C. Diphtheriae. Poor personal and community hygiene are particular risk factors. Lesions are punched out ulcers and appear on extremities. Usual course - acute. Endemic areas - tropics; Pacific Northwest; Southwest USA.

SYNONYMS
- cutaneous diphtheria

CAUSES
- corynebacterium diphtheriae
- skin trauma
- poor hygiene

TREATMENT
- intramuscular diphtheria antitoxin
- penicillin
- erythromycin
- quarantine

ICD-9-CM
032.85 Cutaneous diphtheria

Dubin-Johnson syndrome

DESCRIPTION Rare autosomal recessive disorder characterized by various organic anions as well as bilirubin. The hyperbilirubinemia is conjugated and bile appears in the urine. Rotor syndrome is a variant differentiated by liver histology. Splenomegaly occurs in half of patients and jaundice may occur as early as age 5. Usual course - intermittent.

SYNONYMS
- chronic idiopathic jaundice
- Dubin-Sprinz disease

CAUSES
- impaired intrahepatic bilirubin secretion
- conjugated hyperbilirubinemia

TREATMENT
- decrease bilirubin with phenobarbital

ICD-9-CM
277.4 Disorders of bilirubin excretion

Dyslexia

DESCRIPTION Disparity between intellectual potential and achievement in reading and spelling. Characteristics - normal, intelligent child 2 years behind expected reading level for his grade. Affects children in all socioeconomic levels. Affects more boys than girls.
Signs and symptoms include:
- ◊ Confusion in orientation of letters
- ◊ Reading from right to left
- ◊ Letter and word reversals
- ◊ Omitting words
- ◊ Losing place on a page
- ◊ Images appear blurred
- ◊ Frustration symptoms - behavioral problems, delinquency, withdrawal
- ◊ Cognitive abilities may take over by age 7 or 8 years in some children

SYNONYMS
- congenital word blindness
- primary reading disability

CAUSES
- unknown

TREATMENT
- remedial, corrective, compensatory education. Balance child's academic difficulties with enjoyable successful activities.

ICD-9-CM
784.61 Alexia and dyslexia

Ebola virus hemorrhagic fever

DESCRIPTION Ebola is caused by a virus with an unknown natural source, but transmitted between humans (and infected monkeys). Symptoms occur 4-16 days after infection with fever, chills, headache, myalgia, and anorexia. Vomiting, diarrhea, abdominal pain, sore throat, chest pain, and impaired blood coagulation occur later. Approximately 600 fatalities have been reported (in Africa) since the initial outbreak in 1976. (10)

CAUSES
- Filovirus (RNA virus)

TREATMENT
- Supportive

ICD-9-CM
079.89 Other specified viral infection

Echinococcosis of the lung

DESCRIPTION Infection of the lung with hydatid cysts of the larvae of small tapeworms of the family Taeniidae. Usual course - progressive; 5-20 year latency. Endemic areas - Middle East; Australia; South Africa; South America; Central Europe.

CAUSES
- larval echinococcus granulosus
- canine fecal contamination
- childhood ingestion of contaminated material

TREATMENT
- surgical cystectomy

ICD-9-CM
122.1 Echinococcus granulosus infection of lung

Ecthyma

DESCRIPTION An ulcerative pyoderma usually caused by group A beta-hemolytic streptococcal infection at the site of minor trauma, predominantly of the shins and feet. Healing is with variable scar formation. Usual course - acute; progression of vesiculopustule to crusts to ulceration.

CAUSES
- bacterial infection (streptococcal, staphylococcal)
- poor hygiene
- minor injuries

TREATMENT
- antibiotics
- good hygiene
- proper nutrition

ICD-9-CM
686.8 Other specific local infections of skin & subcutaneous tissue

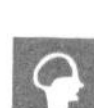

Ectrodactyly, ectodermal dysplasia, clefting syndrome

DESCRIPTION A congenital ectodermal dysplasia. Characteristics - lobster claw deformity, cleft lip, cleft palate, decreased hair growth, photophobic ectrodactyly, syndactyly. Usual course - chronic; progressive.

SYNONYMS
- EEC syndrome

CAUSES
- unknown

TREATMENT
- oral surgery
- ophthalmologic surgery
- orthopedic surgery

ICD-9-CM
757.31 Congenital ectodermal dysplasia

Ehlers-Danlos syndrome

DESCRIPTION A group of inherited disorders of the connective tissue occurring in many types based on clinical, genetic and biochemical evidence, varying in severity from mild to lethal. Transmitted as autosomal recessive, autosomal dominant, or X-linked recessive traits. The major manifestations include hyperextensibility of skin and joints, easy bruising, friability of tissues with bleeding and poor wound healing, calcified subcutaneous spheroids and pseudotumors, and cardiovascular, gastrointestinal, orthopedic, and ocular defects. Usual course: chronic; progressive.

CAUSES
- probable defective cross-linkage of collagen

TREATMENT
- symptomatic
- preventive
- prolonged wound fixation
- conservative surgical repair

ICD-9-CM
756.83 Ehlers-Danlos syndrome

Ehrlichiosis

DESCRIPTION A life-threatening disease, transmitted by ticks, occurring as two distinct clinical entities: HME (Human Monocytic Ehrlichiosis) and HGE (Human Granulocytic Ehrlichiosis). HME occurs primarily in the south-central, southeastern, and mid-Atlantic regions in the U.S. and in Europe and Africa and is transmitted by the Lone Star tick (Amblyomma americanum), while HGE occurs in the upper midwest and northeastern states and is transmitted by ticks of the genus Ixodes. Patients present 1-3 weeks after tick bite with fever, headache, myalgia and other non-specific complaints. Treatment should begin if tick bite is suspected and especially if leukopenia and thrombocytopenia are found. Serologic confirmation is possible during convalescence if antibodies to E. chaffeensis are found.

CAUSES
- Ehrlichia chaffeensis (HME)
- Ehrlichia equi-like organism (HGE)

TREATMENT
- Doxycycline 100 mg BID

ICD-9-CM
082.8 Other specified tick-borne rickettsioses

Elephantiasis, filarial

DESCRIPTION A chronic disease of the tropics due to infection of the lymphatic channels characterized by inflammation and obstruction of the lymphatics and hypertrophy of the skin and subcutaneous tissues. Usual course - acute; chronic; progressive. Endemic areas - South America; Africa; Asia; tropics; subtropics.

SYNONYMS
- Filariasis
- Wuchereriasis
- Lymphatic filariasis

CAUSES
- microfilariae
- Wuchereria bancrofti
- Brugia malayi
- mosquito vector

TREATMENT
- diethylcarbamazine citrate
- plastic surgery
- fulguration
- elastic stockings

ICD-9-CM
125.9 Unspecified filariasis
457.1 Other lymphedema

Empyema

DESCRIPTION Presence of pus in a hollow organ or body cavity, particularly the pleural cavity. Usual course - acute.

CAUSES
- purulent inflammatory exudate of pleural cavity
- pulmonary infection
- thoracic surgery
- esophageal perforation
- hematogenous spread from other sites
- idiopathic
- subphrenic abscess

TREATMENT
- drainage
- antimicrobial therapy

ICD-9-CM
510.9 Empyema without mention of fistula

Encephalitis, Saint Louis

DESCRIPTION A viral disease first observed in Illinois in 1932, closely similar to western equine encephalomyelitis. It occurs in late summer and early fall. Transmitted usually by mosquitoes of the genus Culex. It ranges from an abortive type of infection to severe disease. Endemic areas - Eastern USA; Midwestern USA.

CAUSES
- group B arbovirus
- transmitted by Culex mosquito

TREATMENT
- supportive

ICD-9-CM
062.3 St. Louis encephalitis

Endomyocardial fibrosis, eosinophilic

DESCRIPTION Idiopathic myocardiopathy occurring endemically in various regions of Africa, characterized by cardiomegaly, marked thickening of the endocardium with dense, white fibrous tissue that frequently extends to involve the inner third or half of the myocardium.

SYNONYMS
- Loeffler endomyocardial fibrosis
- Loeffler fibroplastic parietal endocarditis

CAUSES
- unknown
- possibly eosinophil disorder

TREATMENT
- inotropic support
- fluid restriction plus diuretics
- anticoagulants
- immunosuppression
- valve replacement
- Glenn shunt

ICD-9-CM
425.0 Endomyocardial fibrosis

Eosinophilic fasciitis

DESCRIPTION Inflammation of the fascia of the extremities caused by unusual strenuous exercise. Usual course - acute; progressive; relapsing.

CAUSES
- unusual strenuous physical exercise
- inflammatory reaction due to chemotactic collagen breakdown products

TREATMENT
- corticosteroids
- non-steroidal anti-inflammatory drugs

ICD-9-CM
729.4 Fasciitis, unspecified

SEE ALSO
- Scleroderma
- Sjögren syndrome

Eosinophilic gastroenteritis

DESCRIPTION A disorder characterized by infiltration of the mucosa of the small intestine by eosinophils, with edema but without vasculitis. Symptoms include diarrhea, abdominal pain, nausea, fever, malabsorption. The stomach is also frequently involved. This disorder is commonly associated with intolerance to specific foods. Usual course: -chronic; recurrent.

CAUSES
- food allergy
- idiopathic

TREATMENT
- exclusionary diets
- prednisone

ICD-9-CM
558.9 Other and unspecified noninfectious gastroenteritis and colitis

Epithelial mesothelioma

DESCRIPTION A malignant tumor derived from mesothelial tissue of the pleura, with some regions containing spindle-shaped, sarcoma-like cells and other regions showing adenomatous patterns. Usual course - progressive.

CAUSES
- asbestos
- tobacco smoking

TREATMENT
- surgical resection for solitary lesion
- palliative radiotherapy for advanced disease
- palliative chemotherapy for advanced disease
- pleurocentesis for pleural effusion

ICD-9-CM
163.9 Malignant neoplasm of pleura, unspecified

Erythema marginatum

DESCRIPTION Superficial, often asymptomatic, form of gyrate erythema associated with some cases of rheumatic fever. Characterized by presence on the trunk and extensor surfaces of the extremities of a transient eruption of flat to slightly indurated, non-scaling multiple lesions. Usual course - acute.

CAUSES
- rheumatic fever

TREATMENT
- treat underlying disease

ICD-9-CM
695.0 Erythema marginatum

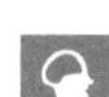

Ewing sarcoma

DESCRIPTION Malignant tumor of bone arising in medullary tissue, occurring more often in cylindrical bones. Prominent symptoms include pain, fever and leukocytosis. Usual course - acute; relapsing probable.

CAUSES
- enchondroma
- aneurysmal bone cyst

TREATMENT
- cyclophosphamide
- possibly surgery
- megavoltage radiotherapy
- vincristine
- actinomycin D
- adriamycin

ICD-9-CM
170.9 Malignant neoplasm of bone and articular cartilage, site unspecified

Fabry disease

DESCRIPTION An x-linked lysosomal storage disease of glycosphingolipid catabolism. Usual course - progressive.

SYNONYMS
- glycosphingolipidosis
- angiokeratoma corporis diffusum
- ceramide trihexoside lipoidosis

CAUSES
- alpha-galactosidase a deficiency
- ceramide trihexosidase deficiency

TREATMENT
- analgesic
- phenytoin
- carbamazepine
- corticosteroid

ICD-9-CM
272.7 Lipidoses

Factor X deficiency

DESCRIPTION Deficiency of Factor X, a storage-stable factor essential to the clotting process that participates both in the intrinsic and extrinsic pathways of blood coagulation. Usually inherited as an autosomal recessive trait, though it can be acquired. It is characterized by defective activity in both the intrinsic and extrinsic pathways, impaired thromboplastin time, and impaired prothrombin consumption. Usual course - chronic; intermittent.

SYNONYMS
- Stuart-Prower factor deficiency

CAUSES
- inherited metabolic abnormality

TREATMENT
- fresh frozen plasma for hemorrhagic episodes

ICD-9-CM
286.3 Congenital deficiency of other clotting factors

SEE ALSO
- Hemophilia

Familial Mediterranean fever

DESCRIPTION Hereditary disease transmitted in an autosomal recessive manner, usually occurring in Armenians and Sephardic Jews. Characteristics include short, recurrent attacks of fever with pain in the abdomen, chest, or joints and erythema resembling that seen in erysipelas. It is sometimes complicated by amyloidosis. Usual course - intermittent.

SYNONYMS
- paroxysmal polyserositis
- familial recurrent polyserositis
- periodic fever
- periodic disease

CAUSES Genetic

TREATMENT
- colchicine

ICD-9-CM
277.3 Amyloidosis

Familial neonatal hyperbilirubinemia

DESCRIPTION Transient familial form of hyperbilirubinemia with onset of jaundice within four days after birth. This form can lead to kernicterus.

SYNONYMS
- transient familial neonatal hyperbilirubinemia

CAUSES
- unknown

TREATMENT
- exchange transfusion

ICD-9-CM
774.6 Unspecified fetal and neonatal jaundice

Fanconi syndrome

DESCRIPTION A general term for a disorder marked by dysfunction of the proximal tubules of the kidney, with generalized hyperaminoaciduria, renal glycosuria, hyperphosphaturia, and water and bicarbonate loss. It occurs in genetic and acquired forms.

CAUSES
- multiple myeloma
- amyloidosis
- Sjogren syndrome
- nephrotic syndrome
- renal transplantation
- vitamin D deficiency
- lead
- mercury
- cadmium
- uranium
- strontium
- tetracycline
- maleic acid
- cystinosis
- Wilson disease
- galactosemia
- hereditary fructose intolerance
- tyrosinemia
- Lowe syndrome

TREATMENT
- no specific treatment
- Shohl's solution
- potassium replacement

ICD-9-CM
270.0 Disturbances of amino-acid transport

Fascioliasis

DESCRIPTION Infection with a trematode worm found in the small intestines of residents in many parts of Asia. Intermediate hosts are snails. Characteristics include nausea, diarrhea, and malabsorption. Usual course - acute; chronic; progressive; 3 month incubation.

CAUSES
- fasciola hepatica

TREATMENT
- praziquantel

ICD-9-CM
121.3 Fascioliasis

Fasciolopsiasis

DESCRIPTION The state of being infected with flukes of the trematode worm genus Fasciolopsis. Characteristics - asymptomatic. Usual course - chronic; progressive. Endemic areas - Southern China; Southeast Asia; Indian subcontinent.

CAUSES
- fasciolopsis buski

TREATMENT
- praziquantel

ICD-9-CM
121.4 Fasciolopsiasis

Fatigue

DESCRIPTION A state of discomfort and decreased efficiency resulting from prolonged or excessive exertion or loss of power (from any cause) to respond appropriately to stimulation.
- Characteristics - closely related to approximately equal terms: Lassitude, tiredness, lethargy, malaise, and ennui

CAUSES Drugs, overexertion, Addison disease, alcohol, anemia, chronic fatigue syndrome (Epstein-Barr virus infection has unclear, possible association), diabetes mellitus, emotional problems (depression, somatization disorder), emphysema, endocarditis, environmental toxins, hepatitis, inadequate nutrition, inadequate rest, infectious mononucleosis, intestinal parasites, malignancies, myasthenia gravis, obesity, poor physical conditioning, rheumatoid arthritis, sedative-hypnotics, systemic lupus erythematosus, thyroid disease, tuberculosis, and others.

TREATMENT
- treat underlying disorder

ICD-9-CM
780.79 Other malaise and fatigue

Favism

DESCRIPTION Hemolytic anemia due to the ingestion of fava beans or after inhalation of pollen from the Vicia fava plant by person with glucose-6-phosphate dehydrogenase deficient erythrocytes. Usual course - acute; chronic; intermittent; relapsing. Endemic areas - malarial endemic areas; worldwide.

CAUSES
- acute hemolysis
- fava bean ingestion
- vicia faba ingestion
- Mediterranean type glucose-6-phosphate dehydrogenase deficiency

TREATMENT
- supportive
- transfusion
- folic acid
- maintain adequate urine output
- alkalinize urine

ICD-9-CM
282.2 Anemias due to disorders of glutathione metabolism

Felty syndrome

DESCRIPTION Chronic rheumatoid arthritis with leukopenia, splenomegaly, pigmented skin spots on the extremities, anemia, and thrombocytopenia. Usual course - chronic.

SYNONYMS
- rheumatoid arthritis-hypersplenism syndrome

CAUSES
- rheumatoid arthritis

TREATMENT
- splenectomy

ICD-9-CM
714.1 Felty syndrome

Fetal alcohol syndrome

DESCRIPTION A syndrome found in infants whose mothers have consumed alcohol during pregnancy. Signs include microcephaly, short palpebral fissures, flat midface, underdeveloped philtrum and thin upper lip. Other, less common signs include low nasal bridge, epicanthal folds, minor ear anomalies, short nose, and micrognathia. Intrauterine or postnatal growth retardation, mental retardation or other neurologic abnormality and two or more of the facial features are needed for the diagnosis.

CAUSES
- Alcohol ingestion during pregnancy. All trimesters have

been associated with abnormalities and no lower limit of alcohol dose is known. Therefore, alcohol consumption during pregnancy should be avoided entirely.

TREATMENT
- Counseling pregnant women
- Patient interventions include behavioral (special education, setting realistic family expectations), surgical (cardiac defects), dental (caries are common), ophthalmic (vision correction), and others as appropriate.

ICD-9-CM
760.71 Fetal alcohol syndrome

REFERENCES

- Lewis DD, Scott WE. Fetal Alcohol Syndrome. American Family Physician. Oct 94:1025-1031.

Filariasis

DESCRIPTION Infection with the filarial worm, Wuchereria bancrofti. The adult worms migrate to the lymphatic system producing recurrent lymphangitis with obstruction and fibrosis. Edema progresses to elephantiasis. Transmitted by mosquitoes, which harbor the larval forms. Usual course - chronic; relapsing; 8-12 month incubation. Endemic areas - Africa; Pacific islands; Southeast Asia; West Indies; Central America; eastern coastal plains of South America.

SYNONYMS
- bancroftian filariasis
- Malayan filariasis
- lymphatic filariasis
- Filarioidea infection

CAUSES
- adult filarial worms
- Wuchereria bancrofti
- Brugia malayi
- Brugia timori
- lymphatic obstruction

TREATMENT
- diethylcarbamazine
- treat hypersensitivity to dying parasite
- aspirin
- antihistamine
- steroids

ICD-9-CM
125.9 Unspecified filariasis

SEE ALSO
- Tropical eosinophilia

First degree AV block

DESCRIPTION P-R interval prolonged to greater than .20 seconds. Normal QRS complex. Usually asymptomatic.

CAUSES
- anterior or inferior myocardial infarction, hypothyroidism, digitalis toxicity, potassium imbalance

TREATMENT
- correct underlying cause
- use caution with use of digitalis

ICD-9-CM
426.11 First degree atrioventricular block

Floppy infant syndrome

DESCRIPTION Congenital myopathy marked by hypotonia and muscle weakness

CAUSES
- CNS diseases, atonic diplegia, congenital cerebellar ataxia, kernicterus, chromosomal defects, oculocerebrorenal syndrome, cerebral lipidoses, Prader-Willi syndrome, spinal cord diseases, spinal cord trauma, Werdnig-Hoffmann disease, peripheral nerve diseases, polyneuritis, familial dysautonomia, congenital sensory neuropathy, neuromuscular junction diseases, myasthenia gravis, infantile botulism, muscle diseases, congenital muscular dystrophy, myotonic dystrophy, glycogen storage disease of muscle and heart, central core disease, nemaline myopathy, mitochondrial myopathies

TREATMENT
- treat underlying disorder

ICD-9-CM
781.99 Other symptoms involving nervous and musculoskeletal systems

SEE ALSO
- Botulism
- Guillain-Barré syndrome
- Kernicterus
- Myasthenia gravis
- Prader-Willi/Angelman syndrome

Forbes-Albright syndrome

DESCRIPTION Galactorrhea-amenorrhea syndrome usually associated with a pituitary tumor. There is no relationship to pregnancy. Usual course - chronic; indolent.

SYNONYMS
- amenorrhea-galactorrhea syndrome
- nonpuerperal galactorrhea

CAUSES
- pituitary prolactinoma

TREATMENT
- bromocriptine
- surgery

ICD-9-CM
253.1 Other and unspecified anterior pituitary hyperfunction

Formaldehyde poisoning

DESCRIPTION Unusual poisoning with formaldehyde due to occupational exposure. Toxic symptoms include gastrointestinal upsets, vascular collapse and coma. 60 mL of 40% formalin can cause fatality. Usual course - acute; chronic; progressive. Endemic areas - occupational exposure.

CAUSES
- cytotoxicity
- conversion to formic acid

TREATMENT
- activated charcoal
- supportive
- bicarbonate infusion
- avoid emetics
- avoid lavage

ICD-9-CM
989.8 Formaldehyde poisoning

Friedreich ataxia

DESCRIPTION Autosomal recessive disease beginning in childhood or youth. Characteristics include sclerosis of the dorsal and lateral columns of the spinal cord. symptoms include ataxia, speech impairment, lateral curvature of the spinal column, peculiar swaying and irregular movements, and paralysis of the muscles of the lower extremities. Usual course - chronic; progressive.

SYNONYMS
- spinocerebellar ataxia
- familial ataxia
- hereditary ataxia of Friedreich
- hereditary spinal ataxia

CAUSES
- usually hereditary

TREATMENT
- surgery for scoliosis
- intervention for heart disease

ICD-9-CM
334.0 Friedreich ataxia

Gardner syndrome

DESCRIPTION An autosomal dominant disorder characterized by familial polyposis of the large bowel, with supernumerary teeth, fibrous dysplasia of the skull, osteomas, fibromas and epithelial cysts. The polyps of the large bowel have malignant potential. Usual course - progressive.

SYNONYMS
- intestinal polyposis III
- polyposis-osteomatosis-epidermoid cyst

CAUSES
- genetic

TREATMENT
- total colectomy

ICD-9-CM
211.3 Benign neoplasm of colon

Gastroenteritis, viral

DESCRIPTION Acute inflammation of the lining of the stomach and intestines accompanied by fever and caused by any one of a number of viruses. Usual course - acute.

SYNONYMS
- epidemic diarrhea
- winter vomiting disease

CAUSES
- rotavirus
- adenovirus
- astrovirus
- Norwalk-like agents
- coxsackievirus
- echovirus

TREATMENT
- fluid replacement
- bismuth subsalicylate

ICD-9-CM
008.69 Other viral enteritis

Gaucher disease

DESCRIPTION Hereditary disorder of glucocerebroside metabolism, usually occurring in infancy, and characterized by mental retardation, bulbar palsy, opisthotonus and enlargement of the spleen and liver. Usual course - acute; progressive.

SYNONYMS
- cerebroside lipoidosis

CAUSES
- beta-glucosidase deficiency
- glucocerebroside accumulation

TREATMENT
- splenectomy for hemorrhage
- orthopedic immobilization
- bone marrow transplantation
- analgesics

ICD-9-CM
272.7 Lipidoses

Geotrichosis

DESCRIPTION An oral, bronchial, pulmonary or intestinal fungal infection. Symptoms include cough, mucopurulent gelatinous sputum (streaked with blood), mouth lesions resembling thrush, fever. Prognosis - uneventful.

CAUSES
- Geotrichum candidum

TREATMENT
- gentian violet
- oral potassium iodide for pulmonary infections

ICD-9-CM
117.9 Other and unspecifed mycoses

Gestational trophoblastic neoplasm

DESCRIPTION A tumor usually arising in the uterus developing from hydatidiform mole,(50%), following abortion (24%), or during normal pregnancy (22%). Usual course - slow onset; curable. Endemic areas - Asia.

SYNONYMS
- choriocarcinoma
- chorioadenoma destruens
- hydatidiform mole

CAUSES
- increasing age

TREATMENT
- hydatidiform mole: removal of mole
- hysterectomy
- stage I: chemotherapy with optional hysterectomy
- stage II: chemotherapy with recommended hysterectomy
- stage III: combination chemotherapy with optional hysterectomy
- stage IV: combination chemotherapy with local radiotherapy plus optional surgery

ICD-9-CM
239.5 Neoplasms of unspecified nature of other genitourinary organs

Giant hypertrophic gastritis

DESCRIPTION Excessive proliferation of the gastric mucosa, producing diffuse thickening of the stomach wall. Frequently associated with inflammatory changes. Usual course - chronic. The presence of diffuse carcinoma; diffuse lymphoma; Zollinger-Ellison syndrome nearly excludes this diagnosis.

SYNONYMS
- Menetrier disease
- protein-losing gastroenteropathy

CAUSES
- idiopathic

TREATMENT
- observation
- H2-receptor blockers
- anticholinergic medications
- vagotomy
- antifibrinolytic medications
- partial gastrectomy

ICD-9-CM
535.20 Gastric mucosal hypertrophy without mention of hemorrhage

Glioblastoma multiforme

DESCRIPTION Astrocytoma of grade III or IV. Characteristics include rapid growth, confinement to the cerebral hemispheres and cell types of a mixture of spongioblasts, astroblasts, and astrocytes. Headache, vomiting, and personality changes comprise prominent symptoms. Most likely in males ages 40-75 years. Usual course - progressive over months.

SYNONYMS
- grade 3 and 4 astrocytoma
- spongioblastoma multiforme

CAUSES Unknown

TREATMENT
- surgical excision plus radiotherapy plus chemotherapy

ICD-9-CM
191.9 Malignant neoplasm of brain, unspecified

Globus hystericus

DESCRIPTION A condition in which the patient has a sense of fullness or lump in the throat. However, no difficulty is encountered when actually swallowing (i.e., not true dysphagia).

CAUSES
- Anxiety disorders

TREATMENT
Antianxiety agents may be needed although simple reassurance is usually sufficient.

ICD-9-CM
300.11 Conversion disorder

SEE ALSO
- Dysphagia

Glomerulonephritis, membranous

DESCRIPTION A disease of the glomerulus manifested clinically by proteinuria, and sometimes by other features of the nephrotic syndrome. Histologically characterized by deposits in the glomerular capillary wall between the epithelial cell and the basement membrane and a thickening of the membrane. Also characteristic are outward projections of the membrane between the epithelial deposits in the form of "spikes". There is some agreement that the deposits are antigen-antibody complexes. Usual course - progressive.

SYNONYMS
- membranous glomerulopathy
- membranous nephropathy
- extramembranous glomerulopathy
- idiopathic membranous glomerulonephritis
- idiopathic membranous nephropathy
- MGN

CAUSES
- idiopathic
- circulating antigen-antibody complexes

TREATMENT
- steroids
- cytotoxic drugs

ICD-9-CM
583.1 Nephritis and nephropathy, not specified as acute or chronic, with lesion of membranous glomerulonephritis

Glomerulonephritis, rapidly progressive

DESCRIPTION Acute glomerulonephritis marked by a rapid progression to end-stage renal failure and, histologically, by profuse epithetical proliferation. The principal signs are anuria, proteinuria, hematuria, and anemia. Usual course - progressive.

SYNONYMS
- extracapillary glomerulonephritis

CAUSES
- idiopathic

TREATMENT
- corticosteroids
- azathioprine
- cyclophosphamide
- anticoagulants
- plasmapheresis
- renal transplantation

ICD-9-CM
583.4 Nephritis and nephropathy, not specified as acute or chronic, with lesion of rapidly progressive glomerulonephritis

Glomerulopathy, membranous

DESCRIPTION A noninflammatory disease of the renal glomerulus. Characteristics - edema, hypertension, subendothelial immune deposits, thickened glomerular basement membrane.

SYNONYMS
- membranous nephropathy

CAUSES
- idiopathic
- drugs
- penicillamine
- gold
- captopril
- hepatitis B
- parasitic infestation
- SLE
- malignancy
- NSAID

TREATMENT
- corticosteroids
- antimetabolites
- antiplatelet drugs
- anticoagulants

ICD-9-CM
583.1 Nephritis and nephropathy, not specified as acute or chronic, with lesion of membranous glomerulonephritis

Glomus jugulare

DESCRIPTION A tumor (nonchromaffin paraganglioma or glomus tympanicum) arising in the temporal bone or the middle ear. Signs including a red, pulsatile mass in the middle ear. Symptoms include tinnitus, hearing loss, and vertigo.

SYNONYMS
- Glomus tympanicum
- Nonchromaffin paraganglioma

CAUSES
- Unknown

TREATMENT
- Excision
- Palliative radiotherapy

ICD-9-CM
194.6 Malignant neoplasm of aortic body and other paraganglia

Glossopharyngeal neuralgia

DESCRIPTION Rare disease of the 9th cranial nerve (glossopharyngeal). Characteristics - paroxysms of sharp, darting pain affecting the posterior pharynx, base of tongue, jaw.

CAUSES Rare tumor (nasopharyngeal or other intracranial tumor), trauma, usually no known cause

TREATMENT
- carbamazepine with or without phenytoin
- surgery

ICD-9-CM
352.1 Glossopharyngeal neuralgia

Glucagonoma

DESCRIPTION Glucagon-secreting tumor of the pancreatic alpha cells characterized by a distinctive rash, weight loss, stomatitis, glossitis, diabetes, hypoaminoacidemia, and normochromic normocytic anemia. Usual course - progressive.

SYNONYMS
- alpha cell tumor
- alpha-cell adenoma

CAUSES
• unknown

TREATMENT
• surgical enucleation to partial pancreatectomy
• fluorouracil plus streptozotocin for unresectable tumor

ICD-9-CM
235.5 Neoplasm of uncertain behavior of other and unspecified digestive organs

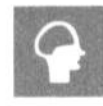

Goodpasture syndrome, pulmonary component

DESCRIPTION Glomerulonephritis associated with pulmonary hemorrhage and circulating antibodies against basement membrane antigens. This condition exists most frequently in young men. It has a course of rapidly progressive renal failure with hemoptysis, pulmonary infiltrates, and dyspnea. Usual course - chronic.

CAUSES Unknown

TREATMENT
• corticosteroids
• cytotoxic agents
• plasmapheresis

ICD-9-CM
446.20 Hypersensitivity angiitis, unspecified

Goodpasture syndrome, renal component

DESCRIPTION Glomerulonephritis occurring most often in young men accompanied by rapidly progressive renal failure. Other characteristics include hemoptysis, dyspnea, and pulmonary infiltrates. Usual course - progressive.

CAUSES
• anti-glomerular basement membrane antibody

TREATMENT
• corticosteroids
• plasmapheresis
• cyclophosphamides
• renal transplantation

ICD-9-CM
446.21 Goodpasture syndrome

Granuloma inguinale

DESCRIPTION Genital ulcers (not to be confused with lymphogranuloma inguinale) caused by Donovania granulomatis; also called donovanosis. Diagnosis is by demonstration of typical intracellular Donovan bodies in crushed-tissue smears. Usual course - acute; progressive; relapsing; indolent. Endemic areas - tropics; subtropics.

SYNONYMS
• donovanosis
• donovania
• granuloma venereum

CAUSES
• sexual transmission
• Calymmatobacterium granulomatous
• fomites
• autoinoculation

TREATMENT
• antibiotics

ICD-9-CM
099.2 Granuloma inguinale

Granulomatous disease of childhood, chronic

DESCRIPTION A group of immunodeficiency of X-linked or autosomal recessive inheritance, caused by failure of the respiratory or metabolic burst resulting in deficient microbicidal activity. Characteristics - patients sustain frequent, severe, and prolonged bacterial and fungal infections. Usual course - chronic.

SYNONYMS
• congenital dysphagocytosis
• familial chronic granulomatosis
• septic progressive granulomatosis

CAUSES
• bacterial infection
• fungal infection
• defective phagocytic cell microbicidal activity
• abnormal oxidative metabolism during phagocytosis

TREATMENT
• antibiotics

ICD-9-CM
686.1 Pyogenic granuloma

HAIR-AN syndrome

DESCRIPTION A multisystem disorder affecting girls and women that consists of hyperandrogenism (HA), insulin resistance (IR) and acanthosis nigricans (AN). Originally thought to be rare, recent studies estimate that insulin resistance and acanthosis nigricans may be present in 1-3% of all hyperandrogenic women. Probably been underdiagnosed because of failure to recognize the characteristic abnormalities of this disorder. Chronic hyperinsulinemia resulting from insulin resistance stimulates the increased ovarian secretion of androgens and the proliferation of the epidermis, which results in hirsutism, virilization, and AN.

CAUSES Insulin resistance and hyperandrogenism are caused by genetic and environmental factors

TREATMENT
• Estrogen-progesterone oral contraceptives
• Antiandrogen therapy alone or in combination with oral contraceptives
• Weight loss helpful

ICD-9-CM
701.2 Acquired acanthosis nigricans

Halitosis

DESCRIPTION Unpleasant odor to the breath. Characteristics - gastrointestinal disorders do not generally cause halitosis, so breath odor does not reflect the state of digestive system or bowel function.

CAUSES
• inhaled substances
• ingested substances
• gingival disease
• dental disease
• food fermentation in mouth
• systemic disease (tonsillitis, pneumonia, bronchiectasis, lung abscess)
• hepatic encephalopathy
• diabetic acidosis
• infectious diseases
• neoplastic disease of the respiratory tract
• hypochondriasis

TREATMENT
• treat any discovered specific cause
• attentive listening
• assurance regarding benign nature (if appropriate)

ICD-9-CM
784.9 Other symptoms involving head and neck

Hallervorden-Spatz disease

DESCRIPTION Autosomal recessive hereditary disorder usually beginning in first or second decade. Characteristics include marked reduction in the number of myelin sheaths of the globus pallidus and substantia nigra, progressive rigidity in legs, dysarthria, choreoathetoid movements, and progressive mental degeneration. Usual course - chronic; progressive.

SYNONYMS
• pigmentary pallidal degeneration syndrome
• progressive pallidal degeneration syndrome
• late infantile neuroaxonal dystrophy

CAUSES
• genetic

TREATMENT
• levodopa
• tryptophan
• megavitamins

ICD-9-CM
333.0 Other degenerative diseases of the basal ganglia

Hand-foot-and-mouth disease

DESCRIPTION Usually mild and self-limited exanthematous eruption most often caused by Coxsackievirus. It occurs primary in preschool children. Characteristics include vesicles on the buccal mucosa, tongue, soft palate, gingivae, and hand and feet, including the palms and soles. Usual course - subacute; chronic; recurrent.

CAUSES
• coxsackie virus

TREATMENT
• symptomatic

ICD-9-CM
074.3 Hand, foot, and mouth disease

Hand-Schuller-Christian syndrome

DESCRIPTION Disseminated, chronic form of Langerhans-cell histiocytosis. May exhibit the classic triad of exophthalmos, diabetes insipidus and bone destruction. Usual course - chronic; remission.

SYNONYMS
• craniohypophyseal xanthoma
• idiopathic chronic xanthomatosis
• multifocal eosinophilic granuloma
• histiocytosis x
• Schueller-Christian Disease

CAUSES
• eosinophilic infiltration

TREATMENT
• chemotherapy
• access to free water

ICD-9-CM
277.89 Other specified disorders of metabolism

SEE ALSO • Letterer-Siwe disease

Hantavirus

DESCRIPTION A genus of the Bunyaviridae family responsible for pneumonia and hemorrhagic fevers. Disease transmission is associated with infected rodents, who manifest no apparent symptoms, but shed virus in feces, urine and saliva. The hantavirus strain that causes disease in Europe and Asia is distinctly different from the hantavirus pulmonary syndrome occurring mainly in southwestern U.S. This syndrome, progressing from flu-like symptoms to respiratory failure, and possibly death is known for its high mortality.

CAUSES
• human infection may occur from inhalation, ingestion (e.g., contaminated food or water), contact with rodent excrement or rodent bites; person-to-person spread or transmission by mosquitos, fleas or other arthropods has not been reported

TREATMENT
• supportive (oxygenation, vital signs monitoring, stabilization of heart rate and blood pressure)
• fluid volume replacement (with caution not to overhy-

drate)
- dopamine or epinephrine for hypotension
- ribavirin

ICD-9-CM
079.81 Hantavirus

Hartnup disease

DESCRIPTION Familial syndrome characterized clinically by a pellagrous rash, cerebellar ataxia, and mental retardation and biochemically by the loss of renal tubular and intestinal transport of neutral amino acids. Usual course - intermittent

CAUSES
- abnormal intestinal amino acid transport
- abnormal renal tubular amino acid transport

TREATMENT
- nicotinamide
- high protein diet

ICD-9-CM
270.0 Disturbances of amino-acid transport

Heat cramp

DESCRIPTION A form of heat exhaustion characterized by muscle spasm attended by pain, dilated pupils, and weak pulse. It occurs in people who lose much salt and water by working intensely in excessive heat. Usual course - acute; intermittent. Endemic areas: tropics; subtropics.

CAUSES
- electrolyte depletion

TREATMENT
- rest
- adequate salt replacement
- isotonic saline solution

ICD-9-CM
992.2 Heat cramps

Hemangioma of the liver

DESCRIPTION Benign tumor made of newly formed blood vessels resulting from malformation of angioblastic tissue of fetal life. Usual course - stable; usually asymptomatic.

SYNONYMS
- cavernous hemangioma of the liver
- cavernoma of the liver

CAUSES
- Unknown

TREATMENT
- none for small asymptomatic lesions
- surgical excision
- radiotherapy has been used for massive hemangiomas

ICD-9-CM
228.04 Hemangioma of intra-abdominal structures

Hemiplegia, acute infantile

DESCRIPTION Hemiparesis, weakness, seizures present at or before birth, due to cerebral thrombosis. Numerous causes for cerebral thrombosis. Usual course - acute.

CAUSES
- cerebral artery embolism
- cerebral artery thrombosis
- vasculitis
- tonsillar infection
- cervical adenitis
- trauma
- arteriosclerosis
- fibromuscular hyperplasia
- sickle cell disease
- lupus
- polyarteritis nodosa
- cyanotic heart disease

TREATMENT
- treat underlying condition
- control seizures
- treat increased intracranial pressure if present

ICD-9-CM
343.4 Infantile hemiplegia

Hemoglobin C disease

DESCRIPTION A disease characterized by compensated hemolysis with a normal hemoglobin level or a mild to moderate anemia. There may be intermittent abdominal discomfort, splenomegaly, and slight jaundice. Hereditary, autosomal recessive. Usual course - chronic.

CAUSES
- point mutation in hemoglobin beta gene

TREATMENT
- supportive
- transfusions
- folate therapy

ICD-9-CM
282.7 Other hemoglobinopathies

Hemosiderosis, pulmonary

DESCRIPTION Rare disease of unknown etiology. Must be distinguished from Goodpasture syndrome and from lung hemorrhage in systemic lupus erythematosus.
- Characteristics - episodes of hemoptysis, hemorrhage into the lung, pulmonary infiltration, secondary iron deficiency anemia. Most common in children. Pathology shows diffuse infiltration with hemosiderin-containing macrophages. Death may occur from massive hemorrhage, although patients may live for several years with pulmonary fibrosis and insufficiency.

CAUSES
- unknown

TREATMENT
- symptomatic and supportive

ICD-9-CM
275.0 Disorders of iron metabolism
516.1 Idiopathic pulmonary hemosiderosis

Hemothorax

DESCRIPTION A collection of blood in the pleural cavity. Characteristic signs and symptoms include chest pain, dyspnea, weakness, tachycardia, and asymmetrical chest movement. Usual course - acute.

CAUSES
- frank bleeding into pleural space
- penetrating chest trauma
- blunt chest trauma
- hematologic disorders

TREATMENT
- drainage by catheter
- thoracotomy if continuous serious bleeding

ICD-9-CM
511.8 Pleurisy with other specified forms of effusion, except tuberculous
860.2 Traumatic hemothorax without mention of open wound into thorax

Hepatic artery aneurysm

DESCRIPTION Aneurysmal dilatation of a portion of the hepatic artery. Characteristics - right upper quadrant pain, bruit in right upper quadrant, jaundice. Usual course - progressive.

CAUSES
- weakening of vessel wall by stone eliciting aneurysmal dilatation

TREATMENT
- surgery

ICD-9-CM
442.84 Other aneurysm of other visceral artery

Hepatic fibrosis, congenital

DESCRIPTION Developmental disorder of the liver characterized by irregular broad bands of fibrous tissue containing multiple cysts formed by disordered terminal bile ducts, chiefly in the portal areas, which leads to portal hypertension. Symptoms include splenomegaly, hepatomegaly, and gastrointestinal bleeding.

CAUSES
- genetic

TREATMENT
- splenectomy
- splenorenal shunt

ICD-9-CM
571.5 Cirrhosis of liver without mention of alcohol

Hepatitis, alcoholic

DESCRIPTION An acute or chronic degenerative and inflammatory lesion of the liver in the alcoholic patient which is potentially progressive or reversible; it does not necessarily include steatosis, fibrosis, or cirrhosis of alcoholics, although it is frequently associated with these conditions. Usual course - acute; chronic.

SYNONYMS
- alcoholic steatonecrosis
- sclerosing hyaline necrosis

CAUSES
- alcoholism

TREATMENT
- well-balanced diet
- intravenous alimentation
- avoid alcohol

ICD-9-CM
571.1 Acute alcoholic hepatitis

SEE ALSO
- Alcohol use disorders

Hereditary angioneurotic edema

DESCRIPTION Inherited C1 inhibitor deficiency. An autosomal dominant disorder characterized by recurrent episodes of edema of the skin, upper respiratory tract, and gastrointestinal tract. Frequently mediated by minor trauma, sudden changes in environmental temperature, and sudden emotional stress. Usual course - acute; intermittent; relapsing.

SYNONYMS
- hereditary angioedema

CAUSES
- No complement C1 esterase inhibitor

TREATMENT
- antifibrinolytic agent
- epsilon-aminocaproic acid

ICD-9-CM
277.6 Other deficiencies of circulating enzymes

Hereditary anhidrotic ectodermal dysplasia

DESCRIPTION A congenital ectodermal defect that is x-linked recessive; autosomal recessive. Only males fully express the condition; female carriers may have mild symptoms in x-linked recessive form; both sexes equally affected in autosomal recessive form. Symptoms: heat intolerance, facial anomalies, anhidrosis, hypotrichosis, short stature, dry skin, no mammary glands, mental retardation. Chronic course.

SYNONYMS
- Christ-Siemens-Touraine syndrome
- Siemens syndrome

CAUSES
- defective ectodermal structures
- inherited disease

TREATMENT
- dental reconstruction

ICD-9-CM
757.31 Congenital ectodermal dysplasia

Hereditary hemorrhagic telangiectasia

DESCRIPTION Autosomal dominant vascular anomaly. Characteristics - multiple small telangiectases of the skin, mucous membranes, gastrointestinal tract and other organs; recurrent episodes of bleeding; gross or occult melena. Usual course - very slowly progressive.

SYNONYMS
- Osler-Weber-Rendu disease

CAUSES
- genetic

TREATMENT
- symptomatic

ICD-9-CM
448.0 Hereditary hemorrhagic telangiectasia

Hernias, external

DESCRIPTION Abnormal protrusion of intra-abdominal tissue through a fascial defect in the abdominal wall. Most often, a hernial mass consists of covering tissues (skin, subcutaneous tissues, etc.), a peritoneal sac, and any contained viscera. Groin hernias (indirect inguinal, direct inguinal, femoral) are the most common (about 75% of cases), followed by incisional and ventral hernias (10%), umbilical (3%), and others (3%). Reducible hernia is one where the contents of the sac may spontaneously or with pressure return to the abdomen. Irreducible (incarcerated) hernia is one whose contents cannot be returned to the abdomen. A strangulated hernia is one where there is compromise to the blood supply of the contents of the sac. Signs and symptoms of a hernia include a heavy feeling in groin, a painful or painless inguinal swelling or lump (may or may not persist with recumbency).

CAUSES
- congenital defect
- postoperative complication (incisional hernia)
- abnormal muscular structures around umbilical cord (umbilical hernia); common in newborns
- weakness in the fascial margin of the internal inguinal ring (indirect inguinal hernia)
- weakness in fascia floor of the inguinal canal (direct inguinal hernia)

TREATMENT
- herniorrhaphy; bowel resection (strangulated or necrotic hernia); elastic corset

ICD-9-CM
553.00 Femoral hernia, unilateral or unspecified (not specified as recurrent)
550.90 Inguinal hernia without mention of obstruction or gangrene, unilateral or unspecified (not specified as recurrent)
550.92 Inguinal hernia without mention of obstruction of gangrene, bilateral (not specified as recurrent)
553.1 Umbilical hernia
553.21 Ventral incisional hernia

Histiocytosis, pulmonary

DESCRIPTION A disorder of the mononuclear phagocyte system caused by tobacco smoking. Characteristics - cough, dyspnea, chest pain, weight loss. No known treatment except to stop smoking. Usual course - chronic; progressive in some cases.

SYNONYMS
- histiocytosis X
- pulmonary eosinophilic granuloma

CAUSES
- disorder of the mononuclear phagocyte system
- tobacco smoking

TREATMENT
- unknown

ICD-9-CM
277.89 Other specified disorders of metabolism

Hutchinson-Gilford syndrome

DESCRIPTION Premature old age. Characteristics - small stature; absence of facial and genital hair; wrinkled skin; gray hair; and appearance, manner, and attitude of old age. Usual course - progressive; fatal. Possibly autosomal recessive.

SYNONYMS
- childhood progeria
- premature senility syndrome

CAUSES
- unknown

TREATMENT
- none

ICD-9-CM
259.8 Other specified endocrine disorders

Hyperbilirubinemia, physiologic neonatal

DESCRIPTION A mild, transient physiological hyperbilirubinemia of unconjugated (indirect) type occurring in the normal neonate.

SYNONYMS
- icterus neonatorum
- hyperbilirubinemia in the newborn

CAUSES
- fetal hemolysis
- inadequate bilirubin conjugation
- prematurity

TREATMENT
- phototherapy

ICD-9-CM
774.6 Unspecified fetal and neonatal jaundice

Hyperhidrosis

DESCRIPTION Excessive perspiration due to over-activity of the sweat glands. Distribution - general or confined to palms, soles, axillas, inframammary region, groin. Symptoms include skin maceration, fissuring, scaling. A bad odor may be produced by decomposition of sweat and cellular debris resulting from yeast and bacteria infection.

CAUSES
- various skin diseases, such as pyogenic or fungal infections, contact dermatitis, fever, hyperthyroidism, central nervous system disorders, psychogenic

TREATMENT
- bromhidrosis (malodorous exudate). Treat with soap containing chlorhexidine. Apply aluminum chlorhydroxy complex after bathing.
- treat any uncovered underlying cause
- localized hyperhidrosis - treat with nighttime applications of aluminum chloride in absolute ethyl alcohol. Cover with polyethylene films if possible. Wash applications away next morning.

ICD-9-CM
780.8 Hyperhidrosis

Hyperthermia, malignant

DESCRIPTION Autosomal inherited condition occurring in patients undergoing general anesthesia. Characteristics - sudden, rapid temperature rise, tachycardia, tachypnea, sweating, cyanosis, muscle rigidity. Usual course - acute.

SYNONYMS
- fulminating hyperpyrexia
- malignant hyperpyrexia

CAUSES
- general anesthesia
- suxamethonium
- succinylcholine
- halothane
- duchenne muscular dystrophy

TREATMENT
- cooling
- cessation of anesthesia
- correct acidosis
- dantrolene
- mannitol

ICD-9-CM
995.86 Malignant hyperthermia

Hyphema

DESCRIPTION Hemorrhage within the anterior chamber of the eye. Usual course - acute; recurrent.

CAUSES
- traumatized iris roof
- traumatized stromal vessels
- spontaneous bleeding

TREATMENT
- strict bed rest
- keep upright
- binocular patching
- mydriatics
- miotics
- antifibrinolytic agents
- surgery
- sedation
- ocular hypotensives

ICD-9-CM
364.41 Hyphema of iris and ciliary body

Hypocalcemia

DESCRIPTION Calcium level of 8.5 mg/dL (2.13 mmol/L) or less (with a normal albumin)
• Characteristics - symptoms include neuromuscular irritability, weakness, weight loss, diarrhea, abdominal cramping, bone pain, paresthesias, headache, seizures, dry skin. Signs include Chvostek's sign and Trousseau's sign.

CAUSES
• Surgically induced hypoparathyroidism, Addison disease, candidiasis, carcinoma of the thyroid, chronic liver disease, hyperphosphatemia, idiopathic, malabsorption, malnutrition, nephrosis, pancreatitis, pernicious anemia, pseudohypoparathyroidism, renal disease, rickets and osteomalacia

TREATMENT
• treat any discovered underlying disorder
• carefully replace calcium

ICD-9-CM
275.41 Hypocalcemia

Hypohidrotic ectodermal dysplasia syndrome

DESCRIPTION Inherited, ectodermal hypoplasia disorder characterized by decreased or no sweating, hairlessness, thin skin, anodontia, mental deficiency, hyperthermia. Usual course - chronic.

CAUSES
• ectodermal hypoplasia

TREATMENT
• cool climate
• water cooling
• dentures
• wig

ICD-9-CM
757.31 Congenital ectodermal dysplasia

Hypophosphatasia

DESCRIPTION Genetic metabolic disorder resulting from serum and bone alkaline phosphatase deficiency leading to ethanolamine phosphaturia and ethanolamine phosphatemia. Clinical characteristics include severe skeletal defects resembling rickets, failure of the calvarium to calcify, dyspnea, cyanosis, and gastrointestinal symptoms, renal calcinosis, failure to thrive. Usual course - chronic; progressive.

SYNONYMS
• juvenile Paget disease
• hyperostosis corticalis juvenilis deformans
• Rathbun syndrome

CAUSES
• unknown

TREATMENT
• symptomatic
• sodium fluoride
• calcitonin
• corticosteroids

ICD-9-CM
275.3 Disorders of phosphorus metabolism

Hypoprothrombinemia

DESCRIPTION Deficiency of prothrombin (coagulation Factor II) in the blood. Characteristics - epistaxis, gingival bleeding, hematuria, melena, excessive bleeding with injury. Usual course - chronic.

SYNONYMS
• prothrombin deficiency
• factor II deficiency

CAUSES
• genetic deficiency
• vitamin K deficiency

TREATMENT
• fresh frozen plasma
• vitamin K

ICD-9-CM
286.3 Congenital deficiency of other clotting factors

Hypospadias

DESCRIPTION A congenital anomaly, occurring in 0.5% of males. The urethra exits at an abnormal position along the ventral midline of the penis.

CAUSES
• Thought to be secondary to an unknown defect in androgen action
• Maternal ingestion of progestational agents in early pregnancy

TREATMENT
Surgical repair.

ICD-9-CM
752.61 Hypospadias (male)

Ichthyosis

DESCRIPTION A symptom in several rare hereditary syndromes - ichthyosis vulgaris; X-linked ichthyosis; lamellar ichthyosis (nonbullous congenital ichthyosiform erythroderma), epidermolytic hyperkeratosis (bullous congenital ichthyosiform erythroderma). Also occurs in several systemic disorders. Xeroderma, the mildest form is neither congenital nor associated with systemic disease. Characteristics - skin is dry, scaling, thick over widespread parts of the body.

SYNONYMS
• Xeroderma
• Dry skin
• Xerosis

CAUSES
• inherited, Refsum syndrome (hereditary mental deficiency and spastic paralysis), Sjögren-Larrson syndrome, leprosy, hypothyroidism, AIDS

TREATMENT
• skin lubricants

ICD-9-CM
757.1 Ichthyosis congenital

SEE ALSO
• Sjögren syndrome

Icterohemorrhagic leptospirosis

DESCRIPTION A severe form of leptospirosis. Characterized by jaundice usually accompanied by azotemia, hemorrhages, anemia, continued fever, and disturbances of consciousness. Usual course - acute; biphasic. Endemic areas: worldwide

SYNONYMS
• Weil syndrome
• leptospiral jaundice
• spirochetal jaundice
• spirochaetosis icterohemorrhagica

CAUSES
• spirochetes of genus leptospira
• systemic infectious disease
• zoonosis
• contact with infected animal tissues
• contact with infected animal urine

TREATMENT
• supportive therapy
• antibiotics

ICD-9-CM
100.0 Leptospirosis icterohemorrhagica

Idiopathic edema

DESCRIPTION Swellings of unknown cause affecting women, occurring intermittently over a period of years. Usually worse during premenstrual phase. Associated with increased aldosterone secretion. Usual course - intermittent; relapsing.

SYNONYMS
• cyclic edema
• periodic edema
• stress edema
• distress edema
• periodic swelling

CAUSES
• unknown
• abnormal albumin metabolism
• hormonal imbalance

TREATMENT
• DECR salt intake
• elastic stockings
• captopril
• bromocriptine
• diuretics

ICD-9-CM
782.3 Edema

IgG heavy chain disease

DESCRIPTION A rare malignant neoplasm of lymphoplasmacytic cells consisting of monoclonal immunoglobulin heavy chains. Usual course - progressive; fatal.

SYNONYMS
• gamma chain disease
• Franklin disease

CAUSES
• secretion of free gamma immunoglobulin chains

TREATMENT
• unresponsive to chemotherapy

ICD-9-CM
273.2 Other paraproteinemias

IgM heavy chain disease

DESCRIPTION Rarest heavy chain disease. Found in patients with chronic lymphocytic leukemia. Characteristics - hepatomegaly, splenomegaly. Usual course - slowly progressive.

SYNONYMS
• mu chain disease

CAUSES
• secretion of free mu chains

TREATMENT
• no specific therapy

ICD-9-CM
273.2 Other paraproteinemias

Interstitial keratitis

DESCRIPTION Chronic, non-ulcerative infiltration of the deep layers of the cornea, rare in the USA. Characteristics - signs and symptoms include photophobia, pain, lacrimation, gradual loss of vision.

CAUSES
• congenital or acquired syphilis; tuberculosis

TREATMENT
• refer to an ophthalmologist for treatment

ICD-9-CM
370.50 Interstitial keratitis, unspecified

Intrahepatic cholestasis due to pregnancy

DESCRIPTION A benign disorder of pregnancy causing jaundice, pruritus, and hepatomegaly that clears upon delivery. Usual course - intermittent.

SYNONYMS
- cholestatic jaundice of pregnancy

CAUSES
- sensitivity to hormones normally produced in pregnancy

TREATMENT
- unnecessary
- cholestyramine for pruritus

ICD-9-CM
646.70 Liver disorders in pregnancy, unspecified

Jaundice

DESCRIPTION A descriptive term implying deposition of bile pigment in the skin and mucous membranes with resulting yellow appearance of the patient. Yellow skin and sclerae appear whenever bilirubin reaches 3 mg/mL. Characteristics - adult jaundice is usually brought about by hemolysis, virus infection, alcoholism, drugs, stones in the bile ducts, cancer of the pancreas or liver.

CAUSES
- preponderance of direct (conjugated) bilirubin:
  - ◊ obstruction - gallstones, common duct stones, tumors, strictures
  - ◊ hepatitis
  - ◊ cirrhosis
  - ◊ drugs
  - ◊ pregnancy (idiopathic cholestatic jaundice of pregnancy)
  - ◊ hereditary
- preponderance of indirect (unconjugated) bilirubin:
  - ◊ hemolysis
  - ◊ neonatal (hepatic immaturity)
  - ◊ drugs
  - ◊ Gilbert syndrome
  - ◊ congestive heart failure

TREATMENT
- according to cause

ICD-9-CM
782.4 Jaundice, unspecified, not of newborn

Jaundice, breast milk

DESCRIPTION Self-limited hyperbilirubinemia in a healthy vigorous neonate. Cause unknown. Usual course - progressive; self-limiting.

CAUSES
- unknown
- possibly maternal estrogen isomer interference with infant bilirubin conjugation

TREATMENT
- interrupt nursing as diagnostic trial

ICD-9-CM
774.30 Neonatal jaundice due to delayed conjugation, cause unspecified

Jet lag

DESCRIPTION The syndrome of jet lag results from transmeridian (East-West) travel between different time zones (North to South travel does not cause jet lag). It is a state of physiological desynchronization (e.g., clock shows that it is lunchtime, but the body says it is the middle of the night). The degree of severity depends on the number of time zones crossed and the direction traveled. Most people find traveling eastward and adapting to a shorter day more difficult than traveling westward and adapting to a longer day. Resulting symptoms include: extreme fatigue, sleep disturbances, loss of concentration, malaise, disorientation, sluggishness, gastrointestinal upset and loss of appetite.

CAUSES
- disturbance in the body's physiological processes (circadian dysrhythmia) that control not only sleep and wakefulness, but also alertness, hunger, digestion, urine production, temperature and hormone secretion

TREATMENT
- no clear evidence that extensive and elaborate prevention programs to avoid jet lag are of value
- short-acting benzodiazepines (e.g., lorazepam) for sleep in transit
- plan destination activities to accommodate for time differences
- the hormone melatonin may be a promising remedy

ICD-9-CM
780.50 Sleep disturbance, unspecified

Juvenile amaurotic familial idiocy

DESCRIPTION Neuronal ceroid lipofuscinosis. Characteristics - loss of vision, onset 5-10 years, death during late adolescence, atypical retinitis pigmentosa, cerebellar ataxia, dementia. Genetics - autosomal recessive. Usual course - progressive.

SYNONYMS
- Spielmeyer-Sjögren chronic neuronal ceroid lipofuscinosis
- Spielmeyer-Vogt disease
- Batten disease

CAUSES
- neuronal accumulation of ceroid
- neuronal accumulation of lipofuscin

TREATMENT
- rehabilitation as needed

ICD-9-CM
330.1 Cerebral lipidoses

Kartagener syndrome

DESCRIPTION An inherited disorder involving a combination of situs inversus, bronchiectasis, and sinusitis. Genetics - familial; autosomal recessive; 1/70 persons of those involved are heterozygous. Usual course - chronic; variable onset.

SYNONYMS
- Kartagener triad

CAUSES
- defective mucociliary clearance

TREATMENT
- chest physiotherapy
- antibiotics
- bronchodilators

ICD-9-CM
759.3 Situs inversus

Kearns-Sayre syndrome

DESCRIPTION Inherited disorder (autosomal dominant with onset before age 15). Characteristics - progressive ophthalmoplegia, pigmentary degeneration of the retina, ataxia, myopathy, cardiac conduction defect. Usual course - progressive; ophthalmic onset at ages 5-20; retinal onset at ages 8-40; cardiac onset at ages 10-40.

SYNONYMS
- oculocraniosomatic neuromuscular disease
- ragged red fiber disease
- ophthalmoplegia-plus
- hereditary external ophthalmoplegia

CAUSES
- unknown

TREATMENT
- folic acid
- coenzyme Q10
- pacemaker

ICD-9-CM
378.55 External ophthalmoplegia

Keratitis, superficial punctate

DESCRIPTION Loss of epithelium from the corneal surface of one or both eyes. Often associated with trachoma, staphylococcus blepharitis, conjunctivitis, or a respiratory tract infection.
- Characteristics - symptoms include photophobia, pain, lacrimation, diminished vision, conjunctival injection

CAUSES ultraviolet light exposure, bacterial infection, viral infection

TREATMENT
- topical antibiotics after positive culture
- for gram-positive organisms: 10-30% sulfacetamide drops every 2 hours and 0.5% erythromycin or 500 u./gm bacitracin ointment tid
- gram-negative organisms: 0.3% gentamicin drops every 2 hours
- use dark glasses
- systemic analgesics for pain

ICD-9-CM
370.21 Punctate keratitis

Keratoconus

DESCRIPTION Degenerative eye disorder characterized by thinning and anterior protrusion of the cornea, usually bilateral, beginning between ages 10 and 20. More frequent in females. Signs and symptoms: blurred vision, myopia, astigmatism.

CAUSES
- transmitted as an autosomal recessive trait

TREATMENT
- hard contact lenses
- glasses with high astigmatic correction
- corneal graft or transplantation

ICD-9-CM
371.60 Keratoconus, unspecified

Kernicterus

DESCRIPTION A condition characterized by high levels of nonconjugated bilirubin in the blood with biliary pigmentation of certain nuclei in the brain and spinal cord and frequently resulting in cerebral palsy, mental retardation, and hearing deficit. It is commonly a sequel to icterus gravis neonatorum. Usual course - acute; progressive; chronic.

SYNONYMS
- bilirubin encephalopathy
- nuclear jaundice

CAUSES
- isoimmunization
- erythrocyte biochemical defects
- erythrocyte structural abnormalities
- infection
- sequestered blood

TREATMENT
- physical therapy

ICD-9-CM
773.4 Kernicterus due to isoimmunization
774.7 Kernicterus not due to isoimmunization

Klinefelter syndrome

DESCRIPTION Congenital disorder. Characteristics - small testes, azoospermia, infertility, increased urinary excretion of gonadotropin, tall long legs, gynecomastia. Associated with an abnormality of the sex chromosomes. Usual course - chronic; manifestations begin at puberty.

SYNONYMS
- seminiferous tubule dysgenesis
- XXY syndrome

CAUSES
- congenital
- supernumerary X chromosome
- mosaicism
- advanced maternal age predisposes

TREATMENT
- mastectomy for disfiguring gynecomastia
- supplemental androgens for delayed secondary sexual characteristics
- supplemental androgens for impotence

ICD-9-CM
758.7 Klinefelter syndrome

Korsakoff psychosis

DESCRIPTION Anterograde and retrograde amnesia with confabulation associated with alcoholic or nonalcoholic polyneuritis. Usual course - subacute; possibly acute; possibly chronic.

SYNONYMS
- alcohol amnestic syndrome

CAUSES
- alcoholism
- thiamine deficiency
- malnutrition

TREATMENT
- parenteral thiamine replacement
- vitamin supplementation

ICD-9-CM
291.1 Alcohol amnestic syndrome

Krabbe leukodystrophy, infantile form

DESCRIPTION Lysosomal storage disease. Characteristics - begins in infancy, fretfulness, rigidity, followed by tonic seizures, convulsions, quadriplegia, deafness, progressive mental deterioration. Usual course - progressive.

SYNONYMS
- globoid cell leukodystrophy; Krabbe disease
- Krabbe brain leukodystrophy
- globoid cell brain sclerosis

CAUSES
- Lysosomal cerebrosidase deficiency

TREATMENT
- none

ICD-9-CM
330.0 Leukodystrophy

Kuru

DESCRIPTION Progressive nervous system disorder of Melanesian tribes of central New Guinea thought to be associated with cannibalism. Usual course - progressive.

CAUSES
- Scrapie PrP (prion)

TREATMENT
- none

ICD-9-CM
046.0 Kuru

SEE ALSO
- Creutzfeldt-Jakob disease

Kyasanur forest disease

DESCRIPTION Severe hemorrhagic fever. Tick-borne arbovirus infection occurring the in the Kyasanur Forest in India. Characteristics - fever, hemorrhagic manifestations and rash. Usual course - recurrent.

CAUSES
- ixodes
- Haemaphysalis spinigera
- tick-borne flavivirus
- rodent hosts
- monkey hosts

TREATMENT
- symptomatic
- fluid replacement
- transfusion

ICD-9-CM
065.2 Kyasanur Forest disease

Lassa fever

DESCRIPTION Acute, possible fatal infectious disease occurring in West Africa. Characteristics - high fever, pharyngitis, vomiting, abdominal pain, dyspnea followed by hemorrhages and shock. Usual course - acute; gradual defervescence.

CAUSES
- lassa virus form of arenavirus found in excreta of wild rodents

TREATMENT
- supportive care
- fluid plus electrolyte therapy

ICD-9-CM
078.89 Other specified diseases due to viruses

Lathyrism

DESCRIPTION A morbid condition resulting from eating leguminous plants (includes many kinds of peas). characteristics - spastic paraplegia, pain, hyperesthesia, paresthesia. Usual course - progressive. Endemic areas - Africa; Asia.

SYNONYMS
- neurolathyrism

CAUSES
- beta-aminopropionitrile ingestion
- sweet peas of species Lathyrus sativus

TREATMENT
- none

ICD-9-CM
988.2 Toxic effect of berries and other plants eaten as food

Laurence-Moon-Biedl syndrome

DESCRIPTION A hereditary syndrome of childhood, transmitted as an autosomal recessive trait, with obesity, retinitis pigmentosa, mental retardation, polydactyly, and hypogonadism as the main features. Usual course - progressive.

SYNONYMS
- Laurence-Moon syndrome
- Bardet-Biedl syndrome

CAUSES
- genetic

TREATMENT
- supportive

ICD-9-CM
759.89 Other specified congenital anomalies

Left ventricular failure, acute

DESCRIPTION Left heart failure. Characteristics - dyspnea, cough, sense of suffocation, frothy sputum, cyanosis, rales, wheezing, tachycardia, Cheyne-Stokes respiration. Usual course - acute.

SYNONYMS
- ventricular failure
- left heart failure

CAUSES
- hypertension
- coronary artery disease
- incompetent mitral valve
- incompetent aortic valve
- myocardial infarction

TREATMENT
- diuretics
- vasodilators
- digitalis

ICD-9-CM
428.1 Left heart failure

Leptospirosis

DESCRIPTION Infection by leptospira organisms transmitted to man from dogs, swine, and rodents or by contact with contaminated water. Characteristics - lymphocytic meningitis, hepatitis, nephritis. Weil's syndrome is severe leptospirosis with jaundice, bleeding and renal failure. Usual course - acute; abrupt; biphasic; relapsing. Endemic areas - Southern USA; tropics.

SYNONYMS
- autumnal fever
- Fort Bragg fever
- mud fever
- pea-picker's disease
- European swamp fever
- Bushy Creek fever
- cane field fever
- swineherd disease

CAUSES
- leptospira interrogans
- spirochete
- contact with infected animal tissues
- contact with infected animal excrement

TREATMENT
- antibiotics, supportive care, fluid replacement, electrolyte therapy, possibly steroids if hepatic coma

ICD-9-CM
100.9 Leptospirosis, unspecified

Lesch-Nyhan syndrome

DESCRIPTION An X-linked disease caused by a deficiency of an enzyme of purine metabolism, hypoxanthine-guanine phosphoribosyl transferase, and characterized by physical and mental retardation, hyperuricemia, self-mutilation, and choreoathetosis.

SYNONYMS
- hypoxanthine-guanine phosphoribosyltransferase deficiency syndrome
- HG-PRT deficiency syndrome

CAUSES
- hypoxanthine-guanine phosphoribosyltransferase deficiency

TREATMENT
- symptomatic and supportive
- protective restraint

ICD-9-CM
277.2 Other disorders of purine and pyrimidine metabolism

Letterer-Siwe disease

DESCRIPTION Acute, disseminated, rapidly progressive form of Langerhans-cell histiocytosis. Genetics - Some familial predisposition. Characteristics include - hemorrhage tendency, eczematoid skin eruption, hepatosplenomegaly, progressive anemia, lymphadenopathy. Usual course - acute; fulminant; progressive; chronic.

SYNONYMS
- acute diffuse histiocytosis
- acute infantile reticuloendotheliosis
- acute reticulosis of infancy
- generalized histiocytosis
- non-lipid reticuloendotheliosis

CAUSES
- nonneoplastic proliferation of langerhans cells

TREATMENT
- irradiation, chemotherapy, steroids, vasopressin replacement, antibiotics

ICD-9-CM
202.50 Letterer-Siwe disease, unspecified site, extranodal and solid organ sites

SEE ALSO
- Histiocytosis, pulmonary

Leukemia, acute monocytic

DESCRIPTION Leukemia in which the predominating leukocytes are identified as monocytes. Characteristics - fever, fatigue, bleeding, lymphadenopathy, hepatosplenomegaly, anemia. Usual course - acute; possibly relapsing.

SYNONYMS
- acute monocytoid leukemia
- monoblastic leukemia
- acute monoblastic leukemia

CAUSES
- chloramphenicol, phenylbutazone, ionizing radiation, benzene, Down syndrome, alkylating agents

TREATMENT
- cytosine arabinoside
- daunorubicin
- 6-thioguanine

ICD-9-CM
206.00 Acute monocytic leukemia without mention of remission

Leukemia, acute myeloblastic

DESCRIPTION An acute non-lymphoblastic leukemia occurs at all ages and is the more common leukemia among adults. Usually associated with irradiation as a causative agent and occurring as a second malignancy following cancer chemotherapy. Characteristics - bleeding, pallor, fever, headaches, vomiting, weakness, lethargy, pallor, joint pain. Usual course - acute; progressive; relapsing.

SYNONYMS
- acute granulocytic leukemia
- acute myelocytic leukemia

CAUSES
- idiopathic
- retroviral infection
- ionizing radiation
- genetic defect
- chemical poisoning

TREATMENT
- chemotherapy
- immunotherapy
- bone marrow transplantation

ICD-9-CM
205.00 Acute myeloid leukemia without mention of remission

Leukemia, acute myelogenous

DESCRIPTION Leukemia arising from myeloid tissue in which the granular, polymorphonuclear leukocytes and their precursors predominate. Characteristics - fever, anorexia, bleeding, hepatosplenomegaly, anemia, lymphadenopathy. Usual course - acute; possibly relapsing.

CAUSES
- Bloom syndrome
- Philadelphia chromosome
- chloramphenicol
- ionizing radiation
- benzene
- Down syndrome
- Fanconi syndrome
- phenylbutazone
- alkylating agents

TREATMENT
- cytosine arabinoside, daunorubicin, 6-thioguanine, prednisone, vincristine, intrathecal methotrexate, cranial radiotherapy

ICD-9-CM
205.00 Acute myeloid leukemia without mention of remission

Leukemia, chronic myelogenous

DESCRIPTION Clonal myeloproliferation caused by malignant transformation of a pluripotent cell. Characteristics - extraordinary overproduction of granulocytes. Usual course - slowly progressive.

SYNONYMS
- chronic granulocytic leukemia

CAUSES
- unknown
- possibly ionizing radiation

TREATMENT
- busulfan, allopurinol, leukophoresis, localized radiotherapy, vincristine, prednisone, cytosine arabinoside, doxorubicin

ICD-9-CM
205.10 Chronic myeloid leukemia without mention of remission

Leukemia, hairy cell

DESCRIPTION A neoplastic disease of the lymphoreticular cells which is considered to be a rare type of chronic leukemia. It is characterized by an insidious onset, splenomegaly, anemia, granulocytopenia, thrombocytopenia, little or no lymphadenopathy, and the presence of "hairy" or "flagellated" cells in the blood and bone marrow. Usual course - chronic; progressive.

SYNONYMS
- leukemic reticuloendotheliosis

CAUSES
- precise cause unknown

TREATMENT
- splenectomy
- interferon

ICD-9-CM
202.40 Leukemic reticuloendotheliosis, unspecified site, extranodal and solid organ sites

Lichen sclerosis of the vulva

DESCRIPTION Thickened skin and accentuated markings affecting the vulva. Characteristics - external genital itching and pain. Usual course - chronic; progressive; may have spontaneous regression.

SYNONYMS
- lichen sclerosis et atrophicus
- lichen albus
- Csillag disease
- white spot disease
- circumscribed scleroderma

CAUSES
- Unknown

TREATMENT
- vitamin A ointment
- intralesional corticosteroids
- topical corticosteroids
- oral estrogen

ICD-9-CM
701.0 Circumscribed scleroderma

Liddle syndrome

DESCRIPTION A rare disease resulting in enhanced sodium loses in the CCD (cortical collecting duct). This results in enhanced sodium delivery distally (along with a non-reabsorbable anion) and subsequent enhanced potassium secretion.

CAUSES Autosomal dominant condition caused by a mutation at the beta subunit of the principal apical sodium channel

TREATMENT
Sodium restriction and amiloride (which inhibits the luminal sodium channel in the CCD)

ICD-9-CM
276.8 Hypopotassemia

SEE ALSO
- Hypokalemia

REFERENCES
- Harrison's Principles of Internal Medicine. McGraw-Hill, 14th edition, 1998

Lipoid nephrosis

DESCRIPTION Nephrosis characterized by edema, albuminuria, changes in lipids and proteins in the blood, accumulation of globules of cholesterol esters in the tubular epithelium of the kidney.

SYNONYMS
- minimal change disease
- foot process disease
- nil disease
- minimal change nephropathy
- minimal change glomerulopathy

CAUSES
- loss of negative charge in glomerular capillary wall

TREATMENT
- steroids
- antibiotics
- cyclophosphamide
- chlorambucil

ICD-9-CM
581.3 Nephrotic syndrome with lesion of minimal change glomerulonephritis

Loiasis

DESCRIPTION A parasitic infection caused by the nematode Loa loa. The vector in the transmission of this infection is the horsefly (Tabanus) or the deerfly or mango fly (Chrysops). The larvae may be seen just beneath the skin or passing through the conjunctiva. Eye lesions are not uncommon. The disease is generally mild and painless. Usual course - chronic; progressive; 10-15 year incubation period. Endemic areas - West Africa; Central Africa.

SYNONYMS
- calabar swellings

CAUSES
• Loa loa filaria

TREATMENT
• diethylcarbamazine

ICD-9-CM
125.2 Loiasis

SEE ALSO
• Filariasis

Ludwig angina

DESCRIPTION Severe form of cellulitis affecting the submandibular, submental, and sublingual spaces. Characteristics - tongue elevation, difficult eating and swallowing, edema of the glottis, fever, tachypnea, and moderate leukocytosis. Usual course - acute.

CAUSES
• oral trauma
• aerobic infection of submandibular space
• anaerobic infection of submandibular space

TREATMENT
• broad-spectrum intravenous antibiotics
• maintain airway
• tracheostomy if necessary

ICD-9-CM
528.3 Cellulitis and abscess of oral soft tissues, excluding lesions specific for gingiva and tongue

Lupus nephritis

DESCRIPTION Glomerulonephritis associated with systemic lupus erythematosus. Characteristics - hematuria, a fulminant or chronic progressive course. Hypertension does not occur until late in the course of the disease. Usual course - relapsing; progressive.

SYNONYMS
• focal glomerulonephritis
• lupus glomerulonephritis

CAUSES
• SLE

TREATMENT
• steroids
• renal transplantation

ICD-9-CM
710.0 Systemic lupus erythematosus
583.81 Nephritis and nephropathy, not specified as acute or chronic, in diseases classified elsewhere

Lymphangitis

DESCRIPTION Inflammation of a lymphatic vessel or vessels. Characteristics - painful subcutaneous streaks along the course of the vessels. Usual course - acute; relapsing.

CAUSES
• beta-hemolytic streptococci
• staphylococcus

TREATMENT
• antibiotics
• drainage
• heat
• moisture

ICD-9-CM
457.2 Lymphangitis

Lymphoma, non-Hodgkin

DESCRIPTION Heterogenous group of malignant lymphomas with absence of giant Reed-Sternberg cells characteristic of Hodgkin disease. Characteristics - widespread disease, painless enlargement of one or more peripheral lymph nodes. Usual course - progressive.

CAUSES
• malignant tumors of lymphoid tissues with the exception of Hodgkin disease

TREATMENT
• radiotherapy
• chemotherapy

ICD-9-CM
202.80 Other malignant lymphomas, unspecified site, extranodal and solid organ sites

Lymphoma, pulmonary

DESCRIPTION Malignant disease of the lung. Characteristics - cough, weight loss, chest pain. Usual course - progressive.

CAUSES
• tumor of the immune system
• Hodgkin lymphoma
• lymphocytic lymphoma

TREATMENT
• radiotherapy
• chemotherapy

ICD-9-CM
202.80 Other malignant lymphomas, unspecified site, extranodal and solid organ sites

Macrocytosis

DESCRIPTION An enlargement of the red blood cells, generally clinically significant when the MCV exceeds 110. Many disorders leading to macrocytosis will also affect other marrow precursors leading to anemia, leukopenia, and/or platelet disorders.

CAUSES
• Vitamin B12 or folate deficiency
• Liver disease (e.g., viral hepatitis, hemochromatosis, primary biliary cirrhosis)
• Hypothyroidism
• Bone marrow disorders and toxins
  ◊ Alcohol overuse
  ◊ Other toxic chemicals/drugs, e.g chemotherapeutic agents
  ◊ Aplastic anemia
  ◊ Myelodysplasia

TREATMENT
Specific treatment depends on the underlying disorder causing the macrocytosis

ICD-9-CM
289.89 Other specified diseases of blood and blood-forming organs

SEE ALSO
• Alcohol use disorders
• Cirrhosis of the liver
• Cirrhosis, primary biliary
• Hepatitis A
• Hepatitis, alcoholic
• Hepatitis B
• Hepatitis C

Magnesium deficiency syndrome

DESCRIPTION Abnormally low magnesium content of the blood plasma. Characteristics - neuromuscular hyperirritability. Usual course - progressive; acute; relapsing.

SYNONYMS
• hypomagnesemia

CAUSES
• dietary deficiency
• decreased absorption
• increased excretion
• alcoholism
• uremia
• diuretics
• parathyroid disease
• eclampsia

TREATMENT
• magnesium

ICD-9-CM
275.2 Disorders of magnesium metabolism

Mallory-Weiss syndrome

DESCRIPTION Mucosal tears usually linear and confined to the esophagogastric junction but may be located in the fundus of the stomach or in the distal esophagus. Upper gastrointestinal bleeding from these lacerations is often precipitated by retching or vomiting. Usual course - acute.

SYNONYMS
• gastroesophageal laceration-hemorrhage syndrome

CAUSES
• retching after alcoholic bout
• hiatus hernia
• atrophic gastritis
• esophagitis
• straining at stool

TREATMENT
• vasopressin
• gastrotomy with sutures

ICD-9-CM
530.7 Gastroesophageal laceration-hemorrhage syndrome

Maple bark stripper disease

DESCRIPTION Granulomatous, interstitial pneumonitis caused by a mold found under the bark of maple logs. Usual course - acute; relapsing.

CAUSES
• hypersensitivity reaction to spores of Cryptostroma corticale

TREATMENT
• eliminate etiological agent

ICD-9-CM
495.6 Maple bark-strippers lung

Maple syrup urine disease

DESCRIPTION Familial cerebral degenerative disease caused by a defect in branched chain amino acid metabolism and characterized by severe mental and motor retardation and urine with a maple-syrup-like odor. Usual course - progressive.

SYNONYMS
• branched chain ketoaciduria

CAUSES
• deficiency of branched chain alpha-ketoacid decarboxylase

TREATMENT
• controlled intake of branched-chain amino acids
• peritoneal and/or hemodialysis

ICD-9-CM
270.3 Disturbances of branched-chain amino-acid metabolism

Marburg virus disease

DESCRIPTION Severe, acute often fatal viral hemorrhagic fever. Characteristics - prostration, fever, pancreatitis, hepatitis. The Marburg virus first infected laboratory workers handling infected African green monkeys. Usual course - acute. Endemic areas: Germany; Yugoslavia; Africa.

SYNONYMS
• green monkey virus disease

CAUSES
• Marburg virus

TREATMENT
- isolation
- treat dehydration
- nasogastric suction
- heparin

ICD-9-CM
078.89 Other specified diseases due to viruses

Marchiafava-Bignami syndrome

DESCRIPTION Progressive degeneration of the corpus callosum. Characteristics - progressive intellectual degeneration, confusion, hallucinations, tremor, rigidity, and convulsions. Usual course - chronic; progressive.

SYNONYMS
- Marchiafava disease
- callosal demyelinating encephalopathy

CAUSES
- chronic alcoholism
- addiction to crude red wine

TREATMENT
- avoid alcohol

ICD-9-CM
341.8 Other demyelinating diseases of central nervous system

Mastocytosis

DESCRIPTION A rare disease characterized by an abnormal increase in mast cells in various body organs and tissues. It can occur in any age group and demonstrates a slight male predominance. Various forms are identified: mastocytoma (a benign cutaneous tumor); urticaria pigmentosa (multiple, small collections of mast cells, salmon or brown color, that may become vesicular or even bullous); and systemic mastocytosis (mast cell infiltrates in the bone marrow, liver, spleen, lymph nodes, gastrointestinal tract, skin and bones). Symptoms include arthralgias, bone pain and anaphylactoid symptoms. Mast cell leukemia is a form of mastocytosis.

SYNONYMS
- cutaneous mastocytosis
- systemic mast cell disease

CAUSES
- exact cause is unknown

TREATMENT
- cutaneous mastocytosis and urticaria pigmentosa seldom require treatment
- systemic mastocytosis:
  ◊ H1 and an H2 antihistamine
  ◊ aspirin therapy (use with caution)
  ◊ oral cromolyn sodium (if GI symptoms are inadequately controlled)
  ◊ surgical excision of mast cells (rare)

ICD-9-CM
757.33 Congenital pigmentary anomalies of skin
202.60 Malignant mast cell tumors, unspecified site, extranodal and solid organ sites

Meckel diverticulum

DESCRIPTION Sacculation or appendage of the ileum derived from an unobliterated yolk stalk. Symptoms of infection may resemble those of appendicitis. Usual course - acute; intermittent; chronic.

CAUSES
- vestigial remnant of omphalomesenteric duct

TREATMENT
- surgery

ICD-9-CM
751.0 Meckel diverticulum

Meigs syndrome

DESCRIPTION Ascites and hydrothorax associated with ovarian fibroma or other pelvic tumors. Usual course - acute; relapsing.

SYNONYMS
- ovarian ascites-pleural effusion syndrome
- Demons-Meigs syndrome

CAUSES
- benign fibroma
- ovarian tumor
- movement of the ascitic fluid across the diaphragm

TREATMENT
- tumor excision

ICD-9-CM
789.5 Ascites

Melioidosis

DESCRIPTION A glanders-like infection of man and animals endemic in SE Asia, NE Queensland Australia, Central, West and Eastern Africa. Likely to be one of the infections seen in patients with AIDS. May be asymptomatic or symptoms can include chills; cough; bloody purulent sputum; abdominal pain; diarrhea.

SYNONYMS
- Stanton disease
- Whitmore disease
- pneumoenteritis
- pseudocholera

CAUSES
- pseudomonas pseudomallei; transmitted by direct contact with infected rodents or infected food, soil, water, excreta; person-to-person transmission possible through use of injection needle

TREATMENT
- trimethoprim-sulfamethoxazole
- ceftazidime

ICD-9-CM
025 Melioidosis

Meningioma

DESCRIPTION Hard, slow growing, vascular tumor arising along the meningeal vessels and superior longitudinal sinus. It invades the dura and skull and leads to thinning and erosion of the skull. Usual course - progressive; surgical cure.

SYNONYMS
- arachnoidal fibroblastoma
- leptomeningioma
- dural endothelioma
- meningeal fibroblastoma

CAUSES
- unknown

TREATMENT
- surgical excision
- radiotherapy for incomplete removal
- radiotherapy for recurrence

ICD-9-CM
225.2 Benign neoplasm of cerebral meninges
225.4 Benign neoplasm of spinal meninges

Mesenteric adenitis, acute

DESCRIPTION Inflammation of lymph glands located in the mesentery. It causes a clinical picture at times that is difficult to differentiate from acute appendicitis.

SYNONYMS
- acute mesenteric lymphadenitis

CAUSES
- yersinia enterocolitica
- yersinia pseudotuberculosis
- streptococcus viridans
- Giardia lamblia
- staphylococcus aureus

TREATMENT
- antibiotics

ICD-9-CM
289.2 Nonspecific mesenteric lymphadenitis

Metachromatic leukodystrophy, late infantile form

DESCRIPTION A form of leukoencephalopathy transmitted autosomal recessive. Characteristics - accumulation of sphingolipid in neural and non-neural tissues with a diffuse loss of myelin in the central nervous system. The infantile form begins in the second year of life with blindness, motor disturbances, mental deterioration. Usual course - progressive.

SYNONYMS
- metachromatic brain leukodystrophy
- metachromatic leukoencephalopathy
- sulfatidosis
- Greenfield disease
- arylsulfatase A deficiency

CAUSES
- arylsulfatase A deficiency

TREATMENT
- none

ICD-9-CM
330.0 Leukodystrophy

Metastatic neoplasm of the liver

DESCRIPTION Progressive form of hepatic cancer that has metastasized from malignancies arising primarily from other locations. Usual course - progressive.

CAUSES
- colon metastases
- rectal metastases
- gastric metastases
- pancreatic metastases
- breast metastases

TREATMENT
- palliative chemotherapy
- palliative radiotherapy
- surgical resection in rare cases

ICD-9-CM
197.7 Secondary malignant neoplasm of liver, specified as secondary

Milker nodules

DESCRIPTION A disease caused by paravaccinia virus, transmitted to humans during milking. Characteristics - purple nodules on fingers or adjacent areas. Lesions break down and crust and heal without scarring. It can be retransmitted to uninfected cows. Usual course - acute; relapsing. Endemic areas - dairy farms.

SYNONYMS
- pseudocowpox
- paravaccinia

CAUSES
- paravaccinia virus of Poxviridae family
- transmitted through direct contact
- cutaneous disease of cow teats
- oral lesions in suckling calves

TREATMENT
- none

ICD-9-CM
051.1 Pseudocowpox
051.9 Paravaccinia, unspecified

Millard-Gubler syndrome

DESCRIPTION Paralysis caused by infarction of the pons involving the 6th and 7th cranial nerves and fibers of the corticospinal tract. Characteristics - crossed paralysis affecting the limbs on one side of the body and the face on the opposite side. Additionally, paralysis of outward movement of the eye. Usual course - acute; chronic; progressive.

SYNONYMS
- alternating inferior hemiplegia
- Gubler paralysis
- abducens-facial syndrome

CAUSES
- basal pontine infarction
- basal pontine tumor

TREATMENT
- supportive plus rehabilitative
- treat underlying cause of infarction

ICD-9-CM
344.89 Other specified paralytic syndrome

Mitral regurgitation due to papillary muscle dysfunction

DESCRIPTION Retrograde blood flow from the left ventricle in the left atrium through an incompetent mitral valve. Characteristics - fatigue, orthopnea, systolic murmur, left ventricular hypertrophy, S3 gallop. Usual course: chronic; progressive; acute (after myocardial infarction).

CAUSES
- coronary artery disease
- infiltrative diseases
- cardiac tumors

TREATMENT
- dental endocarditis prophylaxis
- surgical endocarditis prophylaxis
- nitrates
- calcium channel blockers
- diuretics
- digitalis
- inotropic agents
- afterload reducing agents
- mitral valve replacement

ICD-9-CM
394.9 Other and unspecified mitral valve diseases

SEE ALSO
- Arteriosclerotic heart disease
- Mitral valve prolapse
- Ruptured chordae tendineae

Mitral regurgitation due to rheumatic fever

DESCRIPTION Retrograde blood flow from the left ventricle into the left atrium through an incompetent mitral valve. Characteristics - history of rheumatic fever, fatigue, dyspnea, holosystolic murmur, left ventricular hypertrophy. Usual course - chronic; progressive disability.

CAUSES
- autoimmune cross reaction between streptococcal antigens and heart tissue

TREATMENT
- medical endocarditis prophylaxis
- dental endocarditis prophylaxis
- surgical endocarditis prophylaxis
- afterload reducing agents
- nitrates
- calcium channel blockers
- digitalis
- diuretics
- mitral valve replacement

ICD-9-CM
394.1 Rheumatic mitral insufficiency

SEE ALSO
- Mitral stenosis
- Mitral valve prolapse
- Rheumatic fever

Munchausen syndrome

DESCRIPTION A chronic disorder characterized by habitual presentation for medical care. Often requires hospitalization. The patient gives a plausible and dramatic history, all of which is factitious.
Also, Munchausen by proxy, in which a caregiver creates a history or illness requiring frequent medical care. The caregiver often has a medical background.

SYNONYMS
- chronic factitious disorder with physical symptoms
- hospital-addiction syndrome

CAUSES
- factitious
- external incentives

TREATMENT
- psychotherapy
- behavior modification techniques

ICD-9-CM
301.51 Munchausen syndrome

Mushroom poisoning, Amanita phalloides

DESCRIPTION Characteristics include: nausea, vomiting, abdominal pain, diarrhea, followed by a period of improvement up to 48 hours. Then culminating in severe renal, hepatic, and central nervous system damage. Usual course - acute; progressive. Endemic areas - Western USA; Europe.

CAUSES
- cyclic octapeptide amatoxin
- hepatic cytotoxicity by interference with RNA polymerase
- renal cytotoxicity by interference with RNA polymerase

TREATMENT
- intragastric activated charcoal
- intensive supportive care
- charcoal hemoperfusion
- thioctic (alpha-lipoic acid)

ICD-9-CM
988.1 Toxic effect of mushrooms eaten as food

Mushroom-worker disease

DESCRIPTION Allergic respiratory disease, resembling farmer's lung, developing in persons working with moldy compost prepared for growing mushrooms. Characteristics - fever, dyspnea, dry cough, chills, malaise, myalgia, tachypnea. Usual course - acute; chronic; intermittent; progressive; relapsing.

SYNONYMS
- pulmonary granulomatosis of mushroom pickers

CAUSES
- immunological reaction to inhaled antigens
- Micropolyspora faeni
- thermoactinomyces vulgaris

TREATMENT
- corticosteroids
- eliminate etiological agent

ICD-9-CM
495.5 Mushroom workers lung

Mussel poisoning

DESCRIPTION Food poisoning due to ingestion of toxin from dinoflagellate Gonyaulax. Characteristics - dysesthesias of tongue, lips, fingertips, dysphagia, abdominal cramps, ascending weakness, seizures. Usual course - acute; progressive. Endemic areas - Mid-Pacific coast from May to October; Northeastern seaboard; Western European coast.

SYNONYMS
- mytilotoxism
- paralytic shellfish poisoning

CAUSES
- alkaloid saxitoxin of dinoflagellate gonyaulax catanella
- alkaloid saxitoxin of dinoflagellate gonyaulax tamarensis
- neuromuscular blockade by preventing depolarization
- aerosolized ingestion has been reported

TREATMENT
- emergent gastrointestinal decontamination
- supportive
- mechanical ventilation

ICD-9-CM
988.0 Toxic effect of fish and shellfish eaten as food

Mycetoma

DESCRIPTION Infectious disease of the skin, subcutaneous tissues, and bone, usually affecting the lower extremities, especially the foot. Characterized by chronicity, tumefaction and multiple sinus formation. With early diagnosis, prognosis is good; if identified late in disease, treatment response is limited and amputation may be necessary.

SYNONYMS
- maduromycosis
- Madura foot

CAUSES
- Allescheria boydii or Actinomycetales bacteria; more than 20 species of fungi and bacteria have been implicated

TREATMENT
- penicillin
- tetracycline
- sulfonamides
- streptomycin
- itraconazole
- dapsone
- surgery

ICD-9-CM
039.4 Actinomycotic infections, Madura foot

Myiasis

DESCRIPTION The invasion of living tissues of man and other mammals by dipterous larvae (fly maggots). Usual course - acute. Endemic areas - tropical America; Africa; South America; Mexico; California.

SYNONYMS
- maggot infestation

CAUSES
- ingestion of fly eggs
- eggs deposited in open wounds

TREATMENT
- surgery
- local anesthesia
- mineral oil
- ether bath

ICD-9-CM
134.0 Myiasis

Myringitis, infectious

DESCRIPTION Inflammation, hemorrhage and emission of fluid into the tissue at the end of the external ear canal and the tympanic membrane. Pain is typically sudden in onset and continues for 24 to 48 hours. Bacterial otitis media is suggested if hearing loss and fever are present.

SYNONYMS
bullous myringitis

CAUSES
- bacterial or viral infection

TREATMENT
- analgesics
- antibiotics for secondary infection
- rupture of vesicles with myringotomy knife

ICD-9-CM
384.00 Acute myringitis, unspecified

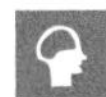

Myxedema heart disease

DESCRIPTION Heart disease associated with primary hypothyroidism. Usual course - acute; progressive.

CAUSES
- decreased thyroid hormone
- congenital developmental defect
- idiopathic
- postablative
- postradiation
- iodine deficiency

TREATMENT
- thyroid hormone replacement

ICD-9-CM
244.9 Unspecified hypothyroidism

Nasopharyngeal cancer

DESCRIPTION This malignancy most often presents with a cervical mass from metastatic spread to a lymph node. Other possible presentations include ipsilateral serous otitis, hearing loss, nasal obstruction, frank epistaxis, purulent or bloody rhinorrhea, and facial neuropathy or facial nerve palsies. Individuals from southern China (in particular, Hong Kong and the province of Guangdong) or Southeast Asia are at particularly high risk.

Stage	5 yr survival
I	65% - 95%
II	50% - 65%
III	30% - 60%
IV	5% - 40%

SYNONYMS
- Cantonese cancer
- Kwangtung tumor

CAUSES Environmental factors, the Epstein-Barr virus and genetic factors have been associated with its development.

TREATMENT
- Radiotherapy
- Chemotherapy

ICD-9-CM
147.9 Malignant neoplasm of nasopharynx, unspecified

SEE ALSO
- Smoking cessation

Necrobiosis lipoidica diabeticorum

DESCRIPTION Degenerative disease of dermal connective tissue. Characteristics - erythematous papules or nodules in the pretibial area that extend to form waxy, yellowish red plaques covered with telangiectatic vessels. The plaques have a red-violet border and depressed atrophic center. Usual course - chronic.

SYNONYMS
- Oppenheim-Urbach disease

CAUSES
- unknown

TREATMENT
- triamcinolone acetonide

ICD-9-CM
250.82 Diabetes with other specified manifestations, type 2 or unspecified type, uncontrolled
709.3 Degenerative skin disorders

SEE ALSO
- Diabetes mellitus, Type 1

Nephropathy, analgesic

DESCRIPTION Kidney damage due to massive intake of analgesics, particularly phenacetin. Usual course - chronic.

CAUSES
- phenacetin
- aspirin
- acetaminophen

TREATMENT
- cessation of analgesic use

ICD-9-CM
965.1 Poisoning by salicylates (aspirin)
965.4 Poisoning by aromatic analgesics, NEC
583.89 Nephritis and nephropathy, not specified as acute or chronic, other

Nephropathy, chronic lead

DESCRIPTION Kidney damage due to lead poisoning. Particularly present in Queensland, Australia. Usual course - chronic.

SYNONYMS
- lead related hyperuricemia
- hyperuricemic nephropathy
- saturnine gout

CAUSES
- lead poisoning
- lead paint ingestion
- lead vapor inhalation
- moonshine alcohol

TREATMENT
- EDTA

ICD-9-CM
984.9 Toxic effect of unspecified lead compound (including fumes)
583.89 Nephritis and nephropathy, not specified as acute or chronic, with other specified pathologic lesion in kidney, other

Nephrosclerosis

DESCRIPTION Hardening of the kidney due to overgrowth and contraction of interstitial connective tissue. Characteristics - edema, headache, hypertension, retinal hemorrhages. Usual course - chronic; progressive.

CAUSES
- unknown
- essential hypertension
- diabetes

TREATMENT
- antihypertensive medication

ICD-9-CM
403.90 Hypertensive renal disease, unspecified without mention of renal failure
403.91 Hypertensive renal disease, unspecified with renal failure

Neuritis/neuralgia

DESCRIPTION Degeneration of peripheral nerves
- Characteristics - insidious onset, muscle weakness with sensory loss, muscle atrophy, decreased tendon reflexes, paresthesias, hyperesthesias in hands and feet. Electromyography shows delayed action potential.

SYNONYMS
- Multiple neuritis
- Peripheral neuropathy
- Polyneuritis

CAUSES
- chronic intoxication (alcohol, arsenic, lead, other drugs)
- infections
- metabolic and inflammatory (diabetes) gout, rheumatoid arthritis, systemic lupus erythematosus
- nutritive (vitamin deficiencies, cachexia)

TREATMENT
- supportive
- physical therapy
- analgesics
- treat underlying specific disorders if possible
- drugs - amitriptyline, carbamazepine, phenytoin (uneven and unpredictable response, but helpful for some)

ICD-9-CM
729.2 Neuralgia, neuritis, and radiculitis, unspecified

Neutropenia, autoimmune

DESCRIPTION Decreased number of neutrophilic leukocytes in the blood due to an autoimmune mechanism. Usual course - acute; chronic; intermittent; progressive; relapsing.

CAUSES
- antineutrophil antibodies

TREATMENT
- antibiotics
- prednisone
- splenectomy
- supportive

ICD-9-CM
288.0 Agranulocytosis

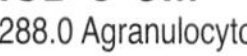

Neutropenia, chronic idiopathic

DESCRIPTION An autosomal dominant, familial disorder with a chronic decrease in number of neutrophilic granulocytes. Characteristics - repeated non-life-threatening infections of skin, oral cavity, and sometimes upper respiratory tract. Usual course - chronic; relapsing.

SYNONYMS
- chronic benign neutropenia

CAUSES
- abnormal homeostasis of mitosis of granulocyte precursors

TREATMENT
- symptomatic

ICD-9-CM
288.0 Agranulocytosis

Neutropenia, cyclic

DESCRIPTION Autosomal dominant disorder of children and young adults characterized by cyclical neutropenia, producing fever, malaise, mouth ulcers and cervical lymphadenopathy. Usual course - relapsing; 21-day cycles.

SYNONYMS
- cyclic agranulocytosis
- periodic neutropenia
- cyclic leukopenia
- periodic myelocytic dysplasia

CAUSES
- defective regulation of hematopoietic cell proliferation

TREATMENT
- glucocorticoids
- androgens
- splenectomy
- antibiotics

ICD-9-CM
288.0 Agranulocytosis

Nevus of Ota

DESCRIPTION A macular lesion on the side of the face (usually lifelong and unilateral), involving the conjunctiva and lids, as well as the adjacent facial skin, sclera, ocular muscles, and periosteum. Histological features vary from those of a mongolian spot to those of a blue nevus. Usual course - chronic.

SYNONYMS
- oculodermal melanocytosis
- nevus fusca-caeruleus ophthalmomaxillaris

CAUSES
- unknown

TREATMENT
- cosmetic cover up

ICD-9-CM
224.3 Benign neoplasm of conjunctiva

Niemann-Pick disease

DESCRIPTION Sphingolipidosis due to sphingomyelinase deficiency with sphingomyelin accumulation in the reticuloendothelial system. There are 5 types (A, B, C, D, and E) with differing ages of onset and differing amounts of CNS involvement and sphingomyelinase activity. Genetics - autosomal recessive. Usual course - acute; chronic; progressive.

SYNONYMS
- sphingomyelin lipidosis
- sphingomyelinase deficiency

CAUSES
- sphingomyelinase deficiency

TREATMENT
- supportive
- splenectomy
- bone marrow transplantation

ICD-9-CM
272.7 Lipidoses

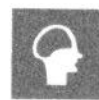

Nitrobenzene poisoning

DESCRIPTION Poisoning due to excessive exposure to nitrobenzene, a benzene derivative used in the manufacture of aniline. Complete recovery from pathologic changes can be expected if survival greater than 24 hours.

SYNONYMS
- nitrobenzol toxicity
- oil of mirbane toxicity

CAUSES
- direct mucous membrane irritation
- methemoglobin formation

TREATMENT
- cutaneous plus gastric decontamination
- oxygen
- 1% methylene blue
- exchange transfusion
- hemodialysis

ICD-9-CM
983.0 Toxic effect of corrosive aromatics

Osteopetrosis

DESCRIPTION Excessive formation of dense trabecular bone leading to pathological fractures, osteitis, splenomegaly with infarct, anemia and extramedullary hemopoiesis. Genetics: malignant form: autosomal recessive; benign form: autosomal dominant. Usual course - progressive; chronic.

SYNONYMS
- marble bone disease
- Albers-Schönberg disease
- osteosclerosis fragilis generalisata

CAUSES
- replacement of marrow space with bone
- no carbonic anhydrase II in erythrocytes
- defective osteoclast function

TREATMENT
- bone marrow transplantation
- calcitriol

ICD-9-CM
756.52 Osteopetrosis

Ovarian mucinous cystadenocarcinoma

DESCRIPTION Carcinoma and cystadenoma of the ovary. Characteristics - multilocular tumor produced by the epithelial cells of the ovary having mucin-filled cavities. Symptoms include abdominal pain and distention, menstrual disturbances, weight loss, dyspareunia, ascites. Clinical findings are the same as those with ovarian serous cystadenocarcinoma.

SYNONYMS
- pseudomucinous ovarian cystadenocarcinoma

CAUSES
- unknown

TREATMENT
- hysterectomy
- stage I: bilateral salpingo-oophorectomy plus omentectomy if high grade
- stage II: add radiotherapy or chemotherapy
- stage III: surgical debulking

ICD-9-CM
183.0 Malignant neoplasm of ovary

Paralysis of the recurrent laryngeal nerve

DESCRIPTION Paralysis may be unilateral or bilateral with many possible underlying causes. Characteristics - dysphagia, stridor, dyspnea, and aphonia. Usual course: acute; insidious.

CAUSES
- innominate artery aneurysm
- right subclavian artery aneurysm
- neck surgery
- thyroid goiter
- trauma
- aortic aneurysm
- left atrial enlargement
- laryngeal tuberculosis

TREATMENT
- treat underlying condition

ICD-9-CM
478.31 Partial unilateral paralysis of vocal cords or larynx

Parapsoriasis

DESCRIPTION A group of slowly evolving erythrodermas. common characteristics: chronicity, resistance to treatment. The group includes chronic and acute lichenoid pityriasis and large and small plaque parapsoriasis. Usual course - chronic; relapsing; benign forms; premalignant forms.

SYNONYMS
- maculopapular erythroderma

CAUSES
- Unknown

TREATMENT
- ultraviolet B light therapy

ICD-9-CM
696.2 Parapsoriasis

Paratyphoid

DESCRIPTION An infection due to any of the salmonella serotypes except S. typhi and salmonellosis. Characteristics - prolonged febrile illness less severe than typhoid fever, frequently follows an attack of salmonella food poisoning.

SYNONYMS
- paratyphoid fever
- enteric fever

CAUSES
- salmonella paratyphi A
- salmonella paratyphi B
- salmonella paratyphi C
- salmonella sendai
- enteric pathogens

TREATMENT
- fluid replacement
- antibiotics in elderly at greatest risk
- antibiotics in infants at greatest risk

ICD-9-CM
002.9 Paratyphoid fever, unspecified

Paroxysmal atrial tachycardia

DESCRIPTION Heart rate greater than 140 beats per minute. May increase up to 250. P waves regular but aberrant. Onset may be sudden. Symptoms include lightheadedness and palpitations.

SYNONYMS
- Premature atrial tachycardia
- Paroxysmal supraventricular tachycardia

CAUSES
- abnormal AV conduction system
- physical or psychological stress
- hypokalemia, hypoxia, caffeine, marijuana, digitalis toxicity, sympathomimetics

TREATMENT
Eliminate known causes; vagal maneuvers; sympathetic blockers (propranolol, quinidine); slow calcium channel blockers (verapamil). Elective cardioversion if unresponsive to drugs.

ICD-9-CM
427.0 Paroxysmal supraventricular tachycardia

Paroxysmal cold hemoglobinuria

DESCRIPTION A rare disease in which blood hemolyzes minutes to hours after exposure to cold (atmospheric, drinking cold water, handwashing in cold water). Usually occurs following a non-specific viral type illness. Usual course - acute; progressive; relapsing.

SYNONYMS
- Donath-Landsteiner hemolytic anemia
- Dressler syndrome
- Harley syndrome

CAUSES
- immune-mediated hemolysis upon rewarming after cold exposure

TREATMENT
- supportive
- transfusion
- oxygen
- maintain adequate urine output
- alkalinize urine
- steroids

ICD-9-CM
283.2 Hemoglobinuria due to hemolysis from external causes

Paroxysmal hemoglobinuria following exercise

DESCRIPTION A benign disorder characterized by red urine, hemoglobinuria, myoglobinuria and abdominal pain. Usual course - acute.

SYNONYMS
- march hemoglobinuria

CAUSES
- strenuous exercise
- running on hard ground
- poorly cushioned shoes

TREATMENT
- unnecessary

ICD-9-CM
283.2 Hemoglobinuria due to hemolysis from external causes

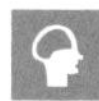

Paroxysmal nocturnal hemoglobinuria

DESCRIPTION Chronic acquired blood cell dysplasia with proliferation of a clone of stem cells producing erythrocytes, platelets, and granulocytes that are abnormally susceptible to lysis by complement. Characteristics - episodic intravascular hemolysis, particularly following infections, and by various thromboses, particularly of the hepatic veins. Usual course - chronic. Genetics - genetic mutation

SYNONYMS
- Marchiafava-Micheli syndrome

CAUSES
- intrinsic erythrocyte defect
- unusual complement sensitivity

TREATMENT
- transfusion
- androgens
- corticosteroids
- anticoagulants

ICD-9-CM
283.2 Hemoglobinuria due to hemolysis from external causes

Pellagra

DESCRIPTION Clinical deficiency syndrome. Characteristics - dermatitis, diarrhea, dementia, inflammation of mucus membranes. Skin lesions appear in area exposed to light and/or trauma. Mental symptoms include depression, irritability, anxiety, confusion, disorientation, delusions and hallucinations. Usual course - progressive. Endemic areas - Southern USA.

SYNONYMS
- niacin deficiency disease

CAUSES
- nicotinic acid deficiency
- tryptophan deficiency
- folic acid deficiency
- carcinoma
- isoniazid

TREATMENT
- nicotinic acid

ICD-9-CM
265.2 Pellagra

Pemphigus, benign chronic familial

DESCRIPTION Benign, persistently recurrent bullous dermatitis (autosomal dominant; 66% positive family history). Characteristics - crops of lesions (may remain localized or become generalized), that rupture, undergo erosion and become thickly crusted. sites: sides of the neck, axillae, groin, and flexural and opposing surfaces of the body. Usual course - intermittent; spontaneous exacerbations with remissions.

SYNONYMS
- Hailey-Hailey disease

CAUSES
- defective intercellular cohesion
- defective tonofilament attachment to desmosomes
- precipitated by infection
- precipitated by trauma

TREATMENT
- antibiotics
- dapsone
- systemic steroids for severe cases
- topical steroids of limited value
- complete excision with split thickness skin graft

ICD-9-CM
694.4 Pemphigus

Pemphigus, Brazilian

DESCRIPTION Progressive and sometimes fatal variant of pemphigus foliaceous endemic in south central Brazil. Most frequently in children and adolescents. Characteristics - flaccid blisters that rupture easily, forming erosions with peripheral rolls of epidermis, associated with a burning sensation. Usual course - progressive; variable. Endemic areas - South Central Brazil.

SYNONYMS
- fogo selvagem

CAUSES
- unknown
- possibly infectious agent

TREATMENT
- topical corticosteroids for localized disease
- systemic corticosteroids for generalized disease

ICD-9-CM
694.4 Pemphigus

Pericholangitis

DESCRIPTION Inflammation of the tissues that surround the bile ducts. Characteristics - fever, mild icterus, hepatomegaly, mild pruritus. Usual course - progressive.

CAUSES
- unknown

TREATMENT
- none

ICD-9-CM
576.9 Unspecified disorder of biliary tract

Perlèche

DESCRIPTION Single or multiple fissures and cracks at corners of the mouth. In advanced stages may extend to lips and cheeks. Usual course - chronic; relapsing; acute.

SYNONYMS
- angulus infectiosus

CAUSES
- poorly fitting dentures
- monilia infection
- dietary deficiency

TREATMENT
- antimonilial drugs
- vitamins
- refit dentures

ICD-9-CM
686.8 Other specific local infections of skin & subcutaneous tissue

Peutz-Jeghers syndrome

DESCRIPTION Multiple pigmented (melanin) macules of the skin and mouth mucosa and multiple polyposis of the small intestine. Usual course - chronic.

SYNONYMS
- intestinal polyposis II
- intestinal polyposis-cutaneous pigmentation syndrome
- periorificial lentiginosis syndrome

CAUSES
- hereditary

TREATMENT
- surgery

ICD-9-CM
759.6 Other hamartoses, NEC

Peyronie disease

DESCRIPTION A disease of unknown etiology producing fibrosis of the sinusoidal spaces of the corpora cavernosa. Patients present with a painful plaque on the dorsum of the penis and may develop penile curvature and erectile failure. Pain generally disappears in 6-12 months.

CAUSES
- Unknown
- Penile trauma on 5-10% of cases

TREATMENT
- Options which may be valuable:
  - ◊ Conservative observation
  - ◊ Surgical correction
  - ◊ Topical verapamil
- Options which may be of little value:
  - ◊ p-aminobenzoic acid
  - ◊ Vitamin E
- Options of little value or hampers subsequent treatments:
  - ◊ Vitamin A
  - ◊ Radiotherapy
  - ◊ orgotein (Peroxinorm) injections
  - ◊ corticosteroid injections

ICD-9-CM
Error: End tag not found. Peyronie disease

SEE ALSO
- Erectile dysfunction

Author(s)
Ira N. Hollander, MD

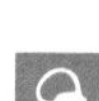

Phlyctenular keratoconjunctivitis

DESCRIPTION Conjunctivitis and keratitis with discrete nodules of inflammation (phlyctenules).
- Characteristics - signs and symptoms include blepharospasm, severe lacrimation, photophobia, and pain

CAUSES
- atopic reaction of a hypersensitive conjunctiva to an unknown allergen, perhaps the protein of staphylococcal, tuberculous or other bacteria

TREATMENT
- Topical corticosteroid and antibiotic combination
- Ophthalmological referral or consultation

ICD-9-CM
370.31 Phlyctenular keratoconjunctivitis

Phosphine poisoning

DESCRIPTION Poisoning by hydrogen phosphide, PH3, a malodorous gas. Usual course - acute; progressive

CAUSES
- acid on phosphorus-contaminated metals
- water on phosphorus-contaminated metals
- acetylene to release phosphine gas
- phosphides to release phosphine gas

TREATMENT
- gastric decontamination
- irrigate eyes
- supportive
- excise sequestered jaw bone

ICD-9-CM
987.8 Toxic effect of other specified gases, fumes, or vapors

Phosphorus poisoning

DESCRIPTION Condition resulting from inhalation or ingestion of phosphorous. Characteristics - garlic breath odor, mandibular necrosis, toothache, anemia, anorexia, weakness, luminescent vomitus. Usual course - acute; progressive.

SYNONYMS
- yellow phosphorous poisoning

CAUSES
- cytotoxicity

TREATMENT
- gastric decontamination
- irrigate eyes
- supportive
- bone excision

ICD-9-CM
983.9 Toxic effect of caustic, unspecified

Pick disease

DESCRIPTION Rare progressive degenerative disease of the brain. Clinically similar to Alzheimer with impaired reasoning, poor insight, memory loss, apathy, amnesia, aphasia, incontinence, and extrapyramidal signs. Pathologically, cortical atrophy is confined to frontal and temporal lobes. Usual course - chronic; progressive.

SYNONYMS
- lobar atrophy
- circumscribed brain atrophy
- presenile dementia

CAUSES
- degenerative disease

TREATMENT
- occupational therapy
- family counseling

ICD-9-CM
331.11 Pick disease

Pickwickian syndrome

DESCRIPTION Extreme obesity with polycythemia, somnolence, hypoventilation, arterial unsaturation and hypercapnia, and pulmonary hypertension. Usual course - chronic; intermittent.

SYNONYMS
- hypoventilation associated with extreme obesity

CAUSES
- marked obesity

TREATMENT
- caloric restriction
- progesterone
- tracheostomy

ICD-9-CM
278.8 Other hyperalimentation

Pilonidal cyst

DESCRIPTION Hair-containing sacrococcygeal dermoid cyst or sinus that opens at a post anal dimple. Usual course - acute; chronic.

SYNONYMS
- pilonidal sinus
- jeep driver's disease
- coccygeal sinus
- piliferous cyst

CAUSES
- ingrown broken hair
- stocky body build
- trauma

TREATMENT
- drainage
- excision

ICD-9-CM
685.1 Pilonidal cyst without mention of abscess

Pituitary basophilic adenoma

DESCRIPTION Small tumor of the anterior lobe whose cells stain with basic dyes and give rise to excessive secretion of ACTH resulting in Cushing syndrome. Characteristics include truncal obesity, hypertension, visual disturbances, menstrual irregularity, impotence, muscle atrophy, osteoporosis, psychic disturbances. Usual course - chronic; progressive.

CAUSES
- unknown

TREATMENT
- transsphenoidal resection
- pituitary irradiation
- bromocriptine

ICD-9-CM
227.3 Benign neoplasms of pituitary gland and craniopharyngeal duct (pouch)

Pituitary chromophobe adenoma

DESCRIPTION Anterior lobe of the pituitary gland tumor. Characteristics - hypopituitarism, headache, lassitude, visual disturbances, galactorrhea, hypogonadism. Usual course - chronic; progressive.

CAUSES
- unknown

TREATMENT
- transsphenoidal resection
- irradiation
- bromocriptine

ICD-9-CM
227.3 Benign neoplasms of pituitary gland and craniopharyngeal duct (pouch)

Pituitary dwarfism

DESCRIPTION Dwarfism caused by hypofunction of the anterior pituitary gland with decreased secretion of growth hormone.

SYNONYMS
- ateliotic dwarfism
- panhypopituitary dwarfism
- hypopituitary dwarfism

CAUSES
- idiopathic
- pituitary tumor
- intrathecal methotrexate
- trauma
- CNS irradiation
- hemochromatosis
- sarcoidosis
- hypothalamic failure
- hypothalamic tumor
- CNS infection
- histiocytosis
- septo-optic dysplasia
- holoprosencephaly
- biologically inactive growth hormone
- growth hormone receptor insensitivity
- deficiency insulin-like growth factor I
- psychosocial dwarfism

TREATMENT
- exogenous growth hormone
- counseling

ICD-9-CM
253.3 Pituitary dwarfism

Pituitary eosinophilic adenoma

DESCRIPTION A tumor of the eosinophilic cells of anterior lobe of the pituitary associated with acromegaly and gigantism Usual course - chronic; progressive.

SYNONYMS
- pituitary acidophilic adenoma

CAUSES
- unknown

TREATMENT
- transsphenoidal resection
- pituitary irradiation
- bromocriptine

ICD-9-CM
227.3 Benign neoplasms of pituitary gland and craniopharyngeal duct (pouch)

SEE ALSO
- Acromegaly

Pituitary gigantism

DESCRIPTION Giantism due to excessive pituitary secretion occurring before puberty and before epiphyses close. May be caused by eosinophilia or chromophobe adenoma. Usual course - insidious.

CAUSES
- somatotropic cell adenoma of the pituitary
- somatotropic cell adenoma of mixed cell
- somatotropic cell adenoma of stem cell
- bronchial adenoma
- pancreatic islet cell tumor
- carcinoid tumor
- ectopic growth hormone production

TREATMENT
- surgery
- irradiation
- bromocriptine

ICD-9-CM
253.0 Acromegaly and gigantism

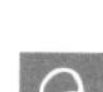

Pituitary hypothyroidism

DESCRIPTION Hypothyroidism caused by deficiency of thyrotropin secretion. Usual course - chronic.

CAUSES
- pituitary irradiation
- pituitary ablative surgery
- failure of anterior pituitary due to infarction

TREATMENT
- thyroid hormone replacement

ICD-9-CM
244.9 Unspecified hypothyroidism

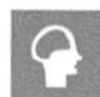

Placental insufficiency syndrome

DESCRIPTION Malnutrition and hypoxia of the fetus due to degenerative changes in the placenta.

CAUSES
- postterm fetus

TREATMENT
- good perinatal care

ICD-9-CM
762.2 Fetus affected by unspecified abnormality of placenta
656.50 Poor fetal growth, unspecified

Pleural malignant mesothelioma

DESCRIPTION Malignant tumor derived from mesothelial tissue. Characteristics - chest pain, dyspnea, weight loss, asthenia, cough, hemoptysis. Usual course - progressive; insidious onset.

CAUSES
- primary tumor of the pleura
- asbestos
- first exposure 20 to 60 years prior to diagnosis

TREATMENT
- surgery
- radiotherapy
- chemotherapy

ICD-9-CM
163.9 Malignant neoplasm of pleura, unspecified

Portal vein thrombosis

DESCRIPTION Clotting of the portal vein of the liver usually from unknown cause. Characteristics - hematemesis, melena splenomegaly, pancytopenia, encephalopathy, portal hypertension. It occurs in pregnancy (especially eclampsia) chronic heart failure, constrictive pericarditis, malignancies. Diagnosis established by angiography. Usual course - chronic; progressive.

CAUSES
- usually idiopathic
- neonatal septicemia
- omphalitis
- hepatocellular cancer
- umbilical vein catheterization for exchange transfusion

TREATMENT
- treat underlying condition
- possible shunt surgery

ICD-9-CM
452 Portal vein thrombosis

SEE ALSO
- Factor V Leiden

Postpartum anxiety/panic disorder

DESCRIPTION This condition is characterized by symptoms of intense anxiety or panic and may involve many somatic symptoms such as cardiac palpitations, tachycardia, tachypnea, dyspnea, hot or cold flashes, chest pain, abdominal pain, dizziness, tremor and feelings of doom and helplessness. Feelings of guilt as well as suicidal thoughts are not present.

CAUSES N/A

TREATMENT
- Relaxation therapy with guided imagery or self-hypnosis
- Individual psychotherapy
- Buspirone or benzodiazepines

ICD-9-CM
648.44 Mental postpartum condition or complication

Author(s)
Moshe S. Torem, MD

Postpartum obsessive compulsive disorder

DESCRIPTION A condition that usually occurs in women who have a previous history or family history of OCD. The patient may have many of the typical symptoms of OCD, however the obsessions and the compulsion are more focused on the baby and the patient's new role and responsibilities of being a mother.

CAUSES N/A

TREATMENT
- Combination of cognitive behavior therapy with pharmacotherapy

ICD-9-CM
648.44 Mental postpartum condition or complication

Author(s)
Moshe S. Torem, MD

Postpartum psychosis

DESCRIPTION This condition is rare and occurs in about 0. 1-0.2% of new mothers. The condition is defined as an atypical psychosis which may begin within the first six months of delivery. Presenting symptoms include severe insomnia, agitation and restlessness, hallucinations, paranoia and delusions focused on the baby. Homicidal and suicidal thought are not uncommon. This condition poses significant danger to the baby's safety and should be managed as a medical emergency requiring hospitalization of the mother.

CAUSES N/A

TREATMENT
- Managed as a medical emergency requiring hospitalization of the mother

ICD-9-CM
648.44 Mental postpartum condition or complication

Author(s)
Moshe S. Torem, MD

Postpoliomyelitis syndrome

DESCRIPTION A slow, progressive muscle weakness and deterioration of function in the previously affected muscles of an individual who had poliomyelitis at least 10 years earlier. The syndrome can appear 30 or more years after a partial or full recovery from the initial polio episode and is noninfectious. It usually involves those muscles most affected by the polio virus, but sometimes affects muscles that are fully recovered or never involved in the initial infection. Other symptoms include fatigue, muscle pain and fasciculations.

SYNONYMS
- polio late effects
- postpoliomyelitis progressive muscular atrophy

CAUSES
- exact cause is unknown

TREATMENT
- physical and occupational therapy
- exercise, e.g., swimming
- consider changes in braces, medication or diet
- weight loss diet, if overweight
- respiratory support, if breathing is affected

ICD-9-CM
138 Late effects of acute poliomyelitis

Prader-Willi/Angelman syndrome

DESCRIPTION A congenital disorder of unknown etiology characterized by mental retardation, muscular hypotonia, obesity, short stature, hypogonadism and frequently developing insulin-resistant diabetes. Genetics - loss of the paternally contributed PWS/AS region on chromosome 15q11-q13; sporadic; risk of inheritance to siblings of an affected child is variable (from <1% to 50%), depending on the specific mechanism of genetic loss. Usual course - progressive. When deletion is inherited from mother the manifestation is called Angelman's syndrome; when the deletion is inherited from father, it is called Prader-Willi.

CAUSES
- hypothalamic dysfunction

TREATMENT
- dietary restrictions
- testosterone
- gastric bypass
- jaw wiring
- progesterone

ICD-9-CM
759.81 Prader-Willi syndrome

Premature atrial contraction (PAC)

DESCRIPTION Premature, abnormal P waves. QRS complexes follow except in very early or blocked PAC. P wave may be buried in the preceding T wave or may be identified in the preceding T wave.

CAUSES
- congestive heart failure, coronary artery disease with ischemia, acute respiratory failure, chronic obstructive pulmonary disease, digitalis toxicity, aminophylline, adrenergic drugs, anxiety, caffeine

TREATMENT
- eliminate known causes

ICD-9-CM
427.61 Supraventricular premature beats

Premature ventricular contraction (PVC)

DESCRIPTION Irregular pulse. Ventricular beat occurs prematurely, followed by a compensatory pause after the premature ventricular contraction. QRS complex is wide and distorted. Most ominous when clustered, multifocal, with R wave on T pattern.

CAUSES
- multiple causes can include psychological stress, physiologic stress, drug toxicity (digitalis, aminophylline, tricyclic antidepressants, beta adrenergics (isoproterenol or dopamine)), caffeine, tobacco, electrolyte imbalances (especially hypokalemia)

TREATMENT
- lidocaine IV bolus and drip infusion
- procainamide IV if induced by digitalis toxicity
- stop digitalis. If caused by hypokalemia, give potassium chloride intravenous drip
- eliminate known causes

ICD-9-CM
427.69 Premature ventricular contraction

Primary lateral sclerosis

DESCRIPTION Degeneration of the lateral columns of the spinal cord. Characteristics - spastic paraplegia, rigidity of limbs, increased tendon reflexes, absence of nutritive and sensory disturbance. Usual course - chronic; slowly progressive.

CAUSES
- unknown
- existence as separate clinical entity questioned

TREATMENT
- none

ICD-9-CM
335.24 Primary lateral sclerosis

Prion diseases

DESCRIPTION A group of degenerative disorders of the central nervous system (and perhaps of peripheral nerves and muscles) caused by proteins, rather than by infectious agents carrying DNA and/or RNA. These disorders affect about 1 person in a million, typically around age 60; 10-15% are inherited. Recognized human disorders in this group include: Kuru, Creutzfeldt-Jakob disease, Gerstmann-Straussler-Scheinker disease, and fatal familial insomnia.

SYNONYMS
- Spongiform encephalopathies

CAUSES Prions (scrapie PrP)

TREATMENT
- None known

ICD-9-CM
046.0 Kuru
046.1 Jakob-Creutzfeldt disease

SEE ALSO
- Creutzfeldt-Jakob disease

REFERENCES
- Prion Diseases of Humans and Animals. Edited by Prusiner SB, Collinge J, Powell J, Anderton B. Ellis Horwood, 1992

Proctalgia fugax

DESCRIPTION Abrupt, sharp or gripping-like pain in the anorectal area. The pain does not radiate. Often the pain wakes the individual in the night. Typically, relief occurs within seconds to minutes, although rare, the pain can be present for hours. The disorder is benign and there is no cure.

SYNONYMS
levator syndrome

CAUSES
- unknown; attributed to spasm of levator ani and coccygeal muscles, sometimes associated with stress or anxiety

TREATMENT
- reassuring patient of benign nature of disease is satisfactory in most cases
- warm baths
- periodic massage
- for severe pain, consider inhaled albuterol, oral clonidine, diltiazem

ICD-9-CM
564.6 Anal spasm

Progressive external ophthalmoplegia

DESCRIPTION Slowly progressive bilateral myopathy affecting the extraocular muscles. Characteristics - weakness of levators of the upper lids, ptosis, followed by total ocular paresis. Usual course - chronic; progressive.

SYNONYMS
- chronic dystrophic ophthalmoplegia

CAUSES
- unknown

TREATMENT
- none

ICD-9-CM
378.72 Progressive external ophthalmoplegia

Progressive hemiatrophy face

DESCRIPTION Atrophy of one half of the face which is usually progressive, but may eventually become stationary.

SYNONYMS
- Romberg disease
- Parry-Romberg syndrome
- progressive hemifacial atrophy

CAUSES
- unknown
- possible lipodystrophy

TREATMENT
- plastic reconstructive surgery
- skin transplantation
- subcutaneous fat transplantation

ICD-9-CM
349.89 Other specified disorders of nervous system, other

Progressive multifocal leukoencephalopathy

DESCRIPTION Serious, usually fatal viral disease. Characteristics - demyelination in white matter of the brain, but may be seen in the brain stem and cerebellum. It occurs secondary to lymphosarcoma and lymphatic myeloid leukemia. Usual course - progressive.

CAUSES
- latent papovavirus

TREATMENT
- cytosine arabinoside

ICD-9-CM
046.3 Progressive multifocal leukoencephalopathy

Prolactinoma

DESCRIPTION A pituitary adenoma which secretes prolactin, leading to increased serum levels of prolactin. Prolactinomas in women are presented with galactorrhea associated with amenorrhea. Though much less common for men, prolactinomas in men rarely produce galactorrhea and are later presented as larger, space-occupying tumors. Usual course - progressive.

SYNONYMS
- prolactin secreting pituitary adenoma
- PRL secreting pituitary adenoma

CAUSES
- prolactin-secreting pituitary microadenoma

TREATMENT
- transsphenoidal resection
- bromocriptine
- irradiation

ICD-9-CM
253.1 Other and unspecified anterior pituitary hyperfunction

SEE ALSO
- Forbes-Albright syndrome
- Multiple Endocrine Neoplasia (MEN)

Pseudocyst pancreas

DESCRIPTION Unilocular cyst of the pancreas. Characteristics - tender mass in left upper quadrant, abdominal pain, weight loss, nausea, anorexia, jaundice. Usual course - acute; progressive.

CAUSES
- acute pancreatitis
- trauma
- pancreatic enzymes released into lesser omentum

TREATMENT
- needle aspiration
- internal drainage surgery
- external drainage

ICD-9-CM
577.2 Cyst and pseudocyst of pancreas

Pulmonary artery thrombosis

DESCRIPTION Blood clot in the pulmonary artery. Characteristics - dyspnea, weakness, chest pain, tachycardia, tachypnea.

CAUSES
- reduction in blood flow of pulmonary artery
- organization of previous embolism
- malignancy
- infection
- trauma
- intrinsic disease

TREATMENT
- anticoagulants

ICD-9-CM
415.19 Pulmonary embolism and infarction, other

Pulmonary hypertension, secondary

DESCRIPTION Increased pressure in the pulmonary circulation above 30 millimeters of mercury systolic, and 12 millimeters of mercury diastolic, secondary to any of the listed causes.

CAUSES
- CHF, left ventricular failure, mitral stenosis, mitral regurgitation, myxoma, pulmonary embolism, interstitial fibrosis, sarcoidosis, asbestosis, radiation, alveolar hypoventilation, chronic obstructive pulmonary disease, chronic bronchitis, emphysema, ventricular septal defect, atrial septal defect, silicosis, anthrasilicosis, tuberculosis, SLE, scleroderma, dermatomyositis, connective tissue disorder, cystic fibrosis

TREATMENT
- corticosteroids, oxygen, cardiac catheterization, nitroprusside, hydralazine, diazoxide, isoproterenol, phentolamine, prazosin, verapamil, nifedipine, captopril

ICD-9-CM
416.8 Other chronic pulmonary heart diseases

Pulmonary infarction

DESCRIPTION Hemorrhagic consolidation of lung parenchyma resulting from thromboembolic pulmonary arterial occlusion. Usual course - acute.

CAUSES
- stasis, vein injury, hypercoagulable state, phlebitis, phlebothrombosis, thrombus, deep vein thrombosis, burn, surgery, oral contraceptives, trauma, hip fracture, immobilization, congestive heart failure, cardiomyopathy, subacute bacterial endocarditis, atrial myxoma, polycythemia rubra vera, sickle cell anemia, pancreatic carcinoma

TREATMENT
- anticoagulation
- heparin
- coumadin
- warfarin
- thrombolytic agent
- urokinase
- streptokinase
- embolectomy
- vena cava clip

ICD-9-CM
415.19 Pulmonary embolism and infarction, other

SEE ALSO
- Pulmonary embolism

Pulmonary interstitial fibrosis, idiopathic

DESCRIPTION Interstitial pneumonia, "nonspecific," or "usual." The term used when etiology leading to pulmonary fibrosis cannot be defined (about 50% of cases). Usual course - chronic; progressive.

SYNONYMS
- alveolocapillary block
- fibrosing alveolitis

CAUSES
- unknown
- loss of functional alveolar-capillary units
- inflammation

TREATMENT
- corticosteroids

ICD-9-CM
516.3 Idiopathic fibrosing alveolitis

Pyogenic abscess liver

DESCRIPTION Bacterial abscess of the liver. Characteristics - fever, abdominal pain, anorexia, jaundice, hepatomegaly, elevated hemidiaphragm. Usual course - acute; relapsing.

CAUSES
- portal vein bacteremia
- systemic bacteremia
- ascending cholangitis
- direct extension
- trauma

TREATMENT
- aspiration
- antibiotics
- surgical drainage

ICD-9-CM
572.0 Abscess of liver

Pyrogenic shock

DESCRIPTION Shock associated with overwhelming infection, most commonly with gram-negative bacteria. Characteristics - fever, tachycardia, chills, myalgia, confusion, tachypnea, hypotension, nausea. Usual course - acute.

SYNONYMS
- septic shock
- endotoxic shock

CAUSES
- inadequate tissue perfusion following bacteremia
- escherichia coli
- klebsiella
- pseudomonas
- serratia
- neisseria meningitidis
- staphylococci; pneumococci; streptococci; bacteroides

TREATMENT
- respiratory support
- fluid replacement
- antibiotics
- vasoactive drugs

ICD-9-CM
785.59 Shock without mention of trauma, other

Q fever

DESCRIPTION Acute, generally self-limited rickettsial infection. Characteristics - fever, chills, headache, myalgia, malaise, rash (rarely), pneumonitis, hepatitis, and endocarditis. No vector involved. Infection by inhalation of dust or aerosols derived from infected domestic animals. Usual course - abrupt; relapsing; chronic; usually mild. Endemic areas - Western USA; Australia; Africa; England; Mediterranean countries.

SYNONYMS
- Australian Q fever
- Balkan grippe
- nine mile fever
- Derrick-Burnet disease
- Query fever

CAUSES
- Coxiella burnetii (rickettsia)
- Aspiration of infected material
- Contaminated raw milk ingestion
- Infected animal conceptional product exposure

TREATMENT
- antibiotics

ICD-9-CM
083.0 Q fever

Ramsay Hunt syndrome, Type 1

DESCRIPTION Ramsay Hunt syndrome Type I, also known as herpes zoster oticus, is a common complication of shingles, a reactivation of the dormant varicella-zoster (chickenpox) virus. The syndrome, caused by the spread of the virus to facial nerves, is characterized by intense ear pain, a rash around the ear, mouth, face, neck, and scalp, and paralysis of facial nerves. Other symptoms may include loss of taste, dry mouth or eyes, hearing loss, vertigo, and tinnitus.
- The prognosis is good. However, in some cases, hearing loss may be permanent. Vertigo may last for days or weeks. Facial paralysis may be temporary or permanent.

SYNONYMS
- Herpes zoster oticus

CAUSES
- Herpes virus

TREATMENT
Some patients require no treatment, although antivirals and/or corticosteroids may be used.

ICD-9-CM
053.11 Geniculate herpes zoster

Ramsay Hunt syndrome, Type 2

DESCRIPTION
- Ramsay Hunt syndrome type 2, also called dyssynergia cerebellaris myoclonica, is a rare, degenerative, neurological disorder characterized by epilepsy, cognitive impairment, myoclonus, and progressive ataxia.
- Symptoms include seizures, tremor, and reduced muscle coordination. Onset of the disorder generally occurs in early adulthood. Tremor may begin in one extremity and later spread to involve the entire voluntary muscular system. Arms are usually more affected than legs. Usual course: progression of the disorder is usually 10 years or longer

SYNONYMS
- Dyssynergia cerebellaris myoclonica

CAUSES
- Unknown

TREATMENTTREATMENT is symptomatic. Myoclonus and seizures may be treated with the valproate.

ICD-9-CM
334.2 Primary cerebellar degeneration

Rat-bite fever, spirillary

DESCRIPTION Infection caused by a rat or mouse bite. Characteristics - wound heals promptly; inflammation recurs at bite site after 10 or more days, accompanied by relapsing fever and regional lymphadenitis; WBC elevated; myalgia, skin rash, chills, malaise, headache. Usual course - relapsing. Endemic areas - Asia; Europe; USA.

SYNONYMS
- sodoku

CAUSES
- spirillum minor-a spirochete
- rodent bite
- rodent scratch
- rodent-ingesting animal bite

TREATMENT
- antibiotics
- rapid bite cleaning

ICD-9-CM
026.0 Rat-bite fever, spirillary

Rat-bite fever, streptobacillary

DESCRIPTION Bacterial infection caused by a rat or mouse bite, although occasionally associated with ingestion of contaminated milk or with the bite of a different rodent. Characteristics (10 or more days following the bite) - abrupt illness with chills, fever, vomiting, headache, arthralgia, backache, elevated WBC, morbilliform petechial skin rash. Usual course - relapsing. Endemic areas - Asia; Europe; USA.

CAUSES
- streptobacillus moniliformis
- rodent bite
- rodent scratch
- contaminated raw milk ingestion

TREATMENT
- antibiotics
- rapid bite cleansing

ICD-9-CM
026.1 Rat-bite fever, streptobacillary

Relapsing fever

DESCRIPTION An acute infectious disease caused by arthropod-borne spirochetes. Clinically characterized by recurrent episodes of fever typically lasting three to five days, headache, arthralgia, myalgia, diarrhea, vomiting, coughing, eye and chest pain, splenomegaly. Two forms of the disease exist: louse-borne and tick-borne. Louse-borne relapsing fever occurs primarily in developing countries and is transmitted by body lice. Tick-borne relapsing fever is less severe and is caused by several species of Borrelia. It is transmitted by soft body ticks of the genus Ornithodoros.

SYNONYMS
- recurrent fever
- tick fever
- famine fever

CAUSES
- body lice
- body ticks

TREATMENT
- tetracyclines
- erythromycin
- penicillin

ICD-9-CM
087.9 Relapsing fever, unspecified

Renal artery stenosis

DESCRIPTION Occlusive disease of the renal arteries. This problem occurs in about 5% of patients with hypertension and is one form of hypertension that is surgically correctable. The disease is most often unilateral. Usual course - progressive.

CAUSES
- atherosclerosis
- fibromuscular dysplasia

TREATMENT
- surgery

- angioplasty
- antihypertensives

ICD-9-CM
440.1 Atherosclerosis of renal artery

Renal infarction

DESCRIPTION Localized area of kidney necrosis caused by either renal arterial or venous occlusion. Characteristics - steady, aching, flank pain, fever, nausea, vomiting, hypertension, leukocytosis, proteinuria, microscopic hematuria. Renal imaging confirms the diagnosis. Usual course - acute.

CAUSES
- renal artery thrombosis
- renal emboli
- arteriosclerosis
- renal artery aneurysm
- fibrous dysplasia
- aortic dissection
- periarteritis nodosa
- vasculitis
- sickle cell disease
- scleroderma
- polycythemia
- trauma
- surgery
- cardiomegaly
- subacute bacterial endocarditis
- atrial myxoma
- rheumatic heart disease

TREATMENT
- surgery
- balloon angioplasty

ICD-9-CM
593.81 Vascular disorders of kidney

Renal vein thrombosis

DESCRIPTION Clotting within the renal vein. Characteristics - lumbar pain; dysuria; enlarged, tender kidney. Usual course - acute; chronic.

CAUSES
- abdominal operation
- CHF
- dehydration
- renal disease
- reduction in renal blood flow
- pregnancy
- constrictive pericarditis
- morbid obesity

TREATMENT
- anticoagulants
- corticosteroids

ICD-9-CM
453.3 Embolism and thrombosis of renal vein

SEE ALSO
- Factor V Leiden

Reticulum cell sarcoma

DESCRIPTION Malignant histiocytic lymphoma made of a substance like embryonic connective tissue. Characteristics - fatigue, anorexia, weight loss, excessive sweating, fever, painless adenopathy, hepatosplenomegaly. Usual course - chronic; progressive; relapsing.

SYNONYMS
- reticulum cell lymphosarcoma
- diffuse histiocytic lymphoma
- reticulosarcoma

CAUSES
- unknown

TREATMENT
- chemotherapy
- radiotherapy
- surgery

ICD-9-CM
200.00 Reticulosarcoma, unspecified site, extranodal and solid organ sites

Retinal vein occlusion

DESCRIPTION One of the causes of sudden unilateral vision loss. Characteristics - extensive retinal hemorrhages; dilated, tortuous retinal veins. Usual course - acute.

SYNONYMS
- central retinal vein occlusion
- CRVO

CAUSES
- Atherosclerosis

TREATMENT
- panretinal photocoagulation

ICD-9-CM
362.35 Central retinal vein occlusion

Retinoblastoma

DESCRIPTION Malignant congenital hereditary blastoma (autosomal dominant with high penetrance). Characteristics - appears in one or both eyes in children under 5 years of age, diagnosed initially by a bright white or yellow pupillary reflex. Usual course - progressive.

SYNONYMS
- glioma retina

CAUSES
- genetic

TREATMENT
- radiotherapy to preserve vision
- photocoagulation to preserve vision
- cryotherapy to preserve vision
- brachytherapy to preserve vision
- enucleation
- palliative radiotherapy for extraocular disease

ICD-9-CM
190.5 Malignant neoplasm of retina

Rhabdomyosarcoma

DESCRIPTION Highly malignant tumor of striated muscle. There are 3 forms - pleomorphic affecting predominantly the extremities of adults; alveolar form, occurring primarily in adolescents and young adults affecting muscles of extremities, trunk, and orbital region; embryonal form, occurring mainly in infants and children, affecting the head and neck, lower genitourinary tract, pelvis and extremities. Usual course - progressive.

SYNONYMS
- rhabdosarcoma

CAUSES
- fetal alcohol syndrome

TREATMENT
- surgical excision
- add radiotherapy in most cases
- group 2: add chemotherapy with vincristine plus dactinomycin
- group 3: add chemotherapy with vincristine plus dactinomycin
- combination chemotherapy for advanced disease

ICD-9-CM
171.9 Malignant neoplasm of connective and soft tissue, site unspecified

Rheumatoid pneumoconiosis

DESCRIPTION Pneumoconiosis associated with rheumatoid arthritis. Characteristics - multiple spherical modular lesions with clearly demarcated borders found throughout both lungs. Usual course: chronic; progressive.

SYNONYMS
- Caplan syndrome
- rheumatoid lung with silicosis
- silicoarthritis

CAUSES
- unknown
- immune mechanism

TREATMENT
- manage complications

ICD-9-CM
714.81 Rheumatoid lung

Rhinosporidiosis

DESCRIPTION Chronic, localized granulomatous infection of mucocutaneous tissues, especially the nose. Characteristics - nasal polyps, tumors, papillomas, or wart-like lesions. Other (rare) areas of infection include the conjunctiva, penis, anus, vagina, ears, pharynx, larynx. Usual course - progressive. Endemic areas - India; Sri-Lanka.

SYNONYMS
- rhinosporosis

CAUSES
- Rhinosporidium seeberi

TREATMENT
- surgery

ICD-9-CM
117.0 Rhinosporidiosis

Rhodococcus infections

DESCRIPTION A recognized animal pathogen which is emerging as a human pathogen, especially in immunocompromised hosts. Necrotizing pneumonia, presumed the result of inhalation inoculation, is the most common type of infection; extra-pulmonary infections usually occur as a result of bacteremic spread from the lungs, especially to the brain.

CAUSES
- Rhodococcus equi, a pleomorphic Gram-positive rod when cultured on solid media, which may also stain acid-fast. (It may have coccus morphology on primary Gram stain from clinical material.) This bacterium is found in nature most commonly in the soil of terrain habituated by grazing animals.

TREATMENT
Antibiotics: particularly macrolides, rifampin, vancomycin, ciprofloxacin, and gentamicin. Successful therapy in immunocompromised persons almost always requires combinations of at least two antibiotics administered for a long duration, not uncommonly in conjunction with "debulking" resection of necrotic, infected tissue. Relapse is common after discontinuation of therapy, and long-term secondary prophylaxis with an oral agent should be considered. Prophylaxis against Mycobacterium avium-complex (MAC) bacteremia in AIDS patients, using rifabutin, clarithromycin, or azithromycin, may also have a prophylactic effect against Rhodococcus equi in those patients.

ICD-9-CM
482.89 Pneumonia due to other specified bacteria

REFERENCES

- Verville TD, Huycke MM, Greenfield RA, Fine DP, Kuhls TL, Slater LN. Rhodococcus equi infections in Humans. Medicine Vol 73, No3, 1994

Author(s)
Leonard N. Slater, MD

Riboflavin deficiency

DESCRIPTION Deficiency of vitamin B2. Deficiency characteristics - cheilosis, photophobia, sore throat, glossitis, fissure tongue, seborrheic dermatitis. Usual course - acute; progressive.

SYNONYMS
- vitamin B2 deficiency
- ariboflavinosis

CAUSES
- inadequate dietary intake
- intestinal malabsorption

TREATMENT
- riboflavin administration

ICD-9-CM
266.0 Ariboflavinosis

Rickettsialpox

DESCRIPTION Mild, self-limited disease transmitted by a mite that is an ectoparasite of the house mouse. Characteristics - eschar-like primary skin lesion, generalize papulovesicular rash, headache, and backache. Usual course - acute; incubation period 10 days to 3 weeks after bite. Endemic areas - USA; Europe; Africa.

CAUSES
- Rickettsia akari
- bite from mite (vector) infected by rodent

TREATMENT
- tetracycline
- chloramphenicol

ICD-9-CM
083.2 Rickettsialpox

Ruptured chordae tendineae

DESCRIPTION Rupture of a tendinous chord that connects each cusp of atrioventricular valves to approximate papillary muscles in the heart ventricles. Characteristics include a dramatic holosystolic apical murmur, precordial thrill, chest pain, dyspnea. Rupture of the chordae of the mitral valve is not uncommon. Usual course - acute; progressive.

CAUSES
- endocarditis
- trauma
- thoracic compression
- myxomatous perforation

TREATMENT
- diuretics
- surgical repair

ICD-9-CM
429.5 Rupture of chordae tendineae

SEE ALSO
- Ruptured mitral papillary muscle

Ruptured mitral papillary muscle

DESCRIPTION Rupture of conical muscular projections from walls of the cardiac ventricles, attached to cusps of the mitral arterioventricular valves by the chordae tendinea. Characteristics - pansystolic murmur, apical thrill, signs and symptoms of congestive heart failure. Usual course - acute; progressive.

SYNONYMS
- papillary muscle rupture

CAUSES
- myocardial infarction
- myocardial necrosis
- trauma

TREATMENT
- diuretics
- surgery

ICD-9-CM
429.6 Rupture of papillary muscle

Schatzki ring

DESCRIPTION Ring-like narrowing of the distal esophagus at the squamocolumnar junction. It is probably congenital and measures 2-4 mm in the submucosa. Characteristics - dysphagia. X-ray with barium swallow confirms the diagnosis by displaying the annular constriction of the lower esophagus. Usual course - chronic; progressive.

SYNONYMS
- esophagogastric ring syndrome
- lower esophageal ring syndrome

CAUSES
- unknown

TREATMENT
- rubber dilatation of ring

ICD-9-CM
530.3 Stricture and stenosis of esophagus
750.3 Congenital tracheoesophageal fistula, esophageal atresia and stenosis

Schistosomiasis, cutaneous

DESCRIPTION Parasitic disease caused by blood flukes of the genus Schistosoma. Fresh and salt water mollusks are intermediate hosts. Characteristics - intense pruritus, stinging, macules, papules, and vesicles. Endemic areas - Hawaii, Florida, Great Lakes area. Usual course - acute; intermittent; relapsing.

SYNONYMS
- swimmer itch
- clam digger's itch

CAUSES
- nonspecific Schistosome cercaria
- snail reservoir
- skin penetration
- abnormal host foreign body reaction

TREATMENT
- antipruritics
- antibiotics for secondary bacterial infections

ICD-9-CM
120.3 Cutaneous schistosomiasis

Schistosomiasis haematobium

DESCRIPTION Parasitic disease caused by blood flukes of the genus Schistosoma haematobium. S. Haematobium causes symptoms in the genitourinary system or lower colon and rectum. Endemic in Africa, India, Middle East, Indian Ocean islands. Usual course - acute; chronic; intermittent; progressive.

SYNONYMS
- endemic hematuria
- urogenital schistosomiasis

CAUSES
- trematode Schistosoma haematobium
- fresh water snail reservoir

TREATMENT
- praziquantel
- metrifonate
- niridazole

ICD-9-CM
120.0 Schistosomiasis due to Schistosoma haematobium

Schistosomiasis japonica

DESCRIPTION Parasitic disease caused by blood flukes of Schistosoma japonica causing disturbances in the small intestine, colon, and rectum. Characteristics - may be asymptomatic, melena, diarrhea, hepatosplenomegaly. Endemic area - Africa, India, Middle East, Indian Ocean islands. Usual course - acute; chronic; intermittent; progressive.

SYNONYMS
- eastern schistosomiasis
- Katayama disease
- Yangtze River disease

CAUSES
- trematode Schistosoma japonica
- fresh water snail reservoir

TREATMENT
- praziquantel
- niridazole
- stibocaptate

ICD-9-CM
120.2 Schistosomiasis due to Schistosoma japonicum

Schistosomiasis mansoni

DESCRIPTION Parasitic disease caused by blood flukes of Schistosoma mansoni causing disturbances in the small intestine, colon, and rectum. Characteristics - diarrhea, weight loss, anorexia, melena, jaundice, hepatosplenomegaly. Endemic areas - Africa, South America, Caribbean, Middle East. May occur in Americans who lived in Puerto Rico. Usual course - acute; chronic; intermittent; progressive.

SYNONYMS
- intestinal bilharziasis
- schistosomal dysentery
- Katayama fever
- Manson schistosomiasis
- Schistosoma mansoni infection
- intestinal schistosomiasis

CAUSES
- trematode Schistosoma mansoni
- fresh water snail reservoir

TREATMENT
- praziquantel
- oxamniquine

ICD-9-CM
120.1 Schistosomiasis due to Schistosoma mansoni

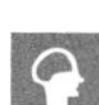

Schistosomiasis of the liver, chronic

DESCRIPTION Parasitic disease caused by blood flukes of the genus Schistosoma that penetrate the skin and develop in the liver, causing fever, eosinophilia, urticaria, hepatosplenomegaly, lymphadenopathy, ascites, esophageal varices. Endemic areas - Africa, Asia, South America, Caribbean Islands.

SYNONYMS
- bilharziasis

CAUSES
- Schistosoma mansoni
- Schistosoma japonicum
- fresh water snails

TREATMENT
- oxamniquine
- praziquantel
- niridazole
- splenorenal anastomosis surgery

ICD-9-CM
120.9 Schistosomiasis, unspecified

Scleredema

DESCRIPTION Diffuse, symmetrical, wooden-like, non-pitting induration of the skin of face, head, shoulders, arms, thorax. Usually preceded by an infectious process. It occurs in association with diabetes mellitus. Resolves in 6 months to 2 years. Usual course - acute; chronic.

SYNONYMS
• scleredema adultorum of Buschke

CAUSES
• unknown
• following streptococcal infection

TREATMENT
• self-limited
• unnecessary

ICD-9-CM
710.1 Systemic sclerosis

Sclerosis of the brain

DESCRIPTION Familial form of leukoencephalopathy occurring in early life and running a slowly progressive course into adolescence or adulthood. Characteristics - nystagmus, ataxia, tremor, choreoathetotic movements, dysarthria, and mental deterioration.

SYNONYMS
• Pelizaeus-Merzbacher disease
• diffuse familial cerebral sclerosis
• aplasia axialis extracorticalis congenita

CAUSES
• genetic

TREATMENT
• supportive

ICD-9-CM
330.0 Leukodystrophy

Scoliosis

DESCRIPTION A lateral curvature of the spine that may be found in the thoracic, lumbar, or thoracolumbar spinal segment. The curve may be convex to the right or to the left. Rotation of the vertebral column around its axis occurs and may cause rib cage deformity. May be associated with kyphosis (humpback) or lordosis (swayback). The most common type is idiopathic (80% of cases), usually begins about ages 8-10, is more common in girls than boys (4-5:1) and is classically asymptomatic.

CAUSES
• structural scoliosis
  ◊ idiopathic (may be transmitted as an autosomal dominant or multifactorial trait)
  ◊ congenital defects of the spine (hemivertebral or unilateral vertebral bridge)
  ◊ paralytic or musculoskeletal (due to polio, cerebral palsy, or muscular dystrophy)
• functional scoliosis
  ◊ poor posture
  ◊ uneven leg length

TREATMENT
• physical therapy and back exercises aimed at strengthening back muscles
• orthopedic back brace (sometimes worn for several years)
• if legs are of unequal length, a shoe lift for the shorter leg
• surgery to correct the deformity (severe cases only)

ICD-9-CM
737.30 Scoliosis (and kyphoscoliosis), idiopathic
754.2 Congenital musculoskeletal deformities of spine

Scurvy, infantile

DESCRIPTION Nutritional disease of children caused by ascorbic acid deficiency. Characteristics - weakness, anemia, spongy gums, mucocutaneous hemorrhages, brawny induration of calves and legs.

SYNONYMS
• vitamin C deficiency
• Barlow disease
• subperiosteal hematoma syndrome

CAUSES
• ascorbic acid deficiency

TREATMENT
• ascorbic acid
• fruit juice

ICD-9-CM
267 Absorbic acid deficiency

Seasonal affective disorder

DESCRIPTION Depression caused by dysfunction of circadian rhythms, that occurs most often in the winter months and is believed to be due to a decrease in exposure to full-spectrum light. In addition to feelings of sadness and anxiety, symptoms include hypersomnia, lethargy, carbohydrate craving and weight gain. Diagnosis usually requires a 2-3 year mood disturbance pattern, with the onset occurring in the autumn, and a remission in the spring. It occurs more commonly in women and among individuals living in the northern latitudes.

SYNONYMS
SAD

CAUSES
• exact cause is unknown; may be linked to amount of melatonin released by the pineal gland

TREATMENT
• phototherapy (light therapy) is preferential treatment
• MAO inhibitor or fluoxetine
• psychotherapy

ICD-9-CM
300.4 Neurotic depression

Second degree AV block

DESCRIPTION Two subtypes:
• Type I or Wenckebach: P-R interval becomes progressively longer with each cycle until a non-conducted atrial beat occurs. After the dropped beat the P-R interval is shorter.
• Type II: Constant P-R intervals preceding a non-conducted atrial beat.
Ventricular rate is irregular. Atrial rhythm is regular.

SYNONYMS
• Mobitz type 1
• Wenckebach period

CAUSES
• inferior wall myocardial infarction, digitalis toxicity, vagal stimulation

TREATMENT
• discontinue digitalis
• atropine if patient is symptomatic.

ICD-9-CM
426.13 Other second degree atrioventricular block

Selective IgA deficiency

DESCRIPTION The most common and mildest immunoglobulin deficiency (<15 mg/dL). IgA is the primary immunoglobulin in human saliva, nasal and bronchial fluids and intestinal secretions. It normally guards against bacterial and viral infections. The deficiency is lifelong and precautions need to be taken to prevent infections.

CAUSES
• autosomal dominant or recessive inheritance
• some drugs may cause transient IgA deficiency
• chromosome 18 abnormalities
• occurs in relatives patients with common variable immunodeficiency

TREATMENT
• no known cure
• treatment for associated diseases
• wear medical alerting identification

ICD-9-CM
279.01 Selective IgA immunodeficiency

Severe acute respiratory syndrome (SARS)

DESCRIPTION SARS is an asymptomatic to severe respiratory illness caused by a novel coronavirus. Symptoms include cough, shortness of breath. Signs include hypoxia, radiographic evidence of pneumonia, fever. Travel within 10 days to an area with known infection (all but 1 U.S. patient had traveled to the Orient).
This illness was first reported in November 2002 from China. The disease spread rapidly away from its original reported site and by May 2003 approximately 8,500 probable cases and 812 deaths had been reported. In the U.S. 45 patients had positive antibody to SARS-CoV or positive RT-PCR on respiratory specimens. None of the U.S. patients died as a result of their infection. The last reported probable case was on June 27, 2003 in Canada.

CAUSES
• Coronavirus (SARS-CoV)

TREATMENT
Primarily supportive

ICD-9-CM
079.82 SARS - associated coronavirus

SEE ALSO
• Pneumonia, viral

Sheehan syndrome

DESCRIPTION Postpartum pituitary necrosis resulting form hypovolemia and shock in the immediate peripartum period. Characteristics - endocrine deficiency syndromes due to loss of anterior lobe pituitary function. Usual course - progressive; acute.

SYNONYMS
• postpartum panhypopituitary syndrome
• postpartum hypopituitarism

CAUSES
• intrapartum hemorrhage
• postpartum hemorrhage
• postpartum infection
• peripheral vascular collapse
• vascular spasm
• DIC

TREATMENT
• hormone replacement therapy
• new pregnancy

ICD-9-CM
253.2 Panhypopituitarism

Shigellosis

DESCRIPTION Acute infection of the bowel. Source of infection: excreta of infected individuals that may be indirectly spread by contaminated food. Incubation period - 1 to 4 days. Characteristics - sudden onset of fever, irritability, drowsiness, anorexia, nausea, vomiting, diarrhea, abdominal pain and distention. Stools show blood, pus and mucus.

CAUSES
• shigella ingestion

TREATMENT
- fluid replacement
- ampicillin
- tetracycline
- sulfamethoxazole-trimethoprim
- chloramphenicol

ICD-9-CM
004.9 Shigellosis, unspecified

Short-bowel syndrome

DESCRIPTION A malabsorption syndrome resulting from massive resection of small bowel. Characteristics - diarrhea, steatorrhea, malnutrition. Usual course - chronic; progressive.

SYNONYMS
- massive bowel resection syndrome

CAUSES
- excessive resection of small bowel

TREATMENT
- parenteral nutrition
- low fat diet
- trace metal replacement
- mineral replacement
- vitamin replacement
- parenteral bile-salt sequestering agent
- H-2 receptor antagonist

ICD-9-CM
579.3 Other and unspecified postsurgical nonabsorption

Shoulder-hand syndrome

DESCRIPTION Clinical disorder of the upper extremity. Characteristics - pain and stiffness in the shoulder with puffy swelling and pain in the ipsilateral hand, sometimes occurring after myocardial infarction. Usual course - chronic; acute exacerbations.

SYNONYMS
- Steinbrocker syndrome
- reflex sympathetic dystrophy syndrome
- coronary-scapular syndrome
- postinfarction sclerodactylia

CAUSES
- reflex sympathetic stimulation
- cerebral vascular accident
- myocardial infarction
- upper extremity trauma

TREATMENT
- physical therapy
- analgesics
- oral steroids
- stellate ganglion block
- steroid injections

ICD-9-CM
337.9 Unspecified disorder of autonomic nervous system

SEE ALSO
- Arthritis, rheumatoid (RA)

Siderosis of the lung

DESCRIPTION Pneumoconiosis due to inhalation of iron particles. X-rays are abnormal, but there is no functional impairment and there are no symptoms. Usual course - chronic; acute; progressive.

SYNONYMS
- silver polisher lung
- welder lung

CAUSES
- inhalation of iron oxide dust

TREATMENT
- unnecessary

ICD-9-CM
503 Pneumoconiosis due to other inorganic dust

Silo filler disease

DESCRIPTION Pulmonary edema caused by nitrogen dioxide intoxication, which may take place among welders or silo fillers. Symptoms may not appear for 12 hours after exposure. Usual course - progressive; acute.

SYNONYMS
- nitrogen dioxide toxicity
- silage gas poisoning
- silo filler pneumoconiosis

CAUSES
- inhalation of nitrogen dioxide

TREATMENT
- bronchodilators
- mechanical ventilation
- supplemental oxygen

ICD-9-CM
506.9 Unspecified respiratory conditions due to fumes and vapors

Silver poisoning

DESCRIPTION Permanent ashen-gray discoloration of the skin, conjunctiva, and internal organs resulting from long over-exposure to silver. Usual course - acute; chronic.

SYNONYMS
- argyria
- argyriasis

CAUSES
- absorption through skin
- inhalation of dust fumes
- accidental ingestion
- abuse of silver nose drops
- mining
- silver plating
- handling of metallic silver

TREATMENT
- emesis
- hydration
- gastric lavage
- activated charcoal

ICD-9-CM
985.8 Toxic effect of other specified metals

Sinding-Larson Johansson disease

DESCRIPTION An inflammatory condition similar to Osgood-Schlatter disease but affecting the distal patellar apophysis and the proximal portion of the patellar tendon. Symptoms include pain and swelling about the distal patella generally aggravated by activity.

SYNONYMS
- Patellar tendinitis

CAUSES

TREATMENT
Conservative measures including rest, ice, NSAIDs, limitation of exacerbating activities. Sinding-Larson Johansson disease may cause more disruption in sporting activities than Osgood-Schlatter disease.

ICD-9-CM
732.4 Juvenile osteochondrosis of lower extremity, excluding foot

Sinoatrial arrest or block

DESCRIPTION Unexpectedly long P-P interval interrupting normal sinus rhythm. Often terminated by a junctional escape beat or return to normal sinus rhythm. QRS complexes uniform, but irregular.

SYNONYMS
- Sinus arrest

CAUSES
- digitalis toxicity, quinidine toxicity, sick sinus syndrome

TREATMENT
- atropine, 0.5 mg intravenously
- Pacemaker for repeated episodes

ICD-9-CM
426.6 Other heart block

Sinus bradycardia

DESCRIPTION Rate of less than 60 beats per minute. A QRS complex follows each P wave.

CAUSES
- sick sinus syndrome, hypothyroidism, mechanical ventilation, inferior myocardial infarction, increased intracranial pressure, increased vagal tone (straining at stool), vomiting, intubation, treatment with beta-blockers and sympatholytic drugs

TREATMENT
- atropine, 0.5 mg every 5 minutes to total of 2.0 mg if needed
- temporary pacemaker if atropine fails

ICD-9-CM
427.81 Sinoatrial node dysfunction

Sinus tachycardia

DESCRIPTION Cardiac rate greater than 100 beats per minute. May rarely increase to exceed 160 beats per minute. Every QRS complex follows a P wave.

CAUSES
- cardiac response to fever, anxiety, vigorous exercise, pain, dehydration, shock, left ventricular heart failure, cardiac tamponade, anemia, hyperthyroidism, hypovolemia, pulmonary embolus, myocardial infarction

TREATMENT
- treat the underlying cause

ICD-9-CM
427.0 Paroxysmal supraventricular tachycardia
785.0 Tachycardia, unspecified

Sjögren syndrome

DESCRIPTION An autoimmune disorder causing decreased function and progressive destruction of the salivary and lacrimal glands.

SYNONYMS
- Sicca syndrome

CAUSES
- Unknown

TREATMENT
- Ocular lubricants

ICD-9-CM
710.2 Sicca syndrome

SEE ALSO
- Arthritis, rheumatoid (RA)

Smallpox

DESCRIPTION An acute infectious disease caused by pox virus. This disease is now extinct worldwide due to successful inoculation. Alastrim, a mild form of the disease is known as variola minor.

SYNONYMS
- variola
- variola major

CAUSES
- double-stranded DNA virus transmitted by inhalation
- rare family transmission

TREATMENT
- isolation, report to health department, meticulous fluid management, skin hygiene, antihistamines, antibiotics for

secondary bacterial infections

ICD-9-CM
050.9 Smallpox, unspecified

Smoking cessation

DESCRIPTION 23 % of U.S. adults smoke and 90% of these are nicotine dependent. Strong correlation exists with history of smoking within 5 minutes of awakening and >25 cigarettes/day. Over 45% of adult smokers attempt to quit annually and 70% have tried to quit at least once. Suspected similarities with noncigarette forms of nicotine/tobacco use such as cigar and pipe smoking, chewing tobacco and snuff.

CAUSES N/A

TREATMENT
Stages
• Precontemplation -does not want to quit - need awareness of smoking/nicotine related diseases. Literature available from American Lung Association, American Cancer Society, and the National Cancer Institute (1-800-4-CANCER)
• Contemplation - wants to quit, but not within month - review prior attempts and identify barriers. Discuss consequences of continued behavior, more education.
• Action - wants to quit or has just quit within 1 month - plan quitting and strategies for relapse. Consider:
◊ Nicotine replacement with transdermal patches, gum, nasal spray or lung inhaler available over the counter
◊ Bupropion (Zyban) 150 mg qd to bid begun 1 week before and continued for 7-12 weeks after smoking cessation. Other antidepressants (eg, nortriptyline) may be effective.
◊ Both nicotine and bupropion
• Maintenance - has quit for > 1 month - deal with relapses immediately, seek cause, and consider nicotine replacement and slow withdrawal
• Relapses - again smoking daily - identify trigger for relapse, develop strategies to deal with triggers, assess stages above, consider adding behavioral modification techniques (eg, classes, hypnosis, acupuncture) or other drugs (eg, clonidine, anxiolytics, nicotine antagonist)
• Physician counseling is critical to patient quitting smoking, doubles success rate
• Parents and teachers: advise children adolescents not to smoke; aid in avoiding addiction

ICD-9-CM
305.1 Tobacco use disorder
292.0 Drug withdrawal syndrome

Author(s)
Edgar A. Lucas, PhD

Somatoform disorders

DESCRIPTION A group of disorders in which there are physical symptoms for which no physical cause can be found. Included in this group are somatization disorder, conversion disorder, and body dysmorphic disorder. Hypochondriasis and chronic pain disorder (somatoform pain disorder) are also classified as somatoform disorders, but are covered in separate topics.
• Somatization disorder: multiple physical symptoms that recur over a period of several years with no medical basis. The patient has usually consulted numerous doctors for treatment and medications. This disorder was previous called hysteria. The symptoms often involve neurological problems (double vision), gynecological problems (painful menstruation) or gastrointestinal problems (abdominal pain).
• Conversion disorder: loss or change of a physical function (paralysis of an arm, blindness, seizures). The symptom is not intentionally produced or faked.
• Body dysmorphic disorder: preoccupation with an imagined defect in a normal-appearing person. The defect may be very minor, but the concern is blown out of proportion. The focus is often on skin wrinkles and blemishes, facial hair, shape of the nose, mouth or jaw.

CAUSES Exact cause is unknown

TREATMENT
• Psychotherapy
• Group therapy
• Family therapy

ICD-9-CM
306.9 Unspecified psychophysiological malfunction

Sotos syndrome

DESCRIPTION A genetic disorder causing physical overgrowth with delayed motor, cognitive, and social development.

SYNONYMS
• cerebral gigantism

CAUSES Unknown

TREATMENT
• Physical therapy
• Speech therapy

ICD-9-CM
253.0 Acromegaly and gigantism

Sparganosis

DESCRIPTION Infection of animals, including fish and man, with a developmental stage of Diphyllobothrium. This stage has recently been referred to as a plerocercoid but the name sparganum has persisted. Therefore, infection of fish or other animals with the plerocercoid larvae is sparganosis. Fish-eating mammals, including man, are the final hosts. Usual course - chronic.

SYNONYMS
• larval diphyllobothriasis

CAUSES
• Spirometra species
• larval diphyllobothrium ingestion from undercooked flesh
• animal flesh poultices

TREATMENT
• surgical excision only

ICD-9-CM
123.5 Sparganosis [larval diphyllobothriasis]

Spinal cord compression

DESCRIPTION Impingement on the spinal cord, usually by an extramedullary neoplasm. Characteristics - local back pain, hyperreflexia, Babinski's sign, weakness of lower extremities, sensory loss, loss of sphincter control. Back pain and weakness may last hours to days, but total loss of function control to the site of compression may take only minutes. Usual course - acute onset; chronic onset; often progressive primary disease.

CAUSES
• carcinoma of the lung
• breast carcinoma
• carcinoma of the prostate
• lymphoma
• neural malignancy
• herniated disk
• extradural abscess
• spinal tuberculosis
• rheumatoid arthritis
• cervical spondylosis

TREATMENT
• high dose corticosteroids
• radiotherapy
• surgery
• chemotherapy for primary tumor

ICD-9-CM
336.9 Unspecified disease of spinal cord

Splenic agenesis syndrome

DESCRIPTION Congenital absence of the spleen, partial situs inversus viscerum accompanied by cardiac defects (right type atria, endocardial cushion defect). This is a familial disorder that is autosomal recessive with sporadic penetrance. Usual course - acute; chronic; progressive.

SYNONYMS
• Ivemark syndrome
• asplenia

CAUSES
• failure of normal asymmetry in morphogenesis

TREATMENT
• antibiotics
• cardiac surgery
• gastrointestinal surgery

ICD-9-CM
759.0 Anomalies of spleen

Squamous cell carcinoma, anterior tongue

DESCRIPTION Malignancy of the oral tongue that does not include the base of the tongue. Characteristics - located on lateral aspects of the undersurface of the tongue.

CAUSES
• unknown

TREATMENT
• surgery plus radiotherapy, depending on staging

ICD-9-CM
141.4 Malignant neoplasm of anterior two-thirds of tongue, part unspecified

Squamous cell carcinoma, anus

DESCRIPTION These malignancies comprise 3-5% of rectal and anal cancers. Characteristics - fungating anal mass, tight sphincter, perineal pain and pressure. Usual course - insidious onset; surgical cure; progressive if untreated.

CAUSES
• condylomata
• rectal fistulae
• rectal fissures
• rectal abscesses
• leukoplakia of the anus
• irradiation

TREATMENT
• surgery
• radiotherapy

ICD-9-CM
154.3 Malignant neoplasm of anus, unspecified

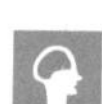

Squamous cell carcinoma, bladder

DESCRIPTION Bladder malignancy frequently associated with parasitic infection or chronic mucosal irritation. Characteristics - highly infiltrative, poor prognosis, gross hematuria, dysuria. Usual course - progressive.

SYNONYMS
• epidermoid bladder carcinoma

CAUSES
• beta-naphthylamine
• 4-aminodiphenyl
• tobacco smoking
• chronic Schistosoma haematobium infection
• aniline dye

TREATMENT
• endoscopic resection

- segmental bladder resection
- total cystectomy
- methotrexate
- cisplatin
- doxorubicin
- intravesical thiotepa
- preoperative radiotherapy
- supervoltage radiotherapy
- intracavitary radium
- interstitial implantations

ICD-9-CM
188.9 Malignant neoplasm of bladder, part unspecified

Squamous cell carcinoma, floor of the mouth

DESCRIPTION These account for 20,000 new cases of oral cancer each year. Appears most often as a red (erythroblastic) lesion at first appearing as an inflammatory lesion. Characteristics - lump in floor of the mouth; chronic, non-healing ulcer; foul breath odor; very few are indurated or raised. Usual course - progressive if not cured.

CAUSES
- tobacco
- alcohol
- poor oral hygiene
- epstein-barr virus
- chronic oral trauma
- plummer-vinson virus
- betel nut chewing

TREATMENT
- surgery plus radiotherapy depending on stage
- surgery plus radiotherapy depending on location

ICD-9-CM
144.9 Malignant neoplasm of floor of mouth, part unspecified

Strabismus

DESCRIPTION Deviation of one eye from parallelism with the other

SYNONYMS
- Squint
- Cross eyes
- Heterotropia

CAUSES
- paralytic (nonconcomitant) strabismus - paralysis of one or more ocular muscles. Nonparalytic (concomitant) - unequal muscle tone.

TREATMENT
- treatment before age 6 years - complete eye exam; corrective lenses or contact lenses; miotics; orthoptic training; surgical restoration of muscle balance

ICD-9-CM
378.9 Unspecified disorder of eye movements

Strongyloidiasis

DESCRIPTION Infection with Strongyloides stercoralis occurring widely in tropical and subtropical countries. Larvae develop in the soil and penetrate the human skin on contact. They travel to the lungs via the bloodstream and thence to the trachea and esophagus and intestines. Usual course - intermittent.

CAUSES
- parasitic infection caused by strongyloides stercorous
- penetration of the skin by larvae
- contaminated food ingestion
- autoinfection

TREATMENT
- thiabendazole

ICD-9-CM
127.2 Strongyloidiasis

Sturge-Weber disease

DESCRIPTION One of the neurocutaneous syndromes. Congenital capillary hemangiomas affect the skin of the face and neck, mucous membranes, meninges, choroid and conjunctiva. Usually unilateral and in trigeminal nerve distribution, hemangiomata can involve the meninges with associated focal brain atrophy, sclerosis, and calcifications. Early onset of seizures is associated with poor outcome of intellectual performance and with neurologic deficits. Course - variable. Complications - seizures, glaucoma, mental retardation, paresis.

SYNONYMS
- Encephalotrigeminal angiomatosis

CAUSES Congenital, but genetics unknown. Occasionally other family members have hemangiomata in non-facial areas to a lesser degree. Incidence: 2/100,000

TREATMENT
- Seizures: Anticonvulsants, neurosurgery
- Monitoring for glaucoma
- Genetic counseling for patient and family

ICD-9-CM
759.6 Other hamartoses, NEC

SEE ALSO
- Ataxia-telangiectasia
- Neurofibromatosis (Types 1 & 2)
- von Hippel-Lindau disease

Author(s)
Nuhad D. Dinno, MD

Subacute combined degeneration

DESCRIPTION The neurologic manifestations of pernicious anemia. Characteristics - peripheral paresthesias, weakness, leg stiffness, unsteadiness, lethargy, fatigue. Usual course - progressive.

SYNONYMS
- subacute combined degeneration of spinal cord
- combined system disease
- posterolateral sclerosis
- ataxic paraplegia
- neuroanemic syndrome
- funicular spinal disease
- Dana syndrome
- Putnam-Dana syndrome
- Lichtheim syndrome

CAUSES
- vitamin B12 deficiency
- pernicious anemia
- no intrinsic factor in gastric secretion

TREATMENT
- intramuscular cobalamin

ICD-9-CM
336.2 Subacute combined degeneration of spinal cord in diseases classified elsewhere

Sulfur dioxide poisoning

DESCRIPTION Irritant gas poisoning as an industrial accident. Characteristics - cough, hemoptysis, wheezing, retching, dyspnea, X-ray findings of diffuse mottled infiltrates indicating pulmonary edema. Usual course - acute; chronic; progressive; relapsing.

CAUSES
- cytotoxicity due to reactions between organic compounds and nitrogen oxides
- oxidation to form sulfuric acid
- occupational exposure
- industrial cleaners

TREATMENT
- supportive
- oxygen
- bronchodilators
- eye dilution plus irrigation
- acid dilution
- analgesia
- corticosteroids
- dilute skin contact
- treat shock
- antibiotics

ICD-9-CM
987.3 Toxic effect of sulfur dioxide

Sunburn

DESCRIPTION
- Characteristics - mild erythema with subsequent scaling, pain, swelling, skin tenderness, blisters, fever, chills, weakness, shock, secondary infections, miliaria-like eruptions, exfoliation

CAUSES
- exposure to sunlight (or other ultraviolet light source) following administration of phototoxicity-producing drugs
- overexposure to ultraviolet rays of UVB (2800 to 3200A); danger increases proportionately to high altitude

TREATMENT
- prophylaxis with sunscreens rated 15 or better
- avoid additional exposure until well
- use tap-water compresses
- avoid topical anesthetic lotions and ointments
- use oral corticosteroids for extensive, severe sunburn (prednisone 10 mg qid for 4-6 days).

ICD-9-CM
692.71 Sunburn

Superior sagittal sinus thrombosis

DESCRIPTION Blood clotting in the superior sagittal sinus, a single venous sinus of the dura mater beginning in front of the crista galli and extending backward in the convex border of the falx cerebri. Characteristics - fever, prostration, headache, obtundation, engorged scalp veins, seizure, aphasia, hemiplegia. Usual course - acute.

SYNONYMS
- superior longitudinal sinus thrombosis

CAUSES
- infection
- extension from osteomyelitis
- dehydration
- trauma
- tumors

TREATMENT
- antimicrobials
- drainage
- surgery

ICD-9-CM
437.6 Nonpyogenic thrombosis of intracranial venous sinus

SEE ALSO
- Factor V Leiden

Syringomyelia

DESCRIPTION Often associated with syringobulbia. Fluid-filled cavity (syrinx) within the substance of the spinal cord or brainstem.

- Characteristics - lack of sensation for noxious stimuli in fingers (painless cut or burn). Cape-like sensory defect over shoulders and back. Spasticity and weakness of the lower extremities. Muscular atrophy and fasciculations. Vertigo, nystagmus

CAUSES
- congenital (50%), intramedullary tumors

TREATMENT
- surgical drainage of the syrinx; plugging obex in 4th ventricle; section of spinal cord at filum terminale

ICD-9-CM
336.0 Syringomyelia and syringobulbia

Tabes dorsalis

DESCRIPTION Parenchymatous neurosyphilis in which there is slowly progressive degeneration of the posterior columns and roots and ganglia of the spinal cord. Occurs 15 to 20 years after initial syphilitic infection. Characteristics - lancinating lightning pains, urinary incontinence, ataxia, impaired position and vibratory sense, optic atrophy, hypotonia, hyporeflexia and trophic joint degeneration (Charcot's joints).

SYNONYMS
- tabetic neurosyphilis
- locomotor ataxia
- Duchenne disease
- spinal cord syphilis

CAUSES
- treponema pallidum

TREATMENT
- penicillin, tetracycline, erythromycin
- anticonvulsants, carbamazepine, phenytoin
- surgery

ICD-9-CM
094.0 Tabes dorsalis
094.89 Other specified neurosyphilis

Takayasu syndrome

DESCRIPTION Pulseless disease. Progressive obliteration of the brachiocephalic trunk and the left subclavian and left common carotid arteries above their origin in the aortic arch. Characteristics - loss of pulse in both arms and carotids; symptoms associated with ischemia of the brain (syncope, transient hemiplegia), eyes (transient blindness), face and arms. Usual course - progressive. Endemic areas - Orient.

SYNONYMS
- pulseless disease
- reverse coarctation
- Martorell syndrome
- brachiocephalic ischemia
- aortic arch syndrome

CAUSES
- unknown; autoimmune; hypersensitivity

TREATMENT
- corticosteroids
- surgery

ICD-9-CM
446.7 Takayasu disease

SEE ALSO
- Subclavian steal syndrome

Tardive dyskinesia

DESCRIPTION A neurological syndrome characterized by involuntary and abnormal movements, usually involving buccal-oral muscles (but any muscle in the body can be affected). The movements include grimacing, sticking out the tongue, smacking and sucking of the lips, and sometimes, rapid movements of the arms and legs (chorea and athetosis). Tardive dyskinesia is associated with long-term use of neuroleptic drugs, usually appears late in the course of drug therapy and may persist indefinitely after discontinuation of the medication.

CAUSES
- up-regulation of dopamine receptors caused by long-term neuroleptic drug use (3 mos to years), prescribed for psychoses, also gastrointestinal and neurologic disorders

TREATMENT
- no effective treatment is available
- when possible, consider discontinuing the neuroleptic drug; some patients may prefer the movements to the possibility of relapse; also, discontinuance of the drug may not reverse tardive dyskinesia

ICD-9-CM
333.82 Orofacial dyskinesia

Thallium poisoning

DESCRIPTION Poisoning due to ingestion of thallium compounds. Characteristics - vomiting, alopecia, neurologic and psychic symptoms, (ataxia, restlessness, delirium, hallucinations, semicoma, blindness), liver and kidney damage. Thallium is commonly found in ant, rat, and roach poisons. Symptoms usually begin approximately 3 weeks after poisoning. Usual course - acute; progressive.

CAUSES
- thallium ingestion

TREATMENT
- gastric decontamination
- potassium ferric hexacyanoferrate
- skin decontamination
- forced diuresis
- hemoperfusion
- hemodialysis
- urine output maintenance
- supportive

ICD-9-CM
985.8 Toxic effect of other specified metals

Thrombocythemia (adult), idiopathic

DESCRIPTION Hemorrhagic thrombocythemia (one of the myeloproliferative syndromes). Characteristics - repeated spontaneous hemorrhages, either external or into the tissues and an extraordinary increase in the number of circulating platelets. Usual course - chronic; progressive.

SYNONYMS
- primary thrombocythemia
- essential thrombocythemia
- primary hemorrhagic thrombocythemia
- essential thrombocytosis
- primary thrombohemorrhagic thrombocytosis

CAUSES
- clonal megakaryocytic disorder

TREATMENT
- chemotherapy
- radiotherapy
- iron replacement
- plateletpheresis
- platelet anti-aggregating agents

ICD-9-CM
238.7 Neoplasm of uncertain behavior of other lymphatic and hematopoietic tissues

Thymoma, malignant

DESCRIPTION Tumor derived from the epithelial or lymphoid elements of the thymus. Characteristics - cough, dyspnea, dysphagia, chest pain, weakness. Usual course - possibly acute; otherwise progressive.

CAUSES
- unknown

TREATMENT
- surgical thymectomy
- radiotherapy for invasive thymoma
- corticosteroids if radiotherapy fails
- chemotherapy for advanced disease

ICD-9-CM
164.0 Malignant neoplasm of thymus

SEE ALSO
- Sjögren syndrome

Thyrotoxic heart disease

DESCRIPTION Heart disease associated with hyperthyroidism. Characteristics - atrial fibrillation, cardiac enlargement, congestive heart failure. Usual course - progressive; relapsing.

SYNONYMS
- hyperthyroid heart disease

CAUSES
- hyperthyroidism

TREATMENT
- treat underlying hyperthyroidism
- radioactive iodine
- surgery
- beta-adrenergic blockers

ICD-9-CM
242.90 Thyrotoxicosis without mention of goiter or other cause without mention of thyrotoxic crisis or storm
425.7 Nutritional and metabolic cardiomyopathy

Thyrotoxic storm

DESCRIPTION Severe thyrotoxicosis accompanied by organ system decompensation. Characteristics - fever, severe tachycardia, dehydration, mental status abnormalities representing dysfunction of the cardiovascular and central nervous systems. Usual course - acute.

SYNONYMS
- thyrotoxicosis
- thyrotoxic crisis
- Basedow crisis

CAUSES
- exacerbation of hyperthyroidism
- thyroid surgery
- infection
- trauma

TREATMENT
- fluids
- propylthiouracil
- iodine
- hydrocortisone
- external cooling
- beta-adrenergic blockers
- oxygen
- treat precipitating factors

ICD-9-CM
242.91 Thytotoxicosis without mention of goiter or other cause with mention of thyrotoxic crisis or storm

Tick paralysis

DESCRIPTION A progressive, ascending paralysis caused by a neurotoxin secreted by a tick who has fed for several days on the host.

CAUSES Neurotoxin in saliva of ticks

TREATMENT
Removal of the tick, including any mouth parts retained in the skin. Complete recovery occurs in about 2 days.

ICD-9-CM
989.5 Toxic effect of venom

Tinea barbae

DESCRIPTION Fungal infection involving the bearded area of the face and neck. Characteristics - kerion-like swellings and nodular swellings with marked crusting. Usual course - acute; chronic.

SYNONYMS
- tinea sycosis
- barber's itch
- beard ringworm

CAUSES
- fungal infection of coarse facial hair
- zoophilic dermatophytes

TREATMENT
- systemic antifungal agents
- systemic steroid added in severe inflammatory infections

ICD-9-CM
110.0 Dermatophytosis of scalp and beard

Tinnitus

DESCRIPTION A very common condition typified by the perception of sound in the absence of an acoustic stimulus. The sound may be of a buzzing, ringing, roaring, whistling or hissing quality or may involve more complex sounds that vary over time. It may be intermittent, continuous or pulsatile (synchronous with the heartbeat).

CAUSES
- damage to inner ear or cochlea
- middle ear infection or result from just about any ear disorder
- aneurysm's
- hardening of the arteries
- several medications

TREATMENT
- treat the underlying cause
- background music
- tinnitus masking device
- hearing aid for associated deafness

ICD-9-CM
388.30 Tinnitus, unspecified

Toluene poisoning

DESCRIPTION A form of poisoning from toluene, a colorless liquid obtainable from coal tar. Toluene is an organic solvent used in rubber, plastic cements, paint removers, etc. Poisoning may result from inhalation or ingestion. Usual course - acute; chronic; progressive.

SYNONYMS
- toluol poisoning
- methylbenzene poisoning
- methylbenzol poisoning
- phenylmethane poisoning

CAUSES
- cytotoxicity

TREATMENT
- supportive; oxygen; bicarbonate
- CPR; gastric decontamination; skin decontamination; eye irrigation
- epinephrine contraindicated

ICD-9-CM
982.0 Toxic effect of benzene and homologues

Toxaphene poisoning

DESCRIPTION Poisoning among agricultural workers using DDT. Characteristics - vomiting, paresthesias, malaise, course tremors, convulsions, pulmonary edema, ventricular fibrillation, respiratory failure. Usual course - acute; chronic; progressive.

SYNONYMS
- chlorinated camphene poisoning

CAUSES
- direct cytotoxicity
- diffuse neuronal excitation

TREATMENT
- gastric decontamination
- skin decontamination
- oxygen
- anticonvulsants
- avoid sympathomimetics
- supportive

ICD-9-CM
989.2 Toxic effect of chlorinated hydrocarbons

Trachoma

DESCRIPTION Chronic infectious disease of the conjunctiva and cornea. Characteristics - photophobia, pain, lacrimation. The organism is a bacterium, Chlamydia trachomatis. Usual course - acute; progressive. Endemic areas - Africa; Middle East; Asia; Central America.

SYNONYMS
- granular conjunctivitis
- Egyptian ophthalmia

CAUSES
- Chlamydia trachomatis
- transmission through birth canal

TREATMENT
- tetracyclines
- erythromycin
- sulfonamides

ICD-9-CM
076.0 Trachoma, initial stage
076.1 Trachoma, active stage
076.9 Trachoma, unspecified

Transposition of the great vessels

DESCRIPTION A congenital heart defect where the great arteries are reversed - the aorta arises from the right ventricle and the pulmonary artery from the left ventricle. This produces two noncommunicating circulatory systems (pulmonary and systemic. It often coexists with other congenital anomalies and affects boys 2 to 3 times more than females. Usual course - acute.

SYNONYMS
- complete dextroposition of the great arteries

CAUSES
- abnormal embryogenesis

TREATMENT
- balloon septostomy
- surgical redirection

ICD-9-CM
745.10 Complete transposition of great vessels

Trench fever

DESCRIPTION Louse-borne disease occurring sporadically in Eastern Europe, Asia, North Africa and Mexico and producing multiple symptoms: fever, weakness, dizziness, severe leg and back pain.

SYNONYMS
- Wolhynia fever
- shin bone fever
- His-Werner disease
- quintana fever

CAUSES
- Rochalimaea quintana transmitted by body lice

TREATMENT
- analgesics
- antipyretics
- delousing

ICD-9-CM
083.1 Trench fever

Trichloroethylene poisoning

DESCRIPTION Trichloroethylene is a widely used industrial solvent and formerly used as an inhalation anesthetic. Poisoning characteristics: dizziness, headache, delirium, vomiting, abdominal pain, jaundice, flush. Usual course - acute; chronic; progressive.

CAUSES
- decomposition to dichloroethylene
- decomposition to phosgene
- decomposition to carbon monoxide
- hepatotoxicity
- renal toxicity

TREATMENT
- supportive
- gastric decontamination
- remove contaminated clothing
- epinephrine contraindicated
- volume expanders
- diuretics for urine output maintenance

ICD-9-CM
982.3 Toxic effect of other chlorinated hydrocarbon solvents

SEE ALSO
- Phosphine poisoning

Trichostrongyliasis

DESCRIPTION Infection by nematodes of the genus Trichostrongylus whose eggs are frequently mistaken for hookworms. Endemic areas - Middle East; Far East; Iran. Usually asymptomatic but may cause cramps and diarrhea. Usual course - acute.

SYNONYMS
- trichostrongyloidiasis

CAUSES
- trichostrongylus larvae ingestion

TREATMENT
- thiabendazole
- pyrantel pamoate

ICD-9-CM
127.6 Trichostrongyliasis

Tricuspid atresia

DESCRIPTION Absence of the orifice between the right atrium and ventricle. Circulation made possible by presence of an atrial septal defect, allowing blood to pass from the right to left atrium and then to the left ventricle and aorta. Intra-atrial communication due to anomalous embryonal development.

- Signs and symptoms include marked underdevelopment, severe cyanosis, clubbing of fingers, prominent jugular A wave, apical heave, pulmonic second sound absent, systolic murmur, enlarged liver, presystolic pulsation. EKG shows left axis deviation, left ventricular hypertrophy, tall P waves. Transposition of great vessels, patent foramen ovale and ventricular septal defect all may accompany tricuspid atresia.

CAUSES
- unknown

TREATMENT
- anticongestive therapy
- surgery to correct condition

ICD-9-CM
746.1 Tricuspid atresia and stenosis, congenital

Tricuspid regurgitation

DESCRIPTION Retrograde blood flow from the right ventricle to the right atrium due to inadequate apposition of the tricuspid valves. Characteristics - low output symptoms plus pulsations in the neck due to high jugular regurgitant waves from the transmitted right ventricular pressure. Usual course - acute; chronic.

SYNONYMS
- tricuspid valve insufficiency

CAUSES
- marked dilatation of right ventricle
- right ventricular failure
- rheumatic heart disease
- cor pulmonale
- congenital heart disease

TREATMENT
- treat underlying condition
- surgery
- tricuspid annuloplasty
- tricuspid valve replacement

ICD-9-CM
424.2 Tricuspid valve disorders, specified as nonrheumatic

Tricuspid stenosis

DESCRIPTION Narrowing of the tricuspid orifice obstructing blood flow from the right atrium to the right ventricle. Characteristics - fatigue, enlarged liver, fluttering discomfort in the neck caused by giant A waves in the jugular pulse. Usual course - chronic; progressive.

SYNONYMS
- tricuspid valve stenosis

CAUSES
- rheumatic fever
- bacterial vegetations
- atrial thrombi
- tumors
- carcinoid heart disease
- fibroelastosis

TREATMENT
- sodium restriction
- digitalization
- diuretics
- surgery
- valvulotomy

ICD-9-CM
397.0 Diseases of tricuspid valve
424.2 Tricuspid valve disorders, specified as nonrheumatic
746.1 Tricuspid atresia and stenosis, congenital

Tropical eosinophilia

DESCRIPTION Subacute or chronic form of filariasis. Characteristics - episodic nocturnal wheezing and coughing, strikingly elevated eosinophilia and lung infiltrations. Usual course - chronic; progressive.

CAUSES
- adult wuchereria bancrofti worms
- adult brugia malayi worms

TREATMENT
- diethylcarbamazine

ICD-9-CM
518.3 Pulmonary eosinophilia

SEE ALSO
- Filariasis

Truncus arteriosus

DESCRIPTION Congenital anomaly in which there is a single arterial trunk arising from the heart, receiving blood from both ventricles and supplying blood to the coronary, pulmonary, and systemic circulations. Frequently co-exists with malformations of other organ systems.
- Characteristics - signs and symptoms begin during the first week of life and include poor development, minimal or absent cyanosis, marked hypertrophy of the heart, loud and clear second sound, harsh systolic murmur at the base and along the left sternal border, continuous bruit over the upper sternum, thrill with maximum intensity over base of the heart, dyspnea, wide pulse pressure.

CAUSES
- unknown

TREATMENT
- surgery
- anticongestive therapy

ICD-9-CM
745.0 Common truncus anomalies

Trypanosomiasis, East African

DESCRIPTION Acute, severe, sometimes fatal form of African trypanosomiasis, transmitted by bites of tsetse flies. Usual course - acute; progressive; lethal within 1 year. Endemic areas - tropical East Africa.

SYNONYMS
- sleeping sickness
- Rhodesian sleeping sickness

CAUSES
- Trypanosoma brucei rhodesiense
- tsetse fly bites
- bushbuck antelope reservoir of infection

TREATMENT
- suramin prior to CNS involvement
- pentamidine prior to CNS involvement
- melarsoprol plus suramin pretreatment for CNS disease

ICD-9-CM
086.4 Rhodesian trypanosomiasis

Trypanosomiasis, West African

DESCRIPTION Chronic, less severe form of African trypanosomiasis. Disease persists for several months or years with central nervous system involvement late in its course. Usual course - chronic; intermittent; relapsing; progressive; delayed onset; successive bouts; intervening latent periods; may persist many years. Endemic areas - tropical West Africa; Central Africa.

SYNONYMS
- sleeping sickness
- Gambian sleeping sickness

CAUSES
- Trypanosoma brucei gambiense
- tsetse fly bites
- transplacental transmission
- human reservoir

TREATMENT
- suramin prior to CNS involvement
- pentamidine prior to CNS involvement
- melarsoprol plus suramin pretreatment for CNS disease

ICD-9-CM
086.3 Gambian trypanosomiasis

Tubular necrosis, acute

DESCRIPTION Acute renal tubular necrosis is a syndrome with multiple causes accounting for 70% of renal failure patients. Types include - stage 1: onset azotemia; stage 2: oliguria; stage 3: diuresis; stage 4: resolving diuresis
Usual course - acute; reversible;

SYNONYMS
- lower nephron nephrosis
- vasomotor nephropathy

CAUSES
- ischemia
- disseminated intravascular coagulation
- nephrotoxins
- trauma
- dehydration
- circulatory insufficiency

TREATMENT
- hemodialysis
- maintain renal perfusion
- maintain euvolemia
- diuretics
- vasopressors
- alkalinization

ICD-9-CM
584.5 Acute renal failure with lesion of tubular necrosis

Uterine bleeding postmenopausal

DESCRIPTION Bleeding from female genital tract beginning one or more years following menopause. Characteristics - may occur from any part of the reproductive tract including uterus, cervix, vagina, vulva; bleeding may be heavy or light.

CAUSES
- Iatrogenic as a result of estrogen replacement therapy
- Infection, atrophy, tumors (benign or malignant), polyps, adnexal pathology. Endometrial carcinoma is the cause of 1/3 of all cases of postmenopausal bleeding.

TREATMENT
- D&C
- discontinue all exogenous estrogens, including creams, etc.
- definitive treatment depends on finding and treating underlying cause

ICD-9-CM
627.1 Postmenopausal bleeding

Ventricular fibrillation

DESCRIPTION Ventricular rhythm rapid and chaotic. QRS complexes wide and irregular.

CAUSES
- myocardial infarction or ischemia, untreated ventricular tachycardia, electrolyte imbalances, digitalis or quinidine toxicity, electric shock, hypothermia

TREATMENT
- if pulse is absent, follow protocol using defibrillation, epinephrine, lidocaine, bretylium. Pronestyl, and sodium bicarbonate as indicated.

ICD-9-CM
427.41 Ventricular fibrillation

Ventricular standstill

DESCRIPTION No QRS complexes. Symptoms include loss of consciousness. No peripheral pulses, blood pressure or respirations. Death.

SYNONYMS
- Asystole

CAUSES
- myocardial infarction or ischemia, untreated ventricular tachycardia, electrolyte imbalances, digitalis or quinidine toxicity, electric shock, hypothermia

TREATMENT
- follow protocol using epinephrine, defibrillation, lidocaine, bretylium. Pronestyl, and sodium bicarbonate as indicated.

ICD-9-CM
427.5 Cardiac arrest

Ventricular tachycardia (VT)

DESCRIPTION Symptoms include chest pain, anxiety, palpitations, dyspnea, shock, coma, death. Ventricular rate usually regular at 140-220 beats per minute. QRS complexes are wide and bizarre.

CAUSES
- myocardial ischemia, infarction, or aneurysm, ventricular catheters, drug toxicity (digitalis or quinidine), hypokalemia, hypercalcemia, anxiety

TREATMENT
- lidocaine bolus if pulse is present. If pulse is absent, follow protocol using defibrillation, epinephrine, lidocaine, bretylium, Pronestyl, and sodium bicarbonate as indicated.

ICD-9-CM
427.1 Paroxysmal ventricular tachycardia

Vernal keratoconjunctivitis

DESCRIPTION Bilateral conjunctivitis associated with corneal epithelial changes. Most likely to occur in spring and fall in males aged 5-20.
• Characteristics - signs and symptoms include tearing; intense itching; redness of the conjunctiva; and a tenacious, mucoid discharge containing numerous eosinophils. Symptoms usually disappear during cold months.

CAUSES
• allergies (probably)

TREATMENT
• topical corticosteroid drops, (e.g., 0.1% dexamethasone drops q 2 h) with supplemental small oral doses if needed
• long-term maintenance treatment with 0.25 prednisolone acetate applied bid
• remember to check ocular pressure if steroids are needed for more than a few weeks

ICD-9-CM
372.13 Vernal conjunctivitis

von Gierke disease

DESCRIPTION An autosomal recessive glycogen storage disease, (Type Ia) Glucose-6-phosphatase deficiency affecting liver and kidneys. Characteristics - hepatomegaly, hypoglycemia, hyperuricemia, xanthomas, bleeding, adiposity. Patients live into adulthood. May lead to symptomatic hypoglycemia. Patients needed added precautions when taking many drugs. Usual course - chronic; progressive.

SYNONYMS
• glucose-6-phosphatase deficiency type Ia
• hepatorenal glycogen storage disease

CAUSES
• genetic enzyme deficiency

TREATMENT
• frequent feeding
• allopurinol

ICD-9-CM
271.0 Glycogenosis

von Hippel-Lindau disease

DESCRIPTION One of the neurocutaneous syndromes (phakomatoses). A familial cancer syndrome with predisposition to ocular and CNS hemangioblastomas, renal cell carcinoma, and pheochromocytomas. Prognosis is variable.

SYNONYMS
• Cerebelloretinal hemangioblastomatosis
• Angiophakomatosis retinae et cerebelli

CAUSES
• Autosomal dominant with gene locus at chromosome region 3p25-3p26

TREATMENT
• Surgery and radiation therapy as indicated
• Genetic counseling of patient and family
• Supportive measures

ICD-9-CM
759.6 Other hamartoses, NEC

Author(s)
Nuhad D. Dinno, MD

von Willebrand disease

DESCRIPTION Group of hemorrhagic disorders in which the von Willebrand factor is either quantitatively or qualitatively abnormal. Usually inherited as an autosomal dominant trait though rare kindreds are autosomal recessive. Symptoms vary depending on severity and disease type but may include prolonged bleeding time, deficiency of factor VIII, and impaired platelet adhesion. Usual course - chronic.

SYNONYMS
• pseudohemophilia
• vascular hemophilia
• angiohemophilia

CAUSES
• no factor VIII associated proteins
• decreased factor VIII associated proteins activity

TREATMENT
• factor VIII replacement
• aminocaproic acid (epsilon-aminocaproic acid)
• Desmopressin (DDAVP)
• oral contraceptives to suppress menses

ICD-9-CM
286.4 Von Willebrand disease

Waldenström macroglobulinemia

DESCRIPTION Malignant neoplasm of cells with lymphocytic, plasmacytic or intermediate morphology which secrete an IgM M component. Usual course - slowly progressive; death 3-10 years. Genetics - slight increased familial incidence.

CAUSES
• IgM M-component secretion

TREATMENT
• chlorambucil
• plasmapheresis for hyperviscosity
• prednisone

ICD-9-CM
273.3 Macroglobulinemia

Werner syndrome

DESCRIPTION Premature senility in an adult. Characteristics - early graying and some hair loss, cataracts, hyperkeratinization, and scleroderma-like changes in the skin of the lower extremities. Usual course - chronic.

SYNONYMS
• adult progeria
• progeria adultorum

CAUSES
• altered glycosaminoglycan turnover
• chromosomal instability

TREATMENT
• symptomatic

ICD-9-CM
259.8 Other specified endocrine disorders

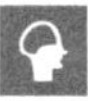

Wernicke encephalopathy

DESCRIPTION Acute, subacute, or chronic neurological disorder. Characteristics - confusion, apathy, drowsiness, atoxic, nystagmus, ophthalmoplegia. Most commonly results from chronic alcohol abuse and accompanied by organic amnesia and other nutritional polyneuropathies. Usual course - acute; subacute; chronic.

SYNONYMS
• Wernicke syndrome
• Wernicke disease
• Gayet-Wernicke syndrome

CAUSES
• thiamine deficiency

TREATMENT
• intravenous thiamine supplementation
• supportive measures

ICD-9-CM
265.1 Other and unspecified manifestations of thiamine deficiency

West Nile fever

DESCRIPTION West Nile virus (WNV) belongs to the Flaviviridae family, similar to the St. Louis encephalitis virus, Japanese encephalitis, and the Murray Valley virus. West Nile fever is endemic in Africa, the Middle East, and West Asia. Occasional outbreaks have been reported in Europe and Australia. The first outbreak of West Nile encephalitis in the United States occurred in the New York City area in 1999. West Nile fever is usually a self-limited disease with influenza-like symptoms. In less than 15% of the cases, especially in the elderly, central nervous system involvement and death may occur. The incubation period is approximately 3-15 days. Most common symptoms are fever, headache, neck pain, vomiting, muscle ache, maculopapular rash, diarrhea, photophobia, altered mental status, and muscle weakness. Recovery is complete for survivors, but muscle weakness may last for several weeks. Many WNV infections may be mistaken for other viral syndromes and may not be reported. All suspected cases should be reported immediately to local health department.

SYNONYMS
• West Nile virus

CAUSES
• Mosquito borne flavivirus

TREATMENT
• No specific treatment available except for supportive therapies

ICD-9-CM
066.3 Other mosquito-borne fever

Whipple disease

DESCRIPTION A malabsorption disorder. Characteristics - diarrhea, steatorrhea, skin pigmentation, arthralgia, arthritis, lymphadenopathy, and central nervous system lesions. Usual course - progressive; curative with treatment.

SYNONYMS
• lipophagic intestinal granulomatosis
• intestinal lipodystrophy
• secondary nontropical sprue

CAUSES
• probable bacterial infection

TREATMENT
• penicillin G
• ampicillin
• tetracycline
• corticosteroids, e.g. prednisone

ICD-9-CM
040.2 Whipple disease

Wilson disease

DESCRIPTION An inherited metabolic disorder characterized by excessive amounts of copper in the liver, brain, kidneys, and corneas. It can lead to tissue necrosis and fibrosis, which in turn can cause hepatic disease and neurologic changes. Without treatment, it leads to fatal hepatic failure. Usual course - chronic.

SYNONYMS
• progressive lenticular degeneration
• Westphal-Struempell pseudosclerosis

CAUSES
• genetic

TREATMENT
• avoid copper-rich foods
• penicillamine, potassium sulfide, pyridoxine, zinc acetate as alternative to penicillamine

ICD-9-CM
275.1 Disorders of copper metabolism

Wolff-Parkinson-White syndrome

DESCRIPTION A form of pre-excitation characterized by a short PR interval and long QRS interval with a delta wave associated with paroxysmal tachycardia (or atrial fibrillation). Usual course - intermittent.

SYNONYMS
- preexcitation syndrome
- anomalous atrioventricular excitation

CAUSES
- accessory atrioventricular pathway
- circus movement conduction due to AV reentrant tachycardia

TREATMENT
- vagal maneuvers
- antiarrhythmic agents
- cardioversion
- electrical pacing
- surgical ablation

ICD-9-CM
426.7 Anomalous atrioventricular excitation

Yaws

DESCRIPTION Non-venereal, infectious, tropical disease usually affecting persons under the age of 15. Spread by direct contact. Characteristics - painless papule that grows into a papilloma. The papule heals, leaving a scar. Late manifestations: deforming lesions of bones, joints, and skin. Usual course - chronic; progressive. Endemic areas - tropical regions.

SYNONYMS
- frambesia
- buba
- pian

CAUSES
- skin contact
- treponema pertenue

TREATMENT
- penicillin

ICD-9-CM
102.9 Yaws, unspecified

Yellow fever

DESCRIPTION An acute infectious disease primarily of the tropics, caused by a virus and transmitted to man by mosquitoes of the genus Aedes and Haemagogus. A live virus vaccine (with few side effects) is effective and should be administered every 10 years. Usual course - acute. Endemic areas - Africa; South America.

CAUSES
- flavivirus
- mosquito bite
- Aedes aegypti

TREATMENT
- fluid replacement
- supportive therapy
- treatment for complications

ICD-9-CM
060.9 Yellow fever, unspecified

Yersinia enterocolitica infection

DESCRIPTION Gram negative, facultatively anaerobic bacteria causing acute gastroenteritis and mesenteric lymphadenitis in children, and arthritis, septicemia, and erythema nodosum in adults. Transmitted through food, water, and person-to-person contact. Usual course - acute.

SYNONYMS
- yersiniosis
- pasteurella pseudotuberculosis infection

CAUSES
- contaminated food ingestion

TREATMENT
- streptomycin
- gentamicin
- tetracycline
- chloramphenicol
- trimethoprim-sulfamethoxazole
- fluid replacement

ICD-9-CM
027.2 Pasteurellosis

Zygomycosis

DESCRIPTION Fungal infection typically seen in immunocompromised or debilitated patients. In healthy individuals, the organisms seldom cause infection. Several forms exist - gastrointestinal, rhinocerebral, disseminated mucormycosis, pulmonary, cutaneous, central nervous system. Prognosis is guarded.

SYNONYMS
- phycomycosis
- mucormycosis

CAUSES
- fungi of the class Zygomycetes

TREATMENT
- Amphotericin B
- surgical removal of necrotic tissue

ICD-9-CM
117.7 Zygomycosis (Phycomycosis or Mucormycosis)

Section 3

U. S. Preventive Services Task Force Recommendations

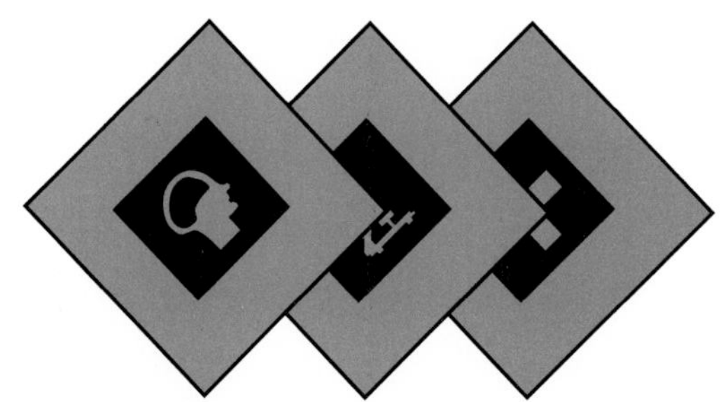

The information in this section was extracted in August 2004 from the web site hosted by the Agency for Healthcare Research and Quality (www.ahcpr.gov/clinic/prevenix.htm). The Practice Guide was added to draw the reader's attention to those recommendations, indicated by (R), which either have good supporting evidence or are strongly recommended for other reasons, and probably should be instituted in many practice settings. The remaining recommendations, indicated by (NR), either have no conclusive evidence or are not indicated in many practice settings.

The reader should be aware that these recommendations relate to screening, counseling, immunizations, or chemoprophylaxis. Do not mistake these preventive measures for the distinct diagnostic measures undertaken when a patient has specific signs or symptoms of a disease process. This section does not apply to a patient presenting with a possible disease process.

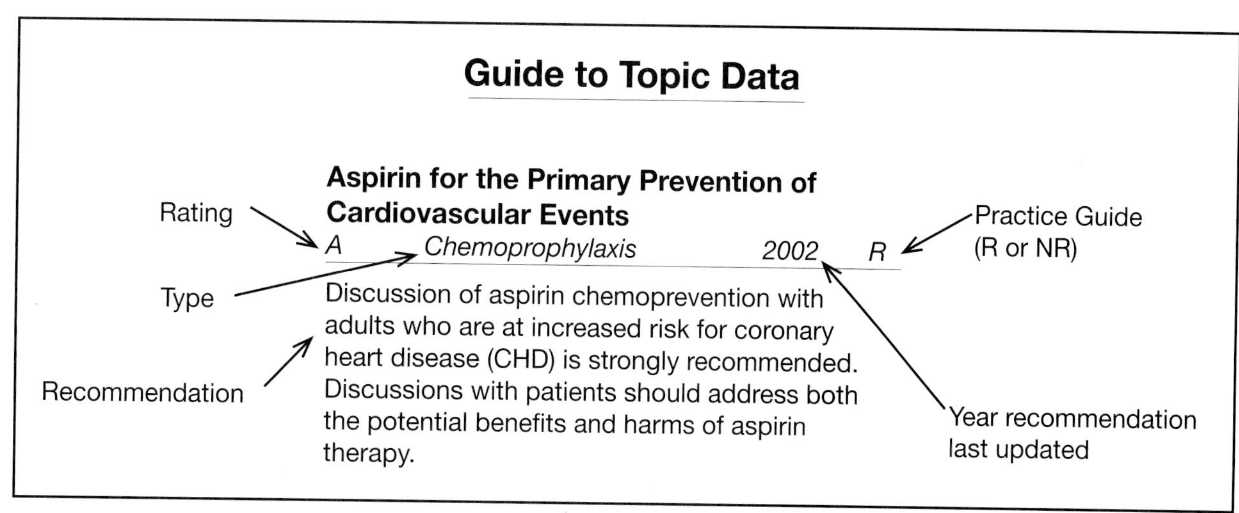

Rating	Interpretation
A	The U.S. Preventive Services Task Force (USPSTF) strongly recommends that clinicians routinely provide [the service] to eligible patients. (The USPSTF found good evidence that [the service] improves important health outcomes and concludes that benefits substantially outweigh harms.)
B	The USPSTF recommends that clinicians routinely provide [the service] to eligible patients. (The USPSTF found at least fair evidence that [the service] improves important health outcomes and concludes that benefits outweigh harms.)
C	The USPSTF makes no recommendation for or against routine provision of [the service]. (The USPSTF found at least fair evidence that [the service] can improve health outcomes but concludes that the balance of the benefits and harms is too close to justify a general recommendation.)
D	The USPSTF recommends against routinely providing [the service] to asymptomatic patients. (The USPSTF found at least fair evidence that [the service] is ineffective or that harms outweigh benefits.)
I	The USPSTF concludes that the evidence is insufficient to recommend for or against routinely providing [the service]. (Evidence that [the service] is effective is lacking, of poor quality, or conflicting and the balance of benefits and harms cannot be determined.)
None	No rating has been applied to this recommendation.

Abdominal Aortic Aneurysm

None *Screening* *1996* *NR*

There is insufficient evidence to recommend for or against routine screening of asymptomatic adults for abdominal aortic aneurysm with abdominal palpation or ultrasound.

Adult Immunizations

None *Immunizations* *1996* *R*

Annual influenza vaccine is recommended for all persons aged 65 and older and persons in selected high-risk groups.

Adult Immunizations

None *Immunizations* *1996* *R*

Pneumococcal vaccine is recommended for all immunocompetent individuals who are age 65 years and older or otherwise at increased risk for pneumococcal disease. There is insufficient evidence to recommend for or against pneumococcal vaccine for high-risk immunocompromised individuals, but recommendations for vaccinating those persons may be made on other grounds.

Adult Immunizations

None *Immunizations* *1996* *R*

The series of combined diphtheria-tetanus toxoids (Td) should be completed for adults who have not received the primary series, and all adults should receive periodic Td boosters.

Adult Immunizations

None *Immunizations* *1996* *R*

Vaccination against measles and mumps should be provided to all adults born after 1956 who lack evidence of immunity. A second measles vaccination is recommended for adolescents and young adults in settings where such individuals congregate (e.g., high schools and colleges).

Alcohol Misuse

B *Screening* *2004* *R*

Screening and behavioral counseling interventions to reduce alcohol misuse by adults, including pregnant women, in primary care settings is recommended.

Alcohol Misuse

I *Screening* *2004* *NR*

There is insufficient evidence to recommend for or against screening and behavioral counseling interventions, in primary care settings, to prevent or reduce alcohol misuse by adolescents.

Aspirin for the Primary Prevention of Cardiovascular Events

A *Chemoprophylaxis* *2002* *R*

Discussion of aspirin chemoprevention with adults who are at increased risk for coronary heart disease (CHD) is strongly recommended. Discussions with patients should address both the potential benefits and harms of aspirin therapy.

Aspirin Prophylaxis in Pregnancy

None *Chemoprophylaxis* *1996* *NR*

There is insufficient evidence to recommend for or against the routine use of aspirin to prevent preeclampsia or intrauterine growth retardation in pregnant women, including those at high risk.

Asymptomatic Bacteriuria

A *Screening* *2004* *R*

Screen all pregnant women for asymptomatic bacteriuria using urine culture at 12-16 weeks gestation.

Asymptomatic Bacteriuria

D *Screening* 2004 NR

Routine screening of men and nonpregnant women for asymptomatic bacteriuria is not recommended.

Asymptomatic Carotid Artery Stenosis

None *Screening* 1996 NR

Insufficient evidence to recommend for or against screening asymptomatic persons for carotid artery stenosis using the physical examination or carotid ultrasound.

For selected high-risk patients, a recommendation to discuss the potential benefits of screening and carotid endarterectomy may be made on other grounds.

Asymptomatic Carotid Artery Stenosis

None *Screening* 1996 R

All persons should be screened for hypertension, and clinicians should provide counseling about smoking cessation.

Back Pain, Low

I *Counseling* 2004 NR

There is insufficient evidence to recommend for or against the routine use of interventions to prevent low back pain in adults in primary care settings.

There is also insufficient evidence to recommend for or against the routine use of educational interventions, mechanical supports, or risk factor modification to prevent low back pain.

Bacterial Vaginosis in Pregnancy

I *Screening* 2001 NR

Insufficient evidence to recommend for or against routinely screening high-risk pregnant women for bacterial vaginosis (BV). (see footnote 2: Counseling to Prevent HIV Infection and Other Sexually Transmitted Diseases)

Rationale: The USPSTF found good-quality studies with conflicting results that screening and treatment of asymptomatic BV in high-risk pregnant women reduces the incidence of preterm delivery. The magnitude of benefit exceeded risk in several studies, but the single largest study reported no benefit among high-risk pregnant women.

Bacterial Vaginosis in Pregnancy

D *Screening* 2001 NR

Routine screening of average-risk asymptomatic pregnant women for BV is not recommended. Rationale: There is good evidence that screening and treatment of BV in asymptomatic women who are not at high risk does not improve outcomes such as preterm labor or preterm birth.

Bladder Cancer

None *Screening* 1996 NR

Routine screening for bladder cancer with urine dipstick, microscopic urinalysis, or urine cytology is not recommended in asymptomatic persons.

Bladder Cancer

None *Screening* 1996 R

All persons who smoke tobacco should be routinely counseled to quit smoking.

Breast Cancer - Chemoprevention

None *Chemoprophylaxis* 2002 NR

Routine use of tamoxifen or raloxifene not recommended for the primary prevention of breast cancer in women at low or average risk for breast cancer.

The USPSTF recommends that clinicians discuss chemoprevention with women at high risk for breast cancer and at low risk for adverse effects of chemoprevention. Clinicians should inform patients of the potential benefits and harms of chemoprevention.

Breast Cancer
B *Screening* *2002* *R*

Screening mammography recommended, with or without clinical breast examination (CBE), every 1-2 years for women aged 40 and older.

Breast Cancer
I *Screening* *2002* *NR*

Insufficient evidence to recommend for or against routine CBE alone to screen for breast cancer.

Breast Cancer
I *Screening* *2002* *NR*

Insufficient evidence to recommend for or against teaching or performing routine breast self-examination (BSE).

Breastfeeding
B *Counseling* *2003* *R*

Structured breastfeeding education recommended and behavioral counseling programs to promote breastfeeding.

Breastfeeding
I *Counseling* *2003* *NR*

Insufficient evidence to recommend for or against the following interventions to promote breastfeeding: brief education and counseling by primary care providers; peer counseling used alone and initiated in the clinical setting; and written materials, used alone or in combination with other interventions.

Cervical Cancer
A *Screening* *2003* *R*

Screening for cervical cancer in women who have been sexually active and have a cervix is strongly recommended.

Cervical Cancer
D *Screening* *2003* *NR*

Routinely screening women older than age 65 for cervical cancer if they have had adequate recent screening with normal Pap smears and are not otherwise at high risk for cervical cancer is not recommended.

Cervical Cancer
D *Screening* *2003* *NR*

Routine Pap smear screening in women who have had a total hysterectomy for benign disease is not recommended.

Cervical Cancer
I *Screening* *2003* *NR*

Insufficient evidence to recommend for or against the routine use of new technologies to screen for cervical cancer.

Cervical Cancer
I *Screening* *2003* *NR*

Insufficient evidence to recommend for or against the routine use of human papillomavirus (HPV) testing as a primary screening test for cervical cancer.

Childhood Immunizations
None *Immunizations* *1996* *R*

All children without established contraindications should receive the following vaccines in accordance with regular schedules:

- Diphtheria-tetanus-pertussis (DTP)
- Oral poliovirus (OPV)
- Measles-mumps-rubella (MMR)
- Conjugate *Haemophilus influenzae* type b
- Hepatitis B
- Varicella

Childhood Immunizations
None Immunizations 1996 R

Hepatitis A vaccine is recommended for children and adolescents at high risk for hepatitis A virus (HAV) infection.

Childhood Immunizations
None Immunizations 1996 R

Pneumococcal vaccine and annual influenza vaccine are recommended for children and adolescents at high risk.

Chlamydial Infection
A Screening 2001 R

Routine screening of all sexually active women aged 25 years and younger, and other asymptomatic women at increased risk for infection, for chlamydial infection is strongly recommended.

Chlamydial Infection
C Screening 2001 NR

No recommendation for or against routinely screening asymptomatic low-risk women in the general population for chlamydial infection.

Chlamydial Infection
B Screening 2001 R

Routine screening of all asymptomatic pregnant women aged 25 years and younger and others at increased risk for infection for chlamydial infection is recommended.

Chlamydial Infection
C Screening 2001 NR

No recommendation for or against routine screening of asymptomatic, low-risk pregnant women aged 26 years and older for chlamydial infection.

Chlamydial Infection
I Screening 2001 NR

Insufficient evidence to recommend for or against routinely screening asymptomatic men for chlamydial infection.

Colorectal Cancer
A Screening 2002 R

Screen men and women 50 years of age or older for colorectal cancer.

Congenital Hypothyroidism
None Screening 1996 R

Screening for congenital hypothyroidism with thyroid function tests on dried-blood spot specimens is recommended for all newborns in the first week of life.

Coronary Heart Disease
D Screening 2004 NR

Recommends against routine screening with resting electrocardiography (ECG), exercise treadmill test (ETT), or electron-beam computerized tomography (EBCT) scanning for coronary calcium for either the presence of severe coronary artery stenosis (CAS) or the prediction of coronary heart disease (CHD) events in adults at low risk for CHD events.

Coronary Heart Disease
I Screening 2004 NR

Insufficient evidence to recommend for or against routine screening with ECG, ETT, or EBCT scanning for coronary calcium for either the presence of severe CAS or the prediction of CHD events in adults at increased risk for CHD events.

Dementia
I Screening 2003 NR

Insufficient evidence to recommend for or against routine screening for dementia in older adults.

Dental and Periodontal Disease
None Counseling 1996 R

The following are suggested:

- Visit a dental care provider on a regular basis.
- Floss daily
- Brush teeth daily with a fluoride-containing toothpaste
- Appropriately use fluoride for caries prevention and chemotherapeutic mouth rinses for plaque prevention

Dental Caries In Preschool Children
B Screening 2004 R

It is recommended that primary care clinicians prescribe oral fluoride supplementation, at currently recommended doses, to preschool children older than 6 months whose primary water source is deficient in fluoride.

Dental Caries In Preschool Children
I Screening 2004 NR

There is insufficient evidence for or against routine risk assessment of preschool children by primary care clinicians for the prevention of dental disease.

Depression
B Screening 2002 R

Screening adults for depression in clinical practices that have systems in place to assure accurate diagnosis, effective treatment, and follow-up is recommended.

Depression
I Screening 2002 NR

Insufficient evidence to recommend for or against routine screening of children or adolescents for depression.

Diabetes Mellitus, Adult Type 2
I Screening 2003 NR

Insufficient evidence to recommend for or against routinely screening asymptomatic adults for type 2 diabetes, impaired glucose tolerance, or impaired fasting glucose.

Diabetes Mellitus, Adult Type 2
B Screening 2003 R

Screen for type 2 diabetes in adults with hypertension or hyperlipidemia.

Down Syndrome
None Screening 1996 R

The offering of amniocentesis or chorionic villus sampling (CVS) for chromosome studies is recommended for pregnant women at high risk for Down syndrome.

The offering of screening for Down syndrome by serum multiple-marker testing is recommended for:

- All low-risk pregnant women
- As an alternative to amniocentesis and CVS for high-risk women

This testing should be offered only to women who are seen for prenatal care in locations that have adequate counseling and follow-up services.

Down Syndrome

None Screening 1996 NR

There is currently insufficient evidence to recommend for or against screening for Down syndrome by individual serum marker testing or ultrasound examination, but recommendations against such screening may be made on other grounds.

Drug Abuse

None Screening 1996 NR

There is insufficient evidence to recommend for or against routine screening for drug abuse with standardized questionnaires or biologic assays. Including questions about drug use and drug-related problems when taking a history from all adolescent and adult patients may be recommended on other grounds.

Drug Abuse

None Screening 1996 R

All pregnant women should be advised of the potential adverse effects of drug use on the development of the fetus.

Clinicians should be alert to the signs and symptoms of drug abuse in patients and refer drug abusing patients to specialized treatment facilities where available.

Elevated Lead Levels in Childhood and Pregnancy

None Screening 1996 R

Screening for elevated lead levels by measuring blood lead at least once at age 12 months is recommended for:

- All children at increased risk of lead exposure
- All children with identifiable risk factors
- All children living in communities in which the prevalence of blood lead levels requiring individual intervention, including residential lead hazard control or chelation therapy, is high or is undefined

Elevated Lead Levels in Childhood and Pregnancy

None Screening 1996 NR

Evidence is currently insufficient to recommend an exact community prevalence below which targeted screening can be substituted for universal screening. Clinicians can seek guidance from their local or state health department.

Elevated Lead Levels in Childhood and Pregnancy

None Screening 1996 NR

There is insufficient evidence to recommend for or against routine screening for lead exposure in asymptomatic pregnant women, but recommendations against such screening may be made on other grounds.

Counseling families about the primary prevention of lead exposure, but recommendations may be made on other grounds.

Family Violence

I Screening 2004 NR

There is insufficient evidence to recommend for or against routine screening of parents or guardians for the physical abuse or neglect of children, of women for intimate partner violence, or of older adults or their caregivers for elder abuse.

Clinicians should be alert to the various presentations of child abuse, spouse and partner abuse, and elder abuse.

Genital Herpes Simplex

None Screening 1996 NR

Routine screening for genital *Herpes simplex* virus (HSV) infection by viral culture is not recommended for asymptomatic persons, including asymptomatic pregnant women.

Genital Herpes Simplex

None Screening 1996 NR

There is insufficient evidence to recommend for or against the examination of pregnant women in labor for signs of active genital HSV lesions, although recommendations to do so may be made on other grounds.

Genital Herpes Simplex

None Screening 1996 R

(see footnote 2: Counseling to Prevent HIV Infection and Other Sexually Transmitted Diseases)

Gestational Diabetes Mellitus

I Screening 2003 NR

Insufficient evidence to recommend for or against routine screening for gestational diabetes.

Glaucoma

None Screening 1996 NR

There is insufficient evidence to recommend for or against routine screening for intraocular hypertension or glaucoma by primary care clinicians.

Glaucoma

None Screening 1996 R

Recommendations to refer high-risk patients for evaluation by an eye specialist may be made on other grounds.

Gonorrhea

None Screening 1996 R

Routine screening for *Neisseria gonorrhoeae* is recommended for:

- Asymptomatic women at high risk of infection
- All high-risk women should be screened during pregnancy

Gonorrhea

None Screening 1996 NR

There is insufficient evidence to recommend for or against screening all pregnant women, or screening asymptomatic men. Recommendations to screen selected high-risk young men may be made on other grounds.

Routine screening is not recommended for the general adult population.

Gonorrhea

None Screening 1996 R

Ocular antibiotic prophylaxis of all newborn infants is recommended to prevent gonococcal opthalmia neonatorum.

Gynecologic Cancers

None Counseling 1996 NR

There is insufficient evidence to recommend for or against routine counseling of women about measures for the primary prevention of gynecologic cancers.

Gynecologic Cancers

None Counseling 1996 R

Clinicians counseling women about contraceptive practices should include information on the potential benefits of the following with respect to gynecologic cancers:

- Oral contraceptives
- Barrier contraceptives
- Tubal sterilization

Clinicians should also promote other practices:

- Maintaining desirable body weight
- Smoking cessation
- Safe sex practices

These measures may reduce the incidence of certain gynecologic cancers and have other proven health benefits.

Healthy Diet

B Counseling 2003 R

Intensive behavioral dietary counseling for adult patients with hyperlipidemia and other known risk factors for cardiovascular and diet-related chronic disease is recommended. Intensive counseling can be delivered by primary care clinicians or by referral to other specialists, such as nutritionists or dietitians.

Hearing Impairment

None Screening 1996 R

Screening for older adults for hearing impairment is recommended through:

- Periodically questioning them about their hearing
- Counseling them about the availability of hearing aid devices
- Making referrals for abnormalities when appropriate

Hearing Impairment

None Screening 1996 NR

There is insufficient evidence to recommend for or against routinely screening asymptomatic adolescents and working-age adults for hearing impairment. Recommendations against such screening, except for those exposed to excessive occupational noise levels, may be made on other grounds.

Hearing Impairment

None Screening 1996 NR

Routine hearing screening of asymptomatic children beyond age 3 years is not recommended.

Hearing Impairment

None Screening 1996 NR

There is insufficient evidence to recommend for or against routine screening of asymptomatic neonates for hearing impairment using evoked otoacoustic emission testing or auditory brainstem response. Recommendations to screen high-risk infants may be made on other grounds.

Hemoglobinopathies

None Screening 1996 R

Neonatal screening for sickle hemoglobinopathies is recommended to identify infants who may benefit from antibiotic prophylaxis to prevent sepsis. Whether screening should be universal or targeted to high-risk groups will depend on:

- The proportion of high-risk individuals in the screening area
- The accuracy and efficiency with which infants at risk can be identified
- Other characteristics of the screening program

Offering screening for hemoglobinopathies to pregnant women at the first prenatal visit is recommended, especially for those at high risk.

Hemoglobinopathies

None Screening 1996 NR

There is insufficient evidence to recommend for or against routine screening for hemoglobinopathies in high-risk adolescents and young adults, but recommendations to offer such testing may be made on other grounds.

Hemoglobinopathies

None Screening 1996 R

All screening efforts must be accompanied by comprehensive counseling and treatment services.

Hepatitis B Virus Infection

A Screening 2004 R

Screening for hepatitis B virus (HBV) infection in pregnant women at their first prenatal visit is strongly recommended.

Hepatitis B Virus Infection

D Screening 2004 NR

Routine screening for hepatitis C virus (HCV) infection in asymptomatic adults who are not at increased risk (general population) for infection is not recommended.

Hepatitis C Virus Infection

D Screening 2004 NR

There is insufficient evidence to recommend routine screening for hepatitis C virus (HCV) infection in asymptomatic adults who are not at increased risk (general population) for infection.

High Blood Pressure

A Screening 2003 R

Screening adults aged 18 and older for high blood pressure strongly recommended.

High Blood Pressure

I Screening 2003 NR

Insufficient evidence to recommend for or against routine screening for high blood pressure in children and adolescents to reduce the risk of cardiovascular disease.

Home Uterine Activity Monitoring

None Screening 1996 NR

Insufficient evidence to recommend for or against home uterine activity monitoring (HUAM) in high-risk pregnancies as a screening test for preterm labor, but recommendations against its use may be made on other grounds.

Home Uterine Activity Monitoring

None Screening 1996 NR

Home uterine activity monitoring (HUAM) is not recommended in normal-risk pregnancies.

Hormone Replacement Therapy

D Chemoprophylaxis 2002 NR

Routine use of estrogen and progestin for the prevention of chronic conditions in postmenopausal women is not recommended.

Hormone Replacement Therapy

I Chemoprophylaxis 2002 NR

Insufficient evidence to recommend for or against the use of unopposed estrogen for the prevention of chronic conditions in postmenopausal women who have had a hysterectomy.

Household and Recreational Injuries

None Counseling 1996 R

Periodic counseling of the parents of children on measures to reduce the risk of unintentional household and recreational injuries is recommended. (see footnote 1: Counseling to Prevent Household and Environmental Injuries)

Household and Recreational Injuries
None Counseling 1996 R

Persons with alcohol or drug problems should be identified, counseled and monitored. Those who use alcohol or illicit drugs should be warned against engaging in potentially dangerous activities while intoxicated.

Household and Recreational Injuries
None Counseling 1996 R

Counseling elderly patients on specific measures to prevent falls is recommended. (see footnote 1: Counseling to Prevent Household and Environmental Injuries)

Human Immunodeficiency Virus Infection
None Screening 1996 R

Clinicians should assess risk factors for human immunodeficiency virus (HIV) infection by obtaining a careful sexual history and inquiring about injection drug use in all patients. Periodic screening for infection with HIV is recommended for all persons at increased risk of infection. (see footnote 2: Counseling to Prevent HIV Infection and Other Sexually Transmitted Diseases)

Human Immunodeficiency Virus Infection
None Counseling 1996 R

All adolescent and adult patients should be advised about risk factors for human immunodeficiency virus (HIV) infection and other sexually transmitted diseases (STDs). (see footnote 2: Counseling to Prevent HIV Infection and Other Sexually Transmitted Diseases)

Human Immunodeficiency Virus Infection
None Screening 1996 R

Screening is recommended for all pregnant women at risk for HIV infection, including all women who live in states, counties, or cities with an increased prevalence of HIV infection. (see footnote 2: Counseling to Prevent HIV Infection and Other Sexually Transmitted Diseases)

Human Immunodeficiency Virus Infection
None Screening 1996 R

Screening infants born to high-risk mothers is recommended if the mother's antibody status is not known.

Human Immunodeficiency Virus Infection
None Screening 1996 NR

There is insufficient evidence to recommend for or against universal screening among low-risk pregnant women in low-prevalence areas, but recommendations to counsel and offer screening to all pregnant women may be made on other grounds.

Idiopathic Scoliosis in Adolescents
D Screening 2004 NR

Routine screening of asymptomatic adolescents for idiopathic scoliosis is not recommended.

Intrapartum Electronic Fetal Monitoring
None Screening 1996 NR

Routine electronic fetal monitoring for low-risk women in labor is not recommended.

There is insufficient evidence to recommend for or against intrapartum electronic fetal monitoring for high-risk pregnant women.

Iron Deficiency Anemia
None Screening 1996 R

Screening for iron deficiency anemia using hemoglobin or hematocrit is recommended for:

- Pregnant women
- High-risk infants

Iron Deficiency Anemia
None Screening 1996 NR

There is insufficient evidence to recommend for or against routine screening for iron deficiency anemia in other asymptomatic persons, but recommendations against screening may be made on other grounds.

Iron Deficiency Anemia
None Screening 1996 R

Encouraging parents to breastfeed their infants and to include iron-enriched foods in the diet of infants and young children is recommended.

Iron Deficiency Anemia
None Screening 1996 NR

There is currently insufficient evidence to recommend for or against the routine use of iron supplements for healthy infants or pregnant women.

Lipid Disorders in Adults
A Screening 2001 R

Routine screening of men aged 35 years and older and women aged 45 years and older for lipid disorders and treating abnormal lipids in people who are at increased risk of coronary heart disease are strongly recommended.

Lipid Disorders in Adults
B Screening 2001 R

Routine screening of younger adults (men aged 20 to 35 and women aged 20 to 45) for lipid disorders if they have other risk factors for coronary heart disease is recommended.

Lipid Disorders in Adults
C Screening 2001 NR

No recommendation is made for or against routine screening for lipid disorders in younger adults (men aged 20 to 35 or women aged 20 to 45) in the absence of known risk factors for coronary heart disease.

Lipid Disorders in Adults
B Screening 2001 R

In screening for lipid disorders measurements including total cholesterol (TC) and high-density lipoprotein cholesterol (HDL-C) are recommended.

Lipid Disorders in Adults
I Screening 2001 NR

Insufficient evidence to recommend for or against triglyceride measurement as a part of routine screening for lipid disorder.

Lung Cancer
I Screening 2004 NR

There is insufficient evidence to recommend for or against screening asymptomatic persons for lung cancer with either low dose computerized tomography (LDCT), chest x-ray (CXR), sputum cytology or a combination of these tests.

Motor Vehicle Injuries
None Counseling 1996 R

The following counseling to all patients, and the parents of young patients, is recommended:

- Use occupant restraints (lap/shoulder safety belts and child safety seats).
- Wear helmets when riding motorcycles.
- Refrain from driving while under the influence of alcohol or other drugs.

Motor Vehicle Injuries
None Counseling 1996 NR

There is currently insufficient evidence to recommend for or against counseling to prevent pedestrian injuries. Related recommendations on the prevention of bicycling injuries are provided in footnote 1: Counseling to Prevent Household and Recreational Injuries.

USPSTF

Neural Tube Defects

None Screening 1996 R

The offering of screening for neural tube defects by maternal serum alpha-fetoprotein (MSAFP) measurement is recommended for all pregnant women who are seen for prenatal care in locations that have adequate counseling and follow-up services available. Screening with MSAFP may be offered as part of multiple-marker screening.

Neural Tube Defects

None Screening 1996 NR

There is insufficient evidence to recommend for or against the offering of screening for neural tube defects by midtrimester ultrasound examination to all pregnant women, but recommendations against such screening may be made on other grounds.

Neural Tube Defects

None Screening 1996 R

Daily multivitamins with folic acid to reduce the risk of neural tube defects are recommended for all women who are planning or capable of pregnancy.

Newborn Hearing

I Screening 2001 NR

Insufficient evidence to recommend for or against routine screening of newborns for hearing loss during the postpartum hospitalization.

Obesity in Adults

B Screening 2003 R

Screen all adult patients for obesity and offer intensive counseling and behavioral interventions to promote sustained weight loss for obese adults.

Obesity in Adults

I Screening 2003 NR

Insufficient evidence to recommend for or against the use of moderate- or low-intensity counseling together with behavioral interventions to promote sustained weight loss in obese adults.

Obesity in Adults

I Screening 2003 NR

Insufficient evidence to recommend for or against the use of counseling of any intensity and behavioral interventions to promote sustained weight loss in overweight adults.

Oral Cancer

I Screening 2004 NR

Insufficient evidence to recommend for or against routinely screening adults for oral cancer.

Osteoporosis

B Screening 2002 R

Screen women aged 65 and older routinely for osteoporosis. Begin routine screening at age 60 for women at increased risk for osteoporotic fractures (e.g., low body weight: < 70kg, Caucasian race, tobacco use, positive family history, low calcium intake, alcohol use, etc.).

Osteoporosis

C Screening 2002 NR

No recommendation for or against routine osteoporosis screening in postmenopausal women who are younger than 60 or in women aged 60-64 who are not at increased risk for osteoporotic fractures.

Ovarian Cancer

D Screening 2004 NR

Routine screening for ovarian cancer is not recommended.

Pancreatic Cancer

D Screening 2004 NR

Routine screening for pancreatic cancer in asymptomatic adults using abdominal palpation, ultrasonography, or serologic markers is not recommended.

Peripheral Arterial Disease

None Screening 1996 NR

Routine screening for peripheral arterial disease in asymptomatic persons is not recommended.

Clinicians should be alert to symptoms of peripheral arterial disease in persons at increased risk, and should evaluate patients who have clinical evidence of vascular disease.

Phenylketonuria

None Screening 1996 R

Screening for phenylketonuria (PKU) by measurement of phenylalanine level on a dried-blood spot specimen is recommended for all newborns prior to discharge from the nursery. Infants who are tested before 24 hours of age should receive a repeat screening test by 2 weeks of age.

Phenylketonuria

None Screening 1996 NR

There is insufficient evidence to recommend for or against routine prenatal screening for maternal PKU, but recommendations against such screening may be made on other grounds.

Physical Activity

I Counseling 2002 NR

Insufficient evidence to recommend for or against behavioral counseling in primary care settings to promote physical activity.

Postexposure Prophylaxis for Selected Infectious Diseases

None Chemoprophylaxis 1996 R

Postexposure prophylaxis should be provided to selected persons with exposure or possible exposure to:

- *Haemophilus influenzae* type b
- Hepatitis A
- Hepatitis B
- Meningococcal pathogens
- Rabies pathogens
- Tetanus pathogens

Preeclampsia

None Screening 1996 R

Screening for preeclampsia with blood pressure measurement is recommended for all pregnant women at the first prenatal visit and periodically throughout the remainder of the pregnancy.

Prostate Cancer

I Screening 2002 NR

Insufficient evidence to recommend for or against routine screening for prostate cancer using prostate specific antigen (PSA) testing or digital rectal examination (DRE).

Rh (D) Incompatibility

A Screening 2004 R

Rh (D) blood typing and antibody testing for all pregnant women during their first visit for pregnancy-related care is strongly recommended.

Rh (D) Incompatibility

B *Screening* *2004* *R*

Repeated Rh (D) antibody testing for all unsensitized Rh (D)-negative women at 24-28 weeksí gestation, unless the biological father is known to be Rh (D)-negative is recommended.

Rubella

None *Screening* *1996* *R*

Routine screening for rubella susceptibility by history of vaccination or by serology is recommended for all women of childbearing age at their first clinical encounter. Susceptible nonpregnant women should be offered rubella vaccination; susceptible pregnant women should be vaccinated immediately after delivery.

An equally acceptable alternative for nonpregnant women of childbearing age is to offer vaccination against rubella without screening.

Rubella

None *Screening* *1996* *NR*

There is insufficient evidence to recommend for or against screening or routine vaccination of young men in settings where large numbers of susceptible young adults of both sexes congregate, such as military bases and colleges.

Routine screening or vaccination of other young men, of older men, and of postmenopausal women is not recommended.

Skin Cancer

I *Screening* *2001* *NR*

Insufficient evidence to recommend for or against routine screening for skin cancer using a total-body skin examination for the early detection of cutaneous melanoma, basal cell cancer, or squamous cell skin cancer.

Skin Cancer

I *Counseling* *2003* *NR*

Insufficient evidence to recommend for or against routine counseling by primary care clinicians to prevent skin cancer.

Suicide Risk

I *Screening* *2004* *NR*

The evidence is insufficient to recommend for or against routine screening by primary care clinicians to detect suicide risk in the general population.

Syphilis

A *Screening* *2004* *R*

It is strongly recommended that clinicians screen persons at increased risk for syphilis infection.

Syphilis

A *Screening* *2004* *R*

It is strongly recommended that clinicians screen all pregnant women for syphilis infection.

Syphilis

D *Screening* *2004* *NR*

Routine screening of asymptomatic persons who are not at increased risk for syphilis infection is not recommended.

Testicular Cancer

D *Screening* *2004* *NR*

Routine screening for testicular cancer in asymptomatic adolescent and adult males is not recommended.

Thyroid Cancer

None Screening 1996 NR

Routine screening for thyroid cancer using neck palpation or ultrasonography is not recommended for asymptomatic children or adults.

There is insufficient evidence to recommend for or against screening persons with a history of external head and neck irradiation in infancy or childhood, but recommendations for such screening may be made on other grounds.

Thyroid Disease

I Screening 2004 NR

Insufficient evidence to recommend for or against routine screening for thyroid disease in adults.

Tobacco Use

A Counseling 2003 R

Screen all adults for tobacco use and provide tobacco cessation interventions for those who use tobacco products.

Tobacco Use

A Counseling 2003 R

Screen all pregnant women for tobacco use and provide augmented pregnancy-tailored counseling to those who smoke.

Tobacco Use

I Counseling 2003 NR

Insufficient evidence to recommend for or against routine screening for tobacco use or interventions to prevent and treat tobacco use and dependence among children or adolescents.

Tuberculous Infection

None Screening 1996 R

Screening for tuberculous infection with tuberculin skin testing is recommended for asymptomatic high-risk persons.

Bacille Calmette-Guérin (BCG) vaccination should be considered only for selected high-risk individuals.

Ultrasonography in Pregnancy

None Screening 1996 NR

Routine third-trimester ultrasound examination of the fetus is not recommended. There is insufficient evidence to recommend for or against routine ultrasound examination in the second trimester in low-risk pregnant women.

Unintended Pregnancy

None Counseling 1996 R

Periodic counseling about effective contraceptive methods is recommended for all women and men at risk for unintended pregnancy. Counseling should be based on information from a careful sexual history and should take into account the individual preferences, abilities, and risks of each patient. (see footnote 2: Counseling to Prevent HIV Infection and Other Sexually Transmitted Diseases)

Visual Impairment

None Screening 1996 R

Vision screening to detect amblyopia and strabismus is recommended once for all children before entering school, preferably between the ages of 3 and 4. Clinicians should be alert for signs of ocular misalignment when examining infants and children.

Visual Impairment
None Screening 1996 R

Screening for diminished visual acuity with the Snellen visual acuity chart is recommended for elderly persons. There is insufficient evidence to recommend for or against screening for diminished visual acuity among other asymptomatic persons, but recommendations against routine screening may be made on other grounds.

Visual Impairment in Children Younger than Age 5
B Screening 2004 R

Screening to detect amblyopia, strabismus, and defects in visual acuity in children younger than age 5 years is recommended.

Vitamin Supplementation to Prevent Cancer and Cardiovascular Disease
I Counseling 2003 NR

Insufficient evidence to recommend for or against the use of supplements of vitamins A, C, or E; multivitamins with folic acid; or antioxidant combinations for the prevention of cancer or cardiovascular disease.

Vitamin Supplementation to Prevent Cancer and Cardiovascular Disease
D Counseling 2003 NR

Beta-carotene supplements, either alone or in combination, for the prevention of cancer or cardiovascular disease is not recommended.

Youth Violence
None Counseling 1996 NR

There is insufficient evidence to recommend for or against clinician counseling of asymptomatic adolescents and adults to prevent morbidity and mortality from youth violence.

Youth Violence
None Counseling 1996 R

Adolescent and adult patients should be screened for problem drinking.

Youth Violence
None Counseling 1996 R

Clinicians should also be alert for symptoms and signs of drug abuse and dependence, the various presentations of family violence, and suicidal ideation in persons with established risk factors.

Footnotes

1 Counseling to Prevent Household and Recreational Injuries

Counseling to prevent household and environmental injuries is recommended for adolscents and adults based on the proven efficacy of risk reduction, although the effectiveness of counseling these patients to prevent injuries has not been adequately evaluated. Persons with alcohol or drug problems should be identified and counseled and their progress monitored. Those who use alcohol or illicit drugs should be warned against engaging in potentially dangerous activities while intoxicated. Counseling elderly patients on specific measures to reduce the risk of falling is recommended based on the fair evidence that these measures reduce the risk of falling, although the effectiveness of counseling elders to prevent falls has not been adequately evaluated. There is insuffecent evidence to recommend for or against the use of external hip protectors to prevent fall injuries, but recommendations for their use in institutionalized elderly may be made on other grounds. More intensive individualized multifactorial intervention is recommended for high-risk elderly patients in settings where adequate resources to deliver such services are available.

2 Counseling to Prevent HIV infection and Other Sexually Transmitted Diseases

All adolescent and adult patients should be advised about risk factors for human immunodeficiency virus (HIV) infection and other sexually transmitted diseases (STDs), and counseled appropriately about effective measures to reduce the risk of infection. Counseling should be tailored to the individual risk factors, needs, and abilities of each patient. This recommendation is based on the proven efficacy of risk reduction, although the effectiveness of clinician counseling in the primary care setting is uncertain.

Individuals at risk for specific STDs should be offered recommendations on screening for:

- Syphilis
- Gonorrhea
- Hepatitis B infection
- HIV infection
- Chlamydial infection

Injection drug users should be advised about measures to reduce their risk and referred to appropriate treatment facilities.

Section 4

Signs & Symptoms: An Algorithmic Approach

Douglas Collins, MD

This Section contains 101 flowcharts (or algorithms) to help the reader in the diagnostic process. The flowcharts are primarily organized by a symptom or sign – the way patients tend to present themselves. The algorithms lead the reader through a series of questions helping to resolve the presenting complaint or finding into a diagnostic entity.

The algorithms are not meant to be complete nor exhaustive lists of diseases. In fact, the physician, in even a brief review, will easily find diseases not represented. However, the clinician will find that following an algorithm through will jog the memory, like running through a pile of leaves, uncovering important questions or bringing back a forgotten case which is relevant today.

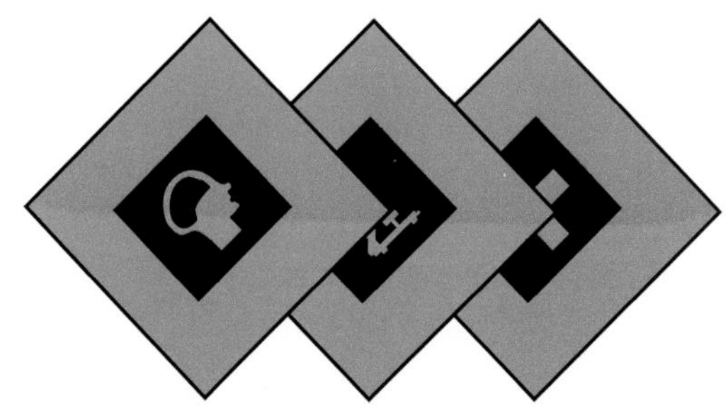

AMENORRHEA

- Pregnancy test positive
  - **Normal gestation**
  - **Ectopic pregnancy**
- Pregnancy test negative
  - Vaginal examination abnormal
    - **Congenital absence of vagina, uterus, or ovaries**
    - **Imperforate hymen**
    - **Ovarian tumor**
    - **Polycystic ovary syndrome**
  - Vaginal examination normal
    - No dwarfism or web-neck
      - Hirsutism or virilism
      - No hirsutism or virilism
        - Weight loss, loss of axillary and pubic hair
          - **Hypopituitarism**
          - **Anorexia nervosa**
        - No weight loss, no loss of axillary or pubic hair
          - Galactorrhea
          - No galactorrhea
    - Dwarfism, web-neck
      - **Turner syndrome**

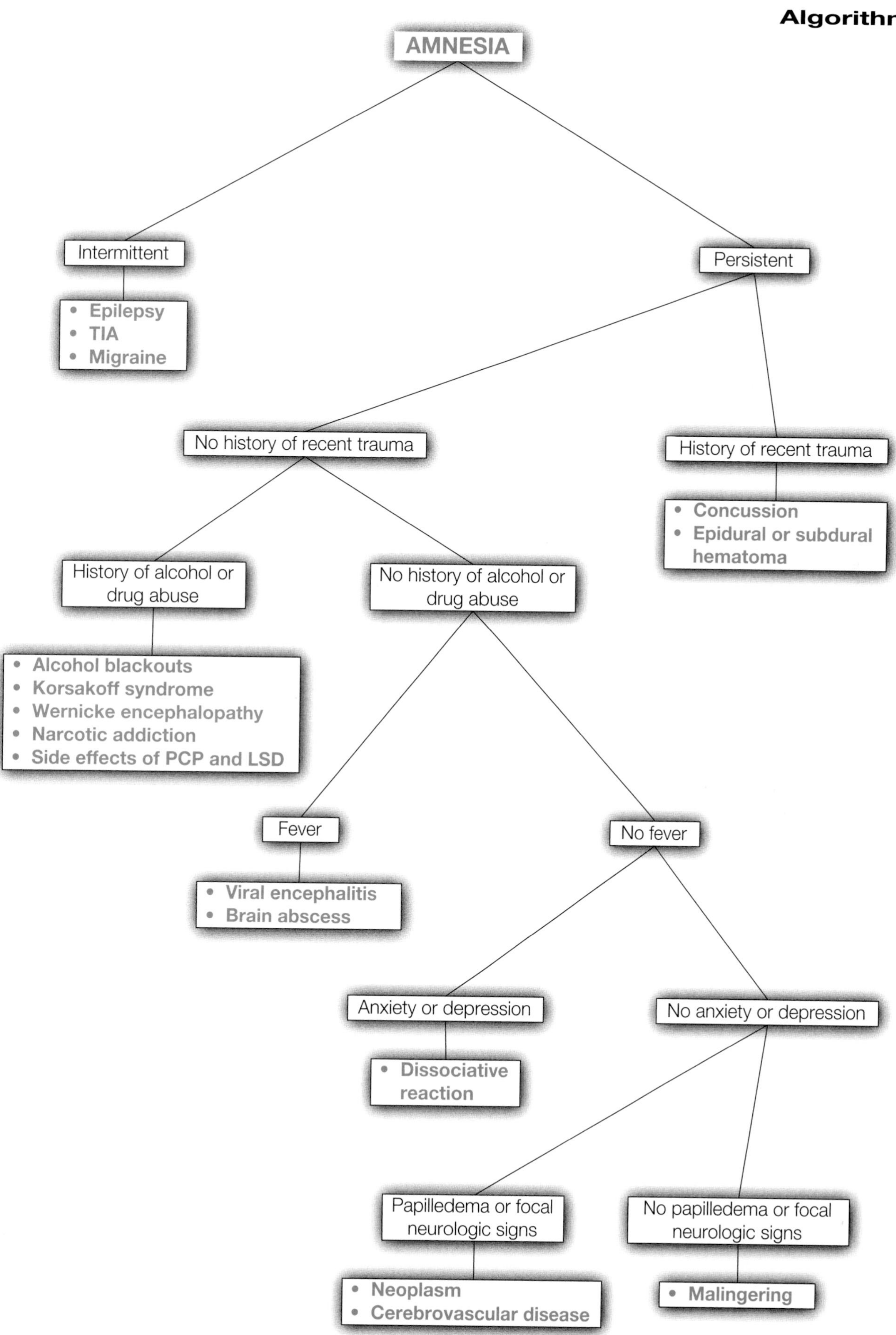
AMNESIA
Intermittent
• Epilepsy
• TIA
• Migraine
Persistent
No history of recent trauma
History of recent trauma
• Concussion
• Epidural or subdural hematoma
History of alcohol or drug abuse
• Alcohol blackouts
• Korsakoff syndrome
• Wernicke encephalopathy
• Narcotic addiction
• Side effects of PCP and LSD
No history of alcohol or drug abuse
Fever
• Viral encephalitis
• Brain abscess
No fever
Anxiety or depression
• Dissociative reaction
No anxiety or depression
Papilledema or focal neurologic signs
• Neoplasm
• Cerebrovascular disease
No papilledema or focal neurologic signs
• Malingering

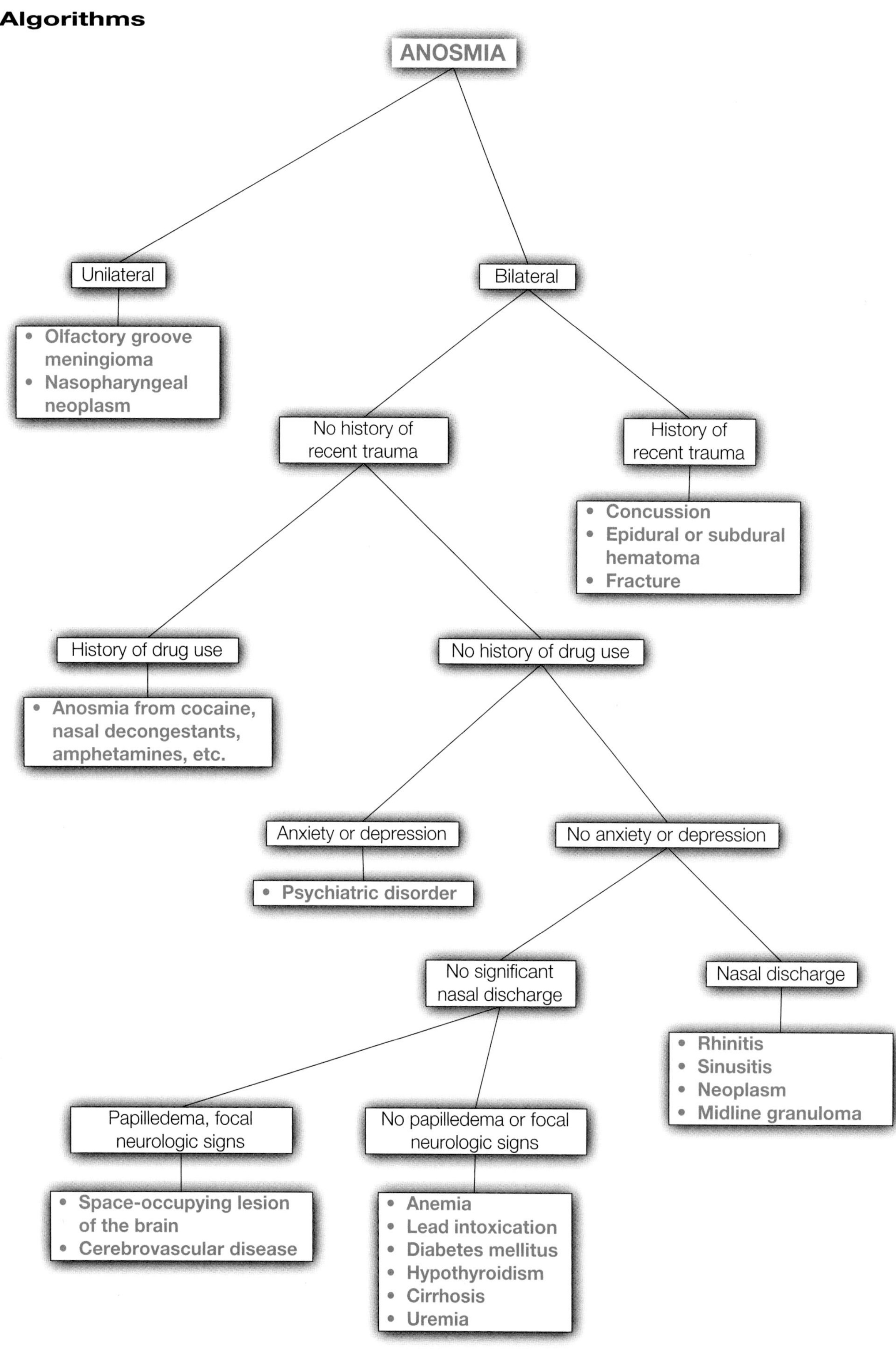
ANOSMIA
Unilateral
Bilateral
• Olfactory groove meningioma
• Nasopharyngeal neoplasm
No history of recent trauma
History of recent trauma
• Concussion
• Epidural or subdural hematoma
• Fracture
History of drug use
No history of drug use
• Anosmia from cocaine, nasal decongestants, amphetamines, etc.
Anxiety or depression
No anxiety or depression
• Psychiatric disorder
No significant nasal discharge
Nasal discharge
• Rhinitis
• Sinusitis
• Neoplasm
• Midline granuloma
Papilledema, focal neurologic signs
No papilledema or focal neurologic signs
• Space-occupying lesion of the brain
• Cerebrovascular disease
• Anemia
• Lead intoxication
• Diabetes mellitus
• Hypothyroidism
• Cirrhosis
• Uremia

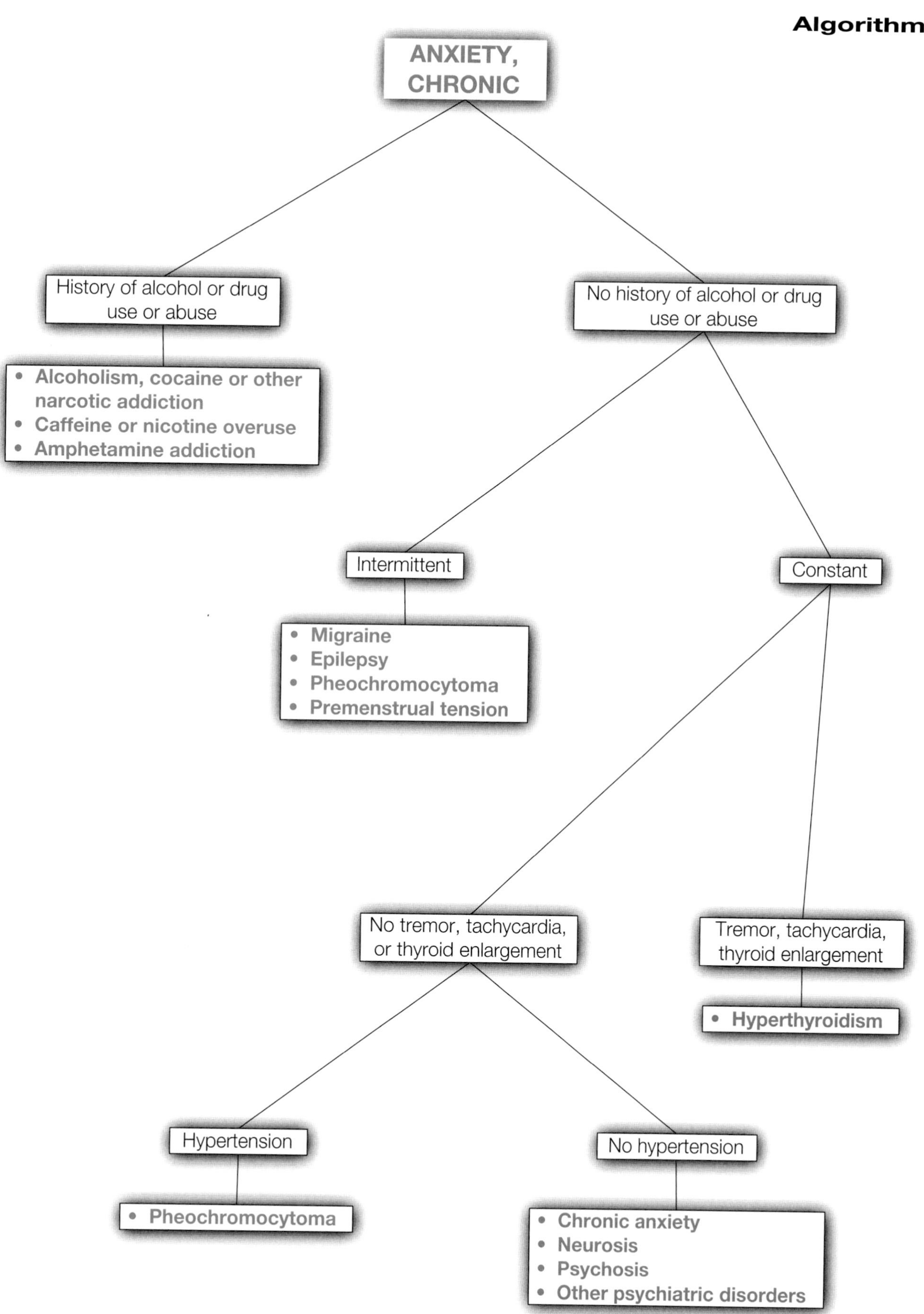
ANXIETY, CHRONIC
History of alcohol or drug use or abuse
• Alcoholism, cocaine or other narcotic addiction
• Caffeine or nicotine overuse
• Amphetamine addiction
No history of alcohol or drug use or abuse
Intermittent
• Migraine
• Epilepsy
• Pheochromocytoma
• Premenstrual tension
Constant
No tremor, tachycardia, or thyroid enlargement
Tremor, tachycardia, thyroid enlargement
• Hyperthyroidism
Hypertension
• Pheochromocytoma
No hypertension
• Chronic anxiety
• Neurosis
• Psychosis
• Other psychiatric disorders

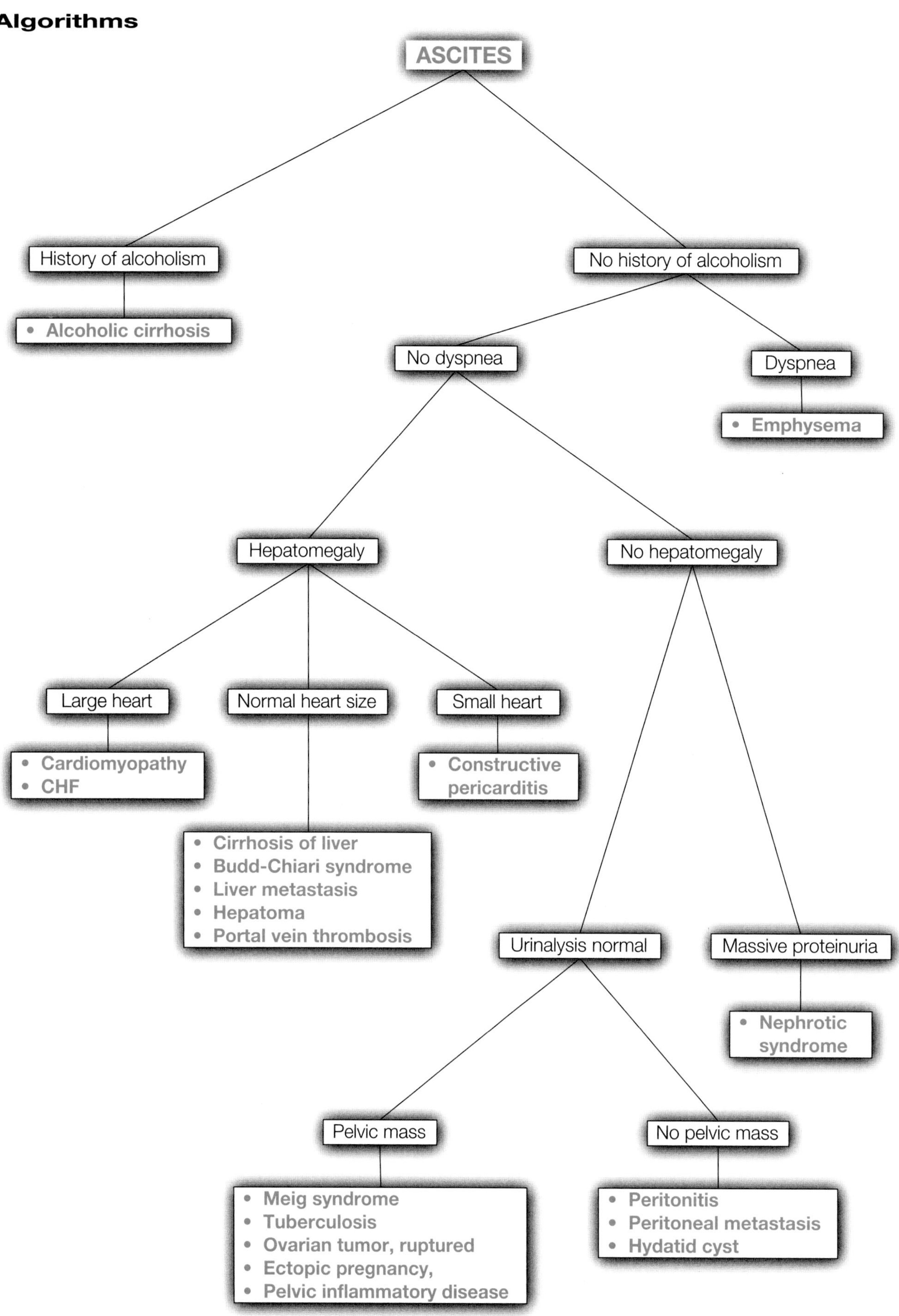
ASCITES
History of alcoholism
• Alcoholic cirrhosis
No history of alcoholism
No dyspnea
Dyspnea
• Emphysema
Hepatomegaly
No hepatomegaly
Large heart
Normal heart size
Small heart
• Cardiomyopathy
• CHF
• Constructive pericarditis
• Cirrhosis of liver
• Budd-Chiari syndrome
• Liver metastasis
• Hepatoma
• Portal vein thrombosis
Urinalysis normal
Massive proteinuria
• Nephrotic syndrome
Pelvic mass
No pelvic mass
• Meig syndrome
• Tuberculosis
• Ovarian tumor, ruptured
• Ectopic pregnancy,
• Pelvic inflammatory disease
• Peritonitis
• Peritoneal metastasis
• Hydatid cyst

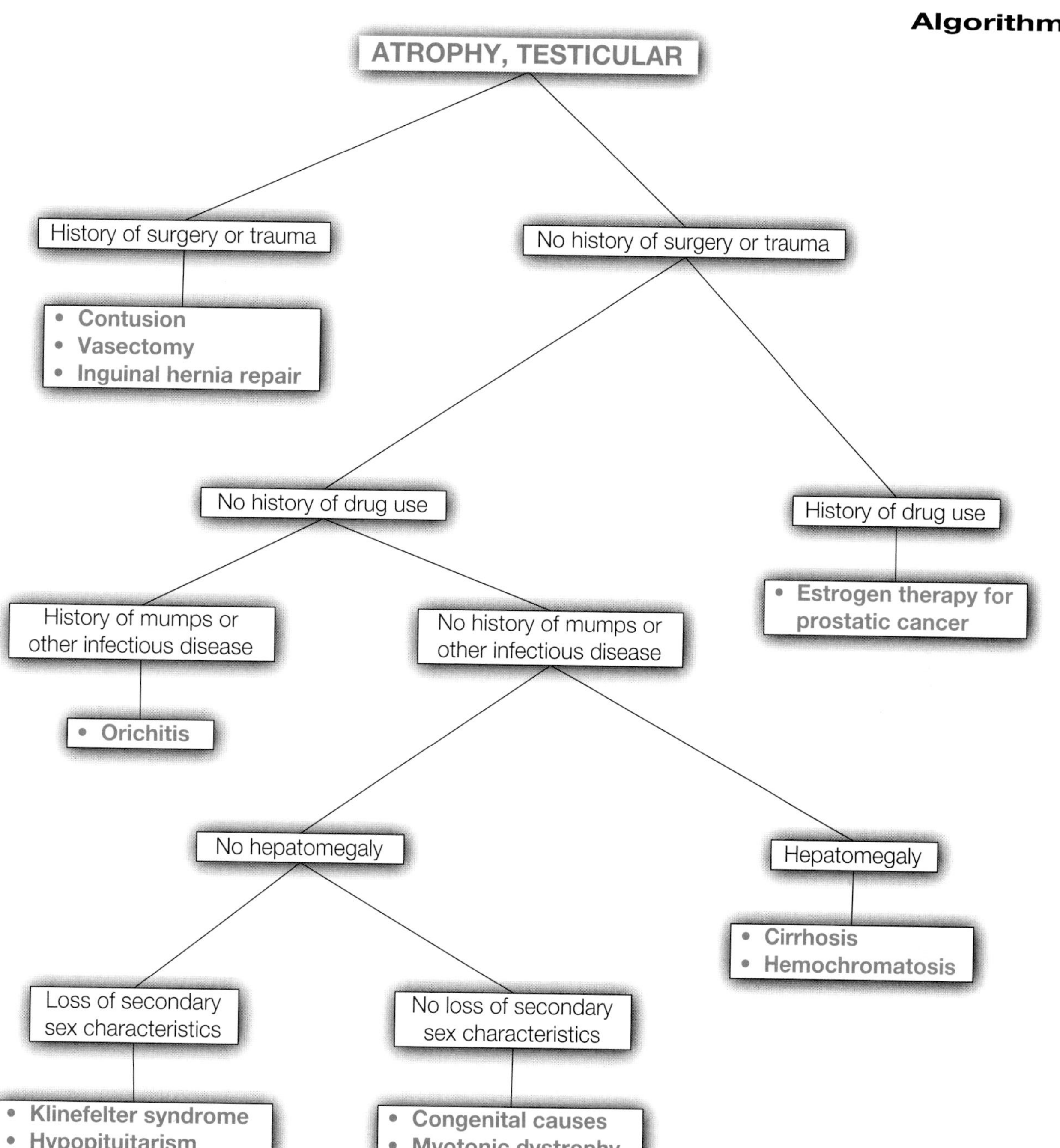
ATROPHY, TESTICULAR
History of surgery or trauma
No history of surgery or trauma
• Contusion
• Vasectomy
• Inguinal hernia repair
No history of drug use
History of drug use
• Estrogen therapy for prostatic cancer
History of mumps or other infectious disease
No history of mumps or other infectious disease
• Orichitis
No hepatomegaly
Hepatomegaly
• Cirrhosis
• Hemochromatosis
Loss of secondary sex characteristics
No loss of secondary sex characteristics
• Klinefelter syndrome
• Hypopituitarism
• Congenital causes
• Myotonic dystrophy

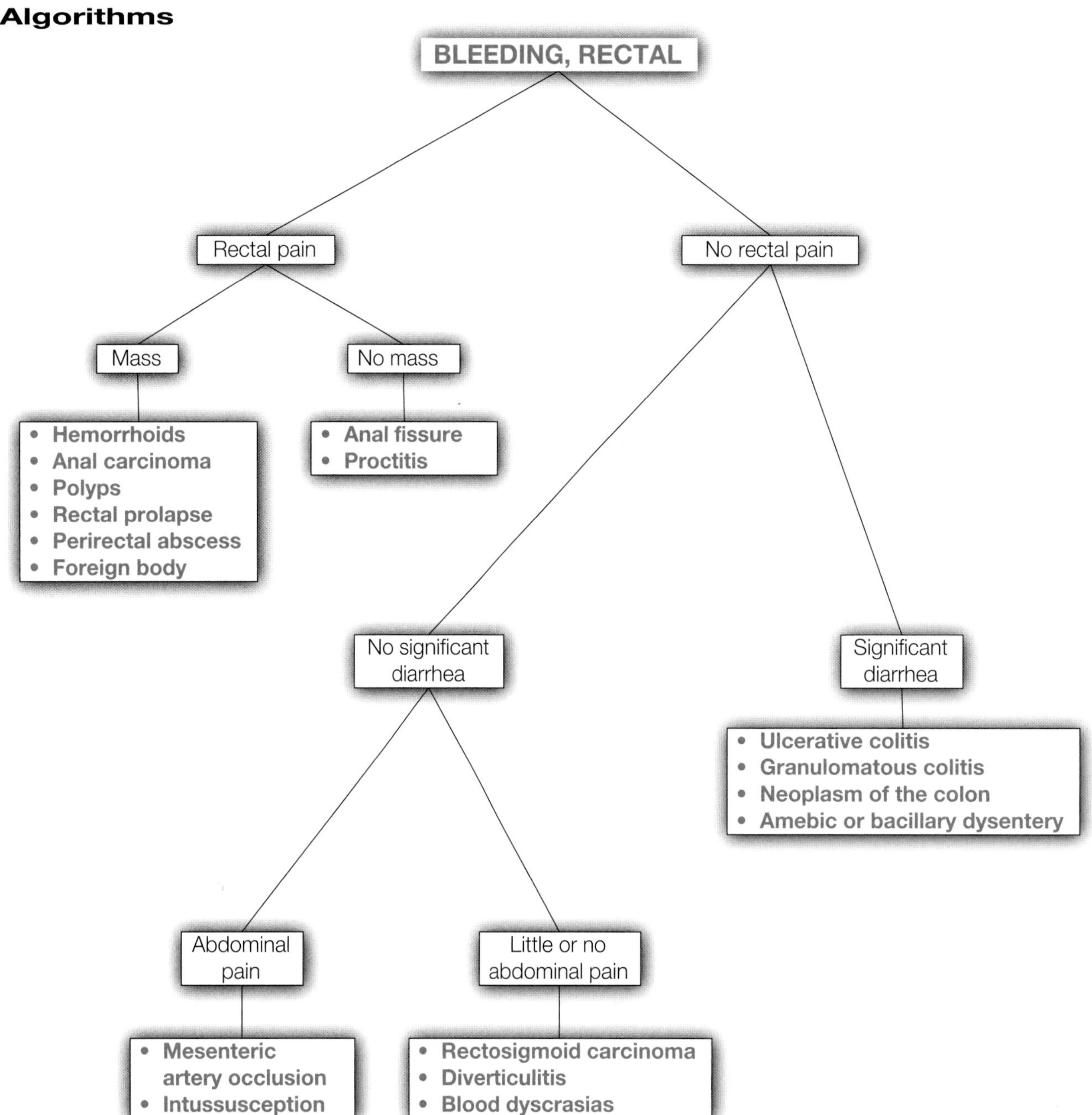
BLEEDING, RECTAL
Rectal pain
No rectal pain
Mass
No mass
• Hemorrhoids
• Anal carcinoma
• Polyps
• Rectal prolapse
• Perirectal abscess
• Foreign body
• Anal fissure
• Proctitis
No significant diarrhea
Significant diarrhea
• Ulcerative colitis
• Granulomatous colitis
• Neoplasm of the colon
• Amebic or bacillary dysentery
Abdominal pain
Little or no abdominal pain
• Mesenteric artery occlusion
• Intussusception
• Rectosigmoid carcinoma
• Diverticulitis
• Blood dyscrasias

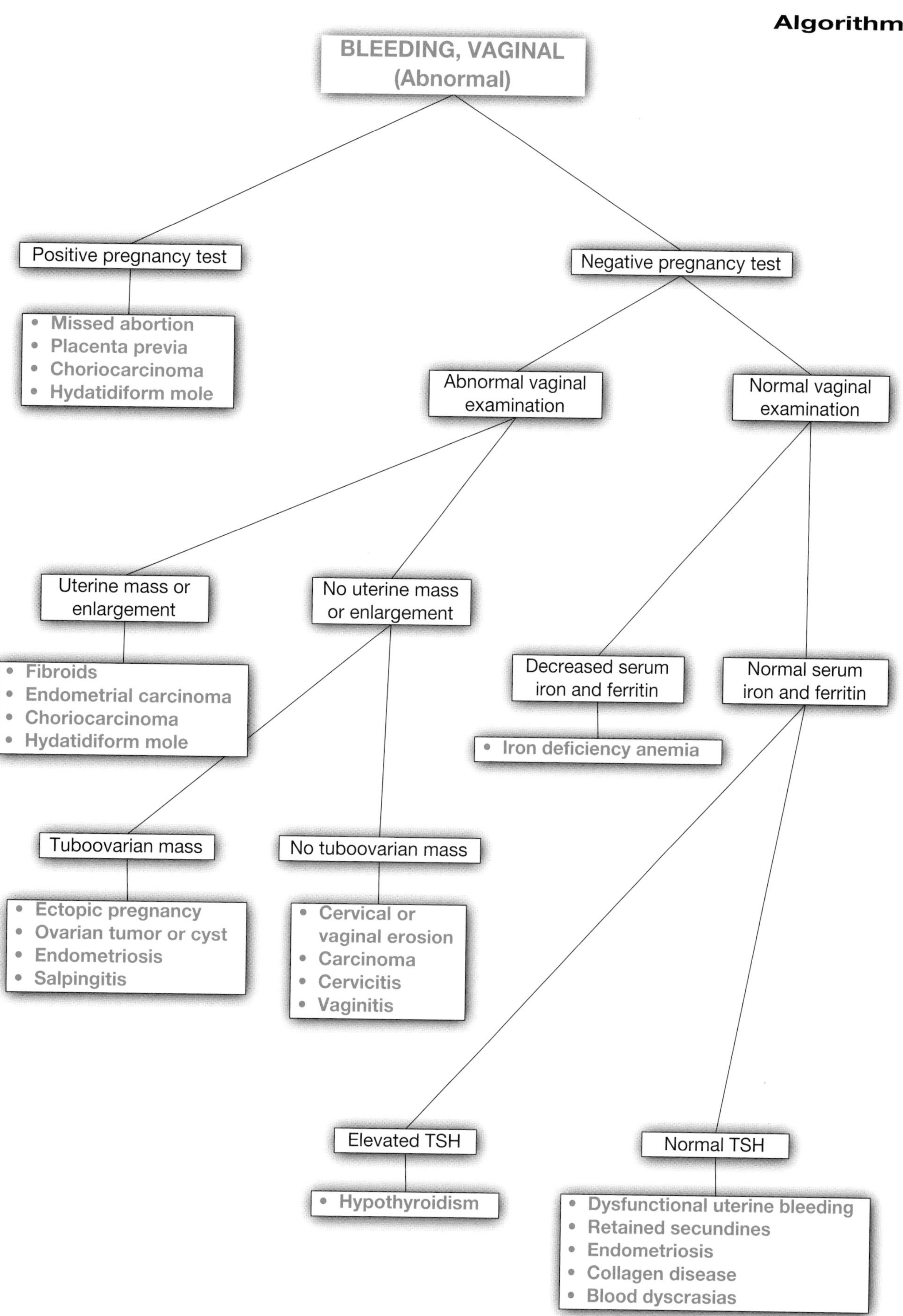
BLEEDING, VAGINAL
(Abnormal)
Positive pregnancy test
• Missed abortion
• Placenta previa
• Choriocarcinoma
• Hydatidiform mole
Negative pregnancy test
Abnormal vaginal examination
Normal vaginal examination
Uterine mass or enlargement
• Fibroids
• Endometrial carcinoma
• Choriocarcinoma
• Hydatidiform mole
No uterine mass or enlargement
Tuboovarian mass
• Ectopic pregnancy
• Ovarian tumor or cyst
• Endometriosis
• Salpingitis
No tuboovarian mass
• Cervical or vaginal erosion
• Carcinoma
• Cervicitis
• Vaginitis
Decreased serum iron and ferritin
• Iron deficiency anemia
Normal serum iron and ferritin
Elevated TSH
• Hypothyroidism
Normal TSH
• Dysfunctional uterine bleeding
• Retained secundines
• Endometriosis
• Collagen disease
• Blood dyscrasias

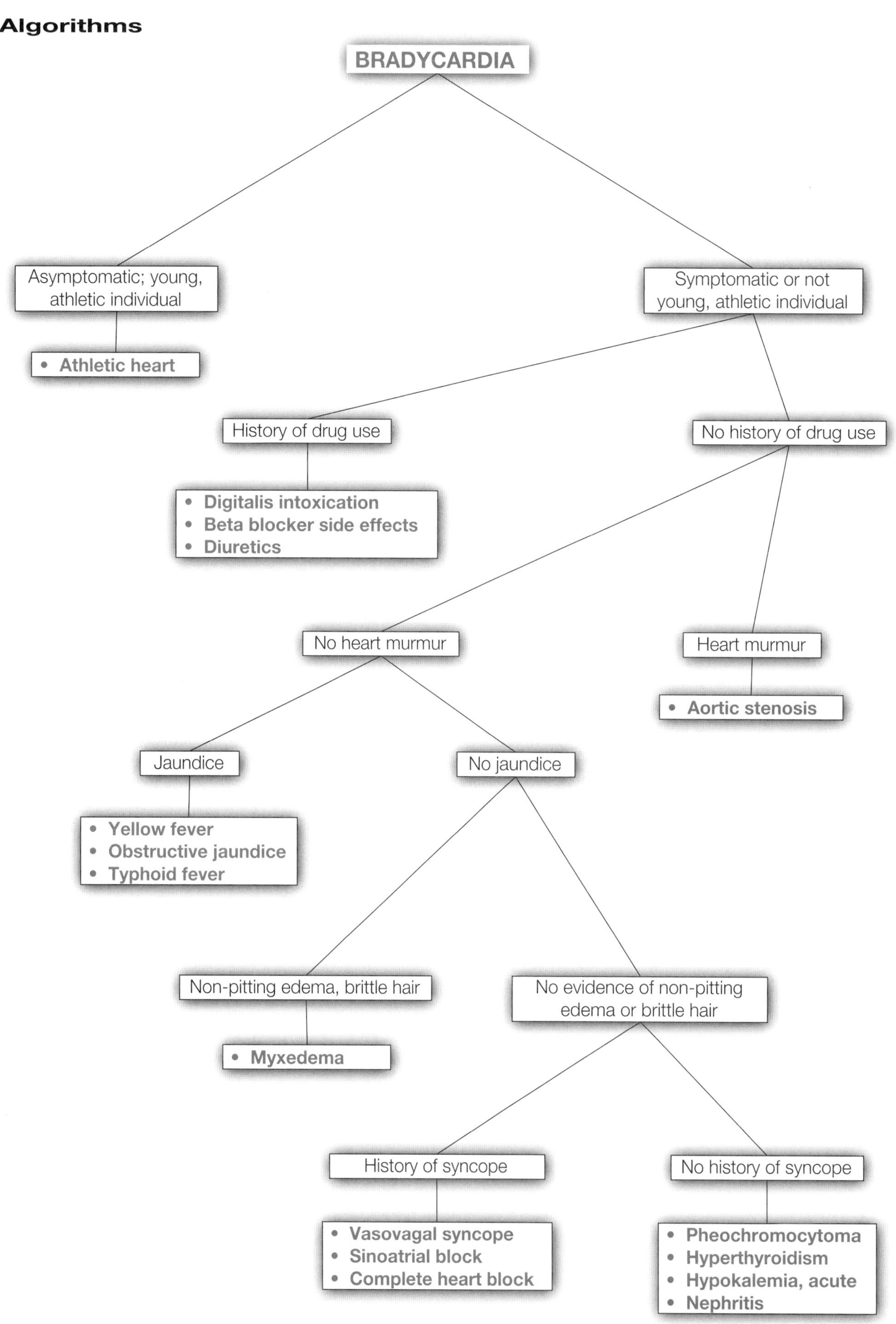
BRADYCARDIA
Asymptomatic; young, athletic individual
• Athletic heart
Symptomatic or not young, athletic individual
History of drug use
• Digitalis intoxication
• Beta blocker side effects
• Diuretics
No history of drug use
No heart murmur
Heart murmur
• Aortic stenosis
Jaundice
• Yellow fever
• Obstructive jaundice
• Typhoid fever
No jaundice
Non-pitting edema, brittle hair
• Myxedema
No evidence of non-pitting edema or brittle hair
History of syncope
• Vasovagal syncope
• Sinoatrial block
• Complete heart block
No history of syncope
• Pheochromocytoma
• Hyperthyroidism
• Hypokalemia, acute
• Nephritis

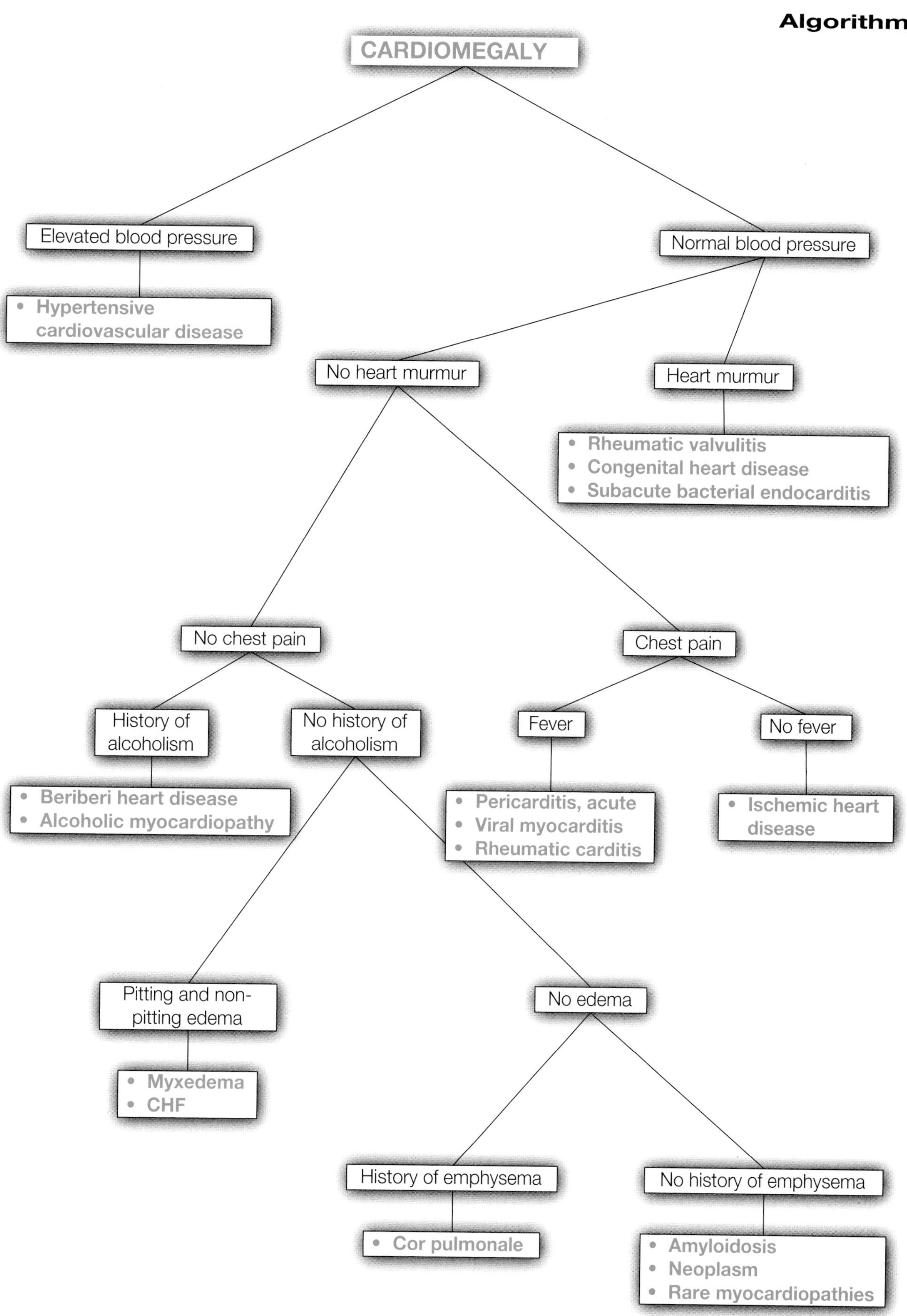
CARDIOMEGALY
Elevated blood pressure
• Hypertensive cardiovascular disease
Normal blood pressure
No heart murmur
Heart murmur
• Rheumatic valvulitis
• Congenital heart disease
• Subacute bacterial endocarditis
No chest pain
Chest pain
History of alcoholism
No history of alcoholism
Fever
No fever
• Beriberi heart disease
• Alcoholic myocardiopathy
• Pericarditis, acute
• Viral myocarditis
• Rheumatic carditis
• Ischemic heart disease
Pitting and non-pitting edema
No edema
• Myxedema
• CHF
History of emphysema
No history of emphysema
• Cor pulmonale
• Amyloidosis
• Neoplasm
• Rare myocardiopathies

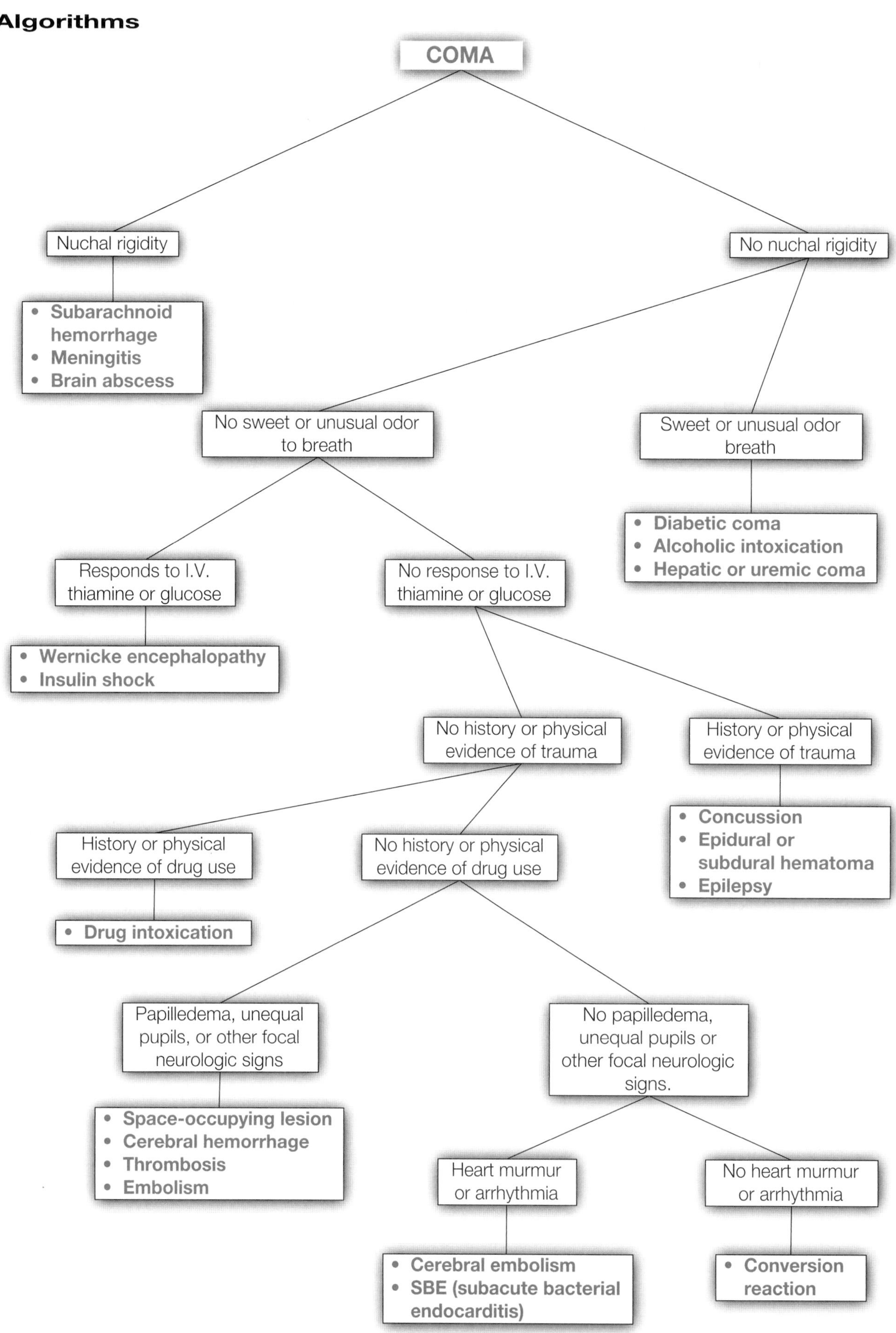
COMA
Nuchal rigidity
• Subarachnoid hemorrhage
• Meningitis
• Brain abscess
No nuchal rigidity
No sweet or unusual odor to breath
Sweet or unusual odor breath
• Diabetic coma
• Alcoholic intoxication
• Hepatic or uremic coma
Responds to I.V. thiamine or glucose
• Wernicke encephalopathy
• Insulin shock
No response to I.V. thiamine or glucose
No history or physical evidence of trauma
History or physical evidence of trauma
• Concussion
• Epidural or subdural hematoma
• Epilepsy
History or physical evidence of drug use
• Drug intoxication
No history or physical evidence of drug use
Papilledema, unequal pupils, or other focal neurologic signs
• Space-occupying lesion
• Cerebral hemorrhage
• Thrombosis
• Embolism
No papilledema, unequal pupils or other focal neurologic signs.
Heart murmur or arrhythmia
• Cerebral embolism
• SBE (subacute bacterial endocarditis)
No heart murmur or arrhythmia
• Conversion reaction

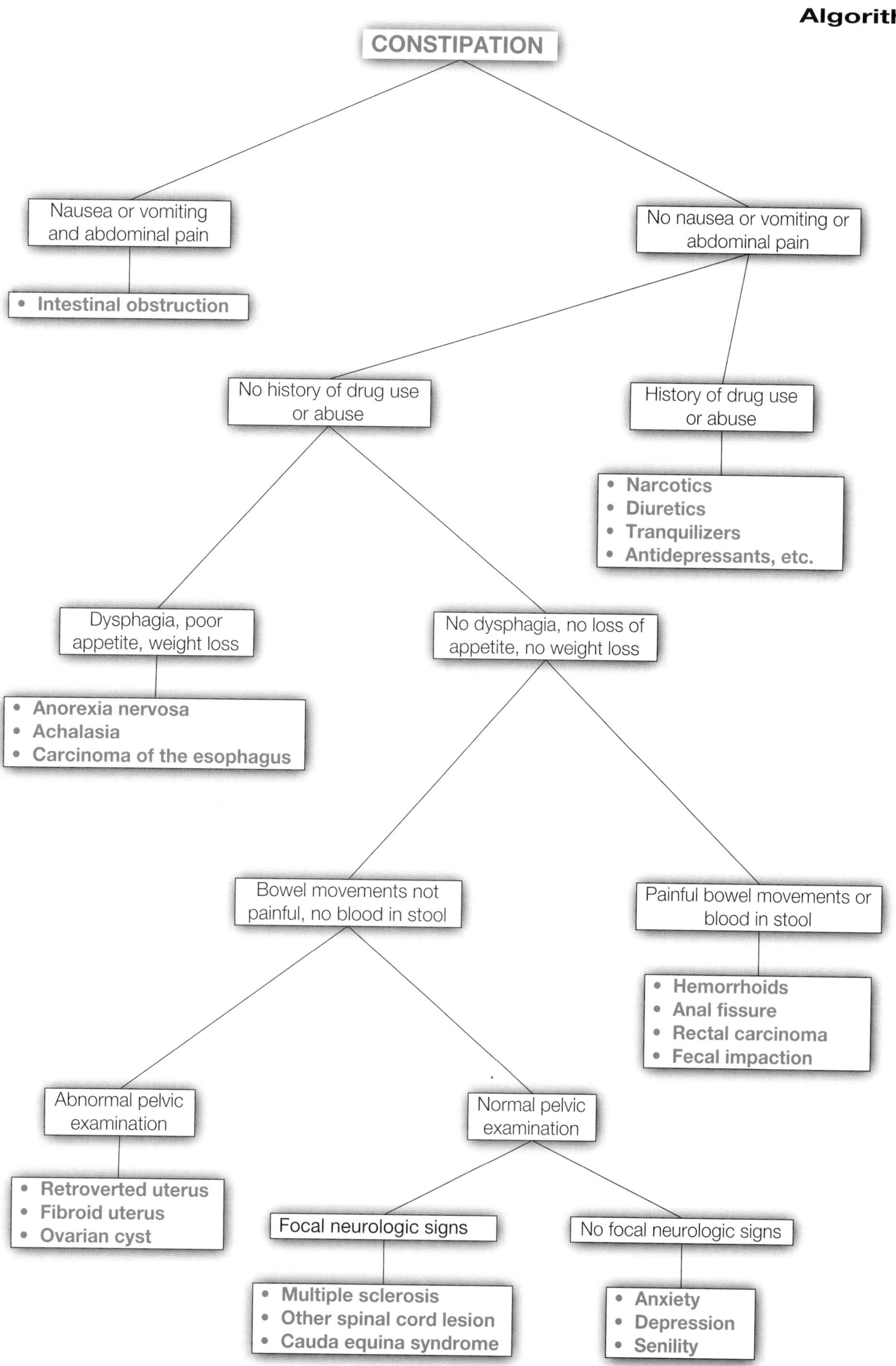
CONSTIPATION
Nausea or vomiting and abdominal pain
• Intestinal obstruction
No nausea or vomiting or abdominal pain
No history of drug use or abuse
History of drug use or abuse
• Narcotics
• Diuretics
• Tranquilizers
• Antidepressants, etc.
Dysphagia, poor appetite, weight loss
• Anorexia nervosa
• Achalasia
• Carcinoma of the esophagus
No dysphagia, no loss of appetite, no weight loss
Bowel movements not painful, no blood in stool
Painful bowel movements or blood in stool
• Hemorrhoids
• Anal fissure
• Rectal carcinoma
• Fecal impaction
Abnormal pelvic examination
• Retroverted uterus
• Fibroid uterus
• Ovarian cyst
Normal pelvic examination
Focal neurologic signs
• Multiple sclerosis
• Other spinal cord lesion
• Cauda equina syndrome
No focal neurologic signs
• Anxiety
• Depression
• Senility

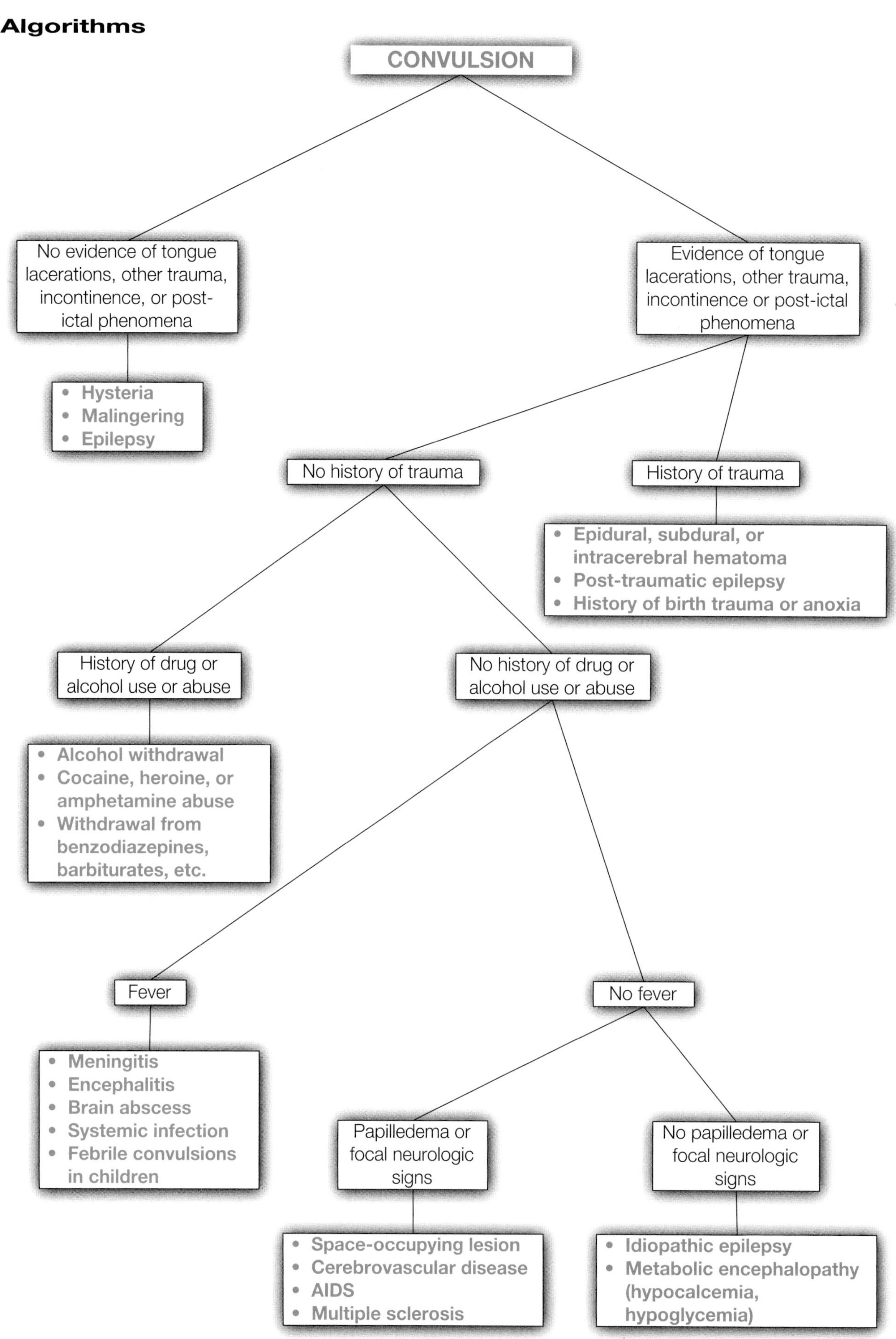
CONVULSION
No evidence of tongue lacerations, other trauma, incontinence, or post-ictal phenomena
• Hysteria
• Malingering
• Epilepsy
Evidence of tongue lacerations, other trauma, incontinence or post-ictal phenomena
No history of trauma
History of trauma
• Epidural, subdural, or intracerebral hematoma
• Post-traumatic epilepsy
• History of birth trauma or anoxia
History of drug or alcohol use or abuse
• Alcohol withdrawal
• Cocaine, heroine, or amphetamine abuse
• Withdrawal from benzodiazepines, barbiturates, etc.
No history of drug or alcohol use or abuse
Fever
• Meningitis
• Encephalitis
• Brain abscess
• Systemic infection
• Febrile convulsions in children
No fever
Papilledema or focal neurologic signs
• Space-occupying lesion
• Cerebrovascular disease
• AIDS
• Multiple sclerosis
No papilledema or focal neurologic signs
• Idiopathic epilepsy
• Metabolic encephalopathy (hypocalcemia, hypoglycemia)

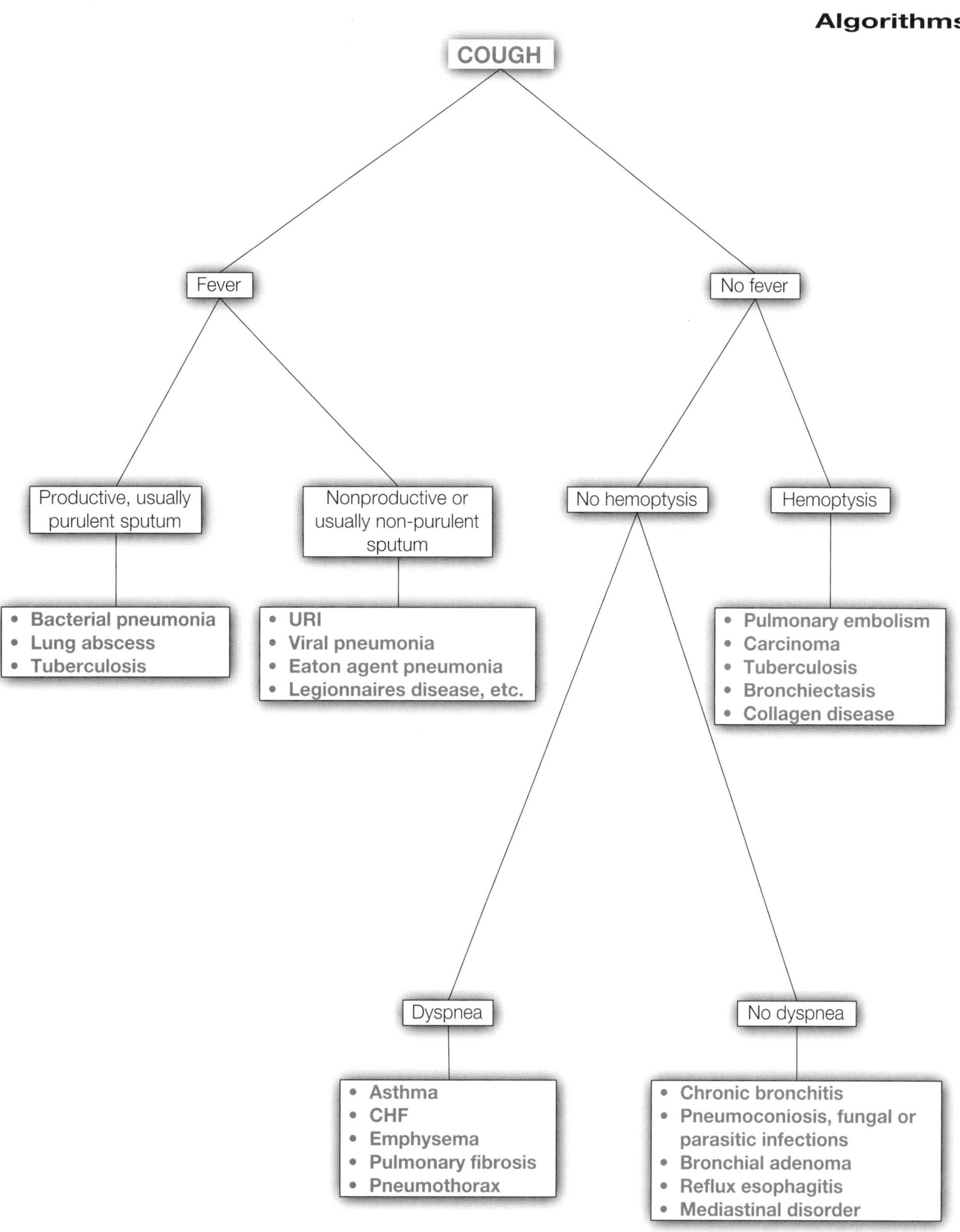
COUGH
Fever
No fever
Productive, usually purulent sputum
Nonproductive or usually non-purulent sputum
No hemoptysis
Hemoptysis
• Bacterial pneumonia
• Lung abscess
• Tuberculosis
• URI
• Viral pneumonia
• Eaton agent pneumonia
• Legionnaires disease, etc.
• Pulmonary embolism
• Carcinoma
• Tuberculosis
• Bronchiectasis
• Collagen disease
Dyspnea
No dyspnea
• Asthma
• CHF
• Emphysema
• Pulmonary fibrosis
• Pneumothorax
• Chronic bronchitis
• Pneumoconiosis, fungal or parasitic infections
• Bronchial adenoma
• Reflux esophagitis
• Mediastinal disorder

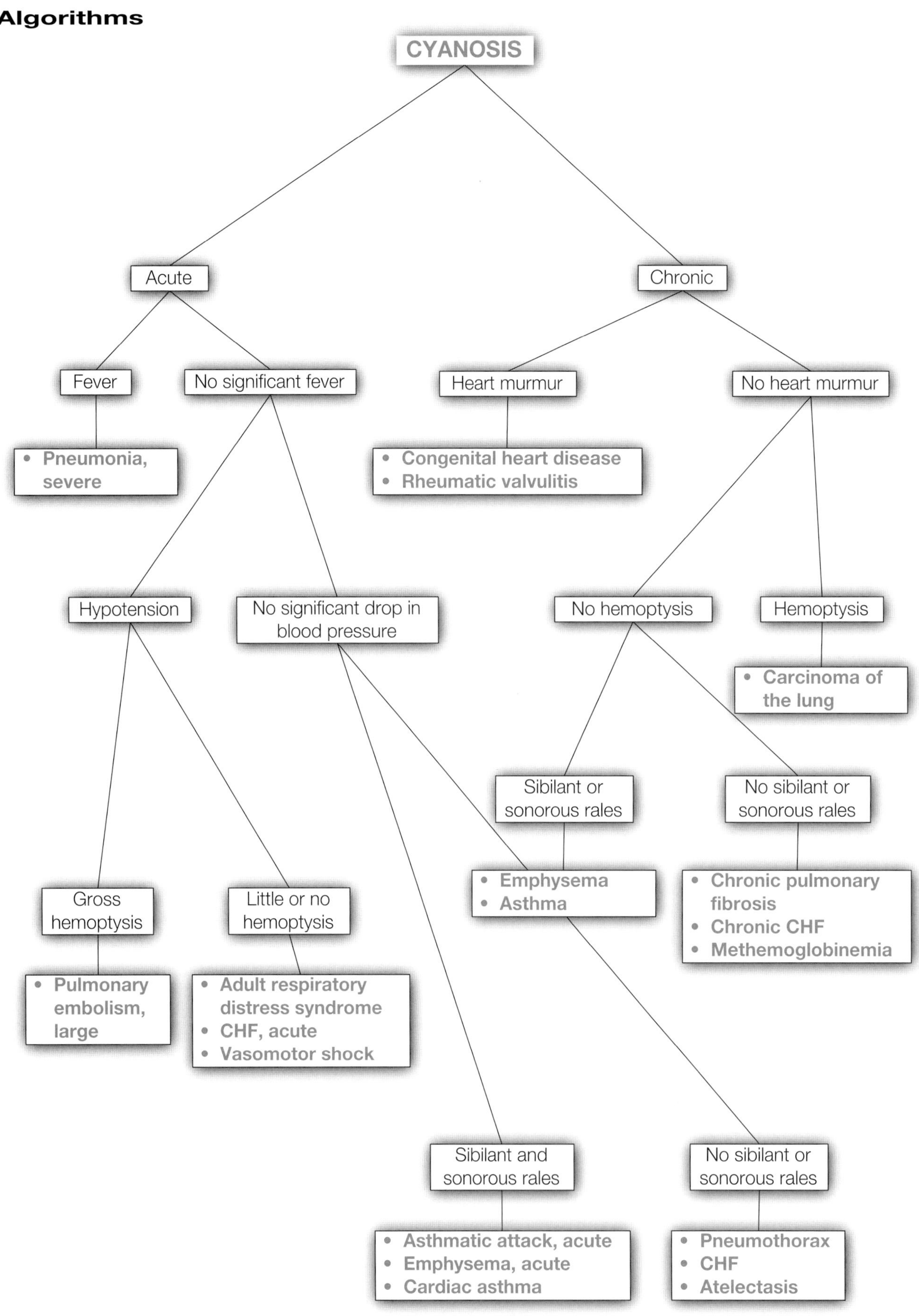
CYANOSIS
Acute
Chronic
Fever
No significant fever
Heart murmur
No heart murmur
• Pneumonia, severe
• Congenital heart disease
• Rheumatic valvulitis
Hypotension
No significant drop in blood pressure
No hemoptysis
Hemoptysis
• Carcinoma of the lung
Sibilant or sonorous rales
No sibilant or sonorous rales
Gross hemoptysis
Little or no hemoptysis
• Emphysema
• Asthma
• Chronic pulmonary fibrosis
• Chronic CHF
• Methemoglobinemia
• Pulmonary embolism, large
• Adult respiratory distress syndrome
• CHF, acute
• Vasomotor shock
Sibilant and sonorous rales
No sibilant or sonorous rales
• Asthmatic attack, acute
• Emphysema, acute
• Cardiac asthma
• Pneumothorax
• CHF
• Atelectasis

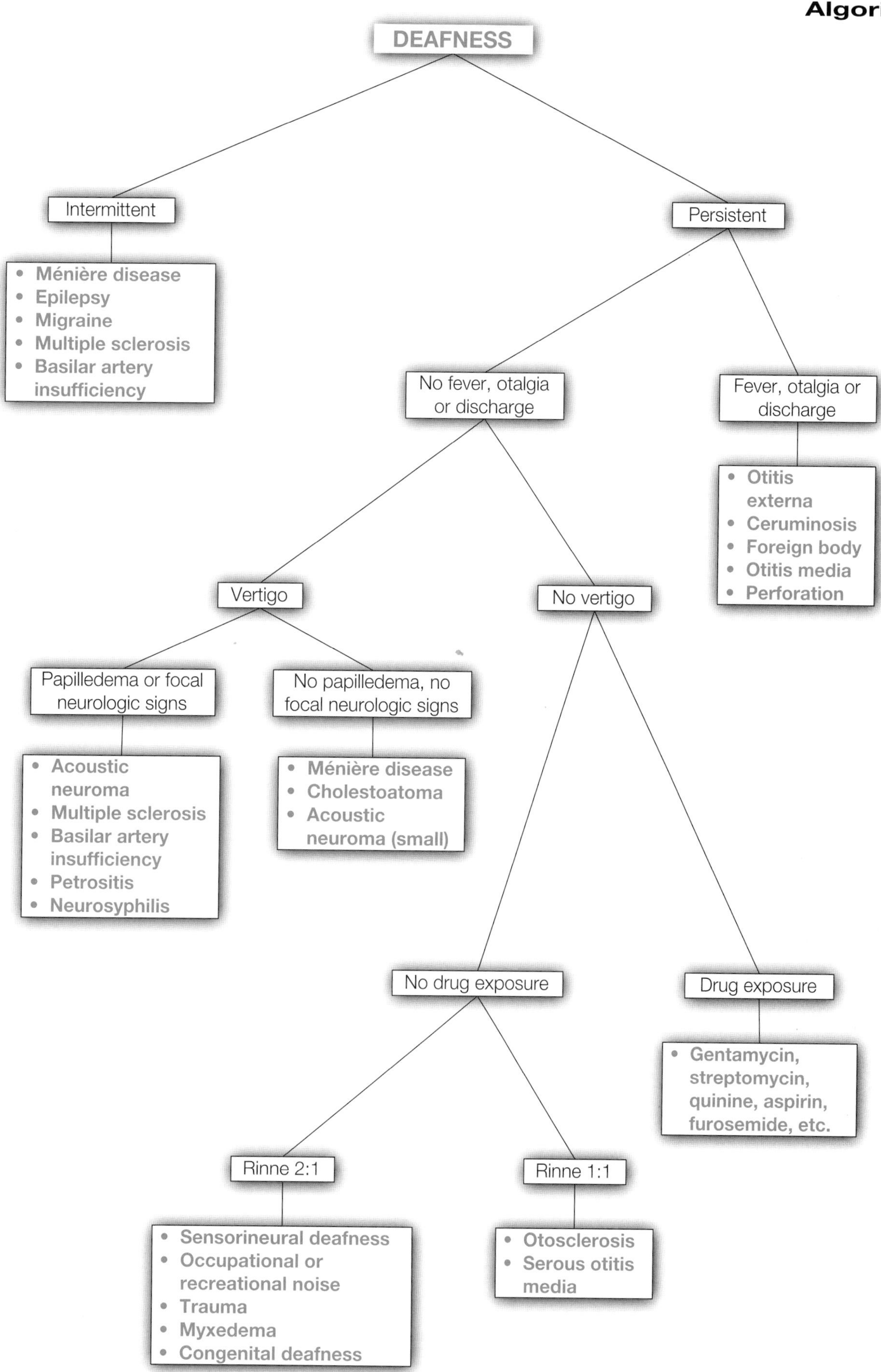
DEAFNESS
Intermittent
• Ménière disease
• Epilepsy
• Migraine
• Multiple sclerosis
• Basilar artery insufficiency
Persistent
No fever, otalgia or discharge
Fever, otalgia or discharge
• Otitis externa
• Ceruminosis
• Foreign body
• Otitis media
• Perforation
Vertigo
No vertigo
Papilledema or focal neurologic signs
No papilledema, no focal neurologic signs
• Acoustic neuroma
• Multiple sclerosis
• Basilar artery insufficiency
• Petrositis
• Neurosyphilis
• Ménière disease
• Cholestoatoma
• Acoustic neuroma (small)
No drug exposure
Drug exposure
• Gentamycin, streptomycin, quinine, aspirin, furosemide, etc.
Rinne 2:1
Rinne 1:1
• Sensorineural deafness
• Occupational or recreational noise
• Trauma
• Myxedema
• Congenital deafness
• Otosclerosis
• Serous otitis media

DEPRESSION

- **Episodic**
  - Psychomotor epilepsy
  - Bipolar disorder
  - Menstruation
- **Not episodic**
  - **History of alcohol or drug use or abuse**
    - Alcoholism
    - Sedative, tranquilizer, or narcotic abuse or chronic use
  - **No history of alcohol or drug use or abuse**
    - **Thyroid mass or nodule**
      - Apathetic hyperthyroidism
      - Hyperparathyroidism
    - **No thyroid mass or nodule**
      - **Hirsutism, obesity, or purple striae**
        - Cushing syndrome
        - Stein-Leventhal syndrome
      - **No hirsutism, obesity, or purple striae**
        - **Papilledema or focal neurologic signs**
          - Space-occupying lesion of the brain
        - **No papilledema or focal neurologic signs**
          - **Cognitive dysfunction**
            - Senile and presenile dementia
            - Cerebral arteriosclerosis
            - Other degenerative disorders of the brain
          - **No cognitive dysfunction**
            - Neurotic or psychotic depression
            - Involutional melancholy

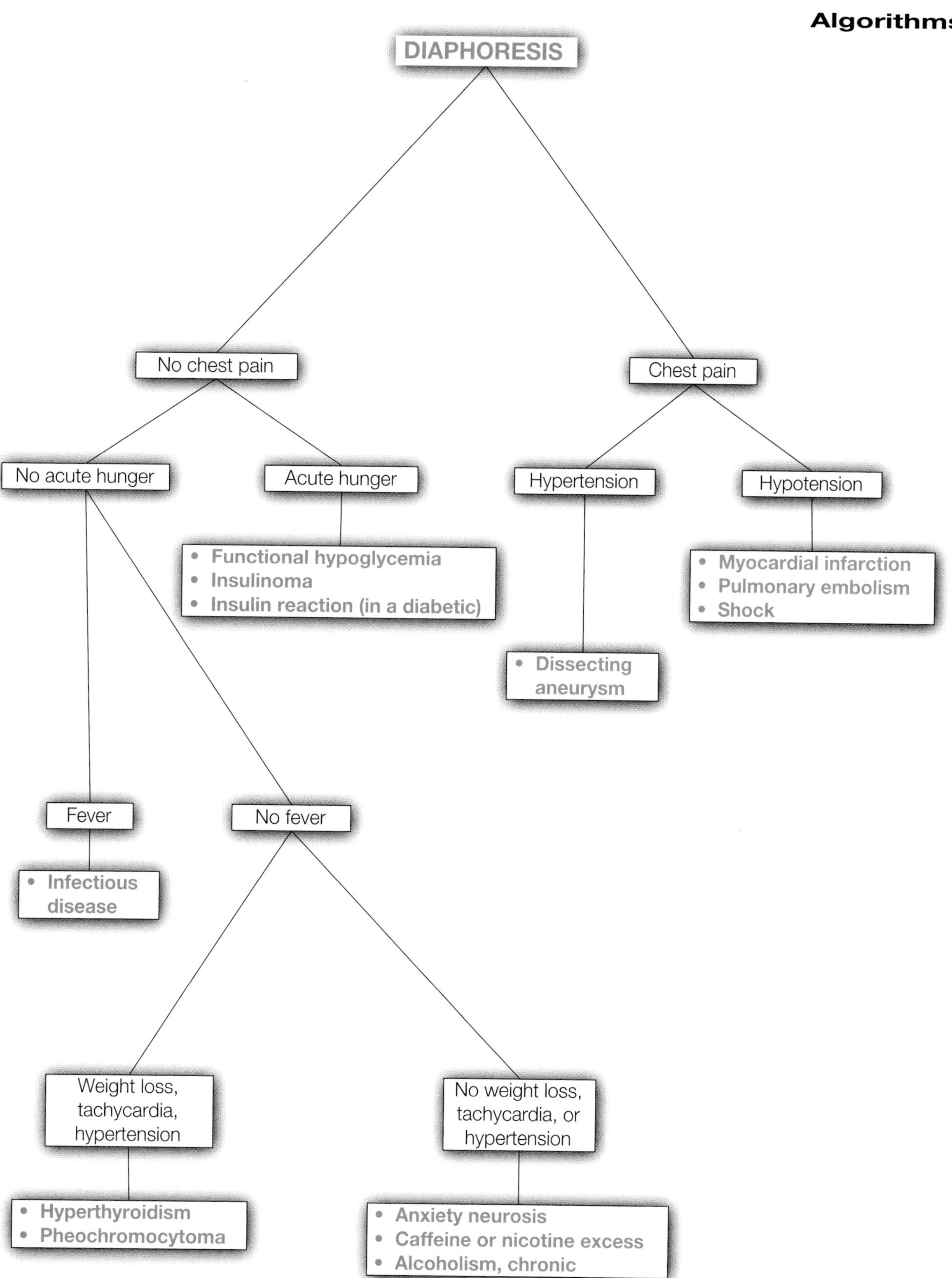
DIAPHORESIS
No chest pain
Chest pain
No acute hunger
Acute hunger
Hypertension
Hypotension
• Functional hypoglycemia
• Insulinoma
• Insulin reaction (in a diabetic)
• Myocardial infarction
• Pulmonary embolism
• Shock
• Dissecting aneurysm
Fever
No fever
• Infectious disease
Weight loss, tachycardia, hypertension
No weight loss, tachycardia, or hypertension
• Hyperthyroidism
• Pheochromocytoma
• Anxiety neurosis
• Caffeine or nicotine excess
• Alcoholism, chronic

DIARRHEA, ACUTE

- **History of drug use**
  - Antibiotics causing pseudomembranous colitis
  - Diarrhea from reserpine, colchine, aspirin, etc.
- **No history of drug use**
  - **History of involvement of other members of family or friends**
    - Botulism
    - Staphylococcal diarrhea
    - Food poisoning
    - Viral gastroenteritis
  - **No history of involvement of other members of family or friends**
    - **Fever**
      - **With blood in stool**
        - Salmonella
        - Shigella
        - Amebiasis
        - Ulcerative colitis
        - Granulomatous colitis
      - **Without blood in stool**
        - Food poisoning
        - Viral gastroenteritis
        - Cholera
    - **No fever**
      - Giardiasis
      - Lactose intolerance
      - Other food intolerance

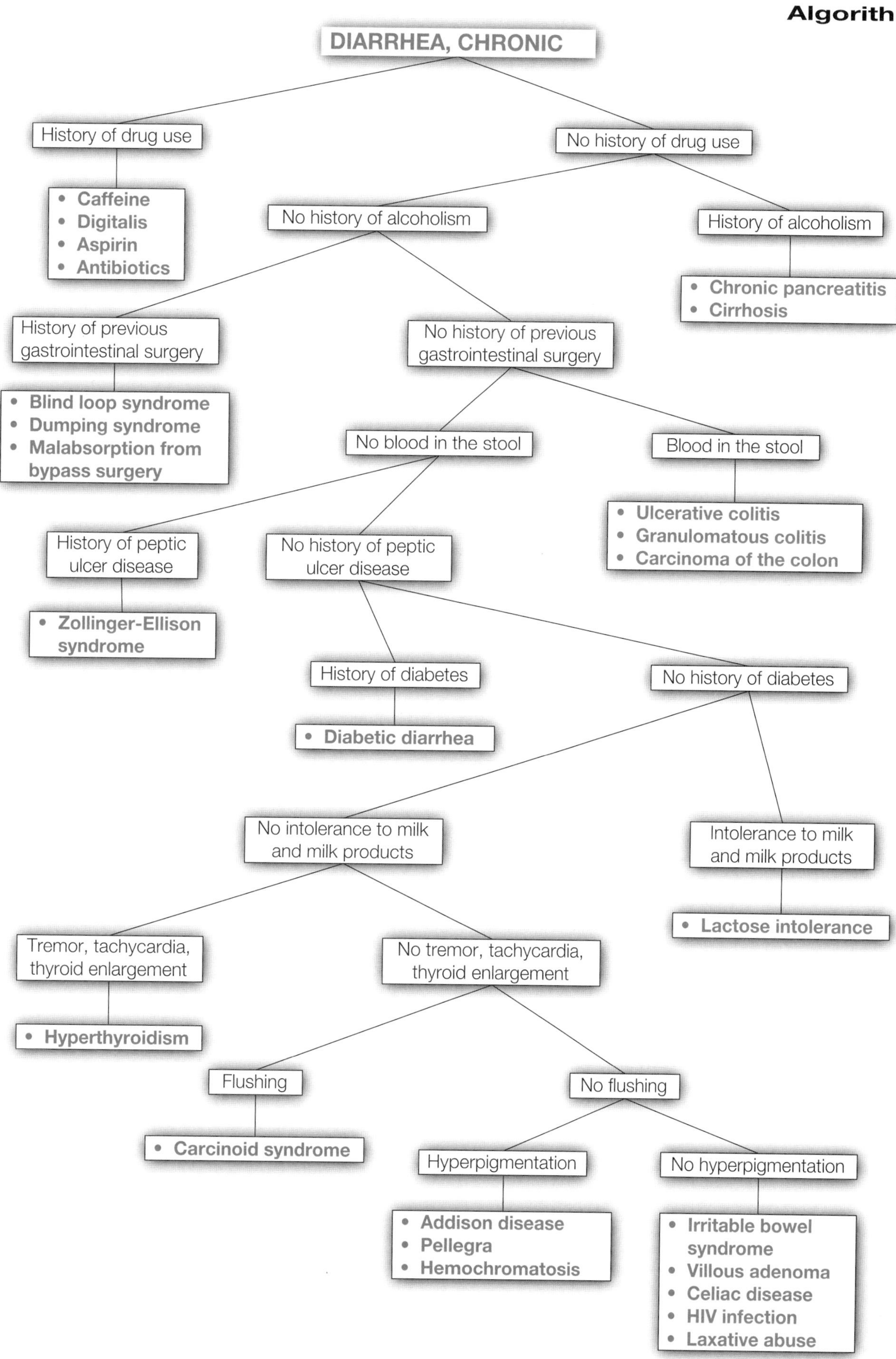
DIARRHEA, CHRONIC
History of drug use
• Caffeine
• Digitalis
• Aspirin
• Antibiotics
No history of drug use
No history of alcoholism
History of alcoholism
• Chronic pancreatitis
• Cirrhosis
History of previous gastrointestinal surgery
• Blind loop syndrome
• Dumping syndrome
• Malabsorption from bypass surgery
No history of previous gastrointestinal surgery
No blood in the stool
Blood in the stool
• Ulcerative colitis
• Granulomatous colitis
• Carcinoma of the colon
History of peptic ulcer disease
• Zollinger-Ellison syndrome
No history of peptic ulcer disease
History of diabetes
• Diabetic diarrhea
No history of diabetes
No intolerance to milk and milk products
Intolerance to milk and milk products
• Lactose intolerance
Tremor, tachycardia, thyroid enlargement
• Hyperthyroidism
No tremor, tachycardia, thyroid enlargement
Flushing
• Carcinoid syndrome
No flushing
Hyperpigmentation
• Addison disease
• Pellegra
• Hemochromatosis
No hyperpigmentation
• Irritable bowel syndrome
• Villous adenoma
• Celiac disease
• HIV infection
• Laxative abuse

DIPLOPIA

- Constant
  - Monocular
    - Marfan disease
    - Congenital double pupil
    - Cataracts
    - Corneal opacities
  - Binocular
    - Fever
      - Cavernous sinus thrombosis
      - Orbital cellulitis
      - Brain abscess
      - Sinusitis
      - Encephalitis
    - No fever
      - No exophthalmos
        - Headache, papilledema, or focal neurologic signs
          - Space-occupying lesion
          - Multiple sclerosis
          - Cerebral aneurysm
          - Migraine
        - No headache, papilledema, or focal neurologic signs
          - Ocular fatigue
      - Exophthalmos
        - Hyperthyroidism
        - A-V aneurysm
        - Orbital tumor or trauma
- Intermittent
  - Myasthenia gravis
  - Ophthalmoplegic migraine

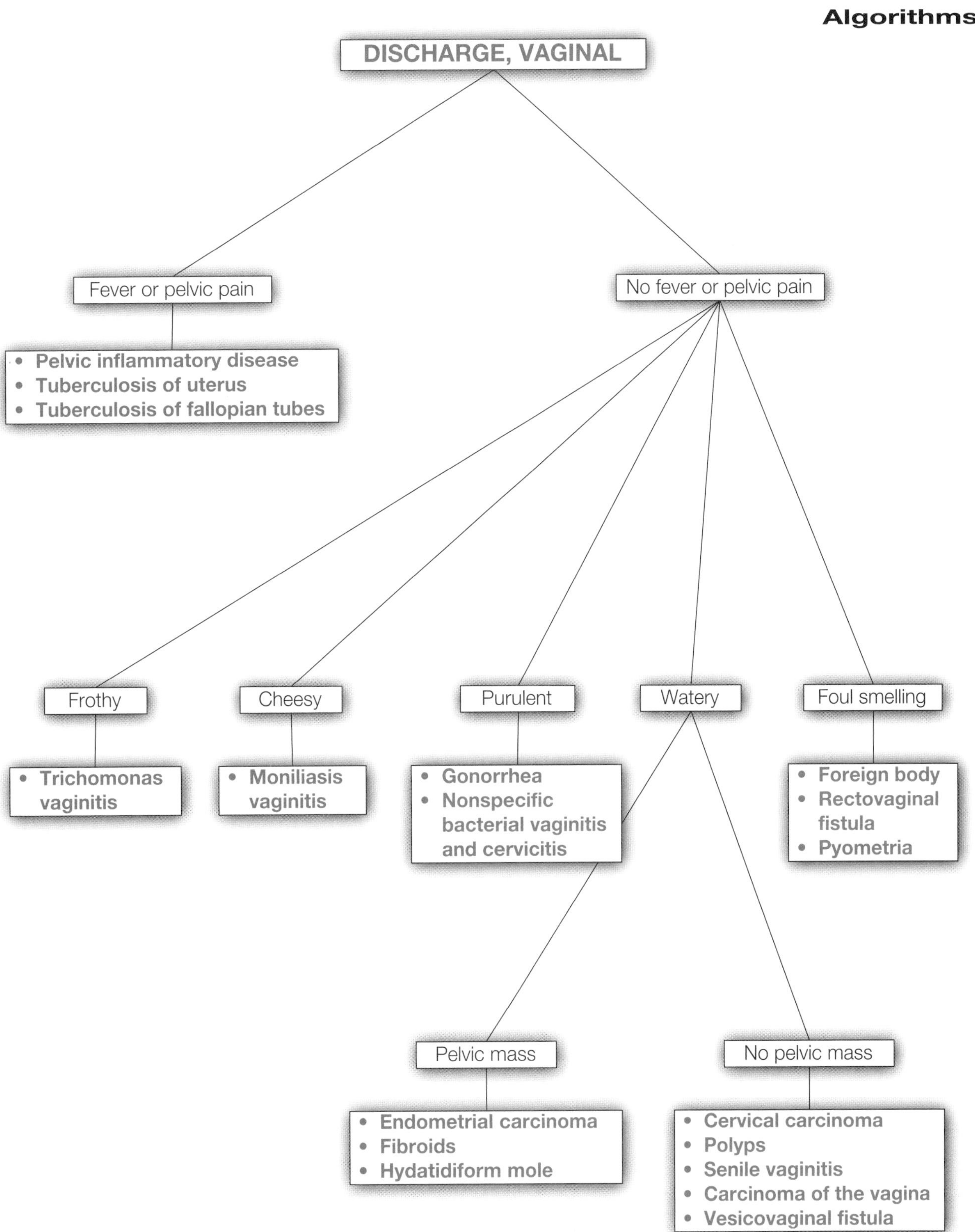
DISCHARGE, VAGINAL
Fever or pelvic pain
No fever or pelvic pain
• Pelvic inflammatory disease
• Tuberculosis of uterus
• Tuberculosis of fallopian tubes
Frothy
Cheesy
Purulent
Watery
Foul smelling
• Trichomonas vaginitis
• Moniliasis vaginitis
• Gonorrhea
• Nonspecific bacterial vaginitis and cervicitis
• Foreign body
• Rectovaginal fistula
• Pyometria
Pelvic mass
No pelvic mass
• Endometrial carcinoma
• Fibroids
• Hydatidiform mole
• Cervical carcinoma
• Polyps
• Senile vaginitis
• Carcinoma of the vagina
• Vesicovaginal fistula

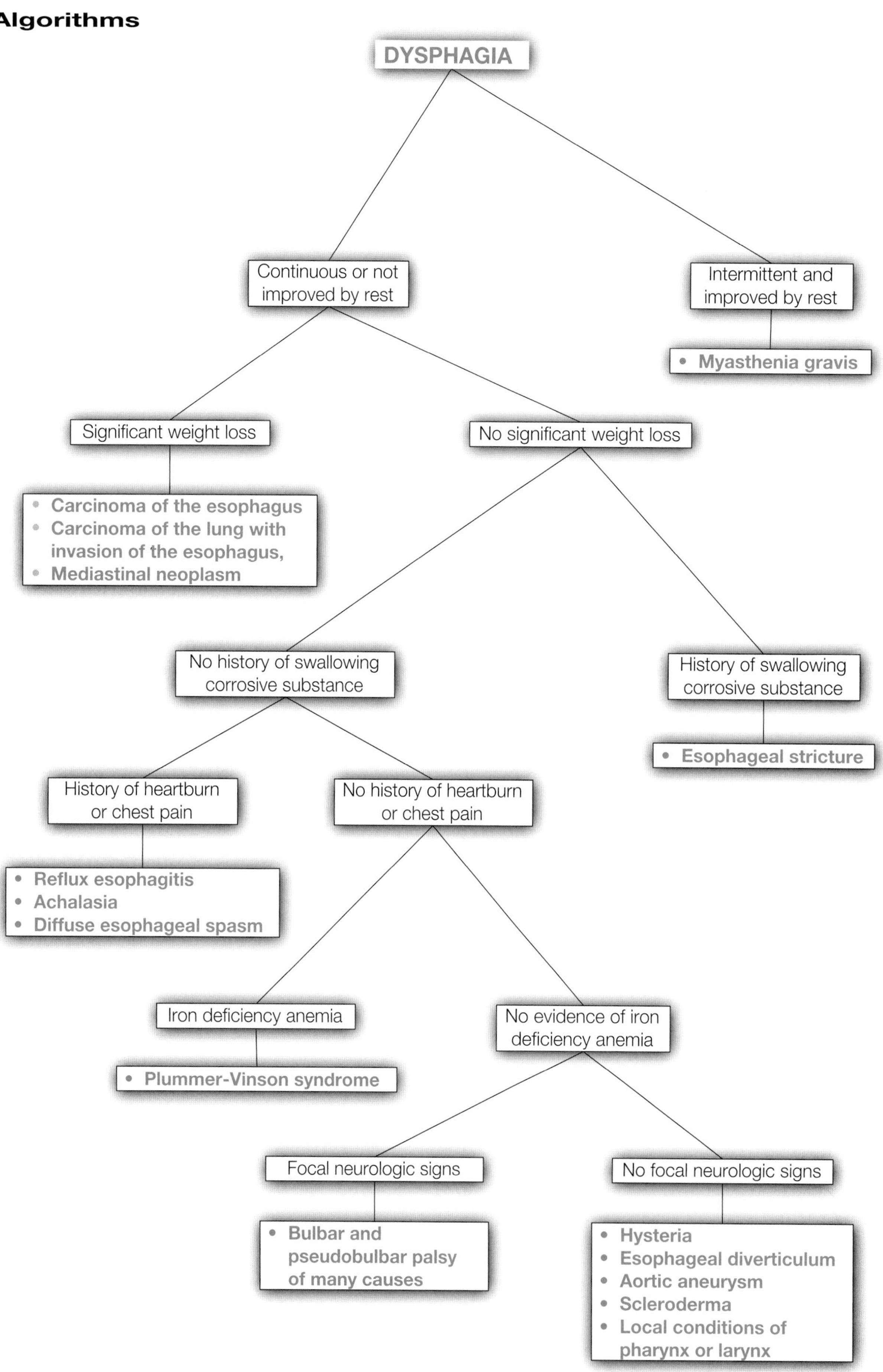
DYSPHAGIA
Continuous or not improved by rest
Intermittent and improved by rest
• Myasthenia gravis
Significant weight loss
No significant weight loss
• Carcinoma of the esophagus
• Carcinoma of the lung with invasion of the esophagus,
• Mediastinal neoplasm
No history of swallowing corrosive substance
History of swallowing corrosive substance
• Esophageal stricture
History of heartburn or chest pain
No history of heartburn or chest pain
• Reflux esophagitis
• Achalasia
• Diffuse esophageal spasm
Iron deficiency anemia
No evidence of iron deficiency anemia
• Plummer-Vinson syndrome
Focal neurologic signs
No focal neurologic signs
• Bulbar and pseudobulbar palsy of many causes
• Hysteria
• Esophageal diverticulum
• Aortic aneurysm
• Scleroderma
• Local conditions of pharynx or larynx

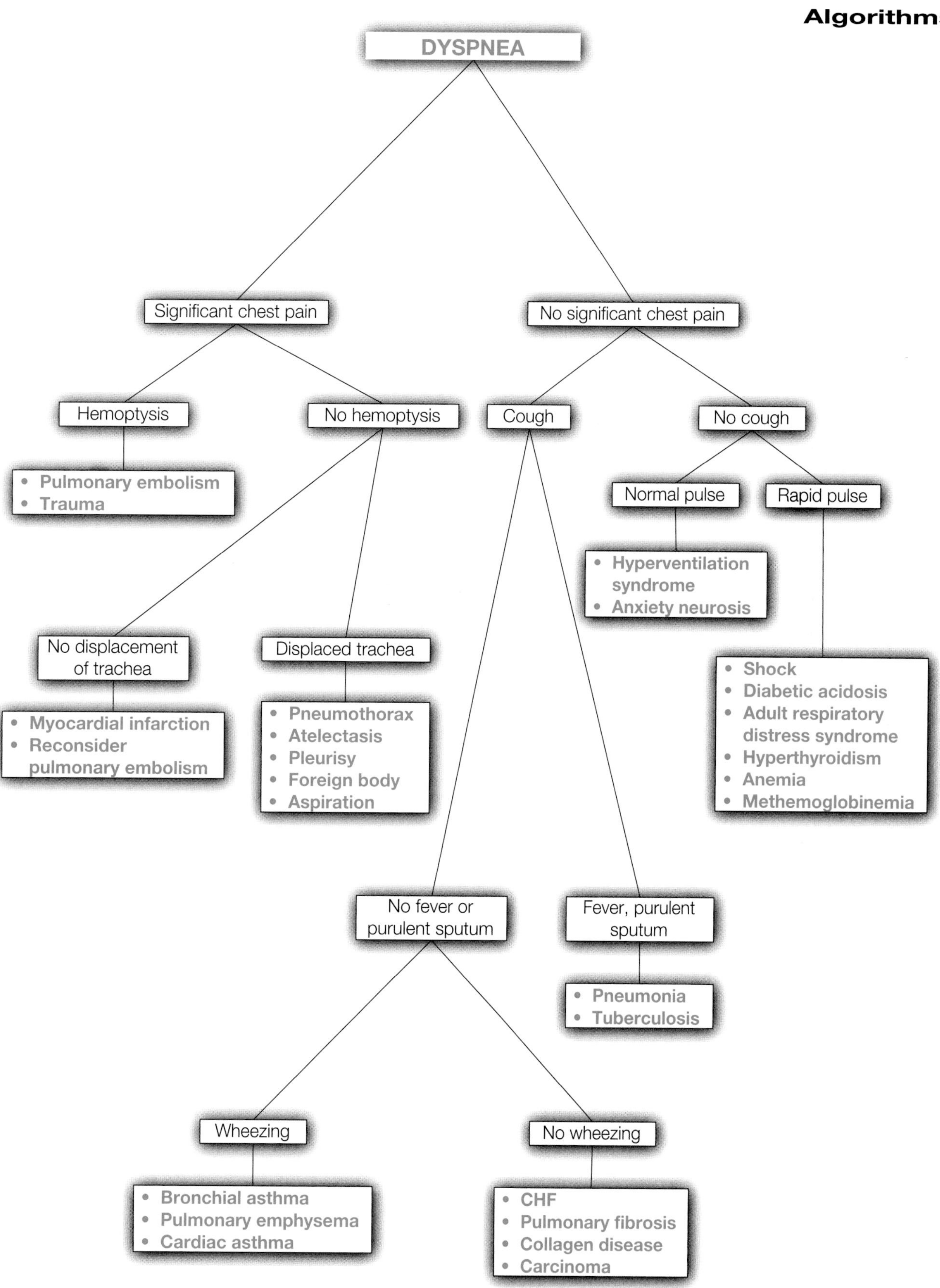
DYSPNEA
Significant chest pain
No significant chest pain
Hemoptysis
No hemoptysis
Cough
No cough
• Pulmonary embolism
• Trauma
Normal pulse
Rapid pulse
• Hyperventilation syndrome
• Anxiety neurosis
No displacement of trachea
Displaced trachea
• Shock
• Diabetic acidosis
• Adult respiratory distress syndrome
• Hyperthyroidism
• Anemia
• Methemoglobinemia
• Myocardial infarction
• Reconsider pulmonary embolism
• Pneumothorax
• Atelectasis
• Pleurisy
• Foreign body
• Aspiration
No fever or purulent sputum
Fever, purulent sputum
• Pneumonia
• Tuberculosis
Wheezing
No wheezing
• Bronchial asthma
• Pulmonary emphysema
• Cardiac asthma
• CHF
• Pulmonary fibrosis
• Collagen disease
• Carcinoma

DYSURIA

- **No fever**
  - **Urethral discharge**
    - Chlamydia or gonococcal urethritis
    - Reiter syndrome
  - **No urethral discharge**
    - **Penile or vulvar lesion, or vaginal discharge**
      - Herpes genitalis
      - Vaginitis
    - **No penile or vulvar lesion, no vaginal discharge**
      - **Hematuria**
        - Cystitis, acute
        - Vesicle calculus
        - Carcinoma of the bladder
        - Tuberculosis
      - **No hematuria**
        - Cystitis, mild-chronic
        - Cystitis, drug-induced
        - Interstitial cystitis, mild
        - Reiter syndrome
        - Irritation (from douche, soap, or spermicidal creams)
- **Fever**
  - Pyelonephritis, acute
  - Prostatitis, acute

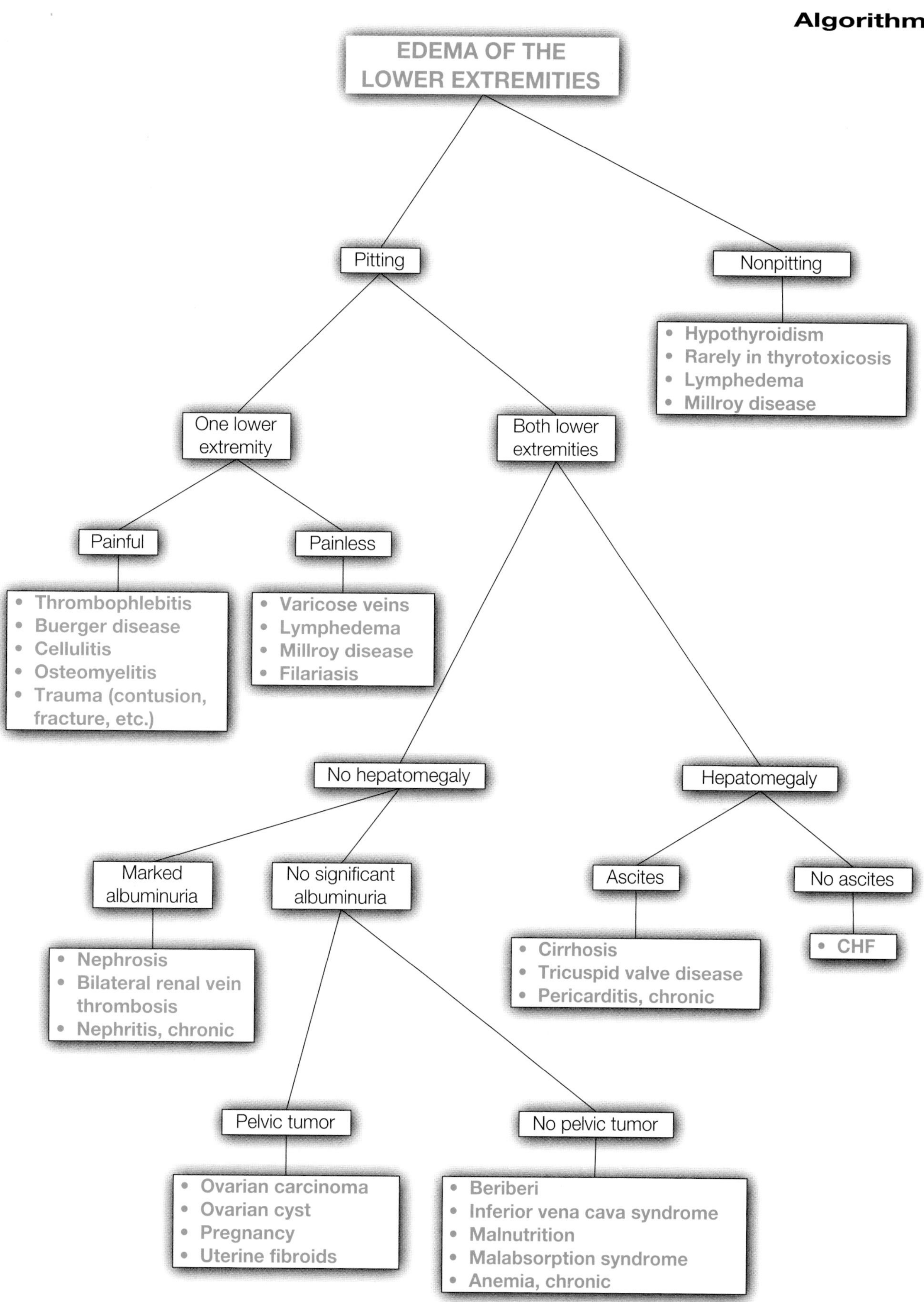
EDEMA OF THE LOWER EXTREMITIES
Pitting
Nonpitting
• Hypothyroidism
• Rarely in thyrotoxicosis
• Lymphedema
• Millroy disease
One lower extremity
Both lower extremities
Painful
Painless
• Thrombophlebitis
• Buerger disease
• Cellulitis
• Osteomyelitis
• Trauma (contusion, fracture, etc.)
• Varicose veins
• Lymphedema
• Millroy disease
• Filariasis
No hepatomegaly
Hepatomegaly
Marked albuminuria
No significant albuminuria
Ascites
No ascites
• Nephrosis
• Bilateral renal vein thrombosis
• Nephritis, chronic
• Cirrhosis
• Tricuspid valve disease
• Pericarditis, chronic
• CHF
Pelvic tumor
No pelvic tumor
• Ovarian carcinoma
• Ovarian cyst
• Pregnancy
• Uterine fibroids
• Beriberi
• Inferior vena cava syndrome
• Malnutrition
• Malabsorption syndrome
• Anemia, chronic
Signs & Symptoms

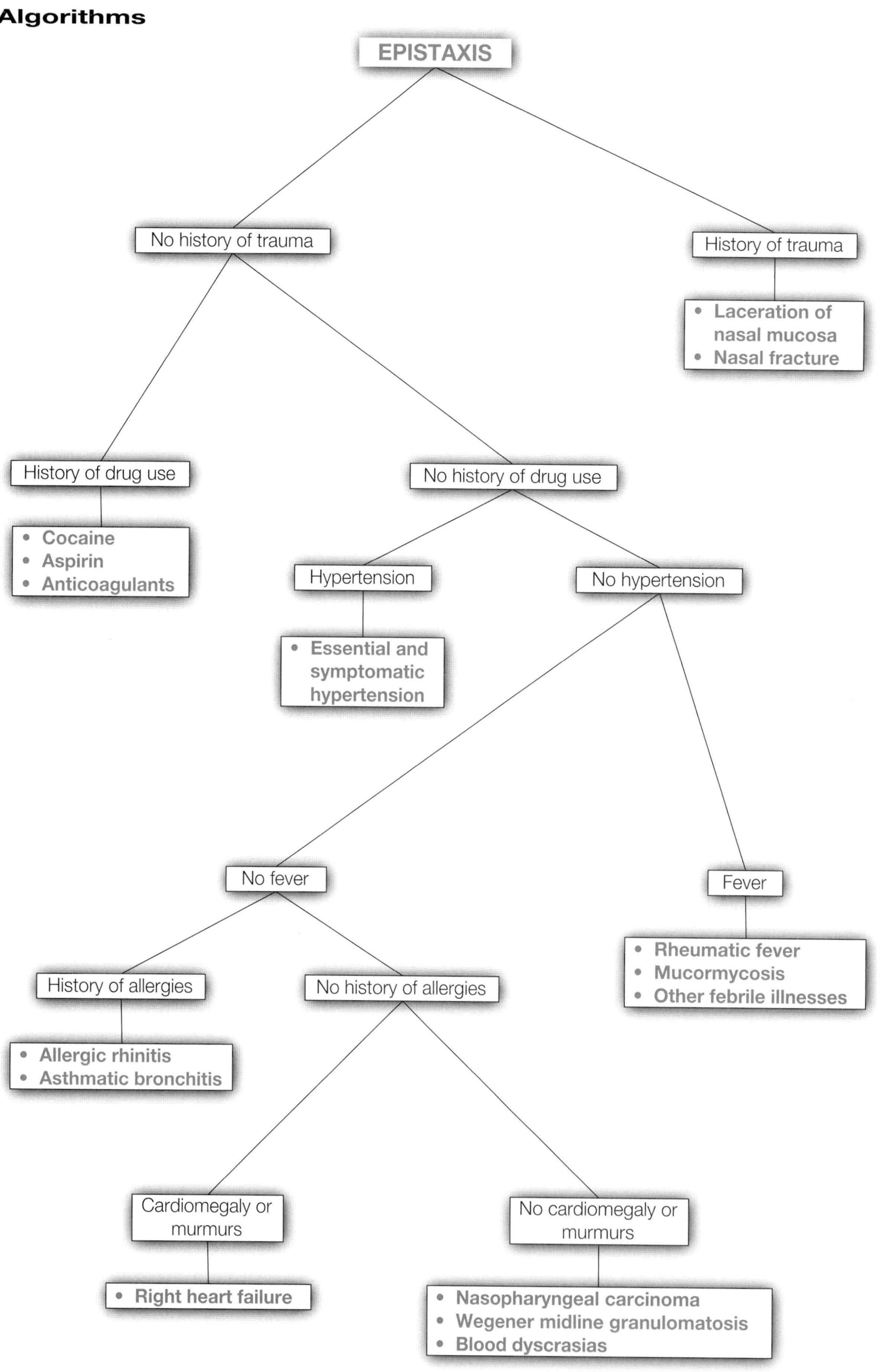
EPISTAXIS
No history of trauma
History of trauma
Laceration of nasal mucosa
Nasal fracture
History of drug use
Cocaine
Aspirin
Anticoagulants
No history of drug use
Hypertension
Essential and symptomatic hypertension
No hypertension
No fever
Fever
Rheumatic fever
Mucormycosis
Other febrile illnesses
History of allergies
Allergic rhinitis
Asthmatic bronchitis
No history of allergies
Cardiomegaly or murmurs
Right heart failure
No cardiomegaly or murmurs
Nasopharyngeal carcinoma
Wegener midline granulomatosis
Blood dyscrasias

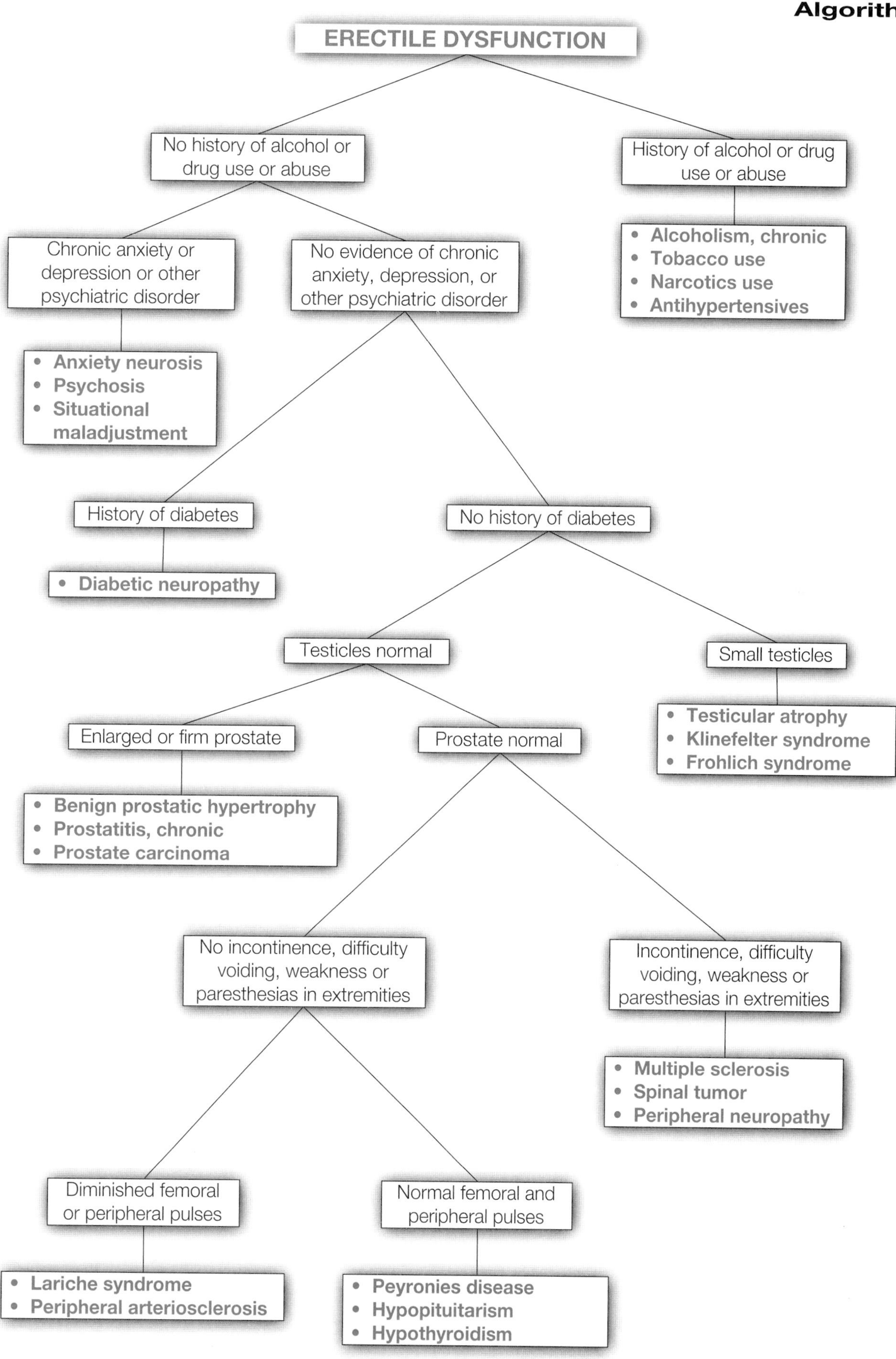
ERECTILE DYSFUNCTION
No history of alcohol or drug use or abuse
History of alcohol or drug use or abuse
• Alcoholism, chronic
• Tobacco use
• Narcotics use
• Antihypertensives
Chronic anxiety or depression or other psychiatric disorder
• Anxiety neurosis
• Psychosis
• Situational maladjustment
No evidence of chronic anxiety, depression, or other psychiatric disorder
History of diabetes
• Diabetic neuropathy
No history of diabetes
Testicles normal
Small testicles
• Testicular atrophy
• Klinefelter syndrome
• Frohlich syndrome
Enlarged or firm prostate
• Benign prostatic hypertrophy
• Prostatitis, chronic
• Prostate carcinoma
Prostate normal
No incontinence, difficulty voiding, weakness or paresthesias in extremities
Incontinence, difficulty voiding, weakness or paresthesias in extremities
• Multiple sclerosis
• Spinal tumor
• Peripheral neuropathy
Diminished femoral or peripheral pulses
• Lariche syndrome
• Peripheral arteriosclerosis
Normal femoral and peripheral pulses
• Peyronies disease
• Hypopituitarism
• Hypothyroidism

EXOPHTHALMOS

- Unilateral
  - No history of trauma
    - Fever
      - Orbital cellulitis
      - Cavernous sinus thrombosis (early)
    - No fever
      - Neoplasm
      - Meningocele
      - Encephalocele
  - History of trauma
    - Orbital bruit
      - Carotid-cavernous fistula
    - No orbital bruit
      - Orbital hemorrhage
      - Fracture
      - Emphysema
- Bilateral
  - No tremor, tachycardia, or enlarged thyroid
    - Associated with fever, chemosis, or ecchymosis
      - Cavernous sinus thrombosis
    - Not associated with fever, chemosis, or ecchymosis
      - Pituitary exophthalmos
      - Congenital exophthalmos
  - Tremor, tachycardia, or enlarged thyroid
    - Hyperthyroidism

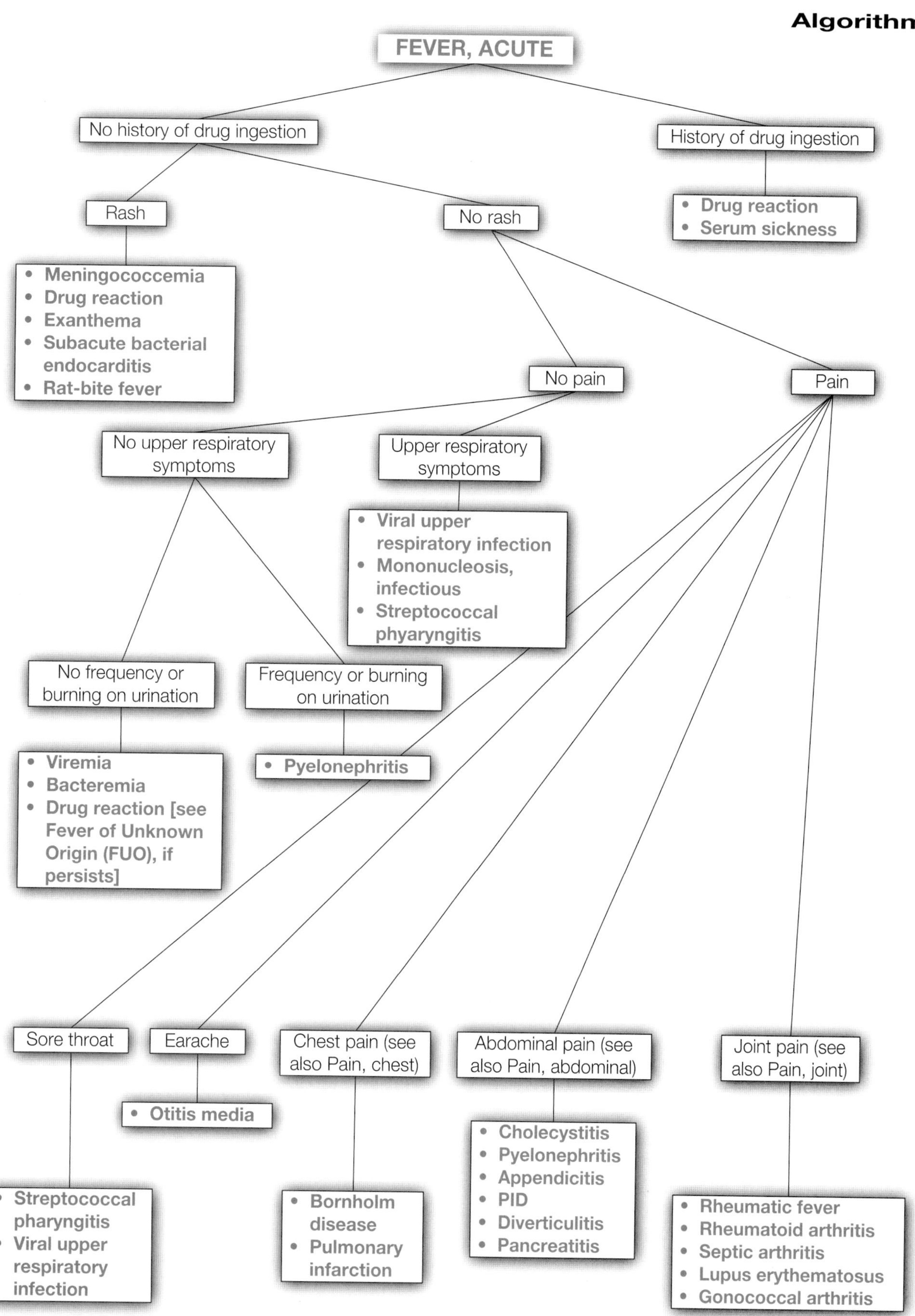
FEVER, ACUTE
No history of drug ingestion
History of drug ingestion
• Drug reaction
• Serum sickness
Rash
No rash
• Meningococcemia
• Drug reaction
• Exanthema
• Subacute bacterial endocarditis
• Rat-bite fever
No pain
Pain
No upper respiratory symptoms
Upper respiratory symptoms
• Viral upper respiratory infection
• Mononucleosis, infectious
• Streptococcal phyaryngitis
No frequency or burning on urination
Frequency or burning on urination
• Viremia
• Bacteremia
• Drug reaction [see Fever of Unknown Origin (FUO), if persists]
• Pyelonephritis
Sore throat
Earache
Chest pain (see also Pain, chest)
Abdominal pain (see also Pain, abdominal)
Joint pain (see also Pain, joint)
• Otitis media
• Streptococcal pharyngitis
• Viral upper respiratory infection
• Bornholm disease
• Pulmonary infarction
• Cholecystitis
• Pyelonephritis
• Appendicitis
• PID
• Diverticulitis
• Pancreatitis
• Rheumatic fever
• Rheumatoid arthritis
• Septic arthritis
• Lupus erythematosus
• Gonococcal arthritis

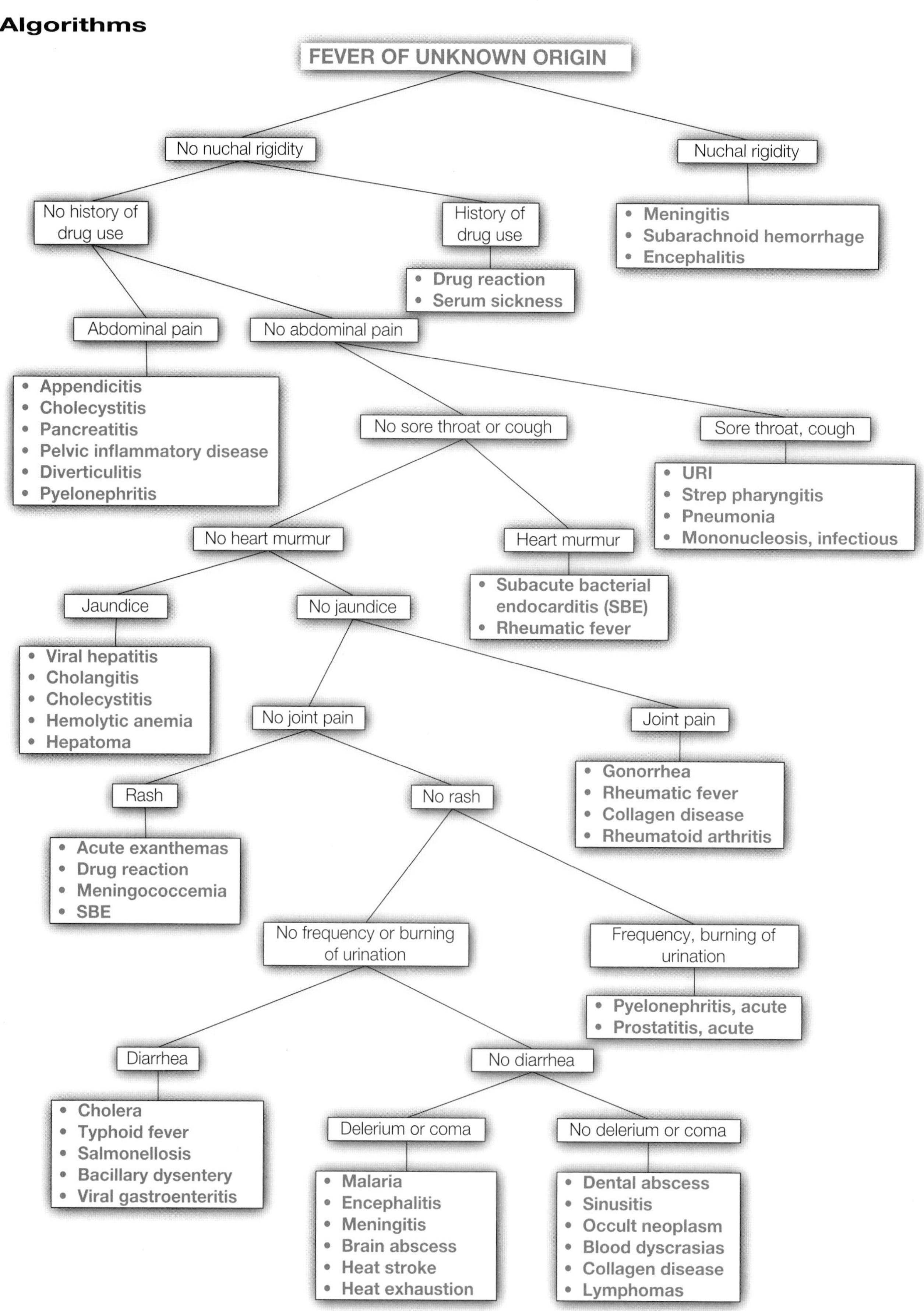
FEVER OF UNKNOWN ORIGIN
No nuchal rigidity
Nuchal rigidity
• Meningitis
• Subarachnoid hemorrhage
• Encephalitis
No history of drug use
History of drug use
• Drug reaction
• Serum sickness
Abdominal pain
No abdominal pain
• Appendicitis
• Cholecystitis
• Pancreatitis
• Pelvic inflammatory disease
• Diverticulitis
• Pyelonephritis
No sore throat or cough
Sore throat, cough
• URI
• Strep pharyngitis
• Pneumonia
• Mononucleosis, infectious
No heart murmur
Heart murmur
• Subacute bacterial endocarditis (SBE)
• Rheumatic fever
Jaundice
No jaundice
• Viral hepatitis
• Cholangitis
• Cholecystitis
• Hemolytic anemia
• Hepatoma
No joint pain
Joint pain
• Gonorrhea
• Rheumatic fever
• Collagen disease
• Rheumatoid arthritis
Rash
No rash
• Acute exanthemas
• Drug reaction
• Meningococcemia
• SBE
No frequency or burning of urination
Frequency, burning of urination
• Pyelonephritis, acute
• Prostatitis, acute
Diarrhea
No diarrhea
• Cholera
• Typhoid fever
• Salmonellosis
• Bacillary dysentery
• Viral gastroenteritis
Delerium or coma
No delerium or coma
• Malaria
• Encephalitis
• Meningitis
• Brain abscess
• Heat stroke
• Heat exhaustion
• Dental abscess
• Sinusitis
• Occult neoplasm
• Blood dyscrasias
• Collagen disease
• Lymphomas

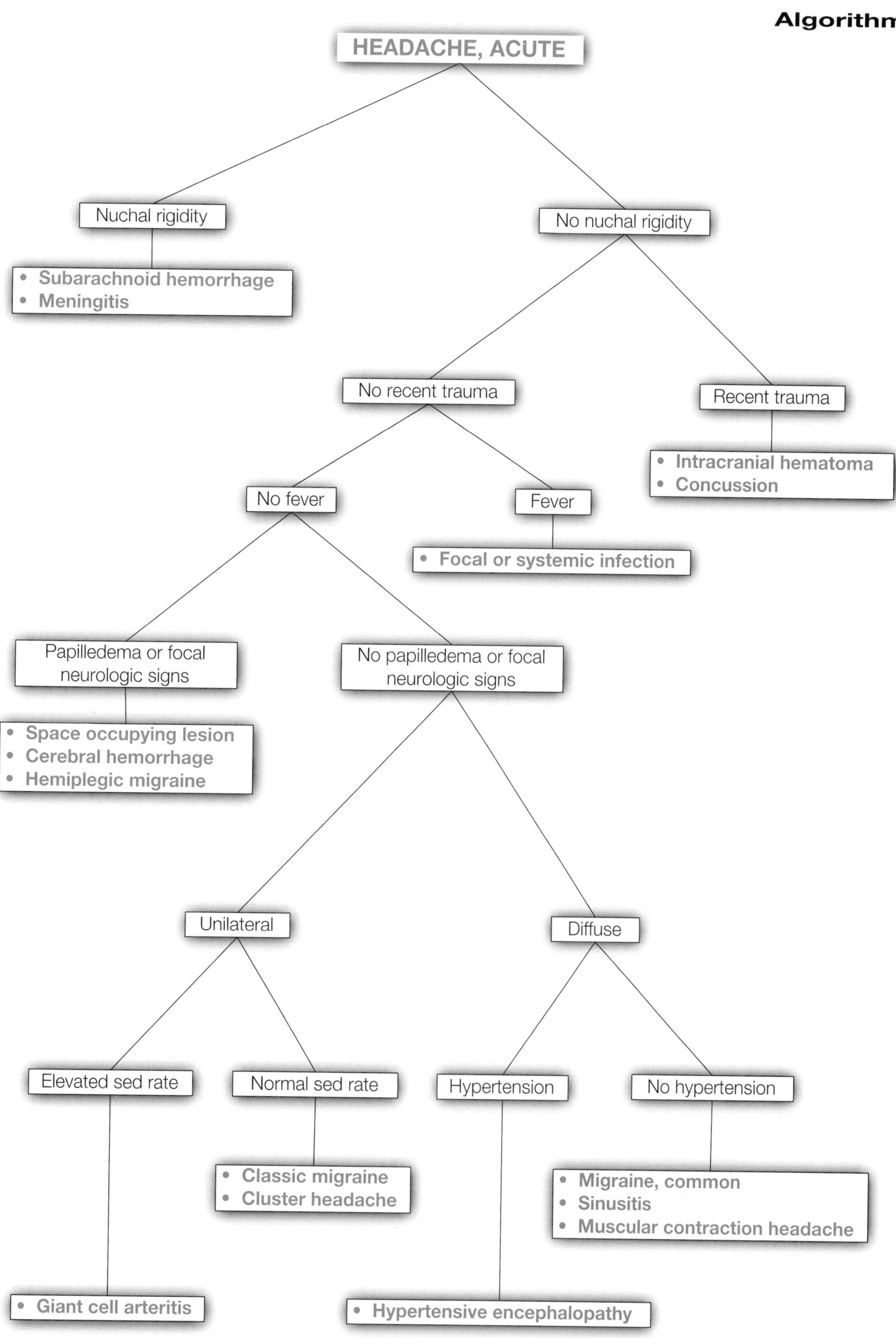
HEADACHE, ACUTE
Nuchal rigidity
• Subarachnoid hemorrhage
• Meningitis
No nuchal rigidity
No recent trauma
Recent trauma
• Intracranial hematoma
• Concussion
No fever
Fever
• Focal or systemic infection
Papilledema or focal neurologic signs
• Space occupying lesion
• Cerebral hemorrhage
• Hemiplegic migraine
No papilledema or focal neurologic signs
Unilateral
Diffuse
Elevated sed rate
Normal sed rate
Hypertension
No hypertension
• Classic migraine
• Cluster headache
• Migraine, common
• Sinusitis
• Muscular contraction headache
• Giant cell arteritis
• Hypertensive encephalopathy

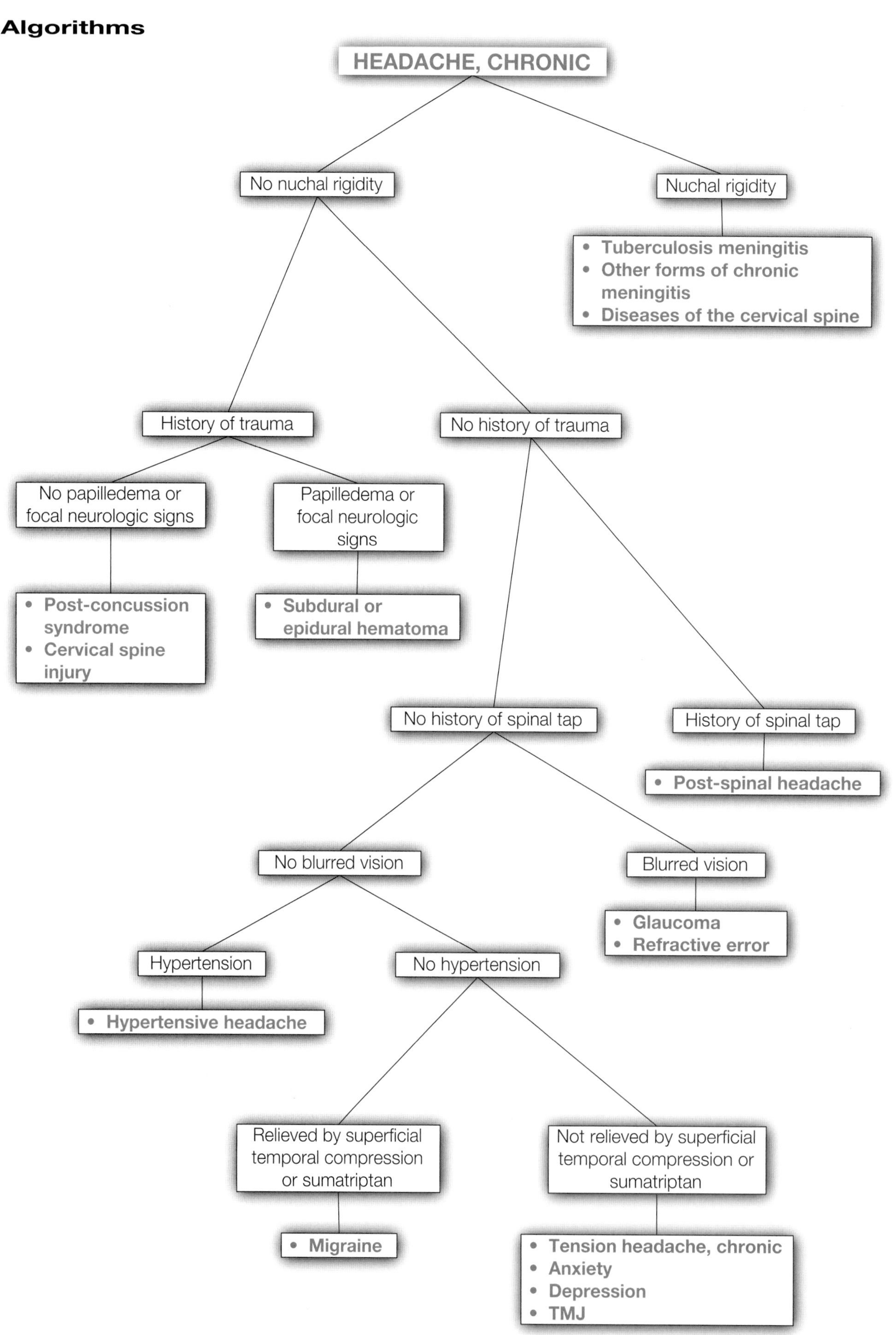
HEADACHE, CHRONIC
No nuchal rigidity
Nuchal rigidity
• Tuberculosis meningitis
• Other forms of chronic meningitis
• Diseases of the cervical spine
History of trauma
No history of trauma
No papilledema or focal neurologic signs
Papilledema or focal neurologic signs
• Post-concussion syndrome
• Cervical spine injury
• Subdural or epidural hematoma
No history of spinal tap
History of spinal tap
• Post-spinal headache
No blurred vision
Blurred vision
• Glaucoma
• Refractive error
Hypertension
No hypertension
• Hypertensive headache
Relieved by superficial temporal compression or sumatriptan
Not relieved by superficial temporal compression or sumatriptan
• Migraine
• Tension headache, chronic
• Anxiety
• Depression
• TMJ

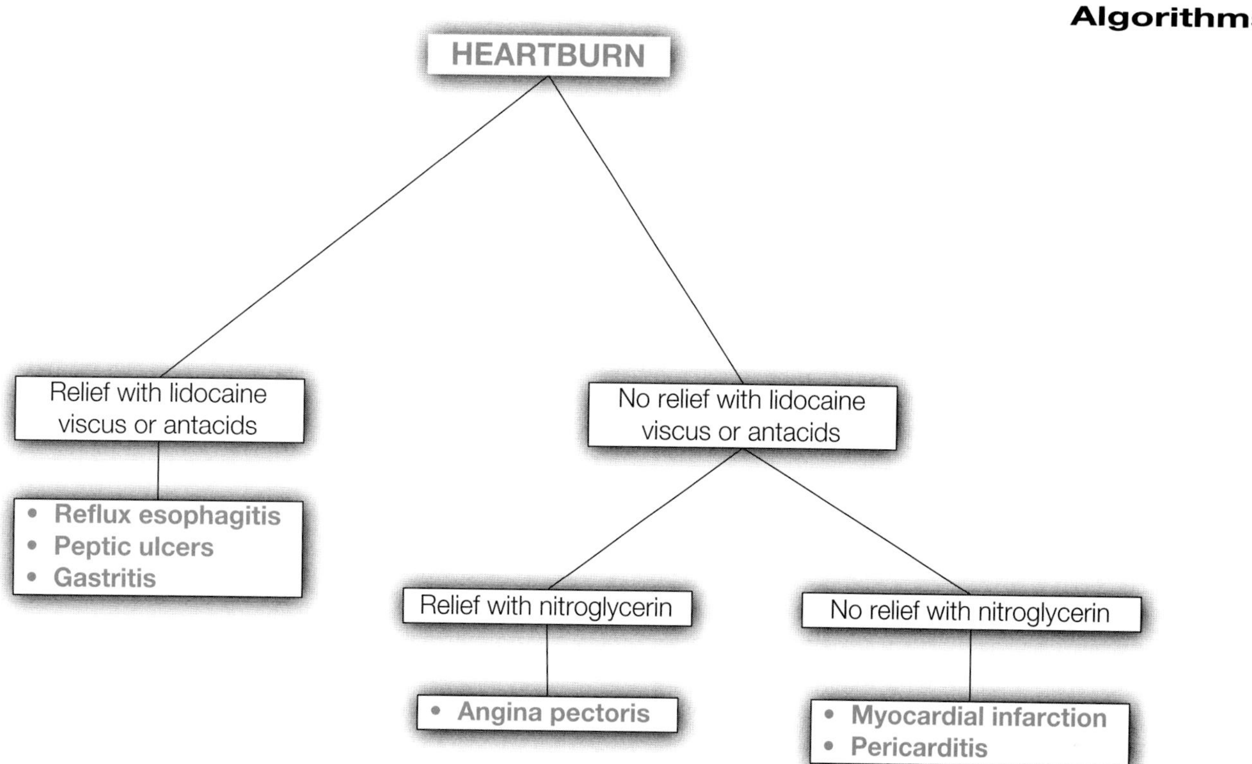
HEARTBURN
Relief with lidocaine viscus or antacids
• Reflux esophagitis
• Peptic ulcers
• Gastritis
No relief with lidocaine viscus or antacids
Relief with nitroglycerin
• Angina pectoris
No relief with nitroglycerin
• Myocardial infarction
• Pericarditis

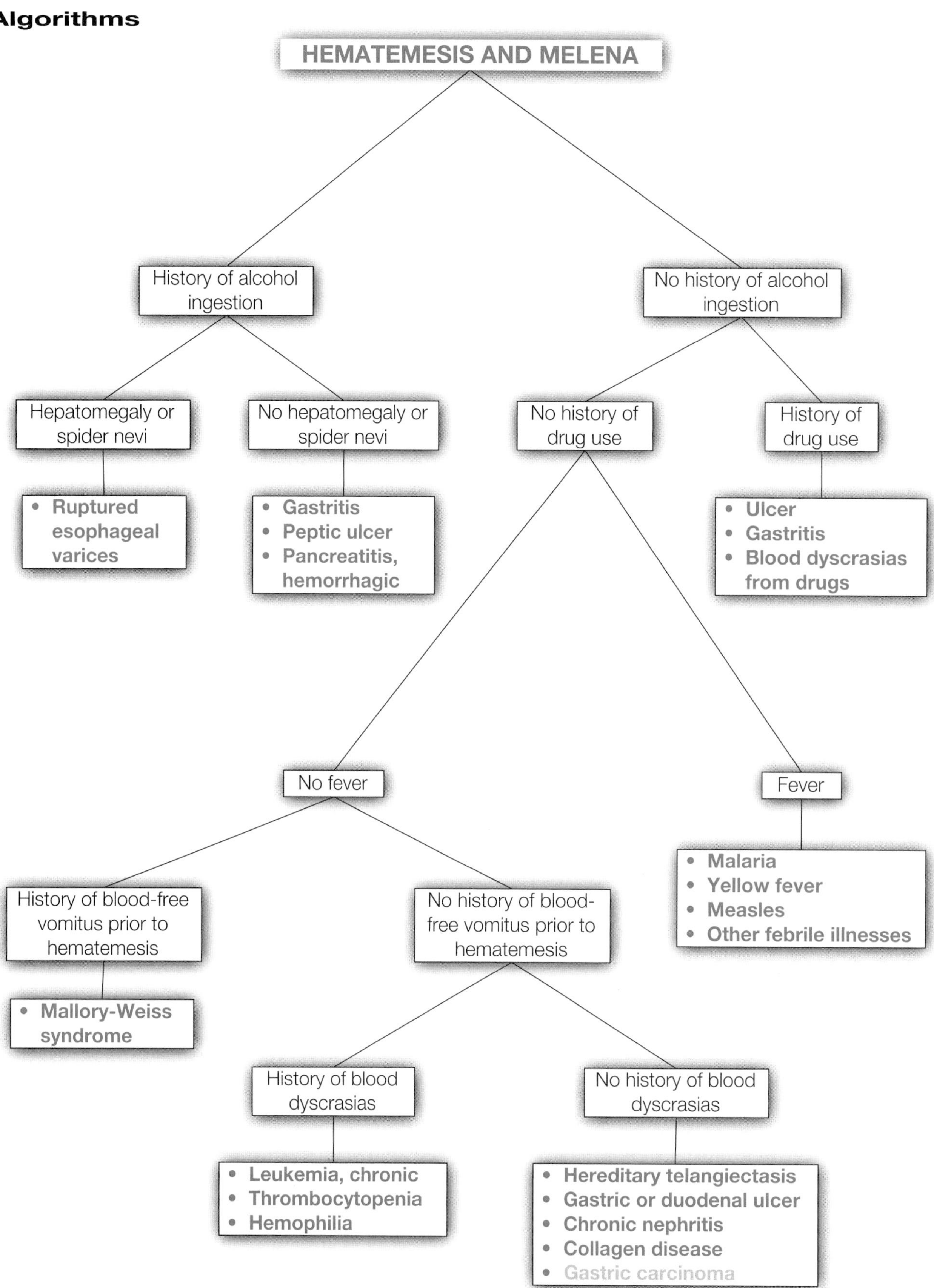
HEMATEMESIS AND MELENA
History of alcohol ingestion
No history of alcohol ingestion
Hepatomegaly or spider nevi
No hepatomegaly or spider nevi
No history of drug use
History of drug use
• Ruptured esophageal varices
• Gastritis
• Peptic ulcer
• Pancreatitis, hemorrhagic
• Ulcer
• Gastritis
• Blood dyscrasias from drugs
No fever
Fever
• Malaria
• Yellow fever
• Measles
• Other febrile illnesses
History of blood-free vomitus prior to hematemesis
No history of blood-free vomitus prior to hematemesis
• Mallory-Weiss syndrome
History of blood dyscrasias
No history of blood dyscrasias
• Leukemia, chronic
• Thrombocytopenia
• Hemophilia
• Hereditary telangiectasis
• Gastric or duodenal ulcer
• Chronic nephritis
• Collagen disease
• Gastric carcinoma

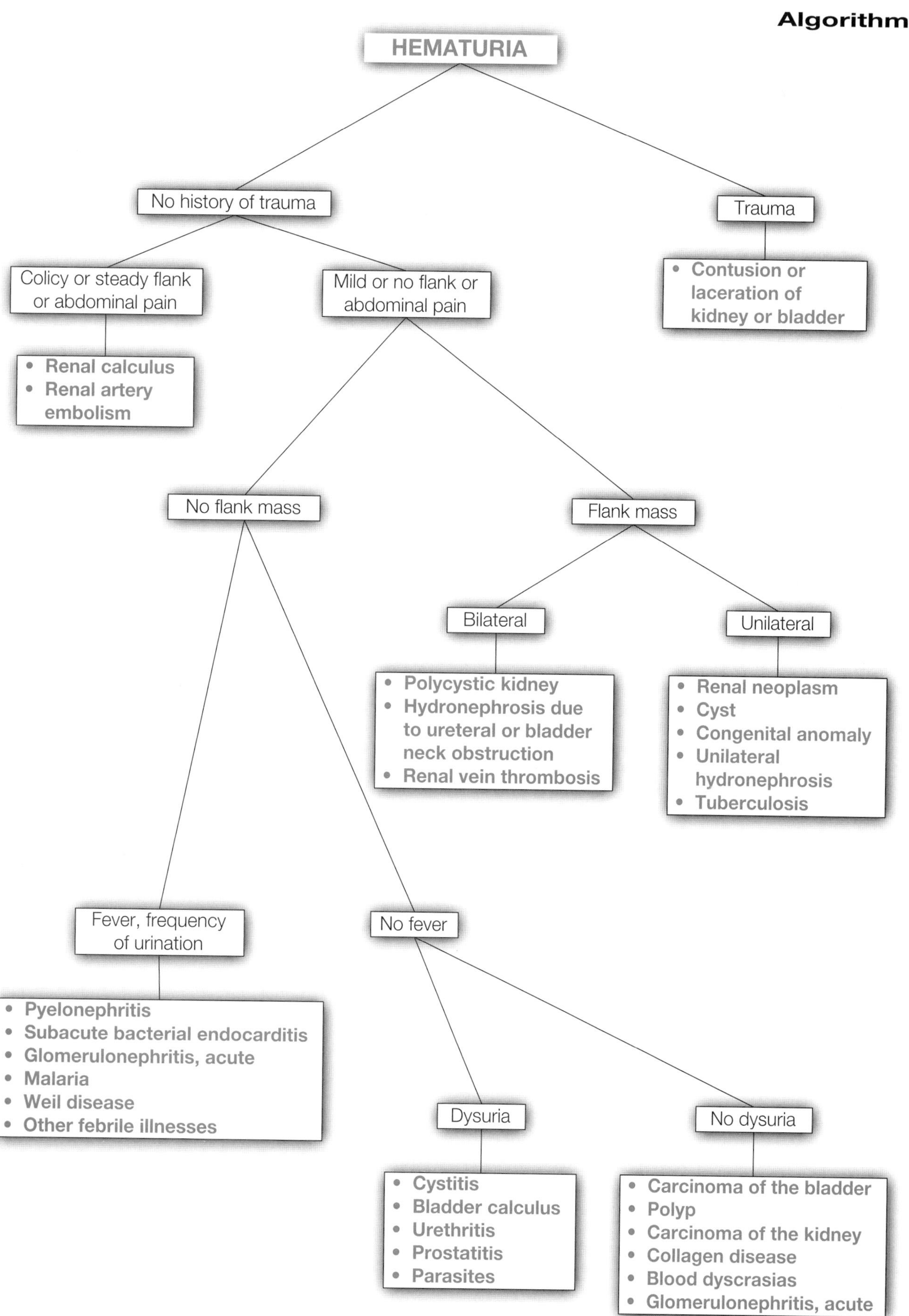
HEMATURIA
No history of trauma
Trauma
Contusion or laceration of kidney or bladder
Colicy or steady flank or abdominal pain
Renal calculus
Renal artery embolism
Mild or no flank or abdominal pain
No flank mass
Flank mass
Bilateral
Polycystic kidney
Hydronephrosis due to ureteral or bladder neck obstruction
Renal vein thrombosis
Unilateral
Renal neoplasm
Cyst
Congenital anomaly
Unilateral hydronephrosis
Tuberculosis
Fever, frequency of urination
Pyelonephritis
Subacute bacterial endocarditis
Glomerulonephritis, acute
Malaria
Weil disease
Other febrile illnesses
No fever
Dysuria
Cystitis
Bladder calculus
Urethritis
Prostatitis
Parasites
No dysuria
Carcinoma of the bladder
Polyp
Carcinoma of the kidney
Collagen disease
Blood dyscrasias
Glomerulonephritis, acute

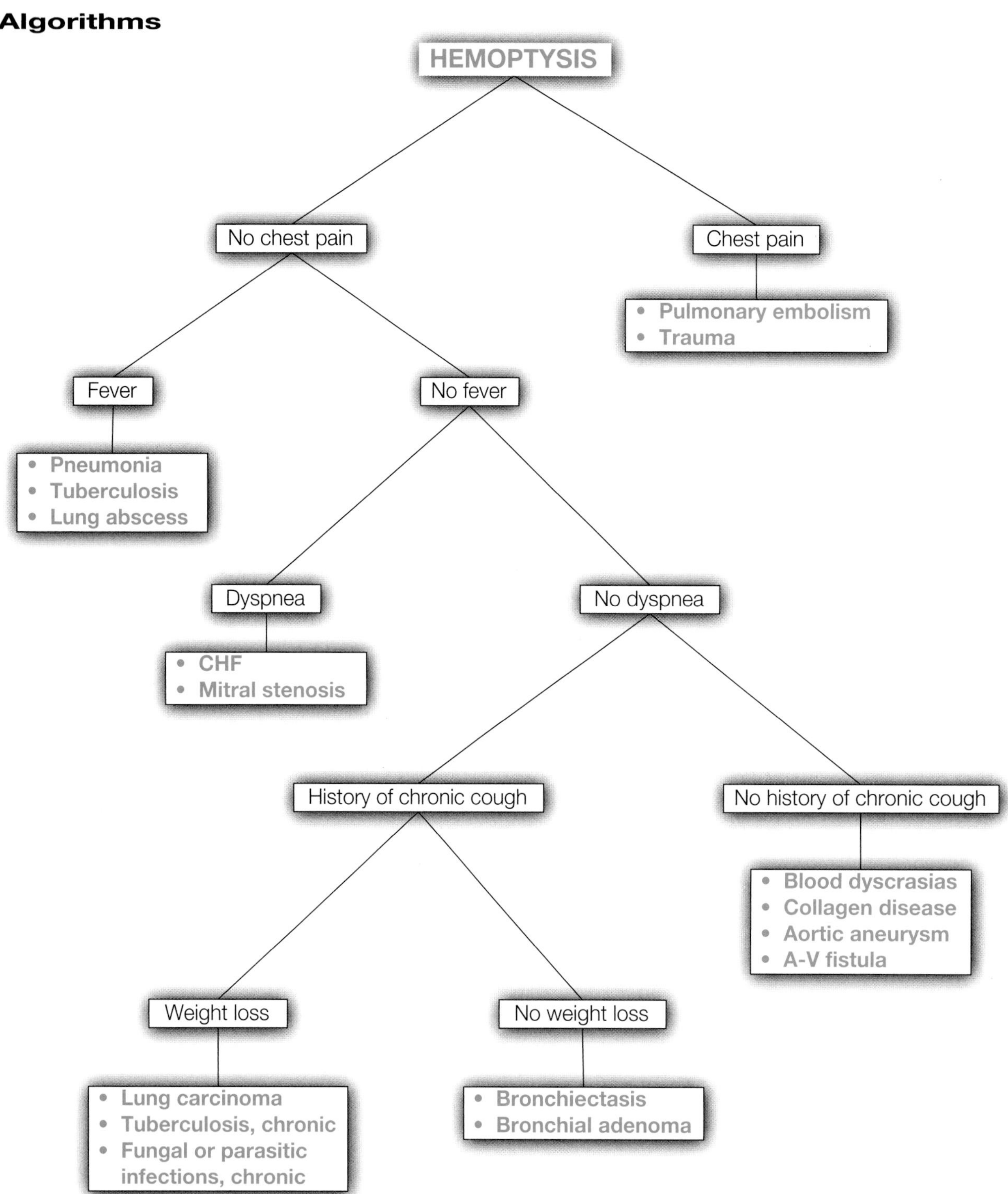
HEMOPTYSIS
No chest pain
Chest pain
• Pulmonary embolism
• Trauma
Fever
No fever
• Pneumonia
• Tuberculosis
• Lung abscess
Dyspnea
No dyspnea
• CHF
• Mitral stenosis
History of chronic cough
No history of chronic cough
• Blood dyscrasias
• Collagen disease
• Aortic aneurysm
• A-V fistula
Weight loss
No weight loss
• Lung carcinoma
• Tuberculosis, chronic
• Fungal or parasitic infections, chronic
• Bronchiectasis
• Bronchial adenoma

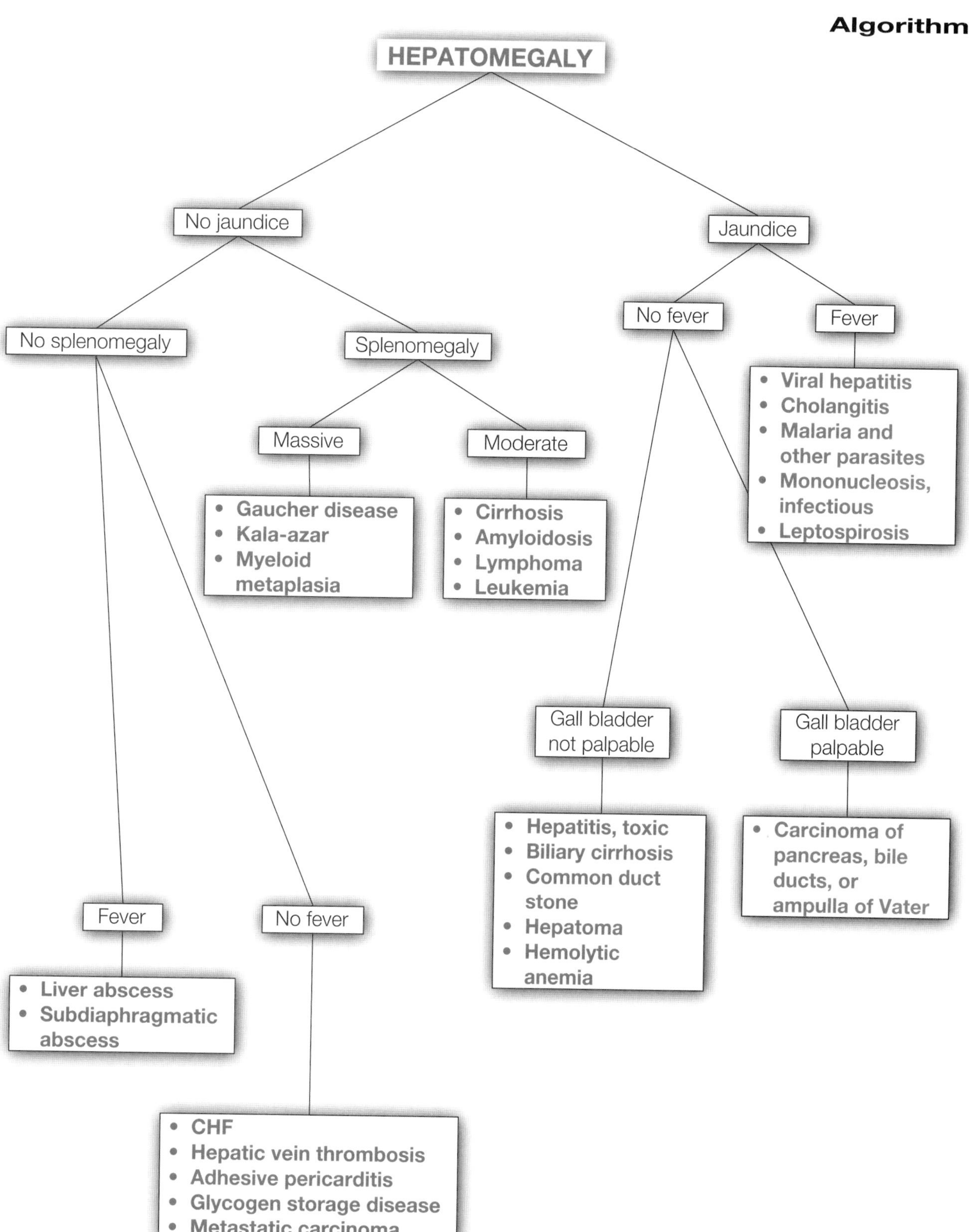
HEPATOMEGALY
No jaundice
Jaundice
No splenomegaly
Splenomegaly
No fever
Fever
Massive
Moderate
• Viral hepatitis
• Cholangitis
• Malaria and other parasites
• Mononucleosis, infectious
• Leptospirosis
• Gaucher disease
• Kala-azar
• Myeloid metaplasia
• Cirrhosis
• Amyloidosis
• Lymphoma
• Leukemia
Gall bladder not palpable
Gall bladder palpable
• Hepatitis, toxic
• Biliary cirrhosis
• Common duct stone
• Hepatoma
• Hemolytic anemia
• Carcinoma of pancreas, bile ducts, or ampulla of Vater
Fever
No fever
• Liver abscess
• Subdiaphragmatic abscess
• CHF
• Hepatic vein thrombosis
• Adhesive pericarditis
• Glycogen storage disease
• Metastatic carcinoma

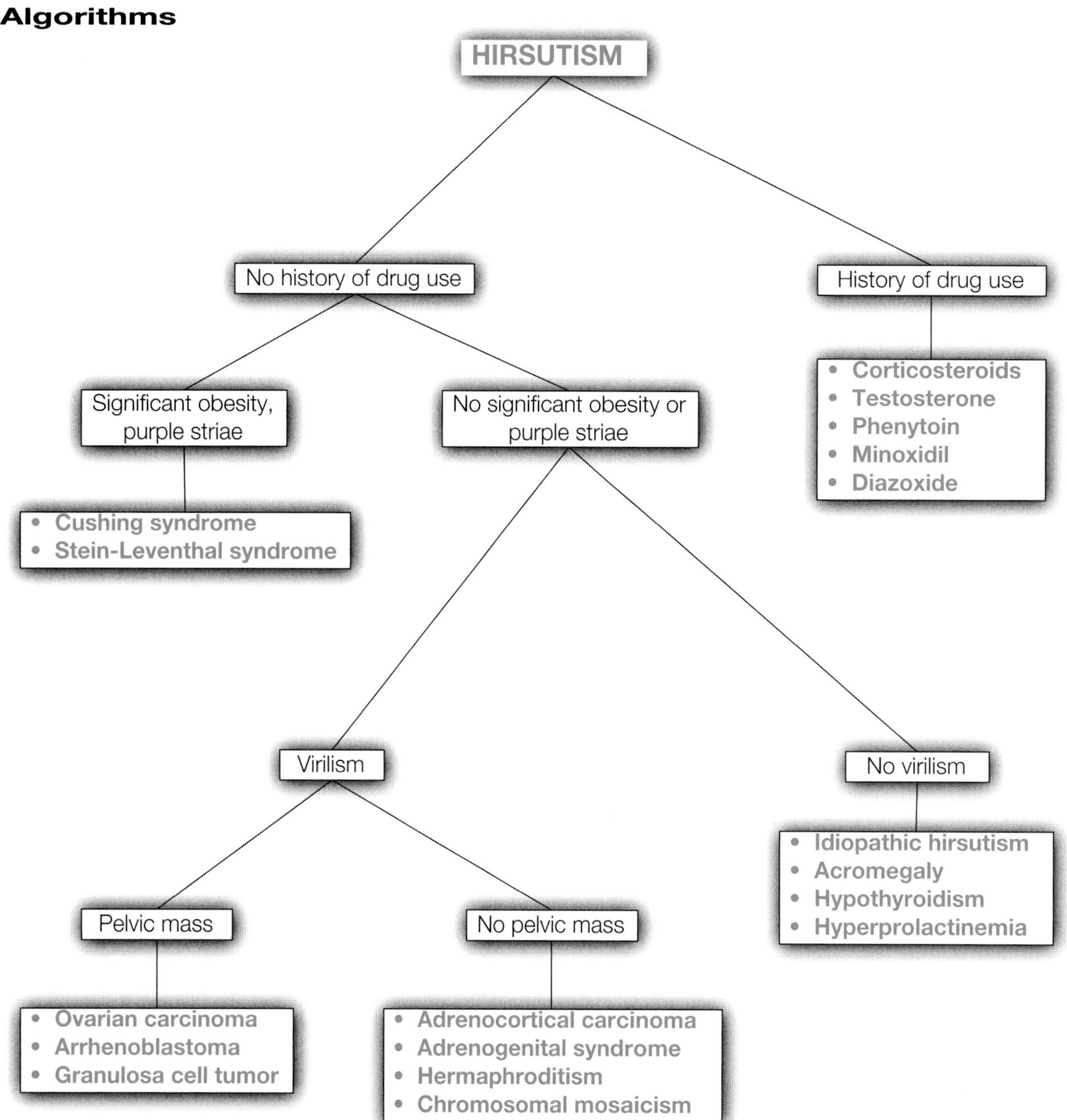
HIRSUTISM
No history of drug use
History of drug use
• Corticosteroids
• Testosterone
• Phenytoin
• Minoxidil
• Diazoxide
Significant obesity, purple striae
No significant obesity or purple striae
• Cushing syndrome
• Stein-Leventhal syndrome
Virilism
No virilism
• Idiopathic hirsutism
• Acromegaly
• Hypothyroidism
• Hyperprolactinemia
Pelvic mass
No pelvic mass
• Ovarian carcinoma
• Arrhenoblastoma
• Granulosa cell tumor
• Adrenocortical carcinoma
• Adrenogenital syndrome
• Hermaphroditism
• Chromosomal mosaicism

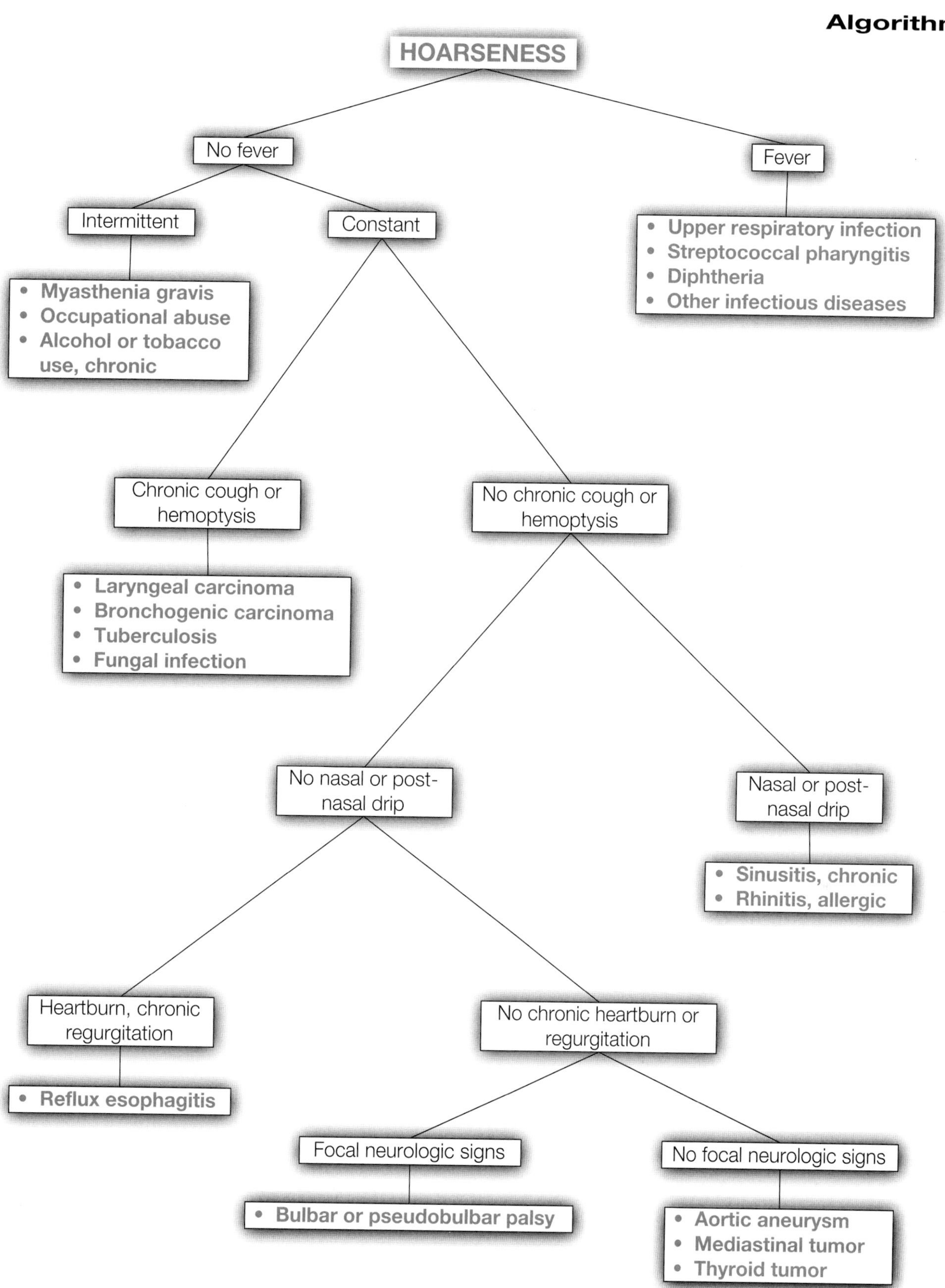
HOARSENESS
No fever
Fever
Intermittent
Constant
• Upper respiratory infection
• Streptococcal pharyngitis
• Diphtheria
• Other infectious diseases
• Myasthenia gravis
• Occupational abuse
• Alcohol or tobacco use, chronic
Chronic cough or hemoptysis
No chronic cough or hemoptysis
• Laryngeal carcinoma
• Bronchogenic carcinoma
• Tuberculosis
• Fungal infection
No nasal or post-nasal drip
Nasal or post-nasal drip
• Sinusitis, chronic
• Rhinitis, allergic
Heartburn, chronic regurgitation
No chronic heartburn or regurgitation
• Reflux esophagitis
Focal neurologic signs
No focal neurologic signs
• Bulbar or pseudobulbar palsy
• Aortic aneurysm
• Mediastinal tumor
• Thyroid tumor

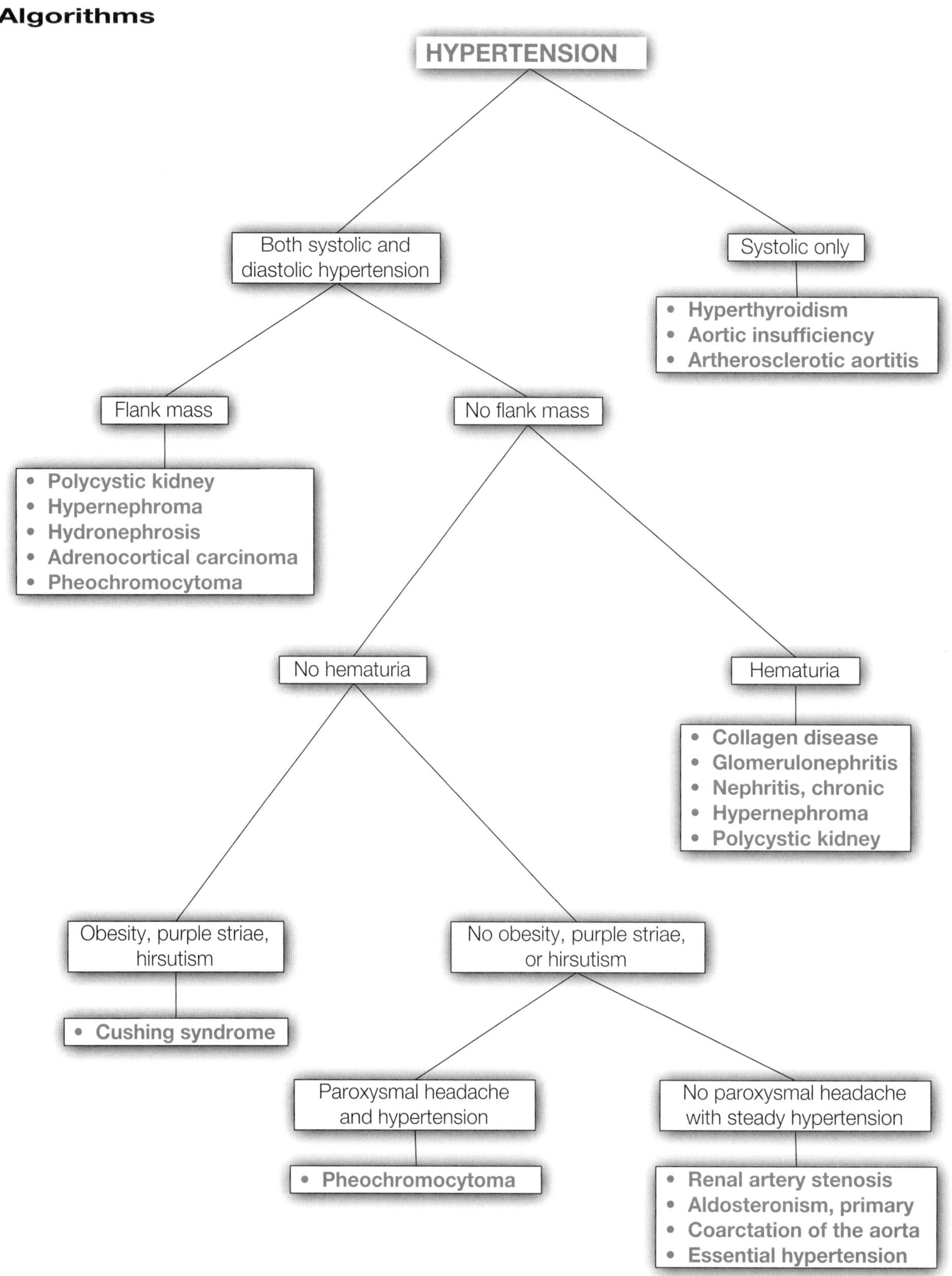
HYPERTENSION
Both systolic and diastolic hypertension
Systolic only
• Hyperthyroidism
• Aortic insufficiency
• Artherosclerotic aortitis
Flank mass
No flank mass
• Polycystic kidney
• Hypernephroma
• Hydronephrosis
• Adrenocortical carcinoma
• Pheochromocytoma
No hematuria
Hematuria
• Collagen disease
• Glomerulonephritis
• Nephritis, chronic
• Hypernephroma
• Polycystic kidney
Obesity, purple striae, hirsutism
No obesity, purple striae, or hirsutism
• Cushing syndrome
Paroxysmal headache and hypertension
No paroxysmal headache with steady hypertension
• Pheochromocytoma
• Renal artery stenosis
• Aldosteronism, primary
• Coarctation of the aorta
• Essential hypertension

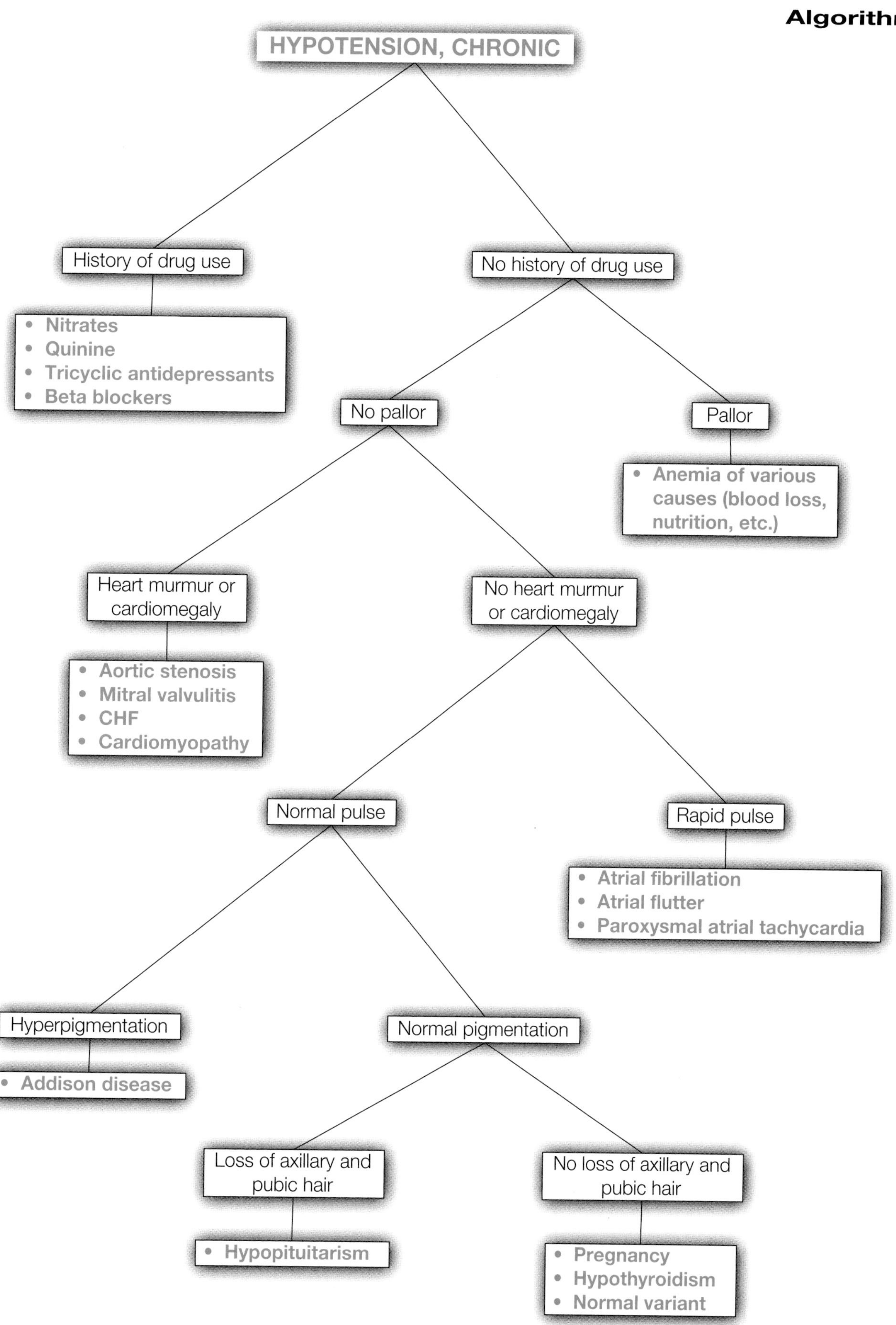
HYPOTENSION, CHRONIC
History of drug use
• Nitrates
• Quinine
• Tricyclic antidepressants
• Beta blockers
No history of drug use
No pallor
Pallor
• Anemia of various causes (blood loss, nutrition, etc.)
Heart murmur or cardiomegaly
• Aortic stenosis
• Mitral valvulitis
• CHF
• Cardiomyopathy
No heart murmur or cardiomegaly
Normal pulse
Rapid pulse
• Atrial fibrillation
• Atrial flutter
• Paroxysmal atrial tachycardia
Hyperpigmentation
• Addison disease
Normal pigmentation
Loss of axillary and pubic hair
• Hypopituitarism
No loss of axillary and pubic hair
• Pregnancy
• Hypothyroidism
• Normal variant

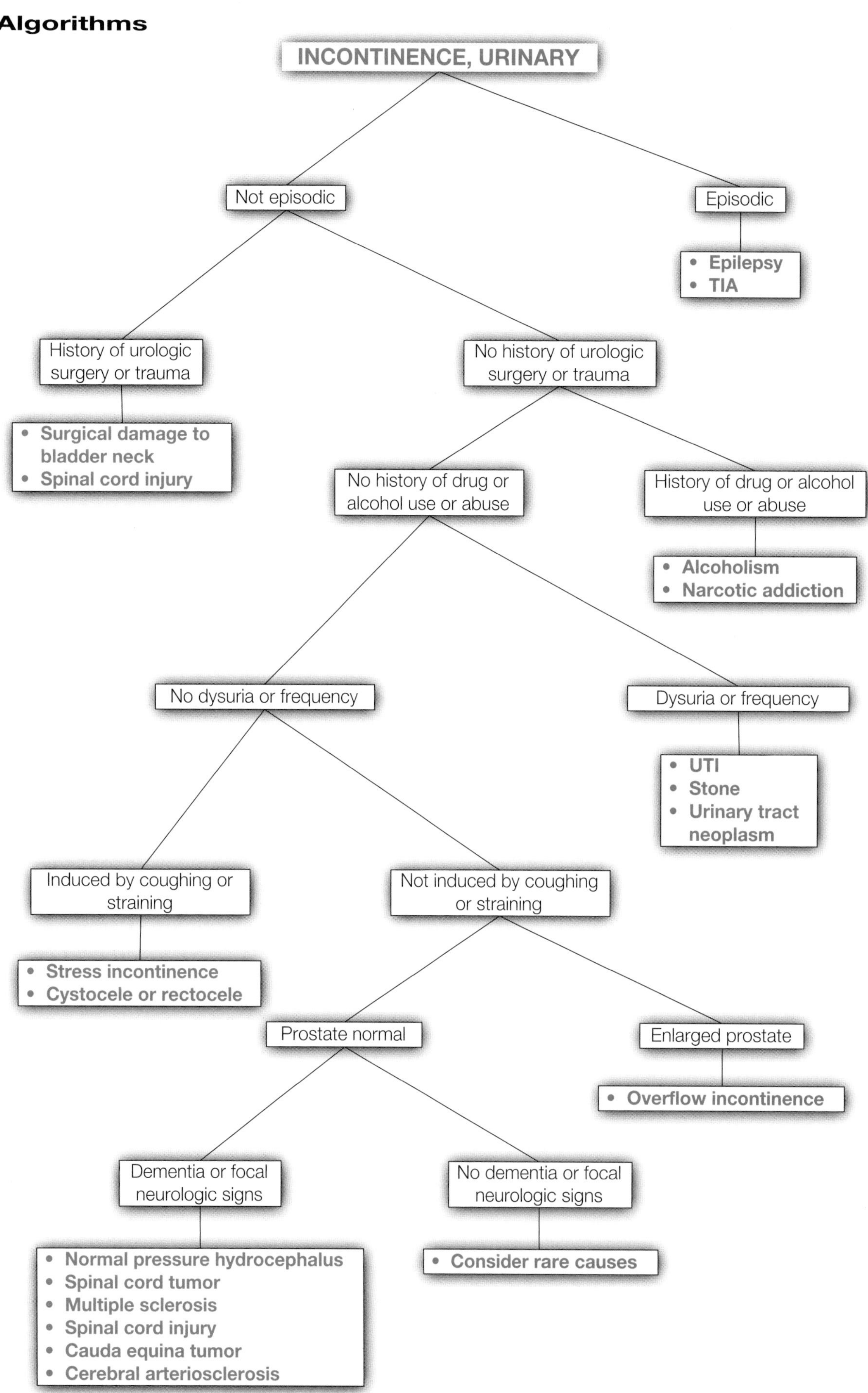
INCONTINENCE, URINARY
Not episodic
Episodic
• Epilepsy
• TIA
History of urologic surgery or trauma
• Surgical damage to bladder neck
• Spinal cord injury
No history of urologic surgery or trauma
No history of drug or alcohol use or abuse
History of drug or alcohol use or abuse
• Alcoholism
• Narcotic addiction
No dysuria or frequency
Dysuria or frequency
• UTI
• Stone
• Urinary tract neoplasm
Induced by coughing or straining
• Stress incontinence
• Cystocele or rectocele
Not induced by coughing or straining
Prostate normal
Enlarged prostate
• Overflow incontinence
Dementia or focal neurologic signs
• Normal pressure hydrocephalus
• Spinal cord tumor
• Multiple sclerosis
• Spinal cord injury
• Cauda equina tumor
• Cerebral arteriosclerosis
No dementia or focal neurologic signs
• Consider rare causes

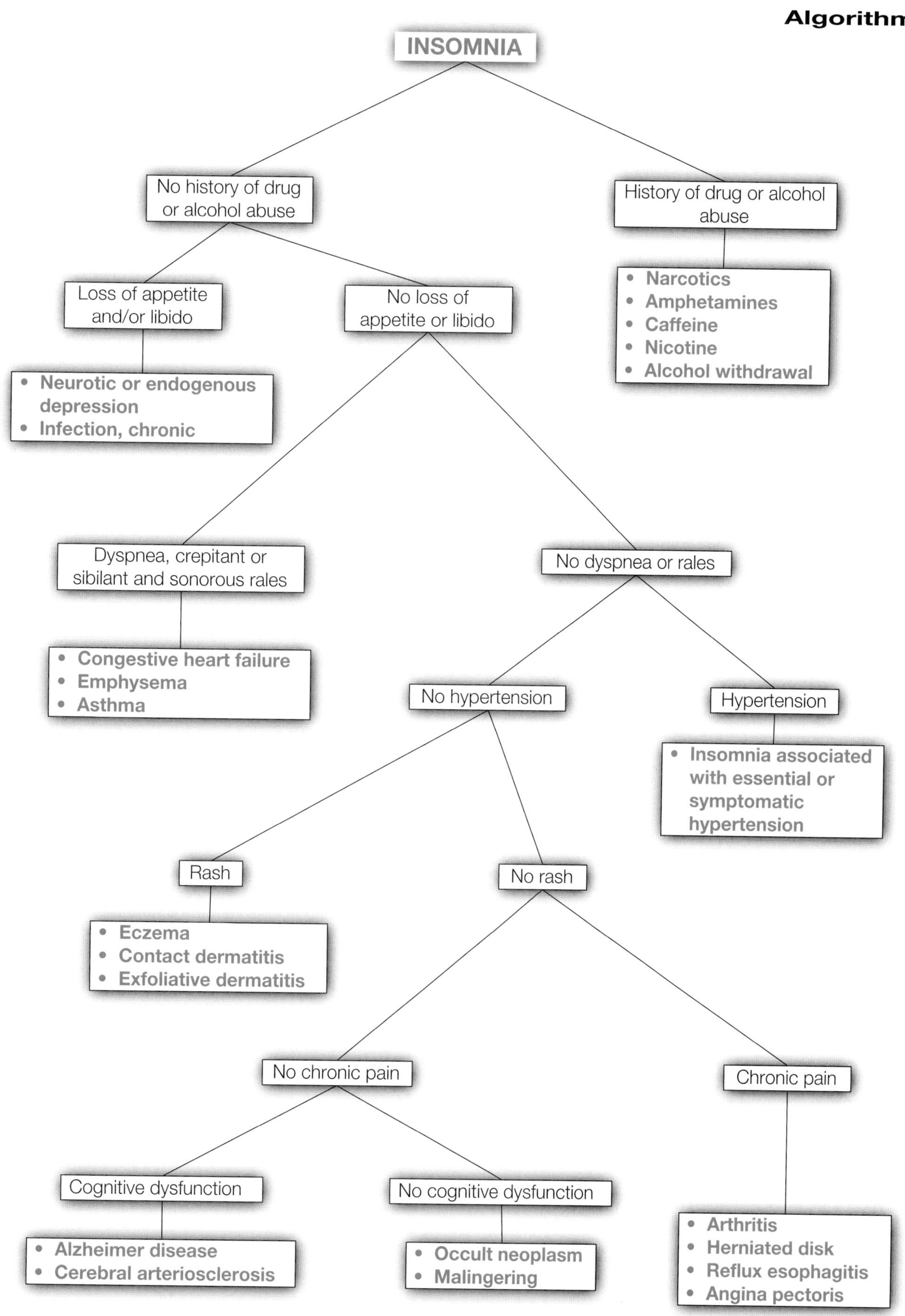
INSOMNIA
No history of drug or alcohol abuse
History of drug or alcohol abuse
• Narcotics
• Amphetamines
• Caffeine
• Nicotine
• Alcohol withdrawal
Loss of appetite and/or libido
• Neurotic or endogenous depression
• Infection, chronic
No loss of appetite or libido
Dyspnea, crepitant or sibilant and sonorous rales
• Congestive heart failure
• Emphysema
• Asthma
No dyspnea or rales
No hypertension
Hypertension
• Insomnia associated with essential or symptomatic hypertension
Rash
• Eczema
• Contact dermatitis
• Exfoliative dermatitis
No rash
No chronic pain
Chronic pain
• Arthritis
• Herniated disk
• Reflux esophagitis
• Angina pectoris
Cognitive dysfunction
• Alzheimer disease
• Cerebral arteriosclerosis
No cognitive dysfunction
• Occult neoplasm
• Malingering

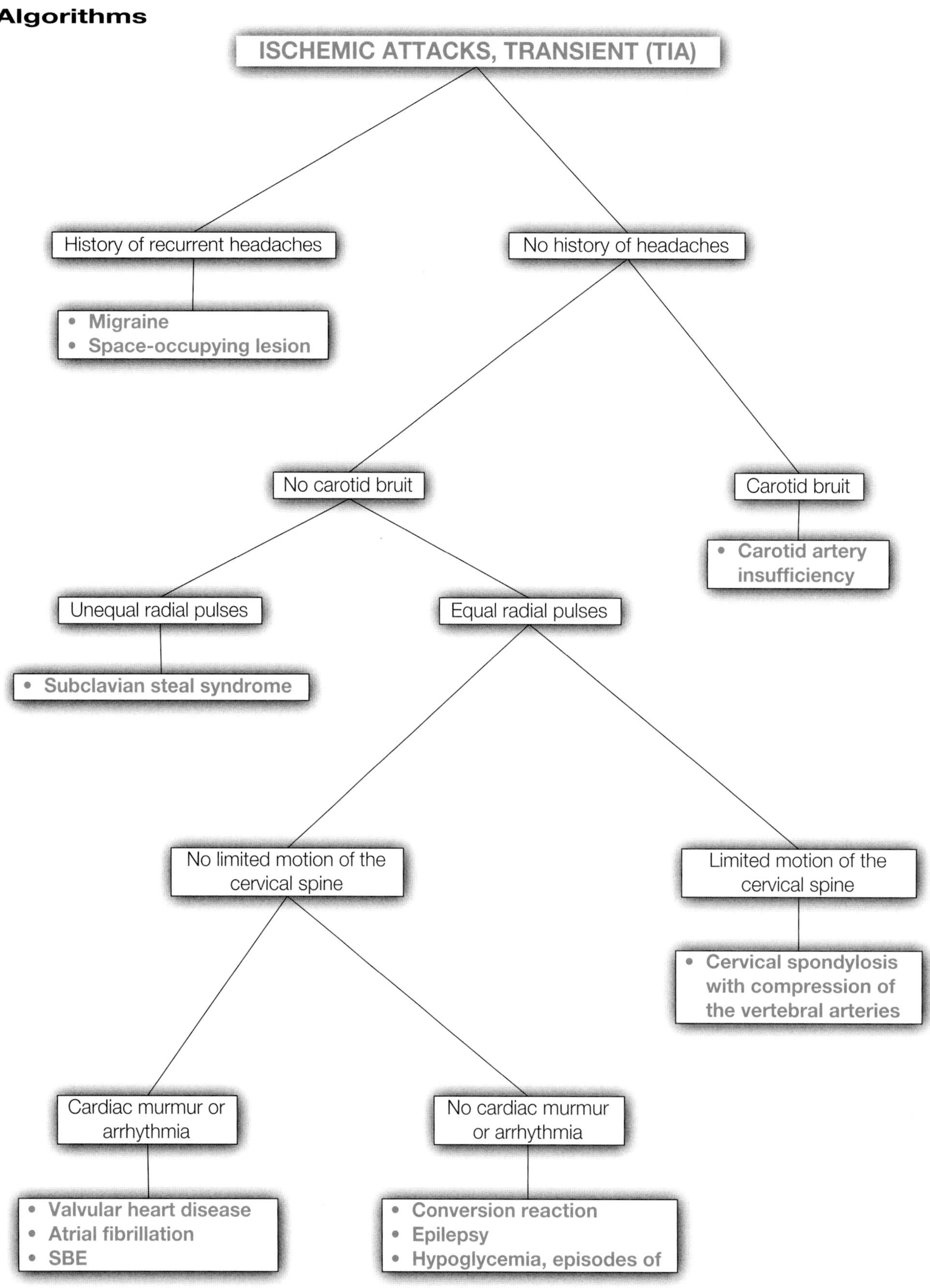
ISCHEMIC ATTACKS, TRANSIENT (TIA)
History of recurrent headaches
• Migraine
• Space-occupying lesion
No history of headaches
No carotid bruit
Carotid bruit
• Carotid artery insufficiency
Unequal radial pulses
• Subclavian steal syndrome
Equal radial pulses
No limited motion of the cervical spine
Limited motion of the cervical spine
• Cervical spondylosis with compression of the vertebral arteries
Cardiac murmur or arrhythmia
• Valvular heart disease
• Atrial fibrillation
• SBE
No cardiac murmur or arrhythmia
• Conversion reaction
• Epilepsy
• Hypoglycemia, episodes of

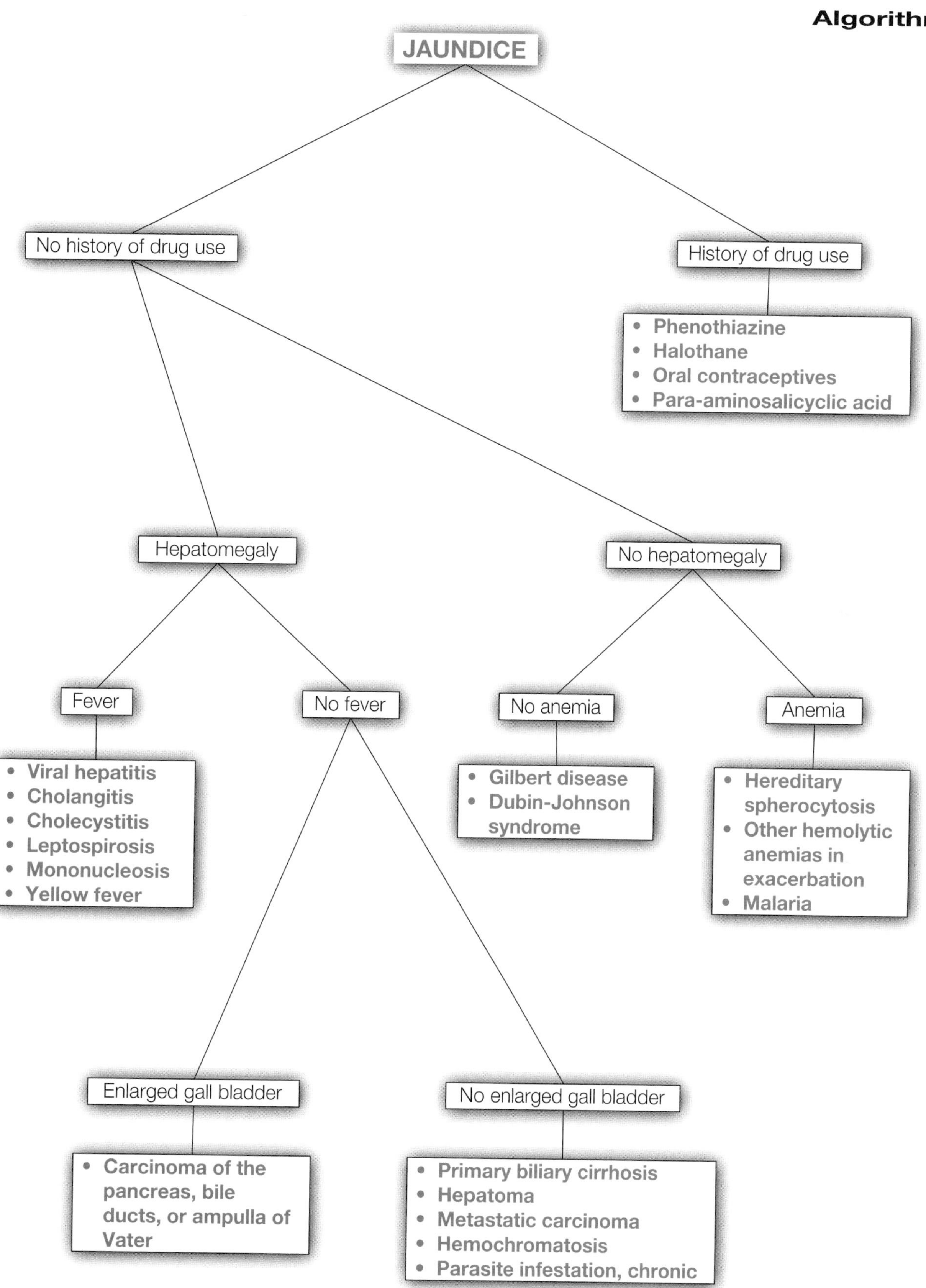
JAUNDICE
No history of drug use
History of drug use
• Phenothiazine
• Halothane
• Oral contraceptives
• Para-aminosalicyclic acid
Hepatomegaly
No hepatomegaly
Fever
No fever
No anemia
Anemia
• Viral hepatitis
• Cholangitis
• Cholecystitis
• Leptospirosis
• Mononucleosis
• Yellow fever
• Gilbert disease
• Dubin-Johnson syndrome
• Hereditary spherocytosis
• Other hemolytic anemias in exacerbation
• Malaria
Enlarged gall bladder
No enlarged gall bladder
• Carcinoma of the pancreas, bile ducts, or ampulla of Vater
• Primary biliary cirrhosis
• Hepatoma
• Metastatic carcinoma
• Hemochromatosis
• Parasite infestation, chronic

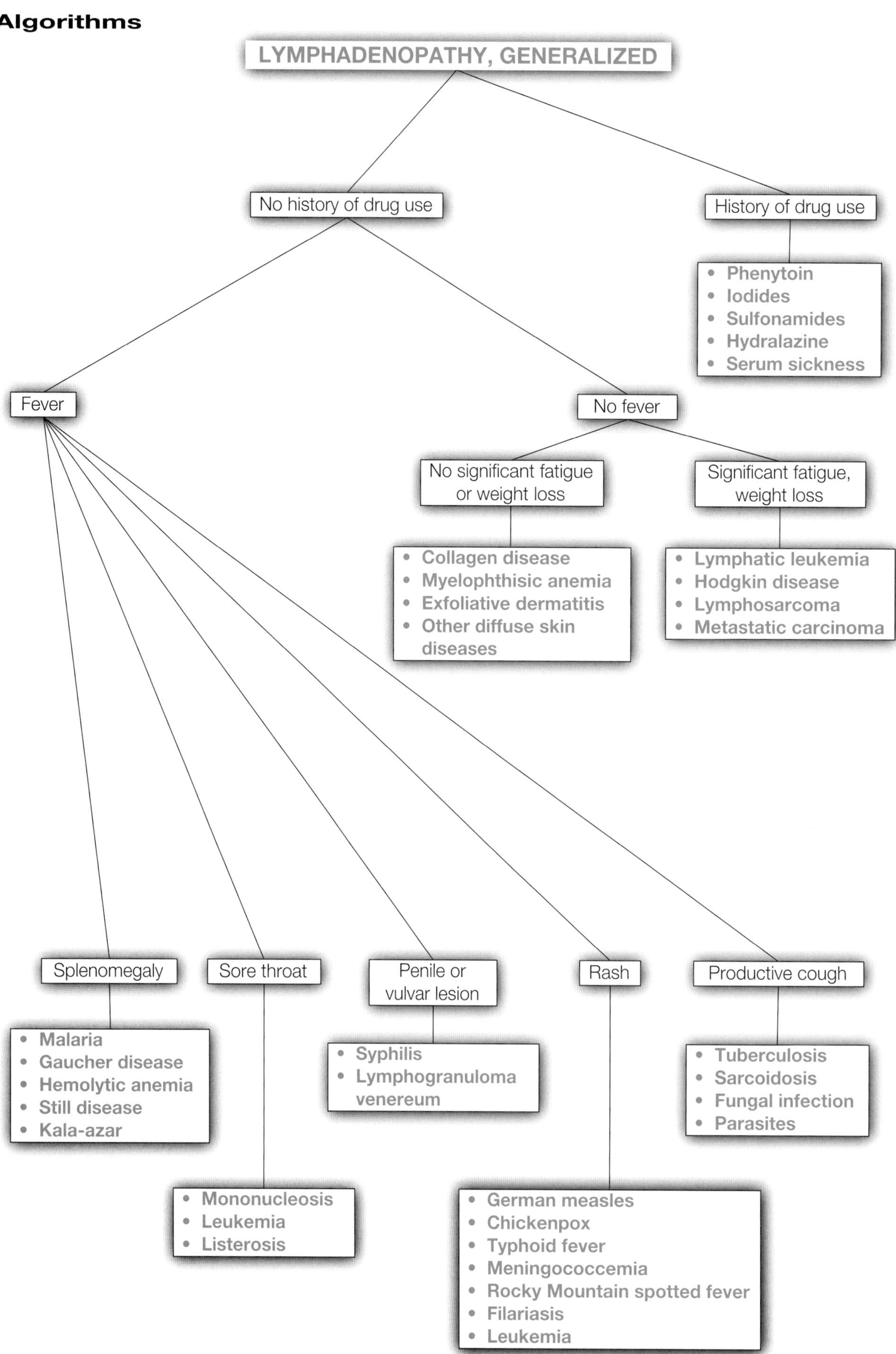
LYMPHADENOPATHY, GENERALIZED
No history of drug use
History of drug use
• Phenytoin
• Iodides
• Sulfonamides
• Hydralazine
• Serum sickness
Fever
No fever
No significant fatigue or weight loss
Significant fatigue, weight loss
• Collagen disease
• Myelophthisic anemia
• Exfoliative dermatitis
• Other diffuse skin diseases
• Lymphatic leukemia
• Hodgkin disease
• Lymphosarcoma
• Metastatic carcinoma
Splenomegaly
Sore throat
Penile or vulvar lesion
Rash
Productive cough
• Malaria
• Gaucher disease
• Hemolytic anemia
• Still disease
• Kala-azar
• Syphilis
• Lymphogranuloma venereum
• Tuberculosis
• Sarcoidosis
• Fungal infection
• Parasites
• Mononucleosis
• Leukemia
• Listerosis
• German measles
• Chickenpox
• Typhoid fever
• Meningococcemia
• Rocky Mountain spotted fever
• Filariasis
• Leukemia

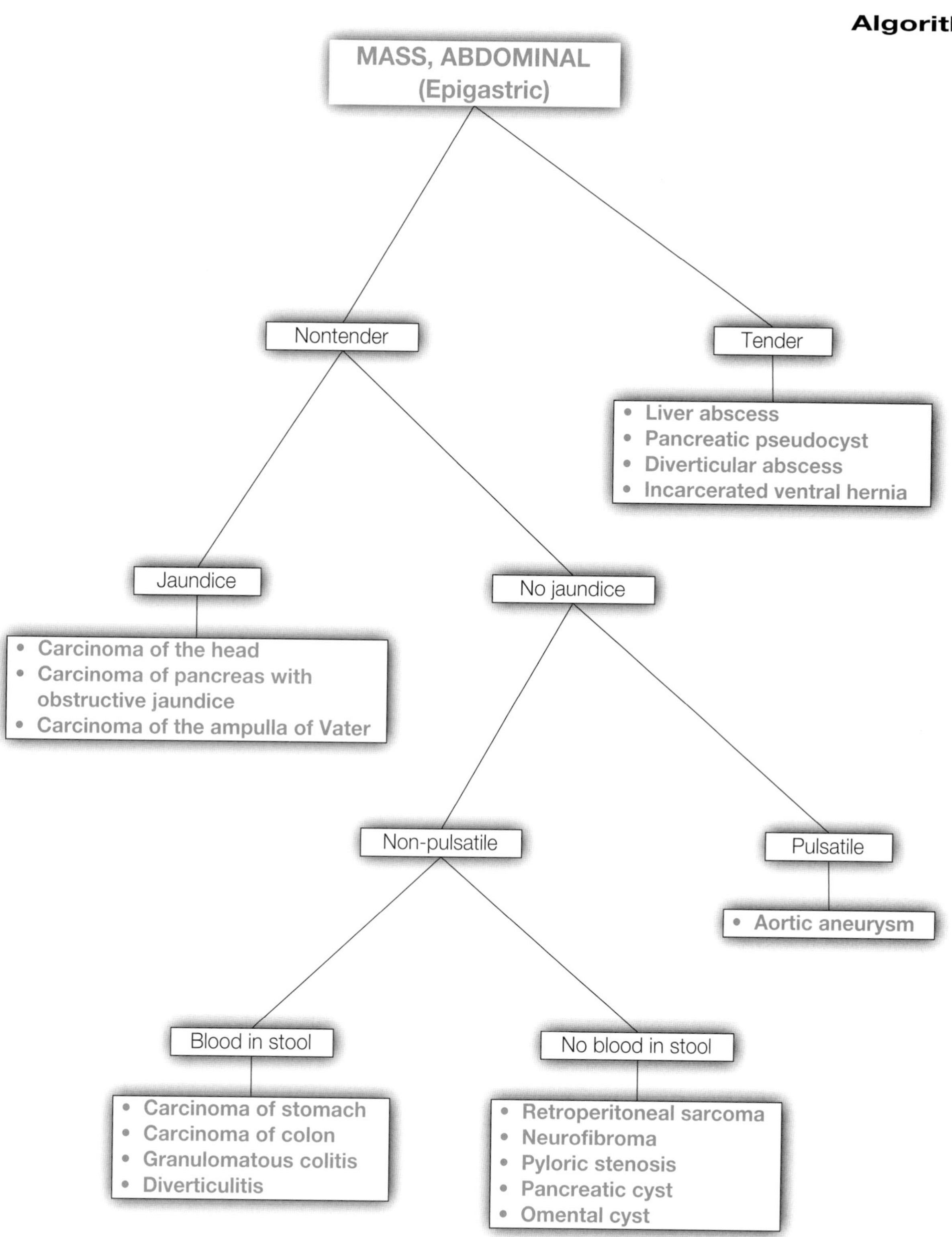
MASS, ABDOMINAL
(Epigastric)
Nontender
Tender
• Liver abscess
• Pancreatic pseudocyst
• Diverticular abscess
• Incarcerated ventral hernia
Jaundice
No jaundice
• Carcinoma of the head
• Carcinoma of pancreas with obstructive jaundice
• Carcinoma of the ampulla of Vater
Non-pulsatile
Pulsatile
• Aortic aneurysm
Blood in stool
No blood in stool
• Carcinoma of stomach
• Carcinoma of colon
• Granulomatous colitis
• Diverticulitis
• Retroperitoneal sarcoma
• Neurofibroma
• Pyloric stenosis
• Pancreatic cyst
• Omental cyst

MASS, ABDOMINAL (Hypogastric)

- Mass disappears on catheterization of bladder
  - Distended bladder
  - Bladder neck obstruction
- Mass remains after catheterization of bladder
  - Pregnancy test positive
    - Normal pregnancy
    - Ectopic pregnancy
  - Pregnancy test negative
    - Mass not reducible
      - Pulsatile
        - Aortic aneurysm
      - Not pulsatile
        - Tender
          - Pyosalpinx
          - Pelvic appendix
          - Diverticulitis
          - Incarcerated hernia
          - Cellulitis
          - Pott disease
        - Non-tender
          - Fibroid uterus
          - Colon carcinoma
          - Ovarian cyst or tumor
          - Endometrial carcinoma
    - Mass is reducible
      - Ventral hernia

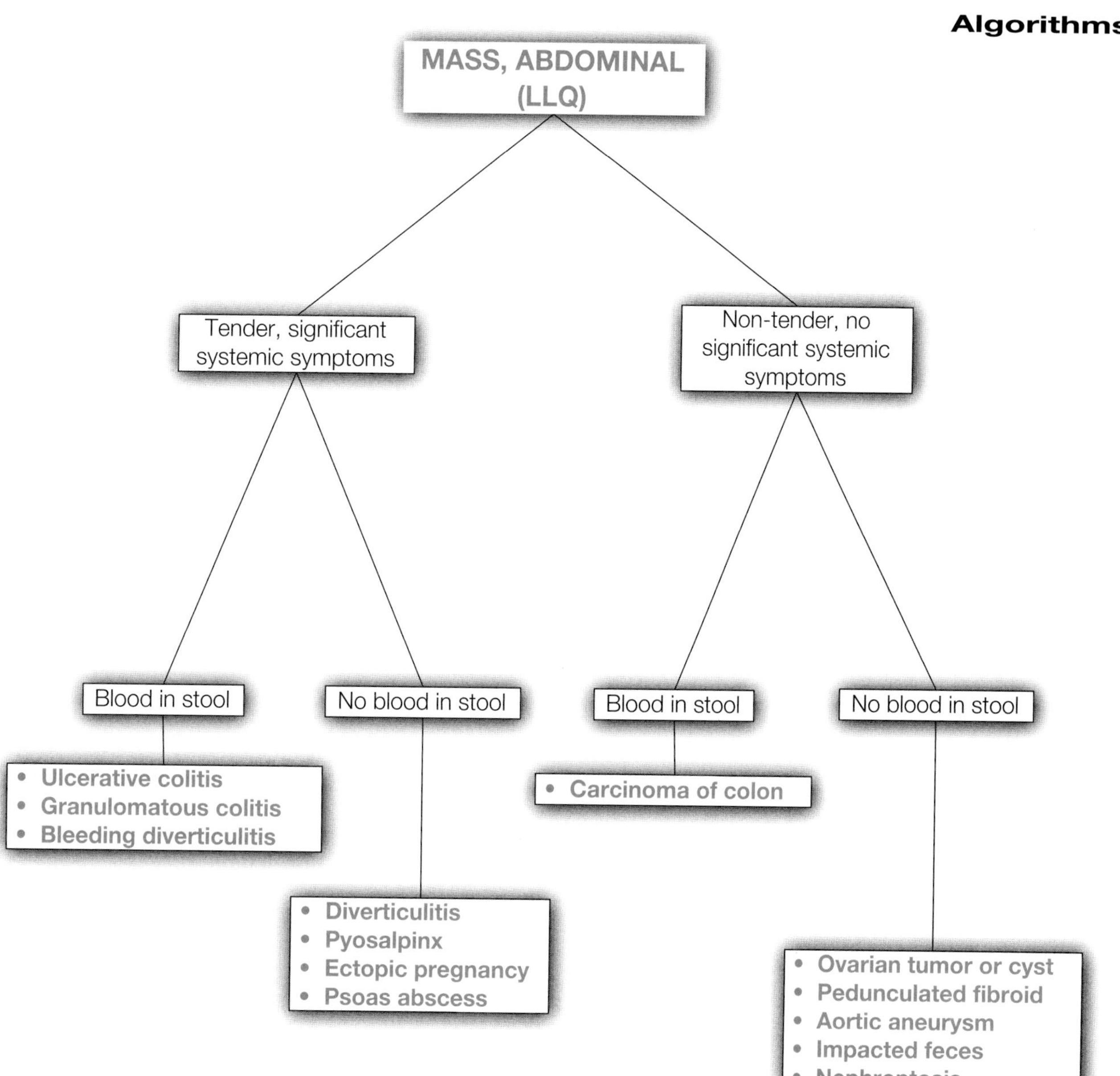
MASS, ABDOMINAL (LLQ)
Tender, significant systemic symptoms
Non-tender, no significant systemic symptoms
Blood in stool
No blood in stool
Blood in stool
No blood in stool
• Ulcerative colitis
• Granulomatous colitis
• Bleeding diverticulitis
• Diverticulitis
• Pyosalpinx
• Ectopic pregnancy
• Psoas abscess
• Carcinoma of colon
• Ovarian tumor or cyst
• Pedunculated fibroid
• Aortic aneurysm
• Impacted feces
• Nephroptosis

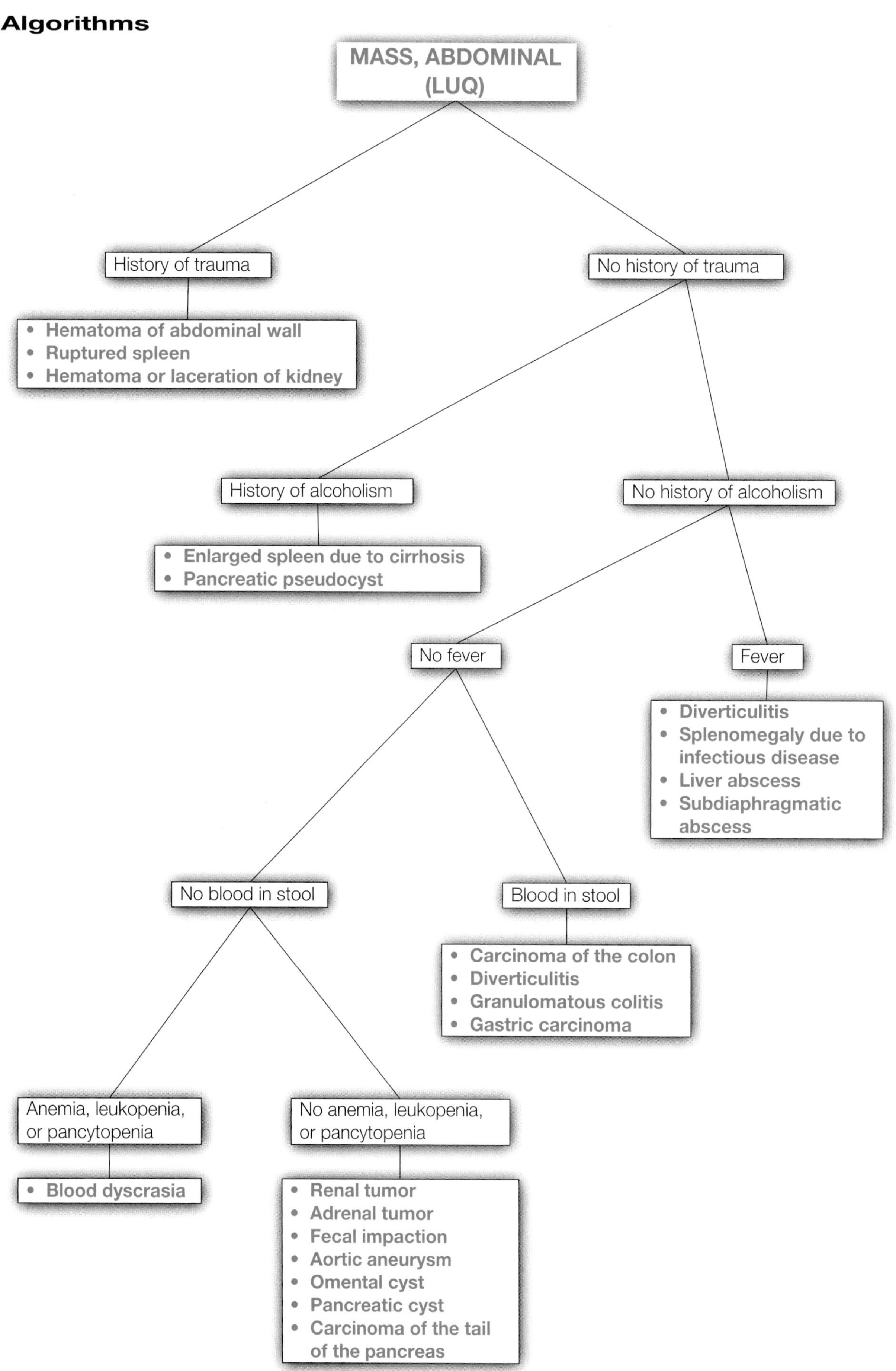
MASS, ABDOMINAL (LUQ)
History of trauma
• Hematoma of abdominal wall
• Ruptured spleen
• Hematoma or laceration of kidney
No history of trauma
History of alcoholism
• Enlarged spleen due to cirrhosis
• Pancreatic pseudocyst
No history of alcoholism
No fever
Fever
• Diverticulitis
• Splenomegaly due to infectious disease
• Liver abscess
• Subdiaphragmatic abscess
No blood in stool
Blood in stool
• Carcinoma of the colon
• Diverticulitis
• Granulomatous colitis
• Gastric carcinoma
Anemia, leukopenia, or pancytopenia
• Blood dyscrasia
No anemia, leukopenia, or pancytopenia
• Renal tumor
• Adrenal tumor
• Fecal impaction
• Aortic aneurysm
• Omental cyst
• Pancreatic cyst
• Carcinoma of the tail of the pancreas

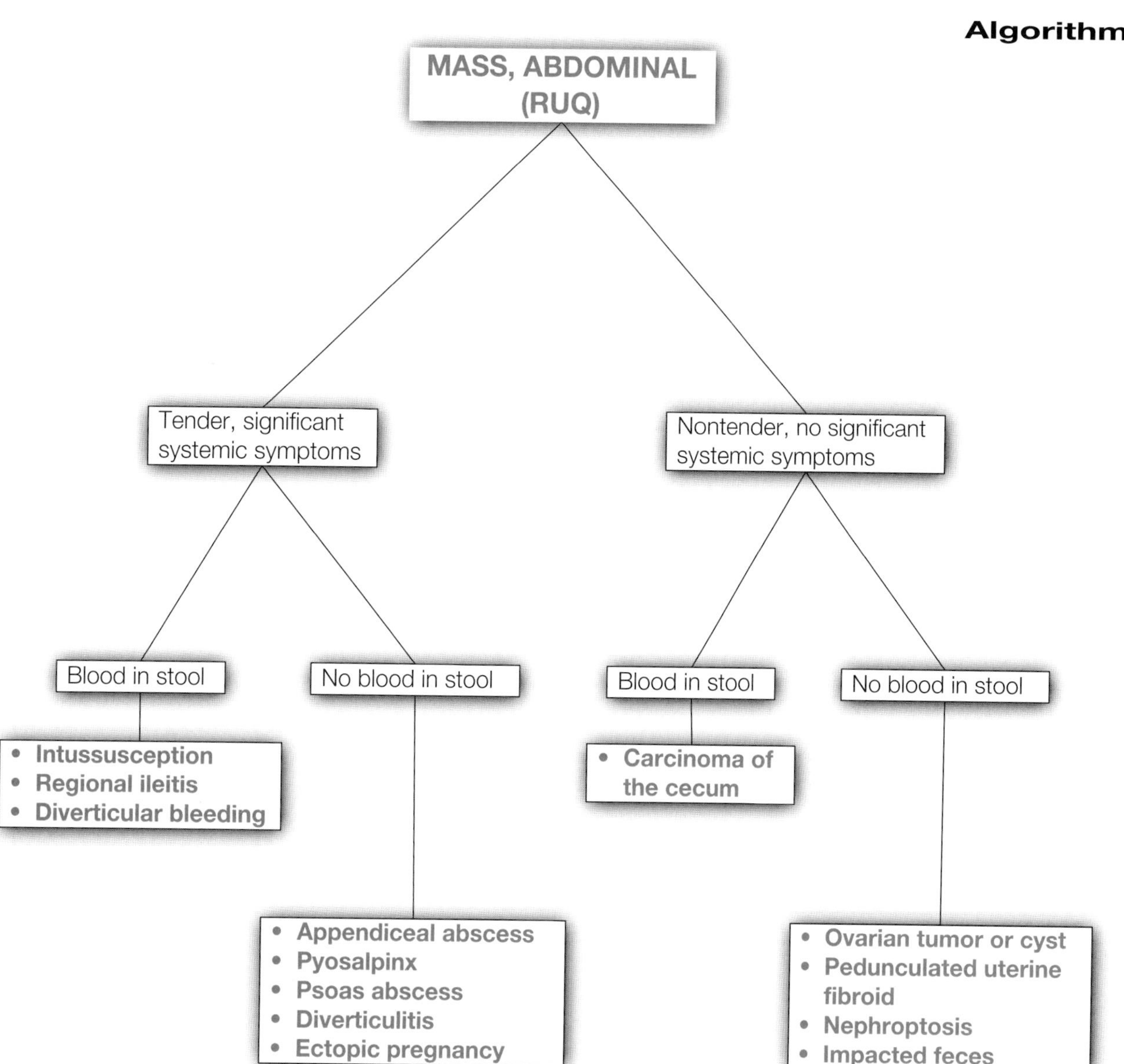
MASS, ABDOMINAL (RUQ)
Tender, significant systemic symptoms
Nontender, no significant systemic symptoms
Blood in stool
No blood in stool
Blood in stool
No blood in stool
• Intussusception
• Regional ileitis
• Diverticular bleeding
• Carcinoma of the cecum
• Appendiceal abscess
• Pyosalpinx
• Psoas abscess
• Diverticulitis
• Ectopic pregnancy
• Ovarian tumor or cyst
• Pedunculated uterine fibroid
• Nephroptosis
• Impacted feces

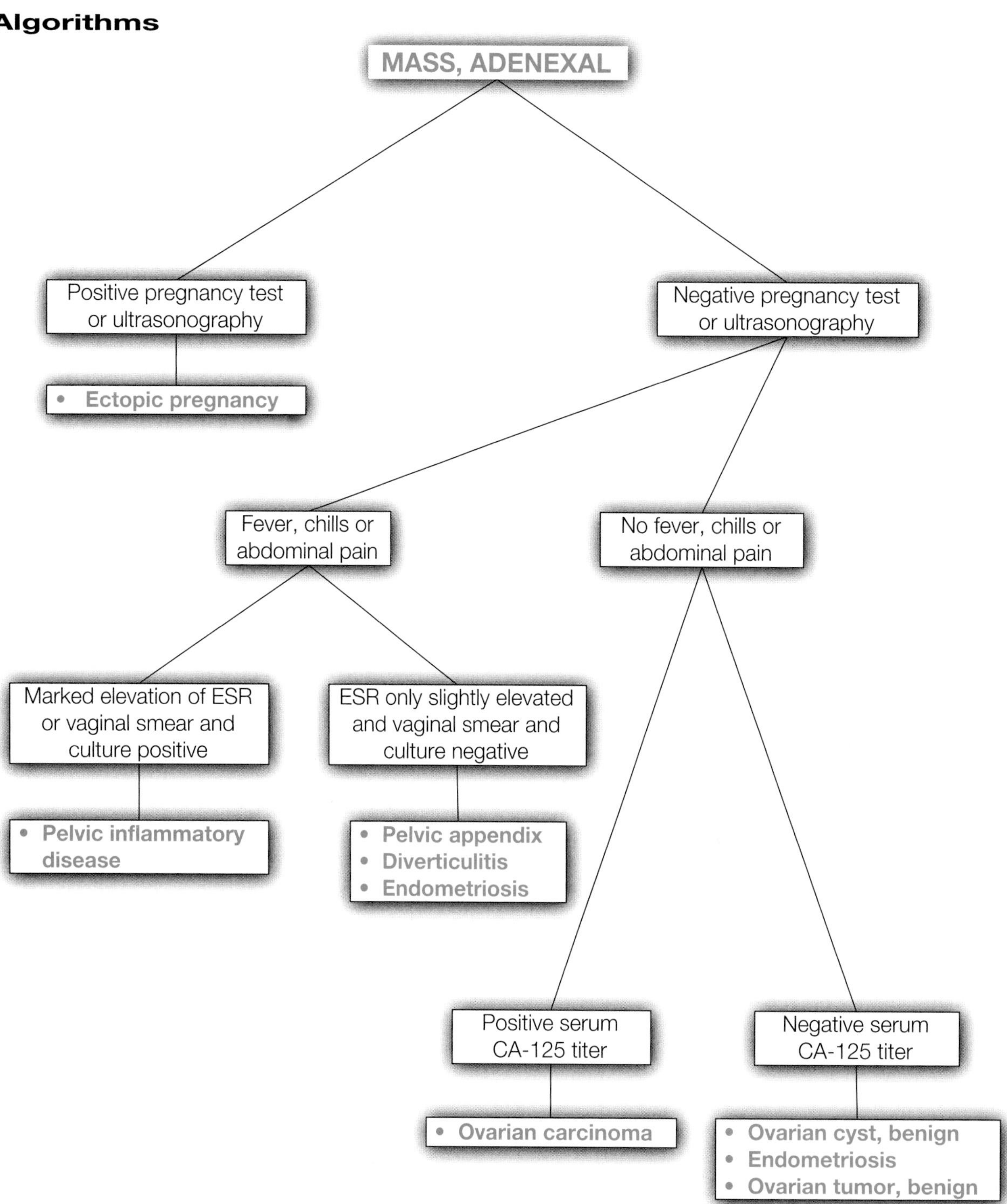
MASS, ADENEXAL
Positive pregnancy test or ultrasonography
• Ectopic pregnancy
Negative pregnancy test or ultrasonography
Fever, chills or abdominal pain
No fever, chills or abdominal pain
Marked elevation of ESR or vaginal smear and culture positive
ESR only slightly elevated and vaginal smear and culture negative
• Pelvic inflammatory disease
• Pelvic appendix
• Diverticulitis
• Endometriosis
Positive serum CA-125 titer
Negative serum CA-125 titer
• Ovarian carcinoma
• Ovarian cyst, benign
• Endometriosis
• Ovarian tumor, benign

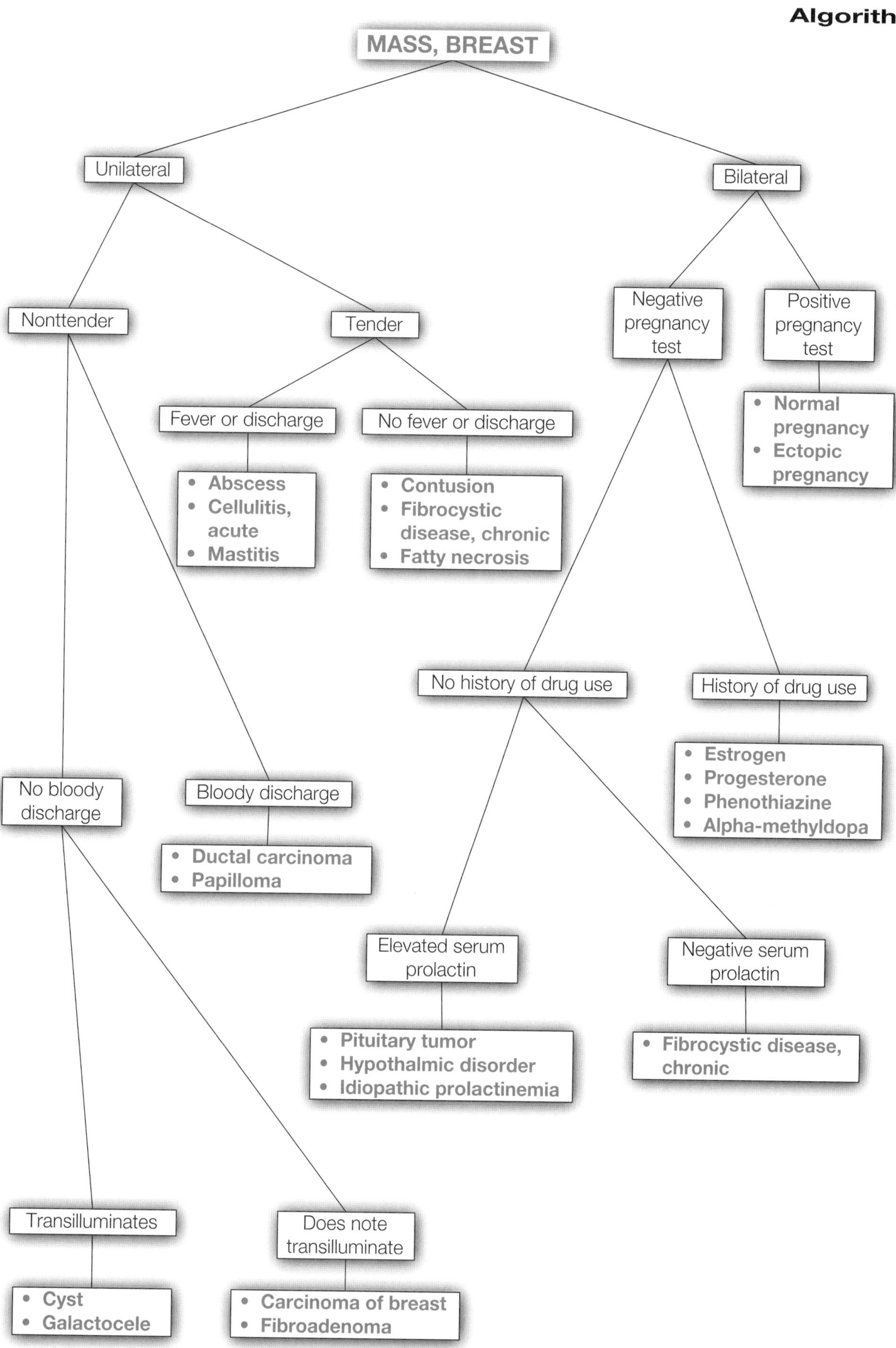
MASS, BREAST
Unilateral
Bilateral
Nonttender
Tender
Negative pregnancy test
Positive pregnancy test
• Normal pregnancy
• Ectopic pregnancy
Fever or discharge
No fever or discharge
• Abscess
• Cellulitis, acute
• Mastitis
• Contusion
• Fibrocystic disease, chronic
• Fatty necrosis
No history of drug use
History of drug use
• Estrogen
• Progesterone
• Phenothiazine
• Alpha-methyldopa
No bloody discharge
Bloody discharge
• Ductal carcinoma
• Papilloma
Elevated serum prolactin
Negative serum prolactin
• Pituitary tumor
• Hypothalmic disorder
• Idiopathic prolactinemia
• Fibrocystic disease, chronic
Transilluminates
Does note transilluminate
• Cyst
• Galactocele
• Carcinoma of breast
• Fibroadenoma

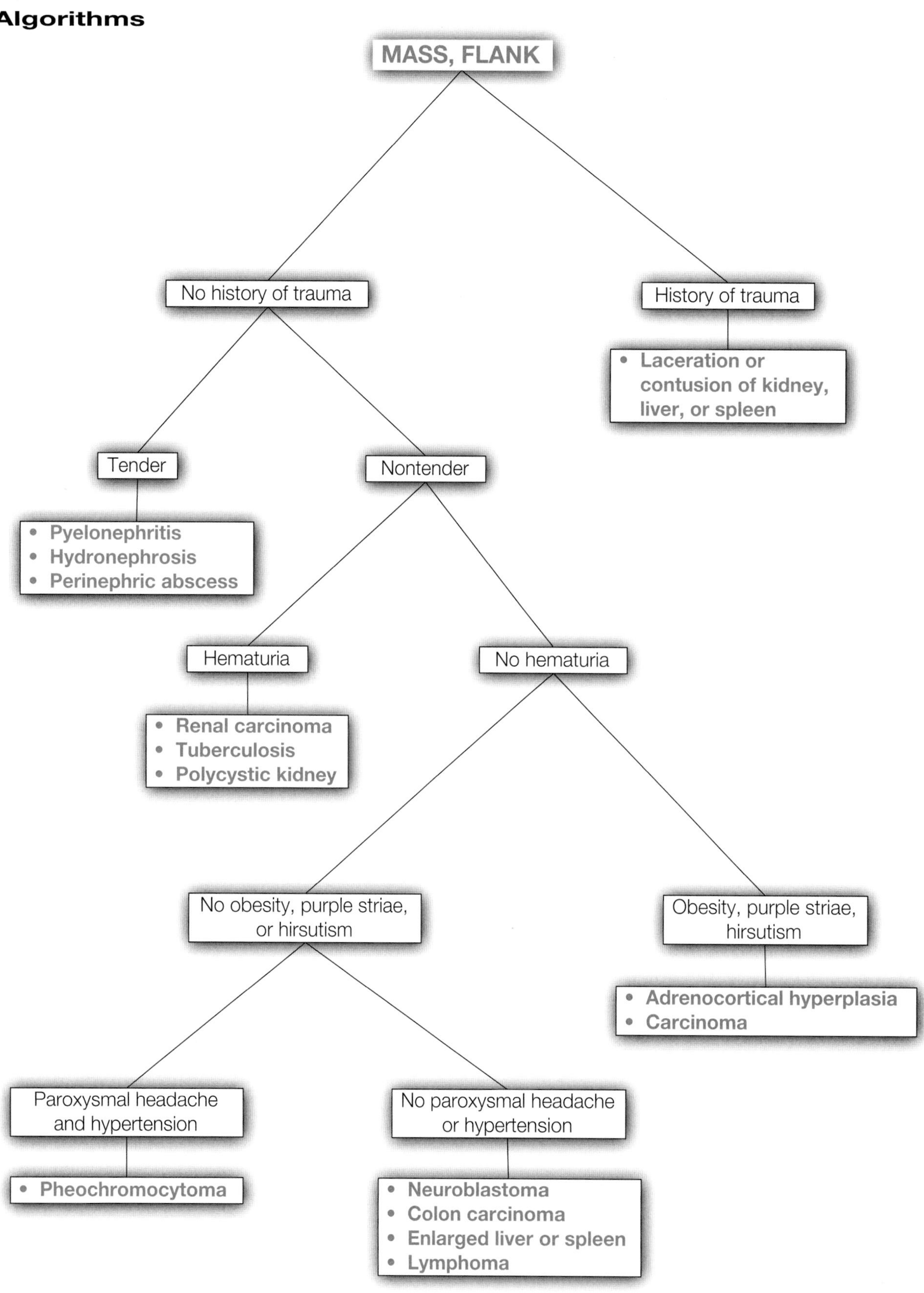
MASS, FLANK
No history of trauma
History of trauma
• Laceration or contusion of kidney, liver, or spleen
Tender
• Pyelonephritis
• Hydronephrosis
• Perinephric abscess
Nontender
Hematuria
• Renal carcinoma
• Tuberculosis
• Polycystic kidney
No hematuria
No obesity, purple striae, or hirsutism
Obesity, purple striae, hirsutism
• Adrenocortical hyperplasia
• Carcinoma
Paroxysmal headache and hypertension
• Pheochromocytoma
No paroxysmal headache or hypertension
• Neuroblastoma
• Colon carcinoma
• Enlarged liver or spleen
• Lymphoma

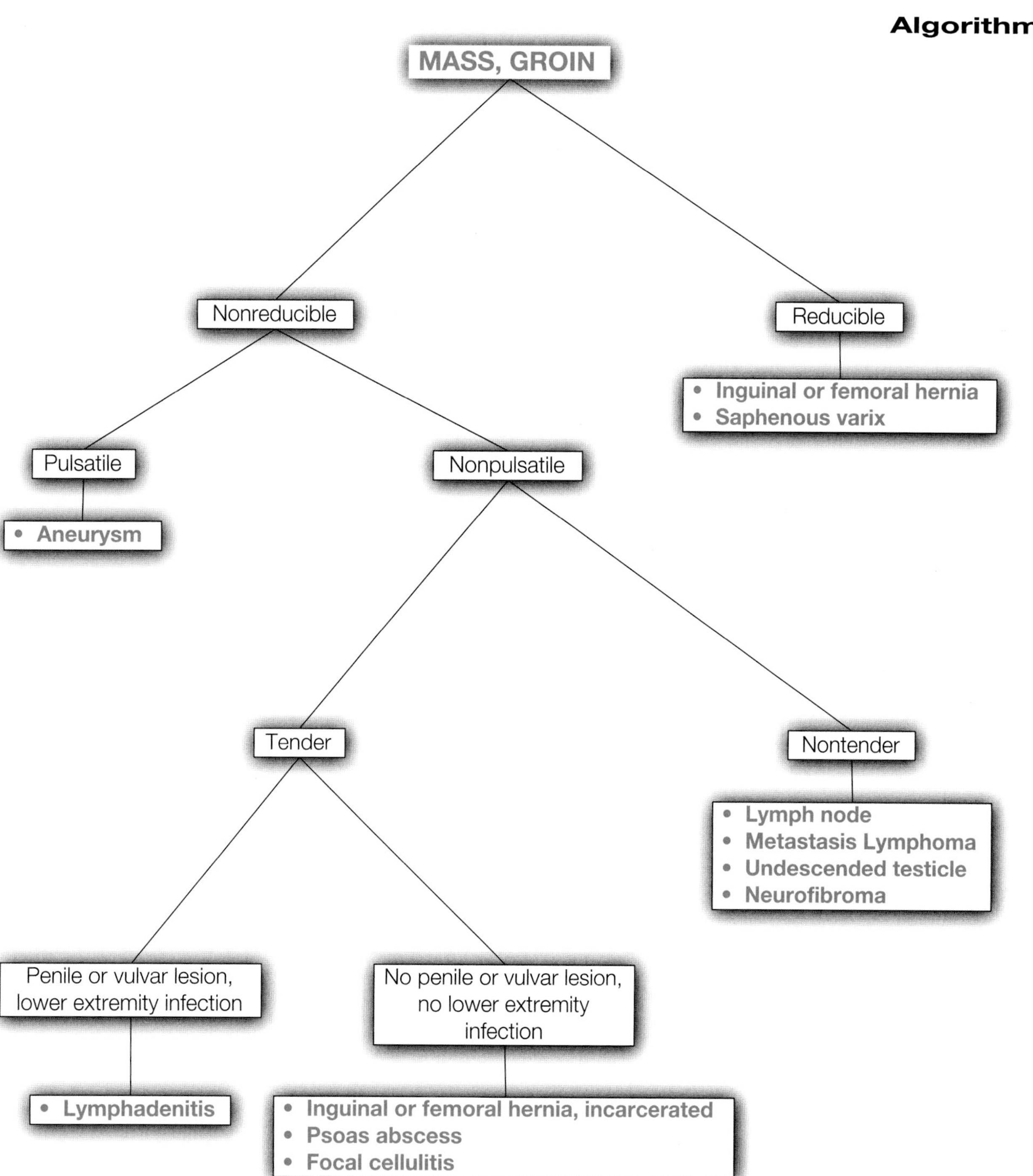
MASS, GROIN
Nonreducible
Reducible
• Inguinal or femoral hernia
• Saphenous varix
Pulsatile
Nonpulsatile
• Aneurysm
Tender
Nontender
• Lymph node
• Metastasis Lymphoma
• Undescended testicle
• Neurofibroma
Penile or vulvar lesion, lower extremity infection
No penile or vulvar lesion, no lower extremity infection
• Lymphadenitis
• Inguinal or femoral hernia, incarcerated
• Psoas abscess
• Focal cellulitis

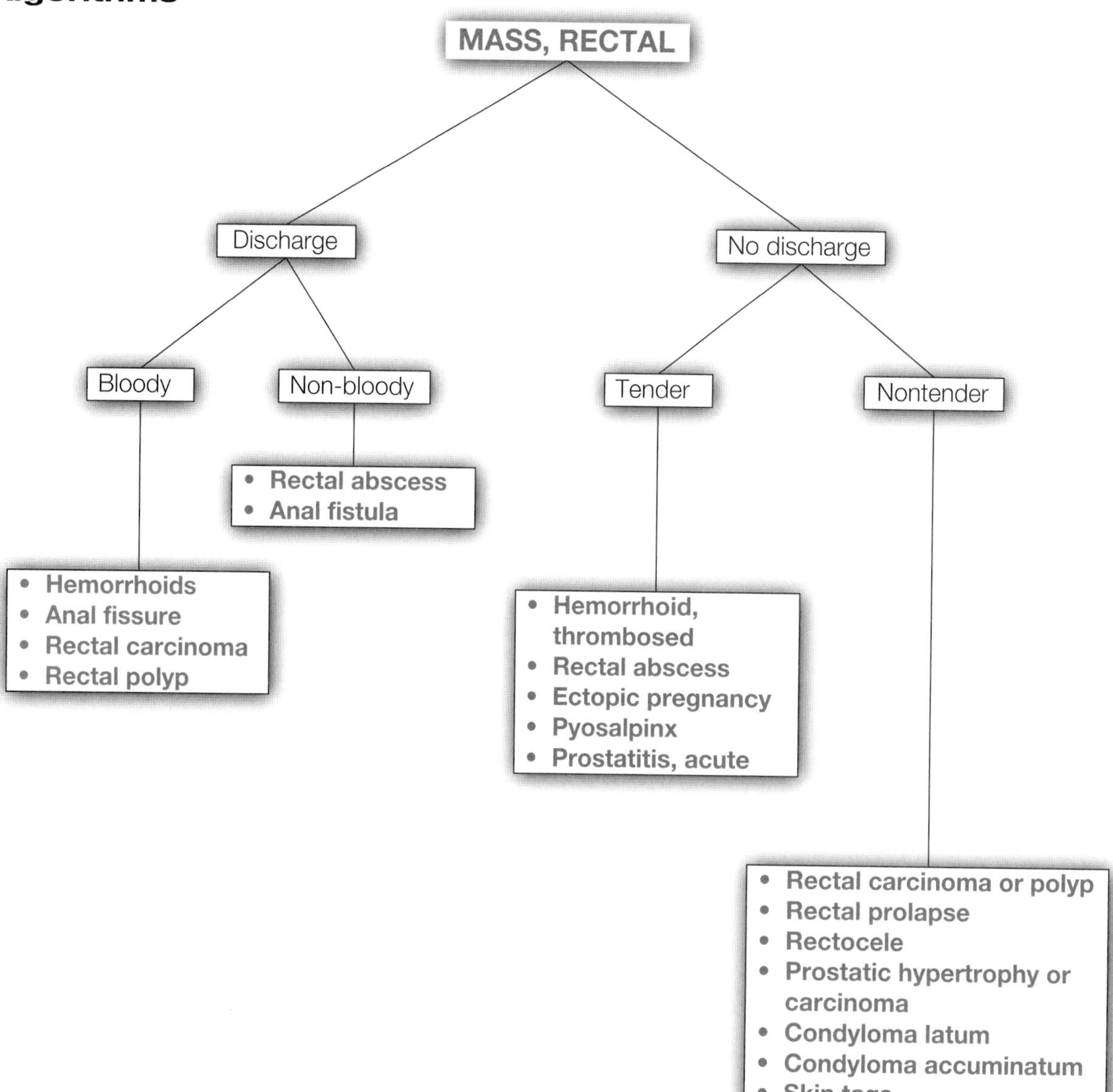
MASS, RECTAL
Discharge
No discharge
Bloody
Non-bloody
Tender
Nontender
• Rectal abscess
• Anal fistula
• Hemorrhoids
• Anal fissure
• Rectal carcinoma
• Rectal polyp
• Hemorrhoid, thrombosed
• Rectal abscess
• Ectopic pregnancy
• Pyosalpinx
• Prostatitis, acute
• Rectal carcinoma or polyp
• Rectal prolapse
• Rectocele
• Prostatic hypertrophy or carcinoma
• Condyloma latum
• Condyloma accuminatum
• Skin tags

MASS, TESTICULAR

- Not reducible
  - Transilluminates
    - Hydrocele
    - Spermatocele
  - Does not transilluminate
    - Tender
      - Retraction and elevation aggravates pain
        - Torsion of the testicle
      - Retraction and elevation does not aggravate the pain
        - Orchitis
        - Epididymitis
        - Inguinal hernia, incarcerated
    - Nontender
      - Testicular tumor
      - Syphilis
- Reducible
  - Inguinal hernia
  - Varicocele

MASS, THYROID

- Diffuse
  - Tremor, tachycardia, or exophthalmos
    - Hyperthyroidism, subacute
    - Thyroiditis
  - No tremor, tachycardia, or exophthalmos
    - Myxedema
      - Hashimoto disease
    - No myxedema (until late)
      - Endemic goiter
      - Riedel struma
      - Carcinoma
      - Sarcoma
- Focal
  - Tremor, tachycardia, or exophthalmos
    - Toxic adenoma
  - No tremor, tachycardia, or exophthalmos
    - Colloid cyst, solitary
    - Adenoma, early
    - Carcinoma
    - Thyroglossal cyst

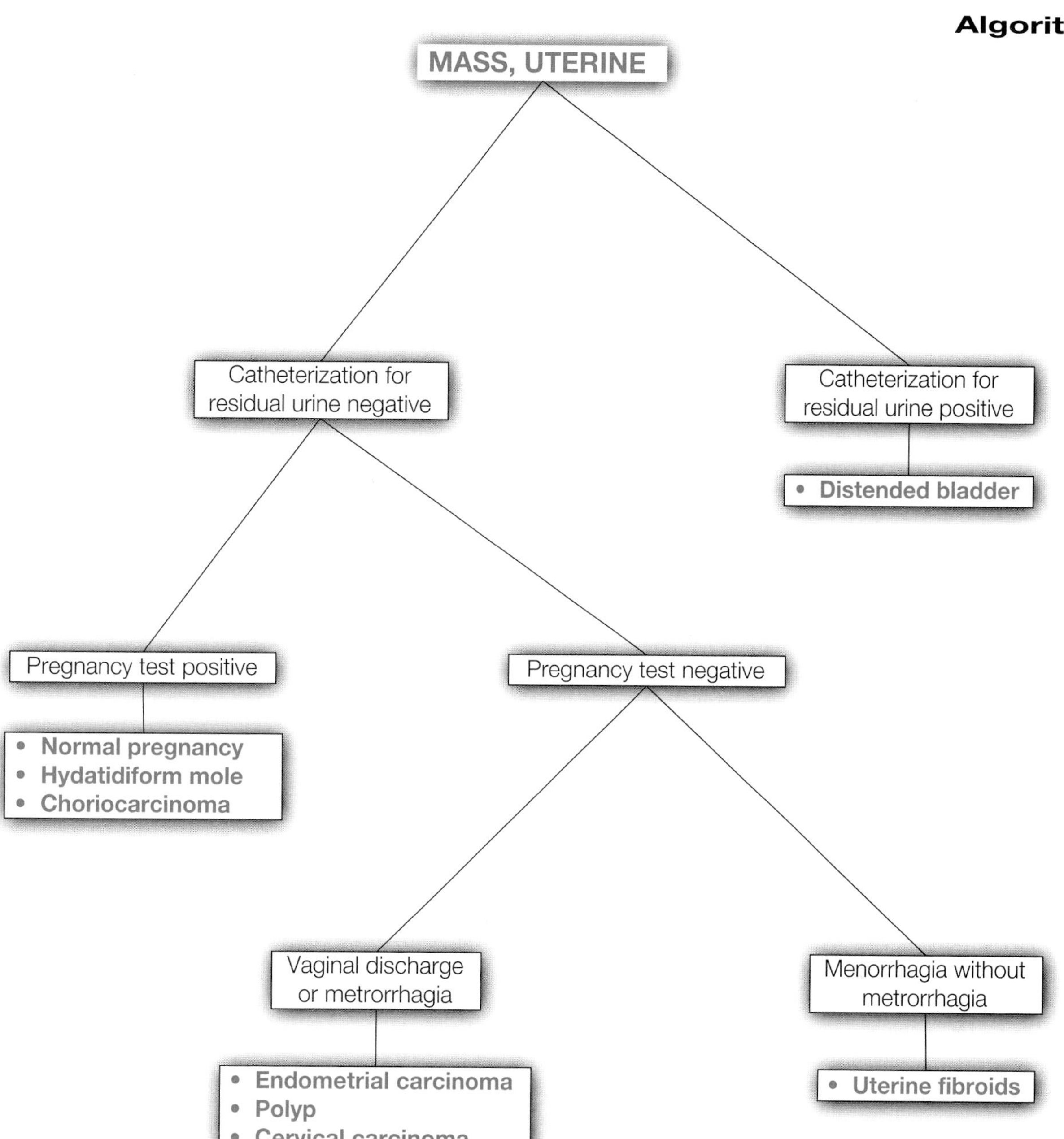
MASS, UTERINE
Catheterization for residual urine negative
Catheterization for residual urine positive
• Distended bladder
Pregnancy test positive
• Normal pregnancy
• Hydatidiform mole
• Choriocarcinoma
Pregnancy test negative
Vaginal discharge or metrorrhagia
• Endometrial carcinoma
• Polyp
• Cervical carcinoma
Menorrhagia without metrorrhagia
• Uterine fibroids

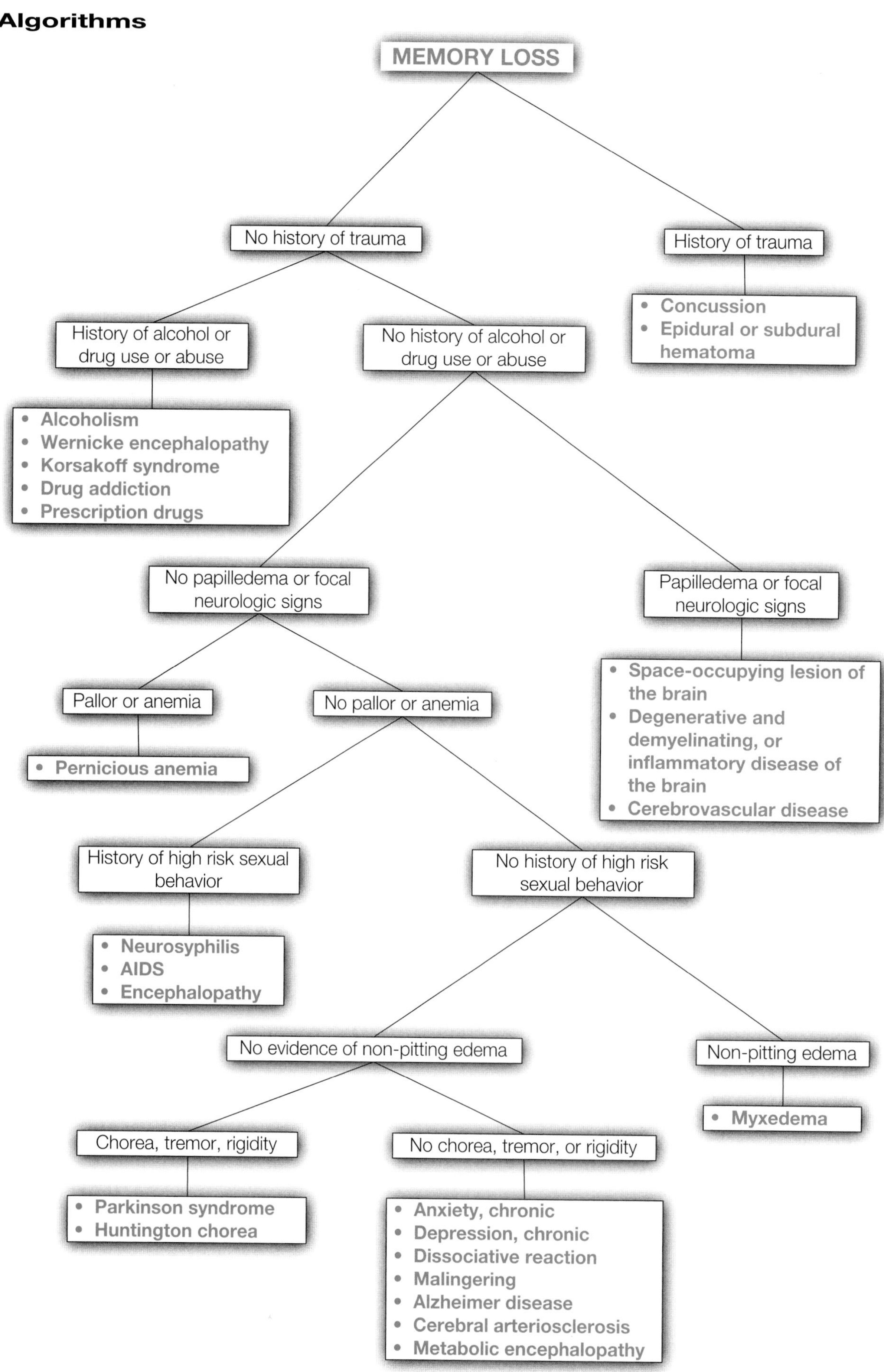
MEMORY LOSS
No history of trauma
History of trauma
• Concussion
• Epidural or subdural hematoma
History of alcohol or drug use or abuse
No history of alcohol or drug use or abuse
• Alcoholism
• Wernicke encephalopathy
• Korsakoff syndrome
• Drug addiction
• Prescription drugs
No papilledema or focal neurologic signs
Papilledema or focal neurologic signs
• Space-occupying lesion of the brain
• Degenerative and demyelinating, or inflammatory disease of the brain
• Cerebrovascular disease
Pallor or anemia
No pallor or anemia
• Pernicious anemia
History of high risk sexual behavior
No history of high risk sexual behavior
• Neurosyphilis
• AIDS
• Encephalopathy
No evidence of non-pitting edema
Non-pitting edema
• Myxedema
Chorea, tremor, rigidity
No chorea, tremor, or rigidity
• Parkinson syndrome
• Huntington chorea
• Anxiety, chronic
• Depression, chronic
• Dissociative reaction
• Malingering
• Alzheimer disease
• Cerebral arteriosclerosis
• Metabolic encephalopathy

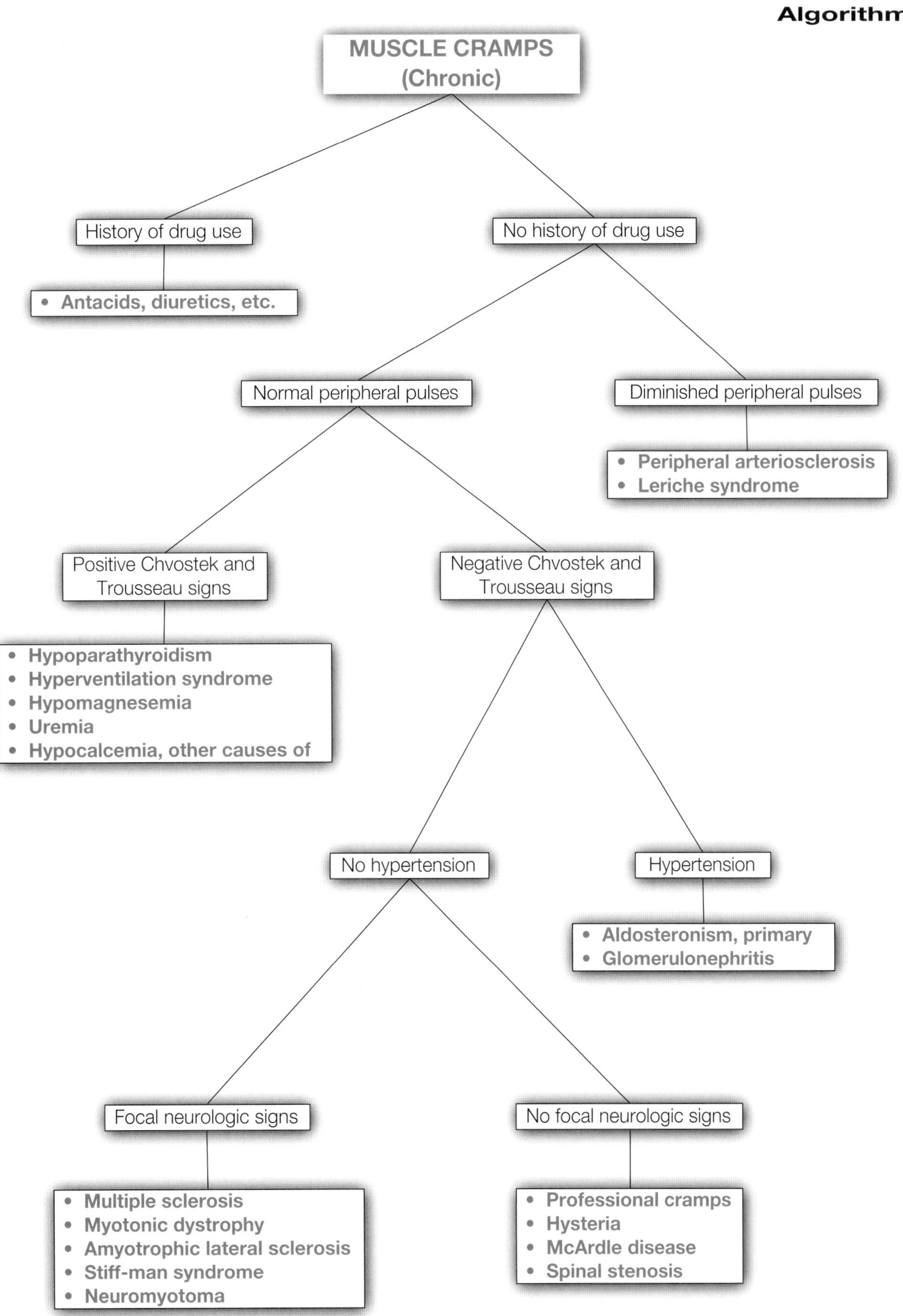
MUSCLE CRAMPS
(Chronic)
History of drug use
• Antacids, diuretics, etc.
No history of drug use
Normal peripheral pulses
Diminished peripheral pulses
• Peripheral arteriosclerosis
• Leriche syndrome
Positive Chvostek and Trousseau signs
• Hypoparathyroidism
• Hyperventilation syndrome
• Hypomagnesemia
• Uremia
• Hypocalcemia, other causes of
Negative Chvostek and Trousseau signs
No hypertension
Hypertension
• Aldosteronism, primary
• Glomerulonephritis
Focal neurologic signs
• Multiple sclerosis
• Myotonic dystrophy
• Amyotrophic lateral sclerosis
• Stiff-man syndrome
• Neuromyotoma
No focal neurologic signs
• Professional cramps
• Hysteria
• McArdle disease
• Spinal stenosis

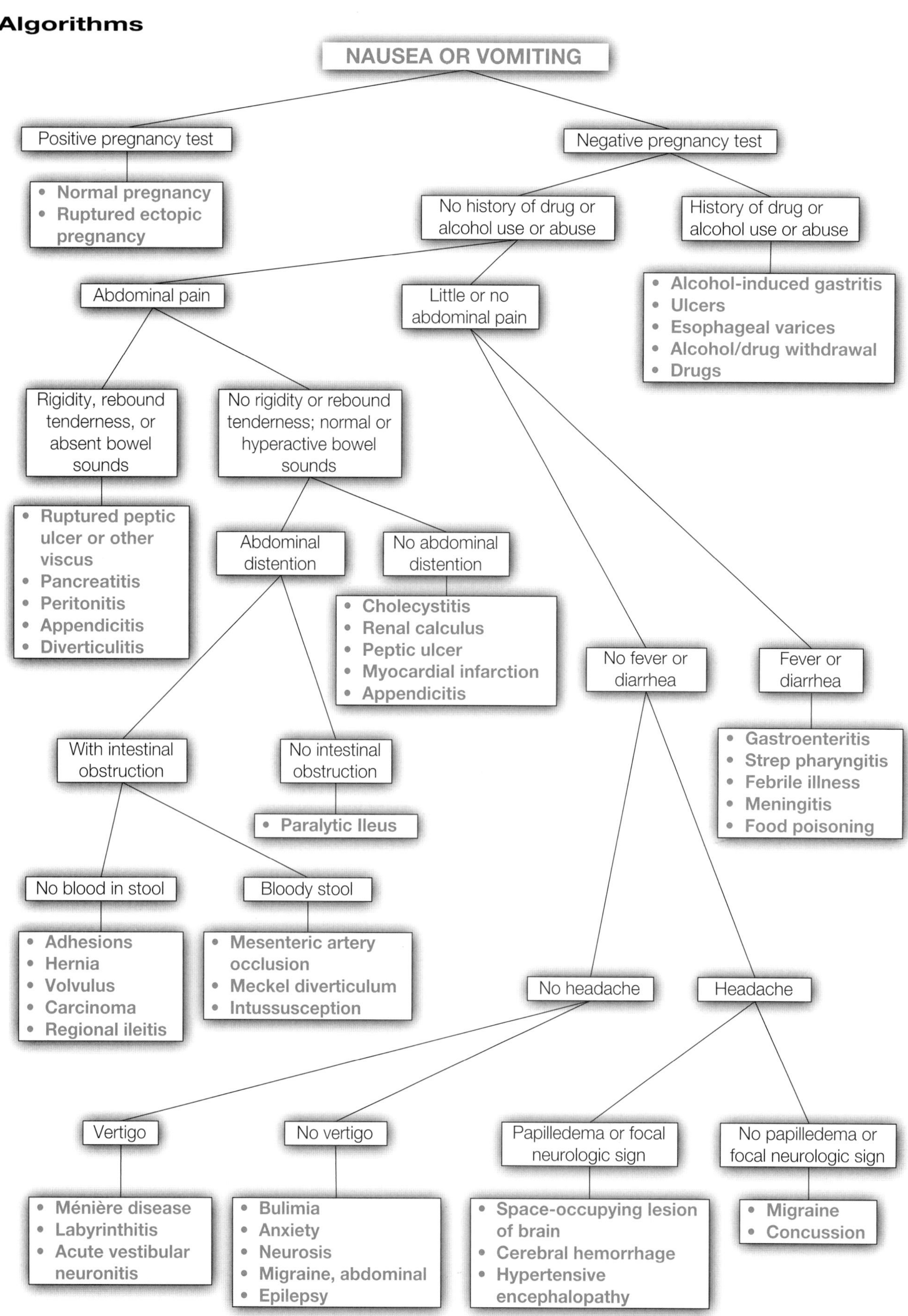
NAUSEA OR VOMITING
Positive pregnancy test
• Normal pregnancy
• Ruptured ectopic pregnancy
Negative pregnancy test
No history of drug or alcohol use or abuse
History of drug or alcohol use or abuse
• Alcohol-induced gastritis
• Ulcers
• Esophageal varices
• Alcohol/drug withdrawal
• Drugs
Abdominal pain
Little or no abdominal pain
Rigidity, rebound tenderness, or absent bowel sounds
No rigidity or rebound tenderness; normal or hyperactive bowel sounds
• Ruptured peptic ulcer or other viscus
• Pancreatitis
• Peritonitis
• Appendicitis
• Diverticulitis
Abdominal distention
No abdominal distention
• Cholecystitis
• Renal calculus
• Peptic ulcer
• Myocardial infarction
• Appendicitis
No fever or diarrhea
Fever or diarrhea
• Gastroenteritis
• Strep pharyngitis
• Febrile illness
• Meningitis
• Food poisoning
With intestinal obstruction
No intestinal obstruction
• Paralytic Ileus
No blood in stool
Bloody stool
• Adhesions
• Hernia
• Volvulus
• Carcinoma
• Regional ileitis
• Mesenteric artery occlusion
• Meckel diverticulum
• Intussusception
No headache
Headache
Vertigo
No vertigo
Papilledema or focal neurologic sign
No papilledema or focal neurologic sign
• Ménière disease
• Labyrinthitis
• Acute vestibular neuronitis
• Bulimia
• Anxiety
• Neurosis
• Migraine, abdominal
• Epilepsy
• Space-occupying lesion of brain
• Cerebral hemorrhage
• Hypertensive encephalopathy
• Migraine
• Concussion

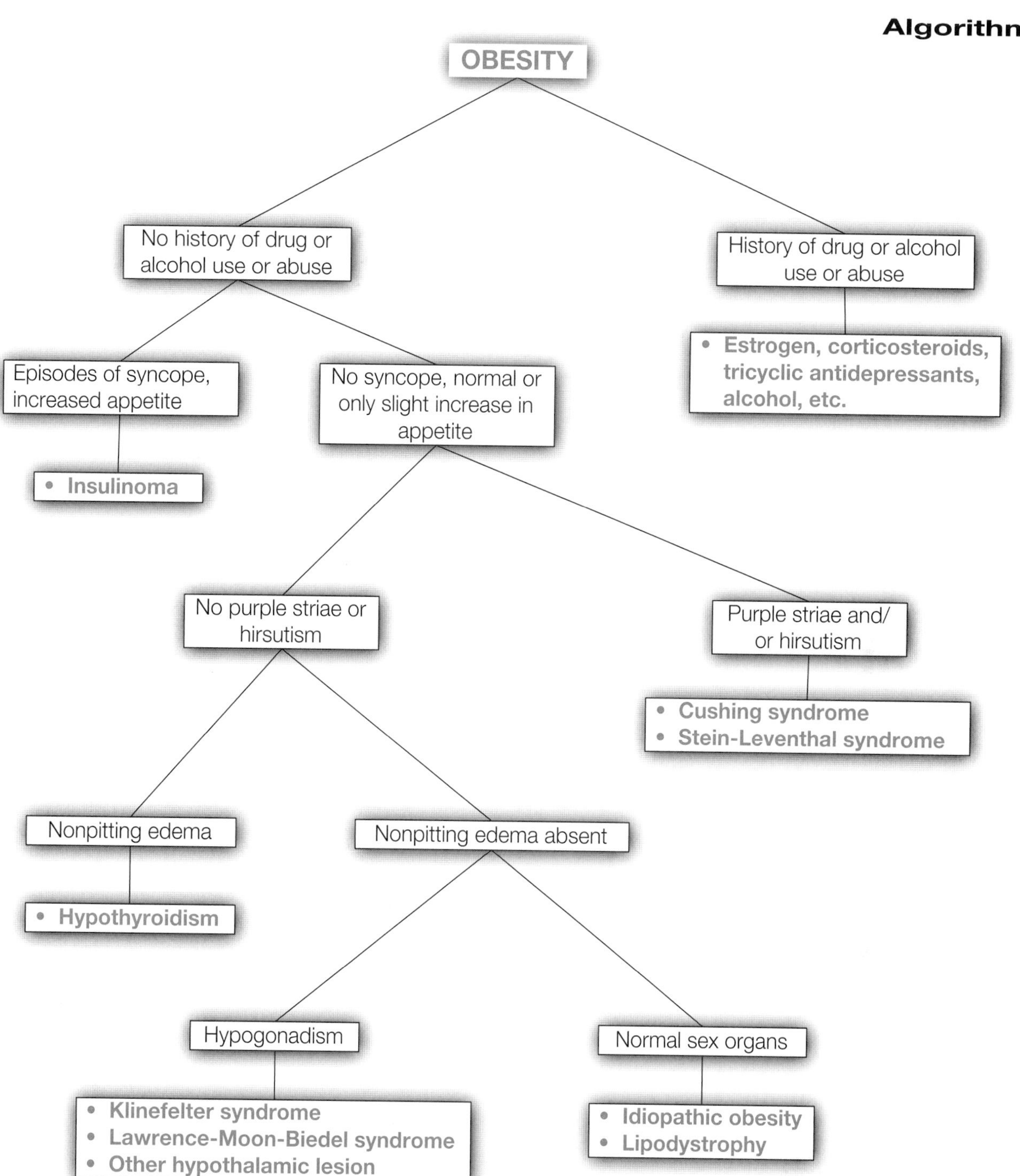
OBESITY
No history of drug or alcohol use or abuse
History of drug or alcohol use or abuse
• Estrogen, corticosteroids, tricyclic antidepressants, alcohol, etc.
Episodes of syncope, increased appetite
• Insulinoma
No syncope, normal or only slight increase in appetite
No purple striae or hirsutism
Purple striae and/ or hirsutism
• Cushing syndrome
• Stein-Leventhal syndrome
Nonpitting edema
• Hypothyroidism
Nonpitting edema absent
Hypogonadism
• Klinefelter syndrome
• Lawrence-Moon-Biedel syndrome
• Other hypothalamic lesion
Normal sex organs
• Idiopathic obesity
• Lipodystrophy

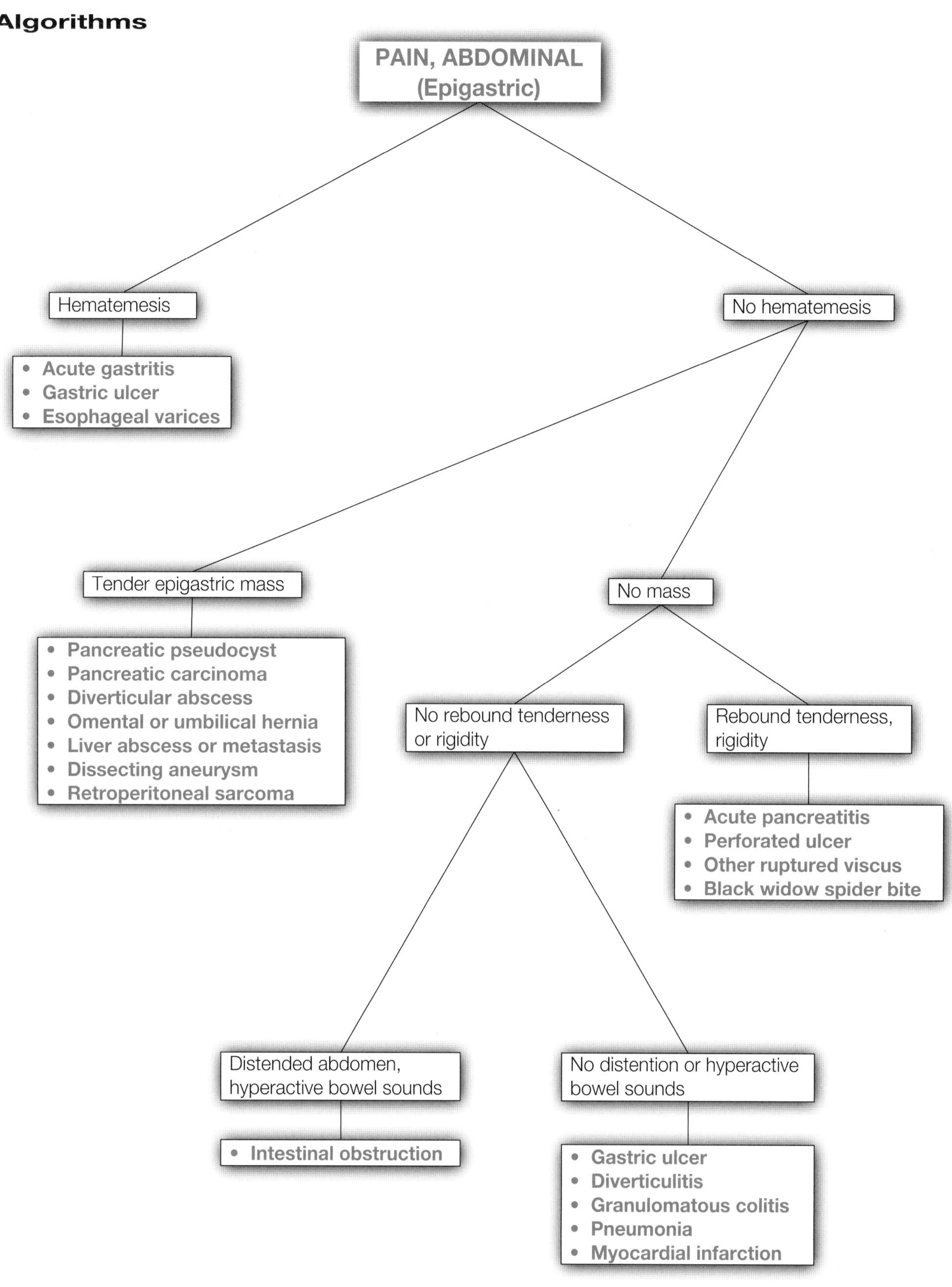
PAIN, ABDOMINAL
(Epigastric)
Hematemesis
• Acute gastritis
• Gastric ulcer
• Esophageal varices
No hematemesis
Tender epigastric mass
• Pancreatic pseudocyst
• Pancreatic carcinoma
• Diverticular abscess
• Omental or umbilical hernia
• Liver abscess or metastasis
• Dissecting aneurysm
• Retroperitoneal sarcoma
No mass
No rebound tenderness or rigidity
Rebound tenderness, rigidity
• Acute pancreatitis
• Perforated ulcer
• Other ruptured viscus
• Black widow spider bite
Distended abdomen, hyperactive bowel sounds
• Intestinal obstruction
No distention or hyperactive bowel sounds
• Gastric ulcer
• Diverticulitis
• Granulomatous colitis
• Pneumonia
• Myocardial infarction

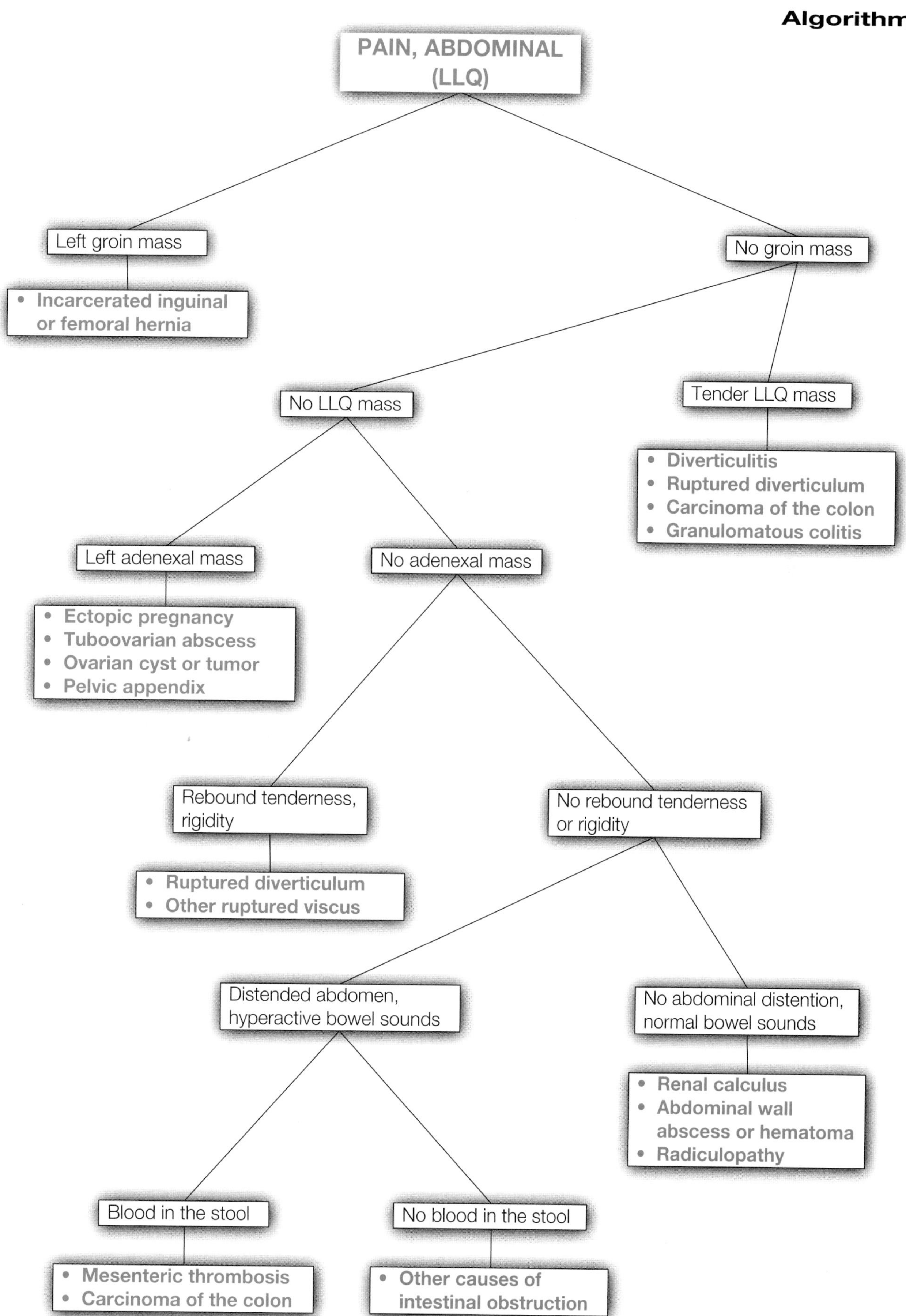
PAIN, ABDOMINAL (LLQ)
Left groin mass
• Incarcerated inguinal or femoral hernia
No groin mass
No LLQ mass
Tender LLQ mass
• Diverticulitis
• Ruptured diverticulum
• Carcinoma of the colon
• Granulomatous colitis
Left adenexal mass
No adenexal mass
• Ectopic pregnancy
• Tuboovarian abscess
• Ovarian cyst or tumor
• Pelvic appendix
Rebound tenderness, rigidity
No rebound tenderness or rigidity
• Ruptured diverticulum
• Other ruptured viscus
Distended abdomen, hyperactive bowel sounds
No abdominal distention, normal bowel sounds
• Renal calculus
• Abdominal wall abscess or hematoma
• Radiculopathy
Blood in the stool
No blood in the stool
• Mesenteric thrombosis
• Carcinoma of the colon
• Other causes of intestinal obstruction

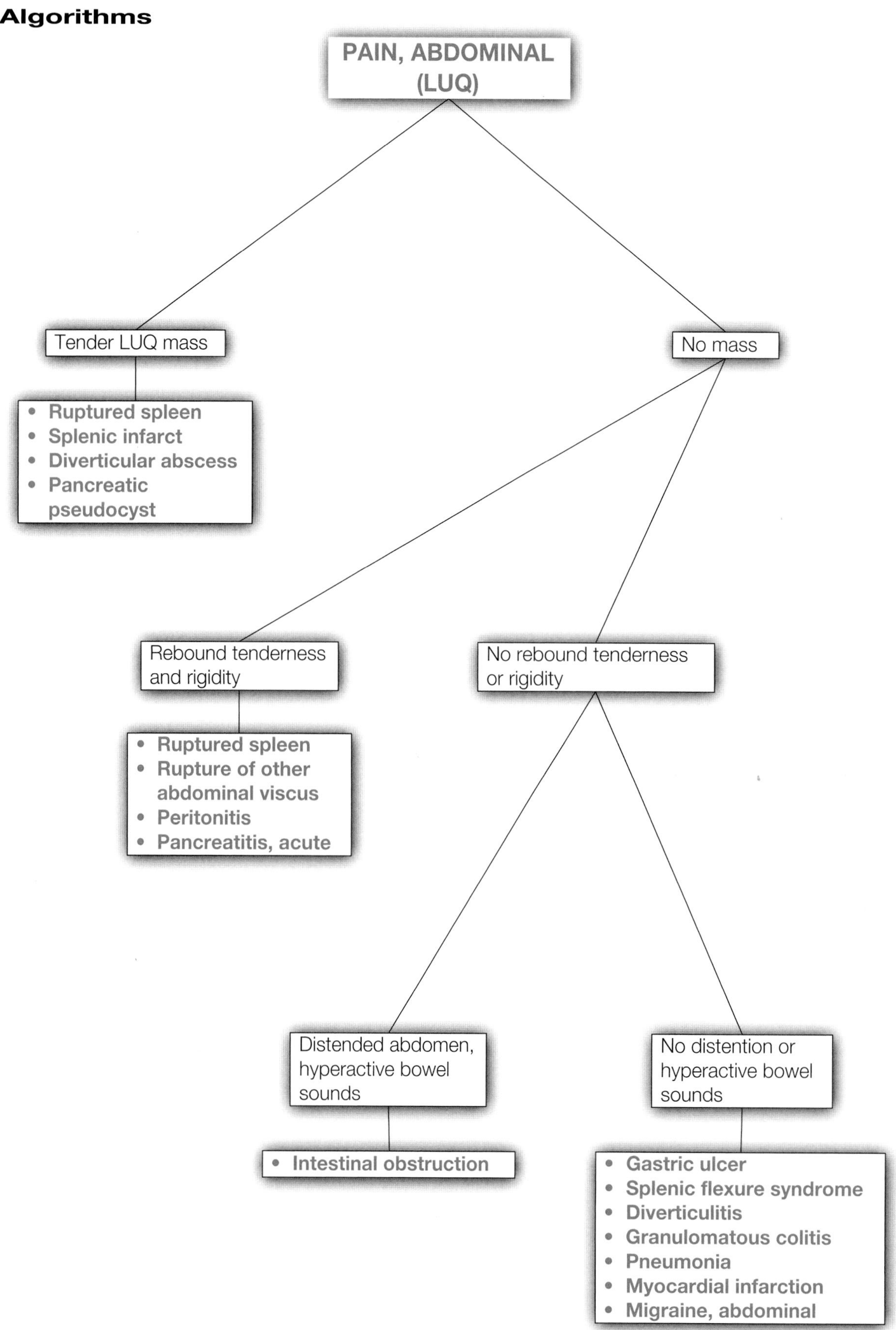
PAIN, ABDOMINAL (LUQ)
Tender LUQ mass
• Ruptured spleen
• Splenic infarct
• Diverticular abscess
• Pancreatic pseudocyst
No mass
Rebound tenderness and rigidity
• Ruptured spleen
• Rupture of other abdominal viscus
• Peritonitis
• Pancreatitis, acute
No rebound tenderness or rigidity
Distended abdomen, hyperactive bowel sounds
• Intestinal obstruction
No distention or hyperactive bowel sounds
• Gastric ulcer
• Splenic flexure syndrome
• Diverticulitis
• Granulomatous colitis
• Pneumonia
• Myocardial infarction
• Migraine, abdominal

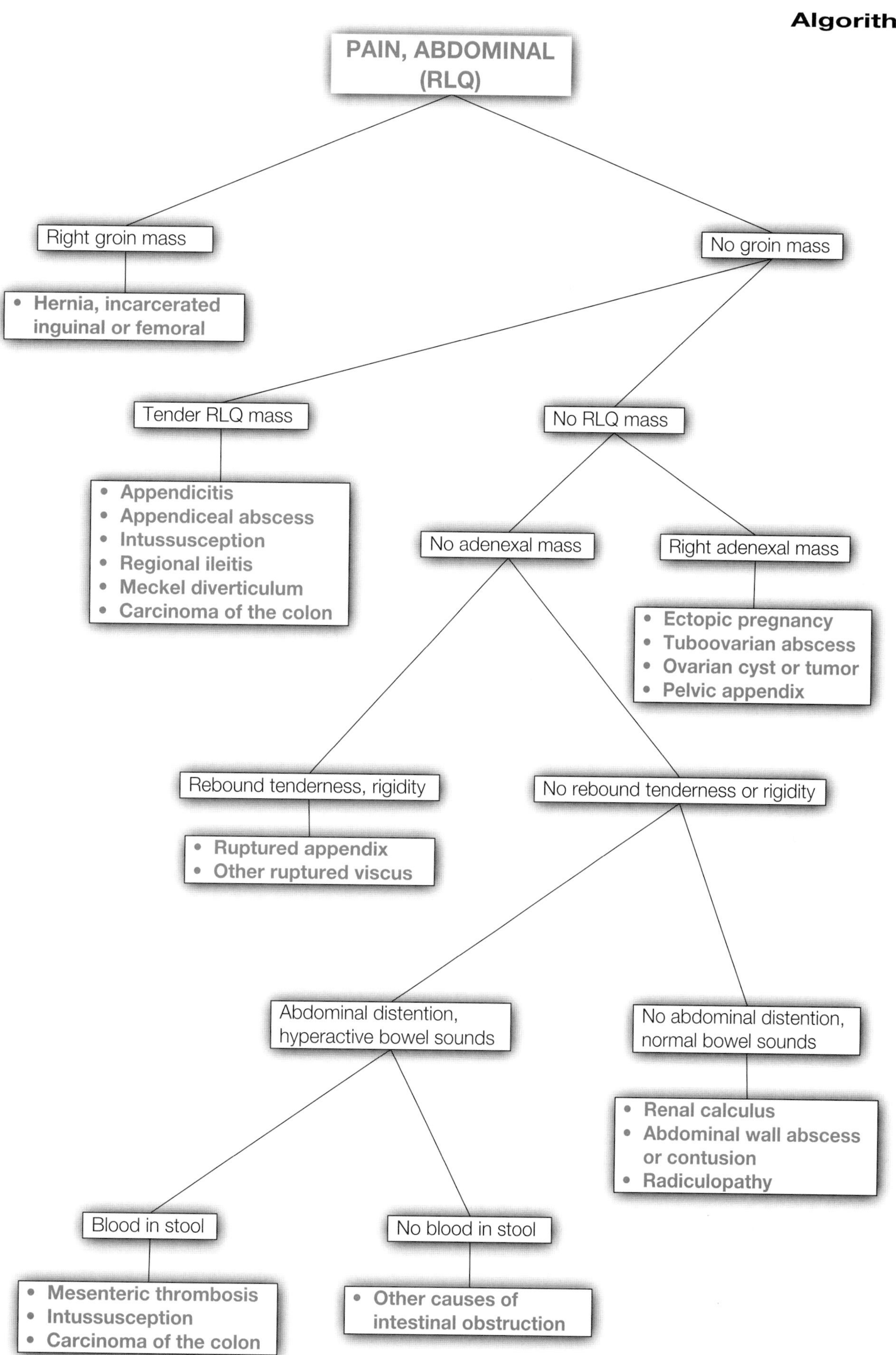
PAIN, ABDOMINAL (RLQ)
Right groin mass
• Hernia, incarcerated inguinal or femoral
No groin mass
Tender RLQ mass
• Appendicitis
• Appendiceal abscess
• Intussusception
• Regional ileitis
• Meckel diverticulum
• Carcinoma of the colon
No RLQ mass
No adenexal mass
Right adenexal mass
• Ectopic pregnancy
• Tuboovarian abscess
• Ovarian cyst or tumor
• Pelvic appendix
Rebound tenderness, rigidity
• Ruptured appendix
• Other ruptured viscus
No rebound tenderness or rigidity
Abdominal distention, hyperactive bowel sounds
No abdominal distention, normal bowel sounds
• Renal calculus
• Abdominal wall abscess or contusion
• Radiculopathy
Blood in stool
• Mesenteric thrombosis
• Intussusception
• Carcinoma of the colon
No blood in stool
• Other causes of intestinal obstruction

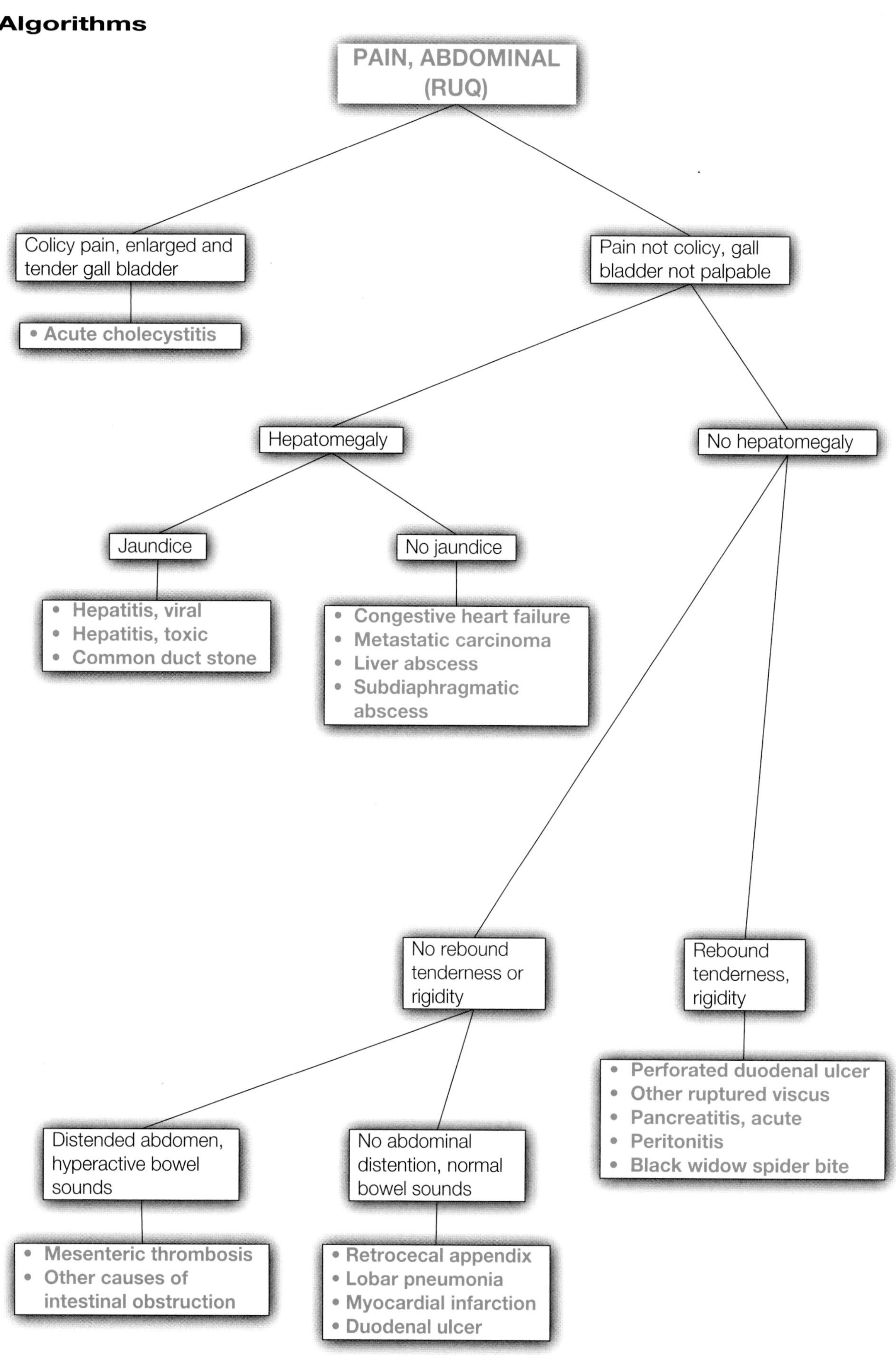
PAIN, ABDOMINAL (RUQ)
Colicy pain, enlarged and tender gall bladder
• Acute cholecystitis
Pain not colicy, gall bladder not palpable
Hepatomegaly
No hepatomegaly
Jaundice
No jaundice
• Hepatitis, viral
• Hepatitis, toxic
• Common duct stone
• Congestive heart failure
• Metastatic carcinoma
• Liver abscess
• Subdiaphragmatic abscess
No rebound tenderness or rigidity
Rebound tenderness, rigidity
• Perforated duodenal ulcer
• Other ruptured viscus
• Pancreatitis, acute
• Peritonitis
• Black widow spider bite
Distended abdomen, hyperactive bowel sounds
No abdominal distention, normal bowel sounds
• Mesenteric thrombosis
• Other causes of intestinal obstruction
• Retrocecal appendix
• Lobar pneumonia
• Myocardial infarction
• Duodenal ulcer

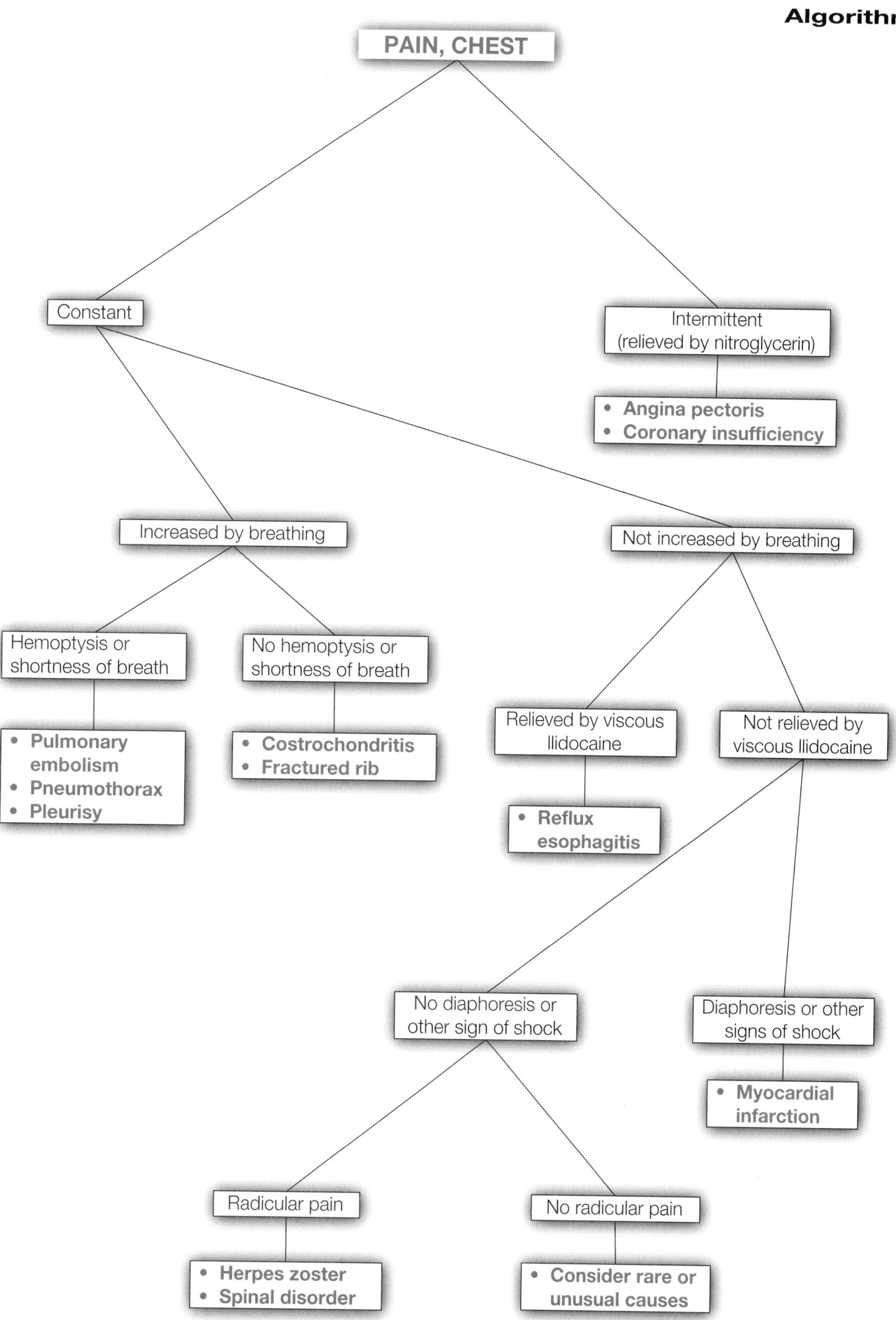
PAIN, CHEST
Constant
Intermittent (relieved by nitroglycerin)
• Angina pectoris
• Coronary insufficiency
Increased by breathing
Not increased by breathing
Hemoptysis or shortness of breath
No hemoptysis or shortness of breath
• Pulmonary embolism
• Pneumothorax
• Pleurisy
• Costrochondritis
• Fractured rib
Relieved by viscous lidocaine
Not relieved by viscous lidocaine
• Reflux esophagitis
No diaphoresis or other sign of shock
Diaphoresis or other signs of shock
• Myocardial infarction
Radicular pain
No radicular pain
• Herpes zoster
• Spinal disorder
• Consider rare or unusual causes

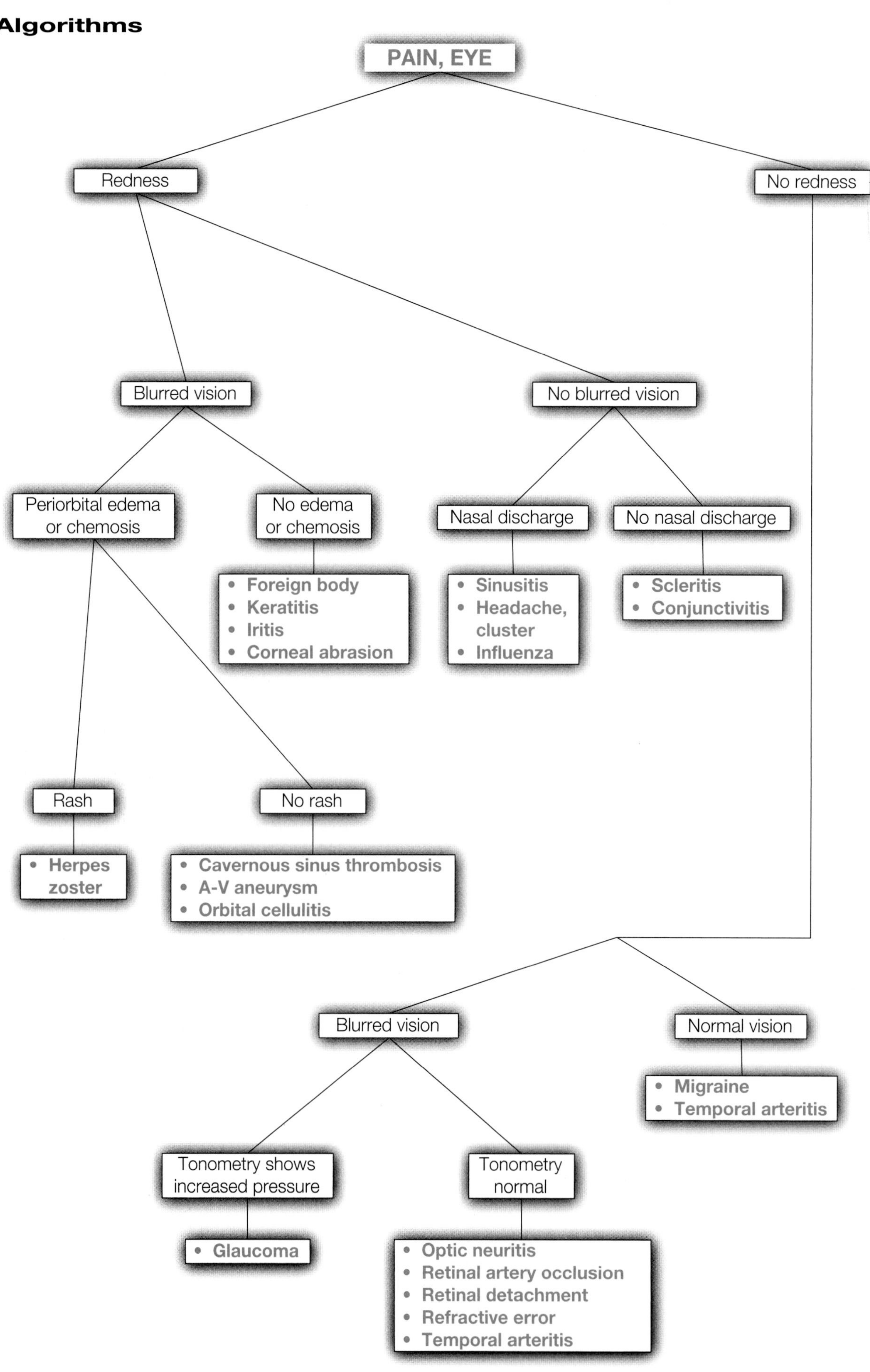
PAIN, EYE
Redness
No redness
Blurred vision
No blurred vision
Periorbital edema or chemosis
No edema or chemosis
Nasal discharge
No nasal discharge
• Foreign body
• Keratitis
• Iritis
• Corneal abrasion
• Sinusitis
• Headache, cluster
• Influenza
• Scleritis
• Conjunctivitis
Rash
No rash
• Herpes zoster
• Cavernous sinus thrombosis
• A-V aneurysm
• Orbital cellulitis
Blurred vision
Normal vision
• Migraine
• Temporal arteritis
Tonometry shows increased pressure
Tonometry normal
• Glaucoma
• Optic neuritis
• Retinal artery occlusion
• Retinal detachment
• Refractive error
• Temporal arteritis

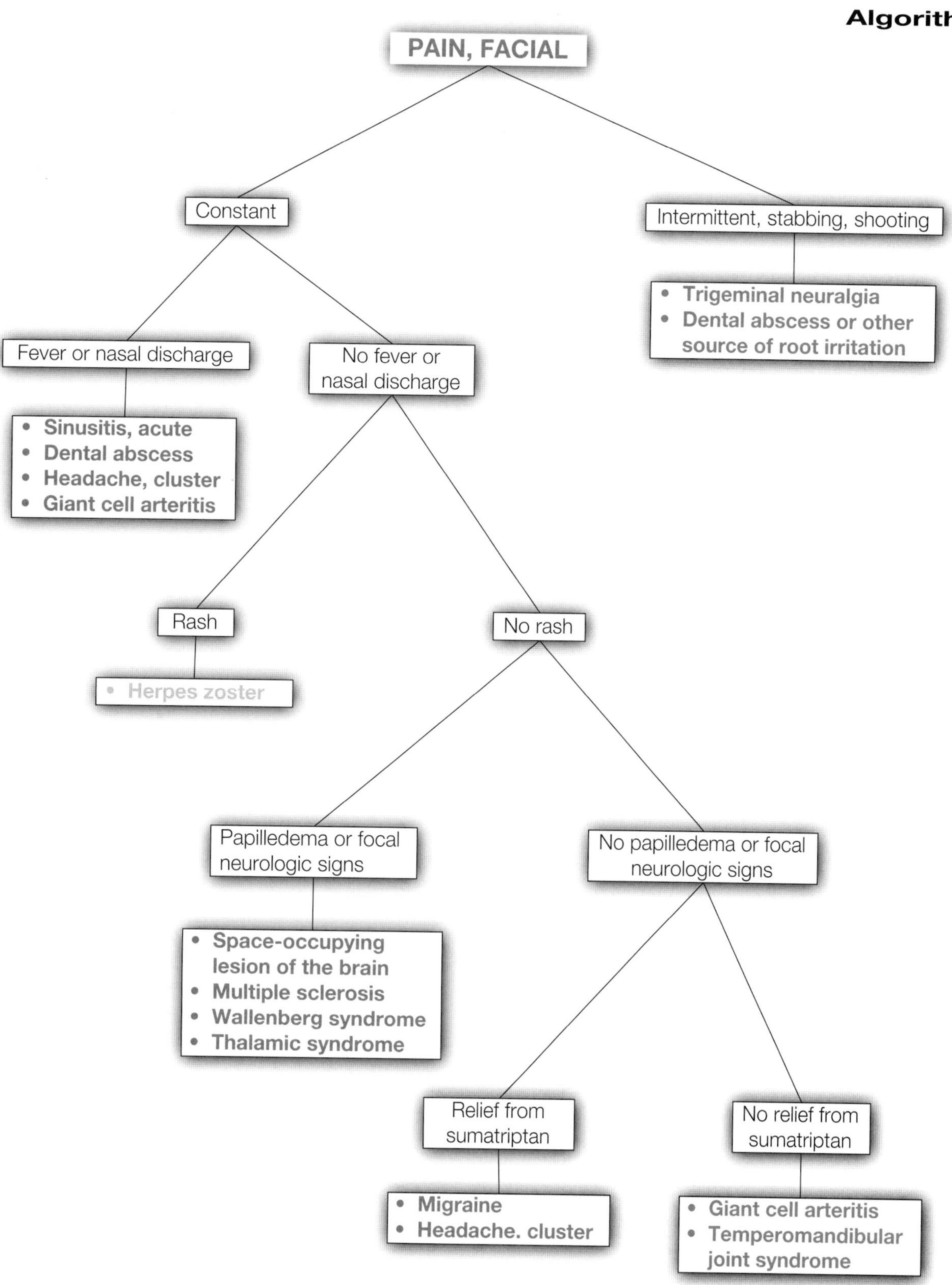
PAIN, FACIAL
Constant
Intermittent, stabbing, shooting
• Trigeminal neuralgia
• Dental abscess or other source of root irritation
Fever or nasal discharge
No fever or nasal discharge
• Sinusitis, acute
• Dental abscess
• Headache, cluster
• Giant cell arteritis
Rash
No rash
• Herpes zoster
Papilledema or focal neurologic signs
No papilledema or focal neurologic signs
• Space-occupying lesion of the brain
• Multiple sclerosis
• Wallenberg syndrome
• Thalamic syndrome
Relief from sumatriptan
No relief from sumatriptan
• Migraine
• Headache. cluster
• Giant cell arteritis
• Temperomandibular joint syndrome

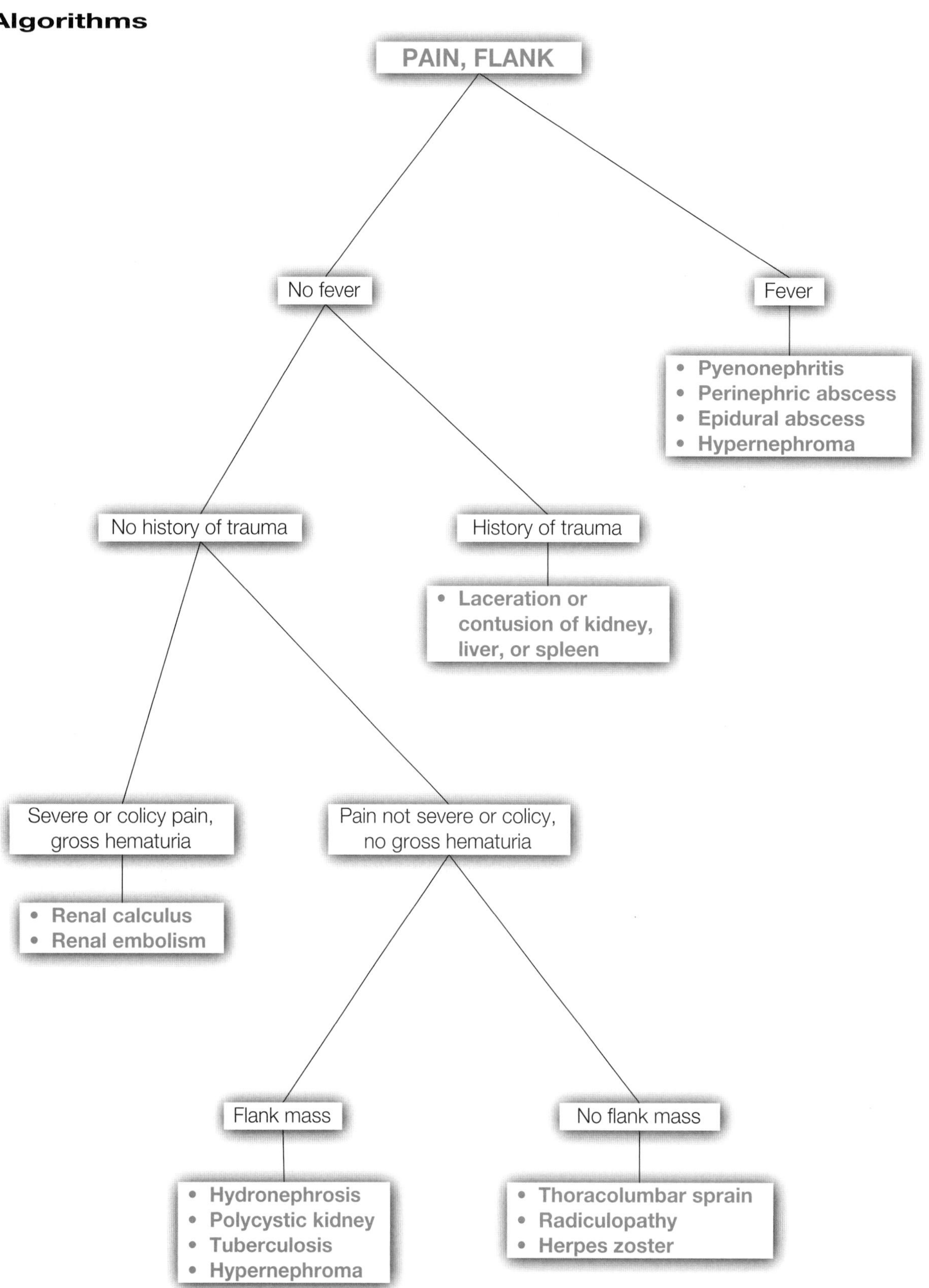
PAIN, FLANK
No fever
Fever
• Pyenonephritis
• Perinephric abscess
• Epidural abscess
• Hypernephroma
No history of trauma
History of trauma
• Laceration or contusion of kidney, liver, or spleen
Severe or colicy pain, gross hematuria
• Renal calculus
• Renal embolism
Pain not severe or colicy, no gross hematuria
Flank mass
• Hydronephrosis
• Polycystic kidney
• Tuberculosis
• Hypernephroma
No flank mass
• Thoracolumbar sprain
• Radiculopathy
• Herpes zoster

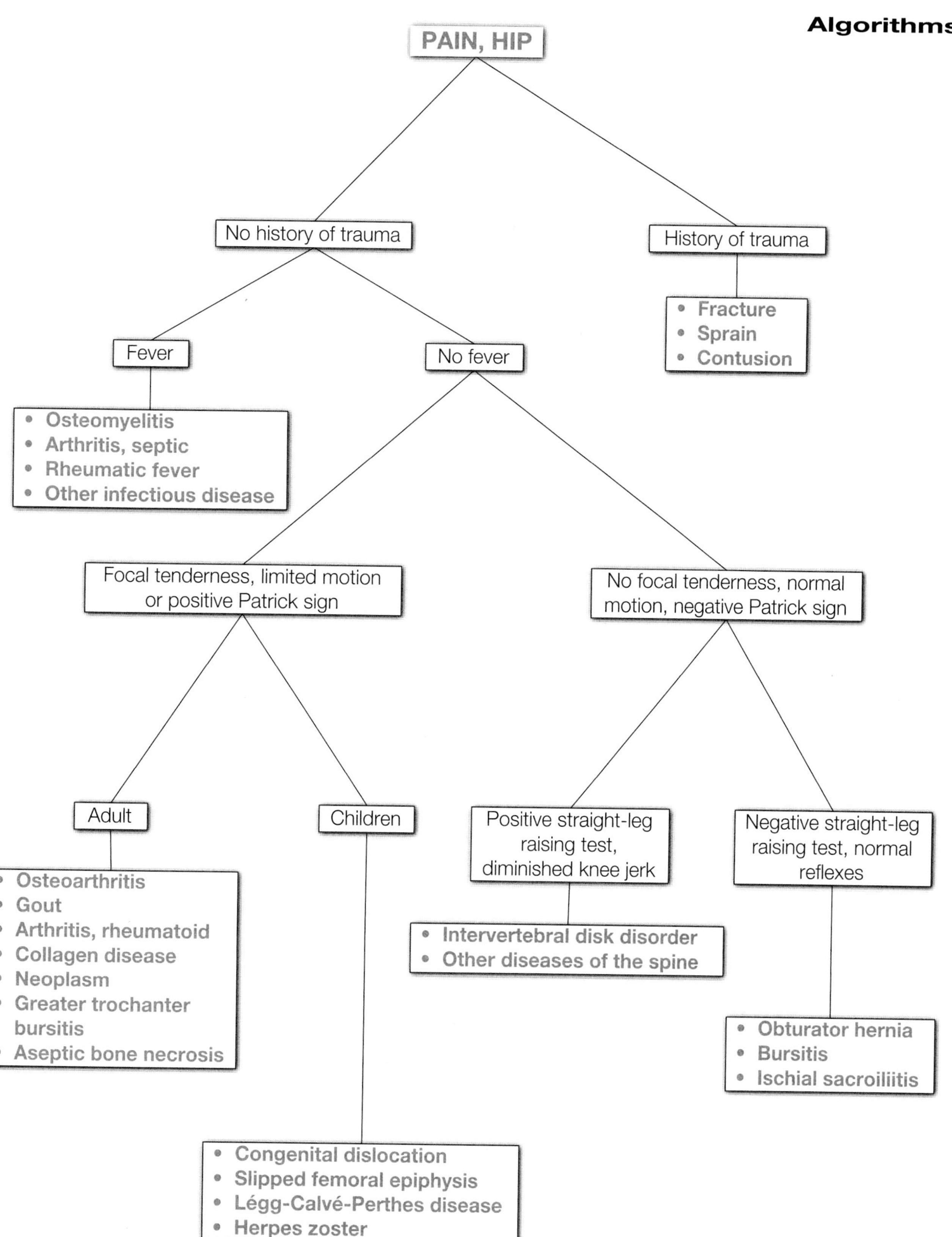
PAIN, HIP
No history of trauma
History of trauma
• Fracture
• Sprain
• Contusion
Fever
No fever
• Osteomyelitis
• Arthritis, septic
• Rheumatic fever
• Other infectious disease
Focal tenderness, limited motion or positive Patrick sign
No focal tenderness, normal motion, negative Patrick sign
Adult
Children
Positive straight-leg raising test, diminished knee jerk
Negative straight-leg raising test, normal reflexes
• Osteoarthritis
• Gout
• Arthritis, rheumatoid
• Collagen disease
• Neoplasm
• Greater trochanter bursitis
• Aseptic bone necrosis
• Intervertebral disk disorder
• Other diseases of the spine
• Obturator hernia
• Bursitis
• Ischial sacroiliitis
• Congenital dislocation
• Slipped femoral epiphysis
• Légg-Calvé-Perthes disease
• Herpes zoster

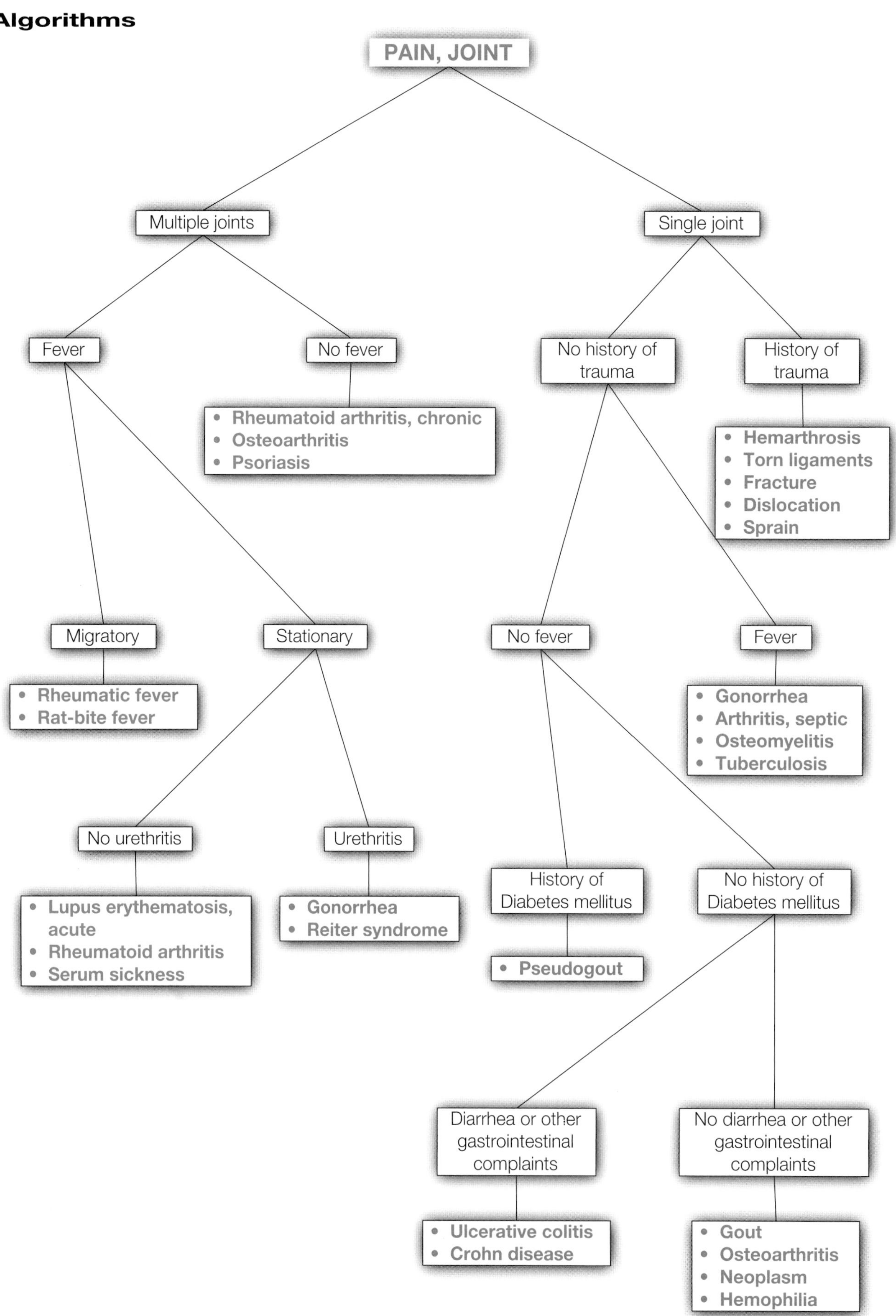
PAIN, JOINT
Multiple joints
Single joint
Fever
No fever
• Rheumatoid arthritis, chronic
• Osteoarthritis
• Psoriasis
No history of trauma
History of trauma
• Hemarthrosis
• Torn ligaments
• Fracture
• Dislocation
• Sprain
Migratory
• Rheumatic fever
• Rat-bite fever
Stationary
No urethritis
• Lupus erythematosis, acute
• Rheumatoid arthritis
• Serum sickness
Urethritis
• Gonorrhea
• Reiter syndrome
No fever
History of Diabetes mellitus
• Pseudogout
No history of Diabetes mellitus
Diarrhea or other gastrointestinal complaints
• Ulcerative colitis
• Crohn disease
No diarrhea or other gastrointestinal complaints
• Gout
• Osteoarthritis
• Neoplasm
• Hemophilia
Fever
• Gonorrhea
• Arthritis, septic
• Osteomyelitis
• Tuberculosis

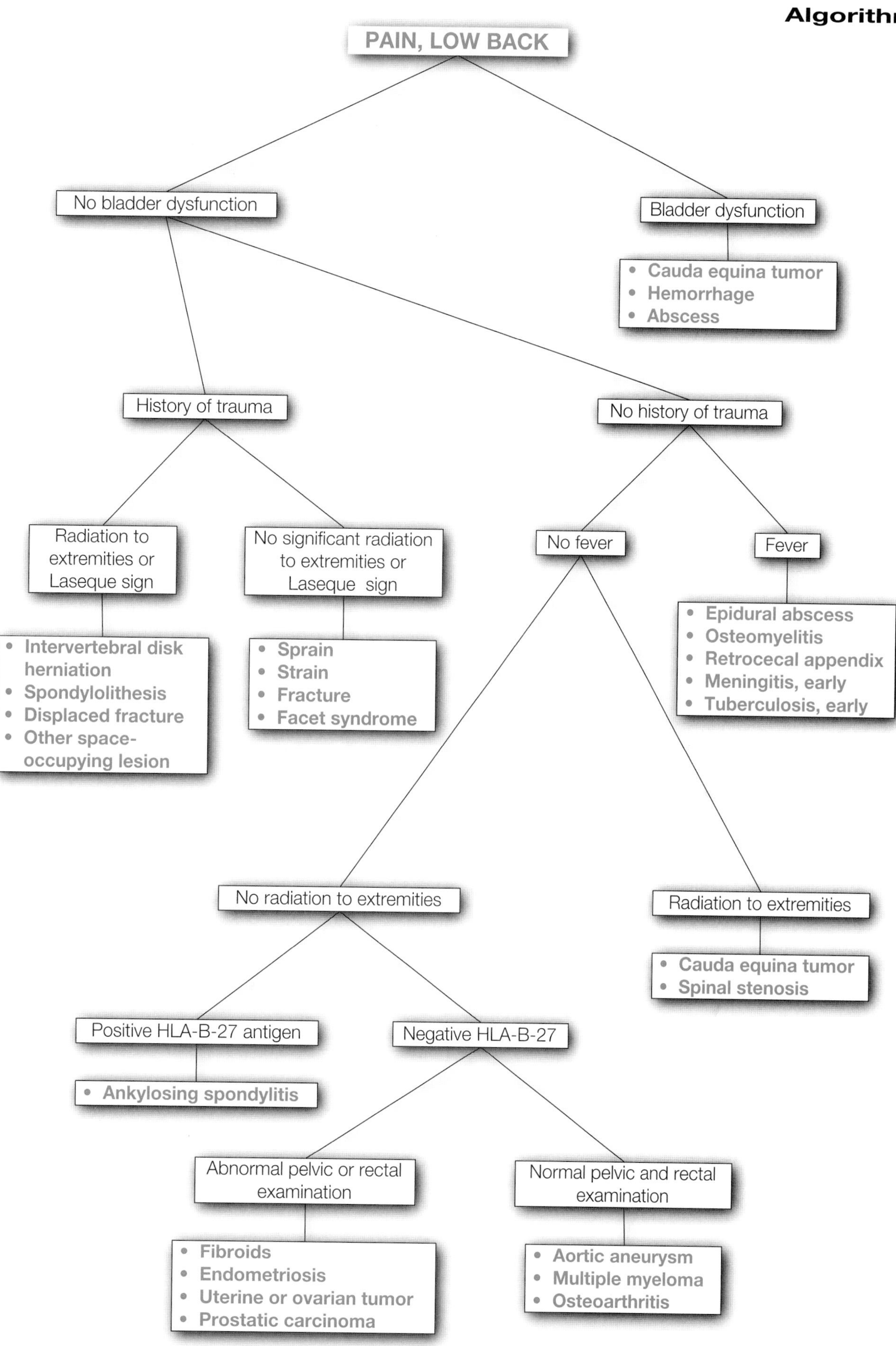
PAIN, LOW BACK
No bladder dysfunction
Bladder dysfunction
• Cauda equina tumor
• Hemorrhage
• Abscess
History of trauma
No history of trauma
Radiation to extremities or Laseque sign
No significant radiation to extremities or Laseque sign
No fever
Fever
• Intervertebral disk herniation
• Spondylolithesis
• Displaced fracture
• Other space-occupying lesion
• Sprain
• Strain
• Fracture
• Facet syndrome
• Epidural abscess
• Osteomyelitis
• Retrocecal appendix
• Meningitis, early
• Tuberculosis, early
No radiation to extremities
Radiation to extremities
• Cauda equina tumor
• Spinal stenosis
Positive HLA-B-27 antigen
Negative HLA-B-27
• Ankylosing spondylitis
Abnormal pelvic or rectal examination
Normal pelvic and rectal examination
• Fibroids
• Endometriosis
• Uterine or ovarian tumor
• Prostatic carcinoma
• Aortic aneurysm
• Multiple myeloma
• Osteoarthritis

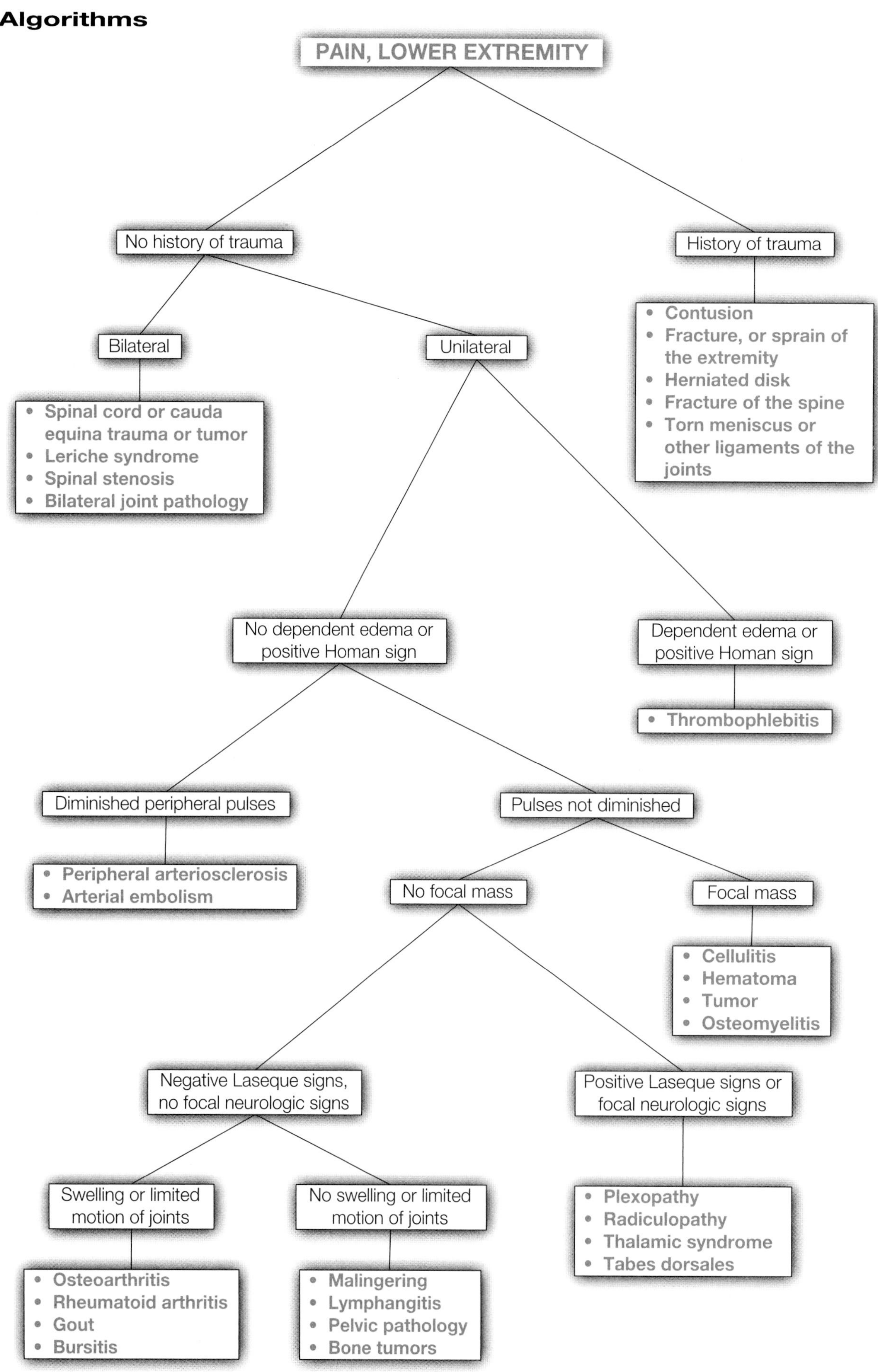
PAIN, LOWER EXTREMITY
No history of trauma
History of trauma
Contusion
Fracture, or sprain of the extremity
Herniated disk
Fracture of the spine
Torn meniscus or other ligaments of the joints
Bilateral
Unilateral
Spinal cord or cauda equina trauma or tumor
Leriche syndrome
Spinal stenosis
Bilateral joint pathology
No dependent edema or positive Homan sign
Dependent edema or positive Homan sign
Thrombophlebitis
Diminished peripheral pulses
Pulses not diminished
Peripheral arteriosclerosis
Arterial embolism
No focal mass
Focal mass
Cellulitis
Hematoma
Tumor
Osteomyelitis
Negative Laseque signs, no focal neurologic signs
Positive Laseque signs or focal neurologic signs
Swelling or limited motion of joints
No swelling or limited motion of joints
Plexopathy
Radiculopathy
Thalamic syndrome
Tabes dorsales
Osteoarthritis
Rheumatoid arthritis
Gout
Bursitis
Malingering
Lymphangitis
Pelvic pathology
Bone tumors

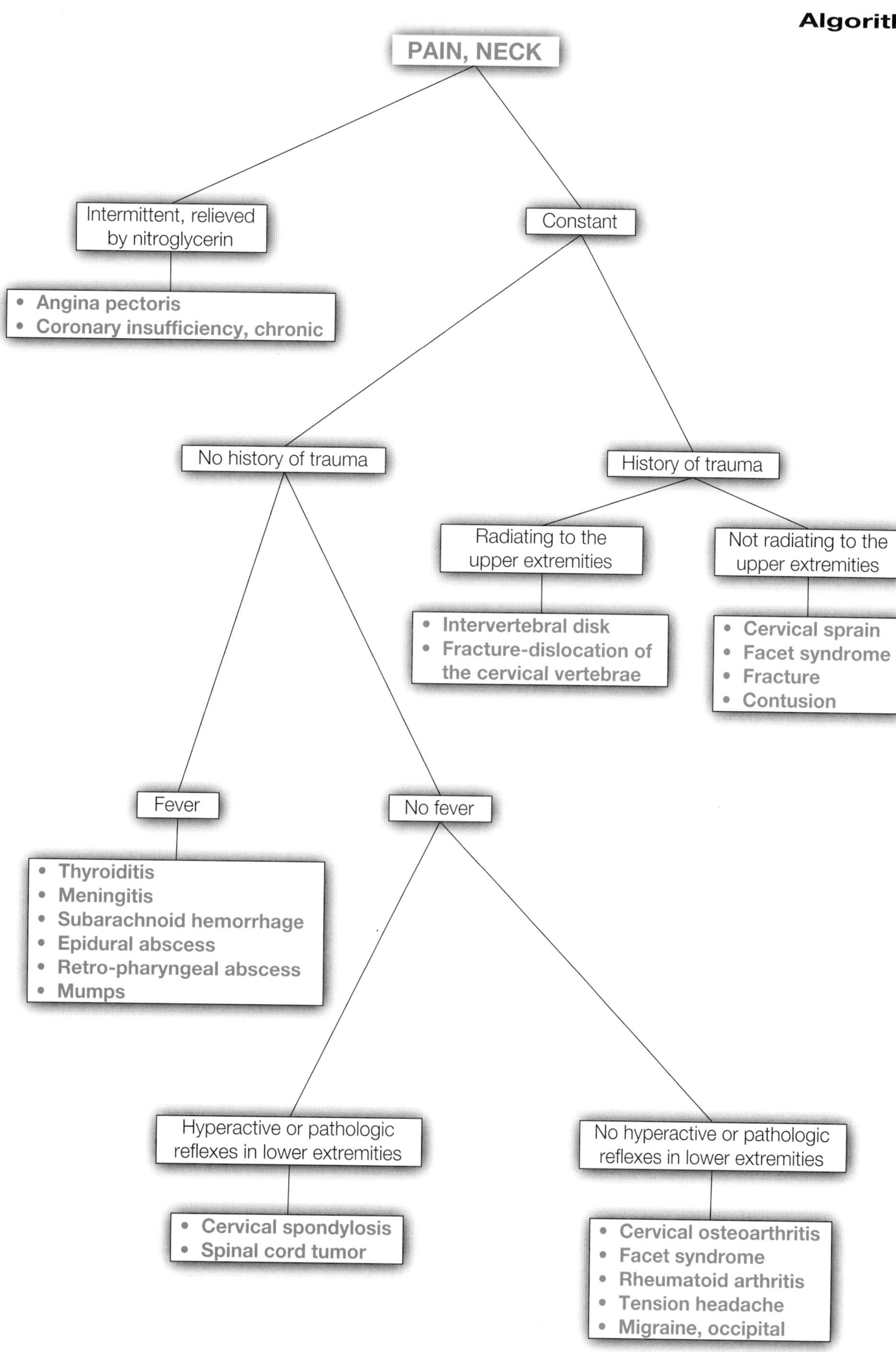
PAIN, NECK
Intermittent, relieved by nitroglycerin
• Angina pectoris
• Coronary insufficiency, chronic
Constant
No history of trauma
History of trauma
Radiating to the upper extremities
• Intervertebral disk
• Fracture-dislocation of the cervical vertebrae
Not radiating to the upper extremities
• Cervical sprain
• Facet syndrome
• Fracture
• Contusion
Fever
• Thyroiditis
• Meningitis
• Subarachnoid hemorrhage
• Epidural abscess
• Retro-pharyngeal abscess
• Mumps
No fever
Hyperactive or pathologic reflexes in lower extremities
• Cervical spondylosis
• Spinal cord tumor
No hyperactive or pathologic reflexes in lower extremities
• Cervical osteoarthritis
• Facet syndrome
• Rheumatoid arthritis
• Tension headache
• Migraine, occipital

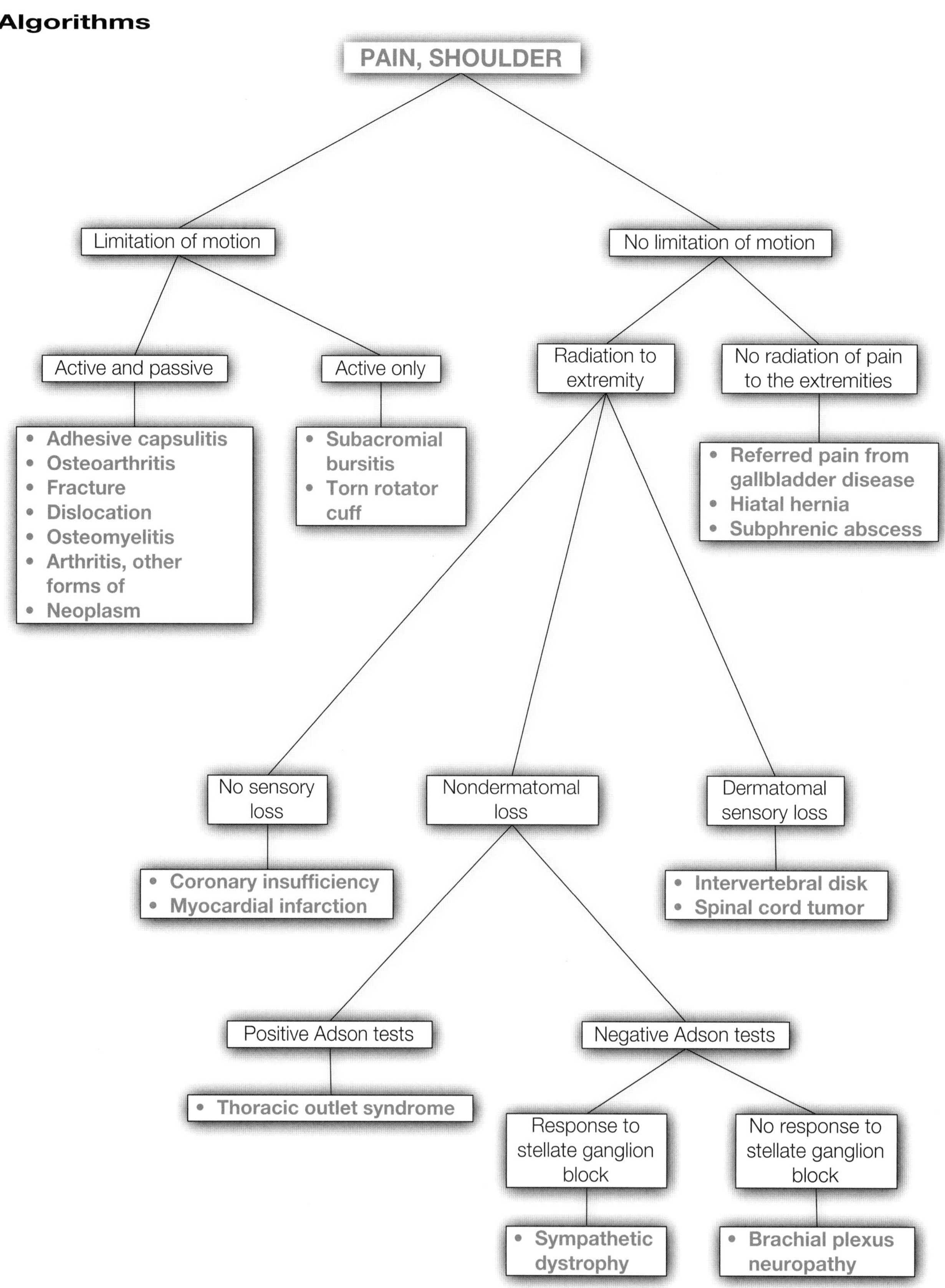
PAIN, SHOULDER
Limitation of motion
No limitation of motion
Active and passive
Active only
Radiation to extremity
No radiation of pain to the extremities
• Adhesive capsulitis
• Osteoarthritis
• Fracture
• Dislocation
• Osteomyelitis
• Arthritis, other forms of
• Neoplasm
• Subacromial bursitis
• Torn rotator cuff
• Referred pain from gallbladder disease
• Hiatal hernia
• Subphrenic abscess
No sensory loss
Nondermatomal loss
Dermatomal sensory loss
• Coronary insufficiency
• Myocardial infarction
• Intervertebral disk
• Spinal cord tumor
Positive Adson tests
Negative Adson tests
• Thoracic outlet syndrome
Response to stellate ganglion block
No response to stellate ganglion block
• Sympathetic dystrophy
• Brachial plexus neuropathy

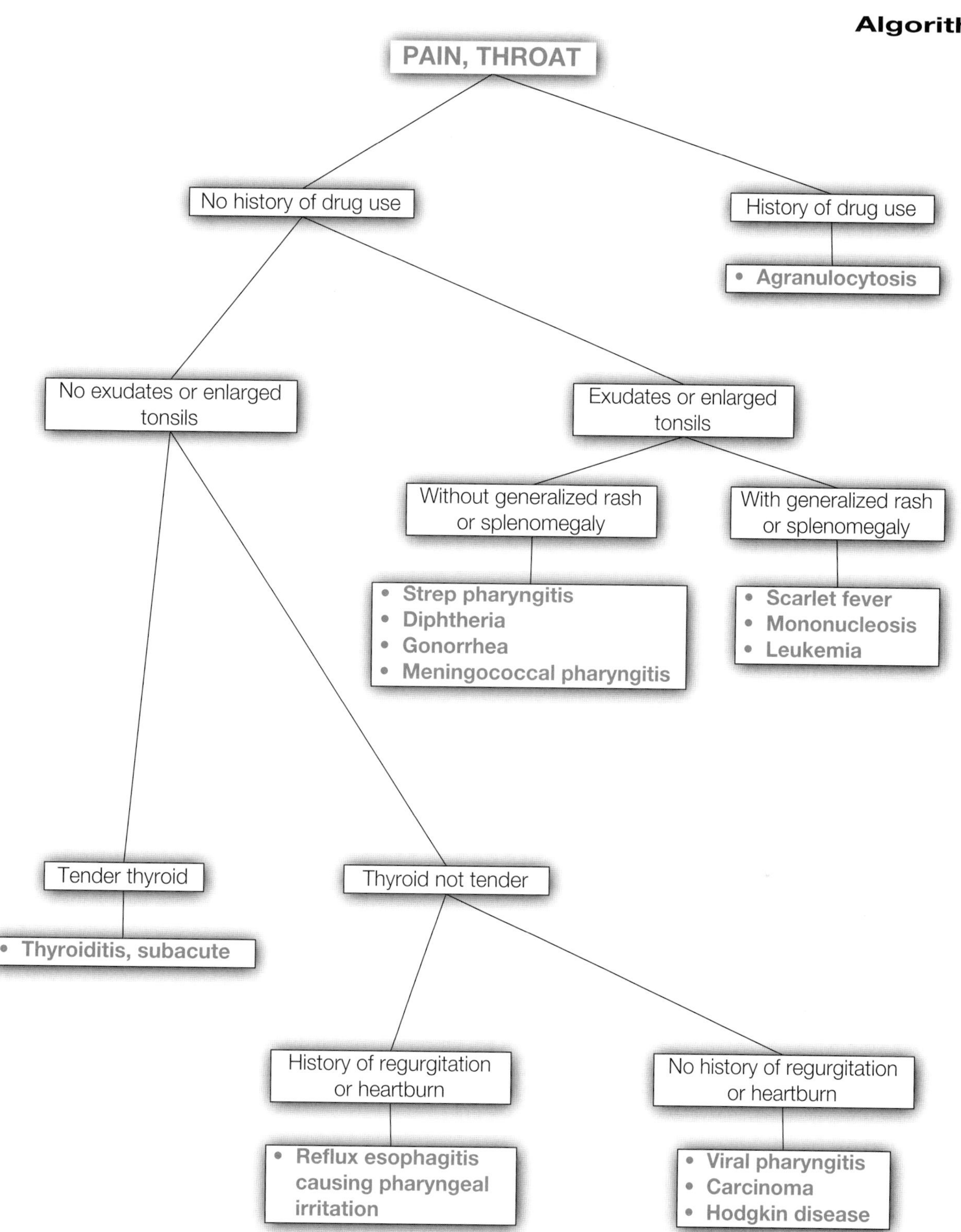
PAIN, THROAT
No history of drug use
History of drug use
• Agranulocytosis
No exudates or enlarged tonsils
Exudates or enlarged tonsils
Without generalized rash or splenomegaly
With generalized rash or splenomegaly
• Strep pharyngitis
• Diphtheria
• Gonorrhea
• Meningococcal pharyngitis
• Scarlet fever
• Mononucleosis
• Leukemia
Tender thyroid
• Thyroiditis, subacute
Thyroid not tender
History of regurgitation or heartburn
No history of regurgitation or heartburn
• Reflux esophagitis causing pharyngeal irritation
• Viral pharyngitis
• Carcinoma
• Hodgkin disease

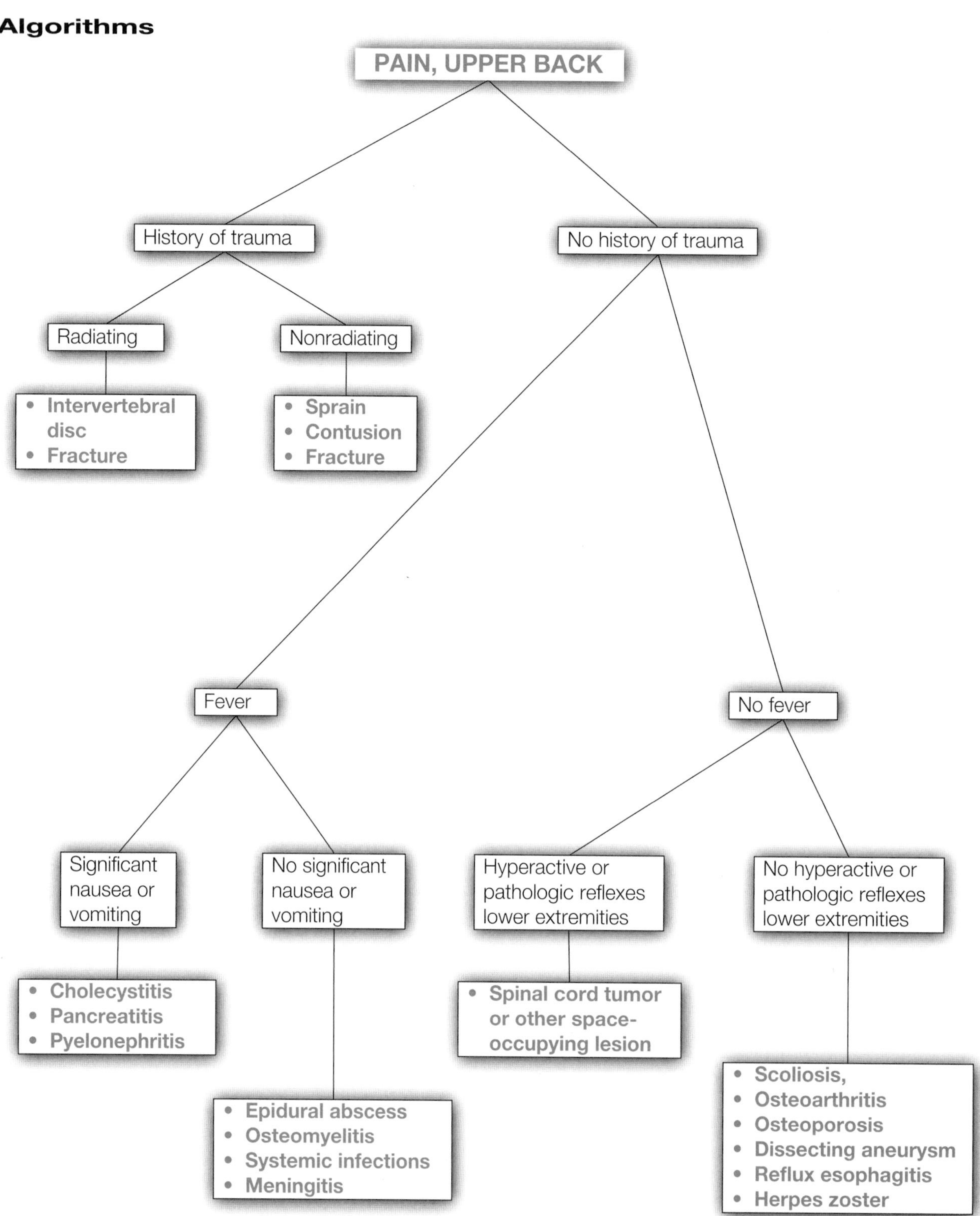
PAIN, UPPER BACK
History of trauma
No history of trauma
Radiating
Nonradiating
• Intervertebral disc
• Fracture
• Sprain
• Contusion
• Fracture
Fever
No fever
Significant nausea or vomiting
No significant nausea or vomiting
Hyperactive or pathologic reflexes lower extremities
No hyperactive or pathologic reflexes lower extremities
• Cholecystitis
• Pancreatitis
• Pyelonephritis
• Spinal cord tumor or other space-occupying lesion
• Epidural abscess
• Osteomyelitis
• Systemic infections
• Meningitis
• Scoliosis,
• Osteoarthritis
• Osteoporosis
• Dissecting aneurysm
• Reflux esophagitis
• Herpes zoster

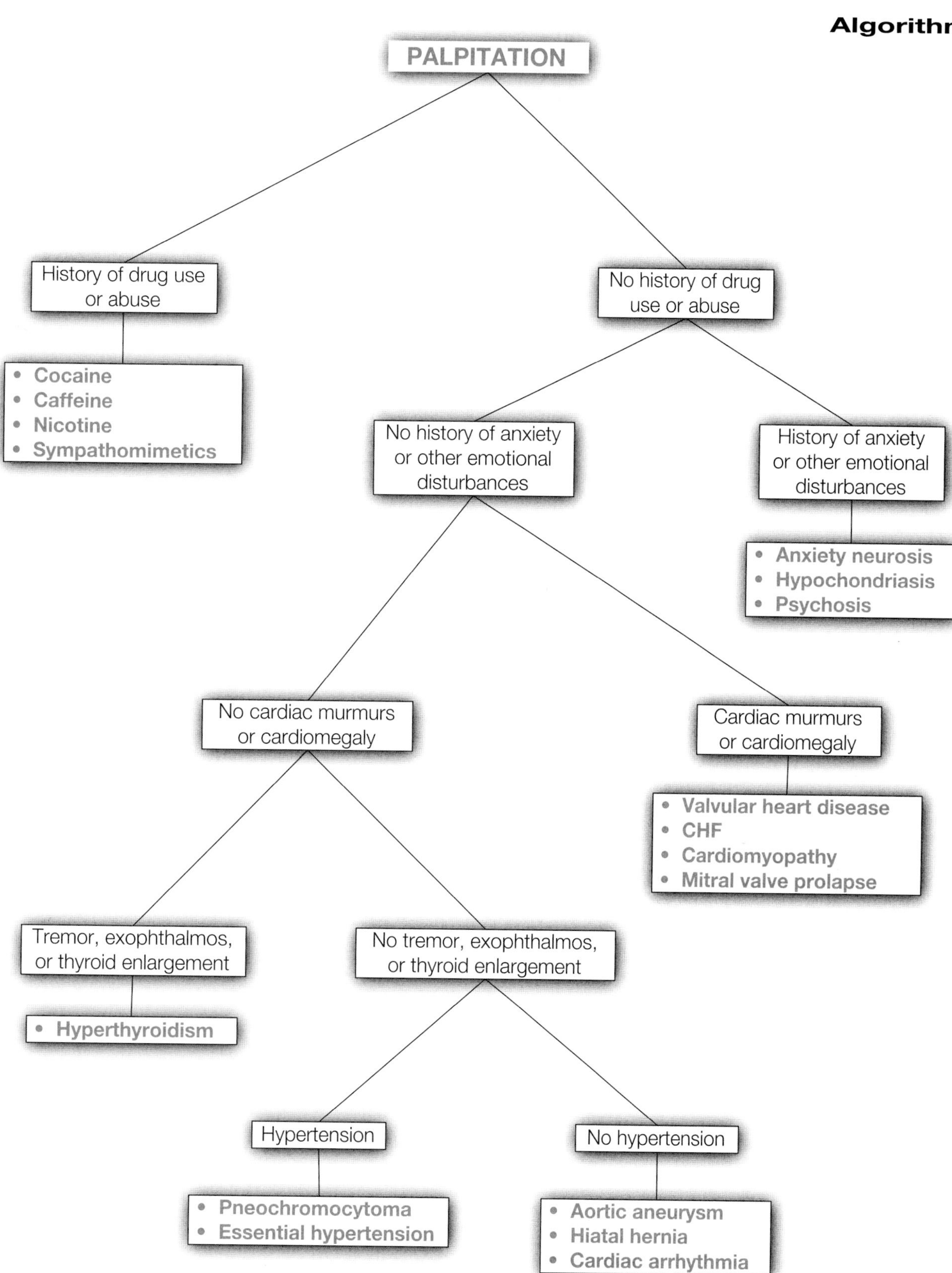
PALPITATION
History of drug use or abuse
• Cocaine
• Caffeine
• Nicotine
• Sympathomimetics
No history of drug use or abuse
No history of anxiety or other emotional disturbances
History of anxiety or other emotional disturbances
• Anxiety neurosis
• Hypochondriasis
• Psychosis
No cardiac murmurs or cardiomegaly
Cardiac murmurs or cardiomegaly
• Valvular heart disease
• CHF
• Cardiomyopathy
• Mitral valve prolapse
Tremor, exophthalmos, or thyroid enlargement
• Hyperthyroidism
No tremor, exophthalmos, or thyroid enlargement
Hypertension
• Pneochromocytoma
• Essential hypertension
No hypertension
• Aortic aneurysm
• Hiatal hernia
• Cardiac arrhythmia

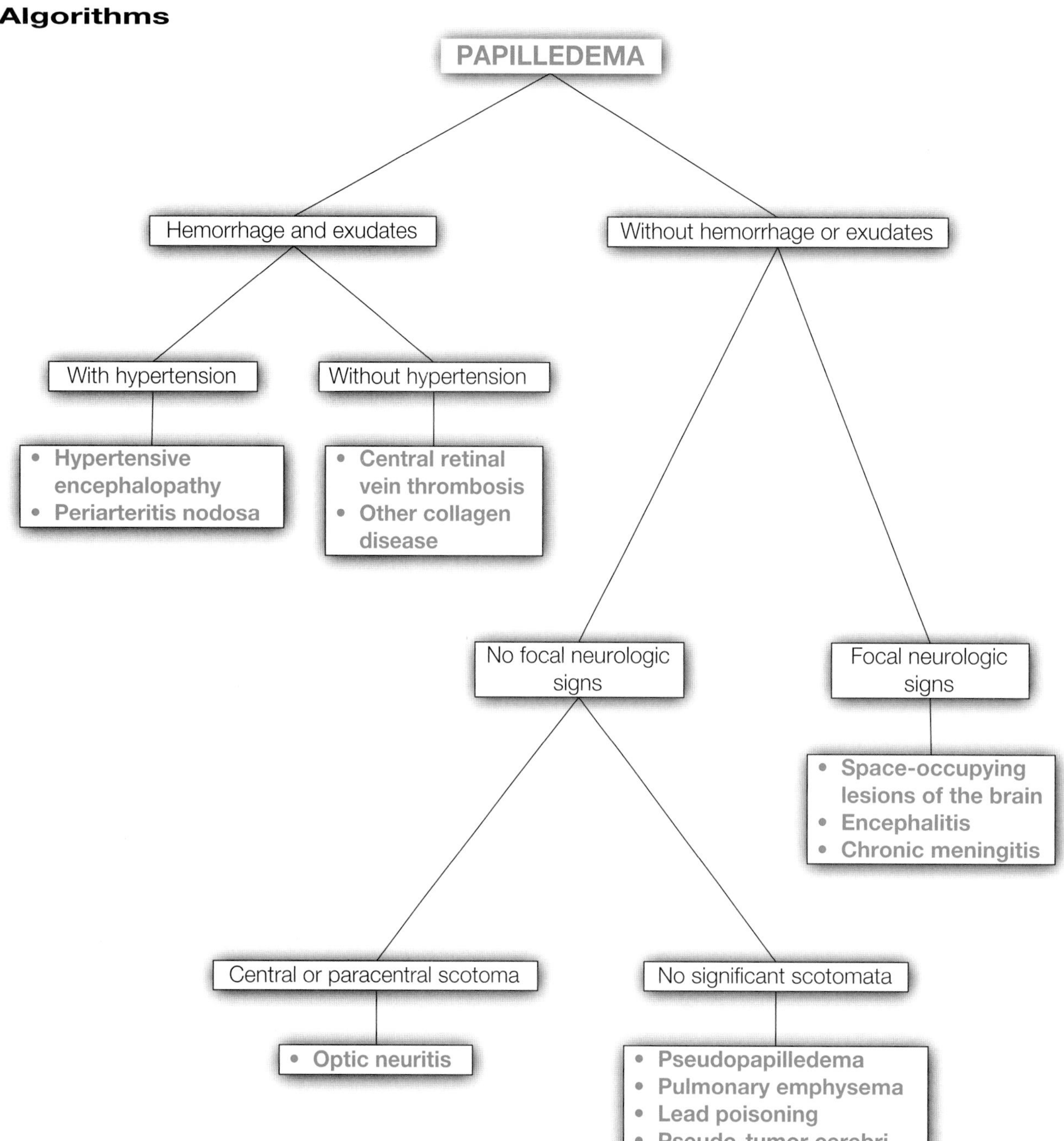
PAPILLEDEMA
Hemorrhage and exudates
Without hemorrhage or exudates
With hypertension
Without hypertension
• Hypertensive encephalopathy
• Periarteritis nodosa
• Central retinal vein thrombosis
• Other collagen disease
No focal neurologic signs
Focal neurologic signs
• Space-occupying lesions of the brain
• Encephalitis
• Chronic meningitis
Central or paracentral scotoma
No significant scotomata
• Optic neuritis
• Pseudopapilledema
• Pulmonary emphysema
• Lead poisoning
• Pseudo-tumor cerebri

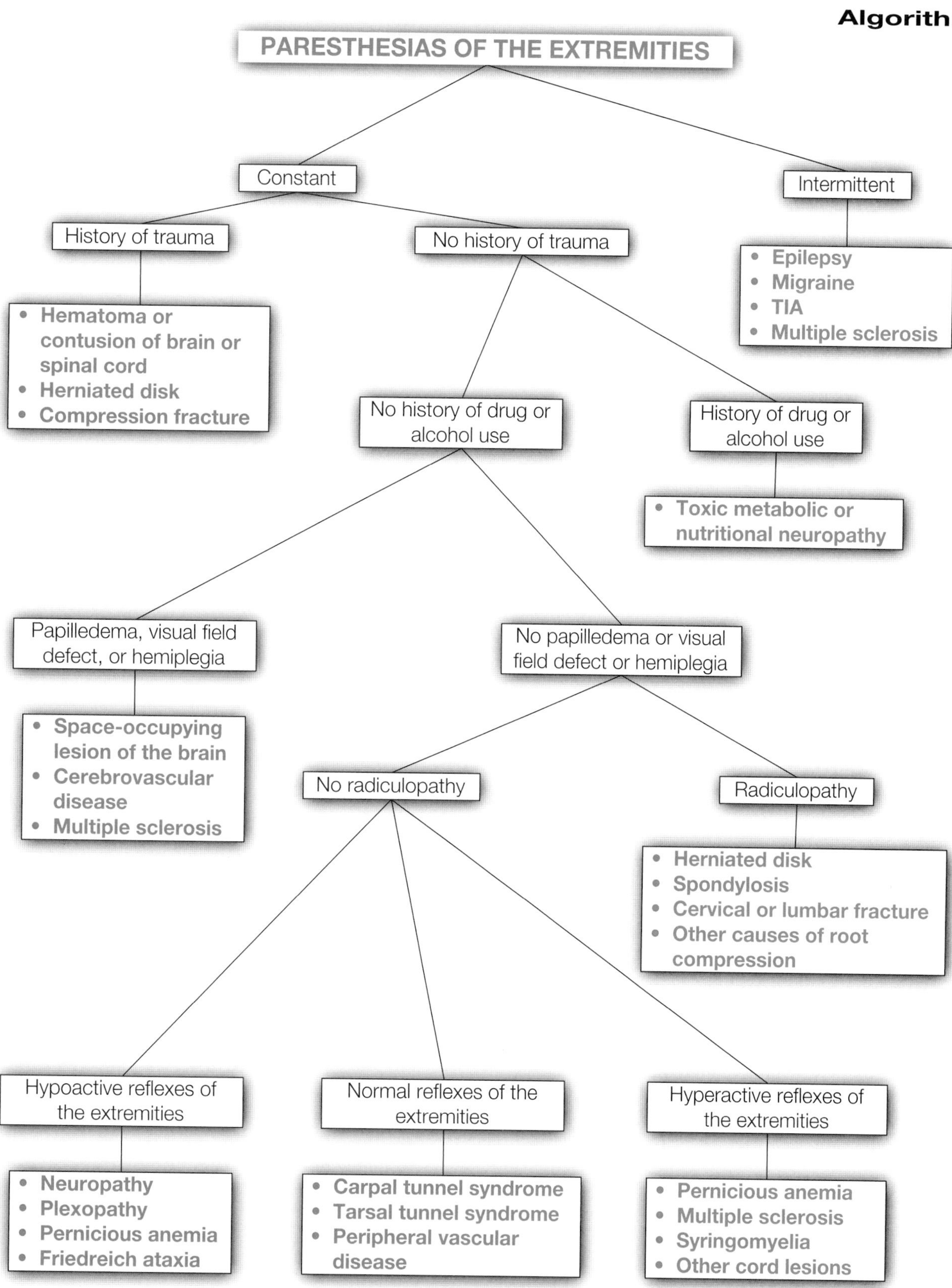
PARESTHESIAS OF THE EXTREMITIES
Constant
Intermittent
History of trauma
No history of trauma
• Hematoma or contusion of brain or spinal cord
• Herniated disk
• Compression fracture
• Epilepsy
• Migraine
• TIA
• Multiple sclerosis
No history of drug or alcohol use
History of drug or alcohol use
• Toxic metabolic or nutritional neuropathy
Papilledema, visual field defect, or hemiplegia
No papilledema or visual field defect or hemiplegia
• Space-occupying lesion of the brain
• Cerebrovascular disease
• Multiple sclerosis
No radiculopathy
Radiculopathy
• Herniated disk
• Spondylosis
• Cervical or lumbar fracture
• Other causes of root compression
Hypoactive reflexes of the extremities
Normal reflexes of the extremities
Hyperactive reflexes of the extremities
• Neuropathy
• Plexopathy
• Pernicious anemia
• Friedreich ataxia
• Carpal tunnel syndrome
• Tarsal tunnel syndrome
• Peripheral vascular disease
• Pernicious anemia
• Multiple sclerosis
• Syringomyelia
• Other cord lesions

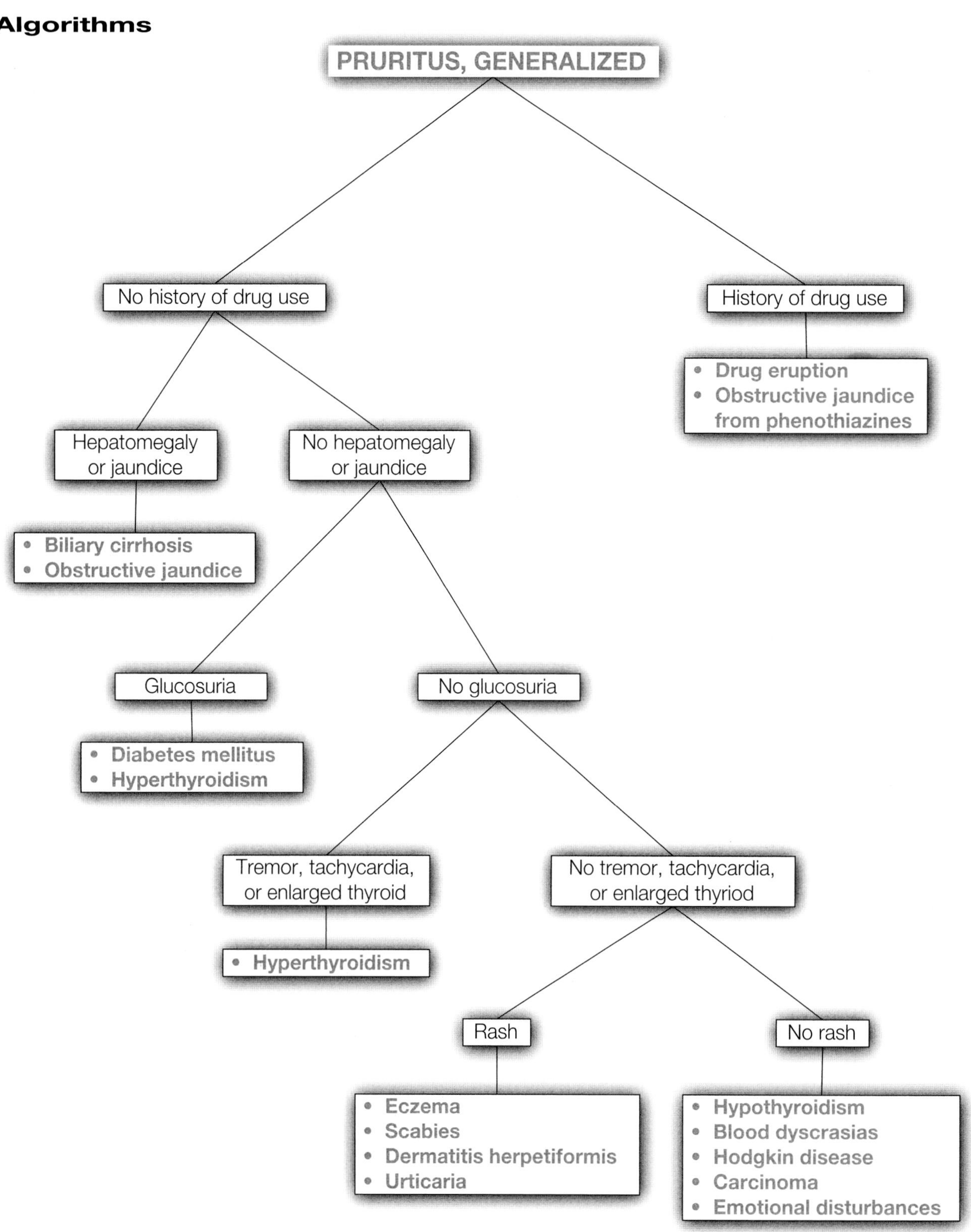
PRURITUS, GENERALIZED
No history of drug use
History of drug use
• Drug eruption
• Obstructive jaundice from phenothiazines
Hepatomegaly or jaundice
No hepatomegaly or jaundice
• Biliary cirrhosis
• Obstructive jaundice
Glucosuria
No glucosuria
• Diabetes mellitus
• Hyperthyroidism
Tremor, tachycardia, or enlarged thyroid
No tremor, tachycardia, or enlarged thyriod
• Hyperthyroidism
Rash
No rash
• Eczema
• Scabies
• Dermatitis herpetiformis
• Urticaria
• Hypothyroidism
• Blood dyscrasias
• Hodgkin disease
• Carcinoma
• Emotional disturbances

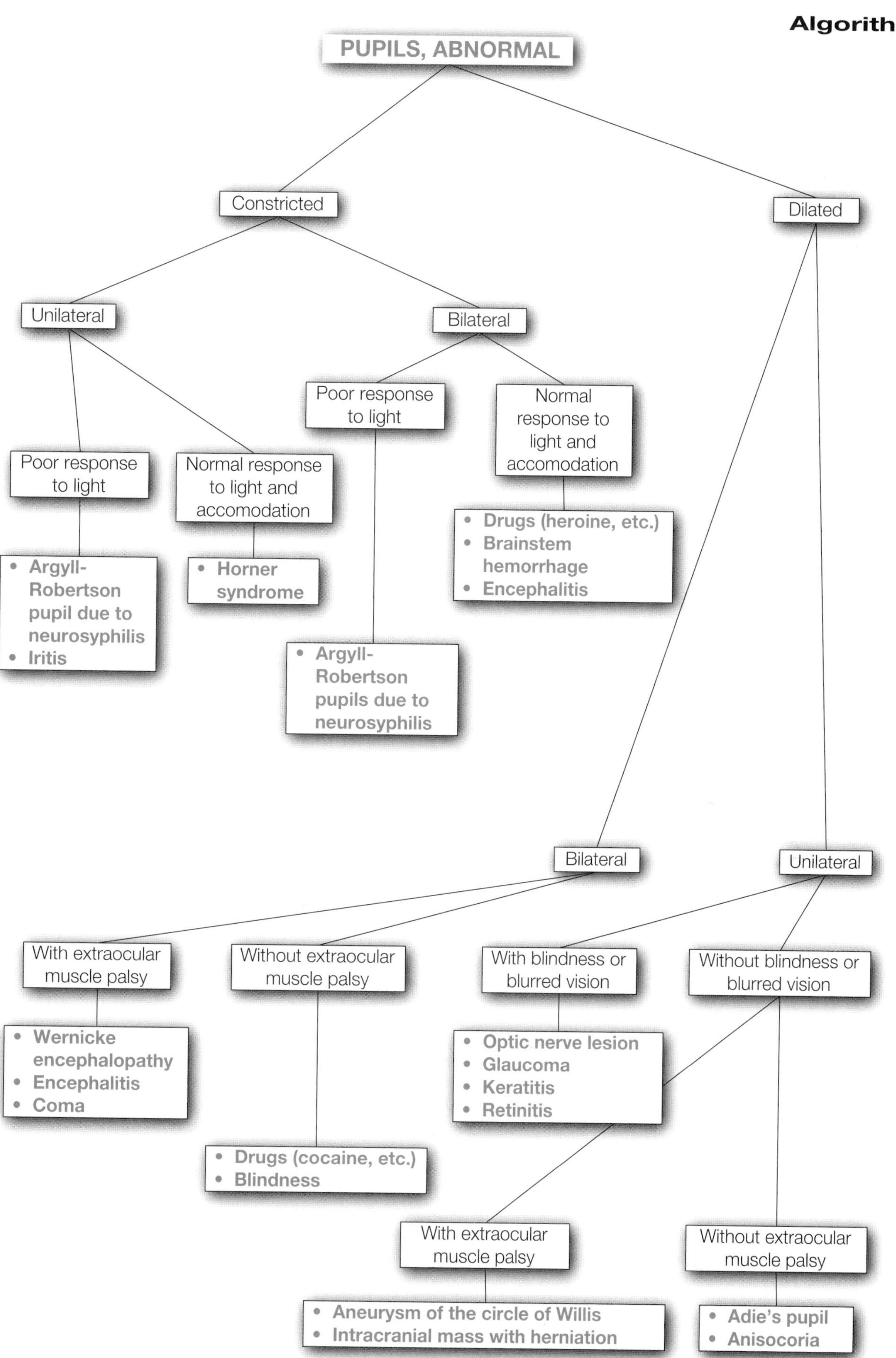
PUPILS, ABNORMAL
Constricted
Dilated
Unilateral
Bilateral
Poor response to light
Normal response to light and accomodation
Poor response to light
Normal response to light and accomodation
• Argyll-Robertson pupil due to neurosyphilis
• Iritis
• Horner syndrome
• Argyll-Robertson pupils due to neurosyphilis
• Drugs (heroine, etc.)
• Brainstem hemorrhage
• Encephalitis
Bilateral
Unilateral
With extraocular muscle palsy
Without extraocular muscle palsy
With blindness or blurred vision
Without blindness or blurred vision
• Wernicke encephalopathy
• Encephalitis
• Coma
• Drugs (cocaine, etc.)
• Blindness
• Optic nerve lesion
• Glaucoma
• Keratitis
• Retinitis
With extraocular muscle palsy
Without extraocular muscle palsy
• Aneurysm of the circle of Willis
• Intracranial mass with herniation
• Adie's pupil
• Anisocoria

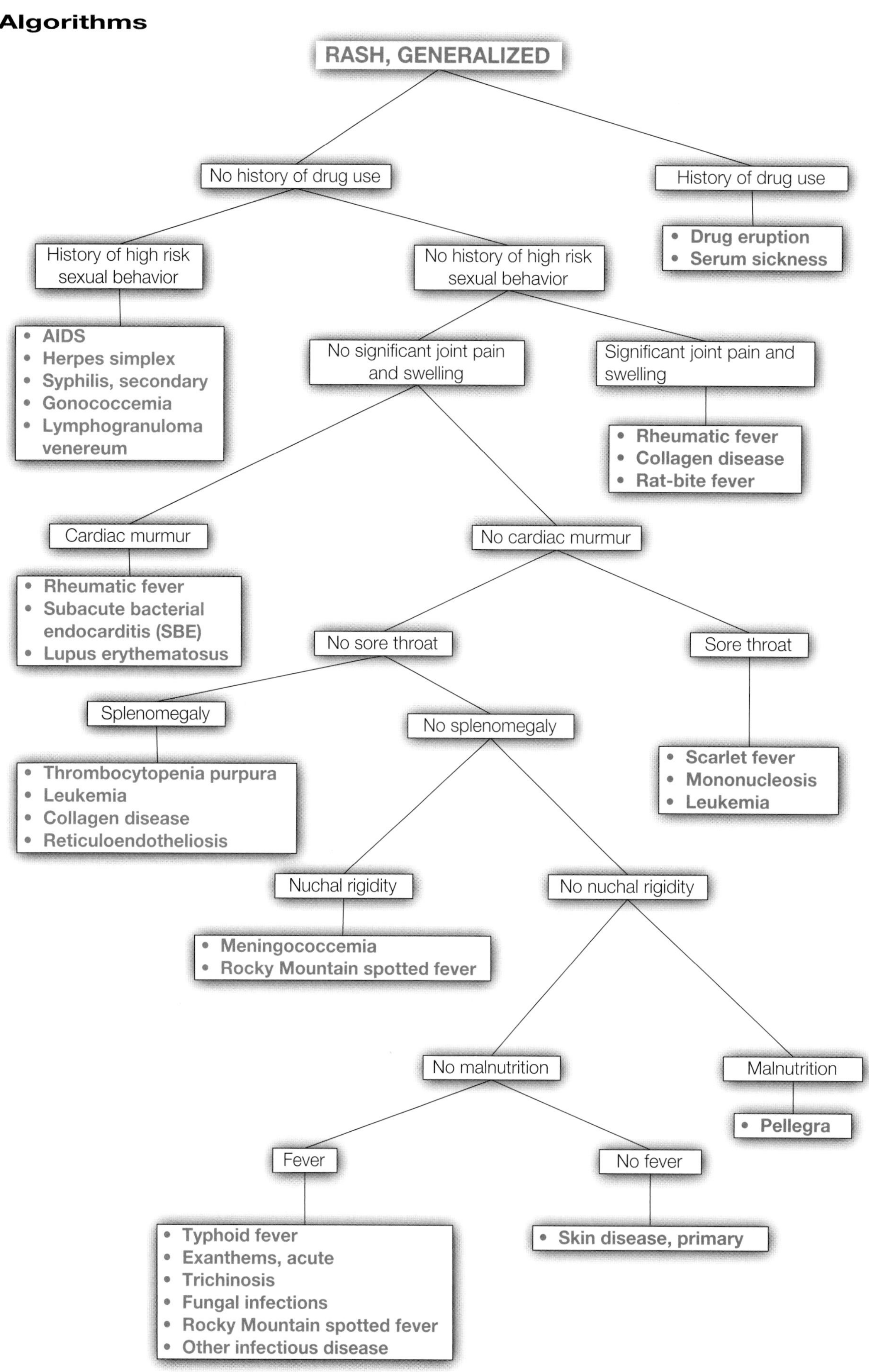
RASH, GENERALIZED
No history of drug use
History of drug use
• Drug eruption
• Serum sickness
History of high risk sexual behavior
• AIDS
• Herpes simplex
• Syphilis, secondary
• Gonococcemia
• Lymphogranuloma venereum
No history of high risk sexual behavior
No significant joint pain and swelling
Significant joint pain and swelling
• Rheumatic fever
• Collagen disease
• Rat-bite fever
Cardiac murmur
• Rheumatic fever
• Subacute bacterial endocarditis (SBE)
• Lupus erythematosus
No cardiac murmur
No sore throat
Sore throat
• Scarlet fever
• Mononucleosis
• Leukemia
Splenomegaly
• Thrombocytopenia purpura
• Leukemia
• Collagen disease
• Reticuloendotheliosis
No splenomegaly
Nuchal rigidity
• Meningococcemia
• Rocky Mountain spotted fever
No nuchal rigidity
No malnutrition
Malnutrition
• Pellegra
Fever
• Typhoid fever
• Exanthems, acute
• Trichinosis
• Fungal infections
• Rocky Mountain spotted fever
• Other infectious disease
No fever
• Skin disease, primary

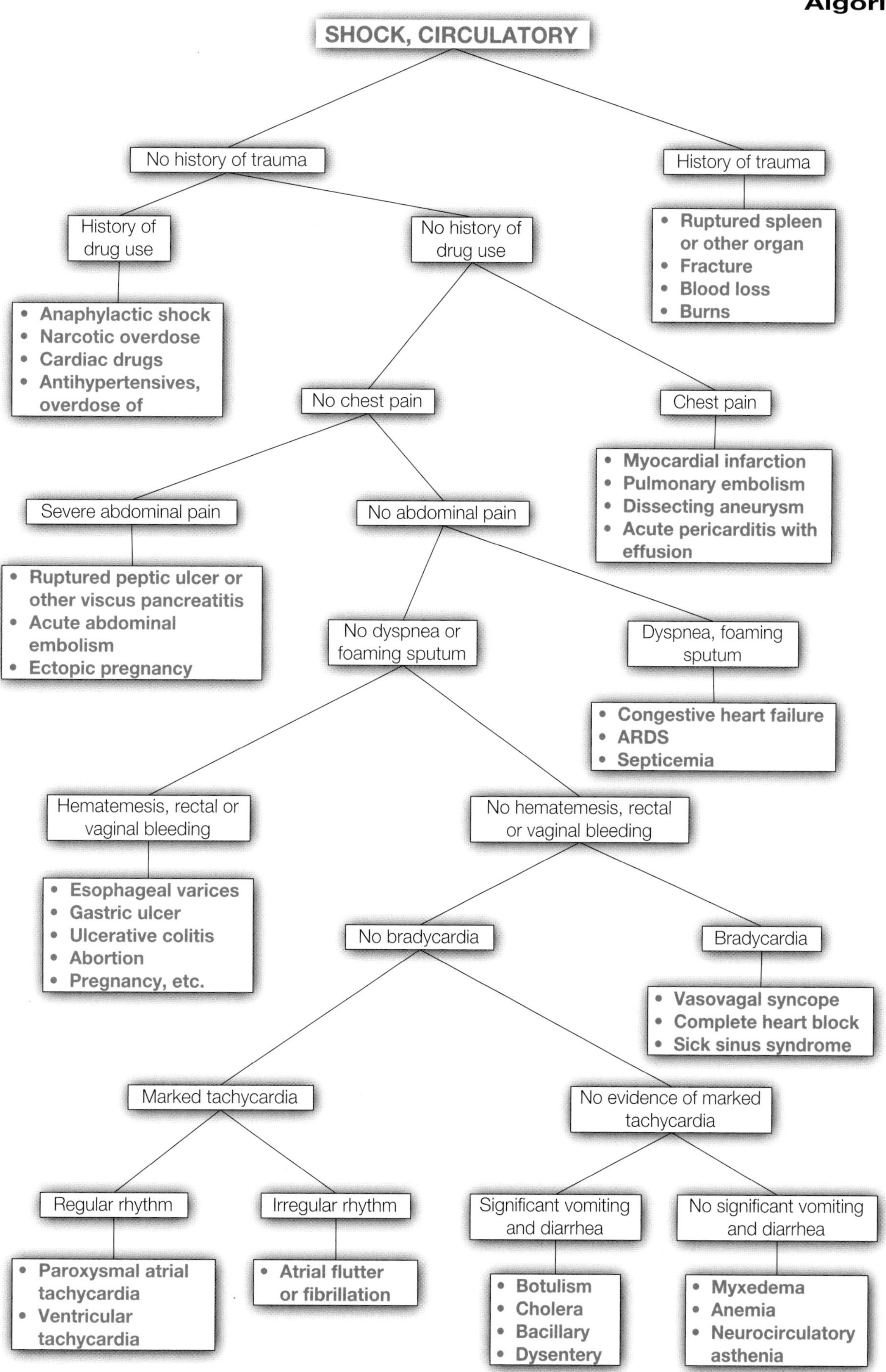

Signs & Symptoms

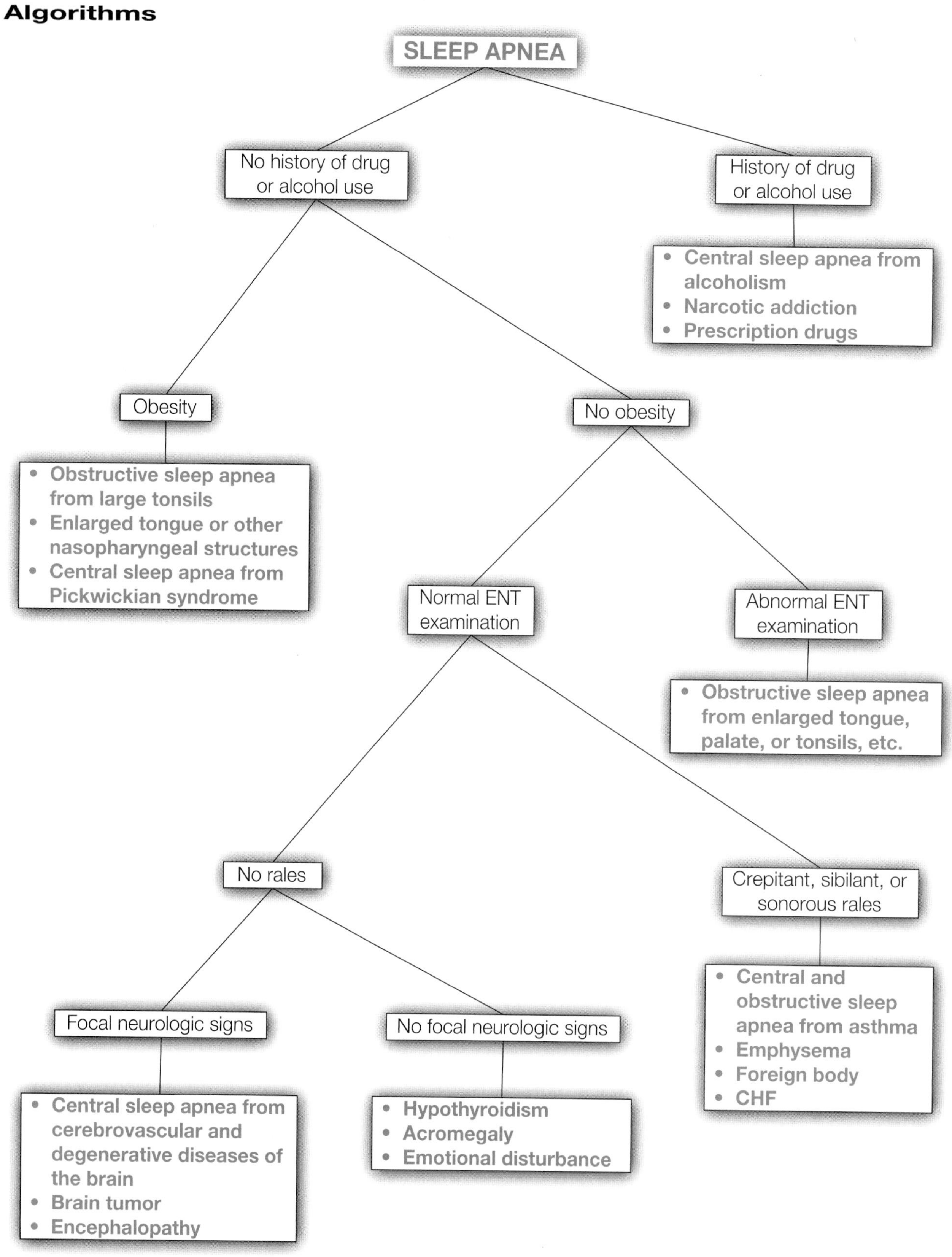
SLEEP APNEA
No history of drug or alcohol use
History of drug or alcohol use
• Central sleep apnea from alcoholism
• Narcotic addiction
• Prescription drugs
Obesity
No obesity
• Obstructive sleep apnea from large tonsils
• Enlarged tongue or other nasopharyngeal structures
• Central sleep apnea from Pickwickian syndrome
Normal ENT examination
Abnormal ENT examination
• Obstructive sleep apnea from enlarged tongue, palate, or tonsils, etc.
No rales
Crepitant, sibilant, or sonorous rales
• Central and obstructive sleep apnea from asthma
• Emphysema
• Foreign body
• CHF
Focal neurologic signs
No focal neurologic signs
• Central sleep apnea from cerebrovascular and degenerative diseases of the brain
• Brain tumor
• Encephalopathy
• Hypothyroidism
• Acromegaly
• Emotional disturbance

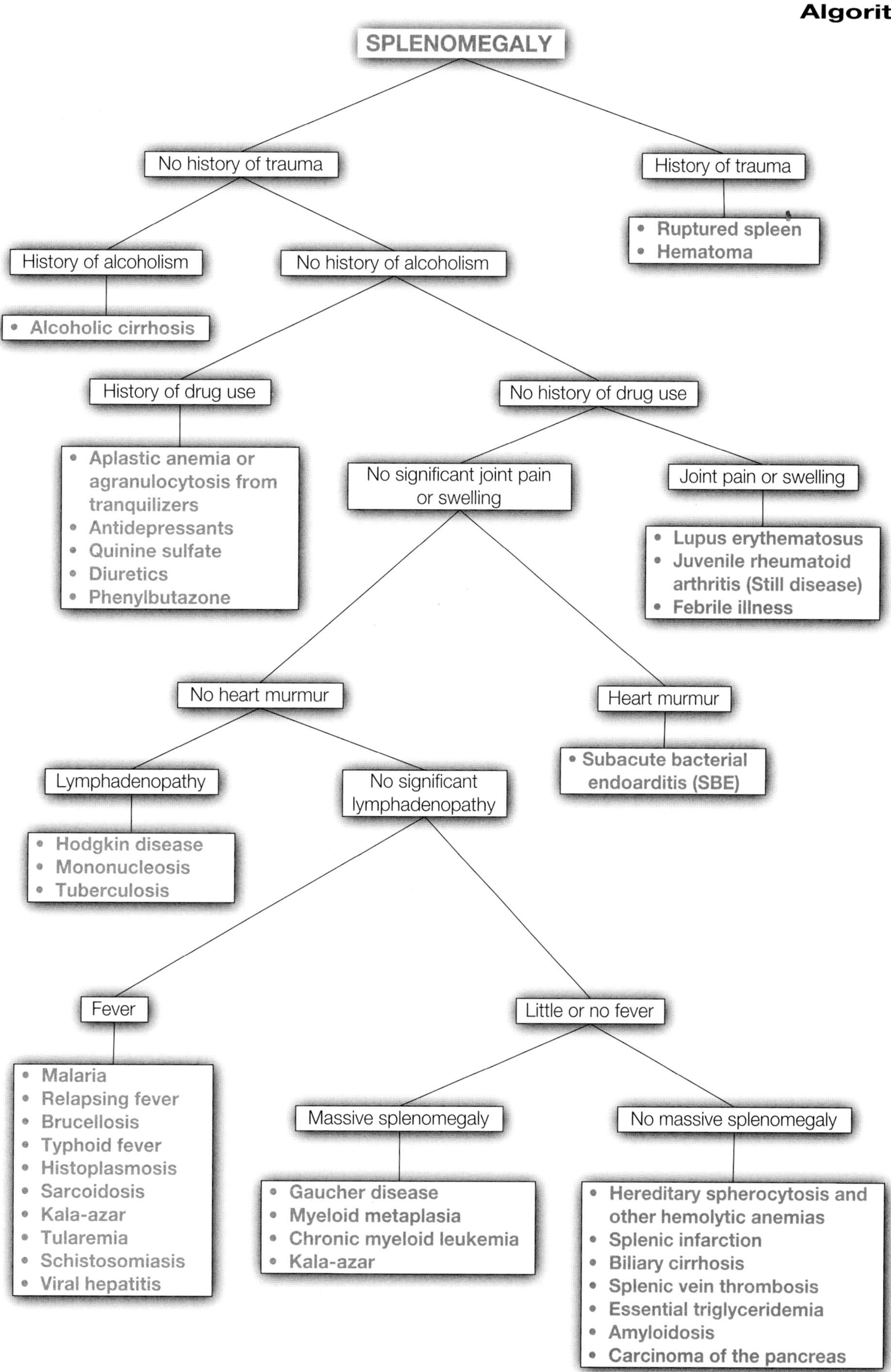
SPLENOMEGALY
No history of trauma
History of trauma
• Ruptured spleen
• Hematoma
History of alcoholism
• Alcoholic cirrhosis
No history of alcoholism
History of drug use
• Aplastic anemia or agranulocytosis from tranquilizers
• Antidepressants
• Quinine sulfate
• Diuretics
• Phenylbutazone
No history of drug use
No significant joint pain or swelling
Joint pain or swelling
• Lupus erythematosus
• Juvenile rheumatoid arthritis (Still disease)
• Febrile illness
No heart murmur
Heart murmur
• Subacute bacterial endoardits (SBE)
Lymphadenopathy
• Hodgkin disease
• Mononucleosis
• Tuberculosis
No significant lymphadenopathy
Fever
• Malaria
• Relapsing fever
• Brucellosis
• Typhoid fever
• Histoplasmosis
• Sarcoidosis
• Kala-azar
• Tularemia
• Schistosomiasis
• Viral hepatitis
Little or no fever
Massive splenomegaly
• Gaucher disease
• Myeloid metaplasia
• Chronic myeloid leukemia
• Kala-azar
No massive splenomegaly
• Hereditary spherocytosis and other hemolytic anemias
• Splenic infarction
• Biliary cirrhosis
• Splenic vein thrombosis
• Essential triglyceridemia
• Amyloidosis
• Carcinoma of the pancreas

SYNCOPE

- **No history of drug use**
  - **History of anxiety, depression, or other emotional disturbances**
    - Hyperventilation syndrome
    - Vasovagal syncope
    - Hysteria
    - Malingering
  - **No history of anxiety, depression, or other emotional disturbances**
    - **Diaphoresis and/or hunger**
      - Insulinoma
      - Insulin reaction
      - Myocardial infarction
    - **No association with diaphoresis or hunger**
      - **No convulsive movements**
        - **Murmur or cardiac arrhythmia**
          - Valvular heart disease
          - Atrial fibrillation
          - Heart block
        - **No murmur or cardiac arrhythmia**
          - **Focal neurologic signs**
            - Stroke
            - TIA
            - Hypoglycemia
          - **No focal neurologic signs**
            - Anemia
            - Heat exhaustion
            - Heat stroke
            - Micturation syncope
            - Cough syncope
            - Carotid sinus syncope
            - Postural hypotension
      - **Convulsive movements**
        - Epilepsy
- **History of drug use**
  - Beta blockers
  - Diuretics
  - Nitrates
  - Hypoglycemic agents

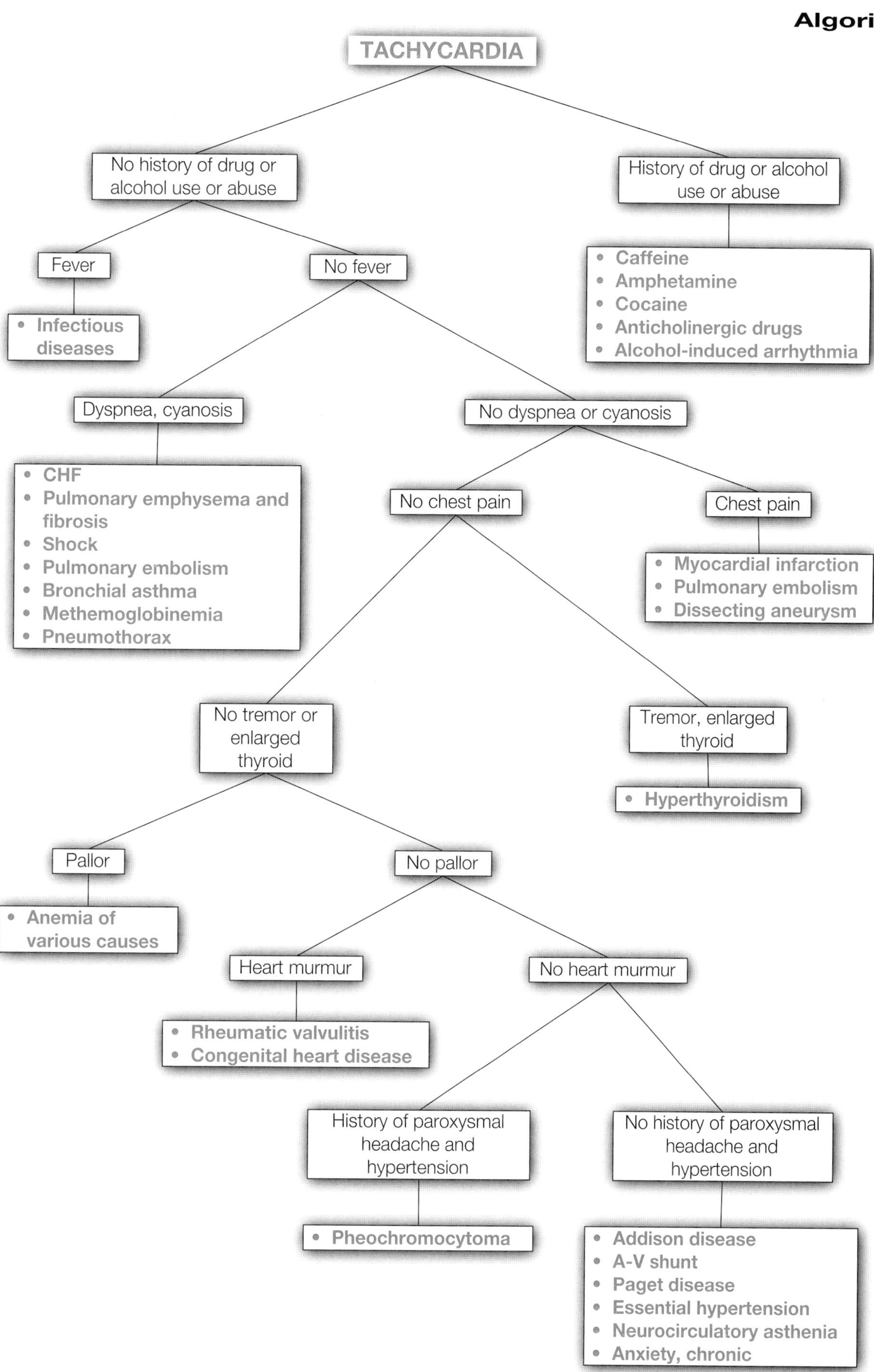
TACHYCARDIA
No history of drug or alcohol use or abuse
History of drug or alcohol use or abuse
• Caffeine
• Amphetamine
• Cocaine
• Anticholinergic drugs
• Alcohol-induced arrhythmia
Fever
• Infectious diseases
No fever
Dyspnea, cyanosis
• CHF
• Pulmonary emphysema and fibrosis
• Shock
• Pulmonary embolism
• Bronchial asthma
• Methemoglobinemia
• Pneumothorax
No dyspnea or cyanosis
No chest pain
Chest pain
• Myocardial infarction
• Pulmonary embolism
• Dissecting aneurysm
No tremor or enlarged thyroid
Tremor, enlarged thyroid
• Hyperthyroidism
Pallor
• Anemia of various causes
No pallor
Heart murmur
• Rheumatic valvulitis
• Congenital heart disease
No heart murmur
History of paroxysmal headache and hypertension
• Pheochromocytoma
No history of paroxysmal headache and hypertension
• Addison disease
• A-V shunt
• Paget disease
• Essential hypertension
• Neurocirculatory asthenia
• Anxiety, chronic

TINNITIS

- **No history of drug use**
  - **Abnormal ENT examination**
    - Cerumen
    - Foreign body
    - Otitis media
    - Perforation
    - Cholesteatoma
  - **Normal ENT examination**
    - **Associated with deafness and/or vertigo**
      - **With focal neurologic signs**
        - Neurosyphilis
        - Tuberculosis
        - Acoustic neuroma, advanced
        - Multiple sclerosis
        - Stroke
        - Vertebrobasilar artery insufficiency
        - Platybasia
        - Brainstem tumor
      - **Without focal neurologic signs**
        - Ménière disease
        - Otosclerosis
        - Syphilis
        - Acute hearing loss syndrome
        - Acoustic neuroma, early
    - **Not associated with significant deafness or vertigo**
      - **Carotid bruit**
        - Carotid stenosis or thrombosis
      - **No bruit**
        - Occupational hazards
        - Migraine
        - Anemia
        - Uremia
- **History of drug use**
  - Toxicity from gentamycin, streptomycin, quinine, aspirin, etc.

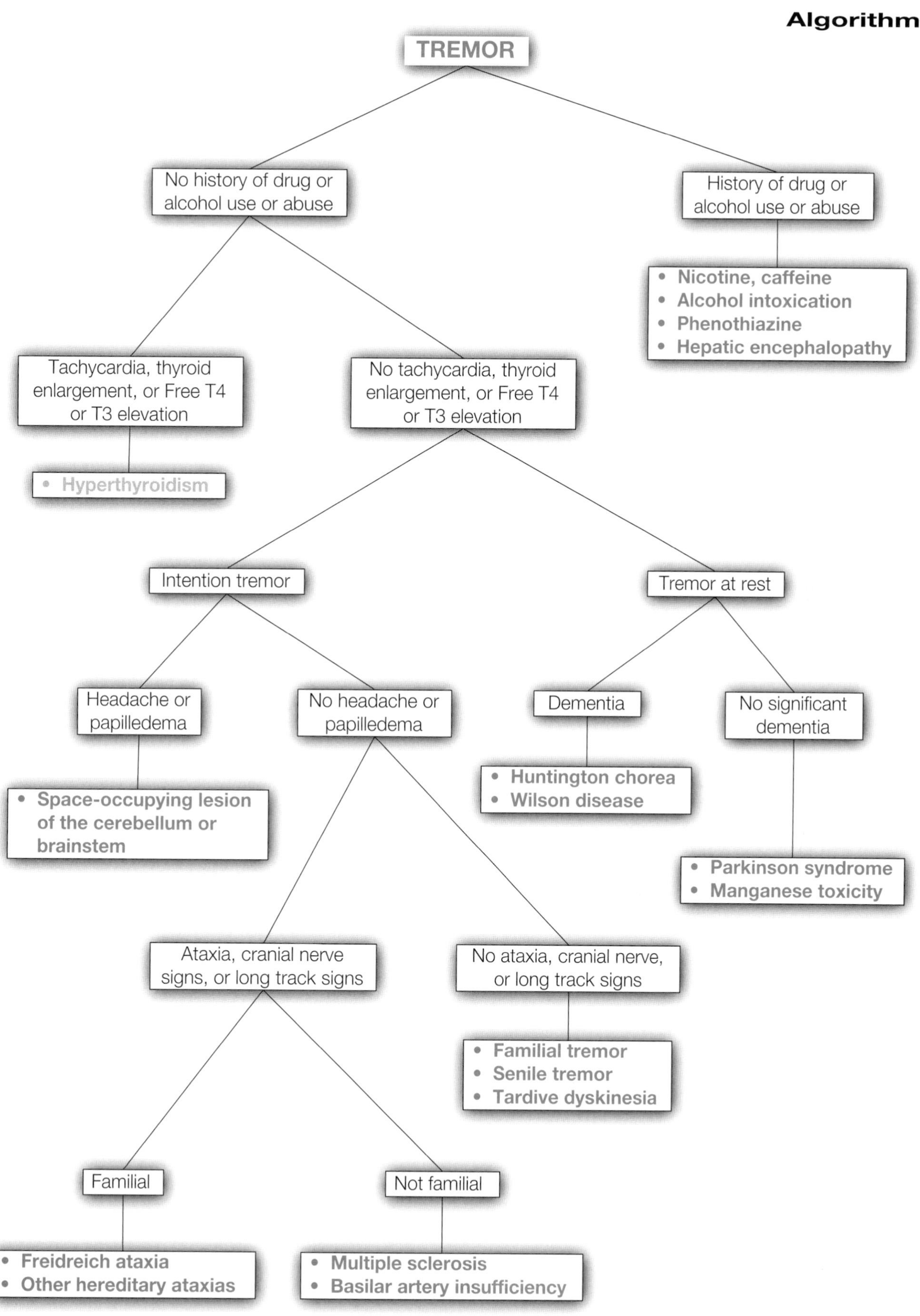

Signs & Symptoms

URINATION, DIFFICULT

- Painless
  - Pelvic or rectal mass
    - Carcinoma of vagina or cervix
    - Ectopic pregnancy
    - Benign prostatic hypertrophy
    - Carcinoma of prostate
    - Rectal carcinoma
    - Foreign body
  - No pelvic or rectal mass
    - Tight anal sphincter or hyperactive reflexes in lower extremities
      - Multiple sclerosis
      - Spinal cord tumor
      - Compression fracture
    - Weak or relaxed rectal sphincter, hypoactive reflexes in lower extremities
      - Cauda equina tumor
      - Hemorrhage or abscess
      - Tabes dorsales
      - Poliomyelitis
      - Diabetic neuropathy
    - Normal sphincter tone and control
      - Bladder neck obstruction
      - Urethral stricture
- Painful
  - Urethral discharge
    - Urethritis, acute
    - Prostatitis, acute
    - Gonorrhea
  - No urethral discharge
    - Cystitis
    - Bladder calculus
    - Urethral carbuncle

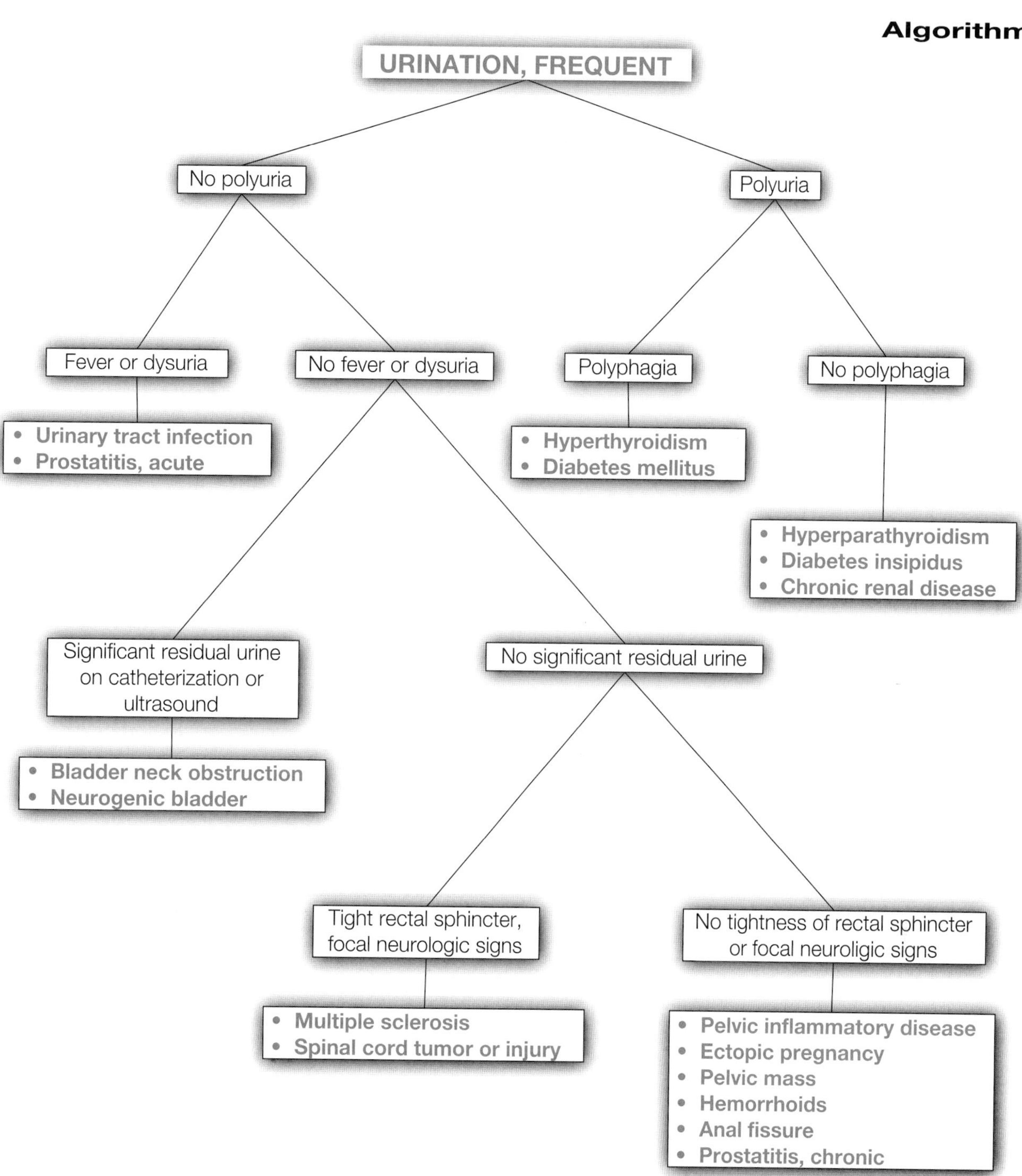
URINATION, FREQUENT
No polyuria
Polyuria
Fever or dysuria
No fever or dysuria
Polyphagia
No polyphagia
• Urinary tract infection
• Prostatitis, acute
• Hyperthyroidism
• Diabetes mellitus
• Hyperparathyroidism
• Diabetes insipidus
• Chronic renal disease
Significant residual urine on catheterization or ultrasound
No significant residual urine
• Bladder neck obstruction
• Neurogenic bladder
Tight rectal sphincter, focal neurologic signs
No tightness of rectal sphincter or focal neuroligic signs
• Multiple sclerosis
• Spinal cord tumor or injury
• Pelvic inflammatory disease
• Ectopic pregnancy
• Pelvic mass
• Hemorrhoids
• Anal fissure
• Prostatitis, chronic

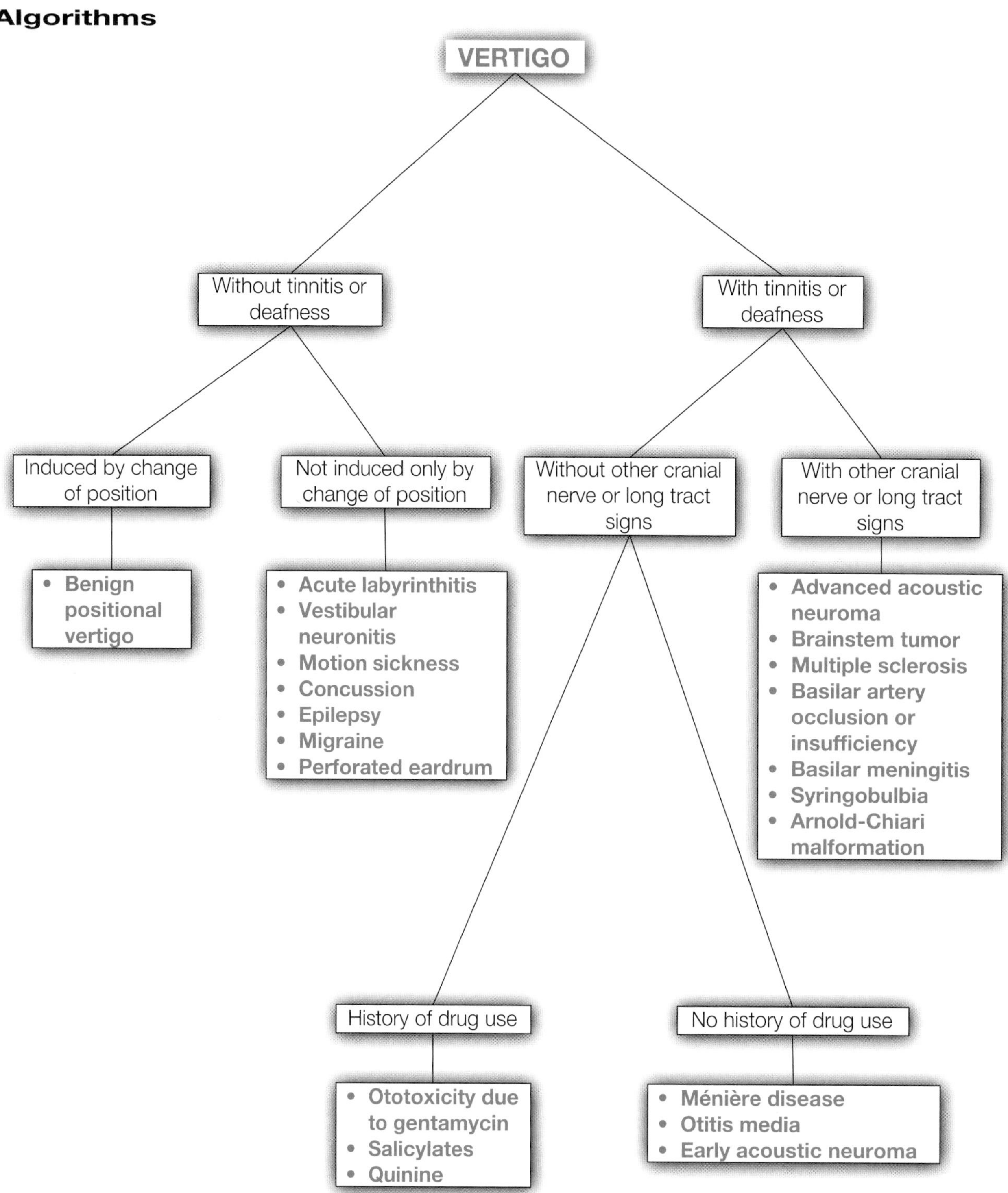
VERTIGO
Without tinnitis or deafness
With tinnitis or deafness
Induced by change of position
Not induced only by change of position
Without other cranial nerve or long tract signs
With other cranial nerve or long tract signs
• Benign positional vertigo
• Acute labyrinthitis
• Vestibular neuronitis
• Motion sickness
• Concussion
• Epilepsy
• Migraine
• Perforated eardrum
• Advanced acoustic neuroma
• Brainstem tumor
• Multiple sclerosis
• Basilar artery occlusion or insufficiency
• Basilar meningitis
• Syringobulbia
• Arnold-Chiari malformation
History of drug use
No history of drug use
• Ototoxicity due to gentamycin
• Salicylates
• Quinine
• Ménière disease
• Otitis media
• Early acoustic neuroma

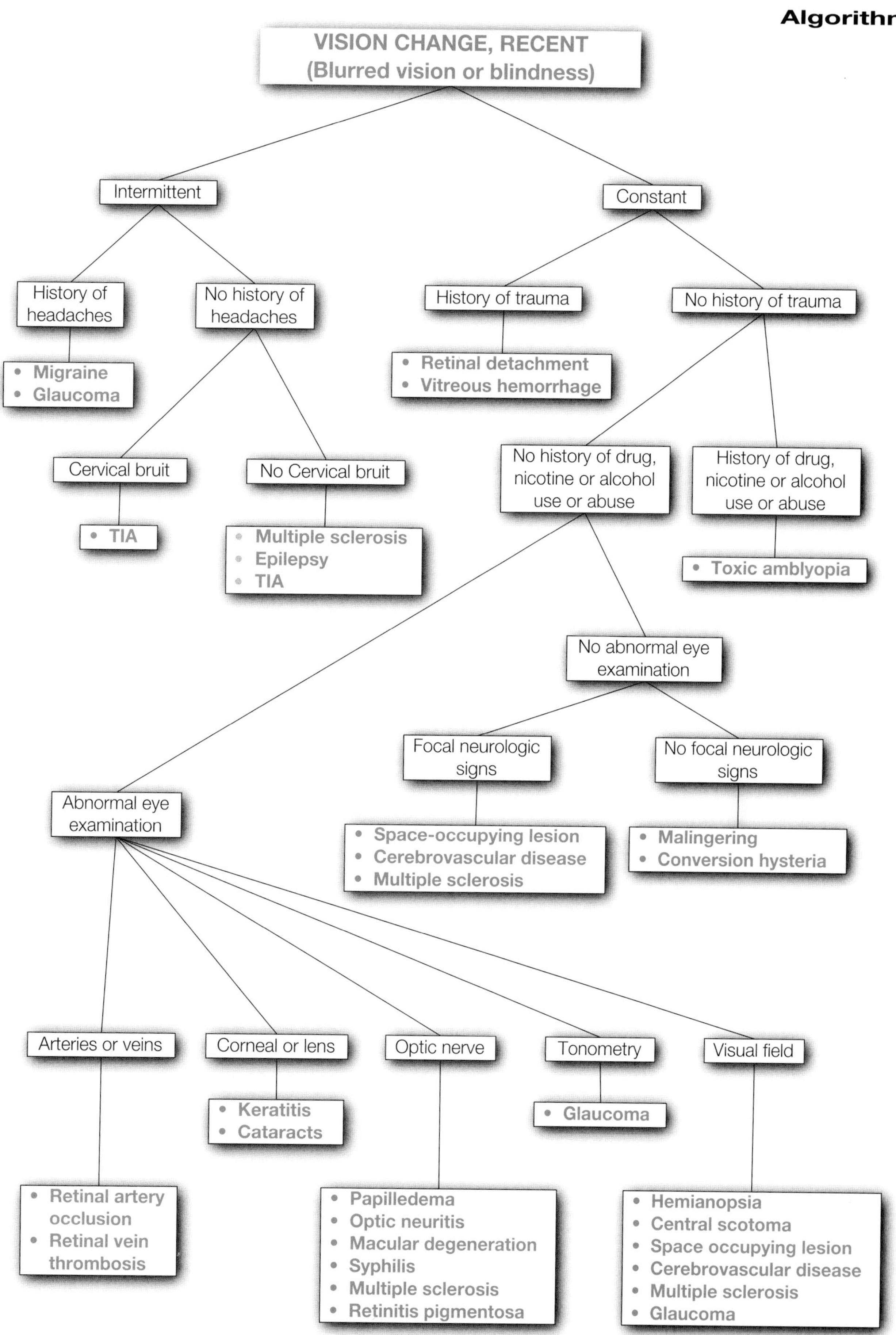
VISION CHANGE, RECENT
(Blurred vision or blindness)
Intermittent
Constant
History of headaches
No history of headaches
History of trauma
No history of trauma
• Migraine
• Glaucoma
• Retinal detachment
• Vitreous hemorrhage
Cervical bruit
No Cervical bruit
No history of drug, nicotine or alcohol use or abuse
History of drug, nicotine or alcohol use or abuse
• TIA
• Multiple sclerosis
• Epilepsy
• TIA
• Toxic amblyopia
No abnormal eye examination
Focal neurologic signs
No focal neurologic signs
Abnormal eye examination
• Space-occupying lesion
• Cerebrovascular disease
• Multiple sclerosis
• Malingering
• Conversion hysteria
Arteries or veins
Corneal or lens
Optic nerve
Tonometry
Visual field
• Keratitis
• Cataracts
• Glaucoma
• Retinal artery occlusion
• Retinal vein thrombosis
• Papilledema
• Optic neuritis
• Macular degeneration
• Syphilis
• Multiple sclerosis
• Retinitis pigmentosa
• Hemianopsia
• Central scotoma
• Space occupying lesion
• Cerebrovascular disease
• Multiple sclerosis
• Glaucoma

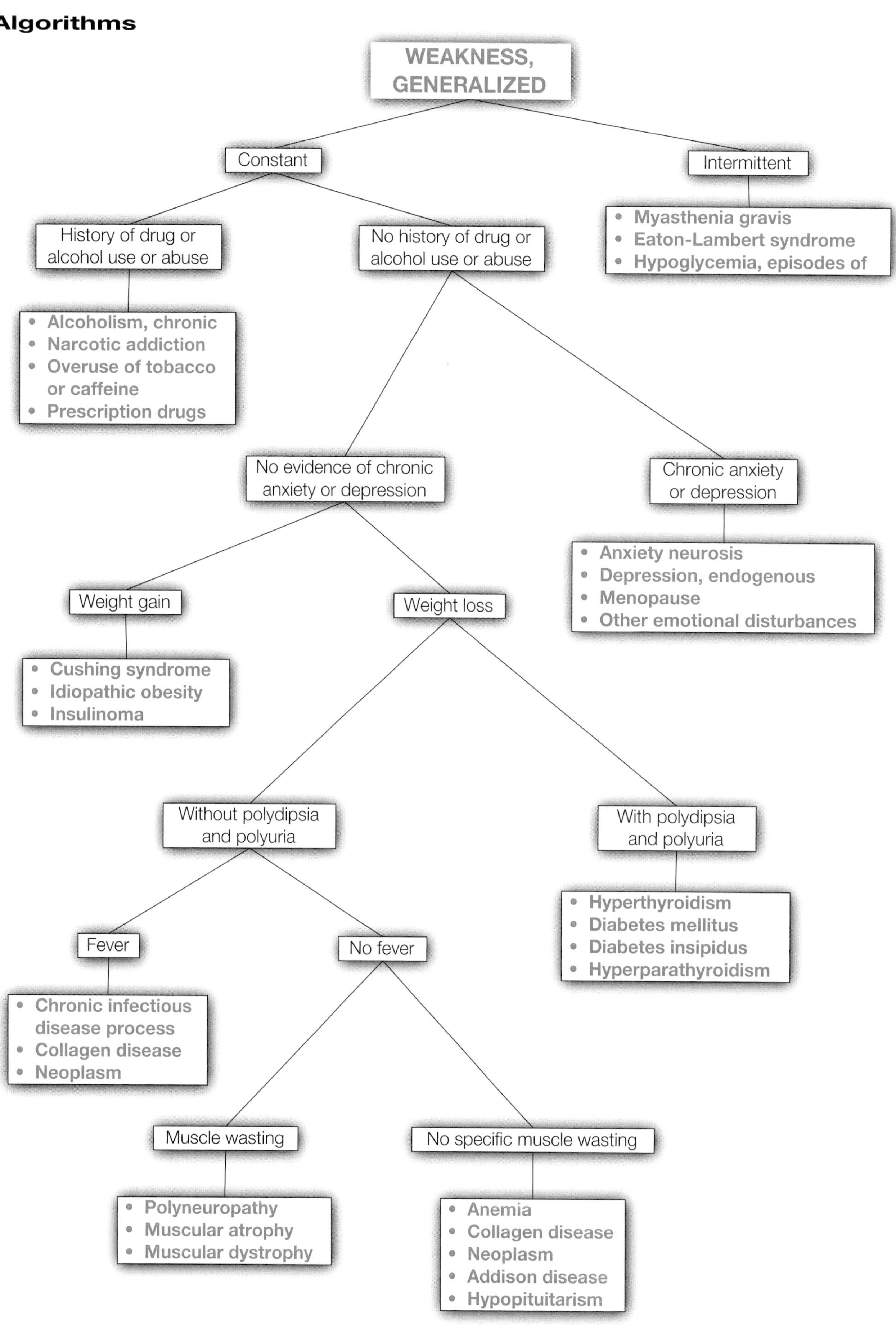
WEAKNESS, GENERALIZED
Constant
Intermittent
• Myasthenia gravis
• Eaton-Lambert syndrome
• Hypoglycemia, episodes of
History of drug or alcohol use or abuse
• Alcoholism, chronic
• Narcotic addiction
• Overuse of tobacco or caffeine
• Prescription drugs
No history of drug or alcohol use or abuse
No evidence of chronic anxiety or depression
Chronic anxiety or depression
• Anxiety neurosis
• Depression, endogenous
• Menopause
• Other emotional disturbances
Weight gain
• Cushing syndrome
• Idiopathic obesity
• Insulinoma
Weight loss
Without polydipsia and polyuria
With polydipsia and polyuria
• Hyperthyroidism
• Diabetes mellitus
• Diabetes insipidus
• Hyperparathyroidism
Fever
• Chronic infectious disease process
• Collagen disease
• Neoplasm
No fever
Muscle wasting
• Polyneuropathy
• Muscular atrophy
• Muscular dystrophy
No specific muscle wasting
• Anemia
• Collagen disease
• Neoplasm
• Addison disease
• Hypopituitarism

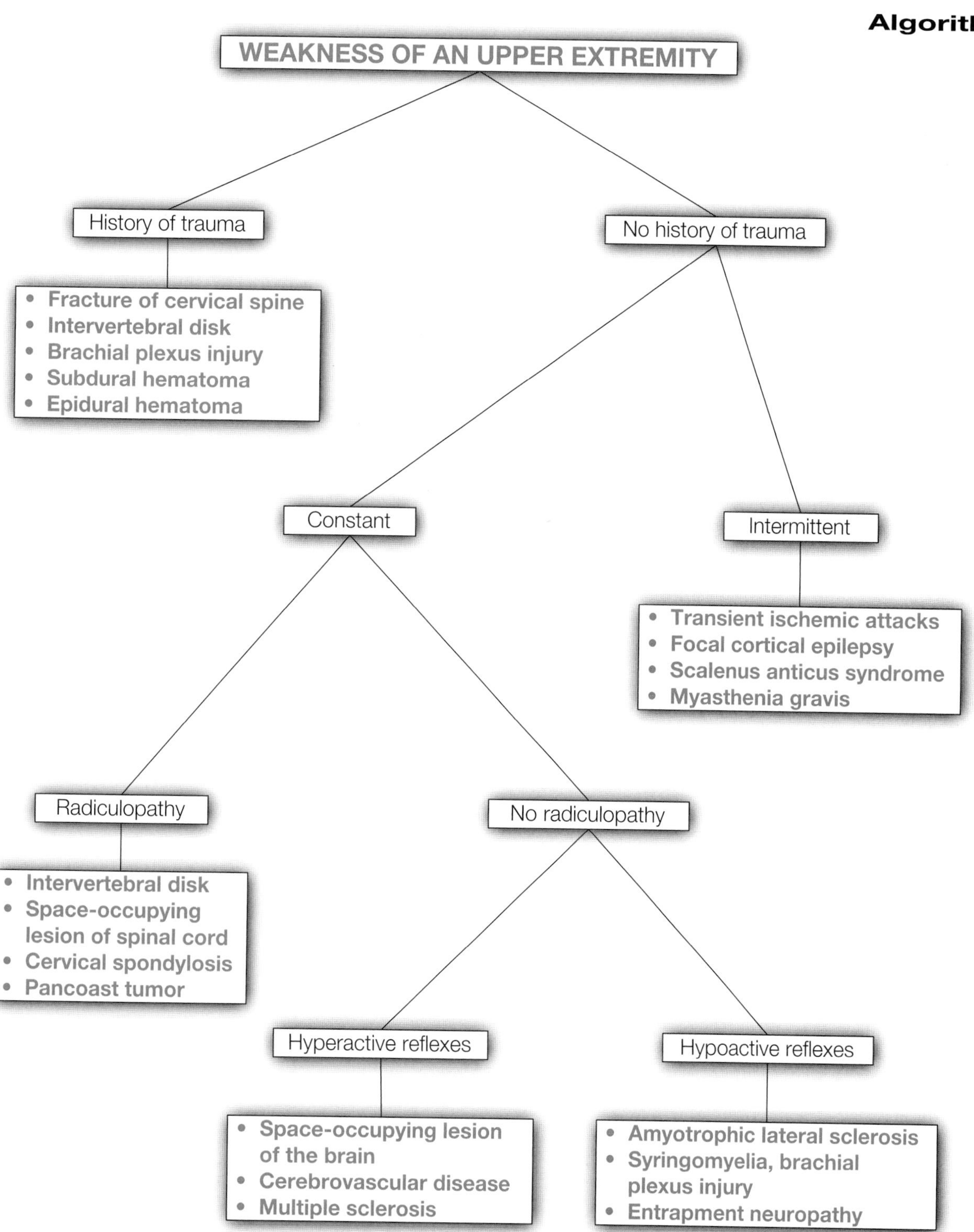
WEAKNESS OF AN UPPER EXTREMITY
History of trauma
• Fracture of cervical spine
• Intervertebral disk
• Brachial plexus injury
• Subdural hematoma
• Epidural hematoma
No history of trauma
Constant
Intermittent
• Transient ischemic attacks
• Focal cortical epilepsy
• Scalenus anticus syndrome
• Myasthenia gravis
Radiculopathy
• Intervertebral disk
• Space-occupying lesion of spinal cord
• Cervical spondylosis
• Pancoast tumor
No radiculopathy
Hyperactive reflexes
• Space-occupying lesion of the brain
• Cerebrovascular disease
• Multiple sclerosis
Hypoactive reflexes
• Amyotrophic lateral sclerosis
• Syringomyelia, brachial plexus injury
• Entrapment neuropathy

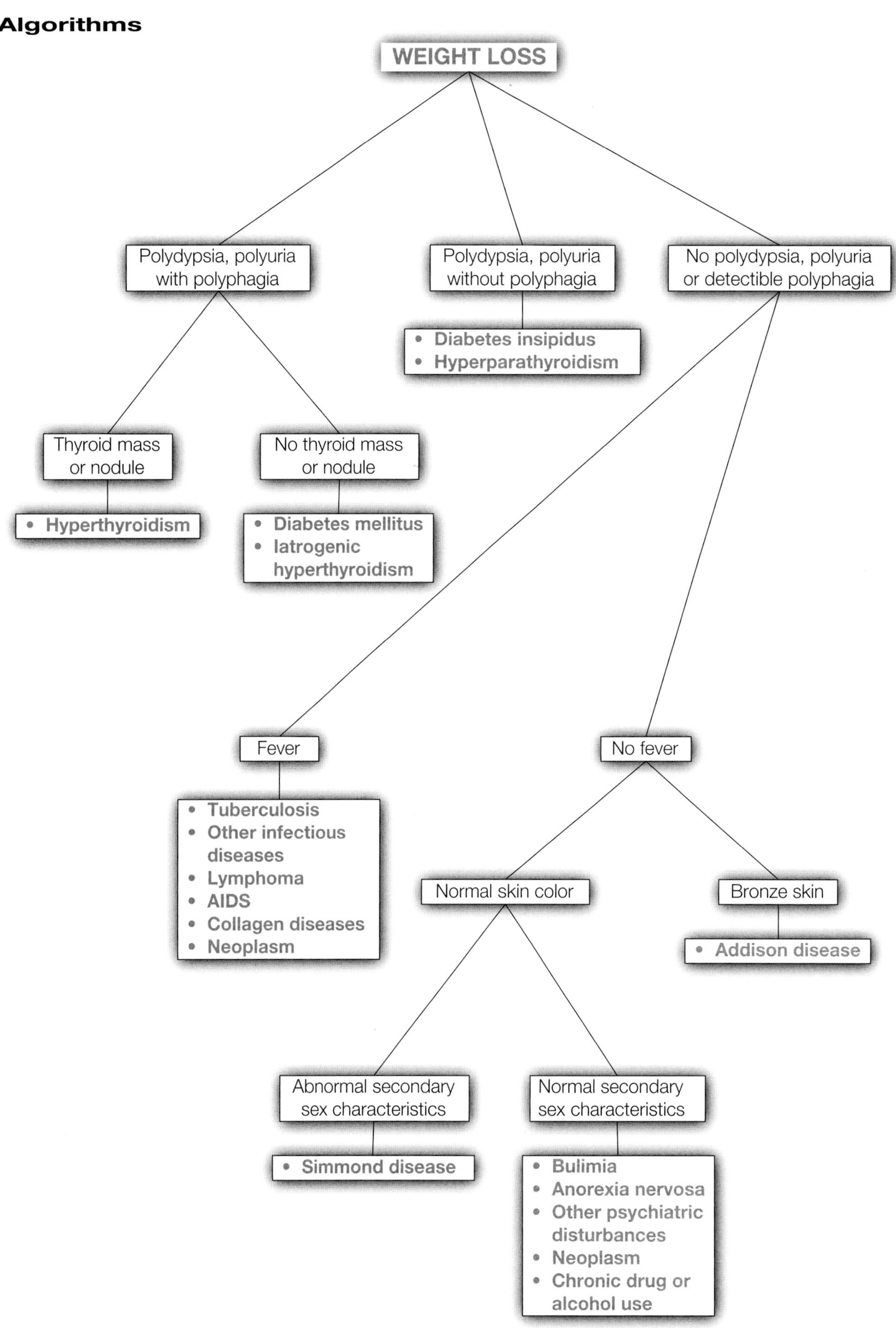
WEIGHT LOSS
Polydypsia, polyuria with polyphagia
Polydypsia, polyuria without polyphagia
No polydypsia, polyuria or detectible polyphagia
• Diabetes insipidus
• Hyperparathyroidism
Thyroid mass or nodule
No thyroid mass or nodule
• Hyperthyroidism
• Diabetes mellitus
• Iatrogenic hyperthyroidism
Fever
No fever
• Tuberculosis
• Other infectious diseases
• Lymphoma
• AIDS
• Collagen diseases
• Neoplasm
Normal skin color
Bronze skin
• Addison disease
Abnormal secondary sex characteristics
Normal secondary sex characteristics
• Simmond disease
• Bulimia
• Anorexia nervosa
• Other psychiatric disturbances
• Neoplasm
• Chronic drug or alcohol use

Section 5

Medication Guide

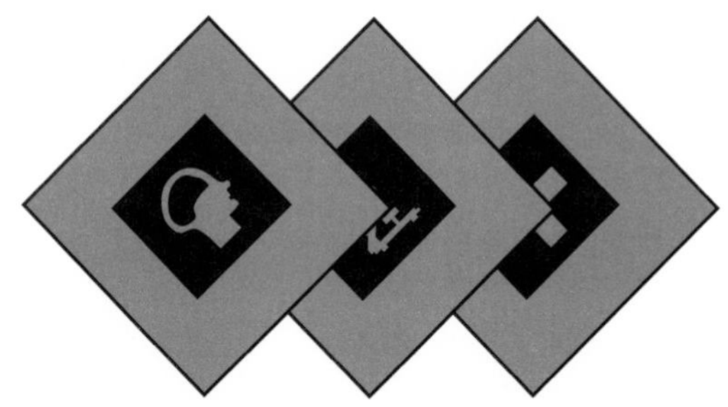

Acarbose

Antidiabetic

Indications: Patients with non-insulin-dependent diabetes mellitus who have failed dietary therapy. May be used alone or in combination with sulfonylureas, insulin, or metformin.

Dose: Adults: PO 25 mg tid with the start of each meal. To minimize GI side effects, some patients may benefit from more gradual dose titration. This may be achieved by initiating treatment at 25 mg daily and increasing the frequency to achieve 25 mg tid. Increase by 25 mg/dose at 4- to 8-wk intervals, according to response, up to a max based on blood glucose response (max, 150/day if no more than 60 kg, 300 mg/day if above 60 kg).

Trade names: Precose Tablets 25 mg

Warnings: Diabetic ketoacidosis; cirrhosis; inflammatory bowel disease; colonic ulceration; intestinal disorders of digestion or absorption; partial or predisposition to intestinal obstruction; conditions that may deteriorate as a result of increased intestinal gas production. Pregnancy Category: [B Insulin is recommended to maintain blood glucose levels during pregnancy]

Interactions: Drugs that produce hyperglycemia (eg, corticosteroids, diuretics, thyroid preparations), phenothiazines, estrogens, oral contraceptives, phenytoin, nicotinic acid, sympathomimetics, calcium channel-blocking drugs, isoniazid: May lead to loss of glucose control.
Intestinal adsorbents (eg, charcoal); digestive enzymes: May lower the efficacy of acarbose.

Acebutolol HCl

Beta-adrenergic blocker

Indications: Management of hypertension and premature ventricular contractions.

Dose: Hypertension:
Adults: PO 400 mg qd initially in single or divided doses; usual response range is 200 to 1200 mg/day.
Elderly: May require lower maintenance doses. Do not exceed 800 mg qd.
Ventricular Arrhythmia:
Adults: PO 400 mg (200 mg bid); may be titrated up to 1200 mg qd.

Trade names: Sectral Capsules 200 mg

Warnings: Hypersensitivity to beta-blockers; persistently severe bradycardia; greater than first-degree heart block; CHF, unless secondary to tachyarrhythmia treatable with beta-blockers; overt cardiac failure; sinus bradycardia; cardiogenic shock. Pregnancy Category: [B]

Interactions: Clonidine: May enhance or reverse acebutolol's antihypertensive effect; potentially life-threatening situations may occur, especially on withdrawal.
NSAIDs: Some agents may impair antihypertensive effect.
Prazosin: May cause increase in orthostatic hypotension.
Verapamil: Effects of both drugs may be increased.

Acetazolamide

Anticonvulsant / Carbonic anhydrase inhibitor

Indications: Prevention or lessening of symptoms associated with acute mountain sickness (tablet only); adjunctive treatment of chronic simple (open-angle) glaucoma and secondary glaucoma; preoperative treatment of acute congestive (closed-angle) glaucoma; adjunctive treatment of 1) edema caused by CHF or drug-induced edema and 2) centrencephalic epilepsies (eg, petit mal, generalized seizures).

Dose: Acute Mountain Sickness:
Adults: PO 500 to 1,000 mg per day in divided doses.
Chronic Simple (Open-Angle) Glaucoma:
Adults: PO 250 mg to 1 g per day, usually in divided doses for amounts above 250 mg.
Diuresis in CHF:
Adults: PO/IV Initially 250 to 375 mg (5 mg/kg) every morning; then give on alternate days or for 2 days alternating with 1 day of rest.
Drug-Induced Edema:
Adults: PO/IV 250 to 375 mg daily for 1 to 2 days, alternating with a day of rest.
Epilepsy:
Adults: PO/IV 8 to 30 mg/kg per day in divided doses; optimum range 375 to 1,000 mg/day. When drug is given in combination with other anticonvulsants, initial dosage is 250 mg daily.
Secondary Glaucoma/Preoperative Treatment of Closed-Angle Glaucoma:
Adults (short-term care): PO 250 mg q 4 hr or 250 mg bid.
Acute care: PO Initially 500 mg; then 125 to 250 mg q 4 hr. IV therapy may be used for rapid relief of increased IOP. Direct IV administration is preferred because IM route is painful.

Trade names: Acetazolamide Tablets 250 mg
Diamox Sequels Capsules, sustained-release 500 mg

Warnings: Hypersensitivity to other sulfonamides; depressed sodium and/or potassium serum levels; marked kidney and liver disease or dysfunction; suprarenal gland failure; hyperchloremic acidosis; adrenocortical insufficiency; severe pulmonary obstruction with increased risk of acidosis; cirrhosis; long-term use in chronic noncongestive angle-closure glaucoma. Sustained release dosage form is not recommended for use as anticonvulsant or for treatment of edema caused by CHF or drug-induced edema. Pregnancy Category: [C]

Interactions: Diflunisal: May cause significant decrease in IOP.
Primidone: Primidone concentrations may be altered.
Quinidine: Quinidine serum levels may be increased.
Salicylates: May cause acetazolamide accumulation and toxicity, including CNS depression and metabolic acidosis.

Acetylcysteine

Respiratory inhalant / Mucolytic

Indications: Reduction of viscosity of bronchopulmonary mucous secretions in patients with chronic or acute lung diseases, pulmonary complications associated with cystic fibrosis, surgery, anesthesia, atelectasis caused by mucous obstruction; diagnostic bronchial studies; prevention or lessening of liver damage after potentially toxic quantity of acetaminophen.
Orphan drug status: IV form for acetaminophen overdose.

Unlabeled indication: Ophthalmic preparation for dry eyes; enema for bowel obstruction.

Dose: Adults: Nebulization (face mask, mouthpiece, tracheostomy) 1 to 10 mL (usually 2 to 5 mL) of 20% solution or 2 to 20 mL (usually 6 to 10 mL) of 10% solution q 2 to 6 hr (usually tid or qid); (nebulization tent) large volumes (up to 300 mL) during treatment period.
Instillation: 1 to 2 mL of 10 to 20% solution as often as q 1 hr.
Diagnostic Bronchograms: 2 to 3 administrations of 1 to 2 mL of 20% solution or 2 to 4 mL of 10% solution q 1 to 4 hr by instillation before procedure.
Acetaminophen Overdose: After appropriate overdose procedures (eg, lavage, induction of emesis), 140 mg/kg as oral loading dose (diluted with soft drink).
Then 70 mg/kg orally 4 hr after loading dose and repeated at 4-hr intervals for total of 17 doses, unless acetaminophen assay indicates otherwise.

Trade names: Mucomyst Solution 10% (as sodium)

Warnings: Standard considerations. Pregnancy

Category: [B]
Interactions: None well documented.
Incompatability: Do not mix with tetracycline, chlortetracycline, oxytetracycline, erythromycin lactobionate, amphotericin B, ampicillin sodium, iodized oil, chymotrypsin, trypsin, or hydrogen peroxide.

Acitretin

Retinoid

Indications: Treatment of severe psoriasis.
Dose: Adults: PO Start with 25 to 50 mg/day given as a single dose with the main meal. Maintenance doses of 25 to 50 mg/day may be given dependent upon the patient's response to initial treatment.
Relapse:
Adults: PO Relapses may be treated as outlined for initial treatment.
Phototherapy:
Adults: PO When used with phototherapy, the phototherapy dose should be decreased by the prescriber based upon the patient's individual response.
Trade names: Soriatane Capsules 10 mg
Warnings: Pregnancy; severe liver or kidney function impairment; chronic abnormal elevation in blood lipid values; concurrent use of methotrexate or tetracyclines; hypersensitivity to other retinoids or any component of the product. Pregnancy Category: [X]
Interactions: Ethanol: Concurrent use of alcohol and acitretin may lead to the formation of etretinate, which increases the duration of teratogenic potential in women.
Glyburide: The glucose-lowering effect of glyburide may be potentiated.
Methotrexate: Because the risk of hepatitis may be increased, concurrent use is contraindicated.
Phenytoin: Protein binding of phenytoin may be reduced.
Progestin 'minipill': Acitretin may interfere with the contraceptive effect.
Tetracyclines: Because acitretin and tetracyclines can cause increased intracranial pressure, concurrent use is contraindicated.
Vitamin A, oral retinoids: Because the risk of hypervitaminosis A is increased, concurrent use is contraindicated.

Acrivastine/ Pseudoephedrine HCl

Antihistamine / Decongestant

Indications: Relief of symptoms associated with seasonal allergic rhinitis.
Dose: Adults and Children (12 yr or older): PO 1 capsule (8 mg acrivastine/60 mg pseudoephedrine) q 4 to 6 hr (up to qid).
Trade names: Semprex-D Capsules 8 mg acrivastine/60 mg pseudoephedrine
Warnings: Hypersensitivity to any ingredient of product; known sensitivity to other alkylamine antihistamines (eg, triprolidine); patients with severe hypertension or coronary artery disease; MAO inhibitor therapy or within 14 days of stopping MAO inhibitor therapy. Pregnancy Category: [B]
Interactions: Acrivastine:
Alcohol; other CNS depressants: Additional decrease in alertness and impairment of CNS performance may occur.
Pseudoephedrine:
Antihypertensive agents that interfere with sympathetic activity (eg, mecamylamine, methyldopa, reserpine, veratrum alkaloids): Antihypertensive effects of these agents may be reduced.
Digitalis: Increased ectopic pacemaker activity may occur.
MAO inhibitors: Contraindicated in patients taking MAO inhibitors and for 14 days after stopping use of an MAO inhibitor.

Acyclovir

Anti-infective / Antiviral

Indications: Parenteral: Treatment of initial or recurrent mucosal and cutaneous herpes simplex viruses (HSV) and varicella zoster (shingles) infections in immunocompromised patients; treatment of herpes simplex encephalitis; treatment of severe initial clinical episodes of genital herpes; treatment of neonatal herpes infections.

Oral: Treatment of initial and recurrent episodes of genital herpes in certain patients; acute treatment of shingles and chickenpox.

Topical: Treatment of initial episodes of herpes genitalis and nonlife-threatening mucotaneous HSV infections in immunocompromised patients (ointment); recurrent herpes labialis (cold sores) (cream).

Unlabeled indication: Treatment of cytomegalovirus and HSV infection after bone marrow or renal transplant; treatment of infectious mononucleosis, varicella pneumonia, chickenpox, and other HSV infections.
Dose: Parenteral: For IV infusion only; rapid or bolus IV must be avoided.
Herpes Simplex Infections in Immunocompromised Patients:
Adults and adolescents 12 yr of age and older: IV 5 mg/kg infused at a constant rate over 1 hr q 8 hr for 7 days.
Children younger than 12 yr of age: IV 10 mg/kg infused at a constant rate over 1 hr q 8 hr for 7 days.
Severe Initial Genital Herpes:
Adults and adolescents 12 yr of age and older: IV 5 mg/kg at a constant rate over 1 hr q 8 hr for 5 days.
Varicella Zoster Infections in Immunocompromised Patients:
Adults and adolescents 12 yr of age and older: IV 10 mg/kg infused at a constant rate over 1 hr q 8 hr for 7 days.
Children younger than 12 yr of age: IV 20 mg/kg infused at a constant rate over 1 hr q 8 hr for 7 days.
Herpes Simplex Encephalitis:
Adults and adolescents 12 yr of age and older: IV 10 mg/kg infused at a constant rate over 1 hr q 8 hr for 10 days.
Children 3 mo to 12 yr of age: IV 20 mg/kg infused at a constant rate over 1 hr q 8 hr for 10 days.
Neonatal Herpes Infections (CDC Recommendations): IV Disseminated and CNS disease: 20 mg/kg q 8 hr for 21 days. Mucocutaneous disease: 20 mg q 8 hr for 14 days.
Oral:
Chickenpox:
Adults and children (greater than 40 kg): PO 800 mg qid for 5 days.
Children 2 yr of age and older (40 kg or less): PO 20 mg/kg qid for 5 days.
Herpes Zoster:
Adults: PO 800 mg q 4 hr 5 times/day for 7 to 10 days.
Initial Genital Herpes:
Adults: PO 200 mg q 4 hr 5 times/day for 10 days.
Suppressive Therapy for Recurrent Genital Herpes:
Adults: PO 400 mg bid for up to 12 mo.
Intermittent Therapy for Recurrent Genital Herpes:
Adults: PO 200 mg q 4 hr 5 times/day for 5 days at earliest sign or symptom of recurrence.
Topical:
Initial Genital Herpes and Herpes Simplex Infections in Immunocompromised Patients:
Adults: Ointment Apply sufficient quantity to cover all lesions q 3 hr, 6 times/day, for 7 days.
Recurrent Herpes Labialis (Cold Sores):
Adults and children 12 yr of age and older: Cream Apply to lesion 5 times/day for 4 days.
Trade names: Acyclovir Injection 50 mg/mL (as

sodium)
Zovirax Tablets 400 mg
Warnings: Hypersensitivity to acyclovir or valacyclovir. Pregnancy Category: [B]
Interactions: Probenecid: IV acyclovir plasma levels may be increased, and the duration of action prolonged, while the urinary excretion and renal Cl may be reduced.
Zidovudine: Increased propensity for lethargy.
Incompatability: Precipitation may occur with bacteriostatic water. Do not add acyclovir to biologic or colloidal fluids.

Adalimumab

Immunologic agent

Indications: Reduce signs and symptoms and inhibit progression of structural damage in patients with moderate to severe active rheumatoid arthritis who have had an inadequate response to 1 or more disease-modifying antirheumatic drugs.
Dose: Adults: SC 40 mg every other wk. Patients not receiving methotrexate concurrently may benefit from 40 mg every wk.
Trade names: Humira Injection 40 mg/0.8 mL
Warnings: Standard considerations. Pregnancy Category: [B]
Interactions: Immunosuppressive therapy: May increase risk of serious infection.
Live vaccines: Do not give concurrently.
Methotrexate: Reduces apparent Cl of adalimumab; however, adjustments in the dose of either drug do not appear necessary.

Adapalene

Retinoid

Indications: Topical treatment of acne vulgaris.
Dose: Adults and children (12 yr and older): Topical Apply a thin film once daily to affected areas after washing in the evening before bedtime.
Trade names: Differin Cream 0.1%
Warnings: Standard considerations. Pregnancy Category: [C]
Interactions: Potentially irritating topical products (eg, medicated or abrasive soaps and cleansers, soaps and cosmetics that have strong drying effect, products with high concentrations of alcohol, spices or limes), products containing sulfur, resorcinol, or salicylic acid: Because of increased risk of local irritation, use with caution.

Adefovir Dipivoxil

Antiviral Agent

Indications: Treatment of chronic hepatitis B in adults with evidence of active viral replication and evidence of persistent elevations in serum aminotransferases (ALT or AST) or histologically active disease.
Dose: Adults: PO 10 mg qd.
Renal Impairment:
Adults: PO For Ccr 50 mL/min or less, administer 10 mg q 24 hr; for Ccr 20 to 49 mL/min, administer 10 mg q 48 hr; for Ccr 10 to 19 mL/min, administer 10 mg q 72 hr; hemodialysis patients, administer 10 mg q 7 days following dialysis.
Trade names: Hepsera Tablets 10 mg
Warnings: Standard considerations. Pregnancy Category: [C]
Interactions: Ibuprofen, drugs that reduce renal function: May increase plasma concentrations of adefovir.

Adenosine

Antiarrhythmic

Indications: Conversion to sinus rhythm of paroxysmal supraventricular tachycardia (PSVT), including that associated with Wolff-Parkinson-White syndrome.

Unlabeled indication: Noninvasive assessment of patients with suspected coronary artery disease in conjunction with thallium tomography. Used with BCNU for treatment of brain tumors.
Dose: Initial dose (adults): IV 6 mg as rapid IV bolus (over 1 to 2 sec).
Repeat administration (adults): If first dose does not eliminate PSVT within 1 to 2 min, give 12 mg as rapid IV bolus; 12 mg dose may be repeated a second time if necessary. Doses over 12 mg are not recommended.
Trade names: Adenocard Injection 3 mg/mL
Adenoscan Injection 3 mg/mL
Warnings: Second- or third-degree AV block or sick sinus syndrome (except in patients with functioning artificial pacemaker); atrial flutter; atrial fibrillation; ventricular tachycardia. Pregnancy Category: [C]
Interactions: Caffeine, theophylline: Antagonize effects of adenosine; larger doses of adenosine may be needed.
Carbamazepine: May produce higher degrees of heart block.
Dipyridamole: Potentiates effects of adenosine; smaller doses may be adequate.

Albumin Human

Plasma protein fraction

Indications: Symptomatic relief and supportive treatment in management of shock, burns, hypoprothrombinemia, adult respiratory distress syndrome, cardiopulmonary bypass, acute liver failure, acute nephrosis, sequestration of protein-rich fluids, erythrocyte resuspension, hypotension or shock during renal dialysis, hyperbilirubinemia and erythroblastosis fetalis.
Dose: Burns: Initial treatment usually consists of large amounts of crystalloid infusions (eg, normal saline, Lactated Ringer's) with lesser amounts of 5% albumin to maintain adequate plasma volume. After first 24 hr, ratio of albumin and crystalloid should maintain plasma albumin level of about 2.5 g +- 0.5 g/100 mL or total plasma protein level about 5.2 g/100 mL. This is best achieved with albumin 25% solution.
Normal Serum Albumin, 5%:
Shock: Give as rapidly as necessary to improve patient's condition and restore normal blood volume.
Adults: IV Initial dose is 500 mL of 5% albumin given as rapidly as tolerated. If response in 30 min is inadequate, give additional 500 mL. In patients with slightly low or normal blood volume, rate is 2 to 4 mL/min.
Children: IV Rate of administration is 25% to 50% adult rate.
Newborns and infants: IV 10 to 20 mL/kg 5% albumin based on clinical response, BP, and assessment of anemia.
Hypoproteinemia: To replace protein loss, 5% albumin may be given.
Albumin Human, 25%:
Shock:
Adults and children: IV Initial dose is determined by patient's condition and response to treatment. Therapy is guided by degree of venous or pulmonary congestion or Hct measurements.
Hypoproteinemia:
Adults: IV 50 to 75 g/day at rate not exceeding 2 mL/min.
Children: IV 25 g/day at rate not exceeding 2 mL/min.
Acute Nephrosis:
Adults: IV 100 mL 25% albumin in combination with loop diuretic repeated daily for 7 to 10 days.
Renal Dialysis:
Adults: IV Approximately 100 mL 25% albumin.
Hyperbilirubinemia and Erythroblastosis Fetalis:
Newborns and infants: IV 1 g/kg 1 to 2 hr before transfusion.

Trade names: Albuminar-5 Injection 5%
Albuminar-25 Injection 25%
Albunex Injection 5%
Albutein 5% Injection 5%
Albutein 25% Injection 25%
Buminate 5% Injection 5%
Buminate 25% Injection 25%
Plasbumin-5 Injection 5%
Plasbumin-25 Injection 25%

Warnings: Severe anemia; cardiac failure; renal insufficiency; presence of normal or increased intravascular volume; chronic nephrosis; hypoprothrombinemic states associated with chronic cirrhosis; malabsorption; protein-losing enteropathies, pancreatic insufficiency; undernutrition. Pregnancy Category: [C]

Interactions: None well documented.

Alclometasone Dipropionate

Corticosteroid / Topical

Indications: Relief of inflammatory and pruritic manifestations of corticosteroid-responsive dermatoses.

Dose: Adults and Children at least 1 yr of age: Topical Apply thin film to affected area bid to tid.

Trade names: Aclovate Cream 0.05%

Warnings: Standard considerations. Pregnancy Category: [C]

Interactions: None well documented.

Alendronate Sodium

Hormone / Bisphosphonates

Indications: Treatment of osteoporosis in postmenopausal women; prevention of osteoporosis in postmenopausal women at risk of developing osteoporosis; treatment of osteoporosis in men; treatment of glucocorticoid-induced osteoporosis in men and women; treatment of Paget disease of the bone.

Dose: Osteoporosis (Postmenopausal Women):
Adults (treatment): PO 70 mg once weekly or 10 mg once daily.
Adults (prevention): PO 35 mg once weekly or 5 mg once daily.
Osteoporosis (Men):
Adults: PO 10 mg once daily.
Glucocorticoid-Induced Osteoporosis:
Adults: PO 5 mg once daily. For postmenopausal women not receiving estrogen, 10 mg once daily.
Paget Disease:
Adults: PO 40 mg once daily for 6 mo. Retreatment may be considered for patients who relapse after a 6-mo observation period.

Trade names: Fosamax Tablets 5 mg

Warnings: Hypocalcemia. Pregnancy Category: [C]

Interactions: Aspirin: Risk of upper GI adverse effects is increased by concomitant use of aspirin and alendronate doses over 10 mg/day.
Calcium supplements, antacids: Decreased alendronate absorption.
Food: Absorption of alendronate is decreased by food.
Liquids: Beverages other than water decrease absorption.
Ranitidine: Increased alendronate absorption; clinical importance unknown.

Alfuzosin HCl

Alpha-1-adrenergic blocker

Indications: Treatment of signs and symptoms of benign prostatic hyperplasia.

Dose: Adults: PO 10 mg/day, immediately after the same meal each day.

Trade names: Uroxatral Tablets, extended release 10 mg

Warnings: Patients with moderate or severe hepatic insufficiency; coadministration with potent CYP3A4 inhibitors (eg, itraconazole, ketoconazole, ritonavir); hypersensitivity to any component of the product. Pregnancy Category: [B]

Interactions: Atenolol: Plasma levels may be elevated by alfuzosin, increasing the pharmacologic and adverse effects.
Cimetidine: Alfuzosin levels may be elevated, increasing the pharmacologic and adverse effects.
Moderate CYP3A4 inhibitors (eg, diltiazem): Alfuzosin plasma levels may be elevated, increasing the pharmacologic and adverse effects.
Potent CYP3A4 inhibitors (eg, itraconazole, ketoconazole, ritonavir): Because plasma concentrations of alfuzosin may be increased more than 2-fold, coadministration of these agents is contraindicated.

Alitretinoin

Retinoid

Indications: Topical treatment of cutaneous lesions of AIDS-related Kaposi sarcoma (KS).

Dose: Adults: Topical Start with bid application to KS lesions. Application can be gradually increased to tid or qid or reduced according to individual lesion tolerance or application site toxicity. If severe irritation occurs, application of drug can be temporarily stopped for a few days until symptoms subside. Apply a sufficient amount of gel to cover the lesion with a generous coating. Allow to dry for 3 to 5 min before covering with clothing. A response to KS lesions may be seen as soon as 2 wk; however, some patients have required over 14 wk.

Trade names: Panretin Gel 0.1%

Warnings: Hypersensitivity to retinoids or any component of the product. Pregnancy Category: [D Could cause fetal harm if absorption were to occur in pregnant women]

Interactions: N,N-diethyl-m-toluamide (DEET): Avoid concurrent use of products containing DEET (a common component of insect repellents).

Allopurinol

Analgesic / Gout / Cytoprotective

Indications: Tablets: Treatment of primary or secondary gout, hyperuricemia resulting from chemotherapy for malignancies, recurrent calcium oxalate renal calculi.

Tablets and injections: Management of patients with leukemia, lymphoma, and solid tumor malignancies when concurrently receiving cancer therapy that causes elevations of serum and urinary uric acid levels. Use injection in patients who cannot tolerate oral therapy.

Unlabeled indication: Prevention of fluorouracil-induced stomatitis and fluorouracil-induced granulocyte suppression.

Dose: Control of Gout/Hyperuricemia:
Adults: PO 100 to 800 mg/day. For amounts over 300 mg, give divided doses.
Secondary Hyperuricemia Associated with Malignancies:
Children 6 to 10 yr: PO 300 mg/day.
Children under 6 yr: PO 150 mg/day.
Prevention of Uric Acid Nephropathy in Vigorous Chemotherapy of Neoplastic Disease:
Adults: PO 600 to 800 mg/day for 2 to 3 days.
Reduction of Risk of Acute Gouty Attacks:
Adults (initial dose): PO 100 mg/day, increased by 100 mg at weekly intervals until adequate response is achieved or max recommended dose (800 mg/day) is reached.
Leukemia, Lymphoma, Solid Tumor Malignancies:

Adults: IV 200 to 400 mg/m^2 /day (max 600 mg/day).
Children: IV Starting dose 200 mg/m^2 /day.

Trade names: Aloprim Powder for injection, lyophilized 500 mg
Zyloprim Tablets 100 mg

Warnings: Standard considerations. Pregnancy Category: [C]

Interactions: Aluminum salts, uricosuric agents: May lessen effectiveness of allopurinol.
Ampicillin: May increase incidence of ampicillin-induced skin rash.
Cyclophosphamide: May enhance bone marrow suppression.
Theophyllines: Theophylline clearance may be decreased, leading to toxicity.
Thiopurines (eg, azathioprine, mercaptopurine): Toxicity of these drugs may be increased.
Drugs that are physically incompatible in solution with allopurinol sodium for injection are the following: amikacin; amphotericin B; carmustine; cefotaxime; chlorpromazine; cimetidine; clindamycin; cytarabine; dacarbazine; daunorubicin; diphenhydramine; doxorubicin; doxycycline; droperidol; floxuridine; gentamicin; haloperidol; hydroxyzine; idarubicin; imipenem plus cilastatin; mechlorethamine; meperidine; metoclopramide; methylprednisolone sodium succinate; minocycline; nalbuphine; netilmicin; ondansetron; prochlorperazine edisylate; promethazine; sodium bicarbonate; streptozocin; tobramycin; vinorelbine tartrate.

Almotriptan Malate

Analgesic / Migraine

Indications: Acute treatment of migraine with or without aura.

Dose: Adults: PO 6.25 to 12.5 mg, if headache returns, may repeat dose after 2 hr (max, 2 doses per 24 hr).
Hepatic or Renal Impairment:
Adults: PO 6.25 mg initially (max, 12.5 mg per 24 hr).

Trade names: Axert Tablets 6.25 mg

Warnings: Ischemic heart disease (eg, angina pectoris, history of MI, documented silent ischemia); symptoms or findings consistent with ischemic heart disease, coronary artery vasospasm (including Prinzmetal variant angina); significant underlying CV disease; uncontrolled hypertension; within 24 hr of treatment with another 5-HT$_1$ agonist, or an ergotamine-containing or ergot-type medication; hemiplegic or basilar migraine; hypersensitivity to any component of the product. Pregnancy Category: [C]

Interactions: Ergot-containing drugs (eg, methysergide): May cause prolonged vasospastic reactions; therefore, contraindicated within 24 hr of almotriptan administration.
Other 5-HT-1B/1D agonists (eg, sumatriptan): Contraindicated within 24 hr of each other.
Potent CYP3A4 inhibitors (eg, erythromycin, itraconazole, ketoconazole, ritonavir): Almotriptan plasma levels may be elevated, increasing the risk of side effects.
Selective serotonin reuptake inhibitors (eg, fluoxetine): Weakness, hyperpyrexia, and incoordination have been reported.

Alosetron

5HT-3 receptor antagonist

Indications: Treatment of irritable bowel syndrome (IBS) in women whose predominant bowel syndrome is diarrhea.

Unlabeled indication: Treatment of IBS in men; carcinoid diarrhea.

Dose: Adults: PO 1 mg/day initially. If after 4 wk the 1 mg/day dose is well tolerated but does not adequately control IBS symptoms, the dose can be increased to 1 mg bid.

Trade names: Lotronex Tablets 1.124 mg (equivalent to 1 mg alosetron base)

Warnings: History of chronic or severe constipation or sequelae from constipation; history of intestinal obstruction, stricture, toxic megacolon, GI perforation, or adhesions; history of ischemic colitis; current or history of Crohn disease or ulcerative colitis; active diverticulitis. Do not initiate therapy in patients with constipation (fewer than 3 bowel movements a week, hard or lumpy stools, or straining during a bowel movement). Pregnancy Category: [B]

Interactions: None well documented.

Alprazolam

Antianxiety / Benzodiazepine

Indications: Treatment of panic disorders with or without agoraphobia (Xanax and Xanax XR); management of anxiety disorders or for short-term relief of symptoms of anxiety, including anxiety associated with depression (immediate-release tablets and oral solution).

Unlabeled indication: Treatment of irritable bowel syndrome, depression, PMS, agoraphobia with social phobia.

Dose: Anxiety Disorder (Immediate-Release Tablets and Oral Solution):
Adults: PO Immediate-release tablets: 0.25 to 0.5 mg tid (max, 4 mg/day in divided doses). Extended-release tablets: Start with 0.5 mg qd and gradually increase if needed.
Elderly/Debilitated Patients:
Adults: PO 0.25 mg bid to tid; may increase dose gradually.
Panic Disorder:
Initial dose: PO Immediate-release tablets: 0.5 mg tid; if needed, increase by max 1 mg/day q 3 to 4 day. May require more than 4 mg/day. Extended-release tablets: start with 0.5 to 1 mg qd (suggested daily dose ranges between 3 and 6 mg).

Trade names: Alprazolam Intensol Oral solution 1 mg/mL
Xanax Tablets 0.25 mg
Xanax XR Tablets, extended-release 0.5 mg

Warnings: Hypersensitivity to other benzodiazepines; psychoses; acute narrow-angle glaucoma; patients receiving itraconazole or ketoconazole. Pregnancy Category: [D]

Interactions: Alcohol and other CNS depressants: Produce additive CNS depressant effects.
Cimetidine, oral contraceptives, disulfiram: May increase effects of alprazolam, producing excessive sedation and impaired psychomotor function.
Digoxin: Serum digoxin concentrations may increase.
Diltiazem, fluvoxamine, grapefruit juice, isoniazid, macrolide antibiotics(eg, erythromycin), nefazodone, non-nucleoside reverse transcriptase inhibitors(eg, delavirdine, efavirenz), protease inhibitors (eg, indinavir): May increase alprazolam plasma concentrations.
Itraconazole, ketoconazole: Concurrent use with alprazolam is contraindicated.
Omeprazole: May increase serum levels of alprazolam and enhance alprazolam's effects.
Rifamycins: May decrease alprazolam plasma concentrations.
Theophyllines: May antagonize sedative effects of alprazolam.

Alprostadil

Prostaglandin / Patent ductus arteriosus / Agent for impotence

Indications: Palliative therapy to maintain patency of ductus arteriosus temporarily, until surgery can be performed, in newborns who have congenital heart defects (eg, pulmonary stenosis, tricuspid atresia) and who depend on patent ductus for survival. Treatment of erectile dysfunction caused by neurogenic, vasculogenic, psychogenic, or mixed etiology. Intracavernosal alprostadil (Caverject only) may be useful adjunct to other diagnostic tests in the diagnosis of erectile dysfunction.

Dose: Ductus Arteriosus:
Newborns: IV 0.01 to 0.4 mcg/kg/min. Drug is infused for shortest time and at lowest effective dose.
Impotence (Erectile Dysfunction of Vasculogenic, Psychogenic, or Mixed Etiology): Intracavernosal Initiate dose titration at 2.5 mcg. If there is a partial response, the dose may be increased by 2.5 mcg to a dose of 5 mcg and then in increments of 5 to 10 mcg, depending on erectile response, until the dose that produces an erection suitable for intercourse and not exceeding a duration of 1 hr is reached. If there is no response to the initial 2.5 mcg dose, the second dose may be increased to 7.5 mcg, followed by increments of 5 to 10 mcg. If there is no response, then the next higher dose may be given within 1 hr. If there is a response, then there should be a 1-day interval before the next dose is given.
Erectile Dysfunction of Pure Neurogenic Etiology (Spinal Cord Injury): Initiate dosage titration at 1.25 mcg. The dose may be increased by 1.25 mcg to a dose of 2.5 mcg, followed by an increment of 2.5 mcg to a dose of 5 mcg, and then in 5 mcg increments until the dose that produces an erection suitable for intercourse and not exceeding a duration of 1 hr is reached. If there is no response, then the next higher dose may be given within 1 hr. If there is a response, then there should be at least 1-day interval before the next dose is given.
Maintenance therapy: The first injections of alprostadil must be done at the health care provider's office by medically trained personnel. Self-injection therapy by the patient can be started only after the patient is properly instructed and well-trained in the self-injection technique. The health care provider should make a careful assessment of the patient's skills and competence with the procedure. Intraurethral Administer as needed to achieve an erection. The onset of injection is 5 to 10 min after administration. Duration of effect is approximately 30 to 60 min. Titrate dose under the supervision of health care provider.
Caverject:
Adjunct to Diagnosis of Erectile Dysfunction:
Adults: Intracavernosal Monitor patients for occurrence of an erection after an intracavernosal injection of alprostadil. Extensions of this testing are the use of alprostadil as an adjunct to laboratory investigations (eg, duplex or Doppler imaging) to allow visualization and assessment of penile vasculature. For these tests, use a single dose of alprostadil that induces a rigid erection.

Trade names: Caverject Powder for injection, lyophilized 6.15 mcg (5 mcg/mL)
Edex Powder for injection, lyophilized 6.225 mcg (5 mcg/mL)
Muse Pellet 125 mcg
Prostin VR Pediatric Injection 500 mcg/mL (in 1 mL dehydrated alcohol)

Warnings: Standard considerations. Caverject: Conditions that might predispose patients to priapism (eg, sickle cell anemia or trait, multiple myeloma leukemia); patients with anatomical deformation of the penis (eg, angulation, cavernosal fibrosis, Peyronie disease); patients with penile implants; use in women, children or newborns; use in men for whom sexual activity is inadvisable or contraindicated. Pregnancy Category: [C]

Interactions: Anticoagulants (eg, heparin, warfarin): After intracavernosal injection, risk of bleeding may be increased.

Alteplase, Recombinant

Tissue plasminogen activator

Indications: Lysis of thrombi in management of acute MI or acute massive pulmonary embolism, management of acute ischemic stroke (Activase only). Restoration of function to central venous access device as assessed by the ability to withdraw blood (Cathflo Activase only).

Dose: Acute Ischemic Stroke:
Adults: IV The recommended dose is 0.9 mg/kg (max, 90 mg) infused over 60 min with 10% of the total dose administered as an initial IV bolus over 1 min. The safety and efficacy of this regimen with coadministration of heparin and aspirin during the first 24 hr after symptom onset has not been investigated. Doses 0.9 mg/kg may be associated with an increased incidence of ICH. Do not use doses more than 0.9 mg/kg (max, 90 mg).
Acute MI: Administer as soon as possible after the onset of symptoms. Do not use a dose of 150 mg because it has been associated with an increase in intracranial bleeding.
Accelerated infusion: The recommended dose is based upon patient weight; do not exceed 100 mg. For patients weighing more than 67 kg, the recommended dose administered is 100 mg as a 15 mg IV bolus, followed by 50 mg infused over the next 30 min and then 35 mg infused over the next 60 min. For patients weighing 67 kg or less, the recommended dose is administered as a 15 mg IV bolus, followed by 0.75 mg/kg infused over the next 30 min not to exceed 50 mg and then 0.5 mg/kg over the next 60 min not to exceed 35 mg. (The safety and efficacy of this accelerated infusion of alteplase regimen has only been investigated with coadministration of heparin and aspirin).
3-hr infusion: 100 mg given as 60 mg (34.8 million IU) in the first hour (with 6 to 10 mg given as a bolus over the first 1 to 2 min), 20 mg (11.6 million IU) over the second hour and 20 mg (11.6 million IU) over the third hour. For smaller patients (less than 65 kg), use a dose of 1.25 mg/kg given over 3 hr as described above.
Coadministration: Although the use of anticoagulants during and following alteplase has been shown to be of equivocal benefit, heparin has been given concomitantly for at least 24 hr in more than 90% of patients. Aspirin or dipyridamole has been given during or following heparin treatment.
Pulmonary Embolism:
Adults: IV 100 mg administered over 2 hr. Initiate or reinstate heparin therapy near the end of or immediately following the alteplase infusion when the partial thromboplastin time or thrombin time returns to twice normal or less.
Restoration of Function to Central Venous Catheter (Cathflo Activase only):
Adults: IV Instill into dysfunctional catheter at a concentration of 1 mg/mL. For patients weighing 30 kg or more, use 2 mg/2 mL; for patients weighing 10 kg or more to less than 30 kg, use 110% of the internal lumen volume of the catheter (max, 2 mg/2 mL). If catheter function is not restored in 120 min after 1 dose, a second dose may be instilled.

Trade names: Activase Powder for injection, lyophilized 50 mg (29 million IU)
Cathflo Activase Powder for injection, lyophilized 2 mg

Warnings: Active internal bleeding; history of cerebrovascular accident; intracranial hemorrhage; recent (within 3 mo) intracranial or intraspinal surgery or trauma; recent previous stroke; seizure at the onset of stroke; intracranial neoplasm; arteriovenous malformation or aneurysm; bleeding diathesis; severe uncontrolled hypertension; evidence of intracranial hemorrhage on pretreatment evaluation; suspicion of subarachnoid hemorrhage; uncontrolled hypertension at time of treatment; current use of oral anticoagulants; prothrombin time longer than 15 sec, administration of heparin within 48 hr preceding stroke onset with an elevated activated partial thromboplastin time at presentation; platelet count below 100,000/mm^3. Pregnancy Category: [C]

Interactions: Anticoagulants (eg, warfarin,

heparin), aspirin, drugs affecting platelet function (eg, abciximab, dipyridamole), vitamin K antagonists: May increase the risk of bleeding.
Nitroglycerin: May reduce alteplase concentrations, decreasing the thrombolytic effect.
Incompatability: Do not add other medications to infusion solution.

Amantadine HCl

Antiparkinson / Antiviral

Indications: Symptomatic treatment of several forms of Parkinson disease or syndrome and drug-induced extrapyramidal reactions; prevention and treatment of influenza A viral respiratory illness, especially in high-risk patients.

Dose: Parkinson Disease:
Adults: PO 100 mg bid when used as single agent.
Initial dose: PO 100 mg/day if patient is debilitated or receiving high doses of other antiparkinson drugs. If necessary, dose may be titrated to max of 400 mg/day.
Drug-Induced Extrapyramidal Reactions:
Adults: PO 100 mg bid; up to 300 mg/day may be given in divided doses.
Influenza A Viral Infection (Symptomatic Treatment):
Adults: PO 200 mg/day as single dose or 100 mg bid. If CNS effects develop on a once-daily dosage, split dosage schedule may reduce complaints.
Elderly over 65 yr: PO 100 mg qd.
Children 9 to 12 yr: PO 100 mg bid.
Children 1 to 9 yr: PO 4.4 to 8.8 mg/kg/day; not to exceed 150 mg/day.
Renal Impairment:
Adults: PO Ccr 30 to 50 mL/min: Administer 200 mg first day followed by 100 mg/day thereafter; Ccr 15 to 29 mL/min: Administer 200 mg first day followed by 100 mg on alternate days; Ccr less than 15 mL/min and hemodialysis patients: Administer 200 mg q 7 days.
Influenza A Viral Infection (Prophylaxis): Same dosages as for symptomatic treatment. However, start in anticipation of contact or as soon as possible after exposure. Continue drug administration for at least 10 days after known exposure. When influenza A virus vaccine is unavailable or contraindicated, administer amantadine for up to 90 days. In conjunction with the vaccine, administer amantadine for 2 to 3 wk after vaccination.

Trade names: Symmetrel Tablets 100 mg
Amantadine HCl Capsules 100 mg

Warnings: Standard considerations. Pregnancy Category: [C]

Interactions: Anticholinergic agents, quinidine, quinine, triamterene, thiazide diuretics, trimethoprim-sulfamethoxazole: May increase the effects of amantadine.
CNS stimulants: The effects of the CNS stimulant may be increased by amantadine.

Amifostine

Selective tissue chemoprotectant and radioprotectant

Indications: Prevent or reduce renal damage in patients receiving repeated cisplatin doses for advanced ovarian or non-small cell lung cancer; reduce incidence of moderate to severe xerostomia in patients undergoing radiation of the parotid gland for head and neck cancer.

Unlabeled indication: Prevent or reduce cisplatin-induced neurotoxicity and cyclophosphamide-induced granulocytopenia; prevent or reduce toxicity of radiation therapy to other areas; reduce toxicity of paclitaxel.

Dose: Reduction of Cumulative Renal Toxicity with Chemotherapy:
Adults: IV Amifostine 910 mg/m^2 once daily as a 15 min IV infusion, 30 min before chemotherapy.
Reduction of Moderate to Severe Xerostomia from Radiation of the Head and Neck:
Adults: IV Amifostine 200 mg/m^2 once daily as a 3 min IV infusion, 15 to 30 min prior to standard fraction radiation therapy (1.8 to 2 Gy).

Trade names: Ethyol Powder for injection, lyophilized 500 mg (anhydrous basis)

Warnings: Sensitivity to aminothiol compounds. Pregnancy Category: [C]

Interactions: Antihypertensives: Coadministration of drugs with similar pharmacologic effects may potentiate hypotension or cause additive side effects, including toxicity.

Amikacin Sulfate

Antibiotic / Aminoglycoside

Indications: Treatment of infections caused by susceptible strains of microorganisms, especially gram-negative bacteria.

Dose: Adults, Children, and Infants: IV/IM 15 mg/kg (ideal body weight)/day in 2 or 3 divided doses. Treatment in heavier patients should not exceed 1.5 g/day.
Uncomplicated utis: IV/IM 250 mg bid.
Newborns: IV/IM Loading dose of 10 mg/kg is recommended followed by 7.5 mg/kg q 12 hr. Lower doses may be needed in first 2 wk of life.

Trade names: Amikin Injection 250 mg/mL

Warnings: Generally not indicated for long-term therapy because of ototoxicity and nephrotoxicity. Pregnancy Category: [D]

Interactions: Drugs with nephrotoxic potential (eg, cephalosporins, enflurane, methoxyflurane, vancomycin): May increase risk of nephrotoxicity.
Loop diuretics (eg, furosemide): May increase risk of auditory toxicity.
Neuromuscular blocking agents (eg, tubocurarine): Amikacin may enhance effects of these agents.
Incompatability: Do not mix with betalactam antibiotics (eg, carbenicillin, ticarcillin).

Amiloride HCl

Potassium-sparing diuretic

Indications: Treatment of CHF or hypertension (in combination with thiazide or loop diuretics) and diuretic-induced hypokalemia.

Unlabeled indication: Reduction of lithium-induced polyuria; slowed reduction of pulmonary function in patients with cystic fibrosis (aerosol form).

Dose: Adult: PO 5 to 10 mg/day.
Lithium-Induced Polyuria: PO 10 to 20 mg/day.
Cystic Fibrosis: Dissolve in 0.3% saline and deliver by nebulizer.

Trade names: Midamor Tablets 5 mg

Warnings: Serum potassium more than 5.5 mEq/L; potassium supplementation; impaired renal function: spironolactone or triamterene therapy. Pregnancy Category: [B]

Interactions: Angiotensin-converting enzyme inhibitors: May result in severely elevated serum potassium levels.
Potassium preparations: May severely increase serum potassium levels, possibly resulting in cardiac arrhythmias or cardiac arrest. Do not administer to patients taking potassium preparations.

Amiloride HCl/ Hydrochlorothiazide (HCTZ)

Potassium-sparing diuretic / Thiazide diuretic

Indications: Treatment of hypertension or congestive heart failure in patients who develop hypokalemia when thiazide or other kaliuretic diuretics are used alone, or in patients in whom maintenance of normal serum potassium levels is clinically important (eg, digitalized patients); alone or as adjunctive treatment with other antihypertensive agents.

Dose: Adults: PO 1 to 2 tablets (5 mg amiloride/50 mg hydrochlorothiazide) daily with meals.

Trade names: Moduretic Tablets 5 mg amiloride/50 mg HCTZ

Warnings: Hyperkalemia (serum potassium levels greater than 5.5 mEq/L); concurrently with other potassium-sparing diuretics (eg, spironolactone), potassium supplements (including potassium-rich diet) except in severe or refractory cases of hypokalemia; impaired renal function; sensitivity to any components of product. Pregnancy Category: [B]

Interactions: Amiloride:
ACE inhibitors (eg, captopril): May result in severely elevated potassium levels.
Potassium preparations: May severely increase serum potassium levels, possibly resulting in cardiac arrhythmias or cardiac arrest. Do not coadminister.
Hydrochlorothiazide:
Bile acid sequestrants: May reduce thiazide absorption; give thiazide at least 2 hr before sequestrant.
Diazoxide: May cause hyperglycemia.
Digitalis glycosides: Diuretic-induced hypokalemia and hypomagnesemia may lead to digitalis-induced arrhythmias.
Lithium: Renal excretion of lithium may be reduced.
Loop diuretics (eg, furosemide): Synergistic effects may occur, resulting in profound diuresis and serious electrolyte abnormalities.
Sulfonylureas (eg, chlorpropamide): Hypoglycemic effect of sulfonylurea may be decreased, necessitating an increase in sulfonylurea dosage.

Aminocaproic Acid

Hemostatic

Indications: Treatment of excessive bleeding from systemic hyperfibrinolysis and urinary fibrinolysis.

Unlabeled indication: Prevention of recurrence of subarachnoid hemorrhage; management of amegakaryocytic thrombocytopenia; abortion; or prevention of attacks of hereditary angioneurotic edema.

Dose: Adults: IV/PO 4 to 5 g in first hour; then 1 to 1.25 g/hr for 8 hr or until bleeding is controlled. Dosage over 30 g/24 hr is not recommended.

Trade names: Amicar Injection 250 mg/mL

Warnings: Active intravascular clotting; DIC; administration to newborns. Pregnancy Category: [Category C]

Interactions: Oral contraceptives or estrogens: May lead to increase in clotting factors, producing state of hypercoagulation.

Aminoglutethimide

Adrenal cortex suppressant

Indications: Suppression of adrenal function in patients with Cushing syndrome.

Unlabeled indication: Suppression of adrenal function in advanced breast carcinoma or metastatic prostate carcinoma.

Dose: Cushing Syndrome:
Adults: PO 250 mg q 6 hr. Titrate to adrenal response in increments of 250 mg/day q 1 to 2 wk. Max daily dose is 2000 mg.
Dosage Adjustment:
Adults: PO Dosage reduction may be required for a Ccr less than 10 mL/min; specific guidelines are not established. Discontinue therapy if patient develops severe rash or rash that lasts more than 5 to 8 days. Therapy may be continued at a lower dose after resolution of mild to moderate skin rashes.

Trade names: Cytadren Tablets 250 mg

Warnings: Standard considerations. Pregnancy Category: [D]

Interactions: CNS depressants: Concurrent use with CNS depressants (eg, narcotics, analgesics, alcohol, antiemetics, benzodiazepines, sedatives, tranquilizers) may potentiate CNS effects.
Dexamethasone, digitoxin, medroxyprogesterone, tamoxifen, theophylline, warfarin: Aminoglutethimide increases oxidative metabolism of these drugs. Higher doses of these agents may be required to achieve therapeutic response during concomitant therapy.

Aminophylline

Bronchodilator / Xanthine derivative

Indications: Prevention or treatment of reversible bronchospasm associated with asthma or COPD.

Unlabeled indication: Treatment of apnea and bradycardia of prematurity.

Dose: Dosage is calculated on basis of lean body weight.
Oral/Rectal: Dose is determined by percentage of theophylline content in aminophylline salt. Aminophylline is 79% theophylline.
Loading Dose:
Adults and children: PO/PR 5 mg/kg.
Maintenance Dose:
Healthy nonsmokers: PO/PR 3 mg/kg q 8 hr.
Elderly and patients with cor pulmonale: 2 mg/kg q 8 hr.
CHF patients: 1 to 2 mg/kg q 12 hr.
Children 9 to 16 yr and young adult smokers: 3 mg/kg q 6 hr.
Children 1 to 9 yr: 4 mg/kg q 6 hr.
Parenteral:
Loading Dose:
Adults and children not receiving theophylline: IV 6 mg/kg.
Adults and children receiving theophylline: IV 0.6 to 3.1 mg/kg.
Maintenance Dose:
Healthy nonsmokers: IV 0.5 to 0.7 mg/kg/hr.
Elderly and patients with cor pulmonale: IV 0.3 to 0.6 mg/kg/hr.
CHF patients: IV 0.1 to 0.5 mg/kg/hr.
Children 9 to 16 yr and young adult smokers: IV 0.8 to 1 mg/kg/hr.
Children 1 to 9 yr: IV 1 to 1.2 mg/kg/hr.
Newborns to infants under 6 mo: Not recommended. Weigh benefits against risks.
Infants 26 to 52 wk: Divide into q 6 hr dosing.
Infants under 26 wk: Divide into q 8 hr dosing.
Infants 6 to 52 wk: 24 hr dosage (mg).
Premature infants older than 4 days postnatal: IV 1.5 mg/kg q 12 hr.
Premature infants less than 24 days postnatal: IV 1 mg/kg q 12 hr.

Trade names: Phyllocontin Tablets, controlled-release (12 hr) 225 mg (equiv. to 178 mg theophylline)
Truphylline Suppositories 250 mg (equiv. to 197.5 mg theophylline)

Warnings: Hypersensitivity to xanthines (eg, caffeine, theobromine) or ethylenediamine; peptic ulcer; seizure disorders not treated with medication. Aminophylline suppositories are contraindicated in presence of irritation or infection of rectum or lower colon. Pregnancy Category: [C]

Interactions: Allopurinol, nonselective beta blockers, calcium channel blockers, cimetidine, oral contraceptives, corticosteroids, disulfiram, ephedrine, influenza virus vaccine, interferon, macrolide antibiotics, mexiletine, quinolone antibiotics, thyroid hormones: May increase aminophylline levels.
Aminoglutethimide, barbiturates, hydantoins, ketoconazole, rifampin, smoking (tobacco and marijuana), sulfinpyrazone, sympathomimetics: May decrease aminophylline levels.
Benzodiazepines, propofol: Aminophylline may

antagonize sedative effects.
Beta-agonists: Effects of both drugs may be antagonized.
Carbamazepine, isoniazid, loop diuretics: May increase or decrease aminophylline levels.
Food: Sustained-released medications are taken on empty stomach to avoid rapid drug release. Low-protein, high-carbohydrate diet may increase aminophylline levels. Charcoal-broiled foods or high-protein, low-carbohydrate diet may decrease aminophylline levels.
Halothane: May cause catecholamine-induced arrhythmias.
Ketamine: May result in seizures.
Lithium: Aminophylline may reduce lithium levels.
Nondepolarizing muscle relaxants: May antagonize neuromuscular blockade.
Incompatability: Do not mix with anileridine hydrochloride, ascorbic acid, chlorpromazine, codeine phosphate, dimenhydrinate, dobutamine hydroxide, epinephrine, erythromycin gluceptate, hydralazine, insulin, levorphanol tartrate, meperidine, methadone, methicillin, morphine sulfate, norepinephrine bitartrate, oxytetracycline, penicillin G potassium, phenobarbital, phenytoin, prochlorperazine, promazine, promethazine, tetracycline, vancomycin, verapamil, vitamin B complex with vitamin C.

Amiodarone

Antiarrhythmic

Indications: Oral: Treatment of life-threatening, recurrent ventricular arrhythmias (ie, ventricular fibrillation and hemodynamically unstable ventricular tachycardia) that do not respond to other antiarrhythmic agents. Use only in patients with the indicated life-threatening arrhythmias because its use is accompanied by substantial toxicity.

Parenteral: Initiation of treatment and prophylaxis of frequently recurring ventricular fibrillation and hemodynamically unstable ventricular tachycardia in patients refractory to other therapy; treatment of ventricular tachycardia and fibrillation when oral amiodarone is indicated but patient is unable to take oral medication.

Unlabeled indication: Conversion of atrial fibrillation and maintenance of sinus rhythm; treatment of supraventricular tachycardia; IV amiodarone has been used to treat AV nodal reentry tachycardia.

Dose: Life-Threatening Recurrent Ventricular Arrhythmias:
Loading dose: PO 800 to 1600 mg/day for 1 to 3 wk. Reduce doses of other antiarrhythmic agents gradually. When adequate arrhythmia control is achieved, reduce dose to 600 to 800 mg/day for 1 mo.
Usual maintenance dose: PO 400 mg/day.
Adults: IV Recommended starting dose is approximately 1000 mg over the first 24 hr administered as follows: rapid administration of 150 mg over first 10 min (15 mg/min), followed by 360 mg over next 6 hr (1 mg/min), then 540 mg over remaining 18 hr (0.5 mg/min). After first 24 hr, continue maintenance infusion rate of 0.5 mg/min (720 mg/24 hr).
Paroxysmal Atrial Fibrillation, PSVT, Symptomatic Atrial Flutter:
Adults: PO 600 to 800 mg/day for 7 to 10 days, then 200 to 400 mg/day.
Arrhythmias in Patients with CHF:
Adults: PO 200 mg/day.
IV to Oral Transition:
Adults: Clinical monitoring is recommended when changing from IV to oral therapy. PO 800 to 1600 mg amiodarone if duration of IV infusion less than 1 wk; 600 to 800 mg amiodarone if duration of IV infusion 1 to 3 wk; 400 mg amiodarone if duration of IV infusion more than 3 wk.

Trade names: Cordarone Tablets 200 mg
Pacerone Tablets 200 mg

Warnings: Oral: Severe sinus-node dysfunction, causing marked sinus bradycardia; second- or third-degree atrioventricular (AV) block; when bradycardia produces syncope, unless used with pacemaker; hypersensitivity to the drug. Parenteral: Marked sinus bradycardia; second- and third-degree atrioventricular block unless functioning pacemaker is available; cardiogenic shock. Pregnancy Category: [D]

Interactions: Anticoagulants: Effect of anticoagulant may be increased. Use of product may require 30% to 50% decrease in anticoagulant dose.
Beta-blockers: Increased risk of hypotension and bradycardia as well as increased effect of beta blockers eliminated by hepatic metabolism.
Calcium channel blockers: Increased risk of atrioventricular block with verapamil or diltiazem as well as hypotension with other calcium blockers.
Cisapride, disopyramide, fluoroquinolones (eg, gatifloxacin, moxifloxacin, sparfloxacin): Possible prolongation of the QT interval, increasing the risk of life-threatening cardiac arrhythmias (including torsades de pointes).
Cholestyramine, rifamycins (eg, rifampin): Amiodarone plasma levels may be reduced, decreasing the pharmacologic effect.
Cimetidine, ritonavir: Amiodarone plasma levels may be elevated, increasing the risk of side effects.
Cyclosporine: Elevated plasma concentrations of cyclosporine resulting in elevated creatinine.
Dextromethorphan: Increased dextromethorphan plasma levels.
Digoxin: Serum digoxin levels may be increased.
Fentanyl: Increased risk of hypotension and bradycardia and decreased cardiac output.
Flecainide: Serum levels of flecainide may be increased.
Hydantoins (eg, phenytoin): Serum concentrations of hydantoins may be increased with potential for symptoms of hydantoin toxicity; also, amiodarone levels may be decreased.
Methotrexate, theophylline: Amiodarone may elevate plasma levels of these agents, increasing the risk of toxicity.
Procainamide: Serum levels of procainamide may be increased.
Quinidine: Serum quinidine levels may increase, creating potential for fatal cardiac arrhythmias.

Amlodipine

Calcium channel blocker

Indications: Hypertension; chronic stable angina; vasospastic (Prinzmetal or variant) angina.

Dose: Adults: PO 5 to 10 mg qd.
Elderly: PO Initially 2.5 mg qd.
Hepatic Impairment: PO Initially 2.5 mg qd.

Trade names: Norvasc Tablets 2.5 mg

Warnings: Sick sinus syndrome; second- or third-degree atrioventricular (AV) block, except with a functioning pacemaker. Pregnancy Category: [Category C]

Interactions: Beta-blockers: May cause increased adverse cardiac effects as a result of myocardial depression.
Fentanyl: Severe hypotension or increased fluid volume requirements have occurred with similar drug.

Amlodipine/Benazepril HCl

Calcium channel blocker / Antihypertensive / ACE inhibitor

Indications: Treatment of hypertension.

Dose: Adults: PO 1 capsule (2.5 to 10 mg amlodipine/10 to 20 mg benazepril)/day.

Trade names: Lotrel Capsule 2.5 mg amlodipine/10 mg benazepril

Warnings: Hypersensitivity to amlodipine,

benazepril, or any other ACE inhibitor. Pregnancy Category: [D (second and third trimester); C (first trimester) ACE inhibitors (eg, benazepril) can cause injury or death to fetus if used during second or third trimester When pregnancy is detected, discontinue as soon as possible]

Interactions: Diuretics: Increased risk of excessive reduction of blood pressure after initiation of amlodipine/benazepril therapy.
Potassium supplements, potassium-sparing diuretics (eg, spironolactone): Increased risk of hyperkalemia.
Lithium: Plasma levels of lithium may be elevated, increasing the risk of toxicity.

Amoxapine

Tricyclic antidepressant

Indications: Relief of symptoms of depression.

Unlabeled indication: Management of chronic pain associated with migraine, chronic tension headache, diabetic neuropathy, phantom limb pain, tic douloureux, cancer pain, peripheral neuropathy, postherpetic neuralgia, and arthritic pain.

Dose: Adults: PO Initial dose: 200 to 300 mg/day; may be given in single daily dose at bedtime once effective dosage is established. Divided doses are given for amounts more than 300 mg/day. Hospitalized patients refractory to antidepressant therapy and with no history of seizures may be cautiously titrated to 600 mg/day in divided doses.
Maintenance: Single daily dose of 300 mg or less at bedtime.
Elderly: PO Initially 25 mg bid or tid. If well tolerated, may be increased to 50 mg bid or tid. Some patients may need up to 300 mg/day.

Trade names: Asendin Tablets 25 mg

Warnings: Hypersensitivity to tricyclic antidepressants; not recommended for use during acute recovery phase of MI. Do not use drug concomitantly with MAOIs except under close medical supervision. Pregnancy Category: [C]

Interactions: Barbiturates, charcoal: May decrease amoxapine blood levels.
Cimetidine, fluoxetine: May increase amoxapine blood levels.
Clonidine: May result in hypertensive crisis.
CNS depressants: Depressant effects may be additive.
MAOIs: May cause serious and possibly fatal hypertensive crisis.

Amprenavir

Antiretroviral / Protease inhibitor

Indications: Treatment of HIV-1 infections in combination with other antiretroviral agents.

Dose: Adults and children 13 to 16 yr: PO (capsules) 1200 mg bid in combination with other antiretroviral agents.
Adults and Children 13 to 16 yr with weight 50 kg or more: PO 1400 mg bid.
Children 4 to 12 yr or 13 to 16 yr with weight less than 50 kg: PO (capsules) 20 mg/kg bid or 15 mg/kg tid (max, 2400 mg/day) in combination with other antiretroviral agents.
Children 4 to 12 yr or 13 to 16 yr with weight less than 50 kg: PO (oral solution) 22.5 mg/kg (1.5 mL/kg) bid or 17 mg/kg (1.1 mL/kg) tid (max, 2800 mg) in combination with other antiretroviral agents.

Trade names: Agenerase Capsules 50 mg

Warnings: Concomitant therapies with cisapride, dihydroergotamine, ergotamine, ergonovine, methylergonovine, or pimozide; midazolam and triazolam; drugs that are highly dependent on CYP3A4 for clearance and for which elevated plasma levels are associated with serious or life-threatening events; when administered in combination with ritonavir, flecainide, and propafenone are contraindicated; hypersensitivity to any component of the product; because of the propylene glycol content, the oral solution is contraindicated in infants and children under 4 yr, pregnant women, patients with renal or hepatic failure, and patients treated with disulfiram or metronidazole. Pregnancy Category: [C]

Interactions: Abacavir, aldesleukin, azole antifungal agents (eg, itraconazole), cimetidine, clarithromycin, delavirdine, dexamethasone, didanosine, erythromycin, ethanol, indinavir, itraconazole, ritonavir, zidovudine: May increase amprenavir plasma levels.
Alprazolam, clorazepate, diazepam, flurazepam, midazolam, triazolam: Amprenavir may increase blood levels of these drugs, which may produce extreme sedation and respiratory depression.
Amiodarone, bepridil, cisapride, ergot derivatives, lidocaine (systemic), quinidine, rifabutin, sildenafil, tricyclic antidepressants: Amprenavir may elevate blood levels of these drugs, which may increase the risk of arrhythmias, hematologic abnormalities, seizures, or other potential serious adverse effects.
Amlodipine, atorvastatin, cerivastatin, carbamazepine, clozapine, cylcosporine, dapsone, diltiazem, erythromycin, felodipine, fentanyl, isradipine, itraconazole, ketoconazole, loratadine, lovastatin, nicardipine, nifedipine, nimodipine, oral contraceptives, pimozide, pravastatin, sildenafil, simvastatin, tacrolimus, tricyclic antidepressants (eg, amitriptyline), verapamil, zidovudine: May have their plasma concentrations increased, which could increase activity or toxicity.
Antacids, carbamazepine, efavirenz, methadone, oral contraceptives, phenobarbital, phenytoin, rifabutin, rifampin, St. John's wort: May decrease plasma levels of amprenavir, which may reduce antiviral activity.
Cisapride, dihydroergotamine, disulfiram, ergotamine, ergonovine, methylergonovine, midazolam, pimozide, triazolam: Use with amprenavir is contraindicated.
Ritonavir: Plasma levels may be decreased by amprenavir.
Warfarin: Risk of bleeding may be increased.

Amyl Nitrite

Antianginal

Indications: Relief of angina pectoris.

Dose: Adult: Inhalation 0.3 mL prn. 1 to 6 inhalations from 1 capsule are usually sufficient. May be repeated in 3 to 5 min.

Trade names: Amyl Nitrite Aspirols Inhalant 0.3 mL
Amyl Nitrite Vaporole Inhalant 0.3 mL

Warnings: Hypersensitivity to nitrates; pregnancy; severe anemia; closed-angle glaucoma; orthostatic hypotension; head trauma; cerebral hemorrhage. Pregnancy Category: [X]

Interactions: Alcohol: Severe hypotension and cardiovascular collapse may occur.
Aspirin: Increased nitrate concentration and actions may occur.
Calcium channel blockers: Symptomatic orthostatic hypotension may occur.
Heparin: Effects of heparin may be decreased.

Anagrelide

Antiplatelet agent

Indications: Thrombocythemia caused by myeloproliferative disorders to reduce platelet count and risk of thrombotic events and to relieve associated symptoms.

Dose: Thrombocythemia:
Adults (initial dose): PO 0.5 mg 4 qid or 1 mg bid for at least 7 days. Titrate to minimum effective dose required to maintain platelet count less than 600,000 cells/mm^3, or within normal range. Avoid dosage increases more than 0.5 mg/day in any 1-wk period. The max recommended dose is 10 mg/day or 2.5 mg/dose.

Trade names: Agrylin Capsules 0.5 mg and

1 mg
Warnings: Standard considerations. Pregnancy Category: [C]
Interactions: Sucralfate: May reduce the oral absorption of anagrelide.

Anakinra

Immunomodulator
Indications: Reduction in signs and symptoms of moderately to severely active rheumatoid arthritis; slowing the progression of structural damage in patients who have failed at least 1 disease-modifying antirheumatic drug.
Dose: Adults: SC 100 mg/day.
Trade names: Kineret Solution 100 mg
Warnings: Hypersensitivity to *E. coli* -derived proteins, anakinra, or any component of product. Pregnancy Category: [B]
Interactions: None well documented.

Apraclonidine

Sympathomimetic
Indications: 1% solution: Control or prevent postsurgical elevations in IOP that occur in patients after argon laser trabeculoplasty or iridotomy.

0.5% solution: Short-term adjunctive therapy in patients on maximally tolerated medical therapy who require additional IOP reduction.
Dose: 0.5% solution: Ophthalmic Instill 1 to 2 drops in affected eye(s) 3 times daily. Apraclondine 0.5% will be used with other ocular glaucoma therapies, use approximately 5 min interval between instillation of each medication to prevent washout of previous dose.
1% solution: Ophthalmic Instill 1 drop in scheduled operative eye 1 hr before initiating anterior segment laser surgery. Instill second drop into same eye immediately upon completion of surgery.
Trade names: lopidine Solution 0.5%
Warnings: Hypersensitivity to any component of this medication or to clonidine; concurrent monoamine oxidase inhibitor therapy. Pregnancy Category: [C]
Interactions: Drugs that may interact include cardiovascular agents and MAOIs. May potentiate effects on pulse and blood pressure.

Aripiprazole

Antipsychotic agent
Indications: Treatment of schizophrenia.
Dose: Usual Dose:
Adults: PO Start with 10 or 15 mg/day on a qd schedule. The effective dose range is 10 to 30 mg/day. Do not increase dosage before 2 wk.
Concurrent Use of CYP3A4 (eg, ketoconazole) or CYP2D6 Inhibitors (eg, fluoxetine, quinidine):
Adults: PO Reduce the usual dose of aripiprazole 50%. Increase the dose when the CYP3A4 or CYP2D6 inhibitor is discontinued.
Concurrent Use of CYP3A4 Inducers (eg, carbamazepine):
Adults: PO Double the usual dose of aripiprazole (to 20 to 30 mg). Additional increases should be based on clinical evaluation. Decrease the dose (to 10 to 15 mg) when the CYP3A4 inducer is discontinued.
Maintenance: No evidence is available from controlled trials; however, it is generally agreed that treatment for acute schizophrenia should be continued for up to 6 mo or more.
Trade names: Abilify Tablets 5 mg
Warnings: Standard considerations. Pregnancy Category: [C]
Interactions: Alcohol: Avoid while using aripiprazole.
CYP2D6 inhibitors (eg, fluoxetine, paroxetine, quinidine), CYP3A4 inhibitors(eg, ketoconazole): May elevate aripiprazole plasma levels, increasing the adverse effects.
CYP2D6 inducers (eg, carbamazepine): May reduce aripiprazole plasma levels, decreasing the therapeutic effect.

Asparaginase

Enzyme
Indications: Adult: Combination therapy for acute lymphocytic leukemia. Do not use as the sole induction agent unless combination therapy is deemed inappropriate.

Pediatric: Acute lymphocytic leukemia. Do not use as the sole induction agent unless combination therapy is deemed inappropriate.
Dose: Acute Lymphocytic Leukemia:
Pediatric: IV Give over 30 min through the side arm of an already running infusion of Sodium Chloride Injection or 5% Dextrose Injection. The drug has little tendency to cause phlebitis when given IV.
Pediatric: IM Limit the volume at a single injection site to 2 mL. For a volume greater than 2 mL, use 2 injection sites.
Acute Lymphocytic Leukemia Induction Regimens:
Pediatric: One of the following combination regimens is recommended for acute lymphocytic leukemia in children.
Acute Lymphocytic Leukemia Induction Regimen I:
Pediatric:
Prednisone: 40 mg/m^2 /day PO in 3 divided doses for 15 days, followed by tapering of the dosage as follows: 20 mg/m^2 for 2 days, 10 mg/m^2 for 2 days, 5 mg/m^2 for 2 days, 2.5 mg/m^2 for 2 days, and then discontinue.
Vincristine sulfate: 2 mg/m^2 IV once weekly on days 1, 8, and 15. The maximum single dose should not exceed 2 mg.
Asparaginase: 1000 IU/kg/day IV for 10 successive days beginning on day 22. When remission is obtained, institute appropriate maintenance therapy. Do not use asparaginase as part of a maintenance regimen. Asparaginase has been used in other combination regimens. Administering the drug IV concurrently with or immediately before a course of vincristine and prednisone may be associated with increased toxicity.
Acute Lymphocytic Leukemia Induction Regimen II:
Pediatric:
Prednisone: 40 mg/m^2 /day PO in 3 divided doses for 28 days (the total daily dose to the nearest 2.5 mg), then gradual discontinuation over 14 days.
Vincristine sulfate: 1.5 mg/m^2 IV weekly for 4 doses, on days 1, 8, 15, and 22. The maximum single dose should not exceed 2 mg.
Asparaginase: 6000 IU/m^2 IM on days 4, 7, 10, 13, 16, 19, 22, 25, and 28. When remission is obtained, institute appropriate maintenance therapy. Do not use asparaginase as part of a maintenance regimen
Acute Lymphocytic Leukemia Single Agent Induction Therapy:
Adult/Pediatric: IV Use asparaginase as the sole induction agent only when a combined regimen is inappropriate because of toxicity or other specific patient-related factors, or in cases refractory to other therapy. Administer 200 IU/kg/day IV for 28 days. Complete remissions are of short duration, 1 to 3 mo.
Trade names: Elspar Powder for injection, lyophilized 10,000 international units
Warnings: Anaphylactic reactions to asparaginase; pancreatitis or a history of pancreatitis. Pregnancy Category: [C]
Interactions: Methotrexate: Asparaginase may diminish or abolish methotrexate's effect on malignant cells. Do not use methotrexate with, or following asparaginase, while asparagine levels are below normal. Asparaginase may augment corticosteroid-induced hyperglycemia.
Vincristine and prednisone: IV administration may be associated with increased toxicity.

Atazanavir Sulfate

Antiviral

Indications: In combination with other antiretroviral agents for the treatment of HIV-1 infection.

Dose: When coadministered with efavirenz, it is recommended that atazanavir 300 mg and ritonavir 100 mg be given with efavirenz 600 mg (all as a single dose with food). Atazanavir without ritonavir should not be coadministered with efavirenz.
Adults: PO 400 mg qd with food.
Hepatic Impairment:
Adults: PO Use with caution in patients with mild to moderate hepatic insufficiency. Consider a dose reduction to 300 mg qd in patients with moderate hepatic insufficiency. Do not use in patients with severe hepatic impairment.

Trade names: Reyataz Capsules 100 mg

Warnings: Drugs (eg, cisapride, ergot derivative, midazolam, pimozide, triazolam) that are highly dependent on CYP3A for Cl and for which elevated plasma levels are associated with serious and/or life-threatening events; hypersensitivity to any component of the product. Pregnancy Category: [B]

Interactions: Antacids and buffered medications (eg, didanosine buffered preparation), efavirenz, H_2-receptor antagonists, proton pump inhibitors (eg, omeprazole), rifampin, St. John's wort: May reduce atazanavir plasma levels, decreasing the therapeutic effect. Coadministration of proton pump inhibitors, rifampin, or St. John's wort with atazanavir is not recommended. Atazanavir without ritonavir should not be coadministered with efavirenz.
Antiarrhythmic agents (eg, amiodarone, quinidine, systemic lidocaine), calcium channel blockers (eg, bepridil, felodipine, nicardipine, verapamil), HMG-CoA reductase inhibitors (ie, atorvastatin, lovastatin, simvastatin), immunosuppressive agents (ie, cyclosporine, sirolimus, tacrolimus), irinotecan, oral contraceptives (eg, ethinyl estradiol and norethindrone), phenytoin, rifabutin, sildenafil, tricyclic antidepressants, warfarin: Atazanavir may increase plasma levels of these agents, increasing the risk of toxicity and, in some instances, life-threatening reactions. Coadministration of bepridil is not recommended. Up to a 75% reduction in the rifabutin dose is recommended. A 50% reduction in the dose of diltiazem should be considered and titrate the dose of other calcium channel blockers. Sildenafil should be used with caution and at a reduced dose of 25 mg q 48 hr and monitor for adverse reactions.
Clarithromycin: Plasma levels of clarithromycin may be elevated by atazanavir, which may result in QTc prolongation. A 50% reduction in clarithromycin dose should be considered. In addition, levels of the active metabolite (14-OH clarithromycin) may be reduced. Use alternative therapy for indications other than *Mycobacterium avium* complex.
Cisapride, ergot derivatives (eg, ergotamine), midazolam, pimozide, triazolam: Coadministration with atazanavir is contraindicated because of serious or life-threatening adverse effects.
H_2-receptor antagonists (eg, cimetidine): Atazanavir plasma levels may be reduced, decreasing the therapeutic effect and increasing the development of resistance.
Indinavir: Coadministration is not recommended because of the increased risk of indirect hyperbilirubinemia.

Atenolol

Beta-adrenergic blocker

Indications: Treatment of hypertension (used alone or in combination with other drugs), angina pectoris resulting from coronary atherosclerosis, acute MI.

Unlabeled indication: Migraine prophylaxis, alcohol withdrawal syndrome, ventricular arrhythmias, supraventricular arrhythmias or tachycardias, esophageal varices rebleeding, anxiety.

Dose: Hypertension:
Adults: PO 50 to 100 mg/day.
Angina Pectoris: PO May require up to 200 mg/day.
Acute MI:
Adults: IV 5 mg over 5 min; second IV follow with 5 mg dose 10 min later.
Adults: PO 50 to 100 mg/day.

Trade names: Tenormin Tablets 25 mg

Warnings: Hypersensitivity to beta-blockers; sinus bradycardia; greater than first-degree heart block; CHF unless secondary to tachyarrhythmia treatable with beta-blockers; overt cardiac failure; cardiogenic shock. Pregnancy Category: [D]

Interactions: Aluminum salts, ampicillin, calcium salts: Plasma levels and pharmacologic effects may be decreased.
Clonidine: May add to or reverse antihypertensive effects; potentially life-threatening situations may occur, especially on withdrawal.
Diltiazem: Pharmacologic effects of atenolol may be increased; symptomatic bradycardia may occur.
Nifedipine, verapamil: Effects of both drugs may be increased.
NSAIDs: Some agents may impair antihypertensive effect.
Prazosin: May increase orthostatic hypotension.
Quinidine: Pharmacologic effects of atenolol may be increased.

Atenolol/Chlorthalidone

Antihypertensive

Indications: Treatment of hypertension.

Dose: Adults: PO 50 mg atenolol/25 mg chlorthalidone or 100 mg atenolol/ 25 mg chlorthalidone once daily.

Trade names: Tenoretic-50 Tablets 50 mg atenolol/25 mg chlorthalidone
Tenoretic-100 Tablets 100 mg atenolol/25 mg chlorthalidone

Warnings: Hypersensitivity to sulfonamide-derived drugs, sinus bradycardia, heart block greater than first degree, cardiogenic shock, overt cardiac failure, anuria. Not for initial therapy of hypertension. Pregnancy Category: [Category D]

Interactions: Clonidine: Beta blockers may exacerbate rebound hypertension associated with clonidine withdrawal. Atenolol/chlorthalidone should be tapered and withdrawn several days before gradual withdrawal of clonidine.
Digitalis glycosides: Diuretic-induced hypokalemia may potentiate digitalis toxicity.
Lithium: May increase therapeutic and toxic effects of lithium; avoid concomitant use.
Nondepolarizing muscle relaxants: May increase effects of these agents.
Norepinephrine: May decrease arterial responsiveness to norepinephrine.
Other antihypertensive agents: May increase antihypertensive effects.
Sulfonylureas: May decrease hypoglycemic effects.

Atomoxetine

Psychotherapeutic

Indications: Treatment of attention-deficit/ hyperactivity disorder (ADHD).

Dose: Adults and Children (over 70 kg): PO Start with 40 mg/day and increase the dose after a minimum of 3 days to a target total daily dose of approximately 80 mg. After 2 to 4 additional wk, the dose may be increased to a max of 100 mg/day in patients who have not achieved an optimal response. In children over 70 kg receiving a strong CYP2D6 inhibitor (eg, fluoxetine), increase the 40 mg/day dose to the target dose of 80 mg/day if symptoms fail to improve after 4 wk and

the initial dose is well-tolerated.
Children (up to 70 kg): PO Start with 0.5 mg/kg/day and increase the dose after a minimum of 3 days to a target total dose of approximately 1.2 mg/kg/day (max, 1.4 mg/kg or 100 mg/day, whichever is less).
In children up to 70 kg receiving a strong CYP2D6 inhibitor (eg, fluoxetine), increase the 0.5 mg/kg/day dose to the target dose of 1.2 mg/kg/day if symptoms fail to improve after 4 wk and the initial dose is well-tolerated.
Impaired hepatic function: PO Moderate hepatic function impairment (Child-Pugh Class B), reduce initial and target doses to 50% of the normal dose; severe hepatic function impairment (Child-Pugh Class C), reduce initial and target doses to 25% of normal.
Trade names: Strattera Capsules 10 mg (as base)
Warnings: Narrow angle glaucoma; MAO inhibitors or within 2 weeks after discontinuing an MAO inhibitor; hypersensitivity to any component of the product. Pregnancy Category: [C]
Interactions: Albuterol: Use with caution, the cardiovascular effects of albuterol may be potentiated.
CYP2D6 inhibitors (eg, fluoxetine, quinidine): The area under the plasma concentration-time curve and peak plasma level of atomoxetine may be increased.
MAO inhibitors (eg, isocarboxazid): Coadministration is contraindicated.
Pressor agents: Possible increased effects of BP.

Atorvastatin Calcium

Antihyperlipidemic / HMG-CoA reductase inhibitor

Indications: Elevated serum triglyceride: As an adjunct to diet for the treatment of patients with elevated serum triglyceride levels (Fredrickson type IV).

Heterozygous familial hypercholesterolemia in pediatric patients: Adjunct to diet to reduce total and LDL cholesterol and apolipoprotein B levels in boys and postmenarchal girls 10 to 17 yr if, after an adequate trial of diet therapy, and LDL remains 160 mg/dL or higher and there is a positive family history of premature CV disease or 2 or more other CV risk factors present.

Homozygous familial hypercholesterolemia: To reduce total cholesterol and LDL cholesterol in patients with homozygous familial hypercholesterolemia as an adjunct to other lipid-lowering treatments or if such treatments are unavailable.

Hypercholesterolemia: Adjunct to diet to reduce elevated total cholesterol, LDL cholesterol, apolipoprotein B, and triglyceride levels and to increase HDL cholesterol.

Type III familial hyperlipoproteinemia: To treat patients with primary dysbetalipoproteinemia (Fredrickson type III) who do not respond adequately to diet.
Dose: Adults: PO 10 to 80 mg/day.
Heterozygous Familial Hypercholesterolemia:
Children (10 to 17 yr): PO Start with 10 mg/day (max, 20 mg/day).
Trade names: Lipitor Tablets 10 mg
Warnings: Active liver disease or unexplained persistent elevation of serum transaminases; pregnancy; lactation; hypersensitivity to any component of the product. Pregnancy Category: [X]
Interactions: Antacids: Coadministration may decrease atorvastatin levels.
Azole antifungal agents (eg, itraconazole), cyclosporine, macrolide antibiotics (eg, erythromycin), gemfibrozil, grapefruit juice, niacin, protease inhibitors (eg, ritonavir), verapamil: Severe myopathy or rhabdomyolysis may occur.
Contraceptives, oral: Coadministration increases AUC for norethindrone and ethinyl estradiol.
Digoxin: Elevated digoxin levels may occur.

Auranofin

Analgesic / Antirheumatic / Gold compound

Indications: Relief of symptoms of active adult rheumatoid arthritis poorly controlled with other therapies.

Unlabeled indication: Treatment of pemphigus and psoriatic arthritis.
Dose: Adults: PO 6 mg/day or 3 mg bid. If no response by 6 mo, dose may be increased to 3 mg tid. Parenteral route may be used when control cannot be achieved by oral form.
Children: Auranofin is not recommended for children; safety and efficacy have not been established. If prescribed, however, the following doses have been recommended. 0.1 mg/kg/day (initial dose); 0.15 mg/kg/day (maintenance dose); 0.2 mg/kg/day (max dose).
Trade names: Ridaura Capsules 3 mg
Warnings: Standard considerations. Pregnancy Category: [C]
Interactions: None well documented.

Azathioprine

Immunosuppressive

Indications: Adjunct for prevention of rejection in renal homotransplantation; treatment in adults for severe, active, erosive rheumatoid arthritis not responsive to conventional management.

Unlabeled indication: Treatment of chronic ulcerative colitis, Crohn disease, myasthenia gravis and Behcet syndrome.
Dose: Renal Transplantation:
Adults and children: IV/PO Initiate with 3 to 5 mg/kg/day as single daily dose. Maintenance levels are 1 to 3 mg/kg/day.
Rheumatoid Arthritis:
Adults: PO Initial dose is 1 mg/kg given as single dose or twice daily. Dose is increased by 0.5 mg/kg/day at 6 to 8 wk, then q 4 wk if there are no serious toxicities and if initial response is unsatisfactory. Max dose is 2.5 mg/kg/day. IV Reserved for patients unable to tolerate oral medications.
Trade names: Azasan Tablets 25 mg
Imuran Tablets 50 mg
Warnings: Pregnancy in patients with rheumatoid arthritis. Pregnancy Category: [D]
Interactions: Allopurinol: Decreases metabolism of azathioprine. Dose of azathioprine is reduced to approximately one-third to one-fourth usual dose when used concomitantly.
Nondepolarizing muscle relaxants (eg, tubocurarine, pancuronium): Azathioprine may resist or reverse neuromuscular blockade.

Azelaic Acid

Topical Anti-infective

Indications: Topical treatment of mild to moderate inflammatory acne vulgaris (cream); topical treatment of papules and pustules of mild to moderate rosacea.
Dose: Adults and Children 12 yr and older: Topical After washing and patting dry, gently but thoroughly massage a thin film of cream or gel into the affected areas bid, in the morning and evening. In the majority of patients with inflammatory lesions, improvement of the condition occurs within 4 wk.
Trade names: Azelex Cream 20%
Finacea Gel 15%
Warnings: Standard considerations. Pregnancy Category: [B]
Interactions: None well documented.

Azithromycin

Antibiotic / Macrolide

Indications: Adults: Treatment of infections of the respiratory tract, chronic obstructive pulmonary disease (COPD), community-acquired pneumonia, *Mycobacterium avium* complex, pelvic inflammatory disease, skin and skin structure, and sexually-transmitted diseases caused by susceptible organisms.

Children: Treatment of acute otitis media caused by susceptible organisms; community-acquired pneumonia, treatment of pharyngitis/tonsillitis caused by *Streptococcus pyogenes* in patients who cannot use first-line therapy.

Dose: Acute Otitis Media:
Children 6 mo and older: PO 30 mg/kg given as a single dose or 10 mg/kg once daily for 3 days or 10 mg/kg as a single dose on the first day (not to exceed 500 mg/day) followed by 5 mg/kg on days 2 through 5 (not to exceed 250 mg/day).
Bacterial Infections:
Adults: PO 500 mg as single dose on first day, then 250 mg/day on days 2 through 5.
Community-Acquired Pneumonia:
Adults and children 16 yr and older: PO 500 mg as a single dose on the first day followed by 250 mg once daily on days 2 through 5.
Adults: IV 500 mg as a single daily dose for greater than or equal to 2 days. Follow IV therapy by the oral route at a single daily dose of 500 mg to complete 7- to 10-day course of therapy.
Children 6 mo and older: PO 10 mg/kg as a single dose on the first day (not to exceed 500 mg/day), followed by 5 mg/kg on days 2 through 5 (not to exceed 250 mg/day).
Gonorrhea:
Adults: PO Single 2 g dose.
Mild to Moderate COPD:
Adults and children 16 yr and older: PO 500 mg/day for 3 days or 500 mg as a single dose on the first day followed by 250 mg once daily on days 2 through 5.
Mycobacterium avium Complex:
Adults: PO Prevention: 1.2 g taken weekly. Treatment: 600 mg/day in combination with ethambutol (15 mg/kg).
Pelvic Inflammatory Disease:
Adults: IV 500 mg as a single daily dose for 1 to 2 days. Follow IV therapy by the oral route at a single daily dose of 250 mg to complete a 7-day course of therapy.
Pharyngitis/Tonsillitis:
Adults and children 16 yr and older: PO 500 mg as a single dose on the first day followed by 250 mg once daily on days 2 through 5.
Children at least 2 yr: PO 12 mg/kg/day for 5 days, not to exceed 500 mg/day.
Genital Ulcer Disease caused by H. ducreyi (chancroid), Nongonococcal Urethritis/Cervicitis caused by C. trachomatis:
Adults: PO Single 1 g dose.
Uncomplicated Skin and Skin Structure Infections:
Adults and children 16 yr and older: PO 500 mg as a single dose on the first day followed by 250 mg once daily for 4 days.

Trade names: Zithromax Tablets 250 mg (as dihydrate)

Warnings: Hypersensitivity to azithromycin, erythromycin, or to any macrolide antibiotic. Pregnancy Category: [B]

Interactions: HMG-CoA reductase inhibitors (eg, lovastatin): Increased risk of myopathy and rhabdomyolysis.
Tacrolimus: Increased tacrolimus plasma levels with increased risk of toxicity.
Warfarin: The anticoagulant effect may be increased, increasing the risk of hemorrhage.

Aztreonam

Antibiotic / Monobactam

Indications: Treatment of infections of urinary tract, lower respiratory tract, skin and skin structure, intra-abdominal infections, gynecologic infections, surgical infections, and septicemia caused by susceptible microorganisms.

Unlabeled indication: Treatment of acute, uncomplicated gonorrhea in patients with penicillin-resistant gonococci.

Dose: Urinary Tract Infection:
Adults: IM/IV 500 mg or 1 g q 8 to 12 hr.
Systemic Infections:
Adults: IM/IV 1 to 2 g q 6 to 12 hr.
Children: IM/IV 30 to 50 mg/kg q 4 to 8 hr.
Acute Uncomplicated Gonorrhea:: IM 1 g. Max recommended dosage is 8 g/day.

Trade names: Azactam Powder for injection (lyophilized cake) 500 mg (with approximately 780 mg L-arginine per gram aztreonam)

Warnings: Standard considerations. Pregnancy Category: [B]

Interactions: Beta-lactamase-inducing antibiotics (eg, cefoxitin, imipenem): May antagonize activity of aztreonam and should not be used concurrently.
Incompatability: Nafcillin sodium, cephradine, metronidazole: Incompatible in admixture.

Baclofen

Skeletal muscle relaxant / Centrally acting

Indications: Oral: Treatment of reversible spasticity resulting from multiple sclerosis. May be of some value in patients with spinal cord injuries and other spinal cord diseases.

Intrathecal: Treatment of severe spasticity of spinal cord origin in patients who are unresponsive to or cannot tolerate oral baclofen therapy. Used intrathecally in single bolus test doses; chronic use requires implantable pump.

Unlabeled indication: Oral: Therapy for trigeminal neuralgia (tic douloureux); tardive dyskinesia.

Intrathecal: Cerebral palsy spasticity in children.

Dose: Adults:
Initial dose: PO 5 mg tid; may be increased by 5 mg/dose q 3 days prn to max 80 mg/day (20 mg qid). Intrathecal Refer to manufacturer's manual for implantable pump.
Screening:
Adults: 1 mL of 50 mcg/mL dilution is administered into the intrathecal space by barbotage over 1 min and patient is observed for 4 to 8 hr; may be repeated 24 hr later with 75 mcg/1.5 mL and 48 hr later with 100 mcg/2 mL. Do not give implantable pump to patients not responding to 100 mcg bolus.
Children: The starting screening dose for pediatric patients is the same as in adult patients (eg, 50 mcg). However, for very small patients, a screening dose of 25 mcg may be tried first.
Postimplant Dose Titration Period: To determine the initial total daily dose of baclofen following implant, double the screening dose that gave a positive effect and administer over a 24-hr period.
Spasticity of Spinal Cord Origin:
Adults: Intrathecal After the first 24 hr, increase the daily dosage slowly in 10% to 30% increments and only once q 24 hr, until desired effect is achieved.
Spasticity of Cerebral Origin:
Adults: Intrathecal After the first 24 hr, increase the daily dose slowly 5% to 15% once q 24 hr, until desired clinical effect is achieved.
Children: After the first 24 hr, increase the daily dose slowly 5% to 15% only once q 24 hr, until the desired

effect is achieved.
Maintenance Therapy for Spasticity of Spinal Cord Origins: Very often the maintenance dose needs to be adjusted during the first few months of therapy while patients adjust to changes in life-style because of the alleviation of spasticity.
Adults: Intrathecal During periodic refills of the pump, the daily dose may be increased 10% to 40%, but no more than 40%, to maintain adequate symptom control. Maintenance dose for long-term continuous infusion has ranged from 12 to 2003 mcg/day, with most patients adequately maintained on 300 to 800 mcg/day.
Maintenance Therapy for Spasticity of Cerebral Origin: Very often the maintenance dose needs to be adjusted during the first few months of therapy while patients adjust to changes in life-style because of the alleviation of spasticity.
Adults: Intrathecal During the periodic refills of the pump, the daily dose may be increased 5% to 20%, but no more than 20%. Ranges from 22 to 1400 mcg/day, with most patients adequately maintained on 90 to 703 mcg/day.
Children less than 12 yr: Average daily dose 274 mcg/day. Requires individual titration. Use the lowest dose with an optimal response.
Children at least 12 yr: Same as adult. Determination of the optimal dose requires individual titration. Use the lowest dose with an optimal response.
Trade names: Lioresal Tablets 10 mg
Warnings: Treatment of spasms from rheumatic disorders, stroke, cerebral palsy and Parkinson disease; use of intrathecal form via IV, IM, SC, or epidural routes. Pregnancy Category: [C]
Interactions: CNS depressants: May cause increased sedative effects.
Morphine (epidural): May cause hypotension and dyspnea.

Beclomethasone Dipropionate

Corticosteroid
Indications: Oral inhalation: QVAR: Maintenance prophylactic treatment of asthma in patients 5 yr and older; asthma patients requiring systemic corticosteroid administration in which adding an inhaled corticosteroid may reduce or eliminate need for systemic corticosteroids.
Dose: Bronchial Asthma:
Adults and children (12 yr and older): PO QVAR: If previous therapy consisted of bronchodilators alone, start with 40 or 80 mcg bid (max dose, 320 mcg bid); if previous therapy consisted of inhaled corticosteroids, start with 40 to 160 mcg bid (max dose, 320 mcg bid).
Children (5 to 11 yr): Aerosol actuation QVAR: If previous therapy consisted of bronchodilators alone or inhaled corticosteroids, start with 40 mcg bid (max dose, 80 mcg bid).
Trade names: QVAR Aerosol 40 mcg/actuation
Warnings: Oral inhalation: Primary treatment of status asthmaticus or acute episodes of asthma; systemic fungal infections; positive sputum cultures of Candida albicans or Aspergillus niger. Pregnancy Category: [C]
Interactions: None well documented.

Benazepril HCl

Antihypertensive / ACE inhibitor
Indications: Treatment of hypertension.
Dose: Adults:
Initial dose: PO 10 mg qd for patients not receiving a diuretic. In patients taking diuretics that cannot be discontinued, give initial dose of 5 mg.
Maintenance: PO 20 to 40 mg/day as single dose or in 2 divided doses; doses up to 80 mg have been used.
Renal function impairment: Initial dose is 5 mg qd for patients with Ccr less than 30 mL/min. Dosage may be titrated upward until BP is controlled or to a total max daily dose of 40 mg.
Trade names: Lotensin Tablets 5 mg
Warnings: Hypersensitivity to ACE inhibitors. Pregnancy Category: [D (second and third trimester); C (first trimester) When pregnancy is detected, discontinue ACE inhibitors as soon as possible]
Interactions: Antacids: May decrease bioavailability of benazepril; separate administration by 1 to 2 hr.
Diuretics: May cause symptomatic hypotension after initial dose of benazepril.
Lithium: May increase lithium levels and symptoms of lithium toxicity.
Potassium preparations, potassium-sparing diuretics: May increase serum potassium levels.
Salicylates (eg, aspirin): May reduce effects of benazepril, especially in low-renin or volume-dependent hypertensive patients.

Benazepril HCl/ Hydrochlorothiazide

Antihypertensive
Indications: Treatment of hypertension. This fixed combination drug is not intended for the initial therapy of hypertension.
Dose: Adults: PO Combination therapy with qd doses of 5 to 20 mg benazepril and 6.25 to 25 mg of hydrochlorothiazide.
Trade names: Lotensin HCT Tablets 20 mg benazepril, 25 mg hydrochlorothiazide
Warnings: Anuric patients; patients hypersensitive to benazepril or any other ACE inhibitor; hydrochlorothiazide or other sulfonamide derivative. Pregnancy Category: [D (second and third trimester); C (first trimester) ACE inhibitors (eg, benazepril) can cause injury or death to fetus if used during second or third trimester When pregnancy is detected, discontinue as soon as possible]
Interactions: Cholestyramine, colestipol: May impair the absorption of hydrochlorothiazide.
Insulin: In diabetic patients, requirements of insulin may be increased, decreased, or unchanged.
Lithium: Plasma levels of lithium may be elevated, increasing the risk of toxicity.
Potassium supplements, potassium-sparing diuretics (eg, spironolactone): Increased risk of hyperkalemia.
Tubocurarine: Effects may be increased.

Benztropine Mesylate

Antiparkinson / Anticholinergic
Indications: Treatment of all forms of parkinsonism; control of extrapyramidal disorders (except tardive dyskinesia) caused by neuroleptic drugs.
Dose: Parkinsonism:
Adults: PO 1 to 2 mg/day; range, 0.5 to 6 mg. Individualize dosage.
Idiopathic Parkinsonism:
Adults: PO Initially 0.5 to 1 mg at bedtime; 4 to 6 mg/day may be required.
Postencephalitic Parkinsonism:
Adults: PO 2 mg/day in 1 or more doses; some patients may require initial dose of 0.5 mg.
Drug-Induced Extrapyramidal Disorders:
Adults: 1 to 4 mg qd or bid.
Acute Dystonic Reactions:
Adults: PO/IM/IV Initial dose is IM/IV 1 to 2 mg; then PO 1 to 2 mg bid.
Trade names: Cogentin Tablets 0.5 mg
Warnings: Angle-closure glaucoma; myasthenia gravis; pyloric or duodenal obstruction; stenosing peptic ulcer; prostatic hypertrophy or bladder neck obstructions; megacolon; tardive dyskinesia; children under 3 yr. Pregnancy Category: [C]
Interactions: Amantadine: May increase

anticholinergic effects.
Digoxin: May increase digoxin serum levels, especially with slow-dissolution oral digoxin tablets.
Haloperidol: May worsen schizophrenic symptoms; may decrease haloperidol serum levels; tardive dyskinesia may develop.
Phenothiazines: May decrease action of phenothiazines. May increase incidence of anticholinergic effects.

Beractant

Lung surfactant

Indications: Prevention and treatment ('rescue') of neonatal respiratory distress syndrome (RDS) in premature infants.

Dose: Newborns and infants: Intratracheal
Prevention: 25 mg/kg/instillation for 4 instillations (total dose of 100 mg/kg is administered in 4 quarter doses); dose is started within 15 min of birth.
Rescue: 25 mg/kg/instillation for 4 instillations (total dose 100 mg/kg). May be repeated for continued or progressive RDS.

Trade names: Survanta Suspension 25 mg phospholipids per mL suspended in 0.9% sodium chloride solution. With 0.5 to 1.75 mg triglycerides, 1.4 to 3.5 mg free fatty acids, and less than 1 mg protein per mL.

Warnings: Standard considerations. Pregnancy Category: []

Interactions: None well documented.

Betaxolol HCl

Beta-adrenergic blocker

Indications: Hypertension.
Ophthalmic preparation: Lowering IOP; ocular hypertension; chronic open-angle glaucoma.

Dose: Hypertension:
Adults: PO 10 to 20 mg/day.
Elderly: PO Reduce initial dose to 5 mg/day.
Glaucoma:
Adults: Ophthalmic 1 to 2 drops bid in affected eye(s). Consider concomitant therapy if IOP is not at satisfactory level.

Trade names: Betoptic Solution 5.6 mg (equivalent to 5 mg base) per mL (0.5%)
Betoptic S Suspension 2.8 mg (equivalent to 2.5 mg base) per mL (0.25%)
Kerlone Tablets 10 mg

Warnings: Hypersensitivity to beta-blockers; sinus bradycardia; greater than first-degree heart block; CHF unless secondary to tachyarrhythmia treatable with beta-blockers; overt cardiac failure; cardiogenic shock. Pregnancy Category: [C]

Interactions: Clonidine: May enhance or reverse antihypertensive effect; potentially life-threatening situations may occur, especially on withdrawal.
NSAIDs: Some agents may impair antihypertensive effect.
Prazosin: May increase postural hypotension.
Verapamil: May increase effects of both drugs.

Bethanechol Chloride

Urinary tract product / Cholinergic stimulant

Indications: Treatment of acute postoperative and postpartum nonobstructive urinary retention and neurogenic atony of the urinary bladder with retention.

Unlabeled indication: Diagnosis and treatment of reflux esophagitis.

Dose: Adults: PO 10 to 50 mg tid to qid on empty stomach. SC 2.5 to 5 mg at 15 to 30 min intervals for max of 4 doses; then minimum effective dose may be repeated tid to qid prn.

Trade names: Urecholine Tablets 5 mg
Duvoid Tablets 10 mg
Myotonachol Tablets 10 mg

Warnings: Hyperthyroidism; peptic ulcer; latent or active asthma; pronounced bradycardia; AV conduction defects; vasomotor instability; coronary artery disease; epilepsy; parkinsonism; coronary occlusion; hypotension; hypertension; bladder neck obstruction; spastic GI disturbances; acute inflammatory lesions of the GI tract; peritonitis; marked vagotonia. Not used when strength or integrity of GI or bladder wall is in question or in presence of mechanical obstruction, when increased muscular activity of GI tract or urinary tract may prove harmful (eg, after recent urinary bladder surgery, GI resection and anastomosis, possible GI obstruction). Pregnancy Category: [C]

Interactions: Cholinergic agents: Possible toxicity because of additive effects.
Ganglionic blocking compounds: Severe hypotension, usually preceded by severe abdominal symptoms.
Quinidine or procainamide: Antagonism of anticholinergic effects of bethanechol.

Bexarotene

Retinoids

Indications: Refractory cutaneous T-cell lymphoma (CTCL).

Dose: Refractory CTCL:
Adults: PO
Initial dose: 300 mg/m^2 /day as a single daily dose. An initial dose of 150 to 225 mg also has been used.
Maintenance dose: Increase dose to 400 mg/m^2 /day if no tumor response after 8 wk. A target maintenance dose of 450 to 525 mg also has been used. Continue therapy as response is favorable. See manufacturer product information for specific body surface area dosing.
Adults: Topical Apply topical gel to cutaneous lesions qod initially. Increase application at weekly intervals (eg, qd, bid, tid) up to target dose of qid as tolerated. Onset of response ranges from 4 to 56 wk. Continue therapy as long as response is favorable. Consider reducing frequency or discontinuing application if severe skin irritation occurs. Resume therapy after several days.
Dosage Adjustment (Oral Therapy):
Adults: PO Adverse reactions requiring dosage adjustment include AST, ALT, or bilirubin greater than 3 times the ULN, leukopenia or neutropenia, or hypertriglyceridemia unresponsive to therapy. Reduce dose to 200 mg/m^2 /day. If reaction does not resolve, decrease to 100 mg/m^2 /day or temporarily discontinue. Bexarotene is metabolized extensively by hepatic cytochrome P450 3A4 isoenzymes. Dosage adjustment in hepatic insufficiency is warranted; however, there are not specific guidelines.

Trade names: Targretin Gelatin capsules for oral use 75 mg

Warnings: Pregnancy; hypersensitivity to bexarotene or other product components. Pregnancy Category: [X]

Interactions: Antidiabetic agents (eg, insulin sulfonylureas, insulin-sensitizers): May enhance antidiabetic agents, resulting in hypoglycemia.
Contraceptives, oral: Potentially can induce metabolic enzymes and thereby theoretically reduce plasma concentrations of hormonal contraceptives. It is strongly recommended that 2 reliable forms of contraception be used concurrently, 1 of which should be nonhormonal.
CYP450 inducers (eg, rifampin, phenytoin, phenobarbital, primidone): May reduce plasma bexarotene concentrations.
CYP450 inhibitors (eg, ketoconazole, itraconazole, erythromycin, grapefruit juice): May increase plasma bexarotene concentrations.
DEET: For topical use, the absorption of DEET increases when used concomitantly with bexarotene gel, resulting in increased toxicity of DEET.
Gemfibrozil: Resulted in substantial increases in

plasma concentrations of bexarotene.
Tamoxifen: Coadministration of bexarotene capsules and tamoxifen resulted in a modest decrease in plasma tamoxifen concentrations, possibly through an induction of cytochrome P450 3A4.
Vitamin A: Bexarotene is a member of the retinoids. Limit vitamin A supplements to avoid potential additive toxic effects (up to 15,000 IU/day).

Bicalutamide

Antiandrogen / Antineoplastic hormone

Indications: Advanced prostate cancer in combination with a luteinizing hormone releasing hormone (LHRH) analog. Safety and efficacy not established.

Dose: Advanced Prostate Cancer:
Adults: PO 50 mg (1 tablet) once daily at the same time of day with or without food.

Trade names: Casodex Tablets for oral use 50 mg.

Warnings: Standard considerations. Pregnancy Category: [X]

Interactions: Warfarin: Prothrombin time may increase when bicalutamide is initiated in patients stabilized on chronic warfarin therapy.

Bisacodyl

Laxative

Indications: Short-term treatment of constipation; evacuation of colon for rectal and bowel evaluations; preparation for delivery or surgery.

Dose: Oral:
Adults: PO 10 to 15 mg.
Preparation of Lower GI Tract: Up to 30 mg.
Children over 6 yr: PO 5 to 10 mg (0.3 mg/kg).
Suppository:
Adults: PR 10 mg.
Children over 2 yr: PR 10 mg.
Children under 2 yr: PR 5 mg.

Trade names: Dulcolax Tablets, enteric-coated 5 mg
Fleet Laxative Tablets, enteric-coated 5 mg
Modane Tablets, enteric-coated 5 mg
Women's Gentle Laxative Tablets, enteric-coated 5 mg
Bisac-Evac Tablets, enteric-coated 5 mg
Caroid Tablets, enteric-coated 5 mg
Correctol Tablets, enteric-coated 5 mg
Feen-a-mint Tablets, enteric-coated 5 mg
Reliable Gentle Laxative Tablets, enteric-coated and delayed-release 5 mg
Bisacodyl Uniserts Suppositories 10 mg

Warnings: Nausea, vomiting, or other symptoms of appendicitis; acute surgical abdomen; fecal impaction; intestinal obstruction; undiagnosed abdominal pain; ulcerative lesions of colon; rectal fissures; ulcerative hemorrhoids. Pregnancy Category: [B]

Interactions: Milk or antacids: May cause enteric coating of tablets to dissolve, resulting in gastric lining irritation or gastric indigestion.

Bisoprolol Fumarate/ Hydrochlorothiazide

Antihypertensive

Indications: Management of hypertension.

Dose: Adults: PO Start with 2.5 mg bisoprolol/ 6.25 mg hydrochlorothiazide daily, increasing the dose in 14-day intervals until optimal response is obtained (max recommended dose 20 mg bisoprolol/12.5 mg hydrochlorothiazide).

Trade names: Ziac Tablets 6.25 mg hydrochlorothiazide/2.5 mg bisoprolol fumarate

Warnings: Cardiogenic shock; overt cardiac failure; second or third degree AV block; marked sinus bradycardia; anuria; hypersensitivity to either component of product or other sulfonamide derivatives. Pregnancy Category: [C]

Interactions: Bisoprolol:
Antiarrhythmic agents (eg, disopyramide), diphenylalkylamine calcium antagonists (eg, verapamil), benzothiazepine calcium antagonists (eg, diltiazem): Use with caution.
Antihypertensives: Actions of other antihypertensive agents may be potentiated.
Beta-blockers: Do not combine with other beta-blockers.
Catecholamine-depleting agents (eg, guanethidine, reserpine): Sympathetic action may be considerably reduced.
Clonidine: If discontinuing clonidine after coadministration with bisoprolol/hydrochlorothiazide, discontinue bisoprolol/hydrochlorothiazide several days before withdrawal of clonidine.
Hydrochlorothiazide:
Alcohol, barbiturates, narcotics: Increased risk of orthostatic hypotension.
Antidiabetic agents: Dose adjustments in antidiabetic agent may be needed.
Antihypertensives: Actions of other antihypertensive agents may be potentiated.
Cholestyramine, colestipol resins: Absorption of hydrochlorothiazide may be impaired.
Adrenocorticotropic hormone, corticosteroids: Increased risk of electrolyte depletion (eg, hypokalemia).
Pressor amines (eg, norepinephrine): Decreased response to pressor amine.
Nondepolarizing skeletal muscle relaxants (eg, tubocurarine): Responsiveness to muscle relaxant may be increased.
Lithium: Plasma levels of lithium may be elevated, increasing the risk of toxicity.
NSAIDs: The antihypertensive, diuretic, and natriuretic effect of hydrochlorothiazide may be reduced.

Bitolterol Mesylate

Bronchodilator / Sympathomimetic

Indications: Prevention and treatment of reversible bronchospasm associated with asthma or other obstructive pulmonary diseases.

Dose: Acute Bronchospasm:
Adults and Children over 12 yr: Oral inhalation 2 inhalations at interval of 1 to 3 min, followed by third inhalation if necessary.
Prevention of Bronchospasm:
Adults and Children over 12 yr: Oral inhalation 2 inhalations q 8 hr, not to exceed 3 inhalations q 6 hr or 2 inhalations q 4 hr.
Solution for Inhalation: Administer during a 10- to 15-min period.
Continuous flow nebulization: 1.5 to 3.5 mg (0.75 to 1.75 mL volume) 3 to 4 times/day with an interval of at least 4 hr between treatments. Max daily dose, 14 mg.
Intermittent flow nebulization: 0.5 to 1.5 mg (0.25 to 0.75 mL volume) 3 to 4 times/day with an interval of at least 4 hr between treatments. Max daily dose, 8 mg.

Trade names: Tornalate Aerosol 0.8% (delivers 0.37 mg/actuation)

Warnings: Standard considerations. Pregnancy Category: [C]

Interactions: None well documented.

Bleomycin Sulfate

Antitumor antibiotic

Indications: Lymphomas (Hodgkin and non-Hodgkin), testicular carcinoma (eg, embryonal cell, choriocarcinoma, teratocarcinoma), germ cell tumors; sclerosis of malignant pleural effusions (eg, treatment, prevention); palliative treatment of squamous cell carcinomas (eg, head, neck).

Unlabeled indication: Mycosis fungoides, osteosarcoma, AIDS-related Kaposi sarcoma.

Dose: Test Dose:
Adults: IV, IM, or SC Because of the possibility of anaphylactoid reaction, treat lymphoma patents with 2 units or less for the first 2 doses. If no acute reaction occurs, follow the regular dosage schedule.
Squamous Cell Carcinoma, Lymphosarcoma, Reticular Cell Sarcoma, Testicular Carcinoma:
Adults: IV, IM, SC 10 to 20 units/m^2 1 or 2 times/wk. Response is usually seen within 3 wk.
Hodgkin Disease:
Adults: IV, IM, SC 10 to 20 units/m^2 1 or 2 times/wk. After a 50% regression of tumor size, a maintenance dose of 1 unit/day or 5 units/wk can be given IV or IM. Response is usually seen within 2 wk. Squamous cell cancers respond more slowly, sometimes requiring 3 wk for improvement. To minimize the risk of pulmonary toxicity, the maximum cumulative dose should not exceed 400 units. When bleomycin is used in combination with other antineoplastic agents, pulmonary toxicities may occur at lower doses.
Pleural Effusions:
Adults: Thoracotomy tube 50 to 60 units diluted with 50 to 100 mL 0.9% Sodium Chloride or 5% Dextrose is instilled into chest via a thoracotomy tube following drainage of excess pleural fluid and confirmation of complete lung expansion. The amount of drainage from the chest tube should be as minimal as possible prior to installation of bleomycin. The thoracotomy tube is then clamped. The patient is moved from the supine to the left and right lateral positions several times during the next 4 hr. The clamp is then removed and suction re-established. It is generally accepted that chest tube drainage should be below 100 mL in a 24-hr period prior to sclerosis. However, bleomycin instillation may be appropriate when drainage is between 100 and 300 mL under clinical conditions that necessitate sclerosis therapy.

Trade names: Blenoxane Sterile powder for reconstitution 15 unit vial (15 units = 15 mg) and 30 unit vial (30 units = 30 mg).

Warnings: Standard considerations. Pregnancy Category: [D]

Interactions: Digoxin and phenytoin: Bleomycin may decrease serum concentrations of digoxin and phenytoin.

Bosentan

Vasodilator / Endothelin receptor antagonist

Indications: Treatment of pulmonary arterial hypertension in patients with WHO Class III and IV symptoms, to improve exercise ability and decrease the rate of clinical worsening.

Dose: Adults and Children over 12 yr:
Initial dose: PO 62.5 mg bid for 4 wk; then increase to maintenance dose of 125 mg bid. If bosentan therapy is reintroduced, it should be at the starting dose.
Patients under 40 kg but over 12 yr:
Initial and maintenance dose: PO 62.5 mg bid. If bosentan therapy is reintroduced, it should be at the starting dose.

Trade names: Tracleer Tablets 62.5 mg

Warnings: Pregnancy; coadministration of cyclosporine or glyburide; hypersensitivity to bosentan or any component of the product. Pregnancy Category: [X Pregnancy must be excluded before starting bosentan]

Interactions: Cyclosporine: Bosentan trough concentrations may be increased, while cyclosporine plasma levels may be decreased; coadministration is contraindicated.
Glyburide: Plasma concentrations of both glyburide and bosentan may be decreased; coadministration is contraindicated.
Ketoconazole: Plasma concentrations of bosentan may be increased.
Hormonal contraceptives (ie, oral, injectable, implantable), HMG-CoA reductase inhibitors (eg, simvastatin), warfarin: Plasma concentrations of these agents may be decreased.

Botulinum Toxin Type A

Botulinum toxins / Ophthalmic surgical adjunct

Indications: Treatment of cervical dystonia in adults to decrease severity of abnormal head position and neck pain associated with cervical dystonia; treatment of strabismus and blepharospasm associated with dystonia, including benign essential blepharospasm or VII nerve disorder; for temporary improvement in appearance of moderate to severe glabellar lines associated with corrugator or procerus muscle activity in patients 65 yr of age or younger.

Unlabeled indication: Treatment of hemifacial spasms, spasmodic torticollis, oromandibular dystonia, spasmodic dysphonia, and other dystonias.

Dose: Blepharospasm:
Adults and children at least 12 yr of age: Initially, inject 1.25 to 2.5 units (0.05 to 0.1 mL volume at each site) into the medial and lateral pretarsal orbicularis oculi of the upper lid and into the lateral pretarsal orbicularis oculi of the lower lid.
Cervical Dystonia:
Adults and children at least 16 yr of age: In patients with known history of tolerance, tailor dosing in initial and sequential treatments to the individual patient based on patient's head and neck position, localized pain, muscle hypertrophy, patient response, and adverse event history. In patients without prior use, use lower dose than in patients with known history of tolerance, adjusting subsequent doses based on individual response.
Glabellar Lines (Botox Cosmetic only):
Adults (65 yr of age or younger): IM Total treatment dose is 20 units in 0.5 mL at intervals no more frequent than q 3 mo (duration of activity of botulinum toxin type A is approximately 3 to 4 mo).
Strabismus:
Adults and children at least 12 yr of age: Inject between 0.05 to 0.15 mL per muscle into extraocular muscles utilizing electrical activity recorded from tip of injection needle as guide to placement within target muscle.

Trade names: Botox Powder for injection 100 units vacuum-dried *Clostridium botulinum* toxin type A neurotoxin complex
Botox Cosmetic Powder for injection 100 units vacuum-dried *Clostridium botulinum* toxin type A neurotoxin complex

Warnings: Infection at the proposed injection site(s). Pregnancy Category: [C]

Interactions: Aminoglycosides, drugs interfering with neuromuscular transmission: The effects of botulinum toxin may be potentiated.

Bretylium Tosylate

Antiarrhythmic

Indications: Prophylaxis and treatment of ventricular fibrillation; treatment of life-threatening ventricular arrhythmia that has failed to respond to first-line antiarrhythmic agents.

Unlabeled indication: Second-line therapy (following lidocaine) for the treatment of ventricular arrhythmia during advanced cardiac life support in CPR.

Dose: Life-Threatening Ventricular Arrhythmias:
Adults:
Initial dose: IV 5 to 10 mg/kg (undiluted) by rapid IV injection; if arrhythmia persists, adjust dosage as necessary.
Maintenance (for continuous suppression): IV Infuse diluted solution at 1 to 2 mg/min. Alternately, infuse diluted solution at 5 to 10 mg/kg over more than 8 min q 6 hr.

Children: IV 5 mg/kg/dose followed by 10 mg/kg at 10 to 30 min intervals (max total dose, 30 mg/kg).
Maintenance: 5 to 10 mg/kg/dose q 6 hr.
Other Ventricular Arrhythmias:
Adults: IV 5 to 10 mg/kg (diluted) over 8 min; if arrhythmia persists, give subsequent doses q 1 to 2 hr.
Maintenance: Administer same dose q 6 hr or infuse 1 to 2 mg/min. IM 5 to 10 mg/kg (undiluted); if arrhythmia persists, give subsequent doses at 1 to 2 hr intervals. Maintain same dosage q 6 to 8 hr.
Children: 5 to 10 mg/kg/dose q 6 hr.

Trade names: Bretylium Tosylate in 5% Dextrose Injection 2 mg/mL (500 mg/vial)
Bretylium Tosylate Injection 50 mg/mL

Warnings: Standard considerations. Pregnancy Category: [C]

Interactions: Antihypertensives: May cause severe hypotension.
Catecholamines: Enhance pressor effects of catecholamines.
Digoxin: May aggravate arrhythmias caused by digitalis toxicity.

Brimonidine Tartrate

Antiglaucoma / Alpha-2 adrenergic agonist

Indications: Lowers IOP in open-angle glaucoma or ocular hypertension.

Dose: Adults and children 2 yr and older: Ophthalmic Instill 1 drop into affected eye(s) tid (approximately 8 hr apart).

Trade names: Alphagan Solution 0.2%
Alphagan P Solution 0.15%

Warnings: Coadministration of MAO inhibitors. Pregnancy Category: [B]

Interactions: Antihypertensives, beta blockers, cardiac glycosides: Brimonidine may reduce pulse and BP; use with caution.
CNS depressants (eg, alcohol, anesthetics, barbiturates, opiates, sedative): Additive or potentiating CNS depressant effect.
MAO inhibitors: Concurrent use contraindicated.
Tricyclic antidepressants: May decrease the effect of brimonidine by altering the metabolism and uptake of circulating amines.

Bromocriptine Mesylate

Antiparkinson

Indications: Treatment of hyperprolactinemia-associated disorders (eg, amenorrhea with or without galactorrhea, infertility, hypogonadism) in patients with prolactin-secreting adenomas; therapy for female infertility associated with hyperprolactinemia; treatment of acromegaly; therapy for Parkinson disease (idiopathic or postencephalitic).

Unlabeled indication: Treatment of hyperprolactinemia associated with pituitary adenomas; therapy for neuroleptic malignant syndrome; treatment of cocaine addiction.

Dose: Hyperprolactinemia-Associated Disorders:
Initial dose: PO 1.25 to 2.5 mg/day; 2.5 mg may be added as tolerated q 3 to 7 days until optimum response. (Dosage range, 2.5 to 15 mg/day).
Acromegaly:
Initial dose: PO 1.25 to 2.5 mg for 3 days at bedtime; may be increased by 1.25 to 2.5 mg as tolerated q 3 to 7 days until optimum response occurs. Dosage range, 20 to 30 mg/day, not to exceed 100 mg/day.
Parkinson Disease:
Initial dose: PO 1.25 mg bid titrated individually. Dosage range, 10 to 40 mg/day, not to exceed 100 mg/day.

Trade names: Parlodel Tablets 2.5 mg (as mesylate)

Warnings: Sensitivity to ergot alkaloids; severe ischemic heart disease or peripheral vascular disease; pregnancy. Pregnancy Category: [Pregnancy category undetermined]

Interactions: Dopamine antagonists (eg, phenothiazines, butyrophenones, metoclopramide): May reduce bromocriptine efficacy.
Erythromycin: May increase bromocriptine serum levels.

Budesonide

Corticosteroid

Indications: Intranasal: Management of seasonal and perennial allergic rhinitis symptoms in adults and children (Rhinocort Aqua).

Oral inhalation: For the maintenance treatment of asthma as prophylactic therapy in adults and children and for patients requiring oral corticosteroid therapy for asthma (inhaler).

Inhalation suspension: Maintenance treatment of asthma and prophylactic therapy in children 12 mo to 8 yr of age.

Oral capsule: Crohn disease.

Dose: Nasal Spray:
Adult and Children at least 12 yr of age: Spray Start with 64 mcg/day administered as 1 spray in each nostril daily.
Maintenance: Spray Titrate to minimum effective dose (max, 256 mcg/day administered as 4 sprays in each nostril daily).
Adult and Children 6 to under 12 yr of age: Spray Start with 64 mcg/day administered as 1 spray in each nostril daily.
Maintenance: Spray Titrate to minimum effective dose (max, 128 mcg/day administered as 2 sprays in each nostril daily).
Aerosol, Turbuhaler:
Adults: Oral inhaler 200 to 400 mcg bid (max, 800 mcg bid).
Children at least 6 yr of age: Oral inhaler 200 mcg bid (max, 400 mcg bid).
Respules:
Children 12 mo to 8 yr of age: Inhalation suspension Administer by inhaled route via jet nebulizer connected to air compressor.
Children receiving bronchodilators alone: 0.5 mg/day administered daily or bid in divided doses (max, 0.5 mg/day).
Children receiving inhaled corticosteroids: 0.5 mg/day administered daily or bid in divided doses (max, 1 mg/day).
Children receiving oral corticosteroids: 1 mg/day administered as 0.5 mg bid or 1 mg daily (max, 1 mg/day).
Oral Capsules:
Adults: PO 9 mg daily in the morning for up to 8 wk (Crohn disease); can be tapered to 6 mg daily for 2 wk prior to complete cessation.

Trade names: Entocort EC Capsules 3 mg budesonide (micronized)
Pulmicort Turbuhaler Powder 200 mcg (each actuation delivers approximately 160 mcg)/metered dose
Pulmicort Respules Inhalation suspension 0.25 mg per 2 mL
Rhinocort Aqua Nasal spray 32 mcg budesonide/spray

Warnings: Untreated localized infections involving the nasal mucosa; relief of acute bronchospasm; primary treatment of status asthmaticus or other acute episodes of asthma when intensive measures are required; hypersensitivity to the drug or drug compound of the product. Not recommended for treatment of nonallergic rhinitis because of lack of data. Pregnancy Category: [B (inhalation) C (oral, intranasal)]

Interactions: Grapefruit juice, CYP3A4 inhibitors (eg, ketoconazole, ritonavir): May increase budesonide plasma levels, increasing the pharmacologic and adverse effects.

Bumetanide

Loop diuretic

Indications: Treatment of edema associated with CHF, hepatic cirrhosis, and renal disease.

Unlabeled indication: Relief of adult nocturia.

Dose: Adults: PO 0.5 to 2 mg/day as single dose. If inadequate response, give second or third dose at 4 to 5 hr intervals up to max 10 mg/day. IM/IV 0.5 to 1 mg/day over 1 to 2 min. May repeat at 2- to 3-hr intervals, up to max 10 mg/day. Reserve parenteral route for situations in which GI absorption is impaired or when oral administration is not practical; replace with oral therapy as soon as possible.

Trade names: Bumex Tablets 0.5 mg

Warnings: Hypersensitivity to other loop diuretics or to sulfonylureas; anuria; hepatic coma or states of severe electrolyte depletion until condition is improved or corrected. Pregnancy Category: [C]

Interactions: Aminoglycosides: Increased auditory toxicity.
Cisplatin: Additive ototoxicity.
Digitalis glycosides: Electrolyte disturbances may predispose to digitalis-induced arrhythmias.
Lithium: Increased plasma lithium levels and toxicity.
NSAIDs: Decreased effects of bumetanide.
Salicylates: Impaired diuretic response in patients with cirrhosis and ascites.
Thiazide diuretics: Synergistic effects that may result in profound diuresis and serious electrolyte abnormalities.

Bupropion HCl

Antidepressant / Smoking deterrent

Indications: Treatment of depression; aid to smoking cessation treatment.

Dose: Antidepressant:
Adults: PO 100 mg bid initially; may increase to 100 mg tid after 3 days (max daily dose, 450 mg; max single dose, 150 mg).
Sustained/extended-release: 150 mg/day initially; may increase to 150 mg bid or qd (Wellbutrin XL) as early as day 4 (max daily dose, 400 mg or 450 mg [Wellbutrin XL]; max single dose, 200 mg).
Hepatic Function Impairment (Severe Hepatic Cirrhosis):
Adults: PO Do not exceed 75 mg qd.
Sustained/extended-release: Do not exceed 100 mg qd or 150 mg qod.
Mild to moderate cirrhosis: Use with caution; consider reduced dose and/or frequency.
Renal Function Impairment:
Adults: PO Use with caution; consider reduced dose and frequency.
Smoking Deterrent:
Adults: PO
Initial dose: 150 mg for first 3 days, increasing to 150 mg bid. Do not give doses greater than 300 mg/day. Initiate treatment while patient is still smoking. Patient should set target date to quit smoking within the first 2 wk of treatment; continue treatment for 7 to 12 wk.
Maintenance: Clinical data not available regarding long-term treatment (more than 12 wk) for smoking cessation. Whether to continue treatment must be determined for individual patients.
Combination treatment: Combination treatment with bupropion and nicotine transdermal system may be prescribed for smoking cessation.

Trade names: Wellbutrin Tablets 75 mg
Wellbutrin SR Tablets, sustained-release 100 mg
Wellbutrin XL Tablets, extended-release 150 mg
Zyban Tablets, sustained-release 150 mg

Warnings: Seizure disorder; current or prior diagnosis of bulimia or anorexia nervosa; concurrent treatment with or within 14 days of discontinuation of MAO inhibitors; concurrent treatment with multiple bupropion products (eg, coadministration of Zyban for smoking cessation and Wellbutrin for depression); abrupt discontinuation of alcohol or sedatives. Hypersensitivity to buproprion or any other component of the product. Pregnancy Category: [B]

Interactions: Alcohol: Adverse neuropsychiatric events or reduced alcohol tolerance may occur.
Amantadine, levodopa: Incidence of bupropion side effects may be increased.
Antidepressants, antipsychotics, systemic steroids, theophylline: May lower seizure threshold.
Carbamazepine: May decrease bupropion serum concentrations.
MAO inhibitors, selegiline: May increase risk of acute bupropion toxicity. Discontinue MAO inhibitors at least 14 days before starting bupropion.
Ritonavir: Plasma levels of bupropion may be elevated, increasing the risk of toxicity.
Tricyclic antidepressants (TCAs): TCA plasma concentrations may be elevated.

Buspirone HCl

Antianxiety

Indications: Treatment of anxiety disorders; short-term relief of anxiety symptoms.

Unlabeled indication: Reduction of symptoms of PMS.

Dose: Adults:
Initial dose: PO 7.5 mg bid; may increase by 5 mg/day q 2 to 3 days prn (max, 60 mg/day in divided doses).

Trade names: BuSpar Tablets 5 mg (4.6 mg as base)

Warnings: Standard considerations. Pregnancy Category: [B]

Interactions: Diazepam: Dizziness, headache, and nausea can occur.
Fluoxetine: Buspirone effects may be decreased. Paradoxical worsening of OCD may occur.
Haloperidol: Buspirone may increase haloperidol plasma levels.
Inducers of CYP3A4 (eg, carbamazepine, dexamethasone, phenobarbital, phenytoin, rifampin): May reduce buspirone plasma levels, decreasing the therapeutic effect.
Inhibitors of CYP3A4 (eg, diltiazem, erythromycin, grapefruit juice, itraconazole, ketoconazole, nefazodone, ritonavir, verapamil): May elevate buspirone plasma levels, increasing the pharmacologic and adverse effects.
MAO inhibitors (eg, isocarboxazid): Risk of elevated BP may be increased.
Nefazadone: If used with buspirone, a low dose (eg, 2.5 mg/day) is recommended.
Trazodone: ALT may be elevated.

Busulfan

Alkylating agent / Alkyl sulfonates

Indications: Palliative treatment of chronic myelogenous leukemia (CML) (oral); allogeneic bone marrow transplantation for CML (IV).
Pediatric: Palliative treatment of CML (oral).

Unlabeled indication: Severe thrombocytosis, polycythemia vera, myelofibrosis; bone marrow transplantation (oral).

Dose: Remission Induction of CML:
Adults: PO 4 to 8 mg/day (60 mcg/kg or 1.8 mg/m^2 /day). When the total leukocyte count is less than 15,000/mm^3, withhold drug. During remission, treatment is resumed when a monthly WBC reaches 50,000/mm^3.
Pediatric: PO 60 to 120 mcg/kg or 1.8 to 4.6 mg/m^2 once daily. When total leukocyte count is less than 15,000/mm^3, withhold drug. During remission, treatment is resumed when a monthly WBC reaches 50,000/mm^3.

Medications

Bone Marrow Ablation:
Adults: PO 1 mg/kg q 6 hr for 16 doses (for a total dose of 16 mg/kg over 4 days) in combination with other agents. An alternate regimen is busulfan 0.4375 to 0.5 mg/kg q 6 hr for 16 doses (total dose of 7 to 8 mg/kg, respectively, over 4 days) alone or in combination with other chemotherapy agents.
Adults: IV 0.8 mg/kg q 6 hr for 16 doses (for a total dose of 12.8 mg/kg over 4 days). Base dose on ideal body weight or actual body weight, whichever is lower. For obese patients, base dosage on adjusted body weight.
Dosage Adjustment:
Pediatric: PO Reduce dose 50% for WBC between 30,000 to 40,000/mm^3. Discontinue therapy if WBC count falls to 20,000/mm^3 or less.
Trade names: Myleran Tablets 2 mg
Warnings: Tablets: Do not use unless a diagnosis of CML has been adequately established. Contraindicated in patients whose disease has demonstrated prior resistance to the drug without a diagnosis of CML. Busulfan is of no value in chronic lymphocytic leukemia, acute leukemia, or in the 'blastic crisis' of CML. Injection: Hypersensitivity to any of its components. Pregnancy Category: [D]
Interactions: Acetaminophen: May decrease busulfan clearance.
Itraconazole: Decreases busulfan clearance 25%, increasing serum levels and effects.
Phenytoin: Increases busulfan clearance at least 15%, reducing serum levels and effects.
Thioguanine: Long-term, concomitant use has resulted in hepatotoxicity and esophageal varices.

Butenafine HCl
Antifungal agent
Indications: Interdigital tinea pedis (athlete's foot); tinea corporis (ringworm); tinea cruris (jock itch); tinea (pityriasis) versicolor caused by susceptible organisms.
Dose: Tinea Pedis:
Adults and Children 12 yr and older: Topical Apply to affected and surrounding area(s) bid for 7 days or qd for 4 wk.
Tinea Corporis, Tinea Cruris, and Tinea (Pityriasis) Versicolor:
Adults and Children 12 yr and older: Topical Apply qd for 2 wk.
Trade names: Lotrimin Ultra Cream 1%
Mentax Cream 1%
Warnings: Standard considerations. Pregnancy Category: [B]
Interactions: None well documented.

Butoconazole Nitrate
Topical / Antifungal
Indications: Local treatment of vulvovaginal candidiasis (moniliasis).
Dose: Nonpregnant Women: Intravaginal 1 applicator (about 5 g) at bedtime for 3 days; may continue up to 6 days if needed.
Pregnant Women: Intravaginal Use only during second or third trimester, 1 applicator (about 5 g) at bedtime for 6 days.
Trade names: Femstat 3 Vaginal cream 2%
Warnings: Hypersensitivity to imidazoles. Pregnancy Category: [C]
Interactions: None well documented.

Butorphanol Tartrate
Narcotic agonist-antagonist analgesic
Indications: Parenteral/Nasal: Management of pain, including postoperative and migraine.

Parenteral: Preoperative or preanesthetic medication (to supplement balanced anesthesia); relief of pain during labor.
Dose: Pain:
Adults: IV 0.5 to 2 mg q 3 to 4 hr prn. IM 1 to 4 mg q 3 to 4 hr prn. Single doses should not exceed 4 mg. Nasal 1 mg (1 spray in 1 nostril). If no relief in 30 to 90 min, may repeat as 1 mg dose. For severe pain, initial dose of 2 mg can be used if patient can remain lying down. Do not repeat for 3 to 4 hr.
Elderly: IV/IM 1/2 normal dose at twice normal interval. Titrate subsequent doses to response. Nasal Initial dose is 1 mg. Wait 90 to 120 min before giving second 1 mg dose.
Preoperative/Preanesthetic:
Adults:
Usual dose: IM 2 mg 60 to 90 min before surgery.
Labor:
Adults: IV/IM 1 to 2 mg in early labor at term; repeat after 4 hr.
Kidney or Liver Impairment:
Adults: IM/IV Increase dosing interval to q 6 to 8 hr initially. Titrate subsequent doses to response.
Trade names: Stadol Injection 1 mg/mL (1 mg of tartrate salt is equal to 0.68 mg base)
Stadol NS Nasal spray 10 mg/mL
Warnings: Standard considerations. Pregnancy Category: [C]
Interactions: Barbiturate anesthetics: Increased CNS and respiratory depression.
CNS depressants (eg, tranquilizers, sedatives, alcohol): Additive CNS depression.

Calcipotriene
Antipsoriatic / Synthetic vitamin D-3
Indications: Ointment and cream: Treatment of plaque psoriasis.

Scalp solution: Topical treatment of chronic, moderately severe psoriasis of the scalp.
Dose: Ointment:
Adults: Topical Apply a thin layer to the affected skin once or twice daily; rub in gently and completely.
Cream:
Adults: Topical Apply a thin layer to the affected skin twice daily; rub in gently and completely.
Scalp solution:
Adults: Topical Comb the hair to remove scaly debris and, after suitably parting, apply twice daily only to the lesions and rub in gently and completely, taking care to prevent the solution from spreading onto the forehead.
Trade names: Dovonex Ointment 0.005%
Warnings: Standard considerations; patients with acute psoriatic eruptions; patients with hypercalcemia or vitamin D toxicity. Pregnancy Category: [C]
Interactions: None well documented.

Calcitonin-Salmon
Hormone
Indications: Treatment of moderate to severe Paget disease, postmenopausal osteoporosis, hypercalcemia. Nasal spray for treatment of symptomatic Paget disease.
Dose: Paget Disease:
Adults:
Initial dose: SC/IM 100 IU/day.
Maintenance dose: SC/IM 50 IU/day or qod is usually sufficient.
Postmenopausal Osteoporosis:
Adults: SC/IM 100 IU/day with supplemental calcium and adequate vitamin D intake. Intranasal 200 IU/day, alternating nostrils.
Hypercalcemia:
Adults:
Starting dose: SC/IM 4 IU/kg q 12 hr. Titrate gradually on basis of response to maximum dose of 8 IU/kg q 6 hr.
Trade names: Calcimar Injection 200 IU/mL
Miacalcin Injection 200 IU/mL

Osteocalcin Injection 200 IU/mL
Salmonine Injection 200 IU/mL
Warnings: Standard considerations. Pregnancy Category: [C]
Interactions: None well documented.

Calcitriol

Fat-soluble vitamin

Indications: Dialysis (Oral, IV): Hypocalcemia and resultant metabolic bone disease in patients on chronic renal dialysis.

Predialysis (Oral): Secondary hyperparathyroidism and resultant metabolic bone disease in patients with moderate to severe chronic renal failure (Ccr 15 to 55 mL/min) not yet on dialysis.

Hypoparathyroidism (Oral): Hypocalcemia in patients with postsurgical hypoparathyroidism, idiopathic hypoparathyroidism, and pseudohypoparathyroidism.

Unlabeled indication: Decreased severity of psoriatic lesions with an initial oral dose of 0.25 mcg bid and topically 0.1 to 0.5 mcg/g petrolatum.
Dose: Dialysis: PO 0.25 mcg/day. Unsatisfactory response, increase dose by 0.25 mcg/day at 4- to 8-wk intervals. Obtain serum calcium levels at least twice weekly during this titration. Normal or only slightly reduced calcium levels may respond to doses of 0.25 mcg every other day. IV 0.02 mcg/kg (1 to 2 mcg) 3 times/wk, every other day. May increase 0.5 to 1 mcg, q 2 to 4 wk. During this titration, obtain serum calcium levels twice weekly.
Hypoparathyroidism: PO Initial dose is 0.25 mcg/day in the morning. Unsatisfactory response, increase dose at 2- to 4-wk intervals. During this titration, obtain serum calcium levels 2 times/wk.
Adults and children (6 yr of age and over): PO 0.5 to 2 mcg daily.
Children (1 to 5 yr of age): PO Have usually been given 0.25 to 0.75 mcg daily. Discontinue if hypercalcemia or serum calcium times phosphate product (Ca x P) totals more than 70.
Predialysis: PO Initial dose is 0.25 mcg/day in adults and pediatric patients over 3 yr of age. Dosage may be increased up to 0.5 mcg/day. In patients under 3 yr of age, dosage is 10 to 15 ng/kg/day.
Trade names: Calcijex Injection 1 mcg/mL
Rocaltrol Capsules 0.25 mcg
Calcitriol Injection Injection 2 mcg/mL
Warnings: Hypercalcemia or patients with vitamin D toxicity; hypersensitivity to any component of this product. Pregnancy Category: [C]
Interactions: Calcium supplements: Avoid uncontrolled intake of additional calcium-containing preparations.
Cholestyramine: May reduce intestinal absorption of fat soluble vitamins.
Ketoconazole: May reduce endogenous calcitriol concentrations.
Magnesium: Magnesium-containing products may cause hypermagnesemia and should be avoided during calcitriol administration to patients on chronic renal dialysis.
Phenytoin/Phenobarbital: Inhibits endogenous synthesis of calcitriol, therefore may require higher doses if given simultaneously.
Phosphate-binding agents: Because phosphate transport in the intestine, kidneys, and bones may be affected, the dosage of phosphate-binding agents must be adjusted based on serum phosphate concentration.
Thiazides: Known to induce hypercalcemia by the reduction of calcium excretion.
Vitamin D: To avoid possible additive effects and hypercalcemia, withhold pharmacologic doses of vitamin D and its derivatives.

Candesartan Cilexetil

Antihypertensive / Angiotensin II antagonist

Indications: Treatment of hypertension.
Dose: Adults: PO Initial dose: 16 mg/day; consider lower dose if volume-depleted. Total daily doses range from 8 to 32 mg in 1 or 2 doses.
Trade names: Atacand Tablets 4 mg
Warnings: Standard considerations. Pregnancy Category: [D (second and third trimester); C (first trimester) Can cause injury or death to fetus if used during second or third trimester]
Interactions: Lithium: Plasma concentrations may be increased by candesartan, resulting in an increase in the pharmacologic and adverse effects of lithium.

Candesartan Cilexetil/ Hydrochlorothiazide

Antihypertensive / Angiotensin II antagonist / Thiazide diuretic

Indications: Treatment of hypertension.
Dose: Adults: PO Atacand HCT may be substituted for previously titrated individual components. The daily dose range for Atacand HCT tablets is candesartan 16 mg combined with HCTZ 12.5 mg to candesartan 32 mg combined with HCTZ 25 mg.
Trade names: Atacand HCT Tablets 16 mg candesartan, 12.5 mg hydrochlorothiazide
Warnings: Any component of product; patients with anuria or hypersensitivity to sulfonamide-derived drugs. Pregnancy Category: [D (second and third trimester)
C (first trimester) Can cause injury and death to fetus if used during second or third trimester]
Interactions: Candesartan:
Alcohol, barbiturates, narcotics: Increased risk of orthostatic hypotension.
Antidiabetic agents (oral and insulin agents): Dosage adjustment of antidiabetic agent may be necessary.
Corticosteroids, ACTH: Increased electrolyte depletion, increasing risk of hypokalemia.
Non-steroidal anti-inflammatory agents: The diuretic, natriuretic, and hypertensive effects of loop, potassium-sparing, and thiazide diuretics may be reduced.
Pressor amines (eg, norepinephrine): Decreased responsiveness of the pressor amine.
Skeletal muscle relaxants, nondepolarizing (eg, tubocurarine): Increased responsiveness of the muscle relaxant.
HCTZ:
Bile acid sequestrants: May reduce HCTZ absorption; give HCTZ at least 2 hr before sequestrant.
Diazoxide: May cause hyperglycemia.
Digitalis glycosides: Diuretic-induced hypokalemia and hypomagnesemia may lead to digitalis-induced arrhythmias.
Lithium: Because renal excretion of lithium may be reduced, avoid use if possible.
Loop diuretics (eg, furosemide): Synergistic effects may occur, resulting in profound diuresis and serious electrolyte abnormalities.
Sulfonylureas (eg, chlorpropamide): Hypoglycemic effect of sulfonylurea may be decreased, necessitating an increase in sulfonylurea dosage.

Capreomycin

Anti-infective / Antitubercular

Indications: Treatment of tuberculosis concomitantly with other antituberculous agents.
Dose: Adults: IV/IM 1 g/day (max, 20 mg/kg/day) for 60 to 120 days, followed by 1 g IV or IM 2 or 3 times weekly.
Trade names: Capastat Sulfate Powder for injection 1 g (as sulfate)/vial

Warnings: Standard considerations. Pregnancy Category: [C]
Interactions: Aminoglycosides (eg, streptomycin): May increase the risk of respiratory paralysis and renal dysfunction.
Nondepolarizing neuromuscular blocking agents (eg, tubocurarine): Neuromuscular blockade may be enhanced.

Capsaicin

Topical / Analgesic
Indications: Temporary relief of pain from rheumatoid arthritis and osteoarthritis; relief of neuralgias (eg, pain after shingles, diabetic neuropathy).

Unlabeled indication: Temporary relief of pain of psoriasis, vitiligo, intractable pruritus, postmastectomy and postamputation neuroma (phantom limb syndrome), vulvar vestibulitis, apocrine chromidrosis, reflex sympathetic dystrophy.
Dose: Adults and Children 2 yr and over: Apply to affected area 3 to 4 times/day or less. Wash hands immediately after application.
Trade names: Capsin Lotion 0.025%
Capzasin•P Cream 0.025%
Dolorac Cream 0.25% in emollient base
No Pain-HP Roll-On 0.075%
Pain Doctor Cream 0.025%
Pain-X Gel 0.05%
R-Gel Gel 0.025%
Zostrix Cream 0.025% in emollient base
Zostrix-HP Cream 0.075% in emollient base
Warnings: Standard considerations. Pregnancy Category: [Safety undetermined]
Interactions: None well documented.

Captopril

Antihypertensive / ACE inhibitor
Indications: Treatment of hypertension, CHF, left ventricular dysfunction after MI, diabetic nephropathy.

Unlabeled indication: Treatment of hypertensive crisis, neonatal and childhood hypertension, rheumatoid arthritis, diagnosis of anatomic renal artery stenosis and primary aldosteronism, treatment of hypertension related to scleroderma renal crisis and Takayasu disease, idiopathic edema, Bartter and Raynaud syndromes, asymptomatic left ventricular dysfunction after MI.
Dose: Diabetic Nephropathy:
Adults: PO 25 mg tid.
Heart Failure:
Adults:
Initial dose: PO 6.25 to 12.5 mg tid; then titrate to usual daily dosage within next several days. Generally to be used in conjunction with a diuretic and digitalis.
Hypertension:
Adults:
Initial dose: PO 25 mg bid to tid; gradually increase q 1 to 2 wk if satisfactory effect is not achieved. Usual dose: 25 to 150 mg bid to tid. Usual dose does not exceed 50 mg tid. Max daily dose is 450 mg.
Left Ventricular Dysfunction after MI:
Adults: PO 6.25 mg 3 days after MI; then 12.5 mg tid and 25 mg tid for next several days.
Target dose: 50 mg tid over next several weeks.
Trade names: Capoten Tablets 12.5 mg
Warnings: Hypersensitivity to ACE inhibitors. Pregnancy Category: [D (second and third trimester); C (first trimester) ACE inhibitors can cause injury or death to fetus if used during second or third trimester When pregnancy is detected, discontinue ACE inhibitors as soon as possible]
Interactions: Food: Reduces bioavailability of captopril.
Indomethacin, salicylates (eg, aspirin): Hypotensive effects may be reduced, especially in low-renin or volume-dependent hypertensive patients.
Lithium: Increased lithium levels and symptoms of lithium toxicity may occur.
Potassium preparations, potassium-sparing diuretics: May increase serum potassium levels.

Captopril/ Hydrochlorothiazide

Antihypertensive / Thiazide diuretic
Indications: Treatment of hypertension.
Dose: Adults: PO Capozide may be substituted for previously titrated individual components. Alternatively, therapy may be started with a single Capozide tablet (25 mg captopril combined with 15 mg HCTZ) qd. For patients not responding sufficiently, the dose may be titrated upward, usually at 6-wk intervals. Maximum daily dose should not exceed 150 mg of captopril or 50 mg of HCTZ.
Trade names: Capozide 50/25 Tablets 50 mg captopril and 25 mg hydrochlorothiazide
Capozide 25/25 Tablets 25 mg captopril and 25 mg hydrochlorothiazide
Capozide 50/15 Tablets 50 mg captopril and 15 mg hydrochlorothiazide
Capozide 25/15 Tablets 25 mg captopril and 15 mg hydrochlorothiazide
Warnings: Anuric patients; patients hypersensitive to captopril or any other ACE inhibitor, HCTZ, or other sulfonamide derivative. Pregnancy Category: [D (second and third trimester); C (first trimester) ACE inhibitors (eg, captopril) can cause injury or death to fetus if used during second or third trimester When pregnancy is detected, discontinue as soon as possible]
Interactions: Alcohol, barbiturates (eg, phenobarbital), narcotics: Orthostatic hypotension may be potentiated.
Anticoagulants (eg, warfarin): Anticoagulant effect may be decreased.
Antidiabetic agents (eg, insulin, sulfonylureas): Dosage adjustment may be necessary because of possible HCTZ-induced elevation in blood glucose levels.
Antigout agents (eg, probenecid): Dosage adjustment may be necessary because of possible HCTZ-induced elevation in blood uric acid levels.
Cardiac glycosides (eg, digoxin): Possible digitalis toxicity associated with hypokalemia.
Cholestyramine, colestipol: May impair the absorption of HCTZ.
Food: Reduces bioavailability of captopril.
Lithium: Plasma levels of lithium may be elevated, increasing the risk of toxicity.
NSAIDs: May reduce the natriuretic and antihypertensive effect of HCTZ.
Potassium supplements, potassium-sparing diuretics (eg, spironolactone): Increased risk of hyperkalemia.
Nondepolarizing muscle relaxants (eg, tubocurarine): Effects may be increased.

Carbamazepine

Anticonvulsant
Indications: Treatment of epilepsy (eg, partial seizures with complex symptoms, generalized tonic-clonic seizures [grand mal], mixed seizure patterns, other partial or generalized seizures) in patients refractory to or intolerant of other agents. Treatment of pain associated with trigeminal neuralgia.

Unlabeled indication: Treatment of certain psychiatric disorders; management of alcohol withdrawal; relief of restless legs syndrome; treatment of postherpetic neuralgia.
Dose: Epilepsy:
Adults and children over 12 yr of age:
Initial dose: PO 200 mg bid (tablets) or 100 mg qid (suspension). Increase weekly by up to 200 mg per

day in 2 divided doses for extended-release or 3 to 4 divided doses for other formulations to reach minimum effective dose (max, 1,000 mg per day in children 12 to 15 yr of age; 1,200 mg per day in children above 15 yr of age; 1,600 mg per day in adults).
Maintenance: 800 to 1,200 mg per day.
Adults and children over 12 yr of age (extended-release):
Initial dose: PO 200 mg bid.
Children 6 to 12 yr of age:
Initial dose: PO 100 mg bid (tablets) or 50 mg qid (suspension). Increase weekly by 100 mg per day in 3 to 4 divided doses (extended-release formulations use a bid regimen) to reach minimum effective dose (max, 1,000 mg per day).
Maintenance: 400 to 800 mg per day in 3 to 4 divided doses.
Children 6 yr of age and younger:
Initial dose: PO 10 to 20 mg/kg per day in 2 or 3 divided doses (tablet) or 10 to 20 mg/kg per day in 4 divided doses (suspension). Increase weekly to achieve optimal clinical response when administered in 3 or 4 divided daily doses (max, 35 mg/kg per day).
Maintenance: Less than 35 mg/kg per day.
Trigeminal Neuralgia:
Adults:
Initial dose: PO 100 mg bid (tablets) or 50 mg qid (suspension). May increase by up to 200 mg per day in 3 to 4 divided doses (tablets: 100 mg increments q 12 hr; suspension: 50 mg qid) prn (max, 1,200 mg per day).
Maintenance: Usually 400 to 800 mg per day. Use minimum effective dose or discontinue drug once q 3 mo.
Adults (extended-release):
Initial dose: PO 100 mg bid (tablets) or 200 mg once daily (capsules).

Trade names: Carbatrol Capsules, extended-release 100 mg
Epitol Tablets 200 mg
Tegretol Tablets, chewable 100 mg
Tegretol XR Tablets, extended-release 100 mg

Warnings: Hypersensitivity to tricyclic antidepressants or carbamazepine; history of bone marrow depression; concomitant use of MAO inhibitors. Discontinue MAO inhibitors at least 14 days before administration of carbamazepine. Pregnancy Category: [D]

Interactions: Acetaminophen, benzodiazepines (eg, midazolam), bupropion, clozapine, cyclosporine, olanzapine, succinimides (eg, ethosuximide), tiagabine, topiramate, ziprasidone: Levels may be reduced by carbamazepine.
Anticoagulants: May decrease anticoagulant effects.
Azole antifungal agents, diltiazem, verapamil, danazol, propoxyphene, macrolide antibiotics (except azithromycin): May increase carbamazepine levels and may result in toxicity.
Barbiturates: May result in decreased carbamazepine serum concentrations, possibly leading to decreased effectiveness.
Charcoal, activated: May reduce absorption of carbamazepine.
Cimetidine: May result in carbamazepine toxicity.
Contraceptives, oral: Causes breakthrough bleeding and reduces effectiveness of contraceptives.
Doxycycline hyclate: May decrease doxycycline hyclate levels.
Felbamate: May decrease concentrations of felbamate or carbamazepine.
Felodipine: May decrease effects of felodipine.
Haloperidol: May decrease effects of haloperidol.
Hydantoins (eg, phenytoin): May decrease carbamazepine levels; may alter hydantoin levels.
Isoniazid: May result in toxicity of isoniazid, carbamazepine, or both.
Lamotrigine: Lamotrigine levels may be decreased, while levels of the active metabolite of carbamazepine may be increased.
Lithium: May cause adverse CNS effects regardless of drug levels.
MAO inhibitors, voriconazole: Coadministration with carbamazepine is contraindicated.
Nondepolarizing muscle relaxants: May make these agents less effective.
Primidone: Decreased carbamazepine levels. Primidone's active metabolite (phenobarbital) may be increased.
Protease inhibitors (eg, indinavir): Carbamazepine levels may be elevated, while protease inhibitor levels may be decreased, resulting in antiretroviral treatment failure.
Selective serotonin reuptake inhibitors (eg, fluoxetine, fluvoxamine): Increased carbamazepine levels with possible toxicity.
Theophylline: May reduce effects of theophylline and carbamazepine. Theophylline levels may be increased or decreased.
Tricyclic antidepressants: May increase carbamazepine levels; may decrease tricyclic antidepressant levels.
Valproic acid: May decrease valproic acid levels; may alter carbamazepine levels.

Carbenicillin Indanyl Sodium

Antibiotic / Penicillin

Indications: Treatment of acute and chronic infections of the upper and lower urinary tract, prostatitis, and asymptomatic bacteriuria caused by susceptible microorganisms.

Dose: Adults: PO 382 to 764 mg qid.

Trade names: Geocillin Tablets 382 mg carbenicillin (118 mL indanyl sodium ester)

Warnings: Hypersensitivity to penicillins, cephalosporins, or imipenem. Do not treat severe pneumonia, empyema, bacteremia, pericarditis, meningitis, and purulent or septic arthritis with oral carbenicillin during acute stage. Pregnancy Category: [B]

Interactions: Contraceptives, oral: May reduce efficacy of oral contraceptives. Use nonhormonal form of contraception during carbenicillin therapy.
Tetracyclines: May impair bactericidal effects of carbenicillin.

Carboplatin

Alkylating agent

Indications: Adult: Ovarian carcinoma. Secondary treatment for palliative treatment of patients with ovarian carcinoma recurrent after prior chemotherapy.

Unlabeled indication: Small cell and nonsmall cell lung, head and neck squamous cell, and testicular cancer; Wilm tumor.

Dose: Ovarian Carcinoma (Single-Agent Therapy):
Adults: IV 360 mg/m^2 on day 1 q 4 wk if neutrophil count is at least 2000/mm^3 and the platelet count is at least 100,000/mm^3.
Ovarian Carcinoma (Combination Therapy with Cyclophosphamide):
Adults: IV Carboplatin 300 mg/m^2 plus cyclophosphamide 600 mg/m^2, both on day 1 q 4 wk for 6 cycles. Do not repeat intermittent courses of the combination until the neutrophil count is at least 2000/mm^3 and the platelet count is at least 100,000/mm^3.
Calvert Formula Dosing:
Adults: IV Carboplatin may be dosed to achieve a target AUC based on the patient's glomerular filtration rate (GFR) using the calvert formula. The desired target AUC depends on the disease and the patient's treatment status. The Calvert formula calculates the carboplatin dose in mg as follows: Total dose (mg) = target AUC (mg/mL/min) x (GFR [mL/min] + 25).
Dosage Adjustments Based on Lowest Posttreatment Blood Counts:

Adults: IV If platelets above 100,000/mm³ and neutrophils above 2000/mm³, then give 125% of adjusted dose from prior course. If platelets are 50,000 to 100,000/mm³ and neutrophils are 500 to 2000/mm³, no dosage adjustment is necessary. If platelets below 50,000/mm³ and neutrophils below 500/mm³, then give 75% of adjusted dose from prior course. Doses above 125% of the starting dose are not recommended.
Renal Function Impairment (Dosage Adjustment):
Adults: IV Baseline Ccr is 41 to 59 mL/min, the recommended dose on day 1 is 250 mg/m²; 16 to 40 mL/min is 200 mg/m²; no more than 15 mL/min, data too limited to permit a recommendation for treatment.

Trade names: Paraplatin Lyophilized powder for injection 50 mg vial

Warnings: History of severe allergic reactions to cisplatin or other platinum compounds or mannitol; severe bone marrow depression; significant bleeding. Pregnancy Category: [D]

Interactions: Aminoglycosides: Concomitant use may increase risk of nephrotoxicity or ototoxicity.
Phenytoin: Serum concentrations may be decreased, resulting in a loss of therapeutic effect.

Carmustine

Alkylating agent / Nitrosoureas

Indications: Brain tumors, multiple myeloma, Hodgkin and non-Hodgkin lymphomas; adjunct to surgery and radiation in newly diagnosed high-grade malignant glioma patients and as an adjunct in recurrent glioblastoma multiforme patients (wafer).

Unlabeled indication: Mycosis fungoides.

Dose: Brain Tumors, Multiple Myeloma, Hodgkin and Non-Hodgkin Lymphomas (Single Agent in Previously Untreated Patients):
Adults: IV 150 to 200 mg/m² q 6 wk, as a single dose or divided into 2 successive daily infusions.
Dosage Reduction:
Adults: IV Compromised bone marrow function or therapy with other myelosuppressive drugs requires a reduction in dose. Do not administer repeat courses until acceptable leukocyte and platelet counts have recovered (usually greater than 4000/mm³ and 100,000/mm³, respectively). Subsequent doses are determined by the clinical and hematologic tolerance of the previous dose. The following leukocyte and platelet counts refer to the levels reached at nadir after prior dose. Give 100% of the prior dose given if the leukocytes are greater than 3000 cells/mm³ and the platelets are greater than 75,000 cells/mm³. Give 70% of the prior dose given if the leukocytes are 2000 to 2999 cells/mm³ and the platelets are 25,000 to 74,999 cells/mm³. Give 50% of the prior dose given if the leukocytes are less than 2000 cells/mm³ and the platelets are less than 25,000 cells/mm³.
Adjunct To Surgery And Radiation In Newly Diagnosed High-Grade Malignant Glioma Patients And As An Adjunct In Recurrent Glioblastoma Multiforme Patients:
Adults: Wafer for implantation 8 wafers placed in the resection cavity, for a total dose of 61.6 mg. If the cavity size and shape will not accommodate this, use the greatest number of wafers that will fit.

Trade names: BiCNU Powder for injection 100 mg
Gliadel Wafer 7.7 mg

Warnings: Standard considerations. Pregnancy Category: [D]

Interactions: Cimetidine: Cimetidine may enhance the myelosuppressive effects of carmustine.
Digoxin, phenytoin: Digoxin and phenytoin serum levels may be reduced by carmustine.

Carvedilol

Alpha-adrenergic blocker / Beta-adrenergic blocker

Indications: Management of essential hypertension; treatment of mild to severe heart failure of ischemic or cardiomyopathic origin. Reduce cardiovascular mortality in clinically stable patients who have survived the acute phase of MI and have a left ventricular ejection fraction of 40% or less.

Unlabeled indication: Angina pectoris.

Dose: Individualize dose and monitor during up-titration.
Essential Hypertension:
Adults: PO Start with 6.25 mg bid, then if tolerated (based on standing BP about 1 hr after dosing), maintain the dose for 7 to 14 days; then increase to 12.5 mg bid, if tolerated, maintain the dose for 7 to 14 days; then increase to 25 mg bid if tolerated and needed (max, 50 mg/day).
CHF:
Adults: PO Start with 3.125 mg bid for 14 days, then, if tolerated, dose may be increased to 6.25 mg bid; dosing may be doubled q 2 wk to the highest amount tolerated by patient (max, 25 mg bid/patients less than 85 kg [187 lbs]; 50 mg bid/patients over 85 kg).
Left Ventricular Dysfunction Following MI:
Adults: PO Start treatment once patient is stable and fluid retention is minimized. The recommended starting dose is 6.25 mg bid and increased to 12.5 mg bid after 3 to 10 days, based on tolerability. The dose may be increased again to the target dose of 25 mg bid. A lower starting dose may be used (3.125 mg bid) and/or, the rate of up-titration may be slowed if clinically indicated (eg, because of low BP, heart rate, or fluid retention). Patients may be maintained at lower dose if higher doses are not tolerated. The recommended dosing regimen need not be altered in patients receiving treatment with an IV or oral beta-blocker during the acute phase of the MI.

Trade names: Coreg Tablets 3.125 mg

Warnings: Decompensated cardiac failure requiring use of IV inotropic therapy; bronchial asthma or related bronchospastic conditions; second- or third-degree AV block; sick sinus syndrome (unless a permanent pacemaker is in place); cardiogenic shock; severe bradycardia; hypersensitivity to the drug. Pregnancy Category: [C]

Interactions: Antidiabetic agents (insulin and oral agents): Blood glucose-lowering effect may be enhanced.
Calcium channel blockers (eg, diltiazem): Conduction disturbances may occur and BP may be altered.
Catecholamine-depleting agents (eg, reserpine): Monitor for hypotension or severe bradycardia.
Clonidine: Heart rate and BP-lowering effects may be potentiated.
Cyclosporine, digoxin: Plasma levels may be elevated by carvedilol, increasing the therapeutic and adverse effects.
Inhibitors of CYP2D6 (eg, fluoxetine, paroxetine, propafenone, quinidine), poor metabolizers of debrisoquine: Expected to increase carvedilol blood levels.
Rifampin: May reduce carvedilol plasma levels, decreasing the pharmacologic effect.

Caspofungin Acetate

Anti-infective / Antifungal

Indications: Treatment of invasive aspergillosis in patients refractory to or intolerant of other antifungal therapies.

Dose: Adults: IV
Loading dose: 70 mg given by slow infusion of about 1 hr on day 1.
Maintenance dose: 50 mg daily by slow infusion of about 1 hr thereafter.

Trade names: Cancidas Powder for injection, lyophilized 50 mg

Warnings: Standard considerations. Pregnancy Category: [C]

Interactions: Cyclosporine: Avoid concurrent

use if possible because caspofungin levels may be elevated, increasing the risk of side effects.
Inducers or mixed inducers/inhibitors of drug clearance (eg, carbamazepine, dexamethasone, efavirenz, nelfinavir, nevirapine, phenytoin, rifampin): Caspofungin blood levels may be decreased, reducing the efficacy.
Tacrolimus: Tacrolimus blood levels may be decreased, reducing the efficacy.
Incompatability: Do not mix or coinfuse with other medications.

Cefaclor

Antibiotic / Cephalosporin

Indications: Treatment of infections of respiratory tract, urinary tract, skin and skin structures; treatment of otitis media caused by susceptible strains of specific microorganisms.

Dose: Adults: PO 250 to 500 mg q 8 hr.
Children: PO 20 to 40 mg/kg/day in divided doses q 8 hr (for otitis media and pharyngitis, q 12 hr) (max 1 g/day).
Acute Bacterial Exacerbations of Chronic Bronchitis:
Adults:
Extended-release: PO 500 mg/day for 7 days.
Secondary Bacterial Infection of Acute Bronchitis:
Adults: PO 500 mg/12 hr for 7 days.
Pharyngitis or Tonsillitis:
Adults: PO 375 mg/12 hr for 10 days.
Uncomplicated Skin and Skin Structure Infections:
Adults: PO 375 mg/12 hr for 7 to 10 days.

Trade names: Ceclor Powder for Oral Suspension 125 mg/5 mL
Ceclor Pulvules Capsules 250 mg

Warnings: Hypersensitivity to cephalosporins. Pregnancy Category: [B]

Interactions: Probenecid: Inhibition of renal excretion of cefaclor.

Cefadroxil

Antibiotic / Cephalosporin

Indications: Treatment of infections of urinary tract, skin and skin structures; treatment of pharyngitis and tonsillitis caused by susceptible strains of specific microorganisms.

Dose: Adults: PO 1 to 2 g/day in single dose or 2 divided doses.
Children: PO 30 mg/kg/day in single dose or 2 divided doses.

Trade names: Duricef Capsules 500 mg (as monohydrate)

Warnings: Hypersensitivity to cephalosporins. Pregnancy Category: [B]

Interactions: Probenecid: Inhibition of renal excretion of cefadroxil.

Cefazolin Sodium

Antibiotic / Cephalosporin

Indications: Treatment of infections of respiratory tract, genitourinary tract, skin and skin structures, biliary tract, bone and joint; perioperative prophylaxis; treatment of septicemia and endocarditis caused by susceptible strains of specific microorganisms.

Dose: Adults: IV/IM 250 mg to 1.5 g q 6 to 12 hr (severe infections: up to 12 g/day).
Children over 1 mo: IV/IM 25 to 50 mg/kg/day in 3 to 4 equal divided doses q 6 to 8 hr (severe infections: up to 100 mg/kg/day).
Perioperative Prophylaxis:
Adults: IV/IM 1 g 30 min to 1 hr prior to surgery; 0.5 to 1 g at appropriate intervals (at least 2 hr) during surgery; 0.5 to 1 g q 6 to 8 hr for 24 hr (up to 5 days) after surgery.
Children over 1 mo: IV/IM 25 to 50 mg/kg/day divided into 3 to 4 equal doses; (max, 100 mg/kg/day).

Trade names: Ancef Injection 500 mg (2.1 mEq sodium/g)
Zolicef Powder for Injection 500 mg (2.1 mEq sodium/g)

Warnings: Hypersensitivity to cephalosporins. Pregnancy Category: [B]

Interactions: Aminoglycosides: May increase risk of nephrotoxicity.
Probenecid: Inhibition of renal excretion of cefazolin.
Incompatability:
Aminoglycosides: Do not add aminoglycosides to cefazolin solutions because inactivation of both drugs may result; administer at separate sites if concurrent therapy is indicated.

Cefepime

Antibiotic / Cephalosporin

Indications: Treatment of pneumonia and infections of the skin and skin structures and urinary tract caused by susceptible strains of specific microorganisms. Treatment of empiric therapy for febrile neutropenic patients as monotherapy. Treatment for complicated intra-abdominal infections in combination with metronidazole.

Dose: Mild to Moderate Uncomplicated or Complicated Urinary Tract Infections:
Adults: IV/IM 0.5 to 1 g q 12 hr for 7 to 10 days.
Severe Uncomplicated or Complicated Urinary Tract Infections:
Adults: IV 2 g q 12 hr for 10 days.
Moderate to Severe Pneumonia:
Adults: IV 1 to 2 g q 12 hr for 10 days.
Moderate to Severe Uncomplicated Skin and Skin Structure Infections:
Adults: IV 2 g q 12 hr for 10 days
Children under 40 kg: 50 mg/kg/dose q 12 hr (q 8 hr for febrile neutropenic patients) for 7 to 10 days. Do not exceed the recommended adult dose.
Renal Impairment (Children): Data not available; however, changes in dosing regimen similar to those in adults are recommended.

Trade names: Maxipime Powder for Injection 500 mg

Warnings: Hypersensitivity to cephalosporins, penicillins, or other beta-lactam antibiotics. Pregnancy Category: [B]

Interactions: Aminoglycosides: Increased risk of nephrotoxicity and ototoxicity.
Incompatability: Metronidazole, vancomycin, gentamicin, tobramycin, netilmicin, aminophylline, and ampicillin (greater than 40 mg/mL).

Cefixime

Antibiotic / Cephalosporin

Indications: Treatment of uncomplicated UTIs, otitis media, pharyngitis, tonsillitis, acute bronchitis, acute exacerbations of chronic bronchitis, and uncomplicated gonorrhea caused by susceptible strains of specific organisms.

Dose: Infection:
Adults and Children (weighing more than 50 kg or older than 12 yr of age): PO 400 mg daily.
Children 6 mo to 12 yr of age: PO 8 mg/kg/day as a single daily dose or in 2 divided doses of 4 mg/kg q 12 hr.
Uncomplicated Gonorrhea:
Adults: PO 400 mg as a single dose.
Dose Adjustment for Renal Function Impairment: Ccr between 21 to 60 mL/min or on hemodialysis, give 75% of dose (300 mg/day). Ccr less than 20 mL/min or on continuous peritoneal dialysis, give 50% of dose (200 mg/day).

Trade names: Suprax Oral suspension 100 mg per 5 mL

Warnings: Allergy to cephalosporin group of antibiotics. Pregnancy Category: [B]

Interactions: Carbamazepine: Plasma concentrations may be elevated by cefixime, increasing

Medications

the risk of side effects.
Warfarin: Increased PT, with and without bleeding, may occur.

Cefoperazone Sodium

Antibiotic / Cephalosporin

Indications: Treatment of infections of respiratory tract, urinary tract, skin and skin structures; treatment of pelvic inflammatory disease, endometritis, and other female genital tract infections; treatment of septicemia and peritonitis caused by susceptible microorganisms.

Dose: Adults: IV/IM 2 to 4 g/day in equally divided doses q 12 hr (severe infections: 6 to 12 g/day in equally divided doses [1.5 to 4 g/dose] q 6, 8, or 12 hr).

Trade names: Cefobid Powder for Injection 1 g (1.5 mEq sodium/g. Also may contain dextrose hydrous.)

Warnings: Hypersensitivity to cephalosporins. Pregnancy Category: [B]

Interactions: Alcohol: May cause acute alcohol intolerance (disulfiram-like reaction); reaction may occur up to 3 days after last dose of cefoperazone.
Aminoglycosides: May increase risk of nephrotoxicity.
Anticoagulants, oral: May increase anticoagulant effect; bleeding complications may occur.
Incompatability:
Aminoglycosides: Do not add aminoglycosides to cefoperazone solutions because inactivation of both drugs may result; administer at separate sites if concurrent therapy is indicated.

Cefotaxime Sodium

Antibiotic / Cephalosporin

Indications: Treatment of infections of lower respiratory tract including pneumonia, urinary tract, skin and skin structures, bone and joints; treatment of bacteremia/septicemia, CNS infections, intra-abdominal infections and gynecological infections including pelvic inflammatory disease, endometritis and pelvic cellulitis caused by susceptible strains of specific microorganisms; perioperative prophylaxis.

Dose: Infection:
Adults: IV/IM Up to 12 g/day in divided doses (from q 4 hr for septicemia to q 12 hr for uncomplicated infection) usually for 7 to 10 days. IV route is preferable for severe infections.
Children 1 mo to 12 yr: IV/IM 50 to 180 mg/kg/day in 4 to 6 divided doses.
Infants 1 to 4 wk: IV 50 mg/kg q 8 hr.
Newborns under 1 wk: IV 50 mg/kg q 12 hr.
Gonorrhea:
Adults: IM 1 g as single dose.
Perioperative Prophylaxis:
Adults: IV/IM 1 g 30 to 90 min prior to surgery.
Cesarean Section:
Adults: IV 1 g as soon as umbilical cord is clamped; second and third dose IV/IM at 6- and 12-hr intervals after first dose.

Trade names: Claforan Powder for Injection 500 mg (2.2 mEq sodium/g)

Warnings: Hypersensitivity to cephalosporins. Pregnancy Category: [B]

Interactions: Aminoglycosides: Increased risk of nephrotoxicity.
Incompatability: Do not add aminoglycosides to cefotaxime solutions because inactivation of both drugs may result; administer at separate sites if concurrent therapy is indicated.

Cefotetan Disodium

Antibiotic / Cephalosporin

Indications: Treatment of infections of urinary tract, lower respiratory tract, skin and skin structures, bone and joint; treatment of gynecological infections; treatment of intra-abdominal infections caused by susceptible strains of specific microorganisms; perioperative prophylaxis.
Concomitant antibiotic therapy: If cefotetan and an aminoglycoside are to be used concomitantly, carefully monitor renal function, especially if higher dosages of the aminoglycoside are to be administered or if therapy is to be prolonged, because of the potential nephrotoxicity and ototoxicity of aminoglycosides.

Dose: Infection:
Adults: IV/IM 1 to 2 g q 12 hr (life-threatening infections: up to 3 g q 12 hr) for 7 to 10 days.
Urinary Tract Infection:
Adults: IV/IM 500 mg q 12 hr, 1 or 2 g q 24 hr, 1 or 2 g ever 12 hr.
Perioperative Prophylaxis:
Adults: IV 1 to 2 g 30 to 60 min prior to surgery. In Cesarean section, give dose as soon as umbilical cord is clamped.

Trade names: Cefotan Powder for Injection 1 g (3.5 mEq sodium/g)

Warnings: Hypersensitivity to cephalosporins. Pregnancy Category: [B]

Interactions: Alcohol: Acute alcohol intolerance (disulfiram-like reaction) may occur up to 3 days after last dose of cefotetan.
Aminoglycosides: Increased risk of nephrotoxicity.
Anticoagulants, oral: Increased anticoagulant effect; bleeding complications may occur.
Incompatability:
Aminoglycosides: Do not add aminoglycosides to cefotetan solutions because inactivation of both drugs may result; administer at separate sites if concurrent therapy is indicated.

Cefoxitin Sodium

Antibiotic / Cephalosporin

Indications: Treatment of infections of lower respiratory tract, urinary tract, skin and skin structures, bone and joint; treatment of intra-abdominal infections, gynecological infections, and septicemia caused by susceptible microorganisms; perioperative prophylaxis. Many infections caused by gram-negative bacteria resistant to some cephalosporins and penicillins respond to cefoxitin.

Dose: Infection:
Adults: IV/IM 1 to 2 g q 6 to 8 hr.
Children 3 mo and over: IV/IM 80 to 160 mg/kg/day in divided doses q 4 to 6 hr (max, 12 g/day).
Surgical Prophylaxis:
Adults: IV/IM 2 g just prior to surgery, then 2 g q 6 hr for 24 hr.
Children 3 mo and over: IV/IM 30 to 40 mg/kg just prior to surgery, then 30 to 40 mg/kg q 6 hr for 24 hr.

Trade names: Mefoxin Powder for Injection 1 g (2.3 mEq sodium/g)

Warnings: Hypersensitivity to cephalosporins. Pregnancy Category: [B]

Interactions: Aminoglycosides: May increase risk of nephrotoxicity.
Probenecid: Inhibition of renal excretion of cefoxitin.
Incompatability:
Aminoglycosides: Do not add aminoglycosides to cefoxitin solutions because inactivation of both drugs may result; administer at separate sites if concurrent therapy is indicated.

Cefpodoxime Proxetil

Antibiotic / Cephalosporin

Indications: Treatment of infections of respiratory tract, urinary tract, skin and skin structures; treatment of sexually transmitted diseases caused by susceptible strains of specific microorganisms.

Dose: Adults: PO 100 to 400 mg q 12 hr.
Children 6 mo to 12 yr: PO 10 mg/kg/day in divided doses q 12 hr (max 200 mg/dose).

Trade names: Vantin Tablets 100 mg

Warnings: Hypersensitivity to cephalosporins. Pregnancy Category: [B]

Interactions: Probenecid: Inhibition of renal excretion of cefpodoxime.

Ceftazidime

Antibiotic / Cephalosporin

Indications: Treatment of infections of lower respiratory tract, skin and skin structures, urinary tract, bone and joint; treatment of gynecological infections; treatment of intra-abdominal infections; treatment of septicemia and CNS infections including meningitis caused by susceptible strains of specific microorganisms; concomitant antibiotic therapy.

Dose: Adults: IV/IM 250 mg to 2 g q 8 to 12 hr.
Children 1 mo to 12 yr: IV 30 to 50 mg/kg q 8 hr (max, 6 g/day).
Newborns under 4 wk: IV 30 mg/kg q 12 hr.

Trade names: Ceptaz Powder for Injection 1 g (as pentahydrate w/ L-arginine)
Fortaz Powder for Injection 500 mg (2.3 mEq sodium/g)
Tazicef Powder for Injection 1 g (2.3 mEq sodium/g)
Tazidime Powder for Injection 500 mg (as pentahydrate w/ L-arginine)

Warnings: Hypersensitivity to cephalosporins.
Pregnancy Category: [B]

Interactions: Aminoglycosides: Increased risk of nephrotoxicity.
Incompatability:
Aminoglycosides: Do not add aminoglycosides to ceftazidime solutions because inactivation of both drugs may result; administer at separate sites if concurrent therapy is indicated.
Sodium bicarbonate: Do not dilute ceftazidime with sodium bicarbonate.

Ceftizoxime Sodium

Antibiotic / Cephalosporin

Indications: Treatment of infections of lower respiratory tract, urinary tract, skin and skin structures, bone and joint; treatment of intra-abdominal infections, pelvic inflammatory disease, gonorrhea, septicemia, and meningitis caused by susceptible microorganisms.

Dose: Adults: IV/IM 1 to 2 g q 8 to 12 hr (life-threatening infections: IV up to 2 g q 4 hr or 3 to 4 g q 8 hr).
Children over 6 mo: IV/IM 50 mg/kg q 6 to 8 hr up to 200 mg/kg/day (max, 12 g/day).

Trade names: Cefizox Powder for Injection 500 mg (2.6 mEq sodium/g)

Warnings: Hypersensitivity to cephalosporins.
Pregnancy Category: [B]

Interactions: Aminoglycosides: Increased risk of nephrotoxicity.
Probenecid: Inhibition of renal excretion of ceftizoxime.
Incompatability:
Aminoglycosides: Do not add aminoglycosides to ceftizoxime solutions because inactivation of both drugs may result; administer at separate sites if concurrent therapy is indicated.

Ceftriaxone Sodium

Antibiotic / Cephalosporin

Indications: Treatment of infections of lower respiratory tract, skin and skin structures, bone and joint, urinary tract; treatment of pelvic inflammatory disease, intra-abdominal infections, gonorrhea, meningitis, and septicemia caused by susceptible microorganisms; preoperative prophylaxis.

Unlabeled indication: Treatment of Lyme disease in patients refractory to penicillin G.

Dose: Infection:
Adults: IV/IM 1 to 2 g/day or in equally divided doses q 12 hr (max, 4 g/day).
Children: IV/IM 50 to 75 mg/kg/day in equally divided doses q 12 hr (max, 2 g/day).
Uncomplicated Gonococcal Infections:
Adults: IM 250 mg as single dose.
Surgical Prophylaxis:
Adults: IV/IM 1 g as single dose 30 min to 2 hr before surgery.
Pediatric Meningitis:
Children: IV/IM 75 mg/kg as loading dose then 100 mg/kg/day in divided doses q 12 hr (max, 4 g/day).

Trade names: Rocephin Powder for Injection 250 mg (3.6 mEq sodium/g)

Warnings: Hypersensitivity to cephalosporins.
Pregnancy Category: [B]

Interactions: Aminoglycosides: Increased risk of nephrotoxicity.
Incompatability: Other antimicrobial drugs.

Cefuroxime

Antibiotic / Cephalosporin

Indications: Oral form: Treatment of infections of lower respiratory tract, urinary tract, skin and skin structures; treatment of uncomplicated gonorrhea, otitis media, pharyngitis, and tonsillitis caused by susceptible strains of specific microorganisms. Treatment of early Lyme disease, pharyngitis/tonsillitis, and impetigo.

Parenteral form: Treatment of infections of lower respiratory tract, urinary tract, skin and skin structures, bone and joint; preoperative prophylaxis; treatment of septicemia, gonorrhea, and meningitis caused by susceptible strains of specific microorganisms.

Dose: Infection:
Adults and Children 12 yr and over: PO 125 to 500 mg bid. IV/IM 750 mg to 1.5 g q 8 hr.
Children under 12 yr: PO 125 to 250 mg bid.
Infants and Children over 3 mo: IV/IM 50 to 150 mg/kg/day (not to exceed adult dose) in equally divided doses q 6 to 8 hr.
Bacterial Meningitis:
Adults and Children 12 yr and over: IV/IM Up to 3 g q 8 hr.
Infants and Children 3 mo to 12 yr: IV/IM 200 to 240 mg/kg/day in divided doses q 6 to 8 hr.
Uncomplicated Gonorrhea:
Adults and Children 12 yr and over: PO 1 g as single dose. IM 1.5 g as single dose.
Preoperative Prophylaxis:
Adults: IV/IM 1.5 g 30 min to 1 hr before surgery then 750 mg q 8 hr for duration of surgery.

Trade names: Ceftin Tablets 125 mg
Zinacef Powder for Injection 750 mg (2.4 mEq sodium/g)

Warnings: Hypersensitivity to cephalosporins.
Pregnancy Category: [B]

Interactions: Aminoglycosides: Increased risk of nephrotoxicity with parenteral cefuroxime.
Probenecid: Inhibition of renal excretion of cefuroxime.
Incompatability:
Aminoglycosides: Do not add aminoglycosides to cefuroxime solutions because inactivation of both drugs may result; administer at separate sites if concurrent therapy is indicated.

Celecoxib

COX-2 inhibitor

Indications: Relief of symptoms of osteoarthritis; relief of symptoms of rheumatoid arthritis in adults; management of acute pain in adults; treatment of primary dysmenorrhea; reduction of the number of adenomatous colorectal polyps in familial adenomatous polyposis (FAP), as an adjunct to usual care (eg, endoscopic surveillance, surgery).

Dose: Osteoarthritis:
Adults: PO 200 mg/day administered as a single dose or as 100 mg bid.
Rheumatoid Arthritis:
Adults: PO 100 to 200 mg bid.
Acute Pain, Primary Dysmenorrhea:

Adults: PO 400 mg initially followed by an additional 200 mg dose on day 1, if needed, then 200 mg twice daily as needed.
FAP:
Adults: PO Continue usual medical care for FAP patients while on celecoxib. To reduce the number of adenomatous colorectal polyps in patients with FAP, the recommended dose is 400 mg (2 x 200 mg capsules) bid. Take with food.
Trade names: Celebrex Capsules 100 mg
Warnings: Allergy to celecoxib or any of its ingredients; allergy to sulfonamides; aspirin triad (eg, asthma, nasal polyps, allergy to aspirin); previous allergic reactions following aspirin or other NSAID use (eg, asthma, hives, rash). Pregnancy Category: [C]
Interactions: ACE inhibitors: NSAIDs may diminish the antihypertensive effect of ACE inhibitors.
Aspirin: Coadministration with celecoxib may result in an increased rate of GI ulceration or other complications.
Fluconazole: Increase in celecoxib plasma concentration may occur because of inhibition of celecoxib metabolism.
Furosemide: NSAIDs can reduce the natriuretic effect of furosemide and thiazides in some patients.
Lithium: Mean steady-state lithium plasma levels increased about 17% in subjects receiving lithium with celecoxib.
P450 2C9 inhibitors: There is a potential for an in vivo drug interaction with drugs that are metabolized by P450 2D6.
Warfarin: Monitor anticoagulant activity, particularly in the first few days, after initiating or changing celecoxib therapy in patients receiving warfarin or similar agents because these patients are at an increased risk of bleeding complications.

Cephalexin

Antibiotic / Cephalosporin
Indications: Treatment of infections of respiratory tract, urinary tract, skin and skin structures and bone; treatment of otitis media caused by susceptible strains of specific microorganisms.
Dose: Adults: PO 1 to 4 g/day in divided doses (max, 4 g/day).
Children: PO (cephalexin monohydrate only) 25 to 100 mg/kg/day in divided doses.
Trade names: Biocef Capsules 500 mg
Keflex Capsules 250 mg
Keftab Tablets 500 mg (as HCl monohydrate)
Warnings: Hypersensitivity to cephalosporins. Pregnancy Category: [B]
Interactions: Probenecid: Inhibition of renal excretion of cephalexin.

Cephradine

Antibiotic / Cephalosporin
Indications: Treatment of infections of respiratory tract, urinary tract, skin and skin structure; treatment of otitis media caused by susceptible strains of microorganisms.
Dose: Adults: PO 250 mg to 1 g q 6 to 12 hr.
Children: PO 25 to 100 mg/kg/day in equally divided doses q 6 to 12 hr (max, 4 g/day).
Trade names: Velosef Capsules 250 mg
Warnings: Hypersensitivity to cephalosporins. Pregnancy Category: [B]
Interactions: Probenecid: Inhibition of renal excretion of cephradine.

Cetirizine

Antihistamine
Indications: Symptomatic relief of symptoms (eg, nasal, nonnasal) associated with seasonal and perennial allergic rhinitis; treatment of uncomplicated skin manifestations of chronic idiopathic urticaria.
Dose: Adults and children 6 yr and over: PO 5 or 10 mg/day.
Children 2 to 5 yr: PO 2.5 mg qd (max, 5 mg/day as 5 mg qd or 2.5 mg q 12 hr).
Children 6 mo to less than 2 yr: PO 2.5 mg qd. The dose in 12 to 23 mo may be increased to a max dose of 5 mg qd, or 2.5 mg q 12 hr.
Hepatic Impairment: PO 5 mg/day (do not administer to children under 6 yr with hepatic impairment).
Renal Impairment:
Ccr (11 to 31 mL/min or hemodialysis): PO 5 mg/day. (Do not administer to children under 6 yr with renal impairment.)
Trade names: Zyrtec Tablets 5 mg
Warnings: Standard considerations. Pregnancy Category: [B]
Interactions: None well documented.

Charcoal, activated

Antidote
Indications: Emergency treatment of poisoning by most drugs and chemicals.

Unlabeled indication: Treatment of diarrhea, stomach gas, and excessive flatulence.
Dose: Acute Intoxication: PO/Gavage tube 30 to 100 g (or 1 g/kg or about 5 to 10 times amount of poison ingested) as suspension (mixed with 6 to 8 oz water).
GI Dialysis: PO/Gavage tube 20 to 40 q 6 hr for 1 to 2 days; alternate aqueous suspension and sorbitol suspension.
Trade names: Actidose-Aqua Liquid 208 mg/mL
Actidose with Sorbitol Liquid 208 mg/mL
CharcoAid Suspension 15 g
CharcoAid 2000 Liquid 15 g
Liqui-Char Liquid 208 mg/mL
Warnings: None known. Ineffective for poisonings by cyanide, mineral acids and alkalis. Not particularly effective for poisonings by ethanol, methanol, and iron salts. Pregnancy Category: [Pregnancy category undetermined]
Interactions: Food (eg, milk, ice cream, sherbet): Decrease the absorptive capacity of drug.
Other medications: May have decreased effectiveness because of absorption by activated charcoal (eg, oral acetylcysteine used as antidote for acetaminophen overdose).
Syrup of ipecac: Inactivated because of absorption by activated charcoal. Do not administer together.

Chloral Hydrate

Sedative / Hypnotic / Nonbarbiturate
Indications: Management of short-term insomnia; sedation; adjunctive to anesthesia, analgesia; prevention or suppression of alcohol withdrawal symptoms (rectal).

Unlabeled indication: Conscious sedation in pediatric dentistry.
Dose: Insomnia:
Adults: PO/PR 500 mg to 1 g 15 to 30 min before bedtime.
Children: PO/PR 50 mg/kg/day (up to 1 g per dose) for sleep.
Premedication:
Adults: PO 500 mg to 1 g 30 min before surgery.
Sedation:
Adults: PO 250 mg tid after meals.
Children: PO/PR 25 mg/kg/day; may be given in divided doses.
Dental Sedation:
Children: 75 mg/kg; supplementation with nitrous oxide may provide better sedation than manufacturer's recommended dosage.
Trade names: Aquachloral Supprettes Suppositories 324 mg

Warnings: Hypersensitivity to chloral derivatives; severe renal or hepatic impairment; gastritis (oral forms); severe cardiac disease. Pregnancy Category: [C]
Interactions: Alcohol and other CNS depressants: May produce additive CNS depression.
Furosemide (IV): Administration within 24 hr of chloral hydrate may lead to diaphoresis, hot flashes, tachycardia, and hypertension.
Oral anticoagulants: Anticoagulant effects may be increased, especially during first 2 wk.
Phenytoin: May reduce effects of phenytoin.

Chlorambucil

Alkylating agent / Nitrogen mustard
Indications: Chronic lymphocytic leukemia, lymphomas.

Unlabeled indication: Ovarian and testicular carcinoma, polycythemia vera.
Dose: Chronic Lymphocytic Leukemia Remission Induction:
Adults: PO 0.1 to 0.2 mg/kg/day (4 to 10 mg/day) for 3 to 6 wk.
Chronic Lymphocytic Leukemia Maintenance:
Adults: PO Doses should not exceed 0.1 mg/kg/day and may be as low as 0.03 mg/kg/day. Doses of 2 to 4 mg/day are typical.
Pulse Dosing for Chronic Lymphocytic Leukemia:
Adults: PO Initial single dose of 0.4 mg/kg. Doses are then given at biweekly or monthly intervals, increasing by 0.1 mg/kg increments until lymphocytosis is controlled or toxicity occurs. Subsequent doses are modified to produce mild hematologic toxicity.
Dosage Reduction:
Adults: PO Dosage reductions are required if the patient has received full-dose radiation or myelotoxic drugs within the last month or has a low leukocyte or platelet count. Do not exceed 0.1 mg/kg/day when lymphocytic infiltration of bone marrow is present, or bone marrow is hypoplastic.
Trade names: Leukeran Tablets 2 mg
Warnings: Standard considerations. Pregnancy Category: [D]
Interactions: None well documented.

Chloramphenicol

Antibiotic
Indications: Treatment of infections caused by susceptible strains of specific microorganisms; serious systemic infections for which less potentially dangerous drugs are ineffective or contraindicated.
Dose: Systemic Infections:
Adults: IV 50 mg/kg/day in divided doses q 6 hr; may require up to 100 mg/kg/day initially for infections caused by moderately resistant organisms.
Children: IV 50 mg/kg/day in 4 doses q 6 hr; 50 to 100 mg/kg/day for severe infections (eg, bacteremia, meningitis).
Infants and Children with immature metabolic processes: IV 25 mg/kg/day.
Newborns: IV Usually 25 mg/kg/day in 4 doses q 6 hr.
Newborns over 14 days (over 2 kg): IV up to 50 mg/kg/day in 4 doses q 6 hr.
Newborns under 2 kg and birth to 14 days (over 2 kg): IV 25 mg/kg qd.
Trade names: Chloromycetin Sodium Succinate Powder for Injection 100 mg/mL (as base) when reconstituted
Warnings: Trivial infections (eg, colds, influenza, throat infections) or infections other than indicated; prophylaxis of systemic bacterial infections; hypersensitivity to product. Pregnancy Category: [C]
Interactions: Agents that suppress bone marrow: Risk or severity of bone marrow suppression may be increased.
Anticoagulants: May enhance anticoagulation action.
Barbiturates: May reduce effectiveness of chloramphenicol while barbiturate effects may be enhanced; effects may last days after barbiturates are withdrawn.
Ferrous salts: May increase serum iron levels.
Hydantoins (eg, phenytoin): May increase serum hydantoin levels, with possible toxicity; chloramphenicol levels may increase or decrease.
Rifampin: May reduce chloramphenicol serum levels; effect may last days after rifampin is withdrawn.
Sulfonylureas: May cause clinical manifestations of hypoglycemia.
Vitamin B-12: May decrease hematologic effects of vitamin B -12 in patients with pernicious anemia.

Chlorhexidine Gluconate

Antiseptic / Germicide
Indications: Surgical scrub; skin cleanser; preoperative skin preparation; skin wound cleanser; hand rinse; oral rinse for gingivitis; an adjunct to scaling and root planning procedures for reduction of pocket depth in adults with periodontitis.

Unlabeled indication: Treatment of acne vulgaris. Amelioration of oral mucositis associated with cytoreductive therapy for bone marrow transplant candidates.
Dose: Skin Use: 5 mL is applied to skin and worked into lather.
Periodontitis: 2.5 mg (1 chip) inserted into periodonted pocket with probing depth at least 5 mm.
Oral Rinse for Gingivitis: 15 mL (1 capful) bid for 30 sec, morning and evening after brushing teeth. Expectorate after rinsing; do not swallow.
Trade names: Bactoshield Solution 4% with 4% isopropyl alcohol
Bactoshield 2 Solution 2% with 4% isopropyl alcohol
Betasept Liquid 4% with 4% isopropyl alcohol
Dyna-Hex 2 Skin Cleanser Liquid 2% with 4% isopropyl alcohol
Dyna-Hex Skin Cleanser Liquid 4% with 4% isopropyl alcohol
Exidine-2 Scrub Solution 2% with 4% isopropyl alcohol
Exidine-4 Scrub Care Solution 4% with 4% isopropyl alcohol
Exidine Skin Cleanser Liquid 4% with 4% isopropyl alcohol
Hibiclens Sponge/Brush 4% with 4% isopropyl alcohol
Hibiclens Antiseptic/Antimicrobial Skin Cleanser Liquid 4% with 4% isopropyl alcohol
Hibistat Germicidal Hand Rinse Rinse 0.5% with 70% isopropanol and emollients
Hibistat Towelettes Wipes 0.5% with 70% isopopranolol
Peridex Oral Rinse 0.12%
PerioChip Chip 2.5 mg
PerioGard Oral Rinse 0.12%
Warnings: Standard considerations. Pregnancy Category: [B (oral rinse) Pregnancy category undetermined for skin use]
Interactions: None well documented.

Chloroquine

Anti-infective / Antimalarial
Indications: Prophylaxis and treatment of acute attacks of malaria caused by Plasmodium vivax, P. malariae, P. ovale, and susceptible strains of P. falciparum; extraintestinal amebiasis.

Unlabeled indication: Treatment of rheumatoid arthritis, systemic and discoid lupus erythematosus, porphyria cutanea tarda, scleroderma, pemphigus, lichen planus, polymyositis and sarcoidosis.
Dose: Doses are listed in base equivalents. (Chloroquine phosphate, 500 mg equals 300 mg base; chloroquine HCl, 50 mg equals 40 mg base.)
Acute Malaria:
Chloroquine Phosphate:
Adults: PO Initial dose is 600 mg, then 300 mg 6 hr

later and 300 mg qd for 2 days.
Children: PO Initial dose is 10 mg/kg, then 5 mg/kg 6 hr later and 5 mg/kg qd for 2 days.
Chloroquine HCl:
Adults: IM Initial dose is 160 to 200 mg; repeat dose in 6 hr if needed (max, 800 mg base total dose in first 24 hr).
Children: 5 mg/kg/dose; repeat dose in 6 hr (max, 10 mg base/kg/24 hr; do not exceed 5 mg/kg as single parenteral dose).
Malaria Suppression:
Adults: PO 300 mg base.
Children: 5 mg/kg/dose (max 300 mg base) weekly. Begin 1 to 2 wk prior to exposure and continue for 4 wk after leaving endemic area. If suppressive therapy is not begun prior to exposure, double initial loading dose and give in 2 divided doses 6 hr apart.
Extraintestinal Amebiasis:
Chloroquine Phosphate:
Adults: PO 600 mg base/day for 2 days, then 300 mg base/day for 2 to 3 wk.
Chloroquine HCl:
Adults: IM 4 to 5 mL (160 to 200 mg base)/day for 10 to 12 days.

Trade names: Aralen Phosphate Tablets 500 mg (equivalent to 300 mg base)
Aralen HCl Injection 50 mg (equivalent to 40 mg base)/mL

Warnings: Retinal or visual field changes.
Pregnancy Category: [D]

Interactions: Cimetidine: May increase chloroquine serum concentration.
Kaolin aluminum or magnesium trisilicate antacids: May decrease GI absorption of chloroquine.
Rabies vaccine: Concomitant administration of intradermally administered rabies vaccine and chloroquine may result in diminished antibody response to vaccine. In this situation CDC recommends administering rabies vaccine IM.

Chlorothiazide

Thiazide diuretic

Indications: Adjunctive treatment in edema associated with CHF, hepatic cirrhosis, and corticosteroid and estrogen therapy; edema caused by various forms of renal dysfunction such as nephrotic syndrome, acute glomerulonephritis, and chronic renal failure (oral and IV); management of hypertension (oral).

Dose: Diuresis and Control of Hypertension:
Children younger than 6 mo (see Precautions): PO 30 mg/kg in 2 divided doses may be required.
Children 6 mo to 2 yr (see Precautions): PO 10 to 20 mg/kg/day in single or 2 divided doses (max, 375 mg/day).
Children 2 to 12 yr (see Precautions): PO 1 g/day.
Edema:
Adults: PO 500 to 1000 mg qd or bid. Many patients respond to intermittent therapy (alternate day therapy or administration on 3 to 5 days each wk). IV Should be reserved for patients unable to take oral medication or for emergency situations. Individualize dosage according to patient response, using the smallest dosage necessary.
Hypertension:
Adults: PO 500 to 1000 mg as a single or divided dose. Increase or decrease dose according to BP response. Rarely, some patients may require up to 2 g/day in divided doses.

Trade names: Diuril Tablets 250 mg
Diurigen Tablets 500 mg

Warnings: Anuria, hypersensitivity to sulfonamide-derived drugs or any component of this product.
Pregnancy Category: [C]

Interactions: Alcohol, barbiturates, narcotics: May potentiate orthostatic hypotension.
Bile acid sequestrants: May reduce thiazide absorption; give thiazide at least 2 hr before bile acid sequestrants.
Diazoxide: May cause hyperglycemia.
Digitalis glycosides: Diuretic-induced hypokalemia and hypomagnesemia may precipitate digitalis-induced arrhythmias.
Lithium: May decrease renal excretion of lithium.
Loop diuretics: Synergistic effects may result in profound diuresis and serious electrolyte abnormalities.
Sulfonylureas, insulin: May decrease hypoglycemic effect of sulfonylureas. Because chlorothiazide may elevate blood glucose levels, may need to increase dosage of sulfonylureas or insulin.

Chlorpromazine HCl

Antipsychotic / Phenothiazine / Antiemetic

Indications: Management of manic phase of manic-depressive disorder; treatment of schizophrenia; relief of anxiety and restlessness prior to surgery; adjunct in treatment of tetanus; management of acute intermittent porphyria, severe behavioral and conduct disorders in children; control of nausea and vomiting; relief of intractable hiccoughs.

Unlabeled indication: Treatment of migraine headaches (IM or IV forms).

Dose: Adults:
Psychiatric (outpatient): IM 25 mg for prompt control; may repeat in 1 hr. PO 25 to 50 mg tid after initial regimen. May initiate oral dosing with 10 mg tid to qid or 25 mg bid or tid.
Psychiatric (inpatient): PO 25 mg tid; increase prn; usually 400 mg/day. IM 25 mg initially; may give additional 25 to 50 mg in 1 hr. Increase gradually until controlled. Up to 2000 mg/day may be needed but generally not for extended periods.
Acute Intermittent Porphyria: PO 25 to 50 mg tid or qid; IM 25 mg tid to qid.
Tetanus: IM 25 to 50 mg tid to qid; IV 25 to 50 mg diluted to greater than or equal to 1 mg/mL and administered at rate of 1 mg/min.
Nausea and Vomiting: PO 10 to 25 mg q 4 to 6 hr prn. PR 100 mg q 6 to 8 hr prn. IM 25 mg. If no hypotension, may give 25 to 50 mg q 4 to 6 hr prn.
During surgery: IM 12.5 mg; repeat in 0.5 hr if necessary and if no hypotension. IV 2 mg per fractional injection, at 2-min intervals (max, 25 mg). Dilute to 1 mg/mL (1 mL [25 mg]) mixed with 24 mL of saline.
Presurgical apprehension: PO 25 to 50 mg 2 to 3 hr prior to surgery. IM 12.5 to 25 mg 1 to 2 hr before surgery.
Intractable Hiccoughs: PO 25 to 50 mg tid to qid. IM May give 25 to 50 mg if symptoms persist 2 to 3 days. IV May use slow infusion if hiccoughs persist.
Children over 6 mo:
Psychiatric (Outpatient): PO 0.5 mg/kg q 4 to 6 hr prn; PR 1 mg/kg q 6 to 8 hr prn; IM 0.5 mg/kg q 6 to 8 hr prn.
Psychiatric (Inpatient): PO Start low and increase gradually; 50 to 100 mg/day may be needed in severe cases or 200 mg/day or more in older children. IM Up to 5 yr: Do not exceed 40 mg/day. 5 to 12 yr: Do not exceed 75 mg/day if possible.
Tetanus: IM/IV 0.5 mg/kg q 6 to 8 hr. When giving IV, dilute to at least 1 mg/mL and administer at rate of 1 mg/2 min. In children 23 kg or under, do not exceed 40 mg/day; 23 to 45 kg, do not exceed 75 mg/day if possible.
Nausea and Vomiting: PO 0.55 mg/kg q 4 to 6 hr. PR 1.1 mg/kg q 6 to 8 hr prn. IM 0.55 mg/kg q 6 to 8 hr prn. Do not exceed 40 mg/day if under 5 yr or 75 mg/day if 5 to 12 yr.
Presurgical apprehension: PO 0.55 mg/kg 2 to 3 hr before surgery. IM 0.55 mg/kg 1 to 2 hr before surgery.

Trade names: Chlorpromazine HCl Tablets 10 mg
Thorazine Tablets 25 mg

Warnings: Comatose or severely depressed states; allergy to product or other phenothiazines;

presence of large amounts of other CNS depressants. Pregnancy Category: [Safety not established]

Interactions: Alcohol and other CNS depressants: May cause increased CNS depression and may precipitate extrapyramidal reaction.
Anticholinergics: May reduce therapeutic effects of and increase anticholinergic effects of chlorpromazine; may lead to tardive dyskinesia.
Barbiturate anesthetics: May increase frequency and severity of neuromuscular excitation and hypotension.
Beta-blockers: May result in increased plasma levels of beta-blocker and chlorpromazine.
Cisapride, sparfloxacin: The risk of life-threatening cardiac arrhythmias, including torsades de pointes, may be increased.
Epinephrine, norepinephrine: Actions of these drugs may be decreased or reversed.
Guanethidine: The hypotensive effect of guanethidine may be inhibited.
Lithium: May cause disorienting unconsciousness and extrapyramidal effects.
Meperidine: May result in excessive sedation and hypotension.
Metrizamide: Risk of seizure may increase.
Paroxetine: Plasma levels of chlorpromazine may be elevated, increasing the risk of side effects.

Chlorpropamide

Antidiabetic / Sulfonylurea

Indications: Adjunct to diet to lower blood glucose in patients with non-insulin-dependent diabetes mellitus (type II) whose hyperglycemia cannot be controlled by diet alone.

Unlabeled indication: Control of neurogenic diabetes insipidus.

Dose: Adults:
Initial dose: PO 250 mg/day in single dose.
Elderly:
Initial dose: PO 100 to 125 mg/day in single dose.
Maintenance: PO 100 to 250 mg/day in single dose.
Severely Diabetic Adults: PO up to 500 mg/day; avoid doses above 750 mg/day.

Trade names: Diabinese Tablets 100 mg

Warnings: Hypersensitivity to sulfonylureas; diabetes complicated by ketoacidosis with or without coma; sole therapy for insulin-independent (type I) diabetes mellitus; diabetes when complicated by pregnancy. Pregnancy Category: [C Insulin is recommended to maintain blood glucose levels during pregnancy Prolonged severe neonatal hypoglycemia can occur if sulfonylureas are administered at time of delivery If administering to pregnant patient, discontinue 2 days to 4 wk before expected date of delivery]

Interactions: Androgens, anticoagulants, chloramphenicol, clofibrate, fenfluramine, methyldopa, MAO inhibitors, phenylbutazone, probenecid, salicylates, sulfonamides, tricyclic antidepressants, urinary acidifiers: May increase hypoglycemic effect.
Beta-blockers, corticosteroids, diazoxide, hydantoins, rifampin, thiazide diuretics, urinary alkalinizers: May decrease hypoglycemic effect.

Chlorthalidone

Thiazide diuretic

Indications: Reduction of edema associated with CHF, hepatic cirrhosis, renal dysfunction, corticosteroid and estrogen therapy; management of hypertension.

Unlabeled indication: Treatment of calcium nephrolithiasis, osteoporosis, diabetes insipidus.

Dose: Edema:
Adults: PO 50 to 200 mg daily or on alternate days.
Hypertension:
Adults: PO 25 to 100 mg daily. Doses above 25 mg/day potentiate potassium excretion but do not benefit sodium excretion or BP reduction.

Trade names: Hygroton Tablets 25 mg
Thalitone Tablets 15 mg

Warnings: Hypersensitivity to thiazides, related diuretics, or sulfonamide-derived drugs; anuria; renal decompensation. Pregnancy Category: [B]

Interactions: Allopurinol: Concurrent use may increase incidence of hypersensitivity reactions to allopurinol.
Amphotericin B, corticosteroids: May intensify potassium depletion.
Anticholinergics: May increase chlorthalidone absorption.
Anticoagulants: May diminish anticoagulant effects.
Bile acid sequestrants: May reduce chlorthalidone absorption. Give chlorthalidone at least 2 hr before bile acid sequestrant.
Calcium salts: Hypercalcemia may develop.
Diazoxide: May cause hyperglycemia.
Digitalis glycosides: Diuretic-induced hypokalemia and hypomagnesemia may precipitate digitalis-induced arrhythmias.
Lithium: May decrease renal excretion of lithium.
Loop diuretics: Synergistic effects may result in profound diuresis and serious electrolyte abnormalities.
Methenamines, NSAIDs: May decrease effectiveness of chlorthalidone.
Sulfonylureas, insulin: May decrease hypoglycemic effect of sulfonylureas.

Cholestyramine

Antihyperlipidemic / Bile acid sequestrant

Indications: Reduction of serum cholesterol in patients with primary hypercholesterolemia; relief of pruritus associated with partial biliary obstruction.

Unlabeled indication: Treatment of antibiotic-induced pseudomembranous colitis, bile salt-mediated diarrhea and digitalis toxicity.

Dose: Adults: PO 4 g 1 to 6 times/day; generally given 3 to 4 times/day.

Trade names: LoCHOLEST Powder for Suspension 4 g anhydrous cholestyramine resin/9 g powder
LoCHOLEST Light Powder for Suspension 4 g anhydrous cholestyramine resin/5.7 g powder
Prevalite Powder 4 g (as anhydrous cholestyramine resin)/5.5 g powder
Questran Powder for Suspension 4 g anhydrous cholestyramine resin/9 g powder
Questran Light Powder 4 g (as anhydrous cholestyramine resin)/5 g powder

Warnings: Hypersensitivity to bile acid sequestering resins; complete biliary obstruction. Pregnancy Category: [Safety not established]

Interactions: Acetaminophen, amiodarone, corticosteroids, digitalis glycosides, HMG-CoA reductase inhibitors (eg, fluvastatin), methotrexate, some NSAIDs (eg, piroxicam), propranolol, thiazide diuretics, ursodiol, warfarin, and other drugs: Cholestyramine may interfere with the absorption of many drugs, especially those listed.
Fats and fat-soluble vitamins A, D, E, and K: Cholestyramine may interfere with normal fat absorption and digestion; consider supplementation with these vitamins and with folic acid.
Iopanoic acid: Coadministration may result in abnormal cholecystography.

Chorionic Gonadotropin

Sex hormones / Ovulation stimulant

Indications: Prepubertal cryptorchidism not caused by anatomical obstruction; selected cases of hypogonadotropic hypogonadism (eg, hypogonadism secondary to pituitary deficiency) in men; induction of ovulation in anovulatory, infertile women in whom

Medications

the cause of anovulation is secondary and not caused by primary ovarian failure and who have been appropriately pretreated with human menotropins.

Dose: Prepubertal Cryptorchidism:
Children (4 yr and older):
Various authorities have advocated the following regimens: IM (1) 4000 USP U 3 times/wk for 3 wk, (2) 5000 USP U qod for 4 injections, (3) 15 injections of 500 to 1000 USP U over a period of 6 wk, or (4) 500 USP U 3 times/wk for 4 to 6 wk (if not successful, another course is begun 1 mo later using 1000 USP U/injection).
Hypogonadotropic Hypogonadism in Men:
Adults:
Various authorities have advocated the following regimens: IM 500 to 1000 USP U 3 times/wk for 3 wk, followed by same dose twice a week for 3 wk, or 4000 USP U 3 times/wk for 6 to 9 mo, following which the dosage may be reduced to 2000 USP U 3 times/wk for an additional 3 mo.

Trade names: Chorex-10 Powder for injection 10,000 units/vial with 10 mL diluent (to make 1000 units/mL)
Chorionic Gonadotropin Powder for injection 5000 units/vial with 10 mL diluent (to make 500 units/mL)
Novarel Powder for injection 10,000 units/vial with 10 mL diluent (to make 1000 units/mL)
Pregnyl Powder for injection 10,000 units/vial with 10 mL diluent (to make 1000 units/mL)
Profasi Powder for injection 5000 units/vial with 10 mL diluent (to make 500 units/mL)

Warnings: Precocious puberty; prostatic carcinoma or other androgen-dependent neoplasm; prior allergic reaction to hCG. Pregnancy Category: [C]

Interactions: None well documented.

Ciclopirox

Topical anti-infective / Antifungal

Indications: Loprox: Shampoo/Gel: Topical treatment of seborrheic dermatitis of the scalp in adults.

Gel: Interdigital tinea pedis and tinea corporis caused by T. rubrum, T. mentagroyphytes, or E. floccosum.

Cream/Suspension: Tinea pedis (athlete's foot), tinea cruris (jock itch), and tinea corporis (ringworm) caused by T. rubrum, T. mentagrophytes, E. floccosum, and M. canis; cutaneous candidiasis (moniliasis) caused by C. albicans; tinea (pityriasis) versicolor caused by M. furfur.

Penlac: As a component of a comprehensive management program for topical treatment in immunocompetent patients with mild to moderate onychomycosis of fingernails and toenails without lunula involvement, caused by T. rubrum.

Dose: Loprox shampoo:
Adults and children 16 yr and older: Topical Wet hair and apply approximately 1 tsp (5 mL) to the scalp. Up to 2 tsp (10 mL) may be used for long hair. Lather and leave on hair and scalp for 3 min. Rinse off. Repeat treatment 2 times/wk for 4 wk, with a minimum of 3 days between applications. If no improvement after 4 wk of treatment, reevaluate the diagnosis.
Loprox cream/suspension:
Adults and children 10 yr and older: Topical Gently massage cream into the affected and surrounding skin areas bid, morning and evening. If no improvement after 4 wk of treatment, reevaluate the diagnosis.
Loprox gel:
Adults and children 16 yr and older: Topical Gently massage gel into affected skin areas of scalp areas bid, morning and evening. If no improvement after 4 wk of treatment, reevaluate the diagnosis.
Penlac:
Adults: Topical Apply qd, at bedtime or 8 hr before washing, to all affected nails with the provided applicator. Apply evenly over the entire nail plate. If possible, apply to nail bed, hyponychium, and the under surface of the nail plate when it is free of the nail bed (eg, onycholysis). Do not remove product on a daily basis. Make daily applications over the previous coat and remove with alcohol q 7 days, repeating this cycle throughout the duration of therapy. As a comprehensive management program for onychomycosis, removal of the unattached, infected nail, as frequently as monthly, by a health care professional, weekly trimming by the patient, and daily application of the medication are integral parts of therapy.

Trade names: Loprox Cream 0.77%
Penlac Nail Lacquer Solution, topical 8%

Warnings: Standard considerations. Pregnancy Category: [B]

Interactions: None well documented.

Cidofovir

Anti-infective / Antiviral

Indications: Treatment of CMV retinitis in patients with AIDS.

Dose: Adult:
Induction: IV 5 mg/kg once weekly for 2 consecutive weeks.
Maintenance dose: IV 5 mg/kg once q 2 wk.
Nephrotoxicity: Reduce the dose of cidofovir to 3 mg/kg for increases in serum creatinine (0.3 to 0.4 mg/dL).
Probenecid: Administer probenecid orally with each dose of cidofovir. Probenecid 2 g given 3 hr prior to the cidofovir dose and 1 g administered 2 hr and again at 8 hr after completion of the cidofovir infusion.

Trade names: Vistide Injection 75 mg/mL

Warnings: History of clinically severe hypersensitivity to probenecid or other sulfa-containing medications; direct intraocular injection. Patients receiving agents with a nephrotoxic potential must discontinue use of such agents at least 1 wk prior to beginning therapy. Initiation of therapy in patients with a serum creatinine greater than 1.5 mg/dL, a calculated Ccr of less than or equal to 55 mL/min, or a urine protein at least 100 mg/dL. Pregnancy Category: [C]

Interactions: Nephrotoxic agents (eg, aminoglycosides, amphotericin B, foscarnet, IV pentamidine): Risk of nephrotoxicity is increased.

Cilostazol

Antiplatelet

Indications: Reduction of symptoms of intermittent claudication as indicated by an increased walking distance.

Dose: Intermittent Claudication: PO 100 mg twice daily, taken at least 30 min before or 2 hr after breakfast and dinner. Consider a dose of 50 mg twice daily during coadministration of such inhibitors of CYP3A4 and CYP2C19.

Trade names: Pletal Tablets 50 mg

Warnings: CHF of any severity; hypersensitivity to any components of the product. Cilostazol and several of its metabolites are inhibitors of phosphodiesterase III. Several drugs with this pharmacologic effect have caused decreased survival compared with placebo in patients with class III to IV CHF. Pregnancy Category: [C]

Interactions: Aspirin: Short-term (up to 4 days) coadministration of aspirin with cilostazol showed a 23% to 35% increase in inhibition of ADP-induced ex vivo platelet aggregation compared with aspirin alone.
Diltiazem: Diltiazem increased cilostazol plasma concentrations by about 53%. Initiate therapy at half the recommended dose.
Macrolides: Erythromycin increased cilostazol C_{max} by 47% and AUC by 73%. Other macrolide antibiotics would be expected to have similar effects. Initiate therapy at half the recommended dose.
Omeprazole: Coadministration of omeprazole did not

significantly affect the metabolism of cilostazol, but the systemic exposure to 3,4-dehydro-cilostazol was increased by 69%, probably the result of omeprazole's potent inhibition of CYP2C19. Initiate therapy at half the recommended dose.
P450 system: Cilostazol could have pharmacokinetic interactions because of effects of other drugs on its metabolism by CYP3A4 or CYP2C19.
Platelet function inhibitors: Cilostazol could have pharmacodynamic interactions with other platelet function inhibitors.

Cimetidine

Histamine H_2 antagonist

Indications: Management of duodenal ulcer; treatment of gastroesophageal reflux disease (GERD), including erosive esophagitis; therapy for benign gastric ulcer; treatment of pathologic hypersecretory conditions; prevention of upper GI bleeding.

Unlabeled indication: Prevention of aspiration pneumonia and stress ulcers; herpes virus infection; chronic idiopathic urticaria; anaphylaxis (relieves dermatologic symptoms only); dyspepsia; used before anesthesia to prevent aspiration pneumonitis; treatment of hyperparathyroidism and control of secondary hyperparathyroidism in chronic hemodialysis patient; treatment of chronic viral warts in children.

Dose: Duodenal Ulcer (Active):
Adults: PO 800 mg at bedtime for 4 to 6 wk.
Alternate regimens: PO 300 mg qid with meals and at bedtime or 400 mg bid.
Maintenance Therapy: PO 400 mg at bedtime.
Active Benign Gastric Ulcer:
Adults: PO 800 mg at bedtime.
GERD:
Adults: PO 1600 mg daily in divided doses (800 mg or 400 mg) for 12 wk, although some patients may require chronic therapy.
Pathologic Hypersecretory Conditions:
Adults: PO 300 mg qid w/meals and at bedtime. If needed, 300 mg doses may be given more often (max, 2400 mg/day).
Prevention of Upper GI Bleeding:
Adults: Continuous IV infusion of 50 mg/hr. For hospitalized patients with pathologic hypersecretory conditions or intractable ulcers, or patients unable to take PO medication.
Usual dose: IM/IV 300 mg q 6 h to 8 h (max 2400 mg/day).

Trade names: Tagamet Tablets 200 mg
Tagamet HB Tablets 100 mg

Warnings: Hypersensitivity to cimetidine or other H -2 antagonists. Pregnancy Category: [B]

Interactions: Antacids, anticholinergics, metoclopramide: May decrease absorption of cimetidine.
Benzodiazepines, caffeine, calcium channel blockers, carbamazepine, chloroquine, labetalol, lidocaine, metoprolol, metronidazole, moricizine, pentoxifylline, phenytoin, propranolol, quinidine, quinine, sulfonylureas, theophyllines, triamterene, tricyclic antidepressants, warfarin: Cimetidine may reduce metabolism and increase serum concentration and pharmacologic/toxic effects of these drugs.
Carmustine: Bone marrow toxicity may be enhanced.
Cigarette smoking: Reversed cimetidine's effects on suppression of nocturnal gastric secretion.
Ferrous salts, indomethacin, fluconazole, ketoconazole, tetracyclines: Cimetidine may decrease absorption of these drugs.
Hydantoins: Hydantoin levels may increase.
Narcotic analgesics: Toxic effects (eg, respiratory depression) may be increased.
Procainamide: Levels of procainamide and its active metabolite may increase.
Tocainide: Cimetidine may decrease the pharmacologic effects of tocainide.

Cisplatin

Alkylating agent

Indications: Metastatic testicular or ovarian tumors, advanced bladder cancer.

Unlabeled indication: Squamous cell carcinoma of the head and neck and of the cervix; lung carcinomas, osteogenic sarcoma, brain tumors; advanced esophageal, adrenal cortex, breast, endometrial, and liver carcinoma, bone marrow transplantation.

Dose: Metastatic Testicular Tumors:
Adults: IV Cisplatin 20 mg/m^2 /day IV for 5 days q 3 wk for 3 courses (combination regimen). Single doses of cisplatin up to 120 mg/m^2 in combination with other antineoplastics have been used.
Metastatic Ovarian Tumors (Cyclophosphamide Combination Therapy):
Adults: IV Cisplatin 75 to 100 mg/m^2 once q 4 wk. Cyclophosphamide 600 mg/m^2 once q 4 wk (day 1).
Metastatic Ovarian Tumors (Single Agent Therapy):
Adults: IV Administer as a single agent of 100 mg/m^2 IV/cycle once q 4 wk.
Advanced Bladder Cancer:
Adults: IV Administer as a single agent. Give 50 to 70 mg/m^2 once q 3 to 4 wk, depending on prior radiation therapy or chemotherapy. For heavily pretreated patients, give an initial dose of 50 mg/m^2 /cycle repeated q 4 wk.
Repeat Courses:
Adults: IV Do not give a repeat course until serum creatinine is below 1.5 mg/dL or BUN is below 25 mg/dL or until circulating blood elements are at an acceptable level (platelets at least 100,000/mm^3, WBC at least 4000/mm^3). Do not give subsequent doses until an audiometric analysis indicates that auditory acuity is within normal limits.
Renal Impairment:
Adults: IV The manufacturer does not recommend the use of cisplatin in patients with renal impairment. Some clinicians recommend not giving cisplatin to patients with a Ccr below 30 mL/min.

Trade names: Platinol AQ Solution for injection 1 mg/mL

Warnings: Pre-existing renal impairment; myelosuppression; hearing impairment; history of allergic reactions to cisplatin or other platinum-containing compounds. Pregnancy Category: [D]

Interactions: Aminoglycosides: Potentiation of nephrotoxicity is possible.
Lithium: Cisplatin may transiently decrease lithium serum levels.
Loop diuretics (eg, furosemide): Potentiation of ototoxicity is possible.
Paclitaxel: Paclitaxel clearance decreases when cisplatin is given immediately prior to paclitaxel, resulting in increased hematologic toxicity.
Phenytoin: Cisplatin may decrease absorption or increase metabolism, resulting in lower serum levels of phenytoin.

Citalopram

Antidepressant / Selective serotonin reuptake inhibitor

Indications: Treatment of major depression as defined in the DSM-III and DSM-III-R category of major depressive disorders.

Dose: Adults: PO Initiate with 20 mg once daily and titrate up to 40 mg/day; max, 60 mg/day.
Elderly: PO Initiate with 20 mg once daily; titrate up to 40 mg/day, if needed.
Hepatic Impairment:
Adults: PO Initiate with 20 mg once daily; titrate up to 40 mg/day, if needed.
Maintenance: Periodically reevaluate long-term usefulness if used for extended periods.
MAO Inhibitor Therapy: Allow at least 14 days between starting or stopping either agent.

Medications

Trade names: Celexa Tablets 20 mg
Warnings: Standard considerations; concomitant use of MAO inhibitors. Pregnancy Category: [C]
Interactions: Beta Blockers (ie, carvedilol, metoprolol, propranolol): Inhibition of metabolism of the beta blocker may occur, resulting in excessive beta blockade (eg, bradycardia).
Cimetidine: Serum levels of citalopram may be increased 40%.
Cyproheptadine: May decrease the pharmacologic effect of citalopram.
Lithium: Lithium may enhance the serotonergic effects of citalopram; use caution if coadministered.
MAO inhibitors: Do not administer with citalopram.
Sumatriptan: Rare postmarketing reports of weakness, hyperreflexia, and incoordination following coadministration.
Metoprolol: Coadministration with citalopram has increased plasma levels of metoprolol 2-fold.

Cladribine

Antimetabolite / Pyrimidine
Indications: Adult: Hairy cell leukemia.

Unlabeled indication: Chronic lymphocytic leukemia, non-Hodgkin lymphoma, acute myeloid leukemia.
Dose: Hairy Cell Leukemia:
Adults: Continuous IV infusion 0.09 mg/kg/day for 7 days, single course. For patients weighing more than 85 kg, preparation of a single dose for administration over 7 days is not advised because solutions may be inadequately preserved because of increased dilution of benzyl alcohol.
Trade names: Leustatin Solution for injection 1 mg/mL, 10 mL single-use vials
Warnings: Standard considerations. Pregnancy Category: [D]
Interactions: None well documented.

Clemastine Fumarate

Antihistamine / Ethanolamine
Indications: Relief of symptoms associated with allergic rhinitis or other upper respiratory allergies, such as sneezing, rhinorrhea, pruritus, and lacrimation; relief of mild, uncomplicated allergic skin manifestation of urticaria and angioedema.
Dose: Adults and Children over 12 yr: PO 1.34 mg bid to 2.68 mg tid (max, 8.04 mg/day).
Children 6 to 12 yr: PO (syrup only) 0.67 to 1.34 mg bid (max, 4.02 mg/day).
Trade names: Dayhist-1 Tablets 1.34 mg as fumarate (equiv. to 1 mg clemastine)
Tavist Allergy Tablets 1.34 mg as fumarate (equiv. to 1 mg clemastine)
Clemastine Fumarate Tablets 2.68 mg (equiv. to 2 mg clemastine)
Warnings: Hypersensitivity to antihistamines; narrow-angle glaucoma; stenosing peptic ulcer; symptomatic prostatic hypertrophy; asthmatic attack; bladder neck obstruction; pyloroduodenal obstruction; MAO inhibitor therapy; use in newborn or premature infants and in nursing women. Pregnancy Category: [B]
Interactions: Alcohol, CNS depressants: May cause additive CNS depressant effects.
MAO Inhibitors: May increase anticholinergic effects of clemastine fumarate.

Clindamycin

Antibiotic / Lincosamide
Indications: Treatment of serious infections caused by susceptible strains of specific microorganisms; treatment of acne vulgaris (topical use); treatment of bacterial vaginosis (vaginal use).
Dose: Adults: PO 150 to 450 mg q 6 hr. IM/IV 0.6 to 2.7 g/day divided into 2 to 4 equal doses. For more serious infections, these doses may need to be increased. Do not use more than 600 mg in single IM injection.
Children:
Clindamycin HCl: PO 8 to 20 mg/kg/day divided into 3 to 4 doses.
Clindamycin palmitate HCl: PO 8 to 25 mg/kg/day divided into 3 to 4 doses.
Children over 1 mo of age: IM/IV 20 to 40 mg/kg/day divided into 3 to 4 equal doses.
Newborns under 1 mo of age: IM/IV 15 to 20 mg/kg/day divided into 3 to 4 equal doses.
Acne:
Adults: Topical Apply thin film to affected area bid.
Acute Pelvic Inflammatory Disease:
Adults: IV 900 mg q 8 hr with gentamicin loading dose 2 mg/kg IV or IM, followed by 1.5 mg/kg 8 hr. Parenteral therapy may be discontinued after 24 hr. After discharge from hospital, continue with doxycycline 100 mg bid for 10 to 14 days or oral clindamycin 450 mg qid for 10 to 14 days.
Vaginosis:
Adults: Intravaginal cream 1 applicatorful, preferably at bedtime, for 3 or 7 consecutive days in nonpregnant patients and 7 days in pregnant patients. Intravaginal suppositories Insert 1 suppository per day, preferably at bedtime, for 3 consecutive days.
Trade names: Cleocin Vaginal ovules 100 mg
Cleocin T Gel 1%
Clindets Suspension, topical 1%
ClindaMax Gel 1%
ClindaMax Lotion Suspension, topical 1%
Clindagel Gel 1%
Cleocin Phosphate Injection 150 mg (as phosphate) per mL
Cleocin Capsules 75 mg (as HCl)
Cleocin Pediatric Granules for Oral Solution 75 mg per 5 mL (as palmitate)
Warnings: Hypersensitivity to lincosamides or any product component; history of regional enteritis, ulcerative colitis, or antibiotic-associated colitis. Pregnancy Category: [B Clindamycin does cross the placenta]
Interactions: Erythromycin: May cause antagonism.
Kaolin-pectin antidiarrheals: May delay absorption of clindamycin.
Nondepolarizing neuromuscular blockers: May enhance actions of neuromuscular blocking agents.
Incompatability: Ampicillin, phenytoin sodium, barbiturates, aminophylline, magnesium sulfate, calcium gluconate.

Clobetasol Propionate

Corticosteroid / Topical
Indications: Relief of inflammatory and pruritic manifestations of corticosteroid-responsive dermatoses; moderate to severe plaque-type psoriasis (Olux foam, Clobex lotion, Temovate E cream).
Dose: Adults and Children over 12 yr of age: Topical Apply thin film to affected area bid. When using the foam, apply directly to the affected area. Treatment (except psoriasis) should be limited to 2 consecutive wk and less than 50 g/wk or 50 mL/wk. In psoriasis, no more than 4 consecutive wk and less than 50 g/wk.
Trade names: Clobex Lotion 0.05%
Cormax Ointment 0.05%
Embeline Cream 0.05%
Embeline E Cream 0.05%
Olux Foam 0.05%
Temovate Cream 0.05%
Temovate Emollient Cream 0.05%
Warnings: Primary scalp infections (scalp application formulation). Standard considerations. Pregnancy Category: [C]
Interactions: None well documented.

Clomiphene Citrate

Ovulation stimulant

Indications: Treatment of ovulatory failure in women desiring pregnancy when partner is fertile and potent.

Unlabeled indication: Treatment of male infertility.

Dose: Initial Therapy: PO 50 mg/day for 5 days. Second and Third Courses: PO 100 mg/day for 5 days.

Trade names: Clomid Tablets 50 mg
Milophene Tablets 50 mg
Serophene Tablets 50 mg

Warnings: Liver disease; history of liver dysfunction; abnormal bleeding of undetermined origin; pregnancy. Pregnancy Category: [X]

Interactions: None well documented.

Clomipramine HCl

Tricyclic antidepressant

Indications: Relief of obsessive-compulsive disorder.

Unlabeled indication: Treatment of panic disorder or chronic pain (eg, migraine, chronic tension headache, diabetic neuropathy, tic douloureux, cancer pain, peripheral neuropathy, postherpetic neuralgia, arthritic pain).

Dose: Adults:
Initial dose: PO 25 mg/day; gradually increase dose to 100 mg/day during first 2 wk. Dose may then be gradually increased to max of 250 mg/day.
Children (10 yr and under):
Initial dose: PO 25 mg/day; gradually increase dose to 3 mg/kg/day or 100 mg/day (whichever is less) during first 2 wk; then slowly increase dose to max 3 mg/kg/day or 200 mg/day (whichever is less).

Trade names: Anafranil Capsules 25 mg

Warnings: Hypersensitivity to any tricyclic antidepressant. Not to be given in combination with or within 14 days of treatment with MAO inhibitors. Not to be given during acute recovery phases of MI. Pregnancy Category: [C Neonatal withdrawal symptoms have been reported]

Interactions: Anticholinergics: Effects may be increased.
Barbiturates, charcoal: May increase effects of clomipramine.
Cimetidine, fluoxetine, haloperidol, phenothiazine antipsychotics, oral contraceptives: May increase effects of clomipramine.
Clonidine: May result in hypertensive crisis.
CNS depressants: Depressant effects may be additive.
Guanethidine: Antihypertensive effects may be decreased.
MAO inhibitors: Sweating, convulsions, and death may occur.

Clonazepam

Anticonvulsant / Benzodiazepine

Indications: Treatment of Lennox-Gastaut syndrome; management of akinetic and myoclonic seizures and absence seizures unresponsive to succinimides; panic disorders.

Unlabeled indication: Treatment of restless legs syndrome, parkinsonian dysarthria, acute manic episodes of bipolar affective disorder, multifocal tic disorders and neuralgias; adjunctive therapy for schizophrenia.

Dose: Panic Disorder:
Adults: PO Start with 0.25 mg bid. An increase to the target dose for most patients of 1 mg/day may be made after 3 days. Dose may be increased in increments of 0.125 to 0.25 mg bid q 3 days until panic disorder is controlled or side effects make further increases undesired (max, 4 mg/day).
Seizure Disorders:
Adults:
Initial dose: PO 1.5 mg/day in 3 divided doses. Increase by 0.5 to 1 mg q 3 days until seizures are adequately controlled (max, 20 mg/day).
Infants and Children (10 yr or younger; 30 kg or less):
Initial dose: PO 0.01 to 0.03 mg/kg/day in 2 to 3 divided doses. Increase by 0.25 to 0.5 mg q 3 days until maintenance dose of 0.1 to 0.2 mg/kg has been reached.

Trade names: Klonopin Tablets 0.5 mg

Warnings: Hypersensitivity to benzodiazepines; psychoses; acute narrow-angle glaucoma; significant liver disease; shock; coma; acute alcohol intoxication. Pregnancy Category: [D]

Interactions: Alcohol and CNS depressants: May cause additive CNS depressant effects.
Carbamazepine, phenytoin, rifampin: May reduce clonazepam serum concentrations, decreasing the clinical effect.
Cimetidine, oral contraceptives, disulfiram: May cause effects of clonazepam to increase, with excessive sedation and impaired psychomotor function.
Digoxin: May increase serum digoxin concentrations.
Theophyllines: May antagonize sedative effects.

Clonidine HCl

Antihypertensive / Antiadrenergic / Centrally acting analgesic

Indications: Management of hypertension. Used in combination with opiates for epidural use for relief of cancer pain.

Unlabeled indication: Treatment of constitutional growth delay in children; diabetic diarrhea; Gilles de la Tourette syndrome; hypertensive urgencies; menopausal flushing; postherpetic neuralgia; diagnosis of pheochromocytoma; ulcerative colitis; reduction of allergen-induced inflammatory reactions in patients with extrinsic asthma; facilitation of smoking cessation; alcohol withdrawal; methadone/opiate detoxification.

Dose: Hypertension:
Adults:
Initial dose: PO 0.1 mg bid; maintenance dose: increase by increments of 0.1 to 0.2 mg/day until desired response is achieved (max, 2.4 mg/day in divided doses). SL 0.2 to 0.4 mg/day. Transdermal 0.1 mg patch weekly initially; titrate to determine best response. Dosage greater than two 0.3 mg patches does not improve efficacy.
Children: PO 5 to 25 mcg/kg/day in divided doses given q 6 hr; increase dose as necessary at 5 to 7 day intervals.
Pain Relief:
Adults: Epidural infusion 30 mcg/hr as starting dose. Dosage may be titrated up or down depending on pain relief and occurrence of adverse events. Experience with dosage rates greater than 40 mcg/hr is limited.

Trade names: Catapres Tablets 0.1 mg
Catapres-TTS-1 Transdermal System 2.5 mg
Catapres-TTS-2 Transdermal System 5 mg
Catapres-TTS-3 Transdermal System 7.5 mg
Duraclon Injection 100 mcg/mL

Warnings: Hypersensitivity to clonidine or any component of adhesive layer of transdermal system. Injection: In the presence of an injection site infection; patients on anticoagulant therapy; patients with a bleeding diathesis; administration above the C4 dermatome because there are not adequate safety data to support such use. Pregnancy Category: [C]

Interactions: Alcohol, CNS depressants: Clonidine may enhance depressant effects.
Beta-adrenergic blocking agents: May increase potential for rebound hypertension when clonidine therapy is discontinued.
Local anesthetics: Epidural clonidine may prolong the duration of pharmacologic effects of epidural local anesthetics, including sensory and motor blockade.

Narcotic analgesics: May potentiate the hypotensive effects of clonidine.
Tricyclic antidepressants: May reduce effect of clonidine.

Clonidine HCl/ Chlorthalidone

Antihypertensive / Diuretic

Indications: Treatment of hypertension; not indicated for initial therapy.

Dose: Adults: PO Once or twice/day from a minimum dose of 0.1 mg clonidine plus 15 mg chlorthalidone to a maximum dose of 0.6 mg clonidine plus 30 mg chlorthalidone.

Trade names: Clorpres Tablets 0.1 mg clonidine and 15 mg chlorthalidone

Warnings: Known hypersensitivity to any component of product or sulfonamide derived drugs. Pregnancy Category: [C]

Interactions: Alcohol, barbiturates, other sedatives: CNS depressive effects may be enhanced with clonidine.
Antihypertensive agents: Action may be increased or potentiated by chlorthalidone.
Insulin, sulfonylureas (eg, chlorpropamide): Hypoglycemic effect may be decreased by chlorthalidone, necessitating an increase in dosage.
Lithium: Because renal excretion of lithium may be reduced, avoid use if possible.
Norepinephrine: Arterial responsiveness to norepinephrine may be decreased.
Tricyclic antidepressants: Effects on clonidine may be reduced.

Clopidogrel

Antiplatelet / Aggregation Inhibitor

Indications: Reduction of atherosclerotic events (eg, MI, stroke, vascular death) in patients with atherosclerosis documented by recent stroke, recent MI, or established peripheral arterial disease. Treatment of acute coronary syndrome (unstable angina/non-Q-wave MI) including patients managed medically and those managed with percutaneous coronary intervention (with or without stent) or coronary artery bypass graft.

Dose: Recent MI, Recent Stroke, or Established Peripheral Arterial Disease: PO 75 mg once daily with or without food.
Acute Coronary Syndrome (Unstable Angina/Non-Q-Wave MI):
Adults: PO Start with a 300 mg loading dose, then continue at 75 mg once daily, initiating and continuing aspirin (75 to 325 mg/day) in combination with clopidogrel.

Trade names: Plavix Tablet 75 mg (as base)

Warnings: Hypersensitivity to the drug; active pathological bleeding such as peptic ulcer or intracranial hemorrhage. Pregnancy Category: [B]

Interactions: Clopidogrel inhibits P450 2C9. Accordingly, clopidogrel may interfere with the metabolism of phenytoin, tamoxifen, tolbutamide, warfarin (prolongs bleeding time), torsemide, fluvastatin, and many NSAIDs, but there are no data with which to predict the magnitude of these interactions. Use with caution when administering clopidogrel with any of these drugs.

Clorazepate Dipotassium

Antianxiety / Benzodiazepine

Indications: Management of anxiety disorders; relief of acute alcohol withdrawal symptoms; adjunctive therapy in management of partial seizures.

Unlabeled indication: Treatment of irritable bowel syndrome.

Dose: Acute Alcohol Withdrawal:
Adults:
Day 1: PO Initial dose is 30 mg, then 30 to 60 mg in divided doses.
Day 2: 45 to 90 mg in divided doses.
Day 3: 22.5 to 45 mg in divided doses.
Day 4: 15 to 30 mg in divided doses. Then gradually reduce to 7.5 to 15 mg/day; discontinue when patient is stable.
Anxiety:
Adults: PO 15 to 60 mg/day in divided doses.
Single bedtime dosing: PO Initial dose is 15 mg.
Elderly or Debilitated Patients:
Initial dose: PO 7.5 to 15 mg/day.
Maintenance:
Adults: PO 22.5 mg/day as single dose alternative once patient is stabilized with 7.5 mg tid; do not use 22.5 mg in single dose to initiate therapy. The 11.25 mg tablet may be given as single dose q 24 hr.
Partial Seizures:
Adults and Children over 12 yr:
Maximum initial dose: 7.5 mg tid; increase by no more than 7.5 mg/wk (max, 90 mg/day).
Children 9 to 12 yr:
Maximum initial dose: 7.5 mg bid; increase by no more than 7.5 mg/wk (max, 60 mg/day).

Trade names: Tranxene T-tab Tablets 3.75 mg
Tranxene-SD Tablets 11.25 mg
Tranxene-SD Half Strength Tablets, extended-release 11.25 mg

Warnings: Hypersensitivity to benzodiazepines; psychoses; acute narrow-angle glaucoma. Pregnancy Category: [D]

Interactions: Alcohol and CNS depressants: Possible additive CNS depressant effects.
Azole antifungal agents (eg, itraconazole, ketoconazole), fluvoxamine, isoniazid, macrolide antibiotics (eg, erythromycin), nefazodone, non-nucleoside reverse transcriptase inhibitors (eg, delavirdine, efavirenz), protease inhibitors(eg, indinavir): May increase diazepam plasma concentrations.
Cimetidine, oral contraceptives, disulfiram: May increase effects of clorazepate, with excessive sedation and impaired psychomotor function.
Digoxin: May increase serum digoxin concentrations.
Omeprazole: May increase clorazepate serum levels and enhance effects.
Rifamycins: May decrease diazepam plasma concentrations.
Theophyllines: May antagonize sedative effects of clorazepate.

Clotrimazole

Topical / Antifungal

Indications: Topical use: Treatment of tinea pedis (athlete's foot), tinea cruris (jock itch), tinea corporis (ringworm), candidiasis, and tinea versicolor.

Oral use (troche): Treatment of oropharyngeal candidiasis; prophylaxis of oropharyngeal candidiasis in specific groups of immunocompromised patients.

Vaginal use: Treatment of vulvovaginal candidiasis.

Dose: Oropharyngeal Candidiasis:
Adults and Children over 3 yr: PO One 10 mg troche (lozenge) dissolved slowly in the mouth 5 times/day for 14 days.
Prophylaxis: PO One 10 mg troche dissolved slowly in the mouth tid.
Dermal Infections: Topical cream Apply thin layer to affected and surrounding areas bid in the morning and evening. Topical lotion Apply thin layer to affected areas bid.
Vaginal Infections:
Women and Girls over 12 yr: Intravaginal Insert 1 applicatorful (5 g) of cream or one suppository at bedtime for 7 to 14 days (treatment for 14 days may yield higher cure rate).

Gyne-Lotrimin Combination Pack: Insert suppository intravaginally at bedtime for 7 consecutive days. Apply topical cream to affected areas bid (morning and evening) for 7 consecutive days.
Mycelex 7 Combination Pack: Insert suppository intravaginally at bedtime for 7 consecutive days. Apply topical cream to affected area bid (morning and evening) for 7 consecutive days.
Trade names: Cruex Cream 1%
Desenex Cream 1%
Gyne-Lotrimin 3 Vaginal suppositories 200 mg
Gyne-Lotrimin 3 Combination Pack Vaginal suppositories 200 mg
Gyne-Lotrimin 7 Vaginal cream 1%
Lotrimin AF Cream 1%
Mycelex Troches 10 mg
Mycelex-7 Vaginal cream 1%
Mycelex-7 Combination Pack Vaginal suppositories 100 mg
Warnings: Standard considerations. Pregnancy Category: [C (troches); B (topical and vaginal use)]
Interactions: None well documented.

Clozapine

Antipsychotic

Indications: Management of severely and chronically mentally ill schizophrenic patients who have not responded to or cannot tolerate standard antipsychotic drug treatment. Reduce risk of recurrent suicidal behavior in patients with schizophrenia or schizoaffective disorder who are judged to be at chronic risk for reexperiencing suicidal behavior.
Dose: Cautious titration and divided dosage schedules are recommended.
Adults:
Initial dose: PO 12.5 mg qd or bid; increase by 25 to 50 mg/day up to 300 to 450 mg/day within 2 wk. May then increase dose in increments not to exceed 100 mg once or twice a week.
Usual dosage: 300 to 600 mg/day (max, 900 mg/day).
Trade names: Clozapine Tablets 12.5 mg
Clozaril Tablets 25 mg
Warnings: History of clozapine-induced agranulocytosis or severe granulocytopenia; myeloproliferative disorders; simultaneous administration with other agents known to cause bone marrow suppression; severe CNS depression or comatose states; uncontrolled epilepsy; hypersensitivity to product. Pregnancy Category: [B]
Interactions: Agents that suppress bone marrow: Risk or severity of bone marrow suppression may be increased.
Anticholinergics: Anticholinergic effects may be potentiated.
Antihypertensives: Hypotensive effects may be potentiated.
Barbiturates (eg, phenobarbital), phenytoin, nicotine, rifampin: May decrease blood levels of clozapine.
Caffeine, cimetidine, erythromycin, ritonavir, serotonin reuptake inhibitors(eg, fluoxetine): May increase blood levels of clozapine.
CNS drugs (eg, carbamazepine, benzodiazepines, TCAs): Use with caution because of CNS effects of clozapine.
Type 1C antiarrhythmics (eg, propafenone, flecainide): Use with caution.

Colesevelam HCl

Antihyperlipidemic / Bile acid sequestrant

Indications: Adjunctive therapy to diet and exercise given alone or with an HMG-CoA reductase inhibitor for the reduction of elevated LDL cholesterol in patients with primary hypercholesterolemia (Fredrickson type IIa).
Dose: Adults:
Monotherapy: PO 1875 mg (3 tablets) bid with meals or 3750 mg (6 tablets) qd with a meal. Depending upon the desired effect the dose can be increase to 4375 mg/day (7 tablets).
Combination therapy: PO 2500 to 3750 mg (4 to 6 tablets) qd.
Trade names: Welchol Tablets 625 mg
Warnings: Bowel obstruction; hypersensitivity to any component of the product. Pregnancy Category: [B]
Interactions: None well documented.

Colestipol HCl

Antihyperlipidemic / Bile acid sequestrant

Indications: Reduction of cholesterol in patients with primary hypercholesterolemia who do not respond adequately to diet.

Unlabeled indication: Treatment of digitalis toxicity.
Dose: Adults:
Tablets: PO 2 to 16 g/day given once or in divided doses. Start with 2 g once or twice daily and increase in amounts of 2 g once or twice daily at 1- or 2-mo intervals.
Granules: PO 5 to 30 g/day given once or in divided doses. Start with 5 g once or twice daily and increase in amounts of 5 g daily over 1 to 2 mo intervals.
Trade names: Colestid Tablets 1 g
Warnings: Hypersensitivity to bile acid sequestering resins; complete biliary obstruction. Pregnancy Category: [Category undetermined]
Interactions: Digitalis glycosides, furosemide, gemfibrozil, hydrocortisone, penicillin G, phosphate supplements, propanolol, tetracyclines, thiazide diuretics, fat soluble vitamins (ie, A, D, E, K): Absorption of these drugs may be decreased.

Cromolyn Sodium

Respiratory inhalant

Indications: Inhalation: Prophylaxis of severe bronchial asthma; prevention of exercise-induced asthma; prevention of acute bronchospasm induced by environmental pollutants and known antigens.

Nasal solution: Prevention and treatment of allergic rhinitis.

Oral: Treatment of mastocytosis.

Ophthalmic: Treatment of vernal keratoconjunctivitis, vernal conjunctivitis, and vernal keratitis.

Unlabeled indication: Oral: Symptoms of food allergies; eczema; dermatitis; ulceration; urticaria pigmentosa; chronic urticaria; hay fever; and postexercise bronchospasm.
Dose: Bronchial Asthma:
Adults and Children (5 yr or under for capsules, at least 2 yr for solution): Nebulization Initially 20 mg inhaled qid at regular intervals.
Adults and Children (over 5 yr): Aerosol 2 metered sprays (1600 mcg) inhaled qid at regular intervals.
Prevention of Acute Bronchospasm:
Adults: 2 metered dose sprays or 20 mg via inhaled capsule or nebulizer (10 to 15 min but no longer than 60 min) before exposure to precipitating factor.
Seasonal or Perennial Rhinitis:
Adults and Children (over 6 yr): Nasal solution with spray device Begin treatment prior to contact with allergen and continue throughout exposure period.
One spray (5.2 mg) in each nostril 3 to 6 times/day at regular intervals.
Mastocytosis:
Adults: PO 200 mg qid 30 min before meals and at bedtime.
Children (2 to 12 yr): PO 100 mg qid 30 min before meals and at bedtime (max, 40 mg/kg/day). Dosage

Medications

maintenance levels are decreased gradually, except with major complication. Abrupt withdrawal may result in increased asthma symptoms.
Term infants to 2 yr: PO 20 mg/kg/day in 4 divided doses (max, 20 mg/kg/day).
Premature to term infants: Not recommended.
Vernal Keratoconjunctivitis, Vernal Conjunctivitis, and Vernal Keratitis:
Adults: Solution 1 or 2 drops in each eye 4 to 6 times/day at regular intervals.
Trade names: Crolom Solution, ophthalmic 4%
Gastrocrom Oral concentrate 5 mg/100 mL
Intal Solution 20 mg/amp (for nebulizer only)
Nasalcrom Nasal Solution 40 mg/mL (each actuation delivers 5.2 mg)
Warnings: Standard considerations. Pregnancy Category: [B]
Interactions: None well documented.

Crotamiton

Scabicide

Indications: Eradication of scabies (Sarcoptes scabiei) and symptomatic treatment of pruritic skin.
Dose: Scabies:
Adults: Topical Thoroughly massage into the skin of whole body from chin down, paying particular attention to all folds and creases. A second application is advisable 24 hr later. Change clothing and bed linen the next morning. A cleansing bath should be taken 48 hr after last application.
Pruritus:
Adults: Topical Massage gently into affected areas until medication is completely absorbed. Repeat as needed.
Trade names: Eurax Cream 10%
Warnings: Primary irritation response to topical medications; hypersensitivity to any component of the product. Pregnancy Category: [C]
Interactions: None well documented.

Cyclobenzaprine HCl

Skeletal muscle relaxant / Centrally acting

Indications: Relief of muscle spasms associated with acute painful musculoskeletal conditions.

Unlabeled indication: Treatment of fibrositis.
Dose: Adults: PO 10 mg tid (max, 60 mg/day). Do not use longer than 3 wk.
Trade names: Flexeril Tablets 5 mg
Warnings: Use of MAO inhibitors or within 14 days of their discontinuation; acute recovery phase of MI; arrhythmias; heart block or conduction disturbances; CHF; hyperthyroidism. Pregnancy Category: [B]
Interactions: Alcohol and other CNS depressants: May cause additive CNS depression.
MAO inhibitors: May cause hyperpyretic crisis, severe convulsions, and death.

Cyclopentolate HCl/ Phenylephrine HCl

Anticholinergic / Decongestant / Mydriatic

Indications: For production of mydriasis.
Dose: Adults and children: Ophthalmic 1 drop each eye q 5 to 10 min.
Trade names: Cyclomydril Solution 0.2% cyclopentolate HCl, 1% phenylephrine HCl
Warnings: Untreated narrow-angle glaucoma; untreated anatomically narrow angles; hypersensitivity to any component of product. Pregnancy Category: [C]
Interactions: Carbachol, pilocarpine, ophthalmic cholinesterase inhibitors: Cyclopentolate may interfere with antihypertensive action of these agents.

Cyclophosphamide

Alkylating agent / Nitrogen mustard

Indications: Adult: Lymphomas, multiple myeloma, leukemias, disseminated neuroblastoma, ovarian adenocarcinoma, retinoblastoma, breast carcinoma, mycosis fungoides.

Pediatric: Lymphomas, multiple myeloma, leukemias, disseminated neuroblastoma, ovarian adenocarcinoma, retinoblastoma, breast carcinoma, mycosis fungoides.

Unlabeled indication: Bronchogenic, small-cell lung, cervical, endometrial, prostate, and testicular carcinomas; sarcomas, bone marrow transplantation; systemic lupus erythematosus, vasculitis, rheumatoid arthritis, and other autoimmune diseases.
Dose: Lymphomas, Multiple Myeloma, Leukemias, Disseminated Neuroblastoma, Ovarian Adenocarcinoma, Retinoblastoma, Breast Carcinoma, Mycosis Fungoides:
Adults: PO/IV Dosage regimens that include cyclophosphamide are too numerous to list. Usual doses range from 500 to 1500 mg/m^2 per course of therapy. In myelosuppressed patients, reduce initial loading dose by 33% to 50%. PO 60 to 120 mg/m^2 /day for initial and maintenance therapy.
Dosage Adjustment (Hepatic Dysfunction Reduction):
Adults: PO/IV If LFTs show bilirubin 3.1 to 5 mg/dL or AST greater than 180 units/L, administer 75% of dose. If bilirubin is greater than 5 mg/dL, no dose is to be given.
Lymphomas, Multiple Myeloma, Leukemias, Ovarian Adenocarcinoma, Retinoblastoma, Breast Carcinoma, Mycosis Fungoides:
Pediatric: PO/IV Doses are similar to those used in adult regimens and calculated based on BSA. Usual doses range from 500 to 1500 mg/m^2 per course of therapy. Follow dosage adjustment guidelines recommended for adults. PO 60 to 120 mg/m^2 /day for initial and maintenance therapy.
Neuroblastoma:
Pediatric: IV 3000 mg/m^2 /day for 2 days or 2000 mg/m^2 /day for 3 consecutive days.
Trade names: Cytoxan Lyophilized powder for injection 100 mg
Neosar Dry powder for injection 100 mg
Warnings: Previous hypersensitivity to the drug; continued use in severely depressed bone marrow function. Pregnancy Category: [D]
Interactions: Anticoagulants: Increased hypoprothrombinemic effect may occur.
Barbiturates, other enzyme inducers: May increase the rate of active cyclophosphamide metabolite formation and possibly increase neutropenic effects.
Chloramphenicol, other enzyme inhibitors: May inhibit cyclophosphamide's antineoplastic activity by decreasing rate of active metabolite formation.
Digoxin: May cause decreased serum levels of digoxin.
Oral quinolone antibiotics: May cause decreased GI absorption of quinolone antibiotics.
Succinylcholine and possibly mivacurium: Prolongation of neuromuscular blockade by cyclophosphamide's inhibition of pseudocholinesterase may occur.

Cycloserine

Anti-infective / Antitubercular

Indications: Treatment of active pulmonary and extrapulmonary tuberculosis when organisms are susceptible (after failure of adequate treatment with primary medications); treatment of UTIs caused by susceptible bacteria when conventional therapy has failed; treatment of Gaucher disease.
Dose: Adults: PO 250 to 500 mg q 12 hr; start with 250 mg q 12 hr for first 2 wk (max, 1 g/day).
Children: PO 15 to 20 mg/kg/day administered in 2 equally divided doses (max, 1 g/day).
Trade names: Seromycin Pulvules Capsules

250 mg
Warnings: Epilepsy; depression; severe anxiety or psychosis; severe renal insufficiency; excessive concurrent use of alcohol. Pregnancy Category: [C]
Interactions: Alcohol: Increases possibility and risk of epileptic episodes. Do not use together.
Isoniazid: May increase cycloserine CNS side effects (eg, dizziness).

Cyclosporine

Immunosuppressive
Indications: Prophylaxis of organ rejection in kidney, liver, and heart allogeneic transplants in conjunction with adrenal corticosteroid therapy; treatment of chronic rejection in patients previously treated with other immunosuppressive agents. Increase tear production in patients whose tear production is presumed to be suppressed because of ocular inflammation associated with keratoconjunctivitis sicca (ophthalmic emulsion).

Unlabeled indication: Prophylaxis in other transplant procedures; treatment of aplastic anemia, atopic dermatitis, Behcet disease, biliary cirrhosis, Crohn disease, rheumatoid arthritis, severe psoriasis, nephrotic syndrome, pulmonary sarcoidosis, pyoderma gangrenosum, ulcerative colitis, alopecia areata.
Dose: Adults and Children: PO 15 mg/kg/day (range, 14 to 18 mg/kg/day) beginning 4 to 12 hr before transplantation. Continue for 1 to 2 wk postoperatively, then taper dose by 5%/wk to maintenance level of 5 to 10 mg/kg/day. Lower doses may be used on basis of patient response, rejection rate, and cyclosporine plasma concentrations. IV 5 to 6 mg/kg/day as single IV dose starting 4 to 12 hr before transplantation. Switch to oral form as soon as patient can tolerate.
Trade names: Sandimmune Capsules, soft gelatin 25 mg
Neoral Capsules, soft gelatin, for microemulsion 25 mg
SangCya Oral solution 100 mg/mL
Warnings: Hypersensitivity to polyoxyethylated castor oil, which is present in concentrate for injection. Active ocular infections (ophthalmic emulsion). Pregnancy Category: [C]
Interactions: Aminoglycosides, amphotericin B, NSAIDs, trimethoprim-sulfamethoxazole, melphalan, quinolones: Additive nephrotoxicity possible.
Amiodarone, diltiazem, fluconazole, imipenem-cilastatin, ketoconazole, macrolide antibiotics (eg, erythromycin), nicardipine: May increase cyclosporine concentrations.
Azathioprine, corticosteroids, cyclophosphamide, verapamil: May cause additive immunosuppression, increasing risk of infection and malignancy.
Carbamazepine, hydantoins, phenobarbital, rifampin, rifabutin: May decrease cyclosporine effects.
Digoxin: May cause elevated digoxin concentrations and toxicity.
Etoposide: May increase etoposide concentrations.
Lovastatin: May cause severe myopathy or rhabdomyolysis; avoid concurrent use.
Metoclopramide: Increases absorption of cyclosporine.
Potassium-sparing diuretics: Causes hyperkalemic effects; avoid concomitant use.

Cyproheptadine HCl

Antihistamine
Indications: Symptomatic relief of perennial and seasonal allergic rhinitis, vasomotor rhinitis, allergic conjunctivitis; amelioration of allergic reactions to blood or plasma; management of allergic pruritic symptoms, mild skin manifestations of uncomplicated urticaria and angioedema, and cold urticaria.
Dose: Adults: PO 4 mg q 8 hr then 4 to 20 mg/day; not to exceed 0.5 mg/kg/day.
Children 7 to 14 yr: PO 4 mg bid or tid (max, 16 mg/day).
Children 2 to 6 yr: PO 2 mg bid or tid (max, 12 mg/day). (PO Total daily dosage 0.25 mg/kg or 8 mg/m^2.)
Trade names: Periactin Tablets 4 mg
Warnings: Hypersensitivity to antihistamines; newborn or premature infants; nursing mothers; narrow-angle glaucoma; stenosing peptic ulcer; symptomatic prostatic hypertrophy; asthmatic attack; bladder neck obstruction; pyloroduodenal obstruction; MAO therapy. Pregnancy Category: [B]
Interactions: Alcohol, CNS depressants: May cause additive CNS depressant effects.
Fluoxetine: Effects of fluoxetine may be reversed.
MAO inhibitors: Anticholinergic effects of cyproheptadine may increase.

Dacarbazine

Alkylating agent / Triazine
Indications: Metastatic malignant melanoma, combination therapy of Hodgkin disease.

Unlabeled indication: Soft-tissue sarcomas.
Dose: Malignant Melanoma:
Adults: IV Dacarbazine 250 mg/m^2 /day for 5 days; may repeat at 3-wk intervals.
Hodgkin Lymphoma (Combination Therapy):
Adults: IV Dacarbazine 150 mg/m^2 /day for 5 days; may be repeated at 4-wk intervals. Alternative regimen is 375 mg/m^2 IV on day 1; repeated q 15 days.
Adjustment in Renal or Hepatic Insufficiency:
Adults: IV Dosage adjustment in hepatic or renal insufficiency is warranted; however, there are no specific guidelines.
Trade names: DTIC-Dome Powder for injection 10 mg/mL
Warnings: Standard considerations. Pregnancy Category: [C]
Interactions: None well documented.

Dactinomycin

Antineoplastic antibiotic
Indications: Adults: Wilms tumor, rhabdomyosarcoma, metastatic nonseminomatous testicular carcinoma, Ewing sarcoma, sarcoma botryides, trophoblastic tumor, metastatic and nonmetastatic choriocarcinoma; radiation therapy.

Pediatric: Wilms tumor, rhabdomyosarcoma, metastatic nonseminomatous testicular carcinoma, Ewing sarcoma, sarcoma botryides, trophoblastic tumor, metastatic choriocarcinoma.

Unlabeled indication: Osteosarcoma, malignant melanoma, Paget disease of the bone.
Dose: Adults: IV Administer the drug in short courses. Base dose on BSA in obese or edematous patients. Dose should not exceed 15 mcg/kg or 400 to 600 mcg/m^2 /day for 5 days. Repeat in 3 wk if necessary. Usual dose is 500 mcg/day for a max of 5 days.
Pediatric: IV Administer the drug in short courses. Base dose on BSA in obese or edematous patients. Do not exceed 15 mcg/kg/day or 400 to 600 mcg/m^2 /day for 5 days. Repeat in 3 to 4 wk if necessary. Usual dose is 0.015 mg/kg/day for 5 days. Alternative schedule is a total dosage of 2.5 mg/m^2 over 1 wk.
Trade names: Cosmegen Lyophilized powder for reconstitution 500 mcg vial with 20 mg of mannitol.
Warnings: If given at or about the time of infection with chicken pox or herpes zoster, a severe generalized disease may occur, which could result in death. Pregnancy Category: [C]
Interactions: No specific drug interactions reported.

Dalteparin Sodium

Anticoagulant

Indications: Prophylaxis of deep vein thrombosis (DVT), which may lead to pulmonary embolism, in patients undergoing hip replacement surgery or in patients undergoing abdominal surgery who are at risk for thromboembolic complications; prophylaxis of ischemic complications in unstable angina and non-Q-wave MI in patients on aspirin therapy.

Dose: DVT Prophylaxis (Abdominal Surgery):
Adults: SC 2500 units starting 1 to 2 hr before surgery and continuing qd for 5 to 10 days. Do not give IM.
DVT Prophylaxis (Hip Replacement Surgery):
Adults: SC If started postoperatively, 2500 units within 4 to 8 hr after surgery, followed by 5000 units/day for 5 to 10 days; if started preoperatively on day of surgery, 2500 units within 2 hr before surgery, followed by 2500 units 4 to 8 hr after surgery and continued at 5000 units/day for 5 to 10 days; if started preoperatively on the evening before surgery, 5000 units 10 to 14 hr before surgery, followed by 5000 units 4 to 8 hr after surgery and continued at 5000 units/day for 5 to 10 days.
Unstable Angina/Non-Q-Wave MI:
Adults: SC 120 units/kg of body weight (max, 10,000 units) q 12 hr with aspirin (75 to 165 mg/day, unless contraindicated) therapy. Continue treatment until patient is clinically stabilized, usually 5 to 8 days.

Trade names: Fragmin Injection 2500 IU (16 mg/0.2 mL)

Warnings: Active major bleeding, thrombocytopenia, hypersensitivity to heparin or pork products; patients undergoing regional anesthesia for unstable angina or non-Q-wave MI. Pregnancy Category: [B]

Interactions: Anticoagulants; platelet inhibitors: Increased risk of bleeding.

Danazol

Hormone

Indications: Treatment of endometriosis; symptomatic treatment of fibrocystic breast disease; prevention of attacks of hereditary angioedema.

Unlabeled indication: Treatment of precocious puberty, gynecomastia, and menorrhagia; treatment of idiopathic immune thrombocytopenia, lupus-associated thrombocytopenia, and autoimmune hemolytic anemia.

Dose: Endometriosis:
Adults: PO 800 mg/day in 2 divided doses.
Fibrocystic Breast Disease:
Adults: PO 100 to 400 mg/day in 2 divided doses.
Hereditary Angioedema:
Adults: PO 200 mg bid to tid.

Trade names: Danocrine Capsules 50 mg

Warnings: Pregnancy; lactation; undiagnosed abnormal genital bleeding; markedly impaired hepatic, renal, or cardiac function. Pregnancy Category: [X]

Interactions: Anticoagulants: May increase anticoagulant effects.
Carbamazepine: May increase carbamazepine concentration.
Cyclosporine: May increase cyclosporine levels, thus increasing risk of nephrotoxicity.
Insulin: Diabetic patients may need increased insulin doses.

Dantrolene Sodium

Skeletal muscle relaxant/direct acting

Indications: Control of spasticity associated with spinal cord injury, stroke, cerebral palsy or multiple sclerosis; prophylaxis, treatment and postcrisis therapy of malignant hyperthermia.

Unlabeled indication: Management of exercise-induced muscle pain, neuroleptic malignant syndrome, heat stroke.

Dose: Chronic Spasticity:
Adults: PO Initial dose 25 mg q day; increase at 4 to 7 day intervals to 25 mg bid to qid, up to max 100 mg bid to qid if necessary.
Children: PO Initial dose 0.5 mg/kg bid; increase to 0.5 mg/kg tid to qid, then by increments of 0.5 mg/kg, up to 3 mg/kg bid to qid, if necessary. Max 100 mg qid.
Malignant Hyperthermia:
Adults and Children:
Preoperative prophylaxis: PO 4 to 8 mg/kg/day in 3 or 4 divided doses for 1 or 2 days prior to surgery with last dose given 3 to 4 hr before surgery or IV 2.5 mg/kg approximately 75 min before anesthesia. Infused over 1 hr. May repeat during surgery, if needed.
Treatment: IV 1 mg/kg by continuous rapid push; evaluate and repeat as needed until cumulative total dose is up to 10 mg/kg.
Postcrisis follow-up: PO 4 to 8 mg/kg/day in 4 divided doses for 1 to 3 days to prevent recurrence. If IV route must be utilized, start with at least 1 mg/kg, as needed.

Trade names: Dantrium Capsules 25 mg
Dantrium Intravenous Powder for Injection 20 mg/vial (approximately 0.32 mg/mL after reconstitution)

Warnings: Active hepatic disease; muscle spasm resulting from rheumatic disorders; where spasticity is used to sustain upright posture and balance in locomotion or to obtain or maintain increased function. Pregnancy Category: [C (parenteral)]

Interactions: Clofibrate: Plasma protein binding of dantrolene reduced.
Estrogens: Women receiving these may be at increased risk for hepatotoxicity.
Verapamil: Hyperkalemia and myocardial depression possible.
Warfarin: Plasma protein binding of dantrolene reduced.

Dapsone

Anti-infective / Leprostatic

Indications: Treatment of dermatitis herpetiformis; leprosy.

Dose: Dermatitis Herpetiformis:
Adults and Children: PO Start with 50 mg/day in adults and correspondingly smaller doses in children. If full control is not achieved with 50 to 300 mg/day, higher doses may be tried. Reduce dose to minimum maintenance level as soon as possible. The time for dosage reduction is 8 mo (range 4 mo to 21/2 yr) and for dosage elimination 29 mo (range 6 mo to 9 yr).
Leprosy:
Adults and Children: PO 100 mg/day in adults and correspondingly smaller doses in children without interruption in therapy with at least 1 antileprosy drug.

Trade names: Dapsone Tablets 25 mg

Warnings: Standard considerations. Pregnancy Category: [C]

Interactions: Didanosine: Absorption of dapsone may be decreased, resulting in a loss of efficacy.
Trimethoprim: Plasma concentrations of both dapsone and trimethoprim may be elevated, increasing the pharmacologic and toxic effects.

Delavirdine Mesylate

Antiretroviral / Non-nucleoside reverse transcriptase inhibitor

Indications: Treatment of HIV-1 infection in combination with appropriate antiretroviral agents when therapy is warranted.

Dose: Adults and Children older than 16 yr: PO 400 mg tid in combination with appropriate antiretroviral therapy.

Trade names: Rescriptor Tablets 100 mg

Warnings: Standard considerations. Pregnancy Category: [C]

Interactions: Antacids: Antacids reduce

absorption of delavirdine. Separate doses by at least 1 hr.
Anticonvulsants (eg, carbamazepine, phenobarbital, phenytoin): Induce hepatic metabolism of delavirdine resulting in decreased plasma concentrations.
Benzodiazepines (eg, alprazolam, midazolam, triazolam): Delavirdine may increase blood levels of these drugs, which may produce extreme sedation and respiratory depression.
Cisapride, dapsone, ergot derivatives, quinidine, rifabutin, warfarin: Delavirdine may elevate blood levels of these drugs, which may increase the risk of arrhythmias or other potentially serious side effects.
Clarithromycin: Coadministration may increase blood levels of delavirdine or clarithromycin.
Didanosine: Separate administration of didanosine and delavirdine by at least 1 hr; coadministration results in a 20% reduction in systemic exposure of both drugs.
Dihydropyridine calcium channel blockers (eg, nifedipine): Delavirdine may elevate blood levels, which may increase toxicity.
Fluoxetine, ketoconazole: Increased delvirdine plasma concentrations.
H_2 antagonists (eg, cimetidine): Concurrent use may reduce absorption of delavirdine. Chronic use of these drugs with delavirdine is not recommended.
Indinavir: Delavirdine inhibits metabolism of indinavir. Consider indinavir dosage reduction if coadministered with delavirdine.
Rifabutin, rifampin: Induce hepatic metabolism of delavirdine resulting in decreased plasma concentrations. These agents should not be coadministered with delavirdine.
Saquinavir: Delavirdine inhibits metabolism of saquinavir. Monitor hepatocellular enzymes frequently if coadministered.

Demeclocycline

Antibiotic / Tetracycline

Indications: Treatment of infections caused by susceptible strains of gram-positive and gram-negative microorganisms.

Dose: Adults: PO 150 mg qid or 300 mg bid.
Children older than 8 yr: PO Usual dose is 7 to 13 mg/kg/day divided into 2 to 4 doses (max, 600 mg/day).
Gonorrhea:
Adults: PO 600 mg followed by 300 mg q 12 hr for 4 days (total 3 g).

Trade names: Declomycin Tablets 150 mg

Warnings: Hypersensitivity to any tetracycline and any component of the product. Pregnancy Category: [D]

Interactions: Antacids containing aluminum, calcium, or magnesium, iron-containing products, dairy products: May decrease the absorption of demeclocycline.
Anticoagulants: Effect of anticoagulant may be enhanced, necessitating a downward adjustment in dosage.
Methoxyflurane: Increased potential for life-threatening renal toxicity.
Oral contraceptives: May reduce the effectiveness of oral contraceptives.
Penicillins: The bactericidal action may be decreased by tetracyclines.

Denileukin Diftitox

Biologic response modifier

Indications: Cutaneous T-cell lymphoma.

Dose: Cutaneous T-Cell Lymphoma:
Adults: IV 1 treatment cycle is 9 or 18 mcg/kg/day administered for 5 consecutive days q 21 days. Infuse over at least 15 min.
Pretreatment Regimen:
Adults: Give acetaminophen 650 mg (PO or rectal) and diphenhydramine 25 to 50 mg (PO or IV) 30 to 60 min before administering denileukin diftitox.
Dosage Adjustments:
Adults: Delay therapy in patients with serum albumin below 3 g/dL.

Trade names: Ontak Frozen, solution for injection 150 mcg/mL

Warnings: Standard considerations. Pregnancy Category: [C]

Interactions: Beta blockers, other antihypertensives: May exacerbate denileukin diftitox-induced hypotension.

Desipramine HCl

Tricyclic antidepressant

Indications: Relief of symptoms of depression.

Unlabeled indication: Facilitation of cocaine withdrawal; treatment of panic and eating disorders (eg, bulimia nervosa).

Dose: Adults: PO 100 to 300 mg/day. May be given in divided doses or once daily at bedtime.
Elderly and Adolescent Patients: PO 25 to 150 mg/day.

Trade names: Norpramin Tablets 10 mg

Warnings: Hypersensitivity to any tricyclic antidepressant. Not to be given in combination with or within 14 days of treatment with an MAOI; cross-sensitivity may occur across the dibenzazepines.
Do not give during acute recovery phases of MI.
Pregnancy Category: [C]

Interactions: Barbiturates, carbamazepine, charcoal: May decrease desipramine effects.
Cimetidine, fluoxetine, haloperidol, quinidine, oral contraceptives, phenothiazine antipsychotics: May increase desipramine effects.
Clonidine: May result in hypertensive crisis.
CNS depressants: CNS and respiratory effects may be increased.
MAOIs: Hyperpyretic crises, severe convulsions and death may occur if administered together or within 14 days of each other.

Desmopressin Acetate

Posterior pituitary hormone

Indications: Control of primary nocturnal enuresis; control of central cranial diabetes insipidus; maintenance of hemostasis in patients with hemophilia A and type I von Willebrand disease during surgery and postoperatively.

Unlabeled indication: Treatment of chronic autonomic failure.

Dose: Central Cranial Diabetes Insipidus:
Adults and Children 12 yr and older: Intranasal 0.1 to 0.4 qd. IV/SC 0.5 to 1 mL qd in 2 divided doses.
PO 0.05 mg bid adjusted for adequate diurnal rhythm (range 0.1 to 1.2 mg/day divided).
Children 3 Mo to 12 yr: Intranasal 0.05 to 0.3 mL qd, either as a single dose or 2 divided doses. PO Begin dosing with 0.05 mg. Careful fluid intake restrictions in children is required to prevent hyponatremia and water intoxification.
Hemophilia A, Type I von Willebrand Disease:
Adults and Children: IV Administer 0.3 mcg/kg diluted in sterile physiologic saline infused slowly over 15 to 30 min. In patients weighing more than 10 kg, use 50 mL diluent; in children weighing up to 10 kg, use 10 mL.
Intranasal Administer by nasal insufflation, 1 spray per nostril, to provide a total dose of 300 mcg. In patients weighing less than 50 kg, 150 mcg administered as a single spray provided the expected effect on Factor VIII coagulant activity, Factor VIII ristocetin cofactor activity, and skin bleeding time.
Primary Nocturnal Enuresis:
Adults and Children 6 yr and older: Intranasal 20 mcg (0.2 mL) at bedtime.

Trade names: DDAVP Tablets 0.1 mg
Stimate Nasal Solution 1.5 mg/mL

Warnings: Standard considerations. Pregnancy Category: [B]

Interactions: Carbamazepine; chlorpropamide: May potentiate antidiuretic effects of desmopressin.

Desonide

Corticosteroid / Topical

Indications: Relief of inflammatory and pruritic manifestations of corticosteroid-responsive dermatoses.

Dose: Adults and Children: Topical Apply sparingly to affected area bid to tid.

Trade names: DesOwen Cream 0.05%
Tridesilon Cream 0.05%

Warnings: Hypersensitivity to other corticosteroids; monotherapy in primary bacterial infections; ophthalmic use. Pregnancy Category: [C]

Interactions: None well documented.

Desoximetasone

Corticosteroid / Topical

Indications: Relief of inflammation and pruritic manifestations of corticosteroid-responsive dermatoses.

Dose: Adults and Children older than 10 yr of age: Topical Apply sparingly to affected areas bid.

Trade names: Topicort Ointment 0.25%
Topicort LP Cream 0.05%

Warnings: Hypersensitivity to other corticosteroids; monotherapy in primary bacterial infections; ophthalmic use. Pregnancy Category: [C]

Interactions: None well documented.

Diazepam

Antianxiety / Benzodiazepine / Anticonvulsant

Indications: Management of anxiety disorders; relief of acute alcohol withdrawal symptoms; relief of preoperative apprehension and anxiety and reduction of memory recall; treatment of muscle spasms, convulsive disorders (used adjunctively), and status epilepticus.

Unlabeled indication: Treatment of irritable bowel syndrome; relief of panic attack.

Dose: Individualize dosage; increase cautiously.
Adults and Children: Usual recommended dose IM/IV 2 to 20 mg, depending on indication and severity. In acute conditions injection may be repeated within 1 hr, but q 3 to 4 hr is usually satisfactory. Dosage and route vary with indication and age.
Children 6 mo and older: Usual daily dose PO 1 to 2.5 mg tid or qid initially; increase gradually as needed and tolerated.
Acute Alcohol Withdrawal:
Adults: PO 10 mg tid to qid first 24 hr, then 5 mg tid to qid prn. IM/IV 10 mg initially, then 5 to 10 mg in 3 to 4 hr if needed.
Anticonvulsant Adjunct:
Adults: PO 2 to 10 mg bid to qid.
Elderly or Debilitated Patients: PO Initial dose 2 to 2.5 mg qd to bid; increase gradually.
Anxiety:
Adults: PO 2 to 10 mg bid to qid. IM/IV 2 to 10 mg; repeat in 3 to 4 hr if needed.
Cardioversion (Anxiety and Tension):
Adults: IM/IV 5 to 15 mg 5 to 10 min before procedure.
Endoscopic Procedures: IM/IV 10 to 20 mg IV or 5 to 10 mg IM approximately 30 min prior to procedure.
Preoperative (Anxiety and Tension):
Adults: IM 10 mg before surgery.
Sedation/Muscle Relaxation:
Adults: IM/IV 2 to 10 mg/dose q 3 to 4 hr prn.
Children 6 mo and older: PO 0.12 to 0.8 mg/kg/day in divided doses. IM/IV 0.04 to 0.2 mg/kg/dose q 2 to 4 hr (max, 0.6 mg/kg in 8-hr period).
Skeletal Muscle Spasm:
Adults: PO 2 to 10 mg tid to qid. IM/IV 5 to 10 mg initially, then 5 to 10 mg in 3 to 4 hr if needed. Larger doses may be necessary in tetanus.
Status Epilepticus and Severe Recurrent Convulsive Disorders:
Adults: IM/IV (IV preferred) 5 to 10 mg initially; then 5 to 10 mg at 10 to 15 min intervals (max total dose, 30 mg). If needed, repeat in 2 to 4 hr.
Children 5 yr and older: IM/IV 1 mg q 2 to 5 min (max total dose, 10 mg). If needed, repeat in 2 to 4 hr.
Infants and Children 1 mo to 5 yr: IM/IV 0.2 to 0.5 mg slowly q 2 to 5 min (max total dose, 5 mg).
Tetanus:
Children 5 yr and older: IM/IV 5 to 10 mg; repeat q 3 to 4 hr prn.
Infants and Children 1 mo to 5 yr: IM/IV 1 to 2 mg slowly; repeat q 3 to 4 hr prn.
Rectal Gel:
Children 2 to 5 yr: Rectal 0.5 mg/kg.
Children 6 to 11 yr: Rectal 0.3 mg/kg.
Adults and Children 12 yr and older: Rectal 0.2 mg/kg. A second dose, when required, may be given 4 to 12 hr after the first dose.

Trade names: Diastat Gel, rectal 2.5 mg (pediatric)
Diazepam Solution, oral 1 mg/mL
Diazepam Intensol Solution (intensol) 5 mg/mL
Valium Tablets 2 mg

Warnings: Hypersensitivity to benzodiazepines; psychoses; acute narrow-angle glaucoma; use in children younger than 6 mo; lactation. Pregnancy Category: [D Avoid drug especially during first trimester because of possible increased risk of congenital malformations]

Interactions: Azole antifungal agents (eg, itraconazole, ketoconazole), diltiazem, fluvoxamine, isoniazid, macrolide antibiotics (eg, erythromycin), nefazodone, non-nucleoside reverse transcriptase inhibitors (eg, delavirdine, efavirenz), protease inhibitors (eg, indinavir): May increase diazepam plasma concentrations.
Cimetidine, oral contraceptives, disulfiram: May increase effects of diazepam with excessive sedation and impaired psychomotor function.
Digoxin: May increase serum digoxin concentrations.
Omeprazole: May increase diazepam levels and enhance effects.
Rifamycins: May decrease diazepam plasma concentrations.
Theophyllines: May antagonize sedative effects of diazepam.
Incompatability: Diazepam interacts with plastic containers and IV tubing, significantly decreasing availability of drug delivered. Do not mix or dilute with other solutions or drugs in a syringe or infusion container.

Dicloxacillin Sodium

Antibiotic / Penicillin

Indications: Treatment of infections caused by penicillinase-producing staphylococcal infection; initial therapy of suspected staphylococcal infection.

Dose: Adults and children weighing greater than 40 kg: PO 125 to 250 mg q 6 hr.
Children weighing less than 40 kg: PO 12.5 to 25 mg/kg/day divided in equal doses q 6 hr.

Trade names: Dicloxacillin Sodium Capsules 250 mg

Warnings: Hypersensitivity to penicillins. Pregnancy Category: [B]

Interactions: Contraceptives, oral: May reduce efficacy of oral contraceptives.
Food: Antibacterial action may be reduced.
Tetracyclines: May impair bactericidal effects of dicloxacillin.

Dicyclomine HCl

Anticholinergic / Antispasmodic

Indications: Treatment of functional bowel/irritable bowel syndrome (eg, irritable colon, spastic colon, mucous colitis).

Unlabeled indication: Intestinal colic in children older than 6 mo.

Dose: Adults: PO 80 mg/day in 4 equally divided doses. Increase to 160 mg/day in 4 equally divided doses. IM 80 mg/day in 4 divided doses.

Trade names: Antispas Injection 10 mg/mL
Bemote Capsules 10 mg
Bentyl Capsules 10 mg
Byclomine Capsules 10 mg
Dibent Injection 10 mg/mL
Dilomine Injection 10 mg/mL
Di-Spaz Capsules 10 mg
Or-Tyl Injection 10 mg/mL

Warnings: Narrow angle glaucoma; adhesions between iris and lens; obstructive uropathy; obstructive disease of GI tract; paralytic ileus; intestinal atony of elderly or debilitated patient; severe ulcerative colitis; toxic megacolon complicating ulcerative colitis; hepatic or renal disease; tachycardia; myocardial ischemia; unstable cardiovascular status in acute hemorrhage; myasthenia gravis; infants younger than 6 mo. Pregnancy Category: [B]

Interactions: Amantadine, tricyclic antidepressants: May cause increased anticholinergic side effects.
Atenolol, digoxin: May increase pharmacologic effects of these drugs.
Phenothiazines: May reduce antipsychotic effectiveness.

Didanosine

Antiretroviral / Nucleoside reverse transcriptase inhibitor

Indications: Didanosine (Videx): Treatment of HIV-1 infection in combination with other antiretrovirals.

Didanosine EC (Videx EC): In combination with other antiretroviral agents for the treatment of HIV-1 infection in adults who require once-daily administration of didanosine or an alternative didanosine formulation.

Dose: Didanosine EC (Videx EC) has not been studied in pediatric patients. Children's dosage recommendations are for didanosine (Videx).
Adults less than 60 kg: PO 125 mg (as 2 tablets) or 167 mg (powder for suspension) q 12 hr or 250 mg qd (capsules).
Adults more than 60 kg: PO 200 mg (as 2 tablets) or 250 mg (powder for suspension) q 12 hr or 400 mg qd (capsules).
Children: PO 120 mg/m^2 bid.

Trade names: Videx Tablets, buffered, chewable/dispersible 25 mg
Videx EC Capsules, delayed-release (with enteric-coated beadlets) 125 mg

Warnings: Standard considerations. Pregnancy Category: [B]

Interactions: Allopurinol: Because allopurinol may cause increased didanosine plasma levels, do not coadminister.
Antacids: Aluminum or magnesium containing antacids may potentiate adverse events associated with the antacid component of didanosine chewable or dispersible tablets and pediatric powder.
Antiretroviral agents: Antiretroviral agents have caused fatal lactic acidosis in women when coadministered with didanosine.
Delavirdine, indinavir: Administer 1 hr prior to didanosine to avoid decreasing plasma levels of delavirdine or indinavir.
Drugs that cause peripheral neuropathy or pancreatitis: Increased risk of these toxicities.
Food: Reduces absorption of didanosine by as much as 50%.
Fluoroquinolones, tetracyclines: Do not administer within 2 hr of didanosine.
Ganciclovir: When coadministered with didanosine, an increase in didanosine plasma levels and a decrease in ganciclovir concentrations may occur.
Itraconazole, ketaconazole, dapsone, and other drugs whose absorption can be affected by gastric acidity: Administer at least 2 hr before didanosine.
Methadone: May decrease didanosine plasma levels.

Diflorasone Diacetate

Anti-inflammatory agent / Corticosteroid / Topical

Indications: Relief of the anti-inflammatory and pruritic manifestations of corticosteroid responsive dermatoses.

Dose: Occlusive dressings may be used for certain conditions.
Cream:
Adult: Topical Apply sparingly to affected area 1 to 3 times/day
Ointment:
Adult: Topical Apply sparingly to affected area 1 to 4 times/day

Trade names: Psorcon E Cream 0.05%

Warnings: Standard considerations. Pregnancy Category: [C]

Interactions: None well documented.

Digoxin

Cardiac glycoside

Indications: Treatment of CHF, atrial fibrillation, atrial flutter, paroxysmal atrial tachycardia, cardiogenic shock.

Dose: Rapid digitalization with loading dose: Adults: IV 0.4 to 0.6 mg or PO tablets 0.5 to 0.75 mg or capsules 0.4 to 0.6 mg in previously undigitalized patients; additional doses may be given cautiously at 6 to 8 hr intervals (IV 0.1 to 0.3 mg or PO tablets 0.125 to 0.375 mg or capsules 0.1 to 0.3 mg) until clinical response is achieved; thereafter adjust dosage based on levels (usual range 0.125 to 0.5 mg/day as single daily dose). In previously digitalized patients, adjust dosage in proportion to ratio of desired vs current serum levels.
Infants and children: Individualize dosage. Usual pediatric doses are listed at end of section.

Trade names: Digitek Tablets 0.125 mg
Lanoxicaps Capsules 0.05 mg
Lanoxin Tablets 0.125 mg

Warnings: Ventricular fibrillation; ventricular tachycardia except in certain cases; digitalis toxicity; beriberi heart disease; hypersensitivity to digoxin; some cases of hypersensitive carotid sinus syndrome. Pregnancy Category: [C]

Interactions: Amiodarone, anticholinergics, bepridol, benzodiazepines, ACE inhibitors, clarithromycin, cyclosporine, diltiazem, erythromycin, indomethacin, itraconazole, propafenone, quinidine, quinine, tetracycline, verapamil: May increase digoxin serum levels.
Antacids, antineoplastics, cholestyramine, colestipol, kaolin/pectin, metoclopramide: May decrease absorption and effect of digoxin.
Penicillamine: May decrease effect of digoxin.
Potassium-sparing diuretics: May alter effect of digoxin.
Thiazide or loop diuretics: May increase effect of digoxin.
St. John's wort, thyroid hormones, thioamines: May decrease effect of digoxin.

Dihydroergotamine Mesylate

Analgesic / Migraine / Ergotamine derivative

Indications: Acute treatment of migraine headaches with or without aura; acute treatment of cluster headache episodes (injection).

Dose: Adults: Intranasal 1 spray (0.5 mg) in each nostril; administer an additional spray (0.5 mg) in each nostril 15 min later for a total dosage of 4 sprays (2 mg). IM / IV / SC Administer 1 mL (1 mg); repeat dose as needed at 1-hr intervals to a total dose of 3 mL (3 mg) for IM or SC administration or 2 mL (2 mg) for IV administration in a 24-hr period (max, 6 mL/wk).

Trade names: D.H.E. 45 Injection 1 mg/mL
Migranal Spray, nasal 4 mg/mL. With 10 mg caffeine and 50 mg dextrose.

Warnings: Hypersensitivity to ergot alkaloids; hepatic or renal impairment; severe pruritus; coronary artery disease; uncontrolled peripheral vascular disease; hypertension; sepsis; use during pregnancy, lactation or in women who may become pregnant; concurrent vasoconstrictor therapy. CYP3A4 inhibitors (eg, macrolide antibiotics [eg, erythromycin], protease inhibitors [eg, ritonavir]). Pregnancy Category: [X]

Interactions: Beta-blockers, vasoconstrictors (eg, epinephrine): Can increase peripheral ischemia, cyanosis, and numbness caused by ergot alkaloids.
CYP3A4 inhibitors (eg, macrolide antibiotics [eg, erythromycin], protease inhibitors [eg, ritonavir]): May increase the risk of life-threatening peripheral ischemia.
Nitrates (eg, nitroglycerin): May oppose effects of nitrates.

Diltiazem HCl

Calcium channel blocker

Indications: Oral: Treatment of angina pectoris caused by coronary artery spasm; chronic stable angina (classic effort-associated angina); essential hypertension (extended- and sustained-release forms only).

Parenteral: Treatment of atrial fibrillation or flutter; paroxysmal supraventricular tachycardia.

Dose: Dosage regimens should be individualized.
Angina:
Adults: PO
Immediate release: Start with 30 mg qid before meals and at bedtime. Gradually increase dosage at 1- to 2-day intervals until optimum response (average optimum dose range 180 to 360 mg/day).
Extended release: Start with 120 to 180 mg once daily. Some patients may respond to doses up to 480 mg once daily. When necessary, titrate the dose over 7 to 14 days.
Cardizem CD and Cartia XT: Start with 120 to 180 mg once daily. Some patients may respond to doses up to 480 mg once daily. When necessary, titrate the dose over 7 to 14 days.
Dilacor XR and Diltia XT: Start with 120 mg once daily. Some patients may respond to doses up to 480 mg once daily. When necessary, titrate the dose over 7 to 14 days.
Tiazac: Start with 120 to 180 mg once daily. Some patients may respond to doses up to 540 mg once daily. When necessary, titrate the dose over 7 to 14 days.
Hypertension:
Adults: PO
Extended release: Start with 60 to 120 mg bid or 180 to 240 mg once daily. Maximum antihypertensive effect usually occurs by 14 days of chronic therapy (optimum dose range 240 to 360 mg once daily but some patients respond to lower doses or higher doses up to 480 mg once daily).
Cardizem CD and Cartia XT: 180 to 240 mg once daily; however, some patients may respond to lower doses. Maximum effect is usually achieved by 14 days of chronic therapy. Usual range is 240 to 360 mg once daily.
Dilacor XR and Diltia XT: 180 to 240 mg once daily (usual dose range 180 to 480 mg once daily. Individual patients, particularly those 60 yr and older, may respond to lower doses of 120 mg once daily. Some patients may require doses up to 540 mg once daily.
Tiazac: Start with 120 to 240 mg once daily. Maximum effect is usually achieved by 14 days of chronic therapy. Usual dose range is 120 to 540 mg once daily.
Sustained release:
Cardizem SR: Start with 60 to 120 mg twice daily. When a maximum antihypertensive effect is achieved (usually about 14 days), adjust dosage (optimum dosage range is 240 to 360 mg/day). Parenteral
Direct IV single bolus injection: Initial dose is 0.25 mg/kg as a bolus administered over 2 min (reasonable dose is 20 mg for average patient). If response is inadequate after 15 min, administer as a second 0.35 mg/kg over 2 min (reasonable dose is 25 mg for average patient). Individualize subsequent IV doses. Dose low body weight patients on a mg/kg basis. Although the duration of action may be shorter, some patients may respond to an initial dose of 0.15 mg/kg.
Continuous IV infusion: For continued reduction of heart rate (up to 24 hr) in patients with atrial fibrillation or atrial flutter, IV infusion may be administered. Immediately following administration of a bolus dose of 20 mg (0.25 mg/kg) or 25 mg (0.35 mg/kg) and reduction of heart rate, begin an IV infusion. The recommended initial infusion rate is 10 mg/hr; however, some patients may maintain response to an initial rate of 5 mg/hr. The infusion rate may be increased in 5 mg/hr increments up to 15 mg/hr as needed, if further reduction in heart rate is necessary. The infusion may be maintained for up to 24 hr (max, 24 hr and 15 mg/hr).

Trade names: Cardizem Tablets 30 mg
Cardizem CD Capsules, extended-release 120 mg
Cardizem SR Capsules, sustained-release 60 mg
CartiaXT Capsules, extended-release 120 mg
Dilacor XR Capsules, extended-release 120 mg
Dilacor XT Capsules, extended-release 120 mg
Tiazac Capsules, extended-release 120 mg

Warnings: Sick sinus syndrome; second- or third-degree AV block; except with functioning pacemaker; hypotension with systolic pressure less than 90 mm Hg; acute MI; pulmonary congestion. Pregnancy Category: [C]

Interactions: Beta-blockers: May have additive negative inotropic and chronotropic effects.
Carbamazepine: Carbamazepine levels may increase.
Cimetidine, ranitidine: Diltiazem levels may be increased.
Cyclosporine: Cyclosporine levels and toxicity may increase.
Encainide: Encainide levels may increase.
Other antihypertensive agents: May have additive effects.
Incompatability: Do not mix with furosemide.

Dimenhydrinate

Antiemetic / Antivertigo / Anticholinergic

Indications: Prevention and treatment of motion sickness, dizziness, nausea, vomiting.

Unlabeled indication: Treatment of Meniere disease, nausea and vomiting of pregnancy, postoperative nausea, and vomiting.

Dose: Motion Sickness:
Adults: PO 50 to 100 mg 30 min prior to travel, followed by 50 to 100 mg q 4 to 6 hr (max 400 mg/day). IM 50 mg prn. IV 50 mg in 10 mL of Sodium Chloride for Injection administered over 2 min.
Children (6 to 12 yr): PO 25 to 50 mg q 6 to 8 hr (max 150 mg/day). IM 1.25 mg/kg qid (max 300 mg/day).

Children (2 to 6 yr): PO Up to 12.5 to 25 mg q 6 to 8 hr (max 75 mg/day). IM 1.25 mg/kg qid (max 300 mg/day).
Trade names: Calm-X Tablets 50 mg
Children's Dramamine Liquid 12.5 mg/5 mL
Dimetabs Tablets 50 mg
Dinate Injection 50 mg/mL
Dramamine Liquid 15.62mg/5 mL
Dramanate Injection 50 mg/mL
Dymenate Injection 50 mg/mL
Hydrate Injection 50 mg/mL
Triptone Tablets 50 mg/mL
Warnings: Use in newborns; allergic reactions to diphenhydramine. Pregnancy Category: [B]
Interactions: Alcohol, CNS depressants: Enhances CNS depressant effects.
Aminoglycosides: May mask signs of aminoglycoside-related ototoxicity.
Anticholinergic drugs: Causes additive anticholinergic effects.
Incompatability: Ammonium chloride, amobarbital, butorphanol, chlorpromazine, glycopyrrolate, heparin, hydrocortisone, hydroxyzine, midazolam, pentobarbital, phenobarbital, phenytoin, prednisolone, prochlorperazine, promethazine, tetracycline, theophylline, thiopental, trifluoperazine.

Diphenhydramine HCl

Antihistamine / Ethanolamine

Indications: Symptomatic relief of perennial and seasonal allergic rhinitis, vasomotor rhinitis and allergic conjunctivitis; temporary relief of runny nose and sneezing caused by common cold; relief of allergic and nonallergic pruritic symptoms; treatment of urticaria and angioedema; amelioration of allergic reactions to blood or plasma; adjunct to epinephrine and other standard measures in anaphylaxis; relief of uncomplicated allergic conditions of immediate type when oral therapy is impossible or contraindicated (parenteral form); treatment and prophylactic treatment of motion sickness; nighttime sleep aid; management of parkinsonism (including drug-induced) in elderly who are intolerant of more potent agents, in mild cases in other age groups and in combination with centrally acting anticholinergics; control of cough from colds or allergy (syrup formulations).
Dose: Hypersensitivity Reactions, Type 1/ Antiparkinsonism/Motion Sickness:
Adults: PO 25 to 50 mg q 4 to 6 hr (max, 300 mg/day). IV/IM 10 to 100 mg (rate not exceeding 25 mg/min or deep IM; max, 400 mg/day).
Children (6 to under 12 yr): PO 12.5 to 25 mg q 4 to 6 hr (max, 150 mg). IV/IM 5 mg/kg/day or 150 mg/m^2 /day (max, 300 mg divided into 4 doses at a rate not exceeding 25 mg/min or deep IM).
Nighttime Sleep Aid:
Adults: PO 50 mg at bedtime.
Cough Suppressant (Syrup):
Adults: PO 25 mg q 4 hr (max, 150 mg/24 hr).
Children (6 to 12 yr): PO 12.5 mg q 4 hr (max, 75 mg/24 hr).
Children (2 to 6 yr): PO 6.25 mg q 4 hr (max, 25 mg/24 hr).
Trade names: 40 Winks Tablets 50 mg
Allergy Medication Liquid 12.5 mg/5 mL
AllerMax Tablets 50 mg
AllerMax Allergy and Cough Formula Liquid 6.25 mg/5 mL
Banophen Capsules 25 mg
Benadryl Injection 50 mg/mL
Benadryl Allergy Capsules, soft-gels 25 mg
Benadryl Allergy Ultratabs Tablets 25 mg
Benadryl Dye Free Liquid 12.5 mg/5 mL
Benadryl Dye Free Allergy Liqui Gels Capsules, soft gels 25 mg
Bydramine Cough Syrup 12.5 mg/5 mL
Compoz Gel Caps Capsules 25 mg
Compoz Nighttime Sleep Aid Tablets 50 mg
Diphen AF Liquid 6.25 mg/5 mL
Diphen Cough Syrup 12.5 mg/5 mL
Diphenhist Solution 12.5 mg/5 mL
Diphenhist Captabs Tablets 25 mg
Dormin Tablets 25 mg
Genahist Liquid 12.5 mg/5 mL
Hyrexin-50 Injection 50 mg/mL
Maximum Strength Nytol Tablets 50 mg
Maximum Strength Sleepinal Capsules and Soft Gels Capsules 50 mg
Maximum Strength Unisom SleepGels Capsules 50 mg/mL
Midol PM Tablets 50 mg
Miles Nervine Tablets 25 mg
Nighttime Sleep Aid Tablets 50 mg
Nytol Tablets 25 mg
Scot-Tussin Allergy DM Liquid 12.5 mg/5 mL
Siladryl Elixir 12.5 mg/5 mL
Silphen DM Syrup 10 mg/5 mL
Sleep-Eze 3 Tablets 25 mg
Sleepwell 2-nite Tablets 25 mg
Snoozefast Tablets 50 mg
Sominex Tablets 25 mg
Sylphen Cough Syrup 12.5 mg/5 mL
Tusstat Syrup 12.5 mg/5 mL
Twilite Tablets 50 mg
Uni-Bent Cough Syrup 12.5 mg/5 mL
Warnings: Hypersensitivity to antihistamines; narrow-angle glaucoma; stenosing peptic ulcer; symptomatic prostatic hypertrophy; asthmatic attack; bladder neck obstruction; pyloroduodenal obstruction; MAOI therapy; history of sleep apnea; use in newborn or premature infants and in nursing women. Pregnancy Category: [B]
Interactions: Alcohol, CNS depressants: May cause additive CNS depression.
MAOIs: May increase anticholinergic effects.
Incompatability: Injectable form is incompatible with dexamethasone sodium phosphate, furosemide, iodipamide meglumine, parenteral barbiturates, and phenytoin.

Dipivefrin Hydrochloride

Sympathomimetic

Indications: Control of IOP in chronic open-angle glaucoma.
Dose: Adults: Ophthalmic 1 gtt in affected eye(s) q 12 hr.
Trade names: Propine Solution 0.1%
Warnings: Narrow-angle glaucoma; hypersensitivity to any component of the product. Pregnancy Category: [B]
Interactions: None well documented.

Disopyramide

Antiarrhythmic

Indications: Suppression and documented prevention of ventricular arrhythmias considered to be life threatening.

Unlabeled indication: Treatment of paroxysmal supraventricular tachycardia.
Dose: Adults: PO 400 to 800 mg/day in 4 divided, evenly spaced doses.
Children (12 to 18 yr): PO 6 to 15 mg/kg/day in divided doses.
Children (4 to 12 yr): PO 10 to 15 mg/kg/day in divided doses.
Children (1 to 4 yr): PO 10 to 20 mg/kg/day in divided doses.
Children (younger than 1 yr): PO 10 to 30 mg/kg/day in divided doses.
Severe Refractory Ventricular Tachycardia: May give PO up to 400 mg q 6 hr.
With Cardiomyopathy or Cardiac Decompensation: Limit to PO 100 mg q 6 to 8 hr initially.
Renal/Hepatic Impairment:

Adults: PO 100 mg q 6 hr; increase to q 8 to 24 hr for patients with deteriorating renal function.
Trade names: Norpace Capsules 100 mg
Norpace CR Capsules, extended-release 100 mg
Warnings: Cardiogenic shock; pre-existing second- or third-degree atrioventricular block (if no pacemaker present); congenital QT prolongation; sick sinus syndrome. Pregnancy Category: [C]
Interactions: Antiarrhythmic agents: May cause widened QRS and prolonged QT.
Erythromycin: May cause increased disopyramide plasma levels.
Hydantoins: May decrease disopyramide serum levels, half-life, and bioavailability.
Rifampin: May decrease disopyramide serum levels.

Disulfiram

Antialcoholic agent

Indications: Aid in management of alcoholism in selected patients who want to remain in state of enforced sobriety.
Dose: Adults: PO
Initial dose: 500 mg qd (single dose) initially for 1 to 2 wk.
Maintenance dose: 125 to 500 mg qd (max, 500 mg/day).
Trade names: Antabuse Tablets 250 mg
Warnings: Hypersensitivity to thiuram derivatives used in pesticides and rubber vulcanization; severe myocardial disease or coronary occlusion; psychoses; patients receiving or who have recently received metronidazole, paraldehyde, alcohol, or alcohol-containing products. Pregnancy Category: [C]
Interactions: Alcohol: Causes severe alcohol-intolerance reaction. Symptoms include flushing, throbbing in head and neck, respiratory difficulty, nausea, vomiting, sweating, thirst, chest pain, palpitations, shortness of breath, tachycardia, hypotension, syncope, weakness, vertigo, blurred vision, and confusion. In severe reactions, there may be respiratory depression, cardiovascular collapse, unconsciousness, convulsions, and death.
Anticoagulants: Disulfiram may increase anticoagulant effect.
Antidepressants, tricyclic: May produce acute organic brain syndrome.
Benzodiazepines: Disulfiram decreases plasma clearance of benzodiazepines metabolized by oxidation, possible increase in CNS side effects.
Chlorzoxazone: CNS side effects of chlorzoxazone may be increased.
Cocaine: CV side effects of cocaine may be increased.
Hydantoins: Disulfiram may increase serum hydantoin levels.
Isoniazid: Acute behavioral and coordination changes.
Metronidazole: May cause patients to exhibit acute toxic psychosis or confusional state. One or both agents may need to be discontinued.
Theophyllines: Disulfiram may inhibit metabolism and increase effect of theophyllines.

Dobutamine

Vasopressor

Indications: Treatment of cardiac decompensation caused by organic heart disease or cardiac surgical procedures.

Unlabeled indication: Congenital heart disease in children undergoing diagnostic cardiac catheterization.
Dose: Adults: IV infusion 2.5 to 10 mcg/kg/min; titrate to desired response; increase in heart rate more than 10% may develop in rate greater than 20 mcg/kg/min; rates up to 40 mcg/kg/min are rarely used. Duration of therapy up to 72 hr without decrease in clinical effectiveness may be used.
Trade names: Dobutrex Injection 12.5 mg/mL
Warnings: Idiopathic hypertrophic subaortic stenosis. Pregnancy Category: [Safety not established]
Interactions: Beta-blockers: May antagonize beta receptor-stimulating activity of dobutamine.
Furazolidone, methyldopa, rauwolfia alkaloids: Hypertension may result.
Guanethidine: May increase pressor response.
Halogenated hydrocarbon anesthetics: May increase risk of arrhythmias by sensitizing cardiac tissue to sympathomimetic agents.
Tricyclic antidepressants: May potentiate effect of dobutamine; use combination with caution.
Incompatability: Chemically incompatible with sodium bicarbonate or other alkaline solutions.

Docetaxel

Mitotic inhibitor

Indications: Locally advanced or metastatic breast cancer; locally advanced or metastatic non-small cell lung cancer.

Unlabeled indication: Ovarian cancer.
Dose: Locally Advanced or Metastatic Breast Cancer:
Adults: IV 60 to 100 mg/m^2 administered over 1 hr q 3 wk.
Dosage Adjustment for Breast Cancer:
Adults:
Initial dose (100 mg/m-2): Adjust dose to 75 mg/m^2 in patients who experience febrile neutropenia, neutrophils less than 500 cells/mm^3 for longer than 1 wk, severe or cumulative cutaneous reactions, or severe peripheral neuropathy. If reactions continue, decrease the dosage to 55 mg/m^2 or discontinue treatment.
Initial dose (60 mg/m-2): Patients who do not experience these symptoms may tolerate higher doses. Discontinue docetaxel treatment entirely if patients develop at least grade 3 peripheral neuropathy.
Locally Advanced or Metastatic Non-Small Cell Lung Cancer:
Adults: IV 70 mg/m^2 administered over 1 hr q 3 wk.
Dosage Adjustments for Non-Small Cell Lung Cancer:
Adults:
Initial dose (75 mg/m-2): Withhold treatment in patients who experience febrile neuropenia, neutrophils less than 500 cells/mm^3 for longer than 1 wk, severe or cumulative cutaneous reactions, or other grade 3 and 4 nonhematological toxicities during treatment until resolution of the toxicity, and then resume at 55 mg/m^2. Discontinue docetaxel treatment entirely if patients develop at least grade 3 peripheral neuropathy.
Locally Advanced or Metastatic Non-Small Cell Lung Cancer Not Previously Treated with Chemotherapy:
Adults: IV Docetaxel 75 mg/m^2 over 1 hr immediately followed by cisplatin 75 mg/m^2 over 30 to 60 min q 3 wk. In patients who are dosed initially at 75 mg/m^2 of docetaxel in combination with cisplatin, and whose nadir platelet count during the previous course of therapy is less than 25,000 cells/mm^3, in patients who experience febrile neutropenia, and in patients with serious nonhematologic toxicities, reduce the docetaxel dose to 65 mg/m^2 in subsequent cycles. In patients who require a further dose reduction, a dose of 50 mg/m^2 is recommended. For cisplatin dosage adjustments, see manufacturer's prescribing information.
Dosage Adjustments in Hepatic Dysfunction:
Adults: IV Avoid use in patients with bilirubin above the upper limit of normal, AST or ALT greater than 1.5 times the upper limit of normal concomitant with alkaline phosphatase greater than 2.5 times the upper limit of normal.
Pretreatment Regimen: To reduce the severity of hypersensitivity reactions and fluid retention, premedicate with 8 mg dexamethasone orally twice daily for 3 days starting the day before docetaxel administration.
Trade names: Taxotere Injection 20 mg
Warnings: History of severe hypersensitivity

reactions to docetaxel or to other drugs formulated with polysorbate 80; neutrophil counts of less than 1500 cells/mm^3. Pregnancy Category: [D]

Interactions: CYP450: Docetaxel is metabolized by cytochrome P450 3A. Potential exists for significant drug interactions between docetaxel and agents that inhibit or induce cytochrome P450 enzymes (eg, rifampin, phenobarbital, erythromycin, ketoconazole).

Dofetilide

Antiarrhythmic

Indications: Maintenance of normal sinus rhythm (delay in time to recurrence of atrial fibrillation/atrial flutter [AF/AFl]) in patients with AF/AFl of more than 1 wk duration who have been converted to normal sinus rhythm; conversion of AF/AFl to normal sinus rhythm.

Unlabeled indication: Ventricular arrhythmias.

Dose: Adults: PO The dose must be individualized according to calculated Ccr and QTc. Use the QT interval if the heart rate is less than 60 bpm. There are no data on use if the heart rate is less than 50 bpm. The usual recommended dose is 500 mcg bid, as modified by the dosing algorithm described in the manufacturer's prescribing information.

Trade names: Tikosyn Capsules 125 mcg

Warnings: Hypersensitivity to drug; congenital or acquired long QT syndromes; baseline QT interval of QTc greater than 440 msec (500 msec in patients with ventricular conduction abnormalities); severe renal impairment (Ccr less than 20 mL/min); concurrent use of cimetidine, ketoconazole, trimethoprim (alone or in combination with sulfamethoxazole), or verapamil; concomitant use of known inhibitors of renal cation transport (eg, megestrol, prochlorperazine). Pregnancy Category: [C]

Interactions: Cimetidine, inhibitors of renal cationic exchange (eg, megestrol, phenothiazines), ketoconazole, trimethoprim (alone or in combination with sulfamethoxazole), verapamil: Are contraindicated.
Drugs actively secreted by renal cationic secretion (eg, amiloride, metformin, triamterene), inhibitors of CYP3A4 isozymes (eg, amiodarone, azole antifungal agents, cannabinoids, diltiazem, grapefruit juice, macrolide antibiotics, nefazodone, norfloxacin, protease inhibitors, quinine, serotonin reuptake inhibitors, zafirlukast): May increase dofetilide levels; use with caution.
Class I (eg, quinidine) or Class III (eg, sotalol) antiarrhythmics: Withhold for at least 3 half-lives prior to dosing with dofetilide.
Drugs that prolong the QT interval (eg, bepridil, cisapride, phenothiazines, tricyclic antidepressants, erythromycin): Concurrent use not recommended.

Donepezil

Reversible cholinesterase inhibitor

Indications: Treatment of mild to moderate dementia of the Alzheimer type.

Dose: Adults: PO 5 mg once daily. May increase to 10 mg qd after 4 to 6 wk.

Trade names: Aricept Tablets 5 mg

Warnings: Hypersensitivity to donepezil or piperidine derivatives. Pregnancy Category: [C]

Interactions: Anticholinergic drugs: Possible reduction of anticholinergic effects.
Cholinesterase inhibitors/Cholinomimetics: Synergistic effects may occur.

Dopamine HCl

Vasopressor

Indications: Correction of hemodynamic imbalances present in shock syndrome after MI, trauma, endotoxic septicemia, surgery and renal failure or imbalances in conditions of chronic refractory cardiac decompensation (eg, CHF).

Dose: Adults: IV Initial dose 2 to 5 mcg/kg/min with incremental changes of 5 to 10 mcg/kg/min at 10 to 15 min intervals until adequate response is noted. Most patients are maintained at less than 20 mcg/kg/min. If dosage exceeds 50 mcg/kg/min, assess renal function frequently.

Trade names: Dopamine HCl Injection 40 mg/mL
Dopamine HCl in 5% Dextrose Injection 80 mg/100 mL (0.8 mg/mL)

Warnings: Pheochromocytoma; uncorrected tachyarrhythmias; ventricular fibrillation. Pregnancy Category: [C]

Interactions: Furazolidone, methyldopa, rauwolfia alkaloids: Hypertension may result.
Guanethidine: Antihypertensive effects of guanethidine may be negated.
MAOIs: May greatly increase pressor response from dopamine.
Phenytoin: Severe hypotension and bradycardia may result after concomitant administration with dopamine.
Tricyclic antidepressants: May decrease pressor response from dopamine.
Incompatability: Chemically incompatible with alkaline solutions (drug is inactivated).

Dornase Alfa

Respiratory inhalant/enzyme

Indications: Treatment of cystic fibrosis.

Dose: Adults and Children older than 5 yr: Inhalation 2.5 mg once daily by oral inhalation via nebulizer; patients older than 21 yr and those with baseline forced vital capacity more than 85% benefit from 2.5 mg bid.

Trade names: Pulmozyme Solution for inhalation 1 mg/mL

Warnings: Hypersensitivity to Chinese hamster ovary cell products. Pregnancy Category: [B]

Interactions: None well documented.

Doxazosin Mesylate

Antihypertensive / Antiadrenergic, peripherally acting

Indications: Treatment of hypertension, alone or in combination with other agents; treatment of benign prostatic hyperplasia (BPH).

Dose: Hypertension:
Adults: PO
Initial dose: 1 mg qd.
Maintenance: Based on standing BP response, may increase to 2 mg and thereafter to 4, 8, and 16 mg.
Benign Prostatic Hyperplasia:
Adults: PO
Initial dose: 1 mg/day.
Maintenance: Increase to 2 mg, and thereafter to 4 and 8 mg qd, which is the max dose for BPH. Recommended titration interval is 1 to 2 wk.

Trade names: Cardura Tablets 1 mg

Warnings: Hypersensitivity to doxazosin, prazosin, or terazosin. Pregnancy Category: [C]

Interactions: Cimetidine: 10% increase in mean AUC of doxazosin.

Doxepin HCl

Antianxiety / Tricyclic antidepressant

Indications: Treatment of psychoneurotic patients with depression and/or anxiety; depression and/or anxiety associated with alcoholism (not to be taken concomitantly with alcohol); depression and/or anxiety associated with organic disease (the possibility of drug interaction should be considered if the patient is receiving other drugs concomitantly); psychotic depressive disorders with associated anxiety including involutional depression and manic-depressive disorders; moderate pruritus with atopic dermatitis or lichen simplex chronicus (topical).

Unlabeled indication: Neurogenic pain, peptic ulcer disease.

Dose: Depression and/or Anxiety:
Adults: PO Initial dose 75 mg/day, increasing as tolerated (max, 300 mg/day). May be given qd or on a divided dosage schedule. If given qd, the max recommended dose is 150 mg/day.
For Mild Cases with Organic Diseases: PO 25 to 50 mg/day.
Pruritus:
Adults: Topical Apply thin film qid with at least 3 to 4 hr between applications. Not recommended for more than 8 days.

Trade names: Sinequan Capsules 10 mg
Zonalon Cream 5%

Warnings: Hypersensitivity to tricyclic antidepressants; use during acute recovery phase after MI; glaucoma; risk of urinary retention; concomitant use with MAO inhibitor; dibenzoxepines may produce cross-sensitivity. Pregnancy Category: [C (oral form); B: (topical)]

Interactions: Alcohol/CNS depressants: CNS and respiratory depression may be potentiated.
Cimetidine: May inhibit metabolism of doxepin, leading to increased concentrations.
Clonidine: Concurrent use may lead to loss of BP control and possibly dangerous increases in BP.
Guanethidine: Hypotensive action may be inhibited.
MAO inhibitors: Concurrent use may lead to severe seizures, hyperpyretic crisis, and fatal reactions. Generally, allow 7 to 10 days between discontinuation of 1 drug and start of another.
SSRIs (eg, fluoxetine): May increase serum concentrations of doxepin; effect may occur up to 5 wk after discontinuation of fluoxetine.
Sympathomimetics (eg, dopamine, epinephrine): Pressor response may increase or decrease; arrhythmias may occur.
Type IC antiarrhythmics (eg, propafenone, flecainide): May inhibit metabolism of doxepin, leading to increased concentrations.

Doxycycline

Antibiotic / Tetracycline

Indications: Treatment of infections caused by susceptible strains of gram-positive and gram-negative bacteria (eg, *Rickettsia*, *Mycoplasma pneumoniae*); treatment of trachoma and susceptible infections when penicillins are contraindicated; treatment of acute intestinal amebiasis; uncomplicated gonorrhea in adults; prophylaxis of malaria caused by Plasmodium falciparum; anthrax (including inhalational anthrax); severe acne.
Periodontitis: Tablet: Adjunct treatment to scaling and root planing to promote attachment level gain and reduce pocket depth.

Subgingival injection: For chronic adult periodontitis for a gain in clinical attachment, reduction in probing depth, and reduction in bleeding on probing.

Dose: Acute Epididymo-Orchitis Caused by Neisseria Gonorrhoeae or Chlamydia Trachomatis:
Adults: PO 100 mg bid for at least 10 days.
Chlamydia Infections:
Adults and Children 8 yr of age and older: PO 100 mg bid for 7 days.
Epididymitis Most Likely Caused by Gonococcal or Chlamydial Infection:
Adults: PO 100 mg bid for 10 days plus a single dose of 250 mg ceftriaxone IM.
Infection:
Adults and children older than 8 yr of age and weighing more than 45 kg: PO 200 mg on the first day (100 mg q 12 hr) then 100 mg/day. For more severe infections (particularly chronic UTI), administer 100 mg q 12 hr. IV 200 mg on the first day (as 1 or 2 infusions) then 100 to 200 mg/day, depending upon the severity of infections, with 200 mg administered in 1 or 2 infusions.
Children older than 8 yr of age and weighing 45 kg or less: PO 4.4 mg/kg divided into 2 doses on day 1 followed by 2.2 mg/kg/day as a single dose or divided into 2 doses on subsequent day. For more severe infections, 4.4 mg/kg may be used. IV 4.4 mg/kg on day 1 (in 1 or 2 infusions) followed with 2.2 to 4.4 mg/kg given as 1 or 2 infusions, depending on the severity of the infection.
Lymphogranuloma Venereum and Granuloma Inguinale:
Adults: PO 100 mg bid for at least 21 days.
Malaria Prophylaxis:
Adults: PO 100 mg daily, beginning 1 to 2 days before travel and continuing for 4 wk after leaving area.
Children older than 8 yr of age: PO 2 mg/kg daily up to 100 mg per day. Begin 1 to 2 days before travel and continue for 4 wk after leaving area.
Nongonococcal Urethritis:
Adults: PO 100 mg bid for 7 days.
Pelvic Inflammatory Disease:
Adults: PO/IV 100 mg q 12 hr plus 2 g cefotetan IV q 12 hr or 2 g cefoxitin IV q 6 hr. Parenteral therapy may be discontinued after 24 hr; continue oral therapy with doxycycline for a total of 14 days.
Periodontitis (Periostat, Atridox):
Adults: PO 20 mg bid as an adjunct following scaling and root planing for up to 9 mo. Administer tablets at least 2 hr before or after meals.
Adults: Subgingival Injection Variable dose, depending on the size, shape, and number of pockets being treated (see product information for preparation and administration).
Sexual Assault Prophylaxis:
Adults: PO 100 mg bid for 7 days plus ceftriaxone and metronidazole.
Syphilis:
Early (except Adoxa, Doryx, Monodox): PO 100 mg bid for 14 days.
More than 1 yr duration (except Adoxa, Doryx, Monodox): 100 mg bid for 28 days.
Primary and secondary (Adoxa, Doryx, Monodox): 300 mg/day in divided doses for at least 10 days.
Uncomplicated Gonococcal Infection (Except Anorectal Infections in Men):
Adults: PO 100 mg bid for at least 7 days. Single visit dose: 300 mg immediately followed with 300 mg in 1 hr.
Uncomplicated Urethral, Endocervical, or Rectal Infections Caused by C. Trachomatis:
Adults: PO 100 mg bid for at least 7 days.
Inhalation Anthrax (Post-exposure):
Adults and children (100 lb [45 kg] or more): PO 100 mg bid for 60 days.
Children (less than 100 lb [45 kg]): PO 2.2 mg/kg bid for 60 days.

Trade names: Adoxa Tablets 50 mg (as monohydrate)
Atridox Injection 42.5 mg (as hyclate, 10%)
Doryx Capsules, coated pellets 75 mg (as hyclate)
Doxy 100 Powder for Injection, lyophilized 100 mg (as hyclate)
Doxy 200 Powder for Injection, lyophilized 200 mg (as hyclate)
Monodox Capsules 50 mg (as monohydrate)
Periostat Tablets 20 mg (as hyclate)
Vibramycin Capsules 50 mg (as hyclate)
Vibra-Tabs Tablets 100 mg (as hyclate)

Warnings: Hypersensitivity to tetracyclines; nursing mothers, infants, and children (Periostat). Pregnancy Category: [D]

Interactions: Antacids (containing aluminum, calcium, or magnesium), bismuth salts, divalent/trivalent cations, zinc salts: May decrease oral absorption of doxycycline.
Barbiturates, carbamazepine, hydantoins: May increase metabolism of and decrease effect of doxycycline.
Cholestyramine, colestipol: May decrease absorption of doxycycline.

Digoxin: May increase digoxin serum levels.
Iron salts: May decrease absorption of doxycycline.
Isotretinoin: Because the risk of pseudotumor cerebri may be increased, avoid isotretinoin administration shortly before, during, or after doxycycline therapy.
Methoxyflurane: Increased potential for nephrotoxicity exists; do not use together.
Milk and dairy products: Although the effects of milk and dairy products on doxycycline absorption are less than observed with other tetracycline derivatives, avoid the administration of milk or dairy products with all tetracycline derivatives.
Oral contraceptives: May decrease contraceptive efficacy.
Penicillins: May interfere with bactericidal action of penicillins.
Warfarin: Anticoagulant effect may be increased; dose may need to be decreased.

Dronabinol

Antiemetic / Antivertigo / Appetite stimulant

Indications: Control of chemotherapy-induced nausea and vomiting unresponsive to other antiemetics; appetite stimulation in AIDS cachexia.

Dose: Antiemetic:
Adults and Children: PO 5 mg/m^2 1 to 3 hr before chemotherapy and q 2 to 4 hr after chemotherapy. Can give 4 to 6 doses/day and increase by 2.5 mg/m^2 /dose; do not exceed 15 mg/m^2 /dose.
Appetite Stimulation:
Adults: PO 2.5 mg bid. Can give single daily dose of 2.5 mg to patients in whom adverse effects develop. Can increase by 2.5 mg/day; do not exceed 20 mg/day.

Trade names: Marinol Capsules, gelatin 2.5 mg

Warnings: Hypersensitivity to marijuana or sesame oil. Pregnancy Category: [B]

Interactions: Amphetamines, cocaine, sympathomimetics: Hypertension; tachycardia.
CNS depressants: Increased CNS adverse effects.

Droperidol

General anesthetic

Indications: Reduction of incidence of nausea and vomiting in surgical and diagnostic procedures.

Unlabeled indication: Antiemetic in cancer chemotherapy.

Dose: Adults: IM or slow IV 2.5 mg max recommended initial dose; additional 1.25 mg doses may be administered to achieve desired effect.
Children (2 to 12 yr): IM / IV 0.1 mg/kg max recommended initial dose, taking into account age and other clinical factors.

Trade names: Inapsine Injection 2.5 mg/mL

Warnings: Known or suspected QT prolongation (ie, QTc interval greater than 440 msec for men or greater than 450 msec for women), including patients with congenital long QT syndrome. Hypersensitivity to butyrophenones. Pregnancy Category: [C]

Interactions: CNS depressants: Additive CNS depression may result.
Diuretics, drugs known to increase the QT interval (eg, cisapride, pimozide): Risk of life-threatening arrhythmias, including torsades de pointes, may be increased.
Incompatability: Barbiturates are physically incompatible with droperidol.

Drotrecogin Alfa (Activated)

Thrombolytic agent / Recombinant human activated protein C

Indications: Reduction of mortality in adult patients with severe sepsis who have a high risk of death.

Dose: Adults: IV 24 mcg/kg/hr for a total infusion duration of 96 hr. If infusion is interrupted, restart at the 24 mcg/kg/hr infusion rate.

Trade names: Xigris Powder for infusion, lyophilized 5 mg

Warnings: Patients with the following situations in whom bleeding could be associated with a high risk of death or important morbidity: active internal bleeding; recent (within 3 mo) hemorrhagic stroke; recent (within 2 mo) intracranial or intraspinal surgery or severe head trauma; trauma with an increased risk of life-threatening bleeding; presence of an epidural catheter; intracranial neoplasm, mass lesion, or evidence of cerebral herniation. Hypersensitivity to drotrecogin alfa (activated) or any component of the product.
Pregnancy Category: [C]

Interactions: Aspirin, oral anticoagulants (eg, warfarin), glycoprotein IIb/IIIa inhibitors: Increased risk of bleeding.
Incompatability: Administer through a dedicated line or dedicated lumen of a multilumen central venous catheter. Only 0.9% Sodium Chloride for Injection, Lactated Ringer's injection, dextrose, or dextrose and saline mixtures can be administered through the same line as drotrecogin alfa (activated).

Dutasteride

Androgen hormone inhibitor

Indications: Treatment of symptomatic benign prostatic hyperplasia in men with an enlarged prostate.

Dose: Adults: PO 0.5 mg once daily.

Trade names: Avodart Capsules 0.5 mg

Warnings: Women; children; hypersensitivity to 5-alpha-reductase inhibitors or any component of the product. Pregnancy Category: [X]

Interactions: Cytochrome P450 3A4 inhibitors (eg, cimetidine, ciprofloxacin, diltiazem, ketoconazole, ritonavir, verapamil): Plasma concentrations of dutasteride may be elevated, increasing the risk of side effects.

Econazole Nitrate

Topical / Antifungal

Indications: Treatment of tinea pedis (athlete's foot), tinea cruris (jock itch), tinea corporis (ringworm), cutaneous candidiasis, tinea versicolor.

Dose: Tinea Pedis, Tinea Cruris, Tinea Corporis, and Tinea Versicolor:
Adults and Children: Topical Apply sufficient quantity to cover affected areas qd. Treat tinea versicolor, tinea cruris, and tinea corporis for 2 wk and tinea pedis for 1 mo.
Cutaneous Candidiasis:
Adults and Children: Topical Apply bid morning and evening for 2 wk.

Trade names: Spectazole Cream 1%

Warnings: Standard considerations. Pregnancy Category: [C]

Interactions: None well documented.

Edetate Calcium Disodium

Antidote

Indications: Treatment of acute and chronic lead poisoning and lead encephalopathy.

Dose: Asymptomatic Adults: IV 5 mL ampule diluted with 250 to 500 mL normal saline or D5W. Administer dilution over 1 hr or more bid for up to 5 days. Interrupt therapy for 2 days; follow with 5 additional days if needed (max 50 mg/kg/day).
Symptomatic Adults: IV 5 mL ampule diluted with 250 to 500 mL normal saline or D5W. Administer dilution over 2 hr. Give second daily infusion 6 hr or more after first.
Children and Patients With Overt or Incipient Lead Encephalopathy: IM 35 mg/kg bid q 8 to 12 hr for 3 to 5

days; give second course no sooner than 4 days later. Procaine or lidocaine may be added (for concentration of up to 0.5%) to minimize pain on injection.

Trade names: Calcium Disodium Versenate Injection 200 mg/mL

Warnings: Anuria; active renal disease; hepatitis. Pregnancy Category: [Safety not established]

Interactions: None well documented.

Efavirenz

Antiretroviral / Non-nucleoside reverse transcriptase inhibitor

Indications: Treatment of HIV-1 infection in combination with other antiretroviral agents.

Dose: Adults: PO 600 mg/day in combination with other antiretroviral agents.
Children 10 to less than 15 kg: PO 200 mg/day in combination with other antiretroviral agents.
Children 15 to less than 20 kg: PO 250 mg/day in combination with other antiretroviral agents.
Children 20 to less than 25 kg: PO 300 mg/day in combination with other antiretroviral agents.
Children 25 to less than 32.5 kg: PO 350 mg/day in combination with other antiretroviral agents.
Children 32.5 to less than 40 kg: PO 400 mg/day in combination with other antiretroviral agents.
Children at least 40 kg: PO 600 mg/day in combination with other antiretroviral agents.

Trade names: Sustiva Capsules 50 mg

Warnings: Concomitant use with cisapride, ergot derivatives, midazolam, or triazolam; hypersensitivity to product. Pregnancy Category: [C]

Interactions: Alprazolam, midazolam, triazolam: May increase blood levels of these drugs, which may produce extreme sedation and respiratory depression. Do not administer concurrently.
Clarithromycin, indinavir, methadone, saquinavir: Efavirenz may decrease plasma concentrations, which could reduce activity of these agents.
Cisapride, ergot derivatives: May elevate levels of these drugs, which may increase the risk of arrhythmias, hematologic abnormalities, or other potentially serious adverse effects. Do not coadminister.
Ethinyl estradiol, nelfinavir, ritonavir: Efavirenz may increase plasma concentrations, which could increase activity or toxicity of these agents.
Phenytoin, carbamazepine, phenobarbital: Plasma concentrations of the anticonvulsant or efavirenz may decrease.
Rifampin: May decrease plasma levels of efavirenz, which may reduce antiviral activity.
Ritonavir: May increase efavirenz plasma level, which could increase side effects.
St. John's wort: May reduce efavirenz plasma concentrations, which may decrease the clinical efficacy.
Warfarin: Plasma concentrations may be increased or decreased.

Eletriptan Hydrobromide

Analgesic / Migraine

Indications: Acute treatment of migraine with or without aura.

Dose: Adults: PO 20 to 40 mg single dose. If required, a second dose may be taken at least 2 hr after the initial dose (max, 80 mg/day).

Trade names: Relpax Tablets 24.2 mg

Warnings: Ischemic heart disease (eg, angina pectoris); symptoms or findings consistent with ischemic heart disease; coronary artery vasospasm (including Prinzmetal variant angina); significant underlying CV disease; cerebrovascular syndromes (including strokes of any type or transient ischemic attacks); peripheral vascular disease (including ischemic bowel disease); uncontrolled hypertension; hemiplegic or basilar migraine; severe hepatic impairment; hypersensitivity to any component of the product; within 24 hr of treatment with another 5-HT_1 agonist or an ergotamine-containing or ergot-type medication (eg, methysergide). Pregnancy Category: [C]

Interactions: Ergot derivatives (eg, dihydroergotamine): Risk of vasospastic reactions may be increased. Concomitant use within 24 hr of eletriptan is not recommended.
Other 5-HT-1 agonists: Concomitant use of other 5-HT_1 agonists within 24 hr of eletriptan is not recommended.
Potent cytochrome P450 3A4 inhibitors (eg, clarithromycin, itraconazole, ketoconazole, nefazodone, nelfinavir, ritonavir, troleandomycin): Eletriptan should not be used within 72 hr of drugs that are potent CYP3A4 inhibitors.

Emtricitabine

Antiviral

Indications: In combination with other antiretroviral agents for the treatment of HIV-1 infections in adults.

Dose: Adults: PO 200 mg qd.
Renal impairment:
Adults: PO Ccr at least 50 mL/min administer 200 mg q 24 hr; Ccr 30 to 49 mL/min administer 200 mg q 48 hr; Ccr 15 to 29 mL/min administer 200 mg q 72 hr; Ccr less than 15 mL/min (including hemodialysis patients) 200 mg q 96 hr (if dosing on day of dialysis, give dose after dialysis).

Trade names: Emtriva Capsule 200 mg

Warnings: Standard considerations. Pregnancy Category: [B]

Interactions: None well documented.

Enalapril Maleate

Antihypertensive / ACE inhibitor

Indications: Treatment of hypertension and symptomatic CHF in combination with diuretics and digitalis and asymptomatic left ventricular dysfunction.

Unlabeled indication: Treatment of diabetic nephropathy, childhood hypertension, hypertension related to scleroderma, and renal crisis scleroderma.

Dose: Heart Failure:
Adults: PO Initial dose: 2.5 mg bid. Usual dose: 2.5 to 20 mg/day in 2 divided doses (max, 40 mg/day). Titrate doses upward as tolerated over a period of a few days or weeks. The max daily dose is 40 mg in divided doses.
High-Risk Patients:
Adults: IV Hypertensive patients at risk (eg, those with heart failure, hyponatremia, high-dose diuretic therapy, recent intensive diureses or increase in diuretic dose, renal dialysis, or severe volume or salt depletion of any etiology) have potential for extremely hypotensive response. Initiate therapy under very close medical supervision. The starting dose should be 0.625 mg or less administered IV over a period of 5 min or more and preferably longer (up to 1 hr).
Hypertension:
Adults: PO Initial dose: 2.5 to 5 mg/day. Titrate to desired BP control. Usual maintenance dose: 10 to 40 mg/day in single or twice daily doses. IV 1.25 mg over a 5-min period q 6 hr. For patients with Ccr of 30 mL/min or less, the dose is 0.625 mg. Dose may be repeated if after 1 hr the clinical response is inadequate. Additional doses of 1.25 mg may be administered at 6-hr intervals. For dialysis patients, the initial dose is 0.625 mg or less given over 5 min or preferably longer (up to 1 hr).
Children: PO Initial dose: 0.08 mg/kg (up to 5 mg) qd. Adjust dose according to BP response. Doses above 0.58 mg/kg (or in excess of 40 mg) have not been studied in pediatric patients.
Left Ventricular Dysfunction:

Adults: PO Initial dose: 2.5 mg bid. Titrate to targeted daily dose of 20 mg in divided doses.
Renal Function Impairment:
Adults: PO Titrate dosage upward until BP is controlled or until a max dosage of 40 mg/day is reached. Use an initial dosage of 5 mg/day in normal renal function and mild impairment (Ccr more than 30 mL/min); 2.5 mg/day in moderate to severe renal impairment (Ccr 30 mL/min or less); and 2.5 mg on the day of dialysis in dialysis patients (adjust dosage on nondialysis days based on BP response).
Trade names: Vasotec Tablets 2.5 mg
Vasotec IV Injection 1.25 mg enalaprilat/mL
Warnings: History of angioedema related to previous treatment with an ACE inhibitor and in patients with hereditary or idiopathic angioedema; hypersensitivity to ACE inhibitors. Pregnancy Category: [D (second, third trimester); C (first trimester)]
Interactions: Allopurinol: Greater risk of hypersensitivity possible with coadministration.
Antacids: Enalapril bioavailability may be decreased. Separate administration times by 1 to 2 hr.
Capsaicin: Cough may be exacerbated.
Digoxin: May increase or decrease plasma levels of digoxin.
Indomethacin, salicylates (eg, aspirin): Hypotensive effects may be reduced, especially in low-renin or volume-dependent hypertensive patients.
Lithium: Increased lithium levels and symptoms of lithium toxicity may occur.
Phenothiazines: May increase pharmacologic effect of enalapril.
Potassium preparations, potassium-sparing diuretics: May increase serum potassium levels.
Rifampin: Pharmacologic effects of enalapril may be decreased.

Enalapril Maleate/ Felodipine

Antihypertensive combinations
Indications: Hypertension: Not indicated for initial treatment of hypertension.
Dose: Adult: PO 1 tablet qd for patients whose BP is not adequately controlled with felodipine or enalapril monotherapy. If inadequate BP control persists beyond 1 to 2 wk, increase to 2 tablets/day.
Trade names: Lexxel Extended-release tablets enalapril maleate 5 mg/felodipine 2.5 mg
Warnings: History of angioedema. Pregnancy Category: [C (first trimester); D (second and third trimesters)]
Interactions: Allopurinol: Enalapril may increase risk of hypersensitivity.
Antacids: Enalapril bioavailability may be decreased. Separate administration times by 1 to 2 hr.
Barbiturates: Effects of felodipine may be decreased.
Capsaicin: Enalapril-induced cough may be exacerbated.
Carbamazepine: Plasma levels of felodipine may be decreased, reducing effect.
CYP3A4 inhibitors (eg, erythromycin): Increased effect of felodipine.
Diuretics: Excessive reduction in BP may occur.
Food: Effects of felodipine may increase if given with grapefruit juice.
Hydantoins: Serum felodipine levels may be decreased, reducing effects.
Indomethacin: Hypotensive effects may be reduced, especially in low-renin or volume-dependent hypertensive patients.
Lithium: Increased lithium levels and symptoms of lithium toxicity may occur.
Phenothiazine: Enalapril may increase pharmacological effect of phenothiazines.
Potassium preparations, potassium-sparing diuretics: Enalapril may increase serum potassium levels.
Rifampin: Pharmacologic effects of enalapril may be decreased.

Enalapril Maleate/ Hydrochlorothiazide

Antihypertensive
Indications: Treatment of hypertension.
Dose: Adults: PO 1 to 2 tablets (each containing 10 mg enalapril maleate and 25 mg hydrochlorothiazide) per day.
Trade names: Vaseretic 5-12.5 Tablets 12.5 mg hydrochlorothiazide, 5 mg enalapril maleate
Vaseretic 10-25 Tablets 25 mg hydrochlorothiazide, 10 mg enalapril maleate
Warnings: Hypersensitivity to any component or to other sulfonamide-derived drugs; history of angioedema related to previous treatment with ACE inhibitor; anuria. Pregnancy Category: [D (second, third trimester); C (first trimester)]
Interactions: Cholestyramine and colestipol resins: May bind to hydrochlorothiazide and decrease its bioavailability.
Diazoxide: Hyperglycemia may occur.
Digitalis glycosides: Arrhythmias may occur.
Indomethacin: Hypotensive effects may be reduced.
Lithium: Toxicity risk is greater; avoid use.
Loop diuretics: Synergistic effects may cause profound diuresis and electrolyte abnormalities.
Potassium preparations, potassium-sparing diuretics: May increase serum potassium levels.
Sulfonylureas: May require dose adjustment.

Enoxaparin Sodium

Anticoagulant
Indications: Prevention of deep vein thrombosis (DVT), which may lead to pulmonary embolism (PE) in patients undergoing hip or knee replacement surgery or abdominal surgery; in conjunction with warfarin sodium for inpatient treatment of acute DVT with and without PE or outpatient treatment of acute DVT without PE; prevention of ischemic complications of unstable and non-Q-wave MI when coadministered with aspirin. In medical patients who are at risk for thromboembolic complications due to severely restricted mobility during acute illness.
Dose: Hip or Knee Replacement Surgery:
Adults: SC 30 mg bid, with initial dose given within 12 to 24 hr postoperatively, provided hemostasis has been established. Average duration of administration is 7 to 10 days, up to 14 days. For hip replacement surgery, 40 mg qd, given initially 9 to 15 hr prior to surgery; continue prophylaxis for 3 wk.
Abdominal Surgery:
Adults: SC 40 mg/day with the initial dose given 2 hr prior to surgery. Usual duration of administration is 7 to 10 days; up to 12 days.
Acute Illness:
Adults: SC 40 mg qd for 6 to 11 days, up to 14 days, in patients at risk for thromboembolic complications caused by severely restricted mobility during acute illness.
DVT/PE Treatment:
Outpatient: SC 1 mg/kg q 12 hr.
Inpatient: SC 1 mg/kg q 12 hr or 1.5 mg/kg qd (same time each day).
Outpatient and inpatient: Initiate warfarin therapy when appropriate (usually within 72 hr of enoxaparin). Continue enoxaparin for a minimum of 5 days and until a therapeutic anticoagulant effect has been achieved. The average duration is 7 days; up to 17 days has been well tolerated.
Unstable Angina/Non-Q-Wave MI:
Adults: SC 1 mg/kg q 12 hr in conjunction with oral aspirin therapy (100 to 325 mg qd); usual duration of treatment is 2 to 8 days, up to 12.5 days.
Thromboembolic Recurrence/Prophylaxis:
Adults: SC 40 mg qd.

Trade names: Lovenox Injection 30 mg/0.3 mL
Warnings: Hypersensitivity to enoxaparin, heparin, or pork products; active major bleeding; thrombocytopenia associated with positive in vitro test for antiplatelet antibody in presence of enoxaparin. Pregnancy Category: [B]
Interactions: Anticoagulants, NSAIDs, platelet inhibitors: Use enoxaparin with care because of increased risk of hemorrhagic reactions.
Incompatability: Do not mix enoxaparin with other injections or infusions.

Ephedrine

Vasopressor / Decongestant
Indications: IM/IV/SC: Treatment of acute hypotensive states; treatment of Adams-Stokes syndrome with complete heart block; stimulation of CNS to combat narcolepsy and depressive states; treatment of acute bronchospasm; treatment of enuresis; treatment of myasthenia gravis; allergic disorders, such as bronchial asthma.

Nasal: Treatment of nasal congestion; promotion of nasal or sinus drainage; relief of eustachian tube congestion.

PO: Temporary relief of shortness of breath, tightness of chest, and wheezing caused by bronchial asthma. Eases breathing for asthma patients by reducing spasms of bronchial muscles.
Dose: Asthma:
Adults and children 12 yr and older: PO 12.5 to 25 mg q 4 hr, not to exceed 150 mg in 24 hr.
Adults: SC/IM/IV 25 to 50 mg SC or IM, or 5 to 25 mg administered by slow IV, repeated q 5 to 10 min, if necessary.
Children: SC/IM 0.5 to 0.75 mg/kg or 16.7 to 25 mg/m^2 q 4 to 6 hr.
Hypotension:
Adults: SC 25 to 50 mg. (IM/IV if rapid effect is needed) 10 to 25 mg may be given by IV push; may give additional doses at 5 to 10 min intervals (max, 150 mg/24 hr).
Children: IV/SC 3 mg/kg/day or 25 to 100 mg/m^2 /day in 4 to 6 divided doses.
Labor:
Adults: SC/IV/IM prn to maintain BP 130/80 mm Hg or less.
Nasal Congestion:
Adults: Nasal Dose is product specific. See labeling.
Trade names: Pretz-D Solution 0.25% ephedrine sulfate
Warnings: Angle-closure glaucoma; patients anesthetized with cyclopropane or halothane; cases in which vasopressor drugs are contraindicated (eg, thyrotoxicosis, diabetes mellitus, hypertension of pregnancy); MAOI therapy; narrow-angle glaucoma; nonanaphylactic shock during general anesthesia with halogenated hydrocarbons or cyclopropane. Pregnancy Category: [C Parenteral administration of ephedrine to maintain BP during low or other spinal anesthesia for delivery can cause acceleration of fetal heart rate Do not use in obstetrics when maternal BP exceeds 130/80]
Interactions: Alpha-adrenergic blockers (eg, phentolamine): Vasoconstricting and hypertensive effects are antagonized.
Diuretics: Vascular response may be decreased.
General anesthetics (eg, halothane, cyclopropane), cardiac glycosides: The potential for the myocardium to be sensitized to the effects of sympathomimetic amines is increased. Arrhythmias may result with coadministration and may respond to beta blockers.
Guanethidine: May negate antihypertensive effects.
MAOIs: Increases pressor response from vasopressors significantly; hypertensive crisis and intracranial hemorrhage are possible.
Rauwolfia alkaloids, methyldopa, furazolidone: May result in hypertension.
Tricyclic antidepressants: May potentiate pressor response.
Urinary acidifiers: May increase elimination of ephedrine.
Urinary alkalinizers: May decrease elimination of ephedrine.
Incompatability: Ephedrine is chemically incompatible with sodium bicarbonate; avoid admixture.

Epirubicin HCl

Antineoplastic antibiotic / Anthracycline
Indications: Breast cancer with axillary node involvement.

Unlabeled indication: Small-cell lung cancer, non-small-cell lung cancer, Hodgkin lymphoma, non-Hodgkin lymphoma.
Dose: Breast Cancer, Combination Therapy:
Adults: IV 100 mg/m^2 /day on day 1 of each 21-day cycle. An alternate regimen is 60 mg/m^2 /day IV on day 1 and day 8 of a 28-day cycle (for a total dose of 120 mg/m^2 during each cycle). Give a total of 6 cycles.
Renal Function Impairment: If bilirubin is 1.2 to 3 mg/dL or AST 2 to 4 times upper limit of normal (ULN), use 50% of recommended starting dose; if bilirubin is more than 3 mg/dL or AST more than 4 times ULN, use 25% of recommended starting dose.
Hepatic Function Impairment: If serum creatinine is more than 5 mg/dL, consider reducing dose 50%.
Lifetime Cumulative Doses of Epirubicin Above which Frequency of Cardiotoxicity Increases:
Adults: 900 mg/m^2 or less.
Adults who have received mediastinal radiation or treatment with other anthracyclines: 650 mg/m^2 or less.
Trade names: Ellence Preservative-free solution for injection 2 mg/mL
Warnings: Baseline neutrophil count less than 1500 cells/mm^3; severe myocardial insufficiency or recent MI; previous treatment with anthracyclines up to the max cumulative dose; hypersensitivity to epirubicin, other anthracyclines, or anthracenediones; severe hepatic dysfunction. Pregnancy Category: [D]
Interactions: Cimetidine: Cimetidine increases the AUC of epirubicin by 50%. Stop cimetidine treatment during treatment with epirubicin.

Erythromycin Ethylsuccinate/ Sulfisoxazole

Anti-infective
Indications: Treatment of acute otitis media in children caused by susceptible strains of *Haemophilus influenzae*.
Dose: Children: PO 50 mg/kg/day erythromycin and 150 mg/kg/day (max 6 gm/day) sulfisoxazole in equally divided doses qid for 10 days.
Trade names: Eryzole Granules for oral suspension Erythromycin ethylsuccinate (equivalent to 200 mg erythromycin activity) and sulfisoxazole acetyl (equivalent to 600 mg sulfisoxazole)per 5 mL when reconstituted
Pediazole Granules for oral suspension Erythromycin ethylsuccinate (equivalent to 200 mg erythromycin activity) and sulfisoxazole acetyl (equivalent to 600 mg sulfisoxazole)per 5 mL when reconstituted
Warnings: Hypersensitivity to chemically related drugs (eg, sulfonylureas, thiazide and loop diuretics, carbonic anhydrase inhibitors, sunscreens containing PABA, local anesthetics) or salicylates; patients taking terfenadine or astemizole; porphyria; use in infants younger than 20 mo, pregnant women at term and women nursing infants younger than 2 mo. Pregnancy Category: [C]
Interactions: Anticoagulants: May increase anticoagulant effects.

Antihistamines, non-sedating (eg, astemizole, terfenadine): Erythromycin significantly alters metabolism of terfenadine. Rare cases of serious cardiovascular events including death have been reported.
Astemizole, bromocriptine, carbamazepine, disopyramide, hexobarbital, methylprednisolone, phenytoin: May cause decreased metabolism and increased concentrations of these drugs.
Cyclosporine: Erythromycin may interfere with metabolism while sulfonamides may decrease cyclosporine levels; both increase risk of nephrotoxicity.
Digoxin: May increase digoxin levels.
Lovastatin: Severe myopathy or rhabdomyolysis may occur.
Methotrexate: Sulfonamides can displace methotrexate from protein-binding sites and increase free methotrexate levels.
Sulfonylureas: Sulfisoxazole may potentiate hypoglycemic effects.
Theophyllines: May increase theophylline plasma concentrations.
Thiopental: May enhance anesthetic effects of thiopental.

Escitalopram Oxalate

Antidepressant / Selective serotonin reuptake inhibitor

Indications: Treatment of major depressive disorders as defined in DSM-IV.

Dose: Adults: PO Start with 10 mg once daily. The dose may be increased to 20 mg after 1 wk. However, 20 mg has not shown a clinical benefit over 10 mg.

Trade names: Lexapro Tablets 5 mg

Warnings: Standard consideration; concurrent use of MAO inhibitors or within 14 days of discontinuing MAO inhibitor treatment. Pregnancy Category: [C]

Interactions: Alcohol: May potentiate the effects of alcohol; use of alcohol is not recommended.
Carbamazepine: Consider possibility of decreased escitalopram serum concentrations and reduced efficacy.
Cimetidine: Serum levels may be increased by cimetidine.
CNS drugs: Use with caution.
Cyproheptadine: May decrease the pharmacologic effect of escitalopram.
Lithium: Serotonergic effects of escitalopram may be enhanced; use with caution.
MAO inhibitors: Do not use in patients receiving MAO inhibitor therapy or within 14 days of stopping such treatment.
Metoprolol: Serum levels may be increased by escitalopram.
Sumatriptan: Rare postmarketing reports of weakness, hyperreflexia, and incoordination following coadministration with selective serotonin reuptake inhibitors have been reported.

Esmolol HCl

Beta-adrenergic blocker

Indications: Short-term management of supraventricular tachyarrhythmias and noncompensatory sinus tachycardia.

Unlabeled indication: Treatment of caffeine toxicity; attenuation of cardiovascular responses to electroconvulsive therapy or induction of anesthesia; adjunct therapy for acute MI and unstable angina; treatment of thyroid storm.

Dose: Adults: Usual: IV 500 mcg/kg/min for 1 min; then infusion of 50 to 200 mcg/kg/min, which has been titrated to desired endpoint (eg, heart rate, BP) in 50 mcg/kg/min increments.

Trade names: Brevibloc Injection 10 mg/mL

Warnings: Sinus bradycardia; second- or third-degree heart block; CHF unless secondary to tachyarrhythmia treatable with beta-blockers; overt cardiac failure; cardiogenic shock. Pregnancy Category: [C]

Interactions: Clonidine: May enhance or reverse antihypertensive effect; potentially life-threatening increases in BP may occur, especially on withdrawal.
NSAIDs: Some agents may impair antihypertensive effect.
Prazosin: Potential for and degree of orthostatic hypotension may be increased.
Verapamil: Effects of both drugs may be increased.
Incompatability: 5% Sodium Bicarbonate Injection.

Esomeprazole Magnesium

Gastrointestinal / Proton Pump Inhibitor

Indications: Treatment of heartburn and other symptoms of gastroesophageal reflux disease (GERD); short-term treatment in healing and symptomatic resolution of erosive esophagitis; maintain symptom resolution and healing of erosive esophagitis; in combination with amoxicillin and clarithromycin for treatment of Helicobacter pylori infection and duodenal ulcer disease to eradicate *H. pylori*.

Dose: Healing of Erosive Esophagitis:
Adults: PO 20 or 40 mg once daily for 4 to 8 wk.
Maintenance of Healing of Erosive Esophagitis:
Adults: PO 20 mg once daily.
Symptomatic GERD:
Adults: PO 20 mg once daily for 4 wk.
H. pylori Eradication to Reduce Risk of Duodenal Ulcer Recurrence:
Adults: PO 40 mg once daily for 10 days in combination with amoxicillin 1000 mg bid and clarithromycin 500 mg bid for 10 days.

Trade names: Nexium Capsules, delayed-release 20 mg

Warnings: Standard considerations. Pregnancy Category: [B]

Interactions: Drugs dependent on gastric pH for bioavailability (eg, ketoconazole, iron salts, digoxin): Absorption of these drugs may be affected.

Estropipate

Estrogens

Indications: Management of moderate to severe vasomotor symptoms associated with menopause; female hypogonadism, female castration, primary ovarian failure, and atrophic conditions caused by deficient endogenous estrogen production; prevention and treatment of osteoporosis.

Dose: Dosage is calculated as estrone sulfate.
Vasomotor Symptoms:
Adults: PO 0.625 to 5 mg/day given cyclically.
Female Hypogonadism, Female Castration, Primary Ovarian Failure:
Adults: PO 1.25 to 7.5 mg/day for 3 wk followed by 8 to 10 day drug-free period.
Osteoporosis:
Adults: PO 0.625 mg/day for 25 days of 31-day cycle.
Atrophic Vaginitis, Kraurosis Vulvae:
Adults: PO 0.625 to 5 mg/day. Give cyclically.
Intravaginal 2 to 4 g/day. Give cyclically.

Trade names: Ogen Tablets 0.625 mg
Ortho-Est Tablets 0.625 mg

Warnings: Breast cancer; estrogen-dependent neoplasia; undiagnosed abnormal genital bleeding; thrombophlebitis or thromboembolic disorders associated with previous estrogen use; known or suspected pregnancy. Pregnancy Category: [X]

Interactions: Antidepressants, tricyclic: Estrogens may alter effects and increase toxicity of these agents.
Barbiturates, modafinil, rifampin, St. John's wort, topiramate: May decrease estropipate concentration.
Corticosteroids: An increase in the pharmacologic and toxicologic effects of corticosteroids may occur.
Hydantoins: Loss of seizure control or decreased

estrogenic effects may occur.

Etanercept

Immunomodulator

Indications: Reducing signs and symptoms and inhibiting the progression of structural damage in moderately to severely active rheumatoid arthritis; reducing signs and symptoms of moderately to severely active polyarticular-course juvenile rheumatoid arthritis (JRA) in patients responding inadequately to 1 or more disease-modifying antirheumatic drugs; reducing signs and symptoms of psoriatic arthritis; reducing signs and symptoms in patients with active ankylosing spondylitis. May be used in combination with methotrexate (MTX) in patients who do not respond adequately to MTX alone in the treatment of rheumatoid or psoriatic arthritis.

Unlabeled indication: Psoriasis; treatment of Wegener granulomatosis (orphan status).

Dose: Adults: SC 50 mg/wk, given as two 25 mg injections at separate sites on the same day or 3 or 4 days apart.
Children (4 to 17 yr): SC 0.8 mg/kg (max, 50 mg) per wk given. For patients weighing more than 31 kg, give the weekly dose as 2 injections, either on the same day or separated by 3 or 4 days.

Trade names: Enbrel Powder for injection, lyophilized 25 mg

Warnings: Sepsis; hypersensitivity to etanercept or to any of its components. Pregnancy Category: [B]

Interactions: None well documented. However, a 7% rate of serious infections was observed in a 24-wk study with patients receiving etanercept and anakinra therapy.

Ethacrynic Acid

Loop diuretic

Indications: Treatment of edema associated with CHF, hepatic cirrhosis, or renal disease; treatment of ascites, congenital heart disease, nephrotic syndrome.

Unlabeled indication: Treatment of glaucoma; treatment of nephrogenic diabetes insipidus, hypercalcemia.

Dose: Adults: PO 50 to 200 mg qd. IV 50 mg (0.5 to 1 mg/kg) qd.
Children: PO 25 mg qd.

Trade names: Edecrin Tablets 25 mg
Edecrin Sodium Powder for injection 50 mg (as ethacrynate sodium) per vial

Warnings: Anuria; infants; increasing azotemia; severe diarrhea; dehydration; electrolyte imbalance; hypotension. Pregnancy Category: [B]

Interactions: Aminoglycosides: May increase auditory toxicity.
Cisplatin: May cause additive ototoxicity.
Digitalis glycosides: Electrolyte disturbances may predispose to digitalis-induced atrial and ventricular arrhythmias.
Lithium: May increase plasma lithium levels and toxicity.
NSAIDs: May decrease effects of ethacrynic acid.
Salicylates: May impair diuretic response in patients with cirrhosis and ascites.
Thiazide diuretics: Synergistic effects may result in profound diuresis and serious electrolyte abnormalities.

Ethambutol HCl

Anti-infective / Antitubercular

Indications: Treatment of pulmonary tuberculosis in combination with 1 or more other antituberculous agents.

Dose: Adults and Children (13 yr and older): PO
In patients not previously treated with antituberculous therapy, administer 15 mg/kg as a single dose every 24 hr. In patients who have received previous antituberculous treatment, administer 25 mg/kg as a single dose every 24 hr.

Trade names: Myambutol Tablets 100 mg

Warnings: Patients with known optic neuritis; hypersensitivity to any component of the product. Pregnancy Category: [B]

Interactions: Aluminum salts (eg, aluminum hydroxide): The absorption of ethambutol may be delayed or reduced; separate the administration times by several hours.

Ethinyl Estradiol/ Levonorgestrel

Contraceptive / Hormone

Indications: Prevention of pregnancy in women after known or suspected contraceptive failure or unprotected intercourse.

Dose: Adult and postpubertal females: Pregnancy test is used to verify presence or absence of pregnancy. Medication is not given if the patient is already pregnant. PO 2 tablets as soon as possible but within 72 hr of unprotected intercourse. Repeat with the remaining 2 tablets in 12 hr. May be used at any time during the menstrual cycle.

Trade names: Preven Tablets Ethinyl estradiol 0.05 mg; levonorgestrel 0.25 mg

Warnings: The following contraindications for daily cyclical oral contraceptives may or may not apply to emergency contraception: known or suspected pregnancy; current or history of pulmonary embolism; current or history of ischemic heart disease; history of cerebrovascular accidents; valvular heart disease with complications; severe hypertension; diabetes mellitus with vascular involvement; headaches with focal neurological symptoms; major surgery with prolonged immobilization; known or suspected carcinoma of the breast or personal history of breast cancer; benign or malignant liver tumors; or active liver disease. Pregnancy Category: [No significant effects on fetal development associated with long-term use before pregnancy or when taken inadvertently during early pregnancy]

Interactions: None well documented.

Ethionamide

Anti-infective / Antitubercular

Indications: Treatment of tuberculosis, in combination with other agents, in patients with *Mycobacterium tuberculosis* resistant to isoniazid or rifampin, or when there is intolerance to other antituberculous agents.

Dose: Adults: PO 15 to 20 mg/kg taken once daily (max, 1 g/day). To reduce GI intolerance, initiate therapy with 250 mg/day and titrate to optimal dose as tolerated (eg, 250 mg/day for 1 or 2 days, followed by 250 mg bid for 1 or 2 days, subsequently increasing the dose to 1 g in 3 or 4 divided doses).
Children 12 yr and older: PO 10 to 20 mg/kg/day in 2 to 3 divided doses given after meals or 15 mg/kg q 24 hr as a single daily dose.

Trade names: Trecator-SC Tablets 250 mg

Warnings: Severe hepatic impairment; hypersensitivity to any component of the product. Pregnancy Category: [C]

Interactions: Antituberculous agents (eg, cycloserine): Adverse effects may be potentiated.
Cycloserine: Risk of occurrence of adverse effects or convulsions may be increased.
Ethanol: Risk of occurrence of psychotic reactions may be increased.
Isoniazid: Transient increases in isoniazid serum levels may occur.

Ethosuximide

Anticonvulsant / Succinimide

Indications: Control of absence (petit mal) seizures.

Dose: Adults and Children 6 yr and older: PO 500 mg/day. Optimal dose for most children is 20 mg/kg/day. Maintenance therapy: Individualize dose. Increase daily dose slowly by 250 mg q 4 to 7 days until control is achieved with minimal side effects. Administered doses exceeding 1.5 g/day in divided doses under strict medical supervision.
Children 3 to 6 yr: Initial dose: PO 250 mg/day.

Trade names: Zarontin Capsules 250 mg

Warnings: Hypersensitivity to succinimides. Pregnancy Category: [Anticonvulsant drugs have been observed to increase the incidence of birth defects]

Interactions: Hydantoins: May increase serum hydantoin levels.
Primidone: Lower primidone and phenobarbital levels may occur.

Etidronate Disodium

Hormone / Biphosphonates

Indications: Treatment of symptomatic Paget disease; prevention and treatment of heterotopic ossification; treatment of hypercalcemia of malignancy.

Unlabeled indication: Treatment of postmenopausal osteoporosis.

Dose: Paget Disease:
Adults: PO Initial treatment is 5 to 10 mg/kg/day (not to exceed 6 mo) or 11 to 20 mg/kg/day (not to exceed 3 mo). Reserve doses greater than 10 mg/kg/day for specific situations. For retreatment, initiate only after etidronate-free period of at least 90 days and if there is evidence of active disease.
Heterotopic Ossification from Spinal Cord Injury:
Adults: PO 20 mg/kg/day for 2 wk followed by 10 mg/kg/day for 10 wk; total treatment period is 12 wk.
Heterotopic Ossification Complicating Total Hip Replacement:
Adults: PO 20 mg/kg/day for 1 mo preoperatively followed by 20 mg/kg/day for 3 mo postoperatively.
Hypercalcemia:
Adults: IV 7.5 mg/kg/day for 3 successive days given by slow infusion (over a period of at least 2 hr). Retreatment may be needed; wait at least 7 days between courses. Adjust dose for renal impairment. Regimen of oral etidronate (20 mg/kg/day for 30 days) may be started after last infusion.

Trade names: Didronel Tablets 200 mg
Didronel IV Injection 30 mg/mL

Warnings: Hypersensitivity to biphosphonates; patients with class Dc and higher renal functional impairment (serum creatinine greater than 5 mg/dL). Pregnancy Category: [C]

Interactions: None well documented.

Etoposide

Podophyllotoxin derivative

Indications: Refractory testicular tumors, small-cell lung cancer.

Unlabeled indication: Bladder carcinoma, lymphomas, leukemias, Ewing sarcoma, Kaposi sarcoma, brain tumors, gestational trophoblastic tumors, ovarian germ cell tumors, refractory breast tumors, rhabdomyosarcomas, Wilms tumor, bone marrow transplantation.

Dose: Testicular Cancer:
Adults: IV 50 to 100 mg/m^2 /day for 3 to 5 days every 3 to 4 wk.
Small-Cell Lung Cancer:
Adults: IV 35 to 50 mg/m^2 /day IV for 4 to 5 days every 3 to 4 wk. PO 2 times the IV dose, rounded to nearest 50 mg, given orally for 21 days. Alternately, 50 mg/m^2 /day orally for 21 days has been given. Repeat regimen after a 1- to 2-wk rest period. Oral bioavailability of the capsules is erratic, averaging 50% (range, 25% to 75%).
Dosage Adjustment:
Adults: Hold etoposide if the platelet count is less than 50,000/mm^3 or the absolute neutrophil count is less than 500/mm^3.
Adjustment in Hepatic Insufficiency:
Adults: Dosage reduction may be warranted; specific guidelines are not available.
Adjustment in Renal Insufficiency:
Adults: For patients with Ccr of 16 to 50 mL/min, give 75% of the usual dose. Consider further dose reduction for those with Ccr 15 mL/min or less.

Trade names: VePesid Concentrate for injection 20 mg/mL
Toposar Concentrate for injection 20 mg/mL
Etopophos Powder for injection 100 mg vial

Warnings: Standard considerations. Pregnancy Category: [D]

Interactions: Warfarin: Etoposide may increase the hypoprothrombinemic effects of warfarin.

Ezetimibe

Antihyperlipidemic

Indications: Administration alone or with HMG-CoA reductase inhibitors as adjunctive therapy to diet for reduction of elevated total cholesterol, low density lipoprotein cholesterol (LDL), and apolipoprotein in patients with primary hypercholesterolemia; with atorvastatin or simvastatin for the reduction of elevated total cholesterol and LDL levels in patients with homozygous familial hypercholesterolemia as an adjunct to other lipid-lowering treatments or if such treatments are unavailable; as adjunctive therapy to diet for the reduction of elevated sitosterol and campesterol levels in patients with homozygous familial sitosterolemia.

Dose: Adults and children over 10 yr: PO 10 mg once daily.

Trade names: Zetia Tablets 10 mg

Warnings: Ezetimibe is contraindicated in combination with HMG-CoA reductase inhibitors in patients with active liver disease or unexplained persistent elevations in serum transaminases; hypersensitivity to any component of the product. Pregnancy Category: [C]

Interactions: Antacids: Aluminum- and magnesium-containing antacids decrease the peak concentration of ezetimibe but not the AUC.
Cholestyramine: The AUC of ezetimibe may be decreased.
Cyclosporine, fibric acid derivatives (eg, fenofibrate, gemfibrozil): Concentrations of ezetimibe may be increased.

Factor IX Concentrates

Antihemophilic

Indications: Management of Factor IX deficiency (hemophilia B, Christmas disease), bleeding episodes in patients with inhibitors to Factor VIII; reversal of coumarin anticoagulant hemorrhage; prevention or control of bleeding in patients with Factor VII deficiency (Proplex T only).

Dose: Adults and Children: IV Dose based on patient condition, degree of deficiency and desired level of Factor IX to be achieved.
Dosing guideline: 1 U/kg times body weight (kg) times desired increase (% of normal).
Factor VII deficiency: 0.5 U/kg times body weight (kg) times desired increase (% of normal), repeated q 4 to 6 h prn.
Hemarthroses: In hemophiliacs with inhibitors to Factor VIII, IV 75 IU/kg.
Maintenance: Usually, IV 10 to 20 IU/kg/day.
Hemophilia A patients with inhibitors to Factor VIII: IV

75 IU/kg as single dose followed by second dose in 12 hr if necessary.
Prophylaxis: In patients with hemophilia B, IV 10 to 20 IU/kg 1 to 2 times/wk.

Trade names: AlphaNine SD Concentrate Dried plasma fraction of Factors II, VII, IX, and X
Konyne 80 Concentrate Dried plasma fraction of coagulation Factors II, VII, IX, and X
Profilnine SD Concentrate Dried plasma fraction of coagulation Factors II, VII, IX, and X
Proplex T Concentrate Dried plasma fraction of coagulation Factors II, VII, IX, and X
BeneFix Concentrate Nonpyrogenic lyophilized powder preparation. Purified protein produced by recombinant DNA for use in therapy of Factor IX deficiency.
Hemonyne Concentrate Dried plasma fraction of coagulation Factors II, VII, IX, and X
Mononine Concentrate 100 IU Factor IX with non-detectable levels of Factors II, VII, and X per mL when reconstituted

Warnings: Treatment of Factor VII deficiency (except for Proplex T); liver disease with signs of intravascular coagulation or fibrinolysis. Pregnancy Category: [C]

Interactions: Aminocaproic acid: May increase risk of thrombosis.

Famciclovir

Anti-infective / Antiviral

Indications: Treatment of acute herpes zoster; treatment or suppression of recurrent genital herpes in immunocompetent patients; treatment of recurrent mucocutaneous herpes simplex infections in HIV-infected patients.

Dose: Herpes zoster:
Adults: PO 500 mg q 8 hr for 7 days. Initiate treatment immediately after diagnosis.
Herpes Simplex:
Adults:
Recurrent Genital Herpes: PO 125 mg bid for 5 days. Initiate treatment at the first sign of recurrence.
Adults:
Suppression Of Recurrent Genital Herpes: PO 250 mg bid for up to 1 year.
HIV-Infected Patients:
Adults:
Recurrent orolabial or genital herpes: PO 500 mg bid for 7 days.
Renal Impairment:
Adults:
Herpes Zoster: Ccr 60 mL/min or more - 500 mg q 8 hr; Ccr 40 to 59 mL/min - 500 mg q 12 hr; Ccr 20 to 39 mL/min - 500 mg q 24 hr; Ccr less than 20 mL/min - 250 mg q 24 hr.
Adults:
Recurrent Genital Herpes: Ccr 40 or more - 125 mg q 12 hr; Ccr 20 to 39 - 125 mg q 24 hr; Ccr less than 20 - 125 mg q 24 hr.

Trade names: Famvir Tablets 125 mg

Warnings: Hypersensitivity to famciclovir, other components of the formulation, or penciclovir cream. Pregnancy Category: [B]

Interactions: Digoxin: Famciclovir may increase digoxin serum concentration.
Probenecid or other drugs significantly eliminated by active renal tubular secretion: May increase famciclovir (penciclovir) serum concentrations.

Famotidine

Histamine H_2 antagonist

Indications: Short-term treatment and maintenance therapy for duodenal ulcer, gastroesophageal reflux disease (GERD, including erosive or ulcerative disease), benign gastric ulcer, treatment of pathologic hypersecretory conditions.

Unlabeled indication: Treatment of upper GI bleeding; prevention of stress ulcers; prior to anesthesia for prevention of pulmonary aspiration of gastric acid.

Dose: Duodenal Ulcer (Active): PO 40 mg at bedtime or 20 mg bid for 6 to 8 wk.
Maintenance: 20 mg at bedtime.
Benign Gastric Ulcer (Acute): PO 40 mg at bedtime.
GERD:
Adults: 20 mg bid (max 6 wk). For esophagitis and accompanying symptoms caused by GERD, 20 to 40 mg bid (max 12 wk).
Pathologic Hypersecretory Conditions:
Adults: Start at 20 mg q 6 hr, continued as clinically indicated; doses up to 160 mg q 6 hr have been used.
Moderate or Severely Impaired Renal Function: (Ccr less than 10 mL/min) May need to reduce to half the dose or increase dosing interval to 36 to 48 hr.
For Hospitalized Patients with Pathologic Hypersecretory Conditions or Intractable Ulcers, or Patients Unable to Take Orally:
Parenteral: 20 mg IV q 12 hr. Parenteral use in GERD not established.

Trade names: Pepcid Tablets 20 mg
Pepcid AC Tablets, chewable 10 mg
Pepcid AC Tablets 10 mg
Pepcid AC Gelcaps 10 mg
Pepcid RPD Tablets, orally disintegrating 20 mg

Warnings: Hypersensitivity to other H -2 antagonists. Pregnancy Category: [B]

Interactions: Ketoconazole: Effects of ketoconazole may be decreased.

Felbamate

Anticonvulsant

Indications: Monotherapy or adjunctive therapy in treatment of partial seizures with and without generalization in epileptic adults. Adjunctive therapy in treatment of partial and generalized seizures associated with Lennox-Gastaut syndrome in children.

Dose: Because of reports of aplastic anemia, it has been recommended to stop use of this drug unless health care provider decides that withdrawal would cause greater risk.
Initial Monotherapy:
Adults and Adolescents 14 yr and older: PO 1200 mg/day in 3 or 4 divided doses; increase in 600 mg increments q 2 wk to 2400 mg/day and then 3600 mg/day if indicated.
Conversion to Monotherapy:
Adults and Adolescents 14 yr and older:
Initial dose: PO 1200 mg/day in 3 or 4 divided doses, reducing dose of other antiepileptic drugs by 1/3. At wk 2, increase felbamate to 2400 mg/day and at week 3, increase to 3600 mg/day; continue to reduce dose of other antiepileptic drugs as indicated.
Adjunctive Therapy:
Adults and adolescents 14 yr and older:
Initial dose: PO 1200 mg/day in 3 or 4 divided doses; reduce original dose of other antiepileptic drugs by 20% to 33% for 1 wk. At week 2, increase felbamate to 2400 mg/day and at week 3, increase to 3600 mg/day if needed; reduce dosage of other antiepileptic drugs as clinically indicated.
Children 2 to 14 yr with Lennox-Gastaut Syndrome: PO 15 mg/kg/day in 3 or 4 divided doses while reducing other antiepileptic drugs at least 20%. Increase felbamate by 15 mg/kg/day increments at weekly intervals up to 45 mg/kg/day; continue to reduce dosage of other antiepileptic drugs as needed.

Trade names: Felbatol Tablets 400 mg

Warnings: Hypersensitivity to felbamate or ingredients of this product; hypersensitivity reactions to other carbamates; history of any blood dyscrasia or hepatic dysfunction. Pregnancy Category: [C]

Interactions: Antiepileptic drugs: Felbamate may increase blood levels of phenytoin and valproic acid and decrease blood levels of carbamazepine. Phenytoin or carbamazepine may increase clearance of felbamate.

Felodipine

Calcium channel blocker

Indications: Treatment of hypertension.

Dose: PO 2.5 to 10 mg once daily. Max 20 mg once daily. Elderly rarely require more than 10 mg qd.

Trade names: Plendil Tablets, extended release 2.5 mg

Warnings: Sick sinus syndrome; second- or third-degree AV block except with functioning pacemaker; hypotension with systolic BP less than 90 mm Hg. Pregnancy Category: [C]

Interactions: Barbiturates: Effects of felodipine may be decreased.
Carbamazepine: Plasma levels of felodipine may be decreased, reducing effect.
Food: Effects of felodipine may increase if given with grapefruit juice.
Histamine H_2 -antagonists: Cimetidine may increase effects of felodipine.
Hydantoins: Serum felodipine levels may be decreased, reducing effects.
Other antihypertensive agents: May have additive effects.

Fenofibrate

Antihyperlipidemic

Indications: Adjunctive therapy to diet for treatment of hypertriglyceridemia in adult patients with type IV or V hyperlipidemia who are at risk of pancreatitis; adjunctive therapy to diet for the reduction of HDL cholesterol, total cholesterol, triglycerides, and apolipoprotein B, and to increase HDL cholesterol in adults with primary hypercholesterolemia or mixed dyslipidemia (Fredrickson types IIa and IIb).

Dose: Primary Hypercholesterolemia/Mixed Hyperlipidemia:
Adults: PO Initial dose is 160 mg/day.
Hypertriglyceridemia:
Adults: PO Start with 54 to 160 mg/day (max, 160 mg/day).

Trade names: Tricor Capsules 67 mg

Warnings: Hepatic or severe renal dysfunction including primary biliary cirrhosis; patients with unexplained persistent liver function abnormality; pre-existing gallbladder disease. Pregnancy Category: [C]

Interactions: Bile acid sequestrants (eg, cholestryramine): Reduces absorption of fenofibrate.
Cyclosporine (eg, Sandimmune): Increases risk of nephrotoxicity.
HMG-CoA reductase inhibitors (eg, lovastatin): Increased risk of severe myopathy, rhabdomyolysis, and acute renal failure.
Oral anticoagulants (eg, warfarin): Anticoagulant effect may be increased.

Fenoprofen Calcium

Analgesic / NSAID

Indications: Symptomatic relief for rheumatoid arthritis, osteoarthritis, mild to moderate pain.

Unlabeled indication: Symptomatic relief for juvenile rheumatoid arthritis; migraine prophylaxis and treatment.

Dose: Rheumatoid Arthritis/Osteoarthritis: PO 300 to 600 mg tid to qid; do not exceed 3.2 g/day.
Mild/Moderate Pain: PO 200 mg q 4 to 6 h prn.

Trade names: Nalfon Pulvules Capsules 200 mg

Warnings: Sensitivity to aspirin or other NSAIDs; preexisting renal disease. Pregnancy Category: [B]

Interactions: Anticoagulants: May increase risk of bleeding caused by gastric erosion.
Methotrexate: May increase methotrexate levels.
Phenobarbital: Phenobarbital, an enzyme inducer, may decrease fenoprofen half-life. Dosage adjustments of fenoprofen may be required if phenobarbital is added or withdrawn.

Filgrastim

Colony-stimulating factor

Indications: Decrease incidence of infection, manifested by febrile neutropenia, in patients with nonmyeloid malignancies receiving myelosuppressive anticancer drugs; cancer patients receiving myelosuppressive chemotherapy; cancer patients receiving bone-marrow transplant; patients with severe chronic neutropenia (SCN); peripheral blood progenitor cell (PBPC) collection and therapy in cancer patients.

Unlabeled indication: Filgrastim may be beneficial in AIDS, drug-induced and congenital agranulocytosis, alloimmune neonatal neutropenia.

Dose: Myelosuppressive chemotherapy: IV/SC 5 mcg/kg/day as a single daily injection; may increase in increments of 5 mcg/kg for each chemotherapy cycle.
Bone marrow transplant: IV/SC 10 mcg/kg/day given as an IV infusion of 4 or 24 hr or as a continuous 24 hr SC infusion.
Severe chronic neutropenia:
Congenital neutropenia:
Starting dose: 6 mcg/kg twice daily SC qd.
Idiopathic or cyclic neutropenia:
Starting dose: 5 mcg/kg as a single injection SC qd.
Dose adjustments: Chronic daily administration is required to maintain clinical benefit. Do not use ANC as the sole indication of efficacy. Individually adjust the dose based on the patients' clinical course as well as ANC. In the Phase III study, the target ANC was 1500 to 10,000/mm^3. However, patients may experience clinical benefit with ANCs below this target range. Reduce the dose if the ANC is persistently more than 10,000/mm^3.

Trade names: Neupogen Injection 300 mcg/mL

Warnings: Hypersensitivity to Escherichia coli-derived proteins. Pregnancy Category: [C]

Interactions: Drugs that may potentiate the release of neutrophils, such as lithium, should be used with caution.
Incompatability: Precipitate may form if diluted with saline.

Finasteride

Androgen hormone inhibitor

Indications: Treatment of symptomatic benign prostatic hyperplasia (BPH).

Unlabeled indication: Adjuvant monotherapy following radical prostatectomy; prevention of progression of first-stage prostate cancer; treatment of male-pattern baldness, acne, and hirsutism.

Dose: Adults: PO 5 mg qd.

Trade names: Proscar Tablets 5 mg
Propecia Tablets 1 mg

Warnings: Use during pregnancy or lactation and use in children. Pregnancy Category: [X]

Interactions: None well documented.

Flavoxate

Urinary tract antispasmodic / Alkalinizer

Indications: Symptomatic relief of dysuria, urgency, nocturia, suprapubic pain, frequency and incontinence associated with cystitis, prostatitis, urethritis, urethrocystitis/urethrotrigonitis.

Dose: Adults and Children (more than 12 yr): PO 100 to 200 mg 3 to 4 times/day.

Trade names: Urispas Tablets 100 mg

Warnings: Pyloric or duodenal obstruction; obstructive intestinal lesions or ileus; achalasia; GI hemorrhage; obstructive uropathies of lower urinary tract. Pregnancy Category: [B]

Interactions: None well documented.

Flecainide Acetate

Antiarrhythmic

Indications: Prevention of paroxysmal atrial fibrillation/flutter (PAF) associated with disabling symptoms; paroxysmal supraventricular tachycardias (PSVTs); prevention of documented life-threatening ventricular arrhythmias.

Dose: PSVT, PAF:
Adults:
Initial dose: PO 50 mg q 12 hr, increasing by 50 mg bid q 4 days until efficacy is achieved.
Max PSVT: 300 mg/day.
Sustained Ventricular Tachycardia:
Adults:
Initial dose: PO 100 mg q 12 hr, increasing to 150 mg bid if needed.
Max: 400 mg/day.

Trade names: Tambocor Tablets 50 mg

Warnings: Preexisting second- or third-degree AV block; right bundle branch block when associated with a left hemiblock (unless a pacemaker is present); recent MI; presence of cardiogenic shock. Pregnancy Category: [C]

Interactions: Amiodarone: Increased flecainide plasma levels.
Cimetidine: Increased bioavailability and clearance of flecainide.
Digoxin: Increased digoxin plasma levels.
Propranolol: Levels of either drug may be increased; additive negative inotropic effects.
Smoking: Increased dosage may be required.
Urinary acidifiers: Effects of flecainide may be decreased.
Urinary alkalinizers: Effects of flecainide may be increased.

Fluconazole

Anti-infective / Antifungal

Indications: Oropharyngeal and esophageal candidiasis; vaginal candidiasis; prevention of candidiasis in bone marrow transplant; Cryptococcal meningitis.

Dose: Candidemia and Disseminated Candida Infections:
Children: PO/IV 6 to 12 mg/kg/day.
C. meningitis: 12 mg/kg on first day, followed by 6 mg/kg/day (or 12 mg/kg/day based on medical judgment of patient's response). Recommended duration is 10 to 12 wk after CSF becomes culture negative.
Newborns: Experience is limited to pharmacokinetic studies in premature newborns. Prolonged $t_{1/2}$ has been noted. These children, in the first 2 wk of life, should receive the same mg/kg dosage as other children, but administered q 72 hr. After the first 2 wk, dose qd.
Cryptococcal Meningitis:
Adults: PO/IV 400 mg first day, followed by 200 mg qd thereafter (400 mg may be used) for 10 to 12 wk after CSF culture is negative for initial meningitis; 200 mg qd for suppression of relapse of cryptococcal meningitis.
Oropharyngeal or Esophageal Candidiasis:
Adults: PO/IV 200 mg first day, followed by 100 mg qd thereafter for minimum of 2 wk for oropharyngeal candidiasis, or for 3 wk and at least 2 wk following resolution of symptoms for esophageal candidiasis.
Children: PO/IV 6 mg/kg on first day, followed by 3 mg/kg qd thereafter for minimum of 2 wk for oropharyngeal candidiasis or 3 wk (at least 2 wk after symptom resolution) for esophageal candidiasis.
Prevention of Candidiasis in Bone Marrow Transplant:
Adults: PO/IV 400 mg qd; in patients with anticipated severe granulocytopenia (less than 500 neutrophils/mm^3), start fluconazole several days before anticipated onset and continue 7 days after neutrophil count rises more than 1000 cells/mm^3.
Systemic Candida Infections:
Adults: Optimal therapeutic dosage and duration not established; however, in noncomparative studies of small numbers of patients, doses up to 400 mg/day have been used.
UTIs and Peritonitis:
Adults: Daily doses of 50 to 200 mg have been used in open, noncomparative studies of small numbers of patients.
Vaginal Candidiasis:
Adults: PO 150 mg single dose.

Trade names: Diflucan Tablets 50 mg

Warnings: Coadministration of cisapride; hypersensitivity to any component of the product. Pregnancy Category: [C]

Interactions: Alfentanil, benzodiazepines (eg, midazolam), buspirone, corticosteroids(eg, prednisone), losartan, nisoldipine, sulfonylureas (eg, glyburide), tacrolimus, theophylline, tricyclic antidepressants, vinca alkaloids (eg, vincristine), zidovudine, zolpidem: Levels may be elevated by fluconazole, increasing the risk of side effects and toxicity.
Anticoagulants (eg, warfarin): Anticoagulant effect may be increased.
Cimetidine, rifamycins (eg, rifampin): Fluconazole plasma levels may be reduced, decreasing therapeutic effects.
Cisapride: Contraindicated; increased cisapride plasma levels with cardiotoxicity may occur.
Cyclosporine: Increased cyclosporine concentrations.
Hydantoins (eg, phenytoin): Increased hydantoin levels.
Hydrochlorothiazide: May increase fluconazole levels, increasing side effects.

Flucytosine

Anti-infective / Antifungal

Indications: Treatment of serious infections caused by susceptible strains of Candida or Cryptococcus.

Unlabeled indication: Treatment of chromomycosis.

Dose: Adults and Children more than 50 kg: PO 50 to 150 mg/kg/day in divided doses q 6 hr.

Trade names: Ancobon Capsules 250 mg

Warnings: Standard considerations. Pregnancy Category: [C]

Interactions: Amphotericin B: Increased therapeutic action and toxicity of flucytosine.
Cytosine: Inactivates antifungal activity of flucytosine.

Fludarabine Phosphate

Purine antimetabolite

Indications: Refractory or progressive chronic B-cell lymphocytic leukemia.

Unlabeled indication: Leukemias, non-Hodgkin's lymphoma.

Dose: Chronic Lymphocytic Leukemia:
Adults: IV 25 to 30 mg/m^2 /day in single daily doses for 5 consecutive days. Repeat course of therapy q 21 to 28 days for 3 additional courses after maximal response is achieved.
Adjustment in Renal Insufficiency:
Adults: IV May require dosage reduction. No specific guidelines published.

Trade names: Fludara Powder for injection 50 mg

Warnings: Standard considerations. Pregnancy Category: [D]

Interactions: Pentostatin: Concomitant therapy may cause severe or fatal pulmonary toxicity.

Fludrocortisone Acetate

Mineralocorticoid

Indications: Partial replacement therapy for primary and secondary adrenocortical insufficiency in Addison disease; treatment of salt-losing adrenogenital syndrome.

Unlabeled indication: Treatment of severe orthostatic hypotension.

Dose: Addison Disease:
Adults: PO 0.05 to 0.1 mg/day (range, 0.1 mg 3 times/wk to 0.2 mg/day).
Salt-Losing Adrenogenital Syndrome:
Adults: PO 0.1 to 0.2 mg/day.

Trade names: Florinef Acetate Tablets 0.1 mg

Warnings: Systemic fungal infections. Pregnancy Category: [C]

Interactions: Amphotericin, potassium-losing diuretics: May increase potassium loss.
Anticholinesterase agents (eg, neostigmine): May antagonize the effects of anticholinesterase agents in myasthenia gravis.
Anticoagulants (eg, warfarin): Dose requirement of anticoagulant may be reduced or effect opposed.
Barbiturates, hydantoins (eg, phenytoin), rifampin: Decreased fludrocortisone activity.
Salicylates: Serum levels may be reduced by corticosteroids, decreasing the effectiveness; in addition, the ulcerogenic effects of both agents may be increased.

Flumazenil

Antidote

Indications: Complete or partial reversal of sedative effects of benzodiazepines where general anesthesia induced or maintained with benzodiazepines, where sedation produced with benzodiazepines for diagnostic or therapeutic procedures, and for the management of benzodiazepine overdose.

Dose: Reversal of Conscious Sedation or in General Anesthesia:
Adults: IV 0.2 mg over 15 sec. If desired level of consciousness is not achieved in 45 sec, additional 0.2 mg doses can be administered at 60 sec intervals (max, 1 mg). In event of resedation, repeat doses (0.2 mg/min to max 1 mg) at 20 min intervals as needed (max, 3 mg/hr).
Management of Suspected Benzodiazepine Overdose:
Adults: IV 0.2 mg over 30 sec. If desired level of consciousness is not achieved in 30 sec, an additional dose of 0.3 mg over 30 sec can be administered. Further doses of 0.5 mg over 30 sec can be administered at 1 min intervals as needed (max, 3 mg).

Trade names: Romazicon Injection 0.1 mg/mL

Warnings: Hypersensitivity to flumazenil or benzodiazepines; in patients given benzodiazepines for control of a potentially life-threatening condition (eg, status epilepticus); in patients showing signs of serious cyclic antidepressant overdose. Pregnancy Category: [C Labor and delivery: Not recommended
Effects on newborn are unknown.

Interactions: Toxic effects of other drugs taken in toxic doses may emerge with reversal of benzodiazepine effect.

Flunisolide

Corticosteroid

Indications: Inhalation: Maintenance treatment of asthma for patients requiring chronic treatment with corticosteroids.

Intranasal: Symptoms of perennial or seasonal rhinitis.

Dose: Adults and Children 6 to 15 yr of age:
Inhalation 2 inhalations (500 mcg) bid.
Adults: Do not exceed 4 inhalations bid (2 mg/day).
Children: Do not exceed 2 inhalations bid (1 mg/day).
Adults:
Initial dose: Intranasal 2 sprays (50 mcg) in each nostril bid (200 mcg/day).
Max: 8 sprays in each nostril daily (400 mcg/day).
Children 6 to 14 yr of age:
Initial dose: Intranasal 1 spray (25 mcg) in each nostril tid or 2 sprays in each nostril bid.
Max: 4 sprays in each nostril daily (200 mcg/day).

Trade names: AeroBid Aerosol approximately 250 mcg/actuation
AeroBid-M Aerosol approximately 250 mcg/actuation
Nasarel Nasal spray 0.025% (25 mcg/actuation)

Warnings: Primary treatment of status asthmaticus or acute asthma when intensive measures are required (inhalation use); untreated local infection of the nasal mucosa (intranasal use); hypersensitivity to any component of the product. Pregnancy Category: [C]

Interactions: None well documented.

Fluocinonide

Corticosteroid

Indications: Relief of inflammatory and pruritic manifestations of corticosteroid-responsive dermatoses.

Dose: Apply to the affected area as a thin film 2 to 4 times/day depending on the severity of the condition.

Trade names: Lidex Cream 0.05%
Lidex-E Cream 0.05%

Warnings: Standard considerations. Pregnancy Category: [C]

Interactions: None well documented.

Fluorouracil

Pyrimidine antimetabolite

Indications: Colon, rectum, breast, gastric, and pancreatic carcinoma (injection); multiple actinic or solar keratoses, superficial basal cell carcinoma (topical).

Unlabeled indication: Ovarian, cervical, bladder, hepatic, islet cell, prostate, endometrial, esophageal, and head and neck carcinoma.

Dose: Colon, Rectum, Breast, Gastric, and Pancreatic Carcinomas:
Adults: IV Individualize dosage based on actual body weight. Use lean body weight if patient is obese or has abnormal fluid retention.
Initial dose: 12 mg/kg/day for 4 days. Do not exceed 800 mg/day. If no toxicity is observed, give 6 mg/kg on days 6, 8, 10, and 12. No therapy is given on days 5, 7, 9, or 11. Discontinue at end of day 12, even with no apparent toxicity.
In poor risk patients and those with inadequate nutritional status: 6 mg/kg/day for 3 days. If no toxicity is observed, give 3 mg/kg on days 5, 7, and 9. Give no therapy on days 4, 6, or 8. Do not exceed 400 mg/day.
Maintenance therapy: Start maintenance therapy 30 days after the last dose. If no toxicity is observed with the first course of therapy, repeat that dose of fluorouracil at 30-day intervals. If toxicity is observed with the first course of therapy, after the patient has recovered from initial toxicity, use a single weekly dose of 10 to 15 mg/kg. Do not exceed a weekly maintenance dose of 1000 mg. Poor risk patients may require a reduced maintenance dose.
Multiple Actinic or Solar Keratoses:
Adults: Topical Apply enough medication to cover affected areas bid for 2 to 6 wk. Complete healing may not occur until 1 to 2 mo after therapy is stopped. Continue medication until the inflammatory response reaches the erosion stage.
Carac: The 0.5% cream is only indicated for the face and anterior scalp areas. Using fingertips, apply qd to cover lesions with a thin film. Do not apply near eyes, nostrils, or mouth. Apply 10 min after thoroughly washing, rinsing, and drying the entire area. After application, wash hands thoroughly. Continued treatment up to 4 wk results in greater lesion reduction.
Superficial Basal Cell Carcinoma (5% Strength Only):
Adults: Topical Apply a sufficient amount to cover the lesions bid for 3 to 6 wk. Treatment may be required for

10 to 12 wk.
Trade names: Adrucil Injection 50 mg/mL
Carac Cream 0.5%
Efudex Cream 5%
Fluoroplex Cream 1%
Warnings: Poor nutritional status; depressed bone marrow function; potentially serious infections; hypersensitivity to fluorouracil or product components; pregnancy (topical); dihydropyrimidine dehydrogenase enzyme (DPD) deficiency (Carac). Pregnancy Category: [D (injection) X (topic)]
Interactions: Cimetidine: May increase serum concentrations of fluorouracil and potentially increase toxicity.
Leucovorin: Leucovorin may enhance GI toxicity of fluorouracil. Fatalities have occurred because of severe toxic enterocolitis.

Fluphenazine

Antipsychotic / Phenothiazine
Indications: Fluphenazine HCl: Management of psychotic disorders.

Fluphenazine decanoate: Long-acting parenteral depot products for long-term antipsychotic therapy.

Unlabeled indication: Nausea/vomiting.
Dose: Fluphenazine HCl:
Adults: PO Initially, 2.5 to 10 mg/day in divided doses at 6 to 8 hr intervals. When symptoms are controlled, gradually reduce dosage to 1 to 5 mg/day.
Fluphenazine Decanoate:
Adults: IM/SC
Initial dose: 12.5 to 25 mg. Do not exceed 100 mg/dose.
Usual dosing interval: 1 to 4 wk and as long as 6 wk in some patients.
Trade names: Fluphenazine HCl Tablets 1 mg
Prolixin Decanoate Injection 25 mg/mL
Warnings: Allergy to any phenothiazine; comatose or severely depressed states; concurrent use of large doses of other CNS depressants; bone marrow depression or blood dyscrasias; liver damage; cerebral arteriosclerosis; coronary artery disease; severe hypotension or hypertension; subcortical brain damage. Pregnancy Category: [Pregnancy category undetermined]
Interactions: Alcohol and other CNS depressants: Increased CNS depression; may precipitate extrapyramidal reaction.
Anticholinergics: Reduced therapeutic effects and increased anticholinergic side effects of fluphenazine; may lead to tardive dyskinesia.
Barbiturate anesthetics: Increased frequency and severity of neuromuscular excitation and hypotension.
Beta-blockers: Increased plasma levels of both drugs.
Bromocriptine: Effectiveness of bromocriptine may be reduced.
Cisapride, sparfloxacin: The risk of life-threatening cardiac arrhythmias, including torsades de pointes, may be increased.
Guanethidine: Hypotensive action may be inhibited.
Hydantoins (eg, phenytoin): Increase or decrease in phenytoin levels.
Lithium: May result in disorientation, unconsciousness, and extrapyramidal symptoms.
Metrizamide: Increased seizure risk.
Paroxetine: Plasma levels of fluphenazine may be elevated, increasing the risk of side effects.

Flurazepam Hydrochloride

Sedative and hypnotic / Benzodiazepine
Indications: Treatment of insomnia.
Dose: Adults: PO 15 to 30 mg at bedtime.
Elderly: PO 15 mg until individual response is determined.
Debilitated patients: PO 15 mg until individual response is determined.
Trade names: Dalmane Capsules 15 mg
Warnings: Hypersensitivity to benzodiazepines; pregnancy. Pregnancy Category: [Contraindicated]
Interactions: Alcohol, other CNS depressants: Additive CNS depressant effects; may continue several days after discontinuation.
Cimetidine, disulfiram, oral contraceptives, isoniazid, omeprazole: Increased effects of flurazepam.
Digoxin: Serum digoxin concentrations may increase.
Phenytoin: Serum concentrations may be increased.
Rifampin: Decreased effects of flurazepam.
Theophyllines: May antagonize sedative effects.

Flutamide

Antiandrogen / Antineoplastic hormone
Indications: Metastatic prostate cancer, combination therapy with a luteinizing hormone-releasing hormone (LHRH) analog (eg, goserelin, leuprolide).

Unlabeled indication: Treatment of hirsutism in women (250 mg/day).
Dose: Prostate Cancer:
Adults: PO 250 mg (2 capsules) q 8 hr.
Stage B-2-C Prostatic Carcinoma:
Adults: PO Start treatment at 8 wk prior to initiating radiation therapy and continue during radiation therapy.
Stage D-2 Metastatic Carcinoma:
Adults: PO Initiate flutamide capsules with the LHRH agonist and continue until progression.
Trade names: Eulexin Capsules for oral use 125 mg
Warnings: Patients with severe hepatic impairment. Pregnancy Category: [D]
Interactions: Prothrombin time may increase when flutamide therapy is initiated in patients stabilized on chronic warfarin therapy.

Fluticasone Propionate/ Salmeterol

Respiratory Inhalant Combination
Indications: Long-term, maintenance treatment of asthma.
Dose: Advair Diskus is available in 3 strengths, containing 100, 250, and 500 mcg of fluticasone propionate each in combination with 50 mcg of salmeterol.
Adults and Children 12 yr and older: Inhalation 1 inhalation bid (morning and evening, approximately 12 hr apart). For patients not currently on an inhaled corticosteroid, the recommended starting dose is fluticasone/salmeterol 100/50 bid. For patients on an inhaled corticosteroid, the recommended starting dose of fluticasone/salmeterol varies from 100/50 to 500/50 bid depending on the concomitant inhaled corticosteroid and the dose.
Trade names: Advair Diskus Powder for inhalation 100 mcg fluticasone propionate, 50 mcg salmeterol
Warnings: Primary treatment of status asthmaticus or other acute episodes of asthma in which intensive measures are required; hypersensitivity to any component of the product. Pregnancy Category: [C]
Interactions: Beta-adrenergic blocking agents (eg, propranolol): May block the pulmonary effect of salmeterol.
Inhibitors of cytochrome P450 3A4 (eg, ketoconazole): Plasma levels of fluticasone may be increased and plasma cortisol AUC may be reduced.
Long-acting beta-2-agonists: Since this product already contains salmeterol, do not use other long-acting inhaled beta -2 -agonists for prevention of exercise-induced bronchospasm or maintenance treatment of asthma.

Loop diuretics (eg, furosemide), thiazide diuretics (eg, hydrochlorothiazide): ECG changes and hypokalemia may be worsened.
MAO inhibitors (eg, isocarboxazid), tricyclic antidepressants (eg, amitriptyline): Use with extreme caution in patients receiving these agents or within 2 wk of discontinuation.

Fluvastatin

Antihyperlipidemic / HMG-CoA reductase inhibitor

Indications: Atherosclerosis: To slow the progression of coronary atherosclerosis.

Hypercholesterolemia: Reduction of elevated total cholesterol, LDL, apo-B, and triglyceride cholesterol levels and to increase HDL levels.

Secondary prevention of coronary events: To reduce the risk of undergoing coronary revascularization procedures in patients with coronary heart disease.

Dose: Adults: PO 20 to 80 mg qd.

Trade names: Lescol Capsules 20 mg
Lescol XL Tablets, extended-release 80 mg

Warnings: Active liver disease or unexplained persistent elevations of LFTs; pregnancy; lactation. Pregnancy Category: [X]

Interactions: Azole antifungal agents (eg, fluconazole), cyclosporine, gemfibrozil, macrolide antibiotics (eg, erythromycin), niacin: Severe myopathy or rhabdomyolysis may occur with coadministration.
Cholestyramine: Reduced absorption of fluvastatin if taken with or up to 4 hr after cholestyramine.
Cimetidine, ranitidine, omeprazole: Fluvastatin serum levels may be increased.
Diclofenac, digoxin, glyburide, hydantoins: Serum levels of these agents may be increased.
Rifampin: Fluvastatin serum levels may be reduced.
Warfarin: Anticoagulant effect of warfarin may be increased.

Fluvoxamine Maleate

Antidepressant / Selective serotonin inhibitor

Indications: Treatment of obsessive-compulsive disorder as defined in DSM-III-R.

Dose: Adults: PO 50 mg as a single dose at bedtime initially.
Usual range: 100 to 300 mg/day. Increase dose in 50-mg increments q 4 to 7 days, as tolerated, until max therapeutic benefit is achieved (max, 300 mg/day). Give total daily doses more than 100 mg in 2 divided doses; if doses are unequal, give larger dose at bedtime.
Maintenance: Dosage is adjusted to maintain patient on lowest effective dosage. Periodically reassess need to continue treatment.
Children (8 to 17 yr): PO Start with 25 mg as a single daily dose at bedtime.
Usual range: 50 to 200 mg/day. Increase dose in 25-mg increments q 4 to 7 days, as tolerated, until max therapeutic benefit is achieved (max, 200 mg/day). Give total daily doses of more than 50 mg in 2 divided doses; if doses are unequal, give larger dose at bedtime.

Trade names: Luvox Tablets 25 mg

Warnings: Do not use within 14 days of starting or stopping MAO inhibitors or in combination with cisapride or pimozide. Pregnancy Category: [C]

Interactions: 5-HT-1 agonists (eg, naratriptan, rizatriptan, sumatriptan, zolmitriptan): Weakness, hyperreflexia, and incoordination have been reported rarely.
Cisapride, pimozide: Increased plasma concentrations of cisapride cause QT prolongation and have been associated with sometimes fatal torsades de pointes-type ventricular tachycardia.
Cyproheptadine: May antagonize the effects of fluvoxamine.
Lithium, tryptophan: May enhance serotonergic effects of fluvoxamine.
MAO inhibitors: Similar selective serotonin inhibitors can cause serious (sometimes fatal) reactions. Do not give fluvoxamine in combination with MAO inhibitors or less than 14 days of discontinuation of MAO inhibitors. After stopping fluvoxamine, wait at least 2 wk before starting MAO inhibitors.
Smoking: Increases metabolism of fluvoxamine.
Sympathomimetics (eg, amphetamine), St. John's wort: May increase the risk of serotonin syndrome.
Warfarin, clozapine, tricyclic antidepressants, benzodiazepines (eg, alprazolam, diazepam, midazolam, triazolam), carbamazepine, methadone, metoprolol, propranolol, theophylline, tacrine, cyclosporine: Plasma levels of these drugs may be increased.

Formoterol Fumarate

Bronchodilator / Sympathomimetic

Indications: Long-term maintenance treatment of asthma; prevention of bronchospasms; prevention of exercise-induced bronchospasm; concomitant therapy with short-acting beta -2 -agonists, inhaled or systemic corticosteroids, and theophylline therapy; long-term administration in the maintenance of bronchoconstriction in patients with chronic obstructive pulmonary disease (COPD), including chronic bronchitis and emphysema.

Dose: Maintenance Treatment of Asthma:
Adults and Children at least 5 yr: Inhalation 12 mcg q 12 hr.
Prevention of Exercise-Induced Bronchospasm:
Adults and Children at least 12 yr: Inhalation 12 mcg 15 min prior to exercise given on an occasional, as-needed basis.
Maintenance Treatment of COPD:
Adults: Inhalation 12 mcg q 12 hr (max, 24 mcg/24 hr).

Trade names: Foradil Aerolizer Inhalation powder in capsules 12 mcg (as fumarate)

Warnings: Standard considerations. Pregnancy Category: [C]

Interactions: Diuretics, steroids, xanthine derivatives: May potentiate the hypokalemic effect of formoterol.
Nonpotassium sparing diuretics (eg, loop or thiazide diuretics): ECG changes and hypokalemia may be worsened by formoterol.
MAOIs, tricyclic antidepressants, drugs known to prolong the QT-c interval: Formoterol may potentiate these agents, increasing the risk of cardiac arrhythmia.
Beta blockers: Effects of both agents may be inhibited.

Foscarnet Sodium

Anti-infective / Antiviral

Indications: Treatment of CMV retinitis in patients with AIDS; treatment of acyclovir-resistant mucocutaneous HSV infections in immunocompromised patients; combination therapy with ganciclovir for patients who have relapsed after monotherapy with either drug.

Dose: CMV Retinitis:
Adults: IV
Initial dose: 60 mg/kg/dose at constant rate over at least 1 hr q 8 hr for 2 to 3 wk. Adjust for clinical response and renal function.
Maintenance dose: 90 mg/kg/day infused over 2 hr, individualized; max maintenance dose is 120 mg/kg/day.
HSV Infections:
Adults: IV
Initial dose: 40 mg/kg/dose (min, 1 hr infusion) q 8 or 12 hr for 2 to 3 wk or until healed.
Maintenance: 90 mg/kg/day given as an IV infusion over 2 hr, individualized; max maintenance dose is 120 mg/kg/day.

Trade names: Foscavir Injection 24 mg/mL
Warnings: Standard considerations. Pregnancy Category: [C]
Interactions: Nephrotoxic drugs: Elimination of foscarnet may be impaired by drugs that inhibit renal tubular secretion. Increased potential for nephrotoxicity with aminoglycosides, amphotericin B, and IV pentamidine.
Pentamidine: Concomitant IV pentamidine may cause hypocalcemia.
Zidovudine: Increased risk of anemia.
Incompatability: Do not give other drugs or supplements via same IV catheter.

Fosinopril Sodium

Antihypertensive / ACE inhibitor

Indications: Hypertension; heart failure.
Dose: Heart Failure:
Adults: PO
Initial dose: 10 mg qd. Increase over several weeks. Usual range is 20 to 40 mg/day. Do not exceed 40 mg/day.
Hypertension:
Adults: PO
Initial dose: 10 mg qd.
Maintenance dose: 20 to 80 mg/day; if inadequate response, consider dividing into 2 doses.
Children (weighing more than 50 kg): PO 5 to 10 mg qd as monotherapy.
Trade names: Monopril Tablets 10 mg
Warnings: Hypersensitivity to ACE inhibitor; history of angioedema related to previous treatment with an ACE inhibitor and in patients with hereditary or idiopathic angioedema. Pregnancy Category: [D (second, third trimester); C: (first trimester)]
Interactions: Allopurinol: Increased risk of hypersensitivity reactions.
Antacids: May decrease effects of fosinopril.
Capsaicin: Cough may be exacerbated.
Digoxin: May increase or decrease levels of digoxin.
Indomethacin, salicylates (eg, aspirin): Hypotensive effects may be reduced, especially in low-renin or volume-dependent hypertensive patients.
Lithium: Increased lithium levels and symptoms of lithium toxicity may occur.
Phenothiazines: May increase pharmacologic effect of fosinopril.
Potassium preparations, potassium-sparing diuretics: May increase serum potassium levels.

Fosphenytoin

Anticonvulsant / Hydantoin

Indications: Short-term parenteral administration when other means of phenytoin administration are unavailable, inappropriate, or less advantageous; treatment of generalized convulsive status epilepticus; prevention and treatment of seizures occurring during neurosurgery; short-term substitution for oral phenytoin.
Dose: To avoid the need to perform molecular weight-based adjustments when converting between fosphenytoin and phenytoin sodium, the fosphenytoin dose is expressed as phenytoin sodium equivalents (PE).
Status Epilepticus:
Adults: IV
Initial/Loading dose: 15 to 20 mg PE/kg.
Maintenance and Non-Emergent Dose:
Adults: IV/IM
Loading dose: 10 to 20 mg PE/kg
Maintenance dose: 4 to 6 PE/kg/day.
Trade names: Cerebyx Injection 150 mg (100 mg phenytoin sodium)
Warnings: Hypersensitivity to phenytoin or other hydantoins; patients with sinus bradycardia, sino-atrial block, second- and third-degree AV block, and Adams-Stokes syndrome. Pregnancy Category: [D]
Interactions: Amiodarone, benzodiazepines, chloramphenicol, cimetidine, disulfiram, estrogens, felbamate, fluconazole, fluoxetine, isoniazid, oxyphenbutazone, phenacemide, phenylbutazone, succinimides, sulfonamides: May increase phenytoin serum concentrations and effects.
Antineoplastic drugs, carbamazepine, diazoxide, enteral nutritional therapy, rifabutin, rifampin, sucralfate: May decrease serum phenytoin concentrations and effects.
Corticosteroids, coumarin anticoagulants, doxycycline, estrogens, felodipine, levodopa, loop diuretics, methadone, oral contraceptives, mexiletine, quinidine, rifabutin, rifampin: The effects of these agents may be impaired.
Cyclosporine: Cyclosporine concentrations may be decreased.
Disopyramide: Disopyramide concentrations and bioavailability may be decreased, while anticholinergic actions may be enhanced.
Divalproex sodium, phenobarbital, sodium valproate, valproic acid: May increase or decrease phenytoin concentrations and effects.
Folic acid: May cause folic acid deficiency.
Itraconazole: Effects of itraconazole may be decreased, while those of phenytoin may be increased.
Metyrapone: Phenytoin may cause subnormal response to metyrapone.
Non-depolarizing muscle relaxants: May cause these agents to have shorter duration or decreased effects.
Primidone: May increase concentrations of primidone and metabolites, increasing the effects.
Sympathomimetics (eg, dopamine): May cause profound hypotension and possibly cardiac arrest.
Theophyllines: Effects of either agents may be decreased.
Incompatability: Do not mix with other drugs.

Frovatriptan Succinate

Analgesic / Migraine

Indications: Acute treatment of migraine attacks with or without aura in adults.
Dose: Adults: PO 2.5 mg with fluids; if headache recurs after initial relief, a second 2.5-mg tablet may be taken provided the interval is at least 2 hr between doses (max, three 2.5 mg tablets/day).
Trade names: Frova Tablets 2.5 mg (as base)
Warnings: Patients with ischemic heart disease (eg, angina pectoris, history of MI, documented silent ischemia); history of symptoms or findings consistent with ischemic heart disease, coronary artery vasospasm, including Prinzmetal variant angina or other underlying CV disease; cerebrovascular syndromes (eg, strokes of any type, transient ischemic attacks); peripheral vascular disease (eg, ischemic bowel disease); uncontrolled hypertension; hemiplegic or basilar migraine; within 24 hr of another 5-HT_1 agonist, and ergotamine-containing or ergot-type medication (eg, dihydroergotamine); hypersensitive to frovatriptan or any inactive ingredient in the tablet. Pregnancy Category: [C]
Interactions: Contraceptives, oral and propranolol: May increase frovatriptan plasma concentrations.
Ergotamine-containing or ergot-type drugs (eg, methysergide): May reduce frovatriptan plasma levels; additive prolonged vasospastic reactions may occur.
Other 5-HT-1 agonists (eg, sumatriptan): Contraindicated within 24 hr of frovatriptan administration.
SSRIs (eg, fluoxetine): May cause weakness, hyperreflexia, and incoordination when given concurrently.

Furosemide

Loop diuretic

Indications: Treatment of edema associated with CHF, hepatic cirrhosis, and renal disease;

hypertension.
Dose: Edema:
Adults: PO 20 to 80 mg/day as a single dose; may titrate up to 600 mg/day. IV/IM 20 to 40 mg qd or bid.
Hypertension:
Adults: PO 40 mg bid.
Max dose: 6 mg/kg.
CHF and Chronic Renal Failure:
Adults: PO Up to 2 to 2.5 g/day. IV Up to 2 to 2.5 g/day.
Max IV bolus: 1 g/day over 30 min.
Acute Pulmonary Edema:
Adults: IV 40 mg (over 1 to 2 min). If response not satisfactory within 1 hr, increase to 80 mg.
Infants and Children: PO
Usual dose: 0.5 to 2 mg/kg qd or bid.
Max dose: 6 mg/kg. IV/IM
Usual dose: 1 mg/kg
Max dose: 6 mg/kg.
Trade names: Lasix Tablets 20 mg
Warnings: Hypersensitivity to sulfonylureas; anuria. Pregnancy Category: [C]
Interactions: Aminoglycosides: May increase auditory toxicity.
Charcoal: May reduce absorption of furosemide.
Cisplatin: May cause additive ototoxicity.
Digitalis glycosides: Electrolyte disturbances may predispose to digitalis-induced arrhythmias.
Lithium: May increase plasma lithium levels and toxicity.
NSAIDs: May decrease effects of furosemide.
Phenytoin: May reduce diuretic effects of furosemide.
Salicylates: May impair diuretic response in patients with cirrhosis and ascites.
Thiazide diuretics: Synergistic effects that may result in profound diuresis and serious electrolyte abnormalities.
Incompatability: Gentamicin, milrinone, or netilmicin in D5W or NS: Do not add to furosemide solution; precipitate forms. Highly acidic solutions of pH less than 5.5: Do not mix with furosemide solution.

Gabapentin

Anticonvulsant

Indications: Adjunctive therapy in treatment of partial seizures with or without secondary generalization in patients above 12 yr with epilepsy; adjunctive therapy for partial seizures in children 3 to 12 yr; management of postherpetic neuralgia in adults.
Dose: Epilepsy:
Adults and children above 12 yr: PO 900 to 1800 mg/day in divided doses tid. Initial dose: 300 mg on day 1 and titrate upward rapidly. To minimize CNS side effects, administer initial dose on day 1 at bedtime.
Children 3 to 12 yr: PO Initiate therapy at 10 to 15 mg/kg/day in divided doses (ie, tid) and titrate dose upward over a period of about 3 days to the effective dose.
Children at least 5 yr: PO The effective dose is 25 to 35 mg/kg/day in divided doses (ie, tid).
Children 3 to 4 yr: PO The effective dose is 40 mg/kg/day in divided doses (ie, 3 times/day).
Postherpetic Neuralgia:
Adults: PO Start with a single 300 mg dose on day 1, 600 mg on day 2 (divided bid), and 900 mg on day 3 (divided tid). Subsequently, titrate the dose upward as needed for pain relief to a daily dose of 1800 mg (divided tid).
Trade names: Neurontin Capsules 100 mg
Warnings: Standard considerations. Pregnancy Category: [C]
Interactions: Antacids: May reduce bioavailability of gabapentin.
Cimetidine: Reduces renal clearance of gabapentin.

Galantamine Hydrobromide

Cholinesterase inhibitor

Indications: Treatment of mild to moderate dementia of the Alzheimer type.
Dose: Adults: PO 4 mg bid. May increase to 8 mg bid after 4 wk. A further increase to 12 mg bid may be attempted after min 4 wk at previous dose.
Trade names: Reminyl Tablets 4 mg (as base)
Warnings: Standard considerations. Pregnancy Category: [B]
Interactions: Bethanechol, succinylcholine: May act synergistically with galantamine.
Erythromycin; ketoconazole; paroxetine: May elevate galantamine levels, increasing the risk of side effects.

Gallium Nitrate

Hypocalcemic agent

Indications: Treatment of symptomatic, cancer-related hypercalcemia unresponsive to adequate hydration.
Dose: Adults: IV 100 to 200 mg/m^2 /day for 5 consecutive days.
Trade names: Ganite Injection 25 mg/mL
Warnings: Severe renal impairment (serum creatinine more than 2.5 mg/dL). Pregnancy Category: [C]
Interactions: Nephrotoxic drugs (eg, aminoglycosides, amphotericin B): May increase risk for development of renal insufficiency.

Ganciclovir

Anti-infective / Antiviral

Indications: IV: Treatment of CMV retinitis in immunocompromised patients, including patients with AIDS; prevention of CMV disease in organ transplant patients at risk for CMV.

Oral: Alternative to the IV formulation for maintenance treatment of CMV retinitis in immunocompromised patients, including patients with AIDS, in whom retinitis is stable following appropriate induction therapy and for whom the risk of more rapid progression is balanced by the benefit associated with avoiding daily IV infusions; prevention of CMV disease in solid organ transplant recipients and in individuals with advanced HIV infection at risk for developing CMV disease.

Unlabeled indication: Treatment of other CMV infections (eg, pneumonitis, gastroenteritis, hepatitis) in some immunocompromised patients.
Dose: CMV Retinitis:
Adults: IV Induction: 5 mg/kg over 1 hr q 12 hr for 14 to 21 days. Maintenance: 5 mg/kg over 1 hr qd or 6 mg/kg over 1 hr/day 5 days/wk (max 6 mg/kg over 1 hr).
PO Following induction treatment, the recommended maintenance dose of oral ganciclovir is 1000 mg 3 times/day with food. Alternatively, the dosing regimen of 500 mg 6 times/day q 3 hr with food, during waking hours, may be used.
CMV Prevention in Transplant Recipients:
Adults: IV 5 mg/kg over 1 hr q 12 hr for 7 to 14 days, followed by 5 mg/kg once daily 7 days/wk or 6 mg/kg once daily 5 days/wk. PO 1000 mg 3 times/day with food.
CMV Prevention in Advanced HIV Infection:
Adults: PO 1000 mg 3 times daily with food.
Decreased Renal Function:
Adults: IV Induction: 5 mg/kg q 12 hr (Ccr at least 70 mL/min); 2.5 mg/kg q 12 hr (Ccr 50 to 69 mL/min); 2.5 mg/kg q 24 hr (Ccr 25 to 49 mL/min); 1.25 mg/kg q 24 hr (Ccr 10 to 24 mL/min); 1.25 mg/kg 3 times a week following hemodialysis (Ccr less than 10 mL/min).
Maintenance: 5 mg/kg q 24 hr (Ccr at least 70 mL/min); 2.5 mg/kg q 24 hr (Ccr 50 to 69 mL/min); 1.25 mg/kg q 24 hr (Ccr 25 to 49 mL/min); 0.625 mg/kg q 24 hr (Ccr 10 to 24 mL/min); 0.625 mg/kg 3 times a week following hemodialysis (Ccr less than 10 mL/min). PO 1000 mg tid or 500 mg q 3 h, 6 times/day (Ccr at least 70 mL/min); 1500 mg qd or 500 mg tid (Ccr 50 to 69 mL/min); 1000 mg qd or 500 mg bid (Ccr 25 to 49 mL/

min); 500 mg qd (Ccr 10 to 24); 500 mg 3 times/wk, following hemodialysis (less than 10 mL/min).
Trade names: Cytovene Capsules 250 mg
Vitrasert Implant 4.5 mg
Warnings: Hypersensitivity to acyclovir. Pregnancy Category: [C]
Interactions: Amphotericin B, cyclosporine, nephrotoxic drugs: May increase serum creatinine.
Cytotoxic drugs: May cause added toxicity.
Didanosine: Ganciclovir may increase didanosine plasma levels. Ganciclovir levels may be decreased when administered 2 hr after didanosine but not when given simultaneously.
Imipenem-cilastatin: May cause generalized seizures.
Probenecid: May reduce renal clearance and increase serum levels of ganciclovir.
Zidovudine: Zidovudine and ganciclovir can cause granulocytopenia; combination therapy at full dose may not be tolerated.
Incompatability: Do not mix with other drugs.

Gatifloxacin

Antibiotic / Fluoroquinolone

Indications: For treatment of bacterial infections, including chronic bronchitis; acute sinusitis; community-acquired pneumonia; uncomplicated and complicated UTIs; pyelonephritis; uncomplicated urethral and cervical gonorrhea; uncomplicated skin and skin structure infections; uncomplicated rectal infections in women; bacterial conjunctivitis (ophthalmic).

Unlabeled indication: Atypical pneumonia; chronic prostatitis.
Dose: Acute Bacterial Exacerbation of Chronic Bronchitis: PO/IV 400 mg q 24 hr for 5 days.
Acute Pyelonephritis: PO/IV 400 mg q 24 hr for 7 to 10 days.
Acute Sinusitis: PO/IV 400 mg q 24 hr for 10 days.
Bacterial Conjunctivitis: Ophthalmic Days 1 and 2, instill 1 drop in affected eye(s) q 2 hr while awake, up to 8 times/day. Days 3 through 7, instill 1 drop up to qid while awake.
Complicated UTIs: PO/IV 400 mg q 24 hr for 7 to 10 days.
Community-Acquired Pneumonia: PO/IV 400 mg q 24 hr for 7 to 14 days.
Uncomplicated Skin and Skin Structure Infections: PO/IV 400 mg q 24 hr for 7 to 10 days.
Hemodialysis; Continuous Peritoneal Dialysis: PO/IV 400 mg initial dose then subsequent dose of 200 mg PO/IV q 24 hr (on day 2 of dosing).
Renal Impairment:
Adults:
Ccr more than 40 mL/min: PO/IV 400 mg initial dose then subsequent dose of 400 mg. PO/IV q 24 hr (on day 2 of dosing).
Ccr less than 40 mL/min: PO/IV 400 mg initial dose then subsequent dose of 200 mg. PO/IV q 24 hr (on day 2 of dosing).
Uncomplicated Urethral Gonorrhea in Men; Endocervical and Rectal Gonorrhea in Women: PO/IV 400 mg q 24 hr in a single dose.
Uncomplicated UTIs (Cystitis): PO/IV 400 or 200 mg q 24 hr. Single dose for 3 days.
Trade names: Tequin Tablets 200 mg
Zymar Ophthalmic solution 3 mg/mL
Warnings: Standard considerations. Pregnancy Category: [C]
Interactions: Aluminum- and magnesium-containing antacids, didanosine-buffered tablets, iron, or zinc salts: May decrease the bioavailability of gatifloxacin.
Antiarrhythmic agents (ie, class IA [eg, procainamide, quinidine], class III [eg, amiodarone, sotalol]), antipsychotics, cisapride, erythromycin, tricyclic antidepressants, any other drug known to prolong the QTc interval: May increase the risk of life-threatening cardiac arrhythmias, including torsades de pointes.
Digoxin: Plasma level of digoxin may be elevated, increasing the risk of toxicity.
NSAIDs: Coadministration may increase the risks of CNS stimulation and convulsions.
Probenecid: Renal clearance of gatifloxacin may be decreased, prolonging the $t_{1/2}$ and increasing plasma levels of gatifloxacin.
Incompatability: Amphotericin B; amphotericin B cholesteryl sulfate; cefoperazone sodium; cefonicid; cefozitin sodium; diazepam; furosemide; heparin sodium; mezlocillin disodium; phenytoin sodium; piperacillin sodium/tazobactam sodium; potassium phosphates; vancomycin in 5% dextrose injection.

Gemcitabine HCL

Nucleoside analog

Indications: Locally advanced or metastatic pancreatic adenocarcinoma in patients previously treated with 5-fluorouracil; locally advanced or metastatic non-small cell lung cancer.

Unlabeled indication: Bladder cancer; biliary cancer; metastatic breast cancer; relapsed or refractory testicular cancer; squamous cell carcinoma of the head and neck; ovarian cancer.
Dose: Pancreatic Adenocarcinoma:
Adults: IV
Cycle 1: 1000 mg/m^2 once weekly for 7 wk followed by 1 wk of rest.
Subsequent cycles: Give the same dose once weekly for 3 consecutive wk followed by 1 wk of rest. After at least 7 doses (1 cycle), the dose may be increased to 1250 mg/m^2 once weekly for 3 wk, followed by 1 wk of rest, if the following criteria are met:
• Nonhematologic toxicity is no greater than WHO Grade 1,
• Platelet nadirs are greater than 100,000 x 10 -6 /L,
• The absolute neutrophil count nadir is more than 1500 x 10 -6 /L. If the patient still meets the above criteria after receiving 3 doses of the higher regimen, the gemcitabine dose may be increased to 1500 mg/m^2 IV once weekly for 3 wk, followed by 1 wk of rest.
Non-Small Cell Lung Cancer:
Adults: IV In combination with cisplatin, 1000 mg/m^2 gemcitabine on days 1, 8, and 15 of each 28-day cycle. Alternatively, 1250 mg/m^2 gemcitabine may be given IV on days 1 and 8 of a 21-day cycle.
Dosage Adjustment:
Adults: Reduce or delay the gemcitabine dose in patients with neutropenia or thrombocytopenia on the day of treatment. On the day of the scheduled dose, if the absolute granulocyte count is 500 to 99 x 10 - 6 /L or the platelet count is 50,000 to 99,999 x 10 -6 /L, then give 75% of the prior dose. If the absolute granulocyte count is less than 500 x 10 -6 /L or the platelet count is less than 50,000 x 10 -6 /L, then hold dose. For grade 3 or 4 nonhematologic toxicity, hold gemcitabine or reduce the dose by 50% in patients with non-small cell lung cancer. Dosage reduction is not required for severe alopecia or nausea and vomiting. Dosage reduction may be necessary in impaired renal or hepatic function. Use additional caution in these patients.
Trade names: Gemzar Lyophilized powder for injection 200 mg
Warnings: Standard considerations. Pregnancy Category: [D]
Interactions: No specific drug interactions have been reported.

Gemfibrozil

Antihyperlipidemic

Indications: Treatment of hypertriglyceridemia in adult patients with type IV or V hyperlipidemia that presents risk of pancreatitis and does not respond to diet; reduction of coronary heart disease risk in type IIb patients who have low HDL levels (in addition to elevated LDL and triglycerides) and have not

responded to other measures.
Dose: Adults: PO 600 mg bid 30 min before morning and evening meals.
Trade names: Lopid Tablets 600 mg
Warnings: Hepatic or severe renal dysfunction, including primary biliary cirrhosis; preexisting gallbladder disease. Pregnancy Category: [B]
Interactions: Lovastatin: Increases risk of rhabdomyolysis.
Oral anticoagulants (eg, warfarin): Anticoagulant effect may be increased.

Glimepiride

Antidiabetic / Sulfonylurea
Indications: Adjunct to diet and exercise in type 2 diabetic patients whose hyperglycemia cannot be controlled by diet and exercise alone; in combination with insulin for type 2 diabetic patients with secondary failure to oral sulfonylureas.
Dose: Adults: PO 1 to 2 mg qd with breakfast or the first main meal of the day. Increase by 1 to 2 mg/dose. Titrate at 1 to 2 wk intervals based on blood glucose response. Maintenance: 1 and 4 mg daily (max, 8 mg/day). Combination therapy with insulin is appropriate for secondary failure to oral sulfonylureas. The same dosing recommendations apply.
Trade names: Amaryl Tablets 1 mg
Warnings: Hypersensitivity to sulfonylureas; diabetic ketoacidosis with or without coma. Pregnancy Category: [C Insulin is recommended to maintain blood glucose levels during pregnancy Prolonged severe neonatal hypoglycemia can occur if sulfonylureas are administered at time of delivery]
Interactions: Alcohol: Produces disulfiram-like reaction (eg, facial flushing, headache, breathlessness).
Chloramphenicol, clofibrate, fenfluramine, histamine H2 antagonists, miconazole, monoamine oxidase inhibitors, probenecid, salicylates, sulfinpyrazone, sulfonamides, tricyclic antidepressants, urinary acidifiers: May increase hypoglycemic effect.
Beta-blockers, cholestyramine, diazoxide, rifampin, thiazide diuretics, urinary alkalinizers: May decrease hypoglycemic effect.

Glucagon

Glucose elevating agent
Indications: Treatment of severe hypoglycemic reactions in diabetic patients when glucose administration is not possible or during insulin shock therapy in psychiatric patients; diagnostic aid in radiologic examination of stomach, duodenum, small bowel, and colon when diminished intestinal motility would be advantageous.

Unlabeled indication: Treatment of propranolol overdose, cardiovascular emergencies, and GI disturbances associated with spasms.
Dose: Hypoglycemia:
Adults and Children more than 20 kg: SC/IM/IV 1 mg (1 unit). Do not use glucagon at concentrations above 1 mg/mL (1 unit/mL).
Children less than 20 kg: SC/IM/IV 0.5 mg (0.5 unit) or a dose equivalent to 20 to 30 mcg/kg.
Insulin Shock Therapy:
Adults: SC/IM/IV 0.5 to 1 mg after 1 hr of coma (larger doses have been used to reverse coma). Patient will usually awaken in 10 to 25 min. If no response, may repeat dose.
Diagnostic Aid:
Adults and Children: IM/IV 0.25 to 2 mg depending on procedure and desired length of smooth muscle relaxation.
Trade names: Glucagon Emergency Kit Powder for Injection 1 mg (1 unit)
Glucagon Diagnostic Kit Powder for Injection 1 mg (1 unit)
Warnings: Standard considerations. Pregnancy Category: [B]
Interactions: Anticoagulants, oral: May increase hypoprothrombinemic effects, possibly with bleeding.

Glycopyrrolate

Anticholinergic / Antispasmodic
Indications: Oral: Adjunctive treatment of peptic ulcer.

Parenteral: Preoperative administration for reduction of salivary, tracheobronchial and pharyngeal secretions, reduction of volume and acidity of gastric secretions, and blockade of cardiac vagal inhibitory reflexes before and during induction of anesthesia and intubation; intraoperatively for counteraction of drug-induced or vagal traction reflexes with associated arrhythmias.
Dose: Peptic Ulcer:
Adults and Children older than 12 yr: PO 1 to 2 mg bid or tid. IM/IV 0.1 to 0.2 mg tid or qid.
Preanesthetic Medication:
Adults: IM 0.004 mg/kg 20 min to 1 hr prior to anesthesia.
Children younger than 12 yr: IM 0.0044 to 0.0088 mg/kg.
Children younger than 2 yr: IM up to 0.0088 mg/kg.
Intraoperative Medication:
Adults: IV 0.1 mg. May repeat at 2 to 3 min intervals.
Children: IV 0.004 mg/kg (max 0.1 mg in single dose); may repeat at 2 to 3 min intervals.
Reversal of Neuromuscular Blockade:
Adults and Children: IV 0.2 mg for each 1 mg neostigmine or 5 mg pyridostigmine. Administer simultaneously.
Trade names: Robinul Tablets 1 mg
Robinul Forte Tablets 2 mg
Warnings: Narrow angle glaucoma; adhesions between iris and lens; obstructive uropathy; obstructive disease of GI tract; paralytic ileus; intestinal atony of elderly or debilitated patients; severe ulcerative colitis; toxic megacolon complicating ulcerative colitis; hepatic or renal disease; tachycardia; myocardial ischemia; unstable cardiovascular status in acute hemorrhage; myasthenia gravis. Pregnancy Category: [B]
Interactions: Haloperidol: May cause decreased serum haloperidol levels, worsened schizophrenic symptoms, and tardive dyskinesia.
Incompatability: Because stability of glycopyrrolate is questionable above pH of 6, do not combine in same syringe with methohexital sodium, chloramphenicol sodium succinate, dimenhydrinate, pentobarbital sodium, thiopental sodium, secobarbital sodium, sodium bicarbonate, diazepam, dexamethasone sodium phosphate, or buffered solution of Lactated Ringer's solution.

Gold Sodium Thiomalate

Anti-inflammatory / Antirheumatic / Gold compound
Indications: Symptomatic relief of active adult and juvenile rheumatoid arthritis not adequately controlled by other therapies.

Unlabeled indication: Treatment of pemphigus and psoriatic arthritis.
Dose: Adults: IM As weekly injections: First wk, 10 mg; second wk, 25 mg; third and following wks, 25 to 50 mg until major clinical improvement or toxicity occurs. If cumulative dose reaches 1 g without improvement, re-evaluate use of gold therapy. Once improvement occurs, dose may be decreased or dosing interval increased. Maintenance therapy: 25 to 50 mg every other wk for 2 to 20 wk. On basis of response, dosage interval may be increased to every third and subsequently fourth wk (maximum dose per injection: 100 mg).
Children: After test dose of 10 mg, give 1 mg/kg

(maximum dose per injection: 50 mg). Dosage schedule similar to that for adults.
Trade names: Aurolate Injection 50 mg/mL
Warnings: Previous severe reaction to gold compounds or other heavy metals; uncontrolled diabetes mellitus or CHF; severe debilitation; kidney disease; liver disease; severe hypertension; agranulocytosis or bleeding disorder; recent radiation exposure; systemic lupus erythematosus; urticaria; eczema. Pregnancy Category: [C]
Interactions: Antimalarials, penicillamine: Safety of combination antirheumatic therapy is unknown. Cytotoxic drugs, immunosuppressives (except steroids), phenylbutazone: May increase risk of blood dyscrasias.

Goserelin Acetate

Gonadotropin-releasing hormone
Indications: Alternative to orchiectomy or estrogen therapy in palliative treatment of advanced carcinoma of prostate; palliative treatment of advanced breast cancer in pre- and postmenopausal women; treatment of endometriosis.
Dose: Adults: SC 3.6 mg implant q 28 days into upper abdominal wall by sterile technique under health care provider's supervision. SC 10.8 mg implant q 12 wk into upper abdominal wall by sterile technique under health care provider's supervision.
Trade names: Zoladex Implant 3.6 mg
Warnings: Hypersensitivity to GnRH, GnRH agonist analogs, LHRH, LHRH-agonist analogs, D,L-lactic and glycolic acid polymer or acetic acid; pregnancy; breastfeeding or lactation; nondiagnosed vaginal bleeding. Pregnancy Category: [D (breast cancer); X (endometriosis, endometrial thinning)]
Interactions: None well documented.

Griseofulvin

Anti-infective / Antifungal
Indications: Treatment of ringworm infections of skin, hair, and nails caused by susceptible fungi.
Dose: Adults: PO 500 to 1000 mg microsize (330 to 750 mg ultramicrosize) in single or divided doses. May need to give for several weeks.
Children: PO 11 mg microsize/kg/day (125 to 500 mg) or 7.3 mg ultramicrosize/kg/day (82.5 to 330 mg).
Trade names: Grifulvin V Tablets 250 mg (as microsize)
Grisactin 500 Tablets 500 mg (as microsize)
Grisactin 250 Capsules 250 mg (as microsize)
Fulvicin P/G Tablets 125 mg (as ultramicrosize)
Gris-PEG Tablets 125 mg (as ultramicrosize)
Grisactin Ultra Tablets 250 mg (as ultramicrosize)
Warnings: Porphyria; hepatic disease. Pregnancy Category: [C]
Interactions: Alcohol: Effects of alcohol may be potentiated with tachycardia and flushing.
Anticoagulants: Anticoagulant effect may be decreased.
Barbiturates: May depress griseofulvin serum levels.
Contraceptives, oral: May cause loss of contraceptive effectiveness.

Guanabenz Acetate

Antihypertensive / Antiadrenergic, centrally acting
Indications: Treatment of hypertension alone or with a thiazide diuretic.
Dose: Adults: PO 4 mg bid initially; may increase by 4 to 8 mg daily q 1 to 2 wk; max dose 32 mg bid.
Trade names: Wytensin Tablets 4 mg
Warnings: Standard considerations. Pregnancy Category: [C]
Interactions: CNS depressants: Increased sedation.

Guanadrel

Antihypertensive / Antiadrenergic, peripherally acting
Indications: Treatment of hypertension in patients not responding adequately to thiazide-type diuretics.
Dose: Adults: PO 10 mg/day (5 mg bid) initially. Maintenance dose: PO 20 to 75 mg/day, usually in 2 divided doses; tid or qid dosing may be needed. In patients with renal impairment, dosage adjustment may be necessary.
Trade names: Hylorel Tablets 10 mg
Warnings: Pheochromocytoma; concurrent use or use within 1 wk of MAOIs; frank CHF. Pregnancy Category: [B]
Interactions: Alpha-blockers, beta-blockers, reserpine: Effects of guanadrel may be potentiated, resulting in excessive orthostatic hypotension and bradycardia.
Indirect-acting sympathomimetics (eg, ephedrine): Reverse antihypertensive effect.
MAOIs, phenothiazines, tricyclic antidepressants: Inhibit antihypertensive effect.

Guanethidine Monosulfate

Antihypertensive / Antiadrenergic, peripherally acting
Indications: Treatment of moderate and severe hypertension and renal hypertension, including that secondary to pyelonephritis, renal amyloidosis, and renal artery stenosis.

Unlabeled indication: Reflex sympathetic dystrophy and causalgia.
Dose: Adults:
Ambulatory: PO 10 mg qd initially; may increase by about 10 mg at 5 to 7 days; increase only if no decrease in standing BP is observed. Maintenance dose: 25 to 50 mg qd.
Hospitalized: PO 25 to 50 mg initially; increase by 25 or 50 mg/day or qod until desired response is obtained.
Loading dose (for severe hypertension): Give at 6 hr intervals over 1 to 3 days, omitting nighttime dose.
Children: PO 0.2 mg/kg/24 hr (6 mg/m^2 /24 hr) as single oral dose initially; increase by increment of 0.2 mg/kg/24 hr q 7 to 10 days. Max: 3 mg/kg/24 hr.
Trade names: Ismelin Tablets 10 mg
Warnings: Known or suspected pheochromocytoma; frank CHF not related to hypertension; use of MAOIs. Pregnancy Category: [C]
Interactions: Anorexiants: May reverse hypotensive effect of drug.
MAOIs: May decrease effectiveness of guanethidine; discontinue MAOIs more than 1 wk before starting guanethidine therapy.
Phenothiazines: May inhibit hypotensive effect.
Sympathomimetics (eg, ephedrine, epinephrine): May reverse hypotensive effect of guanethidine; guanethidine may potentiate effects of sympathomimetics.
Tricyclic antidepressants: May inhibit hypotensive effect of drug.

Guanfacine HCl

Antihypertensive / Antiadrenergic, centrally acting
Indications: Treatment of hypertension.

Unlabeled indication: Amelioration of heroin withdrawal symptoms.
Dose: Adults: PO 1 mg daily at bedtime; may increase gradually up to 3 mg daily.
Trade names: Tenex Tablets 1 mg
Warnings: Standard considerations. Pregnancy Category: [B]
Interactions: Alcohol, CNS depressants:

Increased CNS depression.
Barbiturates, phenytoin: Decreased guanfacine levels with loss of antihypertensive effect.

Halcinonide

Corticosteroid / Topical

Indications: Relief of inflammation and pruritus caused by corticosteroid-responsive dermatoses.

Dose: Adults and Children: Topical Apply thin film to affected area bid to tid.

Trade names: Halog Ointment 0.1%
Halog-E Cream 0.1%

Warnings: Standard considerations. Pregnancy Category: [C]

Interactions: None well documented.

Halobetasol Propionate

Corticosteroid / Topical

Indications: Relief of inflammatory and pruritic manifestations of corticosteroid-responsive dermatoses.

Dose: Adults and Children (older than 12 yr): Topical Apply to affected area once or twice daily. Not recommended for more than 2 consecutive wk or more than 50 g/wk.

Trade names: Ultravate Cream 0.05%

Warnings: Standard considerations. Pregnancy Category: [C]

Interactions: None well documented.

Haloperidol

Antipsychotic / Butyrophenone

Indications: Management of psychotic disorders; control of Tourette disorder in children and adults; management of severe behavioral problems in children; short-term treatment of hyperactive children. Long-term antipsychotic therapy (haloperidol decanoate).

Unlabeled indication: Treatment of phencyclidine (PCP) psychosis; antiemetic; hiccoughs.

Dose: Psychotic disorders:
Adults: PO Moderate symptoms, geriatric or debilitated patients: 0.5 to 2 mg bid to tid. Severe symptoms, chronic or resistant patients: 3 to 5 mg bid to tid. Dosages up to 100 mg/day may be necessary in some patients. IM 2 to 5 mg for prompt control of acutely agitated schizophrenic patients with moderately severe to very severe symptoms. Depending on response, subsequent doses may be needed within 60 min; although 4 to 8 hr intervals may be satisfactory.
Children 3 to 12 yr (weight 15 to 40 kg): PO Initial dose 0.5 mg/day. If needed, increase in 0.5 mg increments at 5 to 7 day intervals up to 0.15 mg/kg/day or until therapeutic effect is obtained. The dose may be divided and given bid to tid. IM Safety and efficacy not established in children.
Tourette disorder:
Adults: PO Start with 0.5 to 1.5 mg tid (max, 10 mg/day).
Children 3 to 12 yr (weight 15 to 40 kg): PO 0.05 to 0.075 mg/kg/day. Severely disturbed psychotic children may require higher doses.
Behavioral disorders/hyperactivity:
Children 3 to 12 yr (weight 15 to 40 kg): PO 0.05 to 0.075 mg/kg/day. Severely disturbed psychotic children may require higher doses. In severely disturbed, nonpsychotic children or in hyperactive children with conduct disorder, short-term administration may suffice. There is little evidence to support dosages greater than 6 mg/day.
Haloperidol decanoate injection: The dose should be individualized under close supervision during initiation and stabilization of therapy. The recommended interval between doses is monthly or q 4 wk, but variations in patient response may dictate a need for adjustments in dose or dosing interval.
Adults: IM (deep injection) Initial dose should not exceed 100 mg. If conversion from oral haloperidol to IM haloperidol decanoate requires more than 100 mg as an initial dose, administer that dose in 2 injections (max, 100 mg initially followed by balance in 3 to 7 days). In patients stabilized on low oral doses (10 mg or less/day), the initial recommended dose of haloperidol decanoate is 10 to 15 times the daily dose. In patients stabilized on higher oral doses, the recommended dose is 20 times the daily dose. Maintenance dosages should be titrated upward or downward based on therapeutic response.

Trade names: Haldol Tablets 0.5 mg
Haldol Decanoate 50 Injection 50 mg (as 70.5 decanoate)/mL
Haldol Decanoate 100 Injection 100 mg (as 141.04 mg decanoate)/mL

Warnings: Severe, toxic CNS depression or comatose states from any cause; Parkinson disease; hypersensitive to any component of the product. Pregnancy Category: [C: Safety not established Haloperidol decanoate]

Interactions: Anesthetics, opiates, alcohol: May increase CNS depressant effects.
Anticholinergics: May increase anticholinergic effects. May worsen schizophrenic symptoms, decrease haloperidol serum concentrations, and lead to tardive dyskinesia.
Azole antifungal agents (eg, itraconazole): Plasma levels of haloperidol may be elevated, increasing the risk of side effects.
Carbamazepine: May decrease effects of haloperidol.
Lithium: May induce disorientation, unconsciousness, and extrapyramidal symptoms.
Rifamycins (eg, rifampin): Plasma levels of haloperidol may be reduced, decreasing the clinical effectiveness.

Heparin

Anticoagulants

Indications: Prophylaxis and treatment of venous thrombosis and its extensions, pulmonary embolism (PE), peripheral arterial embolism, and atrial fibrillation with embolization; diagnosis and treatment of acute and chronic consumption coagulopathies (DIC); prevention of postoperative deep venous thrombosis (DVT), and PE.

Unlabeled indication: Prophylaxis of left ventricular thrombi and cerebrovascular accidents post-MI; treatment of myocardial ischemia; prevention of cerebral thrombosis in evolving strokes; adjunctive treatment of coronary occlusion with acute MI.

Dose: Adults: SC 10,000 to 20,000 U as initial dose followed by 8000 to 20,000 U q 8 to 12 hr. Intermittent IV 10,000 U as initial dose followed by 5000 to 10,000 U q 4 to 6 hr. IV infusion 20,000 to 40,000 U/day.
Children: Intermittent IV 50 U/kg as initial dose followed by 100 U/kg q 4 hr. IV infusion 50 U/kg as initial dose followed by 20,000 U/m^2 /24 hr.
Low-dose Prophylaxis: SC 5000 U 2 hr before surgery and q 8 to 12 hr thereafter for 7 days or until patient is fully ambulatory, whichever is longer.
Surgery of Heart and Blood Vessels:
Adults: 300 to 400 U/kg.
Blood Transfusion: Add 400 to 600 U/100 mL of whole blood.
Clearing Intermittent Infusion Sets: 10 to 100 U/mL.
Laboratory Samples: Add 70 to 150 U/10 to 20 mL of whole blood.

Trade names: Heparin Sodium Injection 1000 units/mL
Hep-Lock Injection 10 units/mL
Hep-Lock U/P Injection 10 units/mL

Warnings: Severe thrombocytopenia; uncontrolled bleeding (except because of DIC); patients in whom suitable blood coagulation tests cannot be performed. Pregnancy Category: [C]

Interactions: Dipyridamole, hydroxychloroquine,

NSAIDs, salicylates: May cause increased risk of bleeding.
Incompatability: Heparin is acidic and incompatible with many drugs.

Hepatitis B Immune Globulin (HBIG)

Immune serum

Indications: For passive, transient prevention of hepatitis B infection after viral exposure via needlestick or mucous membrane contact; prevention of hepatitis B in infants born to HBsAg-positive mothers. Most effective when used within 7 days of exposure.

Dose: Adults and Children: IM 0.06 mL/kg (usually 3 to 5 mL). Administer as soon as possible after exposure and repeat 28 to 30 days later.
Newborns of HBsAg-Positive Mothers: IM 0.5 mL. Administer first HBIG dose as soon as possible, preferably less than 12 hr after birth. Also give hepatitis B vaccine. If hepatitis B vaccine is declined, repeat HBIG at 3 and 6 mo.

Trade names: BayHep B Injection 217 IU/mL
Nabi-HB Injection 312 IU/mL

Warnings: None well documented. Pregnancy Category: [C]

Interactions: Anticoagulants: Give HBIG with caution to people receiving anticoagulant therapy.
Vaccines: To avoid inactivating vaccines containing live viruses (except measles vaccine) or bacteria, give live vaccines 3 mo after HBIG.

Hydralazine HCl

Antihypertensive / Vasodilator

Indications: Treatment of essential hypertension (oral form). Treatment of severe essential hypertension (parenteral form).

Unlabeled indication: Reduction of overload in treatment of CHF, severe aortic insufficiency, and after valve replacement.

Dose: Adjust individually.
Adults: PO Begin with 10 mg qid for 2 to 4 days; then 25 mg qid for 3 to 5 days; then 50 mg qid (max, 300 mg/day). IV/IM 20 to 40 mg repeated prn.
Children: PO 0.75 mg/kg/day in 4 divided doses initially; increase gradually over 3 to 4 wk to max 7.5 mg/kg/day or 200 mg/day. IV/IM 0.1 to 0.2 mg/kg/dose q 4 to 6 hr prn.

Trade names: Apresoline Tablets 25 mg

Warnings: Coronary artery disease; mitral valvular rheumatic heart disease. Pregnancy Category: [C]

Interactions: Beta-blockers: May increase effect of hydralazine or effect of beta-blockers.
NSAIDs: Effects of hydralazine may be decreased.

Hydrochlorothiazide

Thiazide diuretic

Indications: Adjunctive therapy for edema associated with CHF, hepatic cirrhosis, renal dysfunction, and corticosteroid and estrogen therapy; treatment of hypertension.

Unlabeled indication: Prevention of formation and precurrence of calcium nephrolithiasis; therapy for nephrogenic diabetes insipidus.

Dose: Edema:
Adults: PO 25 to 100 mg/day. Rarely patients may require 200 mg/day.
Hypertension:
Adults: PO 25 to 50 mg/day as single dose or 2 divided doses.
Children (2 to 12 yr): PO 37.5 to 100 mg/day in 2 doses.
Infants (6 mo to 2 yr): PO 12.5 to 37.5 mg/day in 2 doses.
Infants (younger than 6 mo): PO Up to 3.3 mg/kg/day in 2 doses.

Trade names: Esidrix Tablets 25 mg
Ezide Tablets 50 mg
Hydro-Par Tablets 25 mg
Hydro-DIURIL Tablets 25 mg
Microzide Capsules 12.5 mg
Oretic Tablets 25 mg

Warnings: Hypersensitivity to thiazides, related diuretics, or sulfonamide-derived drugs; anuria; renal decompensation. Pregnancy Category: [B]

Interactions: Bile acid sequestrants: May reduce thiazide absorption; give thiazide at least 2 hr before resin.
Diazoxide: May cause hyperglycemia.
Digitalis glycosides: Diuretic-induced hypokalemia and hypomagnesemia may precipitate digitalis-induced arrhythmias.
Lithium: May decrease renal excretion of lithium.
Loop diuretics: Synergistic effects may result in profound diuresis and serious electrolyte abnormalities.
Sulfonylureas, insulin: May decrease hypoglycemic effect of sulfonylureas. May need to increase dosage of sulfonylureas or insulin.

Hydrochlorothiazide/ Lisinopril

Antihypertensive combination

Indications: Hypertension; combination not indicated for initial treatment of hypertension.

Dose: Adults: PO Lisinopril 10 to 80 mg; hydrochlorothiazide 6.25 to 50 mg once daily.

Trade names: Prinzide Tablets 10 mg lisinopril/12.5 mg hydrochlorothiazide
Zestoretic Tablets 10 mg lisinopril/12.5 mg hydrochlorothiazide

Warnings: History of angioedema related to an ACE inhibitor; anuria; hypersensitivity to other sulfonamide-related drugs. Pregnancy Category: [C (first trimester); D (second and third trimesters) ACE inhibitors can cause fetal and neonatal morbidity and death when administered during pregnancy]

Interactions: Alcohol, barbiturates, narcotics: Potentiation of orthostatic hypotension may occur.
Antacids: Lisinopril bioavailability may be decreased. Separate administration times by 2 hr.
Bile acid sequestrants: May reduce thiazide absorption; give thiazide 2 hr before resin.
Capsaicin: Lisinopril-induced cough may be exacerbated.
Diazoxide: Hydrochlorothiazide may have additive effects; hyperglycemia.
Digitalis glycosides: Hydrochlorothiazide-induced hypokalemia and hypomagnesemia may precipitate digitalis-induced arrhythmias.
Indomethacin: Reduced hypotensive effects, especially in low-renin or volume-dependent hypertensive patients.
Lithium: Hydrochlorothiazide may decrease renal excretion of lithium, increasing blood levels. Lisinopril may increase lithium levels and induce symptoms of lithium toxicity.
Loop diuretics: Synergistic effects with hydrochlorothiazide may result in profound diuresis and serious electrolyte abnormalities.
Potassium-sparing diuretics, potassium preparations: Lisinopril may increase serum potassium levels.
Skeletal muscle relaxants, depolarizing: May increase responsiveness to muscle relaxant.
Sulfonylureas, insulin: Hydrochlorothiazide may decrease hypoglycemic effect of sulfonylureas. May need to increase dosage of sulfonylureas or insulin.

Hydrochlorothiazide/ Triamterene (HCTZ/ Triamterene)

Diuretic combination

Indications: Treatment of edema or hypertension in patients who have or are at risk of developing hypokalemia.

Dose: Adults: PO 1 to 2 tablets or capsules daily.

Trade names: Maxzide-25MG Tablets 37.5 mg triamterene/25 mg hydrochlorothiazide
Dyazide Capsules 37.5 mg triamterene/25 mg hydrochlorothiazide
Maxzide Tablets 75 mg triamterene/50 mg hydrochlorothiazide

Warnings: Anuria; renal decompensation; severe hepatic disease; hypersensitivity to thiazides, triamterene, or sulfonamide-derived drugs; patients receiving spironolactone, amiloride, or potassium supplements; hyperkalemia; metabolic or respiratory acidosis. Pregnancy Category: [C]

Interactions: Angiotensin-converting enzyme inhibitors: May result in severely elevated serum potassium levels.
Allopurinol: May increase incidence of hypersensitivity reactions to allopurinol.
Amantadine: May increase amantadine plasma levels and risk for adverse effects.
Anticoagulants: May diminish anticoagulant effects.
Bile acid sequestrants: May reduce thiazide absorption; give thiazide at least 2 hr before sequestrant.
Diazoxide: May cause hyperglycemia.
Digitalis glycosides: Diuretic-induced hypokalemia and hypomagnesemia may precipitate digitalis-induced arrhythmias.
Indomethacin: May cause rapid progression into acute renal failure.
Lithium: May decrease renal excretion of lithium; monitor lithium levels.
Loop diuretics: May cause synergistic effects that may result in profound diuresis and serious electrolyte abnormalities.
Methenamines, NSAIDS: May decrease effectiveness of thiazide.
Potassium preparations: May severely increase serum potassium levels, possibly resulting in cardiac arrhythmias or cardiac arrest. Monitor serum potassium closely if potassium is coadministered.
Sulfonylureas, insulin: May decrease hypoglycemic effect of sulfonylureas. May need to adjust dosage of sulfonylureas or insulin.

Hydrocortisone Acetate/ Pramoxine Hydrochloride

Corticosteroid / Anesthetic

Indications: Topical relief of the inflammatory and pruritic manifestations of corticosteroid-responsive dermatoses.

Dose: Topical: Apply to the affected area as a thin film tid or qid, depending on severity of the condition. Administration of topical corticosteroids to children should be limited to the least amount compatible with an effective therapeutic regimen.

Trade names: Analpram HC Cream 1% hydrocortisone acetate/1% pramoxine HCl
Enzone Cream 1% hydrocortisone acetate/1% pramoxine HCl
Pramosone Ointment 1% hydrocortisone acetate/1% pramoxine HCl
ProctoCream HC Cream 1% hydrocortisone acetate/1% pramoxine HCl
ProctoFoam-HC Aerosol Foam 1% hydrocortisone acetate/1% pramoxine HCl
Zone-A Forte Lotion 2.5% hydrocortisone acetate/1% pramoxine HCl

Warnings: History of hypersensitivity to any component of the product. Pregnancy Category: [C]

Interactions: None well documented.

Hydroxychloroquine Sulfate

Anti-infective / Antimalarial / Antirheumatic

Indications: Prophylaxis and treatment of acute attacks of malaria caused by Plasmodium vivax, Plasmodium malariae, Plasmodium ovale, and susceptible strains of Plasmodium falciparum. Treatment of chronic discoid and systemic lupus erythematosus (SLE) and acute or chronic rheumatoid arthritis in patients not responding to other therapies.

Dose: Suppression of Malaria:
Adults: PO 400 mg (310 mg of base) weekly on same day each week.
Children: PO 5 mg/kg of base weekly on same day each week, up to max 400 mg (310 mg of base). Begin 1 to 2 wk prior to exposure; continue for 8 wk after leaving area.
Acute Attack of Malaria:
Adults:
Initial dose: PO 800 mg (620 mg of base).
Children:
Initial dose: PO 10 mg/kg (base), up to adult dose; give half of initial dose 6 hr later and on days 2 and 3.
Rheumatoid Arthritis:
Adults:
Initial dose: PO 400 to 600 mg/day (310 to 465 mg of base) with food or milk.
Maintenance: PO After good response (usually 4 to 12 wk), reduce dosage 50% and continue at 200 to 400 mg/day (155 to 310 mg of base).
Children: Although experience with hydroxychloroquine in children for rheumatoid arthritis or lupus erythematosus is limited, its use may be warranted in some cases. A dose of 3 to 5 mg/kg/day, up to a max 400 mg/day (given once or twice daily) has been recommended. Do not exceed a dose of 7 mg/kg/day.
Lupus Erythematosus:
Adults: PO Initially 400 mg/day or bid. For prolonged therapy, reduce to 200 to 400 mg/day (155 to 310 mg of base).

Trade names: Plaquenil Sulfate Tablets 200 mg (equivalent to 155 mg base)

Warnings: Retinal or visual field changes caused by any 4-aminoquinoline compound; hypersensitivity to 4-aminoquinoline compounds; long-term therapy in children. Pregnancy Category: [C]

Interactions: Digoxin: May increase serum digoxin levels.
Hepatotoxic drugs: May increase potential for hepatotoxicity.

Hydroxyurea

Antisickling / Substituted ureas / Antimetabolite

Indications: Reduce frequency of painful crises and need for blood transfusion in adults with sickle cell anemia with recurrent moderate to severe painful crises; treatment of melanoma; resistant chronic myelocytic leukemia (CML); recurrent, metastatic, or inoperable carcinoma of ovary; as an adjunct to irradiation in local control of primary squamous cell carcinomas of head and neck, excluding lip.

Unlabeled indication: Thrombocythemia; HIV; psoriasis; cervical carcinoma; polycythemia vera.

Dose: Base dosage on patient's actual or ideal weight, whichever is less.
Sickle Cell Anemia:
Adults:
Initial dose: PO 15 mg/kg/day as a single dose. If blood counts are acceptable levels, dose may be increased by 5 mg/kg/day q 12 wk until max tolerated dose

(highest dose not producing toxic blood counts over 24 consecutive wk), or 35 mg/kg/day is reached. Dose is not increased if blood counts are between acceptable and toxic levels. If blood counts are considered toxic, discontinue hydroxyurea until hematologic recovery, then resume therapy after reducing dose by 2.5 mg/kg/day from dose associated with hematologic toxicity. Then, titrate dose up or down q 12 wk in 2.5 mg/kg/day increments until patient is at a stable dose that does not result in hematologic toxicity for 24 wk. Any dose that produces hematologic toxicity twice should not be given again.
Solid Tumors:
Adults:
Intermittent therapy: PO 80 mg/kg (2000 to 3000 mg/m^2) as a single dose every third day.
Continuous therapy: PO 20 to 30 mg/kg as a single daily dose. Hold the dose if WBC decreases to less than 2500/mm^3 or platelet count less than 100,000/mm^3.
Concomitant Irradiation Therapy (Carcinoma of Head and Neck):
Adults: PO 80 mg/kg as a single dose every third day, beginning at least 7 days before initiation of irradiation and continue during radiotherapy and indefinitely afterwards, provided patient is adequately observed and exhibits no unusual or severe reactions.
Resistant CML:
Adults: PO Continuous therapy of 20 to 30 mg/kg as a single daily dose.
Trade names: Droxia Capsules 200 mg
Hydrea Capsules 500 mg
Mylocel Tablets 1000 mg
Warnings: Marked bone marrow suppression; severe anemia; hypersensitivity to product. Pregnancy Category: [D]
Interactions: Antiretroviral agents (eg, didanosine, indinavir, stavudine): Hepatotoxicity, fatal hepatic failure, and severe neurotoxicity reported with concomitant use in HIV-positive patients.
Didanosine: Pancreatitis, occasionally resulting in death, reported with concomitant use in HIV-positive patients.
Fluorouracil: Coadministration may cause neurotoxicity.
Uricosuric agents (eg, probenecid): Hydroxyurea may increase serum uric acid levels.

Hydroxyzine

Antipsychotic / Antihistamine
Indications: Symptomatic relief of anxiety and tension associated with psychoneurosis; adjunct therapy in organic disease states with anxiety; management of pruritus caused by allergic conditions; sedative before and after general anesthesia (PO, IM).
IM route only: Relief of anxiety in acutely disturbed or hysterical patient; treatment of alcoholic delirium tremens or anxiety withdrawal symptoms; preoperative, postoperative, prepartum, and postpartum adjunctive medication to permit reduction in narcotic dosage; alleviation of anxiety; control of emesis; adjunctive therapy in asthma.
Dose: Anxiety:
Adults: PO / IM 50 to 100 mg qid.
Children over 6 yr: PO 50 to 100 mg/day in divided doses.
Children less than 6 yr: PO 50 mg/day in divided doses.
Nausea, Vomiting, and Analgesia (Adjunct):
Adults: IM 25 to 100 mg.
Children: IM 1.1 mg/kg.
Preoperative and Postoperative Administration:
Adults: IM 25 to 100 mg.
Children: IM 1.1 mg/kg.
Prepartum and Postpartum Administration:
Adults: IM 25 to 100 mg.
Pruritus:
Adults: PO / IM 25 mg tid to qid.
Children over 6 yr: PO 50 to 100 mg/day in divided doses.
Children less than 6 yr: PO 50 mg/day in divided doses.
Psychiatric and Emotional Emergencies (ie, acute alcoholism):
Adults: IM 50 to 100 mg stat and q 4 to 6 hr prn.
Sedation:
Adults: PO/IM 50 to 100 mg.
Children: PO/IM 0.6 mg/kg.
Trade names: Atarax Tablets 10 mg
Atarax 100 Tablets 100 mg
Vistaril Capsules 25 mg
Warnings: Standard considerations. Pregnancy Category: [Safety not established; avoid use]
Interactions: Alcohol and CNS depressants: CNS depressant effects may be increased.

Ibutilide Fumarate

Antiarrhythmic
Indications: Rapid conversion of recent onset atrial fibrillation or atrial flutter to sinus rhythm.
Dose: Adults: IV Initial infusion: At least 60 kg (at least 132 lbs) 1 mg (1 vial) infused over 10 min; less than 60 kg (less than 132 lbs) 0.01 mg/kg (0.1 mL/kg) infused over 10 min. If the arrhythmia does not terminate within 10 min after the end of the initial infusion, a second 10 min infusion of equal strength may be administered 10 min after completion of the first infusion.
Trade names: Corvert Solution 0.1 mg/mL
Warnings: Standard considerations. Pregnancy Category: [C]
Interactions: Concomitant Class Ia and III antiarrhythmic agents (eg, amiodarone, disopyramide, procainamide, quinidine, sotalol): Do not give concurrently. Withhold for 5 half-lives prior to and for 4 hr after ibutilide infusion.
Medications that prolong the QT interval (eg, phenothiazines, tricyclic and tetracyclic antidepressants): Potential for proarrhythmia may be increased.
Digoxin: Cardiotoxicity (supraventricular arrhythmia) due to excessive digoxin concentrations may be masked.

Idarubicin

Antineoplastic antibiotic / Anthracycline
Indications: Acute myelocytic leukemia.

Unlabeled indication: Pediatric: Acute lymphocytic anemia; acute nonlymphocytic anemia.
Dose: Acute Myelogenous Leukemia:
Adults: IV Induction therapy in combination with other chemotherapeutic drugs: Idarubicin 12 mg/m^2 /day for 3 days by slow (10 to 15 min) IV injection in combination with cytarabine; may give second course if needed. Reduce dosage of subsequent courses 25% in patients experiencing severe mucositis. Delay therapy until recovery from mucositis occurs.
Acute Lymphocytic Leukemia, Acute Nonlymphocytic Leukemia:
Pediatric: IV Induction therapy in combination with other chemotherapeutic drugs: Idarubicin 10 to 12 mg/m^2 /day for 3 days during each treatment course. Delay therapy until recovery from mucositis occurs. Follow dosage adjustment guidelines recommended for adults.
Solid Tumors:
Pediatric: IV Idarubicin 5 mg/m^2 /day for 3 days during each treatment course. Follow dosage adjustment guidelines recommended for adults.
Trade names: Idamycin Powder for injection 5 mg
Idamycin PFS Solution for injection 1 mg/mL
Warnings: Standard considerations. Pregnancy Category: [D]
Interactions: None well documented.

Idoxuridine

Ophthalmic / Antiviral

Indications: Treatment of herpes simplex keratitis.

Dose: Adults: Ophthalmic solution Instill 1 gtt into infected eye(s) q hr during day and q 2 hr during night. Alternate schedule: Instill 1 gtt q 1 min for 5 min; repeat q 4 hr night and day. Ointment Apply ointment to infected conjunctival sac q 4 hr (5 applications daily).

Trade names: Herplex Solution 0.1%

Warnings: Standard considerations. Pregnancy Category: [C]

Interactions: Boric acid-containing solution: May cause irritation; do not coadminister.

Ifosfamide

Alkylating agent / Nitrogen mustard

Indications: Germ cell testicular cancer.

Unlabeled indication: Soft-tissue, Ewing and osteogenic sarcomas; non-Hodgkin lymphomas; small cell lung, pancreatic, bladder, cervical, and ovarian carcinoma.

Dose: Germ Cell Testicular Cancer:
Adults: IV 1200 mg/m^2 /day for 5 days, repeating this course q 3 wk. Delay further courses until platelets are are least 100,000/mm^3 and WBC at least 4000/mm^3.
Germ Cell Testicular Cancer, Other Regimens:
Adults: IV Other regimens use ifosfamide 2000 mg/m^2 /day on days 1 through 3 (MAID regimen, total dose is 6000 mg/m^2 over 72 hr), or doses as high as 5000 mg/m^2 continuous infusion for 24 hr in combination with other antineoplastics.

Trade names: Ifex Powder for injection 1000 mg

Warnings: Continued use in patients with severely depressed bone marrow function; hypersensitivity to ifosfamide. Pregnancy Category: [D]

Interactions: Ifosfamide may increase the hypoprothrombinemic effect of warfarin.

Imatinib

Tyrosine kinase inhibitor antineoplastic

Indications: Treatment of CML in accelerated phase, blast crisis, or interferon-refractory chronic phase, metastatic GI stromal tumors (GISTs).

Dose: CML Treatment in Accelerated Phase, Blast Crisis, or Interferon-Refractory Chronic Phase:
Adults: PO Continue imatinib as long as response is favorable. Assess therapeutic response after at least 3 mo of continued therapy.
Chronic Phase CML:
Adults: PO 400 mg/day initially. Increase to 600 mg/day, as tolerated, in patients with disease progression, inadequate response to initial dose, or loss of previous hematologic response.
CML in Accelerated Phase or Blast Crisis:
Adults: PO 600 mg/day initially. Increase to 400 mg bid, as tolerated, in patients with disease progression, inadequate response to initial dose, or loss of previous hematologic response.
GISTs:
Adults: PO 400 or 600 mg/day.
Patients with Chronic Phase CML:
Adults: PO If ANC at least 1000 cells/mm^3, continue at present dose. If ANC less than 1000 cells/mm^3 - First occurrence: Discontinue imatinib until ANC at least 1500 cells/mm^3 and platelets at least 75,000 cells/mm^3, then resume treatment at 400 mg/day. Second occurrence: Discontinue imatinib until ANC at least 1500 cells/mm^3 and platelets at least 75,000 cells/mm^3, then resume treatment at 300 mg/day. If platelet count at least 50,000 cells/mm^3, continue at present dose. If platelet count less than 50,000 cells/mm^3 - First occurrence: Discontinue imatinib until platelets at least 75,000 cells/mm^3 and ANC at least 1500 cells/mm^3, then resume treatment at 400 mg/day. Second occurrence: Discontinue imatinib until platelets at least 75,000 cells/mm^3 and ANC at least 1500 cells/mm^3, then resume treatment at 300 mg/day.
Patients with Accelerated Phase CML and Blast Crisis (if Hematologic Toxicity Occurs After at Least 1 Mo of Therapy):
Adults: PO If ANC at least 500 cells/mm^3, continue at present dose. If ANC less than 500 cells/mm^3 - Initial response: Perform marrow aspirate or biopsy. Reduce dose to 400 mg/day if neutropenia is unrelated to leukemia. Recheck counts in 2 wk. Persistent neutropenia for 2 wk: Reduce dose to 300 mg/day and recheck counts in 2 additional weeks. Persistent neutropenia for 4 wk: Perform marrow aspirate or biopsy. If neutropenia is unrelated to leukemia, discontinue imatinib until ANC is at least 1000 cells/mm^3 and platelets are at least 20,000 cells/mm^3, then resume therapy with 300 mg/day. If platelet count is at least 10,000 cells/mm^3, continue at present dose. If platelet count is less than 10,000 cells/mm^3 - Initial response: Perform marrow aspirate or biopsy. Reduce dose to 400 mg/day if thrombocytopenia is unrelated to leukemia. Recheck counts in 2 wk. Persistent thrombocytopenia for 2 wk: Reduce dose to 300 mg/day and recheck counts in 2 additional weeks. Persistent thrombocytopenia for 4 wk: Perform marrow aspirate or biopsy. If thrombocytopenia is unrelated to leukemia, discontinue imatinib until platelet count at least 20,000 cells/mm^3 and ANC at least 1000 cells/mm^3, then resume therapy with 300 mg/day.
Hepatotoxicity:
Adults: PO If serum bilirubin is up to 3 times the upper limit of normal (ULN), continue at present dose. If serum bilirubin is greater than 3 times the ULN, discontinue imatinib until bilirubin is less than 1.5 times the ULN, then resume treatment at next lower dose level (reduce daily dose from 800 to 600 mg, from 600 to 400 mg, or from 400 to 300 mg, as appropriate). If serum transaminases are up to 5 times the ULN, continue at present dose. If serum transaminases are greater than 5 times the ULN, discontinue imatinib until serum transaminases are less than 2.5 times the ULN, then resume treatment at next lower dose level.

Trade names: Gleevec Gelatin Capsules for oral use 100 mg

Warnings: Standard considerations. Pregnancy Category: [D]

Interactions: Acetaminophen: Increased risk of hepatotoxicity.
Drugs that induce CYP3A4 (eg, aminoglutethimide, barbiturates, carbamazepine, dexamethasone, griseofulvin, modafinil, nafcillin, phenytoin, primidone, rifabutin, rifampin, St. John's wort): Decreased imatinib concentrations and antineoplastic efficacy.
Drugs that inhibit CYP3A4 (eg, clarithromycin, diltiazem, erythromycin, itraconazole, ketoconazole, verapamil): Increased imatinib concentrations and toxicity.
Drugs that are metabolized by CYP2C9 (eg, fluvastatin, glimepiride, glipizide, glyburide, phenytoin, warfarin, some NSAIDs): Imatinib may reduce metabolism, resulting in increased concentrations and toxicity.
Drugs that are metabolized by CYP2D6 (eg, propafenone, tricyclic antidepressants, some beta-adrenergic blockers, some SSRIs): Imatinib may reduce metabolism, resulting in increased concentrations and toxicity.
Drugs that are metabolized by CYP3A4 (eg, atorvastatin, triazolobenzodiazepines): Imatinib may reduce metabolism, resulting in increased concentrations and toxicity.

Imipenem-Cilastatin

Anti-infective / Carbapenem

Indications: Treatment of serious infections of lower respiratory tract and urinary tract, intra-abdominal and gynecologic infections, bacterial septicemia, bone and joint infections, skin and skin structure infections, endocarditis, and polymicrobic infections due to

susceptible microorganisms.
Dose: Adults: IV 125, 250, or 500 mg dose over 20 to 30 min. Infuse a 750 mg or 1 g dose over 40 to 60 min. If nausea develops, slow the infusion rate. Max: 50 mg/kg/day or 4 g/day, whichever is lower.
Adults: IM 500 to 750 mg q 12 hr. Max: 1500 mg/day.
Children less than 40 kg: IM 60 mg/kg/day.
Children at least 40 kg: IM Adult dose.
Premature Infants (at least 36 wk Gestational Age): IM 20 mg/kg q 12 hr.
Trade names: Primaxin IV Powder for Injection 250 mg imipenem equivalent and 250 mg cilastatin equivalent. Contains 0.8 mEq sodium.
Primaxin IM Powder for Injection 500 mg imipenem equivalent and 500 mg cilastatin equivalent. Contains 1.4 mEq sodium.
Warnings: IM use with hypersensitivity to local anesthetics of amide type or with severe shock or heart block. IV use with patients with meningitis (safety and efficacy have not been established). Pregnancy Category: [C]
Interactions: Cyclosporine: CNS side effects (eg, myoclonia, seizures) may be increased.
Ganciclovir: Generalized seizures may occur; avoid use.
Probenecid: Minimal increases in imipenem levels and half-life; do not give probenecid concurrently.
Incompatability: Do not physically mix imipenem-cilastatin with other antibiotics.

Imipramine HCl

Tricyclic antidepressant

Indications: Relief of symptoms of depression; treatment of enuresis in children 6 yr and older.

Unlabeled indication: Treatment of chronic pain, panic disorder, eating disorders (bulimia nervosa), and facilitation of cocaine withdrawal.
Dose: Depression: Use parenterally only in patients who are not able or not willing to take oral medication. Give via IM route. Do not administer IV. Up to 100 mg/day in divided doses may be given IM. Switch to oral as soon as possible.
Adults: PO 100 to 300 mg/day, in divided doses or once daily at bedtime.
Elderly & Adolescents: PO 30 to 40 mg/day; may increase up to 100 mg/day.
Children: PO 1.5 mg/kg/day in divided doses; up to maximum of 5 mg/kg/day.
Childhood Enuresis (6 yr): PO 25 mg/day given 1 hr before bedtime; if response unsatisfactory after 1 wk, may increase to 50 mg in children younger than 12 yr. Children older than 12 yr may receive 75 mg/night. Do not exceed 2.5 mg/kg/day.
Trade names: Tofranil Tablets 10 mg
Tofranil-PM Capsules 75 mg
Warnings: Hypersensitivity to any tricyclic antidepressant. Generally not to be given in combination with or within 14 days of treatment with MAO inhibitor or during acute recovery phase of MI; cross-sensitivity may occur among the dibenzazepines. Pregnancy Category: [D]
Interactions: Carbamazepine: Carbamazepine levels may increase; imipramine levels may decrease.
Cimetidine, fluoxetine: May cause increased imipramine blood levels and effects.
Clonidine: May result in hypertensive crisis.
CNS depressants: Depressant effects may be additive.
Dicumarol: Anticoagulant actions may increase.
Guanethidine: Hypotensive action may be inhibited.
MAO inhibitors: May cause hyperpyretic crises, severe convulsions, and death when given with imipramine.
Sympathomimetics: Pressor response may be decreased by indirect-acting sympathomimetics and increased by direct-acting ones.

Imiquimod

Immunomodulator

Indications: Treatment of external genital and perianal warts/condyloma acuminata.
Dose: Adults and Children 12 yr and older: Topical 3 times/wk (eg, Monday, Wednesday, Friday) and leave on skin for 6 to 10 hr. Remove cream by washing treated area with mild soap and water. Continue treatment until there is total clearance of genital/perianal warts or for a max of 16 wk. A rest period of several days may be taken if needed because of discomfort or severity of local skin reaction. Treatment may be resumed after reaction subsides.
Trade names: Aldara Cream 5%
Warnings: Standard considerations. Pregnancy Category: [B]
Interactions: None well documented.

Indapamide

Thiazide diuretic

Indications: Treatment of edema associated with CHF, hepatic cirrhosis, renal dysfunction, and corticosteroid or estrogen therapy; management of hypertension.

Unlabeled indication: Treatment of calcium nephrolithiasis, osteoporosis, or diabetes insipidus.
Dose: Adults: PO 1.25 to 5 mg q morning. Maximum 5 mg/day.
Trade names: Lozol Tablets 1.25 mg
Warnings: Hypersensitivity to thiazides, related diuretics, or sulfonamide-derived drugs; anuria. Pregnancy Category: [B]
Interactions: Bile acid sequestrants: May reduce thiazide absorption; give thiazide at least 2 hr before resin.
Diazoxide: Hyperglycemia may occur.
Digitalis glycosides: Diuretic-induced hypokalemia and hypomagnesemia may precipitate digitalis-induced arrhythmias.
Lithium: May decrease renal excretion of lithium; monitor lithium levels.
Loop diuretics: May result in synergistic effects and result in profound diuresis and serious electrolyte abnormalities.
Sulfonylureas, insulin: May decrease hypoglycemic effect of sulfonylureas. May need to adjust dosage of sulfonylureas or insulin.

Indinavir Sulfate

Antiretroviral / Protease inhibitor

Indications: Treatment of HIV infection in adults when antiretroviral therapy is warranted.
Dose: Adults: PO 800 mg (two 400 mg capsules) q 8 hr.
Trade names: Crixivan Capsules 200 mg
Warnings: Concomitant therapy with amiodarone, cisapride, ergot derivatives, midazolam, pimozide, or triazolam; hypersensitivity to any component of product. Pregnancy Category: [C]
Interactions: Cisapride, midazolam, triazolam: Concomitant use is contraindicated.
Delavirdine: Serum levels of indinavir may be increased; consider a dose reduction of indinavir to 600 mg q 8 hr when administering delavirdine 400 mg bid.
Didanosine: Separate administration by at least 1 hr. The buffers in didanosine preparations may interfere with indinavir's absorption.
Efavirenz: Serum levels of indinavir may be decreased; consider a dose increase of indinavir to 1000 mg q 8 hr.
Fentanyl: Indinavir may elevate plasma levels and prolong the half-life of fentanyl, increasing the risk of side effects.
Itraconazole: Serum levels of indinavir may be

increased; consider a dose reduction of indinavir to 600 mg q 8 hr when administering ketoconazole.
Interleukins, ritonavir, sildenafil: Serum indinavir concentrations may be increased. Consider decreasing indinavir's dose.
Rifabutin: Serum concentrations of rifabutin may be increased. A 50% reduction in rifabutin dosage is recommended by the manufacturer.
Rifampin: May induce enzymes that metabolize indinavir; concomitant use not recommended.
Sildenafil: Ritonavir may elevate sildenafil plasma levels, increasing the risk of adverse effects, including hypotension and visual changes.
St. John's wort: Serum levels of indinavir may be decreased, reducing the clinical effect.

Indomethacin

Analgesic / NSAID

Indications: Indomethacin: Symptomatic treatment of rheumatoid arthritis, osteoarthritis, ankylosing spondylitis, gouty arthritis, acute painful shoulder.

Indomethacin sodium trihydrate (IV): Closure of patent ductus arteriosus.

Unlabeled indication: Treatment of primary dysmenorrhea; migraine prophylaxis; treatment of cluster headache, polyhydramnios, sunburn; cystoid macular edema.

Dose: Rheumatoid Arthritis, Osteoarthritis, Ankylosing Spondylitis:
Adults: PO 25 mg bid or tid up to maximum of 200 mg/day (or 75 mg sustained-release form 1 to 2 times daily)
Gouty Arthritis:
Adults: PO/PR 50 mg tid; do not use sustained-release form.
Acute Painful Shoulder:
Adults: PO 75 to 150 mg/day in divided doses for 7 to 14 days.
Patent Ductus Arteriosus: IV 3 doses total.
Infants younger than 2 Days: IV 0.2 mg/kg followed by 2 doses of 0.1 mg/kg 12 to 24 hr apart.
Infants 2 to 7 Days: 3 doses of 0.2 mg/kg separated by 12 to 24 hr.
Infants older than 7 Days: 0.2 mg/kg followed by 2 doses of 0.25 mg/kg separated by 12 to 24 hr.

Trade names: Indocin Capsules 25 mg
Indocin SR Capsules, sustained-release 75 mg
Indocin IV Injection 1 mg

Warnings: Hypersensitivity to aspirin, iodides, or any NSAID. IV form is also contraindicated in the following cases: proven or suspected untreated infection, bleeding, thrombocytopenia, coagulation defects, necrotizing enterocolitis, significant renal impairment, congenital heart disease when patency of ductus arteriosus is necessary for satisfactory blood flow. Suppositories contraindicated in recent bleeding or proctitis history. Pregnancy Category: [Safety not established]

Interactions: Anticoagulants: May increase risk of gastric erosion and bleeding.
Beta-blockers, ACE inhibitors: Antihypertensive effects may be decreased.
Diflunisal: Diflunisal may decrease the renal clearance and significantly increase indomethacin plasma concentrations that may produce toxicity.
Digoxin: May increase digoxin levels.
Lithium: May decrease lithium clearance.
Loop diuretics: May decrease diuretic effects.
Methotrexate: May increase methotrexate levels.
Penicillamine: Indomethacin may increase the bioavailability of penicillamine.
Potassium-sparing diuretics: Effects of potassium-diuretics may be decreased. Concomitant administration may increase serum potassium levels.
Sympathomimetics: Indomethacin and phenylpropanolamine coadministration may result in increased blood pressure.

Infliximab

Monoclonal antibody

Indications: Reduce signs and symptoms and induce and maintain clinical remission of moderate to severe Crohn disease; reduce number of draining enterocutaneous and rectovaginal fistulas and maintain fistula closure in Crohn disease; in combination with methotrexate to reduce signs and symptoms, inhibit progression of structural damage, and improve physical function in patients with moderately to severely active rheumatoid arthritis who have had inadequate response to methotrexate.

Unlabeled indication: Treatment of plaque psoriasis, ankylosing spondylitis, ulcerative colitis, psoriatic arthritis, psoriasis, Behcet syndrome, uveitis, and juvenile arthritis.

Dose: Rheumatoid Arthritis:
Adults: IV 3 mg/kg infusion followed by additional 3 mg/kg doses at 2 and 6 wk after the first infusion, then q 8 wk thereafter in combination with methotrexate. For patients with incomplete response, may give up to 10 mg/kg or treat as often as q 4 wk.
Moderate to Severe or Fistulizing Crohn Disease:
Adults: IV 5 mg/kg as an induction regimen at 0, 2, and 6 wk, followed by a maintenance regimen of 5 mg/kg q 8 wk. In patients who respond and then lose their response, consider treatment with 10 mg/kg.

Trade names: Remicade Powder for Injection 100 mg (500 mg sucrose)

Warnings: Hypersensitivity to murine proteins or other components of product; moderate or severe CHF. Pregnancy Category: [B]

Interactions: Vaccines: Do not administer live vaccines concurrently.
Incompatability: Do not infuse concomitantly with other agents in the same IV line.

Influenza Virus Vaccine

Vaccine, inactivated virus

Indications: Induction of active immunity against the specific influenza viruses corresponding to strains in current-year vaccine formula; prophylaxis for people at least 6 mo of age at increased risk of complications or exposure to influenza. Fluvirin is not indicated for children under 4 yr.

Dose: Fluzone/Fluvirin:
Adults and Children at least 9 yr: IM 0.5 mL 1 dose.
Children 3 to 8 yr (Fluvirin is indicated only in children 4 yr and older): IM 0.5 mL 1 dose; however, if previously unvaccinated, give 2 doses at least 1 mo apart, administering the second dose before December if possible.
Children 6 to 35 mo (Fluvirin is indicated only in children 4 yr and older): IM 0.25 mL 1 dose; however, if previously unvaccinated, give 2 doses at least 1 mo apart, administering the second dose before December if possible.
FluMist (nasal inhalational only):
Children and adults 9 through 49 yr: Nasal 0.5 mL/season.
Children 5 through 8 yr: Nasal 0.5 mL/season if previously vaccinated with FluMist; 2 doses of 0.5 mL/season, each 60 days apart, if not previously vaccinated with FluMist.

Trade names: FluMist Intranasal spray 10-6.5-7.5 $TCID_{50}$ (median tissue culture infectious dose) each of A/Panama/2007/99(H3N2) (A/Moscow/10/99-like), A/New/Caledonia/20/99(H1N1), and B/Hong Kong/330/2001 per 0.5 mL
Fluvirin Injection (purified split-virus) 15 mcg each: A/Panama/2007/99 (H3N2) (A/Moscow/10/99[H3N2]-like), A/New Caledonia/20/99 (H1N1)-like, and B/Hong Kong/330/2001-like per 0.5 mL.

Fluzone Injection (purified split-virus) 15 mcg each: A/Panama/2007/99 (H3N2) (A/Moscow/10/99[H3N2]-like), A/New Caledonia/20/99 (H1N1)-like, and B/Hong Kong/330/2001-like per 0.5 mL.

Warnings: Immediate hypersensitivity to product or other components; hypersensitivity to eggs or egg products; delayed immunization is recommended for people with active neurologic disorder characterized by changing neurologic findings; defer immunization during acute respiratory disease or other active infection or during acute febrile illness; known or suspected immune deficiency diseases. FluMist: Do not administer parenterally; do not administer to children or adolescents 5 to 17 yr receiving aspirin; do not administer to patients with altered or compromised immune status as a consequence of treatment with systemic corticosteroids, alkylating drugs, antimetabolites, radiation, or other immunosuppressive therapies. Pregnancy Category: [C]

Interactions: Anticoagulants: As with other IM drugs, give with caution to patients receiving anticoagulant therapy.
Antivirals: Do not administer FluMist until 48 hr after cessation of antiviral therapy, and do not administer antivirals until 14 days after giving FluMist, unless medically indicated.
Aspirin: Contraindicated in children or adolescents receiving FluMist.
Immunosuppressant drugs (eg, high-dose corticosteroids), radiation therapy: May result in inadequate response to immunization.
Other vaccines: Do not administer FluMist concurrently with other vaccines.
Pertussis vaccine: In order to attribute causality of adverse reactions, do not give influenza vaccine within 3 days of pertussis vaccination.
Theophylline: Theophylline levels may be increased during first 24 hr following vaccination.

Ipecac Syrup

Antidote

Indications: Treatment of drug overdose and certain poisonings.

Dose: Adults: PO 15 to 30 mL followed by 3 to 4 glasses of water. May repeat dose within 20 min if vomiting does not occur.
Children younger than 1 yr: PO 5 to 10 mL followed by 1/2 glass of water.
Children 1 to 12 yr: PO 15 mL followed by 1 to 2 glasses of water.

Trade names: Available as generic only Syrup Ipecac, USP

Warnings: Do not use in semiconscious, unconscious, pregnant, or lactating persons; do not use if strychnine, corrosives (eg, alkalis, strong acids), or petroleum distillates have been ingested. Pregnancy Category: [C]

Interactions: Activated charcoal: Will absorb ipecac syrup. Give activated charcoal only after ipecac syrup has produced vomiting.
Milk or carbonated beverages: Do not administer with ipecac syrup.

Irbesartan

Antihypertensive / Angiotensin II antagonist

Indications: Treatment of hypertension; nephropathy in type 2 diabetes.

Dose: Hypertension:
Adults: PO Start with 150 mg qd; then titrate to 300 mg qd as necessary.
Children (13 to 16 yr): PO Start with 150 mg qd; then titrate patients requiring a further reduction in BP to 300 mg qd.
Children (6 to 12 yr): PO Start with 75 mg qd; then titrate patients requiring a further reduction in BP to 150 mg qd.
Nephropathy in Type 2 Diabetes:
Adults: PO Titrate dose to 300 mg qd.
Volume- and Salt-Depleted Patients: PO Start with 75 mg.

Trade names: Avapro Tablets 75 mg

Warnings: Standard considerations. Pregnancy Category: [C (first trimester); D (second and third trimesters)]

Interactions: Lithium: Plasma concentrations may be increased by irbesartan, resulting in an increase in the pharmacologic and adverse effects of lithium.

Irinotecan

Topoisomerase I inhibitor

Indications: Metastatic cancer of the colon or rectum after standard treatment with fluorouracil.

Unlabeled indication: Cervical cancer, lung cancer (small cell or non-small cell), ovarian cancer.

Dose: Colon or Rectal Cancer:
Adults: IV Cycle 1: Irinotecan 125 mg/m^2 once weekly for 4 wk followed by 2 wk of rest. Subsequent cycles: Give irinotecan once weekly for 4 wk, followed by 2 wk of rest. Based on response and adverse effects, the dose may be adjusted in 25 to 50 mg/m^2 increments. The weekly dose may be increased to a max of 150 mg/m^2 or decreased to a min of 50 mg/m^2.
Alternate schedule: Irinotecan 350 mg/m^2 IV once q 21 days. Give an initial dose of irinotecan 300 mg/m^2 IV q 21 days in patients at least 70 yr, patients with prior pelvic or abdominal radiation, or patients with a performance status of 2. Based on adverse effects, the dose may be decreased in 50 mg/m^2 increments to a min of 200 mg/m^2 (max, 350 mg/m^2).
Dosage Adjustment for Hepatic Dysfunction:
Adults: IV Once-daily regimen: Dosage should be 125 mg/m^2 if serum bilirubin is less than 1 mg/dL. If bilirubin concentration is 1 to 2 mg/dL, dosage should be 100 mg/m -3. Irinotecan is not recommended if bilirubin is more than 2 mg/dL. Every 21-day regimen: Dosage should be 350 mg/m^2 if serum bilirubin is less than 1 mg/dL. If bilirubin concentration is 1 to 2 mg/dL, dosage should be 300 mg/m^2. Irinotecan is not recommended if bilirubin is more than 2 mg/dL.

Trade names: Camptosar Injection 20 mg/mL, containing sorbitol 45 mg

Warnings: Standard considerations. Pregnancy Category: [D]

Interactions: Antineoplastics: Irinotecan adverse effects (eg, myelosuppression, diarrhea) would possibly be exacerbated by other antineoplastics having similar adverse effects.
Dexamethasone: It is possible that coadministration of dexamethasone and irinotecan may enhance the likelihood of lymphocytopenia. Dexamethasone given as emetic prophylaxis can contribute to hyperglycemia in some patients.
Laxatives: Laxative therapy during irinotecan therapy may increase the severity of diarrhea, but this has not been studied.
Prochloperazine: The incidence of akathesia in clinical trials was greater (8.5%) when prochlorperazine was administered on the same day as irinotecan than when these drugs were given on separate days (1.3%).
Diuretics: The health care provider may wish to withhold diuretics during irinotecan dosing during periods of active vomiting or diarrhea because of the potential risk of dehydration secondary to irinotecan-induced vomiting and diarrhea.

Isometheptene Mucate/ Dichloralphenazone/ Acetaminophen

Migraine

Indications: Relief of tension and vascular

headaches. FDA has classified drug as possibly effective in treatment of migraine headaches.
Dose: Migraine Headache:
Adults: PO 2 capsules at once, followed by 1 capsule q hr until headache is relieved (max, 5 capsules in 12 hr period).
Tension Headache:
Adults: PO 1 to 2 capsules q 4 hr (max, 8 capsules/day).
Trade names: Isocom Capsules 65 mg isometheptene mucate, 100 mg dichloralphenazone, 325 mg APAP
Isopap Capsules 65 mg isometheptene mucate, 100 mg dichloralphenazone, 325 mg APAP
Midchlor Capsules 65 mg isometheptene mucate, 100 mg dichloralphenazone, 325 mg APAP
Midrin Capsules 65 mg isometheptene mucate, 100 mg dichloralphenazone, 325 mg APAP
Migratine Capsules 65 mg isometheptene mucate, 100 mg dichloralphenazone, 325 mg APAP
Warnings: Glaucoma; severe cases of renal disease; hypertension; organic heart disease; hepatic disease; MAO inhibitor therapy. Pregnancy Category: [Pregnancy category undetermined]
Interactions: MAO inhibitors: May result in severe headache, hypertension, hyperpyrexia, and possible hypertensive crisis.

Isoniazid

Anti-infective / Antitubercular
Indications: Treatment of all forms of tuberculosis.

Unlabeled indication: Improvement of severe tremor in multiple sclerosis.
Dose: Tuberculosis:
Adults: PO/IM 5 mg/kg/day as single daily dose (max, 300 mg/day) or 15 mg/kg 2 to 3 times/wk (max, 900 mg).
Infants and Children: PO/IM 10 to 20 mg/kg/day in single daily dose (max, 300 mg/day) or 20 to 40 mg/kg 2 or 3 times/week (max, 400 mg).
Trade names: Nydrazid Injection 100 mg/mL
Isoniazid Tablets 300 mg
Warnings: Previous isoniazid-associated hepatic injury, drug fever, chills, or arthritis; acute liver disease. Pregnancy Category: [Safety undetermined]
Interactions: Aluminum salts: May reduce oral absorption of isoniazid; give isoniazid 1 to 3 hr before aluminum salts.
Carbamazepine: May result in carbamazepine toxicity or isoniazid hepatotoxicity. Monitor carbamazepine concentrations and liver function.
Disulfiram: May result in increased incidence of CNS effects (eg, coordination difficulties, confusion, irritability, aggressiveness).
Enflurane: May result in high-output renal failure in rapid acetylators. Monitor renal function.
Hydantoins: May increase serum hydantoin levels.
Rifampin: May result in higher rate of hepatotoxicity.

Isoproterenol

Bronchodilator / Sympathomimetic
Indications: Management of bronchospasm during anesthesia; adjunctive treatment for shock.
Dose: Bronchospasm during anesthesia:
Adults: IV 0.01 to 0.02 mg. Repeat as necessary.
Shock and hypoperfusion:
Adults: IV 0.5 mcg to 5 mcg/min. Rates over 30 mcg/min have been used in advanced stages of shock.
Heart block, Adams-Stokes attacks, and cardiac arrest:
Adults: Bolus IV 0.02 mg to 0.06 mg initial dose with subsequent dose range of 0.01 mg to 0.2 mg; IV infusion 5mcg/min initial dose; IM 0.2 mg initial dose with a subsequent dose rang of 0.02 mg to 1 mg; SC 0.2 mg initial dose of 0.2 mg with subsequent dose range of 0.15 mg to 0.2 mg; Intracardiac 0.02 mg initial dose. Subsequent dosage and administration method depend on ventricular rate and rapidity with which cardiac pacemaker can take over when drug is withdrawn.
Trade names: Isuprel Injection (1:5000 solution) 0.2 mg/mL isoproterenol HCl
Isoproterenol Hydrochloride Injection (1:5000 solution) 0.2 mg/mL isoproterenol HCl
Medihaler-ISO Aerosol Delivers 80 mcg isoproternol sulfate/actuation
Warnings: Cardiac arrhythmias associated with tachycardia; tachycardia or heart block caused by digitalis intoxication; angina; ventricular arrhythmias requiring inotropic therapy. Pregnancy Category: [C]
Interactions: Cardiac glycosides: Arrhythmias may result with coadministration.
General anesthetics (eg, halothane, cyclopropane): Arrhythmias may result with coadministration.
Ergot alkaloids: Coadministration may result in additive peripheral vasoconstriction.

Isosorbide Dinitrate

Antianginal
Indications: Treatment and prevention of angina pectoris.
Dose: Angina Pectoris:
Adults: SL (sublingual tablets) 2.5 to 5 mg; PO (chewable tablets) 5 mg; PO (oral tablets) 5 to 40 mg q 6 hr; PO (sustained release tablets) 40 to 80 mg q 8 to 12 hr.
Acute Prophylaxis:
Adults: PO (sublingual or chewable tablets) 5 to 10 mg q 2 to 3 hr.
Trade names: Dilatrate-SR Capsules, sustained-release 40 mg
Isordil Tablets, sublingual 2.5 mg
Isordil Tembids Tablets, sustained-release 40 mg
Isordil Titradose Tablets 5 mg
Sorbitrate Tablets 5 mg
Warnings: Hypersensitivity to nitrates; severe anemia; closed-angle glaucoma; orthostatic hypotension; head trauma or cerebral hemorrhage. Pregnancy Category: [C]
Interactions: Alcohol: Severe hypotension and cardiovascular collapse.
Aspirin: Increased nitrate concentration and actions.
Dihydroergotamine: Increased systolic blood pressure and decreased antianginal effects.

Isosorbide Mononitrate

Antianginal
Indications: Prevention of angina pectoris.
Dose: Adults: PO 20 mg bid, given 7 hr apart. Extended-release tablets are given as 30 (1/2 of 60 mg tablet) or 60 mg once daily. After several days dosage may be increased to 120 mg (given as two 60 mg tablets) once daily. Rarely, 240 mg may be required.
Trade names: ISMO Tablets 20 mg
Imdur Tablets, extended-release 30 mg
Monoket Tablets 10 mg
Isotrate ER Tablets, extended-release 60 mg
Warnings: Hypersensitivity to nitrates; severe anemia; closed-angle glaucoma; orthostatic hypotension; head trauma or cerebral hemorrhage. Pregnancy Category: [C]
Interactions: Alcohol: Severe hypotension and cardiovascular collapse may occur.
Aspirin: Increased nitrate concentration and actions.
Calcium channel blockers: Symptomatic orthostatic hypotension.
Dihydroergotamine: Increased systolic BP and decreased antianginal effects may develop.

Isotretinoin

Acne
Indications: Treatment of severe recalcitrant

cystic acne.

Unlabeled indication: Treatment of keratinization disorders, cutaneous T-cell lymphoma, leukoplakia; prevention of skin cancer in patients with xeroderma pigmentosum.

Dose: Adults: PO 0.5 to 1 mg/kg/day divided into 2 doses with food for 15 to 20 wk. For severe cases, dose adjustments up to 2 mg/kg/day may be needed.

Trade names: Accutane Capsules 10 mg
Claravis Capsules 10 mg

Warnings: Hypersensitivity to parabens; pregnancy. Pregnancy Category: [X There is an extremely high risk of deformity to the infant if pregnancy occurs while taking this drug in any amount, even for short periods Potentially, all exposed fetuses can be affected Presently, there are no accurate means of determining after isotretinoin exposure which fetus has or has not been affected]

Interactions: Vitamin A: May increase toxic effects; do not take with isotretinoin.
Tetracycline/Minocycline: Have been associated with pseudotumor cerebri or papilledema in isotretinoin patients.
Carbamazepine: Coadministration has resulted in reduced carbamazepine plasma level.
Drug/Food interactions: When taken with food, the absorption of isotretinoin has increased.

Isradipine

Calcium channel blocker

Indications: Treatment of hypertension.

Dose: Adults: PO 2.5 to 10 mg/day in 2 divided doses (max dose 20 mg/day).

Trade names: DynaCirc Capsules 2.5 mg
DynaCirc CR Tablets, controlled-release 5 mg

Warnings: Standard considerations. Pregnancy Category: [C]

Interactions: None well documented.

Itraconazole

Anti-infective / Antifungal

Indications: Injection: Treatment of aspergillosis, blastomycosis, febrile neutropenia, and histoplasmosis.

Capsules: Treatment of aspergillosis, blastomycosis, histoplasmosis, and onychomycosis.

Oral solution: Treatment of oropharyngeal or esophageal candidiasis and empiric treatment of febrile neutropenia.

Unlabeled indication: Treatment of other fungal infections (superficial mycoses [eg, dermatophytoses]; systemic mycoses [eg, candidiasis, cryptococcus]; and miscellaneous fungal infections [eg, SC mycoses, cutaneous Leishmaniasis]).

Dose: Blastomycosis, Aspergillosis, Histoplasmosis:
Adults: PO 200 to 400 mg/day. Give doses over 200 mg in 2 divided doses. IV 200 mg bid for 4 doses, followed by 200 mg/day. Infuse over 1 hr. Continue IV for 14 days followed by PO for 3 mo or more and until clinical parameters and laboratory tests indicate active fungal infection has subsided. An inadequate treatment period may lead to recurrence.
Empiric Therapy in Febrile, Neutropenic Patients with Suspected Fungal Infections:
Adults: IV 200 mg bid infused over 60 min for 4 doses, followed by 200 mg qd for up to 14 days; continue PO oral solution 200 mg bid until resolution of clinically important neutropenia (safety and efficacy over 28 days not established.)
Esophageal Candidiasis:
Adults: PO 100 mg/day for a minimum of 3 wk. Continue treatment for 2 wk following resolution of symptoms. Doses up to 200 mg/day may be used based on medical judgment of the patient's response. Vigorously swish solution in mouth (10 mL at a time) for several seconds and swallow.
Onychomycosis, Fingernails Only:
Adults: PO 2 treatment pulses separated by a 3-wk period without itraconazole. Each pulse consisting of 200 mg bid for 1 wk.
Onychomycosis, Toenails With or Without Fingernail Involvement:
Adults: PO 200 mg/day for 12 wk.
Oropharyngeal Candidiasis:
Adults: PO, oral solution 200 mg (20 mL)/day for 1 to 2 wk. Vigorously swish solution in mouth for several seconds and swallow.

Trade names: Sporanox Capsules 100 mg

Warnings: Coadministration with pimozide, quinidine, triazolam, or oral midazolam, HMG-CoA reductase inhibitors metabolized by the P450 3A enzyme system (eg, lovastatin, simvastatin); not for treatment of onychomycosis in pregnant women or women contemplating pregnancy; ventricular dysfunction such as CHF or history of CHF. Pregnancy Category: [C]

Interactions: Alfentanil, carbamazepine, corticosteroids, haloperidol, protease inhibitors, rifamycins (eg, rifampin), sirolimus, tacrolimus, tolterodine, vinca alkaloids, warfarin, zolpidem: Levels may be elevated by itraconazole, increasing the risk of adverse effects.
Alprazolam, midazolam (oral), triazolam: Elevated plasma levels of these drugs; may potentiate and prolong their hypnotic and sedative effects. Sedative effects of parenteral midazolam may be prolonged.
Amphotericin B, oral contraceptives: Efficacy may be reduced by itraconazole.
Antacids, H_2-antagonists, nevirapine, phenobarbital, proton pump inhibitors: Reduced plasma itraconazole levels.
Buspirone, busulfan, docetaxel, dofetilide, haloperidol, itraconazole, methylprednisolone, trimetrexate: May elevate plasma concentrations. Adjust dose as needed.
Calcium blockers (eg, amlodipine, felodipine, nifedipine): Edema has occurred with concomitant dihydropyridine calcium blockers.
Cisapride, dofetilide, pimozide, quinidine: Increased levels may result in life-threatening cardiac dysrhythmias and death. Do not use with itraconazole.
Cyclosporine plus HMG-CoA reductase inhibitors: There are rare reports of rhabdomyolysis in renal transplant patients receiving this drug combination. Increased cyclosporine levels may occur. Monitor cyclosporine levels; reduce cyclosporine dose 50% when using itraconazole doses over 100 mg/day.
Didanosine: May decrease therapeutic effects of itraconazole. Administer itraconazole 2 hr or more before didanosine.
Digoxin: Increased digoxin levels. Monitor frequently.
Hypoglycemic agents: Hypoglycemia may occur. Monitor blood glucose.
Indinavir, ritonavir: Plasma levels of itraconazole may be decreased.
Macrolide antibiotics (eg, erythromycin): Plasma levels of itraconazole may be increased.
Phenytoin: Reduced plasma itraconazole levels; altered phenytoin metabolism.
Sulfonylurea: Hypoglycemia may occur.

Kanamycin Sulfate

Antibiotic / Aminoglycoside

Indications: Parenteral: Short-term treatment of serious infections caused by susceptible strains of microorganisms, especially gram-negative bacteria.

Oral: Short-term adjunctive therapy for suppression of intestinal bacteria; treatment of hepatic coma.

Dose: Infection:
Adults and Children: IM/IV 15 mg/kg/day in 2 to 4 divided doses. Do not exceed 1.5 g/day.
Suppression of Intestinal Bacteria:

Adults: PO 1 g qh for 4 hr, then 1 g q 6 hr for 36 to 72 hr.
Tuberculosis:
Adults and children: IM/IV 15 to 30 mg/kg/day (max, 1 g/day).
Hepatic Coma:
Adults: PO 8 to 12 g/day in divided doses.
Trade names: Kantrex Capsules 500 mg
Warnings: Hypersensitivity to aminoglycosides; intestinal obstruction (oral). Generally not indicated for long-term therapy (more than 14 days) because of ototoxicity and nephrotoxicity. Pregnancy Category: [D]
Interactions: Beta-lactam antibiotics (eg, cephalosporins, penicillins): Do not mix in IV solutions.
Digoxin, methotrexate, vitamin A, vitamin K: Oral kanamycin may decrease absorption of these drugs.
Drugs with nephrotoxic potential (eg, amphotericin, cephalosporins, enflurane, methoxyflurane, vancomycin): Increased risk of nephrotoxicity.
Loop diuretics: Increased auditory toxicity.
Neuromuscular blocking agents: Enhanced effects of these agents.
Polypeptide antibiotics: Increased risk of respiratory paralysis and renal dysfunction.

Ketamine HCl

General anesthetic

Indications: Diagnostic and surgical procedures that do not require skeletal muscle relaxation; induction of anesthesia; supplementation of low-potency agents, such as nitrous oxide.
Dose: Adults and Children: induction of anesthesia: IV Initial: 1 to 4.5 mg/kg via slow infusion (over 60 sec); usual dose for 5 to 10 min anesthesia: 2 mg/kg. Maintenance: One-half to full induction dose, repeated as needed. Alternatively IV 0.1 to 0.5 mg/min infusion, augmented with diazepam IV 2 to 5 mg. IM Initial: 6.5 to 13 mg/kg. Maintenance: One-half to full induction dose, repeated as needed.
Trade names: Ketalar Injection 10 mg/mL
Warnings: Patients in whom significant BP elevation would be a serious hazard; hypersensitivity to the drug. Pregnancy Category: [B]
Interactions: Halothane: Decreased cardiac output, BP, and pulse.
Tubocurarine and other nondepolarizing muscle relaxants: Increased neuromuscular effects, resulting in prolonged respiratory depression.
Incompatability: Ketamine is physically incompatible with diazepam and barbiturates.

Ketoconazole

Anti-infective / Antifungal

Indications: Treatment of susceptible systemic and cutaneous fungal infections.
Topical: Seborrheic dermatitis; tinea corporis; tinea cruris; tinea pedis; tinea versicolor.
Dose: Adults: PO 200 to 400 mg qd.
Children older than 2 yr: PO 3.3 to 6.6 mg/kg/day. Treatment may last from 1 wk to 6 mo, depending on infection.
Adults: Topical Apply to affected and immediate surrounding area qd for 2 to 4 wk.
Trade names: Nizoral Tablets 200 mg
Warnings: Fungal meningitis. Pregnancy Category: [C]
Interactions: Antacids: Increased gastric pH may inhibit ketoconazole absorption; separate administration by 2 hr or more.
Benzodiazepines (eg, midazolam): Plasma levels of benzodiazepines may be increased and prolonged.
Corticosteroids: Increased bioavailability and decreased clearance of corticosteroid.
Cyclosporine: Increased cyclosporine concentrations.
Didanosine, histamine H_2 -receptor antagonists (eg, cimetidine), proton pump inhibitors (eg, omeprazole): May decrease ketoconazole absorption.
Dofetilide: Elevated plasma levels of dofetilide may increase the risk of life-threatening cardiac arrhythmia.
Nisoldipine, protease inhibitors (eg, indinavir), tacrolimus, tolterodine: Plasma levels may be elevated by ketoconazole, increasing the risk of side effects.
Rifampin: Decreased serum levels of either drug; avoid concomitant use.
Theophylline: Decreased theophylline serum concentrations.
Warfarin: Increased anticoagulant effect.

Ketoprofen

Analgesic / NSAID

Indications: Treatment of rheumatoid arthritis, osteoarthritis, mild to moderate pain, primary dysmenorrhea.
Sustained-release form only: Treatment of rheumatoid arthritis and osteoarthritis.

OTC Use: Temporary relief of minor aches and pains associated with common cold, headache, toothache, muscular aches, backache, minor arthritis pain, menstrual cramps, and reduction of fever.

Unlabeled indication: Treatment of juvenile rheumatoid arthritis, sunburn, migraine prophylaxis.
Dose: Rheumatoid or Osteoarthritis:
Adults: PO 75 mg tid or 50 mg qid; do not exceed 300 mg/day. Maintenance dose: Reduce initial dosage to 75 to 150 mg/day in elderly or disabled patients or patients with renal impairment. Sustained-release capsule: 200 mg once daily can be used in patients already stabilized on that dose.
Mild to Moderate Pain, Primary Dysmenorrhea:
Adults: PO 25 to 50 mg q 6 to 8 hr prn; do not exceed 300 mg/day.
Mild-To-Severe Renal Function Impairment: PO Maximum recommended total daily dose is 150 mg. In patients with a more severe renal impairment (GFR less than 25 mL/min or end-stage renal impairment), the max total daily dose should not exceed 100 mg.
Hepatic Function Impairment: PO For patients with impaired liver function and serum albumin concentration less than 3.5 g/dL, the max initial total daily dose should be 100 mg.
OTC Use:
Adults: PO 12.5 mg with a full glass of liquid q 4 to 6 hr. If pain or fever persists after 1 hr, follow with 12.5 mg. Do not exceed 25 mg in a 4- to 6-hr period or 75 mg in a 24-hr period. Use the smallest effective dose.
Children: PO Do not give to those younger than 16 yr unless directed by a health care provider.
Trade names: Orudis Capsules 25 mg
Orudis KT Tablets 12.5 mg
Oruvail Capsules, extended-release 100 mg
Warnings: Patients in whom aspirin, iodides, or any NSAID have caused allergic-type reactions. Pregnancy Category: [B]
Interactions: Anticoagulants: Increased risk of gastric erosion and bleeding.
Aspirin: Additive GI toxicity.
Cyclosporine: Nephrotoxicity of both agents may be increased.
Lithium: Serum lithium levels may be increased.
Methotrexate: Increased methotrexate levels.

Ketorolac Tromethamine

Analgesic / NSAID

Indications: Oral and IM forms: Short-term management of moderately severe, acute pain.

Ophthalmic form: Relief of ocular itching caused by seasonal allergic conjunctivitis; treatment of postoperative inflammation in patients who have undergone cataract extraction.
Dose: Multiple Dose:
Adults: IM Younger than 65 yr: 30 mg q 6 hr. Do not

exceed 120 mg/day; older than 65 yr, renal impairment, or weight under 50 kg (110 lbs): 15 mg q 6 hr. Do not exceed 60 mg/day.
Single Dose:
Adults: IM Younger than 65 yr: 60 mg; older than 65 yr, renal impairment, or weight under 50 kg (110 lbs): 30 mg. IV younger than 65 yr: 30 mg; older than 65 yr, renal impairment, or weight under 50 kg (110 lbs): 15 mg.
Children: IM 1 mg/kg up to 30 mg max. IV 0.5 mg/kg up to 15 mg max.
Transition from IV/IM to Oral:
Adults: Younger than 65 yr: 20 mg as a first oral dose for patients who received 60 mg IM single dose, 30 mg IV single dose, or 30 mg multiple dose IV/IM, followed by 10 mg q 4 to 6 hr, not to exceed 40 mg/24 hr. Older than 65 years old, renal impairment, or weight under 50 kg (110 lbs): 10 mg as a first oral dose for patients who received a 30 mg IM single dose, 15 mg IV single dose, or 15 mg multiple dose IV/IM, followed by 10 mg q 4 to 6 hr, not to exceed 40 mg/24 hr.
Ophthalmic: 1 gtt (0.25 mg) qid. For treatment of postoperative inflammation after cataract surgery, continue through first 2 wk of postoperative period.

Trade names: Acular Solution 0.5%
Acular LS Solution 0.4%
Toradol Tablets 10 mg

Warnings: Patients in whom aspirin, iodides, or any NSAID have caused allergic-type reactions; active peptic ulcer disease, recent GI bleeding or perforation; advanced renal impairment and in patients at risk for renal failure because of volume depletion; suspected or confirmed cerebrovascular bleeding; hemorrhagic diathesis, incomplete hemostasis, and those at high risk of bleeding; as prophylactic analgesia before any major surgery and intraoperatively when hemostasis is critical; for intrathecal or epidural administration because of its alcohol content; in labor and delivery; in lactation; in concomitant use with aspirin or other NSAIDs; concomitant use with probenecid. Ophthalmic use: Soft contact lens use. Pregnancy Category: [C]

Interactions: Anticoagulants: May increase risk of gastric erosion and bleeding.
Cyclosporine: Nephrotoxicity of both agents may be increased.
Lithium: Serum lithium levels may be increased.
Methotrexate: May increase methotrexate levels.
Salicylates: May cause additive GI toxicity.

Labetalol HCl

Alpha-adrenergic blocker / Beta-adrenergic blocker

Indications: Management of hypertension.

Unlabeled indication: Treatment of pheochromocytoma; management of clonidine-withdrawal hypertension.

Dose: Adults: PO 100 mg bid initially; maintenance dose usually 200 to 400 mg bid. IV 20 mg over 2 min; then 40 to 80 mg q 10 min up to max of 300 mg. Infusions of 2 mg/min can be initiated and titrated to response.

Trade names: Normodyne Tablets 100 mg
Trandate Tablets 100 mg

Warnings: Severe bradycardia; second- and third-degree heart block; heart failure; cardiogenic shock; bronchial asthma. Pregnancy Category: [C]

Interactions: Beta-adrenergic agonists: Blunted bronchodilator effect.
Cimetidine: Increased bioavailability of labetalol.
Indomethacin: Impaired antihypertensive effect of labetalol.
Inhalation anesthetics: May exaggerate hypotension.
Nitroglycerin: Increased hypotension.
Incompatability: Injection not compatible with 5% Sodium Bicarbonate.

Lactulose

Laxative

Indications: Treatment of constipation; prevention and treatment of portal-systemic encephalopathy, including stages of hepatic precoma and coma.

Dose: Constipation (Chronulac, Constilac, Duphalac):
Adults: PO 15 to 30 mL (10 to 20 g lactulose) daily; may increase to 60 mL/day.
Portal-Systemic Encephalopathy (Cephulac, Cholac, Enulose):
Adults: PO 30 to 45 mL tid to qid. Adjust dosage to produce 2 to 3 soft stools/day. Hourly doses of 30 to 45 mL may be used for rapid laxation initially; once achieved, reduce to recommended daily dose. PR 300 mL with 700 mL water or physiologic saline solution via rectal balloon catheter; retain for 30 to 60 min. May repeat q 4 to 6 hr.
Older Children and Adolescents: PO 40 to 90 mL/day in divided doses to produce 2 to 3 soft stools/day.
Infants: PO 2.5 to 10 mL/day in divided doses to produce 2 to 3 soft stools/day.

Trade names: Cephulac Solution 10 g lactulose/15 mL (less than 1.6 g galactose, less than 1.2 g galactose, and up to 1.2 g of other sugars)
Cholac Solution 10 g lactulose/15 mL (less than 1.6 g galactose, less than 1.2 g galactose, and up to 1.2 g of other sugars)
Chronulac Solution 10 g lactulose/15 mL (less than 1.6 g galactose, less than 1.2 g galactose, and up to 1.2 g of other sugars)
Constilac Solution 10 g lactulose/15 mL (less than 1.6 g galactose, less than 1.2 g galactose, and up to 1.2 g of other sugars)
Constulose Solution 10 g lactulose/15mL (less than 1.6 g galactose, less than 1.2 g galactose, and up to 1.2 g of other sugars)
Duphalac Solution 10 g lactulose/15 mL (less than 1.6 g galactose, less than 1.2 g galactose up to 1.2 g of other sugars)
Enulose Solution 10 g lactulose per 15 mL (less than 1.6 g galactose, less than 1.2 g galactose, and up to 1.2 g of other sugars)

Warnings: Use in patients who require low-galactose diet. Pregnancy Category: [B]

Interactions: Neomycin, other anti-infectives: May interfere with desired degradation of lactulose and prevent acidification of colonic contents.
Nonabsorbable antacids: May inhibit colonic acidification.

Lamotrigine

Anticonvulsant

Indications: Bipolar disorder: Maintenance treatment of bipolar I disorder to delay the time to occurrence of mood episodes in patients treated for acute mood episodes with standard therapy.

Epilepsy: Adjunctive therapy in the treatment of partial seizures in adults and as adjunctive therapy in the generalized seizures of Lennox-Gastaut syndrome in pediatric and adult patients. Conversion to monotherapy in adults with partial seizures who are receiving treatment with a single enzyme-inducing AED (EIAED).

Unlabeled indication: May be useful in adults with generalized tonic-clonic, absence, atypical absence, and myoclonic seizures.

Dose: As Add-On Therapy For Epilepsy:
Lamotrigine Plus AED Regimen Containing Valproic Acid:
Children 2 to 12 yr: PO Wk 1 and 2: 0.15 mg/kg/day in 1 to 2 divided doses. Wk 3 and 4: 0.3 mg/kg/day in 1 to 2 divided doses.
Maintenance dose:: 1 to 5 mg/kg/day (max, 200 mg/day in 1 to 2 divided doses).

Adults older than 12 yr: PO Wk 1 and 2: 25 mg every other day. Wk 3 and 4: 25 mg/day.
Maintenance dose:: 100 to 400 mg/day in 1 to 2 divided doses. To achieve, escalate dose by 25 to 50 mg/day q 1 to 2 wk. In patients receiving valproic acid alone, maintenance doses as high as 200 mg/day have been used.
Lamotrigine Plus EIAEDs without Valproic Acid:
Children 2 to 12 yr: PO Wk 1 and 2: 0.6 mg/kg/day in 2 divided doses. Wk 3 and 4: 1.2 mg/kg/day in 2 divided doses.
Maintenance dose:: 5 to 15 mg/kg/day (max, 400 mg/ day in 2 divided doses).
Adults older than 12 yr: PO Wk 1 and 2: 50 mg/day. Wk 3 and 4: 100 mg/day in 2 divided doses.
Maintenance dose:: 300 to 500 mg/day in 2 divided doses. To achieve, escalate dose by 100 mg/day q 1 to 2 wk. Patients receiving multidrug regimens employing EIAEDs without valproic acid can have a maintenance dose of lamotrigine as high as 700 mg/day.
Conversion from a Single EIAED to Monotherapy with Lamotrigine:
Adults and children at least 16 yr: PO 500 mg/day given as 2 divided doses. Begin conversion by titrating lamotrigine to the target dose (500 mg in 2 divided doses) while maintaining the dose of the EIAED at a fixed level, then withdraw concomitant EIAED by 20% decrements each wk over a 4-wk period.
Escalation Regimen for Patients with Bipolar Disorder:
Patients Not Taking Carbamazepine (or Other Enzyme-Inducing Drugs)or Valproic Acid:
Adults (at least 18 yr): PO Wk 1 and 2: 25 mg/day. Wk 3 and 4: 50 mg/day. Wk 5: 100 mg/day. Wk 6 and 7: 200 mg/day.
Patients Taking Valproic Acid:
Adults (at least 18 yr): PO Wk 1 and 2: 25 mg every other day. Wk 3 and 4: 25 mg/day. Wk 5: 50 mg/day. Wk 6 and 7: 100 mg/day.
Patients Taking Carbamazepine (or Other Enzyme-Inducing Drugs) and Not Taking Valproic Acid:
Adults (at least 18 yr): PO Wk 1 and 2: 50 mg/day. Wk 3 and 4: 100 mg/day in divided doses. Wk 5: 200 mg/ day in divided doses. Wk 6: 300 mg/day in divided doses. Wk 7: up to 400 mg/day in divided doses.
Lamotrigine Dosing Adjustments for Patients with Bipolar Disorder Following Discontinuation of Psychotropics:
After Discontinuation of Valproic Acid (Current Lamotrigine Dose 100 mg/day):
Adults (at least 18 yr): PO Wk 1: 150 mg/day. Wk 2: 200 mg/day. Wk 3 and onward: 200 mg/day.
After Discontinuation of Carbamazepine or Other Enzyme-Inducing Drugs(Current Lamotrigine Dose 400 mg/day):
Adults (at least 18 yr): PO Wk 1: 400 mg/day. Wk 2: 300 mg/day. Wk 3 and onward: 200 mg/day.
Trade names: Lamictal Tablets 25 mg
Lamictal Chewable Dispersible Tablets, chewable 2 mg
Warnings: Standard considerations. Pregnancy Category: [C]
Interactions: Acetaminophen, carbamazepine, hydantoins (eg, phenytoin), oral contraceptives, oxcarbazepine, phenobarbital, primidone, progestins, rifamycins (eg, rifampin), succinimides (eg, methsuximide): Lamotrigine plasma levels may be reduced by these agents, decreasing the therapeutic effect.
Carbamazepine: The risk of carbamazepine toxicity may be increased.
Folate Inhibitors: Lamotrigine is an inhibitor of dihydrofolate reductase. Use caution with other agents that inhibit folate metabolism.
Valproic acid: Plasma levels may be reduced by lamotrigine, decreasing the therapeutic effect.
Valproate increases lamotrigine levels.

Latanoprost

Ophthalmic prostaglandin agonist

Indications: For reduction of elevated IOP in patients with open-angle glaucoma or ocular hypertension.
Dose: 1 drop (1.5 mcg) in the affected eye(s) qd in the evening.
Trade names: Xalatan Ophthalmic solution 0.005% (50 mcg/mL)
Warnings: Standard considerations. Pregnancy Category: [C]
Interactions: Thimerosal: Precipitation occurs when eye drops containing thimerosal are mixed with latanoprost. If such drugs are used, administer with an interval of at least 5 min between applications.

Leflunomide

Antirheumatic agent

Indications: Treatment of active rheumatoid arthritis (RA) to reduce signs and symptoms and to retard structural damage.
Dose: Loading dose: PO 100 mg qd for 3 days.
Maintenance therapy: PO 20 mg qd. If dosing at 20 mg/day is not well-tolerated, the dose may be decreased to 10 mg/day.
Trade names: Arava Tablet 10 mg
Warnings: Pregnancy; standard considerations. Pregnancy Category: [X]
Interactions: Cholestyramine and charcoal: Decrease plasma leflunomide.
Hepatotoxic drugs: May potentiate the hepatotoxicity of leflunomide.
NSAIDs and tolbutamide: Free-fraction serum concentrations were increased by leflunomide.
Rifampin: May increase leflunomide serum levels.

Leucovorin Calcium

Folic acid derivative

Indications: Oral and parenteral: Treatment to diminish toxicity and counteract effect of overdosage of folic acid antagonists.

Parenteral: Treatment of megaloblastic anemia caused by folic acid deficiency when oral therapy is not feasible.
Dose: Colorectal Cancer:
Adults: IV Either 200 mg/m^2 followed by 5-fluorouracil (5-FU) 370 mg/m^2 or 20 mg/m^2 followed by 5-FU 425 mg/m^2 qd for 5 days.
Leucovorin Rescue:
Adults: PO / IV / IM 10 mg/m^2 q 6 hr for 10 doses.
Megaloblastic Anemia Caused by Folic Acid Deficiency:
Adults: IV / IM 1 mg/day.
Trade names: Wellcovorin Tablets 5 mg
Warnings: Pernicious anemia and other megaloblastic anemias secondary to vitamin B -12 deficiency. Pregnancy Category: [C]
Interactions: Barbiturates, hydantoins (eg, phenytoin), primidone: May decrease anticonvulsant activity.
Fluorouracil: Enhances toxicity of fluorouracil.
Methotrexate: May decrease efficacy of intrathecal methotrexate.

Leuprolide Acetate

Gonadotropin-releasing hormone

Indications: Palliative treatment of advanced prostatic cancer (alone or in combination with flutamide); management of endometriosis in women over 18 yr (depot preparation); treatment of children with central precocious puberty (CPP [pediatric injection or depot pediatric]); uterine leiomyomata (depot preparation).

Unlabeled indication: Breast and ovarian carcinoma.
Dose: Advanced Prostate Cancer:
Adults: SC 1 mg/day. IM 7.5 mg q mo (depot preparation).
CPP:

Adults: SC Starting dose: 50 mcg/kg/day as single injection. Individualize dosage and titrate to response.
Adults: IM Starting dose: 0.3 mg/kg q 4 wk (minimum, 7.5 mg) as single injection (depot preparation). Must be administered by health care provider or designated health care provider.
Endometriosis:
Adults: IM 3.75 mg as single monthly injection or 11.25 mg IM q 3 mo (depot preparation).
Uterine Leiomyomata:
Adults: IM 3.75 mg as a single monthly injection or 11.25 mg IM q 3 mo.
Trade names: Lupron Depot Microspheres for injection, lyophilized 3.75 mg
Lupron Depot-3 Month Microspheres for injection, lyophilized 11.25 mg
Lupron Depot-4 Month Microspheres for injection, lyophilized 30 mg
Lupron Depot-Ped Microspheres for injection, lyophilized 7.5 mg
Lupron for Pediatric Use Injection 5 mg/mL
Viadur Implant 72 mg
Warnings: Pregnancy; lactation; hypersensitivity to GnRH, GnRH agonist analogs, or product components; undiagnosed vaginal bleeding. Pregnancy Category: [X Use a nonhormonal method of contraception]
Interactions: None well documented.

Levalbuterol HCl

Bronchodilator / Sympathomimetic
Indications: Treatment or prevention of bronchospasm in patients with reversible obstructive airway disease.
Dose: Adults and children at least 12 yr of age: Inhalation solution Usual starting dose is 0.63 mg tid (q 6 to 8 hr) by nebulization. Patients with more severe asthma or patients who do not respond adequately to the 0.63 mg dose may benefit from 1.25 mg tid.
Children 6 through 11 yr of age: Inhalation solution Recommended dose is 0.31 mg tid by nebulization (max, 0.63 mg tid).
Trade names: Xopenex Solution for inhalation 0.31 mg levalbuterol per 3 mL
Warnings: Hypersensitivity to levalbuterol or racemic albuterol. Pregnancy Category: [C]
Interactions: Beta-blockers (eg, propranolol): Severe bronchospasms may be produced in asthmatic patients taking levalbuterol.
Digoxin: Plasma digoxin levels may be decreased.
Diuretics (eg, loop [eg, furosemide] and thiazide [hydrochlorothiazide]): ECG changes and hypokalemia associated with diuretic therapy may be worsened by levalbuterol administration.
MAO inhibitors (eg, phenelzine), tricyclic antidepressants (eg, amitriptyline): The action of levalbuterol on the vascular system may be potentiated.

Levetiracetam

Anticonvulsant
Indications: Adjunctive therapy in partial onset seizures in adults with epilepsy.
Dose: Adults: PO Initiate therapy with 500 mg bid; dose may be increased by 1,000 mg/day q 2 wk to a max daily dose of 3,000 mg.
Dosage Adjustment for Renal Impairment: For mild renal impairment (Ccr 50 to 80 mL/min), give 500 to 1,000 mg q 12 hr. For moderate impairment (Ccr 30 to 50 mL/min), give 250 mg to 750 mg q 12 hr. For severe impairment (Ccr less than 30 mL/min), give 250 to 500 mg q 12 hr. For patients on dialysis, give 500 to 1,000 mg q 12 hr (following dialysis, a 250 to 500 mg supplemental dose is recommended.
Trade names: Keppra Tablets 250 mg
Warnings: Standard considerations. Pregnancy Category: [C]
Interactions: None well documented.

Levobunolol

Ophthalmic / Glaucoma / Beta-adrenergic blocker
Indications: Treatment of IOP in chronic open-angle glaucoma or ocular hypertension.
Dose: Adults: Topical 1 drop in affected eye(s) qd or bid.
Trade names: AK-Beta Solution 0.25%
Betagan Liquifilm Solution 0.25%
Warnings: Bronchial asthma; severe COPD; sinus bradycardia; second- and third-degree AV block; cardiac failure; cardiogenic shock. Pregnancy Category: [C]
Interactions: Beta blockers, oral: Additive effects on systemic beta blockade.
Epinephrine, ophthalmic: Hypertension caused by unopposed alpha-adrenergic stimulation.

Levofloxacin

Antibiotic / Fluoroquinolone
Indications: Treatment of acute maxillary sinusitis, acute bacterial exacerbation of chronic bronchitis, nosocomial pneumonia, community-acquired pneumonia, skin and skin structure infections, chronic bacterial prostatitis, UTI, and acute pyelonephritis caused by susceptible strains of specific microorganisms.
Ophthalmic use: Treatment of conjunctivitis caused by susceptible strains of aerobic gram-positive and aerobic gram-negative microorganisms.
Dose: Acute Bacterial Exacerbation of Chronic Bronchitis:
Adults: PO / IV 500 mg q 24 hr for 7 days.
Acute Maxillary Sinusitis:
Adults: PO / IV 500 mg q 24 hr for 10 to 14 days.
Bacterial Conjunctivitis:
Adults and children at least 1 yr:
Days 1 and 2: Topical Instill 1 to 2 gtt in affected eye(s) q 2 hr while awake, up to 8 times daily.
Days 3 through 7: Topical Instill 1 to 2 gtt in affected eye(s) q 4 hr while awake, up to qid.
Chronic Bacterial Prostatitis:
Adults: PO / IV 500 mg q 24 hr for 28 days.
Community-Acquired Pneumonia:
Adults: PO / IV 500 mg q 24 hr for 7 to 14 days.
Complicated Skin and Skin Structure Infections; Nosocomial Pneumonia:
Adults: PO / IV 750 mg q 24 hr for 7 to 14 days.
Complicated UTIs; Acute Pyelonephritis:
Adults: PO / IV 250 mg q 24 hr for 10 days.
Uncomplicated Skin and Skin Structure Infections:
Adults: PO / IV 500 mg q 24 hr for 7 to 10 days.
Uncomplicated UTIs:
Adults: PO / IV 250 mg q 24 hr for 3 days.
Trade names: Levaquin Tablets 250 mg
Quixin Solution, ophthalmic 0.5% (5 mg/mL)
Warnings: Hypersensitivity to fluoroquinolones, quinolone antibiotics, or any product component. Pregnancy Category: [C]
Interactions: Antacids, iron salts, sucralfate, zinc salts; didanosine chewable buffered tablets, multivitamins (oral only): May decrease oral absorption of levofloxacin. Stagger administration times.
Antiarrhythmic agents (class Ia [eg, quinidine] and class III [eg, amiodarone]): Because of increased risk of life-threatening cardiac arrhythmias, including torsades de pointes, avoid coadministration of levofloxacin.
Antidiabetic agents: Hyperglycemia or hypoglycemia may occur.
NSAIDs: May increase risk of CNS stimulation and convulsive seizures.

Levothyroxine Sodium

Thyroid hormone

Indications: Replacement or supplemental therapy in hypothyroidism; TSH suppression (in thyroid cancer, nodules, goiters, and enlargement in chronic thyroiditis).

Dose: Individualize dosage.
Infants and Children: In infants with congenital or acquired hypothyroidism, institute therapy with full doses as soon as diagnosis is made. In children with chronic or severe hypothyroidism, an initial oral 25 mcg/day dose is recommended with increments of 25 mcg q 2 to 4 wk until desired effect is achieved. The following guidelines are recommended:
Children more than 12 yr (growth/puberty complete): PO 1.7 mcg/kg/day.
Children more than 12 yr (growth/puberty incomplete): PO 2 to 3 mcg/kg/day.
Children 6 to 12 yr: PO 4 to 5 mcg/kg/day.
Children 1 to 5 yr: PO 5 to 6 mcg/kg/day.
Children 6 to 12 mo: PO 6 to 8 mcg/kg/day.
Children 3 to 6 mo: PO 8 to 10 mcg/kg/day.
Children 0 to 3 mo: PO 10 to 15 mcg/kg/day. Consider a lower starting dose (eg, 25 mcg/day) in infants at risk for cardiac failure, increasing the dose in 4- to 6-wk intervals based on clinical and laboratory response.
Hypothyroidism in Adults and Children in Whom Growth and Puberty are Complete:
Adults and Children: PO Average full replacement dose is approximately 1.7 mcg/kg/day (eg, 100 to 125 mcg/day for 70 kg adult). Older patients may require less than 1 mcg/kg/day. Doses greater than 200 mcg/day are seldom required. For most patients older than 50 yr or patients younger than 50 yr with underlying cardiac disease, an initial starting dose of 25 to 50 mcg/day is recommended, with gradual increments in dose at 6- to 8-wk intervals, as needed. The recommended starting dose in elderly patients with cardiac disease is 12.5 to 25 mcg/day, with gradual dose increments at 4- to 6-wk intervals.
Severe Hypothyroidism:
Adults: PO Recommended starting dose is 12.5 to 25 mcg/day with increases of 25 mcg/day q 2 to 4 wk, accompanied by clinical and laboratory assessment, until TSH level in normalized. IV/IM May be substituted for oral form when oral ingestion is precluded for long periods of time. Initial parenteral dosage should be approximately 50% the previously established oral dosage. A daily maintenance dose of 50 to 100 mcg parenterally should maintain the euthyroid stat once established. Monitor the patient and adjust the dosage as needed.
Subclinical Hypothyroidism:
Adults: PO If treated, a lower dose (eg, 1 mcg/kg/day) than that used for full replacement may be adequate to normalize serum TSH level.
Myxedema Coma:
Adults: IV In myxedema coma or stupor, without concomitant severe heart disease, 200 to 500 mcg may be administered as a solution containing 100 mcg/mL. Full therapeutic effect may not be evident until the following day. An additional 100 to 300 mcg or more may be given on the second day if evidence of significant and progressive improvements has not occurred.
TSH Suppression in Well-Differentiated Thyroid Cancer and Thyroid Nodules:
Adults: PO TSH suppression to less than 0.1 mU/L usually requires a levothyroxine dose greater than 2 mcg/kg/day; however, in patients with high-risk tumors, the target TSH suppression level may be less than 0.01 mU/L. In treatment of benign nodules and nontoxic multinodular goiter, TSH generally is suppressed to a higher target (eg, 0.1 to 0.5 mU/L or 1 mU/L) than that used for treatment of thyroid cancer.

Trade names: Levothroid Tablets 0.025 mg
Levoxyl Tablets 0.025 mg
Synthroid Tablets 0.025 mg

Warnings: Acute MI and thyrotoxicosis uncomplicated by hypothyroidism; coexistence of hypothyroidism and hypoadrenalism (Addison disease) unless treatment of hypoadrenalism with adrenocortical steroids precedes initiation of thyroid therapy.
Pregnancy Category: [A]

Interactions: Anticoagulants, oral: May increase anticoagulant effects.
Cholestyramine, colestipol: May decrease thyroid hormone efficacy.
Digitalis glycosides: May reduce effects of glycosides.
Fasting: Increases absorption from GI tract.
Iron salts: May decrease efficacy of levothyroxine, resulting in hypothyroidism.
Theophyllines: Hypothyroidism; may cause decreased theophylline Cl; Cl may return to normal when euthyroid state is achieved.

Lindane

Scabicide / Pediculicide

Indications: Lotion: Treatment of Sarcoptes scabiei (scabies) in patients who have failed to respond to adequate doses or are intolerant of other approved therapies.

Shampoo: Treatment of Pediculus capitis (head lice) and Pediculus pubis (crab lice) and their ova in patients who have failed to respond to adequate doses or are intolerant of other approved therapies.

Dose: Provide a patient medication guide each time lindane is dispensed.
Lotion: Apply a thin layer over all skin from neck down. Wash hands immediately after applying or use gloves. One ounce is sufficient for an average adult. Do not prescribe more than 2 oz for larger adults. Apply only once. Wash off in 8 to 12 hr (max, 12 hr). Do not retreat. Do not cover areas where medication is applied.
Shampoo: Apply shampoo directly to dry hair without adding water. Work thoroughly into hair and allow to remain in place for 4 min only. Special attention should be given to the fine hairs along the neck. After 4 min, add small quantities of water to hair until a good lather forms. Immediately rinse all lather away. Avoid unnecessary contact of lather with other body surfaces. Most patients will require only 1 oz; do not prescribe more than 2 oz for larger adults. Do not retreat.

Trade names: Lindane Lotion 1%

Warnings: Premature neonates because their skin may be more permeable than full-term infants, and neonates' liver enzymes may not be sufficiently developed; patients with known seizure disorders; hypersensitivity to any component of the product.
Pregnancy Category: [C]

Interactions: Drugs that may lower seizure threshold (eg, antipsychotics, antidepressants, centrally acting anticholinesterases): Because seizure threshold may be lowered, use with caution.
Oils: Oils may enhance absorption; therefore, avoid oil treatments and oil-based hair dressings or conditioners immediately before or after application of lindane shampoo.

Linezolid

Anti-infective / Antibiotic

Indications: Treatment of vancomycin-resistant Enterococcus faecium infections; treatment of nosocomial pneumonia, complicated and uncomplicated skin and skin structure infections, and community-acquired pneumonia caused by susceptible strains of specific organisms.

Dose: No dosage adjustment is necessary when switching from IV to PO. Administer IV infusion over a period of 30 to 120 min.
Vancomycin-Resistant E. faecium Infections, Including Concomitant Bacteremia:
Adults and children 12 yr and older: PO or IV 600 mg q

12 hr for 14 to 28 days.
Children (birth through 11 yr): PO or IV 10 mg/kg q 8 hr for 14 to 28 days. Most preterm neonates younger than 7 days should start with 10 mg/kg q 12 hr. A dose of 10 mg/kg q 8 hr may be considered in neonates with a suboptimal response.
Nosocomial Pneumonia, Complicated Skin and Skin Structure Infections, Community-Acquired Pneumonia, Including Concomitant Bacteremia:
Adults and children 12 yr and older: PO or IV 600 mg q 12 hr for 10 to 14 days.
Children birth through 11 yr: PO or IV 10 mg/kg q 8 hr for 10 to 14 days. Most preterm neonates less than 7 days should start with 10 mg/kg q 12 hr. A dose of 10 mg/kg q 8 hr may be considered in neonates with a suboptimal response.
Uncomplicated Skin and Skin Structure Infections:
Adults and children 12 yr and older: PO 400 mg q 12 hr for 10 to 14 days.
Children 5 to 11 yr: PO 10 mg/kg q 12 hr for 10 to 14 days.
Children younger than 5 yr: PO 10 mg/kg q 8 hr for 10 to 14 days. Most preterm neonates younger than 7 days should start with 10 mg/kg q 12 hr. A dose of 10 mg/kg q 8 hr may be considered in neonates with a suboptimal response.

Trade names: Zyvox Tablets 400 mg (sodium content is 1.95 mg/400 mg tablet [0.1 mEq/tablet])

Warnings: Standard considerations. Pregnancy Category: [C]

Interactions: Adrenergic agents (eg, dopamine, epinephrine): Effects may be enhanced by linezolid.
Serotonergic agents (eg, fluoxetine): Possible increased risk of serotonin syndrome.

Liothyronine Sodium

Thyroid hormone

Indications: Replacement or supplemental therapy in hypothyroidism; TSH suppression for treatment or prevention of euthyroid goiters (eg, thyroid nodules, multinodular goiters, enlargement in chronic thyroiditis); diagnostic agent in suppression tests to differentiate suspected hyperthyroidism from euthyroidism; treatment of myxedema coma/precoma (IV).

Dose: Individualize dosage.
Hypothyroidism:
Adults: PO 25 mcg/day initially, increase by up to 25 mcg q 1 to 2 wk if needed.
Children: PO 5 mcg/day initially, increase by 5 mcg/day at 2 wk intervals, if needed.
Congenital Hypothyroidism:
Children: PO 5 mcg/day initially; increase by 5 mcg/day every 3 to 4 days until desired response achieved. Infants a few mo of age may require only 20 mcg/day for maintenance; at 1 yr, 50 mcg/day may be required; and, above 3 yr, full adult dosage may be required.
Simple (Nontoxic) Goiter:
Adults: PO 5 mcg/day initially, increase by 5 to 10 mcg q 1 to 2 wk. When 25 mcg/day is reached, increase by 12.5 to 25 mcg q 1 to 2 wk if needed.
Children: PO 5 mcg/day initially, increase by 5 mcg/day at 2-wk intervals, if needed.
Myxedema:
Adults: PO 5 mcg/day initially, increase by 5 to 10 mcg q 1 to 2 wk. When 25 mcg/day is reached, increase by 12.5 to 25 mcg q 1 to 2 wk if needed.
Children: PO 5 mcg/day initially, increase by 5 mcg/day at 2-wk intervals, if needed.
Myxedema Coma/Precoma:
Adults: IV 25 to 50 mcg initially. In patients with known or suspected cardiovascular disease, an initial dose of 10 to 20 mcg is suggested; however, base doses on continuous monitoring of the condition and response to therapy.
TSH Suppression Test:
Adults: PO 75 to 100 mcg/day for 7 days.

Trade names: Cytomel Tablets 5 mcg
Triostat Injection 10 mcg/mL

Warnings: Acute MI and thyrotoxicosis uncomplicated by hypothyroidism; coexistence of hypothyroidism and hypoadrenalism (Addison disease), unless treatment of hypoadrenalism with adrenocortical steroids precedes initiation of thyroid therapy.
Pregnancy Category: [A]

Interactions: Anticoagulants, oral: May increase anticoagulant effects.
Beta blockers: May reduce effects of beta blockers.
Cholestyramine, colestipol: May decrease thyroid hormone efficacy.
Digitalis glycosides: May reduce effects of glycosides.
Theophyllines: Hypothyroidism; may cause decreased theophylline clearance; Cl may return to normal when euthyroid state is achieved.

Lisinopril

Antihypertensive / ACE inhibitor

Indications: Treatment of hypertension; treatment of heart failure not responding to diuretics and digitalis; treatment of acute MI within 24 hr in hemodynamically stable patients.

Dose: CHF:
Adults:
Initial dose: PO 5 mg qd with diuretics and digitalis; reduce concomitant diuretic dose, if possible, to minimize hypovolemia. In patients with hyponatremia, initiate with 2.5 mg qd.
Usual dose: PO 5 to 20 mg/day.
Hypertension:
Adults:
Initial dose: PO 10 mg qd.
Maintenance: PO 20 to 40 mg/day; may add diuretic if needed and decrease dose.
Children (6 yr and older): PO Start with 0.07 mg/kg qd (up to 5 mg). Adjust dose according to BP response. Doses above 0.61 mg/kg (or in excess of 40 mg) have not been studied.
MI:
Adults:
Initial dose: PO 5 mg, then 5 mg after 24 hr, then 10 mg after 48 hr.
Maintenance: PO 10 mg/day for 6 wk. Patients should receive, as appropriate, the standard recommended treatments, such as thrombolytics, aspirin, and beta-blockers.

Trade names: Prinivil Tablets 2.5 mg
Zestril Tablets 2.5 mg

Warnings: Hypersensitivity to ACE inhibitors and in patients with hereditary or idiopathic angioedema. Pregnancy Category: [D (second and third trimester); C (first trimester) Can cause injury or death to fetus if used during second or third trimester]

Interactions: Antacids: Lisinopril bioavailability may be decreased. Separate administration times by 1 to 2 hr.
Capsaicin: Cough may be exacerbated.
Digoxin: May increase or decrease plasma digoxin levels.
Indomethacin, salicylates (eg, aspirin): Reduced hypotensive effects, especially in low-renin or volume-dependent hypertensive patients.
Lithium: Increased lithium levels and symptoms of lithium toxicity.
Phenothiazines: May increase pharmacological effect of lisinopril.
Potassium-sparing diuretics, potassium preparations: May increase serum potassium levels.

Lisinopril/ Hydrochlorothiazide

Antihypertensive combination

Indications: Treatment of hypertension.

Dose: Adults: PO Using qd doses of lisinopril/HCTZ combination therapy in lisinopril doses of 10 to 80 mg and HCTZ doses of 6.25 to 50 mg, the antihypertensive response rates generally increase with increasing doses of either component. Do not use dosage higher than lisinopril 80 mg and HCTZ 50 mg.

Trade names: Prinzide 10/12.5 mg Tablets 10 mg lisinopril and 12.5 mg hydrochlorothiazide
Prinzide 20/12.5 mg Tablets 20 mg lisinopril and 12.5 mg hydrochlorothiazide
Prinzide 20/25 mg Tablets 20 mg lisinopril and 25 mg hydrochlorothiazide
Zestoretic Tablets 12.5 mg hydrochlorothiazide and 10 mg lisinopril

Warnings: History of angioedema related to previous treatment with an angiotensin converting enzyme inhibitor; hereditary or idiopathic angioedema; anuria; hypersensitivity to sulfonamide-derived drugs, hypersensitivity to any component of the product.
Pregnancy Category: [D (second and third trimesters) C (first trimester)]

Interactions: HCTZ:
Alcohol, barbiturates, narcotics: Increased risk of orthostatic hypotension.
Antidiabetic agents (oral agents and insulin): Dosage adjustment of antidiabetic agent may be necessary.
Antihypertensive agent: Additive or potentiation of effects.
Cholestyramine, colestipol resins: Impaired absorption of HCTZ.
Corticosteroids, ACTH: Increased electrolyte depletion, increasing the risk of hypokalemia.
Lithium: Renal clearance of lithium may be reduced, increasing the risk of lithium toxicity.
Nondepolarizing skeletal muscle relaxants (eg, tubocurarine): Increased effect of the muscle relaxant.
Nonsteroidal anti-inflammatory agents: The diuretic, natriuretic, and antihypertensive effects of loop, potassium-sparing, and thiazide diuretics may be reduced.
Pressor amines (eg, norepinephrine): Decreased responsiveness to the pressor amine.
Lisinopril:
Diuretic therapy: Excessive reduction in BP after starting lisinopril therapy.
Nonsteroidal anti-inflammatory agents: Worsening of renal function in patients with compromised renal function; antihypertensive effects of lisinopril may be diminished.
Agents increasing serum potassium (eg, potassium-sparing diuretics[eg, spironolactone], potassium supplements, potassium-containing salt substitutes): May lead to increases in serum potassium.
Lithium: Because of possible increased sodium elimination, the risk of lithium toxicity is increased.

Lithium

Antipsychotic / Antimanic

Indications: Management of bipolar disorder and manic episodes of manic-depressive illness.

Unlabeled indication: Treatment of neutropenia; unipolar depression; schizoaffective disorder; prophylaxis of cluster headaches; premenstrual tension; tardive dyskinesia; hyperthyroidism; SIADH, postpartum affective psychosis; corticosteroid-induced psychosis.

Dose: Adults: PO 900 to 1800 mg/day in 2 to 4 divided doses. Give regular capsules tid or qid; slow-release tablets bid or tid. Max dose, 2400 mg/day.
Children at least 12 yr: 15 to 20 mg/kg/day in 2 to 3 divided doses.

Trade names: Eskalith Capsules 300 mg lithium carbonate (8.12 mEq lithium)
Eskalith CR Tablets, controlled-release 450 mg lithium carbonate (12.8 mEq lithium)
Lithobid Tablets, slow-release 300 mg lithium carbonate (8.12 mEq lithium)
Lithonate Capsules 300 mg lithium carbonate (8.12 mEq lithium)
Lithotabs Tablets 300 mg lithium carbonate (8.12 mEq lithium)

Warnings: History of leukemia. Pregnancy Category: [D]

Interactions: Acetazolamide, osmotic diuretics, theophyllines, urinary alkalinizers: Increased renal excretion of lithium.
ACE inhibitors, fluoxetine, loop diuretics, NSAIDs, thiazide diuretics: Increased lithium serum levels.
Carbamazepine, haloperidol, methyldopa: Increased neurotoxic effects despite therapeutic serum levels and normal dosage range.
Iodide salts: Increased risk of hypothyroidism.
Neuromuscular blocking agents, tricyclic antidepressants: Increased pharmacological effects of additive drug.
Phenothiazines: Neurotoxicity, decreased phenothiazine concentrations, or increased lithium concentrations may occur.
Verapamil: Reductions in lithium levels and lithium toxicity have occurred.

Lomustine

Alkylating agent / Nitrosoureas

Indications: Adults and children: Brain tumors, Hodgkin disease.

Dose: Brain Tumors, Hodgkin Disease:
Adults: PO 100 to 130 mg/m^2 administered as a single dose q 6 wk. Do not administer repeat doses of lomustine until leukocyte and platelet counts have recovered to acceptable levels (usually 4000/mm^3 and 100,000/mm^3, respectively). Reduce lomustine dose if administered with other myelosuppressive drugs. Give 100 mg/m^2 to patients with compromised bone marrow function. Some clinicians advocate dosage reductions of 25% when platelet nadirs are 50,000 to 74,999/mm^3, 50% when platelet nadirs are 25,000 to 49,999/mm^3, and 75% when platelet nadirs are less than 25,000/mm^3.
Pediatric: PO 75 to 150 mg/m^2 administered as a single dose q 6 wk. Do not administer repeat doses of lomustine until leukocyte and platelet counts have recovered to acceptable levels (usually 4000/mm^3 and 100,000/mm^3, respectively). Follow dosage adjustment guidelines recommended for adults.
Suggested Lomustine Dose Following Initial Dose:
Adults: PO Give 100% of the prior dose if the leukocytes are greater than 3000 cells/mm^3 and the platelets are greater than 75,000 cells/mm^3. Give 70% of the prior dose if the leukocytes are 2000 to 2999 cells/mm^3 and the platelets are 25,000 to 74,999 cells/mm^3. Give 50% of the prior dose if the leukocytes are less than 2000 cells/mm^3 and the platelets less than 25,000 cells/mm.

Trade names: CeeNU Capsules 10 mg

Warnings: Standard considerations. Pregnancy Category: [D]

Interactions: Alcohol: Lomustine is soluble in alcohol. Some sources recommend avoidance of alcohol on days that lomustine is administered to avoid possible effects on the absorption of lomustine, although there is no documentation of an interaction.

Loperamide HCl

Antidiarrheal

Indications: Control and symptomatic relief of acute nonspecific or chronic diarrhea; reduction in volume of ileostomy output.

Dose: Acute Diarrhea:
Adults: PO 4 mg followed by 2 mg after each unformed stool, not to exceed 16 mg/24 hr.
Children 8 to 12 yr (greater than 30 kg): 2 mg tid.
Children 6 to 8 yr (20 to 30 kg): 2 mg bid.
Children 2 to 5 yr (13 to 20 kg):
First day: 1 mg tid. May decrease to adjust for nutritional and hydration status after 24 hr; usually 0.1 mg/kg after each loose stool but do not exceed total first day dosing recommendations on any day.

Medications

Chronic Diarrhea:
Adults: PO 4 to 8 mg qd or bid.
Trade names: Diar-aid Tablets 2 mg
Imodium Capsules 2 mg
Imodium A-D Tablets 2 mg
Kaopectate II Caplets Tablets 2 mg
Neo-Diaral Capsules 2 mg
Pepto Diarrhea Control Liquid 1 mg/ mL
Warnings: Pseudomembranous colitis caused by antibiotic use; acute diarrhea associated with organisms that penetrate intestinal wall (eg, toxigenic Escherichia coli, Salmonella, Shigella); conditions in which constipation should be avoided; bloody diarrhea; fever; acute ulcerative colitis (potential for toxic megacolon). Pregnancy Category: [B]
Interactions: None well documented.

Lorazepam

Antianxiety / Benzodiazepine
Indications: Treatment of anxiety, anxiety associated with depression (oral); preanesthetic medication for sedation/anxiety and decreased recall, status epilepticus (IV).

Unlabeled indication: Relief of chemotherapy-induced nausea and vomiting; acute alcohol withdrawal; psychogenic catatonia.
Dose: Antianxiety:
Adults: PO Usual dose: 2 to 6 mg/day (range, 1 to 10 mg/day) in divided doses; largest dose at bedtime.
Elderly/Debilitated patients:
Initial dose: 1 to 2 mg/day in divided doses; increase gradually.
Insomnia Caused By Anxiety or Transient Situational Stress:
Adults: PO 2 to 4 mg at bedtime.
Preanesthesia:
Adults: IM 0.05 mg/kg at least 2 hr before procedure (max, 4 mg).
Initial dose: IV 2 mg total or 0.044 mg/kg, whichever is smaller. Do not exceed in patients over 50 yr.
For increased lack of recall: 0.05 mg/kg (max, 4 mg), 15 to 20 min before procedure.
Status epilepticus:
Adults: IV Recommended dose 4 mg given at rate of 2 mg/min. If seizures continue or recur after a 10- to 15-min observation period, an additional 4 mg IV may be administered slowly.
Trade names: Ativan Injection 2 mg/mL
Lorazepam Tablets 0.5 mg
Lorazepam Intensol Oral Solution, Concentrated 2 mg/mL
Warnings: Acute narrow-angle glaucoma; intra-arterial administration (injection); hypersensitivity to benzodiazepines. Pregnancy Category: [D Avoid use, especially during first trimester because of possible increased risk of congenital malformations Advise women of childbearing age to use effective contraceptive method Not recommended during labor and delivery]
Interactions: Alcohol/CNS depressants: Additive CNS depressant effects.
Digoxin: Increased serum digoxin concentrations.
Oral contraceptives: Cl rate of lorazepam may be increased.
Rifampin: Pharmacologic effect of lorazepam may be decreased.
Scopolamine: May result in increased incidence of hallucinations, irrational behavior, and sedation.
Theophyllines: May antagonize sedative effects.

Losartan Potassium

Antihypertensive / Angiotensin II antagonist
Indications: Treatment of hypertension; nephropathy in type 2 diabetic patients; reduce risk of stroke in patients with hypertension and left ventricular hypertrophy.
Dose: Hypertension:
Adults:
Initial dose: PO 50 mg qd; 25 mg qd if volume depleted or history of hepatic impairment.
Maintenance: PO 25 to 100 mg/day.
Nephropathy in Type 2 Diabetes:
Adults:
Initial dose: PO 50 mg qd; the dose may be increased to 100 mg qd based on BP response.
Hypertension in Patients with Left Ventricular Hypertrophy:
Adults: PO 50 mg qd; add hydrochlorothiazide 12.5 mg/day and/or increase the dose of losartan to 100 mg/day followed by an increase in hydrochlorothiazide to 25 mg qd based on BP response.
Trade names: Cozaar Tablets 25 mg
Warnings: Standard considerations. Pregnancy Category: [D (second and third trimester); C (first trimester)]
Interactions: Fluconazole: Losartan plasma levels may be elevated, increasing the antihypertensive and adverse effects.
Indomethacin: The antihypertensive effect of losartan may be blunted.
Lithium: Plasma concentrations may be increased by losartan, resulting in an increase in the pharmacologic and adverse effects of lithium.
Potassium supplement: Concomitant use of potassium-sparing diuretics, potassium supplements, or salt substitutes containing potassium may lead to increases in serum potassium.

Losartan Potassium/ Hydrochlorothiazide

Antihypertensive
Indications: Hypertension.
Dose: Adults: PO 50 mg losartan/12.5 mg hydrochlorothiazide once daily is usual dose (max, 100 mg losartan/25 mg hydrochlorothiazide daily).
Trade names: Hyzaar Tablets 12.5 mg hydrochlorothiazide/50 mg losartan potassium
Warnings: Anuria; hypersensitivity to other sulfonamide-derivatives or any component of product. Pregnancy Category: [C (first trimester); D (second and third trimester)]
Interactions: Losartan potassium:
Fluconazole: Losartan plasma levels may be elevated, increasing the antihypertensive and adverse effects.
Lithium: Plasma levels of lithium may be elevated, increasing the pharmacologic and adverse effects.
Rifamycins (eg, rifampin): Losartan plasma levels may be reduced, decreasing the antihypertensive effects.
Potassium-sparing diuretics (eg, spironolactone), potassium supplements, salt substitutes containing potassium: May lead to increased serum potassium.
Hydrochlorothiazide:
Alcohol, barbiturates, narcotics: Increased risk of orthostatic hypotension.
Antidiabetic agents: Dose adjustments of antidiabetic agent may be needed.
Antihypertensives: Actions of other antihypertensive agents may be potentiated.
Cholestyramine, colestipol resins: Absorption of hydrochlorothiazide may be impaired.
ACTH, corticosteroids: Increased risk of electrolyte depletion (eg, hypokalemia).
Pressor amines (eg, norepinephrine): Decreased response to pressor amine.
Nondepolarizing skeletal muscle relaxants (eg, turbocurarine): Responsiveness to muscle relaxant may be increased.
Lithium: Plasma levels of lithium may be elevated, increasing the risk of toxicity.
NSAIDs: Antihypertensive, diuretic, and natriuretic effects of hydrochlorothiazide may be reduced.

Lovastatin

Antihyperlipidemic / HMG-CoA reductase inhibitor

Indications: To reduce elevated cholesterol and LDL cholesterol levels in patients with primary hypercholesterolemia (types IIa and IIb [immediate-release only]); to slow progression of coronary atherosclerosis in patients with coronary heart disease; to reduce risk of MI, unstable angina, and coronary revascularization procedures; as an adjunct to diet to reduce total and LDL cholesterol and apolipoprotein B levels in adolescent boys and girls (who are at least 1 yr postmenarche) 10 to 17 yr with heterozygous familial hypercholesterolemia (immediate-release only). As an adjunct to diet for reduction of elevated total and LDL cholesterol, apolipoprotein B, and triglycerides and to increase HDL cholesterol in patients with primary hypercholesterolemia (heterozygous familial and nonfamilial) and mixed dyslipidemia (Fredrickson types IIa and IIb) when response to diet restricted in saturated fat and cholesterol and to nonpharmacological measures alone has been inadequate (extended-release only).

Dose: Adults:
Immediate-release: PO 10 to 80 mg/day in a single dose with evening meal or 2 divided doses.
Extended-release: PO 10 to 60 mg/day as a single dose in the evening at bedtime. Individualize dose according to recommended goal of therapy. For patients requiring a small reduction in cholesterol level, a starting dose of 10 mg may be considered.
Heterozygous Familial Hypercholesterolemia:
Adolescents (10 to 17 yr):
Immediate-release: PO 10 to 40 mg/day (max, 40 mg/day).

Trade names: Altocor Tablets, extended-release 10 mg
Mevacor Tablets 10 mg

Warnings: Active liver disease or unexplained persistent elevations of LFTs; pregnancy; lactation. Pregnancy Category: [X]

Interactions: Azole antifungal agents (eg, itraconazole), cyclosporine, danazol, gemfibrozil, grapefruit juice, macrolide antibiotics (eg, erythromycin), niacin, verapamil: Severe myopathy or rhabdomyolysis may occur with coadministration.
Isradipine: May increase the clearance of lovastatin and its metabolites by increasing hepatic blood flow.
Warfarin: Enhanced anticoagulant effect.

Magnesium Citrate

Laxative

Indications: Short-term treatment of constipation; evacuation of colon for rectal and bowel evaluations.

Dose: Adults: PO 1 glassful (approximately 240 mL) prn.
Children (6 to 12 yr): PO 50 to 100 mL. Repeat if necessary.
Children (2 to 6 yr): PO 4 to 12 mL.

Trade names: Citrate of Magnesia
Citro-Nesia

Warnings: Hypersensitivity to any ingredient; nausea, vomiting or other symptoms of appendicitis; acute surgical abdomen; fecal impaction; intestinal obstruction; undiagnosed abdominal pain; intestinal bleeding; renal disease. Pregnancy Category: [Pregnancy category undetermined]

Interactions: Nitrofurantoin: Reduced anti-infective action.
Penicillamine: Reduced action of penicillamine.
Tetracyclines: Impaired absorption of tetracyclines.

Magnesium Sulfate

Anticonvulsant / Electrolyte / Laxative

Indications: Parenteral: Seizure prevention and control in severe preeclampsia or eclampsia without deleterious CNS depression in mother, fetus, or newborn; replacement therapy in magnesium deficiency, especially in acute hypomagnesemia accompanied by signs of tetany similar to those observed in hypocalcemia; corrects or prevents hypomagnesemia by addition to total parenteral nutrition admixture.

Unlabeled indication: Control of hypertension, encephalopathy, and convulsions in children with acute nephritis; inhibition of premature labor; treatment of life-threatening ventricular arrhythmias; prevention and treatment of nutritional magnesium deficiency; laxative (oral).

Dose: Eclampsia: IM/IV 10 to 14 g of magnesium sulfate (as a combination of IM and IV administration) appropriately diluted.
Hyperalimentation:
Adults: TPN Maintenance dose ranges from 8 to 24 mEq (1 to 3 g) daily.
Infants: TPN Maintenance dose ranges from 2 to 10 mEq (0.25 to 1.25 g) daily.
Laxative: Usually 1-time dose.
Adults: PO 10 to 15 g.
Children: PO 5 to 10 g.
Magnesium Deficiency:
Mild magnesium deficiency: IM Usual dose is 1 g, equivalent to 8.12 mEq magnesium (2 mL of 50% solution) injected q 6 hr for 4 doses, equivalent to a total of 32.5 mEq of magnesium per 24 hr.
Severe hypomagnesemia: As much as 250 mg (approximately 2 mEq) per kg (0.5 mL of the 50% solution) may be given within a period of 4 hr if necessary. Alternatively, 5 g (approximately 40 mEq) can be added to 1 L of 5% dextrose injection, or 0.9% sodium chloride injection, for slow IV infusion over a 3-hr period. Use caution so as not to exceed the renal excretion capacity.
Seizures Associated with Epilepsy, Glomerulonephritis, or Hypothyroidism:
Adults: IM/IV 1 g.

Trade names: Epsom Salt Granules see care instructions
Magnesium sulfate Injection 4% (0.325 mEq/mL)

Warnings: Toxemia of pregnancy during 2 hr preceding delivery; MI; myocardial damage; heartblock. Pregnancy Category: [A]

Interactions: Cardiac glycosides (eg, digoxin): Administer magnesium sulfate with extreme caution because of serious changes in cardiac conduction, which can result in heart block, may occur if administration of calcium is required to treat magnesium toxicity.
CNS depressants (eg, barbiturates, narcotics): Possible additive CNS depressant effects.
Neuromuscular blocking agents: Potentiation of neuromuscular blockade.
Nitrofurantoin: Decreased absorption of nitrofurantoin (oral magnesium).
Penicillamine: Reduced penicillamine effects (oral magnesium).
Tetracyclines: Decreased absorption of tetracyclines (oral magnesium).
Incompatability: Alcohol (in high concentrations), alkali carbonates and bicarbonates, alkali hydroxides, arsenates, barium, calcium, clindamycin phosphate, heavy metals, hydrocortisone sodium succinate, phosphates, polymyxin B sulfate, procaine hydrochloride, salicylates, streptomycin, strontium, tartrates, tetracycline, tobramycin.

Maprotiline HCl

Tetracyclic antidepressant

Indications: Depression; anxiety associated with depression.

Unlabeled indication: Relief of chronic neurogenic pain.

Dose: Adults:

Initial dose: PO 25 to 75 mg/day as single dose or divided doses. May be increased to 150 mg/day (outpatient) or 225 mg/day (inpatient).

Trade names: Ludiomil Tablets 25 mg

Warnings: Hypersensitivity to tricyclic antidepressants; MI acute recovery period; seizure disorder; concomitant use with MAO inhibitors. Pregnancy Category: [B]

Interactions: Alcohol, CNS depressants: Additive CNS effects possible.
MAO inhibitors: May precipitate hypertensive crisis and convulsions with possibly fatal results. Discontinue at least 14 days before starting maprotiline.

Measles, Mumps and Rubella Vaccine, Live

Vaccine / Live virus

Indications: Vaccination of individuals known to be susceptible to measles, mumps, or rubella; prevention of occurrence of congenital rubella syndrome (CRS) among offspring of women who contract rubella during pregnancy. Preferred immunizing agent for most children and many adults.

Dose: Adults and Children: SC 0.5 mL. Optimal schedule: Give first dose at 12 to 15 mo; revaccinate routinely at 5 to 6 yr or 11 to 12 yr.

Trade names: M-M-R-II Powder for Injection
Mixture of 3 viruses: at least 1000 measles $TCID_{50}$ (tissue culture infectious doses), at least 20,000 mumps $TCID_{50}$ and at least 1000 rubella $TCID_{50}$ per 0.5 mL dose

Warnings: Pregnancy; moderate to severe hypersensitivity reaction to eggs; immunosuppressive therapy; blood dyscrasia, leukemia, lymphoma of any type or other malignant neoplasms affecting the bone marrow or lymphatic systems; primary or acquired immunodeficiency; active untreated tuberculosis; family history of congenital or hereditary immunodeficiency, until immune competence of potential vaccine recipient is demonstrated. Exception: Vaccinate asymptomatic children with HIV infection. Pregnancy Category: [C (contraindicated)]

Interactions: Human antibody products: To avoid inactivating vaccine, give MMR 2 to 4 wk before or 3 to 11 mo after AGIV, depending on dose. Susceptible postpartum women who received blood products or Rho(D) immune globulin may receive rubella vaccine prior to discharge, provided that rubella titer is measured 6 to 8 wk after vaccination to ensure seroconversion.
Immunosuppressants, interferon, meningococcal vaccine: May inhibit response to MMR vaccine.

Mebendazole

Antihelminthic

Indications: Treatment of pinworm (*Enterobius vermicularis*), round worm (*Ascaris lumbricoides*), common hookworm (*Ancylostoma duodenale*), American hookworm (*Necator americanus*), and whipworm (*Trichuris trichiura*) in single or mixed parasitic infections.

Dose: Trichuriasis, Ascariasis, and Hookworm Infection:
Adults and Children: PO 100 mg tablet AM and PM on 3 consecutive days.
Ascaris Infection:
Adults and Children:
Alternative dose: PO 500 mg as single dose.
Enterobiasis:
Adults and Children: PO 100 mg as single dose.

Trade names: Vermox Tablets, chewable 100 mg

Warnings: Standard considerations. Pregnancy Category: [C]

Interactions: Carbamazepine; hydantoins (eg, phenytoin): Pharmacological effects of mebendazole may be decreased.

Mechlorethamine HCl

Alkylating agent / Nitrogen mustard

Indications: Hodgkin disease, lymphosarcoma, chronic myelocytic or lymphocytic leukemia, polycythemia vera, mycosis fungoides (topical), bronchogenic carcinoma; palliative treatment of malignant effusion (intrapleural, intraperitoneal, or intrapericardial use only).

Dose: Lymphosarcoma, Chronic Myelocytic or Lymphocytic Leukemia, Polycythemia Vera, Bronchogenic Carcinoma; Palliative Treatment of Malignant Effusion (Intrapleural, Intraperitoneal, or Intrapericardial Use Only):
Adults: IV Total dose of 0.4 mg/kg of body weight for each course (as single dose or divided doses of 0.1 to 0.2 mg/kg/day). Dose based on ideal dry body weight. May repeat courses at 3- to 6-wk intervals.
Advanced Hodgkin Disease:
Adults: IV When used in MOPP regimen, dose is 6 mg/m^2 /day on days 1 and 8 of a 28-day cycle. The dose should be decreased 50% if leukocyte count is 3000 to 3999/mm^3, and 75% if the count is between 1000 and 2999/mm^3 or platelets between 50,000 and 100,000/mm^3. On later cycles, do not administer if leukocyte count is less than 1000/mm^3 or platelets are less than 50,000/mm^3.
Mycosis Fungoides:
Adults: Topical Apply compounded solutions or ointments to the entire body surface qd for 6 to 12 mo. If the lesions do not reappear, continue to apply q 2 to 7 days for a total of 3 yr.

Trade names: Mustargen Powder for injection 10 mg

Warnings: Infectious disease; previous anaphylactic reactions to the drug. Pregnancy Category: [D]

Interactions: None well documented.

Meclizine

Antiemetic / Antivertigo / Anticholinergic

Indications: Prevention and treatment of nausea, vomiting, and dizziness of motion sickness; possibly effective treatment for vertigo of vestibular dysfunction origin.

Dose: Motion Sickness:
Adults: PO 25 to 50 mg 1 hr before travel; may repeat q 24 hr during travel.
Vertigo:
Adults: PO 25 to 100 mg/day in divided doses.

Trade names: Antivert Tablets 12.5 mg
Antrizine Tablets 12.5 mg
Bonine Tablets, chewable 25 mg
Dramamine Less Drowsy Tablets 25 mg
Meni-D Capsules 25 mg
Vergon Capsules 25 mg

Warnings: Hypersensitivity to cyclizine; asthma; glaucoma; emphysema; chronic pulmonary disease; shortness of breath; difficulty breathing; urinary retention caused by enlarged prostate. Pregnancy Category: [B]

Interactions: Alcohol, CNS depressants: Additive CNS effects.

Mefenamic Acid

Analgesic / NSAID

Indications: Relief of moderate pain lasting less than 1 wk; treatment of primary dysmenorrhea.

Unlabeled indication: Treatment of sunburn, migraine (acute attack), PMS.

Dose: Acute Pain:
Adults and Children (14 yr and older): PO 500 mg, followed by 250 mg q 6 hr prn. Usually not used more than 1 wk.
Primary Dysmenorrhea:
Adults and Children (14 yr and older): PO 500 mg,

followed by 250 mg q 6 hr starting with onset of bleeding and associated symptoms.
Trade names: Ponstel Capsules 250 mg
Warnings: Patients in whom aspirin, iodides, or any NSAID has caused allergic-type reactions; preexisting renal disease; active ulceration or chronic inflammation of GI tract. Pregnancy Category: [C]
Interactions: Anticoagulants: Increased risk of gastric erosion and bleeding.
Cyclosporine: Nephrotoxicity of both agents may be increased.
Cytochrome P450: Exercise caution when coadministering mefenamic acid with drugs known to inhibit the isoenzyme 2C9.
Lithium: Serum lithium levels may be increased.
Methotrexate: Increased methotrexate levels.
Salicylates: Additive GI toxicity.

Mefloquine HCl

Antimalarial

Indications: Treatment of mild to moderate malaria caused by mefloquine-susceptible strains of Plasmodium falciparum or P. vivax. Prevention of malaria caused by P. falciparum or P. vivax. Patients with acute P. vivax need subsequent treatment with 8-aminoquinolone to prevent relapse.
Dose: Treatment of Malaria:
Adults: PO 5 tablets (1250 mg) as a single dose with food and at least 240 mL of water.
Children: PO 20 to 25 mg/kg as a single dose or split into 2 doses 6 to 8 hr apart with food and at least 240 mL of water.
Prevention of Malaria:
Adults: PO 250 mg once weekly starting 1 wk before exposure and continuing 4 wk after with food and at least 240 mL of water.
Children: PO 3 to 5 mg/kg once weekly starting with 1 wk before exposure and continuing 4 wk after. Take with food and at least 240 mL of water.
Weight up to 19 kg: PO 1/4 tablet.
Weight 20 to 30 kg: PO 1/2 tablet.
Weight 31 to 45 kg: PO 3/4 tablet.
Weight more than 45 kg: PO 1 tablet.
Trade names: Mefloquine HCl Tablets 250 mg
Lariam Tablets 250 mg
Warnings: Acute depression; history of psychosis or convulsions; hypersensitivity to the drug or related compounds (eg, quinine, quinidine). Pregnancy Category: [C]
Interactions: Anticonvulsants: Reduced seizure control.
Drugs known to alter cardiac conduction (eg, antiarrhythmic, beta-adrenergic blockers, CCB, antihistamines, H_2 blockers, tricyclic antidepressants, phenothiazines): Potential for QTc interval prolongation.
Halofantrine: Concurrent use can cause potentially fatal QTc interval prolongation.
Related compounds (eg, quinine, quinidine, chloroquine): Increased risk of seizures and ECG abnormalities.
Typhoid vaccines, live: Reduced effectiveness.

Megestrol Acetate

Progestin

Indications: Palliative treatment of advanced inoperable, recurrent, or metastatic carcinoma of breast or endometrium.

Unlabeled indication: Appetite stimulation in HIV-related cachexia.
Dose: Breast Cancer:
Adults: PO 40 mg qid.
Endometrial Cancer:
Adults: PO 40 to 320 mg/day in divided doses.
Trade names: Megace Suspension 40 mg/mL
Warnings: Hypersensitivity to progestins; as diagnostic test for pregnancy. Pregnancy Category: [D]
Interactions: None well documented.

Melphalan

Alkylating agent / Nitrogen mustard

Indications: Palliative therapy of multiple myeloma (oral and IV) and non-resectable epithelial carcinoma of the ovary (oral).

Unlabeled indication: Breast carcinoma, testicular carcinoma, bone marrow transplantation.
Dose: Multiple Myeloma:
Adults: PO 6 mg/day for 2 to 3 wk as a single daily dose. Resume therapy with 2 mg/day after a rest period at no more than 4 wk and increase dose as necessary.
Alternate regimens: PO 0.25 mg/kg/day for 4 to 7 days or 0.15 mg/kg/day for 7 days. Either regimen can be repeated at 4- to 6-wk intervals after toxicity has resolved. Continuous daily dosing may increase the risk of severe bone marrow depression and secondary malignancy.
Adults: IV 16 mg/m^2 q 2 wk for 4 doses, then as tolerated q 4 wk. The dose should be decreased 50% in patients with BUN at least 30 mg/dL (or serum creatinine at least 1.5 mg/dL).
Epithelial Ovarian Cancer:
Adults: PO 0.2 mg/kg/day for 5 days q 4 to 5 wk.
Dosage Adjustments:
Adults: PO/IV All doses should be adjusted based on hematological parameters at nadir. If WBC is at least 4000 $cells/mm^3$ and platelet count is at least 100,000 $cells/mm^3$, administer 100% of prior dose. If WBC is at least 3000 $cells/mm^3$ and platelet count is at least 75,000 $cells/mm^3$, administer 75% of prior dose. If WBC is at least 2000 $cells/mm^3$ and platelet count is at least 50,000 $cells/mm^3$, administer 50% of prior dose. If WBC is less than 2000 $cells/mm^3$ and platelet count is at least 50,000 $cells/mm^3$, no prior dose is to be given. The manufacturer recommends discontinuing drug for leukocyte count is less than $3000/mm^3$ or platelet count is less than $100,000/mm^3$.
Trade names: Alkeran Tablets 2 mg
Warnings: Standard considerations. Pregnancy Category: [D]
Interactions: Carmustine: Melphalan may increase the likelihood of carmustine pulmonary toxicity.
Cimetidine and interferon alfa: May decrease serum concentrations of melphalan.
Cisplatin: May alter melphalan clearance, resulting in renal dysfunction.
Cyclosporine: Bone marrow transplant patients receiving melphalan followed by cyclosporine had a high frequency of severe renal dysfunction in 1 study.

Memantine HCl

NMDA receptor antagonist

Indications: Treatment of moderate to severe dementia of the Alzheimer type.

Unlabeled indication: Treatment of vascular dementia.
Dose: Adults: PO Start with 5 mg qd. The dose should be increased in 5 mg increments to 5 mg bid, 15 mg/day (5 and 10 mg as separate doses), and 10 mg bid. The minimum recommended interval between dose increases is 1 wk.
Trade names: Namenda Tablets 5 mg
Warnings: Standard considerations. Pregnancy Category: [B]
Interactions: Drugs eliminated via renal mechanisms (eg, cimetidine, hydrochlorothiazide, nicotine, quinidine, ranitidine, triamterene): Plasma concentrations of both drugs may be altered.
Urinary alkalinizers (eg, carbonic anhydrase inhibitors, sodium bicarbonate): Renal Cl of memantine is reduced about 80% under alkaline urine conditions at pH 8.

Menotropins

Sex hormones / Ovulation stimulant

Indications: Women: In conjunction with human chorionic gonadotropin (hCG), for multiple follicular development and ovulation induction in patients who have previously received pituitary suppression.

Men: In conjunction with hCG for stimulation of spermatogenesis in primary or secondary hypogonadotropic hypogonadism caused by a congenital factor or prepubertal hypophysectomy and in secondary hypogonadotropic hypogonadism caused by hypophysectomy, craniopharyngioma, cerebral aneurysm, or chromophobe adenoma.

Dose: Follicular Development and Ovulation Induction:
Adult (women):
Repronex: SC/IM Start with 150 IU for 5 days, then based on patient response, adjust dose. Do not make adjustments more frequently than once q 2 days and do not exceed 75 to 150 IU per adjustment (max, 450 IU/day). Do not dose beyond 12 days. If response is appropriate, give hCG 5000 to 10,000 U 1 day following the last dose of menotropins. Withhold hCG if serum estradiol is greater than 2000 pg/mL.
Pergonal: IM Start with 75 IU FSH/75 IU luteinizing hormone (LH) daily for 7 to 12 days, followed by 5000 to 10,000 U hCG 1 day after the last dose of menotropins. Do not exceed 12 days of menotropins administration.
Repeat dose: IM If there is evidence of ovulation, but no pregnancy, repeat the regimen for at least 2 more courses before increasing the dose to 150 IU FSH/150 IU LH/day for 7 to 12 days, followed by 5000 to 10,000 U hCG 1 day after the last dose of menotropins. If there is evidence of ovulation, but no pregnancy, repeat the same dose for 2 more courses.
Stimulation of Spermatogenesis:
Adults (men): IM Pretreat with hCG alone (5000 U 3 times/wk). Continue hCG for a period sufficient to achieve serum testosterone levels within normal range and masculinization (ie, appearance of secondary sex characteristics), which may take 4 to 6 mo.
Adults (men):
Pergonal: IM 75 IU FSH/75 IU LH 3 times/wk and hCG 2000 U twice weekly for at least 4 mo to ensure spermatozoa in ejaculate. If patient has not responded with increased spermatogenesis at the end of 4 mo continue treatment with 75 IU FSH/75 IU LH 3 times/wk or increase the dose to 150 IU FSH/150 IU LH 3 times/wk, with the hCG dose unchanged.

Trade names: Pergonal Powder or pellet for injection, lyophilized 75 IU FSH activity, 75 IU LH activity
Repronex Powder or pellet for injection, lyophilized 150 IU FSH activity, 150 IU LH activity

Warnings: Women who have high follicle stimulating hormone (FSH) level indicating primary ovarian failure; uncontrolled thyroid and adrenal dysfunction; organic intracranial lesion (eg, pituitary tumor); presence of any cause of infertility other than anovulation unless patient is candidate for in vitro fertilization; abnormal bleeding of undetermined origin; ovarian cysts or enlargement not caused by polycystic ovary syndrome; pregnancy; prior hypersensitivity to menotropins. Men (Pergonal) who have normal gonadotropin levels indicating normal pituitary function; elevated gonadotropin levels indicating primary testicular failure; infertility disorders other than hypogonadotropic hypogonadism. Pregnancy Category: [X]

Interactions: None well documented.

Meperidine HCl

Narcotic analgesic

Indications: Oral and parenteral: Relief of moderate to severe pain.

Parenteral: Preoperative sedation; support of anesthesia; obstetrical analgesia.

Dose: Pain:
Adults: IM/SC/PO 50 to 150 mg q 3 to 4 hr prn. If IV administration is required, reduce dose and administer slowly.
Children: IM/SC/PO 1 to 1.8 mg/kg (up to adult dose) q 3 to 4 hr prn.
Preoperative Sedation:
Adults: IM/SC 50 to 100 mg 30 to 90 min before anesthetic.
Children: IM/SC 1 to 2 mg/kg (0.5 to 1 mg/lb), up to adult dose, 30 to 90 min before beginning anesthesia.
Support of Anesthesia:
Adults: IV Repeated doses diluted to 10 mg/mL by slow injection or by continuous infusion diluted to 1 mg/mL.
Obstetrical Analgesia:
Adults: IM/SC 50 to 100 mg q 1 to 3 hr prn when pains become regular.

Trade names: Demerol HCl Tablets 50 mg

Warnings: Upper airway obstruction; acute asthma; diarrhea due to poisoning or toxins; patients who are receiving or have received MAO inhibitor within last 14 days. Pregnancy Category: [Pregnancy category undetermined Safety not established]

Interactions: CNS depressants (eg, tranquilizers, sedatives, alcohol): Additive CNS depression.
Cimetidine: Monitor for increased respiratory and CNS depression.
Hydantoins: Hydantoins may decrease the pharmacologic effects of meperidine, possibly because of increased hepatic metabolism of the narcotic.
MAO inhibitors, furazolidone: Potentially fatal reactions can occur if meperidine is used in patients within 14 days of receiving MAO inhibitor or furazolidone.
Phenothiazines: Excessive sedation and hypotension.
Incompatability: Do not co-infuse with solutions of soluble barbiturates, aminophylline, heparin, morphine, methicillin, phenytoin, sodium bicarbonate, iodine, sulfadiazine and sulfisoxazole.

Mercaptopurine

Purine antimetabolite

Indications: Adult: Acute lymphoblastic leukemias.

Pediatric: Acute lymphoblastic leukemias.

Unlabeled indication: Acute myeloblastic leukemias (adults).

Dose: Acute Lymphocytic Leukemia, Remission Induction:
Adults: PO Initiate therapy with 2.5 mg/kg/day, rounded to the nearest 25 mg. If no response after 4 wk of therapy, may increase dose to no more than 5 mg/kg/day. An alternative regimen is to initiate therapy with 80 to 100 mg/m^2 /day, rounded to the nearest 25 mg.
Pediatric: PO Initiate therapy with 2.5 mg/kg/day, rounded to the nearest 25 mg. If no response after 4 wk of therapy, may increase dose to no more than 5 mg/kg/day. An alternative regimen is to initiate therapy with 70 to 100 mg/m^2 /day, rounded to the nearest 25 mg.
Acute Lymphocytic Leukemia, Maintenance:
Adults: PO Usual range is 1.5 to 2.5 mg/kg/day as a single dose.
Pediatric: PO Usual range is 1.5 to 2.5 mg/kg/day as a single dose. An alternative regimen is 75 mg/m^2 /day, rounded to the nearest 25 mg.

Trade names: Purinethol Tablets 50 mg

Warnings: Prior resistance to this drug. Pregnancy Category: [D]

Interactions: Allopurinol: Inhibition of mercaptopurine metabolism; coadministration may cause increased toxicity.
Co-trimoxazole: Potentiates bone marrow suppression associated with mercaptopurine.

Methotrexate: May increase oral bioavailability of mercaptopurine.
Warfarin: Mercaptopurine may decrease the hypoprothrombinemic effect of warfarin; monitor and adjust warfarin therapy as necessary.

Meropenem

Anti-infective / Carbapenem

Indications: Treatment of intra-abdominal infections in adults and children at least 3 mo and meningitis in children at least 3 mo when caused by susceptible microorganisms.

Dose: Intra-Abdominal Infections:
Adults: IV 1 g IV q 8 hr.
Children (at least 3 mo): IV 20 mg/kg q 8 hr.
Max dose: 2 g q 8 hr.
Meningitis:
Children (at least 3 mo): IV 40 mg/kg q 8 hr.
Max dose: 2 g q 8 hr.

Trade names: Merrem Powder for Injection 500 mg

Warnings: Hypersensitivity to any component of this product or to other drugs in the same class or in patients who have demonstrated anaphylactic reactions to B-lactarus. Pregnancy Category: [B]

Interactions: Probenecid: Inhibits renal excretion of meropenem. Coadministration is not recommended.
Incompatability: Do not physically mix with solutions containing other drugs.

Mesalamine

Intestinal anti-inflammatory / Aminosalicylic acid derivative

Indications: Treatment of active, mild to moderate distal ulcerative colitis, proctosigmoiditis, or proctitis.

Unlabeled indication: Treatment of Crohn disease.

Dose: Controlled-Release Tablets or Capsules:
Adults: PO 800 mg tid for total of 2.4 g/day for 6 wk.
Suppositories:
Adults: PR 500 mg suppository bid for up to 6 wk. Retain suppository in rectum for at least 1 to 3 hr to achieve max benefit.
Suspension enema:
Adults: PR 4 g in 60 mL as rectal instillation q day for up to 6 wk, preferably at bedtime, retained for 8 hr.

Trade names: Asacol Tablets, delayed release 400 mg
Pentasa Capsules, controlled release 250 mg
Rowasa Suppositories 500 mg

Warnings: Hypersensitivity to salicylates. Pregnancy Category: [B]

Interactions: None well documented.

Mesna

Uroprotectant

Indications: Prevention of ifosfamide-induced hemorrhagic cystitis.

Unlabeled indication: Prevention of cyclophosphamide-induced hemorrhagic cystitis.

Dose: Prevention of Ifosfamide-Induced Hemorrhagic Cystitis:
Adults: IV Mesna dose is given as bolus injections in a dosage equal to 20% of ifosfamide dose at time of administration, 4 hr after, and 8 hr after each ifosfamide dose (eg, for ifosfamide 1,200 mg/m^2, give mesna 240 mg/m^2 at 0, 4, and 8 hr after each ifosfamide dose). The total daily dose of mesna is 60% of the ifosfamide dose. Repeat this dosing schedule on each day that ifosfamide is administered. When the dosage of ifosfamide is adjusted, modify the dose of mesna accordingly.
Adults: PO Following the initial IV mesna dose (20% of ifosfamide dose), the oral mesna dose is 40% of ifosfamide dose 2 and 6 hr after each ifosfamide dose.

Trade names: Mesnex Tablets 400 mg

Warnings: Standard considerations. Pregnancy Category: [B]

Interactions: None well documented.

Metaproterenol Sulfate

Bronchodilator / Sympathomimetic

Indications: Treatment of bronchial asthma and reversible bronchospasm associated with bronchitis and emphysema; control of acute asthma attacks in children at least 6 yr (inhalation solution only).

Dose: Aerosol:
Adults and Children (at least 12 yr): Inhalation 2 to 3 inhalations q 3 to 4 hr, not to exceed 12 inhalations/ day.
Hand Nebulizer:
Adults and Children (at least 12 yr): Inhalation 5 to 15 inhalations q 4 hr prn.
Intermittent Positive Pressure Breathing Apparatus:
Adults and Children (at least 12 yr): Inhalation 0.2 to 0.3 mL of 5% solution in 2.5 mL of diluent q 4 hr prn.
Nebulizer:
Adults and Children (at least 12 yr): Inhalation 0.1 to 0.2 mL in saline to a total volume of 3 mL.

Trade names: Alupent Syrup 10 mg/5 mL

Warnings: Cardiac arrhythmias associated with tachycardia. Pregnancy Category: [C]

Interactions: MAO inhibitors, tricyclic antidepressants: Pressor effects may be potentiated.

Metaraminol

Vasopressor

Indications: Prevention and treatment of acute hypotensive state occurring with spinal anesthesia; adjunctive treatment of hypotension due to hemorrhage, reactions to medications, surgical complications and shock associated with brain damage due to trauma or tumor. Probably effective as adjunct in hypotension due to cardiogenic shock or septicemia.

Dose: Prevention of Hypotension:
Adults: SC/IM 2 to 10 mg; wait at least 10 min before readministering.
Children: SC/IM 0.1 mg/kg.
Treatment of Hypotension:
Adults: IV 15 to 100 mg in 250 to 500 mL of normal saline or D5W; adjust rate to response; may concentrate further in fluid-restricted states.
Children: SC/IM 0.1 mg/kg.
Treatment of Severe Shock:
Adults: IV Push 0.5 to 5 mg followed by infusion of 15 to 100 mg in 500 mL of normal saline or D5W.
Children: IV 0.01 mg/kg as single dose or via infusion of 1 mg/25 mL in normal saline or D5W.

Trade names: Aramine Injection 10 mg/mL (1%, as bitartrate)

Warnings: Use with cyclopropane or halothane anesthesia unless essential. Pregnancy Category: [C]

Interactions: Guanethidine: Antihypertensive effects of guanethidine may be negated.
MAO inhibitors, furazolidone, rauwolfia alkaloids, methyldopa: May significantly increase pressor response, possibly resulting in hypertensive crisis and intracranial hemorrhage.
Tricyclic antidepressants: May decrease pressor response.
Incompatability: Metaraminol is incompatible with many drugs; consult reference prior to admixture.

Methadone HCl

Narcotic analgesic

Indications: Management of severe pain; detoxification and temporary maintenance treatment of narcotic addiction.

Dose: Pain:
Adults: IM/SC/PO 2.5 to 10 mg q 3 to 4 hr prn. May

need higher doses in patients with severe pain or tolerance.
Detoxification:
Adults: PO 15 to 20 mg initially to suppress withdrawal symptoms. Additional doses may be needed.
Patients Physically Dependent on High Doses of Narcotics: PO 40 mg/day may be given for 2 to 3 days; decrease dose q 1 to 2 days.
Maintenance: PO 20 to 40 mg initially to suppress withdrawal symptoms in patients who are heavy heroin users. Additional 10 mg doses can be given prn. Adjust dose as tolerated and required, up to 120 mg/day.
Trade names: Dolophine HCl Tablets 5 mg
Methadose Tablets 5 mg
Warnings: Standard considerations. Pregnancy Category: [Pregnancy category undetermined Methadone use has been associated with low infant birthweight]
Interactions: Barbiturate anesthetics: Drug actions may be additive.
Cimetidine, protease inhibitors: Monitor for increased respiratory and CNS depression.
CNS depressants (eg, tranquilizers, sedatives, alcohol): Additive CNS depression.
Fluvoxamine: Monitor for increased CNS depression when taken with methadone. Monitor for signs and symptoms of withdrawal when fluvoxamine is discontinued.
Hydantoins, rifampin, barbiturates: May decrease effectiveness of methadone.
Urinary acidifiers: May increase renal clearance of methadone.

Methazolamide

Carbonic anhydrase inhibitor

Indications: Treatment of ocular conditions where lowering IOP is likely to be of therapeutic benefit (eg, chronic open-angle glaucoma, secondary glaucoma, preoperatively in acute angle-closure glaucoma).
Dose: Adults: PO 50 to 100 mg bid or tid.
Trade names: Methazolamide Tablets 25 mg
Warnings: Situations in which sodium and/or potassium serum levels are depressed; in cases of marked kidney or liver disease or dysfunction, in adrenal gland failure, and in hyperchloremic acidosis; in patients with cirrhosis (may precipitate hepatic encephalopathy); long-term administration in patients with angle-closure glaucoma. Pregnancy Category: [C]
Interactions: Aspirin (high-dose): Anorexia, tachypnea, lethargy, coma, and death have been reported.
Steroids: Use with caution because of risk of developing hypokalemia.

Methimazole

Antithyroid

Indications: Long-term therapy of hyperthyroidism; amelioration of hyperthyroidism in preparation for subtotal thyroidectomy or radioactive iodine therapy.
Dose: Adults:
Initial dose: PO 15 to 60 mg/day in 3 equal doses at approximately 8-hr intervals.
Maintenance: PO 5 to 15 mg/day.
Children:
Initial dose: PO 0.4 mg/kg/day.
Maintenance: PO Approximately 1/2 initial dose. Alternately, children may be given 0.5 to 0.7 mg/kg/day in 3 divided doses as initial therapy and 1/3 to 2/3 of initial dose for maintenance.
Trade names: Tapazole Tablets 5 mg
Warnings: Use in nursing women. Pregnancy Category: [D]
Interactions: Anticoagulants: May decrease or increase anticoagulant action.
Beta blockers: May increase effects of beta blockers, resulting in toxicity.
Digoxin: May cause increase in effects of digitalis glycosides, including toxicity.
Theophyllines: May alter theophylline clearance in hyperthyroid or hypothyroid patients.

Methotrexate

Antineoplastic / Antimetabolite / Antipsoriatic / Antiarthritic

Indications: Antineoplastic chemotherapy for treatment of gestational choriocarcinoma, chorioadenoma destruens, hydatidiform mole; treatment and prophylaxis of acute (meningeal) lymphocytic leukemia; treatment of breast cancer, epidermoid cancers of head and neck, advanced mycosis fungoides, and lung cancer; in combination therapy in advanced-stage non-Hodgkin lymphoma; as adjunct in high doses followed by leucovorin rescue in nonmetastatic osteosarcoma (postsurgically); symptomatic control of severe psoriasis and severe rheumatoid arthritis; polyarticular-course juvenile rheumatoid arthritis (JRA).
Dose: Choriocarcinoma and Thromboplastic Diseases:
Adults: PO/IM 15 to 30 mg for 5 days. Repeat courses 3 to 5 times as required, with rest periods of more than 1 wk between courses.
Leukemia:
Adults and Children:
Induction: PO/IM 3.3 mg/m^2 /day in combination with prednisone 60 mg/m^2 /day usually for 4 to 6 wk.
Postremission maintenance therapy (usually in combination with other drugs): PO/IM 2 times/wk in total weekly doses of 30 mg/m^2 or IV 2.5 mg/kg q 14 days.
Meningeal Leukemia:
Adults: Intrathecal 12 mg/m^2 (max, 15 mg). Administer q 2 to 5 days until cell count of CSF returns to normal, then give 1 additional dose. Dose reduction may be required in elderly patients because of differences in CSF volume.
Children at least 3 yr: Intrathecal 12 mg. Administer q 2 to 5 days until CSF cell count returns to normal.
Children 2 yr: Intrathecal 10 mg.
Children 1 yr: Intrathecal 8 mg.
Children younger than 1 yr: Intrathecal 6 mg.
Lymphoma (Burkitt Lymphoma, Stages 1 and 2):
Adults: PO 10 to 25 mg/day for 4 to 8 days. Provide 7- to 10-day rest period between courses.
Stage 3 Lymphosarcoma As Part of Combination Therapy:
Adults: PO 0.625 to 2.5 mg/kg/day.
Mycosis Fungoides:
Adults: PO 2.5 to 10 mg/day for 1 wk to 1 mo (based on clinical response or hematologic function). IM 25 mg twice/wk or 50 mg/wk.
Osteosarcoma: Complex high dose with leucovorin rescue and other chemotherapeutic agents. Starting dose for high-dose methotrexate is 12 g/m^2.
Rheumatoid Arthritis:
Adults:
Initial therapy: PO 7.5 mg/wk in single dose or 2.5 mg q 12 hr for 3 doses each wk. Gradually adjust dosage to max response; do not exceed 20 mg/wk.
Polyarticular-Course JRA: PO start with 10 mg/m^2 /wk.
Psoriasis: Individualize dosage. Administer 5 to 10 mg parenteral test dose 1 wk prior to therapy.
Adults: IM/IV/PO 10 to 25 mg/wk (max, 30 mg/wk).
Adults: PO 2.5 mg q 12 hr for 3 doses q wk (max, 30 mg/wk).
Trade names: Methotrexate LPF Sodium Injection 25 mg/mL
Methotrexate Sodium Injection 25 mg/mL
Methotrexate Sodium Powder for injection 20 mg
Rheumatrex Dose Pack Tablets 2.5 mg
Trexall Tablets 5 mg
Warnings: Use in nursing mothers. In patients with psoriasis or rheumatoid arthritis, methotrexate

is contraindicated in pregnancy, alcoholism, alcoholic liver disease, chronic liver disease, overt or laboratory evidence of immunodeficiency syndrome, and preexisting blood dyscrasias (eg, leukopenia, thrombocytopenia); hypersensitivity to the drug. Pregnancy Category: [X (for rheumatoid arthritis and psoriasis); D (other uses)]

Interactions: Charcoal, folic acid: May reduce methotrexate efficacy.
Digoxin: May reduce serum digoxin levels and actions.
Etretinate, NSAIDs, penicillins, probenecid, salicylates, sulfonamides, tetracyclines: May increase methotrexate blood levels and toxicity.
Hydantoins: May reduce plasma levels.
Theophylline: Methotrexate decreases Cl of theophylline.
Trimethoprim: May increase risk of methotrexate-induced bone marrow suppression and megaloblastic anemia.

Methoxsalen

Psoralen

Indications: Symptomatic control of severe, recalcitrant, disabling psoriasis not responsive to other forms of therapy and when diagnosis supported by biopsy (Oxsoralen-Ultra, 8-MOP capsule); use in conjunction with long wave UV radiation for repigmentation of idiopathic vitiligo (8-MOP capsule, Oxsoralen lotion); with long wave UV radiation of white blood cells (photopheresis) with the UVAR Photopheresis System in the palliative treatment of skin manifestations of cutaneous T-cell lymphoma in people not responsive to other forms of treatment (8-MOP capsule, Oxsoralen lotion); extracorporeal administration with UVAR Photopheresis System in the palliative treatment of skin manifestation of cutaneous T-cell lymphoma that is unresponsive to other forms of treatment (Uvadex solution).

Dose: Vitiligo:
Adults:
8-MOP: PO Take 20 mg daily in 1 dose with milk or food 2 to 4 hr prior to UV exposure. Take on alternate days and never on 2 consecutive days. Sun exposure is based on basic skin color. Initial sun exposure should be 15 min for light skin, 20 min for medium-colored skin, and 25 min for dark skin. The second, third, and fourth exposures may be increased by 5 min/each exposure (if basic skin color is light, the second exposure can be increased to 20 min, the third exposure to 25 min, and the fourth exposure to 30 min). Subsequent exposures may gradually be increased based on erythema and tenderness of amelanotic skin (max, 0.6 mg/kg).
Oxsoralen lotion: Apply lotion to a small, well-defined, vitiliginous lesion, then expose this area to UVA light. Initial exposure time must not exceed one half the minimal erythema dose. Regulate treatment intervals by erythema response (once weekly or less, depending on the results). Pigmentation may begin after a few weeks; significant repigmentation may take up to 6 to 9 mo. Periodic treatment may be needed to retain the new pigmentation.
Psoriasis:
Adults:
Oxsoralen-Ultra: PO Take with food or milk 1.5 to 2 hr prior to UVA exposure.
8-MOP: PO Take with food or milk 2 hr prior to UVA exposure. Take according to the following recommendations: Generally, elderly patients should be started at the low end of the dose recommended according to body weight and closely monitored during PUVA therapy. No treatments should be given more often than once every other day because the full extent of phototoxic reactions may not be evident until 48 hr after each exposure. Dosage may be increased by 10 mg after the fifteenth treatment. Patients weighing:
- Less than 30 kg take 10 mg
- 30 to 50 kg take 20 mg
- 51 to 65 kg take 30 mg
- 66 to 80 kg take 40 mg
- 81 to 90 kg take 50 mg
- 91 to 115 kg take 60 mg
- Greater than 115 kg take 70 mg

Cutaneous T-Cell Lymphoma:
Adults:
Uvadex: Extracorporeal with the UVAR Photopheresis System only. (Not for parenteral administration.) Normal treatment schedule: Treatment is given on 2 consecutive days q 4 wk for a minimum of 7 treatment cycles (6 mo). Accelerated treatment schedule: If assessment of the patient during the fourth treatment cycle (approximately 3 mo) reveals an increased skin score from the baseline score, the frequency of treatment may be increased to 2 consecutive treatments q 2 wk. If a 25% improvement in the skin score is attained after 4 consecutive wk, the regular treatment schedule may be resumed (max, 20 cycles). Consult UVAR Photopheresis System Operator's Manual before using this product. Treatment involves collection of leukocytes, photoactivation, and reinfusion of photoactivated cells. During each photopheresis treatment, 200 mcg (10 mL) of Uvadex is injected directly into photoactivation bag during the first buffy coat collection cycle. At the end of 6 cycles, a total of 740 mL (240 mL of buffy coat, 300 mL of plasma, and 200 mL of normal saline priming fluid) is collected and mixed with the 200 mcg of Uvadex present in the photoactivation bag. After photoactivation, the cells are reinfused.

Trade names: 8-MOP Capsules 10 mg
Oxsoralen-Ultra Capsules, soft gelatin 10 mg
Oxsoralen Lotion 1% (10 mg/mL)
Uvadex Solution 20 mcg/mL

Warnings: Patients exhibiting idiosyncratic reactions to psoralen compounds; specific history of light-sensitive disease states should not initiate methoxsalen therapy (eg, lupus erythematosus, porphyria cutanea tarda, erythropoietic protoporphyria, variegate porphyria, xeroderma pigmentosum, albinism); patients exhibiting melanoma or possessing a history of melanoma; patients exhibiting invasive squamous cell carcinomas; patients with aphakia, because of increased risk of retinal damage caused by absence of lenses. Pregnancy Category: [C: 8-MOP (Oxsoralen-Ultra);D: Uvadex]

Interactions: Known photosensitizers (eg, anthralin, coal tar, coal tar derivatives, fluoroquinolone antibiotics, griseofulvin, halogenated salicylanilides, nalidixic acid, organic staining dyes [eg, methylene blue, methyl orange, rose bengal, toluidine blue], phenothiazines, sulfonamides, tetracyclines, thiazide diuretics): Exercise care when using these agents and methoxsalen concurrently.

Methyldopa and Methyldopate HCl

Antihypertensive / Antiadrenergic, centrally acting

Indications: Treatment of hypertension.

Dose: Adults: PO 250 mg bid to tid in the first 48 hr initially, then 500 mg to 2 g/day in 2 to 4 divided doses. Adjust doses at intervals of not less than 2 days until adequate response is achieved. IV 250 to 500 mg q 6 hr prn (max, 1 g q 6 hr).
Children: PO 10 mg/kg/day in 2 to 4 doses (max, 65 mg/kg/day or 3 g/day, whichever is less). IV 20 to 40 mg/kg/day in divided doses every 6 hr (max, 65 mg/kg/day or 3 g/day, whichever is less).

Trade names: Aldomet Tablets 125 mg methyldopa
Warnings: Active hepatic disease or previous hepatic disease associated with methyldopa therapy; coadministration with MAO inhibitors. Pregnancy Category: [B (methyldopa) C (methyldopate HCl)]

Interactions: Anesthetics: May require reduced doses of anesthetics.

Medications

Barbiturates: Actions of methyldopa may be reduced.
Beta blockers: May cause paradoxical hypertension (rare).
Ferrous sulfate or gluconate: May decrease methyldopa absorption.
Haloperidol: May result in dementia or sedation.
Levodopa: BP lowering effects of methyldopa may be potentiated. Central effects of levodopa in Parkinson disease may be potentiated.
Lithium: May precipitate lithium toxicity.
MAO inhibitors: May lead to excessive sympathetic stimulation.
Phenothiazines: Serious elevations in BP may occur.
Sympathomimetics: May potentiate pressor effects of sympathomimetics and lead to hypertension.
Tolbutamide: Enhanced hypoglycemic effects may occur.
Tricyclic antidepressants: Reversal or attenuation of the hypotensive effects of methyldopa.

Methylphenidate Hydrochloride

Psychotherapeutic / CNS stimulant

Indications: Treatment of attention-deficit hyperactivity disorder (ADHD); treatment of narcolepsy (Ritalin, Ritalin SR, Metadate ER, Methylin).

Dose: Adults: PO 10 to 60 mg/day in 2 to 3 divided doses.
Children (6 yr and older): PO 5 mg before breakfast and lunch initially; increase by increments of 5 to 10 mg/wk up to 60 mg/day. Give sustained-release (SR) tablets at 8-hr intervals.
Concerta:
Adults and Children (6 yr and older): PO In patients new to methylphenidate, start with 18 mg qd in the morning, then adjust dose in 18 mg increments at weekly intervals (max, 54 mg qd in the morning).
In patients being converted from methylphenidate regimens to Concerta, start with 18 mg of Concerta every morning in patients receiving methylphenidate 5 mg bid or tid or 20 mg SR; start with 36 mg of Concerta every morning in patients receiving methylphenidate 10 mg bid or tid or 40 mg SR; start with 54 mg of Concerta every morning for patients receiving methylphenidate 15 mg bid or tid or 60 mg SR. The dose of Concerta may be adjusted in 18 mg increments at weekly intervals (max, 54 mg qd in the morning).
Metadate CD:
Adults and Children (6 yr and older): PO Start with 20 mg once daily in the morning before breakfast, then adjust dose in 20 mg increments at weekly intervals (max, 60 mg qd in the morning).
Ritalin LA:
Adults and Children (6 yr and older): PO In patients new to methylphenidate, start with 20 mg qd in the morning, then adjust dose in 10 mg increments at weekly intervals (max, 60 mg qd in the morning). In patients currently using methylphenidate immediate-release or sustained-released, start with 20 mg of Ritalin LA qd in patients receiving 10 mg bid or 20 mg SR; start with 30 mg of Ritalin LA qd in patients receiving 15 mg bid; start with 40 mg of Ritalin LA qd in patients receiving 20 mg bid or 40 mg SR; start with 60 mg of Ritalin LA qd in patients receiving 30 mg bid or 60 mg SR.

Trade names: Ritalin Tablets 5 mg
Metadate ER Tablets, extended-release 10 mg
Methylin Tablets 5 mg
Methylin ER Tablets, extended-release 10 mg
Concerta Tablets, extended-release 18 mg
Ritalin-SR Tablets, sustained-release 20 mg
Metadate CD Capsules, extended-release 10 mg
Ritalin LA Capsules, extended-release 20 mg

Warnings: Marked anxiety, agitation, and tension; glaucoma; motor tics; family history or diagnosis of Tourette syndrome; concurrent treatment with MAO inhibitors and within a minimum of 14 days following discontinuation of a MAO inhibitor. Pregnancy Category: [C]

Interactions: Anticonvulsants (eg, phenobarbital, phenytoin, primidone), selective serotonin reuptake inhibitors (eg, fluoxetine), tricyclic antidepressants(eg, imipramine), coumarin anticoagulants: Plasma levels of these agents may be increased by methylphenidate, increasing the risk of side effects.
Guanethidine: The antihypertensive effects of guanethidine may be decreased.
MAO inhibitors (eg, phenelzine): Because of the risk of hypertensive crisis, methylphenidate is contraindicated in patients receiving MAO inhibitors and for a minimum of 14 days after discontinuation of a MAO inhibitor.

Methylprednisolone

Corticosteroid

Indications: Replacement therapy in primary or secondary adrenal cortex insufficiency; adjunctive therapy for short-term administration in rheumatic disorders; exacerbation or maintenance therapy in collagen diseases; treatment of dermatologic diseases; control of allergic states or allergic and inflammatory ophthalmic processes; management of respiratory diseases; treatment of hematologic disorders; palliative management of neo-plastic diseases; management of cerebral edema associated with primary or metastatic brain tumor, craniotomy or head injury; induction of diuresis in edematous states (from nephrotic syndrome); management of critical exacerbations of GI diseases; management of acute exacerbations of multiple sclerosis; treatment of tuberculous meningitis; management of trichinosis with neurologic or myocardial involvement.
Intra-articular or soft tissue administration: Adjunctive therapy for short-term administration in synovitis of osteoarthritis, rheumatoid arthritis, bursitis, acute gouty arthritis, epicondylitis, acute nonspecific tenosynovitis and posttraumatic osteoarthritis.

Intralesional administration: Management of keloids; treatment of localized hypertrophic, infiltrated, inflammatory lesions of lichen planus, psoriatic plaques, granuloma annulare, lichen simplex chronicus; treatment of discoid lupus erythematosus, necrobiosis lipoidica diabeticorum, alopecia areata and cystic tumors of aponeurosis or tendon.

Topical administration: Treatment of inflammatory and pruritic manifestations of corticosteroid-responsive dermatoses.

Unlabeled indication: Reduction of mortality in severe alcoholic hepatitis; prevention of respiratory distress syndrome; treatment of septic shock; improvement of neurologic function in acute spinal cord injury.

Dose: Methylprednisolone:
Adults: PO 4 to 48 mg/day.
Methylprednisolone Sodium Succinate:
Adults: IV/IM 10 to 40 mg administered over 1 to several min. In severe condition, 30 mg/kg infused over 30 min; may repeat q 4 to 6 hr for 48 to 72 hr.
Infants and Children: IV/IM Not less than 0.5 mg/kg/24 hr.
Methylprednisolone Acetate:
Adults: IM 40 to 120 mg q wk for 1 to 4 wk. Intra-articular/intralesional 4 to 80 mg into joints or lesions.
Topical Apply sparingly to affected areas bid to qid.

Trade names: Medrol Tablets 2 mg
A-Methapred Powder for injection 125 mg per vial
Solu-Medrol Powder for injection 125 mg per vial
depMedalone 40 Injection 40 mg/mL suspension
depMedalone 80 Injection 80 mg/mL suspension
Depo-Medrol Injection 20 mg/mL suspension
Depopred-40 Injection 40 mg/mL suspension
Depopred-80 Injection 80 mg/mL suspension
Duralone-40 Injection 40 mg/mL suspension
Duralone-80 Injection 80 mg/mL suspension
Medralone 40 Injection 40 mg/mL suspension

Medralone 80 Injection 80 mg/mL suspension
Warnings: Systemic fungal infections; idiopathic thrombocytopenic purpura (IM administration); administration of live virus vaccines; topical monotherapy in primary bacterial infections; topical use on face, groin or axilla; use in premature infants (sodium succinate salt). Pregnancy Category: [Pregnancy category undetermined (systemic use); C (topical use)]
Interactions: Anticholinesterases: May antagonize anticholinesterase effects in myasthenia gravis.
Barbiturates: May decrease pharmacologic effect of methylprednisolone.
Hydantoins, rifampin: May increase clearance and decrease efficacy of methylprednisolone.
Ketoconazole: May decrease clearance of methylprednisolone.
Macrolide antibiotics: Significantly decreases methylprednisolone clearance; may need to decrease dose.
Salicylates: May reduce serum levels and efficacy of salicylates.

Methysergide Maleate

Analgesic / Migraine
Indications: Prevention or reduction of intensity of severe and frequent (once weekly or more) vascular headaches; prophylaxis of vascular headache. Not for management of acute attack.
Dose: Adults: PO 4 to 8 mg/day with meals. There must be drug-free interval of 3 to 4 wk after 6 mo of treatment.
Trade names: Sansert Tablets 2 mg
Warnings: Pregnancy; peripheral vascular disease; severe arteriosclerosis; severe hypertension; coronary artery disease; phlebitis or cellulitis in lower limbs; pulmonary disease; collagen disease or fibrotic processes; impaired liver or renal function; valvular heart disease; debilitated states; serious infections. Pregnancy Category: [Contraindicated in pregnancy because of oxytocic properties]
Interactions: Beta blockers: May result in peripheral ischemia, manifested by cold extremities with possible peripheral gangrene.

Metoclopramide

Dopamine antagonist antiemetic agent
Indications: PO: Relief of symptoms associated with acute and recurrent diabetic gastroparesis; short-term therapy of symptomatic, documented gastroesophageal reflux disease in adults who fail to respond to conventional therapy.

Parenteral: Prevention of nausea and vomiting associated with emetogenic cancer chemotherapy; prophylaxis of postoperative nausea and vomiting when nasogastric suction is undesirable; facilitation of small bowel intubation when tube does not pass pylorus with conventional maneuvers.

Unlabeled indication: Treatment of hiccoughs, migraines, postoperative gastric bezoars, improvement in lactation, radiation-induced emesis.
Dose: Nausea and Vomiting Caused by Highly Emetogenic Chemotherapy:
Adults: IV 2 mg/kg by infusion for 2 doses; give the first dose 30 min before chemotherapy, the second dose 2 hr later. If vomiting persists, 3 additional doses of 2 mg/kg may be given q 3 hr. If vomiting is controlled, 3 additional doses of 1 mg/kg may be given q 3 hr. PO 2 mg/kg 1 hr before chemotherapy, followed by 3 more doses at 2-hr intervals. If vomiting persists, 2 additional doses may be given q 3 hr (total daily dose of 12 mg/kg).
Nausea and Vomiting with Less Emetogenic Chemotherapy:
Adults: IV 1 mg/kg by infusion 30 min before chemotherapy, repeated q 2 hr for 3 doses.
Prevention of Delayed Nausea and Vomiting Caused by Chemotherapy:
Adults: PO 0.5 mg/kg qid for 4 days beginning 16 to 24 hr after chemotherapy given, in combination with dexamethasone. May be given IV in patients unable to take PO.
Adjustment in Renal Insufficiency: Reduce initial dose 50% in patients with Ccr less than 40 mL/min. Titrate subsequent doses based on patient response.
Trade names: Maxolon Tablets 10 mg (as monohydrochloride monohydrate)
Octamide Tablets 10 mg (as monohydrochloride monohydrate)
Octamide PFS Injection 5 mg/mL (as monohydrochloride monohydrate)
Reglan Tablets 5 mg (as monohydrochloride monohydrate)
Warnings: Patients in whom increase in GI motility could be harmful (eg, in presence of GI hemorrhage, mechanical obstruction, perforation); pheochromocytoma; epilepsy; patients receiving drugs likely to cause extrapyramidal reactions. Pregnancy Category: [B]
Interactions: Acetaminophen, cyclosporine, ethanol, levodopa, tetracycline: Metoclopramide may increase oral bioavailability or absorption of these drugs.
Anticholinergic, opioid analgesics, levodopa: May decrease effect of metoclopramide on gastric emptying.
Cefprozil, cimetidine, digoxin: Metoclopramide may decrease oral absorption of these drugs.
CNS depressants (eg, alcohol, anesthetics, barbiturates, opiates): May potentiate CNS depressant effects of metoclopramide.
Succinylcholine and possibly mivacurium: By inhibiting plasma cholinesterase metoclopramide may prolong neuromuscular blocking effects such as respiratory depression and paralysis.
Incompatability: Cephalothin, chloramphenicol, sodium bicarbonate.

Metolazone

Thiazide-like diuretic
Indications: Treatment of edema and hypertension.

Unlabeled indication: Prevention of calcium nephrolithiasis; reduction of postmenopausal osteoporosis; reduction of urine volume in diabetes insipidus.
Dose: Adults: PO 0.5 to 1 mg/day (Mykrox) or 2.5- to 20 mg/day (Zaroxolyn). Do not interchange Mykrox with Zaroxolyn. Mykrox is absorbed more rapidly and completely than Zaroxolyn.
Trade names: Zaroxolyn Tablets 2.5 mg
Mykrox Tablets 0.5 mg
Warnings: Anuria; renal decompensation; hepatic coma or precoma. Pregnancy Category: [B]
Interactions: Cholestyramine, colestipol: May decrease effects of metolazone by decreasing absorption.
Diazoxide: Concurrent use may produce severe hyperglycemia.
Digitalis glycosides (eg, digoxin): Urinary loss of potassium and magnesium may predispose patient to digitalis-induced arrhythmia.
Lithium: Metolazone may decrease renal elimination of lithium, resulting in toxicity.
Loop diuretics (eg, furosemide): Concurrent use may produce profound diuresis and electrolyte abnormalities.
Sulfonylureas (eg, tolbutamide): Metolazone may decrease hypoglycemic effect of sulfonylureas by increasing blood glucose.

Metoprolol

Beta-adrenergic blocker

Indications: Used alone or in combination with other antihypertensive agents, for management of hypertension, long-term management of angina pectoris, MI (immediate-release tablets and injection), treatment of stable, symptomatic (NYHA class II or III) heart failure of ischemic, hypertensive, or cardiomyopathic origin (Toprol-XL 25 mg only).

Dose: Hypertension:
Adults:
Initial: PO 100 mg/day in single or divided doses. Give 50 to 100 mg/day in a single dose, extended-release tablet.
Maintenance: PO 100 to 450 mg/day.
Angina:
Adults:
Initial: PO 100 mg/day in 2 divided doses. 100 mg/day in a single dose, extended-release tablet.
Maintenance: PO 100 to 400 mg/day.
MI:
Adults: IV bolus injection 5 mg slowly; may repeat q 2 min up to 15 mg. If tolerated, give PO 50 mg q 6 hr beginning 15 min after last IV dose; continue for 48 hr followed by PO 100 mg bid for 1 to 3 yr. If patient is intolerant of full IV dose, give PO 25 to 50 mg q 6 hr starting 15 min after last IV dose.
CHF:
Adults:
Extended-release tablet: PO Start with 25 mg qd for 2 wk in patients with NYHA class II heart failure and 12.5 mg qd in patients with more severe heart failure; then double the dose q 2 wk to highest dosage tolerated by patient (max, 200 mg).

Trade names: Lopressor Tablets 50 mg
Toprol XL Tablets, extended release 25 mg (23.75 mg metoprolol succinate equivalent to 25 mg metoprolol tartrate)

Warnings: Greater than first-degree heart block; CHF unless secondary to tachyarrhythmia treatable with beta-blockers; overt or moderate to severe cardiac failure; sinus bradycardia; cardiogenic shock; hypersensitivity to beta-blockers; systolic BP below 100 mm Hg; MI in patients with heart rate less than 45 bpm.
Pregnancy Category: [C]

Interactions: Barbiturates: Bioavailability of metoprolol may decrease.
Cimetidine: May increase metoprolol levels.
Clonidine: May enhance or reverse antihypertensive effect; potentially life-threatening situations may occur, especially on abrupt withdrawal of clonidine.
Hydralazine: Serum levels of both drugs may increase.
Lidocaine: Lidocaine levels may increase, leading to toxicity.
NSAIDs: Some agents may impair antihypertensive effect.
Prazosin: Orthostatic hypotension may increase.
Methimazole, propafenone, propylthiouracil, quinidine: Effects of metoprolol may increase.
Rifampin: May decrease effects of metoprolol.
Verapamil: Effects of both drugs may be increased.

Metronidazole

Anti-infective

Indications: Treatment of serious infections caused by susceptible anaerobic bacteria; prophylaxis of postoperative infection in patients undergoing colorectal surgery; treatment of amebiasis; treatment of trichomoniasis and asymptomatic partners of infected patients; bacterial vaginosis (Flagyl ER only).
Topical: Treatment of inflammatory papules, pustules, and erythema of acne rosacea.

Vaginal: Treatment of bacterial vaginosis.

Unlabeled indication: Treatment of hepatic encephalopathy, Crohn disease, antibiotic-associated pseudomembranous colitis, Helicobacter pylori infections.

Dose: Amebiasis:
Adults: PO
Flagyl 375 capsules: Acute amebic dysentery and amebic liver abscess: 750 mg tid for 5 to 10 days.
Flagyl 250 mg tablets: Acute amebic dysentery: 750 mg tid for 5 to 10 days. Amebic liver abscess: 500 or 750 mg tid for 5 to 10 days.
Children: PO
Flagyl 375, Flagyl 250 mg tablets: 35 to 50 mg/kg per 24 hr divided into 3 daily doses for 10 days.
Anaerobic Bacterial Infections: Give IV initially when treating most serious anaerobic infections.
Adults: IV 15 mg/kg loading dose infused over 1 hr (approximately 1 g for a 70 kg adult); then a maintenance dose of 7.5 mg/kg infused over 1 hr q 6 hr (approximately 500 mg for a 70 kg adult). The first maintenance dose should be given 6 hr following initiation of loading dose. Do not exceed 4 g in 24 hr. May follow with similar oral dose. For prophylaxis, loading dose is to be completed 1 hr before surgery, followed by maintenance dose 6 and 12 hr later.
Duration: The usual duration is 7 to 10 days; however, infections of the bone, joint, lower respiratory tract, and endocardium may require longer treatment.
Adults: PO
Flagyl 375, Flagyl 250 mg tablets: Usual dosage is 7.5 mg/kg (approximately 500 mg for a 70 kg adult) q 6 hr (max, 4 g per 24 hr) for 7 to 10 days; however, infections of the bone, joint, lower respiratory tract, and endocardium may require longer treatment.
Bacterial Vaginosis:
Adults: PO 750 mg (Flagyl ER) daily for 7 consecutive days. Vaginal 1 applicator-full (approximately 37.5 mg metronidazole) intravaginally once or twice a day for 5 days; for daily dosing, administer at bedtime
Inflammatory Papules and Pustules of Rosacea:
Adults: Topical Apply thin layer once daily (1% cream) or bid to entire affected areas after washing. Use morning and evening or as directed by health care provider. Avoid application close to eyes.
Trichomoniasis: Individualize treatment for women and men.
Adults: PO
Flagyl 375 capsules: Women: 375 mg bid for 7 consecutive days. When a repeat course is required, a lapse of 4 to 6 wk between courses is recommended.
Flagyl 250 mg tablets: 250 mg tid for 7 consecutive days.
One-day treatment: 2 g as a single dose or in 2 divided doses of 1 g each given on the same day.
Children: PO 5 mg/kg/dose tid for 7 days.

Trade names: Flagyl Tablets 250 mg
Flagyl ER Tablets, extended-release 750 mg
Flagyl 375 Capsules 375 mg
Flagyl I.V. Powder for Injection, lyophilized 500 mg
Flagyl I.V. RTU Injection 5 mg/mL
Metric 21 Tablets 250 mg
MetroCream Cream 0.75%
MetroGel Gel 0.75%
MetroGel-Vaginal Gel 0.75%
MetroLotion Lotion 0.75%
Noritate Cream 1%
Protostat Tablets 250 mg

Warnings: Hypersensitivity to nitroimidazole derivatives or any component of the products; first trimester of pregnancy in patients with trichomoniasis.
Pregnancy Category: [B]

Interactions: Anticoagulants: Anticoagulant effect may be increased.
Barbiturates, phenytoin: Therapeutic failure of metronidazole may occur.
Cimetidine: May prolong the $t_{1/2}$ and decrease plasma Cl of metronidazole.
Disulfiram: Concurrent use may result in acute psychosis or confusional state. Do not give metronidazole to patients who have taken disulfiram within last 2 wk.

Ethanol: Disulfiram-like reaction including flushing, palpitations, tachycardia, nausea, and vomiting may occur with concurrent use.
Lithium: Plasma levels may be elevated by metronidazole, increasing the risk of lithium toxicity.
Incompatability: Do not use aluminum-containing equipment with metronidazole because solution will turn orange/rust color.

Mexiletine HCl

Antiarrhythmic

Indications: Treatment of documented life-threatening ventricular arrhythmias such as sustained ventricular arrhythmias.

Unlabeled indication: Prevention of ventricular arrhythmias in acute phase of MI; reduction of pain, dysesthesia and paresthesia associated with diabetic neuropathy.

Dose: Ventricular Arrhythmias:
Adults: PO 200 mg q 8 hr initially, increasing up to 400 mg q 8 hr if necessary (max, 1200 mg/day). Adjust dose by 50 to 100 mg increments q 2 to 3 days. For rapid control of ventricular arrhythmias, give loading dose of 400 mg followed by 200 mg in 8 hr. With dose no more than 300 mg q 8 hr, may give total daily dose q 12 hr (max, 450 mg q 12 hr).

Trade names: Mexitil Capsules 150 mg

Warnings: Preexisting second- or third-degree atrioventricular block (if pacemaker is not present); cardiogenic shock. Pregnancy Category: [C]

Interactions: Aluminum-magnesium hydroxide, atropine, narcotics: May slow absorption.
Cimetidine: May increase or decrease mexiletine plasma levels.
Hydantoins, rifampin: May increase mexiletine clearance.
Metoclorpramide: May accelerate absorption.
Theophylline: May increase serum theophylline levels.

Mezlocillin Sodium

Antibiotic / Penicillin

Indications: Treatment of infections of lower respiratory tract, urinary tract, skin or skin structure; intra-abdominal infections; uncomplicated gonorrhea; gynecological infections; septicemia; streptococcal infections; severe infections; and Pseudomonas infections caused by susceptible strains of specific microorganisms and prophylaxis.

Dose: Adults: IM/IV 200 to 300 mg/kg/day in 4 to 6 divided doses. Usual doses are 3 g q 4 hr or 4 g q 6 hr. IM Doses should not exceed 2 g/injection.
Children (older than 1 mo to younger than 12 yr): IM/IV 50 mg/kg q 4 hr.
Newborns: IV 75 mg/kg q 6 to 12 hr.

Trade names: Mezlin Powder for injection 1 g (as sodium; contains 1.85 mEq sodium/g)

Warnings: Hypersensitivity to penicillins. Pregnancy Category: [B]

Interactions: Contraceptives, oral: May reduce efficacy of oral contraceptives.
Tetracyclines: May impair bactericidal effects of mezlocillin.
Incompatability: Parenteral aminoglycosides may inactivate aminoglycosides in vitro; do not mix in same IV solution.

Miconazole

Anti-infective / Antifungal

Indications: Parenteral form: Treatment of severe systemic fungal infections.

Vaginal form: Local treatment of vulvovaginal candidiasis (moniliasis).

Topical form: Treatment of topical fungal infections, including tinea infections and candidiasis.

Dose: Systemic Infections:
Adults: IV 200 to 3600 mg/day. May divide into 3 doses. Treatment of meningitis is supplemented by intrathecal injections of 20 mg/dose. Treatment of bladder infections is supplemented by bladder instillations of 200 mg per dose.
Children (1 to 12 yr): IV 20 to 40 mg/kg/day (max, 15 mg/kg/dose).
Children (younger than 1 yr): IV 15 to 30 mg/kg/day (max, 15 mg/kg/dose).
Vaginal Infections:
Adults: Intravaginal 1 suppository (200 mg) at bedtime for 3 days or 1 suppository (100 mg) for 7 days or 1 applicatorful at bedtime for 7 days.
Topical Infections:
Adults: Topical Apply to infected area bid.

Trade names: Absorbine Antifungal Foot Powder Powder 2%
Breezee Mist Antifungal Powder 2%
Femizol-M Vaginal Cream 2%
Fungoid Cream Cream 2%
Fungoid Tincture Solution 2%
Lotrimin AF Spray Liquid 2%
M-Zole 3 Combination Pack Vaginal Suppositories 200 mg
M-Zole 7 Dual Pack Vaginal Suppositories 100 mg
Maximum Strength Desenex Antifungal Cream 2%
Micatin Cream 2%
Monistat 3 Vaginal Suppositories 200 mg
Monistat 7 Vaginal Suppositories 100 mg
Monistat 7 Combination Pack Vaginal Suppositories 100 mg
Monistat-Derm Topical Cream 2%
Monistat Dual-Pak Vaginal Suppositories 200 mg
Only-Clear Spray 2%
Prescription Strength Desenex Spray powder 2%
Tetterine Ointment 2%
Zeasorb-AF Powder 2%

Warnings: Hypersensitivity to imidazoles. Pregnancy Category: [C]

Interactions: Anticoagulants, oral: May cause increased anticoagulant effect.
Antihistamines, nonsedating type (eg, astemizole, terfenadine): Cardiotoxicity, including arrhythmias and death, has occurred when agents of this type were used together with azole-type antifungals.

Midazolam hydrochloride

General anesthetic / Benzodiazepine

Indications: Preoperative sedative; conscious sedation prior to diagnostic, therapeutic or endoscopic procedures; induction of general anesthesia; supplement to nitrous oxide and oxygen for short surgical procedures; infusion for sedation of intubated and mechanically ventilated patients as a component of anesthesia or during treatment in critical care setting.

Unlabeled indication: Treatment of epileptic seizures; alternative for the termination of refractory status epilepticus.

Dose: Preoperative Sedative:
Adults: IM 0.07 to 0.08 mg/kg approximately 1 hr before surgery.
Conscious Sedation:
Adults: IV 1 to 2.5 mg as 1 mg/mL dilution over 2 min. Increase by small increments to total dose of no more than 5 mg in at least 2 min intervals; use less if patient is premedicated with other CNS depressants.
Children: IM 0.1 to 0.15mg/kg. Doses up to 0.5 mg/kg have been used for more anxious patients. Total dose usually does not exceed 10 mg.
Children (younger than 6 mo): IV Titrate in small increments to clinical effect and monitor carefully.
Children (6 mo to 5 yr): IV 0.05 to 0.1 mg/kg. Total dose up to 0.6 mg/kg may be necessary. Do not exceed 6 mg.
Children (6 to 12 yr): IV 0.025 to 0.05 mg/kg. Total dose up to 0.4 mg/kg. Do not exceed 10 mg.

Children (12 to 16 yr): IV Dose as adults.
Induction of General Anesthesia:
Unpremedicated Adults: IV 0.3 to 0.35 mg/kg as 1 mg/mL dilution over 20 to 30 sec, allowing 2 min for effect; may use increments of approximately 25% of initial dose.
Premedicated Adults: IV 0.15 to 0.35 mg/kg over 20 to 30 sec.
Continuous Infusion:
Adults:
Loading dose: 0.01 to 0.05 mg/kg given slowly over several minutes. May be repeated at 10- to 15-min intervals until adequate sedation is achieved.
Maintenance: 0.02 to 0.1 mg/kg/hr (1 to 7 mg/hr).
Pediatric (non-neonatal): IV 0.05 to 0.2 mg/kg over at least 2 to 3 min in patients whose trachea is intubated. Loading dose may be followed by continuous IV infusion at 0.06 to 0.12 mg/kg/hr (1 to 2 mcg/kg/min). Increase or decrease approximately 25% of the initial infusion rate or subsequent infusion rate.
Intubated preterm and term newborns (younger than 32 wk): 0.03 mg/kg/hr (0.5 mcg/kg/min).
Intubated preterm and term newborns (younger than 32 wk): 0.06 mg/kg/hr (1 mcg/kg/min).
Maintenance Of Anesthesia: IV Increments of approximately 25% of induction dose in response to signs of lightening of anesthesia and repeat as necessary.

Trade names: Versed Syrup 2 mg/mL

Warnings: Hypersensitivity to benzodiazepines; uncontrolled pain; existing CNS depression; shock; acute narrow-angle glaucoma; acute alcohol intoxication; coma. Pregnancy Category: [D]

Interactions: Anesthetics, inhalation: Inhalation anesthetics may need to be reduced if midazolam is used as an induction agent. IV administration decreases minimum alveolar concentration of halothane required for general anesthesia.
Azole antifungal agents: Serum concentration of certain benzodiazepines may be increased and prolonged, producing enhanced CNS depression and prolonged effects.
Barbiturates, alcohol, other CNS depressants: May prolong effect and increase risk of underventilation or apnea.
Cimetidine: May increase midazolam levels.
Contraceptives, oral: Coadministration may result in prolongation of benzodiazepine $t_{1/2}$.
Droperidol, narcotics, secobarbital: May accentuate hypnotic effect of midazolam.
Ethanol: Increased CNS effects with acute ethanol ingestion.
Fluvoxamine: Reduced clearance, prolonged $t_{1/2}$ and increased serum concentrations of certain benzodiazepines may occur. Sedation or ataxia may be increased.
Indinavir: Possibly severe sedation and respiratory depression.
Propofol: Pharmacologic effects of propofol may be increased.
Rifamycins: Pharmacokinetic parameters of benzodiazepines may be altered.
Ritonavir: Possibly severe sedation and respiratory depression.
Theophyllines: Sedative effects of benzodiazepines may be antagonized.
Thiopental: Moderate reduction in induction dosage requirements has been noted following use of IM midazolam for premedication.
Valproic acid: Pharmacokinetic parameters of benzodiazepines may be increased. Liver metabolism may be decreased.
Verapamil: Effects of certain benzodiazepines may be increased, producing increased CNS depression and prolonged effects.
Incompatability: Dimenhydrinate, pentobarbital, perphenazine, prochlorperazine, ranitidine.

Miglitol

Antidiabetic / Alpha-glucosidase inhibitor

Indications: Patients with NIDDM who have failed dietary therapy. May be used alone or in combination with sulfonylureas.

Dose: Adults: PO 25 mg tid at the start of each meal. After 4 to 8 wk can increase to 50 mg/dose for 3 mo. If glycosylated hemoglobin level not acceptable after 3 mo can increase at 100 mg tid (max dose).

Trade names: Glyset Tablets 25 mg

Warnings: Diabetic ketoacidosis; inflammatory bowel disease; colonic ulceration; intestinal disorders of digestion or absorption; partial or predisposition to intestinal obstruction; conditions that may deteriorate as a result of increased intestinal gas production. Pregnancy Category: [B]

Interactions: Intestinal absorbents (eg, charcoal), digestive enzymes: May lower efficacy of miglitol.
Drugs that produce hyperglycemia (eg, corticosteroids, diuretics, thyroid preparations): May lead to loss of glucose control.
Ranitidine: Reduced ranitidine bioavailability.
Propranolol: Reduced propranolol bioavailability.

Milrinone Lactate

Cardiovascular

Indications: Short-term treatment of CHF.

Dose: Adults:
Loading dose: IV 50 mcg/kg over 10 min; adjust infusion rate according to hemodynamic and clinical response.

Trade names: Primacor Injection 1 mg/mL

Warnings: Standard considerations. Pregnancy Category: [C]

Interactions: None well documented.
Incompatability: Precipitate forms if furosemide is injected into same IV line as milrinone; do not administer both in same IV line.

Minocycline

Antibiotic / Tetracycline

Indications: Treatment of periodontitis as an adjunct to scaling and root planing. Treatment of infections caused by susceptible strains of gram-positive and gram-negative bacteria, *Rickettsia* and *Mycoplasma pneumonia*, and trachoma; treatment for susceptible infections when penicillins are contraindicated; adjunctive treatment of acute intestinal amebiasis; treatment of asymptomatic carriers of *Neisseria meningitidis* to eliminate meningococci from nasopharynx, chlamydia, inflammatory acne, syphilis, gonorrhea.

Dose: Inflammatory Acne:
Adults: PO 50 mg 1 to 3 times per day.
Meningococcal Carrier State:
Adults: PO 100 mg q 12 hr for 5 days.
Mycobacterium Marinum Infections:
Adults: PO 100 mg q 12 hr for 6 to 8 wk, although optimal doses have not been established.
Periodontitis:
Adults: Subgingival 1 mg microspheres are to be inserted by an oral health care professional.
Primary/Secondary Syphilis:
Adults: PO 200 mg initially then 100 mg q 12 hr for 10 to 15 days.
Renal Impairment: Do not exceed 200 mg per 24 hr.
Susceptible Infections:
Adults: PO/IV 200 mg initially, then PO/IV 100 mg q 12 hr or PO 50 mg qid (max, parenteral 400 mg per 24 hr).
Children older than 8 yr of age: PO/IV 4 mg/kg initially, then 2 mg/kg q 12 hr (max, usual adult dose).
Uncomplicated Gonococcal Infections Except Urethritis and Anorectal Infections in Men:
Adults: PO 200 mg initially followed with 100 mg q 12 hr for at least 4 days, with posttherapy cultures within 2

to 3 days.
Uncomplicated Gonococcal Urethritis in Men:
Adults: PO 100 mg q 12 hr for 5 days.
Uncomplicated Urethral, Endocervical, or Rectal Infections in Adults Caused by C. Trachomatis or Ureaplasma Urealyticum:
Adults: PO 100 mg q 12 hr for at least 7 days.
Trade names: Arestin Microspheres, sustained-release 1 mg (as hydrochloride)
Dynacin Tablets 50 mg (as hydrochloride)
Minocin Capsules, pellet-filled 50 mg (as hydrochloride)
Warnings: Standard considerations. Pregnancy Category: [D]
Interactions: Antacids (containing aluminum, calcium, magnesium, zinc), bismuth salts, divalent or trivalent cations: May decrease oral absorption of minocycline.
Anticoagulants, oral: Increased anticoagulant activity.
Contraceptives, oral: May reduce effect of oral contraceptives.
Digoxin: May increase digoxin serum levels.
Insulin: Increases hypoglycemic potential.
Iron salts: May decrease absorption of minocycline.
Isotretinoin: Because the risk of pseudotumor cerebri may be increased, avoid isotretinoin administration shortly before, during, or after minocycline therapy.
Methoxyflurane: Increased potential for nephrotoxicity exists; do not coadminister.
Milk and dairy products: Although the effects of milk and dairy products on minocycline absorption are less than observed with other tetracycline derivatives, it would be prudent to avoid the administration of milk or dairy products with all tetracycline derivatives.
Penicillins: May interfere with bactericidal action of penicillins.
Urinary alkalinizers, zinc salts: May decrease serum minocycline levels.
Incompatability: Do not mix before or during administration with adrenocorticotropic hormone, aminophylline, amobarbital sodium, amphotericin B, bicarbonate infusion mixtures, calcium gluconate or chloride, carbenicillin, cephalothin sodium, cefazolin sodium, chloramphenicol succinate, colistin sulfate, heparin sodium, hydrocortisone sodium succinate, iodine sodium, methicillin sodium, novobiocin, penicillin, pentobarbital, phenytoin sodium, polymyxins, prochlorperazine, sodium ascorbate, sulfadiazine, sulfisoxazole, thiopental sodium, vitamin K (sodium bisulfate or sodium salt), whole blood.

Minoxidil

Antihypertensive / Topical hair growth
Indications: Oral form: Management of severe hypertension associated with target organ damage in patients who have failed to respond to max doses of a diuretic plus 2 other antihypertensive drugs.

Topical form: Treatment of androgenic alopecia.

Unlabeled indication: Treatment of alopecia areata (topical).
Dose: Adults and children (older than 12 yr): PO 5 mg/day initially. If necessary, can increase to 10, 20, and then 40 mg/day in single or divided doses (max, 100 mg/day).
Children (younger than 12 yr): PO 0.2 mg/kg/day as single dose initially. May increase in 50% to 100% increments until optimal BP control is achieved (usually 0.25 to 1 mg/kg/day; max, 50 mg/day).
Adults: Topical Apply 1 mL to affected scalp areas morning and evening (max, 2 mL/day).
Trade names: Loniten Tablets 2.5 mg
Monoxidil Tablets 2.5 mg
Minoxidil for Men Topical Solution 2%
Rogaine Solution 2%
Warnings: Pheochromocytoma; standard considerations. Pregnancy Category: [C]
Interactions: Guanethidine: May result in profound orthostatic hypotensive effects; discontinue guanethidine before minoxidil therapy.
Topical corticosteroids or retinoids, petrolatum: May enhance cutaneous drug absorption of topically applied minoxidil.

Mirtazapine

Tetracyclic antidepressant
Indications: Treatment of depression.
Dose: Adults:
Initial dose: PO 15 mg/day as single dose. May be increased to 45 mg/day. For acute episodes, continue therapy of depression for at least 6 mo.
Trade names: Remeron Tablets 15 mg
Warnings: Hypersensitivity to maprotiline or mirtazapine; concomitant use with MAO inhibitors. Pregnancy Category: [C]
Interactions: Alcohol, CNS depressants: Additive CNS effects.
MAO inhibitors: May precipitate hypertensive crisis and convulsions with possible fatal results. Do not use mirtazapine in combination with an MAO inhibitors, or within 14 days of starting or stopping therapy with an MAO inhibitors.

Mitomycin

Antineoplastic antibiotic
Indications: Palliative treatment of disseminated adenocarcinoma of stomach or pancreas.

Unlabeled indication: Bladder, colorectal, or breast cancer; squamous cell carcinoma of head and neck, lungs, or cervix; pterygium.
Dose: Mitomycin 0.02% Eye Drops for Pterygium:
Adults: Reconstitute 5 mg vial of mitomycin with 10 mL sterile water for injection for a concentration of 0.5 mg/mL. Transfer 6 mL (3 mg) to a sterile 15 mL eye dropper bottle. Add 9 mL of sterile water for injection for a final concentration of 0.2 mg/mL (0.02% solution). This solution is stable for 1 wk at room temperature (59° to 86°F) and 2 wk refrigerated.
Mitomycin 0.2 mg/mL Ophthalmic Solution for Intraoperative Use:
Adults: Reconstitute 5 mg vial of mitomycin with 10 mL sterile water for injection. Transfer the contents of the vial to a 30 mL sterile vial. Add 15 mL of sterile water for injection for a final volume of 25 mL (0.2 mg/mL). This solution is stable for 52 wk frozen, 2 wk under refrigeration, and 24 hr at room temperature (59° to 86°F).
Palliative Treatment of Disseminated Adenocarcinoma of Stomach or Pancreas:
Adults and Pediatrics:
Initial dose: 10 to 20 mg/m^2, q 6 to 8 wk. Fully reevaluate patients after each course of therapy. Do not exceed 20 mg/m^2. Give an additional course of therapy only after the leukocyte and platelet counts have recovered. Subsequent doses of mitomycin may be adjusted according to the following schedule.
For dosage adjustments of mitomycin, nadir after prior dose (cells/mm-3): 100% of prior dose to be given to more than 3000 leukocytes and more than 75,000 platelets; 70% of prior dose to be given to 2000 to 2999 leukocytes and 25,000 to 74,999 platelets; 50% of prior dose to be given to less than 2000 leukocytes and less than 25,000 platelets. If disease progression continues after 2 courses, discontinue therapy.
Trade names: Mutamycin Powder for injection 5 mg (10 mg mannitol) vials
Warnings: Primary therapy as a single agent; to replace surgery or radiotherapy; hypersensitivity or idiosyncratic reaction to mitomycin; thrombocytopenia; coagulation disorder; increase in bleeding tendency caused by other causes. Pregnancy Category: [Safety for use during pregnancy has not been established Teratological changes have been noted in animal studies]

Interactions: Use of vinca alkaloids in patients who have previously or simultaneously received mitomycin has resulted in acute shortness of breath and severe bronchospasm.

Mitotane

Adrenal cortex suppressant

Indications: Inoperable adrenal cortical carcinoma.

Dose: Inoperable Adrenal Cortical Carcinoma:
Adults: PO Initially 2 to 6 g/day in divided doses, tid or qid. Titrate at least 9 to 10 g/day until adverse effects occur. The max tolerated dose ranges from 2 to 16 g/day. Doses as high as 18 to 19 g/day have been used.

Trade names: Lysodren Tablets 500 mg

Warnings: Standard considerations. Pregnancy Category: [C]

Interactions: CNS depressants (eg, narcotics, analgesics, alcohol, antiemetics, benzodiazepines, sedatives, tranquilizers): Potentiation of CNS effects with mitotane.
Corticosteroids: May increase corticosteroid metabolism, requiring higher corticosteroid doses with long-term mitotane therapy.
Spironolactone: May block the adrenolytic effects of mitotane.
Warfarin: Increases warfarin metabolism; increased warfarin doses may be required.

Mitoxantrone

Antineoplastic antibiotic

Indications: Adult acute nonlymphocytic leukemia (ANLL) as adjunctive therapy; advanced hormone-refractory prostate cancer (in combination with corticosteroids); secondary (chronic) progressive, progressive-relapsing, or worsening relapsing-remitting MS.

Unlabeled indication: Breast cancer, non-Hodgkin lymphoma, autologous bone marrow transplantation.

Dose: MS:
Adults: IV The recommended dosage of mitoxantrone is 12 mg/m^2 given as a short (approximately 5 to 15 min) IV infusion q 3 mo. Do not administer to MS patients who have received a cumulative lifetime dose of 140 mg/m^2 or more, or those with either LVEF of less than 50% or a clinically significant reduction in LVEF.
Prostate Cancer:
Adults: IV Recommended dosage of mitoxantrone is 12 to 14 mg/m^2 given as a short IV infusion q 21 days.
Combination Initial Therapy for ANLL:
Adults: IV For induction, give 12 mg/m^2 /day on days 1 to 3, and give 100 mg/m^2 of cytarabine for 7 days as a continuous 24-hr infusion on days 1 to 7. A second induction course may be given. Give mitoxantrone for 2 days and cytarabine for 5 days using the same daily dosage levels.

Trade names: Novantrone Sterile solution for injection 2 mg/mL

Warnings: Standard considerations. Pregnancy Category: [D]

Interactions: Quinolone antibiotics: Mitoxantrone may decrease oral absorption of quinolone antibiotics.
Topoisomerase II inhibitors and other antineoplastic agents: Have been associated with the development of acute leukemia.

Modafinil

CNS stimulant / Analeptic

Indications: Improve wakefulness in patients with excessive daytime sleepiness associated with narcolepsy.

Dose: Adults and Children (16 yr and older): PO 200 mg/day as a single morning dose.
Hepatic impairment: A dose reduction of 50% is recommended.

Trade names: Provigil Tablets 100 mg

Warnings: Standard considerations. Pregnancy Category: [C]

Interactions: Certain tricyclic antidepressants (eg, clomipramine, desipramine): Plasma levels of certain tricyclic antidepressants may be increased.
Clomipramine: Plasma levels may be increased by modafinil.
Contraceptives, oral: Efficacy may be decreased by modafinil, increasing the risk of unintended pregnancy.
Cyclosporine: Blood levels may be decreased by modafinil.
MAO inhibitors (eg, isocarboxazid): Use with caution.
Methylphenidate: May delay the absorption of modafinil.
Phenytoin: Increased risk of phenytoin toxicity.
Warfarin: Monitor prothrombin times.

Montelukast Sodium

Leukotriene receptor antagonist

Indications: Prophylaxis and chronic treatment of asthma in patients 12 mo and older; relief of symptoms of seasonal allergic rhinitis in patients 2 yr and older.

Dose: Adults and Children (at least 15 yr): PO 10 mg once daily in the evening.
Children (6 to 14 yr): PO 5 mg chewable tablet once daily in the evening.
Children (2 to 5 yr): PO 4 mg chewable tablet once daily in the evening.
Children (12 to 23 mo): PO 1 packet of 4 mg granules daily in the evening.

Trade names: Singulair Tablets 10 mg

Warnings: Standard considerations. Pregnancy Category: [B]

Interactions: Phenobarbital, rifampin: Decreased montelukast levels.

Morphine Sulfate

Narcotic analgesic

Indications: Relief of moderate to severe acute and chronic pain; relief of pain in patients who require opioid analgesics for more than a few days (sustained-release only); management of pain not responsive to nonnarcotic analgesics; dyspnea associated with acute left ventricular failure and pulmonary edema; preoperative sedation; adjunct to anesthesia; analgesia during labor.

Dose: Adults: PO 10 to 30 mg q 4 hr prn. SC/IM 5 to 20 mg/70 kg q 4 hr prn. IV 2.5 to 15 mg/70 kg in 4 to 5 mL Water for Injection over 5 min prn. IV (open-heart surgery) 0.5 to 3 mg/kg. IV (MI pain) 8 to 15 mg; for very severe pain, additional smaller doses may be given q 3 to 4 hr. PR 10 to 20 mg q 4 hr prn. Epidural Initial injection of 5 mg may provide pain relief for up to 24 hr; if pain is not controlled within 1 hr, give incremental doses of 1 to 2 mg. Do not exceed 10 mg/24 hr. Intrathecal Usual dose is 10% of epidural dose. Single injection of 0.2 to 1 mg may provide pain relief for 24 hr. Do not inject more than 2 mL of 5 mg/10 mL ampul or 1 mL of 10 mg/10 mL ampul. Repeat injections not recommended.
Children: SC/IM 0.1 to 0.2 mg/kg q 4 hr.
Max dose: 15 mg.

Trade names: Astramorph PF Injection 0.5 mg/mL
Duramorph Injection 0.5 mg/mL
Infumorph Injection 10 mg/mL
Kadian Capsules, sustained-release 20 mg
MS Contin Tablets, controlled-release 15 mg
MSIR Tablets 15 mg
Oramorph SR Tablets, controlled-release 15 mg
OMS Concentrate Solution 20 mg/mL
RMS Rectal Suppositories 5 mg
Roxanol Solution 20 mg/mL
Roxanol Rescudose Solution 10 mg/2.5 mL
Roxanol 100 Solution 100 mg/5 mL
Roxanol T Solution 20 mg/mL

Roxanol UD Solution 10 mg/ 2.5 mL

Warnings: Hypersensitivity to opiates; upper airway obstruction; acute asthma; diarrhea caused by poisoning or toxins. Injection: Heart failure secondary to chronic lung disease; cardiac arrhythmias; brain tumor; acute alcoholism; delirium tremens; idiosyncrasy to the drug; convulsive states (eg, status epilepticus, tetanus, strychnine poisoning). Immediate-release oral solution: Respiratory insufficiency; severe CNS depression; heart failure secondary to chronic lung disease; cardiac arrhythmias; increased intracranial or cerebrospinal pressure; head injuries; brain tumor; acute alcoholism; delirium tremens; convulsive disorders; after biliary tract surgery; suspected surgical abdomen; surgical anastomosis; idiosyncrasy to the drug; concomitantly with MAO inhibitors or within 14 days of such treatment. Intrathecal/epidural: Infection at injection site; anticoagulation; bleeding condition; parenteral corticosteroids within past 2 wk; any other drug or condition that would contraindicate intrathecal/epidural therapy. Pregnancy Category: [C]

Interactions: Acyclovir, barbiturates, furosemides, heparin, sargramostim, sodium bicarbonate: Precipitation of IV solutions.
Antihistamines, chloral hydrate, glutethimide, methocarbamol: Depressant effects of morphine may be enhanced.
Cimetidine: Monitor for increased respiratory and CNS depression. Concomitant administration of cimetidine and morphine has been reported to precipitate apnea, confusion, and muscle twitching in an isolated report.
Clomipramine, nortriptyline, amitriptyline: Monitor for increased CNS and respiratory depression when administered with morphine.
CNS depressants (eg, alcohol, sedatives, tranquilizers): Additive CNS depression.

Moxifloxacin HCl

Antibiotic / Fluoroquinolone

Indications: Treatment of acute bacterial sinusitis, acute bacterial exacerbation of chronic bronchitis, community-acquired pneumonia, uncomplicated skin and skin structure infections, and conjunctivitis caused by susceptible organisms.

Dose: Acute Bacterial Exacerbation of Chronic Bronchitis:
Adults: IV / PO 400 mg/day for 5 days.
Acute Bacterial Sinusitis:
Adults: IV / PO 400 mg/day for 10 days.
Community-Acquired Pneumonia:
Adults: IV / PO 400 mg/day for 7 to 14 days.
Conjunctivitis:
Adults and children at least 1 yr: Ophthalmic Instill 1 drop in affected eye(s) tid for 7 days.
Uncomplicated Skin and Skin Structure Infections:
Adults: IV / PO 400 mg/day for 7 days.

Trade names: Avelox Tablets 400 mg
Avelox IV Injection (premix) 400 mg
Vigamox Solution, ophthalmic 0.5% (5 mg/mL)

Warnings: Standard considerations. Pregnancy Category: [C]

Interactions: Antacids containing aluminum, calcium, or magnesium; drug formulations containing divalent or trivalent cations (eg, some didanosine formulations);metal cations (eg, iron); multivitamins containing iron or zinc; sucralfate: May decrease the absorption of moxifloxacin.
Cisapride; class IA antiarrhythmic agents (eg, procainamide, quinidine);class III antiarrhythmic agents (eg, amiodarone, sotalol); erythromycin; pentamidine;p henothiazines; tricyclic antidepressants; any other drug known to prolong the QTc interval: Increased risk of torsades de pointes or other ventricular arrhythmias.

Mupirocin

Topical / Anti-infective

Indications: Treatment of impetigo caused by *Staphylococcus aureus* and *Streptococcus pyogenes* (topical ointment); treatment of secondarily infected traumatic skin lesions (up to 10 cm in length or 100 cm^2 in area) caused by susceptible strains of *S. aureus* and *S. pyogenes* (topical cream); eradication of nasal colonization with methicillin-resistant *S. aureus* in adult patients and health care workers (nasal).

Dose: Adults and Children: Topical ointment Apply small amount to affected area tid. Reevaluate lesions not showing a response in 3 to 5 days. Topical cream Apply small amount to affected area tid for 10 days. Reevaluate lesions not showing a response in 3 to 5 days.
Adults and Children 12 yr and older: Nasal Divide approximately one-half of the ointment from a single-use tube between the nostrils and apply morning and evening for 5 days.

Trade names: Bactroban Ointment 2%
Bactroban Nasal Ointment 2%

Warnings: Standard considerations. Pregnancy Category: [B]

Interactions: None well documented.

Mycophenolate Mofetil

Immunosuppressive

Indications: In combination with cyclosporine and corticosteroids for prophylaxis of organ rejection in patients receiving allogenic renal or cardiac transplants.

Dose: Renal Transplantation:
Adults: PO/IV 1 g administered over at least 2 hr bid (daily dose of 2 g).
Cardiac Transplantation:
Adults: PO/IV 1.5 g administered over at least 2 hr bid (daily dose of 3 g).

Trade names: CellCept Capsules 250 mg

Warnings: Hypersensitivity to the drug, mycophenolic acid, or any component of the drug product; persons with a sensitivity to polysorbate 80 (Tween) (IV only). Pregnancy Category: [C]

Interactions: Acyclovir: Possible increased plasma concentrations of both drugs.
Antacids containing magnesium and aluminum hydroxides: Decreased absorption of mycophenolate; do not administer simultaneously.
Azathioprine: Avoid use due to lack of clinical studies.
Cholestyramine: Decreased mycophenolate plasma concentrations; do not give mycophenolate with cholestyramine or other agents that may interfere with enterohepatic recirculation.
Ganciclovir: Possible increased plasma concentrations of both drugs.
Phenytoin: MPA decreased protein binding of phenytoin and may, therefore, increase free phenytoin levels.
Probenecid: May increase plasma concentrations of mycophenolate.
Salicylates: Coadministration increased the free fraction of MPA.
Theophylline: MPA decreased protein binding of theophylline and may, therefore, increase free theophylline levels.

Nadolol

Beta-adrenergic blocker

Indications: Management of hypertension and angina pectoris.

Dose: Hypertension:
Adults: PO Initiate with 40 mg/day; titrate in 40 to 80 mg increments to desired response.
Maintenance: PO 40 to 320 mg/day.
Angina:
Adults: PO Initiate with 40 mg/day; titrate in 40 to 80 mg increments at 3- to 7-day intervals to desired response.
Maintenance: PO 40 to 240 mg/day. Dosage intervals may need to be altered in patients with decreased renal

function.
Trade names: Corgard Tablets 20 mg
Warnings: Hypersensitivity to beta-blockers; greater than first-degree heart block; CHF unless secondary to tachyarrhythmia treatable with beta-blockers or untreated hypotension; overt cardiac failure; sinus bradycardia; cardiogenic shock; bronchial asthma or bronchospasm, including severe COPD. Pregnancy Category: [C]
Interactions: Clonidine: May enhance or reverse antihypertensive effect; potentially life-threatening situations may occur, especially on withdrawal.
Epinephrine: Initial hypertensive episode followed by bradycardia may occur.
Ergot derivatives: Peripheral ischemia, manifested by cold extremities and possible gangrene, may occur.
Insulin: Prolonged hypoglycemia with masking of symptoms may occur.
Lidocaine: Lidocaine levels may increase, leading to toxicity.
NSAIDs: Some agents may impair antihypertensive effect.
Prazosin: Orthostatic hypotension may be increased.
Verapamil: Effects of both drugs may be increased.

Nafarelin Acetate

Gonadotropin-releasing hormone

Indications: Treatment of endometriosis, central precocious puberty in children of both sexes.
Dose: Endometriosis:
Adults: Intranasal 400 mcg/day (200 mcg [1 spray] in 1 nostril in morning and 200 mcg [1 spray] in other nostril in evening. For long-term suppression, 800 mcg/day (1 spray in each nostril bid) may be necessary.
Central Precocious Puberty:
Children: Intranasal 1600 mcg/day (400 mcg [2 sprays] in each nostril in morning and 400 mcg [2 sprays] in each nostril in evening). In some patients 1800 mcg/day (3 sprays in alternating nostrils tid) may be necessary.
Trade names: Synarel Nasal solution 2 mg/mL (as nafarelin base)
Warnings: Hypersensitivity to gonadotropin-releasing hormone (GnRH); or GnRH-agonist analogs; undiagnosed abnormal vaginal bleeding; pregnancy; lactation. Pregnancy Category: [X]
Interactions: None well documented.

Nafcillin Sodium

Penicillinase-resistant penicillin

Indications: Treatment of infections caused by penicillinase-producing staphylococci.
Dose: Adults: IV Usual, 500 mg q 4 hr. Severe infections, 1 g q 4 hr. Infuse over at least 30 to 60 min.
Trade names: Nafcillin Sodium Injection 1 g (as base)
Warnings: Standard considerations. Pregnancy Category: [B]
Interactions: Cyclosporine: May reduce blood levels of cyclosporine.
Disulfiram: May increase nafcillin levels.
Probenecid: May increase nafcillin levels.
Tetracycline: May reduce effectiveness of nafcillin.
Warfarin: May increase warfarin effects.

Naproxen

Analgesic / NSAID

Indications: Rx: Management of mild to moderate pain, symptoms of rheumatoid or osteoarthritis, bursitis, tendonitis, ankylosing spondylitis, primary dysmenorrhea, acute gout. Naproxen (not naproxen sodium) also indicated for treatment of juvenile rheumatoid arthritis. Delayed-release naproxen is not recommended for initial treatment of acute pain because absorption is delayed compared to other naproxen formulations.

OTC: Temporary relief of minor aches and pains associated with the common cold, headache, toothache, muscular aches, backache, minor arthritis pain, pain of menstrual cramps, and reduction of fever.

Unlabeled indication: Sunburn, migraine, PMS.
Dose: Naproxen:
Rheumatoid Arthritis, Osteoarthritis, Ankylosing Spondylitis:
Adults: PO 250 to 500 mg bid; max dose of 1.5 g/day should be used short term only.
Delayed-release: PO 375 to 500 mg bid.
Controlled release: PO 750 to 1000 mg qd.
Individualize dosage. Do not exceed 1500 mg/day.
Suspension: PO 250 mg (10 mL), 375 mg (15 mL), or 500 mg (20 mL) bid.
Pain, Dysmenorrhea, Bursitis, Tendinitis:
Adults: PO 500 mg initially, then 250 mg q 6 to 8 hr. Do not exceed 1250 mg/day.
Juvenile Rheumatoid Arthritis:
Children: PO 10 mg/kg/day in 2 divided doses. For children requiring suspension, 2.5 mL bid can be given for weights of at least 13 kg; 5 mL bid for weights of at least 25 kg, or 7.5 mL bid for weights of at least 38 kg.
Acute Gout:
Adults: PO 750 mg, followed by 250 mg q 8 hr until the attack subsides.
Naproxen Sodium:
Rheumatoid Arthritis, Osteoarthritis, Ankylosing Spondylitis:
Adults: PO 275 to 550 mg bid. May increase to 1.65 g for limited periods.
Acute Gout:
Adults: PO 825 mg initially, then 275 mg q 8 hr prn.
Controlled-release: PO 1000 to 1500 mg once daily on the first day, then 1000 mg once daily until attack has subsided.
Pain, Dysmenorrhea, Tendinitis, Bursitis:
Adults: PO 500 mg initially, then 275 mg q 6 to 8 hr prn. Do not exceed 1375 mg/day.
Controlled release: PO 750 to 1000 mg once daily. Individualize dosage. Do not exceed 1500 mg/day.
Trade names: EC Naprosyn Tablets, delayed-release 375 mg
Naprosyn Tablets 250 mg
Aleve Tablets 200 mg (220 mg naproxen sodium)
Anaprox Tablets 250 mg (275 mg naproxen sodium)
Anaprox DS Tablets 500 mg (550 mg naproxen sodium)
Naprelan Tablets, controlled-release 375 mg (412.5 mg naproxen sodium)
Warnings: Allergy to aspirin, iodides or any NSAID; patients in whom aspirin or other NSAIDs induce symptoms of asthma, rhinitis or nasal polyps. Pregnancy Category: [B]
Interactions: Anticoagulants: May increase effect of anticoagulants because of decreased plasma protein binding. May increase risk of gastric erosion and bleeding.
Lithium: May decrease lithium clearance.
Methotrexate: May increase methotrexate levels.

Naratriptan

Analgesic / Migraine

Indications: Treatment of acute migraine attacks with or without aura.
Dose: Adults: PO 1 or 2.5 mg with onset of migraine headache. Dose is individualized based on response and side effects. The dose may be repeated once after 4 hr if partial response or if the headache returns. The max daily dose is 5 mg in 24 hr.
Trade names: Amerge Tablets 1 mg (as hydrochloride)
Warnings: Patients with history, signs, or symptoms of ischemic heart disease (eg, angina, including Prinzmetal variant, MI, silent myocardial ischemia), cerebrovascular or peripheral vascular

syndromes, uncontrolled hypertension, severe renal or hepatic insufficiency, patients with hemiplegic or basilar migraine, or hypersensitivity to any component of the product. Naratriptan is contraindicated within 24 hr of use with other serotonin agonists, ergotamine compounds, or methysergide. Pregnancy Category: [C]

Interactions: 5-HT-1 agonists (eg, sumatriptan): Increased risk of vasospastic reactions; therefore, coadministration of two 5-HT_1 agonists within 24 hr of each other is contraindicated.
Ergot-containing drugs: May cause additive, prolonged vasospasm.
Selective serotonin reuptake inhibitors (eg, citalopram, fluoxetine, fluvoxamine, paroxetine, sertraline): Weakness, hyperreflexia, and incoordination have been rarely reported.
Sibutramine: Serotonin syndrome, including CNS irritability, motor weakness, shivering, myoclonus, and altered consciousness may occur.

Nateglinide

Antidiabetic

Indications: As monotherapy to lower blood glucose in patients with type 2 diabetes mellitus (noninsulin dependent diabetes mellitus) whose hyperglycemia cannot be adequately controlled by diet and exercise and who have not been chronically treated with other antidiabetic agents; in combination with metformin, but not substituted for metformin, in patients whose hyperglycemia is not adequately controlled with metformin alone.

Dose: Adults: PO 120 mg tid, 1 to 30 min before meals, alone or in combination with metformin. The 60 mg dose of nateglinide may be used, alone or in combination with metformin, in patients near goal glycosylated hemoglobin when treatment is initiated.

Trade names: Starlix Tablets 60 mg

Warnings: Type 1 diabetes; diabetic ketoacidosis. Pregnancy Category: [C]

Interactions: Corticosteroids, sympathomimetics, thiazide diuretics, thyroid products: May reduce the hypoglycemic effects of nateglinide.
MAO inhibitors, nonselective beta-adrenergic blocking agents, NSAIDs, salicylates: May potentiate the hypoglycemic effects of nateglinide.

Nedocromil Sodium

Respiratory inhalant

Indications: Maintenance of mild to moderate bronchial asthma; treatment of itching caused by allergic conjunctivitis.

Dose: Symptomatic adults and children (older than 12 yr): Aerosol inhalation 2 inhalations qid at regular intervals to provide 14 mg/day. May attempt lower frequency of doses in well-controlled patients.

Trade names: Alocril Solution, ophthalmic 2% (20 mg/mL)
Tilade Aerosol 1.75 mg/actuation

Warnings: Standard considerations. Pregnancy Category: [B]

Interactions: None well documented.

Nefazodone HCl

Antidepressant

Indications: Treatment of depression.

Dose: Adults: PO 100 mg bid initially; increase by 100 to 200 mg increments q wk (max, 600 mg/day).
Elderly and Debilitated Patients: PO 50 mg bid initially; increase by 100 mg increments q wk (max, 600 mg/day).

Trade names: Serzone Tablets 50 mg

Warnings: Coadministration with carbamazepine, cisapride, or pimozide; hypersensitivity to nefazodone or other phenylpiperazine antidepressants (eg, trazodone). Pregnancy Category: [C]

Interactions: Benzodiazepines: Increased plasma concentrations and effects of alprazolam and triazolam.
Buspirone: Elevated buspirone concentrations and decreased buspirone metabolite plasma concentrations.
Carbamazepine: Elevated serum carbamazepine concentrations with possible increase in side effects may occur.
Cisapride: Increased cisapride plasma concentrations with cardiotoxicity may occur.
Digoxin: Increased plasma levels of digoxin.
Haloperidol: Decreased haloperidol clearance; may need to adjust haloperidol dose.
HMG-CoA reductase inhibitors (eg, simvastatin): The risk of rhabdomyolysis occurrence may be increased.
MAO inhibitors: Do not use nefazodone concurrently or within 14 days of discontinuing a MAO inhibitors; do not start MAO inhibitors within 1 wk of stopping nefazodone.
Pimozide: Increased plasma concentrations of pimozide may occur associated with QT prolongation and rare cases of serious cardiovascular adverse events, including death, principally caused by ventricular tachycardia of the torsades de pointes type.
Propranolol: Nefazodone may decrease propranolol serum concentration; propranolol may interfere with nefazodone metabolism.
St. John's wort: Increased sedative-hypnotic effects may occur.
Sibutramine, sumatriptan, trazodone: Serotonin syndrome, including irritability, increased muscle tone, shivering, myoclonus, and altered consciousness may occur.

Nelfinavir Mesylate

Antiretroviral / Protease inhibitor

Indications: Treatment of HIV infection in combination with other antiretroviral agents.

Dose: Adults and Children (older than 13 yr): PO 1250 mg bid or 750 mg tid in combination with nucleoside analogs.
Children (2 to 13 yr): PO 20 to 30 mg/kg/dose tid.

Trade names: Viracept Tablets 250 mg

Warnings: Hypersensitivity to nelfinavir or any component of the product. Concomitant therapy with amiodarone, ergot derivatives, quinidine, lovastatin, midazolam, pimozide, simvastatin, and triazolam. Pregnancy Category: [B]

Interactions: Alprazolam, clorazepate, diazepam, estazolam, flurazepam, midazolam, triazolam, zolpidem: Nelfinavir may increase blood levels of these drugs, which may produce extreme sedation and respiratory depression. Do not coadminister.
Amiodarone, cisapride, cyclosporine, lovastatin, pimozide, quinidine, rifabutin, sildenafil, simvastatin, sirolimus, tacrolimus: Nelfinavir may elevate blood levels of these drugs, which may increase the risk of arrhythmias or other potential serious adverse effects.
Carbamazepine, phenobarbital, St. John's wort: May decrease nelfinavir plasma concentrations.
Indinavir: Nelfinavir may increase indinavir blood levels.
Indinavir, ritonavir: May increase nelfinavir plasma concentrations.
Methadone: May decrease methadone concentration.
Oral contraceptives: Concentrations of ethinyl estradiol, a component of oral contraceptives, may be reduced.
Phenytoin: Nelfinavir may decrease blood levels of phenytoin.
Rifabutin: May increase rifabutin concentration and decrease nelfinavir concentration.
Rifampin: May decrease plasma concentrations of nelfinavir.

Neostigmine

Cholinergic muscle stimulant / Anticholinesterase

Indications: Neostigmine bromide (oral) and

methylsulfate (injection): Diagnosis of myasthenia gravis; symptomatic control of myasthenia gravis; antidote for nondepolarizing neuromuscular blocking agents after surgery.

Neostigmine methylsulfate: Prevention and treatment of postoperative distention and urinary retention.

Dose: Diagnosis of Myasthenia gravis:
Adults: IM 0.022 mg/kg.
Children: IM 0.04 mg/kg.
Control of Myasthenia Gravis:
Adults: PO 15 to 375 mg/day; SC/IM 1 mL of 1:2000 solution (0.5 mg); individualize subsequent doses.
Children: IM / IV / SC 0.01 to 0.04 mg/kg dose q 2 to 3 hr prn.
Antidote:
Adults: IV 0.5 to 2 mg by slow infusion repeated as needed, preceded by 0.6 to 1.2 mg of atropine sulfate. May be repeated prn up to total dose of 5 mg.
Children: IV 0.07 to 0.08 mg/kg/dose preceded by 0.008 to 0.025 mg/kg/dose atropine sulfate.
Prevention of Postoperative Urinary Distention and Retention:
Adults: SC / IM 1 mL of 1:4000 solution (0.25 mg) after surgery; repeat q 4 to 6 hr for 2 or 3 days.
Treatment of Postoperative Distention:
Adults: SC / IM 1 mL of 1:2000 solution (0.5 mg), as required.
Treatment of Urinary Retention:
Adults: SC / IM 1 mL of 1:2000 solution (0.5 mg) after bladder is emptied; continue 0.5 mg injection q 3 hr for at least 5 injections.

Trade names: Prostigmin Tablets 15 mg

Warnings: Hypersensitivity to anticholinesterases and bromides; mechanical intestinal or urinary obstruction; peritonitis. Pregnancy Category: [C]

Interactions: Corticosteroids: May antagonize anticholinesterases in myasthenia gravis, producing profound muscular depression.
Succinylcholine: Neuromuscular blockade produced by succinylcholine may be either prolonged or antagonized.

Nevirapine

Antiretroviral / Non-nucleoside reverse transcriptase inhibitor

Indications: In combination with other antiretroviral agents for treatment of HIV-1 infection.

Dose: Adults:
Initial therapy: PO 200 mg daily for 14 days. Total daily dose not to exceed 400 mg.
Maintenance therapy: PO 200 mg bid in combination with other antiretroviral agents.
Children (2 mo to 8 yr of age): PO 4 mg/kg daily for 14 days followed by 7 mg/kg bid. Total daily dose not to exceed 400 mg.
Children (at least 8 yr of age): PO 4 mg/kg daily for 14 days followed by 4 mg/kg bid. Total daily dose not to exceed 400 mg.

Trade names: Viramune Tablets 200 mg

Warnings: Standard considerations. Pregnancy Category: [C]

Interactions: Clarithromycin: Clarithromycin concentrations may be reduced, while concentrations of the active metabolite of clarithromycin may be increased.
Contraceptives, oral: Lower hormone levels and potential contraceptive failure.
Efavirenz, methadone: Concentrations of these agents may be decreased by nevirapine.
Fluconazole: Nevirapine concentrations may be increased.
Ketoconazole: Coadministration resulted in significant reduction in ketoconazole plasma concentrations. Do not coadminister ketoconazole and nevirapine.
Protease inhibitors: Lower protease inhibitor plasma levels.
Rifabutin: Rifabutin concentrations may be increased.
Rifampin, rifabutin: Lower nevirapine plasma levels.
St. John's wort: May reduce nevirapine concentrations, resulting in loss of virologic response and possible resistance to nevirapine and the class of non-nucleoside reverse transcriptase inhibitors.
Warfarin: Plasma concentrations of warfarin may be altered, resulting in potential increases in coagulation time.

Niacin

Vitamin / Antihyperlipidemic

Indications: Prevention and treatment of niacin deficiency or pellagra; treatment of hyperlipidemia (types IV and V); adjunct to diet for the reduction of elevated total and LDL levels in patients with primary hypercholesterolemia when the response to diet and other nonpharmacologic measures alone has been inadequate.

Dose: Pellagra:
Adults: PO Up to 500 mg/day in divided doses.
Adults: Slow IV / SC / IM When oral route is not possible.
Dietary Supplementation:
Adults: PO RDA is 15 to 20 mg/day for adult men and 13 to 15 mg/day for adult women. Increase niacin to 17 to 20 mg/day during pregnancy and lactation.
Children: PO RDA is 5 to 20 mg/day.
Hyperlipidemia:
Adults:
Extended release: PO 500 mg at bedtime for 1 to 4 wk, then 1000 mg at bedtime during wk 5 to 8. If response is inadequate and patient tolerates dose, the dose may be increased by no more than 500 mg in a 4-wk period (max, 2000 mg/day).
Immediate release: PO Initiate therapy at 250 mg with evening meal. The frequency of dose and total daily dose can be increased q 4 to 7 days until a dose of 1.5 to 2 g/day (in divided doses) is reached. If hyperlipidemia is not adequately controlled after 2 mo, increase dosage at 2- to 4-wk intervals to 1 g tid (max, 6 g/day).

Trade names: Slo-Niacin Tablets, controlled-release 250 mg
Niaspan Tablets, extended-release 500 mg

Warnings: Significant liver disease; active peptic ulcer; severe hypotension; arterial hemorrhaging. Pregnancy Category: [A (C if used in doses above RDA)]

Interactions: Adrenergic-blocking agent: May potentiate hypotensive effect.
HMG-CoA reductase inhibitors: Increased risk of myopathy and rhabdomyolysis.

Nicardipine Hydrochloride

Calcium channel blocker

Indications: Treatment of chronic stable (effort-associated) angina (immediate-release capsules); management of hypertension (immediate- and sustained-release capsules; IV when oral therapy not feasible or desirable).

Dose: Angina (Immediate-Release Only):
Adults: PO Usual initial dose 20 mg tid (range, 20 to 40 mg tid).
Hypertension:
Adults:
Immediate-release: PO Usual dose 20 mg tid (range, 20 to 40 mg tid).
Sustained-release: PO Start with 30 mg bid (range, 30 to 60 mg bid). IV Individualize dosage based on severity of hypertension and response of patient during dosing.

Trade names: Cardene Capsules 20 mg
Cardene I.V. Injection 2.5 mg/mL
Cardene SR Capsules, sustained-release 30 mg

Warnings: Sick sinus syndrome; second- or third-degree atrioventricular (AV) block except with functioning pacemaker; advanced aortic stenosis. Pregnancy Category: [C]

Interactions: Cyclosporine: May cause increased cyclosporine levels with possible toxicity.
Other hypertensive agents: May have additive effects.

Nifedipine

Calcium channel blocker

Indications: Treatment of vasospastic (Prinzmetal's or variant) angina, chronic stable angina, hypertension (sustained-release tablets only).

Dose: Capsules:
Adults: PO 10 mg tid (usual dose range, 10 to 20 mg tid); swallow whole. Some patients (eg, coronary artery spasm) respond only to higher doses administered more frequently (eg, 20 to 30 mg tid to qid; max, 180 mg/day). In hospitalized patients, under close observation, dose may be increased in 10 mg increments throughout 4- to 6-hr periods as required to control pain and arrhythmias caused by ischemia. A single dose rarely exceeds 30 mg.
Extended-release tablets:
Adults:
Procardia XL and Nifedical XL: PO 30 or 60 mg once daily, titrated over 7- to 14-day period (max, 120 mg/day).
Adalat CC (hypertension): PO Start with 30 mg/day and titrate dose over 7- to 14-day period (max, 90 mg/day).

Trade names: Adalat Capsules 10 mg
Adalat CC Tablets, extended-release 30 mg
Afeditab CR Tablets, extended-release 30 mg
Nifedical XL Tablets, extended-release 30 mg
Procardia Capsules 10 mg
Procardia XL Tablets, extended-release 30 mg

Warnings: Sick sinus syndrome; second- or third-degree AV block, except with functioning pacemaker. Pregnancy Category: [C]

Interactions: Barbiturates, rifampin: May reduce nifedipine levels, decreasing the therapeutic effect.
Cimetidine: May increase bioavailability of nifedipine.
Cisapride, diltiazem: May elevate nifedipine levels, increasing the risk of side effects.
Fentanyl, parenteral magnesium: Hypotension may occur.
Melatonin: May interfere with the antihypertensive effects of nifedipine.
Tacrolimus: Tacrolimus trough concentrations may be elevated, increasing the risk of toxicity.
Other hypertensive agents: May have additive effects.

Nilutamide

Antiandrogen

Indications: Metastatic prostate cancer in combination with surgical castration.

Dose: Prostate Cancer:
Adults:
Initial dose: PO 300 mg (6 tablets) once daily for 30 days.
Maintenance dose: PO 150 mg (3 tablets) once daily.

Trade names: Nilandron Tablets 50 mg

Warnings: Severe hepatic impairment; severe respiratory insufficiency; hypersensitivity to nilutamide or any component of this preparation. Pregnancy Category: [C]

Interactions: Inhibits hepatic cytochrome P450 enzymes. May alter the elimination of other agents metabolized by the cytochrome P450 system. Monitor patients for increased serum levels and toxicity during concomitant therapy with warfarin, phenytoin, or theophylline.

Nimodipine

Calcium channel blocker

Indications: Improvement of neurologic deficits caused by vasospasm after subarachnoid hemorrhage from ruptured congenital intracranial aneurysms.

Unlabeled indication: Treatment of common and classic migraine and chronic cluster headache.

Dose: Subarachnoid Hemorrhage:
Adults: PO/Nasogastric 60 mg q 4 hr for 21 consecutive days. Initiate therapy within 96 hr of subarachnoid hemorrhage.
Headaches:
Adults: PO 30 mg tid.

Trade names: Nimotop Capsules, liquid 30 mg

Warnings: Standard considerations. Pregnancy Category: [C]

Interactions: Beta-blockers: May cause increased adverse effects because of myocardial contractility or atrioventricular (AV) conduction depression.
Fentanyl: May cause severe hypotension or increased fluid requirements.
Other hypertensive agents: May have additive effects.

Nitroglycerin

Antianginal

Indications: Treatment of acute angina (SL, translingual, IV, transmucosal); prophylaxis of angina (SL, transmucosal, translingual, sustained release, transdermal, topical); control of BP in perioperative or intraoperative hypertension (IV); CHF associated with MI (IV).

Unlabeled indication: Reduce cardiac workload in patients with MI and in refractory CHF (SL, topical, oral, IV); adjunctive treatment of Raynaud disease (topical); treatment of hypertensive crisis (IV).

Dose: Perioperative Hypertension:
Adults: IV 5 mcg/min using nonperipheral vein catheter (PVCP) IV administration set initially; titrate to response.
Angina:
Adults: PO 2.5 or 2.6 mg (sustained-release form) tid to qid initially; titrate to response. SL 0.15 to 0.6 mg dissolved under tongue or in buccal pouch at first sign of acute angina attack; repeat q 5 min (do not exceed 3 tablets in 15 min). Topical 1 to 2 inches q 8 hr up to 4 to 5 inches spread over 3 x 4 inch area and cover with plastic wrap to prevent staining of clothes or application q 4 hr prn. Allow a nitrate-free period of 10 to 12 hr/day. Transdermal 0.2 to 0.4 mg/hr patch initially applied once daily; titrate dose to response. Translingual 1 to 2 sprays onto or under tongue at first onset of attack. Transmucosal 1 mg q 3 to 5 hr during waking hours; tablet placed between lip or cheek and gum.
Refractory Angina, CHF Secondary to Acute MI:
Adults: IV 5 mcg/min initially; titrate according to hemodynamic readings (eg, BP, heart rate, pulmonary capillary wedge pressure).

Trade names: Deponit Transdermal systems 16 mg
Minitran Transdermal systems 9 mg
Nitrek Transdermal systems 22.4 mg
Nitro-Bid Ointment, topical 2% in a lanolin-petrolatum base
Nitro-Bid IV Injection, IV 5 mg/mL
Nitro-Dur Transdermal systems 20 mg
Nitro-Time Capsules, sustained-release 2.5 mg
Nitrodisc Transdermal systems 16 mg
Nitrogard Tablets, buccal, controlled-release (transmucosal) 2 mg
Nitroglyn Capsules, sustained-release 2.5 mg
Nitrol Ointment, topical 2% in a lanolin-petrolatum base
Nitrolingual Aerosol spray, translingual 0.4 mg/metered dose
Nitrong Tablets, sustained-release 2.6 mg
NitroQuick Tablets, sublingual 0.3 mg
Nitrostat Tablets, sublingual 0.3 mg
Transderm-Nitro Transdermal systems 12.5 mg

Warnings: Hypersensitivity to nitrates; severe anemia; closed-angle glaucoma; orthostatic hypotension; early MI; pericarditis or pericardial

tamponade; head trauma or cerebral hemorrhage; allergy to adhesives (transdermal); hypotension or uncorrected hypovolemia (IV); increased intracranial pressure or decreased cerebral perfusion (IV). Pregnancy Category: [C]
Interactions: Alcohol: Severe hypotension and cardiovascular collapse may occur.
Calcium channel blockers: Symptomatic orthostatic hypotension may occur.
Dihydroergotamine: May increase systolic BP and decrease antianginal effects.
Heparin: May decrease anticoagulation effect when used in conjunction with IV nitroglycerin.

Nitroprusside Sodium

Agent for hypertensive emergencies

Indications: Immediate reduction of BP in hypertensive crisis; production of controlled hypotension to reduce bleeding during surgery; for acute congestive heart failure.

Unlabeled indication: Has been used alone or with dopamine in acute MI.
Dose: Give by IV infusion using infusion pump, preferably volmetric pump.
Adults and Children: IV 0.3 mcg/kg/min initially; titrate upward gradually every few minutes to desired effect. Do not exceed 10 mcg/kg/min. Do not use maximum rate for more than 10 min. Average rate of infusion is 3 mcg/kg/min; some patients require much lower doses, especially if other hypotensive agents are used.
Trade names: Nitropress Powder for injection 50 mg/vial
Warnings: Treatment of compensatory hypertension, in which primary hemodynamic lesion is aortic coarctation or arteriovenous shunting; to produce hypotension during surgery in patients with known inadequate cerebral circulation or in moribund patients (A.S.A. Class 5E) coming to emergency surgery; patients with congenital (Leber's) optic atrophy or with tobacco amblyopia; acute CHF associated with reduced peripheral vascular resistance. Pregnancy Category: [C]
Interactions: Antihypertensives, ganglionic blocking agents, volatile anesthetics(eg, enflurane, halothane): Additive hypotensive effects.

Nizatidine

Histamine H_2 antagonist

Indications: Treatment and maintenance of duodenal ulcer, gastroesophageal reflux disease (GERD, including erosive or ulcerative disease) and benign gastric ulcer. Prevention of heartburn, acid indigestion and sour stomach brought on by consuming food and beverages.
Dose: Duodenal Ulcer (Active):
Adults: PO 300 mg at bedtime or 150 mg bid for up to 8 wk.
Maintenance: PO 150 mg at bedtime.
Benign Gastric Ulcer (Acute):
Adults: PO 300 mg at bedtime or 150 mg bid.
GERD:
Adults: PO 150 mg bid.
Moderate to Severe Renal Insufficiency: Dosage adjustment recommended.
Acid Reduction:
Adults: PO 75 mg with water 30 min to 1 hr before consuming food and beverages that may cause symptoms.
Trade names: Axid AR Tablets 75 mg
Axid Pulvules Capsules 150 mg
Warnings: Hypersensitivity to H -2 antagonists. Pregnancy Category: [B]
Interactions: Aspirin: Increased salicylate levels in patients taking very high doses of aspirin (3.9 g/day).
Ketoconazole: Effects of ketoconazole may be reduced.

Norepinephrine

Vasopressor

Indications: Restoration of BP in certain acute hypotensive states; adjunct in treatment of cardiac arrest and profound hypotension.
Dose: Acute Hypotensive States:
Adults: IV 2 to 3 mL/min of 4 mcg base/mL solution (8 to 12 mcg/min); adjust to response. Higher concentration (up to 16 mcg/mL) may be used in fluid-restricted patients. Usual maintenance dose is 2 to 4 mcg/min, but higher doses and prolonged therapy may be needed.
Trade names: Levophed Injection 1 mg (as bitartrate)/mL
Warnings: Hypovolemic states, except temporarily until blood volume replacement is accomplished; mesenteric or peripheral vascular thrombosis, unless essential; generally contraindicated during cyclopropane and halothane anesthesia; profound hypoxia or hypercarbia. Pregnancy Category: [D]
Interactions: Blood or plasma: Chemically incompatible with norepinephrine.
Furazolidone, guanethidine, MAO inhibitors, methyldopa, rauwolfia alkaloids: May increase pressor response, resulting in severe hypertension.
Normal saline: Norepinephrine may lose potency in normal saline solution.
Oxytocic drugs: May cause severe, persistent hypertension.
Phenothiazines (eg, chlorpromazine): May decrease pressor effect.
Tricyclic antidepressants: May increase pressor response.

Norfloxacin

Antibiotic / Fluoroquinolone

Indications: Oral treatment of urinary tract infections (UTIs) caused by susceptible organisms; treatment of STDs caused by Neisseria gonorrhoeae; ocular solution for treatment of superficial ocular infections due to strains of susceptible organisms; prostatitis caused by *E. coli*.
Dose: UTIs:
Adults: PO 400 mg q 12 hr for 3 to 21 days.
STDs:
Adults: PO 800 mg as single dose.
Ocular Infections:
Adults and Children:
Acute infection: Topical 1 to 2 gtt q 15 to 30 min
Moderate infection: Topical 1 to 2 gtt 4 to 6 times/day.
Prostatitis Caused By *E. coli*:
Adults: PO 400 mg q 12 h for 28 days.
Trade names: Chibroxin Solution 3 mg/mL
Noroxin Tablets 400 mg
Warnings: Hypersensitivity to fluoroquinolones, quinolones, or any component; tendonitis or tendon rupture associated with quinolone use. Ophthalmic use: Epithelial herpes simplex keratitis; fungal disease of ocular structure; mycobacterial infections of eye; vaccinia; varicella. Pregnancy Category: [C]
Interactions: Antacids, iron salts, zinc salts, sucralfate, didanosine: May decrease oral absorption of norfloxacin.
Antineoplastic agents: Serum norfloxacin levels may be decreased.
Cyclosporine: Elevated serum cyclosporine levels.
Theophylline: Decreased clearance and increased plasma levels of theophylline may result in toxicity.

Nortriptyline HCl

Tricyclic antidepressant

Indications: Relief of symptoms of depression.

Unlabeled indication: Treatment of panic disorder, premenstrual depression, dermatologic disorders (eg, chronic urticaria, angioedema, nocturnal pruritus in

atopic eczema).
Dose: Adults: PO 25 mg tid to qid. Doses more than 150 mg/day are not recommended.
Elderly and Adolescents: PO 30 to 50 mg/day in divided doses.
Trade names: Aventyl HCl Solution 10 mg base/5 mL
Aventyl HCl Pulvules Capsules 10 mg
Pamelor Capsules 10 mg
Warnings: Hypersensitivity to any tricyclic antidepressant. Generally, not to be given in combination with or within 14 days of treatment with MAO inhibitors or during acute recovery phases of MI. Pregnancy Category: [D Safety not established Limb reduction anomalies have been reported with nortriptyline]
Interactions: Anticoagulants: Dicumaral actions may increase.
Carbamazepine: Carbamazepine levels may increase; nortriptyline levels may decrease.
Cimetidine, fluoxetine: Coadministration may increase nortriptyline blood levels and effects.
CNS depressants: Depressant effects may be additive.
Clonidine: May result in hypertensive crisis.
Guanethidine: Hypotensive action may be inhibited.
MAO Inhibitors: Hyperpyretic crisis, convulsions and death may occur.
Sympathomimetics: Pressor response may decrease.

Octreotide Acetate

Hormone

Indications: Symptomatic treatment of diarrhea associated with carcinoid tumors; treatment of profuse watery diarrhea associated with vasoactive intestinal peptide tumors (VIPoma); to reduce blood levels of growth hormone and IGF-1 in acromegaly patients who have had inadequate response to or cannot be treated with resection, pituitary irradiation and bromocriptine at maximally tolerated doses.

Unlabeled indication: To reduce output from GI fistulas; for variceal bleeding; for relief of diarrhea associated with a variety of conditions; to reduce output from pancreatic fistulas; to treat irritable bowel syndrome; to treat dumping syndrome; to treat the following conditions: Enteric fistula; pancreatitis; pancreatic surgery; glucagonoma; insulinoma; gastrinoma (Zollinger-Ellison syndrome); intestinal obstruction; local radiotherapy; chronic pain management; antineoplastic therapy; decrease insulin requirements in diabetes mellitus; thyrotropin- and TSH-secreting tumors.
Dose: Carcinoid Tumors:
Adults: SC 100 to 600 mcg/day in 2 to 4 divided doses, adjusting to response.
VIPoma:
Adults: SC 200 to 300 mcg/day in 2 to 4 divided doses, adjusting to response.
Acromegaly:
Adults: SC 50 mcg to 500 mcg/tid. Most common dose is 100 mcg/tid; doses more than 300 mcg/day seldom result in additional benefit.
Trade names: Sandostatin Injection 0.05 mg/mL
Sandostatin LAR Depot Injection 10 mg/5 mL
Warnings: Standard considerations. Pregnancy Category: [B]
Interactions: Cyclosporine: May decrease plasma levels of cyclosporine.
Incompatability: Parenteral nutrition solutions.

Ofloxacin

Antibiotic / Fluoroquinolone

Indications: Treatment of acute bacterial exacerbations of chronic bronchitis, community acquired pneumonia, uncomplicated skin and skin structure infections, acute uncomplicated urethral and cervical gonorrhea, nongonococcal urethritis, cervicitis, acute pelvic inflammatory disease, uncomplicated cystitis, complicated UTI, prostatitis caused by Escherichia coli.
Ophthalmic: Treatment of conjunctivitis and corneal ulcer infections caused by susceptible organisms.

Otic: Treatment of otitis externa, chronic suppurative otitis media in patients with perforated tympanic membranes, and acute otitis media in pediatric patients with tympanostomy tubes.
Dose: Acute Otitis Media in Pediatric Patients with Tympanostomy Tubes:
Children 1 to 12 yr: OTIC 5 gtt (0.25 mL, 0.75 mg ofloxacin) instilled into affected ear bid for 10 days.
Acute Pelvic Inflammatory Disease:
Adults: PO/IV 400 mg q 12 hr for 10 to 14 days.
Acute Uncomplicated Urethral and Cervical Gonorrhea:
Adults: PO/IV 400 mg as single dose.
Bacterial Conjunctivitis:
Adults and Children 1 yr or older: Ophthalmic Days 1 and 2 instill 1 to 2 gtt q 2 to 4 hr in affected eye(s). Days 3 through 7 instill 1 to 2 gtt qid.
Bacterial Corneal Ulcer:
Adults and Children 1 yr or older: Ophthalmic Days 1 and 2 instill 1 to 2 gtt into affected eye q 30 min while awake, awaken at approximately 4 to 6 hr after retiring and instill 1 to 2 gtt; days 3 through 7 to 9 instill 1 to 2 gtt q hr while awake; days 7 to 9 instill 1 to 2 gtt qid.
Cervicitis/Urethritis:
Adults: PO/IV 300 mg q 12 hr for 7 days.
Chronic Bronchitis, Community-Acquired Pneumonia, Uncomplicated Skin and Skin Structure Infections:
Adults: PO/IV 400 mg q 12 hr for 10 days.
Chronic Suppurative Otitis Media with Perforated Tympanic Membranes:
Adults and children 12 yr and older: OTIC 10 gtt (0.5 mL, 1.5 mg ofloxacin) instilled into affected ear bid for 10 days.
Complicated UTI:
Adults: PO/IV 200 mg q 12 hr for 10 days.
Epididymitis:
Adults: PO 300 mg bid for 10 days.
Otitis Externa:
Adults and children 12 yr and older: OTIC 10 gtt (0.5 mL, 1.5 mg ofloxacin) instilled into affected ear bid for 10 days.
Children 1 to 12 yr: OTIC 5 gtt (0.25 mL, 0.75 mg ofloxacin) instilled into affected ear bid for 10 days.
Prostatitis:
Adults: PO/IV 300 mg q 12 hr for 6 wk.
Uncomplicated Cystitis Caused by *E. coli* or Klebsiella Pneumoniae:
Adults: PO/IV 200 mg q 12 hr for 3 days.
Uncomplicated Cystitis Caused by Other Pathogens:
Adults: PO/IV 200 mg q 12 hr for 7 days.
Trade names: Floxin Tablets 200 mg
Ocuflox Ophthalmic Solution 3 mg/mL
Warnings: Standard considerations. Ophthalmic: Epithelial herpes simplex keratitis; vaccinia; varicella; fungal disease of ocular structure; mycobacterial infections of the eye. Pregnancy Category: [C]
Interactions: Antacids, didanosine, iron salts, sucralfate, zinc salts: May decrease oral absorption of ofloxacin.
Antineoplastic agents: Serum ofloxacin levels may be decreased.
NSAIDs: Coadministration with ofloxacin may increase risk of CNS stimulation and seizures.
Procainamide: Plasma levels of procainamide may be elevated, increasing the risk of toxicity.
Theophylline: Decreased Cl and increased plasma levels of theophylline may result in toxicity.

Olsalazine Sodium

Intestinal anti-inflammatory / Aminosalicylic acid derivative

Indications: Maintenance of remission of ulcerative colitis in patients intolerant of sulfasalazine.

Dose: Adults: PO 500 mg bid (2 capsules) (total of 1 g/day).
Trade names: Dipentum Capsules 250 mg
Warnings: Hypersensitivity to salicylates or any product component. Pregnancy Category: [C]
Interactions: None well documented.

Omalizumab

Monoclonal antibody

Indications: Treatment of moderate to severe persistent asthma in patients who have a positive skin test or in vitro reactivity to a perennial aero-allergen and whose symptoms are inadequately controlled with inhaled corticosteroids.

Unlabeled indication: Seasonal allergic rhinitis.
Dose: Adults and children 12 yr and older:
SC 150 to 375 mg q 2 or 4 wk. Doses (mg) and dosing frequency are determined by serum total immunoglobulin E (IgE) level (U/mL), measured before the start of treatment, and body weight (kg). Doses greater than 150 mg are divided among more than 1 injection site in order to limit injections to not more than 150 mg/site.
Dosage adjustments: Because total IgE levels are elevated during treatment and remain elevated for up to 1 yr after discontinuation of treatment, retesting of IgE levels during omalizumab treatment cannot be used as a guide for dose determination. Base dose determination after treatment interruptions lasting less than 1 yr on serum IgE levels obtained at the initial dose determination. If treatment is interrupted for 1 yr or more, IgE levels may be retested for dose determination. Adjust doses for significant changes in body weight.
Trade names: Xolair Powder for Injection, lyophilized 202.5 mg (150 mg/1.2 mL after reconstitution)
Warnings: Standard considerations. Pregnancy Category: [B]
Interactions: None well documented.

Omeprazole

GI

Indications: Short-term treatment of active duodenal ulcer, gastroesophageal reflux disease (GERD), including erosive esophagitis and symptomatic GERD; long-term treatment of pathologic hypersecretory conditions (eg, Zollinger-Ellison syndrome, multiple endocrine adenomas, systemic mastocytosis); to maintain healing of erosive esophagitis; in combination with clarithromycin to eradicate *H. pylori*, use clarithromycin and amoxicillin in combination with omeprazole in patients with a 1-yr history of duodenal ulcers or active duodenal ulcers to eradicate *H. pylori*; short-term treatment of active benign gastric ulcer.

Unlabeled indication: Posterior laryngitis; enhanced efficacy of pancreatin for treatment of steatorrhea in cystic fibrosis.
Dose: Active Duodenal Ulcer:
Adults: PO 20 mg/day for 4 to 8 wk.
Erosive Esophagitis:
Adults: PO 20 mg/day for 4 to 8 wk. For maintenance treatment, give 20 mg/day.
Pathologic Hypersecretory Conditions:
Adults: PO For initial dose, give 60 mg/day. Doses up to 120 mg tid have been given. Divide daily doses more then 80 mg.
H. pylori:
Adults (triple therapy): PO 20 mg omeprazole plus clarithromycin 500 mg plus amoxicillin 1000 mg each given bid for 10 days; continue omeprazole 20 mg/day for an additional 18 days if an ulcer is present at start of therapy.
Adults (dual therapy): PO 40 mg omeprazole once daily plus clarithromycin 500 mg tid for 14 days; continue omeprazole 20 mg/day for an additional 14 days if an ulcer is present at start of therapy.
Gastric ulcer:
Adults: PO 40 mg once daily for 4 to 8 wk.
GERD:
Adults (without esophageal lesions): PO 20 mg/day for 4 wk.
Adults (with erosive esophagitis): PO 20 mg/day for 4 to 8 wk.
Trade names: Prilosec Capsules, delayed-release 10 mg
Warnings: Standard considerations. Pregnancy Category: [C]
Interactions: Benzodiazepines: Clearance of benzodiazepines may be decreased.
Cilostazol: Plasma levels may be increased by omeprazole, increasing the therapeutic and adverse effects.
Clarithromycin: Serum concentrations of clarithromycin and omeprazole may be increased.
Drugs depending on gastric pH for bioavailability (eg, ketoconazole, iron salts, ampicillin): Absorption of these drugs may be affected.
Phenytoin: Decreased plasma clearance and increased phenytoin half-life.
Warfarin: Prolonged warfarin elimination.

Ondansetron HCl

Antiemetic / Antivertigo

Indications: Parenteral and oral: Prevention of nausea and vomiting with initial and repeat courses of emetogenic cancer chemotherapy, including high-dose cisplatin; prevention of postoperative nausea or vomiting.

Oral: Prevention of nausea and vomiting associated with radiotherapy in patients receiving either total body irradiation, single high-dose fraction to the abdomen, or daily fractions to the abdomen; prevention of nausea and vomiting associated with highly emetogenic cancer chemotherapy, including cisplatin 50 mg/m^2 or more.

Unlabeled indication: Treatment of nausea and vomiting associated with acetaminophen poisoning or prostacyclin therapy; treatment of acute levodopa-induced psychosis (visual hallucinations); reduction in bulimic episodes due to bulimia nervosa; treatment of spinal or epidural morphine-induced pruritus; management of social anxiety disorder.
Dose: Prevention of Chemotherapy-Induced Nausea and Vomiting:
Adults: IV 0.15 mg/kg infused over 15 min beginning 30 min before emetogenic chemotherapy with 2 additional 0.15 mg/kg doses 4 and 8 hr after the first dose.
Alternatively, infuse 32 mg over 15 min, starting 30 min prior to emetogenic chemotherapy.
Adults and children 12 yr and older: PO (moderately emetogenic cancer chemotherapy) 8 mg bid, administering the first dose 30 min prior to starting emetogenic chemotherapy and the second dose 8 hr after the first dose; subsequent 8 mg doses may be given q 12 hr for 1 to 2 days after completion of chemotherapy.
Children 4 to 11 yr: PO 4 mg tid, starting 30 min prior to chemotherapy, with subsequent doses 4 and 8 hr after the first dose; give 4 mg q 8 hr for 1 to 2 days after completion of chemotherapy.
Prevention of Radiotherapy-Induced Nausea and Vomiting:
Adults: PO 8 mg tid.
Total Body Irradiation:
Adults: PO 8 mg 1 to 2 hr prior to each fraction of radiotherapy administered each day.
Single High-Dose Fraction Radiotherapy to the Abdomen:
Adults: PO 8 mg 1 to 2 hr prior to radiotherapy, with subsequent doses q 8 hr after the first dose for 1 to 2

days after completion of radiotherapy.
Daily Fractionated Radiotherapy to the Abdomen:
Adults: PO 8 mg 1 to 2 hr prior to radiotherapy, with subsequent doses q 8 hr after the first dose for each day radiotherapy is given.
Prevention of Postoperative Nausea and Vomiting:
Adults: IV 4 mg (undiluted) over 30 sec (preferably over 2 to 5 min) or IM 4 mg (undiluted) as a single injection. PO 16 mg as a single dose 1 hr prior to induction of anesthesia.
Children (2 to 12 yr weighing 40 kg or less): IV 0.1 mg/kg
Children (more than 40 kg): IV 4 mg single dose. Administer over 30 sec or longer, preferably over 2 to 5 min.
Prevention of Nausea and Vomiting due to Highly Emetogenic Cancer Chemotherapy:
Adults: PO 24 mg given 30 min prior to start of single-day highly emetogenic chemotherapy, including 50 mg/m^2 or more cisplatin.
Trade names: Zofran Tablets 4 mg (as HCl dihydrate)
Zofran ODT Tablets, orally-disintegrating 4 mg (as base)
Warnings: Standard considerations. Pregnancy Category: [B]
Interactions: Rifamycins (eg, rifampin): Plasma levels of ondansetron may be reduced, decreasing the antiemetic effect.
Incompatability: Alkaline solutions.

Oseltamivir Phosphate

Anti-infective / Antiviral

Indications: Treatment of uncomplicated acute illness caused by influenza infection in patients older than 1 yr who have been symptomatic for 2 days or less; prophylaxis of influenza in patients 13 yr and older.
Dose: Influenza Prophylaxis:
Adults and adolescents 13 yr and older: PO 75 mg qd for 7 days or more, starting within 2 days of exposure.
Renal impairment (Ccr 10 to 30 mL/min): PO 75 mg qod or 30 mg of oral suspension qd.
Treatment of Influenza:
Adults and adolescents 13 yr and older: PO 75 mg bid for 5 days, starting within 2 days of onset of symptoms.
Renal impairment (Ccr 10 to 30 mL/min): PO 75 mg qd for 5 days.
Adults and children 1 yr and older (who cannot swallow capsules): Suspension PO 15 kg or less (33 lbs or less) administer 30 mg (2.5 mL) bid; 16 to 23 kg (34 to 51 lbs) administer 45 mg (3.8 mL) bid; 24 to 40 kg (52 to 88 lbs) administer 60 mg (5 mL) bid; more than 40 kg (more than 88 lbs) administer 75 mg (6.2 mL) bid.
Trade names: Tamiflu Capsules 75 mg
Warnings: Standard considerations. Pregnancy Category: [C]
Interactions: None well documented.

Oxacillin Sodium

Antibiotic / Penicillin

Indications: Treatment of infections caused by penicillinase-producing staphylococci; initial therapy of suspected staphylococcal infection.
Dose: Adults: PO / IV / IM 250 mg to 1 g q 4 to 6 hr.
Children (less than 40 kg): PO / IV / IM 50 to 100 mg/kg/day in divided doses q 4 to 6 hr.
Premature/Neonates: IV / IM 25 mg/kg/day.
Trade names: Oxacillin Sodium Powder for oral solution 250 mg/5 mL
Warnings: Hypersensitivity to penicillins. Do not treat severe pneumonia, empyema, bacteremia, pericarditis, meningitis and purulent or septic arthritis with oral oxacillin during acute state. Pregnancy Category: [B]
Interactions: Contraceptives, oral: Reduced efficacy of oral contraceptives.
Probenecid: Increased oxacillin levels.
Tetracyclines: Impaired bactericidal effects of oxacillin.
Incompatability: Aminoglycosides.

Oxazepam

Antianxiety / Benzodiazepine

Indications: Control of anxiety, anxiety associated with depression; control of anxiety, tension, agitation, and irritability in elderly; treatment of alcoholic patients with acute tremulousness, inebriation, or anxiety associated with alcohol withdrawal.
Dose: Mild to Moderate Anxiety with Associated Tension, Irritability, and Agitation:
Adults: PO 10 to 15 mg tid to qid.
Severe Anxiety Syndromes, Agitation or Anxiety Associated with Depression, Alcoholics with Acute Inebriation and Tremulousness, or Anxiety on Withdrawal:
Adults: PO 15 to 30 mg tid to qid.
Elderly: PO 10 mg tid; increase cautiously up to 15 tid to qid.
Trade names: Serax Tablets 15 mg
Warnings: Hypersensitivity to benzodiazepines; psychoses. Pregnancy Category: [D]
Interactions: Alcohol, CNS depressants: Additive CNS depressant effects.
Digoxin: Increased serum digoxin concentrations.
Theophyllines: May antagonize sedative effects of oxazepam.

Oxcarbazepine

Antiepileptic

Indications: As monotherapy or adjunctive therapy in the treatment of partial seizures in patients with epilepsy.
Dose: Adjunctive Therapy:
Adults: PO Initial dose of 300 mg bid; may be increased by a max of 600 mg/day at weekly intervals; recommended daily dose is 1200 mg/day.
Children 4 to 16 yr: PO Initial dose of 8 to 10 mg/kg generally not to exceed 600 mg/day, given bid; target maintenance dose should be achieved over 2 wk and is dependent upon patient's weight (900 mg/day for 20 to 29 kg; 1200 mg/day for 29.1 to 39 kg; 1800 mg/day for over 39 kg).
Conversion to Monotherapy:
Adults: PO Initial dose of 300 mg bid while simultaneously initiating the reduction of the dose of the concomitant antiepileptic drugs (AEDs). These should be completely withdrawn over 3 to 6 wk while the max dose of the oxcarbazepine should be reached in 2 to 4 wk. Oxcarbazepine may be increased 600 mg/day at weekly intervals; recommended daily dose is 2400 mg/day.
Children 4 to 16 yr: PO Initial dose of 8 to 10 mg/kg/day given in 2 divided doses while simultaneously reducing the dose of concomitant AEDs. The AEDs can be completely withdrawn over 3 to 6 wk while oxcarbazine may be increased by a max increment of 10 mg/kg/day at weekly intervals.
Initiation of Monotherapy:
Adults: PO Initial dose of 300 mg bid; increase dose q 3 days by 300 mg/day to a dose of 1200 mg/day.
Children 4 to 16 yr: PO Initial dose of 8 to 10 mg/kg/day given in 2 divided doses. The dose may be increased by 5 mg/kg/day q 3 days to the maintenance dose based on the following body weights.
- Weight 20 kg: daily dose 600 to 900 mg/day.
- Weight 25 to 30 kg: daily dose 900 to 1200 mg/day.
- Weight 35 to 40 kg: daily dose 900 to 1500 mg/day.
- Weight 45 kg: daily dose 1200 to 1500 mg/day.
- Weight 50 to 55 kg: daily dose 1200 to 1800 mg/day.
- Weight 60 to 65 kg: daily dose 1200 to 2100 mg/day.
- Weight 70 kg; daily dose 1500 to 2100 mg/day.

Renal function impairment: (Ccr less than 30 mL/min): Initiate therapy at 50% of the starting dose; titrate more slowly until the desired response is achieved.

Trade names: Trileptal Tablets 150 mg
Warnings: Standard considerations. Pregnancy Category: [C]
Interactions: May inhibit CYP2C19 and induce CYP3A4/5.
Carbamazepine: May decrease oxcarbazepine's active metabolite (MHD).
Contraceptives, oral: May decrease ethinyl estradiol and levonorgestrel AUC.
Felodipine: May decrease felodipine AUC.
Lamotrigine: Levels may be reduced by oxcarbazine.
Phenobarbital: May decrease MHD and may increase phenobarbital AUC.
Phenytoin: May decrease MHD and may increase phenytoin AUC.
Valproic acid: May decrease oxcarbazepine AUC.
Verapamil: May decrease MHD.

Oxybutynin Chloride

Urinary tract product / Antispasmodic
Indications: Treatment of symptoms of bladder instability associated with voiding in patients with uninhibited and reflex neurogenic bladder (eg, urinary leakage, dysuria). Treatment of overactive bladder with symptoms of urge urinary incontinence, urgency, and frequency (ER tablet).
Dose: Adults (immediate-release tablet or syrup): PO 5 mg bid to tid (max, 5 mg qid).
Children over 5 yr: PO 5 mg bid (max, 5 mg tid).
Adults (ER tablet): PO 5 mg qd adjusted in 5 mg increments at weekly intervals (max, 30 mg/day).
Transdermal system:
Adults: Transdermal 3.9 mg/day applied twice/wk (q 3 or 4 days) to dry, intact skin on abdomen, hip, or buttock, selecting a new application site with each system and avoiding using the same site within 7 days.
Trade names: Ditropan Tablets 5 mg
Ditropan XL Tablets, extended-release 5 mg
Oxytrol Transdermal system 36 mg of oxybutinin delivering 3.9 mg of oxubutinin/day.
Warnings: Untreated angle-closure glaucoma; untreated narrow anterior chamber angles; GI obstruction; paralytic ileus; intestinal atony of elderly or debilitated patients; toxic megacolon complicating ulcerative colitis; severe colitis; obstructive uropathy; myasthenia gravis; unstable cardiovascular status in acute hemorrhage. Pregnancy Category: [B]
Interactions: Anticholinergic drugs (eg, amantadine): Increased risk of anticholinergic side effects.
Beta-blockers (eg, atenolol): Atenolol plasma levels may be elevated, increasing the risk of side effects.
Digoxin: Increased plasma levels of slow-dissolution oral tablets may be increased.
Haloperidol: Worsening of schizophrenic symptoms; tardive dyskinesia; decreased serum haloperidol concentrations, reducing therapeutic effect.
Phenothiazines: Decreased therapeutic effects of phenothiazines; increased incidence of anticholinergic side effects.

Oxytetracycline Hydrochloride/Polymyxin B Sulfate

Ophthalmic Antibiotic
Indications: Treatment of superficial ocular infections involving the conjunctiva and/or cornea caused by susceptible organisms.
Dose: Ophthalmic Approximately 1/2 inch of ointment squeezed from the tube onto the lower lid of the infected eye bid to qid.
Trade names: Terak with Polymyxin B Sulfate Ophthalmic Ointment 10,000 units/g polymyxin B sulfate and 5 mg/g oxytetracycline HCl
Terramycin with Polymyxin B Sulfate Ophthalmic Ointment 10,000 units/g polymyxin B sulfate and 5 mg/g oxytetracycline HCl
Warnings: Standard considerations. Pregnancy Category: []
Interactions: None well documented.

Oxytocin

Oxytocic hormone
Indications: Initiation or improvement of uterine contractions to achieve early vaginal delivery for maternal or fetal reasons (IV); management of inevitable or incomplete abortion (IV); stimulation of uterine contractions during third stage of labor (IV); stimulation reinforcement of labor, as in selected cases of uterine inertia (IV). Control of postpartum bleeding or hemorrhage (IV, IM); initiation of milk let-down (nasal).

Unlabeled indication: Antepartum fetal heart rate testing; relief of breast engorgement.
Dose: Induction or Stimulation of Labor:
Adults: IV 1 to 2 mU/min; adjust by no more than 1 to 2 mU/min at 15 to 30 min intervals until contraction pattern similar to normal labor is obtained.
Control of Postpartum Uterine Bleeding: IV infusion 10 to 40 U in 1000 mL diluent to run as infusion at rate necessary to control uterine atony. IM 10 U (1 mL) after delivery of placenta.
Treatment of Incomplete or Inevitable Abortion: IV infusion 10 to 20 mU/min.
Initial Milk Let-Down: Nasal 1 spray into one or both nostrils 2 to 3 min before nursing or pumping of breasts.
Trade names: Pitocin Injection, parenteral 10 units/mL
Syntocinon Injection, parenteral 10 units/mL
Warnings: Significant cephalopelvic disproportion; inadequate, undeliverable fetal position; obstetric emergencies in which surgical intervention is preferred; cases of fetal distress in which delivery is not imminent; prolonged use in uterine inertia or severe toxemia; hypertonic or hyperactive uterine patterns; when adequate uterine activity fails to achieve satisfactory response; induction or augmentation of labor when vaginal delivery is not indicated (eg, prolapse); pregnancy (nasal product only). Pregnancy Category: [No indication for use in first trimester unless related to spontaneous or induced abortion]
Interactions: Cyclopropane anesthesia:
May cause maternal hypotension, bradycardia and abnormal atrioventricular rhythms.
Parenteral sympathomimetics (eg, methoxamine, dopamine): Increased pressor effect, possibly resulting in postpartum hypertension.
Incompatability: Sodium bicarbonate. Oxytocin is rapidly decomposed in the presence of sodium bisulfite.

Paclitaxel

Mitotic inhibitor
Indications: Advanced ovarian carcinoma, breast cancer, AIDS-related Kaposi's sarcoma, non-small lung cancer.

Unlabeled indication: Squamous cell head and neck cancer, small-cell lung cancer, bladder cancer.
Dose: Usual Dose:
Adults: IV Usual dose ranges from 135 mg/m^2 to 250 mg/m^2 per course of therapy.
Repeat Doses:
Adults: IV After the initial course, hold further courses of therapy until neutrophil count is at least 1500/mm^3 and platelet count is no less than 100,000/mm^3. Reduce dose 20% for subsequent courses in patients who develop severe neutropenia or severe neuropathy. Hold therapy until neutrophil count is at least 1000/mm^3 in AIDS patients.
Ovarian Carcinoma:
Adults: IV infusion For single agents, use 135 to

175 mg/m^2 over 3 hr q 3 wk. When combined with other agents, use 135 mg/m^2 by IV infusion over 24 hr q 3 wk.
Breast Cancer:
Adults: IV infusion 175 mg/m^2 over 3 hr q 3 wk.
Non-Small Cell Lung Cancer:
Adults: IV infusion When combined with other agents, use 135 mg/m^2 over 24 hr q 3 wk.
Kaposi's Sarcoma:
Adults: IV infusion 135 mg/m^2 over 3 hr q 3 wk. As an alternate regiment, use 100 mg/m^2 by IV infusion over 3 hr q 2 wk.
Pretreatment Regimen:
Adults: PO or IV Reduce incidence of hypersensitivity reactions. Premedicate with each of the following:
Corticosteroid: Dexamethasone 20 mg PO or IV 12 and 6 hr before paclitaxel administration. Reduce each dexamethasone dose to 10 mg in AIDS patients. Some clinicians give a third dexamethasone dose immediately prior to paclitaxel.
Diphenhydramine: 50 mg IV 30 to 60 min before paclitaxel.
Histamine H_2 antagonist: Cimetidine 300 mg, ranitidine 50 mg, or famotidine 20 mg IV 30 to 60 min before paclitaxel administration.

Trade names: Taxol Solution for injection 6 mg/mL

Warnings: Hypersensitivity reactions to paclitaxel or other drugs formulated in Cremophor EL (polyoxyethylated castor oil) or polyoxyl 35 castor oil; patients with solid tumors who have baseline neutrophil count of fewer than 1500 cells/mm^3 or in patients with AIDS-related Kaposi's sarcoma with baseline neutrophil counts of less than 1000 cells/mm^3. Pregnancy Category: [D]

Interactions: Cisplatin: Paclitaxel clearance may decrease when given after cisplatin, resulting in increased hematologic toxicity.
CYP450 inducers: May induce the metabolism of paclitaxel.
CYP450 inhibitors: May decrease the metabolism of paclitaxel.
Doxorubicin: Paclitaxel may increase plasma concentrations of doxorubicin and its active metabolite, doxorubicinol.
Ketoconazole: Ketoconazole may inhibit paclitaxel metabolism.

Palivizumab

Monoclonal antibody

Indications: Prevention of serious lower respiratory tract disease caused by RSV in pediatric patients at high risk of RSV disease.

Dose: Pediatrics: IM 15 mg/kg monthly, preferably in anterolateral aspect of thigh. Give doses greater than 1 mL in divided doses.

Trade names: Synagis Powder for injection, lyophilized 50 mg

Warnings: Standard considerations. Pregnancy Category: [C]

Interactions: None well documented.

Pamidronate Disodium

Hormone / Bisphosphonate

Indications: Treatment of moderate to severe hypercalcemia associated with malignancy with or without bone metastases; treatment of Paget disease of bone; treatment of osteolytic bone lesions of multiple myeloma in conjunction with standard antimyeloma chemotherapy.

Unlabeled indication: Treatment of postmenopausal osteoporosis; control of bone metastases from breast cancer; treatment of hyperparathyroidism; prevention of glucocorticoid-induced osteoporosis; management of immobilization-related hypercalcemia.

Dose: Moderate to Severe Hypercalcemia of Malignancy:
Adults: IV For moderate, give 60 to 90 mg as an initial single-dose infusion over 2 to 24 hr. For severe, give 90 mg given as an initial single-dose infusion over 2 to 24 hr. For retreatment, same as initial therapy, on or after 7 days.
Osteolytic Bone Metastases of Breast Cancer:
Adults: IV 90 mg as a 2-hr infusion q 3 to 4 wk.
Osteolytic Bone Lesions of Multiple Myeloma:
Adults: IV 90 mg as a 4-hr infusion on a monthly basis.
Paget Disease:
Adults: IV 30 mg/day as a 4-hr infusion on 3 consecutive days for a total dose of 90 mg. For retreatment, same as initial therapy, when clinically indicated.

Trade names: Aredia Powder for injection, lyophilized 30 mg

Warnings: Hypersensitivity to bisphosphonates. Pregnancy Category: [D]

Interactions: None well documented.
Incompatability: Calcium-containing infusion solutions (eg, Ringer's solution). Do not mix.

Pancuronium Bromide

Nondepolarizing neuromuscular blocker

Indications: Adjunct to general anesthesia for induction of skeletal muscle relaxation; facilitation of management of patients undergoing mechanical ventilation; facilitation of tracheal intubation.

Dose: Surgical Procedures:
Adults and Children greater than 1 mo: IV 0.04 to 0.1 mg/kg initially. For maintenance therapy, use incremental doses q 25 to 60 min beginning with 0.01 mg/kg.
Newborns (less than 1 mo): IV For test dose, use 0.02 mg/kg.
Endotracheal Intubation:
Adults and Children: IV 0.06 to 0.1 mg/kg.
Newborns: IV For test dose, use 0.02 mg/kg.

Trade names: Pavulon Injection 1 mg/mL
Warnings: Hypersensitivity to bromides. Pregnancy Category: [C do not use in early pregnancy]

Interactions: Aminoglycosides, bacitracin, clindamycin, colymycin, polymyxin B, inhalational anesthetics, ketamine, lincomycin, magnesium salts, quinidine, quinine, succinylcholine, vancomycin: May augment action of pancuronium.
Azathioprine, mercaptopurine: May cause reversal of neuromuscular blocking effects of pancuronium.
Carbamazepine, hydantoins: May decrease duration and effect of pancuronium.
Theophyllines: May cause possible resistance to, or reversal of, effects of pancuronium; cardiac arrhythmias may occur.
Trimethaphan: May cause prolonged apnea.

Pantoprazole Sodium

GI

Indications: Oral: Short-term (no more than 8 wk) treatment in the healing and symptomatic relief of erosive esophagitis associated with gastroesophageal reflux disease (GERD); long-term treatment of pathological hypersecretory conditions, including Zollinger-Ellison syndrome; maintenance of healing of erosive esophagitis.

IV: Short-term (7- to 10-day) treatment of GERD, as an alternative to oral therapy in patients unable to continue oral pantoprazole; hypersecretory conditions associated with Zollinger-Ellison syndrome or other neoplastic conditions.

Dose: Maintenance of Healing of Erosive Esophagitis:
Adults: PO 40 mg/day.
Treatment of Erosive Esophagitis:
Adults: PO 40 mg/day for up to 8 wk; an additional 8-wk course of treatment may be considered in patients

who have not healed after 8 wk.
Adults: IV 40 mg/day for 7 to 10 days.
Pathological Hypersecretion Associated with Zollinger-Ellison Syndrome:
Adults: IV 80 mg q 12 hr; based upon individual patient needs, the dose may be increased to 80 mg q 8 hr.
Trade names: Protonix Tablets, delayed-release 40 mg
Protonix IV Powder for Injection 40 mg/vial
Warnings: Standard considerations. Pregnancy Category: [B]
Interactions: None well documented.

Paromomycin Sulfate

Anti-infective / Amebicide / Aminoglycoside

Indications: Treatment of acute and chronic intestinal amebiasis. Adjunctive therapy in management of hepatic coma.

Unlabeled indication: Treatment of other parasitic infections.

Dose: Intestinal Amebiasis:
Adults and Children: PO 25 to 35 mg/kg/day in 3 divided doses with meals for 5 to 10 days.
Hepatic Coma:
Adults: PO 4 g/day in divided doses at regular intervals for 5 to 6 days.
Trade names: Humatin Capsules 250 mg
Warnings: Intestinal obstruction; extraintestinal amebiasis; hypersensitivity to aminoglycosides. Pregnancy Category: [D]
Interactions: Digoxin: May reduce rate and extent of digoxin absorption; this may be offset by decreased digoxin metabolism.
Methotrexate: Decreased absorption of methotrexate.
Neuromuscular blockers: Increased action of both depolarizing and nondepolarizing neuromuscular blocking agents, may prolong need for respiratory support.
Neurotoxic, nephrotoxic, or ototoxic medications (eg, polypeptide antibiotics): Additive adverse effects may occur with concurrent or sequential administration of medications with similar toxic profiles.

Paroxetine HCl

Antidepressant

Indications: Panic disorder or social anxiety disorder, as defined in the DMS-IV; major depressive disorder, as defined in DMS-III (immediate release) or DMS-IV (controlled release).
Immediate release only: Obsessive-compulsive disorder (OCD); generalized anxiety disorder; posttraumatic stress disorder (PTSD), as defined in the DSM-IV.

Controlled release only: Premenstrual dysphoric disorder (PMDD), as defined in the DSM-IV.

Dose: Depression:
Adults: PO
Immediate release: 20 mg/day initially; may increase by 10 mg/day at intervals of at least 7 days (max, 50 mg/day). Administer as single daily dose, usually in morning.
Controlled release: 25 mg/day as a single dose, usually in the morning (usual dose range, 25 to 62.5 mg/day). The dose may be increased in increments of 12.5 mg/day at intervals of at least 1 wk (max, 62.5 mg/day).
Elderly, Debilitated, or Patients with Severe Renal or Hepatic Impairment: PO
Immediate release: 10 mg/day initially; do not exceed 40 mg/day.
Controlled release: 12.5 mg/day initially; do not exceed 50 mg/day.
Generalized Anxiety Disorder/Posttraumatic Stress Disorder:
Adults: PO
Immediate release: 20 mg/day administered as a single dose with or without food, usually in the morning. May increase dose by 10 mg/day at intervals of 1 wk. Usual range, 20 to 50 mg/day.
Controlled release: 12.5 mg/day initially; do not exceed 50 mg/day.
Elderly, Debilitated, or Patients with Severe Renal or Hepatic Impairment: PO 10 mg/day initially; increases may be made if indicated (max, 40 mg/day).
OCD:
Adults: PO
Immediate release: 20 mg/day initially; recommended dose is 40 mg/day. May increase dose by 10 mg/day at intervals of at least 7 days (max, 60 mg/day). Administer as single daily dose, usually in morning.
Panic Disorder:
Adults: PO
Immediate release: 10 mg/day initially; recommended dose is 40 mg/day. May increase dose by 10 mg/day at intervals of at least 7 days (max, 60 mg/day). Administer as single daily dose, usually in morning.
Controlled release: 12.5 mg/day as a single dose, usually in the morning. The dose may be increased in increments of 12.5 mg/day at intervals of at least 1 wk (max, 75 mg/day).
Elderly, debilitated, or patients with severe renal or hepatic impairment: PO
Controlled release: 12.5 mg/day initially; do not exceed 50 mg/day.
PMDD:
Adults: PO
Controlled release: 12.5 mg/day initially, usually in the morning; change doses at intervals of at least 1 wk; usual range is 12.5 to 25 mg/day.
PTSD:
Adults: PO
Immediate release: 20 mg/day initially, usually in the morning; change doses in increments of 10 mg/day and at intervals of at least 1 wk. Usual range, 20 to 50 mg/day.
Social Anxiety Disorder:
Adults: PO
Immediate release: 20 mg/day administered as a single daily dose with or without food, usually in the morning. Usual range is 20 to 60 mg/day.
Controlled release: 12.5 mg initially, usually in the morning. Usual range is 12.5 to 37.5 mg/day. The dose may be increased in increments of 12.5 mg/day at intervals of at least 1 wk (max, 37.5 mg/day).
Elderly, Debilitated, or Patients with Severe Renal or Hepatic Impairment: PO 10 mg/day initially; increase if indicated (max, 40 mg/day).
Trade names: Paxil Tablets 10 mg
Paxil CR Tablets, controlled-release 12.5 mg
Warnings: Standard considerations. Concomitant use in patients taking MAO inhibitors or thioridazine. Pregnancy Category: [C]
Interactions: 5-HT-1 agonists (eg, naratriptan, sumatriptan, zolmitriptan): Weakness, hyperreflexia, and incoordination reported rarely.
Alcohol: Causes additive CNS effects; concurrent use is not recommended.
Cimetidine: May increase paroxetine concentrations.
Cyclosporine: Concentrations of cyclosporine may be elevated, increasing the risk of toxicity.
Cyproheptadine: Pharmacologic effects of paroxetine may be decreased or reversed.
CYP2D6 system: Approach coadministration with other drugs metabolized by cytochrome P450 2D6 (eg, certain antidepressants, phenothiazines, type IC antiarrhythmics) or drugs that inhibit this enzyme (eg, quinidine) with caution.
Digoxin: May decrease digoxin levels.
MAO inhibitors: Can cause serious, sometimes fatal reactions. Do not use concomitantly or within 14 days of each other.
Phenobarbital, phenytoin: May decrease paroxetine concentration; may reduce phenytoin concentration.
Procyclidine: Reduction of procyclidine dose may be

necessary if anticholinergic effects (dry mouth, blurred vision, urinary retention) occur.
Sibutramine: The risk of occurrence of serotonin syndrome may be increased.
St. John's wort: Sedative-hypnotic effects may be increased.
Sympathomimetics (eg, amphetamine): Sensitivity of sympathomimetics and risk of serotonin syndrome may be increased.
Theophylline: Elevated theophylline levels have occurred with paroxetine. Monitor theophylline levels when coadministered.
Thioridazine: May increase thioridazine levels leading to an increased risk of QTc prolongation, ventricular arrhythmias, and death.
Tryptophan: May cause headache, nausea, sweating, and dizziness.
Warfarin: Increased risk of bleeding.
Zolpidem: The effect of zolpidem may be increased.

Pemoline

Psychotherapeutic

Indications: Treatment of attention-deficit hyperactivity disorder (ADHD).

Unlabeled indication: Treatment of narcolepsy and excessive daytime sedation.

Dose: Adults and Children 6 yr and older: PO 37.5 mg/day as a single dose in the morning initially; increase by increments of 18.75 mg weekly until desired response is obtained (max daily dose, 112.5 mg/day).

Trade names: Cylert Tablets 18.75 mg

Warnings: Hepatic insufficiency. Pregnancy Category: [B]

Interactions: None well documented.

Penciclovir

Topical anti-infective / Antiviral

Indications: Treatment of recurrent herpes labialis (cold sores) in adults.

Dose: Adults: Topical Apply to lesions q 2 hr while awake for 4 days. Start treatment as early as possible, during the prodrome or when lesions first appear.

Trade names: Denavir Cream 10 mg/g

Warnings: Standard considerations. Pregnancy Category: [B]

Interactions: None well documented.

Penicillamine

Cystine-depleting agents

Indications: Treatment of Wilson disease; cystinuria; and severe, active rheumatoid arthritis.

Dose: Cystinuria:
Adults: PO Initially, 250 mg/day, and increasing gradually to the requisite amount. Range 1 to 4 g/day. Daily dose should be divided into 4 doses.
Children: PO 30 mg/kg/day divided into 4 doses. If 4 equal doses are not feasible, give the larger portion at bedtime.
Rheumatoid Arthritis:
Adults: PO Start with a single daily dose of 125 to 250 mg/day. The dose may be increased at 1- to 3-mo intervals by 125 to 250 mg/day, as patient response and tolerance indicate. Continue dosage associated with satisfactory remission. If there is no improvement or no signs of potentially serious toxicity after 2 to 3 mo of treatment with 500 to 750 mg/day, increases of 250 mg/day at 2- to 3-mo intervals may be continued until satisfactory remission or signs of toxicity develop. If there is no discernible improvement after 3 or 4 mo of treatment with 1000 to 1500 mg/day, penicillamine should be discontinued.
Maintenance therapy: Many patients respond satisfactorily to dosage within the 500 to 750 mg/day range.
Duration: If a patient has been in remission for 6 mo or more, a gradual, stepwise dosage reduction in decrements of 125 or 250 mg at about 3-mo intervals may be attempted.
Wilson Disease:
Adults: PO 0.25 mg to 2 g/day. Optimal dosage can be determined by measurement of urinary copper excretion and determination of free copper in the serum.

Trade names: Cuprimine Capsules 125 mg
Depen Tablets, titratable 250 mg

Warnings: Pregnancy (except in treatment of Wilson disease or certain cases of cystinuria); penicillamine-related aplastic anemia or agranulocytosis; rheumatoid arthritis patients with a history of renal insufficiency; breastfeeding. Pregnancy Category: [X: Contraindicated in pregnancy]

Interactions: Aluminum salts (eg, aluminum carbonate, sucralfate): GI absorption of penicillamine may be reduced.

Penicillin G Benzathine/ Penicillin G Procaine

Antibiotic / Penicillin

Indications: Treatment of moderately severe infections caused by penicillin-G susceptible microorganisms that are susceptible to serum levels common to this particular dosage form; moderately severe to severe infections of the upper respiratory tract, scarlet fever, erysipelas, and skin and soft-tissue infections caused by susceptible streptococci; moderately severe pneumonia and otitis media caused by susceptible organisms. Severe pneumonia, empyema, bacteremia, pericarditis, meningitis, peritonitis, and arthritis of pneumococcal etiology are better treated with penicillin G sodium or potassium during the acute stage. When high, sustained serum levels are required, penicillin G sodium or potassium, either IM or IV, should be used. This drug should not be used in the treatment of venereal diseases, including syphilis, gonorrhea, yaws, bejel, and pinta.

Dose: Streptococcal Infections Group A (upper-respiratory tract, skin and soft-tissue infections, scarlet fever, and erysipelas):
Adults and Children over 60 lbs: IM 2,400,000 units.
Children 30 to 60 lbs: IM 900,000 to 1,200,000 units.
Children under 30 lbs: IM 600,000 units.
Pneumococcal Infections (except pneumococcal meningitis):
Adults: IM 1,200,000 units repeated q 2 or 3 days until temperature is normal for 48 hr.
Children: IM 600,000 units repeated q 2 or 3 days until temperature is normal for 48 hr.

Trade names: Bicillin C-R Injection 600,000 units/dose (300,000 units each penicillin G benzathine and penicillin G procaine)
Bicillin C-R 900/300 Injection 1,200,000 units/dose (900,000 units penicillin G benzathine and 300,000 units penicillin G procaine)

Warnings: Hypersensitivity to any penicillin or to procaine. Pregnancy Category: [B]

Interactions: Probenecid: Increases and prolongs serum penicillin levels.
Tetracycline: May antagonize the bactericidal effect of penicillin.

Penicillin V

Antibiotic / Penicillin

Indications: Treatment of upper respiratory tract infections; treatment of pneumococcal, streptococci, and staphylococcal infections and fusospirochetosis (Vincent's infection) of oropharynx caused by susceptible microorganisms.

Unlabeled indication: Prophylactic treatment of sickle cell anemia in children; treatment of anaerobic infections; treatment of Lyme disease (Borrelia

Medications

burgdorferi).
Dose: Adults and children over 12 yr: PO 125 to 500 mg qid.
Trade names: Beepen-VK Tablets 250 mg
Pen-Vee K Tablets 250 mg
Penicillin VK Tablets 250 mg
Veetids Tablets 250 mg
Veetids '250' Powder for oral solution 250 mg/5 mL
Warnings: Hypersensitivity to penicillins. Do not treat severe pneumonia, empyema, bacteremia, pericarditis, meningitis, and purulent or septic arthritis with oral penicillin V during acute stage. Pregnancy Category: [B]
Interactions: Beta-blockers: May potentiate anaphylactic reactions of penicillin.
Contraceptives, oral: May reduce efficacy of oral contraceptives.
Erythromycin: May cause synergism or antagonism to develop.
Tetracyclines: May impair bactericidal effects of penicillin V.

Pentamidine Isethionate

Anti-infective / Antiprotozoal

Indications: Parenteral form: Treatment of Pneumocystis carinii pneumonia (PCP).

Inhalation: Prevention of PCP in high risk HIV-infected patients.

Unlabeled indication: Treatment of trypanosomiasis and visceral leishmaniasis.

Dose: Adults and Children: IM / IV 4 mg/kg qd for 14 days.
Adults: Inhalation 300 mg once q 4 wk administered via Respirgard II nebulizer.
Trade names: NebuPent Aerosol 300 mg
Pentacarinat Injection 300 mg
Pentam 300 Injection 300 mg
Warnings: Parenteral form: Once diagnosis of PCP is made, there are no absolute contraindications.
Inhalation: History of anaphylactic reaction to pentamidine. Pregnancy Category: [C]
Interactions: Incompatability: Do not reconstitute with saline solutions. Do not mix with other drugs.

Pentazocine

Narcotic agonist-antagonist analgesic

Indications: Oral and parenteral forms: Management of moderate to severe pain.

Parenteral form: Preoperative or preanesthetic medication; supplement to surgical anesthesia.

Dose: Labor:
Adults: IM 30 mg as single dose; alternatively, when contractions are regular, IV 20 mg for 2 to 3 doses given q 2 to 3 hr.
Pentazocine:
Moderate to Severe Pain:
Adults: IM / SC / IV 30 mg q 3 to 4 hr prn (max, 360 mg/day). Doses greater than 30 mg IV or 60 mg SC / IM are not recommended.
Adults: PO 50 mg q 3 to 4 hr; increase to 100 mg if necessary (max, 600 mg/day).
Pentazocine 12.5 mg With Aspirin 325 mg (Talwin Compound):
Moderate to Severe Pain:
Adults: PO 2 tablets tid to qid.
Pentazocine 25 mg With Acetaminophen 650 mg (Talacen):
Moderate to Severe Pain:
Adults: PO 1 tablet q 4 hr (max, 6 tablets/day).
Trade names: Talacen Tablets 25 mg pentazocine (as HCl)/650 mg acetaminophen
Talwin Injection 30 mg/mL (as lactate)
Talwin Compound Tablets 12.5 mg pentazocine (as HCl)/325 mg aspirin
Talwin NX Tablets 50 mg pentazocine (as HCl)/0.5 naloxone
Warnings: Hypersensitivity to naloxone (in Talwin NX) or sulfites. Pregnancy Category: [C Neonatal abstinence syndrome may develop]
Interactions: Alcohol: Causes additive CNS depression.
Barbiturate anesthetics and any other CNS depressants (eg, benzodiazepines, antidepressants): Causes increased CNS and respiratory depression.
Incompatability:
Barbiturates: Do not mix in the same syringe with pentazocine; precipitation will occur.

Pentobarbital Sodium

Sedative and hypnotic / Barbiturate, Short-acting / Anticonvulsant

Indications: Sedation; short-term treatment of insomnia; preanesthesia; emergency control of convulsions (parenteral form).
Dose: Insomnia:
Adults: PO / IV 100 mg (max IV rate, 50 mg/min). IM / PR 120 to 200 mg (max IM dose, 500 mg or 5 mL volume regardless of concentration).
Sedation:
Adults: PO / PR 20 to 30 mg bid to qid.
Children: PO / IM 2 to 6 mg/kg (max, 100 mg). IV 50 mg.
Convulsions:
Adults: IV Use minimum dose to avoid compounding depression. Administer slowly to allow time for drug to penetrate the blood-brain barrier. Do not exceed 50 mg/min.
Pediatric Patients Unable to Take Orally or by Injection:
Children 12 to 14 yr (36.4 to 50 Kg): PR 60 or 120 mg.
Children 5 to 12 yr (18.2 to 36.4 kg): PR 60 mg.
Children 1 to 4 yr (9 to 18.2 Kg): PR 30 or 60 mg.
Children 2 mo to 1 yr (4.5 to 9 kg): PR 30 mg.
Trade names: Nembutal Sodium Capsules 50 mg
Warnings: Hypersensitivity to barbiturates; manifest or latent porphyria. Pregnancy Category: [D]
Interactions: Alcohol, CNS depressants: May produce additive depressant effects.
Anticoagulants, beta-blockers, calcium-channel blockers (eg, nifedipine, verapamil), theophylline: Activity of these drugs may be reduced.
Anticonvulsants: Serum concentrations of carbamazepine, valproic acid and succinimides may be reduced. Valproic acid may increase barbiturate serum levels.
Corticosteroids: Effectiveness may be reduced.
Estrogen, estrogen-containing oral contraceptives: May cause decreased contraceptive and estrogen effect.
Griseofulvin: Decreased griseofulvin levels.

Pentosan Polysulfate Sodium

Urinary Analgesic

Indications: For relief of bladder pain or discomfort associated with interstitial cystitis.
Dose: Adults: PO 100 mg tid.
Trade names: Elmiron Capsules 100 mg
Warnings: Standard considerations. Pregnancy Category: [B]
Interactions: Anticoagulants, antiplatelet agents, thrombolytics: Pentosan has weak anticoagulant properties and may potentiate the pharmacological action of other anticoagulants, antiplatelet, or thrombolytic drugs.

Pentoxifylline

Hemorheologic

Indications: Intermittent claudication on basis of chronic occlusive arterial disease of limbs.

Unlabeled indication: Treatment of psychopathological symptoms in patients with cerebrovascular insufficiency; treatment of diabetic angiopathies; reduction of incidence of stroke in patients with recurrent TIAs.

Dose: Adults: PO 400 mg tid with meals for greater than or equal to 8 wk. If GI and CNS side effects occur, decrease to 400 mg bid. If side effects persist, discontinue.

Trade names: Trental Tablets, controlled-release 400 mg

Warnings: Intolerance to methylxanthines (ie, caffeine, theophylline); recent cerebral or retinal hemorrhage. Pregnancy Category: [C]

Interactions: Antihypertensives: Small decreases in blood pressure possible with patients receiving pentoxifylline while using antihypertensive drugs. Monitor blood pressure. If indicated, reduce dosage of the antihypertensive.
Cimetidine: Effects of pentoxifylline may be increased.
Theophylline: Concomitant administration with pentoxifylline leads to increased theophylline levels and possible toxicity in some patients. Monitor and adjust closely.
Warfarin: Bleeding and prolonged prothrombin time possible in patients.

Pergolide Mesylate

Antiparkinson

Indications: Adjunctive treatment to levodopa-carbidopa in management of Parkinson disease.

Dose: Administer in divided doses tid.
Adults: PO 0.05 mg/day first 2 days. Gradually increase dose by 0.1 to 0.15 mg/day q 3 days over next 12 days. Dose may then be increased by 0.25 mg/day q 3 days until optimum therapeutic dosage is achieved (mean therapeutic dose is 3 mg/day; max, 5 mg/day). During titration cautiously decrease levodopa-carbidopa (average daily concurrent dose is 650 mg/day of levodopa).

Trade names: Permax Tablets 0.05 mg

Warnings: Hypersensitivity to ergot derivatives or any component of the product. Pregnancy Category: [B]

Interactions: Dopamine antagonists (eg, butyrophenones, metoclopramide, neuroleptics, phenothiazines, thioxanthenes): May diminish effectiveness of pergolide.

Permethrin

Scabicides / Pediculicides

Indications: Cream: Treatment of scabies (Sarcoptes scabiei) infestation.

Lotion/Cream rinse: Treatment of infestation with head lice (Pediculus humanus capitis) and its nits (eggs).

Liquid: Treatment of infestation with Pediculus humanus var. capitis (head louse) and its nits (eggs).

Dose: Scabies: Cream Massage 30 g into the skin from head to soles of feet. Massage into hairline, neck, temple, and forehead of infants and geriatric patients. Remove cream by shower or bath after 8 to 14 hr. One application is generally curative.
Head Lice: Lotion/Cream rinse Apply to hair after washing with shampoo; rinse with water and towel dry. Apply a sufficient amount to saturate hair and scalp, especially behind the ears and nape of neck. Leave on hair for no longer than 10 min, then rinse with water. If lice are observed within 7 days after application, apply a second treatment. Remove remaining nits with nit comb provided.

Trade names: Acticin Cream 5%
Elimite Cream 5%
Permethrin Lotion 1%
Nix Cream Rinse Liquid 1%

Warnings: Standard considerations. Pregnancy Category: [B]

Interactions: None well documented.

Phenelzine Sulfate

Antidepressant / MAO inhibitor

Indications: Treatment of 'atypical' ('nonendogenous' or 'neurotic') depression; management of depression in patients unresponsive to other antidepressant drugs.

Unlabeled indication: Treatment of bulimia; treatment of cocaine addiction; control of panic disorder with agoraphobia.

Dose: Adults: PO 15 mg tid initially; may titrate up to 90 mg/day. Elderly should receive no more than 60 mg/day. After max benefit is achieved, dose can be slowly decreased over several weeks to maintenance dose. Doses as low as 15 mg qod may be used for maintenance.

Trade names: Nardil Tablets 15 mg (as sulfate)

Warnings: Hypersensitivity to MAO inhibitors; pheochromocytoma; CHF; abnormal liver function; history of liver disease; severe renal impairment; cerebrovascular defect; concurrent use of dextromethorphan or CNS depressants (eg, alcohol); sympathomimetic drugs (eg, amphetamine, dopamine, norepinephrine) or related drugs (eg, methyldopa); cardiovascular disease. Pregnancy Category: [C]

Interactions: Amine-containing foods: May cause severe hypertension or hemorrhagic strokes.
Anorexiants: May cause exaggerated pharmacologic effects (eg, severe headaches, hypertension, hyperpyrexia) of anorexiants (amphetamines and related compounds).
CNS depressants: May enhance CNS effects.
Dextromethorphan: Concurrent use has been associated with severe reactions (eg, hyperpyrexia, hypotension, death).
Fluoxetine, paroxetine, sertraline, trazodone: Although data are limited, interactions comparable to those of the tricycle antidepressants and phenelzine may occur.
Guanethidine: MAO inhibitors may antagonize the antihypertensive effect.
Insulin, sulfonylureas: May enhance hypoglycemic action.
Levodopa: May cause hypertensive reactions.
Meperidine: May lead to severe reactions, including hypotension, convulsions, respiratory depression, and vascular collapse.
Sympathomimetics: May cause severe headache, hypertensive crisis, and hyperpyrexia.
Tricyclic antidepressants, buspirone, cyclobenzaprine, carbamazepine, maprotiline, guanethidine, CNS stimulants, tyramine: May lead to potentially fatal reactions, including seizures and hypertensive crisis; mental status changes, hyperthermia.

Phenoxybenzamine HCl

Antihypertensive / Agent for pheochromocytoma

Indications: Control of episodes of hypertension and sweating in patients with pheochromocytoma.

Unlabeled indication: Treatment of micturition disorders resulting from neurogenic bladder; treatment of functional outlet obstruction and partial prostatic obstruction.

Dose: Adults: PO 10 mg bid initially. Usual dosage range is 20 to 40 mg bid to tid.
Children: PO 1 to 2 mg/kg/day in 3 to 4 divided doses.

Trade names: Dibenzyline Capsules 10 mg

Warnings: Conditions in which fall in BP may be undesirable. Pregnancy Category: [Safety not established]

Interactions: Epinephrine: Exaggerated

hypotensive response and tachycardia may occur when epinephrine, or other agents that stimulate both alpha- and beta-receptors, are given concomitantly with phenoxybenzamine.

Phentolamine

Antihypertensive / Agent for pheochromocytoma

Indications: Prevention or control of hypertensive episodes in patients with pheochromocytoma; pharmacologic test for pheochromocytoma (not method of choice); prevention and treatment of dermal necrosis and sloughing following IV administration or extravasation of norepinephrine or dopamine.

Unlabeled indication: Control of hypertensive crises secondary to MAO inhibitor-sympathomimetic amine interactions or withdrawal of clonidine, propranolol or other antihypertensives; in conjunction with papaverine as intracavernous injection for impotence.

Dose: Hypertensive Episodes in Pheochromocytoma:
Adults: IM / IV 5 mg 1 to 2 hr before surgery. Repeat if necessary. During surgery, IV 5 mg as indicated.
Children: IM / IV 1 mg 1 to 2 hr before surgery. During surgery, IV 1 mg as indicated.
Prevention of Dermal Necrosis and Sloughing:
Adults: IV Add 10 mg/1 L of solution containing norepinephrine.
Treatment of Dermal Necrosis or Sloughing After Norepinephrine Extravasation:
Adults: 5 to 10 mg in 10 mL saline solution in area of extravasation within 12 hr.
Children: Infiltrate area 0.1 to 0.2 mg/kg (max, 10 mg).
Diagnosis of Pheochromocytoma:
Adults: IM / IV 2.5 to 5 mg.
Children: IV 1 mg or IM 3 mg.

Trade names: Phentolamine Mesylate Powder for Injection 5 mg (as mesylate)/vial

Warnings: Hypersensitivity to phentolamine or related compounds; MI, coronary insufficiency, angina, or other evidence suggestive of coronary artery disease. Pregnancy Category: [C]

Interactions: Epinephrine, ephedrine: Vasoconstrictive and hypertensive effects of epinephrine and ephedrine are antagonized by phentolamine.

Phenytoin

Anticonvulsant / Hydantoin

Indications: Control of grand mal and psychomotor seizures; prevention and treatment of seizures occurring during or after neurosurgery; control of grand mal type of status epilepticus (parenteral administration).

Unlabeled indication: Control of arrhythmias, (particularly cardiac glycoside-induced arrhythmias); control of convulsions in severe preeclampsia; treatment of trigeminal neuralgia (tic douloureux), recessive dystrophic epidermolysis bullosa and junctional epidermolysis bullosa.

Dose: Individualize dose within clinically effective therapeutic serum level of 10 to 20 mcg/mL.
Seizures:
Adults: PO 100 mg (or 125 mg of suspension) tid initially.
Maintenance: 300 to 400 mg/day (max, 600 mg/day). Sometimes initial 1 g loading dose is divided into 3 doses (400, 300, and 300 mg) and is given at 2-hr intervals. Once seizure control is established, extended-release form (300 mg) may be administered for once-a-day dosing.
Children: PO 5 mg/kg/day in 2 to 3 divided doses initially.
Maintenance: 4 to 8 mg/kg/day (max, 300 mg/day).
Status Epilepticus:
Adults: IV Loading dose of 10 to 15 mg/kg via slow IV. Then PO/IV 100 mg q 6 to 8 hr.
Children: IV Loading dose of 15 to 20 mg/kg at rate not exceeding 1 to 3 mg/kg/min.
Neurosurgery Prophylaxis:
Adults: IM 100 to 200 mg at 4-hr intervals during surgery and postoperatively.

Trade names: Dilantin Infatab Tablets, chewable 50 mg
Dilantin-125 Suspension, oral 125 mg/5 mL
Dilantin Injection 50 mg/mL (46 mg phenytoin)
Dilantin Kapseals Capsules 30 mg (27.6 mg phenytoin)

Warnings: Hypersensitivity to phenytoin or other hydantoins; sinoatrial block; sinus bradycardia; second- and third-degree atrioventricular block; Adams-Stokes syndrome. Pregnancy Category: [Pregnancy category undetermined Consult health care provider Possible risk of birth defects must be considered along with risk of seizures to fetus in untreated epileptic mothers]

Interactions: Acetaminophen: May increase hepatotoxicity potential with chronic phenytoin use.
Amiodarone, chloramphenicol, disulfiram, estrogens, felbamate, fluconazole, isoniazid, cimetidine, trimethoprim, phenylbutazone, oxyphenbutazone, phenacemide, sulfonamides: May increase phenytoin serum levels.
Carbamazepine, sucralfate, antineoplastic agents, rifampin, rifabutin: May decrease phenytoin serum levels.
Corticosteroids, coumarin anticoagulants, doxycycline, estrogens, levodopa, felodipine, methadone, loop diuretics, oral contraceptives, quinidine, rifampin, rifabutin: May impair effects of these agents.
Cyclosporine: May reduce cyclosporine levels.
Disopyramide: May cause decreased disopyramide levels and bioavailability and may enhance anticholinergic actions.
Enteral nutritional therapy: May reduce phenytoin concentrations.
Folic acid: May cause folic acid deficiency.
Metyrapone: Phenytoin may cause subnormal response to metyrapone.
Mexiletine: May decrease mexiletine levels and effects.
Nondepolarizing muscle relaxants: May cause these agents to have shorter duration or decreased effects.
Phenobarbital, sodium valproate, valproic acid: May increase or decrease phenytoin levels. Phenytoin may increase phenobarbital and decrease valproic acid levels.
Primidone: May increase concentrations of primidone and metabolites.
Sympathomimetics (eg, dopamine): May cause profound hypotension and possibly cardiac arrest.
Theophyllines: Effects of either agent may be decreased.
Incompatability: Do not mix with other drugs in syringe.

Pilocarpine

Ophthalmic / Antiglaucoma / Mouth and throat product

Indications: Ophthalmic: Treatment of chronic simple glaucoma, chronic angle-closure glaucoma, acute angle-closure glaucoma, pre- and postoperative management of intraocular tension, treatment of mydriasis.

PO: Treatment of xerostomia in patients with malfunctioning salivary glands because of radiotherapy for cancer of head and neck, relieve dry mouth in patients with Sjogren syndrome.

Unlabeled indication: Relief of dry mouth in patients with graft-vs-host disease (PO).

Dose: Solution:
Adults: Instill 1 to 2 drops of 1% or 2% solution in affected eye(s) 6 times or less/day. More concentrated solutions are sometimes used.
Gel:

Adults: Apply 0.5-inch ribbon in lower conjunctival sac of affected eye(s) once daily at bedtime.
Ocular Therapeutic System:
Adults: Place system into conjunctival cul-de-sac of affected eye(s) at bedtime. Replace each unit q 7 days.
PO 5 mg tid; may titrate 10 mg or less tid.
PO:
Adults: PO Titrate dosage based on therapeutic response and tolerance. To reduce the incidence and severity of side effects, use the lowest effective dose. Do not exceed a maximum of 10 mg/dose.
Radiation-induced Xerostomia:
Adults: PO 5 mg tid. If no response, increase dose to 10 mg tid. Continue uninterrupted for at least 12 wk before assessing for full therapeutic benefit.
Sjogren Syndrome:
Adults: PO 5 mg qid. Continue uninterrupted for at least 6 wk before assessing for full therapeutic benefit.

Trade names: Adsorbocarpine Solution 1%
Akarpine Solution 1%
Isopto-Carpine Solution 0.35%
Pilocar Solution 0.5%
Piloptic-1/2 Solution 0.5%
Piloptic-1 Solution 1%
Piloptic-2 Solution 2%
Piloptic-3 Solution 3%
Piloptic-4 Solution 4%
Piloptic-6 Solution 6%
Pilopine HS Gel 4%
Pilostat Solution 0.5%
Salagen Tablets 5 mg
Ocusert Pilo-20 Ocular therapeutic system Releases 20 mcg/hr for 1 wk
Ocusert Pilo-40 Ocular therapeutic system Releases 40 mcg/hr for 1 wk

Warnings: Hypersensitivity; conditions in which cholinergic effects such as constriction are undesirable. Oral use also contraindicated in uncontrolled asthma, acute iritis, narrow-angle glaucoma, acute inflammatory disease of anterior segment of eye. Pregnancy Category: [C]

Interactions: Anticholinergics: May antagonize action of pilocarpine (PO, ophthalmic).
Beta-blockers: Potential for cardiac conduction disturbances with oral pilocarpine.
Parasympathomimetics: Additive pharmacologic effects and increased toxicity possible.

Pimecrolimus

Topical Immunomodulator

Indications: Short-term and intermittent long-term treatment of mild to moderate atopic dermatitis in nonimmunocompromised patients.

Dose: Adults and children 2 yr and older: Topical Apply a thin layer to the affected skin bid and rub in gently and completely. Re-evaluate patient if symptoms persist beyond 6 wk of treatment.

Trade names: Elidel Cream 1%

Warnings: Standard considerations. Pregnancy Category: [C]

Interactions: None well documented.

Pimozide

Antipsychotic

Indications: Suppression of motor and phonic tics in patients with Tourette syndrome who fail to respond satisfactorily to standard treatment.

Dose: Adults: PO For the initial dose, give 1 to 2 mg/day in divided doses, increasing the dose every other day. For the maintenance dose, give less than 0.2 mg/kg/day or 10 mg/day, whichever is less. Doses greater than 0.2 mg/kg/day or 10 mg/day are not recommended.
Children (at least 12 yr): PO For the initial dose, give 0.05 mg/kg/day (preferably at bedtime); increasing the dose every third day (max, 0.2 mg/kg, not to exceed 10 mg/day).

Trade names: Orap Tablets 1 mg

Warnings: Treatment of simple tics or tics other than those associated with Tourette syndrome; drug-induced motor and phonic tics (eg, amphetamine, methylphenidate, pemoline) until it is determined whether the tics are caused by drugs or Tourette syndrome; patients with congenital long QT syndrome, history of cardiac arrhythmias; administration with other drugs that prolong the QT interval; patients receiving aprepitant or the azole antifungal agents itraconazole, ketoconazole, and voriconazole; patients receiving the macrolide antibiotics azithromycin, clarithromycin, dirithromycin, erythromycin, and troleandomycin; patients receiving protease inhibitors (eg, amprenavir, atazanavir, indinavir, nelfinavir, ritonavir, saquinavir); coadministration of nefazodone, sertraline, zileuton, or ziprasidone; severe toxic CNS depression or comatose states from any cause; hypersensitivity to pimozide. Pregnancy Category: [C]

Interactions: CNS depressants (eg, analgesics, sedatives, anxiolytics): Pimozide may potentiate effects.
Drugs that may cause motor and phonic tics (eg, amphetamine, methylphenidate, pemoline): Coadministration of these agents with pimozide is contraindicated.
Drugs that prolong the QT interval (eg, aprepitant, azole antifungal agents [eg, ketoconazole], macrolide antibiotics [eg, erythromycin], nefazodone, phenothiazines [eg, thioridazine], protease inhibitors [eg, indinavir], sertraline, tricyclic antidepressants [eg, amitriptyline], voriconazole, zileuton, ziprasidone): Increased risk of life-threatening cardiac arrhythmias, including torsades de pointes. Coadministration of these agents with pimozide is contraindicated.
Grapefruit juice: May increase pimozide concentrations, increasing the pharmacologic and adverse effects. Avoid grapefruit juice.

Pindolol

Beta-adrenergic blocker

Indications: Management of mild to moderate hypertension.

Dose: Adults: PO 5 mg bid. May be increased by 10 mg q 3 to 4 wk until desired response; max dose is 60 mg/day.

Trade names: Visken Tablets 5 mg

Warnings: Greater than first-degree heart block; CHF unless secondary to tachyarrhythmia treatable with beta-blockers; overt cardiac failure; sinus bradycardia; cardiogenic shock; hypersensitivity to beta-blockers; bronchial asthma or bronchospasm, including severe COPD. Pregnancy Category: [B]

Interactions: Clonidine: May enhance or reverse antihypertensive effect; potentially life-threatening situations may occur, especially on withdrawal.
Epinephrine: Initial hypertensive episode followed by bradycardia may occur.
Ergot derivatives: Peripheral ischemia, manifested by cold extremities and possible gangrene, may occur.
Insulin: Prolonged hypoglycemia with masking of symptoms may occur.
Lidocaine: Lidocaine levels may increase, leading to toxicity.
NSAIDs: Some agents may impair antihypertensive effect.
Prazosin: Orthostatic hypotension may be increased.
Theophyllines: Elimination of theophylline may be reduced. Also, effects of both drugs may be reduced by pharmacologic antagonism.
Verapamil: Effects of both drugs may be increased.

Pioglitazone

Antidiabetic / Thiazolidinedione

Indications: Type 2 diabetes, as an adjunct to diet and exercise; also may be used in conjunction with a sulfonylurea, metformin, or insulin when diet, exercise, and a single agent alone does not result in adequate glycemic control in patients with type 2 diabetes mellitus.

Dose: Monotherapy: PO Initially, 15 or 30 mg/day, up to 45 mg/day. If monotherapy is inadequate, consider combinations using same starting dose and adjust accordingly. May be given without regard to meals.
Sulfonylureas:
Combination Therapy:
Adults: PO In combination with sulfonylureas, the recommended dose of pioglitazone is 15 or 30 mg qd. If patient reports hypoglycemia, decrease the pioglitazone dose.
Metformin:
Combination Therapy:
Adults: PO In combination with metformin, pioglitazone may be initiated at 15 or 30 mg qd.
Insulin:
Combination Therapy:
Adults: PO In combination with insulin, the recommended dose of pioglitazone is 15 or 30 mg qd. If the patient reports hypoglycemia or if plasma glucose concentrations decrease to less than 100 mg/dL, it is recommended that the insulin dose be decreased 10% to 25%. Individualize further adjustment based on glucose lowering response.

Trade names: Actos Tablet 15 mg

Warnings: Standard considerations. Pregnancy Category: [C]

Interactions: Contraceptives, oral: Oral contraceptives may decrease both hormone components about 30%, potentially reducing contraceptive effectiveness.
P450 system: Cytochrome P450 isoform CYP3A4 is partially responsible for pioglitazone metabolism; therefore, other drugs affected by or affecting this system may interact.

Pirbuterol Acetate

Bronchodilator / Sympathomimetic

Indications: Prevention and treatment of reversible bronchospasm associated with asthma or other obstructive pulmonary diseases.

Dose: Adults and Children 12 yr and older: Inhalation 1 to 2 inhalations q 4 to 6 hr; not to exceed 12 inhalations/day.

Trade names: Maxair Autohaler Aerosol 0.2 mg/actuation

Warnings: Hypersensitivity to drug components; cardiac arrhythmias associated with tachycardia. Pregnancy Category: [C]

Interactions: MAO inhibitors, tricyclic antidepressants: May increase the effects of pirbuterol.

Piroxicam

Analgesic / NSAID

Indications: Treatment of acute or long-term use of rheumatoid arthritis and osteoarthritis.

Unlabeled indication: Symptomatic relief of primary dysmenorrhea, pain, sunburn, juvenile rheumatoid arthritis.

Dose: Rheumatoid Arthritis, Osteoarthritis:
Adults: PO Initiate and maintain at 20 mg/day in 1 to 2 divided doses.

Trade names: Feldene Capsules 10 mg

Warnings: Known allergy or hypersensitivity to aspirin, iodides, or any NSAID, including piroxicam. Pregnancy Category: [C]

Interactions: Alcohol: May augment risk of GI bleeding.
Anticoagulants: May increase effect of anticoagulants because of decreased plasma protein binding and inhibition of platelet aggregation. May increase risk of gastric erosion and bleeding.
Beta-blockers: Antihypertensive effect may be decreased.
Cholestyramine: Effects of piroxicam may be decreased.
Lithium: May decrease lithium clearance.
Methotrexate: May increase methotrexate levels and toxicity.
Ritonivir: May increase concentrations and possibly the toxicity of piroxicam by inhibiting its metabolism.

Pneumococcal 7-Valent Conjugate Vaccine

Vaccine, bacterial

Indications: Active immunization of infants and toddlers against *Streptococcus pneumoniae*; active immunization of infants and toddlers against otitis media caused by serotypes included in the vaccine.

Dose: Preferred sites of IM injection are the anterolateral aspect of the thigh in infants or deltoid muscle of the upper arm in toddlers and young children.
Vaccination schedule:
Children at least 24 mo through 9 yr: IM 3 doses of 0.5 mL each, at approximately 2-mo intervals, followed by a fourth dose of 0.5 mL at 12 to 15 mo of age. Usually the first dose is at 2 mo of age; however, it can be given as young as 6 wk. The recommended dosing interval is 4 to 8 wk. Administer the fourth dose at least 2 mo after the third dose.
Previously Unvaccinated Older Infants and Children Beyond Age of Routine Infant Schedule:
Children at least 24 mo through 9 yr: IM 1 dose of 0.5 mL.
Children 12 to 23 mo: IM 2 doses of 0.5 mL at least 2 mo apart.
Children 7 to 11 mo: IM 3 doses of 0.5 mL, administer 2 doses at least 4 wk apart and the third dose after the 1-yr birthday, separated from the second dose by at least 2 mo.

Trade names: Prevnar Injection 2 mcg each of 6 polysaccharide isolates; 4 mcg of 1 polysaccharide isolate per 0.5 mL dose

Warnings: Severe or moderate febrile illness; hypersensitivity to any component of the product. Pregnancy Category: [C]

Interactions: Immunosuppressive agents (large amounts of corticosteroids, antimetabolites, alkylating agents, cytotoxic agents): Children may not respond optimally to active immunization.

Poliovirus Vaccine, Live, Oral, Trivalent

Vaccine, live virus

Indications: Prevention of poliomyelitis. Infants as young as 6 to 12 wk and all unimmunized children and adolescents up to 18 yr are usual candidates for routine OPV prophylaxis. OPV is also recommended for control of epidemic poliomyelitis. If less than 4 wk remain before protection is needed, single dose of OPV is recommended, with remaining vaccine doses given later if person remains at increased risk. Immunization with IPV may be indicated for unimmunized parents and those in other special situations in which protection may be needed. In household with immunocompromised member or other close contacts or in household with unimmunized adult, use only IPV for all those requiring poliovirus immunization.
Adults: Primary immunization with inactivated polio vaccine is recommended whenever feasible for unimmunized adults subject to increased risk of exposure, such as by travel to or contact with epidemic or endemic areas (eg, developing countries) and for those employed in medical and sanitation facilities.

Dose: Older Children, Adolescents and Adults: PO 0.5 mL. Give 2 doses no less than 6 wk apart (or 8 wk apart or less) followed by third dose 6 to 12 mo later. Infants: PO 0.5 mL. Administer at 2, 4, and 15 to 18 mo. A fourth dose is given when child begins school if third dose of primary series was administered before child's fourth birthday. OPV may be administered with any of following: distilled water, chlorinated tap water, simple syrup, milk, bread, sugar cube, cake.

Trade names: Orimune Suspension, oral Mixture of 3 viruses (Types 1, 2, and 3) propagated in monkey kidney tissue culture

Warnings: Do not administer OPV to any person with immunosuppression or to any household member of immunodeficient person. This includes combined immunodeficiency, hypogammaglobulinemia, agammaglobulinemia, thymic abnormalities, leukemia, lymphoma, generalized malignancy, and lowered resistance to infection from therapy with corticosteroids, alkylating drugs, antimetabolites, or radiation. Advise vaccine recipients to avoid contact with such persons for at least 6 to 8 wk. Do not give OPV to member of household in which there is family history of immunodeficiency until immune status of intended recipient and other children in family is determined to be normal. IPV is preferred for immunizing all persons in these circumstances. Pregnancy Category: [C Use OPV in pregnancy if exposure is imminent and immediate protection is needed]

Interactions: Immune globulin (IG) does not interfere with immunity following OPV. However, do not administer OPV less than 7 days after IG administration unless unavoidable, such as unexpected travel to or contact with epidemic or endemic areas or persons. If OPV is given within 1 wk after IG, the OPV dose should probably be repeated 3 mo later, if immunity is still needed. Like all live viral vaccines, administration to patients or contacts of patients receiving immunosuppressant drugs, including steroids or radiation may predispose patients to disseminated infections or insufficient response to immunization. They may remain susceptible despite immunization. Several routine pediatric vaccines may safely and effectively be administered simultaneously at separate injection sites (eg, DTP, MMR, IPV, Hib, hepatitis B, influenza). National authorities recommend simultaneous immunization at separate sites as indicated by age or health risk. Live virus vaccines may cause delayed-hypersensitivity skin test results (eg, tuberculin, histoplasmin) to appear falsely negative. Effect may persist for several weeks after vaccination. Give tuberculin tests either prior to live-virus vaccination, simultaneously with it, or at least 6 wk after vaccination.

Polyethylene Glycol-Electrolyte Solution

Laxative

Indications: Bowel cleansing prior to GI examination.

Unlabeled indication: Management of acute iron overdose in children.

Dose: Adults: PO/Nasogastric 4 L prior to GI examination. Give orally as 240 mL q 10 min or via NG tube as 1.2 to 1.8 L/hr until 4 L are consumed or until rectal effluent is clear. Via nasogastric (NG) tube, use rate of 1.2 to 1.8 L/hr.

Trade names: CoLyte Powder for oral solution 1 gal: 227.1 g PEG 3350, 21.5 g sodium sulfate, 6.36 g sodium bicarb, 5.53 g NaCl, 2,82 g KCl
GoLYTELY Powder for oral suspension 236 g PEG 3350, 22.74 g sodium sulfate, 6.74 g sodium bicarb, 5.86 g NaCl, 2.97 g KCl
NuLYTELY Powder for reconstitution 420 g PEG 3350, 5.72 g sodium bicarb, 11.2 g NaCl, 1.48 g KCl
OCL Oral solution 146 mg NaCl, 168 mg sodium bicarb, 1.29 g sodium sulfate decahydrate, 75 mg KCl, 6 g PEG 3350, 30 mg polysorbate 80/100 mL

Warnings: GI obstruction; gastric retention; bowel perforation; toxic colitis; toxic megacolon or ileus. Pregnancy Category: [C]

Interactions: Oral medication given within 1 hr of starting therapy: Medication may be flushed from GI tract and not absorbed.

Potassium Citrate/Sodium Citrate/Citric Acid

Systemic alkalinizer/Urinary alkalinizer

Indications: Treatment of chronic metabolic acidosis, particularly when caused by renal tubular acidosis; conditions when long-term maintenance of an alkaline urine is desirable, in treatment of patients with uric acid and cystine calculi of the urinary tract and in conjunction with uricosurics in gout therapy to prevent uric acid nephropathy.

Dose: Adults: PO 3 to 6 tsp (15 to 30 mL), diluted with water, qid after meals and at bedtime, or as directed by health care provider.
Children: PO 1 to 3 tsp (5 to 15 mL), diluted with water qid after meals and at bedtime, or as directed by health care provider.

Trade names: Polycitra Syrup 550 mg potassium citrate, 500 mg sodium citrate, 334 mg citric acid/5 mL (1 mEq K, 1 mEq Na/mL; equiv. to 2 mEq bicarbonate)
Polycitra-LC Solution 550 mg potassium citrate, 500 mg sodium citrate, 334 mg citric acid/5 mL (1 mEq K, 1 mEq Na/mL; equiv. to 2 mEq bicarbonate)

Warnings: Severe renal impairment with oliguria; azotemia; untreated Addison disease; severe myocardial damage; certain situations when patients are on a sodium- or potassium-restricted diet. Pregnancy Category: [Undetermined]

Interactions: Potassium-containing medication, potassium-sparing diuretics (eg, spironolactone), ACE inhibitors (eg, captopril), or cardiac glycosides (eg, digoxin): Concurrent use may lead to toxicity.

Pramipexole Dihydrochloride

Antiparkinson / Non-ergot dopamine receptor agonist

Indications: Treatment of the signs and symptoms of idiopathic Parkinson disease. May be used in conjunction with L-dopa.

Dose: Individualize by careful titration.
Adults: PO Initial dose is 0.125 mg tid. For the maintenance dose, dosage may be increased q 5 to 7 days to max dose of 4.5 mg/day.

Trade names: Mirapex Tablets 0.125 mg

Warnings: Standard considerations. Pregnancy Category: [C]

Interactions: Drugs eliminated via cationic renal secretion (eg, cimetidine, ranitidine, diltiazem, triamterene, verapamil, quinidine, quinine): May reduce oral clearance of pramipexole. Pramipexole dosage adjustment may be needed if therapy with any of these agents is started or stopped during treatment with pramipexole.
Dopamine antagonists (eg, butyrophenones, metoclopramide, phenothiazines, thioxanthenes): May reduce effectiveness of pramipexole.

Pravastatin Sodium

Antihyperlipidemic / HMG-CoA reductase inhibitor

Indications: As an adjunct to diet for reduction of elevated total and LDL cholesterol, apolipoprotein B, and triglyceride levels and to increase HDL cholesterol in patients with primary hypercholesterolemia and mixed dyslipidemia (Frederickson types IIa and IIb); as adjunctive therapy to diet for treatment of patients with elevated serum triglyceride levels (Frederickson type IV); treatment of primary dysbetalipoproteinemia (Frederickson type III) who do not respond adequately to diet; in hypercholesterolemic patients without clinically evident coronary heart disease (CHD) to reduce risk of MI or cardiovascular mortality with no increase in death from noncardiovascular causes; in patients with clinically evident CHD, to reduce risk of total mortality by reducing coronary death, MI, undergoing myocardial revascularization procedures, stroke, and stroke/transient ischemic attack and slow progression of coronary arteriosclerosis.

Dose: Adults: PO 10 to 40 mg/day
Children (8 to 13 yr): PO 20 mg once daily.
Children (14 to 18 yr): PO 40 mg once daily.

Trade names: Pravachol Tablets 10 mg

Warnings: Active liver disease or unexplained persistent elevations of LFTs; pregnancy; lactation. Pregnancy Category: [X]

Interactions: Bile acid sequestrants: Large decrease in pravastatin bioavailability.
Cyclosporine, gemfibrozil: Severe myopathy or rhabdomyolysis; decreased urinary excretion and protein binding of pravastatin.
Protease inhibitors (eg, ritonavir): Pravastatin plasma levels may be reduced, decreasing the efficacy.

Praziquantel

Anti-infective / Antihelminthic

Indications: Infections caused by *Schistosoma mekongi*, *S. japonicum*, *S. mansoni*, *S. hematobium*, liver flukes, *Clonorchis sinensis*, and *Opisthorchis viverrini*.

Unlabeled indication: Treatment of neurocysticercosis, tissue flukes (opisthorchis, felineus, *Paragonimus westermani*, *Fasciola hepatica*), intestinal flukes (Heterophyes heterophyes, *Fascilopsis buski*), and intestinal cestodes (*Diphyllobothrium latum*, *Taenia saginata*, *T. solium*, *Dipylidium caninum*, Hymenolepsis nana), and schistosomiasis (in concurrent use with oxamniquine).

Dose: Schistosomiasis:
Adults and Children at least 4 yr: PO 60 mg/kg in 3 equally divided doses q 4 to 6 hr for 1 day.
Clonorchiasis and Opisthorchiasis:
Adults: PO 75 mg/kg in 3 equally divided doses q 4 to 6 hr for 1 day.

Trade names: Biltricide Tablets 600 mg

Warnings: Ocular cysticercosis. Pregnancy Category: [B]

Interactions: Cimetidine: Plasma levels of praziquantel may be elevated, increasing the pharmacologic and adverse effects.

Prazosin

Antihypertensive / Antiadrenergic, peripherally acting

Indications: Treatment of hypertension.

Dose: Adults:
Initial dose: PO 1 mg bid to tid.
Maintenance: PO 6 to 20 mg/day in divided doses (max, 40 mg/day).
Children: PO 0.5 to 7 mg tid has been suggested.

Trade names: Minipress Capsules 1 mg

Warnings: Hypersensitivity to doxazosin, prazosin, or terazosin. Pregnancy Category: [C]

Interactions: Alcohol: Increased risk of hypotension.
Beta-blockers: Enhanced acute orthostatic hypotensive reaction after first dose of prazosin.
Verapamil: Increased serum prazosin levels and increased sensitivity to orthostatic hypotension.

Prednisone

Corticosteroid

Indications: Endocrine disorders; rheumatic disorders; collagen diseases; dermatologic diseases; allergic states; allergic and inflammatory ophthalmic processes; respiratory diseases; hematologic disorders; neoplastic diseases; edematous states (because of nephrotic syndrome); GI diseases; multiple sclerosis; tuberculous meningitis; trichinosis with neurologic or myocardial involvement.

Unlabeled indication: COPD; Duchenne muscular dystrophy; Graves ophthalmopathy.

Dose: Adults: PO 5 to 60 mg/day.
COPD:
Adults: PO 30 to 60 mg/day for 1 to 2 wk, then taper.
Duchenne Muscular Dystrophy:
Adults: PO 0.75 to 1.5 mg/kg/day.
Graves Ophthalmopathy:
Adults: PO 60 mg/day; taper to 20 mg/day.

Trade names: Deltasone Tablets 2.5 mg
Liquid Pred Syrup 5 mg/5 mL
Meticorten Tablets 1 mg
Orasone Tablets 1 mg
Panasol-S Tablets 1 mg
Prednicen-M Tablets 5 mg
Prednisone Intensol Concentrate Oral solution 5 mg/mL
Sterapred Tablets 5 mg
Sterapred DS Tablets 10 mg

Warnings: Systemic fungal infections; administration of live virus vaccines. Pregnancy Category: [C]

Interactions: Anticholinesterases: Antagonizes anticholinesterase effects in myasthenia gravis.
Anticoagulants, oral: Alters anticoagulant dose requirements.
Barbiturates, hydantoins (eg, phenytoin), rifampin: Decreased pharmacologic effect of prednisone.
Cyclosporine: Enhanced cyclosporine toxicity.
Estrogens, ketoconazole, oral contraceptives: Decreased clearance of prednisone.
Nondepolarizing muscle relaxants: May potentiate, counteract, or have no effect on neuromuscular blocking action.
Salicylates: Reduced serum levels and efficacy of salicylates.
Somatrem: Inhibition of growth-promoting effects of somatrem.
Theophylline: Alterations in pharmacologic activity of either agent.

Primaquine Phosphate

Anti-infective / Antimalarial

Indications: Radical cure or prevention of relapse in vivax malaria; after termination of chloroquine phosphate suppressive therapy in areas where vivax malaria is endemic.

Unlabeled indication: With clindamycin, treatment of Pneumocystis carinii pneumonia associated with AIDS.

Dose: Begin therapy during last 2 wk of or after course of suppression with chloroquine or comparable drug.
Adults: PO 26.3 mg (15 mg base) for 14 days.
Children: PO 0.5 mg/kg/day (0.3 mg/kg/day of base) for 14 days (max, 15 mg/day of base).

Trade names: Available as generic only Tablets 26.3 mg (equiv. to 15 mg base)

Warnings: Concomitant administration of quinacrine and primaquine; acutely ill patient with systemic disease manifested by granulocytopenia (eg, rheumatoid arthritis, lupus erythematosus); concurrent administration of other potentially hemolytic or bone marrow depressant medications. Pregnancy Category: [Pregnancy category undetermined]

Interactions: Quinacrine: May potentiate toxicity of antimalarial compounds that are structurally related to primaquine.

Primidone

Anticonvulsant

Indications: Control of grand mal, psychomotor, or focal epileptic seizures; may control grand mal seizures refractory to other anticonvulsants.

Unlabeled indication: Treatment of benign familial tremor (essential tremor).

Dose: Adults and Children over 8 yr of age: If no previous treatment, initiate as follows: PO For days 1 to 3, give 100 to 125 mg at bedtime; days 4 to 6, give 100 to 125 mg bid; days 7 to 9, give 100 to 125 mg tid; and day 10 through maintenance dose, give 250 mg tid or qid. May increase to 250 mg 5 to 6 times/day, but do not exceed 500 mg qid (2 g/day).
Children under 8 yr of age: PO For days 1 to 3, give 50 mg at bedtime; days 4 to 6, give 50 mg bid; days 7 to 9, give 100 mg bid; and day 10 through maintenance dose, give 125 to 250 mg tid or 10 to 25 mg/kg/day in divided doses.
Patients Already Taking Anticonvulsants: Initiate at 100 to 125 mg at bedtime, gradually increasing dose to maintenance level as other drug is gradually decreased. Complete switch to primidone should occur over more than 2 wk.

Trade names: Mysoline Tablets 50 mg

Warnings: Hypersensitivity to barbiturates; porphyria. Pregnancy Category: [D Consult health care provider regarding anticonvulsant use during pregnancy]

Interactions: Anticoagulants: Decreased anticoagulant effects.
Beta-blockers: Effects of beta-blockers may be reduced.
Carbamazepine: Decreased primidone levels; increased concentrations of carbamazepine.
Corticosteroids: Decreased effect of corticosteroids.
Doxycycline: Decreased doxycycline serum levels.
Estrogens, oral contraceptives: Contraceptive failure has been reported.
Ethanol: Additive CNS suppression.
Felodipine: Decreased effect of felodipine.
Griseofulvin: Decreased serum griseofulvin levels.
Hydantoins, valproic acid: Increased primidone serum levels.
Methadone: Plasma concentrations may be reduced by primidone, leading to opiate withdrawal.
Methoxyflurane: Enhanced renal toxicity may occur.
Metronidazole: Therapeutic failure of metronidazole.
Nifedipine: Decreased nifedipine levels.
Quinidine: Decreased quinidine serum levels.
Succinimides: Decreased primidone levels.
Theophyllines: Decreased theophylline levels.

Procainamide HCl

Antiarrhythmic

Indications: Treatment of documented ventricular arrhythmias that are life threatening.

Dose: Adults: PO 50 mg/kg/day in divided doses (q 3 hr for regular release; q 6 to 12 hr for sustained release, depending on the formulation). IV 20 mg/min for 25 to 30 min as loading dose, then 2 to 6 mg/min for maintenance. IM 50 mg/kg/day in divided doses q 3 to 6 hr until oral therapy is possible.
Children: Safety not established. Following doses have been used: PO 15 to 50 mg/kg/day in divided doses q 3 to 6 hr, max of 4 g/day; IM 20 to 30 mg/kg/day in divided doses q 4 to 6 hr, max 4 g/day; IV 3 to 6 mg/kg/dose over 5 min for loading dose, then 20 to 80 mcg/kg/min continuous infusion (max, 100 mg/dose or 2 g/day).

Trade names: Procanbid Tablets, sustained-release 500 mg
Pronestyl Tablets 250 mg
Pronestyl-SR Tablets, sustained-release 500 mg

Warnings: Complete heart block; idiosyncratic hypersensitivity; lupus erythematosus; torsades de pointes. Pregnancy Category: [C]

Interactions: Amiodarone, cimetidine, trimethoprim: May increase procainamide and NAPA concentrations.
Cisapride, quinolone antibiotics (eg, gatifloxacin), thioridazine, ziprasidone: May increase the risk of life-threatening cardiac arrhythmias, including torsades de pointes.
Group 1a antiarrhythmic agents (eg, quinidine): Coadministration with procainamide is contraindicated.

Procarbazine

Alkylating agent

Indications: Adult and Pediatric: Advanced Hodgkin disease (stage III and IV) as part of the MOPP (nitrogen mustard, vincristine, procarbazine, prednisone) regimen.

Unlabeled indication: Non-Hodgkin lymphoma, brain tumors, small cell lung cancer (adult use).

Dose: Base dosages on patient's actual weight. The following doses are for administration of procarbazine as a single agent. When used in combination with other anticancer drugs, appropriately reduce procarbazine dosage. In the MOPP regimen, the dose is 100 mg/m^2 daily for 14 days.
Hodgkin Disease:
Adults: PO To minimize nausea and vomiting, give single or divided doses of 2 to 4 mg/kg/day for the first wk. Maintain daily dosage at 4 to 6 mg/kg/day until the WBC falls below 4000/mm^3 or the platelets fall below 100,000/mm^3, or until max response is obtained. Upon evidence of hematologic toxicity, discontinue the drug until there has been satisfactory recovery. Resume treatment at 1 to 2 mg/kg/day. When max response is obtained, maintain the dose at 1 to 2 mg/kg/day.
Pediatric: PO Individualize dosage. The dosage schedule is a guideline only: 50 mg/m^2 /day for the first week. Maintain daily dosage at 100 mg/m^2 until leukopenia or thrombocytopenia occurs or max response is obtained. When max response is attained, maintain the dose at 50 mg/m^2 /day. Upon evidence of hematologic or other toxicity, discontinue drug until there has been satisfactory recovery.

Trade names: Matulane Capsules 50 mg

Warnings: Hypersensitivity to procarbazine. Inadequate marrow reserve demonstrated by bone marrow aspiration. Pregnancy Category: [D]

Interactions: Alcohol: Alcohol consumption may cause a disulfiram-like reaction in patients on procarbazine.
CNS depressants (eg, narcotics, analgesics, alcohol, antiemetics, benzodiazepines, sedatives, and tranquilizers): Concurrent use may potentiate CNS effects.
Digitalis glycosides: May result in a decrease in digoxin plasma levels, even several days after stopping chemotherapy.
High-tyramine foods (eg, wine, yogurt, ripe cheese, bananas), OTC antihistamines, and sympathomimetics: Avoid known high-tyramine foods, OTC antihistamines, and sympathomimetics. Procarbazine is a weak MAO inhibitor.
Levodopa: Flushing and a significant rise in BP may result within 1 hr of levodopa administration.
Methotrexate: May increase methotrexate-induced nephrotoxicity.
Radiation or other chemotherapy: May depress bone marrow activity.
Sympathomimetics (indirect-acting): May cause an abrupt increase in BP, resulting in a potentially fatal hypertensive crisis.
Tricyclic antidepressants: Severe toxic and fatal reactions including excitability, fluctuations in BP, convulsions, and coma may occur.

Prochlorperazine

Antipsychotic / Phenothiazine / Antiemetic

Indications: Treatment of schizophrenia; short-term treatment of generalized nonpsychotic anxiety; control of severe nausea and vomiting.

Unlabeled indication: Treatment of migraines (IV).

Dose: Individualize dosage. SC administration is not advised because of local irritation.
Nonpsychotic Anxiety:
Adults: PO 5 mg tid to qid; 15 mg (sustained-release formulation) in morning or 10 mg (sustained-release formation) q 12 hr. Do not exceed 20 mg/day or give for more than 12 wk.
Schizophrenia:
Adults: IM Start with 10 to 20 mg for immediate control of schizophrenic patients with severe symptomatology; if necessary, repeat initial dose q 2 to 4 hr to gain control of patient. More than 3 or 4 doses are seldom necessary. If IM therapy is needed for a prolonged period, give 10 to 20 mg q 4 to 6 hr.
Mild conditions: PO 5 to 10 mg tid or qid.
Moderate to severe conditions: PO 10 mg tid qid, increasing dosage gradually (q 2 or 3 days) until symptoms are controlled or side effects become bothersome. Some patients respond satisfactorily on 50 to 75 mg/day; in more severe disturbances, the optimum dosage is usually 100 to 150 mg/day.
Children 2 to 12 yr: PO / PR 2.5 mg bid or tid. Do not exceed 10 mg the first day.
Children 2 to 5 yr: PO / PR Do not exceed 20 mg/day.
Children 6 to 12 yr: PO / PR Do not exceed 25 mg/day.
IM For children under 12 yr, calculate each dose on the basis of 0.03 mg/kg given by deep IM injection.
Nausea and Vomiting:
Adults: PO 5 or 10 mg tablet tid to qid; 15 mg (sustained-release formulation) on arising or 10 mg q 12 hr. PR 25 mg bid. IM 5 to 10 mg. May repeat q 3 to 4 hr. Do not exceed 40 mg/day. IV 2.5 to 10 mg by slow IV or infusion at a rate not to exceed 5 mg/min (single dose not to exceed 10 mg; max, 40 mg/day).
Children: Adjust according to patient response and severity of symptoms.
Children 18 to 38.5 kg: PO / PR 2.5 mg tid or 5 mg bid; do not exceed 15 mg/day. IM 0.03 mg/kg given by deep IM injection.
Children 13.6 to 17.6 kg: PO / PR 2.5 mg given bid to tid; do not exceed 10 mg/day. IM 0.03 mg/kg given by deep IM injection.
Children 9 to 13 kg: PO / PR 2.5 mg given qd or bid; do not exceed 7.5 mg/day. IM 0.03 mg/kg given by deep IM injection.
Nausea and Vomiting (Surgery):
Adults: IM 5 to 10 mg 1 to 2 hr prior to induction of anesthesia (may repeat once in 30 min) or to control acute symptoms during and after surgery (may repeat once).
Adults: IV injection or infusion 5 to 10 mg 15 to 30 min before induction of anesthesia or to control acute symptoms during or after surgery. Repeat once if necessary. Rate of administration should not exceed 5 mg/min and a single dose should not exceed 10 mg.

Trade names: Compazine Tablets 5 mg (as maleate)
Compro Suppositories 25 mg

Warnings: Coma or severely depressed states; allergy to any phenothiazine; presence of large amounts of other CNS depressants; pediatric patients under 2 yr of age or less than 20 lb; surgery in pediatric patients. Pregnancy Category: [Undetermined]

Interactions: Alcohol or other CNS depressants: May result in increased CNS depression and may precipitate dystonic reactions.
Anticholinergics: May reduce therapeutic effects of prochlorperazine and worsen anticholinergic effects.
Barbiturate anesthetics: Frequency and severity of neuromuscular excitation and hypotension may be increased.
Beta-blockers: May result in increased plasma levels of beta-blocker and prochlorperazine.
Cisapride, sparfloxacin: The risk of life-threatening cardiac arrhythmias, including torsades de pointes, may be increased.
Guanethidine: Hypotensive action of guanethidine may be inhibited.
Metrizamide: Possibility of seizure may be increased when subarachnoid metrizamide injection is used.
Paroxetine: Plasma levels of prochlorperazine may be elevated, increasing the risk of side effects.
Incompatability: Do not mix prochlorperazine injection with other agents in syringe. Do not dilute with any diluent containing parabens as preservative.

Progesterone

Progestin

Indications: Treatment of amenorrhea and functional uterine bleeding; intrauterine contraception in women who have had at least one child.

Unlabeled indication: Treatment of PMS (suppository), premature labor in late stages of pregnancy and menorrhagia (intrauterine).

Dose: Amenorrhea:
Adults: IM 5 to 10 mg/day for 6 to 8 days.
Functional Uterine Bleeding:
Adults: IM 5 to 10 mg/day for 6 days.
Contraceptive: Intrauterine 1 intrauterine system inserted into uterine cavity once yearly.
PMS:
Adults: Intravaginal / PR Insert suppository 200 to 400 mg bid.

Trade names: Crinone Vaginal gel 4% (45 mg)
Prometrium Capsules 100 mg (micronized progesterone)
Progesterone in Oil Injection 50 mg/mL

Warnings: IM, suppository, intrauterine: Hypersensitivity to progestins; thrombophlebitis, thromboembolic disorders, cerebral hemorrhage (or history of these disorders); impaired liver function; breast cancer; undiagnosed vaginal bleeding; missed abortion; diagnostic test for pregnancy; pregnancy or suspected pregnancy. Intrauterine: Previous ectopic pregnancy; presence or history of PID; IV drug abuse. Pregnancy Category: [X]

Interactions: Anticoagulants: Use intrauterine system with caution in patients receiving anticoagulant therapy.

Propafenone

Antiarrhythmic

Indications: Treatment of documented life-threatening ventricular arrhythmias (eg, sustained ventricular tachycardia).

Unlabeled indication: Treatment of supraventricular tachycardias including atrial fibrillation and flutter and arrhythmias associated with Wolff-Parkinson-White syndrome.

Dose: Individually titrate dose based on response and tolerance.
Adults: PO 150 mg q 8 hr initially, increasing at a min of 3- to 4-day intervals to 225 mg q 8 hr and, if necessary, to 300 mg q 8 hr.

Trade names: Rythmol Tablets 150 mg

Warnings: Uncontrolled CHF; cardiogenic shock; sinoatrial, atrioventricular and intraventricular disorders of impulse generation and conduction (eg, sick sinus node syndrome, atrioventricular block) in the absence of an artificial pacemaker; bradycardia; marked hypotension; bronchospastic disorders; manifest electrolyte imbalance; coadministration of cisapride; and known hypersensitivity to the drug. Pregnancy Category: [C]

Interactions: Cimetidine, quinidine, ritonavir:

May increase propafenone plasma concentrations, potentially increasing pharmacologic and adverse effects.
Cisapride: Contraindicated because of increase risk of life-threatening cardiac arrhythmias.
Cyclosporine, desipramine, digoxin, metoprolol, propranolol, theophylline, warfarin: Propafenone may increase plasma concentrations of these agents, increasing the risk of side effects and toxicity.
Local anesthetics: May increase the risk of CNS side effects.
Rifamycins (ie, rifabutin, rifapentine): May decrease propafenone plasma concentrations, decreasing the therapeutic effect.

Propantheline Bromide

Anticholinergic / Antispasmodic

Indications: Adjunctive therapy in treatment of peptic ulcer.

Unlabeled indication: Treatment of secretory and spastic disorders of GI tract, biliary tract, urinary tract, and bladder.

Dose: Peptic Ulcer:
Adults: PO 15 mg 30 min before meals and 30 mg at bedtime.
Patients with Mild Manifestations, Elderly Patients or Those of Small Stature: PO 7.5 mg tid.
Secretory Disorders:
Adults: PO 1.5 mg/kg/day in 3 to 4 divided doses.
Spastic Disorders:
Adults: PO 2 to 3 mg/kg/day in divided doses q 4 to 6 hr and at bedtime.

Trade names: Pro-Banthine Tablets 7.5 mg

Warnings: Hypersensitivity to anticholinergic drugs; narrow-angle glaucoma; adhesions between iris and lens; obstructive uropathy; obstructive disease of GI tract; paralytic ileus; intestinal atony of elderly or debilitated patient; severe ulcerative colitis; toxic megacolon complicating ulcerative colitis; hepatic or renal disease; tachycardia; myocardial ischemia; unstable cardiovascular status in acute hemorrhage; myasthenia gravis. Pregnancy Category: [C]

Interactions: Antacids: Decrease absorption of propantheline if given together.
Drugs with anticholinergic effects (eg, antihistamines, antiparkinson drugs, tricyclic antidepressants): Additive peripheral anticholinergic side effects.
Haloperidol: May cause decreased serum haloperidol levels, worsened schizophrenic symptoms and tardive dyskinesia.
Phenothiazines: May decrease antipsychotic effectiveness of phenothiazines; may produce additive anticholinergic effects.

Propofol

General anesthetic

Indications: Induction and maintenance of anesthesia in adults; induction anesthesia in children at least 3 yr; maintenance anesthesia in pediatric patients at least 2 mo; initiation and maintenance of monitored anesthesia care sedation in adults; sedation in intubated or respiratory-controlled adult ICU patients.

Dose: Anesthesia:
Adults under 55 yr: IV Induction 40 mg q 10 sec until onset. Usual dose is 2 to 2.5 mg/kg total. For maintenance infusion, titrate to 100 to 200 mcg/kg/min (6 to 12 mg/kg/hr). For maintenance intermittent bolus, use 25 to 50 mg increments, as needed.
Elderly, Debilitated, or ASA III/IV: (American Society of Anesthesiologists classification of heart disease, cardiac function, angina, and physical status used to assign risk for anesthesia.) IV 20 mg q 10 sec until onset. Usual dose is 1 to 1.5 mg/kg. For maintenance infusion, titrate to 50 to 100 mcg/kg/min (3 to 6 mg/kg/hr).
Neurosurgical patients: IV Induction 20 mg q 10 sec until onset. Usual dose is 1 to 2 mg/kg. For maintenance infusion, use 100 to 200 mcg/kg/min (6 to 12 mg/kg/hr).
Children at least 3 yr: IV Induction 2.5 to 3.5 mg/kg over 20 to 30 sec. For maintenance infusion (at least 2 mo), use 200 to 300 mcg/kg/min immediately following the induction dose, then, after the first 30 min of maintenance, use infusion rates of 125 to 150 mcg/kg/min titrated to achieve the desired clinical effect, are typically needed.
Sedation:
Adults under 55 yr: IV Initiation 100 to 150 mcg/kg/min (6 to 9 mg/kg/hr) for 3 to 5 min (preferred method) or slow injection of 0.5 mg/kg over 3 to 5 min; follow by maintenance infusion. For maintenance, use 25 to 75 mcg/kg/min (1.5 to 4.5 mg/kg/hr) (preferred method) or incremental bolus doses of 10 to 20 mg.
Elderly, Debilitated, or ASA III/IV: IV Initiation Same as adults; not as rapid bolus. For maintenance, use 20% reduction of adult dose; avoid rapid bolus doses.
ICU Sedation:
Adults: IV Initiation 5 mcg/kg/min (0.3 mg/kg/hr) for at least 5 min; increments of 5 to 10 mcg/kg/min (0.2 to 0.6 mg/kg/hr) over 5 to 10 min may be used until desired level of sedation is achieved. For maintenance, use 5 to 50 mcg/kg/min (0.3 to 3 mg/kg/hr) or higher may be required; use minimum dose required for sedation.

Trade names: Diprivan Injection 10 mg/mL

Warnings: Situations in which general anesthesia or sedation are contraindicated. Pregnancy Category: [B]

Interactions: CNS depressants (eg, barbiturates, benzodiazepines, narcotics): Increased CNS depression.
Incompatability: For IV, do not mix with other therapeutic agents prior to administration. Avoid mixing blood or plasma in same IV catheter.

Propranolol HCl

Beta-adrenergic blocker

Indications: Treatment of hypertension; angina pectoris; hypertrophic subaortic stenosis; MI; pheochromocytoma; migraine prophylaxis; essential tremor; some ventricular and supraventricular arrhythmias.

Unlabeled indication: Treatment of alcohol withdrawal syndrome; esophageal varices rebleeding in portal hypertension; anxiety; thyrotoxicosis symptoms.

Dose: Hypertension:
Adults: PO The initial dose is 40 mg bid initially or 80 mg sustained-release medication/day; titrate to response. The maintenance dose is 120 to 240 mg/day in 2 to 3 divided doses or 120 to 160 mg/day sustained-release medication. Do not exceed 640 mg/day.
Children: PO 0.5 mg/kg bid; titrate q 3 to 5 days to max dose of 16 mg/kg/day.
Angina:
Adults: PO 80 to 320 mg/day in 2 to 4 divided doses or 160 mg/day of sustained-release medication (max, 320 mg/day).
Arrhythmias:
Adults: PO 10 to 30 mg 3 to 4 times/day before meals and at bedtime.
Hypertrophic Aortic Stenosis:
Adults: PO 20 to 40 mg 3 to 4 times/day before meals and at bedtime or 80 to 160 mg sustained-release medication 1 time/day.
MI:
Adults: PO 180 to 240 mg/day in 3 to 4 divided doses up to 240 mg/day.
Pheochromocytoma:
Adults: PO 60 mg/day for 3 days prior to surgery, given with alpha-blocker.
Migraine:
Adults: PO 80 mg in divided doses daily or once daily (sustained release); titrate to response (max dose, 240 mg/day); discontinue after 6 wk if no response.

Arrhythmias (Life-Threatening):
Adults: IV 1 to 3 mg at rate of 1 mg/min; may repeat after 2 min; give subsequent doses q 4 hr.
Essential Tremor:
Adults: PO 40 mg bid initially; titrate to response. The maintenance dose is 120 to 320 mg/day in 2 to 3 divided doses (max, 320 mg/day).
Trade names: Betachron E-R Capsules, extended-release 60 mg
Inderal Tablets 10 mg
Inderal LA Capsules, sustained-release 60 mg
InnoPran XL Capsules, extended-release 80 mg
Propranolol Intensol Solution, concentrated oral 80 mg/mL
Warnings: Hypersensitivity to beta-blockers; greater than first-degree heart block; CHF unless secondary to tachyarrhythmia or untreated hypertension treatable with beta-blockers; overt cardiac failure; sinus bradycardia; cardiogenic shock; untreated bronchial asthma or bronchospasm, including severe COPD. Pregnancy Category: [C]
Interactions: Barbiturates: Decreased bioavailability of propranolol.
Cimetidine: Increased propranolol levels.
Clonidine: Attenuation or reversal of antihypertensive effect; potentially life-threatening increases in BP, especially on withdrawal.
Epinephrine: Initial hypertensive episode followed by bradycardia.
Ergot derivatives: Peripheral ischemia, manifested by cold extremities and possible gangrene.
Hydralazine: Increased serum levels of both drugs.
Insulin: Prolonged hypoglycemia with masking of symptoms.
Lidocaine: Increased lidocaine levels, leading to toxicity.
NSAIDs: Some agents may impair antihypertensive effect.
Phenothiazines: Increased effects of either drug.
Prazosin: Increased orthostatic hypotension.
Methimazole, propafenone, propylthiouracil, quinidine: Increased effects of propranolol.
Rifabutin, rifampin: Decreased effects of propranolol.
Theophylline: Reduces elimination of theophylline; pharmacologic antagonism.
Verapamil: Increased effects of both drugs.

Propranolol HCl/ Hydrochlorothiazide (HCTZ)

Antihypertensive combination

Indications: Management of hypertension.
Dose: The fixed combination is not indicated for initial therapy. The combination may be substituted for the titrated components.
Adults: PO HCTZ can be given at 12.5 to 50 mg/day when used alone. The initial propranolol dose is 80 mg/day and may be increased gradually until optimal BP control is achieved. The usual effective dose when used alone is 160 to 480 mg/day. One Inderide tablet bid can be used to administer up to 160 mg propranolol and 50 mg HCTZ. For propranolol doses greater than 160 mg, the combination products are inappropriate because their use would lead to excessive doses of HCTZ.
Trade names: Inderide Tablets 40 mg propranolol/25 mg HCTZ
Warnings: Cardiogenic shock; sinus bradycardia and greater than first-degree block; bronchial asthma; CHF (unless failure is secondary to a tachy-arrhythmia treatable with propranolol); anuria; hypersensitivity to sulfonamide-derived drugs or any component of this product. Pregnancy Category: [C]
Interactions: Propranolol:
Aluminum hydroxide: May decrease intestinal absorption of propranolol.
Antipyrine, lidocaine: May reduce the clearance of propranolol.
Calcium-channel blocking agent (eg, verapamil): May have additive of synergistic effects with propranolol, depressing myocardial contractility or atrioventricular conduction.
Catecholamine-depleting drugs (eg, reserpine): May produce excessive reduction of resting sympathetic nervous activity, which may result in hypotension, marked bradycardia, vertigo, syncopal attacks, or orthostatic hypotension.
Chlorpromazine: Increased plasma concentrations of both chlorpromazine and propranolol.
Cimetidine: May decrease the metabolism of propranolol, delaying elimination and increasing the blood level.
Ethanol: May slow the rate of propranolol absorption.
Haloperidol: Hypotension and cardiac arrest have been reported with concurrent use of propranolol.
Phenobarbital, phenytoin, rifampin: May increase the rate of propranolol elimination.
Theophylline: Plasma levels may be increased by propranolol; in addition, propranolol may antagonize the effect of theophylline.
Thyroxine: May result in lower T -3 concentrations when used concomitantly with propranolol.
HCTZ:
Alcohol, barbiturates, narcotics: Increased risk of orthostatic hypotension.
Antidiabetic agents (oral agents and insulin): Dosage adjustment of antidiabetic agent may be necessary.
Antihypertensive agent: Additive or potentiation of effects.
Cholestyramine, colestipol resins: Impaired absorption of HCTZ.
Corticosteroids, ACTH: Increased electrolyte depletion, increasing the risk of hypokalemia.
Lithium: Renal clearance of lithium may be reduced, increasing the risk of lithium toxicity.
Nondepolarizing skeletal muscle relaxants (eg, tubocurarine): Increased effect of the muscle relaxant.
Nonsteroidal anti-inflammatory agents: The diuretic, natriuretic, and antihypertensive effects of loop, potassium-sparing, and thiazide diuretics may be reduced.
Pressor amines (eg, norepinephrine): Decreased responsiveness to the pressor amine.

Propylthiouracil

Antithyroid

Indications: Long-term therapy of hyperthyroidism; amelioration of hyperthyroidism in preparation for subtotal thyroidectomy or radioactive iodine therapy; when thyroidectomy is contraindicated or not advisable.

Unlabeled indication: Management of alcoholic liver disease.
Dose: Adults: PO The initial dose is 300 mg/day in 3 equal doses q 8 hr. In patients with severe hyperthyroidism or very large goiters, initial dose is usually 400 mg/day, occasionally up to 600 to 900 mg/ day. The maintenance dose is 100 to 150 mg/day in divided doses q 8 hr.
Children over 10 yr: PO The initial dose is 150 to 300 mg/day in divided doses q 8 hr. The maintenance dose is determined by response.
Children 6 to 10 yr: PO The initial dose is 50 to 150 mg/day in divided doses q 8 hr.
Alternate Dosing for Children: PO The initial dose is 5 to 7 mg/kg/day in divided doses q 8 hr. The maintenance dose is 1/3 to 2/3 initial dose, beginning when patient is euthyroid.
Trade names:
Warnings: Hypersensitivity to antithyroid drugs; lactating women. Pregnancy Category: [D]
Interactions: Anticoagulants: Altered anticoagulant action.
Beta blockers: Increased effects of beta blockers.

Digitalis glycosides: Increased digitalis levels, resulting in toxicity.
Theophylline: Altered theophylline clearance in hyperthyroid or hypothyroid patients.

Protriptyline HCl

Tricyclic antidepressant

Indications: Relief of symptoms of mental depression in patients who are under close medical supervision.

Unlabeled indication: Treatment of obstructive sleep apnea and panic disorder.

Dose: Adults: PO 15 to 60 mg/day in divided doses. The maintenance dose may be given as a single dose.
Elderly and Adolescents: PO The initial dose is 5 mg tid. Increase slowly if needed.

Trade names: Vivactil Tablets 5 mg

Warnings: Hypersensitivity to tricyclic antidepressants. Generally not to be given in combination with or within 14 days of treatment with MAO inhibitors, nor during acute recovery phases of MI. Pregnancy Category: [Pregnancy category undetermined]

Interactions: Cimetidine, fluoxetine: Increased protriptyline blood levels and effects.
CNS depressants: Additive depressant effects.
Clonidine: Hypertensive crisis.
Dicumarol: Increased anticoagulant actions.
Guanethidine: Inhibition of hypotensive action by guanethidine.
MAO inhibitors: Hyperexcitability, hyperthermia, convulsions, and death may occur.
Sympathomimetics, direct-acting (eg, norepinephrine, phenylephrine): Increased pressor response.
Sympathomimetics, indirect-acting (eg, dopamine, ephedrine): Decreased pressor response.

Pseudoephedrine HCl/Guaifenesin/ Dextromethorphan HBr

Decongestant / Expectorant / Antitussive

Indications: Temporary relief of nasal congestion and cough associated with respiratory tract infections and related conditions, such as sinusitis, pharyngitis, bronchitis, and asthma, when these conditions are complicated by tenacious mucus or mucus plugs and congestion.

Dose: Adults and Children over 12 yr: PO 1 or 2 tablets q 12 hr (max, 4 tablets in 24 hr) or up to 2 tsp of syrup 3 to 4 times daily.
Children 6 to 12 yr: PO 1 tablet q 12 hr (max, 2 tablets in 24 hr) or up to 1 tsp 3 to 4 times daily, not to exceed 4 mg per kilogram of body weight of pseudoephedrine in 24 hr.

Trade names: PanMist-DM Syrup 15 mg dextromethorphan HBr, 100 mg guaifenesin, 40 mg pseudoephedrine HCl per 5 mL

Warnings: Hypertension; severe coronary artery disease; MAO inhibitor therapy; pregnancy; nursing; hypersensitivity to any component of product or idiosyncrasy to sympathomimetic amines, which may manifest as insomnia, dizziness, weakness, tremor, or arrhythmias. Pregnancy Category: [C]

Interactions: Digitalis: Ectopic pacemaker activity may be increased by pseudoephedrine.
Guanethidine, mecamylamine, methyldopa, reserpine, veratrum alkaloids: Antihypertensive effects may be reduced by pseudoephedrine.
Kaolin: May increase pseudoephedrine absorption.
MAO Inhibitors (eg, isocarboxazid): May increase the effects of pseudoephedrine. Dextromethorphan is contraindicated with MAO inhibitors.

Pyrazinamide

Anti-infective / Antitubercular

Indications: Initial treatment of active tuberculosis in adults and selected children when combined with other antituberculosis agents.

Dose: Adults: PO 15 to 30 mg/kg qd (max, 2 g/day) or 50 to 70 mg/kg 2 times/week (max, 4 g/dose) or 50 to 70 mg/kg 3 times/wk (max, 3 g).
Children: PO 15 to 30 mg/kg qd (max, 2 g/day) or 50 to 70 mg/kg 2 times/wk (max, 4 g) or 50 to 70 mg/kg 3 times/wk (max, 3 g).

Trade names: Pyrazinamide Tablets 500 mg

Warnings: Severe hepatic damage; acute gout. Pregnancy Category: [C]

Interactions: None well documented.

Pyridostigmine Bromide

Cholinergic muscle stimulant / Anticholinesterase

Indications: Treatment of myasthenia gravis; reversal agent or antagonist to nondepolarizing muscle relaxants such as curariform drugs and gallamine triethiodide (IV only).

Dose: Adults: PO Individualize dosage to meet the needs of the patients.
Syrup/Conventional tablet: Average dose is ten 5 mL tsp (60 mg/5 mL) daily or ten 60 mg tablets spaced to provide max relief when max strength is needed (range is usually 1 to 25 tablets or tsp/day).
Extended-release tablets: One to three 180 mg tablets, qd or bid with at least 6 hr between doses.
IV To supplement oral dosage preoperatively and postoperatively during labor and postpartum, during myasthenic crisis, or when oral therapy is impractical, give approximately 1/30 the oral dose, either IM or very slow IV.
Neonates: IV Neonates of myasthenic mothers may have transient difficulty in swallowing, sucking, and breathing. Injectable pyridostigmine may be indicated (by symptoms and use of the edrophonium test) until syrup can be taken. Dosage requirements range from 0.05 to 0.15 mg/kg IM.
Reversal of Nondepolarizing Muscle Relaxants:
Injection: Give atropine sulfate (0.6 to 1.2 mg) IV immediately prior to pyridostigmine to minimize side effects. Pyridostigmine 10 or 20 mg IV is usually sufficient. Full recovery usually occurs in no more than 15 min but at least 30 min may be required.

Trade names: Mestinon Tablets 60 mg

Warnings: Mechanical intestinal or urinary obstruction; hypersensitivity to anticholinesterase agents. Pregnancy Category: [C]

Interactions: Atropine: May mask signs of overdosage, leading to inadvertent induction of cholinergic crisis.
Corticosteroids: The therapeutic effects of pyridostigmine may be antagonized.
Succinylcholine: Neuromuscular blockade produced by succinylcholine may be prolonged or antagonized.

Quetiapine Fumarate

Antipsychotic

Indications: Treatment of schizophrenia; short-term treatment of acute manic episodes associated with bipolar I disorder.

Dose: Acute Bipolar Mania:
Adults: PO Start with 100 mg/day in bid divided doses on day 1, increase to 400 mg/day on day 4 in increments of up to 100 mg/day in bid divided doses. Further dosage adjustments up to 800 mg/day by day 6 should be in increments no greater than 200 mg/day. Safety of doses greater than 800 mg/day has not been evaluated.
Schizophrenia:
Adults: PO 25 mg bid initially; may increase by 25 to 50 mg bid to tid on the second and third day to

target range of 300 to 400 mg/day by the fourth day. Therapeutic dose range is 150 to 750 mg/day.
With Hepatic Impairment:
Adults: PO Start with 25 mg/day; increase in daily increments of 25 to 50 mg/day to an effective dose.
Trade names: Seroquel Tablets 25 mg
Warnings: Standard considerations. Pregnancy Category: [C]
Interactions: Antihypertensive agents: Hypotensive effects may be enhanced.
Alcohol, CNS-acting drugs: Possible additive CNS depressant effects; use with caution.
Dopamine agonists (eg, ropinirole, pramipexole), levodopa: Quetiapine may antagonize therapeutic effects of dopamine agonists and levodopa.
Hepatic enzyme inducers (eg, carbamazepine, barbiturates, phenytoin, rifampin, glucocorticoids): May decrease the effects of quetiapine; increased doses of quetiapine may be necessary to maintain control of psychotic symptoms.
Inhibitors of CYP3A (eg, ketoconazole, itraconazole, fluconazole, erythromycin): May increase the effects of quetiapine; use with caution.
Lorazepam: Quetiapine increases the effects of lorazepam.
Thioridazine: May decrease the effects of quetiapine.

Quinidine

Antiarrhythmic

Indications: Treatment of premature atrial, atrioventricular junctional, and ventricular contractions; treatment of paroxysmal supraventricular tachycardia, paroxysmal atrioventricular junctional rhythm, atrial flutter, paroxysmal and chronic atrial fibrillation, and paroxysmal ventricular tachycardia not associated with complete heart block; maintenance therapy after electrical conversion of atrial fibrillation or flutter.
Quinidine gluconate (IV administration): Treatment of life-threatening Plasmodium falciparum malaria.
Dose: The following oral doses are expressed as quinidine sulfate salt:
Premature Atrial and Ventricular Contractions:
Adults: PO 200 to 300 mg tid/qid.
Children: PO 30 mg/kg/day or 900 mg/m^2 /day in 5 divided doses.
Paroxysmal Supraventricular Tachycardia:
Adults: PO 400 to 600 mg q 2 to 3 hr until event is abated.
Atrial Flutter: Administer after digitalization and individualize dose.
Conversion of Atrial Fibrillation:
Adults: PO 200 mg q 2 to 3 hr for 5 to 8 doses, then maintain with 200 to 300 mg tid to qid (immediate-release tablets) or 300 to 600 mg bid to tid (sustained-release tablets); do not exceed 3 to 4 g/day.
Quinidine Gluconate:
Adults: PO 324 to 648 mg (1 to 2 tablets) q 8 to 12 hr.
Quinidine Polygalacturonate:
Adults: PO Maintenance dose: 275 mg q 8 to 12 hr.
Parenteral Quinidine Gluconate:
Acute Tachycardia:
Adults: IM 600 mg initially, then 400 mg prn up to q 2 hr.
Children: IV 2 to 10 mg/kg/dose q 3 to 6 hr prn.
P. falciparum Malaria:
Adults: IV 15 mg/kg infused over 4 hr initially, then 7.5 mg/kg over 4 hr q 8 hr for 7 days or until oral therapy can be instituted or 10 mg/kg over 1 to 2 hr initially, then 0.02 mg/kg/min for up to 72 hr or until oral therapy can be instituted.
Trade names: Quinidex Extentabs Tablets, sustained-release 300 mg
Quinora Tablets 300 mg
Quinaglute Dura-Tabs Tablets, sustained-release 324 mg
Quinalan Tablets, sustained-release 324 mg
Cardioquin Tablets 275 mg (equiv. to 200 mg sulfate)
Warnings: Myasthenia gravis; history of thrombocytopenic purpura associated with quinidine administration; digitalis intoxication; complete heart block; left bundle branch block; complete atrioventricular (AV) block with AV nodal or idioventricular pacemaker; aberrant ectopic impulses and abnormal rhythms because of escape mechanisms; history of drug-induced torsade de pointes; history of long QT syndrome. Pregnancy Category: [C]
Interactions: Amiodarone, antacids, cimetidine, verapamil: May increase quinidine levels.
Anticoagulants: May increase effect of anticoagulant; may cause hemorrhage.
Barbiturates, nifedipine, primidone, sucralfate: May decrease quinidine levels.
Beta-blockers: May increase effect of beta-blocker.
Dextromethorphan: May increase plasma dextromethorphan concentrations.
Digitoxin, digoxin: May increase digoxin plasma levels.
Hydantoins: May reduce therapeutic effect of quinidine.
Nondepolarizing neuromuscular blocking agents, succinylcholine: May increase neuromuscular blockade effect.
Propafenone: Increased propafenone levels.
Rifampin: May increase quinidine metabolism.

Quinine Sulfate

Anti-infective / Antimalarial

Indications: Treatment of chloroquine-resistant falciparum malaria; alternative treatment for chloroquine-sensitive strains of *P. falciparum*, *P. malariae*, *P. ovale*, and *P. uivae*.

Unlabeled indication: Prevention and treatment of nocturnal recumbency leg cramps.
Dose: Chloroquine-resistant *P. falciparum* Malaria:
Adults: PO 650 mg q 8 hr for 5 to 7 days.
Children: PO 25 mg/kg/day in divided doses q 8 hr for 5 to 7 days.
Chloroquine-Sensitive Malaria:
Adults: PO 600 mg q 8 hr for 5 to 7 days.
Children: PO 10 mg/kg q 8 hr for 5 to 7 days.
Nocturnal Leg Cramps:
Adults: PO 260 to 300 mg at bedtime.
Trade names: Quinine sulfate Capsules 200 mg
Warnings: G-6-PD deficiency; optic neuritis; tinnitus; history of blackwater fever and thrombocytopenic purpura associated with previous quinine ingestion; pregnancy. Pregnancy Category: [X]
Interactions: Aluminum-containing antacids: Causes delayed or decreased quinine absorption.
Anticoagulants, oral: May cause depression of hepatic enzyme system that synthesizes vitamin K-dependent clotting factors and may enhance action of oral anticoagulants.
Cimetidine: May reduce quinine's clearance and prolong its half-life in body.
Digoxin: May cause increased digoxin serum concentration.
Mefloquine: May cause ECG abnormalities or cardiac arrest and may increase risk of convulsions. Do not use concurrently. Delay administration 12 hr after last dose of quinine.
Neuromuscular blocking agents: May potentiate neuromuscular blockade and may result in respiratory difficulties.
Urinary alkalinizers: May increase quinine serum concentrations and potentiate toxicity.

Quinapril HCl

Antihypertensive / Angiotensin-converting enzyme (ACE) inhibitor

Indications: Treatment of hypertension; adjunctive therapy of CHF.
Dose: CHF:
Adults: PO 5 mg bid initially; may increase dose

weekly for clinical control, usually 20 to 40 mg in 2 equally divided doses.
Renal Function Impairment: Initial dose is 5 mg with Ccr more than 30 mL/min or 2.5 mg with Ccr 10 to 30 mL/min. If well tolerated, it may be given the following day as a bid regimen. In the absence of excessive hypotension or significant deterioration of renal function, the dose may be increased at weekly intervals based on clinical and hemodynamic response.
Hypertension:
Adults: PO 10 or 20 mg qd initially; adjust dosage at intervals of at least 2 wk.
Adults (maintenance): PO 20, 40, or 80 mg/day as single dose or 2 equally divided doses.
Elderly: PO 10 mg qd followed by titration to the optimal response.
Renal Function Impairment: Initial dose varies based on Ccr: more than 60 mL/min is 10 mg; 30 to 60 mL/min is 5 mg; 10 to 30 mL/min is 2.5 mg.

Trade names: Accupril Tablets 5 mg

Warnings: Hypersensitivity to ACE inhibitors; history of angioedema related to previous treatment with an ACE inhibitor. Pregnancy Category: [D (second, third trimester); C (first trimester) Avoid use in pregnant patients and discontinue drug as soon as pregnancy is detected
closely observe infants with histories of in utero exposure]

Interactions: Antacids: Quinapril bioavailability may be decreased. Separate administration times by 1 to 2 hr.
Capsaicin: Cough may be exacerbated.
Digoxin: May cause increased or decreased digoxin levels.
Diuretics: Increased risk of hypotension.
Food: Food (especially fat) reduces bioavailability of quinapril.
Indomethacin, salicylates (eg, aspirin): May reduce hypotensive effects, especially in low renin or volume-dependent hypertensive patients.
Lithium: May cause increased lithium levels and symptoms of lithium toxicity.
Loop diuretics: Effects of loop diuretics may be decreased.
Phenothiazines: Enhanced hypotensive effect.
Potassium supplements and potassium-sparing diuretics: Hyperkalemia.
Tetracycline: Decreased tetracycline absorption.

Quinapril HCl/ Hydrochlorothiazide (HCTZ)

Antihypertensive combination

Indications: Treatment of hypertension.

Dose: The fixed combination is not indicated for initial therapy. The combination may be substituted for the titrated components.
Adults: PO Quinapril monotherapy is an effective treatment of hypertension over a dose range of 10 to 80 mg/day administered qd. HCTZ is effective in doses of 12.5 to 50 mg qd. Patients whose BP is not adequately controlled with quinapril monotherapy may be given quinapril/HCTZ (10/12.5 or 20/12.5). Further increases in dose of either or both components depend on the clinical response. Generally, the dose of HCTZ should not be increased until 2 to 3 wk have elapsed.
Renal Function Impairment:
Adults: No adjustment required as long as Ccr is greater than 30 mL/min; in severe renal impairment, loop diuretics are preferred to thiazides.

Trade names: Accuretic Tablets 10 mg quinapril/12.5 mg HCTZ

Warnings: Patients with a history of angioedema related to previous treatment with an ACE inhibitor; patients with anuria; hypersensitivity to sulfonamide-derived drugs or any component of the product. Pregnancy Category: [D (second and third trimester); C (first trimester) ACE inhibitors (eg, quinapril) can cause injury or death to fetus if used during second or third trimester When pregnancy is detected, discontinue as soon as possible]

Interactions: ACTH, corticosteroids: Electrolyte depletion may be intensified, especially hypokalemia.
Alcohol, barbiturates (eg, phenobarbital), narcotics: Orthostatic hypotension may be potentiated.
Anticoagulants (eg, warfarin): Anticoagulant effect may be decreased.
Antidiabetic agents (eg, insulin, sulfonylureas), antigout agents (eg, probenecid): Dosage adjustment may be necessary because of possible HCTZ-induced elevation in blood glucose levels.
Cardiac glycosides (eg, digoxin): Possible digitalis toxicity associated with hypokalemia.
Cholestyramine, colestipol: May impair the absorption of HCTZ.
Insulin: In diabetic patients, requirements of insulin may be increased, decreased, or unchanged.
Lithium: Plasma levels of lithium may be elevated, increasing the risk of toxicity.
NSAIDs: May reduce the natriuretic and antihypertensive effect of HCTZ.
Potassium supplements, potassium-sparing diuretics (eg, spironolactone): Increased risk of hyperkalemia.
Nondepolarizing muscle relaxants (eg, tubocurarine): Effects may be increased.
Pressor amines (eg, norepinephrine): Response to pressor amines may be decreased.
Tetracycline and other drugs that interact with magnesium: Because of the magnesium content in quinapril, absorption of tetracycline may be reduced, decreasing the therapeutic effect.

Rabeprazole Sodium

Gastrointestinal / Proton Pump Inhibitor

Indications: Short-term treatment in healing and symptomatic relief of duodenal ulcers and erosive or ulcerative gastroesophageal reflux disease (GERD); maintaining healing and reducing relapse rates of heartburn symptoms in patients with GERD; treatment of daytime and nighttime heartburn and other symptoms associated with GERD; long-term treatment of pathological hypersecretory conditions, including Zollinger-Ellison syndrome in combination with amoxicillin and clarithromycin to eradicate *H. pylori*.

Dose: Treatment of Erosive or Ulcerative GERD:
Adults: PO 20 mg/day for 4 to 8 wk, an additional 8 wk may be considered for patients who do not heal.
Maintenance of Erosive or Ulcerative GERD:
Adults: PO 20 mg/day.
Healing of Duodenal Ulcers:
Adults: PO 20 mg/day after the morning meal for 4 wk, additional therapy may be required for some patients.
Treatment of Pathological Hypersecretory Conditions:
Adults: PO 60 mg/day. Doses up to 100 mg qd or 60 mg bid have been administered.
H. pylori Eradication to Reduce Risk of Duodenal Ulcer Recurrence:
Adults: PO 20 mg rabeprazole plus amoxicillin 1000 mg plus clarithromycin 500 mg bid for 7 days with morning and evening meals.

Trade names: Aciphex Tablets, delayed-release 20 mg

Warnings: Known hypersensitivity to substituted benzimidazoles. Pregnancy Category: [B]

Interactions: Drugs dependent on gastric pH for absorption (eg, digoxin, ketoconazole): Plasma levels of digoxin may be increased, while ketoconazole concentrations may be decreased.

Rabies Immune Globulin, Human

Immune serum

Indications: Passive, transient postexposure prevention of rabies infection in susceptible individuals.

Dose: Adults and children: IM 20 IU/kg (0.133 mL/kg) as soon as possible after exposure, preferably with first dose of vaccine.

Trade names: Hyperab Injection 150 IU/mL
Imogam Injection 150 IU/mL

Warnings: Repeated doses once vaccine treatment has been initiated. RIG may theoretically be contraindicated in people who have had life-threatening reactions to human IgG antibody products or any RIG components. Previous complete immunization with rabies vaccine and presence of adequate antibody titer.
Pregnancy Category: [C]

Interactions: Measles, mumps, polio, or rubella live vaccines: Other antibodies in RIG preparation may interfere with response to these live vaccines.

Raloxifene Hydrochloride

Selective estrogen receptor modulator

Indications: For the prevention and treatment of osteoporosis in postmenopausal women.

Dose: Adult women: PO 60 mg qd.

Trade names: Evista Tablets 60 mg

Warnings: Women who are or may become pregnant; women with active or history of venous thromboembolic events, including deep venous thrombosis, pulmonary embolism, and retinal vein thrombosis; allergy to raloxifene or other constituents of the tablet; coadministration of cholestyramine.
Pregnancy Category: [X]

Interactions: Cholestyramine: Major reduction in absorption and enterohepatic cycling of raloxifene; avoid concurrent use.
Highly protein-bound drugs (eg, clofibrate, indomethacin, naproxen, ibuprofen, diazepam, diazoxide): May displace raloxifene from protein-binding sites, increasing the effects of raloxifene.
Warfarin: Raloxifene may decrease anticoagulant effect.

Ramipril

Antihypertensive / Angiotensin converting enzyme (ACE inhibitor)

Indications: Treatment of hypertension; for stable patients who have demonstrated clinical signs of CHF within the first few days after sustaining acute MI; reduce risk of MI, stroke, or death from CV causes in patients at high risk.

Dose: Heart Failure Post-MI:
Adults: PO 2.5 mg bid. Switch to 1.25 mg bid if hypotension occurs. Titrate to target dose of 5 mg bid.
Hypertension:
Adults: PO Initial dose is 2.5 mg qd initially. Maintenance dose is 2.5 to 20 mg/day as single dose or in 2 equally divided doses.
Patients with Renal Impairment: PO 1.25 mg qd in patients with Ccr below 40 mL/min (serum creatinine higher than 2.5 mg/dL; max, 5 mg/day).
Reduction in Risk of MI, Stroke, and Death from CV Causes:
Adults: PO Initial dose is 2.5 mg qd for 1 wk, 5 mg qd for 3 wk, then increase the dose as tolerated to maintenance dose. Maintenance dose is 10 mg qd or in divided doses if patient is hypertensive or recently post-MI.

Trade names: Altace Capsules 1.25 mg
Warnings: Hypersensitivity to ACE inhibitors (particularly history of angioedema). Pregnancy Category: [D (second, third trimester); C (first trimester) Discontinue use in pregnant patients; fetal/neonatal injury and death have occurred Closely observe infants with histories of in utero exposure]

Interactions: Antacids: Ramipril bioavailability may be decreased. Separate administration times by 1 to 2 hr.
Capsaicin: May exacerbate cough.
Digoxin: Increased or decreased digoxin levels.
Diuretics: Increased risk of hypotension.
Indomethacin, salicylates (eg, aspirin): May reduce hypotensive effects, especially in low-renin or volume-dependent hypertensive patients.
Lithium: May cause increased lithium levels and symptoms of lithium toxicity.
Loop diuretics: Effects of loop diuretics may be decreased.
Phenothiazines: Enhanced hypotensive effects.
Potassium supplements, potassium-sparing diuretics: May cause increased potassium serum levels.

Repaglinide

Antidiabetic / Meglitinide

Indications: Adjunct to diet and exercise to lower blood glucose in patients with non-insulin dependent diabetes mellitus (type 2) whose hyperglycemia cannot be controlled by diet and exercise alone. Can be used with metformin or thiazolidinediones (eg, rosiglitazone) when hyperglycemia cannot be controlled by exercise, diet, and either agent alone.

Dose: No fixed dosage regimen; periodically monitor blood glucose to determine minimum effective dose.
Patients Not Previously Treated or Whose $HbA1_C$ is Less Than 8%:
Adults: PO Initial dose is 0.5 mg with each meal.
Patients Previously Treated or Whose $HbA1_C$ is More Than 8%:
Adults: PO Initial dose 1 to 2 mg with each meal.
Combination therapy:
Adults: PO The starting dose and dosage adjustments for combination therapy are the same as repaglinide monotherapy.

Trade names: Prandin Tablets 0.5 mg

Warnings: Insulin-dependent (type 1) diabetes; diabetic ketoacidosis with or without coma; hypersensitivity to repaglinide or its ingredients.
Pregnancy Category: [C Insulin is recommended to maintain blood glucose levels during pregnancy]

Interactions: Barbiturates, carbamazepine, rifampin, troglitazone: May increase repaglinide metabolism.
Erythromycin, ketoconazole, miconazole: May inhibit repaglinide metabolism.
Protein bound drugs (eg, NSAIDs, salicylates, sulfonamides, probenecid, MAO inhibitors, beta-adrenergic blocking agents): May potentiate hypoglycemic effect of repaglinide.

Reserpine/Hydralazine Hydrochloride/ Hydrochlorothiazide

Antihypertensive / Vasodilator / Thiazide diuretic

Indications: Treatment of hypertension.

Dose: Adults: PO Dosage should be determined by individual titration (max, 0.25 mg reserpine/day).

Trade names: Hydrap-ES Tablets 15 mg hydrochlorothiazide, 0.1 mg reserpine, and 25 mg hydralazine HCl
Ser-Ap-Es Tablets 15 mg hydrochlorothiazide, 0.1 mg reserpine, and 25 mg hydralazine HCl

Warnings: Hypersensitivity to any components of product; hypersensitivity to sulfonamide-derived drugs; mental depression or history of mental depression; active peptic ulcer; ulcerative colitis; patients receiving electroconvulsive therapy; coronary artery disease; mitral valvular rheumatic heart disease; anuria.
Pregnancy Category: [C]

Interactions: Reserpine:
Digoxin, quinidine: Risk of cardiac arrhythmias may be increased.
Direct- (eg, epinephrine) and indirect- (eg, amphetamines) acting amines: The effects of direct-acting amines may be prolonged while the effects of indirect-acting amines may be inhibited.

MAO inhibitors: Avoid concurrent use or use with extreme caution.
Tricyclic antidepressants: Antihypertensive effects of reserpine may be decreased.
Hydralazine:
MAO inhibitors: Use with caution.
Potent parenteral antihypertensive agents (eg, diazoxide): Profound hypotensive episodes may occur.
Hydrochlorothiazide:
Insulin: Insulin requirements may be increased, decreased, or unchanged.
Lithium: Renal clearance of lithium may be decreased, increasing the risk of toxicity.
Methyldopa: The risk of hemolytic anemia may be increased.
Norepinephrine: Arterial responsiveness may be decreased by hydrochlorothiazide.
NSAIDs (eg, indomethacin): The diuretic, natriuretic, and antihypertensive effect of hydrochlorothiazide may be reduced.
Tubocurarine: Responsiveness to tubocurarine may be decreased.

Reteplase, Recombinant

Tissue plasminogen activator

Indications: Management of acute MI, to reduce incidence of CHF and mortality associated with an acute MI.

Dose: Adults: IV 10 + 10 U double-bolus injection, each bolus given over 2 min. The second bolus given 30 min after initiation of the first.

Trade names: Retavase Powder for injection, lyophilized 10.4 U (18.1 mg)

Warnings: Active internal bleeding; history of cerebrovascular accident; recent intracranial or intraspinal surgery or trauma; intracranial neoplasm, arteriovenous malformation or aneurysm; bleeding diathesis or severe uncontrolled hypertension because thrombolytic therapy increases the risk of bleeding. Pregnancy Category: [C]

Interactions: Abciximab, aspirin, dipyridamole, heparin, vitamin K antagonists: May increase the risk of bleeding.
Incompatability:
Heparin: Do not add other medications to the same IV.

Riboflavin

Vitamin

Indications: Prevention and treatment of riboflavin deficiency.

Dose: Supplement:
Adults: PO 1.4 to 1.8 mg (men), 1.2 to 1.3 mg (women), 1.6 to 1.8 mg (pregnant or lactating women).
Children: PO 0.8 to 1.2 mg/day.
Treatment of Deficiency:
Adults: PO 5 to 10 mg/day.
Children: PO 2 to 10 mg/day.

Trade names: Riboflavin Tablets 50 mg

Warnings: None well documented. Pregnancy Category: [A (C in doses that exceed the RDA)]

Interactions: None well documented.

Rifabutin

Anti-infective / Antitubercular

Indications: Prevention of disseminated *Mycobacterium avium* complex (MAC) disease in patients with advanced HIV infection.

Dose: Adults: PO 300 to 450 mg once daily.
Infants and Children: PO Up to 5 mg/kg/day.

Trade names: Mycobutin Capsules 150 mg

Warnings: Hypersensitivity to rifabutin or other rifamycins; active tuberculosis. Pregnancy Category: [B]

Interactions: Azole antifungal agents, benzodiazepines, beta blockers, buspirone, chloramphenicol, clarithromycin, clozapine, oral contraceptives, corticosteroids, cyclosporine, delavirdine, digitoxin, disopyramide, doxycycline, erythromycin, estrogens, haloperidol, hydantoins, indinavir, losartan, methadone, mexiletine, morphine, nelfinavir, ondansetron, oral anticoagulants, quinidine, quinine, ritonavir, sulfonylureas, tacrolimus, tamoxifen, theophyllines, tocainide, toremifene, tricyclic antidepressants, troleandomycin, verapamil, zolpidem: Therapeutic efficacy may be decreased because of liver enzyme-inducing properties of rifabutin.
Indinavir, itraconazole, ritonavir: May elevate rifabutin plasma levels, increasing the risk of side effects.
Ketoconazole: May reduce rifabutin plasma levels, decreasing the therapeutic effects.
Zidovudine: May decrease plasma levels of zidovudine.

Rifampin

Anti-infective / Antitubercular

Indications: Adjunctive treatment of tuberculosis; short-term management to eliminate meningococci from nasopharynx in *Neisseria meningitidis* carriers.

Unlabeled indication: Treatment of infections caused by *Staphylococcus aureus* and *Staphylococcus epidermidis*; treatment of gram-negative bacteremia in infancy; treatment of *Legionella*; management of leprosy; prophylaxis of *Haemophilus influenzae* meningitis.

Dose: Tuberculosis: IV dosage form is for initial treatment or retreatment when drug cannot be taken by mouth.
Adults: PO/IV 10 mg/kg/day (max, 600 mg/day) or 10 mg/kg 2 or 3 times/wk (max, 600 mg).
Children: PO/IV 10 to 20 mg/kg/day (max, 600 mg/day) or 10 to 20 mg/kg 2 to 3 times/wk (max, 600 mg).
Meningococcal Carriers:
Adults: PO/IV 600 mg qd for 4 consecutive days.
Children 1 mo or older: PO/IV 10 mg/kg q 12 hr for 2 consecutive days.
Children younger than 1 mo: 5 mg/kg q 12 hr for 2 consecutive days.

Trade names: Rifadin Capsules 150 mg
Rimactane Capsules 300 mg

Warnings: Hypersensitivity to any rifamycin. Pregnancy Category: [C]

Interactions: Azole antifungal agents, benzodiazepines, beta-blockers, buspirone, chloramphenicol, clarithromycin, clozapine, oral contraceptives, corticosteroids, cyclosporine, delavirdine, digitoxin, disopyramide, doxycycline, erythromycin, estrogens, haloperidol, hydantoins, indinavir, losartan, methadone, mexiletine, morphine, nelfinavir, ondansetron, oral anticoagulants, quinidine, quinine, ritonavir, sulfonylureas, tacrolimus, tamoxifen, theophyllines, tocainide, toremifene, tricyclic antidepressants, troleandomycin, verapamil, zolpidem: Therapeutic efficacy may be decreased because of liver enzyme-inducing properties of rifampin.
Digoxin: May decrease digoxin serum concentrations.
Enalapril: May significantly increase BP.
Halothane: Hepatotoxicity and hepatic encephalopathy have been reported with coadministration.
Isoniazid: May result in higher rate of hepatotoxicity.
Ketoconazole: May cause treatment failure of either ketoconazole or rifampin.
Probenecid: Elevates rifampin levels.

Rifapentine

Anti-infective / Antitubercular

Indications: Treatment of pulmonary tuberculosis in conjunction with 1 or more other antituberculosis drug to which the isolate is susceptible.

Dose: Adults and Children (12 yr or older): PO Intensive phase: 600 mg twice weekly (with an interval of 3 days or more) for 2 mo. Continuation phase: 600 mg once weekly for 4 mo.

Trade names: Priftin Tablets 150 mg
Warnings: Hypersensitivity to any of the rifamycins (rifabutin, rifampin). Pregnancy Category: [C]
Interactions: Amitriptyline, azole antifungal agents, barbiturates, buspirone, chloramphenicol, clarithromycin, clofibrate, clozapine, oral contraceptives, corticosteroids, cyclosporine, dapsone, delavirdine, diazepam, digitalis glycosides, disopyramide, doxycycline, erythromycin, fluconazole, fluoroquinolones, haloperidol, indinavir, itraconazole, ketoconazole, levothyroxine, losartan, methadone, mexiletine, morphine, nelfinavir, nifedipine, nortriptyline, ondansetron, phenytoin, progestins, quinidine, quinine, ritonavir, saquinavir, sildenafil, sulfonylureas, tacrolimus, tamoxifen, theophylline, tocainide, toremifene, tricyclic antidepressants, troleandomycin, verapamil, warfarin, zidovudine, zolpidem: Has same interaction potential as rifampin. Potent inducer of hepatic drug metabolizing enzymes. Reduced levels and efficacy of target drugs may occur.
Ketoconazole: May reduce rifapentine plasma levels, decreasing the therapeutic effects.

Riluzole

Neuroprotective

Indications: Treatment of patients with amyotrophic lateral sclerosis (ALS; Lou Gehrig disease).
Dose: Adults: PO 50 mg q 12 hr.
Trade names: Rilutek Tablets 50 mg
Warnings: Standard considerations. Pregnancy Category: [C]
Interactions: Caffeine, theophylline, amitriptyline, quinolones: May reduce riluzole elimination.
Cigarette smoke, rifampin, omeprazole: May enhance riluzole elimination.

Rimantadine HCl

Anti-infective / Antiviral

Indications: Adults: Prophylaxis and treatment of infection caused by various strains of influenza A virus.

Children: Prophylaxis against influenza A virus.
Dose: Prophylaxis and Treatment:
Adults: PO 100 mg bid.
Elderly Nursing Home Patients, Hepatic and Renal Impairment (Ccr less than 10 mL/min): Reduce to 100 mg/day.
Prophylaxis:
Children 10 yr or older: PO 100 mg bid.
Children younger than 10 yr: PO 5 mg/kg/day (max, 150 mg/dose).
Trade names: Flumadine Syrup 50 mg/5 mL
Warnings: Hypersensitivity to drugs of adamantine class including rimantadine and amantadine. Pregnancy Category: [C]
Interactions: Acetaminophen, aspirin: Decreased peak serum concentration of rimantadine.
Cimetidine: Increased serum concentration caused by decreased clearance.

Risedronate Sodium

Hormone / Bisphosphonate

Indications: Treatment of osteoporosis in postmenopausal women; prevention of osteoporosis in postmenopausal women at risk of developing osteoporosis; prevention and treatment of glucocorticoid-induced osteoporosis in men and women; treatment of Paget disease of the bone.
Dose: Paget Disease:
Adults: PO 30 mg once daily for 2 mo.
Treatment and Prevention of Postmenopausal Osteoporosis; Glucocorticoid-Induced Osteoporosis:
Adults: PO 5 mg/day.
Trade names: Actonel Tablets 30 mg
Warnings: Hypocalcemia. Pregnancy Category: [C]
Interactions: Antacids, calcium supplements, oral medicines containing divalent cations: Decrease risedronate absorption, which may decrease activity.

Risperidone

Antipsychotic / Benzisoxazole

Indications: Treatment of schizophrenia; bipolar mania (oral only).
Dose: Bipolar Mania:
Adults: PO 2 to 3 mg per day on a once daily schedule. Adjust dose at intervals of no less than 24 hr in increments of 1 mg daily (max, 6 mg daily). No data to support acute treatment beyond 3 wk.
Schizophrenia:
Adults: PO 1 mg bid on first day, 2 mg bid on second day, and 3 mg bid on third day. Dosage adjustment thereafter should occur at intervals of at least 1 wk in increments of 1 mg bid. Max effect generally occurs in a range of 4 to 8 mg/day (max, 16 mg/day). IM 25 mg q 2 wk (max, 50 mg q 2 wk). Oral risperidone should be given with the first injection and continued for 3 wk to ensure adequate plasma concentrations. Do not make upward dosage adjustments more frequently than q 4 wk.
Special Populations:
Elderly and patients with renal or hepatic impairment who can tolerate at least 2 mg of oral risperidone: IM 25 mg q 2 wk.
Elderly or debilitated patients with severe renal or hepatic impairment and patients predisposed to hypotension or for whom hypotension would pose a risk: PO 0.5 mg bid initially; increase in 0.5 mg increments bid thereafter. Increases above 1.5 mg bid should generally occur at intervals of at least 1 wk.
Trade names: Risperdal Tablets 0.25 mg
Risperdal Consta Powder for Injection 25 mg
Risperdal M-TAB Tablets, orally disintegrating 0.5 mg
Warnings: Standard considerations. Pregnancy Category: [C]
Interactions: Alcohol, CNS depressants: May cause additive CNS depressant effects.
Antihypertensives: Risperidone may enhance hypotensive effects of some antihypertensives.
Carbamazepine: May decrease risperidone plasma levels.
Clozapine, fluoxetine, paroxetine: May increase risperidone plasma levels.
Levodopa and other dopamine agonists: The effects of levodopa and other dopamine agonists may be antagonized.

Ritodrine Hydrochloride

Uterine relaxant

Indications: Management of preterm labor in suitable patients.
Dose: Adults: IV 0.05 mg/min initially, increasing by 0.05 mg/min q 10 min until desired result is obtained. The usual effective dose is between 0.15 to 0.35 mg/min, continued for at least 12 hr after uterine contractions cease.
Trade names: Ritodrine HCl in 5% Dextrose Injection 0.3 mg/mL
Yutopar Injection 10 mg/mL
Warnings: Before 20th wk of pregnancy and when continuation of pregnancy is hazardous to mother or fetus; hypersensitivity; pre-existing maternal conditions that would be seriously affected by pharmacologic properties of beta-mimetic agent. Pregnancy Category: [Contraindicated before 20th wk of pregnancy; otherwise, B]
Interactions: Atropine: Systemic hypertension may be exaggerated.
Beta-adrenergic blockers: Effects are antagonistic; avoid coadministration.
Corticosteroids: Concomitant use may lead to

pulmonary edema.
Magnesium sulfate; diazoxide; meperidine; general anesthetics: Cardiovascular effects of ritodrine may be potentiated.
Sympathomimetics: Effects may be additive or potentiated.

Rituximab

Monoclonal antibody

Indications: Relapsed or refractory low-grade or follicular, CD-20 positive, B-cell non-Hodgkin lymphoma.

Dose: Non-Hodgkin Lymphoma:
Adults: IV infusion Initial therapy: 375 mg/m² given once weekly for 4 or 8 doses.
Retreatment: Patients who subsequently develop progressive disease may be safely retreated with rituximab 375 mg/m² once weekly for 4 doses. Currently, there are limited data concerning more than 2 courses.
Pretreatment Regimens:
Adults: Give acetaminophen 650 mg (PO or rectal) and diphenhydramine 25 to 50 mg (PO or IV) 30 to 60 min before administering rituximab.

Trade names: Rituxan Solution for injection 10 mg/mL

Warnings: IgE-mediated hypersensitivity or anaphylactic reactions to murine proteins or to any component of this product. Pregnancy Category: [C]

Interactions: No specific drug interactions have been reported. Coadministration of drugs with similar pharmacologic effects may cause additive side effects, including toxicity.

Rivastigmine Tartrate

Cholinesterase inhibitor

Indications: Treatment of mild to moderate dementia of the Alzheimer type.

Dose: Adults: PO 1.5 mg twice daily initially, then the dose may be increased by increments of 1.5 mg twice daily at intervals of 2 wk or more (max, 6 mg twice daily).

Trade names: Exelon Capsules 1.5 mg (as base)

Warnings: Hypersensitivity to rivastigmine or carbamate derivatives. Pregnancy Category: [B]

Interactions: Anticholinergic drugs: Possible reduction in anticholinergic effects.
Cholinesterase inhibitors, cholinomimetics: Synergistic effects may occur.

Rizatriptan

Analgesic / Migraine

Indications: Treatment of acute migraine attacks with or without aura.

Dose: Adults: PO 5 or 10 mg tablet with the onset of migraine headache. Individualize dose based on response and side effects. Doses may be repeated after a minimum of 2 hr as needed with a max dose of 30 mg in a 24-hr period. Patients taking propanolol should receive the 5 mg dose with a max of 3 doses (15 mg) in a 24-hr period. The MLT formulation is a rapidly disintegrating tablet that may be taken without water. It is placed on the tongue where it rapidly breaks apart and can then be swallowed with normal saliva production.

Trade names: Maxalt Tablets 5 mg
Maxalt-MLT Tablets, orally disintegrating 5 mg

Warnings: Patients with ischemic heart disease (eg, angina, MI history, silent ischemia, coronary artery vasospastic disease, uncontrolled hypertension, basal or hemiplegic migraine). Rizatriptan is contraindicated within 24 hr of use with other serotonin agonists, ergotamine compounds, or methysergide, or concurrent treatment with MAO inhibitors or within 14 days following discontinuation of an MAO inhibitor.
Pregnancy Category: [C]

Interactions: 5-HT-1 agonists (eg, sumatriptan): Increased risk of vasospastic reactions; therefore, coadministration of two 5-HT_1 agonists within 24 hr of each other is contraindicated.
Ergot-containing drugs: Additive and prolonged vasospasm.
MAO inhibitors: Use of rizatriptan with MAO inhibitors or within 14 days following discontinuation of an MAO inhibitor is contraindicated.
Propanolol: Increased rizatriptan plasma concentrations.
Selective serotonin reuptake inhibitors (eg, citalopram, fluoxetine, fluvoxamine, sertraline): Weakness, hyperreflexia, and incoordination have been rarely reported.
Sibutramine: Serotonin syndrome, including CNS irritability, motor weakness, shivering, myoclonus, and altered consciousness may occur.

Rocuronium Bromide

Nondepolarizing Neuromuscular Blocking Agent

Indications: As an adjunct to general anesthesia for inpatients and outpatients to facilitate both rapid sequence and routine tracheal intubation and to provide skeletal muscle relaxation during surgery or mechanical ventilation.

Dose: Use of a peripheral nerve stimulator is recommended to monitor drug response and determine the need for additional relaxant and adequacy of spontaneous recovery or antagonism.
Continuous Infusion:
Adults: IV 0.01 to 0.012 mg/kg per min initiated only after early evidence of spontaneous recovery from the intubating dose.
Individualization of Dosage:
Children: IV 0.6 mg/kg as an initial dose in children under halothane anesthesia produces excellent to good intubating conditions within 1 min.
Maintenance dose: 0.075 to 0.125 mg/kg administered at 25% recovery of control T_1 provides relaxation for 7 to 10 min.
Elderly (65 yr of age and older): IV exhibited slightly prolonged median clinical duration under opioid/nitrous oxide/oxygen anesthesia following doses of 0.6, 0.9, and 1.2 mg/kg, respectively.
Maintenance dose: 0.1 to 0.15 mg/kg administered at 25% recovery of T_1.
Maintenance:
Adults: IV 0.1, 0.15, and 0.2 mg/kg administered at 25% recovery of control T_1 (defined as 3 twitches of train-of-four).
Rapid Sequence Intubation:
Adults: IV 0.6 to 1.2 mg/kg provides excellent to good intubating conditions in most patients in less than 2 min.
Tracheal Intubation:
Adults: IV 0.6 mg/kg as a recommended initial dose. Good intubation conditions usually occur within 2 min.

Trade names: Zemuron Injection 10 mg/mL

Warnings: Standard considerations. Pregnancy Category: [C]

Interactions: Antibiotics (eg, aminoglycoside antibiotics [eg, kanamycin], bacitracin, clindamycin, lincomycin, polymyxins, sodium colistimethate, tetracyclines), lithium, local anesthetics, magnesium salts, procainamide, quinidine: May enhance the neuromuscular blocking action of rocuronium.
Carbamazepine, phenytoin: Resistance to neuromuscular blocking action of rocuronium may occur.
Nitrous oxide/oxygen with either enflurane or isoflurane: May prolong the clinically effective duration of action of initial and maintenance doses of rocuronium and decrease the required infusion rate.
Succinylcholine: Time of onset of max block following rocuronium may be faster with prior administration of

Medications

succinylcholine.
Incompatability: Should not be mixed with alkaline solutions (eg, barbiturates) in the same syringe or administered simultaneously during IV infusion through the same needle.

Rofecoxib

Analgesic / NSAID

Indications: Relief of signs and symptoms of osteoarthritis and rheumatoid arthritis; treatment of primary dysmenorrhea; management of acute pain in adults.

Dose: Osteoarthritis:
Adults: PO 12.5 to 25 mg once daily.
Rheumatoid Arthritis:
Adults: PO 25 mg once daily (max, 25 mg/day).
Primary Dysmenorrhea and Management of Acute Pain:
Adults: PO 50 mg once daily.

Trade names: Vioxx Tablets 12.5 mg

Warnings: History of asthma, urticaria, or allergic-type reactions to aspirin or other NSAIDs. Pregnancy Category: [C Avoid in late pregnancy because rofecoxib may cause premature closure of ductus arteriosus]

Interactions: ACE inhibitors: Antihypertensive effects may be decreased.
Aspirin: Risk of GI complications (eg, ulceration) may be increased.
Lithium, methotrexate: Rofecoxib may increase plasma levels of these drugs, which may increase activity and adverse effects.
Loop diuretics, thiazide diuretics: Diuretic effects may be decreased.
Rifampin: May decrease rofecoxib plasma levels, which may cause a decrease in activity.
Warfarin: The risk of bleeding may be increased.

Ropinirole Hydrochloride

Antiparkinson / Non-ergot dopamine receptor agonist

Indications: Treatment of the signs and symptoms of idiopathic Parkinson disease. May be used in conjunction with L-dopa.

Dose: Individualize by careful titration.
Adults: PO 0.25 mg tid initially. Then dosage may be increased weekly by 0.75 mg/day until taking 3 mg/day, then by 1.5 mg/day until taking 9 mg/day, then by 3 mg/day to total dose of 24 mg/day.

Trade names: Requip Tablets 0.25 mg

Warnings: Standard considerations. Pregnancy Category: [C]

Interactions: Estrogen: May reduce clearance of ropinirole. Ropinirole dosage adjustments may be needed if estrogen therapy is started or stopped during treatment with ropinirole.
CYP1A2 inducers (eg, smoking, omeprazole): May increase metabolic clearance of ropinirole.
CYP1A2 inhibitors (eg, cimetidine, ciprofloxacin, diltiazem, enoxacin, erythromycin, fluvoxamine, mexiletine, norfloxacin, tacrine): May decrease metabolic clearance of ropinirole. Ropinirole dosage adjustment may be needed if CYP1A2 inhibitor is started or stopped during treatment with ropinirole.
Dopamine antagonists (eg, butyrophenones, metoclopramide, phenothiazines, thioxanthenes): May reduce effectiveness of ropinirole.

Rosuvastatin Calcium

Antihyperlipidemic / HMG-CoA reductase inhibitor

Indications: As an adjunct to diet to reduce elevated total cholesterol (C), LDL-C, nonHDL-C, ApoB, and TG levels and to increase HDL-C in patients with primary hypercholesterolemia and mixed dyslipidemia; as an adjunct to diet for the treatment of patients with elevated serum TG levels; to reduce LDL-C, total-C, and ApoB in patients with homozygous familial hypercholesterolemia as an adjunct to other lipid-lowering treatments or if such treatments are not available.

Dose: Hypercholesterolemia and Mixed Dyslipidemia:
Adults: PO 5 to 40 mg once daily, based on goal of therapy and response.
Homozygous, Familial Hypercholesterolemia:
Adults: PO Start with 20 mg once daily (max, 40 mg/day).
Concurrent Cyclosporine Therapy:
Adults: PO Limit dose of rosuvastatin to 5 mg/day.
Concurrent Lipid-Lowering Therapy:
Adults: PO Effect of rosuvastatin may be enhanced with bile acid-binding resin. Limit dose of rosuvastatin to 10 mg/day in patients receiving gemfibrozil.
Renal Insufficiency:
Adults: PO In patients with severe renal impairment (Ccr less than 30 mL/min/1.73 m^2) not on hemodialysis, start with 5 mg once daily (max, 10 mg once daily).

Trade names: Crestor Tablets 5 mg

Warnings: Pregnancy; breastfeeding; patients with active liver disease or with unexplained persistent elevations of serum transaminases; hypersensitivity to any component of the product. Pregnancy Category: [X]

Interactions: Cyclosporine, gemfibrozil: Plasma concentrations of rosuvastatin may be elevated, increasing the risk of side effects.
Warfarin: Anticoagulant effect of warfarin may be enhanced, increasing the risk of bleeding.

Saquinavir Mesylate

Antiretroviral / Protease inhibitor

Indications: Treatment of advanced HIV infection. Saquinavir is given in combination with nucleoside analogs (eg, zidovudine).

Dose: Adults and Children at least 16 yr: PO Three 200 mg capsules (600 mg) tid within 2 hr after a full meal.

Trade names: Fortovase Capsules 200 mg
Invirase Capsules 200 mg (as mesylate)

Warnings: Coadministration with cisapride, ergot derivatives, midazolam, triazolam. Pregnancy Category: [B]

Interactions: Aldesleukin, cyclosporine, grapefruit juice: May increase saquinavir serum levels.
Carbamazepine, dexamethasone, nevirapine, phenobarbital, phenytoin, rifabutin, rifampin, rifapentine, St. John's wort, other cytochrome P450 3A4 inducers: May increase metabolism of saquinavir and decrease serum levels.
Cisapride, cyclosporine, ergot derivatives, fentanyl, midazolam, triazolam, other drugs metabolized by cytochrome P450 3A4: Serum levels of these drugs may be elevated, increasing the risk of toxicity.
Clarithromycin, delavirdine, indinavir, ketoconazole, nelfinavir, ritonavir: May decrease metabolism of saquinavir and increase serum levels.
Clarithromycin, nelfinavir, sildenafil: Saquinavir may increase levels of these drugs.
Warfarin: The anticoagulant effect may be decreased.

Selegiline HCl

Antiparkinson

Indications: Adjunct to levodopa/carbidopa in idiopathic Parkinson's disease, postencephalitic parkinsonism/symptomatic parkinsonism.

Dose: Adults: PO 10 mg/day as divided dose of 5 mg each taken at breakfast and lunch. Do not exceed 10 mg/day. After 2 to 3 days of treatment, try reducing levodopa/carbidopa dose by 10% to 30%. Further reductions may be possible during continued selegiline therapy.

Trade names: Carbex Tablets 5 mg
Eldepryl Capsules 5 mg

Warnings: Standard considerations. Pregnancy Category: [C]
Interactions: Fluoxetine: May produce a 'serotonin' syndrome (CNS irritability, increased muscle tone, altered consciousness).
Meperidine: Could result in agitation, seizures, diaphoresis, and fever, which may progress to coma, apnea, and death. Reactions may occur several weeks following withdrawal of selegiline.

Senna

Laxative

Indications: Short-term treatment of constipation; preoperative and preradiographic bowel evacuation for procedures involving GI tract.
Dose: Adults: PO 2 tablets, 1 tsp of granules or 10 to 15 mL of syrup, usually at bedtime. PR 1 suppository at bedtime; may repeat in 2 hr.
Children: Generally, for children 6 to 12 yr or more than 60 lb, give (at bedtime) 1 tablet or 1/2 tsp granules PO or 1/2 suppository PR. Liquid dose ranges from 1.25 to 15 mL depending on age and product formulation.
Trade names: Agoral Liquid 25 mg
Black-Draught Granules 20 mg/5 mL
ex•lax Tablets 15 mg
ex•lax chocolate Tablets 15 mg
Fletcher Castoria Liquid 33.3 mg/mL
Senexon Tablets 8.5 mg
Senna-Gen Tablets 8.6 mg
Senokot Granules 15 mg/5 mL
SenokotXTRA Tablets 17 mg
Warnings: Nausea, vomiting, or other symptoms of appendicitis; acute surgical abdomen; fecal impaction; intestinal obstruction; undiagnosed abdominal pain. Pregnancy Category: [C]
Interactions: None well documented.

Sertraline HCl

Antidepressant

Indications: Treatment of major depression; treatment of obsessions and compulsions in patients with obsessive-compulsive disorder (OCD), as defined in the DSM-III-R; treatment of panic disorder with or without agoraphobia, as defined in DSM-IV; posttraumatic stress disorder (PTSD); treatment of premenstrual dysphoric disorder, treatment of social anxiety disorder (social phobia).
Dose: Major Depressive Disorders:
Adults: PO 50 mg qd (max, 200 mg/day). Dose changes should not occur at intervals of less than 1 wk.
OCD:
Adults and Children 13 to 17 yr: PO 50 mg qd (max, 200 mg/day). Dose changes should not occur at intervals of less than 1 wk.
Children 6 to 12 yr: PO 25 mg qd (max, 200 mg/day). Dose changes should not occur at intervals of less than 1 wk.
Panic Disorder, Social Anxiety Disorder, and PTSD:
Adults: PO 25 mg qd; the dose may be increased to 50 mg qd after 1 wk (max, 200 mg/day). Dose changes should not occur at intervals of less than 1 wk.
Premenstrual Dysphoric Disorder:
Adults: PO 50 mg/day, either daily throughout the menstrual cycle or limited to the luteal phase of the menstrual cycle, depending on physician assessment. Patients not responding to 50 mg/day may benefit from increases (at 50 mg increments/menstrual cycle) up to 150 mg/day when dosing throughout the menstrual cycle, or 100 mg/day when dosing during the luteal phase of the menstrual cycle. If a 100 mg/day dose has been established with luteal dosing, use a 50 mg/day titration step for 3 days at the beginning of each luteal phase dosing period.
Switching patients to or from MAOIs: At least 14 days should elapse between discontinuation of an MAOI and initiation of therapy with sertraline.
Trade names: Zoloft Tablets 25 mg
Warnings: Hypersensitivity to any components; concomitant use in patients taking monoamine oxidase inhibitors (MAOIs), pimozide, disulfiram (due to alcohol content in oral concentrate). Pregnancy Category: [C]
Interactions: 5-HT-1 agonists (eg, naratriptan, rizatriptan, sumatriptan, zolmitriptan): Weakness, hyperreflexia, and incoordination reported rarely.
Alcohol, CNS depressants: May enhance CNS depressant effects.
Cimetidine: Increased sertraline AUC (50%), C_{max} (24%), and $t_{1/2}$ (26%). Clinical significance is unknown.
Clozapine: Elevated serum clozapine levels occurred. Closely monitor patients on coadministration.
Hydantoins (eg, phenytoin): Plasma levels may be increased by sertraline, increasing the pharmacologic and adverse effects.
MAO inhibitors: May cause serious, even fatal reactions. Discontinue MAO inhibitors at least 14 days before starting sertraline.
Pimozide: Increase in pimozide AUC and C_{max} of about 40%; concomitant administration is contraindicated.
St. John's wort: Sedative-hypnotic effects of sertraline may be increased.
Sympathomimetics (eg, amphetamine, fenfluramine): Increased sensitivity to sympathomimetics; increased risk of 'serotonin syndrome.'
Tolbutamide: Sertraline significantly decreased the Cl of tolbutamide (16%). Clinical significance is unknown.
Tricyclic antidepressants (eg, amitriptyline): Pharmacologic and toxic effects may be increased by sertraline; 'serotonin syndrome' has been reported.
Type 1C antiarrhythmics (eg, propafenone, flecainide): Plasma levels may be increased. Monitor cardiac function.
Zolpidem: Onset of action of zolpidem may be shortened and the effect increased.

Sildenafil Citrate

Agent for impotence

Indications: Treatment of impotence related to erectile dysfunction of the penis.
Dose: Adults: PO 50 mg once 0.5 to 4 hr prior to sexual activity. Titration to a 25- or a 100-mg dose may be used based on tolerability or efficacy. The max recommended use is once daily.
Dosage Adjustments:
Adults: PO Consider a starting dose of 25 mg in patients older than 65 yr or in patients with hepatic impairment, severe renal impairment, or concurrent use of potent cytochrome P450 3A4 inhibitors (eg, erythromycin, ketoconazole, itraconazole, saquinavir).
Protease inhibitors: Do not exceed a max single dose of 25 mg sildenafil in a 48-hr period.
Alpha-blockers: Do not take 50 or 100 mg doses of sildenafil within 4 hr of alpha-blocker administration; however, a 25 mg dose of sildenafil may be taken at any time.
Trade names: Viagra Tablets 25 mg
Warnings: Patients using any type of organic nitrates (eg, nitroglycerin, isosorbide mono, dinitrate): Enhanced effects leading to prolonged hypotension. Pregnancy Category: [B]
Interactions: Amlodipine, alpha-blockers (eg, doxazosin): Administration may result in an additional decrease in BP.
Cimetidine, erythromycin, ketoconazole, itraconazole, tacrolimus: Increased sildenafil levels potentially leading to increased adverse effects.
Nitrates: Hypotension (see Contraindications).
Protease inhibitors (eg, ritonavir, saquinavir): Sildenafil plasma concentration may be increased, requiring a modification in sildenafil dosage.
Inducers of CYP3A4 (eg, rifampin): May decrease sildenafil levels.

Simethicone

Antiflatulent

Indications: Relief of painful symptoms and pressure of excess gas in digestive tract. Adjunct in treatment of many conditions in which gas retention may be problem, such as postoperative gaseous distention and pain, endoscopic examination, air swallowing, functional dyspepsia, peptic ulcer, spastic or irritable colon, diverticulosis.

Unlabeled indication: Treatment of infant colic.

Dose: Capsules:
Adults: PO 125 mg qid after meals and at bedtime.
Tablets:
Adults: PO 40 to 125 mg qid after meals and at bedtime.
Liquid (Drops):
Adults: PO 40 to 80 mg qid (up to 500 mg/day).
Children 2 to 12 yr: PO 40 mg qid.
Children less than 2 yr: PO 20 mg qid (up to 240 mg/day).

Trade names: Degas Tablets, chewable 80 mg
Extra Strength Gas-X Capsules, softgel 125 mg
Flatulex Drops 40 mg/0.6 mL
Genasyme Tablets, chewable 80 mg
Genasyme Drops Drops 40 mg/0.6 mL
Gas-X Tablets, chewable 80 mg
Maalox Anti-Gas Tablets, chewable 80 mg
Mylanta Gas Tablets, chewable 40 mg
Maximum Strength Mylanta Gas Tablets, chewable 125 mg
Mylicon Drops 40 mg/0.6 mL
Phazyme Drops 40 mg/0.6 mL
Phazyme 95 Tablets, chewable 95 mg
Phazyme 125 Tablets, chewable 125 mg

Warnings: Standard considerations. Pregnancy Category: []

Interactions: None well documented.

Simvastatin

Antihyperlipidemic / HMG-CoA reductase inhibitor

Indications: Adjunct to diet for reducing elevated total cholesterol and LDL cholesterol levels in patients with primary hypercholesterolemia (types IIa and IIb) when response to diet and other nonpharmacologic measures alone are inadequate; to reduce the risk of stroke or transient ischemic attack.

Unlabeled indication: Lower elevated cholesterol levels in patients with heterozygous familial hypercholesterolemia, familial combined hyperlipidemia, diabetic dyslipidemia in noninsulin-dependent diabetic patients, hyperlipidemia secondary to nephrotic syndrome, and homozygous familial hypercholesterolemia in patients who have defective, rather than absent, LDL receptors.

Dose: Adults: PO 5 to 40 mg/day in evening.

Trade names: Zocor Tablets 5 mg

Warnings: Active liver disease or unexplained persistent elevations of liver function values; pregnancy; lactation. Pregnancy Category: [X Use a reliable form of birth control]

Interactions: Azole antifungal agents (eg, ketoconazole), cyclosporine, macrolide antibiotics (eg, erythromycin), gemfibrozil, grapefruit juice, niacin, protease inhibitors (eg, ritonavir), verapamil: Severe myopathy or rhabdomyolysis may occur.
Rifamycins (eg, rifampin): May reduce simvastatin plasma levels, decreasing the pharmacologic effect.

Sodium Bicarbonate

Urinary tract product / Alkalinizer / Electrolyte / Antacid

Indications: Treatment of metabolic acidosis; promotion of gastric, systemic, and urinary alkalinization; replacement therapy in severe diarrhea; used to reduce incidence of chemical phlebitis (used as neutralizing additive solution).

Dose: Adults and Children greater than 2 yr: IV Administration performed in concentrations ranging from 1.5% (isotonic) to 8.4% depending on clinical condition and requirements of patient. SC After dilution to isotonicity (1.5%). The dose depends on the clinical condition and requirements of the patient (including age and weight). PO 325 mg to 2 g 1 to 4 times daily (patients less than 60 yr, max dose 16 g/day; patients greater than 60 yr max dose 8 g/day).
Infants up to 2 yr: IV 4.2% solution at rate up to 8 mEq/kg/day.

Trade names: Bell/ans Tablets 520 mg
Neut Neutralizing additive solution 4% (0.48 mEq/mL)
Sodium Bicarbonate Injection 4.2% (0.5 mEq/mL)

Warnings: Loss of chloride from vomiting or continuous GI suction when patient is receiving diuretics known to produce hypochloremic alkalosis; metabolic and respiratory alkalosis; hypocalcemia in which alkalosis may produce tetany, hypertension, convulsions, or CHF; when administration of sodium could be clinically detrimental. Pregnancy Category: [C]

Interactions: Amphetamine, dextroamphetamine, ephedrine, flecainide, mecamylamine, methamphetamine, pseudoephedrine, quinidine: Sodium bicarbonate can decrease elimination of these drugs, thus increasing their therapeutic effects.
Chlorpropamide, lithium, methotrexate, salicylates, tetracyclines: Sodium bicarbonate can increase elimination of these drugs, thus decreasing their therapeutic effect.
Ketoconazole: PO sodium bicarbonate may decrease the dissolution of ketoconazole in the GI tract, reducing the effectiveness.
Incompatability: Do not mix with IV solutions containing catecholamines, such as dobutamine, dopamine, and norepinephrine.

Sodium Iodide I 131

Radiopharmaceuticals

Indications: Thyroid carcinoma, hyperthyroidism.

Dose: Thyroid Carcinoma, Hyperthyroidism:
Adults: PO Individualize dosage. Usual dose for ablation of normal thyroid tissue: 50 mCi, with subsequent therapeutic doses usually 100 to 150 mCi.

Trade names: Iodotope Capsules 1 to 50 mCi
Sodium Iodide I 131 Capsules 0.75 to 100 mCi

Warnings: Preexisting vomiting and diarrhea; women who are or may become pregnant. Pregnancy Category: [X]

Interactions: Iodine, thyroid, and antithyroid agents: Uptake of iodine 131 will be affected by recent intake of stable iodine in any form, or by use of thyroid, antithyroid, and certain other drugs.

Sodium Polystyrene Sulfonate

Potassium-removing resin

Indications: Treatment of hyperkalemia.

Dose: Adults: PO or via NG tube 15 g 1 to 4 times/day. PR 30 to 50 g q 6 hr has been given as daily enema.
Children: PO Calculate children's dose by exchange ratio of 1 mEq potassium per gram of resin. (1 g/kg q 6 hr has been recommended.)

Trade names: Kayexalate Powder Finely powdered sodium polystyrene sulfonate. Sodium content approximately 100 mg (4.1 mEq)/g
SPS Suspension 15 g/60 mL. Sodium content 1.5 g (65 mEq)

Warnings: Hypokalemia. Pregnancy Category: [C]

Interactions: Digitalis: If hypokalemia occurs, likelihood of toxic effects of digoxin may be increased.
Nonabsorbable cation donating antacids and laxatives

(eg, aluminum carbonate, magnesium hydroxide): Systemic alkalosis has occurred. Potassium exchange capability of sodium polystyrene sulfonate may be reduced. Intestinal obstruction due to concretions of aluminum hydroxide when used in combination has occurred.

Sodium Sulfacetamide/ Sulfur

Antibacterial / Sulfonamide / Keratolytic agent

Indications: Topical control of acne vulgaris, acne rosacea, and seborrheic dermatitis.

Dose: Adults and children 12 yr and older: Topical Apply a thin film to affected areas qd to tid with light massaging to blend in each application.

Trade names: Avar Cleanser 10% sodium sulfacetamide and 5% sulfur
Clenia Cream 10% sodium sulfacetamide and 5% sulfur
Rosula Gel 10% sodium sulfacetamide and 5% sulfur
Sulfacet-R Lotion 10% sodium sulfacetamide and 5% sulfur
Zetacet Topical suspension 10% sodium sulfacetamide and 5% sulfur

Warnings: Kidney disease; known hypersensitivity to sulfonamides, sulfur, or any component of the product. Pregnancy Category: [C]

Interactions: None well documented.

Sotalol HCl

Beta-adrenergic blocker

Indications: Betapace: Management or prevention of life-threatening ventricular arrhythmias.

Betapace AF: Maintenance of normal sinus rhythm in patients with highly symptomatic atrial fibrillation/atrial flutter (AFIB/AFL) (Betapace AF).

Dose: Do not substitute Betapace for Betapace AF because of significant differences in labeling (eg, patient package insert, dosing administration, safety information).
Ventricular Arrhythmias:
Betapace:
Adults: PO 80 mg twice daily; may increase up to 320 mg/day in 2 or 3 divided doses. Patients with a history of symptomatic AFIB/AFL currently receiving Betapace should be transferred to Betapace AF because of the significant differences in labeling.
Betapace AF: Therapy with Betapace AF must be initiated and, if necessary, titrated in a setting that provides continuous ECG monitoring and in the presence of personnel trained in the management of serious ventricular arrhythmias. Monitor patients in this way for a minimum of 3 days on the maintenance dose and do not discharge within 12 hr of electrical or pharmacological conversion to normal sinus rhythm.
Adults: PO Initiate therapy at 80 mg bid if Ccr is greater than 60 mL/min, and 80 mg once daily if the Ccr is 40 to 60 mL/min. Begin continuous ECG monitoring with QT interval measurements 2 to 4 hr after each dose. If the 80 mg dose level is tolerated and QT interval remains less than 500 msec after at least 3 days, the patient may be discharged. Alternatively, during hospitalization, if 80 mg level does not reduce the frequency of relapse of AFIB/AFL and is tolerated without excessive QT interval prolongation (ie, greater than 520 msec), after following the patient for 3 days, the dose level may be increased to 120 mg (once or twice daily depending on Ccr). The max recommended dose in patients with Ccr greater than 60 mL/min is 160 mg bid.

Trade names: Betapace Tablets 80 mg
Betapace AF Tablets 80 mg

Warnings: Betapace: Hypersensitivity to beta-blockers; greater than first-degree heart block; CHF unless secondary to tachyarrhythmia treatable with beta-blockers; overt cardiac failure; sinus bradycardia; cardiogenic shock; bronchial asthma or bronchospasm, including severe COPD; congenital or acquired long QT syndromes. Betapace AF: Sinus bradycardia (less than 50 bpm during waking hours); sick sinus syndrome or second and third degree AV block (unless a functioning pacemaker is present); congenital or acquired QT syndromes; baseline QT interval greater than 450 msec; cardiogenic shock; uncontrolled heart failure; hypokalemia (less than 4 mEq/L); Ccr less than 40 mL/min; bronchial asthma; previous evidence of hypersensitivity to sotalol. Pregnancy Category: [B]

Interactions: Amiodarone, disopyramide, procainamide, quinidine: May prolong cardiac refractoriness.
Calcium channel blockers: Increased risk of hypotension; possible increased effect on atrioventricular conduction or ventricular function.
Clonidine: May enhance or reverse antihypertensive effects; may enhance clonidine rebound hypertension.
Gatifloxacin, moxifloxacin, sparfloxacin: Do not use in patients receiving sotalol because of increased risk of life-threatening cardiac arrhythmias.
Guanethidine, reserpine: Increased hypotension or bradycardia.
Insulin, oral sulfonylurea hypoglycemic agents: Hyperglycemia; symptoms of hypoglycemia may be masked.
NSAIDs: Some agents may impair antihypertensive effect.

Spironolactone

Potassium-sparing diuretic

Indications: Short-term preoperative treatment of primary hyperaldosteronism; long-term maintenance therapy for idiopathic hyperaldosteronism; management of edematous conditions in CHF, cirrhosis of liver and nephrotic syndrome; management of essential hypertension; treatment of hypokalemia.

Unlabeled indication: Treatment of hirsutism; relief of PMS symptoms; short-term treatment of familial male precocious puberty; and short-term treatment of acne vulgaris.

Dose: Diagnosis of Primary Hyperaldosteronism:
Adults: PO 400 mg/day for 4 days (short test) or 3 to 4 wk (long test).
Maintenance Therapy for Hyperaldosteronism:
Adults: PO 100 to 400 mg daily in single or divided doses.
Edema:
Adults: PO 25 to 200 mg/day in single or divided doses.
Children: PO 3.3 mg/kg/day in single or divided doses.
Essential Hypertension:
Adults: PO 50 to 100 mg/day in single or divided doses.
Children: PO 1 to 2 mg/kg bid.
Diuretic-Induced Hypokalemia:
Adults: PO 25 to 100 mg/day when oral potassium or other potassium-sparing regimens are inappropriate.

Trade names: Aldactone Tablets 25 mg
Spironolactone Tablets 25 mg

Warnings: Anuria; acute renal insufficiency; impaired renal excretory function; hyperkalemia. Pregnancy Category: [D]

Interactions: ACE inhibitors: May result in severely elevated serum potassium levels.
Digitalis glycosides: May decrease digoxin clearance, resulting in increased serum digoxin levels and toxicity; may attenuate inotropic action of digoxin.
Mitotane: May decrease therapeutic response to mitotane.
Potassium preparations: May severely increase serum potassium levels, possibly resulting in cardiac arrhythmias or cardiac arrest. Do not take with potassium preparations.

Salicylates: May result in decreased diuretic effect.

Spironolactone/ Hydrochlorothiazide

Diuretic combination

Indications: Edematous conditions for patients with CHF, cirrhosis of the liver accompanied edema or ascites, nephrotic syndrome, or essential hypertension.

Dose: Edema (CHF, hepatic cirrhosis, nephrotic syndrome):
Adults: PO Usual maintenance dose is 100 mg each of spironolactone and hydrochlorothiazide daily, administered in a single dose or divided doses, ranging from 25 to 200 mg of each component daily, depending on the response to the initial titration.
Essential Hypertension:
Adults: PO Varies depending on titration of individual ingredients; however, many patients have an optimal response to 50 to 100 mg each of spironolactone and hydrochlorothiazide daily, given in a single dose or divided doses.

Trade names: Aldactazide Tablets 25 mg spironolactone and 25 mg hydrochlorothiazide

Warnings: Patients with anuria; acute renal insufficiency, significant impairment of renal excretory function; severe hepatic failure; hyperkalemia; hypersensitivity to any component of product or sulfonamide-derived drugs. Pregnancy Category: [C]

Interactions: ACE inhibitors (eg, captopril): Severe hyperkalemia may occur.
Alcohol, barbiturates, narcotics: Orthostatic hypotension may be potentiated.
Antidiabetic agents (oral and insulin): May require dosage adjustment of antidiabetic agent.
Corticosteroids, ACTH: Electrolyte depletion, particularly hypokalemia, may occur.
Digoxin: The t1/2 of digoxin may be prolonged and serum levels may be elevated, increasing the risk of toxicity.
Lithium: Renal clearance of lithium may be decreased, increasing the risk of toxicity.
Nondepolarizing skeletal muscle relaxants (eg, tubocurarine): Unresponsiveness to muscle relaxant may occur.
NSAIDs (eg, indomethacin): The diuretic, natriuretic, and antihypertensive effect of hydrochlorothiazide may be reduced.
Pressor amines (eg, norepinephrine): The vascular response to norepinephrine may be reduced.

Streptokinase

Thrombolytic enzyme

Indications: Acute MI, lysis of intracoronary thrombi, improvement of ventricular function, and reduction of mortality associated with acute MI (IV or intracoronary route); reduction of infarct size and CHF associated with acute MI (IV); lysis of objectively diagnosed (eg, angiography) pulmonary emboli (involving obstruction of blood flow to a lobe or multiple segments, with or without unstable hemodynamics); lysis of objectively diagnosed (eg, ascending venography), acute, extensive thrombi of the deep veins (eg, those involving the popliteal vessels); lysis of acute arterial thrombi and emboli; alternative to surgical revision for clearing totally or partially occluded arteriovenous cannulae when acceptable flow cannot be achieved.

Dose: Acute Evolving Transmural MI:
Adults: IV infusion Administer as soon as possible after symptom onset (greatest benefit when administered within 4 hr, but benefit has been reported up to 24 hr). Infuse a total dose of 1,500,000 IU within 60 min. Intracoronary infusion Administer 20,000 IU by bolus followed by 2000 IU/min for 60 min (total dose, 140,000 IU).
Pulmonary Embolism, Deep Vein Thrombosis (DVT), Arterial Thrombosis, or Embolism:
Adults: IV infusion Administer as soon as possible after onset of thrombolic event, preferably within 7 days. A loading dose of 250,000 IU infused into a peripheral vein over 30 minutes has been found appropriate in over 90% of patients. If thrombin time or any parameter of lysis after 4 hr of therapy is not significantly different from the normal control level, discontinue streptokinase because excessive resistance is present. Dose and duration of therapy (following the loading dose of 250,000 IU/30 min): pulmonary embolism 100,000 IU/hr for 24 hr (72 hr if concurrent DVT is suspected); DVT 100,000 IU/hr for 72 hr; arterial thrombosis or embolism 100,000 IU/hr for 24 to 72 hr.
Arteriovenous Cannulae Occlusion: Slowly instill 250,000 in 2 mL of solution into each occluded limb of the cannula. Clamp off cannula limb(s) for 2 hr. Closely observe patient for adverse effects. After treatment, aspirate contents of infused cannula limb(s) and flush with saline before reconnecting cannula.

Trade names: Streptase Powder for Injection 250,000 IU

Warnings: Active internal bleeding; recent cerebrovascular accident (within 2 mo); intracranial or intraspinal surgery; intracranial neoplasm; severe uncontrolled hypertension. Pregnancy Category: [C]

Interactions: Anticoagulants, agents that alter platelet function (eg, aspirin, other NSAIDs, dipyridamole), other thrombolytic agents, agents that alter coagulation: May increase the risk of bleeding.
Incompatability: Do not add other medication to the streptokinase container.

Streptomycin Sulfate

Anti-infective / Antitubercular

Indications: Treatment of moderate to severe infections caused by susceptible strains of *Mycobacterium tuberculosis* and nontuberculosis infections.

Dose: Tuberculosis:
Adults: IM 15 mg/kg/day (max, 1 g) or 25 to 30 mg/kg 2 or 3 times weekly (max, 1.5 g).
Children: IM 20 to 40 mg/kg/day (max, 1 g) or 25 to 30 mg/kg 2 or 3 times weekly (max, 1.5 g).
Tularemia: IM 1 to 2 g/day in divided doses for 7 to 14 days until patient is afebrile for 5 to 7 days.
Plague: IM 2 g/day in 2 divided doses for minimum of 10 days.
Bacterial Endocarditis:
Streptococcal: IM 1 g bid for 1 wk then 0.5 g bid for the second week in combination with penicillin. In patients over 60 yr, give 0.5 g bid for the entire 2 wk period.
Enterococcal: IM 1 g bid for 2 wk and 0.5 g bid for 4 wk in combination with penicillin.
Concomitant Use with Other Agents:
Adults: IM 1 to 2 g in divided doses q 6 to 12 hr for moderate to severe infections (max, 2 g/day).
Children: IM 20 to 40 mg/kg/day in divided doses q 6 to 12 hr, avoiding excessive doses.

Trade names: Streptomycin Sulfate Injection 400 mg/mL

Warnings: Hypersensitivity to aminoglycosides or any component of the product. Pregnancy Category: [D Crosses the placenta and may cause fetal harm]

Interactions: Ethacrynic acid, furosemide, mannitol, possibly other diuretics: May potentiate the ototoxic effects of streptomycin.
Neurotoxic or nephrotoxic agents (eg, colistin, cyclosporine, gentamicin, kanamycin, neomycin, paromomycin, polymyxin B, tobramycin): May increase the risk of neuro- or nephrotoxicity and should be avoided.

Streptozocin

Alkylating agent / Nitrosoureas

Indications: Adult/Pediatric: Symptomatic or progressive metastatic islet cell carcinoma of the pancreas.

Dose: Pancreatic Islet Cell Carcinoma:
Adult: IV 500 mg/m^2 /day for 5 days q 4 to 6 wk; or 1000 mg/m^2 once a week for the first 2 wk, increased to a max of 1500 mg/m^2 if necessary. Do not give more than 1500 mg/m^2 in a single dose because of dose-related nephrotoxicity. Median total dose to maximal response is 4000 mg/m^2.
Pediatric: IV No pediatric dosing information is available.
Adjustment in Renal Insufficiency:
Adult: IV If Ccr is more than 50 mL/min, administer 100% of usual dose. If Ccr is 10 to 50 mL/min, administer 75% of usual dose. If Ccr is less than 10 mL/min, administer 50% of usual dose.
Trade names: Zanosar Powder for injection 1 g
Warnings: Standard considerations. Pregnancy Category: [C]
Interactions: Nephrotoxic agents: Because streptozocin is nephrotoxic, do not use in combination with other nephrotoxic agents.

Succimer

Detoxification / Chelating agent
Indications: Treatment of lead poisoning in children with blood levels above 45 mcg/dL.

Unlabeled indication: Treatment of heavy metal poisonings (mercury, arsenic); however, further study is needed.
Dose: Children 12 mo and older: PO Start with 10 mg/kg or 350 mg/m^2 q 8 hr for 5 days. Reduce frequency of administration to 10 mg/kg or 350 mg/m^2 q 12 hr for an additional 14 days. A course of treatment lasts 19 days. Repeated courses may be necessary if indicated by weekly monitoring of lead blood concentration. A minimum of 14 days between courses is recommended unless lead blood levels indicate the need for more prompt treatment. In young children unable to swallow capsules, the contents of the capsule can be sprinkled on a small amount of soft food or placed on a spoon and followed with fruit drink.
Trade names: Chemet Capsules 100 mg
Warnings: Standard considerations. Pregnancy Category: [C]
Interactions: Chelating therapy: Coadministration with other chelation therapy is not recommended.

Sucralfate

Gastrointestinal
Indications: Short-term treatment of duodenal ulcer; maintenance therapy of duodenal ulcer (tablets only).

Unlabeled indication: Treatment of gastric ulcers; reflux and peptic esophagitis; treatment of NSAID- or aspirin-induced GI symptoms and mucosal damage; prevention of stress ulcers and GI bleeding in critically ill patients; treatment of oral and esophageal ulcers caused by radiation, chemotherapy, and sclerotherapy; treatment of oral ulcerations and dysphagia in patients with epidermolysis bullosa.
Dose: Active Duodenal Ulcer:
Adults: PO 1 g qid on empty stomach (1 hr before meals and at bedtime) for 4 to 8 wk.
Maintenance (tablets only): 1 g bid.
Trade names: Carafate Tablets 1 g
Warnings: Standard considerations. Pregnancy Category: [B]
Interactions: Aluminum-containing antacids: May increase total body burden of aluminum.
Cimetidine, ciprofloxacin (and other quinolone antibiotics), diclofenac, digoxin, hydantoins (eg, phenytoin), ketoconazole, levothyroxine, penicillamine, quinidine, ranitidine, tetracycline, theophylline: Oral absorption and pharmacologic action of these agents may be reduced if given with sucralfate. Administer 2 hr apart from sucralfate.

Sulfadiazine

Anti-infective / Sulfonamide
Indications: Treatment of chancroid, trachoma, inclusion conjunctivitis, nocardiosis, UTI, toxoplasmosis encephalitis, malaria, meningococcal meningitis, acute otitis media; prophylaxis against meningococcal meningitis and recurrences of rheumatic fevers; with streptomycin as adjunctive therapy for Haemophilus influenza meningitis.
Dose: Adults: PO 2 to 4 g, divided into 3 to 6 doses, q 24 hr.
Children older than 2 mo of age: PO Initially, one-half the 24-hr dose.
Maintenance: 150 mg/kg or 4 g/m^2, divided into 4 to 6 doses, q 24 hr.
Rheumatic Fever Prophylaxis: Under 30 kg give 500 mg q 24 hr; over 30 kg give 1 g q 24 hr.
Trade names: Sulfadiazine Tablets 500 mg
Warnings: Hypersensitivity to sulfonamides; infants less than 2 mo of age (except as adjunctive therapy with pyrimethamine in treating congenital toxoplasmosis); pregnancy at term; nursing period. Pregnancy Category: [C]
Interactions: Anticoagulants, hydantoins (eg, phenytoin), methotrexate, sulfonylureas, thiazide diuretics, uricosuric agents: Effects of these agents may be enhanced by sulfadiazine.
Indomethacin, probenecid, salicylates: May increase free sulfadiazine plasma levels, increasing the pharmacologic and adverse effects.

Sulfasalazine

Anti-infective / Sulfonamide
Indications: Treatment of ulcerative colitis; rheumatoid arthritis and juvenile rheumatoid arthritis (enteric-coated tablets).

Unlabeled indication: Treatment of ankylosing spondylitis, collagenous colitis, Crohn disease, psoriasis, psoriatic arthritis.
Dose: Ulcerative Colitis:
Adults: PO 3 to 4 g/day in evenly divided doses. More than 4 g/day is associated with higher incidence of side effects. May begin with 1 to 2 g/day to lessen GI effects.
Maintenance: 2 g/day in 4 divided doses.
Children at least 2 yr: PO 40 to 60 mg/kg/24 hr initially in 3 to 6 divided doses.
Maintenance: 20 to 30 mg/kg/day in 4 divided doses. Max, 2 g/day.
Rheumatoid Arthritis:
Adults: PO Enteric-coated: 2 g/day in 2 evenly divided doses. May initiate therapy with a lower dosage (eg, 0.5 to 1 g/day) to reduce possible GI intolerance.
Children at least 6 yr: PO Enteric-coated: 30 to 50 mg/kg/day in 2 evenly divided doses. Initiate therapy with 25% to 33% of the planned maintenance dose to lessen GI effects; increase weekly until reaching maintenance dose at 1 mo. Max, 2 g/day.
Trade names: Azulfidine Tablets 500 mg
Azulfidine EN-tabs Tablets, delayed-release 500 mg
Warnings: Hypersensitivity to sulfonamides or chemically related drugs (eg, sulfonylureas, thiazide and loop diuretics, carbonic anhydrase inhibitors, sunscreens containing PABA, local anesthetics); pregnancy at term; lactation; infants less than 2 mo; porphyria; hypersensitivity to salicylates; intestinal or urinary obstruction. Pregnancy Category: [B]
Interactions: Folic acid: Signs of folate deficiency have occurred, but specific symptoms related to deficiency have not been reported.
Methotrexate: Risk of methotrexate-induced bone marrow suppression may be enhanced.
Sulfonylureas: Increased sulfonylurea half-lives and hypoglycemia have occurred.

Sulfinpyrazone

Uricosuric / Gout

Indications: Treatment of chronic and intermittent gouty arthritis. Not intended for relief of acute attack of gout.

Unlabeled indication: Post MI treatment (within 1 to 6 mo of acute MI) to decrease incidence of sudden cardiac death. May also be used to reduce frequency of systemic embolism in rheumatic mitral stenosis.

Dose: Adults: PO Initial: 200 to 400 mg daily in 2 divided doses with meals or milk, gradually increasing to full maintenance dosage in 1 wk. Maintenance: 200 to 800 mg daily, given in 2 divided doses; may increase or decrease after serum urate level is controlled. In case of acute exacerbations, administer concomitant treatment with indomethacin (or another NSAID) or colchicine.

Trade names: Anturane Capsules 200 mg

Warnings: Active peptic ulcer or symptoms of GI inflammation or ulceration; hypersensitivity to phenylbutazone or other pyrazoles; blood dyscrasias. Pregnancy Category: [Use only when clearly needed]

Interactions: Acetaminophen: Increased hepatotoxicity and reduced efficacy of acetaminophen may occur.
Anticoagulants, sulfonylureas (eg, tolbutamide): Blood levels and toxicity of these agents may increase.
Salicylates: Uricosuric action of sulfinpyrazone may be reduced.
Verapamil: Reduced efficacy of verapamil may occur.

Sulindac

Analgesic / NSAID

Indications: Treatment of acute and chronic rheumatoid and osteoarthritis, ankylosing spondylitis, acute gouty arthritis, acute painful shoulder, tendonitis, bursitis.

Unlabeled indication: Treatment of juvenile rheumatoid arthritis and sunburn.

Dose: Osteoarthritis, Rheumatoid Arthritis, Ankylosing Spondylitis:
Adults: PO 150 mg bid.
Acute Painful Shoulder, Acute Gouty Arthritis:
Adults: PO 200 mg bid for 7 to 14 days. Max, 400 mg/day.

Trade names: Clinoril Tablets 150 mg

Warnings: Hypersensitivity to aspirin, iodides, or any NSAID. Pregnancy Category: [Pregnancy category undetermined]

Interactions: Anticoagulants: May increase effect of anticoagulants because of decreased plasma protein binding. May increase risk of gastric erosion and bleeding.
Cimetidine: Sulindac has increased cimetidine bioavailability.
Dimethyl sulfoxide: DMSO may decrease formation of active metabolite of sulindac, possibly resulting in decreased therapeutic effect. Also, topical DMSO with sulindac has resulted in severe peripheral neuropathy.
Lithium: May decrease lithium clearance.
Loop diuretics: Decreased diuresis may result.
Methotrexate: May increase methotrexate levels.
Ranitidine: Sulindac has increased ranitidine bioavailability.

Sumatriptan

Analgesic / Migraine

Indications: Acute treatment of migraine attacks with/without aura; treatment of acute cluster headaches (injection only).

Dose: Adults: PO Recommended dose is up to 100 mg taken with fluids. Doses of 100 mg have not been proven to provide a greater effect than 50 mg. If headache returns, a single additional dose may be taken after 2 hr up to a max of 200 mg per day. If headache returns following an initial dose with the injection, additional doses of single tablets (up to 100 mg per day) may be given with an interval of at least 2 hr between tablet doses. Subcutaneous Administer as soon as symptoms appear. Max single adult dose is 6 mg. Max dose per 24 hr is two 6 mg injections separated by at least 1 hr. Available in auto-injection prefilled syringe devices that deliver 6 mg for easy use; however, lower doses should be used in patients who have side effects at usual dose. Intranasal Administer a single dose of 5, 10, or 20 mg in 1 nostril. A 10 mg dose can be achieved by the administration of a single 5 mg dose in each nostril. If headache returns, the dose may be repeated once after 2 hr. Do not exceed a total daily dose of 40 mg.
Hepatic Function Impairment: Maximum single dose is up to 50 mg.

Trade names: Imitrex Injection 6 mg per 0.5 mL (as succinate)

Warnings: IV use (causes coronary vasospasm); patients with history, signs or symptoms of ischemic heart disease (eg, angina, including Prinzmetal variant, MI, silent myocardial ischemia), cerebrovascular or peripheral vascular syndromes; uncontrolled hypertension; concurrent use or within 24 hr of ergotamine-containing preparations; management of hemiplegic or basilar migraine; concurrent MAO inhibitor therapy or within 2 wk of discontinuing an MAO inhibitor; severe hepatic impairment; hypersensitivity to any component of the product. Pregnancy Category: [C]

Interactions: 5-HT-1 agonists (eg, naratriptan): Increased risk of vasospastic reactions; therefore, coadministration of two 5-HT_1 agonists within 24 hr of each other is contraindicated.
Ergot-containing drugs: May cause additive prolonged vasospastic reactions. Avoid use within 24 hr of each other.
MAO inhibitors: Use of sumatriptan with MAO inhibitors or within 14 days following discontinuation of an MAO inhibitor is contraindicated.
Selective serotonin reuptake inhibitors (eg, citalopram, fluoxetine, fluvoxamine, paroxetine, sertraline): Weakness, hyperreflexia, and incoordination have been reported rarely.
Sibutramine: Serotonin syndrome, including CNS irritability, motor weakness, shivering, myoclonus, and altered consciousness may occur.

Tacrolimus

Immunosuppressive

Indications: PO and IV: Prophylaxis of organ rejection in patients receiving allogenic liver or kidney transplants. Used in conjunction with adrenal corticosteroids.

Topical: Atopic dermatitis.

Unlabeled indication: Prophylaxis of rejection for patients receiving kidney, bone marrow, cardiac, pancreas, pancreatic island cell, and small bowel transplantation.

Dose: Prophylaxis of Organ Rejection Liver Transplants:
Adults: PO 0.1 to 0.15 mg/kg/day in 2 divided daily doses q 12 hr no sooner than 6 hr after transplantation. IV 0.03 to 0.05 mg/kg/day as continuous infusion.
Children: PO 0.15 to 0.2 mg/kg/day in 2 divided daily doses q 12 hr. IV 0.03 to 0.05 mg/kg/day as continuous infusion.
Prophylaxis of Organ Rejection Kidney Transplants:
Adults: PO 0.2 mg/kg/day in 2 divided daily doses q 12 hr, starting within 24 hr of transplantation but delayed until renal function is recovered (eg, serum creatinine of 4 mg/dL or less). Black patients may require higher doses to achieve comparable blood concentration.
Topical Dermatitis:

Adults: Topical Apply thin layer of 0.03% or 0.1% to affected skin areas bid and rub in gently and completely; continue for 1 wk after clearing of atopic dermatitis.
Children (at least 2 yr): Topical Apply thin layer of 0.03% to affected skin areas bid and rub in gently and completely; continue for 1 wk after clearing of atopic dermatitis.

Trade names: Prograf Capsules 0.5 mg
Protopic Ointment 0.03%

Warnings: Hypersensitivity to polyoxyl 60 hydrogenated castor oil, which is present in the injection, or any component of the product. Pregnancy Category: [C]

Interactions: Azole antifungal agents (eg, fluconazole, ketoconazole), calcium channel blockers (eg, diltiazem, nifedipine), clotrimazole, macrolide antibiotics(eg, erythromycin): Tacrolimus plasma levels may be elevated, increasing the risk of toxicity.
Cyclosporine: Additive nephrotoxicity.
Hydantoins (eg, phenytoin): Tacrolimus plasma levels may be reduced, while hydantoin concentrations may be increased.
Mycophenolate mofetil: Plasma levels of mycophenolate mofetil may be elevated.
Rifamycins (eg, rifampin, St. John's wort): Tacrolimus plasma levels may be reduced, increasing the risk of rejection.

Tadalafil

Agent for impotence

Indications: Treatment of erectile dysfunction.

Dose: Adults: PO 10 mg prior to anticipated sexual activity. The dose may be titrated to 5 or 20 mg based on efficacy and tolerability. The max recommended frequency is qd for most patients.
Renal Insufficiency:
Adults: PO Mild renal insufficiency: No dosage adjustment is required. Moderate renal insufficiency (Ccr 31 to 50 mL/min): Start with 5 mg not more than qd (max, 10 mg q 48 hr). Severe renal insufficiency (Ccr less than 30 mL/min) on hemodialysis: Max recommended dose is 5 mg.
Hepatic Impairment:
Adults: PO Mild to moderate hepatic impairment: Dose should not exceed 10 mg qd. Severe hepatic impairment: Use is not recommended.

Trade names: Cialis Tablets 5 mg

Warnings: Administration with nitrates and nitric oxide donors, alpha-blockers (except 0.4 mg/day tamsulosin); hypersensitivity to any component of the product. Pregnancy Category: [B]

Interactions: Alpha-blockers (eg, terazosin), nitrates: Coadministration of these agents with tadalafil is contraindicated (except 0.4 mg/day tamsulosin).
CYP3A4 inducers (eg, carbamazepine, phenytoin, rifampin): Plasma levels may be decreased, reducing tadalafil exposure; however, no dosage adjustment is warranted.
CYP3A4 inhibitors (eg, ketoconazole, ritonavir): Plasma levels of tadalafil may be elevated, increasing the risk of side effects and necessitating dosage adjustment. Do not exceed 10 mg once every 72 hr.

Talc, Sterile Powder

Sclerosing agent

Indications: Decrease or prevent recurrence of malignant pleural effusions.

Dose: Adults: Intrapleural Powder 5 g dissolved in 50 to 100 mL sodium chloride injection is recommended. Aerosol Single 4 to 8 g dose delivered from spray canister (1 to 2 cans), which delivers talc at a rate of 0.4 g/sec.

Trade names: Sclerosol Aerosol 4 g talc
Sterile Talc Powder Powder 5 g talc

Warnings: Standard considerations. Pregnancy Category: [B]

Interactions: None well documented.

Tamoxifen Citrate

Antiestrogen hormone

Indications: Breast carcinoma in women; metastatic breast carcinoma in men and women; reduction in risk of breast cancer in high-risk women; lower risk of invasive breast cancer in women with ductal carcinoma in situ (DCIS).

Unlabeled indication: Mastalgia; decreasing the size and pain of gynecomastia; McCune-Albright syndrome in female pediatric patients (in combination with other agents).

Dose: Tamoxifen Alone as Adjunct to Surgery:
Adults: PO 20 mg/day in 1 to 2 divided doses. Duration of therapy of more than 2 yr is most effective.
Combination Chemotherapy as Adjunct to Surgery:
Adults: PO 10 mg bid in postmenopausal women or women greater than 50 yr with positive axillary nodes for 5 yr.
Advanced Breast Carcinoma in Postmenopausal Women:
Adults: PO 10 to 20 mg bid. Response to therapy should occur within 4 to 10 wk.
Prevention of Breast Cancer in High-Risk Women:
Adults: PO 20 mg/day in 1 to 2 divided doses. Continue for 5 yr.

Trade names: Nolvadex Tablets 10 mg

Warnings: Hypersensitivity to drug; women who require concomitant coumarin-type anticoagulant therapy; women with a history of deep vein thrombosis or pulmonary embolus (reduction in breast cancer incidence and DCIS indications). Pregnancy Category: [D]

Interactions: Aminoglutethimide, phenobarbital: Tamoxifen concentrations may be reduced.
Bromocriptine: Tamoxifen concentrations may be increased.
Rifamycins (eg, rifampin): Tamoxifen plasma levels may be reduced, decreasing the antiestrogenic effect.
Tacrolimus, other drugs metabolized by cytochrome P450 3A4 (eg, amitriptyline, carbamazepine, cyclosporine, lovastatin, sertraline, verapamil): Coadministration may result in reduced clearance and increased serum concentrations of these agents.
Warfarin: Increased hypoprothrombinemic effect.

Tamsulosin HCl

Antiadrenergic, peripherally acting

Indications: Treatment of signs and symptoms of benign prostatic hyperplasia.

Dose: Adults: PO 0.4 mg/day, administered approximately 30 min following the same meal each day. If the patient fails to respond after 2 to 4 wk, the dose may be increased to 0.8 mg/day.

Trade names: Flomax Capsules 0.4 mg

Warnings: Standard considerations. Pregnancy Category: [B]

Interactions: Cimetidine: Concomitant use may decrease tamsulosin clearance and increase the AUC. Use with caution.

Tazarotene

Retinoid

Indications: Treatment of acne (Tazorac cream and gel), psoriasis (Tazorac gel); as an adjunctive agent in mitigation of facial fine wrinkling, facial mottled hyper- and hypopigmentation, and benign facial lentigines in patients who use comprehensive skin care and sunlight avoidance programs (Avage).

Dose: Acne:
Adults and Children (12 yr and older): Topical After gently cleansing and drying the face, apply a thin film (2 mg/cm^2) once daily in the evening where acne lesions appear.

Psoriasis:
Adults (18 yr and older): Topical Apply once a day in the evening to psoriatic lesions, using enough (2 mg/ cm^2) to cover only the lesion with a thin film.
Wrinkling, Hyper- and Hypopigmentation, Lentigines:
Adults (18 yr and older): Topical Apply pea-sized amount once daily at bedtime to lightly cover the entire face including the eyelids if desired.

Trade names: Avage Cream 0.1%
Tazorac Cream 0.05%

Warnings: Pregnancy; hypersensitivity to any component of the product. Pregnancy Category: [X]

Interactions: None well documented.

Telmisartan

Antihypertensive / Angiotensin II antagonist

Indications: Treatment of hypertension.

Dose: Adults: PO 20 to 80 mg/day; usual starting dose, 40 mg/day.

Trade names: Micardis Tablets 20 mg

Warnings: Standard considerations. Pregnancy Category: [C (first trimester); D (second and third trimester)]

Interactions: Digoxin: May increase plasma levels of digoxin, that may increase toxicity.
Lithium: Plasma concentrations may be increased by telmisartan, resulting in an increase in the pharmacologic and adverse effects of lithium.

Telmisartan/ Hydrochlorothiazide

Antihypertensive combination

Indications: Treatment of hypertension.

Dose: The fixed combination is not indicated for initial therapy. The combination may be substituted for the titrated components.
Adults: PO Telmisartan may be used over a dose range of 20 to 80 mg/day, administered qd. HCTZ is effective in doses of 12.5 to 50 mg qd. The dose may be titrated up to 160 mg telmisartan plus 25 mg of HCTZ, if necessary.

Trade names: Micardis HCT Tablets 40 mg telmisartan and 12.5 mg hydrochorothiazide

Warnings: Patients with anuria; hypersensitivity to sulfonamide-derived drugs or any component of this product. Pregnancy Category: [D (second and third trimester); C (first trimester), drugs that act directly on the renin-angiotensin system can cause injury and even death to the developing fetus]

Interactions: Telmisartan:
Digoxin: Peak and trough plasma levels may be elevated by telmisartan.
HCTZ:
Alcohol, barbiturates, narcotics: Increased risk of orthostatic hypotension.
Antidiabetic agents (oral agents and insulin): Dosage adjustment of antidiabetic agent may be necessary.
Antihypertensive agent: Additive or potentiation of effects.
Cholestyramine, colestipol resins: Impaired absorption of hydrochlorothiazide.
Corticosteroids, ACTH: Increased electrolyte depletion, increasing the risk of hypokalemia.
Lithium: Renal Cl of lithium may be reduced, increasing the risk of lithium toxicity.
Nondepolarizing skeletal muscle relaxants (eg, tubocurarine): Increased effect of the muscle relaxant.
Nonsteroidal anti-inflammatory agents: The diuretic, natriuretic, and antihypertensive effects of loop, potassium-sparing, and thiazide diuretics may be reduced.
Potassium supplements: Salt substitutes containing potassium or potassium supplements should not be used without consulting the prescribing physician.
Pressor amines (eg, norepinephrine): Decreased responsiveness to the pressor amine.

Temazepam

Sedative / Hypnotic / Benzodiazepine

Indications: Short-term management of insomnia.

Dose: Adults: PO 7.5 to 30 mg at bedtime; individualize.
Elderly or Debilitated Patients: PO 15 mg until individual response is determined.

Trade names: Restoril Capsules 7.5 mg

Warnings: Hypersensitivity to benzodiazepines; pregnancy. Pregnancy Category: [X]

Interactions: Alcohol, other CNS depressants: Additive CNS depressant effects.
Digoxin: Serum digoxin concentrations may increase.
Theophylline: May antagonize sedative effects.

Teniposide

Podophyllotoxin derivative

Indications: Adult: Refractory childhood acute lymphoblastic leukemia.

Pediatric: Refractory acute lymphoblastic leukemia.

Unlabeled indication: Adult acute lymphocytic leukemia, non-Hodgkin's lymphoma.

Dose: Acute Lymphoblastic Leukemia:
Adults: IV 165 mg/m^2 on days 1, 4, 8, and 11 during consolidation on the 'Linker' regimen. Dosage adjustment: Reduce dose 50% during the first treatment course in patients with Down's syndrome and leukemia. Higher doses may be administered during subsequent courses, depending on the degree of myelosuppression.
Acute Lymphoblastic Leukemia, Combination Therapy:
Pediatric: IV 165 mg/m^2 /dose twice weekly for 8 to 9 doses; or 250 mg/m^2 /dose once a week for 4 to 8 wk in combination with other chemotherapeutic drugs. Dosage adjustment: Reduce dose 50% for the initial course of therapy. Depending on the degree of myelosuppression and mucositis which occur, higher doses may be given during subsequent courses.

Trade names: Vumon Injection concentrate 50 mg/5 mL

Warnings: Hypersensitivity to teniposide or Cremophor EL (polyoxyethylated castor oil). Pregnancy Category: [D]

Interactions: Methotrexate: Plasma clearance of methotrexate may be slightly increased.
Phenytoin: May increase clearance of teniposide, resulting in decreased therapeutic effects.
Tolbutamide, sodium salicylate, and sulfamethizole: May displace protein bound teniposide.

Tenofovir Disoproxil Fumarate

Antiretroviral / Nucleotide analog reverse transcriptase inhibitor

Indications: Treatment of HIV-1 infection in combination with other antiretroviral agents.

Dose: Adults: PO 300 mg/day with a meal. When taking concurrently with didanosine, take tenofovir 2 hr before or 1 hr after didanosine.

Trade names: Viread Tablets 300 mg (equivalent to 245 mg tenofovir disoproxil)

Warnings: Standard considerations. Pregnancy Category: [B]

Interactions: Didanosine: Plasma concentrations of didanosine may be increased.
Indinavir, lopinavir/ritonavir: May increase tenofovir plasma levels. Indinavir plasma concentrations may be decreased by tenofovir.

Terazosin

Antihypertensive / Antiadrenergic, peripherally acting

Indications: Management of hypertension and symptomatic benign prostatic hyperplasia.

Dose: Hypertension:
Adults: PO Initial: 1 mg at bedtime. (Do not exceed this as initial dose to avoid severe hypotensive effects; reinstitute at this dose if drug is discontinued for several days). Maintenance: 1 to 5 mg q day; may consider bid dosing (max, 20 mg/day).
Benign Prostatic Hyperplasia:
Adults: PO.
Initial: 1 mg at bedtime. (Do not exceed this as initial dose); increase dose in step-wise fashion.
Usual maintenance: 10 mg q day for minimum of 4 to 6 wk (max, 20 mg/day).

Trade names: Hytrin Capsules 1 mg

Warnings: Hypersensitivity to doxazosin or prazosin. Pregnancy Category: [C]

Interactions: None well documented.

Terbinafine

Anti-infective / Antifungal

Indications: Treatment of onychomycosis of the toenail or fingernail caused by dermatophytes.
Topical: Interdigital tinea pedis, tinea cruris, or tinea corporis caused by *E. floccosum*, *T. mentagrophytes*, or *T. rubrum*.

Unlabeled indication: Cutaneous candidiasis, pityriasis (tinea) versicolor (topical).

Dose: Adults: PO 250 mg/day for 6 wk for fingernail onychomycosis; 250 mg/day for 12 wk for toenail onychomycosis. Topical Apply to affected areas and surrounding skin once or twice daily.

Trade names: Lamisil Tablets 250 mg
Lamisil AT Cream 1%

Warnings: Preexisting liver disease or renal impairment (Ccr up to 50 mL/min). Pregnancy Category: [B]

Interactions: Caffeine: Terbinafine decreases the clearance of IV caffeine 19%.
Cimetidine: Terbinafine clearance is decreased 33% by cimetidine.
Cyclosporine: Terbinafine increases the clearance of cyclosporine 15%.
Dextromethorphan: Plasma dextromethorphan concentrations may be elevated, increasing the pharmacologic and adverse effects. Terbinafine inhibits dextromethorphan metabolism via the cytochrome P450 2D6 enzyme.
Rifampin: Terbinafine clearance is increased 100% by rifampin.

Terbutaline Sulfate

Bronchodilator / Sympathomimetic

Indications: Treatment of reversible bronchospasm associated with asthma, bronchitis, and emphysema.

Dose: Adults and Children over 15 yr: PO 2.5 to 5 mg at 6 hr intervals, tid during waking hours. Do not exceed 15 mg in 24 hr.
Children 12 to 15 yr: PO 2.5 mg tid. Do not exceed 7.5 mg in 24 hr. SC 0.25 mg given in lateral deltoid area. May repeat in 15 to 30 min. Do not exceed 0.5 mg in 4 hr.

Trade names: Brethaire Aerosol 0.2 mg/ actuation
Brethine Tablets 2.5 mg
Bricanyl Tablets 2.5 mg

Warnings: Cardiac arrhythmias associated with tachycardia. Pregnancy Category: [B]

Interactions: Beta-blockers: Block bronchodilator effect of terbutaline.
MAOIs: Hypertension may occur.
Tricyclic antidepressants: Cardiovascular effects of terbutaline may be enhanced.

Terconazole

Topical / Antifungal

Indications: Local treatment of vulvovaginal candidiasis.

Dose: Adults: Intravaginal 1 suppository at bedtime for 3 days or 1 applicatorful of 0.4% cream at bedtime for 7 days or 1 applicatorful of 0.8% cream for 3 days.

Trade names: Terazole 3 Vaginal cream 0.8%
Terazole 7 Vaginal cream 0.4%

Warnings: Standard considerations. Pregnancy Category: [C Avoid during first trimester because of absorption possibility]

Interactions: None well documented.

Testosterone Cypionate/ Estradiol Cypionate

Androgen/Estrogen combination

Indications: Treatment of moderate to severe vasomotor symptoms associated with menopause.

Dose: Adults: IM Use the lowest dose and regimen that will control symptoms and discontinue medication as promptly as possible. Usual dose is 1 mL (2 mg estradiol and 50 mg testosterone) at 4-wk intervals. Attempt to discontinue or taper medication at 3- to 6-mo intervals.

Trade names: Depo-Testadiol Injection 2 mg/mL estradiol, 50 mg/mL testosterone

Warnings: Known or suspected pregnancy; undiagnosed abnormal genital bleeding; known or suspected cancer of the breast except in appropriately selected patients being treated for metastatic disease; known or suspected estrogen-dependent neoplasm; active thrombophlebitis or thromboembolic disorder. Pregnancy Category: [X]

Interactions: Acetaminophen, ascorbic acid: Estrogen plasma levels may be elevated, increasing the risk of side effects.
Anticoagulants: Anticoagulant effects may be increased, requiring a dosage reduction.
Insulin: Insulin requirements may be reduced by the anabolic effects of testosterone.

Tetanus Immune Globulin

Immune serum

Indications: Passive, transient protection against tetanus in any person that may be contaminated with tetanus spores when: (1) patient's personal history of immunization with tetanus toxoid is unknown or uncertain, (2) person received less than 2 prior doses of tetanus toxoid, or (3) person received 2 prior doses of tetanus toxoid, but delay of more than 24 hr occurred between time of injury and initiation of tetanus prophylaxis.

Unlabeled indication: Treatment of clinical tetanus.

Dose: Adults:
Prophylactic dose: IM 250 U. Give 500 U if wounds are severe or treatment is delayed. Dosage may be increased to 1000 to 2000 U. For therapy of tetanus, give 500 to 3000 or 6000 U. Give deep IM, preferably in upper outer quadrant of gluteal muscle.
Children: IM Dose is calculated on basis of body weight (4 U/kg); however, it may be advisable to administer 250 U regardless of the size of the child. The same amount of toxin is produced by the bacteria in adults and children.

Trade names: Baytet Solution 250 units/syringe

Warnings: Hypersensitivity to human antibody product, thimerosal, or other components; circulating anti-IgA antibodies. Pregnancy Category: [C]

Interactions: There is no significant interaction

between TIG and tetanus toxoid if given at different injection sites. To avoid inactivating vaccines containing live viruses or bacteria, give live vaccines 2 to 4 wk before or 12 wk after TIG.

Thalidomide

Leprostatic

Indications: Acute treatment of cutaneous manifestations of moderate to severe erythema nodosum leprosum (ENL); maintenance therapy for prevention and suppression of cutaneous manifestations of ENL recurrence.

Dose: Adults: PO Initial dose 100 to 300 mg daily, preferably 1 hr after the evening meal. Give 400 mg daily at bedtime or in divided doses at least 1 hr after meals to patients with severe cutaneous ENL reaction or to those who have previously required higher doses to control reaction.
Tapering Schedule: Dosing should continue until signs and symptoms have subsided, usually for at least 2 wk. Taper in 50 mg decrements q 2 to 4 wk. Patients requiring prolonged maintenance treatment to prevent recurrence or who flare during tapering, decrease medication q 3 to 6 mo in decrements of 50 mg q 2 to 4 wk.

Trade names: Thalomid Capsules 50 mg

Warnings: Pregnancy. Pregnancy Category: [X]

Interactions: Barbiturates, chlorpromazine, ethanol, reserpine: The sedative effect of these drugs may be enhanced.

Theophylline

Bronchodilator / Xanthine derivative

Indications: Prevention or treatment of reversible bronchospasm associated with asthma or chronic obstructive pulmonary disease.

Unlabeled indication: Treatment of apnea and bradycardia of prematurity; reduction of essential tremor.

Dose: Dosage based on lean body weight.
Acute Therapy in Patients Not Currently Receiving Theophylline: Loading dose:
Adults and Children: PO 5 mg/kg.
Maintenance:
Children 9 to 16 yr and Young Adult Smokers: PO 3 mg/kg q 6 hr.
Children 1 to 9 yr: PO 4 mg/kg q 6 hr.
Elderly and Cor Pulmonale Patients: PO 2 mg/kg q 8 hr.
Patients With CHF: PO 1 to 2 mg/kg q 12 hr.
Nonsmoking Adults: PO 3 mg/kg q 8 hr.
Acute Therapy in Patients Receiving Theophylline: Each 0.5 mg/kg theophylline administered as a loading dose will increase serum theophylline concentration approximately 1 mcg/mL. If a serum theophylline concentration can be obtained rapidly, defer the loading dose. If this is not possible, clinical judgment must be exercised, using close monitoring. Maintenance doses as per above.
Chronic Therapy: Slow clinical titration preferred.
Initial dose: 16 mg/kg/24 hr or 400 mg/24 hr, whichever is less.
Increasing dose: Increase the above dosage 25% increments at 3-day intervals as long as the drug is tolerated or until the following maximum dose is reached (not to exceed 900 mg, whichever is less).
Maximum Dose (Where Serum Concentration Is Not Measured): Do not attempt to maintain any dose that is not tolerated.
Adults and Children over 16 yr: 13 mg/kg/day.
Children 12 to 16 yr: 18 mg/kg/day.
Children 9 to 12 yr: 24 mg/kg/day.
Children 1 to 9 yr: 24 mg/kg/day.
Adjustments Based on Serum Theophylline Concentrations (Recommended for Final Adjustments in Dosage): If serum theophylline concentration is within the desired range (10 to 20 mcg/mL), maintain dosage if tolerated. If too high (20 to 25 mcg/mL) decrease doses by approximately 10% and recheck in 3 days; (25 to 30 mcg/mL) skip the next dose, decrease subsequent doses by about 25% and recheck after 3 days; (over 30 mcg/mL) skip the next 2 doses, decrease subsequent doses by approximately 50% and recheck in 3 days. If too low (less than 10 mcg/mL) increase dosage 25% at 3-day intervals until either the desired clinical response or serum concentration is achieved.
Infant Guidelines:
Infants 26 to 52 wk: Dosing interval is q 6 hr.
Infants 26 wk or younger: Dosing interval is q 8 hr.
Infants 6 to 52 wk: PO 24 hr dose in mg [(0.2 x age in wk) + 5] x weight in kg.
Premature Infants over 24 days: PO 1.5 mg/kg q 12 hr.
Premature Infants 24 days and younger: PO 1 mg/kg q 12 hr. Final dosage guided by serum concentration after steady state is achieved.

Trade names: Accurbron Syrup 150 mg/15 mL (50 mg/5 mL)
Aquaphyllin Syrup 80 mg/15 mL (26.7 mg/5 mL)
Asmalix Elixir 80 mg/15 mL (26.7 mg/5 mL)
Bronkodyl Capsules 100 mg
Elixomin Elixir 80 mg/15 mL (26.7 mg/5 mL)
Elixophyllin Capsules 100 mg
Lanophyllin Elixir 80 mg/15 mL (26.7 mg/5 mL)
Quibron-T Dividose Tablets 300 mg
Quibron-T/SR Dividose Tablets, timed-release (8 to 12 hours) 300 mg
Respbid Tablets, timed-release (8 to 12 hours) 250 mg
Slo-bid Gyrocaps Capsules, timed-release (8 to 12 hours) 100 mg
Slo-Phyllin Tablets 100 mg
Slo-Phyllin Gyrocaps Capsules, timed-release (8 to 12 hours) 60 mg
Sustaire Tablets, timed-release (8 to 12 hours) 100 mg
T-Phyl Tablets, timed-release (8 to 12 hours) 200 mg
Theo-24 Capsules, timed-release (24 hours) 100 mg
Theo-Dur Tablets, timed-release (8 to 24 hours) 100 mg
Theo-Sav Tablets, timed-release (8 to 24 hours) 100 mg
Theo-X Tablets, controlled-release 100 mg
Theobid Duracaps Capsules, timed-release (12 hours) 260 mg
Theochron Tablets, extended-release 100 mg
Theoclear-80 Syrup 80 mg/15 mL (26.7 mg/5 mL)
Theoclear L.A. Capsules, timed-release (12 hours) 130 mg
Theolair Tablets 125 mg
Theolair-SR Tablets, timed-release (8 to 12 hours) 200 mg
Theovent Capsules, timed-release (12 hours) 125 mg
Uni-Dur Tablets, extended-release (24 hours) 400 mg
Uniphyl Tablets, timed-release (24 hours) 400 mg

Warnings: Hypersensitivity to xanthines; seizure disorders not adequately controlled with medication.
Pregnancy Category: [C]

Interactions: Allopurinol, nonselective beta-blockers, calcium channel blockers, cimetidine, oral contraceptives, corticosteroids, disulfiram, ephedrine, influenza virus vaccine, interferon, macrolide antibiotics (eg, erythromycin), mexiletine, quinolone antibiotics (eg, ciprofloxacin), thyroid hormones: Increase theophylline levels.
Aminoglutethimide, barbiturates, hydantoins, ketoconazole, rifampin, smoking (cigarettes and marijuana), sulfinpyrazone, sympathomimetics: Decrease theophylline levels.
Benzodiazepines and propofol: Theophylline may antagonize sedative effects.
Beta-agonists: Cardiovascular adverse effects may be additive. However, may be used together for additive beneficial effects.
Carbamazepine, isoniazid, and loop diuretics: May increase or decrease theophylline levels.
Halothane: Coadministration has caused catecholamine-induced arrhythmias.

Ketamine: Coadministration may result in seizures.
Lithium: Theophylline may reduce lithium levels.
Nondepolarizing muscle relaxants: Theophylline may antagonize neuromuscular blockade.
Incompatability: Do not mix following solutions with theophylline in IV fluids: ascorbic acid; chlorpromazine; corticotropin; dimenhydrinate; epinephrine HCl; erythromycin gluceptate; hydralazine; hydroxyzine HCl; insulin; levorphanol tartrate; meperidine; methadone; methicillin sodium; morphine sulfate; norepinephrine bitartrate; oxytetracycline; papaverine; penicillin G potassium; phenobarbital sodium; phenytoin sodium; procaine; prochlorperazine maleate; promazine; promethazine; tetracycline; vancomycin; vitamin B complex with C.

Thiabendazole

Anti-infective / Anthelmintic

Indications: Treatment of strongyloidiasis (threadworm infection), cutaneous larva migrans (creeping eruption), and visceral larva migrans alone or in conjunction with enterobiasis (pinworm). Secondary therapy for uncinariasis (hookworm: *Necator americanus* and *Ancylostoma duodenale*), trichuriasis (whipworm), and ascariasis (large roundworm); alleviation of symptoms of trichinosis during invasive phase.

Dose: Adults at least 150 lb (68 kg): PO 1.5 g/dose bid (max, 3 g/day).
Adults and Children 30 to 150 lb (13.6 to 68 kg): PO 10 mg/lb/dose (22 mg/kg/dose) (max, 3 g/day).
Strongyloidiasis, Ascariasis, Uncinariasis, Trichuriasis, Cutaneous larva migrans: Two doses daily for 2 successive days (may repeat for some indications).
Trichinosis: Two doses daily for 2 to 4 successive days.
Visceral larva migrans: Two doses daily for 7 successive days.

Trade names: Mintezol Tablets, chewable 500 mg

Warnings: Standard considerations. Pregnancy Category: [C]

Interactions: Xanthines: Thiabendazole may increase serum concentrations of theophylline to potentially toxic levels.

Thioguanine

Purine antimetabolite

Indications: Adult/Pediatric: Acute nonlymphocytic leukemia.

Unlabeled indication: Chronic myelogenous leukemia.

Dose: Acute Nonlymphocytic Leukemia, Remission Induction, Single Agent Therapy:
Adults: PO 2 mg/kg/day, rounded to nearest 20 mg, as a single daily dose. If no clinical improvement in 4 wk, may slowly increase the dose to 3 mg/kg/day.
Children 3 yr and older: PO 2 mg/kg/day, rounded to nearest 20 mg, as a single daily dose. If no clinical improvement in 4 wk, may slowly increase the dose to 3 mg/kg/day.
Acute Nonlymphocytic Leukemia, Remission Induction, Combination Therapy:
Adults: PO 75 to 200 mg/m^2 /day, rounded to the nearest 20 mg, in 1 or 2 divided doses for 5 to 7 days in each course of therapy until remission occurs.
Acute Nonlymphocytic Leukemia, Maintenance Therapy:
Adults: PO 2 mg/kg/day, rounded to the nearest 20 mg. Alternatively, 75 to 400 mg/m^2 /day PO, titrated to response.
Acute Nonlymphocytic Leukemia, Induction, Combination Therapy:
Infants and children under 3 yr: PO 3.3 mg/kg/day in 2 divided doses for 4 days in each course of therapy until remission occurs.
Acute Leukemia, Remission Induction, Combination Therapy:
Children 3 yr and older: PO 75 to 200 mg/m^2 /day, rounded to the nearest 20 mg, in 1 or 2 divided doses for 5 to 7 days in each course of therapy until remission occurs.
Maintenance Therapy:
Children 3 yr and older: PO 2 mg/kg/day, rounded to the nearest 20 mg. Alternatively, 50 mg/m^2 /day, titrated to response.

Trade names: Thioguanine Tablets 40 mg

Warnings: Prior resistance to this drug. There is usually complete cross-resistance between mercaptopurine and thioguanine. Pregnancy Category: [D]

Interactions: Busulfan: Concomitant therapy may increase risk of hepatotoxicity, esophageal varices, and portal hypertension.

Thiopental Sodium

General anesthetic / Barbiturate

Indications: Induction of anesthesia; supplementation of other anesthetic agents; IV anesthesia for short surgical procedures with minimal painful stimuli; induction of hypnotic state; control of convulsions and increased intracranial pressure (IV administration); induction of preanesthetic sedation or basal narcosis (PR administration).

Dose: Test Dose:
Adults: IV 25 to 75 mg; observe for 60 sec.
Anesthesia:
Adults: IV 50 to 75 mg slowly q 20 to 40 sec until anesthesia is established then 25 to 50 mg prn or continuous infusion of 0.2% or 0.4%.
Children: IV 5 to 6 mg/kg then 1 mg/kg prn.
Infants: IV 5 to 8 mg/kg then 1 mg/kg prn.
Newborns: IV 3 to 4 mg/kg then 1 mg/kg prn.
Convulsive States:
Adults: IV 75 to 125 mg; may need 125 to 250 mg over 10 min.
Children: IV 2 to 3 mg/kg/dose; repeat prn.
Increased Intracranial Pressure:
Adults: IV 1.5 to 3.5 mg/kg.
Children: IV 1.5 to 5 mg/kg/dose; repeat prn.
Psychiatric Disorders:
Adults: IV 100 mg/min slowly with patient counting backwards or as infusion of 50 mL/min of 0.2% solution.
Preanesthetic Sedation:
Adults: PR 1 g/34 kg (30 mg/kg).
Basal Narcosis:
Adults: PR 1 g/22.5 kg (44 mg/kg) (max, 3 to 4 g for adults weighing over 90 kg).
Children over 3 mo: PR 25 mg/kg/dose; if not sedated within 15 to 20 min, may repeat with single dose of 15 mg/kg/dose (max, 1.15 g for children over 34 kg).
Children under 3 mo: PR 15 mg/kg/dose; if not sedated within 15 to 20 min, may repeat with single dose of less than 7.5 mg/kg/dose.

Trade names: Pentothal Powder for Injection 2% (20 mg/mL)

Warnings: Hypersensitivity to barbiturates; variegate or acute intermittent porphyria; absence of suitable veins for IV administration; status asthmaticus. Rectal administration: Patients undergoing rectal surgery; lesions of bowel. Pregnancy Category: [C readily crosses placental barrier]

Interactions: Narcotics: May cause additive barbiturate effects and increase risk of apnea.
Phenothiazines: May increase frequency and severity of neuromuscular excitation and hypotension.
Probenecid: May extend barbiturate effects or effects may be achieved at lower doses.
Sulfisoxazole: May enhance barbiturate effects.
Incompatability: Tubocurarine, succinylcholine, or other acid pH solutions.

Thioridazine HCl

Antipsychotic / Phenothiazine

Indications: Management of schizophrenia.

Dose: Adults: PO Start with 50 to 100 mg tid, increasing the dose gradually in increments (max, 800 mg/day). Total daily dose ranges from 200 to 800 mg divided into 2 to 4 doses.
Children: PO Start with 0.5 mg/kg/day in divided doses, increasing the dose gradually until optimal therapeutic effect is obtained (max, 3 mg/kg/day).
Trade names: Mellaril Tablets 15 mg
Thioridazine HCl Tablets 10 mg
Warnings: Congenital QT interval prolongation; concurrent drugs that prolong the QT interval; history of cardiac arrhythmias; comatose or severely depressed states; allergy to this or any phenothiazine; presence of large amounts of other CNS depressants; severe hypotension or hypertension. Pregnancy Category: [Safety not established]
Interactions: Alcohol and other CNS depressants: May result in increased CNS depression and may precipitate extrapyramidal reaction.
Anticholinergics: May reduce therapeutic effects of thioridazine and worsen anticholinergic effects of thioridazine. May lead to tardive dyskinesia.
Barbiturate anesthetics: Frequency and severity of neuromuscular excitation and hypotension may increase.
Beta-blockers: May result in increased plasma levels of beta-blocker and thioridazine.
Drugs that prolong the QT interval (eg, cisapride), drugs that inhibit CYP2D6 (eg, fluoxetine, paroxetine): May increase the risk of life-threatening cardiac arrhythmias, including torsades de pointes. Coadministration of these agents is contraindicated.
Drugs that reduce the clearance of thioridazine by other mechanisms(eg, fluvoxamine, propranolol, pindolol): May elevate plasma levels of thioridazine, increasing the risk of side effects including life-threatening cardiac arrhythmias. Avoid coadministration of these agents.
Epinephrine: May antagonize effects of epinephrine.
Lithium: May cause disorientation, unconsciousness, and extrapyramidal effects.

Thiotepa

Alkylating agent / Ethylenimines / Methylmelamines

Indications: Bladder cancer, palliative therapy of breast and ovarian carcinoma.

Unlabeled indication: Prevention of pterygium recurrence after postoperative beta-irradiation, autologous bone marrow transplantation.
Dose: Breast and Ovarian Carcinoma:
Adults: IV 0.3 to 0.4 mg/kg every 1 to 4 wk. Alternative regimens, 0.2 mg/kg/day for 4 to 5 days every 2 to 4 wk; or 6 mg/m^2 /day for 4 to 5 days every 2 to 4 wk.
Bladder Tumors:
Adults: Intravesically 30 to 60 mg instilled (in 60 mL of sterile water) once weekly for 4 wk. Retain fluid in bladder for 2 hr. If patient cannot retain for 2 hr, dilute successive doses in 30 mL of sterile water instead of 60 mL. It may be necessary to repeat course of therapy or give maintenance therapy with 30 to 60 mg intravesically once monthly for up to 1 yr. After local resection or fulguration of bladder tumors, prophylaxis with thiotepa 30 to 60 mg has been used.
Trade names: Thioplex Powder for Injection 15 mg
Warnings: History of hypersensitivity reaction, hepatic disease, renal disease, or bone marrow toxicity. Administer reduced doses if therapy is necessary in these patients. Pregnancy Category: [D]
Interactions: Pancuronium: Prolonged apnea and paralysis because of pancuronium occurred in a patient who received thiotepa.
Succinylcholine: Prolonged apnea because of succinylcholine occurred in a patient who had received thiotepa and other antineoplastics.

Thiothixene

Antipsychotic / Thioxanthene

Indications: Management of schizophrenia.
Dose: Mild Conditions:
Adults and children 12 yr and older: PO Start with 2 mg tid, an increase to 15 mg/day is often effective if needed.
Severe Conditions:
Adults and children 12 yr and older: PO Start with 5 mg bid. The usual optimal dose is 20 to 30 mg/day. If indicated, an increase to 60 mg/day may be effective. Doses above 60 mg/day rarely increase the beneficial response.
Trade names: Navane Capsules 1 mg
Warnings: Comatose or severely depressed states; circulatory collapse; CNS depression from any cause; bone marrow depression; blood dyscrasias. Pregnancy Category: [Pregnancy category undetermined]
Interactions: Alcohol, other CNS depressants: May cause additive CNS depressant effects.
Anticholinergics: May reduce therapeutic effects and increase anticholinergic effects of thiothixene; may lead to tardive dyskinesia.
Guanethidine: May inhibit hypotensive effect of guanethidine.

Tiagabine Hydrochloride

Anticonvulsant

Indications: Adjunctive treatment in treatment of partial seizures.
Dose: Adults: PO Initial dose 4 mg qd. Increase by 4 to 8 mg at weekly intervals until response achieved or total of 56 mg/day.
Adolescents 12 to 18 yr: PO Initial dose 4 mg qd. Increase dose by 4 mg after 1 wk and thereafter by 4 to 8 mg at weekly intervals until response achieved or total of 32 mg/day.
Trade names: Gabitril Filmtabs Tablets 4 mg
Warnings: Standard considerations. Pregnancy Category: [C]
Interactions: Enzyme-inducing antiepileptic drugs (eg, carbamazepine, phenytoin, primidone, phenobarbital): Increased tiagabine clearance.

Ticlopidine HCl

Antiplatelet

Indications: Reduction of risk of thrombotic stroke in patients who have experienced stroke precursors and in patients who have had completed thrombotic stroke. Reserved for patients intolerant to aspirin because of greater risk of adverse reactions.

Unlabeled indication: Improved walking distance in intermittent claudication; vascular improvement in chronic arterial occlusion; reduced incidence of neurologic deficit in subarachnoid hemorrhage; reduced incidence of vascular occlusion in uremic patients with arteriovenous shunts or fistulas; control of platelet count in open heart surgery; decreased graft occlusion in coronary artery bypass grafts; reduced degree of proteinuria and hematuria in primary glomerulonephritis; reduced incidence, duration, and severity of infarctive crises in sickle cell disease.
Dose: Adults: PO 250 mg bid with food.
Trade names: Ticlid Tablets 250 mg
Warnings: Presence of hematopoietic disorders (eg, neutropenia, thrombocytopenia); history of thrombotic thrombocytopenic purpura (TTP); presence of hemostatic disorder or active pathologic bleeding (eg, bleeding, peptic ulcer, intracranial bleeding, hemophilia, other coagulation defects); severe liver impairment. Pregnancy Category: [B]
Interactions: Antacids: May reduce ticlopidine absorption.

Aspirin: Increased effect of aspirin on collagen-induced platelet aggregation.
Cimetidine: Elevated ticlopidine levels with possible increase in therapeutic and toxic effects.
Theophylline: Elevated serum theophylline concentrations, increasing risk of toxicity.
Phenytoin: Elevated phenytoin plasma levels with associated somnolence and lethargy have been reported. Exercise caution when administering with ticlopidine.

Timolol Maleate

Beta-adrenergic blocker

Indications: Treatment of hypertension, alone or in combination with other agents; reduction of risk of reinfarction post-MI; migraine prophylaxis; treatment of elevated IOP in chronic open-angle glaucoma, ocular hypertension, aphakic glaucoma patients, patients with secondary glaucoma, and in patients with elevated IOP who need ocular pressure lowering.

Dose: Hypertension:
Adults: PO 10 mg bid, titrate to response q 7 days (max, 60 mg/day).
MI Prophylaxis:
Adults: PO 10 mg bid.
Migraine Prophylaxis:
Adults: PO 10 mg bid (max, 30 mg/day); if no response in 6 wk then discontinue.
Glaucoma:
Adults: Ophthalmic 1 gtt 0.25% to 0.5% solution in affected eye(s) bid.

Trade names: Betimol Solution 0.25%
Blocadren Tablets 5 mg
Timoptic Solution 0.25%
Timoptic Ocudose Solution 0.25%
Timoptic-XE Solution, gel-forming 0.25%

Warnings: Hypersensitivity to beta-blockers; greater than first-degree heart block; CHF unless secondary to tachyarrhythmia treatable with beta-blockers; overt cardiac failure; sinus bradycardia; cardiogenic shock; bronchial asthma or bronchospasm, including severe COPD. Pregnancy Category: [C]

Interactions: Clonidine: May enhance or reverse antihypertensive effect; potentially life-threatening situations may occur, especially on withdrawal.
Epinephrine: Initial hypertensive episode followed by bradycardia may occur.
Ergot derivatives: Peripheral ischemia, manifested by cold extremities and possible gangrene, may occur.
Insulin: Prolonged hypoglycemia with masking of symptoms may occur.
NSAIDs: Some agents may impair antihypertensive effect.
Prazosin: Orthostatic hypotension may be increased.
Theophyllines: Elimination of theophylline may be reduced. Effects of both drugs may be reduced.
Verapamil: Effects of both drugs may be increased.

Tinzaparin Sodium

Anticoagulants

Indications: Treatment of acute symptomatic deep vein thrombosis with or without pulmonary embolism when administered with warfarin.

Dose: Adults: SC 175 anti-Xa IU/kg once daily for more than 6 days and until patient is adequately anticoagulated with warfarin.

Trade names: Innohep Injection 20,000 IU/mL

Warnings: Active major bleeding, heparin-induced thrombocytopenia, hypersensitivity to heparin, sulfites, benzyl alcohol, or pork products. Pregnancy Category: [B]

Interactions: Anticoagulants, platelet inhibitors (eg, dipyridamole, NSAIDs, salicylates): Use with caution because of increased risk of bleeding.

Tizanidine HCl

Skeletal muscle relaxant / Centrally acting

Indications: Acute and intermittent management of increased muscle tone associated with spasticity.

Dose: Adults: PO Initiate therapy with a 4 mg dose, increasing the dose gradually in 2 to 4 mg increments to optimum effect. The dose can be repeated at 6- to 8-hr intervals as needed (max, 3 doses in 24 hr not to exceed 36 mg/day).

Trade names: Zanaflex Tablets 2 mg

Warnings: Standard considerations. Pregnancy Category: [C]

Interactions: Alcohol: Plasma levels of tizanidine may be elevated, increasing the side effects.
Antihypertensive agents: Use with caution; do not administer with other $alpha_2$-adrenergic agonists (eg, clonidine).
Oral contraceptives: Clearance of tizanidine may be reduced; decrease the dosage requirement.

Tolazamide

Antidiabetic / Sulfonylurea

Indications: Adjunct to diet to lower blood glucose in patients with non-insulin-dependent diabetes mellitus (type 2) whose hyperglycemia cannot be controlled by diet alone.

Unlabeled indication: Temporary adjunct to insulin therapy in selected patients with non-insulin-dependent diabetes mellitus to improve diabetic control.

Dose: Adults: PO 100 to 250 mg/day with breakfast or first main meal. If fasting blood sugar (FBS) is less than 200 mg/dL, initial dose is 100 mg/day or if FBS is greater than 200 mg/dL, initial dose is 250 mg/day. In malnourished, underweight, elderly patients use 100 mg/day. May adjust dose by 100 to 250 mg/wk as needed to a maximum of 1000 mg/day. If more than 500 mg/day is required, give in divided doses bid. Doses greater than 1 g/day are not likely to improve control.
Maintenance dose: PO Usual dose is 100 to 1000 mg/day with the average 250 to 500 mg/day. Following initiation of therapy, dosage adjustment is made in increments of 100 to 250 mg at weekly intervals based on patient's blood glucose response.

Trade names: Tolinase Tablets 100 mg

Warnings: Hypersensitivity to sulfonylureas; diabetes complicated by ketoacidosis, with or without coma; sole therapy of insulin-dependent (type 1) diabetes mellitus; gestational diabetes. Pregnancy Category: [C]

Interactions: Androgens, anticoagulants, azole antifungals, chloramphenicol, clofibrate, fenfluramine, fluconazole, gemfibrozil, histamine H_2 antagonists, magnesium salts, methyldopa, MAO inhibitors, phenylbutazone, probenecid, salicylates, sulfinpyrazone, sulfonamides, tricyclic antidepressants, urinary acidifiers: Increased hypoglycemic effect.
Beta-blockers, calcium channel blockers, cholestyramine, corticosteroids, diazoxide, estrogens, hydantoins, isoniazid, nicotinic acid, oral contraceptives, phenothiazines, rifampin, sympathomimetics, thiazide diuretics, thyroid agents, urinary alkalinizers: Decreased hypoglycemic effect.
Charcoal: Charcoal can reduce the absorption; depending on clinical situation, this will reduce sulfonylureas efficacy or toxicity.
Digitalis glycosides: Coadministration may result in increased digitalis serum levels.

Tolbutamide

Antidiabetic / Sulfonylurea

Indications: Oral form: Adjunct to diet to lower blood glucose in patients with non-insulin-dependent diabetes mellitus (type 2) whose hyperglycemia cannot be controlled by diet alone.

IV form (tolbutamide sodium): Aid in diagnosis of pancreatic islet cell adenoma.

Dose: Adults: PO Usually 1 to 2 g/day (range, 0.25 to 3 g) in 1 to 2 divided doses.
For Diagnostic Purposes:
Adults: IV 1 g over 2 to 3 min.

Trade names: Orinase Tablets 500 mg
Orinase Diagnostic Powder for injection 1 g (as sodium)/vial

Warnings: Hypersensitivity to sulfonylureas; diabetes complicated by ketoacidosis with or without coma; sole therapy of insulin-dependent (type 1) diabetes mellitus; diabetes occurring during pregnancy. Pregnancy Category: [C Insulin is recommended to control elevated blood glucose levels during pregnancy]

Interactions: Androgens, anticoagulants, azole antifungals, chloramphenicol, clofibrate, dicumarol, fenfluramine, fluconazole, gemfibrozil, histamine H_2 antagonists, magnesium salts, methyldopa, MAO inhibitors, phenylbutazone, probenecid, salicylates, sulfinpyrazone, sulfonamides, tricyclic antidepressants, urinary acidifiers: May increase hypoglycemic effect.
Beta-blockers, calcium channel blockers, cholestyramine, corticosteroids, diazoxide, estrogens, hydantoins, isoniazid, nicotinic acid, oral contraceptives, phenothiazines, rifampin, sympathomimetics, thiazide diuretics, thyroid agents, urinary alkalinizers: May decrease hypoglycemic effect.
Charcoal: Charcoal can reduce the absorption of sulfonylureas; depending on the clinical situation, this will reduce their efficacy or toxicity.
Digitalis glycosides: Coadministration may result in increased digitalis serum levels.
Digoxin: May cause increased digoxin serum concentrations.
Ethanol: May cause disulfiram-like reaction.

Tolcapone

Antiparkinson

Indications: As an adjunct to levodopa/carbidopa for the management of signs and symptoms of Parkinson's disease.

Dose: Adults: PO 100 or 200 mg tid. The maximum recommended dose is 600 mg/day.

Trade names: Tasmar Tablets 100 mg

Warnings: Hypersensitivity to the drug or its ingredients; patients with liver disease; patients who were withdrawn from tolcapone because of evidence of tolcapone-induced hepatocellular injury; patients with a history of non-traumatic rhabdomyolysis or hyperpyrexia and confusion possibly related to medication. Pregnancy Category: [C]

Interactions: None well documented.

Tolmetin Sodium

Analgesic / NSAID

Indications: Treatment of chronic and acute rheumatoid arthritis and osteoarthritis and juvenile rheumatoid arthritis.

Dose: Osteoarthritis/Rheumatoid Arthritis:
Adults: PO 400 mg tid initially; titrate to 600 to 1600 mg/day for osteoarthritic patients or 600 to 1800 mg/day in divided doses for rheumatoid arthritis patients. Daily doses exceeding 1800 mg/day are not recommended.
Juvenile Rheumatoid Arthritis:
Children 2 yr or older: PO 20 mg/kg/day in 3 to 4 divided doses initially; titrate to 15 to 30 mg/kg/day (max, 30 mg/kg/day).

Trade names: Tolectin 200 Tablets 200 mg (as sodium)
Tolectin 600 Tablets 600 mg (as sodium)
Tolectin DS Capsules 400 mg (as sodium)

Warnings: Hypersensitivity to aspirin, iodides, or any NSAID. Pregnancy Category: [C]

Interactions: Anticoagulants: May increase effect of anticoagulants due to decreased plasma protein binding. May increase risk of gastric erosion and bleeding.
Cyclosporine: May potentiate nephrotoxicity of both agents.
Methotrexate: May increase methotrexate levels.

Tolnaftate

Topical / Antifungal

Indications: Treatment and prophylaxis of tinea pedia (athlete's foot); treatment of tinea cruris (jock itch) or tinea corporis (ringworm) caused by specific fungi; treatment of onchomycosis, chronic scalp infections, palm and sole infections with kerion formation; treatment of tinea versicolor.

Dose: Adults and Children: Topical Apply small amount of ointment, cream, or powder or 1 to 3 gtt of solution to affected area bid for 2 to 3 wk (6 wk if skin is thickened); continue treatment to maintain remission. Reserve powder for mild infections.

Trade names: Absorbine Athlete's Foot Cream Cream 1%
Absorbine Footcare Spray liquid 1%
Aftate for Athlete's Foot Gel 1%
Aftate for Jock Itch Gel 1%
Blis-To-Sol Liquid Liquid 1%
Genaspor Cream 1%
NP-27 Liquid 1%
Quinsana Plus Foot Powder Powder 1%
Tinactin Cream 1%
Tinactin for Jock Itch Cream 1%
Ting Cream 1%

Warnings: Standard considerations. Pregnancy Category: [Undetermined]

Interactions: None well documented.

Tolterodine Tartrate

Urinary tract product / Muscarinic antagonist

Indications: Treatment of overactive bladder with symptoms of urinary frequency, urgency, or urge incontinence.

Dose: Immediate-Release:
Adults: PO 1 to 2 mg daily.
Extended-Release: PO 2 to 4 mg daily.

Trade names: Detrol Tablets 1 mg
Detrol LA Capsule, extended-release 2 mg

Warnings: Urinary retention; gastric retention; uncontrolled narrow-angle glaucoma. Pregnancy Category: [C]

Interactions: Clarithromycin, erythromycin, itraconazole, ketoconazole, miconazole(and other cytochrome P450 3A4 inhibitors): May increase tolterodine plasma levels, which may increase activity and side effects.
Fluoxetine: Plasma levels of tolterodine may be decreased while the AUC of the active 5-hydroxymethyl metabolite may be increased; requires no dosage adjustment.

Topiramate

Anticonvulsant

Indications: Adjunctive therapy for partial onset seizures; primary generalized tonic-clonic seizures; seizures associated with Lennox-Gastaut syndrome.

Dose: Adults 17 yr of age and older: PO 200 to 400 mg daily in 2 divided doses in adults with partial seizures and 400 mg daily in 2 divided doses in adults with primary, generalized, tonic-clonic seizures. Initiate therapy at 25 to 50 mg daily and titrate to an effective dose in increments of 25 to 50 mg weekly. Doses over 400 mg have not been shown to improve response.
Children 2 to 16 yr of age: PO 5 to 9 mg/kg per day in 2

divided doses. Initiate therapy at 25 mg or less (based on range of 1 to 3 mg/kg per day) nightly for first wk and titrate to an effective dose at 1- to 2-wk intervals by increments of 1 to 3 mg/kg per day in 2 divided doses.
Renal Function Impairment (Ccr 70 mL per min or less): Dosage adjustment of 50% of the usual adult dose is recommended.
Trade names: Topamax Tablets 25 mg
Warnings: Standard considerations. Pregnancy Category: [C]
Interactions: Alcohol, CNS depressants: CNS depression and side effects may be increased.
Carbamazepine: Effects of topiramate may be decreased.
Carbonic anhydrase inhibitors (eg, acetazolamide): Increased risk of renal stone formation.
Oral contraceptives: Efficacy of oral contraceptives may be decreased and possible increased breakthrough bleeding.
Phenytoin: Effects of phenytoin may be increased while those of topiramate may decrease.
Valproic acid: Effects of valproic acid and topiramate may both be decreased.

Topotecan HCl

Topoisomerase I inhibitor

Indications: Metastatic carcinoma of the ovary after failure of initial or subsequent chemotherapy; small cell lung cancer sensitive disease after failure of first-line chemotherapy.
Dose: Dosage Adjustment:
Adults: IV If neutropenia develops (defined as absolute neutrophil count less than 1500/mm^3), reduce the dose by 0.25 mg/m^2 for subsequent doses. Alternately, a course of filgrastim may be started on day 6 of each subsequent cycle; give the first filgrastim dose 24 hr after the final topotecan dose.
Ovarian or Small-Cell Lung Cancer:
Adults: IV Topotecan 1.5 mg/m^2 /day over 30 min daily for 5 consecutive days starting on day 1 of a 21-day cycle. Tumor response may be delayed; administer at least 4 cycles provided the tumor is not progressing. Before giving each dose, the patient should have a neutrophil count greater than 1500/mm^3 and a platelet count greater than 100,000/mm^3.
Renal Function Impairment:
Adults: IV Dosage adjustment is recommended in patients with moderate renal impairment (Ccr of 20 to 39 mL/min); give 50% of usual dose. For Ccr less than 20 mL/min, reduce dose; specific recommendations not available.
Trade names: Hycamtin Powder for Injection 4 mg
Warnings: Hypersensitivity to topotecan or to any of its ingredients; pregnancy or breastfeeding; severe bone marrow depression. Pregnancy Category: [D]
Interactions: Cisplatin: Myelosuppression is more severe when topotecan is given in combination with cisplatin.
Filgrastim: Coadministration can prolong the duration of neutropenia. If filgrastim is used, do not initiate until day 6 of the course of therapy, 24 hr after completion of treatment with topotecan.

Torsemide

Loop diuretic

Indications: Management of edema associated with CHF, hepatic cirrhosis, and renal disease; treatment of hypertension.
Dose: Adults: PO/IV 5 to 20 mg once daily. Titrate dose upward until desired response is obtained. Single doses greater than 200 mg have not been studied.
Trade names: Demadex Tablets 5 mg
Warnings: Hypersensitivity to sulfonylureas; anuria; severe electrolyte depletion. Pregnancy Category: [B]
Interactions: Aminoglycosides: May increase ototoxicity.
Anticoagulants: May enhance anticoagulant activity.
Cisplatin: May cause additive ototoxicity.
Digitalis glycosides: Electrolyte disturbances may predispose to digitalis-induced arrhythmias.
Lithium: May increase plasma lithium levels and toxicity.
Nondepolarizing muscle relaxants: May antagonize or potentiate response to muscle relaxants.
NSAIDs: May decrease effects of torsemide.
Probenecid: May reduce action of torsemide.
Salicylates: May impair diuretic response in patients with cirrhosis and ascites.
Sulfonylureas: May decrease glucose tolerance, resulting in need for increased sulfonylurea dose.
Thiazide diuretics: May cause synergistic effects that may result in profound diuresis and serious electrolyte abnormalities.

Trazodone HCl

Antidepressant

Indications: Treatment of depression.

Unlabeled indication: Treatment of neurogenic pain, aggression, panic disorder, cocaine withdrawal.
Dose: Adults: PO 150 mg/day in divided doses initially; increase in 50 mg increments up to maximum of 400 mg/day (outpatients) or 600 mg/day (inpatients).
Elderly patients: PO Start with 75 mg/day in divided doses.
Trade names: Desyrel Tablets 50 mg
Desyrel Dividose Tablets 150 mg
Warnings: Hypersensitivity to trazodone; initial recovery phase of MI. Pregnancy Category: [C]
Interactions: Alcohol, barbiturates, CNS depressants: CNS depressant effects may be additive.
Carbamazepine: Plasma concentrations of trazodone and its active metabolite may be decreased, producing a decrease in therapeutic effect.
Fluoxetine: May increase trazodone serum levels.
Hypotensive agents: May cause additive hypotensive effects.
MAO inhibitors: It is unknown whether interactions may take place. Initiate trazodone therapy cautiously if patient is currently taking or has recently stopped taking MAO inhibitors.
Phenothiazines: Elevated trazodone serum concentrations have occurred, increasing the pharmacologic and toxic effects.
SSRIs: A serotonin syndrome, including irritability, increased muscle tone, shivering, myoclonus, and altered consciousness may occur.

Tretinoin

Retinoids

Indications: Topical treatment of acne vulgaris; as an adjunctive agent for use in the mitigation of fine wrinkles, mottled hyperpigmentation, and tactile roughness of facial skin. PO treatment for acute promyelocytic leukemia.

Unlabeled indication: Treatment of skin cancer; various dermatologic conditions including lamellar ichthyosis, warts, and Darier disease.
Dose: Treatment of Acne:
Adults and Pediatric: Topical Apply lightly to affected area qd before bedtime.
Treatment of Fine Wrinkles, Hyperpigmentation, and Tactile Roughness of Facial Skin:
Adult: Topical Apply lightly to affected area. Use smallest amount possible.
Acute Myelocytic Leukemia:
Adult and Pediatric (more than 1 yr): PO 45 mg/m^2 /day in 2 divided doses. Continue therapy for a max duration of 90 days or for 30 days after achieving complete remission, whichever is shorter.

Trade names: Avita Cream 0.025%
Renova Cream 0.02%
Retin-A Cream 0.025%
Retin-A Micro Gel 0.04%
Vesanoid Capsules 10 mg
Warnings: Do not use if sunburned or have eczema, highly sensitive to the sun, or with skin irritation (Renova only). Pregnancy Category: [C (topical) D (PO)]
Interactions: Benzoyl peroxide, cosmetics with drying effects, resorcinol, salicylic acid, soaps, or sulfur: May result in significant skin irritation.
CYP450: Elimination may be altered by agents that inhibit or induce CYP450 enzymes.
Photosensitizers (eg, fluoroquinolones, phenothiazines, tetracyclines, thiazide diuretics, sulfonamides): May augment photosensitivity.

Triamterene

Potassium-sparing diuretic
Indications: Treatment of edema associated with CHF, hepatic cirrhosis, and nephrotic syndrome; treatment of steroid-induced edema, idiopathic edema, and edema caused by secondary hyperaldosteronism; management of hypertension in patient with diuretic-induced hypokalemia or at risk of hypokalemia.
Dose: Adults: PO 100 mg bid after meals (max, 300 mg/day).
Children: PO 2 to 4 mg/kg/day given in 1 dose or 2 divided doses (max, 300 mg/day).
Trade names: Dyrenium Capsules 50 mg
Warnings: Treatment with spironolactone or amiloride; anuria; severe hepatic disease; hyperkalemia; severe or progressive kidney disease or dysfunction, with exception of nephrosis. Pregnancy Category: [B]
Interactions: ACE inhibitors: May result in severely elevated serum potassium levels.
Indomethacin: May cause rapid progression into acute renal failure.
Potassium preparations and salt substitutes: May severely increase serum potassium levels, possibly resulting in cardiac arrhythmias or cardiac arrest. Do not take with potassium preparations.

Triazolam

Sedative and hypnotic / Benzodiazepine
Indications: Treatment of insomnia.
Dose: Adults: PO 0.125 to 0.5 mg at bedtime.
Elderly or debilitated patients: Initiate with 0.125 mg until individual response is determined.
Trade names: Halcion Tablets 0.125 mg
Warnings: Hypersensitivity to benzodiazepines; pregnancy. Pregnancy Category: [X]
Interactions: Alcohol, CNS depressants (eg, narcotic sedatives): May cause additive CNS depressant effects.
Cimetidine, disulfiram, omeprazole, oral contraceptives: Triazolam effects may increase.
Digoxin: Serum digoxin concentrations may be increased.
Theophylline: May antagonize sedative effects.

Trifluoperazine HCl

Antipsychotic / Phenothiazine
Indications: Management of schizophrenia; short-term treatment (less than 12 wk) of nonpsychotic anxiety.
Dose: Individualize dose.
Schizophrenia:
Adults: PO 2 to 5 mg bid initially. Maintenance: 15 to 20 mg/day in single or divided doses. Few patients may require 40 mg/day or more.
Children: Individualize dosage based on weight of child and severity of symptoms.
Children 6 to 12 yr: PO 1 mg qd or bid initially.
Maintenance: Rarely over 15 mg/day in single or divided doses.
Nonpsychotic Anxiety:
Adults: PO 1 to 2 mg bid (max, 6 mg/day).
Trade names: Trifluoperazine HCl Tablet 1 mg
Warnings: Sensitivity to phenothiazines; comatose or severely depressed states; presence of large amounts of other CNS depressants; bone marrow depression or blood dyscrasias; liver disease. Pregnancy Category: [Undetermined]
Interactions: Alcohol and other CNS depressants (eg, narcotics, sedatives): May result in increased CNS depression and may precipitate dystonic reactions.
Anticholinergics: May reduce therapeutic effects of trifluoperazine and worsen anticholinergic effects of trifluoperazine. May lead to tardive dyskinesia.
Barbiturate anesthetics: May increase frequency and severity of neuromuscular excitation and hypotension.
Beta-blockers: May result in increased plasma levels of beta-blocker and trifluoperazine.
Cisapride, sparfloxacin: The risk of life-threatening cardiac arrhythmias, including torsades de pointes, may be increased.
Guanethidine: May inhibit hypotensive action of guanethidine.
Metrizamide: Possibility of seizure may be increased when subarachnoid metrizamide injection is used.
Paroxetine: Plasma levels of trifluoperazine may be elevated, increasing the risk of side effects.

Trihexyphenidyl HCl

Antiparkinson / Anticholinergic
Indications: Adjunct in treatment of all forms of parkinsonism (postencephalitic, arteriosclerotic, and idiopathic); adjuvant therapy with levodopa for control of drug-induced extrapyramidal disorders.
Sustained-release: Maintenance therapy after patients have been stabilized on tablets or elixir.
Dose: Parkinsonism:
Adults: PO 1 or 2 mg first day; increase by 3 mg increments at intervals of 3 to 5 days, until 6 to 10 mg given daily in divided doses. Some postencephalitic patients may require total daily dose of 12 to 15 mg. Usually given tid at mealtimes. High doses may be taken qid, at mealtimes and at bedtime.
Concomitant use with other anticholinergics: Gradually initiate trihexyphenidyl with progressive reduction of other anticholinergic.
Drug-Induced Extrapyramidal Disorders: Amount and frequency is individualized. Start with single 1 mg dose. If symptoms are not controlled in few hr, progressively increase until controlled. Daily dosage usually ranges 5 to 15 mg in divided doses.
Sustained-Release: Not for initial therapy. Once patient is stabilized, may switch on equipotent daily basis. Give as single dose after breakfast or in bid doses 12 hr apart.
Trade names: Artane Tablets 2 mg
Artane Sequels Capsules, sustained-release 5 mg
Trihexy-2 Tablets 2 mg
Trihexy-5 Tablets 5 mg
Warnings: Standard considerations. Pregnancy Category: [C]
Interactions: Haloperidol: Schizophrenic symptoms may worsen; haloperidol levels may decrease and tardive dyskinesia may develop.
Phenothiazines: Actions of phenothiazines may be decreased.

Trimetrexate Glucuronate

Folic acid antimetabolite / Anti-infective / Antiprotozoal
Indications: As alternative therapy, with concurrent leucovorin administration, for treatment of moderate-to-severe Pneumocystis carinii pneumonia in immunocompromised patients in whom trimethoprim-sulfamethoxazole cannot be used.

Unlabeled indication: Treatment of non-small cell lung, prostate, and colorectal cancer.
Dose: Adults: IV 45 mg/m^2 q/day by IV infusion over 60 to 90 min for 21 days. Leucovorin may be administered IV at dose of 20 mg/m^2 over 5 to 10 min q 6 hr for total daily dose of 80 mg/m^2 or PO at dose of 20 mg/m^2 q 6 hr for 24 days. Adjust dose of trimetrexate and leucovorin according to hematologic toxicity. Interruption of therapy may be necessary for hematologic, hepatic, renal, or mucosal toxicity or for uncontrolled fever. See manufacturer's recommendations.
Trade names: Neutrexin Powder for injection, lyophilized 25 mg
Warnings: Clinically significant sensitivity to trimetrexate, leucovorin, or methotrexate. Pregnancy Category: [D]
Interactions: Hepatic enzyme inducers (eg, phenobarbital, phenytoin, carbamazepine, rifampin, rifabutin): Decreased trimetrexate concentrations and reduced efficacy are possible.
Hepatic enzyme inhibitors (eg, ketoconazole, itraconazole, macrolides, cimetidine): Increased trimetrexate concentrations and increased toxicity are possible.
Hepatotoxic drugs (eg, NSAIDs, etretinate, ethanol, methotrexate, asparaginase): Increased risk of hepatotoxicity may occur.
Nephrotoxic drugs (eg, aminoglycosides, amphotericin B, cisplatin, co-trimoxazole, cyclosporine, ganciclovir, melphalan, NSAIDs): Increased risk of nephrotoxicity may occur.
Pneumococcal vaccine: Reduced vaccine efficacy may occur.
Pyrimethamine, trimethoprim: Increased antifolate effects and increased toxicity may occur.
Yellow fever vaccine, other live vaccines: Increased risk of infection (ie, vaccine toxicity).
Zidovudine: Zidovudine should be discontinued during trimetrexate therapy to allow for full therapeutic doses of trimetrexate.
Incompatability: Do not mix with solutions containing either chloride ion (eg, sodium chloride) or leucovorin, because precipitation occurs instantly.

Trimipramine Maleate

Tricyclic antidepressant
Indications: Relief of symptoms of depression.
Dose: Adolescents and Elderly: PO Initially, 50 mg/day, with gradual incremental increases up to 100 mg/day, depending on response and tolerance.
Hospitalized Patients:
Adults: PO Initially, 100 mg/day. This may be gradually increased in a few days to 200 mg/day, depending on response and tolerance. If improvement does not occur in 2 to 3 wk, the dose may be increased to a max of 250 to 300 mg/day.
Outpatients and Office Patients:
Adults: PO Initially, 75 mg/day in divided doses, increased to 150 mg/day. Dosages over 200 mg/day are not recommended. Maintenance therapy ranges from 50 to 150 mg/day.
Trade names: Surmontil Capsules 25 mg
Warnings: Hypersensitivity to any tricyclic antidepressant; not to be given with or within 14 days of treatment with an MAO inhibitor; during acute recovery phase following an MI; cross-sensitivity may occur among the dibenzazepines. Pregnancy Category: [C]
Interactions: Alcohol, CNS depressants: Depressant effects may be additive.
Catecholamines/anticholinergics: Effects of the catecholamine may be potentiated.
Cimetidine: May cause increased trimipramine blood levels.
Drugs inhibiting CYP2D6 (amiodarone, fluoxetine, quinidine): Trimipramine blood levels may be elevated, increasing the pharmacologic and adverse effects.
MAO inhibitors: May cause hyperpyretic crisis, severe convulsions, and death when given with trimipramine.

Trypsin/Balsam Peru/ Castor Oil

Topical Enzyme
Indications: In acute and chronic conditions such as varicose ulcers, decubital ulcers, eschar, dehiscent wounds and sunburn, relieves pain and promotes healing; debrides eschar and necrotic tissue; stimulates vascular bed; improves epithelization; reduces odor from necrotic wounds.
Dose: Topical: Aerosol Shake well and hold upright approximately 12 inches from the area to be treated. Apply bid or as often as necessary. To remove, wash gently with water.
Trade names: Granulex Aerosol 0.12 mg trypsin/ 87 mg balsam peru/788 mg castor oil per g
Warnings: Standard considerations. Pregnancy Category: []
Interactions: None well documented.

Tuberculin, Purified Protein Derivative

Diagnostic skin test
Indications: Detection of delayed hypersensitivity to *Mycobacterium tuberculosis*; aid in diagnosis of infection with M. tuberculosis; routine testing for tuberculosis; testing individuals suspected of having contact with active tuberculosis; follow-up verification testing in individuals who have had reactions to tuberculin multipuncture devices used as screening test.
Dose: Adults and Children: Intradermal 0.1 mL of 5 TU/0.1 mL concentration (Mantoux test) or multiple puncture device.
Highly sensitized people: Intradermal 0.1 mL of 1 TU/0.1 mL concentration.
Individuals who fail to react to previous injection of 5 TU: Intradermal 0.1 mL of 250 TU/0.1 mL concentration.
Routine Tuberculin Screening:
Children: Perform at 12 mo, 4 to 6 yr, and 14 to 16 yr.
Trade names: Aplitest Injection 5 TU activity/test
Tine Test PPD Injection 5 TU activity/test
Aplisol Injection 5 TU/0.1 mL
Tubersol Injection 1 TU/0.1 mL
Warnings: People known to be tuberculin-positive reactors. Pregnancy Category: [C Use if needed Unrecognized tuberculosis places infant in grave danger of tuberculosis and tuberculous meningitis No adverse effects on fetus from tuberculin have been reported]
Interactions: BCG vaccine, previous: May result in positive PPD test (see Precautions).
Corticosteroids or other immunosuppressive drugs: May suppress reactivity to any tuberculin test.
Recent immunization with live virus vaccines (including influenza, measles, mumps, rubella, polio virus, smallpox, yellow fever): May suppress reactivity to any tuberculin test. If tuberculin skin testing is indicated, perform it either before or simultaneous with immunization or 4 to 6 wk after immunization.

Urokinase

Thrombolytic enzyme
Indications: Lysis of acute massive pulmonary emboli (defined as obstruction of blood flow to a lobe or multiple segments); lysis of pulmonary emboli accompanied by unstable hemodynamics (ie, failure to maintain BP without supportive measures).
Dose: Adults: IV Loading dose of 2000 IU/lb (4400 IU/kg) admixture (0.9% sodium chloride injection, or 5% dextrose injection) instituted soon after onset of

pulmonary embolism and infused at a rate of 90 mL/hr over 10-min period, followed by continuous infusion of 2000 IU/lb/hr (4400 IU/kg/hr) at a rate of 15 mL/hr for 12 hr. Flush tubing with solution (0.9% sodium chloride injection, or 5% dextrose injection) approximately equal to the volume of the tubing in the infusion set. The pump should be set to administer the flush solution at the rate of 15 mL/hr.

Trade names: Abbokinase Injection 250,000 IU

Warnings: Active internal bleeding; recent cerebrovascular accidents (eg, within 2 mo); recent intracranial or intraspinal surgery (eg, within 2 mo); recent trauma including cardiopulmonary resuscitation; intracranial neoplasm, arteriovenous malformation, or aneurysm; known bleeding diatheses; severe uncontrolled arterial hypertension; known hypersensitivity to any component of the product. Pregnancy Category: [B]

Interactions: Anticoagulants, agents that alter platelet function (eg, aspirin, other NSAIDs, dipyridamole), other thrombolytic agents, agents that alter coagulation: May increase the risk of serious bleeding.
Incompatability: Do not use bacteriostatic water for injection; do not add any other medication to urokinase solution.

Valacyclovir HCl

Anti-infective / Antiviral

Indications: Treatment of herpes zoster (shingles); treatment or suppression of genital herpes; treatment of herpes labialis (cold sores).

Dose: Herpes Zoster:
Adults: PO 1 g tid for 7 days (initiate therapy within 48 hr of onset of rash).
Genital Herpes:
Adults:
Initial Episodes: PO 1 g bid for 10 days (initiate therapy within 48 to 72 hr of onset of signs and symptoms).
Recurrent Episodes: PO 500 mg bid for 3 days (initiate therapy within 24 hr of onset of signs or symptoms).
Suppressive Therapy: PO 1 g once daily. If history of recurrence up to 9 recurrences/yr, 500 mg/day may be administered.
HIV-Infected Patients:
Adults: PO 500 mg bid for HIV-infected patients with CD4 cell count of at least 100 cells/mm^3 (efficacy beyond 6 mo of therapy has not been established).
Herpes Labialis:
Adults: PO 2 g bid for 1 day approximately 12 hr apart, initiated at earliest symptoms of cold sore (eg, tingling, burning, itching).

Trade names: Valtrex Tablets 500 mg

Warnings: Hypersensitivity or intolerance to valacyclovir, acyclovir, or any component of the formulation. Pregnancy Category: [B]

Interactions: Cimetidine, probenecid: Increased acyclovir serum concentrations.

Valdecoxib

Analgesic / NSAID

Indications: Relief of signs and symptoms of osteoarthritis and adult rheumatoid arthritis; treatment of primary dysmenorrhea.

Dose: Osteoarthritis, Rheumatoid Arthritis:
Adults: PO 10 mg once daily.
Primary Dysmenorrhea:
Adults: PO 20 mg bid as needed.

Trade names: Bextra Tablets 10 mg

Warnings: Asthma; urticaria; allergic-type reactions after taking aspirin or NSAIDs; sensitivity to valdecoxib. Pregnancy Category: [C]

Interactions: ACE inhibitors: Antihypertensive effect may be decreased.
Aspirin: Risk of GI complications (eg, ulceration) may be increased.
Dextromethorphan: Plasma levels may be reduced by valdecoxib, decreasing the pharmacologic effect.
Fluconazole, ketoconazole, lithium: Plasma levels may be elevated by valdecoxib, increasing the pharmacologic and adverse effects.
Loop diuretics (eg, furosemide): Diuretic effect may be decreased.
Warfarin: Risk of bleeding may be increased.

Valproic Acid and Derivatives

Anticonvulsant

Indications: Sole and adjunctive therapy in simple (petit mal) and complex absence seizures; adjunctive therapy in multiple seizure types, including absence seizures; monotherapy and adjunctive therapy in complex partial seizures that occur in isolation or with other seizure types; manic episodes associated with bipolar disorder (divalproex sodium delayed-release tablets); prophylaxis of migraine headaches (divalproex sodium delayed-release and extended-release [ER] tablets).

Unlabeled indication: Treatment of atypical absence, myoclonic, and tonic-clonic (grand mal) seizures and atonic, elementary partial, and infantile spasm seizures; prevention of recurrent pediatric febrile seizures; intractable status epilepticus in patients who have not responded to other therapies; treatment of minor incontinence after ileoanal anastomosis (subchronic administration); management of anxiety disorders and panic attacks.

Dose: Therapeutic serum levels for most patients with seizures range from 50 to 100 mcg/mL; however, a good correlation has not been established between daily dose, serum level, and therapeutic effect.
Complex Partial Seizures:
Adults and children 10 yr of age and older:
Monotherapy: PO/IV Start at 10 to 15 mg/kg daily and increase by 5 to 10 mg/kg per wk to achieve optimal clinical response, which usually occurs below 60 mg/kg daily.
Conversion to monotherapy: PO/IV Start at 10 to 15 mg/kg daily and increase by 5 to 10 mg/kg per wk to achieve optimal clinical response, which usually occurs below 60 mg/kg daily. Concomitant antiepilepsy drug dosage can usually be reduced approximately 25% q 2 wk. The reduction may be started at initiation of therapy or delayed by 1 to 2 wk if there is a concern that reductions may result in seizures. If the total daily dose exceeds 250 mg, administer in divided doses.
Adjunctive therapy: PO/IV Divalproex sodium or valproic acid may be added to the patient's regimen at a dosage of 10 to 15 mg/kg daily. The dosage may be increased by 5 to 10 mg/kg per wk to achieve optimal response, which usually occurs below 60 mg/kg daily. If the total daily dose exceeds 250 mg, administer in divided doses.
Conversion from Depakote to Depakote ER:
Adults and children 10 yr of age and older: Patients with epilepsy previously receiving Depakote should be administered Depakote ER daily using a dose that is 8% to 20% higher than the daily dose of Depakote. For patients whose Depakote total daily dose cannot be directly converted to Depakote ER, consideration may be given, at the clinician's discretion, to an increase in the patient's Depakote total daily dose to the next higher dosage before converting to the appropriate total daily dose of Depakote ER.
Mania (Divalproex Sodium Delayed-Release Tablets):
Adults: PO 750 mg daily in divided doses. Increase dose as rapidly as possible to achieve the lowest therapeutic dose that produces the desired clinical effect (max, 60 mg/kg daily).
Migraine (Divalproex Sodium):
Divalproex sodium delayed-release tablets: PO Start with 250 mg bid (max, 1,000 mg daily).
Divalproex sodium ER tablets: PO Start with 500 mg

daily for 1 wk, thereafter increasing to 1,000 mg daily. Simple and Complex Absence Seizures: PO/IV Start at 15 mg/kg daily, increasing at 1-wk intervals by 5 to 10 mg/kg daily until seizures are controlled or side effects preclude further increases (max, 60 mg/kg daily). If the total daily dose exceeds 250 mg, administer in divided doses.

Trade names: Depakene Capsules 250 mg (as valproic acid)
Depacon Injection 100 mg/mL
Depakote Tablets, delayed-release 125 mg
Depakote ER Tablets, extended-release 250 mg

Warnings: Hepatic disease dysfunction; known urea cycle disorders; hypersensitivity to the drug. Pregnancy Category: [D]

Interactions: Alcohol, CNS depressants: Enhanced CNS depression.
Amitriptyline/Nortriptyline, barbiturates, diazepam, ethosuximide: May increase levels and actions of these drugs.
Carbamazepine, hydantoins: May result in increased levels of these drugs and reduced efficacy of valproic acid.
Charcoal, cholestyramine: May reduce absorption of valproic acid.
Chlorpromazine, cimetidine, erythromycin, rifampin, salicylates: May increase valproic acid levels.
Clonazepam: May increase risk of absence status in patients with history of absence-type seizures.
Felbamate: Increased valproic acid levels.
Lamotrigine: Decreased valproic acid levels; increased lamotrigine levels.
Meropenem: May decrease valproic acid levels.
Zidovudine: Increased AUC of zidovudine.

Valsartan

Antihypertensive / Angiotensin II antagonist

Indications: Treatment of hypertension either alone or in combination with other antihypertensive drugs; heart failure.

Dose: Hypertension:
Adults:
Initial dose: PO 80 mg qd.
Maintenance: PO 80 to 320 mg qd.
Heart Failure:
Adults:
Initial dose: PO 40 mg bid; titration to 80 and 160 mg bid should be done to the highest dose, as tolerated by the patient.

Trade names: Diovan Capsules 80 mg

Warnings: Standard considerations. Pregnancy Category: [D (second and third trimester); C (first trimester)]

Interactions: Lithium: Plasma concentrations may be increased by valsartan, resulting in an increase in the pharmacologic and adverse effects of lithium.

Valsartan/ Hydrochlorothiazide

Antihypertensive combination

Indications: Treatment of hypertension.

Dose: Dosage must be individualized. The fixed combination is not indicated for initial therapy. The combination may be substituted for the titrated components.
Adults: PO Valsartan may be used over a dose range of 80 to 320 mg/day, administered qd. HCTZ is effective in doses of 12.5 to 50 mg qd. There are no studies evaluating doses of valsartan greater than 160 mg in combination with HCTZ 25 mg.
Renal Impairment (Ccr greater than 30 mL/min): Loop diuretics are preferred to thiazides.

Trade names: Diovan HCT Tablets 12.5 mg hydrochlorothiazide and 80 mg valsartan

Warnings: Hypersensitivity to any component of this product; anuria; hypersensitivity to sulfonamide-derived drugs (HCTZ). Pregnancy Category: [D (second and third trimester); C (first trimester) Drugs that act directly on the renin-angiotensin system can cause injury and death to the developing fetus]

Interactions: Valsartan:
Lithium: Plasma concentrations may be elevated by valsartan, increasing the pharmacologic and toxic effects of lithium.
HCTZ:
Alcohol, barbiturates, narcotics: Increased risk of orthostatic hypotension.
Anticholinergic agents (eg, atropine, biperiden): May increase bioavailability of thiazide-type diuretics.
Antidiabetic agents (oral agents and insulin): Dosage adjustment of antidiabetic agent may be necessary.
Antihypertensive agent: Additive or potentiation of effects.
Cholestyramine, colestipol resins: Impaired absorption of HCTZ.
Corticosteroids, ACTH: Increased electrolyte depletion, increasing the risk of hypokalemia.
Cyclosporin: Concomitant use may increase risk of hyperuricemia and gout-type complications.
Digoxin: Thiazide-induced electrolyte disturbances may predispose to digitalis-induced arrhythmias.
Lithium: Renal Cl of lithium may be reduced, increasing the risk of lithium toxicity.
Methyldopa: Reports of hemolytic anemia occurring with concomitant use.
Nondepolarizing skeletal muscle relaxants (eg, tubocurarine): Increased effect of the muscle relaxant.
Nonsteroidal anti-inflammatory agents: The diuretic, natriuretic, and antihypertensive effects of loop, potassium-sparing, and thiazide diuretics may be reduced.
Potassium supplements: Do not use salt substitutes containing potassium or potassium supplements without consulting the prescribing physician.
Pressor amines (eg, norepinephrine): Decreased responsiveness to the pressor amine.
Vitamin D/Calcium salts: May potentiate rise in serum calcium.

Vancomycin

Anti-infective / Antibiotic

Indications: Parenteral: Treatment of serious or severe infections due to susceptible bacteria not treatable with other antimicrobials (eg, staphylococcus).

Oral: Treatment of pseudomembranous colitis caused by *Clostridium difficile*; treatment of staphylococcal enterocolitis.

Unlabeled indication: IV prophylaxis against bacterial endocarditis in penicillin-allergic patients.

Dose: Adults: PO 500 mg to 2 g/day in 3 or 4 divided doses for 7 to 10 days.
Children: PO 40 mg/kg/day (up to 2 g/day) in 3 or 4 divided doses for 7 to 10 days.
Newborns: PO 10 mg/kg/day in divided doses.
Adults: IV 500 mg by IV infusion q 6 hr or 1 g q 12 hr.
Children: IV 10 mg/kg/dose q 6 hr.
Infants & Newborns: IV 15 mg/kg initially, followed by 10 mg/kg q 12 hr for newborns in first week of life, and q 8 hr for ages up to 1 mo.

Trade names: Lyphocin Powder for Injection, lyophilized 500 mg
Vancocin Pulvules 125 mg
Vancoled Powder for Injection 500 mg

Warnings: Standard considerations. Pregnancy Category: [C]

Interactions: Aminoglycosides: May increase risk of nephrotoxicity.
Neurotoxic and nephrotoxic agents: May give additive toxicity.
Nondepolarizing muscle relaxants: Neuromuscular blockade may be enhanced.

Incompatability: IV solution is incompatible with alkaline injections.

Vardenafil HCl

Agent for impotence

Indications: Treatment of erectile dysfunction.

Dose: Adults: PO Recommended starting dose is 10 mg approximately 60 min prior to sexual activity. Depending on efficacy and side effects, the dose may be decreased to 5 mg or increased to 20 mg.
Geriatric (65 yr and older): PO A 5 mg starting dose is recommended.
Hepatic Impairment:
Adults: PO A 5 mg starting dose is recommended in patients with moderate hepatic impairment (max, 10 mg). Do not use in severe hepatic impairment.
Concomitant Therapy:
Adults: PO In patients receiving ritonavir, do not exceed a single 2.5 mg dose in a 72-hr period. In patients receiving indinavir, itraconazole (400 mg/day), or ketoconazole (400 mg/day), do not exceed a single 2.5 mg dose in a 24-hr period. In patients receiving erythromycin, itraconazole (200 mg/day), or ketoconazole (200 mg/day), do not exceed a single 5 mg dose in a 24-hr period.

Trade names: Levitra Tablets 2.5 mg

Warnings: Administration with nitrates, nitric oxide donors, or alpha blockers; hypersensitivity to any component of the product. Pregnancy Category: [B]

Interactions: Alpha blockers (eg, terazosin), nitrates: Coadministration of these agents with vardenafil is contraindicated.
Class IA (eg, quinidine, procainamide), class III (eg, amiodarone, sotalol) antiarrhythmic agents: Patients with congenital QT prolongation and those receiving these agents should avoid use of vardenafil.
Cytochrome P450 3A4/5 and CYP2C9 (eg, erythromycin, indinavir, itraconazole, ketoconazole, ritonavir): Plasma levels of vardenafil may be elevated, increasing the risk of side effects and necessitating dosage adjustment.

Vasopressin

Posterior pituitary hormone

Indications: Treatment of neurogenic diabetes insipidus; prevention and treatment of postoperative abdominal distention; facilitation of abdominal roentgenography.

Unlabeled indication: Treatment of bleeding esophageal varices.

Dose: Diabetes Insipidus:
Adults: IM/SC 5 to 10 U 2 or 3 times daily as needed. Intranasal injection solution may be given as an individualized dosage intranasally on cotton pledgets, by nasal spray, or dropper.
Children: Reduce dosage proportionally.
Abdominal Distention:
Adults: IM 5 U initially; subsequent injections q 3 to 4 hr prn. May increase the dose to 10 U if necessary.
Abdominal Roentgenography:
Adults: IM/SC 2 injections of 10 U each administered 2 hr and 30 min before films are exposed.
Bleeding Esophageal Varices:
Adults: IV Infuse initially at 0.2 to 0.4 U/min and increase to 0.9 U/min if necessary.

Trade names: Pitressin Injection 20 pressor units/mL

Warnings: Standard considerations. Pregnancy Category: [C]

Interactions: Alcohol, demeclocycline, heparin, lithium, norepinephrine: May decrease the antidiuretic effect of vasopressin.
Carbamazepine, chlorpropamide, clofibrate, fludrocortisone, tricyclic antidepressants, urea: May potentiate antidiuretic effect of vasopressin.
Ganglionic blocking agents: May markedly increase sensitivity to vasopressin pressor effects.

Vecuronium Bromide

Nondepolarizing neuromuscular blocker / Muscle relaxant / Anesthetic adjunct

Indications: Adjunct to general anesthesia to facilitate endotracheal intubation and provide skeletal muscle relaxation during surgery or mechanical ventilation.

Dose: Adults & Children younger than 10 yr: IV Initial dose: for inhalation 0.08 to 0.1 mg/kg. Reduce initial dose by 15% (0.06 to 0.85 mg/kg) if inhalation agents are already in use. If intubation is performed using succinylcholine, reduce initial dose to 0.04 to 0.06 mg/kg with inhalation anesthesia and 0.05 to 0.06 mg/kg with balanced anesthesia. Maintenance: IV bolus 0.01 to 0.015 mg/kg within 25 to 40 min of initial dose, then q 12 to 15 min. IV infusion: 1 mg/kg/min initially beginning 20 to 40 min after IV bolus. Titrate to desired clinical response.
Children 1 to 10 yr: IV Slightly higher initial doses and more frequent supplementation.
Infants 7 wk to 1 yr: IV Slightly lower doses and 1.5 times less frequent.

Trade names: Norcuron Powder for Injection 10 mg

Warnings: Hypersensitivity to vecuronium or bromides. Pregnancy Category: [C]

Interactions: Aminoglycosides, verapamil, inhalation anesthetics (eg, enflurane, isoflurane), lincosamides (eg, clindamycin, lincomycin), magnesium salts, polypeptide antibiotics (eg, bacitracin, polymyxin B): May enhance action of vecuronium (eg, respiratory depression).
Hydantoins, carbamazepine: May cause vecuronium to have shorter duration or decreased effectiveness.
Quinidine, quinine: Recurrent paralysis may occur with injection of quinidine during recovery from use of other muscle relaxants.
Theophyllines: Dose-dependent reversal of neuromuscular blockade is possible.
Thiopurines (eg, mercaptopurine): May decrease or reverse vecuronium action.
Trimethaphan: May cause prolonged apnea.

Venlafaxine

Antidepressant

Indications: Treatment of depression; generalized anxiety disorder (Effexor ER).

Dose: Depression:
Adults (immediate release): PO 75 mg/day in 2 or 3 divided doses; titrate to clinical effect, adding up to 75 mg/day at intervals of at least 4 days (max, 375 mg/day).
Adults (extended release): PO 75 mg/day administered in single dose either in morning or evening at approximately same time qd. Some patients may need to start at 37.5 mg/day for 4 to 7 days before increasing to 75 mg/day. Make dose increases in increments of up to 75 mg/day prn and at intervals of at least 4 days.
Generalized Anxiety Disorder:
Adults (extended release): PO The usual dosage is 75 to 225 mg/day. Some patients may need to start with 37.5 mg/day to avoid overstimulation.

Trade names: Effexor Tablets 25 mg
Effexor XR Capsules, extended-release 37.5 mg

Warnings: Concomitant use with MAO inhibitors. Pregnancy Category: [C]

Interactions: Desipramine, haloperidol: Plasma levels of these drugs may be elevated by venlafaxine, increasing the risk of adverse effects.
MAO inhibitors: MAO inhibitors have produced serious, even fatal, reactions when given concomitantly with venlafaxine. Do not use venlafaxine together with MAO inhibitors or within 14 days of MAO inhibitor use. Wait at least 7 days after stopping venlafaxine before using MAO inhibitors.

St. John's wort: Increased sedative-hypnotic effects may occur.
Sibutramine, sumatriptan, trazodone: Serotonin syndrome, including irritability, increased muscle tone, shivering, myoclonus, and altered consciousness may occur.

Verapamil HCl

Calcium channel blocker

Indications: Oral: Treatment of vasospastic (Prinzmetal's variant), chronic stable (classic effort-associated), and unstable (crescendo, preinfarction) angina; adjunctive treatment with digitalis to control ventricular rate at rest and during stress in atrial flutter or fibrillation; prophylaxis of repetitive paroxysmal supraventricular tachycardia (PSVT); management of essential hypertension. Sustained-release: Management of essential hypertension.

Parenteral: Rapid conversion of PSVTs to sinus rhythm; temporary control of rapid ventricular rate in atrial flutter or fibrillation.

Unlabeled indication: Treatment of migraine and cluster headaches; treatment of hypertrophic cardiomyopathy.

Dose: Adults: PO 40 to 160 mg tid. Do not exceed 480 mg/day. Sustained release: PO 120 to 480 mg/day. Lower doses are given once daily; larger doses divided into 2 doses.
Adults: IV 5 to 10 mg bolus over 2 min. May repeat with 10 mg, 30 min after first dose. Give slower (over at least 3 min) in older patients.
Children 1 to 15 yr: IV 0.1 to 0.3 mg/kg (not to exceed 5 mg) over at least 2 min. May repeat in 30 min.
Children less than 1 yr: IV 0.1 to 0.2 mg/kg (usual range, 0.75 to 2 mg) bolus over 2 min with continuous ECG monitoring.

Trade names: Calan Tablets 40 mg
Calan SR Tablets, sustained release 120 mg
Covera-HS Tablets, extended release 180 mg
Isoptin Tablets 40 mg
Isoptin SR Tablets, sustained release 120 mg
Verelan Capsules, sustained release 120 mg
Verelan PM Capsules, sustained release 100 mg
Verapamil Injection 2.5 mg/mL

Warnings: Hypersensitivity to verapamil; sick sinus syndrome or second- or third-degree atrioventricular (AV) block except with functioning pacemaker; hypotension (less than 90 mm Hg systolic); severe left ventricular dysfunction; cardiogenic shock and severe CHF, unless secondary to supraventricular tachycardia amenable to verapamil; patients with atrial flutter or fibrillation and accessory bypass tract. IV verapamil should not be used concomitantly (within few hours) of IV beta-adrenergic blocking agents or in ventricular tachycardia. Pregnancy Category: [C]

Interactions: Other antihypertensive agents: Additive hypotension.
Beta blockers: May result in increased hypotension and adverse effects because of additive depressant effects on myocardial contractility or AV conduction.
Buspirone: Pharmacologic and adverse effects may be increased by verapamil.
Calcium salts: Clinical effects and toxicities of verapamil may be reversed.
Carbamazepine: Increased carbamazepine serum levels.
Cyclosporine: Increased cyclosporine levels may result.
Dofetilide: Risk of life-threatening ventricular arrhythmias, including torsades de pointes, may be increased. Coadministration with verapamil is contraindicated.
Digitalis glycosides: Increased serum digoxin or digitoxin levels may occur.
Disopyramide: Do not use 48 hr before or 24 hr after verapamil.
Flecainide: May prolong AV conduction.
Nondepolarizing muscle relaxants: Enhanced muscle relaxant effects and prolonged respiratory depression may occur.
Prazosin: Increased prazosin serum levels may result.
Quinidine: Hypotension, bradycardia, ventricular tachycardia, AV block, and pulmonary edema may occur.
Rifampin: Loss of effectiveness of oral verapamil may occur.
Simvastatin: Plasma levels may be elevated by verapamil, increasing the risk of toxicity (eg, rhabdomyolysis).
Incompatability: Do not mix with sodium lactate in polyvinyl chloride bags, albumin, amphotericin B, hydralazine, aminophylline, sodium bicarbonate, nafcillin, or trimethoprim-sulfamethoxazole. Do not mix in solution with pH greater than 6.

Vinblastine Sulfate

Vinca alkaloid

Indications: Adult: Hodgkin's disease, non-Hodgkin's lymphoma, mycosis fungoides, advanced testicular carcinoma, Kaposi's sarcoma, choriocarcinoma, breast cancer.

Pediatric: Hodgkin's disease, non-Hodgkin's lymphoma, mycosis fungoides, Letterer-Siwe disease, choriocarcinoma.

Unlabeled indication: Non-small cell lung carcinoma, bladder cancer, cervical cancer, refractory idiopathic thrombocytopenic purpura, autoimmune hemolytic anemia.

Dose: Initial:
Adults: IV Initially 3.7 mg/m^2 as a single dose/wk. Then increase at weekly intervals in 1.8 mg/m^2 increments until the leukocyte count decreases to about 3000/mm^3. The maximum weekly dose is 18.5 mg/m^2.
Pediatric: IV Initially 2.5 mg/m^2 as a single dose/wk. Then increase at weekly intervals in 1.25 mg/m^2 increments until the leukocyte count decreases to about 3000/mm^3. The maximum weekly dose is 12.5 mg/m^2.
Maintenance:
Adults: IV The maintenance dose is 1.8 mg/m^2 less than the dose required to produce a leukocyte count of 3000/mm^3 every 7 to 14 days. The optimum weekly dose is normally 5.5 to 7.4 mg/m^2. Maintenance doses should not be given until the WBC reaches 4000/mm^3. For an adequate trial, vinblastine must be continued for at least 4 to 6 wk.
Pediatric: IV The maintenance dose is 1.25 mg/m^2 less than the dose required to produce a leukocyte count of 3000/mm^3 every 7 to 14 days. Maintenance doses should not be given until the WBC reaches 4000/mm^3. For an adequate trial, vinblastine must be continued for at least 4 to 6 wk.
Adjustment in Hepatic Insufficiency:
Adults: IV Reduce the dose 50% in patients with a direct serum bilirubin exceeding 3 mg/dL.

Trade names: Vinblastine Sulfate Injection 10 mg

Warnings: Leukopenia; presence of bacterial infection (infections must be under control prior to initiating therapy); significant granulocytopenia unless it is a result of the disease being treated. Pregnancy Category: [D]

Interactions: CYP450 inhibitors: Vinblastine elimination may be reduced by cytochrome P450 enzyme inhibitors.
Erythromycin: Erythromycin may decrease metabolism of vinblastine causing increased toxicity.
Mitomycin: Acute shortness of breath and severe bronchospasm have occurred following concomitant or previous use of mitomycin.
Phenytoin: May reduce phenytoin plasma concentration.

Vincristine Sulfate

Vinca alkaloid

Indications: Adult/Pediatric: Acute lymphocytic leukemia, lymphomas, rhabdomyosarcoma, neuroblastoma, Wilms tumor.

Unlabeled indication: Small-cell lung carcinoma, brain tumors, multiple myeloma, Kaposi sarcoma, chronic lymphocytic and myelocytic leukemias, autoimmune hemolytic anemia, idiopathic thrombocytopenic purpura.

Dose: Acute Lymphocytic Leukemia, Lymphomas, Rhabdomyosarcoma, Neuroblastoma, Wilms Tumor:
Adult: IV 1.4 mg/m^2 weekly (typical dose, 2 mg).
Children weighing more than 10 kg (or body surface area at least 1 m-2): IV 1.4 to 2 mg/m^2 weekly for 3 to 8 wk. Do not exceed a max of 2 mg/dose.
Children weighing up to 10 kg (or body surface area less than 1 m-2): IV 0.05 mg/kg weekly initially. Titrate dose as tolerated, up to a max of 2 mg/dose. Continue therapy for 3 to 8 wk.
Adjustment in Hepatic Insufficiency:
Adult: IV A 50% reduction in dose is recommended for patients having a direct serum bilirubin value more than 3 mg/dL.
Neuroblastoma, Combination Therapy:
Children weighing more than 10 kg (or body surface area at least 1 m-2): IV Vincristine 1 mg/m^2 /day by continuous infusion over 24 hr for 3 days (total dose of 3 mg/m^2 over a 3-day period).

Trade names: Oncovin Solution for Injection 1 mg/mL

Warnings: Patients with demyelinating form of Charcot-Marie-Tooth syndrome. Pregnancy Category: [D Can cause fetal harm when administered to pregnant women]

Interactions: CYP450 inhibitors: Vincristine elimination may be reduced by cytochrome P450 enzyme inhibitors.
Digoxin: May decrease digoxin plasma concentration.
Itraconazole: Vincristine neurotoxicity has occurred during coadministration.
L-asparaginase: Vincristine clearance may decrease when L-asparaginase is given prior to vincristine. Give vincristine 12 to 24 hr prior to L-asparaginase.
Mitomycin: Acute shortness of breath and severe bronchospasm have occurred following concomitant or previous use of mitomycin.
Phenytoin: May reduce phenytoin plasma concentration.
Quinolone antibiotics: Vincristine may decrease oral absorption of quinolone antibiotics.

Vinorelbine Tartrate

Vinca alkaloid

Indications: Unresectable, advanced non-small cell lung cancer.

Unlabeled indication: Breast cancer, cisplatin-resistant ovarian cancer, Hodgkin lymphoma.

Dose: Unresectable, Advanced Non-Small Cell Lung Cancer:
Adults: IV 30 mg/m^2 once weekly until either disease progression or dose-limiting toxicity occur.
Dosage Adjustment for Hematologic Toxicity:
Granulocyte counts should be at least 1000 cells/mm^3 prior to the administration of vinorelbine. Base dosage adjustments on granulocyte counts. See manufacturer's recommendations.
Dosage Adjustment in Hepatic Dysfunction:
Adults: IV Reduce dose 50% if total bilirubin is 2.1 to 3 mg/dL. Reduce dose 25% if total bilirubin is more than 3 mg/dL.

Trade names: Navelbine Solution for Injection 10 mg/mL

Warnings: Pretreatment granulocyte counts less than 1000 cells/mm^3. Pregnancy Category: [D]

Interactions: Cisplatin: Incidence of granulocytopenia increases when vinorelbine is used in combination with cisplatin.
Cytochrome P450 3A enzyme inhibitors (eg ketoconazole, itraconazole, macrolides): May increase vinorelbine serum levels and toxicity.
Mitomycin: Acute pulmonary reactions were noted when vinca alkaloids were given with mitomycin.
Paclitaxel: Monitor for signs and symptoms of neuropathy with concomitant use of vinorelbine and paclitaxel.
Radiation: Radiation recall reactions may occur.

Voriconazole

Anti-infective / Antifungal

Indications: Treatment of invasive aspergillosis; treatment of *Scedosporium apiospermum* and *Fusarium spp.*, including *Fusarium solani*, in patients intolerant of or refractory to other therapy.

Dose: Adults and children (12 yr and older): IV Loading dose of 6 mg/kg q 12 hr for 2 doses, followed by a maintenance dose of 4 mg/kg q 12 hr. If patients are unable to tolerate treatment, reduce the IV maintenance dose to 3 mg/kg q 12 hr.
Adults and children (12 yr and older): PO Once an oral dose can be tolerated, patients weighing more than 40 kg should receive 200 mg q 12 hr. If response is inadequate, the oral dose may be increased to 300 mg q 12 hr. If patients are unable to tolerate oral treatment, reduce the oral dose by 50 mg increments to a minimum of 200 mg q 12 hr. Patients weighing less than 40 kg should receive 100 mg q 12 hr. If the response is inadequate, the oral dose may be increased to 150 mg q 12 hr. If patients weighing less than 40 kg are unable to tolerate oral treatment, reduce the oral dose by 50 mg increments to a minimum of 100 mg q 12 hr.
Hepatic Insufficiency:
Adults and children (12 yr and older): IV or PO It is recommended that the standard loading dose regimens be used but that the maintenance dose be halved in patients with mild to moderate hepatic cirrhosis.

Trade names: Vfend Tablets 50 mg
Vfend IV Powder for injection, lyophilized 10 mg/mL

Warnings: Hypersensitivity to voriconazole or any of it excipients, coadministration of carbamazepine, cisapride, ergot derivatives (eg, ergotamine, dihydroergotamine), long-acting barbiturates, pimozide, quinidine, rifabutin, rifampin, sirolimus. Pregnancy Category: [D]

Interactions: Benzodiazepines (eg, alprazolam), cyclosporine, dihydropyridine calcium channel blockers (eg, felodipine), HMG-CoA reductase inhibitors (eg, lovastatin), NNRT (eg, efavirenz), omeprazole, phenytoin, protease inhibitors (eg, ritonavir), sulfonylurea hypoglycemic agents (eg, glipizide), tacrolimus, vinca alkaloids(eg, vinblastine), warfarin: Plasma exposure to these agents may be increased by voriconazole, increasing the pharmacologic and adverse effects.
Carbamazepine, cisapride, ergot derivatives (eg, ergotamine, dihydroergotamine), long-acting barbiturates, pimozide, quinidine, rifabutin, rifampin, sirolimus: Coadministration of these agents with voriconazole is contraindicated.
Non-nucleoside reverse transcriptase (NNRT) inhibitors (eg, efavirenz), phenytoin: May decrease voriconazole plasma levels, reducing the pharmacologic effect.
NNRT inhibitors (eg, efavirenz), Protease inhibitors (eg, ritonavir): May elevate voriconazole plasma levels, increasing the pharmacologic and adverse effect.
Incompatability: Aminofusin 10%. Do not infuse voriconazole into the same line or cannula with other drug infusions, including parenteral nutrition; do not infuse with blood products or electrolyte supplementations; do not dilute with 4.2% sodium bicarbonate infusion.

Warfarin

Anticoagulants

Indications: Prophylaxis and treatment of venous thrombosis and its extension; prophylaxis and treatment of atrial fibrillation with embolization; prophylaxis and treatment of pulmonary embolism; adjunct in prophylaxis of systemic embolism after MI.

Unlabeled indication: Prevention of recurrent transient ischemic attacks and reduction of risk of recurrent MI; adjunctive treatment of small cell carcinoma of lung.

Dose: Adults: PO 2 to 5 mg/day initially for 2 to 4 days; adjust daily dose according to PT or INR determinations. Usual maintenance dose is PO 2 to 10 mg/day.
Elderly: Lower dosages are recommended.
Adults: IV Provides an alternative administration route for patients who cannot receive oral drugs. The IV dosages would be the same as those that would be used orally. Administer as a slow bolus injection over 1 to 2 min in a peripheral vein.

Trade names: Coumadin Tablets 1 mg

Warnings: Pregnancy; hemorrhagic tendencies; hemophilia; thrombocytopenic purpura; leukemia; recent or contemplated surgery of eye or CNS, major regional lumbar block anesthesia, or surgery resulting in large, open surfaces; patients bleeding from GI, respiratory, or GU tract; threatened abortion; aneurysm; ascorbic acid deficiency; history of bleeding diathesis; prostatectomy; continuous tube drainage of small intestine; polyarthritis; diverticulitis; emaciation; malnutrition; cerebrovascular hemorrhage; eclampsia and preeclampsia; blood dyscrasias; severe uncontrolled or malignant hypertension; severe renal or hepatic disease; pericarditis and pericardial effusion; subacute bacterial endocarditis; visceral carcinoma; following spinal puncture and other diagnostic or therapeutic procedures (eg, IUD insertion) with potential for uncontrollable bleeding; history of warfarin-induced necrosis. Pregnancy Category: [X]

Interactions: Aminoglutethimide, azathioprine, barbiturates, carbamazepine, cholestyramine, ethchlorvynol, ginseng, glutethimide, griseofulvin, mercaptopurine, rifabutin, rifampin, St. John's wort, trazodone, ubiquinone, and vitamin K: Decreased anticoagulant effect of warfarin.
Androgens, amiodarone, cefamandole, cefazolin, cefoperazone, cefotetan, cefoxitin, ceftriaxone, chloramphenicol, cimetidine, clofibrate, danshen, dextrothyroxine, disulfiram, dong quai, erythromycin, fluconazole, glucagon, methimazole, metronidazole, miconazole, moxalactam, nalidixic acid, NSAIDs, phenylbutazone, propylthiouracil, quinidine, quinine, salicylates, sulfinpyrazone, sulfonamides, thyroid hormones, tricyclic antidepressants, and vitamin E: Increased anticoagulant effect of warfarin.
Hydantoins: Serum hydantoin concentration may be elevated, increasing risk of toxicity.

Zafirlukast

Leukotriene receptor antagonist

Indications: Prophylaxis and chronic treatment of asthma in adults and children 5 yr of age and older.

Dose: Adults and Children 12 yr of age or older: PO 20 mg bid.
Children 5 to 11 yr of age: PO 10 mg bid.

Trade names: Accolate Tablets 10 mg

Warnings: Standard considerations. Pregnancy Category: [B]

Interactions: Aspirin: Increased zafirlukast plasma levels.
Erythromycin, theophylline: Lowered zafirlukast plasma concentrations.
Warfarin: Zafirlukast potentiates the hypoprothrombinemic effect of warfarin. Significant increase in the PT may result.

Zalcitabine

Antiretroviral / Nucleoside reverse transcriptase inhibitor

Indications: Combination therapy: For the treatment of selected patients with advanced HIV infection.

Dose: Combination therapy:
Adults and Adolescents more than 13 yr: PO 0.75 mg (coadministered with other antiviral agents) q 8 hr (total daily dose 2.25 mg zalcitabine).

Trade names: Hivid Tablets 0.375 mg

Warnings: Standard considerations. Pregnancy Category: [C]

Interactions: Aminoglycosides, amphotericin, foscarnet: May increase risk of peripheral neuropathy and other zalcitabine toxicities caused by decreased clearance of zalcitabine.
Chloramphenicol, cisplatin, dapsone, disulfiram, ethionamide, glutethimide, gold, hydralazine, iodoquinol, isoniazid, metronidazole, nitrofurantoin, phenytoin, ribavirin, vincristine: May increase risk of peripheral neuropathy.
Drugs associated with pancreatitis (eg, pentamidine): Fatal pancreatitis has occurred, possibly related to zalcitabine and IV pentamidine given concurrently.

Zaleplon

Sedative and hypnotic

Indications: Short-term treatment of insomnia.

Dose: Adults: PO 5 to 20 mg at bedtime.
Elderly/Debilitated Patients: PO 5 to 10 mg at bedtime.
Hepatic Impairment (Mild to Moderate): PO 5 mg at bedtime.

Trade names: Sonata Capsules 5 mg

Warnings: Standard considerations. Pregnancy Category: [C]

Interactions: Alcohol, other CNS depressants: Additive or potentiation of CNS depressant effects.
Cimetidine: May elevate zaleplon plasma levels, increasing the therapeutic and adverse effects.
Rifampin: May reduce zaleplon plasma levels, reducing the effectiveness.

Zanamivir

Antiviral Agent

Indications: Uncomplicated acute illness caused by influenza A and B virus in adults and pediatric patients at least 7 yr of age who have been symptomatic for no longer than 2 days.

Dose: Adults/pediatrics at least 7 yr: Oral inhalation 2 inhalations (one 5 mg blister per inhalation). Give bid (approximately 12 hr apart) for 5 days.

Trade names: Relenza Blisters of powder for oral inhalation 5 mg

Warnings: Standard considerations. Pregnancy Category: [C]

Interactions: None well documented.

Ziprasidone

Antipsychotic / Benzisoxazole

Indications: Treatment of schizophrenia; treatment of acute agitation in schizophrenic patients (injection only).

Dose: Adults: PO 20 to 80 mg bid.
Adults: IM 10 to 20 mg/day (max, 40 mg/day).

Trade names: Geodon Capsules 20 mg (as HCl)

Warnings: Drugs known to prolong the QT interval (eg, quinidine, pimozide, sotalol); patients with a history of QT prolongation; recent acute MI; uncompensated heart failure; known hypersensitivity to the product. Pregnancy Category: [C]

Interactions: Alcohol, CNS-acting drugs: May cause additive CNS effects.
Amiodarone, dofetilide, dolasetron, droperidol,

levomethadyl, moxifloxacin, pimozide, quinidine, sotalol, sparfloxacin, tacrolimus, thioridazine, any other drug known to prolong the QT interval: Contraindicated because of increased risk of torsades de pointes or other malignant ventricular arrhythmias.
Antihypertensive agents: Hypotensive effects may be enhanced.
Carbamazepine: May reduce ziprasidone levels, decreasing the effectiveness.
Ketoconazole, other inhibitors of cytochrome P450 3A4 metabolism: May elevate ziprasidone levels, increasing the risk of toxicity.
Dopamine agonists, levodopa: Effects may be antagonized.

Zolmitriptan

Analgesic / Migraine

Indications: Short-term treatment of migraine attacks with/without aura.

Dose: Adults: PO Initial recommended dose is up to 2.5 mg (eg, 1/2 tablet) with fluids; max recommended single dose is 5 mg. If headache returns, the dose may be repeated after 2 hr, not to exceed 10 mg within a 24-hr period. The effectiveness of a second dose, if the initial dose is ineffective, has not been determined.
Adults: Intranasal One dose of 5 mg for acute migraine. If headache returns, dose may be repeated after 2 hr (max, 10 mg per 24 hr). Response is individual. Doses lower than 5 mg can only be achieved through the use of an oral formulation. Make the choice of dose and route of administration on an individual basis.

Trade names: Zomig Tablets 2.5 mg
Zomig Spray, nasal 5 mg
Zomig ZMT Tablets, orally disintegrating 2.5 mg

Warnings: Ischemic heart disease or in patients with Prinzmetal angina; symptoms consistent with possible ischemic heart disease; uncontrolled hypertension; symptomatic Wolff-Parkinson-White syndrome; use within 24 hr of treatment with another 5-HT agonist or an ergotamine-containing or ergot-like medication; coadministration of, or within 2 wk of discontinuation of, an MAO inhibitor, management of hemiplegic or basilar migraines. Pregnancy Category: [C]

Interactions: 5-HT-1 agonists (eg, sumatriptan): Avoid use within 24 hr of each other.
Cimetidine: Zolmitriptan levels and $t_{1/2}$ may be increased.
Ergot-containing or ergot-type drugs (eg, methysergide): May cause additive prolonged vasospastic reactions. Avoid use within 24 hr of each other.
MAO inhibitors (eg, phenelzine): Do not use zolmitriptan concurrently or within 2 wk of discontinuation of a MAO inhibitor.
Selective serotonin reuptake inhibitors (eg, fluoxetine): Combined use may cause weakness, hyperreflexia, and incoordination.
Sibutramine: Serotonin syndrome, including CNS irritability, motor weakness, shivering, myoclonus, and altered consciousness, may occur.

Zolpidem Tartrate

Sedative and hypnotic

Indications: Short-term treatment of insomnia.

Dose: Adults: PO 10 mg immediately before bedtime.
Elderly, debilitated, or hepatic insufficient patients: An initial 5 mg dose is recommended. Max dose, no more than 10 mg.

Trade names: Ambien Tablets 5 mg

Warnings: Standard considerations. Pregnancy Category: [B]

Interactions: Food: Reduces absorption of zolpidem.
Ritonavir: Possible severe sedation and respiratory depression.

Section 6

ICD-9-CM Index

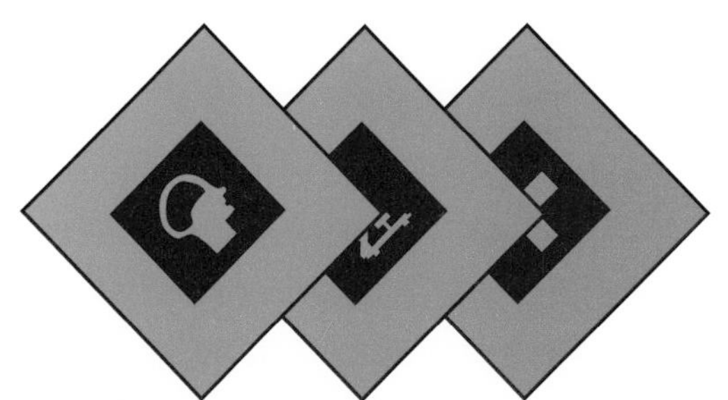

001.9 Cholera, unspecified
Cholera

002.0 Typhoid fever
Typhoid fever

002.9 Paratyphoid fever, unspecified
Paratyphoid
Typhoid fever

003.0 Salmonella gastroenteritis
Food poisoning, bacterial
Salmonella infection

004.0 Shigella dysenteriae
Food poisoning, bacterial

004.9 Shigellosis, unspecified
Food poisoning, bacterial
Shigellosis

005.0 Staphylococcal food poisoning
Food poisoning, bacterial

005.1 Botulism
Botulism
Food poisoning, bacterial

005.9 Food poisoning, unspecified
Diarrhea, acute
Diarrhea, chronic
Food poisoning, bacterial

006.0 Acute amebic dysentery without mention of abscess
Amebiasis

006.3 Amebic liver abscess
Amebiasis

006.4 Amebic lung abscess
Amebiasis

006.5 Amebic brain abscess
Amebiasis
Amebic meningoencephalitis

006.6 Amebic skin ulceration
Amebiasis

006.8 Amebic infection of other sites
Amebiasis

006.9 Amebiasis, unspecified
Amebiasis

007.0 Balantidiasis
Balantidiasis

007.1 Giardiasis
Giardiasis

007.5 Cyclosporiasis
Cyclosporiasis

008.00 Intestinal infection due to Escherichia coli, unspecified
Food poisoning, bacterial

008.43 Intestinal infections due to Campylobacter
Campylobacter infections

008.45 Intestinal infections due to Clostridium difficile
Pseudomembranous colitis

008.69 Other viral enteritis
Gastroenteritis, viral

011.90 Pulmonary tuberculosis, unspecified
Tuberculosis

013.0 Tuberculous meningitis
Tuberculosis, CNS

013.0 TBM
Tuberculosis, CNS

013.2 Tuberculoma of brain
Tuberculosis, CNS

013.4 Tuberculoma of spinal cord
Tuberculosis, CNS

020.0 Bubonic plague
Plague

020.2 Septicemic plague
Plague

020.3 Primary pneumonic plague
Plague

020.4 Secondary pneumonic plague
Plague

020.5 Unspecified pneumonic plague
Plague

021.9 Unspecified tularemia
Tularemia

022.0 Cutaneous anthrax
Anthrax of the skin

022.1 Pulmonary anthrax
Anthrax of the lung

022.2 Gastrointestinal anthrax
Anthrax of the intestine

023.9 Brucellosis, unspecified
Arthritis, infectious, granulomatous
Brucellosis

025 Melioidosis
Melioidosis

026.0 Rat-bite fever, spirillary
Rat-bite fever, spirillary

026.1 Rat-bite fever, streptobacillary
Rat-bite fever, streptobacillary

027.0 Listeriosis
Listeriosis

027.2 Pasteurellosis
Yersinia enterocolitica infection

030.9 Leprosy, unspecified
Leprosy

031.8 Other specified mycobacterial diseases
Arthritis, infectious, granulomatous

031.9 Unspecified diseases due to mycobacteria
Atypical mycobacterial infection

032.0 Faucial diphtheria
Diphtheria

032.1 Nasopharyngeal diphtheria
Diphtheria

032.2 Anterior nasal diphtheria
Diphtheria

032.3 Laryngeal diphtheria
Diphtheria

032.81 Conjunctival diphtheria
Diphtheria

032.82 Diphtheritic myocarditis
Diphtheria

032.83 Diphtheritic peritonitis
Diphtheria

032.84 Diphtheritic cystitis
Diphtheria

032.85 Cutaneous diphtheria
Diphtheria
Diphtheria of the skin

032.89 Other specified diphtheria, other
Diphtheria

032.9 Diphtheria, unspecified
Diphtheria

033.9 Whooping cough, unspecified organism
Pertussis

034.0 Streptococcal sore throat
Pharyngitis

034.1 Scarlet fever
Pharyngitis
Scarlet fever

035 Erysipelas
Erysipelas

036.0 Meningococcal meningitis
Meningococcemia

036.2 Meningococcemia
Meningococcemia

037 Tetanus
Tetanus

038.9 Unspecified septicemia
Sepsis

039.1 Actinomycotic infections, pulmonary
Actinomycosis of the thorax

039.2 Actinomycotic infections, abdominal
Actinomycosis of the kidney

039.4 Actinomycotic infections, Madura foot
Mycetoma

039.9 Actinomycotic infections of unspecified site
Nocardiosis

040.0 Gas gangrene
Anaerobic & necrotizing infections

040.2 Whipple disease
Whipple disease

040.82 Toxic shock syndrome
Toxic shock syndrome

042 Human immunodeficiency virus (HIV) disease
HIV infection & AIDS

045.1 Acute poliomyelitis with other paralysis
Poliomyelitis

046.0 Kuru
Kuru
Prion diseases

046.1 Jakob-Creutzfeldt disease
Creutzfeldt-Jakob disease
Prion diseases

046.3 Progressive multifocal leukoencephalopathy
Progressive multifocal leukoencephalopathy

047.9 Unspecified viral meningitis
Encephalitis, viral
Meningitis, viral

049.9 Unspecified non-arthropod-borne viral diseases of central nervous system
Encephalitis, viral

050.9 Smallpox, unspecified
Smallpox

051.1 Pseudocowpox
Milker nodules

051.9 Paravaccinia, unspecified
Milker nodules

052.9 Varicella without mention of complication
Chickenpox

053.11 Geniculate herpes zoster
Ramsay Hunt syndrome, Type 1

053.29 Herpes zoster (HZV) with ophthalmic complications, other
Herpes eye infections

053.9 Herpes zoster without mention of complication
Herpes zoster

054.0 Eczema herpeticum
Herpes simplex

054.10 Genital herpes, unspecified
Herpes, genital

054.2 Herpetic gingivostomatitis
Stomatitis

054.40 Herpes simplex with unspecified ophthalmic complication
Herpes eye infections

054.9 Herpes simplex without mention of complication
Herpes simplex

055.9 Measles without mention of complication
Measles, rubeola

056.9 Rubella without mention of complication
Measles, rubella

057.0 Erythema infectiosum (fifth disease)
Parvovirus B19 infection

057.8 Other specified viral exanthemata
Roseola

060.9 Yellow fever, unspecified
Yellow fever

061 Dengue
Dengue fever

062.3 St. Louis encephalitis
Encephalitis, Saint Louis

065.2 Kyasanur Forest disease
Kyasanur forest disease

066.1 Tick-borne fever
Colorado tick fever

066.3 Other mosquito-borne fever
Chikungunya
West Nile fever

070 Viral hepatitis
Hepatitis B
Hepatitis C
Hepatitis A

071 Rabies
Rabies

072.9 Mumps without mention of complication
Mumps

073.9 Ornithosis, unspecified
Psittacosis

074.0 Herpangina
Herpangina

074.3 Hand, foot, and mouth disease
Hand-foot-and-mouth disease

075 Infectious mononucleosis
Epstein-Barr virus infections
Mononucleosis

076.0 Trachoma, initial stage
Trachoma

076.1 Trachoma, active stage
Trachoma

076.9 Trachoma, unspecified
Trachoma

077.99 Unspecified diseases of conjunctiva due to viruses
Conjunctivitis, acute

078.0 Molluscum contagiosum
Molluscum contagiosum

078.10 Viral warts, unspecified
Warts

078.11 Condyloma acuminata
Condyloma acuminata

078.19 Other specified viral warts
Warts, plantar

078.3 Cat-scratch disease
Bartonella infections

078.5 Cytomegaloviral disease
Cytomegalovirus inclusion disease

078.88 Other specified diseases due to Chlamydiae
Chlamydia pneumoniae

078.89 Other specified diseases due to viruses
Lassa fever
Marburg virus disease

079.0 Adenovirus
Adenovirus infections

079.81 Hantavirus
Hantavirus

079.82
SARS - associated coronavirus
Severe acute respiratory syndrome (SARS)

079.88 Chlamydia infection
Cervicitis

079.89 Other specified viral infection
Ebola virus hemorrhagic fever

080 Louse-borne [epidemic] typhus
Typhus fevers

081.0 Murine [endemic] typhus
Typhus fevers

081.1 Brill disease
Brill disease
Typhus fevers

082.0 Spotted fevers
Rocky Mountain spotted fever

082.1 Boutonneuse fever
Boutonneuse fever

082.8 Other specified tick-borne rickettsioses
Ehrlichiosis

083.0 Q fever
Q fever

083.1 Trench fever
Bartonella infections
Trench fever

083.2 Rickettsialpox
Rickettsialpox

083.8 Other Bartonella-related diagnoses, including BA/BP
Bartonella infections

084.0 Falciparum malaria (malignant tertian)
Malaria

084.1 Vivax malaria (benign tertian)
Malaria

084.2 Quartan malaria
Malaria

084.3 Ovale malaria
Malaria

084.5 Mixed malaria
Malaria

084.6 Malaria, unspecified
Malaria

084.8 Blackwater fever
Malaria

084.9 Other pernicious complications of malaria
Malaria

085.0 Leishmaniasis, visceral (kala-azar)
Leishmaniasis

085.9 Leishmaniasis, unspecified
Leishmaniasis

086.2 Chagas disease without mention of organ involvement
Chagas disease

086.3 Gambian trypanosomiasis
Trypanosomiasis, West African

086.4 Rhodesian trypanosomiasis
Trypanosomiasis, East African

087.1 Tick-borne relapsing fever
Boutonneuse fever

087.9 Relapsing fever, unspecified
Relapsing fever

088.0 Bartonellosis
Bartonella infections

088.81 Lyme disease
Lyme disease

088.82 Babesiosis
Babesiosis

094.0 Tabes dorsalis
Charcot joint
Tabes dorsalis

094.89 Other specified neurosyphilis
Tabes dorsalis

097.9 Syphilis, unspecified
Syphilis

098.0 Acute gonoccal infection of lower genitourinary tract
Gonococcal infections
Urethritis

098.15 Acute gonococcal cervicitis
Cervicitis

098.2 Chronic gonococcal infection of lower genitourinary tract
Urethritis

099.0 Chancroid
Chancroid

099.1 Lymphogranuloma venereum
Lymphogranuloma venereum

099.2 Granuloma inguinale
Granuloma inguinale

099.3 Reiter disease
Reiter syndrome
Urethritis

099.40 Other nongonococcal urethritis (NGU), unspecified
Urethritis

099.41 Chlamydia trachomatis
Urethritis

099.49 Other nongonococcal urethritis (NGU), other specified organism
Urethritis

099.53 Other venereal diseases due to Chlamydia trachomatis, lower genitourinary sites
Cervicitis

099.8 Other specified venereal diseases
Balanitis

100.0 Leptospirosis icterohemorrhagica
Icterohemorrhagic leptospirosis

100.9 Leptospirosis, unspecified
Leptospirosis

101 Vincent angina
Stomatitis

102.9 Yaws, unspecified
Yaws

110.0 Dermatophytosis of scalp and beard
Alopecia
Tinea barbae
Tinea capitis

110.1 Dermatophytosis of nail
Onychomycosis

110.3 Dermatophytosis of groin and perianal area
Tinea cruris

110.4 Dermatophytosis of foot
Tinea pedis

110.5 Dermatophytosis of the body
Tinea corporis

111.0 Pityriasis versicolor
Tinea versicolor

112.0 Candidiasis of mouth
Candidiasis, mucocutaneous

112.1 Candidiasis of vulva and vagina
Candidiasis, mucocutaneous
Vulvovaginitis, candidal

112.2 Candidiasis of other urogenital sites
Balanitis

112.3 Candidiasis of skin and nails
Onychomycosis
Paronychia

112.5 Candidiasis, disseminated
Candidiasis

112.9 Candidiasis of unspecified site
Candidiasis
Candidiasis, mucocutaneous

114.9 Coccidioidomycosis, unspecified
Coccidioidomycosis

115.90 Histoplasmosis, unspecified without mention of manifestation
Histoplasmosis

115.99 Histoplasmosis, unspecified other
Arthritis, infectious, granulomatous
Histoplasmosis

116.0 Blastomycosis
Blastomycosis

117.0 Rhinosporidiosis
Rhinosporidiosis

117.1 Sporotrichosis
Sporotrichosis

117.2 Chromoblastomycosis
Chromomycosis

117.3 Aspergillosis
Aspergillosis

117.5 Cryptococcosis
Cryptococcosis

117.7 Zygomycosis (Phycomycosis or Mucormycosis)
Zygomycosis

117.9 Other and unspecifed mycoses
Geotrichosis
Sinusitis

120.0 Schistosomiasis due to Schistosoma haematobium
Schistosomiasis haematobium

120.1 Schistosomiasis due to Schistosoma mansoni
Schistosomiasis mansoni

120.2 Schistosomiasis due to Schistosoma japonicum
Schistosomiasis japonica

120.3 Cutaneous schistosomiasis
Schistosomiasis, cutaneous

120.9 Schistosomiasis, unspecified
Schistosomiasis of the liver, chronic

121.3 Fascioliasis
Fascioliasis

121.4 Fasciolopsiasis
Fasciolopsiasis

122.1 Echinococcus granulosus infection of lung
Echinococcosis of the lung

122.9 Echinococcosis, other and unspecified
Tapeworm infestation

123.5 Sparganosis [larval diphyllobothriasis]
Sparganosis

123.8 Other specified cestode infection
Tapeworm infestation

123.9 Cestode infection, unspecified
Tapeworm infestation

124 Trichinosis
Trichinosis

125.2 Loiasis
Loiasis

125.9 Unspecified filariasis
Elephantiasis, filarial
Filariasis

127.0 Ascariasis
Roundworms, intestinal
Roundworms, tissue

127.2 Strongyloidiasis
Strongyloidiasis

127.4 Enterobiasis
Pinworms

127.6 Trichostrongyliasis
Trichostrongyliasis

129 Intestinal parasitism, unspecified
Intestinal parasites

130.9 Toxoplasmosis, unspecified
Toxoplasmosis

131.00 Urogenital trichomoniasis, unspecified
Trichomoniasis

131.01 Trichomonal vulvovaginitis
Trichomoniasis

131.02 Trichomonal urethritis
Urethritis

131.9 Trichomoniasis, unspecified
Trichomoniasis

132.9 Pediculosis, unspecified
Pediculosis

133.0 Scabies
Scabies

134.0 Myiasis
Myiasis

135 Sarcoidosis
Sarcoidosis

136.0 Ainhum
Ainhum

136.1 Behçet syndrome
Behçet syndrome

136.3 Pneumocystosis
Pneumonia, Pneumocystis (PCP)

136.9 Unspecified infectious and parasitic diseases
Anaerobic & necrotizing infections
Cryptosporidiosis

138 Late effects of acute poliomyelitis
Postpoliomyelitis syndrome

141.4 Malignant neoplasm of anterior two-thirds of tongue, part unspecified
Squamous cell carcinoma, anterior tongue

142.0 Malignant neoplasm of parotid gland
Salivary gland tumors

142.1 Malignant neoplasm of submandibular gland
Salivary gland tumors

142.2 Malignant neoplasm of sublingual gland
Salivary gland tumors

142.9 Malignant neoplasm of salivary gland, unspecified
Salivary gland tumors

144.9 Malignant neoplasm of floor of mouth, part unspecified
Squamous cell carcinoma, floor of the mouth

145.9 Malignant neoplasm of mouth, unspecified
Oral cavity neoplasms

147.9 Malignant neoplasm of nasopharynx, unspecified
Nasopharyngeal cancer

150.9 Malignant neoplasm of esophagus, unspecified
Esophageal tumors

151.0 Malignant neoplasm of stomach, cardia
Gastric malignancy

151.1 Malignant neoplasm of stomach, pylorus
Gastric malignancy

151.2 Malignant neoplasm of stomach, pyloric antrum
Gastric malignancy

151.3 Malignant neoplasm of fundus of stomach
Gastric malignancy

151.4 Malignant neoplasm of body of stomach
Gastric malignancy

151.5 Malignant neoplasm of lesser curvature of stomach, unspecified
Gastric malignancy

151.6 Malignant neoplasm of greater curvature of stomach, unspecified
Gastric malignancy

151.8 Malignant neoplasm of other specified sites of stomach
Gastric malignancy

151.9 Malignant neoplasm of stomach, unspecified
Gastric malignancy

153.9 Malignant neoplasm of colon, unspecified
Adenocarcinoma of the colon

154.0 Malignant neoplasm of rectosigmoid junction
Colorectal malignancy

154.1 Malignant neoplasm of the rectum
Adenocarcinoma of the rectum

154.3 Malignant neoplasm of anus, unspecified
Squamous cell carcinoma, anus

155.0 Malignant neoplasm of liver, primary
Hepatoma

156.0 Malignant neoplasm of gallbladder
Adenocarcinoma of the gallbladder

157.0 Malignant neoplasm of head of pancreas
Pancreatic cancer

157.4 Malignant neoplasm of Islets of Langerhans
Insulinoma

157.9 Malignant neoplasm of pancreas, part unspecified
Pancreatic cancer

161.9 Malignant neoplasm of larynx, unspecified
Laryngeal cancer

162.9 Malignant neoplasm of bronchus and lung, unspecified
Lung, primary malignancies

163.9 Malignant neoplasm of pleura, unspecified
Epithelial mesothelioma
Pleural malignant mesothelioma

164.0 Malignant neoplasm of thymus
Thymoma, malignant

170.9 Malignant neoplasm of bone and articular cartilage, site unspecified
Bone tumor, primary malignant
Ewing sarcoma

171.8 Malignant neoplasm of other specified sites of connective and other soft tissue
Neuroblastoma

171.9 Malignant neoplasm of connective and soft tissue, site unspecified
Rhabdomyosarcoma

172.9 Melanoma of skin, site unspecified
Melanoma

173.3 Other malignant neoplasm of skin of other and unspecified parts of face
Basal cell carcinoma
Cutaneous squamous cell carcinoma

173.4 Other malignant neoplasm of scalp and skin of neck
Basal cell carcinoma
Cutaneous squamous cell carcinoma

173.5 Other malignant neoplasm of skin of trunk, except scrotum
Basal cell carcinoma
Cutaneous squamous cell carcinoma

173.6 Other malignant neoplasm of skin of upper limb, including shoulder
Basal cell carcinoma
Cutaneous squamous cell carcinoma

173.7 Other malignant neoplasm of skin of lower limb, including hip
Basal cell carcinoma
Cutaneous squamous cell carcinoma

173.9 Other malignant neoplasm of skin, site unspecified
Basal cell carcinoma
Cutaneous squamous cell carcinoma

174.0 Malignant neoplasm of female breast, nipple and areola
Paget disease of the breast

174.9 Malignant neoplasm of female breast, unspecified
Breast cancer
Paget disease of the breast

175.9 Malignant neoplasm of male breast, other and unspecified sites
Breast cancer

176.0 Kaposi sarcoma of skin
Kaposi sarcoma

180.0 Malignant neoplasm of body of cervix uteri, endocervix
Cervical malignancy
Uterine corpus malignancy

182.0 Malignant neoplasm of corpus uteri, except isthmus
Adenocarcinoma of the endometrium
Uterine corpus malignancy

182.1 Malignant neoplasm of body of uterus, isthmus
Uterine corpus malignancy

182.8 Malignant neoplasm of other specified sites of body of uterus
Uterine corpus malignancy

183.0 Malignant neoplasm of ovary
Ovarian cancer
Ovarian mucinous cystadenocarcinoma

184.0 Malignant neoplasm of vagina
Vaginal malignancy

184.4 Malignant neoplasm of vulva, unspecified
Vulvar malignancy

185 Malignant neoplasm of prostate
Prostatic cancer

186.0 Malignant neoplasm of undescended testis
Testicular malignancies

186.9 Malignant neoplasm of testis, other and unspecified
Testicular malignancies

188.9 Malignant neoplasm of bladder, part unspecified
Adenocarcinoma of the bladder
Bladder tumors
Squamous cell carcinoma, bladder

189.0 Malignant neoplasm of kidney, except pelvis
Renal cell carcinoma
Wilms tumor

190.5 Malignant neoplasm of retina
Retinoblastoma

191.9 Malignant neoplasm of brain, unspecified
Astrocytoma
Glioblastoma multiforme

193 Malignant neoplasm of thyroid gland
Thyroid malignant neoplasia

194.0 Malignant neoplasm of adrenal gland
Neuroblastoma
Pheochromocytoma

194.6 Malignant neoplasm of aortic body and other paraganglia
Glomus jugulare

195.1 Malignant neoplasm of thorax
Neuroblastoma

197.2 Secondary malignant neoplasm of pleura
Pleural effusion

197.7 Secondary malignant neoplasm of liver, specified as secondary
Metastatic neoplasm of the liver

198.89 Secondary malignant neoplasm of other specified sites, other
Oral cavity neoplasms
Thyroid malignant neoplasia

200.00 Reticulosarcoma, unspecified site, extranodal and solid organ sites
Reticulum cell sarcoma

200.20 Burkitt tumor or lymphoma, unspecified site, extranodal and solid organ sites
Lymphoma, Burkitt

201.90 Hodgkin disease, unspecified, unspecified site, extranodal and solid organ sites
Hodgkin disease

202.40 Leukemic reticuloendotheliosis, unspecified site, extranodal and solid organ sites
Leukemia
Leukemia, hairy cell

202.50 Letterer-Siwe disease, unspecified site, extranodal and solid organ sites
Letterer-Siwe disease

202.60 Malignant mast cell tumors, unspecified site, extranodal and solid organ sites
Mastocytosis

202.80 Other malignant lymphomas, unspecified site, extranodal and solid organ sites
Cutaneous T cell lymphoma
Lymphoma, non-Hodgkin
Lymphoma, pulmonary

203.00 Multiple myeloma without mention of remission
Multiple myeloma

204.00 Acute lymphoid leukemia without mention of remission
Leukemia
Leukemia, acute lymphoblastic in adults (ALL)

204.01 Acute lymphoid leukemia in remission
Leukemia, acute lymphoblastic in adults (ALL)

204.10 Chronic lymphoid leukemia
Leukemia

205.00 Acute myeloid leukemia without mention of remission
Leukemia
Leukemia, acute myeloblastic
Leukemia, acute myelogenous

205.10 Chronic myeloid leukemia without mention of remission
Leukemia
Leukemia, chronic myelogenous
Myeloproliferative disorders

205.11 Chronic myeloid leukemia in remission
Myeloproliferative disorders

206.00 Acute monocytic leukemia without mention of remission
Leukemia
Leukemia, acute monocytic

210.4 Benign neoplasm of other and unspecified parts of mouth
Oral cavity neoplasms

211.3 Benign neoplasm of colon
Gardner syndrome

211.7 Benign neoplasm of Islets of Langerhans
Insulinoma

212.7 Benign neoplasm of heart
Atrial myxoma

213.9 Benign neoplasm of bone and articular cartilage, site unspecified
Chondroma

218.0 Submucous leiomyoma of uterus
Uterine myomas

220 Benign neoplasm of ovary
Ovarian tumor, benign

224.3 Benign neoplasm of conjunctiva
Nevus of Ota

225.1 (M9560/0) Benign neoplasm of cranial nerves
Acoustic neuroma

225.2 Benign neoplasm of cerebral meninges
Meningioma

225.4 Benign neoplasm of spinal meninges
Meningioma

227.0 Benign neoplasm of adrenal gland
Pheochromocytoma

227.3 Benign neoplasms of pituitary gland and craniopharyngeal duct (pouch)
Chromophobe adenoma of the pituitary
Pituitary basophilic adenoma
Pituitary chromophobe adenoma
Pituitary eosinophilic adenoma

228.04 Hemangioma of intra-abdominal structures
Hemangioma of the liver

230.0 Carcinoma in situ of lip, oral cavity and pharynx
Oral cavity neoplasms

235.1 Neoplasm of uncertain behavior of lip, oral cavity and pharynx
Oral cavity neoplasms

235.5 Neoplasm of uncertain behavior of other and unspecified digestive organs
Glucagonoma

237.0 Neoplasm of uncertain behavior of pituitary gland and craniopharyngeal duct
Craniopharyngioma

237.70 Neurofibromatosis, unspecified
Neurofibromatosis (Types 1 & 2)

238.4 Polycythemia vera
Polycythemia vera

238.7 Neoplasm of uncertain behavior of other lymphatic and hematopoietic tissues
Myelodysplastic syndromes (MDS)
Myeloproliferative disorders
Thrombocythemia (adult), idiopathic

238.9 Neoplasm of uncertain behavior, site unspecified
Carcinoid tumor

239.2 Neoplasms of unspecified nature of bone, soft tissue, and skin
Bowen disease

239.5 Neoplasms of unspecified nature of other genitourinary organs
Gestational trophoblastic neoplasm

242.00 Toxic diffuse goiter without mention of thyrotoxic crisis or storm
Hyperthyroidism

242.01 Toxic diffuse goiter with mention of thyrotoxic crisis or storm
Hyperthyroidism

242.90 Thyrotoxicosis without mention of goiter or other cause without mention of thyrotoxic crisis or storm
Hyperthyroidism
Thyrotoxic heart disease

242.91 Thytotoxicosis without mention of goiter or other cause with mention of thyrotoxic crisis or storm
Hyperthyroidism
Thyrotoxic storm

244.0 Postsurgical hypothyroidism
Hypothyroidism, adult

244.2 Iodine hypothyroidism
Hypothyroidism, adult

244.8 Other specified acquired hypothyroidism
Hypothyroidism, adult

244.9 Unspecified hypothyroidism
Hypothyroidism, adult
Myxedema heart disease
Pituitary hypothyroidism

245.0 Acute thyroiditis
Thyroiditis

250.00 Diabetes mellitus without mention of complication, type 2 or unspecified type, not stated as uncontrolled
Diabetes mellitus, Type 1
Diabetes mellitus, Type 2

250.01 Diabetes mellitus without mention of complication, type 1, not stated as uncontrolled
Diabetes mellitus, Type 1

250.02 Diabetes mellitus without mention of complication, type 2 or unspecified type, uncontrolled
Diabetes mellitus, Type 2

250.12 Diabetes with ketoacidosis, type 2 or unspecified type, uncontrolled
Diabetic ketoacidosis (DKA)

250.82 Diabetes with other specified manifestations, type 2 or unspecified type, uncontrolled
Hypoglycemia, diabetic
Necrobiosis lipoidica diabeticorum

251.0 Hypoglycemic coma
Hypoglycemia, nondiabetic

251.1 Other specified hypoglycemia
Hypoglycemia, nondiabetic

251.2 Hypoglycemia, unspecified
Hypoglycemia, nondiabetic

251.5 Abnormality of secretion of gastrin
Zollinger-Ellison syndrome

252.0 Hyperparathyroidism
Hyperparathyroidism

252.1 Hypoparathyroidism
Hypoparathyroidism

253.0 Acromegaly and gigantism
Acromegaly
Pituitary gigantism
Sotos syndrome

253.1 Other and unspecified anterior pituitary hyperfunction
Forbes-Albright syndrome
Prolactinoma

253.2 Panhypopituitarism
Hypopituitarism
Sheehan syndrome

253.3 Pituitary dwarfism
Pituitary dwarfism

253.5 Diabetes insipidus
Diabetes insipidus

253.6 Syndrome of inappropriate secretion of antidiuretic hormone
Inappropriate secretion of antidiuretic hormone

255.0 Cushing syndrome
Cushing disease and syndrome

255.10 Primary aldosteronism
Aldosteronism, primary

255.13 Bartter syndrome
Bartter syndrome

255.2 Adrenogenital disorders
Acquired adrenogenital syndrome

255.4 Corticoadrenal insufficiency
Addison disease

256.4 Polycystic ovaries
Polycystic ovarian disease

258.0 Polyglandular activity in multiple endocrine adenomatosis
Multiple endocrine neoplasia (MEN)

259.2 Carcinoid syndrome
Carcinoid syndrome

259.3 Ectopic hormone secretion, NEC
Hyperparathyroidism

259.8 Other specified endocrine disorders
Hutchinson-Gilford syndrome
Werner syndrome

259.9 Unspecified endocrine disorder
Hyperprolactinemia

260 Kwashiorkor
Malnutrition, protein-calorie

261 Nutritional marasmus
Malnutrition, protein-calorie

263.9 Unspecified protein-calorie malnutrition
Malnutrition, protein-calorie

264.9 Unspecified vitamin A deficiency
Vitamin deficiency

265.0 Beriberi
Beriberi heart disease
Beriberi nervous system syndrome

265.1 Other and unspecified manifestations of thiamine deficiency
Vitamin deficiency
Wernicke encephalopathy

265.2 Pellagra
Pellagra

266.0 Ariboflavinosis
Riboflavin deficiency
Vitamin deficiency

266.1 Vitamin B6 deficiency
Vitamin deficiency

266.2 Other B-complex deficiencies
Vitamin deficiency

266.9 Unspecified vitamin B deficiency
Vitamin deficiency

267 Absorbic acid deficiency
Scurvy, infantile
Vitamin deficiency

268.2 Osteomalacia, unspecified
Osteomalacia & rickets

268.9 Unspecified vitamin D deficiency
Vitamin deficiency

269.0 Deficiency of vitamin K
Vitamin deficiency

269.1 Deficiency of other vitamins
Vitamin deficiency

269.2 Unspecified vitamin deficiency
Vitamin deficiency

269.3 Mineral deficiency, NEC
Zinc deficiency

270.0 Disturbances of amino-acid transport
Blue diaper syndrome
Fanconi syndrome
Hartnup disease
Renal tubular acidosis (RTA)

270.2 Other disturbances of aromatic amino acid metabolism
Alcaptonuria

270.3 Disturbances of branched-chain amino-acid metabolism
Maple syrup urine disease

270.6 Disorders of urea cycle metabolism
Argininosuccinicaciduria
Hypernatremia

270.9 Unspecified disorder of amino-acid metabolism
Aminoaciduria

271.0 Glycogenosis
von Gierke disease

271.3 Intestinal disaccharidase deficiencies and disaccharide malabsorption
Lactose intolerance

272.0 Pure hypercholesterolemia
Hypercholesterolemia
Hypertriglyceridemia

272.1 Pure hypertriglyceridemia
Hypertriglyceridemia

272.2 Mixed hyperlipidemia
Hypertriglyceridemia

272.3 Hyperchylomicronemia
Hypertriglyceridemia

272.4 Other and unspecified hyperlipidemia
Hypertriglyceridemia

272.7 Lipidoses
Fabry disease
Gaucher disease
Niemann-Pick disease

273.2 Other paraproteinemias
IgG heavy chain disease
IgM heavy chain disease

273.3 Macroglobulinemia
Waldenström macroglobulinemia

274.0 Gouty arthropathy
Gout

274.10 Gouty nephropathy, unspecified
Gout
Nephropathy, urate

274.11 Uric acid nephrolithiasis
Gout
Nephropathy, urate

274.81 Gouty tophi of ear
Gout

275.0 Disorders of iron metabolism
Hemochromatosis
Hemosiderosis, pulmonary

275.1 Disorders of copper metabolism
Wilson disease

275.2 Disorders of magnesium metabolism
Magnesium deficiency syndrome

275.3 Disorders of phosphorus metabolism
Hypophosphatasia

275.40 Unspecified disorder of calcium metabolism
Hypercalcemia associated with malignancy

275.41 Hypocalcemia
Hypocalcemia

275.42 Hypercalcemia
Hypercalcemia associated with malignancy

276.1 Hyposmolality and/or hyponatremia
Hyponatremia

276.5 Volume depletion
Dehydration

276.7 Hyperpotassemia
Hyperkalemia

276.8 Hypopotassemia
Hypokalemia
Liddle syndrome

276.9 Electrolyte and fluid disorders NEC
Inappropriate secretion of antidiuretic hormone

277.00 Cystic fibrosis without mention of meconium ileus
Cystic fibrosis

277.01 Cystic fibrosis with meconium ileus
Cystic fibrosis

277.1 Disorders of porphyrin metabolism
Porphyria

277.2 Other disorders of purine and pyrimidine metabolism
Lesch-Nyhan syndrome

277.3 Amyloidosis
Amyloidosis
Familial Mediterranean fever

277.4 Disorders of bilirubin excretion
Crigler-Najjar syndrome
Dubin-Johnson syndrome
Gilbert disease

277.6 Other deficiencies of circulating enzymes
Angioedema
Hereditary angioneurotic edema

277.89 Other specified disorders of metabolism
Hand-Schuller-Christian syndrome
Histiocytosis, pulmonary

278.00 Obesity, unspecified
Obesity

278.01 Morbid obesity
Obesity

278.8 Other hyperalimentation
Pickwickian syndrome

279.01 Selective IgA immunodeficiency
Selective IgA deficiency

279.06 Common variable immunodeficiency
Agammaglobulinemia, acquired

279.11 DiGeorge syndrome
DiGeorge syndrome

279.12 Wiskott-Aldrich syndrome
Wiskott-Aldrich syndrome

279.3 Unspecified immunity deficiency
Immunodeficiency diseases

280.9 Iron deficiency anemia, unspecified
Iron deficiency anemia

281.0 Pernicious anemia
Anemia, pernicious

281.1 Other vitamin B12 deficiency anemia
Anemia, pernicious

281.2 Folate-deficiency anemia
Anemia due to folate deficiency

282.2 Anemias due to disorders of glutathione metabolism
Favism

282.49 Other thalassemia
Thalassemia

282.60 Sickle cell disease, unspecified
Anemia, sickle cell

282.7 Other hemoglobinopathies
Hemoglobin C disease

282.9 Hereditary hemolytic anemia, unspecified
Anemia, hemolytic

283.0 Autoimmune hemolytic anemias
Anemia, autoimmune hemolytic

283.2 Hemoglobinuria due to hemolysis from external causes
Paroxysmal cold hemoglobinuria
Paroxysmal hemoglobinuria following exercise
Paroxysmal nocturnal hemoglobinuria

283.9 Acquired hemolytic anemia, unspecified
Anemia, hemolytic

284.9 Aplastic anemia, unspecified
Anemia, aplastic

285.0 Sideroblastic anemia
Anemia, acquired sideroblastic

285.8 Other specified anemias
Anemia, myelophthisic

285.9 Anemia, unspecified
Anemia due to chronic disease

286.0 Congenital factor VIII disorder
Hemophilia

286.1 Congenital factor IX disorder
Hemophilia

286.3 Congenital deficiency of other clotting factors
Afibrinogenemia, congenital
Factor X deficiency
Hypoprothrombinemia

286.4 Von Willebrand disease
von Willebrand disease

286.6 Defibrination syndrome
Disseminated intravascular coagulation (DIC)

286.9 Other and unspecified coagulation defects
Antithrombin deficiency
Protein C deficiency
Protein S deficiency
Prothrombin 20210 (Mutation)

287.0 Allergic purpura
Henoch-Schönlein purpura

287.3 Primary thrombocytopenia
Idiopathic thrombocytopenic purpura (ITP)

288.0 Agranulocytosis
Agranulocytosis
Agranulocytosis, infantile genetic
Neutropenia, autoimmune
Neutropenia, chronic idiopathic
Neutropenia, cyclic

289.2 Nonspecific mesenteric lymphadenitis
Mesenteric adenitis, acute

289.81 Primary hypercoagulable state
Factor V Leiden
Thrombosis, deep vein (DVT)

289.82 Secondary hypercoagulable state
Thrombosis, deep vein (DVT)

289.89 Other specified diseases of blood and blood-forming organs
Macrocytosis
Myeloproliferative disorders

290.0 Senile dementia, uncomplicated
Alzheimer disease
Dementia

290.10 Presenile dementia, uncomplicated
Alzheimer disease
Dementia

290.11 Presenile dementia with delirium
Delirium

290.3 Senile dementia with delirium
Delirium

290.40 Arteriosclerotic dementia, uncomplicated
Dementia

291.0 Alcohol withdrawal delirium
Delirium tremens
Delirium

291.1 Alcohol amnestic syndrome
Korsakoff psychosis
Delirium

291.81 Alcohol Withdrawal
Alcohol use disorders

292.0 Drug withdrawal syndrome
Smoking cessation
Delirium

292.81 Drug-induced delirium
Delirium

293.0 Acute delirium
Delirium

293.1 Subacute delirium
Delirium

293.89 Other specified transient organic mental disorders, other
Delirium

293.9 Unspecified transient organic mental disorder
Post-traumatic stress disorder (PTSD)

295.90 Unspecified schizophrenia, unspecified
Schizophrenia

305.60 Cocaine abuse, unspecified
Substance use disorders

305.90 Other, mixed, or unspecified drug abuse, unspecified
Laxative abuse

306.1 Physiological malfunction arising from mental factors, respiratory
Chronic cough

306.51 Psychogenic vaginismus
Vaginismus

306.59 Physiological malfunction arising from mental factors, genitourinary, other
Ejaculatory disorders

306.8 Other specified psychophysiological malfunction
Bruxism

306.9 Unspecified psychophysiological malfunction
Chronic pain disorder
Somatoform disorders

307.1 Anorexia nervosa
Anorexia nervosa

307.23 Gilles de la Tourette disorder
Tourette syndrome

307.51 Bulimia
Bulimia nervosa

307.6 Enuresis
Enuresis

307.81 Tension headache
Headache, tension

308.3 Other acute reactions to stress
Post-traumatic stress disorder (PTSD)

310.2 Postconcussion syndrome
Post-concussive syndrome

311 Depressive disorder, not elsewhere classified
Depression

314.00 Attention deficit disorder without mention of hyperactivity
Attention deficit/Hyperactivity disorder

314.01 ADD with hyperactivity
Attention deficit/Hyperactivity disorder

317 Mild mental retardation
Mental retardation

318.0 Moderate mental retardation
Mental retardation

318.1 Severe mental retardation
Mental retardation

318.2 Profound mental retardation
Mental retardation

319 Unspecified mental retardation
Mental retardation

320.9 Meningitis due to unspecified bacterium
Meningitis, bacterial

324.0 Intracranial abscess
Brain abscess

325 Phlebitis and thrombophlebitis of intracranial venous sinuses
Cavernous sinus thrombosis

330.0 Leukodystrophy
Adrenoleukodystrophy
Krabbe leukodystrophy, infantile form
Metachromatic leukodystrophy, late infantile form
Sclerosis of the brain

330.1 Cerebral lipidoses
Juvenile amaurotic familial idiocy

331.0 Alzheimer disease
Alzheimer disease
Dementia

331.11 Pick disease
Pick disease

331.81 Reye syndrome
Reye syndrome

332.0 Paralysis agitans
Parkinson disease

333.0 Other degenerative diseases of the basal ganglia
Hallervorden-Spatz disease

333.1 Essential and other specified forms of tremor
Benign essential tremor syndrome

333.4 Huntington disease
Huntington disease

333.82 Orofacial dyskinesia
Tardive dyskinesia

333.83 Spasmodic torticollis
Torticollis

333.99 Other and unspecified extrapyramidal diseases and abnormal movement disorders, other
Restless legs syndrome

334.0 Friedreich ataxia
Friedreich ataxia

334.2 Primary cerebellar degeneration
Ramsay Hunt syndrome, Type 2

334.8 Other spinocerebellar diseases
Ataxia-telangiectasia

334.9 Spinocerebellar disease, unspecified
Ataxia-telangiectasia

335.20 Amyotrophic lateral sclerosis
Amyotrophic lateral sclerosis

335.24 Primary lateral sclerosis
Primary lateral sclerosis

335.29 Motor neuron disease, other
Amyotrophic lateral sclerosis

336.0 Syringomyelia and syringobulbia
Syringomyelia

336.2 Subacute combined degeneration of spinal cord in diseases classified elsewhere
Subacute combined degeneration

336.9 Unspecified disease of spinal cord
Spinal cord compression

337.0 Idiopathic peripheral autonomic neuropathy
Carotid sinus syndrome

337.21 Reflex sympathetic dystrophy of the upper limb
Complex regional pain syndrome

337.22 Reflex sympathetic dystrophy of the lower limb
Complex regional pain syndrome

337.9 Unspecified disorder of autonomic nervous system
Horner syndrome
Shoulder-hand syndrome

340 Multiple sclerosis
Multiple sclerosis

341.8 Other demyelinating diseases of central nervous system
Marchiafava-Bignami syndrome

343.4 Infantile hemiplegia
Hemiplegia, acute infantile

343.9 Infantile cerebral palsy, unspecified
Cerebral palsy

344.60 Cauda equina syndrome without mention of neurogenic bladder
Cauda equina syndrome

344.61 Cauda equina syndrome with neurogenic bladder
Cauda equina syndrome

344.89 Other specified paralytic syndrome
Brown-Sequard syndrome
Millard-Gubler syndrome

345.10 Generalized convulsive epilepsy without mention of intractable epilepsy
Seizure disorders

345.2 Epilepsy, petit mal status
Status epilepticus

345.3 Epilepsy, grand mal status
Brain injury - post acute care issues
Status epilepticus

345.71 Epilepsia partialis continua, with intractable epilepsy, so stated
Status epilepticus

346.00 Classical migraine without mention of intractable migraine
Migraine

346.20 Variants of migraine without mention of intractable migraine
Headache, cluster

346.21 Variants of migraine with intractable migraine, so stated
Headache, cluster
Migraine

346.90 Migraine, unspecified without mention of intractable migraine
Migraine

347 Cataplexy and narcolepsy
Narcolepsy

349.89 Other specified disorders of nervous system, other
Progressive hemiatrophy face

350.1 Trigeminal neuralgia
Trigeminal neuralgia

351.0 Bell palsy
Bell palsy

352.1 Glossopharyngeal neuralgia
Glossopharyngeal neuralgia

353.0 Brachial plexus lesions
Thoracic outlet syndrome

354.0 Carpal tunnel syndrome
Carpal tunnel syndrome

354.4 Causalgia of upper limb
Complex regional pain syndrome

355.6 Lesion of plantar nerve
Morton neuroma (interdigital neuroma)

355.71 Causalgia of lower limb
Complex regional pain syndrome

356.1 Peroneal muscular atrophy
Charcot-Marie-Tooth disease

357.0 Acute infective polyneuritis
Guillain-Barré syndrome

358.00 Myasthenia gravis without acute exacerbation
Myasthenia gravis

358.01 Myasthenia gravis with acute exacerbation
Myasthenia gravis

359.0 Congenital hereditary muscular dystrophy
Muscular dystrophy

359.1 Hereditary progressive muscular dystrophy
Muscular dystrophy

359.2 Myotonic disorders
Muscular dystrophy

359.3 Familial periodic paralysis
Hypokalemic periodic paralysis

361.00 Retinal detachment with retinal defect, unspecified
Retinal detachment

361.2 Serous retinal detachment
Retinal detachment

361.30 Retinal defect, unspecified
Retinal detachment

361.81 Traction detachment of retina
Retinal detachment

362.01 Background diabetic retinopathy
Retinopathy, diabetic

362.02 Proliferative diabetic retinopathy
Retinopathy, diabetic

362.21 Retrolental fibroplasia
Retinopathy of prematurity

362.34 Transient arterial occlusion
Amaurosis fugax

362.35 Central retinal vein occlusion
Retinal vein occlusion

362.51 Nonexudative senile macular degeneration
Macular degeneration, age-related (ARMD)

362.52 Exudative senile macular degeneration
Macular degeneration, age-related (ARMD)

362.57 Drusen (degenerative)
Macular degeneration, age-related (ARMD)

362.63 Lattice degeneration of retina
Retinal detachment

362.74 Pigmentary retinal dystrophy
Retinitis pigmentosa

362.76 Dystrophies primarily involving the retinal pigment epithelium
Amaurosis, congenital

364.3 Unspecified iridocyclitis
Uveitis

364.41 Hyphema of iris and ciliary body
Hyphema

365.00 Preglaucoma, unspecified
Glaucoma, primary open-angle

365.02 Borderline glaucoma, anatomical narrow angle
Glaucoma, primary angle-closure

365.11 Primary open angle glaucoma
Glaucoma, primary open-angle

365.12 Low tension glaucoma
Glaucoma, primary open-angle

365.20 Primary angle-closure glaucoma, unspecified
Glaucoma, primary angle-closure

366.19 Other and combined forms of senile cataract
Cataract

367.0 Hypermetropia
Refractive errors

367.1 Myopia
Refractive errors

367.21 Regular astigmatism
Refractive errors

367.4 Presbyopia
Refractive errors

368.00 Amblyopia, unspecified
Amblyopia

370.00 Corneal ulcer, unspecified
Corneal ulceration

370.21 Punctate keratitis
Keratitis, superficial punctate

370.31 Phlyctenular keratoconjunctivitis
Phlyctenular keratoconjunctivitis

370.50 Interstitial keratitis, unspecified
Interstitial keratitis

371.60 Keratoconus, unspecified
Keratoconus

372.13 Vernal conjunctivitis
Vernal keratoconjunctivitis

372.14 Other chronic allergic conjunctivitis
Conjunctivitis, acute

372.50 Conjunctival degeneration, unspecified
Conjunctivitis, acute

373.00 Blepharitis, unspecified
Blepharitis
Hordeolum (stye)

373.11 Hordeolum externum
Hordeolum (stye)

373.2 Chalazion
Hordeolum (stye)

375.11 Dacryops
Lacrimal disorders

375.15 Tear film insufficiency, unspecified
Lacrimal disorders

376.01 Orbital cellulitis
Cellulitis, periorbital & orbital

376.03 Orbital osteomyelitis
Osteomyelitis

377.10 Optic atrophy, unspecified
Optic atrophy

377.14 Glaucomatous atrophy (cupping) of optic disc
Glaucoma, primary open-angle

377.30 Optic neuritis, unspecified
Optic neuritis

378.55 External ophthalmoplegia
Kearns-Sayre syndrome

378.72 Progressive external ophthalmoplegia
Progressive external ophthalmoplegia

378.9 Unspecified disorder of eye movements
Strabismus

379.00 Scleritis, unspecified
Scleritis

379.21 Vitreous degeneration
Retinal detachment

380.10 Infective otitis externa, unspecified
Otitis externa

380.4 Impacted cerumen
Hearing loss

381.00 Acute nonsuppurative otitis media, unspecified
Otitis media

382.00 Acute suppurative otitis media without spontaneous rupture of ear drum
Hearing loss
Otitis media

382.01 Acute suppurative otitis media with spontaneous rupture of ear drum
Hearing loss

382.9 Unspecified otitis media
Otitis media

383.00 Acute mastoiditis without complications
Mastoiditis

383.01 Subperiosteal abscess of mastoid
Bezold abscess
Mastoiditis

383.02 Acute mastoiditis with other complications
Mastoiditis

383.1 Chronic mastoiditis
Mastoiditis

383.9 Unspecified mastoiditis
Mastoiditis

384.00 Acute myringitis, unspecified
Myringitis, infectious

385.00 Tympanosclerosis, unspecified as to involvement
Hearing loss

386.00 Meniere disease, unspecified
Ménière disease

386.30 Labyrinthitis, unspecified
Labyrinthitis

387.9 Otosclerosis, unspecified
Hearing loss
Otosclerosis (otospongiosis)

388.30 Tinnitus, unspecified
Tinnitus

390 Rheumatic fever without mention of heart involvement
Rheumatic fever

394.0 Mitral stenosis
Mitral stenosis
Mitral valve prolapse

394.1 Rheumatic mitral insufficiency
Mitral regurgitation due to rheumatic fever
Mitral valve prolapse

394.2 Mitral stenosis with insufficiency
Mitral valve prolapse

394.9 Other and unspecified mitral valve diseases
Mitral regurgitation due to papillary muscle dysfunction
Mitral valve prolapse

397.0 Diseases of tricuspid valve
Tricuspid stenosis

401.0 Essential hypertension, malignant
Hypertensive emergencies

401.1 Essential hypertension, benign
Hypertension, essential

403.90 Hypertensive renal disease, unspecified without mention of renal failure
Nephrosclerosis

403.91 Hypertensive renal disease, unspecified with renal failure
Nephrosclerosis

405.01 Secondary malignant renovascular hypertension
Hypertensive emergencies

410.00 Acute myocardial infarction of anterolateral wall, episode of care unspecified
Myocardial infarction

410.90 Acute myocardial infarction of unspecified site, episode of care unspecified
Myocardial infarction

411.1 Intermediate coronary syndrome
Angina

413 Angina pectoris
Angina

413.1 Prinzmetal angina
Angina

413.9 Other and unspecified angina pectoris
Angina

414.00 Coronary atherosclerosis of unspecified type of vessel, native or graft
Arteriosclerotic heart disease
Atherosclerosis

415.0 Acute cor pulmonale
Cor pulmonale

415.19 Pulmonary embolism and infarction, other
Pulmonary artery thrombosis
Pulmonary embolism
Pulmonary infarction
Thrombosis, deep vein (DVT)

416.0 Primary pulmonary hypertension
Primary pulmonary hypertension

416.8 Other chronic pulmonary heart diseases
Pulmonary hypertension, secondary

416.9 Chronic pulmonary heart disease, unspecified
Cor pulmonale

420.91 Acute idiopathic pericarditis
Pericarditis

420.99 Other acute pericarditis
Pericarditis

421.0 Acute and subacute bacterial endocarditis
Endocarditis, infective

421.9 Acute endocarditis, unspecified
Endocarditis, infective

423.9 Unspecified disease of pericardium
Cardiac tamponade

424.0 Mitral valve disorders
Mitral valve prolapse

424.1 Aortic valve disorders
Aortic regurgitation

424.2 Tricuspid valve disorders, specified as nonrheumatic
Tricuspid regurgitation

444.21 Arterial embolism and thrombosis of arteries of upper extremity
Arterial embolus & thrombosis
Atherosclerotic occlusive disease

444.22 Arterial embolism and thrombosis of arteries of lower extremity
Arterial embolus & thrombosis
Atherosclerotic occlusive disease

444.81 Arterial embolism and thrombosis of iliac artery
Arterial embolus & thrombosis

444.9 Arterial embolism and thrombosis of unspecified artery
Arterial embolus & thrombosis

446.0 Polyarteritis nodosa
Polyarteritis nodosa

446.1 Acute febrile mucocutaneous lymph node syndrome [MCLS]
Kawasaki syndrome

446.20 Hypersensitivity angiitis, unspecified
Goodpasture syndrome, pulmonary component

446.21 Goodpasture syndrome
Goodpasture syndrome, renal component

446.4 Wegener granulomatosis
Wegener granulomatosis

446.5 Giant cell arteritis
Giant cell arteritis

446.7 Takayasu disease
Takayasu syndrome

448.0 Hereditary hemorrhagic telangiectasia
Hereditary hemorrhagic telangiectasia

451.0 Phlebitis and thrombophlebitis of superficial vessels of lower extremities
Thrombophlebitis, superficial

451.19 Phlebitis and thrombophlebitis of deep vessels of lower extremities, other
Thrombosis, deep vein (DVT)

451.2 Phlebitis and thrombophlebitis of deep vessels of lower extremities, unspecified
Thrombophlebitis, superficial

452 Portal vein thrombosis
Portal vein thrombosis

453.0 Budd-Chiari syndrome
Budd-Chiari syndrome

453.3 Embolism and thrombosis of renal vein
Renal vein thrombosis

453.8 Embolism and thrombosis of other specified veins
Thrombosis, deep vein (DVT)

454.1 Varicose veins of lower extremities with inflammation
Dermatitis, stasis
Varicose veins

455.6 Unspecified hemorrhoids without mention of complication
Hemorrhoids

456.0 Esophageal varices with bleeding
Esophageal varices

456.1 Esophageal varices without mention of bleeding
Esophageal varices

457.1 Other lymphedema
Elephantiasis, filarial

457.2 Lymphangitis
Lymphangitis

459.2 Compression of vein
Superior vena cava syndrome

459.81 Venous (peripheral) insufficiency, unspecified
Dermatitis, stasis

460 Acute nasopharyngitis (common cold)
Common cold

461.0 Acute maxillary sinusitis
Sinusitis

461.1 Acute frontal sinusitus
Sinusitis

461.2 Acute ethmoidal sinusitis
Sinusitis

461.3 Acute sphenoidal sinusitus
Sinusitis

461.8 Other acute sinusitis
Sinusitis

461.9 Acute sinusitis, unspecified
Sinusitis

462 Acute pharyngitis
Adenovirus infections
Pharyngitis

463 Acute tonsillitis
Pharyngitis

464.00 Acute laryngitis without mention of obstruction
Laryngitis

464.01 Acute laryngitis with obstruction
Laryngitis

464.10 Acute tracheitis without mention of obstruction
Tracheitis, bacterial

464.11 Acute tracheitis with obstruction
Tracheitis, bacterial

464.20 Acute laryngotracheitis without mention of obstruction
Laryngotracheobronchitis
Tracheitis, bacterial

464.21 Acute laryngotracheitis with obstruction
Laryngotracheobronchitis
Tracheitis, bacterial

464.30 Acute epiglottitis without mention of obstruction
Epiglottitis

464.31 Acute epiglottitis with obstruction
Epiglottitis

466.0 Acute bronchitis
Bronchitis, acute

466.11 Acute bronchiolitis due to respiratory syncytial virus
Bronchiolitis

466.19 Acute bronchiolitis due to other infectious organisms
Bronchiolitis

472.1 Chronic pharyngitis
Pharyngitis

473.0 Chronic maxillary sinusitis
Sinusitis

473.9 Unspecified sinusitis (chronic)
Sinusitis

474.00 Chronic tonsillitis
Pharyngitis

474.12 Hypertrophy of adenoids alone
Adenoid hyperplasia

475 Peritonsillar abscess
Peritonsillar abscess

476.0 Chronic laryngitis
Laryngitis

476.1 Chronic laryngotracheitis
Laryngotracheobronchitis

477.9 Allergic rhinitis, cause unspecified
Rhinitis, allergic

478.31 Partial unilateral paralysis of vocal cords or larynx
Paralysis of the recurrent laryngeal nerve

480.0 Pneumonia due to adenovirus
Adenovirus infections

480.1 Pneumonia due to respiratory syncytial virus
Respiratory syncytial virus (RSV) infection

480.9 Viral pneumonia, unspecified
Pneumonia, viral

481 Pneumococcal pneumonia [Streptococcus pneumoniae pneumonia]
Pneumonia, bacterial

482.83 Pneumonia due to other gram-negative bacteria
Legionnaires disease

482.84 Legionnaires disease
Legionnaires disease

482.89 Pneumonia due to other specified bacteria
Rhodococcus infections

483.0 Mycoplasma pneumoniae
Pneumonia, mycoplasma

486 Pneumonia, organism unspecified
Pneumonia, bacterial

487.0 Influenza with pneumonia
Influenza

487.1 Influenza with other respiratory manifestations
Influenza

491.0 Simple chronic bronchitis
Chronic cough

491.8 Other chronic bronchitis
Bronchiolitis obliterans & organizing pneumonia

492.8 Other emphysema
Chronic obstructive pulmonary disease & emphysema

493.00 Extrinsic asthma, unspecified
Asthma

493.10 Intrinsic asthma, unspecified
Asthma

493.90 Asthma, unspecified
Asthma

494.0 Bronchiectasis without acute exacerbation
Bronchiectasis

494.1 Bronchiectasis with acute exacerbation
Bronchiectasis

495.5 Mushroom workers lung
Mushroom-worker disease

495.6 Maple bark-strippers lung
Maple bark stripper disease

495.8 Other specified allergic alveolitis and pneumonitis
Cheese-worker lung
Psittacosis

495.9 Unspecified allergic alveolitis and pneumonitis
Hypersensitivity pneumonitis

496 Chronic airway obstruction, NEC
Chronic obstructive pulmonary disease & emphysema

500 Coal workers pneumoconiosis
Anthracosis

501 Asbestosis
Asbestosis

502 Pneumoconiosis due to other silica or silicates
Silicosis

503 Pneumoconiosis due to other inorganic dust
Siderosis of the lung

504 Pneumonopathy due to inhalation of other dust
Byssinosis

506.9 Unspecified respiratory conditions due to fumes and vapors
Silo filler disease

510.9 Empyema without mention of fistula
Empyema

511.1 Pleurisy with effusion, with mention of a bacterial cause other than tuberculosis
Pleural effusion

511.8 Pleurisy with other specified forms of effusion, except tuberculous
Hemothorax

511.9 Unspecified pleural effusion
Pleural effusion

512.0 Spontaneous tension pneumothorax
Pneumothorax

512.1 Iatrogenic pneumothorax
Pneumothorax

512.8 Other spontaneous pneumothorax
Pneumothorax

513.0 Abscess of lung
Lung abscess

516.0 Pulmonary alveolar proteinosis
Alveolar proteinosis of the lung

516.1 Idiopathic pulmonary hemosiderosis
Hemosiderosis, pulmonary

516.3 Idiopathic fibrosing alveolitis
Pulmonary interstitial fibrosis, idiopathic

518.0 Pulmonary collapse
Atelectasis

518.3 Pulmonary eosinophilia
Eosinophilic pneumonias
Tropical eosinophilia

518.4 Acute edema of lung, unspecified
Pulmonary edema

518.5 Pulmonary insufficiency following trauma and surgery
Near drowning
Respiratory distress syndrome, adult

518.82 Other pulmonary insufficiency, NEC
Respiratory distress syndrome, adult

518.89 Other diseases of lung, NEC
Broncholithiasis

520.7 Teething syndrome
Teething

522.6 Chronic apical periodontitis
Granuloma, pyogenic

523.1 Chronic gingivitis
Gingivitis

524.60 Temporomandibular joint disorders, unspecified
Temporomandibular joint (TMJ) syndrome

526.4 Inflammatory conditions of jaws
Osteomyelitis

527.2 Sialadenitis
Sialadenitis

527.5 Sialolithiasis
Salivary gland calculi

528.0 Stomatitis
Stomatitis

528.2 Oral aphthae
Stomatitis

528.3 Cellulitis and abscess of oral soft tissues, excluding lesions specific for gingiva and tongue
Ludwig angina

528.6 Leukoplakia of oral mucosa, including tongue
Leukoplakia, oral

528.9 Other and unspecified diseases of the oral soft tissues
Granuloma, pyogenic

529.0 Glossitis
Glossitis

530.0 Achalasia and cardiospasm
Cardiospasm

530.10 Esophagitis, unspecified
Brain injury - post acute care issues
Gastroesophageal reflux disease

530.3 Stricture and stenosis of esophagus
Schatzki ring

530.5 Dyskinesia of esophagus
Diffuse esophageal spasm

530.7 Gastroesophageal laceration-hemorrhage syndrome
Mallory-Weiss syndrome

531.90 Gastric ulcer, unspecified as acute or chronic, without mention of hemorrhage, perforation, or obstruction
Peptic ulcer disease

532.90 Duodenal ulcer, unspecified as acute or chronic, without mention of hemorrhage, perforation, or obstruction
Peptic ulcer disease

535.20 Gastric mucosal hypertrophy without mention of hemorrhage
Giant hypertrophic gastritis

535.50 Unspecified gastritis and gastroduodenitis without mention of hemorrhage
Gastritis

536.8 Dyspepsia and other specified disorders of function of stomach
Dyspepsia, functional

537.0 Acquired hypertrophic pyloric stenosis
Pyloric stenosis

540.0 Acute appendicitis with generalized peritonitis
Appendicitis, acute

540.9 Acute appendicitis without mention of peritonitis
Appendicitis, acute

550.90 Inguinal hernia without mention of obstruction or gangrene, unilateral or unspecified (not specified as recurrent)
Hernias, external

550.92 Inguinal hernia without mention of obstruction of gangrene, bilateral (not specified as recurrent)
Hernias, external

553.00 Femoral hernia, unilateral or unspecified (not specified as recurrent)
Hernias, external

553.1 Umbilical hernia
Hernias, external

553.21 Ventral incisional hernia
Hernias, external

555.0 Regional enteritis of small intestine
Crohn disease

555.1 Regional enteritis of large intestine
Crohn disease

555.9 Regional enteritis of unspecified site
Crohn disease

556.9 Ulcerative colitis, unspecified
Ulcerative colitis

558.2 Toxic gastroenteritis and colitis
Diarrhea, acute
Diarrhea, chronic

558.9 Other and unspecified noninfectious gastroenteritis and colitis
Diarrhea, acute
Diarrhea, chronic
Eosinophilic gastroenteritis

560.0 Intussusception
Intestinal obstruction
Intussusception

560.30 Impaction of intestine, unspecified
Intestinal obstruction

560.39 Impaction of intestine, other
Fecal impaction

560.9 Unspecified intestinal obstruction
Intestinal obstruction

562.10 Diverticulosis of colon (without mention of hemorrhage)
Diverticular disease

562.11 Diverticulitis of colon (without mention of hemorrhage)
Diverticular disease

564.00 Constipation, unspecified
Constipation

564.1 Irritable bowel syndrome
Irritable bowel syndrome

564.2 Postgastric surgery syndromes
Dumping syndrome

564.6 Anal spasm
Proctalgia fugax

564.7 Megacolon, other than Hirschsprung
Constipation

564.89 Other functional disorders of intestine
Constipation

565.0 Anal fissure
Anorectal fissure

565.1 Anal fistula
Anorectal fistula

566 Abscess of anal and rectal regions
Anorectal abscess

567.2 Other suppurative peritonitis
Peritonitis, acute

567.9 Unspecified peritonitis
Peritonitis, acute

569.1 Rectal prolapse
Rectal prolapse

569.49 Other specified disorders of rectum and anus, other
Proctitis

571.0 Alcoholic fatty liver
Fatty liver syndrome

571.1 Acute alcoholic hepatitis
Hepatitis, alcoholic

571.2 Alcoholic cirrhosis of liver
Cirrhosis of the liver

571.5 Cirrhosis of liver without mention of alcohol
Cirrhosis of the liver
Cirrhosis, cardiac
Cirrhosis, macronodal
Hepatic fibrosis, congenital

571.6 Biliary cirrhosis
Cirrhosis, primary biliary

571.8 Other chronic nonalcoholic liver disease
Fatty liver syndrome

572.0 Abscess of liver
Pyogenic abscess liver

572.2 Hepatic coma
Hepatic encephalopathy

572.3 Portal hypertension
Portal hypertension

572.4 Hepatorenal syndrome
Hepatorenal syndrome

573.2 Hepatitis in other infectious diseases classified elsewhere
Malaria

574.00 Calculus of gallbladder with acute cholecystitis, without mention of obstruction
Cholecystitis
Cholelithiasis

574.01 Calculus of gallbladder with acute cholecystitis, with obstruction
Cholelithiasis
Cholecystitis

574.10 Calculus of gallbladder with other cholecystitis, without mention of obstruction
Cholelithiasis

574.11 Calculus of gallbladder with other cholecystitis, with obstruction
Cholecystitis

574.20 Calculus of gallbladder without mention of cholecystitis, without mention of obstruction
Cholelithiasis

574.30 Calculus of bile duct with acute cholecystitis, without mention of obstruction
Choledocholithiasis

574.50 Calculus of bile duct without mention of cholecystitis, without mention of obstruction
Choledocholithiasis

575.0 Acute cholecystitis
Cholecystitis
Cholelithiasis

575.10 Cholecystitis, unspecified
Cholecystitis
Cholelithiasis

576.1 Cholangitis
Cholangitis (acute)

576.9 Unspecified disorder of biliary tract
Pericholangitis

577.0 Acute pancreatitis
Pancreatitis

577.1 Chronic pancreatitis
Pancreatitis

577.2 Cyst and pseudocyst of pancreas
Pseudocyst pancreas

579.0 Celiac disease
Celiac disease

579.1 Tropical sprue
Tropical sprue

579.3 Other and unspecified postsurgical nonabsorption
Hypoglycemia, diabetic
Short-bowel syndrome

580.9 Acute glomerulonephritis with unspecified pathological lesion in kidney
Glomerulonephritis, acute

581.3 Nephrotic syndrome with lesion of minimal change glomerulonephritis
Lipoid nephrosis

581.9 Nephrotic syndrome with unspecified pathological lesion in kidney
Nephrotic syndrome

582.89 Nephritis, interstitial, chronic
Balkan nephritis syndrome

583.1 Nephritis and nephropathy, not specified as acute or chronic, with lesion of membranous glomerulonephritis
Glomerulonephritis, membranous
Glomerulopathy, membranous

583.4 Nephritis and nephropathy, not specified as acute or chronic, with lesion of rapidly progressive glomerulonephritis
Glomerulonephritis, rapidly progressive

583.81 Nephritis and nephropathy, not specified as acute or chronic, in diseases classified elsewhere
Lupus nephritis

583.89 Nephritis and nephropathy, not specified as acute or chronic, with other specified pathologic lesion in kidney, other
Nephropathy, analgesic
Nephropathy, chronic lead

584.5 Acute renal failure with lesion of tubular necrosis
Tubular necrosis, acute

584.9 Acute renal failure, unspecified
Renal failure, acute (ARF)

585 Chronic renal failure
Renal failure, chronic

588.8 Other specified disorder resulting from impaired renal function
Hyperparathyroidism
Renal tubular acidosis (RTA)

590.00 Chronic pyelonephritis without lesion of renal medullary necrosis
Pyelonephritis

590.01 Chronic pyelonephritis with lesion of renal medullary necrosis
Pyelonephritis

590.10 Acute pyelonephritis without lesion of renal medullary necrosis
Pyelonephritis

590.11 Acute pyelonephritis with lesion of renal medullary necrosis
Pyelonephritis

590.80 Pyelonephritis, unspecified
Pyelonephritis

591 Hydronephrosis
Hydronephrosis

592.0 Calculus of kidney
Renal calculi

592.9 Urinary calculus, unspecified
Urolithiasis

593.81 Vascular disorders of kidney
Renal infarction

595.0 Acute cystitis
Urinary tract infection in females
Urinary tract infection in males

595.1 Chronic interstitial cystitis
Interstitial cystitis
Urinary tract infection in males

595.2 Other chronic cystitis
Urinary tract infection in males

596.9 Unspecified disorder of bladder
Bladder injury

597.80 Urethritis, unspecified
Urethritis

597.81 Urethral syndrome NOS
Urethritis

599.7 Hematuria
Hematuria

600.90 Hyperplasia of prostate, unspecified, without urinary obstruction
Prostatic hyperplasia, benign (BPH)

600.91
Hyperplasia of prostate, unspecified, with urinary obstruction
Prostatic hyperplasia, benign (BPH)

601.0 Acute prostatitis
Prostatitis

601.1 Chronic prostatitis
Prostatitis

603.9 Hydrocele, unspecified
Hydrocele

604.90 Orchitis and epididymitis, unspecified
Epididymitis

605 Redundant prepuce and phimosis
Phimosis & paraphimosis

606.9 Male infertility, unspecified
Fertility problems

607.1 Balanitis
Balanitis

607.3 Priapism
Priapism

607.84 Impotence of organic origin
Erectile dysfunction

607.85 Peyronie disease
Peyronie disease

608.2 Torsion of testis
Testicular torsion

608.89 Other specified disorders of male genital organs, other
Dyspareunia
Ejaculatory disorders

610.1 Diffuse cystic mastopathy
Fibrocystic breast disease

611.0 Inflammatory disease of breast
Breast abscess

611.1 Hypertrophy of breast
Gynecomastia

611.6 Galactorrhea not associated with childbirth
Hyperprolactinemia

611.71 Mastodynia
Mastalgia

614.9 Unspecified inflammatory disease of female pelvic organs and tissue
Gonococcal infections
Pelvic inflammatory disease (PID)

615.9 Unspecified inflammatory disease of uterus, except cervix
Chlamydial sexually transmitted diseases

616.0 Cervicitis and endocervicitis
Cervicitis
Cervicitis, ectropion & true erosion
Chlamydial sexually transmitted diseases

616.10 Vaginitis and vulvovaginitis, unspecified
Chlamydial sexually transmitted diseases
Vulvovaginitis, bacterial
Vulvovaginitis, estrogen deficient
Vulvovaginitis, prepubescent

617.0 Endometriosis of uterus
Endometriosis

617.3 Endometriosis of pelvic peritoneum
Endometriosis

618.1 Uterine prolapse without mention of vaginal wall prolapse
Uterine prolapse

618.4 Uterovaginal prolapse, unspecified
Uterine prolapse

618.9 Unspecified genital prolapse
Uterine prolapse

621.0 Polyp of corpus uteri
Menorrhagia

621.3 Endometrial cystic hyperplasia
Menorrhagia

621.8 Other specified disorders of uterus, NEC
Menorrhagia

622.1 Dysplasia of cervix (uteri)
Abnormal Pap smear
Cervical dysplasia

622.7 Mucous polyp of cervix
Cervical polyps

625.0 Dyspareunia
Dyspareunia

625.3 Dysmenorrhea
Dysmenorrhea

625.4 Premenstrual tension syndromes
Premenstrual syndrome (PMS)

626.0 Absence of menstruation
Amenorrhea

626.2 Excessive or frequent menstruation
Menorrhagia

626.3 Puberty bleeding
Menorrhagia

626.4 Irregular menstrual cycle
Menorrhagia

626.6 Metrorrhagia
Menorrhagia

626.8 Disorders of menstruation and other abnormal bleeding from female genital tract, other
Dysfunctional uterine bleeding (DUB)
Menorrhagia

627.0 Premenopausal menorrhagia
Menopause
Menorrhagia

627.1 Postmenopausal bleeding
Menorrhagia
Uterine bleeding postmenopausal

627.2 Symptomatic menopausal or female climacteric states
Menopause

627.4 Symptomatic states associated with artificial menopause
Menopause

628.0 Female infertility associated with anovulation
Polycystic ovarian disease

628.4 Female infertility of cervical or vaginal origin
Artificial insemination

628.9 Female infertility of unspecified origin
Fertility problems

629.9 Unspecified disorder of female genital organs
Abortion, spontaneous

630 Hydatidiform mole
Vaginal bleeding during pregnancy

632 Missed abortion
Abortion, spontaneous

633.90 Unspecified ectopic pregnancy without intrauterine pregnancy
Ectopic pregnancy
Vaginal bleeding during pregnancy

634.90 Spontaneous abortion without mention of complication, unspecified
Vaginal bleeding during pregnancy

634.91 Spontaneous abortion without mention of complication, incomplete
Abortion, spontaneous

634.92 Spontaneous abortion without mention of complication, complete
Abortion, spontaneous

640.03 Threatened abortion, antepartum condition or complication
Abortion, spontaneous

641.00 Placenta previa without hemorrhage, unspecified
Placenta previa

641.10 Hemorrhage from placenta previa, unspecified
Placenta previa
Vaginal bleeding during pregnancy

641.20 Premature separation of placenta, unspecified
Abruptio placentae
Placenta previa
Vaginal bleeding during pregnancy

642.40 Mild or unspecified pre-eclampsia, unspecified
Eclampsia (toxemia of pregnancy)
Preeclampsia

642.50 Severe pre-eclampsia, unspecified
Eclampsia (toxemia of pregnancy)
Preeclampsia

642.60 Eclampsia, unspecified
Eclampsia (toxemia of pregnancy)

642.90 Unspecified hypertension complicating pregnancy, childbirth, or the puerperium, unspecified
Eclampsia (toxemia of pregnancy)
Hypertensive emergencies

643.00 Mild hyperemesis gravidarum, unspecified
Hyperemesis gravidarum

643.1 Hyperemesis gravidarum with metabolic disturbance, unspecified
Hyperemesis gravidarum

644.20 Early onset of delivery, unspecified as to episode of care or not applicable
Premature labor

644.21 Early onset of delivery, delivered with or without mention of antepartum condition
Premature labor

646.70 Liver disorders in pregnancy, unspecified
Intrahepatic cholestasis due to pregnancy
Fatty liver syndrome

646.80 Other specified complications of pregnancy, unspecified
Herpes gestationis

646.83 Other specified complications of pregnancy, antepartum condition or complication
Herpes gestationis

648.44 Mental postpartum condition or complication
Baby blues
Postpartum anxiety/panic disorder
Postpartum depression
Postpartum obsessive compulsive disorder
Postpartum psychosis

652.20 Breech presentation without mention of version, unspecified
Breech birth

656.10 Rh isoimmunization in pregnancy, unspecified
Rh incompatibility

656.20 Isoimmunization in pregnancy from other and unspecified blood-group incompatibility, unspecified
Rh incompatibility

656.50 Poor fetal growth, unspecified
Placental insufficiency syndrome

659.20 Pyrexia of unknown origin during labor
Fever of unknown origin (FUO)

670.04 Major puerperal infection, postpartum condition or complication
Puerperal infection

672.0 Pyrexia of unknown origin during puerperium
Fever of unknown origin (FUO)

675.1 Puerperal, postpartum
Breast abscess

676.60 Galactorrhea associated with childbirth, unspecified
Chiari-Frommel syndrome
Galactorrhea

680.9 Carbuncle and furuncle, unspecified site
Furunculosis

681.02 Onychia and paronychia of finger
Paronychia

682.9 Cellulitis and abscess at unspecified site
Anaerobic & necrotizing infections
Cellulitis

684 Impetigo
Impetigo

685.1 Pilonidal cyst without mention of abscess
Pilonidal cyst

686.1 Pyogenic granuloma
Granuloma, pyogenic
Granulomatous disease of childhood, chronic

686.8 Other specific local infections of skin & subcutaneous tissue
Acrodermatitis enteropathica
Ecthyma
Perlèche
Zinc deficiency

690.10 Seborrheic dermatitis, unspecified
Dermatitis, seborrheic

691.0 Diaper or napkin rash
Dermatitis, diaper

691.8 Other atopic dermatitis and related conditions
Dermatitis, atopic

692.0 Contact dermatitis and other eczema due to detergents
Dermatitis, contact

692.5 Contact dermatitis and other eczema due to food in contact with skin
Food allergy

692.71 Sunburn
Sunburn

692.79 Other dermatitis due to solar radiation
Photodermatitis

692.89 Contact dermatitis and other eczema due to other specified agents, other
Id reaction

692.9 Contact dermatitis and other eczema due to unspecified cause
Dermatitis, contact
Photodermatitis

693.0 Dermatitis due to drugs or medicines taken internally
Cutaneous drug reactions

693.1 Dermatitis due to food taken internally
Food allergy

694.0 Dermatitis herpetiformis
Dermatitis, herpetiformis

694.4 Pemphigus
Pemphigus vulgaris
Pemphigus, benign chronic familial
Pemphigus, Brazilian

694.5 Pemphigoid
Pemphigoid, bullous

695.0 Erythema marginatum
Erythema marginatum

695.1 Erythema multiforme
Erythema multiforme
Stevens-Johnson syndrome

695.2 Erythema nodosum
Erythema nodosum

695.3 Rosacea
Acne rosacea

695.4 Lupus erythematosus
Lupus erythematosus, discoid

695.89 Other specified erythematous conditions, other
Dermatitis, exfoliative
Granuloma annulare

696.0 Psoriatic arthropathy
Arthritis, psoriatic

696.1 Other psoriasis
Psoriasis

696.2 Parapsoriasis
Parapsoriasis
Psoriasis

696.3 Pityriasis rosea
Pityriasis rosea

696.5 Other and unspecified pityriasis
Pityriasis alba

697.0 Lichen planus
Lichen planus

698.0 Pruritus ani
Pruritus ani

698.1 Pruritus of genital organs
Pruritus vulvae

698.3 Lichenification and lichen simplex chronicus
Neurodermatitis

701.0 Circumscribed scleroderma
Lichen sclerosis of the vulva

701.2 Acquired acanthosis nigricans
Acanthosis nigricans
HAIR-AN syndrome

701.4 Keloid scar
Keloids

702.0 Actinic keratosis
Keratosis, actinic

704.00 Alopecia, unspecified
Alopecia

704.01 Alopecia areata
Alopecia

704.09 Diseases of hair and hair follicles, other
Alopecia

704.1 Hirsutism
Hirsutism

704.8 Other specified diseases of hair and hair follicles
Folliculitis
Pseudofolliculitis barbae

705.0 Anhidrosis
Anhidrosis

705.1 Prickly heat
Miliaria rubra

705.81 Dyshidrosis
Dyshidrosis

705.83 Hidradenitis
Hidradenitis suppurativa

706.1 Other acne
Acne vulgaris

707.0 Decubitus ulcer
Brain injury - post acute care issues
Pressure ulcer

708.8 Other specified urticaria
Urticaria

709.00 Dyschromia, unspecified
Chloasma
Vitiligo

709.3 Degenerative skin disorders
Necrobiosis lipoidica diabeticorum

710.0 Systemic lupus erythematosus
Lupus nephritis
Systemic lupus erythematosus (SLE)

710.1 Systemic sclerosis
Scleredema
Scleroderma

710.2 Sicca syndrome
Sjögren syndrome

710.3 Dermatomyositis
Polymyositis/dermatomyositis

710.4 Polymyositis
Polymyositis/dermatomyositis

711.00 Pyogenic arthritis, site unspecified
Arthritis, infectious, bacterial

712.10 Chondrocalcinosis due to dicalcium phosphate crystals, site unspecified
Pseudogout (CPPD)

712.20 Chondrocalcinosis due to pyrophosphate crystals, site unspecified
Pseudogout (CPPD)

712.30 Chondrocalcinosis, unspecified, site unspecified
Pseudogout (CPPD)

713.5 Arthropathy associated with neurological disorders
Charcot joint

714.0 Rheumatoid arthritis
Arthritis, rheumatoid (RA)

714.1 Felty syndrome
Arthritis, rheumatoid (RA)
Felty syndrome

714.30 Polyarticular juvenile rheumatoid arthritis, chronic or unspecified
Arthritis, juvenile rheumatoid (JRA)

714.31 Polyarticular juvenile rheumatoid arthritis, acute
Arthritis, juvenile rheumatoid (JRA)

714.32 Pauciarticular onset JRA
Arthritis, juvenile rheumatoid (JRA)

714.33 Monoarticular onset JRA
Arthritis, juvenile rheumatoid (JRA)

714.81 Rheumatoid lung
Rheumatoid pneumoconiosis

715.90 Osteoarthrosis, unspecified whether generalized or localized, site unspecified
Arthritis, osteo

716.30 Climacteric arthritis, site unspecified
Menopause

719.20 Villonodular synovitis, site unspecified
Synovitis, pigmented villonodular

720.0 Ankylosing spondylitis
Ankylosing spondylitis

721.0 Cervical spondylosis without myelopathy
Cervical spondylosis

721.1 Cervical spondylosis with myelopathy
Cervical spondylosis

722.10 Displacement of lumbar intervertebral disc without myelopathy
Lumbar (intervertebral) disk disorders

752.49 Other congenital anomalies of cervix, vagina, and external female genitalia
Vaginal adenosis

752.51 Undescended testis
Cryptorchidism

752.61 Hypospadias (male)
Hypospadias

753.12 Polycystic kidney, unspecified type
Polycystic kidney disease

753.13 Polycystic kidney, autosomal dominant
Polycystic kidney disease

753.14 Polycystic kidney, autosomal recessive
Polycystic kidney disease

753.20 Unspecified obstructive defect of renal pelvis and ureter
Hydronephrosis

754.1 Certain congenital musculoskeletal deformities of sternocleidomastoid muscle
Torticollis

754.2 Congenital musculoskeletal deformities of spine
Scoliosis

755.55 Acrocephalosyndactyly
Apert syndrome

756.52 Osteopetrosis
Osteopetrosis

756.54 Polyostotic fibrous dysplasia of bone
Albright syndrome with precocious puberty

756.83 Ehlers-Danlos syndrome
Ehlers-Danlos syndrome

757.1 Ichthyosis congenital
Ichthyosis

757.31 Congenital ectodermal dysplasia
Ectrodactyly, ectodermal dysplasia, clefting syndrome
Hereditary anhidrotic ectodermal dysplasia
Hypohidrotic ectodermal dysplasia syndrome

757.33 Congenital pigmentary anomalies of skin
Mastocytosis

757.39 Other specified congenital anomalies of skin, other
Bloom syndrome

758.0 Down syndrome
Down syndrome

758.6 Gonadal dysgenesis
Turner syndrome

758.7 Klinefelter syndrome
Klinefelter syndrome

758.9 Conditions due to anomaly of unspecified chromosome
Fragile X syndrome
Williams syndrome

759.0 Anomalies of spleen
Splenic agenesis syndrome

759.2 Congenital anomalies of other endocrine glands
Thyroglossal duct cyst

759.3 Situs inversus
Kartagener syndrome

759.5 Tuberous sclerosis
Tuberous sclerosis complex

759.6 Other hamartoses, NEC
Cowden syndrome
Peutz-Jeghers syndrome
Sturge-Weber disease
von Hippel-Lindau disease

759.81 Prader-Willi syndrome
Prader-Willi/Angelman syndrome

759.82 Marfan syndrome
Marfan syndrome

759.89 Other specified congenital anomalies
Beckwith-Wiedemann syndrome
Cornelia de Lange syndrome
Laurence-Moon-Biedl syndrome

760.71 Fetal alcohol syndrome
Fetal alcohol syndrome

762.1 Premature separation of placenta (when causing newborn complications)
Placenta previa

762.2 Fetus affected by unspecified abnormality of placenta
Placental insufficiency syndrome

763.0 Breech delivery and extraction
Breech birth

763.4 Cesarean delivery
Breech birth

770.89 Other respiratory problems after birth
Respiratory distress syndrome, neonatal

771.0 Congenital rubella
Measles, rubella

771.2 Other congenital infections
Herpes simplex
Malaria
Toxoplasmosis

773.0 Rh hemolytic disease in fetus or newborn
Erythroblastosis fetalis
Rh incompatibility

773.1 ABO hemolytic disease in fetus or newborn
Erythroblastosis fetalis
Rh incompatibility

773.2 Other hemolytic disease in fetus or newborn
Erythroblastosis fetalis
Rh incompatibility

773.3 Isoimmune hydrops fetalis
Erythroblastosis fetalis
Rh incompatibility

773.4 Kernicterus due to isoimmunization
Erythroblastosis fetalis
Kernicterus
Rh incompatibility

773.5 Isoimmune late anemia
Erythroblastosis fetalis
Rh incompatibility

774.30 Neonatal jaundice due to delayed conjugation, cause unspecified
Jaundice, breast milk

774.6 Unspecified fetal and neonatal jaundice
Familial neonatal hyperbilirubinemia
Hyperbilirubinemia, physiologic neonatal

774.7 Kernicterus not due to isoimmunization
Kernicterus

775.0 Syndrome of "infant of a diabetic mother"
Hypoglycemia, diabetic

775.6 Neonatal hypoglycemia
Hypoglycemia, diabetic

776.0 Hemorrhagic disease of newborn
Vitamin deficiency

778.2 Cold injury syndrome of newborn
Hypothermia

778.3 Other hypothermia of newborn
Hypothermia

778.4 Other disturbances of temperature regulation of newborn
Fever of unknown origin (FUO)

779.0 Convulsions in newborn
Seizure disorders

780.09 Alterations of consciousness, other
Delirium

780.2 Syncope and collapse
Syncope

780.31 Febrile convulsions
Seizures, febrile

780.39 Other convulsions
Eclampsia (toxemia of pregnancy)
Seizure disorders

780.50 Sleep disturbance, unspecified
Insomnia
Jet lag

780.51 Insomnia with sleep apnea
Insomnia

780.52 Other insomnia
Insomnia

780.57 Other and unspecified sleep apnea
Sleep apnea, obstructive

780.6 Fever
Fever of unknown origin (FUO)

780.71 Chronic fatigue syndrome
Chronic fatigue syndrome

780.79 Other malaise and fatigue
Fatigue

780.8 Hyperhidrosis
Hyperhidrosis

780.99 Hypothermia not associated with low environmental temperature
Hypothermia

781.99 Other symptoms involving nervous and musculoskeletal systems
Floppy infant syndrome

782.3 Edema
Idiopathic edema

782.4 Jaundice, unspecified, not of newborn
Jaundice

783.40 Lack of normal physiological development, unspecified
Failure to thrive (FTT)

784.0 Headache
Headache, cluster
Migraine

784.61 Alexia and dyslexia
Dyslexia

784.7 Epistaxis
Epistaxis

784.9 Other symptoms involving head and neck
Halitosis

785.0 Tachycardia, unspecified
Sinus tachycardia

785.4 Gangrene
Anaerobic & necrotizing infections

785.50 Shock, unspecified
Shock, circulatory

785.51 Cardiogenic shock
Shock, circulatory

785.59 Shock without mention of trauma, other
Pyrogenic shock
Shock, circulatory

786.09 Dyspnea and respiratory abnormalities, other
Respiratory distress syndrome, adult

786.2 Cough
Chronic cough

786.8 Hiccough
Hiccups

787.1 Heartburn
Brain injury - post acute care issues
Gastroesophageal reflux disease

787.2 Dysphagia
Dysphagia

787.6 Incontinence of feces
Encopresis

787.91 Diarrhea
Diarrhea, acute
Diarrhea, chronic

788.30 Urinary incontinence, unspecified
Enuresis
Urinary incontinence

789.0 Abdominal pain
Colic, infantile

789.5 Ascites
Ascites
Ascites, chylous
Meigs syndrome

795.5 Non-specific reaction to tuberculin skin test without active tuberculosis (PPD positive)
Tuberculosis, latent

798.0 Sudden infant death syndrome
Sudden infant death syndrome (SIDS)

799.2 Nervousness
Restlessness

800.00 Fracture of vault of skull, closed without mention of intracranial injury, unspecified state of consciousness
Brain injury, traumatic

820. Fracture of neck of femur (use appropriate modifier)
Hip fracture

848.9 Sprain and strain, site unspecified
Sprains & strains

850.9 Concussion, unspecified
Brain injury, traumatic

851.xx Cerebral laceration or contusion
Brain injury, traumatic

852.00 Subarchnoid hemorrhage following injury without mention of open intracranial wound, unspecified state of consciousness
Brain injury, traumatic
Subarachnoid hemorrhage

852.30 Subdural hemorrhage following injury with open intracranial wound, unspecified state of consciousness
Subdural hematoma

854.00 Intracranial injury of other and unspecified nature, without mention of intracranial wound, unspecified state of consciousness
Brain injury, traumatic

860.2 Traumatic hemothorax without mention of open wound into thorax
Hemothorax

873.40 Open wound of face without mention of complications, unspecified site
Animal bites

879.8 Open wound(s) of unspecified site(s) without mention of complications
Animal bites

882.0 Open wound of hand except finger(s) alone without mention of complication
Animal bites

910.8 Other and unspecified superficial injury of face, neck, and scalp except eye, without mention of infection
Insect bites & stings

938 Foreign body in digestive system, unspecified
Bezoar

940.2 Alkaline chemical burn of cornea and conjunctival sac
Ocular chemical burns

940.3 Acid chemical burn of cornea and conjunctival sac
Ocular chemical burns

940.9 Unspecified burn of eye and adnexa
Burns

941.00 Unspecified degree burn of face and head, unspecified site
Burns

942.00 Unspecified degree burn of trunk, unspecified site
Burns

948.0 Burn, any degree <10% of BSA (fifth digit can indicate BSA involved in 3rd degree burn)
Burns

949.0 Unspecified burn, unspecified degree
Burns

949.1 Unspecified burn, erythema [first degree]
Burns

949.2 Unspecified burn, blisters, epidermal loss [second degree]
Burns

949.3 Unspecified burn, full thickness skin loss [third degree NOS]
Burns

952.00 Cervical spinal cord injury without evidence of spinal bone injury, C1-C4 level with unspecified spinal cord injury
Cervical hyperextension injuries
Cervical spine injury

958.0 Air embolism
Arterial gas embolism

959.19 Other injury of other sites of trunk
Rape crisis syndrome

959.9 Injury, unspecified site
Rape crisis syndrome

962.3 Poisoning by insulins and antidiabetic agents
Hypoglycemia, diabetic

964.0 Poisoning by iron and its compounds
Iron toxicity, acute

965.1 Poisoning by salicylates (aspirin)
Nephropathy, analgesic
Salicylate poisoning

965.4 Poisoning by aromatic analgesics, NEC
Acetaminophen poisoning
Nephropathy, analgesic

972.1 Poisoning by cardiotonic glycosides and drugs of similar action
Digitalis toxicity

980.1 Methanol poisoning
Methanol poisoning

982.0 Toxic effect of benzene and homologues
Toluene poisoning

982.3 Toxic effect of other chlorinated hydrocarbon solvents
Trichloroethylene poisoning

983.0 Toxic effect of corrosive aromatics
Nitrobenzene poisoning

983.9 Toxic effect of caustic, unspecified
Phosphorus poisoning

984.9 Toxic effect of unspecified lead compound (including fumes)
Gout
Lead poisoning
Nephropathy, chronic lead

985.1 Toxic effect of arsenic and its compounds
Arsenic poisoning

985.8 Toxic effect of other specified metals
Silver poisoning
Thallium poisoning

986 Toxic effect of carbon monoxide
Carbon monoxide poisoning

987.3 Toxic effect of sulfur dioxide
Sulfur dioxide poisoning

987.7 Toxic effect of hydrocyanic acid gas
Cyanide poisoning

987.8 Toxic effect of other specified gases, fumes, or vapors
Phosphine poisoning

988.0 Toxic effect of fish and shellfish eaten as food
Mussel poisoning

988.1 Toxic effect of mushrooms eaten as food
Mushroom poisoning, Amanita phalloides

988.2 Toxic effect of berries and other plants eaten as food
Lathyrism

989.0 Toxic effect of hydrocyanic acid and cyanides
Cyanide poisoning

989.2 Toxic effect of chlorinated hydrocarbons
Toxaphene poisoning

989.5 Toxic effect of venom
Insect bites & stings
Snake envenomations: Crotalidae
Snake envenomations: Elapidae
Tick paralysis

989.8 Formaldehyde poisoning
Formaldehyde poisoning

990 Radiation effects, unspecified
Radiation sickness

991.0 Frostbite of face
Frostbite

991.1 Frostbite of hand
Frostbite

991.2 Frostbite of foot
Frostbite

991.3 Frostbite of other and unspecified sites
Frostbite

991.6 Hypothermia
Hypothermia

992.0 Heat stroke and sun stroke
Heat exhaustion & heat stroke

992.2 Heat cramps
Heat cramp

992.5 Heat exhaustion, unspecified
Heat exhaustion & heat stroke

993.0 Barotrauma, otitic
Barotitis media

993.1 Barotrauma, sinus
Barotitis media

993.2 Other and unspecified effects of high altitude
Altitude illness

993.3 Caisson disease
Decompression sickness

994.1 Drowning and nonfatal submersion
Near drowning

994.6 Motion sickness
Motion sickness

995.0 Other anaphylactic shock
Anaphylaxis

995.1 Angioneurotic edema
Angioedema

995.50 Child abuse, unspecified
Child abuse

995.60 Anaphylactic shock or reaction due to unspecified food
Food allergy

995.86 Malignant hyperthermia
Hyperthermia, malignant

995.89 Other specified adverse effects, NEC, Other
Hypothermia

996.61 Infection and inflammatory reaction due to cardiac device, implant, and graft
Endocarditis, infective

997.4 Digestive system complications, NEC
Hepatorenal syndrome

998.59 Other postoperative infection
Subphrenic abscess

999.5 Other serum reaction
Serum sickness

999.8 Other transfusion reaction
Transfusion reaction, hemolytic

999.9 Other and unspecified complications of medical care, NEC
Milk-alkali syndrome

E860.2 Accidental methanol poisoning
Methanol poisoning

E947.8 Adverse effects in therapeutic use of other drugs and medicinal substances
Anaphylaxis

E947.9 Adverse effects in therapeutic use of unspecified drug or medicinal substance
Anaphylaxis

E950.5 Suicide and self-inflicted poisoning by unspecified drug or medicinal substance
Suicide

E950.9 Suicide attempt
Methanol poisoning

E980.9 Undetermined methanol poisoning
Methanol poisoning

V01.5 Rabies exposure
Rabies

V04.5 Need for prophylactic vaccination and inoculation against rabies
Rabies

V05.9 Need for prophylactic vaccination and inoculation against unspecified single disease
Immunizations

V41.7 Problems with sexual function
Erectile dysfunction

V71.5 Observation following alleged rape or seduction
Rape crisis syndrome

Topic Index

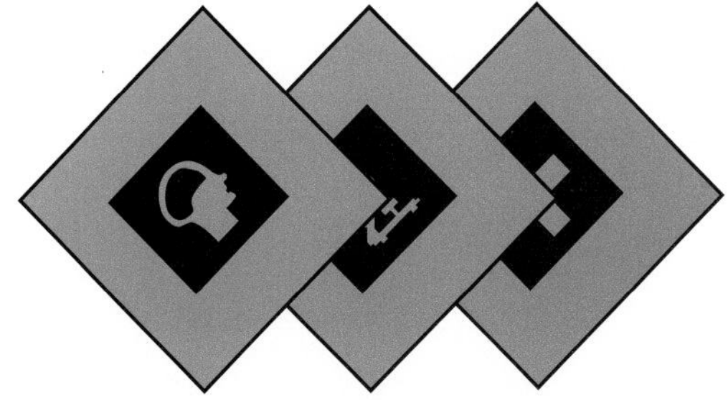

Index

INDEX

- B -

- C -

- D -

- E -

- F -

- G -

- H -

- I -

- J -

- K -

- L -

- M -

- N -

- O -

- P -

- S -

- T -

- U -

- V -

- W -

- X -

- Y -

- Z -